Tth - Thermus Thermophalis
    Both a DNA & RNA Polymerase

Taq Thermus Aquatacus
    Just a DNA Polymerase

LABORATORY ANIMAL
MEDICINE

THIRD EDITION

American College of Laboratory Animal Medicine Series

Steven H. Weisbroth, Ronald E. Flatt, and Alan L. Kraus, eds.:
The Biology of the Laboratory Rabbit, 1974

Joseph E. Wagner and Patrick J. Manning, eds.:
The Biology of the Guinea Pig, 1976

Edwin J. Andrews, Billy C. Ward, and Norman H. Altman, eds.:
Spontaneous Animal Models of Human Disease, Volume 1, 1979; Volume II, 1979

Henry J. Baker, J. Russell Lindsey, and Steven H. Weisbroth, eds.:
The Laboratory Rat, Volume I: Biology and Diseases, 1979; Volume II: Research Applications, 1980

Henry L. Foster, J. David Small, and James G. Fox, eds.:
The Mouse in Biomedical Research, Volume I: History, Genetics, and Wild Mice, 1981; Volume II: Diseases, 1982; Volume Ill: Normative Biology, Immunology, and Husbandry, 1983; Volume IV: Experimental Biology and Oncology, 1982

James G. Fox, Bennett J. Cohen, and Franklin M. Loew, eds.:
Laboratory Animal Medicine, 1984

G. L. Van Hoosier, Jr., and Charles W McPherson, eds.:
Laboratory Hamsters, 1987

Patrick J. Manning, Daniel H. Ringler, and Christian E. Newcomer, eds.:
The Biology of the Laboratory Rabbit, 2nd Edition, 1994

B. Taylor Bennett, Christian R. Abee, and Roy Henrickson, eds.:
Nonhuman Primates in Biomedical Research, Volume I: Biology and Management, 1995; Volume II: Diseases, 1998

Dennis F. Kohn, Sally K. Wixson, William J. White, and G. John Benson, eds.:
Anesthesia and Analgesia in Laboratory Animals, 1997

James G. Fox, Lynn C. Anderson, Franklin M. Loew and Fred W. Quimby, eds.:
Laboratory Animal Medicine, 2nd Edition, 2002

Mark A. Suckow, Steven H. Weisbroth and Craig L. Franklin, eds.:
The Laboratory Rat, 2nd Edition, 2006

James G. Fox, Muriel T. Davisson, Fred W. Quimby, Stephen W. Barthold, Christian E. Newcomer and Abigail L. Smith, eds.:
The Mouse in Biomedical Research, 2nd Edition, Volume I: History, Wild Mice, and Genetics, 2007; Volume II: Diseases, 2007; Volume III: Normative Biology, Husbandry, and Models, 2007; Volume IV: Immunology, 2007

David Backer, ed:
Flynn's Parasites of Laboratory Animals, 2007 (Wiley)

Richard E. Fish, Marilyn J. Brown, Peggy J. Danneman and Alicia Z. Karas, eds.:
Anesthesia and Analgesia in Laboratory Animals, 2nd Edition, 2008

Jack R. Hessler and Noel D.M. Lehner, eds.:
Planning and Designing Animal Research Facilities, 2009

Mark A. Suckow, Karla A. Stevens, and Ronald P. Wilson, eds.:
The Laboratory Rabbit, Guinea Pig, Hamster and other Rodents, 2011

J. Harkness, P Turner, S VandeWoude, C Wheler, eds:
Biology and Medicine of Rabbits and Rodents, 5th Ed, 2012 (Wiley)

Christian R. Abee, Keith Mansfield, Suzette Tardif and Timothy Morris, eds.:
Nonhuman Primates in Biomedical Research, 2nd Edition, Volume I: Biology and Management, 2012; Volume II: Diseases, 2012

Kathryn Bayne and Patricia V. Turner, eds.:
Laboratory Animal Welfare, 2013

James G. Fox and Robert P. Marini eds.:
Biology and Diseases of the Ferret, 2E, 2014 (Wiley)

M. Michael Swindle, ed.:
Swine in the Laboratory: Surgery, Anesthesia, Imaging and Experimental Techniques, 3E, 2015 (Taylor & Francis)

LABORATORY ANIMAL MEDICINE

THIRD EDITION

Edited by

JAMES G. FOX (EDITOR-IN-CHIEF)
Division of Comparative Medicine, Massachusetts Institute of Technology, Cambridge, MA, USA

LYNN C. ANDERSON
Global Animal and Comparative Medicine, Covance Laboratories Inc., Madison, WI, USA

GLEN M. OTTO
Animal Resources Center, University of Texas at Austin, Austin, TX, USA

KATHLEEN R. PRITCHETT-CORNING
Harvard University, Faculty of Arts and Sciences, and
Department of Comparative Medicine, University of Washington, Cambridge, MA, USA

MARK T. WHARY
Division of Comparative Medicine, Massachusetts Institute of Technology, Cambridge, MA, USA

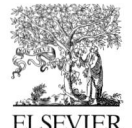

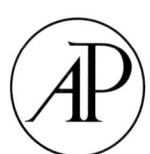

AMSTERDAM • BOSTON • HEIDELBERG • LONDON
NEW YORK • OXFORD • PARIS • SAN DIEGO
SAN FRANCISCO • SINGAPORE • SYDNEY • TOKYO
Academic Press is an imprint of Elsevier

ELSEVIER

Academic Press is an imprint of Elsevier
125, London Wall, EC2Y 5AS.
525 B Street, Suite 1800, San Diego, CA 92101-4495, USA
225 Wyman Street, Waltham, MA 02451, USA
The Boulevard, Langford Lane, Kidlington, Oxford OX5 1GB, UK

Third edition 2015

Library of Congress Cataloging-in-Publication Data
A catalog record for this book is available from the Library of Congress

British Library Cataloguing-in-Publication Data
A catalogue record for this book is available from the British Library

ISBN: 978-0-12-409527-4

For information on all Academic Press publications,
visit our website at http://store.elsevier.com

Typeset by MPS Limited, Chennai, India
www.adi-mps.com

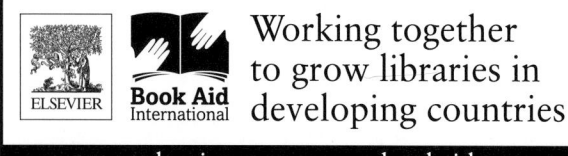

Working together
to grow libraries in
developing countries

www.elsevier.com • www.bookaid.org

Acquisition Editor: Janice Audet
Editorial Project Manager: Mary Preap
Production Project Manager: Karen East and Kirsty Halterman
Designer: Alan Studholme

Printed and bound in China

Contents

8. The Laboratory Woodchuck (Marmota monax)

CHRISTINE A. BELLEZZA, SANDRA SEXTON, LESLIE I. CURTIN,
PATRICK W. CONCANNON, BETTY H. BALDWIN, LOU ANN
GRAHAM, WILLIAM E. HORNBUCKLE, LOIS ROTH AND BUD
C. TENNANT

9. Biology and Diseases of Chinchillas

CHARLIE C. HSU, MAIA M. CHAN AND COLETTE L. WHELER

10. Biology and Diseases of Rabbits

MEGAN H. NOWLAND, DAVID W. BRAMMER, ALEXIS GARCIA
AND HOWARD G. RUSH

11. Microbiological Quality Control for Laboratory Rodents and Lagomorphs

WILLIAM R. SHEK, ABIGAIL L. SMITH AND
KATHLEEN R. PRITCHETT-CORNING

12. Biology and Diseases of Dogs

JEAN A. NEMZEK, PATRICK A. LESTER, A. MARISSA WOLFE,
ROBERT C. DYSKO AND DANIEL D. MYERS, JR.

13. Biology and Diseases of Cats

TANYA BURKHOLDER, CARMEN LEDESMA FELICIANO,
SUE VANDEWOUDE AND HENRY J. BAKER

14. Biology and Diseases of Ferrets

JOERG MAYER, DR. ROBERT P. MARINI AND JAMES G. FOX

15. Biology and Diseases of Ruminants (Sheep, Goats, and Cattle)

WENDY J. UNDERWOOD, RUTH BLAUWIEKEL,
MARGARET L. DELANO, ROSE GILLESBY, SCOTT A. MISCHLER
AND ADAM SCHOELL

16. Biology and Diseases of Swine

KRISTI L. HELKE, PAULA C. EZELL, RAIMON DURAN-STRUUCK
AND M. MICHAEL SWINDLE

17. Nonhuman Primates

ELIZABETH R. MAGDEN, KEITH G. MANSFIELD,
JOE H. SIMMONS AND CHRISTIAN R. ABEE

List of Reviewers

Christian R. Abee University of Texas MD Anderson, Houston, TX, USA

Lotus Altholtz Patterson Veterinary, New York, NY, USA

Lynn C. Anderson Covance, Madison, WI, USA

Jessica Ayers Colorado State University, Fort Collins, CO, USA

Kathryn Bayne AAALAC International, Frederick, MD, USA

Bonnie V. Beaver Texas Veterinary Medical Center, Texas A&M University, College Station, TX, USA

David Besselsen University of Arizona, Tempe, AZ, USA

John Bradfield Senior Director, AAALAC International, Frederick, MD, USA

Rosemary Broome Independent Consultant, San Francisco Bay Area, CA, USA

Margaret L. Casal University of Pennsylvania, Philadelphia, PA, USA

Thomas B. Clarkson Wake Forest School of Medicine, Winston Salem, NC, USA

Leigh Ann Clayton National Aquarium, Baltimore, MD, USA

J. Mark Cline Wake Forest School of Medicine, Winston-Salem, NC, USA

Susan R. Compton Yale University School of Medicine, New Haven, CT, USA

Tim Cooper Penn State College of Medicine, Hershey, PA, USA

Graham Crawshaw Toronto Zoo, Toronto, Ontario, Canada

Jennifer Criley Illinois University, Urbana, IL, USA

Dale DeNardo Arizona State University, Tempe, AZ, USA

David Diamond Massachusetts Institute of Technology, Cambridge, MA, USA

Raimon Duran-Struuck Columbia University School of Medicine, New York, NY, USA

Courtney Ek Boston Children's Hospital, Boston, MA, USA

Sanford Feldman University of Virginia, Charlottesville, VA, USA

Sherril Green Stanford University, Stanford, CA, USA

F. Claire Hankenson Michigan State University, East Lansing, MI, USA

Hilda Holcombe Massachusetts Institute of Technology, Cambridge, MA, USA

Michael Kent Oregon State University, Corvallis, OR, USA

James I. Kim Massachusetts General Hospital, Boston, MA, USA

Hilton Klein Fox Chase Cancer Center, Philadelphia, PA, USA

Carlisle P. Landel Transposagen Pharmaceuticals, Lexington, KY, USA

David Lee-Parritz Tufts Cummings School of Veterinary Medicine, North Grafton, MA, USA

Karen Lencioni California Institute of Technology, Pasadena, CA, USA

Lillian Maggio-Price University of Washington School of Medicine, Seattle, WA, USA

Robert P. Marini Massachusetts Institute of Technology, Cambridge, MA, USA

James O. Marx University of Pennsylvania, Philadelphia, PA, USA

LaVonne D. Meunier GlaxoSmithKline Pharmaceuticals, King of Prussia, PA, USA

Christian Newcomer AAALAC International, Frederick, MD, USA

Roger P Orcutt Dunkirk, NY, USA

Dorcas P O'Rourke East Carolina University, Greenville, NC, USA

Mary M. Patterson Massachusetts Institute of Technology, Cambridge, MA, USA

Stacy Pritt University of Texas Southwestern Medical Center, Dallas, TX, USA

George Sanders University of Washington, Seattle, WA, USA

James Sheets University of Iowa, Iowa City, IA, USA

Jerald Silverman University of Massachusetts Medical School, Worcester, MA, USA

Gerald Smith Eli Lilly & Co, Indianapolis, IN, USA

Stephen A. Smith Dept of Biomedical Sciences and Pathobiology, Virginia Tech, Blacksburg, VA, USA

Mark Suckow University of Notre Dame, Notre Dame, IN, USA

Pat Turner University of Guelph, Ontario, Canada

Wendy J. Underwood Dept of Veterinary Resources, Eli Lilly & Co, Indianapolis, IN, USA

James Weed National Institutes of Health, Bethesda, MD, USA

William White Charles River Laboratories, Wilmington, MA, USA

Michael Wiles The Jackson Laboratory, Bar Harbor, ME, USA

Christina L. Winnicker Charles River Laboratories, Wilmington, MA, USA

Jeffrey D. Wyatt University of Rochester, Rochester, NY, USA

List of Contributors

Christian R. Abee DVM, MS, DACLAM   Department of Veterinary Sciences, Michale E. Keeling Center for Comparative Medicine and Research, The University of Texas MD Anderson Cancer Center, Bastrop, TX, USA

Walter Akers DVM, PhD   Department of Radiology, Washington University School of Medicine, St. Louis, Missouri, USA

Lynn C. Anderson   Global Animal and Comparative Medicine, Covance Laboratories Inc., Madison, WI, USA

Keith M. Astrofsky DVM   Novartis Institutes for Biomedical Research, Cambridge, MA, USA

Janet Baer DVM   California Institute of Technology, Pasadena, CA, USA

David G. Baker DVM, PhD, MS, MPA, DACLAM   Division of Laboratory Animal Medicine, Louisiana State University, School of Veterinary Medicine, Baton Rouge, LA, USA

Henry J. Baker DVM, DACLAM   Scott-Ritchey Research Center, College of Veterinary Medicine, Auburn University, AL

Betty H. Baldwin BS, MS   Department of Clinical Sciences, College of Veterinary Medicine, Cornell University, Ithaca, NY, USA

Stephen W. Barthold DVM, PhD, Diplomate ACVP   EmeritusPathology, Microbiology & Immunology School of Veterinary Medicine, University of California, Davis, CA, USA

Nicole Baumgarth DVM, PhD   Microbiology and Immunology Center for Comparative Medicine, University of California Davis, Davis, CA, USA

Kathryn Bayne   Association for Assessment and Accreditation of Laboratory Animal Care International, Frederick, MD, USA

Kathryn A.L. Bayne MS, PhD, DVM, DACLAM, DACAW, CAAB   AAALAC International, Corporate Dr., Suite #203, Frederick, MD, USA

Bonnie V. Beaver DVM, MS, DSc (hon), DPNAP, DACVB, DACAW   Department of Small Animal Clinical Sciences, College of Veterinary Medicine, Texas A&M University, College Station, TX, USA

Christine A. Bellezza DVM   Office of Research Integrity and Assurance, Office of the Vice Provost for Research, Cornell University, Ithaca, NY, USA

B. Taylor Bennett DVM, PhD   Management Consultant, Hinsdale, IL, USA

Ingrid Bergin VMD, MS, DACLAM, DACVP   Unit for Laboratory Animal Medicine Pathologist, In Vivo Animal Core, University of Michigan, Ann Arbor, Michigan, USA

Ruth Blauwiekel DVM, PhD, DACLAM   University of Vermont, Hills Building, Carrigan Drive, Burlington, VT, USA

David W. Brammer DVM, DACLAM   University of Houston, Animal Care Operations, Houston, TX, USA

Marilyn J. Brown DVM, MS, DACLAM, DECLAM   Global Animal Welfare, Department of Animal Welfare, Charles River Laboratories, Wilmington, MA, USA

Tanya Burkholder DVM, DACLAM   Veterinary Medicine Branch, ORS/DVR, National Institutes of Health, Bethesda, MD, USA

Calvin B. Carpenter DVM, DACLAM   Animal Resources, Alcon Research Ltd., South Freeway, Fort Worth, TX, USA

Maia M. Chan DVM, MS   Seattle Children's Research Institute, Seattle, WA, USA

Kimberly Cheng   The University of British Columbia, Faculty of Land and Food Systems, Avian Research Centre, Vancouver, BC, Canada

Thomas B. Clarkson DVM, DACLAM   Pathology/Comparative Medicine, Wake Forest School of Medicine, Winston-Salem, NC, USA

Charles B. Clifford DVM, PhD, DACVP   Pathology and Technical Services (Retired), Charles River Laboratories Inc., San Diego, CA, USA

J. Mark Cline DVM, PhD, DACVP   Pathology/Comparative Medicine, Wake Forest School of Medicine, Winston-Salem, NC, USA

Lesley A. Colby DVM, DACLAM   Department of Comparative Medicine, University of Washington, Seattle, WA, USA

Patrick W. Concannon MS, PhD   Cornell University, Department of Biomedical Sciences, Ithaca, NY, USA

Lisa A. Conti DVM, MPH, Dipl ACVPM, CPM, CEHP   Global Health Solutions, Tallahassee, FL, USA

Leslie I. Curtin DVM   Laboratory Animal Services, Roswell Park Cancer Institute, Buffalo, NY, USA

Margaret L. Delano MS, DVM   Eli Lilly and Company, Indianapolis, Indiana, USA

Thomas M. Donnelly BVSc, DACLAM, DABVP, DECZM   French National Veterinary School of Alfort, du General de Gaulle, Maisons-Alfort, France

Raimon Duran-Struuck DVM, PhD, DACLAM Columbia Center of Translational Immunology, Department of Surgery; Institute of Comparative Medicine; Columbia University Medical Center, New York, NY, USA

Robert C. Dysko DVM, DACLAM Unit for Laboratory Animal Surgery, University of Michigan, Ann Arbor, MI, USA

Melissa C. Dyson DVM, DACLAM Unit for Laboratory Animal Medicine, University of Michigan, Ann Arbor, MI, USA

Michael Y. Esmail VMD Division of Comparative Medicine, Massachusetts Institute of Technology, Cambridge, MA, USA

Paula C. Ezell DVM, DACLAM Intuitive Surgical, Inc., Norcross, GA, USA

Michale S. Fee PhD Department of Brain and Cognitive Sciences, McGovern Institute, Massachusetts Institute of Technology, Cambridge, MA, USA

Carmen Ledesma Feliciano DVM Comparative Medicine Resident, Laboratory Animal Medicine, Colorado State University, Fort Collins, CO, USA

Paul Flecknell MA, VetMB, PhD, DECLAM, DLAS, DECVA, (Hon) DACLAM, (Hon) FRCVS Comparative Biology Medicine, Newcastle University, Newcastle Upon Tyne, UK

James G. Fox DVM, MS, DACLAM Division of Comparative Medicine, Massachusetts Institute of Technology, Cambridge, MA, USA

Craig L. Franklin DVM, PhD, DACLAM Department of Veterinary Pathobiology, University of Missouri, Columbia, MO, USA

Alexis Garcia DVM, BS Massachusetts Institute of Technology, Division of Comparative Medicine, Cambridge, MA, USA

Rose Gillesby DVM Veterinary Services and Biocontainment Research, Animal Research Support, Zoetis, Richland, MI, USA

Lou Ann Graham Department of Clinical Sciences, College of Veterinary Medicine, Cornell University, Ithaca, NY, USA

F. Claire Hankenson DVM, MS, DACLAM Michigan State University, Campus Animal Resources, East Lansing, MI, USA

John E. Harkness DVM, MS, MEd, Dipl, ACLAM College of Veterinary Medicine, Mississippi State University Mississippi State, MS, USA

Kristi L. Helke DVM, PhD, DACVP Departments of Comparative Medicine and Pathology and Laboratory Medicine, Medical University of South Carolina, Charleston, SC, USA

Hilda Holcombe DVM, PhD, DACLAM Massachusetts Institute of Technology Cambridge, MA, USA

William E. Hornbuckle DVM, BS Department of Clinical Sciences, College of Veterinary Medicine, Cornell University, Ithaca, NY, USA

Charlie C. Hsu VMD, PhD, DACLAM Department of Comparative Medicine, University of Washington, Seattle, WA, USA

Melanie Ihrig DVM, MS, DACLAM Comparative Medicine, Houston Methodist Research Institute, Houston, TX, USA

Carlisle P. Landel PhD Department of Microbiology, Immunology and Molecular Genetics, Transposagen Biopharmaceuticals Inc., University of Kentucky, Lexington, KY, USA

Rusty Lansford PhD Children's Hospital Los Angeles, Keck School of Medicine at USC, Saban Research Institute, Department of Radiology, Los Angeles, CA, USA

Christian Lawrence MS Aquatic Resources Program, Boston Children's Hospital, Boston, USA

Steven L. Leary DVM, DACLAM Veterinary Affairs, Division of Comparative Medicine, Washington University School of Medicine, St. Louis, MO, USA

Rafael Y. Lefkowitz MD, MPH Yale Occupational and Environmental Medicine Program, Yale University School of Medicine, New Haven, CT, USA

Kvin Lertpiriyapong DVM, PhD East Carolina University, The Brody School of Medicine, Moye Blvd, Greenville, NC, USA

Patrick A. Lester DVM, MS, DACLAM Unit for Laboratory Animal Surgery, University of Michigan, Ann Arbor, MI, USA

Neil S. Lipman VMD, DACLAM Center of Comparative Medicine and Pathology, Memorial Sloan Kettering Cancer Center and the Weill Medical College of Cornell University, New York, NY, USA; Veterinary Affairs, Division of Comparative Medicine, Washington University School of Medicine, St. Louis, MO, USA

Jennifer L.S. Lofgren DVM, MS, DACLAM Unit for Laboratory Animal Medicine, University of Michigan Medical School, Ann Arbor, MI, USA

Elizabeth R. Magden DVM, MS, DACLAM, cVMA Department of Veterinary Sciences, Michale E. Keeling Center for Comparative Medicine and Research, The University of Texas MD Anderson Cancer Center, Bastrop, TX, USA

Rachel D. Malcolm MS, BA The Jackson Laboratory, Diagnostic & GQC Laboratories, Bar Harbor, ME, USA

Keith G. Mansfield DVM, DACVP Discovery and Investigative Pathology, Novartis Institutes for Biomedical Research, Cambridge, MA, USA

Robert P. Marini DVM Division of Comparative Medicine, Massachusetts Institute of Technology, Cambridge, Massachusetts, MA, USA

Robert R. Marini DVM Division of Comparative Medicine, Massachusetts Institute of Technology, Cambridge, Massachusetts, MA, USA

Kirk J. Maurer DVM, PhD, ACLAM Center For Comparative Medicine and Research, Dartmouth College Lebanon, NH, USA

Joerg Mayer, Dr. med.vet., MSc, Dipl. ACZM, Dipl. ECZM (small mammal), Dipl. ABVP (ECM) College of Veterinary Medicine, University of Georgia Athens, Georgia

Joy A. Mench DPhil Department of Animal Science and Center for Animal Welfare, University of California, Davis, CA, USA

Marian G. Michaels MD, MPH Professor of Pediatrics and Surgery Children's Hospital of Pittsburgh of UPMC, Division of Infectious Diseases, Pittsburgh, PA, USA

Emily L. Miedel VMD University of Pennsylvania, University Laboratory Animal Resources, Philadelphia, PA, USA

Scott A. Mischler DVM, PhD, DACLAM Worldwide Comparative Medicine, Pfizer Inc., Middletown Rd., Pearl River, NY, USA

Daniel D. Myers DVM, MPH, DACLAM Unit for Laboratory Animal Surgery, University of Michigan, Ann Arbor, MI, USA

Jean A. Nemzek DVM, MS, DACVS Unit for Laboratory Animal Surgery, University of Michigan, Ann Arbor, MI, USA

Steven M. Niemi DVM, DACLAM Harvard University Faculty of Arts and Sciences, Cambridge, MA, USA

Megan H. Nowland DVM, BS, DACLAM University of Michigan, Unit for Laboratory Animal Medicine, Ann Arbor, MI, USA

Dorcas P. O'Rourke DVM, MS, DACLAM Department of Comparative Medicine, East Carolina University, The Brody School of Medicine, Moye Blvd, Greenville, NC, USA

Glen M. Otto DVM, DACLAM Animal Resources Center, University of Texas at Austin, Austin, TX, USA

Mary M. Patterson MS, DVM, DACLAM Division of Comparative Medicine, Massachusetts Institute of Technology, Cambridge, MA, USA

Kathleen R. Pritchett-Corning DVM, DACLAM, MRCVS Harvard University, Faculty of Arts and Sciences, and Department of Comparative Medicine, University of Washington, Cambridge, MA, USA

Fred W. Quimby VMD, PhD, ACLAM Rockefeller University, New Durham, NH, USA

Peter M. Rabinowitz MD, MPH University of Washington Center for One Health Research, Department of Environmental and Occupational Health Sciences, University of Washington School of Public Health, Seattle, WA, USA

Richard J. Rahija DVM, PhD, DACLAM Animal Resources Center, St. Jude Children's Research Hospital, Memphis, TN, USA

Carrie A. Redlich MD, MPH Yale Occupational and Environmental Medicine Program, Yale University School of Medicine, New Haven, CT, USA

Laura G. Reinholdt PhD The Jackson Laboratory, Bar Harbor, ME, USA

Matthew D. Rosenbaum DVM, MS, DACLAM National Jewish Health, Biological Resource Center, Denver, CO, USA

Lois Roth DVM, PhD, DACVP Department of Pathology, MSPCA Angell Memorial, Boston, MA, USA

Howard G. Rush DVM, MS, DACLAM University of Michigan, Unit for Laboratory Animal Medicine, Ann Arbor, MI, USA

Trenton R. Schoeb DVM, PhD, DACVP Department of Genetics, Comparative Pathology Laboratory, Animal Resources Program, UAB Gnotobiotic Facility, University of Alabama at Birmingham, Birmingham, AL, USA

Adam Schoell DVM, DACLAM Zoetis, Portage St, Kalamazoo, MI, USA

Fabrizio C. Serluca PhD, BSc Novartis Institutes for Biomedical Research, Cambridge, MA, USA

Sandra Sexton DVM, DACLAM Laboratory Animal Services, Roswell Park Cancer Institute, Buffalo, NY, USA

William R. Shek DVM, PhD Research Animal Diagnostics, Charles River Laboratories, Wilmington, MA, USA

Nirah H. Shomer DVM, PhD, DACLAM Laboratory Animal Resources, Merck Research Laboratories, Boston, MA, USA

Joe H. Simmons DVM, PhD, DACLAM Insight Diagnostics & Consulting, Pearland, TX, USA

Abigail L. Smith MPH, PhD Department of Pathobiology, University of Pennsylvania School of Veterinary Medicine, Philadelphia, PA, USA

Michael K. Stoskopf DVM, PhD, DACZM Department of Clinical Sciences and Director of the Environmental Medicine Consortium, College of Veterinary Medicine, North Carolina State University, William Moore Dr. Raleigh, NC, USA

Marjorie C. Strobel PhD JAX Mice & Clinical Research Services, The Jackson Laboratory, Bar Harbor, ME, USA

James R. Swearengen DVM, DACLAM, DACVPM National Biodefense Analysis and Countermeasures Center, Research Plaza, Fort Detrick, MD, USA

M. Michael Swindle DVM, DACLAM, DECLAM Medical University of South Carolina, Department of Comparative Medicine and Department of Surgery, Charleston, SC, USA

Michael R. Talcott Division of Comparative Medicine, Veterinary Surgical Services, Washington University School of Medicine, St. Louis, Missouri, USA

Bud C. Tennant DVM, DACVIM Department of Clinical Sciences, College of Veterinary Medicine, Cornell University, Ithaca, NY, USA

Wendy J. Underwood DVM, MS, DACVIM Eli Lilly and Company, Indianapolis, Indiana, USA

Sue VandeWoude DVM, DACLAM Department of Micro-, Immuno- and Pathology, College of Veterinary Medicine and Biomedical Sciences, Colorado State University, Fort Collins, CO, USA

Benjamin J. Weigler DVM, MPH, PhD Washington National Primate Research Center, University of Washington, Seattle, Washington, USA

Mark T. Whary DVM, PhD, DACLAM Division of Comparative Medicine, Massachusetts Institute of Technology, Cambridge, MA, USA

Colette L. Wheler BSc, DVM, MVetSc VIDO-InterVac, University of Saskatchewan, Saskatoon, SK, Canada

Ronald P. Wilson VMD, MS Penn State College of Medicine, Department of Comparative Medicine, Hershey, PA, USA

Christina Winnicker DVM, MPH, DACLAM Enrichment & Behavioral Medicine, Department of Animal Welfare, Charles River Laboratories, Wilmington, MA, USA

A. Marissa Wolfe DVM Department of Comparative Medicine, Medical University of South Carolina, Charleston, SC, USA

Preface to the Third Edition

The American College of Laboratory Animal Medicine (ACLAM) was founded in 1957 to encourage education, training, and research in laboratory animal medicine and to recognize veterinary medical specialists in the field by certification and other means. Continuing education has been an important activity in ACLAM from its inception. The third edition of this teaching text, *Laboratory Animal Medicine* (first edition published in 1984 and the second edition in 2002), reflects the College's continuing effort to foster education. It is, in part, an updated distillation for teaching purposes of a series of volumes on laboratory animals developed by ACLAM over the past four decades: *The Biology of the Laboratory Rabbit* published in 1974, with a second edition in 1994, *The Biology of the Guinea Pig* in 1976, and a two-volume work, *Biology of the Laboratory Rat* in 1979 and 1980, and a second edition in 2006. The publication *Laboratory Hamsters* appeared in 1987. In 1979, the college published a two-volume text on *Spontaneous Animal Models of Human Disease*. In 1981–1983, four volumes of *The Mouse in Biomedical Research* were published, followed by four updated volumes in 2007. A two-volume treatise on *Nonhuman Primates in Biomedical Research* was published in 1995 (Vol. 1) and 1998 (Vol. 2), a second edition in 2012, and a text *Anesthesia and Analgesia in Laboratory Animals* in 1997 followed by a second edition in 2008. *Flynn's Parasites of Laboratory Animals* came out in 2007. *Planning and Design of Research Animal Facilities* was published in 2009; *Biology and Medicine of Rabbits and Rodents, 5th Edition* was published in 2010, *The Laboratory Rabbit, Guinea Pig, Hamster and Other Rodents* was published in 2012, *Laboratory Animal Welfare* in 2013; and most recently, the third edition of *Biology and Diseases of the Ferret* was published in 2014. Finally, the newest in the series, *Swine in the Laboratory: Surgery, Anesthesia, Imaging, and Experimental Techniques, 3E*, is expected in 2015.

Most major advances in biology and medicine in one way or another have depended on the study of animals. During the past generation, the health, genetic integrity, and environmental surroundings of the animals have been recognized as important factors to be taken into account in planning animal studies. The ultimate responsibility for ensuring the validity of scientific results, together with humane and scientifically appropriate animal care, resides with two categories of scientists: veterinarians responsible for the acquisition, care, nutrition, anesthesia, and other aspects of humane animal use and scientific investigators, their staff and students, who use animals as subjects of study. This book therefore is intended for these individuals and others in the fields of biology and medicine who utilize animals in biomedical research. The editors and contributors are particularly hopeful that the text will prove useful in introducing students and scientists embarking on their careers to important concepts related to animals in research.

The contents of this third edition have been greatly expanded and are presented in 39 chapters that provide information on the diseases and biology of the major species of laboratory animals used in biomedical research. The history of laboratory animal medicine, legislation affecting laboratory animals, experimental methods and techniques, design and management of animal facilities, zoonoses, biohazards, and animal models are also covered. Reflective of the ever-increasing use and ease of constructing of genetically engineered animals, chapters include transgenic and knockout mice and genetic monitoring. Rodent and lagomorph surveillance and quality assurance are also included. Also added are chapters dealing with the emerging interest in fish, bird, amphibian, and reptile biology and diseases. The editors acknowledge and thank the contributors' outstanding efforts to follow the guidelines on content and accept sole responsibility for any significant omissions.

As with all volumes of the ACLAM series texts, the contributors and editors of this book have donated publication royalties to the ACLAM to foster continuing education in laboratory animal science. It could not have been completed without the support and resources of the editors' parent institutions. Special thanks are also extended to the reviewers of each chapter, whose excellent and thoughtful suggestions helped the authors and editors present the material in a meaningful and concise manner. We acknowledge and thank Lucille Wilhelm and Alyssa Terestre for their excellent secretarial assistance. The assistance of the staff of Elsevier, particularly Mary Preap, also is greatly appreciated and acknowledged.

James G. Fox, Lynn C. Anderson, Glen Otto,
Kathleen Pritchett-Corning and Mark T. Whary

CHAPTER

1

Laboratory Animal Medicine: Historical Perspectives

*James G. Fox, DVM, MS, DACLAM[a] and
B. Taylor Bennett, DVM, PhD[b]*

[a]Division of Comparative Medicine, Massachusetts Institute of Technology, Cambridge, MA, USA
[b]Management Consultant, Hinsdale, IL, USA

I. INTRODUCTION

Five key terms identify the fields or activities that relate to the care and use of animals in research, education, and testing. *Animal experimentation* refers to the scientific study of animals, usually in a laboratory, for the purpose of gaining new biological knowledge or solving specific medical, veterinary medical, dental, or biological problems. Most commonly, such experimentation is carried out by or under the direction of persons holding research or professional degrees. *Laboratory animal care* is the application of veterinary medicine and animal science to the acquisition

Laboratory Animal Medicine, Third Edition
DOI: http://dx.doi.org/10.1016/B978-0-12-409527-4.00001-8

1

of laboratory animals and to their management, nutrition, breeding, and diseases. The term also relates to the care that is provided to animals as an aid in managing pain and distress. Laboratory animal care is usually provided in scientific institutions under veterinary supervision or guidance. *Laboratory animal medicine* is recognized by the American Veterinary Medical Association as the specialty field within veterinary medicine that is concerned with the diagnosis, treatment, and prevention of diseases in animals used as subjects in biomedical activities. Laboratory animal medicine also encompasses the methods of minimizing and preventing pain or distress in research animals and identifying complicating factors in animal research. *Comparative medicine* is "the study of the nature, cause and cure of abnormal structure and function in people, animals and plants for the eventual application to and benefit of all living things" (Bustad *et al.*, 1976). *Laboratory animal science* is the body of scientific and technical information, knowledge, and skills that bears on both laboratory animal care and laboratory animal medicine and that is roughly analogous to *animal science* in the agricultural sector.

Laboratory animal medicine has grown rapidly because of its inherent scientific importance and because good science and the public interest require the best possible care for laboratory animals. In this chapter, we trace briefly the historical evolution of laboratory animal medicine and consider its relationship to other areas of biology and medicine.

II. ORIGINS OF ANIMAL EXPERIMENTATION

The earliest references to animal experimentation are to be found in the writings of Greek philosopher-physicians of the fourth and third centuries BC. Aristotle (384–322 BC), characterized as the founder of biology, was the first to conduct dissections that revealed internal differences among animals (Wood, 1931). Erasistratus (304–250 BC) was probably the first to perform experiments on living animals, as we understand them today. He established in pigs that the trachea was an air tube

and the lungs were pneumatic organs (Fisher, 1881). Later, Galen (AD 130–200) performed anatomical dissections of pigs, monkeys, and many other species (Cohen and Drabkin, 1948; Cohen, 1959a). He justified experimentation as a long, arduous path to the truth, believing that uncontrolled assertion that was not based on experimentation could not lead to scientific progress. Dogma replaced experimentation in the dark centuries following Galen's lifetime. Whereas anatomical dissection of dead animals and people had been among the earliest types of experimentation, in medieval times this practice was prohibited by ecclesiastical authorities who wanted to prevent acquisition of knowledge about the natural world that could be considered blasphemous. Not until the 1500s was there a reawakening of interest in science. Andreas Vesalius (1514–1564), the founder of modern anatomy, used dogs and pigs in public anatomical demonstrations (Saunders and O'Malley, 1950) (Fig. 1.1). This *vivisection* led to great leaps in the understanding of anatomy's correspondence with physiology. In 1628, Sir William Harvey published his great work on the movement of the heart and blood in animals (Harvey, 2001; Singer, 1957). By the early 1700s, Stephen Hales, an English clergyman, reported the first measurement of blood pressure, using as his subject a horse "fourteen hands high, and about fourteen years of age, [and with] a fistula on her withers" (Hoff *et al.*, 1965) (Fig. 1.2). During the 1800s, France became a primary center of experimental biology and medicine. Scientists, such as François Magendie (1783–1855) and Claude Bernard (1813–1878) (Fig. 1.3) in experimental physiology and Louis Pasteur (1822–1895) in microbiology, contributed enormously to the validation of the scientific method, which included the use of animals. Bernard (1865) commented:

> ... it is proper to choose certain animals which offer favorable anatomical arrangements or special susceptibility to certain influences. For each kind of investigation we shall be careful to point out the proper choice of animals. This is so important that the solution of a physiological or pathological problem often depends solely on the appropriate choice of the animal for the experiment so as to make the result clear and searching.

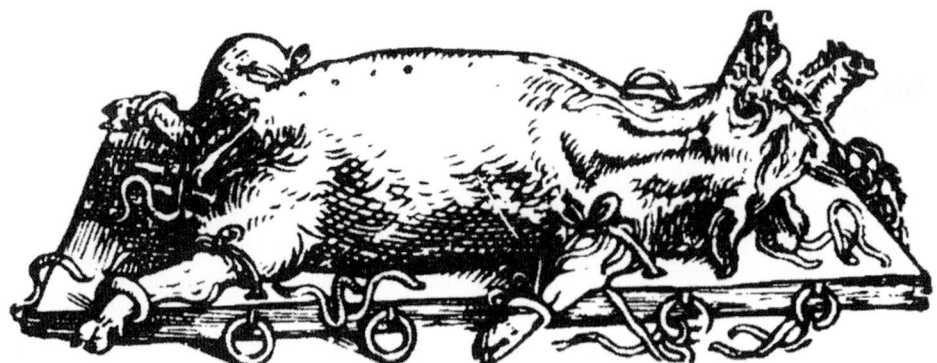

FIGURE 1.1   Illustration by Andreas Vesalius. Pig tied to dissection board *for the administration of vivisections. From Saunders and O'Malley, 1950.*

Statical ESSAYS:

CONTAINING

HÆMASTATICKS;

OR,

An Account of fome HYDRAULICK and HYDROSTATICAL Experiments made on the Blood and Blood-Veffels of Animals.

ALSO

An Account of fome Experiments on Stones in the Kidneys and Bladder; with an Enquiry into the Nature of thofe anomalous Concretions.

To which is added,

An *APPENDIX*,

CONTAINING

OBSERVATIONS and EXPERIMENTS relating to feveral Subjects in the firft Volume. The greateft Part of which were read at feveral Meetings before the Royal Society.

With an INDEX to both VOLUMES.

VOL. II.

Defideratur Philofophia Naturalis vera & aƈtiva cui Medicinæ Scientia inedificetur.
Fran. de Verul. Inftaur. Magna.

By *STEPHEN HALES*, B.D. F.R.S.
Reƈtor of *Farringdon*, *Hampfhire*, and Minifter of *Teddington*, *Middlefex*.

LONDON:

Printed for W. INNYS and R. MANBY, at the Weft-End of St. *Paul's*;
And T. WOODWARD, at the *Half Moon* between the Temple-Gates, *Fleetftreet*. MDCCXXXIII.

FIGURE 1.2   Title page from "Statical Essays" (Hales, 1740).

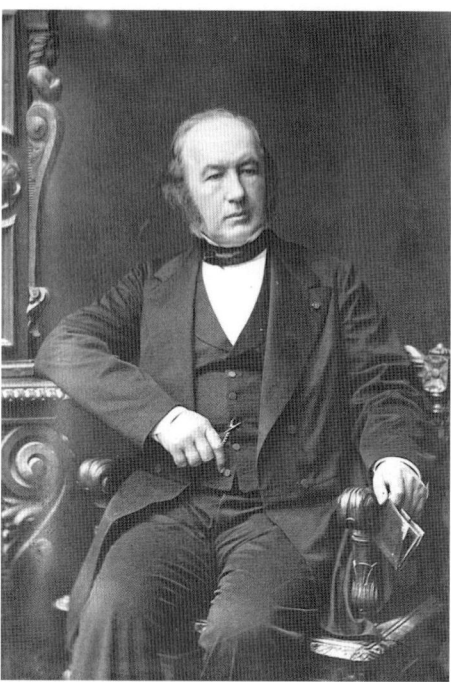

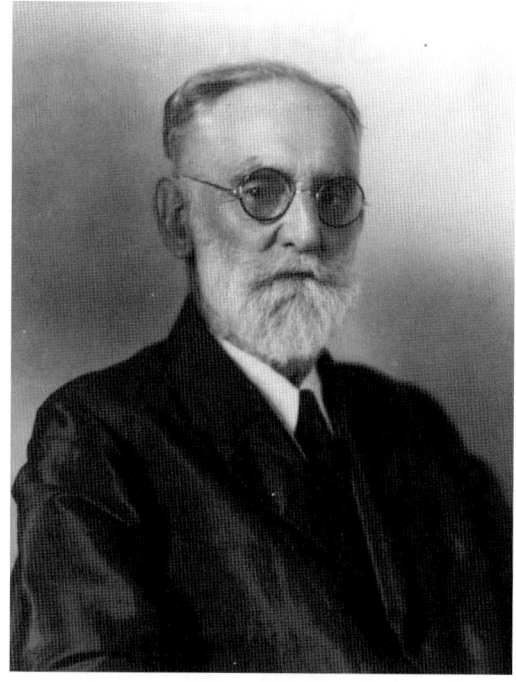

FIGURE 1.3   Claude Bernard, often referred to as the founder of experimental medicine, developed and described highly sophisticated methods of animal research in his laboratory in Paris. *Photograph from Garrison (1929).*

FIGURE 1.4   Dr. Cooper Curtice. Curtice contributed importantly to the demonstration that arthropods can act as carriers of mammalian diseases. *Courtesy of The Nation's Business.*

Pasteur studied infectious diseases in a variety of animals, such as silkworms (*pebrine*), dogs (rabies), and sheep (anthrax). *Pebrine* (pepper) was an economically important disease of silkworms in France when silk was a major fabric; Pasteur and others demonstrated the parasite that caused the disease (Duclaux, 1920). As pathogenic organisms were identified that could be related to specific human diseases, their animal disease counterparts also were studied. Pasteur and others perceived that the study of animal diseases benefited animals and enhanced the understanding of human diseases and pathology. The extraordinary power of the experimental approach, including experiments on animals, led to what has been called the *Golden Age* of scientific medicine. Despite advances in physiological and bacteriological understanding, criticisms of the use of animals in science began, particularly in England (Loew, 1982). The first Society for the Prevention of Cruelty to Animals (SPCA) was established in England, followed in the 1860s by an American SPCA in New York, a Philadelphia SPCA, and a Massachusetts SPCA. Objections to the use of animals in science were part of the concerns of these societies, particularly because Darwin's findings on evolution made *differences* between animals and humans less sure in many persons' minds (Loew, 1982).

Most American and Canadian scientists, physicians, and veterinarians soon applied emerging scientific concepts in their research. D.E. Salmon, recipient of the first

D.V.M. degree awarded in the United States (by Cornell University in 1879), studied bacterial diseases, and the genus *Salmonella*, a ubiquitous human and animal pathogen, was named for him. Cooper Curtice (Fig. 1.4), Theobald Smith, and others first demonstrated the role of arthropod victors in disease transmission in their studies of bovine Texas fever (Schwabe, 1978). The first paper published at the then fledgling Johns Hopkins Hospital and School of Medicine was by the physician William H. Welch, for whom *Clostridium welchii* was named, and was entitled "Preliminary Report of Investigations Concerning the Causation of Hog Cholera" (Welch, 1889). Thus, it became evident that the study of the naturally occurring diseases of animals could illuminate principles applicable to both animals and mankind, and lead to improved understanding of biology in general.

John Call Dalton, M.D. (1825–1889), an American physiologist, spent a year in Bernard's laboratory in Paris around 1850. He was highly impressed with Bernard's instructional methods, which included demonstrations of important physiological principles in living animals. Subsequently, Dr. Dalton included such demonstrations in his teaching at the College of Physicians and Surgeons in New York City (Mitchell, 1895), the forerunner of the *animal labs* in which generations of students in biology and medicine were once trained. When Alexis Carrel received the Nobel Prize in 1912, the citation stated in part: "... you have ...

proved once again that the development of an applied science of surgery follows the lessons learned from animal experimentation" (Malinin, 1979). Thus, starting in ancient times and continuing to the present day, animal experimentation has been one of the fundamental approaches of the scientific method in biological and medical research and education.

III. EARLY VETERINARIANS IN LABORATORY ANIMAL SCIENCE AND MEDICINE

On September 15, 1915, Dr. Simon D. Brimhall (1863–1941; V.M.D., University of Pennsylvania, 1889) (Fig. 1.5) joined the staff of the Mayo Clinic in Rochester, Minnesota, the first veterinarian to fill a position in laboratory animal medicine at an American medical research institution (Cohen, 1959b; Physicians of the Mayo Clinic and the Mayo Foundation, 1937). No such field was recognized at the time, of course; but Dr. Brimhall's activities – management of the animal facilities, development of animal breeding colonies, investigation of laboratory animal diseases (Brimhall and Mann, 1917; Brimhall and Hardenbergh, 1922), and participation in collaborative and independent research (Brimhall *et al.*, 1919–1920) – were the prototype of the present role of *laboratory animal veterinarians* in scientific institutions throughout the world.

The decision to employ a veterinarian at the Mayo Clinic in 1915 appears to have resulted from a unique juxtaposition of institutional needs and personalities. Although the Mayo Clinic was already world renowned, organized research was in only a rudimentary stage of development. Around 1910, an unsuccessful effort was made to convert an old barn, belonging to the chief of surgical pathology, Dr. Louis B. Wilson, for animal experimentation (Braasch, 1969). Then, in 1914, with Dr. William J. Mayo's active encouragement, the Division of Experimental Surgery and Pathology was created, the first real research laboratory at the clinic. Dr. Frank C. Mann, a young medical scientist from Indiana, was invited to head the division, with the primary assignment of developing a first-class animal research laboratory. Dr. Brimhall's employment followed within a year and was accompanied by the planning and ultimate construction of new animal facilities (Figs 1.6 and 1.7). Christopher Graham, M.D., then head of the Division of Medicine, greatly influenced the decision to employ Dr. Brimhall. Perhaps the fact that Dr. Graham was also a veterinarian (V.M.D., University of Pennsylvania, 1892) provided insights into the contributions that veterinary medicine could make to experimental surgery and pathology. Certainly, the concept of mutual support among the professions was not at

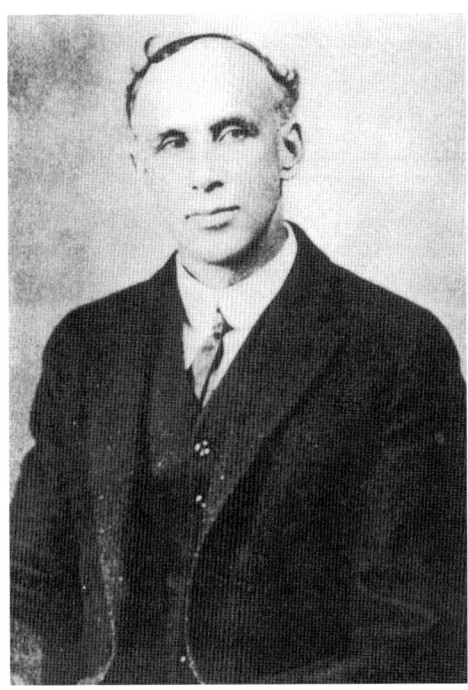

FIGURE 1.5 Simon D. Brimhall, V.M.D., the first veterinarian in laboratory animal medicine at an American medical research institution, worked at the Mayo Clinic from 1915 to 1922. *Courtesy of University of Minnesota Press and Dr. Paul E. Zollman.*

that time widely held; there was, in fact, relatively little interprofessional communication between medicine and veterinary medicine.

Dr. Brimhall retired in 1922 and was succeeded by Dr. John G. Hardenbergh (1892–1963; V.M.D., University of Pennsylvania, 1916). During his 5-year tenure at the Mayo Clinic, Dr. Hardenbergh was an active clinical investigator (Hardenbergh, 1926–1927) as well as animal facility manager. In a stout defense of animal experimentation, he also demonstrated the communication skills in the public arena that were to serve him well later in his career (1941–1958) as executive secretary of the American Veterinary Medical Association (Hardenbergh, 1923).

Dr. Carl F. Schlotthauer (1893–1959; D.V.M., St. Joseph Veterinary College, 1923), who had joined the Mayo Clinic staff in 1924 as assistant in veterinary medicine, succeeded Dr. Hardenbergh in 1927. By this time, the Mayo Foundation was functioning as the graduate medical education and research arm of the Mayo Clinic and had become formally affiliated with the University of Minnesota. Dr. Schlotthauer ultimately became head of the Section of Veterinary Medicine at the Mayo Foundation (1952) and professor of veterinary medicine at the University of Minnesota Graduate School (1945). Thus, he was the first veterinarian to attain a full professorship for laboratory animal medicine-related academic activities. He vigorously opposed antivivisectionist

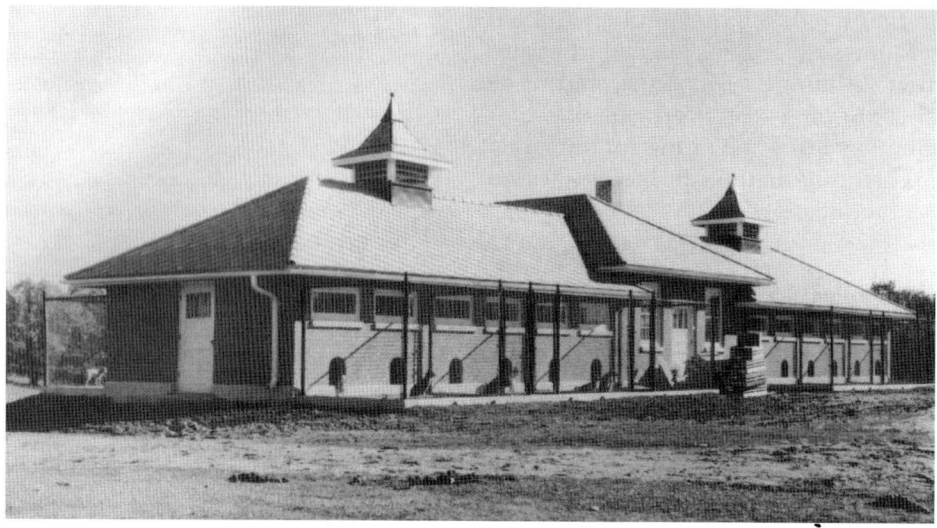

FIGURE 1.6   Dog breeding facility, Institute of Experimental Medicine, Mayo Clinic, constructed in the mid-1920s. *Courtesy of Dr. Paul E. Zollman.*

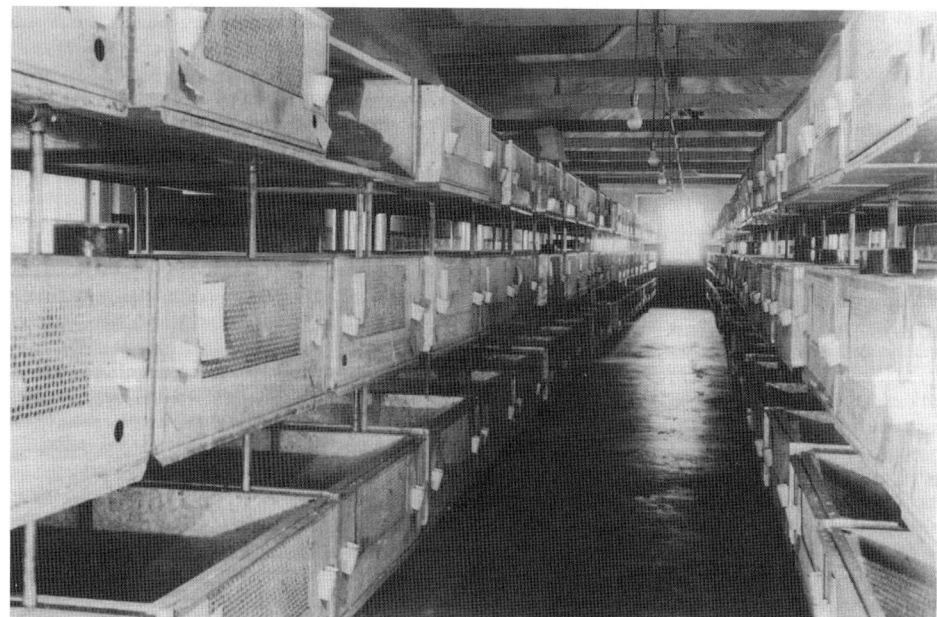

FIGURE 1.7   Interior of guinea pig breeding house, Institute of Experimental Medicine, Mayo Clinic, constructed in the early 1920s. *Courtesy of Dr. Paul E. Zollman.*

attacks on animal research. He was a leader in the state-wide campaign that led to adoption of the Minnesota *pound law* in 1950, i.e., a law authorizing the requisitioning for research and education by approved scientific institutions of impounded, but unclaimed dogs and cats. Dr. Schlotthauer believed that open and honest communication between medical scientists and humane society workers could lead to better public understanding and support of animal research. Consequently, he was also active in humane society activities, serving for many years on the board of directors of the Minnesota Society

for the Prevention of Cruelty to Animals. He also was an important figure in the early years of the American Association for Laboratory Animal Science (AALAS). He was a founding member of its board of directors and presented a paper on animal procurement at its first meeting in 1950 (Schlotthauer, 1950).

Although other veterinarians also held appointments at the Mayo Foundation between 1915 and 1950, Drs. Brimhall, Hardenbergh, and Schlotthauer were the ones most closely associated with activities that today are identified with laboratory animal medicine.

It is noteworthy that the Mayo Clinic/Foundation has maintained a program in animal medicine continuously for more than 95 years, having initiated it long before most medical research institutions were prepared even to consider the possible value of adding veterinarians to their professional staff (P.E. Zollman, personal communication, 1982).

Dr. Karl F. Meyer (1884–1974; D.V.M., University of Zurich, 1924; M.D. [honorary], College of Medical Evangelists, 1936) was an internationally known epidemiologist, bacteriologist, and pathologist. Dr. Meyer was intensely interested in matters related to laboratory animals for most of his professional life. He was the author of an early review of laboratory animal diseases (Meyer, 1928), one of the first publications of its kind in the United States. He was a unique personality (vigorous, dynamic, active); a world traveler on missions related to international health; and a scientist who engendered in his students respect, admiration, love, and fear in varying proportions. Together with his longtime associate Bernice Eddy (Ph.D.), a bacteriologist, Dr. Meyer developed a model animal facility at the George Williams Hooper Foundation at the University of California, San Francisco, during a 30-year tenure as director (1924–1954). Dr. Meyer was often away from the laboratory, and it fell to Dr. Eddy to supervise the animal facility, which she did with great skill and dedication. Dr. Meyer foresaw the need for and was an early advocate of the participation of veterinarians in the operation of institutional laboratory animal colonies (Meyer, 1958). He figured importantly in the planning that led the University of California to create the position of *statewide veterinarian* in 1953, which subsequently was superseded by the appointment of veterinarians at each of the university's major campuses. Among his many honors, Dr. Meyer received the Charles A. Griffin Award of AALAS in 1959.

Dr. Charles A. Griffin (1889–1955; D.V.M., Cornell University, 1913) was a bacteriologist at the New York State Board of Health, Division of Laboratories, Albany, New York, from 1919 to 1954. Dr. Griffin pioneered the concept of the development of *disease-free* animal colonies long before gnotobiotic technology had evolved (Brewer, 1980). In the 1940s, he utilized progeny testing to establish a rabbit colony free of pasteurellosis. Additionally, he showed that *Salmonella* spp. could be transmitted in meat meal (Griffin, 1952). This led feed manufacturers to improve the processing of laboratory animal diets so as to eliminate *Salmonella* contamination. The Charles A. Griffin Award of AALAS was established and named in Dr. Griffin's honor (Table 1.1). He received the award posthumously in 1955, the first recipient of this prestigious award. The Griffin Laboratory at the New York State Board of Health central facility in Albany, New York, also is named in his honor.

Dr. Nathan R. Brewer (1904–2009; D.V.M., Michigan State University, 1937; Ph.D., University of Chicago, 1936) headed the laboratory animal facilities at the University of Chicago from 1945 until his retirement in 1969 (Fig. 1.8). Dr. Brewer's interest in laboratory animals began in the mid-1920s, when he started veterinary school, and continued during his graduate student years in the Department of Physiology at the University of Chicago. Around 1935, Professors Anton J. Carlson (Ingle, 1979) and A.B. Luckhardt first approached Dr. Brewer about managing the University of Chicago animal facilities. They saw merit in the concept of a veterinarian, well grounded in the scientific method, as animal facility manager. They believed this arrangement would contribute to public confidence in the care and treatment of animals in research, and would help to turn aside antivivisection activists. However, many investigators at the university feared that a veterinarian would dictate the conditions of care and use of animals, and they opposed the creation of this position. It was not until 1945 that this opposition was overcome, and Dr. Brewer became supervisor of the Central Animal Quarters. Laboratory animal medicine began its modern evolution in the following years. Dr. Brewer's role was seminal – as a founder of the American Association for Laboratory Animal Science, as the first president of the AALAS (1950–1955), and as a *father figure* for the then youthful group of veterinarians that had been employed by other medical schools and medical research institutions in the Chicago area between 1945 and 1949. Dr. Brewer received the AALAS Griffin Award in 1962. After his retirement in 1969, he remained active and attended local and national AALAS meetings up until his death at the age of 104. To honor his contributions to the field, the AALAS instituted an annual award in 1994, the Nathan Brewer Scientific Achievement Award. In 2005, at the age of 100, the American College of Laboratory Animal Medicine (ACLAM) presented him with a lifetime achievement award, which subsequently became the ACLAM's Nathan R. Brewer Career Achievement Award in 2006.

Dr. Bennett Cohen (1925–1990; D.V.M., Cornell University Veterinary School, 1949; Ph.D., Northwestern Medical School, 1953) was the director of the vivarium at the University of California Medical School in Los Angeles (Fig. 1.9). He was subsequently recruited to the University of Michigan where he founded the Unit for Laboratory Animal Medicine at the University of Michigan and was its director for 23 years. He obtained the rank of Professor of Laboratory Animal Medicine in 1968.

Dr. Cohen was a pioneer and visionary in the field of laboratory animal science for over 40 years. His career of caring for animals used in medical research began at Northwestern University in 1949. A year later, he and veterinary colleagues in the Chicago area founded

TABLE 1.1   Charles A. Griffin Award Recipients

Year	Recipient	Year	Recipient
1956	Charles A. Griffin	1986	Gerald L. Van Hoosier
1957	James A. Reyniers	1987	Orland A. Soave
1958	John B. Nelson	1988	Pravin N. Bhatt
1959	Robert D. Henthorne	1989	Dennis M. Stark
1960	Nathan R. Brewer	1990	Steven H. Weisbroth
1961	Karl Frederich Meyer	1991	Steven P. Pakes
1962	George D. Snell	1992	J. Derrell Clark
1963	C.N. Wentworth Cumming	1993	Robert O. Jacoby
1964	Phillip C. Trexler	1994	Harry Rozmiarek
1965	W.T.S. Thorp	1995	Leo A. Whitehair
1966	Bennett J. Cohen	1996	Henry Baker
1967	James R.M. Innes	1997	Joseph E. Wagner
1968	Robert J. Flynn	1998	Thomas E. Hamm
1969	Melvin M. Rabstein	1999	Steele F. Mattingly
1970	Willard H. Eyestone	2000	Charles A. Montgomery
1971	William I. Gay	2001	Ronald McLaughlin
1972	Lisbeth M. Kraft	2002	Jack R. Hessler
1973	L.R. Christensen	2003	Clarence Reeder and Joseph Mayo
1974	George R. Collins	2004	James E. Corbin
1975	Eleanore E. Storrs	2005	Jerry Fineg
1976	Henry L. Foster	2006	Alvin Moreland
1977	Thomas B. Clarkson	2007	Not presented
1978	Wilhelmina F. Dunning	2008	James G. Fox
1979	John C. Parker	2009	Richard C. Simmonds
1980	Charles W. McPherson	2010	William White
1981	Daniel H. Ringler	2011	Fred Quimby
1982	Charles C. Hunter	2012	Marilyn J. Brown
1983	Jules S. Cass	2013	Steven L. Leary
1984	James R. Ganaway	2014	Mark A. Suckow
1985	Patrick J. Manning		

the Animal Care Panel (ACP), which later became the AALAS. He served as the Association's first secretary, as a member of the board of trustees, and later as president. Three years later, he and a few colleagues saw the need to establish standards of training and experience for veterinarians engaged in laboratory animal medicine. They convinced the American Veterinary Medical Association to accept the veterinary specialty of laboratory animal medicine and establish a specialty certification board. This became the ACLAM. In 2013, there were over 900 board-certified veterinarians in the United States.

In 1963, Dr. Cohen chaired the National Academy of Sciences committee that wrote the first edition of the document that later became *The Guide for Care and Use of Laboratory Animals*. Since then, hundreds of thousands of copies have been distributed, and it has been accepted as a primary reference on laboratory animal care and use. The National Institutes of Health (NIH) now requires that awardee institutions comply with the provisions of the Guide.

Dr. Cohen was the recipient of all of the major national and international awards in laboratory animal

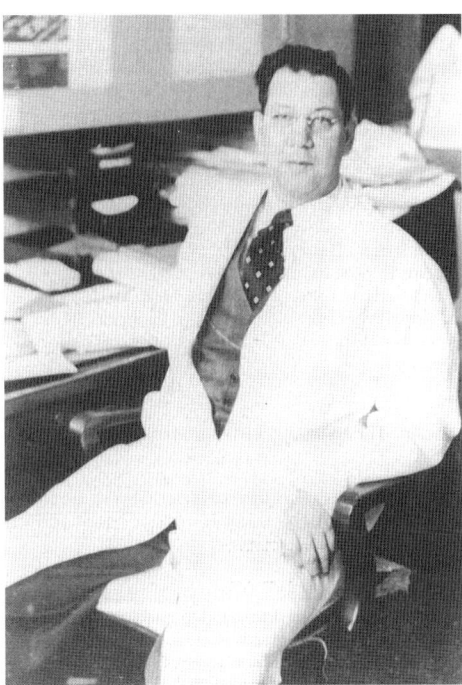

FIGURE 1.8   Dr. Nathan R. Brewer, director of the Central Animal Quarters at the University of Chicago (1945–1969) and first president of the American Association for Laboratory Animal Science. Photograph taken in the late 1940s. *Courtesy of Dr. N. R. Brewer.*

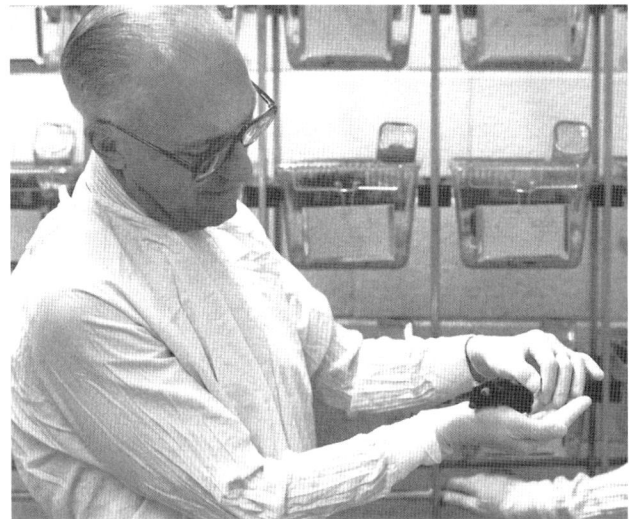

FIGURE 1.9   Dr. Bennett Cohen, a pioneer and visionary in the field of laboratory animal science.

science. In 1966, he received the Griffin Award from the American Association for Laboratory Animal Science. This, the association's highest award, was presented for "Outstanding Accomplishments in the Improvement of Care and Quality of Laboratory Animals." In 1980, he received the Charles River Prize, the highest award of the American Veterinary Medical Association. The inscription reads, "You have been a moving force in laboratory animal science and a major figure in the founding of national organizations that have brought strength, cohesion and credibility to the field." In 1990, the Governing Board of the International Council for Laboratory Animal Science (ICLAS) presented Dr. Cohen with the Council's highest award, the Muhlbock Award, for his work in establishing high standards of laboratory animal care and use worldwide.

In 1991, the Association for Assessment and Accreditation of Laboratory Animal Care International bestowed an award in Dr. Cohen's name, the Bennett J. Cohen Educational Leadership Award. This award recognizes individuals whose activities and attitudes promote the understanding of biomedical research, science education, and public and animal health.

Dr. Cohen also established a national reputation in the field of gerontology. He originated health standards for aging animals and undertook long-term studies of rodent diseases of aging. At the University of Michigan,

he established the Core Facility for Aged Rodents (CFAR) in the Institute of Gerontology and the Gerontology Research and Training Center. The CFAR provided aged rodents for study by scientists campus-wide.

An additional and lasting legacy of Cohen's impact on laboratory animal medicine is the stellar record he achieved in training future generations of specialists in the field. He trained numerous postdoctoral veterinary fellows from 1959 to 1985. Dr. Cohen was originally awarded the NIH training grant while at University of California, Los Angeles (UCLA) in 1960 and transferred the training grant to Ann Arbor when he relocated to the University of Michigan in 1962. It remains recognized internationally for its record of excellence.

Dr. Thomas Clarkson (D.V.M., University of Georgia, 1954) was employed in the pharmaceutical industry for 3 years. He was then recruited to the Wake Forest School of Medicine, then known as Bowman Gray. At Bowman Gray, he directed the vivarium and was an assistant professor of Experimental Medicine (Fig. 1.10). He was promoted to associate professor in 1960 and full professor in 1967. He was chairman of the Department of Comparative Medicine from 1967 to 1979.

Over the course of Dr. Clarkson's 55-year remarkable career as a pioneer in comparative medicine and women's health, Clarkson's research with nonhuman primates moved through a broad range of topics: the effects of cholesterol on atherosclerosis; the effects of social behavior on primate health, especially the influence of stress as a contributor to heart disease; and the study of heart disease in postmenopausal female monkeys. The breadth of Dr. Clarkson's investigations of the relationship among diet, body fat distribution, social factors and hormones on the chronic diseases affecting

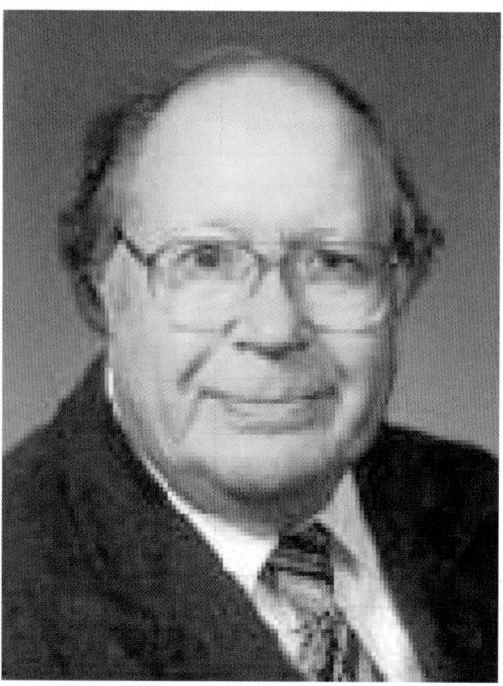

FIGURE 1.10   Dr. Thomas Clarkson, a pioneer in comparative medicine and women's health.

older women is remarkable and a significant legacy to biomedical science.

Dr. Clarkson has served on numerous editorial boards and advisory committees for academia and government. He is the recipient of numerous awards, including the Griffin Award of the American Association for Laboratory Animal Science, the Charles River Prize of the American Veterinary Medical Association, the Albert B. Sabin Heroes of Science Award, and the American College of Laboratory Animal Medicine Mentor Award. Of special note, Dr. Clarkson is one among a few veterinarians who have been elected to the Institute of Medicine of the National Academies of Science.

Dr. Clarkson believed that teaching was central to the mission of academia, and he put the same record of leadership into training others as he did his own research. Importantly, he played a pivotal role in promoting and spearheading formal guidelines for training veterinarians for careers in laboratory animal medicine and biomedical research (Clarkson, 1961b, 1965, 1967). The training program he founded in comparative medicine marked its 53rd consecutive year of NIH funding in 2012, making it the longest continuously supported training program in the nation.

Other personalities that played important roles in the early history of laboratory animal science and medicine have been characterized and their roles assessed by Brewer (1980).

IV. THE ORGANIZATIONS OF LABORATORY ANIMAL SCIENCE

A. Background

Organizations are important in scientific life as a means of implementing the content and activities of the fields they represent. Present-day students of laboratory animal science are confronted with a confusing array of organizational acronyms: AAALAC International, AALAS, ACLAM, ASLAP, APV CALAS, ILAR, ICLAS, NABR, FBR, and so on. It is instructive to examine why organizations such as these came into being and to evaluate their impact on laboratory animal science.

Consider the environment for research in biology and medicine in the United States around 1945. A new national policy was just being initiated to provide increased federal support of science. The use of laboratory animals began to expand rapidly as the funding of medical and biological research increased, and a host of problems as well as challenges accompanied this development. The knowledge base regarding the care and diseases of laboratory animals was small. Published information was scattered and sparse. Few veterinarians were devoting themselves to *laboratory animal care*, which was not yet recognized as a special field. In many institutions, animal facilities and administrative arrangements for operating them were poor. Institutions were ill prepared to accommodate increasingly large animal colonies. Simultaneously, medical scientists were under increasingly vigorous attack from antivivisectionists whose objective was to stop or limit animal research. It became essential for scientists both to confront their persistent critics and to face up to the problems they knew existed.

The Chicago area was a hotbed of antivivisection activity in 1945 (Fig. 1.11). The National Antivivisection Society, based in Chicago, was distributing its literature widely and working for legislative abolition of animal research in Illinois and elsewhere. Orphans of the Storm, a humane society with a strong antivivisection outlook, was headed by its founder, Irene Castle McLaughlin, a famous dancer of the World War I era. Mrs. McLaughlin had been appointed to the Animal Advisory Committee of the Arvey Ordinance. The ordinance permitted the medical schools in Chicago to obtain unclaimed dogs and cats from the public pound. On one occasion, during an inspection of the animal facilities at Northwestern University Medical School, Mrs. McLaughlin deliberately removed a dog from its cage because she felt that the animal was not receiving adequate treatment. She planned to take the dog to her shelter in Winnetka. Dr. Andrew C. Ivy, then professor and chairman of the Department of Physiology, and Dr. J. Roscoe Miller, then dean of the Medical School, were notified. They intercepted Mrs. McLaughlin and the dog at the entrance

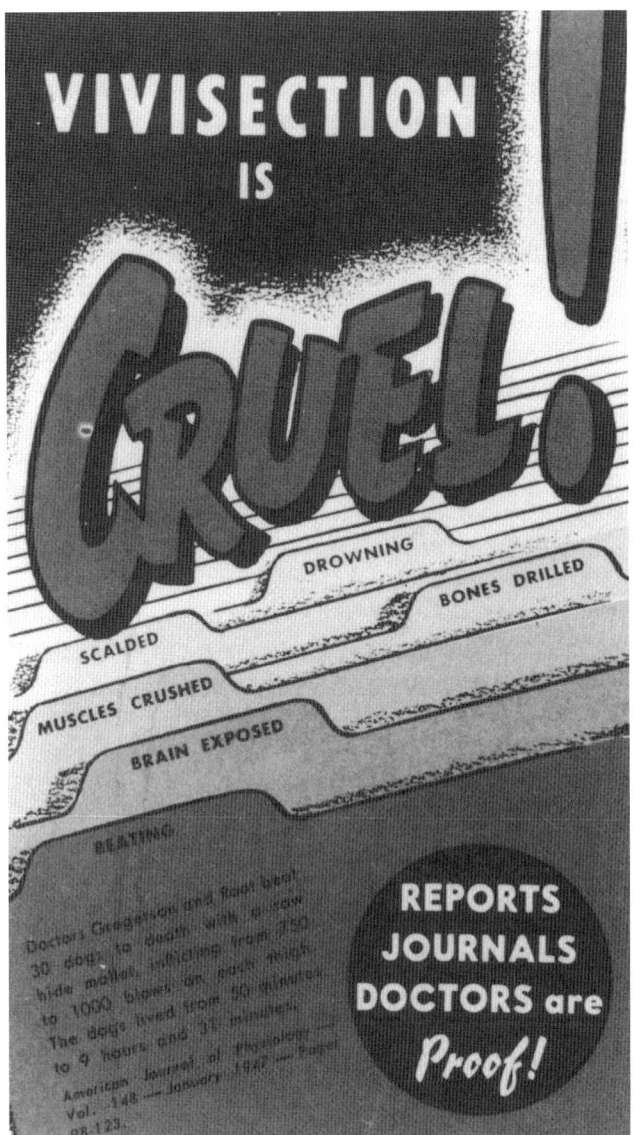

FIGURE 1.11   Cover page of antivivisection brochure, late 1940s.

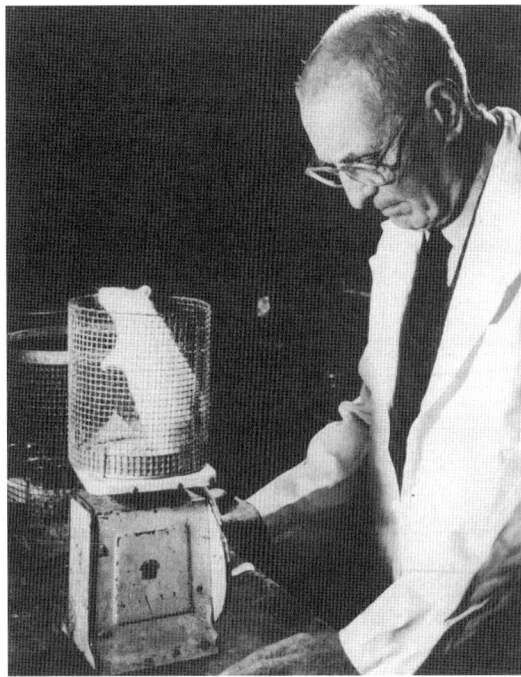

FIGURE 1.12   Dr. Anton J. Carlson, professor of physiology at the University of Chicago and first president of the National Society for Medical Research. *Courtesy of the University of Chicago Archives and Dr. N. R. Brewer.*

of the Medical School. At this point, Mrs. McLaughlin made a citizen's arrest of Dr. Ivy and Dean Miller, and the protagonists proceeded to the Chicago Avenue police station. The dog was returned to the Medical School, and the arrests subsequently were nullified. However, the incident was given wide publicity in the media, especially in the *Chicago Herald-Examiner*, reflecting the antivivisection sentiments of publisher William Randolph Hearst and Mr. Hearst's close friends, Mrs. McLaughlin, and actress Marion Davies. This incident illustrates the flavor of the relationships between animal research scientists and their critics in the mid- and late 1940s. Without realizing it, Mrs. McLaughlin had alerted the scientific community to the significant and determined opposition it faced. An organized response was a clear necessity.

B. The National Society for Medical Research

The National Society for Medical Research (NSMR) was created in 1946 by the Association of American Medical Colleges (AAMC) and about 100 supporting groups (Grafton, 1980). The AAMC had become concerned that progress in medical science could be jeopardized if antivivisectionists were successful in their numerous campaigns to prohibit or restrict animal experimentation. It was deemed essential to establish a separate organization to counter these antiscience activities and, especially, to promote better public understanding of the needs and accomplishments of animal experimentation. Public support of animal research depended upon such understanding. NSMR headquarters were established in Chicago, and Dr. Anton J. Carlson was elected the organization's first president (Fig. 1.12). From its inception, the NSMR contributed importantly to campaigns conducted at the state, city, and county levels to win public support for the use of public pounds as a source of unclaimed dogs and cats for research (Fig. 1.13). Antivivisection efforts to restrict or prohibit animal experimentation were fought successfully in several states. The NSMR also developed educational material about animal research and distributed it throughout the country. In the late 1940s, the NSMR provided legal counsel to several Chicago-area research scientists who had been attacked by the Hearst

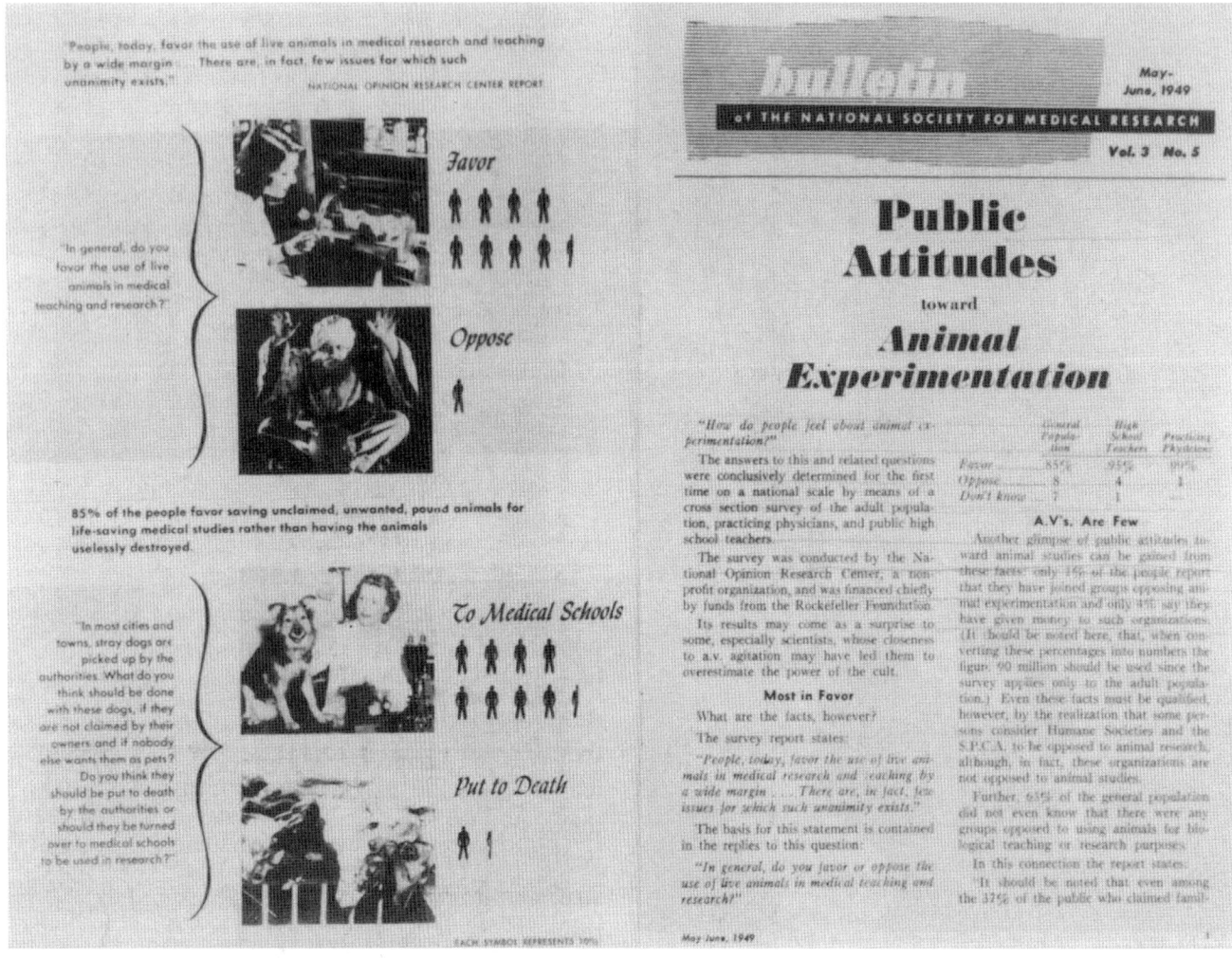

FIGURE 1.13   Inside cover and page 1 of *NSMR Bulletin*, May–June 1949, reporting a national opinion poll on favorable public attitudes toward animal research.

newspapers. Dr. Nathan Brewer was among this group. Libel suits were filed and dragged on for several years, until shortly before William Randolph Hearst's death in 1951. The suits were concluded in favor of the scientists but without significant monetary settlement. The Hearst publications agreed to stop publishing statements tending to damage the reputations of scientists involved in animal research. The suits and Mr. Hearst's death brought to an end the extremist approach of the Hearst publications to the vivisection–antivivisection issue.

In 1952, a *cause célèbre* developed within the American Physiological Society (APS) that also involved other constituent societies of the Federation of American Societies for Experimental Biology (FASEB) and the NSMR. Robert Gesell, M.D., professor and chairman of the Department of Physiology at the University of Michigan from 1923 to 1954 (Fig. 1.14), made the following statement at the APS business meeting on April 15:

The National Society for Medical Research would have us believe that there is an important issue in vivisection versus antivivisection.

To a physiologist there can be no issue on vivisection *per se.*

The real and urgent issue is humanity versus inhumanity in the use of experimental animals.

But the NSMR attaches a stigma of antivivisection to any semblance of humanity.

Antivivisection is their indispensable bogie which must be kept before the public at any cost.

It is their only avenue towards unlimited procurement of animals for unlimited and uncontrollable experimentation.

The NSMR has had but one idea since its organization, namely, to provide an inexhaustible number of animals to an ever growing crowd of career scientists with but little biological background and scant interest in the future of man.

Consider what we are doing in the name of science, and the issue will be clear.

We are drowning and suffocating unanesthetized animals – in the name of science.

We are determining the amount of abuse that life will endure in unanesthetized animals – in the name of science.

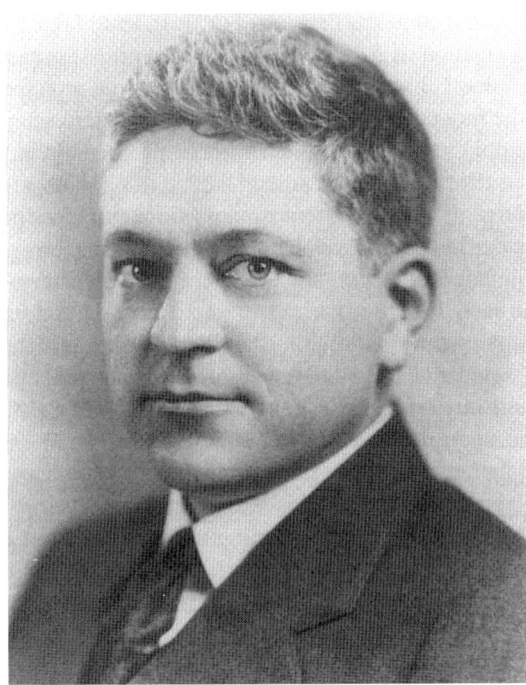

FIGURE 1.14 Dr. Robert Gesell, professor and chairman, 1923–1954, Department of Physiology, University of Michigan. Dr. Gesell's statement at the APS business meeting in 1952 became a *cause célèbre*. Photograph taken in the late 1930s. *Courtesy of the Bentley Historical Library, University of Michigan.*

We are producing frustration ulcers in experimental animals under shocking conditions – in the name of science.

We are observing animals for weeks, months, or even years under infamous conditions – in the name of science.

Yet it is the National Society for Medical Research and its New York satellite that are providing the means to these ends.

And how is it being accomplished?

By undermining one of the finest organizations of our country, THE AMERICAN HUMANE SOCIETY.

With the aid of the halo supplied by the faith of the American people in medical science, the NSMR converts sanctuaries of mercy into animal pounds at the beck and call of experimental laboratories regardless of how the animals are to be used.

What a travesty of humanity!

This may well prove to be the blackest in the history of medical science.

Dr. Gesell had supported the formation of NSMR but subsequently took issue with Dr. Carlson on NSMR involvement in pound legislation. He also was dissatisfied with what he perceived to be a lack of interest by NSMR in promulgating more detailed humane criteria for the care and use of animals than existed at that time. He knew of the formation of the AALAS in 1950 and of the assistance that NSMR provided to AALAS in its formative years. This did not soften his view that NSMR was not constructively dealing with the issue of humane use of animals in research.

Dr. Gesell asked that his statement be made part of the minutes. Vigorous discussion followed. Dr. Ralph Gerard, APS president, explained that it was not APS policy to include all statements by APS members in the minutes. Finally, a motion by Dr. Maurice Visscher, then professor and chairman of the Department of Physiology at the University of Minnesota (later, president of NSMR), was adopted, to be included in the minutes, "that Dr. Gesell had made a statement concerning animal experimentation which criticized physiologists and the NSMR and that the statement had been challenged" (APS minutes, April 15, 1952).

At a second business meeting, on April 17, 1952, the APS adopted the following formal response:

The American Physiological Society reaffirms its sincere belief that the moral justification for humane animal experimentation, for the purpose of furthering biological and medical knowledge, in the interest of both human and animal welfare, is completely established.

The American Physiological Society rejects the sweeping allegations made by Dr. Gesell in a recent business meeting.

The American Physiological Society rejects unequivocally the inference that its members are insensitive to the moral responsibilities which they have in protecting the welfare of man and animals.

The American Physiological Society expresses the hope that in the future all of its members will act in unison in promoting conditions facilitating humane animal experimentation.

Despite efforts by Dr. Gesell to prevent and suppress use of his statement by antivivisection groups, it was distributed widely by these groups in their campaigns for legislative restriction of animal research. After all, it reflected the views of a respected American physiologist. The APS response was not similarly distributed by these groups. Dr. Carlson prepared a lengthy and thoughtful rebuttal of the Gesell statement for members of FASEB, but it too had only a limited distribution (A.J. Carlson, letter to FASEB members, September 17, 1952). After Dr. Gesell's death in 1954, his daughter, Christine Stevens, a founder and the president since 1950 of the Animal Welfare Institute, continued to espouse her father's views and her own strong opinion that too many scientists were insufficiently concerned about humane treatment of animals in research. These views have included critical commentary about NSMR and AALAS (Stevens, 1963, 1976, 1977).

The Gesell–APS–NSMR controversy highlighted issues that, to this day, underlie the difficult relations between the scientific community and the animal rights movement. Perhaps a positive result has been that the controversy also contributed to the climate of opinion that led additional numbers of medical research institutions to employ veterinarians to care for research animals. Ultimately, the controversy raised questions that influenced and should continue to influence all those having a constructive concern for both science and animal welfare. What, if any, are the appropriate limits on scientific freedom in animal research? Who is best qualified to make judgments about the propriety of animal studies? Can *humaneness* be legislated? Is there not a moral imperative to conduct animal studies in the interest of human and animal welfare? How best can refinement of animal studies, reduction in the numbers of animals used, and replacement of animals, where appropriate, best be incorporated into the design of experiments (Russell and Burch, 1959)?

In the 1980s, the National Society for Medical Research merged with the Association for Biomedical Research, which had been organized in 1979, to become the National Association for Biomedical Research (NABR), with Dr. Edward C. Melby as its first president. The NABR advocates for sound public policy in support of ethical and essential animal research. The Scientists' Center for Animal Welfare was formed in 1978 to contribute scientific perspectives to laboratory animal welfare.

C. The American Association for Laboratory Animal Science   ACP ⟶ AALAS

By 1949, veterinarians were managing the laboratory animal facilities at five Chicago-area institutions: the University of Chicago (Nathan R. Brewer), the University of Illinois (Elihu Bond), Northwestern University (Bennett J. Cohen), the Argonne National Laboratory (Robert J. Flynn), and the Hektoen Institute for Medical Research of Cook County Hospital (Robert J. Schroeder). The veterinarians sought one another out to exchange information and experience on the day-to-day problems they were encountering. The group met at least monthly, starting during the summer of 1949. Among the subjects reviewed at these meetings were husbandry and diseases of laboratory animals, the need to develop basic standards of animal care, and the need to counter the strident antivivisection attacks on medical science in the Chicago area. The Chicago veterinarians knew that few other veterinarians elsewhere in the country were engaged in the activity they had begun to identify as *laboratory animal care*. For example, in reviewing the proceedings of a symposium on animal colony maintenance, held under the sponsorship of the New York Academy of Sciences in 1944 (Farris *et al.*, 1945), they noted that not a single veterinarian had presented a paper. Their perception was that the problems of laboratory animal care merited organized attention, and they wondered whether others felt the same way.

Special meetings were arranged when colleagues from other institutions visited Chicago. Among these colleagues were C.F. Schlotthauer, D.V.M., Mayo Clinic; Charles A. Slanetz, Ph.D., director of the Central Animal Facility at the College of Physicians and Surgeons,

Columbia University; Harry Herrlein, Rockland Farms, New City, New York (then a major commercial rodent and rabbit breeding facility); C.N.W. Cumming, Carworth Farms, New City, New York (also a major rodent breeding facility at the time); and W.T.S. Thorp, D.V.M., then chief of the Laboratory Aids Branch, NIH. These meetings were exciting, interesting, and rewarding to the participants. They demonstrated that interest in laboratory animal problems extended well beyond the Chicago area and included individuals who had a broad range of scientific, professional, and technical backgrounds.

In a letter signed by the five Chicago veterinarians and sent in May 1950 to individuals in the United States and Canada thought to have an interest in the care of laboratory animals, the development of a national organization was proposed "to be open to all individuals interested in animal care work on an institutional scale" (Flynn, 1980). The response was overwhelmingly favorable, and the first meeting was convened in Chicago on November 28, 1950, with an attendance of 75. The founding members named the organization the Animal Care Panel (ACP), reflecting their broad concern with the *care* of laboratory animals (Fig. 1.15). *Panel* was used in the name to emphasize the organization's purpose as a forum for the exchange of information on all aspects of animal care. Dr. Brewer was elected the first president, a post he held until 1955. During the early meetings of the ACP, its programs were dominated by papers on animal colony management, design of facilities and equipment,

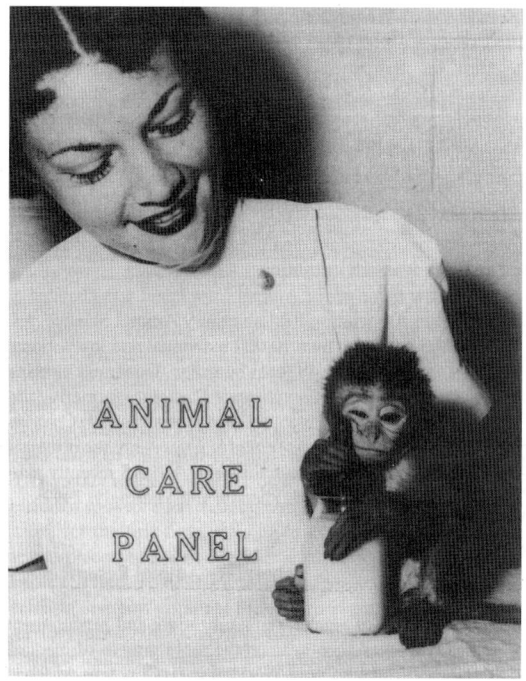

FIGURE 1.15   Cover of early descriptive brochure about the Animal Care Panel, now the American Association for Laboratory Animal Science.

and descriptions of common diseases. This reflected the relatively underdeveloped *state of the art* with respect to the technology of animal care. ACP meetings became more sophisticated with each passing year. By the sixth meeting, in 1955, original research was being presented (Flynn, 1980). In 1963, the annual *Proceedings of the Animal Care Panel* was transformed into the scientific journal *Laboratory Animal Care* and in 1971, renamed *Laboratory Animal Science*. The ACP grew rapidly in its institutional and individual membership, and was characterized by the unique diversity of scientific, professional, and technical backgrounds of its members. By 1960, the ACP was able to employ a full-time executive secretary, Joseph J. Garvey. He had served earlier as assistant executive secretary of the NSMR and, in this position, had assisted with ACP administration, reflecting the support and encouragement the ACP received from the NSMR in its formative years.

From its inception, the ACP also worked to enhance the stature and training of laboratory animal technicians. This activity is exemplified in the career and contributions of George Collins (1917–1974), who served successively as supervisor of the animal facilities at the Argonne National Laboratory, Rockefeller University, the AMA Education and Research Foundation, and the University of Illinois at Chicago (Brewer, 1980). He was a founding member of the AALAS and, in 1963, received the AALAS Animal Technician Award. In 1967, he edited the first edition of the *AALAS Manual for Animal Laboratory Technicians*, a landmark in its time (Collins, 1967).

Development of standards was another early activity of the ACP. Indeed, the first edition of the *Guide for Laboratory Animal Facilities and Care* (Cohen, 1963), now known as the *Guide for the Care and Use of Laboratory Animals* (Moreland, 1978) was prepared under ACP auspices. The guide has become the benchmark standard regarding the care and use of animals in American research institutions.

In 1967, the name of the Animal Care Panel was changed to the AALAS. Today, the AALAS has more than 12,200 individual and institutional members and more than 47 active local branches. Its annual meeting and scientific journals – *Comparative Medicine* and the *Journal of the American Association forLaboratory Animal Science* – are the principal means of scientific exchange in the field. In 1999, the AALAS published its 50-year history (McPherson and Mattingly, 1999).

D. The Institute for Laboratory Animal Research

Many problems of supply, standardization, and procurement of animal resources accompanied the rapid growth of medical and biological research after World War II. Concerns surfaced about these problems within the National Academy of Sciences (NAS). These concerns developed independent of those that led to the formation of the AALAS. The NAS is a private organization with a federal charter. Since 1863, it has been a principal advisor to the federal government on matters related to science and science policy (Seitz, 1967). Election to membership in the NAS or its Institute of Medicine is among the highest honors a scientist can receive. It is a prestigious organization, and therefore, NAS advisory groups, all of which serve without compensation, have a standing and authority they might not otherwise have.

In the early 1950s, organized efforts to improve and standardize animal supply and quality had barely been initiated. Scientific standards for laboratory animal production, genetics, breeding, husbandry, and transportation did not exist. There were no good mechanisms to facilitate information exchange about laboratory animals internationally. Education and training in laboratory animal science were in an undeveloped state, and no guidelines for such training existed. Problems such as these led Dr. Paul Weiss, then chairman of the Division of Biology and Agriculture of the National Research Council (the NAS advisory arm), to appoint a Committee on Animal Resources in 1952. Dr. Weiss appointed Dr. Clarence Cook Little, the eminent geneticist and founder of the Jackson Laboratory (Bar Harbor, Maine), to be chairman. The Committee on Animal Resources recommended establishment of an Institute of Animal Resources (IAR). The IAR commenced full-time operation in July 1953 (Hill, 1980). In 1956, it was renamed Institute of Laboratory Animal Resources. In 1997, it was renamed the Institute for Laboratory Animal Research (ILAR).

Historically, the ILAR office has been headed by an executive secretary (now named the director), with oversight from an advisory council and executive committee that is appointed in accordance with NAS-National Research Council (NRC) procedures. Dr. Orson Eaton, a geneticist from the Bureau of Animal Industry, was the first executive secretary. He was succeeded by the vigorous and energetic Berton F. Hill, who also had a background in genetics. During Hill's tenure (1955–1965), the ILAR became established as the major standards development organization within laboratory animal science. In 1965, Hill was succeeded by Dr. Robert H. Yager, former director of the animal facilities at the Walter Reed Army Institute of Research. Dr. Yager was one of the *founding fathers* of the ILAR, having served on the Committee on Animal Resources in 1952. Among many important ILAR accomplishments during Dr. Yager's tenure were the development of the first guidelines for education and training in laboratory animal medicine (Clarkson, 1967); the publication of an important national survey of animal facilities in the United States (Trum, 1970), following up on the first such survey, during Hill's tenure (Thorp, 1964); and enlargement of the U.S. participation in international laboratory animal activities through support of the ICLAS, known then as the Intentional Committee on Laboratory Animals.

During the formative years of ILAR and AALAS, there were obvious areas of overlap. Both organizations had been involved in standards development, both were holding scientific meetings, and in many other areas their interests coincided. In 1962, the executive committees agreed on a division of responsibility that solidified the ILAR's role in standards development (Garvey and Hill, 1963). This proved to be an important agreement because it enabled ILAR and AALAS to concentrate on the things each could do best. It also was important because of the position that ILAR standards subsequently achieved under the umbrella of the NAS.

The ILAR began publishing a journal, the *ILAR Journal*, in 1990. The *ILAR Journal* is published quarterly and is a peer-reviewed, theme-oriented publication of the ILAR. The journal provides timely information for all those who use, care for, and oversee the use of animals in research. Through the ILAR, expert committee reports, workshops, presentations, and other fora ILAR identifies and disseminates practices for improved animal welfare, and evaluates and encourages the development and validation of non-animal alternatives in research and testing.

E. The American College of Laboratory Animal Medicine

Formal recognition of veterinary medical specialty fields by the American Veterinary Medical Association (AVMA) began in 1951 with the establishment of the American Board of Veterinary Public Health and the American College of Veterinary Pathologists (Grafton, 1974). In 1957, laboratory animal medicine was accorded the same recognition, when the American Board of Laboratory Animal Medicine was incorporated under the laws of the state of Illinois, with 18 *Charter Fellows*. In August 1961, the name was changed to the American College of Laboratory Animal Medicine (ACLAM), and the designation *Fellow* was discontinued in favor of *Diplomat*, a term used by other specialties.

The ACLAM was established to encourage education, training, and research in laboratory animal medicine; to establish standards of training and experience for qualification of specialists; and to certify specialists by examination. These objectives, which today are well understood and accepted, were but a vague concept in the early 1950s. On June 23, 1952, 34 veterinarians assembled in a meeting room at the Ambassador Hotel in Atlantic City, during the AVMA meeting, to consider the role of veterinarians in laboratory animal care. There was a lively discussion about this rapidly developing field, with special emphasis on defining activities that veterinarians were uniquely qualified to pursue (News reports, 1952). Those in attendance noted that medical schools were employing an increasing number of veterinarians and that further growth seemed likely. They felt that more specific definition of this newly developing field was needed. The group organized as the Committee on the Medical Care of Laboratory Animals, with Dr. Nathan R. Brewer as chairman, Dr. Mark Morris as vice chairman, and Dr. W.T.S. Thorp as secretary. The decision was made to organize programs of special interest to laboratory animal veterinarians at future AVMA meetings. During the ensuing 4 years, the term *laboratory animal medicine* came into use to differentiate the activities of veterinarians from other professional or technical people working in the broad area of laboratory animal science. Additionally, within this period, a number of laboratory animal veterinarians were able to establish academic units in their institutions (Clarkson, 1961a), some of which were identified as sections, divisions, or departments of laboratory animal medicine or comparative medicine. With this development, laboratory animal medicine began to establish its separate identity. The committee then proceeded to seek recognition of specialization in the field by the AVMA. Late in 1956, the committee disbanded in favor of the American Board of Laboratory Animal Medicine and the new specialty was born.

F. The American Society of Laboratory Animal Practitioners

The American Society of Laboratory Animal Practitioners (ASLAP) promotes the acquisition and dissemination of knowledge, ideas, and information among veterinarians and veterinary students having an interest in the practice of laboratory animal medicine. The Society does so for the benefit of laboratory animals, other animals, and society in general.

Founded in 1966 as an organization open to all veterinarians with an interested in the practice of laboratory animal medicine, the ASLAP was incorporated in the State of Illinois on July 11, 1967, and was recognized as an ancillary organization of the AVMA. In 1971, the ASLAP attained a sufficient number of members to be recognized as a Constituent Allied Veterinary Organization and to have a seat in the AVMA House of Delegates. In this role, the ASLAP represents laboratory animal practitioners within organized veterinary medicine.

One of the key ASLAP Committees is the Veterinary Student Liaison Committee (VSLC) with a faculty representative at every North American Veterinary School. Veterinary students interested in a career in laboratory animal medicine can obtain career information and learn about ASLAP student memberships from their school's liaison. The VSLC manages the Veterinary Student Award Program, which is intended to increase awareness of the practice of laboratory animal medicine by recognizing students who have demonstrated significant interest and potential in the field.

G. The Association of Primate Veterinarians

The Association of Primate Veterinarian (APV) held its first meeting in 1973 as the Association of Primate Veterinary Clinicians and membership was limited to veterinarians who spent 50% of their time providing direct care for nonhuman primates. Today the association has over 400 members and provides a forum for the dissemination of information relating health and welfare of nonhuman primates and a mechanism for veterinarians to speak collectively on matters affecting nonhuman primates. The APV has published a formulary and guidance documents on subjects such as food restriction, humane endpoints, anesthesia, and analgesia.

H. The International Association of Colleges of Laboratory Animal Medicine

The IACLAM was founded in 2006. The IACLAM is an association of associations and currently includes the ACLAM, the European College of Laboratory Animal Medicine, the Japanese College of Laboratory Animal Medicine, and the Korean College of Laboratory Animal Medicine, and is a member of the World Veterinary Association. The IACLAM promotes and supports training in the specialty of laboratory animal medicine and the development of global standards for the care of laboratory animals. It also supports research through partnerships that promote the Three Rs with an emphasis on the veterinarian's role in refinement.

V. EDUCATION AND TRAINING IN LABORATORY ANIMAL MEDICINE

Veterinarians entering *laboratory animal care* in the 1940s and early 1950s had to be largely self-trained. They relied on their basic education in veterinary medicine and on what they could learn from one another at AALAS and AVMA meetings (Clarkson, 1980). There were no post-D.V.M. training programs. The establishment of the ACLAM in 1957, with its strong commitment to fostering education and training, stimulated more specific discussion of training needs in this new field. At this same time, NIH-supported training programs were being initiated in basic medical science and clinical fields in leading scientific institutions throughout the

country. As mentioned in Section IV-E, by the late 1950s *laboratory animal medicine* was being conducted as an academic program in a few medical schools (Clarkson, 1961a). In such settings, it became possible to consider establishing postdoctoral training. The animal resources program in the Division of Research Resources at the NIH had not yet matured, and the Animal Resources Branch (ARB) did not have training authority. However, with great insight about the underlying significance of laboratory animal medicine, the Physiology Training Committee, within the Division of General Medical Sciences (later to become the National Institute of General Medical Sciences), decided to accept applications to establish a few research training programs in this new field. During the time, this matter was under consideration; Drs. Howard Jenerick and J.H.U. Brown, both physiologists, served as secretaries of the committee. The committee chairmen were Dr. T.C. Ruch, professor and chairman of the Department of Physiology at the University of Washington, and Dr. Wallace O. Fenn, professor and chairman of the Department of Physiology at the University of Rochester. The committee's decision to sponsor such training was of paramount importance, because for the first time, training in laboratory animal medicine was placed on a par with other areas of research training in the medical and biological sciences. In the ensuing years, the specialists that composed the academic core of in the field of laboratory animal medicine were trained in such programs.

The first training program was established in January 1960 at the Bowman Gray Medical School, directed by the then assistant professor of laboratory animal medicine, Thomas B. Clarkson. In July 1960, a second program was started at UCLA Medical School, directed by Bennett J. Cohen, then assistant professor of physiology and director of the vivarium. The program moved with Dr. Cohen to the University of Michigan in 1962. Later, programs were established at other medical schools and universities: Tulane University (1963, Dr. K.F. Burns), Stanford University (1965, Dr. O.A. Soave), the University of Florida (1965, Dr. A.F. Moreland), Johns Hopkins University (1968, Dr. E.C. Melby), and the University of Missouri (1968, Dr. C.C. Middleton). Edgewood Arsenal, Maryland, and Brooks Air Force Base, Texas, became the sites of training programs for military veterinarians. With strong encouragement from Dr. Jules S. Cass, chief veterinary medical officer at the Veterans Administration, a program was established in the mid-1960s at the Hines Veterans Administration Medical Center in the Chicago area. This program was guided initially by Dr. Robert F. Locke.

The *core of knowledge* comprising laboratory animal medicine was not well defined at the time these early programs were started. The curricula of the training programs simply reflected the outlook of the directors and the settings in which they were conducted. Some were formal graduate programs leading to a Master of Science or PhD degree. Others stressed residency training analogous to that of residency programs in the medical specialties. Thus, there were research-oriented programs and others that focused more on the clinical or managerial aspects of laboratory animal medicine (Clarkson, 1961b). By 1964, the need for better definition of the field had become apparent. An ILAR-sponsored workshop held in that year pointed to the need for educational guidelines to be used by all training programs (Clarkson, 1965). The first such guidelines subsequently were published (Clarkson, 1967). A formal process is now in place by the ACLAM that reviews and approves training programs in laboratory animal medicine.

In the mid-1960s, the ARB received training authority, and the training grants in laboratory animal medicine were transferred there. Other aspects of the NIH extramural animal resources program also grew significantly, such as, for example, the laboratory animal science program. Overall, the impact of these programs on laboratory animal medicine has been enormously beneficial. As of 2011, the support for the postdoctoral training comes from the Division of Comparative Medicine within the NIH's Office of Research Infrastructure Programs (ORIP). Training programs supported by the ORIP are designed to train veterinarians for careers in research. The training can be of support of the requirements for an advanced degree. Today many of the training programs recognized by the ACLAM are supported by institutional resources. Post-D.V.M. training is recognized today as necessary for a career in laboratory animal medicine.

VI. ACLAM-SPONSORED TEXTS

In 1969, Dr. Robert Flatt (Iowa State University), Dr. Alan Kraus (University of Rochester), and Dr. Steven Weisbroth (State University of New York) were recruited by the ACLAM to be coeditors of a reference text intended to summarize the current state of knowledge about the laboratory rabbit. The book, *The Biology of the Laboratory Rabbit*, which was the first of 30 ACLAM-sponsored texts centered on the biology and diseases of laboratory animals, was published in 1974 (Weisbroth *et al.*, 1974). The rabbit text, and similar ACLAM-sponsored texts, were designed to collate the salient scientific data available in the literature. At the time, much of the information was out of date and misinformation on the rabbit was appreciable. One example of published misinformation was the case of the rabbit ear mite, *Psoroptes cuniculi.* The earlier texts described at least two ear mites of domestic rabbits, *P. cuniculi* and *Chorioptes cuniculi.* Yet, *C. cuniculi*

has never been described in a research report and has never been observed diagnostically (Weisbroth, 1976). Its appearance in the literature has been traced to the English translation of an obscure German pathology text. Although this mite is mythical, its existence has been dutifully reported in the literature for a full century. *Psoroptes cuniculi* remains the only rabbit mite.

Given the primary orientation of the ACLAM toward laboratory animal medicine, the rabbit, and similar species-oriented ACLAM texts, is biased toward the coverage of disease. For example, chapters in the rabbit book fall into three main groups – those on normative biology, genetics, husbandry, practical feeds and feeding, and physiology; those on the main uses of the rabbit as a laboratory model in teratology, arteriosclerosis, and serogenetics; and those on rabbit diseases. The chapters on disease are organized by etiology, rather than by organ system, with chapters on bacterial disease, viral disease, protozoal disease, arthropod parasites, helminth parasites, neoplastic disease, and inherited disease (Weisbroth, 1976).

From 1974 to 2014, texts were also published on the guinea pig, the hamster, three volumes on the laboratory rat, two volumes on the rabbit, eight volumes on the mouse, four volumes on nonhuman primates, and the third edition on the ferret. Second editions have been published on the rabbit (1974, 1994), rat (1979, 2006), mouse (1982, 2007), and nonhuman primates (1995–98, 2013). A recent publication, *The Laboratory Rabbit*, *Guinea Pig*, *Hamster*, *and Other Rodents*, provides a compilation of information on multiple rodents, as well as the rabbit.

The College also published related texts: in 1979, two volumes of *Spontaneous Animal Models of Human Disease* and *Anesthesia and Analgesia in Laboratory Animals* in 1997 with a second edition in 2012. *Planning and Designing Research Animal Facilities* was published in 2008. *Flynn's Parasites of Laboratory Animals* and *Laboratory Animal Welfare* was published under the auspices of the College in 2010 and 2013, respectively. A text on the clinical chemistry of laboratory animals will be published in 2016.

The text *Laboratory Animal Medicine*, first published in 1984 with a second edition in 2002, and the third edition (this volume) to be published in 2015, reflects the College's effort to foster education and serves as a primary teaching text, and is particularly useful for veterinarians specializing in laboratory animal medicine. A similar text, *Harkness and Wagner's Biology and Medicine of Rabbits and Rodents*, was published under ACLAM auspices in 2010 and is widely used for teaching veterinary students, as well as serving as a ready source of clinical information for veterinary practitioners who see laboratory animal species in general practice.

VII. IMPACT OF LAWS, REGULATIONS, AND GUIDELINES ON LABORATORY ANIMAL MEDICINE

Prior to 1966, no federal law existed in the United States specifically regulating the acquisition or care of research animals. Pressure for federal legislation mounted steadily in the late 1950s and early 1960s. Animal welfare organizations, such as the Humane Society of the United States, the Society for Animal Protective Legislation, and the Animal Welfare Institute, argued for legislation to curb alleged *pet stealing* and abuse of animals in laboratories. They used the media effectively to generate public interest in their causes (e.g., cover headline of *Life*, February 4, 1966: "Concentration Camps for Lost and Stolen Pets: Your Dog Is in Cruel Danger"). Organizations within the scientific community, such as the AALAS, the NSMR, and the FASEB, argued against the proposed legislation. Their position was that the best way to foster the humane use and care of animals was to provide better support of research and training, provide funds to upgrade animal facilities, and strengthen self-regulation through mechanisms such as the newly organized (1965) American Association for Accreditation of Laboratory Animal Care (AAALAC) and institutional committees to assess the adequacy of animal care and use programs (Galton, 1967). In the mid-1990s, the AAALAC assumed a more international role, and in 1996, it renamed itself the Association for Assessment and Accreditation of Laboratory Animal Care International (AAALAC International).

After holding hearings on a series of bills in the House of Representatives and the Senate dealing with the regulation of animal research, the Congress passed the Laboratory Animal Welfare Act in 1966. The principal purposes were to regulate commercial traffic in dogs, cats, monkeys, rabbits, guinea pigs, and hamsters, and to establish standards for their housing and transportation and for *adequate veterinary care*. The act, administered by the U.S. Department of Agriculture (USDA), established a legal requirement for scientific institutions to provide appropriate care for research animals by or under the direction of a veterinarian. Since its initial passage, the act has been broadened and its name changed to Animal Welfare Act (see Chapter 2). For the fiscal year 2012, the number of registered research facilities totaled 1081. The Act has contributed to the betterment of animal care through its requirement for participation of veterinarians in institutional animal medicine programs.

The NIH has long recognized that good research requires animals that are healthy and well cared for. In 1963, it published the first edition of the *Guide for Laboratory Animal Facilities and Care* (Cohen, 1963), as developed by the Standards Committee of the ACP.

Revised several times since 1963 by the ILAR's Committee on Revision of the Guide, it is now the *Guide for the Care and Use of Laboratory Animals*. Since 1979, the NIH and other granting agencies have required scientific institutions to provide assurance of compliance with the standards in the guide as a condition for receiving funds for research. The Guide is also used as the basis for accreditation by the AAALAC. One of the basic requirements established in the guide is for the provision of adequate veterinary medical care, a concept also expressed in the regulations of the Department of Agriculture.

In 1978, the Food and Drug Administration (FDA) promulgated regulations for the conduct of animal experiments relating to new or existing pharmaceutical medicinal substances, food additives, or other chemicals. These regulations, known as the Good Laboratory Practice regulations, also specify the need for adequate diagnosis, treatment, and control of diseases in animals used in such studies. Thus, the standards of the AAALAC, the NIH, the USDA, and the FDA all include specific references to veterinary medical participation in the care of laboratory animals. In fact, these standards provide the basis for implementation of the legal requirement that research animals receive adequate veterinary care.

VIII. REGULATION OF ANIMAL RESEARCH IN THE UNITED KINGDOM AND CANADA

Until 1986, the use of animals in the United Kingdom was governed by the Cruelty to Animals Act of 1876 (French, 1975) (see Chapter 2). The Animals (Scientific Procedures) Act of 1986, as revised in 2013 in response to the European Union Directive 2010/63, is now the governing legislation in the United Kingdom. Major debates about *vivisection* occurred in the Parliament in the late 1860s and early 1870s. Finally, the act was passed with the active support of leading scientists of that time. Antivivisectionists had been working for a law that would have prohibited animal research or regulated it more strictly than called for in the act. The act requires three types of licenses: a personal license for those who carry out procedures on animals; a project license for the program of work; and an establishment license for the place where the work is done. Veterinarians, as such, do not have legal standing under the act that is mandated in the U.S. regulations though each institution must appoint a veterinarian to provide advice on animal health and welfare. In the private sector, the British Laboratory Animals Veterinary Association was organized in 1963 and is affiliated with the British Veterinary Association.

The use of animals in Canada is not specifically regulated by the federal law. However, in 1968, the Canadian Council on Animal Care (CCAC) was established by the major agencies that fund animal research (see Chapter 2). Dr. Harry Rowsell played an instrumental role in the founding of the CCAC and in its operation over the years. The CCAC assesses animal care in Canadian research laboratories based on the standards in the *Guide to the Care and Use of Experimental Animals* (CCAC, 1993). This program has been a major factor in the elevation of animal care standards and the employment of veterinarians in Canadian research laboratories. In addition, 7 of the 10 provinces have laws that apply to the requisition or use of animals in research in those provinces (e.g., Ontario and Alberta).

IX. COMMERCIAL AND ACADEMIC BREEDING OF RODENTS

The development of gnotobiology in the 1950s represented a major conceptual and technological advance in the commercial breeding of healthier rodents for research (Foster, 1958). This advance had been preceded by laboratory research (Trexler and Reynolds, 1957; Reyniers, 1957) and years of attempts to breed animals that would lead to the most unambiguous results in research as possible. With the introduction of genetically engineered mice, academic and industrial animal resource programs have increasingly been engaged in breeding and characterizing numerous lines of mice with unique genetic makeup (see Chapter 3).

X. CONCLUSION

A complete history of the individuals and organizations that have influenced the development of laboratory animal science and medicine would require a separate volume. Some of these topics are as follows: the history of laboratory animal science internationally; the history of the major commercial and institutional animal colonies and of the important genetic stocks and strains of laboratory animals; the evolution of animal technology, including the field of gnotobiology; the contributions of animal technicians to laboratory animal science; the origins of the NIH extramural and intramural laboratory animal science programs; and reviews, in historical perspective, of the major diseases of laboratory animals. Some of these topics are dealt with elsewhere (Cohen, 1979; Foster, 1980; Fox, 1985; Lindsey, 1979; McPherson, 1980; McPherson and Mattingly, 1999). Others must await documentation of the historical record.

Laboratory animal science and medicine are fields of expanding horizons that provide challenging opportunities for satisfying professional careers. The following chapters clearly document the progress that has occurred while pointing to many challenges that lie ahead. It remains for each generation of laboratory animal scientists to build on the base of knowledge established by its predecessors and so determine its own future.

Acknowledgment

We acknowledge the previous contributors, Franklin Loew and Bennett Cohen, for the chapter published in the second edition of *Laboratory Animal Medicine*.

References

Bernard, C., 1865. An Introduction to the Study of Experimental Medicine (trans. H. C. Greene, p. 123. Reprinted by Dover, New York, 1957).

Braasch, W.F., 1969. Early Days of the Mayo Clinic. Thomas, Springfield, Illinois, p. 141.

Brewer, N.R., 1980. Personalities in the early history of laboratory animal science and medicine. Lab. Anim. Sci. 30 (4 Pt. 2), 741–758.

Brimhall, S.D., Hardenbergh, J.G., 1922. A study of so-called kennel lameness: preliminary report. J. Am. Vet. Med. Assoc. 61, 145–154.

Brimhall, S.D., Mann, F.C., 1917. Pathologic conditions noted in laboratory animals. J. Am. Vet. Med. Assoc. 52, 195–204.

Brimhall, S.D., Mann, F.C., Foster, J.P., 1919–1920. The relation of the common bile duct to the pancreatic duct in common domestic and laboratory animals. J. Lab. Clin. Med. 5, 203–206.

Bustad, L.K., Gorham, J.R., Hagreberg, G.A., Padgett, G.A., 1976. Comparative medicine: progress and prospects. J. Am. Vet. Med. Assoc. 169, 90–105.

Canadian Council on Animal Care (CCAC), 1993., second ed. Guide to the Care and Use of Experimental Animals, vol. 1. CCAC, Ottawa, Ontario.

Clarkson, T.B., 1961a. Laboratory animal medicine and the medical schools. J. Med. Educ. 36, 1329–1330.

Clarkson, T.B., 1961b. Graduate and professional training in laboratory animal medicine. Fed. Proc. Fed. Am. Soc. Exp. Biol. 20, 915–916.

Clarkson, T.B., 1965. Laboratory animals. 4. Graduate education in laboratory animal medicine. Proceedings of a workshop. NAS-NRC Publ. 1284, 33. Committee on Professional Education, Institute of Laboratory Animal Resources.

Clarkson, T.B., 1967. A guide to postdoctoral training in laboratory animal medicine. NAS-NRC Publ. 1483, 9. Committee on Professional Education, Institute of Laboratory Animal Resources.

Clarkson, T.B., 1980. Evolution and history of training and academic programs in laboratory animal medicine. Lab. Anim. Sci. 30 (4 Pt. 2), 790–792.

Cohen, B.J., 1959a. The early history of animal experimentation and animal care. 1. Antiquity. Lab. Anim. Sci. 9, 39–45.

Cohen, B.J., 1959b. The evolution of laboratory animal medicine in the United States. J. Am. Vet. Med. Assoc. 135, 161–164.

Cohen, B.J., 1963. Guide for Laboratory Animal Facilities and Care. Anim. Facilities Stand. Comm., Anim. Care Panel, Public Health Serv. Publ. 1024. U.S. Dept. of Health, Education and Welfare, Washington, DC, p. 33.

Cohen, B.J., 1979. ILAR News 22 (2), 26.

Cohen, M.R., Drabkin, I.E., 1948. Sourcebook in Greek Science. McGraw-Hill, New York, p. 479.

Collins, G.R., 1967. Manual for laboratory animal technicians. Animal Technician Training Committee, American Association for Laboratory Animal Science Publ., Joliet, Illinois, 67–3.

DuclauxE., 1920. Pasteur – The History of a Mind (trans. E. F. Smith and F. Hedges), Saunders, Philadelphia, Pennsylvania, p. 363.

Farris, E.J., Carnochan, F.G., Cumming, C.N.W., Farber, S., Hartman, C.G., Hutt, F.B., et al., 1945. Animal colony maintenance. Ann. N.Y. Acad. Sci. 46, 1–126.

Fisher, G.J., 1881. Historical and bibliographical notes. 12. Herophilus and Erasistratus. The medical school of Alexandria, bc 320–250. Ann. Anat. Surg. 4, 28–67.

Flynn, R.J., 1980. The founding and early history of the American association for laboratory animal science. Lab. Anim. Sci. 30 (4 Pt. 2), 765–779.

Foster, H.L., 1958. Large scale production of rats free of commonly occurring pathogens and parasites. Proc. Anim. Care Panel 8, 92–99.

Foster, H.L., 1980. The history of commercial production of laboratory rodents. Lab. Anim. Sci. 30 (4 Pt. 2), 793–798.

Fox, J.G., 1985. Laboratory animal medicine: changes and challenges. Cornell Vet. 75, 159–170.

French, R.D., 1975. Antivivisection and Medical Science in Victorian Society. Princeton University Press, Princeton, New Jersey, p. 425.

Galton, L., 1967. Pain is cruel, but disease is cruel too. N.Y. Times, Sec. 6 (Magazine), February 26, p. 30.

Garrison, F.H., 1929. An Introduction to the History of Medicine, fourth ed. Saunders, Philadelphia, Pennsylvania.

Garvey, J.J., Hill, B.F., 1963. Cooperation for progress. Lab. Anim. Care 13, 179–180.

Grafton, T.S., 1974. The veterinary profession: a review of its progress in the United States and some indications for the future. Vet. Rec. 94, 441–443.

Grafton, T.S., 1980. The founding and early history of the national society for medical research. Lab. Anim. Sci. 30 (4 Pt. 2), 759–764.

Griffin, C.A., 1952. A study of prepared feeds in relation to Salmonella infection in laboratory animals. J. Am. Vet. Med. Assoc. 121, 197–200.

Hales, S., 1740. Statical Essays. Innys and Manby, London.

Hardenbergh, J.G., 1923. The value of animal experimentation to veterinary medicine. J. Am. Vet. Med. Assoc. 62, 731–735.

Hardenbergh, J.G., 1926–1927. Epidemic lymphadenitis with formation of abscess in guinea pigs due to infection with hemolytic streptococcus. J. Lab. Clin. Med. 12, 119–129.

Harvey, W., 2001. On the Motion of the Heart and Blood in Animals. Vol. XXXVIII, Part 3. The Harvard Classics. P.F. Collier & Son, New York, 1909–1914.

Hill, B.F., 1980. The founding and early history of the institute of laboratory animal resources. Lab. Anim. Sci. 30 (4), 780–785.

Hoff, H.E., Geddes, L.A., McCrady, J.D., 1965. The contributions of the horse to knowledge of the heart and circulation. Conn. Med. 29, 795–800.

Ingle, D.J., 1979. Anton J. Carlson: a biographical sketch. Perspect. Biol. Med. 29 (Pt. 2), 114–136.

Lindsey, J.R., 1979. Origin of the laboratory rat. In: Baker, H.G., Lindsey, J.R., Weisbroth, S.H. (Eds.), The Laboratory Rat. Academic Press, New York (Chapter 1), pp. 2–36.

Loew, F.M., 1982. Animal experimentation. Bull. Hist. Med. 56, 123–126.

Malinin, T.I., 1979. Surgery and Life. Harcourt Brace Jovanovich, New York, p. 242.

McPherson, C.W., 1980. The origins of laboratory animal science at the National Institutes of Health. Lab. Anim. Sci. 30 (4 Pt. 2), 786–789.

McPherson, C.W., Mattingly, S.F., 1999. Fifty Years of Laboratory Animal Science. AALAS, Memphis, Tennessee.

Meyer, K.F., 1928. Communicable diseases of laboratory animals. In: Jordan, E.O., Falk, I.S. (Eds.), The Newer Knowledge of Bacteriology and Immunity. Univ. of Chicago Press, Chicago, pp. 607–638.

Meyer, K.F., 1958. Introductory address. Lab. Anim. Sci. 8, 1–5.

Mitchell, S.W., 1895. Memoir of John Call Dalton, 1825–1889. Biographical memoirs. Natl. Acad. Sci. 3, 177.

Moreland, A.M., 1978. Guide for the Care and Use of Laboratory Animals. National Academy of Sciences, National Research Council, Institute of Laboratory Animal Resources, Washington, DC.

News reports, 1952. J. Am. Vet. Med. Assoc. 121, 257.

Physicians of the Mayo Clinic and the Mayo Foundation, 1937. University of Minnesota Press, Minneapolis, Minnesota, p. 184.

Reyniers, J.A., 1957. The control of contamination in colonies of laboratory animals by use of germfree techniques. Proc. Anim. Care Panel 7, 9–29.

Russell, W.M.S., Burch, R.L., 1959. The Principles of Humane Experimental Technique. Methuen, London, p. 238.

Saunders, J.B. de C.M., O'Malley, C.D., 1950. The Illustrations from the Works of Andreas Vesalius of Brussels. World Publ. Co., New York, p. 128.

Schlotthauer, C.F., 1950. Procurement of animals. Lab. Anim. Sci. 1, 20–25.

Schwabe, C.W., 1978. Cattle, Priests, and Progress in Medicine. Univ. of Minnesota Press, Minneapolis, Minnesota, p. 277.

Seitz, F., 1967. The National Academy of Sciences. J. Wash. Acad. Sci. 57, 38–41.

Singer, C., 1957. A Short History of Anatomy and Physiology from the Greeks to Harvey. Dover, New York, p. 209.

Stevens, C. (Ed.), 1963. Letter to the editor. Perspect. Biol. Med. 7 (1) (Autumn), 129–131.

Stevens, C., 1976. Humane considerations for animal models. Animal Models of Thrombosis and Hemorrhagic Diseases. DHEW Publ. (NIH) 76–982, U.S. Dept. of Health and Human Services, National Institutes of Health, Bethesda, Maryland, pp. 151–158.

Stevens, C., 1977. Humane perspectives. The Future of Animals, Cells, Models, and Systems in Research, Development, Education, and Testing. National Academy of Sciences, Washington, DC, pp. 16–24.

Thorp, W.T.S., 1964. ILAR Committee on the Animal Facilities: Survey Animal Facilities in Medical Research, Final Report and Tabular Appendix. National Academy of Sciences, National Research Council, Institute of Laboratory Animal Resources, Washington, DC, p. 157.

Trexler, P.C., Reynolds, L.I., 1957. Flexible film apparatus for the rearing and use of germfree animals. Appl. Microbiol. 5, 406–412.

Trum, B.F., 1970. ILAR committee on laboratory animal facilities and resources survey. Laboratory animal facilities and resources supporting biomedical research. Lab. Anim. Care 20, 795–869.

Weisbroth, S.H., 1976. Writing about rabbits: an editor's reflections. Lab. Anim. 1, 33–37.

Weisbroth, S.H., Flatt, R.E., Kraus, A.L., 1974. The Biology of the Laboratory Rabbit. Academic Press, New York.

Welch, W.H., 1889. Preliminary report of investigations concerning the causation of hog cholera. Johns Hopkins Hosp. Bull. 1 (1), 9–10.

Wood, C.A. (Ed.), 1931. An Introduction to the Literature of Vertebrate Zoology. Oxford Univ. Press, London (Chapter 4).

CHAPTER

2

Laws, Regulations, and Policies
Affecting the Use of Laboratory Animals

Kathryn Bayne, MS, PhD, DVM[a] and
Lynn C. Anderson, DVM, DACLAM[b]

[a]Association for Assessment and Accreditation of Laboratory Animal Care International, Frederick,
MD, USA [b]Global Animal Welfare/Comparative Medicine, Covance Laboratories, Madison, WI, USA

OUTLINE

I. INTRODUCTION

The use of animals in research, testing, and education is subject to a myriad of laws, regulations, policies, and standards. The public's interest in the treatment of laboratory animals and lobbying by animal welfare and antivivisection organizations has led to the passage of many of these laws and regulations during the second half of the 20th century. However, the research community's need for reliable data obtained from laboratory animals in the most humane manner has also helped

ensure a high level of welfare and the ethical use of these animals. Good husbandry practices, veterinary care, animal facility management, and laboratory techniques in the context of the 3Rs (Replacement, Refinement, and Reduction) are all necessary to promote the quality of scientific results.

This chapter provides an overview of the federal laws, regulations, and policies in the U.S. that pertain to laboratory animal care and use. In many instances, these governing principles from different agencies are similar, and, in some cases, they mandate different minimal

Laboratory Animal Medicine, Third Edition
DOI: http://dx.doi.org/10.1016/B978-0-12-409527-4.00002-X

23

requirements. In addition, every state, the District of Columbia, as well as many cities and towns have enacted laws or ordinances pertaining to animal cruelty or the release of pound animals to research facilities.

II. ANIMAL WELFARE

A. U.S. Animal Welfare Act

The first federal legislation in the U.S. to protect animals was the 28-Hour Law enacted in 1873. It required that farm animals be provided food, water, and rest at least once every 28h during transit.

Animals used for research were first protected by federal legislation in 1966, with the passage of the Laboratory Animal Welfare Act (PL-89-544). To help address public concerns over *pet nabbing*, this law required licensing of dealers (individuals or corporations) that bought or sold dogs or cats for research as well as registration of research facilities that used dogs or cats. It also mandated minimum animal care standards for dogs and cats before and after they were used for research; however, the standards did not apply while the animals were being used for an experimental purpose. The law authorized the U.S. Department of Agriculture (USDA) to develop and enforce these regulations. The USDA subsequently established standards for nonhuman primates, rabbits, guinea pigs, and hamsters, in addition to those for dogs and cats. Research facilities that used dogs or cats were required to observe the USDA-specified standards for all of these species. However, facilities that did not use dogs or cats were not required to comply with the regulations for the other species.

The Laboratory Animal Welfare Act was amended in 1970 and renamed the Animal Welfare Act (PL-91–579). The scope of protection was broadened to include animals used for teaching, exhibitions, and the wholesale pet industry. *Animals* included dogs, cats, nonhuman primates, rabbits, guinea pigs, and hamsters and, with certain exceptions, any other warm-blooded animal designated by the U.S. Secretary of Agriculture. Institutions (except primary and secondary schools) that used these species in research, tests, or experiments were required to register as a research facility. For the first time, zoos were required to be licensed. Specifically exempted were horses not used in research and agricultural animals used in food and fiber research, retail pet stores, state and county fairs, rodeos, purebred cat and dog shows, and agricultural exhibitions. The definition of *dealer* was revised to include any person who bought or sold any dog or other animal designated by the USDA for use in research, teaching, or exhibition or as a pet at the wholesale level.

The 1970 amendments also expanded the minimal animal care standards. These standards applied to animals during the course of research, not only before and after experimental use. The Act did not allow the Secretary of Agriculture to establish rules, regulations, or orders with regard to the design or performance of the research. However, it required that every research facility submit an annual report that provided the number of regulated species it used and assurance that it met professionally acceptable standards for the care, treatment, and use of animals, including the appropriate use of anesthetic, analgesic, and tranquilizing drugs.

In 1976, the Animal Welfare Act was amended again (PL-94-279) to include regulation of common carriers and intermediate handlers and to establish transportation standards for animals. Standards were established for shipping conditions and for the containers in which animals were shipped. The amendments also prohibited interstate promotion or shipment of animals for animal fighting ventures.

The Food Security Act of 1985 (PL-99-198) included provisions to amend the Animal Welfare Act, referred to as "The Improved Standards for Laboratory Animal Act." These amendments were based on the following congressional findings:

1. The use of animals is instrumental in certain research and education for advancing knowledge of cures and treatment for diseases and injuries which afflict both humans and animals;
2. Methods of testing that do not use animals are being and continue to be developed which are faster, less expensive, and more accurate than traditional animal experiments for some purposes and further opportunities exist for the development of these methods of testing;
3. Measures which eliminate or minimize the unnecessary duplication of experiments on animals can result in more productive use of federal funds; and
4. Measures which help meet the public concern for laboratory animal care and treatment are important in ensuring that research will continue to progress.

Until 1985, the Animal Welfare Act requirements and USDA regulations were essentially limited to animal care, housing, and transportation standards. The new amendments included specific requirements for research facilities that were related to the experimental use of animals. The law clearly states, however, that nothing in the act should be construed as authorizing the Secretary of Agriculture to promulgate rules, regulations, or orders with regard to the design or performance of research protocols. It also mandates that the USDA may not interrupt the conduct of research during inspections.

The Pet Theft Act of 1990 (PL-101-624) was the fourth amendment to the Animal Welfare Act. It was incorporated in the 1990 Food, Agriculture, Conservation, and

Trade Act, an omnibus farm bill, and was referred to as the "Protection of Pets" legislation. This amendment established a 5-day holding period for dogs and cats held at pounds and shelters (both private and public) before releasing them to dealers. The holding period was designed to allow pet owners and prospective owners the opportunity to claim or adopt animals before they might be sold or used for research. The 1990 Act also allowed the USDA to seek injunctions against any licensed facility found dealing in stolen animals.

In 2002, the Helms amendment to the Farm Security and Rural Investment Act (also known as the 2002 Farm Bill) explicitly excluded rats, mice, and birds used for research from the Act. However, these animals are covered under the act for other purposes (e.g., zoos, aquaria). The rationale for Congress to accept their exclusion from the act was based in large part on the fact that these species are covered by other federal (e.g., PHS Policy) and private (e.g., the Association for Assessment and Accreditation of Laboratory Animal Care (AAALAC) International) systems of oversight, and there are reports that approximately 95% of research using rats and mice is funded by the National Institutes of Health and thus are covered by the Health Research Extension Act/Public Health Service Policy (Bayne *et al.*, 2010).

1. USDA Regulations

The Animal Welfare Act authorizes the USDA, through the Secretary of Agriculture, to develop standards, rules, regulations and orders based on its content. Within the USDA, the Animal Welfare Act is administered through the Animal and Plant Health Inspection Service (APHIS). All rules must be developed in consultation and cooperation with other federal departments and agencies and be reviewed and approved by the Office of Management and Budget. The USDA is required to publish any new regulations or changes in existing regulations in the *Federal Register* and allow a 60-day period during which the public may comment. The final rule on the regulations is published in the *Federal Register*, along with an effective implementation date.

The complete set of USDA regulations and standards are published as the Animal Welfare Regulations in the Code of Regulations (CFR, 1999), Title 9, Animals and Animal Products, Subchapter A, Animal Welfare. Part 1 defines the terms used, Part 2 provides the regulations, Part 3 specifies the standards, and Part 4 includes the rules of practice governing proceedings under the Animal Welfare Act. In addition, the USDA has issued the *Animal Care Policy Manual* to further clarify the intent of the Animal Welfare Act. The principle components of the animal welfare regulations that pertain to research facilities are provided in Part 2, Subparts C and D, which are summarized below.

Regulated Species

The regulated species include any live or dead dog, cat, nonhuman primate, guinea pig, hamster, rabbit, aquatic mammal, or any other warm-blooded animal that is being used or is intended for use in research, teaching, testing, experimentation, or exhibition or as a pet. As noted previously, birds, rats of the genus *Rattus*, and mice of the genus *Mus* bred for use in research, teaching, or testing, and horses and farm animals intended for use as food or fiber or used in studies to improve production and quality of food and fiber, are specifically excluded.

Licensing

Any person operating or desiring to operate as a dealer, broker, exhibitor, or operator of an auction sale must be licensed by the USDA and pay an annual fee. A dealer is any person who, for compensation or profit of more than $500 per year, buys, sells, or negotiates the purchase of, delivers for transportation, or transports a regulated animal for research, teaching, testing, experimentation, or exhibition or for use as a pet or a dog for hunting, security, or breeding purposes. Traditional *bricks and mortar* retail pet stores are exempt unless they sell to a research facility, exhibitor, or wholesale dealer (although the USDA has recently begun requiring federal licensing and inspections for internet-based businesses and others that sell animals sight unseen). Dogs and cats acquired by a dealer or exhibitor must be held for 5 full days, not including the day of acquisition, after acquiring the animal. If the animal was acquired from a contract animal pound or shelter, the animal must be held for at least 10 full days. If the animal is then sold to another dealer, the subsequent dealer is required to hold the animal for a minimum of 24h. Research facilities that obtain dogs and cats from sources other than dealers, exhibitors, and exempt persons must also hold the animals for 5 full days, not including the day of acquisition or time in transit, before the animals are used by the facility.

Registration

Research facilities, intermediate handlers, and common carriers of regulated species must register with the USDA every 3 years; any revisions to the initial registration must be provided at the time of re-registration. Research facilities are defined as any institution, organization, or person that uses live animals in research, testing, or experiments; that purchases or transports live animals; or that receives federal funds for research, tests, or experiments. The Secretary of Agriculture may exempt facilities from registration if they do not use cats, dogs, or a substantial number of other regulated species.

IACUC Responsibilities

To help ensure humane experimental animal use, the 1985 Animal Welfare Act amendments required every animal research facility to establish an Institutional Animal Committee, subsequently designated by the USDA as an Institutional Animal Care and Use Committee (IACUC). Congress mandated that the committee include at least three members appointed by the chief executive officer of the research facility. The members must possess sufficient ability to assess animal care, treatment, and practices in experimental research as determined by the needs of the research facility and shall represent society's concerns regarding the welfare of animal subjects. At a minimum, the IACUC must include one member who is a doctor of veterinary medicine and one member who is not affiliated in any way with the research facility other than as a member of the IACUC. The nonaffiliated member cannot be a member of the immediate family of a person who is affiliated with the facility and is expected to provide representation for general community interests in the proper care and treatment of animals. In instances where the IACUC consists of more than three members, not more than three members can be from the same administrative unit of the facility.

In accordance with the Animal Welfare Regulations, the IACUC has a central role in the oversight of the animal care and use program. The IACUC is responsible for making recommendations to the research facility's administrative representative, designated as the Institutional Official, regarding any aspect of the research facility's animal program, facilities, or personnel training. It is required to review, at least once every 6 months, the research facility's program for humane care and use of animals, based on USDA regulations. The IACUC must also conduct an inspection of all animal study areas and animal facilities at least once every 6 months. Exceptions to the study area inspection requirement may be made by the Secretary of Agriculture if animals are studied in their natural environment or the study area is difficult to access.

After each program review and inspection, the IACUC must file a report of its evaluations with the Institutional Official of the research facility. This report must be signed by a majority of the committee members and must include any minority views expressed by committee members. The report must identify any violation of USDA standards, including any deficiencies in animal care or treatment and any deviations in research practices from originally IACUC-approved proposals. Significant deficiencies, defined as those that threaten animal health or safety, must be distinguished from minor deficiencies. A specific plan and schedule for correcting each deficiency must also be provided in the report. If, however, corrections of significant deficiencies are not implemented, the committee, in consultation with the Institutional Official, must notify the USDA of the deficiencies or deviations. The report must be maintained on file at the research facility for a minimum of 3 years and be made available during inspections by the USDA or any federal funding agency. Federal research facilities are required to have committees with the same composition and responsibilities, except that they are to report deficiencies or deviations to the head of the federal agency conducting the research.

The committee is also charged with reviewing and, if warranted, investigating concerns involving the care and use of research animals. These concerns may be raised by members of the public or laboratory or research personnel or employees who report issues of noncompliance. The committee must also establish a mechanism for addressing such concerns.

In addition, the IACUC is responsible for reviewing and approving all proposed activities or significant changes in activities related to the care and use of animals. IACUC reviewers must have no conflict of interest with the protocol. The IACUC is authorized to require modifications in or withhold approval for these activities; it may also suspend an activity if it determines that the activity is not being conducted in accordance with the IACUC-approved procedures. Any suspended activities must be reported to the USDA. As part of its review, the IACUC must ensure that the activities are in accordance with the regulations unless acceptable justification for a departure is presented in writing.

A proposal to conduct an activity or to make changes in an ongoing activity involving animals must provide the following information: (1) the species and approximate number of animals to be used; (2) a rationale for involving animals and for the appropriateness of the species and numbers of animals to be used; (3) a complete description of the proposed use of the animals; (4) a description of procedures designed to assure that discomfort and pain to animals will be limited to that which is unavoidable for the conduct of scientifically valuable research, including provision for the use of pharmacologic agents to minimize animal discomfort and pain; and (5) a description of any euthanasia method to be used. Review of ongoing protocols must occur no less than annually.

Research protocols submitted to the IACUC must also provide assurance that animal discomfort, distress, or pain will be avoided or minimized. A written, narrative description of the methods and sources used to determine that alternatives are not available is required for procedures that might cause more than momentary or slight pain or distress to the animals. The investigator must also provide written assurance that the activities do not unnecessarily duplicate previous experiments.

For potentially painful procedures, a veterinarian must be consulted. Sedatives, analgesics, or anesthetics must be provided, unless withholding them is scientifically justified in writing and approved by the IACUC. In such instances, the pain-relieving agents may be withheld only for the period of time necessary to meet research objectives. During its review, the committee must also be assured that paralytics will not be used without anesthesia. Animals that would otherwise experience severe or chronic pain or distress that cannot be relieved must be euthanized during or after the procedure. For all research protocols, the method of euthanasia must produce rapid unconsciousness and subsequent death without evidence of pain or distress.

Survival surgical procedures must be performed using aseptic technique and sterile instruments; members of the surgical team must wear surgical gloves and masks. Appropriate preoperative and postoperative care must be provided. Major survival surgery on nonrodents may be conducted only in facilities intended for that purpose and must be maintained under aseptic conditions. An animal may not be used in more than one major operative procedure from which it is allowed to recover, unless the additional procedure is scientifically justified in writing, required as a routine veterinary procedure, or required to protect the health or well-being of the animal. In other special circumstances, requests for exemptions may be made to the administrator of the USDA's APHIS.

The committee must also be assured that the animals' living conditions will be appropriate for their species. The housing, feeding, and nonmedical care of the animals must be directed by a veterinarian or other scientist trained and experienced in the proper care, handling, and use of the species. The IACUC must also be assured that personnel maintaining or studying animals are appropriately qualified and trained.

The Animal Welfare Act addresses one further important topic for the IACUC which is designed to help protect proprietary information within the institution. Specifically, the law stipulates that the research facility is not required to disclose trade secrets or commercial or financial information publicly or to the IACUC. It is unlawful for any member of an IACUC to release any confidential information of the research facility, including trade secrets, processes, operations, style of work, or apparatus. Furthermore, the law protects the identity, confidential statistical data, and amount or source of any income, profits, losses, or expenditures of the research facility. Committee members may not use or attempt to use or reveal to any other person any information that is entitled to protection as confidential information. Failure to comply with these requirements could result in a member being removed from the committee, fined, and imprisoned. Any individual or research facility injured in its business or property by reason of a violation of the confidentiality rules may recover all actual and consequential damages.

Personnel Qualifications

The 1985 Animal Welfare Act amendments also, for the first time, required research facilities to ensure that all scientists, research technicians, animal technicians, and other personnel involved with animal care, treatment, and use are qualified to perform their duties. This responsibility requires each institution to provide training and instruction on the humane methods of animal maintenance and experimentation, including the basic needs and the proper handling and care of each species, pre- and post-procedural care of animals, and methods of aseptic surgery. Personnel must also be instructed about research or testing methods that minimize or eliminate the use of animals or limit animal pain or distress and the utilization of information services that would help them search for alternatives. In addition, they must be informed about the methods whereby deficiencies in animal care and treatment should be reported.

Information Services

To support the required training, the 1985 Animal Welfare Act amendments mandated the Secretary of Agriculture to establish information services at the National Agriculture Library (NAL) to provide: (1) information pertinent to employee training; (2) methods that could prevent unintended duplication of animal experimentation as determined by the needs of the research facility; and (3) improved methods of animal experimentation that could reduce or replace animal use and minimize pain and distress, such as anesthetic and analgesic procedures. The Animal Welfare Information Center, NAL, meets these requirements.

Attending Veterinarian

Each research facility is required to have an attending veterinarian with training or experience in laboratory animal science and medicine who has direct or delegated program responsibility for activities involving animals at the research facility. Part-time or consulting veterinarians must provide a written program of veterinary care and perform regularly scheduled visits to the research facility. The veterinarian is authorized to ensure the provision of adequate veterinary care and to oversee the adequacy of animal care and use. Adequate veterinary care includes the availability of appropriate facilities, personnel, equipment, and services. It also includes the use of appropriate methods to prevent, control, diagnose, and treat diseases and injuries and the provision of emergency veterinary medical care. The veterinarian, through his/her role of oversight of the program of veterinary care must ensure that all animals are observed at least once daily to assess their health and well-being (which can be accomplished by someone other than the attending veterinarian, but communicates directly and frequently to the attending veterinarian). The veterinarian is also responsible for providing guidance to investigators and other personnel regarding the handling, immobilization, anesthesia, analgesia, tranquilization, and euthanasia of animals. Adequate pre- and post-procedural care must be provided in accordance with current established veterinary medical and nursing practices.

Records

The USDA requires records be maintained for each IACUC meeting; each proposed activity involving animals, including any significant changes; the status of IACUC approval for each activity or change; and semi-annual IACUC reports and recommendations. Every research facility must also maintain records concerning any dog or cat purchased, owned, held, transported, euthanized, or sold. These records must document the animal's source and date of acquisition, USDA-designated unique identification tag or tattoo number, species or breed, sex, date of birth or approximate age, and any distinguishing physical characteristics. The transportation, selling, or other disposition of a dog or cat must also be documented, including the name and address of the carrier (if transported) and of the new owner (if sold or donated). With the exception of the source and date of acquisition, these records must accompany any shipment of dogs or cats. A health certificate signed by a licensed veterinarian must accompany all shipments of dogs, cats, and nonhuman primates. Records that relate directly to activities approved by the IACUC must be maintained for the duration of the activity and for an additional 3 years after completion of the activity. A copy of all other records and reports must be maintained for 3 years and shall be available for inspection and copying by authorized APHIS or federal funding agency representatives.

Each research facility must submit an annual report to the USDA on or before December 1 of each calendar year to provide information relevant to the immediately preceding fiscal year (October 1–September 30). The report must ensure: (1) that professionally acceptable standards governing the care, treatment, and use of animals were followed; (2) that each principal investigator has considered alternatives to painful procedures; and (3) that the facility is adhering to the USDA standards and regulations, unless the IACUC has approved exceptions specified and explained by the principal investigator. A summary of any exceptions, including a brief explanation and the species and number of animals affected, must be attached to the annual report. In addition, the report must state the location of all facilities where animals were housed or used in actual research, testing, teaching, or experimentation or were held for these purposes. The common names and the numbers of animals used must be reported in one of three categories: (1) activities involving no pain, distress, or use of pain-relieving drugs; (2) experiments, teaching, research, surgery, or tests where appropriate anesthetic, analgesic, or tranquilizing drugs were used; and (3) painful activities where the use of pain-relieving agents would have adversely affected the procedures, results, or interpretation of the activity. An explanation of the animal procedure(s) conducted in the third category must be attached to the annual report. In addition, the number of animals being bred, conditioned, or held for use, but not yet used, must be listed. The USDA compiles the information contained in the reports from all registered research facilities and submits an annual summary to Congress.

2. USDA Standards

The USDA *Standards* are described in Part 3 of the Animal Welfare Regulations. Dealers, exhibitors, and research facilities are required to meet minimal housing, operating, animal health, husbandry, and transportation standards. These include feeding, watering, sanitation, lighting, ventilation, shelter from extremes of weather and temperatures, adequate veterinary care, and separation by species where the Secretary of Agriculture finds it necessary for the humane handling, care, or treatment of animals. Specific standards, including minimal enclosure space requirements, are provided for dogs, cats, guinea pigs, hamsters, rabbits, nonhuman primates, and marine mammals. The specifications are similar for all species, except marine mammals, and are more detailed for dogs, cats, and nonhuman primates. General standards are also provided for other warm-blooded species, including farm animals used for biomedical research purposes or for testing and production of biologicals for humans or nonagricultural or nonproduction animals. It is beyond the scope of this chapter to provide detailed information regarding these standards. However, several of the most notable aspects, as required by the 1985 amendments to the Animal Welfare Act, are summarized below.

Canine Opportunity for Exercise

Dogs housed in the same primary enclosure must be compatible. Dealers, exhibitors, and research facilities must develop, document, and follow an appropriate plan, approved by the attending veterinarian, to provide dogs over 12 weeks of age with the opportunity for exercise. This rule does not apply to individually housed dogs provided with at least twice the minimum floor space required or to dogs that are group-housed in floor space that meets the minimum space standards for each dog. Bitches with litters and incompatible, aggressive, or vicious dogs are also exempt. The attending veterinarian may also exempt dogs from this program if participation would adversely affect the dog's health or well-being. Such exemptions made by the attending veterinarian must be documented and reviewed at least every 30 days by the veterinarian, unless the condition is permanent. The IACUC may also approve exemptions if the principal investigator determines that it is inappropriate for certain dogs to exercise or be group-housed. This exception must be reviewed annually by the IACUC. Records of these exemptions must be maintained and made available to the USDA or federal funding agency upon request. If a dog is housed without sensory contact with another dog, it must be provided with positive contact with humans at least daily.

Psychological Well-Being of Nonhuman Primates

Dealers, exhibitors, and research facilities must develop, document, and follow an appropriate plan for environmental enhancement adequate to promote the psychological well-being of nonhuman primates. The plan must be in accordance with currently accepted professional standards as cited in appropriate professional journals or reference guides and as directed by the attending veterinarian. At a minimum, the plan must address the social needs of nonhuman primate species known to exist in social groups in nature. Individual animals that are vicious, overaggressive, or debilitated should be individually housed. Nonhuman primates that are suspected of having a contagious disease must be isolated from healthy animals in the colony as determined by the attending veterinarian. Group-housed nonhuman primates must be determined to be compatible in accordance with generally accepted professional practices and actual observations, as directed by the attending veterinarian. Individually housed nonhuman primates must be able to see and hear members of their own or compatible species unless the attending veterinarian determines that this arrangement would endanger their health, safety, or well-being.

Primary enclosures must be enriched by providing means of expressing noninjurious species-typical behavior. Environmental enrichment devices may include perches, swings, mirrors, manipulanda, and foraging or task-oriented feeding methods. Interaction with familiar and knowledgeable personnel is recommended, provided it is consistent with safety precautions. Special attention is required for infant and young juvenile nonhuman primates, those that exhibit signs of psychological distress, those entered in IACUC-approved research protocols that require restricted activity, and individually housed nonhuman primates without sensory contact with nonhuman primates of their own or compatible species. Great apes weighing more than 110 lb must be provided additional opportunities to express species-typical behavior. If a nonhuman primate must be maintained in a restraint device for an IACUC-approved protocol, such restraint must be for the minimum period possible. If the protocol requires more than 12 h of continuous restraint, the nonhuman primate must be provided the daily opportunity for at least 1 continuous hour of unrestrained activity, unless the IACUC approves an exception. Such an exception must be reviewed at least annually. The attending veterinarian may also exempt an individual nonhuman primate from participation in the environmental enhancement plan in consideration of its well-being. However, such an exemption must be documented and reviewed by the attending veterinarian every 30 days. All exemptions must be available for review by the USDA and federal funding agencies upon request and reported in the annual report to the USDA.

3. USDA Enforcement

The USDA is also charged with enforcement of the Animal Welfare Regulations. The Animal Care section of the USDA's Animal and Plant Health Inspection Service (APHIS) is responsible for ensuring compliance of transportation, sale, and handling of animals used in laboratory research. The Act requires the USDA to inspect each research facility at least once each year and, in the case of deficiencies or deviations from the standards promulgated under the act, to conduct follow-up inspections as necessary until all deficiencies or deviations are corrected. APHIS enforces the AWA through unannounced inspections, and investigations may also be conducted as a result of alleged violations of the Animal Welfare Act, in response to public or internal complaints. Animal Care uses a risk-based inspection system which allows inspectors to conduct more frequent and in-depth inspections at problem facilities and fewer (though no less than annual) at facilities that are consistently in compliance. Each research facility is required to permit APHIS officials to enter its place of business; to examine and make copies of the required records; to inspect the facilities, property, and animals; and to document, by taking photographs and other means, conditions, and areas of noncompliance. Should an AWA violation be confirmed, the USDA can take a variety of actions. Many infractions are resolved with an official notice of warning or a stipulation offer, which allow the institution to pay a penalty in lieu of formal administrative proceedings. Should a serious or chronic violation be identified, a Department-level review would occur with the issuance of a formal administrative complaint, which may be resolved by license suspensions, revocations, cease-and-desist orders, civil penalties, or a combination of these penalties through administrative procedures. The Animal Care Information System allows for online searches of inspection reports, including animal inventories, inspection report citations, and the number of animals used in medical research.

B. Public Health Service Policy

The Health Research Extension Act of 1985 (PL-99-158), Section 495, Animals in Research, mandates the Secretary of Health and Human Services, acting through the Director of the National Institutes of Health, to establish guidelines for the proper care and treatment of animals used in biomedical and behavioral research. Any institution receiving support through the U.S. Public Health Service (PHS) for animal research, training, biological testing, or animal-related activities, must provide extensive written assurance of their compliance with the PHS Policy on Humane Care and Use of Laboratory Animals (PHS Policy: OLAW, 2002). The policy applies to all PHS-conducted or -supported activities involving animals regardless of where they are conducted. Most federally supported animal-based biomedical research in the U.S. is funded through the Department of Health and Human Services (DHHS), including the National Institutes of Health (NIH); Centers for Disease Control and Prevention (CDC); Food and Drug Administration (FDA); and Environmental Protection Agency (EPA).

The Office of Laboratory Animal Welfare (OLAW), NIH, is responsible for the implementation, interpretation, and evaluation of compliance with the PHS Policy and for the education of institutions and investigators receiving PHS support. No activity involving animals may be conducted or supported by the PHS unless the institution conducting the activity has an approved written Animal Welfare Assurance on file with OLAW. OLAW may approve or disapprove the assurance or may negotiate a satisfactory assurance with the institution. A new assurance must be submitted at least once every 5 years. The assurance must fully describe the institution's program for the care and use of animals in PHS-conducted or PHS-supported activities. OLAW is also responsible for conducting site visits to selected institutions and for evaluating allegations of noncompliance with PHS Policy. If significant problems are identified and not corrected within a reasonable period of time, the Director of the NIH may suspend or revoke funding to an individual investigator or institution.

The PHS Policy implements the *U.S. Government Principles for the Utilization and Care of Vertebrate Animals Used in Testing, Research, and Training* (IRAC, 1985) developed by the Interagency Research Animal Committee (Table 2.1). OLAW also refers to the NIH Revitalization Act of 1993 (PL-103-43), *Plan for Use of Animals in Research* which requires the Director of the NIH to prepare a plan:

1. For the National Institutes of Health to conduct or support research into
   a. Methods of biomedical research and experimentation that do not require the use of animals;

TABLE 2.1   U.S. Government Principles for the Utilization and Care of Vertebrate Animals Used in Testing, Research, and Training

I.	The transportation, care and use of animals should be in accordance with the Animal Welfare Act (*U.S. Code*, Vol. 7, Secs. 213b *et seq.*) and other applicable Federal laws, guidelines and policies.
II.	Procedures involving animals should be designed and performed with due consideration of their relevance to human or animal health, the advancement of knowledge or the good of society.
III.	The animals selected for a procedure should be of an appropriate species and quality and the minimum number required to obtain valid results. Methods such as mathematical models, computer simulation, and *in vitro* biological systems should be considered.
IV.	Proper use of animals, including the avoidance or minimization of discomfort, distress, and pain when consistent with sound scientific practices, is imperative. Unless the contrary is established, investigators should consider that procedures that cause pain or distress in human beings may cause pain or distress in other animals.
V.	Procedures with animals that may cause more than momentary or slight pain or distress should be performed with appropriate sedation, analgesia, or anesthesia. Surgical or other painful procedures should not be performed on unanesthetized animals.
VI.	Animals that would otherwise suffer severe or chronic pain or distress that cannot be relieved should be painlessly killed at the end of the procedure, or, if appropriate, during the procedure.
VII.	The living conditions of animals should be appropriate for their species and contribute to their health and comfort. Normally the housing, feeding, and care of all animals used for biomedical purposes must be directed by a veterinarian or other scientist trained and experienced in the proper care, handling, and use of the species being maintained or studied. In any case, veterinary care shall be provided as indicated.
VIII.	Investigators and other personnel shall be appropriately qualified and experienced for conducting procedures on living animals. Adequate arrangements shall be made for their in-service training, including the proper and humane care and use of laboratory animals.
IX.	Where exceptions are required in relation to the provisions of these Principles, the decisions should not rest with the investigators directly concerned but should be made, with due regard to Principle II, by an appropriate review group such as the institutional animal research committee. Such exceptions should not be made solely for the purposes of teaching or demonstration.

b. Methods of such research and experimentation that reduce the number of animals used in such research;

c. Methods of such research and experimentation that produce less pain and distress in such animals; and

d. Methods of such research and experimentation that involve the use of marine life (other than marine mammals);

2. For establishing the validity and reliability of the method(s) described in paragraph (1);

3. For encouraging the acceptance by the scientific community of such methods that have been found to be valid and reliable; and

4. For training scientists in the use of such methods that have been found to be valid and reliable.

The Act is one key method by which the 3Rs are implemented in the U.S. research enterprise.

The PHS Policy stipulates that institutions must have an Animal Welfare Assurance approved by OLAW and an IACUC that is responsible for reviewing proposed projects, evaluating the animal care and use program, and inspecting facilities. The IACUC must maintain records of its activities and must report at least annually to OLAW. The Policy also includes the information required for PHS applications or proposals that involve animal use.

In addition to requiring compliance with the Animal Welfare Act, the PHS Policy requires institutions to use the *Guide for the Care and Use of Laboratory Animals* (*Guide*: NRC, 2011a) as the basis for developing and implementing an institutional program for activities involving animals. The *Guide* applies to all live vertebrate animals, including traditional laboratory animals, farm animals, wildlife, and aquatic animals used in research, testing, or teaching. It emphasizes performance standards, which are less prescriptive and more context-specific than rigid engineering standards. The *Guide* also encourages the application of professional judgment and highlights the importance of the Institutional Official, IACUC and Attending Veterinarian to function as a team in the oversight of the animal care and use program.

Recommendations in the *Guide* are based on published data, scientific principles, expert opinion, and experience with methods and practices that are consistent with high-quality, technically and scientifically appropriate, humane animal care and use. The *Guide* provides recommendations for occupational health and safety programs. Numerous relevant references are provided that provide further background to the recommendations of the *Guide*. The PHS Policy also requires that euthanasia of animals be conducted in accordance with the *AVMA Guidelines for the Euthanasia of Animals: 2013 Edition* (American Veterinary Medical Association,

2013). In addition, the PHS Policy recognizes accreditation by the AAALAC International. Institutions that are accredited by AAALAC are assigned *Category 1* assurance status and are not required to submit their most recent semiannual report to OLAW with the assurance statement. Those that are not accredited are awarded *Category 2* assurance status and are required to submit their semiannual report to OLAW.

Unlike the Animal Welfare Act, the PHS Policy requires that the IACUC consist of at least five (not three) members, to include a doctor of veterinary medicine, a practicing scientist with experience in animal research, an individual whose primary concerns are in a nonscientific area, and an individual who is not affiliated with the institution in any way other than as a member of the IACUC. One person may meet more than one of these four requirements, provided there is a minimum of five IACUC members. The IACUC is responsible for reviewing all proposed research projects or proposed significant changes in ongoing research projects in a manner similar to that required by the USDA animal welfare regulations. Whereas the USDA regulations require annual review of ongoing activities, PHS Policy requires the IACUC to conduct a complete review of ongoing activities at least once every 3 years. Records – including the minutes of all IACUC meetings; records of applications, proposals, and proposed significant changes in the care and use of animals and their respective IACUC evaluation; IACUC semiannual program reports and recommendations; and records of accrediting body determinations – must be maintained for at least 3 years. Records related to IACUC-approved activities must be held for 3 years beyond the completion of the activity. All records must be accessible for review and copying by an authorized OLAW or other PHS representative. In other ways, the duties of the IACUC described in the PHS Policy are similar to those in the Animal Welfare Regulations, including conducting semiannual facility inspections and program reviews, providing reports of those evaluations to the Institutional Official, reviewing concerns involving the care and use of animals at the institution, and having the authority to suspend an animal activity.

The PHS requires the IACUC to report to OLAW, through the Institutional Official, at least once every 12 months. This annual report must include any changes in the institution's accreditation status, program for animal care and use, or IACUC membership, as well as the dates of the IACUC's semiannual evaluations of the institution's program and facilities.

C. FDA Good Laboratory Practices

The federal Food, Drug, and Cosmetic Act requires the Food and Drug Administration (FDA), under the

DHHS, to ensure proper procedures for the care and use of laboratory animals, as implemented by the Good Laboratory Practice (GLP) regulations (21 CFR, Part 58) that became effective June 1979 and were most recently amended in 2002 (CFR, 2002). The regulations establish basic standards for conducting and reporting nonclinical safety testing and are intended to ensure the quality and integrity of safety data submitted to the FDA in support of an application for a research or marketing permit. Such permits are required for human and animal drugs, human biological products, medical devices, diagnostic products, food and color additives, and electronic medical products. Basic research studies, clinical or field trials in animals, and human subject trials are not covered by the GLP regulations.

Institutions seeking FDA approval of their products must establish written protocols and standard operating procedures (SOPs); provide adequate facilities, equipment, and animal care; properly identify test substances; and accurately record observations and report results for preclinical studies. The FDA relies heavily on documented adherence to the written protocols and SOPs in judging the acceptability of safety data submitted in support of marketing or clinical research permits. Every study conducted under GLP regulations must have a study director, who is ultimately responsible for the implementation of the protocol and conduct of the study. Each institution must also have a quality-assurance unit that monitors the conduct of studies to ensure that the protocol is being followed and the records are properly maintained.

To help ensure compliance with the GLP regulations, the FDA conducts periodic, routine surveillance inspections and data audits of public, private, and government nonclinical laboratories that may be performing tests on GLP-regulated products. They may also conduct directed inspections to verify the reliability, integrity, and compliance of important or critical safety studies being reviewed in support of pending applications for product research or premarketing approval. In addition, the FDA may conduct inspections to investigate potential noncompliance issues brought to the FDA by *whistleblowers*, the news media, industry complaints, FDA reviewers, other government contacts, or other sources. Inspections of commercial laboratories are conducted without prior notification. Initial inspections of university and government laboratories are initiated only after the facility has been informed in a letter from the Bioresearch Monitoring Program coordinator, Division of Compliance Policy, Office of Enforcement, FDA, of the intent to inspect.

The inspections include a review of the institution's organization and personnel, quality-assurance unit, facilities, equipment, testing facility operations, reagents and solutions, test and control articles, protocols and conduct of nonclinical studies, records, and reports. In addition, the animal care program is evaluated to determine whether the animal care and housing is adequate to preclude stress and uncontrolled influences that could alter the response of the test system to the test article. The inspection includes the animal housing room(s) and SOPs for the environment, housing, feeding, handling, and care of laboratory animals. Newly received animals must be appropriately isolated, identified, and evaluated for health status. Animals of different species, or animals of the same species on different projects, must be separated. Daily logs of animal health observations are randomly reviewed and treatment of animals must be authorized and documented. Cages, racks, and accessory equipment must be cleaned and sanitized, and appropriate bedding must be used. Feed and water samples must be collected at appropriate sources and analyzed periodically, and the analytical documentation must be retained. The pest control program is also reviewed. Copies of the IACUC's SOPs and meeting minutes are reviewed to verify committee operation.

A data audit is also conducted to compare the protocol and amendments, raw data, records, and specimens against the final safety assessment report. This audit is intended to substantiate that protocol requirements were met and that findings were fully and accurately reported. The study methods described in the final report are compared against the protocol and SOPs to confirm that the GLP requirements were met. In addition to reviewing the procedures and methods for animal housing, identification, health observations, and treatment, the audit includes review of the handling of dead or moribund animals and necropsy, histopathology, and pathology procedures. The audit also includes a detailed review of study records and raw data. These data may include animal weight records, food consumption records, and clinical pathology analyses and ophthalmologic examinations.

Inspection reports are classified according to the findings and whether or not objectionable conditions or practices were found during the inspection. If regulatory and/or administrative actions are recommended, the FDA may hold an informal conference, conduct a re-inspection, or issue a warning letter. It may also reject a nonclinical study or studies, disqualify the institution, withhold or revoke a marketing permit, or terminate a permit for preclinical studies.

D. Federal Interagency Cooperation

As part of the Animal Welfare Act, Congress required the Secretary of Agriculture to consult and cooperate with other federal departments and agencies concerned with the welfare of animals used in research. Specifically, the Secretary of Agriculture must consult with the Secretary of Health and Human Services prior to the issuance of regulations. In 1995, authorized representatives of the USDA, NIH, and FDA signed the initial Memorandum of Understanding (MOU) concerning Laboratory Animal Welfare. The MOU was last updated on January 18, 2011, and is valid for 5 years (MOU Number: 225-06-4000, http://grants.nih.gov/grants/olaw/references/finalmou.htm). The cooperating agencies made the following agreements based on mutual concern and interest regarding animal welfare: (1) to share information contained in agency registries, inventories, and listings of organizations that fall under their respective authority; (2) to share information pertaining to significant adverse findings regarding animal care and use and the actions taken by the agency in response to those findings; (3) to share evidence of serious noncompliance with required standards or policies for the care and use of laboratory animals; (4) to coordinate successive evaluations and to avoid redundant evaluations of the same entities; (5) to consult and coordinate with each other on regulatory or policy proposals and significant policy interpretations; (6) to provide each other with resource persons for scientific and educational seminars, speeches, and workshops related to laboratory animal welfare; and (7) to limit dissemination of shared information received to internal agency officials with a need to know and to refer any Freedom of Information Act requests for records provided by another agency to the agency that provided the records. Each agency appoints a liaison to a standing committee which is charged with facilitating implementation of the MOU. The committee is required to meet no less than two times per year to review the effectiveness of the agreement, suggest modifications to the agreement, and to address any urgent issues and specific cases of serious noncompliance.

The NIH has also established an MOU with the U.S. Department of Veterans Affairs (VA), Office of Research Oversight, and Office of Research and Development (http://grants.nih.gov/grants/olaw/references/mou_olaw.htm). The objectives of this MOU are to maintain and enhance agency effectiveness by coordinating efforts and sharing resources and information, especially those related to education and compliance; to avoid duplication of effort in achieving standards for the care and use of laboratory animals; and to promote harmonization among VA-sponsored activities and between VA institutions and other PHS Assured institutions. Many of the specific areas of agreement are patterned after the MOU among the USDA, FDA, and NIH. In addition, the MOU between the NIH and the VA entails: (1) consulting with regard to investigations of noncompliance at VA institutions and sharing information relevant to VA compliance with the PHS Policy; (2) committing OLAW to provide substantive review and consultation of internal VA policies and educational materials to ensure compliance with PHS Policy and to harmonize standards; (3) negotiating Animal Welfare Assurances for VA or VA-affiliated institutions (i.e., more than 75 medical or academic institutions that formally collaborate with the VA in conducting both human and animal research) that do not receive direct PHS support for activities involving live vertebrate animals; and (4) working collaboratively to co-sponsor educational meetings and workshops and to collaborate on online training. The MOU clearly states that interpretation of and determination of noncompliance with PHS Policy remains the exclusive purview of OLAW.

E. EPA Good Laboratory Practices

The EPA regulates chemicals and monitors compliance with environmental laws and regulations designed to reduce pollution to protect public health and the environment. The EPA monitors 44 statutory programs including the Federal Insecticide, Fungicide, and Rodenticide Act (FIFRA), enacted in 1947, which authorizes the administrator of the EPA to register and control the use of pesticides. For the registration of a new pesticide, the EPA conducts a premarket review of its potential health and environmental effects. Animal tests must be conducted according to the EPA's GLPs (CFR 2011), which differ in some respects from the FDA's GLPs. Specifically, the EPA GLPs govern studies related to health effects, environmental effects, and chemical fate testing. Similarities and differences between the FDA and EPA GLPs are described in detail at: http://www.fda.gov/ICECI/EnforcementActions/BioresearchMonitoring/ucm135197.htm.

Since 1976, the Toxic Substances Control Act (TSCA, USC 15) has provided the EPA with authority to require reporting, record-keeping and testing requirements, and restrictions relating to chemical substances and/or mixtures. Certain substances are generally excluded from TSCA, including, among others, food, drugs, cosmetics, and pesticides. TSCA addresses the production, importation, use, and disposal of specific chemicals including polychlorinated biphenyls (PCBs), asbestos, radon, and lead-based paint. According to the final rules published in 1983 (U.S. EPA 1983), TSCA also stipulates the use of GLP standards for conducting chemical studies required by the Act.

F. FWS and NIH Positions on Chimpanzees

After accepting a December 2011 Institute of Medicine (IOM) report, *Chimpanzees in Biomedical and Behavioral Research: Assessing the Necessity* (NRC, 2011b), the NIH convened a Working Group on the Use of Chimpanzees in NIH-Supported Research to advise on the implementation of the IOM report. The report, published in January 2013 contained 28 recommendations and was made available for public comment. In June 2013, the

NIH announced its plans to substantially reduce the use of chimpanzees in NIH-funded research and to retire the majority of chimpanzees it owns.

Specifically, the NIH plans to:

- Retain but not breed up to 50 chimpanzees for future research that meets the IOM principles and criteria (http://iom.edu/Reports/2011/Chimpanzees-in-Biomedical-and-Behavioral-Research-Assessing-the-Necessity.aspx);
- Provide ethologically appropriate facilities (i.e., as would occur in their natural environment) for those chimpanzees as defined by NIH, with space requirements yet to be determined;
- Establish a review panel to consider research projects proposing the use of chimpanzees with the IOM principles and criteria after projects have cleared the NIH peer review process;
- Wind down research projects using NIH-owned or -supported chimpanzees that do not meet the IOM principles and criteria in a way that preserves the research and minimizes the impact on the animals; and
- Retire the majority of the NIH-owned chimpanzees deemed unnecessary for biomedical research to the Federal Sanctuary System contingent upon resources and space availability in the sanctuary system.

In a separate action, in June 2013 the U.S. Fish and Wildlife Service (FWS) proposed classifying captive chimpanzees as endangered. After receipt of a petition in 2010 from a coalition of organizations, including the Jane Goodall Institute, to list all chimpanzees as endangered, the FWS conducted a formal review of the status of the chimpanzee under the Endangered Species Act (ESA). The FWS determined that the ESA does not allow for captive-held animals to be assigned a separate legal status from their wild counterparts. With the classification of the chimpanzee as endangered, certain activities would require a permit, including import and export of chimpanzees into and out of the U.S., *take* (defined by the ESA as harm, harass, kill, injure, etc.) within the U.S., and interstate and foreign commerce. Permits could be issued for scientific purposes or to enhance the propagation or survival of the animals.

G. Professional and Scientific Associations

Many scientific and professional associations have adopted position statements regarding the care and use of laboratory animals. Several of these also provide resources that have made a significant impact on the generally accepted practices for animal facilities.

1. Institute for Laboratory Animal Research

The National Academy of Sciences is a nongovernmental, nonprofit organization chartered by Congress in 1863 to "investigate, examine, experiment, and report upon any subject of science or art... whenever called upon by a federal agency, a group internal to the NRC, or Congress." The Institute for Laboratory Animal Research (ILAR) is a component of the Division on Earth and Life Studies, one of six subject area divisions in the National Research Council (NRC). The NRC is operated jointly by the National Academy of Sciences and the National Academy of Engineering, and is the organizational unit within the National Academies that conducts most policy studies at the request of the federal government.

ILAR is advised by a council of experts in laboratory animal medicine, zoology, genetics, medicine, ethics, and related biomedical sciences. The council provides direction for ILAR's programs. Many of ILAR's reports provide a framework for governmental and institutional animal welfare policies. The most widely distributed publication from ILAR is the *Guide for the Care and Use of Laboratory Animals* (NRC, 2011), which is recognized by the PHS and AAALAC International as a standard reference on laboratory animal care and use programs.

ILAR has published several other standard references that are used to establish and maintain optimal animal care and use programs: *Occupational Health and Safety in the Care and Use of Research Animals* (NRC, 1997); *The Psychological Well-being of Nonhuman Primates* (NRC, 1998); *Recognition and Alleviation of Pain in Laboratory Animals* (NRC, 2009) and its companion report *Recognition and Alleviation of Distress in Laboratory Animals* (NRC, 2008); *Guidance for the Description of Animal Research in Scientific Publications* (NRC, 2011c); and *Animal Models for Assessing Countermeasures to Bioterrorism Agents* (NRC, 2011d). The quarterly *ILAR Journal* (http://dels.nas.edu/global/ilar/Ilar-Journal) publishes contemporary, authoritative articles relevant to laboratory animal medicine, science, and management. ILAR also maintains a large database of commercial and investigator-held unique animal models and an international registry of laboratory registration codes on behalf of the International Committee on Standardized Genetic Nomenclature for Mice.

2. AAALAC International

The AAALAC International is a private, nonprofit organization that promotes the humane treatment of animals in science through a voluntary accreditation program, a program status evaluation service, and educational programs. At the time of this writing, AAALAC International accredits approximately 900 programs in 37 countries. It is a communication-intensive program that stresses application of performance standards and professional judgment, rather than inspection and enforcement of engineering standards. In its assessments of animal care and use programs, AAALAC relies on Three Primary

Standards: the *Guide* (NRC 2011a); the *Guide for the Care and Use of Agricultural Animals in Research and Teaching* (Ag Guide: FASS, 2010); and the *European Convention for the Protection of Vertebrate Animals Used for Experimental and Other Scientific Purposes, Council of Europe* (ETS 123) *1986*. AAALAC International overlays these standards on the laws and regulations for the country in which the institution seeking accreditation is located, and uses other specialty publications to supplement information about specific procedures or techniques related to the care and use of laboratory animals, designated as Reference Resources (http://www.aaalac.org/accreditation/resources.cfm). The use of performance standards allows AAALAC International to evaluate each program independently and to provide guidance appropriate to individual situations. This process helps institutions maintain optimal standards for animal care and use. AAALAC International accreditation is recognized by the PHS.

The on-site assessment is a peer review conducted by a member of AAALAC's Council on Accreditation and at least one *ad hoc* Consultant/Specialist. The Council is comprised of highly accomplished animal care and research professionals from around the globe. AAALAC is governed by a Board of Trustees comprised of representatives of Member Organizations, a select group of prestigious scientific, professional, and educational groups with an interest in advancing biomedical research and animal well-being in science, including the American Association for the Advancement of Science (AAAS), the Federation of American Societies for Experimental Biology, the Society for Neuroscience, Society of Toxicology, and more than 60 other professional scientific, veterinary medical, and patient advocacy organizations.

3. Federation of Animal Science Societies

To help ensure the ethical and humane treatment of farm animals used in agricultural research or teaching, the agricultural community published the *Ag Guide*. The first edition, published in 1988, was revised in 1999 and again in 2010 by the Federation of Animal Science Societies. The third edition of the *Ag Guide* is based on the premise that the housing and management of farm animals do not necessarily change because of the objectives of the research or teaching activity. It includes broad guidelines for institutional policies; agricultural animal health care; husbandry, housing and biosecurity; environmental enrichment; and animal handling and transport. Common agricultural animal species used in research and teaching are handled in more detail in species-specific chapters. The *Ag Guide* is used by AAALAC International for relevant program assessment and accreditation purposes; however, the OLAW has placed some restrictions on the breadth of

applicability of the *Ag Guide* for PHS Assured institutions if the institution's PHS Assurance encompasses all animal research activities at the institution (http://grants.nih.gov/grants/olaw/faqs.htm#instresp_7):

> "The Guide for the Care and Use of Agricultural Animals in Research and Teaching (*Ag Guide*) primarily refers to agricultural animals used in agricultural research for which the scientific objectives are to improve understanding of the animals' use in production agriculture. It is therefore inappropriate to substitute the *Ag Guide* for the Guide based on the species of animal. However, there may be circumstances where it is appropriate to follow the standards of the *Ag Guide* in biomedical research (e.g., transmission studies of avian influenza under poultry production conditions). Information about environmental enrichment, transport, and handling in the *Ag Guide* may be helpful in both agricultural and biomedical research settings. Proposals to conduct such activities should be reviewed on a case-by-case basis and any approval to depart from provisions of the Guide must be based on scientific justifications acceptable to the IACUC."

4. Other Professional Organizations

Several other professional organizations have published guideline documents that either address a particular range of species used in research or fill a gap in existing guidelines. Examples include the American College of Laboratory Animal Medicine (*Medical records for animals used in research, teaching, and testing: Public statement for the American College of Laboratory Animal Medicine* (Field *et al.*, 2007)), the Ornithological Council (*Guidelines to the Use of Wild Birds in Research* (Fair *et al.*, 2010)), the American Society of Mammalogists (*Guidelines of the American Society of Mammalogists for the use of wild mammals in research* (Sikes *et al.*, 2011)), the American Society of Ichthyologists and Herpetologists (*Guidelines for the Use of Live Amphibians and Reptiles in Field and Laboratory Research* (Beaupre *et al.*, 2004)), as well as the Association of Primate Veterinarians (*NHP Food Restriction Guidelines (2014a)* and *Social Housing Guidelines (2014b)*), to name just a few. Such taxon-specific guidelines can provide a useful supplement to the more broadly based guidelines that underpin a high quality animal use program.

H. International Laws and Regulations

It is not the intent of this chapter to provide detailed information on the various international laws and standards governing the care and use of laboratory animals. Because the biomedical research community has become more global, there is increased interest in the harmonization of international standards for the care and use of laboratory animals (Bayne *et al.*, 2014). As a result, the implementation of a legal and regulatory framework for the conduct of animal-based research is becoming increasingly common around the world. Two organizations, in particular, have established guidelines that have global reach:

1. The World Organisation for Animal Health (OIE)

The Office International des Epizooties (OIE) was founded in 1924; in 2003 it was renamed the World Organisation for Animal Health, but the historical acronym was retained. The OIE has a mission of creating a framework of international collaboration and information sharing to improve animal health and welfare. It is comprised of 178 Member Countries and is recognized as a reference organization for the World Trade Organization. The OIE publishes standards (predominantly on animal health and zoonoses) developed by expert groups on terrestrial and aquatic animals. Animal welfare was identified by the OIE as a priority in its 2001–2005 Strategic Plan. Subsequently, the OIE convened a permanent Working Group on Animal Welfare. This Working Group initially focused on standards relating to the long-distance transport of animals, and to the killing of animals for both human consumption and disease control purposes. More recently, laboratory animal welfare was identified as an area of interest. As a result, an *ad hoc* committee of experts in laboratory animal welfare was convened with representation from different geographic regions of the world (the U.S., Canada, Europe, Africa, Asia, South America) to develop baseline standards on laboratory animal care and use. By incorporating these standards in the Terrestrial Animal Health Code (OIE, 2011), the governments of the Member Countries have a responsibility to ensure these standards are reflected in their regulatory frameworks. Standards for laboratory animals appear in Chapter 7.8 of *Use of Animals in Research and Education* (http://web.oie.int/eng/normes/mcode/en_chapitre_1.7.8.htm).

2. Council for International Organizations of Medical Sciences (CIOMS)

CIOMS is an international, non-governmental, non-profit organization established jointly by the World Health Organization (WHO) and the United Nations Educational, Scientific and Cultural Organization (UNESCO) in 1949. It is comprised of 48 international member organizations representing biomedical disciplines and 18 national members representing national academies of sciences and medical research councils. In the laboratory animal medicine and science community, CIOMS is primarily known for its *International Guiding Principles for Biomedical Research Involving Animals* which were first promulgated in 1985. These eleven principles (Table 2.2) served as the basis for the *U.S. Government Principles for the Utilization and Care of Vertebrate Animals Used in Testing, Research, and Training*. The Guiding Principles are designed to assist ethics committees, animal care committees, organizations, societies, and countries in developing programs for the humane care and use of animals in research and education, especially those entities operating without federal or national regulations.

Recently, in collaboration with the International Council for Laboratory Animal Science (ICLAS), the Guiding Principles have been updated to reflect contemporary opinion on the proper use of animals in research (http://grants.nih.gov/grants/olaw/Guiding_Principles_2012.pdf). Like the original 1985 Guiding Principles, the revised Principles (CIOMS-ICLAS, 2012) are intended to be used by the international scientific community to guide institutions in the responsible use of vertebrate animals in scientific and/or educational activities. OLAW has issued a notification that PHS-Assured institutions outside the U.S. are required to implement the revised Guiding Principles (http://grants.nih.gov/grants/guide/notice-files/NOT-OD-13-096.html).

III. IMPORTATION AND EXPORTATION OF ANIMALS AND ANIMAL PRODUCTS

A. U.S. Department of Agriculture

The USDA, APHIS, Veterinary Services (VS), and National Center for Import and Export (NCIE) is charged with (1) facilitating international trade, (2) monitoring the health of animals presented at the border, and (3) regulating the import and export of animals, animal products, and biologics to protect the U.S.'s agricultural resources. It also regulates the import and transport of infectious organisms and vectors of disease agents. This category includes not only animal products and by-products but also biological materials that contain or have been in contact with certain organisms and animal materials (including cell cultures and recombinant products). All imported materials must enter the U.S. through USDA-designated ports of entry. The regulations are set forth in the Code of Federal Regulations (CFR), Title 9, Chapter 1 (CFR 1998a, CFR 1998b).

The individual designated to receive imported material, and who will be responsible for the material, must apply for a USDA permit by submitting a complete VS application form and applicable fee. Importation of cell lines and cell culture products, such as monoclonal antibodies and recombinant proteins, requires an additional form. The information provided must be sufficient for the VS to evaluate disease risk and should include details regarding product processing, production, and nutrient factors.

To protect the health of U.S. livestock and poultry, the USDA requires permits for importation of swine,

TABLE 2.2   CIOMS International Guiding Principles for Biomedical Research (2012)

I.   The advancement of scientific knowledge is important for improvement of human and animal health and welfare, conservation of the environment, and the good of society. Animals play a vital role in these scientific activities and good animal welfare is integral to achieving scientific and educational goals. Decisions regarding the welfare, care, and use of animals should be guided by scientific knowledge and professional judgment, reflect ethical and societal values, and consider the potential benefits and thee impact on the well-being of the animals involved.

II.   The use of animals for scientific and/or educational purposes is a privilege that carries with it moral obligations and responsibilities for institutions and individuals to ensure the welfare of these animals to the greatest extent possible. This is best achieved inn an institution with a culture of care and conscience in which individuals working with animals willingly, deliberately, and consistently act inn an ethical, humane and compliant way. Institutions and individuals using animals have an obligation to demonstrate respect for animals, to be responsible and accountable for their decisions and actions pertaining to animal welfare, care and use, and to ensure that the highest standards of scientific integrity prevail.

III.   Animals should be used only when necessary and only when their u se is scientifically and ethically justified. The principles of the Three Rs – Replacement, Reduction and Refinement – should be incorporated into the design and conduct off scientific and/or educational activities that involve animals. Scientifically sound results and avoidance of unnecessary duplication of animal-based activities are achieved through study and understanding of the scientific literature and proper experimental design. When no alternative methods, such as mathematical models, computer simulation, *in vitro* biological systems, or other non-animal (adjunct) approaches, are available to replace the use of live animals, the minimum number of animals should be used to achieve the scientific or educational goals. Cost and convenience must not take precedence over these principles.

IV.   Animals selected for the activity should be suitable for the purpose and of an appropriate species and genetic background to ensure scientific validity and reproducibility. The nutritional, microbiological, and general health status as well as the physiological and behavioral characteristics of the animals should be appropriate to the planned use as determined by scientific and veterinary medical experts and/or the scientific literature.

V.   The health and welfare of animals should be primary considerations in decisions regarding the program of veterinary medical care to include animal acquisition and/or production, transportation, husbandry and management, housing, restraint, and final disposition of animals, whether euthanasia, rehoming, or release. Measures should be taken to ensure that the animals' environment and management are appropriate for the species and contribute to the animals' well-being.

VI.   The welfare, care, and use of animals should be under the supervision of a veterinarian or scientist trained and experienced in the health, welfare, proper handling, and use of the species being maintained or studied. The individual or team responsible for animal welfare, care and use should be involved in the development and maintenance of all aspects of the program. Animal health and welfare should be continuously monitored and assessed with measures to ensure that indicators of potential suffering are promptly detected and managed. Appropriate veterinary care should always be available and provided as necessary by a veterinarian.

VII.   Investigators should assume that procedures that would cause pain or distress in human beings cause pain or distress in animals, unless there is evidence to the contrary. Thus, there is a moral imperative to prevent or minimize stress, distress, discomfort, and pain in animals, consistent with sound scientific or veterinary medical practice. Taking into account the research and educational goals, more than momentary or minimal pain and//or distress in animals should be managed and mitigated by refinement of experimental techniques and/or appropriate sedation, analgesia, anesthesia, noon-pharmacological interventions, and/or other palliative measures developed in consultation with a qualified veterinarian or scientist. Surgical or other painful procedures should not be performed on unanesthetized animals.

VIII.   Endpoints and timely interventions should be established for both humane and experimental reasons. Humane endpoints and/or interventions should be established before animal use begins, should be assessed throughout the course of the study, and should be applied as early as possible to prevent, ameliorate, or minimize unnecessary and//or unintended pain and/or distress. Animals that would otherwise suffer severe or chronic pain, distress, or discomfort that cannot be relieved and is not part of the experimental design, should be removed from the study and/or euthanized using a procedure appropriate for the species and condition of the animal.

IX.   It is the responsibility of the institution to ensure that personnel responsible for the welfare, care, and use of animals are appropriately qualified and competent through training and experience for the procedures they perform. Adequate opportunities should be provided for on-going training and education in thee humane and responsible treatment of animals. Institutions also are responsible for supervision of personnel to ensure proficiency and the use of appropriate procedures.

X.   While implementation of these Principles may vary from country to country according to cultural, economic, religious, and social factors, a system of animal use oversight that verifies commitment to the Principles should be implemented in each country. This system should include a mechanism for authorization (such as licensing or registering of institutions, scientist,, and/or projects) and oversight which may be assessed at the institutional, regional, and/or national level. The oversight framework should encompass both ethical review off animal use as well as considerations related to animal welfare and care. It should promote a harm–benefit analysis for animal use, balancing the benefits derived from thee research or educational activity with the potential for pain and/or distress experienced by the animal. Accurate records should be maintained to document a system of sound program management, research oversight, and adequate veterinary medical care.

ruminants, other hoof stock, poultry, and other birds (including avian eggs for research purposes, http://www.aphis.usda.gov/import_export/downloads/pro_fer_avian_eggs_research.pdf). Material derived from any animal is potentially subject to USDA regulations and must be cleared by Department of Homeland Security, Customs and Border Protection Agricultural Specialists at the port of arrival before entry into the U.S. is authorized. However, the USDA does not have regulatory authority over the importation of live laboratory animals or laboratory mammal material (including transgenic/knock-out mice and rats, hamsters, gerbils, guinea pigs, rabbits, ferrets, and their blood, tissue, DNA, extracts, antibodies, feces, sera, and antisera for research purposes (blood, sera, antibodies, and antisera is limited to less than 1 liter)) that have not been inoculated with or exposed to any livestock or poultry disease agents exotic to the U.S. and do not originate from facilities where work with exotic disease agents affecting livestock or avian species is conducted. The CDC has jurisdiction over live laboratory mammals and their material. However, the USDA has issued guidelines for importation (see Guidelines for importation #1103, effective October 1998 (USDA, 1998)). Cell lines and other products of cell lines, including monoclonal antibodies, which are not derived from livestock or avian species; are for *in vitro* use; have not been exposed to livestock or avian disease agents exotic to the U.S.; and do not produce antigens or contain genes of livestock or avian disease agents or do not produce monoclonal antibodies directed against livestock or avian disease agents may be imported without a USDA permit. The USDA recommends that each shipment be accompanied by documentation that confirms that animals have not been inoculated with or exposed to any livestock or poultry disease agents exotic to the U.S. In addition, a USDA permit is not required for the importation of material from humans and nonhuman primates that: (1) are not produced in tissue culture, (2) are not actual zoonotic (affects humans and animals) pathogens, and (3) are not potential zoonotic pathogens. APHIS also issues permits for the introduction of genetically engineered organisms that pose a plant pest risk, including insects and microbes.

The USDA, APHIS, and Plant Protection and Quarantine (PPQ) service regulates the importation of plants and other vegetable matter. Feed provided to an animal during transit, such as potatoes or carrots, may be regulated. The importer must consult with the PPQ Permit Office to determine entry requirements. If it cannot be allowed entry, the prohibited vegetable matter must be removed from the cage at the point of entry by a PPQ officer.

B. U.S. Department of Health and Human Services

Under the direction of the U.S. Department of Health and Human Services (DHHS), the PHS, through the Centers for Disease Control and Prevention (CDC), Office of Health and Safety, regulates the importation of nonhuman primates. The DHHS/CDC published a final rule on February 15, 2013 detailing changes to the regulations for the importation of nonhuman primates into the U.S. which became effective 60 days later. The revised regulations (42 CFR 71.53, 2013), effective April 16, 2013, now state that: (1) importers will no longer have to obtain a separate special permit in order to import African green, rhesus macaques, or cynomolgus monkeys into the U.S., but all importers will be required to meet all the standards that were previously listed on the special permit; and (2) any Old World primates that die or are euthanized during the 31-day quarantine period must be tested (antigen capture test) for filovirus infection. Additionally, antibody testing is required for all Old World primates that exhibit signs consistent with a filovirus infection during quarantine; this testing must be done at the end of the quarantine period and before the cohort of primates is released from quarantine. New requirements most pertinent to research are: (1) entry of nonhuman primates into the U.S. is restricted to those ports of entry where CDC Quarantine Stations are located, except in limited circumstances approved in writing in advance by CDC; and (2) quarantine requirements are removed for laboratory-to-laboratory transfers that meet certain criteria. Specifically:

- The laboratory must have both a foreign-based and a U.S.-based facility.
- The nonhuman primates must be part of an ongoing research project that has been approved by an IACUC.
- The recipient laboratory must be registered with CDC and must submit veterinary medical records documenting the primates' current and past health history, including testing for tuberculosis.
- U.S.-based laboratories must be licensed by the USDA; accreditation by the AAALAC International is desirable.
- The foreign-based laboratory must be accredited by a comparable accrediting agency.
- Justification must be provided to the CDC describing the reason a transfer to a U.S. laboratory is necessary (e.g., diagnostic equipment only available in the U.S.-based laboratory).
- A specific and detailed travel itinerary must be submitted to CDC.

Only institutions or individuals registered with the CDC may import nonhuman primates or receive them within a 31-day period of their arrival in the U.S. Under the new provision, importers must have a written worker protection plan for anyone whose duties may result in exposure to nonhuman primates, including procedures for appropriate response measures in the event of an emergency. The proposed protection plan is designed to ensure that individuals who work with or around nonhuman primates are educated on the risks and have the proper personal protective equipment to be safe-guarded from exposure to zoonotic diseases. Importers are registered for a 2-year period and must comply with CDC record-keeping and reporting requirements.

The PHS is also responsible for protecting humans from zoonotic diseases and therefore regulates the importation of other animals that may be infectious to humans. Dogs must have a certificate showing they have been vaccinated against rabies at least 30 days prior to entry into the U.S. Cats are not required to have proof of rabies vaccination for importation into the U.S.; however, some states require vaccination of cats for rabies. The CDC does not regulate snakes or lizards, but does limit imports of small turtles, tortoises, and terrapins, as well as their viable eggs. Turtles with a carapace length of less than 4 inches and turtle eggs may not be imported for any commercial purpose. An individual may import as many as six small turtles or six eggs or any combination totaling six or fewer turtles and turtle eggs for non-commercial purposes. Although the CDC has rescinded its restriction on the importation of birds and bird products, the CDC supports the USDA/APHIS in its ongoing regulations to prohibit or restrict the importation of birds, poultry, and unprocessed birds and poultry products (such as eggs and feathers) from countries where highly pathogenic avian influenza (HPAI H5N1) has been confirmed in poultry.

In addition, the PHS regulates the importation or subsequent distribution of any etiologic agent or any arthropod or animal host or vector of human disease. PHS permits must be obtained for importation and distribution of these materials.

C. U.S. Department of the Interior

The Convention on International Trade in Endangered Species of Wild Fauna and Flora (CITES), established in 1973 and amended in 1979, helps protect wild flora and fauna from extinction by requiring government permits for international trade in threatened wildlife and wildlife products. In the U.S., CITES is enforced by the FWS. It applies to all of the designated vertebrate and invertebrate animal or plant species, whether alive or dead, and any recognizable part of a designated animal. Protection is provided for species in two main categories: (1) those that are most endangered; and (2) other species at serious risk. The most endangered species are listed in Appendix I of the CITES agreement (http://www.cites.org/eng/app/appendices.php). Appendix II includes species that are not currently threatened with extinction but may become so unless trade is subject to strict regulation. Appendix III includes all species that any country identifies as being subject to regulation within its jurisdiction for the purpose of preventing or restricting exploitation and for which the cooperation of other countries is needed. Importation or exportation of these species requires appropriate documents.

The FWS and the Commerce Department's National Marine Fisheries Service jointly administer the Endangered Species Act (ESA), established in 1973 (7 USC §136). The purpose of the ESA is to protect and recover imperiled animal species and their ecosystems. All species of plants and animals are eligible for protection, except pest insects. An endangered species is in danger of extinction while a threatened species is likely to become endangered in the foreseeable future. The law (50 CFR, Chapter IV, Subchapter A, 1973, rev. 2014) prohibits any action, administrative or real, that results in the *taking* of a listed species or adversely affects the habitat of a listed species. Take is defined as "to harass, harm, pursue, hunt, shoot, wound, kill, trap, capture, or collect or attempt to engage in any such conduct." The ESA prohibits import, export, and interstate and foreign commerce of listed species and implements U.S. participation in CITES. A federal permit is required to use listed species for scientific purposes.

The Lacey Act was enacted in 1900 and amended several times, including substantial amendments in 1981 and most recently in the 2008 Farm Bill (though these amendments address the importation of plants). It was enacted to address trafficking in *illegal* wildlife, fish, or plants. The Lacey Act authorizes the FWS to regulate the importation, exportation, transportation, sale, receipt, acquisition, or purchase of fish, wildlife, or plants that may be injurious to humans or to the interests of agriculture, horticulture, forestry, or U.S. wildlife resources. The Lacey Act also provides for effective enforcement of state, federal, American Indian tribal, and foreign conservation laws. In addition, the Lacey Act requires that live wildlife be transported into the U.S. under humane and healthful conditions and that all containers or packages containing wildlife be appropriately labeled when transported in interstate or foreign commerce.

D. Environmental Protection Agency

The Environmental Protection Agency (EPA), which is responsible for enforcing the Federal Insecticide, Fungicide, and Rodenticide Act (FIFRA, 40 CFR, Chapter 1, Subchapter E), considers the potential adverse impact of pesticides on endangered species and their habitats, with the goal of protecting human health and the environment, before licensing the use of pesticides. Under FIFRA, the EPA can issue emergency suspension of the use of certain pesticides or cancel or restrict their use if the environment of an endangered species will be adversely affected. The EPA is authorized to strengthen the pesticide registration process by shifting the burden of proof to the chemical manufacturer. FIFRA also provides federal control of pesticide distribution and sale and requires registration of users (farmers, utility companies, and others) and certification of applicators.

E. Animal Transportation Association and International Air Transport Association

The Animal Transportation Association (ATA) is concerned with the transportation of animals by sea, land, and air. Some of the objectives of the ATA are: (1) to facilitate international and domestic transportation of animals using the most expeditious and economic routes; (2) encourage making live animal cargo a priority for carriers and handlers; (3) encourage the establishment of an animal protection office at principal ports and terminals where live animals are handled that will oversee adequate protection and humane handling of live animal shipments; and (4) encourage research on all phases of animal transportation. The ATA publishes proceedings from its conferences, fact sheets, and industry updates with the goal of informing and improving animal transportation.

The International Air Transport Association (IATA) is the trade association for airlines based around the world and guides the formation of positions on industry and public policy issues. IATA coordinates the Live Animals and Perishables Board (LAPB). The objectives of the LAPB are:

- The adoption of regulations for the acceptance, handling, and loading of live animals in air transport
- The promotion of public awareness and government acceptance of the Live Animals Regulations
- Providing for an open forum for member airlines to exchange and develop information specific to the transport of live animals and perishables
- Promoting an open dialogue with civil aviation authorities and shipping industry.

IATA publishes the Live Animals Regulations (LAR), the global standard for transporting animals by commercial airlines. The LAR addresses the container specification and other transportation requirements for numerous species. IATA has a cooperation agreement with the OIE to enhance veterinary research into animal health during air transport, the development and revision of international standards for air transport of live animals and perishable goods such as biological samples as well as the technical requirements for their international transport.

IV. HAZARDOUS SUBSTANCES

A. Biohazards

The Occupational Safety and Health Act, enacted in 1970, (CFR 1970, revised 2013) is administered and enforced by the Department of Labor and the Occupational Safety and Health Administration (OSHA). The intent is to provide workers with protection against illnesses or injury resulting from unsafe or unsanitary working conditions. The act established the National Institute for Occupational Safety and Health (NIOSH) within the Centers for Disease Control and Prevention. NIOSH plans, directs, and coordinates national programs to develop and establish recommended occupational safety and health standards (29 CFR, Part 1910) and to conduct research, training, and related activities to assure safe and healthful working conditions. These standards address bloodborne pathogens, respiratory protection, occupational noise exposure, hazard communication and other relevant safety measures. Chapter 24, *Control of Biohazards Associated with the Use of Experimental Animals*, provides a comprehensive overview of and references for the programs, facilities, and practices necessary to help assure employee protection against biohazards. These include animal allergies, zoonoses, recombinant DNA, and infectious experimental agents.

B. Chemical Agents

Chapter 21 also addresses the potential hazards of and precautions for working with chemical agents used in experiments. The Toxic Substances Control Act (TSCA), enacted in 1976, authorizes the EPA to require testing of chemical substances entering the environment and to regulate them as necessary. Chemicals used exclusively in pesticides, food, food additives, drugs, and cosmetics are exempt from the TSCA but are regulated by other legislation.

The Drug Enforcement Administration of the Department of Justice is responsible for enforcing the Drug Enforcement Act (PL-93-205). This law requires appropriate security and record management of controlled substances that are considered to be potentially addictive or habituating for human and animal use.

C. Radioactive Materials and Radiation-Emitting Equipment

The Atomic Energy Act of 1954 authorizes the Nuclear Regulatory Commission (NRC) to help ensure that the civilian use of radioactive materials is conducted in a manner consistent with public health and safety, environmental quality, national security, and antitrust laws. In 1974, the NRC became an independent regulatory agency under the provision of the Energy Reorganization Act. The NRC licenses individuals and institutions that use radioactive material and regulates the procurement, use, storage, and disposal of these materials; the facilities, instruments, and equipment used for handling and storing radioactive materials must also meet NRC requirements. Personnel must be provided training in the safe handling and use of ionizing radiation.

The Radiation Control for Health and Safety Act, enacted in 1968, authorizes the Food and Drug Administration, through the Center for Devices and Radiological Health, to regulate the use of products that produce radiation, such as medical diagnostic imaging equipment, irradiators, and electron microscopes. The Safe Medical Devices Act, passed in 1990, updated monitoring of medical devices to require post-market surveillance, and authorizes the FDA to recall devices.

V. NUCLEIC ACID AND NANOMATERIAL RESEARCH GUIDELINES

The NIH/Office of Biotechnology Activities, publishes the *NIH Guidelines for Research Involving Recombinant or Synthetic Nucleic Acid Molecules* (http://osp.od.nih.gov/office-biotechnology-activities/biosafety/nih-guidelines). Recombinant and synthetic nucleic acid molecules are defined as: (1) molecules that (a) are constructed by joining nucleic acid molecules, and (b) can replicate in a living cell (i.e., recombinant nucleic acids); (2) nucleic acid molecules that are chemically or by other means synthesized or amplified, including those that are chemically or otherwise modified but can base pair with naturally occurring nucleic acid molecules (i.e., synthetic nucleic acids); or (3) molecules that result from the replication of those described in (1) or (2). These guidelines apply to any research involving recombinant or synthetic nucleic acids conducted at or sponsored by an institution that receives any of its support from the NIH. If an institution is receiving NIH funding for only research with synthetic nucleic acids, and that research is covered under the amended NIH Guidelines, any research with synthetic nucleic acids or recombinant DNA conducted at the institution, regardless of the source of funding, will need to comply with all of the requirements of the NIH Guidelines. The creation of transgenic animals is covered by the NIH Guidelines. The maintenance of a transgenic rodent colony that can be housed at ABSL1 is exempt from the NIH Guidelines and so does not require Institutional Biosafety Committee (IBC) registration; however, a transgenic rodent colony at ABLS2 or higher and the breeding of all other transgenic animals is subject to the NIH Guidelines and thus requires IBC registration.

NIOSH has published guidelines to assist institutions involved in nanotechnology research. The guidelines, *General Safe Practices for Working with Engineered Nanomaterials in Research Laboratories* (NIOSH, 2012), describe occupational health and safety practices that should be followed during the synthesis, characterization, and research with engineered nanomaterials in the laboratory environment. Key elements described include risk management, hazard identification, exposure assessment, exposure control, and control verification.

References

American Veterinary Medical Association, 2013. AVMA Guidelines for the Euthanasia of Animals: 2013 Edition. <https://www.avma.org/KB/Policies/Pages/Euthanasia-Guidelines.aspx?utm_source=prettyurl&utm_medium=web&utm_campaign=redirect&utm_term=issues-animal_welfare-euthanasia-pdf>.

Animal Welfare Act (PL-91-579), 1970. <http://awic.nal.usda.gov/public-law-91-579-animal-welfare-act-amendments-1970>.

Animal Welfare Act Amendments of 1976 (PL-94-279), 1976. <http://awic.nal.usda.gov/public-law-94-279-animal-welfare-act-amendments-1976>.

Association of Primate Veterinarians, 2014a. Food restriction guidelines for nonhuman primates in biomedical research. <http://www.primatevets.org/Content/files/Public/education/NHPFoodRestrictionGuidelines.pdf> (accessed February 2014).

Association of Primate Veterinarians, 2014b. Social guidelines for nonhuman primates in biomedical research. <http://www.primatevets.org/Content/files/Public/education/APV%20Social%20Housing%20Guidelines%20final.pdf> (accessed February 2014).

Bayne, K., Bayvel, A.C.D., Williams, V., 2014. Laboratory animal welfare: international issues. In: Bayne, K., Turner, P. (Eds.), Laboratory Animal Welfare. Elsevier, New York, pp. 55–76.

Bayne, K., Morris, T., France, M., 2010. Legislation and codes of practice: a global overview. In: Kirkwood, J., Hubrecht, R. (Eds.), Eighth Edition of the UFAW Handbook on the Care and Management of Laboratory Animals and Other Animals Used in Scientific Procedures. Blackwell Publishing, Oxford, UK, pp. 107–123.

Beaupre, S.J., Jacobson, E.R., Lillywhite, H.B., Zamudio, K., 2004. Guidelines for the Use of Live Amphibians and Reptiles in Field and Laboratory Research. American Society of Ichthyologists and Herpetologists. <www.asih.org/files/hacc-final.pdf>.

Code of Federal Regulations (CFR), 1999. Title 9: Animals and Animal Products; Chapter 1: animal and plant health inspection service, department of agriculture; Subchapter A: animal welfare; Parts 1, 2, 3, and 4. Office of the Federal Register, Washington, DC.

CFR, rev. 1998a. Title 9: Animals and Animal Products; Chapter 1: Animal and Plant Health Inspection Service, Department of Agriculture; Subchapter C: Interstate Transportation of Animals (including Poultry) and Animal Products. Office of the Federal Register, Washington, DC.

CFR, rev. 1998b. Title 9: Animals and Animal Products; Chapter 1: Animal and Plant Health Inspection Service, Department of Agriculture; Subchapter D: Exportation and Importation of Animals (Including Poultry) and Animal Products. Office of the Federal Register, Washington, DC.

CFR, rev. 2002. Title 21: Food and Drugs; Chapter 1: Food and Drug Administration, Department of Health and Human Services; Subchapter A: General; Part 58: Good Laboratory Practice for Nonclinical Laboratory Studies. Office of the Federal Register, Washington, DC. <http://cfr.regstoday.com/21cfr58.aspx>.

CFR, 1970, rev. 2013. Title 29: Labor; Chapter 17: occupational safety and health administration; Part 1910: occupational safety and health standards. Office of the Federal Register, Washington, DC.

CFR, 2011, rev. 2003. Title 40: Protection of the Environment; Chapter 1: Environmental Protection Agency; Subchapter E: Pesticide Programs; Part 160: Good Laboratory Practice Standards. Office of the Federal Register, Washington, DC. <http://www.gpo.gov/fdsys/pkg/CFR-2011-title40-vol24/xml/CFR-2011-title40-vol24-part160.xml>.

CFR, 1973, rev. 2014. Title 50: Wildlife and Fisheries; Chapter 1: U.S. Fish and Wildlife, Department of The Interior; Subchap. B: Taking, Possession, Transportation, Sale, Purchase, Barter, Exportation, and Importation of Wildlife and Plants. Office of the Federal Register, Washington, DC.

CFR, rev. 2013. Title 42, Part 71.53. Foreign Quarantine Regulations, Final rule of HHS/CDC Nonhuman Primate Importation Regulations. Office of the Federal Register, Washington, DC. <https://www.federalregister.gov/articles/2013/02/15/2013-03064/control-of-communicable-disease-foreign-requirements-for-importers-of-nonhuman-primates-nhp>.

Council of Europe, 1986. European convention for the protection of vertebrate animals used for experimental and other scientific purposes (ETS 123), Strasbourg. <http://conventions.coe.int/Treaty/en/Treaties/html/123.htm>.

Council of International Medical Science Organizations (CIOMS) – International Council for Laboratory Animal Science (ICLAS), 2012. International guiding principles for biomedical research involving animals. <http://iclas.org/wp-content/uploads/2013/03/CIOMS-ICLAS-Principles-Final1.pdf>.

Fair, J.M., Paul, E., Jones, J. (Eds.), 2010. Guidelines to the Use of Wild Birds in Research, third ed. Ornithological Council <www.nmnh.si.edu/BIRDNET/guide/index.html>.

Farm Security and Rural Investment Act of 2002 (PL-107-171), 2002. Title X, Miscellaneous Subtitle D, Animal Welfare. <http://awic.nal.usda.gov/public-law-107-171-farm-security-and-rural-invest-ment-act-2002>.

Federation of Animal Science Societies, 2010. Guide for the Care and Use of Agricultural Animals in Research and Teaching, third ed. Champaign, IL. <http://www.fass.org/docs/agguide3rd/Ag_Guide_3rd_ed.pdf>.

Field, K., Bailey, M., Foresman, L.L., et al., 2007. Medical records for animals used in research, teaching, and testing: Public statement for the American College of Laboratory Animal Medicine. ILAR J. 48 (1), 37–41.

Food, Agriculture, Conservation, and Trade Act of 1990 (PL-101-624), 1990. Section 2503 – Protection of Pets. <http://awic.nal.usda.gov/public-law-101-624-food-agriculture-conservation-and-trade-act-1990-section-2503-protection-pets>.

Food Security Act (PL-99-198, U.S. Farm Bill of 1985), Subtitle F, Animal Welfare (Improved Standards for Laboratory Animals Act), 1985. <https://awic.nal.usda.gov/public-law-99-198-food-security-act-1985-subtitle-f-animal-welfare>.

Health Research Extension Act of 1985 (PL-99-158), Section 495, Animals in Research, 1985. <http://grants.nih.gov/grants/olaw/references/hrea1985.htm>.

Interagency Research Animal Committee (IRAC), 1985. U.S. Government Principles for Utilization and Care of Vertebrate Animals Used in Testing, Research, and Training. Federal Register, May 20, 1985.

Laboratory Animal Welfare Act of 1966 (PL-89-544), 1966. U.S. Code, vol. 7, Sections. 2131–2157. <http://awic.nal.usda.gov/public-law-89-544-act-august-24-1966>.

National Institute for Occupational Safety and Health (NIOSH), 2012. General Safe Practices for Working with Engineered Nanomaterials in Research Laboratories. DHHS (NIOSH) Publication No. 2012-147. <http://www.cdc.gov/niosh/docs/2012-147/>.

National Institutes of Health Revitalization Act of 1993 (PL-103-43), Plan for Use of Animals in Research, 1993. <http://grants.nih.gov/grants/olaw/pl103-43.pdf>.

National Research Council (NRC), 1997. Occupational Health and Safety in the Care and Use of Research Animals. National Academies Press, Washington, DC.

NRC, 1998. The Psychological Well-Being of Nonhuman Primates. National Academies Press, Washington, DC.

NRC, 2008. Recognition and Alleviation of Distress in Laboratory Animals. National Academies Press, Washington, DC.

NRC, 2009. Recognition and Alleviation of Pain in Laboratory Animals. National Academies Press, Washington, DC.

NRC, 2011a. Guide for the Care and Use of Laboratory Animals. National Academies Press, Washington, DC.

NRC, 2011b. Chimpanzees in Biomedical and Behavioral Research: Assessing the Necessity. National Academies Press, Washington, DC.

NRC, 2011c. Guidance for the Description of Animal Research in Scientific Publications. National Academies Press, Washington, DC.

NRC, 2011d. Animal Models for Assessing Countermeasures to Bioterrorism Agents. National Academies Press, Washington, DC.

Office of Laboratory Animal Welfare (OLAW), 2002. Public Health Service Policy on Humane Care and Use of Laboratory Animals. National Institutes of Health, Department of Health and Human Services, Bethesda, MD.

OIE (World Organisation for Animal Health), 2011. Terrestrial Animal Health Code. <http://web.oie.int/eng/normes/mcode/en_chapitre_1.7.8.htm> (accessed February 2014).

Sikes, R.S., Gannon, W.L., 2011. Animal Care and Use Committee of the American Society of Mammalogists. 2011. Guidelines of the American Society of Mammalogists for the use of wild mammals in research. J. Mammal. 92, 235–253.

Toxic Substances Control Act, USC, Title 15, Chapter 53, 1976. <http://www.epa.gov/oecaagct/lsca.html>.

U.S. Department of Agriculture (USDA), 1998. Guidelines for importation #1103. <http://nvap.aphis.usda.gov/import_export/animals/animal_import/downloads/ilivemam.html>.

U.S. Environmental Protection Agency (EPA), 1983. Toxic substance control: good laboratory practice standards. Federal Register 48, 53922–53944.

3

Biology and Diseases of Mice

Mark T. Whary, DVM, PhD, DACLAM[a], Nicole Baumgarth, DVM, PhD[b], James G. Fox, DVM, MS, DACLAM[a] and Stephen W. Barthold, DVM, PhD, Diplomate ACVP[c]

[a]Division of Comparative Medicine, Massachusetts Institute of Technology, Cambridge, MA, USA
[b]Microbiology and Immunology Center for Comparative Medicine, University of California Davis, Davis, CA, USA [c]EmeritusPathology, Microbiology & Immunology School of Veterinary Medicine, University of California, Davis, CA, USA

I. INTRODUCTION

A. Origin and History

Today's laboratory mouse, *Mus musculus*, has its origins as the 'house mouse' of North America and Europe. Beginning with mice bred by mouse fanciers, laboratory stocks (outbred) derived from *M. musculus musculus* from eastern Europe and *M. m. domesticus* from western Europe were developed into inbred strains (Table 3.1).

Since the mid-1980s, additional strains have been developed from Asian mice (*M.m. castaneus* from Thailand and *M.m. molossinus* from Japan) and from *M. spretus* which originated from the western Mediterranean region.

The laboratory mouse was employed in comparative anatomical studies as early as the 17th century, but accelerated interest in biology during the 19th century, a renewed interest in Mendelian genetics, and the research requirement for a small, economical mammal that was easily housed and bred were instrumental in the

TABLE 3.1   Standardized Abbreviations of Names for Common Inbred Strains

Abbreviation 129	Inbred 129 strains (may include subtype, e.g., 129S6 for 129S6/SvEvTac)
A	A strains
AK	AKR strains
B	C57BL strains
B6	C57BL/6 substrains
B10	C57BL/10 substrains
BR	C57BR strains
C	BALB/c strains
C3	C3H strains
CB	CBA strains
D	DBA strains
D1	DBA/1 substrains
D2	DBA/2 substrains
HR	HRS strains
L	C57L strains
R3	RIIIS strains
J	SJL strains
SW	SWR strains

Note: *The full strain/substrain designation and source should be defined and/or referenced in publications, with abbreviations used after definition thereof.*

development of the 'modern' laboratory mouse. Research use of mice has grown exponentially during the past and current century with the recognition of the power of the mouse for gene and comparative mapping and have made the laboratory mouse, in genetic terms, the most thoroughly characterized mammal on earth (Silver, 1995; Lyon *et al.*, 1996; Morse, 2007a). The current ability to create highly sophisticated, genetically engineered mice by inserting transgenes or targeted mutations into endogenous genes has also made the laboratory mouse the most widely and heavily used experimental animal.

B. Genetic History

Historical reviews have documented the origins of the laboratory mouse, which extend thousands of years into antiquity (Keeler, 1931; Morse, 1978; Silver, 1995). The laboratory mouse belongs within the genus *Mus*, subfamily Murinae, family Muridae, superfamily Muroidea, Order Rodentia, and within the *M. musculus* clade collectively called the 'house mouse' (Lundrigan *et al.*, 2002). Anatomic features of molar teeth and cranial bones were traditionally used by zoologists to identify over 100 different species within the genus, and to differentiate them from other murids. Because of considerable phenotypic

variation within a single *Mus* species, this approach has proven to be inaccurate, and given way to contemporary genetic analysis. The native range of the genus *Mus* is Eurasia and North Africa. Members of this genus are generally classified as aboriginal, consisting of species that live independent of humans, or commensal, which includes taxa that have coevolved and geographically radiated with human civilization since the dawn of agriculture 12,000 years before present (bp). This close association with human agrarian society gave rise to the genus name, derived from Sanskrit, *Mush*: to steal. The commensal group is known as the 'house mouse' clade, consisting of several subspecies of *Mus musculus*, including *M. m. domesticus*, *M. m. musculus*, *M. m. castaneus*, *M. m. bactrianus*, and a lesser known lineage, *M. m. gentilulus* (Prager *et al.*, 1998). The Japanese house mouse, *M. m. molossinus*, is a natural hybrid of *M. m. musculus* and *M. m. castaneus*. The progenitor of the *M. musculus* clade arose in the northern Indian subcontinent and diverged into genetically isolated and distinct species or subspecies due to geographic barriers (mountain ranges). There is debate whether these taxa are species or subspecies, and some have referred to them as 'incipient species,' but their genetic divergence is now blurring as they colonize the world and hybridize.

The native ranges of these taxa are important for understanding the origins of various laboratory mice, whose genomes are mosaics derived from *M. m. domesticus* (~60%), *M. m. musculus* (~30%), and *M. m. castaneus* (~10%) (Wade and Daly, 2005; Wade *et al.*, 2002). It is now apparent that the *M. m. musculus* and *M. m. castaneus* contributions to the laboratory mouse genome were primarily derived from *M. m. molossinus* Japanese fancy mice (Takada *et al.*, 2013). *Mus m. domesticus* is indigenous to western Europe and southwest Asia, *M. m. musculus* to eastern Europe and northern Asia, *M. m. castaneus* to southeast Asia, and *M. m. molossinus* to Japan and the Korean peninsula. The cohabitation of humans with commensal mice gave rise to captive breeding for coat color and behavioral variants in China over 3000 years bp. By the 1700s, mouse 'fanciers' in Asia had created many varieties of fancy mice, as did European fanciers, who subsequently acquired Asian stocks, particularly Japanese fancy mice (*M. m. molossinus*), to mix with European (*M. m. domesticus*) fancy mouse varieties. This genetic mixing for fancy variants was also occurring in the United States, and these mouse lines contributed to many of the major laboratory mice used today. Meanwhile, the European colonial expansion era contributed to the worldwide dissemination of *M. m. domesticus*, which now occupies every continent of the world. It is well documented that wild-caught *M. m. domesticus* also contributed to the genetic composition of fancy and laboratory mice on multiple occasions.

Despite their diverse genetic origins and phenotypic differences, most laboratory mouse strains are closely related, since many were derived from a genetically mixed but small number of fancy mice from a single mouse breeder (Abbie Lathrop's Granby Mouse Farm, Massachusetts) at the beginning of the 20th century. Most inbred laboratory mice share a common maternal mitochondrial genome derived from *M.m. domesticus* (Ferris *et al.*, 1982; Yu *et al.*, 2009), and a common Y chromosome contributed by *M.m. musculus* (Bishop *et al.*, 1985) through its contribution to the genome of *M.m. molossinus* (Nagamine *et al.*, 1992). Thus, the most inclusive name that can be assigned to the genetically mosaic laboratory mouse is *M. musculus*, the over-arching name for the entire commensal clade. There are exceptions, however. C57BL/6 mice contain minor genetic elements derived from *M. spretus* (Hardies *et al.*, 2000), and a number of wild aboriginal species that are not members of the *M. musculus* clade, including *M. spretus, M. caroli,* and others, have been established as inbred lines of mice.

C. Genetics

Genetic mapping in mice began in the early 1900s with a focus on inheritance of coat color. The first autosomal genes, albino and pink-eyed dilution, were linked in 1915 (Haldane *et al.*, 1915). Extensive linkage maps and an impressive array of inbred strains are now available to expedite genetic research (Table 3.1) (Lyon *et al.*, 1996). Mice have 20 pairs of telocentric chromosomes that are differentiated by their size and patterns of transverse bands. The chromosomes are designated by Arabic numbers in order of decreasing size. During the 1970s, chromosome rearrangements were used to assign known genetic linkage groups – identified by Roman numerals – to specific chromosomes and for determining locus order with respect to the centromere. Genes can be located physically on chromosomes by fluorescent *in situ* hybridization (FISH). Development of quantitative trait loci (QTL) methodology for mapping genes and the similarity between mouse and human genomes have made the mouse invaluable for identifying genes and underlying complex traits that are inherent to the most common human genetic diseases (Moore and Nagle, 2000). For more information on comparative genomics, see Chapter 35 *Animal Models in Biomedical Research*, subsection C.

One of the most thoroughly studied genetic systems of the mouse is the *histocompatibility complex.* Histocompatibility (*H*) loci control expression of cell surface molecules that modulate critical immune responses, such as the recognition of foreign tissue. For example, the time, onset, and speed of skin graft rejection are controlled by two groups of *H* loci. The major group is located in the major histocompatibility complex (MHC, *H2*) on chromosome 17. The *H2* complex contains several loci, including K, D, L, I-A, and I-E. Inbred strains of mice, being homozygous, each have unique sets of *H2*

alleles, termed H2 *haplotypes.* For example, the BALB H2 haplotype is $H2^d$ and the C57BL H2 haplotype is $H2^b$. The *International ImMunoGeneTics (IMGT) Information System* provides details on H2 haplotypes for various inbred mice (www.imgt.org/IMGTrepertoireMHC/Polymorphism/haplotypes/mouse/MHC/Mu_haplotypes.html). Minor *H* loci groups are scattered throughout the genome and are responsible for delayed graft rejection. Genes associated with the *H2* complex also control other immunological functions, such as cell–cell interactions in primary immune responses and the level of response to a given antigen. Immune-mediated responses to infectious agents such as viruses and complement activity are influenced directly or indirectly by the *H2* complex (Stuart, 2010). Non-MHC or minor histocompatibility systems also are under active study (Roopenian *et al.*, 2000).

Mouse genomics have accelerated tremendously in the last two decades, heralded by the development of a robust physical map and high-quality genome sequence of the C57BL/6J mouse in 2002 by the *International Mouse Genome Sequencing Consortium* (Waterston *et al.*, 2001). The *Mouse Genomes Project*/Wellcome Trust Sanger Institute is extending this effort to include the genomic sequences of 17 key mouse strains. Completed and evolving sequence data are available through the *European Nucleotide Archive* (www.ebi.ac.uk/ena/home). The burgeoning numbers of inbred mouse strains, natural mutants, induced mutants, transgenic lines, and targeted mutant lines of mice are cataloged in the *Mouse Genome Informatics* (MGI) database: http://www.informatics.jax.org/mgihome). The growing number of mutant mice has fostered the development of a number of mouse repositories, from which specific mice can be located and acquired. In the United States, there are four regional National Institutes of Health (NIH)-supported *Mutant Mouse Regional Resource Centers* (http://www.mmrrc.org), which link to international repositories in Europe, Japan, China, Australia, and Canada, as well as additional resource programs in the United States through the *International Mouse Strain Resource* (IMSR; http://www.informatics.jax.org/imsr/index.jsp) for depositing, archiving, and distributing mutant mouse and embryonic stem cell lines to the scientific community. In addition to numerous mutant mice produced independently by scientists in various academic institutions, three major targeted gene knockout programs, all utilizing C57BL/6N embryonic stem cells, are under way internationally, and funded by the NIH, the European Community, and Genome Canada (Collins *et al.*, 2007; Skarnes *et al.*, 2011). These include the *Knock Out Mouse Project* (KOMP; http://www.knockoutmouse.org), the *European Conditional Mouse Mutagenesis Program* (EUCOMM; http://www.eucomm.org), and the *North American Conditional Mouse Mutagenesis Project* (NorCOMM;http://norcomm.phenogenomics.ca/index.htm). These mouse lines will be available through three distribution centers: the *German Resource Center for Genome Research* (RZPD; http://www.rzpd.de), the KOMP repository (https://komp.org), and the Canadian Mouse Consortium (CMC; http://www.mousecanada.ca/index.htm). The repositories are all linked to the IMSR, and provide access to mice, germplasm, genomic detail, and phenotypic data. Genetic, genomic, and biological data are also available through the *International Mouse Phenotyping Consortium* (IMPC; www.mousephenotype.org) and the *Mouse Genome Database* (MGD; http://www.informatics.jax.org) (Eppig *et al.*, 2012).

D. Breeding Systems

Inbreeding is a fundamental genetic tool applied to the laboratory mouse and detailed information is available on the web (Table 3.2). The first inbred strain (DBA) was developed by C.C. Little in 1909, with the subsequent creation of over 1000 inbred strains and stocks of mice (Festing, 1996). Genetic origins, basic characteristics, references, and breeding performance of inbred strains of mice are available through Michael Festing's online version of *Inbred Strain Characteristics* (http://www.informatics.jax.org/external/festing/mouse/STRAINS.shtml). Overviews of genetic manipulation for the creation of different types of mice are available (Lyon *et al.*, 1996; Silver, 1995).

Inbred mouse lines are termed *strains*, and are achieved by 20 or more brother × sister (filial; F) generations (Table 3.3). Mice within an inbred strain, for practical purposes, are genetically identical (*syngeneic* or *isogenic*) to other mice of the same strain and sex. Because of residual heterozygosity, a strain is not *fully inbred* until after 60 F generations. Most commonly used inbred mouse strains represent 200 or more F generations, providing a high degree of experimental reproducibility. The mouse genome is not static, so when branches of an inbred strain are separated, spontaneous mutations, residual heterozygosity, and retroelement integrations result in genetic differences. Therefore, if branches of an inbred strain are separated before F_{40}, if branches have separated for 100 generations, or if genetic differences arise, the different branches become *substrains*. The same holds true if branches of a substrain diverge, resulting in substrains of the inbred substrain.

When two inbred mouse strains are crossed, the F_1 hybrids are genetically identical to one another (isogenic), but maximally heterozygous (with chromosomes of each chromosomal pair separately contributed by each parental strain), whereas F_2 hybrids are maximally genetically diverse from one another (with chromosomes of both chromosomal pairs containing a mixture of contributions from each parental strain). With each subsequent F generation, mice once again approach inbred status. This technique is used for creating *recombinant inbred* (RI) strains.

RI strains are sets of inbred strains of mice derived from crossing two inbred strains, and developed by single-pair random matings of sibling mice from the F_2 generation, thereby creating separate breeding lines. Each line created is maintained separately, and then propagated by brother–sister matings for 20 generations, with each line becoming a separate inbred strain, but belonging to a set of RI strains. RI mice are useful for mapping phenotypic or quantitative traits that differ between the progenitor strains (Bailey, 1971). RI sets are generally limited to two parental strains. An ongoing international effort has been undertaken to increase allelic diversity among RI strains by creating the *Collaborative Cross* (CC) in which a panel of RI strains are being generated mixing the genomes from eight disparately related inbred (octo-parental) mouse strains, including A/J, C57BL/6J, 129S1/SvImJ, nonobese diabetic (NOD)/ShiLtJ, NZO/HlLtJ, CAST/EiJ, PWK/PhJ, and WSB/EiJ. These eight strains capture nearly 90% of the known genetic variation present among laboratory mice. Future applications of the CC will utilize RI intercrosses of pairs of RI CC lines (Threadgill and Churchill, 2012; Welsh *et al.*, 2012).

Recombinant congenic strains are sets of inbred strains derived in a manner similar to that for RI sets, except that one or more *backcrosses* to one parental strain (designated the *background strain*) are made after the F_1 generation, before inbreeding is begun. The other parental strain is designated as the *donor strain*. The proportion of background and donor genomes is determined by the number of backcrosses preceding inbreeding (Demant and Hart, 1986). *Advanced intercross lines* (AILs) are another type of RI lines. They are made by producing an F_2 generation between two inbred strains and then, in each subsequent generation, intercrossing mice but avoiding sibling matings. The purpose is to increase the possibility of recombination between tightly linked genes.

When a mutation arises spontaneously or is induced within an inbred strain, that mutant mouse becomes *co-isogenic* with the parental inbred strain, being virtually identical except for the single mutant allele. Frequently, a mutation that arose in one inbred strain may be desired within the genetic background of another inbred strain. This can be accomplished by *backcrossing*, in which an F_1 hybrid is created by mating the donor mutant strain to the desired background strain, with subsequent matings to the background strain while retaining the mutant locus. After 10 backcross generations (*N* generations), the mutant mouse line is now *congenic* to the background inbred strain. Backcrossing to create congenic strains of mice has been used extensively when targeted mutations have been induced in 129 embryonic stem cells, with backcrossing onto C57BL/6 inbred mice. Congenic mice are never co-isogenic, as the preserved locus in a congenic mouse is invariably surrounded by flanking DNA, which may significantly influence phenotype (Linder, 2006).

TABLE 3.2   Databases and Websites for Information about Mice

Internet resource	Web address
COMPREHENSIVE DATABASE SITES AND MOUSE SOURCES	
Mouse Genome Database (MGD)	http://www.informatics.jax.org
JAX Mice	http://jaxmice.jax.org/index.shtm
MRC Mammalian Genetics Unit, Harwell, United Kingdom	http://www.mgu.har.mrc.ac.uk
The Whole Mouse Catalog	http://www.rodentia.com/wmc
ORNL Mutant Mouse Database	http://bio.lsd.ornl.gov/mouse
NIH Mutant Mouse Region Resource Center	https://www.mmrrc.org
GENETICALLY ENGINEERED MOUSE SITES AND SOURCES	
Induced Mutant Resource	http://lena.jax.org/resources/documents/imr
TBASE	http://tbase.jax.org
European Mouse Mutant Archive (EMMA)	http://www.emma.rm.cnr.it
BioMedNet Mouse Knockout and Mutation Database	http://research.n.com/mkmd
Cre Transgenic and Floxed Gene Databases	http://www.mshri.on.ca/nagy/cre.htm
University of California Resource of Gene Trap Insertions	http://socrates.berkeley.edu/~skarnes/resource.html
Database of Gene Knockouts	http://www.bioscience.org/knockout/knochome.htm
The Big Blue Web Site	http://eden.ceh.uvic.ca/bigblue.htm
The Mouse Brain Library	http://www.nervenet.org/mbl/mbl.html
MOUSE BIOLOGY	
Mouse Tumor Biology Database (MTB)	http://tumor.informatics.jax.org/cancerlinks.html
The Mammary Transgene Database	http://bcm.tmc.edu/ermb/mtdb/mtdb.html
Gene Expression Database (GXD)	http://www.informatics.jax.org
NetVet and the Electronic Zoo	http://netvet.wustl.edu/vet.htm
The Dysmorphic Human-Mouse Homology Database (DHMHD)	http://www.hgmp.mrc.ac.uk/dhmhd/dysmorph.html
The Mouse Atlas and Gene Expression	http://genex.hgu.mrc.ac.uk
DATABASE PROJECT	
UCD Medpath Transgenic Mouse Searcher 2.0	http://www-mp.ucdavis.edu/personaltgmousel.html
Mouse 2-D PAGE Database	http://biosun.biobase.dk/~pdi/jecelis/mouse_data_select.html
BODY MAP	
Human and Mouse Gene Expression DB	http://bodymap.ims.u-tokyo.ac.jp
UNSW Embryology Mouse Development	http://anatoM.med.unsw.edu.au/cbl/embryo/otheremb/mouse.htm
Dynamic [Embryonic] Development	http://www.acs.ucalgary.ca/~browder/mice.html
Zygote: A Developmental Biology Website	http://zygote.swarthmore.edu/info.html
MOUSE GENOMICS	
Mouse Nomenclature Guidelines and Locus Symbol Registry	http://www.informatics.jax.org/mgihome/nomen
Trans-NIH Mouse Initiative	http://www.nih.gov/science/models/mouse
Gene Dictionary of the Mouse Genome	http://www.nervenet.org/main/dictionary.html
Genetic and Physical Maps of the Mouse Genome	http://www-genome.wi.mit.edu/cgi-bin/mouse/index
Mouse Backcross Service (U.K. HGMP Resource Centre)	http://www.hgmp.mrc.ac.uk/goneaway/mbx.html
The Jackson Laboratory Mapping Panels	http://www.jax.org/resources/documents/cmdata

(Continued)

TABLE 3.2 (Continued)

Internet resource	Web address
WashU GSC Mouse EST Project	http://genome.wustl.edu/est/mouse_esthmpg.html
Japanese Animal Genome Database	http://ws4.niai.affrc.go.jp
NCBI LocusLink	http://www.ncbi.nlm.nih.gov/focuslink
UniGene Mouse Sequences Collection	http://www.ncbi.nlm.nih.gov/unigene/mm.home.html
TIGR Mouse Gene Index	http://www.tigr.org/tdb/mgi/index.html
NIA/NIH Mouse Genomics Home Page	http://lgsun.grc.nia.nih.gov
WICGR Mouse RH Map Home Page	http://www-genome.wi.mit.edu/mouse_rh/index.html
Mammalian Genetics Laboratory, National Institute of Genetics (Japan)	http://www.shigen.nig.ac.jp/mouse/mouse.default.html
CARE AND USE	
Guidelines for Ethical Conduct in the Care and Use of Animals	http://www.apa.org/science/anguide.html
The Ethics of Using Transgenic Animals	http://oslovet.veths.no/transgenics/references.html
Institute for Laboratory Animal Research	http://www4.nationalacademies.org/cls/ilarhome.nsf
Laboratory Registration Code Database	http://www4.nas.edu/cls/afr.nsf/labcodesearch?openform
Research Genetics, Genomic Tools	http://www.resgen.com/index.php3
GENERAL	
American Fancy Rat and Mouse Association	http://www.afrma.org

TABLE 3.3 Kinds of Mice Used in Research[a]

Definition of breeding system	Perpetuation of breeding system	Reference
Random bred stock: Random mating within a large, heterogeneous population	Continue random mating, selection pairs with random numbers method	Poiley (1960) Kimura and Crow (1963)
Inbred strain: Brother-sister mating for more than 20 generations	Continue brother-sister mating	Green (1981a)
F₁ hybrids: Mice from crosses between inbred strains	Cannot be perpetuated	Green (1981a)
Segregating inbred strain: Brother-sister matings system for more than 20 generations with heterozygosity for the mutations forced by (1) backcrossing, (2) intercrossing, (3) crossing and intercrossing, or (4) backcrossing and intercrossing	Continue brother-sister mating with heterozygosity forced by one of the four methods at left or with homozygosity forced by intercrossing homozygotes	Green (1981a)
Coisogenic inbred strains: Occurrence of a mutation within a strain	Perpetuate the mutation by (1) brother-sister mating within strain of origin, (2) backcross or cross-intercross system with strain of origin as parent strain, (3) brother-sister mating with heterozygosity forced by back- or intercrosses, or (4) brother-sister mating between homozygotes	Flaherty (1981) Green (1981a)
Congenic inbred strains: (A) Repeated backcross of mutation-bearing mice for 10 or more generations or (B) cross-intercross system for the equivalent of 20 or more cycles with an inbred parent strain	Perpetuate the transferred mutation by (2), (3), or (4) above. (1) may be used after 10–12 generations of backcrossing with periodic backcrosses to background strain	Flaherty (1981) Green (1981a)
Recombinant inbred strains: Cross between two inbred strains followed by F₁ brother-sister mating for >20 generations to obtain F₂; RI strains are inbred after additional 20 generations of brother-sister matings.	Continue brother-sister matings	Bailey (1971)
Recombinant congenic strains: Same as above except one or more backcrosses of F₁ to one parent strain before beginning brother-sister matings	Continue brother-sister matings	Demant and Hart (1986)
Advanced intercross lines: Nonsibling matings from an F₂ of a cross between two inbred strains	Continue nonsibling matings	

[a]*Modified from Green (1981a)*

In contrast to inbred mice, *outbred* mice are genetically heterogeneous and are maintained by breeding systems that intentionally minimize inbreeding. Outbred mice are called *stocks*, which are defined as a closed population (for at least four generations) of genetically variable mice that are bred to maintain maximal heterozygosity. Outbred mice may be used when high genetic heterogeneity is desired or for experiments requiring large numbers of mice. Outbreeding can be achieved only in a large breeding population using a systematic breeding scheme, or randomized selection of breeders from the population. A small breeding population or passage through the genetic 'bottleneck' of rederivation to improve health status will reduce genetic heterogeneity and lead eventually to some degree of inbreeding. In a population of 25 breeding pairs, e.g., heterozygosity will decrease at 1% per generation with standard randomization techniques. Random breeding involves the statistically random selection of breeders by using a random numbers table or computer program. An outbreeding program that is easy to manage is the circular pair mating system, in which each pair is mated only once. Conceptually, cages are visualized in a circle, and each cage contains one breeding pair in the *n*th generation. Another 'circular' set of cages serves as the breeding nucleus for the *n* + 1 generation. Each mated pair in the *n*th generation contributes one female and one male to the *n* + 1 generation. Outbreeding is accomplished by assigning the female and male derived from each *n*th generation cage to different cages in the *n* + 1 generation.

Most outbred mouse stocks are of 'Swiss' origin, derived from nine mice imported to the United States in 1926, and are therefore quite homogeneous genetically (Chia *et al.*, 2005). Various lines of these mice have been maintained at different institutions, giving rise to numerous closely related stocks. Although considered outbred, they have a high degree of homozygosity, exemplified by the fact that many Swiss mouse stocks are blind due to the homozygous recessive *rd1* allele (Serfilippi *et al.*, 2004b). It is preferable to ensure genetic heterogeneity by intercrossing multiple inbred strains to achieve heterogeneity with known genetic input. In that regard, the *Diversity Outbred* mouse has been developed, which is a heterogeneous stock derived from the same eight founder inbred strains of the CC (Churchill *et al.*, 2012).

Additional types of inbred mice are utilized in research, including *consomic* and *conplastic* strains. Consomic strains, also known as chromosome substitution strains, are inbred mice that are congenic for entire chromosomes, and are useful for studying polygenic traits (Singer *et al.*, 2004). Conplastic mice are inbred mice that are congenic for different mitochondrial genomes (mtDNA) contributed by other inbred strains, other subspecies, or other species of *Mus* (Yu *et al.*, 2009).

E. Induced Mutant Mice (Genetically Engineered Mice)

In addition to spontaneously occurring mutations that are maintained as co-isogenic strains (such as the C57BL/6 beige mouse), mutant lines of mice have been created by radiation mutagenesis, chemical mutagenesis, or transgenesis. Radiation was one of the earlier methods for *in vivo* mutagenesis (Silver, 1995), but *in vitro* radiation of embryonic stem (ES) cells is also performed (Thomas *et al.*, 1998). Chemical mutagenesis involves *in vivo* treatment of male mice or *in vitro* treatment of ES cells with mutagenic chemicals such as ethylmethanesulphonate (EMS) or *N*-ethyl-*N*-nitrosourea (ENU), which induce point mutations in DNA (O'Brien and Frankel, 2003; Justice *et al.*, 1999, 2000).

Technically, a *transgenic* mouse is any mouse in which foreign DNA has been integrated into its genome, regardless of method. However, the term *transgenic* commonly refers to mice that are genetically altered by *additive transgenesis* through microinjection of foreign DNA into the pronucleus of a fertilized egg. Each ensuing embryo results in a genetically different *founder* mouse, since the transgene is integrated in random sites of the genome of each founder mouse. Since the injected DNA is not homologous to the mouse genome and is not an allele, transgenic founders are *hemizygous* (rather than *heterozygous*) for the transgene until the mice carrying the transgene are bred into homozygosity for the transgene. Transgenes typically integrate as tandem repeats, copy numbers affect phenotype of each founder, and may be lost in subsequent generations, thereby changing the phenotype of the mouse line (Tinkle and Jay, 2002). Transgenes are often constructed with an upstream *promoter*, which confers widespread (ubiquitous) or tissue-specific expression of the cDNA, so that the transgene expression pattern reflects the expression pattern of the promoter. Transcriptional regulation of the transgene can be *inducible* by drug-dependent regulatory control, such as the widely used tetracycline (*tet*) regulatory system, in which treatment of mice with tetracycline or doxycycline induces up- or down-regulation of the transgene (Jaisser, 2000).

ES cells are used for the less efficient integration of genetic material by homologous DNA recombination, but allow large-scale screening of ES cell clones for transformation. Integration can be achieved in a random fashion by *gene trapping*, or by *targeted mutation*. Both methods involve homologous DNA recombination. Gene trapping is a high-throughput approach that randomly introduces insertional mutations within the genome. Vectors contain a gene trapping cassette with a promoter-less reporter gene and/or selectable genetic marker flanked by an upstream 3' splice site and a downstream termination sequence. When inserted into an intron of an expressed gene, the gene trap is transcribed from the endogenous promoter of that gene. Gene traps simultaneously inactivate and report the expression of the trapped gene at the insertion site, and provide a DNA tag for the rapid identification of the disrupted gene (Skarnes *et al.*, 2011).

Targeted gene mutations are achieved by homologous recombination of specific sites within the genome of ES cells. Homologous sequences flank the upstream and downstream regions of the targeted gene, and the construct between the flanking sequences may inactivate (*knock out*) or replace (*knock in*) a gene, and typically contains a reporter gene to track the integration. A variation on this approach is site-specific recombinase (SSR) technology. Two of the most common recombinases are Cre from the coliphage P1 and FLP from *Saccharomyces cerevisiae*. Cre and FLP mediate recombination between target sites, termed *loxP* and *FRT*, respectively. For example, Cre *loxP* target sites are engineered to flank the gene target, which can be used in different ways to achieve different outcomes (*conditional mutations*), depending upon the orientation and location of the flanking *loxP* sites. If the *loxP* sites are oriented in opposite directions, Cre recombinase mediates inversion of the floxed segment. If the *loxP* sites are on different chromosomes (*trans*), Cre recombinase mediates a chromosomal translocation. If the *loxP* sites are oriented in the same direction on the same chromosome (*cis*), Cre recombinase mediates deletion of the floxed segment. Once the floxed mutation is created in ES cells, the transformed ES cells are developed into a mouse with the conditional mutation. The conditional mutant mouse is then genetically crossed with a Cre transgenic mouse, in which Cre recombinase is under the control of a ubiquitous or tissue-specific promoter. Wherever and whenever Cre is expressed, Cre recombinase will recognize and recombine the *loxP* sites. This approach can include insertion of reporter genes and selectable markers, and can be under the control of inducible gene expression systems (http://www.eucomm.org/docs/protocols/mouse_protocol_1_Sanger) (Nagy, 2000).

ES cells are pluripotent with the full genetic capacity to develop into mice when implanted into the blastocyst of a developing embryo. Interest in 'embryonal carcinomas' (teratomas) that arose in relatively high frequency in the testes of 129 mice and early gene transfer experiments in the late 1970s and early 1980s led to the development of ES cell lines derived from several different 129 strains. This early emphasis on teratomas prompted creation of 'better' 129 mouse lines that were more prone to development of testicular teratomas, resulting in genetic corruption of the 129 mouse (Simpson *et al.*, 1997; Threadgill *et al.*, 1997). This realization gave rise to the need to revise 129 mouse nomenclature (Festing *et al.*, 1999). This was necessary because genetic variation significantly impacts homologous recombination in order to match genome sequence of the ES cell line with the mouse from which it was derived. ES cells can be created from any mouse strain or hybrid, but 129 ES cell lines have been commonly used. Recent international knockout mouse program efforts use C57BL/6N ES cells.

Transformed ES cells are microinjected into the inner cell mass of recipient blastocysts, which are then implanted into the uteri of pseudopregnant surrogate mothers. The pups that are born are composed of a mixture of cells derived from recipient blastocysts and the transformed ES cells (*chimeras*). The goal is for male chimeric progeny to produce spermatozoa of ES cell origin (containing the mutation), in order to create F_1 progeny by mating the chimera with the desired background strain (http://www.eucomm.org/docs/protocols/mouse_protocol_1_Sanger). For this reason, most ES cell lines are XY, which favors 129 male chimerism. If the ES cells are of 129 (or other) strain origin, the chimeras are often bred to a desired background mouse strain (commonly C57BL/6) and backcrossed for N10 generations, thereby creating *congenic* inbred mouse lines. Recent international knockout mouse efforts utilize C57BL/6N ES cells, so that chimeric males are bred directly with C57BL/6 mice, thereby creating *co-isogenic* lines. The latter approach saves time and money, and creates a more genetically refined mutant mouse. An alternate approach is to allow ES cells to aggregate with a developing embryo to form blastocysts in culture (aggregation chimera), then implant the chimeric blastocysts (Tanaka *et al.*, 2001).

RNA interference (RNAi), which functions through short double-stranded RNA (dsRNA), has also been utilized to produce transgenic mice, known as gene *knockdown* mice (Gao and Zhang, 2007; Peng *et al.*, 2006). The dsRNA is enzymatically processed into small molecules, termed small interfering RNA (siRNA), which find homologous target mRNAs, resulting in interference. This phenomenon is believed to be a self-defense mechanism against viral infection. In order to adapt this approach to generation of transgenic mice, small hairpin RNA (shRNA) can be expressed in the same way as other transgenes in mice, resulting in processing of the shRNA into siRNA with gene-silencing effects. Constructs are introduced into mouse ES cells by electroporation or lentiviral infection. This method can be embellished conditionally, as with other transgenes. Although RNAi knockdown mice are genetically stable, RNAi-mediated transgenesis is never complete, has variable tissue expression, and cannot induce point mutations (Peng *et al.*, 2006).

1. Engineered Endonuclease Technologies

Recent advances in engineered endonuclease (EE) technology, including zinc finger nucleases (ZFNs), transcription activator-like effector nucleases (TALENs), and RNA-guided endonucleases (RGENs), have revolutionized the field of transgenics (Sung *et al.*, 2014; Wijshake *et al.*, 2014; Gaj *et al.*, 2013). ZFNs and TALENs consist of engineered proteins that target DNA fused to the nonspecific endonuclease, Fok1 (Cathomen and Joung, 2008; Joung and Sander, 2013). ZFNs are comprised of three to six tandem zinc finger proteins, each of which targets a specific 3 bp nucleotide sequence. Paired ZFNs are generated, with each half of the pair targeting opposite DNA strands, allowing dimerization of Fok1 which is required for introduction of double-stranded breaks (DSBs) in the DNA of interest (Cathomen and Joung, 2008). TALENs function similarly, but are composed of tandem repeats of 33–35 amino acids, each with nucleotide specificity occurring in two hypervariable amino acids, the 'repeat variable di-residue (RVD)', at positions 12 and 13 (Joung and Sander, 2013).

In contrast to ZFNs and TALENs, clustered regularly interspaced short palindromic repeats (CRISPRs) paired with CRISPR-associated (CRISPR/Cas) systems are RGEN systems that target specific DNA sequences. Cas proteins, rather than Fok1, produce DSB (Hsu *et al.*, 2014).

DSB generated by EE are repaired by host cells by either nonhomologous end joining (NHEJ) or, less commonly, by homologous recombination (HR). NHEJ is an error-prone repair system and results in insertions or deletions (indels) with a relatively high frequency, which can result in gene disruption. HR is a less common repair pathway, but certain manipulations of the engineered nucleases can increase HR efficiency. For example, nucleases can be engineered to generate a break in a single strand of DNA rather than inducing DSB, and the resulting nickases increase the incidence of HR with high fidelity (Gaj *et al.*, 2013; Wijshake *et al.*, 2014). HR allows for the introduction of donor DNA to generate knock-ins, specific point mutations, or for the generation of larger modifications such as insertions of loxP sites (Brown *et al.*, 2013; Wijshake *et al.*, 2014).

Vectors encoding the EE can be injected into mouse embryos by pronuclear injection of DNA, intracytoplasmic injection of RNA, or transfection of mouse ES cells (Sung *et al.*, 2014; Wijshake *et al.*, 2014). One advantage of EE technologies over more traditional transgenic methods is the ability to target DNA and induce mutations in any background strain of mouse negating the need to backcross onto the desired strain. Multiple genes can be targeted with CRISPRs simultaneously, thus avoiding the need to cross single knockout animals (Zhou *et al.*, 2014). In addition, it is possible to obtain bi-allelic mutations in some cases, allowing for the generation of functional gene knockout animals in a single generation (Zhou *et al.*, 2014; Wijshake *et al.*, 2014). Vectors for generating EE are available through plasmid repositories;

websites are available to assist in identifying appropriate DNA sequences to target; and multiple websites post protocols for generating the various types of engineered endonucleases (Xie *et al.*, 2014; Sander *et al.*, 2010; Bae *et al.*, 2014; Reyon *et al.*, 2011; Herscovitch *et al.*, 2012; Wolfson, 2013). CRISPRs tend to be particularly cost effective and easy to design, with minimal restrictions for targeting specific DNA sequences.

F. Nomenclature

There are currently more than 1000 separate outbred stocks and traditional inbred strains, often with multiple substrains (Table 3.4). In addition, there are thousands of induced mutant strains. Therefore, it is critical that strain or stock designations be complete and accurate to avoid semantic and genetic confusion, and to ensure reproducibility of research results. As an example of substrain variation that makes precise nomenclature important, CBA/J mice are homozygous for the retinal degeneration allele (*rd1*), whereas CBA/CaJ mice do not carry this allele. The *International Committee on Standardized Genetic Nomenclature for Mice and Rats*, established in the early 1950s, is responsible for genetic nomenclature rules. The rules are available online at the MGI website (http://www.informatics.jax.org/mgihome/nomen).

Inbred mouse strains are designated by a series of capital letters and/or numbers, which often provide a shorthand description of the origin and history of the strain. The C57BL/6J mouse serves as an example. The inbred strain C57BL originated from Abbie Lathrop's female 57 (and male 52) at the Cold Spring Harbor Laboratory (C), and was the black (BL) line from this female. Early in their history, inbred C57BL mice split into major substrains, e.g., C57BL/6 and C57BL/10. Substrains are identified by appending a forward slash (/) after the inbred strain name. Since 1950, uniform international nomenclature has been built upon these historical names, so that substrains of an inbred strain are now designated using lab codes that are registered in the *International Laboratory Code Registry* maintained at the *Institute for Laboratory Animal Research* (ILAR) of the National Academies (dels.nas.edu/global/ilar/Lab-codes). Laboratory codes are composed of one to five letters that identify an institute, laboratory, or investigator. Each lab code starts with an uppercase letter, followed by lowercase letters if more than one letter is used (such as N, J, Jci, Crl, and Tac). The J in C57BL/6J means it is a substrain maintained at the Jackson Laboratory (J). Another common substrain of C57BL/6 mice is C57BL/6N, which is maintained at NIH (N). Substrains can be cumulative, reflecting the genetic history of the mouse strain. For example, there are a number of C57BL/6J substrains (such as C57BL/6JJci and C57BL/6JJmsSlc), and a number of C57BL/6N substrains (such as C57BL/6NJci, C57BL/6NCrlCrlj,

TABLE 3.4 Examples of Mouse Strain Nomenclature

Strain name	Definition
DBA/2J	Inbred strain named for its characteristic coat color genes (using their original gene symbols), dilute (*d*), brown (*b*), and nonagouti (*a*); it is the second of two sublines separated before 20 generations of brother × sister breeding and is the subline maintained at the Jackson Laboratory (J)
C3H/HeSn-*ash*/+	Co-isogenic segregating inbred mutant strain carrying the ashen (*ash*) mutation, which arose on C3H/HeSn
C57BL/6J-$^{Tyrc-2J}$/+	Co-isogenic segregating inbred mutant strain carrying the albino 2J mutant allele of the cloned tyrosinase gene (*tyr*)
AEJ/GnJ-a^e/A^{w-J}	Inbred strain segregating for two alleles at the agouti gene
AKR.B6-H2b	Congenic inbred strain in which the *b* haplotype at the *H2* complex was transferred from C57BL/6J (B6) to the AKR background
B6.CBA-D4*Mit25*-D4*Mit80*	Congenic strain in which the chromosomal segment between *D4Mit25* and *D4Mit80* was transferred from CBA to B6
B6.Cg m Lepr^{db}/++	Congenic inbred strain in which the linked mutant genes misty (*m*) and diabetes (*Lepr^{db}*) were transferred from multiple, mixed, or unknown genetic backgrounds to B6 and are carried in coupling, i.e., on the same chromosome
B6.Cg-*m* +/+ *Lepr^{db}*	Congenic inbred strain in which the *m* and *Lepr^{db}* mutations are carried in repulsion
BXD-1/Ty	Recombinant inbred (RI) strain number 1 in a set of RI strains derived from a C57BL/6J (B) female mated to a DBA/2J (D) male and made by Taylor (Ty)
CcS1	Recombinant congenic (RC) strain number 1 in a set made by crossing the BALB/c (C) and STS (S) strains, backcrossing one or two times to BALB/c and then inbreeding as with RI strains
CcS1(N4)	Recombinant congenic (RC) strain number 1 in a set made by crossing the BALB/c (C) and STS (S) strains, backcrossing N4 times to BALB/c and then inbreeding as with RI strains
B.A-Chr 1	Chromosome substitution (CSS) or consomic strain in which Chr 1 from A/J has been transferred to the B6 background
C57BL/6J-mt$^{BALB/c}$	Conplastic strain with the nuclear genome of C57BL/6J, and the cytoplasmic genome of BALB/c, developed by crossing male C57BL/6J mice with BALB/c females, followed by repeated backcrossing of female offspring to male C57BL/6J
B6;129-*Cftr^{tm1Unc}*	First targeted mutation of the cystic fibrosis transmembrane regulator gene created at the University of North Carolina, Unc, and carried on a mixed B6 and 129 background
B6.129-*Myf5^{Myod}*	Congenic strain carrying a replacement or 'knock-in' in which the *Myf5* gene was replaced with the *Myod* gene in 129 ES cells and backcrossed onto the B6 genetic background
FVB/N-TgN(MBP) 1Xxx	Transgene in which the human myelin basic protein (*MBP*) gene is inserted into the genome of the National Institutes of Health (N) subline of the FVB strain originally maintained at the National Institutes of Health
FVB/N-*m^{Tg1Zzz}*	Insertional mutation caused by the *Tg1Zzz* transgene made on the FVB/N genetic background
B6C3F1	F$_1$ hybrid made by crossing a C57BL/6 female to a C3H male
B6EiC3-Ts65Dn	Strain maintained by backcrossing mice with the Ts65Dn chromosome aberration to F$_1$ hybrid mice made by crossing females of the Eicher (Ei) subline of C57BL/6 × C3H; note that these mice are not true F$_1$ hybrids, and the F$_1$ designation is omitted
Hsd:ICR	ICR outbred stock maintained at Harlan (Hsd)
Pri:B6, D2-G#	Advanced intercross line (AIL) created at Princeton (Pri) from the inbred strains C57BL/6 × DBA/2; AIL are made similar to RI strains except mice are intercrossed, avoiding sibling matings, to increase the possibility of tightly linked genes recombining

and C57BL/6NTac). Significant differences may exist among these substrains (Mekada *et al.*, 2009). Thus, a string of substrain designations indicate the genetic progression of the substrain, which can be identified when reading the entire strain name. This nomenclature is highly nuanced, as C57BL/6NCrlCrlj mice, whose last letter is a lowercase j, are not a substrain maintained at the Jackson Laboratory (J), but rather at Charles River Japan (Crlj), underscoring the importance of upper- and lowercase lettering in rodent nomenclature. BALB/c mice are another popular inbred strain with numerous substrains. Like the '6' in C57BL/6, the 'c' that follows the '/' in BALB/c is a lowercase letter because of historical precedent. Subsequent substrains follow accepted nomenclature, e.g., BALB/cByJ and BALB/cAnN.

Hybrids of two inbred strains are often used in research, and are particularly common with engineered mutations that are created in 129-derived ES cells, followed by intercrossing the 129 chimeric mice with C57BL/6 or other background strains of mouse. When an F_1 hybrid is created, the female partner is listed first, e.g., a C57BL/6J × 129S2/SvPas hybrid would be designated: C57BL/6J129S2/SvPasF1. RI strain sets that are derived from two parental inbred strains are identified by an X between the two parental strains followed by a hyphen designating the specific RI line, e.g., C57BL/6JXDBA/2J-1, C57BL/6JXDBA/2J-2, etc. CC RI strains do not use the X between the parental strains because they are derived from eight parental strains, so they are designated CC-1, CC-2, etc. In order to simplify the complexity of this nomenclature, abbreviations are used for common inbred strains and substrains of mice (Table 3.4), but it is important to include the full genetic nomenclature in publications. Using the abbreviated nomenclature, C57BL/6J129S2/SvPasF1 mice would be B6129F1 and C57BL/6JXDBA/2J-1 RI mice would be BXD-1. Parental order is an important consideration in nomenclature, as a B6129 mouse is genetically different from a 129B6 mouse due to mitochondrial DNA (from the female) and Y chromosome (from the male) differences.

Mutant genes are designated by a brief abbreviation for the mutation (e.g., *bg* for beige which arose at the Jackson Laboratory, J). The symbol for the parent gene is noted in italics, starting with an uppercase letter (e.g., *Lyst*) and the mutant allele is designated in superscript (e.g., *Lyst^{bgJ}*). Thus, the beige mutation arose in C57BL/6J mice, so that C57BL/6J beige mice, which are co-isogenic with C57BL/6J mice, are designated C57BL/6J-*Lyst^{bgJ}*.

A *transgenic strain* is designated by the strain and substrain name, followed by a symbol for the transgene. Transgene symbols take the form Tg(YYY)#Zzz, where 'Tg' indicates transgenic, YYY defines the transgene as a brief description of the inserted DNA (such as a gene symbol), '#' is the assigned number in the series of events generated using a given construct, and 'Zzz' is the Lab Code. For example, FVB/N-Tg(MMTV-Erb2)1Led mice are inbred FVB/N mice in which the rat *Erb2* gene was introduced under control of the mouse mammary tumor virus (MMTV) LTR promoter (MMTV-Erb2), the first line (1) created in the laboratory of Phil Leder (lab code Led). When a transgene causes an insertional mutation in an identified endogenous gene, the mutant allele of the gene is designated by using the gene symbol and an abbreviation for the transgene as a superscript (-*Abc^{tg1Zzz}*). A targeted mutation, or knockout, is designated by the mutated gene with the identification of the mutational event as a superscript. For example, *Cftr^{tm1Unc}* is a targeted mutation (tm), first line (1) created at the University of North Carolina (lab code Unc) in the cystic fibrosis transmembrane regulator gene (*Cftr*). If the mutant allele was created by gene trap, the superscript would read 'Gt' in lieu of Tg. A gene replacement, or knock-in, uses similar nomenclature; *Myf5^{Myod}* indicates that the *Myf5* gene was replaced by the *Myod* gene.

Congenic mice are often derived from 129 ES cells, backcrossed onto a background strain, such as C57BL/6. Under such circumstances, when the backcross generation is at N10, the '.' symbol is used between the background inbred strain and the donor strain (e.g., C57BL/6N.129P2/OlaHsd-*Abc^{tm1Zzz}*, abbreviated as B6.129- *Abc^{tm1Zzz}*. When backcrossing is incomplete but at the N5 generation, the mouse is an *incipient congenic*, designated with a ';' in lieu of a '.': B6;129- *Abc^{tm1Zzz}*. If the background strain is mixed genetic origin, it is designated STOCK.129- *Abc^{tm1Zzz}*. If the donor strain is mixed origin, it is designated 'Cg'. For example, B6.Cg-*Abc^{tm1Zzz}* outbred stock that meets specific criteria is designated by placing the Lab Code before the stock symbol, separated by a full colon (':'). For example, Hsd:ICR designates an ICR (Swiss) outbred stock maintained by Harlan Sprague Dawley (Hsd).

The above overview covers the nomenclature of commonly encountered types of mice. There are numerous additional specifications for nomenclature of mice. Details are available at the MGI website (http://www.informatics.jax.org/mgihome/nomen).

G. Housing, Husbandry, and Nutrition

1. Housing and Husbandry

Optimum housing conditions and husbandry practices for research mice should be guided by program requirements to ensure biosecurity, occupational health, efficient use of equipment, labor and financial resources, behavioral needs of mice, and investigator needs for consistent colony maintenance, including standardized husbandry practices and nutrition. The emerging interest in the mouse microbiome in combination with the immune competency of diverse genetically engineered mouse strains demands high standards of mouse care. Mouse colonies are optimally maintained as specific-pathogen-free (SPF) which obligates veterinary and facility management to exclude specific organisms. Housing options for SPF immunocompetent mice typically include static or individually ventilated microisolator cages, which differ significantly in cost and labor required to maintain. Severely immunodeficient strains such as NOD.Cg-*Prkdcscid Il2rgtm1Wjl*/SzJ (NSG) mice require staff training, caging systems and husbandry practices that minimize risk for opportunistic infections

(Foreman *et al.*, 2011). Barrier practices and microisolator techniques may include autoclaved or irradiated feed and bedding, autoclaved or acidified water, cage-to-cage transfer of mice using disinfected forceps, positive displacement change hoods, and verified sanitation of caging and equipment through tunnel or rack washers to prevent fomite transmission of infectious agents (Compton *et al.*, 2012). In addition to husbandry staff, it is critical to maintenance of colony health status that investigators who handle cages are also trained in these techniques.

The microenvironment for mice is the cage which will vary in design, size, and composition. Vendors often successfully house production colonies in open-top cages to expedite detection of pathogen transmission should a break occur. End-users usually prefer filter-top microisolator cages which prevent (at least) gross contamination between cages by fecal contamination and aerosolized debris. The objective is to keep mice in an uncrowded, socially compatible, low-odor, dry and clean environment. Ambient temperature should minimize any confounding impact on the animal model and energy expenditure for the mice, while also being suitable for staff and investigators. Shoebox static cages made of polycarbonate, polypropylene, or polystyrene plastic (in order of decreasing cost and durability) with filtered microisolator tops continue to be used for housing and breeding mice. Older cage designs are being rapidly supplanted by individually ventilated caging systems that promote the advantages of increasing housing capacity, decreasing labor costs, and mitigating exposure of mice to noxious gases such as ammonia and exposure of humans to allergens. As more advanced caging systems are developed, the level of biosecurity may be increased but at the cost of increased health surveillance efforts to detect the source of an infectious outbreak (Shek, 2008). Disposable, recyclable polyethylene caging is a recent innovation, particularly for facilities not equipped with a cage wash facility.

Animal care programs should carefully consider the necessity for housing mice on wire-mesh flooring because of injury risk to limbs and thermoregulation issues in neonates and hairless mice which are more difficult to maintain without nesting material. Solid-bottom cages should contain sanitary bedding, such as hardwood chips, paper products, or ground corn cob. Criteria for selecting bedding vary with experimental and husbandry needs. It may be preferable to irradiate or autoclave bedding, but if this is not done, the bedding should be used only after its origin and microbial content have been evaluated (Table 3.5). Germfree and gnotobiotic mice require positive pressure isolators, most usually flexible film, with additional protection provided by sterile air through high-efficiency particulate air (HEPA) filters. This equipment can be negatively pressurized

TABLE 3.5   Tests of Bedding Quality[a]

CHEMICAL PROPERTIES

Pesticides and polychlorinated compounds

Mycotoxins

Nitrosamines

Detergent residues

Ether-extractable substances

Heavy metals

PHYSICAL PROPERTIES

Particle uniformity

Absorptivity

Ammonia evolution

Visible trauma and irritant potential

MICROBIOLOGICAL PROPERTIES

Standard plate count

Yeasts and molds

Coliforms and *Salmonella*

Pseudomonas

[a]*Modified from Kraft (1980).*

when the objective is to contain known or unknown pathogens. Animal care programs should establish enrichment policies which for mice should include social housing when mice are compatible and experiments do not require single housing. Species-specific behaviors are encouraged by nesting material and hiding places such as tubes or shacks.

2. Nutrition

Nutrient requirements for the mouse are influenced by genetic background, disease status, growth rate, pregnancy, lactation, and environmental factors such as ambient temperature. The best current estimate of nutritional requirements is shown in Table 3.6. Nutritional requirements for laboratory mice are also published periodically by the National Research Council and have been reviewed by Knapka and coworkers (Knapka *et al.*, 1974; Knapka, 1983). Feed intake and weight gain data are used to estimate the nutritional needs of a particular stock or strain. Mice consume about 3–5 g of feed per day after weaning, and maintain this intake throughout life. Outbred mice tend to gain weight faster than inbred mice and are heavier at maturity (Figs. 3.1 and 3.2).

Diet is often neglected as a variable in animal-related research. Diet can influence responses to drugs, chemicals, or other factors and lead to biased research results. Therefore, diet must provide a balance of essential

TABLE 3.6   Nutrient Requirements of Mice[a]

Nutrient	Concentration in diet (%)
Protein (as crude protein)	20–25
Fat[b]	5–12
Fiber	2.5
Carbohydrate	45–60

ESTIMATED DIETARY AMINO ACID REQUIREMENT

Amino acid	Natural-ingredient, open-formula diet (%)[c]	Purified diet (%)[d]
Arginine	0.3	—
Histidine	0.2	—
Tyrosine	—	0.12
Isoleucine	0.4	0.2
Leucine	0.7	0.25
Lysine	0.4	0.15
Methionine	0.5	0.3
Phenylalanine	0.4	0.25
Threonine	0.2	0.22
Tryptophan	0.1	0.05
Valine	0.5	0.3

MINERAL AND VITAMIN CONCENTRATIONS OF ADEQUATE MOUSE DIETS

Mineral	Natural-ingredient, open-formula diet[e]	Purified diet[f]	Purified diet[g]	Chemically defined diet[h]
Calcium (%)	1.23	0.52	0.81	0.57
Chloride (%)	—	0.16	—	1.03
Magnesium (%)	0.18	0.05	0.073	0.142
Phosphorus (%)	0.99	0.4	0.42	0.57
Potassium (%)	0.85	0.36	0.89	0.40
Sodium (%)	0.36	0.1	0.39	0.38
Sulfur (%)	—	—	—	0.0023
Chromium (mg/kg)	—	2.0	1.9	4.0
Cobalt (mg/kg)	0.7	—	—	0.2
Copper (mg/kg)	16.1	6.0	4.5	12.9
Fluoride (mg/kg)	—	—	—	2.3
Iodine (mg/kg)	1.9	0.2	36.0	3.8
Iron (mg/kg)	255.50	35.0	299.0	47.6
Manganese (mg/kg)	104.0	54.0	50.0	95.2
Molybdenum (mg/kg)	—	—	—	1.55
Selenium (mg/kg)	—	0.1	—	0.076
Vanadium (mg/kg)	—	—	—	0.25
Zinc (mg/kg)	50.3	30.0	31.0	38.0

(Continued)

TABLE 3.6   (Continued)

Vitamin	Natural-ingredient, open-formula diet[e]	Purified diet[f]	Purified diet[g]	Chemically defined diet[h]
A (IU/kg)	15,000	4000	1100	1730
B_6 (mg/kg)	10	7	22.5	6.0
B_12 (mg/kg)	0.03	0.01	0.023	0.58
D (IU/kg)	5000	1000	1100	1.71
E (IU/kg)	37	50	32	1514
K_1 equiv. (mg/kg)	3	0.05	18	10.7
Biotin (mg/kg)	0.2	0.2	0.2	1
Choline (mg/kg)	2009	1000	750	2375
Folacin (mg/kg)	4	2	0.45	1.43
Inositol (mg/kg)	—	—	—	248
Niacin (mg/kg)	82	30	22.5	35.6
Calcium pantothenate (mg/kg)	21	16	37.5	47.5
Riboflavin (mg/kg)	8	6	7.5	7.1
Thiamin (mg/kg)	17	6	22.5	4.8

[a]Modified from Knapka (1983).
[b]Linoleic acid: 0.6% is adequate.
[c]John and Bell (1976).
[d]Theuer (1971).
[e]Knapka et al. (1974).
[f]Nutrition (1977).
[g]Hurley and Bell (1974).
[h]Pleasants et al. (1973).

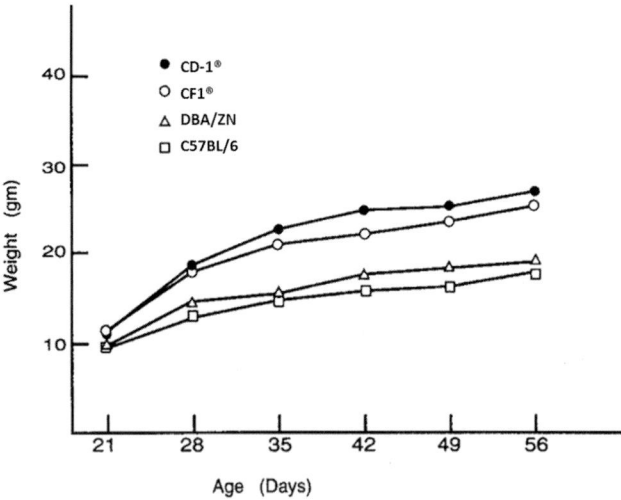
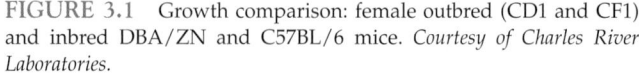

FIGURE 3.1   Growth comparison: female outbred (CD1 and CF1) and inbred DBA/ZN and C57BL/6 mice. *Courtesy of Charles River Laboratories.*

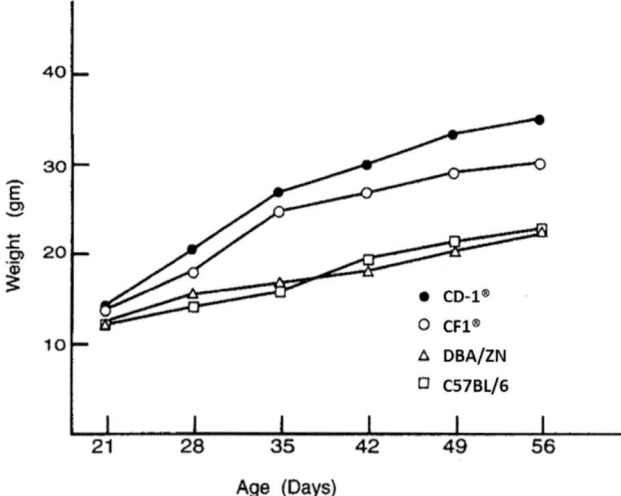

FIGURE 3.2   Growth comparison: male outbred (CD1 and CF1) and inbred DBA/ZN and C57BL/6 mice. *Courtesy of Charles River Laboratories.*

nutrients, and contaminants must be kept to a minimum (see also Chapter 29). Natural-product commercial diets for mice are usually satisfactory for breeding and maintenance. Animal care programs should avoid using fresh produce, grains, fish meal, or other supplements to minimize exposure of colonies to pathogens or harmful chemicals such as pesticide residues or phytoestrogens (Guerrero-Bosagna et al., 2008).

Mouse diets can be purchased as open-formula, fixed-formula, constant nutrition, and closed-formula which are designed to reduce variation in experimental data attributable to diet (reviewed in Barnard *et al.* (2009)). Diets are supplied in standard, irradiated, or autoclavable formulations. Irradiated diets will be virtually free of live microorganisms but have the risk of residual, radio-resistant bacteria. Autoclavable diets are higher in heat-labile nutrient content. Many programs use sterilized mouse chow exclusively to minimize risk of opportunistic infections. Because commercial diets vary in nutrient content, diets should be selected for optimal maintenance of adult mice or for growth and reproduction in breeding colonies.

Mice should have continuous access to potable water even if a high-moisture diet is fed. Water is needed for lubrication of dry food and for hydration. Adult mice drink 6–7 ml of water per day. Decreased water intake will decrease food consumption. Water imbalance may occur immediately post weaning and weanlings on automatic watering systems need extra attention. Water intake will decrease in sick mice. Therefore, dosing mice with medicated water requires careful assessment of hydration and clinical or experimental efficacy of the compound administered.

II. BIOLOGY

A. Physiology and Anatomy

The main reference used to update this section of the 3rd Edition is *Volume III; Normative Biology, Husbandry and Models* in *The Mouse in Biomedical Research*, 2nd Edition, ACLAM Series published by Academic Press. Normative data on the mouse are presented in Table 3.7, and clinical chemistry reference ranges are summarized in Table 3.8.

TABLE 3.7 Normative Data for the Mouse

ADULT WEIGHT

Male	20–40 g
Female	18–35 g

LIFE SPAN

Usual	1–3 years
Maximum reported	4 years
Surface area	0.03–0.06 cm^2
Chromosome number (diploid)	40
Water consumption	6.7 ml/8 weeks age
Food consumption	5.0 g/8 weeks age
Body temperature	98.8°–99.3°F (37°–37.2°C)

(Continued)

TABLE 3.7 (Continued)

PUBERTY

Male	28–49 days
Female	28–49 days
Breeding season	None
Gestation	19–21 days
Litter size	4–12 pups
Birth weight	1.0–1.5 gm
Eyes open	12–13 days
Weaning	21 days
Heart rate	310–840 beats/min

BLOOD PRESSURE

Systolic	133–160 mmHg
Diastolic	102–110 mmHg

BLOOD VOLUME

Plasma	3.15 ml/100 gm
Whole blood	5.85 ml/100 gm
Respiration frequency	163/min
Tidal volume	0.18 (0.09–0.38) ml
Minute volume	24 (11–36) ml/min
Stroke volume	1 μl/g

PLASMA

pH	7.2–7.4
CO_2	21.9 mEq/L
CO_2 pressure	40 ± 5.4 mmHg

LEUKOCYTE COUNT

Total	8.4 (5.1–11.6) × 10^3/μl
Neutrophils	17.9 (6.7–37.2)%
Lymphocytes	69 (63–75)%
Monocytes	1.2 (0.7–2.6)%
Eosinophils	2.1 (0.9–3.8)%
Basophils	0.5 (0–1.5)%
Platelets	600 (100–1000) × 10^3/μl
Packed cell volume	44 (42–44)%
Red blood cells	8.7–10.5 × 10^8/mm^3
Hemoglobin	13.4 (12.2–16.2) g/dl
Maximum volume of single bleeding	5 ml/kg
Clotting time	2–10 min
PTT	55–110 s
Prothrombin time	7–19 s

3. BIOLOGY AND DISEASES OF MICE

TABLE 3.8   Clinical Chemistry Reference Ranges for Adult Mice[a]

Analyte	Units	CD-1		C57BL/6		BALB/cBy	
		M	F	M	F	M	F
Serum							
Glucose	mg/dl	112 ± 38.1	97 ± 39.9	121.7 ± 33.2	134.4 ± 20.3	171.6 ± 57.2	174.9 ± 31.0
Urea nitrogen	mg/dl	38 ± 20.1	37 ± 16	32.7 ± 3.5	23.6 ± 5.3		
Creatinine	mg/dl	1.10 ± 0.45		0.50 ± 0.08	0.84 ± 0.298	0.43 ± 0.14	0.45 ± 0.07
Sodium	mEq/liter	166 ± 8.6	166 ± 4.1	166.7 ± 8.9	160.8 ± 4.40	157.8 ± 5.7	157 ± 6.70
Potassium	mEq/liter	8.0 ± 0.85	7.8 ± 0.75				
Chloride	mEq/liter	125 ± 7.2	130 ± 3.9				
Calcium	mg/dl	8.90 ± 2.06	10.30 ± 1.58			8.10 ± 0.80	
Phosphorus	mg/dl	8.30 ± 1.46	8.00 ± 1.85			5.95 ± 0.63	
Magnesium	mg/dl	3.11 ± 0.37	1.38 ± 0.28				
Iron	μg/dl	474 ± 44	473 ± 16				
Alanine aminotransferase	IU/liter	99 ± 86.3	49 ± 22.6	41.4 ± 16.4	29.3 ± 7.1		
Aspartate aminotransferase	IU/liter	196 ± 132.6	128 ± 60.6	99.5 ± 33.4	73.6 ± 15.3		
Alkaline phosphatase	IU/liter	39 ± 25.7	51 ± 27.3	59 ± 11.4	118 ± 15.9		
Lactate dehydrogenase	IU/liter					378 ± 269	
Protein, total	g/liter	44 ± 11.0	48 ± 8.5	53.9 ± 7.5	63.5 ± 8.8	55.7 ± 8.9	54.6 ± 8.3
Albumin	g/liter			36.7 ± 5.2	46.4 ± 7.0	31.7 ± 4.7	39.3 ± 5.4
Cholesterol	mg/dl	114 ± 56.3	72 ± 20.1	94.8 ± 16.9	92 ± 15.9	150.4 ± 29.9	118.2 ± 36.1
Triglycerides	mg/dl	91 ± 58.5	53 ± 23.6	97 ± 21.1	78 ± 12.2		
Bilirubin	mg/dl	0.4 ± 0.2	0.5 ± 0.35			0.7 ± 0.15	

		Male	Female	Female
Luteinizing hormone	ng/ml	10–40	20–40 (basal)	1500–2000 (proestrus)
Follicle-stimulating hormone	ng/ml	–	80–120 (basal)	250–300 (proestrus/estrus)
Prolactin	ng/ml	<1	10–20	
Growth hormone	ng/ml	–	1–90	–
Thyroid-stimulating hormone	ng/ml	–	300	–
Thyroxine	μg/dl	7.4 ± 0.5 (BALB/c)	–	–
Corticosterone	μg/dl	9 (start of dark period) 5 (start of light period)	40 (middle of dark period)	–
Epinephrine	pg/dl	0–200	–	–
Norepinephrine	pg/dl	30–300	–	–
Progesterone	ng/ml	5 (early proestrus)	35 (late proestrus, estrus)	–
Estradiol	pg/ml	1–5 (basal)	–	–
Testosterone	ng/ml	1.5–2.0	–	–
Urine				
Volume	ml/16 hr	1.6 ± 0.9	1.7 ± 1.1	–
Specific gravity	–	1.0341 ± 0.005	–	–
pH	–	5.011	–	–

(*Continued*)

TABLE 3.8 (Continued)

		Male	Female	Female
Osmolality	Osm/kg	1.06–2.63	–	–
Creatinine	mg/100g/24 hr	2.6 ± 0.91	–	–
Glucose	mg/24 hr	0.53 ± 0.19	–	–
Protein	mg/ml	5	20–30 fold lower	–
Albumin	mg/ml	11.9 ± 0.2	–	–

[a]*Summarized from Loeb and Quimby (1999).*

1. Temperature and Water Regulation

Mice have a relatively large surface area per gram of body weight. This results in dramatic physiologic changes in response to fluctuations in the ambient temperature (T_A). The mouse responds to cold exposure, e.g., by nonshivering thermogenesis. A resting mouse acclimated to cold can generate heat equivalent to triple the basal metabolic rate, a change that is greater than for any other animal. A mouse must generate about $46 \, kcal/m^2$ per 24h to maintain body temperature for each 1°C drop in T_A below the thermoneutral zone. Mice cannot tolerate nocturnal cooling as well as larger animals that have a greater heat sink. Therefore, it is not advisable to conserve energy in animal quarters at night by lowering T_A.

Because of the ratio of evaporative surface to body mass, the mouse has a greater sensitivity than most mammals to water loss. Its biological half-time for turnover of water (1.1 days) is more rapid than for larger mammals. Water conservation is enhanced by cooling of expired air in the nasal passages and by highly efficient concentration of urine.

The conservation of water can preempt thermal stability. If the mouse had to depend on the evaporation of body water to prevent elevations of body temperature, it would go into shock from dehydration. The mouse has no sweat glands, it cannot pant, and its ability to salivate is severely limited. Mice can partially compensate for changes in T_A increases from 20°C to 35°C. It adapts to moderate but persistent increases in environmental temperature by a persistent increase in body temperature, a persistent decrease in metabolic rate, and increased blood flow to the ears to increase heat loss. Its primary means of cooling in the wild is behavioral – retreat into a burrow. In the confinement of a cage, truck, or plane, mice do not survive well in heat and begin to die at an ambient temperature of 37°C or higher. Thus, the mouse is not a true endotherm. In fact, the neonatal mouse is ectothermic and does not have well-developed temperature control before 20 days of age.

The thermoneutral zone for mice varies with strain and with conditioning but is about 29.6–30.5°C, narrower than that of any other mammal measured thus far. Thermoneutrality should not be equated with comfort or physiological economy. Recent data have suggested that mice housed under routine vivarium conditions are chronically cold-stressed. Mice maintained at 21°C were shown to expend more energy compared with mice housed at intermediate (26°C) and a higher temperature (31°C) with an increase in glucose utilization and activation of brown adipose tissue (David *et al.*, 2013). In contrast, other studies report that mice in a T_A range of 21–25°C grow faster, have larger litters, and have more viable pups than those maintained in the thermoneutral zone.

2. Respiratory System

The respiratory tract has three main portions: the anterior respiratory tract consists of nostrils, nasal cavities, and nasopharnyx; the intermediate section consists of larynx, trachea, and bronchi, all of which have cartilaginous support; and the posterior portion of the respiratory tract consists of the lungs. The left lung is a single lobe. The right lung is divided into four lobes: superior, middle, inferior, and postcaval (Cook, 1983) (Fig. 3.3).

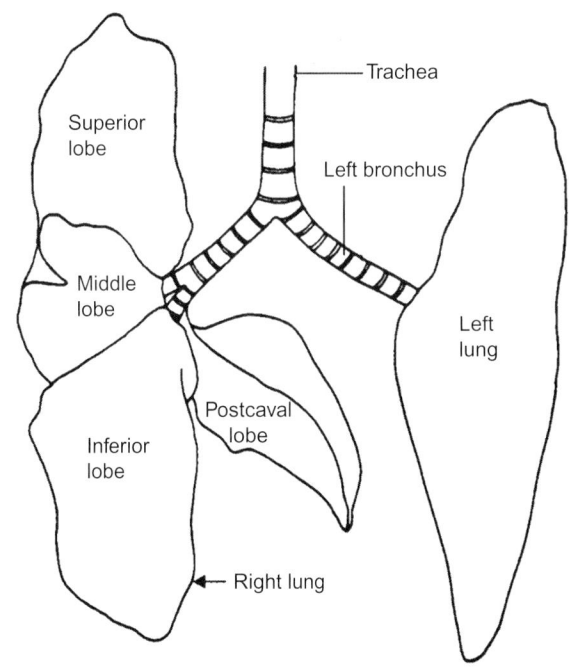

FIGURE 3.3 The five lobes of the lung. *From Cook (1983).*

A mouse at rest uses about 3.5 ml $O_2/g/h$, which is about 22 times more $O_2/g/h$ than is used by an elephant. To accommodate for this high metabolic rate, the mouse has a high alveolar P_{O_2}; a rapid respiratory rate; a short air passage; a moderately high erythrocyte (RBC) concentration; high RBC hemoglobin and carbonic anhydrase concentrations; a high blood O_2 capacity; a slight shift in the O_2-dissociation curve, enabling O_2 to be unloaded in the tissue capillaries at a high P_{O_2}; a more pronounced Bohr effect, i.e., the hemoglobin affinity for O_2 with changes in pH is more pronounced; a high capillary density; and a high blood sugar concentration.

3. Urinary System

The kidneys, ureters, urinary bladder, and urethra form the urinary system. The paired kidneys lie against the dorsal body wall of the abdomen on either side of the midline. The right kidney is normally located anterior to the left kidney. Kidneys from males of many inbred strains are consistently heavier than kidneys from females. The glomeruli of mice are small, about 74 μm in diameter, or about half the size of glomeruli in rats. There are, however, 4.8 times as many glomeruli in the mouse, and the filtering surface per gram of tissue is twice that of the rat.

Mice excrete only a drop or two of urine at a time, and it is highly concentrated (Table 3.8). The high concentration is made possible by long loops of Henle and by the organization of giant vascular bundles (*vasa recta*) associated with the loops of Henle in the medulla. The mouse can concentrate urine to 4300 mOsm/l, whereas humans can concentrate to a maximum of 1160 mOsm/l.

Mice normally excrete large amounts of protein in the urine. Taurine is always present in mouse urine, whereas tryptophan is always absent. Creatinine is also excreted in mouse urine, a trait in which mice differ from other mammals. The creatinine/creatine ratio for fasting mice is about 1:1.4. Mice excrete much more allantoin than uric acid.

4. Gastrointestinal Tract

The submaxillary salivary gland, a mixed gland in most animals, secretes only one type of saliva (seromucoid) in the mouse. The tubular portion of the gastrointestinal (GI) tract consists of esophagus, stomach, small intestine, cecum, and colon. The esophagus of the mouse is lined by a thick cornified squamous epithelium, making gavage a relatively simple procedure. The proximal portion of the stomach is also keratinized, whereas the distal part of the stomach is glandular. Gastric secretion continues whether or not food is present.

The gastrointestinal flora consists of (at least) 1000 species of bacteria that begin to colonize the alimentary canal selectively shortly after birth. The ceca of normal mice contain up to 10^{11} bacteria/g of feces. The bacteria throughout the gastrointestinal tract form a complex ecosystem that provides beneficial effects, such as an increase in resistance to certain intestinal pathogens, production of essential vitamins, and homeostasis of important physiological functions.

Gnotobiotic animals colonized with known microbiota have been used to great advantage as models for biomedical research (see Chapter 39). For certain studies, it is desirable to colonize germfree mice with a defined microbiota. In the mid-1960s, Schaedler was the first to colonize germfree mice with selected bacteria isolated from normal mice (Schaedler and Orcutt, 1983). He subsequently supplied animal breeders with this group of microorganisms. These defined bacteria included aerobic bacteria and some less oxygen-sensitive anaerobic organisms. The so-called extremely oxygen-sensitive (EOS) fusiform bacteria, which make up the majority of the normal microbiota of rodents, were not included, because of technical difficulties in isolation and cultivation. Of the defined microbiotas later used for gnotobiotic studies, the one known as the 'Schaedler flora' was the most popular. In 1978, the National Cancer Institute (NCI) decided to revise the Schaedler flora, or 'cocktail' consisting of eight bacteria, in order to standardize the microbiota used to colonize germfree rodents. The new defined microbiota, now known as the 'altered Schaedler flora' (ASF), consisted of four members of the original Schaedler flora (two lactobacilli, *Bacteroides distasonis*, and the EOS fusiform bacterium), a spiral-shaped bacterium, and three new fusiform EOS bacteria. Studies have quantified the regional colonization of the ASF strains along the gastrointestinal tract (Sarma-Rupavtarm *et al.*, 2004) (Fig. 3.4). Individual strain abundance was dependent on oxygen sensitivity, with microaerotolerant *Lactobacillus murinus* ASF361 present at 10^5–10^7 cells/g of tissue in the upper gastrointestinal tract and obligate anaerobic ASF strains being predominant in the cecal and colonic flora at 10^8–10^{10} cells/g of tissue.

It is difficult to monitor a gnotobiotic mouse colony with a defined microbiota. It is necessary to demonstrate that microorganisms of the specified microbiota are present and that adventitious microorganisms are absent. In the past, monitoring relied on bacterial morphology, limited evaluation of biochemical traits, and growth characteristics. With the advent of polymerase chain reaction (PCR) technology, the eight ASF strains were identified taxonomically by 16S rRNA sequence analysis (Dewhirst *et al.*, 1999). Three strains were previously identified as *Lactobacillus acidophilus* (strain ASF 360), *L. salivarius* (strain ASF 361), and *Bacteroides distasonis* (strain ASF 519), based on phenotypic criteria. 16S rRNA analysis and genome sequencing indicated that each of the strains differed from its presumptive identity (Wannemuehler *et al.*, 2014). The 16S rRNA sequence of strain ASF 361 is essentially identical to the 16S rRNA sequences of the type strains of *L. murinus* and *L. animalis* (both isolated

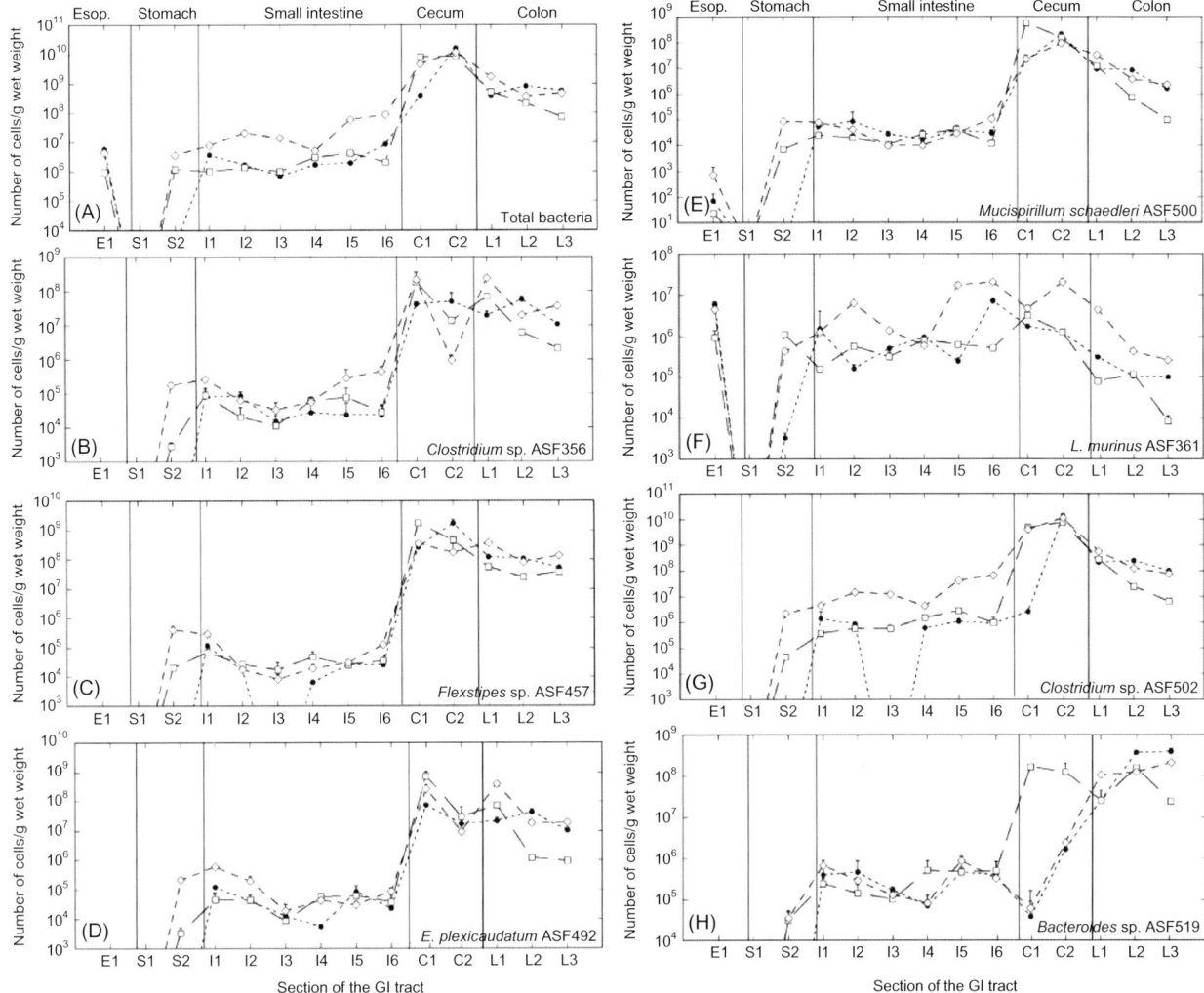

FIGURE 3.4 Distribution of ASF strains in different sections of the gastrointestinal (GI) tracts of three defined flora C.B-17 mice. The number of total bacterial cells of ASF strains (A), ASF356 (B), ASF457 (C), ASF492 (D), ASF500 (E), ASF361 (F), ASF502 (G), and ASF519 (H) in mouse 1 (solid circles), mouse 2 (open squares), and mouse 3 (open diamonds) is shown. The sections are taken from the esophagus (Esop.) (section E1), stomach (sections S1 and S2), small intestine (sections I1 to I6), ileocecal junction and apical cecum (sections C1 and C2, respectively), and colon (sections L1 to L3). *From Sarma-Rupavtarm et al. (2004).*

from mice), and all of these strains probably belong to a single species. Strain ASF 360 is a novel lactobacillus that clusters with *L. acidophilus* and *L. lactis*. Strain ASF 519 is a *Parabacteroides* sp. The spiral-shaped strain, strain ASF 457, is in the *Flexistipes* phylum, exhibits sequence identity with rodent isolates of Robertson, and has been formally named, *Mucispirillum schaedleri* (Robertson *et al.*, 2005). The remaining four ASF strains, which are EOS fusiform bacteria, group phylogenetically with the low-G + C content gram-positive bacteria (*Firmicutes*, *Bacillus-Clostridium* group) (ASF 492 – *Eubacterium plexicaudatium*; ASF 500 – *Firmicutes* bacterium; ASF 502 and ASF 356 – *Clostridium* sp.) (Fig. 3.5). The 16S rRNA sequence information was determined by Dewhirst *et al.* (1999) and draft genome sequences for each member

of ASF were recently published (Wannemuehler *et al.*, 2014). This genetic data will permit detailed analysis of the interactions of ASF organisms during development of intestinal disease in mice that are coinfected with a variety of pathogenic microorganisms.

5. Lymphoreticular System

The lymphatic system consists of lymph vessels, thymus, lymph nodes, spleen, solitary peripheral nodes (Fig. 3.6), and intestinal Peyer's patches. Mouse lymph nodes are numerous but typically are small, reaching only a few millimeters. The typical lymph node is bean-shaped and consists of a cortex and a medulla. The cortex is divided into B lymphocyte domains, called primary follicles, and T lymphocyte domains, known

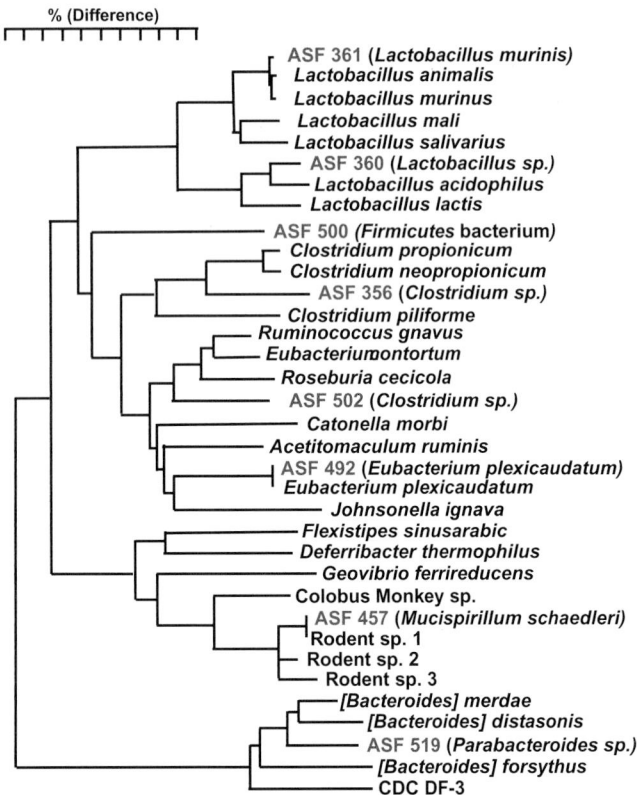

FIGURE 3.5 Phylogenetic relationships of ASF strains. From Dewhirst *et al.* (1999). Draft genome sequences of the ASF (Wannemuehler *et al.*, 2014) have identified ASF356 as *Clostridum* sp., ASF360 as *Lactobacillus* sp., ASF361 as *Lactobacillus murinus*, ASF457 as *Mucispirillum schaedleri*, ASF492 as *Eubacterium plexicaudatum*, ASF500 as *Firmicutes* bacterium, ASF502 as *Clostridum* sp., and ASF519 as *Parabacteroides* sp.

as the diffuse cortex. The mouse does not have palatine or pharyngeal tonsils. The spleen lies adjacent to the greater curvature of the stomach. Different strains of mice have varying degrees of accessory splenic tissue. Age, strain, sex, and health status can affect the size, shape, and appearance of the spleen. Male spleens, e.g., may be 50% larger than those of females. Most lymphocytes enter and leave the spleen in the bloodstream. The so-called white pulp of the spleen is organized along the central arteriole and is subdivided into T- and B-cell zones. The periarteriolar sheath is composed mainly of CD4+ and CD8+ T cells, and lymph follicles, which often contain germinal centers, are located at the periphery. The red pulp consists of sinusoids and hemoreticular tissue. Cellular and humoral components of immunity are distributed to the bloodstream and tissues by efferent lymphatic vessels and lymphatic ducts, which empty into the venous system.

The thymus is a bilobed lymphoid organ lying in the anterior mediastinum. It reaches maximum size around the time of sexual maturity and involutes between 35 and 80 days of age. The thymus plays a major role in maturation and differentiation of T lymphocytes. This function is not complete in newborn mice. Thymectomy is routinely performed in immunological research for experimental manipulation of the immune system. Thymectomy of newborn mice causes a decrease in circulating lymphocytes and marked impairment of certain immune responses, particularly cellular immune responses. Thymectomy in adult mice produces no immediate effect, but several months later mice may develop a progressive decline of circulating lymphocytes and impaired cellular immune responses. The mutant athymic nude mouse is a powerful experimental tool in the study of the thymus in immune regulation (Fogh, 1982).

The mucosa-associated lymph tissue (MALT) contains more lymphoid cells and produces greater amounts of immunoglobulin than both the spleen and the lymph nodes. The term *MALT* designates all peripheral lymphoid tissues connecting to cavities communicating with the external milieu. They include the Peyer's patches, the cecal lymphoid tissue, and the lymphoid tissue in upper and lower respiratory tract, as well as the respiratory and genitourinary system. Lymphatics drain these lymphoid-rich areas, thus providing a direct link with lymph nodes and the bloodstream.

6. Blood and Reticuloendothelial System

Bone marrow and splenic red pulp produce erythrocytic, granulocytic, and megakaryocytic precursors over the life of the mouse. Bone marrow is located in the protected matrix of cancellous bone and is sustained by reticular tissue rich in blood vessels and adipose cells (Pastoret *et al.*, 1998). Normal hematologic values are listed in Table 3.7.

Bone marrow-derived mononuclear phagocytes remove particulate antigens and act as antigen-presenting cells for lymphocytes. Tissue macrophages, which often function in a similar way, are found in many tissues, including peripheral lymphoid tissues, lung, liver, intestine, and skin.

7. Cardiovascular System

The cardiovascular system of mice is reviewed extensively by Hoyt *et al.* in the 2nd Edition of *Volume III; Normative Biology, Husbandry and Models* in the ACLAM Series *The Mouse in Biomedical Research* (Hoyt, 2007). The heart consists of four chambers, the thin-walled atria and the thick-walled ventricles (Fig. 3.7). Mice conditioned to a recording apparatus have mean systolic blood pressures ranging from 84 to 105 mmHg. An increase in body temperature does not lead to an increase in blood pressure. Heart rate, cardiac output, and the width of cardiac myofibers are related to the size of the animal. Heart rates from 310 to 840/min have been recorded for mice, and there are wide variations in rates and blood pressure among strains.

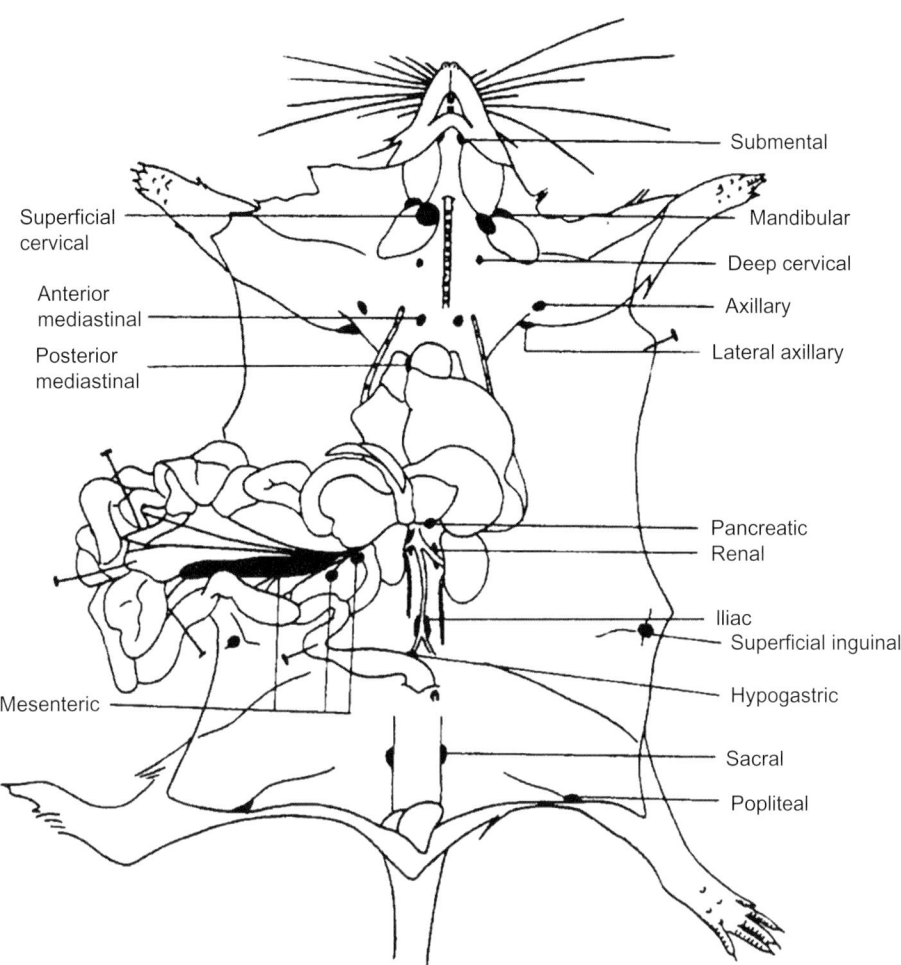

FIGURE 3.6   Lymph nodes. *Modified from Cook (1983).*

8. Musculoskeletal System

The skeleton is composed of two parts: the axial skeleton, which consists of the skull, vertebrae, ribs, and sternum, and the appendicular skeleton, which consists of the pectoral and pelvic girdles and the paired limbs. The normal vertebral formula for the mouse is C7T13L6S4C28, with some variations among strains, especially in the thoracic and lumbar regions.

Normal mouse dentition consists of an incisor and three molars in each quadrant. These develop and erupt in sequence from front to rear. The third molar is the smallest tooth in both jaws; the upper and lower third molar may be missing in wild mice and in some inbred strains. The incisors grow continuously and are worn down during mastication.

9. Nervous System

The mouse brain has a typical mammalian structure as documented by a detailed study of the neuroanatomy of the C57BL/6J mouse (Sidman *et al.*, 1971). More recently, gene expression patterns have been used to study the functional anatomy of the mouse brain (Bohland *et al.*, 2010). Use of wild-type and genetically modified mice in behavior, learning, and memory paradigms has exponentially increased over the last decade.

10. Genital System

The male reproductive organs consist of paired testes, urethra, penis, prostate and associated ducts and glands (Fig. 3.8). The female reproductive organs consist of paired ovaries and oviducts, uterus, cervix, vagina, clitoris, and paired clitoral glands (Fig. 3.9). The clitoral glands are homologous to the male preputial glands and secrete a sebaceous substance through ducts entering the lateral wall of the clitoral fossa. The female mouse normally has five pairs of mammary glands, three in the cervicothoracic region and two in the inguinoabdominal region (Fig. 3.10). The mammary glands are often not appreciated for how far they extend over the cervical, axillary, and inguinoabdominal flank regions which become

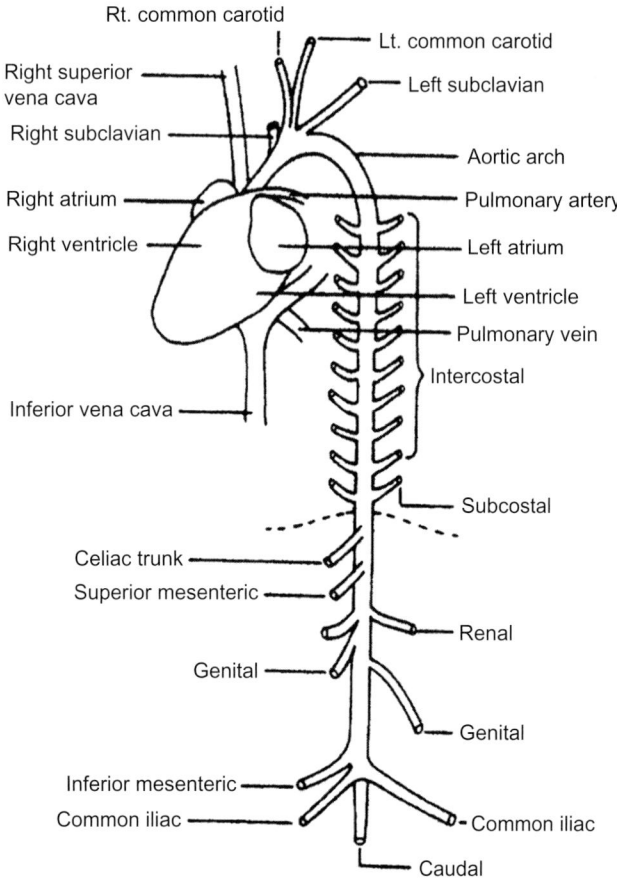

FIGURE 3.7   Heart and major vessels. *Modified from Cook (1983).*

evident when mammary neoplasia develops. Detailed techniques for manipulating gametes and embryos have been developed (Gama Sosa *et al.*, 2010).

B. Reproduction

The following section summarizes normal reproduction in the mouse. The reader is referred to a more comprehensive text in the ACLAM Series (Pritchett and Taft, 2007) and online resources such as The Jackson Laboratories publication of *The Biology of the Laboratory Mouse* (http://jaxmice.jax.org/jaxnotes/509/509j.html). External influences, such as noise, vibration, diet, light cycle, and cage density, and intrinsic factors, such as health status, genetics, and parity impact reproductive success by directly or indirectly influencing the hypothalamic–pituitary axis for hormonal control of ovarian and testicular function. Genotype also dramatically affects the reproductive performance of the mouse. Coincident with the explosion in the number of mouse strains, each with unique induced or spontaneous mutations, a sound breeding program must include training of care staff to recognize anticipated and unanticipated breeding performance and strain or stock characteristics.

In the new age of genomics, older methods of confirming genetic purity of mouse lines are being replaced with formal genetic monitoring by comparing strain-specific panels of single-nucleotide polymorphisms (SNPs).

1. Sexual Maturation

Follicle-stimulating hormone promotes gametogenesis in both sexes. Luteinizing hormone promotes the secretion of estrogen and progesterone in the female and androgen in the male. Prolactin promotes lactation and development of the ovary during pregnancy. These gonadal hormones also ensure proper maintenance of the reproductive tract and modulate behavior to promote successful mating. The hypophysis is usually responsive to hormonal influence by day 6 in the male and day 12 in the female. Ovarian follicle development begins at 3 weeks of age and matures by 30 days. Rising levels of gonadotropins evoke signs of sexual maturity at about the same age. In the female, estrogen-dependent changes such as cornification of vaginal epithelium at the vaginal opening can occur as early as 24–28 days. Puberty is slightly later in the male (up to 2 weeks). Sexual maturation varies among strains and stocks of mice and is subject to seasonal and environmental influences. Mating behavior and the ability to conceive and carry fetuses to parturition are under complex hormonal control mediated by the anterior pituitary.

2. Estrous Cycle

The mouse is polyestrous and cycles every 4–5 days. In the first two phases (proestrus and estrus), active epithelial growth in the genital tract culminates in ovulation. Degenerative epithelial changes occur during the third phase, followed by diestrus, a period of quiescence or slow cell growth. The cycle can be followed by changes in the vaginal epithelium that are often used to determine optimum receptivity of the female for mating and fertilization (Table 3.9). Patency of the vaginal orifice and swelling of the vulva are useful signs of proestrus and estrus (Fig. 3.11). Irregularities of the estrous cycle occur during aging. Seasonal and dietary factors, such as estrogenic substances found in a variety of feeds, and genetic backgrounds also influence estrous cycles.

Estrus is routinely observed in mice at about 14–24 h after parturition (postpartum estrus). However, cornification of the vagina is not complete, and fertile matings are not as frequent compared with normal estrus. Mice are spontaneous ovulators. Ovulation does not accompany every estrus, and estrus may not coincide with every ovulation, because estrus is dependent on gonadal hormones, whereas ovulation is responsive to gonadotropin. The cyclicity of estrus and ovulation is controlled by the diurnal rhythm of the photoperiod. Mating, estrus, and ovulation most often occur during the dark phase of the photoperiod. Reversing the timing

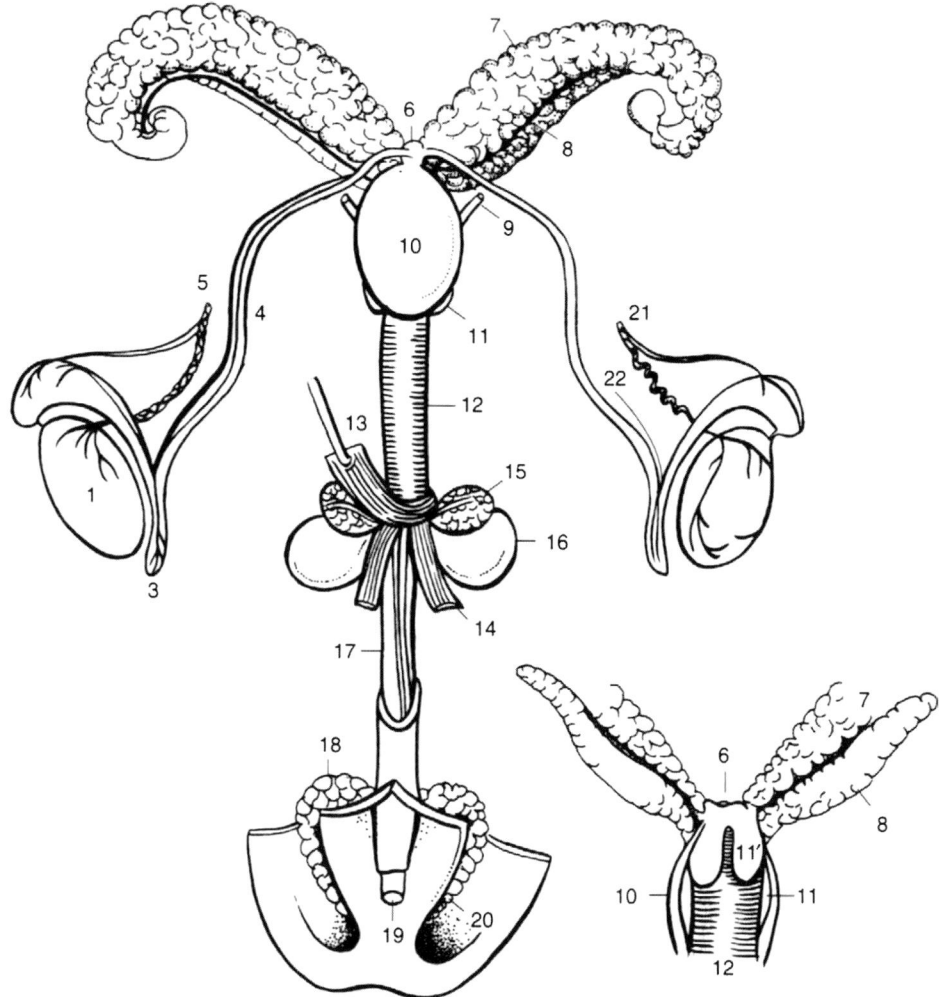

FIGURE 3.8   Reproductive anatomy of male mice. (1) testis, (2) head of epididymitis, (3) caudal epididymitis, (4) vas deferens, (5) testicular vein, (6) ampullary gland, (7) seminal vesicle, (8) anterior prostate, (9) ureter, (10) bladder, (11) ventral prostate, (11') dorsal prostate, (12) urethra, (13) bulbourethral muscle, (14) ischiocavernosus, (15) bulbourethral gland, (16) diverticulum of bulbourethral gland, (17) penis, (18) preputial gland, (19) glans penis, (20) prepuce, (21) testicular artery, and (22) vas deferens artery. *Adapted from (Komarek, 2007).*

of the light–dark cycle reverses the time of estrus, ovulation, and mating.

Pheromones (Table 3.10) and social environment also affect the estrous cycle. For example, estrus may be suppressed in group-housed female mice and reentry into estrus can be synchronized by exposure to pheromones in male mouse urine ('Whitten effect'). Once exposed to male urine, most female mice will be in estrus within 3 days with a second estrus in about 11 days. Hence, estrus can be synchronized by group-housing females prior to pairing with males. In contrast, pheromones from a strange male mouse, particularly of a different strain, may prevent implantation or pseudopregnancy in recently bred females and is known as the 'Bruce effect'. See Section II.C on Behavior for more detail on the effect of pheromones on mouse reproductive behavior.

3. Mating

Mating is normally detected by formation of a vaginal plug (a mixture of the secretions of the vesicular and coagulating glands of the male) whose prevalence is highly strain dependent. The plug usually fills the vagina from cervix to vulva (Fig. 3.11). Plug detection is often coupled with vaginal cytology to evaluate fertility and conception.

When the cervix and vagina are stimulated physically during estrus, prolactin is released from the anterior pituitary to enable the corpus luteum to secrete progesterone. Secretion continues for about 13 days. If fertilization has occurred, the placenta takes over progesterone production. If fertilization does not occur, a pseudopregnant period ensues, during which estrus and ovulation do not occur. Fertilization usually takes place

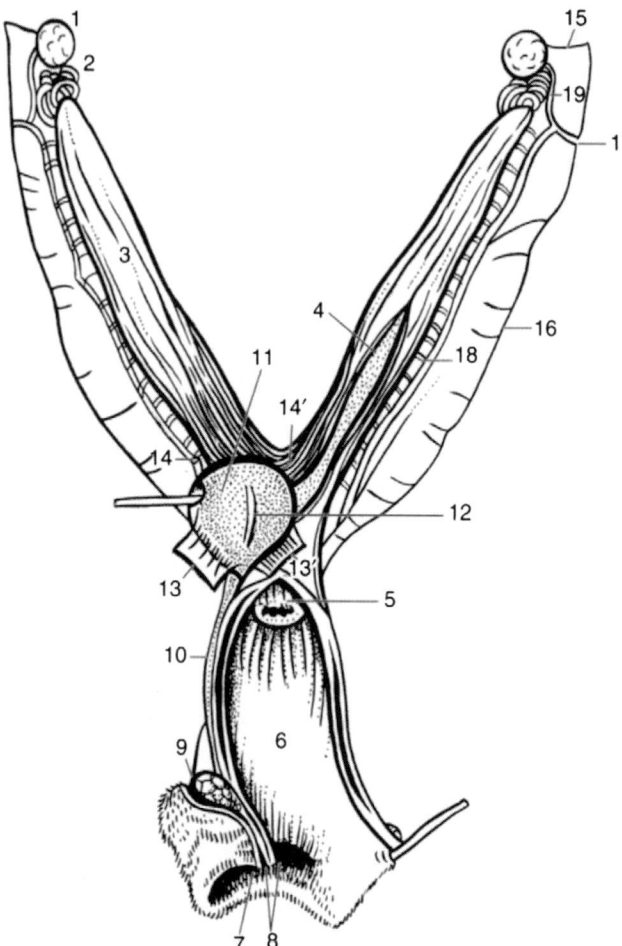

FIGURE 3.9 Reproductive anatomy of female mice. (1) ovary, (2) fallopian tube, (3) uterine horn, (4) endometrium, (5) cervix, (6) vagina, (7) vaginal vestibulum, (8) clitoris, (9) clitoral gland, (10) urethra, (11) bladder, (12) medial ligament of bladder, (13) lateral ligament of bladder, (14) left ureter, (14') right ureter, (15) mesovarium, (16) mesometrium, (17) ovarian artery, (18) uterine horn artery, and (19) ovarian artery and vein. *Adapted from (Komarek, 2007).*

in the ampulla or the upper portion of the oviduct. Ova can be fertilized to produce normal embryos for 10–12 h after ovulation.

4. Gestation

Gestation is usually 19–21 days. Because of postpartum estrus, lactation and gestation can occur simultaneously. Lactation can delay gestation because of delayed

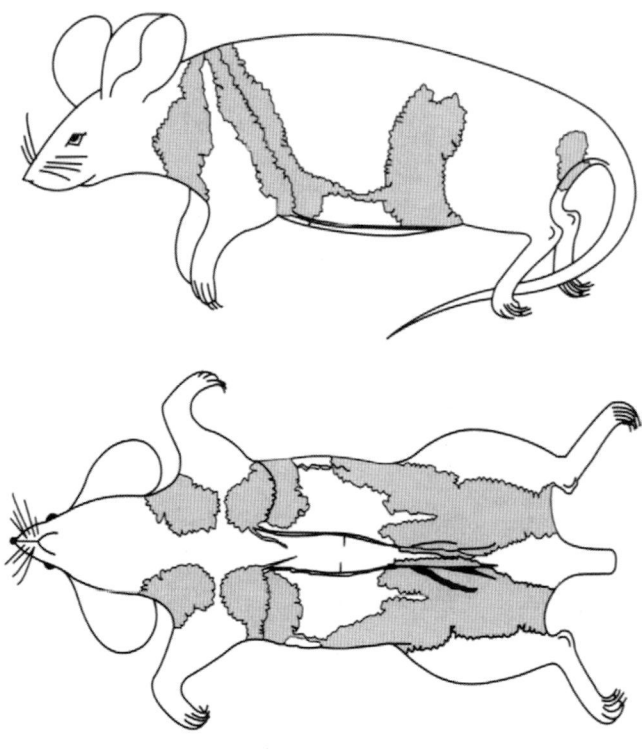

FIGURE 3.10 Distribution of mammary tissue in female mice *Adapted from Komarek (2007).*

TABLE 3.9   Changes in the Reproductive Organs of the Mouse during the Estrous Cycle[a]

Stage	Smear[b]	Uterus	Ovary and oviduct
Proestrus	Epithelial cells to epithelial–cornified cells or epithelial–cornified cells; leukocytes to epithelial cells	Hyperemia and distension increase. Active mitoses in epithelium, few leukocytes	Follicles enlarged and distended with considerable liquor folliculi. Few mitoses in germinal epithelium and in follicular cells
Estrus	Epithelial-cornified cells to cornified + cells	Distension and activity are maximal during estrus and then decrease. No leukocytes	Ovulation occurs, followed by distension of the upper end of oviduct. Active mitoses in germinal epithelium and in follicular cells
Metestrus	Cornified ++ cells, epithelial cells, leukocytes++	Distension decreased. Leukocytes in epithelium. Walls collapsed. Epithelium degenerates. Mitoses rare	Follicles undergoing atresia. Growing corpora lutea. Eggs in oviduct. Few mitoses in germinal epithelium and in follicular cells
Diestrus	Epithelial cells, leukocytes, more or less mucus	Pale in appearance, walls collapsed. Epithelium healthy but contains many leukocytes. Some secretion by uterine glands	Follicles begin rapid growth toward the end of period

[a]*Adapted from Bronson et al. (1996).*
[b] *+ indicates many cells; ++ indicates very many cells; – indicates transition from epithelial to cornified. The descriptions for smears are typical; there is considerable variation.*

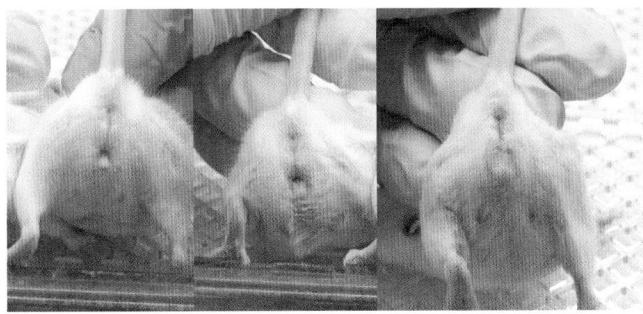

FIGURE 3.11 The female mouse on the left would likely be unreceptive to a male. The mouse in the middle is in proestrus or estrus as evidenced by erythema and edema of the vulva. The female on the right has a vaginal plug as evidence of mating the prior night. *Courtesy of the Division of Comparative Medicine.*

TABLE 3.10 Select Pheromone Effects in Mice

Initiator	Effect
Male-specific major urinary protein MUP20 (darcin)	Rewarding and attractive to females[a]; intermale aggression[a]; area avoidance[b]
Male lacrimal protein ESP1	Lordosis in female mice[a]
Exocrine-gland (lacrimal) secreting peptide 22 (ESP22) produced by juvenile male mice	Inhibitory on older adult male mating behavior[c]

[a]*Martin-Sanchez et al. (2015).*
[b]*Roberts et al. (2012).*
[c]*Ferrero et al. (2013).*

implantation. This may cause prolongation of gestation for up to 12–13 days in certain inbred strains.

The effective reproductive life of some inbred strains approaches 2 years where optimum environmental conditions are maintained, but litter size usually decreases as the female ages. Therefore, females are usually retired by 6 months of age. Average litter size is strain dependent and commonly ranges from 1 to 12 pups.

5. Postnatal Development and Weaning

Maternal care can account for about 70% of the variation in body weight of neonatal mice. Nursing females usually lactate for 3 weeks. Milk production increases up to 12 days postpartum and then declines until weaning at 21 days. Interestingly, oxytocin is required for nursing but is not essential for parturition or reproductive behavior (Nishimori *et al.*, 1996).

Some transmission of humoral immunity from dam to progeny occurs *in utero*, but the majority of antibody is transferred through colostrum. Transmission of passive immunity by colostral antibodies has been demonstrated to a wide variety of antigens, including viruses, bacteria, and parasites. Antibodies continue to be secreted in the milk throughout lactation. Decay of maternally acquired immunity occurs within several months after weaning. Loss of maternal immunity increases susceptibility to infection and warrants continued care of weaned mice under barrier conditions.

C. Behavior

Mice are socially gregarious animals with strong family bonds who communicate through complex olfactory, auditory, tactile, and visual signals. Wild mice aggregate into groups called *demes* with low exchange of individuals between different groups. Each deme consists of kin-related members with a high degree of natural inbreeding,

higher mutation rates compared to other mammals, and a wide range of developmental flexibility based on early life experience, which all contribute to their remarkably successful environmental adaptability. The deme is composed of a dominant breeding male, a hierarchy of females, subordinate males, and juveniles. Wild mice occupy territories measuring just a few square meters when food is abundant to several square kilometers. Mice are crepuscular (active during the twilight hours of dawn and dusk), strongly territorial, and omnivorous. Coprophagy contributes to approximately one-third of their ingesta as an essential nutritional activity. Aside from territoriality, social interactions, breeding, burrowing (when conducive substrates are available), and nest building are major activities. In managing laboratory mice, it is important to understand the complex behavioral biology of their free-living counterparts (Latham and Mason, 2004).

Chemo-olfactory communication is mediated through extremely diverse chemical factors that trigger innate (non-learned) social responses among conspecifics, known as *pheromones* (Table 3.10). Pheromones have been traditionally divided into two broad categories: *releaser* pheromones, which elicit an immediate behavioral response, and *primer* pheromones, which mediate a slowly developing and longer-lasting endocrine response. This original definition of pheromone categories has been expanded to another category, termed *signaler* pheromones, which convey individual or group identity, as well as mediating parent–offspring recognition and mate choice. The biology and genetics of pheromone signaling is being extensively studied in the mouse as a model of mammalian pheromone communication (Brennan and Zufall, 2006; Rodriguez and Boehm, 2009).

Mouse pheromones are excreted in the urine, as well as plantar, salivary, lacrimal, preputial, and mammary glands. In the urine, *major urinary proteins* (Mups), small peptides, MHC class I peptides, volatile chemicals, and sex hormones all contribute to chemosignals that communicate dominance, kinship, diversity, and gender. Wild mice possess a great deal of individual variations of these elements, providing a 'bar code' that distinguishes individuals. Inbreeding of laboratory mice has reduced individual variation, but each inbred strain possesses a characteristic array of signals, and to a certain extent, unique signals exist among individuals within a strain (Sharrow et al., 2001; Sturm et al., 2013). Pheromones are detected by sensory neurons in the vomeronasal organ, the olfactory epithelium, and the lesser known septal organ of Masera within the olfactory epithelium, and the Gruenberg ganglion, which is located at the anterior end of the nasal cavity (Breer et al., 2006; Chamero et al., 2012; Liberles and Buck, 2006; Restrepo et al., 2004). Neuronal signals are transmitted to the ganglion layer of the olfactory bulb, and thence to the brain.

Mups are important components of chemosensory communication in mice, and also an important occupational hazard to human handlers. Chromosome 4 contains a cluster of 21 Mup genes, plus a number of pseudogenes. Mups are small soluble proteins known as lipocalins, which bind small organic chemicals (pheromones) with high affinity, and function as pheromone transporters and stabilizers (thereby contributing to slow release), but also act as protein pheromones themselves. They are synthesized in the liver and excreted in the urine, as well as nasal mucosa, lacrimal glands, and salivary glands. Their endogenous role on metabolic activity is not yet understood. Male mice excrete significantly more Mups in the urine than females. One well-characterized Mup is 'darcin', named after Fitzwilliam Darcy, the romantic hero in Pride and Prejudice. As its name implies, it is a female attractant. Mups also act as kairomones, which function as chemical signals between species. For example, cat and rat Mups invoke fear in mice. Mups are important in the laboratory animal management context, as they are excreted in copious amounts (1–5 mg/ml in urine) and are potent allergens for humans, particularly Mus m 1 (Ag1 or MA1), which is encoded by the Mup 17 gene (Sharrow et al., 2001).

Chemosensory communication has numerous behavioral effects that influence mouse social interactions. One of the most studied behavioral effects is the Bruce effect, or pregnancy block, which is a complex physiologic response in which recently conceived females resorb fetuses during early pregnancy in the presence of an unrelated male, particularly a dominant male. The continued presence of the original mate protects the female from this effect (Bruce, 1959). The Vandenbergh effect results in acceleration of puberty of juvenile females in response to male urine (Vandenbergh, 1973). The Lee–Boot effect occurs among group-housed females that are isolated from males, in which there is suppression of estrus cyclicity (Van Der Lee and Boot, 1955). The Whitten effect results in synchronization of estrus among a group of females in response to a male (Whitten et al., 1968). The Lee–Boot and Whitten effects are utilized in the laboratory to assist in induction of synchronized timed pregnancy, but the Bruce effect can have deleterious consequences on breeding colonies when foreign males are introduced to a breeding colony, as pheromone communication can occur in the absence of direct contact.

The above effects are well-defined pheromone-driven behavioral responses, but chemosensory communication has a myriad of other effects. Estrus, pregnant, or lactating females also accelerate puberty among juvenile females. Females use odor cues to avoid parasite-laden males, males prefer odors of estrus females, and estrus females prefer odors of dominant males. Mice have strong mating and social preferences based upon MHC proteins, which indicate genetic relatedness. Maternal recognition of young is also MHC-related, and pups prefer nest odors of maternal and sibling pups based upon MHC relatedness. Male aggression against unrelated males is also a strong MHC-related phenomenon. MHC haplotypes determine not only MHC proteins in the urine, and MHC-specific olfactory receptors, but also the composition of volatile chemicals in the urine (Kelliher and Wersinger, 2009).

The complexity of social communication extends to auditory stimuli as well. Male mice utilize ultrasonic 'birdsong' to vocally communicate and attract females. Mouse vocalization patterns are largely genetically innate and unique to each strain of mouse, but they can also be modified, or learned, to a limited extent (Arriaga et al., 2012).

The behavioral biology of the mouse is highly complex, and depends upon genetic, physiologic, social, and environmental variables, which all impact on how laboratory mice can best be managed in captivity. It is clear that this rich complexity cannot be fully addressed under laboratory conditions, but that does not mean that basic needs, such as nest building, burrowing, foraging, and olfactory environments, cannot be provided. For example, intermale aggression, which is particularly apparent in some strains of mice such as BALB/c and Swiss-origin stocks and strains, can be minimized by maintaining males from infancy as sibling groups, since adult siblings tend not be aggressive to one another. This sibling bond, however, can be easily broken by short-term separation. Environmental enrichment often features provision of plastic houses, which may make vivarium managers feel good, but maximal enrichment can be provided by provision of nesting material, which includes structural scaffolding, such as crinkled cardboard, which facilitates construction of three-dimensional nests. Mouse nests are replete with 'appeasement' pheromones, thereby contributing to harmony within the cage, whereas introduction of dirty bedding has the opposite effect. Frequent cage changing, including removal of established nests, is highly stressful and disruptive to social harmony within a cage. Provision of appropriate and adequate amounts of bedding material that is conducive to burrowing is desirable. It is important to remember that mice are socially gregarious, and that mouse welfare is optimally enriched by other mice within a socially harmonious deme (Latham and Mason, 2004; Van Loo *et al.*, 2003).

A laboratory mouse ethogram, defined as an operationalized list of mouse behaviors, arranged by their adaptive meaning to the animal, is available on the web: www.mousebehavior.org. Behavioral phenotyping, particularly of transgenic mice, is used extensively in genomic research. A wide variety of standardized test batteries and approaches are used, depending upon the focus of research (reviewed in Crawley 2008). Initial behavioral evaluations include general health, body weight, body temperature, appearance of the fur and whiskers, and neurological reflexes assessment. Specific tests include observations of home cage behaviors, righting reflex, acoustic startle, eye blink, pupil constriction, vibrissae reflex, pinna reflex, Digiscan open field locomotion, rotarod motor coordination, hanging wire, footprint pathway, visual cliff, auditory threshold, pain threshold, and olfactory acuity.

Novel and complex environmental enrichment in animal housing conditions facilitates enhanced sensory and cognitive stimulation as well as physical activity. Environmental enrichment and exercise have beneficial effects such as cognitive enhancement, delayed disease onset, enhanced cellular plasticity, and associated molecular processes in animal models of brain disorders (Pang and Hannan, 2013).

D. Immunology

The immune system of the mouse is very similar to that of humans. The availability of inbred mouse strains, in which each individual animal expresses identical MHC alleles so that tissues and cells can be transplanted without tissue rejection, greatly simplifies and indeed enables functional analyses of immune system components not possible with any other outbred mammalian species. In addition, the ability to genetically manipulate the mouse genome, adding to, altering, and deleting existing genes, enables unprecedented *in vivo* analysis of immune cell functions. It is for these reasons that the mouse is the primary animal model for immunology research.

1. Tissues of the Immune System

The immune system is an unusual organ system in that it consists of both solid tissues and various migrating cell populations. The bone marrow and thymus are considered primary lymphoid organs, as sites of hematopoiesis and B- and T-lymphocyte development, respectively. Lymph nodes, spleen, and intestinal Peyer's patches are considered secondary lymphoid tissues, as sites of immune response initiation. Lymph nodes and spleen are analyzed frequently for studies of immune responses and as organs for immune cell isolation. Tertiary lymphoid tissue sites are those that form in

other solid organs in response to an insult or microbial exposure. Among them are the lymphoid cell aggregates of the gastrointestinal and respiratory tract, also called 'gut-associated lymphoid tissue' (GALT) and bronchus-associated lymphoid tissues (BALT).

2. Cells of the Immune System

Leukocytes are classified as belonging to the innate or adaptive immune system. The innate immune system responds rapidly to an antigen insult via recognition of pathogen-associated molecular patterns (PAMPs), such as lipopolysaccharide, bacterial flagellin, single (s)- and double-stranded (ds) RNA, and non-methylated DNA, via extracellular or intracellular pattern recognition receptors (PRRs). Receptors include the Toll-like receptors (TLRs), such as TLR4 (recognizing LPS), TLR3/7 (ss and dsRNA) and TLR9 (DNA), NOD-like receptors (NOD1/2), and RIG-like receptors (RIG-I, MDA-5) among others (Takeuchi and Akira, 2010). Cells of the innate immune system are monocytes/macrophages, granulocytes and dendritic cells as well as innate-like lymphocyte populations (ILC) 1, 2 and 3, which include natural killer (NK) cells (Spits *et al.*, 2013). Cells of the adaptive immune system (T and B lymphocytes) express a highly antigen-specific receptor that has arisen through gene rearrangement (T-cell and B-cell receptors, respectively). B cells of the B-1 lineage and $\gamma\delta$ T cells are regarded as innate-like cells, as they express a rearranged antigen receptor but seem to respond in an innate-like manner.

Leukocytes are identified and classified by sets of monoclonal antibodies (mAb) against uniquely expressed surface receptors, typically measured by flow cytometry. Identification of a unique receptor by one or more mAb of the same specificity leads to the assignment of a receptor name, as a 'cluster of differentiation (CD)'. For example, T cells are differentiated into two subsets based on their expression of either CD4 or CD8. CD4$^+$ T cells (T helper cells) recognize peptides presented in MHC class II and promote B-lymphocyte activation and activate and regulate cellular immune responses via secretion of differing cytokines (see below). CD8$^+$ T cells recognize antigenic peptides presented in MHC class I and serve as cytotoxic cells during the cell-mediated immune response where they can destroy infected cells (e.g., against cells containing infectious agents).

3. Secreted Products of the Immune System
Immunoglobulins

The major function of B cells is to respond to an encounter with an antigen/pathogen with the production of highly antigen-specific immunoglobulins (Ig; antibodies), which can bind to and inactivate pathogens and toxins. Activation of B cells can lead to their differentiation to plasma cells, which produce large amounts of Ig. Five classes or Ig 'isotypes' can be distinguished, which differ in effector function: IgM, IgG, IgA, IgE, and IgD. The latter is expressed only on the surface of B cells in mice. The IgG class, the most abundant antibody class in the serum, is further divided into subtypes: IgG_1, $IgG_{2a/c}$, IgG_{2b}, and IgG_3. Polymorphisms exist on the Ig locus such that some strains of mice produce the IgG2a subtype (e.g., BALB/c), whereas others produce IgG2c (e.g., C57BL/6) (Zhang et al., 2012). Additional allelic polymorphisms of the locus also exist. For example, BALB/c and 129SV mice express the Igh-a allotype, whereas C57BL/6 mice express the Igh-b allotype. Recombinant inbred strains of mice exist for both BALB/c and C57BL/6, which harbor the reciprocal Igh locus (i.e., Igh-b for BALB/c and Igh-a for C57BL/6 mice). These mice are useful tools for tracking B cells following adaptive cell transfer via allotype-specific mAb (see below).

Immunoglobulin isotype production varies according to the type of immunogen used to evoke the response. IgM is secreted short term after initial exposure to an antigen, followed by the other Ig isotypes. In viral and intracellular bacterial infections, $IgG_{2a/c}$ is dominant, whereas in extracellular bacterial infections IgG_1 dominates the response. IgG_{2b} and IgG_3 are usually induced to carbohydrate or lipid antigens. IgE is linked to parasitic infections and to allergy. Serum antibodies specific for an immunogen can often be measured for the life of the animal. While serum IgA levels are low, IgA is the highest produced Ig in mice. IgA production, however, occurs in plasma cells lodged in the lamina propria of mucosal tissues, from where the IgA is actively transported in dimeric form onto the luminal surface of mucosal tissues as 'secretory' IgA (Brandtzaeg, 2009).

Cytokines and Chemokines

Cytokines are secreted signaling molecules involved in cell–cell communication in a complex biological system (Table 3.11). These include the large family of interleukins (ILs, currently IL-1 to IL-37), tumor necrosis factors (TNFs), interferons (Type I, II, and III) and growth factors such as granulocyte-macrophage colony-stimulating factor (GM-CSF) and stem cell factor (SCF). Cytokine secretion often occurs in response to recognition of antigen via PRR or TCR. Because of their importance in modulating immunity to antigenic stimuli, mice with specific deletions or overexpression of individual cytokines have been made and have contributed to a detailed understanding of many of their often pleotropic functions (Akdis et al., 2011).

Chemokines are a similarly large group of small, secreted molecules that regulate cell trafficking to sites of antigen encounter but also facilitate cell–cell contact by acting as chemoattractants. Chemokines are grouped according to the number of cysteines and disulfide bonds in the molecule into C-X-C-, C-C, C, and CX_3Cl

Chemokine ligands (L) and receptors (R) and designated accordingly as CXCR1-7/CXCL1-16 and CCR1-10/CCL 1-28 (Allen et al., 2007).

4. Polarization of the Immune Response

Immune responses must be coordinated to provide the most appropriate effector functions for the type of pathogen/antigen encountered. Immune effector responses differ depending on the life cycle (facultative or obligate intracellular, extracellular, localized, systemic, etc.) and antigen types displayed by the encountered antigen/pathogen, because this affects the type of PRR engaged and activated. PRR engagement leads to cytokine and chemokine responses by the first responders, i.e., epithelial cells, local macrophage populations and other innate cells. The type of cytokines and chemokines produced then dictates the types of cells recruited to the site of infection and their subsequent differentiation and functions. The PRR engagement also leads to antigen uptake, activation and migration of dendritic cells (DCs) from the site of insult to the regional lymph nodes, where DCs present antigen peptides on MHC molecules to T cells. In addition, the DCs secrete cytokines induced by the initial PRR activation, which cause the differentiation of CD4 T cells towards a particular effector response. For example, secretion of IL-12 in response to activation of TLR2 or 4 will result in the induction of interferon-gamma (IFN-γ) production by CD4 T cells, whereas IL-6 and TGF-β production by DC will induce CD4 T cells to secrete IL-17 (Kara et al., 2014). Because the DC translates signals from PRR at the site of infection into differentiation signals for T cells in the lymph tissues, these cells are regarded as a 'bridge' between the innate and adaptive immune systems.

The specific Ig isotype secreted in response to a pathogen depends to a large degree on the type of cytokine produced by CD4 T cells that provide 'T-cell help' for B cells. T cells that interact with B cells are identified as a discrete subset termed 'T follicular helper cells (T_{FH})' and it is their cytokine profile that directs B cells to secrete a particular Ig isotype (Kara et al., 2014). The classic T_H1/T_H2 dichotomy outlined above was in part shaped by the observation that IFN-γ production will lead to switching of B cells to secrete IgG2a/c, whereas production of IL-4 leads to the secretion of IgG1.

Interestingly, it appears that the cytokine profile induced by the effector T-cell population is mirrored by the innate immune response. Innate-like lymphocytes also have effector phenotypes that correspond to those of CD4 T cells and are induced by the same signals and transcriptional regulators (Spits et al., 2013) and the same appears to be true also for macrophages and other innate immune cells (Sica and Mantovani, 2012). While initial studies identified two particular antagonistic effector response types (termed T_H1 and T_H2 and classified by

TABLE 3.11   Major Sources, Cellular Targets, and *In Vivo* Effects of Select Mouse Cytokines[a]

Cytokine	Cell source	Cell targets	Function
IFN-α, IFN-β	Macrophages, B and T cells, fibroblasts, epithelial cells	Many cell types	Antiviral, antiproliferative, stimulate NK activity and macrophage functions
IFN-γ	T cells, NK cells	Macrophages, lymphocytes, NK cells	Proinflammatory, promotes Th1 immune responses/secretion of Th1-associated cytokines
IL-1α, IL-1β	Macrophages, endothelial cells, keratinocytes, lymphocytes, fibroblasts, osteoblasts	Many cell types	Proinflammatory, stimulates fibroblasts and bone catabolism, neuroendocrine effects (fever, sleep, anorexia, corticotropin release)
IL-2	Activated T cells	Macrophages, T and B cells, NK cells	T-cell growth factor, stimulates NK activity
IL-3	T cells, mast cells	Mast cells, hematopoietic progenitors	Promotes proliferation and differentiation of mast cell and hematopoietic cell lineages (granulocytic, monocytic, megakaryocytic)
IL-4	T cells, basophils, mast cells, bone marrow stromal cells	B and T cells, mast cells, macrophages, hematopoietic progenitors	Proliferation and differentiation of B cells (Ig switching to IgG$_1$ and IgE) and Th2 cells (anti-inflammatory by inhibiting Th1 immune responses)
IL-5	T cells, mast cells	Eosinophils, B cells	Stimulates eosinophilia, growth and differentiation of B-cells, Ig switching
IL-6	Fibroblasts, macrophages, endothelial cells, T cells	B and T cells, thymocytes, hepatocytes, neurons	Differentiation of myeloid cells, induction of acute phase proteins, tropic for neurons
IL-7	Thymic and bone marrow stromal cells	B and T cells	Growth factor for B and T cells
IL-8	Monocytes, neutrophils, fibroblasts, endothelial cells, keratinocytes, T cells	Neutrophils, basophils, T cells	Proinflammatory, activates neutrophils, enhances keratinocyte growth
IL-9	T cells	CD4$^+$ T cells, mast cells	Enhances hematopoiesis
IL-10	Macrophages, T and B cells, mast cells, keratinocytes	Macrophages, T and B cells	Anti-inflammatory Th2 immune responses, inhibits Th1 responses
IL-11	Stromal cells	Hematopoietic progenitor cells	Hematopoiesis
IL-12	T cells	T cells, macrophages	Proinflammatory; promotes NK and cytotoxic lymphocyte activity; induces IFN-γ, which in turn promotes Th1 immune responses
IL-13	T cells	B cells	Activation of Ig transcription, key mediator in asthma
IL-14	Endothelial cells, lymphocytes	B cells	B cell growth factor
IL-15	Fibroblasts, keratinocytes, endothelial cells, and macrophages	T and B cells, NK cells, monocytes, eosinophils, neutrophils	Enhances neutrophil chemokine production, cytoskeletal rearrangements, phagocytosis; delays apoptosis
IL-16	Epithelial cells, mast cells, CD4$^+$ and CD8$^+$ cells, eosinophils	CD4$^+$	CD4$^+$ T-cell growth factor; proinflammatory; enhances lymphocyte chemotaxis, adhesion molecule and IL-2 receptor and *HLA-DR* expression
IL-17	Human memory T cells, mouse αβ TCR$^+$ CD4$^-$ CD8$^-$ thymocytes	Fibroblasts, keratinocytes, epithelial and endothelial cells	Secretion of IL-6, IL-8, PGE2, MCP-1 and G-CSF, induces *ICAM-1* expression, T-cell proliferation
IL-18	Macrophages, keratinocytes, microglial cells	T cells; NK cells; myeloid, monocytic, erythroid, and megakaryocytic cell lineages	Proinflammatory, induces IFN-γ and other Th1 cytokines, promotes Th1 development and NK activity
GM-CSF	Macrophages, stromal cells, fibroblasts, endothelial cells, lymphocytes	Hematopoietic stem cells, neutrophils, macrophages	Growth and differentiation of granulocytes, macrophages
TNF	Macrophages, T and B cells, NK cells	Many cell types	Proinflammatory, fever, neutrophil activation, bone resorption, anticoagulant, tumor necrosis
TGF-β	Platelets, macrophages, T and B cells, placenta, hepatocytes, thymocytes	Many cells types	Anti-inflammatory; promotes wound healing, angiogenesis; suppresses hematopoiesis, lymphopoiesis, Ig production, NK activity; promotes Ig switching to IgA

[a]IFN, interferon; IL, interleukin; GM-CSFs, granulocyte-macrophage colony-stimulating factors; NK, natural killer; TNF, tumor necrosis factor; TGF, tumor growth factor.

T-cell production of IFN-γ and IL-4, respectively), more recent studies now demonstrate a much wider array of effector responses in which innate and adaptive immunity acts together to reinforce an immune response phenotype as well as modulate its size by induction of T regulatory cells (T_{regs}) that generate inhibitory cytokines (Kara *et al.*, 2014; Sica and Mantovani, 2012; Spits *et al.*, 2013). The use of cytokine-deficient and reporter mice that enabled the identification of cytokine-producing cells via expression of a fluorescent reporter was particularly valuable for the development of this more nuanced view of the quality of immune responses.

5. Experimental Approaches to Study Immune System Components

Spontaneous mouse models of immune deficiencies have been used extensively in research. Their use, plus the expanding number of knockout, transgenic, and dominant negative mouse mutants, has advanced understanding of human immune deficiency diseases as well as basic understanding of the immune system (Table 3.12). Interbreeding of multiple immune-deficient mice has allowed the development of 'humanized' mice in which immune cells of the mouse are replaced with those of humans. While many challenges remain to fully

TABLE 3.12   Common Mouse Models of Immunodeficiency

Model	Immunodeficiency	Phenotype	Major uses
Nude mouse	Defective transcription factor gene controlling thymic epithelial cell differentiation	Athymic and hairless (unrelated but linked gene defect) No T-cell functions	Tumor and xenograft studies
SCID mouse	Defective DNA-dependent kinase that recombines gene segments coding for T (TcR) and B (Ig) cell receptors	Hypoplastic lymphoid tissues No Ig or T cell responses Sensitive to ionizing radiation because of defective DNA break repair	V (D)J recombination studies Tumor and xenograft transplantation Lymphocyte subset transfer studies Reconstitution of human hematopoietic system (Hu-PBL-SCID)
Rag-1 and Rag-2 mice	Defective recombinase enzymes (Rag-1 and/or Rag-2), preventing formation of functional B α (Ig) and T (TcR) cell receptors	Hypoplastic lymphoid tissues No Ig or T-cell responses	V (D)J recombination studies Tumor and xenograft transplantation Lymphocyte subset transfer studies
NOD/SCID/IL-2Rγ$^{-/-}$	Multiple immunodeficiencies derived from NOD and SCID mice with loss of IL-2 receptor gamma chain[1]	No T-, B-, or NK-cell activity Decreased complement Impaired macrophage and dendritic cell functions	Model for efficient engraftment of human lymphoid cells
XID mouse	Defect in Bruton's tyrosine kinase gene affecting signal transduction in B cells	Decreased B cell numbers, low IgM Impaired response to polysaccharide antigens	Model for human X-lined agammaglobulinemia
Moth-eaten mouse	Defective phosphatase, impairing signal transduction from cell receptors	Deficient humoral and cellular immunity Lack cytotoxic T and NK cells Moth-eaten pelage secondary to folliculitis Autoimmune syndromes Hypergammaglobulinemia	Apoptosis studies Autoimmune syndromes
Beige mouse	Mutation on chromosome 13 affects pigment granules (coat, retina) and lysosomal granules of type II pneumocytes, mast cells, and NK cells	Diluted coat color Lysosomal storage disease Impaired chemotaxis, bactericidal activity of neutrophils, decreased NK activity	Model for Chediak–Higashi syndrome Crossed onto nude or SCID backgrounds for multiple
1pr and gld mice	Impaired apoptosis from Fas (1pr) or Fas ligand (gld) defect	Generalized lymphoproliferative disease (gld), autoimmunity, immunodeficiency	Immune deficiencies Apoptosis studies Autoimmune syndromes
Cytokine KO mice (IL-2, IL-10, IFN-γ, TNF-β, others)	Genetically engineered disruption (knockout) of cytokine gene	Anemia (IL-2), wasting (IL-2, IL-10), and inflammatory bowel disease (IL-2, IL-10) when housed conventionally	Physiological role of cytokines in immune response and inflammation
Receptor KO mice (TcR, Ig, cytokine, MHC, adhesion molecules, integrins)	Genetically engineered disruption (knockout) of receptor gene	Lack functional response to signal of interest, variable immune compromise Inflammatory bowel disease common in TcR KO	Physiological role of receptors in immune response and inflammation

replenish mice with components of the human immune system, the use of immune-deficient NOD/severe combined immunodeficient (SCID)/IL-2Rγ$^{-/-}$ recipients for transfer of human peripheral blood lymphocytes, cord-blood or bone marrow-derived CD34+ stem cells with human liver and thymus (BLT-mice) is yielding promising results (Akkina, 2013).

Investigators using genetically engineered mice are constantly reminded that phenotypic analysis of these animals must be done cautiously because the immune system may be profoundly affected and in ways that are not always anticipated. This may make it difficult to determine whether a given gene product is directly involved or may be secondary to a more global dysregulation of the immune system. As with other biological systems, compensation mechanisms also may mask the phenotype.

Experimental approaches are being increasingly used to refine the knockout technology by restricting a specific genetic deficiency to a particular tissue of interest using the Cre-lox system, in which tissue-specific or temporal restricted expression of the Cre recombinase induces the deletion of a 'floxed' gene (Mak *et al.*, 2001). Transgenic mice are available that restrict Cre expression to various hematopoietic cells or tissue or drive Cre recombination following injection of tamoxifen. Other approaches are the generation of 'bone marrow irradiation' chimeras. Here, inbred wild-type mice or mice deficient in certain immune cells (Table 3.12) are lethally irradiated by exposure to a gamma-irradiation source to deplete the hematopoietic stem cells. These are then replaced by transfer of bone marrow cells to the irradiated mice. Reconstitution of the hematopoietic system is usually achieved within about 6 weeks, during which time mice are provided with antibiotic-containing drinking water to avoid infections of these temporarily immune-compromised animals. Transfer of bone marrow from a congenic knockout restricts the genetic defect to the hematopoietic system.

A mix of bone marrow from two sources is also often used to generate tissue-specific knockouts. For example, mixing a bone marrow from T-cell-deficient mice (75%) with that of a gene knockout (25%) generates 'mixed bone marrow chimeras' in which all T cells only develop from the knockout, thus lack the gene of interest, whereas most of the other cells T from the wild-type source, effectively constraining the genetic defect to the T-cell population. Sets of congenic mice with defined allotypic differences are often used to confirm the source of individual cells. Such markers include the gene locus CD45.1/CDC45.2 or CD90.1/CD90.2 (Thy1.1/Thy1.2). Alternatively, cells may express a fluorescent transgene, such as green-fluorescent protein (GFP). Identification is usually performed by flow cytometry, or less commonly by immunofluorescence or immunohistochemistry.

Generation of bone marrow chimeras circumvents the time-consuming breeding of Cre recombinase-expressing flx/flx mice. However, numerous controls are needed to exclude off-target effects due to irradiation damage.

Repeat injection of antibodies targeting specific cell populations is another rapid approach that avoids the potential for irradiation damage and allows short-term depletion of individual cell subsets. Its main disadvantage is the need to identify mAb that bind to surface receptors uniquely expressed by a cell subset of interest and the verification of the efficacy of the depletion. Frequently used is antibody treatment for the short-term depletion of T-cell subsets using mAb against CD4 or CD8 as well as individual cytokines.

III. DISEASES

Contemporary knowledge about diseases of laboratory mice has developed primarily from examining the effects of disease on traditional strains and stocks. The widespread use of genetically engineered mice is likely to modify current concepts because of novel or unpredictable interactions among genetic alterations, the genetic backgrounds on which they are expressed, and exogenous factors, such as infectious agents. Because the number of combinations is extraordinarily high, clinical and laboratory diagnosticians should be alert to the potential for altered disease expression in genetically engineered mice and not be misled by unexpected signs, lesions, and epizootiology.

A. Infectious Diseases

1. Microbiological Surveillance and Diagnostics

Many microbial agents have the potential to cause disease in mice or interfere with mouse-based research. Housing and husbandry in microbiologically sheltered environments are designed to reduce the risks of disruptive infection, especially among immunologically dysfunctional mice, but must be accompanied by effective microbiological surveillance. Surveillance should encompass resident mice *and* mouse products (serum, cell lines, transplantable tumors) procured from external sources. Because surveillance strategies will vary with research needs and operating conditions, it is prudent to consult a number of sources, such as the Federation of European Laboratory Animal Science Associations (FELASA) (Nicklas *et al.*, 2002) and commercial laboratories, for guidance. Detailed discussion of microbial quality control is provided in Chapter 10. There are also recommendations regarding specific agents in following sections. Diagnostic methods involve gross and microscopic pathology, parasitology, microbial isolation and culture, serology, and PCR. Serology is particularly important for viral surveillance, and now relies principally on enzyme-linked immunosorbent assay (ELISA), multiplex fluorescent immunoassay (MFI) for simultaneous detection of antibodies to multiple agents (Hsu *et al.*, 2007), indirect fluorescent antibody (IFA) assay, or hemagglutination inhibition (HAI), with the latter two methods generally used for confirmation (Livingston and Riley, 2003; Pritchett-Corning *et al.*, 2009). Mouse antibody production (MAP) testing has been historically used for testing biological materials for contamination by infectious agents. PCR panels for murine infectious agents are now commercially available and have cost and time-saving advantages as well as improved assay sensitivity and specificity. Beyond the classic bacterial and viral murine infections, PCR assays are now available for endo- and ectoparasites (see Chapter 11).

2. Viral Diseases

a. Mousepox (Buller and Fenner, 2007; Esteban and Buller, 2005; Fenner, 1948b, 1949a, b)

Etiology Mousepox is caused by *Ectromelia virus* (ECTV), an orthopoxvirus that is antigenically and genetically closely related to a number of other poxviruses, including vaccinia, variola, and cowpox viruses. The original isolate of ECTV, known as the Hampstead strain, was discovered by J. Marchal in 1930 (Marchal, 1930) as the cause of epizootic disease among laboratory mice in England. The disease featured amputation of extremities, which Marchal termed *ectromelia* (from the Greek, *ectro*, amputation and *melia*, limb). Other strains of the virus include Moscow, NIH-79, Washington University, St. Louis 69, Beijing 70, Ishibahsi I–III, and Naval (NAV) strains, which vary in virulence, but are essentially indistinguishable genetically and serologically, suggesting a common origin. Virus can be isolated from infected tissues by inoculation of cell cultures (BS-C-1, HeLa, L cells) or embryonated eggs. The natural host (and original source of infection of laboratory mice) of ECTV remains unknown.

Clinical Signs The expression of clinical signs reflects an interplay among virus-related factors, including virus strain, dose and portal of entry, and host-related factors, including age, genotype, immunological competence, and gender (Brownstein *et al.*, 1991a). During natural epizootics, it was observed that A, BC, DBA/1, DBA/2, and CBA strains developed acute fatal infections, whereas C57BL/6 mice were resistant to severe disease (Briody, 1966). Experimental studies have shown that all strains of mice are susceptible to infection, but BALB/c, A, DBA/2, and C3H/He mice were highly susceptible, AKR and SJL mice were moderately susceptible, and C57BL/6 mice were highly resistant to lethal

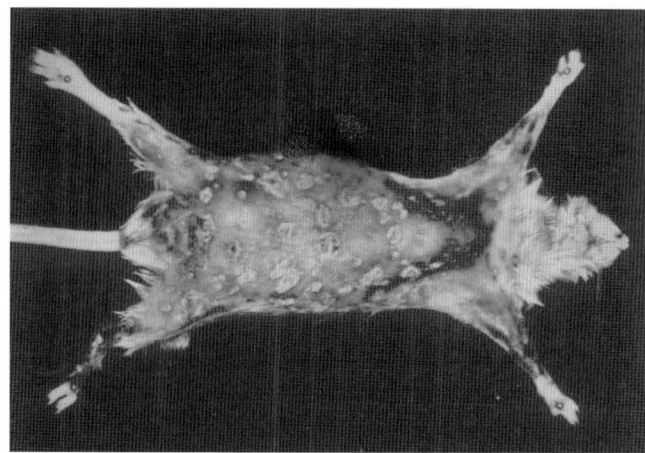

FIGURE 3.12   Mouse after depilation to reveal the rash associated with mouse pox. *From Fenner (1948a).*

infection (Bhatt and Jacoby, 1987c; Wallace and Buller, 1985). The mechanisms of genetic resistance are not fully understood but appear to reflect multiple genes, some of which appear to be expressed through lymphoreticular cells, including NK cells (Brownstein *et al.*, 1991a; Jacoby *et al.*, 1989). The nuances of cytokine and cellular immune responses to ECTV infection have received recent attention (reviewed in Buller and Fenner (2007) and Esteban and Buller (2005)). Outbreaks among susceptible mice are often volatile, with variable morbidity and high mortality in susceptible strains of mice. Clinical signs such as ruffled fur or prostration may occur for only a few hours before death. Mice that survive acute infection may develop chronic disease characterized by a focal or generalized rash anywhere on the body (Fig. 3.12). Conjunctivitis also may occur. Skin lesions usually recede within several weeks, but hairless scars may remain. Additionally, severe viral infection of the feet and tail during the rash syndrome can lead to necrosis and amputation.

Epizootiology Mousepox is not a common disease. Outbreaks occur sporadically and recent outbreaks have been traced to the importation of contaminated mice or mouse products. For example, contaminated mouse serum was responsible for recent outbreaks in the United States (Dick *et al.*, 1996; Lipman *et al.*, 2000). Natural exposure is thought to occur through direct contact and skin abrasions. Cage-to-cage transmission is low and can be virtually nil if filter-topped cages are used (Bhatt and Jacoby, 1987b). Ectromelia virus is highly stable at room temperature, especially under dry conditions, leading to the potential for prolonged environmental contamination in infected colonies (Bhatt and Jacoby, 1987d). Aerogenic exposure is not a major factor in natural outbreaks, and arthropod-borne transmission does not appear to occur. Virus-free progeny can be obtained from immune dams (Bhatt and Jacoby, 1987b). However, intrauterine infection and fetal deaths, albeit rare, have been reported.

Natural transmission is facilitated by intermediately resistant mice, which survive long enough to develop skin lesions that can shed virus for relatively long periods of time. The risks for transmission are further increased by persistence of infectious virus in excreta and exfoliated scabs. Although virus excretion typically lasts for about 3 weeks, virus has been found in scabs and/or feces for up to 16 weeks. Resistant mouse strains also are dangerous because they can shed virus during subclinical infections. However, infections in resistant mice tend to be short-lived. Highly susceptible mice are a relatively small hazard for dissemination of infection, if properly discarded, because they die before virus shedding becomes prominent. Thus, juxtaposition of resistant or intermediately resistant infected mice with highly susceptible mice can provoke explosive outbreaks. Infant and aged mice are usually more susceptible to lethal infection than young adult mice. Maternal immunity among enzootically infected breeding mice may perpetuate infection by protecting young mice from death, but not from infection. Such mice may subsequently transmit infection by contact exposure.

Pathology The classic descriptions of ECTV pathogenesis by Fenner remain timely, including the frequently cited and reproduced figure summarizing the pathogenesis of infection (Fig. 3.13) (Fenner, 1948b). Interest in smallpox has renewed the interest in ECTV as a model of host response to infection (Esteban and Buller, 2005). ECTV multiplies in the cell cytoplasm and produces two types of inclusion bodies. The A type (Marchal body) is well demarcated and acidophilic in histological sections. It is found primarily in epithelial cells of skin (Fig. 3.14) or mucous membranes and can also be found in intestinal mucosa. The B type of inclusion is basophilic and can be found in all ectromelia-infected cells. However, it is difficult to visualize unless cells are stained intensely with hematoxylin. ECTV antigen can be readily visualized by immunohistochemistry on formalin-fixed, paraffin-embedded tissue sections (Esteban and Buller, 2005; Jacoby and Bhatt, 1987).

Following skin invasion, viral multiplication occurs in the draining lymph node and a primary viremia ensues. Splenic and hepatic involvement begin within 3–4 days, whereupon larger quantities of virus are disseminated in blood to the skin. This sequence takes approximately 1 week and, unless mice die of acute hepatosplenic infection, ends with the development of a primary skin lesion at the original site of viral entry. The primary lesion is due to the development of antiviral cellular immunity.

Severe hepatocellular necrosis occurs in susceptible mice during acute stages of mousepox. White spots

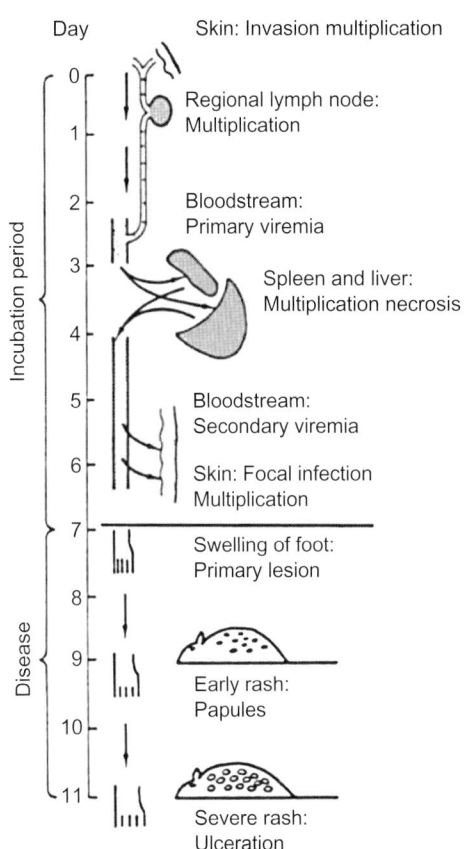

FIGURE 3.13   Diagram illustrating the pathogenesis of mousepox. *From Fenner (1948b).*

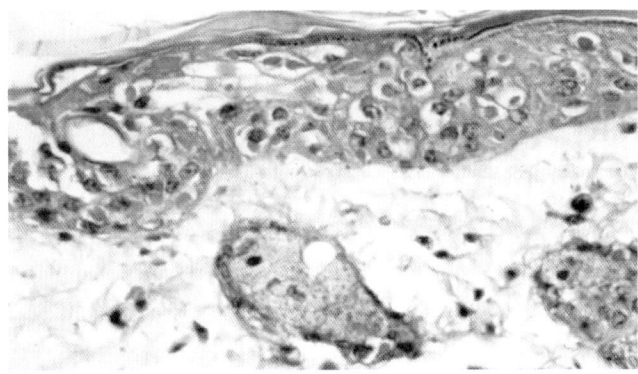

FIGURE 3.14   Skin from a mouse infected with ectromelia virus. Note intracytoplasmic inclusions. *Courtesy of S.W. Barthold.*

indicative of necrosis develop throughout the liver (Fig. 3.15). In nonfatal cases, regeneration begins at the margins of necrotic areas, but inflammation is variable. Splenic necrosis in acute disease commonly precedes hepatic necrosis but is equally or more severe. Necrosis and scarring of red and white pulp can produce a macroscopic 'mosaic' pattern of white and red–brown (Fig. 3.16). Necrosis of thymus, lymph nodes, Peyer's

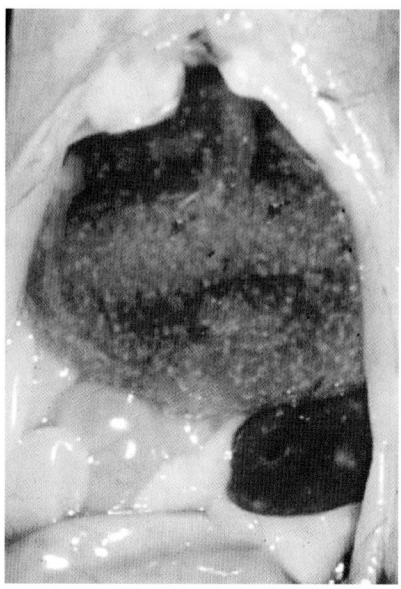

FIGURE 3.15 Multifocal necrotizing hepatitis and splenitis in a mouse during the acute phase of a natural infection with ectromelia virus. *From Percy and Barthold (2007), with permission from Nina Hahn.*

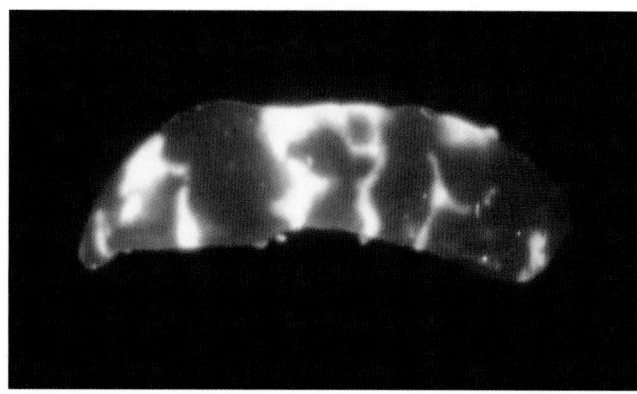

FIGURE 3.16 'Mosaic spleen' from a mouse that survived acute mousepox. The pale bands are due to fibrotic scarring following severe necrosis.

patches, intestinal mucosa, and genital tract also have been observed during acute infection, whereas resistant or convalescent mice can develop lymphoid hyperplasia. Severe intestinal infection may be accompanied by hemorrhage.

The primary skin lesion, which occurs 6–10 days after exposure, is a localized swelling that enlarges from inflammatory edema. Necrosis of dermal epithelium provokes a surface scab and heals as a deep, hairless scar. Secondary skin lesions (rash) develop 2–3 days later as the result of viremia. They are often multiple and widespread and can be associated with conjunctivitis, with blepharitis, and, in severe cases, with buccal and lingual ulcers. The skin lesions also can ulcerate and scab before scarring.

Diagnosis Mousepox can be diagnosed from clinical signs, lesions, serological tests, and demonstration of virus or viral antigen in tissues. Observation of characteristic intracytoplasmic eosinophilic inclusions aids detection of infection. Several serological tests are available to detect mousepox. Historically, the standard test was HAI, using vaccinia antigen as a source of hemagglutinin. ELISA is more sensitive and specific and has replaced HAI for serological monitoring among nonvaccinated mice (Buller *et al.*, 1983). ECTV infection also can be detected by IFA (Buller *et al.*, 1983) and PCR. Serological differentiation of mousepox from vaccinia infection in vaccinated mice is based on the lack of hemagglutinin in the vaccine strain of virus. Thus, serum from vaccinated mice may react by ELISA but should not react by HAI.

Differential Diagnosis Mousepox must be differentiated from other infectious diseases associated with high morbidity and high mortality. These include Sendai pneumonia, mouse hepatitis, and Tyzzer's disease. The latter two can be expressed by acute necrosis in parenchymal organs, but they can be differentiated by morphological, serological, and virological criteria. The skin lesions of chronic mousepox must be differentiated from other skin diseases caused by opportunistic or pathogenic bacteria, ascariasis, and bite wounds.

Prevention and Control Mousepox is a dangerous disease because of its virulence for susceptible mice. Therefore, infected colonies should be quarantined immediately. Depopulation has been used as a primary means for control, but confirmation of infection should be obtained before exposed mice are destroyed. Tissues, supplies, instruments, or other items that have had potential contact with infected mice should be disinfected by heat or chemicals such as formalin, sodium hypochlorite, or chlorine dioxide. Materials should be autoclaved or, preferably, incinerated. Disinfected rooms should be challenged with susceptible sentinel animals that are observed for clinical signs and tested for seroconversion after several weeks. Depopulation and disinfection must be carried out vigorously. Because modern housing and husbandry methods based on the use of microbarrier caging are effective for containing infection, testing and culling properly isolated mice is a potential alternative, especially for irreplaceable breeding mice. Such mice can be quarantined along with cessation of breeding to permit resolution of infection (Bhatt and Jacoby, 1987b). Sequential testing with contact-exposed sentinels should be employed with this option. Additionally, maternal immunity from fully recovered dams can protect mice from infection, thereby enhancing opportunities to derive virus-free mice from previously infected dams, received considerable attention as a model of human CMV infection.

MOUSE CYTOMEGALOVIRUS INFECTION

Etiology Mouse cytomegalovirus (MCMV) is a mouse-specific betaherpesvirus. It can, however, replicate in cell cultures from several species, including mouse (fibroblasts and 3T3 cells), hamster, rabbit, sheep, and nonhuman primate. Cocultivation may be required to rescue latent virus.

Clinical Signs MCMV causes subclinical infection in adult immunocompetent mice, but experimental inoculation of neonates can cause lethal disease due to multisystemic necrosis and inflammation.

Epizootiology The prevalence of MCMV in laboratory mice is probably uncommon but undefined, since infection is clinically silent and serological surveillance is not widely practiced. Wild mice are commonly infected and serve as a natural reservoir for infection, which implies that the entry of virus into a modern vivarium is most likely to occur from contaminated animal products.

Persistence is a central feature of nonlethal infection. Persistently infected mice excrete virus in saliva, urine, and tears for many months, resulting in horizontal transmission through mouse-to-mouse contact. Virus also can infect prostate, testicle, and pancreas, implicating other modes of excretion. Vertical transmission does not appear to be a common factor in natural infection. Further, maternal immunity protects sucklings from infection.

Pathology Mouse cytomegalovirus can replicate in many tissues, and viremia commonly occurs. Lesions are not remarkable during natural infection and may be limited to occasional enlarged cells (megalocytosis) containing eosinophilic intranuclear and/or cytoplasmic inclusions associated with lymphoplasmacytic interstitial inflammation, especially in the cervical salivary glands. Susceptibility to experimental infection varies with age, dose, route, virus strain, and host genotype. Infection can occur in young and adult mice. However, the pathogenicity of MCMV for mice decreases with age. Neonates are highly susceptible to lethal infection, but resistance to disease develops by the time mice are weaned. Immunodeficient mice, however, remain susceptible to pathogenic infection as adults. Persistent infection often affects the salivary glands and pancreas. The persistence of salivary gland infection appears to be dose dependent. There is experimental evidence that MCMV can produce latent infection of B cells, probably T cells as well as aforementioned tissues. Persistent infection may lead to immune complex glomerulonephritis. Latent persistent infection can be reactivated by lymphoproliferative stimuli and by immunosuppression.

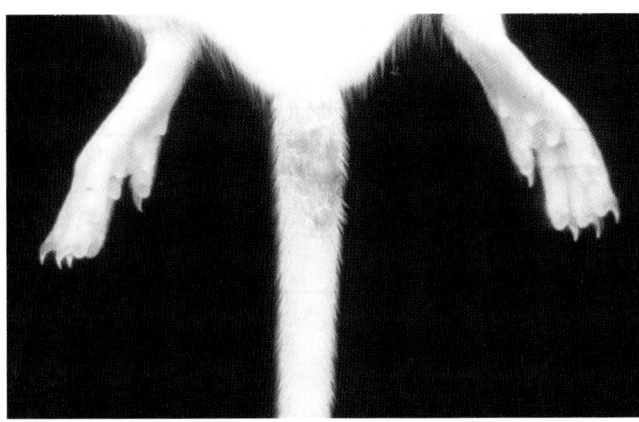

FIGURE 3.17 Vaccination 'take' in a mouse vaccinated by scarification of the tail base with the IHD-T vaccinia virus. *From Jacoby et al. (1983).*

with the caveat that progeny will be transiently seropositive with maternally derived antibody.

Vaccination can control or prevent clinically apparent mousepox. The hemagglutinin-deficient strain of vaccinia virus (IHD-T) is used to scarify skin on the dorsum of the tail. 'Takes' should occur in previously uninfected mice by 6–10 days, but not in infected mice (Bhatt and Jacoby, 1987a) (Fig. 3.17). Infected mice should be quarantined separately or eliminated. Vaccination may not prevent infection, although infection in vaccinated mice is often transient. Furthermore, vaccinia virus can be shed from scarification sites for at least several days. Therefore, other preventive measures, such as strict controls on the entry of mice or mouse products, combined with periodic serological monitoring, should not be relaxed until diagnostic testing has confirmed the elimination of vaccinia and ectromelia virus. Additionally, seroconversion evoked by vaccination must be taken into account in serological monitoring of vaccinated colonies. Finally, vaccinia virus is a human pathogen, so vaccination procedures should include personnel protective measures to prevent exposure.

Research Complications The primary threat from mousepox is mortality in susceptible mice. The loss of time, animals, and financial resources can be substantial.

b. Herpesvirus Infections (Shellam, 2007, 96) *enveloped*

Mice are naturally susceptible to two herpesviruses from the subfamily Betaherpesvirinae and in the genus *Muromegalovirus*, the two species *Murid herpesvirus 1* (of which one of the members is mouse cytomegalovirus (MCMV)) and *Murid herpesvirus 3* (of which one of the members is mouse thymic virus (MTV)). They are species-specific viruses and distinct from each other and from other rodent herpesviruses. MCTV has

Diagnosis MCMV antigens appear to be weak stimuli for humoral antibody production, which is consistent with the fact that cellular immunity is critical for protection against infection. Neutralizing antibody titers are low during acute infection and difficult to find during chronic infection. Serology and PCR-based diagnosis are available, but neither is widely used because of assumptions that infection has a very low prevalence. Detection of enlarged cells with intranuclear inclusions, especially in salivary glands, is diagnostic, if they are present. *In situ* hybridization can be used as an adjunct to routine histopathology.

Differential Diagnosis MCMV infection must be differentiated from infection with MTV. The latter virus can produce necrosis of thymic and peripheral lymphoid tissue when infant mice are experimentally inoculated. Lytic lesions of lymphoid tissues are not a hallmark of MCMV. The viruses can also be distinguished from each other serologically. Sialoadenitis with inclusions can occur during infection with mouse polyoma virus. Like MCMV, MTV infects the salivary gland as its primary target organ.

Prevention and Control Control measures for MCMV have not been established, because it has not been considered an important infection of laboratory mice. Cage-to-cage transmission has not been demonstrated, but horizontal infection from contaminated saliva must be considered. The exclusion of wild mice is essential.

Research Complications MCMV can suppress immune responses. Apart from the potential for interfering with immunology research, it can exacerbate the pathogenicity of opportunistic organisms such as *Pseudomonas aeruginosa.*

MOUSE THYMIC VIRUS INFECTION (Morse, 1989)

Etiology Mouse thymic virus (MTV) is a herpesvirus (murid herpesvirus 3) that is antigenically distinct from MCMV. No suitable *in vitro* method for cultivation has been developed; therefore, viral propagation depends on mouse inoculation.

Clinical Signs Natural infections are subclinical.

Epizootiology The prevalence of MTV is thought to be low. Mice can be infected at any age, although lesions develop only in mice infected perinatally. Mice infected as infants or adults can develop persistent infection of the salivary glands lasting several months or more. Excretion of virus in saliva is considered the primary factor in transmission. Seroconversion occurs in adults but does not eliminate infection. Infection in neonates may not elicit seroconversion, rendering such mice serologically negative carriers. The mode of infection is obscure, but virus is excreted in saliva, suggesting that transmission from infected dams to neonatal mice occurs by ingestion. MTV also has been isolated from the mammary tissue of a lactating mouse, suggesting

the potential for transmission during nursing. Prenatal transmission has not been found.

Pathology MTV causes severe, diffuse necrosis of the thymus and lymphoid tissue with tropism for CD4$^+$ T cells in mice inoculated within approximately 1 week after birth. The severity of thymic and lymph node necrosis can be mouse strain-dependent. Grossly, the thymus is smaller than normal. Infected thymocytes display MTV-positive intranuclear inclusions. Necrosis is followed by granulomatous inflammation and syncytium formation. Reconstitution of lymphoid organs takes 3–8 weeks.

Diagnosis Thymic necrosis associated with intranuclear viral inclusions is the hallmark lesion. Viral antigen can be detected by immunohistochemistry. Serologic detection is effective, but generally not utilized, and is potentially negative in neonatally exposed mice. Suspicion of infection in seronegative mice can be tested by inoculation of virus-free neonatal mice with homogenates of salivary gland or with saliva. Inoculated mice should be examined for thymic necrosis 10–14 days later. PCR or the mouse antibody production (MAP) test can also be used to detect infection.

Differential Diagnosis Reduction of thymus mass can occur in severe mouse coronavirus infection, during epizootic diarrhea of infant mice, or following stress.

Prevention and Control Because MTV induces persistent salivary infection, rederivation or restocking should be considered if infection cannot be tolerated as a research variable.

Research Complications MTV transiently suppresses cellular and humoral immune responses because of its destructive effects on neonatal T lymphocytes.

c. Parvovirus Infections (Jacoby and Ball-Goodrich, 2007; Besselsen *et al.*, 2006)

Parvoviruses are among the most common viral infections in contemporary laboratory mouse populations (Livingston *et al.*, 2002) (Pritchett-Corning *et al.*, 2009), and pose major challenges to both detection and control. The mouse parvoviruses are composed of two antigenically and genetically distinct but related groups, including minute virus of mice (MVM) and mouse parvovirus (MPV), with each group containing a number of strains. The International Committee on Taxonomy of Viruses classifies MPV, MVM, and several other rodent parvoviruses into one genus, *Protoparvovirus*, and species, *Rodent protoparvovirus 1*, but these viruses will be treated separately herein.

MINUTE VIRUS OF MICE

Etiology Minute virus of mice (MVM) is a small (5-kb) single-stranded DNA virus. The prototypic strain is designated MVMp. An allotropic variant with immunosuppressive properties *in vitro* is named MVMi, and additional named strains include MVMc and MVMm. The genome encodes two nonstructural proteins, NS-1 and NS-2, which are highly conserved among the rodent parvoviruses and account for prominent cross-reactivity in serological assays that utilize whole virus antigen. The viral capsid proteins, VP-1 and VP-2, are virus-specific and form the basis for serological differentiation of MVM from MPV. MVM has a broad *in vitro* host range. It replicates in monolayer cultures of mouse fibroblasts (A9 cells), C6 rat glial cells, SV40 (simian virus 40)-transformed human newborn kidney (324K cells), T-cell lymphomas (EL4), and rat or mouse embryo cells, producing cytopathic effects that can include the development of intranuclear inclusions.

Clinical Signs   Natural MVM infections are subclinical. Neonatal mice of some inbred strains are experimentally susceptible to lethal renal and/or intestinal hemorrhage during MVMi infection, but this syndrome has not been reported in natural outbreaks. Experimental inoculation of adult C.B-17-*Prkdc*^scid (SCID) mice with MVMi results in lethal infection (Lamana *et al.*, 2001; Segovia *et al.*, 1999), and similar severe illness has been noted in naturally infected B-cell-deficient NOD.Cg-*H2H4-Igh6* null mice (Naugler *et al.*, 2001).

Epizootiology   MVM is a common virus that naturally infects laboratory mice, but appears to be less common than MPV (Besselsen *et al.*, 2006; Livingston *et al.*, 2002).

MVM is moderately contagious for mice, its only known natural host. Virus can infect the gastrointestinal tract and is excreted in feces and urine. The resistance of rodent parvoviruses to environmental inactivation increases the risks of transmission after virus is excreted. Therefore, contamination of caging, bedding, food, and clothing must be considered a risk for the spread of infection. Transmission occurs by oronasal exposure, but viral contamination of biologicals used for experimental inoculation, such as transplantable tumors, also can be a source of infection. Continuous contact exposure to infected animals or soiled bedding usually induces a humoral immune response within 3 weeks, but limited exposure may delay seroconversion. Young mice in enzootically infected colonies are protected by maternal antibody, but actively acquired immunity develops from infection sustained after the decay of maternal immunity. MVM, in contrast to MPV, is not thought to cause persistent infection; infection in immunocompetent adult mice usually lasts less than 3 weeks (Smith, 1983; Smith and Paturzo, 1988). Infection appears to last less than 1 month, even in oronasally inoculated neonatal mice, but immunodeficient mice may be persistently infected. There is no evidence that MVM is transmitted *in utero*.

Pathology   Natural infections or experimental inoculation of adult mice appears to be nonpathogenic. Contact-exposed neonates have been reported to develop cerebellar lesions, but these are very rare. Experimental infection of neonatal BALB/c, SWR, SJL, CBA, and C3H

mice with MVMi can cause renal hemorrhage and infarction (Brownstein *et al.*, 1991b). DBA/2 mice also developed intestinal hemorrhages and accelerated involution of hepatic hematopoiesis. C57BL/6 neonates are resistant to vascular disease. This lesion has been attributed to viral infection of endothelium. Infection of immunodeficient mice, including SCID and B-cell-deficient mice, results in lethal damage to granulomacrophagic, megakaryocytic, and erythrocytic hematopoietic tissue with severe leukopenia (Lamana *et al.*, 2001; Naugler *et al.*, 2001; Segovia *et al.*, 1999). Intranuclear viral inclusions and viral antigen have been observed in splenic mononuclear cells of B-cell deficient mice (Naugler *et al.*, 2001).

Diagnosis   Serology is the primary method of detecting infection, which utilizes recombinant MVM and MPV major capsid viral proteins (VP2) as antigens, which discriminate between the two groups of mouse parvoviruses. In contrast, the conserved nonstructural protein, NS1 can be used to detect antibody to both groups, but is less sensitive than VP2 assays (Livingston *et al.*, 2002). MVM infection also can be detected by PCR, *in situ* hybridization, and immunohistochemistry. PCR assays can be used to detect MVM- or MPV-specific VP2 or all rodent parvovirus group specific NS1 exons (Besselsen, 1998; Besselsen *et al.*, 2006). MVM can be isolated from the spleen, kidney, intestine, and other tissues by inoculation of the C6 rat glial cell line. It also can be detected by the mouse antibody production test.

Prevention and Control   Because MVM does not persist in immunocompetent mice, control and elimination should exploit quarantine combined with thorough disinfection of the environment, because parvoviruses are resistant to environmental inactivation. MPV has been shown to be successfully eliminated by a cage-by-cage test (serology and fecal PCR) and cull approach, although there are no published reports confirming the success of this strategy for eliminating MVM (Macy *et al.*, 2011). Cesarean rederivation or embryo transfer may also be used to rederive virus-free progeny. Prevention of MVM infection depends on strict barrier husbandry and regular surveillance of mice and mouse products destined for use *in vivo*.

Research Complications   MVM contamination of transplantable neoplasms can occur; therefore, infection can be introduced to a colony through inoculation of contaminated cell lines. Failure to establish long-term cell cultures from infected mice or a low incidence of tumor 'takes' should alert researchers to the possibility of MVM contamination. MVMi has the potential to inhibit the generation of cytotoxic T cells in mixed lymphocyte cultures.

MOUSE PARVOVIRUS   NON-ENV

Etiology   Mouse parvovirus (MPV) is among the more common viruses detected within contemporary mouse colonies, and is more common than MVM (Livingston *et al.*, 2002; Livingston and Riley, 2003; Pritchett-Corning *et al.*, 2009). MPV was initially isolated following its detection as a lymphocytotropic contaminant in *in vitro* assays for cellular immunity. The virus grew lytically in a CD8⁺ T-cell clone designated L3 and inhibited the proliferation of cloned T cells stimulated with antigen or interleukin 2 (IL-2) (McKisic *et al.*, 1993). Molecular analysis of MPV indicates that regions encoding the NS proteins are similar to those of MVM (and other rodent parvoviruses). However, they differ significantly in regions encoding the capsid proteins, accounting for their antigenic specificity. The prototype isolate was first called an 'orphan' parvovirus of mice because its biology and significance were obscure, but it has subsequently been named mouse parvovirus (MPV). Immortalized T cells (L3) are the only cells found thus far to support replication of MPV. There are three genetically distinct variants of MPV, including MPV-1, MPV-2, and MPV-3. MPV-1 includes a number of closely related variants, including MPV-1a, MPV-1b, and MPV-1c. In addition, a hamster parvovirus isolate is closely related to MPV-3, which is infectious to mice and likely to be of mouse origin (Besselsen *et al.*, 2006; Christie *et al.*, 2010).

Clinical Signs MPV infection is clinically silent in infant mice and adult immunocompetent or immunodeficient mice (Besselsen *et al.*, 2007). Immunologic perturbations are the most likely signs of infection (McKisic *et al.*, 1993).

Epizootiology MPV causes persistent infection in infant and adult mice, a property that differentiates it from MVM. *In situ* hybridization has identified the small intestine as a site of viral entry and early replication, but respiratory infection cannot be excluded. Experimental studies following inoculation of neonatal BALB/c and C.B-17-*Prkdc^scid* (SCID) mice revealed that BALB/c mice shed high levels of virus for 3 weeks, with transmission to sentinels exposed during the first 2 weeks of infection. Thereafter, BALB/c mice shed extremely low virus intermittently. In contrast, SCID mice shed high levels of virus until weaning, but lower levels at 6 weeks of age, yet they effectively transmitted infection to sentinels at all stages of infection (Besselsen *et al.*, 2007). Others have shown that transmission of MPV by Sencar mice inoculated as infants was intermittent up to 6 weeks, whereas transmission by mice inoculated as weanlings occurred during the first 2 weeks of infection (Smith *et al.*, 1993). Transmission to BALB/c progeny from infected dams was shown to occur, but embryo transfer rederivation was found to be successful in experimentally infected SCID mice (Besselsen *et al.*, 2008). Humoral (e.g., passively or maternally acquired) immunity can protect against MPV infection. However, immunity to MVM may not confer cross-immunity to MPV (Hansen *et al.*, 1999).

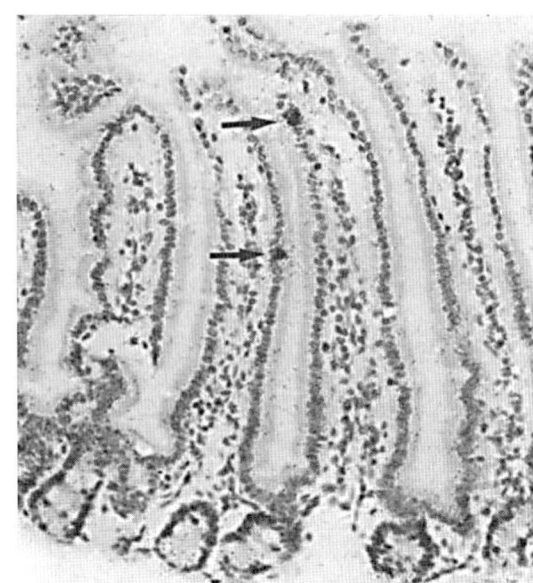

FIGURE 3.18 Mouse parvovirus (arrows) in the intestine after oronasal inoculation of an adult mouse. *In situ* hybridization.

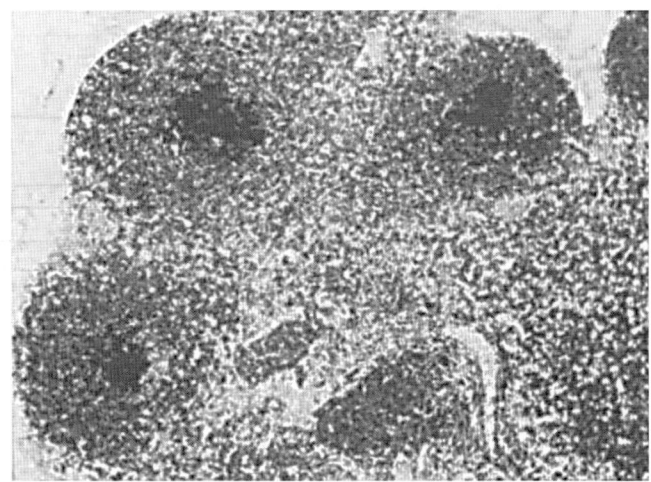

FIGURE 3.19 Mouse parvovirus in the mesenteric lymph node of a persistently infected mouse. *In situ* hybridization localizes the virus to the germinal centers.

Pathology MPV appears to enter through the intestinal mucosa, which is a site of early virus replication (Fig. 3.18). Acute infection is widespread but mild, involving the lung, kidney, liver, and lymphoid organs. Histological lesions are not discernible. Lymphocytotropism is a characteristic of acute and persistent MPV infection in infant and adult mice. During acute infection, virus is dispersed within lymph nodes, but during persistent infection virus localizes in germinal centers (Fig. 3.19).

Diagnosis Because infected mice do not manifest signs or lesions and the virus is very difficult to propagate in cell culture, detection and diagnosis rely on serology and molecular methods. Serology that utilizes MPV VP2 as antigen is a sensitive and specific assay that differentiates MPV from MVM (Livingston et al., 2002). The MAP test also can be used to detect parvovirus infections but is relatively time-consuming and expensive.

As noted for MVM, PCR for murine parvoviruses, using nucleoprotein gene sequences that are conserved among murine parvoviruses, can be used as a screening test. PCR also can be used to detect MPV-specific sequences in the VP2 gene. Although diagnostic PCR is sensitive and specific, it is effective only in actively infected animals. It can be used on feces to detect virus shedding, or applied to tissues, such as mesenteric lymph nodes, obtained at necropsy.

Differential Diagnosis   MPV infection must be differentiated from MVM infection. Because both viruses are enterotropic and lymphocytotropic, serology and PCR must be used to distinguish between them.

Prevention and Control   The persistence of MPV in individual mice, its potential for provoking immune dysfunction, and the resistance of murine parvoviruses to environmental inactivation favor active control and prevention of MPV infection. Quarantine of infected rooms is appropriate. Elimination (depopulation) of infected mice should be considered if they are an immediate threat to experimental or breeding colonies and can be replaced, but a cage-by-cage test and cull approach has been shown to be successful under natural conditions (Macy et al., 2011). For mice that are not easily replaced, virus persistence in the absence of transplacental transmission favors cesarean rederivation or embryo transfer as relatively rapid options to eliminate infection. Control of infection also should include environmental decontamination. Chemical disinfection of suspect animal rooms and heat sterilization of caging and other housing equipment are prudent steps. Prevention is based on sound serological monitoring of mice and surveillance of biologicals destined for inoculation of mice. With the increasing use of mouse germplasm, it is important to note that mouse sperm, oocytes, ovarian tissue, and preimplantation embryos from enzootically MPV-infected mouse colonies may have a high prevalence of MPV contamination, based upon PCR (Agca et al., 2007).

Research Complications   Murine parvoviruses can distort biological responses that depend on cell proliferation. For MPV, such effects are seen on immune function and include augmentation or suppression of humoral and cellular immune responses.

d. Murine Adenovirus Infection (Percy and Barthold, 2007; Spindler et al., 2007)

Etiology   Adenoviruses are nonenveloped DNA viruses that produce intranuclear inclusions *in vitro*

and *in vivo*. Two adenovirus species in the genus *Mastadenovirus* have been associated with mice: *Murine mastadenovirus A* (with the representative strain being MAV-1 or FL) and *Murine mastadenovirus B* (with the representative strain being MAV-2 or K87). Both strains replicate in mouse kidney tissue culture but are antigenically distinct.

Clinical Signs   MAV-1 can cause severe clinical disease after experimental inoculation of infant mice. Signs include scruffiness, lethargy, stunted growth, and often death within 10 days. MAV-2 virus is enterotropic and is responsible for virtually all naturally occurring infections in contemporary mouse populations. Infection is usually subclinical in immunocompetent mice, with the possible exception of transient runting among infant mice. Wasting disease can occur in athymic mice infected with MAV-1.

Epizootiology   The prevalence of adenovirus infection in mouse colonies is low, particularly MAV-1 (Livingston and Riley, 2003, Pritchett-Corning et al., 2009). Transmission occurs by ingestion. Adult mice experimentally infected with MAV-1 may remain persistently infected and excrete virus in the urine for prolonged periods. Adult mice experimentally infected with MAV-2 excrete virus in feces for at least 3 weeks but eventually recover. Athymic mice can shed MAV-2 for at least 6 weeks and episodically for at least 6 months.

Pathology   Infection with MAV-1 causes multisystemic disease characterized by necrosis. Infant mice are especially susceptible to rapidly fatal infection characterized by necrosis of brown fat, myocardium, adrenal cortex, salivary gland, and kidney, with the development of intranuclear inclusions. More mature mice usually develop subclinical infection leading to seroconversion; however, athymic and SCID mice can develop intestinal hemorrhage and wasting, with fatal disseminated infection (Lenaerts et al., 2005). Infection with MAV-2 produces amphophilic, intranuclear inclusions in intestinal epithelium, especially in the distal small intestine (Fig. 3.20). Inclusions are easier to detect in infant mice than in adults. Infection of C.B-17-*Prkdc*^scid mice with MAV-2 results in enteric infection, but also hepatic lesions resembling Reye's syndrome (Pirofski et al., 1991).

Diagnosis   Although MAV strains can be isolated in tissue culture, routine diagnosis depends on detection of infection by serological assay and/or demonstration of adenoviral inclusions, most commonly in the intestinal mucosa. Cross-neutralization tests have revealed that antiserum to MAV-2 neutralizes both strains, but antiserum to MAV-1 neutralizes MAV-2 weakly at best. Therefore, MAV-2 antigen should be used for the serological detection of adenovirus infection irrespective of the assay employed. MAV also can be detected by PCR.

Differential Diagnosis   Intranuclear adenoviral inclusions in intestinal epithelium are pathognomonic

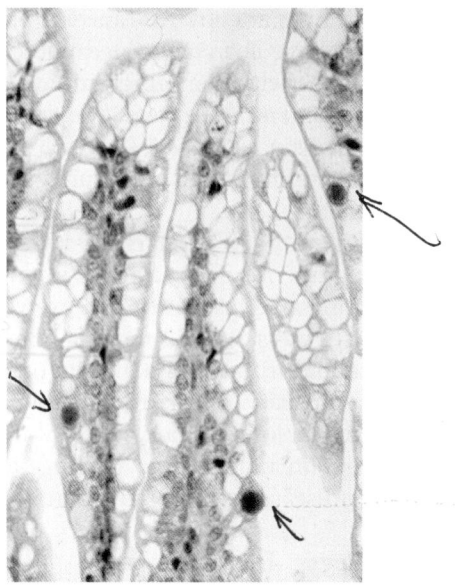

FIGURE 3.20 Intranuclear adenoviral inclusions in the small intestine of an infant mouse naturally infected with mouse adenovirus (MAV B). Enterocytes are also vacuolated, typical of the normal neonatal mouse bowel. *Percy and Barthold (2007).*

and differentiate MAV-2 infection from other known viral infections of mice. Infection may resemble rotavirus infection, with runting and abdominal bloating in infant mice.

Prevention and Control Prevention requires serological monitoring of mice and examination for contamination of animal products such as transplantable tumors. Because MAV-2 infection appears to be transient in individual mice, segregation of infected colonies may be effective for control. However, rederivation coupled with subsequent barrier housing is a more conservative approach.

Research Complications MAV infection is unlikely to affect research using immunocompetent mice. However, it has the potential for pathogenicity in immunodeficient mice.

e. Polyomavirus Infections (Benjamin, 2007)

Mice can incur natural infection with two polyomaviruses: polyoma virus (PyV) and K virus. These viruses belong to the family Polyomaviridae. K virus belongs to the genus *Polyomavirus* and the species *Murine pneumotropic virus*, while the classical polyoma virus belongs to the species *Murine polyomavirus*.

POLYOMA VIRUS

Etiology Polyoma virus (PyV) is a small DNA virus that derives its name 'polyoma' (many tumors) from its ability to experimentally induce multiple types of tumors in mice experimentally infected as neonates. Its

primary importance stems from use in murine models of experimental oncogenesis, with natural infection being rare. The transformative activity is mediated by 'T' (tumor) antigens, encoded by large T, middle T, and small T genes, with middle T (MT) being considered the major viral oncogene, and as a result has been used extensively in transgenic constructs.

Clinical Signs Natural infections in immunocompetent mice are usually subclinical. However, tumor induction, neurological disease, and wasting can occur in naturally exposed immunodeficient mice (McCance *et al.*, 1983; Sebesteny *et al.*, 1980).

Epizootiology Modern husbandry and health care have essentially eliminated natural exposure in laboratory mice. PyV is used for experimental studies and thus can inadvertently be introduced to mouse colonies. Inoculation of mice with contaminated biologicals or cell cultures is a potential source of entry and spread.

Natural transmission occurs via the respiratory route. Exposure of neonatal mice results in persistent infection and shedding of the virus in urine, feces, and saliva, thereby contaminating the environment for spread to other mice. Infection of adult mice is transient, with minimal virus shedding, although PCR has revealed infection lasting up to 5 months in CBA mice inoculated with virus as adults (Berke and Dalianis, 1993). Maternal antibody is highly effective at preventing infection of newborn mice, but as maternal antibody wanes, mice are partially susceptible, with transient virus shedding. Thus, the natural cycle of transmission in enzootically infected populations requires contamination of bedding and nesting material in order to infect and be inefficiently transmitted, which is readily precluded by modern husbandry. Intrauterine infection also can occur, and persistent renal infection, contracted neonatally, can be reactivated during pregnancy. As in immunologically immature neonatal mice, PyV infection can persist in adult immunodeficient mice.

Pathology PyV-induced tumors are essentially a laboratory phenomenon, optimized by virus strain and mouse strain, with AKR, C3H, C58, CBA, SWR, and others being most susceptible, and C57BL/6 being among the most resistant to PyV oncogenesis. Intranasal inoculation of neonatal mice results in initial replication in pulmonary respiratory epithelium (Gottlieb and Villarreal, 2000) followed by viremic dissemination and acute, lethal disease. Tumors appear 2–12 months after inoculation of surviving mice. Tumors of both epithelial and mesenchymal origin arise in multiple organs, particularly mammary carcinomas, basal cell tumors of the skin, carcinomas of salivary glands, thymomas, and various types of sarcomas. Athymic mice can develop cytolytic and inflammatory lesions, followed by multisystemic tumor formation. Intranuclear inclusions may be present in cytolytic lesions. Demyelinating disease and skeletal tumors have been reported in experimentally inoculated and naturally exposed athymic mice, and myeloproliferative disease has been reported in experimentally inoculated C57BL/6-*scid* mice (Szomolanyi-Tsuda *et al.*, 1994).

Diagnosis   PyV can be isolated in mouse fibroblast cell lines, but infection is ordinarily detected serologically. Additionally, PCR and immunohistochemistry can be used.

Differential Diagnosis   Wasting in athymic mice can be caused by other infectious agents, including coronaviruses, Sendai virus (SV), and *Pneumocystis.* Intranuclear inclusions can occur in infections caused by mouse adenovirus, mouse cytomegalovirus, and K virus.

Prevention and Control   Control depends on elimination of infected mice and material, together with prevention of airborne spread. Biological material destined for mouse inoculation should be tested for PyV by the MAP test or molecular diagnostics.

Research Complications   PyV infection can affect experiments by inadvertent contamination of cell lines or transplantable tumors, leading to infection of inoculated mice and the potential for epizootic spread.

K Virus Infection   K virus has historical importance, and is apparently absent from contemporary mouse populations (Livingston and Riley, 2003; Pritchett-Corning *et al.*, 2009), but it continues to be tested for, adding to the expense of infectious disease surveillance. Oral inoculation of neonatal mice results in initial infection of capillary endothelium in the intestine, followed by viremic spread. Vascular endothelium is the primary target in affected tissues, which often include the lung, liver, spleen, and adrenal glands. Dyspnea occurs from pulmonary infection because of edema and hemorrhage. Infection of immunocompetent adult mice is subclinical and results in a vigorous immune response. However, both adults and infant mice develop persistent infection. The primary organ for persistence is the kidney, with shedding of virus from tubular epithelium, and shedding can be reactivated by immunosuppression (Greenlee *et al.*, 1991). Additionally, infection of athymic mice can lead to clinical signs and lesions akin to those described for neonatally inoculated mice. Gross lesions are limited to pulmonary hemorrhage and edema. Histologically, intranuclear inclusions, which are visualized more easily using immunohistochemistry, are present in vascular endothelium of infected tissues. Mild hepatitis with hepatocyte degeneration also may develop. Infection can be detected by serology or PCR. Prevention and control measures, if ever to be found within a mouse population, are similar to those described for PyV.

f. Lactate Dehydrogenase–Elevating Virus Infection (Coutelier and Brinton, 2007)

Etiology   Lactate dehydrogenase–elevating virus (LDV) is a mouse-specific small enveloped RNA virus belonging to the family Arteriviridae. Infected mice are persistently viremic, resulting in increased concentration of several serum enzymes, most notably lactate dehydrogenase (LDH). Infection is common among wild mice, but is now rare in contemporary laboratory mouse populations. However, surveys of biologic material indicate that LDV may be a common contaminant of biologic materials (Nicklas *et al.*, 1993).

Clinical Signs   Infection is subclinical. However, poliomyelitis has occurred in immunosuppressed C58 and AKR mice inoculated with LDV, and has recently been observed in ICR-*scid* mice following inoculation with contaminated biologic material (Carlson-Scholz *et al.*, 2011).

Epizootiology   The primary mode of mouse-to-mouse transmission is mechanical transfer from aggressive behavior (e.g., bite wounds). Inoculation of mice with contaminated animal products such as cell lines, transplantable tumors, or serum is probably the most common source of induced infection. It is important to note, with respect to mechanical transmission, that infection induces lifelong viremia. Natural transmission between cagemates or between mother and young is rare even though infected mice may excrete virus in feces, urine, milk, and probably saliva.

Pathology   Viremia peaks within 1 day after inoculation, then persists at a diminished level. The elevation of enzyme levels in blood is thought to result primarily from viral interference with clearance functions of the reticuloendothelial system. LDV selectively targets mature F4/F8-positive macrophages, which are continually produced by uninfected progenitor cell populations, thereby maintaining persistent infection. Virus also escapes immune clearance by evolution of neutralizing antibody-resistant quasi-species. No lesions are seen in naturally infected mice. The only significant lesion that can arise from experimental infection is poliomyelitis. This syndrome requires a combination of immunosuppression (due to age, genetics or induced means), mouse strain (C58, AKR, C3H/Fg, and PL), neurotropic LDV strains, and endogenous ecotropic murine leukemia virus. The mouse strain-dependent element is homozygosity for the $Fv\text{-}1^n$ allele, which permits replication of endogenous N-tropic ectotropic murine leukemia virus. Mice develop spongiosis, neuronal necrosis, and astrocytosis of the ventral spinal cord and brain stem, with axonal degeneration of ventral roots. Lesions contain both LDV and retrovirus. Although this syndrome is largely experimentally induced, a natural outbreak of poliomyelitis has been reported in *Fv-1* homozygous ICR-*scid* mice following inoculation with contaminated biologic material (Carlson-Scholz *et al.*, 2011).

Diagnosis   Plasma LDH levels are elevated, a response that is used to detect and titrate LDV infectivity. Of the five isoenzymes of LDH in mouse plasma, only

LDH-V is elevated. SJL/J mice in particular show spectacular increases in LDH levels (15–20 times normal), a response controlled by a recessive somatic gene. LDV is detected by measuring LDH levels in mouse plasma before and 4 days after inoculation of specific pathogen-free (SPF) mice with suspect material. It is important to use nonhemolyzed samples because hemolysis will produce falsely elevated readings. Plasma enzyme levels are measured in conventional units/ml, 1 conventional unit being equivalent to 0.5 International Units (IU). Normal plasma levels are 400–800 IU, whereas in LDV infection, levels as high as 7000 IU can occur. LDV also interferes with the clearance of other serum enzymes and results in their elevation in serum. In a recent survey, 6000 serum samples were tested by serum LDH enzyme assays, among which 10% were deemed potentially positive. However, PCR revealed that all were false-positives (Pritchett-Corning *et al.*, 2009), emphasizing the inaccuracy of traditional enzyme assays.

Infection provokes a modest humoral antibody response, but it is difficult to detect because of formation of virus–antibody immune complexes. Molecular diagnostics also can be used to diagnose infection in mouse tissues and serum and biologic materials. However, inhibitory factors in cells and serum may cause false-negative results in PCR testing, so appropriate quality control measures are essential if this method is used (Lipman and Henderson, 2000).

Prevention and Control Transplantable tumors have been a common source of LDV historically. Therefore, tumors or cell lines destined for mouse inoculation should be monitored for LDV contamination. Although LDV can contaminate tumor cell lines, it does not replicate in the tumor cells. Therefore, one can attempt to free tumors of virus by passaging them through athymic nude rats, which are not nonpermissive to LDV but are permissive to xenografts.

Research Complications LDV has numerous potential effects on immunological function. It may reduce autoantibody production, cause transient thymic necrosis and lymphopenia, suppress cell-mediated immune responses, and enhance or suppress tumor growth.

g. Lymphocytic Choriomeningitis Virus Infection (Barthold and Smith, 2007)

Etiology The house mouse is the natural host for lymphocytic choriomeningitis virus (LCMV), an Old World member of the Arenaviridae family that has spread worldwide along with *M. musculus*. LCMV virions are pleomorphic, containing single-stranded RNA, and bud from the cell membrane. Disease associated with infection is due to host immune response to the otherwise non-cytolytic virus. Its name is derived from the immune-mediated inflammation resulting from the intracerebral inoculation of virus into immunologically

competent mice. LCMV is a zoonotic virus that may cause a variety of clinical manifestations in humans, including meningitis. It has been extensively studied as an experimental model of virus-induced immune injury, using a number of closely related strains, including ones that have been selected for their relative neurotropism or viscerotropism. LCMV can be propagated in a variety of mammalian, avian, and even tick cell lines, with minimal cytopathic effect. These characteristics favor its propensity to persistently and silently contaminate biologic products, such as tumor cell lines.

Clinical Signs Natural infection in immunocompetent adult mice is usually self-limiting and subclinical. During enzootic infection of a mouse population, LCMV is transmitted *in utero* from persistently infected dams to their fetuses or to neonates, which are persistently infected and immunologically tolerant to LCMV. Since LCMV is non-cytolytic in and of itself is minimally pathogenic, congenitally infected mice grow into adulthood, reproduce, and therefore transmit infection to the next generation. However, with age, immune tolerance breaks down, and mice develop a syndrome known as 'late disease' in which mice will progressively lose weight and die. *In utero* infection results in a low level of fetal mortality and maternal cannibalism of infected pups. The immune tolerance to LCMV is virus-specific, with the mice capable of eliciting effective immune responses against other agents.

Clinical signs following experimental inoculation of LCMV vary with age and strain of mouse, route of inoculation, and strain of virus. When virus is inoculated intracerebrally into immunocompetent adult mice, mice develop immune-mediated lymphocytic choriomeningitis, characterized by illness beginning 5–6 days after inoculation. Sudden death may result or subacute illness associated with one or more of the following signs may develop: ruffled fur, hunched posture, motionlessness, and neurological deficits. Mice suspended by the tail display coarse tremors of the head and extremities, culminating in clonic convulsions and tonic extension of the rear legs. Spontaneous convulsions also can occur. Animals usually die or recover in several days. A visceral form of infection can occur in adult mice inoculated by peripheral routes with 'viscerotropic' strains. It can be subclinical or lead to clinical signs, including ruffled fur, conjunctivitis, ascites, somnolence, and death. If mice survive, recovery may take several weeks. Surviving mice may have immune exhaustion due to consumption of lymphoid tissue, in contrast to immune tolerance that occurs when mice are infected *in utero* or as neonates. Runting and death from LCMV infection may occur in neonatally infected mice and can lead to transient illness or to death. Clinical signs are nonspecific, recovery is slow, and survivors may remain runted. This early form of disease is attributed to endocrine dysfunction caused

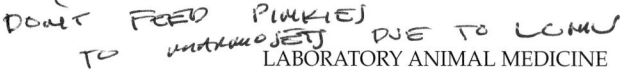

amplifier

by LCMV infection. Late-onset disease can occur in previously subclinical carrier mice that develop immune complex glomerulonephritis. It is usually the result of prenatal or neonatal infection and occurs in persistently infected mice when they are 9–12 months old. Clinical signs are nonspecific and include ruffled fur, hunched posture, weight loss, proteinuria, and ascites.

Epizootiology LCMV is distributed widely in wild *M. musculus* throughout the world. Among common laboratory species, mice, hamsters, guinea pigs, and nonhuman primates are susceptible to infection, but only the mouse and the hamster are known to transmit virus. LCMV infection is rare in laboratory mice produced and maintained in modern quarters (Livingston and Riley, 2003; Pritchett-Corning *et al.*, 2009). Infection is usually introduced through inoculation of virus-infected biologicals, such as transplantable tumors, or by feral mice. Wild mice are a natural reservoir of infection and a potential threat to research colonies if they gain entry inadvertently. Naturally infected carrier mice can have persistently high concentrations of virus in many organs, thereby facilitating virus excretion in saliva, nasal secretions, and urine. Persistently infected neonates usually reach breeding age and can perpetuate infection in a breeding colony. Thus introduction of a single LCMV carrier mouse to a breeding colony can eventually result in a high prevalence of persistently infected mice. Infection in adult mice, in contrast, is often acute because of the onset of effective immunity, and the spread of virus is halted. Horizontal spread of infection is enhanced by close contact, but rapid horizontal spread is not characteristic. Mice can transmit LCMV to hamsters, which can remain viremic and viruric for many months, even if they contract infection as adults. Infected hamsters can transmit virus to other hamsters and mice and are the primary source of human LCMV infection. Persistent infection in immunodeficient mice may carry greater risks for viral excretion and zoonotic transmission.

Pathology LCMV disease is a prototype for virus-induced, T-lymphocyte-mediated immune injury, noncytolytic endocrine dysfunction, and immune complex disease. However, lesions comparable to experimentally induced disease are rare during natural infection. Intracerebral inoculation of virus into immunocompetent adult mice induces nonsuppurative leptomeningitis, choroiditis, and focal perivascular lymphocytic infiltrates. Host tissues are damaged during the course of the cellular immune response to the virus. The character of visceral lesions depends on virus strain and mouse strain; the ratio of cytolytic to proliferative responses in lymphoid organs is mouse strain-dependent. In severe infection, nonsuppurative inflammation can occur in many tissues. The severity of accompanying cytolytic lesions seems to parallel the intensity of cellular immunity. Liver lesions can include hepatocyte necrosis accompanied by nodular infiltrates of lymphoid cells and Kupffer cells, activated sinusoidal endothelium, an occasional granulocyte or megakaryocyte, and fatty metamorphosis. Cytolysis, cell proliferation, and fibrinoid necrosis can develop in lymphoid organs. Necrosis of cortical thymocytes can lead to thymic involution. Lesions of late-onset disease are characterized by formation of immune complexes and associated inflammation. Renal glomeruli and the choroid plexus are most severely affected, but complexes may also be trapped in synovial membranes, blood vessel walls, and skin. Lymphoid nodules can form in various organs. Lesions associated with early deaths in neonatally infected mice have not been thoroughly described but include hepatic necrosis.

The lesions of acute and persistent LCMV infection reflect separate immunopathologic processes. In adult mice with acute LCMV infection, virus multiplies in DCs, B cells, and macrophages, whereas T cells are resistant. Internal viral epitopes induce humoral immune responses, but surface epitopes elicit cell-mediated immunity and neutralizing antibodies. Thus, elimination of virus and virus-associated immunological injury are both T-cell-mediated. This apparent paradox has been explained by the view that prompt cellular immunity limits viral replication and leads to host survival, whereas slower cellular immune responses permit viral spread and increase the number of virus-infected target cells subject to attack once immunity is fully developed. Antibody can be detected by 1 week after infection but does not play a significant role in eliciting acute disease. Lesions of LCMV infection appear to develop from direct T-cell-mediated damage to virus-infected cells and may involve humoral factors released from immune effector T cells. LCMV also can suppress humoral and cellular immunity in acutely infected mice.

Persistent infection commonly evolves from exposure early in pregnancy, and virus has been demonstrated in the ovaries of carrier mice. Prenatal or neonatal infection induces immunological tolerance to LCMV, which can then replicate to high titer in many tissues. Nevertheless, persistently infected mice develop humoral antibody to LCMV. Antibody can complex with persistent virus to elicit complement-dependent inflammation in small vessels. Immune complex glomerulonephritis exemplifies this process, as noted above.

Diagnosis LCMV infection can be diagnosed serologically. Whereas immunocompetent adult mice will normally seroconvert after exposure, carrier mice may develop poor humoral immune responses. Therefore, testing must avoid false-negative results. Employment of adult contact sentinel mice is a useful strategy for detecting LCMV infection by seroconversion. Tissues, including biologic products and cell lines, can be tested by PCR. A traditional method for detection involved collection of small blood samples from persistently infected live suspects, which are often viremic, and using them to inoculate cultured cells or adult and neonatal mice. Intracerebral inoculation of LCMV-positive tissues should elicit neurological signs in adult mice within 10 days, whereas infant mice should remain subclinical. Histological examination of brains from affected adults may reveal nonsuppurative inflammation, but lesions may be minimal in mice infected with viscerotropic isolates. Immunohistochemistry can be used to detect viral antigen in brains of suckling and adult mice. Intraperitoneal inoculation of adult mice may yield short-lived infection with seroconversion, i.e., the MAP test. Virus can be grown and quantified in several continuous cell lines, including mouse neuroblastoma (N-18) cells, BHK-21 cells, and L cells. Application of immunofluorescence staining to detect LCMV antigen in inoculated cultured cells yields results more quickly than animal inoculation. Of course, all diagnostic procedures involving potential contact with live virus should be carried out under strict containment conditions to avoid infection of laboratory personnel (see Chapter 29). The use of *in vitro* detection has the added advantage, in this regard, of reducing biohazardous exposure and the use of live animals for testing.

Differential Diagnosis Neurological signs must be differentiated from those due to mouse hepatitis virus, mouse encephalomyelitis virus, and meningoencephalitis from bacterial infection. Trauma, neoplasia, and toxicities also must be ruled out in neurological disease with low prevalence. Late-onset disease is associated with characteristic renal lesions, including deposition of viral antigen in tissues. Early-onset disease must be differentiated from other causes of early mortality, such as mouse hepatitis virus, ectromelia virus, reovirus 3 infection, Tyzzer's disease, or husbandry-related insults.

Prevention and Control Adequate safeguards for procurement and testing of animals and animal products are essential to prevent entry. Because mouse-to-mouse spread is slow, selective testing and culling for seropositive or carrier mice is possible. If mice are easily replaced, however, depopulation is a safer and more reliable option. Valuable stock can be rederived, but progeny must be tested to preclude *in utero* transmission. Because infected hamsters can excrete large quantities of virus, exposed hamsters should be destroyed and hamsters should not be housed with mice. Infection of immunodeficient mice poses similar risk. LCMV can be transmitted to human beings, who can contract flu-like illness or severe CNS disease. More frequently, human infection is subclinical. The zoonotic potential of LCMV infection makes it especially important to detect and eliminate carrier animals and other potentially contaminated sources, such as cell cultures, transplantable

neoplasms, and vaccines to prevent human exposure. Serum banking and periodic serological testing of high-risk human populations, such as those working with LCMV experimentally, are recommended.

Research Complications LCMV may stimulate or suppress immunological responses *in vivo* and *in vitro*, and it can replicate in cells used as targets or effectors for immunological studies. Introduction of immune cells to a carrier animal may elicit an immunopathological response. Immune complex disease can complicate long-term experiments and morphological interpretations. Illness and death in mice and zoonotic risk to humans are obvious research-related hazards.

h. SV Infection (Brownstein, 2007)

Etiology SV is a paramyxovirus that is antigenically related to human parainfluenza virus 1. Viral particles are pleomorphic, contain single-stranded RNA, and have a lipid solvent-sensitive envelope that contains glycoproteins with hemagglutinating, neuraminidase, and cell fusion properties. SV grows well on embryonated hens' eggs and in several mammalian cell lines (e.g., monkey kidney, baby hamster kidney [BHK-21], and mouse fibroblast [L]). Virus replicates in the cytoplasm and by budding through cell outer membranes. Once common in laboratory rodent populations, SV is now rare or absent (Livingston and Riley, 2003; Pritchett-Corning *et al.*, 2009).

Clinical Signs Clinically affected adult mice often assume a hunched position and have an erect hair coat. Rapid weight loss and dyspnea occur, and there may be chattering sounds and crusting of the eyes. Although highly susceptible adults may die, lethal infection is more common in suckling mice. Sex differences in susceptibility have not been found. Genetically resistant mice usually have subclinical infection. Athymic mice and immunodeficient mice are at high risk for development of a wasting syndrome. They develop illness later than their immunocompetent counterparts, since clinical signs in immunocompetent mice are related to immune-mediated destruction of respiratory epithelium. Opportunistic infections can complicate the clinical presentation. For example, secondary bacterial infections of the ear can cause vestibular signs.

Epizootiology SV is transmitted by aerosol and is highly contagious. Morbidity in infected colonies is commonly 100%, and mortality can vary from 0% to 100%, partly because strains of mice vary greatly in their susceptibility to lethal SV infection. For example, C57BL/6 mice are highly resistant to clinically apparent infection, whereas DBA/2 mice are highly susceptible. Aerogenic infection is promoted by high relative humidity and by low air turnover. Prenatal infection does not occur. Enzootic infection is commonly detected in postweaned mice (5–7 weeks old) and is associated with seroconversion within 7–14 days and the termination of infection. Therefore, entrenched infection is perpetuated by the introduction of susceptible animals. There is no evidence for persistent infection in immunocompetent mice, but prolonged infection is common in immunodeficient mice. Maternally acquired immunity protects young mice from infection, and actively acquired immunity is thought to be long-lived. Rats, hamsters, and guinea pigs also are susceptible to SV infection. Therefore, bidirectional cross-infection is a risk during outbreaks.

Pathology Viral replication is nominally restricted to the respiratory tract and peaks by the first week after infection. Gross lesions feature partial to complete consolidation of the lungs (Fig. 3.21). Individual lobes are meaty and plum-colored, and the cut surface may exude a frothy serosanguinous fluid. Pleural adhesions or lung abscesses caused by secondary bacterial infection are seen occasionally, and fluid may accumulate in the pleural and pericardial cavities.

SV targets airway epithelium and type II pneumocytes. Type I pneumocytes are less severely affected. Histologically, the pattern of pneumonia is influenced by mouse genotype. Susceptible mice usually have significant bronchopneumonia and interstitial pneumonia, whereas the interstitial component may be less prominent in resistant mice. Typical changes begin with inflammatory edema of bronchiolar lamina propria, which may extend to alveolar ducts, alveoli, and perivascular spaces. Necrosis and exfoliation of bronchiolar epithelium ensue, frequently in a segmental pattern (Fig. 3.22). Alveolar epithelium also may desquamate, especially in severe disease, and necrotic cell debris and inflammatory cells can accumulate in airways and alveolar spaces. Alveolar septae are usually infiltrated by leukocytes to produce interstitial pneumonia (Fig. 3.23). Lymphoid cells also invade peribronchiolar and perivascular spaces. The lymphocytic response to SV infection reflects the fact that cellular immunity contributes both to lesions and to recovery. Local immunoglobulin synthesis by infiltrating cells also occurs. The extent of inflammatory cell infiltration corresponds to the level of genetic resistance expressed by the infected host, with clinically susceptible hosts mounting a more florid immune response than resistant hosts. Additionally, strain-related differences in the severity of infection may reflect differences in airway mucociliary transport. Multinucleated syncytia are occasionally seen in affected sucklings and SCID mice, and inclusion bodies have been reported in infected athymic mice.

Regeneration and repair begin shortly after the lytic phase and are characterized by hyperplasia and squamous metaplasia of bronchial epithelium, which may extend into alveolar septae. Proliferation of cuboidal

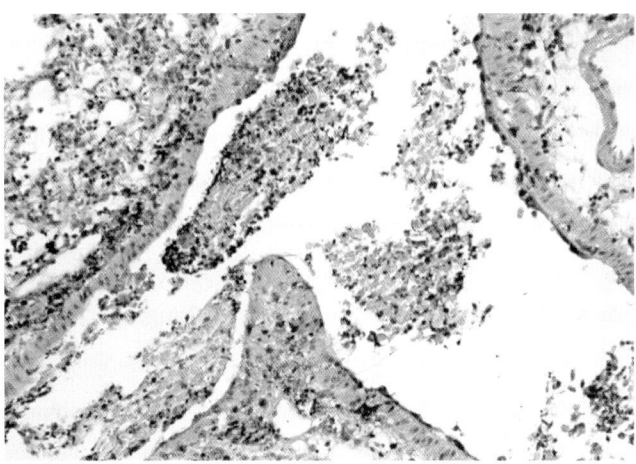

FIGURE 3.22   Necrotizing bronchiolitis in a DBA mouse infected with SV. *Courtesy of S.W. Barthold.*

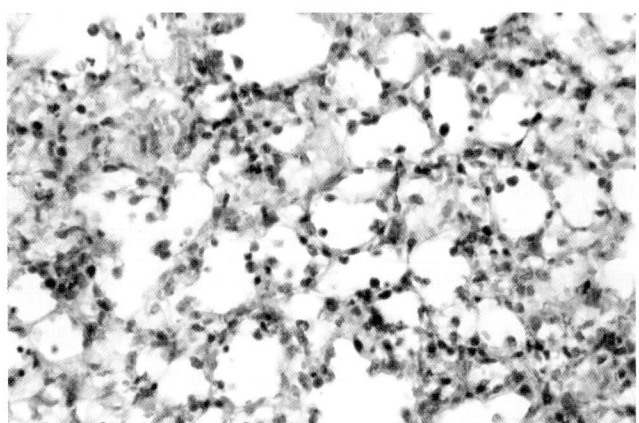

FIGURE 3.23   Interstitial pneumonia in a DBA mouse infected with SV. *Courtesy of S.W. Barthold.*

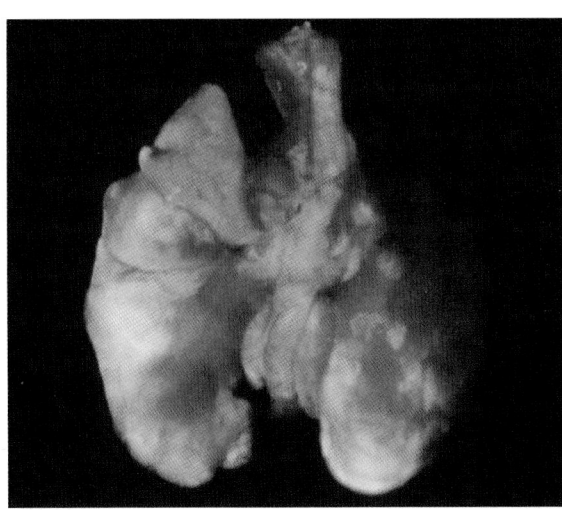

FIGURE 3.21   Lungs from a DBA mouse infected with SV. Note consolidation of lung tissue at the hilus. *Percy and Barthold (2007).*

MEATY   PLUM   COLORED   LUNGS

epithelium may give terminal bronchioles an adenoma-toid appearance. Repair of damaged lungs is relatively complete in surviving mice, but lymphocytic infiltrates, foci of atypical epithelium, and mild scarring can persist. Acute phase lesions are prolonged in immunodeficient mice, which can lead to wasting and death. Aged mice also have a prolonged recovery phase accompanied by focal pulmonary fibrosis (Jacoby et al., 1994).

Diagnosis   SV is notable for its ability to cause epi-zootics of acute respiratory distress in adult genetically susceptible strains. Serology is an effective means to detect infection in all strains of immunocompetent mice. Antibody can be detected by 7 days postinfection and coincides with development of clinical signs related to the immune-mediated necrotizing bronchiolitis and alveoli-tis. Repeated serologic sampling over several weeks can help stage infection within a population. Alternatively, sentinel animals can be added to seropositive colonies to detect active infection. Irrespective of serologic results, histopathology, immunohistochemistry (which can be performed on formalin-fixed, paraffin-embedded sec-tions), and, where possible, virus isolation should be used to confirm infection. Virus can be isolated from the respiratory tract for up to 2 weeks, with peak titers occurring at about 9 days postinfection. Nasopharyngeal washings or lung tissue homogenates are most reliable and should be inoculated into embryonated hens' eggs or BHK-21 cell monolayer cultures. SV infection of cul-tured cells is non-cytolytic, so erythrocyte agglutination or antigen detection methods must be used. RT-PCR also can be used to detect virus in infected lungs.

Differential Diagnosis   Respiratory infection caused by pneumonia virus of mice (PVM) is generally milder or subclinical. Histologically, necrosis of airway epithelium is less severe. Bacterial pneumonias of mice, including murine respiratory mycoplasmosis, are spo-radic and can be differentiated morphologically and by isolation of causative organisms. Because SV pneumonia may predispose the lung to opportunistic bacterial infec-tions, the presence of bacteria should not deter evalua-tion for a primary viral insult.

Control and Prevention   SV infection is self-lim-iting in surviving immunocompetent mice. Suckling mice from immune dams are protected from infection by maternal antibody until after weaning. Control and eradication measures must eliminate exposure of sus-ceptible animals, so that infection can 'burn out.' This is most easily accomplished by a quarantine period of 4–6 weeks wherein no new animals are introduced either as adults or through breeding. Control also is aided by the fact that SV is highly labile. Barrier housing is preferred for prevention and for control of transmis-sion. Vaccination with formalin-killed virus can provide short-term protection of valuable mice but is not com-monly used for prevention.

Research Complications   SV can cause immuno-suppression and can inhibit growth of transplantable tumors. This effect has been attributed to virus-induced modification of tumor cell surface membranes. Pulmonary changes during SV pneumonia can compro-mise interpretation of experimentally induced lesions and may lead to opportunistic infections by other bac-teria. They also have been associated with breeding dif-ficulties in mice. This sign is thought to be an indirect effect due to stress, fever, or related changes during acute infection.

i. Murine Pneumonia Virus Infection (Brownstein, 2007; Dyer *et al.*, 2012)

Etiology   Murine pneumonia virus (PVM) is an enveloped RNA virus in the genus *Pneumovirus* and spe-cies *Murine pneumonia virus* of the Paramyxoviridae fam-ily. All isolates appear to have similar physicochemical, biological, and antigenic properties, but virulent strains have been selectively developed for experimental use. The virus agglutinates erythrocytes of several rodent species, including mice. It replicates well *in vitro* in BHK-21 cells but, as with SV, is non-cytolytic in cultured cells.

Clinical Signs   Natural PVM infection in mice is subclinical. Therefore, its name is clinically misleading, being derived from pneumonic illness that occurred after serial passage of the agent in mice. However, dysp-nea, listlessness, and wasting may develop in immu-nodeficient mice infected with PVM (Weir *et al.*, 1988). PVM is used experimentally as a model to study acute respiratory infection, using highly pathogenic strains of the virus (Dyer *et al.*, 2012).

Epizootiology   PVM causes natural infections of mice, rats, hamsters, and probably other rodents and may be infectious for rabbits. Serological data indicate that PVM was once common, but is now relatively uncommon (Livingston and Riley, 2003; Pritchett-Corning *et al.*, 2009). PVM appears to spread less rap-idly than SV. Intimate contact between mice is probably required for effective transmission. This characteristic may reflect the fact that environmental inactivation of virus occurs rapidly. Infection is acute and self-limiting in immunocompetent mice but may persist in immuno-deficient mice.

Pathology   PVM replicates exclusively in the res-piratory tract and reaches peak titers in the lung 6–8 days after infection. Although pulmonary consolidation can occur in experimentally infected mice, gross lesions are rare during natural infection. Histological lesions can occur in the upper and lower respiratory tract. They con-sist of mild necrotizing rhinitis, necrotizing bronchiolitis, and interstitial pneumonia, which usually occur within 2 weeks after exposure to virus and are largely resolved by 3 weeks. The predominant inflammatory infiltrate is comprised of mononuclear cells, but some neutrophils

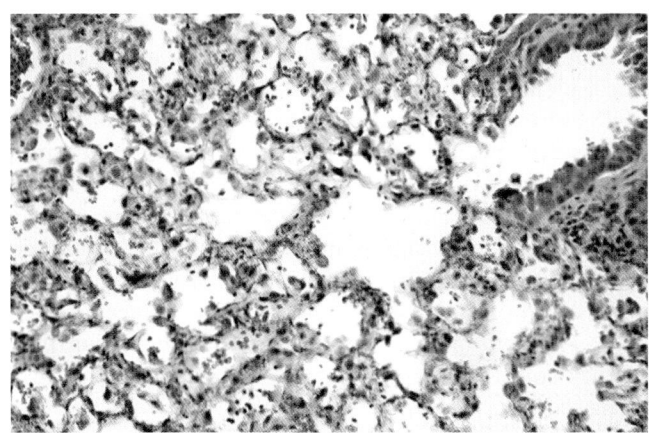

FIGURE 3.24 Severe interstitial pneumonia in an athymic mouse chronically infected with pneumonia virus of mice (MPnV). *Courtesy of S.W. Barthold.*

are usually present. Immunohistochemistry on paraffin-embedded tissues can be used to detect viral antigen in bronchiolar epithelium, alveolar macrophages, and alveolar epithelium during acute infection. Residual lesions include nonsuppurative perivasculitis, which can persist for several weeks after acute infection has ceased. Severe progressive pneumonia, with wasting, can occur in immunodeficient mice. It is characterized by generalized pulmonary consolidation that reflects severe interstitial pneumonia with desquamated alveolar pneumocytes and leukocytes filling alveolar spaces (Fig. 3.24).

Diagnosis Diagnosis is based primarily on serological detection that can be supplemented by histopathology, immunohistochemistry, *in situ* hybridization, and virus isolation. Virus replication in BHK-21 cells is detected by immunofluorescence or other antigen detection methods. Virus also can be detected in tissues by RT-PCR.

Differential Diagnosis Because PVM is antigenically distinct from other murine viruses, serology is the most useful method to separate PVM infection from other respiratory infections of mice. However, in immunodeficient mice, where clinical signs and lesions are typical, it must be differentiated from other pneumonias, especially those due to SV and *Pneumocystis*. Additionally, PVM can coexist with and exacerbate *Pneumocystis* infection in immunodeficient mice (Bray *et al.*, 1993).

Prevention and Control PVM infection is acute and self-limiting in immunocompetent mice, but persistent in immunodeficient mice. Seropositive mice should be viewed as either immune or in the final stages of acute infection. Therefore, control and prevention follows guidelines applicable to SV infection.

Research Complications PVM can exacerbate pneumocystosis, as noted above.

j. Reovirus Infections (Ward *et al.*, 2007) NON-EHV ✓

Two members of the family Reoviridae infect laboratory mice: reovirus *per se* (species: *Mammalian orthoreovirus*) and murine rotavirus (species: *Rotavirus A*), also known as epizootic diarrhea of infant mice (EDIM) virus.

MAMMALIAN ORTHOREOVIRUS (REOVIRUS 1, 2, AND 3)

Etiology Reoviruses of mammals, although taxonomically considered one type species, have been divided into three cross-reacting prototypic serotypes: reovirus 1, 2 and 3, which can be differentiated by cross-serum neutralization. Mice can be infected with any serotype, but reovirus 3 is emphasized because it has been associated with naturally occurring disease. Natural infections in mice are usually not caused by pure serotypes, because reoviruses actively recombine. A number of wild-type and laboratory strains have been characterized, and related viruses have been recovered from virtually every mammal tested, as well as birds, reptiles, and insects. The virion contains segmented, double-stranded RNA and is relatively heat stable. Reoviruses replicate well in BHK-21 cells and other continuous cell lines, as well as in primary monolayer cultures from several mammals.

Clinical Signs Clinical disease is rare and age dependent. Acute disease affects sucklings at about 2 weeks of age, whereas adults have subclinical infection. Signs in sucklings include emaciation, abdominal distension, and oily, matted hair due to steatorrhea. Icterus may develop and is most easily discerned as discoloration in the feet, tail, and nose. Incoordination, tremors, and paralysis occur just before death. Convalescent mice are often partially alopecic and are typically runted. Alopecia, runting, and icterus may persist for several weeks, even though infectious virus can no longer be recovered. Infants born to immune dams are protected from disease by maternal immunity.

Epizootiology The prevalence of reovirus 3 infection in contemporary mouse colonies is rare (Livingston and Riley, 2003; Pritchett-Corning *et al.*, 2009). Reoviruses are highly contagious among infant mice and can be transmitted by the oral–fecal or aerosol routes, but mechanical transmission by arthropods has also been documented. Additionally, virus may be carried by transplantable neoplasms and transmitted inadvertently by injection. Transmission is inefficient among adult mice. There is no evidence that vertical transmission is important or that genetic resistance or gender influence expression of disease. Infection in immunocompetent mice appears to be self-limiting, lasting up to several weeks but terminating with the development of host immunity. The course of infection in immunodeficient mice should be considered prolonged, but the duration has not been determined.

Pathology Reovirus 3 can cause severe pantropic infection in infant mice. After parenteral inoculation, virus can be recovered from the liver, brain, heart, pancreas, spleen, lymph nodes, and blood vessels. Following ingestion, reoviruses gain entry by infecting intestinal epithelial cells (M cells) that cover Peyer's patches. Virus can be carried to the liver in leukocytes, where it is taken up by Kupffer cells prior to infecting hepatocytes.

In acute disease, livers may be large and dark, with yellow foci of necrosis. The intestine may be red and distended, and, in infants, intestinal contents may be bright yellow. Myocardial necrosis and pulmonary hemorrhages have been reported. Myocardial edema and necrosis are especially prominent in papillary muscles of the left ventricle. The brain may be swollen and congested. Central nervous system lesions have a vascular distribution, and are most prevalent in the brain stem and cerebral hemispheres. Neuronal degeneration and necrosis are followed quickly by meningoencephalitis and satellitosis. Severe encephalitis may evoke focal hemorrhage. In the chronic phase, wasting, alopecia, icterus, and hepatosplenomegaly may persist. Orally infected suckling mice can develop multifocal hepatocyte necrosis, which may include the accumulation of dense eosinophilic structures resembling Councilman bodies. Hepatocytomegaly, Kupffer cell hyperplasia, and intrasinusoidal infiltrates of mononuclear cells and neutrophilic leukocytes also can develop. In experimentally inoculated mice, necrotic foci can persist in the liver for at least 4 weeks. Chronic active hepatitis may develop after acute infection and result in biliary obstruction. Acinar cells of the pancreas and salivary glands can undergo degeneration and necrosis. Because pancreatic duct epithelium is susceptible to infection, parenchymal lesions in the pancreas may be caused by obstruction rather than by viral invasion of parenchyma. Pulmonary hemorrhage and degeneration of skeletal muscles also have been observed. Both humoral and cellular immunity seem to participate in host defenses, but it is unclear how host immunity may influence the course of chronic infection.

Oronasal inoculation of infant mice with reovirus 1 results in a similar distribution but significantly milder lesions compared to reovirus 3. In contrast, reovirus 2 is highly enterotropic, inducing mild enteritis without lesions in other tissues, similar to Epizootic Diarrhea of Infant Mice (EDIM) (Barthold *et al.*, 1993).

Diagnosis Serology uses reovirus 3 as antigen, which detects seroconversion to all serotypes, and viral RNA can be detected by RT-PCR. A presumptive diagnosis of reovirus infection is aided clinically by detection of the oily hair effect, accompanied by jaundice and wasting. The presence histologically of multisystemic necrosis is consistent with severe reovirus 3 infection but should be confirmed by immunohistochemistry or virus isolation.

Differential Diagnosis Reovirus infection must be differentiated from other diarrheal diseases of infant mice, including those caused by mouse coronaviruses, EDIM virus, *Salmonella* spp., or *Clostridium piliforme*.

Prevention and Control Although surviving mice appear to recover completely from infection, the potential for a carrier state is unresolved. Therefore, it may be necessary, after adequate testing for the continued presence of virus by the use of sentinels, MAP testing, or other appropriate means, to rederive or replace infected stock. Prevention depends on adequate barrier husbandry coupled with adequate serological monitoring.

Research Complications Reovirus 3 infection can interfere with research in several ways. Infections in breeding colonies can result in high mortality among sucklings from nonimmune dams. Virus has been commonly recovered from transplantable neoplasms and is suspected of being oncolytic. The potential exists for interference with hepatic, pancreatic, cardiovascular, or neurological research.

ROTAVIRUS (Barthold, 1997a; Ward et al., 2007)

Etiology Rotaviruses are double-stranded, segmented RNA viruses that have a wheel-like ultrastructural appearance. EDIM virus is a group A rotavirus that replicates in differentiated epithelial cells of the small intestine by budding into cisternae of endoplasmic reticulum. Currently, only a single antigenic strain is recognized, but antigenically distinct variants may exist. EDIM virus shares an inner capsid antigen with rotaviruses of rabbits, fowl, nonhuman primates, human beings, and domestic and companion animals. These agents tend to be species-specific under natural conditions and can be differentiated by serum neutralization tests. Cultivation of EDIM virus requires the presence of proteolytic enzymes to cleave an outer capsid polypeptide.

Clinical Signs Clinical signs occur in infant mice less than 2 weeks old. This age-related susceptibility also applies to infection in immunodeficient mice. Furthermore, clinical signs occur only in offspring of nonimmune dams, because maternal immunity protects infants until they have outgrown susceptibility to clinical disease. The cardinal signs are bloated abdomens with fecal soiling of the perineum, which may extend to the entire pelage in severe cases. Despite high morbidity, mortality is low because affected mice continue to nurse. Transient weight loss does occur, and there may be a delay in reaching adult weight. Recovery from infection usually occurs in about 2 weeks and, once weight is regained, is clinically complete.

Epizootiology EDIM virus appears to be infectious only for mice and occurs episodically in mouse colonies, and infection is probably widespread geographically (Livingston and Riley, 2003; Pritchett-Corning *et al.*, 2009). All ages and both sexes can be infected, but genetic resistance and susceptibility have not been determined. The virus is highly contagious and is transmitted by the oral–fecal route. Subclinically infected adult mice can shed virus in feces for at least 17 days, an interval that may be extended in immunodeficient mice. After oral inoculation, virus is essentially restricted to the gastrointestinal tract, although small amounts of virus may be present in the liver, spleen, kidney, and blood. Nursing dams can contract infection from their litters. Transplacental transmission has not been demonstrated.

Pathology   Gross lesions occur primarily in the gastrointestinal tract, but thymic involution can result from infection-related stress. The intestine is often distended, flaccid, and filled with gray–green gaseous liquid or mucoid fecal material that soils the pelage. The stomach contains curdled milk, except in terminal cases with anal impaction due to caking of dried feces. Virus preferentially infects terminally differentiated enterocytes in the small and large intestines, which accounts for the age-related susceptibility to disease; the number of such cells decreases as the intestinal tract matures. Characteristic histological lesions are often very subtle, but are most easily discerned in the small intestine in mice less than 2 weeks old. They consist of vacuolation of villar epithelial cells with cytoplasmic swelling, which give villi a clubbed appearance (Fig. 3.25). The vacuoles must be differentiated from normal absorption vacuoles in nursing mice. The lamina propria may be edematous, but necrosis and inflammation are not prevalent.

Diagnosis   EDIM virus infection is readily detected serologically. Clinical disease is diagnosed from signs and typical histological lesions in the intestine, which can be confirmed by immunohistochemical or ultrastructural demonstration of virus in the intestine or in intestinal filtrates or smears. Rotavirus antigen can be detected in feces by ELISA, but certain dietary ingredients can cause false-positive reactions. Infection can also be diagnosed by RT-PCR.

Differential Diagnosis   EDIM virus infection must be differentiated from other diarrheal diseases of suckling mice such as intestinal coronavirus (mouse hepatitis virus) infection, reovirus 3 infection, Tyzzer's disease, and salmonellosis. The presence of milk in the stomach can be helpful in differentiating EDIM virus infection from more severe enteric infections, such as those caused by pathogenic coronaviruses, during which cessation of nursing often occurs. The possibility of dual infections must also be considered. Thymic necrosis in EDIM virus-infected mice, although nonspecific, must be differentiated from that due to mouse thymic virus (MTV) infection or other stressors.

Prevention and Control   The spread of EDIM can be controlled effectively by the use of microbarrier cages and good sanitation. Because infection appears to be acute and self-limiting, cessation of breeding for 4–6 weeks to allow immunity to build in adults while preventing access to susceptible neonates also is recommended. Alternatively, litters with diarrhea can be culled, in combination with the use of microbarrier cages. The duration of infection in immunodeficient mice has not been determined, but it is reasonable to assume that chronic infection occurs. Therefore, such animals should be eliminated. Litters from immune dams are more resistant to infection. If EDIM virus is allowed to become enzootic within a colony, clinical signs will disappear within the population, which may be an appropriate management approach in conventional colonies. Prevention of EDIM virus infection depends on maintenance of sanitary barrier housing with adequate serological surveillance.

Research Complications   The research complications of EDIM infection pertain to clinical illness with diarrhea and retarded growth. Transient thymic necrosis may perturb immunological responses.

k. Murine Coronavirus (Mouse Hepatitis Virus) Infection (Barthold, 1997a,b)

Etiology   Coronaviruses are large, pleomorphic, enveloped RNA viruses with radially arranged peplomers (spikes). In mice, early clinical and laboratory investigations emphasized their potential to induce hepatitis, so their original designation, which is still used actively, is mouse hepatitis virus (MHV). During that time, enteritis in infant mice was recognized as a separate entity caused by an uncharacterized virus, known as Lethal Intestinal Virus of Infant Mice (LIVIM). Subsequent studies revealed that hepatitis-causing MHV and

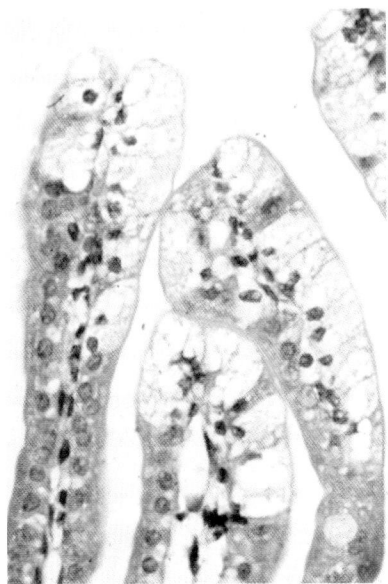

FIGURE 3.25   Mouse rotavirus (EDIM) infection. Note swelling of enterocytes at the tips of villi. *Percy and Barthold (2007).*

enteritis-causing L̲I̲V̲I̲M̲ w̲e̲r̲e̲ c̲l̲o̲s̲e̲l̲y̲ r̲e̲l̲a̲t̲e̲d̲ coronaviruses, now collectively termed MHV. MHV isolates dif-
fer in biologic behavior according to their organ tropism
into two biotypes: *enterotropic* strains, which infect primarily the intestinal tract, and *polytropic* strains, which
initially infect the respiratory tract but may progress
to multisystemic dissemination, including the liver and
brain. These differences are often reflected in their cell
tropism *in vitro*. However, natural isolates may contain
features of both biotypes.

Several prototype polytropic strains have been extensively studied as experimental models of hepatitis and
encephalitis. They include JHM (MHV4), MHV-1, MHV-
3, MHV-S, and MHV-A59. Numerous additional strains
have been identified that differ in virulence, tissue tropism, and antigenicity. Differentiation by strain, particularly under natural conditions, is irrelevant, since
mutation is common among coronaviruses, and even
named prototype strains differ significantly depending upon passage history. Although MHV isolates and
strains share internal antigens (M and N), they can be
distinguished by neutralization tests that detect strain-
specific spike (S) antigens. MHV shares antigens with the
coronaviruses of rats, a finding that has been exploited
to develop heterologous antigens for serological tests.
MHV also is related to human coronavirus OC43.

A number of established cell lines may be used for
propagating polytropic MHV strains *in vitro*. However,
field isolates are difficult to maintain *in vitro*. NCTC
1469 mouse liver cells are useful for growing many
polytropic strains. MHV can also be grown in mouse
macrophages, cells that have been used for genetic
studies of resistance and susceptibility to infection.
Enterotropic strains, because of their tendency to be
strictly enterotropic, have been grown in CMT-93 cells
derived from a rectal carcinoma in a C57BL mouse,
but are generally difficult to propagate in cell culture.
Irrespective of cellular substrate used for isolation or
propagation, syncytium formation is emblematic of
MHV infection (Fig. 3.26).

Clinical Signs   Clinical signs depend primarily on
the age, strain, and immunological status of infected
mouse and strain and tropism of virus. As with many
murine viruses, infection is often clinically silent among
immunologically competent mature mice. Clinical morbidity is most often associated with s̲u̲c̲k̲l̲i̲n̲g̲ m̲i̲c̲e̲ l̲e̲s̲s̲
t̲h̲a̲n̲ 2̲ w̲e̲e̲k̲s̲ o̲l̲d̲ or with immunodeficient mice. Suckling
mice infected with enterotropic MHV d̲e̲v̲e̲l̲o̲p̲ inappe-
t̲e̲n̲c̲e̲, d̲i̲a̲r̲r̲h̲e̲a̲, a̲n̲d̲ d̲e̲h̲y̲d̲r̲a̲t̲i̲o̲n̲, o̲f̲t̲e̲n̲ t̲e̲r̲m̲i̲n̲a̲t̲i̲n̲g̲ i̲n̲
d̲e̲a̲t̲h̲ (Fig. 3.27). Epizootics of enterotropic MHV have
been known to result in 100% mortality among neonatal
mice in a breeding colony. Older mice (2–3 weeks of age)
may have ruffled pelage and runting. Neurotropic strains
such as MHV-JHM may induce flaccid paralysis of the
hindlimb, but this sign is rarely encountered alone during

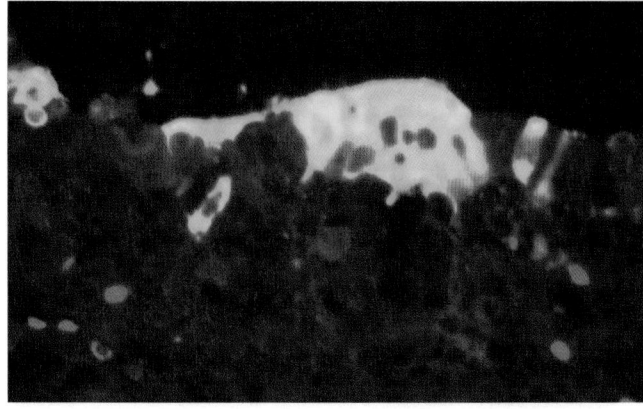

FIGURE 3.26 Immunofluorescent staining of MHV-infected
intestinal mucosa. Note the syncytium in the center, typical of MHV.
Courtesy of S.W. Barthold.

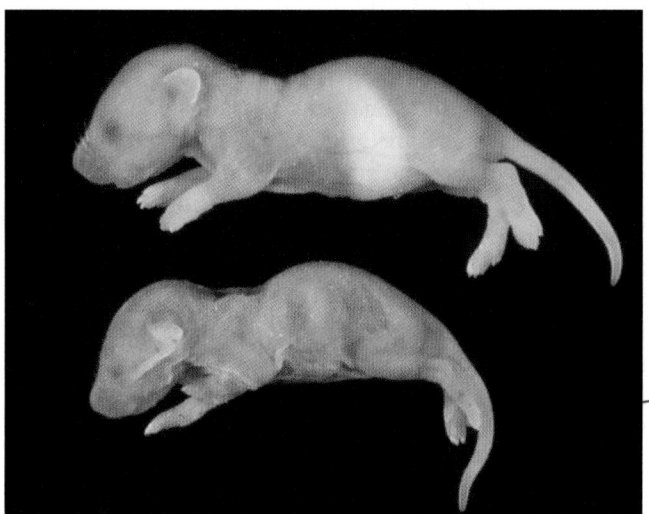

FIGURE 3.27   Infant mice with enterotropic MHV infection. Upper
mouse appears normal and has a milk-filled stomach. Lower mouse
is runted and dehydrated and has an empty stomach. *From Barthold
et al.* (1982).

natural infection. Conjunctivitis, convulsions, and circling may be seen occasionally. Enterotropic strains may
not cause acute disease in athymic mice when exposed
as adults, whereas mildly pathogenic polytropic strains
can cause a progressive wasting syndrome that may be
accompanied by progressive paralysis.

Epizootiology   MHV infection, despite constant
surveillance and preventive programs, continues to
be a common threat to laboratory mouse populations
(Livingston and Riley, 2003; Pritchett-Corning *et al.*,
2009). There are no reports of natural transmission from
mice to other species, but suckling rats have been found
to develop necrotizing rhinitis after intranasal inoculation with MHV-S. MHV is highly contagious, with natural transmission occurring by respiratory or oral routes.

CYSTERM H *— SYSTEMIC*

Enterotropic biotypes predominate in natural infections in contemporary laboratory animal facilities, since they tend to be the most contagious due to copious excretion of virus in feces, whereas polytropic strains generally spread by direct respiratory contact. Natural vertical transmission has not been demonstrated. Introduction of MHV through injection of contaminated biologicals can be an important factor in epizootics, especially because some isolates infect B lymphocytes and, by implication, hybridomas nonlytically.

Infection in immunocompetent mice is self-limiting. Immune-mediated clearance of virus associated with seroconversion usually begins about a week after infection, and mice recover fully within 3–4 weeks. Humoral and cellular immunity participate in host defenses to infection, and T-cell-dependent immunity is an absolute requirement. Thus, age-related resistance to MHV correlates with maturation of lymphoreticular tissues, but intestinal proliferative kinetics are critical determinants of disease susceptibility with enterotropic MHV. Enzootic infection had been construed to include persistent infection in individual mice. Current evidence suggests, however, that enzootic infection results either from the fresh and continuous introduction of immunologically naive or deficient mice or from the recurrent infection of immune mice with MHV variants that arise by natural mutation. Mutation is favored by immune pressure in enzootically infected colonies as well as missteps during natural replication, which include copying errors and recombination. Thus, mice that have developed immunity to one strain of MHV can remain susceptible to one or more genetically and antigenically divergent strains, resulting in reinfection. This caveat has practical importance for breeding colonies. Maternal immunity protects suckling mice against homologous MHV strains but not against antigenically variant strains. However, maternal immunity, even to homologous strains, depends on the presence of maternally acquired antibody in the lumen of the intestine. Therefore, the susceptibility of young mice to infection increases significantly at weaning.

Strain differences in resistance and susceptibility to polytropic MHV can be inherited as an autosomal dominant trait. For example, DBA/2 mice are highly susceptible to MHV-3 and die acutely even as adults, whereas A/J mice develop resistance to lethal infection shortly after weaning. However, genetic resistance is also virus strain-dependent. Therefore, mice resistant to one strain of MHV may be susceptible to another strain. It also is worth noting that the expanded use of genetically altered mice with novel or unanticipated deficits in antiviral responses may alter the outcome of virus–host interactions unpredictably. This pertains to MHV as well as other agents. For example, MHV infection has presented as granulomatous peritonitis and pleuritis in interferon-gamma (IFN-γ) knockout mice (France et al., 1999).

Pathology Polytropic strains replicate initially in the nasal mucosa, where necrotizing rhinitis may occur. Viremic dissemination can follow if virus gains access to regional blood vessels and lymphatics. Thus, viremia leads to secondary infection of vascular endothelium and parenchymal tissues in multiple organs including liver, brain, lymphoid organs, and other sites. Mice also may develop central nervous system disease by direct extension of infection from the olfactory mucosa along olfactory tracts. At necropsy, yellow–white foci indicative of necrosis can occur in multiple tissues, with the involvement of the liver as the classical lesion. Liver involvement may be accompanied by icterus and peritonitis. Histologically, necrosis can be focal or confluent and may be infiltrated by inflammatory cells (Fig. 3.28). Syncytia commonly form at the margin of necrotic areas and, in mild infections, may develop in the absence of frank necrosis. Syncytia formation is a hallmark of infection in many tissues, including the intestine (Fig. 3.26), lung, liver, lymph nodes, spleen, thymus, brain, and bone marrow and in vascular endothelium in general. Although syncytia are transient in immunocompetent mice, they are a persistent feature in chronically infected, immunodeficient mice (Fig. 3.29). Neurotropic variants cause acute necrotizing encephalitis or meningoencephalitis in suckling mice, with demyelination in the brain stem and in peri-ependymal areas secondary to viral invasion of oligodendroglia. Convalescent mice may have residual mononuclear cell infiltrates around vessels or as focal lesions in the liver. Immunodeficient mice can develop progressive necrotic lesions in the liver and elsewhere. Compensatory splenomegaly may occur because of expansion of hematopoietic tissue.

Enterotropic strains infect primarily the intestine and associated lymphoid tissues, although some may also

GUT

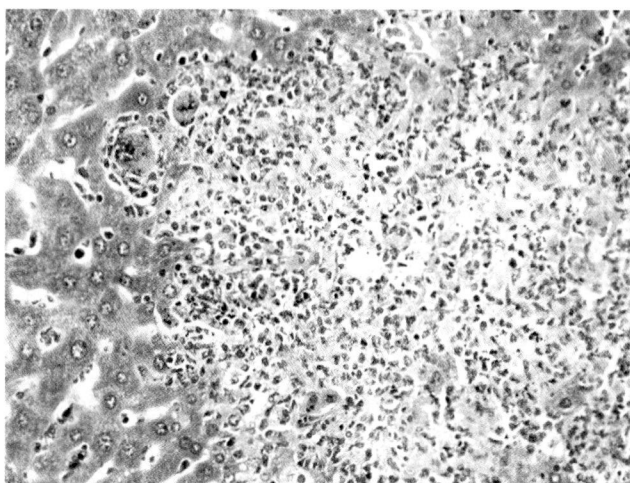

FIGURE 3.28 Necrosis, inflammation, and syncytium in the liver of a mouse infected with MHV. *Courtesy of S.W. Barthold.*

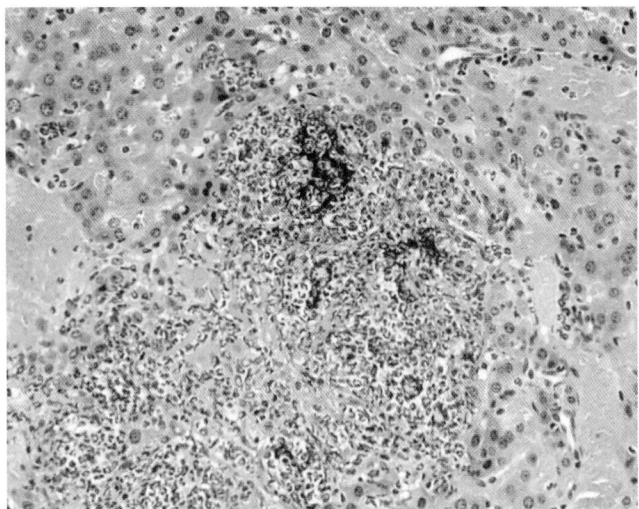

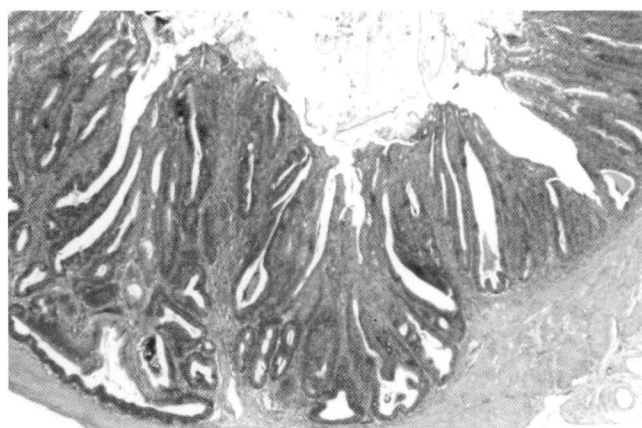

FIGURE 3.31 Proliferative colitis in an athymic mouse chronically infected with enterotropic MHV. *Courtesy of S.W. Barthold.*

FIGURE 3.29 Hepatitis and syncytia in the liver of an SCID mouse. Note the much more obvious syncytia in this liver due to absence of immune response, compared to liver of an infected immunocompetent mouse in Figure 3.28. *Courtesy of S.W. Barthold.*

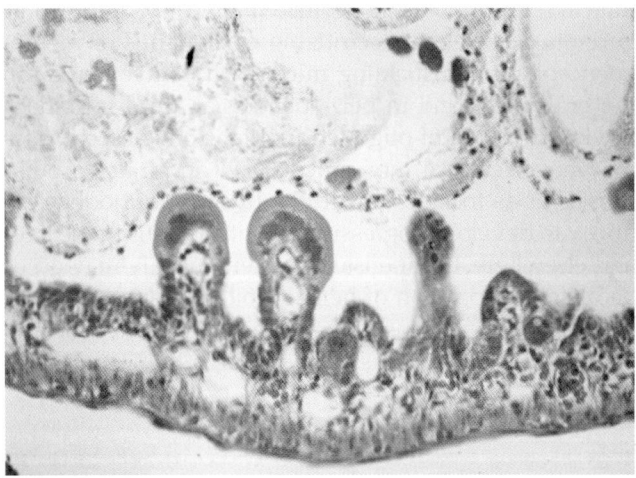

FIGURE 3.30 Small intestine of neonatal mouse infected with enterotropic MHV. Villi are markedly attenuated and there are prominent syncytia at the tips of villi. Percy and Barthold (2007).

cause systemic lesions, especially in the liver and brain. The most common sites are terminal ileum, cecum, and proximal colon. The severity of disease is age-related, and dependent upon intestinal proliferative kinetics, similar to EDIM, with young infants being at highest risk for lethal infection. Pathogenic strains can cause lesions ranging from villus attenuation to fulminant necrotizing enterotyphlocolitis, which can kill suckling mice within a few days (Fig. 3.27). The stomach is often empty, and the intestine is filled with watery to mucoid yellowish, sometimes gaseous contents. Syncytia are a

consistent feature in viable mucosa (Fig. 3.30) and not only are formed in intestine but also may be present in mesenteric lymph nodes and endothelium of mesenteric vessels. Enterocytes may contain intracytoplasmic inclusions, but they are not diagnostic. Surviving mice develop compensatory mucosal hyperplasia, which eventually recedes, but may contribute to clinical signs due to osmotic, secretory, and malabsorptive diarrhea. Older mice are equally susceptible to infection, but are resistant to severe disease due to their mature (more rapid) intestinal proliferative kinetics. Pathology may be subtle, consisting of transient syncytia without necrotic lesions. In adult mice, syncytia can be found most often in the surface mucosal epithelium of the ascending colon. The exception occurs in immunodeficient mice, such as athymic and SCID mice, which can develop chronic proliferative bowel disease of varying severity with MHV antigen in mucosal epithelium (Figs. 3.31 and 3.32). This may not always be present, as athymic nude mice exposed as adults may only manifest a few enterocytic syncytia without hyperplasia.

Diagnosis   Because MHV infection is often subclinical, serological testing is the most reliable diagnostic tool. Many animal resources rely on sentinel mouse protocols for continuous serological surveillance. Serology is well established, sensitive, and reliable. Neutralization tests are used to differentiate individual virus strains in the research laboratory but are inappropriate for routine use, because of cost, technical complexity, and serologic identification *per se* does not predict biological behavior, including virulence or tissue tropism. Serology also can be used in the context of MAP testing in which adult mice are inoculated with suspect tissues to elicit seroconversion. RT-PCR protocols to detect virus in tissues or excreta are available. The detection of syncytia augmented, when possible, by immunohistochemistry to

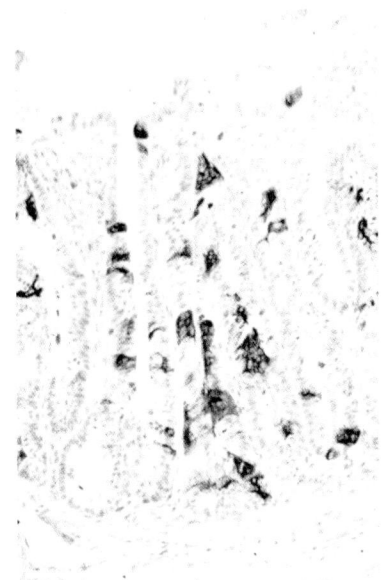

FIGURE 3.32   MHV antigen in colonic mucosa of an athymic mouse chronically infected with enterotropic MHV. *Courtesy of S.W. Barthold.*

detect MHV antigen is a useful and practical means to confirm infection. This strategy should attempt to select mice that are in early stages of infection, because necrosis in infant mice or seroconversion in older mice may reduce the chances of detecting syncytia or viral antigens. The option of using immunodeficient mice as sentinels can be considered, because they sustain prolonged infection. However, they should be securely confined because they also amplify virus loads. If properly controlled, amplification in immunodeficient mice can, however, facilitate subsequent virus isolation in tissue culture.

Differential Diagnosis   MHV infection must be differentiated from other infectious diseases that cause diarrheal illness, runting, or death in suckling mice and wasting disease in immunodeficient mice. These include EDIM, mousepox, reovirus 3 infection, Tyzzer's disease, and salmonellosis. Neurological signs or demyelinating lesions must be differentiated from mouse encephalomyelitis virus infection or noninfectious CNS lesions, such as neoplasms, including polyoma virus-induced tumors in athymic mice.

Prevention and Control   Control and prevention of MHV infection can be difficult because of the numerous variables that influence its expression. Perhaps the most important factor is the duration of infection in individual mice and in mouse colonies. There is evidence that infection in an individual immunocompetent mouse is acute and self-limiting. Such mice can be expected to develop immunity and eliminate virus within 30 days. Therefore, selective quarantine at the cage (not room) level with the temporary cessation of

breeding can be used effectively to eliminate infection. Quarantine at the room basis is likely to fail, since mutations arise and continually reinfect the mouse population. Additionally, maternally derived immunity can protect infant mice from infection until they are weaned and moved to uncontaminated quarters. Careful testing with sentinel mice should be used to assess the effectiveness of quarantine or 'natural rederivation,' as just described. Immunodeficient mice, in contrast, are susceptible to chronic infection and viral excretion. Mice with unrecognized or unanticipated immune dysfunction or with selective immune dysfunction may impact on MHV infection and its control. Such colonies, which may contain highly valuable or irreplaceable mice, may be rescued by cesarean rederivation or embryo transfer if vertical transmission of MHV infection is subsequently ruled out. Although rodent coronaviruses are not viable for extended periods in the environment, excreted virus may remain infectious for up to several days, so proper sanitation and disinfection of caging and animal quarters as well as stringent personal sanitation are essential to eliminate infection.

The prevention of MHV requires procurement of animals from virus-free sources and maintenance under effective barrier conditions monitored by a well-designed quality assurance program. Control of feral mouse populations, proper husbandry and sanitation, and strict monitoring of biological materials that may harbor virus (e.g., transplantable neoplasms, cell lines) are also important strategies to prevent adventitious infection.

Research Complications   Numerous research complications have been attributed to MHV, and the unpredictable outcome of infection in genetically altered mice is likely to lengthen the list. For example, apart from its clinical impact, MHV may stimulate or suppress immune responses, contaminate transplantable neoplasms, and be reactivated by treatment of subclinically infected animals with several classes of drugs, including immunosuppressive agents, and by intercurrent infections. It also can alter tissue enzyme levels. Additionally, the ubiquitous threat of MHV infection and uncertainty about its potential effects on a given research project provoke concerns that may exceed its true impact. For example, transient infection with a mild enterotropic strain is unlikely to disrupt systemic immune responses, whereas infection with a polytropic strain may be highly disruptive. This is not to say that subclinical or strictly enterotropic infection should be taken lightly but simply to caution against overreaction in assessing the impact of an outbreak.

l. Theiler's Murine Encephalomyelitis Virus Infection (Lipton *et al.*, 2007)   NON-ENV

Etiology   Mice are susceptible to infection by two members of the Cardiovirus genus within the

Picornaviridae family, including a virus in the species *Encephalomyocarditis virus* (EMCV) and Theiler's murine encephalomyelitis virus (TMEV), a virus in the species *Theilovirus*. EMCV has a less selective host range and can infect wild mice, but is not known to infect laboratory mice. TMEV is a small, nonenveloped, RNA virus that was discovered by Max Theiler during experimental studies of yellow fever virus in mice. Established prototype strains include TO (Theiler's original), FA, DA, and GD VII, the last of which is named after George Martine (George's disease), an assistant in Theiler's laboratory. TMEV is rapidly destroyed by temperatures over 50°C and by alcohol but not by ether. It can be cultivated *in vitro* in several continuous cell lines, but BHK-21 cells are routinely used for isolation and propagation. TMEV is antigenically related to EMCV. As with other nonenveloped viruses, TMEV is resistant to environmental inactivation, a factor that must be considered in control and prevention of infection.

Clinical Signs   The development of clinical disease depends on virus strain, mouse strain, and route of exposure, but natural disease is exceedingly rare (estimated at 0.1–0.01% of infected mice). When clinical signs occur, they are expressed as neurological disease. The characteristic sign is flaccid posterior paralysis, which may be preceded by weakness in the forelimbs or hindlimbs, but in mice that are otherwise alert (Fig. 3.33). Some mice may recover, but death frequently ensues, often because of failure to obtain food or water. Furthermore, mice that recover from the paralytic syndrome are disposed to a chronic demyelinating phase, which is expressed as a gait disturbance.

Epizootiology   Infection occurs primarily in laboratory mice with the exception of the MGH strain, which has been isolated from laboratory rats and is pathogenic in mice and rats after experimental inoculation. The prevalence of TMEV in mouse colonies is low, a reflection of the slow rate at which virus is transmitted from mouse to mouse, but it continues to be among the more common viral contaminants of mouse colonies

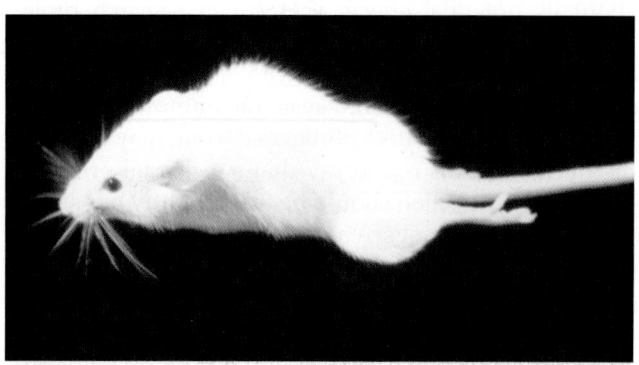

FIGURE 3.33   Posterior paralysis in a mouse naturally infected with mouse encephalomyelitis virus (MEV).

(Livingston and Riley, 2003; Pritchett-Corning *et al.*, 2009). TMEV infection is acquired by ingestion and replicates primarily in the intestinal mucosa. Enteric infection can persist after the development of host immunity and can result in chronic or intermittent excretion of virus in feces over several months (Brownstein *et al.*, 1989). Mice often become infected shortly after weaning, but virus is seldom recovered in mice over 6 months of age. However, neurologic infection can persist in the brain and spinal cord for at least 1 year. Immunity to one strain of TMEV provides cross-protection to other strains. There are no reports of differences in mice with respect to susceptibility to infection under natural conditions. Prenatal transmission has not been found.

Pathology   Intestinal TMEV infection does not cause lesions, but virus can be detected in enterocytes by immunohistochemistry or *in situ* hybridization. Poliomyelitis-like disease, the syndrome that may be encountered during natural infections, is characterized by acute necrosis of ganglion cells and neurons, neuronophagia, and perivascular inflammation, which occur particularly in the ventral horn of the spinal cord gray matter but also can involve higher centers such as the hippocampus, thalamus, and brain stem. During the subsequent demyelinating phase, mononuclear cell inflammation develops in the leptomeninges and white matter of the spinal cord, accompanied by patchy demyelination. The white-matter lesions are due to immune injury. Spontaneous demyelinating myelopathy, affecting the thoracic spinal cord and associated with MEV infection, has also been reported in aged mice. Virulent strains may cause acute encephalitis after experimental inoculation, whereas less virulent isolates produce acute poliomyelitis followed by chronic demyelinating disease.

Diagnosis   Infection is usually detected serologically or by PCR of feces, but virus shedding from infected mice may be intermittent. Clinical signs are striking, if they occur, but are too rare to rely on for routine diagnosis. Histological lesions in the CNS and especially the spinal cord are characteristic when present.

Differential Diagnosis   Neurotropic variants of MHV may, on occasion, cause similar neurological signs. Injury or neoplasia affecting the spinal cord can also produce posterior paralysis. Polyoma virus infection in athymic mice can induce tumors or demyelination in the CNS, which may result in clinical signs resembling those of TMEV infection.

Prevention and Control   Disease-free stocks were originally developed by foster-nursing infant mice. This technique, cesarean rederivation, or embryo transfer can be used successfully to eliminate infection. In either case, foster mothers should be surveyed in advance to ensure their MEV-free status. Selective culling can be considered as an option to eliminate infection, because infection spreads slowly. However, the virus is hardy in the environment and resists chemical inactivation, so it may be prudent to depopulate and disinfect rooms if the presence of infection is unacceptable.

Research Complications The principal hazard from TMEV for research relates to its potential effects on the CNS.

m. Mouse Norovirus Infection
(Wobus *et al.*, 2006)

Noroviruses are nonenveloped RNA viruses that belong to the family Caliciviridae. They are notoriously resistant to environmental inactivation, and cause significant gastrointestinal morbidity in humans. Noroviruses are species-specific, including MNV, which exclusively infects mice. Until the discovery of MNV, replication of noroviruses *in vitro* has not been possible. For this reason, MNV has emerged as an important small animal model of norovirus pathogenesis. MNV was relatively recently discovered in 2003, and subsequent surveillance has revealed that it is the most common adventitious virus infection in laboratory mice (Hsu *et al.*, 2005; Pritchett-Corning *et al.*, 2009). Over 35 MNV isolates have been found in mouse research colonies around the world, which display nearly 90% genetic identity, comprising a single genetic cluster. Although genetically homogeneous, significant biological differences exist among MNV strains (Thackray *et al.*, 2007). MNV effectively replicates in macrophages and dendritic cells, including the mouse macrophage-like RAW264.7 cell line, as well as a microglial cell line (Wobus *et al.*, 2004).

Clinical Signs Clinical signs of infection in immunocompetent mice are usually absent, but infection leads to systemic disease with high mortality in interferon αβγ receptor and STAT1 null mice. Affected mice have loss of body weight, ruffled fur, and hunched posture (Ward *et al.*, 2006). Experimental infection of 129 and C3H mice with MNV-1 caused mild diarrhea (Kahan *et al.*, 2011).

Epizootiology MNV is transmitted by the fecal–oral route, and contaminates the environment as an environmentally resistant virus. For this reason, it can efficiently infect sentinel mice with soiled bedding (Manuel *et al.*, 2008). Duration of infection varies with MNV strain, mouse immunocompetence and mouse genotype. Experimental studies have revealed that several MNV strains persist in various tissues of C57BL/6J, Hsd:ICR, and Jcl:ICR and C.B-17-*Prkdc^scid* mice, with fecal shedding for at least 35–60 days (Goto *et al.*, 2009; Hsu *et al.*, 2006; Thackray *et al.*, 2007). Although not clinically ill, RAG1 null mice are unable to clear infection (Wobus *et al.*, 2006). Comparative studies with MNV-1 and MNV-3 have shown differences in virus replication and shedding (Kahan *et al.*, 2011). MNV has a tropism for macrophages and dendritic cells, and virus can be detected in the intestine, intestinal lymphoid tissue, liver, and spleen (Hsu *et al.*, 2006; Kahan *et al.*, 2011; Wobus *et al.*, 2006).

Pathology Naturally and experimentally infected STAT1 or IFNγR null mice may develop splenomegaly and multifocal pale spots on the liver. Microscopic findings include varying degrees of hepatitis, focal interstitial pneumonia, vasculitis, peritonitis, and pleuritis (Karst *et al.*, 2003; Ward *et al.*, 2006). Encephalitis, cerebral vasculitis, pneumonia, and hepatitis have also been described in intracerebrally infected STAT1 null mice (Karst *et al.*, 2003). Infection of immunocompetent mice may be associated with mild inflammation of the intestine, splenic hypertrophy, and lymphoid hyperplasia of spleen and lymph nodes (Mumphrey *et al.*, 2007).

Diagnosis MNV infection can be detected by serology or RT-PCR. Sentinel mouse surveillance, using soiled bedding, is an effective strategy for detecting MNV (Manuel *et al.*, 2008)

Differential Diagnosis The mild change in fecal consistency associated with MNV in adult mice may mimic rotavirus, coronavirus, *Helicobacter* spp., *Citrobacter rodentium*, or other enteric diseases. Disseminated lesions in STAT1 or IFNγR null mice must be differentiated from other polytropic viral diseases in immunodeficient mice, including MHV.

Prevention and Control Depopulation and decontamination has been shown to be effective at eliminating MNV from an enzootically infected colony, whereas test-and-removal of positive mice was found to be ineffective (Kastenmayer *et al.*, 2008). Embryo transfer and cesarean rederivation are also effective (Goto *et al.*, 2009; Perdue *et al.*, 2007). Neonatal mice are resistant to infection, so that cross-fostering neonates onto uninfected dams is another effective means of rederivation MNV-free mice (Artwohl *et al.*, 2008; Compton, 2008).

Research Complications The tropism of MNV for macrophages and dendritic cells is likely to modify immune responses, and MNV infection may interfere with studies involving enteric disease.

n. Hantavirus Infection (MacLachlan and Dubovi, 2011)

Hantaviruses are RNA viruses belonging to the very large Bunyaviridae family. They differ from other members of this family by not being arthropod-borne. Each hantavirus is antigenically distinct and maintained within single or at most a few rodent or insectivore hosts, but are infectious for other hosts. Infection is lifelong, and virus is transmitted by shedding of virus in urine, feces, and saliva. Several hantaviruses are zoonotic and may cause severe disease in humans. Although there is overlap, hantaviruses in Asia and Europe cause *hemorrhagic fever with renal syndrome* (HFRS) in humans, a multisystem disease with significant renal involvement, and hantaviruses that are endemic in the Americas cause *hantavirus pulmonary syndrome* (HPS) in humans, which is a multisystem disease with pulmonary involvement. Among the better-known Old World HFRS hantaviruses are Hantaan, Seoul, Puumala, and Dobrava–Belgrade viruses. Sin Nombre virus is the best known New World PHS hantavirus, among many others. Most notably from the perspective of laboratory animal medicine, the Norway rat, *Rattus norvegicus*, serves as a reservoir host for hantavirus in the wild, but infection has also been associated with laboratory rats. In addition to being endemic in wild rats in Asia, it has been found to be endemic in wild rats in the eastern United States and associated with human cases of HFRS (Childs *et al.*, 1988; LeDuc *et al.*, 1984; Tsai *et al.*, 1985). Over 120 cases of hantavirus infection have been transmitted to humans from laboratory rats in Japan, Belgium, and the United Kingdom (Desmyter *et al.*, 1983; Kawamata *et al.*, 1987; Lloyd *et al.*, 1984; Umenai *et al.*, 1979). *M. musculus* is not considered to be a primary reservoir host, but hantavirus infection has been documented serologically in conventional and barrier-maintained laboratory mice and rats in Korea (Won *et al.*, 2006), infection of wild *M. musculus* has been documented in the United States (Baek *et al.*, 1988), and infection of wild mice in Europe has been associated with human exposure (Diglisic *et al.*, 1994). Hantaviruses are difficult to culture *in vitro*. Infection in rodents is subclinical and is detected by serology or RT-PCR. The main research complication from natural infection is the zoonotic risk and potentially subclinical effects on the immune response associated with viral defenses such as $CD8^+$ T cell (Taruishi *et al.*, 2007) and NK function as demonstrated in human studies (Braun *et al.*, 2014).

o. Retrovirus Infection (Mammary Tumor Viruses and Mouse Leukemia Viruses) (Coffin *et al.*, 1997; MacLachlan and Dubovi, 2011; Morse, 2007b)

The mouse is host to a number of enveloped RNA viruses of the family Retroviridae, subfamily Orthovirinae, including the two type species (and their variants) *mouse mammary tumor virus* (MMTV) and *murine leukemia virus* (MLV). These viruses belong to a diverse assemblage of related mobile DNA elements that are integrated into the host genome, and collectively termed 'retroelements', which include retrovirus-related elements and nonviral elements. During cell division, retroelements are transcribed into RNA, and subsequently reverse-transcribed into DNA copies that become integrated into a new location within the genome. This process utilizes reverse transcriptase, which is encoded by the retroelement. Over millennia, retroelements have been repeatedly integrated within the genome in large numbers, comprising approximately 40% of the mammalian genome. Various families of mouse retroelements share sequence similarity, despite their random distribution throughout the mouse genome, and the

majority of them are truncated, mutated, and methylated to become incapable of infectivity. Nevertheless, many of them continue to be mobile within the genome. Noninfectious retrovirus-related retroelements include IAP, VL30, MusD, and ETn elements.

Replication-competent retroviruses represent the pinnacle of the retroelement constellation and are best considered as the most evolutionarily recent members. These include MMTV and MLV. MTV and MLV share similar genetic structure, except that the long terminal repeat (LTR) region of the MMTV genome encodes an additional superantigen (*Sag*). Both MMTV and MLV include *exogenous* viruses, which are horizontally transmitted, replication-competent viruses, and *endogenous* viruses, which are closely related to exogenous viruses, encoded within the mouse genome, and transmitted by Mendelian inheritance. Exogenous MMTV and MLV exist in wild mouse populations, but have been eliminated from contemporary laboratory mice. However, they may continue to be used experimentally, including Bittner MMTV, and Gross, Friend, Moloney, and Rauscher MLVs. In particular, mouse colonies may be purposely infected with MMTV for mammary cancer research and are termed 'MMTV-positive', reflecting their exogenous virus status, even though the mice may also carry endogenous MMTV.

The genomes of all inbred strains of mice encode one or more (over 50 in some mouse strains) endogenous MMTV loci, the distribution of which is unique to each inbred strain of mouse. Most MMTV genomic loci do not encode infectious virus or are transcriptionally inactive, except for mouse strains (DBA, C3H, GRS) that carry *Mtv1 or Mtv2* loci. These loci encode infectious virus, which can be visualized as B-type particles by electron microscopy. Likewise, all mouse strains carry endogenous MLV loci within their genome, but not all mice carry replication-competent MLV sequences. Some endogenous MLVs encode infectious virus, which can be visualized as C-type particles by electron microscopy. Mice have often evolved mechanisms to counter the deleterious effects of retroviruses by preventing reentry or replication of virus into other cells. If an endogenous retrovirus is still infectious to other mouse cell targets, it is termed *ecotropic*, whereas if it is no longer infectious for mouse cells, but can infect cells of other species, it is termed *xenotropic*. Viruses capable of infecting cells of mice as well as other species are termed *polytropic*. The combinations of endogenous replication-competent MLVs and cell tropism factors are a reflection of selective breeding of mouse strains for susceptibility to various types of cancer.

Clinical Signs   Mice were originally inbred for specific phenotypes, including mammary tumors and lymphomas. Thus, some strains of mice were genetically selected for unique combinations of endogenous MMTV and MLV in concert with susceptibility factors that favored their expression and disease manifestations. In addition, noninfectious retroelements continue to reintegrate randomly within the genome during cell division as retro transposons. These ongoing integrations contribute to genetic drift, spontaneous mutations, and well-recognized mouse strain phenotypes, including the athymic nude allele, the hairless allele, and the rodless retina allele, among others.

Epizootiology Exogenous MMTV and MLV are horizontally transmissible, primarily through the milk of lactating females. Endogenous retroviruses and retroelements are inherited through the genome. Replication-competent endogenous MMTVs and MLVs are also transmissible like their exogenous counterparts, but differ by being integrated within the genome of the mouse.

Pathology Replication-competent MMTV and MLV, regardless of their exogenous or endogenous origin, are usually clinically silent. Their ability to cause neoplasia is a reflection of genetic selection for susceptibility factors that are genetically encoded within individual mouse strain genomes. MMTV derives its name from its association with induction of mammary carcinomas in mammary cancer-susceptible strains of mice. MLV is associated with lymphomas, the pattern of which is mouse strain specific. For example, AKR mice develop 100% prevalence of thymic lymphoma between 6 and 12 months of age, whereas aging BALB/c mice commonly develop multicentric lymphoma. In these strains of mice, multiple endogenous MLVs are coexpressed in tissues and undergo recombination events that allow them to target and transform cells into neoplasia. Despite its name, MMTV can induce lymphomas in some strains of mice, such as SJL mice which develop lymphomas arising from enteric lymphoid tissue and mesenteric lymph nodes.

Diagnosis Exogenous retroviruses have been eliminated from contemporary mouse populations, unless purposely introduced for experimental purposes. Because endogenous retroviruses and retroelements are encoded within the genome, and reflect the unique genetic composition of each strain of mouse, they are not targets of diagnostic pursuit.

Differential Diagnosis Patterns of some types of neoplasia within individual inbred strains of mice are a reflection of their endogenous retroviral integration.

Prevention and Control Exogenous retroviruses have been eliminated from laboratory mice by cesarean rederivation and foster nursing. MMTV-S, the 'Bittner agent', continues to be purposely maintained in some mouse breeding populations, but can be eliminated by foster-nursing or other means. Caution is advised when re-deriving such mouse colonies for other purposes, as elimination of exogenous MMTV will be an unintended consequence.

Research Complications Endogenous retroviruses and retroelements influence the life span of individual strains of mice, and random integrations during cell division can give rise to spontaneous mutations and genetic drift. It is estimated that significant mutations may arise due to mobile retroelement integrations every 50 generations.

p. Astrovirus Infection (Akkina, 2013; Yokoyama et al., 2012, Farkas et al., 2012)

Astroviruses are small, nonenveloped, single-stranded RNA viruses that have been associated with human gastroenteritis and detected in association with other enteric pathogens. The viral family Astroviridae is split into two genuses: *Avastrovirus* for those astroviruses infecting avians and *Mamastrovirus* for those infecting mammals. Astrovirus infection has been detected in research mice (MuAstV) using metagenomic analyses and appears to have a wide geographical, institutional, and host strain distribution.

Clinical Signs None reported.

Epizootiology PCR screening has found MuAstV infection in up to 22% of a variety of mouse strains housed in vendor and academic facilities in the United States and Japan. The virus has been detected most commonly in immunocompromised mice (NSG, NOD-SCID, NSG-3GS, C57BL6-Timp-3$^{-/-}$, and uPA-NOG), but also in immuncompetent strains (B6J, ICR, Bash2, and BALB/c). Both immunodeficient and immunocompetent mice are susceptible to MuAstV, but adaptive immunity is required to clear the virus. Based on human epidemiology indicating children are at highest risk for infection, the virus may preferentially infect young mice.

Pathology Immunodeficient mice showed no sign of pathology based on histopathology.

Diagnosis PCR data has indicated that MuAstV causes a systemic, chronic infection in immunocompromised mice, indicating samples from most tissues will be PCR positive. Yokoyama *et al.* (2012) detected high viral load (up to 10^9 genome copies) per fecal pellet from immunocompetent mice.

Differential Diagnosis None, in the absence of lesions and clinical disease.

Prevention and Control Because immunocompetent mice clear the infection, quarantine may be successful but lack of routine screening for MuAstV in laboratory mice will allow for uncontrolled spread of the infection.

Research Complications Based on limited surveys, MuAstV may have a high prevalence in laboratory mice. The impact of infection on both innate and adaptive immune responses warrants further investigation to assess the potential for confounding research data.

3. Bacterial Diseases

This section briefly describes the etiology, clinical signs, epizootiology, pathology, diagnosis, differential diagnoses, prevention and control, and research complications of the most common bacterial diseases encountered in research colonies of mice. As sequencing technology becomes more available, the number and genus/species classification of bacteria potentially responsible for infections, in particular, opportunistic infections, will grow (Benga *et al.*, 2014). Potential candidates include members of Pasteurellaceae, *Bordetella hinzii*, *Streptococcus danielae*, *Acinetobacter* spp., and others, for which little is currently known about their pathogenic potential.

a. *Lawsonia Intracellularis*

Etiology *Lawsonia intracellularis*, an obligate intracellular bacterium and the causative agent of proliferative enteropathy, is not a pathogen encountered in research colonies of mice but has been reported to infect wild mice and rats in close contact with infected livestock (Collins *et al.*, 2011).

Clinical Signs None reported but should consider *Lawsonia* as a differential in necropsy cases with gross or histologic evidence of proliferative lower bowel lesions.

Epizootiology Although mice are experimentally susceptible to infection and develop classic lesions of hyperplastic ileitis and typhlocolitis (Murakata *et al.*, 2008), susceptibility varied with mouse strain and source of inoculum from rabbits or swine, suggesting important differences in *L. intracellularis* strains.

Pathology Lawsonia infection may result in hyperplastic ileitis, typhlitis and/or colitis, and hemorrhagic intestines may be noted (Percy and Barthold, 2007).

Diagnosis *Lawsonia* spp. has been diagnosed using a variety of techniques, including PCR, immunohistochemistry, *in situ* hybridization, and Warthin–Starry silver stains.

Differential Diagnosis Bacterial infections associated with hyperplastic intestinal epithelium, including *C. rodentium* and enterohepatic helicobacter species in susceptible (typically immunodeficient) mouse strains.

Prevention and Control Species separation from hosts more commonly associated with natural infection (hamsters, ferrets, pigs).

Research Complications None reported.

b. Mycoplasmosis (Cassell *et al.*, 1986; Lindsey *et al.*, 1982, 1991i; Percy and Barthold, 2007)

The following section describes infection due to *Mycoplasma pulmonis* and summarizes infections associated with other murine mycoplasmas including *M. arthritidis*, *M. neurolyticum*, *M. collis*, and *M. muris*. Antigenic cross-reactivity among these species, and especially between *M. pulmonis* and *M. arthritidis*, mandates that reliable diagnostic strategies incremental to serology (ELISA, IFA, MFIA) such as culture (often false negative) and PCR be employed to distinguish potentially pathogenic infections. When screening cell lines

for opportunistic pathogens, PCR is the most efficient method to discriminate between *M. pulmonis* and mycoplasma contaminants associated with cell culture.

MYCOPLASMA PULMONIS

Etiology *M. pulmonis* is a pleomorphic, gram-negative bacterium that lacks a cell wall and has a single outer limiting membrane. It causes murine respiratory mycoplasmosis (MRM).

Clinical Signs Mice are relatively resistant to florid MRM; thus, subclinical infection is more common. When clinical signs occur, they reflect suppurative rhinitis, otitis media, and chronic pneumonia. Affected mice may display inactivity, weight loss, and ruffled hair coat, but the most prominent signs are 'chattering' and dyspnea, due to rhinitis and purulent exudate in nasal passages. Otitis media may cause a head tilt, whereas suppurative inflammation in the brain and spinal cord, although rare, can cause flaccid paralysis. Experimental infection of the genital tract can cause oophoritis, salpingitis, and metritis, which may lead to infertility or fetal deaths. Experimental inoculation of SCID mice has caused systemic infection accompanied by severe arthritis (Evengard *et al.*, 1994).

Epizootiology MRM historically was a common infectious disease of mice, but improved housing, husbandry, and health surveillance have reduced its prevalence dramatically. Serologic data from a large diagnostic laboratory indicated *M. pulmonis* infection affects about 0.01% of conventionally housed mouse colonies in the United States and 0.16% in Europe (Pritchett-Corning *et al.*, 2009). *M. pulmonis* infection is contracted by inhalation and can occur in suckling and adult mice. Therefore, infection should be considered highly contagious. Mice injected with cells harvested from *M. pulmonis* contaminated cell cultures may develop disease. *M. pulmonis* can also be transmitted venerally; *in utero* infection has been demonstrated in rats but not in mice. Because transplacental infection occurs in rats, the same route may be possible in mice, particularly immunocompromised strains. Concomitant viral pneumonia (SV, mouse coronavirus) or elevated environmental ammonia concentrations may increase susceptibility to MRM. *M. pulmonis* also infects rats, hamsters, guinea pigs, and rabbits. Among these species, only rats are significant reservoirs of infection for mice.

Pathology *M. pulmonis* is an extracellular organism that colonizes the apical cell membranes of respiratory epithelium. Attachment occurs anywhere from the anterior nasal passages to the alveoli and may be mediated by surface glycoproteins. The organism may injure host cells through competition for metabolites such as carbohydrates and nucleic acids or by release of toxic substances such as peroxides. Ciliostasis, reduction in the number of cilia, and ultrastructural changes leading to cell death have also been described. Detrimental effects on ciliated epithelium can lead to disrupted mucociliary transport, which exacerbates pulmonary disease.

Experimental infection of MRM is dose dependent. Doses of 10^4 colony-forming units (CFUs) or less cause mild, transient disease involving the upper respiratory tract and middle ears, whereas higher doses often lead to acute, lethal pneumonia. Additionally, *M. pulmonis* strains can differ in virulence. Survivors of severe infection may develop chronic bronchopneumonia with bronchiectasis and spread infection to other mice. Intravenous inoculation of *M. pulmonis* can cause arthritis in mice, but arthritis is not a significant feature of natural infection.

Host genotype also is a major factor in the outcome of infection, with resistance being expressed phenotypically through the bactericidal efficiency of alveolar macrophages. Strains derived from a C57BL background appear to be resistant to pathogenic infection, whereas BALB/c, C3H, DBA/2, SWR, AKR, CBA, SJL, and other strains have varying degrees of increased susceptibility (Cartner *et al.*, 1996; Lai *et al.*, 1993).

The initial lesion of MRM is suppurative rhinitis, which may involve the trachea and major airways. Early inflammatory lesions, if not quickly resolved, progress to prominent squamous metaplasia. Transient hyperplasia of submucosal glands may occur, and lymphoid infiltration of the submucosa can persist for weeks. Syncytia can sometimes be found in nasal passages, in association with purulent exudate (Fig. 3.34). Affected mice also develop suppurative otitis media and chronic laryngotracheitis with mucosal hyperplasia and lymphoid cell infiltrates. Pulmonary lesions are typified by bronchopneumonia, which spreads from the hilus. Lymphoid cells and plasma cells accumulate around bronchi which often contain neutrophils in their lumen. Chronic lung disease features suppurative bronchitis, bronchiolitis, and alveolitis (Fig. 3.35). Chronicity also increases the prevalence of bronchiectasis and abcessation.

Diagnosis Accurate diagnosis should exploit the complementary use of clinical, serological, microbiological, molecular, and morphological methods. Clinical signs are variable but can be characteristic when they occur. Serology is sensitive but although antibodies do not clear the infection, seroconversion may be weak or take months and may not accurately differentiate between *M. pulmonis* infection and *M. arthriditis* infection (Cassell *et al.*, 1981). Therefore samples for culture and PCR of the upper respiratory tract should be obtained to confirm diagnosis. Buffered saline or *Mycoplasma* broth should be used to lavage the trachea, larynx, pharynx, and nasal passages. Specimens for culture from the genital tract are warranted if this site is suspected. *Mycoplasma* spp. may be difficult to grow, so it is prudent to confirm that the relevant expertise and quality control exist in the diagnostic laboratory. Speciation can be accomplished by immunofluorescence or immunoperoxidase staining or by growth inhibition. Immunohistochemistry should be considered to supplement basic histopathologic examination. Immunofluorescence and immunoperoxidase techniques are available to identify mycoplasma antigens in tissue sections or in cytological preparations of tracheobronchial or genital tract lavages (Brunnert *et al.*, 1994). PCR assays for *M. pulmonis* at veterinary diagnostic laboratories and PCR kits to screen cell cultures for mycoplasma are readily available.

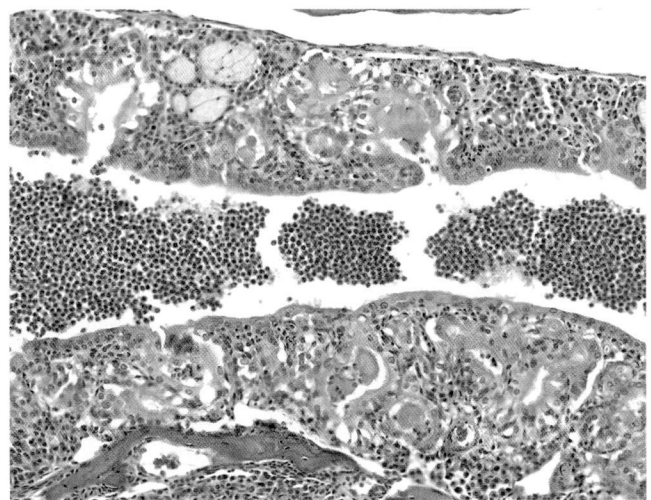

FIGURE 3.34 *Mycoplasma pulmonis*-induced rhinitis in a mouse. The turbinate mucosa contains accumulations of plasma cells and lymphocytes, the epithelium is decreased in thickness and has lost most cilia, and the lumen contains neutrophilic exudate. *Courtesy of Trenton Schoeb.*

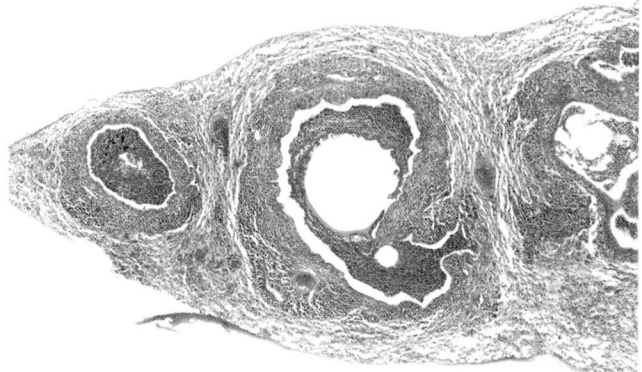

FIGURE 3.35 *Mycoplasma pulmonis*-induced bronchiolitis and bronchiolectasis in a mouse. The bronchioles are dilated, contain neutrophilic exudate, and are surrounded by accumulations of plasma cells and lymphocytes, and the mucosa is infiltrated with inflammatory cells. *Courtesy of Trenton Schoeb.*

Differential Diagnosis MRM must be differentiated from bronchopneumonia associated with cilia-associated respiratory (CAR) bacillus. Silver stains may reveal CAR bacilli adherent to the respiratory epithelium. SV also can cause bronchopneumonia in mice but can be detected by serology and immunohistochemistry. Other causes of respiratory infection include PVM, corynebacteriosis and, in immunodeficient mice, *Pneumocystis murina* infection. Combined infections with known pathogens or secondary opportunists also must be considered.

Prevention and Control Mice mount an effective immune response to *M. pulmonis*, as measured by their recovery from mild infection and their resistance to infection after active or passive immunization (Cartner et al., 1998). Antibodies of various classes are produced locally and systemically, but clearance of the infection has been attributed to innate immune responses (Love et al., 2010; Sun et al., 2013). There is some evidence that antibody may facilitate phagocytosis of *M. pulmonis*. T-cell responses, however, appear to exacerbate *M. pulmonis* in mice, because immunity cannot be transferred with immune cells. In addition, athymic and neonatally thymectomized mice are not more susceptible than immunocompetent mice to *M. pulmonis* pneumonia. Nude and SCID mice develop less severe respiratory disease than immunocompetent mice but infection becomes systemic and they may develop suppurative disease in multiple organs and joints (arthritis).

Host immunity aside, effective control and prevention of MRM depend primarily on maintenance of *Mycoplasma*-free colonies under barrier conditions supported by careful surveillance for infection by serology, microbiology, PCR, and histopathology. Cesarean or embryo rederivation may eliminate infection, although vertical transmission may occur in immunocompromised mice. Treatment with tetracycline suppresses clinical disease but does not eliminate infection. Earlier interest in developing DNA-based vaccines against *M. pulmonis* has not achieved clinical application (Lai et al., 1997).

Research Complications *M. pulmonis* can interfere with research by causing clinical disease or death. Experiments involving the respiratory tract, such as inhalation toxicology, can be compromised by chronic progressive infection. Additionally, affected mice are at greater risk during general anesthesia. *M. pulmonis* may alter immunological responsiveness. For example, it is mitogenic for T and B lymphocytes and can increase NK cell activity. Perhaps one of the most important complications of *Mycoplasma* infection is contamination of cell lines and transplantable tumors.

Other Murine Mycoplasmas Cell lines are often contaminated with mycoplasma species such as *M. arginini*, *M. hyorhinis*, *M. orale*, or *M. fermentans* that can distort the results of *in vitro* assays (Garner et al.,

2000). Initial evidence of a contamination is often by PCR evidence of mycoplasma at the genus level when cell lines are PCR screened for opportunistic murine pathogens prior to use in mice. Other than *M. pulmonis*, these mycoplasmas are not normally considered mouse pathogens in immunocompetent mice. In contrast, injection of mycoplasma contaminated cells into immunodeficient mice (e.g., xenografts) may result in clinical disease or confounding effects on immune responses (Peterson, 2008). Mycoplasma contamination of murine embryonic stem cells has adversely affected germline transmission and postnatal health of chimeric progeny (Markoullis et al., 2009).

Mycoplasma arthritidis is antigenically related to *M. pulmonis*. Therefore, serological evidence of mycoplasma infection must be supplemented by other diagnostic tests, as outlined above, to differentiate between these agents. Differentiation is important because *M. arthritidis*, though arthritogenic in mice after intravenous inoculation, is nonpathogenic during natural infection. *Mycoplasma collis* has been isolated from the genital tract of mice but does not appear to cause natural disease.

Mycoplasma neurolyticum is the etiological agent of rolling disease, a rare syndrome which occurs within hours after intravenous inoculation of *M. neurolyticum* exotoxin. Characteristic clinical signs include spasmodic hyperextension of the head and the raising of one foreleg followed by intermittent rolling on the long axis of the body. The rolling becomes more constant, but mice occasionally leap or move rapidly. After 1–2h of rolling, animals become comatose and usually die within 4h. All published reports of rolling disease are associated with experimental inoculation of *M. neurolyticum* or exotoxin. Large numbers of organisms are needed to produce disease, and there is no indication that, under natural conditions, organisms replicate in the brain to concentrations required for the induction of these signs. Because animals are frequently inoculated with biological materials by parenteral routes, contamination with *M. neurolyticum* may induce rolling disease inadvertently. Diagnosis can be made from the appearance of typical clinical signs, astrocytic swelling, and isolation of the causative organism. Clinical signs must be differentiated from rolling associated with *Pseudomonas*- and *P. pneumotropica*-caused otitis. *M. pulmonis* has been recovered from the brain of mice but does not seem to cause overt neurological disease.

Hemotropic Mycoplasmas Ribosomal RNA sequencing has reclassified *Hemobartonella muris* and *Eperythrozoon coccoides* as *Mycoplasma hemomuris* and *Mycoplasma coccoides*, respectively (Neimark et al., 2005; Percy and Barthold, 2007). Distinct from the mycoplasmas just discussed, these agents are trophic for red blood cells and cause anemia and hemolytic disease. These infections could be encountered in wild mice but are rarely found in research mice. Diagnosis is by morphologic assessment of blood smears and PCR.

Clinical Signs Mice infected with *M. coccoides* may remain clinically normal or develop febrile, hemolytic anemia and splenomegaly, which can be fatal. Hepatocellular degeneration and multifocal necrosis have been recorded in acute infections. Hemotropic mycoplasma infections are long-lived and are expressed clinically in one of two ways: acute febrile anemia and latent or subclinical infection that can be reactivated by splenectomy. The carrier state may be lifelong.

Epizootiology The primary natural vector of *M. coccoides*, historically, is the mouse louse, *Polyplax serrata*. Infection was associated with primitive housing and husbandry conditions that no longer occur in modern vivaria. Although the risks for infection have been reduced substantially by modern animal care procedures, *M. coccoides* can be transmitted to mice from contaminated biological products such as transplantable tumors or blood plasma.

Diagnosis Splenectomy or inoculation of test material into splenectomized mice is the most sensitive means of detecting *M. coccoides* infection. These procedures provoke mycoplasmemia, usually within 2–4 days. Because mycoplasmemia may be transient, blood smears stained by the Romanowsky or indirect immunofluorescence procedures of the blood should be prepared every 6 h, beginning at 48 h after splenectomy of index animals or inoculation of test specimens into splenectomized animals to ensure that mycoplasmemia is not missed.

Prevention and Control Treatment of *M. coccoides* infection is not practical. Control is based on culling or rederivation of infected stock. If replacement animals are readily available, euthanasia is a more prudent course. Suspect biological materials destined for animal inoculation should be screened for mycoplasma contamination by inoculation of splenectomized mice.

Research Complications Subclinical infection can be reactivated by irradiation, immunosuppressive therapy, or intercurrent disease. Conversely, *M. coccoides* may potentiate coincident viral infections in mice. This effect has been clearly demonstrated for mouse coronavirus and has been suspected for lymphocytic choriomeningitis virus and LDV. Active infection also may suppress interferon production.

c. CAR Bacillus Infection

Etiology CAR bacillus is a slender, gram-negative, non-spore-forming bacillus, which, in rats, produces clinical disease and lesions that closely resemble those of MRM (see Chapter 4).

Clinical Signs Chronic respiratory disease has been produced in mice by experimental inoculation, but natural clinical disease is rare (Griffith *et al.*, 1988;

Pritchett-Corning *et al.*, 2009). Furthermore, putative natural cases were reported in mice that were seropositive for SV and pneumonia virus of mice. Therefore, CAR bacillus may exacerbate respiratory disease as an opportunist rather than as a primary pathogen. On balance, it is assumed that mice contract natural infection, but attributing severe chronic respiratory disease in mice solely to CAR bacillus should be supported by screening for other respiratory pathogens.

Epizootiology CAR bacillus is transmitted by direct contact; dirty bedding transfer to sentinel mice may not reflect colony infection status.

Pathology Lung lesions are typically mild in mice and are similar to respiratory mycoplasmosis. Uncomplicated CAR bacillus infection results in peribronchiole cuffing with lymphocytes and plasma cells. Severe bronchiolitis and pneumonia are possible (Fig. 3.36). Fatal bronchopneumonia was reported in OB/OB mice (Griffith *et al.*, 1988).

Diagnosis An ELISA for serological screening is routinely used; PCR and histology are used for definitive diagnosis. In active infection, histologic assessment using Warthin–Starry or similar stains will reveal argyrophilic bacilli adherent to the apical membranes of bronchial respiratory epithelium along with the presence of peribronchial lymphocytes (Fig. 3.37). Alternatively, immunohistochemistry assays have also been used successfully to detect infection. Recovery of CAR bacillus requires cell culture or culture in embryonated eggs.

Differential Diagnosis Respiratory mycoplasmosis, Bordetella (avium, hinzii).

Prevention and Control Given CAR bacillus does not form spores, disinfection of the environment should be effective. Treatment using sulfamerazine (500 mg/l)

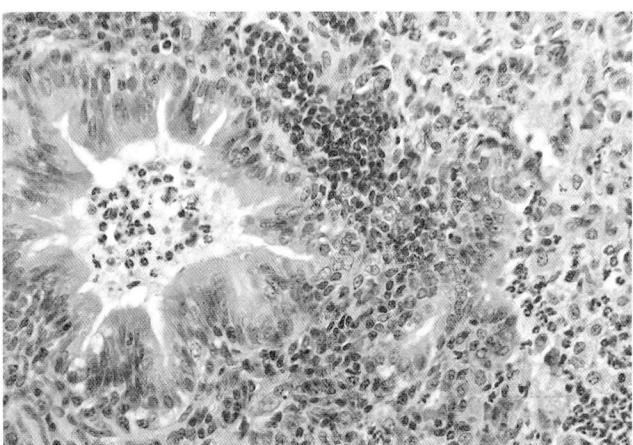

FIGURE 3.36 CAR bacillus-induced bronchiolitis and pneumonia in a mouse. The bronchiole is surrounded by lymphocytes, the lumen contains neutrophilic exudate, and the epithelium is hyperplastic. Adjacent alveoli contain neutrophils and macrophages. *Courtesy of Trenton Schoeb.*

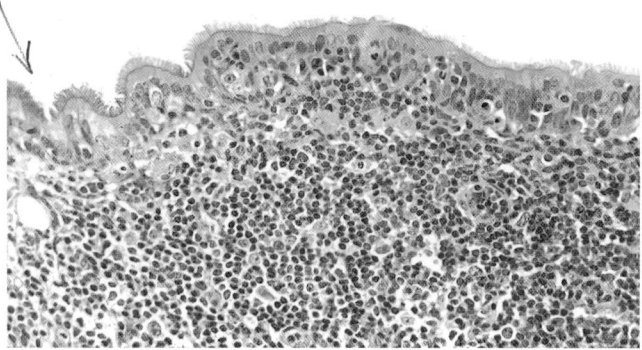

FIGURE 3.37 CAR bacillus-induced rhinitis in a mouse. The epithelium is infiltrated by neutrophils and lymphocytes, and the underlying lymphoid tissue is hyperplastic. Basophilic CAR bacilli are visible among the cilia at left. *Courtesy of Trenton Schoeb.*

in drinking water may eradicate infection (Matsushita and Suzuki, 1995) but culling or embryo rederivation is recommended.

Research Complications Infection is most often subclinical, but like other infectious agents for mice, may confound studies particularly when mice are immunocompromised (Griffith *et al.*, 1988).

d. Transmissible Murine Colonic Hyperplasia

Etiology The causative agent of transmissible murine colonic hyperplasia, *C. rodentium* (formerly *Citrobacter freundii* strain 4280), is a nonmotile, gram-negative rod that ferments lactose but does not utilize citrate or does so marginally (Barthold, 1980; Schauer *et al.*, 1995).

Clinical Signs *C. rodentium* infection can be a self-limiting colitis with sterilizing immunity or lead to severe colitis with life-threatening dehydration. Clinically apparent infection is characterized by retarded growth, ruffled fur, soft feces or diarrhea, rectal prolapse, and moderate mortality in older suckling or recently weaned mice (Barthold *et al.*, 1978).

Epizootiology *C. rodentium* is not detected in the gastrointestinal flora of normal mice, and therefore, there is not a carrier state. It is thought to be introduced by contaminated mice, food, or bedding, from which it spreads by contact or additional fecal contamination. *C. rodentium* shares several pathogenic mechanisms, such as attaching and effacing lesions mediated by the intimin receptor, with select *Escherichia coli* (reviewed in Collins *et al.* (2014)). *C. rodentium* is used experimentally to model colitis caused by enteropathogenic (EPEC) and enterohemorrhagic *E. coli* (EHEC) in humans (Mallick *et al.*, 2012; Collins *et al.*, 2014). Host genotype can influence the course and severity of disease (Barthold *et al.*, 1977). For example, DBA, NIH Swiss, and C57BL mice are relatively resistant to mortality, whereas C3H/HeJ mice are relatively susceptible both as sucklings and as adults. Interestingly, C57BL mice obtained from different

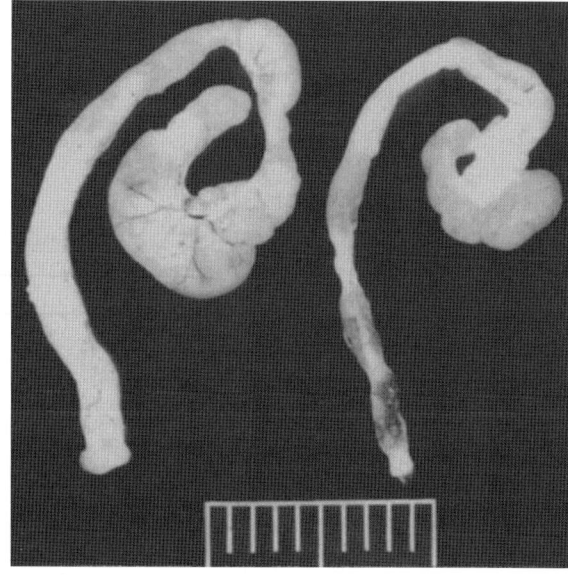

FIGURE 3.38 Colons of a normal mouse (right) and of a mouse with transmissible murine colonic hyperplasia (left). The descending colon is thickened and opaque because of mucosal hyperplasia. *From Barthold et al.* (1978).

commercial sources have varying susceptibility to *C. rodentium* (ostensibly due to the presence or absence of segmented filamentous bacteria). Diet also can modulate infection, but specific dietary factors responsible for this effect have not been identified.

Pathology *C. rodentium* attaches to the mucosa of the descending colon and displaces the normal flora. Attachment is accompanied by effacement of the microvillus border and formation of pedestal-like structures (attaching and effacing lesions) (Schauer and Falkow, 1993; Newman *et al.*, 1999). Colonization results in prominent mucosal hyperplasia, by unknown mechanisms. The characteristic gross finding is severe thickening of the descending colon, which may extend to the transverse colon and lasts for 2–3 weeks in surviving animals (Fig. 3.38). Affected colon segments are rigid and either are empty or contain semiformed feces. Histologically, accelerated mitotic activity results in a markedly hyperplastic mucosa, which may be associated with secondary inflammation and ulceration (Fig. 3.39). Lesions subside after several weeks. Intestinal repair is rapid and complete in adults but slower in sucklings.

Diagnosis Diagnosis depends on clinical signs, characteristic gross and histological lesions, and isolation of *C. rodentium* from the gastrointestinal tract or feces. The organism can be cultured on MacConkey's agar during early phases of infection, whereas the intestine may be free of *C. rodentium* during later stages of the disease. *C. rodentium* also can be detected by molecular hybridization (Schauer *et al.*, 1995).

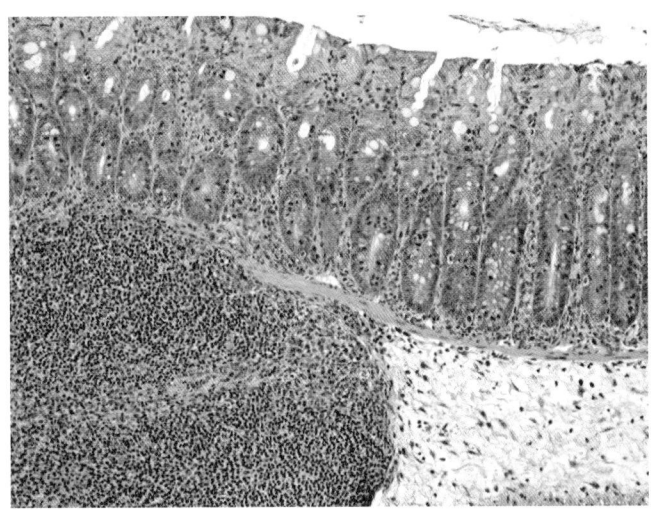

FIGURE 3.39 Colonic inflammation, edema, mild hyperplasia of the epithelium, and significant development of mucosa-associated lymphoid tissue (MALT) caused by *C. rodentium* infection. *Courtesy of Suresh Muthupalani.*

Differential Diagnosis Transmissible murine colonic hyperplasia must be differentiated from other diarrheal diseases of mice, including infections caused by coronavirus, rotavirus, adenovirus, reovirus, *Salmonella*, *C. piliforme*, and *Helicobacter* spp.

Prevention and Control Some success in curtailing epizootics has been achieved by adding antimicrobials to the drinking water (Barthold, 1980; Silverman *et al.*, 1979). Because *C. rodentium* may contaminate food, bedding, or water, proper disinfection of such materials is prudent before they are used for susceptible animals. Additionally, the employment of microbarrier caging can reduce transmission. Surveillance for *C. rodentium* should be incorporated into quality-assurance programs, and the organism screened for during quarantine of incoming mice from atypical sources.

Research Complications The potential effects on research of colonic hyperplasia as a clinically severe disease are obvious. Colonic hyperplasia has been shown to increase the sensitivity of colonic mucosa to chemical carcinogens and to decrease the latent period between administration of carcinogen and the appearance of focal atypical cell growth (Barthold and Beck, 1980). *C. rodentium* infection has been incriminated in immune dysfunction, poor reproductive performance, and failure to thrive in T-cell receptor transgenic mice (Maggio-Price *et al.*, 1998). Immunocompromised mice infected with *C. rodentium* will die from sepsis.

e. Pseudomoniasis (Lindsey *et al.*, 1991b; Percy and Barthold, 2007)

Etiology *Pseudomonas aeruginosa* is a motile, gram-negative rod.

Clinical Signs *P. aeruginosa* infections are almost always silent, but immunologically compromised animals are prone to septicemia (Brownstein, 1978). *P. aeruginosa* can, e.g., cause severe or lethal infections in athymic and SCID mice. Sick mice may have equilibrium disturbances, conjunctivitis, serosanguinous nasal discharge, edema of the head, weight loss, and skin infections. Immunosuppressed mice may also develop gastrointestinal ulcers. Generalized infection is associated with severe leukopenia, especially neutropenia. Neurologic signs are rare, but there are reports of central nervous system infection. Chronic proliferative inflammation in the cochlea and vestibular apparatus with dissolution of surrounding bone may cause torticollis.

Epizootiology *P. aeruginosa* is not considered a component of the normal flora. However, it is an opportunist that inhabits moist, warm environments such as water and skin. Once established in a host, it may be found chronically in the nasopharynx, oropharynx, and gastrointestinal tract, all sites from which additional environmental contamination or direct transmission to susceptible mice can occur.

Pathology Pathogenic infection is most common in immunodeficient mice. Organisms enter at the squamocolumnar junction of the upper respiratory tract and, in some cases, the periodontal gingiva. Bacteremia is followed by necrosis or abscess formation in the liver, spleen, or other tissues. If otitis media occurs, the tympanic bullae may contain green suppurative exudate. The bowel may be distended with fluid, and gastrointestinal ulceration has been reported.

Diagnosis Infection is diagnosed on the basis of history (e.g., immune dysfunction or recent immunosuppression), clinical signs, lesions, and isolation of *P. aeruginosa* from affected mice. Carrier mice can be detected either by nasal culture or by placing bottles of sterile, nonacidified, nonchlorinated water on cages for 24–48 h and then culturing the sipper tubes. *P. aeruginosa* can also be cultured from feces.

Differential Diagnosis Pseudomoniasis must be differentiated from other bacterial septicemias that may occur in immunodeficient mice. These include, but are not limited to, corynebacteriosis, salmonellosis, colibacillosis, staphylococcosis, and Tyzzer's disease.

Prevention and Control Infection can be prevented by acidification or hyperchlorination of the drinking water (Homberger *et al.*, 1993). These procedures will not, however, eliminate established infections. Entry of infected animals can be prevented by surveillance of commercially procured colonies. Maintenance of *Pseudomonas*-free animals usually requires barrier-quality housing and husbandry. *P. aeruginosa* has a long history in the literature of antibiotic resistance and resistance to quaternary amine disinfectants.

2.5-3.5 pH
10-15 ppm Chlorine

Research Complications *P. aeruginosa* infection is not a substantial threat to immunocompetent mice but can complicate experimental studies by causing fatal septicemia in immunodeficient mice. Viral infections that alter host defense mechanisms, such as MCMV may enhance susceptibility to pseudomoniasis.

f. Pasteurella Pneumotropica Infection (Lindsey et al., 1991a; Percy and Barthold, 2007)

Etiology   *Pasteurella pneumotropica* is a short, gram-negative rod.

Clinical Signs   Many early observations concerning the pathogenicity of *P. pneumotropica* are questionable because they were made on colonies of mice with varying levels of bacterial and viral contamination. Infection is usually subclinical. Therefore, *P. pneumotropica* is most properly viewed as an opportunistic pathogen. Studies of experimental *P. pneumotropica* suggest that it may complicate pneumonias due to *Mycoplasma pulmonis* or SV. It has also been associated with suppurative or exudative lesions of the eye, conjunctiva, skin, mammary glands, and other tissues, especially in immunodeficient mice or in mice with a predisposing primary infection.

Epizootiology   *P. pneumotropica* is a ubiquitous inhabitant of the skin, upper respiratory tract, and gastrointestinal tract of mice. Litters from infected dams can become infected during the first week after birth.

Pathology   Infections can cause suppurative inflammation, which may include abcessation. Dermatitis, conjunctivitis, dacryoadenitis, panophthalmitis, mastitis, and infections of the bulbourethral glands have been attributed to *P. pneumotropica*. Preputial and orbital abscesses also occur, especially in athymic mice (Fig. 3.40). Its role in metritis is unclear, but it has been cultured from the uterus, and there is some evidence that it may cause abortion or infertility. Cutaneous lesions can occur without systemic disease. They include suppurative lesions of the skin and subcutaneous tissues of the shoulders and trunk.

Diagnosis   Diagnosis requires isolation of the organism on standard bacteriological media. Although infection can be detected serologically by ELISA (Wullenweber-Schmidt *et al.*, 1988; Boot *et al.*, 1995a, b), subclinical carriers often do not seroconvert. PCR assays also are available (Dole *et al.*, 2010) and have shown that *P. pneumotropica* did not transmit from infected mice to contact or dirty bedding sentinels (Ouellet *et al.*, 2011; Dole *et al.*, 2013).

Differential Diagnosis   Suppurative lesions in mice may be caused by other bacteria, including *Staphylococcus, Streptococcus, Corynebacterium, Klebsiella,* and *Mycoplasma.*

Treatment   Antibiotic sensitivity testing *in vitro* indicated *P. pneumotropica* was significantly more sensitive than *P. aeruginosa* to enrofloxacin (Sasaki *et al.*, 2007). Enrofloxacin in the drinking water at 85 mg/kg daily for 7 days eliminated clinical signs and infection in a closed breeding colonic of transgenic mice and after 14 days of treatment there were no detectable carriers when the colony was screened 4 weeks later (Matsumiya and Lavoie, 2003).

Prevention and Control   Because *P. pneumotropica* is an opportunistic organism, it should be excluded from colonies containing immunodeficient mice and from breeding colonies. Achieving this goal will normally require barrier housing supported by sound microbiological monitoring. Rederivation should be considered to eliminate infection in circumstances where infection presents a potential threat to animal health or experimentation.

Research Complications   Clinically severe infection in immunodeficient mice is the major complication. Although clinically silent, experimental evidence has shown that *P. pneumotropica* infection in immunocompetent mice (C57BL/6) stimulated transcription of multiple proinflammatory cytokines for at least 7 days with residual elevation detectable 28 days later (Patten *et al.*, 2010).

g. Helicobacteriosis

Pioneering studies conducted in the 1990s first linked a novel microaerobic bacterium, *Helicobacter hepaticus*, with chronic active hepatitis and hepatic tumors in A/JCr mice (Fox *et al.*, 1994, 2011; Ward *et al.*, 1994). The organism could be visualized by electron microscopy in the bile canaliculi of the liver in susceptible mouse strains (Fig. 3.41). Subsequently, it was associated with inflammatory bowel disease in several murine models (Table 3.13) which were further developed to examine the role of immune cell subsets, such as T regulatory cells, in the pathogenesis of inflammatory bowel disease (IBD) and colon cancer (Fig. 3.42). Helicobacteriosis is

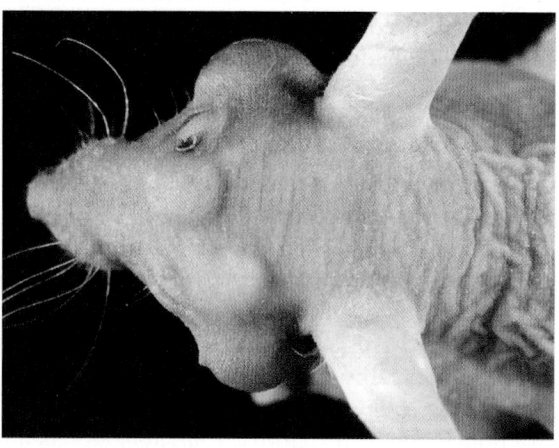

FIGURE 3.40   Multiple abscesses (head, orbita) in a nude mouse caused by *P. pneumotropica*.

now appreciated to be a common infection of laboratory mice. It is caused by a growing list of *Helicobacter* spp. that vary in clinical, pathologic, and epidemiologic significance (Whary and Fox, 2004; Fox *et al.*, 2011). Because recognition and investigation of helicobacteriosis continues to evolve, many important questions about the impact of this infection on mice remain unresolved.

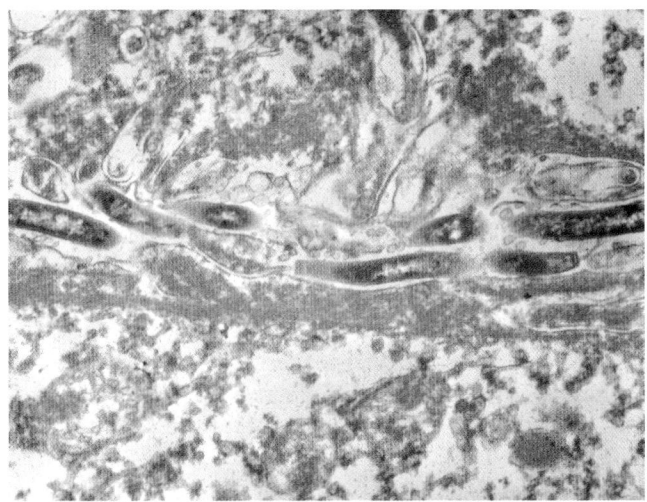

FIGURE 3.41 Electron micrograph of *H. hepaticus* in the hepatic biliary canaliculi of an SCID mouse.

H. hepaticus infection is emphasized here, because it is among the most prevalent causes of helicobacteriosis and has been studied more extensively than other murine enterohepatic *Helicobacter* spp. (EHS) (Fox *et al.*, 1994, 2011; Ward *et al.*, 1994; Suerbaum *et al.*, 2003). However, current information about other murine helicobacters is summarized in the concluding section.

Etiology *Helicobacter* spp. are gram-negative, microaerophilic, curved to spiral-shaped organisms that have been isolated from the gastrointestinal mucosa of many mammals, including humans and mice (Fox *et al.*, 2000; Whary and Fox, 2004). To date, the genus includes 20 formally named *Helicobacter* spp. assigned on the basis of 16S rRNA analysis, complemented by biochemical, molecular, and morphological characteristics. The organisms can be grown on freshly prepared antibiotic impregnated blood agar or in broth supplemented with fetal bovine serum in a microaerobic atmosphere (5% CO_2, 80% N_2, 10% H_2).

There are currently 11 formally named *Helicobacter* species have been isolated from laboratory mice, as well as several other novel *Helicobacter* spp. awaiting formal naming. Species isolated from mice include *H. hepaticus*, *H. bilis* (which also infects rats), *H. muridarum*, *H. rappini*, and *H. rodentium*, *H. ganmani*, *H. mastomyrinus*, *H. magdeburgensis*, *and H. typhlonius*, each of which

TABLE 3.13   *H. hepaticus-* and *H. bilis-*Associated IBD and Colon Cancer in Mice[a]

Genetic status of mice	Type of defect	Pathology	References
CD45RB (high)-reconstituted ICR defined flora *scids*	Reconstitution with naïve CD4[+] T cells	Typhlocolitis	Cahill *et al.* (1997)
TCRα, β mutants	Defective T-receptors	Typhlocolitis	Chin *et al.* (2000)
Scid ICR-defined flora[b]	T- and B-cell deficient	Typhlocolitis	Shomer *et al.* (1998), Shomer *et al.* (1997)
C57BL/IL-10[−/−c]	Lacks IL-10	Typhlocolitis	Burich *et al.* (2001), Kullberg *et al.* (2001), Kullberg *et al.* (2006), Kullberg *et al.* (2002)
C57BLRag2[−/−]	T- and B-cell deficient	Typhlocolitis	Burich *et al.* (2001)
129SvEv/Rag2[−/−]	T- and B-cell deficient	Typhlocolitis, colon cancer	Erdman *et al.* (2003a, 2009), Knutson *et al.* (2013), Mangerich *et al.* (2012)
IL-7[−/−]/RAG-2[−/−]	IL7, T and B cell deficiency	None	von Freeden-Jeffry *et al.* (1998)
A/JCr	Normal	Typhlitis	Fox *et al.* (1996a)
Swiss Webster gnotobiotic	Monoassociated	Enterocolitis	Fox *et al.* (1996b)
129SvEv/NF-κβ (p50[−/−]p65[+/−])	Defective NF-κβ pathway	Typhlocolitis	Erdman *et al.* (2001)
mdrla[−/−d]	Lack P-glycoprotein	Typhlocolitis	Maggio-Price *et al.* (2002)
SMAD3[−/−d]	Defective TGF-β pathway	Typhlocolitis, colon cancer	Maggio-Price *et al.* (2006)

[a]*In mice of the same genetic status which had* H. hepaticus *(or other* Helicobacter *spp.)-negative microflora, no intestinal disease was noted.*
[b]*Mice infected with* H. bilis *also developed IBD (Shomer et al., 1997).*
[c]*IBD also developed in C57Bl/IL-10[−/−] mice experimentally infected with a novel urease-negative* Helicobacter *spp. (Fox et al., 1999) now named* H. typhlonius *(Franklin et al., 2001); also IBD produced with* H. trogontum *(Whary et al., 2006) and* H. cinaedi *(Shen et al., 2009).*
[d]H. bilis *produces IBD (Maggio-Price et al., 2002, 2006) and colon cancer (Maggio-Price et al., 2006).*

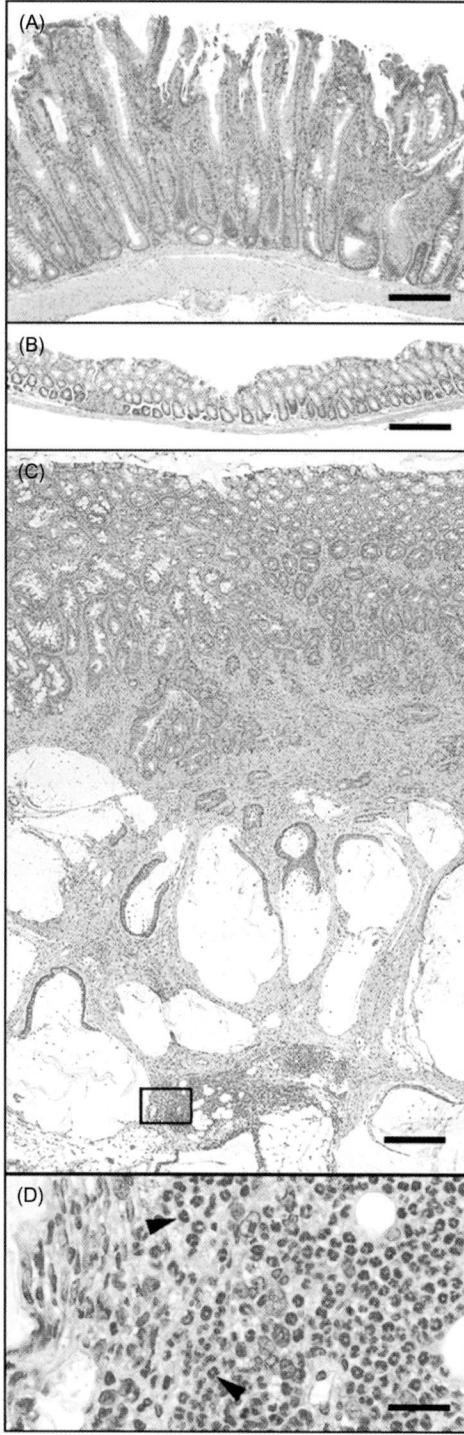

FIGURE 3.42 Regulatory cells lacking IL-10 did not suppress inflammation or dysplasia when transferred either before or after *H. hepaticus* infection. (A) Infected untreated mice developed moderate to severe inflammation, hyperplasia, and dysplasia in the cecum and colon at 4 months after infection. (B) Inflammation and dysplasia were significantly suppressed after transfer of wild-type regulatory cells. (C) Regulatory cells lacking IL-10 were unable to suppress inflammation or dysplasia. Mice receiving IL-10$^{-/-}$ regulatory cells had an increased frequency of mucinous cancer. (D) Dense inflammatory infiltrate in the mucinous tumor (inset of C) composed mainly of neutrophils (arrowheads) and a few macrophages. A–C: bar = 250 μm; D: bar = 25 μm.

have been formally named (except for *H. rappini*) (Fox and Lee, 1997; Franklin *et al.*, 1999; Whary and Fox, 2004). Most recently, *Helicobacter pullorum*, a human pathogen, has been isolated from commercial, barrier-maintained mice (Boutin *et al.*, 2010). These EHS are most commonly urease-, catalase-, and oxidase-positive. However, *H. rodentium*, *H. typhlonicus*, and another novel *Helicobacter* sp. are urease-negative.

Clinical Signs   Helicobacteriosis in adult immuno-competent mice is usually asymptomatic. Liver enzymes are elevated in *H. hepaticus*-infected A/JCr mice (Fox *et al.*, 1996a). Infection of immune-dysregulated mice with *H. hepaticus* can cause inflammatory bowel disease, which may present as rectal prolapse and/or diarrhea (Miller *et al.*, 2014).

Epizootiology   Recent surveys and anecdotal evidence suggest that helicobacteriosis is widespread among conventional and barrier-maintained mouse colonies (Shames *et al.*, 1995; Fox *et al.*, 1998b; Taylor *et al.*, 2007; Lofgren *et al.*, 2011). Furthermore, *H. hepaticus* (and probably other helicobacters) can persist in the gastrointestinal tract, particularly the cecum and colon, and is readily detected in feces. These results indicate that transmission occurs primarily by the fecal–oral route and imply that carrier mice can spread infection chronically in enzootically infected colonies.

Pathology   *Helicobacter* spp. colonize the crypts of the lower bowel, where, depending on host genotype, the organisms can be pathogenic or nonpathogenic. *H. hepaticus* and *H. bilis*, e.g., can cause inflammation in the gastrointestinal tract, which is expressed as IBD and colon cancer in immunodeficient mice or typhlitis in A/JCr mice infected with *H. hepaticus* (Ward *et al.*, 1996; Knutson *et al.*, 2013; Shomer *et al.*, 1997; Erdman *et al.*, 2003b; Nguyen *et al.*, 2013). Thickening of the cecum and large bowel develops because of proliferative typhlitis, colitis, proctitis, and lower bowel carcinoma. These lesions can occur without coincident hepatitis. Indeed, *Helicobacter* spp. induced IBD and colon carcinoma are increasingly popular models to study pathogenesis of the disease in humans (Table 3.13).

Helicobacter spp. also can cause liver disease. Bacterial translocation is thought to occur and results in colonization of the liver and progressive hepatitis. It is characterized by angiocentric nonsuppurative hepatitis and hepatic necrosis (Fig. 3.43). Inflammation originates in portal triads and spreads to adjacent hepatic parenchyma. Hepatic necrosis also may occur adjacent to intralobular venules, which can contain microthrombi. Additionally, phlebitis may affect central veins. This lesion has been linked to the presence of organisms in bile canaliculi by silver stains and electron microscopy. Age-related hepatocytic proliferation can develop in infected livers, a response that is more pronounced in male mice than in female mice (Fox *et al.*, 1996a). This lesion may

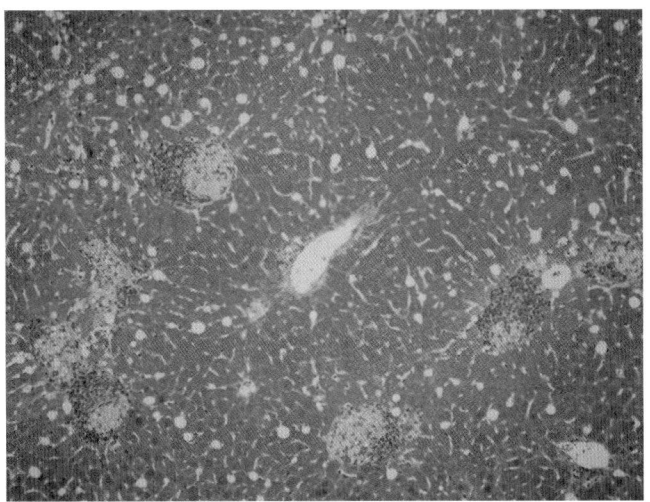

FIGURE 3.43 *H. bilis*-induced nonsuppurative hepatitis and hepatic necrosis. Inflammation originates in portal triads and spreads to adjacent hepatic parenchyma.

increase susceptibility to hepatomas and hepatocellular carcinomas among aged male A/JCr and B6C3F1 mice from infected colonies. An increased incidence of hepatic hemangiosarcoma also has been noted in *H. hepaticus*-infected male B6C3F1 mice. In this context, A/JCr, C3H/HeNCr, and SJL/NCr mice are susceptible to hepatitis, whereas C57BL/6 mice are resistant (Ward *et al.*, 1994). The finding of severe liver disease and tumor induction in B6C3F1 mice infected with *H. hepaticus* infers that genetic susceptibility to *H. hepaticus*-induced neoplasia has a dominant pattern of inheritance. Studies with *H. hepaticus* in recombinant inbred mice also indicate that disease susceptibility has multigenetic properties (Hailey *et al.*, 1998; Fox and Lee, 1997; Ihrig *et al.*, 1999; Franklin, 2006; Hillhouse *et al.*, 2011).

Diagnosis Rapid generic diagnosis can be accomplished by PCR detection of the highly conserved 16S rRNA region of the *Helicobacter* genome in feces or tissues, using suitable oligonucleotide primers (Fox *et al.*, 1998a; Shames *et al.*, 1995; Beckwith *et al.*, 1997). However, genus-specific PCR does not differentiate among different *Helicobacter* spp. Molecular speciation can be accomplished by 16S rRNA sequencing, restriction fragment length polymorphism analysis of the PCR product or use of species-specific PCR assays. This procedure requires suitable skill and experience to avoid technological pitfalls and should be performed by qualified laboratories. An IgG ELISA using the outer membrane protein as the antigen has been proposed for serological diagnosis, but shared antigens among EHS create lack of specificity for the assay. As noted above, helicobacters can be isolated on antibiotic-impregnated blood agar under microaerobic conditions and can then be speciated biochemically, and by *Helicobacter* species-specific PCR. Isolation of

H. hepaticus and from other *Helicobacter* spp. with spiral to curved morphology from feces should be preceded by passing slurried samples through a 0.45-μm filter before plating. If infection with larger fusiform helicobacters (*H. bilis*, *H. rappini*) is suspected, filtration at 0.65 μm is preferred. Helicobacters grow slowly and require prolonged incubation of cultures (up to 3 weeks) before they can be deemed negative. Signs (rectal prolapse) and lesions (hepatitis, typhlocolitis), depending on host genotype, can be suggestive of infection. Histopathological examination should include silver stains, especially of liver, to attempt to visualize spiral or curved organisms (Whary and Fox, 2004).

Differential Diagnosis Clinically apparent helicobacteriosis must be differentiated from other gastrointestinal or hepatic infections of mice. Coronavirus infection, *Clostridium piliforme*, and *Salmonella* spp. can cause enterocolitis and/or hepatitis. *C. rodentium* also causes colonic hyperplasia, which can present as rectal prolapse.

Infections Caused by Other Helicobacters of Mice *H. bilis* has been isolated from the livers and intestines of aged mice and experimentally induces IBD in SCID mice as does *H. hepaticus*. *H. bilis* also experimentally produces lower bowel cancer in immunocompromised mice (Nguyen *et al.*, 2013). *Helicobacter muridarum* colonizes the ileum, cecum, and colon. It appears to be nonpathogenic, although it can colonize the stomach of mice and induce gastritis under certain circumstances. *H. 'rappini'* has been isolated from the feces of mice without clinical signs. *H. rodentium* also colonizes the intestine and may be a component of normal flora. A dual infection of *H. bilis* and *H. rodentium* was noted in a natural outbreak of IBD in immunocompromised mice (Shomer *et al.*, 1998). A novel urease negative helicobacter, which has been named *H. typhlonius*, causes IBD in IL-10$^{-/-}$ and SCID mice (Franklin *et al.*, 1999, 2001; Fox *et al.*, 1999). Decreased reproductive efficiency has been reported in IL10 knockout mice infected with *H. rodentium* and/or *H. typhlonius* (Sharp *et al.*, 2008).

Prevention and Control Eradication of infection from small numbers of mice, such as quarantine groups, can be achieved by standard rederivation or intensive antibiotic therapy. The best results have been obtained by triple therapy with amoxicillin, metronidazole, and bismuth given for 2 weeks (Del Carmen Martino-Cardona *et al.*, 2010). This strategy requires repeated daily gavage rather than administration in drinking water, but it has successfully eliminated *H. hepaticus* from naturally infected mice. Antibiotic impregnated wafers have been used to eradicate *Helicobacter* spp. in mouse colonies (Kerton and Warden, 2006). Wide-scale, eradication of enzootic helicobacteriosis can be expensive and time-consuming, without guarantee of success. Careful husbandry procedures can limit infection within a colony (Whary *et al.*, 2000). Therefore, strategies have to be weighed carefully against risks of enzootic infection for the health and use of mice. In contrast, infection should be avoided in immunodeficient mice, including genetically engineered mice with targeted or serendipitous immune dysfunction. Lastly, the outcome of opportunistic helicobacteriosis has not been thoroughly examined. This condition could occur during simultaneous infection with two or more *Helicobacter* species or during combined infection with an intestinal virus (e.g., coronavirus) and *Helicobacter* spp. If highly valuable animals are exposed, antibiotic therapy or rederivation may be warranted.

Research Complications   Chronic inflammation of the liver and or gastrointestinal tract may be injurious to health. Additionally, it may impede the development and assessment of noninfectious disease models, such as IBD models in mice with targeted deletions in T-lymphocyte receptors (Fox *et al.*, 2011). *H. hepaticus* infections provoke a strong Th1 proinflammatory response, which may perturb other immunological responses. *H. hepaticus* infection also has been incriminated as a cofactor or promoter in the development of hepatic neoplasia in A/ JCr, B6C3F1, AB6F1, B6AF1, and CARKO mice (Hailey *et al.*, 1998; Fox *et al.*, 1998a; Garcia *et al.*, 2008, 2011).

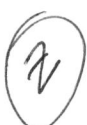

h. Salmonellosis (Ganaway, 1982; Lindsey *et al.*, 1991c; Percy and Barthold, 2007)

Etiology   The genus *Salmonella* contains two species, *S. bongori* which infects mainly poikilotherms and rarely, humans, and *S. enterica* which includes approximately 2500 serovars and are a major cause of food-borne illness in humans (Fookes *et al.*, 2011). The salmonella of historical importance in mice that are now rare include *S. enterica* subsp. *enterica* serovar Typhimurium (aka *S. Typhimurium*) and serovar Enteritidis (*S. Enteritidis*). *S. Enteritidis* is a motile, gram-negative rod that rarely ferments lactose. The genomes of many strains have been sequenced. Virulence factors carried on pathogenicity islands and plasmids include antimicrobial resistance genes, type III secretion systems, Vi antigen, lipopolysaccharide and other surface polysaccharides, flagella, and factors essential for a intracellular life cycle in macrophages (de Jong *et al.*, 2012). Pathogen-associated molecular patterns (PAMPs) unique to salmonella interact with TLRs and NOD-like receptors (NLRs) which recruit neutrophils and macrophages leading to inflammasome formation and release of pro-inflammatory IL-6, IL-1β, TNF-α, and IFN-γ.

Clinical Signs   Acute infection is especially severe in young mice (Casebolt and Schoeb, 1988). It is characterized by anorexia, weight loss, lethargy, dull coat, humped posture, and occasionally conjunctivitis. Gastroenteritis is a common sign, but feces may remain formed. Subacute infection can produce distended abdomens from hepatomegaly and splenomegaly. Chronic disease is expressed as anorexia and weight loss. Enzootic salmonellosis in a breeding colony can produce episodic disease with alternating periods of quiescence and high mortality. The latter can be associated with diarrhea, anorexia, weight loss, roughened hair coat, and reduced production.

Epizootiology   *S. Typhimurium* is commonly used experimentally and cross-contamination in a mouse facility is a risk. Modern production and husbandry methods have reduced the importance of salmonellosis as a natural infection of mice. However, the organisms are widespread in nature. Therefore, cross-infection from other species or from feral mice remains a potential hazard. Salmonellas are primarily intestinal microorganisms that can contaminate food and water supplies. Infection occurs primarily by ingestion. Salmonella have a broad host range and vermin, birds, feral rodents, and human carriers are potential sources of infection. Other common laboratory species such as nonhuman primates, dogs, and cats also can serve as carriers. Conversely, murine salmonellosis presents a zoonotic hazard to humans.

The induction and course of infection are influenced by the virulence and dose of the organism, route of infection, host sex and genetic factors, nutrition, and intercurrent disease. Suckling and weanling mice are more susceptible to disease than mature mice. Immune deficiency, exposure to heavy metals, and environmental factors such as abnormal ambient temperatures can increase the severity of disease. Nutritional iron deficiency has an attenuating effect on *Salmonella* infection in mice, whereas iron overload appears to promote bacterial growth and enhance virulence. Resistance to natural infection is increased by the presence of normal gastrointestinal microflora. Resistance to infection also can be an inherited trait among inbred strains. Among the most important considerations is that mice that recover from acute infection can become subclinical carriers and a chronic source of contamination from fecal shedding.

Pathology   The virulence of *S. Enteritidis* depends on its ability to penetrate intestinal walls, enter lymphatic tissue, multiply, and disseminate. Organisms reach Peyer's patches within 12 h after inoculation and spread quickly to the mesenteric lymph nodes. Bacteremia results in spread to other lymph nodes, spleen, and liver within several days. In chronic infections, organisms persist in the spleen and lymph nodes as well as in the liver and gallbladder and from the latter are discharged into the intestinal contents. Bacteria reaching the intestine can reinvade the mucosa and can be shed intermittently in the feces for months. *S. Enteritidis* infection also has been associated with chronic arthritis.

Acute deaths may occur without gross lesions, but visceral hyperemia, pale livers, and catarrhal enteritis are more common. If mice survive for up to several weeks, the intestine may be distended and reddened, whereas the liver and spleen are enlarged and contain yellow–gray foci of necrosis. Affected lymph nodes are also enlarged, red, and focally necrotic. Focal inflammation can develop in many organs, including the myocardium (Percy and Barthold, 2007).

Histologic lesions reflect the course of disease and the number of bacteria in affected tissues. During acute infection, necrotic foci are found in the intestine, mesenteric lymph nodes, liver, and spleen. Neutrophilic leukocytes and histiocytes accumulate in lymphoid tissues. Thrombosis from septic venous embolism may occur, especially in the liver. Granulomatous lesions are particularly characteristic of chronic salmonellosis, especially in the liver.

Diagnosis Diagnosis is based on isolation of salmonellas together with documentation of compatible clinical signs and lesions. In mice with systemic disease, bacteria may persist in the liver and spleen for weeks. During acute stages, bacteria can also be isolated from the blood. Subclinically infected animals can be detected by fecal culture using selective enrichment media (Selenite F broth plus cystine followed by streaking on brilliant green agar). Culture of the mesenteric lymph nodes may be more reliable, because fecal shedding can be intermittent. Isolates can be speciated with commercial serotyping reagents. Alternatively, isolates can be sent to a reference laboratory for confirmation. Antibodies to salmonellas can be detected in the serum of infected mice by an agglutination test. However, this method is not entirely reliable, because serological cross-reactivity is common even among bacteria of different genera. PCR-based assays are also available.

Differential Diagnosis Salmonellosis must be differentiated from other bacterial diseases, including Tyzzer's disease, *Helicobacter* spp., pseudomoniasis, corynebacteriosis, *C. rodentium*, and pasteurellosis. Viral infections that cause enteritis or hepatitis must also be considered, especially infections caused by coronavirus, ectromelia virus, and reoviruses. Among noninfectious conditions, mesenteric lymphadenopathy is an aging-associated lesion in mice and is not indicative of chronic salmonellosis.

Prevention and Control Salmonellosis can be prevented by proper husbandry and sanitation. Contact between mice and potential carriers, such as nonhuman primates, dogs, and cats, should be prevented. Diets should be cultured periodically to check for inadvertent contamination. Contaminated colonies should be replaced to eliminate infection and its zoonotic potential.

Research Complications Apart from the clinical manifestations, the zoonotic potential for salmonellosis is a major concern. This includes transmission among laboratory species, but especially between mice and the personnel working with them.

i. Streptobacillosis (Lindsey *et al.*, 1991e; Percy and Barthold, 2007)

Etiology *Streptobacillus moniliformis* is a nonmotile, gram-negative, pleomorphic rod that can exist as a nonpathogenic L-phase variant *in vivo*. However, it can revert to the virulent bacillus form.

Clinical Signs Streptobacillosis generally has an acute phase with high mortality, followed by a subacute phase and finally a chronic phase that may persist for months. Signs of acute disease include a dull, damp hair coat and keratoconjunctivitis. Variable signs include anemia, diarrhea, hemoglobinuria, cyanosis, and emaciation. Cutaneous ulceration, arthritis, and gangrenous amputation may occur during chronic infection. The arthritis can leave joints deformed and ankylosed. Hindlimb paralysis with urinary bladder distention, incontinence, kyphosis, and priapism may occur if vertebral lesions impinge on motor nerves. Breeding mice may have stillbirths or abortions.

Epizootiology Streptobacillosis has historical importance as a disease of rats and mice, but modern husbandry, production, and health surveillance strategies have reduced its impact dramatically (Wullenweber, 1995). Subclinical, persistently infected rats are the most likely source of dissemination to mice, but mouse-to-mouse transmission then ensues. Transmission may occur from aerogenic exposure, bite wounds, or contaminated equipment, feed, or bedding. *S. moniliformis* is also pathogenic for humans, causing rat bite fever (Haverhill fever).

Pathology During acute disease, necrotic lesions develop in thoracic and abdominal viscera, especially in the liver, spleen, and lymph nodes. Histological lesions include necrosis, septic thrombosis of small vessels, acute inflammation, fibrin deposition, and abscesses. Chronically infected mice may develop purulent polyarthritis because of the organism's affinity for joints.

Diagnosis Diagnosis depends on clinical and pathological evidence of septicemia and isolation of the organism on blood agar. The organism has been recovered from joint fluid as long as 26 months after infection. Isolation from chronic lesions requires serum-enriched medium. *S. moniliformis* as a cause of septic joints in humans has been diagnosed using PCR and electrospray-ionization followed by mass spectrometry (Mackey *et al.*, 2014).

Differential Diagnosis Clinical signs must be differentiated from septicemic conditions, including mousepox, Tyzzer's disease, corynebacteriosis, salmonellosis, mycoplasmosis, pseudomoniasis, and traumatic lesions.

Prevention and Control Control is based on exclusion of wild rodents or carrier animals such as latently infected laboratory rats. Bacterins and antibiotic therapy are not adequately effective. The potential for cross-infection is a reason not to house rats and mice in the same room.

Research Complications   Infection can be disabling or lethal in mice and has zoonotic potential for humans.

j. Corynebacteriosis (Lindsey *et al.*, 1982; Weisbroth, 1994; Percy and Barthold, 2007)

Etiology   Corynebacteria are short gram-positive rods. *Corynebacterium kutscheri* is the cause of pseudotuberculosis in mice and rats. *Corynebacterium bovis* has been associated with hyperkeratosis, especially in immunodeficient mice (Clifford *et al.*, 1995; Scanziani *et al.*, 1998; Dole *et al.*, 2013).

Clinical Signs   *C. kutscheri* infection is often subclinical in otherwise healthy mice. Active disease is precipitated by immunosuppression or environmental stresses and is expressed as an acute illness with high mortality or a chronic syndrome with low mortality. Clinical signs include inappetence, emaciation, rough hair coat, hunched posture, hyperpnea, nasal and ocular discharge, cutaneous ulceration, and arthritis. *C. bovis* infection causes hyperkeratotic dermatitis characterized by scaly skin, which is accompanied by alopecia in haired mice. Severe infection may cause death. Corynebacterial keratoconjunctivitis has been reported in aged C57BL/6 mice (McWilliams *et al.*, 1993).

Epizootiology   Subclinically infected animals harbor *C. kutscheri* in the upper alimentary tract, colon, respiratory tract, regional lymph nodes, middle ear, and preputial gland. *C. bovis* colonizes skin and is shed in feces. Therefore, transmission is by direct contact, fecal–oral contact, and aerosol. Resistance to infection appears to be under genetic control in some mouse strains. Rats are susceptible to *C. kutscheri*, so cross-infection to mice may occur.

Pathology   Lesions caused by *C. kutscheri* develop from hematogenous spread to various internal organs and appear as gray–white nodules in the kidney, liver, lung, and other sites. Cervical lymphadenopathy and arthritis of the carpometacarpal and tarsometatarsal joints also may occur. Septic, necrotic lesions often contain caseous material or liquefied exudate. Histologic lesions are characterized by coagulative or caseous necrosis bordered by intense neutrophilic infiltration. Colonies of gram-positive organisms with 'Chinese letter' configurations can usually be demonstrated using tissue Gram stains of caseous lesions. Mucopurulent arthritis of carpal, metacarpal, tarsal, and metatarsal joints are related to bacterial colonization of synovium accompanied by necrosis, cartilage erosion, ulceration, and eventually ankylosing pan arthritis. *C. kutscheri* is not a primary skin pathogen, but skin ulcers or fistulas follow bacterial embolization and infarction of dermal vessels. Subcutaneous abscesses have also been reported.

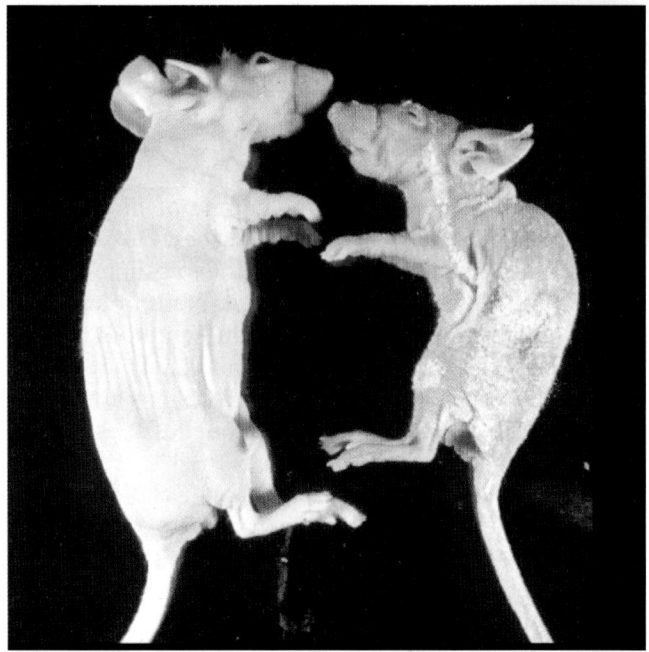

FIGURE 3.44   Hyperkeratosis associated with *C. bovis* infection.

"CHINESE LETTER" BACTERIA

Hyperkeratotic dermatitis caused by *C. bovis* is characterized grossly by skin scaliness and alopecia. Microscopically, skin lesions consist of prominent acanthosis and moderate hyperkeratosis accompanied by mild nonsuppurative inflammation (Fig. 3.44). Hyperkeratosis is typically more severe in glabrous athymic mice than in haired mice. Organisms can be demonstrated in hyperkeratotic layers by Gram stain.

Diagnosis   *C. kutscheri* is usually diagnosed by culture and tissue Gram stains on lesions from clinically apparent cases. Agglutination serology is available, and immunofluorescence, immunodiffusion, and ELISA tests have been reported (Boot *et al.*, 1995a). PCR of skin swabs or feces is a sensitive and specific method for the detection of *C. bovis* infection in mice (Dole *et al.*, 2013).

Differential Diagnosis   The caseous nature of *C. kutscheri*-induced lesions helps separate them from necrotic changes or abscesses caused by other infectious agents of mice. Thus, they can be differentiated from streptococcosis, mycoplasmosis, and other septicemic bacterial infections in which caseous necrosis does not occur. Because mice can sustain natural infections with *Mycobacterium avium*, histochemical techniques for acid-fast bacilli and appropriate culture methods for mycobacteria should be considered if nodular inflammatory lesions of the lung are detected. Diffuse scaling dermatitis in athymic nude mice is classic for *C. bovis* infection; however, in one case report *Staphylococcus xylosus* was instead isolated in high numbers from the skin lesions (Russo *et al.*, 2013). Hyperkeratotic dermatitis caused by

C. bovis must be differentiated from scaly skin caused by low humidity in glabrous mice.

Prevention and Control *C. kutscheri* infection occurs sporadically and infected colonies should be culled or rederived into an SPF facility as treatment is not curative and control is difficult.

C. bovis can be endemic in athymic nude mouse colonies. Prevention and control are difficult because both immunocompetent and athymic mice as well as humans can carry *C. bovis* on the skin and in the upper respiratory system, respectively. *C. bovis* readily contaminates the environment as aerosolization within a class II biosafety cabinet was shown to spread the bacterium during cage-change procedures (Burr *et al.*, 2012). Antibiotic treatment has been unrewarding (Burr *et al.*, 2011)

Research Complications Corynebacteriosis can cause morbidity and mortality, especially among immunodeficient mice. Dermatologic disease in suckling mice can be fatal but is less severe and transient in weanling mice.

k. Staphylococcosis (Lindsey *et al.*, 1991d; Shimizu, 1994; Percy and Barthold, 2007; Besch-Williford and Franklin, 2007)

Etiology Staphylococci are gram-positive organisms that commonly infect skin and mucous membranes of mice and other animals. The two most frequently encountered species are *Staphylococcus aureus*, which can be highly pathogenic, and *S. epidermidis*, which is generally nonpathogenic. Species subtypes are identified by phage typing and biochemistry profiles. Pathogenic staphylococci are typically coagulase-positive, although *S. xylosus* has caused serious infections and is coagulase-negative (Gozalo *et al.*, 2010).

Clinical Signs Staphylococcosis causes suppurative conjunctivitis, periorbital and retroorbital abscesses, preputial adenitis, and pyoderma in mice, particularly in immunocompromised strains such as nude mice. Some evidence suggests that staphylococci can produce primary cutaneous infections, but they are more likely opportunistic organisms that induce lesions after contamination of skin wounds. Eczematous dermatitis develops primarily on the face, ears, neck, shoulders, and forelegs and can progress to ulcerative dermatitis, abscessation (including botryomycotic granulomas), and cellulitis. Because lesions are often pruritic, scratching causes additional trauma and autoinoculation. Staphylococcal infection in the genital mucosa of males may produce preputial gland abscesses. These occur as firm, raised nodules in the inguinal region or at the base of the penis and may rupture to spread infection to surrounding tissues. Male mice also may develop septic balanoposthitis secondary to penile self-mutilation. Retrobulbar abscesses caused by *S. aureus* are frequently

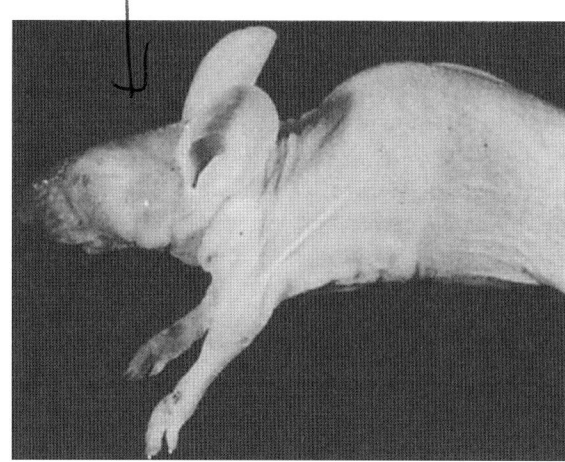

FIGURE 3.45　Furunculosis in an athymic mouse.

noted in athymic mice. SJL mice, which are NK cell deficient, are prone to necrotic dermatitis on the tail secondary to *S. xylosus* infection.

Epizootiology Staphylococci are ubiquitous and can be carried on the skin and in the nasopharynx and gastrointestinal tract. They also can be cultured from cages, room surfaces, and personnel. The prevalence of staphylococcal dermatitis appears to be influenced by host genotype, the overall health of the animal, and the degree of environmental contamination with *Staphylococcus* spp. C57BL/6, C3H, DBA, and BALB/c mice are among the most susceptible strains. Age may also influence susceptibility, with young mice being more susceptible than adults. Immunodeficient mice (e.g., athymic mice) contaminated with staphylococci often develop abscesses or furunculosis (Fig. 3.45). As noted above, behavioral dysfunction resulting in self-mutilation, including scratching and trichotillomania, is a likely predisposing factor. Once virulent staphylococci contaminate the environment, colonization of the gastrointestinal tract can occur and produce a carrier state. Phage typing can help to determine the source of infection. Human phage types of staphylococci can infect mice, but the zoonotic importance of this connection is not clear.

Pathology Gross lesions are typified by suppurative, ulcerative and necrotic dermatitis involving the head and neck but may extend to the shoulders and forelegs (Percy and Barthold, 2007). Superficial or deep abscesses may occur in conjunction with dermatitis or separately, as, e.g., in the external male genitalia. Histologically, acute skin infections result in ulceration with neutrophils in the dermis and subcutis. Chronic lesions contain lymphocytes, macrophages, and fibroblasts. Deep infections appear as coalescing botryomycotic pyogranulomas with necrotic centers containing bacterial colonies. Infected athymic mice may develop

"BUNCH of GRAPES"

furunculosis of the muzzle and face accompanied by regional lymphadenitis.

Diagnosis Diagnosis is made by documenting gross and histological lesions, including Gram staining of suspect tissues, complemented by isolation of gram-positive, coagulase-positive (*S. aureus*), or coagulase-negative *Staphylococcus* species.

Differential Diagnosis Staphylococcosis must be differentiated from other suppurative infections of mice, including pasteurellosis, streptococcosis, corynebacteriosis, and pseudomoniasis. Ectoparasitism, fight wounds, and self-mutilation *per se* should also be considered.

Prevention, Control, and Treatment Removal of affected animals, sterilization of food and bedding, and frequent changing of bedding may limit or reduce transmission. In affected animals, nail trimming can reduce self-inflicted trauma. Conditions that facilitate aggressive or self-mutilating behavior should be avoided.

Research Complications Staphylococcosis can cause illness and disfigurement in mice. Immunodeficient mice are at increased risk.

l. Streptococcosis (Lindsey *et al.*, 1991f; Nakayama and Weyant, 1994; Percy and Barthold, 2007; Besch-Williford and Franklin, 2007)

Etiology Streptococci are ubiquitous commensal gram-positive organisms and in some cases, primary pathogens. Pathogenic streptococcal infections in laboratory mice are caused by β-hemolytic organisms in Lancefield's group C, but epizootics caused by group A streptococci have occurred, and group G organisms have been isolated occasionally. Group D has been reclassified as an *Enterococcus*. Alpha-hemolytic streptococci can cause systemic disease in SCID mice, and group B *Streptococcus* sp. infection has been reported to cause meningoencephalitis in athymic mice (Schenkman *et al.*, 1994). Additionally, *Streptococcus dysgalactiae* subsp. *equisimilis* has Lancefield group G or C antigens and was isolated from visceral abscesses of immunocompetent mice (Greenstein *et al.*, 1994).

Clinical Signs Cutaneous infections can cause ulcerative dermatitis over the trunk, which may appear gangrenous, whereas systemic infections may be expressed as conjunctivitis, rough hair coat, hyperpnea, somnolescence, and emaciation.

Epizootiology Mice can carry streptococci subclinically in their upper respiratory tracts. Lethal epizootics can occur, but factors leading to clinical disease are unknown, although some infections may be secondary to wound contamination.

Pathology Systemic lesions reflect hematogenous dissemination and include abscessation, endocarditis, splenomegaly, and lymphadenopathy (Percy and Barthold, 2007). Streptococcal cervical lymphadenitis can lead to fistulous drainage to the neck complicated by

ulcerative dermatitis. Infection with α-hemolytic streptococci can cause inflammatory lesions affecting kidney and heart.

Diagnosis Diagnosis and differential diagnosis depend on isolation of organisms from infected tissues, combined with histopathologic confirmation.

Differential Diagnosis Streptococcosis must be differentiated from other suppurative infections of mice, including staphylococcosis, pasteurellosis, corynebacteriosis, and pseudomoniasis.

Prevention and Control Removal of affected animals, sterilization of food and bedding, and frequent changing of bedding may limit or reduce transmission.

Research Complications Immunodeficient mice are at increased risk for streptococcosis.

m. Colibacillosis (Percy and Barthold, 2007)

Etiology *E. coli* is a small gram-negative rod that is a normal inhabitant of the mouse intestine.

Epizootiology Infection is considered nonpathogenic in immunocompetent mice. However, hyperplastic typhlocolitis resembling transmissible murine colonic hyperplasia has been reported in SCID mice infected with a non-lactose-fermenting *E. coli* (Waggie *et al.*, 1988; Arthur *et al.*, 2012).

Clinical Signs Affected mice develop lethargy and fecal staining.

Pathology Gross lesions consist of segmental thickening of the colon or cecum, which may contain blood-tinged feces. Microscopically, affected mucosa is hyperplastic and may be inflamed and eroded.

Diagnosis Diagnosis depends on demonstrating lesions and isolating non-lactose-fermenting *E. coli*.

Differential Diagnosis This condition must be differentiated from proliferative and inflammatory intestinal disease caused by *Lawsonia intracellularis*, *C. rodentium*, or enterotropic mouse hepatitis virus, especially in immunodeficient mice. Colibacillosis provides an example of the morbidity associated with a nominally innocuous organism when it affects an immunocompromised host.

Prevention and Control Removal of affected animals and disinfection of caging and equipment will limit or reduce transmission.

Research Complications Clinical illness may develop in immunodeficient mice.

n. Klebsiellosis

Historically, *Klebsiella pneumoniae* is a ubiquitous gram-negative organism that is a natural inhabitant of the mouse alimentary tract. Most commercial vendors have excluded it from their barriers. It can be pathogenic for the respiratory and urinary tract of mice after experimental inoculation but is not a significant cause of naturally occurring disease.

Etiology   *Klebsiella oxytoca* is an opportunistic pathogen implicated in various clinical diseases in animals and humans.

Epizootiology   *K. oxytoca* also is purported to be an etiological agent of antibiotic-associated hemorrhagic colitis (AAHC) in adult humans and adolescents. In animals, *K. oxytoca* has been isolated from apparently healthy sentinel rodents being monitored for pathogens in health surveillance programs and from utero-ovarian infections including suppurative endometritis, salpingitis, perioophoritis, and peritonitis in aged B6C3F1 mice (Davis *et al.*, 1987; Rao *et al.*, 1987). A model of AAHC has been developed in rats by administering amoxicillin-clavulanate followed by orally infecting rats with a strain of *K. oxytoca* cultured from a patient with AAHC. Studies in humans suggest that *K. oxytoca* exerts its pathogenicity in part through a cytotoxin. Recently, authors have showed that several animal isolates of *K. oxytoca*, including clinical isolates, produced secreted products in bacterial culture supernatant that display cytotoxicity on HEp-2 and HeLa cells, indicating the ability to produce cytotoxin. Using mass spectroscopy techniques, they also confirmed tilivalline as the cytotoxin present in animal *K. oxytoca* strains. Tilivalline may serve as a biomarker for *K. oxytoca*-induced cytotoxicity (Darby *et al.*, 2014).

Clinical Signs   *K. oxytoca* has been cultured from cases of suppurative otitis media, urogenital tract infections, and pneumonia in C3H/HeJ and NMRI-Foxn1 (*nu*) mice (Bleich *et al.*, 2008). Additionally, *K. oxytoca* was recently cultured from three breeding colonies of NOD. Cg-Prkdc^scid^ Il2rg^tm1Wjl^/SzJ (NSG) mice with chronic renal inflammation and ascending urinary tract infections (Foreman *et al.*, 2011).

Differential Diagnosis   Other bacterial infections capable of causing suppurative lesions, including staphylococci, streptococci, *Pasteurella* sp., and *E. coli*, among others are considered a differential diagnosis.

Research Complications   Morbidity and mortality from spontaneous infections can affect ongoing research.

o. Clostridium Infections

CLOSTRIDIUM DIFFICILE

Etiology   *Clostridium difficile* was identified as the etiology of antimicrobial-associated pseudomembranous colitis in humans and currently a considerable cause of morbidity in hospitalized patients who acquire nosocomial infections. In the early 2000s, an increased interest in *C. difficile* infection (CDI) resulted from the emergence of a hyper-virulent strain (NAP1/BI/027) associated with frequent recurrences and more severe clinical disease (Abou Chakra *et al.*, 2014; McFarland, 2009; Kuijper *et al.*, 2006). *C. difficile* has also been implicated in antibiotic-associated colitis in Syrian hamsters (Bartlett *et al.*, 1977), guinea pigs (Lowe *et al.*, 1980), rabbits (Thilsted *et al.*,

1981; Ryden *et al.*, 1991), prairie dogs (Muller *et al.*, 1987), ostriches (Frazier *et al.*, 1993), and horses (Diab *et al.*, 2013). *C. difficile* is a rod-shaped strict anaerobe. Cycloserine-cefoxitin-fructose agar (CCFA) is a commonly used selective medium for *C. difficile*. Cultures are incubated under anaerobic conditions at 35–37°C. When grown on blood agar, *C. difficile* colonies are nonhemolytic and gray, and have a slightly raised umbonate profile with filamentous edges and a ground-glass appearance. Colonies grown on blood agar have fluorescence under ultraviolet light. *C. difficile* forms acid from glucose and fructose, but is negative on lactose, maltose, and sucrose. Two closely related exotoxins, Toxin A and Toxin B, are produced by *C. difficile*. Recent taxonomic classification support placement of *C. difficile* and its close relatives within the family Peptostreptococcaceae. The authors suggested renaming it *Peptoclostridium difficile* (Yutin and Galperin, 2013).

Epizootiology   It is estimated that *C. difficile* spores germinate and establish infection less than 10h after ingestion. Spores rapidly transit through the upper gastrointestinal tract and colonize the colon and cecum. Spore shedding begins less than 2h postingestion. When C57BL mice were challenged with 10^8 CFU of *C. difficile* spores, severe CDI signs developed and all mice were clinically affected by 48h postchallenge (Chen *et al.*, 2008).

Specific methods to control and prevent *C. difficile* infections in mice have not been described. Given the method of transmission of *C. difficile* and *C. perfringens* are via ingestion or spores, these clostridia can probably be excluded from mouse colonies by maintaining strict husbandry practices, robust sanitation, and use of autoclaved feed, bedding, cages, and cage accessories. Sudden dietary changes should be avoided and antibiotics should be used judiciously to minimize disruption of the normal gut microbiota of mice.

Diagnosis of *C. difficile*-associated disease is generally based on detection of cytotoxin using a tissue culture cytotoxicity assay. PCR assays for detection of both *C. difficile* and its cytotoxins have been developed (Eastwood *et al.*, 2009). There are no published regimens specifically for the treatment of natural *C. difficile* infections in mice. Oral doses given twice daily of 2mg vancomycin for 7 days to experimentally infected gnotobiotic mice caused a 2- to 3-log decrease in vegetative bacterial cell count and no detectable cytotoxin. Bacterial counts and cytotoxin levels returned to previous levels after treatment was discontinued.

Clinical Signs   Untreated mice are relatively resistant to infection with *C. difficile* and do not develop fatal infections, although these mice can become asymptomatic carriers that persistently shed low numbers of spores (Lawley *et al.*, 2009). Susceptibility of mice to infection must be induced by disrupting the microbiota through antibiotic treatment. Brief exposure to environmental spore contamination is sufficient for transmission of *C. difficile* to naïve but susceptible mice. The CDI transmission model has been used to demonstrate that clindamycin treatment of asymptomatic carriers of *C. difficile* can inadvertently trigger the excretion of high levels of spores (Lawley *et al.*, 2009). A C57BL mouse model of recurrence/relapse CDI has been reported (Sun *et al.*, 2011). The primary bout of CDI induced little or no protective antibody response against *C. difficile* toxins and mice continued shedding *C. difficile* spores. Antibiotic treatment of surviving mice induced a second episode of diarrhea. A simultaneous reexposure of mice to *C. difficile* bacteria or spores elicited a full clinical spectrum of CDI similar to that of the primary infection. Immunosuppressive agents resulted in more severe and fulminant recurrent disease. Vancomycin treatment only delayed disease recurrence; however, neutralizing polysera against both TcdA and TcdB completely protected mice against CDI relapse (Sun *et al.*, 2011). A recent study in C57BL mice demonstrated that antibiotic-mediated alteration of the gut microbiome favors a global metabolic profile, and therefore increases susceptibility to *C. difficile* clinical diseases (Theriot *et al.*, 2014).

C. difficile is not tissue invasive and only toxigenic strains are associated with disease. Experimental *C. difficile* infections include diarrhea, cecitis, polymorphonuclear cell infiltration of the lamina propria, inflammation, pseudomembrane formation, and death.

Differential Diagnosis *C. difficile*-induced diarrhea is most often associated with antibiotic treatment. Other clostridial diseases in mice must be ruled out as well as other enteric pathogens in mice causing diarrhea and mortality. *Salmonella* spp. and *C. rodentium* should be considered in the differential diagnosis.

CLOSTRIDIUM PERFRINGENS

Etiology *Clostridium perfringens* is associated with a number of diseases in domestic animals and humans. *C. perfringens* is a nonmotile, rod-shaped, encapsulated, anaerobic bacterium measuring 4–8 µm in length and 0.8–1.5 µm in diameter (Murray *et al.*, 2002). *C. perfringens* grow rapidly on blood agar, and colonies are smooth, round, and grayish in color, and are surrounded by a double zone of hemolysis. *C. perfringens* is grouped into five types based on the production and secretion of four major toxins. *C. perfringens* produces a number of other virulence-enhancing toxins and hydrolytic enzymes. The most significant of these is probably enterotoxin, released with the bacterial spore after cell lysis.

Epizootiology *C. perfringens* is most likely acquired by the ingestion of spores that originated in the soil or in the intestinal tract of a carrier animal. The organism can be a member of the normal microbiota in human and domestic animals. Factors that have been associated with the proliferation of the organism of these species include poor

husbandry and sudden dietary changes (Quinn *et al.*, 2002). Methods to control and prevent *C. perfringens* infections have not been evaluated in mice. Because the bacterium is most likely acquired by the ingestion of spores, it can probably be excluded from mouse colonies by maintaining good sanitation and sterilizing feed, bedding, cages, and cage accessories. Sudden dietary changes have also been associated with proliferation of the organism and should be avoided if possible (Quinn *et al.*, 2002).

Clinical Signs Only a few reports in the literature exist describing clinical disease associated with *C. perfringens* infection in mice (Matsushita and Matsumoto, 1986; Rozengurt and Sanchez). Disease has been observed in mice of both sexes, from 2 to 32 days old, and in female mice of breeding age. Clinical signs have included hunched posture, ruffled hair coat, enlarged painful abdomen, soft or impacted feces, hindquarter paralysis, and dyspnea. Sudden death without premonitory signs has also been reported. The toxin types of *C. perfringens* isolated from these cases were reported to be non-type A (Matsushita and Matsumoto, 1986), type B (Rozengurt and Sanchez, 1999), and type D (Clapp and Graham, 1970). Mucosal necrosis in both the large and small intestine is a consistent finding on microscopic examination of tissues from mice with clinically apparent *C. perfringens* infections.

Differential Diagnosis *C. perfringens* produces a number of major and minor toxins. Different types of the bacterium produce different toxins which account for different disease outcomes. *C. perfringens* type A is a constituent of the normal microbiota of the intestine of humans and other animal species. Bacterial culture should be obtained from live or recently dead animals, and placed in anaerobic transfer medium for transport to a microbiology laboratory and should be cultured soon after their arrival. A presumptive diagnosis for *C. perfringens* can be based on the presence of large gram-positive rods in fecal smears or in histologic sections of intestines (Quinn *et al.*, 2002). Definitive diagnosis is based on toxin identification.

Mice treated with chlortetracycline hydrochloride in drinking water at a level of 11 mg/l for 2 weeks have eliminated *C. perfringens*-associated disease (Matsushita and Matsumoto, 1986). Penicillin G in the diet or changing the diet has also been reported to be effective in disease remission. *C. perfringens* treatments in domestic species include ampicillin, amoxicillin-clavulanate, tylosin, clindamycin, metronidazole, and bacitracin (Marks, 2013; McGorum *et al.*, 1998). Commercially available bacterins for use in mice were not effective in controlling the disease (Clapp and Graham, 1970).

Research Complications Clostridia are large, rod-shaped, gram-positive anaerobic bacteria. Naturally occurring clostridial infection in mice is rare. Epizootics of *C. perfringens* type D infection with high mortality have been reported in a barrier colony where heavy mortality occurred in 2- to 3-week-old suckling mice. Clinical signs included scruffy hair coats, paralysis of the hindquarters, and diarrhea or fecal impaction. However, attempts to reproduce the disease experimentally with clostridia isolated from naturally infected animals were unsuccessful. *C. perfringens* also has been isolated from sporadic cases of necrotizing enteritis in recently weaned mice.

CLOSTRIDIUM PILIFORME – *TYZZER'S DISEASE*
(Fujiwara and Ganaway, 1994; Ganaway, 1982; Ganaway et al., 1971; Percy and Barthold, 2007)

Etiology Tyzzer's disease is named for Ernest Tyzzer, who first described it in a colony of Japanese Waltzing mice. The causative organism, *C. piliforme* (formerly *Bacillus piliformis*), is a long, thin, gram-negative spore-forming bacterium that appears to require living cells for *in vitro* growth. It has not been grown successfully on cell-free media, but it can be propagated by inoculation of susceptible vertebrates, in select cell lines, the yolk sac of embryonated eggs, or hepatocyte cell cultures obtained from mice (Ganaway *et al.*, 1985; Kawamura *et al.*, 1983).

Clinical Signs Clinical disease occurs as unexpected deaths that may be preceded by diarrhea and inactivity. Although outbreaks can be explosive and mortality is usually high, morbidity varies. Additionally, subclinical infections can occur, accompanied by the development of antibodies to *C. piliforme*. Stresses, such as overcrowding, high temperature and humidity, moist food, and immunosuppression, and young age, may predispose mice to Tyzzer's disease. Susceptibility and resistance also are influenced by host genotype. It has been shown, e.g., that C57BL/6 mice are more resistant than DBA/2 mice to Tyzzer's disease (Waggie *et al.*, 1981). Resistance to severe infection appears to be due, in part, to B-lymphocyte function. The role of T cells in resistance is not clear, because susceptibility among athymic mice appears to vary (Livingston *et al.*, 1996). However, the involvement of T cells can be inferred by the fact that several interleukins modulate resistance and susceptibility. Depletion of neutrophils or NK cells also increases susceptibility to infection.

Epizootiology Current prevalence rates, reservoirs of infection, carrier states, and the mechanism of spread remain speculative. Tyzzer's disease occurs in many species of laboratory animals and in domestic and free-living species. Some strains appear capable of cross-infecting mice, rats, and hamsters, whereas others have a more restricted host range (Franklin *et al.*, 1994). Therefore, the risks for cross-infection depend on the strain causing a given outbreak. Although the vegetative form of *C. piliforme* is unstable, spores can retain infectivity at room temperature for at least 1 year and should be viewed as the primary means of spread. Natural infection is probably due to ingestion of organisms, which are subsequently shed in feces. Feces-contaminated food and soiled bedding are the most likely sources of environmental contamination. Prenatal infection can be induced by intravenous inoculation of pregnant mice, but its importance in the natural transmission of infection has not been determined.

Pathology Infection begins in the gastrointestinal tract, followed by bacteremic spread to the liver and, to a smaller extent, the heart. The lesions are characterized by necrosis in these tissues and in the mesenteric lymph nodes. Grossly, segments of the ileum, cecum, and colon may be red and dilated, with watery, fetid contents, whereas the liver, mesenteric lymph nodes, and heart often contain gray–white foci. Histologically, intestinal lesions include necrosis of mucosal epithelium, which may be accompanied by acute inflammation and hemorrhage. In the liver, foci of coagulation necrosis are generally distributed along branches of the portal vein, a finding compatible with embolic infection from the intestine. Peracute lesions are largely free of inflammation, but neutrophils and lymphocytes may infiltrate less fulminant lesions. Myocardial necrosis is sporadic in natural infection.

Diagnosis Tyzzer's disease is diagnosed most directly by the demonstration of characteristic intracellular organisms in tissue sections of liver and intestine. Bundles of long, slender rods occur in the cytoplasm of viable cells bordering necrotic foci, especially in the liver (Fig. 3.46) and intestine. They are found more easily during early stages of infection. Organisms in tissue sections do not stain well with hematoxylin–eosin stain. Silver stains, Giemsa stains, or periodic acid-Schiff stains are usually required for visualization of the organism. PCR and serologic assays are readily available at diagnostic laboratories. Older supplemental procedures included inoculation of cortisonized mice or embryonated eggs

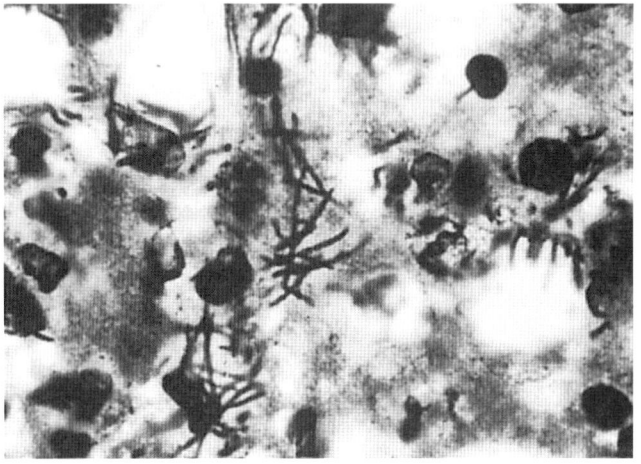

FIGURE 3.46 *C. piliforme* in the liver on a mouse with Tyzzer's disease (Warthin–Starry stain).

" PICK—UP STICKS"

with suspect material, followed by histological or immunocytochemical demonstration of organisms in tissues.

Differential Diagnosis The histological detection of organisms is essential for differentiating Tyzzer's disease from other infections that can produce similar signs and lesions, especially mousepox, coronaviral hepatitis, reoviral hepatitis, helicobacteriosis, and salmonellosis. It also is important not to misconstrue extracellular rods as *C. piliforme.*

Prevention and Control Barrier housing and husbandry that incorporate sanitation measures to avoid the introduction or buildup of spores in the environment are the bases for control or prevention of Tyzzer's disease. If infection occurs, spore formation will make control or elimination by antibiotic therapy problematic. Therefore, strict quarantine, followed by replacement of affected or exposed stock, must be considered. Rederivation by embryo transfer or cesarean section should take the potential for prenatal transmission of infection into account in housing and testing offspring. Thorough decontamination of the environment with an oxidizing disinfectant must be included in any control program. Additionally, procurement of food and bedding from suppliers with thorough quality assurance and vermin control programs is essential for both prevention and control. Husbandry supplies should be stored in vermin-proof quarters, and the option of heat sterilization of food and bedding should be considered.

Research Complications Research complications stem from clinical morbidity and mortality. Mice with immune dysfunction are at increased risk. There is recent evidence that infection causes elevations in selected cytokines (Van Andel *et al.*, 2000).

p. Mycobacteriosis

Etiology Two mycobacteria are known to be pathogenic for laboratory mice: *Mycobacterium avium-intracellulare* and *M. lepraemurium.* Both are acid-fast, obligate intracellular bacteria.

Epizootiology Mycobacteria are widespread in water and soil. Their presence in laboratory mice would indicate a significant break in husbandry practices. Infection with *M. avium-intracellulare* should be considered extremely rare, with the only published report describing an episode in a breeding colony of C57BL/6 mice (Waggie *et al.*, 1983). The source of the outbreak was presumed to be drinking water. *Mycobacterium lepraemurium* has been isolated from healthy laboratory mice and can persist as a latent infection, but its significance is primarily historical, as a model for human leprosy. It is highly unlikely to encounter this infection in a modern, well-managed mouse colony.

Clinical Signs *M. avium-intracellulare* infection is typically subclinical but mice have developed granulomatous pneumonia (Waggie *et al.*, 1983).

Pathology Lesions are classically a chronic granulomatous disease with granulomas, Langhans giant cells, and concurrent presence of acid-fast bacteria in various organs including the lungs, liver, spleen and lymph nodes. *M. lepraemurium* may cause alopecia, thickening of skin, subcutaneous swellings, and ulceration of the skin. Disease can lead to death or clinical recovery. Gross lesions are characterized by nodules in subcutaneous tissues and in reticuloendothelial tissues and organs (lung, spleen, bone marrow, thymus, and lymph nodes). Lesions can also occur in the lung, skeletal muscle, myocardium, kidneys, nerves, and adrenal glands. The histologic hallmark is perivascular granulomatosis with accumulation of large, foamy epitheloid macrophages (lepra cells) packed with acid-fast bacilli.

Diagnosis Acid-fast bacilli in lesions are the hallmark of presumptive diagnosis of mycobacteriosis. Definitive diagnosis results from positive culture which takes days to weeks to rule out or positive PCR assays which are more time-efficient but require associated expertise.

Differential Diagnosis Other bacterial species that cause granulomatous lesions in mice.

Research Complications Natural infection is very rare.

q. Proteus Infection

Etiology *Proteus mirabilis* is a ubiquitous gram-negative organism that can remain latent in the respiratory and intestinal tracts of normal mice (Percy and Barthold, 2007).

Epizootiology *Proteus mirabilis* colonizes the intestinal tract of most humans and is commonly found in research mice unless specifically excluded.

Clinical Signs Clinical disease can occur following stress or induced immunosuppression. Immunodeficient mice have a heightened susceptibility to pathogenic infection.

Pathology *Proteus* has been associated with ulcerative lesions in the gastrointestinal tract of immunodeficient mice. Infected animals lose weight, develop diarrhea, and die within several weeks. If septicemia develops, suppurative or necrotic lesions, including septic thrombi, may be found in many organs, but the kidney is commonly affected. *Proteus* pyelonephritis is characterized by abscessation and scarring. Ascending lesions may occur following urinary stasis, but hematogenous spread cannot be ruled out. *Proteus mirabilis* and *Pseudomonas aeruginosa* have been isolated concomitantly from cases of suppurative nephritis or pyelonephritis. Infection in immunodeficient mice is typified by splenomegaly and focal necrotizing hepatitis. Pulmonary lesions include edema and macrophage activation. Septic thrombi can occur, however, in many tissues.

Diagnosis Culture recovery of *Proteus mirabilis* as a predominant or single isolate confirms an opportunistic local or systemic infection.

Differential Diagnosis Gram-negative bacterial infections.

Research Complications Natural infections are typically isolated cases.

r. Leptospirosis (Percy and Barthold, 2007)

Etiology Leptospirosis remains one of the most common zoonoses transmissible from rodents (Desvars *et al.*, 2011) but is exceedingly rare in laboratory mice. Infection with *Leptospira interrogans* serovar *ballum* has been reported on several occasions (see Chapter 29).

Epizootiology *Leptospira* are gram-negative organisms that, after a septicemic phase, establish persistent infection in the renal tubules and are periodically excreted in the urine.

Clinical Signs Natural infection is subclinical and causes no significant lesions. Experimental infections can result in severe vascular, hepatic and renal lesions dependent on serovar, mouse strain and immunocompetency.

Diagnosis Diagnosis requires isolation of organisms in kidney culture. Serological testing should be used with caution because neonatal exposure can lead to persistent infection without seroconversion. Histologic examination of kidney using silver stains can also be attempted. PCR assays are reliable for preliminary diagnosis.

Differential Diagnosis Not applicable in research colonies.

Research Complications Persistent murine infections associated with active shedding present a zoonotic hazard for humans; therefore, infected mice should be culled. Elimination of infection from highly valuable mice requires rederivation.

4. Chlamydial Diseases (Percy and Barthold, 2007)

a. Chlamydia Infection

Etiology *Chlamydia trachomatis* is an intracellular organism that produces glycogen-positive intracytoplasmic inclusions (elementary bodies). *C. trachomatis* causes ocular and urogenital disease in humans. However, at least one strain historically referred to as the 'Nigg agent' after Clara Nigg, is most recently classified as *Chlamydia muridarum* and is used experimentally to model human chlamydia infection.

Epizootiology Mice are susceptible to natural infection and experimental infection with *C. trachomatis* and *Chlamydophila psittaci*, especially immunodeficient mouse strains.

Clinical Signs Natural infections are typically subclinical but persistent.

Pathology *C. muridarum* is also known as the 'mouse pneumonitis agent' due to severe acute infection which is characterized by ruffled fur, hunched posture, and labored respiration due to interstitial pneumonitis and death in 24h. Mice with more chronic infections may develop progressive emaciation and cyanosis of the ears and tail. Experimental infections to model human venereal chlamydia infections will develop hydrosalpinx, cervical, and vaginal infections in female mice and urethritis in male mice.

Diagnosis *Chlamydia* can be diagnosed by impression smears stained with Giemsa or Macchiavello stains, cell culture, or inoculation of embryonated eggs. PCR and sequencing can be used to speciate the type of chlamydia.

Differential Diagnosis *C. muridarum, C. trachomatis,* and *C. psittaci* are included in the differential diagnosis.

Research Complications *Chlamydia* is a rare spontaneous infection in research mice; its potential significance is low.

5. Mycotic Diseases

a. Pneumocystosis

Etiology *Pneumocystis murina* (*Pm*) is a common opportunistic organism of laboratory mice and other mammals. When first described by Chagas in 1909, *P. carinii* was misidentified as *Trypanosoma cruzi* and was considered a protozoan (Chagas, 1909). It was renamed as a new species, *P. carinii*, when observed in a rat in 1912 (Delanoë, P. and Delanoë, M. 1912). *P. carinii*, however, has now been grouped taxonomically with the fungi based on DNA analysis and the homology of *P. murina* housekeeping genes with those found in fungi (Edman *et al.*, 1989; Stringer *et al.*, 2002; Wakefield *et al.*, 1992). These DNA studies and apparent differences of host susceptibility prompted a new name, *P. jiroveci*, for pneumocystis isolated from humans (Stringer *et al.*, 2002; Frenkel, 1999). *P. carinii* is now used to name the organism in rats and *P. murina*, the organism in mice.

Clinical Signs *Pm* infection is subclinical in immunocompetent mice. However, it can be clinically severe in immunodeficient mice, because an adequate complement of functional T lymphocytes is required to suppress infection (Roths *et al.*, 1990; Shultz and Sidman, 1987; Walzer *et al.*, 1989; Weir *et al.*, 1986). B cells have also been shown to be critical to clearance of infection and the mechanism appears only partially related to IgG and has a more important role in promoting activation and expansion of T cells (Lund *et al.*, 2003). B cells may also protect early hematopoietic progenitor activity during systemic responses to pneumocystis infection (Hoyt *et al.*, 2014). Infection proceeds slowly, but relentlessly in immunodeficient mice leading to clinical signs of pneumonia, usually within several months. Primary signs include dyspnea and hunched posture, which may be accompanied by wasting and scaly skin. Severe cases, such as those that occur in advanced disease in SCID mice, may be fatal.

Epizootiology *Pm* is known to infect a number of mammalian hosts, including ferrets, rats, mice, and humans. *Pm* is a ubiquitous organism that is often present as a latent infection. Although firm prevalence data are not available, because detection methods are not simple to apply, infection is assumed to be present in mouse colonies unless ruled out by extensive surveillance. Although these organisms appear morphologically similar, there are antigenic and genetic differences among *P. murina* isolated from different hosts (Weinberg and Durant, 1994; Cushion, 1998). Furthermore, studies indicate that *P. carinii* isolated from one host species is unable to survive and replicate after inoculation into a different immunodeficient host species (Gigliotti *et al.*, 1993b).

Pm infection also occurs in human beings, but transmission between rodents and human beings has not been documented. *Pm* is transmitted by aerosol and establishes persistent, quiescent infection in the lungs of immunocompetent mice. Prenatal infection has not been demonstrated.

Pathology *Pm* is normally not pathogenic but can be activated by intercurrent immunosuppression. Activation fills the lung with trophic and cystic forms. Gross lesions occur in the lungs, which are often rubbery and fail to deflate (Fig. 3.47). Histopathological changes are characterized by interstitial alveolitis with thickening of alveolar septa from proteinaceous exudate and infiltration with mononuclear cells (Fig. 3.48) (Roths *et al.*, 1990). Alveolar spaces may contain vacuolated

eosinophilic material and macrophages. Special stains are required to visualize *Pm*. Silver-based stains reveal round or partially flattened 3- to 5-mm cysts in affected parenchyma (Fig. 3.49). In florid cases, alveolar spaces may be filled with cysts, but cysts may be sparse in mild cases. Disease can be especially severe when subclinically infected immunodeficient mice are reconstituted with competent immune cells that subsequently promote pneumonitis.

Diagnosis Respiratory distress in immunodeficient mice should elicit consideration of pneumocystosis. Pathologic examination of the lung, including silver

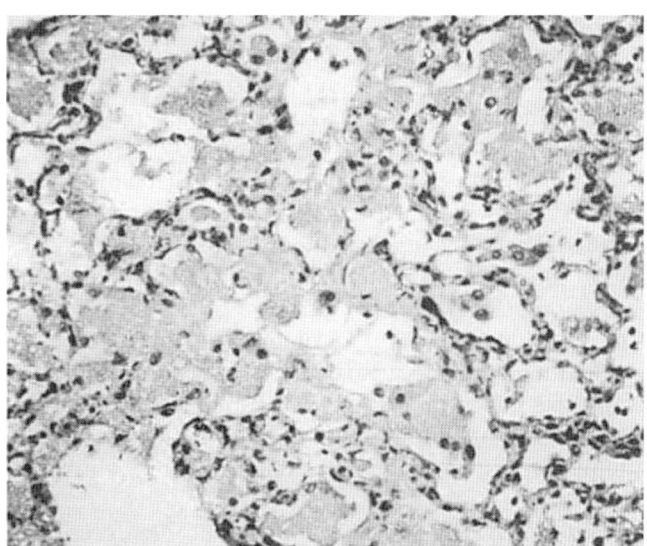

FIGURE 3.48 *Pneumocystis* pneumonia, illustrating hypercellular alveolar septa and alveoli containing proteinaceous exudate and macrophages.

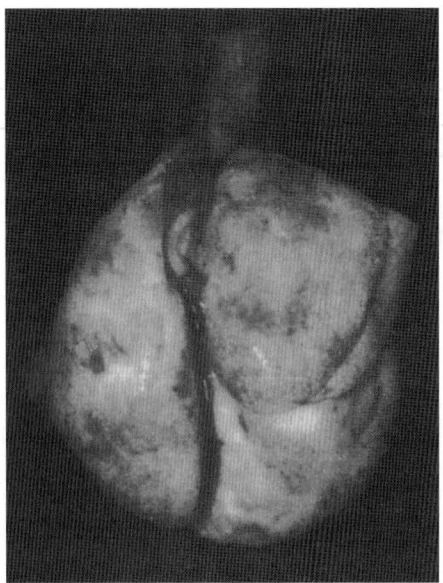

FIGURE 3.47 Lung from a mouse with *Pneumocystis* pneumonia that has failed to collapse after removal.

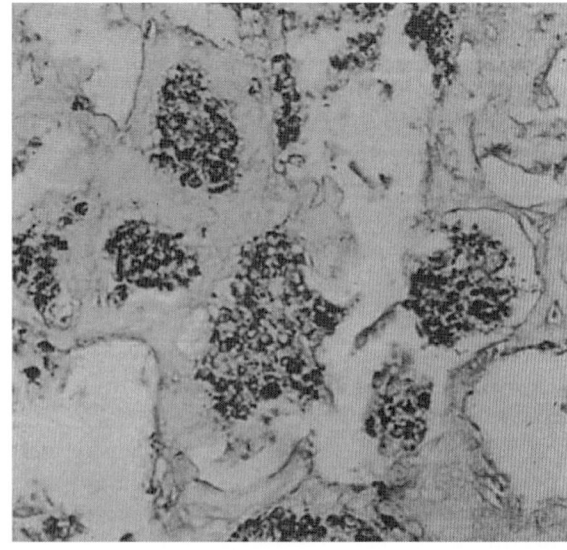

FIGURE 3.49 *Pneumocystis* pneumonia, illustrating *Pneumocystis* cysts in alveoli (Gomori methenamine–silver stain).

methenamine staining, is essential to confirm a presumptive clinical diagnosis. Past infections of immunocompetent mice also can be detected by ELISA (Furuta et al., 1985). PCR can be used to detect active infection (Gigliotti et al., 1993a; Reddy et al., 1992) and is particularly useful for screening immunodeficient mice.

Differential Diagnosis Pneumocystosis must be differentiated from viral pneumonias of mice. It is worth noting, in this regard, that pneumonia virus of mice has been shown to accelerate the development of pneumocystosis in SCID mice (Bray et al., 1993; Roths et al., 1993).

Prevention and Control Pm infection is a significant disease threat to immunodeficient mice. Its widespread distribution strongly suggests that susceptible mice should be protected by microbarrier combined, where possible, with macrobarrier housing. Husbandry procedures should include proper sterilization of food, water, and housing equipment and the use of HEPA-filtered change stations. Infected colonies can be rederived by embryo transfer or cesarean methods, because infection does not appear to be transmitted *in utero*.

Research Complications Pneumonia in immunodeficient mice is the major complication of Pm infection.

b. Dermatomycosis (Ringworm) (Godfrey, 2007)

Trichophyton mentagrophytes is the most common fungal agent of mice. However, infection rarely causes clinical disease. Clinical signs include sparse hair coats or well-demarcated crusty lesions, with a chalky surface on the head, tail, and legs (favus or ringworm). Skin lesions are composed of exfoliated debris, exudate, mycelia, and arthrospores with underlying dermatitis. Invasion of hair shafts is not characteristic. Diagnosis depends on effective specimen collection. Hairs should be selected from the periphery of the lesion, and hairless skin should be scraped deeply to obtain diagnostic specimens. *T. mentagrophytes* rarely fluoresces under ultraviolet light, and hyphae must be differentiated from bedding fibers, food particles, and epidermal debris. Histological sections should be stained with a silver stain or Schiff's reagent to reveal organisms. *Trichophyton* also can be cultured on Sabouraud agar. Plates are incubated at room temperature (22–30°C), and growth is observed at 5–10 days.

Ringworm is not easily eradicated from laboratory mice. The use of antifungal agents to treat individual mice is time-consuming, expensive, and variably effective. Rederivation is a more prudent course. Cages and equipment should be sterilized before reuse. Concurrent infection with ectoparasites also must be considered during eradication steps.

Candida albicans and other systemic mycoses are not important causes of disease in mice, but they can be opportunistic pathogens in immunodeficient mice.

6. Parasitic Diseases

a. Protozoal Diseases (Wasson, 2007)

GIARDIASIS

Etiology Giardia muris is a pear-shaped, flagellated organism with an anterior sucking disk. It inhabits the duodenum of young and adult mice, rats, and hamsters.

Clinical Signs Infection is often subclinical, unless organisms proliferate extensively, and can cause weight loss, a rough hair coat, sluggish movement, and abdominal distension, usually without diarrhea. Additionally, immunodeficient mice may die during heavy infestation.

Epizootiology The contemporary prevalence of affected mouse colonies is not well documented, but surveys during the 1980s found the rates exceeding 50%. Transmission occurs by the fecal–oral route. Cross-infection between mice and hamsters after experimental inoculation of organisms has been demonstrated, whereas rats were resistant to isolates from mice and hamsters (Kunstyr et al., 1992). C3H/He mice are particularly susceptible to giardiasis, whereas BALB/c and C57BL/10 mice are more resistant. Additionally, female mice appear to be more resistant to infection than male mice (Daniels and Belosevic, 1995). C57BL/6 females, e.g., have lower trophozoite burdens and for a shorter interval than male mice. Females also shed cysts later than male mice. These differences may be related to a more potent humoral immune response to *Giardia* in female mice.

Pathology Gross lesions are limited to the small intestine, which may contain yellow or white watery fluid. Histopathology reveals organisms in the lumen that often adhere to microvilli of enterocytes or reside in mucosal crevices or mucus. The crypt/villus ratio may be reduced, and the lamina propria may have elevated numbers of inflammatory cells.

Diagnosis Diagnosis is based on detection of trophozoites in the small intestine or in wet mounts of fecal material. Organisms can be recognized in wet preparations by their characteristic rolling and tumbling movements. Ellipsoidal cysts with four nuclei also may be detected in feces. Infection also can be detected by serology (Daniels and Belosevic, 1994) and by PCR (Mahbubani et al., 1991).

Treatment, Prevention, and Control Murine giardiasis can be treated by the addition of 0.1% dimetridazole to drinking water for 14 days. Prevention and control depend on proper sanitation and management, including adequate disinfection of contaminated rooms.

Research Complications Accelerated cryptal cell turnover and suppression of the immune response to sheep erythrocytes have been observed in infected mice. The potential for severe or lethal infection in immunodeficient mice was noted previously.

SPIRONUCLEOSIS

Etiology *Spironucleus muris* is an elongated, pear-shaped, bilaterally symmetrical flagellated protozoan that commonly inhabits the duodenum, usually in the crypts of Lieberkühn. It is smaller than *Giardia muris* and lacks an anterior sucking disk.

Clinical Signs *S. muris* infection is usually subclinical in normal adult mice. It is more pathogenic, however, for young, stressed, or immunocompromised mice (Kunstyr *et al.*, 1977). Additionally, clinical morbidity may indicate an underlying primary infection with an unrelated organism. Clinically affected mice can have a poor hair coat, sluggish behavior, and weight loss. Mice at 3–6 weeks of age are at notably higher risk for clinically evident infection. They can develop dehydration, hunched posture, abdominal distension, and diarrhea. Severe infections can be lethal.

Epizootiology Transmission occurs by the fecal–oral route and can occur between hamsters and mice as well as between mice. It does not appear to be transmitted between mice and rats (Schagemann *et al.*, 1990). The most recent surveys, which are somewhat dated, indicated that prevalence rates exceeded 60% among domestic mouse colonies in the mid-1980s. There is some evidence that inbred strains vary in their susceptibility to infection and their rate of recovery (Baker *et al.*, 1998; Brett and Cox, 1982).

Pathology Gross findings associated with infection include watery, red–brown, gaseous intestinal contents. However, it is essential to rule out primary or coinfection by other organisms before attributing these lesions to spironucleosis. Microscopically, acute disease is associated with distension of crypts and intervillous spaces by pear-shaped trophozoites and inflammatory edema of the lamina propria. Organisms can be visualized more easily with periodic acid-Schiff staining, which may reveal invasion of organisms between enterocytes and in the lamina propria. Chronic infection is associated with lymphoplasmacytic infiltration of the lamina propria and occasional intracryptal inflammatory exudate.

Diagnosis Diagnosis is based on identification of trophozoites in the intestinal tract. They can be distinguished from *Giardia muris* and *Tritrichomonas muris* by their small size, horizontal or zigzag movements, and the absence of a sucking disk or undulating membrane. PCR-based detection also is available (Rozario *et al.*, 1996). It is not clear whether duodenitis is a primary pathogenic effect of *S. muris* or represents opportunism secondary to a primary bacterial or viral enteritis. Therefore, it is prudent to search for underlying or predisposing infections.

Treatment, Prevention, and Control Treatment consists of adding 0.1% dimetridazole to drinking water for 14 days, as described for giardiasis. Prevention and control require good husbandry and sanitation.

Research Complications As with giardiasis, infection can accelerate enterocytic turnover in the small intestine. There is some evidence that infected mice may have activated macrophages that kill tumor cells nonspecifically and that infection can diminish responses to soluble and particulate antigens. Additionally, infected mice also have increased sensitivity to irradiation. Such effects should, however, be interpreted cautiously in order to rule out intercurrent viral infections.

Tritrichomoniasis *T. muris* is a nonpathogenic protozoan that occurs in the cecum, colon, and small intestine of mice, rats, and hamsters. No cysts are formed, and transmission is by ingestion of trophozoites passed in the feces. It can be detected by microscopy or by PCR (Viscogliosi *et al.*, 1993).

Coccidiosis *Eimeria falciformis* is a pathogenic coccidian that occurs in epithelial cells of the large intestines of mice. It was common in European mice historically but is seldom observed in the United States. Heavy infection may cause diarrhea and catarrhal enteritis.

Klosiella muris causes renal coccidioisis in wild mice but is rare in laboratory mice. Mice are infected by ingestion of sporulated sporocysts. Sporozoites released from the sporocysts enter the bloodstream and infect endothelial cells lining renal arterioles and glomerular capillaries, where schizogony occurs. Mature schizonts rupture into Bowman's capsule to release merozoites into the lumen of renal tubules. Merozoites can enter epithelial cells lining convoluted tubules, where the sexual phase of the life cycle is completed. Sporocysts form in renal tubular epithelium and eventually rupture host cells and are excreted in the urine, but oocysts are not formed. Infection is usually nonpathogenic and subclinical. Gray spots may occur in heavily affected kidneys and are the result of necrosis, granulomatous inflammation, and focal hyperplasia. Destruction of tubular epithelium may impair renal physiology. Diagnosis is based on detection of organisms in tissues. Prevention and control require proper sanitation and management techniques. There is no effective treatment.

Cryptosporidiosis *Cryptosporidium muris* is a sporozoan that adheres to the gastric mucosa. It is uncommon in laboratory mice and is only slightly pathogenic. *Cryptosporidium parvum* inhabits the small intestine and is usually nonpathogenic in immunocompetent and athymic mice (Ozkul and Aydin, 1994; Taylor *et al.*, 1999). Athymic mice may develop cholangitis and hepatitis, however, if organisms gain access to the biliary tract.

Entamoebiasis *Entamoeba muris* is found in the cecum and colon of mice, rats, and hamsters throughout the world. Organisms live in the lumen, where they feed on particles of food and bacteria. They are considered nonpathogenic.

Encephalitozoonosis *Encephalitozoon cuniculi* is a gram-positive microsporidian that infects rabbits, mice, rats, guinea pigs, dogs, nonhuman primates, humans, and other mammals. Infection is extremely rare among laboratory mice. The life cycle of the organism is direct, and animals are infected by ingesting spores or by cannibalism. Spore cells are disseminated in the blood to the brain and other sites. Infection can last more than 1 year, and spores shed in the urine serve as a source of infection. Vertical transmission has not been confirmed in mice. *E. cuniculi* is an obligate intracellular parasite, but infection usually elicits no clinical signs of disease. Organisms proliferate in peritoneal macrophages by asexual binary fission. They have a capsule that accepts Giemsa and Goodpasture stains but is poorly stained by hematoxylin. Fulminating infection can cause lymphocytic meningoencephalitis and focal granulomatous hepatitis. In contrast to encephalitozoonosis in rabbits, affected mice do not develop interstitial nephritis. Infection is diagnosed by cytological examination of ascitic fluid smears, histopathologic examination of brain tissues stained with Goodpasture stain, and ELISA serology. No effective treatment has been reported. Prevention and control require rigid testing and elimination of infected colonies and cell lines. PCR-based assays may also be useful.

Toxoplasmosis *Toxoplasma gondii* is a ubiquitous gram-negative coccidian parasite for which the mouse serves as a principal intermediate host. However, the prevalence of natural infection is negligible because laboratory mice no longer have access to sporulated cysts shed by infected cats, which were historically the major source for cross-infection. Toxoplasmosis can cause necrosis and granulomatous inflammation in the intestine, mesenteric lymph nodes, eyes, heart, adrenals, spleen, brain, lung, liver, placenta, and muscles. Diagnosis is based on ELISA serology, histopathology, and PCR. Control and prevention depend largely on precluding access of mice to cat feces or to materials contaminated with cat feces. Oocytes are very resistant to adverse temperatures, drying, and chemical disinfectants; therefore, thorough cleaning of infected environments is required.

b. Cestodiasis (Pritchett, 2007; Baker, 2007)

HYMENOLEPIS (RODENTOLEPIS) NANA (DWARF TAPEWORM) INFESTATION

Etiology *Hymenolepis (Rodentolepis) nana*, the dwarf tapeworm, infects mice, rats, and humans although the zoonotic risk has been questioned (Macnish *et al.*, 2002). Adults are extremely small (25–40 mm) and have eggs with prominent polar filaments and rostellar hooks (Fig. 3.50).

Clinical Signs Young adult mice are most frequently infected. Signs and lesions include weight loss and focal enteritis, but clinical disease is rare unless infestation is severe.

Epizootiology The life cycle may be direct or indirect (*R. nana* is the only cestode known that does not require an intermediate host). The indirect cycle utilizes arthropods as intermediate hosts. Liberated oncospheres penetrate intestinal villi and develop into a cercocystis stage before reemerging into the intestinal lumen 10–12 days later. The scolex attaches to the intestinal mucosa, where the worm grows to adult size in 2 weeks. The cycle from ingestion to patency takes 20–30 days.

Pathology Cysticerci are found in the lamina propria of the small intestine and sporadically in the mesenteric lymph nodes, whereas adults, which have a serrated profile, are found in the lumen. Inflammation is not a feature of infection.

Diagnosis Infection can be diagnosed by demonstrating eggs in fecal flotation preparations or by opening the intestine in Petri dishes containing warm tap water to facilitate detection of adults. *R. nana* can be differentiated from another species of rodent tapeworm, *H. diminuta*, by the fact that *R. nana* has rostellar hooks and eggs with polar filaments. However, *H. diminuta* requires an intermediate arthropod host, so it is rarely found in contemporary mouse colonies.

Treatment, Prevention, and Control Drugs recommended for treatment and elimination include praziquantel (0.05% in the diet for 5 days), albendazole, mebendazole, and thiabendazole. Although the benzimidazoles have an excellent activity against cestodes and nematodes in rats, they have not been tested extensively in mice. The potential for successful treatment is high, however, because eggs do not survive well outside the host and because the prevalence of infestation is low in caged mice kept in properly sanitized facilities. Because *R. nana* can directly infect humans, proper precautions should be taken to avoid oral contamination during handling of rodents (see Chapter 28).

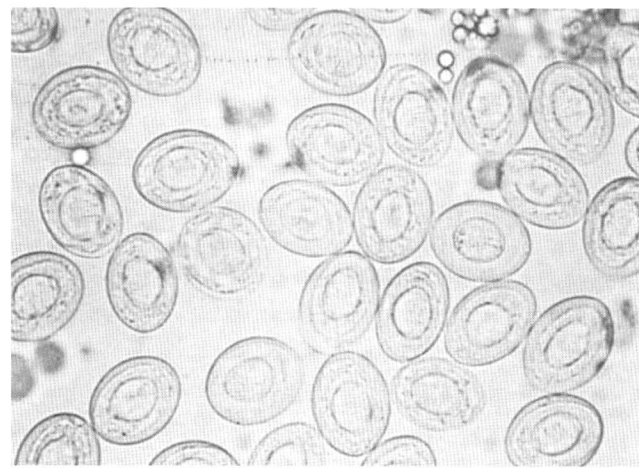

FIGURE 3.50   Eggs of *Hymenolepis (Rodentolepsis) nana*.

Hymenolepis microstoma is found in the bile ducts of rodents and could be confused with *R. nana* in the mouse. However, the location of the adult as well as the large size of *H. microstoma* eggs compared with those of *R. nana* make differential diagnosis relatively simple. The mouse and the rat are intermediate hosts of the cestode *Taenia taeniaformis*. The definitive host is the cat. This parasite should not be found in laboratory mice housed separately from cats.

c. Nematodiasis (Wescott, 1982)

SYPHACIA OBVELATA (MOUSE PINWORM) INFESTATION

Etiology   *Syphacia obvelata*, the common mouse pinworm, is a ubiquitous parasite of wild and laboratory mice. The rat, gerbil, and hamster are also occasionally infected. Female worms range from 3.4 to 5.8 mm in length, and male worms are smaller (1.1–1.5 mm). Eggs are flattened on one side and have pointed ends (Fig. 3.51). The nucleus fills the shell and is frequently at a larval stage when eggs are laid.

Clinical Signs   Infestation is usually subclinical, although heavily infested mice can occasionally sustain intestinal lesions, including rectal prolapse, intussusception, enteritis, and fecal impaction.

Epizootiology   Pinworm infestation is one of the most commonly encountered problems in laboratory mice. A national survey revealed that more than 30% of barrier colonies and about 70% of conventional colonies were affected (Jacoby and Lindsey, 1997; Carty, 2008). *Syphacia obvelata* infestation can occur unexpectedly in commercial barrier murine colonies, resulting in widespread dissemination of the parasite into academic mouse colonies. The epizootiological impact of pinworm infestation is increased by the airborne dissemination of eggs, which can remain infectious even after drying. The life-cycle is direct and completed in 11–15 days. Females deposit their eggs on the skin and hairs of the perianal region. Ingested eggs liberate larvae in the small intestine and they migrate to the cecum within 24 h. Worms remain in the cecum for 10–11 days, where they mature and mate. The females then migrate to the large intestine

to deposit their eggs as they leave the host. There is unconfirmed speculation that larvae may reenter the rectum. Infestation usually begins in young mice and can recur, but adult mice tend to be more resistant. *Syphacia* infestation often occurs in combination with *Aspiculuris tetraptera*. Because the life cycle of *Syphacia* is much shorter than that of *Aspiculuris*, the number of mice that are apt to be infected with *S. obvelata* is correspondingly greater. There is evidence that resistance to infestation may be mouse strain-specific (Derothe *et al.*, 1997).

Pathology   Gross lesions are not prevalent, aside from the presence of adults in the lumen of the intestine.

Diagnosis   Infestation is diagnosed by demonstrating reniform-shaped eggs in the perianal area or adult worms in the cecum or large intestine. Four- to 5-week-old mice should be examined because the prevalence is higher in this age group than in older mice. Because most eggs are deposited outside the gastrointestinal tract, fecal examination is not reliable. Eggs are usually detected by pressing cellophane tape to the perineal area and then to a glass slide that is examined by microscopy. *Aspiculuris tetraptera* eggs are not ordinarily found in tape preparations and are easily differentiated from eggs of *S. obvelata* (see below). Adult worms can be found in cecal or colonic contents diluted in a Petri dish of warm tap water. They are readily observed with the naked eye or with a dissecting microscope. An ELISA also is available to detect serum antibodies to *S. obvelata* somatic antigens (Sato *et al.*, 1995). PCR assays are increasingly being used to augment traditional diagnostic methods and to discriminate between pinworm species (Dole *et al.*, 2011). PCR panels for pinworm detection using fecal pellets are available from commercial diagnostic laboratories.

Treatment, Prevention, and Control   Pinworm infestation can be treated effectively by a number of regimens, which include the use of anthelmintics such as piperazine, ivermectin, and benzimidazole compounds alone or in combination (Klement *et al.*, 1996; Le Blanc *et al.*, 1993; Lipman *et al.*, 1994; Flynn *et al.*, 1989; Wescott, 1982; Zenner, 1998). Because some of the recommended therapies have the potential for toxicity, it is prudent to keep mice under close clinical observation during treatment (Davis *et al.*, 1999; Skopets *et al.*, 1996; Toth *et al.*, 2000). Fenbendazole diets can be fed with 1 week on/1 week off rotation with normal chow although the potential impact on experimental data must be considered (Duan *et al.*, 2012; Gadad *et al.*, 2010; Landin *et al.*, 2009). Prevention of reinfestation requires strict isolation because *Syphacia* eggs become infective as soon as 6 h after they are laid, and they survive for weeks, even in dry conditions. Strict sanitation, sterilization of feed and bedding, and periodic anthelmintic treatment are required to control infestation. The use of microbarrier cages can reduce the spread of infective eggs.

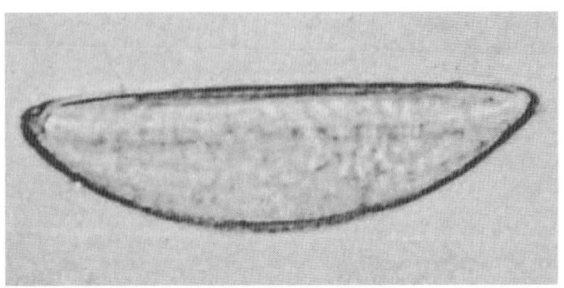

FIGURE 3.51   *Syphacia obvelata* egg.

Research Complications Unthriftiness and perturbation of host immune responses are the primary complications of pinworm infection.

Syphacia muris is the common rat pinworm. It can potentially infest mice but is not found in well-managed colonies. It can be differentiated from *S. obvelata* because *S. muris* eggs are smaller. Treatment is the same as for pinworms of mice.

ASPICULURIS TETRAPTERA (MOUSE PINWORM) INFECTION

Etiology *Aspiculuris tetraptera* is the other major oxyurid of the mouse and may coinfect mice carrying *S. obvelata*. Females are 2.6–4.7 mm long, and males are slightly smaller. The eggs are ellipsoidal (Fig. 3.52).

Clinical Signs Ingested eggs hatch, and larvae reach the middle colon, where they enter crypts and remain for 4–5 days. They move to the proximal colon about 3 weeks after infection of the host. Because the life cycle is 10–12 days longer than in *S. obvelata*, infestations appear in somewhat older mice; heaviest infestation is expected in 5–6 weeks after initial exposure. Infection is usually subclinical, but heavy loads can produce signs similar to those discussed for *S. obvelata*. Light to moderate loads do not produce clinical disease.

Epizootiology As noted under *S. obvelata*, pinworm infestation is highly prevalent and contagious in laboratory mice. The life cycle is direct and takes approximately 23–25 days. Mature females inhabit the large intestine, where they survive from 45 to 50 days and lay their eggs. The eggs are deposited at night and are excreted in a mucous layer, covering fecal pellets. They require 6–7 days at 24°C to become infective and can survive for weeks outside the host.

Pathology See *S. obvelata* (Section III, A,5,c).

Diagnosis *Aspiculuris tetraptera* eggs can be detected in the feces, and adult worms are found in the large intestine. Eggs are not deposited in the perianal area; therefore, cellophane tape techniques are not useful.

Treatment, Prevention, and Control Measures for treatment, prevention, and control are similar to those described for *S. obvelata*. Because *A. tetraptera* takes longer to mature and because eggs are deposited in feces rather than on the host, adult parasites are more amenable to treatment by frequent cage rotations. Immune expulsion of parasites and resistance to reinfection are hallmarks of *A. tetraptera* infection.

Research Complications See *S. obvelata* (Section III, A,5,c).

d. Acariasis (Mite Infestation) (Baker, 2007)

Several species of mites infest laboratory mice. They include *Myobia musculi*, *Radfordia affinis*, *Myocoptes musculinus*, and, less commonly, *Psorergates simplex*. The common murine mites are described below, while less frequently encountered species are listed in Table 3.14. These include the mouse mite *Trichoecius romboutsi*, which resembles *Myocoptes* and *Ornithonyssus bacoti*, the tropical rat mite, which can infect laboratory mice. Characteristics of specific infestations are described after a general introductory section.

Clinical Signs Mites generally favor the dorsal anterior regions of the body, particularly the top of

TABLE 3.14 Ectoparasites of Laboratory Mice of the Order Acarina

Suborder	Genus	Species	Common name
Mesostigmata	*Ornithonyssus*	*bacoti*	Tropical rat mite
	Ornithonyssus	*sylviarum*	Northern fowl mite
	Liponyssoides	*sanguineus*	House mouse mite
	Haemogamasus	*pontiger*	
	Eulaelaps	*stabularis*	
	Laelaps	*echidninus*	Spiny rat mite
	Haemolaelaps	*glasgowi*	
	Haemolaelaps	*casalis*	
Prostigmata			
Family Myobiidae Subfamily Myobiinae	*Myobia*	*musculi*	Fur mite
	Radfordia	*affinis*	Fur mite
Family Psorergatidae	*Psorergates*	*simplex*	Hair follicle mite
Family Sarcoptidae	*Notoedres*	*musculi*	
Family Demodicidae	*Demodex*	*musculi*	
Astigmata			
Family Myocoptidae	*Myocoptes*	*musculinus*	
	Trichoecius	*romboutsi*	

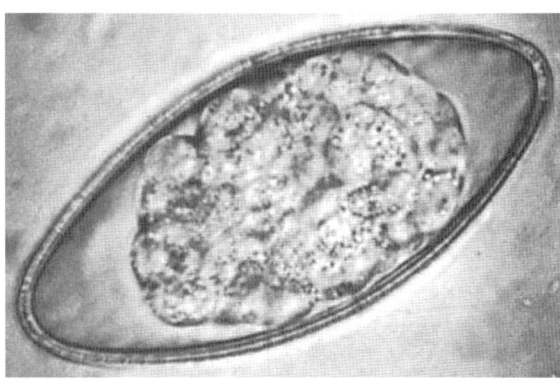

FIGURE 3.52 *Aspiculuris tetraptera* egg.

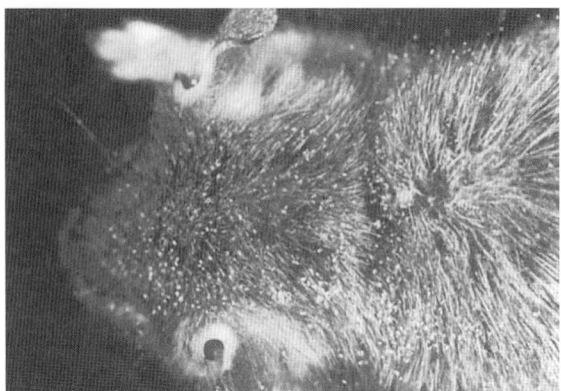

FIGURE 3.53   *Acariasis.*

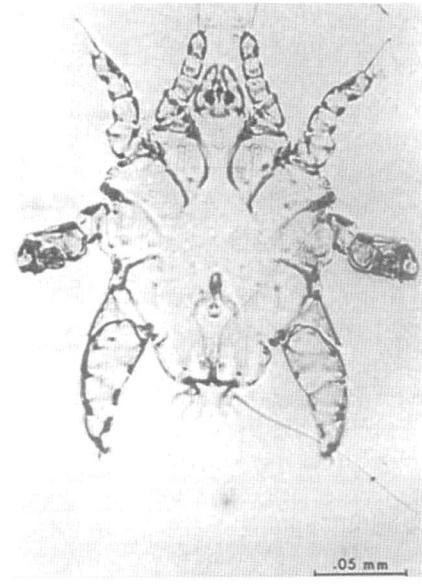

FIGURE 3.54   *M. musculinus* male. *From Weisbroth (1982).*

the head, neck, and withers (areas least amenable to grooming), but in severe cases, all areas of skin can be infested (Fig. 3.53). Skin lesions of acariasis include pruritis, scruffiness, patchy hair loss, and, in severe cases, ulceration and pyoderma initiated or compounded by self-inflicted trauma.

Epizootiology Ectoparasitism in mice is dominated by acariasis. A 1997 survey (Jacoby and Lindsey, 1997; Carty, 2008) reported mite infestations in 40% of colonies. Acarids spend their entire lives on the host. Populations are limited by factors such as self-grooming, mutual grooming, the presence of hair, and immunological responses, which tend to produce hypersensitivity dermatitis. Inherited resistance and susceptibility also affect clinical expression of acariasis. Mite populations, e.g., vary widely among different stocks and strains of mice housed under similar conditions.

Pathology Gross lesions include scaly skin, regional hair loss, abrasions, and ulcerations. Histologically, hyperkeratosis, acanthosis, and chronic dermatitis may occur. Long-standing infestation provokes chronic inflammation, fibrosis, and proliferation of granulation tissue. Ulcerative dermatitis associated with acariasis may have an allergic pathogenesis but often results in secondary bacterial infections. Lesions resemble allergic acariasis in other species and are associated with mast cell accumulations in the dermis.

Diagnosis Classic methods of detection include direct observation of the hair and skin of dead or anesthetized mice. Hairs are parted with pins or sticks and examined with a dissecting microscope. Examination of young mice, prior to the onset of immune-mediated equilibrium, is likely to be more productive. Alternatively, recently euthanized mice can be placed on a black paper, and double-sided cellophane tape can be used to line the perimeter to contain the parasites. As the carcass cools, parasites will vacate the pelage and crawl onto the paper. Sealed Petri dishes can also be used. Cellophane tape also can be pressed against areas of the pelt of freshly

euthanized mice and examined microscopically. Skin scrapings made with a scalpel blade can be macerated in 10% KOH/glycerin or immersion oil and examined microscopically. This method has the disadvantage of missing highly motile species and low-level populations of slower moving immature forms. It is important to remember that mite infestations may be mixed, so the identification of one species does not rule out the presence of others.

Detecting mites in sentinels exposed to dirty bedding from colony animals has been reported to be unreliable (Lindstrom *et al.*, 2011). Thus, PCR assays offered by commercial diagnostic laboratories are increasingly being used to augment traditional diagnostic methods and to test individual animals or equipment using a swabbing technique; samples can be pooled to decrease cost (Jensen *et al.*, 2013).

Gross anatomical features facilitate differentiation of intact mites. *Myocoptes* has an oval profile with heavily chitinized body, pigmented third and fourth legs, and tarsal suckers (Fig. 3.54). *Myobia* and *Radfordia* have a similar elongated profile, with bulges between the legs. *Myobia* has a single tarsal claw on the second pair of legs (Fig. 3.55), whereas *Radfordia* has two claws of unequal size on the terminal tarsal structure of its second pair of legs (Fig. 3.56). Histopathological examination of skin is helpful for diagnosing unique forms of acariasis, such as the keratotic cysts associated with *Psorergates simplex* infestation.

Treatment, Prevention, and Control Ivermectin can be used topically, in drinking water or as a medicated feed and often is the first-choice approach for attempting eradication although cost and potential toxicity are concerns. Because of potential differences in

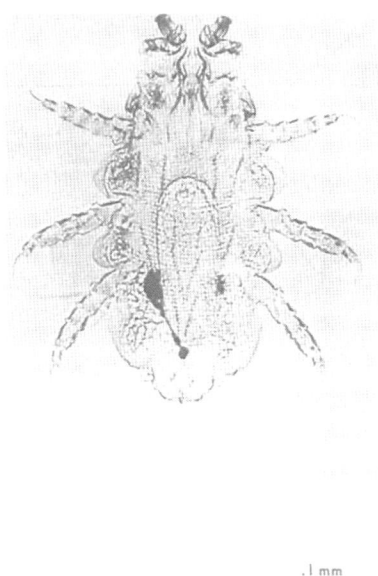

FIGURE 3.55   *M. musculi* female. *From Weisbroth (1982).*

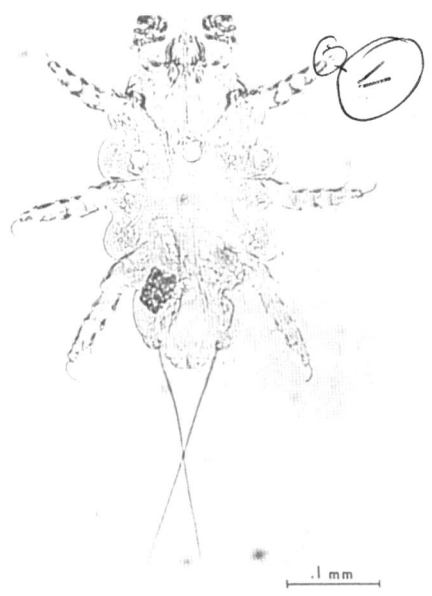

FIGURE 3.56   *R. affinis* female. *From Weisbroth (1982).*

blood–brain barrier permeability to ivermectin, pilot treatments should be evaluated. For large facilities, ivermectin medicated feed may be an attractive option (Ricart Arbona *et al.*, 2010). For valuable lines of mice, rederivation may be cost- and time-effective. Control and prevention programs should be carried out on a colony-wide basis, which includes thorough sanitation of housing space and equipment to remove residual eggs.

Research Complications   Hypersensitivity dermatitis has the potential to confound immunological studies (Jungmann *et al.*, 1996), especially those involving

skin, and has been shown to elevate serum IgE (Morita *et al.*, 1999). Heavy mite infestations can cause severe skin lesions and have been associated with weight loss, infertility, and premature deaths. Chronic acariasis also may provoke secondary amyloidosis due to long-standing dermatitis.

ADDITIONAL CHARACTERISTICS OF MURINE ACARIASIS

Myocoptes Musculinus   This is the most common ectoparasite of the laboratory mouse but frequently occurs in conjunction with *Myobia musculi*. The life cycle includes egg, larva, protonymph, tridonymph, and adult stages. Eggs hatch in 5 days and are usually attached to the middle third of the hair shaft. The life cycle may range from 8 to 14 days. Transmission requires direct contact, for mice separated by wire screens do not contract infestations from infested hosts. Bedding does not seem to serve as a vector. Neonates may become infested within 4–5 days of birth, and parasites may live for 8–9 days on dead hosts.

Myocoptes appears to inhabit larger areas of the body than *Myobia* and tends to displace *Myobia* during heavy infestations. It has some predilection for the skin of the inguinal region, abdominal skin, and back, but it will also infest the head and neck. It is a surface dweller that feeds on superficial epidermis. Infestation can cause patchy thinning of the hair, alopecia, or erythema. Lesions can be pruritic, but ulceration has not been reported. Chronic infestations induce epidermal hyperplasia and nonsuppurative dermatitis.

Myobia Musculi   This is a common mite of laboratory mice. The life cycle of *Myobia* can be completed in 23 days and includes an egg stage, first and second larval stages, protonymph, deutonymph, and adult. Eggs attach at the base of hair shafts and hatch in 7–8 days. Larval forms last about 10 days, followed by nymphal forms on day 11. Adults appear by day 15 and lay eggs within 24 h.

Myobia are thought to feed on skin secretions and interstitial fluid but not on blood. They are transmitted primarily by contact. Mite populations increase during new infestations, followed by a decrease to equilibrium in 8–10 weeks. The equilibrated population can be carried in colonies for long periods (up to years). Population fluctuations may represent waves of egg hatchings. Because mites are thermotactic, they crawl to the end of hair shafts on dead hosts, where they may live for up to 4 days. Infestation may result in hypersensitivity dermatitis, to which C57BL mice are highly susceptible. Clinical signs vary from ruffled fur and alopecia to pruritic ulcerative dermatitis. Therefore, lesions can be exacerbated by self-inflicted trauma.

Radfordia Affinis   *Radfordia* is thought to be common in laboratory mice, but it closely resembles *Myobia* and may occur as a mixed infestation. Therefore, its true prevalence is conjectural. Additionally, its life cycle has not been described. It does not appear to cause clinical morbidity.

Psorergates Simplex This species has not been reported as a naturally occurring infection in well-managed colonies for several decades, but it is unique in that it inhabits hair follicles. Its life cycle is unknown, but developmental stages from egg to adult may be found in a single dermal nodule. Transmission is by direct contact. Invasion of hair follicles leads to development of cyst-like nodules, which appear as small white nodules in the subcutis. Histologically, they are invaginated sacs of squamous epithelium, excretory products, and keratinaceous debris. There is usually no inflammatory reaction, but healing may be accompanied by granulomatous inflammation. Diagnosis is made by examining the subcuticular surface of the pelt grossly or by histological examination. Sac contents also can be expressed by pressure with a scalpel blade or scraped and mounted for microscopic exam.

Mesostigmoid Mites Rarely, blood-sucking *Ornithonyssus bacoti* and *Laelaps echidnina*, normally limited to wild rodents, can also infect laboratory rodent colonies (Watson, 2008; Fox, 1982). These mites may also transiently bite humans and can transmit zoonotic infections (see Chapter 29). Unlike the more common rodent fur mites, mesostigmoid mites live off the host and can travel a long distance in search of a blood meal. They access research colonies via contaminated supplies or wild rats and mice gaining access to the facility.

e. Pediculosis (LICE) (Percy and Barthold, 2007)

Polyplax serrata, the mouse louse, is encountered in wild mice but no longer is a significant issue in research colonies. Eggs are deposited at the base of hair shafts and nymph stages and adults can be found principally on the dorsum. *P. serrata* causes pruritus with associated dermatitis, anemia and debilitation and historically is the vector for *Mycoplasma coccoides*.

B. Metabolic and Nutritional Diseases

1. Amyloidosis

Amyloidosis is caused by the deposition of insoluble (polymerized), mis-folded amyloid protein fibrils in organs and/or tissues. Primary amyloidosis is a naturally occurring disease in mice, associated with the deposition of amyloid proteins consisting primarily of immunoglobulin light chains. Secondary amyloidosis is associated with antecedent and often chronic inflammation. It results from a complex cascade of reactions involving release of multiple cytokines that stimulate amyloid synthesis in the liver (Falk and Skinner, 2000).

Primary amyloidosis is common among aging mice (Lipman *et al.*, 1993) but also may occur in young mice

of highly susceptible strains such as A and SJL or somewhat older C57BL mice. Other strains, such as BALB/c and C3H are highly resistant to amyloidosis (Percy and Barthold, 2007). Secondary amyloidosis is usually associated with chronic inflammatory lesions, including dermatitis resulting from prolonged acariasis. It can be induced experimentally, however, by injection of casein and may occur locally in association with neoplasia or in ovarian corpora lutea in the absence of other disease. In reactive amyloid A (AA) amyloidosis, serum AA (SAA) protein forms deposits in mice, domestic and wild animals, and humans that experience chronic inflammation. AA amyloid fibrils are abnormal β-sheet-rich forms of the serum precursor SAA, with conformational changes that promote fibril formation. Similar to prion diseases, recent findings suggest that AA amyloidosis could be transmissible in mice and other species (Murakami *et al.*, 2014). Amyloid fibrils induce a seeding-nucleation process that may lead to development of AA amyloidosis. Amyloidosis can shorten the life span of mice and can be accelerated by stress from intercurrent disease.

Amyloid appears histologically as interstitial deposition of a lightly eosinophilic, acellular material in tissues stained with hematoxylin and eosin. However, it is birefringent after staining with Congo Red when viewed with polarized light. Deposition patterns vary with mouse strain and amyloid type. Although virtually any tissue may be affected, the following sites are common: hepatic portal triads, periarteriolar lymphoid sheaths in spleen, renal glomeruli and interstitium (which can lead to papillary necrosis), intestinal lamina propria, myocardium (and in association with atrial thrombosis), nasal submucosa, pulmonary alveolar septa, gonads, endocrine tissues, and great vessels (Fig. 3.57).

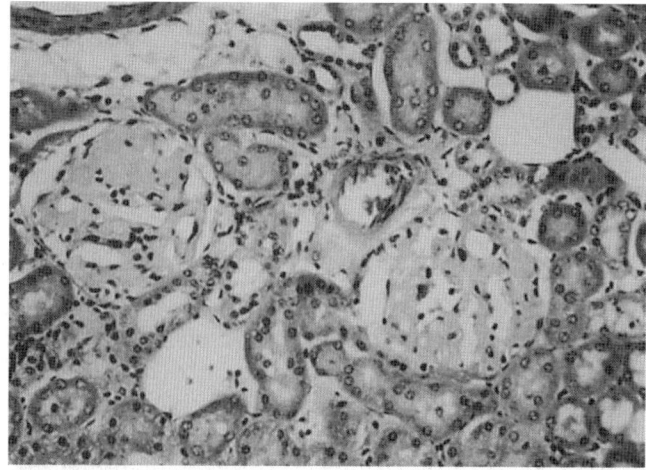

FIGURE 3.57 Renal amyloidosis with prominent amyloid deposition in glomeruli.

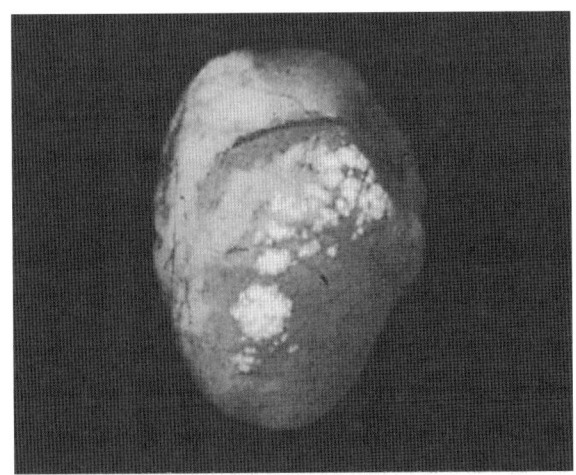

FIGURE 3.58   Epicardial mineralization.

Damn Bad Calcinosis

2. Soft Tissue Mineralization

Naturally occurring mineralization of the myocardium and epicardium and other soft tissues is a common finding at necropsy in some inbred strains of mice. Although this condition is usually an incidental finding at necropsy, interference with organ function such as the heart cannot be ruled out if lesions are severe. It occurs in BALB/c, C3H, and especially DBA mice (Eaton *et al.*, 1978; Brownstein, 1983; Brunnert *et al.*, 1999). It is found in the myocardium of the left ventricle (Fig. 3.58), in the intraventricular systems, and in skeletal muscle, kidneys, arteries, and lung and may be accompanied by fibrosis and mononuclear inflammatory infiltrates. DBA mice also can develop mineralization in the tongue and cornea.

Dietary, environmental, disease-related, and endocrine-related factors are thought to influence the prevalence of this lesion. Ectopic mineralization is associated clinically with skin and vascular connective tissue conditions in humans and mouse models have been developed to study metastatic and dystrophic tissue mineralization (Li and Uitto, 2013). Pseudoxanthoma elasticum (PXE), a heritable ectopic mineralization disorder in humans, is caused by mutations in the ABCC6 gene. Knockout Abcc6$^{-/-}$ mice model the histopathologic and ultrastructural features of PXE, notably with mineralization of the vibrissae dermal sheath, serving as a biomarker of tissue mineralization (Benga *et al.*, 2014). Other inbred mouse strains, including KK/HlJ and 129S1/SvImJ, also develop vibrissae dermal mineralization and have an SNP (rs32756904) in the Abcc6 gene associated with low levels of ABCC6 protein expression in the liver. DBA/2J and C3H/HeJ mice have the same polymorphism and low ABCC6 protein levels; however, these mice only develop tissue mineralization when fed an experimental diet enriched in phosphate and low in magnesium.

3. Reye's-Like Syndrome

A Reye's-like syndrome has been reported in BALB/cByJ mice (Brownstein *et al.*, 1984). The etiology is unknown; however, antecedent viral infection may be involved. Affected mice rapidly become lethargic and then comatose. They also tend to hyperventilate. High mortality ensues within 6–18h, but some mice may recover. Lesions are characterized grossly by swollen, pale liver and kidneys. The major histopathological findings include swollen hepatocytes with fatty change and nuclear swelling among astrocytes in the brain. Hepatic lesions resembling changes in Reye's syndrome have been reported in SCID mice infected with MAdV-1 (Pirofski *et al.*, 1991).

4. Vitamin, Mineral, and Essential Fatty Acid Deficiencies (Tobin et al., 2007)

Vitamin deficiencies in mice have not been thoroughly described. Unfortunately, much of the information that does exist reflects work carried out 30–50 years ago; thus, the reliability and specificity of some of these syndromes is questionable. Vitamin A deficiency may produce tremors, diarrhea, rough hair coat, keratitis, poor growth, abscesses, hemorrhages, and sterility or abortion. Vitamin A is recognized for its importance in development of the immune system (Ross, 2012) and knockout mouse models have been used to demonstrate genetic polymorphisms in humans that negatively regulate intestinal β-carotene absorption and conversion to retinoids in response to vitamin A requirements for growth and reproduction (von Lintig, 2012). Vitamin E deficiency can cause convulsions and heart failure, as well as muscular dystrophy and hyaline degeneration of muscles. Two knockout mouse models of severe vitamin E deficiency were independently developed and lack α-tocopherol transfer protein (α-TTP), a gene that controls plasma and tissue α-tocopherol concentrations by exporting α-tocopherol from the liver. *Ttpa*$^{-/-}$ mice have very low to undetectable levels of α-tocopherol and are infertile. The phenotype includes neuronal degeneration associated with progressive ataxia and age-related behavioral defects (Yu and Schellhorn, 2013). Deficiency of B complex vitamins produces nonspecific signs such as alopecia, decreased feed consumption, poor growth, poor reproduction and lactation, as well as a variety of neurological abnormalities. Choline deficiency produces fatty livers and nodular hepatic hyperplasia, as well as myocardial lesions, decreased conception, and decreased viability of litters. Folic acid-deficient diets cause marked decreases in red and white cell blood counts and the disappearance of megakaryocytes and nucleated cells from the spleen. Pantothenic acid deficiency is characterized by nonspecific signs, such as weight loss, alopecia, achromotrichia, and posterior paralysis, as well as other neurological abnormalities. Thiamin deficiency is associated with neurological signs, such as violent convulsions, cartwheel movements, and decreased food consumption. Dietary requirements for ascorbic acid have not been shown in mice, and mouse diets are generally not fortified with ascorbic acid. The gulonolactone oxidase knockout mouse ($Gulo^{-/-}$) on the C57BL/6 background requires vitamin C supplementation although the plasma ascorbate concentration of $Gulo^{-/-}$ mice fed a vitamin C-deficient diet is maintained at 15% of wild-type concentrations, suggesting an uncharacterized pathway to generate a small amount of ascorbate (Yu and Schellhorn, 2013). The $Gulo^{-/-}$ mouse has become the model of choice in studying the role of vitamin C in complex diseases. Vitamin C production has been successfully restored in $Gulo^{-/-}$ mice using adenovirus vectors, making it possible to robustly manipulate physiological ascorbate concentrations in an inbred mouse.

Mineral deficiencies have been described only for several elements, and the consequences of the deficiencies are similar to those observed for other species. For example, iodine-deficient diets produce thyroid goiters; magnesium-deficient diets may cause fatal convulsions; manganese deficiency may cause congenital ataxia from abnormal development of the inner ear; and zinc deficiency may cause hair loss on the shoulders and neck, emaciation, decreased liver and kidney catalase activity, and immunosuppression.

Chronic essential fatty acid deficiency may cause hair loss, dermatitis with scaling and crusting of the skin, and occasional diarrhea. Infertility has also been associated with this syndrome. Mice have an absolute requirement for a dietary source of linoleic and/or arachidonic acid.

5. Alopecia and Chronic Ulcerative Dermatitis in Black Mice (Sundberg, 1994; Ward, 2000)

The significant syndrome of ulcerative dermatitis (UD) is a common idiopathic skin lesion that causes morbidity and early euthanasia losses in C57BL/6 and related lines of mice. Significant pruritus leads to skin trauma associated with opportunistic bacterial infection and deep dermal ulcerations. Initial signs include alopecia and papular dermatitis, which usually occur over the dorsal trunk (Fig. 3.59). Progressive inflammation can be halted, sometimes reversed, by nail trimming and therapy with a wide spectrum of topical or systemic antibiotics, steroids, and other drugs such as Vitamin E and aloe, all of which speak to the frustrating search for a primary etiology. Treatment should be based on microbiological culture and sensitivity and screening for ectoparasites as hypersensitivity to acariasis has been proposed. Seasonal fluctuation in the incidence of disease suggests that environmental factors may play a role. The incidence appears to increase during periods of significant seasonal changes in temperature and humidity, i.e., the onset of winter and early spring. There is some

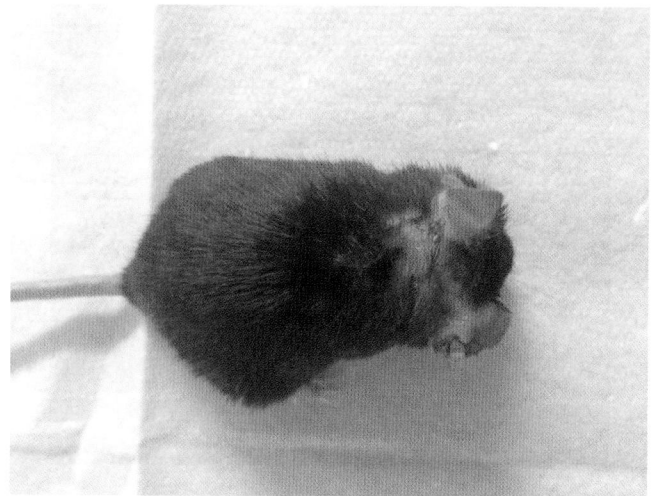

FIGURE 3.59 Dorsal chronic ulcerative dermatitis in a C57BL/6. *Courtesy of Abigail Powell.*

evidence that incidence is related to dietary fat with mice on high fat or *ad libitum* diets being more susceptible than those on restricted diets (Neuhaus *et al.*, 2012).

6. Postpartum Ileus

Ileus associated with high mortality has been reported to occur in primiparous female mice during the second week of lactation (Kunstyr, 1986). This disorder has been described as acute intestinal pseudo-obstruction (IPO) in C57BL/6 mice free of known pathogens (Feinstein *et al.*, 2008). Lactating mice are either found dead or becoming moribund. Segments of the small intestine become distended with fluid contents and histologically there is apoptosis of the villus epithelium of the small intestine and superficial epithelial cells of the large intestine. The enteric nervous system appears morphologically normal but necrotic enterocytes, mucosal erosions, and acute mucosal inflammation are commonly observed. There is no strong evidence for metabolic issues such as hypocalcemia or low blood glucose. The direct cause is unknown but death probably results from sepsis secondary to loss of barrier function reflected in apoptosis of the gut epithelium during peak lactation.

C. Environmental, Behavioral, and Traumatic Disorders

Environmental variables can affect responses of mice in experimental situations. Changes in respiratory epithelial physiology and function from elevated levels of ammonia, effects of temperature and humidity on metabolism, effects of light on eye lesions and retinal function, and effects of noise on neurophysiology are examples of complications that can vary with the form of insult and the strain of mouse employed.

1. Temperature-Related Disorders

Mice do not easily acclimatize to sudden and dramatic changes in temperature. Therefore, they are susceptible to both hypothermia and hyperthermia. Mice also are susceptible to dehydration. Poorly functioning automatic watering system valves or water bottles, resulting in spills (hypothermia) or obstructed sipper tubes (dehydration), are a significant cause of husbandry-related morbidity. Shipping mice between facilities, irrespective of distance, warrants institutional guidelines to minimize exposure to temperature extremes. Reheat coils should be designed to fail in the closed position to avoid overheating holding rooms.

2. Ringtail

Ringtail is a condition associated with low relative humidity. Clinical signs include annular constriction of the tail and occasionally of the feet or digits, resulting in localized edema that can progress to dry gangrene (Fig. 3.60). It should be differentiated from dryness and gangrene that may occur in hairless mice exposed to low temperatures and perhaps other environmental or nutritional imbalances. Necrosis of legs, feet, or digits also can occur in suckling mice because of disruption of circulation by wraps of stringy nesting material such as cotton wool.

3. Corneal Opacities

Corneal opacities can result from acute or chronic keratitis, injury (unilateral) and developmental defects; the latter may occur in combination with inherited microphthalmia in C57 black mice (Koch and Gowen, 1939). There is some evidence that the buildup of ammonia in mouse cages may contribute to inflammatory keratitis, because it can be controlled by increasing the frequency of cage cleaning. Corneal opacities and anterior polar cataracts are a developmental defect in inbred C57 black mice (Pierro and Spiggle, 1967). Corneal opacity may be associated with keratolenticular adhesions involving a persistent epithelial stalk of the lens vesicle, which normally disappears around day 11 of gestation (Koch and Gowen, 1939).

4. Malocclusion

Typically noted in runted or cachectic mice soon after weaning, malocclusion of the open-rooted, continually growing incisor teeth is an inherited trait expressed as poorly aligned incisors, especially of the lower incisors causing osteomyelitis, soft tissue abscesses, or necrosis in the lips or oral cavity. The incidence of inherited malocclusion varies with mouse strain (Petznek *et al.*, 2002). Malocclusion in older mice may be the result of trauma or oral neoplasia. Overgrown molar teeth have been associated with trauma to developing tooth buds.

5. Skin Trauma

Skin lesions can be caused by fighting, tail biting, and overgrooming such as whisker chewing. Barbering of facial hair and whiskers in subordinate mice by a dominant cagemate is common and may be solved by removing the dominant, normally haired mouse.

Hair or whisker chewing (barbering) has long been interpreted to be a manifestation of social dominance. Apparent dominant animals retain whiskers, whereas cagemates have 'shaved faces' (Fig. 3.61). Chronic hair chewing can produce histological abnormalities such as poorly formed or pigmented club hairs. Once chewing has ceased, many mice regrow previously lost hair in

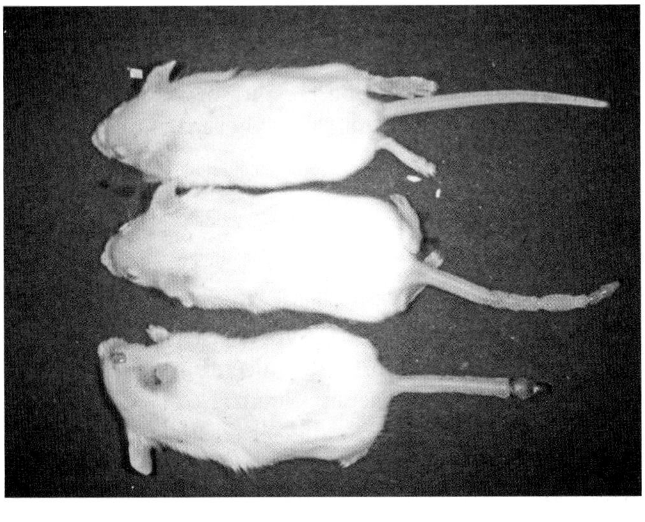

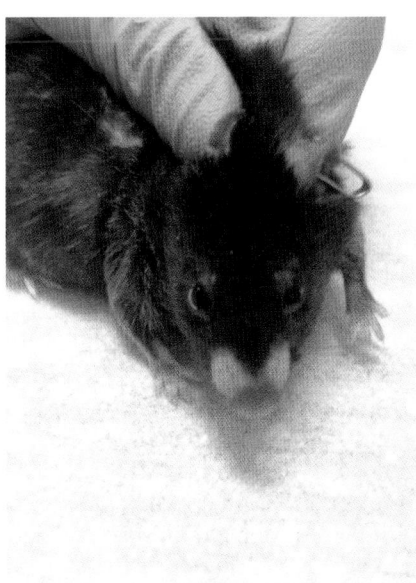

FIGURE 3.60   Ringtail, an idiopathic annular constriction around the tail of mice associated with low relative humidity.

FIGURE 3.61   Barbering of the whiskers. *Courtesy of Abigail Powell.*

several weeks. Both sexes may engage in this activity, and sometimes females may be dominant. Barbering of whiskers and fur-plucking behavior in mice has been suggested to model human trichotillomania (compulsive hair plucking) because of similarities including elevated serotonin levels (Dufour et al., 2010), 'barbers' predominately pluck hair from the scalp and around the eyes and the genitals; the behavior is female biased, and begins during puberty and is impacted by genetic background (Garner et al., 2004).

Fighting is more common in male mice and more aggressive in some strains (SJL, FVB, BALB/c) with bite wounds typically located on the head, neck, shoulders, perineal area, and tail. Often one mouse in the cage is free of lesions and is the likely aggressor. Removal of the unaffected male may end the fighting or simply reorder the dominance order. Removing males for breeding and then regrouping them often results in fighting. For programs that produce sentinel mice in-house, castration is an option to reduce aggression in group-housed male sentinels (Lofgren et al., 2012). Regional alopecia, especially around the muzzle, may result from abrasion against cage surfaces. Improperly diluted disinfectants may also cause regional hair loss. Ear tags used for identification may cause pruritis and self-induced trauma. Hair removal products or clipping prior to imaging or application of experimental compounds to the skin may cause pruritus and can augment lesions that interfere with test results. Dermatophytosis, ectoparasitism, or idiopathic hair loss must be considered in the differential diagnoses for muzzle or body alopecia.

D. Congenital, Aging-Related, and Miscellaneous Disorders (Burek et al., 1982; Percy and Barthold, 2007)

Common idiopathic lesions in aging mice include cardiomyopathy (with or without mineralization or arteritis), chronic nephropathy (frequently with mineralization), myelofibrosis (fibrotic change in the bone marrow) especially in female mice, melanosis in the meninges, ovarian atrophy (with or without hyaline material), pigment (ceroid-lipofuscin), tubular or stromal hyperplasia, cystic endometrial hyperplasia, testicular tubular degeneration or mineralization, prostate atypical epithelial hyperplasia, gastric glandular epithelial hyperplasia, pancreatic islet cell hyperplasia, dental dysplasia of incisor teeth, pituitary hyperplasia of pars intermedia and pars distalis, cataracts, increased extramedullary hematopoiesis in spleen, and lymphocytic infiltrates or other inflammatory changes in various tissues, including Harderian gland, salivary gland, kidney, liver, gall bladder, nasal, trachea, thyroid, periovarian fat, epididymis, and urinary bladder. Lymphoma is also very common (Haines et al., 2001).

1. Cardiovascular System

Spontaneous atrial thrombosis is rare in mice (<1% in 2-year-old mice) and appears to be strain-related, with a high prevalence in RFM mice. It also is more common in aged mice affected by kidney disease and amyloidosis. Organizing thrombi will be found usually in an enlarged, hyperemic left atrium and auricle and may be accompanied by amyloidosis. Affected mice may display signs of heart failure, particularly severe dyspnea. Induction of atrial thrombosis in B6C3F1 mice has been used to assess cardiovascular risk of chemical exposures (Yoshizawa et al., 2005). Myocardial and epicardial mineralization is described above (Section III,B,2). Periarteritis, also known as arteritis, polyarteritis, or systemic arteritis, impacts older mice and lesions may be observed in multiple tissues, including the spleen, heart, tongue, uterus, testes, kidney, and urinary bladder. The media of the affected vessels is homogenous and intensely eosinophilic with hematoxylin and eosin stain. Fibrosis and mononuclear cells infiltrate the vessel wall. Experimental coronary arteritis with cardiac hypertrophy has been model in DBA/2 and other strains by intraperitoneal administration of mannoprotein–beta-glucan complex isolated from C. albicans (Nagi-Miura et al., 2006).

2. Respiratory Tract

Hyperplasia of alveolar or bronchial epithelium occurs in old mice and must be differentiated from pulmonary tumors. Pulmonary histiocytosis, acidophilic macrophage pneumonia, and acidophilic crystalline pneumonia are synonymous morphologic descriptions of an idiopathic lung lesion that can be incidental or the cause of significant morbidity. Incidence varies with mouse strain or stock, with C57BL, 129S4/SvJae and Swiss mice and older mice in general particularly susceptible. Histologically, alveoli and bronchioles are filled with varying quantities of macrophages containing eosinophilic crystalline material (Ward et al., 2001). The crystalline material consists of YM1 and/or YM2 chitanases and can be found in other tissues including the upper respiratory tract, stomach, gall bladder, and bone marrow where it is described as hyalinosis (Nio et al., 2004).

3. Alimentary Tract
a. Stomach

Gastric lesions include crypt dilatation, submucosal fibrosis, adenomatous gastric hyperplasia, mineralization, and erosion or ulceration. Gastric ulcers have been induced by cold stress, food restriction (Rehm et al., 1987), chemical injury (Yadav et al., 2013), and gastritis and gastric tumors by helicobacter infection (Fox et al., 2003). Germfree mice have reduced muscle tone in the intestinal tract. Cecal volvulus is a common cause of death in germfree mice and is caused by rotation of the large, thin-walled cecum.

b. Liver

Age-associated lesions are common in the livers of mice. Cellular and nuclear pleomorphism, including binucleated and multinucleated cells, are detectable by 6 months. Mild focal necrosis occurs with or without inflammation, but an association of mild focal hepatitis with a specific infectious disease is often hard to confirm. Other geriatric hepatic lesions include biliary hyperplasia with varying degrees of portal hepatitis, hepatocellular vacuolization, amyloid deposition (especially in periportal areas), strangulated or herniated lobes, hemosiderosis, lipofuscinosis, and fibrosis. Extramedullary hematopoiesis occurs in young mice and in response to anemia.

c. Pancreas

Exocrine pancreatic insufficiency has been reported in CBA/J mice. Acinar cell atrophy is common but is strain- and sex-dependent.

4. Lymphoreticular System

Blood-filled mesenteric lymph nodes may occur in aged mice, especially C3H mice. This condition is an incidental finding and should not be confused with infectious lymphadenopathy such as that associated with salmonellosis. Aggregates, or nodules of mononuclear cells, are found in many tissues of aged mice, including the salivary gland, thymus, ovary, uterus, mesentery and mediastinum, urinary bladder, and gastrointestinal tract. These nodules should not be mistaken for lymphosarcomas. Grossly observable black pigmentation in the spleen of C57BL/6 is normal and is melanosis caused by melanin deposition (Weissman, 1967). The spleen is subject to amyloidosis and hemosiderin deposition. Lipofuscin deposition is common, especially in older mice. The thymus undergoes age-associated atrophy.

A variety of genetic immunodeficiencies have been described in mice, many of which increase susceptibility to infectious diseases. Perhaps the most widely known of these is the athymic nude mouse that lacks a significant hair coat and, more importantly, fails to develop a thymus and thus has a severe deficit of T-cell-mediated immune function. Additionally, SCID mice, which lack both T and B lymphocytes, are used widely and are highly susceptible to opportunistic agents such as *Pneumocystis murina*. Specific immune deficits have become excellent models for studying the ontogeny and mechanisms of immune responsiveness (Table 3.12).

5. Musculoskeletal System

Age-associated osteoporosis or senile osteodystrophy can occur in some mice. It is not associated with severe renal disease or parathyroid hyperplasia. Nearly all strains of mice develop some form of osteoarthrosis. It is generally noninflammatory, affects articulating surfaces, and results in secondary bone degeneration.

6. Urinary Tract

Glomerulonephritis is a common kidney lesion of mice. It is more often associated with persistent viral infections or immune disorders rather than with bacterial infections. Its prevalence in some strains approaches 100%. NZB and NZB × NZW F_1 hybrid mice, e.g., develop immune complex glomerulonephritis as an autoimmune disease resembling human lupus erythematosus, whereas glomerular disease is relatively mild in NZB mice (NZB mice have a high incidence of autoimmune hemolytic anemia). Renal changes occur as early as 4 months of age, but clinical signs and severe disease are not present until 6–9 months. The disease is associated with wasting and proteinuria, and lesions progress until death intervenes. Histologically, glomeruli have proteinaceous deposits in the capillaries and mesangium. Later, tubular atrophy and proteinaceous casts occur throughout the kidney. Immunofluorescence studies show deposits of immunoglobulin and the third component of complement, which lodge as immune complexes with nuclear antigens and antigens of murine leukemia virus in glomerular capillary loops. Mice infected with LCMV or with retroviruses can also develop immune complex glomerulonephritis.

Mice also can develop chronic glomerulopathy characterized by progressive thickening of glomerular basement membrane by PAS-positive material that does not stain for amyloid. This lesion can be accompanied by proliferation of mesangial cells; local, regional, or diffuse mononuclear cell infiltration; and fibrosis. Advanced cases may lead to renal insufficiency or failure.

Interstitial nephritis can be caused by bacterial or viral infections but may also be idiopathic. Typical lesions include focal, regional, or diffuse interstitial infiltration of tubular parenchyma by mononuclear cells, but glomerular regions also may be involved. Severe lesions can be accompanied by fibrosis, distortion of renal parenchyma, and intratubular casts, but not by mineralization. If renal insufficiency or failure ensues, it can lead to ascites.

Some strains of mice, such as BALB/c, can develop polycystic kidney disease, which, if severe, can compromise normal renal function.

Urinary tract obstruction occurs as an acute or chronic condition in male mice. Clinical signs usually include wetting of the perineum from incontinence. In severe or chronic cases, wetting predisposes to cellulitis and ulceration. At necropsy, the bladder is distended, and proteinaceous plugs are often found in the neck of the bladder and proximal urethra. In chronic cases the urine may be cloudy, and calculi may develop in the bladder. Additionally, cystitis, urethritis, prostatitis, balanoposthitis, and hydronephrosis may develop. This condition must be differentiated from infectious cystitis or pyelonephritis and from the agonal release of secretions from accessory sex glands, which is not associated with an inflammatory response. Hydronephrosis also may occur without urinary tract obstruction. Ascending pyelitis occurs in mice secondary to urinary tract infection.

7. Genital Tract

a. Female

Parvovarian cysts are observed frequently and may be related to the fact that mouse ovaries are enclosed in membranous pouches. Amyloidosis is also common in the ovaries of old mice. Cystic endometrial hyperplasia may develop unilaterally or bilaterally and may be segmental. In some strains, the prevalence in mice older than 18 months is 100%. Endometrial hyperplasia is often associated with ovarian atrophy. Mucometra is relatively common in adult female mice. The primary clinical sign is abdominal distension resembling pregnancy among mice that do not whelp.

b. Male

Testicular atrophy, sperm granulomas, and tubular mineralization occur with varying incidence. Preputial glands, especially of immunodeficient mice, can become infected with opportunistic or pathogenic bacteria. Spontaneous lesions in prostate, coagulating gland (anterior prostatic lobe), seminal vesicles, and ampullary glands were described in control B6C3F1 mice from 12 National Toxicology Program 2-year carcinogenicity and toxicity studies conducted in one of four different laboratories (Suwa et al., 2002). Lymphocytic infiltration, inflammation, edema, epithelial hyperplasia, mucinous cyst, mucinous metaplasia, adenoma, adenocarcinoma, granular cell tumor, and glandular atrophy were variously observed in accessory sex glands.

8. Endocrine System

Accessory adrenal cortical nodules are found in periadrenal and perirenal fat, especially in females. These nodules have little functional significance other than their potential effect on failures of surgical adrenalectomy. Lipofuscinosis, subcapsular spindle cell hyperplasia, and cystic dilatation of cortical sinusoids are found in the adrenal cortices of aged mice.

Some inbred strains have deficiencies of thyrotropic hormone, resulting in thyroid atrophy. Thyroid cysts lined by stratified squamous epithelium and generally of ultimo-branchial origin may be seen in old mice. Amyloid can be deposited in the thyroid and parathyroid glands as well as in the adrenal glands. Spontaneous diabetes mellitus occurs in outbred swiss mice and genetic

variants of several strains such as NOD mice (Lemke et al., 2008).

High levels of estrogen in pregnancy may influence postpartum hair shedding. Various endocrine effects on hair growth have also been described. Abdominal and thoracic alopecia have been reported in B6C3F1 mice.

9. Nervous System

Symmetrical mineral deposits commonly occur in the thalamus of aged mice. They may also be found in the midbrain, cerebellum, and cerebrum and are particularly common in A/J mice. Lipofuscin accumulates in the neurons of old mice. Age-associated peripheral neuropathy with demyelination can be found in the nerves of the hindlimbs in C57BL/6 mice. Deposits of melanin pigment occur in heavily pigmented strains, especially in the frontal lobe. A number of neurologically mutant mice have been described. They commonly have correlative anatomical malformations or inborn errors of metabolism. A seizure syndrome in FVB mice has been described (Goelz et al., 1998) and can be spontaneous or associated with tail tattooing, fur clipping, and fire alarms. Mice are most often female with a mean age of 5.8 months (range, 2–16 months) and can exhibit facial grimace, chewing automatism, ptyalism with matting of the fur of the ventral aspect of the neck and/or forelimbs, and clonic convulsions that may progress to tonic convulsions and death. Ischemic neuronal necrosis was consistently observed in these mice and is consistent with status epilepticus in humans.

10. Organs of Special Sense

a. Eye (Also See Corneal Opacities)

Unilateral and bilateral microphthalmia and anophthalmia are frequent (as high as 12%) developmental defects in inbred and congenic strains of C57BL mice, especially impacting the right eye and female mice. These conditions may first be recognized due to ocular infections, secondary to inadequate tear drainage. Other common findings include central corneal opacities, iridocorneal and corneal-lenticular adhesions, abnormal formation of the iris and ciliary body, cataracts, extrusion of lens cortical material with dispersion throughout the eye, failure of vitreous development, and retinal folding. These syndromes can be reproduced by exposure to alcohol at critical stages of embryogenesis when the optic cup and lens vesicle are developing and impacting normal development of other ocular structures, including the iris, ciliary body, vitreous, and retina (Smith et al., 1994).

Retinal degeneration can occur as either an environmental or a genetic disorder (Chang et al., 2007) in mice. Nonpigmented mice, both inbred and outbred, can develop retinal degeneration from exposure to light, with the progression of blindness being related to light intensity and duration of exposure. Mouse genetics have been shown to be more important than potential light associated tissue injury (Serfilippi *et al.*, 2004a). Other strains such as C3H, CBA, and FVB are genetically predisposed to retinal degeneration because they carry the *rd* gene, which leads to retinal degeneration within the first few weeks of life and has been used extensively as a model for retinitis pigmentosa (Farber and Danciger, 1994). Presence of the *rd* gene in some mouse strains highlights that impaired vision must be a consideration when selecting strains for behavioral assays that rely on visual clues (Garcia *et al.*, 2004). Blindness does not interfere with health or reproduction and blind mice cannot be distinguished from non-blind mice housed in standard caging. Cataracts can occur in old mice and have a higher prevalence in certain mutant strains.

b. Ear

Vestibular syndrome associated with head tilt, circling, or imbalance can result from infectious otitis or from necrotizing vasculitis of unknown etiology affecting small and medium-sized arteries in the vicinity of the middle and inner ears.

E. Neoplastic Diseases (Jones *et al.*, 1983–1993; Maronpot *et al.*, 1999; Percy and Barthold, 2007)

1. Lymphoreticular and Hematopoietic Systems

Neoplasms of lymphoid and hematopoietic tissues are estimated to have a spontaneous prevalence of 1–2%. There are, however, some strains of mice that have been specifically inbred and selected for susceptibility to spontaneous tumors. Leukemogenesis in mice may involve viruses and chemical or physical agents. Viruses associated with lymphopoietic and hematopoietic neoplasia belong to the family Retroviridae (type C oncornaviruses) and contain RNA-dependent DNA polymerase (reverse transcriptase). These viruses are generally noncytopathogenic for infected cells, and mice appear to harbor them as normal components of their genome. Although they may be involved in spontaneous leukemia, they are not consistently expressed in this disease. Recombinant viruses have recently been discovered that can infect mouse cells and heterologous cells and are associated with spontaneous leukemia development in high leukemia strains such as AKR mice. Their phenotypic expression is controlled by mouse genotype. Endogenous retroviruses are transmitted vertically through the germ line. Horizontal transmission is inefficient but can occur by intrauterine infection or through saliva, sputum, urine, feces, or milk. The leukemia induced by a given endogenous virus is usually of a single histopathological type. Loss of function in nucleic acid-recognizing, TLR3, TLR7, and TLR9 can result in

spontaneous retroviral viremia and acute T-cell lymphoblastic leukemia (Yu *et al.*, 2012). Chemical carcinogens, such as polycyclic hydrocarbons, nitrosoureas, and nitrosamines, and physical agents such as X-irradiation can also induce hematological malignancies in mice.

a. Lymphoblastic Lymphoma (Thymic Lymphoma, B-Cell Lymphoma)

The most common hematopoietic malignancy in the mouse is lymphocytic leukemia that originates in the thymus. Disease begins with unilateral atrophy and then enlargement of one lobe of thymus as tumor cells proliferate. Cells can spread to the other lobe and then to other hematopoietic organs, such as the spleen, bone marrow, liver, and peripheral lymph nodes. Clinical signs include dyspnea and ocular protrusion. The latter sign is due to compression of venous blood returning from the head. Tumor cells spill into the circulation late in disease. Most of these tumors originate from T lymphocytes or lymphoblasts, but there are leukemias of B-lymphocyte or null cell lineage. In the last two syndromes, the lymph nodes and spleen are often involved, but the thymus is generally normal.

b. Reticulum Cell Sarcoma (Histiocytic Lymphoma, Follicular Center Cell Lymphoma)

Reticulum cell sarcomas are common in older mice, especially in inbred strains such as C57BL/6 and SJL. Primary tumor cell types have been divided into several categories based on morphological and immunohistochemical features. Histiocytic sarcomas correspond to the older Dunn classification as type A sarcomas and are composed primarily of reticulum cells. The tumor typically causes splenomegaly and nodular lesions in other organs, including the liver, lung, kidney, and the female reproductive tract. Follicular center cell lymphomas correspond to Dunn type B sarcomas. They originate from B-cell regions (germinal centers) of peripheral lymphoid tissues, including the spleen, lymph nodes, and Peyer's patches. Typical tumor cells have large vesiculated, folded, or cleaved nuclei and ill-defined cytoplasmic borders. Tumors also often contain small lymphocytes. Type C reticulum cell tumors often involve one or several lymph nodes rather than assuming a wide distribution. They consist of reticulum cells with a prominent component of well-differentiated lymphocytes.

c. Myelogenous Leukemia

Myelogenous leukemia is uncommon in mice and is associated with retrovirus infection. Disease begins in the spleen, resulting in marked splenomegaly, but leukemic spread results in involvement of many tissues including the liver, lung, and bone marrow. Leukemic cells in various stages of differentiation can be found in peripheral blood. In older animals, affected organs may appear green because of myeloperoxidase activity, giving rise to the term chloroleukemia. The green hue fades on contact with air. Affected mice are often clinically anemic and dyspneic.

d. Erythroleukemia

Erythroleukemia is rare in mice. The major lesion is massive splenomegaly, which is accompanied by anemia and polycythemia. Hepatomegaly can follow, but there is little change in the thymus or lymph nodes. Erythroleukemia can be experimentally induced in mice by Friend spleen focus-forming virus (SFFV) which initially activates the erythropoietin (Epo) receptor and the receptor tyrosine kinase sf-Stk in erythroid cells, resulting in proliferation, differentiation, and survival. In a second stage, SFFV activates the myeloid transcription factor PU.1, blocking erythroid cell differentiation, and in conjunction with the loss of p53 tumor suppressor activity, results in the outgrowth of malignant cells (Cmarik and Ruscetti, 2010).

e. Mast Cell Tumors

Mast cell tumors are also very rare in mice. They are found almost exclusively in old mice and grow slowly. They should not be confused with mast cell hyperplasia observed in the skin following painting with carcinogens or X-irradiation.

f. Plasma Cell Tumors

Natural plasma cell tumors are infrequent in the mouse. They can, however, be induced by intraperitoneal inoculation of granulomatogenic agents such as plastic filters, plastic shavings, or a variety of oils, particularly in BALB/c mice. Mineral oil-induced plasmacytomas in BALB/c mice produce large amounts of endogenous retroelements such as ecotropic and polytropic murine leukemia virus and intracisternal A particles. Associated inflammation may promote retroelement insertion into cancer genes, thereby promoting tumors (Knittel *et al.*, 2014). Similar to other spontaneous cancers, plasmacytoma development in mice is inhibited by innate immune responses of NK cells which when activated by viruses will release γINF (Thirion *et al.*, 2014).

2. Mammary Gland

Mammary tumors can be induced or modulated by a variety of factors, including viruses, chemical carcinogens, radiation, hormones, genetic background, diet, and immune status. Certain inbred strains of mice, such as C3H, A, and DBA/2, have a high natural prevalence of mammary tumors. Other strains, such as BALB/c, C57BL, and AKR, have a low prevalence.

Among the most important factors contributing to the development of mammary tumors are mammary tumor viruses. Several major variants are known. The

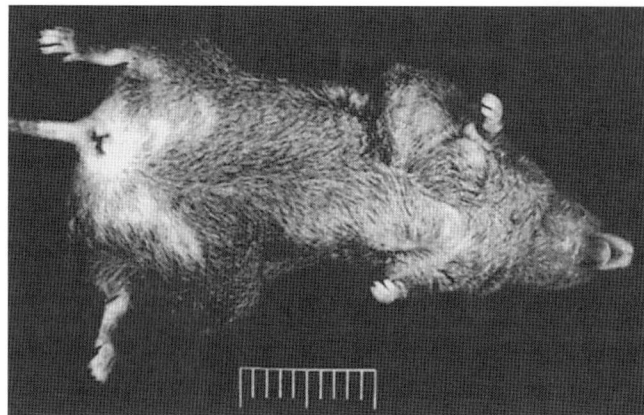

FIGURE 3.62   Mammary tumors in a C3H mouse.

primary tumor virus MMTV-S (Bittner virus) is highly oncogenic and is transmitted through the milk of nursing females. Infected mice typically develop a precursor lesion, the hyperplastic alveolar nodule, which can be serially transplanted.

Spontaneous mammary tumors metastasize with high frequency, but this property is somewhat mouse strain dependent. Metastases go primarily to the lung. Some mammary tumors are hormone dependent, some are ovary dependent, and others are pregnancy dependent. Ovary-dependent tumors contain estrogen and progesterone receptors, whereas pregnancy-dependent tumors have prolactin receptors. Ovariectomy will dramatically reduce the incidence of mammary tumors in C3H mice. If surgery is done in adult mice 2–5 months of age, mammary tumors will develop, but at a later age than normal.

Grossly, mammary tumors may occur anywhere in the mammary chain. They present as one or more firm, well-delineated masses, which are often lobular and maybe cystic (Fig. 3.62). Histologically, mammary tumors have been categorized into three major groups: carcinomas, carcinomas with squamous cell differentiation, and carcinosarcomas. The carcinomas are divided into adenocarcinoma types A, B, C, Y, L, and P. Most tumors are type A or B. Type A consists of adenomas, tubular carcinomas, and alveolar carcinomas. Type B tumors have a variable pattern with both well-differentiated and poorly differentiated regions. They may consist of regular cords or sheets of cells or papillomatous areas. These two types are locally invasive and may metastasize to the lungs. Type C tumors are rare and are characterized by multiple cysts lined by low cuboidal to squamous epithelial cells, and they have abundant stroma. Type Y tumors, which are also rare, are characterized by tubular branching of cuboidal epithelium and abundant stroma. Adenocarcinomas with a lacelike morphology (types L and P) are hormone dependent and have a branching tubular structure.

The control or prevention of mammary neoplasms depends on the fact that some strains of mammary tumor virus are transmitted horizontally, whereas others are transmitted vertically. Although horizontally transmitted virus such as MMTV-S can be determined by cesarean rederivation or by foster nursing, endogenous strains of tumor virus may remain. Fortunately, these latter tumor viruses have generally low oncogenicity relative to the Bittner virus. Mammary tumors are increased in frequency in C57BL Apc$^{+/-}$ female mice infected with *H. hepaticus* (Rao *et al.*, 2007).

3. Liver

Mice develop an assortment of liver changes as they age, including proliferative lesions which can progress from hyperplastic foci to hepatomas to hepatocellular carcinomas. Almost all strains of mice have a significant prevalence of hepatic tumors, some of which appear to result from dietary contamination or deficiency and *H. hepaticus* infections in susceptible strains of mice such as the A/JCr male mouse (Fox *et al.*, 1994; Ward *et al.*, 1994). The prevalence of spontaneous liver tumors in B6C3F$_1$ hybrids is increased by feeding choline-deficient diets or when infected with *H. hepaticus* (Hailey *et al.*, 1998). Tumors also can develop in mice exposed to environmental chemicals, many of which are carcinogenic or potentially carcinogenic (Hoenerhoff *et al.*, 2009).

Spontaneous liver tumors in mice occur grossly as gray to tan nodules or large, poorly demarcated dark-red masses. They are usually derived from hepatocytes, whereas cholangiocellular tumors are rare. Hepatomas are well circumscribed and well differentiated, but they compress adjacent liver tissue as they develop. Hepatocellular carcinomas are usually invasive and display histopathological patterns ranging from medullary to trabecular. Large carcinomas also may contain hemorrhage and necrosis. Carcinomas also may metastasize to the lungs.

4. Lung

Primary respiratory tumors of mice occur in relatively high frequency. It has been estimated that more than 95% of these tumors are pulmonary adenomas that arise either from type 2 pneumocytes or from Clara cells lining terminal bronchioles. Pulmonary adenomas usually appear as distinct whitish nodules that are easily detected by examination of the lung surface. Malignant alveologenic tumors are infrequent and consist of adenocarcinomas and squamous cell carcinomas. They invade pulmonary parenchyma and are prone to metastasize. The prevalence of spontaneous respiratory tumors is mouse strain-dependent. For example, the prevalence is high in aging A strain mice but low in aging C57BL mice. The number of tumors per lung is also higher in susceptible mice.

Pulmonary tumors often occur as well-defined gray nodules. Microscopically, adenomas of alveolar origin consist of dense ribbons of cuboidal to columnar cells with sparse stroma. Adenomas of Clara cell origin are usually associated with bronchioles. They have a tubular to papillary architecture consisting of columnar cells with basal nuclei. Pulmonary adenocarcinomas, though comparatively rare, are locally invasive. They often form papillary structures and have considerable cellular pleomorphism.

5. Neoplasms of Other Organ Systems

Given the rapid development of mouse strains genetically predisposed to neoplasia, the Mouse Tumor Biology Database maintained by Jackson Laboratory is a valuable centralized resource for the most current tumor descriptions. The database contains information on more than 4400 strains and substrains, 348 tissues and organs, over 42,000 tumor frequency records, and nearly 4800 histopathological images and descriptions.

References

Abou Chakra, C.N., Pepin, J., Sirard, S., Valiquette, L., 2014. Risk factors for recurrence, complications and mortality in *Clostridium difficile* infection: a systematic review. PLoS One 9, e98400.

Agca, Y., Bauer, B.A., Johnson, D.K., Critser, J.K., Riley, L.K., 2007. Detection of mouse parvovirus in *Mus musculus* gametes, embryos, and ovarian tissues by polymerase chain reaction. Comp. Med. 57, 51–56.

Akdis, M., Burgler, S., Crameri, R., Eiwegger, T., Fujita, H., Gomez, E., et al., 2011. Interleukins, from 1 to 37, and interferon-gamma: receptors, functions, and roles in diseases. J. Allergy Clin. Immunol. 127, 701–721, e1–70.

Akkina, R., 2013. New generation humanized mice for virus research: comparative aspects and future prospects. Virology 435, 14–28.

Allen, S.J., Crown, S.E., Handel, T.M., 2007. Chemokine: receptor structure, interactions, and antagonism. Annu. Rev. Immunol. 25, 787–820.

Arriaga, G., Zhou, E., Jarvis, E.D., 2012. Of mice, birds, and men: the mouse ultrasonic song system has some features similar to humans and song-learning birds. PLoS One 7, e46610.

Arthur, J.C., Perez-Chanona, E., Muhlbauer, M., Tomkovich, S., Uronis, J.M., Fan, T.J., et al., 2012. Intestinal inflammation targets cancer-inducing activity of the microbiota. Science 338, 120–123.

Artwohl, J.E., Purcell, J.E., Fortman, J.D., 2008. The use of cross-foster rederivation to eliminate murine norovirus. J. Am. Assoc. Lab. Anim. Sci. 47, 19–24.

Bae, S., Park, J., Kim, J.S., 2014. Cas-OFFinder: a fast and versatile algorithm that searches for potential off-target sites of Cas9 RNA-guided endonucleases. Bioinformatics 30, 1473–1475.

Baek, L.J., Yanagihara, R., Gibbs, C.J.J., Miyazaki, M., Gajdusek, D.C., 1988. Leaky virus: a new hantavirus isolated from *Mus musculus* in the United States. J. Gen. Virol. 69, 3129–3132.

Bailey, D.W., 1971. Recombinant-inbred strains: an aid to finding identity, linkage, and function of histocompatibility and other genes. Transplantation 11.

Baker, D.G., 2007. Parasites of rats and mice. In: Baker, D.G. (Ed.), Flynn's Parasites of Laboratory Animals. Blackwell Publishing, Ames, IA.

Baker, D.G., Malineni, S., Taylor, H.W., 1998. Experimental infection of inbred mouse strains with *Spironucleus muris*. Vet. Parasitol. 77, 305–310.

Barnard, D.E., Lewis, S.M., Teter, B.B., Thigpen, J.E., 2009. Open- and closed-formula laboratory animal diets and their importance to research. J. Am. Assoc. Lab. Anim. Sci. 48, 709–713.

Barthold, S.W., 1980. The microbiology of transmissible murine colonic hyperplasia. Lab. Anim. Sci. 30, 167–173.

Barthold, S.W., 1997a. Mouse hepatitis virus infection, intestine, mouse. In: Jones, T.C., Popp, J.A., Mohr, U. (Eds.), Monographs on Pathology of Laboratory Animals. Digestive System, second ed. Springer, Washington, DC.

Barthold, S.W., 1997b. Mouse hepatitis virus infection, liver, mouse. In: Jones, T.C., Popp, J.A., Mohr, U. (Eds.), Monographs on Pathology of Laboratory Animals. Digestive System. Springer, Washington, DC.

Barthold, S.W., 1997c. Murine rotavirus infection, intestine, mouse. In: Jones, T.C., Popp, J.A., Mohr, U. (Eds.), Monographs on Pathology of Laboratory Animals: Digestive System, second ed. Springer, Washington, DC.

Barthold, S.W., Beck, D., 1980. Modification of early dimethylhydra-zine carcinogenesis by colonic mucosal hyperplasia. Cancer Res. 40, 4451–4455.

Barthold, S.W., Smith, A.L., 2007. Lymphocytic choriomeningitis virus. In: Fox, J.G., Barthold, S.W., Davisson, M.T., Newcomer, C.E., Quimby, F., Smith, A.L. (Eds.), The Mouse in Biomedical Research. II. Diseases. Elsevier, London.

Barthold, S.W., Osbaldiston, G.W., Jonas, A.M., 1977. Dietary, bacterial, and host genetic interactions in the pathogenesis of transmissible murine colonic hyperplasia. Lab. Anim. Sci. 27, 938–945.

Barthold, S.W., Coleman, G.L., Jacoby, R.O., Livestone, E.M., Jonas, A.M., 1978. Transmissible murine colonic hyperplasia. Vet. Pathol. 15, 223–236.

Barthold, S.W., Smith, A.L., Lord, P.F., Bhatt, P.N., Jacoby, R.O., Main, A.J., 1982. Epizootic coronaviral typhlocolitis in suckling mice. Lab. Anim. Sci. 32, 376–383.

Barthold, S.W., Smith, A.L., Bhatt, P.N., 1993. Infectivity, disease patterns, and serologic profiles of reovirus serotypes 1, 2, and 3 in infant and weanling mice. Lab. Anim. Sci. 43, 425–430.

Bartlett, J.G., Onderdonk, A.B., Cisneros, R.L., Kasper, D.L., 1977. Clindamycin-associated colitis due to a toxin-producing species of Clostridium in hamsters. J. Infect. Dis. 136, 701–705.

Beckwith, C.S., Franklin, C.L., Hook Jr., R.R., Besch-Williford, C.L., Riley, L.K., 1997. Fecal PCR assay for diagnosis of Helicobacter infection in laboratory rodents. J. Clin. Microbiol. 35, 1620–1623.

Benga, L., Benten, W.P., Engelhardt, E., Kohrer, K., Gougoula, C., Sager, M., 2014. 16S ribosomal DNA sequence-based identification of bacteria in laboratory rodents: a practical approach in laboratory animal bacteriology diagnostics. Lab. Anim 48 (4), 305–12.

Benjamin, T.L., 2007. Polyoma viruses. In: Fox, J.G., Barthold, S.W., Davisson, M.T., Newcomer, C.E., Quimby, F., Smith, A.L. (Eds.), The Mouse in Biomedical Research. II. Diseases. Elsevier, London.

Berke, Z., Dalianis, T., 1993. Persistence of polyomavirus in mice infected as adults differs from that observed in mice infected as newborns. J. Virol. 67, 4369–4371.

Besch-Williford, C., Franklin, C.L., 2007. Aerobic Gram-positive organisms. In: Fox, J.G., Barthold, S.W., Davisson, M.T., Newcomer, C.E., Quimby, F., Smith, A.L. (Eds.), The Mouse in Biomedical Research. II. Diseases. Elsevier, London.

Besselsen, D.G., 1998. Detection of rodent parvoviruses by PCR. Methods Mol. Biol. 92, 31–37.

Besselsen, D.G., Romero, M.J., Wagner, A.M., Henderson, K.S., Livingston, R.S., 2006. Identification of novel murine parvovirus strains by epidemiological analysis of naturally infected mice. J. Gen. Virol. 87, 1543–1556.

Besselsen, D.G., Becker, M.D., Henderson, K.S., Wagner, A.M., Banu, L.A., Shek, W.R., 2007. Temporal transmission studies of mouse parvovirus 1 in BALB/c and C.B-17/Icr-Prkdc(scid) mice. Comp. Med. 57, 66–73.

Besselsen, D.G., Romero-Aleshire, M.J., Munger, S.J., Marcus, E.C., Henderson, K.S., Wagner, A.M., 2008. Embryo transfer rederivation of C.B-17/Icr-Prkdc(scid) mice experimentally infected with mouse parvovirus 1. Comp. Med. 58, 353–359.

Bhatt, P.N., Jacoby, R.O., 1987a. Effect of vaccination on the clinical response, pathogenesis, and transmission of mousepox. Lab. Anim. Sci. 37, 610–614.

Bhatt, P.N., Jacoby, R.O., 1987b. Mousepox in inbred mice innately resistant or susceptible to lethal infeciton with ectromelia virus. III. Experimental transmission of infection and derivation of virus-free progeny from previously infected dams. Lab. Anim. Sci. 37, 23–27.

Bhatt, P.N., Jacoby, R.O., 1987c. Mousepox in inbred mice innately resistant or susceptible to lethal infection with ectromelia virus. I. Clinical responses. Lab. Anim. Sci. 37, 11–15.

Bhatt, P.N., Jacoby, R.O., 1987d. Stability of ectromelia virus strain NIH-79 under various laboratory conditions. Lab. Anim. Sci. 37, 33–35.

Bishop, C.E., Boursot, P., Baron, B., Bonhomme, F., Hatat, D., 1985. Most classical Mus musculus domesticus laboratory mice carry a Mus musculus musculus Y chromosome. Nature 315, 70–72.

Bleich, A., Kirsch, P., Sahly, H., Fahey, J., Smoczek, A., Hedrich, H.J., et al., 2008. Klebsiella oxytoca: opportunistic infections in laboratory rodents. Lab. Anim. 42, 369–375.

Bohland, J.W., Bokil, H., Pathak, S.D., Lee, C.K., Ng, L., Lau, C., et al., 2010. Clustering of spatial gene expression patterns in the mouse brain and comparison with classical neuroanatomy. Methods 50, 105–112.

Boot, R., Thuis, H., Bakker, R., Veenema, J.L., 1995a. Serological studies of Corynebacterium kutscheri and coryneform bacteria using an enzyme-linked immunosorbent assay (ELISA). Lab. Anim. 29, 294–299.

Boot, R., Thuis, H.C., Veenema, J.L., Bakker, R.G., 1995b. An enzyme-linked immunosorbent assay (ELISA) for monitoring rodent colonies for Pasteurella pneumotropica antibodies. Lab. Anim. 29, 307–313.

Boutin, S.R., Shen, Z., Roesch, P.L., Stiefel, S.M., Sanderson, A.E., Multari, H.M., et al., 2010. Helicobacter pullorum outbreak in C57BL/6NTac and C3H/HeNTac barrier-maintained mice. J. Clin. Microbiol. 48, 1908–1910.

Brandtzaeg, P., 2009. Mucosal immunity: induction, dissemination, and effector functions. Scand J. Immunol. 70, 505–515.

Braun, M., Bjorkstrom, N.K., Gupta, S., Sundstrom, K., Ahlm, C., Klingstrom, J., et al., 2014. NK cell activation in human hantavirus infection explained by virus-induced IL-15/IL15Ralpha expression. PLoS Pathog. 10, e1004521.

Bray, M.V., Barthold, S.W., Sidman, C.L., Roths, J., Smith, A.L., 1993. Exacerbation of Pneumocystis carinii pneumonia in immunodeficient (SCID) mice by concurrent infection with a pneumovirus. Infect. Immun. 61, 1586–1588.

Breer, H., Fleischer, J., Strotmann, J., 2006. The sense of smell: multiple olfactory subsystems. Cell Mol. Life Sci. 63, 1465–1475.

Brennan, P.A., Zufall, F., 2006. Pheromonal communication in vertebrates. Nature 444, 308–315.

Brett, S.J., Cox, F.E., 1982. Immunological aspects of Giardia muris and Spironucleus muris infections in inbred and outbred strains of laboratory mice: a comparative study. Parasitology 85 (Pt 1), 85–99.

Briody, B.A., 1966. The natural history of mousepox. Natl. Cancer Inst. Monogr. 20, 105–116.

Bronson, F.H., Dagg, C.P., Snell, G.D., 1966. Reproduction. In: Green, E.L. (Ed.), Biology of the Laboratory Mouse, second ed. McGraw-Hill, New York, pp. 187–204.

Brown, A.J., Fisher, D.A., Kouranova, E., Mccoy, A., Forbes, K., Wu, Y., et al., 2013. Whole-rat conditional gene knockout via genome editing. Nat. Methods 10, 638–640.

Brownstein, D.G., 1978. Pathogenesis of bacteremia due to Pseudomonas aeruginosa in cyclophosphamide-treated mice and potentiation of virulence of endogenous streptococci. J. Infect Dis. 137, 795–801.

Brownstein, D.G., 1983. Genetics of dystrophic epicardial mineralization in DBA/2 mice. Lab. Anim. Sci. 33, 247–248.

Brownstein, D.G., 2007. Sendai virus and pneumonia virus of mice (PVM). In: Fox, J.G., Barthold, S.W., Davisson, M.T., Newcomer, C.E., Quimby, F., Smith, A.L. (Eds.), The Mouse in Biomedical Research. II. Diseases. Elsevier, London.

Brownstein, D.G., Johnson, E.A., Smith, A.L., 1984. Spontaneous Reye's-like syndrome in BALB/cByJ mice. Lab. Invest. 51, 386–395.

Brownstein, D.G., Bhatt, P.N., Ardito, R.B., Paturzo, F.X., Johnson, E.A., 1989. Duration and patterns of transmission of Theiler's mouse encephalomyelitis virus infection. Lab. Anim. Sci. 39, 299–301.

Brownstein, D.G., Bhatt, P.N., Gras, L., Jacoby, R.O., 1991a. Chromosomal locations and gonadal dependence of genes that mediate resistance to ectromelia (mousepox) virus-induced mortality. J. Virol. 65, 1946–1951.

Brownstein, D.G., Smith, A.L., Jacoby, R.O., Johnson, E.A., Hansen, G., Tattersall, P., 1991b. Pathogenesis of infection with a virulent allotropic variant of minute virus of mice and regulation by host genotype. Lab. Invest. 65, 357–364.

Bruce, H.M., 1959. An exteroceptive block to pregnancy in the mouse. Nature 184, 105.

Brunnert, S.R., Dai, Y., Kohn, D.F., 1994. Comparison of polymerase chain reaction and immunohistochemistry for the detection of Mycoplasma pulmonis in paraffin-embedded tissue. Lab. Anim. Sci. 44, 257–260.

Brunnert, S.R., Shi, S., Chang, B., 1999. Chromosomal localization of the loci responsible for dystrophic cardiac calcinosis in DBA/2 mice. Genomics 59, 105–107.

Buller, R.M., Bhatt, P.N., Wallace, G.D., 1983. Evaluation of an enzyme-linked immunosorbent assay for the detection of ectromelia (mousepox) antibody. J. Clin. Microbiol. 18, 1220–1225.

Buller, R.M.L., Fenner, F., 2007. Mousepox. In: Fox, J.G., Barthold, S.W., Davisson, M.T., Newcomer, C.E., Quimby, F., Smith, A.L. (Eds.), The Mouse in Biomedical Research, second ed. Academic Press/Elsevier, New York.

Burek, J.D., Melello, J.A., Warner, S.D., 1982. Selected non-neoplastic diseases. In: Foster, H.L., Small, J.D., Fox, J.G. (Eds.), The Mouse in Biomedical Research. Academic Press, New York.

Burich, A., Hershberg, R., Waggie, K., Zeng, W., Brabb, T., Westrich, G., et al., 2001. Helicobacter-induced inflammatory bowel disease in IL-10- and T cell-deficient mice. Am. J. Physiol. Gastrointest Liver Physiol. 281, G764–G778.

Burr, H.N., Lipman, N.S., White, J.R., Zheng, J., Wolf, F.R., 2011. Strategies to prevent, treat, and provoke Corynebacterium-associated hyperkeratosis in athymic nude mice. J. Am. Assoc. Lab. Anim. Sci. 50, 378–388.

Burr, H.N., Wolf, F.R., Lipman, N.S., 2012. Corynebacterium bovis: epizootiologic features and environmental contamination in an enzootically infected rodent room. J. Am. Assoc. Lab. Anim. Sci. 51, 189–198.

Cahill, R.J., Foltz, C.J., Fox, J.G., Dangler, C.A., Powrie, F., Schauer, D.B., 1997. Inflammatory bowel disease: an immunity-mediated condition triggered by bacterial infection with Helicobacter hepaticus. Infect. Immun. 65, 3126–3131.

Carlson-Scholz, J.A., Garg, R., Compton, S.R., Allore, H.G., Zeiss, C.J., Uchio, E.M., 2011. Poliomyelitis in MuLV-infected ICR-SCID mice after injection of basement membrane matrix contaminated with lactate dehydrogenase-elevating virus. Comp. Med. 61, 404–411.

Cartner, S.C., Simecka, J.W., Briles, D.E., Cassell, G.H., Lindsey, J.R., 1996. Resistance to mycoplasmal lung disease in mice is a complex genetic trait. Infect. Immun. 64, 5326–5331.

Cartner, S.C., Lindsey, J.R., Gibbs-Erwin, J., Cassell, G.H., Simecka, J.W., 1998. Roles of innate and adaptive immunity in respiratory mycoplasmosis. Infect. Immun. 66, 3485–3491.

Carty, A.J., 2008. Opportunistic infections of mice and rats: Jacoby and Lindsey revisited. ILAR J. 49, 272–276.

Casebolt, D.B., Schoeb, T.R., 1988. An outbreak in mice of salmonellosis caused by Salmonella enteritidis serotype enteritidis. Lab. Anim. Sci. 38, 190–192.

Cassell, G.H., Lindsey, J.R., Davis, J.K., Davidson, M.K., Brown, M.B., Mayo, J.G., 1981. Detection of natural Mycoplasma pulmonis infection in rats and mice by an enzyme linked immunosorbent assay (ELISA). Lab. Anim. Sci. 31, 676–682.

Cathomen, T., Joung, J.K., 2008. Zinc-finger nucleases: the next generation emerges. Mol. Ther. 16, 1200–1207.

Chagas, C., 1909. Uber eine neue Trypoanosomiasis des Menschen. Mem. Inst. Oswaldo Cruz 3, 1–218.

Chamero, P., Leinders-Zufall, T., Zufall, F., 2012. From genes to social communication: molecular sensing by the vomeronasal organ. Trends Neurosci. 35, 597–606.

Chang, B., Hawes, N.L., Pardue, M.T., German, A.M., Hurd, R.E., Davisson, M.T., et al., 2007. Two mouse retinal degenerations caused by missense mutations in the beta-subunit of rod cGMP phosphodiesterase gene. Vision Res. 47, 624–633.

Chen, X., Katchar, K., Goldsmith, J.D., Nanthakumar, N., Cheknis, A., Gerding, D.N., et al., 2008. A mouse model of Clostridium difficile-associated disease. Gastroenterology 135, 1984–1992.

Chia, R., Achilli, F., Festing, M.F.W., Fisher, E.M.C., 2005. The origins and uses of mouse outbred stocks. Nat. Genet. 37, 1181–1186.

Childs, J.E., Glass, G.E., Korch, G.W., Arthur, R.R., Shah, K.V., Glasser, D., et al., 1988. Evidence of human infection with a rat-associated Hantavirus in Baltimore, Maryland. Am. J. Epidemiol. 127, 875–878.

Chin, E.Y., Dangler, C.A., Fox, J.G., Schauer, D.B., 2000. Helicobacter hepaticus infection triggers inflammatory bowel disease in T cell receptor alphabeta mutant mice. Comp. Med. 50, 586–594.

Christie, R.D., Marcus, E.C., Wagner, A.M., Besselsen, D.G., 2010. Experimental infection of mice with hamster parvovirus: evidence for interspecies transmission of mouse parvovirus 3. Comp. Med. 60, 123–129.

Churchill, G.A., Gatti, D.M., Munger, S.C., Svenson, K.L., 2012. The diversity outbred mouse population. Mamm. Genome 23, 713–718.

Clapp, H.W., Graham, W.R., 1970. An experience with Clostridium perfringens in cesarean derived barrier sustained mice. Lab. Anim. Care 20, 1081–1086.

Clifford, C.B., Walton, B.J., Reed, T.H., Coyle, M.B., White, W.J., Amyx, H.L., 1995. Hyperkeratosis in athymic nude mice caused by a coryneform bacterium: microbiology, transmission, clinical signs, and pathology. Lab. Anim. Sci. 45, 131–139.

Cmarik, J., Ruscetti, S., 2010. Friend spleen focus-forming virus activates the tyrosine kinase sf-Stk and the transcription factor PU.1 to cause a multi-stage erythroleukemia in mice. Viruses 2, 2235–2257.

Coffin, J.M., Hughes, S.H., Varmus, H.E., 1997. Retroviruses. Cold Spring Harbor Laboratory Press, New York.

Collins, A.M., Fell, S., Pearson, H., Toribio, J.A., 2011. Colonisation and shedding of Lawsonia intracellularis in experimentally inoculated rodents and in wild rodents on pig farms. Vet. Microbiol. 150, 384–388.

Collins, F.S., Rossant, J., Wurst, W., Consortium, T.I.M.K.O., 2007. A mouse for all reasons. Cell 128, 9–13.

Collins, J.W., Keeney, K.M., Crepin, V.F., Rathinam, V.A., Fitzgerald, K.A., Finlay, B.B., et al., 2014. Citrobacter rodentium: infection, inflammation and the microbiota. Nat. Rev. Microbiol. 12, 612–623.

Compton, S.R., 2008. Prevention of murine norovirus infection in neonatal mice by fostering. J. Am. Assoc. Lab. Anim. Sci. 47, 25–30.

Compton, S.R., Paturzo, F.X., Smith, P.C., Macy, J.D., 2012. Transmission of mouse parvovirus by fomites. J. Am. Assoc. Lab. Anim. Sci. 51, 775–780.

Cook, M.J., 1983. Anatomy. In: Foster, H.L., Small, J.D., Fox, J.G. (Eds.), The Mouse in Biomedical Research. Academic Press, New York.

Coutelier, J.-P., Brinton, M.A., 2007. Lactate dehydrogenase-elevating virus. In: Fox, J.G., Barthold, S.W., Davisson, M.T., Newcomer, C.E., Quimby, F., Smith, A.L. (Eds.), The Mouse in Biomedical Research. II. Diseases. Elsevier, London.

Crawley, J.N., 2008. Behavioral phenotyping strategies for mutant mice. Neuron 57, 809–818.

Cushion, M.T., 1998. Genetic heterogeneity of rat-derived pneumocystis. FEMS Immunol. Med. Microbiol. 22, 51–58.

Daniels, C.W., Belosevic, M., 1994. Serum antibody responses by male and female C57Bl/6 mice infected with Giardia muris. Clin. Exp. Immunol. 97, 424–429.

Daniels, C.W., Belosevic, M., 1995. Comparison of the course of infection with Giardia muris in male and female mice. Int. J. Parasitol. 25, 131–135.

Darby, A., Lertpiriyapong, K., Sarkar, U., Seneviratne, U., Park, D.S., Gamazon, E.R., et al., 2014. Cytotoxic and pathogenic properties of Klebsiella oxytoca isolated from laboratory animals. PLoS One 9 (7), in press.

David, J.M., Chatziioannou, A.F., Taschereau, R., Wang, H., Stout, D.B., 2013. The hidden cost of housing practices: using noninvasive imaging to quantify the metabolic demands of chronic cold stress of laboratory mice. Comp. Med. 63, 386–391.

Davis, J.K., Gaertner, D.J., Cox, N.R., Lindsey, J.R., Cassell, G.H., Davidson, M.K., et al., 1987. The role of Klebsiella oxytoca in utero-ovarian infection of B6C3F1 mice. Lab. Anim. Sci. 37, 159–166.

Davis, J.A., Paylor, R., Mcdonald, M.P., Libbey, M., Ligler, A., Bryant, K., et al., 1999. Behavioral effects of ivermectin in mice. Lab. Anim. Sci. 49, 288–296.

De Jong, H.K., Parry, C.M., Van Der Poll, T., Wiersinga, W.J., 2012. Host–pathogen interaction in invasive Salmonellosis. PLoS Pathog. 8, e1002933.

Delanoë, P., Delanoë, M., 1912. Sur les rapports des kystes de Carini du poumon des rats avec le Trypanosoma lewisi. Comptes rendus de "l'Academie des sciences 155, 658–661.

Del Carmen Martino-Cardona, M., Beck, S.E., Brayton, C., Watson, J., 2010. Eradication of Helicobacter spp. by using medicated diet in mice deficient in functional natural killer cells and complement factor D. J. Am. Assoc. Lab. Anim. Sci. 49, 294–299.

Demant, P., Hart, A.A.M., 1986. Recombinat congenic strains – a new tool for analyzing genetic traits by more than one gene. Immunogenetics 24, 416–422.

Derothe, J.M., Loubes, C., Orth, A., Renaud, F., Moulia, C., 1997. Comparison between patterns of pinworm infection (Aspiculuris tetraptera) in wild and laboratory strains of mice, Mus musculus. Int. J. Parasitol. 27, 645–651.

Desmyter, J., Leduc, J.W., Johnson, K.M., Brasseur, F., Deckers, C., Van Ypersele De Strihou, C., 1983. Laboratory rat associated outbreak of haemorrhagic fever with renal syndrome due to Hantaan-like virus in Belgium. Lancet 11, 445–448.

Desvars, A., Cardinale, E., Michault, A., 2011. Animal leptospirosis in small tropical areas. Epidemiol. Infect. 139, 167–188.

Dewhirst, F.E., Chien, C.C., Paster, B.J., Ericson, R.L., Orcutt, R.P., Schauer, D.B., et al., 1999. Phylogeny of the defined murine microbiota: altered Schaedler flora. Appl. Environ. Microbiol. 65, 3287–3292.

Diab, S.S., Songer, G., Uzal, F.A., 2013. Clostridium difficile infection in horses: a review. Vet. Microbiol. 167, 42–49.

Dick, E.J.J., Kittell, C.L., Meyer, H., Farrar, P.L., Ropp, S.L., Esposito, J.J., et al., 1996. Mousepox outbreak in a laboratory mouse colony. Lab. Anim. Sci. 46, 602–611.

Diglisic, G., Xiao, S.-Y., Gligic, A., Obradovic, M., Stojanovic, R., Velimirovic, D., et al., 1994. Isolation of a Puumala-like virus from Mus musculus captured in Yugoslavia and its association with severe hemorrhagic fever with renal syndrome. J. Infect. Dis. 169, 204–207.

Dole, V.S., Banu, L.A., Fister, R.D., Nicklas, W., Henderson, K.S., 2010. Assessment of rpoB and 16S rRNA genes as targets for PCR-based identification of Pasteurella pneumotropica. Comp. Med. 60, 427–435.

Dole, V.S., Zaias, J., Kyricopoulos-Cleasby, D.M., Banu, L.A., Waterman, L.L., Sanders, K., et al., 2011. Comparison of traditional and PCR methods during screening for and confirmation of Aspiculuris tetraptera in a mouse facility. J. Am. Assoc. Lab. Anim. Sci. 50, 904–909.

Dole, V.S., Henderson, K.S., Fister, R.D., Pietrowski, M.T., Maldonado, G., Clifford, C.B., 2013. Pathogenicity and genetic variation of 3 strains of Corynebacterium bovis in immunodeficient mice. J. Am. Assoc. Lab. Anim. Sci. 52, 458–466.

Duan, Q.W., Liu, Y.F., Booth, C.J., Rockwell, S., 2012. Use of Fenbendazole-Containing therapeutic diets for mice in experimental cancer therapy studies. J. Am. Assoc. Labor. Anim. Sci. 51, 224–230.

Dufour, B.D., Adeola, O., Cheng, H.W., Donkin, S.S., Klein, J.D., Pajor, E.A., et al., 2010. Nutritional up-regulation of serotonin paradoxically induces compulsive behavior. Nutr. Neurosci. 13, 256–264.

Dyer, K.D., Garcia-Crespo, K.E., Glineur, S., Domachowske, J.B., Rosenberg, H.F., 2012. The pneumonia virus of mice (MPnV) model of acute respiratory infection. Viruses 4, 3494–3510.

Eastwood, K., Else, P., Charlett, A., Wilcox, M., 2009. Comparison of nine commercially available Clostridium difficile toxin detection assays, a real-time PCR assay for C. difficile tcdB, and a glutamate dehydrogenase detection assay to cytotoxin testing and cytotoxigenic culture methods. J. Clin. Microbiol. 47, 3211–3217.

Eaton, G.J., Custer, R.P., Johnson, F.N., Stabenow, K.T., 1978. Dystrophic cardiac calcinosis in mice: genetic, hormonal, and dietary influences. Am. J. Pathol. 90, 173–186.

Edman, J.C., Edman, U., Cao, M., Lundgren, B., Kovacs, J.A., Santi, D.V., 1989. Isolation and expression of the Pneumocystis carinii dihydrofolate reductase gene. Proc. Natl. Acad. Sci. USA 86, 8625–8629.

Eppig, J.T., Blake, J.A., Bult, C.J., Kadin, J.A., Richardson, J.E., Group, T.M.G.D., 2012. The Mouse Genome Database (MGD): comprehensive resource for genetics and genomics of the laboratory mouse. Nucl. Acids Res. 40, D881–D886.

Erdman, S., Fox, J.G., Dangler, C.A., Feldman, D., Horwitz, B.H., 2001. Typhlocolitis in NF-kappa B-deficient mice. J. Immunol. 166, 1443–1447.

Erdman, S.E., Poutahidis, T., Tomczak, M., Rogers, A.B., Cormier, K., Plank, B., et al., 2003a. CD4+ CD25+ regulatory T lymphocytes inhibit microbially induced colon cancer in Rag2-deficient mice. Am. J. Pathol. 162, 691–702.

Erdman, S.E., Rao, V.P., Poutahidis, T., Ihrig, M.M., Ge, Z., Feng, Y., et al., 2003b. CD4(+)CD25(+) regulatory lymphocytes require interleukin 10 to interrupt colon carcinogenesis in mice. Cancer Res. 63, 6042–6050.

Erdman, S.E., Rao, V.P., Poutahidis, T., Rogers, A.B., Taylor, C.L., Jackson, E.A., et al., 2009. Nitric oxide and TNF-alpha trigger colonic inflammation and carcinogenesis in Helicobacter hepaticus-infected, Rag2-deficient mice. Proc. Natl. Acad. Sci. USA 106, 1027–1032.

Esteban, D., Buller, R., 2005. Ectromelia virus: the causative agent of mousepox. J. Gen. Virol. 86, 2645–2659.

Evengard, B., Sandstedt, K., Bolske, G., Feinstein, R., Riesenfelt-Orn, I., Smith, C.I., 1994. Intranasal inoculation of Mycoplasma pulmonis in mice with severe combined immunodeficiency (SCID) causes a wasting disease with grave arthritis. Clin. Exp. Immunol. 98, 388–394.

Falk, R.H., Skinner, M., 2000. The systemic amyloidoses: an overview. Adv. Intern. Med. 45, 107–137.

Farber, D.B., Danciger, M., 1994. Inherited retinal degenerations in the mouse. In: Wright, A.F., Jay, B. (Eds.), Molecular Genetics of Inherited Eye Disorders. Harwood, Chur, Switzerland.

Farkas, T., Fey, B., Hargitt 3rd, E., Parcells, M., Ladman, B., Murgia, M., et al., 2012. Molecular detection of novel picornaviruses in chickens and turkeys. Virus Genes 44, 262–272.

Feinstein, R.E., Morris, W.E., Waldemarson, A.H., Hedenqvist, P., Lindberg, R., 2008. Fatal acute intestinal pseudoobstruction in mice. J. Am. Assoc. Lab. Anim. Sci. 47, 58–63.

Fenner, F., 1948a. The epizootic behaviour of mouse-pox (infectious ectromelia). Brit. J. Exp. Path. 29, 69–91.

Fenner, F., 1948b. The pathogenesis of acute exanthema. An interpretation based on experimental investigations with mouse-pox (infectious ectromelia of mice). Lancet 2, 915–920.

Fenner, F., 1949a. Studies in mousepox, infectious ectromelia of mice; a comparison of the virulence and infectivity of three strains of ectromelia virus. Aust. J. Exp. Biol. Med. Sci. 27, 31–43.

Fenner, F., 1949b. Studies in mousepox, infectious ectromelia of mice; the effect of age of the host upon the response to infection. Aust. J. Exp. Biol. Med. Sci. 27, 45–53.

Ferrero, D.M., Moeller, L.M., Osakada, T., Horio, N., Li, Q., Roy, D.S., et al., 2013. A juvenile mouse pheromone inhibits sexual behaviour through the vomeronasal system. Nature 502, 368–371.

Ferris, S.D., Sage, R.D., Wilson, A.C., 1982. Evidence from mtDNA sequences that common laboratory strains of inbred mice are descended from a single female. Nature 295, 163–165.

Festing, M.F.W., 1996. Origins and characteristics of inbred strains of mice. In: Lyon, M.F., Rastan, S., Brown, S.D.M. (Eds.), Genetic Variants and Strains of the Laboratory Mouse. Oxford University Press, Oxford.

Festing, M.F.W., Simpson, E.M., Davisson, M.T., Mobraaten, L.E., 1999. Revised nomenclature for strain 129 mice. Mamm. Genome 10, 836.

Flaherty, L., 1981. Congenic strains. In: Foster, H.L., Small, J.D., Fox, J.G. (Eds.), The Mouse in Biomedical Research. Academic Press, New York.

Flynn, B.M., Brown, P.A., Eckstein, J.M., Strong, D., 1989. Treatment of Syphacia obvelata in mice using ivermectin. Lab. Anim. Sci. 39, 461–463.

Fogh, J. (Ed.), 1982. The Nude Mouse in Experimental and Clinical Research. Academic Press, New York.

Fookes, M., Schroeder, G.N., Langridge, G.C., Blondel, C.J., Mammina, C., Connor, T.R., et al., 2011. Salmonella bongori provides insights into the evolution of the Salmonellae. PLoS Pathog. 7, e1002191.

Foreman, O., Kavirayani, A.M., Griffey, S.M., Reader, R., Shultz, L.D., 2011. Opportunistic bacterial infections in breeding colonies of the NSG mouse strain. Vet. Pathol. 48, 495–499.

Fox, J.G., 1982. Outbreak of tropical rat mite dermatitis in laboratory personnel. Arch. Dermatol. 118, 676–678.

Fox, J.G., Lee, A., 1997. The role of Helicobacter species in newly recognized gastrointestinal tract diseases of animals. Lab. Anim. Sci. 47, 222–255.

Fox, J.G., Dewhirst, F.E., Tully, J.G., Paster, B.J., Yan, L., Taylor, N.S., et al., 1994. Helicobacter hepaticus sp. nov., a microaerophilic bacterium isolated from livers and intestinal mucosal scrapings from mice. J. Clin. Microbiol. 32, 1238–1245.

Fox, J.G., Li, X., Yan, L., Cahill, R.J., Hurley, R., Lewis, R., et al., 1996a. Chronic proliferative hepatitis in A/JCr mice associated with persistent Helicobacter hepaticus infection: a model of helicobacter-induced carcinogenesis. Infect. Immun. 64, 1548–1558.

Fox, J.G., Yan, L., Shames, B., Campbell, J., Murphy, J.C., Li, X., 1996b. Persistent hepatitis and enterocolitis in germfree mice infected with Helicobacter hepaticus. Infect. Immun. 64, 3673–3681.

Fox, J.G., Dewhirst, F.E., Shen, Z., Feng, Y., Taylor, N.S., Paster, B.J., et al., 1998a. Hepatic Helicobacter species identified in bile and gallbladder tissue from Chileans with chronic cholecystitis. Gastroenterology 114, 755–763.

Fox, J.G., Macgregor, J.A., Shen, Z., Li, X., Lewis, R., Dangler, C.A., 1998b. Comparison of methods of identifying Helicobacter hepaticus in B6C3F1 mice used in a carcinogenesis bioassay. J. Clin. Microbiol. 36, 1382–1387.

Fox, J.G., Gorelick, P.L., Kullberg, M.C., Ge, Z., Dewhirst, F.E., Ward, J.M., 1999. A novel urease-negative Helicobacter species associated with colitis and typhlitis in IL-10-deficient mice. Infect. Immun. 67, 1757–1762.

Fox, J.G., Dangler, C.A., Schauer, D.B., 2000. Inflammatory bowel disease in mouse models: role of gastrointestinal microbiota as proinflammatory modulators. In: Ward, J.M., Mahler, J., Maronpot, R.R., Sundberg, J.P., Frederickson, R. (Eds.), Pathology of Genetically Engineered Mice. Iowa State University Press, Ames, IA.

Fox, J.G., Wang, T.C., Rogers, A.B., Poutahidis, T., Ge, Z., Taylor, N., et al., 2003. Host and microbial constituents influence Helicobacter pylori-induced cancer in a murine model of hypergastrinemia. Gastroenterology 124, 1879–1890.

Fox, J.G., Ge, Z., Whary, M.T., Erdman, S.E., Horwitz, B.H., 2011. Helicobacter hepaticus infection in mice: models for understanding lower bowel inflammation and cancer. Mucosal Immunol. 4, 22–30.

France, M.P., Smith, A.L., Stevenson, R., Barthold, S.W., 1999. Granulomatous peritonitis in interferon-gamma gene knockout mice naturally infected with mouse hepatitis virus. Aust. Vet. J. 77, 600–604.

Franklin, C., 2006. Microbial considerations in genetically engineered mouse research. ILAR J. 47, 141–155.

Franklin, C.L., Motzel, S.L., Besch-Williford, C.L., Hook Jr., R.R., Riley, L.K., 1994. Tyzzer's infection: host specificity of Clostridium piliforme isolates. Lab. Anim. Sci. 44, 568–572.

Franklin, C.L., Riley, L.K., Livingston, R.S., Beckwith, C.S., Hook Jr., R.R., Besch-Williford, C.L., et al., 1999. Enteric lesions in SCID mice infected with 'Helicobacter typhlonicus,' a novel urease-negative Helicobacter species. Lab. Anim. Sci. 49, 496–505.

Franklin, C.L., Gorelick, P.L., Riley, L.K., Dewhirst, F.E., Livingston, R.S., Ward, J.M., et al., 2001. Helicobacter typhlonius sp. nov., a novel murine urease-negative Helicobacter species. J. Clin. Microbiol. 39, 3920–3926.

Frazier, K.S., Herron, A.J., Hines 2nd, M.E., Gaskin, J.M., Altman, N.H., 1993. Diagnosis of enteritis and enterotoxemia due to Clostridium difficile in captive ostriches (Struthio camelus). J. Vet. Diagn. Invest. 5, 623–625.

Frenkel, J.K., 1999. Pneumocystis pneumonia, an immunodeficiency-dependent disease (IDD): a critical historical overview. J. Eukaryot. Microbiol. 46, 89S–92S.

Fujiwara, K., Ganaway, J.R., 1994. Bacillus piliformis. In: Waggie, K.S., Kagayima, N., Allen, A.M., Nomura, T. (Eds.), Manual of Microbiological Monitoring of Laboratory Animals. National Institutes of Health Publication, Bethesda, MD, pp. 94–2498.

Furuta, T., Fujiwara, K., Yamanouchi, K., Ueda, K., 1985. Detection of antibodies to Pneumocystis carinii by enzyme-linked immunosorbent assay in experimentally infected mice. J. Parasitol. 71, 522–523.

Gadad, B.S., Daher, J.P.L., Hutchinson, E.K., Brayton, C.F., Dawson, T.M., Pletnikov, M.V., et al., 2010. Effect of Fenbendazole on three behavioral tests in male C57BL/6N mice. J. Am. Assoc. Lab. Anim. Sci. 49, 821–825.

Gaj, T., Gersbach, C.A., Barbas 3rd, C.F., 2013. ZFN, TALEN, and CRISPR/Cas-based methods for genome engineering. Trends Biotechnol. 31, 397–405.

Gama Sosa, M.A., De Gasperi, R., Elder, G.A., 2010. Animal transgenesis: an overview. Brain Struct. Funct. 214, 91–109.

Ganaway, J.R., 1982. Bacterial and mycotic diseases of the digestive system. In: Foster, H.L., Small, J.D., Fox, J.G. (Eds.), The Mouse in Biomedical Research. Academic Press, New York.

Ganaway, J.R., Allen, A.M., Moore, T.D., 1971. Tyzzer's disease. Am. J. Pathol. 64, 717–730.

Ganaway, J.R., Spencer, T.H., Waggie, K.S., 1985. Propagation of the etiologic agent of Tyzzer's disease (Bacillus piliformis) in cell culture. Contribution of Laboratory Animal Science to the Welfare of Man and Animals: Past, Present, and Future. Eighth Symposium of ICLAS/CALAS (1983). John Wiley & Sons Inc.

Gao, X., Zhang, P., 2007. Transgenic RNA interference in mice. Physiology 22, 161–166.

Garcia, A., Ihrig, M.M., Fry, R.C., Feng, Y., Xu, S., Boutin, S.R., et al., 2008. Genetic susceptibility to chronic hepatitis is inherited codominantly in *Helicobacter hepaticus*-infected AB6F1 and B6AF1 hybrid male mice, and progression to hepatocellular carcinoma is linked to hepatic expression of lipogenic genes and immune function-associated networks. Infect. Immun. 76, 1866–1876.

Garcia, A., Zeng, Y., Muthupalani, S., Ge, Z., Potter, A., Mobley, M.W., et al., 2011. *Helicobacter hepaticus*-induced liver tumor promotion is associated with increased serum bile acid and a persistent microbial-induced immune response. Cancer Res. 71, 2529–2540.

Garcia, M.F., Gordon, M.N., Hutton, M., Lewis, J., Mcgowan, E., Dickey, C.A., et al., 2004. The retinal degeneration (rd) gene seriously impairs spatial cognitive performance in normal and Alzheimer's transgenic mice. Neuroreport 15, 73–77.

Garner, C.M., Hubbold, L.M., Chakraborti, P.R., 2000. Mycoplasma detection in cell cultures: a comparison of four methods. Br. J. Biomed. Sci. 57, 295–301.

Garner, J.P., Weisker, S.M., Dufour, B., Mench, J.A., 2004. Barbering (fur and whisker trimming) by laboratory mice as a model of human trichotillomania and obsessive-compulsive spectrum disorders. Comp. Med. 54, 216–224.

Gigliotti, F., Haidaris, P.J., Haidaris, C.G., Wright, T.W., Van Der Meid, K.R., 1993a. Further evidence of host species-specific variation in antigens of *Pneumocystis carinii* using the polymerase chain reaction. J. Infect. Dis. 168, 191–194.

Gigliotti, F., Harmsen, A.G., Haidaris, C.G., Haidaris, P.J., 1993b. *Pneumocystis carinii* is not universally transmissable between mammalian species. Infect. Immun. 61, 2886–2890.

Godfrey, V.L., 2007. Fungal diseases in laboratory mice. In: Fox, J.G., Barthold, S.W., Davisson, M.T., Newcomer, C.E., Quimby, F., Smith, A.L. (Eds.), The Mouse in Biomedical Research. II. Diseases. Elsevier, London.

Goelz, M.F., Mahler, J., Harry, J., Myers, P., Clark, J., Thigpen, J.E., et al., 1998. Neuropathologic findings associated with seizures in FVB mice. Lab. Anim. Sci. 48, 34–37.

Goto, K., Hayashimoto, N., Yasuda, M., Ishida, T., Kameda, S., Takakura, A., et al., 2009. Molecular detection of murine norovirus from experimentally and spontaneously infected mice. Exp. Anim. 58, 135–140.

Gottlieb, K., Villarreal, L.P., 2000. The distribution and kinetics of polyomavirus in lungs of intranasally infected neonatal mice. Virology 266, 52–65.

Gozalo, A.S., Hoffmann, V.J., Brinster, L.R., Elkins, W.R., Ding, L., Holland, S.M., 2010. Spontaneous Staphylococcus xylosus infection in mice deficient in NADPH oxidase and comparison with other laboratory mouse strains. J. Am. Assoc. Lab. Anim. Sci. 49, 480–486.

Green, E.L., 1981. Genetics and Probability in Animal Breeding Experiments. Macmillan, New York.

Greenlee, J.E., Phelps, R.C., Stroop, W.G., 1991. The major site of murine K papovavirus persistence and reactivation is the renal tubular epithelium. Microb. Pathog. 11, 237–247.

Greenstein, G., Drozdowicz, C.K., Nebiar, F., Bozik, R., 1994. Isolation of *Streptococcus equisimilis* from abscesses detected in specific pathogen-free mice. Lab. Anim. Sci. 44, 374–376.

Griffith, J.W., White, W.J., Danneman, P.J., Lang, C.M., 1988. Cilia-associated respiratory (CAR) bacillus infection of obese mice. Vet. Pathol. 25, 72–76.

Guerrero-Bosagna, C.M., Sabat, P., Valdovinos, F.S., Valladares, L.E., Clark, S.J., 2008. Epigenetic and phenotypic changes result from a continuous pre and post natal dietary exposure to phytoestrogens in an experimental population of mice. BMC Physiol. 8, 17.

Hailey, J.R., Haseman, J.K., Bucher, J.R., Radovsky, A.E., Malarkey, D.E., Miller, R.T., et al., 1998. Impact of *Helicobacter hepaticus* infection in B6C3F1 mice from twelve National Toxicology Program two-year carcinogenesis studies. Toxicol. Pathol. 26, 602–611.

Haines, D.C., Chattopadhyay, S., Ward, J.M., 2001. Pathology of aging B6;129 mice. Toxicol. Pathol. 29, 653–661.

Haldane, J.B.S., Sprunt, A.D., Haldane, N.M., 1915. Reduplication in mice. J. Genet. 5, 133–135.

Hansen, G.M., Paturzo, F.X., Smith, A.L., 1999. Humoral immunity and protection of mice challenged with homotypic or heterotypic parvovirus. Lab. Anim. Sci., 49380–49384.

Hardies, S.C., Wang, L., Zhou, L., Casavant, C., Huang, S., 2000. LINE-1 (L1) lineages in the mouse. Mol. Biol. Evol. 17, 616–628.

Herscovitch, M., Perkins, E., Baltus, A., Fan, M., 2012. Addgene provides an open forum for plasmid sharing. Nat. Biotechnol. 30, 316–317.

Hillhouse, A.E., Myles, M.H., Taylor, J.F., Bryda, E.C., Franklin, C.L., 2011. Quantitative trait loci in a bacterially induced model of inflammatory bowel disease. Mamm. Genome 22, 544–555.

Hoenerhoff, M.J., Hong, H.H., Ton, T.V., Lahousse, S.A., Sills, R.C., 2009. A review of the molecular mechanisms of chemically induced neoplasia in rat and mouse models in National Toxicology Program bioassays and their relevance to human cancer. Toxicol. Pathol. 37, 835–848.

Homberger, F.R., Pataki, Z., Thomann, P.E., 1993. Control of *Pseudomonas aeruginosa* infection in mice by chlorine treatment of drinking water. Lab. Anim. Sci. 43, 635–637.

Hoyt, T.R., 2007. Mouse phyisology. In: Fox, J.G., Barthold, S.W., Davisson, M.T., Newcomer, C.E., Quimby, F.W., Smith, A.L. (Eds.), Normative Biology, Husbandry and Models in the Mouse in Biomedical Research, second ed. Academic Press, San Diego, CA.

Hoyt, T.R., Dobrinen, E., Kochetkova, I., Meissner, N., 2014. B cells modulate systemic responses to Pneumocystis lung infection and protect on-demand hematopoiesis via T cell-independent, innate mechanism when type-I-IFN-signaling is absent. Infect. Immun.

Hsu, C.C., Wobus, C.E., Steffen, E.K., Riley, L.K., Livingston, R.S., 2005. Development of a microsphere-based serologic multiplexed fluorescent immunoassay and a reverse transcriptase PCR assay to detect murine norovirus 1 infection in mice. Clin. Diag. Lab. Immunol. 12, 1145–1151.

Hsu, C.C., Riley, L.K., Wills, H.M., Livingston, R.S., 2006. Persistent infection with and serologic cross-reactivity of three novel murine noroviruses. Comp. Med. 56, 247–251.

Hsu, C.C., Franklin, C.L., Riley, L.K., 2007. Multiplex fluorescent immunoassay for the simultaneous detection of serum antibodies to multiple rodent pathogens. Lab. Anim. (NY) 36, 36–38.

Hsu, P.D., Lander, E.S., Zhang, F., 2014. Development and applications of CRISPR-Cas9 for genome engineering. Cell 157, 1262–1278.

Hurley, L.S., Bell, L.T., 1974. Genetic influence on response to dietary manganese deficiency in mice. J. Nutr. 104, 133–137.

Ihrig, M., Schrenzel, M.D., Fox, J.G., 1999. Differential susceptibility to hepatic inflammation and proliferation in AXB recombinant inbred mice chronically infected with *Helicobacter hepaticus*. Am. J. Pathol. 155, 571–582.

Jacoby, R.O., Ball-Goodrich, L., 2007. Parvoviruses. In: Fox, J.G., Barthold, S.W., Davisson, M.T., Newcomer, C.E., Quimby, F., Smith, A.L. (Eds.), The Mouse in Biomedical Research. II. Diseases. Elsevier, London.

Jacoby, R.O., Bhatt, P.N., 1987. Mousepox in inbred mice innately resistant or susceptible to lethal infection with ectromelia virus. 2. Pathogenesis. Lab. Anim. Sci. 37, 16–22.

Jacoby, R.O., Bhatt, P.N., Johnson, E.A., Paturzo, F.X., 1983. Pathogenesis of vaccinia (IHD-T) virus infection in BALB/cAnN mice. Lab. Anim. Sci. 33, 435–441.

Jacoby, R.O., Bhatt, P.N., Brownstein, D.G., 1989. Evidence that NK cells and interferon are required for genetic resistance to infection with ectromelia virus. Arch. Virol. 108, 49–58.

Jacoby, R.O., Bhatt, P.N., Barthold, S.W., Brownstein, D.G., 1994. Sendai virus pneumonia in aged BALB/c mice. Exp. Gerontol. 29, 89–100.

Jacoby, R.O., Lindsey, J.R., 1997. Health care for research animals is essential and affordable. FASEB J. 11, 609–614.

Jaisser, F., 2000. Inducible gene expression and gene modification in transgenic mice. J. Am. Soc. Nephrol. 11, S95–S100.

Jensen, E.S., Allen, K.P., Henderson, K.S., Szabo, A., Thulin, J.D., 2013. PCR testing of a ventilated caging system to detect murine fur mites. J. Am. Assoc. Lab. Anim. Sci. 52, 28–33.

John, A.M., Bell, J.M., 1976. Amino acid requirements of the growing mouse. J. Nutr. 106, 1361–1367.

Jones, T.C., Mohr, U., Hunt, R.D., 1983-1993. Monographs on Pathology of Laboratory Animals. Springer, Berlin, Germany; New York.

Joung, J.K., Sander, J.D., 2013. TALENs: a widely applicable technology for targeted genome editing. Nat. Rev. Mol. Cell Biol. 14, 49–55.

Jungmann, P., Freitas, A., Bandeira, A., Nobrega, A., Coutinho, A., Marcos, M.A., et al., 1996. Murine Acariasis. II. Immunological Dysfunction and evidence for chronic activation of Th-2 lymphocytes. Scand. J. Immunol. 43, 604–612.

Justice, M.J., Noveroske, J.K., Weber, J.S., Zheng, B., Bradley, A., 1999. Mouse ENU mutagenesis. Hum. Mol. Genet. 8, 1955–1963.

Justice, M.J., Carpenter, D.A., Favor, J., Neuhauser-Klaus, A., Hrabe De Angelis, M., Soewarto, D., et al., 2000. Effects of ENU dosage on mouse strains. Mamm. Genome 11, 484–488.

Kahan, S.M., Liu, G., Reinhard, M.K., Hsu, C.C., Livingston, R.S., Karst, S.M., 2011. Comparative murine norovirus studies reveal a lack of correlation between intestinal virus titers and enteric pathology. Virology 421, 202–210.

Kara, E.E., Comerford, I., Fenix, K.A., Bastow, C.R., Gregor, C.E., Mckenzie, D.R., et al., 2014. Tailored immune responses: Novel effector helper T cell subsets in protective immunity. PLoS Pathog. 10, e1003905.

Karst, S.M., Wobus, C.E., Lay, M., Davidson, J., Virgin, H.W.I., 2003. STAT1-dependent innate immunity to a Norwalk-like virus. Science 299, 1575–1578.

Kastenmayer, R.J., Perdue, K.A., Elkins, W.R., 2008. Eradication of murine norovirus from a mouse barrier facility. J. Am. Assoc. Lab. Anim. Sci. 47, 26–30.

Kawamata, J., Yamanouchi, T., Dohmae, K., Miyamoto, H., Takahaski, M., Yamanishi, K., et al., 1987. Control of laboratory acquired hemorrhagic fever with renal syndrome (HFRS) in Japan. Lab. Anim. Sci. 37, 431–436.

Kawamura, S., Taguchi, F., Ishida, T., Nakayama, M., Fujiwara, K., 1983. Growth of Tyzzer's organism in primary monolayer cultures of adult mouse hepatocytes. J. Gen. Microbiol. 129, 277–283.

Keeler, C.E., 1931. The Laboratory Mouse. Its Origin, Heredity, and Culture. Harvard University Press, Cambridge.

Kelliher, K., Wersinger, S., 2009. Olfactory regulation of the sexual behavior and reproductive physiology of the laboratory mouse: effects and neural mechanisms. ILAR J. 50, 28–42.

Kerton, A., Warden, P., 2006. Review of successful treatment for Helicobacter species in laboratory mice. Lab. Anim. 40, 115–122.

Kimura, M., Crow, J.F., 1963. On the maximum avoidance of inbreeding. Genet. Res. 4, 399–415.

Klement, P., Augustine, J.M., Delaney, K.H., Klement, G., Weitz, J.I., 1996. An oral ivermectin regimen that eradicates pinworms (Syphacia spp.) in laboratory rats and mice. Lab. Anim. Sci. 46, 286–290.

Knapka, J.J., 1983. Nutrition. In: Foster, H.L., Small, J.D., Fox, J.G. (Eds.), The Mouse in Biomedical Research. Academic Press, New York.

Knapka, J.J., Smith, K.P., Judge, F.J., 1974. Effect of open and closed formula rations on the performance of three strains of laboratory mice. Lab. Anim. Sci. 24, 480–487.

Knittel, G., Metzner, M., Beck-Engeser, G., Kan, A., Ahrends, T., Eilat, D., et al., 2014. Insertional hypermutation in mineral oil-induced plasmacytomas. Eur. J. Immunol. 44, 2785–2801.

Knutson, C.G., Mangerich, A., Zeng, Y., Raczynski, A.R., Liberman, R.G., Kang, P., et al., 2013. Chemical and cytokine features of innate immunity characterize serum and tissue profiles in inflammatory bowel disease. Proc. Natl. Acad. Sci. USA 110, E2332–E2341.

Koch, Gowen, 1939. Arch. Pathol. Lab. Med. 28.

Komarek, V., 2007. Gross anatomy. In: Fox, J.G., Barthold, S.W., Davisson, M.T., Newcomer, C.E., Quimby, F., Smith, A.L. (Eds.), The Mouse in Biomedical Research. III. Normative Biology, Husbandry, and Models. Elsevier, London.

Kraft, L.M., 1980. The manufacture, shipping and receiving and quality control of rodent bedding materials. Lab. Anim. Sci. 30, 366–376.

Kuijper, E.J., Coignard, B., Tull, P., 2006. Emergence of Clostridium difficile-associated disease in North America and Europe. Clin. Microbiol. Infect. 12 (Suppl. 6), 2–18.

Kullberg, M.C., Rothfuchs, A.G., Jankovic, D., Caspar, P., Wynn, T.A., Gorelick, P.L., et al., 2001. Helicobacter hepaticus-induced colitis in interleukin-10-deficient mice: cytokine requirements for the induction and maintenance of intestinal inflammation. Infect. Immun. 69, 4232–4241.

Kullberg, M.C., Jankovic, D., Gorelick, P.L., Caspar, P., Letterio, J.J., Cheever, A.W., et al., 2002. Bacteria-triggered CD4(+) T regulatory cells suppress Helicobacter hepaticus-induced colitis. J. Exp. Med. 196, 505–515.

Kullberg, M.C., Jankovic, D., Feng, C.G., Hue, S., Gorelick, P.L., Mckenzie, B.S., et al., 2006. IL-23 plays a key role in Helicobacter hepaticus-induced T cell-dependent colitis. J. Exp. Med. 203, 2485–2494.

Kunstyr, I., 1986. Paresis of peristalsis and ileus lead to death in lactating mice. Lab. Anim. 20, 32–35.

Kunstyr, I., Ammerpohl, E., Meyer, B., 1977. Experimental spironucleosis (hexamitiasis) in the nude mouse as a model for immunologic and pharmacologic studies. Lab. Anim. Sci. 27, 782–788.

Kunstyr, I., Schoeneberg, U., Friedhoff, K.T., 1992. Host specificity of Giardia muris isolates from mouse and golden hamster. Parasitol. Res. 78, 621–622.

Lai, W.C., Linton, G., Bennett, M., Pakes, S.P., 1993. Genetic control of resistance to Mycoplasma pulmonis infection in mice. Infect. Immun. 61, 4615–4621.

Lai, W.C., Pakes, S.P., Ren, K., Lu, Y.S., Bennett, M., 1997. Therapeutic effect of DNA immunization of genetically susceptible mice infected with virulent Mycoplasma pulmonis. J. Immunol. 158, 2513–2516.

Lamana, M.L., Albella, B., Bueren, J.A., Segovia, J.C., 2001. In vitro and in vivo susceptibility of mouse megakaryocytic progenitors to strain i of parvovirus minute virus of mice. Exp. Hematol. 29, 1303–1309.

Landin, A.M., Frasca, D., Zaias, J., Van Der Put, E., Riley, R.L., Altman, N.H., et al., 2009. Effects of fenbendazole on the murine humoral immune system. J. Am. Assoc. Lab. Anim. Sci. 48, 251–257.

Latham, N., Mason, G., 2004. From house mouse to mouse house: the behavioral biology of free-living Mus musculus and its implications in the laboratory. Appl. Anim. Behav. Sci. 86, 261–289.

Lawley, T.D., Clare, S., Walker, A.W., Goulding, D., Stabler, R.A., Croucher, N., et al., 2009. Antibiotic treatment of Clostridium difficile carrier mice triggers a supershedder state, spore-mediated transmission, and severe disease in immunocompromised hosts. Infect. Immun. 77, 3661–3669.

Le Blanc, S.A., Faith, R.E., Montgomery, C.A., 1993. Use of topical ivermectin treatment for Syphacia obvelata in mice. Lab. Anim Sci. 43, 526–528.

Leduc, J.W., Smith, G.A., Johnson, K.M., 1984. Hantaan-like viruses from domestic rats captured in the United States. Am. J. Trop. Med. Hyg. 33, 992–998.

Lemke, L.B., Rogers, A.B., Nambiar, P.R., Fox, J.G., 2008. Obesity and non-insulin-dependent diabetes mellitus in Swiss-Webster mice associated with late-onset hepatocellular carcinoma. J. Endocrinol. 199, 21–32.

Lenaerts, L., Verbeken, E., Declercq, E., Naesens, L., 2005. Mouse adenovirus type 1 infection in SCID mice: an experimental model for antiviral therapy of systemic adenovirus infections. Antimicrob. Agents Chemother. 49, 4689–4699.

Li, Q., Uitto, J., 2013. Mineralization/anti-mineralization networks in the skin and vascular connective tissues. Am. J. Pathol. 183, 10–18.

Liberles, S.D., Buck, L.B., 2006. A second class of olfactory chemosensory receptors in the olfactory epithelium. Nature 442, 645–650.

Linder, C.C., 2006. Genetic variables that influence phenotype. ILAR J. 47, 132–140.

Lindsey, J.R., Cassell, G.H., Davidson, M.K., 1982. Mycoplasma and other bacterial diseases of the respiratory system In: Foster, H.L. Small, J.D. Fox, J.G. (Eds.), The Mouse in Biomedical Research, vol. 2. Academic Press, New York. pp. 21–41.

Lindsey, J.R., Boorman, G.A., Collins, M.J., Hsu, C.K., Van Hoosier, G.L., Wagner, J.E., 1991a. Pasteurella pneumotropica. In: Council, N.R. (Ed.), Infectious Diseases of Mice and Rats. National Academy Press, Washington, DC.

Lindsey, J.R., Boorman, G.A., Collins, M.J., Hsu, C.K., Van Hoosier, G.L., Wagner, J.E., 1991b. Pseudomonas aeruginosa. In: Council, N.R. (Ed.), Infectious Diseases of Mice and Rats. National Academy Press, Washington, DC.

Lindsey, J.R., Boorman, G.A., Collins, M.J., Hsu, C.K., Van Hoosier, G.L., Wagner, J.E., 1991c. Salmonella enteritidis. In: Council, N.R. (Ed.), Infectious Diseases of Mice and Rats. National Academy Press, Washington, DC.

Lindsey, J.R., Boorman, G.A., Collins, M.J., Hsu, C.K., Van Hoosier, G.L., Wagner, J.E., 1991d. Staphylococcus aureus. In: Council, N.R. (Ed.), Infectious Diseases of Mice and Rats. National Academy Press, Washington, DC.

Lindsey, J.R., Boorman, G.A., Collins, M.J., Hsu, C.K., Van Hoosier, G.L., Wagner, J.E., 1991e. Streptobacillus moniliformis. In: Council, N.R. (Ed.), Infectious Diseases of Mice and Rats. National Academy Press, Washington, DC.

Lindsey, J.R., Boorman, G.A., Collins, M.J., Hsu, C.K., Van Hoosier, G.L., Wagner, J.E., 1991f. Streptococcus pneumoniae. In: Council, N.R. (Ed.), Infectious Diseases of Mice and Rats. National Academy Press, Washington, DC.

Lindstrom, K.E., Carbone, L.G., Kellar, D.E., Mayorga, M.S., Wilkerson, J.D., 2011. Soiled bedding sentinels for the detection of fur mites in mice. J. Am. Assoc. Lab. Anim. Sci. 50, 54–60.

Lipman, N.S., Henderson, K., 2000. False negative results using RT-PCR for detection of lactate dehydrogenase-elevating virus in a tumor cell line. Comp. Med. 50, 255–256.

Lipman, N.S., Dalton, S.D., Stuart, A.R., Arruda, K., 1994. Eradication of pinworms (Syphacia obvelata) from a large mouse breeding colony by combination oral anthelmintic therapy. Lab. Anim. Sci. 44, 517–520.

Lipman, N.S., Perkins, S., Nguyen, H., Pfeffer, M., Meyer, H., 2000. Mousepox resulting from use of ectromelia virus-contaminated, imported mouse serum. Comp. Med. 50, 426–435.

Lipman, R.D., Gaillard, E.T., Harrison, D.E., Bronson, R.T., 1993. Husbandry factors and the prevalence of age-related amyloidosis in mice. Lab. Anim. Sci. 43, 439–444.

Lipton, H.L., Manoj-Kumar, A.S., Hertzler, S., 2007. Cardioviruses: encephalomyocarditis virus and Theiler's murine encephalitis virus. In: Fox, J.G., Barthold, S.W., Davisson, M.T., Newcomer, C.E., Quimby, F., Smith, A.L. (Eds.), The Mouse in Biomedical Research. II. Diseases, second ed. Elsevier, London.

Livingston, R.S., Riley, L.K., 2003. Diagnostic testing of mouse and rat colonies for infectious agents. Lab. Anim. 32, 44–51.

Livingston, R.S., Franklin, C.L., Besch-Williford, C.L., Hook Jr., R.R., Riley, L.K., 1996. A novel presentation of Clostridium piliforme infection (Tyzzer's disease) in nude mice. Lab. Anim. Sci. 46, 21–25.

Livingston, R.S., Besselsen, D.G., Steffen, E.K., Besch-Williford, C.L., Franklin, C., Riley, L.K., 2002. Serodiagnosis of mice minute virus and mouse parvovirus infections in mice by enzyme-linked immunosorbent assay with baculovirus-expressed recombinant VP2 proteins. Clin. Diag. Lab. Immunol. 9, 1025–1031.

Lloyd, G., Bowen, E.T.W., Jones, N., Pendry, A., 1984. HFRS outbreak associated with laboratory rats in UK. Lancet 1, 175–176.

Loeb, W., Quimby, F., 1999. The Clinical Chemistry of Laboratory Animals. Taylor & Francis, Philadelphia, PA.

Lofgren, J.L., Whary, M.T., Ge, Z., Muthupalani, S., Taylor, N.S., Mobley, M., et al., 2011. Lack of commensal flora in Helicobacter pylori-infected INS-GAS mice reduces gastritis and delays intraepithelial neoplasia. Gastroenterology 140, 210–220.

Lofgren, J.L., Erdman, S.E., Hewes, C., Wong, C., King, R., Chavarria, T.E., et al., 2012. Castration eliminates conspecific aggression in group-housed CD1 male surveillance mice (Mus musculus). J. Am. Assoc. Lab. Anim. Sci. 51, 594–599.

Love, W., Dobbs, N., Tabor, L., Simecka, J.W., 2010. Toll-like receptor 2 (TLR2) plays a major role in innate resistance in the lung against murine Mycoplasma. PLoS One 5, e10739.

Lowe, B.R., Fox, J.G., Bartlett, J.G., 1980. Clostridium difficile-associated cecitis in guinea pigs exposed to penicillin. Am. J. Vet. Res. 41, 1277–1279.

Lund, F.E., Schuer, K., Hollifield, M., Randall, T.D., Garvy, B.A., 2003. Clearance of Pneumocystis carinii in mice is dependent on B cells but not on P-carinii-specific antibody. J. Immunol. 171, 1423–1430.

Lundrigan, B.L., Jansa, S.A., Tucker, P.I., 2002. Phylogenetic relationships in the Genus Mus, based on paternally, maternally, and biparentally inherited characteristics. Syst. Biol. 51, 410–431.

Lyon, M.F., Rastan, S., Brown, S.D.M., 1996. Genetic Variants and Strains of the Laboratory Mouse. Oxford University Press, Oxford.

Mackey, J.P., Vazquez Melendez, E.L., Farrell, J.J., Lowery, K.S., Rounds, M.A., Sampath, R., et al., 2014. Direct detection of indirect transmission of Streptobacillus moniliformis rat bite fever infection. J. Clin. Microbiol. 52(6), 2259–61.

Maclachlan, N.J., Dubovi, E.J., 2011. Fenner's Veterinary Virology. Elsevier, New York.

Macnish, M.G., Morgan, U.M., Behnke, J.M., Thompson, R.C., 2002. Failure to infect laboratory rodent hosts with human isolates of Rodentolepis (=Hymenolepis) nana. J. Helminthol. 76, 37–43.

Macy, J.D., Cameron, G.A., Smith, P.C., Ferguson, T.A., Compton, S.R., 2011. Detection and control of mouse parvovirus. J. Am. Assoc. Lab. Anim. Sci. 50, 516–522.

Maggio-Price, L., Nicholson, K.L., Kline, K.M., Birkebak, T., Suzuki, I., Wilson, D.L., et al., 1998. Diminished reproduction, failure to thrive, and altered immunologic function in a colony of T-cell receptor transgenic mice: possible role of Citrobacter rodentium. Lab. Anim. Sci. 48, 145–155.

Maggio-Price, L., Shows, D., Waggie, K., Burich, A., Zeng, W., Escobar, S., et al., 2002. Helicobacter bilis infection accelerates and H. hepaticus infection delays the development of colitis in multiple drug resistance-deficient (mdr1a −/−) mice. Am. J. Pathol. 160, 739–751.

Maggio-Price, L., Treuting, P., Zeng, W., Tsang, M., Bielefeldt-Ohmann, H., Iritani, B.M., 2006. Helicobacter infection is required for inflammation and colon cancer in SMAD3-deficient mice. Cancer Res. 66, 828–838.

Mahbubani, M.H., Bej, A.K., Perlin, M., Schaefer 3rd, F.W., Jakubowski, W., Atlas, R.M., 1991. Detection of Giardia cysts by using the polymerase chain reaction and distinguishing live from dead cysts. Appl. Environ. Microbiol. 57, 3456–3461.

Mak, T.W., Penninger, J.M., Ohashi, P.S., 2001. Knockout mice: a paradigm shift in modern immunology. Nat. Rev. Immunol. 1, 11–19.

Mallick, E.M., Mcbee, M.E., Vanguri, V.K., Melton-Celsa, A.R., Schlieper, K., Karalius, B.J., et al., 2012. A novel murine infection model for Shiga toxin-producing Escherichia coli. J. Clin. Invest. 122, 4012–4024.

Mangerich, A., Knutson, C.G., Parry, N.M., Muthupalani, S., Ye, W., Prestwich, E., et al., 2012. Infection-induced colitis in mice causes dynamic and tissue-specific changes in stress response and DNA damage leading to colon cancer. Proc. Natl. Acad. Sci. USA 109, E1820–E1829.

Manuel, C.A., Hsu, C.C., Riley, L.K., Livingston, R.S., 2008. Soiled-bedding sentinel detection of murine norovirus 4. J. Am. Assoc. Lab. Anim. Sci. 47, 31–36.

Marchal, J., 1930. Infectious ectromelia. A hitherto undescribed virus disease of mice. J. Pathol. Bacteriol. 33(3), 713–728.

Markoullis, K., Bulian, D., Holzlwimmer, G., Quintanilla-Martinez, L., Heiliger, K.J., Zitzelsberger, H., et al., 2009. Mycoplasma contamination of murine embryonic stem cells affects cell parameters, germline transmission and chimeric progeny. Transgenic Res. 18, 71–87.

Marks, S.L., 2013. Clostridium perfringens and Clostridium difficile-associated diarrhea. In: Greene, C.E. (Ed.), Infectious Diseases of the Dog and Cat, fourth ed. Elsevier Saunders, St. Louis, MO.

Maronpot, R.R., Boorman, G.A., Gaul, B., 1999. Pathology of the Mouse. Cache River Press, Vienna, IL.

Martin-Sanchez, A., Mclean, L., Beynon, R.J., Hurst, J.L., Ayala, G., Lanuza, E., et al., 2015. From sexual attraction to maternal aggression: when pheromones change their behavioural significance. Horm. Behav. 68., 65–76.

Matsumiya, L.C., Lavoie, C., 2003. An outbreak of Pasteurella pneumotropica in genetically modified mice: treatment and elimination. Contemp. Top. Lab. Anim. Sci. 42, 26–28.

Matsushita, S., Matsumoto, T., 1986. Spontaneous necrotic enteritis in young RFM/Ms mice. Lab. Anim. 20, 114–117.

Matsushita, S., Suzuki, E., 1995. Prevention and treatment of cilia-associated respiratory bacillus in mice by use of antibiotics. Lab. Anim. Sci. 45, 503–507.

Mccance, D.J., Sebesteny, A., Griffen, B.E., Balkwill, F., Tilly, R., Gregson, N.A., 1983. A paralytic disease in nude mice associated with polyomavirus infection. J. Gen. Virol. 64, 57–67.

Mcfarland, L.V., 2009. Renewed interest in a difficult disease: Clostridium difficile infections – epidemiology and current treatment strategies. Curr. Opin. Gastroenterol. 25, 24–35.

Mcgorum, B.C., Dixon, P.M., Smith, D.G., 1998. Use of metronidazole in equine acute idiopathic toxaemic colitis. Vet. Rec. 142, 635–638.

Mckisic, M.D., Lancki, D.W., Otto, G., Padrid, R., Snook, S., Cronin, D.C., et al., 1993. Identification and propogation of a putative immunosuppressive orphan parvovirus in cloned T cells. J. Immunol. 150, 419–428.

Mcwilliams, T.S., Waggie, K.S., Luzarraga, M.B., French, A.W., Adams, R.J., 1993. Corynebacterium species-associated keratoconjunctivitis in aged male C57BL/6J mice. Lab. Anim. Sci. 43, 509–512.

Mekada, K., Abe, K., Murakami, A., Nakamura, S., Nakata, H., Moriwaki, K., et al., 2009. Genetic differences among C57BL/6 substrains. Exp. Anim. 58, 141–149.

Miller, C.L., Muthupalani, S., Shen, Z., Fox, J.G., 2014. Isolation of Helicobacter spp. from Mice with Rectal Prolapses. Comp. Med. 64, 171–178.

Moore, K.J., Nagle, D.L., 2000. Complex trait analysis in the mouse: the strengths, the limitations, and the promise yet to come. Annu. Rev. Genet. 34, 653–686.

Morita, E., Kaneko, S., Hiragun, T., Shindo, H., Tanaka, T., Furukawa, T., et al., 1999. Fur mites induce dermatitis associated with IgE hyperproduction in an inbred strain of mice, NC/Kuj. J. Dermatol. Sci. 19, 37–43.

Morse, H.C.I., 1978. Origins of Inbred Mice: Proceedings of a Workshop. Academic Press.

Morse, H.C.I., 2007a. Building a better mouse: one hundred years of genetics and biology. In: Fox, J.G., Barthold, S.W., Davisson, M.T., Newcomer, C.E., Quimby, F., Smith, A.L. (Eds.), The Mouse in Biomedical Research. 2. Diseases. Elsevier, London.

Morse, H.C.I., 2007b. Retroelements in the mouse. In: Fox, J.G., Barthold, S.W., Davisson, M.T., Newcomer, C.E., Quimby, F., Smith, A.L. (Eds.), The Mouse in Biomedical Research. 2. Diseases. Elsevier, London.

Morse, S.S., 1989. A mammalian herpesvirus cytolytic for CD4+ (L3T4+) T lymphocytes. J. Exp. Med. 169, 591–596.

Muller, E.L., Pitt, H.A., George, W.L., 1987. Prairie dog model for antimicrobial agent-induced Clostridium difficile diarrhea. Infect. Immun. 55, 198–200.

Mumphrey, S.M., Changotra, H., Moore, T.N., Heimann-Nichols, E.R., Wobus, C.E., Reilly, M.J., et al., 2007. Murine norovirus 1 infection is associated with histopathological changes in immunocompetent hosts, but clinical disease is prevented by STAT1-dependent interferon responses. J. Virol. 81, 3251–3263.

Murakami, T., Ishiguro, N., Higuchi, K., 2014. Transmission of systemic AA Amyloidosis in animals. Vet. Pathol. 51, 363–371.

Murakata, K., Sato, A., Yoshiya, M., Kim, S., Watarai, M., Omata, Y., et al., 2008. Infection of different strains of mice with Lawsonia intracellularis derived from rabbit or porcine proliferative enteropathy. J. Comp. Pathol. 139, 8–15.

Murray, P.R., Rosenthal, K.S., Kobayashi, G.S., Pfaller, M.A., 2002. Clostridium Medical Microbiology. Mosby, St. Louis, MO.

Nagamine, C.M., Nishioka, Y., Moriwaki, K., Boursot, P., Bonhomme, F., Lau, Y.F., 1992. The musculus-type Y chromosome of the laboratory mouse is of Asian origin. Mamm. Genome 3, 84–91.

Nagi-Miura, N., Harada, T., Shinohara, H., Kurihara, K., Adachi, Y., Ishida-Okawara, A., et al., 2006. Lethal and severe coronary arteritis in DBA/2 mice induced by fungal pathogen, CAWS, Candida albicans water-soluble fraction. Atherosclerosis 186, 310–320.

Nagy, A., 2000. Cre recombinase: the universal reagent for genome tailoring. Genesis 26, 99–109.

Nakayama, M., Weyant, R.S., 1994. Streptococcus pneumoniae. In: Waggie, K.S., Kagayima, N., Allen, A.M., Nomura, T. (Eds.), Manual of Microbiological Monitoring of Laboratory Animals. National Institutes of Health Publication, Bethesda, MD, pp. 94–2498.

Naugler, S.L., Myles, M.H., Bauer, B.A., Kennett, M.J., Besch-Williford, C.L., 2001. Reduced fecundity and death associated with parvovirus infection in B-lymphocyte deficient mice. Contemp. Top. Lab. Anim. Sci. 40.

Neimark, H., Peters, W., Robinson, B.L., Stewart, L.B., 2005. Phylogenetic analysis and description of Eperythrozoon coccoides, proposal to transfer to the genus Mycoplasma as Mycoplasma coccoides comb. nov. and request for an opinion. Int. J. Syst. Evol. Microbiol. 55, 1385–1391.

Neuhaus, B., Niessen, C.M., Mesaros, A., Withers, D.J., Krieg, T., Partridge, L., 2012. Experimental analysis of risk factors for ulcerative dermatitis in mice. Exp. Dermatol. 21, 712–713.

Newman, J.V., Zabel, B.A., Jha, S.S., Schauer, D.B., 1999. Citrobacter rodentium espB is necessary for signal transduction and for infection of laboratory mice. Infect. Immun. 67, 6019–6025.

Nguyen, D.D., Muthupalani, S., Goettel, J.A., Eston, M.A., Mobley, M., Taylor, N.S., et al., 2013. Colitis and colon cancer in WASP-deficient mice require Helicobacter species. Inflamm. Bowel Dis. 19, 2041–2050.

Nicklas, W., Kraft, V., Meyer, B., 1993. Contamination of transplantable tumors, cell lines, and monoclonal antibodies with rodent viruses. Lab. Anim. Sci. 43, 296–300.

Nicklas, W., Baneux, P., Boot, R., Decelle, T., Deeny, A., Fumanelli, M., et al., 2002. Recommendations for the health monitoring of rodent and rabbit colonies in breeding and experimental units. Lab. Anim. 36, 20–42.

Nio, J., Fujimoto, W., Konno, A., Kon, Y., Owhashi, M., Iwanaga, T., 2004. Cellular expression of murine Ym1 and Ym2, chitinase family proteins, as revealed by in situ hybridization and immunohistochemistry. Histochem. Cell Biol. 121, 473–482.

Nishimori, K., Young, L.J., Guo, Q., Wang, Z., Insel, T.R., Matzuk, M.M., 1996. Oxytocin is required for nursing but is not essential for parturition or reproductive behavior. Proc. Natl. Acad. Sci USA 93, 11699–11704.

Nutrition, A.I.O., 1977. Report of the American institute of nutrition ad hoc committee on standards for nutritional studies. J. Nutr. 107, 1340–1348.

O'brien, T.P., Frankel, W.N., 2003. Moving forward with chemical mutagenesis in the mouse. J. Physiol. 554, 13–21.

Ouellet, M., Cowan, M., Laporte, A., Faubert, S., Heon, H., 2011. Implementation of a PCR assay of Pasteurella pneumotropica to accurately screen for contaminated laboratory mice. Lab. Anim. (NY) 40, 305–312.

Ozkul, I.A., Aydin, Y., 1994. Natural Cryptosporidium muris infection of the stomach in laboratory mice. Vet. Parasitol. 55, 129–132.

Pang, T.Y., Hannan, A.J., 2013. Enhancement of cognitive function in models of brain disease through environmental enrichment and physical activity. Neuropharmacology 64, 515–528.

Pastoret, P.P., Brazin, P.G.H., Govaerts, A. (Eds.), 1998. Handbook of Vertebrate Immunology. Academic Press, Boston.

Patten Jr., C.C., Myles, M.H., Franklin, C.L., Livingston, R.S., 2010. Perturbations in cytokine gene expression after inoculation of C57BL/6 mice with Pasteurella pneumotropica. Comp. Med. 60, 18–24.

Peng, S., York, J., Zhang, P., 2006. A transgenic approach for RNA interference-based genetic screening in mice. Proc. Natl. Acad. Sci. USA 103, 2252–2256.

Percy, D.H., Barthold, S.W., 2007. Mouse Pathology of Laboratory Rodents and Rabbits. Blackwell, Oxford, 3–124.

Perdue, K.A., Green, K.Y., Copeland, M., Barron, E.L., Mandel, M., Faucette, L.J., et al., 2007. Naturally occurring murine norovirus infection in a large research institution. J. Am. Assoc. Lab. Anim. Sci. 46, 39–46.

Peterson, N.C., 2008. From bench to cageside: risk assessment for rodent pathogen contamination of cells and biologics. ILAR J. 49, 310–315.

Petznek, H., Kappler, R., Scherthan, H., Muller, M., Brem, G., Aigner, B., 2002. Reduced body growth and excessive incisor length in insertional mutants mapping to mouse Chromosome 13. Mamm. Genome 13, 504–509.

Pierro, L.J., Spiggle, J., 1967. Congenital eye defects in the mouse. I. Corneal opacity in C57black mice. J. Exp. Zool. 166, 25–33.

Pirofski, L., Horwitz, M.S., Scharff, M.D., Factor, S.M., 1991. Murine adenovirus infection of SCID mice induces hepatic lesions that resemble human Reye syndrome. Proc. Natl. Acad. Sci. USA 88 (10), 4358–4362.

Pleasants, J.R., Wostmann, B.S., Reddy, B.S., 1973. Improved lactation in germfree mice following changes in the amino acid and fat components of a chemically defined diet. In: Heneghan, J.B. (Ed.), Germfree Research. Academic Press, New York.

Poiley, S.M., 1960. A systematic method of breeder rotation for non-inbred laboratory animal colonies. Proc. Anim. Care Panel 10, 159–166.

Prager, E.M., Orrego, C., Sage, R.D., 1998. Genetic variation and phylogeography of central Asian and other house mouse mice, including a major new mitochondrial lineage in Yemen. Genetics 150, 835–861.

Pritchett, K., Taft, R., 2007. Reproductive biology of the laboratory mouse. In: Jg, F., Sw, B., Mt, D., Ce, N., Fw, Q., Al, S. (Eds.), The Mouse in Biomedical Research; Normative Biology, Husbandry and Models, second ed. Elsevier Academic Press.

Pritchett, K.R., 2007. Helminth Parasites of Laboratory Mice. In: Fox, J.G., Barthold, S.W., Davisson, M.T., Newcomer, C.E., Quimby, F., Smith, A.L. (Eds.), The Mouse in Biomedical Research. II. Diseases. Elsevier, London.

Pritchett-Corning, K.R., Cosentino, J., Clifford, C.B., 2009. Contemporary prevalence of infectious agents in laboratory mice and rats. Lab. Anim. 43, 165–173.

Quinn, P.J., Markey, B.K., Carter, M.E., Donnelly, W.J.C., Leonard, F.C., Maghire, D., 2002. Clostridium species. Veterinary Microbiology and Microbial Disease. Blackwell Science, Oxford.

Rao, G.N., Hickman, R.L., Seilkop, S.K., Boorman, G.A., 1987. Utero-ovarian infection in aged B6C3F1 mice. Lab. Anim. Sci. 37, 153–158.

Rao, V.P., Poutahidis, T., Fox, J.G., Erdman, S.E., 2007. Breast cancer: should gastrointestinal bacteria be on our radar screen? Cancer Res. 67, 847–850.

Reddy, L.V., Zammit, C., Schuman, P., Crane, L.R., 1992. Detection of Pneumocystis carinii in a rat model of infection by polymerase chain reaction. Mol. Cell Probes. 6, 137–143.

Rehm, S., Sommer, R., Deerberg, F., 1987. Spontaneous nonneoplastic gastric lesions in female Han:NMRI mice, and influence of food restriction throughout life. Vet. Pathol. 24, 216–225.

Restrepo, D., Arellano, J., Oliva, A.M., Schaefer, M.L., Lin, W., 2004. Emerging views on the distinct but related roles of the main and accessory olfactory systems in responsiveness to chemosensory signals in mice. Horm. Behav. 46, 247–256.

Reyon, D., Kirkpatrick, J.R., Sander, J.D., Zhang, F., Voytas, D.F., Joung, J.K., et al., 2011. ZFNGenome: a comprehensive resource for locating zinc finger nuclease target sites in model organisms. BMC Genomics 12, 83.

Ricart Arbona, R.J., Lipman, N.S., Wolf, F.R., 2010. Treatment and eradication of murine fur mites: III. Treatment of a large mouse colony with ivermectin-compounded feed. J. Am. Assoc. Lab. Anim. Sci. 49, 633–637.

Roberts, S.A., Davidson, A.J., Mclean, L., Beynon, R.J., Hurst, J.L., 2012. Pheromonal induction of spatial learning in mice. Science 338, 1462–1465.

Robertson, B.R., O'rourke, J.L., Neilan, B.A., Vandamme, P., On, S.L., Fox, J.G., et al., 2005. Mucispirillum schaedleri gen. nov., sp. nov., a spiral-shaped bacterium colonizing the mucus layer of the gastrointestinal tract of laboratory rodents. Int. J. Syst. Evol. Microbiol. 55, 1199–1204.

Rodriguez, I., Boehm, U., 2009. Pheromone sensing in mice. Results Probl. Cell Differ. 47, 77–96.

Roopenian, D.C., Simpson, E., Eds., 2000. Minor Histocompatibility Antigens: From the Laboratory to the Clinic. Landes Bioscience, Austin, TX.

Ross, A.C., 2012. Vitamin A and retinoic acid in T cell-related immunity. Am. J. Clin. Nutr. 96, 1166S–1172S.

Roths, J.B., Marshall, J.D., Allen, R.D., Carlson, G.A., Sidman, C.L., 1990. Spontaneous Pneumocystis carinii pneumonia in immunodeficient mutant scid mice. Natural history and pathobiology. Am. J. Pathol. 136, 1173–1186.

Roths, J.B., Smith, A.L., Sidman, C.L., 1993. Lethal exacerbation of Pneumocystis carinii pneumonia in severe combined immunodeficiency mice after infection by pneumonia virus of mice. J. Exp. Med. 177, 1193–1198.

Rozario, C., Morin, L., Roger, A.J., Smith, M.W., Muller, M., 1996. Primary structure and phylogenetic relationships of glyceraldehyde-3-phosphate dehydrogenase genes of free-living and parasitic diplomonad flagellates. J. Eukaryot. Microbiol. 43, 330–340.

Rozengurt, N., Sanchez, S., 1999. Duodenal adenomas in Balb/-c mice monoinfected with Clostridium perfringens. J. Comp. Pathol. 121, 217–225.

Russo, M., Invernizzi, A., Gobbi, A., Radaelli, E., 2013. Diffuse scaling dermatitis in an athymic nude mouse. Vet. Pathol. 50, 722–726.

Ryden, E.B., Lipman, N.S., Taylor, N.S., Rose, R., Fox, J.G., 1991. Clostridium difficile typhlitis associated with cecal mucosal hyperplasia in Syrian hamsters. Lab. Anim. Sci. 41, 553–558.

Sander, J.D., Maeder, M.L., Reyon, D., Voytas, D.F., Joung, J.K., Dobbs, D., 2010. ZiFiT (Zinc Finger Targeter): an updated zinc finger engineering tool. Nucl. Acids Res. 38, W462–W468.

Sarma-Rupavtarm, R.B., Ge, Z., Schauer, D.B., Fox, J.G., Polz, M.F., 2004. Spatial distribution and stability of the eight microbial species of the altered schaedler flora in the mouse gastrointestinal tract. Appl. Environ. Microbiol. 70, 2791–2800.

Sasaki, H., Kawamoto, E., Kunita, S., Yagami, K., 2007. Comparison of the in vitro susceptibility of rodent isolates of Pseudomonas aeruginosa and Pasteurella pneumotropica to enrofloxacin. J. Vet. Diagn. Invest. 19, 557–560.

Sato, Y., Ooi, H.K., Nonaka, N., Oku, Y., Kamiya, M., 1995. Antibody production in *Syphacia obvelata* infected mice. J. Parasitol. 81, 559–562.

Scanziani, E., Gobbi, A., Crippa, L., Giusti, A.M., Pesenti, E., Cavalletti, E., et al., 1998. Hyperkeratosis-associated coryneform infection in severe combined immunodeficient mice. Lab. Anim. 32, 330–336.

Schaedler, R.W., Orcutt, R.P., 1983. Gastrointestinal microflora. In: Foster, H.L., Small, J.D., Fox, J.G. (Eds.), The Mouse in Biomedical Research. Academic Press, New York.

Schagemann, G., Bohnet, W., Kunstyr, I., Friedhoff, K.T., 1990. Host specificity of cloned *Spironucleus muris* in laboratory rodents. Lab. Anim. 24, 234–239.

Schauer, D.B., Falkow, S., 1993. The eae gene of *Citrobacter freundii* biotype 4280 is necessary for colonization in transmissible murine colonic hyperplasia. Infect. Immun. 61, 4654–4661.

Schauer, D.B., Zabel, B.A., Pedraza, I.F., O'hara, C.M., Steigerwalt, A.G., Brenner, D.J., 1995. Genetic and biochemical characterization of *Citrobacter rodentium* sp. nov. J. Clin. Microbiol. 33, 2064–2068.

Schenkman, D.I., Rahija, R.J., Klingenberger, K.L., Elliott, J.A., Richter, C.B., 1994. Outbreak of group B streptococcal meningoencephalitis in athymic mice. Lab. Anim. Sci. 44, 639–641.

Sebesteny, A., Tilly, R., Balkwill, F., Trevan, D., 1980. Demylination and wasting associated wigh polyomavirus infection in nude (*nu/nu*) mice. Lab. Anim. Sci. 14, 337–345.

Segovia, J.C., Gallego, J.M., Bueren, J.A., Almendral, J.M., 1999. Severe leukopenia and dysregulated erythropoiesis in SCID mice persistently infected with the parvovirus minute virus of mice. J. Virol. 73, 1774–1789.

Serfilippi, L.M., Pallman, D.R., Gruebbel, M.M., Kern, T.J., Spainhour, C.B., 2004a. Assessment of retinal degeneration in outbred albino mice. Comp. Med. 54, 69–76.

Serfilippi, L.M., Stackhouse-Pallman, D.R., Gruebbel, M.M., Kern, T.J., Spainhour, C.B., 2004b. Assessment of retinal degeneration in outbred albino mice. Comp. Med. 54, 69–76.

Shames, B., Fox, J.G., Dewhirst, F., Yan, L., Shen, Z., Taylor, N.S., 1995. Identification of widespread *Helicobacter hepaticus* infection in feces in commercial mouse colonies by culture and PCR assay. J. Clin. Microbiol. 33, 2968–2972.

Sharp, J.M., Vanderford, D.A., Chichlowski, M., Myles, M.H., Hale, L.P., 2008. *Helicobacter* infection decreases reproductive performance of IL10-deficient mice. Comp. Med. 58, 447–453.

Sharrow, S.D., Vaughn, J.L., Zidek, L., Novotny, M.V., Stone, M.J., 2001. Pheromone binding by polymorphic mouse major urinary proteins. Prot. Sci. 11, 2247–2256.

Shek, W.R., 2008. Role of housing modalities on management and surveillance strategies for adventitious agents of rodents. ILAR J. 49, 316–325.

Shellam, G.R., Redwood, A.J., Smith, L.M., Gorman, S., 2007. Murine cytomegalovirus and other herpesviruses In: Fox, J.G. Barthold, S.W. Davisson, M.T. Newcomer, mC.E. Quimby, F.W. Smith, A.L. (Eds.), The Mouse in Biomedical Research. II. Diseases, vol. II. Elsevier, London. pp. 1–48.

Shen, Z., Feng, Y., Rogers, A.B., Rickman, B., Whary, M.T., Xu, S., et al., 2009. Cytolethal distending toxin promotes *Helicobacter cinaedi*-associated typhlocolitis in interleukin-10-deficient mice. Infect. Immun. 77, 2508–2516.

Shimizu, A., 1994. Staphylococcus aureus. In: Waggie, K.S., Kagayima, N., Allen, A.M., Nomura, T. (Eds.), Manual of Microbiological Monitoring of Laboratory Animals. National Institutes of Health Publication, Bethesda, MD, pp. 94–2498.

Shomer, N.H., Dangler, C.A., Schrenzel, M.D., Fox, J.G., 1997. *Helicobacter bilis*-induced inflammatory bowel disease in SCID mice with defined flora. Infect. Immun. 65, 4858–4864.

Shomer, N.H., Dangler, C.A., Marini, R.P., Fox, J.G., 1998. *Helicobacter bilis/Helicobacter rodentium* co-infection associated with diarrhea in a colony of scid mice. Lab. Anim. Sci. 48, 455–459.

Shultz, L.D., Sidman, C.L., 1987. Genetically determined murine models of immunodeficiency. Annu. Rev. Immunol. 5, 367–403.

Sica, A., Mantovani, A., 2012. Macrophage plasticity and polarization: in vivo veritas. J. Clin. Invest. 122, 787–795.

Sidman, R.L., Angevine, J.B., Pierce, E.T., 1971. Atlas of the Mouse Brain and Spinal Cord. Harvard University Press, Cambridge, MA.

Silver, L.M., 1995. Mouse Genetics: Concepts and Applications. Oxford University Press, Oxford.

Silverman, J., Chavannes, J.M., Rigotty, J., Ornaf, M., 1979. A natural outbreak of transmissible murine colonic hyperplasia in A/J mice. Lab. Anim. Sci. 29, 209–213.

Simpson, E.M., Linder, C.C., Sargent, E.E., Davisson, M.T., Mobraaten, L.E., Sharp, J.J., 1997. Genetic variation among 129 mouse substrains and its importance for targeted mutagenesis in mice. Nat. Genet. 16, 19–27.

Singer, J.B., Hill, A.E., Burrage, L.C., Olszens, K.R., Song, J., Justice, M.J., et al., 2004. Genetic dissection of complex traits with chromosome substitution strains of mice. Science 304, 445–448.

Skarnes, W.C., Rosen, B., West, A.P., Koutsourakis, M., Bushell, W., Iyer, V., et al., 2011. A conditional knock out resource for the genome-wide study of mouse gene function. Nature 474, 337–344.

Skopets, B., Wilson, R.P., Griffith, J.W., Lang, C.M., 1996. Ivermectin toxicity in young mice. Lab. Anim. Sci. 46, 111–112.

Smith, A.L., 1983. Response of weanling random-bred mice to inoculation with minute virus of mice. Lab. Anim. Sci. 33, 37–39.

Smith, A.L., Paturzo, F.X., 1988. Explant cultures for detection of minute virus of mice in infected mouse tissue. J. Tissue Cult. Methods 11, 45–47.

Smith, A.L., Jacoby, R.O., Johnson, E.A., Paturzo, F.X., Bhatt, P.N., 1993. In vivo studies with an 'orphan' parvovirus. Lab. Anim. Sci. 43, 175–182.

Smith, R.S., Roderick, T.H., Sundberg, J.P., 1994. Microphthalmia and associated abnormalities in inbred black mice. Lab. Anim. Sci. 44, 551–560.

Spindler, K.R., Moore, M.L., Cauthen, A.N., 2007. Mouse adenoviruses. In: Fox, J.G., Barthold, S.W., Davisson, M.T., Newcomer, C.E., Quimby, F., Smith, A.L. (Eds.), The Mouse in Biomedical Research. II. Diseases, second ed. Elsevier, London.

Spits, H., Artis, D., Colonna, M., Diefenbach, A., Di Santo, J.P., Eberl, G., et al., 2013. Innate lymphoid cells – a proposal for uniform nomenclature. Nat. Rev. Immunol. 13, 145–149.

Stringer, J.R., Beard, C.B., Miller, R.F., Wakefield, A.E., 2002. A new name (*Pneumocystis jiroveci*) for Pneumocystis from humans. Emerg. Infect. Dis. 8, 891–896.

Stuart, P.M., 2010. Major histocompatibility complex (MHC): mouse. *eLS*.

Sturm, T., Leinders-Zufall, T., Macek, B., Walzer, M., Jung, S., Pommer, B., et al., 2013. Mouse urinary peptides provide a molecular basis for genotype discrimination by nasal sensory neurons. Nat. Commun. 41, 1616.

Suerbaum, S., Josenhans, C., Sterzenbach, T., Drescher, B., Brandt, P., Bell, M., et al., 2003. The complete genome sequence of the carcinogenic bacterium *Helicobacter hepaticus*. Proc. Natl. Acad. Sci. USA 100, 7901–7906.

Sun, X., Wang, H., Zhang, Y., Chen, K., Davis, B., Feng, H., 2011. Mouse relapse model of *Clostridium difficile* infection. Infect. Immun. 79, 2856–2864.

Sun, X., Jones, H.P., Dobbs, N., Bodhankar, S., Simecka, J.W., 2013. Dendritic cells are the major antigen presenting cells in inflammatory lesions of murine Mycoplasma respiratory disease. PLoS One 8, e55984.

Sundberg, J.P., 1994. Chronic ulcerative dermatitis in black mice. In: Sundberg, J.P. (Ed.), Handbook of Mouse Mutations with Skin and Hair Abnormalities: Animal Models and Biomedical Tools. CRC Press, Boca Raton, FL.

Sung, Y.H., Jin, Y., Kim, S., Lee, H.W., 2014. Generation of knockout mice using engineered nucleases. Methods.

Suwa, T., Nyska, A., Haseman, J.K., Mahler, J.F., Maronpot, R.R., 2002. Spontaneous lesions in control B6C3F1 mice and recommended sectioning of male accessory sex organs. Toxicol. Pathol. 30, 228–234.

Szomolanyi-Tsuda, E., Dundon, P.L., Joris, I., Schultz, L.D., Woda, B.A., Welsh, R.M., 1994. Acute, lethal, natural killer cell-resistant myeloproliferative disease induced by polyomavirus in severe combined immunodeficient mice. Am. J. Pathol. 144.

Takada, T., Ebata, T., Noguchi, H., Keane, T.M., Adams, D.J., Narita, T., et al., 2013. The ancestor of extant Japanese fancy mice contributed to the mosaic genomes of classical inbred strains. Genome Res. 23 (8), 1329–1338.

Takeuchi, O., Akira, S., 2010. Pattern recognition receptors and inflammation. Cell 140, 805–820.

Tanaka, M., Hadjantonakis, A.K., Nagy, A., 2001. Aggregation chimeras: combining ES cells, diploid and tetraploid embryos. Methods Mol. Biol. 158, 135–154.

Taruishi, M., Yoshimatsu, K., Araki, K., Okumura, M., Nakamura, I., Kajino, K., et al., 2007. Analysis of the immune response of Hantaan virus nucleocapsid protein-specific CD8+ T cells in mice. Virology 365, 292–301.

Taylor, M.A., Marshall, R.N., Green, J.A., Catchpole, J., 1999. The pathogenesis of experimental infections of *Cryptosporidium muris* (strain RN 66) in outbred nude mice. Vet. Parasitol. 86, 41–48.

Taylor, N.S., Xu, S., Nambiar, P., Dewhirst, F.E., Fox, J.G., 2007. Enterohepatic *Helicobacter* species are prevalent in mice from commercial and academic institutions in Asia, Europe, and North America. J. Clin Microbiol. 45, 2166–2172.

Thackray, L.B., Wobus, C.E., Chachu, K.A., Liu, B., Alegre, A.R., Henderson, K.S., et al., 2007. Murine noroviruses comprising a single genogroup exhibit biological diversity despite limited sequence divergence. J. Virol. 81, 10460–10474.

Theriot, C.M., Koenigsknecht, M.J., Carlson Jr., P.E., Hatton, G.E., Nelson, A.M., Li, B., et al., 2014. Antibiotic-induced shifts in the mouse gut microbiome and metabolome increase susceptibility to *Clostridium difficile* infection. Nat. Commun. 5, 3114.

Theuer, R.C., 1971. Effect of essential amino acid restriction on the growth of female C57BL mice and their implanted BW10232 adenocarcinomas. J. Nutr. 101, 223–232.

Thilsted, J.P., Newton, W.M., Crandell, R.A., Bevill, R.F., 1981. Fatal diarrhea in rabbits resulting from the feeding of antibiotic-contaminated feed. J. Am. Vet. Med. Assoc. 179, 360–362.

Thirion, G., Saxena, A., Hulhoven, X., Markine-Goriaynoff, D., Van Snick, J., Coutelier, J.P., 2014. Modulation of the host microenvironment by a common non-oncolytic mouse virus leads to inhibition of plasmacytoma development through Nk cell activation. J. Gen. Virol. 95 (pt 7), 1504–1509.

Thomas, J.W., Lamantia, C., Magnuson, T., 1998. X-ray-induced mutations in mouse embryonic stem cells. Proc. Natl. Acad. Sci. USA 95, 1114–1119.

Threadgill, D.W., Churchill, G.A., 2012. Ten years of the Collaborative Cross. G3: Genes/Genomics/Genetics 2.

Threadgill, D.W., Yee, D., Matin, A., Nadeau, J.H., Magnuson, T., 1997. Geneology of the 129 inbred strains: 129/SvJ is a contaminated inbred strain. Mamm. Genome. 8, 390–393.

Tinkle, B.T., Jay, G., 2002. Molecular biology, analysis, and enabling technologies: analysis of transgene integration. In: Pinkert, C.A. (Ed.), Transgenic Animal Technology: A Laboratory Handbook. Academic Press, New York.

Tobin, G., Stevens, K.A., Russell, R.J., 2007. Nutrition. In: Fox, J.G., Barthold, S.W., Davisson, M.T., Newcomer, C.E., Quimby, F., Smith, A.L. (Eds.), The Mouse in Biomedical Research. III. Normative Biology, Husbandry, and Models. Elsevier, London.

Toth, L.A., Oberbeck, C., Straign, C.M., Frazier, S., Rehg, J.E., 2000. Toxicity evaluation of prophylactic treatments for mites and pinworms in mice. Contemp. Top. Lab. Anim. Sci. 39, 18–21.

Tsai, T.F., Bauer, S.P., Sasso, D.R., Whitfield, S.G., Mccormick, J.B., Caraway, T.C., et al., 1985. Serological and virological evidence of Hantaan virus-related enzootic in the United States. J. Infect. Dis. 152.

Umenai, T., Lee, H., Lee, P., Saito, T., Toyoda, T., Hongo, M., et al., 1979. Korean hemorrhagic fever in staff in an animal laboratory. Lancet 1, 314–316.

Van Andel, R.A., Franklin, C.L., Besch-Williford, C.L., Hook, R.R., Riley, L.K., 2000. Prolonged perturbations of tumour necrosis factor-alpha and interferon-gamma in mice inoculated with Clostridium piliforme. J. Med. Microbiol. 49, 557–563.

Vandenbergh, J.G., 1973. Acceleration and inhibition of puberty in female mice by pheromones. J. Reprod. Fertil. Suppl. 19, 411–419.

Van Der Lee, S., Boot, L.M., 1955. Spontaneous pseudopregnancy in mice. Acta Physiol. Pharm. N 4, 442–444.

Van Loo, P., Van Zutphen, L., Baumans, V., 2003. Male management: coping with aggression problems in male laboratory mice. Lab. Anim. 37, 300–313.

Viscogliosi, E., Philippe, H., Baroin, A., Perasso, R., Brugerolle, G., 1993. Phylogeny of trichomonads based on partial sequences of large subunit rRNA and on cladistic analysis of morphological data. J. Eukaryot. Microbiol. 40, 411–421.

Von Freeden-Jeffry, U., Davidson, N., Wiler, R., Fort, M., Burdach, S., Murray, R., 1998. IL-7 deficiency prevents development of a non-T cell non-B cell-mediated colitis. J. Immunol. 161, 5673–5680.

Von Lintig, J., 2012. Provitamin A metabolism and functions in mammalian biology. Am. J. Clin. Nutr. 96, 1234S–1244S.

Wade, C.M., Daly, M.J., 2005. Genetic variation in laboratory mice. Nat. Genet. 37, 1175–1180.

Wade, C.M., Kulbokas, E.J.I., Kirby, A.W., Zody, M.C., Mullikin, J.C., Lander, E.S., et al., 2002. The mosaic structure of variation in the laboratory mouse genome. Nature 420, 574–578.

Waggie, K.S., Hansen, C.T., Ganaway, J.R., Spencer, T.S., 1981. A study of mouse strains susceptibility to *Bacillus piliformis* (Tyzzer's disease): the association of B-cell function and resistance. Lab. Anim. Sci. 31, 139–142.

Waggie, K.S., Wagner, J.E., Lentsch, R.H., 1983. A naturally occurring outbreak of Mycobacterium avium-intracellulare infections in C57BL/6N mice. Lab. Anim. Sci. 33, 249–253.

Waggie, K.S., Hansen, C.T., Moore, T.D., Bukowski, M.A., Allen, A.M., 1988. Cecocolitis in immunodeficient mice associated with an enteroinvasive lactose negative E. coli. Lab Anim. Sci. 38, 389–393.

Wakefield, A.E., Peters, S.E., Banerji, S., Bridge, P.D., Hall, G.S., Hawksworth, D.L., et al., 1992. *Pneumocystis carinii* shows DNA homology with the ustomycetous red yeast fungi. Mol. Microbiol. 6, 1903–1911.

Wallace, G.D., Buller, R.M., 1985. Kinetics of ectromelia virus (mousepox) transmission and clinical response in C57BL/6J, BALB,cByJ and AKR inbred mice. Lab. Anim. Sci. 35, 41–46.

Walzer, P.D., Kim, C.K., Linke, M.J., Pogue, C.L., Huerkamp, M.J., Chrisp, C.E., et al., 1989. Outbreaks of *Pneumocystis carinii* pneumonia in colonies of immunodeficient mice. Infect. Immun. 57, 62–70.

Wannemuehler, M.J., Overstreet, A.-M., Ward, D.V., Phillips, G.J., 2014. Draft genome sequences of the altered Schaedler flora, a defined bacterial community from gnotobiotic mice. Genome Announcements 2, e00287–e00314.

Ward, J.M., 2000. Pathology of Genetically Engineered Mice. Iowa State University Press, Ames, IA.

Ward, J.M., Fox, J.G., Anver, M.R., Haines, D.C., George, C.V., Collins Jr., M.J., et al., 1994. Chronic active hepatitis and associated liver tumors in mice caused by a persistent bacterial infection with a novel *Helicobacter* species. J. Natl. Cancer Inst. 86, 1222–1227.

Ward, J.M., Anver, M.R., Haines, D.C., Melhorn, J.M., Gorelick, P., Yan, L., et al., 1996. Inflammatory large bowel disease in immunodeficient mice naturally infected with *Helicobacter hepaticus*. Lab. Anim. Sci. 46, 15–20.

Ward, J.M., Yoon, M., Anver, M.R., Haines, D.C., Kudo, G., Gonzalez, F.J., et al., 2001. Hyalinosis and Ym1/Ym2 gene expression in the stomach and respiratory tract of 129S4/SvJae and wild-type and CYP1A2-null B6, 129 mice. Am. J. Pathol. 158, 323–332.

Ward, J.M., Wobus, C.E., Thackray, L.B., Erexson, C.R., Faucette, L.J., Belliot, G., et al., 2006. Pathology of immunodeficient mice with naturally occurring murine norovirus infection. Toxicol. Path. 34, 708–715.

Ward, R.L., Mcneal, M.M., Farone, M.B., Farone, A.L., 2007. Reoviridae. In: Fox, J.G., Barthold, S.W., Davisson, M.T., Newcomer, C.E., Quimby, F., Smith, A.L. (Eds.), The Mouse in Biomedical Research. II. Diseases. Elsevier, London.

Wasson, K., 2007. Protozoa. In: Fox, J.G., Barthold, S.W., Davisson, M.T., Newcomer, C.E., Quimby, F., Smith, A.L. (Eds.), The Mouse in Biomedical Research. II. Diseases. Elsevier, London.

Waterston, R.H., et al., 2001. Initial sequencing and comparative analysis of the mouse genome. Nature.

Watson, J., 2008. New building, old parasite: Mesostigmatid mites – an ever-present threat to barrier facilities. ILAR J. 49, 303–309.

Weinberg, G.A., Durant, P.J., 1994. Genetic diversity of *Pneumocystis carinii* derived from infected rats, mice, ferrets, and cell cultures. J. Eukaryot. Microbiol. 41, 223–228.

Weir, E.C., Brownstein, D.G., Barthold, S.W., 1986. Spontaneous wasting disease in nude mice associated with *Pneumocystis carinii* infection. Lab. Anim. Sci. 36, 140–144.

Weir, E.C., Brownstein, D.G., Smith, A.L., 1988. Respiratory disease and wasting in athymic mice infected with pneumonia virus of mice. Lab. Anim. Sci. 38, 133–137.

Weisbroth, S.H., 1982. Arthropods. In: Foster, H.L., Small, J.D., Fox, J.G. (Eds.), The Mouse in Biomedical Research. Academic Press, New York.

Weisbroth, S.H., 1994. Corynebacterium kutscheri. In: Waggie, K.S., Kagayima, N., Allen, A.M., Nomura, T. (Eds.), Manual of Microbiological Monitoring of Laboratory Animals. National Institutes of Health Publication, Bethesda, MD, pp. 94–2498.

Weissman, I., 1967. Genetic and histochemical studies on mouse spleen black spots. Nature 215, 315.

Welsh, C.E., Miller, D.R., Manly, K.F., Wang, J., Mcmillan, L., Morahan, G., et al., 2012. Status and acces to the Collaborative Cross population. Mamm. Genome 23, 706–712.

Wescott, S.H., 1982. Helminths. In: Foster, H.L., Small, J.D., Fox, J.G. (Eds.), The Mouse in Biomedical Research. Academic Press, New York.

Whary, M.T., Fox, J.G., 2004. Natural and experimental *Helicobacter* infections. Comp. Med. 54, 128–158.

Whary, M.T., Cline, J.H., King, A.E., Hewes, K.M., Chojnacky, D., Salvarrey, A., et al., 2000. Monitoring sentinel mice for *Helicobacter hepaticus*, *H rodentium*, and *H bilis* infection by use of polymerase chain reaction analysis and serologic testing. Comp. Med. 50, 436–443.

Whary, M.T., Danon, S.J., Feng, Y., Ge, Z., Sundina, N., Ng, V., et al., 2006. Rapid onset of ulcerative typhlocolitis in B6.129P2-IL10tm1Cgn (IL-10−/−) mice infected with *Helicobacter trogontum* is associated with decreased colonization by altered Schaedler's flora. Infect. Immun. 74, 6615–6623.

Whitten, W.K., Bronson, F.H., Greenstein, J.A., 1968. Estrus-inducing pheromone of male mice. Transport by movement of air. Science 161, 584–585.

Wijshake, T., Baker, D.J., Van De Sluis, B., 2014. Endonucleases: new tools to edit the mouse genome. Biochim. Biophys. Acta 1842 (10), 1942–1950.

Wobus, C.E., Karst, S.M., Thackray, L.B., Chang, K.O., Sosnovtsev, S.V., Belliot, G., et al., 2004. Replication of a norovirus in cell culture reveals a tropism for dendritic cells and macrophages. PLoS Biol. 2, e432.

Wobus, C.E., Thackray, L.B., Virgin, H.W.I., 2006. Murine norovirus: a model system to study norovirus biology and pathogenesis. J. Virol. 80, 5104–5112.

Wolfson, W., 2013. Addgene: the bank that gives points for (plasmid) deposits. Chem. Biol. 20, 857–858.

Won, Y.-S., Jeong, E.-S., Park, H.-J., Lee, C.-H., Nam, K.-H., Kim, H.-C., et al., 2006. Microbiological contamination of laboratory mice and rats in Korea from 1999 to 2003. Exp. Anim. 55, 11–16.

Wullenweber, M., 1995. *Streptobacillus moniliformis* – a zoonotic pathogen. Taxonomic considerations, host species, diagnosis, therapy, geographical distribution. Lab. Anim. 29, 1–15.

Wullenweber-Schmidt, M., Meyer, B., Kraft, V., Kaspareit, J., 1988. An enzyme-linked immunosorbent assay (ELISA) for the detection of antibodies to *Pasteurella pneumotropica* in murine colonies. Lab. Anim. Sci. 38, 37–41.

Xie, S., Shen, B., Zhang, C., Huang, X., Zhang, Y., 2014. sgRNAcas9: a software package for designing CRISPR sgRNA and evaluating potential off-target cleavage sites. PLoS One 9, e100448.

Yadav, S.K., Adhikary, B., Bandyopadhyay, S.K., Chattopadhyay, S., 2013. Inhibition of TNF-alpha, and NF-kappaB and JNK pathways accounts for the prophylactic action of the natural phenolic, allylpyrocatechol against indomethacin gastropathy. Biochim. Biophys. Acta 1830, 3776–3786.

Yokoyama, C.C., Loh, J., Zhao, G., Stappenbeck, T.S., Wang, D., Huang, H.V., et al., 2012. Adaptive immunity restricts replication of novel murine astroviruses. J. Virol. 86, 12262–12270.

Yoshizawa, K., Kissling, G.E., Johnson, J.A., Clayton, N.P., Flagler, N.D., Nyska, A., 2005. Chemical-induced atrial thrombosis in NTP rodent studies. Toxicol. Pathol. 33, 517–532.

Yu, P., Lubben, W., Slomka, H., Gebler, J., Konert, M., Cai, C., et al., 2012. Nucleic acid-sensing Toll-like receptors are essential for the control of endogenous retrovirus viremia and ERV-induced tumors. Immunity 37, 867–879.

Yu, R., Schellhorn, H.E., 2013. Recent applications of engineered animal antioxidant deficiency models in human nutrition and chronic disease. J. Nutr. 143, 1–11.

Yu, X., Gimsa, U., Wester-Rosenlof, L., Kanitz, E., Otten, W., Kunz, M., et al., 2009. Dissecting the effects of mtDNA variations on complex traits using mouse conplastic strains. Genome Res. 19, 159–165.

Yutin, N., Galperin, M.Y., 2013. A genomic update on clostridial phylogeny: gram-negative spore formers and other misplaced clostridia. Environ. Microbiol. 15, 2631–2641.

Zenner, L., 1998. Effective eradication of pinworms (Syphacia muris, Syphacia obvelata and Aspiculuris tetraptera) from a rodent breeding colony by oral anthelmintic therapy. Lab. Anim. 32, 337–342.

Zhang, Z., Goldschmidt, T., Salter, H., 2012. Possible allelic structure of IgG2a and IgG2c in mice. Mol. Immunol. 50, 169–171.

Zhou, J., Shen, B., Zhang, W., Wang, J., Yang, J., Chen, L., et al., 2014. One-step generation of different immunodeficient mice with multiple gene modifications by CRISPR/Cas9 mediated genome engineering. Int. J. Biochem. Cell Biol. 46, 49–55.

4

Biology and Diseases of Rats

Glen M. Otto, DVM, DACLAM[a], Craig L. Franklin, DVM, PhD, DACLAM[b] and Charles B. Clifford, DVM, PhD, DACVP[c]

[a]Animal Resources Center, University of Texas at Austin, Austin, TX, USA [b]Department of Veterinary Pathobiology, University of Missouri, Columbia, MO, USA [c]Pathology and Technical Services (Retired), Charles River Laboratories Inc., San Diego, CA, USA

OUTLINE

I. INTRODUCTION

A. Major Taxonomic and Historical Considerations

The laboratory rat, *Rattus norvegicus*, is within the order Rodentia and family Muridae. The genus *Rattus* contains at least 56 species (retrieved January 28, 2014, from the Integrated Taxonomic Information System online database http://www.itis.gov); however, the Norway rat, *R. norvegicus*, and the black rat, *R. rattus*, are the two species most commonly associated with the genus. *Rattus rattus* preceded *R. norvegicus* in migration from Asia to Europe and the Americas by several hundred years. The former species reached Europe in the 12th century, and the Americas in the 16th century; whereas, *R. norvegicus* emerged in the 18th century in Europe and in the 19th century in the Western Hemisphere. Globally, the Norway rat has largely displaced the black rat, probably because of the Norway rat's larger size and aggressiveness. The domestication and introduction of the albino *R. norvegicus* is rooted by its use in Europe and America in the 1800s as prey for a sport (rat baiting) in which individuals would wager on which terrier dog would most swiftly kill the largest number of rats confined to a pit. Because of the large numbers of rats needed for this sport, wild rats were purpose-bred, and albinos were selected out by some people as a hobby (Robinson, 1965; Mayhew, 1851).

Early experimental use of the rat was reviewed by Hedrich (Hedrich, 2000). Early experiments using rats in nutrition research date back to at least 1828, when rats were starved as part of fasting studies (McCay, 1973). Savory used them in 1863 in protein studies (Savory, 1863), and J.M. Philipeaux, reported on the effects of adrenalectomy in albino rats in 1856 (Philipeaux, 1856). Rats were used in experiments only sporadically in Europe and North America until about 1890. Pivotal to the development of the rat for use in research were Henry H. Donaldson, and Milton Greenman at the Wistar Institute in the early 20th century, who did much to produce and define early stocks of laboratory rats (Lindsey, 1979).

B. Uses in Research

The rat is second only to the mouse as the most frequently used mammal in biomedical and behavioral research. Characteristics such as a short gestation and a relatively short life span, docile behavior, and ready availability of animals with well-defined health and genetic backgrounds are responsible for the importance of the rat as a laboratory animal. The rat is a standard species for toxicological, teratological, and carcinogenesis testing by the pharmaceutical industry and governmental regulatory agencies. Its early use in behavioral, neurological, nutritional, and endocrinology studies continues today. The size of the rat enables it to be used for surgical procedures, varying from organ transplantation to vascular techniques. Although the number of commonly used inbred strains is dwarfed by those of the mouse, inbred rat strains do represent an important repertoire of disease models (Table 4.1).

C. Summary of Laboratory Management and Husbandry

1. Macroenvironment

Rooms in which rats are to be housed should meet the guidelines of the *Guide for the Care and Use of Laboratory Animals* (National Research Council, 2011). Wall, ceiling, and floor surfaces should be made of materials that allow for effective sanitation and that resist damage from normal use and manipulation of equipment. The environment of the room should be well controlled, to ensure animal well-being and to help limit variables to those of the experimental design. Although rats, like most other species, can adapt to changes in temperature and humidity, room temperatures within a range of 70–76°F and with a relative humidity of 30–70% are typically accepted as being appropriate. Twenty-four-hour temperature/humidity recorders, either located in animal rooms or as a

TABLE 4.1 Commonly Used Rat Strains

Inbred strains	Usefulness as models
ACI	Congenital genitourinary anomalies, prostatic adenocarcinomas
BB/Wor	Juvenile insulin-dependent diabetes mellitus
BN (Brown Norway)	Inducible, transplantable myeloid leukemia, hydronephrosis, bladder carcinoma
BUF (Buffalo)	Spontaneous autoimmune thyroiditis, host for transplantable Morris hepatoma
COP (Copenhagen)	Prostate adenocarcinoma
F-344 (Fischer 344)	Inbred rat model for National Toxicology Program's Carcinogen Bioassay Program and the National Institute on Aging
LEW (Lewis)	Multiple sclerosis, various experimentally induced autoimmune diseases
LOU/C	Myeloma, production of IgG autoantibody
SHR (spontaneous hypertensive rat)	Hypertension, cardiovascular research
WF (Wistar-Furth)	Mononuclear cell leukemia
Zucker	Obesity

Mutant strains	Characteristics
Brattleboro	Diabetes insipidus (autosomal recessive)
Gunn	Jaundice, kernicterus (autosomal recessive)
Nude	T cell deficient (autosomal recessive)
Obese SHR	Type 4 hyperlipoproteinemia (autosomal recessive)

component of an electronic environmental management system, are useful in detecting changes in environmental conditions. Practice over many years has shown that, in general, ventilation rates of 10–15 air changes/hour of fresh air are sufficient to compensate for heat load and the generation of NH_3 and CO_2 from animals. A stable photoperiod is necessary to avoid changes in reproductive behavior, food intake, and weight gain. A cycle of 12–14h light and 10–12h dark is typically used for rats. Rats are particularly susceptible to phototoxic retinopathy. There is evidence to indicate that light intensity at cage level should be between 130 and 325 lux to prevent retinopathy (National Research Council, 2011). Management precautions such as not having exposed cages on the top shelves of tall racks should be considered.

Prevention and control of infectious diseases are partially a function of the location, size, and environmental conditions of a rat housing room. Strategies for limiting the transfer of pathogens will vary according to the potential impact that infectious agents may have on a particular group of rats and the study in which they are being used. For instance, an appropriate-sized room or cubicle may reflect the space necessary to separate rats by such criteria as pathogen status, immunological status, vendor, protocol, or investigator. Modifications such as the incorporation of Class 100 flexible wall enclosures may be useful to help ensure the specific pathogen status of rats over an extended period of time. Because of stress produced by noise, rat rooms should be located distant from mechanical rooms, cage-washing centers, and species that are apt to produce noise (National Research Council, 2011).

2. Primary Enclosures

The amount of cage space needed for rats, whether group or individually housed, is a function of animal weight, age and sex, as well as the specific physiological or protocol requirements of the animal(s) (National Research Council, 2011). Unless there is an experimental need, rats should be housed in solid-bottom rather than in wire-bottom cages. This will help prevent pododermatitis and injuries that are more frequently associated with wire floors, and bedding within solid-bottom cages provides some minimum environmental enrichment. However, enrichment enhances animal well-being by providing stimulation of natural species behavior. The resulting psychological benefits to the animal also result in a more robust biological model system and can improve the quality of scientific data derived form those animals (National Research Council, 2011). The most frequently used materials for solid-bottom cages are polycarbonate and polypropylene. The former plastic is often preferred because it may be repeatedly autoclaved without damage and because its translucency allows for observation of animals. Various contact bedding materials are appropriate for rats (e.g., hardwood chips, ground corncob, cellulose sheets).

3. Sanitation

Solid-bottom cages should typically be sanitized at a frequency of 1–2 times per week. A less frequent cycle may be appropriate if cage density is very low, if there are perinatal considerations, or if ventilated cages are used; and a more frequent cycle, if cage density is high or if pathophysiological considerations exist (e.g., diabetes) which increase the rate of soiling of the bedding. A detailed description of appropriate sanitation for rodent housing is given in *The Guide* (National Research Council, 2011).

II. BIOLOGY

A. Morphophysiology

This section provides a summary of some of the morphophysiological characteristics of the rat that may be useful to the reader. For more comprehensive descriptions, see the references cited in this section.

1. General Appearance

The Norway rat has small, thick ears and a tail that is about 85% of the length of the body (in contrast, *R. rattus* has larger ears and a tail that is distinctly longer than the body). The hair coat is composed of two classes – long and short hair shafts, with the former being more sparse. Hair growth in the young rat is cyclic, with the resting period and the growing period each being 17 days. In the female, there are usually 12 teats, with three pairs in the pectoral and three pairs in the abdominal region (Greene, 1963). Body weights and growth rates are dependent on the stock, strain, and source of rats. Of the two most commonly used outbred stocks, the Sprague-Dawley is larger than the Wistar, and the inbred Fischer 344 rat is smaller than either of the outbreds.

2. Sensory Organs

Rat eyes are exophthalmic, which increases the risk of injury from trauma and drying during anesthesia. The eyelids are well developed, and only the cornea is visible. The cornea is moistened by secretions from the lacrimal glands and the Harderian gland, which is located medially to the orbit. When a rat is stressed (e.g., because of malnutrition, dehydration, disease, or environmental factors) there can be an excessive secretion of Harderian gland products containing porphyrins, which is termed chromodacryorrhea. This results in a reddish secretion or crust located periorbitally and at the nares that may be a useful indicator of an illness or a husbandry problem (Moore, 1995). Interestingly, the porphyrins in these secretions will fluoresce, and it has been suggested that the Harderian gland may have a function as a modulator of light-mediated responses (Cui *et al.*, 2003). The orbital venous plexus has a slightly different anatomy than the orbital sinus observed in the mouse, but it is a useful site for blood collection in the anesthetized animal (Timm, 1979; Sharma *et al.*, 2014). Rats do not have robust color vision and their ability to discriminate based on color is difficult to demonstrate. It does, however, appear that they do have dichromatic color vision with two types of cones, one of which is responsive to ultraviolet (UV) wavelengths with a response centered around 359 nm (Koolhass, 1999; Jacobs *et al.*, 2001). This shift to the UV as compared to human vision is accompanied by a relative insensitivity of rat vision to longer wavelengths, since both the long-wavelength cone pigment and rod pigment have a peak sensitivity around 505–509 nm. This can be exploited by the use of dim red lighting (peak wavelengths greater than ~625 nm) generated using red bulbs or transparent red films/filters to view rats during their dark cycle, but it must be understood that intense red light (e.g., a bulb positioned close to the cage) can be perceived by the animals, and also that even dim red light can affect their photoperiodic physiology (McCormack and Sontag, 1980). Olfactory signals are strong determinants for behavior in the rat. Male rats recognize the social status of other males, females in estrus, and kinship by olfactory cues. Rats also detect alarm pheromones from other rats (Koolhass, 1999). The vomeronasal organ is critical for many pheromone responses (Liman, 1996).

The hearing range of rats extends from 250 Hz to nearly 80 kHz (Sales and Milligan, 1992), with the most sensitive hearing in the range of 8–32 kHz. Except for the rat's high-frequency sensitivity, its hearing capability corresponds closely to that of other mammals (Kelly and Masterton, 1977). The ultrasonic range of hearing and vocalization in the 22- to 80-kHz range is used for a variety of positive and negative communications, such as those emitted by pups left alone by their dam, or by adults during sexual and aggressive behavior (Koolhass, 1999; Portfors, 2007). Because frequencies that are disruptive to rats may not even be audible to humans, it is important to minimize ultrasonic noise in animal facilities. Monitoring equipment capable of detecting ultrasound should be utilized when screening rodent housing or use areas for noise contamination, and care must be taken when selecting equipment to avoid those known to emit ultrasound including some models of occupancy sensors (Weigler et al., 2007) and some types of energy-efficient high-frequency electronic ballasts that are used to drive linear fluorescent lamps (personal experience; author G.O.).

An extremely important sensory organ for touch in the rat is the array of sensitive vibrissae that are used to sample the environment in a variety of ways (Hartmann, 2011).

3. Skeleton

The skull is composed of the following bones: paired nasal, premaxillary, maxillary, zygoma, palatine, lacrimal, frontal, parietal, squamosal, periotic capsule, tympanic bulla, and mandible; six auditory ossicles; four turbinates; and single vomer, ethmoid, basisphenoid, presphenoid, occipital, interparietal, and hyoid bones.

The vertebral column consists of seven cervical, 13 thoracic, six lumbar, four sacral, and 27–30 caudal vertebrae. The ribs consist of ventral calcified and dorsal ossified segments without true costal cartilages. The humerus, ulna, and radius are similar to those of other mammalian species. The carpus consists of nine bones. The pelvis is formed by two ossa coxae, which articulate with the first two sacral vertebrae. The bones of the hindlimb are the femur, the tibia, and the fibula, which articulates proximally with the tibia but is fused distally. The tarsus is composed of eight bones (Greene, 1963).

4. Digestive System

The dental formula of the rat is 2(I 1/1, C 0/0, PM 0/0, M 3/3). Incisors grow continuously. If the incisors are not worn evenly or are misaligned due to gingivitis or congenital defects, the resulting malocclusion may lead to nonfunctional, spiral elongation of the incisors, injury to the palate, and reduced food intake. The salivary glands are paired and consist of the parotid, the submandibular, and the smaller sublingual glands. The parotid gland is serous and consists of three or four lobes located ventrolaterally from the caudal border of the mandible to the clavicle. The submandibular glands are mixed glands situated ventrally between the caudal border of the mandibles and the thoracic inlet. The sublingual glands are mucous and located at the rostral pole of the submandibular glands. Multilocular adipose tissue, referred to as brown fat or the hibernating gland, is located in the ventral and lateral portions of the neck and can be confused with salivary glands. Figure 4.1 depicts the location of the salivary glands, cervical lymph nodes, and associated muscles and blood vessels (Constantinescu, 2011).

The stomach is divided into two parts: the forestomach, or cardiac portion, which is nonglandular; and the corpus, or pyloric portion, which is glandular. A structure referred to as the limiting ridge (margo plicatus) separates the two portions, with the esophagus entering at the lesser curvature of the stomach through a fold of the ridge. This anatomical configuration is sometimes mentioned as a reason that rats cannot vomit, but this is somewhat simplistic, since rats, along with other rodents, do not possess many of the anatomical and neurological components that are required for a functional vomiting reflex (Horn et al., 2013).

The small intestine of the adult rat consists of the duodenum (8 cm), jejunum (80 cm), and ileum (3 cm). The comma-shaped cecum is thin-walled, with a prominent mass of lymphoid tissue in its apical portion. The colon consists of the ascending colon, with prominent oblique mucosal ridges, and the transverse and descending portions, with longitudinal mucosa folds.

The liver has four lobes: the median, which has a deep fissure for the hepatic ligament; the right lateral, which is partially divided; the left, which is large; and the caudate, which is small and surrounds the esophagus. The rat does not have a gallbladder, and bile ducts from each lobe form the common bile duct, which enters the duodenum about 25 mm from the pyloric sphincter.

The pancreas is a very diffuse and lobulated organ that can be differentiated from adjacent adipose tissue by its darker color and firm consistency. Numerous excretory ducts fuse into two to eight large ducts, which empty into the common bile duct (Bivin et al., 1979). Figure 4.2 depicts the abdominal and thoracic viscera in situ (Greene, 1963).

5. Respiratory System

The rat has a maxillary recess (sinus) located between the maxillary bone and the lateral lamina of the ethmoid bone. The recess contains the lateral nasal gland (Steno's gland), which has morphologic similarities to a serous

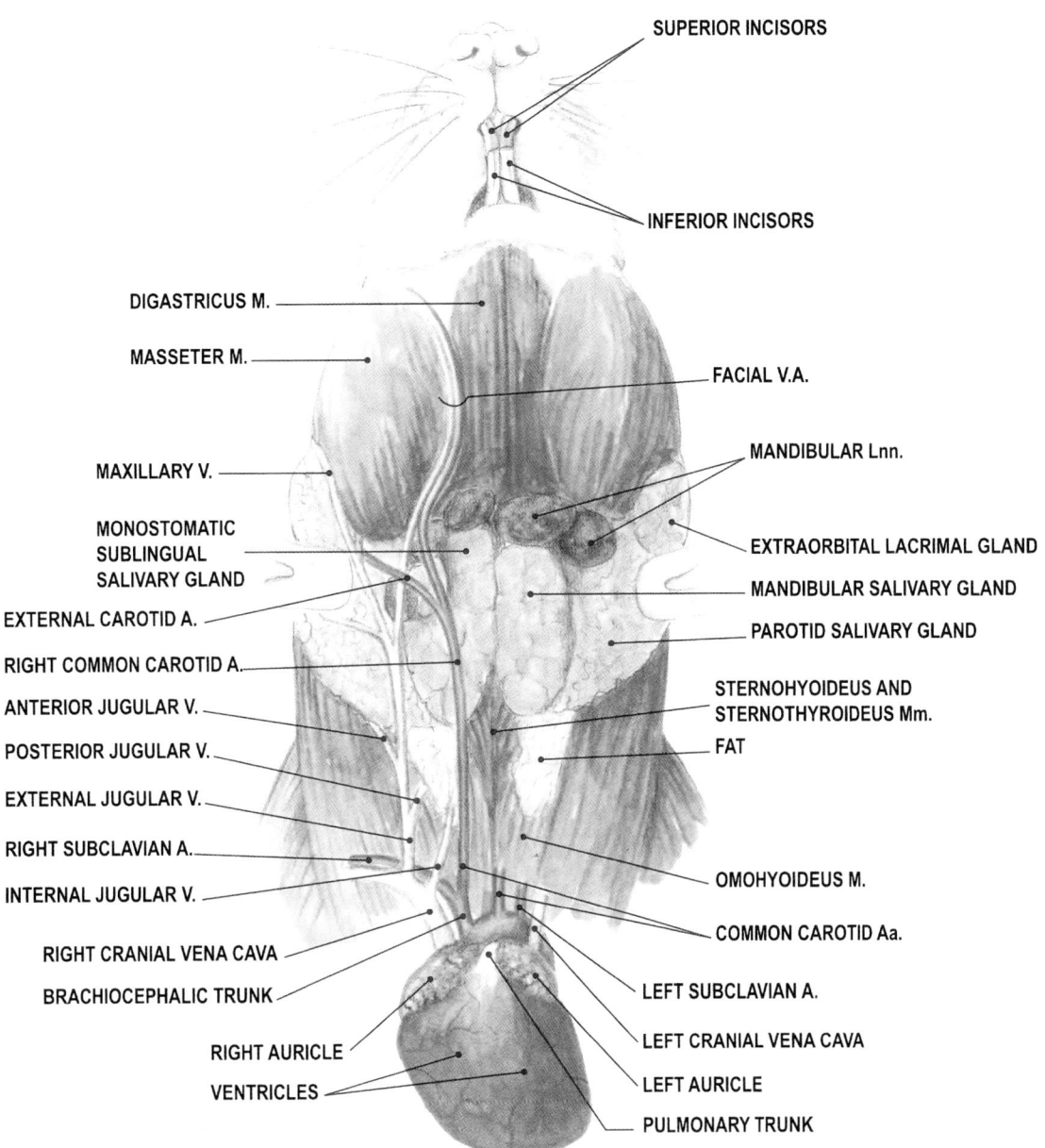

FIGURE 4.1 Anatomy of the superficial ventral cervical area including muscles, salivary glands, major vessels, and lymph nodes. *From Constantinescu (2011).*

salivary gland and secretes a watery product discharged at the rostral end of the nasal turbinate. It has been postulated that this secretion may act to regulate the viscosity of the mucous layer overlying the nasal epithelium.

The lungs consist of the left lung, which is single-lobed, and the right lung, which is divided into the cranial, middle, accessory, and caudal lobes. The pulmonary vein has cardiac striated muscle fibers within its wall that are contiguous with those in the heart. The rat does not have an adrenergic nerve supply to the bronchial musculature, and bronchoconstriction is controlled by vagal tone (Bivin *et al.*, 1979).

6. Genitourinary System

The male rat has a number of highly developed accessory sex glands (Fig. 4.3). The paired bulbourethral glands (Cowper's glands) at the base of the penis open into the dorsal surface of the urethral flexure. Within the abdominal cavity and surrounding the bladder are the large vesicular glands (seminal vesicles) and the prostate gland, which is composed of the dorsocranial (coagulation gland), ventral, and dorsolateral lobes. The female rat has a bicornate uterus, and although the uterine horns appear fused distally, there are two distinct ossa uteri and cervices.

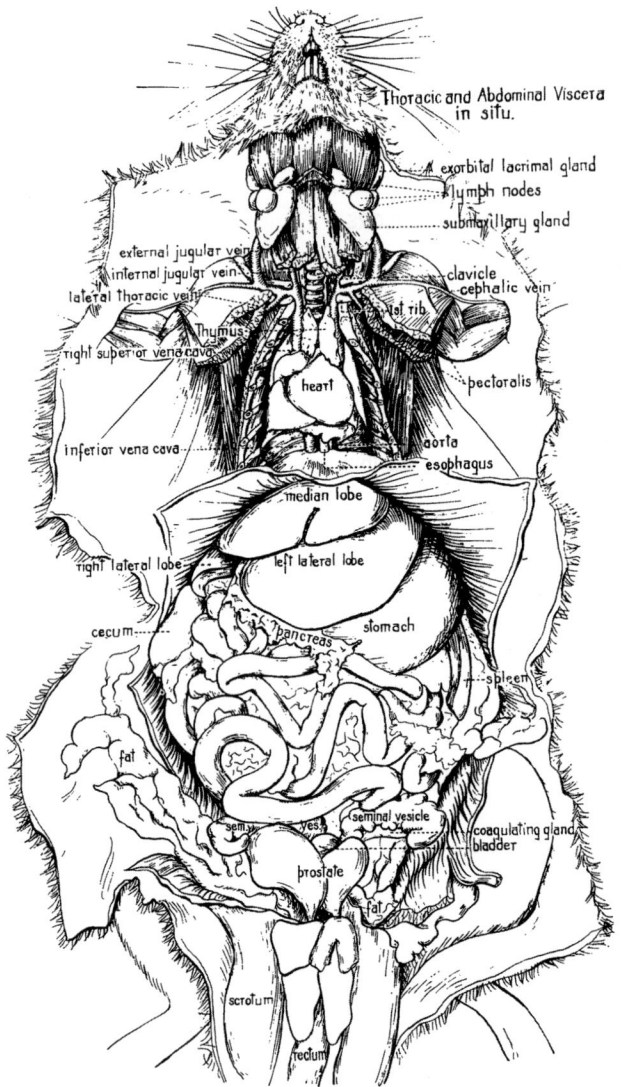

FIGURE 4.2   Abdominal and thoracic viscera *in situ. From Greene (1963).*

The right kidney is more craniad than the left and has its cranial edge at the L1 vertebra and its caudal edge at the level of L3. Like the kidneys of other rodents, the rat kidney is unipapillate, making the rat useful for studies in which cannulization of the kidney is done. The rat is also widely used as a model for investigating nephron transport in an *in vivo* micropuncture system, because of the presence of superficial nephrons in the renal cortex (Vallon, 2009).

7. Central Nervous System

The brain is characterized by large olfactory bulbs, a lissencephalic (smooth) cerebrum, and the two parafloccular lobes of the cerebellum, which lie in deep sockets of the periotic capsule of the skull. The hypophysis (pituitary gland) lies behind the optic chiasma and is attached to the base of the brain by a thin hollow stalk, the infundibulum. The ventricular system is similar to that of other animals, but the rat lacks a foramen of Magendie. The spinal cord ends at the fourth lumbar vertebra, with the filum terminale ending at the level of the tail beyond the third caudal nerves (Greene, 1949).

8. Cardiovascular System

The heart is located on a midline in the thorax, with its apex near the diaphragm and its lateral aspects bounded mainly by the lungs. The heart is exposed to the left thoracic wall between the third and fifth ribs, making it a useful site for cardiac blood collection that for humane reasons is generally perfumed as a sedated, nonsurvival procedure. The blood supply to the atria of the rat, unlike that of higher mammals, is largely extracoronary from branches of the internal mammary and subclavian arteries.

B. Normal Physiological Values

Many of the normal values determined for a specific group of rats may be accurate for only that source and stock/strain. Other factors such as age, pathogen status, sample collection methods, and husbandry conditions of the colony are also important variables (Suber and Kodell, 1985; Dameron *et al.*, 1992; Perez *et al.*, 1997). Selected physiological, clinical chemistry, and hematological values are listed in Tables 4.2–4.5. *Note*: the values provided in these tables are meant to be representative examples useful for educational purposes. Laboratory-specific normal ranges and/or strain, sex and age-matched control data should be used for research and diagnostic purposes.

C. Nutrition

Rats are categorized as omnivores, and nutritionally adequate diets are readily available from commercial sources. However, the refinement of ingredients within diet formulations may vary according to classifications of commercially available products. The three classifications of diets are (1) natural-ingredient, (2) purified, and (3) chemically defined. The most commonly used type for most research applications is the natural-ingredient diet, composed of agricultural products and by-products. This class of diet can be either an open-formula diet, in which the information on the amount of each ingredient is available, or a closed-formula diet, in which such information is held confidential by the producer. The nutrient composition of ingredients in natural-ingredient diets varies from batch to batch because of various factors (e.g., relative costs of grains, weather conditions, harvesting and storage conditions, and concentrations of contaminants). Certified, natural-ingredient diets

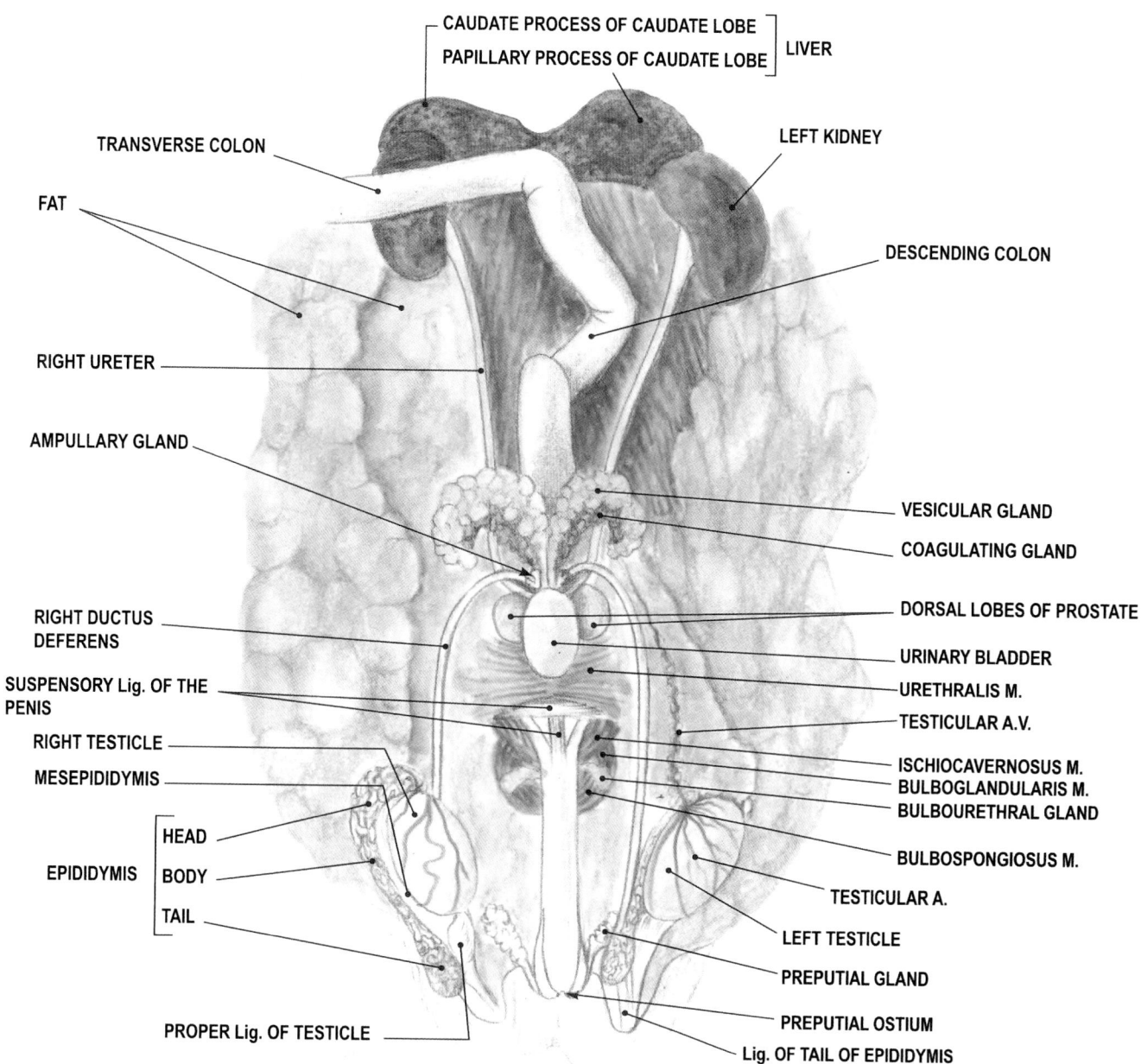

CAUDATE PROCESS OF CAUDATE LOBE
PAPILLARY PROCESS OF CAUDATE LOBE] LIVER

TRANSVERSE COLON

FAT

LEFT KIDNEY

DESCENDING COLON

RIGHT URETER

AMPULLARY GLAND

VESICULAR GLAND

COAGULATING GLAND

RIGHT DUCTUS DEFERENS

DORSAL LOBES OF PROSTATE

URINARY BLADDER

SUSPENSORY Lig. OF THE PENIS

URETHRALIS M.

TESTICULAR A.V.

RIGHT TESTICLE

MESEPIDIDYMIS

ISCHIOCAVERNOSUS M.
BULBOGLANDULARIS M.
BULBOURETHRAL GLAND

HEAD

EPIDIDYMIS BODY

BULBOSPONGIOSUS M.

TAIL

TESTICULAR A.

LEFT TESTICLE

PREPUTIAL GLAND

PROPER Lig. OF TESTICLE

PREPUTIAL OSTIUM

Lig. OF TAIL OF EPIDIDYMIS

FIGURE 4.3   Male urogenital system. *From Constantinescu (2011).*

are used for toxicological and other Good Laboratory Practice (GLP) studies because each lot is assayed and certified not to exceed established maximum concentrations of a set list of contaminants (e.g., pesticides, heavy metals, mycotoxins, and estrogens) that could influence study results.

The nutrient concentrations in purified diets are less variable because defined ingredients, each composed of a single nutrient or nutrient class (e.g., casein, sugar, starch, vegetable oil, cellulose), are used in their formulation. A frequently used purified diet for rats is AIN-76. The downside of this class of diets is that they are more expensive and often less palatable. Chemically defined diets are formulated with very basically defined ingredients (e.g., specific amino acids, sugars, triglycerides, and essential fatty acids). These diets are costly and tend to lack palatability (National Research Council, 1996). A comprehensive description of the nutrient requirements of rats is available (National Research Council, 1995). Phytoestrogens are being increasingly recognized as a dietary variable that can have significant effects in both female and male rats (Boettger-Tong *et al.*, 1998; Weber *et al.*, 2001).

In most instances, rats are fed *ad libitum*. However, there are numerous reports that demonstrate that unlimited

TABLE 4.2   Selected Normative Data for the Rat[a]

ADULT

Weight	
Male	300–500 g
Female	250–300 g
Life span	2.5–3 years
Body temperature	37.5°C
Basal metabolism rate (400-g rat)	35 kcal/24 h
Chromosome number (diploid)	42
Puberty	50 ± 10 days
Gestation	21–23 days
Litter size	8–14
Birth weight	5–6 g
Eyes open	10–12 days
Weaning	21 days
Food consumption/24 h	5 g/100 g body weight
Water consumption/24 h	8–11 ml/100 g body weight

CARDIOVASCULAR

Arterial blood pressure	
Mean systolic	116 mmHg
Mean diastolic	90 mmHg
Heart rate	300–500 beats/min
Cardiac output	50 ml/min
Blood volume	6 ml/100 g body weight

RESPIRATORY

Respirations/min	85
Tidal volume	1.5 ml
Alveolar surface area (400 g rat)	7.5 m^2

RENAL

Urine volume/24 h	5.5 ml/100 g body weight
Na$^+$ excretion/24 h	1.63 mEq/100 g body weight
K$^+$ excretion/24 h	0.83 mEq/100 g body weight
Urine osmolarity	1659 mOsm/kg of H_2O
Urine pH	7.3–8.5
Urine specific gravity	1.04–1.07

[a]Data from Baker (1979) and Bivin et al. (1979).

feeding of rats on long-term carcinogenesis and toxicological studies reduces longevity and increases the incidence of neoplasia relative to rats fed at 70–80% of the ad libitum food amount. These effects have been found in Sprague-Dawley, Wistar, and F-344 rats and have caused increased variability among 2-year carcinogenicity and safety assessment studies, compromising the usefulness of bioassays in risk assessment (Keenan et al., 1996). For instance, Wistar rats fed 80% of ad libitum beginning at 16 weeks of age had very significant reductions in the incidence of lung, mammary, pancreatic islet cell, and pituitary tumors relative to controls fed ad libitum. The overall incidence of malignant tumors was 16% in the feed-limited group and 37% in the ad libitum group, even though the feed-limited group had a greater longevity. There was also a reduction in chronic inflammation and fibrosis of the heart, acute inflammation of the prostate, radiculoneuropathy, and acinal hyperplasia of the mammary gland in feed-limited animals (Roe et al., 1995). Four pathways have been implicated as potentially mediating the caloric restriction effect. These are the insulin-like growth factor (IGF-1)/insulin signaling pathway, the sirtuin pathway, the adenosine monophosphate (AMP)-activated protein kinase (AMPK) pathway, and the target of rapamycin (TOR) pathway (Speakman and Mitchell, 2011).

D. Reproduction

1. Reproductive Physiology

In the rat, the vagina is closed at birth by compact epithelium, referred to as the vaginal plate (Del Vecchio, 1992). This begins to degenerate and cornify at 20–35 days of age and is completely open between 40 and 80 days of age. Persistence of the vaginal plate can result in a fully imperforate vagina or in the presence of a vaginal septum, anomalies that may be associated with infertility or metritis (Lezmi et al., 2011). Vaginal opening can be used as an external indicator of impending puberty in female rats, and a similar phenomenon, preputial separation, occurs in male rats (Korenbrot et al., 1977). A study in Wistar rats documented vaginal opening in control females at approximately 36 days of age and balano-preputial separation in control males at approximately 46 days of age (Engelbregt et al., 2000). Puberty is defined as the onset of sexual maturity indicated by the ability to bear viable young, and it occurs before full body size and weight are attained. As in most species, puberty occurs in females earlier than in males and also varies with stock or strain. Puberty most often occurs at 2–3 months of age in the rat (Fox and Laird, 1970), although considerable variation exists in reported values. Kohn and Barthold (1984) report 40–60 days, Bennett and Vickery (1970) report 50–72 days, and Ayala et al. (1998) report 45–47 days. Estrus, which should be distinguished from puberty, begins before full reproductive competency is reached and has been reported to occur at 36 days in the Wistar rat (Eckstein et al., 1973). However, some authors report successfully breeding Wistar BH rats at 35 days of age (Rosen et al., 1987).

TABLE 4.3 Clinical Chemistry Reference Ranges for Adult Rats[a]

Analyte	Units	Sprague-Dawley[b]		Fisher 344[d]	
		M	F	M	F
SERUM					
Glucose	mg/dl	115 ± 16.9	111 ± 17.2	115 ± 12.5[c]	
Urea nitrogen	mg/dl	19 ± 2.2	21 ± 3.4	15 ± 2.5[c]	
Creatinine	mg/dl	0.70 ± 0.11	0.70 ± 0.13		
Sodium	mEq/l	150 ± 3.4	148 ± 3.5	149 ± 3.0[c]	
Potassium	mEq/l	7.00 ± 0.65	6.1 ± 0.67	4.80 ± 0.35[c]	
Chloride	mEq/l	103.0 ± 1.90	104.0 ± 2.4	106 ± 3.0[c]	
Calcium	mg/dl	12.0 ± 0.94	12.1 ± 0.71	10.5 ± 0.50[c]	
Phosphorus	mg/dl	7.30 ± 1.5	5.80 ± 1.10		
Magnesium		3.12 ± 0.41[e]	2.60 ± 0.21[e]		
Iron	μg/dl	152 ± 70	220 ± 130 (19–21 weeks)		
Total iron-binding capacity	μg/dl	368[c]			
Alanine aminotransferase	IU/l	49 ± 24.1	69 ± 44.9	78 ± 11	49 ± 8
Aspartate aminotransferase	IU/l	95 ± 31.7	99 ± 54.5		
Alkaline phosphatase	IU/l	130 ± 43.7	117 ± 41.7	49.5 ± 9.25[c]	
Lactate dehydrogenase	IU/l	275 ± 112		650 ± 75	650 ± 75 (20 weeks)
Sorbitol dehydrogenase	IU/l	20 ± 5[c] (32 weeks)		20.0 ± 7.5[c]	
γ-Glutamyl transpeptidase	IU/l	2.5 ± 1.25[c]			
Creatinine kinase	IU/l	275 ± 112.5[c]		400 ± 50[c]	
Protein, total	g/l	70 ± 5.0	75 ± 5	70.5 ± 4.75[c]	
Albumin	g/l	34 ± 2.0	40 ± 2.5	42.5 ± 3.75[c]	
Cholesterol	mg/dl	119 ± 51.3	119 ± 29.0	96.5 ± 14.25	130 ± 10.0
Triglycerides	mg/dl	266 ± 121.4	249 ± 159.7	122 ± 21.25	62.5 ± 11.25
Bilirubin	mg/dl	0.3 ± 0.16	0.4 ± 0.27	0.3 ± 0.1[c]	
Bile acids	μmol/l	40 ± 10[c] (20 weeks)		30 ± 10[c]	
Uric acid	mg/dl	1.52 ± 0.30	1.25 ± 0.36		
URINE					
Volume	ml/16h			9.5 ± 4.0	9.3 ± 5.6
	ml/22h	15.7 ± 6.7	11.0 ± 5.0		
Specific gravity				1.022 ± 0.007	1.017 ± 0.007
Osmolality	mOsm/kg	943 ± 327	995 ± 367		
pH		7.8 ± 0.5	7.7 ± 0.5	6.0–6.5[c]	
Chloride	mmol/l	148 ± 36	151 ± 51		

(Continued)

TABLE 4.3   (Continued)

Analyte	Units	Sprague-Dawley[b]		Fisher 344[d]	
		M	F	M	F
Sodium	mmol/l	31 ± 11	50 ± 22		
Potassium	mmol/l	121 ± 31	110 ± 45		
Phosphorus	mg/dl	142 ± 34	156 ± 62		
Creatinine	mg/dl	136 ± 40	116 ± 41	80 ± 28	54 ± 25
Glucose	mg/dl			9.9 ± 3.9	5.5 ± 2.3
Protein	mg/dl			98.8 ± 54.4	11.2 ± 5.5
Alkaline phosphatase	IU/l			152 ± 61	73 ± 37
Lactate dehydrogenase	IU/l			28 ± 15	16 ± 8
N-Acetyl-β-glucosaminidase	IU/l			12.2 ± 7.8	5.9 ± 2.7
Aspartate aminotransferase				14.4 ± 6.5	3.6 ± 2.5
γ-Glutamyl transpeptidase	IU/l			4964 ± 780	1873 ± 215
Insulin clearance	μl/min/100 g	857 ± 178			
Glomerular filtration rate	μl/min	275 ± 33[c]			
Urine flow	μl/min/100 g	5.2 ± 2.0			

[a]Values are for 12-month-old animals, unless noted otherwise, as summarized from Loeb and Quimby (1999).
[b]6–18 months old.
[c]Gender not specified.
[d]58–l 12 weeks old.
[e]Wistar strain.

TABLE 4.4

Hormone[b]	Units	Male	Female
Luteinizing hormone	ng/ml	0.16–0.64	0.32–0.64 (basal)
			24.6–32.8 (late proestrus)
Follicle stimulating hormone	ng/ml	5.56–11.1 (light period)	2.22–4.44 (basal)
		11.1–20.0 (dark period)	8.85–13.3 (preovulatory, estrus)
Prolactin	ng/ml	28.6 (dark period)	5.4–10.7 (basal)
		1.8–10.7 (light period)	71.4–107 (late proestrus)
		71.4 (after coitus)	
Growth hormone	ng/ml	0.4–80[a]	
Thyroid stimulating hormone	ng/ml	2.27–3.4	0.57 (basal)
			1.14 (early light period)
Adrenocorticotropic hormone	pg/ml	30–100	
Vasopressin	pg/ml	1–8[a]	
Oxytocin	pg/ml	4–10.5[a]	
Thyroxine (T$_4$)	μg/dl	5.1 ± 0.4	4.9 ± 0.1 (Long-Evans)
Triiodothyronine (T$_3$)	ng/dl	66 ± 3.5	83 ± 3 (Long-Evans)
Free T$_4$	ng/dl	2.212 ± 0.055[a]	
Free T$_3$	pg/dl	208.49 ± 8.55[a]	

(Continued)

TABLE 4.4 (Continued)

Hormone[b]	Units	Male	Female
Calcitonin	pg/ml	200–1000[a] (F-344/9 months)	
Parathyroid hormone	pg/ml	140–180	<50–400 (Sprague-Dawley)
1,25-Dihydroxy vitamin D	pg/ml	120 ± 24	96 ± 17 (Wistar)
Corticosterone	μg/dl	15–23 (late light period)	70 (late light period)
		1–6 (late dark period)	17 (late dark period)
Aldosterone	ng/dl	12–35 (late light period)	25–35 (9–10 a.m.)
		4–11 (middle light period)	
Epinephrine	pg/dl	253 ± 30[a] (awake, undisturbed; Sprague-Dawley)	
		460 ± 60[a] (handled)	
		180 ± 24[a] (asleep)	
Norepinephrine	pg/dl	710 ± 110[a] (awake, undisturbed; Sprague-Dawley)	
		830 ± 130[a] (handled)	
		460 ± 80[a] (asleep)	
Progesterone	ng/ml		1–5 (early proestrus)
			40–50 (estrus)
			20–30 (first diestrus day)
Estradiol	pg/ml		<10 (basal)
			20–30 (2nd diestrus day)
			40–50 (proestrus)
Testosterone	ng/ml	3 (1330–1600 h)	
		<1 (2130 h)	
	pg/ml		500–600 (proestrus)
			100 (estrus)

[a]Gender not specified.
[b]Strain not specified.

The estrous cycle of rats is most often 4–5 days in length and occurs throughout the year, as well as postpartum. Seasonal variation is not observed in laboratory colonies. For a 4-day estrous cycle, approximately 1 day is spent in each of the four stages: estrus, metestrus, diestrus, and proestrus. However, cycles of up to 6 days are not uncommon, with the additional time in diestrus or proestrus (Peluso, 1992). In proestrus, the uterus can appear 'ballooned' with fluid, especially in a peripubertal rat; this condition should not be mistaken for hydrometra.

Ovulation occurs approximately 8–11 h after the onset of estrus, usually between midnight and 2 a.m. (Peluso, 1992), although this would obviously depend on timing of the light cycle. Ova remain viable for approximately 10–12 h (Fox and Laird, 1970).

Testes descend from the abdomen into the scrotum at approximately 15 days of age (Russell, 1992). Sperm are first produced at about 45–46 days of age, but fertility (puberty) does not occur until approximately 62–65 days of age, and sperm production is not maximal until 75 days of age (Russell, 1992). Interestingly, on histologic examination of young rat testes, more degenerate germ cells are noted prior to 75 days of age than afterward, indicative of the poor efficiency of spermatogenesis at early ages in the rat (Russell et al., 1987). Male sexual behavior is, in part, dependent on age and experience. Prepubertal males have no preference for females in estrus, and female-oriented sexual behavior is reported to decrease after 150 days of age (Matuszczyk et al., 1994; Smith et al., 1992). Decreased serum testosterone may be partially responsible for age-related decreases in mating

TABLE 4.5 Hematological Parameters in the Rat[a]

Parameter (units)	Stock/Strain					
	Crl:CD(SD)		Crl:LE		F344/DuCRL	
	Male	Female	Male	Female	Male	Female
WBC (K/μl)	11 (4.0–18)	9.5 (2.4–18)	9.8 (5.6–14)	8.7 (4.9–13)	6.7 (2.1–9.6)	7.4 (1.9–12)
Neutrophils (K/μl)	3.4 (1.0–6.7)	2.6 (0.7–5.9)	4.0 (2.2–6.5)	3.2 (1.7–5.4)	2.5 (0.7–3.9)	2.4 (0.5–4.4)
Lymphocytes(K/μl)	6.5 (2.2–12)	6.1 (1.5–11.5)	5.0 (2.5–7.9)	4.6 (2.6–7.9)	3.6 (1.0–5.7)	4.4 (1.2–7.5)
Monocytes (K/μl)	0.7 (0.2–1.4)	0.6 (0.1–1.2)	0.7 (0.3–1.2)	0.7 (0.3–1.3)	0.5 (0.1–1.0)	0.5 (0.1–1.0)
Eosinophils (K/μl)	0.1 (0–0.5)	0.1 (0–0.5)	0.1 (0–0.5)	0.2 (0–0.8)	0.1 (0–0.3)	0.1 (0–0.5)
Basophils (K/μl)	0.03 (0–0.2)	0.03 (0–0.2)	0.03 (0–0.1)	0.04 (0–0.3)	0.02 (0–0.1)	0.03 (0–0.1)
Neutrophils (%)	32 (16–54)	28 (14–55)	41 (30–51)	38 (25–51)	37 (25–53)	32 (19–47)
Lymphocytes (%)	61 (38–79)	63 (37–81)	51 (41–63)	53 (38–65)	54 (40–67)	59 (42–74)
Monocytes (%)	6.3 (3–11)	6.5 (3–11)	6.6 (3–10)	7.4 (4–12)	7.6 (7.7–12)	6.8 (2.9–12)
Eosinophils (%)	1.2 (0.1–4.3)	1.4 (0.2–4.8)	1.2 (0.1–4.1)	1.6 (0.1–7.3)	0.9 (0–3.7)	1.6 (0.1–5.5)
Basophils (%)	0.3 (0–1.7)	0.3 (0–1.6)	0.3 (0–1.6)	0.4 (0–2.4)	0.4 (0–1.1)	0.4 (0–1.3)
RBC (M/μl)	7.7 (5.8–10)	7.4 (5.5–9.8)	7.6 (6.0–9.4)	7.6 (6.7–8.6)	8.3 (7.1–9.7)	8.1 (6.6–9.4)
Hemoglobin (g/dl)	17 (13–23)	16 (13–22)	16 (13–20)	16 (14–18)	16 (14–19)	16 (13–18)
Hematocrit (%)	51 (39–69)	48 (37–64)	52 (43–62)	51 (43–60)	54 (47–62)	54 (44–62)
MCV (fl)	67 (58–77)	66 (58–75)	69 (63–76)	67 (61–75)	65 (60–69)	67 (63–70)
MCH (pg)	22 (17–25)	22 (18–25)	21 (19–24)	21 (20–23)	20 (17–22)	20 (17–22)
MCHC (g/dl)	33 (27–38)	33 (27–38)	31 (29–33)	31 (29–43)	31 (27–34)	30 (26–32)
RDW (%)	16 (14–18)	15 (13–17)	16 (13–17)	14 (12–15)	15 (14–17)	13 (12–15)
Platelets (M/μl)	1.6 (0.8–2.6)	1.6 (0.8–2.4)	1.4 (0.7–1.9)	1.3 (0.6–1.7)	1.1 (0.8–1.6)	1.1 (0.7–1.5)
MPV (fl)	7.4 (5.9–10)	7.3 (5.8–9.6)	8.0 (6.7–9.2)	8.1 (5.8–9.5)	6.9 (5.8–8.2)	6.8 (5.7–8.1)

[a]Derived from vendor data (Charles River Research Models) on animals 8–10 weeks of age; mean (95% confidence interval).

behavior, but this does not appear to completely explain the phenomenon.

Coitus occurs more frequently during dark periods than light periods, and more frequently during the latter portion of the dark cycle than during the early portion (Mercier *et al.*, 1987). Multiple intromissions (5–15), each lasting 0.3–0.6 s and with two to nine pelvic thrusts (Bennett and Vickery, 1970), precede the first ejaculation, which lasts about 1 s. This first series of intromissions is called the ejaculatory latency and lasts about 10 min, followed by a refractory period (Dewsbury, 1970). A single ejaculation with fewer intromissions is less likely to impregnate the female. Multiple series of intromissions and ejaculations occur, usually about seven, with increasing refractory periods between successive episodes. Coitus can be confirmed in rats by detection of spermatozoa on a vaginal smear, by observation of a vaginal plug (the pale coagulum formed by seminiferous fluid visible in the vagina), or by direct observation of sexual behavior.

Implantation of the blastocyst into the endometrium occurs between 5 and 7 days after fertilization and actually represents a process that requires 12–24 h for completion (Peluso, 1992; Enders, 1970; Garside *et al.*, 1996). Parturition occurs 21–23 days after the time of coitus, although it can occur as early as 19 days (Bennett and Vickery, 1970; Baker, 1979). Pregnant rats whose time of coitus is known are therefore of known gestational stage and are referred to as timed pregnant.

2. Detection of Estrus and Pregnancy

Several methods can be used to determine if a rat is in estrus, which is useful in production of timed pregnant rats. Rats in estrus often exhibit specific behavior, including ear quivering when the back or head are stroked, and lordosis ('sway-back' posture) when the pelvic area is stimulated (Blandau *et al.*, 1941). Additionally, the vulva becomes swollen, and the vaginal wall appears dry in estrus, instead of the moist pink appearance during metestrus or diestrus. This is due to cornification of the vaginal epithelium during estrus (Baker, 1979). These changes in the vaginal epithelium can be assessed by cytologic examination of vaginal smears (Montes and Luque, 1988). In estrus, 25–100% of the epithelial cells are cornified (Bennett and Vickery, 1970). Changes in vaginal fluids and cytology also lead to changes in the electrical impedance in the vagina during estrus. This has been widely exploited as an alternative method of estrus detection (Koto et al., 1987a, b) using a device referred to as an impedance meter in which an electrical probe is inserted into the vagina. However, when compared to cytology, impedance measurement provides less information regarding the specific phase of estrus, and the physical stimulation of the probe may induce pseudopregnancy (Singletary et al., 2005).

Pregnancy is difficult to detect early in gestation, but conception rates of 85% or more are often observed for outbred rat stocks, somewhat less in inbred strains. After approximately 10 days, careful palpation can detect the developing fetuses; this is especially accurate after 12 days of gestation. Transabdominal real-time ultrasonography can begin to detect pregnancy at 9–10 days and is quite accurate thereafter, with fetal heartbeat detectable by Doppler by day 12 (Ypsilantis et al., 2009). By 14 days of gestation, mammary gland and nipple development are evident (Bennett and Vickery, 1970).

3. Husbandry Needs

Inbred rats are generally bred monogamously or in trios, with one male and two females in each cage. Outbred rats may also be bred monogamously but are more often bred polygamously by commercial breeders for reasons of economy. Pregnant females are removed and placed into separate cages a few days before parturition to minimize cannibalism or abandonment of litters.

A number of variables have been identified that may influence the husbandry requirements of a reproducing population of laboratory rats. Despite the lack of seasonal variation in estrous cycles in the rat, both ovarian function and the estrous cycle are influenced by light cycles. Continuous light has been reported to cause persistent estrus and cystic follicles in the ovaries, without formation of corpora lutea (Fox and Laird, 1970). Chronic exposure to even low-intensity light during the dark cycle has been reported to result in earlier vaginal opening and ovarian atrophy (Beys et al., 1995; Fox and Laird, 1970). Caloric restriction, a 15–30% decrease from ad libitum caloric intake, may cause cessation of estrous cycles and delayed sexual maturation (Fox and Laird, 1970).

High ambient temperatures can result in male infertility (Pucak et al., 1977) by causing irreversible degeneration of the seminiferous epithelium. Significantly, the damage may occur in rats as young as 4 days and in rats with prolonged exposure to temperatures as low as 26.6°C.

4. Parturition

Female rats increase nest-building activity approximately 5 days prepartum and continue through lactation (Bennett and Vickery, 1970). Nesting behavior adequate for successful reproduction can be expressed using typical hardwood chip bedding in solid-bottomed cages. Supplemental materials may be used by breeding females, but this behavior may be more learned than innate in laboratory rats (Van Loo and Baumans, 2004). Approximately 1.5–4h before the first pup is born, clear mucoid fluid discharges from the vagina. In early labor, the female walks about the cage and stretches. This behavior becomes more exaggerated as events progress; then the female will lie on her abdomen with rear legs extended off the cage floor. As pups are born, the female pulls the placenta from the birth canal and eats it. Parturition averages 1–3.5h, varying with litter size. Nursing usually begins only after all pups are born.

Litter size varies with stock, strain, source, and maternal age. The following are examples of the effect of maternal age. Wistar BH rats had an average of 1.69 more pups (11.80 vs. 10.11) when first mated at 105 days than when first mated at 35 days of age (Rosen et al., 1987). The second litter is usually the largest (Bennett and Vickery, 1970). After 9 months of age, litter size is further decreased, and the pregnancy rate declines after 12 months of age (Niggeschulze and Kast, 1994). Loss of fetuses, termed pregnancy wastage, occurs as a function of age (Mattheij and Swarts, 1991), with less than 5% wastage in 4-month-old rats, 30% in 9-month-old rats, and 65% at 11 months of age. Wastage is primarily due to preimplantation and early postimplantation mortality. In contrast to the decremental effects of aging on litter size, maternal behavior in virgin rats is enhanced at 19–20 months, when compared with those at 3–4 months of age (Gonzalez and Deis, 1990). In addition, at least some maternal stressors can lead to fetal wastage. An increase in fetal wastage was reported to be due to an earthquake that occurred when the dams were at 7, 8, or 9 days of gestation, although no difference was noted in the number of live births, fetal weight, or incidence of runts (Fujinaga et al., 1992). This raises the possibility of similar fetal loss when rats are shipped at this stage of gestation, although such has not been documented in the peer-reviewed literature. Strenuous maternal exercise, i.e., running on a treadmill, has also been reported to result in decreased litter size and decreased fetal weight (Mottola et al., 1992). Dystocia is rare in rats. Cannibalism is not frequently encountered and is an indicator of maternal stress.

5. Early Development of the Newborn

Rat pups are altricial and nidicolous; they are hairless and blind, with poorly developed limbs, short tails, and closed ear canals (Baker, 1979). There is an inverse relationship between fetal or birth weight and litter size (Romero *et al.*, 1992). This phenomenon is significant for the reproductive toxicologist because the tendency of a test substance to cause decreased fetal weight may be masked if it also causes fetal loss. Other factors also influence birth weight and weaning weight, including the age of the dams. Pups of dams mated at 105 days of age weighed more at weaning than pups of dams mated at 35 or 70 days (Rosen *et al.*, 1987). The external acoustic meati open between 2.5 and 3.5 days of age. Internally, the cochlea and organ of Corti are immature at birth but develop rapidly to approximately adult morphology by the time of weaning. Rats appear to first be able to hear at about 9 days of age, although they are able to vocalize from the time of birth (Feldman, 1992). Incisors erupt at 6–8 days of age, although molars do not erupt until 16 (molar 1), 18 (molar 2), and 32–34 days of age (molar 3) (Brown and Leininger, 1992). The retina is poorly developed at birth, equivalent to a human fetus of 4–5 months. The eyelids open at about 14–17 days of age, although the retina does not fully mature until 30–40 days of age, and the final components in the angle of the anterior chamber are not fully formed until 60 days of age (Weisse, 1992). Some hairs may be present on the trunk at birth, usually associated with touch domes, indicating that they are guard hairs (English and Munger, 1992). Pups are considered fully haired at about 7–10 days of age. Maternal antibody is transferred passively across the yolk sac *in utero* (Laliberte *et al.*, 1984). Antibody can also be transferred across the intestinal mucosa from maternal colostrum and milk in the suckling rat. This transfer occurs at low rates shortly after birth, reaches maximal rates at day 14, and ceases by the 21 days, when gut closure is said to be complete (Martin *et al.*, 1997).

6. Sexing

Sex is readily determined in mature rats by direct observation of the perineal region. Males have a distinct scrotum located between the anus and the preputial opening. The penis is often visible and is larger than the urethral papilla of the female. In addition the distance between the anus and the genital opening, called the anogenital distance, is greater in the male than in the female.

Sex discrimination is more difficult in prepubertal rats but is possible even in neonates. Comparative evaluation will reveal that neonatal males have a greater anogenital distance than their female littermates, although the distinction is more subtle than in adults. A technique for sex determination of preblastocyst embryos has also been described (Utsumi *et al.*, 1991). Male embryos ceased development in the presence of antibody to the HY antigen, and resumed development only after the antibody was washed off. In contrast, 80% of the embryos that developed into blastocysts in the presence of the HY antibody produced female pups after the blastocysts were implanted. Polymerase

chain reaction (PCR) primers constructed from sequences found in the male sex determining region Y (SRY) have been used to determine the sex of embryonic tissues during postmortem analysis (Miyajima *et al.*, 2009).

7. Weaning

Rats are weaned at 20–21 days of age, although they may be weaned successfully as early as 17 days. The micturition reflex does not fully mature in rat pups until after day 15, prior to which the animals may not be fully capable of urination without maternal stimulation (Maggi *et al.*, 1986). As is the case with some other species, orphaned pups or those subjected to very early weaning for experimental purposes may require perianal stimulation to avoid urinary distension and possible urinary tract disease.

8. Synchronization of Estrus

Synchronization of estrus for timed pregnancy matings, or to prepare recipients in embryo transfer, can be performed by administering 40 µg of luteinizing hormone releasing hormone agonist (LHRH) to mature female rats (Borjeson *et al.*, 2014). Treated females can be bred four days later. Synchronization of estrus in the rat has also been accomplished by administration of 40 mg methoxyprogesterone in the drinking water for 6 days (in 200 ml ethanol/liter water, prepared fresh daily), followed by intramuscular injection with 1 IU of pregnant mare's serum (Baker, 1979). Although synchronization of estrus may be useful in the production of large numbers of timed pregnant rats, estrus staging via the use of vaginal cytology or an impedance meter, as described above, may be more practical in most circumstances.

9. Sperm Collection, Artificial Insemination, and Embryo Transfer

Electroejacuation of rats is possible, but the use of sperm collected in this fashion for artificial insemination (AI) in rats is complicated by the rapid coagulation of semen, especially when the semen is obtained by electroejaculation, due to the contributions of the coagulating glands and seminal vesicles (Bennett and Vickery, 1970). For this reason, electroejaculation may have more practicality as a method for evaluation of reproductive soundness in male rats (McCoy *et al.*, 2013). For artificial insemination or sperm cryopreservation, epididymal sperm is most commonly collected during a terminal dissection. Sperm harvested from the proximal portion (head) of the cauda epididymis are reported to have greater fertility than sperm for the middle (body) or caudal (tail) portions (Moore and Akhondi, 1996). Once collected, sperm may be surgically introduced directly into the uterus of estrous females (Nakatsukasa *et al.*, 2003). An essential step in ensuring the success of AI is the induction of pseudopregnancy in the recipient female by prior mating with a vasectomized male, by mechanical stimulation of the vagina, or by electrical stimulation of the cervix (Bennett and Vickery, 1970; Rouleau et al., 1993).

Embryo transfer in rats is used as an alternative to cesarean rederivation in order to eliminate pathogens from breeding lines. Embryo transfer can also be used as a research technique to investigate whether specific characteristics are due to, or modified by, the uterine environment, in contrast to being solely determined by genetic factors (Kubisch and Gomez-Sanchez, 1999; Rouleau et al., 1993). Cryopreservation techniques allow harvested embryos to be stored for long periods prior to subsequent implantation. Hormonal superovulation of rats is commonly performed using pregnant mare serum gonadotropin (PMSG) followed by human chorionic gonadotropin (HCG) in a fashion similar to that used in mice, although other methods involving follicle stimulating hormone (FSH) with or without luteinizing hormone (LH) have also been utilized (Corbin and McCabe, 2002). For embryo manipulation, depending on the development stage required, embryos are collected 1–5 days after the females are bred. When embryo transfer is being used as a rederivation method, embryos are then suspended in PBS with BSA and fetal calf serum and surgically transferred into the uterus or oviduct of the pseudopregnant recipient (Kubisch and Gomez-Sanchez, 1999; Rouleau et al., 1993). Nonsurgical implantation of embryos through the cervix, using an otoscope, has also been reported (Bennett and Vickery, 1970) but has not found wide use. In vitro fertilization (IVF) is performed in the rat but is used primarily as a research tool for events in fertilization and early development rather than as a colony management tool (Gaddum-Rosse et al., 1984; Vanderhyden et al., 1986). Microinsemination of individual oocytes via intracytoplasmic sperm injection (ICSI) is a specific IVF technique that has the potential for being used to rescue or maintain strains that do not produce motile spermatozoa, as it has been used in mice (Tanemura et al., 1997; Songsasen and Leibo, 1998). By adding exogenous DNA to the process, it can also be exploited as a method for producing transgenic rats (Hirabayashi et al., 2005).

10. Cryopreservation

Cryopreservation has not been performed in rats as often as it has in mice, but the technique is becoming more widespread, for the same reasons that it is used widely in mice (Tada et al., 1995). Cryopreservation can be an efficient method of maintaining the potential of raising live mice of the thousands of genetically modified genotypes currently available (Songsasen and Leibo, 1998). It can serve as a fail-safe measure, should a strain become genetically contaminated. In addition to being used for murine reproductive purposes, frozen embryos are also used to test culture reagents and environments for human IVF (Meyer et al., 1997). Although embryos, two-cell through morula, are most frequently cryopreserved, the techniques for cryopreservation of mouse sperm have been developed (Songsasen and Leibo, 1998; Tanemura et al., 1997). Sperm cryopreservation has been successful in rats. Offspring can be obtained with thawed sperm using direct intrauterine insemination (Nakatsukasa et al., 2003) or via IVF using cryopreserved sperm (Seita et al., 2009).

E. Behavior

Aspects of rat behavior relevant to experimental design and disease status may be considered in two broad and overlapping categories: normal behavior, and stressors and stress responses. Only a few examples will be cited here.

Laboratory rats of all stocks and strains have been selected for many years for a variety of traits, among which is docility. Nonetheless, strain differences exist. Rats from a Sprague-Dawley background (such as the CD and SD stocks) and Lewis rats are generally more docile than Brown Norway or F-344 rats. Frequent gentle handling will increase docility, which not only reduces the likelihood of occupational injury for animal workers but also avoids stress for the rats. Infrequent or rough handling will evoke fear responses and is used as a stressor in research projects. The presence or absence of acclimation to handling of both pre- and postweaning animals can modulate subsequent handling-induced stress and lead to altered responses in behavioral studies in animals (Hirsjarvi and Valiaho, 1995; Shalev et al., 1998) and 'playful' handling can be a refinement to reduce stress when performing procedures such as injections (Cloutier et al., 2014). Handling also leads to vocalizations, often in the range of 22kHz, typical for rat alarm calls (Brudzynski, 2009). Stress-induced vocalization from rats in one cage can make handling more difficult or have an effect on the behavior of other rats within hearing range (Brudzynski and Chiu, 1995). An additional interesting fact regarding rat vocalization, illustrative of its importance in rat behavior, is that rat pups vocalize in the ultrasonic range, probably to signal their mothers, even before their ears are sufficiently developed for them to be capable of hearing (Feldman, 1992).

Rats are most active at night but will also move and feed some during the day; they are also more active in the mornings than in afternoons (Saibaba et al., 1996). This circadian rhythm is relevant to a broad range of behavioral measurements. For example, pain threshold is often determined in a tail flick test. Female rats have shorter tail flick response times in the middle of the dark period, as well as during estrus and metestrus (Martinez-Gomez et al., 1994).

Rats, like other rodents, are coprophagic and vary considerably between individuals in the percentage of feces consumed. This may be of significance when fasting rats for gastric procedures, quantifying fecal output volume or measuring intestinal absorption of some agents.

Rats may be housed singly or in groups. In general, male rats are less likely to fight when housed together than are male mice, but they also do well when housed singly, as is the norm in many toxicology and safety assessment studies. Although historical experience has shown that laboratory rats appear to adapt well to single housing, there are demonstrable physiological and behavioral differences between rodents maintained in a social housing as compared to cage isolation (Gonder and Laber, 2007). The 2011 revision of the Guide for the Care and Use of Laboratory Animals strongly recommends that members of social species such as rats be housed in compatible groups whenever possible (National Research Council, 2011). However, as the emphasis on group housing begins to change the way institutions care for their animals, it needs to be recognized that a shift from single to group housing can function as a significant variable in a broad range of experimental studies. Such changes should be discussed with all groups involved so that the potential effects on the research study can be explored proactively by consulting the relevant literature, and also so that unanticipated effects can be recognized and evaluated retrospectively.

When afforded the choice, rats have shown preferences for solid flooring, bedding consisting of large particles of aspen wood chips, and nest boxes (Manser et al., 1995a, b, 1998a, b; Blom et al., 1995), although the consequences of being deprived of the preferred housing factors have not been reported. When provided with objects as part of an environmental enrichment program, rats will chew on inanimate objects such as wooden blocks and nylon bones and balls (Watson, 1993; Chmiel and Noonan, 1996). The provision of environmental enrichment is an important part of providing high-quality research animal care, but as is the case with social housing, it can significantly change the baseline behavior and experimental responses (Simpson and Kelly, 2011). As a result, when changes are made, it must be carefully considered as a research variable with the potential for unintended effects.

III. DISEASES

A. Infectious Diseases

1. Bacterial, Mycoplasmal, and Rickettsial Infections

Although substantial evidence supports a salubrious role for a complex microflora in laboratory rodents, including contributions to gastrointestinal and immunologic development and function, endocrine and nervous systems, as well as metabolism, this section will be limited to detrimental, or potentially so, host–bacterial interactions, i.e., infection (Treuting et al., 2012; Rohde et al., 2007). Discussion of bacterial disease in laboratory rats is also compounded by changes in pathogen prevalence across North America, Europe, and Japan, such that many of the 'classical' pathogens of rats such as Corynebacterium kutscheri and Mycoplasma pulmonis are very rare (Pritchett-Corning et al., 2009; Livingston and Riley, 2003). However, they should not be forgotten, as they not only persist in wild populations and pet rodents, but there are many other regions of the bioresearch world where pathogen prevalence profiles cannot be assumed. Thus, we will briefly mention some bacteria which are primarily of historical interest in many areas of the world, as well as others likely to be of health or research significance to laboratory rats only in special situations or to individual rats, not to entire groups.

a. Streptococcal Pulmonary Disease

Etiology Pneumonia caused by S. pneumoniae has historically been referred to as streptococcosis. However, because the term streptococcosis could be used to describe any streptococcal infection, it is inherently nonspecific and should be avoided. Several species of Streptococcus are opportunistic pathogens in rats (i.e., they can cause clinical disease under at least some circumstances). Streptococcus pneumoniae, which is α-hemolytic, is the Streptococcus species of most historic concern in the rat.

Epizootiology and Transmission Streptococcus pneumoniae is rare in commercially obtained rats and for more than 20 years has been considered to be a pathogen of low significance in laboratory animals (National Research Council, 1991). Numerous serotypes of S. pneumoniae exist; disease is predominantly associated with infection by more pathogenic serotypes, especially 2, 3, 8, 16, and 19 (Fallon et al., 1988). Humans are the natural host of S. pneumoniae, with both adults and children frequently colonized. Streptococcus pneumoniae is transmitted primarily via aerosol, although fomites may play a minor role.

Clinical Signs Disease due to S. pneumoniae has been infrequently reported in rats, but infection is usually asymptomatic and results in colonization of the nasopharynx. No reports could be found of disease due to S. pneumoniae in laboratory rats in the last 20 years, and infection also appears to be rare (Pritchett-Corning et al., 2009). It is possible that older reports may have been confounded by concomitant infection with other respiratory pathogens such as Pneumocystis carinii, which was not recognized at that time as a cause of disease in immunocompetent rats. The rat, however, is used as an experimental model of human S. pneumoniae infection, although immunosuppression, neutropenia, or other special techniques are usually necessary to induce disease (Chiavolini et al., 2008).

Pathology Reports of disease associated with *S. pneumonia* in rats resembles that in both human and nonhuman primates, characterized by suppurative inflammation in the upper respiratory tract, which spreads to the lung to cause bronchopneumonia (Kohn and Barthold, 1984) and sometimes fibrinosuppurative pleuritis. Affected rats may become bacteremic and may develop fibrinopurulent inflammation of other serous surfaces (e.g., peritoneum, synovium) and other tissues.

Diagnosis and Differential Diagnosis Monitoring for *S. pneumoniae* infection is often conducted by nasopharyngeal culture onto blood agar. Differentiation of *S. pneumoniae* from other α-hemolytic streptococci is most often performed by the optochin inhibition test. Optochin inhibition is greater for most *S. pneumoniae* strains than for other α-hemolytic streptococci. PCR is also commercially available to detect *S. pneumoniae* in samples from the nasopharynx or lung. However, because of the occurrence of nonpathogenic isolates (Fallon et al., 1988), detection of *S. pneumoniae* in rats, even if a respiratory problem is present in the colony, does not necessarily provide a diagnosis without corroborating histopathology, nor does isolation of *S. pneumoniae* from asymptomatic rats necessarily indicate a colony health threat.

Prevention and Control Contamination with this agent is rare in contemporary colonies, and since there may be nonpathogenic strains, action to eliminate *S. pneumoniae* is only indicated in the presence of characteristic lesions or detection of known pathogenic serotypes. Depopulation can be performed, followed by restocking with animals from a clean source that are maintained to remain SPF via the use of standard exclusion techniques.

Research Complications Animals affected by pneumonia or septicemia would be poor subjects for research, but physiologic variability associated with asymptomatic carriage have not been reported.

b. Other Streptococcal Species

β-Hemolytic streptococci are also detected in laboratory rats but rarely cause disease. β-Hemolytic streptococci are divided into groups based on Lancefield antigens, with Lancefield groups B and G most commonly isolated from rats. Some of these organisms have been used in experimental infections in rats, but only once have they been associated with naturally occurring disease. In this single report, Group B streptococci were linked to myocarditis and abscesses found in a few 21- to 24-day old pups of a Munich Wistar–Frömter line transgenic for human diphtheria toxin (Shuster et al., 2013). Exclusion of β-hemolytic streptococci from most rat colonies is neither necessary nor practical, for humans are often carriers. *Enterococcus* spp., which are not truly streptococci, are often considered together with *Streptococcus* spp. So-called streptococcal enteropathy is actually due to nonhemolytic (γ-hemolytic) Lancefield group D enterococci, including *Enterococcus hirae, E. faecium-durans* 2, and *E. faecalis* 2 (Barthold, 1997). Streptococcal enteropathy is a disease that affects only suckling rats, not postweaning animals. Affected litters develop diarrhea or soft stools, with bright yellow pasty feces. Mortality can be high. Microscopically, the villi of the small intestine are carpeted with gram-positive cocci. Disease is clearly associated with some strains of enterococci and not with others, but the factors determining the pathogenic potential have not been elucidated. They may, however, involve the ability of pathogenic isolates to adhere to the surface of the microvilli. Control of *Streptococcus* spp. and *Enterococcus* spp. is problematic, because the organisms are widespread, including being cultivable in a high percentage of the human population (Del Vecchio, 1992). Some *Enterococcus* spp. have even been considered autochthonous flora of the rat (Savage, 1971). Streptococci can be excluded by aseptic microisolator technique or by use of isolators (Pleasants, 1974), yet the low incidence of disease may not warrant the additional time, expense, or other resources that such housing techniques would require.

c. Pseudotuberculosis

Etiology *Corynebacterium kutscheri* is a gram-positive coryneform (club-shaped) bacterium which can be found in soil, sewage, and marine environments, and has been explored for possible utility of bioremediation of oil spills (Oyetibo et al., 2013). In rats, mice, guinea pigs, and hamsters, *C. kutscheri* is the cause of pseudotuberculosis, although in the last two species, there is only bacteriological evidence, i.e., no disease has been reported.

Epizootiology and Transmission Transmission is probably through direct contact or oronasal exposure.

Clinical Sign Infections with *C. kutscheri* are rare (Pritchett-Corning et al., 2009; Livingston and Riley, 2003) and usually clinically silent (Suzuki et al., 1988; Amao et al., 1995). Nonspecific clinical signs may be observed in advanced disease, such as ruffled fur, hunched posture, dyspnea and rales, porphyria, mucopurulent ocular and nasal discharges, lethargy, and lameness. These are usually followed by death in 1–7 days.

Pathology Gross lesions of *C. kutscheri* infection consist of solitary or multiple randomly distributed abscesses in the lung, liver, kidney, skin, and joints. The lesions are due to septic emboli becoming trapped in organs and tissues that contain an extensive capillary network. In the rat, the lung is the organ most frequently involved (Fig. 4.4). Suppurative inflammation may also be found in the preputial gland and tympanic bullae. Histopathologically, the lesions are generally as expected from the gross findings. Interstitial inflammation in the

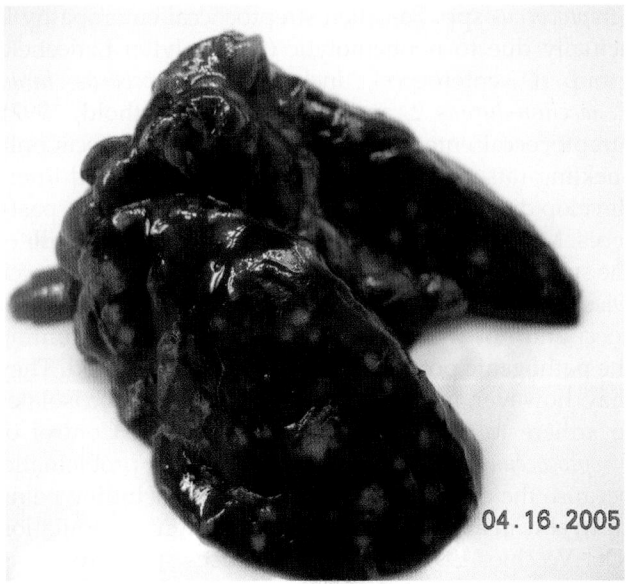

04.16.2005

FIGURE 4.4   Multiple abscesses in a rat lung caused by *C. kutscheri*. *Courtesy of Joanne Bella Hodges.*

lung is due to the hematogenous seeding of the lung with bacteria, although bronchi and bronchioles may also contain suppurative exudate. Caseous necrosis is often prominent, and epithelioid macrophages and multinucleated giant cells may be present in areas of abscessation. Large areas of caseous necrosis may also be present in the liver. Septic embolic glomerulitis may be present in the kidneys, as may abscesses with or without pyelonephritis. Abscesses and caseous necrosis may also be observed in virtually any tissue.

Diagnosis   In infected colonies, *C. kutscheri* will typically cause latent infections and may be detected by PCR or cultured from submaxillary (cervical) lymph nodes, oropharynx and nasopharynx, middle ears, and preputial glands of feces (Amao *et al.*, 1995, 2002, 2008). Latent infections may be triggered to become clinical by a variety of stressors that can cause immunosuppression in the host. These include poor husbandry, overcrowding, shipping, malnutrition, intercurrent infections, irradiation, and treatment with immunosuppressive drugs (Barthold and Brownstein, 1988). As with other persistent infections, such as mycoplasmosis, disease is more frequent in older animals. Definitive diagnosis is accomplished by bacteriologic culture (Fox *et al.*, 1987) or PCR (Jeong *et al.*, 2013). The best site, other than lesions, to culture is probably the submandibular (cervical) lymph nodes. The oral cavity, cecum, colon, and rectum may also harbor the organism. As feces have been identified in mice as a suitable culture site, they may also be a suitable sample for PCR, although this has not been confirmed in rats. Microscopic evaluation of lesions may reveal the characteristic irregularly branching arrays of

gram-positive rods in tissue sections (Brown and Brenn stain) or impression smears (Gram's stain). However, if possible, histopathology should always be confirmed by bacteriology or PCR. Serology has also been widely employed for detection of *C. kutscheri* infection in immunocompetent rats (Fox *et al.*, 1987; Boot *et al.*, 1995). As with other serologic assays, especially serologic assays for agents more antigenically complex than viruses, false positives and false negatives occasionally occur, so positive results should always be confirmed by culture or PCR.

Differential Diagnosis   Differential diagnosis for the presence of multiple abscesses in rats should include streptococcosis, streptobacillosis, mycoplasmosis (pulmonary abscesses), Cilia-associated respiratory (CAR) bacillus infection (pulmonary abscesses), or other miscellaneous bacteria. Of these, only mycoplasmosis and CAR bacillus infection would be found predominantly in older animals. PCR may be helpful in these situations as it can be performed on fresh, frozen, or formalin-fixed paraffin-embedded tissue, although the first two are preferable to the last.

Prevention and Control   Typical rederivation and bioexclusion techniques can be used to maintain colonies free of the agent.

Research   Complications   Morbidity/mortality from clinical disease can disrupt ongoing studies and is most likely to occur should the bacteria contaminate immunocompromised rats.

d. Tyzzer's Disease

Etiology   Tyzzer's disease, first discovered by Tyzzer in Japanese Waltzing mice (Tyzzer, 1917), is caused by *Clostridium piliforme* (Duncan *et al.*, 1993), formerly known as *Bacillus piliformis*. The host range is protean among mammals, including numerous rodent species, rabbits, carnivores, horses, and both nonhuman and human primates (DeLong and Manning, 1994; Skelton *et al.*, 1995).

Epizootiology and Transmission   *Clostridium piliforme* is transmitted horizontally in rats by spores through fecal–oral contamination. The spores are highly resistant to desiccation and some disinfectants (Ganaway, 1980). The delicate vegetative form, however, survives only inside of cells. After being ingested, *C. piliforme* spores produce a vegetative form, which is actively phagocytosed by mucosal epithelial cells covering the gut-associated lymphoid tissue, or Peyer's patches (Tyzzer, 1917; Duncan *et al.*, 1993).

Clinical Signs   *Clostridium piliforme* infection is usually clinically silent (Motzel and Riley, 1992; Hansen *et al.*, 1992b). Overt disease in rats, as in other species, is most likely to be observed in young, recently weaned animals. In these, the clinical signs are nonspecific (anorexia, lethargy, emaciation, ruffled fur) and may include acute death without clinical signs. Diarrhea may be noted and may contain mucus and blood. Particularly in the rat, a distended abdomen has been observed in weanlings with Tyzzer's disease, albeit at a very low incidence (Hansen *et al.*, 1992a).

Pathology Grossly, in the minority of cases which produce disease, multiple, pale foci, pinpoint or larger, of necrosis are often visible on the surface of and within the liver. Megaloileitis – a greatly dilated, flaccid, and hyperemic ileum – may be present. Hyperemia, edema, hemorrhage, and ulceration may affect any part of the intestine, especially the terminal ileum, cecum, and colon. Secondary to intestinal involvement, mesenteric lymph nodes may be enlarged, hyperemic, and edematous. In the heart, pale circumscribed areas may be visible on the epicardium. Myocardial necrosis due to Tyzzer's disease may also appear as pale linear streaks or areas in the heart, especially near the apex. Histopathologically, characteristic lesions may be observed in the liver, ileum, cecum, and colon, and, less frequently, the heart. In the intestinal tract, there may be necrotizing enteritis, typhlitis, and colitis. Coagulative necrosis in the liver is the hallmark lesion and is often accompanied by a moderate leukocytic infiltrate, usually neutrophils and mononuclear cells, at the periphery of the lesions. Acute lesions may be hemorrhagic, and mineralization may occur with time. In the heart, myocardial degeneration and necrosis occurs in a minority of cases, often with a mixed leukocytic infiltrate and dystrophic calcification.

Diagnosis Diagnosis of clinical disease depends on demonstration of the organism in tissue. Histopathologic evaluation is diagnostic if the characteristic bacilli are observed (Tyzzer, 1917; Duncan *et al.*, 1993). The vegetative form of the organism is a filamentous bacillus, 8–20 μm long and 0.3–0.5 μm wide. Bacilli are intracellular, are often numerous, and may appear as either a jumbled array (pickup stick) or parallel arrangement, as dictated by the shape of the cell. The vegetative form may rarely be visible in hepatocytes in tissue sections stained with hematoxylin and eosin, but usually special stains are necessary, including Warthin–Starry silver (best), Giemsa, and methylene blue stains. Although gram-negative, *C. piliforme* stains very poorly with gram stains. Tissue smears may facilitate rapid diagnosis; Giemsa-stained smears of suspicious liver lesions are especially useful (Percy and Barthold, 2007). In the liver, the organisms are most often observed in surviving hepatocytes at the periphery or within lesions. In the intestine, normal gut flora within mucosal crypts and superimposed upon the mucosal epithelial cells may complicate evaluation. Organisms may also occasionally be observed in cardiac myocytes or myocytes of the tunica muscularis of the intestine. Colony screening for latent infection is problematic. Serologic screening is rapid and technically simple (Motzel and Riley, 1992)

but is subject to false positives, yielding results that can be difficult to put into context, as has been recently reported in rabbits (Pritt *et al.*, 2010). Disease provocation tests, or stress tests, to exacerbate latent infections are sometimes used as a follow-up test when serologic positive results are obtained. However, there is some doubt as to efficacy of stress tests that rely on chemical immunosuppression, usually with cyclophosphamide (Boivin *et al.*, 1990), followed by histopathologic evaluation. The doubt arises because test animals may have already cleared the *C. piliforme* infection and therefore may no longer be susceptible to activation of 'latent' infection. Alternatively, sentinel animals can be placed on soiled bedding, but this may require sentinels to be of the same species (to avoid species specificity causing false negatives), for not even gerbils are susceptible to all strains of *C. piliforme* (Motzel and Riley, 1992; Franklin *et al.*, 1994). PCR is also useful, as it is a sensitive and specific method to detect DNA from the organism. Thus, it can be used on fecal samples (Furukawa *et al.*, 2002), but will only detect animals which have not cleared infection. It can be used on ileum, cecum or colon, but only during the period when organisms are present. PCR is useful for screening grossly observed liver lesions for *C. piliforme*, and can additionally be used on paraffin-embedded tissues as a confirmatory test following histopathologic evaluation.

Differential Diagnosis Differential diagnoses for necrotizing hepatitis in the rat should include other bacterial septicemias, such as *Corynebacterium kutscheri*, as well as infection with rat virus.

Prevention and Control As is the case with the other bacterial diseases described in this section, control in contemporary colonies is through the use of exclusion techniques. However, the fact the organism produces spores suggests that (1) cross-contamination from conventional or wild-caught colonies could be more likely, and (2) very thorough decontamination would be indicated after an outbreak.

Research Complications Interference of *Clostridium piliforme* with research has primarily been attributed to the morbidity and mortality, although effects on coagulation and leukokines have also been reported in mice with subclinical *C. piliforme* infection (Van Andel *et al.*, 2000).

e. Pasteurellosis

Etiology *Pasteurella pneumotropica* is a gram-negative coccobacillus. It grows aerobically on sheep blood agar without producing hemolysis, producing smooth, gray or occasionally yellow translucent colonies (Carter, 1984; Nicklas, 2007). It has been isolated from numerous mammalian species, including humans, and has long been considered to be of low significance in immunocompetent rats (National Research Council, 1991).

Epizootiology and Transmission *Pasteurella pneumotropica* has a high prevalence in infected colonies and is most often isolated from the nasopharynx, cecum, vagina, uterus, and conjunctiva during routine monitoring (National Research Council, 1991).

Clinical Signs and Pathology The vast majority of animals are asymptomatic, with only rare instances of conjunctivitis, metritis, and mastitis (Percy and Barthold, 2007). Histologically, any lesions that occur are characterized by necrosuppurative inflammation.

Diagnosis and Differential DiagnosiS Screening for *P. pneumotropica* may be conducted by either culture or PCR. Culture is best conducted on the sites mentioned above, although feces, oral swabs, or even dust that has accumulated in animal air spaces, such as within the plenum of some individually ventilated caging systems, are all suitable for PCR (Henderson *et al.*, 2013).

Prevention and Control Control of the agent may not be necessary in immunocompetent rats, because of the rarity of *P. pneumotropica*-induced disease. Treatment with enrofloxacin has been described for the mouse (Goelz *et al.*, 1997). Rederivation by either cesarean section or embryo transfer will also eliminate the agent (Nicklas, 2007). Offspring should also be held in strict isolation – i.e., not mixed in with a breeding colony – until confirmed negative for *P. pneumotropica*. *Pasteurella pneumotropica* is not transmitted to a significant degree by fomites, does not persist or multiply in the environment, and only very rarely colonizes humans. Therefore, once a colony is free of the agent, there is relatively little risk of reinfection except through introduction or incursion of infected animals.

Research Complications Studies that involve tissues and organs affected by the associated inflammation would be affected.

f. Salmonellosis

Etiology Salmonellosis is the disease caused by bacteria of the genus *Salmonella*. The taxonomic classification and subdivision of the genus remain somewhat controversial and, like much taxonomy, subject to change. All salmonellas that one is likely to encounter in rats belong to *S. enterica* which comprises more than 2500 serovars (Tindall *et al.*, 2005; Timme *et al.*, 2013). These vary greatly in pathogenicity and geographic distribution, which makes serovar classification useful in epizootiologic investigations. For simplicity sake, however, this discussion will treat *S. enterica* as a single entity.

Epizootiology and Transmission Salmonellosis may be virtually nonexistent in laboratory rats in the United States, but because infection is thought to be prevalent among many other species of vertebrates, including wild rodents, the potential for introduction remains. *Salmonella enterica* is transmitted by ingestion of contaminated materials, including feed, bedding, or water. Incursion of wild or feral rodents into a laboratory facility poses a further risk.

Clinical Signs As in most species, clinical signs of infection with S. enterica in rats are rare but may include a hunched posture, ruffled fur, lethargy, weight loss, and conjunctivitis. Soft stools and diarrhea may also be observed, usually in less than 20% of animals.

Pathology In rats with subclinical infections, gross and microscopic lesions will usually be absent. Rats with clinical disease may have evidence of gastrointestinal involvement and septicemia, including mural thickening and mucosal ulcers in the cecum and ileum, as well as splenomegaly. Microscopically, enteric lesions are characterized by edema of the lamina propria, leukocyte infiltration in areas of ulceration, and reactive hyperplasia of crypt epithelial cells. Lymphoid hyperplasia, with focal necrosis and neutrophil infiltration, may be observed in Peyer's patches, as well as in the spleen and mesenteric lymph nodes. Septicemic rats will have necrosis in the spleen and liver, with emboli composed of fibrin, bacteria, and debris present in liver, spleen, and lymph nodes (Percy and Barthold, 2007).

Diagnosis Colony screening is most often conducted on fecal samples by microbiologic culture or by PCR. Suspected cases of salmonellosis may also be tested by culture or PCR of feces, mesenteric lymph nodes, liver, spleen, or blood. Material is placed in enrichment broth and then inoculated onto selective growth medium. Although symptomatic animals should be culture-positive, an infected colony may have only a low incidence of asymptomatic carriers, perhaps less than 5%. Detection of *S. enterica* in these colonies may require repeated testing of significant numbers of samples. It is unknown at this time if PCR would find a higher rate of carriage than detected by culture.

Differential Diagnosis Differential diagnoses for diarrheal disease in rats include Tyzzer's disease, rotavirus infection, enterococcal enteropathy, cryptosporidiosis, and problems with feed and/or water.

Prevention and Control Salmonellosis is prevented by rigorous pest control and by ensuring that food and bedding are not contaminated. Good personal hygiene of employees will prevent them from serving as a source of *Salmonella* or other enteric pathogens to the colony. Once *S. enterica* is detected in a colony, all animals are usually destroyed, and all surfaces and materials either sterilized or safely discarded. Strict quarantine of a small group of animals may be practical in some situations, prior to rederivation by embryo transfer or cesarian section. This may be most feasible in a flexible film or semirigid isolator. Treatment is not recommended, because a chronic carrier state may result and there is the potential for zoonotic disease.

Research Complications Rats infected with *S. enterica* should not be used in research, because of the zoonotic potential and the risk they animals pose to other animals.

g. Pseudomoniasis

Etiology Pseudomoniasis refers to clinical disease caused by *Pseudomonas aeruginosa*, a gram-negative bacillus of the order Eubacteriales, family Pseudomonadaceae.

Epizootiology and Transmission *Pseudomonas aeruginosa* is motile, aerobic, oxidase-positive, and widely distributed in water, soil, sewage, and the skin and gastrointestinal tract of many animals. It is considered as part of the common commensal flora of humans, domestic animals, and laboratory rodents and isolation frequency increases in animals and humans receiving antibiotics (Kiska and Gilligan, 1999).

Clinical Signs and Pathology Despite its near ubiquity, *P. aeruginosa* is rarely implicated in disease except in mammals with specific and severe host defense deficits, particularly hosts or tissues deficient in functional phagocytes (i.e., macrophages and neutrophils, and their serum opsonins). Thus, athymic nude mice are not subject to a high incidence of pseudomoniasis unless irradiated or treated with myelosuppressive agents. In general, pseudomoniasis is considered to be of low significance in rats (National Research Council, 1991) but should be suspected when rats that are irradiated or treated with radiomimetic agents die earlier than expected (Percy and Barthold, 2007). In particular, pseudomoniasis has been reported as a consequence of infection of indwelling jugular catheters (Wyand and Jonas, 1967). Signs were those of septicemia. Necropsy findings included vegetative valvular endocarditis and multifocal hemorrhagic pneumonia. Histologically, fibrin emboli, leukocytes, and gram-negative bacteria were observed in the heart, lung, and occasionally other organs.

Diagnosis Pseudomoniasis is diagnosed by either cultural identification of the organism or by PCR. However, caution should be exercised in attributing observed morbidity and mortality to an organism as nearly ubiquitous as *P. aeruginosa*. Although *Pseudomonas* will grow on blood agar, isolation is enhanced by the use of selective media, such as *Pseudomonas* isolation agar, or *Pseudomonas* agar P. The use of selective media is particularly recommended when screening clinically healthy animals, because only low numbers of organisms may be harbored in the common sites for isolation, the cecum, and nasopharynx.

Prevention and Control Exclusion of *P. aeruginosa* is rarely justified in a research setting as it requires gnotobiotic methods and sterilization of all water reaching the animals, as well as sterilization of cages, feed, and bedding. Animals must be maintained in isolators or microisolators and must be routinely monitored. All possible sources of contamination from human skin or any wet surface must be strictly prohibited. Control of *P. aeruginosa* infection often begins with the watering system. *Pseudomonas aeruginosa* is one of many bacteria that form biofilms, layers of bacteria, usually with reduced metabolic activity, embedded in a dense glycocalyx. Bacteria in a biofilm are extraordinarily resistant to chlorine (150- to 3000-times more resistant than free-floating bacteria) and monochloramine (2- to 100-fold; LeChevallier *et al.*, 1988) and may be inaccessible to antibiotics. Nonetheless, chlorination (10–13 ppm) or acidification (pH 2.5–3.0) can significantly reduce the colonization of mice with *P. aeruginosa* but will not eliminate infection. Rederivation by cesarian section or embryo transfer is required to eliminate *P. aeruginosa* from an infected colony. Treatment with gentamycin in the animal drinking water, at 1 g/l, has been reported to eliminate the infection in mice but is probably not practical for large groups of rats (Urano *et al.*, 1977).

Research Complications As mentioned above, infection of indwelling catheters has been reported, and disease caused by the organism could interfere with radiation studies or those using strains with specific immune deficits.

h. Streptobacillosis

One cause of rat-bite fever, *Streptobacillus moniliformis* is primarily of historic interest in laboratory rats. This zoonotic agent is virtually nonexistent in modern laboratory animals but nonetheless bears brief mention because of the potentially serious consequences of infection (Anderson *et al.*, 1983; Wullenweber, 1995). The agent is a gram-negative pleomorphic bacillus, which will grow nonhemolytically on sheep blood agar, although trypticase soy agar enriched with 20% horse serum is preferred (Weisbroth, 1982; Savage, 1984).

Streptobacillus moniliformis is commensal in wild rats, inhabiting the nasopharynx, middle ear, and respiratory tract. It is present in blood and urine of infected rats and is transmitted to humans by bite wounds, aerosols, and fomites (Will, 1994). The organism is nonpathogenic in rats. Clinical signs in humans follow a 3- to 10-day incubation period and include fever, vomiting, arthralgia, and rash. Disease is treated with antibiotics, and mortality is low.

Colonies of laboratory rats are monitored by PCR or by culture of blood and nasopharyngeal swabs for *Streptobacillus moniliformis*, and any colony in which the organism is confirmed should immediately be terminated. Because wild rats are the reservoir for *S. moniliformis*, detection of this delicate bacterium in a laboratory rat colony would indicate close-range exposure to infected wild rats.

i. Helicobacteriosis

Etiology A number of enterohepatic *Helicobacter* spp. have been found as natural infections of rats. *Helicobacter muridarum*, one of the first helicobacters identified in rodents, was initially reported in 1992 (Lee *et al.*, 1992). *H. trogontum* has now been identified as the most prevalent of the naturally occurring intestinal helicobacters (Mendes *et al.*, 1996) in rats, and *H. bilis* has been reported from the large bowel of immunodeficient rats (Haines *et al.*, 1998). More recently, *H. pullorum* was isolated from a breeding colony of inbred Brown Norway rats housed in the same room as an infected mouse colony. Persistent infection of Brown Norway rats was also established by oral inoculation (Cacioppo *et al.*, 2012b). A similar inoculum resulted in persistent infection of four of 10 Sprague-Dawley rats; none of eight other Sprague-Dawley rats receiving dirty bedding from infected Brown Norway rats became infected (Cacioppo *et al.*, 2012a). No lesions were attributed to *Helicobacter* in any of the rats. All currently identified helicobacters of laboratory rats are microaerophilic, gram-negative flagellated bacteria that may be spiral, slightly curved, or straight. Coccoid forms have also been described for *H. bilis* and *H. pylori* (Fox *et al.*, 1995).

Epizootiology and Transmission The host range of rat *Helicobacter* species is not fully elucidated. Clearly, *H. bilis* has been found in rats and mice, and there is also an additional report of it in a dog (Eaton *et al.*, 1996). *Helicobacter muridarum* has been reported in rats and mice. *H. pullorum* has been reported in mice, rats, chickens, and humans. No host range has been reported for *H. trogontum*. Many other *Helicobacter* species, however, are able to colonize a phylogenetically wide range of mammalian hosts. With the exception of an attempt to transmit *H. pullorum* by soiled bedding, no studies have been published on the transmission of naturally occurring *Helicobacter* infections in rats. In mice, horizontal transmission by soiled bedding, probably fecal–oral transmission, has been demonstrated (Livingston *et al.*, 1998), although it has recently been shown that soiled bedding sentinels will only detect a subset of infected mice (Henderson *et al.*, 2013). Fecal–oral transmission is also presumed in rats.

Clinical Signs Once established, infection by any *Helicobacter* species is typically lifelong. Infection, or colonization, should be distinguished from disease. *Helicobacter muridarum* and *H. trogontum* may be nonpathogenic in rats, although *H. muridarum* has been reported to cause lymphocytic gastritis in aged mice, possibly associated with a loss of parietal cell mass leading to increased gastric pH.

Pathology Key pathogenic factors for *H. pylori* include urease, a vacuolating cytotoxin (*vacA*), and the presence of a pathogenicity island. All of the enterohepatic *Helicobacter* spp. currently identified in rats are urease-positive (Fox and Lee, 1997). Other virulence factors have not been reported. Lesions reported in athymic nude rats infected with *H. bilis* are similar to those reported in immunodeficient mice inoculated with *H. bilis* or *H. hepaticus* and include proliferative and ulcerative typhlitis, colitis, and proctitis (Haines *et al.*, 1998),

although no causal role was confirmed. No lesions due to any naturally occurring *Helicobacter* species have been reported in immunocompetent laboratory rats. The only report of lesions in rats due to natural *Helicobacter* infection involved a small group of 11 male athymic nude rats, 5–8 months of age, infected with *H. bilis* (Haines *et al.*, 1998). In these rats, gross lesions consisted of focal or diffuse thickening of the cecal wall, with normal-appearing colon and rectum. Cystic mesenteric lymph nodes were also noted in eight of the 11 rats. Histologically, all 11 rats had proliferative typhlitis, with eight of the animals also having similar lesions in the colon and rectum. Crypt epithelium was hyperplastic, with cytoplasmic basophilia, increased mitoses, and fewer goblet cells than normally observed. The lamina propria was infiltrated by lymphocytes, plasma cells, and a few eosinophils. Mucosal erosion and ulceration were observed in the cecum of the most severely affected rats. The authors experimentally reproduced many aspects of the disease by intraperitoneal injection of approximately 5×10^8 *H. bilis* bacteria in phosphate-buffered saline. *Helicobacter* infection should, therefore, be a prime differential diagnosis when proliferative lesions of the large bowel are observed in rats. Spontaneous chronic ulcerative colitis has also been reported in athymic nude rats apparently free of *Helicobacter* infection (Thomas and Pass, 1997). The authors were unable to culture *Helicobacter* spp. from affected animals, although no molecular techniques were employed.

Diagnosis Diagnosis of *Helicobacter* infection in laboratory rats is best accomplished by PCR (Riley *et al.*, 1996; Fox and Lee, 1997; Henderson *et al.*, 2013). Samples are most often fecal pellets or fecal dust, although cecal mucosal scrapings or tissue may also be used. *Helicobacter* spp may also be cultured from a variety of sources. Culture from contents of the large intestine is greatly complicated, however, by the rich flora of the site. Fox and Lee (1997) recommend passage of cecal contents through a 0.65-µm filter, then culture on *Brucella* agar with antibiotics (trimethoprim, vancomycin, polymyxin) to suppress growth of unwanted organisms that are not removed by the filter. Culture is generally considered to have less sensitivity for detecting helicobacters, so negative culture results must be interpreted cautiously.

Prevention and Control In general, it is relatively simple to exclude from animal colonies those rodent-specific organisms that do not multiply or survive for long in the environment. However, given the uncertainty as to the full host range of rat helicobacters, the possibility of transmission by humans is difficult to exclude. The usual source of infection for *Helicobacter* infection in rats is nonetheless expected to be contaminated rodents or other laboratory animals. No indication of transmission by feed, bedding, water, or aerosols has been reported, although *Helicobacter* DNA can be detected on surfaces contaminated by dust, presumably fecal in origin, from animal cages.

Once a colony is infected, treatment of small groups of animals may be possible. Several antibiotic regimens have been reported to be successful for mice and might similarly be attempted in rats. These have primarily involved oral dosing with antibiotics by gavage several times each day or incorporation of antibiotics into the diet. Elimination of infection from large groups of rats would be less likely to be 100% effective, even if practical obstacles of dosing could be overcome, because even a single rat retaining any viable *Helicobacter* could lead to reinfection of the entire colony. Cross-fostering pups from infected dams onto nursing uninfected dams has been reported as successful for mice (Singletary *et al.*, 2003), although it has not been reported in rats. Rederivation of infected stocks by caesarian section or embryo transfer is also successful.

Research Complications Research complications due to infection by *Helicobacter* spp. in rats have not been reported.

j. Cilia-Associated Respiratory Bacillus

Etiology Usually referred to as CAR bacillus, the CAR bacillus is not taxonomically classified in the genus *Bacillus*. Rather, it has been tentatively placed in a group of bacteria known as 'gliding bacteria,' based on the fact that they are motile but without visible means for such motility, and may be related to *Flavobacterium* or *Flexispira*, based on 16S rRNA sequencing (Cundiff *et al.*, 1995a; Kawano *et al.*, 2000). Final identification, however, is still pending. CAR bacillus has been identified in rats, mice, and rabbits among common laboratory animals (van Zwieten *et al.*, 1980; MacKenzie *et al.*, 1981; Waggie *et al.*, 1987; Griffith *et al.*, 1988).

Epizootiology and Transmission Transmission is primarily via direct contact with infected animals. Fomites probably do not play a significant role in natural transmission of CAR bacillus, and bedding does not transmit the infection well (Matsushita *et al.*, 1989; Cundiff *et al.*, 1995b). Airborne exposure is not an important means of transmission (Itoh *et al.*, 1987).

Clinical Signs In rats, infection is usually asymptomatic, although nonspecific clinical signs such as weight loss and dyspnea may occur.

Pathology CAR bacillus infection may not always present gross lesions, although translucent gray cystic lesions, representing dilated, mucus-filled airways may be visible on the pleural surface (Itoh *et al.*, 1987). Coinfection with *Mycoplasma pulmonis* or other pathogens may occur, resulting in suppurative bronchopneumonia. Histopathologically, hyperplastic peribronchial and peribronchiolar mononuclear cell cuffs are observed in the lungs (Itoh *et al.*, 1987; Matsushita and Joshima, 1989). A thin basophilic layer may be observed on

the surface of the airway epithelium in hematoxylin–eosin-stained sections, giving the impression that the cilia are more basophilic than normal, but this is not specific and should not be used as a definitive diagnostic feature. With Warthin–Starry or methenamine silver stain, filamentous bacilli are readily observed among cilia of respiratory epithelium from the nasal cavity to the bronchioles (Fig. 4.5). The upper respiratory tract is involved earlier in the course of infection than the lower tract and should be included in histologic examinations for CAR bacillus infection.

Diagnosis Colonies are easily screened for CAR bacillus infection by serologic techniques (Matsushita *et al.*, 1987; Shoji *et al.*, 1988; Lukas *et al.*, 1987). Because

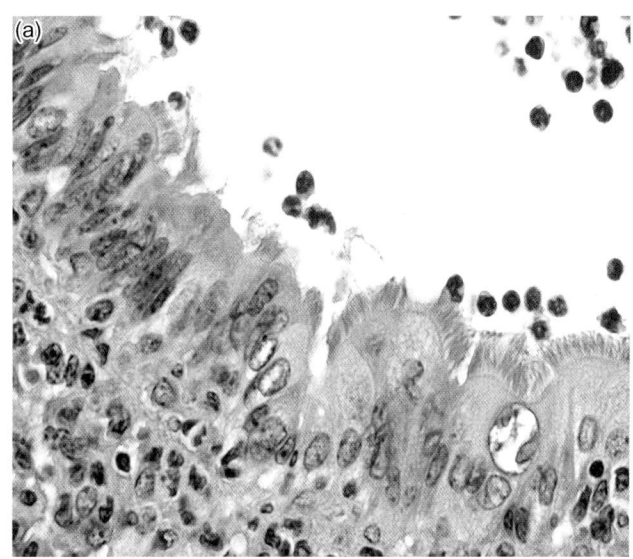
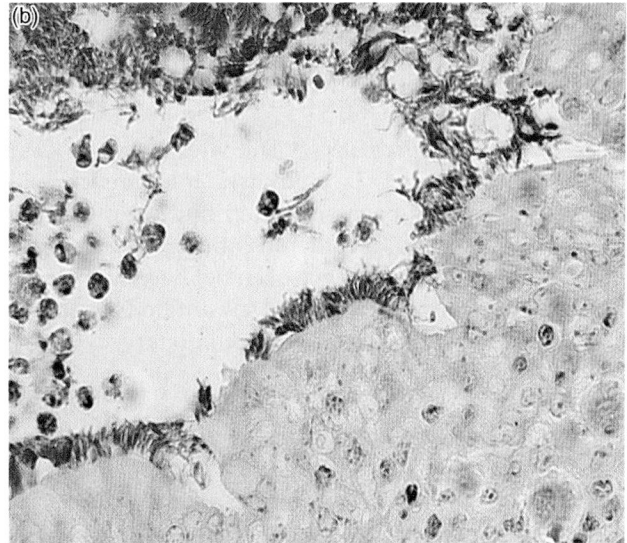

FIGURE 4.5 Rat bronchus stained via H & E (a) and Warthin–Starry (b). Innumerable filamentous bacteria are densely clustered at the ciliated surface of the columnar epithelium. Note the polymorphonuclear cell exudate in the bronchial lumen. Magnification: × 400.

false-positive reactions can occur (Hook *et al.*, 1998), any positive results should be confirmed by a Steiner stain of tracheal mucosal scraping or histopathology with use of special stains, or by PCR. Interestingly, because infection is not readily transmitted by soiled bedding (Cundiff *et al.*, 1995b), many sentinel programs may fail to detect CAR bacillus infection. Infection is lifelong, and the organisms are readily retrievable by tracheal lavage or scraping (Medina *et al.*, 1998). Therefore, CAR bacillus may be readily detected by PCR (Cundiff *et al.*, 1994), which may serve as an important confirmatory test to follow positive serologic results. PCR may be positive prior to serologic conversion, and samples for PCR may be collected as nasal swabs as a nonterminal procedure (Franklin *et al.*, 1999).

Differential Diagnosis CAR bacillus infection should be distinguished from murine respiratory mycoplasmosis, pneumonia due to other bacteria (i.e., *Streptococcus pneumoniae*, *Corynebacterium kutscheri*, etc.), and viruses. Detection of CAR bacillus infection should also raise the suspicion of coinfection with other pathogens, especially *Mycoplasma pulmonis* (van Zwieten *et al.*, 1980; MacKenzie *et al.*, 1981).

Prevention and Control CAR bacillus infection is prevented by exclusion of infected animals. No effective treatment has been described. As an alternative to elimination and rederivation of entire infected colonies, the requirement for direct contact for transmission may possibly be exploited to advantage. If individual animals or cages are monitored by serology, and then negative individuals are monitored by PCR, all rats that are positive (or all cages that have a positive rat) by either test may be eliminated or quarantined. Because the infection is not transmitted well by aerosol or fomites, it may be possible to control the spread of infection. However, the expense, the labor, and the consequences of possible failure would have to be weighed against the value of saving some of the rats.

Research Complications The interference of CAR bacillus with research is unknown. Interference with ciliary function has been suspected but not measured. Effects of CAR bacillus on other respiratory functions and on the immune response have been not been reported in rats, although in mice it incited an antibody response and increased some serum and pulmonary cytokines (Kendall *et al.*, 2000, 2001).

k. Mycoplasmosis

Etiology Murine respiratory mycoplasmosis (MRM), also known as chronic respiratory disease, is caused by *Mycoplasma pulmonis* (Kohn and Kirk, 1969; Lindsey *et al.*, 1971).

Epizootiology and Transmission The infection is rare in North America (Pritchett-Corning *et al.*, 2009). *Mycoplasma pulmonis* is transmitted horizontally by direct contact and aerosol and vertically by *in utero* transmission (Lindsey *et al.*, 1982). Venereal transmission may also be possible.

Clinical Signs Although infection can begin in young rats, clinical signs are usually observed only in older animals; *M. pulmonis* infection is clinically silent in young animals. Clinical signs are nonspecific, referable to the respiratory and auditory involvement, and include rales and dyspnea, snuffling and chattering, and ocular and nasal discharges, as well as chromodacryorrhea, rubbing of eyes, and head tilt. Rats with severe middle ear involvement may spin when held up by the tail. Decreased reproductive efficiency has also been reported in rats (Leader *et al.*, 1970).

Pathology The disease outcome depends on a complex interaction of factors relating to host, pathogen, and environment (Lindsey *et al.*, 1985). Host factors include age, strain (Davis and Cassell, 1982), immune status and lymphoreticular function, and the presence of intercurrent infections such as Sendai virus (Schoeb *et al.*, 1985); host nutritional deficiencies such as vitamin A and E deficiencies may exacerbate disease (Tvedten *et al.*, 1973). *Mycoplasma* isolates may also vary in virulence (Davidson *et al.*, 1988). Environmental factors may include intracage ammonia, temperature, humidity, etc. (Schoeb *et al.*, 1982). *Mycoplasma pulmonis* possibly damages host cells by causing dysfunction and/or loss of cilia (Kohn, 1971), which is a likely cause of the accumulation of exudate, opportunistic bacterial infections, and impaired transport of ova (infertility). *Mycoplasma pulmonis* competes for the host cell nutrients and metabolites (Cassell *et al.*, 1986) and may also produce toxic metabolites, such as peroxides and nonspecific mitogens (Naot *et al.*, 1979a, b). The latter may cause proliferation of autoreactive clones of lymphocytes, leading to the host becoming a victim of its own immune system. *Mycoplasma pulmonis* successfully evades the host's immune defenses, so infection and some lesions (especially those in the upper respiratory tract) are persistent and often progressive. The exact mechanism by which *M. pulmonis* evades the host immune system, however, is unknown.

Gross lesions of MRM (Percy and Barthold, 2007) include suppurative rhinitis, otitis media, laryngitis, and tracheitis in the upper respiratory tract. In the lung, suppurative bronchopneumonia with or without atelectasis, bronchiectasis, and abscesses may occur; widespread bronchiectatic abscesses lead to the appearance referred to as 'cobblestone' lung, primarily seen in adults with endstage disease (Fig. 4.6). This classic lesion of MRM is rare in recent years. Arthritis may rarely be observed. No genital tract lesions are usually observed, but occasionally partially resorbed fetuses and suppurative salpingitis may be found. Histopathologically (Kohn and Kirk, 1969; Percy and Barthold, 2007), airway lesions in

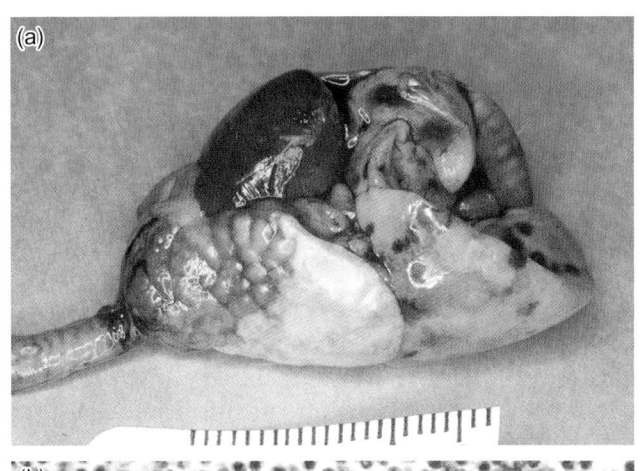

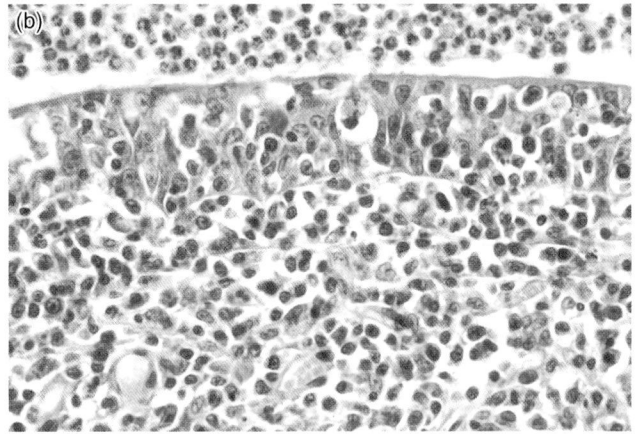

FIGURE 4.6 *M. pulmonis* infection in a rat. Note the 'cobblestone' appearance of the lungs in the gross photograph (a). Histologically, a polymorphonuclear exudate is present in the lumen of the airway while a chronic inflammatory infiltrate is present below the respiratory epithelium. *Courtesy of Dr. T. R. Schoeb.*

the respiratory tract are usually characterized by suppurative exudate, hyperplasia (squamous metaplasia) of mucosal epithelium, and often striking hyperplasia of the bronchial-associated lymphoid tissue (BALT) that could even potentially be confused with lymphoma. Other respiratory tract lesions include pseudoglandular hyperplasia of the nasal epithelium in chronic cases, and hyperplasia of peribronchial alveolar type II pneumocytes. CAR bacillus and/or other secondary bacterial pneumonias also frequently accompany MRM. Lesions in the female genital tract of rats with mycoplasmosis may include suppurative oophoritis and salpingitis, or hydrosalpingitis, and chronic suppurative endometritis or pyometra.

Diagnosis Diagnosis of mycoplasmosis in an individual rat is usually based on cultural isolation (especially exudate in the upper respiratory tract and middle ears) or PCR. Surveillance of infections in colonies, however, is most effectively accomplished by serology (Cassell *et al.*, 1981; Lussier, 1991) or by PCR on respiratory samples. Note that due to the sensitivity of the organism to desiccation, it is doubtful whether soiled bedding would be effective in transmitting it to sentinels. Pathology, including gross examination, and histopathology should not be considered diagnostic by themselves but may provide guidance in selecting more definitive tests such as PCR on deparaffinized tissue.

Differential Diagnosis Differential diagnoses for MRM include other bacterial pneumonias, such as *Corynebacterium kutscheri* infection, streptococcosis, CAR bacillus infection, and (rarely) mycotic pneumonia. All of these infections are considered rare (Pritchett-Corning *et al.*, 2009). Iatrogenic lesions due to gavage errors should also be considered a possibility. Viral infections are less likely to be mistaken for MRM, but intercurrent infections are common, including Sendai virus, pneumonia virus of mice, and others. All of these are also rare in contemporary laboratory rats (Pritchett-Corning *et al.*, 2009; Livingston and Riley, 2003).

Prevention and Control Use of high-quality vendors, careful sanitation practices, segregation of clean colonies from conventional or wild rodents and isolation and testing of rats imported from suspect sources are steps commonly taken to protect research colonies. Antibiotics such as tetracycline have been used historically to minimize symptoms and prolong survival of affected animals in order to salvage long-tern studies, but antimicrobial eradication is unlikely. Depopulation and restocking (or rederivation in the case of unique strains) are indicated to eliminate colony contamination.

Research Complications *Mycoplasma pulmonis* interferes with research by its effects on the immune system, the respiratory system, and the reproductive system and by being a primary cause of early mortality in infected colonies (Cassell *et al.*, 1986; Swing *et al.*, 1995; Lindsey *et al.*, 1971, 1982). It has also confounded the diagnosis of pulmonary lymphoproliferative disease in toxicology safety testing (Schoeb *et al.*, 2009a, b).

l. Mycoplasma Haemomuris (Hemobartonellosis)

Etiology *Mycoplasma haemomuris*, formerly *Haemobartonella muris*, is a gram-negative bacterium parasitizes erythrocytes of rats (Neimark *et al.*, 2001, 2002). It is an obligate parasite and cannot be grown *in vitro*.

Epizootiology and Transmission Because *M. haemomuris* is transmitted by the spiny rat louse, *Polyplax spinulosa*, which is very rare in modern laboratory animal facilities, erythrocytic mycoplasmosis is also correspondingly rare (National Research Council, 1991). However, the potential exists for infection of biological materials, which would provide a route of introduction into rat colonies. In addition, both the agent and the vector are still extant in North America and presumably elsewhere, indicating a continuing, albeit low-level, threat.

Clinical Signs Clinical signs are typically observed only if the normally latent infection is activated by immunosuppression or splenectomy (National Research Council, 1991). Signs are due to erythrocyte destruction and may include weight loss, hemoglobinuria, pallor, and dyspnea. Clinical pathology demonstrates anemia, reticulocytosis, increased coagulation times, decreased plasma proteins, and increased serum immunoglobulins (IgG and IgM).

Pathology Necropsy of rats with *M. haemomuris* infection is unrewarding except in the case of active infections, when anemia, hemoglobinuria, and splenomegaly may be observed. Blood films are likely to show parasitemia only in active infections.

Diagnosis *M. haemomuris* infection should be suspected whenever lice are found in a rat colony or whenever anemia and hemoglobinuria are observed. Diagnosis should be based on detection of the organisms on erythrocytes, where they appear as round (coccoid), elongate (rod), or dumbbell-shaped densities on the erythrocyte surface.

Prevention and Control *M. haemomuris* infection is readily prevented by excluding *Polyplax spinulosa* and controlling biologic materials being introduced into a colony. Once the disease is confirmed in a colony, rederivation by embryo transfer or cesarian section is warranted, although treatment with antirickettsial compounds such as tetracyclines or arsenicals may be appropriate for small groups of rats (Ristic and Kreier, 1984).

Research Complications *M. haemomuris* exerts its effects on research by virtue of its parasitism of erythrocytes. It reduces the half-life of erythrocytes, can alter function of the mononuclear phagocyte system, and can increase rejection of transplantable tumors, as well as interfering with research in other blood-borne parasitic diseases such as malaria and trypanosomiasis.

2. Viral Infections

As with bacteria, many of the 'classical' viral pathogens of rats such as Sendai virus are very rare (Pritchett-Corning *et al.*, 2009; Livingston and Riley, 2003). However, they should not be forgotten as they not only persist in wild populations and pet rodents, but there are many other regions of the bioresearch world where they may possibly persist. Thus, we will briefly mention a few viruses that are primarily of historical interest in many areas of the world.

a. Sendai Virus Infection

Etiology *Sendai virus* is an RNA virus of the family *Paramyxoviridae*, genus and species *Respirovirus*. The species contains strains that are antigenically homologous (Jacoby and Gaertner, 2006).

Epizootiology and Transmission Although Sendai virus was once very prevalent in commercial sources of mice and rats, it is rarely seen in today's colonies (Pritchett-Corning *et al.*, 2009; Liang *et al.*, 2009; Schoondermark-van de Ven *et al.*, 2006; Livingston and Riley, 2003; Mahler and Kohl, 2009, McInnes *et al.*, 2011). Sendai virus is highly contagious, with transmission occurring through the respiratory tract either by aerosol or direct contact.

Clinical Signs Unlike Sendai virus-induced disease in mice, an asymptomatic and self-limiting disease is usually induced by Sendai virus in rats. Clinical signs associated with the virus may include reduced production and litter sizes, as well as retarded growth of young within breeding colonies. Infrequently, clinical respiratory signs occur (Makino *et al.*, 1973). It has been shown in Lewis rats, inoculated intranasally with Sendai virus, that draining lymph nodes of the upper respiratory tract are the initial and major site of antibody production. Development of serum immunoglobulin G (IgG) antibodies coincides with clearance of respiratory tract infection and recovery from viral infection (Liang *et al.*, 1999). Coinfection with other respiratory pathogens such as *Mycoplasma pulmonis*, CAR bacillus, *Pasteurella pneumotropica*, and pneumonia virus of mice (PVM) increases the severity of clinical disease and pulmonary lesions (Besch-Williford *et al.*, 1987; Carthew and Aldred, 1988).

Pathology After exposure, the initial tropism in the upper respiratory tract induces a rhinitis characterized by focal to diffuse necrosis of the epithelial cells, and a leukocytic infiltrate composed of neutrophils, lymphocytes, and plasma cells. Within the lungs there is a hyperplastic to suppurative bronchitis and focal alveolitis. Alveolar septa are hypercellular, with infiltrates of alveolar macrophages, neutrophils, and lymphocytes. Viral replication occurs in bronchial epithelial cells, type I and type II pneumocytes, and alveolar macrophages. Later, there is pronounced perivascular and peribronchial cuffing with a lymphocytic and plasmacytic infiltrate that may remain 7 months after the acute phase of the infection (Burek *et al.*, 1977; Percy and Barthold, 2007). Based upon experimental infection, lesion severity has been shown to be more severe in Brown Norway and LEW rats than in F-344 rats (Liang *et al.*, 1995; Sorden and Castleman, 1991).

Diagnosis Due to the low prevalence of clinical signs, diagnosis is best achieved by detection of antibodies to the virus and demonstration of typical lesions in the respiratory tract. The multiplex fluorescent immunoassay (MFI or MFIA; Hsu *et al.*, 2007; Wunderlich *et al.*, 2011) has replaced ELISA as the test of choice for diagnosis of Sendai virus infections in rats due to improved sensitivity and specificity and the requirement of much lower amounts of serum. In situations where confirmation is desired, IFAs or western blots can be used to confirm or refute MFI results. Moreover, PCR assays are now available for the diagnosis of active infections; trachea and lungs are preferred sites of sample collection.

Prevention and Control Prevention of Sendai virus introduction into an existing colony requires knowledge of the pathogen status of the source and, in some cases, quarantine with serological testing of incoming rats and mice. Regular and periodic serologic testing within colonies of rats and mice should be done to help prevent and control infection within rodent housing facilities. While the prevalence of infection is likely low in wild rats, the latter remain a potential source of infection if not appropriately controlled (Easterbrook *et al.*, 2008). Moreover, the use of Sendai virus as a research tool continues and these studies also serve as a source of potential infection. PCR testing should be done on all transplantable tumors, cell lines, and other biological materials to prevent transmission of Sendai virus from infected materials to recipient animals (Bauer *et al.*, 2004). Of note, Sendai virus is not readily detected in indirect sentinel monitoring of programs of mice (Artwohl *et al.*, 1994; Compton *et al.*, 2004). Thus sentinel programs may fail to detect this infection, but the limited transmission may also prevent inadvertent infection from wild rodents or experimental studies. If Sendai virus is introduced into a rat colony of immunocompetent rats, neutralizing antibody in infected rats renders the infection self-limiting. Accordingly, if antibody-naive rats are not introduced and if pregnant and preweanling rats are killed and breeding is halted, the virus will be eliminated from the colony within 4–8 weeks (Jacoby and Gaertner, 2006). This presumes that either all rats in the colony have been exposed, as might occur where rats are housed in open-top cages, or that all further interindividual transmission is prevented, so that no new infections occur during the clearing, or 'burnout' phase, which could perpetuate the infection.

Research Complications In addition to research complications associated with the respiratory tract tropisms of the virus, it may modulate some immunological responses, e.g., reducing the severity of adjuvant arthritis (Garlinghouse and Van Hoosier, 1978) and depressing T cell and thymocytotoxic autoantibody (Takeichi *et al.*, 1988).

b. Rat Coronavirus Infection

Etiology In the family *Coronaviridae*, the type species of the genus *Betacoronavirus* is *Murine coronavirus*. This species contains several distinct serotypes, including murine hepatitis virus and rat coronaviruses. The two prototype coronaviruses in rats are Parker's rat coronavirus (RCV-P) and sialodacryoadenitis virus (RCV-SDA). In addition to these two coronavirus strains, there are others that have been isolated and found to differ antigenically from either RCV-P or RCV-SDA. Historically, RCV-P and RCV-SDA were considered to induce two rather distinct sets of clinical signs and types of lesions in rats (Jacoby and Gaertner, 2006). More recently, however, the clinical signs, pathogenicity, and histological lesions are considered to be variable but similar for both RCV-P and RCV-SDA, and defining the neutralization group of a new RCV isolate is not useful in predicting its pathogenic potential (Compton *et al.*, 1999). Moreover, because these are highly mutable coronaviruses, field isolates may exhibit additional genetic and antigenic differences, but are likely capable of inducing a similar spectrum of disease. The antigenic differences between RCV-P and RCV-SDA are significant enough to allow cross-infection with either virus. Probably the most important point to be made from a clinical perspective is that neutralizing antibodies to one virus prototype will not offer significant cross protection from the other virus strain, thus allowing viral shedding and recurrence of clinical signs and lesions, albeit diminished (Percy and Barthold, 2007; Jacoby, 1986; Bihun and Percy, 1994; Kojima and Okaniwa, 1991; Weir *et al.*, 1990). However, with the low prevalence of these viruses in contemporary laboratory rat colonies, this scenario is unlikely to occur.

Epizootiology Rat coronaviruses are very contagious, with transfer to susceptible rats by direct contact with infected rats, and indirectly by aerosol and fomites (La Regina *et al.*, 1992). During outbreaks, morbidity is high, but mortality is very low (Percy and Barthold, 2007). Virus is present in target tissues for about 1 week after exposure, at which time heightened antibody levels render the infection self-limiting. However, immunity is not lifelong. Under experimental conditions, it has been shown that rats are susceptible to reinfection with a homologous strain as early as 6 months after initial infection and that such rats are able to transfer infection to naive rats by cage contact. However, the severity of lesions in reinfected rats is minimal compared with those associated with primary infections (Percy *et al.*, 1990; Weir *et al.*, 1990). Differences in pathogenicity have been reported among a few rat strains (Jacoby and Gaertner, 2006; Carthew and Slinger, 1981).

Clinical Signs Rat coronaviruses may induce either asymptomatic infections or transient clinical infections (sialodacryoadenitis) associated with tissue tropisms for the salivary glands, lacrimal glands, Harderian glands, and respiratory epithelium. There are two distinctive types of clinical disease associated with the virus. The first is associated with breeding colonies in which the virus is endemic with mature rats immune to infection, and in which clinical disease is primarily associated with preweanling, nonimmune animals that display ocular signs associated with conjunctivitis. These signs are transient, lasting for a week or less. The second type of clinical picture is associated with a sudden onset of clinical signs in naive postweanling-to-adult rats that have been exposed to infected rats. Signs include cervical swelling due to inflammation and edema of submaxillary salivary glands (Fig. 4.7), nasal and ocular discharges

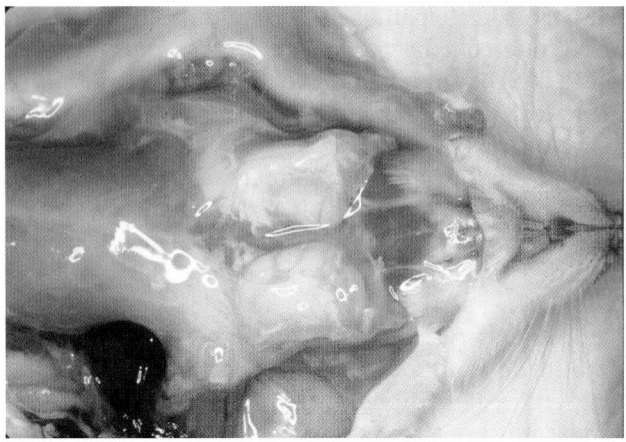

FIGURE 4.7   Edematous, swollen, and pale submaxillary salivary glands caused by coronaviral infection. *Courtesy of Dr. T. R. Schoeb.*

that are usually porphyrin stained, photophobia, corneal opacities, and corneal ulcers. In most animals, the signs last for less than 2 weeks. However, in some animals a chronic keratitis and megaloglobus may persist (Jacoby and Gaertner, 2006).

Pathology   The microscopic changes associated with rhinitis, tracheitis, and focal bronchitis during the acute stage of the disease include a mononuclear and polymorphonuclear cell infiltration, hyperplastic respiratory epithelia with loss of ciliated surfaces, and focal alveolitis. The lesions within the lower respiratory tract abate in about 7–10 days, and those in the nasopharynx remain somewhat longer (Percy and Barthold, 2007). Histological changes associated with sialodacryoadenitis (SDA) in affected salivary and lacrimal glands include coagulation necrosis of ductal and acinar epithelial cells during the acute stages of the disease, followed by squamous metaplasia during the reparative period that begins 7–10 days after infection. There is a mixed leukocyte infiltrate. Regeneration of the epithelial cells occurs in about 4 weeks postinfection. However, focal lesions may persist an additional several weeks in the Harderian glands.

Diagnosis   Once antibodies are produced, about 7 days after infection, diagnosis of rat coronavirus infection is best achieved by serology using the MFI method with confirmatory IFA or western blot testing when desired. During outbreaks, especially prior to seroconversion, histological examination of the Harderian glands and the submaxillary and parotid salivary glands may aid in diagnosis (Percy and Barthold, 2007) and PCR of the infected glands is useful in confirmation of active infections (Besselsen *et al.*, 2002; Compton and Riley, 2001). However, because the disease is often subclinical, typical signs associated with salivary gland and Harderian gland tropisms may not be useful.

Differential   Diagnosis   Differential diagnoses include *Mycoplasma* and Sendai virus infections, and stress-associated factors that induce chromodacryorrhea (Percy and Barthold, 2007). Due to its contagiousness, rat coronavirus is readily detectable by indirect sentinel programs.

Prevention and Control   Preventing transfer of this highly contagious coronavirus to naive colonies is predicated upon preventing entry of infected rats into a facility through knowledge of the pathogen status of vendor colonies and an effective quarantine program. Like most viral agents of rats, the prevalence of RCV in laboratory rats is declining markedly (Liang *et al.*, 2009; Livingston and Riley, 2003; Mahler and Kohl, 2009; McInnes *et al.*, 2011; Pritchett-Corning *et al.*, 2009; Schoondermark-van de Ven *et al.*, 2006). However, in one report, this agent was prevalent in wild rats, so effective control of the latter is of paramount importance (Easterbrook *et al.*, 2008). Control of infection within a colony or facility is based upon the fact that rats shed the virus for only about 1 week, after which they are immune and not latently infected. The virus is not transmitted vertically. Eliminating rat coronavirus from a colony is achieved by allowing the virus to spread quickly to all animals, preventing entry of susceptible rats to the room, and suspension of breeding and removal of preweanlings. The rapidity in which all animals will seroconvert and no longer shed the virus will determine the period of time needed before susceptible animals can be safely introduced or breeding resumed. In most instances, a 6- to 8-week period should be allowed (Jacoby and Gaertner, 2006). Alternatively, if suspension of breeding cannot be done, a method to continue breeding and eliminate SDA is to define a subset of the breeding colony that is seropositive and to relocate these breeding animals to a separate room, allow litters to be born in the original colony until the relocated breeders are in late gestation, and then kill all animals in the original colony (Brammer *et al.*, 1993).

Research Complications   Research complications associated with SDA reflect tropisms for the lacrimal and salivary glands, vomeronasal organ, and respiratory epithelium (Percy and Barthold, 2007). Exposure keratitis may also result from lack of tear production or exophthalmus associated with edema of Harderian glands. Except for long-term ocular lesions, research complications would be expected to be linked to the period of active infection and the 2- to 3-week reparative period. During this period, food intake frequently decreases if cervical swelling occurs. Rat coronavirus infection may also have unanticipated effects on ongoing studies as evidenced by impairment of nerve regeneration that occurred in during a recent outbreak (Yu *et al.*, 2011).

c. Rat Parvovirus Infection

Etiology Parvoviruses are single-stranded DNA viruses that have a predilection for mitotically active host cells. Parvoviruses that infect rats include (Kilham's) rat virus (RV), (Toolan's) H-1 virus, rat parvovirus (RPV), and rat minute virus (RMV). In the nomenclature proposed by the International Committee on Taxonomy of Viruses, all of these viruses, plus minute virus of mice and mouse parvovirus are merged into one species, *Rodent protoparvovirus 1*. The first two viruses were initially isolated from a transplantable tumor (RV) and a tumor cell line passed in rats (H-1). In the 1980s, testing of rat sera indicated the presence a parvovirus that was neither RV nor H-1. This virus, which was initially referred to as rat orphan parvovirus (OPV), is now designated rat parvovirus (RPV; Jacoby *et al.*, 1996). In 2002, three variants of another novel parvovirus, rat minute virus (RMV), were isolated from naturally infected rats (Wan *et al.*, 2002).

Epizootiology and Transmission Rat virus is excreted in urine and milk and is transmitted by aerosol through direct contact or fomites (Jacoby *et al.*, 1996). RV-contaminated bedding, stored at room temperature for up to 5 weeks, is capable of inducing seroconversion of rats for up to 5 weeks (Yang *et al.*, 1995). Rats may harbor and transmit RV long after seroconversion occurs, with the frequency of persistent infection during natural outbreaks (Gaertner *et al.*, 1996) and experimental infections (Ball-Goodrich *et al.*, 2001) being RV strain-dependent. After experimental inoculation of RV into neonatal rats, the virus persists in tissues for up to 14 weeks, and the duration of infectivity to cage contacts up to 10 weeks. Infection of pregnant females also results in persistent infection of progeny; however pups of persistently infected dams are protected, presumably by maternal antibody (Jacoby *et al.*, 2001). If weanling rats are inoculated, the duration of viral recovery and infectivity is decreased to 7 and 3 weeks, respectively (Paturzo *et al.*, 1987; Jacoby *et al.*, 1988). In persistent infections, DNA and antigenic evidence of RV is most likely to be observed in lymphoid tissues, endothelium, vascular muscle tunics, and renal tubular epithelium (Gaertner *et al.*, 1996; Jacoby *et al.*, 1991).

Clinical Signs Clinical signs associated with RV infection occur very sporadically in colonies showing serological evidence of infection and are usually seen only in preweanling animals. In such colonies, reduced litter size, runted litters, and fetal and neonatal death may be observed. Although subclinical infections in postweanling rats are the rule, an outbreak characterized by hemorrhage and necrosis of the brain, testes, and epididymides has been reported in young adult rats (Coleman *et al.*, 1983). The ability of RV to cross the placenta appears to depend on the virus strain, dose, and time of gestation. Resistance to lethal infection develops during the first postpartum week (Gaertner *et al.*, 1996; Jacoby *et al.*, 1988). Serological surveys of rat colonies have indicated that rat parvoviruses, especially RPV (Liang *et al.*, 2009; Livingston and Riley, 2003; Mahler and Kohl, 2009; McInnes *et al.*, 2011; Pritchett-Corning *et al.*, 2009; Schoondermark-van de Ven *et al.*, 2006; Clifford and Watson, 2008) are among the most prevalent viruses of contemporary research rat colonies; however, clinical disease is rarely reported. Natural infectious by H-1, RPV, and RMV have received very little study. To date, none have been associated with naturally occurring clinical disease, suggesting that they are primarily subclinical infections (Ball-Goodrich *et al.*, 1998; Wan *et al.*, 2002; Weisbroth *et al.*, 1998).

Pathology The correlation of age and RV pathogenicity is thought to be due to the decreased complement of target cells in the S-phase of division needed for productive infection. The immune status of the host is also significant to the outcome of RV infection. Immunocompetent adult rats mount a classic Th1 immune response that results in viral clearance (Ball-Goodrich *et al.*, 2002), whereas rat virus in athymic rats induces a more severe and persistent infection than in euthymic rats (Gaertner *et al.*, 1995, 1989).

Diagnosis Diagnosis of RV, RPV, RMV, and H-1 virus can be accomplished by serology. Serologic tests usually include recombinant capsid viral protein (VP2) antigens of each parvovirus along with a recombinant nonstructural protein (NS1) antigen. The latter is shared among parvoviruses so that animals infected with any parvovirus will seroconvert to this antigen. NS1-based tests thus represent a non-specific assay that provides confirmatory testing for the specific VP2-based assays (Besselsen *et al.*, 2008; Kunita *et al.*, 2006; Livingston *et al.*, 2002). PCR assays for RV, H-1, RPV and RMV have also been developed that provide a rapid, specific and sensitive means for detecting viral DNA in tissue (Besselsen *et al.*, 1995a, b), feces or the environment.

Research Complications Research complications induced by RV are associated with its tropism for mitotically active cells of fetuses, neonates, cell cultures, and tumors. Rat virus has been shown to modulate immune function through its tropism for T-cell lymphocytes (McKisic *et al.*, 1995). Rat virus infection in the diabetes-resistant BioBreeding rat increases the expression of macrophage cytokines, leading to an autoimmune diabetes (Chung *et al.*, 1997). The effect of RV on the immune system has been shown to be rat strain dependent for natural killer cell activity. Natural killer cell-mediated cytotoxicity is increased in Brown Norway rats, whereas it is decreased in Wistar–Furth rats (Darrigrand *et al.*, 1984).

The effects, if any, that naturally occurring RPV, H-1 or RMV infections may have on research are unknown.

d. Rat Theilovirus

There has long been suspicion that rats may harbor a host specific cardiovirus as evidenced by seroconversion to the closely related Theiler's murine encephalomyelitis virus (TMEV; genus *Cardiovirus* and species *Theilovirus*). Isolation of the MHG virus (McConnell *et al.*, 1964) and subsequently a virus designated NSG910 (Ohsawa *et al.*, 2003) from rats provided further evidence of distinct rat cardioviruses. In 2008, a novel rat theilovirus (RTV) was isolated from the feces of asymptomatic rats.

In immunocompetent rats, RTV replicates in enterocytes of the small intestine and following experimental inoculation, is shed for 4–8 weeks. No clinical signs have been associated with either experimental inoculation or natural infection, and the virus does not spread beyond the intestinal tract. While experimental intracranial inoculations with the MHG virus resulted in paralysis in suckling rats (McConnell *et al.*, 1964), this finding was not reproduced with RTV (Drake *et al.*, 2011). Differential strain susceptibility has been identified with experimentally infected SD rats from one vendor exhibiting prolonged fecal shedding and higher infectivity and seroconversion when compared to SD rats from another vendor. In contrast to immunocompetent rats, immunodeficient nude rats exhibit persistent fecal shedding and the virus can be found in extraintestinal sites. The latter findings suggest that adaptive immunity is important in elimination of this virus.

Infections with RTV are best diagnosed by serology. In addition, PCR tests are available for detection of active infections, with feces or intestine serving as optimal samples for testing (Drake *et al.*, 2011). Little is known about control of RTV infections, although measures employed for TMEV in mice are likely effective with RTV infections. In one report, a test and cull strategy was shown to be effective in eliminating the virus from a contaminated colony (Dyson, 2010). Serological surveys, including those that previously used TMEV as an antigen suggest that RTV is of low to moderate prevalence in contemporary research rat colonies (Liang *et al.*, 2009; Livingston and Riley, 2003; Mahler and Kohl, 2009; McInnes *et al.*, 2011; Pritchett-Corning *et al.*, 2009; Schoondermark-van de Ven *et al.*, 2006).

e. Pneumonia Virus of Mice Infection

Pneumonia virus of mice (Genus *Pneumovirus* and species *Murine pneumonia virus* (PVM) is a pneumovirus in the family *Paramyxoviridae*. Contrary to the virus's common name, serological evidence indicates infectivity in mice, rats, hamsters, gerbils, guinea pigs, and rabbits. The prevalence of seropositive rat colonies was reported in 1982 to exceed 50%; however, today serological evidence of PVM infection is rare to non-existent in rats (Liang *et al.*, 2009; Livingston and Riley, 2003; Mahler and Kohl, 2009; McInnes *et al.*, 2011; Pritchett-Corning

et al., 2009; Schoondermark-van de Ven *et al.*, 2006). Diagnosis is typically accomplished by serology. PCRs are also available for detection of active infections with trachea or lungs, the sites of infection, serving as optimal samples for testing. The virus does not cause clinical disease, but multifocal, nonsuppurative vasculitis and interstitial pneumonitis with necrosis are prominent lesions seen in the acute phase of the disease. These lesions persist for several weeks. Historically, the virus was considered to be a significant co-pathogen with other respiratory agents such as *Mycoplasma pulmonis*, and cross species transmission is a potential concern (Percy and Barthold, 2007).

f. Group B Rotavirus Infection

Diarrhea in suckling rats has been associated with a virus in the species *Rotavirus B*, from the genus *Rotavirus* and family *Reoviridae* (Eiden *et al.*, 1985). The authors who first reported this disease named it 'infectious diarrhea of infant rats' (Vonderfecht *et al.*, 1984) so it is sometimes referred to by the acronym, IDIR. Affected infant rats excreted feces that varied from liquid to being poorly formed, and the animals displayed erythema and bleeding of the perianal skin. Pathology associated with infection included small intestinal villous atrophy, villous epithelial necrosis, and syncytial cell formation. This same agent was found to be associated with diarrhea in humans and has been shown by enzyme immunoassay inhibition assay to be prevalent in children and adults. Human isolates were shown to induce diarrhea in infant rats (Eiden *et al.*, 1985; Vonderfecht *et al.*, 1985). This suggests that under nonexperimental conditions there may be cross-infectivity between humans and rats. Although the virus is not frequently included in screening panels, commercial serology and PCR assays are available. The prevalence is unknown but generally thought to be low.

g. Hantavirus Infection

Hantaviruses are enveloped RNA viruses of the genus *Hantavirus*, family *Bunyviridae*. Rodents serve as the natural reservoirs for hantaviruses, with each virus in the genus being associated with a specific rodent species. Hantavirus infections in rodents are characterized by being chronic and subclinical, with virus being shed persistently in the feces and urine. Hantaviruses pose as significant zoonotic agents. *Rattus norvegicus* is the natural host for the Seoul Hantavirus, causing hemorrhagic fever with renal syndrome (HFRS) in humans. Hantavirus has been isolated from wild rats in Baltimore and several other cities in the United States. One report cites evidence of human infection with a rat-associated Hantavirus (Childs *et al.*, 1988). Cotton rats, *Sigmodon hispidus*, are reservoirs for a Hantavirus that has induced Hantavirus pulmonary syndrome in individuals living in Florida (Hutchinson *et al.*, 1998). Transmission of Hantavirus from laboratory rats to laboratory personnel has been reported in Japan, Belgium, and the United Kingdom (Desmyter *et al.*, 1983; Lloyd *et al.*, 1984). In both reports, multiple cases occurred that resulted in hemorrhagic fever with renal syndrome.

h. Rat Respiratory Virus

'Rat Respiratory Virus' was a working name given to a putative viral agent thought to be the cause of idiopathic histiocytic pneumonia often seen in rats (Elwell and Mahler, 1997; Gilbert *et al.*, 1997; Slaoui *et al.*, 1998; Riley *et al.*, 1997). It is now known that these lesions are due to *Pneumocystis carinii* infection (Livingston *et al.*, 2011; Henderson *et al.*, 2012; see Section II.A.4. in this chapter).

i. Other Viral Infections

There are several rodent viruses for which there is serological evidence of infection in the rat, but for which there are negligible data demonstrating any clinical or pathological importance. These viruses include mouse adenovirus, reovirus 3, parainfluenza virus 3, and endogenous retroviruses (Kohn and Barthold, 1984; Percy and Barthold, 2007; National Research Council, 1991).

3. Parasitic Infections

a. Protozoa

Protozoa are of little consequence in laboratory rats in recent decades (National Research Council, 1991; Kohn and Barthold, 1984). There are several reasons for this. First, no spontaneous disease due to any naturally occurring enteric protozoa of laboratory rats has been reported. Second, parenteral infections are rare in laboratory rats because of absence of vectors. Third, there is almost universal use of high-quality diets, which are generally subjected to heat disinfection prior to use. The days of giving rats fresh produce have happily slipped into the past. Protozoa of potential significance in rodent facilities include *Encephalitozoon cuniculi* and two enteric flagellates, *Spironucleus muris* and *Giardia muris*, which may contribute to disease and alter immune responses in mice.

Toxoplasmosis is a zoonotic disease caused by *Toxoplasma gondii*. Toxoplasmosis in rats is usually subclinical. The definitive host is the domestic cat and other felids, which shed oocysts in the feces. Rats, like many other vertebrates, serve as intermediate hosts. Transmission to rats is via ingestion of cat feces. Ingestion of infected intermediate hosts might also horizontally transmit the infection, although it would not be expected as a mode of transmission in a well-managed rat colony. Infected rats can transmit *T. gondii* vertically, but only very poorly. Therefore, in order for a rat colony to remain infected with *T. gondii*, cat feces would need to be repeatedly introduced. As a result, *T. gondii* is an organism is of

little current significance in research facilities, and routine monitoring for toxoplasmosis in rats is not commonplace.

Numerous enteric flagellates have been reported in laboratory rats over the years, but none are of known significance. The most commonly seen are in the order Trichmonadida (trichomonads) or of the genera *Chilomastix* or *Hexamastix* (Pritchett-Corning *et al.*, 2009). The life-cycle of all flagellates and another common commensal protozoan, *Entamoeba muris*, is direct (Baker, 2007), with fecal–oral transmission. Trophozoites, the feeding form, are present in the gastroinestinal tract. Reproduction is asexual and produces resistant cyst forms, which are shed in the feces (Kunstyr, 1977).

Spironucleus muris colonizes mice, rats, and hamsters, where it inhabits glandular crypts and the lumen of the small intestine (Gruber and Osborne, 1979; Baker, 2007). Age-infection relationships have not been reported for rats but are probably similar to that of mice, in which animals under 6 weeks of age are more susceptible to infection. Transmission of cloned *S. muris* between rats and mice has been attempted (Schagemann *et al.*, 1990). An isolate from rats was not infective to hamsters, immunocompetent mice, or athymic nude mice. Similarly, rats were not persistently colonized by isolates from mice or hamsters.

Cysts of *S. muris* are resistant to drying (room temperature for 14 days), freezing (−20°C for 6 months), pH 2.2 for 1 day, or 0.1% glutaraldehyde for 1h (Kunstyr and Ammerpohl, 1978). *Spironucleus muris* infection is diagnosed by examination of wet mounts of duodenal scrapings of weanling rats. Phase-contrast microscopy is especially helpful in observing the trophozoites. Identification is usually based on the size, $3–4 \times 10–15\,\mu m$, and characteristic rolling motion of the flagellated trophozoites. Cysts may be observed in wet mounts or in fecal smears. These measure $4 \times 7\,\mu m$ and are reported to have a characteristic banded pattern (Kunstyr, 1977). Recently, a PCR for *S. muris* was developed that has superior sensitivity when compared to wet mounts or fecal smears (Jackson *et al.*, 2013).

Giardia spp. are ancient, with one of the most highly conserved genomes of all eukaryotes (Yu *et al.*, 1996, 1998; 1996). *Giardia* also has its own microbiota, including mycoplasma-like particles and bacteria (Feely *et al.*, 1988) and viruses (Tai *et al.*, 1991, 1996). *Giardia muris* colonizes a wide variety of mammalian hosts, including rats, mice, and hamsters (Baker, 2007). Trophozoites attach to the surface of intestinal epithelial cells via a surface membrane mannose-binding lectin and can occur via any point on the parasite surface (Inge *et al.*, 1988). Cysts stored in liquid feces have remained infective for at least 1 year (Craft, 1982).

No naturally occurring clinical disease has been reported in rats infected with *G. muris*. Experimental infection with *G. lamblia* and *G. duodenalis* has resulted in secretion of specific immunoglobulin A into bile (Loftness et al., 1984; Sharma and Mayrhofer, 1988a).

Giardiasis is diagnosed similarly to spironucleosis. Trophozoites, measuring 7–13 × 5–10 μm, have a characteristic piriform or teardrop shape, with a broad, rounded anterior tapering to a pointed posterior end. The trophozoites have a slight curvature toward the ventral side, which causes the motion of their multiple flagella to impart a rolling motion to the organisms in wet mounts (Baker, 2007). In stained preparations, the darkly stained dual nuclei are prominent. Two small, dark median bodies are also visible, immediately posterior to the nuclei. Cysts may also be identified on fecal smears or with fecal flotation methods. PCR tests with high sensitivity are also available for the diagnosis of G. muris.

Entamoeba muris is a nonpathogenic commensal amoeba of rats, mice, and hamsters (Baker, 2007). Trophozoites, measuring 8–30 μm in length, are found in wet-mount preparations of contents from the cecum and colon, where they feed on bacteria. Cysts 9–20 μm in diameter have eight nuclei and can be observed in feces.

Control measures in rats for all intestinal flagellates and Entamoeba muris are similar. Rederivation, either by cesarean section or by embryo transfer, is effective. Contaminated animal rooms should be thoroughly cleaned, then disinfected with chlorine dioxide solutions or other suitable disinfectants (Weaver and Wickramanayake, 2001), prior to repopulation introduction. All materials brought into the room, which may have had prior exposure to rodents or rodent feces should be autoclaved. All animals should be monitored for infection prior to introduction. This should include examination of rats of appropriate age, i.e., 3–6 weeks.

Treatment of animals to eliminate infection with intestinal flagellates has met with limited success. Metronidazole (Flagyl) or dimetridazole can be added to the drinking water but is ineffective against cysts in the environment. Other authors have reported success in eliminating Giardia spp., using metronidazole in rats and mice (Sharma and Mayrhofer, 1988b). Significantly, however, metronidazole has been shown to be carcinogenic in rats and mice (Koch-Weser and Goldman, 1980).

b. Nematodes

OXYURIASIS

Etiology   Three species of oxyurid nematodes (pinworms) – *Syphacia muris*, *S. obvelata*, and *Aspiculuris tetraptera* – occur in the laboratory rat. Their continued prevalence (Liang et al., 2009; Livingston and Riley, 2003; McInnes et al., 2011, Pritchett-Corning et al., 2009, Schoondermark-van de Ven et al., 2006, Clifford and Watson, 2008), despite the dramatic progress in eliminating viral and bacterial pathogens, is due both to the persistence of the eggs in the environment and to the low degree of attention paid to these parasites.

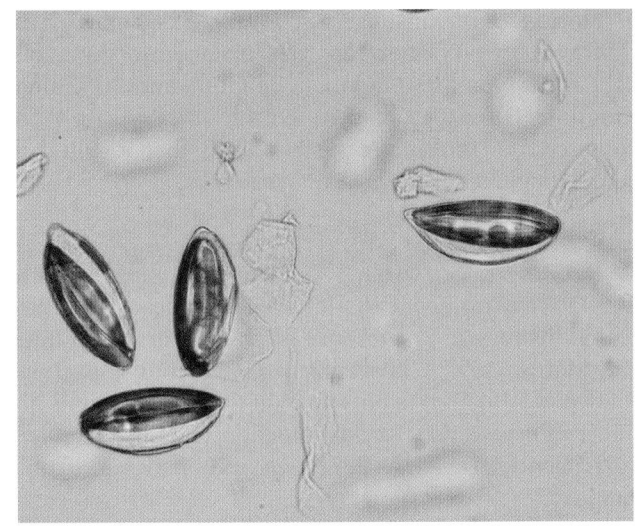

FIGURE 4.8   *Syphacia muris* ova.

Syphacia muris is the most common oxyurid of the rat (Liang et al., 2009; Livingston and Riley, 2003; Pritchett-Corning et al., 2009). *Syphacia obvelata* is more frequently found in mice, hamsters, and gerbils but is also occasionally found in the rat, especially when housed in the same room with infested mice. The morphology of adults of both S. muris and S. obvelata is similar, although S. muris is slightly smaller and the male has a longer tail, measured as a proportion of body width (Baker, 2007). Eggs vary more markedly between the species, with eggs of S. muris being 72–82 × 25–36 μm and those of S. obvelata being 118–153 × 33–55 μm. In addition, the eggs of S. obvelata are almost completely flat along one side, whereas those of S. muris are only slightly flattened on one side (Fig. 4.8).

Adult A. tetraptera are readily recognized by the four alae present at the anterior end of the body (Fig. 4.9). Eggs of A. tetraptera are approximately the same size as S. muris eggs, measuring 89–93 × 36–42 μm, and are bilaterally symmetrical.

Epizootiology and Transmission   Syphacia spp. have a direct life-cycle, requiring 11–15 days for completion (Baker, 2007). Transmission is horizontal via ingestion of eggs. Eggs, which remain viable at room conditions for weeks to months, are deposited around the anus and in the colon and become infective in approximately 6 h. They are ingested during self-cleaning and hatch in the small intestine. The larvae then mature in the cecum in 10–11 days. *Aspiculuris tetraptera* is also transmitted horizontally by ingestion of eggs, which are extremely persistent in the environment (Baker, 2007). The direct life-cycle is longer than that of *Syphacia*, requiring 23–25 days. Also unlike in *Syphacia*, *Aspiculuris* eggs are passed in the feces and are not deposited around the anus.

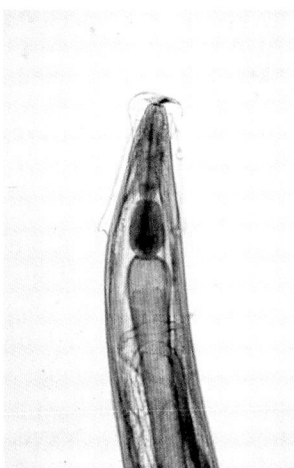

FIGURE 4.9 *Aspiculuris tetraptera* adult pinworm. Note that the prominent cervical alae extend all the way to the level of the pharyngeal bulb.

Clinical Signs and Pathology Rats infected with pinworms are generally asymptomatic. Gross lesions of oxyuriasis are very rare (Baker, 2007), and histologic lesions of oxyuriasis have not been reported.

Diagnosis Diagnosis of oxyuriasis is most practically accomplished by direct examination of macerated cecum and colon under low magnification with a stereomicroscope. This is almost as sensitive as complete direct examination of the large bowel and is significantly less time-consuming. Examination for eggs must be tailored to the infesting species suspected. The perianal tape test is effective only for *Syphacia* spp., and fecal flotation or fecal concentration and centrifugation is effective for *A. tetraptera* (Parkinson *et al.*, 2011). Screening for oxyurid eggs is significantly less sensitive than direct examination of the bowel for the adult helminths (Klement *et al.*, 1996; West *et al.*, 1992), although as a posttreatment diagnostic tool, perianal tape testing was found to be highly sensitive for *S. muris* infection (Hill *et al.*, 2009). For optimal diagnostics, use of more than one diagnostic method is recommended (Effler *et al.*, 2008). Recently, PCR assays have been developed, which add a highly sensitive methodology for detection of these agents (Feldman and Bowman, 2007; Parel *et al.*, 2008; Parkinson *et al.*, 2011). Because pinworm transmission to sentinel animals may be delayed, PCR testing may be particularly amenable to health monitoring programs as it allows for easy testing of colony animals.

Prevention and Control Several anthelmintics, including fenbendazole (Barlow *et al.*, 2005; Coghlan *et al.*, 1993; Huerkamp *et al.*, 2000, 2004), ivermectin (Zenner, 1998; Sueta *et al.*, 2002) new generation avermectins (Oge *et al.*, 2000; Sevimli *et al.*, 2009) and levamisole (Ince *et al.*, 2010) have been shown to eliminate pinworms in mice or rats when administered through a variety of routes (reviewed in Pritchett and Johnston (2002)). However, some treatments such as topical selemectin and diet-delivered moxidectin have been ineffective (Gonenc *et al.*, 2006; Hill *et al.*, 2006; Oge *et al.*, 2000). Fenbendazole-medicated feed is perhaps the most common therapeutic because of its ovacidal, larvacidal, and adulticidal properties and the ease of use; ivermectin is not ovicidal (Pritchett and Johnston, 2002). However, when treating rats for pinworms, consideration should be given to potential effects of the anthelmintic. Ivermectin has known deleterious effects (reviewed in Pritchett and Johnston (2002)) whereas fenbendazole is considered either inconsequential or potentially detrimental to ongoing studies (Barron *et al.*, 2000; Cray *et al.*, 2008, 2013; Duan *et al.*, 2012; Gao *et al.*, 2008; Hunter *et al.*, 2007b; Landin *et al.*, 2009; Vento *et al.*, 2008; Villar *et al.*, 2007). Because ova can readily contaminate and persist in the environment (Lytvynets *et al.*, 2013), decontamination of the latter may also be warranted. Heat, ethylene oxide formaldehyde gas, and chlorine dioxide with or without didecyl di-methyl ammonium chloride have been shown to be effective, while potassium peroxysulphate, alcohol/chlorhexidine, and ultraviolet light were not (Dix *et al.*, 2004). Of note, treatment failures have occurred, but these likely involved lack of consideration of biology and risk factors associated with re-infection (Huerkamp *et al.*, 2004). Oxyuriasis can also be eliminated by rederivation and is readily excluded by proper adherence to modern practices of barrier room technology (Hasslinger and Wiethe, 1987).

Research Complications Numerous research effects of oxyuriasis have been described. In rats, oxyuriasis has been reported to interfere with adjuvant arthritis (Pearson and Taylor, 1975), growth rate (Wagner, 1988), intestinal electrolyte transport (Lubcke *et al.*, 1992), cardiac reactivity to b-adrenergic stimulation (Silveira *et al.*, 2003) and the immune response to allergic sensitization (Demirturk *et al.*, 2007). In other studies, infections have had no deleterious effects (Carlberg and Lang, 2004).

TRICHOSOMOIDES CRASSICAUDA

Etiology This trichurid nematode is found only in the rat (Baker, 2007). Although geographically widespread, *Trichosomoides crassicauda* is virtually nonexistent in barrier-maintained rodents that have been rederived by cesarean section or embryo transfer. Adult females, approximately 10mm long, live in the urinary bladder, either free in the lumen or embedded in the mucosa (Baker, 2007; Antonakopoulos *et al.*, 1991; Cornish *et al.*, 1988). The males are anatomically degenerate and exist symbiotically in the vagina or uterus of the females.

Clinical Signs Infestation with *T. crassicauda*, although persistent, is usually clinically inapparent (Baker, 2007). Usually very few worms, perhaps averaging three in number (Barthold, 1996b), are present in the bladder, where they cause mild uroepithelial hyperplasia (Antonakopoulos *et al.*, 1991; Zubaidy and Majeed, 1981). When found in the renal pelvis, they are associated with mild pyelitis and pyelonephritis.

Epizootiology Embryonated eggs are laid and pass in the urine. Transmission of *T. crassicauda* is via ingestion of these eggs and probably occurs from dam to pups prior to weaning. The eggs hatch in the stomach, where the larvae penetrate the wall and pass through the peritoneal cavity or bloodstream to reach the lungs and other tissues. Most larvae lodge in tissues other than the kidneys and may cause hemorrhages or granulomas. Only those that reach the kidney or bladder survive and develop to maturity. The entire life-cycle is 8–9 weeks, so eggs are not present in the urine until the rats are 8–12 weeks of age.

Pathology Early speculation concerning the possible etiologic role of *T. crassicauda* infestation in causing bladder tumors in a famous study in rats that were administered high doses of saccharin in the diet (Anonymous, 1977; Homburger, 1977) has not been supported by later investigators (Barthold, 1996b). However, proliferative changes in uroepithelium caused by *T. crassicauda* infestation are identical to those produced early in carcinogenesis by chemical compounds such as *N*-methylnitrosourea (MNU) (Pauli *et al.*, 1996).

Diagnosis *Trichosomoides crassicauda* infestation is diagnosed in live rats by filtration of urine and then examination of the filter medium for the eggs. Diagnosis in recently killed rats is by direct examination of the bladder wall, histopathology, scanning electron microscopy, or microscopic examination of cryostat sections stained with acridine orange (Barthold, 1996b; Cornish *et al.*, 1988). The last two methods are purported to be more reliable but are probably not practical for routine, large-scale screening.

Prevention and Control Treatment for *T. crassicauda* infestation has been reported, using a single dose of ivermectin (Summa *et al.*, 1992). Follow-up found that the infestation was not eliminated in one of 30 rats, perhaps because of reinfection. Once a colony is free of this parasite, however, there should be little chance of reintroduction if no infected rats enter the colony.

Research Complications No confirmed research effects of *T. crassicauda* infestation have been reported in the scientific literature, although proliferative changes in the urothelium would render these animals unsuitable for research involving the urinary system (Cohen *et al.*, 1998).

c. Cestodes

Etiology There are only two adult cestodes that are likely to be encountered in laboratory rats: *Rodentolepis nana* (also often referred to as *Hymenolepis nana*) and *Hymenolepis diminuta*. The primary differences of

consequence between the two species are that *R. nana* is zoonotic and can have a direct life-cycle, whereas *H. diminuta* always has an indirect life-cycle, utilizing an intermediate host, and is not zoonotic. Although not uncommon in wild rats (Easterbrook *et al.*, 2008), both are rare in laboratory rats (Livingston and Riley, 2003).

Rodentolepis nana averages 20–40 mm long but can vary greatly. It is slender and less than 1 mm wide. The scolex has four suckers, and a rostellum armed with 20–27 hooks (Fig. 4.10). Mature proglottids are trapezoidal and contain as many as 200 eggs, which are thin-shelled, oval, and colorless and have six visible polar filaments. Within the eggs, the embryo, or oncosphere, has three pairs of hooklets within an inner envelope (Fig. 4.11). The eggs are approximately 30–56 × 44–62 μm and do not persist for long periods outside the host.

Hymenolepis diminuta is larger than *H. nana*, 20–60 mm long and 3–4 mm wide. The scolex of *H. diminuta* also has four suckers but the rostellum is unarmed – it has no hooks. Eggs of *H. diminuta* are 60–88 × 52–81 μm, and the oncosphere has three pairs of hooks, but no polar filaments.

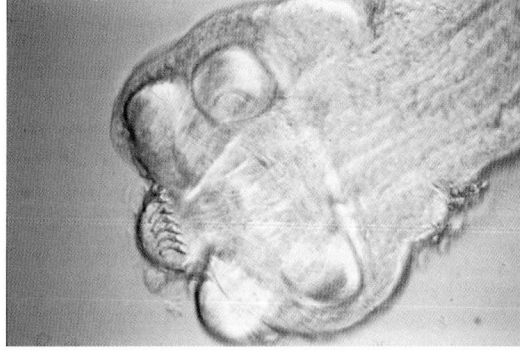

FIGURE 4.10 *Rodentolepis (Hymenolepis) nana* adult tapeworm. Note the rostellum armed with hooks.

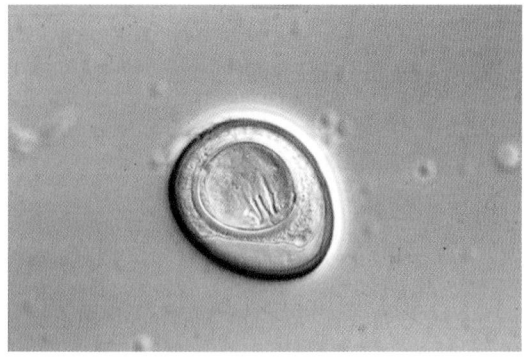

FIGURE 4.11 *Rodentolepis (Hymenolepis) nana* ova. Note the hooklets.

In addition to the adult cestodes, one may occasionally encounter larvae of *Taenia taeniaformis*, also called cysticercus fasciolaris. The cysts are found in the livers of rats, mice, and hamsters and are up to several centimeters in diameter. They are readily identified by the presence in the cyst of a scolex, strobila, and bladder (Hsu, 1979). Although considered nonpathogenic (Baker, 2007), the cyst may be associated with the development of hepatic sarcomas, probably in a mechanism similar to the induction of sarcomas in the rat by a variety of foreign bodies (Altman and Goodman, 1979; Elcock *et al.*, 2001). Because the definitive host is the cat, detection of the cysticercus is evidence that materials in the animals' immediate environment, usually feed, were contaminated with unsterilized feces from an infected cat. Control, therefore, is simple.

Epizootiology   *Rodentolepis nana* lives in the small intestine of rats, mice, hamsters, and primates, including humans. It is primarily the ability to parasitize humans that gives *R. nana* significance, for it causes little damage in rats or mice. Furthermore, it is not clear whether or not human infestations represent infestation with distinct strains, i.e., whether or not the strains of *R. nana* present in rats are infective for humans (Baker, 2007). In the direct life-cycle (Hsu, 1979), which requires 14–16 days, embryonated eggs are ingested and hatch in the small intestine. The oncospheres penetrate villi and develop into cysticercoid larvae in 4–5 days. These larvae reenter the lumen, the scolex evaginates, and they attach to the mucosa. An additional 10–12 days are required before mature proglottids are formed. Adults live only a few weeks. Infection normally results in some level of immunity, which prevents autoinfection. When autoinfection occurs, eggs hatch in the small intestine and develop, without being passed in the feces, and can result in very high worm burdens. In the indirect life-cycle, grain beetles (*Tenebrio molitor* and *T. obscurus*) and fleas (*Pulex irritans*, *Ctenocephalus canis*, *Xenopsylla cheopis*) serve as intermediate hosts. Rats and other definitive hosts are infected by ingesting the intermediate host.

Hymenolepis diminuta has a similar host range: mice, rats, hamsters, and primates, including humans (Hsu, 1979). The life-cycle of *H. diminuta* is always indirect and is similar to the indirect life-cycle of *R. nana*.

Clinical Signs   Both *Rodentolepis nana* and *Hymenolepis diminuta* are pathogenic in rats only in severe infections, where retarded growth, weight loss, impaction, and death have been reported in the older literature (Hsu, 1979), although no recent reports excluding the contributions of other potential pathogens have been published.

Pathology   Although presence of the parasites can be identified during gross examination or microscopically in tissue sections, there are no associated significant lesions.

Diagnosis   Infection is diagnosed by detection of the adult cestodes on direct examination of the small intestine, by observation of the eggs in feces (smear or fecal flotation), or by histopathologic detection of cysticercoids or adults in the small intestine (Hsu, 1979). Infection is most common in recently weaned rats and young adults, probably because of acquired immunity in older animals.

Prevention and Control   *Rodentolepis nana* and *H. diminuta* infection is prevented by purchase of clean stocks of rodents, by adequate disinfection of barrier room supplies, and thorough insect control and exclusion of wild rodents (Baker, 2007). Treatment of infected animals is not generally recommended, because of the zoonotic implications of this disease.

Research Complications   Experimentally, *H. diminuta* has been shown to elicit a host Th2 type immune response (McKay, 2010; Starke and Oaks, 2001; Webb *et al.*, 2007) that may modulate models of intestinal and extraintestinal disease (Graepel *et al.*, 2013; Hunter *et al.*, 2005, 2007a; Reardon *et al.*, 2001). However, inadvertent interference of research has been not been reported likely because of the rarity of hymenolepiasis in rat research colonies.

d. Trematodes

Numerous trematodes have been reported in wild rats, including *Plagiorchis muris*, *P. philippinensis*, and *P. javensis*. Some are zoonotic (Hong *et al.*, 1996), but none are significant in laboratory rats and trematodes are not even addressed in some texts (Baker, 2007).

e. Mites

FUR MITES

Etiology   *Radfordia ensifera* is the fur mite most likely to be encountered in laboratory rats, although other fur mites, such as *Radfordia affinis* or *Myobia musculi*, could possibly be harbored on the pelage (Fig. 4.12).

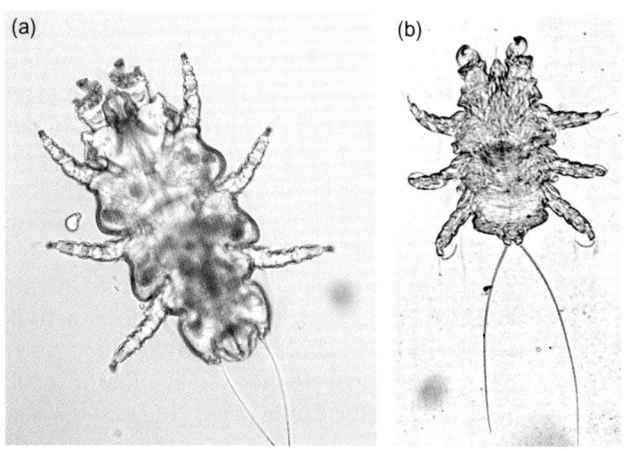

FIGURE 4.12 Adult fur mites. *Radfordia ensifera* (a) and *Myobia musculi* (b).

Epizootiology   Fur mites are transmitted by eggs, which can persist in the environment for long periods. The eggs hatch in 7–8 days, and females can begin to lay eggs after another 16 days.

Clinical Signs   Infestation can result in pruritus, self-excoriation, and secondary bacterial infection.

Diagnosis   A number of diagnostic methods for the detection of fur mites have been developed including fur plucks, tape tests, and skin scrapes which can be used on live animals and examination of cooled rats or pelts using a dissecting microscope; the latter may be aided by placing the animal or pelt on a black background. Because mites or eggs may be found on different parts of the body (Metcalf Pate *et al.*, 2011; Ricart Arbona *et al.*, 2010b), examination of several sites is recommended. Studies comparing sensitivity of various assays have been performed in mice (Metcalf Pate *et al.*, 2011) but are likely applicable to rats. Recently, PCR assays have been developed that show superior sensitivity to traditional techniques (Karlsson *et al.*, 2014; Parkinson *et al.*, 2011; Rice *et al.*, 2013; Weiss *et al.*, 2012; Jensen *et al.*, 2013). These assays are also useful in assessment of posttreatment efficacy although animal environmental samples may remain positive for several weeks (Rice *et al.*, 2013). Of note, detection of fur mites using indirect sentinel monitoring programs has met with mixed success in mice (Lindstrom *et al.*, 2011; Ricart Arbona *et al.*, 2010b).

Prevention and Control   Several fur mite treatments have been developed in mice that are likely applicable to rats. Compounds used include topical selemectin alone (Gonenc *et al.*, 2006) or in conjunction with amitraz- and fipronil-treated nestlets (Bornstein *et al.*, 2006), topical moxidectin (Mook and Benjamin, 2008; Pollicino *et al.*, 2008; Pullium *et al.*, 2005), and ivermectin (administered topically or in food or water) with or without cross fostering (Conole *et al.*, 2003; Huerkamp *et al.*, 2005; Ricart Arbona *et al.*, 2010c). As with pinworm treatment, consideration should be given to possible effects of the treatment. For example, although uncommon, ivermectin has been associated with neurologic clinical signs in mice being treated for mite infestations (Ricart Arbona *et al.*, 2010a). Of note, there are numerous anecdotal reports of infection recurrence, thus animals should be monitored regularly to ensure effective treatment. Infestation can also be eliminated by rederivation and is readily excluded by proper adherence to modern practices of barrier room technology.

Research Complications   In mice, fur mite infestation has been associated with increased mitotic activity in the skin, immunologic alterations, amyloidosis and a Th2 immune response that results in elevation of serum IgE (Pochanke *et al.*, 2006; Roble *et al.*, 2012).

Other Mites   Rats may also be infested with the mesostigmatid mites, *Ornithonyssus bacoti* (the tropical rat mite) and *Laelaps echidnina* (Watson, 2008). Unlike fur mites, these are blood-sucking mites that live in the environment and are only found on the rat during periods of feeding. Clinical signs may range from none to anemia and debility with severe infestations. These mites can also carry a number of rodent pathogens. Moreover, they will bite humans and can carry several zoonotic diseases. Suspicion of mesostigmatid mite infestation often arises when animal care personnel are bitten. Diagnosis may be achieved by direct observation of blood engorged mites on rats or in the environment. Mites may also be found in sticky insect traps, although the latter may lack sensitivity as a sole diagnostic tool (Watson, 2008). Elimination of mites must include treatment of both animals and environment. Treatments reported to be effective include permethrin-impregnated cotton balls for mice and pyrethrin permethrin or dichlorvos treatment of the environment (Cole *et al.*, 2005; Hill *et al.*, 2005; Watson, 2008; Chu and Couto, 2005).

f. Lice

Pediculosis in the laboratory rat is currently rare and is attributed to only one species, *Polyplax spinulosa* (Baker, 2007). *Polyplax spinulosa* females are approximately 0.6–1.5 mm long; females are larger than males. Like all insects, they have six legs (Fig. 4.13). The female lays eggs, called nits, which are cemented to hairs. The eggs have a distinct operculum, with a row of pores near the operculated end. The eggs hatch by a pneumatic mechanism in 5–6 days; the larvae ingest air through the pores, pass it through the body, and then use that pressure to force open the operculum (Owen, 1992). The young nymphs are paler than the yellow–brown adults but are morphologically similar. After three ecdyses, or molts, they become adults. Depending on environmental conditions, the ecdyses require 1–3 weeks. The entire life-cycle is completed in 2–5 weeks. Adults live only 25–28 days. Transmission is by direct contact (Baker, 2007).

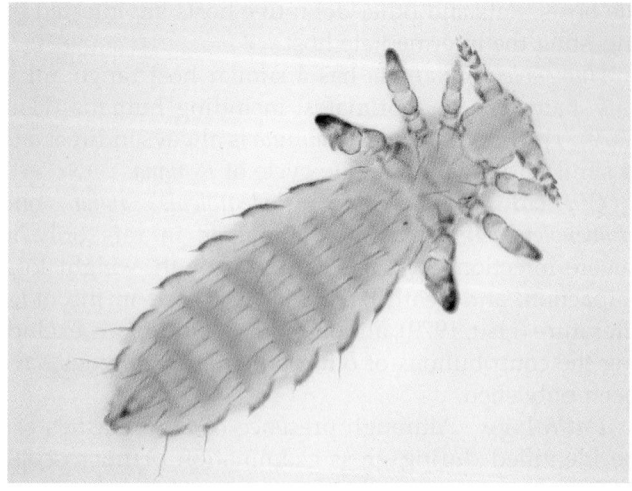

FIGURE 4.13   *Polyplax spinulosa* adult louse.

Pediculosis is usually inapparent, although heavily parasitized animals may appear unthrifty and pruritic. *Polyplax spinulosa* is also the vector of *Mycoplasma haemomuris* and other pathogens (Baker, 2007). Diagnosis is by direct examination of the pelt for adults, nymphs, and eggs (Baker, 2007). Any time that infestation with *P. spinulosa* is detected, blood smears should be screened for *Haemobartonella muris*.

Pediculosis is prevented by introducing only animals free of the condition. Insecticides approved for use in veterinary medicine may be used effectively to treat infestations, as may subcutaneous administration of ivermectin (Baker, 2007), but would probably be advisable only in especially valuable rats in the absence of significant intercurrent infections.

4. Fungal Infections

a. Pneumocystis Carinii

Etiology   *Pneumocystis carinii* is classified as a fungus based upon DNA base sequences in genes encoding ribosomal RNAs (Stringer, 1993). Our understanding of pneumocystosis in rats has changed significantly in the last few years. *P. carinii* causes a host-specific infection (rats only) with two distinct diseases seen in immunodeficient vs. immunocompetent rats.

Epizootiology and Transmission   *Pneumocystis carinii* is naturally acquired by rats through airborne transmission (Hughes, 1982) or possibly by fomites such as soiled bedding (Albers *et al.*, 2009).

Disease Presentation in Immunodeficient Rats   In rats with impaired immunity, such as athymic nude rats, the organism proliferates uncontrolled within the lung, filling alveoli and resulting in dyspnea, wasting and death (Pohlmeyer *et al.*, 1993; Deerberg *et al.*, 1993). In addition to the foamy material comprising trophozoites, phospholipids, macrophages, and debris filling aveoli, the infection in nude rats was also noted to have interstitial and perivascular lymphocytic infiltration. The abundant organisms in these cases are usually easily identified by special stains such as methenamine silver that demonstrate the fungal cysts within the alveoli and bronchioles. Rats which are immunocompromised by various methods are also susceptible to this form of infection and have been used as a model of *P. jirovecii* pneumonitis that occurs in some human patients with uncontrolled HIV infections (Oz and Hughes, 1996).

Disease Presentation in Immunocompetent Rats   *P. carinii* is also prevalent in immunocompetent rats, where it has been shown to cause the interstitial pneumonia that had been previously informally referred to as 'Rat Respiratory Virus, RRV' (Livingston *et al.*, 2011; Henderson *et al.*, 2012). In immunocompetent rats, lesions occur following infection, regardless of the age of the rats. *P. carinii* has a slow doubling time, estimated at 4.5 days (Aliouat *et al.*, 1999), and does not appear to incite a host response until a population density threshold is reached. At that point, lesions begin to be visible and specific antibodies are produced. Thereafter, the population of *P. carinii* diminishes and the infection is eventually cleared. It is noteworthy that even at peak population, the number of organisms present is magnitudes less than the population densities achieved in immunodeficient rats. The lower population density may explain the difficulty in finding *Pneumocystis* cysts using special stains in infected immunocompetent rats, although diligent searching of multiple sections may eventually be fruitful.

Pathology   Gross lesions of *P. carinii* infection become visible in 50% or more of infected rats 4–5 weeks after infection, and have been observed in many strains, suggesting that all strains and stocks of rats are probably susceptible. At necropsy, red–brown or tan lesions are scattered throughout the lung in a pattern typical of interstitial pneumonia. These lesions may be resolved after another 8–12 weeks. Microscopically, the lesions are characteristic enough they were reported as diagnostic for this disease (Albers *et al.*, 2009) and this has been supported by subsequent molecular diagnosis (Henderson *et al.*, 2012). Microscopic lesions will occur in 50–100% of infected rats and are typically characterized as lymphohistiocytic interstitial pneumonia. In *Pneumocystis* interstitial pneumonia in immunocompetent rats, alveolar septa are thickened with macrophages and lymphocytes, and alveoli contain macrophages, lymphocytes, and debris. Multinucleated giant cells may occasionally be present, and slight interstitial hemorrhage is common. Eosinophils and/or neutrophils are occasionally present but not a useful diagnostic criterion. The other hallmark of the histopathologic appearance is perivascular lymphocyte cuffing (Fig. 4.14). Bands, or cuffs, of macrophages

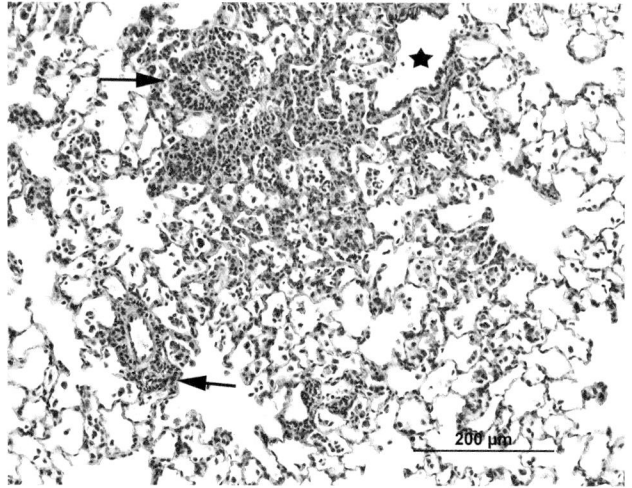

FIGURE 4.14   Photomicrograph of rat lung with interstitial pneumonia due to *Pneumocystis carinii*. Note the bands, or cuffs, of lymphocytes and macrophages encircling interstitial vessels (black arrows). Alveolar septa are thickened. Bronchioles (black star) are much less affected than the vessels.

and lymphocytes encircle interstitial arteries when the first lesions of interstitial pneumonia are observed. Over the next few weeks, lymphocytes come to predominate, and these lymphoid cuffs will persist after the infiltrates in the alveoli and septa have resolved. Increased BALT is not considered to be a major component of the lesions.

Diagnosis The diagnosis in immunocompetent rats may be made provisionally based on the characteristic histologic lesions, although it is recommended to confirm it with PCR on lung tissue. Special stains such as methenamine silver may demonstrate the fungal cysts within the alveoli. Screening of groups of rats for *P. carinii* may be accomplished by serology or by PCR. Rats will produce antibodies by approximately 6–8 weeks after infection and will remain antibody positive for life. Lung tissue is the best sample for PCR, bronchial wash is somewhat less sensitive (perhaps because of the relatively low population density of the fungus), nasal samples may occasionally be positive, and oral swabs are ineffective (Henderson *et al.*, 2012).

Differential diagnosis. The characteristic lymphohistiocytic interstitial pneumonia must be differentiated from bronchial or bronchiolar inflammation as observed with *Mycoplasma pulmonis*, CAR bacillus, Sendai virus and coronavirus.

Research Complications The impact of *P. carinii* infection on research using immunocompetent rats has not been well-explored, although it has been a confounding factor in inhalation studies (Gilbert *et al.*, 1997). In addition, because of its high prevalence and the fact that it results in observable pulmonary inflammation, it might be a differential diagnosis to consider in instances where unexpected pulmonary or cardiopulmonary results are observed.

b. *Encephalitozoon cuniculi*

Etiology *Encephalitozoon cuniculi*, is a microsporidian fungal parasite of a wide variety of mammalian hosts, including rodents, lagomorphs, carnivores, and primates, including humans. It has also been reported in birds (Poonacha *et al.*, 1985; Reetz, 1993). Resistance to infection and the outcome of infection are dependent on T-cell function, which is strain dependent (Liu *et al.*, 1989; Niederkorn *et al.*, 1981). Athymic nude mice, and presumably athymic nude rats, are more susceptible to lethal infection than are euthymic animals. *Encephalitozoon cuniculi* has also been recovered from transplantable ascites tumors in rats (Petri, 1969).

Epizootiology and Transmission Encephalitozoonosis is occasionally found in conventional rabbit colonies, but is rare in rats. It is transmitted by ingestion, and possibly inhalation, of spores shed in urine (Wilson, 1979). Vertical transmission has been proposed in primates, foxes, mice, rabbits, and guinea pigs but not in rats (Boot *et al.*, 1988; Liu *et al.*, 1988).

Clinical Signs Clinical signs and gross lesions of *E. cuniculi* infection are not reported in rats.

Pathology On histopathologic examination (Majeed and Zubaidy, 1982), rats with *E. cuniculi* infection may have nonsuppurative or granulomatous meningoencephalitis in any or all parts of the brain and occasionally the spinal cord. Interstitial nephritis may also be observed. Less frequently, similar lesions may be observed in other tissues. Spores may be observed in, or more frequently adjacent to, any of the lesions. Spores stain poorly with hematoxylin and eosin but are strongly gram-positive.

Diagnosis Diagnosis of *E. cuniculi* infection is usually based on serology (Pakes *et al.*, 1984). Screening of colonies by serology is probably the most efficient method, because infected colonies normally have a high prevalence (Gannon, 1980). As with all serologic assays, positive serologic results should be confirmed by a second method or by repeating the assay on groups of animals to establish a pattern of positive results. Histopathologic observation of the organism is definitive as is the detection of *E. cuniculi* DNA by PCR; kidney, urine and brain are preferred sampling sites for the latter.

Differential Diagnosis The primary histopathologic differential diagnosis for *E. cuniculi* infection in rats is toxoplasmosis, which is very rare. *Encephalitozoon cuniculi* measures $1 \times 2\,\mu m$, stains well with Gram stain and poorly with hematoxylin and eosin. *Toxoplasma gondii* measures $2 \times 4\,\mu m$, stains well with hematoxylin and eosin, and poorly with Gram stain (Wilson, 1979).

Prevention and Control Encephalitozoonosis is controlled by purchasing only animals that are free of *Encephalitozoon* and by maintaining them away from infected animals. There is currently no effective treatment.

Research Complications Research complications of *E. cuniculi* infections have not been reported in rats, although it is potentially a confounding factor if histopathologic evaluation of the central nervous system and kidney is part of the study (Majeed and Zubaidy, 1982).

c. Other Fungal Infections

Other fungal infections in the rat have been infrequently reported and are associated with predisposing factors that reduce immunocompetence. In one report, about one-fifth of Wistar rats on a 2-year carcinogenesis study had chronic rhinitis associated with *Aspergillus fumigatus* (Rehm *et al.*, 1988). The predisposing factor in these animals was thought to be Sendai virus infection; Sendai is currently very rare. Clinical signs included sniffing and nasal exudation. At necropsy, yellowish, friable material was present either unilaterally or bilaterally in the nasal cavities, and in the most severe cases, the nasal cavities were completely blocked. The *A. fumigatus*-induced rhinitis was, in most cases, limited to the naso- and maxilloturbinates. A bronchial abscess containing hyphae and multiple fruiting heads occurred in one rat.

Tracheobronchial aspergillosis was reported in an aged F-344 rat with concomitant large granular-cell leukemia. Immunodeficiency due to the leukemia was thought to be involved with the multifocal, transmural necrotic lesions of the trachea and bronchi (Hubbs et al., 1991).

Royals et al. (Royals et al., 1999) reported two cases of fungal-induced rhinitis in rats that had no known immunosuppression. Corncob and hardwood bedding from two sources were tested to determine if the source of the Aspergillus infection was bedding material. A range of 700–5400 fungal spores per gram of nonautoclaved corncob bedding was found. Six genera of fungi (Cladosporidium, Acremonium, Penicillium, Aspergillus, Fusarium, and Scolobasidium) were isolated from the samples of corncob bedding, whereas only negligible counts were isolated from hardwood bedding samples. The authors suggested that either the use of autoclaved or γ-irradiated corncob bedding should be considered as a means to eliminate fungal contamination of bedding.

Dermatomycosis (ringworm) due to Trichophyton mentagrophytes has been reported in wild and laboratory rats. However, it has not been reported in laboratory rats for many years. In rats, dermatomycosis may be presented clinically by patchy hair loss and scurfy or erythematous papular-pustular lesions (Weisbroth et al., 1998).

B. Noninfectious Diseases

1. Genetic Predisposition to Disease

Traits that may be desirable to one investigator may be undesirable to another. Every stock and strain of laboratory rat has been carefully selected for specific genetic traits for decades. Common among these are albinism, behavioral characteristics, such as docility and willingness to breed in captivity, and certain tumor profiles.

Overt metabolic diseases such as obesity (Zucker rat), diabetes (BB rat), and hypertension (SHR and fawn-hooded and Dahl rats) make these strains valuable models in biomedical research, whereas spontaneous appearance of the same characteristics in outbred stocks may complicate other research studies. More subtle strain-related tendencies, such as immunologic responsiveness characteristics in Brown Norway and Lewis rats, are exploited by researchers in particular areas of research. In recent years, genetic manipulation has allowed further development of specifically tailored metabolic disease to model critical human defects. It is beyond the scope of this chapter to catalog the innumerable genetic traits or strain-related variations that occur in laboratory rats, and the reader is encouraged to consult the literature and genomic databases such as

the NIH-supported Rat Genome Database for specific information on particular genes, strains, and conditions (Laulederkind et al., 2013).

In addition to known and characterized, spontaneous or induced, genetic variation in rats, isolated colonies of breeding rats inevitably experience some degree of genetic drift. Although this may be monitored to some degree in inbred rats by molecular techniques such as restriction fragment length polymorphisms, it is more difficult to assess the degree to which it has occurred in outbred stocks, where expected interindividual variation may obscure intercolony differences. Nonetheless, any two colonies started from the same source will vary increasingly with time unless there is a sufficient and ongoing exchange of breeders between the colonies. Genetic drift within a population can also be reduced by careful adherence to specific outbreeding programs, such as line breeding with systematic exchange of breeders between multiple lines. 'Randomized' breeding is an important tool used to maintain genetic heterogeneity, but this is a carefully planned process that must not be confused with a haphazard approach that simply pairs 'random' animals.

The inevitability of some degree of genetic drift should not, however, blind researchers to the large role played by environmental, husbandry, dietary, and experimental variables in apparent differences between succeeding groups of animals. These extraneous factors can also have a major impact on the expression of underlying genetic traits. An example of modification of lesion prevalence is the impact of ad libitum overfeeding on increasing the incidence of progressive renal disease (Keenan et al., 1996, 1998).

Brown Norway rats have a high incidence of eosinophilic granulomatous pulmonary inflammation, nearing 100% incidence in both males and females at 3–4 months of age. Brown Norway rats from colonies worldwide are affected, including those maintained in isolators. Affected colonies are seronegative for all known agents, and rats of other strains maintained with the Brown Norway rats do not develop lung lesions. The lung lesions are scattered throughout the parenchyma and are characterized by generally well-organized granulomas of Langhans' giant cells, macrophages, and eosinophils. No foreign material, fungi, or bacteria are routinely visible or can be demonstrated by polarized light or special stains. This inbred strain is used for studies of allergy and asthma due to the inherent pulmonary hyperresponsiveness, and it has been hypothesized that the eosinophilic inflammatory lesion seen in this syndrome may be an allergic or reactive response to an environmental insult (Noritake et al., 2007).

Polyarteritis (panarteritis) nodosa is a vascular disease that has been identified in Sprague-Dawley and spontaneously hypertensive rats. Gross lesions are apparent in the large, muscular arteries of the mesentery and visceral organs, which become enlarged and tortuous. Histological changes in the walls of affected arteries include fibrinoid necrosis and muscular hypertrophy. It is often identified as an incidental lesion, but in a study of the disease in rats on an inbred ACI background the rupture of affected arteries was identified as a potential cause of sporadic death (Cohen *et al.*, 2007).

2. Nutritional Diseases

Frank dietary deficiencies are uncommon, probably for several reasons. First, high-quality commercial diets are in almost universal use. Second, rats store fat-soluble vitamins and vitamin B_{12}, manufacture vitamin C, and can fulfill many of their requirements for other B vitamins by coprophagy. However, heat and moisture, such as are associated with autoclaving, can reduce vitamin levels, particularly lysine, vitamin A, vitamin E, riboflavin, and thiamin. Prolonged storage can have similar effects. In addition, diets designed for maintenance of adult rodents may be too low in protein and fat for optimal growth of young animals or successful reproduction. Clinical evidence of dietary insufficiency may include decreased reproductive performance, litter loss, poor growth, and sparse hair coat. Signs of severe deficiencies of specific vitamins are rare. If they occur, they include squamous metaplasia of salivary ducts with hypovitaminosis A, disseminated hemorrhage with hypovitaminosis K, and embryonic death and testicular degeneration with hypovitaminosis E. Nutritional deficiencies can also alter disease susceptibility and severity.

In addition, feed qualities, aside from total levels of calories and specific nutrients, must be considered, including contaminating chemicals, microbes, and the size and hardness of pellets. For example, feeding a powdered diet will result in an increased incidence of malocclusion.

3. Management-Related Diseases

There are a wide variety of health problems that may be caused by suboptimal care and management, including those relating to experimental manipulations. Only a few of the most common will be mentioned. Sanitation of the animal's cage, bedding, water, and feed, as well as of experimental equipment, is critical. High moisture content in bedding leads to rapid growth of bacteria, which can increase the incidence of urinary tract infections and, possibly, mastitis and skin lesions. Bacterial urease production in urine-saturated zones of bedding can increase ammonia levels. High moisture content in food may increase environmental fungal spore contamination through the proliferation of mold. Some softwood bedding materials emit aromatic compounds that may increase hepatic microsomal levels and affect responses to test compounds, although these compounds are usually completely sublimated during the drying phase in

bedding manufacture. Considerations of air quality might also include factors such as ammonia concentration, CO_2 levels, dusts, disinfectant residues, and pollutants.

Rats are sensitive to temperature, humidity, noise, vibration, light, room activity, and other perceptible changes in their environment. Relative humidity of less than 40% has been linked to the poorly characterized condition known as ringtail, although there can be other factors involved (Crippa *et al.*, 2000). Ringtail is primarily a condition of young rats, usually sucklings, characterized by the formation of prominent annular constrictions of the tail and occasionally of the digits. Portions of affected extremities distal to the constrictions often become necrotic and are sloughed. This condition should not be confused with bite wounds or the normal, more subtle annulations of rat tails which develop with age.

Rats, especially albino rats that have no protective iris pigmentation, can be susceptible to retinal degeneration when exposed to ambient light levels above a certain threshold, which can vary depending on the intensity of the light exposure, the duration of the light cycle, and the illumination levels the animals have been exposed to previously (Semple-Rowland and Dawson, 1987). For rats raised under very dim conditions (6 lux), functional and histological damage can occur with as little as 270 lux of irradiation as measured at the cage level with a 12:12 light:dark cycle. Beyond simple retinal injury, exposure to very high light levels of 1600 lux for 12 h each day for 8 days resulted in necrosis in Harderian glands, likely as a result of the photoreactive properties of the porphyrin secretions (Kurisu *et al.*, 1996). Historically recommended room light levels are in the range of 325–400 lux as measured 1 m above the floor (National Research Council, 2011). Note that these recommended levels as measured 1 m above the floor do not necessarily reflect actual light levels to which rats are exposed in individual cages at various levels in racks at varying distances from light fixtures. Light energy exposure from a generating source is a distance-squared function, so the exposure of animals in cages at the top levels of the rack can be greatly increased over those in the lower levels. This should be recognized as a potential study variable, and if retinal function or structure is to be evaluated as part of a study, the rack location of animals in various experimental groups should be randomized at the initiation of the study or uniformly rotated throughout the study. In addition to intensity-related adverse effects, disruption of the light:dark cycle and resulting exposure to constant light may cause anestrus and other breeding problems. Light exposure (contamination) during the dark phase of the light cycle, with light levels as low as 0.21 lux, has been reported to interfere with rat tumor and metabolism studies, and there are design and management strategies that can be utilized to minimize the physiologic disruptions of light leaks during the dark cycle (Dauchy *et al.*, 2011).

4. Traumatic and Iatrogenic Diseases

Traumatic lesions are uncommon in the rat. Rats housed in wire-bottom cages may develop pododermatitis or lesions on their hocks if housed long-term in such caging. Occasionally, wire-grid floors will allow a rat's foot to become entrapped in the wire grid causing severe edema and injury to the foot and leg, a complication which may occur when rats are allowed to recover from anesthesia in a wire-bottom cage. Group housing of rats is much less likely to result in traumatic injuries due to fighting than is seen in mice. Ulcerative dermatitis, associated with *Staphylococcus aureus* and self-induced trauma from scratching, has been reported (Fox *et al.*, 1977; Wagner *et al.*, 1977). In one report (Fox *et al.*, 1977), the skin lesions were observed only in rats originating from two breeding colonies of one commercial vendor, leading to the hypothesis that the lesions may have been associated with specific *Staphylococcus* phage types or host susceptibility factors.

Adynamic ileus, sometimes leading to death, may occur subsequent to intraperitoneal administration of chloral hydrate. This lesion is noteworthy as it may be mistaken for pathology due to Tyzzer's disease in young rats. Clinical signs occur several days after anesthesia and include lethargy, anorexia, and abdominal distension. The most prominent dilatation occurs in the jejunum, ileum, and cecum. The usual anesthetic dose of chloral hydrate is 400 mg/kg; however, the concentration of the drug, not the dosage, appears to be correlated with the induction of ileus (Fleischman *et al.*, 1977). Use of chloral hydrate in contemporary laboratories is rare except for certain neuroscience models, and comparative studies with more commonly used anesthetic agents are ongoing in order to identify acceptable alternatives (Maud *et al.*, 2014).

C. Neoplastic Diseases

The prevalence of neoplastic disease in the rat is well defined because this species has been routinely used for decades in large-scale carcinogenic, aging, and toxicological studies. Stock- and strain-specific differences in the prevalence of some types of tumors are well documented (Boorman and Everitt, 2006). However, the overall prevalence of neoplasia and that of specific tumor types may vary considerably within stocks or strains because of genetic variation, environmental influences, and differences in laboratory methodologies and diagnostic criteria. The age at which rats are surveyed is also important, because most tumors, other than mammary gland fibroadenomas in many stocks and testicular tumors in F-344 rats, occur in animals greater than 18 months old (Kohn and Barthold, 1984). Table 4.6 compares the incidence of the most frequently occurring tumors in Sprague-Dawley and F-344 rats.

TABLE 4.6 Incidence of Most Prevalent Tumors in Two-Year-Old Rats[a]

Organ/tissue	Incidence (%)			
	Sprague-Dawley (Crl:CD(SD))		Wistar Han (Crl:WI(Han))	
	Male	Female	Male	Female
TESTES				
Interstitial cell tumor	4.0	—	1.2	—
UTERUS				
Endometrial stromal polyp	—	1.2	—	6.8
OVARY				
Granulosa cell/theca cell tumor	—	0.8	—	1.1
MAMMARY GLAND				
Fibroadenoma	0.8	32.7	0.2	12.6
Carcinoma	0.2	9.2	0	3.0
LIVER				
Hepatocellular adenoma/carcinoma	2.9	2.2	5.3	2.2
LYMPHORETICULAR				
Lymphocytic leukemia	0.6	0.3	1.2	0.8
Histiocytic sarcoma	1.0	0.6	0.7	0.3
PITUITARY				
Adenoma/carcinoma, pars distalis	60.9	66.1	24.7	45.9
ADRENAL GLAND				
Cortical adenoma	1.8	4.7	1.7	1.2
Pheochromocytoma, benign	12.0	2.5	1.3	0.4
Pheochromocytoma, malignant	1.9	0.1	0.3	0
PANCREAS				
Islet cell adenoma	7.8	3.3	2.1	0.4
Islet cell carcinoma	0.8	0	0.8	0.2
THYROID				
C-cell adenoma	7.8	7.5	6.9	7.0
C-cell carcinoma	0.3	0.6	1.4	1.6
Follicular cell adenoma	0.8	1.1	4.4	2.7
Follicular cell carcinoma	0.2	0	1.0	1.2

[a]*Adapted from: Giknis, M.L.A. and Clifford, C.B. 2011 Neoplastic and Non-Neoplastic Lesions in the Charles River Wistar Hannover [Crl:WI(Han)] Rat. [online] Charles River Laboratories. Available at: <http://www.criver.com/files/pdfs/rms/wistarhan/rm_rm_r_wistar_han_tox_data_2011.aspx>[Accessed 27 March 2014]; and Giknis, M.L.A. and Clifford, C.B. 2013. Compilation of Spontaneous Neoplastic Lesions and Survival in Crl:CD®(SD) Rats From Control Groups. [online] Charles River Laboratories. Available at: <http://www.criver.com/files/pdfs/rms/cd/rm_rm_r_cd_rat_tox_data_2013.aspx> [Accessed 27 March 2014].*

Among the environmental influences, diet has long been known to be an important factor in modulating tumor prevalence (Boorman and Everitt, 2006). Dietary factors may include manipulations of dietary composition (Rogers *et al.*, 1993) such as high fat (Eustis and Boorman, 1985), specific amino acid deficiencies (Nakae, 1999), or even high protein levels. High protein may alter chronic progressive nephropathy (CPN) which can, in turn, alter the development of renal neoplasia (Seely *et al.*, 2002). Overall caloric intake is also a key factor in the age of onset, rate of tumor growth, and types of tumors observed. Rats in two-years studies fed *ad libitum*, will have lower survival and more tumors, especially those tumors such as pancreatic, mammary, and pituitary where endocrine influences play a role (Keenan *et al.*, 1995).

Another environmental influence on the prevalence of tumors is the pathogen or disease status of the rats in a particular report. Data on tumor risk can be significantly influenced by the effect that some infectious diseases may have on longevity, pre-neoplastic or neoplastic changes, and masking of small tumors (Boorman and Everitt, 2006).

1. Mammary Gland

Mammary gland tumors are the most frequently occurring tumors in most stocks and strains of rats. Sprague-Dawley stocks often have an incidence of 50% in aged female animals, whereas F-344 have a lower incidence of about 25–30%, and Wistar Han have an incidence of 30% or less (Boorman *et al.*, 1990b; Giknis and Clifford, 2011, 2013). Most mammary tumors are benign fibroadenomas, with carcinomas occurring less frequently. Both types can occur in aged males; however, the incidence is usually less than 1%. The tumors may arise in mammary tissue at any point from the neck to the inguinal area, and they tend to attain a large size and become ulcerated unless surgically excised. On gross examination, fibroadenomas are freely movable in subcutaneous tissues, circumscribed, firm, and lobulated. Histologically, they are characterized by well-differentiated acinar epithelial components surrounded by inter- and intralobular connective tissue components (Boorman *et al.*, 1990b; Percy and Barthold, 2007).

2. Testicle

Interstitial cell tumors occur in about 80% of F-344 rats by the age of 15 months (Boorman *et al.*, 1990a), whereas they occur at a much lower (Giknis and Clifford, 2011, 2013) frequency in Wistar Han and Sprague-Dawley rats. They are discrete, soft, and yellow to brown, with areas of hemorrhage, and may occur in multiple sites unilaterally or bilaterally. Histologically, their Leydig's cell origin is apparent. Tumors have two cell types that are arranged in solid sheets or in an organoid pattern.

The cell types are (1) polyhedral to elongated cells with granular to vacuolated cytoplasm, and (2) smaller cells with hyperchromatic nuclei and scanty cytoplasm (Boorman and Everitt, 2006; Percy and Barthold, 2007).

3. Pituitary Gland

Pituitary tumors occur frequently in aged rats of many stocks and strains, including Sprague-Dawley, F-344 and Wistar Han rats (Giknis and Clifford, 2011, 2013; Percy and Barthold, 2007). Most pituitary tumors are classified as chromophobe adenomas, originating from the pars distalis. In some reports, the prevalence of pituitary tumors is greater in female F-344 and Sprague-Dawley rats. Carcinomas of the pars distalis are reported with much less frequency; however, their reported prevalence may vary considerably because of differences in classification protocols by pathologists. As was previously noted, caloric restriction significantly reduces the incidence of pituitary tumors in rats.

Chromophobe adenomas vary in size, often reaching 0.5 cm in diameter. Grossly, the tumors are soft and dark red due to prominent hemorrhagic areas. They are well circumscribed and, because of their size, often compress adjacent brain tissue and induce hydrocephalus. Microscopically, they consist of large polygonal cells with prominent vesicular nuclei and eosinophilic cytoplasm. The architecture of the tumors consists of cells arranged in nests, cords, or sheets separated by vascular sinusoids (Boorman and Everitt, 2006).

4. Adrenal Gland

The incidence of cortical adenoma in Sprague-Dawley rats has been recently reported as 2% in males and 5% in females. Pheochromocytoma (approximately 85% benign) was reported to have an incidence of 14% in males and 2% in females of this stock, although as with other tumors, there was tremendous variation between studies. For example, the range of benign pheochromocytoma, reported in all 20 of 20 studies included in the survey, was from 1% to 28%. F-344 rats have a relatively low incidence of adrenal cortical neoplasia; pheochromocytomas occur at a higher rate, and are observed in approximately 32% of males and 5% of females (Table 4.6).

5. Pancreas

Endocrine tumors of the pancreatic islet cells are relatively common in some stocks of rats. A mean control group incidence of 8% has recently been reported in males, and 3% in female Sprague-Dawley rats (Giknis and Clifford, 2013). For Wistar Han, islet tumors were observed in 36 of 1217 males (2%) in control groups in 16 studies, of which 26 were adenomas and 10 were classified as carcinomas (Giknis and Clifford, 2011). Among the 1217 Wistar Han females in control groups in the same set of studies, there were only seven islet cell tumors, five adenomas and two carcinomas. In the F-344 rat, the incidence is similar, 4% in males and 1.5% in females (Boorman and Everitt, 2006). Grossly, islet cell tumors may be either single or multiple and are circumscribed and reddish brown. Islet cell carcinomas are distinguished from adenomas by capsular invasion and metastases. Tumors of the exocrine pancreas are less common (Boorman and Everitt, 2006).

6. Lymphoreticular System

Large granular lymphocytic leukemia is a major cause of death in F-344 rats (Percy and Barthold, 2007), with a reported incidences of up to 50%, with average incidences around 34% in males and 20% in females (Boorman and Everitt, 2006). The initial site of malignancy is thought to be the spleen (Fig. 4.15). The neoplastic cells are transplantable to rats of the same strain. Unlike leukemia in mice, this leukemia in rats is not associated with a retrovirus. Diagnosis is based upon clinical signs of anemia, jaundice, weight loss, and laboratory findings of splenomegaly, elevated leukocyte counts of up to 400,000/ml, and diffuse infiltration of malignant lymphocytes in various organs (Percy and Barthold, 2007). In the Sprague-Dawley rat and most other stocks, the incidence is quite low.

Other lymphoreticular tumors include lymphocytic lymphoma and histiocytic sarcoma, each of having an incidence of approximately 1% in both Sprague-Dawley and Wistar Han rats (Giknis and Clifford, 2011, 2013).

D. Miscellaneous Conditions

1. Congenital/Hereditary Anomalies

It is beyond the scope of this chapter to catalog congenital defects in rats. The incidence of such defects is obviously influenced by administration of mutagenic and teratogenic substances, but it also varies with strain, age of mother, disease status, coincidences of statistics, and human terminology. Rats are susceptible to a wide variety of genetic diseases, some of which make them valuable models and others of which are confounding variables. Only a few spontaneous defects, involving the urinary tract, heart, and central nervous system, will be mentioned here. The growing range of genetically engineered diseases, and their unintentional side effects, will not be addressed. Researchers and supporting animal resource professionals are strongly urged to investigate, with due scientific scrutiny, background information concerning specific stocks and strains, prior to embarking on courses of research involving any laboratory animal. Databases of defects observed in reproductive studies may be available from animal vendors and some contract research organizations.

Hydronephrosis is one of the more commonly reported congenital defects of rats, characterized by unilateral or bilateral dilation of the renal pelvis. Although it may be inherited as a single dominant gene in the Gunn rat, it appears to be polygenic in the Brown Norway and Sprague-Dawley rats (Van Winkle *et al.*, 1988). The right kidney is affected more often than the left. Severity of hydronephrosis can vary from a slight dilation of the renal pelvis to such severe dilation that the kidney appears as a transparent cystic structure. The ureter may also be affected to varying degrees. The normal renal pelvis of young animals may appear to be dilated, however, so some caution is required in identifying hydronephrosis (Maronpot, 1996). Hydronephrosis may also be mistaken for pyelonephritis, in which the material in the dilated pelvis is typically cloudy; for polycystic kidneys; and for renal papillary necrosis. Culture and histopathology of the affected site will distinguish among these conditions.

Congenital lesions of the cardiovascular system are less frequently reported but include ventricular and atrial

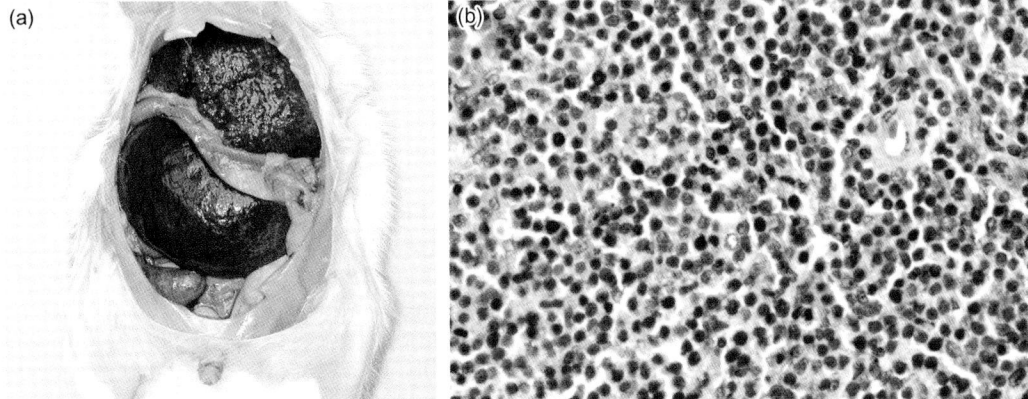

FIGURE 4.15   Splenomegaly and hepatomegaly associated with large granular lymphocytic leukemia in an F344 rat (a). Light micrograph (b) demonstrates the pleomorphic neoplastic cells in an affected spleen. *Courtesy of Dr. T. R. Schoeb.*

septal defects, dextrocardia, and defects of the valves and endocardial cushion, as well as various anomalies of the great vessels. Overall incidence of cardiac defects has been estimated in one colony of Sprague-Dawley rats at 2.3% (Johnson *et al.*, 1993). Interestingly, high rates of cardiac septal defects, resulting in right ventricular hypertrophy, are observed in the Wistar-Kyoto inbred rats used as control for the outbred spontaneous hypertensive rat (SHR) stock (Slama *et al.*, 2002).

Hydrocephalus is an example of a relatively uncommon congenital defect that may arise as a more prevalent anomaly in small, isolated breeding populations. When such situations are recognized, it may be possible to intentionally further increase the prevalence through inbreeding in order to establish a strain that can serve as an animal model for the disease. Selective inbreeding from such a colony resulted in the establishment of breeding lines that had a prevalence of hydrocephalus well over 25% (Kohn *et al.*, 1981). Seizures have also been reported in a variety of stocks and strains of rat but have been reported most frequently in various Wistar stocks (Nunn and Macpherson, 1995). Wistar rats are especially used in investigation of audiogenic seizures (Garcia-Cairasco *et al.*, 1998).

Congenital and genetically determined ocular defects are very common in some strains of rats. Retinal degeneration is an age-related lesion that can be accelerated by exposure to light (Lai *et al.*, 1978). In albino rats, the lack of a pigmented tapetum increases light exposure to the retina and predisposes for the development of retinal atrophy. Fischer rats (F-344) have an incidence of corneal mineralization that varies from 10 to 100%, depending on subline (Bruner *et al.*, 1992; Yoshitomi and Boorman, 1990). This is characterized by deposition of calcium salts, often visible in routinely stained sections as basophilic granules, along the interface of the corneal epithelium and the stroma. Other ocular abnormalities reported in laboratory rats include retinal degeneration, cataracts, osseous and cartilaginous metaplasia of the sclera, and colobomas.

Several abnormalities of the reproductive tract have been reported in laboratory rats, including transverse vaginal septum in female Wistar and Sprague-Dawley (Barbolt and Brown, 1989; De Schaepdrijver *et al.*, 1995; Lezmi *et al.*, 2011). Affected animals are functionally sterile if the septum is complete, and subfertile if the septum only partially prevents spermatozoa from entering the uterus. Pseudohermaphroditism is occasionally observed in rats, most often male pseudohermaphroditism, also known as testicular feminization; i.e., testes are present internally, but the external genitalia are approximately female. Affected rats are karyotypically XY but express the default feminine phenotype. Although mutant strains have been selected for this characteristic (Allison *et al.*, 1965), it is also occasionally observed in other strains

as well. In the testicular-feminized rat (*tfm*), the defect is a lack of androgen receptors due to a point mutation (Yarbrough *et al.*, 1990), although defects in other genes could potentially result in similar syndromes.

2. Age-Related Diseases

Laboratory rats are subject to a wide range of neoplastic and nonneoplastic age-related diseases, as are most aging mammals. Because of the use of rats in 2-year carcinogenicity studies, and as models of gerontology for humans, diseases of the geriatric rat have particular significance to the laboratory animal professional. The type, incidence, and severity of these lesions vary greatly with stock or strain of rat, infectious disease status, experimental manipulation, and husbandry practices, including dietary restriction. Only a few of the most common nonneoplastic conditions will be discussed here, and readers are encouraged to consult the scientific literature, perhaps starting with these excellent reviews for additional information concerning the particular stock or strain with which they are concerned (Boorman *et al.*, 1990; Mohr *et al.*, 1992). In addition, the National Toxicology Program Nonneoplastic Lesion Atlas available on the Internet at <http://ntp.niehs.nih.gov/nnl/> is an excellent resource (Cesta *et al.*, 2014). Neoplastic conditions are afforded a separate section in this chapter.

CPN is an important age-related disease of rat kidneys and is among the most common causes of death in rats in lifetime studies. Synonyms abound, including 'chronic progressive nephrosis' and 'old rat nephropathy'. The condition is more common in males than in females and is progressive, as correctly indicated by its appellation (Hard and Khan, 2004). Gross lesions of CPN are first observed in rats more than 6 months of age and are characterized by pitting of the cortical surface. Because of cortical interstitial fibrosis, removal of the renal capsule may tear the cortical parenchyma. As it becomes more severe in rats more than 1 year of age, the cortical surface becomes increasingly irregular and may develop areas of pallor. Microscopically, glomerular changes are characterized by thickened basement membranes, thickening of the capillary tufts, adhesions to the parietal layer of Bowman's membrane, and segmental glomerulosclerosis (Short and Goldstein, 1992). As the disease advances, numerous tubules in both the cortex and medulla are often dilated and filled with eosinophilic proteinaceous casts. Secondary hyperparathyroidism may occur subsequent to renal functional compromise in advanced cases, resulting in widespread dystrophic mineralization. The etiopathogenesis of CPN is poorly understood and is probably multifactorial. However, several of the major contributing factors have been described (Barthold, 1996a; Percy and Barthold, 2007). First, the reported incidence varies with strain. This indicates probably at least some genetic predisposition for the development of CPN. Sprague-Dawley and F-344 rats have high incidences, whereas Wistar and Long-Evans stocks have a lower incidence. Reported incidences, however, are difficult to interpret, because of geographic variation in use of different stocks and strains (Wistar rats have been used more predominantly in Europe, and Sprague-Dawley rats in the United States), which could lead to other factors, such as housing and diet, actually causing what otherwise appears to be a strain-related change. For example, when many of the reports of the incidence of CPN in European rats were published, rats were housed five per cage, which is known to result in decreased feed consumption and decreased weight gain, relative to single housing. Second, gender is a determining factor in the development of CPN. Male rats have an earlier onset, higher incidence at any given age, and greater severity of lesions than do females. Third, diet is a critical factor and is also the factor that may be the most amenable to management solutions. It is now clear that moderate dietary restriction will greatly reduce the incidence and severity of CPN at any given age, relative to *ad libitum* overfeeding. The mechanism is hypothesized to be that overfeeding results in prolonged increases in renal blood flow and glomerular filtration rate (Gumprecht *et al.*, 1993). This hyperfiltration causes glomerular hypertrophy, leading to macromolecule filtration deficits, mesangial damage, glomerulosclerosis, and protein leakage. Whatever the mechanism, however, 25–30% reduction in caloric intake, relative to *ad libitum*, results in decreased incidence and severity of CPN in female rats, and decreased severity of CPN in male rats, as well as increased survival in both sexes (Keenan *et al.*, 1995).

Nephrocalcinosis is defined as the deposition of calcium phosphate in renal tissue, although a variety of additional terms are sometimes employed to reflect the localization of the mineral in the cortex, medulla, and so on. In contrast to CPN, which is more common in males, nephrocalcinosis is more common in female rats. In addition to gender, the incidence varies with age and strain and may occur in F-344 rats as young as 7 weeks old. The incidence in F-344 rats may reach 50%, whereas the lower incidence of 0–7% is reported in stocks of Sprague-Dawley and Wistar rats (Montgomery and Seely, 1990). An especially high incidence is observed in BDIX rats. The incidence and severity of nephrocalcinosis may be increased by several dietary manipulations, including high levels of calcium, high phosphorus, low calcium/phosphorus ratios, or low magnesium (Percy and Barthold, 2007). However, it is not clear if dietary levels of these minerals are key determining factors in the background incidence of nephrocalcinosis. Histologically (Short and Goldstein, 1992), mineral deposition is observed most frequently at the corticomedullary junction, in cells of the pars recta and thin loops of Henle, as well as in the lumen of these tubules.

Urolithiasis is the formation of mineral deposits within the urine, occasionally observed in the renal pelvis and/or the urinary bladder, more frequently the latter. The incidence of urolithiasis is generally low, but it bears brief discussion for a couple reasons. First, copulatory plugs (Percy and Barthold, 2007), very firm proteinaceous bodies formed by seminal fluids, can often be found in the bladders and urethras of male rats and are occasionally mistaken for uroliths. Copulatory plugs, however, are not considered to be lesions. Second, although uroliths are sporadically observed in aging rats of both sexes, their detection in rats less than six months of age usually indicates bacterial infection, with cystic uroliths most often associated with an ascending *E. coli* infection; renal uroliths, rare in younger rats, are more often associated with an embolic spread of infection. Rats predisposed to urinary tract infection such as the Zucker Diabetic Fatty rat, may have an elevated incidence, as do rats with hydronephrosis. Uroliths are usually calcium phosphate and struvite, although determination of the composition is rarely helpful.

Chronic myocardial disease is a major cause of death in aged male rats of multiple strains, including Sprague-Dawley, when fed *ad libitum* (Keenan *et al.*, 1995). The condition is often known as cardiomyopathy, or chronic progressive cardiomyopathy, and may be observed as early as 3 months of age. Grossly, the heart is enlarged, occasionally with pale streaks visible. Increased weight of the heart correlates well with the degree of damage observed on histologic examination. Microscopically (Lewis, 1992), there is necrosis of myocardial fibers and an interstitial infiltration of mononuclear cells. Later in the course of the disease, fibrosis may be more prominent. Large reactive nuclei are also observed in myofibers. The most commonly affected myocardial sites are the papillary muscles and interventricular septum. As with CPN, the incidence of chronic progressive cardiomyopathy can be dramatically reduced at any age by moderate dietary restriction, i.e., reduction of 25–30% of total caloric intake relative to *ad libitum* overfed rats (Keenan *et al.*, 1995).

Changes in skin and pelage in geriatric laboratory rats are often observed but rarely reported, which may cause concern to the inexperienced observer. The most common change is thinning or loss of hair, especially over the back (Elwell *et al.*, 1990, 1992). This may be observed in any stock or strain but is especially common in the Brown Norway rat. Old albino rats also have a more yellow appearance at times, because of the accumulation of sebum in the skin. The rings of scales covering the tail increase in number with age to 190 at 1 year (English and Munger, 1992). They continue to become more prominent and more yellowed with time after that. The yellowish material which accumulates on the tail and adjacent to the ear also may become black with time, probably from oxidation and/or bacterial action. In addition, male rats accumulate brown-pigmented foci on the skin, termed scales (Tayama and Shisa, 1994). These scales can be detached and can overlay skin of 'normal' color. They are found on the dorsum, with some on the tail and perineum. Scale formation is abrogated by gonadectomy. The nature of the pigment is unclear, but it may be oxidized lipid or amino acids.

Alveolar histiocytosis is a very common incidental finding in the lung of aging rats of many stocks and strains (Dungworth *et al.*, 1992). Grossly, alveolar histiocytosis is visible as white to pale tan foci, usually about 1 mm in diameter, visible on the pleural surface. The foci may extend slightly above the pleural surface in uninflated lung. Microscopically (Boorman and Eustis, 1990), clusters of alveoli, often in a subpleural locations or adjacent to a terminal bronchiole, contain increased numbers of large, pale, foamy-appearing macrophages. Occasionally, cholesterol clefts may be visible in the more dense aggregates of macrophages, and a slight infiltration of lymphocytes may be present around adjacent vessels, probably as a response to proinflammatory mediators released by the macrophages. Alveolar histiocytosis should not be mistaken for any of the viral pneumonias of rats, because affected animals are seronegative, and any lymphoid infiltrate is slight and localized to the areas of macrophage aggregation. The cause of alveolar histiocytosis is not known, but it is not considered to be infectious.

Acknowledgment

The authors acknowledge the conributions of Dennis Kohn to the 2nd Edition.

References

Albers, T.M., Simon, M.A., Clifford, C.B., 2009. Histopathology of naturally transmitted "rat respiratory virus": progression of lesions and proposed diagnostic criteria. Vet. Pathol. 46, 992–999.

Aliouat, E.M., Dujardin, L., Martinez, A., Duriez, T., Ricard, I., Dei-Cas, E., 1999. *Pneumocystis carinii* growth kinetics in culture systems and in hosts: involvement of each life cycle parasite stage. J. Eukaryot. Microbiol. 46, 116S–117S.

Allison, J.E., Stanley, A.J., Gumbreck, L.G., 1965. Sex chromatin and idiograms from rats exhibiting anomalies of the reproductive organs. Anat. Rec. 153, 85–91.

Altman, N.H., Goodman, D.G., 1979. Neoplastic diseases In: Baker, H.J. Lindsey, J.R. Weisbroth, S.H. (Eds.), The Laboratory Rat, vol. 1 Academic Press, New York. Biology and Diseases.

Amao, H., Akimoto, T., Komukai, Y., Sawada, T., Saito, M., Takahashi, K.W., 2002. Detection of *Corynebacterium kutscheri* from the oral cavity of rats. Exp. Anim. 51, 99–102.

Amao, H., Komukai, Y., Akimoto, T., Sugiyama, M., Takahashi, K.W., Sawada, T., et al., 1995. Natural and subclinical *Corynebacterium kutscheri* infection in rats. Lab. Anim. Sci. 45, 11–14.

Amao, H., Moriguchi, N., Komukai, Y., Kawasumi, H., Takahashi, K., Sawada, T., 2008. Detection of *Corynebacterium kutscheri* in the faeces of subclinically infected mice. Lab. Anim. 42, 376–382.

Anderson, L.C., Leary, S.L., Manning, P.J., 1983. Rat-bite fever in animal research laboratory personnel. Lab. Anim. Sci. 33, 292–294.

Anonymous, 1977. Saccharin and cancer. N. Engl. J. Med. 297, 560–561.

Antonakopoulos, G.N., Turton, J., Whitfield, P., Newman, J., 1991. Host–parasite interface of the urinary bladder-inhabiting nematode *Trichosomoides crassicauda*: changes induced in the urothelium of infected rats. Int. J. Parasitol. 21, 187–193.

Artwohl, J.E., Cera, L.M., Wright, M.F., Medina, L.V., Kim, L.J., 1994. The efficacy of a dirty bedding sentinel system for detecting Sendai virus infection in mice: a comparison of clinical signs and seroconversion. Lab. Anim. Sci. 44, 73–75.

Ayala, M.E., Monroy, J., Morales, L., Castro, M.E., Dominguez, R., 1998. Effects of a lesion in the dorsal raphe nuclei performed during the juvenile period of the female rat, on puberty. Brain Res. Bull. 47, 211–218.

Baker, D.E.J., 1979. Biology and diseases In: Baker, H.J. Lindsey, J.R. Weisbroth, S.H. (Eds.), The Laboratory Rat, vol. 1 Academic Press, New York, pp. 153–168.

Baker, D.G., 2007. Flynn's Parasites of Laboratory Animals. Blackwell Publishing, Ames, IA.

Ball-Goodrich, L.J., Hansen, G., Dhawan, R., Paturzo, F.X., Vivas-Gonzalez, B.E., 2002. Validation of an enzyme-linked immunosorbent assay for detection of mouse parvovirus infection in laboratory mice. Comp. Med. 52, 160–166.

Ball-Goodrich, L.J., Johnson, E., Jacoby, R., 2001. Divergent replication kinetics of two phenotypically different parvoviruses of rats. J. Gen. Virol. 82, 537–546.

Ball-Goodrich, L.J., Leland, S.E., Johnson, E.A., Paturzo, F.X., Jacoby, R.O., 1998. Rat parvovirus type 1: the prototype for a new rodent parvovirus serogroup. J. Virol. 72, 3289–3299.

Barbolt, T.A., Brown, G.L., 1989. Vaginal septum in the rat. Lab. Anim. 18, 47–48.

Barlow, S.C., Brown, M.M., Price, H.V., 2005. Eradication of Syphacia muris from food-restricted rats without environmental decontamination. Contemp. Top. Lab. Anim. Sci. 44, 23–25.

Barron, S., Baseheart, B.J., Segar, T.M., Deveraux, T., Willford, J.A., 2000. The behavioral teratogenic potential of fenbendazole: a medication for pinworm infestation. Neurotoxicol. Teratol. 22, 871–877.

Barthold, S.W., 1996a. Chronic progressive nephropathy, rat. In: Jones, T.C., Hard, G.C., Mohr, U. (Eds.), Urinary System Springer, Berlin.

Barthold, S.W., 1996b. *Trichosomoides crassicauda* infection, urinary bladder, rat. In: Jones, T.C., Hard, G.C., Mohr, U. (Eds.), Urinary System. Springer, Berlin, Germany.

Barthold, S.W., 1997. Streptococcal enteropathy, intestine, rat. In: Jones, T.C., Popp, J.A., Mohr, U. (Eds.), Digestive System. Springer-Verlag, Berlin, Germany.

Barthold, S.W., Brownstein, D.G., 1988. The effect of selected viruses on *Corynebacterium kutscheri* infection in rats. Lab. Anim. Sci. 38, 580–583.

Bauer, B.A., Besch-Williford, C.L., Riley, L.K., 2004. Comparison of the mouse antibody production (MAP) assay and polymerase chain reaction (PCR) assays for the detection of viral contaminants. Biologicals 32, 177–182.

Bennett, J.P., Vickery, B.H., 1970. In: Hafez, E.S.E. (Ed.), Reproduction and Breeding Techniques for Laboratory Animals Lea and Febiger, Philadelphia, PA, pp. 299–315.

Besch-Williford, C.L., Wagner, J.E., Templeman, C.C., 1987. Establishment of a commercial production colony of Sprague-Dawley rats free of Sendai virus. Lab. Anim. Sci. 37, 666–667.

Besselsen, D.G., Besch-Williford, C.L., Pintel, D.J., Franklin, C.L., Hook Jr., R.R., Riley, L.K., 1995a. Detection of H-1 parvovirus and Kilham rat virus by PCR. J. Clin. Microbiol. 33, 1699–1703.

Besselsen, D.G., Besch-Williford, C.L., Pintel, D.J., Franklin, C.L., Hook Jr., R.R., Riley, L.K., 1995b. Detection of newly recognized rodent parvoviruses by PCR. J. Clin. Microbiol. 33, 2859–2863.

Besselsen, D.G., Franklin, C.L., Livingston, R.S., Riley, L.K., 2008. Lurking in the shadows: emerging rodent infectious diseases. ILAR J. 49, 277–290.

Besselsen, D.G., Wagner, A.M., Loganbill, J.K., 2002. Detection of rodent coronaviruses by use of fluorogenic reverse transcriptase-polymerase chain reaction analysis. Comp. Med. 52, 111–116.

Beys, E., Hodge, T., Nohynek, G.J., 1995. Ovarian changes in Sprague-Dawley rats produced by nocturnal exposure to low intensity light. Lab. Anim. 29, 335–338.

Bihun, C.G., Percy, D.H., 1994. Coronavirus infections in the laboratory rat: degree of cross protection following immunization with a heterologous strain. Can. J. Vet. Res. 58, 224–229.

Bivin, W.S., Crawford, M.P., Brewer, N.R., 1979. Morphophysiology In: Lindsey, J.R. Baker, H.J. Weisbroth, S.H. (Eds.), The Laboratory Rat, vol. 1 Academic Press, New York, pp. 74–103. Biology and Diseases.

Blandau, R.J., Boling, J.L., Young, W.C., 1941. The length of heat in the albino rat as determined by the copulatory response test. Anat. Rec. 79, 453–463.

Blom, H.J., Van Tintelen, G., Van Vorstenbosch, C.J., Baumans, V., Beynen, A.C., 1996. Preferences of mice and rats for types of bedding material. Lab. Anim. 30, 234–244.

Boettger-Tong, H., Murthy, L., Chiappetta, C., Kirkland, J.L., Goodwin, B., Adlercreutz, H., et al., 1998. A case of a laboratory animal feed with high estrogenic activity and its impact on in vivo responses to exogenously administered estrogens. Environ. Health Perspect. 106, 369–373.

Boivin, G.P., Wagner, J.E., Besch-Williford, C.L., 1990. Use of cyclophosphamide in diagnostic provocation of Tyzzer's disease in hamsters. LAS 40 545–545.

Boorman, G.A., Chapin, R.E., Mitsumori, K., 1990a. Testis and epididymis. In: Boorman, G.A., Eustis, S.L., Elwell, M.R., Montgomery, C.A., Mackenzie, W.F. (Eds.), Pathology of the Fischer Rat: Reference and Atlas. Academic Press, San Diego, CA.

Boorman, G.A., Eustis, S.L., 1990. Lung. In: Boorman, G.A., Eustis, S.L., Elwell, M.R., Montgomery, C.A., Mackenzie, W.F. (Eds.), Pathology of the Fischer Rat: Reference and Atlas. Academic Press, San Diego, CA.

Boorman, G.A., Eustis, S.L., Elwell, M.R., Montgomery, C.A., MacKenzie, W.F. (Eds.), 1990. Pathology of the Fischer Rat. Academic Press, Orlando, FL.

Boorman, G.A., Everitt, J.I., 2006. Neoplastic disease. In: Suckow, M.A., Weisbroth, S.H., Franklin, C.L. (Eds.), The Laboratory Rat, second ed. Elsevier Academic Press, San Diego, CA.

Boorman, G.A., Wildon, J.T., Van Zwieten, M.J., Eustis, S.L., 1990b. Mammary gland. In: Boorman, G.A., Eustis, S.L., Elwell, M.R., Montgomery, C.A., Mackenzie, W.F. (Eds.), Pathology of the Fischer Rat: Reference and Atlas. Academic Press, San Diego, CA.

Boot, R., Thuis, H., Bakker, R., Veenema, J.L., 1995. Serological studies of Corynebacterium kutscheri and coryneform bacteria using an enzyme-linked immunosorbent assay (ELISA). Lab. Anim. 29, 294–299.

Boot, R., Van Knapen, F., Kruijt, B.C., Walvoort, H.C., 1988. Serological evidence for Encephalitozoon cuniculi infection (nosemiasis) in gnotobiotic guineapigs. Lab. Anim. 22, 337–342.

Borjeson, T.M., Pang, J., Fox, J.G., Garcia, A., 2014. Administration of luteinizing hormone releasing hormone agonist for synchronization of estrus and generation of pseudopregnancy for embryo transfer in rats. J. Am. Assoc. Lab. Anim. Sci. 53, 232–237.

Bornstein, D.A., Scola, J., Rath, A., Warren, H.B., 2006. Multimodal approach to treatment for control of fur mites. J. Am. Assoc. Lab. Anim. Sci. 45, 29–32.

Brammer, D.W., Dysko, R.C., Spilman, S.C., Oskar, P.A., 1993. Elimination of sialodacryoadenitis virus from a rat production colony by using seropositive breeding animals. Lab. Anim. Sci. 43, 633–634.

Brown, H.R., Leininger, J.R., 1992. In: Mohr, U. Dungworth, D.L. Capen, C.C. (Eds.), Pathobiology of the Aging Rat, vol. 2 ILSI Press, Washington, DC, pp. 309–322.

Brudzynski, S.M., 2009. Communication of adult rats by ultrasonic vocalization: biological, sociobiological, and neuroscience approaches. ILAR J. 50, 43–50.

Brudzynski, S.M., Chiu, E.M., 1995. Behavioural responses of laboratory rats to playback of 22 kHz ultrasonic calls. Physiol. Behav. 57, 1039–1044.

Bruner, R.H., Keller, W.F., Stitzel, K.A., Sauers, L.J., Reer, P.J., Long, P.H., et al., 1992. Spontaneous corneal dystrophy and generalized basement membrane changes in Fischer-344 rats. Toxicol. Pathol. 20, 357–366.

Burek, J.D., Zurcher, C., Van Nunen, M.C., Hollander, C.F., 1977. A naturally occurring epizootic caused by Sendai virus in breeding and aging rodent colonies. II. Infection in the rat. Lab. Anim. Sci. 27, 963–971.

Cacioppo, L.D., Shen, Z., Parry, N.M., Fox, J.G., 2012a. Resistance of Sprague-Dawley Rats to infection with Helicobacter pullorum. J. Am. Assoc. Lab. Anim. Sci. 51, 803–807.

Cacioppo, L.D., Turk, M.L., Shen, Z., Ge, Z., Parry, N., Whary, M.T., et al., 2012b. Natural and experimental Helicobacter pullorum infection in Brown Norway rats. J. Med. Microbiol. 61, 1319–1323.

Carlberg, K.A., Lang, B.Z., 2004. Infection with pinworms (Syphacia obvelata) does not affect the plasma corticosterone concentration in male, nonpregnant female, and pregnant female rats. Contemp. Top. Lab. Anim. Sci. 43, 46–49.

Carter, G.R., 1984. Pasteurella In: Krieg, N.R. Holt, J.G. (Eds.), Bergey's Manual of Systematic Bacteriology, vol. 1 William and Wilkins, Baltimore, MD.

Carthew, P., Aldred, P., 1988. Embryonic death in pregnant rats owing to intercurrent infection with Sendai virus and Pasteurella pneumotropica. Lab. Anim. 22, 92–97.

Carthew, P., Slinger, R.P., 1981. Diagnosis of sialodacryoadenitis virus infection of rats in a virulent enzootic outbreak. Lab. Anim. 15, 339–342.

Cassell, G.H., Davis, J.K., Simecka, J.W., Lindsey, J.R., Cox, N.R., Ross, S., et al., 1986. Mycoplasmal infections: disease pathogenesis, implications for biomedical research, and control. In: Bhatt, P.N., Jacoby, R.O., Morse, H.C., New, A.E. (Eds.), Viral and Mycoplasmal infections of Laboratory Rodents: Effects on Biomedical Research Academic Press, Orlando, FL.

Cassell, G.H., Lindsey, J.R., Davis, J.K., Davidson, M.K., Brown, M.B., Mayo, J.G., 1981. Detection of natural Mycoplasma pulmonis infection in rats and mice by an enzyme linked immunosorbent assay (ELISA). Lab. Anim. Sci. 31, 676–682.

Cesta, M.F., Malarkey, D.E., Herbert, R.A., Brix, A., Hamlin II, M.H., Singletary, E., et al., 2014. The National Toxicology Program Web-based nonneoplastic lesion atlas: a global toxicology and pathology resource. Toxicol. Pathol. 42, 458–460.

Chiavolini, D., Pozzi, G., Ricci, S., 2008. Animal models of Streptococcus pneumoniae disease. Clin. Microbiol. Rev. 21, 666–685.

Childs, J.E., Glass, G.E., Korch, G.W., Arthur, R.R., Shah, K.V., Glasser, D., et al., 1988. Evidence of human infection with a rat-associated Hantavirus in Baltimore, Maryland. Am. J. Epidemiol. 127, 875–878.

Chmiel, D.J., Noonan, M., 1996. Preference of laboratory rats for potentially enriching stimulus objects. Lab. Anim. 30, 97–101.

Chu, D.K., Couto, M.A., 2005. Arthropod infestation in a colony of mice. Lab. Anim. (NY) 34, 25–27.

Chung, Y.H., Jun, H.S., Kang, Y., Hirasawa, K., Lee, B.R., Van Rooijen, N., et al., 1997. Role of macrophages and macrophage-derived cytokines in the pathogenesis of Kilham rat virus-induced autoimmune diabetes in diabetes-resistant BioBreeding rats. J. Immunol. 159, 466–471.

Clifford, C.B., Watson, J., 2008. Old enemies, still with us after all these years. ILAR J. 49, 291–302.

Cloutier, S., Wahl, K., Baker, C., Newberry, R.C., 2014. The social buffering effect of playful handling on responses to repeated intraperitoneal injections in laboratory rats. J. Am. Assoc. Lab. Anim. Sci. 53, 168–173.

Coghlan, L.G., Lee, D.R., Psencik, B., Weiss, D., 1993. Practical and effective eradication of pinworms (Syphacia muris) in rats by use of fenbendazole. Lab. Anim. Sci. 43, 481–487.

Cohen, J.K., Cai, L.Q., Zhu, Y.S., La Perle, K.M., 2007. Pancreaticoduodenal arterial rupture and hemoabdomen in ACI/SegHsd rats with polyarteritis nodosa. Comp. Med. 57, 370–376.

Cohen, S.M., Anderson, T.A., De Oliveira, L.M., Arnold, L.L., 1998. Tumorigenicity of sodium ascorbate in male rats. Cancer Res. 58, 2557–2561.

Cole, J.S., Sabol-Jones, M., Karolewski, B., Byford, T., 2005. Ornithonyssus bacoti infestation and elimination from a mouse colony. Contemp. Top. Lab. Anim. Sci. 44, 27–30.

Coleman, G.L., Jacoby, R.O., Bhatt, P.N., Smith, A.L., Jonas, A.M., 1983. Naturally occurring lethal parvovirus infection of juvenile and young-adult rats. Vet. Pathol. 20, 49–56.

Compton, S.R., Homberger, F.R., Paturzo, F.X., Clark, J.M., 2004. Efficacy of three microbiological monitoring methods in a ventilated cage rack. Comp. Med. 54, 382–392.

Compton, S.R., Riley, L.K., 2001. Detection of infectious agents in laboratory rodents: traditional and molecular techniques. Comp. Med. 51, 113–119.

Compton, S.R., Smith, A.L., Gaertner, D.J., 1999. Comparison of the pathogenicity in rats of rat coronaviruses of different neutralization groups. Lab. Anim. Sci. 49, 514–518.

Conole, J., Wilkinson, M.J., Mckellar, Q.A., 2003. Some observations on the pharmacological properties of ivermectin during treatment of a mite infestation in mice. Contemp. Top. Lab. Anim. Sci. 42, 42–45.

Constantinescu, G.M., 2011. Comparative Anatomy of the Mouse and the Rat. American Association for Laboratory Animal Science, Memphis, TN.

Corbin, T.J., Mccabe, J.G., 2002. Strain variation of immature female rats in response to various superovulatory hormone preparations and routes of administration. J. Am. Assoc. Lab. Anim. Sci. 41, 18–23.

Cornish, J., Vanderwee, M.A., Findon, G., Miller, T.E., 1988. Reliable diagnosis of Trichosomoides crassicauda in the urinary bladder of the rat. Lab. Anim. 22, 162–165.

Craft, J.C., 1982. Experimental infection with Giardia lamblia in rats. J. Infect. Dis. 145, 495–498.

Cray, C., Villar, D., Zaias, J., Altman, N.H., 2008. Effects of fenbendazole on routine immune response parameters of BALB/c mice. J. Am. Assoc. Lab. Anim. Sci. 47, 32–36.

Cray, C., Watson, T., Zaias, J., Altman, N.H., 2013. Effect of fenbendazole on an autoimmune mouse model. J. Am. Assoc. Lab. Anim. Sci. 52, 286–289.

Crippa, L., Gobbi, A., Ceruti, R.M., Clifford, C.B., Remuzzi, A., Scanziani, E., 2000. Ringtail in suckling Munich Wistar Fromter rats: a histopathologic study. Comp. Med. 50, 536–539.

Cui, Z.J., Zhou, Y.D., Satoh, Y., Habara, Y., 2003. A physiological role for protoporphyrin IX photodynamic action in the rat Harderian gland? Acta Physiol. Scand. 179, 149–154.

Cundiff, D.D., Besch-Williford, C.L., Hook, R.R., Franklin, C.L., Riley, L.K., 1994. Detection of cilia-associated respiratory bacillus by PCR. J. Clin. Microbiol. 32, 1930–1934.

Cundiff, D.D., Besch-Williford, C.L., Hook, R.R., Franklin, C.L., Riley, L.K., 1995a. Characterization of cilia-associated respiratory bacillus in rabbits and analysis of the 16S rRNA gene sequence. Lab. Anim. Sci. 45, 22.

Cundiff, D.D., Riley, L.K., Franklin, C.L., Hook, R.R., Besch-Williford, C.L., 1995b. Failure of a soiled bedding sentinel system to detect Cilia-associated Respiratory bacillus infection in rats. Lab. Anim. Sci. 45, 219–221.

Dameron, G.W., Weingand, K.W., Duderstdt, J.M., Odioso, L.W., Dierckman, T.A., Schwecke, W., et al., 1992. Effect of bleeding site on clinical laboratory testing of rats: orbital venous plexus versus posterior vena cava. Lab. Anim. Sci. 42, 299–301.

Darrigrand, A.A., Singh, S.B., Lang, C.M., 1984. Effects of Kilham rat virus on natural killer cell-mediated cytotoxicity in brown Norway and Wistar Furth rats. Am. J. Vet. Res. 45, 200–202.

Dauchy, R.T., Dupepe, L.M., Ooms, T.G., Dauchy, E.M., Hill, C.R., Mao, L., et al., 2011. Eliminating animal facility light-at-night contamination and its effect on circadian regulation of rodent physiology, tumor growth, and metabolism: a challenge in the relocation of a cancer research laboratory. J. Am. Assoc. Lab. Anim. Sci. 50, 326–336.

Davidson, M.K., Davis, J.K., Lindsey, J.R., Cassell, G.H., 1988. Clearance of different strains of Mycoplasma pulmonis from the respiratory tract of C3H/HeN mice. Infect. Immun. 56, 2163–2168.

Davis, J.K., Cassell, G.H., 1982. Murine respiratory mycoplasmosis in LEW and F344 rats: strain differences in lesion severity. Vet. Pathol. 19, 280–293.

Deerberg, F., Pohlmeyer, G., Wullenweber, M., Hedrich, H.J., 1993. History and pathology of an enzootic Pneumocystis carinii pneumonia in athymic Han:RNU and Han:NZNU rats. J. Exp. Anim. Sci., 1–11. 1993/10/01.

Delong, D., Manning, P.J., 1994. Bacterial diseases. In: Manning, P.J., Ringler, D.H., Newcomer, C.E. (Eds.), The Biology of the Laboratory Rabbit. Academic Press, San Diego, CA.

Del Vecchio, F.R., 1992. Normal development, growth and aging of the female genital tract In: Mohr, U. Dungworth, D.L. Capen, C.C. (Eds.), Pathobiology of the Aging Rat, vol. 1, ILSI Press, Washington, DC.

Demirturk, N., Kozan, E., Demirdal, T., Fidan, F., Aktepe, O.C., Unlu, M., et al., 2007. Effect of parasitosis on allergic sensitization in rats sensitized with ovalbumin: interaction between parasitosis and allergic sensitization. Adv. Ther. 24, 1305–1313.

De Schaepdrijver, L.M., Fransen, J.L., Van Der Eycken, E.S., Coussement, W.C., 1995. Transverse vaginal septum in the specific-pathogen-free Wistar rat. Lab. Anim. Sci. 45, 181–183.

Desmyter, J., Leduc, J.W., Johnson, K.M., Brasseur, F., Deckers, C., Van Ypersele De Strihou, C., 1983. Laboratory rat associated outbreak of haemorrhagic fever with renal syndrome due to Hantaan-like virus in Belgium. Lancet 2, 1445–1448.

Dewsbury, D.A., 1970. Copulatory behavior. In: Hafez, E.S.S. (Ed.), Reproduction and Breeding Techniques for Laboratory Animals Lea and Febiger, Philadelphia, pp. 123–136.

Dix, J., Astill, J., Whelan, G., 2004. Assessment of methods of destruction of Syphacia muris eggs. Lab. Anim. 38, 11–16.

Drake, M.T., Besch-Williford, C., Myles, M.H., Davis, J.W., Livingston, R.S., 2011. In vivo tropisms and kinetics of rat theilovirus infection in immunocompetent and immunodeficient rats. Virus Res. 160, 374–380.

Duan, Q., Liu, Y., Booth, C.J., Rockwell, S., 2012. Use of fenbendazole-containing therapeutic diets for mice in experimental cancer therapy studies. J. Am. Assoc. Lab. Anim. Sci. 51, 224–230.

Duncan, A.J., Carman, R.J., Olsen, G.J., Wilson, K.H., 1993. Assignment of the agent of Tyzzer's desease to Clostridium piliforme comb. nov. on the basis of 16S rRNA sequence analysis. Internat. J. Sys. Bact. 43, 314–318.

Dungworth, D.L., Ernst, H., Nolte, T., Mohr, U., 1992. Nonneoplastic lesions in the lungs In: Mohr, U. Dungworth, D.L. Capen, C.C. (Eds.), Pathobiology of the Aging Rat, vol. 1, ILSI Press, Washington, DC.

Dyson, M.C., 2010. Management of an outbreak of rat theilovirus. Lab. Anim. (NY) 39, 155–157.

Easterbrook, J.D., Kaplan, J.B., Glass, G.E., Watson, J., Klein, S.L., 2008. A survey of rodent-borne pathogens carried by wild-caught

Norway rats: a potential threat to laboratory rodent colonies. Lab. Anim. 42, 92–98.

Eaton, K.A., Dewhirst, F.E., Paster, B.J., Tzellas, N., Coleman, B.E., Paola, J., et al., 1996. Prevalence and varieties of helicobacter species in dogs from random sources and pet dogs: animal and public health implications. J. Clin. Mirobiol. 34, 3165–3170.

Eckstein, B., Golan, R., Shani Mishkinsky, J., 1973. Onset of puberty in the immature female rat induced by 5α-androstane-3β,17β-diol. Endocrinology 92, 941–945.

Effler, J.C., Hickman-Davis, J.M., Erwin, J.G., Cartner, S.C., Schoeb, T.R., 2008. Comparison of methods for detection of pinworms in mice and rats. Lab. Anim. (NY) 37, 210–215.

Eiden, J., Vonderfecht, S., Yolken, R.H., 1985. Evidence that a novel rotavirus-like agent of rats can cause gastroenteritis in man. Lancet 2, 8–11.

Elcock, L.E., Stuart, B.P., Wahle, B.S., Hoss, H.E., Crabb, K., Millard, D.M., et al., 2001. Tumors in long-term rat studies associated with microchip animal identification devices. Exp. Toxicol. Pathol. 52, 483–491.

Elwell, M.R., Mahler, J.F., 1997. "Have you seen this?" Inflammatory lesions on the lungs of rats. Toxicol. Path. 25, 529–531.

Elwell, M.R., Stedham, M.A., Kovatch, R.M., 1990. Skin and subcutis. In: Boorman, G.A., Eustis, S.L., Elwell, M.R., Montgomery, C.A., Mackenzie, W.F. (Eds.), Pathology of the Fischer Rat: Reference and Atlas. Academic Press, San Diego, CA.

Elwell, M.R., Stedham, M.A., Kovatch, R.M., 1992. Skin and subcutis In: Mohr, U. Dungworth, D.L. Capen, C.C. (Eds.), Pathobiology of the Aging Rat, vol. 1, ILSI Press, Washington, DC.

Engelbregt, M.J., Houdijk, M.E., Popp-Snijders, C., Delemarre-Van De WaaL, H.A., 2000. The effects of intra-uterine growth retardation and postnatal undernutrition on onset of puberty in male and female rats. Pediatr. Res. 48, 803–807.

Enders, A.C., 1970. In: Hafez, E.S.E. (Ed.), Reproduction and Breeding Techniques for Laboratory Animals Lea and Febiger, Philadelphia, PA, pp. 137–156.

English, K.B., Munger, B.L., 1992. Normal development of the skin and subcutis of the albino rat In: Mohr, U. Dungworth, D.L. Capen, C.C. (Eds.), Pathobiology of the Aging Rat, vol. 2, ILSI Press, Washington, DC.

Eustis, S.L., Boorman, G.A., 1985. Proliferative lesions of the exocrine pancreas: relationship to corn oil gavage in the National Toxicology Program. J. Natl. Cancer Inst. 75, 1067–1073.

Fallon, M.T., Reinhard, M.K., Gray, B.M., Davis, T.W., Lindsey, J.R., 1988. Inapparent Streptococcus pneumoniae Type 35 infections in commercial rats and mice. Lab. Anim. Sci. 38, 129–132.

Feely, D.E., Chase, D.G., Hardin, E.L., Erlandsen, S.L., 1988. Ultrastructural evidence for the presence of bacteria, viral-like particles, and mycoplasma-like organisms associated with Giardia spp. J. Protozool. 35, 151–158.

Feldman, M.L., 1992. In: Mohr, U. Dungworth, D.L. Capen, C.C. (Eds.), Pathobiology of the Aging Rat, vol. 2, ILSI Press, Washington, DC, pp. 121–147.

Feldman, S.H., Bowman, S.G., 2007. Molecular phylogeny of the pinworms of mice, rats and rabbits, and its use to develop molecular beacon assays for the detection of pinworms in mice. Lab. Anim. (NY) 36, 43–50.

Fleischman, R.W., Mccracken, D., Forbes, W., 1977. Adynamic ileus in the rat induced by chloral hydrate. Lab. Anim. Sci. 27, 238–243.

Fox, J.G., Lee, A., 1997. Special topic overview: the role of helicobacter species in newly recognized gastrointestinal tract diseases of animals. Lab. Anim. Sci. 47, 222–255.

Fox, J.G., Niemi, S.M., Ackerman, J., Murphy, J.C., 1987. Comparison of methods to diagnose an epizootic of Corynebacterium kutscheri pneumonia in rats. Lab. Anim. Sci. 37, 72–75.

Fox, J.G., Niemi, S.M., Murphy, J.C., Quimby, F.W., 1977. Ulcerative dermatitis in the rat. Lab. Anim. Sci. 27, 671–678.

Fox, J.G., Yan, L.L., Dewhirst, F.E., Paster, B.J., Shames, B., Murphy, J.C., et al., 1995. Helicobacter bilis sp. nov., a novel Helicobacter species isolated from the bile, liver, and intestines of aged, inbred mice. J. Clin. Microbiol. 33, 445–454.

Fox, R.R., Laird, C.W., 1970. In: Hafez, E.S.E. (Ed.), Reproduction and Breeding Techniques for Laboratory Animals Lea and Febiger, Philadelphia, PA, pp. 107–122.

Franklin, C.L., Motzel, S.L., Beschwilliford, C.L., Hook, R.R., Riley, L.K., 1994. Tyzzer's infection – Host specificity of Clostridium piliforme isolates. Lab. Anim. Sci. 44, 568–572.

Franklin, C.L., Pletz, J.D., Riley, L.K., Livingston, B.A., Hook Jr., R.R., Besch-Williford, C.L., 1999. Detection of cilia-associated respiratory (CAR) bacillus in nasal-swab specimens from infected rats by use of polymerase chain reaction. Lab. Anim. Sci. 49, 114–117.

Fujinaga, M., Baden, J.M., Mazze, R.I., 1992. Reproductive and teratogenic effects of a major earthquake in rats. Lab. Anim. Sci. 42, 209–210.

Furukawa, T., Furumoto, K., Fujieda, M., Okada, E., 2002. Detection by PCR of the Tyzzer's disease organism (Clostridium piliforme) in feces. Exp. Anim. 51, 513–516.

Gaddum-Rosse, P., Blandau, R.J., Langley, L.B., Battaglia, D.E., 1984. In vitro fertilization in the rat: observations on living eggs. Fertil. Steril. 42, 285–292.

Gaertner, D.J., Jacoby, R.O., Johnson, E.A., Paturzo, F.X., Smith, A.L., 1995. Persistent rat virus infection in juvenile athymic rats and its modulation by immune serum. Lab. Anim. Sci. 45, 249–253.

Gaertner, D.J., Jacoby, R.O., Smith, A.L., Ardito, R.B., Paturzo, F.X., 1989. Persistence of rat parvovirus in athymic rats. Arch. Virol. 105, 259–268.

Gaertner, D.J., Smith, A.L., Jacoby, R.O., 1996. Efficient induction of persistent and prenatal parvovirus infection in rats. Virus Res. 44, 67–78.

Ganaway, J.R., 1980. Effect of heat and selected chemical disinfectants upon infectivity of spores of Bacillus piliformis (Tyzzer's Disease). Lab. Anim. Sci. 30, 192–196.

Gannon, J., 1980. A survey of Encephalitozoon cuniculi in laboratory animal colonies in the United Kingdom. Lab. Anim. 14, 91–94.

Gao, P., Dang, C.V., Watson, J., 2008. Unexpected antitumorigenic effect of fenbendazole when combined with supplementary vitamins. J. Am. Assoc. Lab. Anim. Sci. 47, 37–40.

Garcia-Cairasco, N., Oliveira, J.A., Wakamatsu, H., Bueno, S.T., Guimaraes, F.S., 1998. Reduced exploratory activity of audiogenic seizures in susceptible Wistar rats. Physiol. Behav. 64, 671–674.

Garlinghouse Jr., L.E., Van Hoosier Jr., G.L., 1978. Studies on adjuvant-induced arthritis, tumor transplantability, and serologic response to bovine serum albumin in Sendai virus-infected rats. Am. J. Vet. Res. 39, 297–300.

Garside, D.A., Charlton, A., Heath, K.J., 1996. Establishing the timing of implantation in the Harlan Porcellus Dutch and New Zealand White rabbit and the Han Wistar rat. Regul. Toxicol. Pharmacol. 23, 69–73.

Giknis, M.L.A., Clifford, C.B., 2011. Neoplastic and Non-Neoplastic Lesions in the Charles River Wistar Hannover [Crl:WI(Han)] Rat. Charles River, Wilmington, MA.

Giknis, M.L.A., Clifford, C.B., 2013. Compilation of Spontaneous Neoplastic Lesions and Survival in Crl:CD(SD) Rats from Control Groups. Charles River, Wilmington, MA.

Gilbert, B.E., Black, M.B., Waldrep, J.C., Bennick, J., Montgomery, C., Knight, V., 1997. Cyclosporin A Liposome aerosol: lack of acute toxicity in rats with a high incidence of underlying pneumonitis. Inhal. Toxicol. 9, 717–730.

Goelz, M.F., Thigpen, J.E., Mahler, J., Rogers, W.P., Locklear, J., Wiegler, B.J., et al., 1997. Efficacy of various therapeutic regimens in eliminating Pasteurella pneumotropica from the mouse. Lab. Anim. Sci. 46, 280–285.

Gonder, J.C., Laber, K., 2007. A renewed look at laboratory rodent housing and management. ILAR J. 48, 29–36.

Gonenc, B., Sarimehmetoglu, H.O., Ica, A., Kozan, E., 2006. Efficacy of selamectin against mites (Myobia musculi, Mycoptes musculinus and Radfordia ensifera) and nematodes (Aspiculuris tetraptera and Syphacia obvelata) in mice. Lab. Anim. 40, 210–213.

Gonzalez, D.E., Deis, R.P., 1990. The capacity to develop maternal behavior is enhanced during aging in rats. Neurobiol. Aging 11, 237–241.

Graepel, R., Leung, G., Wang, A., Villemaire, M., Jirik, F.R., Sharkey, K.A., et al., 2013. Murine autoimmune arthritis is exaggerated by infection with the rat tapeworm, Hymenolepis diminuta. Int. J. Parasitol. 43, 593–601.

Greene, E.C., 1949. In: Ferris, E.J., Griffith, J.Q. (Eds.), The Rat in Laboratory Investigation J. B. Lippincott, Hafner Press, New York, pp. 24–50.

Greene, E.C., 1963. Anatomy of the Rat. Hafner Publ. Co., New York.

Griffith, J.W., White, W.J., Danneman, P.J., Lang, C.M., 1988. Cilia-associated respiratory (CAR) bacillus infection of obese mice. Vet. Pathol. 25, 72–76.

Gruber, H.E., Osborne, J.W., 1979. Ultrastructural features of spironucleosis (hexamitiasis) in x-irradiated rat small intestine. Lab. Anim. 13, 199–202.

Gumprecht, L.A., Long, C.R., Soper, K.A., Smith, P.F., Haschek-Hock, W.M., Keenan, K.P., 1993. The early effects of dietary restriction on the pathogenesis of chronic renal disease in Sprague-Dawley rats at 12 months. Toxicol. Pathol. 21, 528–537.

Haines, D.C., Gorelick, P.L., Battles, J.K., Pike, K.M., Anderson, R.J., Fox, J.G., et al., 1998. Inflammatory and large bowel disease in immunodeficient rats naturally and experimentally infected with Helicobacter bilis. Vet. Pathol. 35, 202–208.

Hansen, A.K., Dagnaes-Hansen, F., Mollegaard-Hansen, K.E., 1992a. Correlation between megaloileitis and antibodies to Bacillus piliformis in laboratory rat colonies. Lab. Anim. Sci. 42, 449–453.

Hansen, A.K., Skovgaard-Jensen, H.J., Thomsen, P., Svendsen, O., Dagnaes-Hansen, F., Mollegaard-Hansen, K.E., 1992b. Rederivation of rat colonies seropositive for Bacillus piliformis and the subsequent screening for antibodies. Lab. Anim. Sci. 42, 444–448.

Hard, G.C., Khan, K.N., 2004. A contemporary overview of chronic progressive nephropathy in the laboratory rat, and its significance for human risk assessment. Toxicol. Pathol. 32, 171–180.

Hartmann, M.J., 2011. A night in the life of a rat: vibrissal mechanics and tactile exploration. Ann. N Y Acad. Sci. 1225, 110–118.

Hasslinger, M.A., Wiethe, T., 1987. Oxyurid infestation of small laboratory animals and its control with ivermectin. Tierarztl. Prax. 15, 93–97.

Hedrich, H.J., 2000. History, strains and models. In: Krinke, G.J. (Ed.), The Laboratory Rat. Academic Press, London.

Henderson, K.S., Dole, V., Parker, N.J., Momtsios, P., Banu, L., Brouillette, R., et al., 2012. Pneumocystis carinii causes a distinctive interstitial pneumonia in immunocompetent laboratory rats that had been attributed to "rat respiratory virus." Vet. Pathol. 49, 440–452.

Henderson, K.S., Perkins, C.L., Havens, R.B., Kelly, M.J., Francis, B.C., Dole, V.S., et al., 2013. Efficacy of direct detection of pathogens in naturally infected mice by using a high-density PCR array. J. Am. Assoc. Lab. Anim. Sci. 52, 763–772.

Hill, W.A., Randolph, M.M., Boyd, K.L., Mandrell, T.D., 2005. Use of permethrin eradicated the tropical rat mite (Ornithonyssus bacoti) from a colony of mutagenized and transgenic mice. Contemp. Top. Lab. Anim. Sci. 44, 31–34.

Hill, W.A., Randolph, M.M., Lokey, S.J., Hayes, E., Boyd, K.L., Mandrell, T.D., 2006. Efficacy and safety of topical selamectin to eradicate pinworm (Syphacia spp.) infections in rats (Rattus norvegicus) and mice (Mus musculus). J. Am. Assoc. Lab. Anim. Sci. 45, 23–26.

Hill, W.A., Randolph, M.M., Mandrell, T.D., 2009. Sensitivity of perianal tape impressions to diagnose pinworm (Syphacia spp.) infections in rats (Rattus norvegicus) and mice (Mus musculus). J. Am. Assoc. Lab. Anim. Sci. 48, 378–380.

Hirabayashi, M., Kato, M., Ishikawa, A., Kaneko, R., Yagi, T., Hochi, S., 2005. Factors affecting production of transgenic rats by ICSI-mediated DNA transfer: effects of sonication and freeze-thawing of spermatozoa, rat strains for sperm and oocyte donors, and different constructs of exogenous DNA. Mol. Reprod. Dev. 70, 422–428.

Hirsjarvi, P., Valiaho, T., 1995. Effects of gentling on open-field behaviour of Wistar rats in fear-evoking test situation. Lab. Anim. 29, 380–384.

Homburger, F., 1977. Saccharin and cancer. N. Engl. J. Med. 297, 560–561.

Hong, S.J., Woo, H.C., Chai, J.Y., 1996. A human case of Plagiorchis muris (Tanabe, 1922: Digenea) infection in the Republic of Korea: freshwater fish as a possible source of infection. J. Parasitol. 82, 647–649.

Hook Jr., R.R., Franklin, C.L., Riley, L.K., Livingston, B.A., Besch-Williford, C.L., 1998. Antigenic analyses of cilia-associated respiratory (CAR) bacillus isolates by use of monoclonal antibodies. Lab. Anim. Sci. 48, 234–239.

Horn, C.C., Kimball, B.A., Wang, H., Kaus, J., Dienel, S., Nagy, A., et al., 2013. Why can't rodents vomit? A comparative behavioral, anatomical, and physiological study. PLoS One 8, e60537.

Hsu, C.C., Franklin, C., Riley, L.K., 2007. Multiplex fluorescent immunoassay for the simultaneous detection of serum antibodies to multiple rodent pathogens. Lab. Anim. (NY) 36, 36–38.

Hsu, C.K., 1979. Parasitic diseases In: Baker, H.J. Lindsey, J.R. Weisbrot H, S.H. (Eds.), The Laboratory Rat, vol. I, Academic Press, New York. Biology and Diseases.

Hubbs, A.F., Hahn, F.F., Lundgren, D.L., 1991. Invasive tracheobronchial aspergillosis in an F344/N rat. Lab. Anim. Sci. 41, 521–524.

Huerkamp, M.J., Benjamin, K.A., Webb, S.K., Pullium, J.K., 2004. Long-term results of dietary fenbendazole to eradicate Syphacia muris from rat colonies. Contemp. Top. Lab. Anim. Sci. 43, 35–36.

Huerkamp, M.J., Benjamin, K.A., Zitzow, L.A., Pullium, J.K., Lloyd, J.A., Thompson, W.D., et al., 2000. Fenbendazole treatment without environmental decontamination eradicates Syphacia muris from all rats in a large, complex research institution. Contemp. Top. Lab. Anim. Sci. 39, 9–12.

Huerkamp, M.J., Zitzow, L.A., Webb, S., Pullium, J.K., 2005. Crossfostering in combination with ivermectin therapy: a method to eradicate murine fur mites. Contemp. Top. Lab. Anim. Sci. 44, 12–16.

Hughes, W.T., 1982. Natural mode of acquisition for de novo infection with Pneumocystis carinii. J. Infect. Dis. 145, 842–848.

Hunter, M.M., Wang, A., Hirota, C.L., Mckay, D.M., 2005. Neutralizing anti-IL-10 antibody blocks the protective effect of tapeworm infection in a murine model of chemically induced colitis. J. Immunol. 174, 7368–7375.

Hunter, M.M., Wang, A., Mckay, D.M., 2007a. Helminth infection enhances disease in a murine TH2 model of colitis. Gastroenterology 132, 1320–1330.

Hunter, R.L., Choi, D.Y., Kincer, J.F., Cass, W.A., Bing, G., Gash, D.M., 2007b. Fenbendazole treatment may influence lipopolysaccharide effects in rat brain. Comp. Med. 57, 487–492.

Hutchinson, K.L., Rollin, P.E., Peters, C.J., 1998. Pathogenesis of a North American hantavirus, Black Creek Canal virus, in experimentally infected Sigmodon hispidus. Am. J. Trop. Med. Hyg. 59, 58–65.

Ince, S., Kozan, E., Kucukkurt, I., Bacak, E., 2010. The effect of levamisole and levamisole + vitamin C on oxidative damage in rats naturally infected with Syphacia muris. Exp. Parasitol. 124, 448–452.

Inge, P.M., Edson, C.M., Farthing, M.J., 1988. Attachment of *Giardia lamblia* to rat intestinal epithelial cells. Gut 29, 795–801.

Itoh, T., Kohyama, K., Takakura, A., Takenouchi, T., Kagiyama, N., 1987. Naturally occurring CAR bacillus infection in a laboratory rat colony and epizootiological observations. Exp. Anim. 36, 387–393.

Jackson, G.A., Livingston, R.S., Riley, L.K., Livingston, B.A., Franklin, C.L., 2013. Development of a PCR assay for the detection of *Spironucleus muris*. J. Am. Assoc. Lab. Anim. Sci. 52, 165–170.

Jacobs, G.H., Fenwick, J.A., Williams, G.A., 2001. Cone-based vision of rats for ultraviolet and visible lights. J. Exp. Biol. 204, 2439–2446.

Jacoby, R., 1986. Rat coronavirus. In: Bhatt, P., Jacoby, R., Morse Iii, H., New, A. (Eds.), Viral and Mycoplasmal Infections of Laboratory Rodents Academic Press, Orlando, FL.

Jacoby, R.O., Ball-Goodrich, L., Paturzo, F.X., Johnson, E.A., 2001. Prevalence of rat virus infection in progeny of acutely or persistently infected pregnant rats. Comp. Med. 51, 38–42.

Jacoby, R.O., Ball-Goodrich, L.J., Besselsen, D.G., Mckisic, M.D., Riley, L.K., Smith, A.L., 1996. Rodent parvovirus infections. Lab. Anim. Sci. 46, 370–380.

Jacoby, R.O., Gaertner, D.J., 2006. Viral disease. In: Suckow, M.A., Weisbroth, S.H., Franklin, C.L. (Eds.), The Laboratory Rat. Elsevier, San Diego, CA.

Jacoby, R.O., Gaertner, D.J., Bhatt, P.N., Paturzo, F.X., SmitH, A.L., 1988. Transmission of experimentally-induced rat virus infection. Lab. Anim. Sci. 38, 11–14.

Jacoby, R.O., Johnson, E.A., Paturzo, F.X., Gaertner, D.J., Brandsma, J.L., Smith, A.L., 1991. Persistent rat parvovirus infection in individually housed rats. Arch. Virol. 117, 193–205.

Jensen, E.S., Allen, K.P., Henderson, K.S., Szabo, A., Thulin, J.D., 2013. PCR testing of a ventilated caging system to detect murine fur mites. J. Am. Assoc. Lab. Anim. Sci. 52, 28–33.

Jeong, E.S., Lee, K.S., Heo, S.H., Seo, J.H., Choi, Y.K., 2013. Rapid identification of *Klebsiella pneumoniae, Corynebacterium kutscheri, and Streptococcus pneumoniae* using triplex polymerase chain reaction in rodents. Exp. Anim. 62, 35–40.

Johnson, P.D., Dawson, B.V., Goldberg, S.J., 1993. Spontaneous congenital heart malformations in sprague dawley rats. Lab. Anim. Sci. 43, 183–188.

Karlsson, E.M., Pearson, L.M., Kuzma, K.M., Burkholder, T.H., 2014. Combined evaluation of commonly used techniques, including PCR, for diagnosis of mouse fur mites. J. Am. Assoc. Lab. Anim. Sci. 53, 69–73.

Kawano, A., Nenoi, M., Matsushita, S., Matsumoto, T., Mita, K., 2000. Sequence of 16S rRNA gene of rat-origin cilia-associated respiratory (CAR) bacillus SMR strain. J. Vet. Med. Sci. 62, 797–800.

Keenan, K.P., Laroque, P., Ballam, G.C., Soper, K.A., Dixit, R., Mattson, B.A., et al., 1996. The effects of diet, ad libitum overfeeding, and moderate dietary restriction on the rodent bioassay: the uncontrolled variable in safety assessment. Toxicol. Pathol. 24, 757–768.

Keenan, K.P., Laroque, P., Dixit, R., 1998. Need for dietary control by caloric restriction in rodent toxicology and carcinogenicity studies. J. Toxicol. Environ. Health, Part B 1, 135–148.

Keenan, K.P., Soper, K.A., Hertzog, P.R., Gumprecht, L.A., Smith, P.F., Mattson, B.A., et al., 1995. Diet, overfeeding, and moderate dietary restriction in control Sprague-Dawley rats: II. Effects on age-related proliferative and degenerative lesions. Toxicol. Pathol. 23, 287–302.

Kelly, J.B., Masterton, B., 1977. Auditory sensitivity of the albino rat. J. Comp. Physiol. Psychol. 91, 930–936.

Kendall, L.V., Riley, L.K., Hook Jr., R.R., Besch-Williford, C.L., Franklin, C.L., 2000. Antibody and cytokine responses to the cilium-associated respiratory bacillus in BALB/c and C57BL/6 mice. Infect. Immun. 68, 4961–4967.

Kendall, L.V., Riley, L.K., Hook Jr., R.R., Besch-Williford, C.L., Franklin, C.L., 2001. Differential interleukin-10 and gamma interferon mRNA expression in lungs of cilium-associated respiratory bacillus-infected mice. Infect. Immun. 69, 3697–3702.

Kiska, D.L., Gilligan, P.H., 1999. Pseudomonas. In: Murray, P.R., Baron, E.J., Pfaller, M.A., Tenover, F.C., Yolken, R.H. (Eds.), Manual of Clinical Microbiology. ASM Press, Washington, DC.

Klement, P., Augustine, J.M., Delaney, K.H., Klement, G., Weitz, J.I., 1996. An oral ivermectin regimen that eradicates pinworms (*Syphacia spp.*) in laboratory rats and mice. Lab. Anim. Sci. 46, 286–290.

Koch-Weser, J., Goldman, P., 1980. Drug therapy: metronidazole. N. Engl. J. Med. 303, 1212–1218.

Kohn, D.F., 1971. Bronchiectasis in rats infected with *Mycoplasma pulmonis*: an electron microscopic study. Lab. Anim. Sci. 21, 856–861.

Kohn, D.F., Barthold, S.W., 1984. Biology and disease of rats. In: Fox, J.G., Cohen, B.J., Loew, F.M. (Eds.), Laboratory Animals Medicine. Academic Press, San Diego, CA.

Kohn, D.F., Chinookoswong, N., Chou, S.M., 1981. A new model of congenital hydrocephalus in the rat. Acta Neuropathol. 54, 211–218.

Kohn, D.F., Kirk, B.E., 1969. Pathogenicity of *Mycoplasma pulmonis* in laboratory rats. Lab. Anim. Care 19, 321–330.

Kojima, A., Okaniwa, A., 1991. Antigenic heterogeneity of sialodacryoadenitis virus isolates. J. Vet. Med. Sci. 53, 1059–1063.

Koolhass, J.M., 1999. The laboratory rat The UFAW Handbook on the Care and Management of Laboratory Animals. Blackwell Science Ltd., Malden, MA, pp. 313–330.

Koto, M., Miwa, M., Togashi, M., Tsuji, K., Okamoto, M., Adachi, J., 1987a. A method for detecting the optimum for mating during the 4-day estrous cycle in the rat: measuring the value of electrical impedance of the vagina. Jikken Dobutsu 36, 195–198.

Koto, M., Miwa, M., Tsuji, K., Okamoto, M., Adachi, J., 1987b. Change in the electrical impedance caused by cornification of the epithelial cell layer of the vaginal mucosa in the rat. Jikken Dobutsu 36, 151–156.

Korenbrot, C., Huhtaniemi, I., Weiner, R., 1977. Preputial separation as an external sign of pubertal development in the male rat. Biol. Reprod. 17, 298–303.

Kubisch, H.M., Gomez-Sanchez, E.P., 1999. Embryo transfer in the rat as a tool to determine genetic components of the gestational environment. Lab. Anim. Sci. 49, 90–94.

Kunita, S., Chaya, M., Hagiwara, K., Ishida, T., Takakura, A., Sugimoto, T., et al., 2006. Development of ELISA using recombinant antigens for specific detection of mouse parvovirus infection. Exp. Anim. 55, 117–124.

Kunstyr, I., 1977. Infectious form of *Spironucleus (Hexamita) muris*: banded cysts. Lab. Anim. 11, 185–188.

Kunstyr, I., Ammerpohl, E., 1978. Resistance of faecal cysts of *Spironucleus muris* to some physical factors and chemical substances. Lab. Anim. 12, 95–97.

Kurisu, K., Sawamoto, O., Watanabe, H., Ito, A., 1996. Sequential changes in the harderian gland of rats exposed to high intensity light. Lab. Anim. Sci. 46, 71–76.

Lai, Y.L., Jacoby, R.O., Jonas, A.M., 1978. Age-related and light-associated retinal changes in Fischer rats. Invest. Ophthalmol. Vis. Sci. 17, 634–638.

Laliberte, F., Mucchielli, A., Laliberte, M.F., 1984. Dynamics of antibody transfer from mother to fetus through the yolk-sac cells in the rat. Biol. Cell. 50, 255–261.

Landin, A.M., Frasca, D., Zaias, J., Van Der Put, E., Riley, R.L., Altman, N.H., et al., 2009. Effects of fenbendazole on the murine humoral immune system. J. Am. Assoc. Lab. Anim. Sci. 48, 251–257.

La Regina, M., Woods, L., Klender, P., Gaertner, D.J., Paturzo, F.X., 1992. Transmission of sialodacryoadenitis virus (SDAV) from infected rats to rats and mice through handling, close contact, and soiled bedding. Lab. Anim. Sci. 42, 344–346.

Laulederkind, S.J., Hayman, G.T., Wang, S.J., Smith, J.R., Lowry, T.F., Nigam, R., et al., 2013. The Rat Genome Database 2013—data, tools and users. Brief Bioinform 14, 520–526.

Leader, R.W., Leader, I., Witschi, E., 1970. Genital mycoplasmosis in rate treated with testosterone propionate to produce constant estrus. J. Am. Vet. Med. Assoc. 157, 1923–1925.

Lechevallier, M.W., Cawthon, C.D., Lee, R.G., 1988. Inactivation of biofilm bacteria. Appl. Environ. Microbiol. 54, 2492–2499.

Lee, A., Phillips, M.W., O'Rourke, J.L., Paster, B.J., Dewhirst, F.E., Fraser, G.J., et al., 1992. *Helicobacter muridarum* sp. nov., a microaerophilic helical bacterium with a novel ultrastructure isolated from the intestinal mucosa of rodents. Int. J. Syst. Bacteriol. 42, 27–36.

Lewis, D.J., 1992. Nonneoplastic lesions in the cardiovascular system In: Mohr, U. Dungworth, D.L. Capen, C.C. (Eds.), Pathobiology of the Aging Rat, vol. 1, ILSI Press, Washington, DC.

Lezmi, S., Thibault-Duprey, K., Bidaut, A., Hardy, P., Pino, M., Macary, G.S., et al., 2011. Spontaneous metritis related to the presence of vaginal septum in pregnant Sprague Dawley Crl:CD(SD) rats: impact on reproductive toxicity studies. Vet. Pathol. 48, 964–969.

Liang, C.T., Shih, A., Chang, Y.H., Liu, C.W., Lee, Y.T., Hsieh, W.C., et al., 2009. Microbial contaminations of laboratory mice and rats in Taiwan from 2004 to 2007. J. Am. Assoc. Lab. Anim. Sci. 48, 381–386.

Liang, S.C., Schoeb, T.R., Davis, J.K., Simecka, J.W., Cassell, G.H., Lindsey, J.R., 1995. Comparative severity of respiratory lesions of sialodacryoadenitis virus and Sendai virus infections in LEW and F344 rats. Vet. Pathol. 32, 661–667.

Liang, S.C., Simecka, J.W., Lindsey, J.R., Cassell, G.H., Davis, J.K., 1999. Antibody responses after Sendai virus infection and their role in upper and lower respiratory tract disease in rats. Lab. Anim. Sci. 49, 385–394.

Liman, E.R., 1996. Pheromone transduction in the vomeronasal organ. Curr. Opin. Neurobiol. 6, 487–493.

Lindsey, J.R., 1979. The Laboratory Rat. Academic Press, New York.

Lindsey, J.R., Baker, H.J., Overcash, R.G., Cassell, G.H., Hunt, C.E., 1971. Murine chronic respiratory disease: significance as a research complication and experimental production with *Mycoplasma pulmonis*. Am. J. Pathol. 64, 675–716.

Lindsey, J.R., Cassell, G.H., Davidson, M.K., 1982. Mycoplasmal and other bacterial disease of the respiratory system In: Foster, H.L. Small, J.D. Fox, J.G. (Eds.), The Mouse in Biomedical Research, vol. II, Academic Press, New York.

Lindstrom, K.E., Carbone, L.G., Kellar, D.E., Mayorga, M.S., Wilkerson, J.D., 2011. Soiled bedding sentinels for the detection of fur mites in mice. J. Am. Assoc. Lab. Anim. Sci. 50, 54–60.

Liu, J.J., Greeley, E.H., Shadduck, J.A., 1988. Murine encephalitozoonosis: the effect of age and mode of transmission on occurrence of infection. Lab. Anim. Sci. 38, 675–679.

Liu, J.J., Greeley, E.H., Shadduck, J.A., 1989. Mechanisms of resistance/susceptibility to murine encephalitozoonosis. Parasite Immunol. 11, 241–256.

Livingston, R.S., Besch-Williford, C.L., Myles, M.H., Franklin, C.L., Crim, M.J., Riley, L.K., 2011. *Pneumocystis carinii* infection causes lung lesions historically attributed to rat respiratory virus. Comp. Med. 61, 45–59.

Livingston, R.S., Besselsen, D.G., Steffen, E.K., Besch-Williford, C.L., Franklin, C.L., Riley, L.K., 2002. Serodiagnosis of mice minute virus and mouse parvovirus infections in mice by enzyme-linked immunosorbent assay with baculovirus-expressed recombinant VP2 proteins. Clin. Diagn. Lab. Immunol. 9, 1025–1031.

Livingston, R.S., Riley, L.K., 2003. Diagnostic testing of mouse and rat colonies for infectious agents. Lab. Anim. (NY) 32, 44–51.

Livingston, R.S., Riley, L.K., Besch-Williford, C.L., Hook, R.R., Franklin, C.L., 1998. Transmission of *Helicobacter hepaticus* infection to sentinel mice by contaminated bedding. Lab. Anim. Sci. 48, 291–293.

Lloyd, G., Bowen, E.T., Jones, N., Pendry, A., 1984. HFRS outbreak associated with laboratory rats in UK. Lancet 1, 1175–1176.

Loftness, T.J., Erlandsen, S.L., Wilson, I.D., Meyer, E.A., 1984. Occurrence of specific secretory immunoglobulin A in bile after inoculation of *Giardia lamblia* trophozoites into rat duodenum. Gastroenterology 87, 1022–1029.

Lubcke, R., Hutcheson, F.A., Barbezat, G.O., 1992. Impaired intestinal electrolyte transport in rats infested with the common parasite *Syphacia muris*. Dig. Dis. Sci. 37, 60–64.

Lukas, V., Ruehl, W.W., Hamm, T.E., 1987. An enzyme-linked, immunosorbent assay to intact serum IgG in rabbits naturally exposed to cilia-associated respiratory bacillus. LAS 37 553–553.

Lussier, G., 1991. Detection methods for the identification of rodent viral and mycoplasmal infections. Lab. Anim. Sci. 41, 199–225.

Lytvynets, A., Langrova, I., Lachout, J., Vadlejch, J., 2013. Detection of pinworm eggs in the dust of laboratory animals breeding facility, in the cages and on the hands of the technicians. Lab. Anim. 47, 71–73.

Mackenzie, W.F., Magill, L.S., Hulse, M., 1981. A filamentous bacterium associated with respiratory disease in wild rats. Vet. Pathol. 18, 836–839.

Maggi, C.A., Santicioli, P., Meli, A., 1986. Postnatal development of micturition reflex in rats. Am. J. Physiol. 250, R926–R931.

Mahler, M., Kohl, W., 2009. A serological survey to evaluate contemporary prevalence of viral agents and Mycoplasma pulmonis in laboratory mice and rats in western Europe. Lab. Anim. (NY) 38, 161–165.

Majeed, S.K., Zubaidy, A.J., 1982. Histopathological lesions associated with *Encephalitozoon cuniculi* (nosematosis) infection in a colony of Wistar rats. Lab. Anim. 16, 244–247.

Makino, S., Seko, S., Nakao, H., Mikazuki, K., 1973. An epizootic of Sendai virus infection in a rat colony (author's transl). Jikken Dobutsu 22, 275–280.

Manser, C.E., Elliot, H., Morris, T.H., Broom, D.M., 1995a. The use of a novel operant system to determine the strength of preference for flooring in laboratory rats. Lab. Anim. 30, 1–6.

Manser, C.E., Morris, T.H., Broom, D.M., 1995b. An investigation into the effects of solid or grid cage flooring on the welfare of laboratory rats. Lab. Anim. 29, 353–363.

Manser, C.E., Broom, D.M., Overend, P., Morris, T.H., 1998a. Operant studies to determine the strength of preference in laboratory rats for nest-boxes and nesting materials. Lab. Anim. 32, 36–41.

Manser, C.E., Broom, D.M., Overend, P., Morris, T.H., 1998b. Investigations into the preferences of laboratory rats for nest-boxes and nesting materials. Lab. Anim. 32, 23–35.

Maronpot, R.R., 1996. Spontaneous hydronephrosis. In: Jones, T.C., Hard, G.C., Mohr, U. (Eds.), Urinary System Springer, Berlin, Germany.

Martin, M.G., Wu, S.V., Walsh, J.H., 1997. Ontogenetic development and distribution of antibody transport and Fc receptor mRNA expression in rat intestine. Dig. Dis. Sci. 42, 1062–1069.

Martinez-Gomez, M., Cruz, Y., Salas, M., Hudson, R., Pacheco, P., 1994. Assessing pain threshold in the rat: changes with estrus and time of day. Physiol. Behav. 55, 651–657.

Matsushita, S., Joshima, H., 1989. Pathology of rats intranasally inoculated with the cilia-associated respiratory bacillus. Lab. Anim. 23, 89–95.

Matsushita, S., Joshima, H., Matsumoto, T., Fukutsu, K., 1989. Transmission experiments of cilia-associated respiratory bacillus in mice, rabbits, and guinea pigs. Lab. Anim. 23, 96–102.

Matsushita, S., Kashima, M., Joshima, H., 1987. Serodiagnosis of cilia-associated respiratory bacillus infection by the indirect immunofluorescence assay technique. Lab. Anim. 21, 356–359.

Mattheij, J.A.M., Swarts, J.J.M., 1991. Quantification and classification of pregnancy wastage in 5-day cyclic young through middle-aged rats. Lab. Anim. 25, 30–34.

Matuszczyk, J.V., Appa, R.S., Larsson, K., 1994. Age-dependent variations in the sexual preference of male rats. Physiol. Behav. 55, 827–830.

Maud, P., Thavarak, O., Cedrick, L., Michele, B., Vincent, B., Olivier, P., et al., 2014. Evidence for the use of isoflurane as a replacement for chloral hydrate anesthesia in experimental stroke: an ethical issue. Biomed. Res. Int. 2014, 802539.

Mayhew, H., 1851. Jack Black. London Labour and the London Poor. Stationer's Hall Court: Griffen, Bohn, and Company.

McCay, C.M., 1973. Notes on the History of Nutrition Research. Hans Huber, Berne, Switzerland.

McConnell, S.J., Huxsoll, D.L., Garner, F.M., Spertzel, R.O., Warner Jr., A.R., Yager, R.H., 1964. Isolation and characterization of a neurotropic agent (Mhg Virus) from adult rats. Proc. Soc. Exp. Biol. Med. 115, 362–367.

McCormack, C.E., Sontag, C.R., 1980. Entrainment by red light of running activity and ovulation rhythms of rats. Am. J. Physiol. 239, R450–R453.

McCoy, M.R., Montonye, D., Bryda, E.C., 2013. Electroejaculation of chimeric rats. Lab. Anim. (NY) 42, 203–205.

McInnes, E.F., Rasmussen, L., Fung, P., Auld, A.M., Alvarez, L., Lawrence, D.A., et al., 2011. Prevalence of viral, bacterial and parasitological diseases in rats and mice used in research environments in Australasia over a 5-y period. Lab. Anim. (NY) 40, 341–350.

McKay, D.M., 2010. The immune response to and immunomodulation by Hymenolepis diminuta. Parasitology 137, 385–394.

McKisic, M.D., Paturzo, F.X., Gaertner, D.J., Jacoby, R.O., Smith, A.L., 1995. A nonlethal rat parvovirus infection suppresses rat T lymphocyte effector functions. J. Immunol. 155, 3979–3986.

Medina, L.V., Chladny, J., Ortman, J.D., Artwohl, J.E., Bunte, R.M., Bennett, B.T., 1998. Rapid way to identify the cilia-associated respiratory bacillus: tracheal mucosal scraping with a modified microwave Steiner silver impregnation. Lab. Anim. Sci. 46, 113–115.

Mendes, E.N., Queiroz, D.M., Dewhirst, F.E., Paster, B.J., Moura, S.B., Fox, J.G., 1996. Helicobacter trogontum sp. nov., isolated from the rat intestine. Int. J. Syst. Bacteriol. 46, 916–921.

Mercier, O., Perraud, J., Stadler, J., 1987. A method for routine observation of sexual behaviour in rats. Lab. Anim. 21, 125–130.

Metcalf Pate, K.A., Rice, K.A., Wrighten, R., Watson, J., 2011. Effect of sampling strategy on the detection of fur mites within a naturally infested colony of mice (Mus musculus). J. Am. Assoc. Lab. Anim. Sci. 50, 337–343.

Meyer, T.K., Yurchak, M.R., Pliego, J.F., Wincek, T.J., Dukelow, W.R., Kuehl, T.J., 1997. Cryopreservation of murine zygotes for use in testing culture environments. Lab. Anim. Sci. 47, 496–499.

Miyajima, A., Sunouchi, M., Mitsunaga, K., Yamakoshi, Y., Nakazawa, K., Usami, M., 2009. Sexing of postimplantation rat embryos in stored two-dimensional electrophoresis (2-DE) samples by polymerase chain reaction (PCR) of an Sry sequence. J. Toxicol. Sci. 34, 681.

Mohr, U., Dungworth, D.L., Capen, C.C., 1992. Pathobiology of the Aging Rat. International Life Sciences Institute, Washington, DC.

Montes, G.S., Luque, E.H., 1988. Effects of ovarian steroids on vaginal smears in the rat. Acta Anat. (Basel) 133, 192–199.

Montgomery, C.A., Seely, J.C., 1990. Kidney. In: Boorman, G.A., Eustis, S.L., Elwell, M.R., Montgomery, C.A., MacKenzie, W.F. (Eds.), Pathology of the Fischer Rat. Reference and Atlas Academic Press, San Diego, pp. 127–153.

Mook, D.M., Benjamin, K.A., 2008. Use of selamectin and moxidectin in the treatment of mouse fur mites. J. Am. Assoc. Lab. Anim. Sci. 47, 20–24.

Moore, D.M., 1995. In: Rollin, B.E. Kesel, M.J. (Eds.), The Experimental Animal in Biomedical Research, vol. 2, CRC Press, Boca Raton, FL. Chapter 11.

Moore, H.D., Akhondi, M.A., 1996. Fertilizing capacity of rat spermatozoa is correlated with decline in straight-line velocity measured by continuous computer-aided sperm analysis: epididymal rat spermatozoa from the proximal cauda have a greater fertilizing capacity in vitro than those from the distal cauda or vas deferens. J. Androl. 17, 50–60.

Mottola, M.F., Plust, J.H., Christopher, P.D., Schachter, C.L., 1992. Effects of exercise on maternal glycogen storage patterns and fetal outcome in mature rats. Can. J. Physiol. Pharmacol. 70, 1634–1638.

Motzel, S.L., Riley, L.K., 1992. Subclinical infections and transmission of Tyzzer's disease in rats. Lab. Anim. Sci. 42, 439–443.

Nakae, D., 1999. Endogenous liver carcinogenesis in the rat. Pathol. Int. 49, 1028–1042.

Nakatsukasa, E., Kashiwazaki, N., Takizawa, A., Shino, M., Kitada, K., Serikawa, T., et al., 2003. Cryopreservation of spermatozoa from closed colonies, and inbred, spontaneous mutant, and transgenic strains of rats. Comp. Med. 53, 639–641.

Naot, Y., Merchav, S., Ben-David, E., Ginsburg, H., 1979a. Mitogenic activity of Mycoplasma pulmonis. I. Stimulation of rat B and T lymphocytes. Immunology 36, 399–406.

Naot, Y., Simon-Tou, R., Ginsburg, H., 1979b. Mitogenic activity of Mycoplasma pulmonis. II. Studies on the biochemical nature of the mitogenic factor. Eur. J. Immunol. 9, 149–151.

National Research Council, 1991. Infectious Diseases of Mice and Rats. National Academy Press, Washington, DC.

National Research Council, 1995. Nutritional Requirements of Laboratory Animals, fourth ed. National Academy Press, Washington, DC.

National Research Council, 1996. Laboratory Animal Management—Rodents. National Academy Press, Washington, DC.

National Research Council, 2011. Guide for the Care and Use of Laboratory Animals, eighth ed. The National Academies Press, Washington, DC.

Neimark, H., Johansson, K.E., Rikihisa, Y., Tully, J.G., 2001. Proposal to transfer some members of the genera Haemobartonella and Eperythrozoon to the genus Mycoplasma with descriptions of 'Candidatus Mycoplasma haemofelis', 'Candidatus Mycoplasma haemomuris', 'Candidatus Mycoplasma haemosuis' and 'Candidatus Mycoplasma wenyonii'. Int. J. Syst. Evol. Microbiol. 51, 891–899.

Neimark, H., Johansson, K.E., Rikihisa, Y., Tully, J.G., 2002. Revision of haemotrophic Mycoplasma species names. Int. J. Syst. Evol. Microbiol. 52, 683.

Nicklas, W., 2007. Pasteurellaceae. In: Fox, J.G., Barthold, S.W., Davisson, M.T., Newcomer, C.E., Quimby, F.W., Smith, A.L. (Eds.), The Mouse in Biomedical Research, second ed. Academic Press, Burlington, MA.

Niederkorn, J.Y., Shadduck, J.A., Schmidt, E.C., 1981. Susceptibility of selected inbred strains of mice to Encephalitozoon cuniculi. J. Infect. Dis. 144, 249–253.

Niggeschulze, A., Kast, A., 1994. Maternal age, reproduction, and chromosomal aberrations in Wistar derived rats. Lab. Anim. 28, 55–62.

Noritake, S., Ogawa, K., Suzuki, G., Ozawa, K., Ikeda, T., 2007. Pulmonary inflammation in brown Norway rats: possible association of environmental particles in the animal room environment. Exp. Anim. 56, 319–327.

Nunn, G., Macpherson, A., 1995. Spontaneous convulsions in charles river wistar rats. Lab. Anim. 29, 50–53.

Oge, H., Ayaz, E., Ide, T., Dalgic, S., 2000. The effect of doramectin, moxidectin and netobimin against natural infections of Syphacia muris in rats. Vet. Parasitol. 88, 299–303.

Ohsawa, K., Watanabe, Y., Miyata, H., Sato, H., 2003. Genetic analysis of a Theiler-like virus isolated from rats. Comp. Med. 53, 191–196.

Owen, D.G., 1992. Ectoparasites (Phylum Arthropoda). Parasites of Laboratory Animals. Royal Society of Medicine Services, Ltd, London.

Oyetibo, G.O., Ilori, M.O., Obayori, O.S., Amund, O.O., 2013. Biodegradation of petroleum hydrocarbons in the presence of nickel and cobalt. J. Basic Microbiol. 53, 917–927.

Oz, H.S., Hughes, W.T., 1996. Effect of sex and dexamethasone dose on the experimental host for Pneumocystis carinii. Lab. Anim. Sci. 46, 109–110.

Pakes, S.P., Shadduck, J.A., Feldman, D.B., Moore, J.A., 1984. Comparison of tests for the diagnosis of spontaneous encephalitozoonosis in rabbits. Lab. Anim. Sci. 34, 356–359.

Parel, J.D., Galula, J.U., Ooi, H.K., 2008. Characterization of rDNA sequences from *Syphacia obvelata, Syphacia muris,* and *Aspiculuris tetraptera* and development of a PCR-based method for identification. Vet. Parasitol. 153, 379–383.

Parkinson, C.M., O'Brien, A., Albers, T.M., Simon, M.A., Clifford, C.B., Pritchett-Corning, K.R., 2011. Diagnosis of ecto- and endoparasites in laboratory rats and mice. J. Vis. Exp., e2767.

Paturzo, F.X., Jacoby, R.O., Bhatt, P.N., Smith, A.L., Gaertner, D.J., Ardito, R.B., 1987. Persistence of rat virus in seropositive rats as detected by explant culture. Brief report. Arch. Virol. 95, 137–142.

Pauli, B.U., Gruber, A.D., Weinstein, R.S., 1996. Transitional cell carcinoma, bladder, rat. In: Jones, T.C., Hard, G.C., Mohr, U. (Eds.), Urinary System. Springer, Berlin, Germany.

Pearson, D.J., Taylor, G., 1975. The influence of the nematode *Syphacia oblevata* on adjuvant arthritis in the rat. Immunology 29, 391–396.

Peluso, J.J., 1992. In: Mohr, U., Dungworth, D.L., Capen, C.C. (Eds.), Pathobiology of the Aging Rat. ILSI Press, Washington, DC, pp. 337–349.

Percy, D.H., Barthold, S.W., 2007. Pathology of Laboratory Rodents and Rabbits. Blackwell Publishing, Ames, IA.

Percy, D.H., Bond, S.J., Paturzo, F.X., Bhatt, P.N., 1990. Duration of protection from reinfection following exposure to sialodacryoadenitis virus in Wistar rats. Lab Anim Sci. 40, 144–149.

Perez, C., Canal, J.R., Dominguez, E., Campillo, J.E., Guillen, M., Torres, M.D., 1997. Individual housing influences certain biochemical parameters in the rat. Lab. Anim. 31, 357–361.

Petri, M., 1969. Studies on *Nosema cuniculi* found in transplantable ascites tumours with a survey of microsporidiosis in mammals. Acta Pathol. Microbiol. Scand. Suppl. 204, 1–91.

Philipeaux, J.M., 1856. Note sur le extirpation des capsules suprarenal chez albino rats *(Mus rattus)*. de Medecine at de Chirurgie 43.

Pleasants, J.R., 1974. Gnotobiotics. In: Melby, E.C., Altman, N.H. (Eds.), Handbook of Laboratory Animal Science. CRC Press, Cleveland, OH.

Pochanke, V., Hatak, S., Hengartner, H., Zinkernagel, R.M., Mccoy, K.D., 2006. Induction of IgE and allergic-type responses in fur mite-infested mice. Eur. J. Immunol. 36, 2434–2445.

Pohlmeyer, G., Deerberg, F., England, F., 1993. Nude rats as a model of natural *Pneumocystis carinii pneumonia*: sequential morphological study of lung lesions. J. Comp. Pathol., 217–230. 1993/10/01.

Pollicino, P., Rossi, L., Rambozzi, L., Farca, A.M., Peano, A., 2008. Oral administration of moxidectin for treatment of murine acariosis due to *Radfordia affinis*. Vet. Parasitol. 151, 355–357.

Poonacha, K.B., William, P.D., Stamper, R.D., 1985. Encephalitozoonosis in a parrot. J. Am. Vet. Med. Assoc. 186, 700–702.

Portfors, C.V., 2007. Types and functions of ultrasonic vocalizations in laboratory rats and mice. J. Am. Assoc. Lab. Anim. Sci. 46, 28–34.

Pritchett, K.R., Johnston, N.A., 2002. A review of treatments for the eradication of pinworm infections from laboratory rodent colonies. Contemp. Top. Lab. Anim. Sci. 41, 36–46.

Pritchett-Corning, K.R., Cosentino, J., Clifford, C.B., 2009. Contemporary prevalence of infectious agents in laboratory mice and rats. Lab. Anim. 43, 165–173.

Pritt, S., Henderson, K.S., Shek, W.R., 2010. Evaluation of available diagnostic methods for *Clostridium piliforme* in laboratory rabbits *(Oryctolagus cuniculus)*. Lab. Anim. 44, 14–19.

Pucak, G.J., Lee, C.S., Zaino, A.S., 1977. Effects of prolonged high temperature on testicular development and fertility in the male rat. Lab. Anim. Sci. 27, 76–77.

Pullium, J.K., Brooks, W.J., Langley, A.D., Huerkamp, M.J., 2005. A single dose of topical moxidectin as an effective treatment for murine acariasis due to *Myocoptes musculinus*. Contemp. Top. Lab. Anim. Sci. 44, 26–28.

Reardon, C., Sanchez, A., Hogaboam, C.M., Mckay, D.M., 2001. Tapeworm infection reduces epithelial ion transport abnormalities in murine dextran sulfate sodium-induced colitis. Infect. Immun. 69, 4417–4423.

Reetz, J., 1993. Naturally-acquired microsporidia *(Encephalitozoon cuniculi)* infections in hens. Tierarztl Prax 21, 429–435.

Rehm, S., Waalkes, M.P., Ward, J.M., 1988. Aspergillus rhinitis in Wistar (Crl:(WI)BR) rats. Lab. Anim. Sci. 38, 162–166.

Ricart Arbona, R.J., Lipman, N.S., Riedel, E.R., Wolf, F.R., 2010a. Treatment and eradication of murine fur mites: I. Toxicologic evaluation of ivermectin-compounded feed. J. Am. Assoc. Lab. Anim. Sci. 49, 564–570.

Ricart Arbona, R.J., Lipman, N.S., Wolf, F.R., 2010b. Treatment and eradication of murine fur mites: II. Diagnostic considerations. J. Am. Assoc. Lab. Anim. Sci. 49, 583–587.

Ricart Arbona, R.J., Lipman, N.S., Wolf, F.R., 2010c. Treatment and eradication of murine fur mites: III. Treatment of a large mouse colony with ivermectin-compounded feed. J. Am. Assoc. Lab. Anim. Sci. 49, 633–637.

Rice, K.A., Albacarys, L.K., Metcalf Pate, K.A., Perkins, C., Henderson, K.S., Watson, J., 2013. Evaluation of diagnostic methods for *Myocoptes musculinus* according to age and treatment status of mice *(Mus musculus)*. J. Am. Assoc. Lab. Anim. Sci. 52, 773–781.

Riley, L.K., Franklin, C.L., Hook, R.R., Besch-Williford, C., 1996. Identification of murine helicobacters by PCR and restriction enzyme analysis. J. Clin. Microbiol. 34, 942–946.

Riley, L.K., Simmons, J.H., Purdy, G., Livingston, R.S., Franklin, C.L., Besch-Williford, C.L., 1997. Research update: idiopathic lung lesions in rats. ACLAD Newsletter 20.

Ristic, M., Kreier, J.P., 1984. Family III. Anaplasmatacaea. In: Krieg, I.N.R., Holt, J.G. (Eds.), Bergey's Manual of Systematic Bacteriology. Williams and Wilkins, Baltimore, MD.

Robinson, R., 1965. Genetics of the Norway Rat. Pergamon Press, New York.

Roble, G.S., Boteler, W., Riedel, E., Lipman, N.S., 2012. Total IgE as a serodiagnostic marker to aid murine fur mite detection. J. Am. Assoc. Lab. Anim. Sci. 51, 199–208.

Roe, F.J.C., Lee, P.N., Conybeare, G., Kelly, D., Matter, B., Prentice, D., et al., 1995. The biosure study: influence of composition of diet and food consumption on longevity, degenerative diseases, and neoplasia in Wistar rats studied for up to 30 months post weaning. Food Chem. Toxicol. 33 (Suppl. 1), 1S–100S.

Rogers, A.E., Zeisel, S.H., Groopman, J., 1993. Diet and carcinogenesis. Carcinogenesis 14, 2205–2217.

Rohde, C.M., Wells, D.F., Robosky, L.C., Manning, M.L., Clifford, C.B., Reily, M.D., et al., 2007. Metabonomic evaluation of Schaedler altered microflora rats. Chem. Res. Toxicol. 20, 1388–1392.

Romero, A., Villamayor, F., Grau, M.T., Sacristan, A., Ortiz, J.A., 1992. Relationship between fetal weight and litter size in rats: application to reproductive toxicology studies. Reprod. Toxicol. 6, 453–456.

Rosen, M., Kahan, E., Derazne, E., 1987. The influence of the first-mating age of rats on the number of pups born, their weights, and their mortality. Lab. Anim. 21, 348–352.

Rouleau, A.M., Kovacs, P.R., Kunz, H.W., Armstrong, D.T., 1993. Decontamination of rat embryos and transfer to specific pathogen-free recipients for the production of a breeding colony. Lab. Anim. Sci. 43, 611–615.

Royals, M.A., Getzy, D.M., Vandewoude, S., 1999. High fungal spore load in corncob bedding associated with fungal-induced rhinitis in two rats. Contemp. Top. Lab. Anim. Sci. 38, 64–66.

Russell, L.D., 1992. In: Mohr, U. Dungworth, D.L. Hapen, C.C. (Eds.), Pathobiology of the Aging Rat, vol. 1, ILSI Press, Washington, DC, pp. 395–405.

Russell, L.D., Alger, L.E., Nequin, L.G., 1987. Hormonal control of pubertal spermatogenesis. Endocrinology 120, 1615–1632.

Saibaba, P., Sales, G.D., Stodulski, G., Hau, J., 1996. Behavious of rats in their home cages: daytime variations and effects of routine husbandry procedures analysed by time sampling techniques. Lab. Anim. 30, 13–21.

Sales, G.D., Milligan, S.R., 1992. Ultrasound and laboratory animals. Anim. Technol. 43, 89–98.

Savage, D.C., 1971. Defining the gastrointestinal microflora of laboratory mice. In: National Research Council, Defining the Laboratory Animal. IV Symposium, International Committee on Laboratory Animals, National Academy of Sciences, Washington, DC.

Savage, N., 1984. Genus streptobacillus In: Krieg, I.N.R. Holt, J.G. (Eds.), Bergey's Manual of Systematic Bacteriology, vol. I, William and Wilkins, Baltimore, MD.

Savory, W.S., 1863. Experiments on food, its destination and uses. Lancet 81, 381–383.

Schagemann, G., Bohnet, W., Kunstyr, I., Friedhoff, K.T., 1990. Host specificity of cloned *Spironucleus muris* in laboratory rodents. Lab. Anim. 24, 234–239.

Schoeb, T.R., Davidson, M.K., Lindsey, J.R., 1982. Intracage ammonia promotes growth of *Mycoplasma pulmonis* in the respiratory tract of rats. Infect. Immun. 38, 212–217.

Schoeb, T.R., Kervin, K.C., Lindsey, J.R., 1985. Exacerbation of murine respiratory mycoplasmosis in gnotobiotic F344/N rats by Sendai virus infection. Vet. Pathol. 22, 272–282.

Schoeb, T.R., Mcconnell, E.E., Juliana, M.M., Davis, J.K., Davidson, M.K., Lindsey, J.R., 2009a. *Mycoplasma pulmonis* and lymphoma. Environ. Mol. Mutagen. 50, 1–3. author reply 6–9.

Schoeb, T.R., Mcconnell, E.E., Juliana, M.M., Davis, J.K., Davidson, M.K., Lindsey, J.R., 2009b. *Mycoplasma pulmonis* and lymphoma in bioassays in rats. Vet. Pathol. 46, 952–959.

Schoondermark-Van De Ven, E.M., Philipse-Bergmann, I.M., Van Der Logt, J.T., 2006. Prevalence of naturally occurring viral infections, *Mycoplasma pulmonis* and *Clostridium piliforme* in laboratory rodents in Western Europe screened from 2000 to 2003. Lab. Anim. 40, 137–143.

Seely, J.C., Haseman, J.K., Nyska, A., Wolf, D.C., Everitt, J.I., Hailey, J.R., 2002. The effect of chronic progressive nephropathy on the incidence of renal tubule cell neoplasms in control male F344 rats. Toxicol. Pathol. 30, 681–686.

Seita, Y., Sugio, S., Ito, J., Kashiwazaki, N., 2009. Generation of live rats produced by in vitro fertilization using cryopreserved spermatozoa. Biol. Reprod. 80, 503–510.

Semple-Rowland, S.L., Dawson, W.W., 1987. Retinal cyclic light damage threshold for albino rats. Lab. Anim. Sci. 37, 289–298.

Sevimli, F.K., Kozan, E., Sevimli, A., Dogan, N., Bulbul, A., 2009. The acute effects of single-dose orally administered doramectin, eprinomectin and selamectin on natural infections of *Syphacia muris* in rats. Exp. Parasitol. 122, 177–181.

Shalev, U., Feldon, J., Weiner, I., 1998. Gender- and age-dependent differences in latent inhibition following pre-weaning non-handling: implications for a neurodevelopmental animal model of schizophrenia. Int. J. Dev. Neurosci. 16, 279–288.

Sharma, A.W., Mayrhofer, G., 1988a. Biliary antibody response in rats infected with rodent *Giardia duodenalis* isolates. Parasite Immunol. 10, 181–191.

Sharma, A., Fish, B.L., Moulder, J.E., Medhora, M., Baker, J.E., Mader, M., et al., 2014. Safety and blood sample volume and quality of a refined retro-orbital bleeding technique in rats using a lateral approach. Lab. Anim. (NY) 43, 63–66.

Sharma, A.W., Mayrhofer, G., 1988b. A comparative study of infections with rodent isolates of *Giardia duodenalis* in inbred strains of rats and mice and in hypothymic nude rats. Parasite Immunol. 10, 169–179.

Shoji, Y., Itoh, T., Kagiyama, N., 1988. Enzyme-linked immunosorbent assay for detection of serum antibody to CAR bacillus. Exp. Anim. 37, 67–72.

Short, B.G., Goldstein, R.S., 1992. Nonneoplastic lesions in the kidney In: Mohr, U. Dungworth, D.L. Capen, C.C. (Eds.), Pathobiology of the Aging Rat, vol. 1, ILSI Press, Washington, DC.

Shuster, K.A., Hish, G.A., Selles, L.A., Chowdhury, M.A., Wiggins, R.C., Dysko, R.C., et al., 2013. Naturally occurring disseminated group B streptococcus infections in postnatal rats. Comp. Med. 63, 55–61.

Silveira, A.C., Gilioli, R., Oliveira, E.S., Bassani, R.A., 2003. Subsensitivity to beta-adrenergic stimulation in atria from rats infested with *Syphacia* sp. Lab. Anim. 37, 63–67.

Simpson, J., Kelly, J.P., 2011. The impact of environmental enrichment in laboratory rats—behavioural and neurochemical aspects. Behav. Brain Res. 222, 246–264.

Singletary, K.B., Kloster, C.A., Baker, D.G., 2003. Optimal age at fostering for derivation of Helicobacter hepaticus-free mice. Comp. Med. 53, 259–264.

Singletary, S.J., Kirsch, A.J., Watson, J., Karim, B.O., Huso, D.L., Hurn, P.D., et al., 2005. Lack of correlation of vaginal impedance measurements with hormone levels in the rat. Contemp. Top. Lab. Anim. Sci. 44, 37–42.

Skelton, H., Smith, K., Hilyard, E., Hadfield, T., Tuur, S., Wagner, K., et al., 1995. Bacillus piliformis (Tyzzer's Disease) in an HIV-1+ patient: confirmation with 16S rRNA sequence analysis. J. Invest. Dermatol. 104 687–687.

Slama, M., Susic, D., Varagic, J., Frohlich, E.D., 2002. High rate of ventricular septal defects in WKY rats. Hypertension 40, 175–178.

Slaoui, M., Dreef, H.C., Van Esch, E., 1998. Inflammatory lesions in the lungs of Wistar rats. Toxicol. Pathol. 26, 712–713. discussion 714.

Smith, E.R., Stefanick, M.L., Clark, J.T., Davidson, J.M., 1992. Hormones and sexual behavior in relationship to aging in male rats. Horm. Behav. 26, 110–135.

Songsasen, N., Leibo, S.P., 1998. Live mice derived from cryopreserved embryos derived in vitro with cryopreserved ejaculated spermatozoa. Lab. Anim. Sci. 48, 275–281.

Sorden, S.D., Castleman, W.L., 1991. Brown Norway rats are high responders to bronchiolitis, pneumonia, and bronchiolar mastocytosis induced by parainfluenza virus. Exp. Lung. Res. 17, 1025–1045.

Speakman, J.R., Mitchell, S.E., 2011. Caloric restriction. Mol. Aspects Med. 32, 159–221.

Starke, W.A., Oaks, J.A., 2001. Ileal mucosal mast cell, eosinophil, and goblet cell populations during Hymenolepis diminuta infection of the rat. J. Parasitol. 87, 1222–1225.

Stringer, J.R., 1993. The identity of *Pneumocystis carinii*: not a single protozoan, but a diverse group of exotic fungi. Infect. Agents Dis. 2, 109–117.

Suber, R.L., Kodell, R.L., 1985. The effect of three phlebotomy techniques on hematologic and clinical chemical evaluation in Sprague-Dawley rats. Vet. Clin. Pathol. 14, 23–30.

Sueta, T., Miyoshi, I., Okamura, T., Kasai, N., 2002. Experimental eradication of pinworms (*Syphacia obvelata* and *Aspiculuris tetraptera*) from mice colonies using ivermectin. Exp. Anim. 51, 367–373.

Summa, M.E., Ebisui, L., Osaka, J.T., De Tolosa, E.M., 1992. Efficacy of oral ivermectin against *Trichosomoides crassicauda* in naturally infected laboratory rats. Lab. Anim. Sci. 42, 620–622.

Suzuki, E., Mochida, K., Nakagawa, M., 1988. Naturally occurring subclinical *Corynebacterium kutscheri* infection in laboratory rats: strain and age related antibody response. Lab. Anim. Sci. 38, 42–45.

Swing, S.P., Davis, J.K., Egan, M.L., 1995. In vitro effects of *Mycoplasma pulmonis* on murine natural killer cell activity. Lab. Anim. Sci. 45, 352–356.

Tada, N., Sata, M., Mizorogi, T., Kasai, K., Gawa, S., 1995. Efficient cryopreservation of hairless mutant (bald) and normal Wistar rat embryos by vitrification. Lab. Anim. Sci. 45, 323–325.

Tai, J.H., Chang, S.C., Chou, C.F., Ong, S.J., 1996. Separation and characterization of two related giardiaviruses in the parasitic protozoan *Giardia lamblia*. Virology 216, 124–132.

Tai, J.H., Wang, A.L., Ong, S.J., Lai, K.S., Lo, C., Wang, C.C., 1991. The course of giardiavirus infection in the *Giardia lamblia* trophozoites. Exp. Parasitol. 73, 413–423.

Takeichi, N., Hamada, J., Takimoto, M., Fujiwara, K., Kobayashi, H., 1988. Depression of T cell-mediated immunity and enhancement of autoantibody production by natural infection with microorganisms in spontaneously hypertensive rats (SHR). Microbiol. Immunol. 32, 1235–1244.

Tanemura, K., Wakayama, T., Kuramoto, K., Hayashi, Y., Sato, E., Ogura, A., 1997. Birth of normal young by microinsemination with frozen-thawed round spermatids collected from aged azoospermic mice. Lab. Anim. Sci. 47, 203–204.

Tayama, K., Shisa, H., 1994. Development of pigmented scales on rat skin: relation to age, sex, strain, and hormonal effect. Lab. Anim. Sci. 44, 240–244.

Thomas, D.S., Pass, D.A., 1997. Chronic ulcerative typhlocolitis in CBH- rnu/rnu (Athymic nude) rats. Lab. Anim. Sci. 47, 423–427.

Timm, K.I., 1979. Orbital venous anatomy of the rat. Lab. Anim. Sci. 29, 636–638.

Timme, R.E., Pettengill, J.B., Allard, M.W., Strain, E., Barrangou, R., Wehnes, C., et al., 2013. Phylogenetic diversity of the enteric pathogen *Salmonella enterica* subsp. *enterica* inferred from genome-wide reference-free SNP characters. Genome Biol. Evol. 5, 2109–2123.

Tindall, B.J., Grimont, P.A., Garrity, G.M., Euzeby, J.P., 2005. Nomenclature and taxonomy of the genus *Salmonella*. Int. J. Syst. Evol. Microbiol. 55, 521–524.

Treuting, P.M., Clifford, C.B., Sellers, R.S., Brayton, C.F., 2012. Of mice and microflora. Vet. Pathol., 44–63. Online 49.

Tvedten, H.W., Whitehair, C.K., Langham, R.F., 1973. Influence of Vitamins A and E on gnotobiotic and conventiionally maintained rats exposed to *Mycoplasma pulmonis*. J. Am. Vet. Med. Assoc. 163, 605–612.

Tyzzer, E.E., 1917. A fatal disease of Japanese waltzing mice caused by a spore-forming bacillus (*Bacillus piliformis* N. sp.). J. Med. Res. 37, 307–338.

Urano, T., Maejima, K., Okada, O., Takashina, S., Syumiya, S., Tamura, H., 1977. Control of *Pseudomonas aeruginosa* infection in laboratory mice with gentamicin. Jikken Dobutsu 26, 259–262.

Utsumi, K., Satoh, E., Iritani, A., 1991. Sexing of rat embryos with antisera specific for male rats. J. Exp. Zool. 260, 99–105.

Vallon, V., 2009. Micropuncturing the nephron. Pflugers Arch. 458, 189–201.

Van Andel, R.A., Franklin, C.L., Besch-Williford, C.L., Hook, R.R., Riley, L.K., 2000. Prolonged perturbations of tumour necrosis factor-alpha and interferon-gamma in mice inoculated with *Clostridium piliforme*. J. Med. Microbiol. 49, 557–563.

Van Loo, P., Baumans, V., 2004. The importance of learning young: the use of nesting material in laboratory rats. Lab. Anim. 38, 17–24.

Van Winkle, T.J., Womack, J.E., Barbo, W.D., Davis, T.W., 1988. Incidence of hydronephrosis among several production colonies of outbred Sprague-Dawley rats. Lab. Anim. Sci. 38, 402–406.

Van Zwieten, M.J., Solleveld, H.A., Lindsey, J.R., De Groot, F.G., Zurcher, C., Hollander, C.F., 1980. Respiratory disease in rats associated with a filamentous bacterium: a preliminary report. LAS 30, 215–221.

Vanderhyden, B.C., Rouleau, A., Walton, E.A., Armstrong, D.T., 1986. Increased mortality during early embryonic development after in-vitro fertilization of rat oocytes. J. Reprod. Fertil. 77, 401–409.

Vento, P.J., Swartz, M.E., Martin, L.B., Daniels, D., 2008. Food intake in laboratory rats provided standard and fenbendazole-supplemented diets. J. Am. Assoc. Lab. Anim. Sci. 47, 46–50.

Villar, D., Cray, C., Zaias, J., Altman, N.H., 2007. Biologic effects of fenbendazole in rats and mice: a review. J. Am. Assoc. Lab. Anim. Sci. 46, 8–15.

Vonderfecht, S.L., Huber, A.C., Eiden, J., Mader, L.C., Yolken, R.H., 1984. Infectious diarrhea of infant rats produced by a rotavirus-like agent. J. Virol. 52, 94–98.

Vonderfecht, S.L., Miskuff, R.L., Eiden, J.J., Yolken, R.H., 1985. Enzyme immunoassay inhibition assay for the detection of rat rotavirus-like agent in intestinal and fecal specimens obtained from diarrheic rats and humans. J. Clin. Microbiol. 22, 726–730.

Waggie, K.S., Spencer, T.H., Allen, A.M., 1987. Cilia associated respiratory (CAR) bacillus infection in New Zealand White rabbits. LAS 37 533–533.

Wagner, J.E., Owens, D.R., Laregina, M.C., Vogler, G.A., 1977. Self trauma and Staphylococcus aureus in ulcerative dermatitis of rats. J. Am. Vet. Med. Assoc. 171, 839–841.

Wagner, M., 1988. The effect of infection with the pinworm (*Syphacia muris*) on rat growth. Lab. Anim. Sci. 38, 476–478.

Wan, C.H., Soderlund-Venermo, M., Pintel, D.J., Riley, L.K., 2002. Molecular characterization of three newly recognized rat parvoviruses. J. Gen. Virol. 83, 2075–2083.

Watson, D.S.B., 1993. Evaluation of inanimate objects on commonly monitored variables in preclinical safety studies for mice and rats. Lab. Anim. Sci. 43, 378–380.

Watson, J., 2008. New building, old parasite: mesostigmatid mites—an ever-present threat to barrier facilities. ILAR J. 49, 303–309.

Weaver, L., Wickramanayake, G., 2001. Kinetics of the inactivation of microorganisms. In: Block, S. (Ed.), Disinfection, Sterilization, and Preservation, fifth ed. Lippincott Wiliams & Wilkins, Philadelphia, PA.

Webb, R.A., Hoque, T., Dimas, S., 2007. Expulsion of the gastrointestinal cestode, Hymenolepis diminuta by tolerant rats: evidence for mediation by a Th2 type immune enhanced goblet cell hyperplasia, increased mucin production and secretion. Parasite Immunol. 29, 11–21.

Weber, K.S., Setchell, K.D., Stocco, D.M., Lephart, E.D., 2001. Dietary soy-phytoestrogens decrease testosterone levels and prostate weight without altering LH, prostate 5alpha-reductase or testicular steroidogenic acute regulatory peptide levels in adult male Sprague-Dawley rats. J. Endocrinol. 170, 591–599.

Weigler, B.J., Carte, A.D., Martineau, J.M., Noson, D., Soriano, P., 2007. Motion detectors as the cause of poor reproductibe performance in mice. JAALAS 46, 120–121.

Weir, E.C., Jacoby, R.O., Paturzo, F.X., Johnson, E.A., 1990. Infection of SDAV-immune rats with SDAV and rat coronavirus. Lab. Anim. Sci. 40, 363–366.

Weisbroth, S.H., 1982. Bacterial and mycotic diseases In: Foster, H.L. Small, D. Fox, J.G. (Eds.), The Laboratory Rat, vol. 1, Academic Press, New York. Biology and Diseases.

Weisbroth, S.H., Peters, R., Riley, L.K., Shek, W., 1998. Microbiological assessment of laboratory rats and mice. ILAR J. 39, 272–290.

Weiss, E.E., Evans, K.D., Griffey, S.M., 2012. Comparison of a fur mite PCR assay and the tape test for initial and posttreatment diagnosis during a natural infection. J. Am. Assoc. Lab. Anim. Sci. 51, 574–578.

Weisse, I., 1992. In: Mohr, U. Dung worth, D.L. Capen, C.C. (Eds.), Pathobiology of the Aging Rat, vol. 2, ILSI Press, Washington, DC, pp. 65–119.

West, W.L., Schofield, J.C., Bennett, B.T., 1992. Efficacy of the "micro-dot" technique for administering topical 1% ivermectin for the control of pinworms and fur mites in mice. Contemp. Top. Lab. Anim. Sci. 31, 7–10.

Will, L.A., 1994. Rat-bite fevers. In: Beran, G.W., Steele, J.H. (Eds.), Handbook of Zoonoses, Section A: Bacterial, Rickettsial, Chlamydial and Mycotic, second ed. CRC Press, Boca Raton, FL.

Wilson, J.M., 1979. The biology of *Encephalitozoon cuniculi*. Med. Biol. 57, 84–101.

Wullenweber, M., 1995. *Streptobacillus moniliformis* – a zoonotic pathogen. Taxonomic considerations, host species, diagnosis, therapy, geographical distribution. Lab. Anim. 29, 1–15.

Wunderlich, M.L., Dodge, M.E., Dhawan, R.K., SheK, W.R., 2011. Multiplexed fluorometric immunoassay testing methodology and troubleshooting. J. Vis. Exp. (58), e3715. Available from http://dx.doi.org/10.3791/3715.

Wyand, D.S., Jonas, A.M., 1967. *Pseudomonas aeruginosa* infection in rats following implantation of an indwelling jugular catheter. Lab. Anim. Care 17, 261–267.

Yang, F.C., Paturzo, F.X., Jacoby, R.O., 1995. Environmental stability and transmission of rat virus. Lab. Anim. Sci. 45, 140–144.

Yarbrough, W.G., Quarmby, V.E., Simental, J.A., Joseph, D.R., Sar, M., Lubahn, D.B., et al., 1990. A single base mutation in the androgen receptor gene causes androgen insensitivity in the testicular feminized rat. J. Biol. Chem. 265, 8893–8900.

Yoshitomi, K., Boorman, G.A., 1990. Eye and associated glands. In: Boorman, G.A., Eustis, S.L., Elwell, M.R., Montgomery, C.A., Mackenzie, W.F. (Eds.), Pathology of the Fischer Rat. Reference and Atlas. Academic Press, San Diego, CA.

Ypsilantis, P., Deftereos, S., Prassopoulos, P., Simopoulos, C., 2009. Ultrasonographic diagnosis of pregnancy in rats. J. Am. Assoc. Lab. Anim. Sci. 48, 734–739.

Yu, D.C., Wang, A.L., Botka, C.W., Wang, C.C., 1998. Protein synthesis in Giardia lamblia may involve interaction between a downstream box (DB) in mRNA and an anti-DB in the 16S-like ribosomal RNA. Mol. Biochem. Parasitol. 96, 151–165.

Yu, D.C., Wang, A.L., Wang, C.C., 1996. Amplification, expression, and packaging of a foreign gene by giardiavirus in *Giardia lamblia*. J. Virol. 70, 8752–8757.

Yu, V.M., Mackinnon, S.E., Hunter, D.A., Brenner, M.J., 2011. Effect of sialodacryoadenitis virus infection on axonal regeneration. Microsurgery 31, 458–464.

Zenner, L., 1998. Effective eradication of pinworms (*Syphacia muris*, *Syphacia obvelata* and *Aspiculuris tetraptera*) from a rodent breeding colony by oral anthelmintic therapy. Lab. Anim. 32, 337–342.

Zubaidy, A.J., Majeed, S.K., 1981. Pathology of the nematode *Trichosomoides crassicauda* in the urinary bladder of laboratory rats. Lab. Anim. 15, 381–384.

5

Biology and Diseases of Hamsters

Emily L. Miedel, VMD[a] and F. Claire Hankenson, DVM, MS, DACLAM[b]

[a]University of Pennsylvania, University Laboratory Animal Resources, Philadelphia, PA, USA
[b]Michigan State University, Campus Animal Resources, East Lansing, MI, USA

I. INTRODUCTION

The hamster species used as research models include the Syrian (golden), *Mesocricetus auratus*; the Chinese (striped-back), *Cricetulus griseus*; the Armenian (gray), *C. migratorius*; the European, *Cricetus cricetus*; and the Djungarian, *Phodopus campbelli* (Russian dwarf) and *P. sungorus* (Siberian dwarf). Hamsters are classified as members of the order Rodentia, suborder Myomorpha, superfamily Muroidea, and in family Cricetidae. Animals in this family are characterized by large cheek pouches, thick bodies, short tails, and an excess of loose skin. They have incisors that erupt continuously and cuspidate molars that do not continue to grow ((I 1/1, C 0/0, PM 0/0, M 3/3) × 2

= 16). In 2010, it was reported that approximately 146,000 hamsters were used in research in the United States (United States Department of Agriculture, 2010).

II. SYRIAN HAMSTER

A. Introduction

The reader is referred to the American College of Laboratory Animal Medicine Series reference entitled *The Laboratory Rabbit, Guinea Pig, Hamster and Other Rodents* (Suckow et al., 2012) for a comprehensive source of information on hamster biology and diseases, experimental techniques, and research models.

1. Description

The Syrian or golden hamster (*Mesocricetus auratus*) originated in Syria and naturally resides in the arid, temperate regions of southeast Europe and Asia Minor. In their native environment, hamsters live in deep tunnels that provide cooler temperatures and higher humidity than the general desert environment. They are nocturnal animals in the laboratory, but field research has shown diurnal activity in females in the wild (Gattermann *et al.*, 2008). The adult Syrian hamster usually grows to a length of 6–8 inches (14–19 cm) and weighs between 110 and 140 g. The adult female of this breed tends to be larger than the male. The hamster has a small blunt tail and smooth, short hair. Normal coloration is reddish gold, with a grayish-white ventrum. Hair-coat colors also include cream, albino, piebald, and cinnamon; the length of hair can also vary (Harkness *et al.*, 2010). Hamster ears are pointed, with dark pigmentation, and the eyes are small, dark, and bright. Male hamsters can be identified by prominent flank glands and by large testicles that protrude behind the body on each side of the tail. The normal gross anatomy for the golden hamster has been described in this section (Hoffman *et al.*, 1968; Murray, 2012).

2. Use in Research

Practically all Syrian hamsters now in use as laboratory animals originated from one litter captured in Syria in 1930. The use of the golden hamster as a laboratory animal was initiated by Saul Adler, who sought a laboratory animal susceptible to infection with *Leishmania* (Adler, 1948). Only three littermates, one male and two females, were retained in captivity, and it is the progeny of these animals that were first imported to the United States in 1938. By 1973, the hamster had become the third most commonly used laboratory animal in the United States, behind mice and rats. Hamster use in research has steadily declined by approximately 67% since its peak in the early 1970s; currently hamsters are less frequently used than mice, rats, rabbits, and guinea pigs (United States Department of Agriculture, 2010).

Hamsters have several unique anatomical and physiological features that make them desirable research models. In addition, they are susceptible to a variety of carcinogens and develop certain tumors other animal models do not. Metabolic diseases can be induced in hamsters through dietary manipulation, and they develop a variety of inherited diseases that are similar to human syndromes. Furthermore, hamsters are relatively free of pathogens yet are susceptible to several experimental infectious diseases (Valentine *et al.*, 2012).

Hamsters are used often for carcinogenesis studies; in fact, the hamster cheek-pouch carcinogenesis model is a popular model to study oral tumor formation (Vairaktaris *et al.*, 2007, 2008a, b). They are also used extensively to study pancreatic ductal adenocarcinoma through the administration of nitrosamines (Konishi *et al.*, 1998; Uchida *et al.*, 2008) or via the transplantable cell line, PGHAM-1, which models metastatic pancreatic cancer (Fukuhara *et al.*, 2005; Uchida *et al.*, 2008). The hamster is also susceptible to respiratory tract tumors and can be induced to develop nonsmall cell lung carcinoma through a course of injections of the carcinogen 4-(methylnitrosamino)-1-(3-pyridyl)-1-butanone (NNK), with or without the addition of hyperoxia (Oreffo *et al.*, 1993; Sunday *et al.*, 1995). The role of Simian virus 40 (SV40), a polyomavirus, in human cancers remains controversial (Rollison *et al.*, 2004); however, the hamster remains a valuable model for investigation of this viral disease process. Hamsters injected with SV40 develop a variety of tumors depending on the route of inoculation and the age of hamster when inoculated (Allison *et al.*, 1967; Cicala *et al.*, 1993; Sroller *et al.*, 2008). Additionally, the Syrian hamster is used to study the effects of exogenous estrogenic compounds on tumor development, with 100% of male hamsters developing renal tumors after the administration of estrogens (Li and Li, 1996; Liehr, 1997). Finally, the hamster is one of the few animal models that permit the replication of human adenoviruses, which holds promise as a potential cancer therapeutic (Hjorth *et al.*, 1988; Thomas *et al.*, 2006).

Hamsters, like humans, are highly susceptible to metabolic diseases and present with several related clinical signs and syndromes. The hamster is commonly used as a model for cholesterol cholelithiasis, which can be induced via excess dietary cholesterol or by feeding a sucrose-rich diet (Cohen *et al.*, 1989; Khallou *et al.*, 1991; Trautwein *et al.*, 1999). Hamsters are also susceptible to diabetes mellitus induced by differing methods. Chemical agents such as streptozotocin (STZ) or alloxan can be used; however, STZ may be more effective and reliable than alloxan (Phares, 1980). The addition of nicotinamide (dosed intraperitoneally) at 15 min before STZ injection results in partial protection against the beta-cytotoxic effect of STZ, resulting in partial preservation of insulin stores (Fararh *et al.*, 2002; Masiello *et al.*, 1998). Diabetes mellitus can also be induced via dietary modifications. A high-fat (15%) diet containing modest cholesterol (0.12%) fed for three weeks will induce type 2 diabetes along with related comorbidities such as obesity, hyperinsulinemia, hyperleptinemia, hypercholesterolemia, and hypertriglyceridemia (Van Heek et al., 2001). Syrian hamsters of the albino-panda-albino (APA) strain develop diabetes with nephropathy following STZ injections and also develop coronary lesions (Horiuchi *et al.*, 2005). Syrian hamsters possess similar lipid metabolism to humans and are useful models for atherosclerosis, induced via dietary manipulation (Mitchell and McLeod, 2008; Simionescu *et al.*, 1993; Wissler, 1991).

Syrian hamsters have spontaneous genetic mutations that manifest with conditions resembling human cardiovascular disease. Cardiomyopathy in the Syrian hamster is a naturally occurring, inherited condition and, as such, is an established animal model for both dilated cardiomyopathy (DCM) and hypertrophic cardiomyopathy (HCM). In the hamster, both DCM and HCM are caused by a defect in the sarcoglycan gene, a component of the dystrophin complex (Bajusz et al., 1969; Escobales and Crespo, 2006, 2008; Goineau et al., 2001; Ikeda and Ross, 2000; Lipskaia et al., 2007; Ryoke et al., 1999; Sakamoto et al., 1997). Cardiomyopathic hamster lines include the original polymyopathic line 1.50, as well as BIO 82.62, BIO TO-2, BIO 53, and UMX-7.1. Some strains are characterized by significant cardiac hypertrophy, some by ventricular dilation without hypertrophy, and still other strains show compensatory hypertrophy progressing to left ventricular dilation (Cruz et al., 2007; Goineau et al., 2001; Homburger, 1979; Ikeda and Ross, 2000; Sakamoto et al., 1997).

Syrian hamsters were originally introduced as laboratory animals that could be infected with Leishmania (Adler, 1948). Their susceptibility to experimentally induced infectious diseases continues to make them valuable infectious disease models. Hamsters serve as experimental models of Hantavirus pulmonary syndrome (McElroy et al., 2004; Milazzo et al., 2002; Wahl-Jensen et al., 2007). Hamsters are also susceptible to the coronovirus that leads to severe acute respiratory syndrome (SARS); therefore, they are also useful for efficacy studies for vaccinations and immunotherapy treatments against this virus (Roberts et al., 2005). Hamsters are susceptible to fungal infections, including Histoplasma spp., and are sensitive to small inocula. They then can be involved in refinements for disease diagnosis. Most of the fungi grow in the spleen, lymph nodes, and liver. Hamsters infected with Mycoplasma pneumoniae are used as models of localized infection in the respiratory tract (Brunner, 1997).

Other pathogens to which hamsters are susceptible include Mycobacteria spp., Clostridium difficile (Kokkotou et al., 2008), Treponema pallidum (Kajdacsy-Balla et al., 1993), Toxoplasma spp. (Pavesio et al., 1995), and Babesia spp. (Wozniak et al., 1996). In addition, hamsters can serve as models of leprosy, atypical tuberculosis, and leptospirosis, as well as other protozoal and helminthic infections. Leishmania infantum infection causes polymyositis and may be a new model for inflammatory myopathy (Paciello et al., 2010). Syrian hamsters have historically been valuable for the study of prion disease. Laboratory mice are now the animal model of choice for this research area, yet hamster strains are still occasionally used in the study of prions because of their susceptibility to scrapie, transmissible mink encephalopathy (TME), Creutzfeldt–Jakob disease, and Gerstmann–Staussler syndrome (GSS) (Lowenstein et al., 1990). These prions cause slow, progressive, degenerative diseases in the central nervous system (CNS). Hamsters develop amyloid-like deposits in their brains, which may be similar to extracellular deposits of amyloid found in human Alzheimer's disease (Czub et al., 1986). Scrapie prions replicate to high titers in the brains of several species of hamsters, making it possible to compare the human and hamster forms of the disease in a single host (Lowenstein et al., 1990; Marsh and Hanson, 1978). Further information about the prion diseases can be obtained in reviews by Prusiner (1991) and Trevitt and Collinge (2006).

In addition to the above models, hamsters are preferred for several other experimental uses. Chronic obstructive pulmonary disease (COPD) and emphysema can be induced via a single intratracheal dose of porcine pancreatic elastase (Borzone et al., 2007) or feeding a diet deficient in copper (Soskel et al., 1984). Hamsters are also used to study gastropathy related to administration of nonsteroidal anti-inflammatory drugs (NSAIDs) (Kolbasa et al., 1988; Fitzpatrick et al., 1999).

In 1976, the hamster oocyte was discovered to be penetrable by human spermatozoa (Yanagimachi et al., 1976). Since that time, one of the main uses of Syrian hamsters in the biomedical setting has been to aid in the assessment of human fertility using the zona-free hamster oocyte assay, which analyzes the ability of sperm to capacitate eggs, undergo the acrosome reaction, and fuse with the oocyte (Barros et al., 1978). Results obtained from the assay correlate well with human in vitro fertilization results, but the process is labor-intensive and difficult to standardize. As new techniques are developed to assess male fertility (such as intracytoplasmic sperm injection), the hamster oocyte assay has begun to wane in popularity (Aitken, 2006).

B. Biology

1. Anatomy and Physiology

a. Development

A newborn M. auratus pup weighs 2–3 g. It is hairless, with eyes and ears closed. A unique feature of this rodent pup is that incisor teeth are visible at birth. At approximately day 4–5 of age, the ears will open; at day 9, hair growth is first observed; and between days 14 and 16, the eyes will open (Mulder, 2012). By weaning at day 21 of age, the pup weighs 35–40 g. By maturity at 6–8 weeks, males weigh 85–110 g and females weigh 95–120 g. There may be additional increase in weight with increased age. Male and female hamsters can be identified by comparing the anogenital distances (longer in the male) and by observing mammae on the ventrum of the female or noting the prominence of the posterior scrotum of the male.

The reproductive life span begins around 6–8 weeks and continues until 14 months of age (Mulder, 2012). The total life span averages 2 years, with the potential for aging up to 3 years. It is of interest to note that the average life span of the female golden hamster may be markedly shorter than that of males, depending on strain and source of the animals (Bernfeld *et al.*, 1986). The short life cycle of the Syrian hamster, ranging between 18 and 24 months, makes it an excellent animal for the study of development and the effect of teratogenic agents. The eighth day of pregnancy is the optimal time for teratogenic studies, when hourly development of the fetal pups can be observed (Ferm, 1967). Normative physiological data, such as heart rate and respiration, can be found in Table 5.1. Serum blood chemistry values have been provided in Table 5.2. It should be mentioned that serum chemistry parameters may differ between sexes and strains of hamsters (Maxwell *et al.*, 1985).

b. Oral Cavity

i. CHEEK POUCHES The cheek pouches, bilateral invaginations of the oral mucosa, are found in the lateral buccal walls. Often these highly distensible pouches are used by the hamster for temporary storage of food and bedding materials. These pouches do not contain glands but are rich in mast cells, are highly vascular, and lined with stratified squamous epithelium (deArruda and Montenegro, 1995). Blood supply to the pouches is carried by branches from the external carotid artery (Davis *et al.*, 1986). More specifically, the pouches are supplied by six small arteries in the neck and face that are potentially important in controlling cheek pouch blood flow (Davis *et al.*, 1986). The pouches can easily be everted (Fig. 5.1), with their blood flow intact, and have been used extensively for microvascular studies of inflammation, tumor growth, vascular smooth muscle function, and ischemia reperfusion studies (Svensjo, 1990; Hedqvist *et al.*, 1990; Bertuglia and Reiter, 2007). These pouches lack an intact lymphatic drainage pathway and are therefore described as 'immunologically privileged.' Studies have shown that the surface density of Langerhans cells in the cheek pouches is markedly decreased, which may contribute to the specialized immune status of the tissue (Bergstresser *et al.*, 1980). The pouch tissue will support the long-term survival of transplanted foreign tissue without immunological rejection. As mentioned previously, the Syrian hamster model of carcinogenesis in the cheek pouch is one of the best animal systems for the evaluation of human oral cancer development (Gimenez-Conti and Slaga, 1993).

ii. DENTITION Due to the morphological makeup of their crown teeth, retention of fine food particles often occurs, and Syrian hamsters develop dental caries under defined conditions of diet and oral flora (Krasse, 1966). Studies show that the caries rate in hamsters is influenced not only by the amount of carbohydrate in the diet, but

also by the form of carbohydrate. The presence or absence of vitamins in the diet is also thought to be a contributing factor (Shklar, 1972). Historical reports have suggested that caries may be caused by infectious bacteria and transmissible among rodents via oral routes (Jordan and van Houte, 1972). While hamsters were useful models at one time for studying caries-induced lesions, other rodent models are now more common (Bowen, 2013).

TABLE 5.1 Normative Data – Syrian (Golden) Hamster[a]

Adult weight	
Male	85–140 g
Female	95–120 g
Life-span	
Average	2 years
Maximum expected	3 years
Chromosome number (diploid)	44
Water consumption	30 ml/day
Food consumption	10–15 g/day (adult)
Body temperature	36.2–37.5°C
Puberty	
Male	6–8 weeks (90 g)
Female	8–12 weeks (90–100 g)
Gestation	15–18 days
Litter size	4–12 pups
Birth weight	2–3 g
Eyes open	15 days
Weaning	21 days (35–40 g)
Heart rate	280–412
Respiratory frequency	74 (33–127)
Leukocyte counts	
Total	7.62×10^3/mm
Neutrophils	
Segmented	21.9%
Nonsegmented	8.0%
Lymphocytes	73.5%
Monocytes	2.5%
Eosinophils	1.1%
Basophils	1.1%
Erythrocyte sedimentation rate	1.64 mm/h
Platelets	670.0×10^3/mm (indirect)
Red blood cells	7.50×10^6/mm
Hemoglobin	16.8%

[a]From *Aeromedical Review* (1975).

TABLE 5.2 Mean ± SD Serum Blood Chemistry Values for Adult Syrian Hamsters[a]

Serum analyte	Units	Male	Female
Glucose	mg/dl	84.0 ± 18.5	100.0 ± 16.6
Urea nitrogen	mg/dl	23.2 ± 4.1	27.5 ± 4.6
Creatinine	mg/dl	0.40 ± 0.89	0.50 ± 0.15
Sodium	mEq/l	148.0 ± 3.70	148.0 ± 3.70
Potassium	mEq/l	6.50 ± 0.75	6.40 ± 0.73
Chloride	mEq/l	104.0 ± 3.10	104.0 ± 3.60
Bicarbonate	mEq/l	29.9 ± 2.9[b]	
Calcium	mg/dl	12.6 ± 0.59	13.2 ± 1.38
Phosphorus	mg/dl	5.40 ± 1.00	5.50 ± 1.09
Magnesium	mg/dl	2.50 ± 0.20	2.20 ± 0.10
Alanine aminotransferase	IU/l	44.7 ± 25.9	50.3 ± 18.3
Aspartate aminotransferase	IU/l	61.2 ± 39.1	53.3 ± 22.7
Alkaline phosphatase	IU/l		126 ± 6
Lactate dehydrogenase	IU/l	257 ± 63.6	208 ± 54.7
Creatinine kinase	IU/l	469 ± 174	520 ± 184
Protein, total	g/l	63 ± 3.2	59 ± 3.4
Albumin	g/l	43 ± 2.2	41 ± 2.8
Cholesterol	mg/dl	143 ± 23.5	158 ± 35.3
Triglycerides	mg/dl	209 ± 53.3	212 ± 52.7
Bilirubin, total	mg/dl	0.3 ± 0.09	0.3 ± 0.13
Bile acids	μmol/l		0.9 ± 0.2
Uric acid		4.6 ± 0.5	4.4 ± 0.5
Luteinizing hormone	ng/ml	10–30	20–40 (basal) 1500–2000 (late proestrus)
Follicle stimulating hormone	ng/ml	200–300	100–200 (basal) 400–600 (preovulatory, estrus)
Prolactin	ng/ml	5–10	10–15 (basal) 30 (late proestrus)
Thyroid stimulating hormone	ng/ml	300[b]	
Thyroxine (T$_4$)	μg/dl	3–7[b]	
Triiodothyronine (T$_3$)	ng/dl	30–80[b]	
Cortisol	μg/dl	2.75 ± 0.44	0.33 ± 0.04 (start of light)
Progesterone	ng/ml		1.0 (basal) 10–12 (proestrus) 6–8 (estrus, diestrus)
Estradiol	pg/ml		5–10 (basal) 300–400 (proestrus)
Testosterone	ng/ml	1.5–2.0	

[a]Summarized from Loeb and Quimby (1999).
[b]Gender not specified.

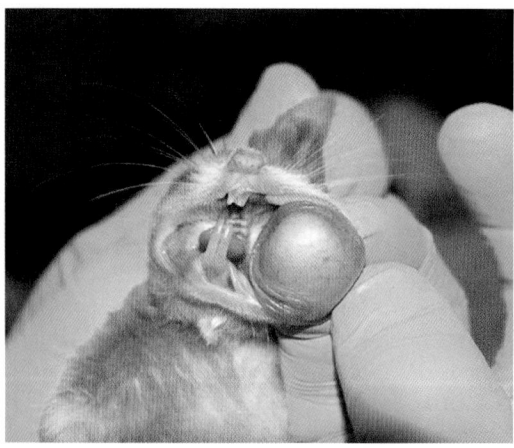

FIGURE 5.1 The cheek pouch has been manually everted for illustrative purposes. Note the vasculature supplying the pouch. *Credit: Jerald Silverman and Academic Press.*

c. Gastrointestinal System

i. STOMACH AND INTESTINES The hamster has a distinctly compartmentalized stomach consisting of two parts: the glandular stomach and the nonglandular forestomach. The forestomach and glandular stomach are separated from each other by the incisurae of the greater and lesser curvatures (Magalhaes, 1968). The nonglandular forestomach is functionally similar to that of ruminants and has an elevated pH level and microflora that contribute to digestion through a fermentation process.

The incidence of neoplasms in Syrian hamsters varies by study. These differences are likely due to age, strain differences, breeding environment, diet, and other unknown factors. Two studies showed high incidences of spontaneous neoplasms in the gastrointestinal tract (Fortner, 1957; Van Hoosier and Trentin, 1979), while other studies do not document such findings (Tanaka et al., 1991). The experimental induction of papillomas and adenocarcinoma in the forestomach and intestines, as well as adenomatous polyps in the colon, historically validated the hamster model of gastrointestinal carcinogenesis (Homburger, 1968).

Syrian hamsters respond predictably to intragastric administration of purified cholera enterotoxin, presenting with intraluminal accumulation of fluid in the small bowel, cecum, and proximal colon. Therefore, this animal was historically used to study pharmacological agents, such as indomethacin, polymyxin B sulfate, glucose electrolyte solutions, and colchicine that may inhibit intestinal fluid secretions (Lepot and Banwell, 1976).

ii. PANCREAS/GALLBLADDER/BILIARY TRACT In the hamster, the major pancreatic ducts join the common bile duct shortly before it enters the duodenum. This anatomical configuration is similar to that of mice and rats, but is distinct from other mammals, including humans. The pancreas of the Syrian hamster is similar in function to that of the mouse and rat.

The Syrian hamster can serve as a model for pancreatic carcinogenesis. Most commonly, pancreatic tumors are induced by the subcutaneous administration of nitrosamines, but the transplantable cell line (PGHAM-1), mentioned previously, can also reproduce metastatic pancreatic cancer (Uchida et al., 2008).

d. Pulmonary System

The conductive airways of the Syrian hamster contain a limited number of glandular structures, primarily in the proximal trachea, which facilitates modeling chronic bronchitis (Hayes et al., 1977). The pulmonary vascular bed is similar to that of humans and hamsters develop pulmonary lesions that resemble human centrilobular emphysema when exposed to intratracheal porcine pancreatic elastase (Borzone et al., 2007, Kleinerman, 1972). Spontaneous bronchiogenic and pulmonary cancers are rare; hence, the Syrian hamster is a good model to study chemical carcinogenesis of the respiratory tract (Homburger, 1968).

e. Genitourinary System

In the Syrian hamster, the reproductive and urogenital tracts develop from the same embryonic germinal ridge, rendering the kidneys highly responsive to estrogen. As a consequence, administration of estrogen to male hamsters leads to renal tumors and represents a critical model for studying the effects of exogenous estrogenic compounds on tumor development (Li et al., 1993). Hamsters are one of the most reliable models for studying the effect of chemical carcinogens on the urinary bladder (Van Hoosier and Ladgies, 1984).

f. Endocrine System

Hamsters are reported to be the first model in which the equivalent of Addisonian adrenal necrosis could be studied (Frenkel, 1956). The adrenal glands show a distinct difference in size by 4 weeks of age, depending on the sex of the animal. Male adrenal glands reportedly have a greater number of reticular cells within the adrenal cortex, accounting for a size double that of female adrenal glands (Militzer et al., 1990).

g. Immunological System

Hamsters have unique immune system characteristics. Hamsters do not reject skin allografts to the same extent as compared to rejection by other laboratory animals, and they have enhanced susceptibility to select infections (Streilein, 1978). Streilein et al. (1980) determined, based upon skin grafting experiments, that the original littermates identified in 1930 had very little alloantigenic variation. In addition, few mutational changes in this defined gene pool have occurred since the introduction of the hamster into biomedical use (Streilein et al., 1980). Many immunological studies have focused on the organization of major histocompatibility complex (MHC) class I genes in hamsters. While diversity exists at the MHC class II locus, the region is likely similar among the strains of Syrian hamsters that are available for research (Hixon et al., 1996).

Related to their short gestation period, the ontogeny of the thymic system and associated cellular immunity in Syrian hamsters is delayed compared to other rodents. In addition, only four of the five immunoglobulin (Ig) classes have been described in the hamster, i.e., IgM, IgG, IgA, and IgE, while IgD remains to be defined, and at least two strains of inbred hamsters are deficient in the sixth component of complement. Another IgG isotype, classified as IgG_3, has been isolated from some strains of inbred Syrian hamsters. This immunoglobulin is differentiated from IgG_1 and IgG_2 by its affinity for protein A (Coe et al., 1995). Immunodeficiency has not been linked to deficiencies in IgG_3.

Structural information for hamster immunoglobulins has been limited; however the first crystal structure of a hamster IgG Fab fragment and the complete cDNA sequence of the stimulatory antibody HL4E10 (which contains the first example of a hamster lambda light chain) has been identified. As the HL4E10 antibody is uniquely costimulatory for $\gamma\delta$ T cells, humanized versions may be of clinical relevance in treating $\gamma\delta$ T cell dysfunction-associated diseases, such as chronic non-healing wounds and cancer (Verdino et al., 2011).

h. Secretory and Sebaceous Glands

i. HARDERIAN GLANDS Harderian glands are pigmented lacrimal glands located posterior to the ocular globes. These secretory glands release a lipid- and porphyrin-rich material that lubricates the eyes and eyelids. Additionally, the harderian gland is a site of immune response, a source of thermoregulatory lipids and pheromones, a photoprotective organ and part of a retinal–pineal axis. Marked sexual dimorphism of these glands in Syrian hamsters was first reported in the 1950s and has not been shown to exist in the Chinese, Armenian, or Djungarian hamster. Female and male Syrian hamsters differ most significantly in the type of lipid droplets secreted by the Harderian glands and in the relative concentration of secreted porphyrin (females secrete up to 10^3-times more porphyrin than males) (Buzzell, 1996). This glandular dimorphism is androgen-dependent and exhibits seasonal variation. A complete histologic description of the gland has been published (Buzzell, 1996).

ii. FLANK GLANDS Coarse hair over darkly pigmented skin can be readily observed in the costovertebral

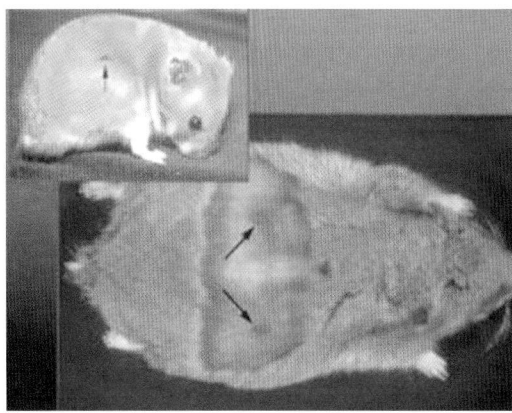

FIGURE 5.2   The flank glands in the male hamster (arrows) are used as sex glands and for olfactory marking. Females also have these glands, although they are less prominent.

area in males (Fig. 5.2). The flank glands of the Syrian hamster are dermal structures composed of sebaceous glands that produce secretions in response to androgens. When the male is sexually excited, hair over these glands becomes wet, and the male may appear pruritic. These glandular secretions are likely used for territorial marking. The female also has dorsal sebaceous glands, but are not as easily identified and the secretions are associated with the estrous cycle (Hamilton and Montagna, 1950).

i. Hibernation

Hibernation is a state of inactivity and metabolic depression in endotherms. This behavior, not exhibited in mice, rats, or guinea pigs, enables hamsters to be used for a variety of unique experimental objectives in behavioral and physiological research (Horwitz et al., 2013; Lyman, 1979; Storey, 2010). Hibernation ability varies among different hamster species and between individual animals; however, exposure to cold stimulates the hamster to gather food, and it will hibernate at a temperature of approximately 5°C (±2°). Unlike the European hamster, which is a true hibernator, the Syrian hamster is not used extensively for hibernation studies since it may not reliably enter hibernation when exposed to cold temperatures and bouts of hibernation may be short (Lyman, 1982). Because cold exposure and hibernation in the hamster are associated with desaturation of white adipose tissue, hamsters are useful for studies of factors controlling the saturation of fat.

2. Genetics

Syrian hamsters have a diploid chromosome number of 44. Numerous mutations have been introduced since the establishment of this animal model in the 1930s (Yoon and Peterson, 1979). Eighteen of the mutations involve coat and eye color; the earliest mutations produced brown, cream, piebald, and white hamsters. Six mutations involve the neuromuscular system, and six are identifiable by quantity or texture of hair. Breeders have also developed inbred strains of hamsters, some of which are of value to researchers because of genetically transmitted diseases or conditions, and unique susceptibility to teratogenic and carcinogenic agents (Homburger, 1972). In 2014, the first successful transgenic hamsters were created, promoting the future use of genetically engineered hamsters as disease models (Gao *et al.*, 2014). Hamster embryonic stem cell lines have also been established (Doetschman *et al.*, 1988).

3. Nutrition

Hamsters can be maintained on standard rodent diets, but relatively little research has been done on specific nutritional requirements of hamsters (Newberne and McConnell, 1979). Nonetheless, commercial rodent feed (intended for mice and rats) is generally used as the basic diet for hamsters, and hamsters placed on these formulations have normal growth and reproduction. Regardless of gender, Syrian hamsters consume approximately the same amount of food daily, between 5.5 and 8.9 g, during growth and development. Although once commonplace, additional supplementation of grains, fruits, and vegetables is unnecessary and, should be discouraged because of the associated risk of exposure to unwanted contaminants (Coates, 1991; Mulder, 2012; Slater, 1972).

Syrian hamsters may have nutritional requirements that differ from other rodents, potentially due to the presence of a nonglandular forestomach and initial digestion via fermentation. For hamsters, unlike other rodents, soybean meal offers better nutritional efficiency than fish meal. Carbohydrates in the diet can induce changes in both the glucose and lipid metabolism in hamsters (Kasim-Karakas *et al.*, 1996). The mineral requirements for zinc, copper, and potassium are increased in the Syrian hamster, although the levels of other minerals are similar to those of the rat (Newberne and McConnell, 1979). Syrian hamsters require sources of many of the B vitamins and also need a source of non-nutritive bulk (Warner and Ehle, 1976). Vitamin E has been reported as essential for preventing myocytolysis in cardiomyopathic hamsters; deficiencies in this vitamin, combined with oxidative stress, may play a role in the pathogenesis of heart disease in hamsters (Sakanashi *et al.*, 1991). In addition, vitamin E can reduce fatty streak accumulation in hypercholesterolemic hamsters (Xu *et al.*, 1998).

For animals used in research, it is imperative that the diet be adequate to ensure that the biological responses obtained are, in fact, related to the experimental procedure (Newberne and Fox, 1980). Studies of hamster nutrition have shown that increased rates of survival for male and female hamsters are linked to long-term diets of 20 g lactalbumin/100 g of food (Birt *et al.*, 1982).

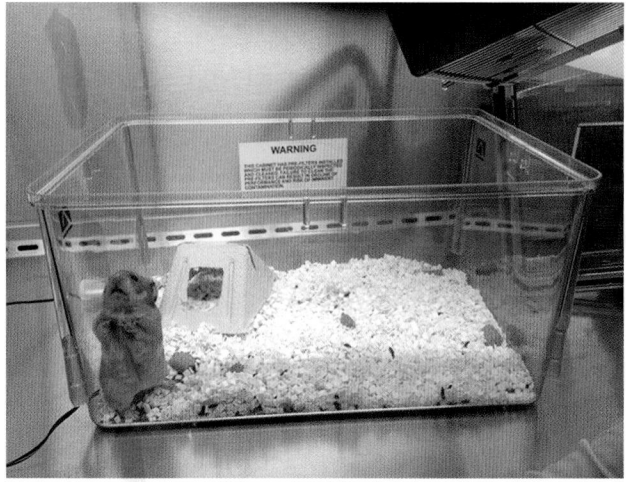

FIGURE 5.3   Shoe-box caging for hamsters. Note the placement of food on the cage bottom.

In addition, variations in dietary components can influence the outcome of spontaneous disease (Birt and Pour, 1985; Birt *et al.*, 1985). Studies have shown that hamsters changed from a diet of rodent chow to semipurified feed are susceptible to colocolic intussusception within 7–10 days of the change to the nutritionally refined diet (Cunnane and Bloom, 1990).

Although it is generally recommended that laboratory animals be fed in a manner that minimizes food contamination with excreta, Syrian hamsters are an exception. If food hoppers are used for hamsters, the feed pellets must be able to fall through the slots to the floor of the cage (Harkness *et al.*, 1977). In a hamster study that began with observations of failing health, decreased conception, and increased cannibalism, the problems were traced to a change in feeders. The feeders that contributed to these problems had 5/16-inch-wide slots that prevented the food from dropping to the cage floor. Because hamsters have a broad muzzle, the animals were forced to bite the food simultaneously from both sides of the individual metal strips of the feeder. The situation resulted in broken teeth and severe weight loss due to starvation.

Placement of the food directly on the floor of the cage, in addition to or in lieu of the use of a feeder, is preferred for adults and young hamsters (Fig. 5.3), who can begin to eat solid dry food at about 7–10 days of age. Like many other rodents, hamsters are naturally coprophagic. The placement of food on the floor of the enclosure is acceptable per federal regulations (Code of Federal Regulations (CFR), 2013). Fluid requirements are approximately 8.5 ml per 100 g body weight, but can vary significantly between genders (National Research Council, 1995), potentially linked to their natural adaptations for water conservation (Committee on Rodents, 1996). The use of a stainless steel sipper tube for drinking

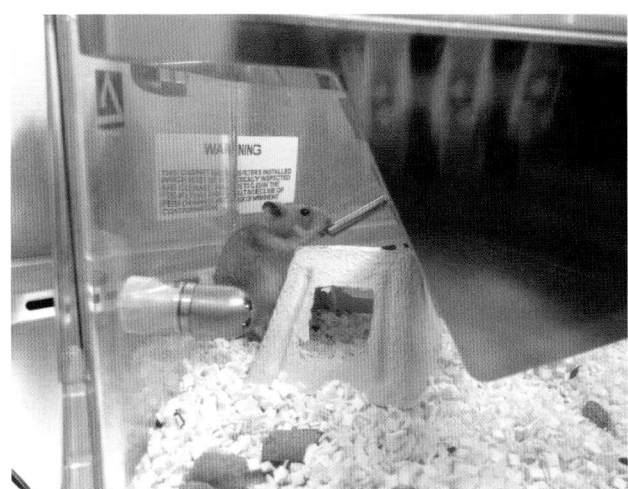

FIGURE 5.4 Syrian hamster drinking from elongated stainless steel sipper tube.

water or administration of other fluids is advised since hamsters can bite or chew through glass or plastic (Fig. 5.4). The location of the sipper tube must be sufficiently low for the smallest animal that is caged, as even nursing pups benefit from fluids, in addition to milk from the dam, to prevent gastrointestinal disturbances.

4. Pharmacology

Hamsters are apparently more sensitive to the metabolic effects of corticosteroids than some other laboratory animals, and are less responsive to histamine. Hamsters are very resistant to morphine; it generally has no sedative or hypnotic effects (Houchin, 1943; Tseng *et al.*, 1979). Hamsters are also susceptible to *Clostridum difficile* overgrowth (discussed in greater detail under Bacterial Infections, Section I.C.1.a) following the administration of several commonly used antibiotics, including lincomycin, clindamycin, ampicillin, vancomycin, erythromycin, cephalosporins, gentamicin, and penicillin (Percy and Barthold, 2007).

5. Mating and Reproduction

The male hamster is sexually mature at approximately 90g body weight. In the female, estrus begins within 6–8 weeks, yet it is recommended that breeding be withheld until the hamster reaches a weight of 90–100g. Copulation activity may begin as early as 4 weeks of age, but it is unusual for pregnancy to occur before 8 weeks of age. For both genders, the ability to reproduce decreases at approximately 14 months of age. However, senescent females can often be successfully bred with younger males, even though there is a notable increase in defective ova and a decrease in number of offspring produced (Slater, 1972). The female has a 4-day estrous cycle that can be assessed by evaluation of the vaginal discharge. The end of ovulation (usually day 2

of the cycle) is marked by the appearance of a copious postovulatory discharge that fills the vagina and may extrude through the vaginal orifice. The discharge is creamy white, opaque, and very viscous, with a distinct odor. The female can be successfully mated in the evening of the third day after this postovulatory discharge.

Hamsters are usually test-mated by trial placement to determine if the female is receptive to the male. All animals should be caged individually for at least 1 week, allowing males to establish cage dominance and the females to cycle normally. On the third day following a post-ovulatory discharge, a female is introduced into a cage with a male approximately 1–2h prior to the start of the dark cycle. It has been reported that the females are receptive to mating for approximately 16h from early evening until mid-afternoon on the following day (Ciaccio and Lisk, 1971). If the female is ready for mating, she will quickly assume a position of lordosis with hindlegs spread and tail erect, and will maintain this position if the male exhibits interest. If mating does not occur within 5min, or if the female is aggressive, she is removed and another female can be presented to the male. If copulation occurs, the pair can be left together until the following light cycle. With a normal dark cycle, ovulation and fertilization generally occur during the early morning hours, and this (the day of separation) is considered day 1 of gestation.

Gestation in the Syrian hamster is from 15 to 18 days in length. Disturbances should be minimized during pregnancy; after mating, the female can be moved to a separate nesting cage for at least 2 days prior to and 10 days after parturition to minimize maternal rejection or cannibalization of the litter. Despite early accounts of successful cross-fostering of pups with nursing mothers (Richards, 1966; Rowell, 1960), there are no recent peer-reviewed published accounts of successful cross-fostering of hamsters, although there are anecdotal comments online. Bottle feeding of newborn hamsters is very difficult and rarely (if ever) successful.

Another breeding mechanism is to trio-breed with one male and two females in the cage for 1–2 weeks, followed by the removal of the females to a separate cage for parturition. Since Syrian female hamsters tend to be aggressive, measures should be taken to reduce chances for injury as a result of fighting. It is recommended that breeding pairs/trios include a male hamster that is older than the female(s). For adequate veterinary care, breeding hamsters should be checked daily for fight wounds.

Female hamsters may undergo pseudopregnancy, usually as a result of an infertile mating. The female hamster can be examined for postovulatory discharge on days 5 and 9 after mating. If the discharge is present, she is exhibiting normal estrous cycles and is not pregnant. A hamster that is pregnant will have a distinct gain in weight, with abdominal distension, approximately 10 days after mating.

Studies have shown that the time of mating and the light–dark cycle under which the animals are housed have effects on the time of parturition (Viswanathan and Davis, 1992). Just prior to parturition, the female becomes restless and alternates between eating, grooming, and nest building. An increase in respiratory rate is also a sign that the litter can be expected to deliver within the next several hours. The most common time for parturition is on the 16th day of gestation, and parturition itself usually lasts for more than 3 h. A change toward maternal behavior occurs abruptly in late gestation for female Syrian hamsters; this differs from the gradual onset of maternal behavior observed throughout gestation in mice and rats (Buntin *et al.*, 1984).

Litters range in size from four to 12 pups, with six to eight pups being the most common size. It is possible to sex the pups at birth by comparing the distance from the external urethral orifice to the anus (greater in males), but it is preferable to leave the litter undisturbed for the first 7–10 days after birth. During this time, fresh food pellets and water are provided for the mother, but no cage changes should be performed. Cannibalism may occur if the mothers are potentially stressed or threatened; alternatively, a mother may put pups into her cheek pouch due to transient stress, but then removes them when she becomes calm. If it is necessary to disturb the litter, the dam should be provided with food pellets on the cage floor with which she can stuff her cheek pouches. This may decrease the likelihood of cannibalism of newborn pups by the mother.

Hamster pups should remain with the dam until they are at least 19 days of age. Normal weaning time is 21–28 days, and the estrous cycle does not usually resume for the mother until 1–8 days following parturition (Battles, 1985). Young from different litters can usually be housed together until 40–50 days of age, when it becomes necessary to separate the females due to aggression. Males from the same litter may be kept together for a longer period of time.

6. Management and Husbandry

a. Caging and Environment

Hamsters can be maintained in colonies; however, mature animals are usually caged separately because of their tendency to fight. Females to be mated must be given some degree of isolation from adult males and other pregnant or lactating females.

A hamster weighing 60 g or less requires about 10 in^2 of space. An animal over 60 g should have 13–19 in^2 depending on body weight. A female with a litter should have approximately 121 in^2. The height of the cage for hamsters must be 6 inches from the cage floor to the cage top (CFR, 2008; Institute of Laboratory Animal Research, 2011).

Caging used for other laboratory rodents is acceptable for hamsters provided it is escape-proof. Hamsters are capable of chewing through thick wood and aluminum. Doors and corners must be close-fitting, and latches must be secure. Plastic shoe-box cages with locking lids are recommended. It is essential to have a solid bottom for nesting females and for their young. Preference testing of hamsters found that solid-floored cages with bedding material were more readily inhabited than wire cages; however, age and/or prior experience may have affected the choice by the animals (Arnold and Estep, 1994).

Recommended bedding materials include processed hardwood chips, sawdust, shavings, corncobs, and certified paper products (Fig. 5.5). It has been shown that, without nesting material, hamsters have a preference for pine shavings over aspen shavings, and corn cob and aspen shavings are preferred over wood pellets. Interestingly these preferences were eliminated when nesting material (paper towel) was provided (Lanteigne and Reebs, 2006). Aromatic hydrocarbons in these materials may induce nonspecific hepatic enzymes in the hamster (Harkness, 1994). Normal urine output is slight, and hamsters tend to consistently use one corner of the cage for elimination. Replacement of bedding materials can be routinely done once or twice weekly, and can be left for up to 10–14 days, particularly when it is desirable to leave a litter undisturbed.

Male and female group-housed hamsters typically fight, but stable groups have been reported when animals were housed together starting at a young age. Use of enrichment devices may reduce aggression between cage mates (Arnold and Westbrook, 1998). Environmental enrichment for hamsters should include some sort of burrow, pipe, tube, or shelter to mimic natural habitats of underground burrows (Fig. 5.5) (Arnold and Westbrook, 1998;

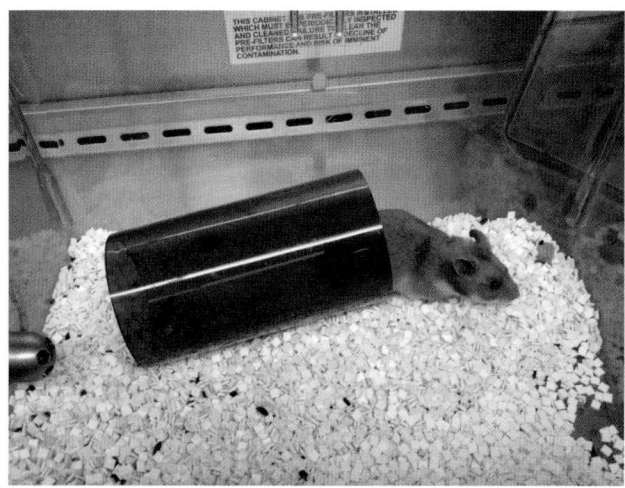

FIGURE 5.5   Example of plastic tube that can be placed in the cage to provide enrichment.

Baumans, 2005). Additionally, nest material (or material that provides ability for nest building) is recommended, as hamsters of both genders make nests (Gattermann et al., 2001; Lanteigne and Reebs, 2006; Richards, 1969). Hamsters that had bedding material 40–80 cm in depth showed significantly less cage-bar chewing and increased burrow construction than hamsters housed in bedding that was only 10 cm deep (Hauzenberger et al., 2006). Hamsters also use running wheels; these devices can be added to the housing cage as a form of environmental enrichment (Beaulieu and Reebs, 2009).

Cages used for housing adult hamsters must be maintained in an environment of approximately 68–79°F with 30–70% humidity (Institute for Laboratory Animal Research, 2011). Hamsters are fairly adaptable to cooler temperatures, with one study showing that pre-hibernation hamsters prefer temperatures around 8°C (46°F), while post-hibernation hamsters show a preference for higher temperatures around 24°C (75°F) (Gumma et al., 1967).

A daily light period of 12–14 h is recommended. The longer 14-h period is required for breeding colonies. A light intensity of 323 lux (30 ft-candles) measured approximately 1 m above the floor has been recommended for rodents (Institute for Laboratory Animal Research, 2011).

b. Handling and Restraint

Hamsters are nocturnal animals, so they tend to be quite inactive during the light cycle in the animal facility. Males are more docile and easier to handle than females. Frequent handling can contribute to reduced aggressiveness, but a startled or awakened hamster is likely to roll on its back and threaten to bite.

To safely manipulate hamsters, place a small cup or container in the cage. The animal will usually enter the container, and the container with the hamster can be quickly moved to another cage. The easiest method of hand restraint is to grasp the hamster around the head and shoulders, approaching the animal carefully from the rear. Another method is to approach the animal in much the same way, but grasp only the skin. With the loose skin bunched securely in the hand, the skin is taut over the thorax and abdomen. As the animal is lifted, the hand holding the hamster is rotated so that the hamster's body is supported (Fig. 5.6). An alternative to this method is to approach from the animal's head, so that the thumb and forefinger are gripping the base of the tail; as before, the loose skin is secured between the fingers and the palmar surface before lifting. Still another method is to approach from the head and enclose the entire body with one hand. The thumb is placed at the base of the rear leg, with the first and second fingers on the opposite side at the base of the tail. The third and fourth fingers restrain the head and forelegs.

C. Diseases

1. Infectious Diseases

a. Bacterial Infections

i. PROLIFERATIVE ENTERITIS (TRANSMISSIBLE ILEAL HYPERPLASIA) Proliferative enteritis is an infectious disease of hamsters that results in high morbidity and mortality. Proliferative enteritis is characterized by diarrhea in weanling hamsters with segmental proliferative lesions in the epithelium of the terminal ileum. This disease has also been refered to as regional enteritis, enzootic intestinal adenocarcinoma, transmissible ileal hyperplasia, and 'wet tail.' While the term 'wet tail' has been used extensively to describe this disease, this terminology can be confusing since it merely denotes a clinical description of diarrhea, and there are several other diseases that cause diarrhea in hamsters (Frisk, 2012).

Etiology While the incidence of proliferative enteritis has decreased since it was first reported in the late 1950s (Cooper and Gebhart, 1998), this disease entity remains a concern in hamster colonies due to its extremely contagious nature and high rates of morbidity and mortality.

The causative organism isolated from hamsters with proliferative enteritis is *Lawsonia intracellularis* (Stills, 1991; Cooper et al., 1997a). *L. intracellularis*, related to *Desulfovibrio desulfuricans*, is a gram-negative, nonspore forming, slightly curved rod (1.5 × 0.35 μm) that is an obligate intracellular bacterium (Fox et al., 1994). In addition, this bacterium is challenging to manipulate or culture in cell lines (Cooper and Gebhart, 1998). It causes proliferative enteropathy in a number of other species including pigs, ferrets, horses, deer, and rabbits (Cooper et al., 1997a,b; Fox et al., 1994).

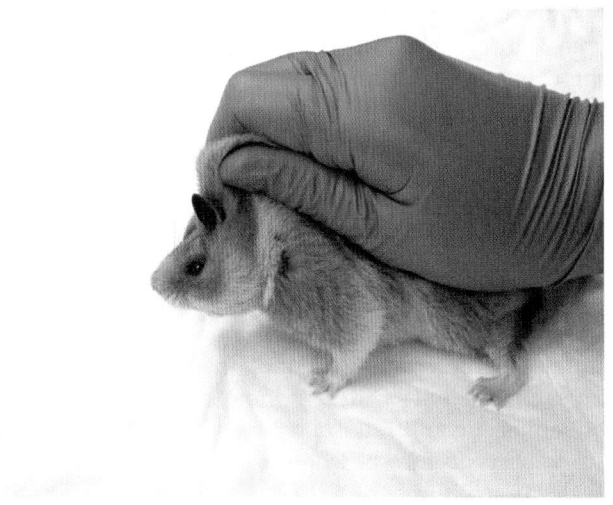

FIGURE 5.6 One-hand restraint of hamsters is demonstrated. The excessive loose skin is gathered tautly around the neck as the animal is lifted. *Credit: Jerald Silverman and Academic Press.*

Clinical Signs Watery diarrhea results in characteristic moist, matted fur on the tail, perineum, and ventral abdomen. Other clinical signs include dehydration, inactivity and a hunched appearance, inferred to be secondary to abdominal pain. Abdominal distention, hypothermia, and convulsions can occur just prior to death. Prolapse of the rectum or intussusception is often noted (Friedman, 1965; Frisk, 2012). Death occurs in 50–90% of cases associated with an outbreak, usually within 48h after onset of clinical signs (Freidman, 1965). Chronic courses of proliferative enteritis have also been observed in hamsters with mild diarrhea and weight loss (Frisk *et al.*, 1977; Jacoby *et al.*, 1975; Lawson and Gebhart, 2000); however, it is important to recognize that the disease may be self-limiting without clinical signs. Jacoby *et al.* (1975) observed hamsters after experimental transmission of proliferative ileitis and divided clinical signs into acute, subacute, and chronic. Acute signs occurred in 10% of hamsters 7–10 days after inoculation, the primary sign being hemorrhagic diarrhea. Subacute signs of delayed growth and diarrhea appeared 21–30 days after transmission. The chronic disease did not produce clinical signs, with those animals showing normal growth rates.

Transmission and Epizootiology Natural transmission most likely occurs by the fecal–oral route, following ingestion of contaminated fecal material. Increased severity and development of disease have been associated with factors such as overcrowding, transport, surgery, limited and purified diets (Decker and Henderson, 1959), transplantation of neoplasms (Lussier and Pavilanis, 1969), and experimental leishmaniasis (Frenkel, 1972). Cross-species transmission has been shown to occur experimentally between infected swine and hamsters (McOrist and Lawson, 1987). Vertical transmission has not been evaluated; however, it is not considered likely that *L. intracellularis* can cross the placenta to infect the fetus. In addition, it is unknown how long *L. intracellularis* can survive in the environment and if this is important in natural infections (Cooper and Gebhart, 1998).

Necropsy Findings Gross lesions can include a segmental thickening and congestion of the ileum, enlargement of the mesenteric lymph nodes, peritonitis, and adhesions, although lesions are not always observed (Fig. 5.7). Histopathologic changes are characterized by hyperplasia of columnar mucosal epithelial cells in the terminal ileum, proliferation of glandular epithelium, and lymphadenitis with lymphoid hyperplasia, edema, and leukocytic infiltration of sinusoids (Frisk *et al.*, 1977). Intestinal crypts may be lengthened, with increased mitosis, decreased numbers of goblet cells, and villar atrophy (Fig. 5.8). Finally, *L. intracellularis* can often be identified, using Warthin–Starry silver stain, in the apical cytoplasm of crypt enterocytes (Cooper and Gebhart, 1998).

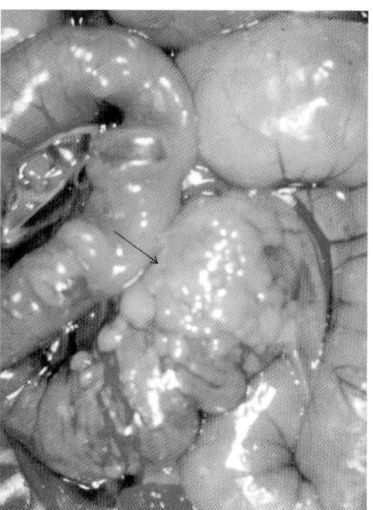

FIGURE 5.7   The abdominal viscera of a hamster with proliferative enteritis. The arrow denotes the thickening of the terminal jejunum and ileum. *Reprinted with permission from J.G. Fox and J.C. Murphy.*

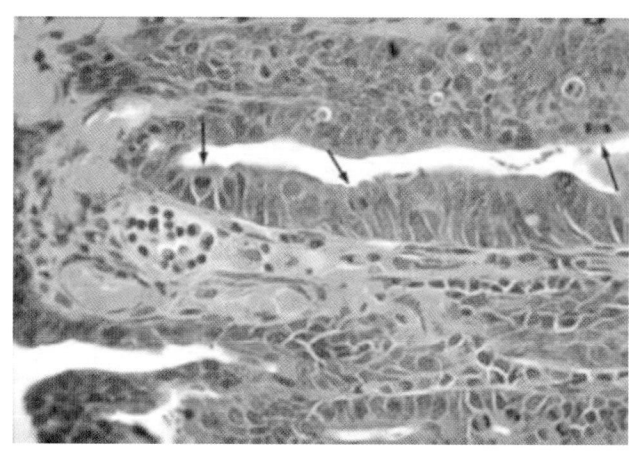

FIGURE 5.8   The crypt epithelium in an animal with proliferative enteritis. There are an increased number of mitotic figures (arrows) coupled with cellular immaturity in the epithelium. *Reprinted with permission from Harold F. Stills Jr.*

Pathogenesis and Diagnosis Weanling hamsters are very susceptible to this disease, but become less susceptible by 6 weeks of age, and resistant to infection by 10 weeks of age (Jacoby and Johnson, 1981). The lesions observed in the ileum develop in two phases following the experimental transmission of the disease (Jacoby, 1978). The initial phase is characterized by hyperplasia, which begins as a focal lengthening of villi. Approximately 3 weeks following transmission, an inflammatory phase begins, associated with focal or segmental necrosis of crypt epithelium. The evolution of the lesions is closely associated with a particulate bacterial antigen that can be detected by immunoperoxidase staining or *in situ* hybridization in the cytoplasm of mucosal epithelial cells. It is not clear what mechanism is utilized by *L. intracellularis* to localize to the gastrointestinal tract; however, cellular receptors or factors in the microenvironment may be important (Cooper and Gebhart, 1998). The proposed model for entry into the crypt epithelial cells involves attachment of the bacteria to the microvillus brush border, ingestion by endocytosis, and release from vacuoles into the cytoplasm of the cell. Released bacteria may then multiply within the epithelial cells prior to cell rupture. Additional bacteria may then attach to neighboring epithelial cells and spread the infection more rapidly (Jasni *et al.*, 1994). Serum antibodies have been detected that are specific for the intracytoplasmic antigen, which may be of diagnostic value (Stills, 1991). Commercially available polymerase chain reaction (PCR) assays are readily available for detection of *L. intracellularis* in fecal samples (Cooper *et al.*, 1997b; Jones *et al.*, 1993).

Differential Diagnosis Other infectious diseases that should be considered for hamsters with diarrhea are Tyzzer's disease (*Clostridium piliforme*), *Clostridium difficile* enterotoxemia, and salmonellosis. Microbiologic and pathologic findings should distinguish between the various possibilities. When observed, the described proliferative changes involving the ileum are pathognomonic for the disease (Frisk, 2012).

Prevention, Control, and Treatment Prior to obtaining hamsters for the biomedical facility, one should review the vendor/supplier history of the animal colonies with regard to enteritis. Animals should be purchased from a colony with minimal disease history, and they should not be mixed with animals from other sources. Hamsters with diarrhea should be separated and isolated from other animals. Treatment should be supportive and aggressive to correct nutritional and electrolyte imbalances. Antibiotic therapy indicated for *L. intracellularis* should be administered, although treatment has only been moderately successful. Tetracycline (10 mg/kg PO q12h for 5–7 days), enrofloxacin (10 mg/kg PO or IM q12h for 5–7 days), and trimethoprim-sulfa combinations (30 mg/kg PO q12h for 5–7 days) have been recommended; these can be added to drinking water to control infections (Donnelly, 1997). Colony depopulation, facility sanitation, and repopulation with uninfected hamsters remain the best way to eliminate proliferative ileitis (Frisk, 2012).

Research Complications Enteritis can be a major problem because of its prevalence, variable morbidity (20–60%), and high mortality (approximately 90%).

ii. TYZZER'S DISEASE This condition was first reported in Japanese Waltzing mice but has since been diagnosed in several other species including rats, rabbits, gerbils, cats, rhesus monkeys, dogs, horses, guinea pigs, and hamsters (Ganaway *et al.*, 1971; Waggie *et al.*,

1987). The disease is caused by *Clostridium piliforme*, a spore-forming intracellular bacterium. Transmission is believed to occur through the oral ingestion of *C. piliforme* spores from the feces of infected animals (Waggie *et al.*, 1987). Although Tyzzer's disease has only been sporadically reported in hamsters, transmission to hamsters is a possibility whenever hamsters are housed near susceptible species (Frisk, 2012). Clinical signs include roughened hair coats, diarrhea, and high mortality in animals that tend to be of weaning age or immunosuppressed (Donnelly, 1997). Reported necropsy lesions include enterocolitis, lymphadenitis, and multifocal necrotizing hepatitis (Fig. 5.9) (Nakayama *et al.*, 1975). The diagnosis depends on the demonstration of the characteristic organism in the affected tissue, particularly in the epithelial and smooth muscle cells of the ileum, cecum, and colon, following special staining with Giemsa or silver techniques (Waggie *et al.*, 1987). In experimental infections, inflammatory lesions may be present within 2 days of inoculation, while foci of liver necrosis occur within 4 days (Waggie *et al.*, 1987). Infection with *C. piliforme* may not always manifest into clinical disease in the hamster. Outbreaks may have lesions localized in the intestines, the liver, or primarily in cardiac muscle, with or without intestinal involvement (Nakayama *et al.*, 1976; Magaribuchi *et al.*, 1977; Zook *et al.*, 1977). The most important factors in the control and prevention of Tyzzer's disease involve improved sanitation and isolation, since elimination of *C. piliforme* spores is critical for containing an outbreak. Treatment is not usually described in reported outbreaks. Oxytetracycline was added to the water of a pet store supplier of hamsters with an outbreak without success (Motzel and Gibson, 1990).

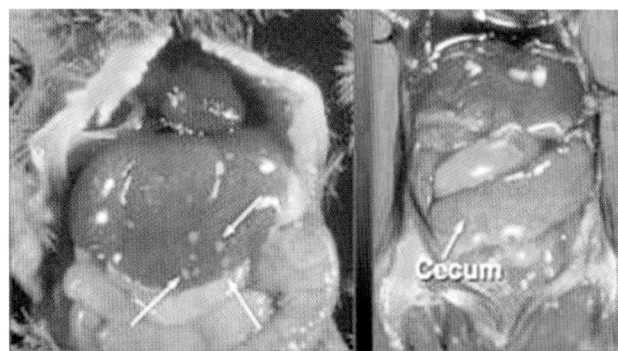

FIGURE 5.9 Gross lesions in Tyzzer's disease include hepatomegaly and multifocal hepatic necrosis (arrows) as seen on the left. Intestinal lesions, seen on the right, involve the ileum through the colon and include loss of tone and serosal edema. In some cases, hyperemia and hemorrhage may occur. *Reprinted with permission from Sherri L. Motzel.*

WHITE SPOTS ON LIVER

iii. **CLOSTRIDIUM DIFFICILE** Enteritis associated with this bacterium has been linked to inappropriate antibiotic administration (i.e., antibiotic-associated enteritis), stress, experimental manipulation, and heavy environmental contamination with *C. difficile* (Ryden *et al.*, 1991; Rehg and Lu, 1982; Blankenship-Paris *et al.*, 1995b). Antibiotics associated with enterocolitis in hamsters include lincomycin, clindamycin, ampicillin, vancomycin, erythromycin, cephalosporins, gentamicin, and penicillin (Percy and Barthold, 2007); *C. difficile* overgrowth subsequently occurs and can cause enterocolitis due to alterations to intestinal microflora (Frisk, 2012). *C. difficile* can also cause disease in hamsters unrelated to antibiotic use. Hamsters may unexpectedly die with or without signs of diarrhea and have lesions of cecitis. Affected hamsters may vary in age from juveniles to adults (Hart *et al.*, 2010). It is postulated that cecal dysbiosis results in cecal hyperplasia, overgrowth of the bacteria, and resultant necrotizing cecitis (Fig. 5.10) (Ryden *et al.*, 1991). A reported outbreak with toxigenic, cytotoxin B-positive *C. difficile* resulted in profuse, watery, and hemorrhagic diarrhea that was highly associated with mortality (Chang and Rohwer, 1991). Histologic findings included typhlitis and colitis in these adult hamsters.

Additionally, hamsters used as models of atherosclerosis and placed on high-fat and -cholesterol diets may be prone to development of enteric disease associated with toxigenic *C. difficile*; necrohemorrhagic typhlitis and cecal mucosal hyperplasia were commonly noted in these hamsters (Blankenship-Paris *et al.*, 1995b). Alterations in diet may be risk factors in disease development due to changes in intestinal microflora, pH, and ability to mount immune responses (Blankenship-Paris *et al.*, 1995a). The development of antibodies against the virulence factors, toxins A and B, has proved useful in preventing disease relapse and subsequent reinfections in hamsters (Kink and Williams, 1998). Control of an

outbreak of *C. difficile*-associated disease may be accomplished by depopulation, decontamination of animal holding rooms with chlorine dioxide, and repopulation (Hart *et al.*, 2010).

Experimental infection with *C. difficile* serves as an important model for studying the human disease. This model has provided valuable information with regard to the role of toxins in the pathogenesis and potential treatments of the disease (Goulding *et al.*, 2009).

iv. **SALMONELLOSIS** The rarity of salmonellosis in hamsters is likely attributable to well-managed facilities, improved quality of animals, regulated diets, and standards of animal care (Percy, 1987). This disease is rare in hamsters, although outbreaks had been reported historically (Innes *et al.*, 1956). At necropsy, multifocal hepatic necrosis without enteritis has been described. Histologically, the disease is characterized by septic thrombi involving the veins and venules, an unusual feature of bacterial infection in hamsters. Preventive procedures, should salmonellosis be suspected, should include the isolation of hamsters from other rodents and quality control procedures to preclude the introduction of contaminated food or bedding. Antibiotic treatment typically is unrewarding (Frisk, 1987).

v. **HELICOBACTER SPP.** *Helicobacter* spp. are motile gram-negative bacteria that are curved to spiral to fusiform in morphology. The hamster intestine is naturally colonized with several *Helicobacter* spp. that are not typically associated with clinical disease. Species identified in the hamster include *H. cinaedi, H. mesocricetorum, H. cholecystus, H. aurati,* and a novel *Helicobacter* species (in the *H. bilis* cluster) (Fox *et al.*, 2009; Patterson *et al.*, 2000a, b; Whary and Fox, 2004). *H. cinaedi* has been isolated from the intestinal tract of hamsters and has not been shown to cause pathological changes in this species (Gebhart *et al.*, 1989). However, it has been shown to cause enteritis, proctocolitis, and rectal infection in humans (Gebhart *et al.*, 1989; Whary and Fox, 2004). Hamsters should be considered a potential source of infection in humans, especially immonocompromised individuals (Fox, 2002). *H. mesocricetorum* has been isolated from the feces of hamsters and is considered a nonpathological commensal of the intestine (Simmons *et al.*, 2000). Its causal association with pancreatic lesions has not been established. *H. cholecystus* has been isolated from hamsters with cholangiofibrosis and centrilobular pancreatitis in hamsters (Franklin *et al.*, 1996). *H. aurati* has been associated with several experimentally induced lesions. Syrian hamsters infected with *H. aurati* had gastritis, chronic and progressive typhlocolitis, intestinal metaplasia, and dysplastic lesions in the large intestine (Patterson *et al.*, 2000a, b). Hamsters showed either no clinical signs or chronic weight loss/poor body

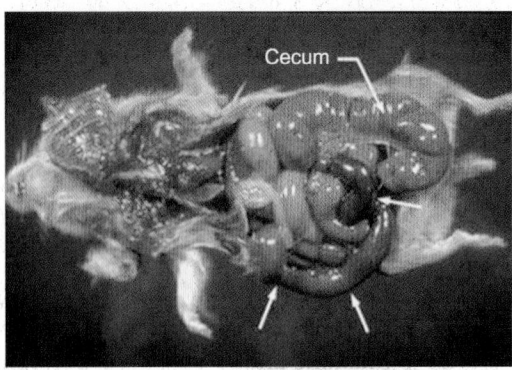

FIGURE 5.10   Lesions of *Clostridium difficile* enterocolitis. Note the distended cecum and markedly hemorrhagic distal small intestine (arrows). *Reprinted with permission from Susan V. Gibson.*

condition. *Helicobacter* spp. were also isolated from a hamster with gastric adenocarcinoma (Nambier *et al.*, 2006; Patterson *et al.*, 2000a, b). A novel *Helicobacter* species was identified, from the livers of aged hamsters, that appears closely related to *H. bilis* and may play a role in hepatobiliary disease: the livers from those hamsters had lesions of chronic hepatitis, hepatic dysplasia, and biliary hyperplasia (Fox *et al.*, 2009).

vi. PNEUMONIA

Etiology and Prevalence A survey originated in 1975 listed pneumonia as the second-most common hamster disease after diarrhea, and implicated *Pasteurella pneumotropica, Streptococcus pneumoniae*, and other *Streptococcus* spp. in the disease process (Renshaw *et al.*, 1975); however, their importance in producing clinical disease of hamsters is unclear. Nonetheless, *Pasteurella* and *Streptococcus* are commonly listed in health reports for hamsters. Infection with *Corynebacterium paulometabulum* has been reported as a suspected cause of acute pneumonia in hamsters (Tansey *et al.*, 1995); however, nasal infections with another strain, *C. kutscheri*, were subclinical in hamsters (Amao *et al.*, 1991).

Clinical Signs Overt manifestations of disease may include depression, anorexia, and nasal and ocular discharges, with 'chattering' and respiratory distress.

Pathogenesis Various causes of stress, including significant variations from recommended environmental temperatures, may be contributing and predisposing factors to respiratory disease in the hamster.

Differential Diagnosis A judicious assessment of clinical signs, lesions, and the results of microbiology laboratory reports is essential to definitively diagnose the etiologic agent (see above) of pneumonia in hamsters.

Prevention, Control, and Treatment Stressful situations should be avoided, and affected animals should be isolated. If treatment is necessary, the use of antibiotics to which the etiologic organism is sensitive may be appropriate. A number of antibiotics are associated with fatal enterocolitis in this species; therefore, careful selection of antimicrobials is imperative.

b. Viral Infections

i. PREVALENCE Current recommendations are that several viral infections should be monitored serologically in hamster breeding units. Most viral infections do not manifest any clinical disease in hamsters, with the exception of hamster polyomavirus (HAPyV) and *Rodent protoparvovirus 1* (a species designation that also contains viral strains such as mouse parvovirus). Viruses for which one should routinely screen include, but are not limited to, lymphocytic choriomeningitis virus (LCMV), the *Protoparvovirus* genus, murine pneumonia virus (MPnV), *Mammalian orthoreovirus* (reovirus type 3; Reo 3), and *Sendai virus* (SV) (Mulder, 2012). Multiple

groups have reported on the presence of antibodies to numerous viruses in Syrian hamsters.

ii. LYMPHOCYTIC CHORIOMENINGITIS VIRUS
The hamster is the most common animal species to transmit LCMV to humans (Cassano *et al.*, 2012); however, the laboratory mouse, *Mus musculus*, is the primary reservoir for the virus.

Etiology The infection is caused by an RNA virus of the arenavirus group.

Clinical Signs Disease manifestation is ultimately dependent on a variety of factors including virus strain, dose of virus administered, route of infection, age of the host, strain of the host, and host immunocompetence (Barthold and Smith, 2007). Clinical signs may vary depending on whether the LCMV infection is natural or experimentally induced. In adult hamsters, natural infection generally causes an acute short-term infection that rarely causes illness. Infections in perinatally exposed animals remain subclinical, despite the fact that hamsters are shedding large amounts of virus during this period. Approximately half of hamsters infected congenitally or as newborns remain persistently infected and may develop chronic, progressive fatal disease characterized by inactivity, weight loss and wasting (Skinner and Knight, 1979). Impaired reproductive performance has been reported for chronically infected female hamsters (Parker *et al.*, 1976).

Transmission The implantation of tumors, unknowingly containing LCMV, has been the principal method of transmission to laboratory hamsters. Transmission in natural infections is primarily due to direct contact, although fomites and aerosols have been implicated in the spread of LCMV (Fox *et al.*, 2002). High concentrations of virus have been found in the blood, organs, urine, and feces of Syrian hamsters. Viral shedding occurs primarily in the urine and saliva, but also in feces, milk, semen, and nasal secretions (Skinner and Knight, 1979). LCMV can be transmitted vertically or horizontally.

Necropsy Findings Histopathology of tissues from animals that were perinatally infected and unable to clear the infection develop chronic disease characterized by lymphocytic infiltration of the liver, lung, pancreas, kidney, spleen, meninges, and brain (Genovesi and Peters, 1987; Oldstone and Dixon, 1969; Parker *et al.*, 1976) as well as a chronic glomerulonephropathy and widespread vasculitis. The progressive glomerulonephritis can be attributed to antigen–antibody complex deposition in the arterioles and glomerular basement membranes of the infected kidney (Buchmeier and Oldstone, 1978; Oldstone and Dixon, 1969).

Pathogenesis The experimental infection of young adult hamsters results in a viremia that decreases in titer over a period of 3 months. Virus excreted in the urine persists longer and is detectable in greater amounts than that found in blood. Complement-fixing antibodies appear by 10 days postinfection, reach peak levels by day 60, and decline slowly thereafter. Some hamsters infected neonatally remain healthy and follow a pattern of infection similar to that of young adults. However, other neonates develop disease with persistent viremia and lower levels of both complement-fixing and neutralizing antibodies. The presence of viral antigen and γ-globulin in the glomeruli of affected hamsters suggests an immune complex mechanism for the glomerulonephropathy, analogous to that reported for LCMV disease in mice (Buchmeier and Oldstone, 1978; Parker *et al.*, 1976).

Differential Diagnosis Other potential causes of wasting disease include graft *versus* host disease and any procedures resulting in suppression of normal immune responses. Possible renal lesions should be differentiated from glomerular amyloidosis.

Prevention, Control, and Treatment A quality-assurance program that includes the regular testing of hamster colonies for antibodies and transplantable tumors for virus, with the elimination of infected animals or tumors, is the principal means of prevention. If dirty-bedding sentinels are used to screen hamster colonies for LCMV, care must be taken when interpreting negative results since LCMV is best transmitted via direct contact and viral transmission through dirty bedding is limited (Ike *et al.*, 2007). Since feral mice may be reservoirs of infection, their direct or indirect contact with experimental animal colonies should be avoided.

Research Complications LCMV is zoonotic and can be transmitted to humans through contact with rodents (see Chapter 28). The spectrum of disease manifested in humans varies from asymptomatic infection to rare cases of severe infection localized to the central nervous system. Studies that utilize LCMV-infected hamsters require Animal Biosafety Level 3 containment (CDCP-NIH, 2009). In a survey of biological contaminants, LCMV was isolated from 28% of hamster transplantable tumors (Nicklas *et al.*, 1993). Humans can be infected either by direct contact or by inhalation of infectious aerosolized rodent excretions or secretions (Amman *et al.*, 2007; Bowen *et al.*, 1975; Skinner and Knight, 1979). In 2005, three human patients died and one became seriously ill after receiving organs from a common infected donor. It was revealed that the donor had recently acquired a pet hamster that was seropositive for LCMV. Furthermore, 3% of the pet hamsters from the rodent distributor implicated in the outbreak were seropositive for the virus (Jay *et al.*, 2005).

iii. SENDAI VIRUS

Etiology Sendai virus is a single-stranded pleomorphic RNA virus and is the type species of the genus *Respirovirus* of the *Paramyxoviridae* family. Although mice are believed to be the natural host and most common laboratory animal affected, rats and hamsters are susceptible to natural infection (Percy and Palmer, 1997). Initial reports of the condition in hamsters were from Sendai, Japan (Matsumoto *et al.*, 1954).

Clinical Signs SV infection may lead to mortality in newborn pups; however, most infections are subclinical in hamsters.

Epizootiology and Transmission An enzootic form of the infection was reported historically at a research facility in association with the periodic, but continuous, introduction of susceptible hamsters from a commercial vendor (Profeta *et al.*, 1969). Transmission studies in mice have indicated that direct contact with infected rodents or contaminated fomites constitutes the primary route of infection. Aerosol inhalation has been successfully used to experimentally infect hamsters (Blandford and Charlton, 1977).

Necropsy Findings Consolidation of the lungs has been described (Profeta *et al.*, 1969). Experimental infections in hamsters have resulted in hyperplasia of the nasal mucosal epithelium, hyperplasia of bronchial epithelium, peribronchial edema, and peribronchial lymphocytic infiltration, which resolves within 2 weeks postinoculation (Percy and Palmer, 1997). These findings concurred with those seen in a SV vaccine study (Tagaya *et al.*, 1995). Lesions and sites of viral replication within the respiratory tract are similar to those reported in strains of laboratory mice (Percy and Palmer, 1997).

Pathogenesis Studies done in the mouse have shown that this agent causes a descending infection that is typically restricted to the mucociliary epithelium of conducting airways, but is capable of spreading to the alveolar epithelium (Brownstein, 2007). In male Syrian hamsters intranasally inoculated with Sendai, viral antigen was present postinoculation day 3 in the respiratory tract epithelium of the nasal passages and trachea. Antigen was present in the bronchioles by day 5, and antibodies were present by day 7, remaining at high levels throughout the 21-day study (Percy and Palmer, 1997).

Differential Diagnosis Additional causes of pneumonia to exclude from the list of differentials include *Corynebacterium* spp. (Tansey *et al.*, 1995), *Streptococcus pneumoniae, Pasteurella pneumotropica*, other *Streptococcus* spp., and MPnV (Renshaw *et al.*, 1975).

Prevention, Control, and Treatment Based on the likelihood that other laboratory animal species are the source of SV infections observed in hamsters, experimental hamsters should be housed in rooms separate from mice, rats, and guinea pigs. Hamsters from different sources should not be housed in the same room unless all sources are known to be free of the virus. In addition, analogous procedures described for mice should be applicable to hamsters (Parker and Richter, 1982). Dirty-bedding sentinels have been shown to be only variably efficacious in detecting SV outbreaks in mice (Compton et al., 2004), therefore, colony surveillance measures may need to be modified. Animal-derived biological products should be screened by PCR or hamster antibody production (HAP) test before use in colony hamsters (Cassano et al., 2012).

Research Complications SV infection may be lethal to suckling hamsters (Profeta et al., 1969). In addition, reports of immunosuppressive effects of the virus in other species may be extrapolated to infection in hamsters (Garlinghouse and Van Hoosier, 1978). Due to effects on the nasal mucosal epithelium, and given the importance of olfactory cues to the hamster, SV infection may complicate studies of behavior and olfactory function in hamsters (Murphy and Schneider, 1970; Percy and Palmer, 1997).

iv. MURINE ADENOVIRUS (MADV) Infections with *Murine adenovirus* have been reported in mice, rats, and other rodents, including hamsters, although no specific hamster adenovirus has been isolated. Hamsters can be experimentally infected with adenoviruses from a variety of other species. Infections are typically subclinical in hamsters unless the animal is stressed or immunocompromised (Richter, 1986). Mice can be naturally infected with two strains, MADV strain FL (now known as MAdV A) and K87 (now known as MAdV B). Hamsters can be serologically positive for antibodies to MAdV A, although reports of adenoviral infections are sporadic (Suzuki et al., 1982). Naturally occurring enteric adenovirus infection in hamsters, closely resembling infection with MAdVB in mice, is not associated with clinical disease and affects animals less than 24 days of age (Gibson et al., 1990). Adenoviral intranuclear inclusion bodies may be found in the intestinal epithelium in young hamsters.

v. HAMSTER POLYOMAVIRUS (HaPyV) Hamster polyomavirus was first described in Germany in association with spontaneous skin epitheliomas from which viral particles were later identified (Graffi et al., 1967). The same virus also causes lymphoma, which is atypical of a polyomavirus (Delmas et al., 1985). HaPyV is a double-stranded, non enveloped DNA virus, and member of the *Polyomaviridae* family in the *Polyomavirus* genus (ICTV, 2013).

Epizootiology The exact origin of HaPyV has not been elucidated. The virus has been isolated from the spleen and kidney of subclinically infected European hamsters, suggesting them as the natural host, with infection transferred to Syrian hamsters inadvertently after species co-mingling (Hannoun et al., 1974; Percy and Barthold, 2007). The virus is likely transmitted

horizontally via ingestion of virions or through contaminated fomites (Ambrose and Coggin, 1975; Coggin et al., 1983). HaPyV is unusual in that it displays tropism for both undifferentiated keratinocytes and also lymphocytes. Due to this variable tissue tropism, it may cause two different disease syndromes. The syndrome observed in an individual hamster depends upon the immunological status of the animal and the age of the hamster when infected. One syndrome occurs in naive juvenile hamsters that manifests as an epizootic multicentric lymphoma involving the mesentery, intestines, liver, kidney, and thymus (Barthold et al., 1987; Graffi et al., 1969; Simmons et al., 2001). Lymphoma may also be induced by injection of virus or viral DNA (Barthold et al., 1987; Graffi et al., 1969, 1970). With the second disease syndrome, hamsters develop trichoepitheliomas on the face, feet, neck, back, flanks, and abdomen. These tumors typically develop in hamsters aged 3 months to 1 year (Coggin et al., 1985; Graffi et al., 1970; Scherneck and Feunteun, 1990). Simultaneous formation of both epitheloimas and lymphomas in a single hamster rarely happens (Barthold et al., 1987). Virus likely persists in the renal tubular epithelium and is shed in urine. Additionally, virus-containing shed keratinocytes or enterocytes released in the feces can be a source of infection (Simmons et al., 2001).

Clinical Signs Hamsters with lymphoma will likely have signs that are dependent on the organ system infiltrated with disease, but generally signs include weight loss, dyspnea, and dehydration. Palpable masses may be found upon examination. Hamsters with trichoepitheliomas present with nodules within the cutis. The tumors may grow gradually and regress spontaneously (Barthold et al., 1987; Coggin et al., 1978).

Prevention and Control Therapy is not recommended. Culling of the entire colony, and decontamination of the facility, has failed to prevent new outbreaks in some facilities. The virus is stable in the environment, but is susceptible to DNase, phenols, and KOH. It has shown resistance to UV light, formaldehyde vapor, RNase, proteinase K, and chlorinated and iodinated disinfectants (Ambrose and Coggin, 1975; Coggin et al., 1983, Manci et al., 1984).

vi. HAMSTER PARVOVIRUS (RODENT PROTOPARVOVIRUS 1 (RPV-1)) Hamster parvovirus (HaPV) was first described in 1982 in a colony of suckling hamsters that experienced high mortality (Gibson, 1983). Hamster parvovirus is a non enveloped single-stranded DNA virus in the family *Parvoviridae*. The virus shares homology with the mouse parvoviruses, including 94.6% homology with mouse parvovirus 1 (MPV-1) and over 98% homology with MPV-3 (Besselsen et al., 1996, 2006). Currently, the International Committee on Viral Taxonomy considers all the rodent parvoviruses

SIMILAR TO MOUSE PARVO

(mouse parvovirus, H-1 parvovirus, Kilham rat virus, minute virus of mice) as one species, *Rodent protoparvovirus 1*, based on similarity of sequenced genomes, although multiple substrains can be identified.

Epizootiology and Pathogenesis There is evidence that the hamster is not the natural host for any strain of RPV-1 because rodent parvoviruses are typically subclinical in their natural host and multiple rodent parvoviruses cause a similar course of disease when inoculated into young hamsters. The mouse is likely the natural host of this strain of RPV-1 due to the fact that MPV-3 is nearly identical to HaPV (Besselsen et al., 2006, 2008; Christie *et al.*, 2010). Furthermore, experimental infection of mice with the hamster-derived strain of RPV-1 had similar pathogenesis to mice infected with the strain MPV-1 (Christie *et al.*, 2010). However, infection of hamsters with MPV-3 has not been demonstrated. HaPV is likely transmitted via ingestion or inhalation of viral particles (Jacoby *et al.*, 1996).

Clinical Disease Infection in adult hamsters is typically subclinical. Young hamsters (2–4 weeks old) are most susceptible to HaPV. Affected hamsters are runted with incisior teeth abnormalites, domed craniums, small testicles, and a potbellied appearance (Gibson, 1983). Hemmorhagic disease has also been reported, causing diarrhea, ataxia, and mortality (Besselsen *et al.*, 1999). Hamsters that survive typically seroconvert within 1–3 weeks, but animals remain persistently infected for several weeks. It has not been determined whether hamsters are shedding viral particles during that time. Humoral immunity prevents re-infection (Jacoby *et al.*, 1996).

Diagnosis, Prevention, and Control Diagnosis can be made with PCR using MPV-3/HaPV specific primers (Besselson et al., 1999, 2006; Christie *et al.*, 2010). Monitoring cell lines, serum, and tumors prior to use in the colony is the primary way to prevent HaPV from being inadvertently introduced. Outbreak management should include quarantine, facility disinfection, and restocking with new hamsters (Jacoby *et al.*, 1996; Cassano *et al.*, 2012).

c. Parasitic Diseases

i. PROTOZOA Fecal smears of Syrian hamsters may contain a large number and variety of organisms. Yet, their etiologic role in enteric disease remains a matter for speculation, as they have been found in comparable numbers in diverse species in both healthy and diseased animals. The presence of *Spironucleus muris* (previously *Hexamita* sp.) has been reported as an incidental finding (Wagner *et al.*, 1974). *Tritrichomonas muris* has been successfully eradicated from the intestinal tract using a regimen of 80 mg of metronidazole administered intragastrically for 6 days (Taylor *et al.*, 1993). This protocol is insufficient for the eradication of *Giardia muris*, which has a high prevalence in hamsters but is not associated

with significant clinical signs or lesions. If removal of *Giardia* is deemed necessary, there have been successful reports of adding dimetridazole to the drinking water to eliminate *Giardia* (Moore, 1990; Sebesteny, 1969).

ii. NEMATODES The hamster has been reported to be susceptible to several species of pinworms, including *Syphacia mesocriceti, Syphacia criceti, Syphacia stroma, Syphacia peromysci, Syphacia obvelata, Syphacia muris, Aspiculuris tetraptera* (in Siberian dwarf hamsters, specifically), and *Dentostomella translucida* (Burr *et al.*, 2012). Mice have been known to transmit *Syphacia obvelata* to Syrian hamsters (Watson, 1946), and Syrian hamsters can become infected with *S. muris*, the rat oxyurid, as a consequence of direct contact with infected rats (Ross *et al.*, 1980). Eradication has been reported by two treatment courses with piperazine citrate (10 mg/ml of drinking water) for 7 days separated by 5 days without treatment (Unay and Davis, 1980). Treatment strategies for mice and rats are well documented, with avermectins and benzimidazoles being the most widely used anthelmintics for pinworm eradication (Pritchett, 2007; Pritchett and Johnston, 2002). Studies detailing treatment strategies in hamsters are limited, but treatment can most likely be adapted from the treatment of other rodents. The pinworm life cycle is direct, and transmission occurs through direct contact and fomites such as dirty cages and bedding material (Wightman *et al.*, 1978).

iii. CESTODES

Etiology (Prevalence, Host Range) Hamsters are susceptible to a number of cestode infections of the family *Hymenolepididae*, including *Rodentolepis nana, Hymenolepis diminuta*, and *Rodentolepis microstoma*. Historically, *Rodentolepis nana*, the dwarf tapeworm, was one of the most important internal parasites found in hamsters (Renshaw *et al.*, 1975); infection has been found in animals from commercial colonies (Pinto *et al.*, 2001). *Rodentolepis nana* ranges in size from 25 to 40 mm in length and is usually found in the small intestine. The host range includes mice, rats, nonhuman primates, and humans, but host-specificity is uncertain. It has been postulated that the human strain of *R. nana* may be noninfective to rodents (Macnish *et al.*, 2002).

Clinical Signs The consequences of infection are usually benign, but the effects depend on the number of parasites and degree of intestinal occlusion, as impactions have been reported with large worm burdens (Soave, 1963).

Epizootiology and Transmission *Rodentolepis nana* is the only known tapeworm with either a direct or an indirect cycle; flour beetles or fleas serve as the intermediate host. The direct cycle predominates and is 14–16 days in length, while the indirect life cycle is variable. Autoinfection can also occur when eggs hatch within the host in which they were produced, rather than being excreted through the feces. Eggs then undergo development into mature worms within the intestinal tract of the original host. Evidence supports autoreinfection as a means for massive clinical infection in humans, as well as potentially causing clinical disease in rodents. Induced immunity through the direct life cycle can prevent autoreinfection (Heyneman, 1961).

Diagnosis   A diagnosis can be made by the demonstration of eggs in the feces or by isolation of the mature worm in the intestines at necropsy. *R. nana* can be distinguished from *H. diminuta* by the presence of hooks on the scolex in the former. Molecular techniques such as PCR-RFLP are also available for identification (Casanova *et al.*, 2001; Macnish *et al.*, 2003).

Prevention, Control, and Treatment   Preventive and control measures include isolation and quarantine of newly acquired animals, effective insect and wild-rodent control, and regular sanitation of cages and ancillary equipment. Praziquantel, thiabendazole, and niclosamide have been reported to be effective and safe (Ronald and Wagner, 1975). A study using *H. diminuta* as the cestode model showed several effective oral single-dose agents including praziquantel, bunamidine, niclosamide, cambendazole, and mebendazole (Ostlind *et al.*, 2004).

Research Complications   Although any infection associated with morbidity and mortality may interfere with research, the primary significance of *R. nana* is its potential transmissibility to humans, despite growing evidence of host-adapted strains. Accordingly, personnel working with infected hamsters should be informed of potential transmission and receive instruction in appropriate hygienic procedures.

iv. MITES
Etiology and Prevalence   Ascariasis in hamsters is predominantly associated with two species of the genus *Demodex* (*D. criceti* and *D. aurati*); *D. cricetuli* infests Armenian hamsters. In addition, infections with ear mites (*Notoedres* sp.), the tropical rat mite (*Ornithonyssus bacoti*), and a nasal mite (*Spleorodens clethrionomys*) have also been reported. Despite high infection rates with *Demodex* spp., clinical signs of skin disease are uncommon.

Clinical Signs   Clinical signs are rare, even with high infestations (Nutting, 1961). Alopecia, predominantly of the rump and back, with dry, scaly skin has been noted in association with *D. aurati* and *D. criceti* (Estes *et al.*, 1971). Notoedric mange in the female hamster usually affects only the ears; however, in males, lesions may also be observed on the nose, genitalia, tail, and feet.

Pathology   Reported cases of demodectic mange were characterized by dilated hair follicles that contained debris and mites, loss of hair shaft, an increase

in thickness of the corneum, and little evidence of inflammation.

Pathogenesis   The direct life cycle takes approximately 24 days to complete. *D. criceti* and *D. aurati* complete their life cycles within different areas of the epidermis, permitting dual-species infection (Nutting, 1961). Males may be more susceptible to infection and disease than females. Clinical disease, when seen, has mostly been associated with immunosuppressive factors, such as underlying disease, advanced age, tumors, etc. (Estes *et al.*, 1971; Tani *et al.*, 2001). Demodectic mange has been observed in hamsters involved in a lymphosarcoma transmission study and a chemical carcinogenesis study, although lesions were apparently more related to increasing age than experimental procedures (Estes *et al.*, 1971).

Diagnosis and Treatment   A diagnosis can be established by the demonstration of mites in skin scrapings, even though the presence of *Demodex* spp. in association with lesions does not necessarily establish a cause-and-effect relationship. Topical amitraz is the standard treatment for demodicosis. Regimes vary from weekly to every 14 days, with treatment length recommended for at least 4 weeks following a negative skin scrape (Hasegawa, 1995; Meredith, 2006). Other drugs reported to be effective are coumaphos and oral ivermectin (Hasegawa, 1995; Tani *et al.*, 2001). While it may be an extreme approach, weekly cleansings with shampoos (selenium sulfide and benzoyl peroxide) can be used in combination with topical treatment (Hasegawa, 1995) for those critical research animals that are particularly affected.

2. Neoplastic Diseases

a. Introduction

The degree of background tumor incidence in Syrian hamsters has been a controversial topic in the literature. Although some reports state that hamsters have a low incidence of naturally occurring tumors, other groups have found the occurrence of spontaneous tumors to be quite high (Homburger, 1983; Pour *et al.*, 1976a). For example, the overall incidence of spontaneous malignant neoplasms in Syrian hamsters has been estimated to be 3.7%, based on 435 tumors found in 11,972 animals (Van Hoosier and Trentin, 1979). Tanaka *et al.* (1991) reported tumor incidences in male hamsters of 10.6% and 11.5% in two cohorts, and Pour *et al.* (1976a, b, c) noted an overall incidence of 32% in one colony *versus* 42% in another. Factors affecting the difference in numbers of tumors reported include the strain, age, and sex distribution of the animals observed; the environmental conditions and source of the colony (i.e., genetic differences between colonies); and the extent to which the animals are examined grossly and microscopically. There is general consensus that tumors occur more frequently in females than in males (Pour *et al.*, 1976a; Van Hoosier and Trentin, 1979).

b. Benign Neoplasms

Reported benign neoplasms of the Syrian hamster include intestinal polyps, adrenal adenomas, splenic hemangiomas, islet cell pancreatic tumors, hepatic adenomas, squamous papillomas of the forestomach, and fibroadenomas of the mammary gland. One report found the incidence of benign tumors to be 10% in males and 13% in females when 200 control animals from the BIO 15.16 line were examined (Homburger, 1983).

c. Malignant Neoplasms

Lymphosarcoma is the most frequently reported malignant tumor of the Syrian hamster. Other malignancies include adrenocortical carcinoma, renal cell carcinoma, and subcutaneous sarcoma (Homburger, 1983).

Of special interest in this regard are the reported outbreaks of horizontally transmitted malignant lymphomas in a hamster colony, with an incidence of 50–90% in young inbred and random-bred animals (Ambrose and Coggin, 1975). The agent associated with the disease is the HaPyV (Coggin *et al.*, 1983; Prokoph *et al.*, 1996). These reports are historically important because the disease poses an epizootic threat to experimental colonies and because the disease condition in hamsters is a valuable model for understanding host–virus relationships in other species.

3. Miscellaneous Diseases

a. Amyloidosis and Associated Nephrotic Syndrome

Amyloidosis, a disease in which normally soluble proteins polymerize as insoluble fibrils, is a principal cause of death in hamsters on long-term experiments. The two components of amyloid are amyloid A (AA), which is derived from amyloid fibrils, and amyloid P (AP), also known as 'female protein' (FP), a member of the pantraxin family of plasma proteins (Tennent *et al.*, 1993). Studies have shown that sex hormones regulate the expression of AP and that levels in females are normally 100- to 200-fold greater than levels in males (Coe *et al.*, 1981). When compared to males, female Syrian hamsters have a distinct predisposition to acquire amyloidosis, with increased severity and earlier onset. Organs involved typically include the liver, kidney, stomach, adrenal, thyroid, and spleen (Coe and Ross, 1990). Testosterone has been linked to the inhibition of hepatic synthesis of AP, which is the homolog of primary importance in the deposition of amyloid (Coe and Ross, 1990). The incidence of nephrotic syndrome due to amyloidosis was reported to be 6% in a colony of Syrian hamsters, with ascites and anasarca observed (Murphy *et al.*, 1984). Affected hamsters can present

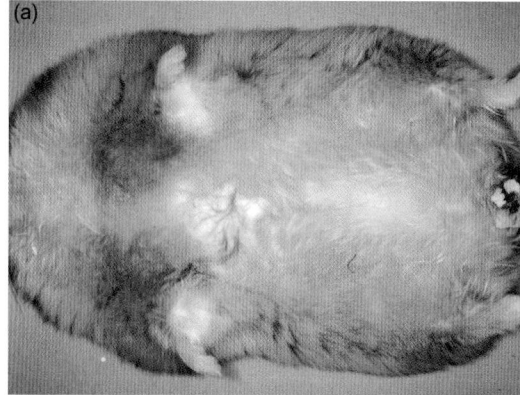
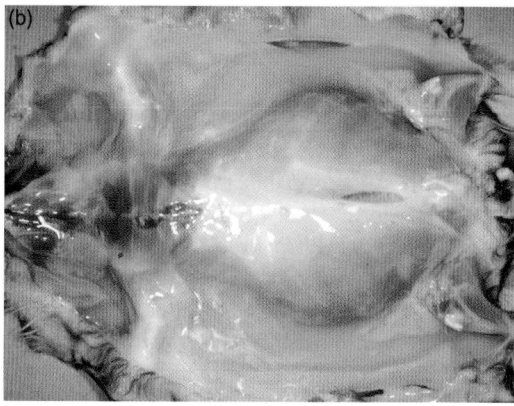

FIGURE 5.11   (A) Male hamster exhibiting nephrotic syndrome: note the distended abdomen indicative of subcutaneous edema and ascites. (B) Skin reflected showing subcutaneous edema. *Reprinted with permission from J.G. Fox and J.C. Murphy.*

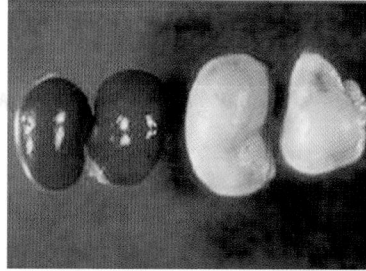

FIGURE 5.12   Classic appearance of amyloidosis in the kidneys on the right. Normal hamster kidneys are shown on the left for comparison. *Reprinted with permission from J. Derrell Clark.*

with extensive subcutaneous edema, ascites and hydrothorax (Fig. 5.11). The primary gross lesions are pale tan, enlarged, and misshapen kidneys (Fig. 5.12). Serum albumin is decreased and the total globulin component is increased in hamsters over 1 year of age. Proteinuria, hypercholesterolemia, triglyceridemia, and high levels of creatinine have been reported (Murphy *et al.*, 1984). Clinical signs and laboratory test findings of low albumin, ascites, and proteinuria are classic for a diagnosis of nephrotic syndrome, as described in humans.

Histologically, characteristic amyloid deposits are present initially in the glomeruli of the kidney and subsequently in a variety of tissues. Because amyloidosis in mice is strain-associated, genetic factors should be considered in the etiology and pathogenesis of the disease in hamsters. Amyloidosis in the Syrian hamster is used as a model to understand the pathogenesis of the same disease in humans, including the form linked to Alzheimer's disease (Coe et al., 1997). Amylodosis can be induced experimentally using casein or lipopolysaccharide (LPS) subcutaneous injections (Hol et al., 1986; Niewold et al., 1987).

b. Polycystic Disease

Polycystic disease is a common postmortem finding in Syrian hamsters, with cysts having been observed in up to 76% of hamsters over 1 year of age (Gleiser et al., 1970). The liver is a common site, but several organs may be affected, including the cecum, kidneys, ovaries, and spleen (Table 5.3). The liver lesions are related to developmental defects of normal ductal structures (i.e., bile ducts), whereas cysts in other organs likely develop from dilations of the lymphatic system. The condition may be associated with distension of the abdomen, but other clinical signs have not been recorded. Typical findings include cysts of variable size that can be unilocular to multilocular (Kaup et al., 1990). At necropsy, the cysts are thin-walled with clear watery fluid varying in color from amber to green. Findings in one study mentioned that the proteinaceous nature of the fluid resulted in white solidified collections within cysts in the cecal walls (Kaup et al., 1990). Reports have found that a higher incidence of intraperitoneal cysts occurs in European compared to Syrian hamsters (Kaup et al., 1990).

c. Chronic Hepatitis

Chronic hepatitis and cirrhosis were first described as an incidental finding during various carcinogen studies (Chesterman and Pomerance, 1965). Disease has been linked to dietary contamination, infection with bacterial pathogens, and immune system abnormalities, yet a common etiology has not been identified (Brunnert and Altman, 1991; Fox et al., 2009). The primary means of diagnosis has been from necropsy, since there are usually no clinical signs of disease, even in cirrhotic animals (Hamilton and Reynolds, 1983). In most strains, females are more commonly affected than males (Homburger, 1972). Significant elevations of both alanine aminotransferase (ALT) and bile acids may be seen on serum clinical chemistries (Brunnert and Altman, 1991).

d. Atrial Thrombosis

Atrial thrombosis is a common finding in aged Syrian hamsters. The exact incidence varies greatly, from 16% reported in one colony to 73% incidence in another (McMartin, 1977; Pour, 1976a). Males and females are equally affected, but females develop the condition at an earlier age. Atrial thrombosis may be most commonly seen in the APA strain of hamster, accompanied by cardiac hypertrophy that develops with age (Doi et al., 1987). Clinical signs are suggestive of heart failure and include tachypnea, tachycardia, and cyanosis (Sichuk et al., 1965). Upon necropsy, thrombi are present, primarily in the left atrium. One study also noted that there was bilateral ventricular hypertrophy in the hearts with thrombosis and myxomatous thickening of the atrioventricular valves. However, the valvular lesions were also found in all aged hamsters, regardless of whether thrombi were present or not (McMartin and Dodds, 1982). Doi et al. (1987) propose that an increase in relative and absolute heart weights seen in older APA hamsters is suggestive of cardiac hypertrophy. It is postulated that thrombi occur as a result of local blood stasis, secondary to heart failure (McMartin and Dodds, 1982).

TABLE 5.3   Frequency of Cysts at Various Sites

Organ systems	Number (%)	
	Syrian hamster[a]	European hamster[b]
Gastrointestinal system		
Esophagus	1/40 (2.5%)	—
Liver	17/40 (42.5%)	54/150 (36.0%)
Cecum	—	18/150 (12.0%)
Colon	—	1/150 (0.7%)
Reproductive system		
Seminal vesicle	4/17 (23.5%)	—
Epididymis	8/17 (47.0%)	—
Uterus	1/23 (4.35%)	—
Ovary	1/23 (4.35%)	13/150 (8.7%)
Endocrine		
Adrenal	1/40 (2.5%)	—
Pancreas	5/40(12.5%)	—
Other		
Kidney	2/40 (5.0%)	7/150 (4.7%)
Spleen	—	2/150(1.3%)

[a]Gleiser et al. (1970).
[b]Kaup et al. (1990).

III. CHINESE HAMSTER

A. Introduction

The Chinese hamster (*Cricetulus griseus*), also known as the striped-back hamster, was first used as a laboratory

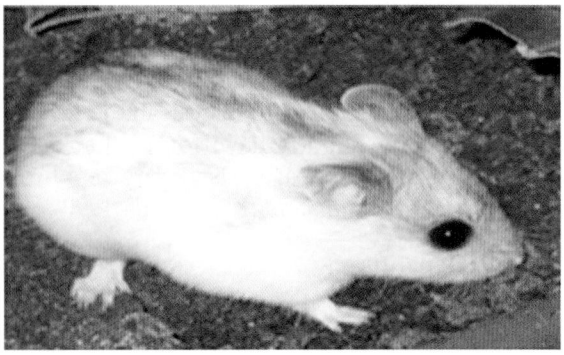

FIGURE 5.13 Appearance of the adult Chinese hamster, *Cricetulus griseus*. Note the dark stripe of fur along the dorsal midline.

TABLE 5.4　Normal Hemogram of the Chinese Hamster[a,b,c]

Parameter	Mean ± SD
Erythrocytes ($10^6/\mu l$)	7.1 ± 0.01
Packed cell volume (%)	42.1 ± 5.6
Hemoglobin (g/dl)	12.4
Leukocytes ($10^3/\mu l$)	5.5
Neutrophils (%)	19.3 ± 2.2
Bands (%)	0.2 ± 0.1
Lymphocytes (%)	76.1 ± 7.8
Monocytes (%)	2.1 ± 0.3
Eosinophils (%)	1.7 ± 0.7
Basophils	0.1 ± 0.04
Sedimentation rate (mm/h)	3.5 ± 1.7
Bleeding time (s)[c]	55

[a]*Table from Feeney (2012) reprinted with permission from Academic Press.*
[b]*From Moore (1966).*
[c]*From Yerganian et al. (1955).*

animal in 1919 (Fig. 5.13) (Yerganian, 1985). Benefits such as small size, polyestrous cycle, short gestation period, and low chromosome number encouraged the use of this specific hamster breed in biomedical research. Today, use of this animal in research is greatly overshadowed by the extensive use of cell lines derived from its ovarian cells. Chinese hamster ovary (CHO) cells are used almost exclusively for cell culturing experiments to obtain heterologous protein products (Oka and Rupp, 1990). Over the last two decades, CHO cells have been used to synthesize a wide array of recombinant therapeutic proteins that have been utilized clinically for the treatment of many human diseases (Jayapal et al., 2007).

The Chinese hamster has been shown to be susceptible to a number of infectious disease agents, such as bacteria, mycobacteria, protozoa, diphtheria, rabies, influenza, and equine encephalitis (Yerganian, 1958). Spontaneous hereditary diabetes mellitus, with similarities to the human disease, has been described (Meier and Yerganian, 1959) as well as susceptibility to experimental induction of stomach and esophageal cancer by oral diethylnitrosamine (Baker et al., 1974).

Chinese hamsters can be purchased commercially and fare well under standardized laboratory housing conditions. Because their size is comparable to that of the laboratory mouse, a similar style of caging is adequate.

B. Biology

The Chinese hamster, like the Syrian hamster, has a cheek pouch that can be utilized as an immunologically privileged site (Yerganian, 1958). Another unique biological feature of this animal is its low chromosome number of ($2n = 22$), which is beneficial for cytogenetic studies. The 10 large pairs of autosomes and two sex chromosomes can be readily differentiated. The constant diploidy maintained in cell culture provides a stable cell system for assessment of agents with known or suspected mutagenic and carcinogenic properties.

Adult animals weigh between 39 and 46 g, and are approximately 9 cm long. Newborns weigh 1.5–2.5 g. The average normal life span under laboratory conditions is 2.5–3.0 years. Adult males have exceptionally large testicles; also, the spleen and brain in both sexes are relatively larger, with respect to overall body size, than those of the Syrian hamster (Festing, 1972). The normal hemogram is shown in Table 5.4 (Moore, 1966).

There appear to be no unique dietary needs for Chinese hamsters. They do very well on standard rodent chow, but wheat germ may be used as a supplement for breeders. The average daily water intake was shown to be 11.4 ml per 100 g body weight for males and 12.9 ml per 100 g body for females (Thompson, 1971).

Early attempts to breed Chinese hamsters under laboratory conditions were unsuccessful until a reversed illumination schedule was employed to establish a production colony (Yerganian, 1958). Sexual maturity is indicated by vaginal opening, with a mucus-like, creamy material frequently secreted at the beginning of estrus. The estrous cycle consists of four phases, with distinct behavioral characteristics associated with vaginal orifice changes (Yerganian, 1958). Routine examinations of the vulva can assist with determining estrus and optimal breeding time. Progesterone levels are significantly different during the estrus cycle and pregnancy. During the 4-day cycle, maximal synthesis of progesterone occurs on day 3, which differs from the low levels found on day 3 of the Syrian hamster cycle (Sato et al., 1984). Normal reproductive data are shown in Table 5.5 (Moore, 1965).

TABLE 5.5   Reproductive Data for the Chinese Hamster

Weaned	21–25 days[a]
Sexually mature	8–12 weeks[a]
Type of estrous cycle	Polyestrus[b]
Duration of estrous cycle	4 days[a]
Length of estrus	6–8 hr[a]
Ovulation time	Immediately before estrus[b]
Copulation	2–4 h after start of dark period[c]
Implantation	5–6 days[b]
Gestation	20.5 days[a]
Average litter size	4.5–5.2[b]
Number of mammae	8[b]
Postpartum estrus	4 days[a]

[a]Yerganian (1958).
[b]Festing (1972).
[c]Moore (1965).

Because females can become very aggressive immediately following mating and even kill the male, hand mating was originally used for breeding purposes. However, selective monogamous breeding with docile females having high fecundity was found to be very successful for establishing breeding colonies (Calland et al., 1986). It has also been shown that Chinese hamsters can be mated in groups (Cisar et al., 1972). Infertility in young female hamsters may be due to an excess growth of hair around the vulva, preventing penile penetration during copulation attempts.

Pregnancy is indicated by a closed vagina with dry, pale, and scaly perineal tissues at day 4 following mating. Progesterone levels in peripheral blood increase through day 12 of pregnancy, stabilize through day 18, peak on day 19, and then dramatically drop prior to parturition (Sato et al., 1984). Dystocia may occur as a result of fetal wedging in the proximal portion of the vagina during parturition attempts. The fetuses can be saved by surgical removal.

Newborn animals have front incisors. Body hair appears at 3–4 days of age, with complete coverage in 7 days. Eyes and ears open within 10–14 days, and testicles descend in males at about 30 days of age. As animals approach sexual maturity, aggressive females may fight until dominance is established.

C. Diseases

1. Infectious Diseases

The Chinese hamster appears to be experimentally susceptible to a number of infectious disease agents; yet, little has been reported concerning spontaneous infections in this species. Tyzzer's disease is similar to that seen in Syrian hamsters. The presence of antibodies against murine viruses has also been reported in Chinese hamsters. Parasitic infections may include persistent intestinal colonization with Trichomonas spp; however, few reports of other infecting endo- and ectoparasites exist in the literature. Despite the identification of Demodex sinocricetuli (Desch and Hurley, 1997) in Cricetulus barabensis (a species considered to be synonymous with C. griseus), there appears to be a very low susceptibility to demodectic mange in Chinese hamsters (Benjamin and Brooks, 1977).

2. Metabolic/Genetic Diseases

a. Diabetes Mellitus

Spontaneous diabetes mellitus was first recognized in 1957 during the course of inbreeding (Meier and Yerganian, 1959). The disease is similar in a number of aspects to insulin-dependent diabetes of humans (Yerganian, 1965).

Etiology   The disease is associated with a degranulation of the β-cells of the pancreatic islets of Langerhans, resulting in a primary defect in the biosynthesis of insulin.

Clinical Signs   Animals can show signs as early as 18 days of age, but the disease may occur at any age. Polydipsia and polyuria develop, with up to 50–70 ml of urine passed in 24 h. Urine staining and scald may develop on the abdomen. At the onset of disease, there may be an initial weight gain, but animals can become lethargic and require close clinical management. Occasionally, hamsters develop blindness and nonspecific conjunctivitis and alopecia may be seen. Animals are very susceptible to mild stress of any kind, and sudden death may be triggered by such procedures as cage transfer and changes in environmental parameters. Diabetic females may be infertile, but hamsters that do become pregnant tend to have increased numbers of abortions and fetal deaths at delivery.

Epizootiology   The disease appears to be transmitted as a recessive factor. When glucosuria was used to characterize diabetes, it was shown that four recessive genes were involved (Butler and Gerritsen, 1970). If any two of the four genes were homozygous, glucosuria could result. Apparently the duration, severity, and constancy of glucosuria is controlled by modifier genes. It has also been shown that 100% of the offspring become diabetic if the parents are ketotic (Gerritsen et al., 1970).

Necropsy Findings   Macroscopic lesions are confined mainly to the kidneys, which are slightly enlarged, spongy, and friable in diabetic animals. The renal pelvis may be dilated. When hydronephrosis is seen, retained urine is clear but odoriferous, and the urinary bladder is usually distended with urine. In some animals, the liver may be moderately enlarged with a yellow to gray color.

Microscopically, the pancreatic islets of Langerhans are decreased in number (Meier and Yerganian, 1959). There is a decrease in the number of β-cells; remaining cells stain lightly basophilic with cytoplasmic granulation and vacuolization. There is periodic acid-Schiff (PAS)-positive material within the cytoplasm that accumulates around pyknotic nuclei. Ultrastructural findings in the pancreas have been characterized (Boquist, 1969). Renal convoluted tubules contain much protein precipitate, and glomeruli are hypocellular with marked sclerosis. Intercapillary homogeneous material can be observed that is PAS positive. Bowman's capsule may be slightly to moderately thickened, and adhesions may be present between the glomerulus and capsule. PAS-positive material is also found in the basement membrane, which may appear wrinkled and slightly thickened. The liver shows an intact lobular arrangement with extensive vacuolization of cells with perinuclear haloes. Intracytoplasmic material is PAS-positive, but negative when stained for fat. PAS-positive material is occasionally found in pericardial adipose tissue.

Pathogenesis   The basic defect is a degranulation of β-cells, which results in a decreased amount of insulin production with a reciprocal increase in glucagon. In highly inbred glucosuric strains with diabetes, there is a greatly reduced level of pancreatic insulin and a significantly elevated level of glucagon in both pancreas and stomach. A decrease in lactate dehydrogenase (LDH) isozymes appears to be associated with severity of the diabetic condition (Chang *et al.*, 1977). A contributing factor to the observed renal pathology may be subnormal levels of specific glycosidases in the kidneys, with a resulting change in turnover of tissue glycoproteins (Chang, 1981).

Differential Diagnosis   Because diabetes mellitus is a spontaneous disease, it should be ruled out whenever a colony illness occurs. If the animals are being used as a model to study diabetes, the experimental protocol will dictate the diagnostic monitoring procedures. Certainly Tyzzer's disease must be considered both in the initial differential phases and also as a secondary complication, since diabetic animals are very susceptible to stress and subsequent immunosuppression.

Treatment and Control   It has been previously suggested that treatment with hypoglycemic drugs may be indicated in breeding females in an attempt to maintain inbred lines (Meier and Yerganian, 1961).

Research Complications   The disease could potentially occur in animals being used in research protocols unrelated to diabetes. Because cellular metabolism is affected, cytogenetic studies could produce unreliable data.

3. Traumatic Diseases

Female littermates can become very aggressive as they reach maturity. Severe bite wounds, especially about the tail and head area, can be inflicted, and death is not an uncommon occurrence. Litters should be separated before fighting becomes a problem. Following attempts at breeding, the female can become quite aggressive to the male, so some means of removing the male must be anticipated.

4. Neoplastic Diseases

In general, Chinese hamsters have a low incidence of spontaneous tumors, with mainly the liver and reproductive organs involved. The rarity of spontaneous and induced leukemias may reflect the absence of innate tumor viruses.

Uterine adenocarcinomas were detected in 30 of 120 females (Ward and Moore, 1969). The growths were firm and white with implantation frequently seen on the visceral and parietal peritoneum. Approximately 10% of affected hamsters had lung metastases. Another report showed 11 of 77 affected with similar characteristics except that no pulmonary metastasis was seen (Benjamin and Brooks, 1977). Vaginal bleeding was the sign most often seen initially. The incidence of ovarian tumors was significantly increased with radiation exposure, but was rarely reported in control animals (Kohn and Gultman, 1964).

Hepatomas were found in 66 of 253 animals (Ward and Moore, 1969). These were benign and most often occurred as multiple nodules. Nodular hyperplasia, a nonneoplastic lesion, was seen in 111 of 157 animals in another survey (Benjamin and Brooks, 1977).

Pancreatic adenocarcinomas were reported in three 3-year-old females that were partially inbred for the development of spontaneous diabetes mellitus (Poel and Yerganian, 1961); however, it is believed that these tumors are rare in nondiabetic animals.

5. Miscellaneous Diseases

a. Cerebral Hemorrhage

Hemorrhage occurred in 20% of both control and experimental animals in a ^{131}I chronic toxicity study, (Ward and Moore, 1969). Deaths occurred at 1–2 years of age. Grossly, the hemorrhage was most evident between the cerebral hemispheres, with blood often in the lateral ventricles. Microscopically, the hemorrhage was shown to be caused by inflammation and necrosis of the anterior cerebral artery. A homogeneous PAS-positive material could be seen within the media of the diseased artery. The vessel wall was greatly thickened in chronic cases. The cause of the cerebral hemorrhage has not been determined but it is postulated to involve an inflammatory or degenerative change in the anterior cerebral artery. The true incidence of cerebral hemorrhage is not known since other reports have not seen cerebral hemorrhage in necropsies of control or naive Chinese hamsters (Benjamin and Brooks, 1977).

b. Periodontitis

This condition was found in a strain of Chinese hamster with hereditary diabetes mellitus (Cohen *et al.*, 1961). The lesion is characterized by absorption of alveolar bone, inflammation, and pocket formation due to splitting of the epithelial attachment. The disease corresponds to that seen in humans with diabetes mellitus.

c. Nephrosclerosis

In a study of 157 animals, 46 had evidence of nephrosclerosis (Benjamin and Brooks, 1977). The pathology was different from the intercapillary glomerulosclerosis associated with diabetes mellitus. Grossly, pitting and a decrease in size were noted in severely affected kidneys. Microscopically, tubular degeneration, mild interstitial fibrosis, and focal atrophy of the cortex were seen early in the disease process. In more advanced conditions, hyaline sclerosis of glomeruli, more severe interstitial fibrosis, and tubular degeneration were noted.

d. Spondylosis

The incidence and extent of spondylosis were increased in hamsters with spontaneous diabetes mellitus compared to nondiabetic control animals (Silberberg and Gerritsen, 1976).

e. Pulmonary Granulomas

Pulmonary granulomas were observed in 54 of 157 animals (Benjamin and Brooks, 1977). Grossly, the lesions appeared as subpleural, yellowish gray foci, measuring 1–3 mm in diameter with variable involvement of the lung parenchyma. Microscopically, lesions consisted of alveolar collections of lipid-filled macrophages, mixed inflammatory cells, septal fibrosis, and occasional cholesterol clefts. Affected animals were housed in both suspended wire cages and plastic shoe box cages with different types of bedding; the etiology remains unknown.

IV. ARMENIAN HAMSTER

A. Introduction

The Armenian hamster (*Cricetulus migratorius*), also known as the gray hamster, was first introduced as a laboratory research animal in the 1960s because of its susceptibility to mutagenic and carcinogenic agents (Fig. 5.14). Cytological features are comparable to those of the Chinese hamster, so this species is also used for cytogenetic studies. Like the Syrian hamster, the Armenian hamster is highly susceptible to oncogenic viruses but has a high tolerance to both homologous and heterologous transplantable tumors. Armenian hamsters are used to study infection with prion diseases.

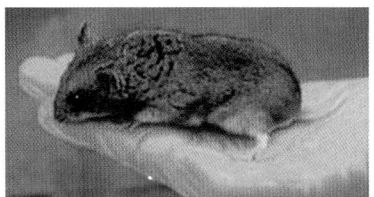

FIGURE 5.14 Armenian hamster (*Cricetulus migratorius*).

B. Biology

Care and management procedures are similar to those of the Chinese hamster. Body size and weight (33–80 g) are also similar. The diploid chromosome number is 22, with the X and Y chromosome of equal size. Captured animals are aggressive, but if reared in the laboratory, they can be bred successfully. Sexual maturity occurs around 50 days of age. The gestation period is 18–19 days, with an average litter size of five to seven pups.

C. Diseases

Reports concerning spontaneous infectious diseases in the Armenian hamster are rare. The expression of spontaneous amyloidosis differs in gender-specific AP expression and susceptibility to AA amyloidosis from that seen in the Syrian hamster (de Beer *et al.*, 1993). Hepatocellular carcinomas have been reported in animals exposed to estrogen (Coe *et al.*, 1990).

Skin lesions have been attributed to mite infestations, which have been identified as *Demodex cricetuli* (Hurley and Desch, 1994). This mite is similar to *D. aurati* of the Syrian hamster and occupies hair follicles, particularly along the face and back.

V. EUROPEAN HAMSTER

A. Introduction

The European hamster (*Cricetus cricetus*) developed some importance as a laboratory model when several wild-caught animals from a West German industrial area were found to have bronchogenic squamous cell carcinoma. It has since been found to be susceptible to *N*-diethylnitrosamine (DEN), with the subsequent development of respiratory tumors (Mohr *et al.*, 1973). The European hamster is believed to be a more suitable model than the Syrian hamster for highly concentrated and prolonged smoke-inhalation studies (Reznik *et al.*, 1975). The Bern Convention of 1979 established the European hamster as a strictly protected species in Appendix II, and later became listed in Appendix IV of the Habitats Directive, therefore being provided strict legal protection in all European countries (Ziomek and

TABLE 5.6   Normal Hemogram of the European Hamster

Hemogram	Silverman and Chavannes (1977)		Emminger et al. (1975)	
	Value	Percentage	Value	Percentage
Leukocytes (10^3/ml)	7.4 ± 2.6		8.3 ± 2.2	
Neutrophils	1.71 ± 0.06	23.2 ± 2.5	2.87 ± 3.74	34.6 ± 17
Lymphocytes	5.47 ± 0.06	74.0 ± 2.3	5.02 ± 0.39	60.0 ± 17.6
Monocytes	0.192 ± 0.015	2.6 ± 0.6	0.083 ± 0.022	1.00 ± 1.00
Eosinophils	0.005 ± 0.002	0.07 ± 0.10	0.093 ± 0.018	1.13 ± 0.83
Basophils	0.001 ± 0.002	0.02 ± 0.07	0	0
Thrombocytes (10^3/ml)			210 ± 32	
RBC (106/ml)	7.64 ± 0.42		7.45 ± 0.49	
PCV (%)	49.2 ± 1.6			
Hemoglobin (g/dl)	18.0 ± 0.7			

Banaszek, 2007). There are no breeding colonies of these animals presently housed in the United States; instead, sources are from European institutional research breeding colonies. They are not widely used research animals, and most of their use in the biomedical field involves studies of hibernation.

B. Biology

European hamsters are nocturnal, and they hibernate during the winter months in the wild. They are the largest hamster species, being minimally three-times the size of a Syrian hamster, with males larger than the females. Their outward appearance consists of white faces and feet, bodies with reddish brown dorsums, cranioventral black patches, and caudolateral white patches. These hamsters tend to be very aggressive, are easily frightened and will attack and bite. Those in captivity through laboratory breeding have become much easier to handle. Each litter develops a defined social order, with the heaviest male being dominant (Reznik-Schuller et al., 1974). The average life span of a research-bred European hamster is 34 months for females and 31 months for males, which may be related to the higher reported incidence of neoplasia in males (Ernst et al., 1989). Their life span is 4–10 years in the wild (Reznik-Schuller et al., 1974). Like the Chinese hamster, the European hamster has a chromosome diploid number of 2n = 22. A normal hemogram is presented in Table 5.6.

Water consumption is 5ml/100g body weight, and average food consumption is 2.9g/100g body weight in summer (August) and 1.8g/100g body weight in winter (November) (Silverman and Chavannes, 1977). These animals are mainly seed eaters, but will readily consume a standard laboratory rodent diet.

TABLE 5.7   Reproductive Data for the European Hamster[a]

Sexual maturity	Females, 80–90 days
	Males, 60 days
Estrus cycle	4–6 days
Gestation	18–21 days (captured)
	15–17 days (laboratory-born)
Litter size	7–9
Weaning	25–28 days

[a]Data from Mohr et al. (1973).

Reproductive data are shown in Table 5.7. Females have a regular four-stage estrus cycle of 4–6 days (Reznik et al., 1979). Proestrus lasts a few hours, estrus lasts 1–2 days, there is a metestrus of 6h, and diestrus lasting 2–4 days (Reznik-Schüller et al., 1974). Estrus is determined by vaginal smears and by test-mating, using a steel mesh divider to keep the pair separated. The female is only receptive to the male for a short period during estrus, and markedly aggressive during the other three stages of the cycle. When no aggressiveness is observed, hamsters may be mated (Mohr et al., 1973). Females tend to bear one to two litters per year, each with six to nine pups (Reznik-Schuller et al., 1974). Newly weaned animals (25 days postpartum) have an average body weight of 75g, with 6-month-old females and males approaching 300 and 400g, respectively (Mohr et al., 1973). Sexual activity is not observed in winter months, during which time females and males are very aggressive toward each other. In the nonbreeding season, the female's vagina is closed and the male's scrotum is decreased in size with the testes situated in the abdominal cavity.

Anatomy of the European hamster has been studied extensively. The exocrine pancreas was described in an attempt to determine the suitability of this animal as a model for pancreatic cancer (Spikermann and Althoff, 1980). The nasal cavity has been fully described, as have comparative analyses of organ weights (Reznik and Jensen, 1979; Reznik et al., 1973).

Photoperiodic regulation of annual cycles has been described in European hamsters (Pevet, 1988). The critical photoperiod, at which time gonadal regression is induced, is between 15 and 15.5 h. Studies have also implicated a circannual rhythm in physiological variations in these animals, including changes in body weight and food intake even under conditions of constant photoperiods (Masson-Pevet et al., 1994; Wollnik and Schmidt, 1995). There is a slight reduction in activity in the winter months. As mentioned previously, these hamsters are true hibernators. Hibernation affects thrombocyte and leukocyte values, but no significant difference in these values has been noted in nonhibernating animals during winter or summer (Reznik et al., 1979).

C. Diseases

Spontaneous neoplasia (bengin or malignant) is common in older European hamsters, with up to a 70% incidence by 2 years of age. Neoplasia is also slightly more prevalent in males than in females. The most frequent tumors in descending order are leukemias and lymphomas, adrenal pheochromocytomas, and granulosa cell tumors in females (Ernst et al., 1989). Thymomas discovered in a small number of examined European hamsters resembled benign human thymomas (Ghadially and Illman, 1965). Thymic tumors were associated with large numbers of mast cells, which are not normally seen in the human form of disease (Ghadially and Illman, 1965). Similar to the Syrian and Chinese hamsters, the European hamster has a very low incidence of spontaneous pulmonary neoplasia (Ernst et al., 1989). In a small group of males (n=8), animals were found to be generally free of endoparasites, ectoparasites, and blood parasites (Silverman and Chavannes, 1977). One outbreak of Spironucleus muris associated with chronic enteritis was reported in seven newly captured European hamsters (Maatthiesen et al., 1976).

European hamsters are prone to developing cysts within the peritoneal cavity, particularly in the liver. Cysts tend to occur more often in females than in males and additional locations for cysts include the cecum, ovaries, spleen, kidney, and colon (Kaup et al., 1990).

Secondary bacterial infections with Corynebacteria, Staphylococcus, Pasteurella pneumotropica, and Pasteurella multicoda have been associated with pathological processes resembling fistulated abscesses in the head and jaws of the European hamster. The development of such disorders as malocclusion, osteomyelitis, and dysplasia appears to increase with age and suggest that the European hamster could be of use in dental research (Kunstyr et al., 1987). These disease processes in the mouth are often complicated by secondary bacterial infections, which may be fatal (Ernst et al., 1989).

VI. DJUNGARIAN HAMSTER

A. Introduction

The Djungarian hamsters are *Phodopus campbelli* (Russian dwarf) and *P. sungorus* (Siberian dwarf) (Fig. 5.15). Initially these animals were assumed to be subspecies; however, they are now believed to be separate species. The two may be confused because the common name 'Djungarian' is often used to denote either species. The most obvious factor to phenotypically differentiate *P. campbelli* from *P. sungorus* is the lack of dramatic coat color change in response to a short photoperiod: *P. sungorus* molts to a pure white haircoat, while *P. campbelli* retains its gray haircoat. Karyotype analysis using G-banding and chromosomal painting with probes from the Syrian and Chinese hamsters has confirmed close phylogenetic relationship between *P. sungorus* and *P. campbelli* (Romanenko et al., 2007). Unique C-banding patterns in *P. sungorus* chromosomes distinguish the karyotype from that of *P. campbelli* (Ross, 1998). The Russian dwarf hamster has been traced to Siberia, China, and Mongolia and is a distant relative of the Syrian hamster (Cooper et al., 1991). The Siberian dwarf hamster is native to the steppes of Kazakhstan, Manchuria, and northern China (Wynne-Edwards and Lisk, 1984). These hamsters range from 50 to 100 mm in body length, with an additional 10 mm of tail. Body weights range from 18 to 25 g, with mature males reaching 40–50 g.

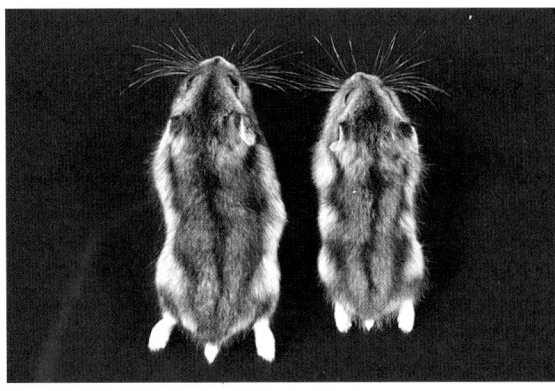

FIGURE 5.15 Dungarian hamsters. Males (left) are larger than females.

The dorsal fur is gray, and a dark stripe runs dorsally along the length of the body. The fur of the ventrum, limbs, and tail tends to be white. Djungarian hamsters generally live for 9–15 months, although survival up to 2 years has been reported (Lawrie and Megahy, 1991). The normal karyotype of the Djungarian species is $2n = 28$ chromosomes. These hamsters have a high incidence of neoplasia and are susceptible to carcinogens, and can be infected with oncogenic viruses, particularly Rous sarcoma virus (RSV), *Human mastadenovirus A* (formerly known as human adenovirus 12), and SV40 (Pogosianz, 1975). The dwarf hamsters are extensively used in behavior and reproductive physiology studies.

B. Biology

Dwarf hamsters have the most compressed reproductive cycle of any eutherian mammal. They can mate on the day of parturition (following an 18-day gestation) and deliver the second litter, while weaning the first, within a 36-day time period (Newkirk *et al.*, 1997). Similar to the Syrian and Chinese hamsters, the two Djungarian hamster species have a 4-day estrus cycle with spontaneous ovulation (Erb *et al.*, 1993). Pregnancy in *Phodopus campbelli* is dependent on continued secretion of progesterone by the corpus luteum through late gestation (Edwards *et al.*, 1995). Prolactin levels in this species are absent during midgestation and resume in late gestation. Possible roles for this reappearance of activity include influences on lactogenesis, mammary gland development, and the regulation of maternal behavior toward newborns (Edwards *et al.*, 1995). Successful reproduction in *P. campbelli* is dependent on monogamous parental care by both males and females (Wynne-Edwards and Lisk, 1984, 1987). In contrast, male *P. sungorus* do not participate in the rearing of offspring. The nonaggressive behavior of females facilitates the maintenance of breeding pairs throughout life, with weaning of offspring occurring at 3 weeks of age. Females can bear between one and 18 litters, with each consisting of one to nine pups, in their reproductive years (Pogosianz, 1975). Reproductive development in females is accelerated when exposed to males of the same species (Reasner and Johnston, 1988). Increased food hoarding has been observed in *P. sungorus* as a behavioral adaptation to provide accessible energy during pregnancy (Bartness, 1997). Endocrinology in *P. sungorus* is similar to that of other rodent species, yet differs from that of *P. campbelli*. This implies that the two species of Djungarian hamsters have undergone evolutionary selection pressures with respect to reproductive endocrinology (Mcmillan and Wynne-Edwards, 1998). As adults, these hamsters are biologically dependent on the critical photoperiod, which is approximately 13h (*versus* 12.5h in the Syrian and 15.5h in the European hamsters)

(Pevet, 1988). Changes in photoperiod influence seasonal changes in breeding activities, thermoregulation, hair-coat growth, and fat metabolism (Pogosianz, 1975; Ebling, 1994). Djungarian hamsters have been widely used in studies of the pineal gland and melatonin secretion in mediating the effects of photoperiod. These hamsters are unusual in that they do not hibernate even when exposed to temperatures below −40°C (Schlenker, 1985). Seasonal acclimation of blood-gas transport during periods of colder temperatures is facilitated by an increased relative heart weight, increased surface area of erythrocytes, and slightly altered hemoglobin content, all of which aid in oxygen transport (Puchalski and Heldmaier, 1986). These animals also decrease their resting metabolic rates and increase their capacity for nonshivering thermogenesis to adapt to inclement temperatures (Schlenker, 1985).

Djungarian hamsters are omnivorous (Sawrey *et al.*, 1984). They can be maintained on the same diet as Syrian hamsters and are less costly to maintain because of their smaller size (Pogosianz, 1975).

C. Diseases

High incidence of neoplasia, particularly of the oral cavity, skin, and mammary glands has been reported in Russian dwarf hamsters, particularly in females (Lawrie and Megahy, 1991). In a study of 30 animals ranging from 6 to 12 months of age, 30% were found to have metastatic tumors that consisted of fibromas ($n = 4$), fibrosarcomas ($n = 2$), mammary adenocarcinomas ($n = 2$), and fibroma with liver cell carcinoma ($n = 1$) (Cooper *et al.*, 1991). The incidence of the tumors has changed over time, with mammary tumors increasing and skin tumors decreasing in frequency; this may reflect genetic alterations linked to further inbreeding (Pogosianz and Sokova, 1982). Affected dwarf hamsters are reported to exhibit rapid weight loss, similar to that seen with disease conditions of bronchopneumonia and incisor malocclusion. Dermatologic conditions of trichophytosis have been reported (Pogosianz, 1975). Other skin problems include alopecia and ventral dermatitis caused by demodectic mites.

Female Russian dwarf hamsters prevented from breeding may develop cystic ovaries, with clinical presentations of swollen abdomens and bloody vaginal discharge (Lawrie and Megahy, 1991).

Hypersensitivity to bedding materials, particularly cedar chips, has been empirically reported. Affected dwarf hamsters may develop alopecia with dry skin and have secondary bacterial infections (McGuire, 1993).

Enteritis with rectal prolapse, although common in other varieties of hamsters, has not been noted in the Russian hamster (Lawrie and Megahy, 1991).

References

Adler, S., 1948. Origin of the golden hamster, Cricetus auratus, as a laboratory animal. Nature 162, 256–257.

Aitken, R.J., 2006. Sperm function tests and fertility. Int. J. Androl. 29, 69–75.

Allison, A.C., Chesterman, F.C., Baron, S., 1967. Induction of tumors in adult hamsters with simian virus 40. J. Natl. Cancer Inst. 38, 567–572.

Amao, H., Akimoto, T., Takahashi, K., Nakagawam, M., Saito, M., 1991. Isolation of Corynebactrium kutscheri from aged Syrian hamsters (Mesocricetus auratus). Lab. Anim. Sci. 41, 265–267.

Ambrose, K.R., Coggin, J.H.J., 1975. An epizootic in hamsters of lymphomas of undetermined origin and mode of transmission. J. Natl. Cancer Inst. 54, 877–879.

Amman, B.R., Pavlin, B.I., Albariño, C.G., Comer, J.A., Erickson, B.R., Oliver, J.B., et al., 2007. Pet rodents and fatal lymphocytic choriomeningitis in transplant patients. Emerg. Infect. Dis. 13, 719.

Arnold, C., Westbrook, R.D., 1998. Enrichment in group-housed laboratory golden hamsters. Anim. Welf. Inf. Cent. Newsl. 8, 22–24.

Arnold, C.E., Estep, D.Q., 1994. Laboratory caging preferences in golden hamsters (Mesocricetus auratus). Lab. Anim. 28, 232–238.

Bajusz, E., Baker, J.R., Nixon, C.W., Homburger, F., 1969. Spontaneous, hereditary myocardial degeneration and congestive heart failure in a strain of Syrian hamsters. Infect. Immun. 56, 105–129.

Baker, J.R., Mason, M.M., Yerganian, G., Weisburger, E.K., Weisburger, J.H., 1974. Induction of tumors of the stomach and esophagus in inbred Chinese hamsters by oral diethylnitrosamine. Proc. Soc. Exp. Biol. Med. 146, 291–293.

Barros, C., Gonzalez, J., Herrera, E., Bustos-Obregon, E., 1978. Fertilizing capacity of human spermatozoa evaluated by actual penetration of foreign eggs. Contraception 17, 87–92.

Barthold, S.W., Bhatt, P.N., Johnson, E.A., 1987. Further evidence for papovavirus as the probable etiology of transmissible lymphoma of Syrian hamsters. Lab. Anim. Sci. 37, 283.

Barthold, S.W., Smith, A.L., 2007. Lymphocytic choriomeningitis virus. In: Fox, J.G., Barthold, S.W., Davisson, M.T., Newcomer, C.E., Quimby, F.W., Smith, A.L. (Eds.), The Mouse in Biomedical Research, second ed. Elsevier, New York, pp. 179–213.

Bartness, T.J., 1997. Food hoarding is increased by pregnancy, lactation, and food deprivation in Siberian hamsters. Am. J. Physiol. 272, R118–R125.

Battles, A.H., 1985. The biology, care, and diseases of the Syrian hamster. Compend. Contin. Educ. Pract. Vet. 7, 815–825.

Baumans, V., 2005. Environmental enrichment for laboratory rodents and rabbits: requirements of rodents, rabbits, and research. ILAR J. 46, 162–170.

Beaulieu, A., Reebs, S.G., 2009. Effects of bedding material and running wheel surface on paw wounds in male and female Syrian hamsters. Lab. Anim. 43, 85–90.

Benjamin, S.A., Brooks, A.L., 1977. Spontaneous lesions in Chinese hamsters. Vet. Pathol. 14, 449–462.

Bergstresser, P.R., Toews, G.B., Gilliam, J.N., Streilein, J.W., 1980. Unusual numbers and distribution of Langerhans cells in skin with unique immunologic properties. J. Invest. Dermatol. 74, 312–314.

Bernfeld, P., Homburger, F., Adams, R.A., Soto, E., Van Dongen, C., 1986. Base-line data in a carcinogen-susceptible first generation hybrid strain of Syrian golden hamsters: FID Alexander. J. Natl. Cancer Inst. 77, 165–171.

Bertuglia, S., Reiter, R.J., 2007. Melatonin reduces ventricular arrhythmias and preserves capillary perfusion during ischemia – reperfusion events in cardiomyopathic hamsters. J. Pineal Res. 42, 55–63.

Besselsen, D.G., Pintel, D.J., Purdy, G.A., Besch-Williford, C.L., Franklin, C.L., Hook, R.R., et al., 1996. Molecular characterization of newly recognized rodent parvoviruses. J. Gen. Virol. 77, 899–911.

Besselsen, D.G., Gibson, S.V., Besch-Williford, C.L., Purdy, G.A., Knowles, R.L., Wagner, J.E., et al., 1999. Natural and experimentally induced infection of Syrian hamsters with a newly recognized parvovirus. Comp. Med. 49, 308–312.

Besselsen, D.G., Romero, M.J., Wagner, A.M., Henderson, K.S., Livingston, R.S., 2006. Identification of novel murine parvovirus strains by epidemiological analysis of naturally infected mice. J. Gen. Virol. 87, 1543–1556.

Besselsen, D.G., Franklin, C.L., Livingston, R.S., Riley, L.K., 2008. Lurking in the shadows: emerging rodent infectious diseases. ILAR J. 49, 277–290.

Birt, D.F., Pour, P.M., 1985. Interaction of dietary fat and protein in spontaneous diseases of Syrian golden hamsters. J. Natl. Cancer Inst. 75, 127–133.

Birt, D.F., Schuldt, G.H., Salmasi, S., 1982. Survival of hamsters fed graded levels of two protein sources. Lab. Anim. Sci. 32, 363–366.

Birt, D.F., Patil, K., Pour, P.M., 1985. Comparative studies on the effects of semipurified and commercial diet on longevity and spontaneous and induced lesions in the Syrian golden hamster. Nutr. Cancer 7, 167–177.

Blandford, G., Charlton, D., 1977. Studies of pulmonary and renal immunopathology after nonlethal primary Sendai viral infection in normal and cyclophosphamide-treated hamsters. Am. Rev. Respir. Dis. 115, 305–314.

Blankenship-Paris, T.L., Chang, J., Dalldorf, F.G., Gilligan, P.H., 1995a. In vivo and in vitro studies of Clostridium difficile-induced disease in hamsters fed an atherogenic, high fat diet. Lab. Anim. Sci. 45, 47–53.

Blankenship-Paris, T.L., Walton, B.J., Hayes, Y.O., Chang, J., 1995b. Clostridium difficile infection in hamsters fed an atherogenic diet. Vet. Pathol. 32, 269–273.

Boquist, L., 1969. Pancreatic islet morphology in diabetic Chinese hamsters. Acta Pathol. Microbiol. Scand. 75, 399–414.

Borzone, G., Liberona, L., Olmos, P., Saez, C., Meneses, M., Reyes, T., et al., 2007. Rat and hamster species differences in susceptibility to elastase-induced pulmonary emphysema relate to differences in elastase inhibitory capacity. Am. J. Physiol. Regul. Integr. Comp. Physiol. 293, R1342–R1349.

Bowen, G.S., Calisher, C.H., Winkler, W.G., Kraus, A.L., Fowler, E.H., Garman, R.H., et al., 1975. Laboratory studies of a lymphocytic choriomeningitis virus outbreak in man and laboratory animals. Am. J. Epidemiol. 102, 233–240.

Bowen, W.H., 2013. Rodent model in caries research. Odontology 101, 9–14.

Brownstein, D.G., 2007. Sendai virus and pneumonia virus of mice (MPNV), second ed. In: Fox, J.G., Barthold, S.W., Davisson, M.T., Newcomer, C.E., Quimby, F.W., Smith, A.L. (Eds.), The Mouse in Biomedical Research, vol. 2 Elsevier, New York, pp. 281–310.

Brunner, H., 1997. Models of mycoplasma respiratory and genital tract infections. Wien Klin Wochenschr. 109, 569–573.

Brunnert, S.R., Altman, N.H., 1991. Laboratory assessment of chronic hepatitis in Syrian hamsters. Lab. Anim. Sci. 41, 559–562.

Buchmeier, M.J., Oldstone, M.B., 1978. Virus-induced immune complex disease: identification of specific viral antigens and antibodies deposited in complexes during chronic lymphocytic choriomeningitis virus infection. J. Immunol. 120, 1297–1304.

Buntin, J.D., Jaffe, S., Lisk, R.D., 1984. Changes in responsiveness to newborn pups in pregnant, nulliparous golden hamsters. Physiol. Behav. 32, 437–439.

Burr, H.N., Paluch, L.R., Roble, G.S., Lipman, N.S., 2012. Parasitic diseases. In: Suckow, M.A., Stevens, K.A., Wilson, R.P. (Eds.), The Laboratory Rabbit, Guinea Pig, Hamster, and Other Rodents, first ed. Academic Press, Waltham, MA, pp. 839–866.

Butler, L., Gerritsen, G.C., 1970. A comparison of the modes of inheritance of diabetes in the Chinese hamster and the KK mouse. Diabetologia 6, 163–167.

Buzzell, G.R., 1996. Sexual dimorphism in the Harderian gland of the Syrian hamster is controlled and maintained by hormones, despite seasonal fluctuations in hormone levels: functional implications. Microsc. Res. Tech. 34, 133–138.

Calland, C.J., Wightman, S.R., Neal, S.B., 1986. Establishment of a Chinese hamster breeding colony. Lab. Anim. Sci. 36, 183–185.

Casanova, J., Santalla, F., Durand, P., Vaucher, C., Feliu, C., Renaud, F., 2001. Morphological and genetic differentiation of Rodentolepis straminea (Goeze, 1752) and Rodentolepis microstoma (Dujardin, 1845) (Hymenolepididae). Parasitol. Res. 87, 439–444.

Cassano, A., Rasmussen, S., Wolf, F.R., 2012. Viral diseases. In: Suckow, M.A., Stevens, K.A., Wilson, R.P. (Eds.), The Laboratory Rabbit, Guinea Pig, Hamster, and Other Rodents Academic Press, Waltham, MA, pp. 821–837.

Centers for Disease Control and Prevention – National Institutes of Health (CDCP-NIH), 2009. Biosafety in Microbiological and Biomedical Laboratories, fifth ed. US Government Printing Office, Washington, DC, HHS Publ. http://www.cdc.gov/biosafety/publications/bmbl5/BMBL.pdf.

Chang, A.Y., 1981. Biochemical abnormalities in the Chinese hamster (Cricetulus griseus) with spontaneous diabetes. Int. J. Biochem. 13, 41–43.

Chang, A.Y., Noble, R.E., Wyse, B.M., 1977. Comparison of highly inbred diabetic and nondiabetic lines in the Upjohn colony of Chinese hamsters. Diabetes 26, 1963–1971.

Chang, J., Rohwer, R.G., 1991. Clostridium difficile infection in adult hamsters. Lab. Anim. Sci. 41, 548–552.

Chesterman, F.C., Pomerance, A., 1965. Cirrhosis and liver tumours in a closed colony of golden hamsters. Br. J. Cancer 19, 802–811.

Christie, R.D., Marcus, E.C., Wagner, A.M., Besselsen, D.G., 2010. Experimental infection of mice with hamster parvovirus: evidence for interspecies transmission of mouse parvovirus 3. Comp. Med. 60, 123–129.

Ciaccio, L.A., Lisk, R.D., 1971. Hormonal control of cyclic estrus in the female hamster. Am. J. Physiol. 221 (3), 936–942.

Cicala, C., Pompetti, F., Carbone, M., 1993. SV40 induces mesotheliomas in hamsters. Am. J. Pathol. 142, 1524–1533.

Cisar, C.F., Gumperz, E.P., Nicholson, F.S., Moore Jr., W., 1972. A practical method for production of breeding of Chinese hamsters (Cricetulus griseus). Lab. Anim. Sci. 22, 725–727.

Coates, M.E., 1991. Nutrition and feeding, seventh ed. In: Poole, T. (Ed.), The UFAW Handbook on the Care and Management of Laboratory Animals, vol. 1 Blackwell Science, Oxford, pp. 45–60.

Code of Federal Regulations (CFR), 2013. Title 9; Animals and Service; Part 3: Standards; Subpart B: Specifications for the Humane Handling, Care, Treatment and Transportation of Guinea Pigs and Hamsters. Office of the Federal Register, Washington, DC.

Coe, J.E., Ross, M.J., 1990. Amyloidosis and female protein in the Syrian hamster. Concurrent regulation by sex hormones. J. Exp. Med. 171, 1257–1267.

Coe, J.E., Margossian, S.S., Slayter, H.S., Sogn, J.A., 1981. Hamster female protein. A new pentraxin structurally and functionally similar to C-reactive protein and amyloid P component. J. Exp. Med. 153, 977–991.

Coe, J.E., Ishak, K.G., Ross, M.J., 1990. Estrogen induction of hepatocellular carcinomas in Armenian hamsters. Hepatology 11, 570–577.

Coe, J.E., Schell, R.F., Ross, M.J., 1995. Immune response in the hamster: definition of a novel IgG not expressed in all hamster strains. Immunology 86, 141–148.

Coe, J.E., Cieplak, W., Hadlow, W.J., Ross, M.J., 1997. Female protein, amyloidosis, and hormonal carcinogenesis in Turkish hamster: differences from Syrian hamster. Am. J. Physiol. 273, R934–R941.

Coggin Jr., J.H., Thomas, K.V., Huebner, R., 1978. Horizontally transmitted lymphomas of Syrian hamsters. Fed. Proc. (United States) 37, 2086–2088.

Coggin, J.H.J., Bellomy, B.B., Thomas, K.V., Pollock, W.J., 1983. B-cell and T-cell lymphomas and other associated diseases induced by an infectious DNA viroid-like agent in hamsters (Mesocricetus auratus). Am. J. Pathol. 110, 254–266.

Coggin, J.H.J., Hyde, B.M., Heath, L.S., Leinbach, S.S., Fowler, E., Stadtmore, L.S., 1985. Papovavirus in epitheliomas appearing on lymphoma-bearing hamsters: lack of association with horizontally transmitted lymphomas of Syrian hamsters. J. Natl. Cancer Inst. 75, 91–97.

Cohen, B.I., Matoba, N., Mosbach, E.H., McSherry, C.K., 1989. Dietary induction of cholesterol gallstones in hamsters from three different sources. Lipids 24, 151–156.

Cohen, M.M., Shklar, G., Yerganian, G., 1961. Periodontal pathology in a strain of Chinese hamster, Cricetulus griseus, with hereditary diabetes mellitus. Am. J. Med. 31, 864–867.

Committee on Rodents, Institute of Laboratory Animal Resources, 1996. Laboratory Animal Management: Rodents. National Academy Press, Washington, DC.

Compton, S.R., Homberger, F.R., Paturzo, F.X., Clark, J.M., 2004. Efficacy of three microbiological monitoring methods in a ventilated cage rack. Comp. Med. 54, 382–392.

Cooper, D.M., Gebhart, C.J., 1998. Comparative aspects of proliferative enteritis. J. Am. Vet. Med. Assoc. 212, 1446–1451.

Cooper, D.M., Swanson, D.L., Barns, S.M., Gebhart, C.J., 1997a. Comparison of the 16S ribosomal DNA sequences from the intracellular agents of proliferative enteritis in a hamster, deer, and ostrich with the sequence of a porcine isolate of Lawsonia intracellularis. Int. J. Syst. Bacteriol. 47, 635–639.

Cooper, D.M., Swanson, D.L., Gebhart, C.J., 1997b. Diagnosis of proliferative enteritis in frozen and formalin-fixed, paraffin-embedded tissues from a hamster, horse, deer and ostrich using a Lawsonia intracellularis specific multiplex PCR assay. Vet. Microbiol. 54, 47–62.

Cooper, J.E., Knowler, C., Pearson, A.J., 1991. Tumours in Russian hamsters (Phodopus sungorus). Vet. Rec. 128, 335–336.

Cruz, N., Arocho, L., Rosario, L., Crespo, M.J., 2007. Chronic administration of carvedilol improves cardiac function in 6-month-old Syrian cardiomyopathic hamsters. Pharmacology 80, 144–150.

Cunnane, S.C., Bloom, S.R., 1990. Intussusception in the Syrian golden hamster. Br. J. Nutr. 63, 231–237.

Czub, M., Braig, H.R., Diringer, H., 1986. Pathogenesis of scrapie: study of the temporal development of clinical symptoms, of infectivity titers and scrapie-associated fibrils in brains of hamsters infected intraperitoneally. J. Gen. Virol. 67, 2005–2009.

Davis, M.J., Ferrer, P.N., Gore, R.W., 1986. Vascular anatomy and hydrostatic pressure profile in the hamster cheek pouch. Am. J. Physiol. 250, H291–H303.

deArruda, M.S.P., Montenegro, M.R., 1995. The hamster cheek pouch: an immunologically privileged site suitable to the study of granulomatous infections. Rev. Inst. Med. Trop. Sao Paulo 37, 303–309.

de Beer, M.C., de Beer, F.C., Beach, C.M., Gonnerman, W.A., Carreras, I., Sipe, J.D., 1993. Syrian and Armenian hamsters differ in serum amyloid A gene expression. Identification of novel Syrian hamster serum amyloid A subtypes. J. Immunol. 150, 5361–5370.

Decker, R.H., Henderson, L.M., 1959. Hydroxyanthranilic acid as a source of niacin in the diets of the chick, guinea pig and hamster. J. Nutr. 68, 17–24.

Delmas, V., Bastien, C., Scherneck, S., Feunteun, J., 1985. A new member of the polyomavirus family: the hamster papovavirus. Complete nucleotide sequence and transformation properties. EMBO J. 4, 1279–1286.

Desch Jr., C.E., Hurley, R.J., 1997. Demodex sinocricetuli: new species of hair follicle mite (Acari: Demodicidae) from the Chinese form of the striped hamster, Cricetulus barabensis (Rodentia: Muridae). J. Med. Entomol. 34, 317–320.

Doetschman, T., Williams, P., Maeda, N., 1988. Establishment of hamster blastocyst-derived embryonic stem (ES) cells. Dev. Biol. 127, 224–227.

Doi, K., Yamamoto, T., Isegawa, N., Doi, C., Mitsuoka, T., 1987. Age-related non-neoplastic lesions in the heart and kidneys of Syrian hamsters of the APA strain. Lab. Anim. 21, 241–248.

Donnelly, T.M., 1997. Disease problems of small rodents. In: Hillyer, E.V., Quesenberry, K.E. (Eds.), Ferrets, Rabbits, and Rodents: Clinical Medicine and Surgery Saunders, Philadelphia, PA, pp. 307–327.

Ebling, F.J.P., 1994. Photoperiodic differences during development in the dwarf hamsters Phodopus sungorus and Phodopus campbelli. Gen. Comp. Endocrinol. 95, 475–482.

Edwards, H.E., Reburn, C.J., Wynne-Edwards, K.E., 1995. Daily patterns of pituitary prolactin secretion and their role in regulating maternal serum progesterone concentrations across pregnancy in the Djungarian hamster (Phodopus campbelli). Biol. Reprod. 52, 814–823.

Emminger, A., Reznik, G., Reznik-Schuller, H., Mohr, U., 1975. Differences in blood values depending on age in laboratory-bred European hamsters (Cricetus cricetus L.). Lab. Anim. 9, 33–42.

Erb, G.E., Edwards, H.E., Jenkins, K.L., Mucklow, L.C., Wynne-Edwards, K.E., 1993. Induced components in the spontaneous ovulatory cycle of the Djungarian hamster (Phodopus campbelli). Physiol. Behav. 54, 955–959.

Ernst, H., Kunstyr, I., Rittinghausen, S., Mohr, U., 1989. Spontaneous tumours of the European hamster (Cricetus cricetus L.). Z. Versuchstierkd. 32, 87–96.

Escobales, N., Crespo, M.J., 2006. Angiotensin II-dependent vascular alterations in young cardiomyopathic hamsters: role for oxidative stress. Vascul. Pharmacol. 44, 22–28.

Escobales, N., Crespo, M.J., 2008. Early pathophysiological alterations in experimental cardiomyopathy: the Syrian cardiomyopathic hamster. P.R. Health Sci. J. 27, 307–314.

Estes, P.C., Richter, C.B., Franklin, J.A., 1971. Demodectic mange in the golden hamster. Lab. Anim. Sci. 21 (6), 825–828.

Fararh, K.M., Atoji, Y., Shimizu, Y., Takewaki, T., 2002. Isulinotropic properties of nigella sativa oil in streptozotocin plus nicotinamide diabetic hamster. Res. Vet. Sci. 73, 279–282.

Feeney, W.P., 2012. The Chinese or Striped-Back Hamster. In: Suckow, M.A., Stevens, K.A., Wilson, R.P. (Eds.), The Laboratory Rabbit, Guinea Pig, Hamster, and Other Rodents. Academic Press, Boston, pp. 907–922.

Ferm, V.H., 1967. The use of the golden hamster in experimental teratology. Lab. Anim. Care 17, 452–462.

Festing, M., 1972. Hamsters. In: University Federation for Animal Welfare, The UFAW Handbook on the Care and Management of Laboratory Animals Churchill-Livingstone, Edinburgh, pp. 242–256.

Fitzpatrick, L.R., Sakurai, K., Le, T., 1999. Effect of naproxen on the hamster gastric antrum: ulceration, adaptation and efficacy of anti-ulcer drugs. Aliment Pharmacol. Ther. 13, 1553–1562.

Fortner, J.G., 1957. Spontaneous tumors, including gastrointestinal neoplasms and malignant melanomas, in the Syrian hamster. Cancer 10, 1152–1156.

Fox, J.G., 2002. The non-H. pylori helicobacters: their expanding role in gastrointestinal and systemic diseases. Gut. 50, 273–283.

Fox, J.G., Dewhirst, F.E., Paster, B.J., Shames, B., Yan, L.L., Murphy, J.C., 1994. Intracellular Campylobacter-like organism from ferrets and hamsters with proliferative bowel disease is a Desulfovibrio sp. J. Clin. Microbiol. 32, 1229–1237.

Fox, J.G., Newcomer, C.E., Rozmiarek, H., 2002. Selected zoonoses. In: Fox, J.G., Cohen, B.J., Loew, F.M. (Eds.), Laboratory Animal Medicine, second ed. Academic Press, New York, pp. 1060–1098.

Fox, J.G., Shen, Z., Muthupalani, S., Rogers, A.R., Kirchain, S.M., Dewhirst, F.E., 2009. Chronic hepatitis, hepatic dysplasia, fibrosis, and biliary hyperplasia in hamsters naturally infected with a novel Helicobacter classified in the H. bilis cluster. J. Clin. Microbiol. 47, 3673–3681.

Franklin, C.L., Beckwith, C.S., Livingston, R.S., Riley, L.K., Gibson, S.V., Besch-Williford, C.L., et al., 1996. Isolation of a novel Helicobacter species, Helicobacter cholecystus sp. nov., from the gallbladders of Syrian hamsters with cholangiofibrosis and centrilobular pancreatitis. J. Clin. Microbiol. 34, 2952–2958.

Frenkel, J.K., 1956. Effects of hormones on the adrenal necrosis produced by Besnoitia jellisoni in golden hamsters. J. Exp. Med. 103 (3), 375–398.

Frenkel, J.K., 1972. Infection and immunity in hamsters. Prog. Exp. Tumor Res. 16, 326–367.

Friedman, M.H., 1965. "Wet-tail disease" of hamsters. Lab. Anim. Dig. 1, 19.

Frisk, C.S., 1987. Bacterial and mycotic diseases. In: van Hoosier, G.L., McPherson, C.W. (Eds.), Laboratory Hamsters Academic Press, Orlando, FL, pp. 111–133.

Frisk, C.S., 2012. Bacterial and fungal diseases. In: Suckow, M.A., Stevens, K.A., Wilson, R.P. (Eds.), The Laboratory Rabbit, Guinea Pig, Hamster, and Other Rodents, first ed. Academic Press, Waltham, MA, pp. 797–820.

Frisk, C.S., Wagner, J.E., Owens, D.R., 1977. Hamster enteritis: a review. Lab. Anim. 11, 79–85.

Fukuhara, M., Uchida, E., Tajiri, T., Aimoto, T., Naito, Z., Ishiwata, T., 2005. Re-expression of reduced VEGF activity in liver metastases of experimental pancreatic cancer. J. Nippon Med. Sch. 72, 155–164.

Ganaway, J.R., Allen, A.M., Moore, T.D., 1971. Tyzzer's disease. Am. J. Pathol. 64, 717–732.

Gao, M., Zhang, B., Liu, J., Guo, X., Li, H., Wang, T., et al., 2014. Generation of transgenic golden Syrian hamsters. Cell Res. 24, 380–382.

Garlinghouse Jr., L.E., Van Hoosier Jr., G.L., 1978. Studies on adjuvant-induced arthritis, tumor transplantability, and serologic response to bovine serum albumin in Sendai virus infected rats. Am. J. Vet. Res. 39, 297–300.

Gattermann, R., Fritzsche, P., Neumann, K., Al-Hussein, I., Kayser, A., Abiad, M., et al., 2001. Notes on the current distribution and the ecology of wild golden hamsters (Mesocricetus auratus). J. Zool. 254, 359–365.

Gattermann, R., Johnston, R.E., Yigit, N., Fritzsche, P., Larimer, S., Özkurt, S., et al., 2008. Golden hamsters are nocturnal in captivity but diurnal in nature. Biol. Lett. 4, 253–255.

Gebhart, C.J., Fennell, C.L., Murtaugh, M.P., Stamm, W.E., 1989. Campylobacter cinaedi is normal intestinal flora in hamsters. J. Clin. Microbiol. 27, 1692–1694.

Genovesi, E.V., Peters, C.J., 1987. Susceptibility of inbred Syrian golden hamsters (Mesocricetus auratus) to lethal disease by lymphocytic choriomeningitis virus. Exp. Biol. Med. 185, 250–261.

Gerritsen, G.C., Needham, L.B., Schmidt, F.L., Dulin, W.E., 1970. Studies on the prediction and development of diabetes in offspring of diabetic Chinese hamsters. Diabetologia 6, 158–162.

Ghadially, F.N., Illman, O., 1965. Naturally occurring thymomas in the European hamster. J. Pathol. Bacteriol. 90, 465–469.

Gibson, S.V., 1983. Mortality in weanling hamsters associated with tooth loss. Lab. Anim. Sci. 33, 497.

Gibson, S.V., Rottinghaus, M.S., Wagner, J.E., Stills, H.F.J., Stogsdill, P.S., Kinden, D.A., 1990. Naturally acquired enteric adenovirus infection in Syrian hamsters (Mesocricetus auratus). Am. J. Vet. Res. 51, 143–147.

Gimenez-Conti, I.B., Slaga, T.J., 1993. The hamster cheek pouch carcinogenesis model. J. Cell Biochem. Suppl. F 17, 83–90.

Gleiser, C.A., Van Hoosier Jr., G.L., Sheldon, W.G., 1970. A polycystic disease of hamsters in a closed colony. Lab. Anim. Care 20, 923–929.

Goineau, S., Pape, D., Guillo, P., Ramee, M.P., Bellissant, E., 2001. Hemodynamic and histomorphometric characteristics of dilated cardiomyopathy of Syrian hamsters (bio TO-2 strain). Can. J. Physiol. Pharmacol. 79, 329–337.

Goulding, D., Thompson, H., Emerson, J., Fairweather, N.F., Dougan, G., Douce, G.R., 2009. Distinctive profiles of infection and pathology in hamsters infected with *Clostridium difficile* strains 630 and B1. Infect. Immun. 77, 5478–5485.

Graffi, A., Schramm, T., Graffi, I., Bierwolf, D., Bender, E., 1967. Virus-associated skin tumors of the Syrian hamster. J. Natl. Cancer Inst. 40, 867–873.

Graffi, A., Bender, E., Schramm, T., Kuhn, W., Schneiders, F., 1969. Induction of transmissible lymphomas in Syrian hamsters by the application of DNA from viral hamster papovavirus-induced tumors and by cell-free filtrates from human tumors. Med. Sci. 64, 1172–1175.

Graffi, A., Bender, E., Schramm, T., Graffi, I., Bierwolf, D., 1970. Studies on the hamster papilloma and the hamster virus lymphoma. Bibl. Haematol. 36, 293.

Gumma, M.R., South, F.E., Allen, J.N., 1967. Temperature preference in golden hamsters. Anim. Behav. 15, 534–537.

Hamilton, J.B., Montagna, W., 1950. The sebaceous glands of the hamster. I. Morphological effects of androgens on integumentary structures. Am. J. Anat. 86, 191–233.

Hamilton, J.M., Reynolds, T., 1983. Cholangiofibrosis in the Syrian golden hamster. Vet. Rec. 112, 359–360.

Hannoun, C., Guillon, J.C., Chatelain, J., 1974. Natural latent infection of the european hamster ("cricetus cricetus," linne) with a papovavirus. I. Isolation of virus in golden hamster and new-born mice (author's transl)]. Ann. Microbiol. (Paris) 125, 215–226.

Harkness, J.E., 1994. Small rodents. Vet. Clin. North Am. Small Anim. Pract. 21, 89–102.

Harkness, J.E., Wagner, J.E., Kusewitt, D.F., Frisk, C.S., 1977. Weight loss and impaired reproduction in the hamster attributable to an unsuitable feeding apparatus. Lab. Anim. Sci. 27, 117–118.

Harkness, J.E., Turner, P.V., VandeWoude, S., Wagner, J.E., 2010. Harkness and Wagner's Biology and Medicine of Rabbits and Rodents. Williams and Wilkins, Media, Pennsylvania, PA.

Hart, M., O'Conner, E., Davis, M., 2010. Multiple peracute deaths in a colony of Syrian hamster. Lab. Anim. Sci. 40, 325–327.

Hasegawa, T., 1995. A case report of the management of demodicosis in the golden hamster. J. Vet. Med. Sci. 57, 337–338.

Hauzenberger, A.R., Gebhardt-Henrich, S.G., Steiger, A., 2006. The influence of bedding depth on behaviour in golden hamsters (*Mesocricetus auratus*). Appl. Anim. Behav. Sci. 100, 280–294.

Hayes, J.A., Christensen, T.G., Snider, G.L., 1977. The hamster as a model of chronic bronchitis and emphysema in man. Lab. Anim. Sci. 27, 762–770.

Hedqvist, P., Raud, J., Dahlen, S.E., 1990. Microvascular actions of eicosanoids in the hamster cheek pouch. Adv. Prostaglandin Thromboxane Leukot. Res. 20, 153–160.

Heyneman, D., 1961. Studies on helminth immunity. III. Experimental verification of autoinfection from cysticercoids of Hymenolepis nana in the white mouse. J. Infect. Dis. 109, 10–18.

Hixon, M.L., Lewis, A.M.J., Levine, A.S., Chattopadhyay, S.K., 1996. Limited diversity in the major histocompatibility complex class II loci of Syrian hamster DNA. Lab. Anim. Sci. 46, 679–681.

Hjorth, R.N., Bonde, G.M., Pierzchala, W.A., Vernon, S.K., Wiener, F.P., Levner, M.H., et al., 1988. A new hamster model for adenoviral vaccination. Arch. Virol. 100, 279–283.

Hoffman, R.A., Robinson, P.F., Magalhaes, H., 1968. The Golden Hamster: Its Biology and Use in Medical Research. Iowa State Univ. Press, Ames, IA.

Hol, P.R., Snel, F.W., Niewold, T.A., Gruys, E., 1986. Amyloid-enhancing factor (AEF) in the pathogenesis of AA-amyloidosis in the hamster. Virchows Arch. B Cell. Pathol. Incl. Mol. Pathol. 52, 273–281.

Homburger, F., 1968. The Syrian golden hamster in chemical carcinogenesis research. Prog. Exp. Tumor Res. 10, 164–237.

Homburger, F., 1972. Disease models in Syrian hamsters. Prog. Exp. Tumor Res. 16, 69–86.

Homburger, F., 1979. Myopathy of hamster dystrophy: history and morphologic aspects. Ann. N Y Acad. Sci. 317, 2–17.

Homburger, F., 1983. Background data on tumor incidence in control animals (Syrian hamsters). Prog. Exp. Tumor Res. 26, 259–265.

Horiuchi, K., Takatori, A., Inenaga, T., Ohta, E., Ishii, Y., Kyuwa, S., et al., 2005. Histopathological studies of aortic dissection in streptozotocin-induced diabetic APA hamsters. Exp. Anim. 54, 363–367.

Horwitz, B.A., Chau, S.M., Hamilton, J.S., Song, C., Gorgone, J., Saenz, M., et al., 2013. Temporal relationships of blood pressure, heart rate, baroreflex function, and body temperature change over a hibernation bout in Syrian hamsters. Am. J. Physiol-Reg. I 305, R759–R768.

Houchin, O.B., 1943. Toxic levels of morphine for the hamster. Exp. Biol. Med. 54, 339–340.

Hurley, R.J., Desch Jr., C.E., 1994. *Demodex cricetuli*: new species of hair follicle mite (Acari: Demodecidae) from the Armenian hamster, *Cricetulus migratorius* (Rodentia: Cricetidae). J. Med. Entomol. 31, 529–533.

ICTV, 2013. ICTV Master Species List 2013 – International Committee on Taxonomy of Viruses. <http://www.ictvonline.org/virusTaxonomy.asp>.

Ike, F., Bourgade, F., Ohsawa, K., Sato, H., Morikawa, S., Saijo, M., et al., 2007. Lymphocytic choriomeningitis infection undetected by dirty-bedding sentinel monitoring and revealed after embryo transfer of an inbred strain derived from wild mice. Comp. Med. 57, 272–281.

Ikeda, Y., Ross Jr., J., 2000. Models of dilated cardiomyopathy in the mouse and the hamster. Curr. Opin. Cardiol. 15, 197–201.

Innes, J.R.M., Wilson, C., Ross, M.A., 1956. Epizootic *Salmonella enteritidis* infection causing septic pulmonary phlebothrombosis in hamsters. J. Infect. Dis. 98, 133–141.

Institute of Laboratory Animal Resources, 2011. Guide for the Care and Use of Laboratory Animals. National Academy Press, Washington, DC.

Jacoby, R.O., 1978. Transmissible ileal hyperplasia of hamsters. I. Histogenesis and immunocytochemistry. Am. J. Pathol. 91, 433–450.

Jacoby, R.O., Johnson, E.A., 1981. Transmissible ileal hyperplasia. In: Hamster Immune Responses in Infectious and Oncologic Diseases, pp. 267–289.

Jacoby, R.O., Osbaldiston, G.W., Jonas, A.M., 1975. Experimental transmission of atypical ileal hyperplasia of hamsters. Lab. Anim. Sci. 25, 465–473.

Jacoby, R.O., Ball-Goodrich, L.J., Besselsen, D.G., McKisic, M.D., Riley, L.K., Smith, A.L., 1996. Rodent parvovirus infections. Lab. Anim. Sci. 46, 370–380.

Jasni, S., McOrist, S., Lawson, G.H.K., 1994. Experimentally induced proliferative enteritis in hamsters: an ultrastructural study. Res. Vet. Sci. 56, 186–192.

Jay, M.T., Glaser, C., Fulhorst, C.F., 2005. The arenaviruses. J. Am. Vet. Med. Assoc. 227, 904–915.

Jayapal, K.P., Wlaschin, K.F., Hu, W., Yap, M.G., 2007. Recombinant protein therapeutics from CHO cells-20 years and counting. Chem. Eng. Progress 103, 40–47.

Jones, G.F., Ward, G.E., Murtaugh, M.P., Lin, G., Gebhart, C.J., 1993. Enhanced detection of intracellular organism of swine proliferative enteritis, ileal symbiont intracellularis, in feces by polymerase chain reaction. J. Clin. Microbiol. 31, 2611–2615.

Jordan, H.V., van Houte, J., 1972. The hamster as an experimental model for odontopathic infections. Prog. Exp. Tumor Res. 16, 539.

Kajdacsy-Balla, A., Howeedy, A., Bagasra, O., 1993. Experimental model of congenital syphilis. Infect. Immun. 61, 3559–3561.

Kasim-Karakas, S.E., Vriend, H., Almario, R., Chow, L.C., Goodman, M.N., 1996. Effects of dietary carbohydrates on glucose and lipid metabolism in golden Syrian hamsters. J. Lab. Clin. Med. 128, 208–213.

Kaup, F.J., Konstyr, I., Drommer, W., 1990. Characteristics of spontaneous intraperitoneal cysts in golden hamsters and European hamsters. Exp. Pathol. 40, 205–212.

Khallou, J., Riottot, M., Parquet, M., Verneau, C., Lutton, C., 1991. Biodynamics of cholesterol and bile acids in the lithasic hamster. Br. J. Nutr. 66, 479–492.

Kink, J.A., Williams, J.A., 1998. Antibodies to recombinant *Clostridium difficile* toxins A and B are an effective treatment and prevent relapse of *C. difficile-associated* disease in a hamster model of infection. Infect. Immun. 66, 2018–2025.

Kleinerman, J., 1972. Some aspects of pulmonary pathology in the Syrian hamster. Prog. Exp. Tumor Res. 16, 287–299.

Kohn, H.I., Gultman, P.H., 1964. Life span, tumor incidence, and intercapillary glomerulosclerosis in the Chinese hamster (*Cricetulus griseus*) after whole-body and partial-body exposure to X-rays. Radiat. Res. 21, 622–643.

Kokkotou, E., Moss, A.C., Michos, A., Espinoza, D., Cloud, J.W., Mustafa, N., et al., 2008. Comparative efficacies of rifaximin and vancomycin for treatment of Clostridium difficile-associated diarrhea and prevention of disease recurrence in hamsters. Antimicrob. Agents Chemother. 52, 1121–1126.

Kolbasa, K.P., Lancaster, C., Olafsson, A.S., Gilbertson, S.K., Robert, A., 1988. Indomethacin-induced gastric antral ulcers in hamsters. Gastroenterology 95, 932–944.

Konishi, Y., Tsutsumi, M., Tsujiuchi, T., 1998. Mechanistic analysis of pancreatic ductal carcinogensis in hamsters. Pancreas 16, 300–306.

Krasse, B., 1966. Human streptococci and experimental caries in hamsters. Arch. Oral Biol. 11 429–IN14.

Kunstyr, I., Ernst, H., Merkt, M., Reichart, P., 1987. Spontaneous pathology of the European hamster (*Cricetus cricetus*). Malocclusion, dysplastic, and inflammatory processes on the jaws. Z. Versuchstierkd. 29, 171–180.

Lanteigne, M., Reebs, S.G., 2006. Preference for bedding material in Syrian hamsters. Lab. Anim. 40, 410–418.

Lawrie, A.M., Megahy, I.W., 1991. Tumours in Russian hamsters. Vet. Rec. 128, 411–412.

Lawson, G.H.K., Gebhart, C.J., 2000. Proliferative enteropathy. J. Comp. Path. 122, 77–100.

Lepot, A., Banwell, J.G., 1976. The Syrian hamster: a reproducible model for studying changes in intestinal fluid secretion in response to enterotoxin challenge. Infect. Immun. 14, 1167–1171.

Li, J.J., Gonzalez, A., Banerjee, S., Banerjee, S.K., Li, S.A., 1993. Estrogen carcinogenesis in the hamster kidney: role of cytotoxicity and cell proliferation. Environ. Health Perspect. 101 (Suppl. 5), 259–264.

Li, J.J., Li, S.A., 1996. Estrogen carcinogenesis in the hamster kidney: a hormone-driven multistep process. Prog. Clin. Biol. Res. 394, 255–267.

Liehr, J.G., 1997. Hormone-associated cancer: mechanistic similarities between human breast cancer and estrogen-induced kidney carcinogenesis in hamsters. Environ. Health Perspect. 105 (Suppl 3), 565–569.

Lipskaia, L., Pinet, C., Fromes, Y., Hatem, S., Cantaloube, I., Coulombe, A., et al., 2007. Mutation of the delta-sarcoglycan is associated with Ca(2+)-dependent vascular remodeling in the Syrian hamster. Am. J. Pathol. 171, 162–171.

The Clinical Chemistry of Laboratory AnimalsLoeb, W., Quimby, F. (Eds.), 1999., second ed. Taylor and Francis, Philadelphia, PA.

Lowenstein, D.H., Butler, D.A., Westaway, D., McKinley, M.P., DeArmond, S.J., Prusiner, S.B., 1990. Three hamster species with different scrapie incubation times and neuropathological features encode distinct prion proteins. Mol. Cell Biol. 10, 1153–1163.

Lussier, G., Pavilanis, V., 1969. Presence of intranuclear inclusion bodies in proliferative ileitis of the hamster (*Mesocricetus auratus*). A preliminary report. Lab. Anim. Care 19, 387.

Lyman, C.P., 1979. Usefulness of the hamster in the study of hibernation. In: Altman, P.L. Dittman Katz, D. (Eds.), Inbred and Genetically Defined Strains of Laboratory Animals, Vol 2 Fed. Am. Soc. Exp. Biol., Bethesda, Maryland, pp. 431.

Lyman, C.P., 1982. Sensitivity to arousal. In: Lyman, C.P. (Ed.), Hibernation and Torpor in Mammals and Birds Academic Press, New York, pp. 77–91.

Maatthiesen, T., Kunstyr, I., Tuch, K., 1976. Hexamita-muris infection in mice and European hamsters in a laboratory animal colony. Z. Versuchstierkd. 18, 113–120.

Macnish, M.G., Morgan, U.M., Behnke, J.M., Thompson, R.C.A., 2002. Failure to infect laboratory rodent hosts with human isolates of *Rodentolepis* (= *Hymenolepis*) *nana*. J. Helminthol. 76, 37–43.

Macnish, M.G., Ryan, U.M., Behnke, J.M., Thompson, R.C.A., 2003. Detection of the rodent tapeworm *Rodentolepis* (= *Hymenolepis*) *microstoma* in humans. A new zoonosis? Int. J. Parasitol. 33, 1079–1085.

Magalhaes, H., 1968. Gross anatomy. In: Hoffman, R.A., Robinson, P.F., Magalhaes, H. (Eds.), The Golden Hamster – Its Biology and Use in Medical Research Iowa State University Press, Ames, IA, pp. 91–109.

Magaribuchi, T., Koshimizu, K., Fujiwara, K., 1977. An outbreak of "wet tail" in hamsters due to the Tyzzer's organism. Exp. Anim. 26, 123–129.

Manci, E.A., Heath, L.S., Leinbach, S.S., Coggin Jr., J.H., 1984. Lymphoma-associated ulcerative bowel disease in the hamster (*Mesocricetus auratus*) induced by an unusual agent. Am. J. Pathol. 116, 1–8.

Marsh, R.F., Hanson, R.P., 1978. The Syrian hamster as a model for the study of slow virus diseases caused by unconventional agents. Fed. Proc. Fed. Am. Soc. Exp. Biol. 37, 2076–2078.

Masiello, P., Broca, C., Gross, R., Roye, M., Manteghetti, M., Hillaire-Buys, D., et al., 1998. Experimental NIDDM: development of a new model in adult rats administered streptozotocin and nicotinamide. Diabetes 47, 224–229.

Masson-Pevet, M., Naimi, F., Canguilhem, B., Saboureau, M., Bonn, D., Pevet, P., 1994. Are the annual reproductive and body weight rhythms in the male European hamster (*Cricetus cricetus*) dependent upon a photoperiodically entrained circannual clock? J. Pineal Res. 17, 151–163.

Matsumoto, T., Nagata, I., Kariya, Y., Ohaski, K., 1954. Studies on a strain of pneumotropic virus of hamster. Nagoya J. Med. Sci. 17, 93–97.

Maxwell, K.O., Wish, C., Murphy, J.C., Fox, J.G., 1985. Serum chemistry reference values in two strains of Syrian hamsters. Lab. Anim. Sci. 35, 67–70.

McElroy, A.K., Smith, J.M., Hooper, J.W., Schmaljohn, C.S., 2004. Andes virus M genome segment is not sufficient to confer the virulence associated with andes virus in Syrian hamsters. Virology 326, 130–139.

McGuire, J., 1993. *Phodopus sungorus* (Russian dwarf hamsters). <http://netvet.wustl.edu>.

McMartin, D.N., 1977. Spontaneous atrial thrombosis in aged Syrian hamsters. I. Incidence and pathology. Thromb. Haemost. 38, 447–456.

McMartin, D.N., Dodds, W.J., 1982. Animal model of human disease: atrial thrombosis in aged Syrian hamsters. Am. J. Pathol. 107, 277.

Mcmillan, H.J., Wynne-Edwards, K.E., 1998. Evolutionary change in the endocrinology of behavioral receptivity: divergent roles for progesterone and prolactin within the genus *Phodopus*. Biol. Reprod. 59, 30–38.

McOrist, S., Lawson, G.H.K., 1987. Possible relationship of proliferative enteritis in pigs and hamsters. Vet. Microbiol. 15, 293–302.

Meier, H., Yerganian, G., 1959. Spontaneous hereditary diabetes mellitus in Chinese hamster (*Cricetulus griseus*). I. pathological findings. Proc. Soc. Exp. Biol. Med. 100, 810–815.

Meier, H., Yerganian, G., 1961. Spontaneous diabetes mellitus in the Chinese hamster (*Cricetulus griseus*). III. Maintenance of a diabetic hamster colony with the aid of hypoglycemic therapy. Diabetes 10, 19–21.

Meredith, A., 2006. Skin diseases and treatment of hamsters. In: Paterson, S. (Ed.), Skin Diseases of Exotic Pets Blackwell Science Ltd, Oxford, pp. 251–263.

Milazzo, M.L., Eyzaguirre, E.J., Molina, C.P., Fulhorst, C.F., 2002. Maporal viral infection in the Syrian golden hamster: a model of hantavirus pulmonary syndrome. J. Infect. Dis. 186, 1390–1395.

Militzer, K., Herberg, L., Buttner, D., 1990. The ontogenesis of skin and organ characteristics in the Syrian golden hamster. II. Body and organ weights as well as blood glucose and plasma levels. Exp. Pathol. 40, 139–153.

Mitchell, P.L., McLeod, R.S., 2008. Conjugated linoleic acid and atherosclerosis: studies in animal models. Biochem. Cell Biol. 86, 293–301.

Mohr, U., Schuller, H., Reznik, G., Althoff, J., Page, N., 1973. Breeding of European hamsters. Lab. Anim. Sci. 23, 799–802.

Moore, G.J., 1990. Giardia and Trichomonas infections in Syrian hamsters: efficacy of dimetridazole therapy and containment of infection. Anim. Tech. 41, 133–136.

Moore Jr., W., 1965. Observations on the breeding and care of the Chinese hamster, Cricetulus griseus. Lab. Anim. Care 15, 95–101.

Moore Jr., W., 1966. Hemogram of the Chinese hamster. Am. J. Vet. Res. 27, 608–610.

Motzel, S.L., Gibson, S.V., 1990. Tyzzer disease in hamsters and gerbils from a pet store supplier. J. Am. Vet. Med. Assoc. 197, 1176–1178.

Mulder, G., 2012. Anatomy, physiology, and behavior. In: Suckow, M.A., Stevens, K.A., Wilson, R.P. (Eds.), The Laboratory Rabbit, Guinea Pig, Hamster, and Other Rodents, first ed. Academic Press, Waltham, MA, pp. 765–777. (2012).

Murphy, J.C., Fox, J.G., Niemi, S.M., 1984. Nephrotic syndrome associated with renal amyloidosis in a colony of Syrian hamsters. J. Am. Vet. Med. Assoc. 185, 1359–1362.

Murphy, M.R., Schneider, G.E., 1970. Olfactory bulb removal eliminates mating behavior in the male golden hamster. Science 167, 302–304.

Murray, K., 2012. Anatomy, physiology, and behavior. In: Suckow, M.A., Stevens, K.A., Wilson, R.P. (Eds.), The Laboratory Rabbit, Guinea Pig, Hamster, and Other Rodents, first ed. Academic Press, Waltham, MA, pp. 753–765.

Nakayama, M., Saegusa, J., Itoh, K., Kiuchi, Y., Tamura, T., Ueda, K., et al., 1975. Transmissible enterocolitis in hamsters caused by Tyzzer's organism. Jpn. J. Exp. Med. 45, 33–41.

Nakayama, M., Machii, K., Goto, Y., Fujiwara, K., 1976. Typhlohepatitis in hamsters infected perorally with the Tyzzer's organism. Jpn. J. Exp. Med. 46, 309–324.

National Research Council, 1995. Nutritional Requirements of Laboratory Animals, fourth ed. National Academy Press, Washington, DC.

Newberne, P.M., Fox, J.G., 1980. Nutritional adequacy and quality control of rodent diets. Lab. Anim. Sci. 30, 352–365.

Newberne, P.M., McConnell, R.G., 1979. Nutrition of the Syrian golden hamster. Prog. Exp. Tumor Res. 24, 127–138.

Newkirk, K.D., Mcmillan, H.J., Wynne-Edwards, K.E., 1997. Length of delay to birth of a second litter in dwarf hamsters (*Phodopus*): evidence for post-implantation embryonic diapause. J. Exp. Zool. 278, 106–114.

Nicklas, W., Kraft, V., Meyer, B., 1993. Contamination of transplantable tumors, cell lines, and monoclonal antibodies with rodent viruses. Lab. Anim. Sci. 43, 296–300.

Niewold, T.A., Hol, P.R., van Andel, A.C., Lutz, E.T., Gruys, E., 1987. Enhancement of amyloid induction by amyloid fibril fragments in hamster. Lab. Invest. 56, 544–549.

Nutting, W.B., 1961. *Demodex aurati* sp. nov. and *D. criceti*, ectoparasites of the golden hamster (*Mesocricetus auratus*). Parasitology 51, 515–522.

Oka, M.S., Rupp, R.G., 1990. Large-scale animal cell culture: a biological perspective. Bioprocess Tech. 10, 71–92.

Oldstone, M.B., Dixon, F.J., 1969. Pathogenesis of chronic disease associated with persistentlymphocytic choriomeningitis viral infection I. Relationship of antibody production to disease in neonatally infected mice. J. Exp. Med. 131, 1–19.

Oreffo, V.I., Lin, H.W., Padmanabhan, R., Witschi, H., 1993. K-ras and p53 point mutations in 4-(methylnitrosamino)-1-(3-pyridyl)-1-butanone-induced hamster lungg tumo. Carcinogenesis 14, 451–455.

Ostlind, D.A., Mickle, W.G., Smith, S.K., Cifelli, S., Ewanciw, D.V., 2004. The *Hymenolepis diminuta*-golden hamster (*Mesocricetus auratus*) model for the evaluation of gastrointestinal anticestode activity. J. Parasitol. 90, 898–899.

Paciello, O., Wojcik, S., Gradoni, L., Oliva, G., Trapani, F., Lovane, V., et al., 2010. Syrian hamster infected with *Leishmania infantum*: a new experimental model for inflammatory myopathies. Muscle Nerve. 41, 355–361.

Parker, J.C., Richter, C.B., 1982. Viral diseases of the respiratory system. In: Foster, H.L., Small, J.D., Fox, J.G. (Eds.), The Biology of the Laboratory Mouse Academic Press, New York, pp. 107–155.

Parker, J.C., Igel, H.J., Reynolds, R.K., Lewis, A.M.J., Rowe, W.P., 1976. Lymphocytic choriomeningitis virus infection in fetal, newborn, and young adult Syrian hamsters. Infect. Immun. 13, 967–981.

Patterson, M.M., Schrenzel, M.D., Feng, Y., Fox, J.G., 2000a. Gastritis and intestinal metaplasia in Syrian hamsters infected with *Helicobacter aurati* and two other microaerobes. Vet. Pathol. 37, 589–596.

Patterson, M.M., Schrenzel, M.D., Feng, Y., Xu, S., Dewhirst, F.E., Paster, B.J., et al., 2000b. *Helicobacter aurati* sp. nov., a urease-positive *Helicobacter* species cultured from gastrointestinal tissues of Syrian hamsters. J. Clin. Microbiol. 38, 3722–3728.

Pavesio, C.E., Chiappino, M.L., Gormley, P., Setzer, P.Y., Nichols, B.A., 1995. Acquired retinochoroiditis in hamsters inoculated with ME 49 strain toxoplasma. Invest. Ophthalmol. Vis. Sci. 36, 2166–2175.

Percy, D.H., 1987. Zoonoses in laboratory animals. Can. Vet. J. 28, 268–269.

Percy, D.H., Palmer, D.J., 1997. Pathogenesis of Sendai virus infection in the Syrian hamster. Lab. Anim. Sci. 47, 132–137.

Percy, D.H., Barthold, S.W., 2007. Hamster. In: Percy, D.H., Barthold, S.W. (Eds.), Pathology of Laboratory Rodents and Rabbits, third ed. Blackwell, Ames, Iowa, pp. 179–204.

Pevet, P., 1988. The role of the pineal gland in the photoperiodic control of reproduction in different hamster species. Reprod. Nutr. Dev. 28, 443–458.

Phares, C.K., 1980. Streptozotocin-induced diabetes in Syrian hamsters: new model of diabetes mellitus. Experientia 36, 681–682.

Pinto, R.M., Goncalves, L., Gomes, DC., Noronha, D., 2001. Helminth fauna of the golden hamster Mesocricetus auratus in Brazil. Contemp. Top. Lab. Anim. Sci. 40, 21–26.

Poel, W.E., Yerganian, G., 1961. Adenocarcinoma of the pancreas in diabetes-prone Chinese hamsters. Am. J. Med. 31, 861–863.

Pogosianz, H.E., 1975. Djungarian hamster—a suitable tool for cancer research and cytogenetic studies. J. Natl. Cancer Inst. 54, 659–664.

Pogosianz, H.E., Sokova, O.I., 1982. Tumours of the Dungarian hamster. IARC Sci. Publ. 34, 451–455.

Pour, P., Kmoch, N., Greiser, E., Mohr, U., Althoff, J., Cardesa, A., 1976a. Spontaneous tumors and common diseases in two colonies of Syrian hamsters. I. Incidence and sites. J. Natl. Cancer Inst. 56, 931–935.

Pour, P., Mohr, U., Althoff, J., Cardesa, A., Kmoch, N., 1976b. Spontaneous tumors and common diseases in two colonies of Syrian hamsters. II. Respiratory tract and digestive system. J. Natl. Cancer Inst. 56, 937–948.

Pour, P., Mohr, U., Althoff, J., Cardesa, A., Kmoch, N., 1976c. Spontaneous tumors and common diseases in two colonies of Syrian hamsters. III. Urogenital system and endocrine glands. J. Natl. Cancer Inst. 56, 949–961.

Pritchett, K.R., 2007. Helminth parasites of laboratory mice. In: Fox, J.G., Barthold, S.W., Davisson, M.T., Newcomber, C.E., Quimby, F.W., Smith, A.L. (Eds.), The Mouse in Biomedical Research, vol. Diseases, second ed. Academic Press, New York, pp. 551–564.

Pritchett, K.R., Johnston, N.A., 2002. A review of treatments for the eradication of pinworm infections from laboratory rodent colonies. Contemp. Top. Lab. Anim. Sci. 41, 36–46.

Profeta, M.L., Lief, F.S., Plotkin, S.A., 1969. Enzootic Sendai infection in laboratory hamsters. Am. J. Epidemiol. 89, 316–324.

Prokoph, H., Arnold, W., Schwartz, A., Scherneck, S., 1996. In vivo replication of hamster polyomavirus DNA displays lymphotropism in hamsters susceptible to lymphoma induction. J. Gen. Virol. 77, 2165–2172.

Prusiner, S.B., 1991. Molecular biology and transgenetics of prion diseases. Crit. Rev. Biochem. Mol. Biol. 26, 397–438.

Puchalski, W., Heldmaier, G., 1986. Seasonal changes of heart weight and erythrocytes in the Djungarian hamster, Phodopus sungorus. Comp. Biochem. Physiol. A 84, 259–263.

Reasner, D.S., Johnston, R.E., 1988. Acceleration of reproductive development in female Djungarian hamsters by adult males. Physiol. Behav. 43, 57–64.

Rehg, J.E., Lu, Y.S., 1982. Clostridium difficile typhlitis in hamsters not associated with antibiotic therapy. J. Am. Vet. Med. Assoc. 181, 1422–1423.

Renshaw, H.W., Van Hoosier Jr., G.L., Amend, N.K., 1975. A survey of naturally occurring diseases of the Syrian hamster. Lab. Anim. 9, 179–191.

Reznik, G., Jensen, K.A., 1979. Anatomy of the nasal cavity of the European hamster (Cricetus cricetus). Z. Versuchstierkd. 21, 321–340.

Reznik, G., Reznik-Schuller, H., Mohr, U., 1973. Comparative studies of organs in the European hamster (Cricetus cricetus L.), the Syrian golden hamster (Mesocricetus auratus W.), and the Chinese hamster (Cricetulus griseus M.). Z. Versuchstierkd. Bd. 15, S272–S282.

Reznik, G., Reznik-Schuller, H., Schostek, H., Deppe, K., Mohr, U., 1975. Comparative studies concerning the suitability of European hamsters and Syrian golden hamsters for investigations on smoke exposure. Arzneimittelforschung 25, 923–926.

Reznik, G., Reznik-Schuller, H., Emminger, A., Mohr, U., 1979. Comparative studies of blood from hibernating and nonhibernating European hamsters (Cricetus cricetus L.). Lab. Anim. Sci. 25, 210–215.

Reznik-Schuller, H., Reznik, G., Mohr, U., 1974. The European hamster (Cricetus cricetus L.) as an experimental animal: breeding methods and observations of their behaviour in the laboratory. Z. Versuchstierkd. 16, S48–S58.

Richards, M.P.M., 1966. Maternal behaviour in the golden hamster: responsiveness to young in virgin, pregnant, and lactating females. Anim. Behav. 14, 310–313.

Richards, M.P.M., 1969. Effects of oestrogen and progesterone on nest building in the golden hamster. Anim. Behav. 17, 356–361.

Richter, C.B., 1986. Mouse adenovirus, K virus, pneumonia virus of mice. In: Bhatt, P.N., Jacoby, R.O., Morse, I.H.C. (Eds.), Viral and Mycoplasmal Infections of Laboratory Rodents Academic Press, New York, pp. 137–192.

Roberts, A., Vogel, L., Guarner, J., Hayes, N., Murphy, B., Zaki, S., et al., 2005. Severe acute respiratory syndrome coronavirus infection of golden Syrian hamsters. J. Virol. 79, 503–511.

Rollison, D.E., Page, W.F., Crawford, H., Gridley, G., Wacholder, S., Martin, J., et al., 2004. Case control study of cancer among US army veterans exposed to simian virus 40-contaminated adenovirus vaccine. Am. J. Epidemiol. 160, 317–324.

Romanenko, S.A., Volobouev, V.T., Perelman, P.L., Lebedev, V.S., Serdukova, N.A., Trifonov, V.A., et al., 2007. Karyotype evolution and phylogenetic relationships of hamsters (Cricetidae, Muroidea, Rodentia) inferred from chromosomal painting and banding comparison. Chromosome Res. 15, 283–298.

Ronald, N.C., Wagner, J.E., 1975. Treatment of Hymenolepis nana in hamsters with yomesan (niclosamide). Lab. Anim. Sci. 25, 219–220.

Ross, C.R., Wagner, J.E., Wrightman, S.R., Dill, S.E., 1980. Experimental transmission of Syphacia muris among rats, mice, hamsters, and gerbils. Lab. Anim. Sci. 30, 35–37.

Ross, P.D., 1998. Phodopus sungorus. Am. Soc. Mammol., 1–9. (Mammalian Species No. 595). Available at: https://kataloge.thulb.uni-jena.de/DB=1/LNG=EN/CLK?IKT=12&TRM=636891429

Rowell, T.E., 1960. Retrieving and other behavior in lactating golden hamsters. Proc. Zool. Soc. 135, 265–282.

Ryden, E.B., Lipman, N.S., Taylor, N.S., Rose, R., Fox, J.G., 1991. Clostridium difficile typhlitis associated with cecal mucosal hyperplasia in Syrian hamsters. Lab. Anim. Sci. 41, 553–558.

Ryoke, T., Gu, Y., Mao, L., Hongo, M., Clark, R.G., Peterson, K.L., et al., 1999. Progressive cardiac dysfunction and fibrosis in the cardiomyopathic hamster and effects of growth hormone and angiotensin-converting enzyme inhibition. Circulation 100, 1734–1743.

Sakamoto, A., Ono, K., Abe, M., Jasmin, G., Eki, T., Murakami, Y., et al., 1997. Both hypertrophic and dilated cardiomyopathies are caused by mutation of the same gene, delta-sarcoglycan, in hamster: an animal model of disrupted dystrophin-associated glycoprotein complex. Proc. Natl. Acad. Sci. USA 94, 13873–13878.

Sakanashi, T., Sako, S., Nozuhara, A., Adachi, K., Okamoto, T., Koga, Y., et al., 1991. Vitamin E deficiency has a pathological role in myocytolysis in cardiomyopathic Syrian hamster (BIO 14.6). Biochem. Biophys. Res. Commun. 181, 145–150.

Sato, T., Komeda, K., Shirama, K., 1984. Plasma progesterone concentrations during the estrous cycle, pregnancy, and lactation in the Chinese hamster, Cricetulus griseus. Jikken Dobutsu 33, 501–508.

Sawrey, D.K., Baumgardner, D.J., Campa, M.J., Ferguson, B., Hodges, A.W., Dewsbury, D.A., 1984. Behavioral patterns of Djungarian hamsters: an adaptive profile. Anim. Learn. Behav. 12, 297–306.

Scherneck, S., Feunteun, J., 1990. The hamster polyomavirus—a brief review of recent knowledge. Arch. Geschwulstforsch. 60, 271–278.

Schlenker, E.H., 1985. Ventilation and metabolism of the Djungarian hamster (Phodopus sungorus) and the albino mouse. Comp. Biochem. Physiol. A 82, 293–295.

Sebesteny, A., 1969. Pathogenicity of intestinal flagellates in mice. Lab. Anim. 3, 71–77.

Shklar, G., 1972. Experimental oral pathology in the Syrian hamster. Prog. Exp. Tumor Res. 16, 518.

Sichuk, G., Bettigole, R.E., Der, B.K., Fortner, J.G., 1965. Influence of sex hormones on thrombosis of left atrium in Syrian (golden) hamsters. Am. J. Physiol. 208, 465–470.

Silberberg, R., Gerritsen, G.C., 1976. Aging changes in intervertebral discs and spondylosis in Chinese hamsters. Diabetes 25, 477–483.

Silverman, J., Chavannes, J.M., 1977. Biological values of the European hamster (Cricetus cricetus). Lab. Anim. Sci. 27, 641–645.

Simionescu, N., Sima, A., Dobrian, A., Tirziu, D., Simionescu, M., 1993. Pathobiochemical changes of the arterial wall at the inception of atherosclerosis. Curr. Top. Pathol. 87, 1–45.

Simmons, J.H., Riley, L.K., Besch-Williford, C.L., Franklin, C.L., 2000. Helicobacter mesocricetorum sp. nov., a novel Helicobacter isolated from the feces of Syrian hamsters. J. Clin. Microbiol. 38, 1811–1817.

Simmons, J.H., Riley, L.K., Franklin, C.L., Besch-Williford, C.L., 2001. Hamster polyomavirus infection in a pet Syrian hamster (Mesocricetus auratus). Vet. Path. 38, 441–446.

Skinner, H.H., Knight, E.H., 1979. The potential role of Syrian hamsters and other small animals as reservoirs of lymphocytic choriomeningitis virus. J. Small Anim. Pract. 20, 145–161.

Slater, G.M., 1972. The care and feeding of the Syrian hamster. Prog. Exp. Tumor. Res. 16, 42–49.

Soave, O.A., 1963. Diagnosis and control of common diseases of hamsters, rabbits, and monkeys. J. Am. Vet. Med. Assoc. 142, 285–290.

Soskel, N.T., Watanabe, S., Sandberg, L.B., 1984. Mechanisms of lung injury in the copper-deficient hamster model of emphysema. CHEST 85 (Suppl. 6), 70S–73S.

Spikermann, V.A.R., Althoff, J., 1980. The fine structure of the exocrine pancreas of the European hamster (Cricetus cricetus L.): electron microscopic investigations. Z. Versuchstierkd. 22, 36–42.

Sroller, V., Vilchez, R.A., Stweart, A.R., Wong, C., Butel, J.S., 2008. Influence of the viral regulatory region on tumor induction by simian virus 40 in hamsters. J. Virol. 82, 871–879.

Stills Jr., H.F., 1991. Isolation of an intracellular bacterium from hamsters (Mesocricetus auratus) with proliferative ileitis and reproduction of the disease with a pure culture. Infect. Immun. 59, 3227–3236.

Storey, K.B., 2010. Out cold: biochemical regulation of mammalian hibernation – a mini-review. Gerontology 56, 220–230.

Streilein, J.W., 1978. Hamster immune responses: experimental models linking immunogenetics, oncogensis, and viral immunity. Fed. Proc. Fed. Am. Soc. Exp. Biol. 37, 2023–2108.

Streilein, J.W., Duncan, W.R., Homburger, F., 1980. Immunogenetic relationships among genetically defined, inbred domestic Syrian hamster strains. Transplantation 30, 358–361.

Suckow, M.A., Stevens, K.A., Wilson, R.P., 2012. The Laboratory Rabbit, Guinea Pig, Hamster, and Other Rodents, first ed. Academic Press, Waltham, MA.

Sunday, M.E., Willett, C.G., Graham, S.A., Oreffo, V.I., Linnoila, R.I., Witschi, H., 1995. Histochemical characterization of non-neuroendocrine lung tumors and neuroendocrine cell hyperplasia induced hamster lung by 4-(methylnitrosamino)-1-(3-pyridyl)-1-butanone with or without hyperoxia. Am. J. Pathol. 147, 740–752.

Suzuki, E., Matsubara, J., Saito, M., Muto, T., Nakagawa, M., Imaizumi, K., 1982. Serological survey of laboratory rodents for infection with Sendai virus, mouse hepatitis virus, reovirus type 3, and mouse adenovirus. Jpn. J. Med. Sci. Biol. 35, 249–254.

Svensjo, E., 1990. The hamster cheek pouch as a model in microcirculation research. Eur. Respir. J. Suppl. 12, 595s–600s.

Tagaya, M., Morie, M.I., Miyadai, T., et al., 1995. Efficacy of temperature-sensitive Sendai virus vaccine in hamsters. Lab. Anim. Sci. 45, 233–238.

Tanaka, A., Hisanaga, A., Ishinishi, N., 1991. The frequency of spontaneously-occurring neoplasms in the male Syrian golden hamster. Vet. Hum.Toxicol. 33, 318–321.

Tani, K., Iwanaga, T., Sonoda, K., Hayashiya, S., Hayashiya, M., Taura, Y., 2001. Ivermectin treatment of demodicosis in 56 hamsters. J. Vet. Med. Sci. 63, 1245–1247.

Tansey, G., Roy, A.F., Bivin, W.S., 1995. Acute pneumonia in a Syrian hamster: isolation of a Corynebacterium species. Lab. Anim. Sci. 45, 366–367.

Taylor, D.M., Farquhar, C.F., Neal, D.L., 1993. Studies on the eradication of intestinal protozoa of Syrian hamsters in quarantine and their transfaunation to mice. Lab. Anim. Sci. 43, 359–360.

Tennent, G.A., Baltz, M.L., Osborn, G.D., Butler, P.J., Noble, G.E., Hawkins, P.N., et al., 1993. Studies of the structure and binding properties of hamster female protein. Immunology 80, 645–651.

Thomas, M.A., Spencer, J.F., La Regina, M.C., Dhar, D., Tollefson, A.E., Toth, K., et al., 2006. Syrian hamster as a permissive immunocompetent animal model for the study of oncolytic adenovirus vectors. Cancer Res. 66, 1270–1276.

Thompson, R., 1971. The water consumption and drinking habits of a few species and strains of laboratory animals. J. Inst. Anim. Tech. 22, 29–36.

Trautwein, E.A., Siddiqui, A., Hayes, K.C., 1999. Characterization of the bile acid profile in developing male and female hamsters in response to dietary cholesterol challenge. Comp. Biochem. Physiol. A Mol. Integr. Physiol. 124, 93–103.

Trevitt, C.R., Collinge, J., 2006. A systematic review of prion therapeutics in experimental models. Brain 129, 2241–2265.

Tseng, L.F., Ostwald, T.J., Loh, H.H., Li, C.H., 1979. Behavioral activities of opioid peptides and morphine sulfate in golden hamsters and rats. Psychopharmacology 64, 215–218.

Uchida, E., Matsushita, A., Yanagi, K., Hiroi, M., Aimoto, T., Nakamura, Y., et al., 2008. Experimental pancreatic cancer model using PGHAM-1 cells: characteristics and experimental therapeutic trials. J. Nippon Med. Sch. 75, 325–331.

Unay, E.S., Davis, B.J., 1980. Treatment of Syphacia obvelata in the Syrian hamster (Mesocricetus auratus) with piperazine citrate. Am. J. Vet. Res. 41, 1899–1900.

United States Department of Agriculture, 2010. Animal Care Annual Report of Activities. United States Department of Agriculture, Animal and Plant Heath Inspection Service. Available at: <http://www.aphis.usda.gov/animal_welfare/efoia/downloads/2010_Animals_Used_In_Research.pdf>.

Vairaktaris, E., Papageorgiou, G., Derka, S., Moulavassili, P., Nkenke, E., Kessler, P., et al., 2007. Expression of ets-1 is not affected by N-ras or H-ras during ral oncogenesis. J. Cancer Res. Clin. Oncol. 133, 227–233.

Vairaktaris, E., Papakosta, V., Derka, S., Vassiliou, S., Nkenke, E., Spyridonidou, S., et al., 2008a. H-ras and c-fos exhibit similar expression patterns during most stages of oral oncogenesis. In Vivo 22, 621–628.

Vairaktaris, E., Spyridonidou, S., Papakosta, V., Vyllliotis, A., Lazaris, A., Perrea, D., et al., 2008b. The hamster model of sequential oral oncogenesis. Oral Oncol. 44, 315–324.

Valentine, H., Daugherity, E.K., Singh, B., Maurer, K.J., 2012. Anatomy, physiology, and behavior. In: Suckow, M.A., Stevens, K.A., Wilson, R.P. (Eds.), The Laboratory Rabbit, Guinea Pig, Hamster, and Other Rodents, first ed. Academic Press, Waltham, MA, pp. 875–906. 2012.

Van Heek, M., Austin, T.M., Faarley, C., Cook, J.A., Tetzloff, G.G., Davis, H.R., 2001. Ezetimibe, a potent cholesterol absorption inhibitor, normalizes combined dyslipidemia in obese hyperinsulinemic hamsters. Diabetes 50, 1330–1335.

Van Hoosier Jr., G.L., Trentin, J.J., 1979. Naturally occurring tumors of the Syrian hamster. Prog. Exp. Tumor Res. 23, 1–12.

Verdino, P., Witherden, D.A., Podshivalova, K., Rieder, S.E., Havran, W.L., et al., 2011. cDNA Sequence and Fab Crystal Structure of HL4E10, a Hamster IgG Lambda Light Chain Antibody Stimulatory for γδ T Cells. PLoS One 6 (5), e19828. http://dx.doi.org/10.1371/journal.pone.0019828

Viswanathan, N., Davis, F.C., 1992. Timing of birth in Syrian hamsters. Biol. Reprod. 47, 6–10.

Waggie, K.S., Thornburg, L.P., Grove, K.J., Wagner, J.E., 1987. Lesions of experimentally induced Tyzzer's disease in Syrian hamsters, guinea pigs, mice, and rats. Lab. Anim. 21, 155–160.

Wagner, J.E., Doyle, R.E., Ronald, N.C., Garrison, R.G., Schmitz, J.A., 1974. Hexamitiasis in laboratory mice, hamsters, and rats. Lab. Anim. Sci. 24, 349–354.

Wahl-Jensen, V., Chapman, J., Asher, L., Fisher, R., Zimmerman, M., Larsen, T., et al., 2007. Temporal analysis of andes virus and sin nombre virus infections of Syrian hamsters. J. Virol. 81, 7449–7462.

Ward, B.C., Moore Jr., W., 1969. Spontaneous lesions in a colony of Chinese hamsters. Lab. Anim. Care 19, 516–521.

Warner, R.G., Ehle, F.R., 1976. Nutritional idiosyncrasies of the golden hamster (Mesocricetus auratus). Lab. Anim. Sci. 26, 670–673.

Watson, J.M., 1946. Helminths infective to man in the Syrian hamster. Brit. Med. J. 2, 578.

Whary, M.T., Fox, J.G., 2004. Natural and experimental Helicobacter infections. Comp. Med. 54, 128–158.

Wightman, S.R., Pilitt, P.A., Wagner, J.E., 1978. *Dentostomella translucida* in the Mongolian gerbil (*Meriones unguiculatus*). Lab. Anim. Sci. 28, 290–296.

Wissler, R.W., 1991. Update on the pathogenesis of atherosclerosis. Am. J. Med. 91, 3S–9S.

Wollnik, F., Schmidt, B., 1995. Seasonal and daily rhythms of body temperature in the European hamster (*Cricetus cricetus*) under semi-natural conditions. J. Comp. Physiol. B 165, 171–182.

Wozniak, E.J., Lowenstine, L.J., Hemmer, R., Robinson, T., Conrad, P.A., 1996. Comparative pathogenesis of human WA1 and babesia microti isolates in a Syrian hamster model. Lab. Anim. Sci. 46, 507–515.

Wynne-Edwards, K.E., Lisk, R.D., 1984. Djungarian hamsters fail to conceive in the presence of multiple males. Anim. Behav. 32, 626–628.

Wynne-Edwards, K.E., Lisk, R.D., 1987. Male–female interactions across the female estrous cycle: a comparison of two species of dwarf hamster (*Phodopus campbelli* and *Phodopus sungorus*). J. Comp. Psychol. 101, 335–344.

Xu, R., Yokoyama, W.H., Irving, D., Rein, D., Walzem, R.L., German, J.B., 1998. Effect of dietary catechin and vitamin E on aortic fatty streak accumulation in hypercholesterolemic hamsters. Atherosclerosis 137, 29–36.

Yanagimachi, R., Yanagimachi, H., Rogers, B.J., 1976. The use of the zona-free animal ova as a test-system for the assessment of the fertilizing capacity of human spermatozoa. Biol. Reprod. 15, 471–476.

Yerganian, G., 1958. The striped-back or Chinese hamster. J. Natl. Cancer Inst. 20, 705–727.

Yerganian, G., 1965. Spontaneous diabetes mellitus in the Chinese hamster, Cricetulus griseus. Int. Cong. Ser. Excerpta Med. 84, 612–627.

Yerganian, G., 1985. The biology and genetics of the Chinese hamster. In: Gottesman, M. (Ed.), Molecular Cell Genetics Wiley, New York, pp. 3–36.

Yerganian, G., Klein, E., Roy, A., 1955. Physiological studies on Chinese hamster, *Cricetulus griseus*. II. A method for study of bleeding time in hamsters. Fed. Proc. Fed. Am. Soc. Exp. Biol. 14, 424.

Yoon, C.H., Peterson, J.S., 1979. Recent advances in hamster genetics. Prog. Exp. Tumor Res. 24, 157–161.

Ziomek, J., Banaszek, A., 2007. The common hamster, *Cricetus cricetus* in Poland: status and current range. Folia Zool. 56, 235–242.

Zook, B.C., Huang, K., Rhorer, R.G., 1977. Tyzzer's disease in Syrian hamsters. J. Am. Vet. Med. Assoc. 171, 833–836.

Biology and Diseases of Guinea Pigs

Nirah H. Shomer, DVM, PhD, DACLAM[a],
Hilda Holcombe, DVM, PhD, DACLAM[b]
and John E. Harkness, DVM, MS, MEd, DACLAM[c]

[a]Laboratory Animal Resources, Merck Research Laboratories, Boston, MA, USA
[b]Massachusetts Institute of Technology, Cambridge, MA, USA [c]College of Veterinary Medicine,
Mississippi State University, Mississippi State, MS, USA

OUTLINE

I. INTRODUCTION

The guinea pig (*Cavia porcellus*), the only New World rodent used commonly in research, has contributed to studies of anaphylaxis, asthma, gnotobiotics, immunology, infectious and nutritional disease, and otology, among others. Several outbred and inbred strains were used historically, but, at present, only outbred pigmented stocks, albino Hartley stocks, and IAF hairless stock are available commercially in the United States (Fig. 6.1). Husbandry considerations include noninjurious housing, appropriate food, prevention of intraspecies aggression, environmental stability, and reproductive aspects, including a long gestation. Although guinea pigs are susceptible to a wide range of diseases, current breeding and housing conditions have reduced the occurrence of many spontaneous infectious diseases in these animals. Diseases of concern that do occur in research colonies include respiratory diseases (especially those caused by *Bordetella, Streptococcus*, and adenovirus), chlamydiosis, pediculosis, dermatophytosis, hypovitaminosis C, pregnancy toxemia, urolithiasis, traumatic lesions, dental malocclusion, ovarian cysts, and antibiotic-induced intestinal dysbiosis.

A. Taxonomy and General Comments

The order Rodentia is subdivided into three suborders: Sciuromorpha (squirrel-like rodents), Myomorpha

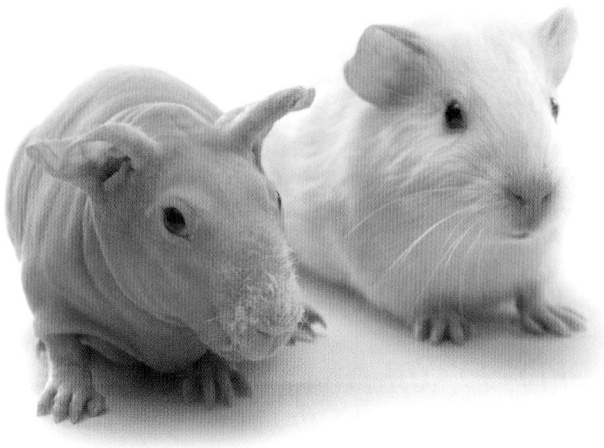

FIGURE 6.1 A Hartley guinea pig typical of the shorthair, English and American varieties (*right*), and an IAF hairless guinea pig (*left*). *Courtesy of Charles River Laboratories.*

(rat-like rodents), and Hystricomorpha (porcupine-like rodents). The domestic guinea pig (*C. porcellus*) is classified as a New World hystricomorph rodent belonging to the family Caviidae (Pritt, 2012). Although recent investigations involving DNA sequencing question the traditional phylogenetic position of the guinea pig, evidence suggesting that the Hystricomorpha reclassified outside Rodentia is controversial and inconclusive. Further work in this area needs to be done (Wolf *et al.*, 1993; Cao *et al.*, 1997; Stephens *et al.*, 2009).

The family Caviidae consists of five genera and approximately 23 species of South American rodents. All Caviidae have four digits on the forefeet and three on the hindfeet. The soles of the feet are hairless, and the nails are short and sharp. Members of the genus *Cavia* have stocky bodies with a large head, short limbs and ears, a single pair of mammae, and a vestigial tail.

Guinea pigs were first domesticated by the Andean Indians of Peru as a food source and as a sacrificial offering to the Incan gods (Morales, 1995). The Dutch introduced guinea pigs to Europe in the sixteenth century, where they were bred by fanciers. There are several color (white, black, brown, red, brindle, and roan) and hair-coat varieties of guinea pigs. They may be mono-, bi-, or tricolored and have short regular hair (shorthair or English), longer hair arranged in whorls (Abyssinian), long straight hair (Peruvian), or medium-length fine hair (silky). These varieties can interbreed (Harkness, 1997).

B. Uses in Research and Biomethodology

Guinea pigs have been used in research for over 200 years, and the term 'guinea pig' has become a synonym for 'experimental subject.' Their gentle temperament, commercial availability, and extensive historical use as a research model make them useful as research

subjects. However, their use has declined sharply in recent decades. Approximately 191,000 were used in 2013 in biomedical research and teaching in the United States (U.S. Department of Agriculture, Animal and Plant Health Inspection Service, 2010), which is down from a high of 599,000 animals in 1985. Publications of research using guinea pigs have decreased from approximately 3500 per year in the 1980s to fewer than 1000 publications in 2011 (MEDLINE). Compared with other rodent models, they more closely model human vitamin C metabolism and some immunological responses, for example, airway reactivity in asthma. However, they have largely been overshadowed by rats and mice, which have a shorter life cycle, larger litters, have been successfully genetically modified, and are subject to fewer regulations in the United States. The guinea pig was the first laboratory animal species derived and maintained in an axenic state (Wagner and Foster, 1976). Guinea pigs have been used in a variety of studies, including anaphylaxis, asthma, delayed hypersensitivity, genetics, gnotobiotics, immunology, infectious disease, nutrition, otology, and pharmacology, and for research in space (Gray, 1998). They are used by the pharmaceutical industry for preclinical testing of cardiac safety of new drugs, and hairless guinea pigs are used for development and testing of topical drug preparations (Hauser *et al.*, 2005.) Guinea pigs are also used extensively in the medical device industry for sensitivity testing (e.g., Beuhler and Kligman tests), and as a source of serum complement in laboratories using the complement fixation test to diagnose infectious disease.

Although guinea pigs are docile and easy to handle, their lack of a tail and their thick skin make blood collection relatively challenging compared with collection from rats and mice. Small volumes (e.g., 100 μl) can be collected by jugular, saphenous, or cephalic venipuncture. Collection of more than a few drops of blood generally requires techniques that require anesthesia, e.g., retro-orbital bleeding, cranial vena cava puncture, or terminal cardiac puncture. Guinea pigs are also challenging to intubate or to dose orally due to their unique pharyngeal anatomy; an elongated soft palate covers the back of the throat, leaving only the small palatal ostium for access to the trachea and esophagus.

C. Availability and Sources

The shorthair albino English or Hartley guinea pig is used commonly in biomedical research, testing, and teaching. Outbred animals are available commercially from several breeders of laboratory animals. Additional types of guinea pigs used in research include outbred pigmented guinea pigs, and a hairless (euthymic) Hartley guinea pig. Two inbred lines (strains 2 and 13) are no longer commercially available, although strain 13 guinea pigs can be obtained from United States Army Medical Research Institute of Infectious Diseases (USAMRIID).

D. Laboratory Management and Husbandry

Commonly used caging systems for guinea pigs housed in research facilities include solid-sided, wire-mesh or solid-floor cages stacked vertically on racks, individual microisolator cages, solid-bottom plastic caging, and solid-bottom plastic caging in a ventilated rack. Wire-mesh flooring may result in injuries to feet and legs and reduced production in breeding animals, and should be avoided unless deemed necessary for experimental purposes. Solid-bottom cages may be bedded with commercially available materials such as ground corncobs, hardwood chips or shavings, and paper products. Guinea pigs given the option of wood shavings versus paper sheets for bedding spent significantly more time during the light cycle in areas of the cage bedded with wood shavings than with paper sheets, yet had a slight preference for paper sheets under dark conditions (Kawakami et al., 2003.) Some bedding materials may interfere in animal test systems involving ascorbic acid depletion because of the presence of low levels of vitamin C in some bedding materials such as cedar shavings (Dunham et al., 1994).

Guinea pigs are social animals and as such should be housed in compatible groups whenever possible in accordance with the Guide for the Care and Use of Laboratory Animals (Guide) (Reinhardt, 1997; National Research Council, 2011). Commercial breeders often use large, solid-bottom, plastic or metal tubs with wire-bar tops to house breeding groups. Cage space requirements differ by country. In the United States, the Guide recommendations for guinea pigs are 60 in^2 of floor space for animals weighing 350 g or less and 101 in^2 for animals weighing more than 350 g. For all animals, the height of the primary enclosure should be at least 7 in. Generally recommended environmental parameters for housing guinea pigs include a dry-bulb macroenvironmental temperature of 20–26°C (68–79°F), relative humidity of 30–70%, ventilation of 10–15 fresh air changes per hour with no draft, and a 12 h light–12 h dark light cycle (National Research Council, 2011).

Feed is usually provided in a J-type feeder, which hangs inside the cage or is built into the cage door. It is important that the feeder provide easy access to feed. Guinea pigs do not adapt readily to changes in the presentation of their feed or water. When changes are necessary, it is important to observe the animals often and closely to ensure that they are eating and drinking. Supplemental feed, such as clean hay, may be placed in a crock or similar feeder and be removed on a regular basis if it is not eaten. Hay and other natural foods have the potential to be contaminated with rodent pathogens. Some facilities autoclave hay before use. Water can be provided in water bottles or by an automatic watering system. Guinea pigs often manipulate their water bottles or lixits, and spill water into their cages.

With solid-bottom, bedded cages it is important to remove soiled, wet bedding and replace it as needed with fresh, dry bedding to help prevent ulcerative pododermatitis and other dermatopathies. Automatic watering valves used in solid-bottom caging systems should be located outside the cage to minimize wet or flooded cages.

Guinea pigs are gentle, docile animals that rarely scratch or bite when handled. When guinea pigs are approached, their first response may be to become immobilized, followed by rapid running, generally preferring the perimeter of the cage. Large guinea pigs should be picked up with two hands. One hand is placed beneath the chest and upper abdomen, and the other hand must support the hindquarters. Two-handed support is especially important to prevent injury of pregnant females and large adults. Rodent restraint devices used for rats and mice are not easily adapted to guinea pigs because of their compact body shape.

Learning in guinea pigs may occur rapidly or progressively over several trials, depending on the learning paradigm (Sansone and Bovet, 1970). Positive reinforcement (operant conditioning) paradigms are recommended for effecting learned behaviors because aversive stimuli that may induce anxiety or fear, such as restraint, inversion, electric shock, or presence of a predator, may induce in the guinea pig a profound somatic and autonomic motor inhibition known as tonic immobility behavior. Tonic immobility, also known as animal hypnosis or feigning death, is mediated by periaqueductal gray matter, the limbic forebrain, and spinal areas. Therefore, tonic immobility should not be used as a means of restraint (Vieira et al., 2011).

II. BIOLOGY

A. Unique Physiologic and Anatomic Characteristics

Several aspects of the anatomy, physiology, and metabolism of the guinea pig are unique among domesticated rodents and are reviewed in detail by Hargaden and Singer (2012).

1. Circulatory and Lymphoreticular Systems

The erythrocytic indices of the guinea pig (red cell count, hemoglobin, and packed cell volume) are relatively low compared with those of other laboratory rodents (Manning et al., 1984). However, the historical erythrocyte values reported were lower than those seen currently in young, specific pathogen-free (SPF) guinea pigs (Table 6.1). The historical mean white count was considerably higher, suggesting that underlying subclinical disease may have contributed to a relative anemia and leukocytosis. Table 6.1 gives both historical values from the literature and values reported in 2008 for young,

TABLE 6.1   Approximate Physiologic Values for Guinea Pigs[a,b,c,d,e,f]

General data

Body weight: adult male	900–1000 g	Thermal neutrality range[i]	2–31°C
Body weight: adult female	700–900 g	Cardiovascular and respiratory systems[l,m,n,o]	
Birth weight	60–115 g	Respiratory rate	42–104/min
Body surface area[d,g,h]	700–830 g: 9.2 (wt in g)$^{2/3}$ cm^2	Tidal volume	2.3–5.3 ml/kg body weight
	200–680 g: 10.1 (wt in g)$^{2/3}$ cm^2	Oxygen use	0.76–0.83 ml/g body weight/h
Rectal temperature[i]	37.2–39.5°C	Plasma CO_2	18–26 mM/l
Diploid number[i,j]	64	CO_2 pressure	21–59 mmHg
Life span: usual	3–4 years	Plasma pH	7.17–7.53
Life span: extreme	6–7 years	Heart rate	230–380/min
50% Survival	60 months	Blood volume	69–75 ml/kg body weight
Food consumption	6 g/100 g body weight/day	Cardiac output[p]	240–300 ml/min/kg body weight
Water consumption	10 ml/100 g body weight/day	Blood pressure	80–94/55–58 mmHg
Gastrointestinal transit time[k]	13–30 h	Upper critical temperature[i]	30°C

Clinical chemistry (serum)

Total protein	4.5–5.9 g/dl	Calcium	9.0–11.3 mEq/dl
Albumin	2.3–3.0 g/dl	Phosphorus	4.2–6.5 mEq/dl
Globulin	1.7–2.6 g/dl	Magnesium	2.1–2.7 mg/dl
Glucose	80–110 mg/dl	Sodium	121–126 mEq/l
Blood urea nitrogen	15.7–31.5 mg/dl	Potassium	4–6 mEq/l
Creatinine	1.0–1.8 mg/dl	Chloride	96–98 mEq/l
Total bilirubin	0.2–0.4 mg/dl	Alanine aminotransferase	31–51 IU/l
Lipids	95–240 mg/dl	Alanine transaminase	32–51 IU/l
Phospholipids	25–75 mg/dl	Alkaline phosphatase	68–71 IU/l
Total triglyceride	28–76 mg/dl	Aspartate aminotransferase	38–57 IU/l
Cholesterol	20–43 mg/dl	Aspartate serum transaminase	38–58 IU/l
Lactate dehydrogenase	37–63 IU/l	Creatine phosphokinase	80–130 IU/l

Blood values

Blood cells[p,q]	Historical values 1974–77[p,q]	8- to 10-week male[r] Hartley (mean 95% interval)
Erythrocytes[s]	5.4 × 10^6/mm^3 ± 12%[s]	5.74 × 10^6/mm^3 (4.41–7.56)
Hematocrit	43 ± 12%	49.0 % (37.3–64.5)
Hemoglobin	13.4 g/dl ± 12%	15.7 g/dl (12.7–21.3)
Mean Cell Volume (MCV)	81 μm^3	85.5 μm^3 (78.8–92)
Mean Cell Hemoglobin (MCH)	25 pg	27.5 pg (20.9–30.2)
Mean Cell Hemoglobin Concentration (MCHC)	30%	32% (24.8–36.2)
Leukocytes	9.9 × 10^3/mm^3 ± 30%	4.2 × 10^3/mm^3 (1.86–7.16)
Neutrophils	28–44%	24–62%
Lymphocytes	39–72%	35–74%

(Continued)

TABLE 6.1   (Continued)

Blood values

Kurloff cells	3–4%	
Monocytes	3–12%	0.3–3%
Basophils	0–3%	0–1.5%
Platelets	$250–850 \times 10^3/\text{mm}^3$	$230–1469 \times 10^3/\text{mm}^3$
Eosinophils	1–5%	0–5%

[a]Loeb and Quimby (1999).
[b]Festing (1976).
[c]Charles River Breeding Laboratories (1982).
[d]White and Lang (1989).
[e]Clifford and White (1999).
[f]Harkness and Wagner (1995).
[g]Hong et al. (1977).
[h]Klaassen and Doull (1980).
[i]Short and Woodnott (1969).
[j]Robinson (1971).
[k]Jilge (1980).
[l]Schalm et al. (1975).
[m]Sisk (1976).
[n]Payne et al. (1976).
[o]Schermer (1967).
[p]Quillec et al. (1977).
[q]Laird (1974).
[r]Charles River Laboratories (2008).
[s]Coefficient of variation.

naïve laboratory guinea pigs; the latter data are probably a better representation of reference ranges in contemporary animal facilities. Lymphocytes are the predominant leukocyte in the peripheral blood. Neutrophils (heterophils or psuedoeosinophils) have distinct eosinophilic granules in the cytoplasm (Schalm *et al.*, 1975; Sanderson and Phillips, 1981). The Foa-Kurloff or Kurloff cell is an estradiol-dependent mononuclear leukocyte unique to the guinea pig. These cells are found primarily in the thymus and in the sinusoids of the spleen, liver, and lung, with increased numbers in the peripheral circulation during pregnancy. Large numbers are seen also in the placenta, where they may have a role in preventing the maternal rejection of the fetal placenta during pregnancy (Marshall *et al.*, 1971). The Kurloff cell (Fig. 6.2) has a large mucopolysaccharide, intracytoplasmic inclusion body, which is metachromatic and periodic acid-Schiff positive, and contains proteoglycans (Landemore *et al.*, 1994) and hydrolytic enzymes (Taouji *et al.*, 1994), similar to the smaller intracytoplasmic granules found in natural killer (NK) cells. The Kurloff cell has NK cytotoxic activity *in vitro* and may be part of cancer resistance in the guinea pig (Debout *et al.*, 1995).

Guinea pigs, like ferrets and primates, are relatively resistant to the effects of steroids, and the numbers of thymic and peripheral lymphocytes are not reduced markedly by corticosteroid injections (Hodgson and Funder, 1978). The guinea pig is an established model for the study of genetic control of the histocompatibility-linked immune response (Chiba *et al.*, 1978). Although

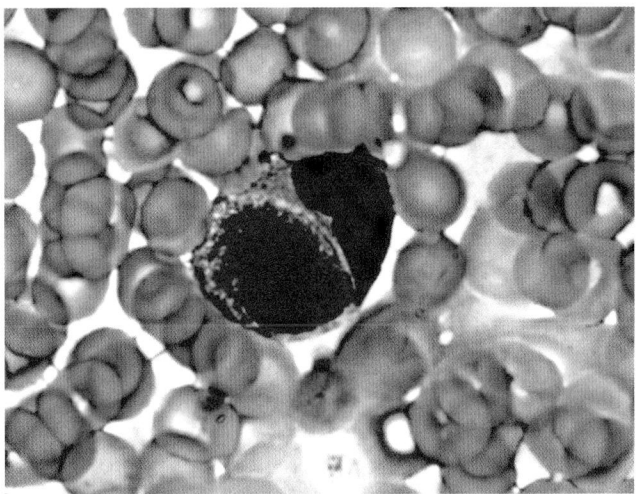

FIGURE 6.2   A Foa-Kurloff cell in a peripheral blood smear of a guinea pig. The intracytoplasmic inclusion body is large and conspicuous.

the thymus of the guinea pig is located in the ventral cervical region and is easy to remove surgically, accessory thymic islets exist in contiguous fascia. The thymus apparently has no afferent lymphatic vessels (Ernström and Larsson, 1967).

2. Gastrointestinal System

The anatomy of the guinea pig has been reviewed by Hargaden and Singer (2012) and Cooper and Schiller (1975). The guinea pig dental formula is 2(I 1/1

C 0/0 PM 1/1 M 3/3) = 20, with a diastema or gap between the incisors and premolars. All teeth are open-rooted and grow continuously (hypsodontic). The incisors are normally white, unlike the yellow to orange incisors of other rodents. The upper incisors are shorter than the lower pair. The oral cavity is small and narrow, and the soft palate covers nearly the entire back of the pharynx, with only the small palatal ostium offering access to the esophagus and trachea. This makes the guinea pig an obligate nasal breather (Nixon, 1974) and makes intubation and oral gavage challenging.

Guinea pigs are monogastric hind-gut fermenters. Unlike that of other rodents, the stomach is undivided and is lined entirely with glandular epithelium. The large cecum can hold up to 65% of the total gastrointestinal content. The gastric emptying time is approximately 2 h. Cecal emptying time is very slow, and total gastrointestinal transit time is approximately 20 h (Manning et al., 1984). With coprophagy, the total transit time can be approximately 60–70 h (Jilge, 1980).

3. Cardiovascular System

Compared with the rat, the guinea pig has both a lower basal coronary blood flow and a lower peak coronary blood flow. The intercoronary collateral network is well developed; therefore, it is difficult to produce a cardiac infarct in the guinea pig by acute coronary artery occlusion (Brewer and Cruise, 1994). Also, compared with the rat, the guinea pig myocardiocytes are not as 'stiff' (Kapel'ko and Navikova, 1993). Brewer and Cruise (1994) provide more details on the comparative aspects of the guinea pig heart. Anesthetised instrumented guinea pigs are used in cardiac safety evaluation of candidate drugs (Hauser et al., 2005, Marks et al., 2012).

4. Respiratory System

The guinea pig has been used as a model of lung-function impairment and bronchial reactions, including airway hyperresponsiveness and reactions that resemble asthma in humans (Nagase et al., 1994; Martin, 1994; Cook et al., 1998). A thorough review of the guinea pig respiratory system with an emphasis on species differences was presented by Brewer and Cruise (1997). Blood-gas parameters, acid–base balance, and hemodynamic and respiratory functions are described in Barzago et al. (1994).

5. The Ear

The large, accessible guinea pig ear is used for several types of auditory studies (McCormick and Nuttall, 1976). The Preyer or pinna reflex, which involves a cocking of the pinnae in response to a sharp sound, may be used in otologic studies as a measurement of hearing function. Advantages of using the guinea pig ear include the large bullae, ease of surgical entry to the

middle and inner ears, and protrusion of the cochlea and blood vessels into the cavity of the middle ear, which allows examination of the microcirculation of the inner ear (Manning et al., 1984). There are two reported mutations causing inner ear malformation and a resulting behavior known as 'waltzing' (Banks, 1989; Ernstson and Ulfendahl, 1998).

6. Pituitary Gland

Pituitary growth hormone is responsible for postnatal growth in vertebrates. Surgical removal of the pituitary gland in most species results in alteration of the growth pattern. However, hypophysectomy does not alter the growth rate of guinea pigs. In addition, supplementation with guinea pig pituitary extract fails to alter the growth rate of both hypophysectomized and normal guinea pigs. Somatomedins insulin-like growth factor I (IGF-I) and IGF-II are responsible for growth in the guinea pig. Unlike other species, the somatomedins in the guinea pig are not growth-hormone dependent. Hypophysectomy does not decrease the level of somatomedins. It is not known what regulates somatomedin expression in the guinea pig (Baumann, 1997).

B. Life Cycle and Physiologic Values

Tables 6.1 and 6.2 list general normative, physiologic, and life cycle data for the guinea pig. Values may vary with age, strain, sex, environment, and method of data

TABLE 6.2　Reproductive Values for Guinea Pigs[a]

First ovulation	4–5 weeks
First ejaculation	8–10 weeks
Breeding onset: male	600–700 g (3–4 months)
Breeding onset: female	350–450 g (2–3 months)
Cycle length	15–17 days
Implantation	6–7 days postovulation
Gestation period	59–72 days
Postpartum estrus	60–80% fertile
Litter size	2–5
Litter interval	96 days
Weaning age	180 g (14–28 days)
Breeding life	18 months to 4 years (4–5 litters)
Young production	0.7–1.3/sow/month
Preweanling mortality	5–15%
Milk composition[b]	3.9% fat, 8.1% protein, 3.0% lactose
Milk yield (maximum)[c]	45–65 ml/kg body weight/day

[a]Phoenix (1970), Gresham and Haines (2012), Sisk (1976), Peplow et al. (1974), Laird (1974), and Festing (1976).
[b]Nelson et al. (1951).
[c]Davis et al. (1979).

collection. For more detailed information regarding the source of the data and method of collection, references should be consulted.

C. Diets, Nutrition, and Feeding

Guinea pigs should receive a feed prepared specifically for the species and containing vitamin C. Previous recommendations were to use commercial guinea pig feeds within 90 days of milling; however, most commercially available laboratory guinea pig chows now contain stabilized vitamin C and can be used for 180 days postmilling. In some situations, additional feedstuff high in vitamin C (e.g., properly cleaned and fresh orange wedges, kale, cabbage) is fed. Commercially available guinea pig chow is pelleted and contains approximately 18–20% crude protein and 9–18% fiber. Diets low in Mg, with incorrect Ca:P ratios, or with inadvertent feeding of diets containing extremely high levels of vitamin D have been associated with increased incidence of metastatic calcification (Maynard, et al., 1958, Galloway et al., 1964, Jensen et al., 2013; Holcombe et al., 2014). Feed should be stored in a cool, dry, dark area.

Guinea pigs are fastidious eaters and do not adapt rapidly to changes in food and water. Because guinea pigs 'imprint' food type (and water taste) early in life, they may not recognize other foods, including powdered diets, water additives, and vegetable supplements. Placing powder in an agar matrix or blending foods during a transition can facilitate food changes. Guinea pigs scatter food and dribble water from sipper tubes, which makes measuring consumption difficult (Harkness et al., 2010).

Diets and nutrition are discussed further in Section III, B. There are comprehensive reviews of guinea pig nutrition by Mannering (1949), Reid and Bieri (1972), Navia and Hunt (1976), and Gresham and Haines (2012). The latter reference includes a tabular summary of estimated nutritional requirements of guinea pigs and signs associated with several deficiency states.

D. Behavior

Reviews of guinea pig behavior include those of Sachser (1998) and Hargaden and Singer (2012). Guinea pig behaviors are also discussed in later husbandry sections. Behaviors in guinea pigs that may affect experimental outcomes or harm animals include hair chewing, skin biting, ear nibbling, trampling of young, boars climbing from pen to pen, and intermale aggression. In mixed-sex groups, a dominant male hierarchy and a less defined female hierarchy develop. Scent marking with urine, anal, and supracaudal gland secretions and vocalization and agonistic displays are used to assert dominance and defend territory. The presence or absence of barbering, ear chewing, wounds, and fighting are evidence of competition and social status. Research and breeding guinea pigs are typically housed in groups of sows only or of one boar with up to five sows. In harem breeding situations, a dominant female may be apparent by her lack of fight wounds or hair loss from barbering. Sexually immature males can be housed together, but mature boars may fight and group housing of adult males is not recommended. Shelters placed in a cage with several males reduce intramale aggression (Agass and Ruffle, 2005; Walters et al., 2012).

Guinea pigs move, rest, and often eat as groups, with activity occurring both day and night (White et al., 1989), although some authors state that guinea pigs are usually nocturnal (Kawakami et al., 2003). In a cage without adequate sheltering sites, guinea pigs align along the cage perimeter, end to end, with pups near the end of the line. They usually avoid the center area. When guinea pigs become stressed, they may, depending on the stressor, vocalize, become immobile or 'freeze,' jump or hop ('pop-corning'), dart, or stampede, even exiting the cage (Mayer, 2003; Donatti and Leite-Panissi, 2009).

Learning in guinea pigs may occur rapidly or progressively over several trials, depending on associated stressors and study paradigm. Because guinea pigs respond to aversive stimuli with immobility or erratic movement, positive reinforcement learning paradigms effect more rapid learning (Agterberg et al., 2010; Hargaden and Singer, 2012).

Guinea pigs may use a dozen or more audible call types, based on sonogram indicators. Situations evoking these sounds include several categories: calls to increase proximity, greeting and proximity-maintaining calls, proximity-regaining calls, distress calls, and alarm calls (Berryman, 1976; Grimsley et al., 2011).

E. Reproduction

Comprehensive descriptions of the reproductive anatomy and physiology of the guinea pig are found in Phoenix (1970), Cooper and Schiller (1975), Sisk (1976), and Gresham and Haines (2012). Reproductive data are summarized in Table 6.2.

1. Reproductive Anatomy and Sexual Maturation

Accessory sex glands in the male guinea pig include large, transparent, smooth seminal vesicles (up to 10 cm in length), prostate, coagulating, bulbourethral, and rudimentary preputial glands. Testes remain in inguinal pouches; inguinal canals are open for life. There is an os penis.

The uterus is bicornate and terminates into a single os cervix. The vagina is sealed by the vaginal closure membrane, an epithelial structure that ruptures just before the onset of estrus and reforms after ovulation (Stockard and Papanicolaou, 1919).

(A)
(B)

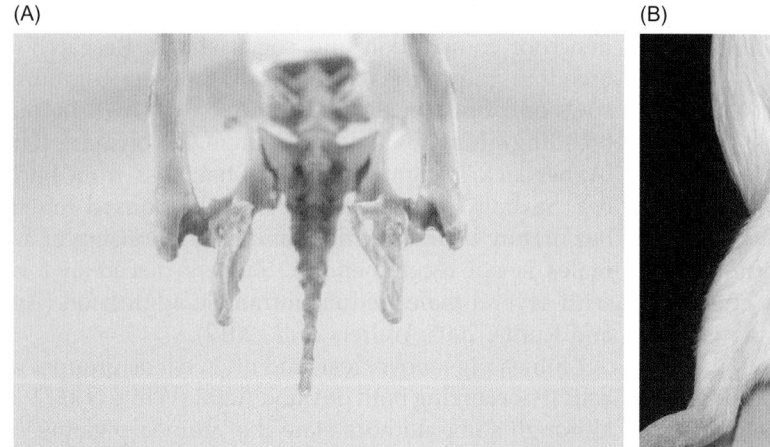
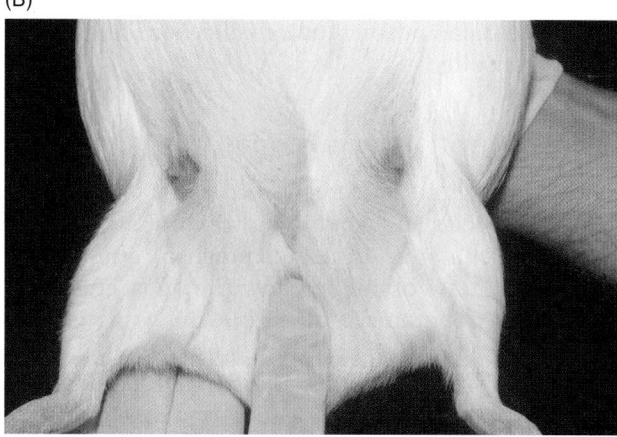

FIGURE 6.3   (A) The pelvis of a pregnant female guinea pig. The pubic symphysis separates up to 3 cm by the day of parturition. (B) The separation of the pubic symphysis is readily palpable during the last week of pregnancy.

Sows should be bred first when they are large enough to bear a litter, but before the calcification of the fibrocartilaginous pubic symphysis. This calcifies and becomes fused between 6 and 9 months of age. Females that give birth for the first time after the pubic symphysis fuses are prone to dystocia. Guinea pig vendors in the United States breed females for the first time when they are between 350–500 g or 5–13 weeks. Boars are first used for breeding at 500–800 g (7–13 weeks).

Guinea pigs are spontaneous ovulators and, under laboratory conditions, polyestrous breeders. Both monogamous and harem breeding systems can be used. With either system, continuous cohabitation allows mating to occur during the sow's fertile postpartum estrus and will result in an average of five litters per sow per year. Heavily bred sows may cease hair growth, resulting in partial (patchy) alopecia.

2. Estrous Cycle

The estrous cycle of the guinea pig lasts approximately 16 days (range of 13–21 days). Proestrus (1–1.5 days) is characterized by vaginal swelling, rupture of the vaginal closure membrane, increased activity, and a vaginal smear of nucleated and cornified epithelial cells (Hennessy and Jenkins, 1994; Stockard and Papanicolaou, 1917). Estrus lasts 8–11 h and is indicated by a swollen congested vulva, a perforate vaginal membrane, and lordosis posture, with rear quarters elevated (Harper, 1968; Phoenix, 1970). Vaginal impedance measurements can be used also to assess the stage of estrous cycle in female guinea pigs (Lilley et al., 1997.) Metestrus (3 days) and diestrus (11–12 days) complete the estrous cycle. A fertile postpartum estrus occurs from 2 to 10 h after parturition (Rowlands, 1949, Sisk, 1976).

There is no conclusive evidence of cycle synchronization among group-housed sows (Donovan and Kopriva, 1965; Harned and Casida, 1972). Estrus can be synchronized with progesterone administered orally or as a subcutaneous implant (Ueda et al., 1998; Gregoire et al., 2012).

3. Mating and Gestation

During copulation, the boar makes one or two intromissions and then ejaculates. Coital completion is indicated by grooming, scooting, and perianal marking by the boar (Manning et al., 1984). A copulatory or vaginal plug may be found in the female or the bedding, but a lack of finding such a plug will provide no indication as to whether copulation occurred. Approximately 60–85% of matings, including postpartum matings, are fertile. The gestation period is an average of 68 days (ranges from 59–72 days). Blastocysts implant on day 6 or 7 of gestation. Placentation is labyrinthine hemomonochorionic, similar to that of humans, which can make the guinea pig a good model for reproductive toxicology studies.

Pregnancy can be detected by gentle palpation of the uterus. At day 15 of gestation, firm, oval swellings of approximately 5 mm in diameter can be felt in the uterine horns. Radiographs and ultrasound have also been used to diagnose pregnancy. Fluid-filled round swellings in the uteri are apparent on the echograph at day 16 of gestation, and diagnosis approaches 100% on day 19 (Inaba and Mori, 1986). During late pregnancy, abdominal distension becomes evident, and the pubic symphysis separates to 3 cm during the last week (Fig. 6.3).

Gestation length is generally inversely proportional to litter size. Relaxin is produced by the placenta, beginning around day 30 of gestation and continuing to about day 63 (Zarrow, 1947). Relaxin is responsible for the loosening of the fibrocartilaginous pelvic symphysis prior to parturition. Sows do not build nests. Young are delivered quickly, with pups being born every 3–7 min and completion of parturition in 30 min. Large litters (3 or more) are associated with a higher incidence of still-births. It is rare for a sow to eat stillborn pups. Dystocia can occur in obese sows, sows bred for the first time after fusion of the pubic symphysis, and sows with large fetuses (Hisaw *et al.*, 1944).

4. Early Development of the Newborn

Pups are born precocious, with the hair, teeth, and open eyes and ears, and are fully mobile. Young pups will begin to eat and drink within hours of birth. The feeder and sipper tube may be lowered to provide access to the smaller animals. Average birth weight ranges from 45 to 115 g. Those pups weighing less than 50 g at birth generally do not survive. Young do not nurse for the first 24 h.

Even though young guinea pigs begin eating solid food and drinking water within hours of birth, pup mortality of up to 50% can be seen if pups are undersized or do not receive milk from a sow during the first 3–4 days of life. Voluntary micturition does not occur until pups are between 7 and 14 days of age. Young can be weaned as early as 14 days, but are typically weaned at 21 days of age.

Sexing guinea pigs is done by examining the anogenital region (Fig. 6.4). In immature males, the penis can be palpated just anterior to the preputial opening or extruded with gentle pressure at its base. Adult boars have large testes in obvious scrotal pouches.

5. Artificial Insemination

Artificial insemination (AI) has been used successfully in guinea pigs. Electroejaculation produces 0.4–0.8 ml of semen, which can be placed through a bulbed pipette into the vagina (Rowlands, 1957; Freund, 1969). In some electroejaculated boars, the ejaculum coagulates in the urethra. Alternatively, sperm can be harvested from the vasa deferentia and epididymides. Intraperitoneal insemination has been reported, with up to 100% incidence of conception when used in conjunction with estrus synchronization (Rowlands, 1957; Ueda *et al.*, 1998). Additonal methods include injection of sperm directly into uterine horns following laparotomy and endoscope-guided transcervical insemination (Yanagimachi and Mahi, 1976). AI with conception has been successful up to 16 h postestrus.

6. Superovulation and Embryo Transfer

Superovulation has been induced in guinea pigs by intraperitoneal administration of human menopausal gonadotropin (hMG) and by active immunization against the inhibin α-subunit (Shi *et al.*, 2000; Dorsch *et al.*, 2008). Embryo recovery increased from an average of 1.73 on day 2.5 post-coitus in untreated animals to an average of seven recovered from guinea pigs treated with hMG

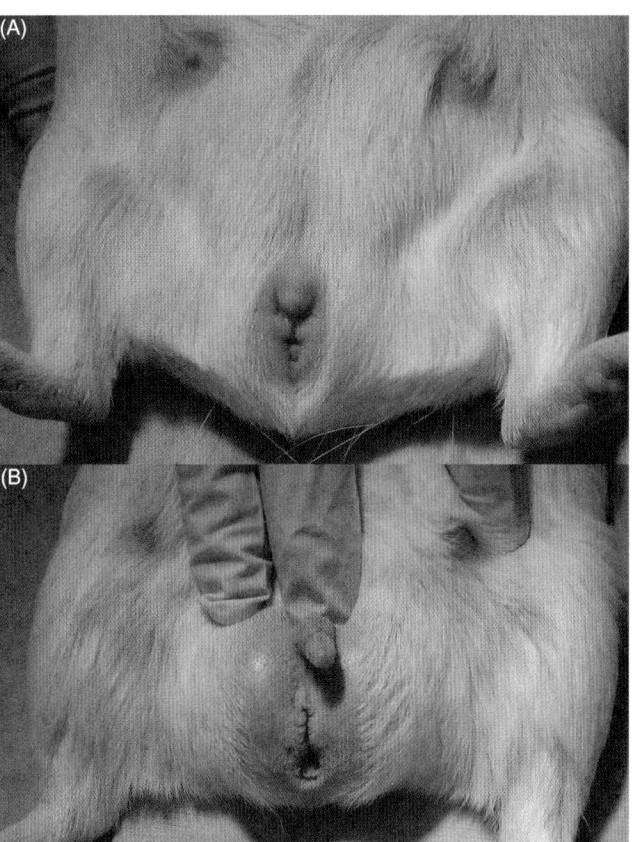

FIGURE 6.4 Sexing guinea pigs. (A) Females have a Y-shaped depression in the perineal tissue. The anus is located at the base of the Y, the membrane-covered vulvar opening is at the intersection of the branches, and the top branches of the Y surround the urethral opening. (B) In immature males, the penis can be palpated just anterior to the preputial opening or extruded with gentle pressure at its base.

(Dorsch *et al.*, 2008). Embryo transfer has been reported rarely in guinea pigs. A method for embryo transfer for the purpose of rederiving a guinea pig colony for eradicating certain pathogens has been described (Parker *et al.*, 2006.) Timed mated females were used as embryo donors and recipients. Embryos were harvested from donors at 1.5 and 2.5 days post-coitus and transferred to pseudopregnant females mated to vasectomized males 1.5–2.5 days earlier. Fifty-nine embryos were transferred into 10 recipients, and two singleton pups were born at 69 and 71 days of gestation.

III. DISEASES

A. Infectious Diseases

Improvements in gnotobiotic derivation, barrier housing, diets, caging, environmental control, routine health surveillance, and information sharing have virtually eliminated most of the disease conditions once prevalent in conventionally housed guinea pigs. Comprehensive reviews of diseases in guinea pigs in research settings are found in Percy and Barthold (2007) and Gresham and Haines (2012). *Staphylococcus aureus* is an opportunistic pathogen that can cause pododermatitis (bumblefoot) in guinea pigs housed on wire bars and in caging with improper sanitation. *Clostridium difficile* and other enteric bacteria have been implicated in antibiotic-associated typhlocolitis. Both ulcerative pododermatitis and antibiotic-associated colitis will be discussed in Section III, D.

Although spontaneous disease is now rare in guinea pig colonies, similarities between human and guinea pig immune systems and the high susceptibility guinea pigs have for many infectious agents continue to make them useful as a model for a number of infectious diseases and for vaccine development. (Padilla-Carlin *et al.*, 2008). Although naturally occurring *Helicobacter* species have not been isolated from guinea pigs, experimental infection with *H. pylori* results in severe gastritis that can persist for at least 5 months, making this a good small animal model for *H. pylori* in humans (Shomer *et al.*, 1998; Sjunnesson *et al.*, 2003). The similarity of the guinea pig pulmonary system to that of humans also makes this species a good model for several bacterial and viral infections, including Legionnaires disease and *Mycobacterium tuberculosis*. (Padilla-Carlin *et al.*, 2008). Guinea pigs are extremely sensitive to infection with tuberculosis and they have been used as sentinels in human hospitals. The guinea pig model of tuberculosis remains the gold standard for testing the potency and standardizing PPD use in humans (Hanif and Garcia-Contreras, 2012).

1. Bacterial and Mycoplasmal Diseases

a. Bordetella bronchiseptica

Etiology   *Bordetella bronchiseptica* is a common commensal organism in many species, including guinea pigs, rats, rabbits, mice, dogs, swine, cats, turkeys, and primates. The organism is a short, gram-negative rod or coccobacillus, aerobic, motile, and non-spore-forming. Growth *in vitro* is best at 30°C but is slow to poor at 37°C, with minute, circular, pearlescent colonies present at 24 h and maximum-sized colonies apparent at 72 h. Colonies embed in the media and are surrounded variably by a zone of β-hemolysis (Boot *et al.*, 1994; Brabb *et al.*, 2012). Immunologic studies (Wullenweber and Boot, 1994) and macrorestriction digestion of DNA techniques, as well as evidence of phenotypic modulation of surface components, provide evidence for serotypic variation within the species. Restriction enzyme analysis of chromosomal DNA demonstrated that diversity among isolates was striking even within a host species (Sacco *et al.*, 2000). The organism variably dissociates in culture (isogenic mutation), and these isolates vary in hemolysin, dermonecrotoxin, proteases, adenylate cyclase, and hemagglutinin production, which may affect host specificity, virulence, and disease manifestation (Griffith *et al.*, 1996).

Clinical Signs   Subclinical infections are encountered more commonly than clinical outbreaks. The epizootic respiratory or septicemic disease can progress rapidly (often within 24–72 h) and produce high mortality; all ages and both sexes are affected. There may also be sporadic deaths in enzootically infected colonies. Clinical signs include inappetence, depression, upper respiratory discharge, dyspnea, cyanosis, and death. A genital form with a 5- to 7-day incubation period causes infertility, stillbirths, and abortions (Brabb *et al.*, 2012).

Epizootiology and Transmission   The organism is found commonly in the respiratory tracts of many species and potentially may be transmitted among these species. The potential for transmission of *Bordetella* sp. from rabbits to guinea pigs is a primary reason these two species should be housed in separate areas. Transmission is by fine particle aerosol onto the respiratory mucosa, by contaminated fomites, or by genital contact (Nakagawa *et al.*, 1971; Trahan *et al.*, 1987). Many guinea pigs carry *Bordetella bronchiseptica* as a commensal resident. Higher morbidity and mortality occur among the young and historically in Strain 2 inbred animals.

Necropsy Findings   Bordetellosis is manifested by various degrees of pulmonary consolidation with respiratory exudation, purulent bronchitis, tracheitis, and otitis media. Consolidated lung areas are dark red or red brown to gray. Peribronchiolar and perivascular inflammatory cells contribute to fibrinous or fibrinopurulent bronchopneumonia. In uterine infections there may be pyosalpinx and dead embryos or fetuses (Brabb *et al.*, 2012).

Pathogenesis   The organism attaches firmly to ciliated respiratory epithelium, where it proliferates rapidly and causes ciliary paralysis, an inflammatory response, antiphagocytic activity, and dermonecrosis, presumably through the action of an intracellular, heat-labile toxin (Quinn *et al.*, 1994).

Differential Diagnosis   Although several bacterial and some viral agents may cause acute bronchopneumonia in guinea pigs, including *Streptococcus pneumoniae*, *S. zooepidemicus*, *Klebsiella pneumoniae*, and adenovirus, *Bordetella* sp. infection has historically been the most common clinical diagnosis, possibly due to its ease of culture. Definitive diagnosis is through swabbing of the lumen of the bronchi or lower trachea and aerobic culture on sheep blood and MacConkey's agar or Smith and Baskerville medium (Smith and Baskerville, 1979). Enzyme-linked immunosorbent assay (ELISA) and indirect immunofluorescence assay (IFA) serologic testing are more sensitive than culture for detecting the organism, but various *Bordetella* antigenic variants should be used in serologic testing because of antigenic variations described earlier (Wullenweber and Boot, 1994).

Prevention, Control, and Treatment Because clinical disease arises often from a preexisting subclinical infection, the reduction or elimination of stressors is essential. Purchasing *Bordetella*-free stock and screening existing colonies for carriers are important diagnostic and preventive measures. Because *B. bronchiseptica* is commonly carried by pet dogs and cats, some vendors and research facilities restrict pet ownership by animal caretakers. Disease is controlled by isolation of animals infected with or susceptible to *B. bronchiseptica* and treatment or removal of the clinically ill. Infected animals may be treated with general supportive care and appropriate antibiotics, e.g., fluoroquinolone or trimethoprim-sulfonamides.

b. *Streptococcus equi* subsp. *zooepidemicus*

Etiology *Streptococcus equi* subsp. *zooepidemicus* is a Lancefield's group C *Streptococcus* (Timoney *et al.*, 1997). The β-hemolytic, gram-positive organism has an antiphagocytic capsule (M-like antigen) and produces several exotoxins, including hyaluronidase, a protease, and a streptokinase. The subspecies *zooepidemicus* survives longer off the host than does the obligate pathogen *S. equi* (Quinn *et al.*, 1994).

Clinical Signs This pyogenic bacterium is associated with suppuration and abscess formation, usually in the cervical lymph nodes (cervical lymphadenitis or 'lumps'), which are evident on observation and careful palpation (Fig. 6.5). Other signs that may be present are torticollis, nasal or ocular discharge, dyspnea and cyanosis, hematuria and hemoglobinuria, cyanotic and swollen mammary glands, abortions, stillbirths, and unexpected deaths, although the presence of enlarged cervical nodes in otherwise healthy guinea pigs is the usual and only sign. There may be inapparent upper respiratory infections (Kohn, 1974).

Epizootiology and Transmission Although transmission from guinea pigs to humans has not been reported, the zoonotic potential of this agent should be considered when working with infected guinea pigs. Guinea pigs of all ages are affected, but the infection may be more common in females. The organism inhabits mucosal surfaces. Transmission of the organism is via aerosol onto respiratory, oropharyngeal, conjunctival, or female genital epithelium. The disease is of low contagion (Murphy *et al.*, 1991).

Necropsy Findings The most common finding on necropsy is one or more abscessed and encapsulated cervical lymph nodes, although the node itself usually is destroyed. The abscesses may be up to several centimeters in diameter and contain a nonodorous, yellow-white to red-gray pus. Other conditions that may be caused by *S. equi* subsp. *zooepidemicus* include pneumonia, generalized lymphadenitis, septicemia (Fig. 6.6), focal hepatitis, otitis media, pleuritis, peri- and myocarditis, nephritis, mastitis, metritis, and arthritis with necrosis and hemorrhage (Kinkler *et al.*, 1976; Harkness *et al.*, 2010; Brabb *et al.*, 2012).

Differential Diagnosis Another organism linked historically to cervical lymphadenitis in guinea pigs is *Streptobacillus moniliformis*, which is carried by wild rats. This organism is seldom involved and is also of low contagion (Aldred *et al.*, 1974). Diagnostic criteria include clinical and necropsy signs and isolation of β-hemolytic streptococci from an abscess margin or heart blood. Chains of streptococci can be seen on Gram stain of exudates from infected guinea pigs (Fig. 6.7). Other organisms that can cause upper respiratory lesions and death in guinea pigs include *S. pneumoniae*, *B. bronchiseptica*, *K. pneumoniae*, adenovirus, and others. Additional

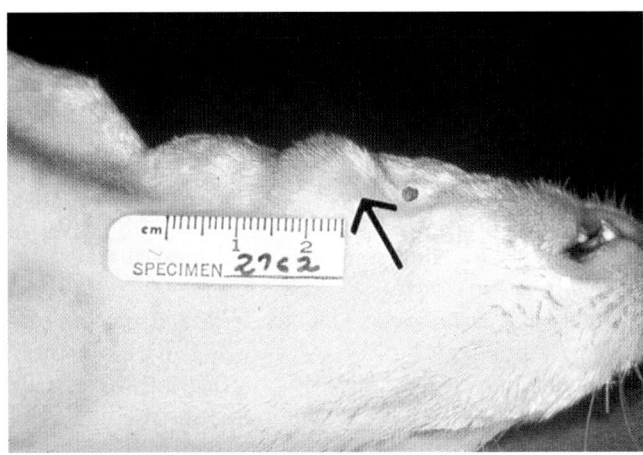

FIGURE 6.5 Swellings in the ventral neck are enlarged lymph nodes infected with *Streptococcus zooepidemicus*, the causal organism of most cases of caseous lymphadenitis.

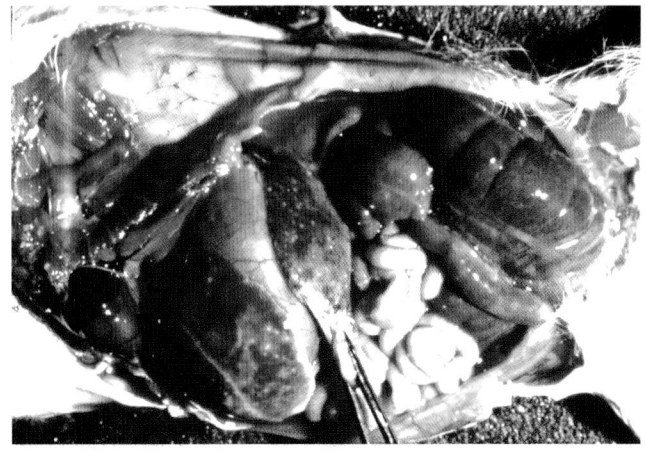

FIGURE 6.6 Septicemia in a guinea pig infected with *Streptococcus zooepidemicus*. Multiple abscesses are evident in the liver and spleen.

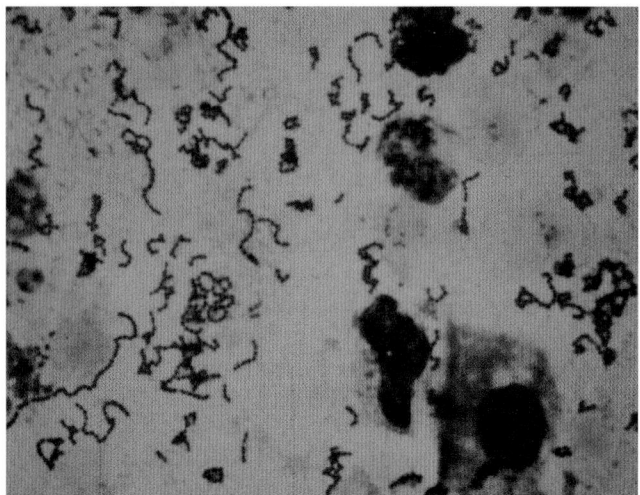

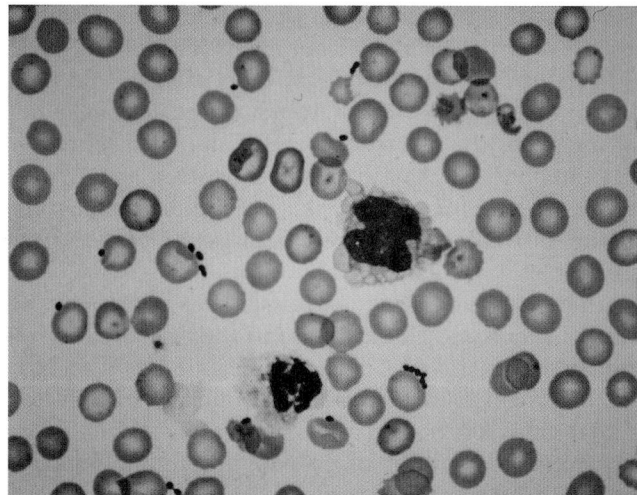

FIGURE 6.7   Gram stain of the peritoneal exudate from a guinea pig infected with *Streptococcus zooepidemicus*. Note the characteristic chains of cocci, 250×.

FIGURE 6.8   Diplococci in the peripheral blood of a guinea pig infected with *Streptococcus pneumoniae*. Wright-giemsa stain, 250×.

rule-outs for masses in the neck include lipomas or lymphoma in aged guinea pigs.

Prevention, Control, and Treatment   Methods of preventing streptococcal cervical lymphadenitis include obtaining disease-free stock, feeding nonabrasive feed (assuming crude fiber may abrade the pharyngeal mucosa), trimming overgrown or broken teeth, and using feeders that do not abrade the skin of the neck. Disease is controlled by removing affected animals from the colony or replacing the entire colony. Treatment usually involves surgical removal of the abscess and its capsule. Antibiotics safe for use in guinea pigs (e.g., fluoroquinolones, trimethoprim-sulfonamides, gentamicin, or chloramphenicol) may be effective.

c. *Streptococcus pneumoniae*

Etiology   *S. pneumoniae* is gram-positive, α-hemolytic, and oval to lancet shaped. It occurs in culture in paired or chain formation (Fig. 6.8). The two serotypes recovered most often from guinea pigs are types 4 and 19F, at least some of which are assumed to be identical with certain human serovars (Parker *et al.*, 1977), although one recent study found that guinea pigs may be a reservoir for a serotype 19F that had an unique allele combination not found in humans (Van der Linden, *et al.*, 2009).

Clinical Signs   Subclinical upper respiratory tract carrier states of *S. pneumoniae* in guinea pigs (and in humans) are high, often over 50% prevalence in some colonies. This high carrier state accounts for sporadic epidemics occurring when animals are stressed or malnourished. Clinical signs, when they do occur, include high mortality or, in less acute cases, depression, anorexia, nasal and ocular discharge, sneezing and coughing, dyspnea, torticollis, or abortion and stillbirths.

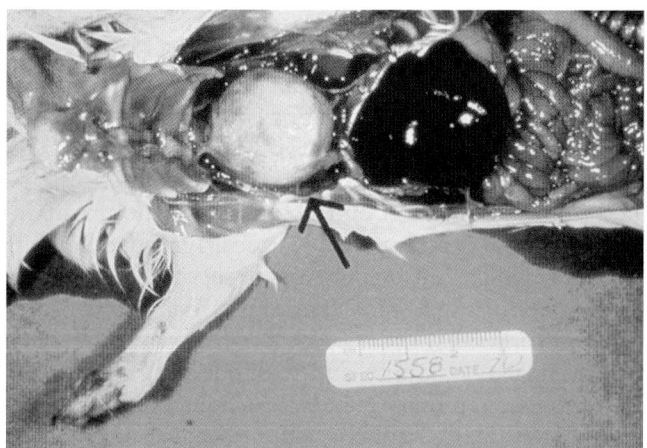

FIGURE 6.9   Fibrinopurulent pericarditis in a guinea pig, caused by *Streptococcus pneumoniae*. The pericardial sac is thickened and opaque (arrow). *From Guinea Pigs: Infectious Disease, Laboratory Animal Medicine and Science, Series II, American College of Laboratory Animal Medicine. Used with permission.*

Epidemiology and Transmission   *S. pneumoniae* infections are rarely reported or detected in research colonies. Transmission is by respiratory aerosol, by direct contact with infected animals (including humans), or vertically during birth.

Necropsy Findings   Lesions seen at necropsy are primarily pyogenic processes occurring in one or more forms: fibrinopurulent pleuritis, pericarditis (Fig. 6.9), peritonitis, suppurative pneumonia, otitis media, endometritis, and arthritis, among others (Boot and Walvoort, 1986; Witt *et al.*, 1988). The pulmonary lesion is an acute, fibrinopurulent bronchopneumonia with thrombosis of pulmonary vessels.

Pathogenesis The organism becomes established in the upper respiratory tract, where it is protected by a polysaccharide capsule and can activate an alternative complement pathway, which initiates some of the pathologic changes associated with the infection.

Differential Diagnosis S. *pneumoniae* can usually be observed on Gram-stained impression smears of infected tissue, or can be cultured on blood agar incubated under 5–10% carbon dioxide. Matsubara *et al.* (1988) developed an ELISA for streptococci. Definitive identification of S. *pneumoniae* requires serotyping among the 83 different capsular polysaccharides. The serotyping test, the Quellung reaction, utilizes a serum pool product or type-specific antisera. The bacterial capsule appears opaque and swollen when the antibody reacts with surface antigens. Differential diagnoses include various respiratory and systemic pathogens including *Bordetella* sp., other streptococci, *Salmonella* spp., *Klebsiella* sp., and adenovirus.

Prevention, Control, and Treatment Guinea pigs free from streptococcal exposure or infection should be purchased for research or teaching. Clinical disease may occur in carrier animals when they are stressed or malnourished. Treatment is more likely to cause reversion to a subclinical, carrier state than eliminate the infection. Clinically affected guinea pigs should be removed from the colony and efforts made to reduce predisposing factors. Antibiotics safe for use in guinea pigs may, in some cases, reverse the pathologic process, but subclinical infections may remain.

d. *Salmonella enterica*

Etiology Salmonellosis, seen rarely in research guinea pigs, is caused by several serovars of the gram-negative bacillus *Salmonella enterica*, subspecies *enterica*; however, serovars *Typhimurium* and *Enteritidis* are encountered most frequently (Brabb *et al.*, 2012).

Clinical Signs In peracute to acute infections the only signs of salmonellosis in an animal or colony may be high morbidity and mortality. Epizootic outbreaks occur more often in late pregnant, weanling, aged, and malnourished guinea pigs (Wagner, 1976; Harkness *et al.*, 2010). In longer term survivors or in sporadic clinical cases in colonies with endemic infection, guinea pigs may exhibit rough hair coats, weakness, conjunctivitis, abortion of small litters, and light-colored feces or intermittent diarrhea (Schaeffer and Donnelly, 1996). Mortality may be as high as 50–100% of the population.

Epizootiology and Transmission Pathogenic *Salmonella* spp. are found worldwide in a variety of vertebrates, and one species or serovar of *Salmonella* may affect a wide variety of animal species. The pattern of infection may be epizootic, enzootic, or subclinical with shedding of infectious organisms. Inapparent

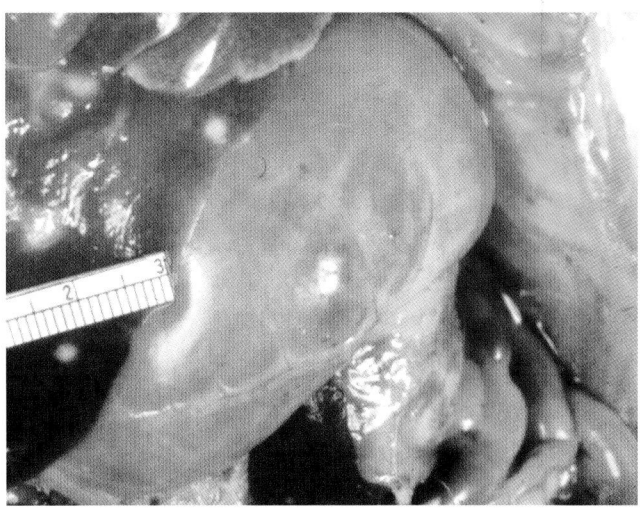

FIGURE 6.10 Multifocal hepatic abscesses in a guinea pig infected with *Salmonella enterica.*

carriers shed the organisms intermittently, which poses a continuing threat to other animals, including humans.

Transmission of salmonellae among animals may be fecal–oral, blood–oral, or tissue–oral, or via the conjunctiva. The organisms are shed in the feces of wild rodents or other animals and contaminate food (e.g., green vegetables, hay) intended for guinea pigs. Guinea pigs are highly susceptible to *Salmonella* spp., and the incubation period is 5–7 days.

Necropsy Findings Gross lesions in guinea pigs dying from salmonellosis may not be present or may include hepatomegaly, splenomegaly, and small yellow necrotic foci throughout the viscera (Fig. 6.10) (Percy and Barthold, 2007).

Pathogenesis Salmonellae enter the body through the gastrointestinal tract or via the conjunctiva and elicit histiocytosis, tissue necrosis, and abscess formation.

Differential Diagnosis Diagnosis requires recovery of the organism from feces, heart, blood, spleen, or other affected organs through enrichment in a broth such as selenite F or tetrathionate, culture on MacConkey's or brilliant green agar, and identification of the organism. Serotyping identifies the serovar (Percy and Barthold, 2007; Brabb *et al.*, 2012.)

Prevention, Control, and Treatment Salmonellosis in guinea pigs is now a rare disease in most research colonies because of the use of barrier-raised stock and improved husbandry and health monitoring. Aging, other diseases, malnutrition, and enviromental stress are predisposing factors. Treatment is not recommended. Antibiotic use may cause an infection to become subclinical and lead to antibiotic resistance. The best control and treatment recommendation for *Salmonella*-infected animals is to euthanize the entire colony, sanitize caging and equipment thoroughly, and restock with animals known to be free of *Salmonella* spp.

e. Other Bacteria

Clostridium piliforme *C. piliforme*, the causative organism of Tyzzer's disease, is a gram-negative, curved rod and an obligate, intracellular anaerobe with subterminal spores that persist for years in the environment. The disease occurs in several species, including rodents, rabbits, cats, dogs, horses, and some nonhuman primates. This disease, reported rarely in guinea pigs, causes emaciation, dehydration, lethargy, diarrhea, and death. The organism causes a necrotizing ileitis, typhlitis, and hepatic necrosis in weanling guinea pigs. Lesions seen at necropsy include multifocal necrosis and inflammation of the ileum, cecum, and colon. Prevention is to avoid stressors and to maintain good sanitation. Diagnosis is through identifying characteristic filamentous bacteria in a Giemsa- or Warthin–Starry-stained section of enterocytes. The organism has not been directly cultured *in vitro*. Reported spontaneous cases have identified an unclassified spirochete occurring along with the Tyzzer's organism and lesions (McLeod *et al.*, 1977; Zwicker *et al.*, 1978; Waggie *et al.*, 1986; Harkness *et al.*, 2010).

Pasteurella multocida Pasteurellosis is rare in guinea pigs in well-managed colonies, and the prevalence of infection is unknown. An epizootic reported by Wright (1936) involved sporadic, unexpected deaths with pulmonary consolidation, fibrinopurulent serositis, and conjunctivitis. Diagnosis is by culture and identification of the characteristic gram-negative coccobacillary rods.

Pseudomonas aeruginosa *Pseudomonas* infections are rare in guinea pigs but have been associated with pulmonary lesions involving lung consolidation and a severe, focal, necrotizing bronchopneumonia (Bostrom *et al.*, 1969). *Pseudomonas* may also cause conjunctivitis and otitis media. Clusters of bacteria surrounded by necrotic debris (grossly, 'sulfur granules') may be present in focal, suppurative lesions. Samii *et al.* (1996) reported a pet guinea pig with an abdomen painful on palpation and containing a 2 × 3 cm mass in the caudal abdomen. Necropsy revealed an enlarged, inflamed, fibrous prostate gland with local extension of the inflammation. *Pseudomonas aeruginosa* was isolated from the gland. *Pseudomonas* is ubiquitous and may be spread in drinking water or in damp bedding or food.

Chlamydophila cavia (Chlamydia cavia) *Chlamydophila caviae*, referred to also as *Chlamydia caviae* historically, formerly *Chlamydia psittaci*, is a gram-negative, obligate intracellular bacterium, and is the causative agent of guinea pig inclusion conjunctivitis

(GPIC) (Schmeer *et al.*, 1985; Cherian and Magee, 1990). Infections may be subclinical. Signs may be limited to mild reddening of the eyelids, or can include conjunctivitis with serous to purulent exudate, rhinitis, and genital tract infections (Deeb *et al.*, 1989). Abortions and lower respiratory tract infections are reported. The clinical disease is self-limiting, with complete recovery in 3–4 weeks. Historically, detection was based on demonstration of intracytoplasmic inclusion bodies in Giemsa- or Macchiavello-stained conjunctival epithelial cells. More sensitive polymerase chain reaction (PCR) assays are available and have been used to detect the organism in guinea pigs and other species (Everett *et al.*, 1999; Lutz-Wohlgroth *et al.*, 2006; Pantchev, *et al.*, 2009) Differential diagnoses include causes of bacterial conjunctivitis in guinea pigs: streptococci, coliforms, *S. aureus*, and *Pasteurella multocida*. The disease is self-limiting and typically does not require treatment. The conjunctival and genital infections in guinea pigs have served as models for the human disease (Rank *et al.*, 1979; Deeb *et al.*, 1989; Rank and Sanders, 1992). The zoonotic potential should be considered and proper protective equipment worn by staff handling potentially infected guinea pigs. When indicated, *Chlamydophila* sp. are sensitive to sulfonamide antimicrobials.

Experimental infection of the guinea pig genital tract with *C. caviae* is a good model for chlamydial genital infections in humans (DeClercq *et al.*, 2013). Disease can be sexually transmitted, and perinatal transmission is possible. Similar to children born to females infected with *C. trachomatis*, guinea pig pups born to sows infected with genital *C. caviae* are prone to conjunctivitis.

Klebsiella pneumoniae *Klebsiella pneumoniae* is a gram-negative, nonmotile bacillus that causes rare epizootics in guinea pigs of all ages and both sexes. Predisposing factors include malnutrition, magnitude of exposure, unsanitary environments, and genetic predisposition (Brabb *et al.*, 2012). Clinical signs of *Klebsiella* infection are anorexia, dyspnea, and death. Necropsy and histologic findings include seropurulent or serofibrinous lesions in the thoracic and abdominal cavities, mastitis, splenomegaly, thrombosis, coagulative necrosis of the liver, granular degeneration of the renal tubule cells, and septicemias. The pulmonary lesion is an acute, necrotizing bronchopneumonia. *Klebsiella* can be isolated from the blood, liver, spleen, peritoneal exudate, and cerebrospinal fluid of infected animals.

Streptobacillus moniliformis *Streptobacillus*, an organism of low contagion carried by wild rats and birds, rarely causes disease in research guinea pig colonies. Lesions include cervical adenitis with abscessation (see also *S. equi* subsp. *zooepidemicus* in Section III, A, 1) and a pyogranulomatous bronchopneumonia (Aldred *et al.*, 1974; Kirchner *et al.*, 1992).

Yersinia pseudotuberculosis *Yersinia pseudotuberculosis* is a gram-negative, nonhemolytic, exotoxin- and enzyme-producing, pleomorphic rod. Optimal incubation temperatures are 20–30°C. Virulent strains may grow within macrophages (Quinn *et al.*, 1994). The organism, which infects both sexes and all ages of guinea pigs and has otherwise a wide host spectrum, can cause (1) an acute, highly fatal septicemia; (2) chronic emaciation, diarrhea, and death within 3–4 weeks; (3) nonfatal lymphadenitis; or (4) a subclinical carrier state, usually following a clinical phase (Ganaway, 1976; Obwolo, 1977). *Yersinia pseudotuberculosis* can infect humans. The zoonotic disease, yersiniosis or pseudotuberculosis, is rare in research guinea pigs in the United States, although guinea pigs are very susceptible to this infection. Because of a persistent carrier state in guinea pigs, euthanasia is advised.

Listeria monocytogenes Listeriosis is rare in guinea pigs, with few literature reports describing infection and actual or possible clinical signs. The causative agent, the gram-positive rod *Listeria monocytogenes*, is widespread in the environment, including in soil and bedding. Clinical signs linked to *Listeria* infection in hairless guinea pigs were unilateral or bilateral keratoconjunctivitis (Colgin *et al.*, 1995) and reproductive disorders (Ganaway, 1976). Prevention and control involve general precautions. Euthanasia instead of treatment is recommended because of the zoonotic potential of the organism.

Mycoplasmas Mycoplasmas (*Mycoplasma caviae*, *M. pulmonis*, and others) and acholeplasmas may occur as latent infections in the reproductive tract, brain, and nasopharynx of guinea pigs (Stalheim and Matthews, 1975; Brabb *et al.*, 2012).

2. Viral Infections

Guinea pigs are susceptible to infection with a number of viruses, and have been used as models of human disease, including influenza transmission (Lowen *et al.*, 2006). However, with the exception of adenovirus and cytomegalovirus, viral infections are no longer common or reported in laboratory guinea pigs. Viral diseases of guinea pigs are reviewed in Brabb *et al.* (2012).

a. Guinea Pig Adenovirus

Etiology Adenoviral respiratory tract infection in guinea pigs is attributed to an adenovirus (GpAV, GAV; DNA, enveloped) with the typical icosahedral symmetry and 252 capsomers. PCR results indicate that the guinea pig adenovirus is genetically distinct from adenoviruses infecting other species (Pring-Åkerblom *et al.*, 1997). GpAV is a separate serotype within the genus *Mastadenovirus* and has the highest level of homology with other animal *Mastadenoviruses* and human subgroups A, C, and F (Feldman *et al.*, 2001).

Clinical Signs The prevalence of the subclinical disease is unknown because of lack of specific serologic tests, but subclinical infections may be common. Clinical disease is rare. Affected animals usually die without prior signs, or they may develop dyspnea, tachypnea, dry rales, crepitations, and lethargy (Eckhoff *et al.*, 1998).

Epizootiology and Transmission Guinea pig adenovirus infection occurs worldwide and may have a higher prevalence than reported. The clinical disease has no age predilection, is sporadic in endemically affected colonies, and is characterized by low morbidity and high mortality (Eckhoff *et al.*, 1998). Transmission is via the respiratory route.

Necropsy Findings Lesions include well-demarcated areas of dark red pulmonary consolidation, compensatory emphysema, and in some cases a catarrhal exudate in air passages. Histologic effects include necrosis and sloughing of bronchiolar, bronchial, and tracheal epithelial cells, which contain large, oval, intranuclear inclusion bodies. The surviving epithelium and underlying lamina propria are underlain with a mixed population of inflammatory cells (Crippa *et al.*, 1997; Eckhoff *et al.*, 1998).

Pathogenesis Factors for predisposition to infection include stress, an immunologically compromised animal, strain and site of replication of the virus, and perhaps anesthetic gas irritation of the respiratory tract. The virus enters the tracheal and bronchial epithelial cells, where replication and cell damage occur. Epithelial erosion, parenchymal inflammation, and exudation in airways follow (Pring-Åkerblom *et al.*, 1997).

Differential Diagnosis Diagnosis of adenovirus disease is by exclusion of other causes and by histologic and electron microscopic examination of air passageway epithelial tissue. There is no specific serologic test available, and the use of the mouse adenovirus strain FL antigen produces excessive false-positive reactions (Pring-Åkerblom *et al.*, 1997). Active disease can be detected by PCR from feces or freshly frozen lungs. Other agents that may infect the respiratory system of guinea pigs are *B. bronchiseptica*, *Streptococcus* sp., *K. pneumoniae*, cytomegalovirus, herpesvirus, and Sendai and parainfluenza viruses (Eckhoff *et al.*, 1998).

Prevention, Control, and Treatment Obtaining guinea pig stocks without a history of clinical adenovirus infection, reduction of stress in a colony, and observation of immunocompromised animals are methods of prevention and control. There is no treatment.

Research Complications Adenoviral vectors are used experimentally for aural gene delivery in guinea pigs in models of hearing loss. Natural infection of study animals with GpAV did not obviously affect the transfection efficiency of human adenoviral vectors expressing GFP (Hankenson, *et al.*, 2010). However, inapparent pulmonary infections may become clinical problems when animals are stressed.

b. Cytomegalovirus

Etiology   *Caviid herpesvirus 2*, also known as guinea pig cytomegalovirus (GPCMV) or the salivary gland virus, is a species-specific pathogen that is detected sporadically in laboratory guinea pigs (Schoondermark-van de Ven, 2006).

Clinical Signs   GPCMV infection is usually subclinical. Strain of host, pregnancy, and an immunocompromised state may predispose to more serious illness. Clinical signs may include weight loss, conjunctivitis, and lymphadenopathy.

Epizoology and Transmission   GPCMV continues to be detected sporadically and is likely dependent in part on housing conditions. Six out of 15 guinea pig facilities located in Europe and screened for various infectious agents between 2000 and 2003 were serologically positive for GPCMV (Schoondermark-van de Ven, 2006). Acute infection is followed by a chronic, persistent infection (Isom and Gao, 1988). Transmission is by exposure to saliva carrying the virus, or transplacental transmission can occur throughout gestation. A preexisting maternal antibody does not prevent transmission to the fetuses. Cesarean section rederivation does not interrupt the transmission, presumably due to transplacental infection.

Necropsy Findings   Experimental introduction of the virus causes more severe signs, but the natural disease in susceptible animals ranges from karyomegaly of salivary gland epithelium (submaxillary gland) to severe interstitial pneumonia, splenomegaly, lymphadenopathy, and fetal meningitis. Congenital neurological abnormalities and deafness can be caused by GPCMV.

Pathogenesis   A viremia within 2 days of exposure results in widespread, systemic dissemination of the virus, and although animals generally remain ostensibly healthy, the salivary gland, hepatic, and renal cells are the primary sites for replication. Many more organs become infected by 10 days. By 12–14 days the viremia ceases and the virus is more difficult to find in visceral organs. By 3 weeks postexposure, inclusion bodies are present in the salivary glands. A chronic, persistent phase continues in the salivary gland and thymus in adults and in the salivary glands and spleen of fetuses (Isom and Gao, 1988).

Differential Diagnosis   Diagnosis of GPCMV is by microscopic identification of large, eosinophilic, usually intranuclear inclusion bodies in the ductal epithelial cells of the submaxillary salivary gland. The inclusions form at 5 days up to 3 weeks postexposure. Inclusion bodies may also be seen in the brain, lung, kidney, spleen, pancreas, thymus, and liver. Indirect fluorescent antibody techniques and histopathology are methods of diagnosis.

Prevention, Control, and Treatment   Prevention and control are by selecting guinea pig stock known free of GPCMV, screening new arrivals, selective necropsy, or serologic testing. There is no treatment.

Research Complications   The natural disease may be unapparent (unless detected by serology or necropsy) but could interfere with studies involving tissues harboring the virus.

c. Poliovirus

The poliovirus affecting guinea pigs is an RNA-containing member of the family Picornaviridae with some antigenic cross-reaction with the GDVII strain of *Theilovirus*. Genetic variants among host guinea pigs may affect predisposition to infection and clinical signs (Van Hoosier and Robinette, 1976). Clinical signs include depression, lameness in one or more limbs, flaccid paralysis, weight loss, and death over 2 weeks. Hansen *et al.* (1997) reported that serologic evidence of this infection is more common in pet store than in laboratory populations. Nevertheless, poliovirus infection remains a possible diagnosis in guinea pigs with lameness.

Clinical signs are rare, and within colonies clinical disease is sporadic, if it exists at all. The transmission route of the virus is not proven, although fecal–oral transmission is common among *Picornaviridae*. In mice and rats the endemic epizootic cycle of *Theilovirus* (formerly *Theiler's murine encephalomyelitis virus*) is by fecal–oral transmission (Lipton and Rozhon, 1986).

Necropsy signs of poliovirus infection are histologic and include meningomyeloencephalitis, perineuronal inflammation, neuronal degeneration, and necrosis of the anterior horn cells of the lumbar spinal cord. In mice the virus replicates presumably in the gray matter of the cortex and progresses into the white matter and upper motor neuron pathways.

Diagnosis is by a positive ELISA using the *Theilovirus* strain GDVII mouse virus antigen combined with histopathologic finding of central nervous system and lumbar spinal cord lesions (Hansen *et al.*, 1997).

Hansen *et al.* (1997) recommended vitamin C for prevention, control, and treatment, given that vitamin C contributes to adrenocorticosteroid production and, presumably, protection of myelin. The infection may complicate research investigations of the central nervous system of the guinea pig.

d. Lymphocytic Choriomeningitis Virus

The RNA arenavirus causing lymphocytic choriomeningitis in mice, dogs, and primates (including humans) is a rare pathogen in guinea pigs. The virus infection in guinea pigs is contracted iatrogenically via inoculation with contaminated biologicals, or possibly through inhalation, ingestion, or through the skin following exposure to biting insects or infected wild mice. Associated signs are central nervous system dysfunction and hindlimb paralysis. The virus may cause a lymphocytic infiltration in meninges, choroid plexi, ependyma, liver, and lungs. The liver is the best site for IFA detection of the virus, and antibodies can be detected by ELISA. The virus causes disease in humans and has many systemic effects in guinea pigs that would interfere with research projects (Van Hoosier and Robinette, 1976).

e. Other Viruses

Overt viral diseases are rare in guinea pigs, but there are many reports of inapparent infections other than those described above. Reviews of these infections are found in Van Hoosier and Robinette (1976), Hsiung *et al.* (1986), and Brabb *et al.* (2012). The viruses include poxviruses, guinea pig retrovirus, parainfluenza viruses, murine pneumonia virus, mammalian orthoreovirus (reovirus 3), simian virus 5, herpesviruses, and Sendai virus.

3. Parasitic Diseases

a. Protozoa

Intestinal protozoa are most often commensal organisms, and clinical signs caused by pathogenic protozoa are rare. Comprehensive descriptions of protozoa of guinea pigs include Ronald and Wagner, 1976, Ballweber and Harkness, 2007, and Brabb *et al.*, 2012.

Eimeria caviae   *Eimeria caviae*, a protozoan of the phylum Apicomplexa, is a moderately pathogenic coccidium with ellipsoidal oocysts without a micropyle. Infection with *E. caviae* in connection with high populations of *Balantidium coli* may occur in the proximal colon, with *Balantidium* as a secondary agent producing clinical disease. Stress also is a significant predisposing factor in the pathogenesis of clinical coccidiosis. Transmission of *E. caviae* occurs with ingestion of sporulated oocysts.

Clinical signs in severely infected weanlings include lethargy, anorexia, and watery to pasty feces lasting 4–7 days. Oocysts may not appear in feces before 10 days postexposure, so a soiled hair coat, diarrhea, and even death may occur before oocysts are detected in feces. In survivors, constipation may follow the diarrhea (Percy and Barthold, 2007). Oocysts in feces require 2–11 days outside the host to develop to an infective stage. Factors affecting maturation include oxygen, heat, and humidity.

Necropsy findings include edema, hyperemia, hemorrhage, and white or yellow plaques in the thickened proximal colon and adjacent cecal wall. Intestinal contents are watery and often contain blood. Histologic examination shows colonic epithelial cell hyperplasia, intracellular coccidian forms, enterocyte sloughing, and edema and congestion of the lamina propria. Ingested, sporulated oocysts invade the mucosal crypts of Liekberkühn of the proximal colon and, during schizogony, damage the epithelium. The prepatent period is 10 or more days (Ellis and Wright, 1961; Hurley *et al.*, 1995).

Diagnosis is by finding oocysts on fecal flotation or by examining mucosal scrapings or a stained tissue section. Other causes of similar signs include pantothenic acid or vitamin C deficiencies, crytosporidiosis, bacterial enteropathies, and coronavirus infection. Prevention is through good sanitation and husbandry, reduction of stress, and provision of fresh, appropriate feed. Treatment involves use of sulfonamides with known anti-*Eimeria* activity and provision of adequate vitamin C.

Cryptosporidium wrairi   *Cryptosporidium wrairi* is a coccidium of guinea pigs that has a prolonged phase of endogenous replication. Subclinical infection may be common. Clinical signs are seen most often in young animals (under 300 g or up to 16 weeks of age), and may be exacerbated by concomitant *Escherichia coli* enterotoxemia. Clinical signs may include weight loss (most common sign), anorexia, potbellied appearance, rectal prolapse, and, uncommonly, diarrhea and death (Lindsey, 1990).

Transmission is fecal–oral. Necropsy findings, especially in the young, are those of a diffuse enteritis from duodenum to the cecum. Infections are patent for 2 weeks and clear by 3–4 weeks postingestion in young and 1–2 weeks in adults (Chrisp *et al.*, 1990). Intestinal signs include hyperemia, edema, atrophy or necrosis of villus tips, lymphocyte infiltration, and hyperplasia of crypt epithelium. Cryptosporidial bodies are seen intracellularly in the brush border epithelium near villus tips and are most numerous in the anterior ileum. The bodies are basophilic and round to oval, 1–4 μm in diameter. Detection of the organism is by identification in mucosal scrapings examined on phase contrast microscopy or on stained tissue sections (Gibson and Wagner, 1986).

Toxoplasma   *Toxoplasma* infections, acquired when guinea pigs ingest feces from infected cats, are rare and primarily subclinical. Clinical signs include vulvar bleeding and abortion (Vetterling, 1976; Green and Morgan, 1991). Markham (1937) reported an encephalitis with associated clinical signs. The asexual stages of the organism, which may survive for up to 5 years, are distributed in most tissues, with tachyzoites in virtually every organ and bradyzoites in the brain, heart, and skeletal muscle, where they may be detected histologically. Modest immune responses occur in the host, and antibodies to *T. gondii* can be identified. Infection of the uterus, placenta, and fetus may be subclinical or cause a blood-filled uterus, fetal deaths, and abortion.

Balantidium caviae   *Balantidium caviae* in guinea pigs is usually a nonpathogenic, ciliated protozoan possessing a micro- and a macronucleus and is transmitted by the fecal–oral route (Ballweber and Harkness, 2007). It inhabits the cecum and colon, and its trophozoites may be an opportunistic pathogen in bacterial enteropathies, following mucosal damage, or with *E. caviae*, a true pathogen present *antemortem* in the intestinal wall

(Krishnan, 1968). The organism is identified histologically in intestinal wall (*postmortem* invasion of the wall occurs also) and in intestinal content and feces.

Klossiella cobayae *Klossiella cobayae* sporocysts are ingested with urine and excyst in the gut. Sporozoites pass via the circulation to renal tubule epithelium, glomerular capillaries, spleen, and lungs. Maturing schizonts contain 8–12 merozoites, which on host cell rupture pass to the proximal tubular epithelium, where second generation schizogony occurs. Large schizonts, containing up to 100 merozoites, can cause significant enlargement of infected epithelial cells. Gametogonous and sporogonous forms occur in the epithelium of the loop of Henle, and schizogonous stages occur in epithelial cells of the proximal convoluted tubules and in the glomeruli. Merozoites in the loop of Henle produce zygotes, which undergo sporogony (Vetterling, 1976). Histologic signs include presence of protozoal forms and inflammatory cell infiltrates.

Clinical and gross necropsy signs are rare except in heavy infections, when the renal surface is irregular with gray mottling caused by proliferation of interstitial fibroblasts, which may cause some renal impairment (Taylor *et al.*, 1979). Prevention involves good sanitation and removal of susceptible animals from exposure to the urine of infected animals.

Other Protozoa Many other protozoa, commensal and potentially pathogenic, have been found in guinea pigs, including *Endolimax caviae*, *Entamoeba caviae*, *Giardia duodenalis*, *Leishmania enrietti*, *Tritrichomonas caviae*, *Sarcocystis caviae*, and *Trypanosoma cruzi* (Milei *et al.*, 1989; Ballweber and Harkness, 2007). *Giardia duodenalis* has caused enteritis, *Leishmania enrietti*, cutaneous nodules and ulcers, and *Trypanosoma cruzi*, a chronic myocarditis.

Prevention and control are by strict sanitation and periodic screening for the organism. Sulfonamides are not an effective treatment.

b. Nematodes

Paraspidodera uncinata *Paraspidodera uncinata*, the cecal worm (and only common helminth) of guinea pigs, inhabits but does not penetrate the cecal and colonic mucosa and is considered nonpathogenic. There is a single report that this agent causes bronchoalveolar eosinophilia (Conder *et al.*, 1989). The worms mature in 45 days, and the ellipsoidal egg to egg life cycle is around 51–66 days. The ova, transmitted in the feces, become infectious 3–9 days after shedding. Removing fresh feces and maintaining good sanitation are essential in infected colonies. Adult male worms are 11–22 mm long, and the females are 16–28 mm (Linquist and Hitchcock, 1950).

Baylisascaris procyonis Paratenic hosts, including guinea pigs, may ingest embryonated ascarid eggs of *Baylisascaris procyonis* present in raccoon feces. Resulting larvae migrate via small intestine, other organs, and the bloodstream throughout the host, often including the central nervous system (thus the name cerebral larva migrans) where they may cause damage and inflammation with associated clinical signs, including torticollis, ataxia, anorexia, opisthotonos, stupor, and hyperexcitability (Craig *et al.*, 1995; Van Andel *et al.*, 1995). Preventive measures include exclusion of raccoon feces contamination and removal of ova from the environment. Humans ingesting eggs may become infected.

c. Cestodes, Acanthocephala, and Pentastomes

Flynn (1973) noted the occurrence of the pentastome *Linguatula serrata* nymphs ('tongue worm') in guinea pigs. Ballweber and Harkness (2007) referenced reports of *Anoplocephala* sp. and *Monoecolestus* sp. in guinea pigs in South America.

d. Trematodes

Fasciola hepatica and *F. gigantica* rarely infect guinea pigs exposed to infectious metacercariae shed from snails. The metacercariae move to a vegetation substrate, lose their tails, and encyst on leafy vegetables that guinea pigs may eat. Adult flukes mature in the host's liver and shed eggs into the small intestine and feces. Eggs require a snail intermediate host to mature. The consequent biliary and hepatic damage may cause anorexia, debilitation, and death (Voge, 1973; Wescott, 1976). Infected guinea pigs may become emaciated, anemic, and possibly paretic due to aberrant parasite migration. Lesions occur primarily in the liver.

e. Arthropods
Mites

Etiology Mites reported to infest guinea pigs include the once common listrophorid fur mite *Chirodiscoides caviae*, the demodex mite *Demodex caviae*, myocoptid *Myocoptes musculinus*, and the sarcoptids *Trixacarus caviae*, *Sarcoptes scabiei*, and *Notoedres muris*. Among these mites, only *Chirodiscoides* and *Trixacarus* are reported commonly, and then usually in pet guinea pigs (Ronald and Wagner, 1976).

Clinical Signs *C. caviae* infestation is usually subclinical, although a dense population of the elongated mites moving on hair shafts is readily apparent. Heaviest infestations occur on the posterior trunk and may cause pruritis, self-trauma, alopecia, and dermatitis. Adult males are often coupled in a noncopulatory position with nymphal females (Wagner *et al.*, 1972; Ronald and Wagner, 1976).

T. caviae, a burrowing, sarcoptidiform mite, can be asymptomatic or can produce an intensely pruritic, generalized dermatitis, with the presence and severity of lesions related to variations in host strain susceptibility and to self-traumatization (Rothwell *et al.*, 1991). Secondary infections may contribute to the severity and distribution of signs. *Trixacarus* lesions occur most often on the trunk, inner thighs, neck, and shoulders, and may be patchy or generalized. Affected skin is dry to oily with alopecia and marked hyperkeratosis.

Heavily infected animals self-mutilate, lose weight, become lethargic or, in response to intense pruritis, run, bump into objects, convulse, and may die (Kummel *et al.*, 1980; Zajac *et al.*, 1980). Less-susceptible guinea pigs show less intense signs and may carry mites while skin lesions heal. The stress of the disease may cause infertility and abortion.

Histologic lesions caused by *Trixacarus* are confined to the stratum corneum and consist of epidermal hyperplasia (or thinning) and orthokeratotic and parakeratotic hyperkeratosis. Folds in the stratum corneum contain mites and eggs. Adult mites are found in short tunnels. Spongiosis and leukocytic and monocytic infiltration occur in the dermis (Dorrestein and VanBronswijk, 1979; Percy and Barthold, 2007). The blood differential count may show heterophilia, eosinophilia, and basophilia (Rothwell *et al.*, 1991).

Demodex caviae, reported rarely, may localize in the conjunctiva and forequarters and cause alopecia and crust, and papule formation. *Myocoptes*, *Sarcoptes*, and *Notoedres* may cause a pruritic dermatitis (Ronald and Wagner, 1976).

Epizootiology and Transmission *C. caviae* was reported first in 1917, and *T. caviae* was reported in the United Kingdom in 1972 and in the United States in 1979. Both genera are distributed widely in North America and Europe and probably occur worldwide. Transmission of mites is by direct contact or via pelage, cage debris, fomites, or bedding. *Trixacarus* has a 10- to 14-day life cycle. Sows pass the mites to weanlings, to naive adults, and cool carcasses pass mites to live, warmer cagemates (Ronald and Wagner, 1976).

Necropsy Findings *Chirodiscoides* causes no abnormal necropsy findings (except for mites and ova on hair shafts) in infested guinea pigs. *Trixacarus*, however, can cause severe cutaneous lesions (Fig. 6.11) and associated loss of body fat, a pale liver, and subcutaneous signs associated with secondary bacterial infection, e.g., staphylococcal pyoderma (Kummel *et al.*, 1980).

Pathogenesis *C. caviae* and its ova attach to hair shafts and do not burrow into the skin. Adult *Trixacarus* burrow into the stratum corneum, and the pruritic response is apparently due to an initial allergic response to mite antigen and consequent inflammation.

Differential Diagnosis Diagnosis of specific mite infestations is by microscopic examination of hair shafts or skin scrapings and identifying the specific mites. *Chirodiscoides* is ovoid and elongated with a triangular anterior (Ronald and Wagner, 1976). The paired adult male and female nymphs are also characteristic of this mite. Coinfections with lice and with other mites may be common in pet guinea pigs.

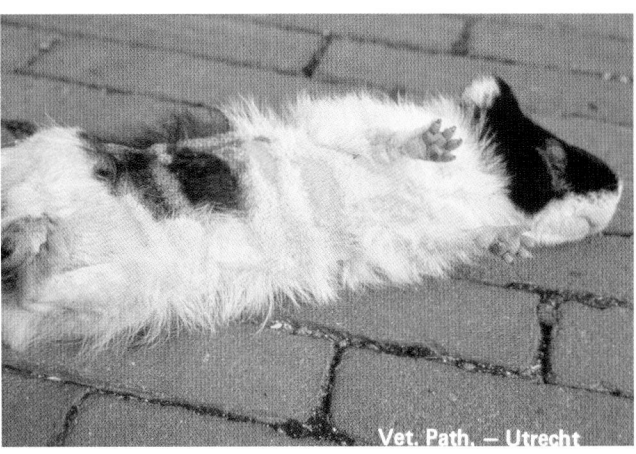

FIGURE 6.11   Severe infestation with *Trixacarus caviae*. *Used with permission: Department of Pathobiology, Veterinary Medicine, University of Utrecht.*

T. caviae infestation is indicated by clinical signs, especially pruritis, and by finding the mites in skin scrapings or in biopsy section. These mites are shorter (135–200 μm) than *S. scabiei* (200–450 μm), and skin and hair may have to be dissolved in 10% potassium hydroxide and then filtered (No. 80 mesh) to retain the mites. Mites occur more often on the lumbar region and on the lateral aspects of the rear legs (Zajac *et al.*, 1980).

Other skin conditions in guinea pigs that may resemble *Trixacarus* lesions include pediculosis, dermatophytosis, barbering, and sarcoptic and notoedric mange.

Prevention and Control Acariasis is more likely to occur in guinea pigs maintained in unsanitary conditions and not provided adequate veterinary care. *Trixacarus* lesions seem to occur in some strains more than others and in stressed animals. Control of an outbreak is by repeated treatment of all animals and thorough cleaning and sanitization of the environment. Larvae and nymphs in the environment may establish new infestations (Collins *et al.*, 1986).

Treatment Treatment of *Chirodiscoides* is by application at a 2-week interval of a diluted (water and propylene glycol) spray of ivermectin, selamectin, or pyrethrin (Harkness and Ballweber, 2007; Brabb *et al.*, 2012). *Trixacarus* is treated with ivermectin 0.2–0.5 mg/kg SC or orally thrice at 7- to 10-day intervals. Treated guinea pigs may be shaved or bathed in a medicated shampoo to loosen and remove cutaneous debris (Henderson, 1973; McKellar *et al.*, 1992). The infestation may persist despite ivermectin treatment (Shipstone, 1997).

Research Complications *T. caviae* can cause transient, pruritic papulovesicular lesions in humans (Kummel *et al.*, 1980). Guinea pigs with untreated, severe acariasis are not useful in research, especially if the study involves cutaneous responses.

Lice

The lice that infect guinea pigs worldwide are members of the suborder Mallophaga, or the chewing or biting lice. *Gliricola porcelli* is a slender louse, and *Gyropus ovalis* is ovoid. *Trimenopan hispidum* and *T. jenningsi* occur also. The lice abrade the skin and ingest fluids (White *et al.*, 2003).

Clinical signs, other than seeing the nits or the 1.0- to 1.5-mm adult lice attached to hair shafts, may be inapparent, but heavy infestations may cause erythema, scratching, alopecia, and scabbing around the ears and nape of the neck (Ronald and Wagner, 1976).

Gliricola is seen more often than *Gyropus*, and mixed infections occur. Laboratory guinea pigs are infested rarely. Transmission is by direct contact with infected host or via contaminated bedding. On death of the host, lice migrate away from the cooling body along the hair shafts.

Diagnosis is by viewing with a hand lens the adult or immature mites. *Gliricola* has a narrow head and body (0.3 mm wide), whereas *Gyropus* is broader (0.5 mm) and ovoid. Lice infestation is prevented by obtaining clean stock and by maintaining good sanitation. Control involves isolation, treatment with dust, dip, or ivermectin, medicated shampoos and shaving, and cleaning the environment.

Fleas and Ticks Ronald and Wagner (1976) report that *Ctenocephalides felis*, the cat (and dog) flea, and *Nosopsyllus fasciatus*, the northern rat flea, can infest *C. porcellus*, but occurrence in laboratory guinea pigs is rare, assuming separation from infested household pets and wild rodents. Signs reported include pruritis, skin crusts, and anemia (White *et al.*, 2003).

C. felis is an intermediate host for the cestode *Dipylidium caninum*, and *N. fasciatus* for the hymenolepid tapeworms. Neither Ronald and Wagner (1976) nor Ballweber and Harkness (2007) mention tick infestations on guinea pigs, but some tick genera, e.g., *Dermacentor*, could possibly affect guinea pigs.

4. Mycoses

a. Dermatophytes

Etiology Dermatophytosis or epizootic ringworm in guinea pigs is caused primarily by the zoophilic filamentous, dermatophyte *Trichophyton mentagrophytes*, an aerobic, ubiquitous, saprophytic, keratinophilic fungus. *Arthroderma benhamiae*, a teleomorph derived from mating strains of the *T. mentagrophytes* complex, *Microsporum* spp., and *Scopulariopsis brevicaulis*, have been isolated from guinea pigs with dermatitis (Sprouse, 1976; Coutinho *et al.*, 2001; Drouots *et al.*, 2008; Brabb *et al.*, 2012). Fungi live in soil, on other animals, or in straw, food, and wood (Medlean and Ristic, 1992; Vangeel *et al.*, 2000).

Clinical Signs Dermatophyte lesions begin on the muzzle and head (Fig. 6.12), hair, and nails and occur

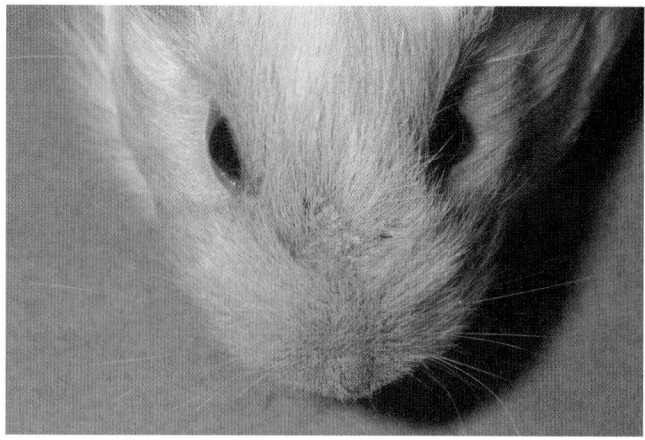

FIGURE 6.12   A facial lesion of dermatomycosis in a guinea pig caused by *Trichophyton mentagrophytes*.

most often in young guinea pigs or in guinea pigs genetically predisposed, stressed, pregnant, malnourished, diseased, or living in unsanitary conditions (Kraemer *et al.*, 2012). Subclinical infections exist. Lesions in 'hairless' guinea pig strains resemble more closely those in human skin (Hänel *et al.*, 1990). The irregularly shaped areas of alopecia, scaling, crusting, and reddening may extend to the back and sides but rarely to the limbs (Valiant and Frost, 1984; Pollock, 2003; Kraemer *et al.*, 2013). Associated with the lesion may be vesicles, pustules, and abscesses attributed to secondary bacterial infection. Lesions are often self-limiting, sometimes pruritic, and can last up to 30 or more days. Severely affected young may die.

Epizootiology and Transmission Dermatophytoses occur in many warm-blooded species, especially in younger animals in close contact. Primates, dogs, cats, horses, swine, ruminants, rodents, and birds are common hosts. Transmission occurs by direct contact with spores either on the animal itself or on fomites, such as bedding. This zoonotic disease has an incubation period of around 9–12 days.

Necropsy Findings Changes in the skin caused by dermatophytes are confined to the superficial keratin layers and structures of the skin and hair follicles. An ultraviolet light source may cause *M. canis* to fluoresce yellow green, but false positive and negative results occur.

Pathogenesis The fungi solubilize keratin with proteases, which produces the scale accumulation on and around the lesion and the loosening and weakening of hair shafts. The dermatophyte penetrates the stratum corneum or invades hair follicles. Growth continues down the hair shaft to the keratogenous zone until the growth inward equals the outward growth rate (Medlean and Ristic, 1992).

Differential Diagnoses Several conditions cause or are related to hair loss in guinea pigs, including protein and caloric deficiency, chewing and barbering, bacterial dermatopathies (e.g., *Staphylococcus* and *Streptococcus*), cystic ovary effects, acariasis, and continuous breeding. Diagnosis is by any of the following: observation of irregularly shaped, nonpruritic, flaky-skin lesions on the head; recovery of the organism from hair and epithelial debris on Sabouraud's dextrose agar or dermatophyte test media; and observation of species-characteristic morphologic features and macroconidia in *Microsporum* (or of microconidia in *Trichophyton*) (McAleer, 1980; Harvey, 1995). Epithelial debris and hair are best obtained by vigorous brushing with a toothbrush. Culture of the fungus is the most reliable diagnostic method, and growth usually occurs within 10 days (Medlean and Ristic, 1992).

Prevention Prevention of dermatophytoses involves selection of nonsusceptible animals, good husbandry, including appropriate feed and clean environment, and alleviation of stress. Dark, moist environments support survival and replication of dermatophytes.

Control Control involves improved sanitation and husbandry, reduction of stressors, and removal of infected animals, and environmental control. Infected hairs must be removed from the environment. The disease is usually self-limiting, but full resolution may take months.

Treatment If treatment of this zoonotic disease is pursued, drugs that may be used include griseofulvin 25 mg/kg PO q24h for 2 weeks past resolution of clinical signs, topical 1.5% griseofulvin in dimethyl sulfoxide solution for 5–7 days, 1% tolnaftate topically, or butenafine topically for 10 days (Post and Saunders, 1979; Valiant and Frost, 1984; Hoppmann and Barron, 2007). Oral griseofulvin is absorbed poorly in the intestine unless given with a high-fat meal, and the drug is teratogenic. Other drugs currently used to treat ringworm include thiabendazole, ketoconazole (with hair clipped), itraconazole, and terbinafine hydrochloride (Ghannoum et al., 2008).

b. *Encephalitozoon cuniculi*

Encephalitozoon cuniculi is a single-cell, intracellular microsporidian (and true fungus) affecting canids, rabbits, rats, mice, nonhuman primates, guinea pigs, and other species. In guinea pigs there are no known clinical signs of infection and few if any gross necropsy signs. The subclinical infection and infrequent use of serologic screening for the organism in guinea pigs suggest that the true prevalence is unknown and could, in fact, be high (Vetterling, 1976; Percy and Barthold, 2007).

Infective spores are disseminated in the urine and then ingested or inhaled. Transplacental transmission has been suspected in several species (Boot et al., 1988). Guinea pigs are relatively resistant to infection, and the source of spores may be exposure to rabbit urine.

Microscopic lesions occur primarily in the brain and kidney. Infected brain may have randomly distributed necrotic foci, microgranulomas, perivascular lymphoplasmacytic cuffs, and lymphocytic meningitis. Renal lesions, which may not occur, are multiple, 2- to 4-mm gray-to-white granulomatous foci seen as indentations or plaques just beneath the renal capsule, lesions that could be confused with nephrosis in older guinea pigs. The histologic lesion is an interstitial, mononuclear nephritis (Wan et al., 1996; Percy and Barthold, 2007), although lesions may occur also in the liver and lungs.

The ingested organism undergoes merogony and then sporogony in the cytoplasm of endothelial cells, peritoneal macrophages, renal tubular epithelium, and oligodendrocytes. Spores are found intracellularly and, after cell rupture, extracellularly. Diagnosis involves characteristic histologic lesions, birefringence of organisms under polarized light, staining with periodic acid-Schiff or Goodpasture-carbol fuchsin stain, and indirect ELISA, fluorescent immunoassay, and Western blot, and other methods. Serologic screening is the preferred method (Wan et al., 1996). Lesions may be confused with those of toxoplasmosis but can be distinguished by Gram stain.

Prevention and control of encephalitozoonosis involves purchase or breeding of seronegative animals, housing away from seropositive rabbits, a regular program of serologic screening and removal of seropositive animals, and strict sanitation. There is no treatment reported for use in guinea pigs, but fenbendazole and albendazole have been used in rabbits with variable results (Wan et al., 1996; Harcourt-Brown and Holloway, 2003).

c. Other Mycoses

Spontaneous infections with *Histoplasma capsulatum* and *Candida albicans* have occurred. *Histoplasma* caused emaciation, lameness, gastroenteritis, and lymphadenopathy (Donnelly and Lackner, 2000). *Candida* infection was associated with occlusive capillary embolism and tissue infarction (Brabb et al., 2012). Other fungal infections have been reported rarely.

Guinea pigs are susceptible to experimental infections with *Cryptococcus neoformans*, *Coccidioides immitis*, *Blastomyces dermatitidis*, and *Aspergillus fumigatus* (Schmidt, 2002). A normal stomach inhabitant, *Torulopsis pintolopesii*, may cause an enteritis (Kunstýř et al., 1980). *Scopulariopsis* sp., *Aspergillus* sp., and *Penicillium* sp. may be part of the fungal microbiota of the guinea pig's haircoat (Couto et al., 2010).

B. Metabolic and Nutritional Diseases

Well-managed colonies of guinea pigs rarely experience primary nutritional deficiencies or excesses,

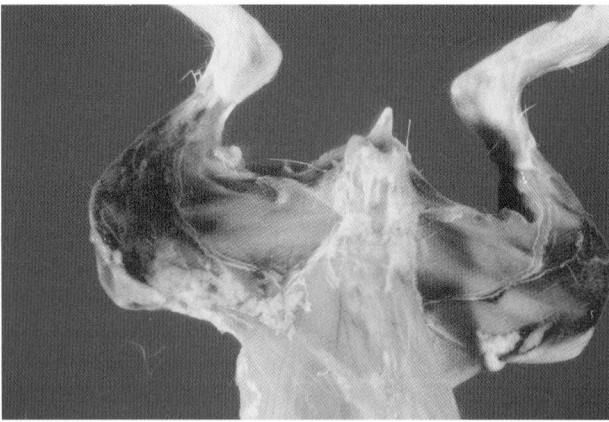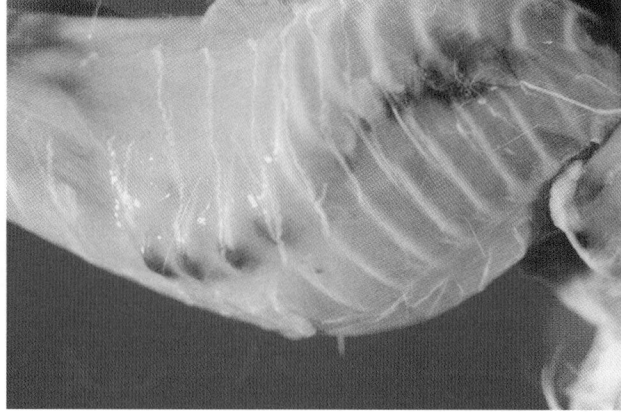

FIGURE 6.13   Scurvy. Limb (*left*) and costochondral (*right*) hemorrhages due to vitamin C deficiency in a guinea pig.

except perhaps after accidental feeding of out-of-date or improperly formulated feed with low levels of vitamin C, feeding rabbit pellets, failing to fill water bottles, or dispensing multivitamin supplement instead of vitamin C only. Malnutrition and its consequences occur more commonly in pet guinea pigs than in research animals. Under certain housing situations, larger guinea pigs can bully younger guinea pigs. This can cause nutritional deficiencies in those younger guinea pigs. This should be considered when group housing guinea pigs of different sizes. Marginal deficiencies, however, do occur in some research colonies, and the consequences are increased susceptibility to infectious disease, especially streptococcal infections and enteropathies. Signs of conjunctivitis or upper respiratory disease should always suggest a marginal vitamin C deficiency, and treatment should include vitamin C supplementation. Signs associated with many specific dietary deficiencies are failure to gain weight, weight loss, rough hair coat, pale mucous membranes, lethargy, anemia, and various signs of opportunistic infectious disease.

1. Hypovitaminosis C

Etiology   Hypovitaminosis C, known also as scorbutus or scurvy, is a multisystemic disease occurring in the small number of species (notably humans, some other primates, guinea pigs, and bats) that lack the genetic code to produce the hepatic enzyme L-gulonolactone oxidase. This enzyme converts L-gulonolactone into the isomers L-ascorbate (AH) and L-dehydroascorbic acid (DHA) (Marcus and Coulston, 1990). Probable primary roles of vitamin C are acting as a cofactor in hydroxylation and amidation reactions by transferring electrons to enzymes that provide reducing equivalents (i.e., protons) and scavenging both intracellular and extracellular superoxide radicals and singlet oxygen, whose activity results in tissue damage (Chakrabarty *et al.*, 1992). Lack of vitamin C results in defective cross-linking of collagen

fibrils characterized by defective wound healing and fragile capillaries.

Clinical Signs   Hypovitaminosis C in laboratory guinea pigs may be subclinical, accompanied by overt signs of an infectious disease (e.g., diarrhea, upper respiratory infection), or a primary vitamin C deficiency. Marginal deficiencies are particularly important in research animals because of an increased susceptibility to infectious disease. Signs of secondary (usually bacterial) infection include unexpected death, diarrhea, weight loss, swollen and reddened orbital margins, dehydration, and dyspnea. The most obvious clinical signs of primary hypovitaminosis C are related to fragility of small blood vessels, which rupture, resulting in painful bruises, reluctance to move, screaming when restrained, and swollen joints (Clarke *et al.*, 1980).

Necropsy Findings   The most common gross necropsy findings include hemorrhage in the subperiosteum, adrenal cortex, skeletal muscles, joints (especially stifles and costochondral junctions, Fig. 6.13), and intestine. The gut may be atonic and hyperemic.

Histologic changes can be extensive and are related in many cases to the absence of hydroxyproline and hydroxylysine elements in connective tissues. Epiphyseal growth centers of long bones are deranged with greatly reduced osteoid formation, degenerating and deranged chondrocytes, decreased bony trabeculae in the marrow cavity, reduced osteoclastic and increased osteoblastic activity, and multiple microfractures. Myofilaments are fragmented and mitochondria swollen (Kim, 1977). Hemorrhage occurs in many tissues.

Pathogenesis   With defects in amino acid (including tyrosine and phenylalanine) metabolism, fibroblasts and osteoprogenitor cells produce defective intracellular architecture and the products dentin, collagen, and osteoid. Junctional defects and cytoplasmic disruption occur between endothelial cells; within the muscle, liver, and connective tissue cells; in pericapillary fibrous tissue;

and in arterial intimae. Subendothelial cholesterol deposition increases, as does lipid peroxidation of cardiac muscle. Iron absorption in the gut and steroidgenesis in the adrenal gland decrease; this may be related to increased macrophage cytotoxicity (Thurnham, 1997). Macrophage migration and heterophil phagocytosis are decreased (Percy and Barthold, 2007). Cholesterol catabolism is slowed, reducing bile acid production and consequently fat-soluble vitamin assimilation, and cholesterol accumulates in the liver.

Differential Diagnosis Weakness, pain, and death in young guinea pigs can be due to infectious disease, osteoarthritis, heat stress, and toxemias. A history of inappropriate feed, decreased prothrombin time, and a serum vitamin C level below 0.55 mg/dl (normal around 2.01 mg/dl) indicate hypovitaminosis C (Kim, 1977).

Control and Prevention Foods providing at least 6 mg vitamin C per day are adequate; a vitamin C level of 250–500 mg/l in the drinking water provides adequate levels if the water is replenished daily (Groves, 1992). Vitamin C 'half-life' in solution in glass bottles is approximately 24 h. In food stored at 72°F, vitamin C has only 33% original activity at 30 days postmilling and 14% at 90 days. Previous recommendations were to use guinea pig chow within 90 days of milling; however, most commercial manufactures of laboratory chow now use stabilized vitamin C and guarantee a shelf life of at least 180 days. Guinea pigs on alcohol consumption studies have an increased need for vitamin C (Zloch and Ginter, 1995). Dietary considerations for vitamin C are discussed earlier in the chapter, but vitamin levels in food must be adequate; lesions develop in 7–10 days with no dietary vitamin C and in approximately 3 weeks on marginally deficient diets. Improper compounding and storage, autoclaving, and feeding food formulated for other species are common errors that lead to vitamin C deficiencies in laboratory guinea pigs. Pregnant guinea pigs may require up to 30 mg/kg daily, but the levels given commonly (e.g., 10 mg/kg daily) probably exceed requirements.

Treatment Treatment of guinea pigs with scorbutus involves parenteral or oral administration of vitamin C daily at levels up to 30 mg/kg. Recovery occurs rapidly over 1–2 weeks.

Research Complications Because hypovitaminosis C causes such profound and extensive changes, including decreased disease resistance, research using scorbutic guinea pigs is compromised in multiple ways.

2. Toxemias of Pregnancy

Etiology There are two conditions similar in many clinical and pathologic aspects but different in primary causation (Percy and Barthold, 2007). Both conditions are referred to as 'pregnancy ketosis,' but are best described separately as (1) preeclampsia, eclamptogenic toxemia,

or the circulatory form; and (2) fasting ketosis or the metabolic–nutritional form (Van Beek and Peeters, 1998). The circulatory form arises from abnormal vascular changes that lead to ischemia of the uteroplacental unit, and the nutritional form progresses from hypoglycemia and hyperlipidemia (Seidl *et al.*, 1979).

Clinical Signs Preeclampsia occurs in late pregnancy (last 2 weeks) and immediately postpartum. It occurs more often in multiparous, obese, stressed sows with a large fetal load, but normal sows may succumb also. Affected animals may die without clinical signs or may be dehydrated, depressed, anorexic, and underweight. Proteinuria, acidic urine (pH 5–6, normal pH 8), ketonuria, elevated serum creatinine, and increased or decreased plasma triglyceride levels occur. Unlike preeclampsia in humans (who also have a labyrinthine hemomonochorionic placentation), guinea pigs exhibit hypertension variably and edema rarely, if ever (Ganaway and Allen, 1971; Golden *et al.*, 1980). The guinea pig placenta is labyrinthine hemomonochorial with maternal blood circulating around a single trophoblastic layer over fetal capillaries.

Fasting ketosis occurs in the last trimester (after 45 days) of pregnancy but occurs more often in the last 1–2 weeks. Affected animals are weak, depressed, and dehydrated, and may die following a 1- to 3-day fast. Urine is acidic and contains ketone bodies, and other abnormal clinical chemistry may include variable plasma glucose levels, hyperlipidemia, and elevated alkaline phosphatase and ornithine carbamyl transferase serum levels (Bergman and Sellers, 1960).

Epizootology Many mammalian species, including humans, nonhuman primates, rabbits, dogs, ruminants, and guinea pigs, exhibit similar conditions in late pregnancy or early lactation, but characteristics vary.

Necropsy Findings Necropsy findings are similar between the two forms, but preeclamptic animals usually exhibit more severe changes. In the preeclamptic or circulatory form, the uterus, placenta, and adrenal cortices show petechial and ecchymotic hemorrhage and focal necrosis. Placental attachment sites, which detach easily, are also affected. Fetuses are dead and decomposing. Livers are enlarged, yellow tan, and have necrotic foci. Kidney lesions include subcapsular hemorrhage. Ketosis can cause gastric ulcers in guinea pigs (Wagner, 1976).

Lesions in fasting ketosis or the metabolic–nutritional form include marked fatty infiltration of the liver, kidney, adrenal glands, and vessel walls (Assali *et al.*, 1960). The uterus and placentae have petechial and ecchymotic hemorrhages, but these organs are not affected as severely as those in preeclamptic animals. In fasting-induced ketosis, livers develop fewer necrotic areas, if any.

Pathogenesis Preeclampsia in guinea pigs has been induced experimentally by constricting the abdominal aorta or severing or ligating arteries supplying the pregnant uterus. Pathogenesis beyond the occurrence of uteroplacental ischemia is poorly defined and only certain elements are similar to what is known of preeclampsia in humans. The proposed course in guinea pigs involves thrombocytopenia, thromoplastin release, alterations in the renin–angiotensin system, vasoconstriction, deposition of fibrin, and disseminated intravascular coagulation.

The initial causes of preeclampsia in humans are multifactorial and involve reduced placental perfusion due to insufficient vascular dilation (uterine vessels in late pregnancy only 40% normal size) and defective trophoblastic replacement of vascular endothelium accompanied by fibrinoid accumulation in and around vessels. This process in turn proceeds to generalized endothelial dysfunction through a maternal response to trophoblast antigens or vasoconstriction and activation of a clotting cascade initiated by oxygen-free radicals, lipid peroxides, and proteases. Triglyceride levels increase within endothelial cells. There is apparently a genetic predisposition to these events (Van Beek and Peeters, 1998).

Differential Diagnosis Clinical signs of depression and death in late pregnancy suggest a diagnosis of pregnancy ketosis. Acidic urine, absence of acute septicemic disease (e.g., salmonellosis, bordetellosis), and poor response to treatment support the diagnosis.

Prevention Pregnant guinea pigs should be fed a nutritious and balanced diet continuously without changes. Guinea pig breeding stock with no history of obesity or deaths during pregnancy should be selected and housed in a reduced stress environment.

Treatment Many treatments for toxemias of pregnancy have been tried, with rare success. Administration of electrolyte fluids, glucose, calcium gluconate, corticosteroids, and various combinations of fruits and vegetables provide no certain disease reversal.

Research Complications Any research project involving breeding or obese guinea pigs, particularly in a stressful environment, can have many sudden animal deaths.

3. Urolithiasis and Cystitis

Etiology The specific cause of mineral crystallization and urolith formation in the urinary tract of guinea pigs is unknown, but probably involves genetic factors, diets with calcium, magnesium, and phosphorus imbalances, cystitis, nephritis, or urinary tract environmental factors. Decreased urine flow, elevated urine pH, and the uroliths themselves may predispose to cystitis. Proteinaceous urethral plugs found occasionally in older male guinea pigs probably originate from seminal vesicle content (Wagner, 1976).

Peng *et al.* (1990) and Okewole *et al.* (1991) identified several bacteria associated with cystitis in guinea pigs, including *Escherichia coli*, *Staphylococcus* sp., and *Streptococcus pyogenes*. Cystitis often accompanies urolithiasis, lower urinary tract infections, immunosuppresion, estrogenic stimulation, or diabetes and may be mild to severe and acute, subacute ulcerative, or chronic (Peng, Griffith, and Lang, 1990).

Clinical Signs Urolithiasis is usually subclinical and occurs in older sows, but when urinary tract blockage or infection occurs, weakness, weight loss, pain on palpation, vocalization, straining, anuria or dysuria, anorexia, a small, thickened bladder, and hematuria may be seen, with some signs progressing over several weeks. Untreated animals may die (Ball *et al.*, 1991). Urine sediment may contain crystals, erythrocytes, and epithelial cells (Mancinelli, 2012).

Epizootiology Urolithiasis in guinea pigs occurs more often in aged (over 30 months) females. Urinary tract blockage by proteinaceous plugs occurs in aged males (Wagner, 1976).

Necropsy Findings In addition to finding unilateral or bilateral uroliths in the bladder, kidneys, ureters, uretra, vagina, or passed in the urine, concretions of up to 2 cm in diameter may occur in the bladder or urethra. With concurrent cystitis, the bladder may be distended with urine and have thickened, hemorrhagic walls with calculi adherent to the mucosa (Peng *et al.*, 1990; Okewole *et al.*, 1991). Proteinaceous plugs occur in the male urethra or bladder.

Continued occlusion of urinary output results in hydroureter, hydrourethra, or hydronephrosis with the fluid containing white to brown mineral sediment or solid masses. On analysis, the stones may be (in order of frequency) calcium carbonate, calcium phosphate, magnesium ammonium phosphate hexohydrate, or calcium oxalate. Individual uroliths may contain a mixture of these crystal types (Hawkins *et al.*, 2009).

Pathogenesis Kok (1997) described a progression of ionic saturation, supersaturation, nucleation, crystallization, and crystal growth in urolith formation. In the bladder, urinary protein may provide a nucleus for crystal formation (Ball *et al.*, 1991).

Differential Diagnosis Diagnosis of urolithiasis is based on clinical signs of cystitis and on detection by radiography or ultrasonography of urinary tract masses (Gaschen *et al.*, 1998). Other conditions causing hematuria or urinary tract blockage in guinea pigs are infection, neoplasia, and trauma to the genitalia.

Prevention and Control Means of prevention include selection of animals known free of urolithiasis, provision of appropriate food and ample water, and immediate clinical care of guinea pigs with cystitis. Alfalfa hay and some of the dark leafy vegetables are high in calcium. Grass hay and other sources of vitamin C may be preferable in order to avoid stone formation.

Treatment Treatment involves provision of fluids and appropriate systemic antibiotics based on culture and sensitivity (e.g., fluoroquinolones), proper diet, and, if indicated, cystoscopic or surgical removal of uroliths (Stuppy *et al.*, 1979; Pizzi, 2009).

4. Malnutrition

a. Protein and Caloric Deprivation

Protein, caloric, and fatty acid deficiencies occur occasionally when feeding is restricted or neglected, or can occur due to malocclusion. The usual consequences of these deficiencies are reproductive impairment, both infertility and death of low weight (under 50 g) neonates, and hair loss. Pregnancy and lactation may cause a negative energy balance and subsequent hair loss in frequently bred sows.

The limiting amino acids for guinea pigs are arginine, methionine, and tryptophan. Guinea pigs can produce niacin from tryptophan, and tryptophan-deficient diets can produce cataract formation (Reid and von Sallman, 1960).

Deficiencies in essential fatty acids result in weight loss, ulcerative dermatitis, hair loss, and visceral abnormalities (Navia and Hunt, 1976).

b. Vitamin Deficiencies and Excesses

Hypovitaminosis C was discussed in Section III, B, 1. Hypovitaminosis A, which is rare in herbivores, leads to poor growth, keratitis, squamous metaplasia, crusty eyelids and pinnae, and loss of organization in tooth-forming elements. Hypervitaminosis A, which can be caused by giving a multivitamin supplement, leads to degeneration of cartilaginous epiphyseal plates in long bones, abnormal bone repair, and teratogenic effects during organogenesis at 14–20 days (Navia and Hunt, 1976).

The effects of vitamins D and K in guinea pigs are not well defined; guinea pigs may synthesize sufficient vitamin K (and most B vitamins) to prevent overt abnormalities. Experimental vitamin D deficiency produces wider epiphyseal cartilage plates (Rummens *et al.*, 2002), enamel hypoplasia, and weight loss. Rickets is not a spontaneous disease in guinea pigs. Hypervitaminosis D caused by accidental dietary misformulation was reported to cause anorexia, weight loss, and death (Jensen *et al.*, 2013).

Thiamin (B_1) deficiency leads to central nervous system disorders, including tremors and imbalance. In B-deficient scorbutic animals, increased muscle weakness occurs in thiamin-deficient guinea pigs. Riboflavin (B_2) deficiency leads to corneal vascularization, skin lesions, and myocardial hemorrhage, as well as the general signs of decreased growth and failure to thrive. Niacin (nicotinic acid) deficiency in young guinea pigs produces anemia and diarrhea. Pyridoxine (B_6) deficiency in young animals causes depression in phagocytic activity of myeloid cells, and folic acid deficiency, again in young animals, causes the general signs as well as profuse salivation and terminal convulsions.

Pantothenic acid deficiency leads to anorexia, weight loss, and intestinal hemorrhage, and, if deficient during weeks 9 and 10 of gestation, causes abortion and sometimes death of dams. Choline deficiency produces poor growth and fatty liver.

Deficiencies of vitamin E or selenium or both cause similar signs in many species. In guinea pigs, primary, distinctive signs are hindlimb weakness through myasthenia or muscular dystrophy, reduced reproductive performance, paralysis, and death (Hill *et al.*, 2003; Percy and Barthold, 2007). Iatrogenic deficiency of selenium and vitamin C was reported to cause skeletal muscle cell death (Hill *et al.*, 2009). Underlying or associated signs include coagulative necrosis of muscle, testicular degeneration, degenerative changes in seminiferous tubules and reduction of spermatozoa and spermatids, and elevated serum creatine phosphokinase. Muscular dystrophy precedes testicular degeneration. Lethargy and conjunctivitis are seen in debilitated animals.

c. Mineral Deprivation and Excesses

Interactions among magnesium, potassium, phosphates, calcium, and hydrogen ions are complex and are well described in guinea pigs (Navia and Hunt, 1976).

Calcium and phosphates in excess increase the requirement for magnesium, which contributes to the problem of metastatic mineralization, described below. Guinea pigs use cation exchange and phosphate anions for removing excess hydrogen ions rather than removing protons by excretion of ammonium ions. Calcium turnover is rapid in guinea pigs.

Phosphate ions are a critical component of the causes of metastatic mineralization. Magnesium supplementation is essential to offset hyperphosphatemia. High phosphate levels lower plasma pH.

Potassium will counteract the adverse effects of excess phosphate by providing an exchange cation to remove excess hydrogen ions. Manganese deficiency produces reproductive disorders and pancreatic hypoplasia, and copper deficiency produces slow growth and myelination failure. Magnesium deficiency leads to poor weight gain, hair loss, and hindlimb weakness.

5. Metastatic Calcification or Mineralization

Multifocal mineralization of skeletal and cardiac muscle fibers may occur in guinea pigs over 1 year of age and is usually subclinical. Gross evidence includes irregular, gray patches on tissue surfaces that grate when cut with a blade. Histologic changes, notable in hindlimb muscles, include mononuclear cell infiltration, mineralization, and fibrosis (King and Alroy, 1996). Clinical signs, if they occur, include poor growth, hair loss, muscle stiffness, bone deformities, nephrosis, and death.

Mineral deposition, however, is not confined to muscles but occurs also in the renal collecting tubules, interstitium, convoluted tubules, and Bowman's capsule, and in other soft tissues, especially around elbows and ribs, and in lungs, trachea, aorta, liver, stomach, uterus, and sclera.

Probable causes of metastatic mineralization include feeding diets with calcium, phosphate, magnesium, and vitamin D imbalances (Sparschu and Christie, 1968 and Holcombe *et al.*, 2014). Mineral deposits are usually calcium phosphates or carbonates combined with other minerals (Jones *et al.*, 1996). Local low tissue pH may also be involved (Navia and Hunt, 1976). Prevention of this disorder is one of the primary reasons that food intended for other species should not be fed to guinea pigs.

6. Diabetes Mellitus

Diabetes mellitus is uncommon in guinea pigs, except in certain inbred colonies or male Abyssinian-Hartley colonies with a genetic predisposition (Glage *et al.*, 2007) or a yet unidentified infectious agent. Clinical signs can be evident at 3–6 months of age, affect both sexes, and include polyuria, weight loss, infertility, cataract formation, variable glycemia, hyperlipemia, glycosuria (over 100–2000 mg/dl), and rare ketonuria (Lang *et al.*, 1977; Williams, 2012). The disease resembles type I diabetes mellitus in humans, with islet hyperplasia, degranulation of beta (β) cells, thickening of basal membranes of peripheral capillaries, fatty infiltration of exocrine cells, and glomerulosclerosis. Spontaneous remissions accelerated by feeding hay and leafy greens occur, and injected insulin is not needed to maintain the animals; however, administration of insulin or an oral hypoglycemic agent has decreased gylcosuria (Vannevel, 1998; McNulty, 1999).

7. Anorexia

Anorexia in guinea pigs is common, especially if feeders or waterers or food (odor, taste, density, texture, form), or water (flavor) is changed. Guinea pigs are neophobic, and by 4 days of age develop food preferences and then may not recognize as food other diets, including powders, vegetables, and supplements. Other factors that may cause inappetence are postsurgical stressors, ketosis, malocclusion, drafts, illness, and water deprivation (Harkness *et al.*, 2010). Treatments include providing preferred or sweetened foods, changing feeder or waterer, treating existing disease, reducing crowding, or reducing obesity (without fasting).

8. Heat Stress

Guinea pigs are sensitive to sudden or extreme environmental changes, and such changes are known predisposing factors to respiratory disease and stress-precipitated illnesses. In addition, guinea pigs, whose ancestors lived at high, cooler altitudes, are heat-stressed easily, even when in direct sunlight at temperatures as low as 70°F. Heat-stressed guinea pigs develop shallow, rapid respiration, weakness, hyperthermia, coma, and death. Timely intervention with cool water baths, corticosteroids, and parenteral fluids may prevent deaths (Schaeffer and Donnelly, 1996).

C. Traumatic Lesions

1. Barbering and Skin Biting

Pulling and ingestion (trichotillomania) of cage mates' hair occurs primarily in group-housed, female guinea pigs. This aggressive activity may be precipitated by stressors or need to displace another guinea pig from a food or water source (Reinhardt, 2005; Hargaden and Singer, 2012).

Chewing of hair (trichophagia) may occur with or without causing bite wounds and lacerations of skin. Self-barbering occurs caudal to the anterior shoulders, but dominance-associated or agonistic trichophagia by conspecifics occurs usually on the rump, back, and ears and around the eyes (Wagner, 1976). Barbering and skin damage occur most often among status seeking adult males with or without a sow present, but they occur also when parents groom young (and nibble around eyes and ears) and when weanlings chew a sow's hair. Particularly severe chewing may occur during intermale competition for food, water, toys, or space, and with adults attacking young. Self-barbering occurs also in areas that the guinea pig can reach and may be ameliorated by feeding hay and dark, leafy greens.

Biting may cause alopecia, skin scratches, lacerations, and deep wounds (King, 1956) or severe preputial dermatitis (Lee *et al.*, 1978). Perineal wounds contaminated with bedding and feces may become infected, extend to the prepuce, and cause bleeding and urine retention, pain during mating, and decreased reproductive activity. Some boars develop a habit of scooting on a solid bottom cage and pushing bedding and material into their prepuce. Bedding adhering to the moist prepuce can cause similar signs.

Prevention of trichophagia involves reduction of environmental stressors, early weaning, separation of boars into individual cages or provision of shelters, and perhaps hay feeding. If this is seen in harem breeding, females should be separated. Females will typically accept young for nursing that are not their own. Treatment involves frequent, thorough cleaning of the wound and placing the guinea pig into a clean cage (Lee *et al.*, 1978). Few topical antimicrobials are effective as a treatment and may, if ingested, precipitate enterotoxemia.

Severe ear chewing, an aggressive behavior in groups of guinea pigs, can interfere with ear notch or tag identification of guinea pigs as research subjects. Severe ear damage may result in infections and partial or complete loss of pinnae.

2. Other Traumatic Injuries

Traumatic injuries in guinea pigs include limbs caught and injured in wire cage walls or floors, bone fractures from improper handling or dropping, diaphragmatic hernia, broken or luxated vertebral column, fracture of the liver capsule, and broken teeth. Guinea pigs may be traumatized when dropped, when leaping from a cage, from improper restraint, or when bitten by another animal.

D. Iatrogenic and Management-Related Disorders

1. Adjuvant-Induced Pulmonary Granulomas

Guinea pigs injected subcutaneously with Freund's complete adjuvant may develop pulmonary granulomas. These lesions may be similar to perivascular lymphoid nodules or focal pneumonia caused by other conditions (Schiefer and Stunzi, 1979).

2. Alopecia

Because of the high metabolic demands of pregnancy in the guinea pig, and probable genetic and metabolic factors, frequently bred sows housed singly or in groups often show hair thinning. Gerold *et al.* (1997) found few fur defects in group-housed breeding sows fed 15.5% crude protein and 19.5% crude fiber supplemented with 200 g hay scattered on the cage floor. Hair loss in breeding groups has been attributed to trichophagia. Hair regrows when breeding ceases or the social dynamic in cages changes (Wagner, 1976). Alopecia in the absence of aggressive grooming and chewing by other guinea pigs may occur also in young animals at weaning, when the hair coat changes character, and when guinea pigs are on low-protein or low-calorie diets, and within social relationships (see Section III, C, 1).

3. Dystocia

Dystocia occurs commonly in guinea pigs and may be due to uterine inertia, pregnancy toxemia, fetuses that are too large to pass through the pelvic canal, or because the os coxae fail to separate, despite relaxin release, to the 2.5–3 cm needed to allow a fetus to pass. Failure of the fibrocartilaginous pelvic joint to separate adequately occurs most often in sows bred for the first time over 7 months of age, after the symphysis usually fuses and becomes resistant to relaxin. Signs of dystocia include a still-narrow symphysis as gestation nears day 73, straining, depression, and vaginal discharge. Prevention involves breeding first before 7 months of age, preventing obesity and fasting while pregnant, and removing animals with a known family history of dystocia. Young guinea pigs involved in a dystocia experience hypoxia, which is often fatal. Treatment involves digital removal of the fetuses from the tract, providing the sow calcium, glucose, and 1–3 units/kg oxytocin (only if public symphysis is confirmed to be open), or cesarean section (Martinho, 2006; Williams, 2012).

4. Ulcerative Pododermatitis (Bumblefoot)

Ulcerative pododermatitis, or bumblefoot, occurs on the volar surfaces of one of more feet and presents with enlarged, firm, ulcerated wounds (Fig. 6.14). Taylor *et al.* (1971) isolated *Staphylococcus* from chronic, ulcerative pododermatitis lesions, which were associated with amyloid accumulation in the liver, adrenal glands, spleen, and pancreatic islets. Prevention and treatment of bumblefoot and hyperkeratosis involve provision of smooth wire or solid-bottom cage floors with bedding, good sanitation, reduction of obesity, and, in severe cases, antibiotic treatment, softening with lotion, and surgical debriding. *S. aureus* can also cause pneumonia, mastitis, conjunctivitis, cheilitis, and osteoarthritis. The bacterium has been associated with an exfoliative dermatitis characterized by alopecia, erythema, scabs, and epidermal cracks (Ishihara, 1980). Staphylococci apparently enter the skin through abrasions. The histologic lesion is parakeratosis with minimal inflammation (Percy and Barthold, 2007). Pododermatitis rapidly progresses to osteomyelitis so quick and effective treatment is essential. Amputation is not an option, even in pet guinea pigs, due to how their body weight is distributed. Some

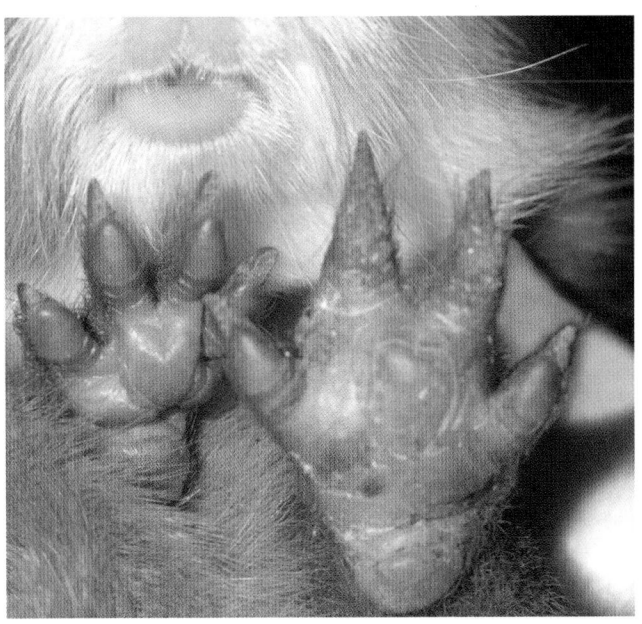

FIGURE 6.14 Pododermatitis due to a chronic *Staphylococcus aureus* infection (left forefoot).

animals die, whereas others recover and hair grows to cover the lesions.

5. *Antibiotic-Associated Typhlocolitis*

Enteropathies and deaths in guinea pigs occurring within 1–5 days of administration of certain antibiotics are assumed to result from (1) antibiotic-induced suppression of resident microflora, perhaps *Bacteriodes*; (2) loss of cecal colonization resistance; and (3) colonization, proliferation, and toxin production by transiting or resident commensals, usually one or more strains of the spore-former *C. difficile.*

Escherichia coli, not a normal intestinal inhabitant in guinea pigs, may proliferate in an antibiotic-caused dysbiosis (Farrar and Kent, 1965; Winter *et al.*, 2013). Antibiotics most often implicated are the aminopenicillins, cephalosporins, clindamycin, streptomycin, and lincomycin (Brophy and Knoop, 1982). Penicillin at dosages as low as 2000 U or ampicillin at dosages over 6 mg/kg q8h for 8 days is known to cause deaths (Lowe *et al.*, 1980; Young *et al.*, 1987).

Signs of antibiotic-associated typhlocolitis vary with drug dose, strain of opportunistic pathogen, and host susceptibility, but may include rapidly progressive lethargy, rough hair coat, diarrhea, and death. Hemorrhagic typhlitis is observed at necropsy, with the cecum distended and containing bloody, liquid feces (Fig. 6.15). Histologically, there is a severe inflammatory reaction in the lamina propria and microulceration of the mucosa with inflammatory cell infiltration.

C. difficile is a common, fecal-borne, anaerobic, gram-positive, commensal organism whose large, subterminal spores persist in the environment. Some strains of *C. difficile* produce protein exotoxins (cytotoxins) A and B, which bind to epithelial cell membrane receptors.

Toxin B is more cytotoxic but requires toxin A (known also as an enterotoxin) to access mucosal cells. Toxin A causes fluid secretion, mucosal damage, and inflammation. Cell death occurs subsequently. Drug prophylaxis is not advised; the preferred drug in treating human cases, metronidazole, may exacerbate toxicosis in guinea pigs (Cleary *et al.*, 1998). Treatment of antibiotic-induced typhlitis in guinea pigs is supportive: fluids, a highly palatable food supplement, and heat.

6. *Other Drug Reactions*

Bendele *et al.* (1990) reported that a single subcutaneous injection of the quinolone nalidixic acid at 350 mg/kg into 6-week-old male guinea pigs caused severe degeneration of middle-zone chondrocytes in weight-bearing joints by 48 h postdosing. Quinolones and fluoroquinolones should, therefore, be used cautiously in immature guinea pigs. Otoconial (inner ear cell) loss in the striola region of both utricle and saccule occurred in adult, mixed-sex guinea pigs following seven intraperitoneal injections of streptomycin at 250 mg/kg per injection (Takumida *et al.*, 1997). Recovery often occurred in 8–10 weeks. Aminoglycosides interfere with calcium uptake into otoconia.

E. Neoplastic Diseases

Neoplasia does occur in guinea pigs, especially in those over 3 years of age, but it is extremely rare in the younger animals found in research colonies. Around 25 different benign and malignant neoplasms have been reported, with fibrosarcomas, lipomas, several types of adenomas, liposarcomas, and leiomyosarcomas occurring occasionally in any of several organs or tissues. Of the hundreds of tumors reported in tens of thousands of guinea pigs necropsied, those of the hemolymphopoietic system are most common, followed by those of the respiratory system, integument (Fig. 6.16), reproductive tract,

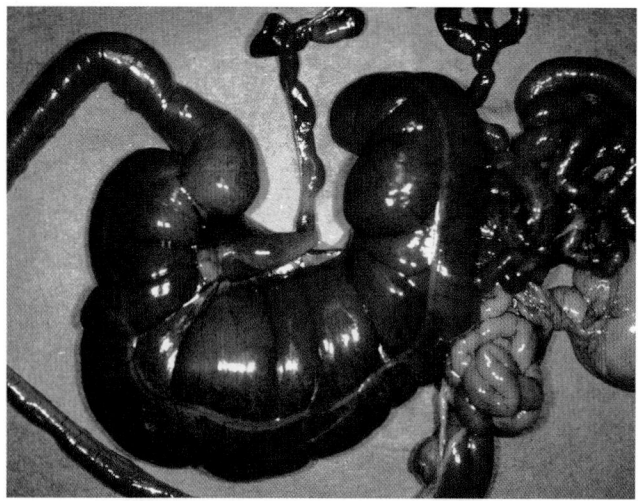

FIGURE 6.15 Antibiotic-associated typhlocolitis in a guinea pig treated with bicillin. The cecum is extremely distended.

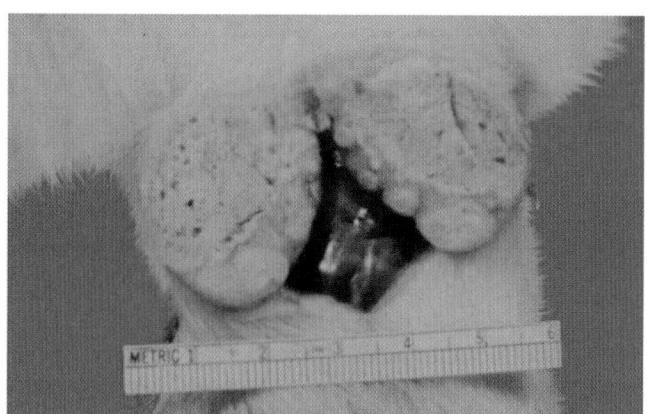

FIGURE 6.16 Trichofolliculoma.

mammary gland, hemopoietic system, cardiovascular system, and endocrine glands. Neoplasias are reviewed in depth in Williams (2012).

F. Miscellaneous Conditions

Several miscellaneous conditions that have occurred in guinea pigs are described in detail in Wagner and Manning (1976) and in Williams (2012).

1. Digestive System

a. Malocclusion

The elodontic and hypsodontic teeth of the herbivorous guinea pig are eroded continuously by abrasive materials in feed, but when malalignment of occlusal surfaces occurs, teeth become malformed and overgrown and do not wear evenly. Malocclusion may occur because of shortness of the maxilla, abnormally narrow mandibular separation (anaesognathism), nutritional deficiency, or broken or deviated teeth because of trauma or periodontal infection (Wagner, 1976; Emily, 1991). Root abscesses may extend into the mandible or maxillary sinus and cause exophthalmos. Premolars and molars are involved most often, but incisors may also be maloccluded.

Clinical signs include inappetance, weight loss, drooling ('slobbers'), oral laceration and bleeding, gaping mouth, and death. Necropsy findings include periodontal disease and overgrown teeth, often with sharp edges and points on the labial side of maxillary and lingual side of rostral mandibular cheek teeth (Jekl et al., 2008). Elongated coronal surfaces may arch, inhibit tongue movement, and force open the mouth (Legendre, 2002).

Diagnosis is by clinical signs and oral examination, which is facilitated with sedation and a penlight or otoscope. Other causes of drooling include folic acid deficiency, chronic fluorosis, heat stress, hypovitaminosis C, and dental abscesses (Harkness and Wagner, 1995). Treatment of overgrowth, which provides relief for several weeks, involves trimming the overgrown teeth to 2–3 mm above the gingiva and then filing sharp points. This can be performed with a high-speed dental bur or rongeurs, and should only be attempted in anesthetized animals. Infected teeth should be removed, the abscess drained, and suitable antibiotic given (Grahn et al., 1995); however, tooth extraction via bucotomy is complicated because of difficulty in access and the relative paucity of alveolar bone in the mandible. Because of a probable inherited component, especially in 2/N and 13/N inbred strains, guinea pigs with malocclusion are undesirable as breeders.

b. Other Gastrointestinal and Hepatic Conditions

Gastric ulcers are probably secondary to other conditions, such as uremia, ketosis, excessive stress, or perhaps *Citrobacter* infection (Wagner, 1976). Acute gastric volvulus and dilation were reported by Lee et al. (1977). Six breeder guinea pigs aged up to 26 months were found dead or with dyspnea, cyanosis, tachycardia, and distended stomachs containing fluid and gas and rotated 180° on the mesenteric axis. The diaphragm was displaced anteriorly. The cause of the volvulus was not apparent.

Wagner (1976) and Vanrobaeys et al. (1998) reported several cases of an acute, usually fatal necrotic typhlitis, or typhlocolitis in guinea pigs of all ages. Strain 13 guinea pigs were involved more commonly than were other strains, and postulated causes were experimental manipulation, antibiotic use, corticosteroid injection, fasting, torsion, or advanced pregnancy. There may be no associated clinical signs except death. Cecal impaction by wood shavings, hair, or inspissated digesta may occur.

Other gastrointestinal conditions include colonic stricture, dilation, cecal torsion, cecal and rectal impactions, rectal prolapse, and circumanal sebaceous accumulations.

Hepatic problems include contusions and focal coagulative hepatic necrosis, perhaps due to agonal hypoxia (Percy and Barthold, 2007) and idiopathic cholangiofibrosis.

2. Cardiovascular System

Rhabdomyomatosis (cardiac rhabdomyoma) is manifested by pale, pink foci or streaks with indistinct margins and is a relatively common finding in the myocardium, usually in the left ventricle, of guinea pigs. Similar lesions occur in dogs, swine, and humans. The streaks represent glycogen accumulation in myofibers or Purkinje fibers (Jacobson et al., 2010) and occur because of a congenital abnormality of glycogen metabolism. The lesions are seen best in alcohol-fixed specimens stained with periodic acid-Schiff stain (Manning, 1976; Kobayashi et al., 2010). There is no apparent cardiac impairment caused by the lesions.

3. Respiratory System

Perivascular and peribronchiolar lymphoid nodules may begin at an early age and continue as a common occurrence in older animals, and perivascular lymphoid nodules, consisting of normal lymphocytes, may be present in the adventitia of the pulmonary arteries and veins. In older guinea pigs, these aggregations reach 0.5 mm in diameter and are visible grossly as pinpoint-sized, subpleural foci. The primary cause for these nodules is unknown, but is likely related to antigenic stimulation, as they are less common in Specific Pathogen Free (SPF) guinea pigs (Wagner, 1976; Percy and Barthold, 2007). Other rarely reported respiratory abnormalities include thickened pulmonary artery musculature, osseous metaplasia in alveolar septa, and foreign body pneumonia.

4. Urogenital System

a. Nephrosclerosis

Chronic renal disease in guinea pigs has no certain cause. Autoimmune, infectious, and vascular disorders may underlie the signs, and a high-protein diet may contribute to the disease (Borkowski et al., 1988). Nephrosclerosis, seen occasionally as an incidental finding in aged guinea pigs, is characterized by weakness, anemia, dilute urine, and increased blood urea nitrogen and creatinine (Baggio et al., 1997). Necropsy signs include a pitted subcapsular renal surface with pale streaks extending into the cortex and even into the medulla. This segmental to diffuse interstitial fibrosis causes the kidney to have an irregular surface. Most glomeruli remain normal, but immune complex deposition occurs in basement membranes (Percy and Barthold, 2007). In guinea pigs, chronic renal failure may predispose to cochlear dysfunction, especially in the hair cells (Ohashi et al., 1999).

b. Ovarian Cysts

In the normal guinea pig, ovaries lie caudal and lateral to the kidneys and are 6–8 mm long and 4–5 mm in diameter (Hargaden and Singer, 2012). The rete ovarii are derived from mesonephric tubules and occur in the hilus of the ovary.

Cysts of the rete ovarii are common in sows between 1.5 and 5 years of age. The cause of the cysts is unknown, as is their overall prevalence in laboratory-housed guinea pigs; however, both androgens and estrogens may be involved in the pathogenesis (Field et al., 1989). Incidence noted at postmortem may range from 76–90% in older sows. Clinical signs include anorexia, depression, abdominal distension, bilateral, symmetric hair loss over flanks and rump, and reproductive failure (Keller et al., 1987). Diagnosis is by careful clinical examination (avoid rupturing the cyst), radiography, or real-time ultrasonographic imaging using a 6.0- or 10.0-MHz mechanical sector transducer (Beregi et al., 1999).

The cysts are up to 7 cm or more in diameter, singular or multilocular, unilateral or bilateral (right more often than left), and may be associated with leiomyomas of the uterine body or horn, cystic endometrial hyperplasia, or endometritis (Schaeffer and Donnelly, 1996). The larger cysts may cause pressure atrophy in adjacent ovarian tissues. Treatment involves surgical removal of the cystic ovaries via median laparotomy (Beregi et al., 1999).

5. Musculoskeletal System

a. Osteoarthrosis

Jimenez et al. (1997) reported spontaneous, progressive osteoarthritis of the stifle and other joints in male Dunkin Hartley guinea pigs. The condition was noted as early as 3 months of age and had become severe by 22 months. Changes in cartilage included increased levels of proteoglycans and decreased collagen. Histologic abnormalities included osteophytes, calcification of collateral ligaments of the joint, and degeneration of weight-bearing, articular surfaces. In addition to genetic predisposition, joint injury, hypovitaminosis C, and obesity may contribute to joint degeneration (Gupta et al., 1972). Wei et al. (1998) studied the pathogenesis of osteoarthrosis in depth and determined that mechanical load and stiffness are significant pathogenic mechanisms.

b. Other Musculoskeletal Abnormalities

Other musculoskeletal abnormalities include scorbutus lesions, fibrous osteodystrophy, nutritional myopathy, and consequences of injections and bites.

6. Sensory and Endocrine Systems

a. Ocular Problems

The eye of the guinea pig has a paurangiotic retina, few vessels near the optic disk, and no tapetum. Pupil dilation is accomplished by using 1% tropicamide drops or, in pigmented animals, one drop each of 1% atropine and 10% phenylephrine given three to four times within a 15-min period (Kern, 1989). Examination of the eye is best accomplished using a 20-diopter (D) or 30-D indirect condensing lens. Fluorescein dye use, exfoliative conjunctival examination, and culture are diagnostic methods.

A common ocular disorder seen in guinea pigs is blepharitis with epithelial flaking, crusting, alopecia, swelling, and reddening of the lids (Kirschner, 1996). These signs, often called 'dull eyes,' are seen usually in guinea pigs with marginal hypovitaminosis C, with subclinical infections, usually of the upper respiratory tract, or with malocclusion or renal disease (Bauck, 1989). Other ocular problems include dermatophytosis of the lids, common bacterial infections, herpesvirus conjunctivitis, and listerial keratoconjunctivitis (Colgin, et al., 1995).

Conjunctivitis in guinea pigs may be caused by chlamydophilae, streptococci, staphylococci, Pasteurella spp., and physical or chemical irritants. Panoophthalmitis is usually due to an infection with Streptococcus equi subsp. zooepidemicus (Kern, 1989). An upper molar root abscess may extend into a maxillary sinus and orbit, causing exophthalmos. Other causes of exophthalmos in guinea pigs are orbital trauma, foreign bodies, sialocele, lacrimal gland cysts or inflammation, and neoplasia (Grahn et al., 1995). Allgoewer et al. (1999) reported conjunctival lesions with lymphosarcoma.

Nodules ('pea eye') protruding from the conjunctival sac of adult guinea pigs may be a portion of a lacrimal gland (Kern, 1989) or a yellow, subconjunctival fat deposit (Bauck, 1989).

Cataracts may result from feeding a diet low in L-tryptophan (under 0.1%) (Reid and von Sallman, 1960). Heritable cataracts have been reported (Bettelheim *et al.*, 1997) in strain 13/N guinea pigs and are due to a single, autosomal, gene deletion of 34 residues that produces a novel zeta-crystallin lens protein. Homozygote lenses are completely opaque, and heterozygote lenses have a well-demarcated opaque nucleus with a normal cortex. Cataracts may also occur in diabetic guinea pigs (Lang *et al.*, 1977).

Other ocular abnormalities include ophthalmitis, ocular dermoid, microphthalmia, corneal dryness, ototoxicity from toxin ingestion, ulceration, osseous metaplasia, and an osseous choristoma of the ciliary body (Griffith *et al.*, 1988; Bauck, 1989).

Treatment of infectious ocular disorders includes topical or systemic antibiotics known safe and effective in guinea pigs, typically fluoroquinolones, chloramphenicol, and the trimethoprim-sulfonamides.

b. Endocrine Disorders

Hyperthyroidism, hyperparathyroidism, and hyperadrenocorticism have been reported in guinea pigs, but the incidence of these conditions is low (Zeugswetter *et al.*, 2007; Brandão *et al.*, 2013).

7. Multisystemic Conditions
a. Amyloidosis

Deposition of amyloid A (AA) in the kidney, liver, spleen, and adrenal glands is associated with aging or chronic inflammatory conditions, such as staphylococcal pododermatitis and osteoarthritis (Taylor *et al.*, 1971; Borkowski *et al.*, 1988), or with multiple casein injections (Skinner *et al.*, 1974). Amyloid is an extracellular deposition of polymerized serum protein subunits that have a role in inflammation (Shtrasburg *et al.*, 2005). The condition is slowly progressive, begins in the renal mesangium, and then extends into subendothelial portions of capillary basement membranes (Jones *et al.*, 1996).

b. Plant and Other Toxicoses

Guinea pigs that eat grasses contaminated with hyphal masses (sclerotia) of *Claviceps purpura*, which produces the alkaloids ergotamine and ergometrine, may develop dry gangrene of the feet. These toxins damage the capillary epithelium and lead to thrombosis and necrosis (Frye, 1994).

References

Agass, K., Ruffle, I., 2005. A refinement in guinea pig housing within the laboratory environment. Anim. Technol. Welfare 4, 51–52.

Agterberg, M.J.H., vander Broek, M., Philippens, I.H.C.H.M., 2010. A less stressful animal model: a conditional avoidance behavior task for guinea pigs. Lab. Anim. 44, 206–210.

Aldred, P., Hill, A.C., Young, C., 1974. The isolation of *Streptobacillus moniliformis* from cervical abscesses of guineapigs. Lab. Anim. 8, 213–221.

Allgoewer, I., Ewingmann, A., Pfleghaar, S., 1999. Multicentric lymphosarcoma and conjunctival manifestations. Vet. Ophthalmol. 2, 117–119.

Assali, N.S., Longo, L.D., Holm, L.W., 1960. Toxemia-like syndromes in animals. Obstet. Gynecol. Surv. 15, 151–181.

Baggio, B., Plebani, M., Gambaro, G., 1997. Pathogenesis of idiopathic calcium nephrolithiasis. Crit. Rev. Clin. Lab. Sci. 35, 153–189.

Ball, R.A., Suckow, M.A., Hawkins, E.C., 1991. Bilateral ureteral calculi in a guinea pig. J. Small Exotic Anim. Med. 1, 60–63.

Ballweber, L., Harkness, J.E., 2007. Parasites of guinea pigs. In: Baker, D.G. (Ed.), Flynn's Parasites of Laboratory Animals. Blackwell Publishing, Ames, IA, pp. 421–449.

Banks, R., 1989. Biology, care, identification, nomenclature, breeding, and genetics. USAMRRID Seminar Series. Retrieved April 3 2015 from <http://netvet.wustl.edu/species/guinea/GUINPIG.TXT>.

Barzago, M.M., Bortolotti, A., Stellari, F.F., Pagoni, C., Marraro, G., Bonati, M., 1994. Respiratory and hemodynamic functions, blood-gas parameters, and acid-base balance of ketamine-xylazine anesthetized guinea pigs. Lab. Anim. Sci. 44, 648–650.

Bauck, L., 1989. Ophthalmic conditions in pet rabbits and rodents. Compend. Contin. Educ. Pract. Vet. 11, 258–268.

Baumann, G., 1997. Growth without a pituitary? Lessons from the guinea pig [editorial comment]. Endocrinology 138, 3575–3576.

Bendele, A.M., Hulman, J.F., Harvey, A.K., Hrubey, P.S., Chandrasekhar, S., 1990. Passive role of articular chondrocytes in quinolone-induced arthropathy in guinea pigs. Toxicol. Pathol. 18, 304–312.

Beregi, A., Zorn, S., Felkai, F., 1999. Ultrasonic diagnosis of ovarian cysts in ten guinea pigs. Vet. Radiol. Ultrasound 40, 74–76.

Bergman, E.N., Sellers, A.F., 1960. Comparison of fasting ketosis in pregnant and non-pregnant guinea pigs. Am. J. Physiol. 198, 1083–1086.

Berryman, T.C., 1976. Guinea pig vocalizations: their structure, causation, and function. Z. Tierpsychol. 41, 80–106.

Bettelheim, F.A., Churchill, A.C., Zigler Jr., J.S., 1997. On the nature of hereditary cataract in strain 13/N guinea pigs. Curr. Eye Res. 16, 917–924.

Boot, R., Walvoort, H.C., 1986. Otitis media in guineapigs: pathology and bacteriology. Lab. Anim. 20, 242–248.

Boot, R., Thuis, H., Wieten, G., 1994. Multifactorial analysis of antibiotic sensitivity of *Bordetella bronchiseptica* isolates from guineapigs, rabbits, and rats. Lab. Anim. 29, 45–49.

Boot, R., Van Knapen, F., Kruijt, B.C., Walvoort, H.C., 1988. Serological evidence for *Encephalitozoon cuniculi* infection (nosemiasis) in gnotobiotic guineapigs. Lab. Anim. 22, 337–342.

Borkowski, G.L., Griffith, J.W., Lang, C.M., 1988. Incidence and classification of renal lesions in 240 guinea pigs. Lab. Anim. Sci. 38, 514.

Bostrom, R.E., Huckins, J.G., Kroe, D.J., Lawson, N.S., Martin, J.F., Ferrell, J.F., et al., 1969. Atypical fatal pulmonary botryomycosis in two guinea pigs due to *Pseudomonas aeruginosa*. J. Am. Vet. Med. Assoc. 155, 1195–1199.

Brabb, T., Newsome, D., Burich, A., Hanes, M., 2012. Infectious diseases. In: Suckow, M.A., Stevens, K.W., Wilson, R.P. (Eds.), The Laboratory Rabbit, Guinea Pig, Hamster, and Other Rodents. Academic Press, Waltham, MA, pp. 575–683.

Brandão, J., Vergneau-Grosset, C., Mayer, J., 2013. Hyperthyroidism and hyperparathyroidism in guinea pigs (*Cavia procellus*). Vet. Clin. Exot. Anim. 16, 407–420.

Brewer, N.R., Cruise, L.J., 1994. The guinea pig heart – some comparative aspects. Contemp. Top. Lab. Anim. Sci. 33, 64–70.

Brewer, N.R., Cruise, L.J., 1997. The respiratory system of the guinea pig: emphasis on species differences. Contemp. Top. Lab. Anim. Sci. 36, 100–108.

Brophy, P.F., Knoop, F.C., 1982. Bacillus pumilus in the induction of clindamycin-associated enterocolitis in guinea pigs. Infect. Immun. 35, 289–295.

Cao, Y., Okada, N., Hasegawa, M., 1997. Phylogenetic position of guinea pigs revisited. Mol. Biol. Evol. 14, 461–464.

Chakrabarty, S., Nandi, A., Mukhopadhyay, C.K., Chatterjee, I.B., 1992. Protective role of ascorbic acid against lipid peroxidation and myocardial injury. Mol. Cell. Biol. 111, 41–47.

Charles River Breeding Laboratories, 1982. Technical Bulletin 1. Charles River Breeding Laboratories, Wilmington, MA.

Charles River Laboratories, 2008. <http://www.criver.com/files/pdfs/rms/guinea-pigs/hartley/rm_rm_r_hartley_guinea_pig_clinical_pathology_data.aspx>.

Cherian, P.V., Magee, W.E., 1990. Monoclonal antibodies to *Chlamydia psittaci* guinea pig inclusion conjunctivitis (GPIC) strain. Vet. Microbiol. 22, 43–51.

Chiba, J., Otokawa, M., Nakagawa, M., Egashira, Y., 1978. Serological studies on the major histocompatibility complex of new inbred strains of the guinea pig. Microbiol. Immunol. 22, 545–555.

Chrisp, C., Reid, W., Rush, H., Suckow, M., Bush, A., Thomann, M., 1990. Cryptosporidiosis in guinea pigs: an animal model. Infect. Immun. 58, 674–679.

Clarke, G.L., Allen, A.M., Small, J.D., Lock, A., 1980. Subclinical scurvy in the guinea pig. Vet. Pathol. 17, 40–44.

Cleary, R.K., Grossman, M.D., Fernandez, F.B., Stull, T.S., Fowler, J.J., Walters, M.R., et al., 1998. Metronidazole may inhibit intestinal colonization with *Clostridium difficile*. Dis. Colon Rectum 41, 464–467.

Clifford, C.B., White, W.J., 1999. The guinea pig. In: Loeb, W.F., Quimby, F.W. (Eds.), The Clinical Chemistry of Laboratory Animals, second ed., pp. 65–70.

Colgin, L.M.A., Nielsen, R.E., Tucker, F.S., Okerberg, C.V., 1995. Case report of listerial keratoconjunctivitis in hairless guinea pigs. Lab. Anim. Sci. 45, 435–436.

Collins, G.H., Pope, S.E., Griffin, D.L., 1986. *Trixacarus caviae.* (Acari: Scarcoptidae): dimensions, population composition and development of infection in guinea pigs. J. Aust. Entomol. Soc. 25, 17–22.

Conder, G.A., Richards, I.M., Jen, L.W., Marbury, K.S., Oostveen, J.A., 1989. Bronchoalveolar eosinophilia in guinea pigs harboring inapparent infections of *Paraspidodera uncinata*. J. Parasitol. 75 (1), 144–146.

Cook, E.B., Stahl, J.L., Lilly, C.M., Haley, K.J., Sanchez, H., Luster, A.D., et al., 1998. Epithelial cells are a major cellular source of the chemokine eotaxin in the guinea pig lung. Allergy Asthma 19, 15–22. Proceedings, Providence, RI.

Cooper, G., Schiller, A.L., 1975. Anatomy of the Guinea Pig. Harvard University Press, Cambridge, MA.

Coutinho, S.D.A., Carvalho, V.M., de, Costa, E.O. da, 2001. Guinea pig ringworm outbreak due to *Trichophyton mentagrophytes* and *Scopulariopsis brevicaulis*. Clin. Vet. 6, 30–32.

Couto, M.S., Pantoga, L.D.M., Mourão, C.L., Paixão, G.C., 2010. Fungal microbiota of the hair coat of laboratory animals. Revista Brasileira do Ciencia Veterinária 17, 52–54.

Craig, S.J., Conboy, G.A., Hanna, P.E., 1995. *Baylisascaris* sp. infection in a guinea pig. Lab. Anim. Sci. 45, 312–313.

Crippa, L., Giusti, A.M., Sironi, G., Cavalletti, E., Scanziani, E., 1997. Asymptomatic adenoviral respiratory tract infection in guinea pigs. Lab. Anim. Sci. 47, 197–202.

Davis, S.R., Mapham, T.B., Lock, K.J., 1979. Relative importance of prepartum and post-partum factors in the control of milk yield in the guinea pig. J. Dairy Res. 46, 613–621.

Debout, C., Taouji, S., Izard, J., 1995. Increase of a guinea pig natural killer cell (Kurloff cell) during leukemogenesis. Cancer Lett. 97, 117–122.

De Clercq, E., Kalmar, I., Vanrompay, D., 2013. Animal models for studying female genital tract infection with Chlamydia trachomatis. Infect. Immun. 81 (9), 3060–3067.

Deeb, B.J., DiGiacomo, R.F., Wang, S.P., 1989. Guineapig inclusion conjunctivitis (GPIC) in a commercial colony. Lab. Anim. 23, 103–106.

Donatti, A.F., Leite-Panissi, C.R., 2009. GABAergic antagonist blocks the reduction of tonic immobility behavior indused by activation of 5-HT₂ receptors in the basolateral nucleus of the amygdala in guinea pigs. Brain Res. Bull. 79, 358–364.

Donnelly, T.M., Lackner, P.A., 2000. Ocular discharge in a guinea pig. Lab. Anim. (NY) 29 (5), 23–25.

Donovan, B.T., Kopriva, P.C., 1965. Effect of removal or stimulation of the olfactory bulbs on the estrous cycle of the guinea pig. Endocrinology 77, 213–217.

Dorrestein, G.M., VanBronswijk, J.E.M.H., 1979. *Trixacarus caviae* Fain, Howell, and Hyatt. 1972 (Acari: Sarcoptidae) as a cause of mange in guinea-pigs and papular urticaria in man. Vet. Parasitol. 5, 389–398.

Dorsch, M.M., Glage, S., Hedrich, H.J., 2008. Collection and cryopreservation of preimplantation embryos of *Cavia porcellus*. Lab. Anim. 42, 489–494.

Drouots, S., Mignon, B., Fratti, M., Rossje, P., Monod, M., 2008. Pets as the main source of two zoonotic species of the *Trichophyton mentagrophytes* in Switzerland, *Arthroderma vanbreuseghemii* and *Arthroderma benhamiae*. Vet. Dermatol. 20, 13–18.

Dunham, W.B., Young, M., Tsao, C.S., 1994. Interference by bedding materials in animal test systems involving ascorbic acid depletion. Lab. Anim. Sci. 44, 283–285.

Eckhoff, G.A., Mann, P., Gaillard, E.T., Dykstra, M.J., Swanson, G.L., 1998. Naturally developing virus-induced lethal pneumonia in two guinea pigs (*Cavia porcellus*). Contemp. Top. Lab. Anim. Sci. 37, 54–57.

Ellis, P.A., Wright, A.E., 1961. Coccidiosis in guinea pigs. J. Clin. Pathol. 14, 394–396.

Emily, P., 1991. Problems peculiar to continually erupting teeth. J. Small Exotic Anim. Med. 1, 56–59.

Ernstson, S.G., Ulfendahl M., 1998. *The German Waltzing guinea pig: a new strain with a new pattern of inner ear degeneration*. Presented at the Association for Research in Otolaryngology, <http://www.aro.org/archives/1998/229.html>.

Ernström, V., Larsson, B., 1967. Export and import of lymphocytes in the thymus during steroid-induced involution and regeneration. Acta Pathol. Microbiol. Scand. 70, 371–374.

Everett, K.D., Bush, R.M., Andersen, A.A., 1999. Emended description of the order Chlamydiales, proposal of Parachlamydiaceae fam. nov. and Simkaniaceae fam. nov., each containing one monotypic genus, revised taxonomy of the family Chlamydiaceae, including a new genus and five new species, and standards for the identification of organisms. Int. J. Syst. Bacteriol. 49 (Pt 2), 415–440.

Farrar, W.E., Kent, T.H., 1965. Enteritis and coliform bacteremia in guinea pigs given penicillin. Am. J. Pathol. 47, 629–642.

Feldman, S.H., Sikes, R., Eckhoff, G., 2001. Comparison of the deduced amino acid sequence of guinea pig adenovirus hexon protein with that of other Mastadenoviruses. Comp. Med. 51 (2), 120–126.

Festing, M.F.W., 1976. The guinea-pig The UFAW Handbook on the Care and Management of Laboratory Animals (Universities Federation for Animal Welfare, ed.), fifth ed. Churchill Livingstone, Edinburgh, pp. 229–247.

Field, J.J., Griffith, J.W., Lang, C.M., 1989. Spontaneous reproductive tract leiomyomas in guinea pigs. J. Comp. Pathol. 101, 287–294.

Flynn, R.J., 1973. Nematodes. In: Flynn, R.J. (Ed.), Parasites of Laboratory Animals. Iowa State University Press, Ames, IA, pp. 226–228.

Freund, M., 1969. Interrelationships among the characteristics of guinea pig semen collected by electro-ejaculation. J. Reprod. Fert. 19, 393–403.

Frye, F.L., 1994. Apparent spontaneous ergot-induced necrotizing dermatitis in a guinea pig. J. Small Exotic Anim. Med. 2, 165–166.

Galloway, J.H., Glover, D., Fox, W.C., 1964. Relationship of diet and age to metastatic calcification in guinea pigs. Lab. Anim. Care 14, 6–12.

Ganaway, J.R., 1976. Bacterial, mycoplasma, and rickettsial diseases. In: Wagner, J.E., Manning, P.J. (Eds.), The Biology of the Guinea Pig. Academic Press, New York, pp. 121–135.

Ganaway, J.R., Allen, A.M., 1971. Obesity predisposes to pregnancy toxemia (ketosis) of guinea pigs. Lab. Anim. Sci. 21, 40–44.

Gaschen, L., Ketz, C., Lang, J., Weber, U., Bacciarini, L., Kohler, I., 1998. Ultrasonographic detection of adrenal gland tumor and ureterolithiasis in a guinea pig. Vet. Radiol. Ultrasound (Raleigh, NC) 39, 43–46.

Gerold, S., Huisinga, E., Iglauer, F., Kurzawa, A., Morankic, A., Reimers, S., 1997. Influence of feeding hay on the alopecia of breeding guinea pigs. Zentralbl. Veterinarmed. Reihe A 44, 341–348.

Ghannoum, M.A., Long, L., Pfister, W.R., 2008. Determination of the efficacy of terbinafine hydrochloride nail solution in the topical treatment of dermatophytosis in a guinea pig model. Mycoses 52, 35–43.

Gibson, S.V., Wagner, J.E., 1986. Cryptosporidiosis in guinea pigs: a retrospective study. J. Am. Vet. Med. Assoc. 189, 1033–1034.

Glage, S., Kamino, K., Jörns, A., Hedrich, H.J., Wedekind, D., 2007. Hereditary hyperglycemia and pancreatic degeneration in guinea pigs. J. Exp. Anim. Sci. 43, 309–317.

Golden, J.G., Hughes, H.C., Lang, C.M., 1980. Experimental toxemia in the pregnant guinea pig (*Cavia porcellus*). Lab. Anim. Sci. 30, 174–179.

Grahn, B., Wolfer, J., Machin, K., 1995. Diagnostic ophthalmology/ Ophthalmologie diagnostique. Can. Vet. J. 36, 59.

Gray, T., 1998. A Brief History of Animals in Space. National Aeronautics and Space Administration. Retrieved 2013–05-26.

Green, L.E., Morgan, K.L., 1991. Toxoplasma abortion in a guinea pig. Vet. Rec. 129, 266–267.

Gregoire, A., Allard, A., Huaman, E., Leon, S., Silva, R.M., Buff, S., et al., 2012. Control of the estrous cycle in guinea-pig (Cavia porcellus). Theriogenology 78, 842–847.

Gresham, V.C., Haines, V.L., 2012. Management, husbandry, and colony health. The Laboratory Rabbit, Guinea Pig, Hamster, and Other Rodents. Elsevier, Waltham, MA, pp. 603–616.

Griffith, J.W., Sassani, J.W., Bowman, T.A., Lang, C.M., 1988. Osseous choristoma of the ciliary body in guinea pigs. Vet. Pathol. 25, 100–102.

Griffith, J.W., Brasky, K.M., Lang, C.M., 1996. Experimental pneumonia virus of mice infection of guineapigs spontaneously infected with *Bordetella bronchiseptica*. Lab. Anim. 31, 52–57.

Grimsley, J.M., Palmer, A.R., Wallace, M.N., 2011. Different representations of tooth chatter and purr call in guinea pig auditory cortex. Neuroreport 22 (12), 613–616.

Groves, M.H., 1992. Hypovitaminosis C in the guinea pig [letter]. Vet. Rec. 131, 40.

Gupta, B.N., Conner, G.H., Meyer, D.B., 1972. Osteoarthritis in guinea pigs. Lab. Anim. Sci. 22, 362–368.

Hänel, H., Braun, B., Löschhorn, K., 1990. Experimental dermatophytosis in nude guinea pigs compared with infections in Pirbright White animals. Mycoses 33, 179–189.

Hanif, S.N., Garcia-Contreras, L., 2012. Pharmaceutical aerosols for the treatment and prevention of tuberculosis. Front. Cell Infect. Microbiol. 2, 118.

Hankenson, F.C., Wathen, A.B., Eaton, K.A., Miyazawa, T., Swiderski, D.L., Raphael, Y., 2010. Guinea pig adenovirus infection does not inhibit cochlear transfection with human adenoviral vectors in a model of hearing loss. Comp. Med. 60, 130–135.

Hansen, A.K., Thomsen, P., Jensen, H.-J.S., 1997. A serological indication of the existence of a guineapig poliovirus. Lab. Anim. 31, 212–218.

Harcourt-Brown, F.M., Holloway, H.K., 2003. *Encephalitozoon cuniculi* in pet rabbits. Vet. Rec. 152, 427–431.

Hargaden, M., Singer, L., 2012. Anatomy, physiology, and behavior. In: Suckow, M.A., Stevens, K.W., Wilson, R.P. (Eds.), The Laboratory Rabbit, Guinea Pig, Hamster, and Other Rodents. Academic Press, Waltham, MA, pp. 575–602.

Harkness, J.E., 1997. Pet rodents – A Guide for Practitioners. AAHA Press, Lakewood, CO.

Harkness, J.E., Wagner, J.E., 1995. The Biology and Medicine of Rabbits and Rodents. Williams & Wilkins, Baltimore, MD.

Harkness, J.E., Ballweber, L.R., 2007. Parasites of guinea pigs. In Flynn's Parasites of Laboratory Animals, second ed. Blackwell Publishing, pp. 421–449.

Harkness, J.E., Turner, R.V., Vandewoude, S., Wheler, C.L., 2010. The Biology and Medicine of Rabbits and Rodents, fifth ed. Blackwell Publishing, Ames, IA.

Harned, M.A., Casida, L.E., 1972. Failure to obtain group synchrony of estrus in the guinea pig. J. Mammal. 53, 223–225.

Harper, L.V., 1968. The effects of isolation from birth on the social behavior of guinea pigs in adulthood. Anim. Behav. 16, 58–64.

Harvey, C., 1995. Rabbit and rodent skin diseases. Semin. Avian Exotic Pet Med. 4, 195–204.

Hauser, D.S., Stade, M., Schmidt, A., Hanauer, G., 2005. Cardiovascular parameters in anaesthetized guinea pigs: a safety pharmacology screening model. J. Pharmacol. Toxicol. Methods. 52 (1), 106–114.

Hawkins, M.G., Ruby, A.L., Drazenovich, T.L., Westropp, J.L., 2009. Composition and characteristics of urinary calculi from guinea pigs. J. Am. Vet. Med. Assoc. 234 (2), 214–220.

Henderson, J.D., 1973. Treatment of cutaneous acariasis in the guinea pig. J. Am. Vet. Med. Assoc. 163, 591–592.

Hennessy, M.B., Jenkins, R., 1994. A descriptive analysis of nursing behavior in the guinea pig (*Cavia porcellus*). J. Comp. Psychol. 108, 23–28.

Hill, K.E., Montine, T.J., Motley, A.K., Li, X., May, J.M., Burk, R.F., 2003. Combined deficiency of vitamins E and C causes paralysis and death in guinea pigs. Am. J. Clin. Nutr. 77 (6), 1484–1488.

Hill, K.E., Motley, A.K., May, J.M., Burk, R.F., 2009. Combined selenium and vitamin C deficiency causes cell death in guinea pig skeletal muscle. Nutr. Res. 29 (3), 213–219.

Hisaw, F.L., Zarrow, M.X., Money, W.L., Talmage, R.V.N., Abramowitz, A.A., 1944. Importance of the female reproductive tract in the formation of relaxin. Endocrinology 34, 122–143.

Hodgson, R.J., Funder, J.W., 1978. Glucocorticoid receptors in the guinea pig. Am. J. Physiol. 235, R115–R120.

Holcombe, H., Parry, N.M., Rick, M., Brown, D.E., Albers, T.M., Refsal, K.R., et al., 2014. Hypervitaminosis D and metastatic calcification in a colony of inbred strain 13 guinea pigs, Cavia porcellus. Vet. Pathol. (Prepublished Oct. 3, 2014 as http://dx.doi.org/10.1177/0300985814551423.)

Hong, C.C., Ediger, R.D., Raetz, R., Djurickovic, S., 1977. Measurement of guinea pig body surface area. Lab. Anim. Sci. 27, 474–476.

Hoppmann, E., Barron, H.W., 2007. Rodent dermatology. J. Exot. Ped. Med 16, 238–255.

Hsiung, G.-D., Griffith, B.P., Bia, F.J., 1986. Herpesvirus and retroviruses of guinea pigs. In: Bhatt, P.N., Jacoby, R.O., Morse III, H.C., New, A.E. (Eds.), Viral and Mycoplasmal Infections of Laboratory Rodents. Academic Press, Orlando, FL, pp. 451–504.

Hurley, R.J., Murphy, J.C., Lipman, N.S., 1995. Diagnostic exercise: depression and anorexia in recently shipped guinea pigs. Lab. Anim. Sci. 45, 305–308.

Inaba, T., Mori, J., 1986. Use of echography in guinea pigs for pregnancy diagnosis. Nihon Juigaku Zasshi 48, 615–618.

Ishihara, C., 1980. An exfoliative skin disease in guinea pigs due to *Staphylococcus aureus*. Lab. Anim. Sci. 30, 552–557.

Isom, H.C., Gao, M., 1988. The pathogenecity and molecular biology of guinea pig cytomegalovirus. In: Darai, G. (Ed.), Virus Diseases in Laboratory and Captive Animals. Martinus Nijhoff Publ., Boston, MA, pp. 247–265.

Jacobson, B., Kreutzer, M., Meemken, D., Baumgärtner, W., Herdem, C., 2010. Proposing the term *purkinjeoma*: protein gene product 9.5 expression in 2 porcine cardiac rhabdomyomes indicates possible purkinje fiber cell origin. Vet. Pathol. 47, 738–740.

Jekl, V., Hauptman, K., Knotek, Z., 2008. Quantitative and qualitative assessments of intraoral lesions in 180 small herbivorous mammals. Vet. Rec. 162 (14), 442–449.

Jensen, J.A., Brice, A.K., Bagel, J.H., Mexas, A.M., Yoon, S.Y., Wolfe, J.H., 2013. Hypervitaminosis D in guinea pigs with α-mannosidosis. Comp. Med. 63 (2), 156–162.

Jilge, B., 1980. The gastrointestinal transit time in the guinea-pig. Z. Versuchstierkd. 22, 204–210.

Jimenez, P.A., Glasson, S.S., Trubetskoy, O.V., Haimes, H.B., 1997. Spontaneous osteoarthritis in Dunkin Hartley guinea pigs: histologic, radiologic, and biochemical changes. Lab. Anim. Sci. 47, 598–600.

Jones, T.C., Hunt, R.D., King, N.W. (Eds.), 1996. Veterinary Pathology. Williams & Wilkins, Baltimore, MD.

Kapel'ko, V.I., Navikova, N.A., 1993. Comparison of functional load in rat and guinea pig hearts. News Physiol. Sci. 8, 157–160.

Kawakami, K., Takeuchi, T., Yamaquchi, S., Ago, A., Nomura, M., Gonda, T., et al., 2003. Preference of guinea pigs for bedding materials: wood shavings versus paper cutting sheet. Exp. Anim. 52, 11–15.

Keller, L.S.E., Griffith, J.W., Lang, C.M., 1987. Reproductive failure associated with cystic rete ovarii in guinea pigs. J. Vet. Pathol. 24, 335–339.

Kern, T.J., 1989. Ocular disorders of rabbits, rodents, and ferrets. In: Kirk, R.W. (Ed.), Current Veterinary Therapy X – Small Animal Practice. Saunders, Philadelphia, PA, pp. 681–685.

Kim, J.C.S., 1977. Ultrastructural studies of vascular and muscular changes in ascorbic acid deficient guineapigs. Lab. Anim. 11, 113–117.

King, J.A., 1956. Social relations of the domestic guinea pigs after living under semi-natural conditions. Ecology 37, 221–228.

King, N.W., Alroy, J., 1996. Intracellular and extracellular depositions: degenerations. In: Jones, T.C., Hunt, R.D., King, N.W. (Eds.), Veterinary Pathology, sixth ed. Williams & Wilkins, Baltimore, MD, pp. 50–55.

Kinkler Jr., R.J., Wagner, J.E., Doyle, R.E., Owens, D.R., 1976. Bacterial mastitis in guinea pigs. Lab. Anim. Sci. 26, 214–217.

Kirchner, B.K., Lake, S.G., Wightman, S.R., 1992. Isolation of *Streptobacillus moniliformis* from a guinea pig with granulomatous pneumonia. Lab. Anim. Sci. 42, 519–521.

Kirschner, S.E., 1996. Ophthalmologic diseases in small mammals. In: Hillyer, E.V., Quesenberry, K.E. (Eds.), Ferrets, Rabbits, and Rodents: Clinical Medicine and Surgery. Saunders, Philadelphia, PA, pp. 339–345.

Klaassen, C.D., Doull, J., 1980. Evaluation of safety: toxicologic evaluation. In: Doull, J., Klaassen, C.D., Amdur, M.O. (Eds.), Casarett and Doull's Toxicology, second ed. Macmillan, New York, pp. 11–27.

Kobayashi, T., Kobayashi, Y., Fakuda, U., Ozeki, Y., Takahashi, M., Fujioka, S., et al., 2010. J. Toxicol. Pathol. 23, 107–110.

Kohn, D.F., 1974. Bacterial otitis media in the guinea pig. Lab. Anim. Sci. 24, 823–825.

Kok, D.J., 1997. Intratubular crystallization events. World J. Urol. 15, 219–228.

Kraemer, A., Mueller, R.S., Werckenthin, C., Straubinger, R.K., Hein, J., 2012. Dermatophytes in pet guinea pigs and rabbits. Vet. Micro. 157, 208–213.

Kraemer, A., Hein, J., Heusinger, A., Mueller, R.S., 2013. Clinical signs, therapy and zoonotic risk of pet guinea pigs with dermatophytosis. Mycoses. 56, 168–172.

Krishnan, R., 1968. Balantidiosis in a guinea pig. Indian Vet. J. 45, 917–920.

Kummel, B.A., Estes, S.A., Arlian, L.G., 1980. *Trixacarus caviae* infestation of guinea pigs. J. Am. Vet. Med. Assoc. 177, 903–908.

Kunstýř, I., Niculescu, E., Naumann, S., Lippert, E., 1980. *Torulopsis pintolopesii*, an opportunistic pathogen in guineapigs? Lab. Anim. 14, 43–45.

Laird, C.W., 1974. Clinical pathology: blood chemistry In: Melby Jr., E.C. Altman, N.H. (Eds.), Handbook of Laboratory Animal Science, vol. 2. CRC Press, Cleveland, OH, pp. 345–436.

Landemore, G., Quillec, M., Letaief, S.E., Izard, J., 1994. The proteoglycan skeleton of the Kurloff body as evidenced by cuprolinic blue staining. Histochem. J. 26, 350–354.

Lang, C.M., Munger, B.L., Rapp, F., 1977. The guinea pig as an animal model of diabetes mellitus. Lab. Anim. Sci. 27, 789–805.

Lee, K.J., Johnson, W.D., Lang, C.M., 1977. Acute gastric dilation associated with gastric volvulus in the guinea pig. Lab. Anim. Sci. 27, 685–686.

Lee, K.J., Johnson, W.D., Lang, C.M., 1978. Preputial dermatitis in male guinea pigs (*Cavia porcellus*). Lab. Anim. Sci. 28, 99.

Legendre, L.F., 2002. Malocclusions in guinea pigs, chinchillas and rabbits. Can. Vet. J. 43 (5), 385–390.

Lilley, K.G., Epping, R.J., Hafner, L.M., 1997. The guinea pig estrous cycle: correlation of vaginal impedance measurements with vaginal cytologic findings. Lab. Anim. Sci. 47, 632–637.

Lindquist, W.D., Hitchcock, D.J., 1950. Studies on infections of a caecal worm, Paraspidoderauncinata, in guinea pigs. J. Parasitol. 36 (6), 37–38.

Lindsey, D.S., 1990. Laboratory models of cryptosporidiosis. In: Fayer, R. (Ed.), Cryptosporidium and Cryptosporidiosis. CRC Press, Boca Raton, FL, pp. 209–223.

Lipton, H.L., Rozhon, E.J., 1986. Theiler's encephalomyelitis viruses. In: Bhatt, P.N., Jacoby, R.O., Morse III, H.C., New, A.E. (Eds.), Viral and Mycoplasmal Infections of Laboratory Rodents. Academic Press, Orlando, FL, pp. 253–275.

Loeb, W.F., Quimby, F.W. (Eds.), 1999. The Clinical Chemistry of Laboratory Animals, second ed. Taylor & Francis, Philadelphia, PA.

Lowe, B.R., Fox, J.G., Bartlett, J.G., 1980. *Clostridium difficile*-associated cecitis in guinea pigs exposed to penicillin. Am. J. Vet. Res. 41, 1277–1279.

Lowen, A.C., Mubareka, S., Tumpey, T.M., García-Sastre, A., Palese, P., 2006. The guinea pig as a transmission model for human influenza viruses. Proc. Natl. Acad. Sci. USA. 103 (26), 9988–9992.

Lutz-Wohlgroth, L., Becker, A., Brugnera, E., Huat, Z.L., Zimmermann, D., Grimm, F., et al., 2006. Chlamydiales in guinea-pigs and their zoonotic potential. J. Vet. Med. A Physiol. Pathol. Clin. Med. 53, 185–193.

Mancinelli, E., 2012. Surgical treatment of urolithiasis in two guinea pigs. Brit. Vet. Zoo. Soc. Proc.

Mannering, G.J., 1949. Vitamin requirements of the guinea pig. Vitam. Horm. (San Diego) (New York) 7, 201–211.

Manning, P.J., Wagner, J.E., Harkness, J.E., 1984. Biology and diseases of guinea pigs. In: Fox, J.G., Cohen, B.J., Loew, F.M. (Eds.), Laboratory Animal Medicine. Academic Press, Orlando, Florida, pp. 150–181.

Marcus, R., Coulston, A.M., 1990. Water soluble vitamins. In: Gilman, A.G., Rall, T.W., Nies, A.S., Taylor, P.I. (Eds.), The Pharmacological Basis of Therapeutics, eighth ed. Pergamon Press, New York, pp. 1530–1552.

Markham, F.S., 1937. Spontaneous toxoplasma encephalitis in the guinea pig. Am. J. Hyg. 26, 193–196.

Marks, L., Borland, S., Philp, K., Ewart, L., Lainée, P., Skinner, M., et al., 2012. The role of the anaesthetised guinea-pig in the preclinical cardiac safety evaluation of drug candidate compounds. Toxicol. Appl. Pharmacol. 263 (2), 171–183.

Marshall, A.H.E., Swettenham, K.V., Vernon-Roberts, B., Revell, P.A., 1971. Studies on the function of the Kurloff cell. Int. Arch. Allergy Appl. Immunol. 40, 137–152.

Martin, J.G., 1994. Animal models of bronchial hyperresponsiveness. Rev. Mal. Respir. 11, 93–99.

Martinho, F., 2006. Dystocia caused by ectopic pregnancy in a guinea pig (Cavia porcellus). Vet. Clin. Exot. Anim. 9, 713–716.

Matsubara, J., Kamiyama, T., Miyoshi, T., Ueda, H., Saito, M., Nakagawa, M., 1988. Serodiagnosis of Streptococcus pneumoniae infection in guinea-pigs by an enzyme-linked immunosorbent assay. Lab. Anim. 22, 304–308.

Mayer, J., 2003. Natural history of the guinea pig (Cavia porcellus). Exot. Mammal Med. Surg. 1.2, 7.

Maynard, L.A., Boggs, D., Fisk, G., Seguin, D., 1958. Dietary mineral interrelations as a cause of soft tissue calcification in guinea pigs. J. Nutr. 64, 85–97.

McAleer, R., 1980. An epizootic in laboratory guinea pigs due to Trichophyton mentagrophytes. Aust. Vet. J. 56, 234–236.

McCormick, J.G., Nuttall, A.L., 1976. Auditory research. In: Wagner, J.E., Manning, P.J. (Eds.), The Biology of the Guinea Pig. Academic Press, New York, pp. 281–303.

McKellar, Q.A., Midgley, D.V., Galbraith, E.A., Scott, E.W., Bradley, A., 1992. Clinical and pharmacological properties of ivermectin in rabbits and guinea pigs. Vet. Rec. 130, 71–73.

McLeod, C.G., Stookey, J.L., Harrington, D.G., White, J.D., 1977. Intestinal Tyzzer's disease and spirochetosis in a guinea pig. Vet. Pathol. 14, 229–235.

McNulty, E., 1999. Polydipsia, polyuria, and glucosuria in a male guinea pig (Cavia porcellus). Lab. Anim. 28, 19–20.

Medlean, L., Ristic, Z., 1992. Diagnosing dermatophytosis in dogs and cats. Vet. Med. (Kansas City, MO) 87, 1086–1104.

Milei, J., Scordo, D., Basombrio, M.A., Beigelman, R.L., Storino, R.A., 1989. Myocardial involvement in Cavia porcellus naturally infected with Trypanosoma cruzi. Medicina (Buenos Aires) 49, 315–319.

Morales, E., 1995. The Guinea Pig: Healing, Food, & Ritual in the Andes. University Arizona Press, Tucson, AZ.

Murphy, J.C., Ackerman, T.I., Marini, R.P., Fox, T.G., 1991. Cervical lymphadenitis in guinea pigs: infection via intact ocular and nasal mucosa by Streptococcus zooepidemicus. Lab. Anim. Sci. 41, 251–254.

Nagase, T., Dallaire, M.J., Ludwid, M.S., 1994. Airway and tissue responses during hyperpnea-induced constriction in guinea pigs. Am. J. Respir. Crit. Care Med. (New York, NY) 149, 1342–1347.

Nakagawa, M., Muto, T., Yoda, H., Nakano, T., Imaizumi, K., 1971. Experimental Bordetella bronchiseptica infection in guinea pigs. Jpn. J. Vet. Sci. 33, 53–60.

National Research Council, 2011. Guide for the Care and Use of Laboratory Animals. National Academy Press, Washington, DC.

Navia, J.M., Hunt, C.E., 1976. Nutrition, nutritional diseases, and nutrition research applications. In: Wagner, J.E., Manning, P.J. (Eds.), The Biology of the Guinea Pig. Academic Press, New York, pp. 235–267.

Nelson, W.L., Kaye, A., Moore, M., Williams, H.H., Harrington, B.L., 1951. Milking techniques and composition of guinea pig milk. J. Nutr. 44, 585–594.

Nixon, J.M., 1974. Breathing patterns in the guinea-pig. Lab. Anim. 8, 71–77.

Obwolo, M.J., 1977. The pathology of experimental yersiniosis in guinea pigs. J. Comp. Pathol. 87, 213–221.

Ohashi, T., Kenmochi, M., Kinoshita, H., Ochi, K., Kikuchi, H., 1999. Cochlear function of guinea pigs with experimental chronic renal failure. Ann. Otol. Rhinol. Laryngol. 108, 955–962.

Okewole, P.A., Odeyemi, P.S., Oladunmade, M.A., Ajagbonna, B.O., Onah, J., Spencer, T., 1991. An outbreak of Streptococcus pyogenes infection associated with calcium oxalate urolithiasis in guineapigs (Cavia porcellus). Lab. Anim. 25, 184–186.

Padilla-Carlin, D.J., McMurray, D.N., Hickey, A.J., 2008. The guinea pig as a model of infectious diseases. Comp. Med. 58 (4), 324–340.

Pantchev, A., Sting, R., Bauerfeind, R., Tyczka, J., Sachse, K., 2009. Detection of all Chlamydophila and Chlamydia spp. of veterinary interest using species-specific real-time PCR assays. Comp. Immunol. Microbiol. Infect. Dis. 33, 473–484.

Parker, G.A., Russell, R.J., De Paoli, A., 1977. Extrapulmonary lesions of Streptococcus pneumoniae infection in guinea pigs. Vet. Pathol. 14, 332–337.

Parker, N.J., Chou S., Mahoney M., Driscoll R., Mendonca D., Conour L., 2006. Embryo transfer as a means of eliminating potential pathogens in the guinea pig (Cavia porcellus). Presented at National AALAS Meeting, Salt Lake City, UT.

Payne, B.J., Lewis, H.B., Murchison, T.E., Hart, E.A., 1976. Hematology of laboratory animals In: Melby Jr., E.C. Altman, N.H. (Eds.), Handbook of Laboratory Animal Science, vol. 3. CRC Press, Cleveland, OH, pp. 383–461.

Peng, X., Griffith, J.W., Lang, C.M., 1990. Cystitis, urolithiasis, and cystic calculi in aging guineapigs. Lab. Anim. 24, 159–163.

Peplow, A.M., Peplow, P.V., Hafez, E.S.E., 1974. Parameters of reproduction In: Melby Jr., E.C. Altman, N.H. (Eds.), Handbook of Laboratory Animal Science, vol. 1. CRC Press, Cleveland, OH, pp. 105–116.

Percy, D.H., Barthold, S.W., 2007. Guinea Pig Pathology of Laboratory Rodents and Rabbits, third ed. Iowa State University Press, Ames, IA.

Phoenix, C.H., 1970. Guinea pigs. In: Hafez, E.S.E. (Ed.), Reproduction and Breeding Techniques for Laboratory Animals. Lea & Febiger, Philadelphia, PA, pp. 244–257.

Pizzi, R., 2009. Cystoscopic removal of a urolith from a pet guinea pig. Vet. Rec. 165, 148–149.

Pollock, C., 2003. Fungal diseases of laboratory rodents. Vet. Clin. North Am. Exot. Anim. Prac. 6, 401–413.

Post, K., Saunders, J.R., 1979. Topical treatment of experimental ringworm in guinea pigs with griseofulvin in dimethylsulfoxide. Can. Vet. J. 20, 45–48.

Pring-Åkerblom, P., Blažek, K., Schramlová, J., Kunstýř, I., 1997. Polymerase chain reaction for detection of guinea pig adenovirus. J. Vet. Diag. Investig. (Columbia, MO) 9, 232–236.

Pritt, S., 2012. Taxonomy and history. In: Suckow, M.A., Stevens, K.W., Wilson, R.P. (Eds.), The Laboratory Rabbit, Guinea Pig, Hamster, and Other Rodents. Academic Press, Waltham, MA, pp. 563–574.

Quillec, M., Debout, C., Izard, J., 1977. Red cell and white cell counts in adult female guinea pigs. Pathol. Biol. 25, 443–446.

Quinn, P.J., Carter, M.E., Markey, B., Carter, G.R., 1994. Clinical Veterinary Microbiology. Wolfe Publ., London.

Rank, R.G., Sanders, M.M., 1992. Pathogenesis of endometritis and salpingitis in a guinea pig model of chlamydial genital infection. Am. J. Pathol. 140, 927–936.

Rank, R.G., White, H.J., Barron, A.L., 1979. Humoral immunity in the resolution of genital infection in female guinea pigs infected with the agent of guinea pig inclusion conjunctivitis. Infect. Immun. 26, 573–579.

Reid, M.E., Bieri, J.G., 1972. Nutrient requirements of the guinea pig 'Nutrient Requirements of Laboratory Animals' (Subcommittee on Laboratory Animal Nutrition). National Academy of Sciences, Washington, DC, pp. 9–19.

Reid, M.E., von Sallman, L., 1960. Nutritional studies with the guinea pig. VI. Tryptophan (with ample dietary niacin). J. Nutr. 70, 329–336.

Reinhardt, V., 1997. Comfortable Quarters for Laboratory Animals, eighth ed. Animal Welfare Institute, Washington, DC, pp. 15–31.

Reinhardt, V., 2005. Hair pulling: a review. Lab. Anim. 39, 361–369.

Robinson, R., 1971. Guinea pig chromosomes. Guinea Pig News 4, 15–18.

Ronald, N.C., Wagner, J.E., 1976. The arthropod parasites of the genus *Cavia*. In: Wagner, J.E., Manning, P.J. (Eds.), The Biology of the Guinea Pig. Academic Press, Orlando, FL, pp. 201–209.

Rothwell, T.L.W., Pope, S.E., Rajczyk, Z.K., Collins, G.H., 1991. Haematological and pathological responses to experimental *Trixacarus caviae* infection in guinea pigs. J. Comp. Path. 104, 179–185.

Rowlands, I.W., 1949. Postpartum breeding in the guinea pig. J. Hyg. 47, 281–287.

Rowlands, I.W., 1957. Insemination of the guinea-pig by intraperitoneal injection. J. Endocrinol. 16, 98–106.

Rummens, K., van Bree, R., Van Herck, E., Zaman, Z., Bouillon, R., Van Assche, F.A., et al., 2002. Vitamin D deficiency in guinea pigs: exacerbation of bone phenotype during pregnancy and disturbed fetal mineralization, with recovery by 1,25(OH)2D3 infusion or dietary calcium-phosphate supplementation. Calcif. Tissue Int. 71 (4), 364–375. Epub 2002 August 29.

Sacco, R.E., Register, K.B., Nordholm, G.E., 2000. Restriction endonuclease analysis discriminates Bordetella bronchiseptica isolates. J. Clin. Microbiol. 38 (12), 4387–4393.

Sachser, N., 1998. Of domestic and wild guinea pigs: studies in sociophysiology, domestication, and social evolution. Naturwissenschaften 85, 307–317.

Samii, V.F., Dumonceaux, G., Nyland, T.G., 1996. Radiographic diagnosis–prostatitis in a guinea pig. Vet. Radiol. Ultrasound (Raleigh, NC) 37, 357–358.

Sanderson, J.H., Phillips, C.G., 1981. An Atlas of Laboratory Animal Haematology. Clarendon, Oxford.

Sansone, M., Bovet, D., 1970. Avoidance learning by guinea pigs. Queensland J. Exper. Psychol. 22, 458–461.

Schaeffer, D.O., Donnelly, T.M., 1996. Disease problems of guinea pigs and chinchillas. In: Hillyer, E.V., Quesenberry, K.E. (Eds.), Ferrets, Rabbits, and Rodents: Clinical Medicine and Surgery. Saunders, Philadelphia, PA, pp. 260–281.

Schalm, O.W., Jain, N.C., Carroll, E.J., 1975. Veterinary Hematology, third ed. Lea & Febiger, Philadelphia, PA.

Schermer, S., 1967. The Blood Morphology of Laboratory Animals. Davis, Philadelphia, PA.

Schiefer, B., Stunzi, H., 1979. Pulmonary lesions in guinea pigs and rats after subcutaneous injection of Freund's complete adjuvant on homologous pulmonary tissue. Zentralbl. Veterinarmed. Reihe A 26, 1–10.

Schmeer, N., Weiss, R., Reinacher, M., Krauss, H., Karo, M., 1985. Course of chlamydia-induced inclusion conjunctivitis in the guinea pig in experimental animal husbandry. Z Versuchstierkd 27, 233–240.

Schmidt, A., 2002. Animal models of aspergillosis - also useful for vaccination strategies? Mycoses 45 (1–2), 38–40.

Schoondermark-van de Ven, E.M., Philipse-Bergmann, I.M., van der Logt, J.T., 2006. Prevalence of naturally occurring viral infections, *Mycoplasma pulmonis* and *Clostridium piliforme* in laboratory rodents in Western Europe screened from 2000 to 2003. Lab. Anim. 40, 137–143.

Seidl, D.C., Hughes, H.C., Bertolet, R., Lang, C.M., 1979. True pregnancy toxemia (preeclampsia) in the guinea pig *(Cavia porcellus)*. Lab. Anim. Sci. 29, 472–478.

Shi, F., Mochida, K., Suzuki, O., Matsuda, J., Ogura, A., Tsonis, C.G., et al., 2000. Development of embryos in superovulated guinea pigs following active immunization against the inhibin alpha-subunit. Endocr. J. 47, 451–459.

Shipstone, M., 1997. *Trixacarus caviae* infection in a guinea pig: failure to respond to ivermectin administration. Aust. Vet. Pract. 27, 143–146.

Shomer, N.H., Dangler, C.A., Whary, M.T., Fox, J.G., 1988. Experimental Helicobacter pylori infection induces antral gastritis and gastric mucosa-associated lymphoid tissue in guinea pigs. Infect. Immun. 66 (6), 2614–2618.

Short, D.J., Woodnott, D.P. (Eds.), 1969. The Institute of Animal Technicians Manual of Laboratory Animal Practice and Techniques. Thomas, Springfield, Illinois.

Shtrasburg, S., Gal, R., Gruys, E., Perl, S., Martin, B.M., Kaplan, B., et al., 2005. An ancillary tool for the diagnosis of amyloid A amyloidosis in a variety of domestic and wild animals. Vet. Pathol. 42, 132–139.

Sisk, D.B., 1976. Physiology. In: Wagner, J.E., Manning, P.J. (Eds.), The Biology of the Guinea Pig. Academic Press, New York, pp. 63–98.

Sjunnesson, H., Sturegard, E., Hynes, S., Willen, R., Feinstein, R., Wadstrom, T., 2003. Five month persistence of Helicobacter pylori infection in guinea pigs. APMIS 111 (6), 634–642.

Skinner, M., Cathcart, E.S., Cohen, A.S., Benson, M.D., 1974. Isolation and identification by sequence analysis of experimentally induced guinea pig amyloid fibrils. J. Exp. Med. 140, 871–876.

Smith, I.M., Baskerville, A.J., 1979. A selective medium facilitating the isolation and recognition of *Bordetella bronchiseptica* in pigs. Res. Vet. Sci. 27, 187–192.

Sparschu, G.L., Christie, R.J., 1968. Metastatic calcification in a guinea pig colony. Lab. Anim. Care 18, 520–527.

Sprouse, R.F., 1976. Mycoses. In: Wagner, J.E., Manning, P.J. (Eds.), The Biology of the Guinea Pig. Academic Press, New York, pp. 153–161.

Stalheim, O.H.V., Matthews, P.J., 1975. Mycoplasmosis in specific-pathogen-free and conventional guinea pigs. Lab. Anim. Sci. 25, 70–71.

Stephens, R.S., Myers, G., Eppinger, M., Bavoil, P.M., 2009. Divergence without difference: phylogenetics and taxonomy of Chlamydia resolved. FEMS Immunol. Med. Microbiol. 55, 115–119.

Stockard, C.R., Papanicolaou, G.N., 1917. The existence of a typical oestrous cycle in the guinea pig – with a study of its histological and physiological changes. Am. J. Anat. 22, 225–283.

Stockard, C.R., Papanicolaou, G.N., 1919. The vaginal closure membrane, copulation, and the vaginal plug in the guinea–pig, with further considerations of the oestrous rhythm. Biol. Bull. 37 (4), 222–245.

Stuppy, D.E., Douglass, P.R., Douglass, P.J., 1979. Urolithiasis and cystotomy in a guinea pig (*Cavia porcellanus*). Vet. Med. Small Anim. Clin. 74, 565–567.

Takumida, M., Zhang, D.M., Yajin, K., Harada, Y., 1997. Effect of streptomycin on the otoconial layer of the guinea pig. J. Oto-Rhino-Laryngol. Relat. Spec. (Basel) 59, 263–268.

Taouji, S., Buat, M.-L., Izard, J., Landemore, G., 1994. Kurloff cell lyso-somal arylsulphatases: presence of both cationic and highly anionic isoforms of the sole B class. Biol. Cell 80, 43–48.

Taylor, J.L., Wagner, T.E., Owens, D.R., Stuhlman, R.A., 1971. Chronic pododermatitis in guinea pigs: a case report. Lab. Anim. Sci. 21, 944–945.

Thurnham, D.I., 1997. Micronutrients and immune function: some recent developments. J. Clin. Pathol. 50, 887–891.

Timoney, J.F., Artiushin, S.C., Boschwitz, J.S., 1997. Comparison of the sequences and functions of *Streptococcus equi* pr-like proteins SeM and SzPSe. Infect. Immun. 65, 3600–3605.

Trahan, C.J., Stephenson, E.H., Ezzell, J.W., Mitchell, W.C., 1987. Airborne-induced experimental *Bordetella bronchiseptica* pneumonia in strain 13 guineapigs. Lab. Anim. 21, 226–232.

Ueda, H., Kosaka, T., Takahashi, K.W., 1998. Intraperitoneal insemination of the guinea pig with synchronized estrus induced by progesterone implant. Exp. Anim. 47, 271–275.

U.S. Department of Agriculture, Animal and Plant Health Inspection Service-Animal Care, 2010. Animal Welfare Report – Fiscal Year 2010. USDA, Washington, DC.

Valiant, M.E., Frost, B.M., 1984. An experimental model for evaluation of antifungal agents in a *Trichophyton mentagrophytes* infection of guinea pigs. Chemotherapy 30, 54–60.

Van Andel, R.A., Franklin, C.L., Besch-Williford, C., Riley, L.K., Hook Jr., R.R., Kazacos, K.R., 1995. Cerebrospinal larva migrans due to

Baylisascaris procyonis in a guinea pig colony. Lab. Anim. Sci. 45, 27–30.

Van Beek, E., Peeters, L.L.H., 1998. Pathogenesis of preeclampsia: a comprehensive model. Obstet. Gynecol. Surv. 53, 233–239.

van der Linden, M., Al-Lahham, A., Nicklas, W., Reinert, R.R., 2009. Molecular characterization of pneumococcal isolates from pets and laboratory animals. PLoS One 4 (12), e8286.

Vangeel, I., Pasmans, F., Vanrobaeys, M., De Herdt, P., Haesebrouck, F., 2000. Prevalence of dermatophytes in asymptomatic guinea pigs and rabbits. Vet. Rec. 146, 440–441.

Van Hoosier Jr., G.L., Robinette, L.R., 1976. Viral and chlamydial diseases. In: Wagner, J.E., Manning, P.J. (Eds.), The Biology of the Guinea Pig. Academic Press, New York, pp. 137–152.

Vannevel, J., 1998. Diabetes mellitus in a 3-year old, intact, female guinea pig. Can. Vet. J. 39, 503.

Vanrobaeys, M., de Herdt, P., Ducatelle, R., Devrise, L.A., Charlier, G., Haesebrouck, F., 1998. Typhlitis caused by intestinal *Serpulina*-like bacteria in domestic guinea pigs (*Cavia porcellus*). J. Clin. Micro. 36, 690–694.

Vetterling, J.M., 1976. Protozoan parasites. In: Wagner, J.E., Manning, P.J. (Eds.), The Biology of the Guinea Pig. Academic Press, New York, pp. 163–196.

Vieira, E.B., Menescal-de-Oliveira, L., Leite-Panissi, C.R.A., 2011. Functional mapping of the periaquaductal gray matter involved in organizing tonic immobility behavior in guinea pigs. Behavioural Brain Res. 216, 94–99.

Voge, M., 1973. Trematodes. In: Flynn, R. (Ed.), Parasites of Laboratory Animals. Iowa State University Press, Ames, IA, pp. 120–154.

Waggie, K.S., Wagner, J.E., Kelley, S.T., 1986. Naturally occurring *Bacillus piliformis* infection (Tyzzer's disease) in guinea pigs. Lab. Anim. Sci. 36, 504–506.

Wagner, J.E., 1976. Miscellaneous disease conditions of guinea pigs. In: Wagner, J.E., Manning, P.J. (Eds.), The Biology of the Guinea Pig. Academic Press, New York, pp. 227–234.

Wagner, J.E., Foster, H.L., 1976. Germfree and specific pathogen free. In: Wagner, J.E., Manning, P.J. (Eds.), The Biology of the Guinea Pig. Academic Press, New York, pp. 21–30.

Wagner, J.E., Manning, P.J. (Eds.), 1976. The Biology of the Guinea Pig. Academic Press, New York.

Wagner, J.E., Al-Rabiai, S., Rings, R.W., 1972. *Chirodiscoides caviae* infestation in guinea pigs. Lab. Anim. Sci. 22, 750–752.

Walters, S.L., Torres-Urbana, C.J., Chichester, L., Rose, R.E., 2012. The impact of huts on physiological stress: a refinement in post-transport housing of male guinea pigs (*Cavia porcellus*). Lab. Anim. 46, 220–224.

Wan, C.-H., Franklin, C., Riley, L.K., Hook Jr., R.R., Besch-Williford, C., 1996. Diagnostic exercise: granulomatous encephalitis in guinea pigs. Lab. Anim. Sci. 46, 228–230.

Wei, L., deBri, E., Lundberg, A., Svensson, O., 1998. Mechanical load and primary guinea pig osteoarthrosis. Acta Orthop. Scand. 69, 351–357.

Wescott, R.B., 1976. Helminth parasites. In: Wagner, J.E., Manning, P.J. (Eds.), The Biology of the Guinea Pig. Academic Press, New York, pp. 197–200.

White, S.D., Bourdeau, P.J., Meredith, A., 2003. Dermatologic problems in guinea pigs. Comp. Cont. Educ. Prac. 25, 690–697.

White, W.J., Lang, C.M., 1989. The guinea pig. In: Loeb, W.F., Quimby, F.W. (Eds.), The Clinical Chemistry of Laboratory Animals. Pergamon Press, New York, pp. 27–30.

White, W.J., Balk, M.W., Lang, C.M., 1989. Use of cage space by guinea pigs. Lab. Anim. 23, 208–214.

Williams, B.H., 2012. Non-infectious diseases. In: Suckow, M.A., Stevens, K.A., Wilson, R.P. (Eds.), The Laboratory Rabbit, Guinea Pig, Hamster, and Other Rodents. Elsevier, Waltham, MA, pp. 685–704.

Winter, S.E., Lopez, C.A., Bäumler, A.J., 2013. The dynamics of gut-associated microbial communities during inflammation. EMBO Rep. 14 (4), 319–327.

Witt, W.M., Hubbard, G.B., Fanton, T., 1988. *Streptococcus pneumoniae* arthritis and osteomyelitis with vitamin C deficiency in guinea pigs. Lab. Anim. Sci. 38, 192–194.

Wolf, B., Reinecke, K., Aumann, K.-D., Brigelius-Flohe, R., Flohe, L., 1993. Taxonomical classification of the guinea pig based on its Cu/Zn superoxide dismutase sequence. Biol. Chem. Hoppe-Seyler 374, 641–649.

Wright, J., 1936. An epidemic of *Pasteurella* infection in guinea pig stock. J. Pathol. Bacteriol. 42, 209–212.

Wullenweber, M., Boot, R., 1994. Interlaboratory comparison of enzyme-linked immunosorbent assay (ELISA) and indirect immunofluorescence for detection of *Bordetella bronchiseptica* antibodies in guinea pigs. Lab. Anim. 28, 335–339.

Yanagimachi, R., Mahi, C.A., 1976. The sperm acrosome reaction and fertilization in the guinea pig: a study in vivo. J. Repord. Fert. 46, 49–54.

Young, J.D., Hust, W.J., White, W.J., Lang, C.M., 1987. An evaluation of ampicillin pharmacokinetics and toxicity in guinea pigs. Lab. Anim. Sci. 37, 652–656.

Zajac, A., Williams, J.F., Williams, C.S.F., 1980. Mange caused by *Trixacarus caviae* in guinea pigs. J. Am. Vet. Med. Assoc. 177, 900–903.

Zarrow, M.X., 1947. Relaxin content of blood, urine, and other tissues of pregnant and postpartum guinea pigs. Proc. Soc. Exp. Biol. Med. 66, 488–491.

Zeugswetter, F., Fenske, M., Hassan, J., Kunzel, F., 2007. Cushing's syndrome in a guinea pig. Vet. Rec. 160, 878–880.

Zloch, Z., Ginter, E., 1995. Moderate alcohol consumption and vitamin C status in the guinea-pig and the rat. Physiol. Res. 44, 173–176.

Zwicker, G.M., Dagle, G.E., Adee, R.R., 1978. Naturally occurring Tyzzer's disease and intestinal spirochetosis in guinea pigs. Lab. Anim. Sci. 28, 193–198.

CHAPTER

7

Biology and Diseases of Other Rodents

Thomas M. Donnelly BVSc, DACLAM, DABVP, DECZM[a],
Ingrid Bergin VMD, MS, DACLAM, DACVP[b]
and Melanie Ihrig DVM, MS, DACLAM[c]

[a]French National Veterinary School of Alfort, du General de Gaulle, Maisons-Alfort, France
[b]Unit for Laboratory Animal Medicine Pathologist, In Vivo Animal Core,
University of Michigan, Ann Arbor, Michigan, USA
[c]Comparative Medicine, Houston Methodist Research Institute, Houston, TX, USA

OUTLINE

I. INTRODUCTION

Although laboratory rats and mice constitute over 90% of all vertebrates used in research, other species also have contributed significantly to innovations in the biomedical sciences. Rodents of other species account for less than 0.5% of rodents used annually; however, they too have been responsible for insights into biological processes and disease pathogenesis. In this chapter some of these less common species are described with respect to their research use, biology, husbandry, and disease susceptibility. The website of the National Research Council's Institute for Laboratory Animal Research contains additional links to online databases for repositories of animal models and less common species (ILAR, 2014).

A. Special Considerations

Before considering each species, there are some general concerns relating to the use of nontraditional rodents in research. These include Institutional Animal Care and Use Committee (IACUC) oversight of field studies, zoonotic disease risk, and the risk of disease transmission from wild-origin rodents to traditional laboratory rodent species.

1. IACUC Issues

The 2011 Guidelines of the American Society of Mammalogists summarizes some of the issues arising from IACUC oversight of field studies using nontraditional rodents (Sikes and Gannon, 2011). While rats of the genus *Rattus* and mice of the genus *Mus* are exempt from the Animal Welfare Act (AWA), other rodents species are not. The AWA indicates that field study "that does not harm, or materially alter the behavior of the animal under study" is exempt from IACUC review (9 CFR 1.1), however this leaves a considerable gray zone depending on how one defines 'harm' or 'altered behavior'. For Public Health Service-funded studies, the use of any vertebrate animal requires IACUC oversight, including those in field studies. Additionally, the requirements under the AWA for USDA reporting are retroactive. Thus, while many 'observation only' or 'live trapping' field studies will fall under USDA pain category C (no or slight pain or distress), if inadvertent injury occurs resulting in pain or necessitating euthanasia, the animal must be reported in the higher pain category (Sikes and Gannon, 2011). These and other issues pertaining to the special circumstances of IACUC oversight of field studies should be understood by both IACUC members and investigators.

2. Occupational Health Issues

The use of nontraditional rodents also raises questions about zoonotic disease risk, particularly in the context of wild-caught animals or in field studies. Clearly the health of researchers and animal husbandry personnel must be paramount. Yet this must be balanced by contextually appropriate consideration of actual disease risk and the impact on an individual's ability to carry out their job. As an example, the CDC-recommended PPE originally recommended for prevention of hantavirus infection in field researchers using *Peromyscus leucopus* (white-footed mouse) included a powered air-purifying respirator (PAPR), a device that restricts mobility and visibility in a field situation, predisposing the wearer to falls (Hafner, 2007). The subsequent update to these guidelines took a more practical and risk assessment-based approach, considering evidence that researchers were far more likely to become infected by living in cabins and other seasonal dwellings chronically inhabited by mice than by trapping or handling mice (Kelt and Hafner, 2010). Thus avoidance or cleaning of contaminated dwellings (with appropriate HEPA filter-respiratory protection) was emphasized and PPE recommendations for field handling of animals were reduced (Kelt and Hafner, 2010). As another example of context affecting disease risk, many zoonoses of wild-caught rodents are spread by fleas or ticks, and thus pose little concern to animal husbandry personnel in a laboratory setting with properly conditioned animals. Depending on the agent, investigators using the same animals may face a small risk in the case of needlestick injuries (Herwaldt, 2001). These examples illustrate that occupational health recommendations and practices must take into account the biology of transmission and a realistic, context-specific risk assessment.

3. Implications for Colony Health

Besides disease transmission to humans, nontraditional rodents in a colony, particularly wild-caught ones, may pose a disease transmission risk to traditional laboratory rodent species. There are few studies looking at disease agents in wild nontraditional rodents that may be infective for laboratory rats and mice. Most studies have investigated the incidence and pathogenicity of mycoplasma strains. Koshimizu *et al.* (1993) isolated *Mycoplasma pulmonis* and *M. arthritidis* from healthy wild *Rattus argentiventer* (rice field rat) and *R. exulans* (Polynesian rat), but did not isolate mycoplasma from *Myodes smithii* (Smith's vole) or *Millardia meltada* (Indian soft-furred rat). The pathogenicity of these mycoplasma isolates to laboratory mice and rats was not investigated. Goto *et al.* (1993) isolated five novel mycoplasma strains from *Suncus murinus* (Asian musk shrew). The mycoplasma strains caused no gross or microscopic lesions in animals from which they were isolated and were not infective for mice and rats. Evans-Davis *et al.* (1998) isolated a new species of mycoplasma, *M. volis*, from healthy field-trapped *Microtus ochrogaster* (prairie vole). Infection of laboratory rats and mice with *M. volis* resulted in seroconversion, development of microscopic lung lesions but no clinical signs. Consequently we know that serological or polymersae chain reaction (PCR)-screening may be used to detect known rodent disease agents. However, novel rodent viruses or other pathogens associated with nontraditional rodents may not be detected and the impact of these agents on traditional rodent species is unknown. Moreover, exposure to novel

rodent agents may arise not only from non-traditional rodents housed in an animal facility but also from wild rodents that inadvertently gain entry to a facility. A study in Michigan suggests that the prevalence of significant laboratory disease agents in wild rodent populations may not be as high as anticipated. Dyson *et al.* (2009) demonstrated that *Helicobacter* spp. were the most commonly detected infection in necropsied wild-caught *Peromyscus leucopus* (white footed mouse). In the same study, serology was negative for 14 viral agents tested. Serum from wild-caught rodents used in serology may be limited in sensitivity, as reliance on cross-reactivity can decrease efficacy of serological testing (Niewiesk and Prince, 2002). This is an important point in designing surveillance programs. Dirty bedding systems with conventional outbred mouse sentinels will remove the concern of wild rodent serum cross-reactivity, but the efficiency of disease agent transfer will vary depending on the infectious agent and the husbandry practices at a given institution. Detection using more direct (and expensive) techniques such as necropsy and histology are not without value in specific circumstances but have limited sensitivity as screening tools because many zoonotic or animal disease agents cause no lesions or nonspecific lesions in the host species. Thus the basic recommendation to prevent disease transmission from wild-caught nontraditional rodents should be based on a case-by-case risk-assessment plan that takes into account what is known about the wild-caught rodent to be housed, the infectious agents with the highest likelihood of occurrence, the biology of these agents, and the available means for disease transmission control. As with control of zoonotic diseases, control of disease transmission to animals must incorporate context-appropriate recommendations that address the concern but do not fall into the trap of intervention disproportionate to risk. Effective prophylaxis against a significant number of known or unknown disease agents can be achieved by standard good husbandry practices. These practices include quarantine and conditioning programs, housing species separately, a sentinel program using standard laboratory mice or rats, and prevention of airspace or fomite interspecies transmission (e.g., proper microisolator technique). Proposed measures for rodent disease control must balance cost, experimental needs, anticipated outcome severity, and the likelihood of disease transmission.

B. Rodent Taxonomy

The order Rodentia is the largest order of living Mammalia with 2277 species placed in 28 families or approximately 42% of worldwide mammalian biodiversity (Carleton and Musser, 2005). They are found worldwide except in Antarctica and on some oceanic islands. Ecologically, they are remarkably diverse. Some species spend their entire lives above the ground in the canopy of rainforests; others rarely emerge from beneath the ground. Some species are highly aquatic, while others are equally specialized for life in deserts. Many rodents are to some degree omnivorous; others are highly specialized, eating, for example, only a few species of invertebrates or fungi.

1. Rodent Anatomy

Despite their morphological and ecological diversity, all rodents share one characteristic: a highly specialized dentition for gnawing (the term rodent is derived from the Latin *rodens* meaning gnawing). Rodents have a single pair of upper and a single pair of lower hypertrophied incisors that are actually retained deciduous second incisors (Taylor and Butcher, 1951). Between each incisor and the first cheek tooth is a toothless interval called the diastema. The incisors are rootless and grow continuously. Enamel is deposited on the anterior and lateral incisor surfaces; the posterior incisor surface is dentin. During gnawing, as the incisors chisel against each other, they wear away the softer dentine, leaving a sharp enamel edge. This 'self-sharpening' system is very effective and is one of the keys to the enormous ecological success of rodents.

Using the incisors together to chisel away at a surface requires muscle that forcefully brings the lower jaw forward. In rodents, this is done primarily by the masseter muscle. The masseter can be divided into three parts: the superficial masseter, the lateral masseter, and the medial masseter. By moving the skeletal attachment or origin of the masseter rostrally, rodents gain both a mechanical advantage and an additional range of lower jaw movement. Mammalogists have traditionally divided rodents into three groups based on how the masseter attachments evolved (Simpson, 1945; Wilson and Reeder, 1993).

In the 'sciuromorphous' condition (from Latin *sciurus* meaning a squirrel), the origin of the lateral masseter moves forward and attaches to the front of the zygomatic arch where it meets the rostrum. The origin of the superficial masseter is also shifted forward, but the origin of the medial masseter does not change much. The front of the zygomatic arch has developed into a large, distinctive zygomatic plate in sciuromorph rodents such as squirrels, beavers, geomyids and heteromyids. In the 'hystricomorphous' condition (from Latin *hystrix* meaning a porcupine), the infraorbital foramen becomes very large. Through it, part of a much-expanded medial masseter passes to originate on the side of the rostrum rostrally to the zygomatic arch. This condition is found in porcupines (both New and Old World families), guinea pigs, and jerboas. The third, 'myomorphous' condition (from Greek *mys* meaning a mouse) probably arose from a sciuromorphous ancestral state. It includes the development of a zygomatic plate and rostral shifting of the lateral masseter, as in sciuromorphs. The infraorbital foramen is also moderately enlarged, and a slip of medial masseter passes through it. The myomorphous

condition is found in true rats and mice (New and Old World Families), hamsters, gerbils, and voles. How these three conditions evolved is widely debated. It is accepted, however, that more than one group of rodents achieved some of them independently.

The morphology of the insertion of the masseter on the lower jaw also differs among groups of rodents. In the 'sciurognathous' jaw, the angular process, which receives most of the masseter, arises almost in a line with the rest of the jaw; that is, it originates in the same vertical plane that also includes the socket of the incisors. In the 'hystricognathous' jaw, the origin of the angular process is distinctly lateral to this plane, and the angular process is often flared laterally. The coronoid process is usually reduced in hystricognathous forms.

2. Rodent Suborders

The classical rodent suborders Sciuromorpha, Myomorpha, and Hystricomorpha originate from Brandt (1855), who based his names on Waterhouse's (1839) characterizations of sciuromorphous, myomorphous, and hystricomorphous zygomasseteric morphologies. Since that time, the question of rodent suborders has become a continuous work-in-progress. The next significant step in rodent characterization was made by Tullberg (Tullberg, 1899) who combined mandibular conformation (sciurognathy vs. hystricognathy) and Brandtian zygomasseteric criteria to describe two major rodent groups, the Sciurognathi (Sciuromorphi and Myomorphi) and Hystricognathi (Bathyergomorphi and Hystricomorphi). Subsequently, most mammalian taxonomists have adopted either the Brandtian trisubordinal (Lavocat, 1978; Wood, 1965) or Tullbergian dual subordinal models (Landry, 1999; Patterson and Wood, 1982).

Other taxonomists have recognized more primary divisions within Rodentia (whether or not called a suborder), anywhere from 5 to 16 (Hartenberger, 1998; McKenna and Bell, 1997). Within each of these classifications, problematic and/or poorly understood groups have been acknowledged by the qualifiers of *'incertae sedis'* or *'suborder indeterminate.'*

In contrast to disagreement over suborders, the number of families of living rodents considered valid has remained fairly stable over the past half-century, at around 30–35 (Anderson and Jones, 1984; Carleton, 1984; Hartenberger, 1985; Simpson, 1945; Wilson and Reeder, 1993). In this chapter, we recognize 33 families (Table 7.1) based on the provisional classification of Carleton and Musser (Carleton and Musser, 2005). Recent molecular studies have generally sustained the monophyletic status of most of these families. Variation of this number of families depends on authors' decisions concerning the rank of certain groups as subfamily *versus* family.

Carleton and Musser list five suborders, Sciuromorpha, Castorimorpha, Myomorpha, Anomaluromorpha, and

TABLE 7.1   Provisional Suprafamilial Classification of Rodentia

ORDER RODENTIA	33 FAMILIES, 481 GENERA, 2277 SPECIES
Suborder Sciuromorpha	61 genera, 307 species
Family Aplodontiidae	Mountain beaver or sewellel
	1 genus, 1 species
Family Sciuridae	Squirrels, chipmunks, marmots, and prairie dogs
	51 genera, 278 species
Family Gliridae	Dormice
	9 genera, 28 species
Suborder Castorimorpha	13 genera, 102 species
Family Castoridae	Beavers
	1 genus, 2 species
Family Heteromyidae	Pocket mice, kangaroo rats, and mice
	6 genera, 60 species
Family Geomyidae	Pocket gophers
	6 genera, 40 species
Suborder Myomorpha	326 genera, 1569 species
Superfamily Dipodoidea	
Family Dipodidae	Jerboas
	16 genera, 51 species
Superfamily Muroidea	
Family Platacanthomyidae	Spiny dormouse and pygmy dormouse
	2 genera, 2 species
Family Spalacidae	Blind mole rats, African mole rats, zokors, and bamboo rats
	6 genera, 36 species
Family Calomyscidae	Mouse-like hamsters
	1 genus, 8 species
Family Nesomyidae	African and Malagasy endemic rats and mice
	21 genera, 61 species
Family Cricetidae	New World rats, mice, voles and hamsters, and relatives
	130 genera, 681 species
Family Muridae	Old World mice and rats, gerbils, voles, and lemmings
	150 genera, 730 species
Suborder Anomaluromorpha	4 genera, 9 species
Family Anomaluridae	Scaly-tailed squirrels
	3 genera, 7 species
Family Pedetidae	Springhare or springhaas
	1 genus, 2 species

(Continued)

TABLE 7.1   (Continued)

ORDER RODENTIA	33 FAMILIES, 481 GENERA, 2277 SPECIES
Suborder Hystricomorpha	77 genera, 290 species
Infraorder Ctenodactylomorphi	
Family Ctenodactylidae	Gundis
	4 genera, 5 species
Infraorder Hystricognathi	
Family Bathyergidae	African mole rats or blesmols
	5 genera, 17 species
Family Hystricidae	Old World porcupines
	3 genera, 11 species
Family Petromuridae	Rock rat or dassie
	1 genus, 1 species
Family Thryonomyidae	Cane rats or grasscutters
	1 genus, 2 species
Family Erethizontidae	New World porcupines
	5 genera, 16 species
Family Chinchillidae	Chinchillas and visachas
	3 genera, 7 species
Family Dinomyidae	Pacarana
	1 genus, 1 species
Family Caviidae	Cavies and Patagonian 'hares' or maras
	6 genera, 18 species
Family Dasyproctidae	Acuchis and agoutis
	2 genera, 13 species
Family Cuniculidae	Pacas
	1 genus, 2 species
Family Ctenomyidae	Tuco-tucos
	1 genus, 60 species
Family Octodontidae	Degus, rock rats, and viscacha rats
	8 genera, 13 species
Family Abrocomidae	Chinchilla rats or chinchillones
	2 genus, 10 species
Family Echimyidae	Spiny rats
	21 genera, 87 species
Family Myocastoridae	Coypu or nutria
	1 genus, 1 species
Family Capromyidae	West Indian hutias
	8 genera, 20 species
Family Heptaxodontidae	Giant hutias (now extinct)
	4 genera, 4 species

Modified after Carleton and Musser (2005).

Hystricomorpha (Table 7.1) for the purpose of organizing hierarchical taxonomic information. They retain Brandt's (1855) names for three of the five suborders (Sciuromorpha, Myomorpha, and Hystricomorpha).[1] In contrast, other rodent authorities have emphatically recommended against using Brandtian descriptions (Landry, 1999; Wood, 1985). They contend that the descriptive meaning of the terms does not strictly agree with the morphologies of included members, and that this contradiction will only continue to cause confusion. Sciuromorpha, Myomopha, and Hystricomorpha have excellent support as monophyletic taxa. However, evidence for Castorimorpha and Anomaluromorpha is less persuasive. Future phylogenetic investigation of these two groups must address the question as to where they belong within one of the other three suborders.

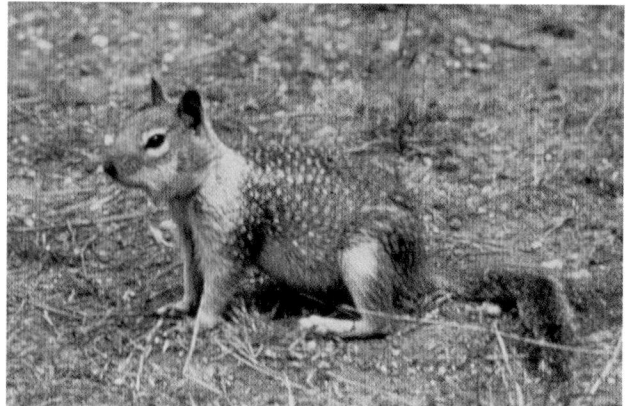

FIGURE 7.1 *Spermophilus beecheyi* – California or Beechey ground squirrel. It is also known as a rock squirrel. Side view. *Photograph by the Audio Visual Office, US Fish and Wildlife Service and the Mammal Images Library of the American Society of Mammalogists.*

II. GROUND SQUIRRELS: *UROCITELLUS, ICTODOMYS,* AND *SPERMOPHILUS*

The ground squirrels were grouped in the genus *Spermophilus* until 2009 when the taxonomy was reviewed based on findings that this genus did not represent a monophyletic grouping. *Spermophila* were then reclassified into eight genera (Helgen *et al.*, 2009). The most common species used in research are *Urocitellus richardsonii* (Richardson's ground squirrel), *Ictodomys tridecemlineatus* (13-lined ground squirrel), *Spermophilus lateralis* (golden-mantled ground squirrel), and *S. beecheyi* (California ground squirrel; Beechey ground squirrel; rock squirrel). Examples of ground squirrels are shown in Figs. 7.1 and 7.2.

A. Introduction

1. Description

The head and body length of ground squirrels is 130–406 mm, the well-furred tail is 38–254 mm long, and weight range is 85–1000 g (Nowak, 1999; Streubel and Fitzgerald, 1978). Their fur is grizzled brownish or yellowish gray, often with fine light spots on the upper parts, and the underparts are whitish or yellow. Ground squirrels have large internal cheek pouches to carry food.

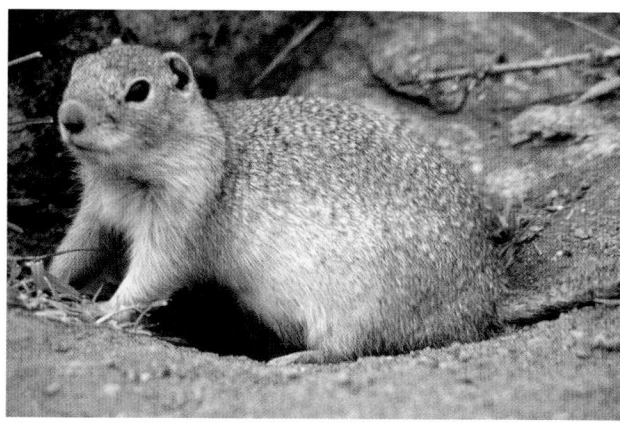

FIGURE 7.2 *Spermophilus elegans* – Wyoming ground squirrel. It is also known as *Urocitellus elegans.* Side view at burrow entrance, Rocky Mountain National Park, Colorado. *Photograph by B.J. Bergstrom and the Mammal Images Library of the American Society of Mammalogists.*

In *I. tridecemlineatus* there is a series of alternating dark and light longitudinal stripes with a row of light spots on each of the dark stripes (Streubel and Fitzgerald, 1978). The name *Citellus* has often been used for this genus, but is not now in general use.

2. Distribution

The native range of ground squirrels as a group includes the Great Plains region of the United States and the south-central region of Canada. *U. richardsonii* inhabits the prairies of central Alberta and western Montana to western Minnesota; *I. armatus* inhabits southwestern Montana, southeastern Idaho, western Wyoming, and northern Utah; *I. tridecemlineatus* occupies central Alberta to Ohio and southern Texas; *S. lateralis* is found in southwestern Canada and from North Dakota to Washington; and *S. beecheyi* extends from southern Washington to northern Baja California (Nowak, 1999).

---

[1] Brandt's names, intended as a suprafamilial rank, do not merit any special consideration as far as the International Code of Zoological Nomenclature, International Commission on Zoological Nomenclature (2012) Amendment of Articles 8, 9, 10, 21, and 78 of the International Code of Zoological Nomenclature, to expand and refine methods of publication (Zookeys 219, 1–10) is concerned. Aside from requirements of formal publication and availability, the Code does not prescribe standard suffices to denote relative rank or stipulate strict adherence to priority for taxa recognized above the family-group.

Their habitat includes prairies and steppes, tundra, rocky country, open woodlands, or desert mountain ranges. They are not found in areas with a dense forest cover.

3. *Habitat*

Most ground squirrels construct burrows with the length and character varying across species (Michener and Koeppl, 1985; Streubel and Fitzgerald, 1978). During warm months Richardson's ground squirrels live in extensive colonies. Males establish territories of about 0.06 hectares, which cover the burrows of three to five females. Within a week after mating, the females establish their own territories, averaging 0.016 hectares, within the male territories (Michener and Koeppl, 1985). Thirteen-lined ground squirrels live in small, scattered groups. They are not highly social and lack territorial activity; although the occupied burrow is defended, the area around it is not (Streubel and Fitzgerald, 1978).

4. *Use in Research*

Ground squirrels continue to be used in the investigation of hibernation (Olson *et al.*, 2013; Storey, 1997; Vucetic *et al.*, 2013). Despite the virtual arrest of physiologic functions and minimal delivery of glucose and oxygen, homeostatic control is maintained. Many researchers have investigated the adaptive hibernation strategies of ground squirrels. For example, cardiac muscle undergoes hypertrophy during hibernation, to maintain cardiac output despite low heart rate. Unlike the pathological condition of hypertrophic cardiomyopathy, there is a higher relative proportion of the alpha isoform of the cardiac myosin heavy chain, which preserves contractile strength (Nelson and Rourke, 2013; Storey, 1997).

Additional interesting work has been done on other aspects of ground squirrel biology. California ground squirrels (*S. beecheyi*) have serum metalloproteinase inhibitors with inhibitory activity against rattlesnake venom (Biardi *et al.*, 2011). This adaptation is beneficial to the animal, as adult Beechey ground squirrels regularly confront northern Pacific rattlesnakes attempting to prey on their pups. It may also have applications to therapies potentially useful in human medicine. Ground squirrels have also been used to investigate hepatitis B infections and hepatocellular carcinoma (Marion *et al.*, 1986; Tennant *et al.*, 1991). The cholesterol-fed Richardson's ground squirrel is an effective animal model for cholesterol gallstone formation (MacPherson and Pemsingh, 1997; MacPherson *et al.*, 1987).

B. Biology

All ground squirrels are diurnal. *U. richardsonii* has three daily activity periods: during the first 2h after dawn, from 10:00 a.m. to 2:00 p.m., and from 4:00 p.m. to sunset (Michener and Koeppl, 1985). For about 7 months

(September or October to April or May) Richardson's ground squirrels hibernate in their burrows. *I. tridecemlineatus* doubles its weight by September and hibernates from October to early April (Streubel and Fitzgerald, 1978). Female ground squirrels are monestrous and normally bear one litter per year; mating takes place shortly after emergence from hibernation. The gestation period is 23–31 days, litter size averages from two to 15 (7.5 in *S. richardsonii*), and females wean their young at 4–6 weeks. By 11 months juveniles have attained full size and sexual maturity (Michener and Koeppl, 1985). Published information on biological reference parameters is limited to one report on serum proteins and transferrins (Nadler, 1968).

C. Husbandry

An excellent recent review of the captive husbandry of 13-lined ground squirrels was published by Merriman *et al.* (2012) at the University of Wisconsin, who maintain an NIH-funded breeding colony of these animals for their own use and for shipping to other investigators. In the wild the diet of ground squirrels consists of seeds, nuts, grains, roots, bulbs, mushrooms, green vegetation, insects and other small invertebrates, and birds' eggs (Schitoskey and Woodmansee, 1978). Although they may store food in their burrows, they do not appear to use it until awakening in spring. In the Merriman review, the animals are maintained on a diet of high protein (≥25%) dog chow supplemented with black sunflower seeds. Carrots, celery, and live mealworms are also used to supplement breeding animals and juveniles (Merriman *et al.*, 2012). In the same facility, supplementation with kitten milk replacer was implemented as a behavior modification to facilitate animal observation and medication administration and as a dietary supplement in cases of inadequate maternal milk production. Of note, the authors report that the animals readily learned to drink the milk replacer directly from a pipette and thus this method did not necessitate handling. Ground squirrels can be maintained in a laboratory at 18–22°C and induced to hibernate in an unlighted room maintained at 5–10°C (Reiter *et al.*, 1983). Ground squirrels will lose considerable weight during hibernation and may die if forced to hibernate much beyond the end of their natural hibernating season (Davis, 1984). Emaciated squirrels should be removed from hibernation at any time to reduce mortality. Enrichment activities for thirteen-lined ground squirrels during captivity and rehabilitation have been described (Cook-Babcook, 1996). Additional husbandry information on other species of ground squirrels may be gleaned from the methods sections in primary literature and from the laboratory websites of researchers working with these species; for example, the laboratory of Gail Michener (2014) at the University of Lethbridge for Richardson's ground squirrels.

D. Diseases

1. Infectious Diseases

A. Bacterial Infections

Gangrenous dermatitis caused by *Corynebacterium ulcerans* has been reported in wild Richardson's ground squirrels (Olson *et al.*, 1988). Six squirrels died of toxemia, but 57 responded to topical and parenteral administration of antibiotics. The epizootic was believed to be associated with bite wounds due to fighting.

Purulent cutaneous and visceral lesions associated with *Staphylococcus aureus* were observed in a colony of commercially supplied golden-mantled ground squirrels and were associated with death in 1/3 of the animals (Campbell *et al.*, 1981).

Infection of wild California ground squirrels with *Yersinia pestis* occurs frequently in plague-endemic areas such as southern California and Alaska (Spano, 1994; Townzen *et al.*, 1996). Transmission of the bacillus is associated with the fleas *Hoplopsyllus anomalus* and *Oropsylla montana*. Ground squirrels become infected with plague following hibernation and again when reoccupying colonial burrows (Davis, 1999).

B. Viral Infections

Ground squirrels infected with ground squirrel hepatitis virus (GSHV) develop a mild, nonprogressive persistent hepatitis (Cullen and Marion, 1996). Histologically there is chronic portal lymphoplasmacytic hepatitis with small aggregates of mononuclear inflammatory cells in the parenchyma. Serum aspartate and alanine transaminases (AST and ALT) are mildly elevated.

Adult Richardson's ground squirrels have been infected experimentally with Western equine encephalomyelitis virus by intranasal instillation (Leung *et al.*, 1978). Highest titers of virus were recovered from the brain, and histopathological changes involving the central nervous system included meningitis, vasculitis, perivascular cuffing, gliosis, neuronophagia, and neuronal degeneration. The virus was also found in a variety of extraneural tissues. The duration and magnitude of viremia were sufficient to provide virus source for arthropods.

Ground squirrels are susceptible to infection with rabies virus, and Russian scientists have shown a prolonged incubation period of rabies virus during hibernation (Botvinkin *et al.*, 1985). In the United States antigenic or genetic variants of rabies viruses from rodents and woodchucks corresponds to the variants associated with the major terrestrial wildlife reservoir within the geographic region of specimen origin (Childs *et al.*, 1997).

C. Parasitic Infections

Richardson's ground squirrels have been infected experimentally with sporocysts of *Sarcocystis campestris*

from badgers (Wobeser *et al.*, 1983). Hepatitis and phlebitis of hepatic veins were present in animals killed between 4 and 8 days. Meronts were found in endothelial cells beginning on day 9 and were most numerous in the lung. Four of 10 squirrels infected died between days 11 and 13. Foci of inflammation were visible in the myocardium and brain of animals killed at 64 days.

The most prevalent intestinal parasites in a large survey of wild Wyoming ground squirrels (*Spermophilus elegans*) were coccidia of the genus *Eimeria* (Stanton *et al.*, 1992). Most ground squirrels harbored two or more species.

An unidentified species of *Demodex* mite was described in the hair follicles and sebaceous gland ducts in the ear canals of seven California ground squirrels from California (Waggie and Marion, 1997). Similar mites were observed in Meibomian glands of the eyelids. Microscopic changes were minimal and no associated clinical signs or macroscopic lesions were observed.

Lethal myiasis of wild Richardson's ground squirrels by the sarcophagid fly *Neobellieria citellivora* has been reported (Michener, 1993).

D. Fungal Infections

Adiaspores of *Emmonsia crescens*, a saprophytic fungus, were detected in lungs of two of 81 (2.5%) *U. richardsonii*, three of 17 (17.6%) *I. tridecemlineatus*, and 35 of 44 (79.5%) *S. franklini* in Saskatchewan. Infection was more common in adults than in young (Leighton and Wobeser, 1978).

2. Metabolic and Nutritional Diseases

Spontaneous diabetes mellitus is described in a captive golden-mantled ground squirrel (Heidt *et al.*, 1984).

3. Neoplastic Diseases

Hepatocellular carcinoma has developed in California ground squirrels infected with the hepadnavirus GSHV (Marion *et al.*, 1986). GSHV is related to the oncogenic hepadnaviruses hepatitis B virus (HBV) and woodchuck hepatitis virus (WHV). Liver carcinoma appeared in two of 28 GSHV-bearing animals studied and in one of 23 squirrels with antibody to the virus. Each animal was 4 years or older when the tumor was detected. In a separate study, hepatocellular carcinoma was observed in six (50%) of 12 Richardson's ground squirrels (Marion *et al.*, 1986). Serological tests for GSHV were uniformly negative. Southern blot analyses of liver cell DNA demonstrated infection with a hepadnavirus related to GSHV.

Single case reports of exophthalmos associated with a Harderian gland adenocarcinoma and a squamous cell skin carcinoma have been reported in two male California ground squirrels (Morrow and Day-Lollini, 1990; Trigo and Riser, 1981).

4. Miscellaneous

Supernumerary teeth are described in Richardson's ground squirrel and hybrid individuals (Goodwin, 1998).

III. PRAIRIE DOGS: CYNOMYS

There are five species of prairie dog of which the most commonly used in research is *Cynomys ludovicianus* (black-tailed prairie dog; Fig. 7.3).

A. Introduction

1. Description

Black-tailed prairie dogs are stout, short-tailed, short-legged squirrels. Their head and body length is 280–330 mm, tail length is 30–115 mm, and weight is 0.7–1.4 kg. Their coat is a grizzled yellow-gray on top, and the underparts are lighter. The tail of *C. ludovicianus* has a black tip and accounts for the common name (Hoogland, 1996).

2. Distribution

C. ludovicianus inhabits open plains and plateaus and is found on the Great Plains from Montana and southern Saskatchewan to extreme northern Mexico (Hoogland, 1996). Their numbers have declined due to habitat encroachment in recent years. From 2003 to 2008, a joint ruling of the FDA and CDC made it illegal to buy, sell, trade, or transport prairie dogs within the United States

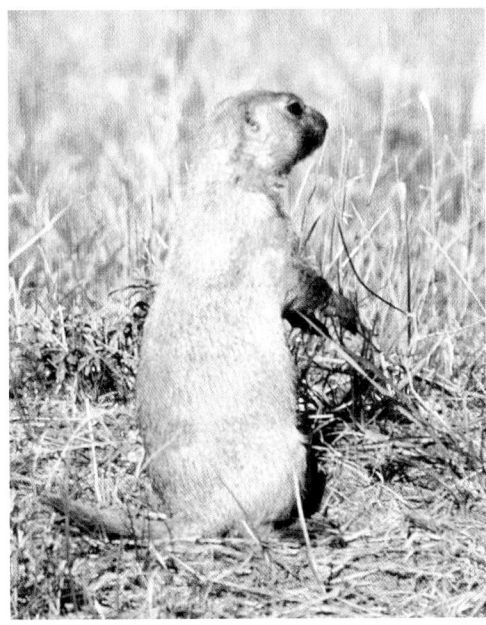

FIGURE 7.3 *Cynomys ludovicianus* – black-tailed prairie dog. Side view, Wind Cave, South Dakota. *Photograph by G.L. Twiest and the Mammal Images Library of the American Society of Mammalogists.*

This ruling was based on the transmission of the exotic zoonotic disease monkeypox to humans from captive populations of prairie dogs that had been co-housed with imported Gambian pouched rats (Azad, 2004; Croft *et al.*, 2007). The ban on domestic commerce or transport of prairie dogs was lifted in 2008 but a ban on import of exotic African rodents for the pet trade remains in place (Hoogland *et al.*, 2009).

3. Habitat

Prairie dogs nest in 300–450 mm chambers within elaborate tunneled burrows up to 34 m long and topped by volcano-shaped cones of soil (Hoogland, 1996). The black-tailed prairie dog is found in large colonies, or 'towns,' that usually cover about 100 hectares. Towns are divided into 'wards,' which are made up of several 'coteries.' Containing an average of 8.5 individuals, the coterie is a discrete social unit typically consisting of a single adult male, three or four adult females, and several 1- to 2-year-old juveniles (Hoogland, 1996). All members of a coterie are socially integrated and display territorial defense toward outsiders (Hoogland, 1979; 1996).

4. Use in Research

Within the field of biomedicine, the black-tailed prairie dog has historically been used to study biliary physiology and the pathophysiology of gallstone formation (Chen *et al.*, 1997; Cohen and Mosbach, 1993; Holzbach, 1984). The anatomy of the prairie dog biliary system has been described in detail (Grace *et al.*, 1988). More recently, the prairie dog has been utilized in the context of infectious disease research. Much of this research pertains to zoonotic diseases such as monkeypox or other orthopoxviruses; *Yersinia pestis*, the causative agent of plague; or *Francisella tularensis*, the causative agent of tularemia) (Azad, 2004).

Prairie dogs were investigated as a model for the human pathogen *Orthopox variola* (smallpox) by investigators at the CDC (Carroll *et al.*, 2013). This investigation was undertaken since there is no known susceptible small animal model for smallpox and prairie dogs were highly susceptible in the 2003 U.S. outbreak of the related *Orthopoxvirus* monkeypox. Unfortunately, prairie dogs experimentally infected with smallpox did not develop clinical disease nor was viral DNA detectable after nasal or intradermal inoculation, although seroconversion was demonstrated.

B. Biology

Black-tailed prairie dogs are diurnal and terrestrial. They become dormant during severe weather but are not deep hibernators (Nowak, 1999). Prairie dogs are very social and reinforce their relationship within a coterie by activities such as nuzzling, grooming, playing together, and vocal communication (Waring, 1970). Female prairie dogs are monestrous and in the wild do not start breeding until 2 years of age (Hoogland, 1998). Mating takes place from early March to late April and gestation lasts 34–37 days (Hoogland, 1997). Each coterie is a cooperative breeding unit in which breeding occurs at the same time, and each adult female produces one litter per year. Offsetting the nepotism and potential detrimental inbreeding, lactating females will then kill offspring of close kin (Hoogland, 1994).

Black-tailed prairie dogs have good low-frequency hearing (as low as 4 Hz), and are more sensitive than any other rodent yet tested at frequencies below 63 Hz (Heffner et al., 1994). In contrast, they are relatively insensitive in their midrange and have poor high-frequency hearing.

Physiologic reference values including serum and chemistry and hematology were reported by Broughton (1992) and more recently by Keckler et al. (2010). Hematology values for adult prairie dogs are listed in Table 7.2. The latter study also included weight, core body temperature, and circadian rhythm parameters. Values were, on the whole, similar to that previously reported in the Broughton study, which used single sampling in older, wild-caught animals, with some exceptions including lower leucocyte, erythrocyte, and hematocrit values. These differences may reflect acclimation, which was not performed for the earlier study, or differences in sampling technique and methodology.

C. Husbandry

In the wild, black-tailed prairie dogs feed on herbs and grasses, maintaining a 'rotating pasture' that causes fast-growing plants to predominate around colonies. They do not store food in their burrows (Hoogland, 1996). Information on captive diets is limited and variable. Keckler et al. (2010) fed a specially formulated high-fiber diet (Exotic Nutrition, Newport News, VA) supplemented with fruit or beet-based treats, sweet potatoes, timothy hay, and monkey biscuits. Hoogland et al. (2009) describe acceptable diet items for privately owned animals including timothy hay, a commercially available prairie dog (Oxbow Animal Health, Murdock, NE) or rabbit diet, and vegetable or cereal treats. They further describe a formula of one part goat's milk, one part pureed sweet potato, and two parts water or Pedialyte for syringe-feeding of unweaned juveniles.

D. Diseases

1. Infectious Diseases

Prairie dogs were the direct vector for human infection in a 2003 U.S. outbreak of monkeypox (Anderson, 1982; Anderson et al., 2003; Azad, 2004; Di Giulio and

Eckburg, 2004; Guarner et al., 2004; Reynolds et al., 2007). The prairie dogs became infected by housing in proximity to infected Gambian pouched rats at a pet distributor. Prairie dogs had a high incidence of clinical disease and mortality. Reported lesions included fibrinonecrotizing bronchopneumonia, enteritis, and lymphadenopathy, sometimes with pulmonary vasculitis. Classical poxvirus intracytoplasmic eosinophilic inclusion bodies were difficult to detect by light microscopy but viral arrays were evident ultrastructurally and virus could be detected by PCR (Langohr et al., 2004). A total of 78 suspected and 32 laboratory-confirmed cases in humans were eventually reported in the U.S. Nineteen patients were hospitalized for clinical disease or quarantine (Di Giulio and Eckburg, 2004; Reynolds et al., 2007). Disease transmission from prairie dogs to humans was believed to be by mucocutaneous and respiratory routes (Guarner et al., 2004). Clinical disease in humans consisted of fever, lymphadenopathy, maculopapular rash, and skin lesions progressing from vesicular to ulcerative and crusting. A minority of patients developed severe systemic complications including pneumonitis and encephalitis (Di Giulio and Eckburg, 2004; Reynolds et al., 2007; Reynolds et al., 2006b). The highest risk factor for infection was direct contact with an infected animal, with veterinary workers and households owning and treating an infected animal at highest risk (Croft et al., 2007; Reynolds et al., 2007). Since prairie dogs were accidental vectors but not the native host for this disease, and the last clinical case in the United States was in 2003, prairie dogs should not currently be considered a high zoonotic risk for monkeypox transmission in the United States.

A more likely, but still uncommon, zoonotic disease of prairie dogs is tularemia, caused by the bacteria Francisella tularensis, which occurs sporadically in wild or wild-caught animals (La Regina et al., 1986). In 2004, tularemia was detected in a group of prairie dogs that became ill at a pet distributor in Texas. These animals were distributed domestically and internationally, with human disease transmission occurring in some cases (Avashia et al., 2004). Positive cultures were obtained from 63 animals (Petersen et al., 2004). Immunohistochemistry was used to demonstrate bacteria in lesions in formalin-fixed tissue (Zeidner et al., 2004). Gross manifestation includes scattered white pinpoint hepatosplenic lesions and massive, purulent bronchopneumonia. Diagnosis was confirmed by direct fluorescent antibody tests and culture of spleen and liver samples. Clinical signs include sudden death or nonspecific signs of systemic illness with hepatic or respiratory involvement. Disease transmission routes to other animals and to humans include mucous membranes (gastrointestinal, conjunctival), biting insects or needlesticks, or respiratory transmission. Because of the risk of aerosolization, necropsy of suspect cases or experimental infections should take place under

TABLE 7.2 Selected Comparative Hematological Values of Adult Rodents[a]

Species and reference	RBC (×10⁶/µl)	Hematocrit (%)	Hb (g/dl)	MCV (fl)	MCH (pg)	MCHC (g/dl)	WBC (×10³/µl)	Neutrophils (×10³/µl)	Lymphocytes (×10³/µl)	Monocytes (×10³/µl)	Eosinophils (×10³/µl)	Basophils (×10³/µl)
Prairie dog Cynomys ludovicianus (Keckler et al., 2010)	4.0 *2-5*	24 *14-36*	8 *4-11*	62 *57-66*	20 *19-22*	32 *29-34*	3 *1-6*	1.6 (granulocytes) *0.8-2.8*	1.2 *0.5-3.0*	0.5 *0.2-0.9*	na	na
Kangaroo rat Dipodomys panamintinus (Scelza and Knoll, 1982)	7.9 *5.8-10*	49.2 *46-52.4*	16.1 *15-17.2*	na	20.5 *16.5-24.5*	33 *31.3-34.7*	4.6 *1.3-7.9*	na	na	na		
Dipodomys merriami (Haley et al., 1960)	8.5 *na*	47.5 *na*	13.1 *na*	na	na	na	7.7 *7.1-8.3*	1 *na*	6.2 *na*	0.3 *na*	na	na
Pack rat Neotoma fuscipes (Weber et al., 2002)	7.7 *5.7-11.2*	37.0 *36.9-48.9*	11.2 *8.2-14*	48.4 *41.7-60.8*	14.7 *12.3-14.9*	30.4 *26.8-32.4*	10.9 *4.2-31.5*	6.3 *1.2-16*	3.6 *0.7-13.9*	0.5 *0.1-1.5*	0.3 *0-1.9*	0.2 *0-0.9*
Grasshopper mouse Onychomys torridus (Swindle et al., 1985)	7.8 *3.2-9*	45 *33-54*	14.5 *11-16.4*	57.7 *50.8-67*	18.4 *16-27.3*	32 *27.3-34.2*	7.4 *2-18.6*	2.3 *0.7-8.9*	4 *1.2-10.3*	0.2 *0-2.9*	0.6 *0-2.1*	0.02 *0-0.4*
Deer mouse Peromyscus leucopus (Wu et al., 1999)	na	44.5 *38-49*	na	na	na	na	6.21 *2.0-12.3*	0.7 *0.1-2.7*	5.1 *1.7-9.5*	0 *0-0.08*	0.1 *0-0.08*	na
Cotton rats (Robel et al., 1996)	5.6	34.6	11.0	62.0	19.5	32.3	11.9	9.2	4.5	0.0	0.3	0.0
Sigmodon hispidus (inbred)	4.8	34.4	10.5	70.3	22.0	31.3	6.7	2.9	3.2	0.1	0.4	0.0
Sigmodon hispidus (captive wild)	6.0	41.9	13.4	71.3	21.1	31.9	10.2	2.9	5.9	0.1	0.1	0.1
Sigmodon hispidus (wild)	na	na	na	na	na	na	na	na	na	na	na	na
White-tailed rats (Cantrell and Padovan, 1987)	5.4	45.7	14.4	na	na	na	9.1	1.5	7.1	0.1	0.4	0
Mystromys albicaudatus (male)	4.4-6.7 *4.6*	41-50 *39.7*	12.6-16.9 *12.9*				5.2-15.7 *9.6*	0.4-4.1 *7.1*	4.1-12.8 *7.1*	0-0.5 *0.1*	0.1-0.9 *0.4*	0
Mystromys albicaudatus (female)	3-5.9	33-45	11.0-16.3				5.5-24.6	3.9-13.0	3.9-13.0	0-0.4	0.1-0.8	0
Gerbils Meriones unguiculates (Mays, 1969)	8.5 *7.0-10.0*	48 *41-52*	15 *12.1-16.9*	56.4 *na*	17.6 *na*	31.2 *na*	11.0 *4.3-21.6*	19.0 *3-41*	78.0 *32-97*	3.0 *0-9*	1.0 *0-4*	0.6 *0-2*
Voles Microtus pinetorum (Harvey et al., 2008)	11.0 *9.0-12.9*	40.8 *32.3-49.4*	15.0 *12.8-17.1*	37.5 *27.5-47.4*	13.7 *11.4-16.0*	36.9 *31.6-42.1*	4.1 *0.7-7.5*	1.1 *0-2.6*	2.8 *0-5.5*	0.2 *0-0.5*	0.03 *0-0.10*	0.02 *0-0.01*
Multimammate rats Mastomys natalensis (Kagira et al., 2005)	7.9 *5.5-9.5*	44.5 *34.4-65.0*	14.8 *10.6-18.3*	55.1 *46.0-64.8*	20.1 *17.3-34.8*	36.9 *30.8-58.4*	11.9 *7.5-20.0*	na	na	na	na	na

[a]Values shown are the mean, with the range or reference interval in italics underneath the mean. Additional values and values for juvenile, captive bred vs. wild may be found in the source publications.

BSL3 (respiratory precautions) conditions, although animal housing and handling of diagnostic materials can be performed at BSL2 (Chosewood and Wilson, 2009).

Wild prairie dog populations are highly susceptible to epizootics of *Yersinia pestis*, the plague bacterium, and are often the subject for field studies of plague epidemiology (Johnson *et al.*, 2011). Although not reported in captive populations, this agent should be a consideration in field studies or when working with wild-caught prairie dogs. Transmission occurs by direct contact, inhalation of aerosolized droplets, or by flea bites. Since the latter is the most common route of human infection, prevention of flea bites or parasite extermination should be implemented into field studies or quarantine procedures. Dusting with deltamethrin, a pyrethrin-type insecticide, was successfully used to control plague in prairie dogs in a field setting during an epizootic outbreak (Jones *et al.*, 2012).

As with many rodent species, prairie dogs are susceptible to *Clostridium difficile* typhlocolitis, which can be induced by administration of the cephalosporin antibiotic cefoxitin (Muller *et al.*, 1987). The disease in prairie dogs has a more chronic course than in other animal models of *C. difficile*-induced diarrhea.

Parasitism is relatively common in prairie dogs. Five species of the intestinal coccidian *Eimeria* were identified in wild-caught black-tailed prairie dogs from Wyoming (Seville, 1997). *Eimeria* spp. appear cross-reactive between prairie dogs and ground squirrels. Central nervous system migration of *Baylisascaris* spp. ('raccoon roundworm') larvae caused ataxia, torticollis, and loss of righting reflex in three prairie dogs maintained at a research facility (Dixon *et al.*, 1988). The infection was transmitted from *Baylisascaris* eggs on the cages, which had previously housed raccoons. Infection occurred despite washing of the cages at 82.2°C (180°F) in a large pass-through cage washer and storage of the cages for up to 6 months. Hepatic cysticercosis (i.e., larval *Taenia* sp. infection), has been described in wild-caught black-tailed (Banks *et al.*, 1995) and white-tailed prairie dogs (*C. leucurus*) (Rockett *et al.*, 1990). In the white-tailed prairie dogs, the cestodes were identified as larval *T. mustelae* but speciation of the *Taenia* in the black-tailed prairie dogs was not possible. In all species, hepatic cysticercosis takes the form of small 1–2 mm diameter, white, fluid-filled cysts containing larval forms of the cestode. Speciation is based on morphological characteristics of the cyst and the larvae. The presence of larval cysts is typical of the intermediate host, either natural or aberrant, and maturation does not occur in this host. The intermediate host is typically a prey species of the definitive host, which acquires infection by ingestion of the intermediate host. Dermatophyte infection causing hair loss was reported in three captive Mexican prairie dogs (*C. mexicanus*) in a Texas zoo. The causative agent was *Microsporum gypseum* (Porter, 1979). Demodicosis has also been reported in association with alopecia and was successfully treated by sponge application of 250 ppm amitraz dips for 3–5 min at 4-day intervals for 2 months (Jekl *et al.*, 2006).

2. Neoplastic Diseases

The two most-reported spontaneous neoplasms in prairie dogs are hepatocellular carcinoma and elodontoma.

Hepatocellular carcinoma was reported in 12 of 61 prairie dogs necropsied, with metastasis to lung, spleen, or heart in five cases (Garner *et al.*, 2004). An attempt to identify viral agents was unsuccessful, although virus-like inclusion bodies have been reported in other clinical case reports (Une *et al.*, 1996).

Proliferative, expansile masses of the incisors previously described as odontomas, but more recently renamed elodontomas, are frequently seen in captive prairie dogs and other members of Sciuromorpha (Boy and Steenkamp, 2006; Smith *et al.*, 2013; Wagner, 1999). Prairie dogs have elodont (continuously growing) incisors and are subject to trauma, insufficient wear, and abnormal growth due to husbandry or nutritional conditions. Elodontomas are essentially hamartomas (benign malformations) and consist of abnormal odontogenic epithelium and alveolar bone at the apex of the maxillary incisors. These are not true neoplasms but rather aberrations of growth. Due to the misdirected but continuous growth, elodontomas of maxillary incisors commonly cause upper respiratory obstruction as they expand into the nasal cavity. Mandibular elodontomas are reported less but have been associated with oropharyngeal obstruction (Smith *et al.*, 2013). A variety of palliative treatments with antibiotics, decongestants, and steroids have been applied. Surgical extraction of the incisors has been utilized but, depending on the disease progression, is challenging and frequently results in fractured incisors. Extraction through the nasal cavity has been advocated to decrease the risk of incisor fracture, but recurrence and incomplete resolution of clinical signs were still common outcomes (Smith *et al.*, 2013). Placement of an earlobe retractor (earlobe 'plug') as a breathing tube via rhinotomy was successfully utilized as a means of treating elodontoma-associated breathing difficulties in one case (Bulliot and Mentre, 2013).

Other neoplasms sporadically reported in this species include a thoracic lipoma, which resulted in death due to respiratory compression (Rogers and Chrisp, 1998), and an epiglottal fibrosarcoma (Suedmeyer and Pace, 1994).

3. Miscellaneous

Respiratory disease either independent of or in association with elodontomas, are common problem in captive prairie dogs. Because this problem is not common in wild or zoo prairie dogs, diet and environmental conditions may be the underlying cause. Griner (1983) found that prairie dogs in the San Diego Zoo become obese and develop severe dermatitis after 2–3 years in captivity.

IV. POCKET GOPHERS: GEOMYIDAE

Geomys (Eastern pocket gophers) includes eight species and *Thomomys* (Western pocket gophers), nine species. Examples of pocket gophers are given in Figs. 7.4–7.8.

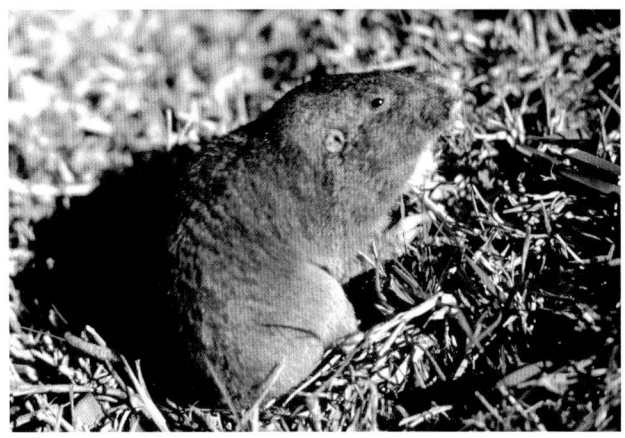

FIGURE 7.6 *Geomys breviceps* – Baird's Pocket Gopher. Side view. *Photograph by G.N. Cameron and the Mammal Images Library of the American Society of Mammalogists.*

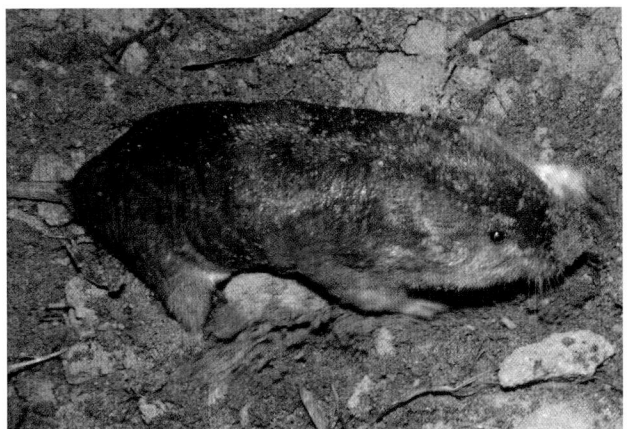

FIGURE 7.4 *Geomys attwateri* – Attwater's Pocket Gopher. Dorsolateral view of adult gopher digging, Welder Wildlife Refuge, San Patricio County, Texas. *Photograph by G.N. Cameron and the Mammal Images Library of the American Society of Mammalogists.*

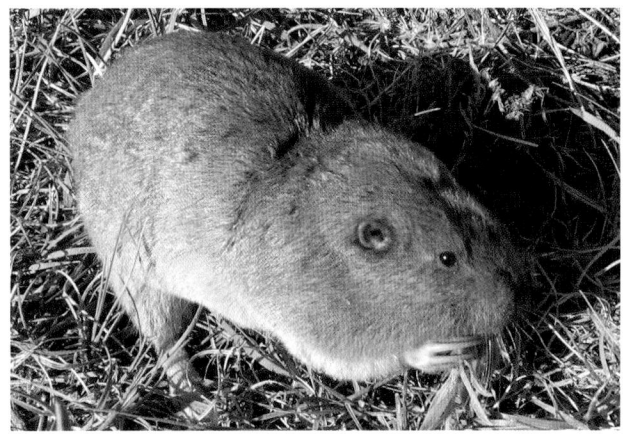

FIGURE 7.7 *Thomomys talpoides* – Northern Pocket Gopher. Quarter view of adult gopher, U.S. Air Force Academy, Colorado Springs, Colorado. *Photograph by D.W. Hale and the Mammal Images Library of the American Society of Mammalogists.*

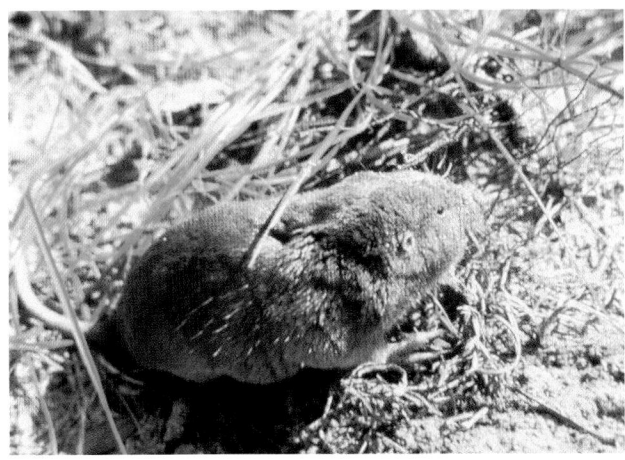

FIGURE 7.5 *Geomys pinetis* – Southeastern Pocket Gopher. Side view of gopher with tail, ears and forefeet visible, Lower Wekiva River State Preserve, Seminole County, Florida. *Photograph by J.D. McMurtray and the Mammal Images Library of the American Society of Mammalogists.*

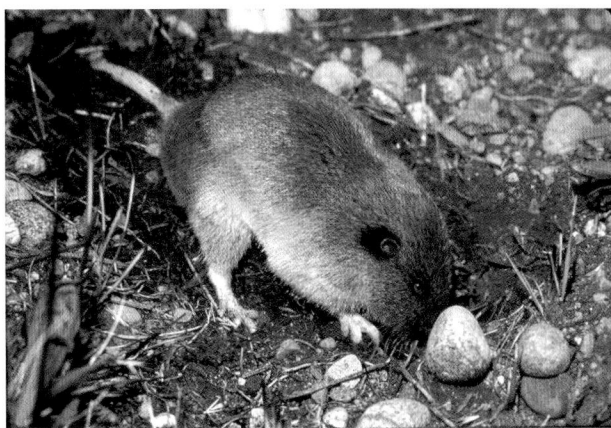

FIGURE 7.8 *Thomomys mazama* – Western Pocket Gopher. Side view of gopher digging, Weir Prairie, Washington. *Photograph by W.P. Leonard and the Mammal Images Library of the American Society of Mammalogists.*

A. Introduction

1. Taxonomy

Species boundaries in the genera *Geomys* and *Thomomys* are poorly defined (Patton and Smith, 1989). Varying degrees of hybridization exist between geographically differentiated pocket gophers, and the distinction between specific or subspecific levels is debatable among authors. Intraspecific genetic diversity appears driven in part by microgeographical habitat restriction and mitochondrial DNA analysis has been used to analyze closely related subspecies of pocket gophers as an example of how geographic restriction affects species divergence (Alvarez-Castaneda and Patton, 2004; Soto-Centeno et al., 2013).

2. Description

The description is adapted from Nowak (1999). Pocket gophers have stout, thickset bodies and large skulls adapted for burrowing. The tail is short, naked, and very sensitive to touch. Ears and eyes are small, and well-developed lacrimal glands supply a thick fluid that cleans the cornea of dirt while the animal is burrowing. The lips can be closed behind the curved incisors, so the animal can gnaw dirt while burrowing. There are two long external fur-lined cheek pouches. The legs are short with powerful forearms and five strong digging claws. Size varies widely, but males are larger than females. Head and body length is 90–300 mm, and tail length is 40–140 mm.

3. Distribution

Western pocket gophers live in deserts, prairies, open forests, and meadows. They are found west of the Rocky Mountains, from southwestern Canada to southern Baja California and central Mexico. Eastern pocket gophers prefer loose, sandy soil in open and sparsely wooded areas. They are found east of the Rocky Mountains, ranging from southern Manitoba and Wisconsin to northeastern Mexico and across to Florida (Hall, 1981).

4. Habitat

Pocket gophers are fossorial and thus spend most of their life underground, surfacing to gather food for storage. They dig two types of tunnels: long, winding, shallow tunnels constructed to obtain food such as roots and tubers from above; and deep tunnels for shelter, with chambers for nests, food storage, and fecal deposits (Hall, 1981).

5. Use in Research

Pocket gophers are principally utilized as animal models for aspects of molecular evolution, including the influence of geographic isolation on speciation and coevolution of parasite–host relationships (Bianco et al.,

1989; Chambers et al., 2009; Hafner et al., 1994; McClellan, 2000; Smith, 1998). Other research uses are as subjects in health and environmental impact studies of heavy metals, radionuclide waste, and other soil contaminants (Budd et al., 2004; Gallegos et al., 2007; Reynolds et al., 2006a). They are considered a sentinel species for this purpose since their fossorial behavior results in high contact and ingestion of soil contaminants.

B. Biology

Most of the information is summarized from Nowak (1999) or Hall (1981). Pocket gophers do not hibernate, although they may become inactive during winter. They are solitary animals. When two adults are placed together, they usually fight viciously. The only exception to this behavior occurs during the breeding season. The mating system of pocket gophers is promiscuous, with female choice at its base (Patton and Smith, 1993). Western pocket gophers are monestrous and produce one litter per year. The gestation ranges from 18 to 19 days, and litter size ranges from one to 10. Species of Eastern pocket gopher in northern regions have one litter per year, but species in southern regions have two litters per year, with smaller average litter sizes. The young are generally weaned at 4–5 weeks and remain in their mother's burrow for 1–2 months. They reach adult weight at 5–6 months and are sexually mature the following breeding season. An exception is *Geomys pinetis* in which females reach sexual maturity at 4–6 months. Virtually no biological reference range material is available save one publication on serum protein patterns (Bongardt et al., 1968).

C. Husbandry

DeVries and Sikes (2009) reviewed captive husbandry practices for Baird's pocket gopher (*G. breviceps*) that could likely be adapted to other related species (DeVries and Sikes, 2009). Captive husbandry of these animals poses challenges owing to their specialized fossorial habitat and behavioral requirements for digging and a varied substrate. Previous attempts at housing these animals in single cages with strictly soil substrate resulted in death from exhaustion due to continuous digging behavior. DeVries and colleagues developed a system of three polycarbonate cages interconnected with PVC piping. The three cages contained pine wood chips, hay, and topsoil, respectively, to provide varied burrowing substrate. Partial covering was used to provide a dark microenvironment. The caging was readily adapted to a large colony yet could be placed on standard laboratory animal racks and was readily deconstructed for sanitizing. Wild pocket gophers feed mainly on the underground parts of plants, especially roots and tubers, but they also eat stems. In captivity, they were fed rodent chow, sweet and russet potatoes, carrots, apples, and bean sprouts (DeVries and Sikes, 2009). Since they reportedly do not drink free-standing water in the wild, no water was provided and water needs were met by washed vegetables. Dietary and environmental adequacy was demonstrated by weight gain and normal molting during the 18-month duration of colony maintenance. Treatment for internal and external parasites by topical insecticide powder and ivermectin injections (doses not specified) during quarantine was cited as an important component of successful health management of this colony.

D. Diseases

Very limited information is available on diseases of pocket gophers. Parasitism is a significant health issue in captive and wild pocket gophers (DeVries and Sikes, 2009; Wilber *et al.*, 1994). Heavy ascarid ('roundworm') infestation was cited as the cause of death during quarantine in one captive pocket gopher (DeVries and Sikes, 2009). Approximately 90% of wild pocket gophers harbor *Eimeria* spp. coccidia (Wilber *et al.*, 1994). Filariid nematodes of the genus *Litomosoides* have been reported in the abdominal and/or thoracic cavities of wild pocket gophers (Brant and Gardner, 2000). One hundred and twenty-two species of biting lice (order Mallophaga) are known to infest pocket gophers and are a model for host–parasite evolutionary co-speciation (Hafner and Page, 1995; Hellenthal and Price, 1994). The lice are highly host-specific. Griner (1983) described malocclusion of the incisor teeth leading to malnutrition in a male pocket gopher and captive management included provision of fruit bark for chewing (DeVries and Sikes, 2009; Griner, 1983).

V. KANGAROO RATS: *DIPODOMYS*

The two species generally studied are *Dipodomys spectabilis* (Bannertail kangaroo rat) and *D. merriami* (Merriam's kangaroo rat). See Figs. 7.9 and 7.10.

A. Introduction

1. *Taxonomy*

The family Heteromyidae contains six genera and 60 species (Nowak, 1999). The genus *Dipodomys* was recently confirmed as a monophyletic division and contains 21 species that live primarily in North America (Alexander and Riddle, 2005; Nowak, 1999).

2. *Description*

The description is adapted from Nowak (1999). Kangaroo rats are highly modified for travel by jumping.

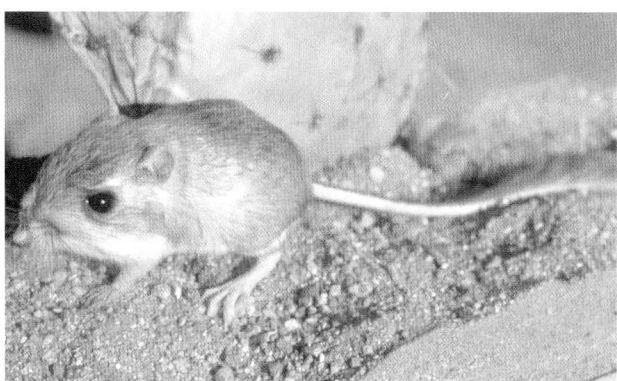

FIGURE 7.9 *Dipodomys merriami* – Merriam's kangaroo rat. Side view, feet and tail visible, Santa Rita Experimental Range, Pima County, Arizona. *Photograph by T.L. Best and the Mammal Images Library of the American Society of Mammalogists.*

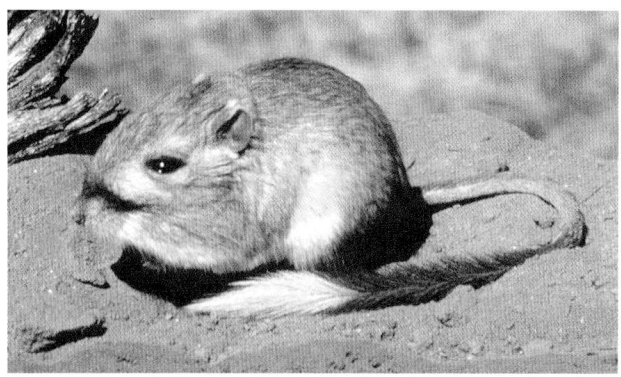

FIGURE 7.10 *Dipodomys spectabilis* – banner-tailed kangaroo rat. Side view, Pedro Armendariz lava field, Socorro County, New Mexico. *Photograph by T.L. Best and the Mammal Images Library of the American Society of Mammalogists.*

The hind legs are long and powerful, and the forelimbs reduced. The tail is longer than the head and body and serves as a balancing organ in locomotion and as a prop when standing. The leaping action of *Dipodomys* is similar to that of kangaroos (*Macropus* spp.), hence their common name of kangaroo rats. As in Geomyidae, all Heteromyidae rodents have external fur-lined cheek pouches. *Dipodomys* are unique in the Heteromyidae because their cheek teeth grow throughout life; the cheek teeth of other genera of Heteromyidae do not. The head and body length is 100–200 mm, tail length is 100–215 mm, and weight range is 35–180 g.

3. *Distribution*

All species of *Dipodomys* are found in North America, including northern Mexico. *D. spectabilis* is found in Arizona, New Mexico, western Texas, and northern Mexico; *D. merriami* is found in the southwestern U.S., northern Mexico, and Baja California (Hall, 1981).

4. Habitat

Kangaroo rats dwell in arid and semiarid country with some brush or grass (Nowak, 1999). They prefer open ground that permits an unobstructed view of the surroundings and is best for their method of locomotion. *Dipodomys* spp. construct burrows in well-drained, easily worked soil. *D. spectabilis* builds a labyrinth of tunnels within a prominent mound that is gradually built up as soil is excavated.

5. Use in Research

Kangaroo rats have been used extensively in the study of renal physiology and water conservation (Issaian et al., 2012; Stallone and Braun, 1988) and behavior (Yoerg and Shier, 1997). They have also been used in investigations looking at disuse osteoporosis (Muths and Reichman, 1996), evolutionary neuroanatomy (Jacobs and Spencer, 1994), decompression sickness (Hills and Butler, 1978), climate change (Moses et al., 2012), and as biosentinels for environmental contamination by mining operations (Espinosa-Reyes et al., 2010).

B. Biology

All species of *Dipodomys* are primarily diurnal (Schroder, 1979). Kangaroo rats seldom drink water, and utilize metabolically derived water from the breakdown of food within the body. They conserve moisture by coming out of their burrows at night when humidity is the highest and concentrating urine within highly efficient kidneys (Hall, 1981). The dorsal gland, a prominent androgen-independent, oil-secreting gland, is present on the back between the shoulders of males and females (Randall, 1986).

Kangaroo rats are highly territorial, and only one adult is found per burrow. Savage battles often take place when two kangaroo rats are placed together (Eisenberg and Isaac, 1963). They are not vocal but are known to produce a thumping or drumming sound with hindfeet. The foot drumming functions as an alarm system against predation by snakes, advertises territory, and repels intruders (Randall, 1986). Intraspecific agonistic behavior and foraging habits have been recently reviewed (Goetze et al., 2008).

Breeding may occur throughout the year. Females are seasonally polyestrous and estrus is correlated to availability of food. Although providing captive kangaroo rats with water for restricted periods mimics abundant seasons, Eisenberg and Isaac (1963) do not recommend *ad libitum* water, as some kangaroo rats become addicted to drinking and develop a diabetes insipidus-like syndrome. Gestation lasts approximately 29–33 days. Litter size ranges from one to six in the wild, with one to eight in *D. spectabilis* and an average of 2.6 in *D. merriami*. Weaning in *Dipodomys* spp. occurs

between 21 and 29 days (Eisenberg and Isaac, 1963). Hematocrits have been reported for *D. panamintinus* (Scelza and Knoll, 1982) and *D. merriami* (Haley et al., 1960). Hematology values for adult kangaroo rats are listed in Table 7.2.

C. Husbandry

Anderson and Jones (1984) contend that *Dipodomys* spp. are difficult to breed in the laboratory because of their aggressive nature toward one another. However, they are not aggressive toward humans (Williams, 1980). Kangaroo rats can be maintained together in an extremely large housing area (Fine et al., 1986). Several researchers have been successful at breeding *Dipodomys* and have produced many litters of kangaroo rats in captivity (Butterworth, 1961; Chew, 1958; Daly et al., 1984; Day et al., 1956). However, the methods required are time-consuming and intensive. During periods of nonreceptivity, female kangaroo rats are extremely aggressive toward males and will frequently attack and sometimes kill cage mates (Fine et al., 1986). The diet in the wild consists of seeds, some fruits, leaves, stems, buds, and insects and other invertebrates. A study of *D. merriami* in Arizona showed that approximately 80% of its food consisted of seeds and 15% consisted of insects (Reichman, 1975). Because of potential shortages caused by drought, kangaroo rats store food in their burrows. The diet in the laboratory is usually grains and seeds with lettuce as a source of water (Williams, 1980). Although kangaroo rats rarely drink in the wild, they will drink if offered water in captivity. Bathing in dust, like chinchillas, is necessary for the welfare of kangaroo rats. When denied dust bathing in captivity, they develop sores on the body and the fur becomes matted from oily secretions on the back (Nowak, 1999).

Kangaroo rats have fragile tails that will break off if used to restrain the animal. The recommended technique of restraining a kangaroo rat is by the skin on the nape of the neck (Fine et al., 1986).

D. Diseases

1. Infectious Diseases

Parasitic diseases have been extensively described in wild-caught kangaroo rats (Ernst and Chobotar, 1978; Fain and Lukoschus, 1978; Gummer et al., 1997; Hill and Best, 1985; Pfaffenberger et al., 1985; Stout and Duszynski, 1983; Thomas et al., 1991). However, there appear to be no cases in laboratory-reared kangaroo rats.

2. Metabolic/Nutritional Diseases

Suckow et al. (1996) described a male, wild-caught kangaroo rat that developed anorexia and wasting due to a gastric trichobezoar. They commented on the lack of information regarding the clinical medicine of this species.

3. Iatrogenic Diseases

Kangaroo rats develop spongiform degeneration of the central auditory system, particularly in the cochlear nucleus and auditory nerve root. The lesions are similar to that seen in the Mongolian gerbil (*Meriones unguiculatus*) (McGinn and Faddis, 1997). Degeneration is more numerous in animals continually exposed to modest levels of low-frequency noise (<75 dB SPL).

4. Neoplastic Diseases

Griner (1983) diagnosed mammary gland adenocarcinoma in a female kangaroo rat from the San Diego Zoo.

VI. PACK RATS: NEOTOMA

Pack rats or wood rats include *Neotoma floridana* (Allegheny wood rat; Fig. 7.11), *N. albigula* (white-throated wood rat), *N. mexicana* (Mexican wood rat), *N. cinerea* (bushy-tailed wood rat), and *N. fuscipes* (dusky-footed wood rat).

A. Introduction

1. Taxonomy

There are 19 species in the genus *Neotoma*. The name 'pack rat' or 'trade rat' comes from their habit of dropping the item they are carrying and taking new material if they find a more attractive object during foraging. They also often pick up shining objects or silverware from camps (Nowak, 1999).

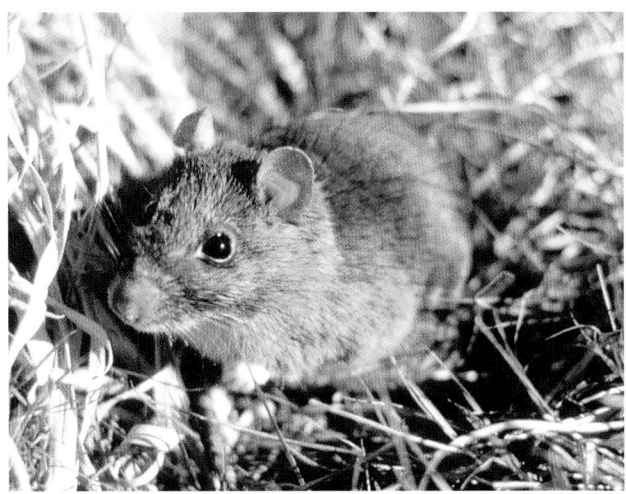

FIGURE 7.11 *Neotoma floridana* – Eastern or Allegheny wood rat. Front view, Riley County, Kansas. *Photograph by D. Post and the Mammal Images Library of the American Society of Mammalogists.*

2. Description

The description is taken from Nowak (1999). Head and body length is 150–230 mm, tail length is 75–240 mm, and weight is 200–450 g. The fur is generally soft and dense, and the color on the back ranges from pale to dark gray; the underparts range from a pure white to pale gray. The ears are large, and bare on the tips or naked. In some species the tail is sparsely haired, but in the bushy-tailed wood rat the tail is well covered.

3. Distribution

Wood rats are found in Central America (Honduras and Nicaragua) and North America. *Neotoma floridana* is found primarily on the eastern coast of the United States (Wiley, 1980); *N. albigula* is found in the southwestern United States to central Mexico; *N. mexicana* ranges from Colorado and southwestern Utah to western Honduras; *N. cinerea* ranges from northwestern Canada to North Dakota and Arizona (Escherich, 1981); and *N. fuscipes* ranges from western Oregon to northern Baja California.

4. Habitat

Wood rats live in a variety of habitats ranging from low, hot, dry deserts to humid jungles and to rocky slopes above the timberline. Some species of wood rats build elaborate dens composed of twigs, stems, foliage, bones, rocks, or whatever material is available. These 'houses' often rest on the ground or are placed against rocks or the base of a tree. Species inhabiting areas where spiny cactus grows build their houses almost entirely over this plant. The dens are placed so that it is almost impossible for a predator to approach without being pierced by thorns. Some species do not build large houses but use crevices among rocky outcrops. They close the openings to the crevices with sticks or other material. Much variation exists between shelters, even within the same species, depending on habitat conditions and availability of materials. Cameron and Rainey (1972) reported all three types of housing for *N. lepida* (Cameron and Rainey, 1972).

5. Use in Research

Wood rats have been used in behavioral and neurological studies (Towe and Harrison, 1993; Williams, 1980). Additionally, their role as reservoirs for a variety of zoonotic disease agents has been examined, including endemic murine typhus (*Rickettsia typhus*) (Worth, 1950), trypanosomiasis (Chagas disease) (Charles *et al.*, 2013), *Bartonella* spp. (Morway *et al.*, 2008), and Leishmaniasis (McHugh *et al.*, 1996). Wood rats have been identified as mammalian hosts for plague (*Yersinia pestis*) in British Columbia and California (Davis *et al.*, 2008; Lewis, 1989; Mian *et al.*, 1996). *N. fuscipes* is an important mammal reservoir of Lyme disease (*Borrelia burgdorferi*) in California and Oregon (Burkot *et al.*, 1999) and of human granulocytic ehrlichiosis (*Ehrlichia phagocytophila*) in certain areas of northern California (Nicholson *et al.*, 1999). Sin nombre virus (hantavirus) has been identified in four species of *Neotoma* from Arizona and Utah (Dearing *et al.*, 1998). Other *Bunyaviridae* (Jamestown Canyon virus and Morro Bay virus) were isolated from the dusky-footed wood rat in California (Fulhorst *et al.*, 1996). One or more indigenous arenaviruses are associated with *Neotoma* spp. in North America (Kosoy *et al.*, 1996; Lele *et al.*, 2003; Milazzo *et al.*, 2013). Some, like Catarina virus, are only believed to affect wood rats (Milazzo *et al.*, 2013). However, Whitewater Arroyo virus has been associated with lethal hemorrhagic fever in humans on rare occasions (Byrd *et al.*, 2000). Recently, dietary influences on gut microbiota and cytochrome P450 patterns were evaluated in *Neotoma* spp. Specifically the microbiota included a preponderance of novel species with cellulolytic and detoxification genes adapted to ingested plant species (Kohl *et al.*, 2011). Experimental feeding of plants with differing endogenous toxin properties influenced cytochrome c P450 expression patterns (Malenke *et al.*, 2012).

An antihemorrhagic factor in the serum of *N. micropus* against western rattlesnake venom has been identified and found similar to that in hispid cotton rat (*Sigmodon hispidus*) and in opossum (*Didelphis virginiana*) sera (Garcia and Perez, 1984).

B. Biology

Wood rats are nocturnal and active throughout the year. They have long or all-year breeding cycles but small litters. In the southern part of the range, female *Neotoma* can breed any time of the year. In the north, females begin breeding in December or January and continue producing litters until August to October (Williams, 1980). The gestation period of *Neotoma* spp. varies from 30–40 days (Olson *et al.*, 2013). The mothers wean the young in about 4 weeks and the pups reach sexual maturity at 7–8 months. The incisor teeth of nursing pups are laterally divergent for the first 2 weeks of life, and the mother's nipple fits into the gap (Hamilton, 1953). The young are then dragged around attached to the mother's teat. Eastern wood rats possess a ventral marking gland that is androgen-dependent (Clarke, 1975). Howell (1926) has made detailed anatomical descriptions of *Neotoma* (Howell, 1926). Normal hematology and serum biochemistry values have been published for the dusky wood rat (*N. fuscipes*) and were comparable to those of the house rat (*Rattus rattus*) (Weber *et al.*, 2002). Hematology values for adult packrats are listed in Table 7.2. Stress-related neutrophilia (stress leukogram) was seen in animals sampled immediately following capture.

C. Husbandry

Researchers have maintained colonies of Eastern wood rats successfully in captivity (Alligood *et al.*, 2011;

Alligood *et al.*, 2009; Dewsbury, 1974; Kinsey, 1976; Knoch, 1968; Smyser and Swihart, 2014; Worth, 1950). Smyser and Swihart (2014) and Alligood *et al.* 2011 developed successful strategies for captive breeding of endangered Allegheny wood rats and Key Largo wood rats, respectively, with eventual re-introduction to the wild. Worth (1950) found *N. floridana* easy to handle, but Dewsbury (1974) used metal mesh gloves. The diet of wood rats in the wild consists of roots, stems, leaves, seeds, and some invertebrates (Birney and Twomey, 1970; Chew, 1958; Harriman, 1974). In captivity, wood rats can be successfully maintained on standard laboratory rat diets (Williams, 1980). Alligood *et al.* (2011) utilized lab rodent diets (Mazuri Rodent pellets 5663, St Louis, MO) supplemented with daily fresh vegetables and forage. Water was provided ad libitum but the authors noted that most water in the wild was obtained from food sources. A variety of bedding materials including hay, palm fronds, wood shavings, and grasses were provided. *Neotoma* spp. are neat, sanitary animals and make good pets if they can overcome their extreme timidity (Nowak, 1999).

Neotoma spp. are generally solitary. In a colony of captive Eastern wood rats, a tyrannical social organization developed in which one animal killed or wounded all others (Kinsey, 1976). In field and laboratory studies, Escherich (1981) found that male *N. cinera* fought ferociously for harems of one to three females (Escherich, 1981). However, Williams (1980) reported that fighting in captivity is uncommon, even in overcrowded or multigenerational cages, and the males do not attack pups (Williams, 1980). Alligood *et al.* (2009) housed Key Largo wood rats individually in custom-designed wire mesh caging with opaque nest boxes. Caging could be joined via wire mesh tubing and effective behavioral markers of breeding receptivity were determined to allow safe pairing of male and female animals for breeding (Alligood *et al.*, 2009).

Blood samples can be obtained in the field by femoral vein puncture in bushy-tailed wood rats that have been injected intramuscularly with ketamine hydrochloride (Frase and Van Vuren, 1989). Dosages ranged from 30 to 110 mg/kg. Alligood *et al.* (2011) utilized isoflurane inhalation anesthesia when handling was necessary.

D. Diseases

1. Infectious Diseases

Wild-caught wood rats are infected with numerous ecto- and endoparasites, including ticks, fleas, and oocysts of host-specific *Eimeria* spp (Wheat and Ernst, 1974) (Charles *et al.*, 2012; Durden *et al.*, 1997; Lang, 1996; Marchiondo and Upton, 1987; Straneva and Gallati, 1980; Wheat and Ernst, 1974). Infection with the raccoon roundworm *Baylisascaris procyonis* has been associated with decimation of wild populations of wood rats, owing to encephalitis from cerebral migration of this parasite in an aberrant host (Page *et al.*, 2012).

Wood rats are important reservoirs of many zoonotic agents (see *Use in Research* – Section VI, A, 5), and suitable precautions must be taken when handling wild-caught animals. Chitin synthetase inhibitors (e.g., lufenuron), delivered via a feed cube have been effectively used to control fleas in wild populations of wood rats in California, as part of efforts to control *Yersinia pestis* (plague) (Davis, 1999). A variety of trypanosomes have been identified in peripheral blood of wood rats, including host-specific species *Trypanosoma neotomae* (Wood, 1936) and *T. kansasensis* (Upton *et al.*, 1989) and the zoonotic agent *Trypanosoma cruzi*, the causative agent of Chagas disease. The likelihood of transmission of *T. cruzi* to humans in a laboratory setting is low as the agent is typically (Charles *et al.*, 2013) spread by the feces of insect vectors (reduviid bug) which contaminate an insect bite. However, direct transmission from blood is also possible (e.g., needlestick injury). Host-specific and zoonotic arenaviruses have been identified in wood rats (Byrd *et al.*, 2000). Wood rats themselves may develop encephalitis associated with the potentially zoonotic arenavirus Whitewater Arroyo virus (Lele *et al.*, 2003). Transmission of arenaviruses to humans or other animals is by contact with fecal, urinary, pharyngeal secretions, or via blood. Laboratory colonies of wood rats should be screened serologically for agents of potential zoonotic concern.

A variety of nonzoonotic diseases have been described in wood rats. These include natural infection with *Brucella neotomae* (nonpathogenic to humans) in the desert wood rat *N. lepida* (Stoenner and Lackman, 1957). Novel *Hepatozoon* spp. were identified in two species of wood rats (Allen *et al.*, 2011). Hepatozoa are intracellular Apicomplexan parasites of red blood cells or other peripheral blood cells. Infection is spread by ingestion of ticks (not by tick bites) or ingestion of intermediate hosts. In some host species, infection is asymptomatic but in others, infection is associated with leukocytosis and/or myositis and proliferative bone lesions (i.e., *H. americanum* in dogs). The pathological potential of *Hepatozoon* spp. in wood rats is unknown. The filarial worm *Dunnifilaria meningica* has been described in *N. micropus* trapped in Mexico (Gutierrez-Pena, 1987). The small adult worms are found in the subarachnoid spaces along the cerebellum and the medulla oblongata. Female worms are approximately 50 mm long, males about 25 mm. Short, sheathed microfilariae are found in the peripheral blood.

Encysted larval *Echinococcus multilocularis* was found in the liver of a bushy-tailed wood rat in Wyoming (Kritsky *et al.*, 1977). Protoscolices and calcareous corpuscles were absent. Besnoitiosis, manifested as subcutaneous cysts, and asymptomatic *Toxoplasma gondii* infection were concurrently identified in a southern plains wood rat from Texas (Charles *et al.*, 2011). Since the wood rat is an intermediate host for both *Echinococcus* and *Toxoplasma*, the zoonotic transmission risk in a laboratory setting is not high, as the typical transmission mode in this instance is ingestion of the intermediate host. There is a small possibility of Toxoplasma transmission via needlestick injury, if sufficient tachy or bradyzoites are present in the blood (Herwaldt, 2001).

Naturally acquired rabies was detected in an Eastern wood rat by fluorescent antibody testing and mouse inoculation (Dowda *et al.*, 1981).

2. Other Diseases

Chronic glomerulonephropathy, manifesting as tubular proteinosis and membranous glomerulonephritis progressing to sclerosis has been described as highly prevalent in aged captive Key Largo wood rats (Terrell *et al.*, 2012). The lesions and progression resembled chronic progressive glomerulopathy of laboratory rats and dietary influences were suspected. Montali (1980) described a uterine adenocarcinoma in a 48-month-old female Eastern wood rat housed at the National Zoological Park in Washington, DC (Montali, 1980).

VII. GRASSHOPPER MICE: ONYCHOMYS

Onychomys torridus and *O. leucogaster* are commonly studied animals (see Figs. 7.12 and 7.13). They are among the most carnivorous of all rodents.

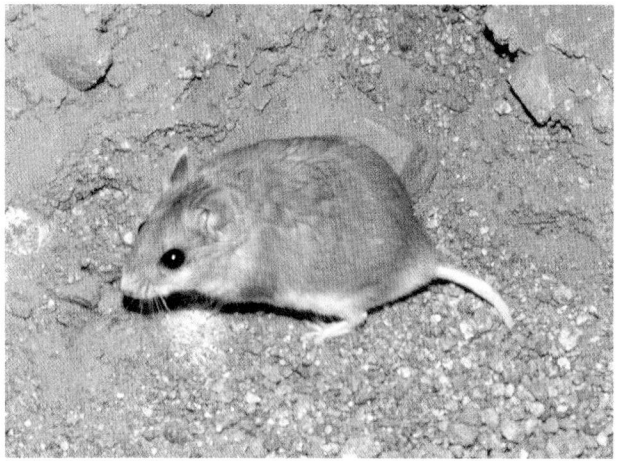

FIGURE 7.12 *Onychomys leucogaster* – Northern grasshopper mouse. Side view, Portal, Chochise, Arizona. *Photograph by R.B. Forbes and the Mammal Images Library of the American Society of Mammalogists.*

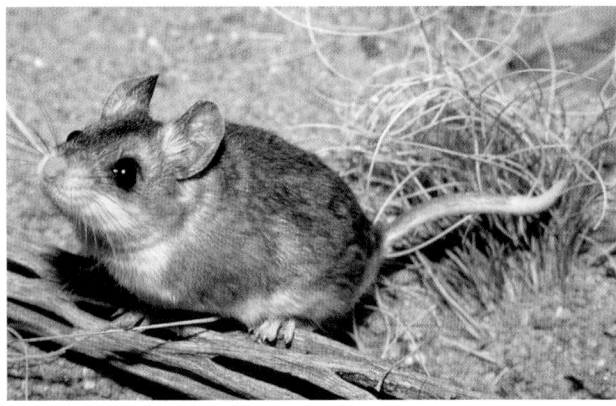

FIGURE 7.13 *Onychomys torridus* – Southern grasshopper mouse. Oblique front view, Portal, Cochise, Arizona. *Photograph by R.B. Forbes and the Mammal Images Library of the American Society of Mammalogists.*

A. Introduction

1. Taxonomy

The genus *Onychomys* contains three species of animals commonly called grasshopper mice. Two of the three species, *O. leucogaster* and *O. torridus*, have been studied more extensively in the laboratory.

2. Description

The head and body length is 90–130 mm, tail length is 30–60 mm, and weight is 30–60 g. The dorsal coat of *O. torridus* is gray and of *O. leucogaster*, brown. Both species have white ventral fur and distal tail tips (McCarty, 1975, 1978). Grasshopper mice are carnivorous and exhibit modifications in the jaw-muscle architecture that promote large bite forces for preying upon large prey (Williams *et al.*, 2009).

3. Distribution

O. torridus is found in the southwestern United States and northern Mexico; *O. leucogaster* is found from eastern Washington and southern Manitoba to extreme northern Mexico (McCarty, 1975, 1978).

4. Habitat

Grasshopper mice inhabit short-grass prairies and desert scrub. They live in any shelter they can find at ground level, although they are good climbers. The nest may be constructed in a burrow taken over from another rodent. Like that of most predators, the population density of grasshopper mice is low (average of 1.8 per hectare), although male–female pairs may associate all year. Their home range is well defined and covers 2–3 hectares. Captive individuals of the same sex are very aggressive to one another, often fighting to the death (McCarty, 1975, 1978).

5. Use in Research

The aggressive nature of grasshopper mice has led to their use in behavior studies. These have included studies on predatory behavior (McCarty *et al.*, 1976); sex differences in behavior, activity, and discrimination learning (Kemble and Enger, 1984); and drug effects on aggression (Cole and Wolf, 1970). Grasshopper mice have also been used to investigate Lyme disease (*Borrelia burgdorferi*) transmission via urine (Czub *et al.*, 1992) and the effect of photoperiod and melatonin on seasonal gonadal cycles (Frost and Zucker, 1983).

Grasshopper mice have been used to examine comparative antibody formation (Lochmiller *et al.*, 1991), cancer induction (Dewsbury and Jansen, 1972; Taylor *et al.*, 1993), and population dynamics using DNA and mitochondrial analysis (Alexander and Riddle, 2005; Riddle *et al.*, 1993; Sullivan *et al.*, 1996).

Grasshopper mice are an alternate host to prairie dogs (*C. ludovicianus*) for the plague bacillus *Yersinia pestis* (Salkeld *et al.*, 2010). In American grasslands, plague sporadically erupts in epizootics that decimate prairie dog colonies, yet the causes of outbreaks and mechanisms for inter epizootic persistence of this disease are poorly understood. Using field data on prairie community ecology, flea behavior, and plague-transmission biology, it has been found that plague can persist in prairie dog colonies for prolonged periods due to the abundance of the grasshopper mouse (*O. leucogaster*) as an alternate host (Franklin *et al.*, 2010; Stapp *et al.*, 2009). These findings offer an alternative perspective on plague's ecology (i.e., disease transmission exacerbated by alternative hosts) and have ramifications for plague dynamics in Asia and Africa, where a single main host has traditionally been considered to drive *Yersinia* ecology (Boone *et al.*, 2009). Abundance thresholds of alternate hosts appear to be a key phenomenon determining outbreaks of disease in many multihost-disease systems.

Grasshopper mice have been widely used in research investigations of reproduction (Dewsbury and Jansen, 1972).

B. Biology

Both *O. torridus* and *O. leucogaster* are nocturnal and active throughout the year. They are largely carnivorous. Grasshopper mice can breed throughout the year, but most reproductive activity in the wild occurs from May to September. Females have a 5- to 7-day estrous cycle, and gestation lasts 26–37 days (Horner, 1968; Pinter, 1970; Taylor, 1968). In the wild they produce several litters per year, although in the laboratory they have been reported to produce up to 12 litters per year (Pinter, 1970). The litter size ranges from one to six, averaging 3.6 in *O. leucogaster* and 2.6 in *O. torridus* (McCarty, 1978).

The young are weaned at 3 weeks, and sexual maturity is reached between 2 and 5 months in *O. leucogaster* and as early as 6 weeks in *O. torridus*. The copulatory behavior of southern grasshopper mice has been described (Dewsbury and Jansen, 1972).

The midventral sebaceous gland is larger in the male than in the female; castration causes an involution of the gland in both sexes. The secretions of the midventral gland are probably used for communications such as territorial marking, advertising of gonadal status, or pup identification (Pinter, 1985). In captivity the northern grasshopper mouse requires dust baths to keep its coat from becoming too oily (Fine *et al.*, 1986). Swindle *et al.* (1985) determined normal hematologic values from a colony of healthy adult *O. torridus*. Hematology values for adult grasshopper mice are listed in Table 7.2.

C. Husbandry

Grasshopper mice eat plant material occasionally in the wild, but the main diet consists of grasshoppers, beetles, and small vertebrates, including other rodents. *Onychomys torridus* prey extensively on scorpions, and are physiologically resistant to scorpion envenomation following natural stings (Rowe and Rowe, 2008). Venom resistance shows intra- and interspecific variability that covaries with scorpion sympatry and allopatry, patterns consistent with the hypothesis that venom resistance in grasshopper mice is an adaptive response to feeding on their neurotoxic prey. In the laboratory they are reported to survive well eating fresh mouse carcasses supplemented with seeds and water *ad libitum* (Fine *et al.*, 1986). Although grasshopper mice are aggressive predators in the wild, it is claimed that they become quite gentle in captivity and make fascinating pets (Nowak, 1999).

Egoscue (1960) successfully maintained and bred a laboratory colony of northern grasshopper mice. The animals were fed commercial mouse ration *ad libitum* that was periodically supplemented with a grain mixture and canned dog food. McCarty (1978) successfully maintained *O. leucogaster* in outdoor pens. In Japan, Matsuzaki *et al.* (1994). established a breeding colony of northern grasshopper mice captured in New Mexico. The rate of pregnancy for this colony was 75% when males and females were caged together for more than 30 days, and 4% when breeding pairs were caged from 1–7 days. Both cases were of monogamous mating. The mean litter size was 3.5 ± 1.2, with a range of one to six. The rate of weaning was 78.8%. The mean gestation period was 27.4 ± 2.0 days, with a range of 25–31. Matsuzaki *et al.* (1994) found it was possible to breed grasshopper mice year-round in a rearing room with fixed temperature and humidity. Southern grasshopper mice can be successfully cross-species fostered on white-footed mice (*Peromyscus leucopus*) (McCarty and Southwick, 1977a).

Harriman (1976) determined taste preferences, using Richter-type drinking tests (test solution opposite distilled water) for northern grasshopper mice. The animals showed strong drinking preferences for all concentrations of sugars above 0.05–0.10 M and hypotonic concentrations of saline. Taste preferences by grasshopper mice for these chemicals were similar to those exhibited by Mongolian gerbils tested with the same items. Grasshopper mice do not hear low frequencies as well as do other desert rodents such as kangaroo rats and gerbils (Heffner and Heffner, 1985).

D. Diseases

1. Infectious Diseases

Swindle *et al.* (1985) evaluated a captive colony of southern grasshopper mice for infectious diseases and parasites. They found no infectious diseases, but tropical rat mites (*Ornithonyssus bacoti*) parasitized the colony twice.

a. Bacterial Infections

Thomas *et al.* (1988) challenged laboratory-born progeny from two geographically distant populations of northern grasshopper mice with *Yersinia pestis* to determine their relative susceptibilities. One of the *O. leucogaster* populations was associated with a known epizootic focus of the disease and was nearly 2000 times more resistant to mortality than were members of another population from an area historically free of plague. In another study, Thomas *et al.* (1989) fed a mouse (*Mus musculus*) inoculated with *Y. pestis* to 20 laboratory-reared *O. leucogaster* from a parental population naturally exposed to plague. Three of the 20 *O. leucogaster* died, four survived with antibody titers against *Y. pestis*, and 13 survived with no titer against *Y. pestis*. In contrast, when 20 *O. leucogaster* from a plague-naive parental population were fed infected prey, seven died and 13 survived with no antibody titer against *Y. pestis*. The results suggested that the carnivorous behavior of *O. leucogaster* appears to promote strong selection for resistance to plague in areas where they are naturally exposed.

Grasshopper mice (and white-footed mice, *Peromyscus leucopus*) experimentally infected and naturally exposed to the Lyme disease spirochete, *Borrelia burgdorferi*, develop cystitis (Czub *et al.*, 1992). The pathologic changes observed in the urinary bladder of infected mice included lymphoid aggregates, vascular proliferation and hypertrophy, and perivascular infiltrates. Grasshopper mice are susceptible to *Coxiella burnetii*, although spontaneous infections have not been described under laboratory conditions (Wallach and Boever, 1983).

b. Viral Infections

Keis and Mitchell (1975) found inclusion bodies typical of cytomegalovirus (CMV) in the submandibular and sublingual glands of southern grasshopper mice. Serologic evaluation of wild-caught grasshopper mice suggests they can be infected with St. Louis equine encephalitis virus (Davis *et al.*, 1981).

c. Parasitic Infections

Pfaffenberger *et al.* (1985) trapped and examined 92 *O. leucogaster* in New Mexico for helminths. The authors found the grasshopper mice infected with two species of nematodes (*Litomosoides carinii, Mastophorus muris*), two species of cestodes (*Hymenolepis citelli* and one unknown), and one species of acanthocephalan (*Moniliformis clarki*). All infections represent new host and distribution records.

Eimeria onychomysis is a coccidian parasite infecting *O. leucogaster* (Upton *et al.*, 1992). Hnida *et al.* (1998) described a new species of *Eimeria* infecting three species of *Onychomys* (*O. arenicola, O. leucogaster,* and *O. torridus*) captured in New Mexico and Arizona. Six of 59 animals (10%) were infected. Isolates recovered from *O. leucogaster* and *O. torridus* were inoculated into *O. leucogaster* and produced infections with a prepatent period of 7 days and a patent period of 7–23 days.

Feral grasshopper mice have numerous parasitic infestations with the flea *Monopsyllus exilis* (Davis *et al.*, 1981). Nutting *et al.* (1973) described an unidentified *Demodex* mite that infected the tongue, esophagus, and oral cavity of *O. leucogaster*. Hughes and Nutting (1981) named the parasite *Demodex leucogasteri* and described its biology and host pathogenesis.

d. Fungal Infections

Grasshopper mice are susceptible to *Coccidioides immitis* although spontaneous infections have not been described under laboratory conditions (Wallach and Boever, 1983).

2. *Idiopathic Diseases*

Convulsive seizures similar to that seen in Mongolian gerbils (*Meriones unguiculatus*) were observed to occur in nine male (*n* = 29) and 23 female (*n* = 50) southern grasshopper mice maintained in captivity (McCarty and Southwick, 1975). The preweaning parental environment has a significant influence on the prevalence of convulsive seizures (McCarty and Southwick, 1977b).

Swindle *et al.* (1985) observed multiple limb defects, including brachydactyly, syndactyly, and hemimelia, in offspring from a colony of *O. torridus* in the United States.

VIII. DEER MICE: *PEROMYSCUS*

A. Introduction

1. *Description*

The genus *Peromyscus* contains seven subgenera and 60 species. The two species most commonly used in

research are *P. maniculatus*, the prairie deer mouse, and *P. leucopus*, the white-footed mouse (see Figs. 7.14 and 7.15). The common name of deer mice derives from the animals' agility at jumping and running in comparison with house mice.

Peromyscus maniculatus ranges from southeastern Alaska throughout Canada and the United States to Mexico; however, it is not found regularly in moist environments (Baker, 1968). In New York, Pennsylvania, and Michigan two morphological and behavioral forms of *P. maniculatus* coexist but occupy different ecologic niches. In the wild, *P. maniculatus* builds nests of leaves and lives with a population density of 1–25 individuals per hectare. It is considered a social animal. *Peromyscus leucopus* lives in population densities of 5–39 per hectare with males and females pair bonding and females excluding other females from their home ranges (0.1 hectare).

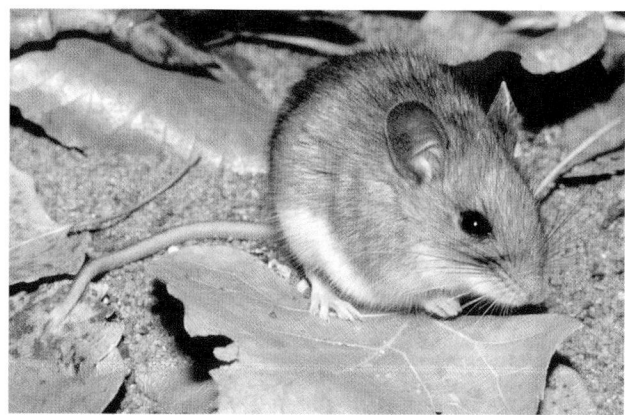

FIGURE 7.14 *Peromyscus leucopus* – white-footed deer mouse. Oblique front view, Bernalillo County, New Mexico. *Photograph by R.B. Forbes and the Mammal Images Library of the American Society of Mammalogists.*

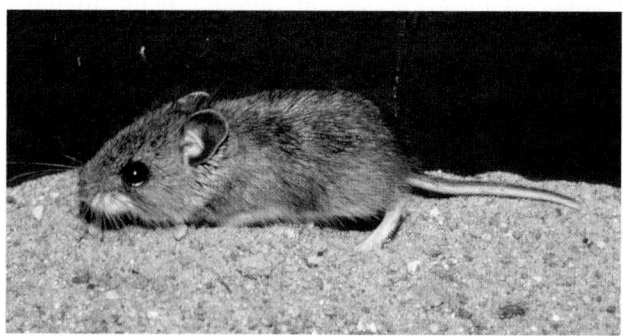

FIGURE 7.15 *Peromyscus maniculatus* – North American deer mouse. Lateral view, Socorro County, New Mexico. *Photograph by R.B. Forbes and the Mammal Images Library of the American Society of Mammalogists.*

2. Use in Research

Both *P. maniculatus* and *P. leucopus* adapt readily to the laboratory environment and have been used extensively for studies in genetics, physiology, aging, cataracts, and behavior (Blanco *et al.*, 2004; Burger and Gochfeld, 1992; Cutler, 1985; Dewsbury, 1984; Harris *et al.*, 2013; Tripathi *et al.*, 1991; Ungvari *et al.*, 2008). *Peromyscus californicus* are genetically susceptible to a heritable hyperlipidemia that is inducible by a high fat diet (Krugner-Higby *et al.*, 2011; Krugner-Higby *et al.*, 2006). This has been used as an experimental model of metabolic syndrome. *Peromyscus* are used in neurological research of epilepsy and refined methods for generating audiogenic seizures have been developed (Veres *et al.*, 2013). Inbred *Peromyscus* with particular genetic or physiological traits have played important roles. Dr. George Smith inbred both species for studies on aging (Fine *et al.*, 1986). *Peromyscus* spp. with varying response to lipopolysaccharide challenge were used to elucidate immunological mechanisms of effective bacterial clearance (Martin *et al.*, 2008). Renewed use in research has centered on their susceptibility to zoonotic diseases. They are well known as the principal vector for North American hantaviruses, including Sin Nombre virus (Luis *et al.*, 2012; MacNeil *et al.*, 2011; Schlegel *et al.*, 2014). Additionally, *Peromyscus* are naturally occurring vectors for numerous other zoonotic diseases either directly or via fleas or ticks. *P. leucopus* is a significant host for *Ixodes scapularis* (the black-legged tick or deer tick). Thus it has been studied for its role in the epidemiology of *Borrelia burgdorferi*, the causative agent of Lyme disease (Schwanz *et al.*, 2011) and as a recipient of potential wildlife oral vaccine strategies to reduce Lyme disease transmission to humans (Schwanz *et al.*, 2011). Ixodid ticks also are host to the blood parasites *Babesia microti* and *Anaplasma phagocytophilum* (formerly *Ehrlichia phagocytophila*) (Magnarelli *et al.*, 2013). The latter is the causative agent of human granulocytic anaplasmosis (formerly granulocytic ehrlichiosis). Other zoonotic diseases found naturally in *Peromyscus* spp. include trypanosomiasis (Anosa and Kaneko, 1984), toxoplasmosis (Rejmanek *et al.*, 2010), tularemia (Wobeser *et al.*, 2007), and potential food and water-borne pathogens such as *Cryptosporidium* and *Giardia* (Kilonzo *et al.*, 2013).

The Peromyscus Genetic Stock Center (PGSC) has been maintained at the University of South Carolina in Columbia, SC, since 1995 (Felder, 2014). It houses colonies of wild-type and mutant *Peromyscus* spp. and serves as a resource for animals and tissues, and genetic and husbandry information (Felder *et al.*, 2012). Assisted reproduction protocols have been developed (Veres *et al.*, 2012). Detailed information is accessible through links on the Stock Center website about the various *Peromyscus* cell lines and embryonic stem cells that are available (Felder, 2014).

B. Biology

Animals vary in color, although most are dark brown to sandy with white or nearly white underparts. Adults molt once a year. Deer mice have large, haired ears and a long tail. They are active throughout the year and generally nocturnal. *Peromyscus maniculatus* may live 8 years under laboratory conditions (Nowak, 1999). *Peromyscus leucopus* is primarily nocturnal but may be active throughout the day. The species conserves water through urine volume reduction. Reproduction, thermoregulation, molting, and nest building all influence melatonin (Hamilton and Whitaker, 1979; Lackey *et al.*, 1985). The dental formula is I 1/1, C 0/0, PM 2/1, M 3/3, and molars are rooted. The separation of cardiac from pyloric portions of the stomach is less distinct than that of Old World rodents. Data for food and water consumption have been published (Lackey *et al.*, 1985). Hematology values have been reported for adult deer mice (Wu *et al.*, 1999) and are listed in Table 7.2.

The natural breeding season for *P. maniculatus* is March to October in the northern portions of its range. *Peromyscus leucopus* is also a seasonal breeder in the northern range but breeds all year in Mexico. Both species breed year-round under laboratory conditions. *Peromyscus maniculatus* females are polyestrous and produce three to four litters per year (in the laboratory they may have as many as 14 litters per year). *Peromyscus leucopus* females have 6-day estrous cycles with spontaneous ovulation and a postpartum estrus. In both species litter size averages five, and the gestation period is 22–23 days in length (Drickamer and Vestal, 1973). The presence of males does not accelerate the onset of puberty nor induce estrous cycle synchrony in females; however, it is critical for cycle regularity (Yasukawa *et al.*, 1978). When males and females are housed together as preweanlings, they show delayed reproduction as adults (Hill, 1974).

C. Husbandry

Reviews of Peromyscus husbandry have been published (Dewey and Dawson, 2001; Joyner *et al.*, 1998). Additional information is available from Heideman (2004) and from the PGSC (Felder, 2014). Both *P. maniculatus* and *P. leucopus* adapt readily to plastic solid-bottom cages. They are frequently housed as breeding pairs, with separation of the male after parturition only required occasionally (Brand and Ryckman, 1968; Dewsbury, 1975; Heideman, 2004). High intercolony variation in reproductive success was reported by Heideman (2004) with some colonies averaging only 50% successful breeding pairs. *Peromyscus leucopus* self-selected a higher room temperature (32.4°C) than did laboratory mice (Lackey *et al.*, 1985). Cages should be equipped with bedding (wood shavings) and separate nest-building material (Dewsbury, 1975, 1974). They are maintained on 16:8h light:dark cycle, and although they move more rapidly than other domesticated rodents, they are easy to handle. Nutrition has not been thoroughly studied. In the wild their diet consists of seeds, nuts, berries, insects, small invertebrates, and carrion. At PGSC, *Peromyscus* are fed commercially available pelleted rodent feed (Harlan Teklad Rodent Diet 8604) without supplementation. Heideman (2004) reports feeding high fat diets to breeding animals to enhance reproduction.

D. Diseases

When *Peromyscus* are brought into an animal facility from the wild, special precautions must be taken to avoid introduction of several zoonotic diseases, including hantavirus and others as mentioned under Uses in Research. Additional zoonotic concerns may include leptospirosis, *Hymenolepis* spp., Rocky Mountain spotted fever, chlamydiosis, Q-fever, Western and Venezuelan equine encephalitis, sylvatic plague, and coccidioidomycosis (Clark, 1984; Davis *et al.*, 1981; Fine *et al.*, 1986; Wallach and Boever, 1983). As discussed in the introduction, the risk to human health must be tempered by a realistic assessment of the actual risk to human handlers. For example, *Borrelia burgdorferi* and *Anaplasma phagocytophila* are two of the most common infections in wild *Peromyscus* but are generally transmitted via an arthropod vector (Davis *et al.*, 1981; Fine *et al.*, 1986; Wallach and Boever, 1983), thus present much less risk of transmission in a laboratory facility. Additionally, while *Peromyscus* are considered a chronically infected 'maintenance host' for *B. burgdorferi* and thus may pose a risk for exposure via needlestick, *Anaplasma* infections are typically transient, owing to a strong immune response that may eliminate infection (Levin and Fish, 2000; Magnarelli *et al.*, 2013). In at least one instance, Lyme disease was transmitted from infected to naive *Peromyscus* by direct contact (Burgess *et al.*, 1986). With respect to *Peromyscus* health, no apparent adverse effects on animal behavior (wheel-running) or peripheral blood counts was detected with experimental *B. burgdorferi* infection (Schwanz *et al.*, 2011). Both ectoparasites and endoparasites (including *Aspicularis, Syphacia, Capillaria, Nippostrongylus, Nematospiroides, Trichuris, Mastophorus, Ricturlaria coloradensis*, and *Acanthocephala clarki*) are common in *Peromyscus*. In a recent small screen of wild *Peromyscus leucopus* caught within a laboratory facility in Michigan, serology and PCR were negative for 12 viral agents of concern for laboratory mice, including MHV, MPV, Sendai, and LCMV (Dyson *et al.*, 2009). *Peromyscus* has been shown to seroconvert but not to develop clinical disease with mouse hepatitis virus (Silverman *et al.*, 1982). In the Michigan screen, *Peromyscus* were

also negative for *Mycoplasma pulmonis* and CAR bacillus, however seven of eight animals screened were PCR positive for *Helicobacter* spp. (Dyson *et al.*, 2009). Other spontaneous diseases in Peromyscus include adiaspiromycosis, (pulmonary fungal infection) which is typically an incidental finding, Tyzzer's disease (*C. piliforme*), associated with high mortality, and ringtail, typically correlated with low humidity (Fine *et al.*, 1986).

IX. RICE RATS: ORYZOMYS

Oryzomys palustris is the most commonly studied species. It is also called the marsh rice rat because it is found in habitats such as swamps and salt marshes. Early American settlers called *O. palustris* rice rats because of their fondness for cultivated rice (Wolfe, 1982). Figure 7.16 shows *Orzymous capito*.

A. Introduction

1. Taxonomy

Within the genus *Oryzomys* are five subgenera and 50 species. *Oryzomys palustris* is the best-known species and most widely studied. Multiple chromosomal polymorphisms within single, natural populations, more than have previously been reported in a mammal, have made many aspects of the systematics of this genus undetermined (Koop *et al.*, 1983; Maia and Hulak, 1981). Polymorphic variation seems stable within a population and is not the result of hybridization, human disturbance, or nonspecific mutagenic agents.

2. Description

Head and body length is 100–200 mm, tail length is 75–250 mm, and the weight is usually 40–80 g (Wolfe, 1982). Williams (1980) states that *Oryzomys* may range

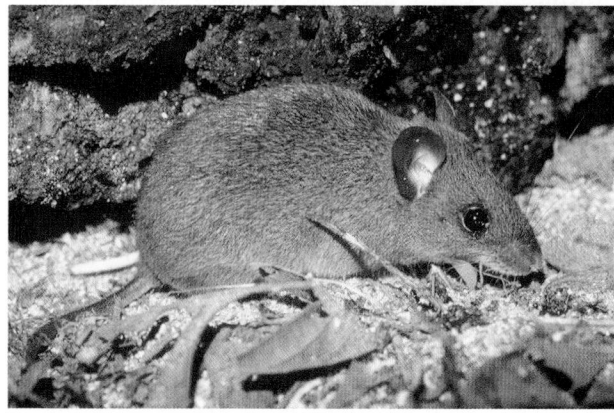

FIGURE 7.16 *Oryzomys capito* – rice rat. Side view, Parque Nacional Guatapo, Miranda, Venezuela. *Photograph by PV August and the Mammal Images Library of the American Society of Mammalogists.*

from 25–150 g. The upperparts are grayish brown to yellow brown, mixed with black; the sides are paler, with less black; the underparts are white to pale buff; and the tail varies from brownish above and white below to uniformly dusky. *Oryzomys palustris* is mouse-like; the pelage is coarse but not bristly or spiny. The tail is usually long, with annulations showing through the sparse hairs (Wolfe, 1982). Rice rats may be confused with cotton rats (*Sigmodon*), but the latter have longer, grizzled fur and a shorter, stouter tail.

3. Habitat

Oryzomys palustris is a semiaquatic North American rodent that occurs in wetland habitats such as swamps and salt marshes. It is found mostly in the eastern and southern U.S., from New Jersey and Kansas south to Florida and northeastern Tamaulipas, Mexico (Wolfe, 1982).

4. Use in Research

The rice rat spontaneously develops periodontal disease (Leonard, 1979a,b), and placing the animal on a high-sucrose diet accelerates the periodontitis (Shklair and Ralls, 1988). Using this animal model, researchers have investigated the effects of pharmacological drugs, dietary vitamin E, and rotational stress on periodontal bone resorption (Cohen and Meyer, 1993; Leonard *et al.*, 1979).

Park (1974a,b,c; Park and Nowosielski-Slepowron, 1974) described the anatomy and histology of the rice rat's teeth, the growth and development of the maxilla and mandible, and the relationship of these processes to tooth eruption and calcification.

Edmonds and Stetson (1993) investigated the effect of photoperiod on reproduction and reproductive development in rice rats. Their work highlighted the role of the pineal gland and its secretion of melatonin on reproduction (Edmonds *et al.*, 1995; Edmonds and Stetson, 1994, 1995). Rice rats have been used to study metal-pollutant uptake and its relationship to genetic damage in South Carolina (Peles and Barrett, 1997).

B. Biology

Eighty-four specimens of *Oryzomys subflavus*, collected in the State of Pernambuco, Brazil, were studied. A Robertsonian chromosome polymorphism, characterized by a varying diploid number of 50, 49, 48, and 46, was found. All specimens showed a chromosome arm number of 56. G-banding patterns in somatic cells allowed identification of the chromosome pairs (2, 3, 5, and 7) involved in centric fusion (Maia and Hulak, 1981).

C. Husbandry

Several papers describe the care in captivity and reproduction of different species of *Oryzomys*. Graeff Teixeira *et al.* (1998) described care in captivity and recommended providing a hollow brick to use as shelter and to reduce stress; Mello (1978) reviewed aspects of the biology, growth, and reproduction of *Oryzomys eliurus* under laboratory conditions. Villela and Alho (1983) described the postnatal development and growth of *O. subflavus* in a laboratory setting; and Worth (1967) reviewed the reproduction, development, and behavior of captive *O. laticeps*.

Park and Nowosielski-Slepowron (1975) examined body growth using weight and length parameters following the introduction of the rice rat to laboratory conditions and described the history of breeding the animals over 15 generations. The same authors surveyed skull development of the rice rat (*O. palustris natator*) covering a period of 21 days to 16 months and involving equal numbers of males and females (*n* = 108) (Park and Nowosielski-Slepowron, 1976).

D. Diseases

The spiny rat louse, *Polyplax spinulosa*, was collected from a wild rice rat in Tennessee (Durden, 1988). This sucking louse is typically parasitic on domestic rats, and the author commented that as most sucking lice are normally host-specific, such cross-familial host infestation is noteworthy. The rice rat is the predominant reservoir host for Bayou virus, a cause of hantavirus pulmonary syndrome (Torrez Martinez *et al.*, 1998). Webster (1987) reported a rice rat found in North Carolina with vertebral column deformity. They believed the kyphosis was probably inherited.

X. CANE MICE: *ZYGODONTOMYS*

Researchers have sometimes described *Zygodontomys brevicauda* (Fig. 7.17) as *Z. microtinus* in the literature.

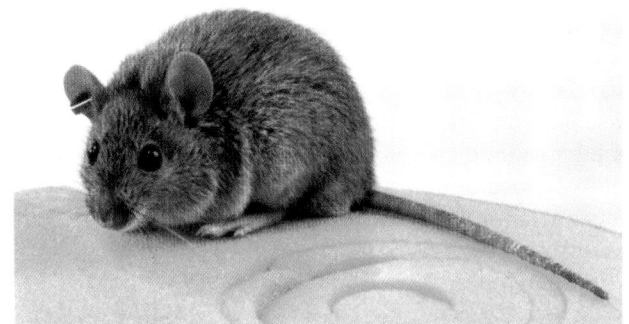

FIGURE 7.17 *Zygodontomys brevicauda* – cane mouse. Side view of captive mouse, The Rockefeller University, New York. *Photograph by TM Donnelly and the Mammal Images Library of the American Society of Mammalogists.*

Older references refer to unrelated species (e.g., *Z. lasiurus* and *Z. pixuna*) that are properly called the genus *Bolomys* (e.g., *lasiurus*, *lenguarum*, and *pixuna*) (Voss, 1991).

A. Introduction

1. Description

Zygodontomys brevicauda is about 100 g or less in body weight with a grizzled brown pelage and a tail about three-fourths the length of its head and body.

2. Distribution

Cane mice are widely distributed in the tropical lowlands of eastern Central America, northern South America, and adjacent continental islands.

3. Habitat

Mainland populations of *Zygodontomys* typically inhabit savannas or weedy areas around human settlements where the species is sometimes an agricultural pest. Cane mice are nocturnal, omnivorous, and terrestrial, seldom or never climbing trees (Voss, 1991).

4. Use in Research

Cane mice are used in comparative studies of mammalian circannual reproductive cycles since this is one of the few tropical species known to lack a reproductive response to photoperiod (Bronson and Heideman, 1992; Heideman and Bronson, 1990). *Zygodontomys brevicauda* is also a good animal model for evolutionary quantitative genetics. Its short generation time, high diploid chromosome numbers, and the availability of F$_1$ and F$_2$ hybrids from crosses between geographically isolated populations make experimental analyses of evolutionary divergence less difficult (Voss, 1992). Virologists have used laboratory colonies of cane mice in studies of arboviruses, such as yellow fever virus (Bates and Weir, 1944); nariva virus, a rodent paramyxovirus (Beare, 1975; Tikasingh *et al.*, 1966); Venezuelan equine encephalomyelitis (Downs *et al.*, 1962); and cocal virus, a rhabdovirus (Jonkers *et al.*, 1964). *Zygodontomys brevicauda* is a natural host of Guanarito virus, the cause of Venezuelan hemorrhagic fever (VHF) (Fulhorst *et al.*, 1999b). Fever, malaise, and a sore throat initially characterize this disease in humans. Abdominal pain, diarrhea, a variety of hemorrhagic manifestations, and convulsions usually follow. Since a VHF emergence in 1989 up until 1997, Venezuelan authorities have reported 220 cases with a fatality rate of 33% (Salas *et al.*, 1998).

B. Biology

Sexual maturation of cane mice is rapid, and litter sizes are moderately large in comparison with those of other New World muroids such as *Peromyscus*. The work of Voss *et al.* (1992) and Aguilera (1985) are in close accord. Females become sexually mature at 21–26 days and males at 40–60 days. Gestation lasts 25 days, with litters usually consisting of four or five young but ranging from 1 to 11. Larger litters consist of smaller neonates, and the young open their eyes at 6–8 days. By day 16 females wean their young. Ovulation in females is spontaneous. Pairing females with males in cages divided by wire partitions that permit limited physical contact, but not copulation, does not accelerate the occurrence of estrus or ovulation. Estrous cycling does not differ between single-housed females and females housed with males in divided cages. Copulatory plugs are formed when animals mate.

C. Husbandry

Voss *et al.* (1992) maintained their colony according to recommendations in the *Guide* for temperature and humidity. However, cages were cleaned only once every 1 or 2 weeks because cane mice urinate and defecate sparingly compared with laboratory mice (*Mus musculus.*) Food consisted of commercial mouse chow, supplemented by dry cat food and chopped frozen vegetables. Lactating females were provided double rations. Cane mice are strong and agile and jump abruptly with slight provocation (Voss *et al.*, 1992; Worth, 1967). Cages should be placed at the bottom of a deep (at least 2.5 feet) box before removing the wire lid to prevent escape. (Voss *et al.*, 1992) found that animals of all ages in their colony were aggressive and leather gloves were necessary for handling. Females became aggressive shortly before parturition and males were removed to prevent injuries. Males rarely injured females, and pairing younger females with older males reduced female aggression. Williams (1980) reported that researchers maintaining two different colonies of *Zygodontomys* found the animals nonaggressive to handlers.

D. Diseases

1. Infectious Diseases

Voss *et al.* (1992) were unable to isolate known bacterial pathogens from seven of eight animals randomly selected for microbiological screening. *Yersinia pseudotuberculosis* was isolated from the nasal cavity of one animal. The major concern with cane mice is their zoonotic potential as the natural host of Guanarito virus (family Arenaviridae), the etiologic agent of VHF (Fulhorst *et al.*, 1999a). Animals developed chronic viremic infections characterized by persistent shedding of infectious virus in oropharyngeal secretions and urine.

Pinworms (*Syphacia* sp.) and the trichomonad intraduodenal protozoan *Hexamita* were found in the colony of Voss *et al.* (1992). Fifty-five species of arthropod ectoparasites are known to infest *Z. brevicauda* in nature, but only the tropical rat mite (*Ornithonyssus bacoti*) appears to persist in laboratory-bred, wild-derived animals (Voss *et al.*, 1992).

XI. COTTON RATS: *SIGMODON*

There are eight species of cotton rats. Of these, *Sigmodon hispidus* (Fig. 7.18) and *S. fulviventer* (Fig. 7.19) are most often used as laboratory animals. However, *S. hispidus* is used far more often than *S. fulviventer*. The term *cotton rat* as used in the text refers to *S. hispidus*.

A. Introduction

1. Description

Sigmodon hispidus is a robust, stocky rodent that weighs 80–130 g with a head-to-body length of 125–200 mm. The

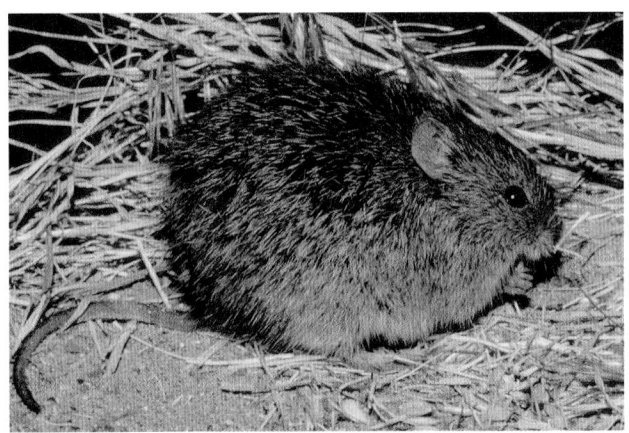

FIGURE 7.18   *Sigmodon hispidus* – hispid cotton rat. Side view, Luna County, New Mexico. *Photograph by R.B. Forbes and the Mammal Images Library of the American Society of Mammalogists.*

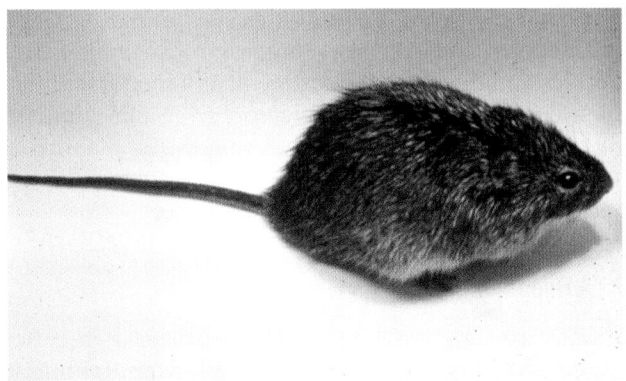

FIGURE 7.19   *Sigmodon fulviventer* – tawny-bellied cotton rat. Dorsolateral view, The Museum, Michigan State University, Michigan. *Photograph by C.S. St. Clair, A.S. Ahl, and the Mammal Images Library of the American Society of Mammalogists.*

tail length is 75–166 mm (Cameron and Spencer, 1981). The fur is coarse, dark brown to black interspersed with yellow or light tan hairs over the back and sides, while the underparts are usually pale to dark gray. The ears are small, and the three central digits of each paw are larger than the other two. All species of cotton rats are similar in appearance although there is wide variation in chromosome number among species (Zimmerman, 1970). Voss (1992) has revised the South American species of *Sigmodon*, but further α-taxonomic studies are needed.

2. Distribution

Sigmodon hispidus occurs in the southern United States to northern Venezuela and northwestern Peru. *Sigmodon fulviventer* occurs in southeastern Arizona and central New Mexico to central Mexico (Nowak, 1999).

3. Habitat

Cotton rats prefer grassy and shrubby areas (Nowak, 1999). They are the most abundant rodents in the southeastern United States, Mexico, and Central America.

4. Use in Research

Cotton rats are an important animal model for viral respiratory tract diseases, particularly those caused by paramyxoviruses (Bem *et al.*, 2011; Green *et al.*, 2013; Niewiesk and Prince, 2002). Respiratory syncytial virus (RSV), a leading cause of respiratory tract infections in human infants (Piazza *et al.*, 1995; Prince *et al.*, 1999); parainfluenza virus 3, the second leading cause of pediatric respiratory disease (Ottolini *et al.*, 1996; Prince and Porter, 1996); and measles virus (Niewiesk, 1999; Niewiesk *et al.*, 1997) replicate well in cotton rats. Cotton rats are particular useful for RSV vaccine studies, as they have been demonstrated to develop the phenomenon of 'enhanced disease' upon challenge in animals that have previously received certain RSV vaccine formulations. As this phenomenon is a known complication of candidate human RSV vaccinations, an animal model that replicates this tendency is highly desirable (Boukhvalova and Blanco, 2013). Cotton rats can also be infected with avian and swine influenza and have been used to test influenza vaccination strategies (Blanco *et al.*, 2004, 2013; Yim *et al.*, 2012). Adenovirus pneumonia in infected animals is similar to that in humans (Prince *et al.*, 1993), and ocular adenovirus infection in cotton rats is the only animal model of epidemic keratoconjunctivitis (Tsai *et al.*, 1992).

The susceptibility of cotton rats to human adenovirus replication has led to their use in studies of adenoviral mediated gene therapy. In this research replication-defective adenoviruses are used as vectors to deliver foreign genes. Researchers have used cotton rats to investigate gene therapy for cystic fibrosis (Yei *et al.*, 1994), erythropoiesis stimulation (Setoguchi *et al.*, 1994), ocular gene transfer (Tsubota *et al.*, 1998), cervical cancer treatment (Billings *et al.*, 2010; Bischoff *et al.*, 1996), and malignant central nervous system tumors (Shine *et al.*, 1997).

Many viral, protozoan, metazoan, and bacterial pathogens can be transmitted to cotton rats. These include *Rickettsia tsutsugamushi*, the causative agent of scrub typhus (Gage *et al.*, 1990), *Leishmania donovani* (Azazy *et al.*, 1994), and *Echinococcus multilocularis* (Kroeze and Tanner, 1985). Cotton rats are naturally infected with the filarial nematode *Litomosoides carinii* and are popular animal models to screen antifilarial drugs (Chatterjee *et al.*, 1989; Kershaw and Storey, 1976). They can be nasally colonized with methicillin-resistant *Staphylococcus aureus* (MRSA) to test interventional strategies (Desbois *et al.*, 2013). Researchers have investigated the role of the wild cotton rat as a natural reservoir of Lyme disease, the hantavirus Black Creek Canal virus, and Venezuelan equine encephalitis (Banks *et al.*, 1998; Billings *et al.*, 2010; Elangbam *et al.*, 1989; Oliver *et al.*, 1995; Rollin *et al.*, 1995; Zarate and Scherer, 1968) and have proposed the cotton rat as a biomonitor to study the impact of environmental pollutants on exposed wildlife.

B. Biology

Wild cotton rats may be active at night or day but they are typically diurnal under laboratory conditions. Their activity patterns may change in the wild or in the laboratory, and nocturnal animals may become diurnal (Johnston and Zucker, 1983). A relative dominance system in which males dominate females and adults dominate juveniles characterizes cotton rat behavior. Cotton rats are solitary animals, with the only prolonged social contact occurring between males and females for reproduction. Aggressive behavior is common, and caged animals will inflict severe bite wounds on cage mates and sometimes fight to the death (Faith *et al.*, 1997; Niewiesk and Prince, 2002).

Gestation in cotton rats is 27 days, and litter size is 1–12 young with an average of five to seven. The young weigh 6.5–8.0 g and open their eyes at 24 h. In wild populations, they may be weaned at 5–7 days. Sexual maturity occurs at 40–60 days (Nowak, 1999). Lifespan in captivity is between 14 months (inbred strains) and 23 months (wild-type) (Niewiesk and Prince, 2002).

Hematological data have been reported for wild and laboratory cotton rats of different ages and sexes (Dotson *et al.*, 1987, 1990; Katahira and Ohwada, 1993; Leveson *et al.*, 1989; Maity and Guru, 1998; McMurry *et al.*, 1995; Robel *et al.*, 1996; Ubelaker *et al.*, 1993; Webb *et al.*, 2003). Hematology values for adult inbred, captive bred and wild caught cotton rats are listed in Table 7.2. The retroorbital route has been previously recommended for blood collection (Niewiesk and Prince, 2002). However, a subzygomatic route has been described that relies on

the presence of a subzygomatic sinus unique to this species (Ayers *et al.*, 2012). Itoh *et al.* (1989) have characterized the gastrointestinal flora of cotton rat.

C. Husbandry

Husbandry has been reviewed (Faith *et al.*, 1997; Juan-Salles *et al.*, 2009; Niewiesk and Prince, 2002). All report that cotton rats will attempt to bite and escape when picked up. Leather garden gloves simplify handling but for inexperienced handlers, a handling device enabling cage transfer without direct contact has been developed (Niewiesck *et al.*, 1997). Cotton rats can be kept housed in standard polycarbonate cages with hardwood-chip or corncob bedding. Animals drink more than standard laboratory rats, thus caretakers may need to change cages twice a week.

Kawase and Satoh (1978) described breeding cotton rats in the laboratory. Niewiesk and Prince (2002) recommended weaning at 2–3 weeks into single sex groups, followed by monogamous pairing of breeding animals by 6 weeks of age. Faith *et al.* (1997) noted that reproductive performance is poor when few animals are kept in the room, but good when it is fully occupied. Niewiesk and Prince (2002) recommend not to separate breeding pairs once they are established.

Cotton rats are omnivorous and feed on vegetation, insects, and other small animals. They will eat eggs and chicks of bobtail quail and become pests by eating sugarcane and sweet potatoes (Nowak, 1999). Nutritional requirements for cotton rats are similar to those of laboratory rats (*Rattus norvegicus*), and standard rodent diets appear suitable for maintenance and reproduction (Cameron and Eshelman, 1996; Niewiesk and Prince, 2002).

Cotton rats are available from some large commercial vendors, namely Harlan Laboratories (Indianapolis, IN) (Niewiesk and Prince, 2002), Sage Labs (St Louis, MO), and Charles River-France (L'Arbresle, France). Inbred cotton rats are available from Harlan Laboratories and Charles River Laboratories (Wilmington, MA). Additionally, the company Sigmovir (Rockville, MD) supplies and develops the cotton rat as a model for infectious disease research. Investigators from this company have been instrumental in increasing the availability of molecular biology and immunology reagents for this model (Blanco *et al.*, 2004).

D. Diseases

There are few incidents of clinical disease in cotton rats. Most lesions in laboratories result from fighting.

1. Infectious Diseases

Literature citations describing infectious disease in the cotton rat are typically referring field surveys. Sentinel programs in laboratory colonies typically concentrate on screening for standard laboratory rodent pathogens (Niewiesk and Prince, 2002).

a. Protozoa

Eimeria spp. and *Isospora* spp. coccidia have been isolated from the feces of wild cotton rats (Barnard *et al.*, 1974; Castro *et al.*, 1998). Elangbam *et al.* (1993) observed cryptosporidia in the large intestine in one of nine cotton rats from Oklahoma.

Dubey and Sheffield (1988) found a novel sarcocyst sp., which they named *S. sigmodontis*, in skeletal muscle of three of four cotton rats from Georgia. The protozoan cysts were not infectious for dogs and cats.

b. Nematodes

Boggs *et al.* (1991) recovered five species of gastrointestinal helminthes: *Longistriata adunca, Syphacia sigmodontis, Strongyloides* sp., *Protospirura muris*, and *Raillietina* sp. Cotton rats infected with *Strongyloides* sp. are reportedly indistinguishable clinically from noninfected hosts (Elangbam *et al.*, 1990). Holliman and Meade (1980) found encapsulated larvae of *Trichinella spiralis* in wild-trapped cotton rats in Virginia.

c. Mites/Lice/Ticks

Durden *et al.* (1993) found eight species of parasitic arthropods on 28 wild cotton rats collected in Florida. The most prevalent parasites were the flea *Polygenis gwyni;* the American dog tick, *Dermacentor variabilis;* and the tropical rat mite, *Ornithonyssus bacoti.*

2. Metabolic/Nutritional Disease

Iglauer *et al.* (1993) reported ringtail in a colony of cotton rats in Scandinavia.

3. Traumatic Injuries

Faith *et al.* (1997) reported that the main lesions they saw in a laboratory colony in Texas resulted from fighting among animals. Cotton rats should not be picked up by the tail, as they spin when picked up and the tail skin easily degloves.

4. Neoplastic Diseases

Kawase and Ishikura (1995) described fundic gastric tubular adenocarcinoma in 61 female and two male cotton rats in a colony of 258 females and 283 males in Japan. In which spontaneously developed adenomatous hyperplasia was described with the lesions. Faith *et al.* (1997) in Texas saw no evidence of neoplasia in their colony of cotton rats.

5. Miscellaneous

Constant and Phillips (1952) described dystrophic calcinosis in cotton rats consuming a partially purified diet with lesions in heart, skeletal muscles, liver, adipose tissues, kidneys, and urinary bladder. Chandra *et al.* (1993) observed cystic epithelial calcification in 37 of 60 wild cotton rat urinary bladders, with no detectable relationship to environmental contaminations.

Sorden and Watts (1996) reported sporadic exophthalmos and heart failure in 3- to 12-month-old cotton rats from an inbred colony. The exophthalmos resulted from orbital venous sinus thrombosis secondary to generalized venous stasis due to right heart failure. Microscopically, there was multifocal cardiac myocyte necrosis, mineralization, and mononuclear inflammatory cell infiltration; cotton rats more than 5 months of age also had foci of interstitial fibrosis and myocyte atrophy. Additional lesions included right ventricular dilatation and unilateral or bilateral atrial thrombosis. The authors attributed the heart failure to a heritable cardiomyopathy. Faith *et al.* (1997) also reported a similar form of degenerative cardiomyopathy accompanied by skeletal muscle degeneration, necrosis, and mineralization. These lesions resemble those induced by vitamin E deficiency and Swensen and Telford (1973) described similar skeletal and myocardial lesions in the experimentally vitamin E-deficient cotton rat. Nevertheless, the potential role of vitamin E or selenium deficiency in spontaneous cardiomyopathy or skeletal muscle degeneration of cotton rats is unknown.

a. Age-Related Disorders

Faith *et al.* (1997) found a condition similar to chronic progressive nephropathy of laboratory rats (*Rattus norvegicus*) in one-third of 18 laboratory-maintained adult cotton rats.

XII. WHITE-TAILED RATS: MYSTROMYS

Mystromys albicaudatus (Fig. 7.20) is the species principally studied. It has fallen out of use as a laboratory animal species, with no primary publications found in major scientific databases within the last 5 years.

A. Introduction

1. Description

The white-tailed rat is the only species in the genus *Mystromys. Mystromys* is in the subfamily Cricetinae (hamsters), which includes *Calomyscus, Phodopus, Cricetus, Cricetulus,* and *Mesocricetus* (Nowak, 1999). It is thick-bodied, is relatively large (13.6–18.4 cm long), has a long white tail (5–8 cm), and weighs 75–185 g. The fur is gray-brown and smooth and the belly is white. The white-tailed rat has un-grooved, yellow incisor teeth; sharp-tipped claws; and no cheek pouches. In addition, it has a two-compartment stomach and a large, ventral

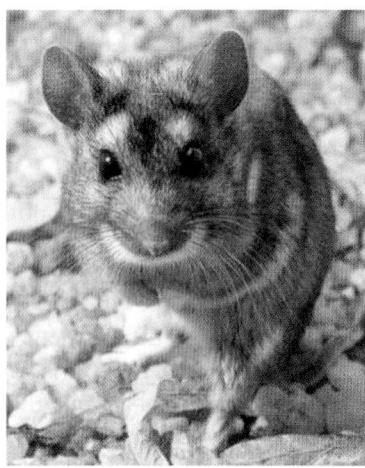

FIGURE 7.20   *Mystromys albicaudatus* – white-tailed rat. Front view. *Photograph from Planet Mammiferes.*

sebaceous gland (Fine *et al.*, 1986). Females have a rudimentary prostate gland (Hall *et al.*, 1967). The ears of *M. albicaudatus* are erect; the eyes are dark; and the animal is alert, inquisitive, and quick.

2. Distribution

This animal is found on the grassy flats and dry, sandy areas of South Africa: Cape Province, Natal, Free State, and Swaziland (Skinner and Chimimba, 2006).

3. Habitat

Mystromys albicaudatus lives underground, often in burrows made by other animals, and is nocturnal (Nowak, 1999). It eats seeds and other vegetable matter.

4. Use in Research

Historically, white-tailed rats were used in diabetes mellitus research where they have been demonstrated to spontaneously develop hyperglycemia, polyuria, glycosuria, ketonuria, and degenerative changes in the islets of Langerhans. The disease is more common in males and is not associated with obesity (Little *et al.*, 1982; Riley *et al.*, 1975). The animals have been used to study diabetic angiopathy and hepatic mitochondrial function in diabetes (Schmidt *et al.*, 1974, 1980).

Mystromys albicaudatus is an excellent model of American cutaneous leishmaniasis (*Leishmania braziliensis*) and has also been used as an experimental host for *L. donovani* and *L. mexicani* (McKinney and Hendricks, 1980; Mikhail and Mansour, 1973; Sayles *et al.*, 1981). It has been used for vaccination studies with *L. braziliensis* (Beacham *et al.*, 1982; Franke *et al.*, 1985). White-tailed rats have been infected experimentally with Crimean–Congo hemorrhagic fever virus (Shepherd *et al.*, 1989). They have also been infected with human *Streptococcus* spp. to investigate caries development (Larson and Fitzgerald,

1968). Other studies using *Mystromys* include chemically induced carcinogenicity (Roebuck and Longnecker, 1979; Yamamoto *et al.*, 1972), thermoregulation (Downs and Perrin, 1995), and digestion (Mahida and Perrin, 1994; Perrin and Maddock, 1983).

B. Biology

1. Physiological Characteristics

Although found in a temperate climate, *M. albicaudatus* has been shown to have thermal characteristics typical of a rodent adapted to a cold temperature regime and consequently has a higher metabolic rate than anticipated (Downs and Perrin, 1995). The growth and development of the stomach, gastric epithelia, and associated microflora have been well documented. The neonatal monogastric stomach with distinct separations into glandular and cornified regions gives way in the infantile period to fornical papillae, which provide microhabitats for colonization by symbiotic anaerobic bacilli. As development continues and ingestion of solid food begins, papillae become colonized by bacilli, which increase in abundance without epithelial damage, suggesting that the bacilli are autochthonous and symbiotic and aid in digestion processes (Maddock and Perrin, 1981; Perrin and Curtis, 1980). The details of chemical reactions mediated by stomach bacteria during ingestion of food have been documented (Perrin and Kokkinn, 1986; Perrin and Maddock, 1983, 1985).

Females have two pairs of inguinal mammae, and males have an os penis.

2. Normal Values

The normal weights of spleen, kidneys, liver, heart, lung, pancreas, brain, and gonads for 53 adult female and 51 adult male white-tailed rats have been published (Becker and Middleton, 1979). Serum chemistry and electrolyte determinations and nonfasted urinalysis results have been reported (Becker *et al.*, 1979; Streett and Highman, 1971). Serum chloride and serum glucose levels were greater and serum sodium levels lower for female rats. An unusually high physiological level of urine protein was detected, and it was determined that standard dipstick methods for determining urine protein levels in this species gave artificially high results. (Cantrell and Padovan, 1987) determined blood values from 90 *Mystromys*, 3–24 months of age, to establish normal values and to evaluate the influence of age and gender. Hematology values for adult white-tailed rats are listed in Table 7.2. Males over 6 months of age had higher red blood cell counts, packed cell volumes, and hemoglobin levels than females of the same age. Age and gender did not cause detectable differences in leukocyte numbers in animals over 6 months old. Intraperitoneal pentobarbital anesthesia (3 mg/50 g) has been recommended (Padovan, 1985). A technique for repeat blood sampling has been described (Stuhlman *et al.*, 1972b).

3. Biology of Reproduction

Females become sexually mature at 146 days and have a gestation period of 38 days (Hallett and Meester, 1971). Breeding pairs should be established at a young age to avoid aggressiveness among adults, and males are removed at parturition. Females give birth to small litters (three) with high survival to weaning (80%). Neonatal survival can be increased to 95% by selecting as breeders dams that do not cannibalize their young (Fine *et al.*, 1986). Newborns attach firmly to the nipples of the dams and are dragged about for 3 weeks (Hall *et al.*, 1967). The life span of white-tailed rats is 6 years (Dean, 1978).

C. Husbandry

Wild *Mystromys* eat seeds, other vegetable matter, and insects (Perrin, 1987). In the laboratory, commercial rodent diet and water are offered *ad libitum*. White-tailed rats are housed as breeding pairs in solid-bottom rodent cages lined with corncob bedding. Standard environmental conditions for temperature (22 ± 2°C), humidity (40–70%) and light (12-h cycles) are satisfactory. Animals are maintained as monogamous lifetime mates (Fine *et al.*, 1986).

White-tailed rats should be picked up around the thorax and never by the tail because it is fragile. Perrin described a system of activity monitor for *M. albicaudatus* (Maddock and Perrin, 1981). Stuhlman *et al.* (1972b) used heat-dilated tail veins to obtain repeated blood samplings for glucose measurements in white-tailed rats. Intraperitoneal pentobarbital (3 mg/50 g) has been used for anesthesia (Padovan, 1985).

D. Diseases

1. Infectious Diseases

Tyzzer's disease has been induced experimentally in immunosuppressed weanling *M. albicauditus* by oral inoculation with *Clostridium piliformis* spores. Focal necrosis was observed in the tunica muscularis of the intestine, periportal region of the liver, the ventricular myocardium, and the brain stem (Waggie *et al.*, 1986).

La Regina *et al.* (1978) described a fatal enteric syndrome with high mortality (59%) in adult *Mystromys*, associated with ingestion of a topically applied antibiotic of bacitracin, neomycin, and polymyxin. Clinical signs included anorexia, depression, and rough hair coat. Predominant necropsy findings were hemorrhagic typhlitis and colitis.

2. Metabolic Diseases

Spontaneous diabetes mellitus in the white-tailed rat is common is more frequent in males than in females (Hallett and Politzer, 1972; Packer *et al.*, 1970). Hyperglycemia (>170 mg/dl) is a consistent finding, whereas polyuria, polydipsia, glycosuria, and ketonuria are less commonly found; obesity is not a characteristic (Stuhlman *et al.*, 1972a, 1974, 1975). The primary lesion is in the islets of Langerhans (Goeken *et al.*, 1972). Elevated glycosylated hemoglobin levels cannot be used to distinguish diabetic from normal white tailed rats measured glycosylated hemoglobin in normal and diabetic white-tailed rats (Little *et al.*, 1982).

In a study of 175 nondiabetic and diabetic white-tailed rats, it was found that glomerulosclerosis is associated with diabetes in this species (Riley *et al.*, 1975). Basement membrane thickness in skeletal muscle capillaries was also determined to be greater in diabetic *versus* normal *M. albicaudatus* (Yesus *et al.*, 1976).

3. Iatrogenic Diseases

A case series report of ringtail in suckling white-tailed rats (<7 days of age) maintained at relative humidity ranging from 12–38% was described by Stuhlman and Wagner (1971). When the relative humidity was increased to 50% no more cases occurred.

4. Neoplastic Diseases

Rantanen and Highman (1970) reported spontaneous tumors in a colony of *M. albicaudatus*. The neoplasms listed were perianal squamous cell carcinoma, adnexal tumor of the skin, osteosarcoma of the scapula, leiomyosarcoma of the uterus, adenocarcinoma of the liver, hepatoma, and pituitary adenoma.

5. Miscellaneous

a. Congenital Disorders

Rodrigues *et al.* (1971) described an inherited condition of partial oculocutaneous albinism with ophthalmic pathology in white-tailed rats. The condition appeared similar to Chediak–Higashi syndrome, a phagocyte bactericidal disorder.

Prieur *et al.* (1979) studied tissues from affected *M. albicaudatus* and found no evidence of cytoplasmic granule enlargement. They concluded that the inherited partially albinic disease is different from the Chediak–Higashi syndrome.

XIII. GERBILS AND JIRDS: *MERIONES*

Gerbils generally studied include *Meriones unguiculatus* (Mongolian gerbil; Fig. 7.21), *M. libycus* (Libyan jird, red-tailed jird), *M. crassus* (desert gerbil), *M. hurrianae*

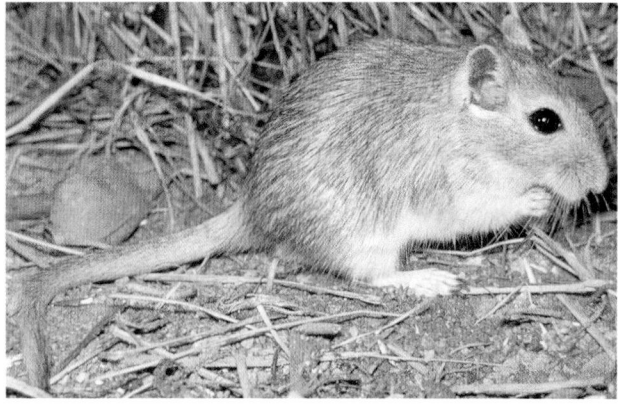

FIGURE 7.21 *Meriones unguiculatus* – Mongolian gerbil or jird. Side view, Prague Zoo, Czechoslovakia. *Photograph by M. Andera and the Mammal Images Library of the American Society of Mammalogists.*

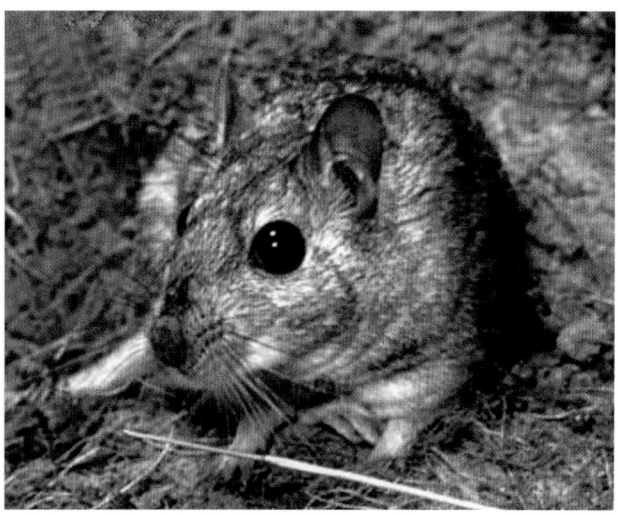

FIGURE 7.22 *Meriones shawi* – Shaw's jird. Front view, Tolworth Laboratory Studio, Surrey, U.K. *Photograph by E.J. Taylor and the Mammal Images Library of the American Society of Mammalogists.*

(Indian desert gerbil), and *M. vinagradovi* (grapevine gerbil). Figure 7.22 shows Shaw's jird (*Meriones shawi*). The common name jird is Arabic for gerbil, and is often used to describe gerbils from Northern Africa and Central Asia.

There are 14 species in four subgenera. The term *gerbil* as used in the text refers to the Mongolian gerbil, *Meriones unguiculatus*. All Mongolian gerbils available for research were derived from 20 pairs trapped in eastern Mongolia in 1935. The animals were taken to the Kitasato Institute, Japan, and later a subcolony was established at Central Laboratories for Experimental Animals, Tokyo. Schwenker imported 11 pairs to the United States from the Tokyo subcolony in 1954 (Marston, 1976).

A. Introduction

1. Description

Externally, gerbils are rat-like. The head and body length is 95–180 mm, and tail length is 100–193 mm. Weight averages 50–55 g in laboratory-raised females and 60 g in males (Norris and Adams, 1972a). The covering of fur on the tail is short near the base and progressively longer toward the tip so that it is slightly bushy. Coloration of upper parts varies from pale, clear yellowish through sandy and gray. The sides of the body are generally lighter than the back.

2. Distribution

Wild *M. unguiculatus* are found in Mongolia, adjacent parts of southern Siberia and northern China, and Manchuria.

3. Habitat

Gerbils inhabit clay and sandy deserts, bush country, and arid steppes. They are terrestrial, and wild *M. unguiculatus* construct simple burrows in soft soil where they spend most of their time. The tunnels are underground, about 2–3 feet in length and 1.3 inches in diameter.

4. Use in Research

The gerbil is highly susceptible to cerebral infarction following unilateral ligation of one common carotid artery and is used in studies of the pathogenesis of stroke (Akai *et al.*, 1995; Somova *et al.*, 2000; Traystman, 2003). Gerbils are used as an animal model for the study and treatment of epilepsy (Bertorelli *et al.*, 1995; Buckmaster *et al.*, 2000). Spontaneous epileptiform seizures mimic those of human idiopathic epilepsy, and both seizure-sensitive and resistant strains have been bred. The gerbil is also used in auditory research (Urquiza *et al.*, 1988). Deafened gerbils have been used in ontogenetic cochlear implant research (Hessel *et al.*, 1997, 1998, 2000).

The gerbil has been used extensively in behavioral investigations, especially those relating to territoriality. A major monograph describing olfactory communication and territorial behavior in the gerbil afforded a detailed study on the neurological and physiological mechanisms that control these functions (Thiessen and Yahr, 1977).

A wide variety of parasitic infections can be transmitted to gerbils. Experimental protozoal infections include *Giardia lamblia* (Belosevic *et al.*, 1983; Faubert *et al.*, 1983) and the cattle piroplasm *Babesia divergens* (Dkhil *et al.*, 2013; Lewis and Williams, 1979; Lewis *et al.*, 1981). Researchers frequently use gerbils to maintain nematode parasites in the laboratory, study the pathogenesis of nematode infections, and investigate anthelmintic drug resistance. Examples of nematodes infecting gerbils are

Strongyloides stercoralis (Nolan *et al.*, 1993), *Ostertagia circumcincta* (Court *et al.*, 1988), *Haemonchus contortus* (Conder *et al.*, 1991), *Nematospiroides dubius* (Jenkins, 1977), *Trichostrongylus colubriformis* (Maclean *et al.*, 1987), *Heligmosomoides kurilensis* (Asakawa, 1987), *Capillaria philippinensis* (Cross *et al.*, 1978), and *Acanthocheilonema viteae* (Maki and Weinstein, 1991).

Gerbils are excellent animal models for studying diseases caused by filarial nematodes (Klei *et al.*, 1997; Nasarre *et al.*, 1997; Storey, 1993). They have been used extensively to investigate serious human diseases such as lymphatic filariasis caused by *Wuchereria bancrofti* (Cross *et al.*, 1981; Zielke, 1979) and *Brugia malayi* (Li *et al.*, 1991; Partono and Purnomo, 1987; Trpis, 1994). *Wuchereria bancrofti* and *B. malayi* are responsible for 90% and 10%, respectively, of the 90 million infections worldwide in Latin America, sub-Saharan Africa, and Southeast Asia. Researchers also use gerbils to study the filarial parasite *Onchocerca volvulus*, a major cause of human blindness in equatorial Africa where the parasite infects more than 20 million persons (Abraham *et al.*, 2002; Bianco *et al.*, 1989). Other filarial nematodes used in gerbils include *B. pahangi* (Nasarre *et al.*, 1997) and *Loa loa*, the African eye worm (Suswillo *et al.*, 1977; Wanji *et al.*, 2002).

Hydatid disease has been investigated in gerbils. Larvae of the tapeworms *Echinococcus granulosus* and *E. multilocularis* are found as cysts in the liver and other organs of rodents, ruminants, and humans. The cysts, though slow-growing, are often proliferative and large, and result in fatal infections. *E. multilocularis* infection is an important zoonotic disease in Asia. Echinococcal infections in gerbils are used to investigate larval parasite proliferation and metastasis (Eckert *et al.*, 1983; Kamiya *et al.*, 1987; Kia, 2003; Ohnishi and Kutsumi, 1995). Gerbils are also used as animal models of cysticercosis and infected with taeniid tapeworms such as *Taenia polyacantha* (Fujita *et al.*, 1991), *T. crassiceps* (Sato *et al.*, 2000), and *T. solium* (Avila *et al.*, 2002; Avila *et al.*, 2006).

Gerbils are infected with digenetic flukes to study diseases caused by parasitic trematodes, such as schistosomiasis, which affects 200 million persons and kills 250,000 annually. Trematodes experimentally infecting gerbils include *Schistosoma japonicum* (Liang *et al.*, 1983); *S. haematobium* (Bayssade-Dufour *et al.*, 1994); *Paragonimus heterotremus*, a cause of pulmonary distomiasis (Asavisanu *et al.*, 1985); and the avian schistosome *Austrobilharzia variglandis*, a cause of marine cercarial dermatitis, or 'swimmer's itch' (Bacha *et al.*, 1982).

The young gerbil is an animal model in which uniformly fatal Rift Valley fever virus-induced encephalitis is produced without significant extraneural lesions (Anderson *et al.*, 1988). Gerbils have been used as a vertebrate host to study the enhancement of arbovirus transmission by concurrent host infection with microfilariae (Turell *et al.*, 1984; Vaughan *et al.*, 2012).

5. Sources

Mongolian gerbils are available from B&K Universal Ltd. (Grimston, Aldbrough, Hull, UK) and from Charles River Laboratories (Wilmington, MA).

B. Biology

Gerbils have a large, ventral, abdominal marking gland that is androgen-dependent. It attains greater size in the male and develops at an earlier age (Thiessen and Yahr, 1977). The adrenal cortex produces nearly equal amounts of corticosterone and 19-hydroxycorticosterone (Drummond *et al.*, 1988). When the adrenal gland weight is compared with the body weight, the gerbil adrenal gland is approximately three-times the size of the adrenal in the rat (Cullen *et al.*, 1971).

Mays (1969), Gattermann (1979), and Termer and Glomski (1978) have reported normal reference ranges for hematological and clinical biochemical parameters in juvenile and adult gerbils. Hematology values for adult gerbils are listed in Table 7.2. General data on organ weights are found in the monograph by Thiessen and Yahr (1977).

Norris and Adams have published extensively on reproduction in the gerbil (Norris and Adams, 1972b, 1974, 1981, 1982). Male gerbils attain sexual maturity by 70–84 days. Vaginal opening in females occurs at 40–60 days, 30 days before sexual maturity occurs. Gerbils tend to pair-bond, and when older females lose their mate, getting them to accept another is often impossible. The gestation period of nonlactating gerbils is 24–26 days, but lactating females always have a prolonged gestation of 27 days. If females are bred in the postpartum period, they delay implantation, and gestation can be as long as 48 days. Mean litter size ranges from three to seven. Young gerbils suckle for about 21 days and begin to eat solid foods at 16 days. In general, researchers consider day 25 to be most suitable for weaning.

C. Husbandry

Gerbils of other species are often used in other countries as research animals. Several papers describe the breeding and care in captivity of these species: *Meriones vinagradovi* (Ismailov and Ismailov, 1981); *M. crassus* (Marafie *et al.*, 1978); M. *hurrianae* (Saibaba *et al.*, 1988); and *M. libycus* (Wisniewski, 1985).

The diet of wild *Meriones* consists of green vegetation, roots, bulb seeds, cereals, fruits, and insects. Zeman (1967) described a semi-purified diet for gerbils, and in the laboratory, gerbils thrive on commercially available pelleted rodent diets. However, because of the fat metabolism of gerbils, they develop high blood cholesterol concentrations on diets containing more than

4% fat (Leach and Holub, 1984; Nicolosi *et al.*, 1981; Temmerman *et al.*, 1988).

Gerbils excrete little urine, and fecal pellets are hard and dry. Their cages require less frequent cleaning than those of other laboratory rodents. Gerbils adapt to a wide range of ambient temperatures but are generally maintained in laboratories at 70–72°F. Due to their propensity to develop nasal dermatitis at relative humidities above 50%, a low humidity is advisable.

Gerbils require sand bathing to keep their coats from becoming oily. Tortora *et al.* (1974) described the effect of sand deprivation on behavior in gerbils. Gerbils often stand erect on their hind limbs, so it is important that cages have a solid bottom and that the floor-to-lid height is tall enough to allow for this behavior.

D. Diseases

1. Infectious Diseases

a. Bacterial/Mycoplasmal/Rickettsial Diseases

Facial eczema, 'sore nose,' and nasal dermatitis all describe a common skin condition seen in gerbils. Clinical lesions next to the external nares appear erythematous initially, progress to localized alopecia, and develop into an extensive moist dermatitis. The cause is believed to be increased Harderian gland secretion of porphyrins similar to chromodacryorrhea in rats, which act as a primary skin irritant. Experimental Harderian gland-adenectomized gerbils do not develop nasal or facial lesions (Bresnahan *et al.*, 1983; Farrar *et al.*, 1988). Various staphylococcal species (*Staphylococcus aureus* and *S. xylosus*) may act synergistically to produce the dermatitis (Solomon *et al.*, 1990). Stress factors such as environmental humidity above 50% or overcrowding cause excessive Harderian gland secretion (Farrar *et al.*, 1988). Bacterial maxillary sinusitis can be detected clinically in the gerbil using magnetic resonance imaging (Allen *et al.*, 1993).

Naturally occurring Tyzzer's disease, an enterohepatic disease caused by the obligately intracellular bacterium *Clostridium piliforme*, is the most frequently described fatal infectious disease of gerbils (Koopman *et al.*, 1980; Motzel and Gibson, 1990; Port *et al.*, 1970; White and Waldron, 1969). Common clinical and pathological findings were sudden death or death after a short period of disease, and the presence of multiple foci of hepatic necrosis. Diarrhea and necrotic lesions in the intestinal tracts were variably present. Experimentally induced Tyzzer's disease has confirmed that gerbils are extremely susceptible to infection (Waggie *et al.*, 1984). An attempt to eradicate *Helicobacter* spp. in gerbils using dietary administration of antibiotics was complicated by the death of some gerbils from *C. difficile* (Bergin *et al.*, 2005). The probable route of infection in naturally occurring

infection is by mouth, as gerbils exposed to infected bedding will contract Tyzzer's disease (Yokomori *et al.*, 1989). Strittmatter (1972) eliminated Tyzzer's disease in the gerbil by fostering offspring to mice.

De la Puente-Redondo *et al.* (1999) describe an epidemic of *Citrobacter rodentium* colitis in Mongolian gerbils. The disease occurred acutely in nine gerbils, six dying less than 48 h after the onset of diarrhea. Microscopically, these animals had a thickening of the colon and rectum with extension into the small intestine. There was intestinal ulceration and goblet cell hyperplasia in the colon. The lesions were similar in appearance to those of transmissible murine colonic hyperplasia (Barthold, 1980). Cultures from abdominal masses and kidney grew pure cultures of *C. rodentium*, and the addition of oxytetracycline (800 mg/l) to the drinking water prevented further disease (de la Puente-Redondo *et al.*, 1999).

The Mongolian gerbil is also susceptible to infection by *Helicobacter pylori*, which causes severe gastritis, gastric ulceration, and intestinal metaplasia (Wang and Fox, 1998). Watanabe *et al.* (1998) described the development of gastric adenocarcinoma in 37% of infected gerbils maintained for 62 weeks. The histological progression of *H. pylori* infection in the gerbil was found to closely resemble that observed in human patients, where early intestinal metaplasia and gastric ulceration are replaced by antral gastric adenocarcinoma.

b. Viral/Chlamydial Diseases

Cowpox virus has been isolated from *M. libycus* in the Eastern European republic of Georgia (Tsanava Sh *et al.*, 1989).

c. Parasitic Diseases

Protozoa Vincent *et al.* (1975) recovered *Tritrichomonas caviae* and a species of entamoeba from experimental animals.

Nematodes Wightman *et al.* (1978a,b) identified *Syphacia obvelata*, the mouse pinworm, and *Dentostomella translucida*, an oxyurid in Mongolian gerbils. An adult gerbil from a research colony and a litter of 5-week-old gerbils from a pet store were found to have pinworms identified as *S. obvelata*. Wightman *et al.* (1978b) caged infected gerbils with uninfected gerbils, and uninfected mice and infected mice with uninfected gerbils. The results of these studies showed that *S. obvelata* can be transmitted from gerbil to gerbil, gerbil to mouse, and mouse to gerbil. *Dentostomella translucida* was found in the small intestine of 39 out of 43 gerbils from a research colony and in five pet gerbils, establishing the gerbil as a new host for the parasite. Wightman *et al.* (1978a) found an average of four parasites per animal and no clinical manifestations of disease associated with the infection. The prepatent period of infection was between 25 and 29 days.

Cestodes Vincent *et al.* (1975) recovered the cestode *Hymenolepis diminuta* from laboratory gerbils, and Lussier and Loew (1970) reported a case of natural *H. nana* infection in gerbils.

Mites Levine and Lage (1984) described *Liponyssoides sanguineus*, the primary vector of *Rickettsia akari*, infesting Mongolian gerbils, mice (*Mus musculus*), and laboratory-reared Egyptian gerbils (*Meriones libycus*), but did not observe any manifestations of disease. They found only a few mites were present on each animal although numerous mites were present in the bedding. Vincent *et al.* (1975) recovered the forage mite *Tyrophagus castellani* from a colony of laboratory gerbils. *T. castellani* is a pest of stored food products and causes 'copra itch' among workers handling copra and a dermatitis in people who handle cheese. Schwarzbrott *et al.* (1974) reported a case of demodicosis in a male laboratory gerbil.

d. Fungal Infections

There have been no reports of naturally occurring or experimental dermatophyte infections in the Mongolian gerbil (Donnelly *et al.*, 2000). Other fungal infections in *Meriones* spp. are exceedingly rare. *Cryptococcus neoformans* was reported in a captive *M. libycus* at the Zoological Society of London (Parsons *et al.*, 1987).

2. Metabolic/Nutritional Diseases

Vincent *et al.* (1979) found that research gerbils develop spontaneous, insidious periodontal disease after 6 months on standard laboratory rodent diets. On the same diets about 10% of the animals became obese, and some showed decreased glucose tolerance, elevated serum immunoreactive insulin, and diabetic changes in the pancreas and other organs. The authors noted that some breeder gerbils exhibited hyperactivity of the adrenal cortex associated with hyperglycemia, hyperlipidemia, and degenerative vascular disease.

3. Traumatic Disorders

Thin skin covers the tail of the gerbil. Unlike rats or mice, if a gerbil is picked up by the tip of its tail, the skin will often slip off, leaving a raw, exposed tail that eventually becomes necrotic and will shed (Donnelly, 1997). If the tail skin is lost, the bare tail must be surgically amputated where the skin ends.

4. Iatrogenic Diseases

A fatal syndrome of acute toxicity was produced in Mongolian gerbils following the injection of a penicillin–dihydrostreptomycin–procaine combination. The toxicity was determined to be due to the dihydrostreptomycin component. Fifty milligrams of dihydrostreptomycin produced 80–100% mortality in 55- to 65-g gerbils (Wightman *et al.*, 1980).

Approximately 20–40% of gerbils develop reflex, stereotypic, epileptiform (clonic–tonic) seizures from around two months of age (Kaplan, 1975; Kaplan and Miezejeski, 1972). Animals seize in response to sensory stimulation and forced exploratory behavior, but the incidence and severity of their seizures are variable; the seizures generally pass in a few minutes, may be mild or severe, and have no lasting effects. Although the incidence and severity of seizures often decrease with age, certain subsets of adult gerbils can be induced to seize following prolonged test regimens with progressive severity (Scotti *et al.*, 1998). The susceptibility is seen in selectively bred lines, inherited and related to a deficiency in cerebral glutamine synthetase (Laming *et al.*, 1989).

Spongiform lesions arise in dendrites and glia in the brain stem of domestic Mongolian gerbils and *M. libycus* (McGinn and Faddis, 1998). The lesions are characterized by the microcysts and vacuolar neuronal degeneration in the absence of astrocytosis. Axonal, dendritic, and neuronal perikarya degeneration accompanied by phagocytosis is often seen (Ostapoff and Morest, 1989). The lesions are bilateral, most pronounced within the cochlear nucleus, and increase in number, size, and extent with age. These spongiform lesions either cause or are associated with significant neural degeneration and appear to be the result of a common excitotoxic mechanism such as low-frequency noise (McGinn and Faddis, 1997). In contrast, feral Mongolian gerbils and their offspring show few spongiform lesions.

Cystic ovaries occur frequently in Mongolian gerbils (Clark, 1978; Jung and Kim, 2005; Norris and Adams, 1972b). Removal of affected ovaries does not significantly affect reproductive performance. Females with one ovary are slightly inferior in fertility compared with normal females; a general decline in fertility may be evident in older females. The mean number of litters, young born, and age at last parturition were 8 ± 4, 37 ± 20, and 462 ± 96 days (two ovaries) compared with 7 ± 4, 30 ± 16, and 417 ± 142 days (one ovary), respectively (Norris and Adams, 1972b). Clark *et al.* (1986) found they could enhance the productivity of gerbil breeding colonies by using only the 40% of females that exhibit vaginal opening before 25 days of age as breeder females. Early-maturing females are more likely to breed successfully on first pairing, and the lifetime fecundity of early-maturing females is more than twice that of their late-maturing littermates. Two-thirds of the early-maturing females that failed to reproduce following a first pairing became pregnant following a second, but only 11% of late-maturing females did so. (Mighell and Baker, 1990) have reported cesarean section for successful treatment of dystocia in a gerbil.

5. Neoplastic Diseases

Major surveys of spontaneous neoplasia in laboratory colonies of Mongolian gerbils are reported (Benitz and

Kramer, 1965; Matsuoka and Suzuki, 1995; Ringler *et al.*, 1972; Rowe *et al.*, 1974; Vincent and Ash, 1978; Vincent *et al.*, 1975). A 24–39% incidence of neoplasia in gerbils usually occurs after 2–3 years of age (Matsuoka and Suzuki, 1995; Vincent *et al.*, 1979). Squamous cell carcinoma of the sebaceous ventral scent gland in males and ovarian granulosa cell tumor in females account for 80% of tumors seen in animals greater than 3 years of age. The ventral marking gland tumors invade locally and can metastasize to lymph nodes and lung (Deutschland *et al.*, 2011; Jackson *et al.*, 1996; Raflo and Diamond, 1980). Adrenocortical tumors, cutaneous squamous cell carcinoma, malignant melanoma, and renal and splenic hemangiomas are the next most commonly reported tumors. Numerous other tumors, including duodenal and cecal adenocarcinoma, hepatic lymphangioma, hemangioma and cholangiocarcinoma, splenic and renal hemangioma, uterine leiomyoma and hemangiopericytoma, ovarian teratoma, testicular teratoma, and malignant melanoma were reported. However, the total incidence of these tumors was less than 5% (Matsuoka and Suzuki, 1995; Meckley and Zwicker, 1979; Vincent and Ash, 1978; Vincent *et al.*, 1975, 1979). Case reports of spontaneously occurring tumors in gerbils include infiltrative craniopharyngioma (Guzman-Silva *et al.*, 1988), granulosa cell tumor (Guzman-Silva and Costa-Neves, 2006), lymphoma (Rembert *et al.*, 2000; Su *et al.*, 2001; Wenzlow *et al.*, 2008), histiocytic sarcoma (Chen *et al.* 1992), systemic mastocytosis (Guzman-Silva, 1997), sebaceous gland adenocarcinoma (Gil da Costa *et al.*, 2007), malignant melanoma (Cramlet *et al.*, 1974; Fabian *et al.*, 2012; Rembert and Johnson, 2001), and astrocytoma (Kroh *et al.*, 1987).

6. Miscellaneous

a. Congenital Disorders

Shakibi and Weiss (1969) found a prevalence of ventricular septal heart disease in newborn gerbils. In a group of 12- to 30-week-old male gerbils, Ninomiya and Nakamura (1987) reported spontaneous hyperplasia in both seminiferous and epididymal tubules. They considered the hyperplasia in young animals as congenital.

b. Age-Related Disorders

In two separate reviews, Bingel (1995) and Vincent *et al.* (1975) reported the pathologic findings in aging Mongolian gerbil colonies. Besides neoplasia, they found a high incidence of chronic interstitial nephritis. Other nonneoplastic lesions included renal cortical retention cysts and liver disease. Calcinosis cutis was also observed in two older male gerbils (Vincent and Ash, 1978). Mongolian gerbils have a remarkable propensity for the development of aural cholesteatoma; canal cholesteatomas develop spontaneously in aged

animals (Fulghum and Chole, 1985; Kim and Chole, 1998; Yamamoto-Fukuda *et al.*, 2011).

XIV. VOLES: *MICROTUS*

The genus *Microtus* (literally 'small ears' from the Greek) is a group of voles found in the Northern hemisphere primarily in Europe and North America. Within the genus *Microtus* there are approximately 67 species commonly referred to as voles or meadow mice (Carleton and Musser, 2005). An alternative hypothesis stresses one or two intercontinental dispersions and extensive regional cladogenesis; such a viewpoint has gained more credence, emerging from studies of allozymes, chromosomes, mitochondrial DNA, and fossils. The most widely used in research include *Microtus californicus* (California vole), *Microtus ochrogaster* (prairie vole), *Microtus pennsylvanicus* (meadow vole), *Microtus montanus* (montane vole), *Microtus oeconomus* (tundra vole), *Microtus pinetorum* (pine vole), and *Microtus arvalis* (common vole). A variety of different species of voles are pictured in Figs. 7.23–7.27.

A. Introduction

1. Description and Distribution

With the exception of *M pinetorum*, which belongs to the subgenus *Pitymys*, the species mentioned above belong to the subgenus *Microtus*. Individuals in the subgenus *Pitymys* are adapted to semifossorial life, showing a reduction of eyes, external ears, and tail and a close, velvety pelage (Nowak, 1999). With the exception

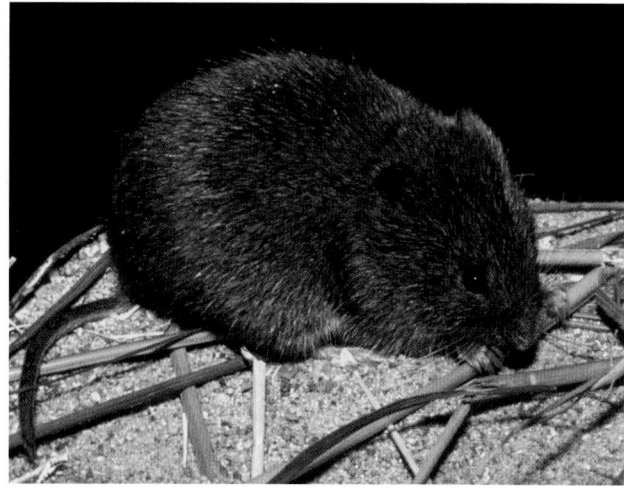

FIGURE 7.23 *Microtus longicaudus* – long-tailed vole. Lateral view of adult, Sandia Mountains, Bernalillo County, New Mexico. *Photograph by R.B. Forbes and the Mammal Images Library of the American Society of Mammalogists.*

of *M. arvalis*, which is found extensively throughout Europe, all others listed above are distributed in North America. In addition, *M. oeconomus* is distributed throughout northern Europe, Siberia, and north-central China. In the past two decades, *M. oeconomus* has become more abundant and more widespread throughout Lithuania, due primarily to changes in land use over that same time period (Balciauskas *et al.*, 2010). *M. pennsylvanicus* is found in the northern United States, Canada, and Alaska (Reich, 1981).

2. Use in Research

Weanling meadow voles have been used in nutrition studies where they serve as bioassay animals for protein content of feeds, the digestibility of forages, and the presence of toxins (Shore and Douben, 1994; Talmage and Walton, 1991). *M. pennsylvanicus* has also been used in studies of the influence of sexually dimorphic spatial learning (Galea *et al.*, 1996), as well as in studies on experimental infection with borrelia and babesia (Anderson *et al.*, 1986; Campbell *et al.*, 1994).

The prairie vole (*M. ochrogaster*) has emerged as a pre-eminent animal model for elucidating the genetic and neurobiological mechanisms governing complex social behavior in vertebrates. Prairie voles have been used extensively to study the physiology of the vomeronasal organ and the ways in which chemosensory cues affect courtship, territorial marking, aggression, and

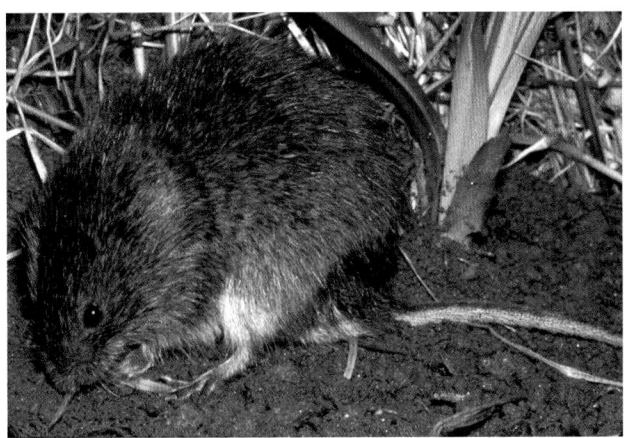

FIGURE 7.24 *Microtus oeconomus* – root vole. Oblique view, Zitny Ostrov, Slovak Republic. *Photograph by M. Andera and the Mammal Images Library of the American Society of Mammalogists.*

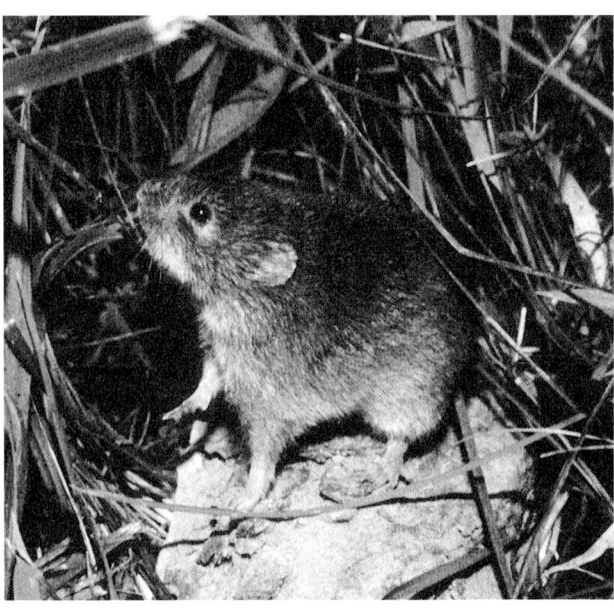

FIGURE 7.26 *Microtus ochrogaster* – prairie vole. Side view, in simulated grassland environment, Illinois. *Photograph by R.B. Forbes and the Mammal Images Library of the American Society of Mammalogists.*

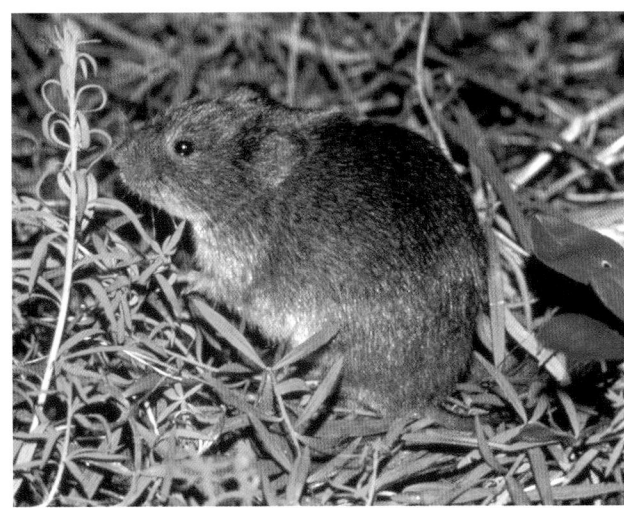

FIGURE 7.25 *Microtus pennsylvanicus* – meadow vole. Side view, Ann Arbor, Michigan. *Photograph by L.L. Master and the Mammal Images Library of the American Society of Mammalogists.*

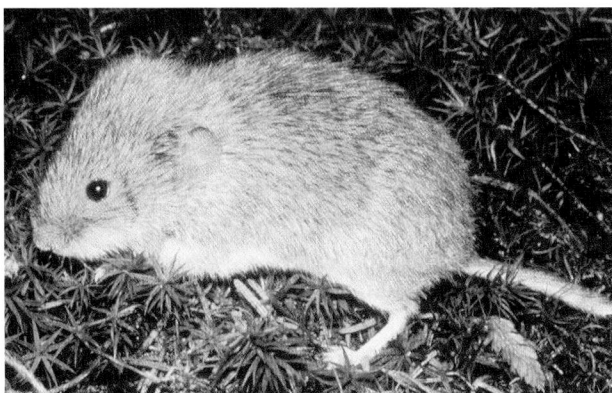

FIGURE 7.27 *Myodes glareolus* – red-backed bank vole. Side view, entire animal in view, Sumava Mountains, Czech Republic. *Photograph by M. Andera and the Mammal Images Library of the American Society of Mammalogists.*

reproduction (Curtis *et al.*, 2001; Hairston *et al.*, 2003; Sun *et al.*, 2014; Taylor *et al.*, 1992). In addition, prairie voles are monogamous, and studies have focused on the neuropeptides oxytocin and vasopressin and their control over such complex behaviors as pair-bonding, paternal care, maternal care, and mate-guarding (Insel and Shapiro, 1992; Young *et al.*, 2011). Often the polygamous and somewhat antisocial *M. pennsylvanicus* serves as a contrasting species in these studies and in investigations of the mu-opioid receptor and neuropeptide Y, which also affect offspring attachment and social bonding behavior between mates (Hostetler *et al.*, 2013; Inoue *et al.*, 2013). Prairie voles have also been used as a model for anxiety and depression. Socially isolating adult females resulted in elevated corticosteroid concentrations, prolonged sensitivity to stress-inducing challenges, and negative cardiovascular effects (Grippo *et al.*, 2009, 2012; Kim and Kirkpatrick, 1996). The prairie vole is an emerging rodent model for investigating the genetics, evolution, and molecular mechanisms of social behavior. McGraw *et al.* (2011) have constructed a genome wide, high-resolution linkage map of the prairie vole to facilitate this research.

The montane vole *(M. montanus)* has been developed as an experimental model for the study of African trypanosomiasis (Frommel *et al.*, 1991; Seed and Hall, 1980). They have also proven sensitive to the effects of plant-derived 6-methoxybenzoxazolinone, which alters the sex ratio of litters (Berger *et al.*, 1987).

The common vole *(M. arvalis)*, has been used as an herbivorous model of chemically induced diabetes mellitus (Arai *et al.*, 1996; Sasaki *et al.*, 1991) and for the evaluation of sex chromosome abnormalities (Zima *et al.*, 1992). The tundra vole *(M. oeconomus)* has been used to study the effect of atherogenic diets (Dieterich and Preston, 1977b, 1979).

3. Sources

A list of vole researchers who breed and supply voles may be found at the Vole Genomics Initiative website of Emory University (Young *et al.*, 2014).

B. Biology

1. Unique Physiologic Characteristics and Attributes

Unlike most rodents, voles have rootless molars, which continue to grow throughout their life. This feature of their teeth allows them to chew large quantities of abrasive grasses, which as herbivores is a major component of their diet (Oxberry, 1975).

Voles are among the most prolific mammals, with reports of female *M. pennsylvanicus* producing as many as 17 litters in a single year (Hamilton and Whitaker,

1979). The common vole *(M. arvalis)*, is sexually mature at 2–3 weeks, and some females mate and conceive at 13–14 days of age. Young grow very fast, reaching 30 g by 40 days of age. Litter size is 4–7 with females capable of having a new litter every 3 weeks (Balaz, 2010).

The prairie vole lives in a monogamous relationship, and the male assists the female in raising offspring. Young remain part of a family group until they are ready to establish their own relationship. Both female and male offspring remain nonproductive into adulthood if maintained in the presence of the dominant male (Stalling, 1990). In contrast, *M. pennsylvanicus* males are promiscuous, and the sexes nest separately (Reich, 1981). Pine voles display a cooperative system of breeding in social groups of two to nine animals in which only one female reproduces but all members of the group participate in the care of newborns (Smolen, 1981). Presence of prairie vole fathers within the group accelerates pup development, whereas the presence of meadow vole fathers hinders development (Jackson, 1997). Pregnancy is often terminated in the pregnant female if urine from an unknown male is introduced. Young from *M. pinetorum* and *M. ochrogaster* cling tenaciously to the teats of the females and can be dragged for considerable distances if the female is frightened. Other species of *Microtus* display this clinging behavior with varying degrees of tenacity.

2. Normal Values

Extensive hematologic and biochemical data has been published on the common vole (Dobrowolska, 1982a,b; Dobrowolska and Gromadzka-Ostrowska, 1983, 1984; Dobrowolska and Gromadzka, 1978; Dobrowolska *et al.*, 1976; Nikodemusz and Imre, 1979; Rewkiewicz-Dziarska, 1975a,b). Normal hematologic values for the pine (Harvey *et al.*, 2008), tundra (Dieterich and Preston, 1977b), and meadow (Bergeron *et al.*, 1986; Dieterich and Preston, 1977a; Knopper and Mineau, 2004) have been described. Seasonal variations in hematological indices are seen in wild voles. Hematology values for adult pine voles are listed in Table 7.2. Plasma chemistry values have also been published for the pine and meadow vole (Bergeron *et al.*, 1986; Harvey *et al.*, 2008).

3. Nutrition

Voles are herbivores and have a high metabolic rate. Meadow voles have evolved such that they subsist on a low-calorie diet and must be fed frequently. This species of vole relies heavily on the breakdown of carbohydrates during fasting. The carbohydrate catabolism results in profound hypoglycemia after only 6 h of fasting (Nagy and Pistole, 1988). In voles on high-fiber diets, cellulolytic bacteria can be isolated from their esophageal sac where gastric fermentation takes place, leading to higher pH and volatile fatty acids compared to those in the fundic or pyloric regions of the stomach (Kudo and

Oki, 1981). Voles are sensitive to the presence of various solutes added to drinking water, which can complicate oral dosing (Jackson, 1997). A complete discussion of the nutrient requirement of voles has been published (National Research Council, 1978). In general, their nutritional needs can be met by feeding standard mouse or rat breeding chow supplemented with hamster food and/or toasted wheat germ. Field voles require 8% or more protein in their diet to prevent retardation of growth and sexual development (Spears and Clarke, 1987).

4. Reproduction

Voles breed from early spring through early autumn. Female voles are polyestrous and usually have multiple litters each year. Breeding of Microtus spp in laboratories is not difficult (Kudo and Oki ,1982). *Microtus pennsylvanicus* has, like most *Microtus* females, eight mammae and produces three to 10 immature young per litter that are weaned by 12 days of age (Reich, 1981). Female *M. ochrogaster* have six mammae and produce one to seven young per litter (average 3.5) (Stalling, 1990). *Microtus pinetorum* females have only four mammae and produce one to four young per litter (average two to six) (Smolen, 1981). The success of females of a particular species becoming pregnant during the postpartum estrus varies from 40–70% (Morrison *et al.*, 1976). Neonatal mortality may be high, especially if the litter is disturbed during the first week.

Female *M. pennsylvanicus* are induced ovulators and can be bred any time. Ovulation occurs 12–18 h after copulation. Species of voles vary in the ability to detect definitive estrous cycle patterns. Despite attempts to elucidate breeding cycles by vaginal cytology, the Japanese field vole (*M. montebelli*) shows no clear pattern; the common vole (*M. arvalis*) shows 6- to 18-day cycles.

Superovulation for the production of transgenic voles was studied in the prairie vole (*M. ochrogaster*) and success varied with age and genetic background. Females 4–16 weeks of age produced an average of 14 embryos (Keebaugh *et al.*, 2012).

C. Husbandry

All species of voles can be bred successfully in solid-bottom cages of varying sizes (Leslie and Ranson, 1940; Morrison *et al.*, 1976; Nelson *et al.*, 1996; Solomon and Vandenbergh, 1994), although a minimum floor space of 1 ft² was recommended for housing a breeding pair (Richmond and Conaway, 1969). Both unsupplemented commercial rabbit feed or supplemented (wheat germ and oats) commercial rodent breeding chow have been used successfully (Cooper, 2010). Water should be offered *ad libitum*, and special care must be taken to provide sufficient water with the diet (Solomon and Vandenbergh, 1994). Voles are generally housed in a

controlled environment: temperature 23–25°C, relative humidity 60–70%, and a 12-h light cycle for maintenance or 14-h light cycle for breeding (Cooper, 2010). Care must be taken to avoid complete cage cleaning during the first week following parturition since this commonly results in cannibalism of an entire litter. Likewise, leaving a small amount of dirty litter in an otherwise cleaned cage helps maintain normal reproductive cycles in female voles.

D. Diseases

1. Infectious Diseases

Wild voles have been hosts for hantaviruses; cowpox virus; *Leptospira* sp.; *Emmonsia* sp.; *Toxoplasma gondii*; *Encephalitozoon cuniculi*; *Neospora caninum*; the larval stages of *Echinococcus multilocularis*; the mites *Echinolaelaps* sp.; and the blood parasites *Babesia microti*, *Haemobartonella microti*, and *Trypanosoma microti*. The latter parasites are not generally associated with clinical signs (Bennett *et al.*, 1997; Cavanagh *et al.*, 2004; Chantrey *et al.*, 2006; Fuehrer *et al.*, 2010; Kuiken *et al.*, 1991). In addition, various dermatomycoses, rabies-like viruses, and *Yersinia pseudotuberculosis* have been isolated from voles (Cox, 1979; Ditrich and Otcenasek, 1982; English and Southern, 1967; Sodja *et al.*, 1982; Zhou *et al.*, 2004). The Acanthocephalan parasites *Moniliformis clarki* and *Cochliomyia hominivorax* have been found to parasitize meadow voles (Wallach and Boever, 1983). *Bordetella bronchiseptica* has been found associated with fatal pulmonary infection of *Microtus montanus* (Jensen and Duncan, 1980). The field vole (*Microtus agrestis*) is a known maintenance host of *Mycobacterium microti* and it has been shown that infected animals develop tuberculosis. Thorough pathological examination of captured diseased animals has shown that voles develop systemic disease with most frequent involvement of spleen and liver, followed by skin, lymph nodes, and lungs. Bacterial shedding occurs from the skin, sputum and saliva (Kipar *et al.*, 2013).

2. Neoplastic Diseases

Adenocarcinoma of the mammary gland has been diagnosed infrequently in colony-raised *M. ochrogaster*, however, lacrimal adenocarcinoma was a common cause of death among colony-reared adult *M. montanus* (Lindsay, 1976).

3. Other Diseases

Malocclusion has been diagnosed in pine, Japanese field (M. montebelli) and long-tailed (M. longicaudus) voles (Harvey *et al.*, 2009; Maser and Hooven, 1970; Sugita *et al.*, 1995). Chronic interstitial nephritis is not uncommon in older colony-bred meadow voles (Dieterich and Preston, 1977a). The etiology is unknown, but the kidneys have histologic evidence of increased interstitial connective tissue with hyaline casts in many tubules. In contrast, older wild meadow moles often have pyelonephritis (Geller and Christian, 1982).

XV. MULTIMAMMATE RATS/MICE: MASTOMYS

A. Introduction

1. Taxonomy

These animals are native to South Africa and also known as multimammate rats or multimammate mice (Hulin and Quinn, 2006; Smit *et al.*, 2001). The common name describes the high number of mammary glands, usually eight to 12 pairs, but there may be as many as 18 pairs. The genus *Mastomys* generates taxonomic confusion. The two most commonly used species in research are *Mastomys natalensis* (Fig. 7.28) and *Mastomys coucha*. These species are morphologically identical and overlap in their native South African habitats (Kneidinger, 2008). The two species differ in chromosome number, some biochemical traits, and sperm morphology (Duplantier *et al.*, 1990; Kneidinger, 2008). Biochemical markers including hepatic glucose phosphate isomerase isoenzymes, hemoglobin subunits, and certain protein markers in muscle have been identified that enable differentiating between the species (Kruppa *et al.*, 1990; Smit *et al.*, 2001). Kruppa *et al.* (1990) indicated that the most commonly used species in research, while typically reported as *M. natalensis*, is actually *M. coucha*. Literature continues to be unclear on this point. (Robbins and van der Straeten, 1989) analyzed all the taxa associated with *Mastomys* but did not allocate any of them to species. The following genus and species names have been used in the past to describe this animal: *M. coucha, Rattus (Praomys) natalensis, R. (Praomys) coucha*, and *R. (Mastomys) natalensis*.

2. Description

The description is taken from Nowak (1999). The head and body length is 60–170 mm, tail length is 60–150 mm, and weight is 20–80 g. The tail is approximately equal in length to the body. Animals have a light gray to brown dorsum and light gray underside. *Mastomys* superficially resembles *Rattus*.

3. Distribution

Originally described as South African species, animals with identical chromosomal features have been found in Tanzania and Senegal in West Africa (Duplantier *et al.*, 1990). Given the confusion with taxonomic status, it probably suffices to state that the multimammate rat is one of the most widely distributed and abundant rodents in Africa.

4. Habitat

Multimammate rats occur in many types of habitat. They may once have been restricted to savannas but can now be found throughout much of sub-Saharan Africa, chiefly in association with people (Nowak, 1999). They do not occupy large towns probably because of competition with *Rattus*. The diet and ecology of *M. natalensis* in their native habitat have been published (Oguge, 1995).

5. Use in Research

Multimammate rats serve as hosts for a wide variety of infectious agents, including some important zoonotic agents. In wild populations, *M. natalensis* is reportedly the natural host of the hemorrhagic fever agent Lassa virus while *M. coucha* is the natural host of bubonic plague (Kneidinger, 2008; Smit *et al.*, 2001). Immunologically, lymphocytes from *M. natalensis* show greater proliferation in response to presentation of *Y. pestis* antigens than lymphocytes from *M. coucha*, which perhaps mediates the greater resistance of *M. natalensis* to plague (Arntzen *et al.*, 1991). They are the subject of field and laboratory-based studies in the pathogenesis and epidemiology of these agents (Fichet-Calvet and Rogers, 2009; Lalis *et al.*, 2012; Lecompte *et al.*, 2006; Makundi *et al.*, 2008). *M. natalensis* has also been studied for the impact of rodent population density on spread of Mopeia virus (Goyens *et al.*, 2013). This is an arenavirus related to Lassa virus that occurs naturally in *M. natalensis* but non-pathogenic to humans, thus rendering it a safer subject for study.

Multimammate rats have been used in field or laboratory studies of other zoonotic agents including leptospirosis, leishmania, and Crimean–Congo hemorrhagic fever virus (Holt *et al.*, 2006; Machang'u *et al.*, 1997, 2004; Nolan and Farrell, 1987; Shepherd *et al.*, 1989). *M. natalensis* has been identified as a reservoir for numerous nontuberculous *Mycobacterium* spp., including *M. intracellulare* complex (Durnez *et al.*, 2008), environmental contaminants that can opportunistically infect

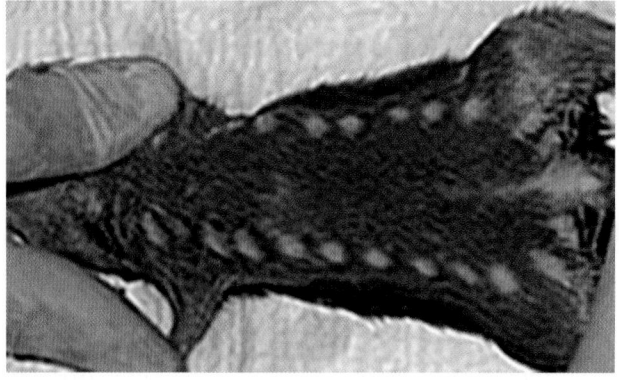

FIGURE 7.28 *Mastomys natalensis* – multimammate mouse. Ventral view of female multimammate mouse showing the large number of mammary glands.

immune-compromised individuals. Experimentally, *M. natalensis* has been used as a model for studying bacterial infection with the water-borne mycobacterium *M. ulcerans* (Singh *et al.*, 1984).

Mastomys natalensis or *M. coucha* have additionally been used to investigate the pathogenesis and treatment of the parasitic agents *Plasmodium berghei*, *Entamoeba histolytica*, and *Trypanosoma brucei rhodesiense* (Khare *et al.*, 1984; Rickman and Kanyangala, 1990; Srivastava and Gupta, 1985); the nematodes *Nippostrongylus brasiliensis*, *Dipetalonema viteae*, *Brugia malayi*, *B. pahangi*, *Litomosoides carinii*, *Acanthocheilonema viteae*, *Wuchereria bancrofti* (Chatterjee *et al.*, 1988; Joseph *et al.*, 2011; Redl and Kassai, 1979; Sangvaranond and Zahner, 1989; Zielke, 1980); and the trematode *Schistosoma mansoni* (Coelho *et al.*, 1980).

Mastomys natalensis spontaneously develops gastric carcinoid and serves as a model for Zollinger Ellison syndrome in humans (Kumazawa *et al.*, 1989; Nilsson *et al.*, 1992; Vigen *et al.*, 2012). The role of hypergastrinemia in tumor production, as well as CCK-A and CCK-B/gastrin receptors on enterochromaffin-like carcinoid cells and their relationship to histamine secretion have been well studied (Kolby *et al.*, 1998; Vigen *et al.*, 2012).

Mastomys natalensis has an endogenous papillomavirus (MnPV) which has been sequenced and shown to produce cutaneous tumors on activation (Schafer *et al.*, 2011; Tan *et al.*, 1994). *M. coucha* has a related papillomavirus (McPV2) that produces anogenital condylomas in this species. Serological markers for detection of these agents and monitoring of tumor development have been developed (Schafer *et al.*, 2010). The morphology of experimentally induced keratoacanthomas and squamous cell carcinomas has been published (Rudolph *et al.*, 1981). *M. natalensis* has also been used as a model for chemical oncogenicity (Hoch-Ligeti *et al.*, 1985; Tajima, 1981; Wayss *et al.*, 1981) as well as general toxicology (Holmes *et al.*, 1995, 1996, 1997).

Multimammate rats have been used to study the role of mucosal anaphylaxis on gastric ulcer formation (Andre and Andre, 1981; Andre *et al.*, 1981), and some individuals spontaneously develop autoimmune thyroiditis (Solleveld *et al.*, 1985).

B. Biology

1. Physiological Characteristics

Several investigations have focused on unique aspects of *M. natalensis* biology. The submaxillary salivary glands of *M. natalensis* are the richest available source of nerve growth factor (Aloe *et al.*, 1981; Matsushima *et al.*, 1990; Sirigu *et al.*, 1985, 1988). Both males and females have a prostate gland (Dixon *et al.*, 1988; Gross and Didio, 1987). As part of the study of various infectious agents, the immune response has been characterized in normal animals (Beucher and Charreire, 1983; Zahner

et al., 1987a,b). Mammary gland growth and response to reproductive hormones have been compared to those in laboratory mice (Nagasawa *et al.*, 1989). Like laboratory rats, the multimammate rat does not have a gallbladder. Renal physiologic parameters have been investigated as a potential differentiating factor between *M. natalensis* and *M. coucha* but were found to be similar between these species (Ntshotsho *et al.*, 2004).

2. Normal Values

The multimammate rat has a life span of 3 years, its weight at birth is 2–3 g, its eyes open at 13–17 days, and it is weaned at 19–21 days. Selected hematologic (Kagira *et al.*, 2005) and serum biochemistry data (Yamamoto *et al.*, 1999) of juvenile and adult multimammate rats have been published. Hematology values for adult multimammate rats are listed in Table 7.2.

3. Reproduction

Multimammate rats reproduce well as monogamous pairs and have litters of six to 12 young, although numbers as high as 22 are reported (Neal, 1977). Birth weight is 2–3 g, young open their eyes at 13–17 days, and they are weaned at 19–21 days. Males and females reach puberty at 55–75 days of age. They breed year-round and will mate at the postparturient estrus. Estrous cycles average 6–8 days, and females have a 23-day gestation period. Life span is approximately 3 years (Williams, 1980).

4. Behavior

While these animals appear almost tame in the wild, Veenstra (1958) claims they are very aggressive when held under laboratory conditions, and care must be taken to avoid being bitten. They keep their bodies well groomed and their cages clean and will attempt to dispose of waste by pushing it through a hole in the cage. In captivity, stereotypic behaviors similar to those of rats, characterized by repetitive sniffing, rearing, licking, exhibiting head movements, and biting have been described (Gulati *et al.*, 1986, 1988).

C. Husbandry

Colonies of *M. natalensis* have been established by many of the scientists that use them, and inbred lines varying in susceptibility to gastric carcinoids have been developed (Kneidinger, 2008; Randeria, 1978; Vigen *et al.*, 2012). Under field conditions *M. natalensis* eats mostly grass and other seeds (Nowak, 1999). In suitable habitats multimammate rats will eat insects. Near human populations *M. natalensis* eats nearly everything humans do. In the laboratory, they have been kept successfully on commercial laboratory rat or mice feed (Jackson and Van Aarde, 2004; Solleveld, 1987; Williams,

1980). *M. natalensis* had a wider tolerance for protein ranges in the diet than *M. coucha*, which had depressed reproductive parameters at protein levels both higher and lower than 10–15% (Jackson and Van Aarde, 2004). No comprehensive reviews of husbandry are available but review of methods in published research involving *Mastomys* shows that most researchers house this species in standard solid-bottom rodent cages with wood-chip bedding and feed commercial laboratory rodent feed with *ad libitum* water.

D. Diseases

1. Infectious Diseases

A number of zoonotic agents, most notably Lassa virus and *Yersinia pestis* have been associated with wild-caught multimammate rats (see Uses in Research); however, these agents should not be problematic in established laboratory colonies. Mastomys also frequently harbor a naturally occurring arenavirus, Mopeia virus that is non-pathogenic to humans. The prevalence of this agent in laboratory colonies of *Mastomys* and its pathogenic potential for *Mastomys* or other rodent species is unknown. MnPV, the papillomavirus responsible for cutaneous tumors in *M. natalensis* and McPV2, the papillomavirus responsible for anal condylomata in *M. coucha* have an unknown prevalence in laboratory colonies, nor is their pathogenicity to other laboratory rodent species known (Pruthi *et al.*, 1983; Schafer *et al.*, 2011; Tan *et al.*, 1994). An enteric *Helicobacter*, *H. mastomyrinus*, was isolated from the liver and cecum of asymptomatic *M. natalensis* and animals with colitis (Shen *et al.*, 2005). *H. mastomyrinus* has been associated with colitis in several strains of genetically engineered mice (Eaton *et al.*, 2011). This illustrates that the potential for agents from wild rodents to cause disease in other laboratory animal species should not be forgotten.

2. Neoplastic Diseases

Lymphosarcomas, parathyroid adenomas, prostatic tumors, reticulum cell sarcomas, adenomas of the glandular stomach, and gastric carcinoids are relatively common (Holland, 1970; Kozima *et al.*, 1970; Kumazawa *et al.*, 1989; Kurokawa *et al.*, 1968; Saito *et al.*, 1977; Snell and Stewart, 1967, 1969, 1975; Stewart and Snell ,1968; Tielemans *et al.*, 1987). Gastric carcinoids are particularly common both as spontaneous and inducible tumors and *M. natalensis* is a model organism for this condition (Fossmark *et al.*, 2011; Vigen *et al.*, 2012). Lymphoepithelial thymoma is common in animals over 2 years of age and is often associated with myositis, atrophy of skeletal muscle, and myocarditis (Kurokawa *et al.*, 1968; Stewart and Snell, 1968). Other less common tumors reported include granulosa cell tumors of ovaries, testicular tumors, adrenal gland adenomas, pituitary adenomas, hepatomas, nephroblastomas, and

adenomas of the pancreas (Hosoda *et al.*, 1976; Jobard *et al.*, 1974; Snell and Hollander, 1972; Snell and Stewart, 1975; Stewart and Snell, 1975).

3. Miscellaneous

a. Aging Lesions

In animals over 2 years of age, many multimammate rats develop osteoarthritis. Degenerative joint disease affects the diarthroses and intervertebral discs, with many peripheral joints involved. Degenerated discs protrude into the vertebral canal at multiple sites along the vertebral column (Snell and Stewart, 1975). A histopathological survey of lesions in aged *Mastomys* has been published (Solleveld *et al.*, 1982).

b. Autoimmune Disease

Autoimmune thyroiditis occurs spontaneously in many individuals (Solleveld *et al.*, 1985). As the animals age, increasing numbers of autoantibodies are found. Membranous or membranoproliferative glomerulonephritis are frequent lesions. In chronic cases, the appearance is that of a classic 'end-stage' kidney, with glomerular changes accompanied by tubular nephrosis, tubular atrophy, protein casts, and interstitial mononuclear inflammation. These kidney lesions are thought to have an autoimmune pathogenesis (Snell and Stewart, 1975).

c. Other Conditions

A relatively high incidence of duodenitis and duodenal ulcer occurs in multimammate rats, and afflicted rats have been used to study cellular regeneration (Smedley *et al.*, 1990).

XVI. DEGUS: OCTODON

A. Introduction

1. Description

The description of *Octodon degus* (Fig. 7.29) is adapted from the review by Woods (1974). The head and body length is 125–195 mm, and tail length is 105–165 mm. Weight varies between 170–300 g for adults. The upper parts are grayish to brown, and underparts are creamy yellow. A black brush at the tip of the tail is prominent and gives rise to their other common name of 'trumpet-tail' rats.

2. Distribution

Degus occur naturally in northern and western Chile, on the west slope of the Andes up to 1200 m.

3. Habitat

Degus are found in open areas near thickets, rocks, or stone walls. They construct an elaborate communal burrow system, with the main section under rocks or shrubs.

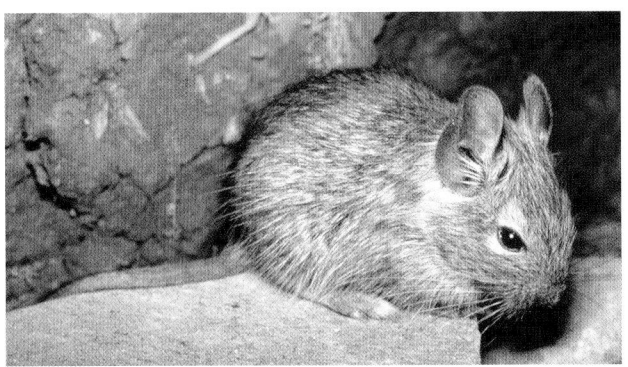

FIGURE 7.29 *Octodon degus* – negu. Oblique view, Prague Zoo, Czechoslovakia. *Photograph by M. Andera and the Mammal Images Library of the American Society of Mammalogists.*

A complex network of tunnels and surface paths leads out to feeding sites. *Octodon degus* live in small colonies with a strong social organization based on group territoriality. The burrow is the center of the defended territory. Females of the same social group often rear their young in a common burrow (Ebensperger *et al.*, 2006, 2007).

4. Use in Research

The unique characteristics of the degu have made it increasingly popular as a laboratory animal. The precocious neonates are animal models used to study neurobiological developmental patterns. It is also a popular model for neurodegenerative conditions of aging, including Alzheimer's disease (Ardiles *et al.*, 2013). Other degenerative conditions of aging, such as diabetes and cancer, are also studied in the degu (Ardiles *et al.*, 2013). The diurnal sleep pattern of the degu, in contrast to that of nocturnal rats and mice, makes it an excellent model to investigate human sleep/wake and circadian behavior (Lee, 2004). Alteration of light cycles, feeding patterns, and/or social organization can create the circadian equivalent of 'jet lag' in degus. Degus are highly social rodents and this feature is useful in determining the effects of altered social structures on behavioral or neurochemical parameters (Colonnello *et al.*, 2011). Researchers have also used the degu to investigate how herbivorous animals match their foraging and digestion to seasonal changes in availability and quality of food (Bozinovic *et al.*, 1997; Kenagy *et al.*, 1999), drug tolerance (Gaule *et al.*, 1990; Letelier *et al.*, 1985), and diabetes development and cataract formation (Barker *et al.*, 1983; Datiles and Fukui, 1989).

B. Biology

The first four digits of degus are well developed with sharp claws for burrowing. The fifth digit is shorter. Females have four pairs of mammary glands, and the testicles of males are intra-abdominal (Bates and Weir, 1944;

Contreras and Bustos-Obregon, 1980; Weir, 1970). The adrenal glands are large compared with those of other rodents on a per body weight basis (Galli and Marusic, 1976). The degu spleen is unusual, with sinusoids lined by endothelial cells having cuboidal morphology that gives the spleen a glandular appearance (Murphy *et al.*, 1980).

Reference values for selected hematologic and serum chemistry values for degus have been published and are similar to values reported for guinea pigs and rats (Murphy *et al.*, 1978; Jekl *et al.*, 2011c). Reference hematologic and serum protein values from normal degus that ranged in age from 3–48 months were similar for both sexes (Murphy *et al.*, 1978).

C. Husbandry

A breeding and experimental degu colony was successfully maintained at the University of Michigan for many years (Ardiles *et al.*, 2013; Colby *et al.*, 2012). Husbandry and biology were recently reviewed and a Cold Spring Harbor Protocol for the use of this species is available based on the University of Michigan colony (Palacios and Lee, 2013).

Laboratory colonies breed throughout the year, and females may have more than one annual litter. Degu social behavior is an important component in their husbandry (Colby *et al.*, 2012; Lee, 2004). Degus fare much better with social housing than individual housing, particularly during the juvenile period (Colby *et al.*, 2012). Animals raised in isolation develop lethargy and behavioral deficits that cannot be remedied by use of running wheels or other enrichment (Colby *et al.*, 2012; Lee, 2004). Short-term individual housing (<4 weeks) followed by re-housing with littermates can be used successfully (Colby *et al.*, 2012). Mature animals in a breeding colony are typically maintained as breeding pairs or as one male with multiple females. Females are induced ovulators and require the presence of a male to induce ovulation (Weir, 1970). Females exhibit considerable social tolerance, and may be housed together without fighting (Davis, 1975; Colby *et al.*, 2012). Males can be pair or group-housed but are less tolerant to re-grouping once they have been individually housed, although they may tolerate housing with a male littermate following individual housing (Colby *et al.*, 2012). Solid-bottom, opaque-sided caging is used with nonadherent bedding (paper or corn cob). Running wheels were provided in this colony as part of the experimental protocol, but which also served as enrichment.

Degu dietary requirements in captivity have been recently evaluated (Colby *et al.*, 2012). Dietary requirements are different for juvenile or lactating animals than for adult animals. Obesity, diabetes, and insulin resistance can be avoided in adult animals by feeding a lower energy, higher fiber diet (e.g., LabDiet 5001;

PMI International, St. Louis, MO) but the same diet in lactating or growing animals will result in poor litter size, growth, and survivability. Thus it is recommended to feed a breeder diet (e.g.., ProLab RMH 2000; PMI International) to breeding animals and juveniles and transition them to the lower energy, higher fiber diet between 10 weeks and 6 months of age. Fresh or dried alfalfa can be provided to breeding females once weekly (Colby *et al.*, 2012). Water is provided *ad libitum*, although degus may not consume much water. Acidification of water is recommended to avoid opportunistic infection by *Pseudomonas* spp. (Najecki and Tate, 1999).

Gestation in degus lasts for 90 days (Weir, 1970). Litters contain one to 10 young with an average of seven pups. The young are precocial, thus are born fully furred with their eyes open within 1 day. They weigh about 14 g at birth, ranging in size from 5 to 6.5 cm from nose to base of tail (Reynolds and Wright, 1979). Pups typically nurse for 4–5 weeks, although they will begin eating solid foods by 2 weeks. Pups in the laboratory are generally weaned at 5–6 weeks into same sex social groups (Colby *et al.*, 2012). The age of sexual maturity has been variably reported between 45 days and 6 months (Weir, 1970) but with optimal diet averages around 3 months (Colby *et al.*, 2012). Breeding maturity in males can be assessed by the presence of penile spines.

Handling animals by the tail is not recommended due to the risk of degloving injury (Woods and Boraker, 1975). Some laboratory colonies use nylon fishnets to transfer and handle degus (Najecki and Tate, 1999). In the wild, degus take dust baths to keep their coats free of oil. Providing a dust bath twice a week has been recommended but other colonies have successfully maintained animals without one (Colby *et al.*, 2012; Palacios and Lee, 2013). Running wheels appear to be preferred enrichment devices, while the animals do not use PVC tubes or nest boxes (Colby *et al.*, 2012).

D. Diseases

The most common diseases reported in a survey of 300 privately owned degus were dental conditions (Jekl *et al.*, 2011d). Most common dental conditions are malocclusion of either the molars or incisors (Jekl *et al.*, 2011a,b,d). Elodontomas, which are non-neoplastic proliferative masses of elodont (continuously erupting) teeth, can also occur in the degu, as in prairie dogs (Jekl *et al.*, 2008). Rigid endoscopes or laryngoscopes have been successfully used to evaluate the degu oral cavity (Jekl and Knotek, 2007).

Other commonly occurring non-infectious diseases include cataracts (Worgul and Rothstein, 1975; Jekl *et al.*, 2011d). Cataract formation may be congenital or acquired as a side-effect of diabetes development. Spontaneous diabetes mellitus is common in the degu and has been associated with feeding guinea pig chow, fresh fruit, or other dietary causes of hyperglycemia (Fox and Murphy, 1979; Najecki and Tate, 1999). A diabetic degu will develop cataracts within four weeks (Datiles and Fukui, 1989). Diabetes has also been associated with islet amyloidosis (Nishi and Steiner, 1990).

Polycystic kidney disease, similar to the congenital condition in humans and mice, was described in an aged female degu in association with chronic renal failure (Cadillac *et al.*, 2003). Cerebral amyloid deposition, similar to that seen in the vascular manifestations of Alzheimer's disease, have been reported as a spontaneous occurrence in the degu and proposed as a model for this disease (van Groen *et al.*, 2011).

Pseudomonas infection is common in degus if acidified water is not used (Colby *et al.*, 2012; Najecki and Tate, 1999). Najecki and Tate (1999) also described fatal diarrhea associated with *Giardia* spp. in adults and pups. Acute suppurative bronchopneumonia, caused by *Klebsiella pneumoniae*, was described in a degu (Murphy *et al.*, 1980).

Traumatic injuries are common in degus (Jekl *et al.*, 2011d). A tibial fracture in a 3-month-old degu was repaired by medullary fixation (Beregi *et al.*, 1994).

Babero and Cattan (1975) described helminth parasites from *O. degus* in Chile, with descriptions of three new species, including a whipworm, *Trichuris bradleyi*.

Anderson *et al.* (1990) diagnosed a primary bronchioloalveolar carcinoma with renal and hepatic metastases in a mature male degu that was found dead in a zoological exhibit. Murphy *et al.* (1980) surveyed 189 degus ranging in age from 2 to 60 months for neoplasia. Few neoplasias were reported – one animal had a reticulum cell sarcoma (histiocytic lymphoma) of a cervical lymph node which resulted in death due to tracheal compression. Two degus had hepatocellular carcinoma with metastasis to lung, kidney, or heart. One of these resembled a mixed hepatocellular and cholangiocarcinoma. Other tumors reported included splenic hemangioma, and a mesenteric lipoma. A single case report of a vaginal leiomyosarcoma has been reported (Soto-Gamboa *et al.*, 2009). Transitional cell carcinoma in the renal pelvis was reported in an aged female degu that also had a choristoma (normal tissue in abnormal location) in the contralateral kidney (Lester *et al.*, 2005). The choristoma consisted of trabecular bone with adipose tissue.

XVII. NAKED MOLE RATS: *HETEROCEPHALUS GLABER*

A. Introduction

1. Description

Naked mole rats belong to the family of African mole rats, Bathyergidae. The taxonomy of this rodent family has been in debate for years, due to the extensive

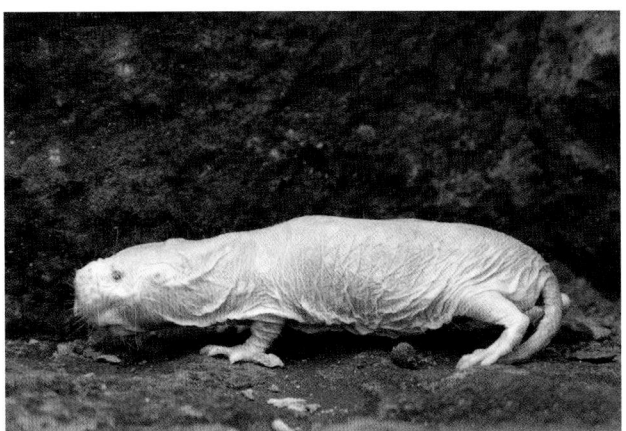

FIGURE 7.30   *Heterocephalus glaber* – naked mole rat. Side view. *Photograph from Cleveland Metro Parks Zoo.*

interspecific and intergeneric evolutionary convergence, as well as the intraspecific polymorphism in size and color patterns, making it difficult to clearly separate genera and species using morphological and morphometric traits. Kock *et al.* (2006) used allozyme, nuclear and mitochondrial DNA markers to clarify the taxonomy and distinguish a new genus (*Fukomys*) from the existing genera. There are at least 30 species in the family comprising six genera, including the newly described *Fukomys*. The naked mole rat (*Heterocephalus glaber*; Fig. 7.30) is the sole representative of the genus *Heterocephalus* (Faulkes and Bennett, 2013; Kock *et al.*, 2006).

2. Distribution

All genera of the Bathyergidae are found exclusively in hot, arid, and semi-arid, regions of sub-Saharan Africa.

3. Habitat

Bathyergidae inhabit a subterranean environment and live in colonies. Naked mole rats construct extensive foraging tunnels that run at root or tuber level and construct a chamber for nesting deeper underground. Naked mole rats were first collected in Ethiopia in 1842 (Ruppel, 1842). They have since been collected throughout their natural habitat, which extends from northeastern Kenya, throughout Somalia, and into the southeastern area of Ethiopia (Brett, 1986).

4. Use in Research

Naked mole rats have a number of interesting characteristics that make them valuable research models. They are one of only two mammalian species exhibiting eusocial behavior. Extensive investigation of this trait has resulted in a body of work describing their eusocial structure and its evolutionary development (Dengler-Crish and Catania, 2007; Faulkes and Bennett, 2013; Jarvis, 1981; O'Riain *et al.*, 1996; Sherman *et al.*, 1991).

Further study of naked mole rats in the laboratory revealed several other traits worthy of investigation. Naked mole rats are the longest living rodent known (Buffenstein, 2005, 2008). Although infant mortality may be high in captivity, upon reaching adulthood they have a life span of up to 30 years. Consequently, they have become an important model for aging research (Buffenstein, 2005; Edrey *et al.*, 2011; Kim *et al.*, 2011). The oxidative stress theory of aging has long been accepted as a credible explanation of aging and death. However, research using naked mole rats has contributed to mounting evidence that there is no direct relationship between reactive oxygen species and longevity (Lewis *et al.*, 2013; Shi *et al.*, 2010).

Despite having an exceptionally long life span, naked mole rats rarely develop cancer with age. Numerous studies have investigated the underlying factors that confer longevity and cancer resistance (Azpurua and Seluanov, 2012; Buffenstein, 2005; Edrey *et al.*, 2011; Kim *et al.*, 2011; Seluanov *et al.*, 2009). Naked mole-rat fibroblasts secrete extremely high-molecular-mass hyaluronan, probably to provide skin elasticity needed for life in underground tunnels. The hyaluronan protects cells from perturbation of the signalling pathways that are sufficient for malignant transformation in other species conferring cancer resistance (Tian *et al.*, 2013).

Naked mole rats have adapted to living with low oxygen and high CO_2 levels with no adverse effects because of the environmental conditions in their subterranean habitat. Mammalian brains deprived of oxygen for even brief periods of time are susceptible to irreversible brain damage. However, brain tissue from naked mole rats is highly resistant to hypoxia and their neurons are able to recover from anoxia lasting 30 min or longer (Larson and Park, 2009). Understanding this resistance to the effects of hypoxia and the underlying mechanisms responsible has implications for the clinical prevention of brain damage in the face of oxygen deprivation.

B. Biology

Naked mole rats are tube-shaped rodents with loose, wrinkled, pink and gray-tinged skin sparsely covered with thick tactile vibrissae-like hairs that are prominent on the face and tail. The mouth closes behind large external incisors that allow naked mole rats to tunnel through dirt using the teeth while keeping the mouth and airway clear. The tail is approximately half the length of the body. Although often described as mouse-sized, great variation exists in the weight of naked mole rats within a colony, within each gender, and even within a single litter. At 11 months of age the weight within a captive-bred litter ranged from 25.7 to 43.4 g and the variation in the weight range between successive litters in the same colony was equally diverse (Jarvis, 1991). A breeding female can weigh as much as 110 g.

Naked mole rats resemble social insects in their behavior. They establish colonies with a single breeding female. The nonbreeding animals are responsible for food collection and distribution, and share the care of young (Jarvis, 1981). When the breeding female dies or is removed from a colony, working females are capable of becoming a breeding female and will compete, at times aggressively, for the position.

C. Husbandry

In nature, naked mole rats live in sealed burrows with narrow tunnels running between chambers. The animals move about in close contact with the earthen walls under conditions of minimal noise and airflow. Consequently, the temperature and humidity in these underground burrows are relatively high, varying between 80 and 90°F (Yahav and Buffenstein, 1991). To simulate this situation in the laboratory, yet allow observation of the animals and maintenance of their housing, a laboratory tunnel system must be transparent, approximately 4–7 cm in diameter, easily cleaned and made of durable material. Circular or square tunnels made of glass or acrylic have been used to achieve these criteria. Several chambers made from standard rodent caging of various sizes, are attached to the tunnels, and serve as feeding, nesting, and toilet chambers (Artwohl et al., 2002; Sherman et al., 1991) Except for the toilet chamber, which may require frequent changing, the system should not be cleaned unless necessary as naked mole rats are easily disturbed and rely on odors to navigate through their burrows. The subterranean habitat of naked mole rats has resulted in an exquisite sensitivity to noise and vibrations. Any such disturbances cause a panic response. Constant background low-intensity white noise can be used to ameliorate the effects of unavoidable noise during routine colony maintenance (Ludwig and Collinar, 2009; Sherman et al., 1991).

Achieving the high temperature and humidity levels found in the naked mole rats natural habitat may be difficult to achieve in the laboratory. Consequently, ventilation may need to be reduced, and the temperature and humidity supplemented with portable units (Artwohl et al., 2002). In the wild, naked mole rats feed on tubers, roots and bulbs that extend into their burrows. In the laboratory they are maintained on a variety of vegetables that are provided daily, and a continual supply of sweet potatoes, squash or apples. No source of water is provided as the water requirements of naked mole rats are met in the food supplied.

The breeding female gives birth every 76–84 days. Naked mole rats are more sensitive to colony disturbances when a new litter is present. Manipulation of the nest chamber during the 2 weeks following parturition may alarm the adults, leading to removal of the pups from the nest chamber. Should this occur, the pups may be trampled and killed. During this critical time it is important to manipulate the colony as little as possible (Sherman et al., 1991).

D. Diseases

Although the naked mole rat has an exceptionally long life span, few diseases have been documented in this species. Furthermore, published surveys of disease in naked mole rats are sparse. A retrospective study by (Delaney et al., 2013) examined the spontaneous histologic lesions in adult naked mole rats in a captive zoological collection colony over a 15-year period. With the exception of chronic renal disease and age-associated heart lesions, the authors found most of the lesions observed were related to diet or behavior. Among the 115 animals reviewed, the lesions seen most often were renal mineralization and hepatic hemosiderosis, which were both assumed to be diet related. Behavior-related trauma and extramedullary hematopoiesis, most probably developed in response to the trauma, were the second most frequent lesions observed. The absence of disease in naked mole rats despite their long life span has generated interest in this species as an exceptional model of aging (Buffenstein, 2008; Edrey et al., 2011).

References

Abraham, D., Lucius, R., Trees, A.J., 2002. Immunity to Onchocerca spp. in animal hosts. Trends Parasitol. 18, 164–171.

Aguilera, M., 1985. Growth and reproduction in Zygodontomys microtinus (Rodentia, Cricetidae) from Venezuela in a laboratory bred colony. Mammalia 49, 75–83.

Akai, F., Maeda, M., Hashimoto, S., Taneda, M., Takagi, H., 1995. A new animal model of cerebral infarction: magnetic embolization with carbonyl iron particles. Neurosci. Lett. 194, 139–141.

Alexander, L.F., Riddle, B.R., 2005. Phylogenetics of the new world rodent family heteromyidae. J. Mammal. 86, 366–379.

Allen, K.E., Yabsley, M.J., Johnson, E.M., Reichard, M.V., Panciera, R.J., Ewing, S.A., et al., 2011. Novel Hepatozoon in vertebrates from the southern United States. J. Parasitol. 97, 648–653.

Allen, K.L., van Bruggen, N., Cooper, J.E., 1993. Detection of bacterial sinusitis in the Mongolian gerbil (Meriones unguiculatus) using magnetic resonance imaging. Vet. Rec. 132, 633–635.

Alligood, C.A., Wheaton, C.J., Daneault, A.J., Carlson, R.C., Savage, A., 2009. Behavioral predictors of copulation in captive Key Largo woodrats (Neotoma floridana smalli). Behav. Processes 81, 337–342.

Alligood, C.A., Daneault, A.J., Carlson, R.C., Dillenbeck, T., Wheaton, C.J., Savage, A., 2011. Development of husbandry practices for the captive breeding of Key Largo woodrats (Neotoma floridana smalli). Zoo Biol. 30, 318–327.

Aloe, L., Cozzari, C., Levi-Montalcini, R., 1981. The submaxillary salivary glands of the African rodent Praomys (mastomys) natalensis as the richest available source of the nerve growth factor. Exp. Cell Res. 133, 475–480.

Alvarez-Castaneda, S.T., Patton, J.L., 2004. Geographic genetic architecture of pocket gopher (Thomomys bottae) populations in Baja California, Mexico. Mol. Ecol. 13, 2287–2301.

Anderson Jr., G.W., Slone Jr., T.W., Peters, C.J., 1988. The gerbil, Meriones unguiculatus, a model for Rift Valley fever viral encephalitis. Arch. Virol. 102, 187–196.

Anderson, J.F., Johnson, R.C., Magnarelli, L.A., Hyde, F.W., Myers, J.E., 1986. Peromyscus leucopus and Microtus pennsylvanicus simultaneously infected with Borrelia burgdorferi and Babesia microti. J. Clin. Microbiol. 23, 135–137.

Anderson, L.C., 1982. The capture and laboratory maintenance of hibernating ground squirrels. Lab. Anim. (NY) 11, 64–65.

Anderson, M.G., Frenkel, L.D., Homann, S., Guffey, J., 2003. A case of severe monkeypox virus disease in an American child: emerging infections and changing professional values. Pediatr. Infect. Dis. J. 22, 1093–1096.

Anderson, S.H., Jones, J.K., 1984. Orders and Families of Recent Mammals of the World. John Wiley & Sons, New York.

Anderson, W.I., Steinberg, H., King, J.M., 1990. Bronchioalveolar carcinoma with renal and hepatic metastases in a degu (Octodon degus). J. Wildl. Dis. 26, 129–131.

Andre, F., Andre, C., 1981. Gastric ulcer disease: gastric ulcer induced by mucosal anaphylaxis in ovalbumin-sensitized Praomys (Mastomys) natalensis. Am. J. Pathol. 102, 133–135.

Andre, F., Gillon, J., Andre, C., Jourdan, G., 1981. Prevention of reaginic antibody production and anaphylactic gastric ulcer by pesticides and by a polychlorinated biphenyl. Environ. Res. 25, 381–385.

Anosa, V.O., Kaneko, J.J., 1984. Pathogenesis of Trypanosoma brucei infection in deer mice (Peromyscus maniculatus). Light and electron microscopic study of testicular lesions. Vet. Pathol. 21, 238–246.

Arai, T., Kaneko, H., Takagi, H., Ogino, T., Sasaki, M., Matsumoto, H., et al., 1996. High sensitivity to streptozotocin in herbivorous voles, Microtus arvalis, compared to mice. Vet. Res. Commun. 20, 215–224.

Ardiles, A.O., Ewer, J., Acosta, M.L., Kirkwood, A., Martinez, A.D., Ebensperger, L.A., et al., 2013. Octodon degus (Molina 1782): a model in comparative biology and biomedicine. Cold Spring Harb. Protoc. 2013, 312–318.

Arntzen, L., Wadee, A.A., Isaacson, M., 1991. Immune responses of two Mastomys sibling species to Yersinia pestis. Infect. Immun. 59, 1966–1971.

Artwohl, J., Hill, T., Comer, C., Park, T., 2002. Naked mole-rats: unique opportunities and husbandry challenges. Lab. Anim. (NY) 31, 32–36.

Asakawa, M., 1987. Genus Heligmosomoides Hall, 1916 (Heligmosomidae: Nematoda) from the Japanese wood mice, Apodemus spp. III. The life cycle of Heligmosomoides kurilensis kobayashii (Nadtochii, 1966) in ICR mice and preliminary experimental infection to jirds. J. Coll. Dairy (Ebetsu) 12, 131–140.

Asavisanu, R., Setasuban, P., Komalamisra, C., 1985. Experimental infection of Paragonimus heterotremus metacercariae to the Mongolian gerbils (Meriones unguiculatus). Southeast Asian J. Trop. Med. Public Health 16, 344–345.

Avashia, S.B., Petersen, J.M., Lindley, C.M., Schriefer, M.E., Gage, K.L., Cetron, M., et al., 2004. First reported prairie dog-to-human tularemia transmission, Texas, 2002. Emerg. Infect. Dis. 10, 483–486.

Avila, G., Aguilar, L., Benitez, S., Yepez-Mulia, L., Lavenat, I., Flisser, A., 2002. Inflammatory responses in the intestinal mucosa of gerbils and hamsters experimentally infected with the adult stage of Taenia solium. Int. J. Parasitol. 32, 1301–1308.

Avila, G., Teran, N., Aguilar-Vega, L., Maravilla, P., Mata-Miranda, P., Flisser, A., 2006. Laboratory animal models for human Taenia solium. Parasitol. Int. (55. Suppl), S99–S103.

Ayers, J.D., Rota, P.A., Collins, M.L., Drew, C.P., 2012. Alternatives to retroorbital blood collection in hispid cotton rats (Sigmodon hispidus). J. Am. Assoc. Lab. Anim. Sci. 51, 239–245.

Azad, A.F., 2004. Prairie dog: cuddly pet or Trojan horse? Emerg. Infect. Dis. 10, 542–543.

Azazy, A.A., Devaney, E., Chance, M.L., 1994. A PEG-ELISA for the detection of Leishmania donovani antigen in circulating immune complexes. Trans. R Soc. Trop. Med. Hyg. 88, 62–66.

Azpurua, J., Seluanov, A., 2012. Long-lived cancer-resistant rodents as new model species for cancer research. Front. Genet. 3, 319.

Babero, B.B., Cattan, P.E., 1975. The helminth fauna of Chile: III. Parasites of the degu rodent, Octodon degus Monina, 1782, with descriptions of three new species. [Spanish] Helmintofauna de Chile: III. Parasitos del roedor degu, Octodon degus Monina, 1782, con la descripcion de tres nuevas especies. Bol. Chil. Parasitol. 30, 68–76.

Bacha Jr., W.J., Roush Jr., R., Icardi, S., 1982. Infection of the gerbil by the avian schistosome Austrobilharzia variglandis (Miller and Northrup 1926; Penner 1953). J. Parasitol. 68, 505–507.

Baker, R.H., 1968. Habitats and distribution. In: King, J.A. (Ed.), Biology of Peromyscus (Rodentia) American Society of Mammalogists, Stillwater, OK, pp. 98–121.

Balaz, I., 2010. Somatic characteristics and reproduction of common vole, Microtus arvalis (Microtus arvalis. Biologia (Bratisl) 65, 1064–1071.

Balciauskas, L., Balciauskiene, L., Baltrunaite, L., 2010. Root vole, Microtus oeconomus, in Lithuania: changes in the distribution range. Folia Zool. Brno. 59, 267–277.

Banks, C.W., Oliver Jr., J.H., Phillips, J.B., Clark, K.L., 1998. Life cycle of Ixodes minor (Acari: Ixodidae) in the laboratory. J. Med. Entomol. 35, 496–499.

Banks, R.E., Coviello, G.M., Bowers, T.M., Sherman, K.E., 1995. Cysticercosis in prairie dogs. Contemp. Top. Lab. Anim. Sci. 34, 96–98.

Barker, S.A., Fish, F.P., Tomana, M., Garner, L.C., Settine, R.L., Prchal, J., 1983. Gas chromatographic/mass spectrometric evidence for the identification of a heptitol and an octitol in human and Octodon degu eye lenses. Biochem. Biophys. Res. Commun. 116, 988–993.

Barnard, W.P., Ernst, J.V., Dixon, C.F., 1974. Coccidia of the cotton rat, Sigmodon hispidus, from Alabama. J. Parasitol. 60, 406–414.

Barthold, S.W., 1980. Diagnostic exercise. Transmissible murine colonic hyperplasia. Lab. Anim. Sci. 30, 641–642.

Bates, M., Weir, J.M., 1944. The adaptation of a cane rat (Zygodontomys) to the laboratory and its susceptibility to the virus of yellow fever. Am. J. Trop. Med. Hyg. 24, 35–37.

Bayssade-Dufour, C., Vuong, P.N., Farhati, K., Picot, H., Albaret, J.L., 1994. Speed of skin penetration and initial migration route of infective larvae of Schistosoma haematobium in Meriones unguiculatus. C. R. Acad. Sci. III 317, 529–533.

Beacham, B.E., Romito, R., Kay, H.D., 1982. Vaccination of the African white-tailed rat, Mystromys albacaudatus, with sonicated Leishmania braziliensis panamensis promastigotes. Am. J. Trop. Med. Hyg. 31, 252–258.

Beare, A.S., 1975. Myxoviruses. Dev. Biol. Stand. 28, 3–17.

Becker, S.V., Middleton, C.C., 1979. Organ weights and organ:body weight ratios of the African white-tailed rat (Mystromys albacaudatus). Lab. Anim. Sci. 29, 44–47.

Becker, S.V., Schmidt, D.A., Middleton, C.C., 1979. Selected biological values of the African white-tailed sand rat (Mystromys albacaudatus). Lab. Anim. Sci. 29, 479–481.

Belosevic, M., Faubert, G.M., MacLean, J.D., Law, C., Croll, N.A., 1983. Giardia lamblia infections in Mongolian gerbils: an animal model. J. Infect. Dis. 147, 222–226.

Bem, R.A., Domachowske, J.B., Rosenberg, H.F., 2011. Animal models of human respiratory syncytial virus disease. Am. J. Physiol. Lung Cell Mol. Physiol. 301, L148–L156.

Benitz, K.F., Kramer Jr., A.W., 1965. Spontaneous tumors in the Mongolian gerbil. Lab. Anim. Care 15, 281–294.

Bennett, M., Crouch, A.J., Begon, M., Duffy, B., Feore, S., Gaskell, R.M., et al., 1997. Cowpox in British voles and mice. J. Comp. Pathol. 116, 35–44.

Beregi, A., Felkai, F., Seregi, J., Sarosi, L., 1994. Medullary fixation of a tibial fracture in a three-month-old degu (Octogon degus). Vet. Rec. 134, 652–653.

Berger, P.J., Negus, N.C., Rowsemitt, C.N., 1987. Effect of 6-methoxy-benzoxazolinone on sex ratio and breeding performance in Microtus montanus. Biol. Reprod. 36, 255–260.

Bergeron, J.M., Jodoin, L., Drapeau, G., 1986. A comparison of blood plasma parameters in wild and laboratory meadow voles (Microtus pennsylvanicus). Lab. Anim. Sci. 36, 698–700.

Bergin, I.L., Taylor, N.S., Nambiar, P.R., Fox, J.G., 2005. Eradication of enteric helicobacters in Mongolian gerbils is complicated by the occurrence of Clostridium difficile enterotoxemia. Comp. Med. 55, 265–268.

Bertorelli, R., Adami, M., Ongini, E., 1995. The Mongolian gerbil in experimental epilepsy. Ital. J. Neurol. Sci. 16, 101–106.

Beucher, F., Charreire, J., 1983. Lymphoid cells from the rodent Praomys (Mastomys) natalensis express antigenic determinants present on mouse and rat lymphocytes. Immunol. Lett. 7, 99–106.

Bianco, A.E., Mustafa, M.B., Ham, P.J., 1989. Fate of developing larvae of Onchocerca lienalis and O. volvulus in micropore chambers implanted into laboratory hosts. J. Helminthol. 63, 218–226.

Biardi, J.E., Ho, C.Y., Marcinczyk, J., Nambiar, K.P., 2011. Isolation and identification of a snake venom metalloproteinase inhibitor from California ground squirrel (Spermophilus beecheyi) blood sera. Toxicon 58, 486–493.

Billings, A.N., Rollin, P.E., Milazzo, M.L., Molina, C.P., Eyzaguirre, E.J., Livingstone, W., et al., 2010. Pathology of Black Creek Canal virus infection in juvenile hispid cotton rats (Sigmodon hispidus). Vector Borne Zoonotic Dis. 10, 621–628.

Bingel, S.A., 1995. Pathologic findings in an aging Mongolian gerbil (Meriones unguiculatus) colony. Lab. Anim. Sci. 45, 597–600.

Birney, E.C., Twomey, S.L., 1970. Effects of sodium chloride on water consumption, weight, and survival in the woodrats, Neotoma micropus and Neotoma floridana. J. Mammal. 51, 372–375.

Bischoff, J.R., Kirn, D.H., Williams, A., Heise, C., Horn, S., Muna, M., et al., 1996. An adenovirus mutant that replicates selectively in p53-deficient human tumor cells. Science 274, 373–376.

Blanco, J.C., Pletneva, L., Boukhvalova, M., Richardson, J.Y., Harris, K.A., Prince, G.A., 2004. The cotton rat: an underutilized animal model for human infectious diseases can now be exploited using specific reagents to cytokines, chemokines, and interferons. J. Interferon Cytokine Res. 24, 21–28.

Blanco, J.C., Pletneva, L.M., Wan, H., Araya, Y., Angel, M., Oue, R.O., et al., 2013. Receptor characterization and susceptibility of cotton rats to avian and 2009 pandemic influenza virus strains. J. Virol. 87, 2036–2045.

Boggs, J.F., McMurry, S.T., Leslie Jr., D.M., Engle, D.M., Lochmiller, R.L., 1991. Influence of habitat modification on the community of gastrointestinal helminths of cotton rats. J. Wildl. Dis. 27, 584–593.

Bongardt, H., Richens, V.B., Howard, W.E., 1968. Serum protein patterns in pocket gophers. J. Mammal. 49, 544–547.

Boone, A., Kraft, J.P., Stapp, P., 2009. Scavenging by mammalian carnivores on prairie dog colonies: implications for the spread of plague. Vector Borne Zoonotic Dis. 9, 185–190.

Botvinkin, A.D., Nikiforova, T.A., Sidorov, G.N., 1985. Experimental rabies in hibernator rodents. Acta Virol. 29, 44–50.

Boukhvalova, M.S., Blanco, J.C., 2013. The cotton rat sigmodon hispidus model of respiratory syncytial virus infection. Curr. Top. Microbiol. Immunol. 372, 347–358.

Boy, S.C., Steenkamp, G., 2006. Odontoma-like tumours of squirrel elodont incisors – elodontomas. J. Comp. Pathol. 135, 56–61.

Bozinovic, F., Novoa, F.F., Sabat, P., 1997. Feeding and digesting fiber and tannins by an herbivorous rodent, Octodon degus (Rodentia:Caviomorpha). Comp. Biochem. Physiol. A Physiol. 118, 625–630.

Brand, L.R., Ryckman, R.E., 1968. Laboratory life histories of Peromyscus eremicus and Peromyscus interparietalis. J. Mammal. 49, 495–501.

Brandt, J.F., 1855. Beiträge zur nähern Kenntniss der säugethiere Russland's, De l'Imprimerie de l'Académie impériale des sciences, St.-Pétersbourg.

Brant, S.V., Gardner, S.L., 2000. Phylogeny of species of the genus Litomosoides (Nematatoda: Onchocercidae): evidence of rampant host switching. J. Parasitol. 86, 545–554.

Bresnahan, J.F., Smith, G.D., Lentsch, R.H., Barnes, W.G., Wagner, J.E., 1983. Nasal dermatitis in the Mongolian gerbil. Lab. Anim. Sci. 33, 258–263.

Brett, R.A., 1986. The ecology and behaviour of the naked mole-rat (Heterocephalus glaber Ruppell): (Rodentia:Bathyergidae). PhD Thesis, University of London.

Bronson, F.H., Heideman, P.D., 1992. Lack of reproductive photoresponsiveness and correlative failure to respond to melatonin in a tropical rodent, the cane mouse. Biol. Reprod. 46, 246–250.

Broughton II, G., 1992. Hematologic and blood chemistry data for the prairie dog (Cynomys ludovicianus). Comp. Biochem. Physiol. Comp. Physiol. 101, 807–812.

Buckmaster, P.S., Jongen-Relo, A.L., Davari, S.B., Wong, E.H., 2000. Testing the disinhibition hypothesis of epileptogenesis in vivo and during spontaneous seizures. J. Neurosci. 20, 6232–6240.

Budd, R.L., Gonzales, G.J., Fresquez, P.R., Lopez, E.A., 2004. The uptake and distribution of buried radionuclides by pocket gophers (Thomomys bottae). J. Environ. Sci. Health A Tox. Hazard. Subst. Environ. Eng. 39, 611–625.

Buffenstein, R., 2005. The naked mole-rat: a new long-living model for human aging research. J. Gerontol. A Biol. Sci. Med. Sci. 60, 1369–1377.

Buffenstein, R., 2008. Negligible senescence in the longest living rodent, the naked mole-rat: insights from a successfully aging species. J. Comp. Physiol. B 178, 439–445.

Bulliot, C., Mentre, V., 2013. Original rhinostomy technique for the treatment of pseudo-odontoma in a prairie dog (Cynomys ludovicianus). J. Exotic. Pet. Med. 22, 76–81.

Burger, J., Gochfeld, M., 1992. Survival and reproduction in Peromyscus leucopus in the laboratory: viable model for aging studies. Growth Dev. Aging 56, 17–22.

Burgess, E.C., Amundson, T.E., Davis, J.P., Kaslow, R.A., Edelman, R., 1986. Experimental inoculation of Peromyscus spp. with Borrelia burgdorferi: evidence of contact transmission. Am. J. Trop. Med. Hyg. 35, 355–359.

Burkot, T.R., Clover, J.R., Happ, C.M., DeBess, E., Maupin, G.O., 1999. Isolation of Borrelia burgdorferi from Neotoma fuscipes, Peromyscus maniculatus, Peromyscus boylii, and Ixodes pacificus in Oregon. Am. J. Trop. Med. Hyg. 60, 453–457.

Butterworth, B.B., 1961. The breeding of Dipodomys deserti in the laboratory. J. Mammal. 42, 413–414.

Byrd, R.G., Cone, L.A., Commess, B.C., Williams-Herman, D., Rowland, J.M., Lee, B., et al., 2000. Fatal illnesses associated with a New World arenavirus - California, 1999–2000. MMWR Morb. Mortal. Wkly. Rep. 49, 709–711.

Cadillac, J.M., Rush, H.G., Sigler, R.E., 2003. Polycystic and chronic kidney disease in a young degu (Octodon degus). Contemp. Top. Lab. Anim. Sci. 42, 43–45.

Cameron, G.N., Eshelman, B.D., 1996. Growth and reproduction of hispid cotton rats (Sigmodon hispidus) in response to naturally occurring levels of dietary protein. J. Mammal. 77, 220–231.

Cameron, G.N., Rainey, D.G., 1972. Habitat utilization by Neotoma lepida in the Mohave desert. J. Mammal. 53, 251–266.

Cameron, G.N., Spencer, S.R., 1981. Sigmodon hispidus. Mamm. Species 158, 1.

Campbell, G.A., Kosanke, S.D., Toth, D.M., White, G.L., 1981. Disseminated staphylococcal infection in a colony of captive ground squirrels (Citellus lateralis). J. Wildl. Dis. 17, 177–181.

Campbell, G.D., Barker, I.K., Johnson, R.P., Shewen, P.E., McEwen, S.A., Surgeoner, G.A., 1994. Response of the meadow vole (Microtus pennsylvanicus) to experimental inoculation with Borrelia burgdorferi. J. Wildl. Dis. 30, 408–416.

Cantrell, C., Padovan, D., 1987. Haematology of Mystromys albicaudatus. Lab. Anim. 21, 326–329.

Carleton, M.D., 1984. Introduction to rodents. In: Anderson, S., Jones, J.K. (Eds.), Orders and Families of Recent Mammals of the World John Wiley & Sons, Inc, New York, pp. 255–265.

Carleton, M.D., Musser, G.G., 2005. Order Rodentia. In: Wilson, D.E., Reeder, D.M. (Eds.), Mammal Species of the World: A Taxonomic and Geographic Reference Johns Hopkins University Press, Baltimore, MD, pp. 745–752.

Carroll, D.S., Olson, V.A., Smith, S.K., Braden, Z.H., Patel, N., Abel, J., et al., 2013. Orthopoxvirus variola infection of Cynomys ludovicianus (North American black tailed prairie dog). Virology 443, 358–362.

Castro, A., Chinchilla, M., Guerrero, O.M., Gonzalez, R., 1998. Eimeria species (Eucoccidida: Eimeriidae) found in the cotton rat Sigmodon hispidus in Costa Rica. Rev. Biol. Trop. 46, 339–340.

Cavanagh, R.D., Lambin, X., Ergon, T., Bennett, M., Graham, I.M., van Soolingen, D., et al., 2004. Disease dynamics in cyclic populations of field voles (Microtus agrestis): cowpox virus and vole tuberculosis (Mycobacterium microti). Proc. Biol. Sci. 271, 859–867.

Chambers, R.R., Sudman, P.D., Bradley, R.D., 2009. A phylogenetic assessment of pocket gophers (Geomys): evidence from nuclear and mitochondrial genes. J. Mammal. 90, 537–547.

Chandra, A.M., Paranjpe, M.G., Qualls Jr., C.W., Lochmiller, R.L., 1993. Calcification of the urinary bladder in the wild cotton rat (Sigmodon hispidus). J. Comp. Pathol. 109, 197–201.

Chantrey, J.C., Borman, A.M., Johnson, E.M., Kipar, A., 2006. Emmonsia crescens infection in a British water vole (Arvicola terrestris). Med. Mycol. 44, 375–378.

Charles, R.A., Ellis, A.E., Dubey, J.P., Barnes, J.C., Yabsley, M.J., 2011. Besnoitiosis in a southern plains woodrat (Neotoma micropus) from Uvalde, Texas. J. Parasitol. 97, 838–841.

Charles, R.A., Kjos, S., Ellis, A.E., Dubey, J.P., Shock, B.C., Yabsley, M.J., 2012. Parasites and vector-borne pathogens of southern plains woodrats (Neotoma micropus) from southern Texas. Parasitol. Res. 110, 1855–1862.

Charles, R.A., Kjos, S., Ellis, A.E., Barnes, J.C., Yabsley, M.J., 2013. Southern plains woodrats (Neotoma micropus) from southern Texas are important reservoirs of two genotypes of Trypanosoma cruzi and host of a putative novel Trypanosoma species. Vector Borne Zoonotic Dis. 13, 22–30.

Chatterjee, R.K., Singh, D.P., Misra, S., 1988. Dipetalonema viteae in Mastomys natalensis: effect of pregnancy and lactation on establishment and course of infection. Trop. Med. Parasitol. 39, 29–30.

Chatterjee, R.K., Fatma, N., Agarwal, V.K., Sharma, S., Anand, N., 1989. Comparative antifilarial efficacy of the N-oxides of diethylcarbamazine and two of its analogues. Trop. Med. Parasitol. 40, 474–475.

Chen, H.C., Slone Jr., T.W., Frith, C.H., 1992. Histiocytic sarcoma in an aging gerbil. Toxicol. Pathol. 20, 260–263.

Chen, Q., De Petris, G., Yu, P., Amaral, J., Biancani, P., Behar, J., 1997. Different pathways mediate cholecystokinin actions in cholelithiasis. Am. J. Physiol. 272, G838–G844.

Chew, R.M., 1958. Reproduction by Dipodomys merriami in captivity. J. Mammal. 39, 597–598.

Childs, J.E., Colby, L., Krebs, J.W., Strine, T., Feller, M., Noah, D., et al., 1997. Surveillance and spatiotemporal associations of rabies in rodents and lagomorphs in the United States, 1985–1994. J. Wildl. Dis. 33, 20–27.

Chosewood, L.C., Wilson, D.E., 2009. Biosafety in Microbiological and Biomedical Laboratories. Centers for Disease Control and Prevention, Washington, DC.

Clark, G.R., 1978. Hydrovarium in a Mongolian gerbil (Meriones unguiculatus). Vet. Med. Small Anim. Clin. 73, 792–793.

Clark, J.D., 1984. Biology and diseases of other rodents. In: Fox, J.G., Cohen, B.J., Loew, F.M. (Eds.), Laboratory Animal Medicine Academic Press, San Diego, CA, pp. 186–206.

Clark, M.M., Spencer, C.A., Galef Jr., B.G., 1986. Improving the productivity of breeding colonies of Mongolian gerbils (Meriones unguiculatus). Lab. Anim. 20, 313–315.

Clarke, J.W., 1975. Androgen control of the ventral scent gland in Neotoma floridana. J. Endocrinol. 64, 393–394.

Coelho, P.M., Gazzinelli, G., Pellegrino, J., 1980. Schistosoma mansoni: host antigen occurrence on worms recovered from laboratory vertebrate animals. Parasitology 81, 349–354.

Cohen, B.I., Mosbach, E.H., 1993. Cholesterol cholelithiasis. Adv. Vet. Sci. Comp. Med. 37, 289–312.

Cohen, M.E., Meyer, D.M., 1993. Effect of dietary vitamin E supplementation and rotational stress on alveolar bone loss in rice rats. Arch. Oral. Biol. 38, 601–606.

Colby, L.A., Rush, H.G., Mahoney, M.M., Lee, T.M., 2012. The degu. In: Suckow, M.A., Stevens, K.A., Wilson, R.P. (Eds.), The Laboratory Rabbit, Guinea Pig, Hamster, and Other Rodents Academic Press, New York, pp. 1032–1054.

Cole, H.F., Wolf, H.H., 1970. Laboratory evaluation of aggressive behavior of the grasshopper mouse (Onychomys). J. Pharm. Sci. 59, 969–971.

Colonnello, V., Iacobucci, P., Fuchs, T., Newberry, R.C., Panksepp, J., 2011. Octodon degus. A useful animal model for social-affective neuroscience research: basic description of separation distress, social attachments and play. Neurosci. Biobehav. Rev. 35, 1854–1863.

Conder, G.A., Johnson, S.S., Guimond, P.M., Geary, T.G., Lee, B.L., Winterrowd, C.A., et al., 1991. Utility of a Haemonchus contortus/jird (Meriones unguiculatus) model for studying resistance to levamisole. J. Parasitol. 77, 83–86.

Constant, M.A., Phillips, P.H., 1952. The occurrence of a calcinosis syndrome in the cotton rat. I. The effect of diet on the ash content of the heart. J. Nutr. 47, 317–326.

Contreras, L., Bustos-Obregon, E., 1980. Anatomy of reproductive tract in Octodon degus Molina: a nonscrotal rodent. Arch. Androl. 4, 115–124.

Cook-Babcook, M.A., 1996. Enrichment activities for thirteen-lined ground squirrels (Spermophilus tridecemlineatus). Wildl. Rehabil. 14, 143–154.

Cooper, J.J., 2010. Voles. In: Hubrecht, R., Kirkwood, J.K. (Eds.), The UFAW Handbook on the Care and Management of Laboratory and other Research Animals Wiley-Blackwell, Oxford, pp. 370–379.

Court, J.P., Lees, G.M., Coop, R.L., Angus, K.W., Beesley, J.E., 1988. An attempt to produce Ostertagia circumcincta infections in Mongolian gerbils. Vet. Parasitol. 28, 79–91.

Cox, F.E.G., 1979. Ecological importance of small mammals as reservoirs of disease. In: Stoddart, D.M. (Ed.), Ecology of Small Mammals Springer, Netherlands, pp. 213–238.

Cramlet, S.H., Toft II, J.D., Olsen, N.W., 1974. Malignant melanoma in a black gerbil (Meriones unguiculatus). Lab. Anim. Sci. 24, 545–547.

Croft, D.R., Sotir, M.J., Williams, C.J., Kazmierczak, J.J., Wegner, M.V., Rausch, D., et al., 2007. Occupational risks during a monkeypox outbreak, Wisconsin, 2003. Emerg. Infect. Dis. 13, 1150–1157.

Cross, J.H., Banzon, T., Singson, C., 1978. Further studies on Capillaria philippinensis: development of the parasite in the Mongolian gerbil. J. Parasitol. 64, 208–213.

Cross, J.H., Partono, F., Hsu, M.Y., Ash, L.R., Oemijati, S., 1981. Further studies on the development of Wuchereria bancrofti in laboratory animals. Southeast Asian J. Trop. Med. Public Health 12, 114–122.

Cullen, J.M., Marion, P.L., 1996. Non-neoplastic liver disease associated with chronic ground squirrel hepatitis virus infection. Hepatology 23, 1324–1329.

Cullen, J.W., Pare, W.P., Mooney, A.L., 1971. Adrenal weight to body weight ratios in the Mongolian gerbil (Meriones unguiculatus). Growth 35, 169–176.

Curtis, J.T., Liu, Y., Wang, Z., 2001. Lesions of the vomeronasal organ disrupt mating-induced pair bonding in female prairie voles (Microtus ochrogaster). Brain Res. 901, 167–174.

Cutler, R.G., 1985. Peroxide-producing potential of tissues: inverse correlation with longevity of mammalian species. Proc. Natl. Acad. Sci. USA 82, 4798–4802.

Czub, S., Duray, P.H., Thomas, R.E., Schwan, T.G., 1992. Cystitis induced by infection with the Lyme disease spirochete, Borrelia burgdorferi, in mice. Am. J. Pathol. 141, 1173–1179.

Daly, M.M., Wilson, I., Behrends, P., 1984. Breeding of captive kangaroo rats, Dipodomys merriami and D. microps. J. Mammal. 65, 338–341.

Datiles III, M.B., Fukui, H., 1989. Cataract prevention in diabetic Octodon degus with Pfizer's sorbinil. Curr. Eye Res. 8, 233–237.

Davis, D.E., 1984. Pitfalls in the use of ground squirrels for research on hibernation. Can. J. Zool. 62, 1656–1658.

Davis, J.W., Karstad, L.H., Trainer, D.O., 1981. Infectious Diseases of Wild Mammals. Iowa State University Press, Ames, IA.

Davis, R.M., 1999. Use of orally administered chitin inhibitor (lufenuron) to control flea vectors of plague on ground squirrels in California. J. Med. Entomol. 36, 562–567.

Davis, R.M., Cleugh, E., Smith, R.T., Fritz, C.L., 2008. Use of a chitin synthesis inhibitor to control fleas on wild rodents important in the maintenance of plague, Yersinia pestis, in California. J. Vector Ecol. 33, 278–284.

Davis, T.M., 1975. Effects of familiarity on agonistic encounter behavior in male degus (Octodon degus). Behav. Biol. 14, 511–517.

Day, B.N., Egoscue, H.J., Woodbury, A.M., 1956. Ord kangaroo rat in captivity. Science 124, 485–486.

Dean, W.R.J., 1978. Conservation of the white-tailed rat in South Africa. Biol. Conservat. 13, 133–140.

Dearing, M.D., Mangione, A.M., Karasov, W.H., Morzunov, S., Otteson, E., St Jeor, S., 1998. Prevalence of hantavirus in four species of Neotoma from Arizona and Utah. J. Mammal. 79, 1254–1259.

Delaney, M.A., Nagy, L., Kinsel, M.J., Treuting, P.M., 2013. Spontaneous histologic lesions of the adult naked mole rat (Heterocephalus glaber): a retrospective survey of lesions in a zoo population. Vet. Pathol. 50, 607–621.

de la Puente-Redondo, V.A., Gutierrez-Martin, C.B., Perez-Martinez, C., del Blanco, N.G., Garcia-Iglesias, M.J., Perez-Garcia, C.C., et al., 1999. Epidemic infection caused by Citrobacter rodentium in a gerbil colony. Vet. Rec. 145, 400–403.

Dengler-Crish, C.M., Catania, K.C., 2007. Phenotypic plasticity in female naked mole-rats after removal from reproductive suppression. J. Exp. Biol. 210, 4351–4358.

Desbois, A.P., Sattar, A., Graham, S., Warn, P.A., Coote, P.J., 2013. MRSA decolonization of cotton rat nares by a combination treatment comprising lysostaphin and the antimicrobial peptide ranalexin. J. Antimicrob. Chemother. 68, 2569–2575.

Deutschland, M., Denk, D., Skerritt, G., Hetzel, U., 2011. Surgical excision and morphological evaluation of altered abdominal scent glands in Mongolian gerbils (Meriones unguiculatus). Vet. Rec. 169, 636.

DeVries, M.S., Sikes, R.S., 2009. Husbandry methods for pocket gophers. Southwest Nat. 54, 363–366.

Dewey, M.J., Dawson, W.D., 2001. Deer mice: the drosophila of North American mammalogy. Genesis 29, 105–109.

Dewsbury, D.A., 1975. Copulatory behavior of white-footed mice (Peromyscus leucopus). J. Mammal. 56, 420–428.

Dewsbury, D.A., 1984. Muroid rodents as research animals. ILAR News 28, 8–15.

Dewsbury, D.A., Jansen, P.E., 1972. Copulatory behavior of southern grasshopper mice (Onychomys torridus). J. Mammal. 53, 267–278.

Dewsbury, D.D., 1974. Copulatory behavior of Neotoma floridana. J. Mammal. 55, 864–866.

Dieterich, R.A., Preston, D.J., 1977a. The meadow vole (Microtus pennsylv anicus) as a laboratory animal. Lab. Anim. Sci. 27, 494–499.

Dieterich, R.A., Preston, D.J., 1977b. The tundra vole (Microtus oeconomus) as a laboratory animal. Lab. Anim. Sci. 27, 500–506.

Dieterich, R.A., Preston, D.J., 1979. Atherosclerosis in lemmings and voles fed a high fat, high cholesterol diet. Atherosclerosis 33, 181–189.

Di Giulio, D.B., Eckburg, P.B., 2004. Human monkeypox: an emerging zoonosis. Lancet Infect. Dis. 4, 15–25.

Ditrich, O., Otcenasek, M., 1982. Microsporum vanbreuseghemii and Trichophyton simii in Czechoslovakia. Czech Mycol. 36, 236–242.

Dixon, D., Reinhard, G.R., Kazacos, K.R., Arriaga, C., 1988. Cerebrospinal nematodiasis in prairie dogs from a research facility. J. Am. Vet. Med. Assoc. 193, 251–253.

Dkhil, M.A., Abdel-Baki, A.S., Al-Quraishy, S., Abdel-Moneim, A.E., 2013. Hepatic oxidative stress in Mongolian gerbils experimentally infected with Babesia divergens. Ticks Tick Borne Dis. 4, 346–351.

Dobrowolska, A., 1982a. Serum γ-globulin concentration in different stages of sexual activity in females of common vole, Microtus arvalis, pall. Comp. Biochem. Physiol. A Comp. Physiol. 71, 465–467.

Dobrowolska, A., 1982b. Variability of hematocrit value, blood serum beta- and gamma-globulin level and body weight in different transferrin genotypes of common vole (Microtus arvalis, Pallas 1779) from natural population. Comp. Biochem. Physiol. A Comp. Physiol. 73, 105–110.

Dobrowolska, A., Gromadzka, J., 1978. Relationship between haematological parameters and progesterone blood concentration in different stages of estrous cycle in common vole, Microtus arvalis. Comp. Biochem. Physiol. Part A Physiol. 61, 483–485.

Dobrowolska, A., Gromadzka-Ostrowska, J., 1983. Influence of photoperiod on morphological parameters, androgen concentration, haematological indices and serum protein fractions in common vole (Microtus arvalis, Pall.). Comp. Biochem. Physiol. A Comp. Physiol. 74, 427–433.

Dobrowolska, A., Gromadzka-Ostrowska, J., 1984. Age and androgen-related changes in morphological parameters, haematological indices and serum protein fraction in common vole (Microtus arvalis Pall.) growing in different photoperiods. Comp. Biochem. Physiol. A Comp. Physiol. 79, 241–249.

Dobrowolska, A., Rewkiewicz-Dziarska, A., Szarska, I., 1976. The effect of exogenic thyroxine on activity of the thyroid gland, blood serum proteins and leukocytes in the common vole Microtus arvalis, Pallas. Comp. Biochem. Physiol. A Comp. Physiol. 53, 323–326.

Donnelly, T.M., 1997. Tail-slip in gerbils – Improper handling. Lab. Anim. (NY) 26, 15–16.

Donnelly, T.M., Rush, E.M., Lackner, P.A., 2000. Ringworm in small exotic pets. Sem. Avian Exotic Pet Med. 9, 82–93.

Dotson, R.L., Leveson, J.E., Marengo-Rowe, A.J., Ubelaker, J.E., 1987. Hematologic and coagulation studies on cotton rats, Sigmodon hispidus. Comp. Biochem. Physiol. A Comp. Physiol. 88, 553–556.

Dotson, R.L., Leveson, J.E., Marengo-Rowe, A.J., Ubelaker, J.E., 1990. Hemostatic parameters of the blood of cotton rats, Sigmodon hispidus, infected with Parastrongylus costaricensis (Metastrongyloidea: Angiostrongylidae). Trans. Am. Microsc. Soc. 109, 399–406.

Dowda, H., DiSalvo, A.F., Redden, S., 1981. Naturally acquired rabies in an eastern wood rat (Neotoma floridana). J. Clin. Microbiol. 13, 238–239.

Downs, C.T., Perrin, M.R., 1995. The thermal biology of the white-tailed rat Mystromys albicaudatus, a cricetine relic in southern temperate African grassland. Comp. Biochem. Physiol. A Physiol. 110, 65–69.

Downs, W.G., Spence, L., Aitken, T.H., 1962. Studies on the virus of Venezuelan equine encephalomyelitis in Trindidad, W. I. III. Reisolation of virus. Am. J. Trop. Med. Hyg. 11, 841–843.

Drickamer, L.C., Vestal, B.M., 1973. Patterns of reproduction in a laboratory colony of Peromyscus. J. Mammal. 54, 523–528.

Drummond, T.D., Mason, J.I., McCarthy, J.L., 1988. Gerbil adrenal 11 beta- and 19-hydroxylating activities respond similarly to inhibitory or stimulatory agents: two activities of a single enzyme. J. Steroid Biochem. 29, 641–648.

Dubey, J.P., Sheffield, H.G., 1988. Sarcocystis sigmodontis n. sp. from the cotton rat (Sigmodon hispidus). J. Parasitol. 74, 889–891.

Duplantier, J.M., Britton-Davidian, J., Granjon, L., 1990. Chromosomal characterization of three species of the genus Mastomys in Senegal. Z Zool. Syst. Evol. Forsch 28, 289–298.

Durden, L.A., 1988. The spiny rat louse, Polyplax spinulosa, as a parasite of the rice rat, Oryzomys palustris, in North America. J. Parasitol. 74, 900–901.

Durden, L.A., Banks, C.W., Clark, K.L., Belbey, B.V., Oliver Jr., J.H., 1997. Ectoparasite fauna of the eastern woodrat, Neotoma floridana: composition, origin, and comparison with ectoparasite faunas of western woodrat species. J. Parasitol. 83, 374–381.

Durden, L.A., Klompen, J.S., Keirans, J.E., 1993. Parasitic arthropods of sympatric opossums, cotton rats, and cotton mice from Merritt Island, Florida. J. Parasitol. 79, 283–286.

Durnez, L., Eddyani, M., Mgode, G.F., Katakweba, A., Katholi, C.R., Machang'u, R.R., et al., 2008. First detection of mycobacteria in African rodents and insectivores, using stratified pool screening. Appl. Environ. Microbiol. 74, 768–773.

Dyson, M.C., Eaton, K.A., Chang, C., 2009. Helicobacter spp. in wild mice (Peromyscus leucopus) found in laboratory animal facilities. J. Am. Assoc. Lab. Anim. Sci. 48, 754–756.

Eaton, K.A., Opp, J.S., Gray, B.M., Bergin, I.L., Young, V.B., 2011. Ulcerative typhlocolitis associated with Helicobacter mastomyrinus in telomerase-deficient mice. Vet. Pathol. 48, 713–725.

Ebensperger, L.A., Hurtado, M.J., Leon, C., 2007. An experimental examination of the consequences of communal versus solitary breeding on maternal condition and the early postnatal growth and survival of degu, Octodon degus, pups. Anim. Behav. 73, 185–194.

Ebensperger, L.A., Hurtado, M.J., Valdivia, I., 2006. Lactating females do not discriminate between their own young and unrelated pups in the communally breeding rodent, Octodon degus. Ethology 112, 921–929.

Eckert, J., Thompson, R.C., Mehlhorn, H., 1983. Proliferation and metastases formation of larval Echinococcus multilocularis. I. Animal model, macroscopical and histological findings. Z Parasitenkd 69, 737–748.

Edmonds, K.E., Rollag, M.D., Stetson, M.H., 1995. Effects of photoperiod on pineal melatonin in the marsh rice rat (Oryzomys palustris). J. Pineal. Res. 18, 148–153.

Edmonds, K.E., Stetson, M.H., 1993. Effect of photoperiod on gonadal maintenance and development in the marsh rice rat (Oryzomys palustris). Gen. Comp. Endocrinol. 92, 281–291.

Edmonds, K.E., Stetson, M.H., 1994. Photoperiod and melatonin affect testicular growth in the marsh rice rat (Oryzomys palustris). J. Pineal. Res. 17, 86–93.

Edmonds, K.E., Stetson, M.H., 1995. Effects of prenatal and postnatal photoperiods and of the pineal gland on early testicular development in the marsh rice rat (Oryzomys palustris). Biol. Reprod. 52, 989–996.

Edrey, Y.H., Hanes, M., Pinto, M., Mele, J., Buffenstein, R., 2011. Successful aging and sustained good health in the naked mole rat: a long-lived mammalian model for biogerontology and biomedical research. ILAR J. 52, 41–53.

Egoscue, H.J., 1960. Laboratory and field studies of the northern grasshopper mouse. J. Mammal. 44, 61–67.

Eisenberg, J.F., Isaac, D.E., 1963. The reproduction of heteromyid rodents in captivity. J. Mammal. 44, 61–67.

Elangbam, C.S., Qualls Jr., C.W., Lochmiller, R.L., Novak, J., 1989. Development of the cotton rat (Sigmodon hispidus) as a biomonitor of environmental contamination with emphasis on hepatic cytochrome P-450 induction and population characteristics. Bull. Environ. Contam. Toxicol. 42, 482–488.

Elangbam, C.S., Qualls Jr., C.W., Lochmiller, R.L., Boggs, J.F., 1990. Strongyloidiasis in cotton rats (Sigmodon hispidus) from central Oklahoma. J. Wildl. Dis. 26, 398–402.

Elangbam, C.S., Qualls Jr., C.W., Ewing, S.A., Lochmiller, R.L., 1993. Cryptosporidiosis in a cotton rat (Sigmodon hispidus). J. Wildl. Dis. 29, 161–164.

English, M.P., Southern, H.N., 1967. Trichophyton persicolor infection in a population of small wild mammals. Sabouraudia 5, 302–309.

Ernst, J.V., Chobotar, B., 1978. The endogenous stages of Eimeria utahensis (Protozoa: Eimeriidae) in the kangaroo rat, Dipodomys ordii. J. Parasitol. 64, 27–34.

Escherich, P.C., 1981. Social Biology of the Bushy-Tailed Woodrat, Neotoma Cinerea. University of California Press, Berkeley, CA.

Espinosa-Reyes, G., Torres-Dosal, A., Ilizaliturri, C., Gonzalez-Mille, D., Diaz-Barriga, F., Mejia-Saavedra, J., 2010. Wild rodents (Dipodomys merriami) used as biomonitors in contaminated mining sites. J. Environ. Sci. Health A Tox. Hazard. Subst. Environ. Eng. 45, 82–89.

Evans-Davis, K.D., Dillehay, D.L., Wargo, D.N., Webb, S.K., Talkington, D.F., Thacker, W.L., et al., 1998. Pathogenicity of Mycoplasma volis in mice and rats. Lab. Anim. Sci. 48, 38–44.

Fabian, A., Halasz, N., Gal, J., 2012. Multiple metastatic melanoma malignum in Mongolian gerbil (Meriones unguiculatus) skin. Case report. [Hungarian] Tobbszoros attetet kepezo melanoma malignum Mongol futoeger (Meriones unguiculatus) boreben. Esetismertetes. Magy Allatorvosok Lapja 134, 126–128.

Fain, A., Lukoschus, F.S., 1978. Dipodomydectes americanus gen. et sp. n. (Acari: Hypoderidae) from the kangaroo rat. J. Parasitol. 64, 137–138.

Faith, R.E., Montgomery, C.A., Durfee, W.J., Aguilar-Cordova, E., Wyde, P.R., 1997. The cotton rat in biomedical research. Lab. Anim. Sci. 47, 337–345.

Farrar, P.L., Opsomer, M.J., Kocen, J.A., Wagner, J.E., 1988. Experimental nasal dermatitis in the Mongolian gerbil: effect of bilateral harderian gland adenectomy on development of facial lesions. Lab. Anim. Sci. 38, 72–76.

Faubert, G.M., Belosevic, M., Walker, T.S., MacLean, J.D., Meerovitch, E., 1983. Comparative studies on the pattern of infection with Giardia spp. in mongolian gerbils. J. Parasitol. 69, 802–805.

Faulkes, C.G., Bennett, N.C., 2013. Plasticity and constraints on social evolution in African mole-rats: ultimate and proximate factors. Philos. Trans. R. Soc. Lond. B Biol. Sci. 368, 20120347.

Felder, M.R., 2014. University of South Carolina, Columbia, SC. Peromyscus Genetic Stock Center, at <http://stkctr.biol.sc.edu/index.html> , (accessed January 2014.).

Felder, M.R., Vrana, P.B., Szalai, G., Shorter, K., Lewandowski, A., 2012. Development of resources for Peromyscus laboratory research. Integr. Comp. Biol. 52, E242.

Fichet-Calvet, E., Rogers, D.J., 2009. Risk maps of Lassa fever in West Africa. PLoS Negl. Trop. Dis. 3, e388.

Fine, J., Quimby, F.W., Greenhouse, D.D., 1986. Annotated bibliography on uncommonly used laboratory animals: mammals. ILAR News 24, 3–38.

Fossmark, R., Qvigstad, G., Martinsen, T.C., Hauso, O., Waldum, H.L., 2011. Animal models to study the role of long-term hypergastrinemia in gastric carcinogenesis. J. Biomed. Biotechnol. 2011, 975479.

Fox, J.G., Murphy, J.C., 1979. Cytomegalic virus-associated insulitis in diabetic Octodon degus. Vet. Pathol. 16, 625–628.

Franke, E.D., McGreevy, P.B., Katz, S.P., Sacks, D.L., 1985. Growth cycle-dependent generation of complement-resistant Leishmania promastigotes. J. Immunol. 134, 2713–2718.

Franklin, H.A., Stapp, P., Cohen, A., 2010. Polymerase chain reaction (PCR) identification of rodent blood meals confirms host sharing by flea vectors of plague. J. Vector Ecol. 35, 363–371.

Frase, B.A., Van Vuren, D., 1989. Techniques for immobilizing and bleeding marmots and woodrats. J. Wildl. Dis. 25, 444–445.

Frommel, T.O., Fujikura, Y., Seed, J.R., 1991. Tissue alterations in Microtus montanus chronically infected with Trypanosoma brucei gambiense. J. Parasitol. 77, 164–167.

Frost, D., Zucker, I., 1983. Photoperiod and melatonin influence seasonal gonadal cycles in the grasshopper mouse (Onychomys leucogaster). J. Reprod. Fertil. 69, 237–244.

Fuehrer, H.P., Bloschl, I., Siehs, C., Hassl, A., 2010. Detection of Toxoplasma gondii, Neospora caninum, and Encephalitozoon cuniculi in the brains of common voles (Microtus arvalis) and water voles (Arvicola terrestris) by gene amplification techniques in western Austria (Vorarlberg). Parasitol. Res. 107, 469–473.

Fujita, O., Oku, Y., Okamoto, M., Sato, H., Ooi, H.K., Kamiya, M., et al., 1991. Early development of larval Taenia polyacantha in experimental intermediate hosts. J. Helminthol. Soc. Wash 58, 100–109.

Fulghum, R.S., Chole, R.A., 1985. Bacterial flora in spontaneously occurring aural cholesteatomas in Mongolian gerbils. Infect. Immun. 50, 678–681.

Fulhorst, C.F., Hardy, J.L., Eldridge, B.F., Chiles, R.E., Reeves, W.C., 1996. Ecology of Jamestown Canyon virus (Bunyaviridae: California serogroup) in coastal California. Am. J. Trop. Med. Hyg. 55, 185–189.

Fulhorst, C.F., Bowen, M.D., Salas, R.A., Duno, G., Utrera, A., Ksiazek, T.G., et al., 1999a. Natural rodent host associations of Guanarito and pirital viruses (Family Arenaviridae) in central Venezuela. Am. J. Trop. Med. Hyg. 61, 325–330.

Fulhorst, C.F., Ksiazek, T.G., Peters, C.J., Tesh, R.B., 1999b. Experimental infection of the cane mouse Zygodontomys brevicauda (family Muridae) with guanarito virus (Arenaviridae), the etiologic agent of Venezuelan hemorrhagic fever. J. Infect. Dis. 180, 966–969.

Gage, K.L., Burgdorfer, W., Hopla, C.E., 1990. Hispid cotton rats (Sigmodon hispidus) as a source for infecting immature Dermacentor variabilis (Acari: Ixodidae) with Rickettsia rickettsii. J. Med. Entomol. 27, 615–619.

Galea, L.A., Kavaliers, M., Ossenkopp, K.P., 1996. Sexually dimorphic spatial learning in meadow voles Microtus pennsylvanicus and deer mice Peromyscus maniculatus. J. Exp. Biol. 199, 195–200.

Gallegos, P., Lutz, J., Markwiese, J., Ryti, R., Mirenda, R., 2007. Wildlife ecological screening levels for inhalation of volatile organic chemicals. Environ. Toxicol. Chem. 26, 1299–1303.

Galli, S.M., Marusic, E.T., 1976. Adrenal steroid biosynthesis by two species of South American Rodents: octodon degus and Abrocoma benetti. Gen. Comp. Endocrinol. 28, 10–16.

Garcia, V.E., Perez, J.C., 1984. The purification and characterization of an antihemorrhagic factor in woodrat (Neotoma micropus) serum. Toxicon 22, 129–138.

Garner, M.M., Raymond, J.T., Toshkov, I., Tennant, B.C., 2004. Hepatocellular carcinoma in black-tailed prairie dogs (Cynomys ludovicianus): tumor morphology and immunohistochemistry for hepadnavirus core and surface antigens. Vet. Pathol. 41, 353–361.

Gattermann, R., 1979. Hematologic and clinical chemical normal ranges of the Mongolian gerbil (Meriones unguiculatus). [German] Hamatologische und klinisch-chemische Normalbereiche der Mongolischen Wustenrennmaus (Meriones unguiculatus). Kurze Mitteilung. Z. Versuchstierkd. 21, 273–275.

Gaule, C., Vega, P., Sanchez, E., Del Villar, E., 1990. Drug metabolism in Octodon degus: low inductive effect of phenobarbital. Comp. Biochem. Physiol. C 96, 217–222.

Geller, M.D., Christian, J.J., 1982. Population dynamics adreno cortical function and pathology in Microtus pennsylvanicus. J. Mammal. 63, 85–95.

Gil da Costa, R.M., Rema, A., Payo-Puente, P., Gartner, F., 2007. Immunohistochemical characterization of a sebaceous gland carcinoma in a gerbil (Meriones unguiculatus). J. Comp. Pathol. 137, 130–132.

Goeken, J.A., Packer, J.T., Rose, S.D., Stuhlman, R.A., 1972. Structure of the islets of Langerhans. Pathological studies in normal and diabetic Mystromys albicaudatus. Arch. Pathol. 93, 123–129.

Goetze, J.R., Nelson, A.D., Stasey, C., 2008. Notes on behavior of the Texas kangaroo rat (Dipodomys elator). Tex. J. Sci. 60, 309–316.

Goodwin, H.T., 1998. Supernumerary teeth in Pleistocene, Recent, and hybrid individuals of the Spermophilus richardsonii complex (Sciuridae). J. Mammal. 79, 1161–1169.

Goto, K., Itoh, T., Ebukuro, S., Kagiyama, N., Harasawa, R., 1993. Characterization of mycoplasma strains isolated from house musk shrews (Suncus murinus) and their infectivity in mice and rats. Jikken Dobutsu 42, 363–369.

Goyens, J., Reijniers, J., Borremans, B., Leirs, H., 2013. Density thresholds for Mopeia virus invasion and persistence in its host Mastomys natalensis. J. Theor. Biol. 317, 55–61.

Grace, P.A., McShane, J., Pitt, H.A., 1988. Gross anatomy of the liver, biliary tree, and pancreas in the black-tailed prairie dog (Cynomys ludovicianus). Lab. Anim. 22, 326–329.

Graeff Teixeira, C., Garrido, C.T., Santos, F.T., Aguiar, L.F.S., 1998. The using of hollow bricks as a shelter for adaptation of wild rodents' colonies in captivity. [Portuguese] Tijolos vazados como abrigo para adaptacao de roedores silvestres em cativeiro. Rev. Soc. Bras. Med. Trop. 31, 319–322.

Green, M.G., Huey, D., Niewiesk, S., 2013. The cotton rat (Sigmodon hispidus) as an animal model for respiratory tract infections with human pathogens. Lab. Anim. (NY) 42, 170–176.

Griner, L.A., 1983. Pathology of Zoo Animals: A Review of Necropsies Conducted Over a Fourteen-Year Period at the San Diego Zoo and San Diego Wild Animal Park. Zoological Society of San Diego, San Diego, CA.

Grippo, A.J., Trahanas, D.M., Zimmerman II, R.R., Porges, S.W., Carter, C.S., 2009. Oxytocin protects against negative behavioral and autonomic consequences of long-term social isolation. Psychoneuroendocrinology 34, 1542–1553.

Grippo, A.J., Moffitt, J.A., Sgoifo, A., Jepson, A.J., Bates, S.L., Chandler, D.L., et al., 2012. The integration of depressive behaviors and cardiac dysfunction during an operational measure of depression: investigating the role of negative social experiences in an animal model. Psychosom. Med. 74, 612–619.

Gross, S.A., Didio, L.J., 1987. Comparative morphology of the prostate in adult male and female Praomys (Mastomys) Natalensis studied with electron microscopy. J. Submicrosc. Cytol. 19, 77–84.

Guarner, J., Johnson, B.J., Paddock, C.D., Shieh, W.J., Goldsmith, C.S., Reynolds, M.G., et al., 2004. Monkeypox transmission and pathogenesis in prairie dogs. Emerg. Infect. Dis. 10, 426–431.

Gulati, A., Srimal, R.C., Dhawan, B.N., 1986. Stereotyped behaviour and striatal dopamine receptors in albino rat and the desert rat (Mastomys natalensis): a comparative study. Indian J. Exp. Biol. 24, 248–251.

Gulati, A., Srimal, R.C., Dhawan, B.N., 1988. An analysis of stereotyped behaviour in Mastomys natalensis. Naunyn Schmiedebergs Arch. Pharmacol. 337, 572–575.

Gummer, D.L., Forbes, M.R., Bender, D.J., Barclay, R.M., 1997. Botfly (Diptera:Oestridae) parasitism of Ord's kangaroo rats (Dipodomys ordii) at Suffield National Wildlife Area, Alberta, Canada. J. Parasitol. 83, 601–604.

Gutierrez-Pena, E.J., 1987. Dunnifilaria meningica sp. n. (Filarioidea: Onchocercidae) from the central nervous system of the wood-rat (Neotoma micropus) in Mexico. Trop. Med. Parasitol. 38, 294–298.

Guzman-Silva, M.A., 1997. Systemic mast cell disease in the Mongolian gerbil, Meriones unguiculatus: case report. Lab. Anim. 31, 373–378.

Guzman-Silva, M.A., Costa-Neves, M., 2006. Incipient spontaneous granulosa cell tumour in the gerbil, Meriones unguiculatus. Lab. Anim. 40, 96–101.

Guzman-Silva, M.A., Rossi, M.I., Guimaraes, J.S., 1988. Craniopharyngioma in the Mongolian gerbil (Meriones unguiculatus): a case report. Lab. Anim. 22, 365–368.

Hafner, M.S., 2007. Field research in mammalogy: an enterprise in peril. J. Mammal. 88, 1119–1128.

Hafner, M.S., Page, R.D., 1995. Molecular phylogenies and host–parasite cospeciation: gophers and lice as a model system. Philos. Trans. R. Soc. Lond. B Biol. Sci. 349, 77–83.

Hafner, M.S., Sudman, P.D., Villablanca, F.X., Spradling, T.A., Demastes, J.W., Nadler, S.A., 1994. Disparate rates of molecular evolution in cospeciating hosts and parasites. Science 265, 1087–1090.

Hairston, J.E., Ball, G.F., Nelson, R.J., 2003. Photoperiodic and temporal influences on chemosensory induction of brain fos expression in female prairie voles. J. Neuroendocrinol. 15, 161–172.

Haley, T.J., Lindberg, R.G., Flesher, A.M., Raymond, K., McKibben, W., Hayden, P., 1960. Response of the kangaroo rat (Dipodomys merriami Mearns) to single whole-body X-irradiation. Radiat. Res. 12, 103–111.

Hall III, A., Persing, R.L., White, D.C., Ricketts Jr., R.T., 1967. Mystromys albicaudatus (the African white-tailed rat) as a laboratory species. Lab. Anim. Care 17, 180–188.

Hall, E.R., 1981. The mammals of North America. John Wiley & Sons, New York.

Hallett, A.F., Meester, J., 1971. Early post natal development of the South African hamster Mystromys albicaudatus. Zool. Afr. 6, 221–228.

Hallett, A.F., Politzer, W.M., 1972. Diabetes mellitus in Mystromys albicaudatus. Arch. Pathol. 93, 178.

Hamilton Jr., W.J., 1953. Reproduction and young of the Florida wood rat Neotoma f. floridana (Ord). J. Mammal. 34, 180–189.

Hamilton, W.J., Whitaker, J.O., 1979. Mammals of the Eastern United States. Comstock Publishing Associates, Ithaca, NY.

Harriman, A.E., 1974. Self–selection of diet by Southern Plains wood rats (Neotoma micropus). J. Gen. Psychol. 90, 53–61.

Harriman, A.E., 1976. Preferences by northern grasshopper mice for solutions of sugars, acids, and salts in Richter-type drinking tests. J. Gen. Psychol. 95, 85–92.

Harris, S.E., Munshi-South, J., Obergfell, C., O'Neill, R., 2013. Signatures of rapid evolution in urban and rural transcriptomes of white-footed mice (Peromyscus leucopus) in the New York metropolitan area. PLoS One 8, e74938.

Hartenberger, J.-L., 1985. The order rodentia: major questions on their evolutionary origin, relationships and suprafamilial systematics. In: Luckett, W.P., Hartenberger, J.-L. (Eds.), Evolutionary Relationships Among Rodents Springer, US, pp. 1–33.

Hartenberger, J.-L., 1998. Description de la radiation des Rodentia (Mammalia) du Paléocène supérieur au Miocène; incidences phylogénétiques. C. R. Acad. Sci. IIA 326, 439–444.

Harvey, S.B., Alworth, L.C., Blas-Machado, U., 2009. Molar malocclusions in pine voles (Microtus pinetorum). J. Am. Assoc. Lab. Anim. Sci. 48, 412–415.

Harvey, S.B., Krimer, P.M., Correa, M.T., Hanes, M.A., 2008. Hematology and plasma chemistry reference intervals for mature laboratory pine voles (Microtus pinetorum) as determined by using the non-parametric rank percentile method. J. Am. Assoc. Lab. Anim. Sci. 47, 35–40.

Heffner, H.E., Heffner, R.S., 1985. Hearing in two cricetid rodents: wood rat (Neotoma floridana) and grasshopper mouse (Onychomys leucogaster). J. Comp. Psychol. 99, 275–288.

Heffner, R.S., Heffner, H.E., Contos, C., Kearns, D., 1994. Hearing in prairie dogs: transition between surface and subterranean rodents. Hear. Res. 73, 185–189.

Heideman, P.D., 2004. Top-down approaches to the study of natural variation in complex physiological pathways using the white-footed mouse (Peromyscus leucopus) as a model. ILAR J. 45, 4–13.

Heideman, P.D., Bronson, F.H., 1990. Photoperiod, melatonin secretion, and sexual maturation in a tropical rodent. Biol. Reprod. 43, 745–750.

Heidt, G.A., Conaway, H.H., Frith, C., Farris Jr., H.E., 1984. Spontaneous diabetes mellitus in a captive golden-mantled ground squirrel, Spermophilus lateralis (Say). J. Wildl. Dis. 20, 253–255.

Helgen, K.M., Cole, F.R., Helgen, L.E., Wilson, D.E., 2009. Generic revision in the holarctic ground squirrel genus Spermophilus. J. Mammal. 90, 270–305.

Hellenthal, R.A., Price, R.D., 1994. Two new subgenera of chewing lice (Phthiraptera: Trichodectidae) from pocket gophers (Rodentia: Geomyidae), with a key to all included taxa. J. Med. Entomol. 31, 450–466.

Herwaldt, B.L., 2001. Laboratory-acquired parasitic infections from accidental exposures. Clin. Microbiol. Rev. 14, 659–688. table of contents.

Hessel, H., Ernst, L.S., Walger, M., von Wedel, H., Dybek, A., Schmidt, U., 1997. Meriones unguiculatus (Gerbil) as an animal model for the ontogenetic cochlear implant research. Am. J. Otol. 18, S21.

Hessel, H., Ernst, S., Mickenhagen, A., Dück, M., von Wedel, H., Walger, M., 2000. Einsatz der mongolischen Wüstenrennmaus (Meriones unguiculatus) als Tiermodell in der ontogenetischen Kochleaimplantatforschung. [German] Using the Mongolian gerbil (Meriones unguiculatus) as an animal model in ontogenetic cochlear implant research. HNO 48, 209–214.

Hessel, H., Walger, M., Ernst, S., Foerst, A., von Wedel, H., Klunter, H.D., et al., 1998. A method for the induction of a cochlea-specific auditory deprivation in the gerbil (Meriones unguiculatus). ORL J. Otorhinolaryngol. Relat. Spec. 60, 61–66.

Hill, J.L., 1974. Peromyscus: effect of early pairing on reproduction. Science 186, 1042–1044.

Hill, T.P., Best, T.L., 1985. Coccidia from California kangaroo rats (Dipodomys spp.). J. Parasitol. 71, 682–683.

Hills, B.A., Butler, B.D., 1978. The kangaroo rat as a model for type I decompression sickness. Undersea. Biomed. Res. 5, 309–321.

Hnida, J.A., Wilson, W.D., Duszynski, D.W., 1998. A new Eimeria species (Apicomplexa: Eimeriidae) infecting Onychomys species (Rodentia: Muridae) in New Mexico and Arizona. J. Parasitol. 84, 1207–1209.

Hoch-Ligeti, C., Wagner, B.P., Deringer, M.K., Stewart, H.L., 1985. Tumor induction in Praomys (Mastomys) natalensis by N,N'–2,7–fluorenylenebisacetamide. J. Natl. Cancer Inst. 74, 909–915.

Holland, J.M., 1970. Prostatic hyperplasia and neoplasia in female Praomys (Mastomys) natalensis. J. Natl. Cancer Inst. 45, 1229–1236.

Holliman, R.B., Meade, B.J., 1980. Native trichinosis in wild rodents in Henrico County, Virginia. J. Wildl. Dis. 16, 205–207.

Holmes, E., Bonner, F.W., Nicholson, J.K., 1995. Comparative studies on the nephrotoxicity of 2-bromoethanamine hydrobromide in the Fischer 344 rat and the multimammate desert mouse (Mastomys natalensis). Arch. Toxicol. 70, 89–95.

Holmes, E., Bonner, F.W., Nicholson, J.K., 1996. Comparative biochemical effects of low doses of mercury II chloride in the F344 rat and the multimammate mouse (Mastomys natalensis). Comp. Biochem. Physiol. C Pharmacol. Toxicol. Endocrinol. 114, 7–15.

Holmes, E., Bonner, F.W., Nicholson, J.K., 1997. 1H NMR spectroscopic and histopathological studies on propyleneimine-induced renal papillary necrosis in the rat and the multimammate desert mouse (Mastomys natalensis). Comp. Biochem. Physiol. C Pharmacol. Toxicol. Endocrinol. 116, 125–134.

Holt, J., Davis, S., Leirs, H., 2006. A model of Leptospirosis infection in an African rodent to determine risk to humans: seasonal fluctuations and the impact of rodent control. Acta. Trop. 99, 218–225.

Holzbach, R.T., 1984. Animal models of cholesterol gallstone disease. Hepatology 4, 191S–198S.

Hoogland, J.L., 1979. Aggression, ectoparasitism, and other possible costs of prairie dog (Sciuridae, Cynomys spp.) coloniality. Behaviour 69, 1–35.

Hoogland, J.L., 1994. Nepotism and infanticide among prairie dogs. In: Parmigiani, S., vom Saal, F.S. (Eds.), Infanticide and Parental Care Harwood Academic Publishers, Chur, Switzerland, pp. 321–337.

Hoogland, J.L., 1996. Cynomys ludovicianus. Mamm. Species 535, 1–10.

Hoogland, J.L., 1997. Duration of gestation and lactation for Gunnison's prairie dogs. J. Mammal. 78, 173–180.

Hoogland, J.L., 1998. Estrus and copulation of Gunnison's prairie dogs. J. Mammal. 79, 887–897.

Hoogland, J.L., James, D.A., Watson, L., 2009. Nutrition, care, and behavior of captive prairie dogs. Vet. Clin. North Am. Exot. Anim. Pract. 12, 255–266. viii.

Horner, B.E., 1968. Gestation period and early development in Onychomys leucogaster brevicaudus. J. Mammal. 49, 513–515.

Hosoda, S., Suzuki, H., Suzuki, M., 1976. Spontaneous tumors and atypical proliferation of pancreatic acinar cells in Mastomys (Praomys) natalensis. J. Natl. Cancer Inst. 57, 1341–1346.

Hostetler, C.M., Hitchcock, L.N., Anacker, A.M., Young, L.J., Ryabinin, A.E., 2013. Comparative distribution of central neuropeptide Y (NPY) in the prairie (Microtus ochrogaster) and meadow (M. pennsylvanicus) vole. Peptides 40, 22–29.

Howell, A.B., 1926. Anatomy of the Wood Rat. The Williams & Wilkins Company, Baltimore, MD.

Hughes, S.E., Nutting, W.B., 1981. Demodex leucogasteri n. sp. from Onychomys leucogaster – with notes on its biology and host pathogenesis. Acarologia 22, 181–186.

Hulin, M.S., Quinn, R., 2006. Wild and black rats Laboratory Rat. Elsevier Academic Press Inc, San Diego, CA, pp. 865–882.

Iglauer, F., Schuler, T., Holub, S., Sachs, R., 1993. Ringtail disorder observed in cotton rats (Sigmodon hispidus). Scand. J. Lab. Anim. Sci. 20, 119–121.

ILAR, 2014. Washington DC. Repositories of Laboratory Animal Models and Strains. at <http://dels.nas.edu/global/ilar/links-repositories> , (accessed January 2014.).

Inoue, K., Burkett, J.P., Young, L.J., 2013. Neuroanatomical distribution of mu-opioid receptor mRNA and binding in monogamous prairie voles (Microtus ochrogaster) and non-monogamous meadow voles (Microtus pennsylvanicus). Neuroscience 244, 122–133.

Insel, T.R., Shapiro, L.E., 1992. Oxytocin receptor distribution reflects social organization in monogamous and polygamous voles. Proc. Natl. Acad. Sci. USA 89, 5981–5985.

International Commission on Zoological Nomenclature, 2012. Amendment of Articles 8, 9, 10, 21 and 78 of the International Code of Zoological Nomenclature to expand and refine methods of publication. Zookeys 219, 1–10.

Ismailov, S.G., Ismailov, M.N., 1981. The breeding of grapevine gerbils in laboratory conditions. [Russian]. Izv. Akad. Nauk. Azerbaid. (Ser Biol Nauk) 1, 69–72.

Issaian, T., Urity, V.B., Dantzler, W.H., Pannabecker, T.L., 2012. Architecture of vasa recta in the renal inner medulla of the desert rodent Dipodomys merriami: potential impact on the urine concentrating mechanism. Am. J. Physiol. Regul. Integr. Comp. Physiol. 303, R748–R756.

Itoh, K., Tamura, H., Mitsuoka, T., 1989. Gastrointestinal flora of cotton rats. Lab. Anim. 23, 62–65.

Jackson, R.K., 1997. Unusual laboratory rodent species: research uses, care, and associated biohazards. ILAR J. 38, 13–21.

Jackson, T.A., Heath, L.A., Hulin, M.S., Medina, C.L., Scarlett, L.M., Rogers, K.L., et al., 1996. Squamous cell carcinoma of the midventral abdominal pad in three gerbils. J. Am. Vet. Med. Assoc. 209, 789–791.

Jackson, T.P., Van Aarde, R.J., 2004. Diet quality differentially affects breeding effort of Mastomys coucha and M. natalensis: implications for rodent pests. J. Exp. Zool. A Comp. Exp. Biol. 301, 97–108.

Jacobs, L.F., Spencer, W.D., 1994. Natural space-use patterns and hippocampal size in kangaroo rats. Brain Behav. Evol. 44, 125–132.

Jarvis, J.U., 1981. Eusociality in a mammal: cooperative breeding in naked mole-rat colonies. Science 212, 571–573.

Jarvis, J.U.M., 1991. Methods for capturing, transporting, and maintaining naked mole-rats in captivity. In: Sherman, P.W., Jarvis, J.U.M., Alexander, R.D. (Eds.), The Biology of the Naked Mole-Rat Princeton University Press, Princeton, NJ, pp. 476–483.

Jekl, V., Knotek, Z., 2007. Evaluation of a laryngoscope and a rigid endoscope for the examination of the oral cavity of small mammals. Vet. Rec. 160, 9–13.

Jekl, V., Hauptman, K., Jeklova, E., Knotek, Z., 2006. Demodicosis in nine prairie dogs (Cynomys ludovicianus). Vet. Dermatol. 17, 280–283.

Jekl, V., Gumpenberger, M., Jeklova, E., Hauptman, K., Stehlik, L., Knotek, Z., 2011a. Impact of pelleted diets with different mineral compositions on the crown size of mandibular cheek teeth and mandibular relative density in degus (Octodon degus). Vet. Rec. 168, 641.

Jekl, V., Hauptman, K., Jeklova, E., Knotek, Z., 2011b. Dental eruption chronology in degus (Octodon degus). J. Vet. Dent. 28, 16–20.

Jekl, V., Hauptman, K., Jeklova, E., Knotek, Z., 2011c. Selected haematological and plasma chemistry parameters in juvenile and adult degus (Octodon degus). Vet. Rec. 169, 71.

Jekl, V., Hauptman, K., Knotek, Z., 2011d. Diseases in pet degus: a retrospective study in 300 animals. J. Small Anim. Pract. 52, 107–112.

Jekl, V., Hauptman, K., Skoric, M., Jeklova, E., Fictum, P., Knotek, Z., 2008. Elodontoma in a degu (Octodon degus). J. Exotic Pet Med. 17, 216–220.

Jenkins, D.C., 1977. Nematospiroides dubius: the course of primary and challenge infections in the jird, meriones unguiculatus. Exp. Parasitol. 41, 335–340.

Jensen, W.I., Duncan, R.M., 1980. Bordetella bronchiseptica associated with pulmonary disease in mountain voles (Microtus montanus). J. Wildl. Dis. 16, 11–14.

Jobard, P., Delbarre, G., Delbarre, B., Aron, E., Ghaly, A.F., 1974. A renal tumour of the nephroblastoma type in Praomys (Mastomys) natalensis. Experientia 30, 416–418.

Johnson, T.L., Cully, J.F., Collinge, S.K., Ray, C., Frey, C.M., Sandercock, B.K., 2011. Spread of plague among black-tailed prairie dogs is associated with colony spatial characteristics. J. Wildl. Manage. 75, 357–368.

Johnston, P.G., Zucker, I., 1983. Lability and diversity of circadian rhythms of cotton rats Sigmodon hispidus. Am. J. Physiol. 244, R338–R346.

Jones, P.H., Biggins, D.E., Eads, D.A., Eads, S.L., Britten, H.B., 2012. Deltamethrin flea-control preserves genetic variability of black-tailed prairie dogs during a plague outbreak. Conserv. Genet. 13, 183–195.

Jonkers, A.H., Spence, L., Downs, W.G., Worth, C.B., 1964. Laboratory studies with wild rodents and viruses native to Trinidad. II. Studies with the Trinidad Caraparu-like agent TRVL 34053-1. Am. J. Trop. Med. Hyg. 13, 728–733.

Joseph, S.K., Verma, S.K., Sahoo, M.K., Dixit, S., Verma, A.K., Kushwaha, V., et al., 2011. Sensitization with anti-inflammatory BmAFI of Brugia malayi allows L3 development in the hostile peritoneal cavity of Mastomys coucha. Acta Trop. 120, 191–205.

Joyner, C.P., Myrick, L.C., Crossland, J.P., Dawson, W.D., 1998. Deer mice as laboratory animals. ILAR J. 39, 322–330.

Juan-Salles, C., Patrício, R., Garrido, J., Garner, M.M., 2009. Disseminated Mycobacterium avium subsp. avium infection in a captive Richardson's ground squirrel (Spermophilus richardsonii). J. Exotic Pet Med. 18, 306–310.

Jung, D.S., Kim, O.J., 2005. [High prevalence of ovarian cysts in Mongolian gerbils with reproductive disorders]. Korean. Lab. Anim. Res. 21, 1–4.

Kagira, J.M., Maina, N.W., Thuita, J.K., Ngotho, M., Hau, J., 2005. Influence of cyclophosphamide on the haematological profile of laboratory bred African soft-furred rats (Mastomys natalensis). Scand. J. Lab. Anim. Sci. 32, 153–158.

Kamiya, M., Ooi, H.K., Oku, Y., Okamoto, M., Ohbayashi, M., Seki, N., 1987. Isolation of Echinococcus multilocularis from the liver of swine in Hokkaido, Japan. Jpn. J. Vet. Res. 35, 99–107.

Kaplan, H., 1975. What triggers seizures in the gerbil, Meriones unguiculatus? Life Sci. 17, 693–698.

Kaplan, H., Miezejeski, C., 1972. Development of seizures in the mongolian gerbil (Meriones unguiculatus). J. Comp. Physiol. Psychol. 81, 267–273.

Katahira, K., Ohwada, K., 1993. Hematological standard values in the cotton rat (Sigmodon hispidus). Jikken Dobutsu 42, 653–656.

Kawase, S., Ishikura, H., 1995. Female-predominant occurrence of spontaneous gastric adenocarcinoma in cotton rats. Lab. Anim. Sci. 45, 244–248.

Kawase, S., Satoh, N., 1978. Breeding of cotton rat in laboratory. [Japanese]. Rep. Hokkaido Inst. Public Health 28, 90–91.

Keckler, M.S., Gallardo-Romero, N.F., Langham, G.L., Damon, I.K., Karem, K.L., Carroll, D.S., 2010. Physiologic reference ranges for captive black-tailed prairie dogs (Cynomys ludovicianus). J. Am. Assoc. Lab. Anim. Sci. 49, 274–281.

Keebaugh, A.C., Modi, M.E., Barrett, C.E., Jin, C., Young, L.J., 2012. Identification of variables contributing to superovulation efficiency for production of transgenic prairie voles (Microtus ochrogaster). Reprod. Biol. Endocrinol. 10, 54.

Keis, A.F., Mitchell, O.G., 1975. Cytomegalovirus in the submandibular and sublingual glands of the southern grasshopper mouse (Onychomys torridus torridus). J. Dent. Res. 54, 626–628.

Kelt, D.A., Hafner, M.S., 2010. Updated guidelines for protection of mammalogists and wildlife researchers from hantavirus pulmonary syndrome (HPS). J. Mammal. 91, 1524–1527.

Kemble, E.D., Enger, J.M., 1984. Sex differences in shock motivated behaviors, activity, and discrimination learning of northern grasshopper mice (Onychomys leucogaster). Physiol. Behav. 32, 375–380.

Kenagy, G.J., Veloso, C., Bozinovic, F., 1999. Daily rhythms of food intake and feces reingestion in the degu, an herbivorous Chilean rodent: optimizing digestion through coprophagy. Physiol. Biochem. Zool. 72, 78–86.

Kershaw, W.E., Storey, D.M., 1976. Host–parasite relations in cotton rat filariasis. I: the quantitative transmission and subsequent development of Litomosoides carinii infections in cotton rats and other laboratory animals. Ann. Trop. Med. Parasitol. 70, 303–312.

Khare, S., Saxena, J.K., Sen, A.B., Ghatak, S., 1984. Erythrocyte membrane-bound enzymes in Mastomys natalensis during Plasmodium berghei infection. Aust. J. Exp. Biol. Med. Sci. 62 (Pt 2), 137–143.

Kia, E.B., 2003. Immunoperoxidase staining of alveolar hydatid cyst from an experimentally infected gerbil. Southeast Asian J. Trop. Med. Public Health 34 (Suppl. 2), 108–109.

Kilonzo, C., Li, X., Vivas, E.J., Jay-Russell, M.T., Fernandez, K.L., Atwill, E.R., 2013. Fecal shedding of zoonotic food-borne pathogens by wild rodents in a major agricultural region of the central California coast. Appl. Environ. Microbiol. 79, 6337–6344.

Kim, E.B., Fang, X., Fushan, A.A., Huang, Z., Lobanov, A.V., Han, L., et al., 2011. Genome sequencing reveals insights into physiology and longevity of the naked mole rat. Nature 479, 223–227.

Kim, H.J., Chole, R.A., 1998. Experimental models of aural cholesteatomas in Mongolian gerbils. Ann. Otol. Rhinol. Laryngol. 107, 129–134.

Kim, J.W., Kirkpatrick, B., 1996. Social isolation in animal models of relevance to neuropsychiatric disorders. Biol. Psychiatry 40, 918–922.

Kinsey, K.P., 1976. Social behavior in confined populations of the Allegheny woodrat, Neotoma floridana magister. Anim. Behav. 24, 181–187.

Kipar, A., Burthe, S.J., Hetzel, U., Rokia, M.A., Telfer, S., Lambin, X., et al., 2013. Mycobacterium microti tuberculosis in its maintenance host, the field vole (Microtus agrestis): characterization of the disease and possible routes of transmission. Vet. Pathol..

Klei, T.R., McVay, C.S., Coleman, S.U., Enright, F.M., Rao, U.R., 1997. Adoptive transfer of granulomatous inflammation to Brugia antigens in jirds. J. Parasitol. 83, 626–629.

Kneidinger, C.M., 2008. Mastomys natalensis and Mastomys coucha: identification, habitat preferences, and population genetics. MSc Thesis, Department of Zoology, University of Johannesburg, South Africa, p. 98.

Knoch, H.W., 1968. The Eastern wood rat, Neotoma floridana osagensis: a laboratory colony. Trans. Kans. Acad. Sci. 71, 361–372.

Knopper, L.D., Mineau, P., 2004. Organismal effects of pesticide exposure on meadow voles (Microtus pennsylvanicus) living in golf course ecosystems: developmental instability, clinical hematology, body condition, and blood parasitology. Environ. Toxicol. Chem. 23, 1512–1519.

Kock, D., Ingram, C.M., Frabotta, L.J., Honeycutt, R.L., Burda, H., 2006. On the nomenclature of Bathyergidae and Fukomys n. gen. (Mammalia: Rodentia). Zootaxa 1142, 51–55.

Kohl, K.D., Weiss, R.B., Dale, C., Dearing, M.D., 2011. Diversity and novelty of the gut microbial community of an herbivorous rodent (Neotoma bryanti). Symbiosis 54, 47–54.

Kolby, L., Wangberg, B., Ahlman, H., Modlin, I.M., Nilsson, O., 1998. Histamine metabolism of gastric carcinoids in Mastomys natalensis. Yale J. Biol. Med. 71, 207–215.

Koop, B.F., Baker, R.J., Genoways, H.H., 1983. Numerous chromosomal polymorphisms in a natural population of rice rats (Oryzomys, Cricetidae). Cytogenet. Cell Genet. 35, 131–135.

Koopman, J.P., Mullink, J.W., Kennis, H.M., van der Logt, J.T., 1980. An outbreak of Tyzzer's disease in Mongolian gerbils (Meriones unguiculatus). Z. Versuchstierkd. 22, 336–341.

Koshimizu, K., Saito, T., Shinozuka, Y., Tsuchiya, K., Cerda, R.O., 1993. Isolation and identification of mycoplasma strains from various species of wild rodents. J. Vet. Med. Sci. 55, 323–324.

Kosoy, M.Y., Elliott, L.H., Ksiazek, T.G., Fulhorst, C.F., Rollin, P.E., Childs, J.E., et al., 1996. Prevalence of antibodies to arenaviruses in rodents from the southern and western United States: evidence for an arenavirus associated with the genus Neotoma. Am. J. Trop. Med. Hyg. 54, 570–576.

Kozima, K., Muroashi, T., Soga, J., Tazawa, K., 1970. Histological and immunohistochemical studies on spontaneous renal lesions of Praomys (Mastomys) natalensis. Acta Pathol. Jpn. 20, 311–325.

Kritsky, D.C., Leiby, P.D., Miller, G.E., 1977. The natural occurrence of Echinococcus multilocularis in the bushy-tailed woodrat, Neotoma cinerea rupicola, in Wyoming. Am. J. Trop. Med. Hyg. 26, 1046–1047.

Kroeze, W.K., Tanner, C.E., 1985. Echinococcus multilocularis: responses to infection in cotton rats (Sigmodon hispidus). Int. J. Parasitol. 15, 233–238.

Kroh, H., Walencik, S., Mossakowski, M.J., Weinrauder, H., 1987. Spontaneous astrocytoma in the Mongolian gerbil (Meriones unguiculatus). Neuropatol. Pol. 25, 329–336.

Krugner-Higby, L., Caldwell, S., Coyle, K., Bush, E., Atkinson, R., Joers, V., 2011. The effects of diet composition on body fat and hepatic steatosis in an animal (Peromyscus californicus) model of the metabolic syndrome. Comp. Med. 61, 31–38.

Krugner-Higby, L., Shelness, G.S., Holler, A., 2006. Heritable, diet-induced hyperlipidemia in California mice (Peromyscus californicus) is due to increased hepatic secretion of very low density lipoprotein triacylglycerol. Comp. Med. 56, 468–475.

Kruppa, T.F., Iglauer, F., Ihnen, E., Miller, K., Kunstyr, I., 1990. Mastomys natalensis or Mastomys coucha. Correct species designation in animal experiments. Trop. Med. Parasitol. 41, 219–220.

Kudo, H., Oki, Y., 1981. Fermentation and VFA production in the esophageal sac of Microtus montebelli fed different rations. Nihon Juigaku Zasshi 43, 299–305.

Kudo, H., Oki, Y., 1982. Breeding and rearing of Japanese field voles (Microtus montebelli Milne-Edwards) and Hungarian voles (Microtus arvalis Pallas) as new herbivorous laboratory animal species. [Japanese]. Jikken Dobutsu 31, 175–183.

Kuiken, T., van Dijk, J.E., Terpstra, W.J., Bokhout, B.A., 1991. The role of the common vole (Microtus arvalis) in the epidemiology of bovine infection with Leptospira interrogans serovar hardjo. Vet. Microbiol. 28, 353–361.

Kumazawa, H., Takagi, H., Sudo, K., Nakamura, W., Hosoda, S., 1989. Adenocarcinoma and carcinoid developing spontaneously in the stomach of mutant strains of Mastomys natalensis. Virchows Arch. A Pathol. Anat. Histopathol. 416, 141–151.

Kurokawa, Y., Fujii, K., Suzuki, M., Sato, H., 1968. Spontaneous tumors of the thymus in mastomys (Rattus natalensis). Gann 59, 145–150.

Lackey, J.A., Huckaby, D.G., Ormiston, B.G., 1985. Peromyscus leucopus. Mamm. Species 247, 1–10.

Lalis, A., Leblois, R., Lecompte, E., Denys, C., Ter Meulen, J., Wirth, T., 2012. The impact of human conflict on the genetics of Mastomys natalensis and Lassa virus in West Africa. PLoS One 7, e37068.

Laming, P.R., Cosby, S.L., O'Neill, J.K., 1989. Seizures in the Mongolian gerbil are related to a deficiency in cerebral glutamine synthetase. Comp. Biochem. Physiol. C 94, 399–404.

Landry, S.O., 1999. A proposal for a new classification and nomenclature for the Glires (Lagomorpha and Rodentia). Mitt Mus Naturkunde Berl. Zoolog Reihe 75, 283–316.

Lang, J.D., 1996. Factors affecting the seasonal abundance of ground squirrel and wood rat fleas (Siphonaptera) in San Diego County, California. J. Med. Entomol. 33, 790–804.

Langohr, I.M., Stevenson, G.W., Thacker, H.L., Regnery, R.L., 2004. Extensive lesions of monkeypox in a prairie dog (Cynomys sp). Vet. Pathol. 41, 702–707.

La Regina, M., Kier, A.B., Wagner, J.E., 1978. A fatal enteric syndrome in Mystromys albicaudatus (white tailed rat) following topical antibiotic treatment. Lab. Anim. Sci. 28, 587–590.

La Regina, M., Lonigro, J., Wallace, M., 1986. Francisella tularensis infection in captive, wild caught prairie dogs. Lab. Anim. Sci. 36, 178–180.

Larson, J., Park, T.J., 2009. Extreme hypoxia tolerance of naked mole-rat brain. Neuroreport 20, 1634–1637.

Larson, R.H., Fitzgerald, R.J., 1968. Caries development in the African white-tailed rat (Mystromys albicaudatus) infected with a streptococcus of human origin. J. Dent. Res. 47, 746–749.

Lavocat, R., 1978. Rodentia and lagomorpha Evolution of African Mammals. Harvard University Press, Cambridge, pp. 66–89.

Leach, A.B., Holub, B.J., 1984. The effect of dietary lipid on the lipoprotein status of the Mongolian gerbil. Lipids 19, 25–33.

Lecompte, E., Fichet-Calvet, E., Daffis, S., Koulemou, K., Sylla, O., Kourouma, F., et al., 2006. Mastomys natalensis and Lassa fever, West Africa. Emerg. Infect. Dis. 12, 1971–1974.

Lee, T.M., 2004. Octodon degus: a diurnal, social, and long-lived rodent. ILAR J. 45, 14–24.

Leighton, F.A., Wobeser, G., 1978. The prevalence of adiaspiromycosis in three sympatric species of ground squirrels. J. Wildl. Dis. 14, 362–365.

Lele, S.M., Milazzo, M.L., Graves, K., Aronson, J.F., West, A.B., Fulhorst, C.F., 2003. Pathology of Whitewater Arroyo viral infection in the white-throated woodrat (Neotoma albigula). J. Comp. Pathol. 128, 289–292.

Leonard, E.P., 1979a. Enzyme histochemistry of periodontal pathogenesis in the rice rat (Oryzomys palustris). Cell Mol. Biol. Incl. Cyto Enzymol. 24, 241–248.

Leonard, E.P., 1979b. Periodontitis. Animal model: periodontitis in the rice rat (Oryzomys palustris). Am. J. Pathol. 96, 643–646.

Leonard, E.P., Reese, W.V., Mandel, E.J., 1979. Comparison of the effects of ethane-1-hydroxy-1,1-diphosphonate and dichloromethylene diphosphonate upon periodontal bone resorption in rice rats (Oryzomys palustris). Arch. Oral. Biol. 24, 707–708.

Leslie, P.H., Ranson, R.M., 1940. The mortality, fertility and rate of natural increase of the vole (Microtus agrestis) as observed in the laboratory. J. Anim. Ecol. 9, 27–52.

Lester, P.A., Rush, H.G., Sigler, R.E., 2005. Renal transitional cell carcinoma and choristoma in a degu (Octodon degus). Contemp. Top. Lab. Anim. Sci. 44, 41–44.

Letelier, M.E., Del Villar, E., Sanchez, E., 1985. Drug tolerance and detoxicating enzymes in Octodon degus and Wistar rats. A comparative study. Comp. Biochem. Physiol. C 80, 195–198.

Leung, M.K., McLintock, J., Iversen, J., 1978. Intranasal exposure of the Richardson's ground squirrel to Western equine encephalomyelitis virus. Can. J. Comp. Med. 42, 184–191.

Leveson, J.E., Marengo-Rowe, A.J., Dotson, R.L., Ubelaker, J.E., 1989. Hematology of cotton rats, Sigmodon hispidus, infected with Parastrongylus costaricensis (Metastrongyloidea: Angiostrongylidae). Trans. Am. Microsc. Soc. 108, 380.

Levin, M.L., Fish, D., 2000. Immunity reduces reservoir host competence of Peromyscus leucopus for Ehrlichia phagocytophila. Infect. Immun. 68, 1514–1518.

Levine, J.F., Lage, A.L., 1984. House mouse mites infesting laboratory rodents. Lab. Anim. Sci. 34, 393–394.

Lewis, D., Williams, H., 1979. Infection of the Mongolian gerbil with the cattle piroplasm Babesia divergens. Nature 278, 170–171.

Lewis, D., Young, E.R., Baggott, D.G., Osborn, G.D., 1981. Babesia divergens infection of the Mongolian gerbil: titration of infective dose and preliminary observations on the disease produced. J. Comp. Pathol. 91, 565–572.

Lewis, K.N., Andziak, B., Yang, T., Buffenstein, R., 2013. The naked mole-rat response to oxidative stress: just deal with it. Antioxid Redox Signal 19, 1388–1399.

Lewis, R.J., 1989. British Columbia. Plague in bushy-tailed woodrats. Can. Vet. J. 30, 596–597.

Li, B.W., Chandrashekar, R., Alvarez, R.M., Liftis, F., Weil, G.J., 1991. Identification of paramyosin as a potential protective antigen against Brugia malayi infection in jirds. Mol. Biochem. Parasitol. 49, 315–323.

Liang, Y.R., Guo, Y.X., Yi, X.Y., Zeng, X.F., Peng, L.X., Zeng, Q.S., 1983. Schistosoma japonicum: a comparison of the development of the parasite and associated pathological changes in mice and jirds (Meriones unguiculatus). Int. J. Parasitol. 13, 531–538.

Lindsay, J.W., 1976. Spontaneous occurrence of tumors in laboratory-reared arvicoline rodents. Cancer Res. 36, 4092–4098.

Little, R.R., Parker, K.M., England, J.D., Goldstein, D.E., 1982. Glycosylated hemoglobin in Mystromys albicaudatus: a diabetic animal model. Lab. Anim. Sci. 32, 44–47.

Lochmiller, R.L., Vestey, M.R., McMurry, S.T., 1991. Primary immune responses of selected small mammal species to heterologous erythrocytes. Comp. Biochem. Physiol. A Comp. Physiol. 100, 139–143.

Ludwig, W., Collinar, M., 2009. Experiences in keeping the Naked mole-rat (Heterocephalus glaberi) at Dresden Zoo. [German] Erfahrungsbericht zur Haltung von Nacktmullen (Heterocephalus glaber) im Zoo Dresden. Zool. Gart. 78, 61–74.

Luis, A.D., Douglass, R.J., Hudson, P.J., Mills, J.N., Bjornstad, O.N., 2012. Sin Nombre hantavirus decreases survival of male deer mice. Oecologia 169, 431–439.

Lussier, G., Loew, F.M., 1970. Case report. Natural Hymenolepis nana infection in mongolian gerbils (Meriones unguiculatus). Can. Vet. J. 11, 105–107.

Machang'u, R.S., Mgode, G., Mpanduji, D., 1997. Leptospirosis in animals and humans in selected areas of Tanzania. Belg. J. Zool. 127, 97–104.

Machang'u, R.S., Mgode, G.F., Assenga, J., Mhamphi, G., Weetjens, B., Cox, C., et al., 2004. Serological and molecular characterization of leptospira serovar Kenya from captive African giant pouched rats (Cricetomys gambianus) from Morogoro Tanzania. FEMS Immunol. Med. Microbiol. 41, 117–121.

Maclean, J.M., Lewis, D., Holmes, P.H., 1987. Studies on the pathogenesis of Trichostrongylus colubriformis in Mongolian gerbils (Meriones unguiculatus). J. Comp. Pathol. 97, 645–652.

MacNeil, A., Ksiazek, T.G., Rollin, P.E., 2011. Hantavirus pulmonary syndrome, United States, 1993–2009. Emerg. Infect. Dis. 17, 1195–1201.

MacPherson, B.R., Pemsingh, R.S., 1997. Ground squirrel model for cholelithiasis: role of epithelial glycoproteins. Microsc. Res. Tech. 39, 39–55.

MacPherson, B.R., Pemsingh, R.S., Scott, G.W., 1987. Experimental cholelithiasis in the ground squirrel. Lab. Invest. 56, 138–145.

Maddock, A.H., Perrin, M.R., 1981. A microscopical examination of the gastric morphology of the white-tailed rat Mystromys albicaudatus (Smith 1834). S. Afr. J. Zool. 16, 237–247.

Magnarelli, L.A., Williams, S.C., Norris, S.J., Fikrig, E., 2013. Serum antibodies to Borrelia burgdorferi, Anaplasma phagocytophilum, and Babesia microti in recaptured white-footed mice. J. Wildl. Dis. 49, 294–302.

Mahida, H., Perrin, M.R., 1994. The effect of different diets on the amount of organic acid produced in the digestive tract of Mystromys albicaudatus. Acta Theriol. (Warsz) 39, 21–27.

Maia, V., Hulak, A., 1981. Robertsonian polymorphism in chromosomes of Oryzomys subflavus (Rodentia, Cricetidae). Cytogenet. Cell Genet. 31, 33–39.

Maity, B., Guru, P.Y., 1998. Age related haematological changes in cotton rats (Sigmodon hispidus). Biol. Mem. 24, 49–53.

Maki, J., Weinstein, P.P., 1991. Transplantation into jirds as a method of assessing the viability and reproductive integrity of adult Acanthocheilonema viteae from culture. J. Parasitol. 77, 749–754.

Makundi, R.H., Massawe, A.W., Mulungu, L.S., Katakweba, A., Mbise, T.J., Mgode, G., 2008. Potential mammalian reservoirs in a bubonic plague outbreak focus in Mbulu District, northern Tanzania, in 2007. Mammalia 72, 253–257.

Malenke, J.R., Magnanou, E., Thomas, K., Dearing, M.D., 2012. Cytochrome P450 2B diversity and dietary novelty in the herbivorous, desert woodrat (Neotoma lepida). PLoS One 7, e41510.

Marafie, E., Nayak, R., Al–Zaid, N., 1978. Breeding and reproductive physiology of the desert gerbil, Meriones crassus. Lab. Anim. Sci. 28, 397–401.

Marchiondo, A.A., Upton, S.J., 1987. Eimeria albigulae and E. ladronensis: new host records from the bushy-tailed woodrat, Neotoma cinerea, from Utah. J. Parasitol. 73, 421–422.

Marion, P.L., Van Davelaar, M.J., Knight, S.S., Salazar, F.H., Garcia, G., Popper, H., et al., 1986. Hepatocellular carcinoma in ground squirrels persistently infected with ground squirrel hepatitis virus. Proc. Natl. Acad. Sci. USA 83, 4543–4546.

Marston, J.H., 1976. The Mongolian gerbil. In: Kirkwood, J.K., Hubrecht, R. (Eds.), The UFAW Handbook on the Care and Management of Laboratory Animals Churchill Livingstone, Edinburgh, pp. 236–274.

Martin, L.B., Weil, Z.M., Nelson, R.J., 2008. Fever and sickness behaviour vary among congeneric rodents. Funct. Ecol. 22, 68–77.

Maser, C., Hooven, E.F., 1970. Dental abnormalities in Microtus longicaudus. Murrelet 51, 11.

Matsuoka, K., Suzuki, J., 1995. Spontaneous tumors in the Mongolian gerbil (Meriones unguiculatus). [Japanese]. Exp. Anim. 43, 755–760.

Matsushima, Y., Ikeno, T., Ikeno, K., Tanaka, S., 1990. An electrophoretic polymorphism in salivary amylases (Amy-1) of mastomys (Praomys coucha). Lab. Anim. 24, 308–312.

Matsuzaki, T., Matsuzaki, K., Yokohata, Y., Ohtsubo, R., Kamiya, M., Yates, T.L., 1994. Breeding of the northern grasshopper mouse (Onychomys leucogaster) as a laboratory animal. Jikken Dobutsu 43, 395–401.

Mays Jr., A., 1969. Baseline hematological and blood biochemical parameters of the Mongolian gerbil (Meriones unguiculatus). Lab. Anim. Care 19, 838–842.

McCarty, R., 1975. Onychomys torridus. Mamm. Species 59, 1–5.

McCarty, R., 1978. Onychomys leucogaster. Mamm. Species 87, 1–6.

McCarty, R., Southwick, C.H., 1975. The development of convulsive seizures in the grasshopper mouse (Onychomys torridus). Dev. Psychobiol. 8, 547–552.

McCarty, R., Southwick, C.H., 1977a. Cross-species fostering: effects on the olfactory preference of Onychomys torridus and Peromyscus leucopus. Behav. Biol. 19, 255–260.

McCarty, R., Southwick, C.H., 1977b. Effects of parental environment on the prevalence of convulsive seizures in Onychomys torridus. Dev. Psychobiol. 10, 359–364.

McCarty, R.C., Whitesides, G.H., Tomosky, T.K., 1976. Effects of p-chlorophenylalanine on the predatory behavior of Onychomys torridus. Pharmacol. Biochem. Behav. 4, 217–220.

McClellan, D.A., 2000. The codon-degeneracy model of molecular evolution. J. Mol. Evol. 50, 131–140.

McGinn, M.D., Faddis, B.T., 1997. Kangaroo rats exhibit spongiform degeneration of the central auditory system similar to that found in gerbils. Hear. Res. 104, 90–100.

McGinn, M.D., Faddis, B.T., 1998. Neuronal degeneration in the gerbil brainstem is associated with spongiform lesions. Microsc. Res. Tech. 41, 187–204.

McGraw, L.A., Davis, J.K., Young, L.J., Thomas, J.W., 2011. A genetic linkage map and comparative mapping of the prairie vole (Microtus ochrogaster) genome. BMC Genet. 12, 60.

McHugh, C.P., Melby, P.C., LaFon, S.G., 1996. Leishmaniasis in Texas: epidemiology and clinical aspects of human cases. Am. J. Trop. Med. Hyg. 55, 547–555.

McKenna, M.C., Bell, S.K., 1997. Classification of Mammals Above the Species Level. Columbia University Press, New York.

McKinney, L.A., Hendricks, L.D., 1980. Experimental infection of Mystromys albicaudatus with Leishmania braziliensis: pathology. Am. J. Trop. Med. Hyg. 29, 753–760.

McMurry, S.T., Lochmiller, R.L., Chandra, S.A., Qualls Jr., C.W., 1995. Sensitivity of selected immunological, hematological, and reproductive parameters in the cotton rat (Sigmodon hispidus) to subchronic lead exposure. J. Wildl. Dis. 31, 193–204.

Meckley, P.E., Zwicker, G.M., 1979. Naturally-occurring neoplasms in the Mongolian gerbil, Meriones unguiculatus. Lab. Anim. 13, 203–206.

Mello, D.A., 1978. Some aspects of the biology of Oryzomys eliurus (Wagner, 1845) under laboratory conditions (Rodentia, Cricetidae). Rev. Bras. Biol. 38, 293–295.

Merriman, D.K., Lahvis, G., Jooss, M., Gesicki, J.A., Schill, K., 2012. Current practices in a captive breeding colony of 13-lined ground squirrels (Ictidomys tridecemlineatus). Lab. Anim. (NY) 41, 315–325.

Mian, L.S., Nwadike, C.N., Hitchcock, J.C., Madon, M.B., Myers, C.M., 1996. Plague activity in San Bernardino County during 1995. Proc. Pap. Annu. Conf. Mosq. Vector Control Assoc. Calif 64, 80–84.

Michener, G.R., 1993. Lethal myiasis of Richardson's ground squirrels by the sarcophagid fly Neobellieria citellivora. J. Mammal. 74, 148–155.

Michener, G.R., 2014. University of Lethbridge, Alberta, Canada. Richardson's ground squirrels., at http://research.uleth.ca/rgs/introduction.cfm, (accessed January 2014.).

Michener, G.R., Koeppl, J.W., 1985. Spermophilus richardsonii. Mamm. Species 243, 1–8.

Mighell, J.S., Baker, A.E., 1990. Caesarean section in a gerbil [letter]. Vet. Rec. 126, 441.

Mikhail, J.W., Mansour, N.S., 1973. Mystromys albicaudatus, the African white-tailed rat, as an experimental host for Leishmania donovani. J. Parasitol. 59, 1085–1087.

Milazzo, M.L., Amman, B.R., Cajimat, M.N., Mendez-Harclerode, F.M., Suchecki, J.R., Hanson, J.D., et al., 2013. Ecology of Catarina virus (family Arenaviridae) in southern Texas, 2001–2004. Vector Borne Zoonotic Dis. 13, 50–59.

Montali, R.J., 1980. An overview of tumors in zoo animals. In: Montali, R.J., Migaki, G. (Eds.), The Comparative Pathology of Zoo Animals Smithsonian Institution Press, Washington, DC, pp. 531–542.

Morrison, P., Dieterich, R., Preston, D., 1976. Breeding and reproduction of fifteen wild rodents maintained as laboratory colonies. Lab. Anim. Sci. 26, 237–243.

Morrow, G.W., Day-Lollini, P.A., 1990. Diagnostic exercise: exophthalmos in a ground squirrel. Lab. Anim. Sci. 40, 411–412.

Morway, C., Kosoy, M., Eisen, R., Montenieri, J., Sheff, K., Reynolds, P.J., et al., 2008. A longitudinal study of Bartonella infection in populations of woodrats and their fleas. J. Vector Ecol. 33, 353–364.

Moses, M.R., Frey, J.K., Roemer, G.W., 2012. Elevated surface temperature depresses survival of banner-tailed kangaroo rats: will climate change cook a desert icon? Oecologia 168, 257–268.

Motzel, S.L., Gibson, S.V., 1990. Tyzzer disease in hamsters and gerbils from a pet store supplier. J. Am. Vet. Med. Assoc. 197, 1176–1178.

Muller, E.L., Pitt, H.A., George, W.L., 1987. Prairie dog model for antimicrobial agent–induced Clostridium difficile diarrhea. Infect. Immun. 55, 198–200.

Murphy, J.C., Niemi, S.M., Hewes, K.M., Zink, M., Fox, J.G., 1978. Hematologic and serum protein reference values of the Octodon degus. Am. J. Vet. Res. 39, 713–715.

Murphy, J.C., Crowell, T.P., Hewes, K.M., Fox, J.G., Shalev, M., 1980. Spontaneous lesions in the degu. In: Montali, R.J., Migaki, G. (Eds.), The Comparative Pathology of Zoo Animals Smithsonian Institution Press, Washington, DC, pp. 437–444.

Muths, E., Reichman, O.J., 1996. Kangaroo rat bone compared to white rat bone after short-term disuse and exercise. Comp. Biochem. Physiol. A Physiol. 114, 355–361.

Nadler, C.F., 1968. The serum proteins and transferrins of the ground squirrel subgenus Spermophilus. Comp. Biochem. Physiol. 27, 487–503.

Nagasawa, H., Koshimizu, U., Watanabe, M., Tokuda, K., Sumita, H., Kano, Y., 1989. Mammary gland growth and response to hormones in mastomys compared with mice. Lab. Anim. Sci. 39, 313–317.

Nagy, T.R., Pistole, D.H., 1988. The effects of fasting on some physiological parameters in the meadow vole, Microtus pennsylvanicus. Comp. Biochem. Physiol. A Comp. Physiol. 91, 679–684.

Najecki, D.L., Tate, B.A., 1999. Husbandry and management of the degu (Octodon degus). Lab. Anim. (NY) 28, 54–62.

Nasarre, C., Coleman, S.U., Rao, U.R., Klei, T.R., 1997. Brugia pahangi: differential induction and regulation of jird inflammatory responses by life-cycle stages. Exp. Parasitol. 87, 20–29.

Neal, B.R., 1977. Reproduction of the multimammate rat, Praomys (Mastomys) natalensis (Smith) in Uganda. Z. Saugetierkd. 42, 221–231.

Nelson, O.L., Rourke, B.C., 2013. Increase in cardiac myosin heavy-chain (MyHC) alpha protein isoform in hibernating ground squirrels, with echocardiographic visualization of ventricular wall hypertrophy and prolonged contraction. J. Exp. Biol. 216, 4678–4690.

Nelson, R.J., Fine, J.B., Demas, G.E., Moffatt, C.A., 1996. Photoperiod and population density interact to affect reproductive and immune function in male prairie voles. Am. J. Physiol. 270, R571–R577.

Nicholson, W.L., Castro, M.B., Kramer, V.L., Sumner, J.W., Childs, J.E., 1999. Dusky-footed wood rats (Neotoma fuscipes) as reservoirs of granulocytic Ehrlichiae (Rickettsiales: Ehrlichieae) in northern California. J. Clin. Microbiol. 37, 3323–3327.

Nicolosi, R.J., Marlett, J.A., Morello, A.M., Flanagan, S.A., Hegsted, D.M., 1981. Influence of dietary unsaturated and saturated fat on the plasma lipoproteins of Mongolian gerbils. Atherosclerosis 38, 359–371.

Niewiesck, S., Volp, F., ter Meulen, V., 1997. A maintenance and handling device for cotton rat. Lab. Anim. (NY) 26, 32–33.

Niewiesk, S., 1999. Cotton rats (Sigmodon hispidus): an animal model to study the pathogenesis of measles virus infection. Immunol. Lett. 65, 47–50.

Niewiesk, S., Eisenhuth, I., Fooks, A., Clegg, J.C., Schnorr, J.J., Schneider-Schaulies, S., et al., 1997. Measles virus-induced immune suppression in the cotton rat (Sigmodon hispidus) model depends on viral glycoproteins. J. Virol. 71, 7214–7219.

Niewiesk, S., Prince, G., 2002. Diversifying animal models: the use of hispid cotton rats (Sigmodon hispidus) in infectious diseases. Lab. Anim. 36, 357–372.

Nikodemusz, E., Imre, R., 1979. Effect of repetitive blood sampling on red cell count, hematocrit and hemoglobin values in the common vole (Microtus arvalis Pallas). Z. Versuchstierkd. 21, 276–280.

Nilsson, O., Wangberg, B., Johansson, L., Modlin, I.M., Ahlman, H., 1992. Praomys (Mastomys) natalensis: a model for gastric carcinoid formation. Yale J. Biol. Med. 65, 741–751. discussion 827–749.

Ninomiya, H., Nakamura, T., 1987. Benign testicular hyperplasia in Mongolian gerbils (Meriones unguiculatus). Jikken Dobutsu 36, 191–194.

Nishi, M., Steiner, D.F., 1990. Cloning of complementary DNAs encoding islet amyloid polypeptide, insulin, and glucagon precursors from a New World rodent, the degu, Octodon degus. Mol. Endocrinol. 4, 1192–1198.

Nolan, T.J., Farrell, J.P., 1987. Experimental infections of the multimammate rat (Mastomys natalensis) with Leishmania donovani and Leishmania major. Am. J. Trop. Med. Hyg. 36, 264–269.

Nolan, T.J., Megyeri, Z., Bhopale, V.M., Schad, G.A., 1993. Strongyloides stercoralis: the first rodent model for uncomplicated and hyperinfective strongyloidiasis, the Mongolian gerbil (Meriones unguiculatus). J. Infect. Dis. 168, 1479–1484.

Norris, M.L., Adams, C.E., 1972a. The growth of the Mongolian gerbil, Meriones unguiculatus, from birth to maturity. J. Zool. 166, 277–282.

Norris, M.L., Adams, C.E., 1972b. Incidence of cystic ovaries and reproductive performance in the Mongolian gerbil, Meriones unguiculatus. Lab. Anim. 6, 337–342.

Norris, M.L., Adams, C.E., 1974. Sexual development in the Mongolian gerbil, Meriones unguiculatus, with particular reference to the ovary. J. Reprod. Fertil. 36, 245–248.

Norris, M.L., Adams, C.E., 1981. Pregnancy concurrent with lactation in the Mongolian gerbil (Meriones unguiculatus). Lab. Anim. 15, 21–23.

Norris, M.L., Adams, C.E., 1982. Lifetime reproductive performance of Mongolian gerbils (Meriones unguiculatus) with 1 or 2 ovaries. Lab. Anim. 16, 146–150.

Nowak, R.M., 1999. Walker's Mammals of the World. The Johns Hopkins University Press, Baltimore, MD.

Ntshotsho, P., van Aarde, R.J., Nicolson, S.W., Jackson, T.P., 2004. Renal physiology of two southern African Mastomys species (Rodentia: Muridae): a salt-loading experiment to assess concentrating ability. Comp. Biochem. Physiol. A Mol. Integr. Physiol. 139, 441–447.

Nutting, W.B., Satterfield, L.C., Cosgrove, G.E., 1973. Demodex sp. infesting tongue, esophagus, and oral cavity of Onychomys leucogaster, the grasshopper mouse. J. Parasitol. 59, 893–896.

O'Riain, M.J., Jarvis, J.U., Faulkes, C.G., 1996. A dispersive morph in the naked mole-rat. Nature 380, 619–621.

Oguge, N.O., 1995. Diet, seasonal abundance and microhabitats of Praomys (Mastomys) natalensis (Rodentia: Muridae) and other small rodents in the Kenyan sub-humid grassland community. Afr. J. Ecol. 33, 211–223.

Ohnishi, K., Kutsumi, H., 1995. Possible formation of new brood capsule by the previously formed brood capsule in Echinococcus multilocularis metacestodes. Southeast Asian J. Trop. Med. Public Health 26, 319–321.

Oliver Jr., J.H., Chandler Jr., F.W., James, A.M., Sanders Jr., F.H., Hutcheson, H.J., Huey, L.O., et al., 1995. Natural occurrence and characterization of the Lyme disease spirochete, Borrelia burgdorferi, in cotton rats (Sigmodon hispidus) from Georgia and Florida. J. Parasitol. 81, 30–36.

Olson, J.M., Jinka, T.R., Larson, L.K., Danielson, J.J., Moore, J.T., Carpluck, J., et al., 2013. Circannual rhythm in body temperature, torpor, and sensitivity to A(1) adenosine receptor agonist in arctic ground squirrels. J. Biol. Rhythms 28, 201–207.

Olson, M.E., Goemans, I., Bolingbroke, D., Lundberg, S., 1988. Gangrenous dermatitis caused by Corynebacterium ulcerans in Richardson ground squirrels. J. Am. Vet. Med. Assoc. 193, 367–368.

Ostapoff, E.M., Morest, D.K., 1989. A degenerative disorder of the central auditory system of the gerbil. Hear. Res. 37, 141–162.

Ottolini, M.G., Porter, D.D., Hemming, V.G., Hensen, S.A., Sami, I.R., Prince, G.A., 1996. Semi-permissive replication and functional aspects of the immune response in a cotton rat model of human parainfluenza virus type 3 infection. J. Gen. Virol. 77 (Pt 8), 1739–1743.

Oxberry, B.A., 1975. An anatomical, histochemical, and autoradiographic study of the ever-growing molar dentition of Microtus with comments on the role of structure in growth and eruption. J. Morphol. 147, 337–353.

Packer, J.T., Kraner, K.L., Rose, S.D., Stuhlman, R.A., Nelson, L.R., 1970. Diabetes mellitus in Mystromys albicaudatus. Arch. Pathol. 89, 410–415.

Padovan, D., 1985. Intraperitoneal pentobarbitone anaesthesia of Mystromys albicaudatus. Lab. Anim. 19, 16–18.

Page, L.K., Johnson, S.A., Swihart, R.K., Kazacos, K.R., 2012. Prevalence of Baylisascaris procyonis in habitat associated with Allegheny woodrat (Neotoma magister) populations in Indiana. J. Wildl. Dis. 48, 503–507.

Palacios, A.G., Lee, T.M., 2013. Husbandry and breeding in the Octodon degu (Molina 1782). Cold Spring Harb. Protoc. 2013, 350–353.

Park, A.W., 1974a. Biology of the rice rat (Oryzomys palustris natator) in a laboratory environment. III. Morphology of dentition. Acta Anat. (Basel) 87, 45–56.

Park, A.W., 1974b. Biology of the rice rat (Oryzomys palustris natator) in a laboratory environment. IV. Mineralisation of the molar teeth. Acta Anat. (Basel) 87, 433–446.

Park, A.W., 1974c. Biology of the rice rat (Oryzomys palustris natator) in a laboratory environment. V. The maxillary and mandibular osteodental fissures. Acta Anat. (Basel) 88, 217–230.

Park, A.W., Nowosielski-Slepowron, B.J., 1974. Biology of the rice rat (Oryzomys palustris natato) in a laboratory environment. VIII. Postweaning body growth. Zentralbl. Veterinarmed. C 3, 364–370.

Park, A.W., Nowosielski-Slepowron, B.J., 1975. Biology of the rice rat (Oryzomys palustris natator) in a laboratory environment. VII. Pre-weaning growth of the body. Acta Anat. (Basel) 91, 500–509.

Park, A.W., Nowosielski-Slepowron, B.J., 1976. Biology of the rice rat (Oryzomys palustris natator) in a laborabory environment. X. Postweaning growth of the skull. Acta Anat. (Basel) 94, 356–368.

Parsons, R.C., Spratt, D.M.J., Kirkwood, J.K., 1987. Cryptococcus neoformans in six species of small mammals at the Zoological Society of London. Erkrankungen Der Zootiere 29, 137–141.

Partono, F., Purnomo, 1987. Periodicity studies of Brugia malayi in Indonesia: recent findings and a modified classification of the parasite. Trans. R. Soc. Trop. Med. Hyg. 81, 657–662.

Patterson, B., Wood, A.E., 1982. Rodents from the Deseadan Oligocene of Bolivia and the relationships of the Caviomorpha. Bull. Mus. Comp. Zool. 149, 371–543.

Patton, J.L., Smith, M.F., 1989. Genetic structure and the genetic and morphologic divergence among pocket gopher species (genus Thomomys). In: Otte, D., Endler, J.A. (Eds.), Speciation and Its Consequences Sinauer Associates, Sunderland, MA, pp. 284–304.

Patton, J.L., Smith, M.F., 1993. Molecular evidence for mating asymmetry and female choice in a pocket gopher (Thomomys) hybrid zone. Mol. Ecol. 2, 3–8.

Peles, J.D., Barrett, G.W., 1997. Assessment of metal uptake and genetic damage in small mammals inhabiting a fly ash basin. Bull. Environ. Contam. Toxicol. 59, 279–284.

Perrin, M.R., 1987. Effects of diet on the gastric papillae and microflora of the rodents Mystromys albicaudatus and Cricetomys gambianus. S. Afr. J. Zool. 22, 67–76.

Perrin, M.R., Curtis, B.A., 1980. Comparative morphology of the digestive system of 19 species of southern African myomorph rodents in relation to diet and evolution. S. Afr. J. Zool. 15, 22–33.

Perrin, M.R., Kokkinn, M.J., 1986. Comparative gastric anatomy of Cricetomys gambianus and Saccostomus campestris (Cricetomyinae) in relation to Mystromys albicaudatus (Cricetinae). S. Afr. J. Zool. 21, 202–210.

Perrin, M.R., Maddock, A.H., 1983. Preliminary investigations of the digestive process of the white-tailed rat Mystromys albicaudatus (Smith 1834). S. Afr. J. Zool. 18, 128–133.

Perrin, M.R., Maddock, A.H., 1985. Comparative gastric morphology of some African rodents. In: Duncker, H.R., Fleischer, G. (Eds.), Functional Morphology in Vertebrates: Proceedings of the 1st International Symposium on Vertebrate Morphology, Giessen, 1983 Gustav Fischer Verlag, Stuttgart, West Germany, pp. 317–324.

Petersen, J.M., Schriefer, M.E., Carter, L.G., Zhou, Y., Sealy, T., Bawiec, D., et al., 2004. Laboratory analysis of tularemia in wild-trapped, commercially traded prairie dogs, Texas, 2002. Emerg. Infect. Dis. 10, 419–425.

Pfaffenberger, G.S., Kemether, K., de Bruin, D., 1985. Helminths of sympatric populations of kangaroo rats (Dipodomys ordii) and grasshopper mice (Onychomys leucogaster) from the high plains of eastern New Mexico. J. Parasitol. 71, 592–595.

Piazza, F.M., Schmidt, H.J., Johnson, S.A., Dotson, D.L., Darnell, M.E., Ottolini, M.G., et al., 1995. A cotton rat model of effectors of immunity to respiratory syncytial virus other than serum antibody. Pediatr. Pulmonol. 19, 355–359.

Pinter, A.J., 1970. Reproduction and growth for two species of grasshopper mice (Onychomys) in the laboratory. J. Mammal. 51, 236–243.

Pinter, A.J., 1985. Effects of hormones and gonadal status on the midventral gland of the grasshopper mouse Onychomys leucogaster. Anat. Rec. 211, 318–322.

Port, C.D., Richter, W.R., Moise, S.M., 1970. Tyzzer's disease in the gerbil (Meriones unguiculatus). Lab. Anim. Care 20, 109–111.

Porter, S.L., 1979. Microsporum gypseum infection in three Mexican prairie dogs. Vet. Med. Small Anim. Clin. 74, 71–73.

Prieur, D.J., Olson, H.M., Young, D.M., 1979. Partial oculocutaneous albinism in Mystromys albicaudatus: nonhomology with the Chediak-Higashi syndrome. Lab. Anim. Sci. 29, 40–43.

Prince, G.A., Porter, D.D., 1996. Treatment of parainfluenza virus type 3 bronchiolitis and pneumonia in a cotton rat model using topical antibody and glucocorticosteroid. J. Infect. Dis. 173, 598–608.

Prince, G.A., Porter, D.D., Jenson, A.B., Horswood, R.L., Chanock, R.M., Ginsberg, H.S., 1993. Pathogenesis of adenovirus type 5 pneumonia in cotton rats (Sigmodon hispidus). J. Virol. 67, 101–111.

Prince, G.A., Prieels, J.P., Slaoui, M., Porter, D.D., 1999. Pulmonary lesions in primary respiratory syncytial virus infection, reinfection, and vaccine-enhanced disease in the cotton rat (Sigmodon hispidus). Lab. Invest. 79, 1385–1392.

Pruthi, A.K., Kharole, M.U., Gupta, R.K., Kumar, B.B., 1983. Occurrence and pathology of intracutaneous cornifying epitheliomas in Mastomys natalensis, the multimammate mouse. Res. Vet. Sci. 35, 127–129.

Raflo, C.P., Diamond, S.S., 1980. Metastatic squamous-cell carcinoma in a gerbil (Meriones unguiculatus). Lab. Anim. 14, 237–239.

Randall, J.A., 1986. Lack of gonadal control of the dorsal gland and sandbathing in male and female bannertail kangaroo rats (Dipodomys spectabilis). Horm. Behav. 20, 95–105.

Randeria, J.D., 1978. The inbreeding of the Y and the Z strains of Praomys natalensis with special reference to the laboratory uses of the Mastomys. J. S. Afr. Vet. Assoc. 49, 197–199.

Rantanen, N.W., Highman, B., 1970. Spontaneous tumors in a colony of Mystromys albicaudatus (African white-tailed rat). Lab. Anim. Care 20, 114–119.

Redl, P., Kassai, T., 1979. The course of primary and secondary Nippostrongylus brasiliensis infection in the multimammate rat (Mastomys natalensis) and albino rat. Parasitol. Hung 12, 71–78.

Reich, L.M., 1981. Microtus pennsylvanicus. Mamm. Species 159, 1–8.

Reichman, O.J., 1975. Relation of desert rodent diets to available resources. J. Mammal. 56, 731–751.

Reiter, R.J., Steinlechner, S., Richardson, B.A., King, T.S., 1983. Differential response of pineal melatonin levels to light at night in laboratory-raised and wild-captured 13-lined ground squirrels (Spermophilus tridecemlineatus). Life Sci. 32, 2625–2629.

Rejmanek, D., Vanwormer, E., Mazet, J.A., Packham, A.E., Aguilar, B., Conrad, P.A., 2010. Congenital transmission of Toxoplasma gondii in deer mice (Peromyscus maniculatus) after oral oocyst infection. J. Parasitol. 96, 516–520.

Rembert, M.S., Johnson, A.J., 2001. What's your diagnosis? Pigmented mass in an experimental gerbil. Spontaneous malignant melanoma. Lab. Anim. (NY) 30, 22–25.

Rembert, M.S., Coleman, S.U., Klei, T.R., Goad, M.E.P., 2000. Neoplastic mass in an experimental Mongolian gerbil. Contemp. Top. Lab. Anim. Sci. 39, 34–36.

Rewkiewicz-Dziarska, A., 1975a. Seasonal changes in hemoglobin and erythrocyte indexes in Microtus arvalis (Pallis, 1779). Bull. Acad. Pol. Sci. Biol. 23, 481–486.

Rewkiewicz-Dziarska, A., 1975b. Seasonal changes in leukocyte indexes in Microtus arvalis (Pallas, 1779). Bull. Acad. Pol. Sci. Biol. 23, 475–480.

Reynolds, K.D., Schwarz, M.S., McFarland, C.A., McBride, T., Adair, B., Strauss, R.E., et al., 2006a. Northern pocket gophers (Thomomys talpoides) as biomonitors of environmental metal contamination. Environ. Toxicol. Chem. 25, 458–469.

Reynolds, M.G., Yorita, K.L., Kuehnert, M.J., Davidson, W.B., Huhn, G.D., Holman, R.C., et al., 2006b. Clinical manifestations of human monkeypox influenced by route of infection. J. Infect. Dis. 194, 773–780.

Reynolds, M.G., Davidson, W.B., Curns, A.T., Conover, C.S., Huhn, G., Davis, J.P., et al., 2007. Spectrum of infection and risk factors for human monkeypox, United States, 2003. Emerg. Infect. Dis. 13, 1332–1339.

Reynolds, T.J., Wright, J.W., 1979. Early postnatal physical and behavioural development of degus (Octodon degus). Lab. Anim. 13, 93–99.

Richmond, M., Conaway, C.H., 1969. Management, breeding, and reproductive performance of the vole, Microtus ochrogaster, in a laboratory colony. Lab. Anim. Care 19, 80–87.

Rickman, R., Kanyangala, S., 1990. A comparative study of the infectivity of T.b. rhodesiense isolates from man to 3 species of small laboratory rodents. East Afr. Med. J. 67, 413–418.

Riddle, B.R., Honeycutt, R.L., Lee, P.L., 1993. Mitochondrial DNA phylogeography in northern grasshopper mice (Onychomys leucogaster) – the influence of Quaternary climatic oscillations on population dispersion and divergence. Mol. Ecol. 2, 183–193.

Riley, T., Stuhlman, R.A., Van Peenen, H.J., Esterly, J.A., Townsend, J.F., 1975. Glomerular lesions of diabetes mellitus in Mystromys albicaudatus. Arch. Pathol. 99, 167–169.

Ringler, D.H., Lay, D.M., Abrams, G.D., 1972. Spontaneous neoplasms in aging gerbillinae. Lab. Anim. Sci. 22, 407–414.

Robbins, C.B., van der Straeten, E., 1989. Comments on the systematics of Mastomys Thomas 1915 with the description of a new West African species. Senckenberg. Biol. 69, 1–14.

Robel, G.L., Lochmiller, R.L., McMurry, S.T., Qualls Jr., C.W., 1996. Environmental, age, and sex effects on cotton rat (Sigmodon hispidus) hematology. J. Wildl. Dis. 32, 390–394.

Rockett, J., Seville, R.S., Kingston, N., Williams, E.S., Thorne, E.T., 1990. A cestode, Taenia mustelae, in the black-footed ferret (Mustela nigripes) and the white-tailed prairie dog (Cynomys leucurus) in Wyoming. J. Helminthol. Soc. Wash. 57, 160–162.

Rodrigues, M., Streett Jr., R.P., Highman, B., 1971. Partial ocular albinism in Mystromys albicaudatus (African white-tailed rat). Arch. Pathol. 92, 212–218.

Roebuck, B.D., Longnecker, D.S., 1979. Response of two rodents, Mastomys natalensis and Mystromys albicaudatus, to the pancreatic carcinogen azaserine. J. Natl. Cancer Inst. 62, 1269–1271.

Rogers, K., Chrisp, C., 1998. Lipoma in the mediastinum of a prairie dog (Cynomys ludovicianus). Contemp. Top. Lab. Anim. Sci. 37, 74–76.

Rollin, P.E., Ksiazek, T.G., Elliott, L.H., Ravkov, E.V., Martin, M.L., Morzunov, S., et al., 1995. Isolation of black creek canal virus, a new hantavirus from Sigmodon hispidus in Florida. J. Med. Virol. 46, 35–39.

Rowe, A.H., Rowe, M.P., 2008. Physiological resistance of grasshopper mice (Onychomys spp.) to Arizona bark scorpion (Centruroides exilicauda) venom. Toxicon 52, 597–605.

Rowe, S.E., Simmons, J.L., Ringler, D.H., Lay, D.M., 1974. Spontaneous neoplasms in aging Gerbillinae. A summary of forty-four neoplasms. Vet. Pathol. 11, 38–51.

Rudolph, R.L., Muller, H., Reinacher, M., Thiel, W., 1981. Morphology of experimentally induced so-called keratoacanthomas and squamous cell carcinomas in 2 inbred-lines of Mastomys natalensis. J. Comp. Pathol. 91, 123–134.

Ruppel, E., 1842. Heterocephalus nov. gen. Uber Saugethiere aus de Ordnung de Nager (1834) Mus Senckenberg 3, 91–116.

Saibaba, P., Urs, Y.L., Desai, B.L., Sanjeevarayappa, K.V., 1988. Breeding and management of Indian desert gerbil (Meriones hurrianae Jerdon) under captivity and seminatural conditions. Indian J. Exp. Biol. 26, 481–482.

Saito, S., Kurokawa, Y., Sato, H., 1977. Effects of various diets on growth, longevity and incidence of spontaneous tumors of Praomys (Mastomys) natalensis. Sci. Rep. Res. Inst. Tohoku Univ. Med. 24, 33–42.

Salas, R.A., de Manzione, N., Tesh, R., 1998. Venezuelan hemorrhagic fever: eight years of observation. [Spanish] Fiebre hemorragica venezolana: ocho anos de observacion. Acta Cient. Venez. 49 (Suppl. 1), 46–51.

Salkeld, D.J., Salathe, M., Stapp, P., Jones, J.H., 2010. Plague outbreaks in prairie dog populations explained by percolation thresholds of alternate host abundance. Proc. Natl. Acad. Sci. USA 107, 14247–14250.

Sangvaranond, A., Zahner, H., 1989. 19s and 7s antibody response of Mastomys natalensis in experimental filarial (Litomosoides carinii, Acanthocheilonema viteae, Brugia malayi, B. pahangi) infections. Zentralbl. Veterinarmed. B 36, 374–384.

Sasaki, M., Arai, T., Usui, T., Oki, Y., 1991. Immunohistochemical, ultrastructural, and hormonal studies on the endocrine pancreas of voles (Microtus arvalis) with monosodium aspartate-induced diabetes. Vet. Pathol. 28, 497–505.

Sato, H., Ihama, Y., Kamiya, H., 2000. Survival of destrobilated adults of Taenia crassiceps in T-cell-depleted Mongolian gerbils. Parasitol. Res. 86, 284–289.

Sayles, P.C., Hunter, K.W., Stafford, E.E., Hendricks, L.D., 1981. Antibody response to Leishmania mexicana in African white-tailed rats (Mystromys albicaudatus). J. Parasitol. 67, 585–586.

Scelza, J., Knoll, J., 1982. Seasonal variation in various blood indices of the kangaroo rat, Dipodomys panamintinus. Comp. Biochem. Physiol. A Comp. Physiol. 71, 237–241.

Schafer, K., Neumann, J., Waterboer, T., Rosl, F., 2011. Serological markers for papillomavirus infection and skin tumour development in the rodent model Mastomys coucha. J. Gen. Virol. 92, 383–394.

Schafer, K., Waterboer, T., Rosl, F., 2010. A capture ELISA for monitoring papillomavirus-induced antibodies in Mastomys coucha. J. Virol. Methods 163, 216–221.

Schitoskey Jr., F., Woodmansee, S.R., 1978. Energy requirements and diet of the California ground squirrel. J. Wildl. Manage. 42, 373–382.

Schlegel, M., Jacob, J., Kruger, D.H., Rang, A., Ulrich, R.G., 2014. Hantavirus emergence in rodents, insectivores and bats what comes next?. In: Johnson, N. (Ed.), Role of Animals in Emerging Viral Diseases Elsevier Academic Press Inc, San Diego, CA, pp. 235–292.

Schmidt, G., Martin, A.P., Stuhlman, R.A., Townsend, J.F., Lucas, F.V., Vorbeck, M.L., 1974. Evaluation of hepatic mitochondrial function in the spontaneously diabetic Mystromys albicaudatus. Lab. Invest. 30, 451–457.

Schmidt, G.E., Martin, A.P., Townsend, J.F., Vorbeck, M.L., 1980. Basement membrane synthesis in spontaneously diabetic Mystromys albicaudatus. Lab. Invest. 43, 217–224.

Schroder, G.D., 1979. Foraging behavior and home range utilization of the bannertial kangaroo rat (Dipodomys spectabilis). Ecology 60, 657–665.

Schwanz, L.E., Voordouw, M.J., Brisson, D., Ostfeld, R.S., 2011. Borrelia burgdorferi has minimal impact on the Lyme disease reservoir host Peromyscus leucopus. Vector Borne Zoonotic Dis. 11, 117–124.

Schwarzbrott, S.S., Wagner, J.E., Frisk, C.S., 1974. Demodicosis in the Mongolian gerbil (Meriones unguiculatus): a case report. Lab. Anim. Sci. 24, 666–668.

Scotti, A.L., Bollag, O., Nitsch, C., 1998. Seizure patterns of Mongolian gerbils subjected to a prolonged weekly test schedule: evidence for a kindling-like phenomenon in the adult population. Epilepsia 39, 567–576.

Seed, J.R., Hall, J.E., 1980. A review on the use of Microtus montanus as an applicable experimental model for the study of African trypanosomiasis. Ann. Soc. Belg. Med. Trop. 60, 341–348.

Seluanov, A., Hine, C., Azpurua, J., Feigenson, M., Bozzella, M., Mao, Z., et al., 2009. Hypersensitivity to contact inhibition provides a clue to cancer resistance of naked mole-rat. Proc. Natl. Acad. Sci. USA 106, 19352–19357.

Setoguchi, Y., Danel, C., Crystal, R.G., 1994. Stimulation of erythropoiesis by in vivo gene therapy: physiologic consequences of transfer of the human erythropoietin gene to experimental animals using an adenovirus vector. Blood 84, 2946–2953.

Seville, R.S., 1997. Eimeria spp. (Apicomplexa: Eimeriidae) from black- and white-tailed prairie dogs (Cynomys ludovicianus and Cynomys leucurus) in central and southeast Wyoming. J. Parasitol. 83, 166–168.

Shakibi, J.G., Weiss, L., 1969. The prevalence rate of congenital heart disease in newborn gerbils (Meriones unguiculatus). A preliminary report. Henry Ford Hosp. Med. J. 17, 241–246.

Shen, Z., Xu, S., Dewhirst, F.E., Paster, B.J., Pena, J.A., Modlin, I.M., et al., 2005. A novel enterohepatic Helicobacter species 'Helicobacter mastomyrinus' isolated from the liver and intestine of rodents. Helicobacter 10, 59–70.

Shepherd, A.J., Leman, P.A., Swanepoel, R., 1989. Viremia and antibody response of small African and laboratory animals to Crimean–Congo hemorrhagic fever virus infection. Am. J. Trop. Med. Hyg. 40, 541–547.

Sherman, P.W., Jarvis, J.U.M., Alexander, R.D. (Eds.), 1991. The Biology of the Naked Mole-Rat. Princeton University Press, Princeton, NJ.

Shi, Y., Buffenstein, R., Pulliam, D.A., Van Remmen, H., 2010. Comparative studies of oxidative stress and mitochondrial function in aging. Integr. Comp. Biol. 50, 869–879.

Shine, H.D., Wyde, P.R., Aguilar-Cordova, E., Chen, S.H., Woo, S.L., Grossman, R.G., et al., 1997. Neurotoxicity of intracerebral injection of a replication-defective adenoviral vector in a semipermissive species (cotton rat). Gene. Ther. 4, 275–279.

Shklair, I.L., Ralls, S.A., 1988. Periodontopathic micro-organisms in the rice rat (Oryzomys palustris). Microbios 55, 25–31.

Shore, R.F., Douben, P.E., 1994. Predicting ecotoxicological impacts of environmental contaminants on terrestrial small mammals. Rev. Environ. Contam. Toxicol. 134, 49–89.

Sikes, R.S., Gannon, W.L., 2011. Guidelines of the American Society of Mammalogists for the use of wild mammals in research. J. Mammal. 92, 235–253.

Silverman, J., Paturzo, F., Smith, A.L., 1982. Effects of experimental infection of the deer mouse (Peromyscus maniculatus) with mouse hepatitis virus. Lab. Anim. Sci. 32, 273–274.

Simpson, G.G., 1945. The principles of classification and a classification of mammals. Bull. Am. Mus. Nat. Hist. 85, 1–350.

Singh, N.B., Srivastava, A., Verma, V.K., Kumar, A., Gupta, S.K., 1984. Mastomys natalensis: a new animal model for Mycobacterium ulcerans research. Indian J. Exp. Biol. 22, 393–394.

Sirigu, P., DiDio, L.J., Gross, S.A., Perra, M.T., 1985. Morphological and histochemical study of the submandibular gland in Praomys (Mastomys) natalensis. Acta Anat. (Basel) 121, 81–83.

Sirigu, P., Gross, S.A., DiDio, L.J., Lantini, M.S., 1988. Histochemical localization of prostaglandin-synthetase in the salivary glands of Praomys (Mastomys) natalensis. Basic Appl. Histochem. 32, 321–325.

Skinner, J.D., Chimimba, C.T., 2006. The Mammals of the Southern African Subregion. Cambridge University Press.

Smedley, F.H., Rimmer, J., Samanidis, A., Wastell, C., 1990. Cell renewal in non-specific duodenitis, ulcer-related duodenitis and duodenal ulcer. Experiments in Mastomys (Praomys natalensis). Digestion 45, 72–79.

Smit, A., van der Bank, H., Falk, T., de Castro, A., 2001. Biochemical genetic markers to identify two morphologically similar South African Mastomys species (Rodentia: Muridae). Biochem. Syst. Ecol. 29, 21–30.

Smith, M., Dodd, J.R., Hobson, H.P., Hoppes, S., 2013. Clinical techniques: surgical removal of elodontomas in the black-tailed prairie dog (Cynomys ludovicianus) and eastern fox squirrel (Sciurus niger). J. Exotic Pet Med. 22, 258–264.

Smith, M.F., 1998. Phylogenetic relationships and geographic structure in pocket gophers in the genus Thomomys. Mol. Phylogenet. Evol. 9, 1–14.

Smolen, M.J., 1981. Microtus pinetorum. Mamm. Species 147, 1–7.

Smyser, T.J., Swihart, R.K., 2014. Allegheny woodrat (Neotoma magister) captive propagation to promote recovery of declining populations. Zoo Biol. 33, 29–35.

Snell, K.C., Hollander, C.F., 1972. Tumors of the testes and seminal vesicles in Praomys (Mastomys) natalensis. J. Natl. Cancer Inst. 49, 1381–1393.

Snell, K.C., Stewart, H.L., 1967. Neoplastic and non-neoplastic renal disease in Praomys (Mastomys) natalensis. J. Natl. Cancer Inst. 39, 95–117.

Snell, K.C., Stewart, H.L., 1969. Hematopoietic neoplasms and related conditions in Praomys (Mastomys) natalensis. J. Natl. Cancer Inst. 42, 175–202.

Snell, K.C., Stewart, H.L., 1975. Spontaneous diseases in a closed colony of Praomys (Mastomys) natalensis. Bull. World Health Organ. 52, 645–650.

Sodja, I., Lim, D., Matouch, O., Seidlova, A., Farnik, J., Svec, J., et al., 1982. Small wild rodents rabies in Czechoslovakia. J. Hyg. Epidemiol. Microbiol. Immunol. 26, 131–140.

Solleveld, H.A., 1987. The multimammate mouse. In: Poole, T.B. (Ed.), The UFAW Handbook on the Care and Management of Laboratory Animals Longman Scientific & Technical, London, pp. 346–359.

Solleveld, H.A., van Zwieten, M.J., Zurcher, C., Hollander, C.F., 1982. A histopathological survey of aged Praomys (mastomys) natalensis. J. Gerontol. 37, 656–665.

Solleveld, H.A., Coolen, J., Haaijman, J.J., Hollander, C.F., Zurcher, C., 1985. Autoimmune thyroiditis. Spontaneous autoimmune thyroiditis in praomys (Mastomys) coucha. Am. J. Pathol. 119, 345–349.

Solomon, H.F., Dixon, D.M., Pouch, W., 1990. A survey of staphylococci isolated from the laboratory gerbil. Lab. Anim. Sci. 40, 316–318.

Solomon, N.G., Vandenbergh, J.G., 1994. Management, breeding, and reproductive performance of pine voles. Lab. Anim. Sci. 44, 613–617.

Somova, L.I., Gregory, M.A., Nxumalo, E.N., 2000. Mongolian gerbil (Meriones unguiculatus) as a model of cerebral infarction for testing new therapeutic agents. Methods Find Exp. Clin. Pharmacol. 22, 203–210.

Sorden, S.D., Watts, T.C., 1996. Spontaneous cardiomyopathy and exophthalmos in cotton rats (Sigmodon hispidus). Vet. Pathol. 33, 375–382.

Soto-Centeno, J.A., Barrow, L.N., Allen, J.M., Reed, D.L., 2013. Reevaluation of a classic phylogeographic barrier: new techniques reveal the influence of microgeographic climate variation on population divergence. Ecol. Evol. 3, 1603–1613.

Soto-Gamboa, M., Gonzalez, S., Hayes, L.D., Ebensperger, L.A., 2009. Validation of a radioimmunoassay for measuring fecal cortisol metabolites in the hystricomorph rodent, Octodon degus. J. Exp. Zool. A Ecol. Genet. Physiol. 311, 496–503.

Spano, R.K., 1994. Ground squirrel management in the Angeles National Forest. Proc. Vertebr. Pest. Conf. 16, 68–71.

Spears, N., Clarke, J.R., 1987. Effect of nutrition, temperature and photoperiod on the rate of sexual maturation of the field vole (Microtus agrestis). J. Reprod. Fertil. 80, 175–181.

Srivastava, R., Gupta, S.K., 1985. Effect of lanosterol on the susceptibility of Mastomys natalensis to Entamoeba histolytica infection. Trans. R. Soc. Trop. Med. Hyg. 79, 422.

Stalling, D.T., 1990. Microtus ochrogaster. Mamm. Species 355, 1–9.

Stallone, J.N., Braun, E.J., 1988. Regulation of plasma antidiuretic hormone in the dehydrated kangaroo rat (Dipodomys spectabilis M.). Gen. Comp. Endocrinol. 69, 119–127.

Stanton, N.L., Shults, L.M., Parker, M., Seville, R.S., 1992. Coccidian assemblages in the Wyoming ground squirrel, Spermophilus elegans elegans. J. Parasitol. 78, 323–328.

Stapp, P., Salkeld, D.J., Franklin, H.A., Kraft, J.P., Tripp, D.W., Antolin, M.F., et al., 2009. Evidence for the involvement of an alternate rodent host in the dynamics of introduced plague in prairie dogs. J. Anim. Ecol. 78, 807–817.

Stewart, H.L., Snell, K.C., 1968. Thymomas and thymic hyperplasia in Praomys (Mastomys) natalensis. Concomitant myositis, myocarditis, and sialodacryoadenitis. J. Natl. Cancer Inst. 40, 1135–1159.

Stewart, H.L., Snell, K.C., 1975. Patterns of neoplastic and nonneoplastic diseases of Praomys (Mastomys) natalensis. Recent Results Cancer Res. 52, 139–144.

Stoenner, H.G., Lackman, D.B., 1957. A new species of Brucella isolated from the desert wood rat, Neotoma lepida Thomas. Am. J. Vet. Res. 18, 947–951.

Storey, D.M., 1993. Filariasis: nutritional interactions in human and animal hosts. Parasitology (107 Suppl), S147–S158.

Storey, K.B., 1997. Metabolic regulation in mammalian hibernation: enzyme and protein adaptations. Comp. Biochem. Physiol. A Physiol. 118, 1115–1124.

Stout, C.A., Duszynski, D.W., 1983. Coccidia from kangaroo rats (Dipodomys spp.) in the western United States, Baja California, and northern Mexico with descriptions of Eimeria merriami sp. n. and Isospora sp. J. Parasitol. 69, 209–214.

Straneva, J.E., Gallati, W.W., 1980. Eimeria strangfordensis sp. n., Eimeria barleyi sp. n., and eimeria antonellii sp. n. from the eastern woodrat (Neotoma floridana) from Pennsylvania. J. Parasitol. 66, 329–332.

Streett Jr., R.P., Highman, B., 1971. Blood chemistry values in normal Mystromys albicaudatus and Osborne-Mendel rats. Lab. Anim. Sci. 21, 394–398.

Streubel, D.P., Fitzgerald, J.P., 1978. Spermophilus tridecemlineatus. Mamm. Species 103, 1–5.

Strittmatter, J., 1972. Elimination of Tyzzer's disease in the Mongolian gerbil (Meriones unguiculatus) by fostering to mice. [German] Eliminierung der Tyzzer's Krankheit bei der Mongolischen Rennmaus (Meriones unguiculatus) durch Ammenaufzucht mit Mausen. Z. Versuchstierkd. 14, 209–214.

Stuhlman, R.A., Wagner, J.E., 1971. Ringtail in Mystromys albicaudatus: a case report. Lab. Anim. Sci. 21, 585–587.

Stuhlman, R.A., Packer, J.T., Doyle, R.E., 1972a. Spontaneous diabetes mellitus in Mystromys albicaudatus. Repeated glucose values from 620 animals. Diabetes 21, 715–721.

Stuhlman, R.A., Packer, J.T., Rose, S.D., 1972b. Repeated blood sampling of Mystromys albicaudatus (white-tailed rat). Lab. Anim. Sci. 22, 268–270.

Stuhlman, R.A., Packer, J.T., Doyle, R.E., Brown, R.V., Townsend, J.F., 1975. Relationship between pancreatic lesions and serum glucose values in Mystromys albicaudatus. Lab. Anim. Sci. 25, 168–174.

Stuhlman, R.A., Srivastava, P.K., Schmidt, G., Vorbedk, M.L., Townsend, J.F., 1974. Characterization of diabetes mellitus in South African hamsters (Mystromys albicaudatus). Diabetologia (10 Suppl), 685–690.

Su, Y.C., Wang, M.H., Wu, M.F., 2001. Cutaneous B cell lymphoma in a Mongolian gerbil (Meriones unguiculatus). Contemp. Top. Lab. Anim. Sci. 40, 53–56.

Suckow, M.A., Terril-Robb, L.A., Grigdesby, C.F., 1996. Gastric trichobezoar in a banner-tailed kangaroo rat (Dipodomys spectabilis). Lab. Anim. 30, 383–385.

Suedmeyer, W.K., Pace, L., 1994. Management of an epiglottal fibrosarcoma in a black-tailed prairie dog (Cynomys ludovicianus). J. Sm. Exot. Anim. Med. 2, 163–164.

Sugita, S., Uchiumi, O., Fujiwara, K., Niida, S., Fukuta, K., 1995. Brain deformation caused by hyperplasia molar teeth (macrodonts) in the Japanese field vole (Microtus montebelli). [Japanese]. Exp. Anim. 43, 769–772.

Sullivan, J., Holsinger, K.E., Simon, C., 1996. The effect of topology on estimates of among-site rate variation. J. Mol. Evol. 42, 308–312.

Sun, P., Smith, A.S., Lei, K., Liu, Y., Wang, Z., 2014. Breaking bonds in male prairie vole: long-term effects on emotional and social behavior, physiology, and neurochemistry. Behav. Brain Res. 265, 22–31.

Suswillo, R.R., Nelson, G.S., Muller, R., McGreevy, P.B., Duke, B.O., Denham, D.A., 1977. Attempts to infect jirds (Meriones unguiculatus) with Wuchereria bancrofti, Onchocerca volvulus, Loa loa loa and Mansonella ozzardi. J. Helminthol. 51, 132–134.

Swensen, S.R., Telford, I.R., 1973. Lipofuscin distribution and histological lesions in the vitamin E deficient cotton rat (Sigmodon hispidus hispidus). Arch. Histol. Jpn. 35, 327–341.

Swindle, M.M., Hulebak, K.L., Yarbrough, B.A., 1985. Haematology and pathology of captive southern grasshopper mice (Onychomys torridus). Lab. Anim. 19, 195–199.

Tajima, K., 1981. A light and electron microscopic study on N-butyl-N-nitroso urethane induced esophageal carcinomas of Mastomys and rats. Acta Med. Biol. (Niigata) 28, 85–117.

Talmage, S.S., Walton, B.T., 1991. Small mammals as monitors of environmental contaminants. Rev. Environ. Contam. Toxicol. 119, 47–145.

Tan, C.H., Tachezy, R., Van Ranst, M., Chan, S.Y., Bernard, H.U., Burk, R.D., 1994. The Mastomys natalensis papillomavirus: nucleotide sequence, genome organization, and phylogenetic relationship of a rodent papillomavirus involved in tumorigenesis of cutaneous epithelia. Virology 198, 534–541.

Taylor, A.C., Butcher, E.O., 1951. The regulation of eruption rate in the incisor teeth of the white rat. J. Exp. Zool. 117, 165–188.

Taylor, G.N., Lloyd, R.D., Mays, C.W., 1993. Liver cancer induction by 239Pu, 241Am, and thorotrast in the grasshopper mouse, Onychomys leukogaster. Health Phys. 64, 141–146.

Taylor, J.M., 1968. Reproductive mechanisms of the female southern grasshopper mouse, Onychomys torridus longicaudus. J. Mammal. 49, 303–309.

Taylor, S.A., Salo, A.L., Dewsbury, D.A., 1992. Estrus induction in four species of voles (Microtus). J. Comp. Psychol. 106, 366–373.

Temmerman, A.M., Vonk, R.J., Niezen-Koning, K., Berger, R., Fernandes, J., 1988. Long-term and short-term effects of dietary cholesterol and fats in the Mongolian gerbil. Ann. Nutr. Metab. 32, 177–185.

Tennant, B.C., Mrosovsky, N., McLean, K., Cote, P.J., Korba, B.E., Engle, R.E., et al., 1991. Hepatocellular carcinoma in Richardson's ground squirrels (Spermophilus richardsonii): evidence for association with hepatitis B-like virus infection. Hepatology 13, 1215–1221.

Termer, E.A., Glomski, C.A., 1978. Cellular blood picture of Mongolian gerbil throughout 1st year of life – longitudinal-study. Exp. Hematol. 6, 499–504.

Terrell, S.P., Origgi, F.C., Agnew, D., 2012. Glomerulonephropathy in aged captive Key Largo woodrats (Neotoma floridana smalli). Vet. Pathol. 49, 710–716.

Thiessen, D.D., Yahr, P., 1977. The Gerbil in Behavioral Investigations: Mechanisms of Territoriality and Olfactory Communication. University of Texas Press, Austin, TX.

Thomas, H.H., Best, T.L., Lydeard, C., 1991. Parasitic and phoretic arthropods of the elephant-eared and the Santa Cruz kangaroo rats. J. Wildl. Dis. 27, 358–360.

Thomas, R.E., Barnes, A.M., Quan, T.J., Beard, M.L., Carter, L.G., Hopla, C.E., 1988. Susceptibility to Yersinia pestis in the northern grasshopper mouse (Onychomys leucogaster). J. Wildl. Dis. 24, 327–333.

Thomas, R.E., Beard, M.L., Quan, T.J., Carter, L.G., Barnes, A.M., Hopla, C.E., 1989. Experimentally induced plague infection in the northern grasshopper mouse (Onychomys leucogaster) acquired by consumption of infected prey. J. Wildl. Dis. 25, 477–480.

Tian, X., Azpurua, J., Hine, C., Vaidya, A., Myakishev-Rempel, M., Ablaeva, J., et al., 2013. High-molecular-mass hyaluronan mediates the cancer resistance of the naked mole rat. Nature 499, 346–349.

Tielemans, Y., Vierendeels, T., Willems, G., 1987. Histochemical and proliferative changes preceding the onset of spontaneous gastric adenocarcinoma in Mastomys natalensis. Virchows Arch. A Pathol. Anat. Histopathol. 411, 275–281.

Tikasingh, E.S., Jonkers, A.H., Spence, L., Aitken, T.H., 1966. Nariva virus, a hitherto undescribed agent isolated from the Trinidadian rat, Zygodontomys b. brevicauda (J. A. Allen & Chapman). Am. J. Trop. Med. Hyg. 15, 235–238.

Torrez Martinez, N., Bharadwaj, M., Goade, D., Delury, J., Moran, P., Hicks, B., et al., 1998. Bayou virus-associated hantavirus pulmonary syndrome in Eastern Texas: identification of the rice rat, Oryzomys palustris, as reservoir host. Emerg. Infect. Dis. 4, 105–111.

Tortora, D.F., Eyer, J.C., Overmann, S.R., 1974. The effect of sand deprivation on sandbathing and marking in Mongolian gerbils (Meriones unguiculatus). Behav. Biol. 11, 403–407.

Towe, A.L., Harrison, T.A., 1993. Cerebral response to pyramidal tract stimulation in wood rats and its relation to laboratory rats. Exp. Brain Res. 97, 311–316.

Townzen, K.-R., Thompson, M.-A., Smith, C.-R., 1996. Investigations and management of epizootic plague at ice house reservoir, Eldorado National Forest, California, 1994 and 1995. Proc. Vertebr. Pest. Conf. 17, 68–74.

Traystman, R.J., 2003. Animal models of focal and global cerebral ischemia. ILAR J. 44, 85–95.

Trigo, F.J., Riser, M., 1981. A squamous cell carcinoma in a California ground squirrel (Spermophilus beecheyi). J. Wildl. Dis. 17, 405–408.

Tripathi, B.J., Tripathi, R.C., Borisuth, N.S., Dhaliwal, R., Dhaliwal, D., 1991. Rodent models of congenital and hereditary cataract in man. Lens. Eye Toxic. Res. 8, 373–413.

Trpis, M., 1994. Aedes (Gymnometopa) mediovittatus (Diptera: Culicidae) as an experimental vector of Brugia pahangi and B. malayi (Spirurida: Filariidae). J. Med. Entomol. 31, 442–444.

Tsai, J.C., Garlinghouse, G., McDonnell, P.J., Trousdale, M.D., 1992. An experimental animal model of adenovirus-induced ocular disease. The cotton rat. Arch. Ophthalmol. 110, 1167–1170.

Tsanava, Sh.A., Marennikova, S.S., Sakvarelidze, L.A., Shelukhina, E.M., Ianova, N.N., 1989. Isolation of cowpox virus from the red-tailed jird. [Russian] Vydelenie virusa ospy korov ot krasnokhvostoi peschanki. Vopr. Virusol. 34, 95–97.

Tsubota, K., Inoue, H., Ando, K., Ono, M., Yoshino, K., Saito, I., 1998. Adenovirus-mediated gene transfer to the ocular surface epithelium. Exp. Eye Res. 67, 531–538.

Tullberg, T., 1899. Ueber das System der Nagethiere: Eine Phylogenetische Studie, Akademische Buchdruckerei, Upsala, MN.

Turell, M.J., Rossignol, P.A., Spielman, A., Rossi, C.A., Bailey, C.L., 1984. Enhanced arboviral transmission by mosquitoes that concurrently ingested microfilariae. Science 225, 1039–1041.

Ubelaker, J.E., Wilkerson, L.D., Leveson, J.E., Marengorowe, A.J., 1993. Blood chemical changes in cotton rats, Sigmodon hispidus, infected with Parastrongylus costaricensis (Nematoda: Angiostrongyloidea). Trans. Am. Microsc. Soc. 112, 217–229.

Une, Y., Tatara, S., Nomura, Y., Takahashi, R., Saito, Y., 1996. Hepatitis and hepatocellular carcinoma in two prairie dogs (Cynomys ludovicianus). J. Vet. Med. Sci. 58, 933–935.

Ungvari, Z., Krasnikov, B.F., Csiszar, A., Labinskyy, N., Mukhopadhyay, P., Pacher, P., et al., 2008. Testing hypotheses of aging in long-lived mice of the genus Peromyscus: association between longevity and mitochondrial stress resistance, ROS detoxification pathways, and DNA repair efficiency. Age (Dordr) 30, 121–133.

Upton, S.J., Fridell, R.A., Tilley, M., 1989. Trypanosoma kansasensis sp. n. from Neotoma floridana in Kansas. J. Wildl. Dis. 25, 410–412.

Upton, S.J., McAllister, C.T., Brillhart, D.B., Duszynski, D.W., Wash, C.D., 1992. Cross-transmission studies with Eimeria arizonensis-like oocysts (Apicomplexa) in New World rodents of the Genera baiomys, Neotoma, Onychomys, Peromyscus, and Reithrodontomys (Muridae). J. Parasitol. 78, 406–413.

Urquiza, R., Rico, F., Figuerola, J.A., 1988. The gerbil (Meriones unguiculatus) in auditory research. [Spanish] El jerbo (Meriones unguiculatus) en investigacion auditiva. Acta Otorrinolaringol. Esp. 39, 227–233.

van Groen, T., Kadish, I., Popovic, N., Popovic, M., Caballero-Bleda, M., Bano-Otalora, B., et al., 2011. Age-related brain pathology in Octodon degu: blood vessel, white matter and Alzheimer-like pathology. Neurobiol. Aging 32, 1651–1661.

Vaughan, J.A., Mehus, J.O., Brewer, C.M., Kvasager, D.K., Bauer, S., Vaughan, J.L., et al., 2012. Theoretical potential of passerine filariasis to enhance the enzootic transmission of West Nile virus. J. Med. Entomol. 49, 1430–1441.

Veenstra, A.J.F., 1958. Behaviour of the multimammate mouse, Rattus (Mastomys) natalensis (A. Smith). Anim. Behav. 6, 195–206.

Veres, M., Duselis, A.R., Graft, A., Pryor, W., Crossland, J., Vrana, P.B., et al., 2012. The biology and methodology of assisted reproduction in deer mice (Peromyscus maniculatus). Theriogenology 77, 311–319.

Veres, M., Payne, S., Fernandes, P., Crossland, J.P., Szalai, G., 2013. Improved technique for induction and monitoring of audiogenic seizure in deer mice. Lab. Anim. (NY) 42, 166–169.

Vigen, R.A., Chen, D., Zhao, C.M., 2012. Pathobiology of gastric carcinoids and adenocarcinomas in rodent models and patients: Studies of gastrocystoplasty, gender-related factors and autophagy. Front. Gastrointest. Res. 30, 202–211.

Villela, O.M.M., Alho, C.J.R., 1983. Postnatal development and growth of Oryzomys subflavus (Rodentia: Cricetidae) in laboratory setting. Rev. Bras. Biol. 43, 321–326.

Vincent, A.L., Ash, L.R., 1978. Further observations on spontaneous neoplasms in the Mongolian gerbil, Meriones unguiculatus. Lab. Anim. Sci. 28, 297–300.

Vincent, A.L., Porter, D.D., Ash, L.R., 1975. Spontaneous lesions and parasites of the Mongolian gerbil, Meriones unguiculatus. Lab. Anim. Sci. 25, 711–722.

Vincent, A.L., Rodrick, G.E., Sodeman Jr., W.A., 1979. The pathology of the Mongolian Gerbil (Meriones unguiculatus): a review. Lab. Anim. Sci. 29, 645–651.

Voss, R.S., 1991. An introduction to the Neotropical muroid rodent genus Zygodontomys. Bull. Am. Mus. Nat. Hist. 210, 1–113.

Voss, R.S., 1992. A revision of the South American species of Sigmodon (Mammalia: Muridae) with notes on their natural history and biogeography. Am. Mus. Novit. 3050, 1–56.

Voss, R.S., Heideman, P.D., Mayer, V.L., Donnelly, T.M., 1992. Husbandry, reproduction and postnatal development of the neotropical muroid rodent Zygodontomys brevicauda. Lab. Anim. 26, 38–46.

Vucetic, M., Stancic, A., Otasevic, V., Jankovic, A., Korac, A., Markelic, M., et al., 2013. The impact of cold acclimation and hibernation on antioxidant defenses in the ground squirrel (Spermophilus citellus): an update. Free Radic. Biol. Med. 65, 916–924.

Waggie, K.S., Marion, P.L., 1997. Demodex sp. in California ground squirrels. J. Wildl. Dis. 33, 368–370.

Waggie, K.S., Ganaway, J.R., Wagner, J.E., Spencer, T.H., 1984. Experimentally induced Tyzzer's disease in Mongolian gerbils (Meriones unguiculatus). Lab. Anim. Sci. 34, 53–57.

Waggie, K.S., Thornburg, L.P., Wagner, J.E., 1986. Experimentally induced Tyzzer's disease in the African white-tailed rat (Mystromys albicaudatus). Lab. Anim. Sci. 36, 492–495.

Wagner, R.A., 1999. Diagnosing odontomas in prairie dogs. Exotic. DVM 1, 7–10.

Wallach, J.D., Boever, W.J. (Eds.), 1983. Diseases of Exotic Animals: Medical and Surgical Management W. B. Saunders, Philadelphia, PA.

Wang, T.C., Fox, J.G., 1998. Helicobacter pylori and gastric cancer: Koch's postulates fulfilled? Gastroenterology 115, 780–783.

Wanji, S., Tendongfor, N., Vuong, P.N., Enyong, P., Bain, O., 2002. The migration and localization of Loa loa infective and fourth-stage larvae in normal and immunosuppressed rodents. Ann. Trop. Med. Parasitol. 96, 823–830.

Waring, G.H., 1970. Sound communications of black-tailed, white-tailed and Gunnison's prairie dogs. Am. Midl. Nat. 83, 167–185.

Watanabe, T., Tada, M., Nagai, H., Sasaki, S., Nakao, M., 1998. Helicobacter pylori infection induces gastric cancer in mongolian gerbils. Gastroenterology 115, 642–648.

Waterhouse, G.R., 1839. Mammalia [With a notice and ranges, by Charles Darwin]. Smith, Elder, London.

Wayss, K., Reyes-Mayes, D., Volm, M., 1981. Chemical carcinogenesis by the two-stage protocol in the skin Mastomys natalensis (Muridae) using topical initiation with 7,12-dimethylbenz(a)anthracene and topical promotion with 12-0-tetradecanoylphorbol-13-acetate. Virchows Arch. B Cell Pathol. Incl. Mol. Pathol. 38, 13–21.

Webb, R.E., Leslie Jr., D.M., Lochmiller, R.L., Masters, R.E., 2003. Immune function and hematology of male cotton rats (Sigmodon hispidus) in response to food supplementation and methionine. Comp. Biochem. Physiol. A Mol. Integr. Physiol. 136, 577–589.

Weber, D.K., Danielson, K., Wright, S., Foley, J.E., 2002. Hematology and serum biochemistry values of dusky-footed wood rat (Neotoma fuscipes). J. Wildl. Dis. 38, 576–582.

Webster, W.D., 1987. Kyphosis in the marsh rice rat (Oryzomys palustris). J. Wildl. Dis. 23, 171–172.

Weir, B.J., 1970. The management and breeding of some more hystricomorph rodents. Lab. Anim. 4, 83–97.

Wenzlow, N., Stanley, R.L., Patterson-Kane, J.C., 2008. B cell lymphoma causing splenomegaly in a Sundevall's jird (Meriones crassus subspecies perpallidus). Vet. Rec. 162, 455–456.

Wheat, B.E., Ernst, J.V., 1974. Eimeria glauceae sp. n. and Eimeria dusii sp. n. (Protozoa: Eimeriidae) from the eastern woodrat, Neotoma floridana, from Alabama. J. Parasitol. 60, 403–405.

White, D.J., Waldron, M.M., 1969. Naturally-occurring Tyzzer's disease in the gerbil. Vet. Rec. 85, 111–114.

Wightman, S.R., Pilitt, P.A., Wagner, J.E., 1978a. Dentostomella translucida in the Mongolian gerbil (Meriones unguiculatus). Lab. Anim. Sci. 28, 290–296.

Wightman, S.R., Wagner, J.E., Corwin, R.M., 1978b. Syphacia obvelata in the Mongolian gerbil (Meriones unguiculatus): natural occurrence and experimental transmission. Lab. Anim. Sci. 28, 51–54.

Wightman, S.R., Mann, P.C., Wagner, J.E., 1980. Dihydrostreptomycin toxicity in the Mongolian gerbil, Meriones unguiculatus. Lab. Anim. Sci. 30, 71–75.

Wilber, P.G., McBee, K., Hafner, D.J., Duszynski, D.W., 1994. A new coccidian (Apicomplexa: Eimeriidae) in the northern pocket gopher (Thomomys talpoides) and a comparison of oocyst survival in hosts from radon-rich and radon-poor soils. J. Wildl. Dis. 30, 359–364.

Wiley, R.W., 1980. Neotoma floridana. Mamm. Species 139, 1–7.

Williams, C.S.F., 1980. Wild rats in research. In: Baker, H.J., Lindsey, J.R., Weisbroth, S.H. (Eds.), The Laboratory Rat. II. Research Applications Academic Press, San Diego, CA, pp. 245–256.

Williams, S.H., Peiffer, E., Ford, S., 2009. Gape and bite force in the rodents Onychomys leucogaster and Peromyscus maniculatus: does jaw-muscle anatomy predict performance? J. Morphol. 270, 1338–1347.

Wilson, D.E., Reeder, D.M., 1993. Mammal Species of the World: A Taxonomic and Geographic Reference. Smithsonian Institution Press, Washington, DC.

Wisniewski, P.J., 1985. The Libyan jird in captivity. Int. Zoo News (IZN) 32, 16–18.

Wobeser, G., Cawthorn, R.J., Gajadhar, A.A., 1983. Pathology of Sarcocystis campestris infection in Richardson's ground squirrels (Spermophilus richardsoni). Can. J. Comp. Med. 47, 198–202.

Wobeser, G., Ngeleka, M., Appleyard, G., Bryden, L., Mulvey, M.R., 2007. Tularemia in deer mice (Peromyscus maniculatus) during a population irruption in Saskatchewan, Canada. J. Wildl. Dis. 43, 23–31.

Wolfe, J.L., 1982. Oryzomys palustris. Mamm. Species 176, 1–5.

Wood, A.E., 1965. Grades and clades among rodents. Evolution 19, 115–130.

Wood, A.E., 1985. The relationships, origin and dispersal of the hystricognathous rodents. In: Luckett, W.P., Hartenberger, J.-L. (Eds.), Evolutionary Relationships Among Rodents. Springer, US, pp. 475–513.

Wood, F.D., 1936. Trypanosoma Neotomae, sp. nov., in the Dusky-Footed Wood Rat and the Wood Rat Flea. University of California Press, Berkeley, CA.

Woods, C.A., Boraker, D., 1975. Octodon degus. Mamm. Species 67, 1–5.

Woods, F.N., 1974. Leptospira interrogans in the Ballum serogroup from a vole, Microtus oeconomus (Pallas) in Alaska. J. Wildl. Dis. 10, 325–326.

Worgul, B.V., Rothstein, H., 1975. Congenital cataracts associated with disorganized meridional rows in a new laboratory animal: the degu (Octodon degus). Biomedicine 23, 1–4.

Worth, C.B., 1950. Observations on the behavior and breeding of captive rice rats and wood rats. J. Mammal. 31, 421–426.

Worth, C.B., 1967. Reproduction, development and behavior of captive Oryzomys laticeps and Zygodontomys brevicauda in Trinidad. Lab. Anim. Care 17, 355–361.

Wu, P.J., Greeley, E.H., Hansen, L.G., Segre, M., 1999. Hematology values from clinically healthy Peromyscus leucopus. J. Zoo Wildl. Med. 30, 589–590.

Yahav, S., Buffenstein, R., 1991. Huddling behavior facilitates homeothermy in the naked mole rat Heterocephalus glaber. Physiol. Zool. 64, 871–884.

Yamamoto-Fukuda, T., Takahashi, H., Koji, T., 2011. Animal models of middle ear cholesteatoma. J. Biomed. Biotechnol. 2011, 11.

Yamamoto, R.S., Kroes, R., Weisburger, J.H., 1972. Carcinogenicity of diethylnitrosamine in Mystromys albicaudatus (African white-tailed rat). Proc. Soc. Exp. Biol. Med. 140, 890–892.

Yamamoto, Y., Noguchi, Y., Noguchi, A., Nakayama, K., Mochida, K., Takano, K., et al., 1999. Serum biochemical values in two inbred strains of mastomys (Praomys coucha). Exp. Anim. 48, 293–295.

Yasukawa, N., Michael, S.D., Christian, J.J., 1978. Estrous cycle regulation in the white-footed mouse (Peromyscus leucopus) with special reference to vaginal cast formation. Lab. Anim. Sci. 28, 46–50.

Yei, S., Mittereder, N., Wert, S., Whitsett, J.A., Wilmott, R.W., Trapnell, B.C., 1994. In vivo evaluation of the safety of adenovirus-mediated transfer of the human cystic fibrosis transmembrane conductance regulator cDNA to the lung. Hum. Gene. Ther. 5, 731–744.

Yesus, Y.W., Esterly, J.A., Stuhlman, R.A., Townsend, J.F., 1976. Significant muscle capillary basement membrane thickening in spontaneously diabetic Mystromys albicaudatus. Diabetes 25, 444–449.

Yim, K., Miles, B., Zinsou, R., Prince, G., Boukhvalova, M., 2012. Efficacy of trivalent inactivated influenza vaccines in the cotton rat Sigmodon hispidus model. Vaccine 30, 1291–1296.

Yoerg, S.I., Shier, D.M., 1997. Maternal presence and rearing condition affect responses to a live predator in kangaroo rats (Dipodomys heermanni arenae). J. Comp. Psychol. 111, 362–369.

Yokomori, K., Okada, N., Murai, Y., Goto, N., Fujiwara, K., 1989. Enterohepatitis in Mongolian gerbils (Meriones unguiculatus) inoculated perorally with Tyzzer's organism (Bacillus piliformis). Lab. Anim. Sci. 39, 16–20.

Young, K.A., Gobrogge, K.L., Liu, Y., Wang, Z., 2011. The neurobiology of pair bonding: insights from a socially monogamous rodent. Front. Neuroendocrinol. 32, 53–69.

Young, L.J., Thomas, J.W. and McGraw, L.A., 2014. Emory University, Atlanta, GA. Vole Genomics Initiative., at <http://www.research.yerkes.emory.edu/Youngcollaborators.html>, (accessed January 2014.).

Zahner, H., Gorkow, C., Soulsby, E.J., Schutze, H.R., Geyer, E., Reiner, G., 1987a. Homocytotropic antibodies of the multimammate rat, Mastomys natalensis. Demonstration and characterization of 2 types classified as IgE and IgG3. Z. Versuchstierkd. 29, 243–256.

Zahner, H., Soulsby, E.J., Weidner, E., Sanger, I., Lammler, G., 1987b. Reaginic and homocytotropic IgG antibody response of Mastomys natalensis in experimental infections of filarial parasites (Litomosoides carinii, Dipetalonema viteae, Brugia malayi, B. pahangi). Parasitol. Res. 73, 271–280.

Zarate, M.L., Scherer, W.F., 1968. Contact-spread of Venezuelan equine encephalomyelitis virus among cotton rats via urine or feces and the naso- or oropharynx. A possible transmission cycle in nature. Am. J. Trop. Med. Hyg. 17, 894–899.

Zeidner, N.S., Carter, L.G., Monteneiri, J.A., Petersen, J.M., Schriefer, M., Gage, K.L., et al., 2004. An outbreak of Francisella tularensis in captive prairie dogs: an immunohistochemical analysis. J. Vet. Diagn. Invest. 16, 150–152.

Zeman, F.J., 1967. A semipurified diet for the Mongolian Gerbil (Meriones unguiculatus). J. Nutr. 91, 415–420.

Zhou, D., Tong, Z., Song, Y., Han, Y., Pei, D., Pang, X., et al., 2004. Genetics of metabolic variations between Yersinia pestis biovars and the proposal of a new biovar, microtus. J. Bacteriol. 186, 5147–5152.

Zielke, E., 1979. Attempts to infect Meriones unguiculatus and Mastomys natalensis with Wuchereria bancrofti from West Africa. Tropenmed. Parasitol. 30, 466–468.

Zielke, E., 1980. On the longevity and behaviour of microfilariae of Wuchereria bancrofti, Brugia pahangi and Dirofilaria immitis transfused to laboratory rodents. Trans. R. Soc. Trop. Med. Hyg. 74, 456–458.

Zima, J., Macholan, M., Misek, I., Sterba, O., 1992. Sex chromosome abnormalities in natural populations of the common vole (Microtus arvalis). Hereditas 117, 203–207.

Zimmerman, E.G., 1970. Karyology, systematics and chromosomal evolution in the rodent genus, Sigmodon. Publ. Mus. Mich. State Univ. Biol. 4, 385–454.

CHAPTER

8

The Laboratory Woodchuck (*Marmota monax*)

Christine A. Bellezza, DVM[a], Sandra Sexton, DVM, DACLAM[b], Leslie I. Curtin, DVM[b], Patrick W. Concannon, MS, PhD[c], Betty H. Baldwin, BS, MS[d], Lou Ann Graham[d], William E. Hornbuckle, DVM, BS[d], Lois Roth, DVM, PhD, DACVP[e] and Bud C. Tennant, DVM, DACVIM[d]

[a]Office of Research Integrity and Assurance, Office of the Vice Provost for Research, Cornell University, Ithaca, NY, USA [b]Laboratory Animal Services, Roswell Park Cancer Institute, Buffalo, NY, USA [c]Cornell University, Department of Biomedical Sciences, Ithaca, NY, USA [d]Department of Clinical Sciences, College of Veterinary Medicine, Cornell University, Ithaca, NY, USA [e]Department of Pathology, MSPCA Angell Memorial, Boston, MA, USA

OUTLINE

© 2015 Elsevier Inc. All rights reserved.

I. INTRODUCTION

A. Major Taxonomic Considerations

The Eastern woodchuck, *Marmota monax*, is in the family Sciuridae of the order Rodentia. Common names include groundhog, whistle-pig, and chuck. Natural distribution includes the Eastern and Midwestern United States, Southeastern Alaska, and Southern Canada. The woodchuck is a large, burrow-digging animal with a thickset body, short legs, long claws, broad flat head, almost no neck, small, round ears, and a short, hairy tail (Fig. 8.1). Adults in captivity reach an average body size of 3–5 kg in males, and 2.5–5 kg in females. Colors vary from a grizzly gray-brown to reddish, with a darker head and black feet. Black as well as white (presumably albino) woodchucks have been reported. The fur consists of a soft dense undercoat and a longer, coarse upper fur.

B. Use in Research

Woodchucks are obligate hibernators in the wild, and have an annual cycle that involves large changes in food intake, body weight, and metabolic state. Body weight increases 25–100% during the spring and summer, and decreases by 15–50% during autumn and winter hibernation. There is a brief breeding season immediately following emergence from hibernation (Hamilton, Jr. 1934; Concannon *et al.*, 1990). Similar changes occur in laboratory maintained woodchucks, even when prevented from entering a deep-hibernation state and constantly maintained in natural photoperiod and at room temperature. Captive and laboratory reared-woodchucks have been used as models to study food intake, obesity, and energy balance (Bailey, 1965; Fall, 1971; Young, 1984; Rawson

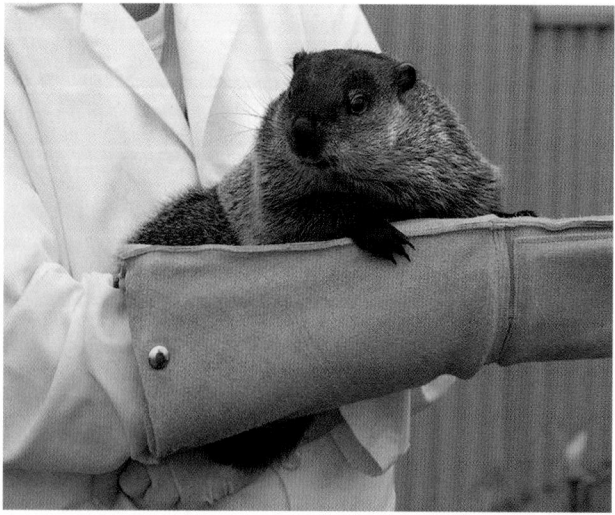

FIGURE 8.1 Laboratory reared woodchuck held with primate restraining glove.

et al., 1998); endogenous circannual cycles (Concannon *et al.*, 1992); photoperiod entrainment of circannual cycles (Concannon *et al.*, 1997a); seasonal breeding (Christian *et al.*, 1972; Baldwin *et al.*, 1985; Concannon *et al.*, 1990); hibernation (Davis, 1977; Spurrier *et al.*, 1987); and viral hepatitis and its sequelae including hepatocellular carcinoma (Popper *et al.*, 1987). There are indigenous populations of woodchucks that have a high incidence of woodchuck hepatitis virus (WHV) infection. The use of the laboratory woodchuck as a model for viral hepatitis has also resulted in the use of hepatitis-positive animals in the evaluation of antiviral compounds.

Laboratory maintained woodchucks typically are not subjected to hibernation-inducing conditions of food withdrawal and cold-room temperatures, except where the goal is to study aspects of hibernation or role of temperature in regulation of circannual cycles. In the absence of such conditions and deep hibernation, the animals nevertheless continue to undergo circannual changes in metabolic and reproductive activity. However, circannual cycles in the laboratory then tend to advance, with animals breeding 2–8 weeks earlier than in the wild (Concannon *et al.*, 1997b). The use of artificial photoperiod to synchronize the circannual cycles of animals in a group or colony is important for reproduction and synchronization of metabolic cycles among animals (Concannon *et al.*, 1996; Concannon *et al.*, 1997a). The possible asynchrony among animals of the circannual changes in metabolic state should be considered with any use of woodchucks as experimental animals. The biology of circannual cycles and seasonal breeding is considered in detail in subsequent sections.

C. Availability and Sources

Woodchucks are easily trapped from the wild (Young and Sims, 1979). Captive animals may be used as breeding stock to form colonies of defined animals adapted to laboratory conditions and free from WHV infection and other diseases common to wild woodchucks. Prior to trapping woodchucks, state laws concerning the capture of animals for research should be investigated. Newly captured woodchucks should be examined for signs of illness or abnormal behavior, tattooed for permanent identification, and dusted with an insecticidal powder. They should be bled periodically, assessed for WHV status, and isolated for 6 months before being introduced to the colony. While it is difficult to accurately age adult woodchucks, it is possible to distinguish juveniles (<1 year) and yearlings from adults (Young and Sims, 1979).

The prevalence of WHV in feral woodchucks is not known. However, several studies have demonstrated a marked dichotomy in the percentage of WHV positive woodchucks between geographical areas (Tyler *et al.*, 1981; Wong *et al.*, 1982; Tennant and Gerin, 1994). Woodchucks from New York and New England may be preferable to woodchucks from the Mid-Atlantic region as foundation animals for breeding colonies. Woodchucks are also commercially available, and it is possible to purchase woodchucks born and bred in captivity, woodchucks infected with WHV, and woodchucks that are certifiably free of the infection.

D. General Laboratory Management and Husbandry

1. Housing

Woodchucks may be housed in metal cages designed for rabbits, dogs or cats. Modifications need to be made because woodchucks have sharp incisors, considerable strength, and climbing ability. They can escape through any hole large enough to admit their heads which requires reducing gaps greater than 1½ inches. Latches may be necessary to secure the corners of the doors. Food and water dishes as well as cage floors must be secured so that woodchucks cannot remove them.

Solid floors are preferable to slatted floors for several reasons. The large, soft feces of woodchucks do not fall through slats into collection pans and thorough cleaning of slatted floors is difficult. Slats are also used as toeholds and may result in toenails being ripped.

Woodchucks may also be housed in large pens or runs. The tops of chain link pens must be enclosed. Woodchucks positive for WHV are housed in Horsfall cages because of the potential biohazard and transmission of WHV to negative woodchucks.

Wooden or metal nest boxes provide a burrow-like environment for woodchucks. Woodchucks typically hide in nestboxes in response to noise or movement making it easier to catch and handle them. The boxes facilitate cleaning cages since woodchucks will usually remain calm inside boxes.

Bedding material such as woodchips should be provided. Woodchucks carry bedding into boxes for nesting, and will use bedding for covering their feces. Most woodchucks are fastidious, defecating in one corner of their cage, and will use food to cover up feces if they are not provided with bedding material.

Water should be supplied *ad libitum*; woodchucks drink large amounts especially during periods of high food consumption. Water can be supplied in large ceramic bowls which are difficult to tip over, or in heavy glass bottles with sipper tubes.

Woodchucks can be successfully maintained at 17–23°C. Woodchucks are sensitive to high environmental temperatures and air conditioners and/or fans should be used, if necessary, to keep them cool in summer or warm climates. Humidity can be maintained at approximately 50% using humidifiers; lower humidity levels have been associated with a ring-tail like syndrome in pups.

Light cycles should approximate normal day length. Light cycles can be adjusted daily, weekly, or monthly to correspond to seasonal changes in day length.

2. Identification

As a temporary means of identification, the fur may be clipped or dyed. Tattoo ink on fur lasts about one week. Hair growth occurs rapidly between late May and October and clipped areas should be rechecked weekly.

Ear tags, ear notches, and tattoos can be used for more permanent identification of woodchucks. Tattooing is preferred because trauma to the ear can cause the tag to be removed or the notch to be altered. Tattoos are best placed on the chest or inner thigh where the hair is thin. The hair over the tattoo must be clipped periodically to maintain visibility. When tattooing, the area should be first clipped and surgically scrubbed and an antibiotic ointment applied after the tattoo. Tattoo needles should be changed between animals and gas sterilized before reuse.

3. Handling and Restraint

Woodchucks have powerful jaws and large incisors and are capable of inflicting serious bite wounds. Using a nest box equipped with a handle facilitates removal of the animal from its cage while minimizing stress, and may be used for short term transportation. Calmer woodchucks can be carried with a gloved hand underneath and supporting the body (Fig. 8.1). Fractious or aggressive woodchucks can be removed from their cage by either grasping the tail and lifting them off the floor of the cage or they can be encouraged to enter a metal, mail box shaped, restraining and transport cage (Fig. 8.2) and the cage closed with a custom-fitted cover (Fig. 8.3). Manual handling and restraint is best accomplished using elk hide elbow-length primate handling gloves.

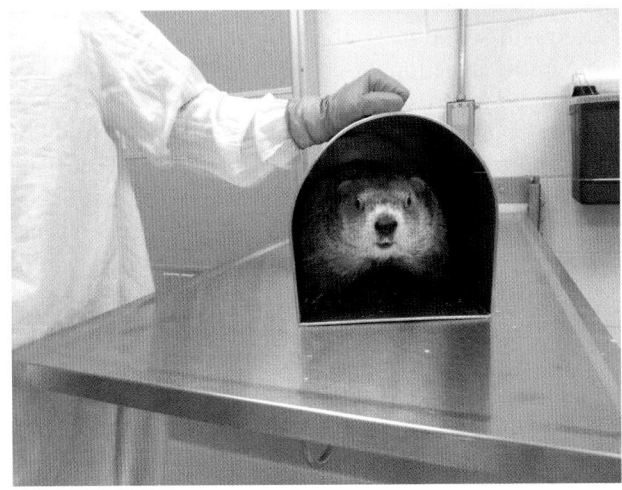

FIGURE 8.2 Laboratory woodchuck after voluntary entry into metal 'mail box' restraining device.

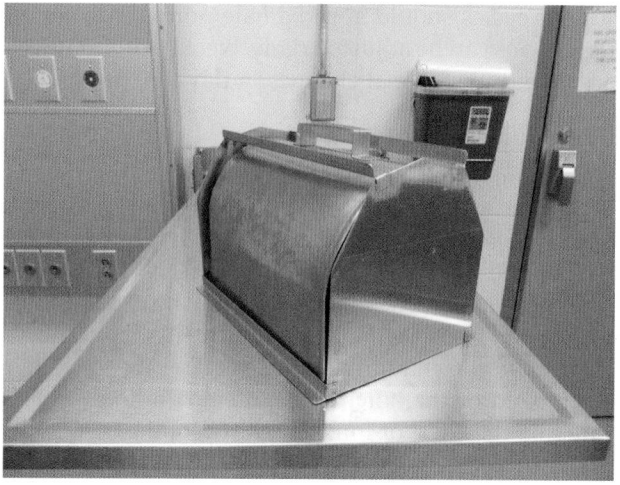

FIGURE 8.3 The door of the metal 'mail box' restraining device has been closed and can be used to transport the woodchuck locally.

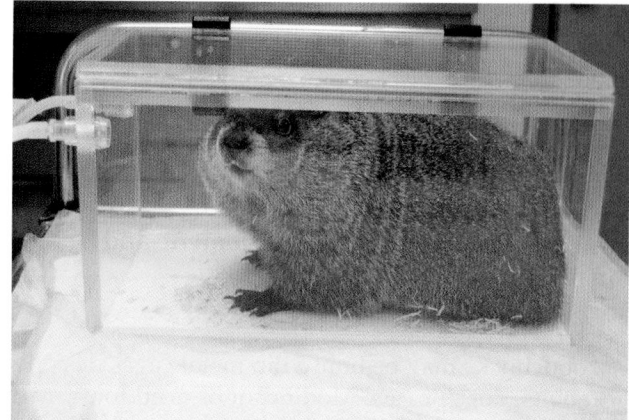

FIGURE 8.4 The transparent plastic box use for induction of anesthesia.

The gloved hand is used to pin the animal's head to the examination table by applying gentle pressure to the back of the neck. The opposite hand then grasps the base of the tail. Once immobilized, most woodchucks calm down, and minor manipulations such as intramuscular injections can be performed. Squeeze boxes have also been used to handle woodchucks (Snyder, 1985), however they can be awkward to use in confined spaces and require additional time and effort.

4. Anesthesia

Chemical restraint is necessary for most manipulations of woodchucks. In the authors' experience, ketamine (50 mg/kg) in combination with xylazine (5 mg/kg) IM has proved to be safe and effective for phlebotomy and short surgical procedures. Lower doses may be effective in animals anesthetized infrequently, but may result in a shorter duration of action. Anesthesia is induced in approximately 5 minutes and lasts up to 20 minutes. If adequate sedation is not achieved within 5 minutes of the initial injection, a second injection of ½ the initial dose can be given.

For woodchucks with compromised liver function, isoflurane tank induction (Fig. 8.4) followed by maintenance on a facemask or endotracheal intubation has proven safe and effective. This anesthetic regimen is also effective for imaging and surgical procedures. Unlike most rodents, woodchucks may vomit while under anesthesia which can result in aspiration pneumonia. For this reason, animals should be monitored closely during tank induction, and pre-anesthetic fasting may be required.

An alternative to inhalation anesthesia is the intravenous administration of sodium pentobarbital. A dosage of 2–6 mg/kg is administered through a previously implanted catheter or into the sublingual vein to prolong the anesthetic state induced by ketamine/xylazine.

Anesthesia lasts on average 20–40 minutes. Other investigators have used Innovar Vet®, 0.35 ml/kg IM (Snyder, 1985). Innovar Vet® can be reversed with naloxone. Regardless of the anesthetic used, it is important to withhold access to water until the animals are fully recovered from anesthesia to prevent accidental drowning.

5. Physical Examination

Woodchucks should first be observed without disturbing them, keeping in mind that when woodchucks are upset, they may chatter, whistle, or make wheezing noises which may be mistaken for evidence of respiratory problems (Young and Sims, 1979). Observations which can be detected without handling the animal include ocular discharge, labored respiration, nasal discharge, discharge or foul odors from the ears, head tilt, or apparent weight loss. On closer examination, folliculitis, bite wounds, or ventral edema etc., may be apparent. Incisors can be examined by enticing the animal to bite on something. With appropriate restraint, auscultation of the heart and lungs, and palpation of the abdomen should be performed. To complete the examination, the woodchuck should be released a distance from its nestbox to observe its ability to ambulate. An unwillingness to move is usually a sign of a serious underlying illness.

Thorough abdominal palpation generally requires anesthesia to reduce abdominal tone. In the authors' experience, palpation of the anesthetized woodchuck is useful in diagnosing pregnancy, in estimating whelping dates, and in detection of organomegaly, including hepatomegaly due to hepatocellular carcinoma (HCC).

6. Clinical Techniques

a. Venipuncture

Venipuncture in woodchucks can be challenging because they lack readily accessible peripheral veins and general anesthesia is usually required. Woodchcucks

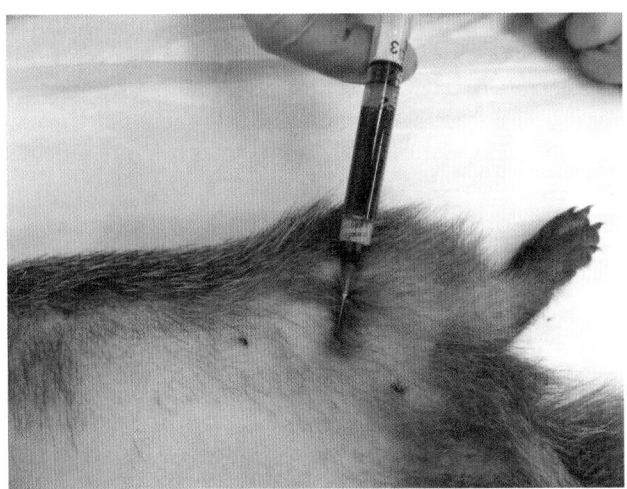

FIGURE 8.5   Bleeding the anesthetized woodchuck from the femoral canal.

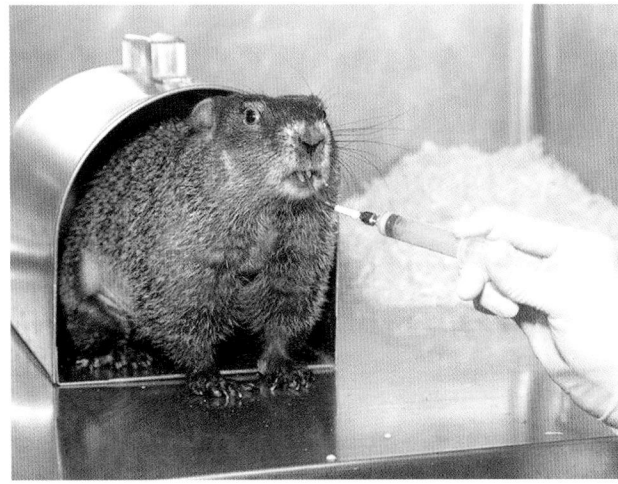

FIGURE 8.7   Laboratory woodchucks after training taking experimental medication suspended in complete liquid diet formulated for woodchucks.

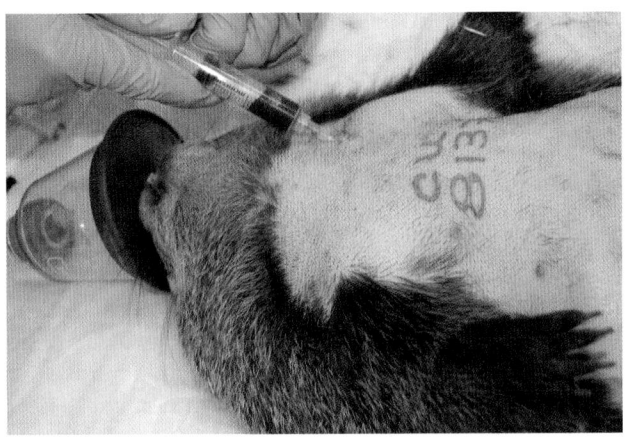

FIGURE 8.6   Bleeding from the anesthetized woodchuck from the linguofacial vein.

can be routinely bled from the femoral vein or artery (Fig. 8.5). Following anesthesia, the venipuncture site is clipped and scrubbed with alcohol and an antiseptic. The femoral pulse is palpated in the inguinal region and is used as a reference point since the vessels are not visible. A vacutainer tube and a 22-gauge, 1" needle may be used. Direct pressure is applied following venipuncture to minimize hematoma formation.

Samples can also be obtained from the maxillary or linguifacial veins (Fig. 8.6) which run in close proximity to the clavicle. Here, the woodchuck is placed on its back, head toward the phlebotomist, and a 22-gauge, 1" needle is directed straight into the notch formed where the clavicle meets the sternum. Care must be taken to avoid entering the thorax. Cardiac puncture has been used and is the easiest and quickest method to obtain large amounts of blood, but complications such as

cardiac tamponade and death may occur. Small amounts of blood can be obtained from the cephalic veins (on the medial aspect of the front legs) or tarsal veins (on the dorsal aspect of the rear feet).

b. Oral Medications

Tablets are crushed and mixed with liquid. Liquids are given PO by dose syringe (Fig. 8.7). Woodchucks can be trained to readily accept oral medications by mixing the medication with or following it with a small amount of a liquid, such as molasses or liquid diet.

c. Injections

Intramuscular injections can be given in the gastrocnemius or quadriceps muscles. While it is easiest for two people to inject woodchucks, it is possible for an experienced technician to accomplish the task alone by holding the tail and allowing the animal to grasp the edge of the cage with its front paws. Repeated injections of large volumes of irritating substances such as ketamine may cause myonecrosis. If frequent injections are unavoidable, the alternation of muscle groups and hind legs is recommended.

d. Cystocentesis

Urine collection may be accomplished by cystocentesis (Fig. 8.8) in anesthetized woodchucks. Large amounts of intra-abdominal fat can make palpation of the bladder difficult. Ultrasound guidance facilitates the collection procedure.

7. Research Techniques

Reported research on woodchucks has involved the use of intravenous catheters, liver biopsies (Mrozek *et al.*, 1994), vascular access ports (Woolf *et al.*, 1989),

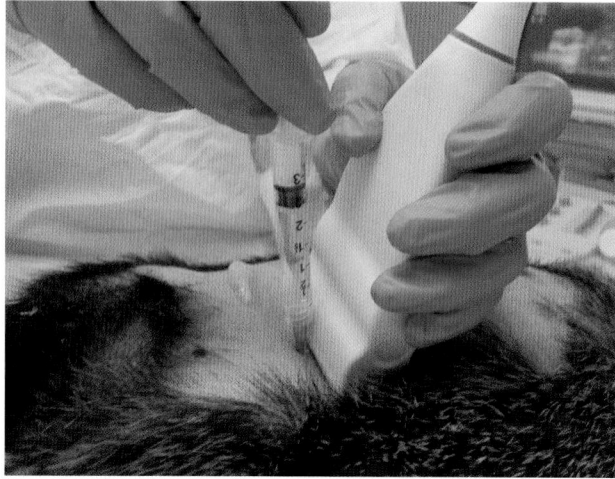

FIGURE 8.8   Urine collection by cystocentesis.

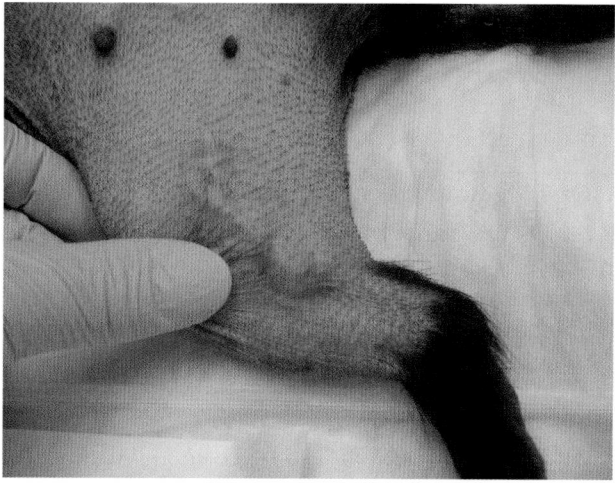

FIGURE 8.9   Vascular access port with catheter surgically placed in the femoral vein. Post-surgical healing is complete and the catheter is ready for use.

embryo collection (Concannon *et al.*, 1997b), and electroejaculation (Concannon *et al.*, 1996) and magnetic resonance imaging (MRI) (McKenzie *et al.*, 2006; Buitrago *et al.*, 2010).

Intravenous catheters may be placed in the cephalic vein but general anesthesia and possible surgical cut down may be required. Vascular access ports (Fig. 8.9). are useful for repeated drug administration, blood sampling, and for the administration of contrast agents associated with imaging.

Repeated live biopsies may be obtained under general anesthesia and ultrasound guidance using 18 gauge 'True-Cut' biopsy needles. Gentle pressure is applied to the biopsy site for 5 minutes following the procedure to reduce post-biopsy hemorrhage.

MR under general anesthesia is a useful modality for noninvasive, long-term, longitudinal monitoring of the progression of HCC and for assessment of antitumor therapy. Contrast agents may be administered through a vascular access port and woodchucks tolerate repeated imaging procedures.

II. BIOLOGY

A. Unique Characteristics and Comparative Physiology

1. Annual Metabolic Cycles

The annual cycle of changes in metabolic state and reproductive function persists in the laboratory, even if animals are not subjected to so called hibernation-inducing conditions of food withdrawal or cold-room temperatures of 5–10°C. However, circannual cycles may become shortened to 11, 10, or 9 months if woodchucks are not subjected to seasonal changes in the daily photoperiod which mimic natural changes (Concannon *et al.*, 1992). Most woodchucks maintained at temperatures of 20–25°C and with food and water constantly available will undergo seasonal periods of reduced body temperature (unpublished observations).

In autumn and early winter, woodchucks may be found with rectal temperatures of 30°C or lower. This period of physiological hypothermia presumably reflects an attempt at hibernation which is part of the normal circannual cycle. This period is associated with low levels of free thyroid hormone despite the presence of moderate to high levels of total thyroid hormone (Concannon *et al.*, 1999). The majority of thyroid hormone at that time appears bound to thyroxine-binding globulin (TBG) and other proteins such that very little free hormone is available to promote mitochondrial activity and basal metabolism (Young, 1984; Rawson *et al.*, 1998). Resting metabolism has been measured, and VO2 was reported to average 4.4 ± 0.3ml/min/kg in early autumn (Rawson *et al.*, 1998).

Despite the low metabolic activity, the gonads slowly regain function, such that they are fully recrudescent at the end of the 'hibernation period' in mid to late winter. Body weight declines in autumn, winter, and early spring as fat stores are utilized for metabolic needs. In one study, weight losses were far greater in females than in males (Snyder, 1985).

In late winter and early spring, metabolic activity increases dramatically, and rectal temperatures are increased to high-normal values; food intake increases if food is available, but body weight gain is small or negligible. These changes are presumably due both to increased pituitary secretion of TSH causing more thyroxine secretion, and to decreased amounts of TBG resulting in increased amounts of free thyroxine. There is also a seasonal increase in prolactin at this time (Concannon *et al.*, 1999). In early spring, resting metabolism is elevated. Average VO2 in early spring was reported to be increased from that of autumn (7.3 *versus* 4.4 ml/min/kg). After the brief breeding season and short 31 day pregnancies of late winter and early spring there is a decline in thyroid hormones in spring and summer. As a result, the animals undergo a transition from minimal weight gain to rapid weight gain. Weight gain consists almost entirely of fat deposits in preparation for hibernation. Increases in body weight of 70–100% over a 3–5 month period can occur. Typical increases from nadir to peak body weight in laboratory woodchucks have been reported to be 45–100% in one study and 40–50% in another (Young and Sims, 1979; Concannon *et al.*, 1993).

In summer, food intake spontaneously declines, often rapidly, several weeks before peak body weight is reached. The signal mechanism is not known, but the result is a brief period of very positive energy balance in summer, followed by a slow protracted decline in body weight in autumn and winter.

Other elements of the circannual cycle that have been less well studied include fur molts in the late summer and late winter, changes in pituitary hormone secretion, and presumably changes in adrenal function (Young and Sims, 1979).

2. Endogenous Circannual Cycles

The annual cycle of metabolic and reproductive activity in woodchucks persists, with changes quantitatively the same, even if the animals are maintained under constant photoperiods. In males maintained in daily photoperiods of 12 hours of light and 12 hours of dark, patterns of gonadal activity had approximately 12-month intervals for 1–3 years before then 'free-running' at circannual intervals of 8–10 months (Concannon *et al.*, 1992). The majority of animals will become asynchronous and free-run after 2–3 years if photoperiod cues simulating those of the natural environment are not provided. In studies using large block changes in the photoperiod, similar to those used in other species, photoperiod was unable to modify the circannual cycles of woodchucks.

3. Photo-Entrainment of Circannual Cycles to 12 Months

The endogenous cycle of woodchucks can be entrained to 12-month intervals by exposure to simulated natural photoperiods. This has been done, using weekly or twice per month or monthly changes in the daily light cycle to approximate that of the outdoors (unpublished observations). However, the preferred and best studied method is to change the daily photo-phase each day, using microprocessor controlled timers for room lights. The simulation of natural, 0–4 minutes-per-day increases and decreases in daily photo-phase is accomplished by changing the time of lights on and the time of lights off each day with the most rapid changes at the times of the vernal and autumnal equinoxes (Concannon *et al.*, 1997a). Similarly produced but Southern Hemisphere photoperiods beginning at 3 months of age or at 15 months of age re-entrained the woodchuck cycle to an austral annual cycle which was 6-months out of phase with the photo-entrained Northern Hemisphere cycles (Concannon *et al.*, 1997a).

4. Hibernation

In the wild, woodchucks immerge into winter burrows in autumn, usually between September 15 and November 1, hibernate for 3–5 months, and emerge in late winter sometime in February or March. Field data suggest that males emerge before females, and adults emerge before yearlings. Natural hibernation involves bouts of torpor (inactivity due to reduced resting metabolism) at 2–4°C above ambient temperature and bouts of arousal (activity associated with transient increases in resting basal metabolism) at varying intervals. Periods of each can range from 1–7 days, with torpor becoming progressively longer and then shorter during the hibernation period. The physiology underlying the associated behavior and alteration in temperature set point is not understood. In the laboratory, a period of deep hibernation can be induced by reducing room temperature to 15°C or lower (Snyder, 1985), and removing food. Others have used temperatures of 6–8°C, removed both food and water, and used constant darkness, but have also observed that most animals will also hibernate in the presence of food and light (Young and Sims, 1979). In the authors' experience, at hibernation-inducing temperatures of 6–8°C, morbidity and mortality may increase unless measures are taken to ensure appropriate preparative weight gains under natural photoperiod. Clearly, consideration must be given to correct timing, humidity, and possible unnatural disturbances.

Without the so-called hibernation-inducing conditions like food withdrawal, water withdrawal, temperature reduction, and darkness, most photo-entrained woodchucks will nevertheless undergo periods of physiological hypothermia, during the expected period of hibernation. Body temperatures may range from euthermic to only 1–2°C above room temperature. In one study, the average rectal temperature of woodchucks maintained at 20°C room temperature was 37°C in early spring, and only 29°C in early autumn (Rawson *et al.*, 1998). The physiological hypothermia presumably reflects a hypothyroid state, reduced metabolism, and the same mechanisms that promote deep hibernation at lower temperatures. As with deep hibernation, spontaneous permanent arousal occurs in late winter. During the period of hibernation, with either deep or mild hypothermia, weight losses of 15–50% are common.

TABLE 8.1   Range of Mean (±Sem) Hematological Values Obtained in 5–10 Studies Each Involving 10–30 Woodchucks in Comparison to Published Mean (±SD) Values

Parameter	Published values[a]	Unpublished values[b]	
		Low mean[c]	High mean[d]
ERYTHROCYTES			
Hematocrit % (HCT)	39 ± 7	35.5 ± 3.4	40.7 ± 4.9
Red cell count (RBC) (×10^6/uL)	5.3 ± 0.8	4.7 ± 0.4	5.2 ± 0.6
Mean corpuscle volume (MCV) (fl)	77 ± 7	73 ± 4	76 ± 4
Mean corpusc. Hb (MCH) (pg)	26 ± 4	24.9 ± 2.1	26.1 ± 1.4
M.C. Hb. conc. (MCHC) (g/dL)	34 ± 3	33.9 ± 0.7	35.9 ± 1.3
Red cell distribution width (RDW) (%)	na	14.0 ± 1.5	17.5 ± 2.5
Nucleated RBC (per 100 WBC)	na	1.5 ± 0.5	3.0 ± 0.5
Hemoglobin (Hb) (g/dL)	13.2 ± 2.6	12.2 ± 1.2	13.4 ± 2.1
% Saturation	na	23 ± 5 n = 5	45 ± 9 n = 5
WHITE BLOOD CELLS			
White cell count (WBC) (×10^3/uL)	10.1 ± 4.0	8.7 ± 2.3	10.4 ± 4.4
Segm. neutrophils (×10^3/uL)	6.4 ± 3.3	5.5 ± 2.1	6.6 ± 2.2
Band neutrophils (×10^3/uL)	0.1 ± 0.1	0.01 ± 0.05	0.03 ± 0.05
N (Eosinophils) (×10^3/uL)	0.4 ± 0.4	0.2 ± 0.2	0.4 ± 0.5
Lymphocytes (×10^3/uL)	2.6 ± 1.3	2.1 ± 0.9	3.1 ± 1.2
Monocytes (×10^3/uL)	0.6 ± 0.6	0.6 ± 0.3	1.1 ± 0.6
HEMOSTASIS			
Platelets (×10^3/uL)	na	451 ± 55	525 ± 91
Mean platelet vol. (fl)	na	6.8 ± 0.6	7.1 ± 0.5
PT (sec)	na	6.5 ± 0.5	7.6 ± 0.6
APTT (sec)	na	26 ± 3	31 ± 6
Fibrinogen (FIB) (mg/dL)	na	193 ± 42	225 ± 30

[a]Graham (1985) mean ± SD reported for 328 observations on 62 adult woodchucks over a 1 year period.
[b]Mean (± sem) values for groups of 12–30 adult woodchucks.
[c]Lowest mean value observed for a study involving a group of 10–30 healthy adult woodchucks.
[d]Highest mean value observed for a study involving a group of 10–33 healthy adult woodchucks.

B. Normal Physiological Values

1. Longevity

The mean age at death for wild woodchucks has been reported to be 14.9 months with 50% surviving only 8 months (Snyder, 1985). The mean age at death for woodchucks captured at 3–5 months of age and maintained in a zoo environment was 4.5 years (Snyder, 1977). Maximum longevity was 10 years. In the authors' laboratory, woodchucks can live for up to 14 years (unpublished data).

2. Hematology

Blood cell parameters in woodchucks appear to fall within the range reported for other rodent species based on published and more recent observations (Table 8.1). Unpublished observations by the authors also suggest that some values may vary with season. However, the time-course of such changes has not been determined. Hematocrit can be higher in autumn (mean, 40%) than in spring (mean, 36%). Likewise, the percent saturation of hemoglobin (40 vs. 25%). The mean values for most other parameters are fairly narrow (Table 8.1) suggesting little seasonal influence.

TABLE 8.2 Range of Mean (± Sem) Serum Chemistry Values in Multiple Unpublished Studies Involving 15–30 Woodchucks Per Study in Comparison to Published Mean (± SD) Values

Parameter	Published values[a]	Unpublished values[b]	
		Low mean[c]	High mean[d]
PROTEINS			
Albumin (g/dL)	3.7 ± 0.8	2.3 ± 0.2	3.4 ± 0.3
A:G Ratio	na	0.7 ± 0.2	1.1 ± 0.3
Globulin (g/dL)	3.2 ± 1.2	3.0 ± 0.5	3.6 ± 0.6
Total protein (g/dL)	6.9 ± 1.2	5.5 ± 0.3	6.9 ± 0.6
ELECTROLYTES AND ACID-BASE			
Sodium (mEq/L)	147 ± 4	143 ± 3	151 ± 3
Potassium (mEq/L)	4.7 ± 0.7	3.7 ± 0.3	4.4 ± 0.4
Sodium/potassium	na	34 ± 3	40 ± 4
Chloride (mEq/L)	97 ± 7	98 ± 3	102 ± 3
Total CO_2 (mEq/L)	na	31 ± 2	34 ± 3
Bicarbonate (mEq/L)	na	30 ± 3	34 ± 4
Anion gap (mEq/L)	na	15 ± 4	20 ± 4
Calcium (mg/dL)	10.1 ± 0.7	9.7 ± 0.5	11.0 ± 0.6
Phosphate (mg/dL)	5.0 ± 1.3	3.8 ± 0.6	5.4 ± 1.9
LIVER AND MUSCLE			
Alanine amino transferase (U/L)	2.0 ± 1.0	1.0 ± 1.0	3.5 ± 2.5
Aspartate amino transferase (U/L)	26 ± 13	21 ± 12	34 ± 21
Creatine kinase (U/L)	600 ± 512	478 ± 350	690 ± 310
Gamma GT (U/L)	1.7 ± 0.9	na	na
Alkaline phosphatase (U/L)	10 ± 9	7.2 ± 2.1	19.3 ± 5.5
Total bilirubin (mg/dL)	0.05 ± 0.05	0.11 ± 0.05	0.32 ± 0.1
Cholesterol (mg/dL)	na	140 + 40	210 ± 50
Glucose (mg/dL)	184 ± 61	186 ± 21	220 ± 40
OTHER SERUM ENZYMES			
Amylase (U/L)	na	2210 ± 648	2645 ± 910
Lipase (U/L)	na	201 ± 62	361 ± 75
RENAL FUNCTION			
Urea nitrogen (mg/dL)	na	13 ± 5	25 ± 6
Creatinine (mg/dL)	na	0.9 ± 0.2	1.5 ± 0.5

[a]*Graham (1985) mean ± SD reported for 345 observations on 62 adult woodchucks over a 1 year period.*
[b]*Mean (± sem) values for groups of 12–30 adult woodchucks.*
[c]*Lowest mean value observed for a study involving a group of 10–30 healthy adult woodchucks.*
[d]*Highest mean value observed for a study involving a group of 10–33 healthy adult woodchucks.*

3. Biochemistry

Serum chemistry results for woodchucks (Table 8.2) can vary among studies, although electrolytes as expected are rather stable parameters. Our unpublished results suggest that some serum enzymes may exhibit changes in concentration related to the annual cycle but timecourses of such changes have not been well characterized. The range of observed mean values for various studies in normal woodchucks suggests potential seasonal effects on alanine amino transferase and alkaline phosphatase, and possibly aspartate amino transferase (Table 8.2). Mean values of other enzymes are less variable and may be less affected by season, including amylase, lipase, and creatine kinase. Mean protein values especially the albumin fraction, can vary considerably, perhaps seasonally. Whether the observed variations in creatinine (0.9–1.5 ug/dl), total bilirubin (0.12–0.30 mg/dl), urea nitrogen (13–25 mg/dl), and cholesterol (140–210 mg/dl) involve seasonal changes remains to be determined.

C. Nutrition

Specific nutritional requirements of woodchucks have not been established. However, the composition of commercially available rabbit food (at least 15% protein) resembles that of the diet of free-ranging woodchucks. In the laboratory, woodchucks have been successfully fed rabbit chow formulated into larger sized blocks (approx. 5.5 cm × 1.5 cm). The large blocks require gnawing which helps to wear down the woodchucks' continually growing incisors. This diet seems adequate in maintaining adults and supporting growth and reproduction. Brittle incisors, increased susceptibility to infection and alopecia, and all problems associated with an inadequate diet (Young and Sims, 1979) have not been observed. A rabbit 'breeder's formulation' diet, which has a higher caloric and protein content (at least 17%) and smaller sized pellets can be successfully fed to pregnant females and pups (unpublished observation).

Significant pup mortality during the periweaning period (30–80 days of age) can occur and may be caused by competition for food. One approach is to provide two large bowls of rabbit pellets per litter, and check the bowls twice daily to ensure that clean, fresh food is always available. These measures have significantly reduced periweaning mortality (unpublished observation).

D. Biology of Reproduction

1. Overview and Breeding Season

Males and females typically have a single, brief 2–4 week winter breeding season in which fertile matings occur, with the female being receptive and the male sexually aggressive. They can produce one litter per year. In the wild, the breeding season begins at or shortly after the emergence from winter hibernation, in late winter. Following gonadal regression in summer, gonadal recrudescence occurs during hibernation, beginning in late autumn or early winter. Peak gonadal activity occurs in late winter. These changes, and the subsequent pattern of gonadal regression during late spring and summer are all part of the endogenous circannual cycle of sequential

changes in endocrine function and tissue metabolism. The endogenous cycle is entrained by photoperiod and hibernation activity in the wild. In the laboratory, without efforts to provide photoperiod entrainment, the breeding seasons of individuals usually become asynchronous after 1 or 2 years, with intervals becoming shorter than 12 months (Snyder, 1985; Concannon et al., 1992). As a result, the breeding season may not be concurrent within breeding pairs or groups. Therefore, laboratory breeding requires considerable attention to photo-entrainment of the circannual cycle, and selection of breeding pairs or breeding groups based on concomitant periods of testis enlargement and vulval swelling.

Even with efforts to photo-entrain cycles, the breeding season in the laboratory typically advances by 1–2 months in the calendar year during the first 1–3 years. Therefore, although the breeding season in the wild is in late February or March, colony-born animals or animals in captivity after 1–2 years may be more likely to breed in late January and early February. Laboratory studies have usually not involved forced hibernation. Whether low-temperature hibernation in the laboratory would have an influence on the timing of the breeding season beyond that provided by photoperiod, perhaps delaying it to the 'normal' time, has not been studied.

Fertility in adults 2 or more years old can approximate 100% in the wild. Pregnancy rates in yearling females are only 50%. Males typically reach sexual maturity and first breed at 22 months of age (Snyder, 1985), but undergo pubertal changes at 10–11 months of age (Concannon et al., 1993). Information on basic woodchuck reproduction has been gleaned from observation in the wild (Hamilton, Jr. 1934; Snyder and Christian, 1960; Christian et al., 1972) and from studies of endocrine, behavioral, gonadal, and genital changes observed in captive and laboratory-raised animals (Concannon et al., 1984; Hikim et al., 1991a,b; Hikim et al., 1992; Concannon et al., 1996; Concannon et al., 1997b).

2. Female Reproduction

During proestrus and estrus there is detectable and measurable vulval swelling (Concannon et al., 1997b). Vulval diameter increases from 5 mm to >7 mm over a 1–3 week period, typically remains near maximal diameters of 7–12 mm for 5–8 days, and then recedes over the next few weeks. Proestrus, the period of swelling before first willingness to copulate, typically lasts 1–2 weeks. The period of fertile estrus following proestrus vulval enlargement has been estimated to be about 1 week. Fertility in females paired with males either before, at, or 1 week after vulval swelling reached 7 mm was similar (55–67%). Pairing between 1 and 2 weeks after obvious swelling was reported to reduce pregnancy rates to 33%. The conclusion was that estrus lasts 5–10 days in most instances (Concannon et al., 1997b).

In general, woodchucks are reflex ovulators, with ovulation being induced by multiple copulations during peak estrus. Mating behavior is difficult to monitor because of the animals' secretive nature. Video-study suggested that estrous females will mate with a sexually aggressive male several times in one day, usually for only one day, but sometimes over a 2–3 day period (Concannon et al., 1997b). However, in woodchucks as in cats, spontaneous ovulations can also occur (Concannon et al., 1997b). The incidence of spontaneous ovulation is presumed to be slight. Following ovulation and fertilization, serum progesterone is elevated during the 31–32 days of gestation, during the 5–8 weeks of lactation and, in many females, for 1–8 weeks post lactation. The only exception is a transient decline in progesterone for an 8–24-hour period before and during parturition. Such a decline appears to be part of the normal mechanism of parturition. The corpora lutea of pregnancy are the source of progesterone in each instance, with the same corpora lutea becoming enlarged post-partum. Litter size can range from 1–10, and typically is 2–7. The average in one study of laboratory woodchucks was 3.8 but varied with age, being 2.9 in yearlings, 3.6 in young adults, and 4.2 in 3–4 year old animals (Concannon et al., 1997b).

In the absence of induced ovulation or pregnancy, signs of estrus subside, and ovarian follicles spontaneously luteinize, and result in moderate to extensive elevations in serum progesterone for several weeks or months. This spontaneous luteinization of follicles in nonbred and in mated but nonpregnant females typically coincides with the time when cohort females are giving birth and suckling young. It is also the period when woodchucks experience a circannual increase in prolactin. The incidence of pseudo pregnancy immediately following infertile matings appears to be small but has not been studied in detail.

Woodchucks have a double cervix and a complete medial septum in the body of the uterus. Therefore, all conceptuses in any one horn are derived from the ipsilateral ovary (Concannon et al., 1984). There has been limited study of serum estrogen levels and vaginal cytology changes during the breeding season (Hikim et al., 1991a; Hikim et al., 1992), of vulval swelling patterns, of embryo collection and homologous surgical transfer (Concannon et al., 1997b), and of behavior during mating (Hikim et al., 1992; Concannon et al., 1997a,b). Following co-housing of estrous female(s) and a fertile male, the intervals to first mating ranged from 6 minutes to 6 hours. Copulation typically lasted from 1–12 minutes. Ejaculation responses of males occurred at 2–7 minutes and were followed by 2–8 minutes of inactive amplexus (Concannon et al., 1997b). Females mate 1–17 times in a 4–8 hour period. Fertility was associated with the number of matings lasting longer than 3 or 5 minutes (but not with the total number of matings, with some matings being very brief).

Blastocysts implant on day 5 or 6 after fertile mating (Concannon et al., 1997b). Initial embryonic attachment and early implantation occur during a decidual reaction of the uterine endometrium at sites in the lumen opposite the region of the uterine mesentery (or mesometrium), away from the mesentery and blood supply. It is therefore termed antimesometrial implantation, a phenomenon that occurs in related species. Soon thereafter, subsequent embryo development and attachment of the discoid placenta is observed to occur on the mesometrial side of the uterus, close to the mesentery and blood supply. Fetal development can be monitored by abdominal palpation from day 10–11 onward, and more readily after day 15 (Concannon et al., 1997b). Ultrasound can also be used but details have not been reported. Parturition occurs at 31 or 32 days after fertile mating during a transient decline in serum progesterone. The young are born with eyes closed. Lactation generally lasts 6–7 weeks if the dam is left to determine the time for weaning.

3. Male Reproduction

Woodchucks have abdominal testes in summer and early autumn. In the wild, testicular recrudescence, scrotal development, and testis descent occur each year during hibernation, and males emerge from hibernation in late winter with peak-size testes and with peak spermatogenesis completed. In laboratory-housed males these changes appear to occur more rapidly in late autumn and early winter, and breeding condition is often reached by midwinter in late January or early February. Testis volumes range from a peak size of 3–5 cm^3 to a nadir size of less than 0.3 cm^3. The male breeding season, while often earlier in the calender year than in the wild, typically coincides with that of females if the animals are photo-entrained. In one study, fertility of males with enlarged scrotal testes was 100% (Concannon et al., 1996). The breeding season of an individual male has been estimated to range from 4–8 weeks and averages 6 weeks. The period of peak fertility may be less, but has not been studied. The annual cycle of spermatogenesis has been studied histologically (Christian et al., 1972), and the onset of testicular recrudescence has been advanced by administration of exogenous gonadotropin (Hikim et al., 1991b). Woodchucks have very prominent Cowper's glands (bulbourethral glands) that are the source of the urethral plugs produced during ejaculation, and are most likely the source of vaginal plugs sometimes observed in females after mating. Stimulation parameters that yield electroejaculation have been reported, as have changes in sperm numbers obtainable by electroejaculation throughout the breeding season (Concannon et al., 1996).

4. Laboratory Breeding and Female Fertility

In one study (Concannon *et al.*, 1997b), 75% of 2–4-year old estrus females became pregnant when housed with males and provided *ad libitum* opportunity to mate. Fertility was lower in yearling females (56%) and in females five years of age or greater (58%), and in females subjected to repeated handling and video observation (37%).

a. Housing

Housing for breeding need not be specialized, in that pregnancies have been obtained in both cages and pens, with either recently or chronically pair-housed animals, or with males housed with a harem of 2–5 females. However, fertility may be improved by single housing or same sex housing until the estimated onset of the breeding season. Pair or harem housing can be initiated in a colony based on calendar date of expected breeding season, on vulval swelling monitored in individual females, on initial vulval swelling in 25% of the females for the colony, and/or on a protocol of starting 2 weeks after enlarged scrotal testes are confirmed in 50% of the males in the colony (unpublished observations). Housing in pens rather than cages seems preferable and may yield higher fertility but data are lacking. Continuing to provide one or more nest boxes provides individual animals with a place of refuge. Harem housing of a male with 2–4 females in a pen is most efficient. When pair housing in cages, results tend to be better if the cage has a solid floor rather than a grate floor.

b. Detection of Estrus

Proestrus can be detected based on serial measurement of vulval diameters, with diameters >7 mm indicating obvious proestrus. Estrus is suggested by attainment of a peak size, which may be variable among females (8–12 mm) (Concannon *et al.*, 1997b). Late estrus is suggested by a softening of the vulva or loss of apparent turgor. Vaginal smears can be obtained by vaginal lavage and examined, with changes reminiscent of those in other laboratory rodents being evident to a smaller or larger degree depending on the individual. Smears can also be obtained by use of a moist cotton-tipped swab. The potential to induce ovulation by vaginal manipulation exists. Typically a moderate degree of cornification is observed in exfoliate cytology. While neutrophils may be present anytime, often a decrease occurs during proestrus and estrus followed by an increase in late estrus or post estrus. Detailed examination of smears in woodchucks has been reported (Hikim *et al.*, 1992).

c. Pregnancy and Pregnancy Diagnosis

Pregnancy has been estimated to range from 30–33 days from observed matings. Pregnancies in 12 animals involved parturitions at 31–32 days after mating (mean 31.9 ± 0.1 days). In that study the mean parturition date was March 13 ± 1 day in females born into a colony in which photoperiod simulated natural changes in photoperiod, and March 17 ± 1 day for captured animals bred in the laboratory and similarly maintained. These dates were earlier than the mean date of April 12 ± 1 days for pregnant females captured in the wild (Concannon *et al.*, 1997b). In that study, pregnancy was diagnosed by abdominal palpation following anesthesia with ketamine and xylazine. Uterine vesicle diameters were approximately 11 mm at day 10, 20 mm at day 15, 27 mm at day 20, and 40 mm at day 25. Palpation can be used to predict parturition date with considerable accuracy and can be done routinely by a trained technician. Fetal heartbeats are detected by ultrasound at mid gestation, but the time of earliest detection has not been determined.

Once pregnancy is confirmed, the female can be removed to a birthing pen or cage, or the male removed, and the female left in the same enclosure. Litters have been successfully raised with a male co-housed with the female(s), but pup survival is sometimes better if the male is removed following pregnancy diagnosis or immediately after birth of the litter. Having two pregnant and/or postpartum females in the same pen does not affect pup survival or growth. Females do better if left undisturbed with a nest box and bedding from mid gestation onward. Nest boxes can be examined daily to confirm the date of parturition and examine pups.

d. Early Development of Newborn

Pups can be examined most readily by 'training' the dam to move into a second box ('refuge box'). The refuge box is placed with its opening placed at the entrance to the main nest box. The lid of the main nest box is opened, and the dam is encouraged to enter the refuge box.

In our experience, normal pup weight at birth typically ranges from 20–40 g, and averages 27 g. At birth, pups have a reddish color, thin translucent smooth skin, and closed eyes (Fig. 8.10). At one day of age, the skin is wrinkled and less red, the eyes are still closed, and the teeth nonerupted. Sex can be determined by ano-genital distance. The umbilical remnant is present and is lost by day 4. Milk, if present, is visible in the stomach through the translucent skin, and is one parameter that can be checked daily to ensure that the dam is caring for her pup. At 4 days, mean bodyweight is 65 g (Fig. 8.11). The skin is graying, but pinkish on the abdomen, and hair growth begins. Transfer of pups 4–21 days of age to foster dams is often successful, and can be used when dams become sick, or perform poorly. At 2 weeks of age, fur has developed (Fig. 8.12). Long muzzle hairs and a grizzled appearance are characteristic. Pinnae are more obvious, and eye slits visible. Teeth erupt at 17–24 days of age. At 3–4 weeks, color varies greatly, male testes are

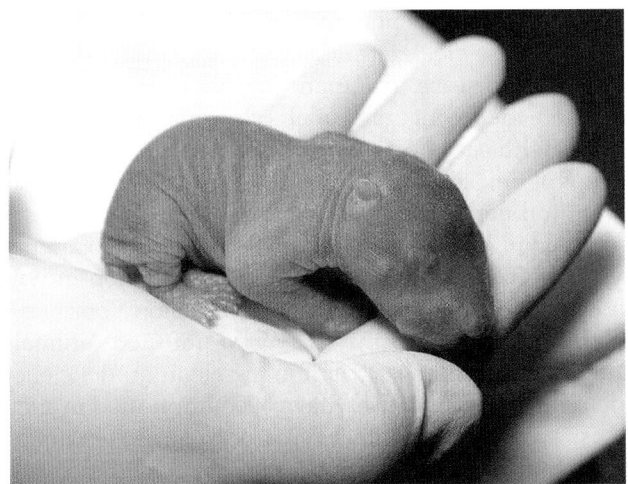

FIGURE 8.10   Newborn woodchuck, 1 day of age.

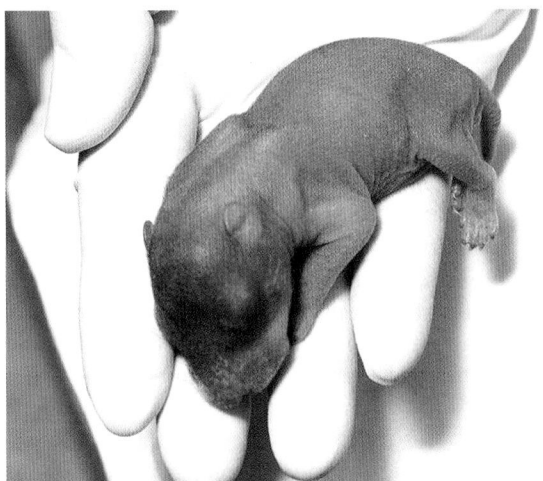

FIGURE 8.11   Newborn woodchuck, 4 days of age.

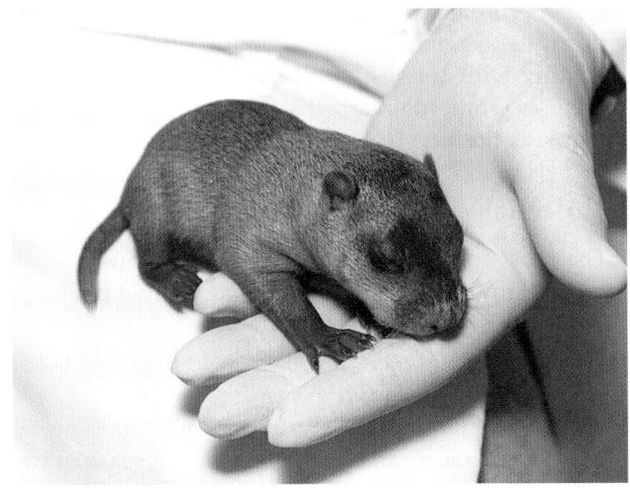

FIGURE 8.12   Newborn woodchuck, 14 days of age.

scrotal, animals respond to sound, and the eyes open. At 3 weeks, weight ranges from 100–220 g, and averages 160 g. At 4 weeks, the physiognomy is more like the adult, upper teeth erupt, the pups are active and ambulatory, but are still suckling.

e. Neonatal Mortality

Pup survival observed by the authors is slightly lower than that reported for some laboratory animals. In our experience, neonatal deaths average 20% in the first week, with most deaths occurring within the first 3 days. Mortality can reach 28% by 4 weeks postpartum. Adoption of a 'runt' pup to another postpartum dam can be successful. Another 1–5% of pups alive at 4 weeks may die before three months of age, possibly due to competition for food. It may help to provide two large bowls of rabbit pellets per litter and check the bowls frequently to ensure that clean, fresh food is always available.

f. Lactation and Weaning

Mother infant contact decreases between the fifth and sixth weeks after birth. Pups will frequently leave the nest box at four weeks of age, and are weaned by the end of the sixth week (unpublished observations). Pups can often be reared in the pen with the dam for 1 year without problems. Pups grow rapidly and reach 2.5–3.5 kg by 4 months. Some readily eat large block-pellets from weaning, but others require softening of such food with water or access to small pellets for several months. Providing small pellets of a breeding rabbit chow for 6–9 months, beginning by 5 weeks of age, works well for all juveniles. More than one bowl of food should be provided to each litter and kept full. Competition for food has resulted in emaciation and death in weanling pups.

For unknown reasons, female woodchucks must be housed individually for several weeks after weaning, or serious fighting will result. Similar problems have not been observed among group-housed females after weaning or in unbred yearling females.

g. Nutrition

Dams do not appear to require a special diet during gestation. They can be transferred to a small-pellet, breeding rabbit chow diet, *ad libitum*, in late gestation. Then food is automatically available later for the weanling pups without further changes.

E. Behavior

Seasonal changes in food intake, activity, and hormone levels result in behavioral changes that may affect research results. In cases of weight loss, body weights for experimental animals should always be compared with those of control animals since weight loss can be normal. Torporous woodchucks may shake and show lethargy and anorexia, and can be difficult to differentiate from sick animals. As a general rule, sick animals may have a slightly decreased body temperature (normal body temperature is 37°C), but the body temperature of torporous animals will approach that of room temperature (as low as 8–10°C) (Beaudoin *et al.*, 1969). Torporous animals become more active within 24 hours following handling and manipulation. Handling animals daily can prevent them from entering natural hypothermia or hibernation, yet may be necessary if animals are studied intensively during the fall and winter months.

Elevated testosterone levels during the breeding season are correlated with an increased incidence of fighting between male woodchucks. Adult males in proximity to females should be housed in individual cages; young males may be housed together through their second spring. Under controlled conditions, adult males can be housed together if introduced to each other outside the breeding season, given additional nest boxes, and isolated from females.

III. DISEASES

A. Colony Health Overview

During the day to day management of colony health, 50–70% of those woodchucks requiring treatment have dermatologic problems, the majority of which have bacterial folliculitis. Tail base dermatitis is observed in woodchucks housed in metal stovepipes. Bite wounds and associated cellulitis are common during the breeding season. Ectoparasites are not a problem because recently acquired wild woodchucks are treated prior to admission to the colony.

Diarrhea is observed in 5% of the colony and in most instances is related to stress and/or transitional changes in food and water intake. Loose stools are commonly observed in woodchucks during the breeding season and just prior to and just after hibernation. Giardiasis is a contributing factor in some individuals with diarrhea but is not believed to be a primary intestinal pathogen in the majority of woodchucks with loose stools. Primary bacterial enterocolitis is not common and salmonellosis is rare. Rectal prolapse, intussusception, and intestinal volvulus are examples of obstructive disorders which occur in some woodchucks with diarrhea.

Fifteen percent of the woodchucks in the colony require diagnostic and/or medical management of ocular lesions, respiratory conditions, dental problems, ear infections, or chronic debilitation. Conjunctivitis attributed to bedding irritants and/or bacterial infections and ocular lesions acquired from fighting are common. Respiratory problems are often associated with diaphragmatic hernias, cardiomyopathy, profound obesity,

and rhinitis and/or pneumonia. Rarely, neoplasms and dental disease are determined to be the cause of obstructive airway disease. Traumatic injuries of teeth are more common than congenital malocclusions. A few woodchucks with ear infections, as discussed later in this section, will develop central nervous system signs.

Central nervous system signs or edema and/or ascites occur in less than 5% of the woodchucks examined by our staff. Cerebral nematodiasis is common in wild woodchucks, otitis media/interna in colony born, and hepatic encephalopathy in WHV infected animals. Cerebral hemorrhage, vitamin E-selenium deficiency, and renal encephalopathy have been implicated in a few cases. Woodchucks with edema and/or ascites invariably have cardiomyopathy or immune mediated glomerulonephritis, the latter of which is associated with WHV infection.

A wide spectrum of miscellaneous problems account for the remaining 5–10% of woodchucks requiring examination and treatment. Toe and/or nail injuries, as well as lameness associated with soft tissue and skeletal lesions, are expected due to the active and aggressive nature of woodchucks. Osteomyelitis is not an uncommon sequelae to bite wounds. Traumatic fractures and dislocations are occasionally diagnosed in young woodchucks and pathologic fractures due to neoplasia are rare. Hematuria occurs in occasional woodchucks and is usually associated with cystitis and cystic calculi. Peripheral arteriovenous fistulas rarely occur and need to be differentiated from abscesses, neoplasms, and *Taenia crassiceps* lesions. Parasitic infections such as *T. crassiceps*, *Ackertia marmota*, and *Baylisascaris* sp. are not a problem in laboratory reared woodchucks.

Because woodchucks hide symptoms of illness as a survival mechanism, diseases are often advanced when diagnosed. Woodchucks are frequently found dead, having displayed no apparent clinical signs. The most common cause of death in WHV positive woodchucks is hepatocellular carcinoma. The most common causes of death in woodchucks negative for WHV are cardiomyopathy with congestive heart failure, aorta rupture, nephritis, glomerulonephritis, pneumonia, and diaphragmatic hernia.

B. Infectious Diseases

The most commonly encountered infectious diseases in captive and laboratory reared woodchucks are bacterial folliculitis, otitis, and pneumonia.

1. Bacterial Diseases

a. Bacterial Folliculitis

Folliculitis is a common bacterial skin disease of captive woodchucks. A review of records in one laboratory revealed that at any given time up to 30% of colony animals had skin lesions (Panic *et al.*, 1992). Cytology taken from intact pustules of exudative lesions usually reveals many gram-positive bacteria (cocci). Mixed cultures of *Staphylococcus aureus* and *Streptococcus* spp. Group A are most commonly obtained; however, pure cultures of the above isolates as well as of *Pasteurella multocida* have also been obtained.

The associated skin lesions, which do not seem pruritic, include erythema, papules, pustules, epidermal collarettes, ulcers, and draining tracts. These lesions are often covered by a patch of matted hair. In later stages, crust, alopecia, hyperpigmentation, and lichenification may be seen. Multiple lesions are usually present, and most frequently involve the dorsal lumbosacral region, the limbs, face, and inguinal areas. Pododermatitis is usually associated with severe erythematous swellings or draining tracts. Folliculitis can be fatal to neonates and, less often, adults if they develop septicemia.

Since folliculitis is rare in feral woodchucks and in woodchucks housed in Horsfall units, husbandry practices may be implicated in causing infections. *Staphylococcus aureus* and *Streptococcus* spp. Group A are common cutaneous florae reported to induce infection in rats and mice in the presence of predisposing factors such as moisture, wounds, crowding, high environmental temperatures, and low dietary protein (Panic *et al.*, 1992). An investigation of predisposing factors for bacterial folliculitis in woodchucks suggested that skin lesions may be associated with the stress involved in transferring animals between facilities, and/or the hormonal fluctuations that occur during the breeding season (Panic *et al.*, 1992). Nutrition does not appear to be a factor. Folliculitis appears to be contagious among woodchucks and can spread to animals in adjacent pens. Preventive measures include individual housing, limiting movement of woodchucks between facilities, and attention to cleaning and disinfection of cages and all materials in contact with animals.

Treatment consists of clipping the hair around the lesion, cleaning the area with diluted solutions of chlorhexidene or povidone-iodine, debriding when necessary, and applying a topical bactericide. Parenteral antibiotic treatment is reserved for animals with deep cellulitis or multiple lesions. Typically, lesions resolve within 10 days, resulting in mild hyperpigmentation and alopecia until subsequent hair growth occurs during the summer.

b. Otitis

Otitis externa, characterized by a discharge from one or both ears (Fig. 8.13) is more common in older woodchucks and occasionally extends to the inner and/or middle ear. External ear disease may lead to otitis media/interna. Signs of inner ear disease include a head tilt toward the affected ear, nystagmus, circling,

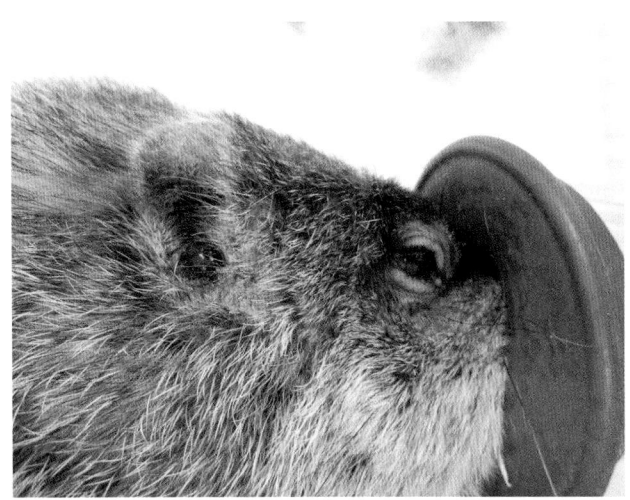

FIGURE 8.13 The external ear of an adult woodchuck showing drainage from *otitis externa*.

rolling, and/or loss of balance. Woodchucks can have otitis media/interna without an otic discharge. Otitis media/interna occasionally develops into meningitis and/or encephalitis, and prolapse of the cerebellum through the foramen magnum has been observed (Roth, 1984). No predominant bacterial organism is responsible for these infections. Organisms cultured from the ear include *Morganella morganii*, *Proteus* sp., *Escherichia coli*, *Citrobacter koseri diversus*, and *Streptococcus* sp.

Treatment for external ear disease involves anesthetizing the woodchuck, culturing the ear canal, examining the canal for foreign bodies, polyps or a ruptured tympanic membrane, flushing with dilute (1:40) chlorhexidene solution, and applying topical antibiotic solution pending culture and sensitivity results. If the tympanic membrane has ruptured or if otitis media/interna is present, the ear should be flushed with warm, sterile saline instead of chlorhexidene, a topical antibiotic/anti-inflammatory drug combination should be used, and systemic antibiotics administered. If the tympanic membrane has not already ruptured in cases of otitis media/interna, doing so is necessary to provide ventilation and drainage.

c. Pneumonia

Lobar or bronchopneumonia and occasionally aspiration pneumonia are important differential diagnoses for respiratory problems. Bacterial pneumonia is more common, either occurring as a primary entity or a complication to some other illness. Severe cases are associated with pulmonary abscesses, suppurative pleuritis, or septicemia. Acute aspiration is rarely a life threatening problem in animals that are being gavaged or dosed orally with liquid medications. Mild, chronic granulomatous reactions to inhaled or aspirated irritants are more typical and affected animals are not usually symptomatic.

Woodchucks with pneumonia can die suddenly with no premonitory signs of illness. Lethargy, inappetence, or weight loss may be nonspecific indications. Respiratory distress may become apparent when woodchucks are restrained for examination and naso-ocular discharges may be evident. Thoracic auscultation and radiography, tracheal culture, and a hemogram are indicated in many cases. The most common bacterial organism cultured from the lungs of woodchucks with pneumonia is β-hemolytic *Streptococcus* sp., but mixed cultures and cultures including *Staphylococcus aureus*, *Pasteurella* sp., *Escherichia coli*, and *Bordetella bronchiseptica* are also common. *Bordetella bronchiseptica* is identified with a unique form of lobar pneumonia which has to be distinguished from pulmonary abscesses or neoplasia. The morbidity and mortality attending cases with suppurative pleuritis and septicemia are high. Early diagnosis and aggressive treatment is required to resolve less serious forms of pneumonia.

d. *Helicobacter marmotae*

Fox *et al.* (1994, 1995) have isolated *Helicobacter hepaticus* and *H. bilis* from mice with hepatitis and primary hepatic neoplasms have been associated with *H. hepaticus* infection (Ward *et al.*, 1994; Hailey *et al.*, 1998). In a cohort of 10 WHV carrier woodchucks with HCC that originated in their native habit, the closely related *H. marmotae* was cultured from the liver of one woodchuck and infection was demonstrated by PCR in the livers of eight others (Fox *et al.*, 2002). Subsequently, A/J mice, known to be susceptible to *H. hepaticus* induced hepatic neoplasia, were successfully infected experimentally with *H. marmotae* and developed hepatitis but hepatic neoplasms were not reported (Patterson *et al.*, 2010). The prevalence of *H. marmotae* infection in laboratory born and reared woodchucks should be determined and compared to that of woodchucks trapped in the native habitat. Experimental *H. marmotae* infection in woodchucks should be investigated further, the possible interaction between WHV and *H. marmotae* studied, and the potential of *H. marmotae* as a co-factor in hepatocarcinogenesis in the woodchuck explored.

2. Viral Diseases

a. Woodchuck Hepatitis Virus

The woodchuck infected with WHV has been shown to be an excellent animal model for the study of hepatitis B virus (HBV) infection of humans (Tennant and Gerin, 1994). WHV and HBV both belong to the family *Hepadnaviridae* (Tennant and Gerin, 1994). Infection in both species can lead to chronic hepatitis and HCC. Because of similarities between the viruses, the woodchuck has been used to study the mechanisms of

hepatocellular injury in acute and chronic viral hepatitis, to assess the oncogenic role of the virus, and to examine possible interactions between hepadnaviruses, diet and/or other environmental factors in hepatocarcinogenesis. Woodchuck studies have also been useful to develop and evaluate antiviral strategies for treating chronic liver disease and preventing HCC as well as to investigate therapeutic treatments for HCC (Tennant and Gerin, 1994).

Experimental neonatal WHV infection results in a chronic carrier rate of 50% or more. Almost all chronic carriers will develop HCC; the median time to HCC in WHV carriers is 29 months (Tennant and Gerin, 1994). Resulting liver tumors can be detected by abdominal palpation of anesthetized woodchucks or by ultrasound examination. Grossly, tumors may range from 1 mm nodules to 10 cm masses (Fig. 8.2). The histological features of these tumors have been described (Tennant and Gerin, 1994), and include tumor cells densely packed in thick, irregular trabeculae, basophilic cytoplasm, large vesicular nuclei, and prominent nucleoli (Fig. 8.3). Elevations in serum α-fetoprotein or serum GGT can be used as a marker of hepatocellular carcinoma (Graham, 1985; Cote *et al.*, 1990). Woodchucks with hepatocellular carcinoma may be asymptomatic or may develop anorexia, weight loss and/or lethargy. Ultimately, HCC will result in death, frequently preceded by an encephalopathic episode associated with elevated blood ammonia and/or hypoglycemia (Curtin *et al.*, 2011).

b. Herpes Virus of Marmots

Herpes virus of marmots (HVM) has been detected in laboratory woodchucks. Persistent infection can approach 20% in laboratory colonies (unpublished observation). No deaths or clinical signs in woodchucks have been attributed to HVM, but lysis of hepatocytes after several days of tissue culture has been reported to be associated with HVM (Schecter *et al.*, 1988). There appears to be no association between HVM status and the outcome of experimental WHV infection (i.e., the rate of chronicity) or in the development of HCC. The virus has been isolated from blood, lymphocytes, saliva, urine, and rectal/genital swabs. Venereal transmission from males to females and transmission from mother to offspring is significant.

c. Rabies

Although rodents are rarely infected with rabies, there has been a steady increase since the 1980s in the incidence of woodchuck rabies particularly in the eastern United States (Childs *et al.*, 1997). Affected woodchucks exhibit central nervous system signs including aggression and can initiate unprovoked attacks, which is not unlike the presentation of woodchucks with cerebrospinal nematodiasis (see *Baylisascaris* sp. section below). Definitive diagnosis of rabies is made by direct immunofluorescent antibody staining of brain tissue. Personnel dealing with wild-caught woodchucks should receive pre-exposure rabies immunizations.

d. Powassan Virus

Woodchucks are reservoirs for Powassan virus, a little known flavivirus that causes encephalitis in humans and can be fatal, especially to children. Powassan virus does not cause clinical disease in woodchucks. One study demonstrated that 80% of woodchucks trapped in Tompkins County, NY, had positive titers to the virus (Fleming, 1978), and the tick, *Ixodes cookei*, is an important vector in transmitting the virus.

3. *Parasitic Disease*

Woodchucks in the wild are known to harbor many parasites (Fleming, 1978). Parasite burdens decline after introduction into captivity. Except for *Giardia* spp., *Entamoeba muris*, and low levels of *Citellina triradiata* infections, colony-born woodchucks rarely have evidence of parasitism. Common parasites of wild woodchucks include *Taenia crassiceps*, *Baylisascaris* sp., *Dicrocoelium dendriticum*, *Ackertia marmotae*, and *Capillaria* spp. Of these, *A. marmotae* and *Capillaria hepatica* are associated with hepatic lesions. External parasites can be completely eradicated from laboratory colonies by dusting with insecticidal powder and manually removing ticks upon admission of woodchucks to the colony.

a. Protozoan

Giardia sp. Woodchucks in captivity are known to harbor *Giardia duodenalis* in their small intestine. Infection rates in colony-born animals can approach 28% (unpublished observations). However, it is unclear whether *Giardia* sp. causes clinical signs since woodchucks with severe diarrhea have shown neither cysts in the feces nor positive ELISA test results. Additionally, well-formed woodchuck feces may have an excess of *Giardia* sp. cysts. It is also unclear whether the *Giardia* sp. which infects woodchucks is transmissible to humans. Diagnosis is made by finding cysts in the feces using the zinc floatation method, trophozoites in fresh fecal smears, or by getting a positive result on an ELISA test for *Giardia* sp. (Alexon® Antigen capture test). Variable treatment success has been achieved with metronidazole (10–25 mg/kg PO once daily for 5 days), albendazole (25 mg/kg BID PO for 4 days) and fenbendazole (50 mg/kg PO once daily for 10 days).

Entamoeba Muris *Entamoeba muris* is a nonpathogenic amoeba of rodents found in approximately 50% of woodchuck fecal samples obtained from the authors' colony. No clinical signs have been observed.

Eimeria sp. Four species of *Eimeria* (*Eimeria monacis*, *E. os*, *E. perforoides*, *E. tuscarorensis*) are found in wild woodchucks but no gross lesions have been attributed to coccidian infections (Fleming, 1978). Low levels of *Eimeria* sp. infection were reported in colony-born woodchucks (Cohn *et al.*, 1986).

Toxoplasma Gondii Woodchucks, like other mammals, are intermediate hosts to *Toxoplasma gondii*. Cats are definitive hosts. Woodchucks become infected by ingesting oocysts in cat feces or by transplacental migration of tachyzoites from their mothers (Georgi, 1985). In one study, 8% of wild woodchucks exhibited antibody response to *Toxoplasma gondii*, but none demonstrated clinical signs or gross lesions (Fleming, 1978).

Sarcocystis sp. *Sarcocystis* sp. bradyzoites in sarcocysts have been found in woodchuck muscle, but no clinical signs or reactions have been reported (Roth, 1984).

b. Nematodes

Wild woodchucks harbor many nematodes, including *Ackertia marmotae*, *Baylisascaris laevis*, *Baylisascaris columnaris*, *Baylisascaris procyonis*, *Capillaria hepatica*, *Capillaria tamiasstriati*, *Citellina triradiata*, *Citellinema bifurcatum*, *Obeliscoides cuniculi*, *Strongyloides* sp., *and Trichostrongylus axei* (Fleming, 1978). No clinical signs or pathological lesions are observed except where woodchucks serve as intermediate hosts (Fleming, 1978).

Ackertia Marmotae *Ackertia marmotae* adults are present in lymphatics of the liver and gallbladder, and rarely in the lung and kidney (Fleming, 1978) and do not appear to cause any inflammation or lesions. Microfilariae in the skin cause microfilarial dermatitis (Panic *et al.*, 1992). The intermediate host for *A. marmotae* is the tick, *Ixodes cookei*. While *A. marmotae* microfilariae can persist in colony woodchucks for at least 39 months, *A. marmotae* infection can be eliminated from colonies by manually removing ticks and using insecticidal powders when woodchucks are first introduced to the colony (Cohn *et al.*, 1986).

Baylisascaris sp. *Baylisascaris procyonis* and *Baylisascaris columnaris*, parasites of the raccoon and skunk, respectively, have been implicated in causing encephalitis due to larval migration in the brains of woodchucks (Roth *et al.*, 1982). Affected woodchucks demonstrate abnormal behavior, including increased tameness or viciousness, head tilt, circling and/or paralysis. Because the differential diagnosis includes rabies, no treatment is recommended, and immunofluorescent antibody staining of a portion of brain tissue for rabies should be performed. Some brain tissue should be saved for histological examination. Definitive diagnosis of cerebrospinal nematodiasis can be made based on the results of histologic examination of brain tissue or examination of Baermannized brain tissue (Roth *et al.*, 1982).

Citellina Triradiata The pinworm, *Citellina triradiata*, which is found in the cecum and large intestine, has been found in colony-born woodchucks, and is transmitted directly. While it is not known to cause any pruritus or clinical signs, sanitation and single housing should reduce the incidence of infection.

Obeliscoides Cuniculi *Obelescoides cuniculi* is a common parasite of wild woodchucks, with one study showing a 92% infection rate (Cohn *et al.*, 1986). *O. cuniculi* is found in the stomach, where it sometimes causes petechiae of the mucosa. The natural host is the wild rabbit. In captive bred woodchucks the infection is short-lived. Fecal egg counts fall rapidly. The nematode has not been found in colony-born animals. The larvae and adult forms do not survive hibernation of the host, and in the wild the infection of woodchucks is probably perpetuated by reinfection from rabbits.

c. Cestodes

Taenia Crassiceps The larval form of *Taenia crassiceps*, a tapeworm of wild canids causes large, fluid-filled masses containing hundreds of cysticerci (Georgi, 1985). Woodchucks ingest the infected eggs and the embryos migrate to their site of development. Replication occurs by budding and results in many cysticerci contained in a single cyst. Masses are most commonly found in the axillary region and the adjacent thoracic wall, but have been found in other subcutaneous locations, in the abdominal and thoracic cavities, and in the liver and lung (Anderson *et al.*, 1990a). Lesions do not seem pruritic or painful or to cause any systemic signs of illness. They can interfere with movement and/or eating depending upon their size and location (Anderson *et al.*, 1990a). Surgical removal of small masses is possible. The tendency for larger lesions to infiltrate the surrounding area with finger-like projections makes excision difficult. Care must be taken to prevent cyst rupture and dissemination of cysticerci.

Taenia Mustelae *Taenia mustelae* cystecerci are found in 4–6 mm cysts on the surface of and in the parenchyma of the liver. The cysts may also contain hard, yellow material that is presumably calcified pus (Fleming, 1978).

d. Trematodes

Dicrocoelium Dendriticum *Dicrocoelium dendriticum*, the lancet liver fluke, is found in the bile ducts of sheep, cattle, pigs, deer, cottontail rabbits, and woodchucks (Georgi, 1985). The fluke eggs are eliminated in the feces of the definitive hosts and are ingested by terrestrial snails. Cercaria develop in the snails, are secreted in mucus, and are ingested by ants. The definitive host then ingests the ants while grazing. The metacercaria migrate up the common bile duct. Scarring of the liver, and histologic lesions typical of perilobular cirrhosis are seen in sheep and woodchucks (Mapes, 1950).

e. External Parasites

Wild woodchucks are hosts to many external parasites (Whitaker and Schmeltz, 1973). Some of the most common are the mite *Androlaelaps fahrenholzi*, the louse *Endeleinellus marmotae*, the tick *Ixodes cookei*, and the flea *Orpsylla arctomys*. *Ixodes cookei* is a vector for *Ackertia marmotae* and the Powassan virus. This tick may also serve as vectors for Rocky Mountain Spotted Fever rickettsiae and *Borrelia burgdorferi*, the spirochete that causes Lyme disease (Magnarelli and Swihart, 1991). External parasites can be eliminated by treating newly captured woodchucks with organophosphate-containing powders and by manually removing ticks before entry into the colony (Cohn *et al.*, 1986).

C. Metabolic/Nutritional

1. Capture Myopathy

A syndrome resembling white muscle disease has been associated with the capture of wild woodchucks. In one study, up to 60% of wild woodchucks captured in traps had lesions of myopathy, while no woodchucks which were shot had any such lesions (Fleming, 1978). Grossly, discrete, pale, white muscle was observed. Histologically, there was swelling, loss of cross striation with hyalinization or fragmentation, and occasionally mineralization. The only clinical sign in any of the affected woodchucks was lethargy. The myopathy was not related to vitamin E/selenium levels and might be similar to steroid myopathy.

2. White Muscle Disease

As in other species, white muscle disease in woodchucks, is a nutritional disease, resulting from insufficient intake or bioavailability of vitamin E and/or selenium. Since nutritional deficiencies rarely occur in the wild, capture myopathy is the suspected cause of myodegeneration in recently trapped woodchucks and nutritional myopathy (white muscle disease) is the suspected cause of these lesions in animals that have been in captivity for at least several weeks. Lesions, indistinguishable from those of capture myopathy most commonly involve the muscles used most often. In woodchucks, the characteristic discrete white, pale streaks are typically seen in the muscles of the upper forelegs, hindlegs, and cranial dorsum (hypaxial and epaxial muscles), as well as the heart. Affected woodchucks demonstrate varying degrees of weakness, dysphagia, and reluctance to move. Histological lesions include swollen, dark pink stained muscle, occasional fragmentation, mineralization, and in chronic cases, muscle atrophy and fibrosis. Profoundly affected woodchucks usually die. Woodchucks with milder manifestations respond to vitamin E/selenium supplementation.

3. *Hepatic Lipidosis*

Hepatic lipidosis resulting in death has been reported in wildcaught woodchucks and was thought to have resulted from a failure of these animals to adapt to laboratory conditions and diet (Roth, 1984). Varying degrees of hepatic lipidosis have been observed in colony woodchucks with inadequate food intake, chronic debilitating illness or exposure to hepatotoxic medications. For example, hepatic lipidosis was a prominent necropsy finding in woodchucks treated with the antiviral drug FIAU (Tennant *et al.*, 1998).

D. Traumatic

Bite wounds are quite common among group-housed colony animals, particularly during the breeding season. These wounds occur most frequently on the head, neck and limbs. While fighting usually results in minor bite wounds, severe wounds including fractured limbs, ruptured eyes, and deep lacerations have been seen. If not treated promptly with topical disinfectants and parenteral antibiotics for deep wounds, systemic infection and/or abscessation will occur. Attention to husbandry issues can reduce serious fighting. Anesthetized woodchucks should be allowed to recover fully from anesthesia before being returned to their cage or serious bite wounds may be inflicted upon the recovering woodchuck.

Traumatic injuries can also result from woodchucks jumping out of cages. Typical injuries include broken incisors and/or fractured limbs. Woodchucks are avid climbers and occasionally get a limb caught in a cage door or bottle bracket, resulting in avulsion or fracture of toes and/or limbs. Broken incisors usually grow back without any complications, but the opposite incisor may need trimming until regrowth is complete. Fractures, if not open or badly displaced, heal well with simple cage confinement.

E. Iatrogenic

Perhaps associated with the high incidence of bacterial skin problems observed in woodchucks, localized infections and septicemia commonly occur following invasive procedures such as venipuncture, intravenous catheterization, and surgery. Careful attention to sterility can minimize these infections. The skin should be clipped and scrubbed with a disinfectant and alcohol. These measures alone are enough to prevent infections associated with venipuncture. Sterile surgical techniques and sterilized instruments, needles, and catheters should be used. Suture materials should be chosen with care. In the authors' experience, the administration of parenteral antibiotics and topical antibiotic ointments to the incision reduces the incidence of infection following surgical procedures and catheterization.

Gait abnormalities can be caused by repeated intramuscular injections and subsequent fibrosing myositis. Rarely, arteriovenous fistulas occur at venipuncture sites particularly in the inguinal area. These fistulas can result in cardiomyopathy and associated heart failure or death due to rupture and hemorrhage. Thrombus formation is a fairly common sequelae to indwelling catheterization, but clinical problems associated with thrombosis are rare.

F. Neoplastic

HCC is the most common neoplasm in the woodchuck because of its association with WHV. The neoplasms are usually extensive in the liver, but metastasis to other organs is rare. The neoplastic cells are usually well differentiated and arranged in sheets, cords, and trabeculae, without portal structures or regard to lobular architecture. While HCC affects virtually all woodchucks chronically infected with WHV, it has occasionally been observed in WHV negative animals. In one study of 128 woodchucks seronegative for WHV, one woodchuck with histological evidence of HCC was reported (Roth *et al.*, 1984). The mass was focal and composed of well differentiated hepatic cells. There were no signs of hepatitis.

Published reports of nonhepatic neoplasms have included testicular teratoma, seminoma, Sertoli cell tumor, testicular lymphosarcoma, interstitial cell tumor and adenoma of the rete testis (Foley *et al.*, 1993), lymphosarcoma (Foley *et al.*, 1993), meningioma (Podell *et al.*, 1988), fibrosarcoma (Young and Sims, 1979), and uterine leiomyoma (Foley *et al.*, 1993). Neoplasms, as in most species, are most common in older woodchucks, and as long-term studies continue, diagnoses of neoplasms increase. In the authors' colony, up to 15% of woodchucks which die or are euthanized have a nonhepatic neoplasm diagnosed at necropsy. The more common neoplasms are lymphoma, seminoma, and interstitial cell tumors of the testicle, and myeloproliferative disease.

G. Miscellaneous

1. *Congenital*

a. Diaphragmatic Hernia

Woodchucks appear to have a natural weakness in the dorsal portion of the diaphragm. Pressure applied to the thorax during manual restraint may enlarge this opening enough to allow omentum and/or abdominal organs to pass. Signs of diaphragmatic hernia include dyspnea, tachypnea, and muffled thoracic auscultation. Definitive diagnosis can be challenging; radiographs and ultrasound examination may or may not show abdominal contents in the chest. Clinical signs usually result from pulmonary atelectasis, and can lead to death.

2. Age-Related

a. Ringtail

A ringtail-like syndrome similar to that seen in rats has been seen in neonatal woodchucks (7–28 days of age). The lesion begins as an annular constriction of the tail which progresses to edema, inflammation, necrosis, and sloughing of the tail distal to the constriction. As in the rat, ringtail appears to be associated with low humidity. In the authors' experience, humidity levels of 50% prevent the problem.

3. Cardiovascular

A high incidence of arteriosclerosis, aortic rupture, and cerebrovascular and cardiovascular disease has been reported in captive woodchucks (Snyder and Ratcliffe, 1969).

a. Cardiomyopathy

Cardiomyopathy, which frequently results in congestive heart failure, is a relatively common finding in woodchucks. Clinical signs include respiratory distress, ascites, subcutaneous edema, muffled heart sounds, heart murmurs, and arrhythmias. Sudden death in the absence of these signs can occur. Thoracic radiography and ultrasonography are useful in diagnosis. At necropsy, a grossly enlarged and dilated heart is observed. In one study, enlarged hearts weighed an average of 32.3 grams ± 5.4 grams whereas normal hearts weighed an average of 11.6 grams ± 2.8 grams (Roth and King, 1986).

b. Aortic Rupture

Aortic rupture (Fig. 8.14) is a common cause of death in wild caught woodchucks (Snyder and Ratcliffe, 1969), as well as in colony-born animals (unpublished observations). In nearly all cases, there are no premonitory signs prior to death. There appears to be no gender bias and the mean age at death is 2 years greater than the mean age at all other natural deaths. No relationship between aortic rupture and hepatocellular carcinoma or chronic WHV infection is detected. Young woodchucks dying from aortic rupture are more likely to have concurrent glomerulonephritis or interstitial nephritis suggesting that systemic hypertension is a predisposing factor (Van Schoick, personal communication). The contributing roles of hypertension, dietary copper and zinc and underlying connective tissue disorders have not been fully investigated.

c. Cerebrovascular

Nearly 7% of captive woodchucks were reported to have evidence of cerebral hemorrhage at death (Snyder and Ratcliffe, 1969). In some, hemorrhage was associated with arteriosclerosis of the brain. Vascular hypertension and atherogenic diets are possible causes (Snyder, 1985). In colony woodchucks fed 16.5% protein and only 2.8% fat, cerebral hemorrhage and arteriosclerosis were only infrequently seen at necropsy (unpublished observations).

Only seven of 350 woodchucks necropsied over 4 years had evidence of cerebral hemorrhage. Six died and one was euthanized because it appeared to be blind.

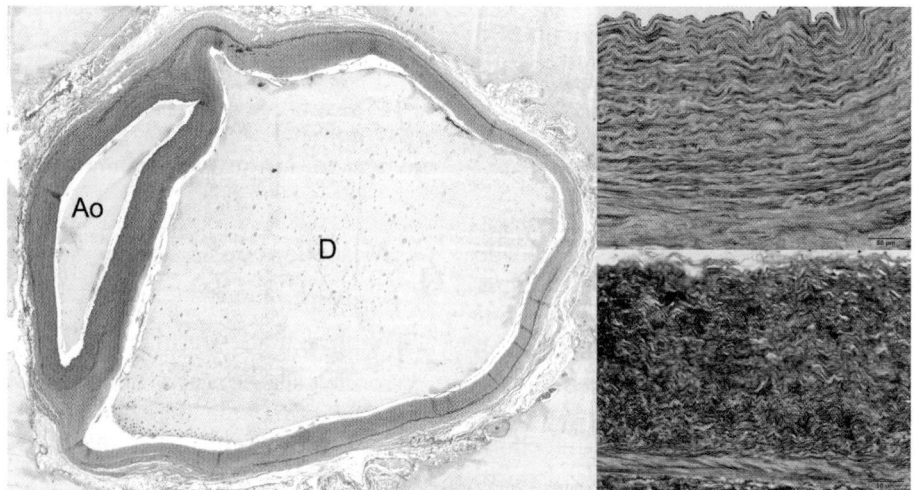

FIGURE 8.14 Left. Large medial dissection of the thoracic aorta in a 5 year old male breeder. There is a large false lumen (D) that dwarfs the aortic lumen (Ao). Right. Movat's pentachrome stain. In the upper right, the normal aortic media has abundant well-organized elastic lamina with smooth muscle cells and scant collagen (lumen at top). In the lower right, the wall of the dissection has a thick collagenous pseudo-intima lacking elastin, with a thin layer of relatively normal outer media. Masson's trichrome. The dissection extended from the aortic arch to caudal to the renal arteries. The dissection had ruptured in the abdomen, resulting in hemoabdomen and death from exsanguination.

In three woodchucks, the cause of death was a ruptured abdominal aorta, two of which had degenerative vascular disease and thrombosis in their brains; one also had renal vascular lesions. Cerebellar hemorrhage was the cause of death in two woodchucks suspected of having vascular disease, one of which had glomerulonephritis and interstitial nephritis. The blind woodchuck which was euthanized had vascular lesions in its brain, heart, and kidney. Systemic hypertension was suspected, but no antemortem blood pressure studies were performed to confirm this same suspicion.

In summary, vascular disease including vessel rupture may be linked to renal disease, vasculitis, and perhaps associated hypertension. Immune complex deposition in glomerular capillaries, as seen in HBV-infected humans, may lead to direct vessel injury. Vascular disease secondary to deposition of HBV antigen/antibody complexes has been demonstrated in humans (Schoen, 1994), and similar mechanisms may lead to vascular disease of woodchucks.

4. Renal Diseases

A 4-year necropsy study involving 390 woodchucks revealed 164 lesions of the urogenital system. A little more than a third (37%) of these lesions had histopathologic features of nonsuppurative interstitial nephritis, 14% had glomerulonephritis, 4% percent had tubular nephrosis, and 3% had pyelonephritis (unpublished observations). The more severe and/or chronic cases sometimes had mixed lesions, varying degrees of fibrosis, and rarely amyloid deposition. Although a few died or were euthanized because of signs attributed to protein-losing nephropathy and/or renal failure, the cause of death was not attributed to renal disease. The majority died of concurrent illnesses such as cardiomyopathy, aortic ruptures, neoplasia, and infections of other organ systems. Histopathologic evidence of renal disease was either coincidental, contributing, or a sequelae to the primary illness.

Clinical signs of renal disease are not easily detected in groups of woodchucks, which necessitates isolation of animals with suspected illness for more critical observation. Lethargy, inappetence and/or weight loss, increased water consumption and excessive soiling of bedding (polydipsia and polyuria), uremic odor which can permeate cage and room, facial swelling and abdominal distension, and neurologic signs (Anderson et al., 1990b) give reason for expanded examinations. Physical examination, clinicopathologic evaluations, and ultrasonography are useful in diagnosis. Anasarca and/or ascites and clinicopathologic evidence of protein-losing nephropathy is typical of glomerulonephritis. Enlarged kidneys occur in occasional woodchucks with glomerulonephritis, tubular nephrosis, hydronephrosis, and

neoplasia. Disparity in kidney size and/or loss of renal mass is often attributed to chronic fibrosing nephritis.

Immune-mediated glomerulonephritis, diagnosed based on the presence of light microscopic lesions and the presence of host immunoglobulin, is associated with WHV infection (Peters et al., 1992). In one study, three types of glomerulonephritis, membranous, mixed membranous and mesangial proliferative, and mesangial proliferative glomerulonephritis, were identified in six of 142 woodchucks with chronic WHV infection (Peters et al., 1992). Several types of glomerulonephritis are also associated with HBV infection in humans. Membranous nephritis is more common in younger individuals in both diseases (Peters et al., 1992). In both humans and woodchucks it is unclear if the types of glomerulonephritis are truly distinct disease forms or represent progression from one form to another. The woodchuck may be a useful animal model for the study of glomerulonephritis associated with HBV infection, particularly for investigating the progression of renal lesions.

5. Gastrointestinal Disease

Nonsuppurative inflammatory bowel disease (IBD) is occasionally observed in histologic sections of the intestinal tract of woodchucks. Lymphocytic plasmacytic enteritis, enterocolitis, enterotyphlocolitis, or colitis infrequently cause overt clinical signs of disease. In a necropsy study of 24 woodchucks with intestinal disease, IBD was a primary finding in two cases, one of which had a protracted history of diarrhea and the second had ascites and lymphangiectasia (unpublished observations). Eosinophilic enterotyphlitis and lymphoplasmacytic colitis were incidental findings in a woodchuck with central nervous system signs. IBD was accompanied by necrotizing enteritis and/or bowel infarction in 10 other woodchucks, only one of which had diarrhea. One of these woodchucks had a colonic-mesenteric volvulus and the death in the remaining woodchucks was attributed to extraintestinal lesions. Necrotizing enteritis and/or infarction were the dominant lesions in 11 woodchucks, many of which exhibited no signs of illness prior to death. Infectious etiology was suspected in three animals with necrotizing enteritis. Of these, *Clostridium difficile* and its endotoxin were isolated from the intestine in one woodchuck and intranuclear inclusion bodies were observed in crypt epithelium in a second. In other species, intranuclear inclusion bodies have been associated with parvovirus enteritis. Additional tests (IFA or examination of tissue by electron microscopy) were not done on this case. Two woodchucks had suppurative gastroenteritis, but no organism was cultured.

Rectal prolapse, sometimes associated with colonic intussusception, is a rare condition seen in young woodchucks, pregnant dams, or dams that have recently whelped. Rectal prolapse and intussusception may result from straining associated with diarrhea or labor. If diagnosed and treated early, a prolapse can be manually reduced and kept in place with a purse string suture. Intussusceptions require surgery.

The ascending colon of the woodchuck consists of a short straight segment that is firmly attached to the body wall by the mesocolon, and two loops that lie free in the abdomen. The two loops occasionally twist upon each other forming an overhand knot which leads to strangulation of the colon. Woodchucks are typically found dead, having shown no prior clinical signs.

Intestinal obstruction can result from entrapment in diaphragmatic hernias or from stricture formation by omental adhesions. A partial obstruction may produce clinical signs such as anorexia, weight loss, and depression whereas a total obstruction may result in sudden, unexpected death.

6. Dental Problems

Dental problems, including broken incisors, abscessed/infected teeth, and long incisors caused by malocclusion are occasionally seen. Neoplasia involving the mouth (squamous cell carcinoma, ameloblastoma, fibrosarcoma) is extremely rare. Dental problems may cause systemic illness or difficulty eating resulting in poor condition.

IV. THE WOODCHUCK AS AN EXPERIMENTAL ANIMAL MODEL FOR HBV RESEARCH

The identification of the Australia antigen (Blumberg et al., 1965, 1967) and the establishment of its relation to the virus of hepatitis B (Dane et al., 1970; Okuchi and Murakami 1968; Prince 1968) are among the most important medical discoveries of the twentieth century. These observations resulted in major advances in knowledge of the natural history of viral infections of the liver and in diagnosis and control (Ganem and Prince, 2004). A small percentage of adults that become infected with HBV become chronically infected but a much larger fraction of infants and young children infected with HBV become chronic carriers. Such HBV carriers may develop chronic hepatitis that progresses to cirrhosis (Alberti et al., 1978, 1979; Dudley et al., 1972; Prince et al., 1970; Ganem and Prince, 2004), and there is convincing epidemiological and molecular evidence that HBV is an etiological factor in the hepatocarcinogenisis (Blumberg and London, 1982; Buendia, 1994; Benhenda et al., 2009; Tan, 2011; Shlomai et al., 2014). Although chimpanzees can be infected with HBV and have been valuable animal models for investigation of viral pathogenesis and in vaccine development, cost and physical limitations

have limited their use and recently revised NIH policies have restricted their use further. The need for readily available animal models for preclinical HBV research has been well recognized.

A. Natural History of WHV Infection

Summers and his colleagues were the first to describe infection of the WHV infection in a colony of woodchucks at the Philadelphia Zoological Gardens with high rates of chronic hepatitis and HCC (Summers et al., 1978). In 15% of the woodchucks, the serum was found to contain viral DNA polymerase activity and viral particles morphologically similar to HBV. It was concluded that WHV was a member of the same family of viruses as HBV (Summers et al., 1978) and WHV subsequently was classified as a member of the genus Orthohepadnavirus, family Hepadnaviridae (Gust et al., 1986; Melnick, 1982; Robinson et al., 1982). The genetic organization of WHV is similar to HBV and to other mammalian hepadnaviruses. Numerous 22-nm spherical particles and related filaments are found in the serum of infected woodchucks composed of the viral envelope proteins (WHsAg). Complete virions are 42–45 nm in diameter and composed of an exterior envelope (WHsAg), the nucleocapsid or core protein (WHcAg), and within the nucleocapsid, the partially double-stranded DNA genome (Tiollais et al., 1985; Ganem and Varmus, 1987; Ganem and Prince, 2004). The replicative cycle of WHV appears to be identical to that of HBV (Summers, 1981; Tiollais et al., 1985; Ganem and Varmus, 1987). The transition of viral DNA to viral RNA during hepadnavirus replication is comparable to that of retroviruses (Ganem and Varmus, 1987; Summers, 1981; Ganem and Prince, 2004; Menne and Cote, 2007). Unlike retroviruses, however, integration of viral DNA into the host genome is not required for replication of hepadnaviruses as is the case with retroviruses. The integration of WHV DNA sequences into host cell genomic DNA appears to have a significant role in hepatocarcinogenesis (described below).

The woodchuck habitat extends from northern Georgia, Alabama, and Mississippi in the southern United States, west to Oklahoma, Kansas, Nebraska, North and South Dakota, north to Quebec and Labrador, and across Canada to British Columbia and the Yukon Territory, including a region in southeastern Alaska. A comprehensive, seroepidemiological study of WHV infection has not been performed, and the prevalence of WHV infection throughout most of this range remains unknown. WHV infection, however, is known to be hyperendemic in the mid-Atlantic states, and the woodchucks originally studied by Summers and colleagues (1978) originated in Pennsylvania. Of the woodchucks from Pennsylvania, New Jersey, and Maryland, 23% were test positive for WHsAg, and an additional 36%

were positive for anti-WHs antibody for prevalence rate of infection of 59% (Tyler *et al.*, 1981). Others have confirmed high rates of WHV infection in the mid-Atlantic states (Wong *et al.*, 1982). In contrast, the prevalence of WHV infection in central New York State has been estimated to be 2% based on the presence of antibody to the WHV surface anitgen; the rate of persistent WH surface antigenemia is less than 0.2% (Wong *et al.*, 1982). Although the number of woodchucks tested is small, no serological evidence of WHV infection has been found in Vermont, Massachusetts, or Iowa (Lutwick *et al.*, 1982; Summers, 1981; Young and Sims, 1979).

Hepatic 'adenomas' that ranged in diameter from 0.3–1.0 cm were described in woodchucks from the Philadelphia Zoological Garden many years ago (Fox, 1912; Ratcliffe, 1933). Two woodchucks were later described with primary hepatic neoplasms, one from the Washington Zoological Park and one trapped in Bethesda, Maryland (Habermann *et al.*, 1954). In addition to woodchucks from Pennsylvania (Snyder and Ratcliffe, 1969), other cases of hepatic neoplasia have been reported in laboratory-maintained woodchucks originally trapped in New York and Maryland (Bond, 1970; Long *et al.*, 1975). The hepatic neoplasms associated with naturally acquired WHV infection characteristically were well-differentiated HCCs with hyperchromatic nuclei and prominent nucleoli (Snyder and Summers, 1980). In most cases, chronic, active hepatitis was present in the nonneoplastic liver, with abundant portal mononuclear cell infiltration extending beyond the limiting plate. There also was scattered parenchymal hepatocellular necrosis, bile duct proliferation, and in some there was evidence of early fibrosis (Popper *et al.*, 1981; Roth *et al.*, 1985; Snyder and Summers, 1980; Snyder *et al.*, 1982). Progression of neoplasia from foci of altered hepatocytes, to small neoplastic nodules and to frank HCC, was described, and some HCCs contained significant numbers of infiltrating hematopoietic cells (Popper *et al.*, 1981; Abe *et al.*, 1988). Trabecular, pseudoglandular, and pelioid histological patterns have been observed in HCCs of woodchucks, similar to that of humans (Roth *et al.*, 1985). Metastasis of HCC outside the liver, which occurs in humans and experimental animal models with some frequency, has not been reported in woodchucks by most investigators, although pulmonary metastases have been observed (Roth *et al.*, 1985).

B. Other Naturally Occurring Hepadnavirus Infections of Animals

Since the description of WHV, closely related hepadnaviruses have been described in several other mammalian and avian species (Table 8.1). The morphology and genetic organization of these hepadnaviruses are similar (Ganem and Varmus, 1987; Tiollais *et al.* 1985; Gerlich, 2013). The ground squirrel hepatitis virus (GSHV 1) was described in California ground squirrels (*Spermophilus beecheyi*) (Marion *et al.*, 1980, 1986; Weiser *et al.*, 1983; Kodama *et al.*, 1985). Persistent GSHV infection is associated with chronic hepatitis and with HCC, although the frequency of HCC is considered to be less than that associated with chronic WHV infection and develops at an older age in California ground squirrels (Marion *et al.*, 1986). A similar hepadnavirus has been described in the arctic ground squirrel (*Spermophilus parryi*) and named the arctic GSHV (AGSHV). Infection with AGSHV was associated with a remarkably high rate of HCC (Testut *et al.*, 1996). Infection with a putative hepadnavirus has been described in Eastern gray squirrels (*Spermophilus carolinensis*) in Pennsylvania (Feitelson *et al.*, 1986). Lesions of hepatitis were reported, but hepatic tumors were not observed. Evidence also has been reported for hepadnavirus infection in Richardson's ground squirrels (*Spermophilus richardsonii*) originating in Alberta (Minuk *et al.*, 1986; Tennant *et al.*, 1991b). The hepatic lesions including HCC were remarkably similar to those described in woodchucks, California ground squirrels, and Arctic ground squirrels.

Infection with the duck HBV (DHBV) was first reported in Pekin ducks (*Anas domesticus*; Mason *et al.*, 1980; Omata *et al.*, 1983, 1984) and DHBV has a worldwide distribution. Much of the current understanding of hepanavirus replication is based on *in vivo* and *in vitro* research involving DHBV (Marion *et al.*, 1987; Beck and Nassal, 2007; Reaiche-Miller *et al.*, 2013). Avihepadnaviruses have been described in a wide variety of wild bird families (Funk *et al.*, 2007). From Germany, avian hepadnaviruses have been described in gray herons (*Ardea cinerea*; heron HBV; Sprengel *et al.*, 1988), and in snow geese (*Anser caerulescens*; snow goose HBV; Chang *et al.*, 1999). Hepatic neoplasms have not been associated with heron HBV infection (Sprengel *et al.*, 1988).

C. Experimental Hepadnavirus Infection of Woodchucks

The original observations of WHV infection were made with woodchucks trapped in the native habitat and subsequently maintained in the laboratory. Such woodchucks in which WHV infection was naturally acquired proved to be valuable sources of virus and hepatic tissue for histological and molecular analyses; however, their limitations for experimental purposes were soon recognized. It was impossible to know when and for how long trapped woodchucks had been infected with WHV or to be certain about their nutritional history and/or exposure to environmental factors, which might have influenced the course of WHV infection. Importantly, hepatic lesions caused by nematodes such as *Ackertia marmotae* and *Capillaria* spp. were common in wild woodchucks (Cohn *et al.*, 1986) and could complicate the interpretation of experimental results.

Summers and colleagues (1980) described the experimental infection of 4–8-month-old woodchucks with serum from chronic WHV carriers. They described successful productive infection, but infection was self-limited, and no woodchucks became chronic carriers. Attempts by others to infect juvenile or adult woodchucks experimentally resulted in acute WHV infection (Millman *et al.*, 1984; Tyler *et al.*, 1986; Wong *et al.*, 1982) but, with one exception, did not cause chronic WHV infection. Morphological and molecular virological studies of the liver have shown that virtually 100% of hepatocytes become infected after experimental WHV inoculation (Kajino *et al.*, 1994). Although replicative forms were cleared rapidly during recovery, covalently closed circular WHV DNA persisted in three of 10 woodchucks after evidence of WHV replication had ceased (Kajino *et al.*, 1994). Clearance of experimental WHV infection in adult woodchucks is associated with robust humoral and cell-mediated immune responses (Guo *et al.*, 2000; Shanmuganathan *et al.*, 1997; Menne and Cote, 2007). Treatment with immune suppressive doses of cyclosporine A significantly increases the rate of chronic WHV infection (Cote *et al.*, 1991, 1992).

When adult humans are infected with HBV, less than 5% become chronic carriers (Seeff *et al.*, 1987; Tassopoulos *et al.*, 1987). HBV infection early in life, however, results in high rates of chronic infection (Blumberg and London, 1982; Ganem and Varmus, 1987; Gerlich, 2013). The high rates of chronic WHV infection observed in woodchucks from hyperendemic areas (Popper *et al.*, 1981; Snyder and Summers, 1980; Tyler *et al.*, 1981) suggested that, as in humans, infection in woodchucks early in life (or possibly *in utero* infection) must be necessary to account for the high WHV carrier rates.

To utilize the advantages of the woodchuck as an experimental animal model, it became necessary to breed and rear woodchucks in laboratory animal facilities. The result allowed knowledge of the experimental woodchucks' genetic background, definition of their diet, and, prevention of possible natural exposure to WHV infection and to other diseases endemic in populations of wild woodchucks. To meet this requirement, a breeding colony of WHV-negative woodchucks was established at Cornell University in 1979. The colony served as the source of woodchucks for experimental studies of WHV pathogenesis and hepatocarcinogenesis. Woodchucks born in the laboratory animal setting are inoculated at birth with diluted serum from standardized infectious pools obtained from chronic WHV carrier woodchucks (Gerin *et al.*, 1989; Popper *et al.*, 1987; Tennant *et al.*, 2004; Menne and Cote, 2007). After inoculation, woodchucks are monitored using specific serological markers of WHV infection (WHV DNA, WHsAg, anti-WH core antibody, and anti-WH surface antibody) (Cote *et al.*, 1993; Wong *et al.*, 1982; Menne and Cote, 2007).

The rate of chronic WHV infection after neonatal inoculation is 60% or greater (Gerin *et al.*, 1989; Popper *et al.*, 1987; Tennant *et al.*, 1988; Tennant, *et al.*, 2004; Menne and Cote, 2007). Survival analyses have been made of chronic WHV carriers experimentally infected at birth with WHV, of woodchucks that recovered from neonatal WHV infection by clearing WH viremia and developing anti-WHs antibody, and of control woodchucks not infected with WHV but born and raised under similar laboratory conditions. All WHV carriers were dead by 56 months of age, and the lifetime risk of HCC was 100% (Gerin *et al.*, 1989; Popper *et al.*, 1987). The median time to death from HCC in WHV carriers was 29 months. In contrast, 42% of the woodchucks with resolved WHV infection and 62% of uninfected controls were alive at 56 months of age. Although the rate of HCC in WHV carriers was significantly higher than that of woodchucks in which WHV infection was resolved, 17% of the woodchucks that recovered from neonatal WHV infection developed HCC (Gerin *et al.*, 1989). HCC was not observed in the uninfected, laboratory-reared, control woodchucks. These results provide compelling direct experimental evidence for the carcinogenicity of WHV and, by analogy, for other mammalian hepadnaviruses (HBV, GSHV, and AGSHV) in which naturally acquired hepadnavirus infection has been associated with HCC (Tennant, *et al.*, 2004). The rate of HCC in woodchucks with experimentally induced chronic WHV infection was similar to that observed in woodchucks with naturally acquired chronic WHV infection (Snyder and Summers, 1980; Popper *et al.*, 1981; Roth *et al.*, 1985; Tennant *et al.*, 2004), and the presence of preneoplastic foci of altered hepatocytes with progressive aneuploid change (Cullen *et al.*, 1994) also was similar (Abe *et al.*, 1988; Toshkov *et al.*, 1990).

In contrast to humans and experimental mice, the sex of experimental woodchucks does not influence the rate of WHV associated HCC (Wands, 2007). This result was unexpected because both in humans infected with HBV and in laboratory rodents in which HCC is induced by chemical hepaticarcinogens, males tend to have higher rates of HCC than females. The explanation may be related to the unusual circannual reproductive cycle of the woodchuck. For at least 8 months of the year, the testicles of male woodchucks are abdominal and produce little or no testosterone, resulting effectively in functional castration (Baldwin *et al.*, 1985). With one exception, diseases caused by WHV infection are confined to the liver. Immune-mediated glomerulonephritis has been reported with increased frequency in woodchucks chronically infected with WHV, and it appears to be similar etiologically to the glomerulonephritis in humans associated with chronic HBV infection (Peters et al., 1992).

Investigation of hepadnavirus replication has been impeded by the limited availability of tissue culture systems. However, full-length clones of the genomes of HBV (Will et al., 1982), WHV (Miller et al., 1990), DHBV (Sprengel et al., 1984), and GSHV (Seeger et al., 1987) have been shown to be infectious, and injection directly into the hepatic parenchyma of the homologous host species results in productive hepadnavirus infection. During transfection experiments to determine the viral gene or genes responsible for host range restriction, it was found that woodchucks could be infected with GSHV (Seeger et al., 1987, 1991). The chipmunk (Eutamias species) also had been shown to be susceptible to GSHV infection (Trueba et al., 1985).

HCC in woodchucks chronically infected with WHV has been reported to occur more frequently (Gerin et al., 1989; Popper et al., 1981, 1987) than in California ground squirrels chronically infected with GSHV. In chronic GSHV infection, HCC also develops at an older age (Marion et al., 1986). Because woodchucks could be infected with both hepadnaviruses, it could be determined whether the apparent differences in oncogenicity between GSHV and WHV in their respective natural hosts were the result of differences in host response or of viral genetic differences. When neonatal woodchucks were experimentally infected with WHV or GSHV, the rates of chronic infection for each virus were similar, and at 2 years of age no difference was noted in the severity of chronic hepatitis (Seeger et al., 1991). By 2 years, hepatic neoplasms had developed in 13 of 16 chronic WHV carriers. In sharp contrast, only one of 16 chronic GSHV carriers at that age had developed a single, grossly identifiable hepatic tumor nodule (5 mm diameter), which was classified as a hepatic adenoma. On the basis of these observations, it was concluded that the difference between GSHV and WHV in oncogenic capacity that had been observed in their respective natural hosts must be due to genetic differences between the viruses, although the additional differences in host factors could not be excluded. It would be useful to infect California ground squirrels with WHV, but this may not be possible. Attempts to transfect California ground squirrels with WHV DNA have not yet been successful (Seeger et al., 1987). It should, however, be possible to assess differences in the viral genetic determinants of oncogenicity using WHV/GSHV chimeric hepadnavirus constructs.

D. Mechanisms of Hepatocarcinogenesis Associated with Hepadnavirus Infection

There are three lines of evidence that now provide compelling evidence indicating that HBV has an important etiological role in human hepatocarcinogenesis. The first came from epidemiological studies. In regions of the world where HBV infection was hyperendemic (Sub-Saharan Africa, Asia) the prevalence of HCC was remarkably increased (Maupas et al., 1975; Szmuness, 1978; Beasley and Lin, 1978). Case control studies demonstrated significantly higher rates of HCC in individuals chronically infected with HBV than in uninfected case controls both in hyperendemic regions of Africa (Blumberg et al., 1975; Maupas et al., 1975; Prince et al., 1975) and Asia (Okuda et al., 1982) and in the United States and Great Britain, where the rates of HBV infection and HCC were relatively low (Tabor et al., 1977; Viola et al., 1981). Finally, compelling evidence came from the now classical prospective epidemiological studies conducted in Taiwan that demonstrated the significant increased relative risk of HCC in individual chronic HBV carriers (Beasley, 1982, 1988; Beasley and Lin, 1978; Beasley et al., 1981). A similarly high relative risk of HCC in HBV carriers also was reported in the United States (Prince and Alcabes, 1982).

The second line of evidence is molecular and comes from the demonstration of covalent integration of truncated HBV DNA sequences in the cellular DNA of hepatic neoplasms from HBV carriers (Brechot et al., 1981; Chen et al., 1982; Shafritz, 1982). These observations suggest that HBV has a direct oncogenic role similar to that of other tumor-producing viruses in which integrated viral DNA or, in the case of retroviruses, proviral DNA causes malignant transformation by insertional mutagenesis (Chen et al., 1982; Shafritz, 1982). Finally, the comparative medical evidence strongly supports an etiological role of hepadnaviruses in hepatocarcinogenesis. At least four members of the family Sciuridae have been described in which persistent hepadnavirus infection has been closely associated with development of HCC (Table 8.1; Summers et al., 1978; Marion et al., 1983, 1986; Testut et al., 1996; and Tennant et al., 2004).

How hepadnaviruses actually cause HCC, however, is not completely understood. Two general mechanisms have been proposed to explain hepadnavirus-associated hepatocarcinogenesis (Tennant, 1992). One hypothesis is that hepadnaviruses have a direct molecular role (Buendia, 1994; Buendia, 1995). In this model, integration of hepadnaviral nucleic acid sequences into host cell DNA is considered a critical mutagenic event, which causes an alteration in expression of genes that regulate the cell cycle (protooncogenes and tumor suppressor genes). Ultimately, these changes result in neoplastic transformation of hepatocytes. Hepadnavirus integration is thought to initiate cell transformation in a manner comparable with that caused by chemical hepatocarcinogens (Farber and Sarma, 1987; Pitot and Dragan, 1991).

Support for the molecular hypothesis comes from detection of integrated hepadnaviral sequences in the cellular DNA of most primary hepatic tumors from HBV carriers (Brechot *et al.*, 1981; Chen *et al.*, 1982; Shafritz, 1982). Similar integrations of viral nucleic acids have been observed in other mammalian cancers caused by DNA tumor viruses (Johnson and Williams, 1982). Integrations in the apparently nonneoplastic hepatic tissue of HBV people suggests integration precedes formation of hepatic neoplasms. Although occasional integrations have been identified in or near a potential oncogene, the large majority of HBV integrations in human HCC appear random.

Integrated WHV sequences also have been found in most HCCs from WHV-infected woodchucks (Korba *et al.*, 1989). Characteristically, only portions of the viral genome are integrated, and the sequences are often rearranged (Ganem and Varmus, 1987; Schadel *et al.*, 1980). Molecular cloning and analyses of integrated WHY DNA and associated flanking sequences of cellular DNA initially demonstrated that integrations occurred at multiple sites within the woodchuck genome (Fuchs *et al.*, 1989; Kaneko *et al.*, 1986; Korba *et al.*, 1989; Mitamura *et al.*, 1982; Ogston *et al.*, 1982; Rogler *et al.*, 1987). Multiple integrations were sometimes observed in a single tumor mass. One explanation for multiple integrations was that several hepadnavirus integrations could have accumulated in a single hepatocyte and been propagated clonally by the transformed hepatocyte. The alternative was that an initial integration of hepadnaviral DNA was followed by secondary rearrangements of integrated viral sequences (Rogler, 1991). Integrations of WHV DNA have been reported in apparently nontumorous liver of woodchucks (Fuchs *et al.*, 1989; Korba *et al.*, 1989; Mitamura *et al.*, 1982; Ogston *et al.*, 1982; Rogler *et al.*, 1987). These reports combined with the unique integration patterns of individual hepatic tumors, suggests that integration occurs early in hepatocarcinogenesis and before clonal expansion. Evidence of integrations in early neoplastic nodules has been described before development of frank HCC (Rogler, 1991; Yang *et al.*, 1993, 1996).

Mammalian hepadnaviruses do not contain oncogenes similar to those found in transforming retroviruses (Ganem and Varmus, 1987; Tiollais *et al.*, 1985). Upregulation of most of the well-characterized protooncogenes has not been demonstrated (Moroy *et al.*, 1986). Increased expression (5–50-fold) of c-*myc* was observed, however, in three of a series of nine woodchuck HCCs (Hsu *et al.*, 1988; Moroy *et al.*, 1986, 1989), and truncation and rearrangement of the gene were demonstrated. In one tumor, no direct linkage between WHV DNA integration and c-*myc* activation was demonstrated. In that case, rearrangement and activation of c-*myc* appeared to be similar to that observed in Burkitt's lymphoma and in acute B and T cell leukemias in which chromosomal translocations are present (Moroy *et al.*, 1986). In the other two integrations, c-*myc* activation was the result

of insertional mutagenesis (Hsu *et al.*, 1988), and WHV DNA insertions interrupted different regions of the c-*myc* locus. The position and orientation of the WHV and c-*myc* sequences and the use of the c-*myc* promoter excluded involvement of the hepadnaviral promoter in c-*myc* activation (i.e., promoter insertion). In both cases, WHV sequences analogous to one of the HBV enhancers were present, suggesting an enhancer insertion mechanism (Hsu *et al.*, 1988). In a large series of woodchuck HCCs, activation of c-*myc* was observed in 10% of the tumors (Dejean and de The, 1990) and Jacob et al. (2004) have shown the size and grade of hepatocelluar carcinomas in WHV carrier woodchucks are directly correlated with viral integrations.

Buendia and her colleagues now have demonstrated that N-myc messenger RNA was overexpressed in 60% of woodchuck HCCs examined, and this transcript was not detected in normal woodchuck liver. Insertions of WHV nucleic acid sequences were located adjacent to cellular N-*myc* sequences in 20% of the tumors studied. Woodchucks have two N-*myc* loci. One N-*myc* locus was homologous to the N-*myc* gene of other mammalian species; the other was an intronless gene with the characteristic structure of a retrotransposon and was identified as N-*myc2* (Fourel *et al.*, 1990). N-*myc2* was mapped to the X chromosome. Expression of N-*myc2* is highly restricted, and the brain is the only normal tissue of the woodchuck in which N-*myc2* RNA was detected (Fourel *et al.*, 1992).

The physiological function, if any, of N-*myc2* remains unknown (Fourel *et al.*, 1992). A distinctive feature of hepatocarcinogenesis in woodchucks with chronic WHV infection appears to be the coupling of viral integration into the *myc* family of protooncogenes. Viral integrations appear to be preferentially associated with the N-*myc2* locus (Flajolet *et al.*, 1997; Wei *et al.*, 1998). Insertion of WHV enhancer sequences either upstream or downstream of the N-myc2 coding domain result in increased transcription either of normal N-myc2 RNA or of a hybrid N-*myc2*/WHV transcript that is initiated at the normal N-*myc2* start site. Transcriptional activation by enhancer insertion appears to be a common mechanism (Wei *et al.*, 1992). A liver-specific regulatory element in the WHV genome has been identified that appears to control cis activation of N-*myc2* (Fourel *et al.*, 1996). Downstream integration of WHV DNA also has been associated with activation of N-*myc2* (Fourel *et al.*, 1994).

Recently, Buendia and colleagues have reported that transgenic mice carrying the N-*myc2* gene under the control of WHV regulatory sequences are highly predisposed to cancer of the liver (Renard *et al.*, 2000). Seventy percent developed either HCC or hepatocellular adenomas. A transgenic founder that carried the unmethylated WHV/N-*myc2* transgene sequence died at the age of 2 months with a large liver tumor, demonstrating the high oncogenic capacity of the woodchuck

N-*myc* retroposon. Mutations or deletions of the catenin gene similar to those of HCCs from humans and mice (De La Coste *et al.*, 1998) were present in 25% of the hepatic tumors of the N-*myc2* transgenic animals, and tumor latency (time to tumor) was significantly reduced (Renard *et al.*, 2000). When N-*myc2* transgenic mice were crossed with *p53* null mice, the absence of one p53 allele markedly accelerated the onset of liver cancer, providing direct experimental evidence for synergy in multistage hepatocarcinogenesis between activation of N-myc2 and diminished expression of *p53* (Renard *et al.*, 2000).

Like the woodchuck, the California ground squirrel possesses a functional, transcriptionally active N-*myc2* locus in the brain (Quignon *et al.*, 1996). However, increased N-*myc2* expression is unusual in HCCs from California ground squirrels infected with GSHV. Amplification of c-*myc* expression, however, is more frequent in ground squirrel hepatic neoplasms than in those of woodchucks (Transy *et al.*, 1992). HCCs from woodchucks experimentally infected either with WHV or with GSHV have been analyzed (Hansen *et al.*, 1993). The propensity for WHV genomic DNA to integrate in or near the N-*myc2* locus in HCCs from chronic WHV carriers was confirmed, whereas in woodchuck HCCs associated with GSHV infection, such integrations were exceptional. Seven of 17 (41%) WHV-induced tumors had rearrangements of the N-*myc2* allele. Only one of 16 GSHV-associated tumors (6%), however, had such N-myc2 rearrangements. Based on the observations in GSHV-induced HCCs from ground squirrels and from woodchucks, it was concluded that the differences in hepadnavirus insertion and in N-*myc* activation between woodchucks and ground squirrels were due primarily to viral genetic differences and not to differences in the respective host species (Hansen *et al.*, 1993). A similar conclusion was reached by Buendia and her colleagues (Quignon *et al.*, 1996).

Transfection of a nonmalignant, SV-40 T antigen-transformed mouse hepatic cell line with HBV DNA produced cells with a malignant phenotype that grew in soft agar and were tumorigenic in nude mice. The HBV X gene (HBX 1) transcript was expressed at a much higher level than that observed *in vivo* (Hohne *et al.*, 1990). In subsequent studies, it was concluded that overexpression of the HBX was required for malignant transformation of the cell line (Seifer *et al.*, 1991). HBX is known to promote hepatocarcinogenesis in c-myc transgenic mice (Terradillos *et al.*, 1997) and may promote hepadnavirus-induced hepatocarcinogenesis (Seeger and Mason, 2000).

The X gene appears to be essential for normal replication of hepadnaviruses *in vivo* (Chen *et al.*, 1993). The woodchuck hepatitis X (WHX 1) protein is coexpressed with WHcAg in the liver of chronic WHV carrier woodchucks (Feitelson *et al.*, 1993; Jacob *et al.*, 1997). Feitelson and colleagues demonstrated that when WHX was cotranslated *in vitro* with p53, WHX/p53 complexes developed, and similar WHX/p53 complexes were demonstrated in the livers of chronic WHV carriers (Feitelson *et al.*, 1997). Combined with observations in HBV transgenic mice (Ghebranious and Sell, 1998; Ueda *et al.*, 1995), the observations of Feitelson *et al.* suggest that binding of WHX to p53 may prevent entry of p53 into the nucleus, diminish tumor suppressor activity, and represent an important mechanism by which the hepadnavirus X-gene product could promote hepatocarcinogenesis (Feitelson *et al.*, 1997). Mutations of p53 also may alter its tumor suppressor activity, but such mutations were found primarily in the less differentiated hepatic tumors, suggesting the mutations altered tumor progression at a later stage of development (Hsia *et al.*, 2000; Ueda *et al.*, 1995).

The second hypothesis regarding the role of hepadnavirus in hepatocarcinogenesis is that hepatic injury caused by viral infection and related hepatocellular regeneration provide an environment that enhances fixation of spontaneous mutations, rearrangements, or chromosomal translocations that are responsible for malignant transformation of hepatocytes. Such a role for hepadnaviruses in hepatocarcinogenesis would be comparable to the processes of promotion and/or progression recognized in multistage chemical hepatocarcinogenesis (Farber and Sarma, 1987; Hanahan and Weinberg, 2000; Pitot and Dragan, 1991; Tennant, 1992).

Support for this model comes from the observation that chronic liver injury associated with cirrhosis frequently precedes the development of HCC in HBV-infected people (Kalayci *et al.*, 1991; Zhou *et al.*, 1999). Chronic hepatitis C virus infection results in progressively severe chronic hepatitis and cirrhosis and is frequently associated with development of HCC. A significant increase in the rate of HCC has been observed in inherited forms of chronic liver disease in humans including hemochromatosis and alpha-1-antitrypsin deficiency (Schafer and Sorrell, 1999). These inherited diseases also are associated with development of progressive hepatocellular injury, regeneration, and cirrhosis that precede development of HCC (Johnson and Williams, 1987).

Experimental evidence supporting the role of hepatic inflammation and hepatocellular injury as a key event in hepadnavirus-associated HCC comes from the work of Chisari and colleagues with transgenic mice described above (Chisari, 2000; Chisari *et al.*, 1989; Dunsford *et al.*, 1990; Moriyama *et al.*, 1990). In the lines of transgenic mice they have studied, a direct relation was found between the expression and retention of HBsAg in hepatocytes and the severity of hepatitis. A close correlation also was observed between the severity of hepatitis in transgenic mice and development of HCC (Chisari *et al.*, 1989; Dunsford *et al.*, 1990; Sell *et al.*, 1991). Increased free radical production within the liver was associated with oxidative DNA damage, similar to that suggested in woodchucks (Bannasch *et al.*, 1995) and that has been observed in other mice (Faux *et al.*, 1992).

Aflatoxin is among the most potent hepatocarcinogens known and is a frequent contaminant of the diets of populations with high incidence rates of HBV infection and HCC. The possible interaction between hepadnavirus infection and aflatoxin has been investigated using the woodchuck model (Bannasch *et al.*, 1995; Rivkina *et al.*, 1996; Tennant *et al.*, 1991a). When administered early in life to woodchucks experimentally infected at birth with WHV, aflatoxin B1 did not appear to increase the rate of chronic WHV infection or the rate of development of HCC (Tennant *et al.*, 1991a). When administered beginning at 1 year of age to established chronic WHV carriers, the time to tumor was moderately but significantly reduced by aflatoxin B1 treatment (Bannasch *et al.*, 1995). A similar synergistic interaction between HBV and aflatoxin has been reported in the tree shrew (Yan *et al.*, 1996).

It has been shown that HBV transgenic mice are more susceptible to chemical hepatocarcinogenesis than controls (Dragani *et al.*, 1990). When transgenic mice that expressed HBsAg were exposed to nitrosodiethylamine (NDMA 1) or aflatoxin, they developed hepatic adenomas and HCC more rapidly and more extensively than unexposed transgenic controls or normal mice receiving either of these hepatocarcinogens. These results demonstrated a significant synergistic interaction between chemical hepatocarcinogens and the chronic hepatocellular injury induced by overexpression of HBsAg in transgenic mice (Sell *et al.*, 1991). A similar synergistic effect of HBX expression in transgenic mice and NDMA in hepatocarcinogenesis has also been reported (Slagle *et al.*, 1996). Another possible hepatocarcinogenic mechanism related to hepatic inflammation has been suggested by studies of nitric oxide (NO) production in chronic viral hepatitis. In the liver, NO biosynthesis from argmme is catalyzed by inducible NO synthetase. Endotoxin, y-interferon, and other cytokines (Billiar *et al.*, 1992a, b; Cullen *et al.*, 1989; Curran *et al.*, 1990, 1991; Geller *et al.*, 1993; Hortellano *et al.*, 1992; Knowles *et al.*, 1990; Wood *et al.*, 1993) can increase the activity of this enzyme significantly. NO under certain circumstances may have a protective effect against experimental hepatic injury (Curran *et al.*, 1991). Under other conditions, hepatic production of NO may contribute to development of the hypotension associated with septic shock (Kilbourn *et al.*, 1990).

Woodchucks chronically infected with WHV excrete more nitrate in the urine and more NDMA than uninfected control woodchucks (Liu *et al.*, 1991). Similar increased nitric oxide (NO) production has been observed in HBV transgenic mice (Chisari, 2000). Nitrate and NDMA are derived from NO produced from L-arginine. Urinary nitrate excretion also is increased in a human patient with chronic HBV infection (Nguyen *et al.*, 1992).

In primary hepatocyte cultures from normal woodchucks, NO synthesis can be induced by endotoxin, and hepatocytes cultured from chronic WHV carriers produce significantly more NO and nitrosamine than hepatocytes from uninfected controls (Liu *et al.*, 1992). SV-40 T antigen transformed woodchuck hepatocyte cell lines have the capacity to produce NO in response to endotoxin (Liu *et al.*, 1993) utilizing the L-arginine–NO pathway and to produce N-nitrosodimethylamine (NDMA). WHsAg purified from woodchuck serum can induce NO production in woodchuck hepatocyte cultures (Liu *et al.*, 1994). NO reacts with oxygen O_2 to produce nitric oxide (NO_2), which exists in equilibrium with dinitrogen trioxide (N_2O_3) and dinitrogen tetroxide (N_2O_4). N_2O_3 and N_2O_4 are potent nitrosating agents capable of reacting with water to form nitrite and nitrate (Marletta *et al.*, 1988) or, in neutral solution, of nitrosating dialkylamines to form nitrosamines. NO could act as a carcinogen indirectly by causing formation of hepatocarcinogenic nitrosamines such as NDMA, which is a strong alkylating agent. Point mutations can be induced by NDMA by methylation of guanine to 7-methyl and to O6-methylguanine, or by methylation of adenine to 3-methyladenine (Archer, 1989; Magee, 1989).

NO also has the capacity to act as a direct mutagen (Wink *et al.*, 1991). *In vitro*, NO can deaminate deoxynucleosides, deoxynucleotides, or intact DNA and contribute to deamination-related mutations. It has been predicted based on studies of the rate of deamination of guanine to xanthine *in vitro* that guanine/cytosine–7 adenine/thymine transitions could be a frequent form of mutation induced by NO. Adenosine deamination to hypoxanthine would be expected to result in adenine/thymine–7 guanine/cytosine transitions, and removal of the xanthine formed by guanine deamination would result in depurination and transversions (Nguyen *et al.*, 1992). The demonstration of increased NO formation in the hepadnavirus-infected liver suggests that NO could have an important role in hepatocarcinogenesis.

E. Use of the Woodchuck Model in Development of Antiviral Therapy

Woodchucks with experimentally induced chronic WHV infection are now frequently used in the preclinical assessment of antiviral drugs being developed for treatment of chronic HBV infection. Nucleoside analogs (Chu *et al.*, 1998; Hostetler *et al.*, 2000; Korba *et al.*, 2000a, b, c) and immune response modifiers have been tested (Gangemi *et al.*, 1996). Before testing in woodchucks, the drugs are screened for antiviral activity against HBV in the 2.2.15 cell system, a HepG2 cell line engineered to produce HBV constitutively (Korba and Gerin, 1992).

Acyclovir and azidothymidine, which had no selectivity in 2.2.15 cells, had no antiviral effect in the woodchuck model of HBV infection. Adenine-5' arabinoside monophosphate, which had moderate antiviral activity *in vitro*, had significant antiviral activity in woodchucks *in vivo*, and activity was increased by specific liver targeting (Enriquez *et al.*, 1995). Most nucleoside analogs with intermediate antiviral activity *in vitro* against HBV had intermediate antiviral activity *in vivo*. One exception was 1-(2-Deoxy-2-fluoro-ß-D-arabinofuranosyl)-5-iodouracil, which had modest *in vitro* activity. In woodchucks, however, 1-(2-Deoxy-2-fluoro-ß-D-arabinofuranosyl)-5-iodouracil had potent antiviral activity but was highly toxic, as had been observed in humans (Tennant *et al.*, 1998). The *in vitro* activity of 1-(2-fluoro-5-methyl, L-arabinofuranosyl) uracil (L-FMAU, clevudine) was only moderate but was highly potent *in vivo* in WHV carrier woodchucks (Chu *et al.*, 1998; Peek *et al.*, 2000). Lobucavir (BMS-180194) also had intermediate *in vitro* activity in the 2.2.15 cell system but, at the dosage studied, had potent antiviral activity against WHV (Tennant *et al.*, 1996). Lamivudine, which had a very high selective index *in vitro*, was a potent antiviral drug in woodchucks with favorable pharmacokinetics (Rajagopalan *et al.*, 1996) and was without toxicity at doses of 5 or 15 mg/kg/day for 28 days (Korba *et al.*, 2000b; Peek *et al.*, 1997). The absence of effect of lamivudine on hepatic cccDNA was postulated to be due to the absence of cell division (Moraleda *et al.*, 1997). Lamivudine has been shown in the woodchuck model to act synergistically both with alpha-interferon (Korba *et al.*, 2000a) and with famciclovir (Korba *et al.*, 2000c). Similarly, high antiviral potency of the closely related emtricitabine has been shown in WHV carrier woodchucks (Korba *et al.*, 2000d). Extended lamivudine treatment of woodchucks with chronic WHV infections delayed the development of HCC and significantly extended survival in one study (Peek *et al.*, 1997; Tennant et al., 2004). In another study, no effect of lamivudine was observed on hepatocarcinogenesis. Although treatment was begun at an older age, the duration of treatment was not as long and the apparent effect of treatment on viral load was not as great (Mason *et al.*, 1998). A very high rate of polymerase gene mutations was detected in both humans and woodchucks after long-term lamivudine therapy (Brechot *et al.*, 1981; Peek *et al.*, 1997; Zhou *et al.*, 1999). Animal models of HBV infection have been valuable in determining the mechanisms of hepadnavirus replication, for studies of pathogenesis, and for investigation of viral hepatocarcinogenesis. The woodchuck also appears to be useful in the discovery and development of antiviral drugs to treat HBV infection and for testing new forms of immunotherapy. In particular, the woodchuck is ideal for studying the impact of antiviral treatment and immunotherapy on the outcome of hepadnavirus infection and on survival. The median life expectancy of experimentally infected chronic WHV carriers is approximately 29 months, and almost all develop

TABLE 8.3   Hepatitis B Viruses (Hepadnaviruses) of Animals

Virus scientific name	Host	
GENUS: ORTHOHEPADNAVIRUS		
Hepatitis B virus (HBV)[a]	Human	*Homo sapiens*
Woodchuck hepatitis virus (WHV)	Woodchuck, groundhog	*Marmota monax*
California ground squirrel hepatitis virus (GSHV)	California ground squirrel	*Spermophilus beecheyi*
Arctic ground squirrel hepatitis virus (AGSHV)	Artic ground squirrel	*Spermophilus parryii*
Wooly monkey hepatitis B virus (WMHBV)	Woolly monkey	*Lagothrix labotricha*
Richardson's ground squirrel virus	Richardson's ground squirrel	*Urocitellus richardsonii*
GENUS: AVIHEPADNAVIRUS		
Duck hepatitis B virus (DHBV)	Domestic Duck	*Anas domesticus*
Heron hepatitis B virus (HHBV)	Gray heron	*Ardea cineria*
Snow goose hepatitis B virus (SGHBV)	Snow goose	*Anser caerulescens*
White stork hepatitis virus (STHBV)	White stork	*Ciconia ciconia*
Crane hepatitis virus (CHBV)	Demoiselle crane	*Anthropoides virgo*
	Gray crowned crane	*Balearica reglorum*
Parrot hepatitis B virus (PHB)	Ring-necked parrot	*Psittacula krameri*

[a]*Naturally acquired HBV infection also has been demonstrated in the chimpanzee, gorilla, gibbon, and orangutan.*

HCC. New types of prophylaxis or therapy, therefore, can be evaluated under controlled experimental conditions in a relevant animal model within a reasonable time frame. It is possible to infect neonatal woodchucks born in the laboratory with standardized inocula and produce a high rate of chronic WHV carriers that are useful for controlled investigations (Tennant and Gerin, 2001; Tennant et al., 2004; Menne and Cote, 2007). WHV has been shown experimentally to cause hepatocellular carcinoma, supporting conclusions based on epidemiological and molecular virological studies that HBV is an important etiological factor in human hepatocarcinogenesis. Chronic WHV carrier woodchucks have become a valuable animal model for the preclinical evaluation of antiviral therapy for HBV infection, providing useful pharmacokinetic and pharmacodynamic results in a relevant animal disease model. It also has been shown that the pattern of toxicity and hepatic injury observed in woodchucks treated with certain fluorinated pyrimidines is remarkably similar to that observed in humans that were treated with the same drugs, suggesting the woodchuck has significant potential for the preclinical assessment of antiviral drug toxicity.

References

Abe, K., Kurata, T., Shikata, T., Tennant, B.C., 1988. Enzyme-altered liver cell foci in woodchucks infected with woodchuck hepatitis virus. Jpn. J. Cancer Res. 79, 466–472.

Alberti, A., Diana, S., Scullard, G.H., Eddleston, W.F., Williams, R., 1978. Full and empty dane particles in chronic hepatitis B virus infection: relation to hepatitis B e antigen and presence of liver damage. Gastroenterology 75, 869–874.

Anderson, W.I., Scott, D.W., Hornbuckle, W.E., King, J.M., Tennant, B.C., 1990a. Taenia crassiceps infection in woodchucks: a retrospective study of 13 cases. Vet. Dermatol. 1, 85–92.

Anderson, W.I., deLahunta, A., Hornbuckle, W.E., King, J.M., Tennant, B.C., 1990b. Two cases of renal encephalopathy in the woodchuck (marmota monax). Lab. Anim. Sci. 40, 86–88.

Archer, M.C., 1989. Mechanisms of action of N-nitroso compounds. Cancer Surv. 8, 241–250.

Bailey, E.D., 1965. Seasonal changes in metabolic activity of non-hibernating woodchucks. Can. J. Zool. 43, 905–909.

Baldwin, B.H., Tennant, B.C., Reimers, T.J., Cowan, R.G., Concannon, P.W., 1985. Circannual changes in serum testosterone concentrations of adult and yearling woodchucks (marmota monax). Biol. Reprod. 32, 804–812.

Bannasch, P., Khoshkou, N.I., Hacker, H.J., Radaeva, S., Mrozek, M., et al., 1995. Synergistic hepatocarcinogenic effect of hepadnaviral infection and dietary aflatoxin Bl in woodchucks. Cancer Res. 55, 3318–3330.

Beasley, R.P., 1982. Hepatitis B virus as the etiologic agent in hepacellular carcinoma – epidemiological considerations. Hepatology 2, 21S–26S.

Beasley, R.P., 1988. Hepatitis B virus. the major etiology of hepatocellular carcinoma. Cancer 61, 1942–1956.

Beasley, R.P., Lin, C.C., 1978. Hepatoma risk among hepatitis B surface antigen carriers. Am. J. Epidemiol. 108, 247.

Beasley, R.P., Hwang, L.Y., Lin, C.C., Chien, C.S., 1981. Hepatocellular carcinoma and hepatitis B virus. A prospective study of 22 707 men in taiwan. Lancet 2, 1129–1133.

Beaudoin, R.L., Davis, D.E., Murrell, K.D., 1969. Antibodies to larval taenia crassiceps in hibernating woodchucks, marmota monax. Exp. Parasitol. 24, 42–46.

Beck, J., Nassal, M., 2007. Hepatitis B virus replication. World J. Gastroenterol. 13, 48–64.

Benhenda, S., Cougot, D., Neuveut, C., Buendia, M.A., 2009. Liver cell transformation in chronic HBV infection. Viruses 1, 630–646.

Billiar, T.R., Curran, R.D., Harbrecht, B.C., Stadler, J., Williams, D.L., et al., 1992a. Association between synthesis and release of cGMP and nitric oxide biosynthesis by hepatocytes. Am. J. Physiol. 262, C1077–C1082.

Billiar, T.R., Hoffman, R.A., Curran, R.D., Langrehr, J.M., Simmons, R.L., 1992b. A role for inducible nitric oxide biosynthesis in the liver in inflammation and in the allogeneic immune response. J. Lab. Clin. Med. 120, 192–197.

Blumberg, B.S., Alter, H.J., Visnich, S., 1965. A 'new' antigen in leukemia sera. JAMA 191, 541–546.

Blumberg, B.S., Gerstley, B.J., Hungerford, D.A., London, W.T., Sutnick, A.I., 1967. A serum antigen (australia antigen) in down's syndrome, leukemia, and hepatitis. Ann. Intern. Med. 66, 924–931.

Blumberg, B.S., Larouze, B., London, W.T., Werner, B., Hesser, J.E., et al., 1975. The relation of infection with the hepatitis Bagent to primary hepatic carcinoma. Am. J. Pathol. 81, 669–682.

Blumberg, B.S., London, W.T., 1982. Hepatitis B virus: pathogenesis and prevention of primary cancer of the liver. Cancer 50, 2657–2665.

Bond, E., 1970. Hepatoma and arteriosclerosis in a woodchuck. J. Wildl. Dis. 6, 418–421.

Brechot, C., Hadchouel, M., Scotto, J., Fonck, M., Potet, F., et al., 1981. State of hepatitis B virus DNA in hepatocytes of patients with hepatitis B surface antigen-positive and -negative liver diseases. Proc. Natl. Acad. Sci. USA 78, 3906–3910.

Buendia, M.A., 1994. Animal models for hepatitis B virus and liver cancer. In: Brechot, C. (Ed.), Primary Liver Cancer: Etiological and Progression Factors CRC Press, Boca Raton, FL, pp. 211–224.

Buendia, M.A., 1995. The complex role of hepatitis B virus in human hepatocarcinogenesis. In: Barbanti-Brodano, G., Bendinelli, M., Friedman, H. (Eds.), DNA Tumor Viruses: Oncogenic Mechanisms Plenum Press, New York, pp. 171–193.

Buitrago, S., Curtin, L.I., Bellezza, C.A., Tennant, B.C., Iyer, R.V., 2010. Repeated dynamic contrast-enhanced magnetic resonance imaging using a vascular access port in the woodchuck, (marmota monax). Am. Assoc. Lab. Anim. Sci. 49, 694.

Chang, S.F., Netter, H.J., Bruns, M., Schneider, R., Frolich, K., et al., 1999. A new avian hepadnavirus infecting snow geese (anser caerulescens) produces a significant fraction of virions containing single-stranded DNA. Virology 262, 39–54.

Chen, H.S., Kaneko, S., Girones, R., Anderson, R.W., Hornbuckle, W.E., et al., 1993. The woodchuck hepatitis virus X gene is important for establishment of virus infection in woodchucks. J. Virol. 67, 1218–1226.

Chen, O.S., Hoyer, B.H., Nelson, J., Purcell, R.H., Gerin, J.L., 1982. Detection and properties of hepatitis B viral DNA in liver tissues from patients with hepatocellular carcinoma. Hepatology 2, 42S–46S.

Childs, J.E., Colby, L., Krebs, J.W., Strine, T., Feller, M., et al., 1997. Surveillance and spatiotemporal associations of rabies in rodents and lagomorphs in the united states, 1985–1994. J. Wildl. Dis. 33, 20–27.

Chisari, F.V., 2000. Viruses, immunity, and cancer: Lessons from hepatitis B. Am. J. Pathol. 156, 1117–1132.

Chisari, F.V., Klopchin, K., Moriyama, T., Pasquinelli, C., Dunsford, H.A., et al., 1989. Molecular pathogenesis of hepatocellular carcinoma in hepatitis B virus transgenic mice. Cell 59, 1145–1156.

Christian, J.J., Steinberger, E., McKinney, T.D., 1972. Annual cycle of spermatogenesis and testis morphology in woodchucks. J. Mammal. 53, 708–716.

Chu, C.K., Boudinot, F.D., Peek, S.F., Hong, J.H., Choi, Y., et al., 1998. Preclinical investigation of L-FMAU as an anti-hepatitis B virus agent. Antivir. Ther. 3, 113–121.

Cohn, D.L., Erb, H.N., Georgi, J.R., Tennant, B.C., 1986. Parasites of the laboratory woodchuck (marmota monax). Lab. Anim. Sci. 36, 298–302.

Concannon, P., Baldwin, B., Tennant, B., 1984. Serum progesterone profiles and corpora lutea of pregnant, postpartum, barren and isolated females in a laboratory colony of woodchucks (marmota monax). Biol. Reprod. 30, 945–951.

Concannon, P., Roberts, P., Baldwin, B., Erb, H., Tennant, B., 1993. Alteration of growth, advancement of puberty, and season-appropriate circannual breeding during 28 months of photoperiod reversal in woodchucks (marmota monax). Biol. Reprod. 48, 1057–1070.

Concannon, P., Roberts, P., Parks, J., Bellezza, C., Tennant, B., 1996. Collection of seasonally spermatozoa-rich semen by electroejaculation of laboratory woodchucks (marmota monax), with and without removal of bulbourethral glands. Lab. Anim. Sci. 46, 667–675.

Concannon, P., Roberts, P., Ball, B., Schlafer, D., Yang, X., et al., 1997a. Estrus, fertility, early embryo development, and autologous embryo transfer in laboratory woodchucks (marmota monax). Lab. Anim. Sci. 47, 63–74.

Concannon, P., Roberts, P., Baldwin, B., Tennant, B., 1997b. Long-term entrainment of circannual reproductive and metabolic cycles by northern and southern hemisphere photoperiods in woodchucks (marmota monax). Biol. Reprod. 57, 1008–1015.

Concannon, P.W., Baldwin, B., Roberts, P., Tennant, B., 1990. Endocrine correlates of hibernation-independent gonadal recrudescence and the limited late-winter breeding season in woodchucks, marmota monax. J. Exp. Zool. Suppl. 4, 203–206.

Concannon, P.W., Parks, J.E., Roberts, P.J., Tennant, B.C., 1992. Persistent free-running circannual reproductive cycles during prolonged exposure to a constant 12L:12D photoperiod in laboratory woodchucks (marmota monax). Lab. Anim. Sci. 42, 382–391.

Concannon, P.W., Castracane, V.D., Rawson, R.E., Tennant, B.C., 1999. Circannual changes in free thyroxine, prolactin, testes, and relative food intake in woodchucks, marmota monax. Am. J. Physiol. 277, R1401–R1409.

Cote, P.J., Pohl, C., Boyd, J., Tennant, B.C., Gerin, J.L., 1990. Alpha-fetoprotein in the woodchuck model of hepadnavirus infection and disease: immunochemical analysis of woodchuck alpha-feto-protein and measurement in serum by quantitative monoclonal radioimmunoassay. Hepatology 11, 824–833.

Cote, P.J., Roneker, C., Cass, K., Schodel, F., Peterson, D., et al., 1993. New enzyme immunoassays for the serologic detection of woodchuck hepatitis virus infection. Viral. Immunol. 6, 161–169.

Cullen, J.M., Marion, P.L., Newbold, J.E., 1989. A sequential histologic and immunohistochemical study of duck hepatitis B virus infection in pekin ducks. Vet. Pathol. 26, 164–172.

Cullen, J.M., Linzey, D.W., Gebhard, D.H., 1994. Nuclear ploidy of normal and neoplastic hepatocytes from woodchuck hepatitis virus - infected and uninfected woodchucks. Hepatology 19, 1072–1078.

Curran, R.D., Billiar, T.R., Steuhr, D.J., Ochoa, J.B., Harbrecht, B.G., et al., 1990. Multiple cytokines are required to induce hepatocyte nitric oxide production and inhibit total protein synthesis. Ann. Surg. 212, 462–469. Discussion 470–471.

Curran, R.D., Ferrari, F.K., Kispert, P.H., Stadler, J., Steuhr, D.J., et al., 1991. Nitric oxide and nitric oxide-generating compounds inhibit hepatocyte protein synthesis. FASEB J. 5, 2085–2092.

Curtin, L.I., Buitrago, S., Tennant, B.C., Iyer, R.V., 2011. Efficient end-point monitoring of hepatitis virus infected hepatocellular carcinoma positive woodchucks (marmota monax) using a handheld glucometer. J. Am. Assoc. Lab. Anim. Sci. 50, 734.

Dane, D.S., Cameron, C.H., Briggs, M., 1970. Virus-like particles in serum of patients with australia-antigen-associated hepatitis. Lancet 1, 695–698.

Davis, D.E., 1977. Role of ambient temperature in emergence of woodchucks (marmota monax) from hibernation. J. Am. Midl. Nat. 97, 224–229.

Dejean, A., deThe, H., 1990. Hepatitis B virus as an insertional mutagene in human hepatocellular carcinoma. Mol. Biol. Med. 7, 213–222.

de La Coste, A., Romagnolo, B., Billuart, P., Renard, C.A., Buendia, M.A., et al., 1998. Somatic mutations of the beta-catenin gene are frequent in mouse and human hepatocellular carcinomas. Proc. Natl. Acad. Sci. USA 95, 8847–8851.

Dragani, T.A., Manenti, G., Farza, H., Della Porta, G., Tiollais, P., Pourcel, C., et al., 1990. Transgenic mice containing hepatitis B virus sequences are more susceptible to carcinogen-induced hepatocarcinogenesis. Carcinogenesis 11, 953–956.

Dudley, F.J., Scheuer, P.J., Sherlock, S., 1972. Natural history of hepatitis-associated antigen-positive chronic liver disease. Lancet 2, 1388–1393.

Dunsford, H.A., Sell, S., Chisari, F.V., 1990. Hepatocarinogenesis due to chronic liver cell injury in hepatitis B virus transgenic mice. Cancer Res. 50, 3400–3407.

Enriquez, P.M., Jung, C., Josephson, L., Tennant, B.C., 1995. Conjugation of adenine arabinoside 5′-monophosphate to arabinogalactan: synthesis, characterization and antiviral activity. Bioconjug. Chem. 6, 195–202.

Fall, M.W., 1971. Seasonal variations in the food consumption of woodchucks (marmota monax). J. Mammal. 52, 370–375.

Farber, E., Sarma, D.S., 1987. Hepatocarcinogenesis: a dynamic cellular perspective. Lab. Invest. 56, 4–22.

Faux, S.P., Francis, J.E., Smith, A.G., Chipman, J.K., 1992. Induction of 8-hydroxydeoxyguanosine in Ah-responsive mouse liver by iron and Aroclor 1254. Carcinogenesis 13, 247–250.

Feitelson, M.A., Millman, I., Blumberg, B.S., 1986. Tree squirrel hepatitis B virus: antigenic and structural characterization. Proc. Natl. Acad. Sci. USA 83, 2994–2997.

Feitelson, M.A., Lega, L., Duan, L.X., Clayton, M., 1993. Characteristics of woodchuck hepatitis X-antigen in the lives and sera from infected animals. J. Hepatol. 17, S24–S34.

Feitelson, M.A., Ranganathan, P.N., Clayton, M.M., Zhang, S.M., 1997. Partial characterization of the woodchuck tumor suppressor, p53, and its interaction with woodchuck hepatitis virus X antigen in hepatocarcinogenesis. Oncogene 15, 327–336.

Flajolet, M., Gegonne, A., Ghysdael, J., Tiollais, P., Buendia, M.A., et al., 1997. Cellular and viral trans-acting factors modulate N-myc2 promoter activity in woodchuck liver tumors. Oncogene 15, 1103–1110.

Fleming, W.J., 1978 Parasites and disease of the woodchuck (marmota monax) in Tompkins County, New York. Ph.D. Thesis. Cornell University. 109pp.

Foley, G.L., Anderson, W.I., Schlafer, D.H., Hornbuckle, W.E., Baldwin, B.H., et al., 1993. Neoplastic and non-neoplastic lesions of the reproductive tract of the woodchuck (marmota monax). J. Zoo Wildl. Med. 24, 475–481.

Fourel, G., Trepo, C., Bougueleret, L., Henglein, B., Ponzetto, A., et al., 1990. Frequent activation of N-myc genes by hepadnavirus insertion in woodchuck liver tumours. Nature 347, 294–298.

Fourel, G., Transy, C., Tennant, B.C., Buendia, M.A., 1992. Expression of the woodchuck N-myc2 retroposon in brain and in liver tumors is driven by a cryptic N-myc promoter. Mol. Cell Biol. 12, 5336–5344.

Fourel, G., Couturier, J., Wei, Y., Apiou, F., Tiollais, P., et al., 1994. Evidence for long-range oncogene activation by hepadnavirus insertion. EMBO J. 13, 2526–2534.

Fourel, G., Ringeisen, F., Flajolet, M., Tronche, F., Pontoglio, M., et al., 1996. The HNF1/HNF4-dependent We2 element of woodchuck hepatitis virus controls viral replication and can activate the N-myc2 promoter. J. Virol. 70, 8571–8583.

Fox, H., 1912. Observations upon neoplasms in wild animals in the philadelphia zoological garden. J. Pathol. Bacteriol. 17, 217–231.

Fox, J.G., Yan, L.L., Dewhirst, F.E., Paster, B.J., Shames, B., et al., 1995. Helicobacter bilis sp. nov., a novel helicobacter species isolated from bile, livers, and intestines of aged, inbred mice. J. Clin. Microbiol. 33, 445–454.

Fox, J.G., Shen, Z., Xu, S., Feng, Y., Dangler, C.A., et al., 2002. *Helicobacter marmotae* sp. nov. isolated from livers of woodchucks and intestines of cats. J. Clin. Microbiol. 40, 2513–2519.

Fuchs, K., Heberger, C., Weimer, T., Roggendorf, M., 1989. Characterization of woodchuck hepatitis virus DNA and RNA in the hepatocellular carcinomas of woodchucks. Hepatology 10, 215–220.

Funk, A., Mhamdi, M., Will, H., Sirma, H., 2007. Avian hepatitis B viruses: molecular and cellular biology, phylogenesis, and host tropism. World J. Gastroenterol. 13, 91–103.

Ganem, D., Prince, A.M., 2004. Hepatitis B virus infection–natural history and clinical consequences. N. Engl. J. Med. 350, 1118–1129.

Ganem, D., Varmus, H.E., 1987. The molecular biology of the hepatitis B viruses. Annu. Rev. Biochem. 56, 651–693.

Gangemi, J.D., Korba, B.E., Tennant, B.C., Ueda, H., Jay, G., 1996. Antiviral and antiproliferative activities of y interferons in experimental hepatitis B virus infection. Antivir. Ther. Suppl. 4, 64–70.

Geller, D.A., Nussler, A.K., Di Silvio, M., Loenstein, C.J., Shapiro, R.A., et al., 1993. Cytokines, endotoxin, and glucocorticoids regulate the expression of inducible nitric oxide synthase in hepatocytes. Proc. Natl. Acad. Sci. USA 90, 522–526.

Georgi, J.R., 1985. Parasitology for Veterinarians. W.B. Saunders Company, Philadelphia, PA.

Gerin, J.L., Cote, P.J., Korba, B.E., Tennant, B.C., 1989. Hepadnavirus-induced liver cancer in woodchucks. Cancer Detect. Prev. 14, 227–229.

Ghebranious, N., Sell, S., 1998. The mouse equivalent of the human p53ser249 mutation p53ser246 enhances aflatoxin hepatocarcinogenesis in hepatitis B surface antigen transgenic and p53 heterozygous null mice. Hepatology 27, 967–973.

Gerlich, W.H., 2013. Medical virology of hepatitis B: how it began and where we are now. Virol. J. 10, 239. –422X–10–239.

Graham, E.S., 1985 Clinicopathological Investigation of Woodchuck Hepatitis Virus Infection. Ph.D. Thesis. Cornell University. 245pp.

Guo, J.T., Zhou, H., Liu, C., Aldrich, C., Saputelli, J., et al., 2000. Apoptosis and regeneration of hepatocytes during recovery from transient hepadnavirus infections. J. Virol. 74, 1495–1505.

Gust, I.D., Burrell, C.J., Coulepis, A.G., Robinson, W.S., Zuckerman, A.J., 1986. Taxonomic classification of human hepatitis B virus. Intervirology 25, 14–29.

Habermann, R.T., Williams Jr, F.P., Eyestone, W.H., 1954. Spontaneous hepatomas in two woodchucks and a carcinoma of the testis in a badger. J. Am. Vet. Med. Assoc. 125, 295–298.

Hailey, J.R., Haseman, J.K., Bucher, J.R., Radovsky, A.E., Malarkey, D.E., et al., 1998. Impact of helicobacter hepaticus infection in B6C3F1 mice from twelve national toxicology program two-year carcinogenesis studies. Toxicol. Pathol. 26, 602–611.

Hamilton, W.J., 1934. The life history of the rufescent woodchuck, *marmota monax rufescens* howell. Ann. Carnegie Mus. 23, 85–178.

Hanahan, D., Weinberg, R.A., 2000. The hallmarks of cancer. Cell 100, 57–70.

Hansen, L.J., Tennant, B.C., Seeger, C., Ganem, D., 1993. Differential activation of myc gene family members in hepatic carcinogenesis by closely related hepatitis B viruses. Mol. Cell Biol. 13, 659–667.

Hikim, A.P., Woolf, A., Bartke, A., Amador, A.G., 1991a. The estrous cycle of captive woodchucks (marmota monax). Biol. Reprod. 44, 733–738.

Hikim, A.P., Hikim, I.S., Amador, A.G., Bartke, A., Woolf, A., et al., 1991b. Reinitiation of spermatogenesis by exogenous gonadotropins in a seasonal breeder, the woodchuck (marmota monax), during gonadal inactivity. Am. J. Anat. 192, 194–213.

Hikim, A.P., Woolf, A., Bartke, A., Amador, A.G., 1992. Further observations on estrus and ovulation in woodchucks (marmota monax) in captivity. Biol. Reprod. 46, 10–16.

Hohne, M., Schaefer, S., Seifer, M., Feitelson, M.A., Paul, D., et al., 1990. Malignant transformation of immortalized transgenic hepatocytes after transfection with hepatitis B virus DNA. EMBO J. 9, 1137–1145.

Hortellano, S., Genaro, A.M., Bosca, L., 1992. Phorbol esters induce nitric oxide synthase activity in rat hepatocytes. J. Biol. Chem. 267, 24937–24940.

Hostetler, K.Y., Beadle, J.R., Hornbuckle, W.E., Bellezza, C.A., Tochkov, I.A., et al., 2000. Antiviral activities of oral 1-0-hexadecyl-propanediol-3-phospho-acyclovir and acyclovir in wood chucks with chronic woodchuck hepatitis virus infection. Antimicrob. Agents Chemother. 44, 1964–1969.

Hsia, C.C., Nakashima, Y., Thorgeirsson, S.S., Harris, C.C., Minemura, M., et al., 2000. Correlation of immunohistochemical staining and mutations of p53 in human hepatocellular carcinoma. Oncol. Rep. 7, 353–356.

Hsu, T.Y., Moroy, T., Etiemble, J., Louise, A., Trepo, C., Tiollais, P., et al., 1988. Activation of c-myc by woodchuck hepatitis virus insertion in hepatocellular carcinoma. Cell 55, 627–635.

Jacob, J.R., Ascenzi, M.A., Roneker, C.A., Toshkov, I.A., Cote, P.J., et al., 1997. Hepatic expression of the woodchuck hepatitis virus X-antigen during acute and chronic infection ad detection of a woodchuck hepatitis virus X-antigen antibody response. Hepatology 26, 1607–1615.

Jacob, J.R., Sterczer, A., Toshkov, I.A., Yeager, A.E., Korba, B.E., et al., 2004. Integration of woodchuck hepatitis and N-myc rearrangement determine size and histologic grade of hepatic tumors. Hepatology 39, 1008–1016.

Johnson, P.J., Williams, R., 1982. Of woodchucks and men: the continuing story of hepatitis B and hepatocellular carcinoma. Br. Med. J. (Clin. Res. Ed.) 284, 1586–1588.

Johnson, P.J., Williams, R., 1987. Cirrhosis and the aetiology of hepatocellular carcinoma. J. Hepatol. 12, 54–59.

Kajino, K., Jilbert, A.R., Saputelli, J., Aldrich, C.E., Cullen, J., et al., 1994. Woodchuck hepatitis virus infections: very rapid recovery after a prolonged viremia and infection of virtually every hepatocyte. J. Virol. 68, 5792–5803.

Kalayci, C., Johnson, P.J., Davies, S.E., Williams, R., 1991. Hepatitis B virus related hepatocellular carcinoma in the non-cirrhotic liver. J. Hepatol. 12, 54–59.

Kaneko, S., Oshima, T., Kodama, K., Aoyama, S., Yoshikawa, H., et al., 1986. Stable integration of woodchuck hepatitis virus DNA in transplanted tumors and established tissue culture cells derived from a woodchuck primary hepatocellular carcinoma. Cancer Res. 46, 3608–3613.

Kilbourn, R.G., Gross, S.S., Jubran, A., Adams, J., Griffith, O.W., et al., 1990. NG-methyl-L-arginine inhibits tumor necrosis factor-induced hypotension: implications for the involvement of nitric oxide. Proc. Natl. Acad. Sci. USA 87, 3629–3632.

Knowles, R.G., Merrett, M., Salter, M., Moncada, S., 1990. Differential induction of brain, lung and liver nitric oxide synthase by endotoxins in the rat. Biochem. J. 270, 833–836.

Kodama, K., Ogasawara, N., Yoshikawa, H., Murakami, S., 1985. Nucleotide sequence of a cloned woodchuck hepatitis virus genome: evolutional relationship between hepadnaviruses. J. Virol. 56, 978–986.

Korba, B.E., Wells, F.V., Baldwin, B., Cote, P.J., Tennant, B.C., et al., 1989. Hepatocellular carcinoma in woodchuck hepatitis virus-infected woodchucks: presence of viral DNA in tumor tissue from chronic carriers and animals serologically recovered from acute infections. Hepatology 9, 461–470.

Korba, B.E., Cote, P., Hornbuckle, W., Schinazi, R., Gangemi, J.D., Tennant, B.C., et al., 2000a. Enhanced antiviral benefit of combination therapy with larnivudine and alpha interferon against WHY replication in chronic carrier woodchucks. Antivir. Ther. 5, 95–104.

Korba, B.E., Cote, P., Hornbuckle, W., Schinazi, R., Gerin, J.L., Tennant, B.C., 2000b. Enhanced antiviral benefit of combination therapy with larnivudine and famciclovir against WHY replication in chronic WHV carrier woodchucks. Antivir. Res. 45, 19–32.

Korba, B.E., Cote, P., Hornbuckle, W., Tennant, B.C., Gerin, J.L., 2000c. Treat ment of chronic woodchuck hepatitis virus infection in the Eastern woodchuck (Mannota monax) with nucleoside analogues is predictive of therapy for chronic hepatitis B virus infection in humans. Hepatology 31, 1165–1175.

Korba, B.E., Gerin, J.L., 1992. Use of a standardized cell culture assay to assess activities of nucleoside analogs against hepatitis B virus replication. Antivir. Res. 19, 55–70.

Korba, B.E., Schinazi, R.F., Cote, P., Tennant, B.C., Gerin, J.L., 2000d. Effect of oral administration of emtricitabine on woodchuck hepatitis virus replication in chronically infected woodchucks. Antimicrob. Agents Chemother. 44, 1757–1760.

Liu, R.H., Baldwin, B., Tennant, B.C., Hotchkiss, J.H., 1991. Elevated formation of nitrate and N- nitrosodimethylamine in woodchucks (Marmota monax) associated with chronic woodchuck hepatitis virus infection. Cancer Res. 51, 3925–3929.

Liu, R.H., Jacob, J.R., Tennant, B.C., Hotchkiss, J.H., 1992. Nitrite and nitrosamine synthesis by hepatocytes isolated from normal woodchucks (Marmota monax) and woodchucks chronically infected with woodchuck hepatitis virus. Cancer Res. 52, 4139–4143.

Liu, R.H., Jacob, J.R., Hotchkiss, J.H., Tennant, B.C., 1993. Synthesis of nitric oxide and nitrosarnine by immortalized woodchuck hepatocytes. Carcinogenesis 14, 1609–1613.

Liu, R.H., Jacob, J.R., Hotchkiss, J.H., Cote, P.J., Gerin, J.L., Tennant, B.C., 1994. Woodchuck hepatitis virus surface antigen induces nitric oxide synthesis in hepatocytes: possible role in hepatocarcinogenesis. Carcinogenesis 15, 2875–2877.

Long, G.G., Terrell, T.G., Stookey, J.L., 1975. Hepatomas in a group of captive woodchucks. J. Am. Vet. Med. Assoc. 167, 589.

Lutwick, L.I., Hebert, M.B., Sywassink, J.M., 1982. Cross-reactions between the hepatitis B and woodchuck hepatitis viruses. In: Szmuness, W., Alter, H.J., Maynard, J.E. (Eds.), Viral Hepatitis Franklin Press Institute, Philadelphia, PA, pp. 711.

Magee, P.N., 1989. The experimental basis for the role of nitroso compounds in human cancer. Cancer Surv. 8, 207–239.

Magnarelli, L.A., Swihart, R.K., 1991. Spotted fever group rickettsiae or borrelia burgdorferi in ixodes cookei (ixodidae) in connecticut. J. Clin. Microbiol. 29, 1520–1522.

Mapes, C.R., 1950. The lancet fluke, a new parasite of the woodchuck. Cornell. Vet. 40, 346–349.

Marion, P.L., Oshiro, L.S., Regnery, D.C., Scullard, G.H., Robinson, W.S., 1980. A virus in beechey ground squirrels that is related to hepatitis B virus of humans. Proc. Natl. Acad. Sci. USA 77, 2941–2945.

Marion, P.L., Knight, S.S., Salazar, F.H., Popper, H., Robinson, W.S., 1983. Ground squirrel hepatitis virus infection. Hepatology 3, 519–527.

Marion, P.L., Van Davelaar, M.J., Knight, S.S., Salazar, F.H., Garcia, G., et al., 1986. Hepatocellular carcinoma in ground squirrels persistently infected with ground squirrel hepatitis virus. Proc. Natl. Acad. Sci. USA 83, 4543–4546.

Marion, P.L., Cullen, J.M., Azcarraga, R.R., Van Davelaar, M.J., Robinson, W.S., 1987. Experimental transmission of duck hepatitis B virus to pekin ducks and to domestic geese. Hepatology 7, 724–731.

Marletta, M., Yoon, P.S., Iyengar, R., Leaf, C.D., Wishnok, J.S., 1988. Macrophage oxidation of L-arginine to nitrite and nitrate: nitric oxide is an intermediate. Biochem. 27, 8706–8711.

Mason, W.S., Seal, G., Summers, J., 1980. Virus of pekin ducks with structural and biological relatedness to human hepatitis B virus. J. Virol. 36, 829–836.

Maupas, P., Werner, B., Larouze, B., Millman, I., London, W.T., et al., 1975. Antibody to hepatitis-B core antigen in patients with primary hepatic carcinoma. Lancet 2, 9–11.

McKenzie, E.J., Jackson, M., Turner, A., Gregorash, L., Harapiak, L., 2006. Chronic care and monitoring of woodchucks (marmota monax) during repeated magnetic resonance imaging of the liver. J. Am. Assoc. Lab. Anim. Sci. 45, 26–30.

Melnick, J.L., 1982. Classification of hepatitis A virus as enterovirus type 72 and of hepatitis B virus as hepadnavirus type 1. Intervirology 18, 105–106.

Menne, S., Cote, P.J., 2007. The woodchuck as an animal model for pathogenesis and therapy of chronic hepatitis B virus infection. World J. Gastroenterol. 13, 104–124.

Miller, R.H., Girones, R., Cote, P.J., Hornbuckle, W.E., Chestnut, T., et al., 1990. Evidence against a requisite role for defective virus in the establishment of persistent hepadnavirus infections. Proc. Natl. Acad. Sci. USA 87, 9329–9332.

Millman, I., Southam, L., Halbherr, T., Simmons, H., Kang, C.M., 1984. Woodchuck hepatitis virus: experimental infection and natural occurrence. Hepatology 4, 817–823.

Minuk, G.Y., Shaffer, E.A., Hoar, D.I., Kelly, J., 1986. Ground squirrel hepatitis virus (GSHV) infection and hepatocellular carcinoma in the canadian richardson ground squirrel (spermophilus richardsonii). Liver 6, 350–356.

Mitamura, K., Hoyer, B.H., Ponzetto, A., Nelson, J., Purcell, R.H., et al., 1982. Woodchuck hepatitis virus DNA in woodchuck (marmota monax) liver tissue. Hepatology 2, 47S–50S.

Moriyama, T., Guilhot, S., Klopchin, K., Moss, B., Pinkert, C.A., et al., 1990. Immunobiology and pathogenesis of hepatocellular injury in hepatitis B virus transgenic mice. Science 248, 361–364.

Moroy, T., Etiemble, J., Bougueleret, L., Hadchouel, M., Tiollais, P., 1989. Structure and expression of her, a locus rearranged with c-myc in a woodchuck hepatocellular carcinoma. Oncogene 4, 59–65.

Moroy, T., Marchio, A., Etiemble, J., Trepo, C., Tiollais, P., et al., 1986. Rearrangement and enhanced expression of c-myc in hepatocellular carcinoma of hepatitis virus infected woodchucks. Nature 324, 276–279.

Mrozek, M., Lehr, B., Zillman, U., Bannasch, P., 1994. A technique for serial liver biopsies in the woodchuck (marmota monax). J. Exp. Anim. Sci. 37, 34–41.

Nguyen, T., Brunson, D., Crespi, C.L., Penman, B.W., Wishnok, J.S., et al., 1992. DNA damage and mutation in human cells exposed to nitric oxide in vitro. Proc. Natl. Acad. Sci. USA 89, 3030–3034.

Ogston, C.W., Jonak, G.J., Rogler, C.E., Astrin, S.M., Summers, J., 1982. Cloning and structural analysis of integrated woodchuck hepatitis virus sequences from hepatocellular carcinomas of woodchucks. Cell 29, 385–394.

Okuchi, K., Murakami, S., 1968. Observations on australia antigen in japanese. Vox Sanguinis 15, 374–385.

Okuda, K., Nakashima, T., Sakamoto, K., Ikari, T., Hidaka, H., et al., 1982. Hepatocellular carcinoma arising in noncirrhotic and highly cirrhotic livers: a comparative study of histopathology and frequency of hepatitis B markers. Cancer 49, 450–455.

Omata, M., Uchiumi, K., Ito, Y., Yokosuka, O., Mori, J., et al., 1983. Duck hepatitis B virus and liver diseases. Gastroenterology 85, 260–267.

Omata, M., Yokosuka, O., Imazeki, F., Matsuyama, Y., Uchiumi, K., et al., 1984. Transmission of duck hepatitis B virus from chinese carrier ducks to japanese ducklings: a study of viral DNA in serum and tissue. Hepatology 4, 603–607.

Panic, R., Scott, D.W., Tennant, B.C., Anderson, W.I., Johnson, M., 1992. Skin disorders of the laboratory woodchuck (marmota monax): a retrospective study of 113 cases (1980–1990). Cornell. Vet. 82, 405–421.

Patterson, M.M., Rogers, A.B., Fox, J.G., 2010. Experimental *Helicobacter marmotae* infection in A/J mice causes enterohepatic disease. J. Med. Microbiol. 59, 1235–1241.

Peters, D.N., Steinberg, H., Anderson, W.I., Hornbuckle, W.E., Cote, P.J., et al., 1992. Immunopathology of glomerulonephritis associated with chronic woodchuck hepatitis virus infection in woodchucks (marmota monax). Am. J. Pathol. 141, 143–152.

Pitot, H.C., Dragan, Y.P., 1991. Facts and theories concerning the mechanisms of carcinogenesis. FASEB J. 5, 2280–2286.

Podell, M., Pokras, M., Gerlach, P., Jakowski, R., 1988. Meningioma in a woodchuck exhibiting central vestibular deficits. J. Wildl. Dis. 24, 695–699.

Popper, H., Shih, J.W., Gerin, J.L., Wong, D.C., Hoyer, B.H., et al., 1981. Woodchuck hepatitis and hepatocellular carcinoma: correlation of histologic with virologic observations. Hepatology 1, 91–98.

Popper, H., Roth, L., Purcell, R.H., Tennant, B.C., Gerin, J.L., 1987. Hepatocarcinogenicity of the woodchuck hepatitis virus. Proc. Natl. Acad. Sci. USA 84, 866–870.

Prince, A.M., 1968. An antigen detected in the blood during the incubation period of serum hepatitis. Proc. Natl. Acad. Sci. USA 60, 814–821.

Prince, A.M., Alcabes, P., 1982. The risk of development of hepatocellular carcinoma in hepatitis B virus carriers in new york: a preliminary estimate using death-records matching. Hepatology 2, 15S–20S.

Prince, A.M., Leblanc, L., Krohn, K., Masseyeff, R., Alpert, M.E., 1970. S.H. antigen and chronic liver disease. Lancet 2, 717–718.

Prince, A.M., Szmuness, W., Michon, J., Demaille, J., Diebolt, G., et al., 1975. A case/control study of the association between primary liver cancer and hepatitis B infection in senegal. Int. J. Cancer 16, 376–383.

Quignon, F., Renard, C.A., Tiollais, P., Buendia, M.A., Transy, C., 1996. A functional N-myc2 retroposon in ground squirrels: implications for hepadnavirus-associated carcinogenesis. Oncogene 12, 2011–2017.

Ratcliffe, H.L., 1933. Incidence and nature of tumors in captive mammals and birds. Am. J. Cancer 17, 116–135.

Rawson, R.E., Concannon, P.W., Roberts, P.J., Tennant, B.C., 1998. Seasonal differences in resting oxygen consumption, respiratory quotient, and free thyroxine in woodchucks. Am. J. Physiol. 274, R963–R969.

Reaiche-Miller, G.Y., Thorpe, M., Low, H.C., Qiao, Q., Scougall, C.A., et al., 2013. Duck hepatitis B virus covalently closed circular DNA appears to survive hepatocyte mitosis in the growing liver. Virology 446, 357–364.

Renard, C.A., Fourel, G., Bralet, M.P., Degott, C., De La Coste, A., et al., 2000. Hepatocellular carcinoma in WHV/N-myc2 transgenic mice: oncogenic mutations of beta-catenin and synergistic effect of p53 null alleles. Oncogene 19, 2678–2686.

Rivkina, M., Cote, P.J., Robinson, W.S., Tennant, B.C., Marion, P.L., 1996. Absence of mutations in the p53 tumor suppressor gene in woodchuck hepatocellular carcinomas associated with hepadnavirus infection and intake of aflatoxin B1. Carcinogensis 17, 2689–2694.

Robinson, W.S., Marion, P.L., Feitelson, M.A., Siddiqui, A., 1982. The hep-DNA virus group: hepatitis B and related viruses. In: Szmuness, W., Alter, H.J., Maynard, J.E. (Eds.), Viral Hepatitis Franklin Institute Press, Philadelphia, PA, pp. 57–68.

Rogler, C.E., 1991. Cellular and molecular mechanisms of hepatocarcinogenesis associated with hepadnavirus infection. Curr. Top. Microbiol. Immunol. 168, 103–140.

Rogler, C.E., Hino, O., Su, C.Y., 1987. Molecular aspect of persistent woodchuck hepatitis virus and hepatitis B virus infection and hepatocellular carcinoma. Hepatology 7, 74S–78S.

Roth, L., 1984. Hepatopathology of the Woodchuck (marmota monax).

Roth, L., King, J.M., 1986. Congestive cardiomyopathy in the woodchuck, marmota monax. J. Wildl. Dis. 22, 533–537.

Roth, L., Georgi, M.E., King, J.M., Tennant, B.C., 1982. Parasitic encephalitis due to baylisascaris sp. in wild and captive woodchucks (marmota monax). Vet. Pathol. 19, 658–662.

Roth, L., King, J.M., Tennant, B.C., 1984. Primary hepatoma in a woodchuck (marmota monax) without serologic evidence of woodchuck hepatitis virus infection. Vet. Pathol. 21, 607–608.

Roth, L., King, J.M., Hornbuckle, W.E., Harvey, H.J., Tennant, B.C., 1985. Chronic hepatitis and hepatocellular carcinoma associated with persistent woodchuck hepatitis virus infection. Vet. Pathol. 22, 338–343.

Schadel, F., Sprengel, R., Weimer, T., Frenholz, D., Schneider, R., et al., 1980. Aminal hepatitis B viruses. Adv. Viral. Oncol. 8, 73–102.

Schecter, E.M., Summers, J., Ogston, C.W., 1988. Characterization of a herpesvirus isolated from woodchuck hepatocytes. J. Gen. Virol. 69, 1591–1599.

Schafer, D.F., Sorrell, M.F., 1999. Hepatocellular carcinoma. Lancet 353, 1253–1257.

Schoen, F.J., 1994. Blood vessels, inflammatory disease – the vasculitides. In: Cotran, R.C., Kumar, V., Robbins, S.L. (Eds.), Pathologic Basis for Disease W.B. Saunders, Philadelphia, PA, pp. 490.

Seeff, L.B., Beebe, G.W., Hoofnagle, J.H., Norman, J.E., Buskell-Bales, Z., et al., 1987. A serologic follow-up of the 1942 epidemic of post-vaccination hepatitis in the united states army. N. Engl. J. Med. 316, 965–970.

Seeger, C., Marion, P.L., Ganem, D., Varmus, H.E., 1987. *In vitro* recombinants of ground squirrel and woodchuck hepatitis viral DNAs produce infectious virus in squirrels. J. Virol. 61, 3241–3247.

Seeger, C., Baldwin, B., Hornbuckle, W.E., Yeager, A.E., Tennant, B.C., et al., 1991. Woodchuck hepatitis virus is a more efficient oncogenic agent than ground squirrel hepatitis virus in a common host. J. Virol. 65, 1673–1679.

Seeger, C., Mason, W.S., 2000. Hepatitis B virus biology. Microbiol. Mol. Biol. Rev. 64, 51–68.

Sell, S., Hunt, J.M., Dunsford, H.A., Chisari, F.V., 1991. Synergy between hepatitis B virus expression and chemical hepatocarcinogens in transgenic mice. Cancer Res. 51, 1278–1285.

Seifer, M., Hohne, M., Schaefer, S., Gerlich, W.H., 1991. *In vitro* tumorigenicity of hepatitis B virus DNA and HBx protein. J. Hepatol. 13 (Suppl 4), S61–S65.

Shafritz, D.A., 1982. Hepatitis B virus DNA molecules in the liver hepatitis B surface antigen carriers: mechanistic considerations in the pathogenesis of hepatocellular carcinoma. Hepatology 2, 35S–41S.

Shanmuganathan, S., Waters, J.A., Karayiannis, P., Thursz, M., Thomas, H.C., 1997. Mapping of the cellular immune responses to woodchuck hepatitis core antigen epitopes in chronically infected woodchucks. J. Med. Virol. 52, 128–135.

Shlomai, A., de Jong, Y.P., Rice, C.M., 2014. Virus associated malignancies: the role of viral hepatitis in hepatocellular carcinoma. Semin. Cancer Biol. 26, 78–88.

Slagle, B.L., Lee, T.H., Medina, D., Finegold, M.J., Butel, J.S., 1996. Increased sensitivity to the hepatocarcinogen diethylnitrosamine in transgenic mice carrying the hepatitis B virus X gene. Mol. Carcinog. 15, 261–269.

Snyder, R.L., 1977. Longevity and disease patterns in captive and wild woodchucks. Am. Assoc. Zool. Parks Aquariums, 535–552.

Snyder, R.L., 1985. The laboratory woodchuck. In: Fox, J.G., Anderson, L.C., Loew, R.M., Quimby, F.W., (Eds.). Laboratory Animal Medicine pp. 20–32.

Snyder, R.L., Christian, J.J., 1960. Reproductive cycle and litter size of the woodchuck. Ecology 41, 647–655.

Snyder, R.L., Ratcliffe, H.L., 1969. Marmota monax: a model for studies of cardiovascular, cerebrovascular and neoplastic disease. Acta Zool. Pathol. Antverp 48, 265–273.

Snyder, R.L., Summers, J.W., 1980. Woodchuck hepatitis virus and hepatocellular carcinoma. In: Essex, M., Todaro, G., zur Hausen, H., (Eds.). Viruses in Naturally Occuring Cancers. Cold Spring Harbor Laboratory, NY: Cold Spring Harbor Conferences on Cell Proliferation. pp. 447–457.

Snyder, R.L., Tyler, G., Summers, J., 1982. Chronic hepatitis and hepatocellular carcinoma associated with woodchuck hepatitis virus. Am. J. Pathol. 107, 422–425.

Sprengel, R., Kuhn, C., Manso, C., Will, H., 1984. Cloned duck hepatitis B virus DNA is infectious in pekin ducks. J. Virol. 52, 932–937.

Sprengel, R., Kaleta, E.F., Will, H., 1988. Isolation and characterization of a hepatitis B virus endemic in herons. J. Virol. 62, 3832–3839.

Spurrier, W.A., Oeltgen, P.R., Myers, R.D., 1987. Hibernation trigger from hibernating woodchucks *marmota-monax* induces physiological alterations and opiate-like responses in the primate macaca-mulatta. J. Thermal. Biol. 12, 139–142.

Summers, J., Smolec, J.M., Snyder, R., 1978. A virus similar to human hepatitis B virus associated with hepatitis and hepatoma in woodchucks. Proc. Natl. Acad. Sci. USA 75, 4533–4537.

Summers, J.W., 1981. Three recently described animal virus models for human hepatitis B virus. Hepatology 1, 179–183.

Summers J.W., Smolec J.M., Werner B.G., Kelly T.J., Tyler G.V., et al., 1980. Hepatitis B virus and woodchuck hepatitis virus are members of a novel class of DNA viruses. In: Essex, M., Todaro, G., zur Hausen, H., (Eds.). Viruses in Naturally Occuring Cancers. Cold Spring Harbor Laboratory, NY: Cold Spring Harbor Conferences on Cell Proliferation. pp. 459–470.

Szmuness, W., 1978. Hepatocellular carcinoma and the hepatitis B virus: evidence for a causal association. Prog. Med. Virol. 24, 40–69.

Tabor, E., Gerety, R.J., Vogel, C.L., Bayley, A.C., Anthony, P.P., et al., 1977. Hepatitis B virus infection and primary hepatocellular carcinoma. J. Natl. Cancer Inst. 58, 1197–1200.

Tan, Y.J., 2011. Hepatitis B virus infection and the risk of hepatocellular carcinoma. World J. Gastroenterol. 17, 4853–4857.

Tassopoulos, N.C., Papaevangelou, G.J., Sjogren, M.H., Roumeliotou-Karayannis, A., Gerin, J.L., et al., 1987. Natural history of acute hepatitis B surface antigen-positive hepatitis in greek adults. Gastroenterology 92, 1844–1850.

Tennant, B.C., 1992. Hepatocarcinogenesis in experiemental woodchuck hepatitis virus infection. In: Sirica, A.E. (Ed.), The Rolle of Cell Types in Hepatocarcinogenesis. CRC Press, London, pp. 323–349.

Tennant, B.C., Gerin, J.L., 1994. The woodchuck model of hepatitis B virus infection. In: Arias, I.M., Boyer, J., Fausto, N., Jakoby, W.B., Schachter, D. (Eds.), The Liver: Biology and Pathobiology. Raven Press, New York, pp. 1455–1466.

Tennant, B.C., Gerin, J.L., 2001. The woodchuck model of hepatitis B virus infection. ILAR J. 42, 89–102.

Tennant, B.C., Hornbuckle, W.E., Baldwin, B.H., King, J.M., Cote, P.J., et al., 1988. Influence of age on the response to experimental woodchuck hepatitis virus infection. In: Zuckerman, A.J., Liss, A.R. (Eds.), Viral Hepatitis and Liver Disease. Alan R. Liss, Inc., New York, pp. 462–464.

Tennant, B.C., Hornbuckle, W.E., Yeager, A.E., Baldwin, B.H., Sherman, W.K., et al., 1991a. Effects of aflatoxin B 1 on experimental woodchuck hepatitis virus infection and hepatocellular carcinoma. In: Hollinger, F.B., Lemon, S.M., Margolis, H. (Eds.), Viral Hepatitis and Liver Disease. Williams & Wilkins, Baltimore, MD, pp. 599–600.

Tennant, B.C., Mrosovsky, N., McLean, K., Cote, P.J., Korba, B.E., et al., 1991b. Hepatocellular carcinoma in richardson's ground squirrels (spermophilus richardsonii): evidence for association with hepatitis B-like virus infection. Hepatology 13, 1215–1221.

Tennant, B.C., Baldwin, B.H., Bellezza, C.A., Cote, P.J., Korba, B.E., et al., 1996. Antiviral activity of BMS-180194 in the woodchuck model of hepatitis B virus infection. Abstracts of the Interscience Conference on Antimicrobial Agents and Chemotherapy. 36: 167.

Tennant, B.C., Baldwin, B.H., Graham, L.A., Ascenzi, M.A., Hornbuckle, W.E., et al., 1998. Antiviral activity and toxicity of fialuridine in the woodchuck model of hepatitis B virus infection. Hepatology 28, 179–191.

Tennant, B.C., Toshkov, I.A., Peek, S.F., Jacob, J.R., Menne, S., et al., 2004. Hepatocellular carcinoma in the woodchuck model of hepatitis B virus infection. Gastroenterology 127, S283–S293.

Terradillos, O., Billet, O., Renard, C.A., Levy, R., Molina, T., et al., 1997. The hepatitis B virus X gene potentiates c-myc induced liver oncogenesis in transgenic mice. Oncogene 14, 395–404.

Testut, P., Renard, C.A., Terradillos, O., Vitvitski-Trepo, L., Tekaia, F., et al., 1996. A new hepadnavirus endemic in arctic ground squirrels in alaska. J. Virol. 70, 4210–4219.

Tiollais, P., Pourcel, C., Dejean, A., 1985. The hepatitis B virus. Nature 317, 489–495.

Toshkov, I., Hacker, H.J., Roggendorf, M., Bannasch, P., 1990. Phenotypic patterns of preneoplastic and neoplastic hepatic lesions in woodchucks infected with woodchuck hepatitis virus. J. Cancer Res. Clin. Oncol. 116, 581–590.

Transy, C., Fourel, G., Robinson, W.S., Tiollais, P., Marion, P.L., Buendia, M.A., 1992. Frequent amplification of c-myc in ground squirrel liver tumors associated with past ongoing infection with hepadnavirus. Proc. Natl. Acad. Sci. USA 89, 3874–3878.

Trueba, D., Phelan, M., Nelson, J., Beck, F., Pecha, B.S., et al., 1985. Transmission of ground squirrel hepatitis virus to homologous and heterologous hosts. Hepatology 5, 435–439.

Tyler, G.V., Summers, J.W., Snyder, R.L., 1981. Woodchuck hepatitis virus in natural woodchuck population. J. Wildl. Dis. 17, 297–301.

Tyler, G.V., Snyder, R.L., Summers, J., 1986. Experimental infection of the woodchuck (marmota monax monax) with woodchuck hepatitis virus. Lab. Invest. 55, 51–55.

Ueda, H., Ullrich, S.J., Gangemi, J.D., Kappel, C.A., Ngo, L., et al., 1995. Functional inactivation but not structural mutation of p53 causes liver cancer. Nat. Genet. 9, 41–47.

Viola, L.A., Barrison, I.G., Coleman, J.C., Paradinas, F.J., Fluker, J.L., et al., 1981. Natural history of liver disease in chronic hepatitis B surface antigen carriers. survey of 100 patients from great britain. Lancet 2, 1156–1159.

Wands, J., 2007. Hepatocellular carcinoma and sex. N. Engl. J. Med. 357, 1974–1976.

Ward, J.M., Fox, J.G., Anver, M.R., Haines, D.C., George, C.V., et al., 1994. Chronic active hepatitis and associated liver tumors in mice caused by a persistent bacterial infection with a novel helicobacter species. J. Natl. Cancer Inst. 86, 1222–1227.

Wei, Y., Fourel, G., Ponzetto, A., Silvestro, M., Tiollais, P., et al., 1992. Hepadnavirus integration: mechanisms of activation of the N-myc2 retrotransposon in woodchuck liver tumors. J. Virol. 66, 5265–5276.

Wei, Y., Tennant, B., Ganem, D., 1998. In vivo effects of mutations in woodchuck hepatitis virus enhancer II. J. Virol. 72, 6608–6613.

Weiser, B., Ganem, D., Seeger, C., Varmus, H.E., 1983. Closed circular viral DNA and asymmetrical heterogeneous forms in livers from animals infected with ground squirrel hepatitis virus. J. Virol. 48, 1–9.

Whitaker Jr, J.O., Schmeltz, L.L., 1973. External parasites of the woodchuck, marmota monax, in indiana. Entomol. News 84, 69–72.

Will, H., Cattaneo, R., Koch, H.G., Darai, G., Schaller, H., et al., 1982. Cloned HBV DNA causes hepatitis in chimpanzees. Nature 299, 740–742.

Wink, D.A., Kasprzak, K.S., Maragos, C.M., Elespuru, R.K., Misra, M., et al., 1991. DNA dearninating ability and genotoxicity of nitric oxide and its progenitors. Science 254, 1001–1003.

Wong, D.C., Shih, J.W., Purcell, R.H., Gerin, J.L., London, W.T., 1982. Natural and experimental infection of woodchucks with woodchuck hepatitis virus, as measured by new, specific assays for woodchuck surface antigen and antibody. J. Clin. Microbiol. 15, 484–490.

Wood, E.R., Berger, H., Sherman, P.A., Lapetina, E.G., 1993. Hepatocytes and macrophages express an identical cytokine inducible nitric oxide synthase gene. Biochem. Biophys. Res. Comm. 191, 767–774.

Woolf, A., Curl, J., Gremillion-Smith, C., 1989. The use of subcutaneous ports in the woodchuck (marmota monax). Lab. Anim. Sci. 39, 620–622.

Yan, R.Q., Su, J.J., Huang, D.R., Gan, Y.C., Yang, C., Huang, G.H., 1996. Human hepatitis B virus and hepatocellular carcinoma. II. Experimental induction of hepatocellular carcinoma in tree shrews exposed to hepatitis B virus and aflatoxin Bl. J. Cancer Res. Clin. Oncol. 122, 289–295.

Yang, D., Alt, E., Rogler, C.E., 1993. Coordinate expression of N-myc 2 and insulin-like growth factor II in precancerous altered hepatic foci in woodchuck hepatitis virus carriers. Cancer Res. 53, 2020–2027.

Yang, D., Faris, R., Hixson, D., Affigne, S., Rogler, C.E., 1996. Insulin-like growth factor II blocks apoptosis of N-myc2-expressing woodchuck liver epithelial cells. J. Virol. 70, 6260–6268.

Young, R.A., 1984. Interrelationships between body weight, food consumption and plasma thyroid hormone concentration cycles in the woodchuck, marmota monax. Comp. Biochem. Physiol. A Comp. Physiol. 77, 533–536.

Young, R.A., Sims, E.A., 1979. The woodchuck, marmota monax, as a laboratory animal. Lab. Anim. Sci. 29, 770–780.

Zhou, T., Saputelli, J., Aldrich, C.E., Deslauriers, M., Condreay, L.E., et al., 1999. Emergence of drug-resistant populations of woodchuck hepatitis virus in woodchucks treated with the antiviral nucleoside lamivudine. Antimicrob. Agents Chemother. 43, 1947–1954.

9

Biology and Diseases of Chinchillas

Charlie C. Hsu, VMD, PhD, DACLAM[a]*, Maia M. Chan, DVM,*
MS[b] *and Colette L. Wheler, BSc, DVM, MVetSc*[c]

[a]Department of Comparative Medicine, University of Washington, Seattle, WA, USA
[b]Seattle Children's Research Institute, Seattle, WA, USA [c]VIDO-InterVac, University of
Saskatchewan, Saskatoon, SK, Canada

I. INTRODUCTION

A. Taxonomy and General Comments

Chinchillas are rodents belonging to the Chinchillidae family in the suborder Hystricognatha and are related to guinea pigs and degus. There are two species of chinchilla, the short-tailed chinchilla, *Chinchilla chinchilla*, and the long-tailed chinchilla, *Chinchilla lanigera* (Figs. 9.1–9.3), which is the species most commonly used in biomedical research (ITIS, 2013). Chinchillas are native to South America, specifically the dry climate of the Andean mountains of Chile, Bolivia, and Peru. They live in colonies in extensive burrow systems (Busso *et al.*, 2012). Both species are listed as critically endangered by the International Union for Conservation of Nature because of a drastic population decline due to illegal hunting for the fur trade and reduction of habitat quality (IUCN, 2013). Most captive chinchillas are descended from 11 animals that were captured in the early 1920s (Richardson, 2003). Early attempts at captive breeding for fur production enjoyed limited success; however, with improvements in colony management, chinchilla fur farms became established. Demand for chinchillas as research animals initially turned to these fur farms, and over time some began supplying chinchillas for research

Laboratory Animal Medicine, Third Edition
DOI: http://dx.doi.org/10.1016/B978-0-12-409527-4.00009-2

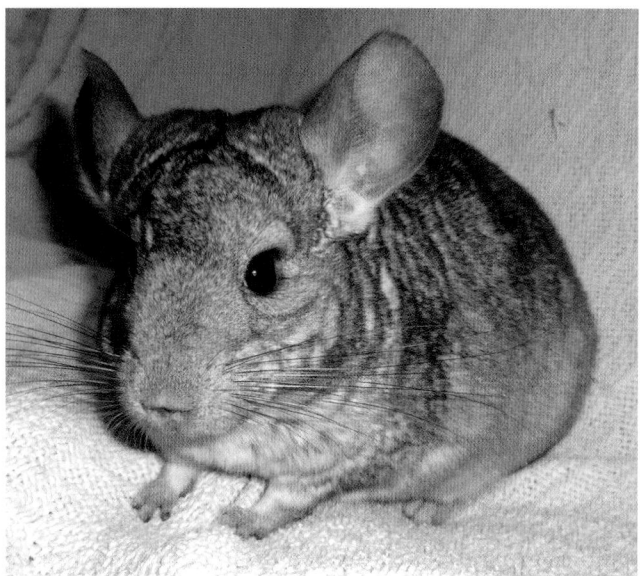

FIGURE 9.1   An adult standard gray *Chinchilla lanigera. Courtesy of Dr. A. Keffer.*

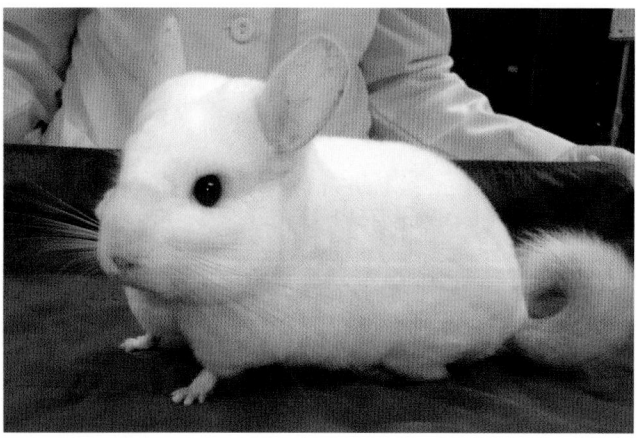

FIGURE 9.2   An adult pink white *Chinchilla lanigera. Courtesy of Dr. A. Keffer.*

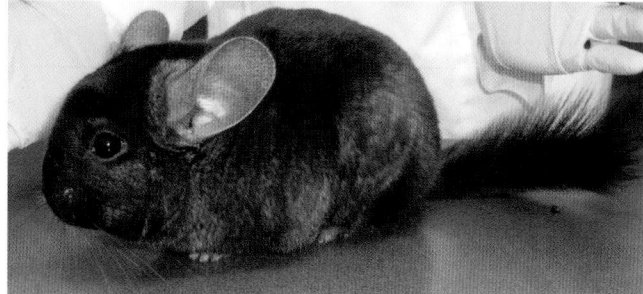

FIGURE 9.3   An adult ebony *Chinchilla lanigera. Courtesy of Dr. A. Keffer.*

(Martin, 2012a). Today, chinchillas are successfully bred in captivity for their fur, for the pet trade, and for biomedical research.

B. Uses in Research

Because of the similarities to the human hearing range, their anatomical size, and the accessibility of their tympanic bullae, chinchillas have been used as an important model in acoustic research since the late 1970s, and research related to the auditory system remains the primary field utilizing chinchillas as experimental models today. Areas of study include otitis media, cholesteatoma, therapeutic treatment of aural disease, noise and chemical-induced hearing loss, Ménière's disease, tinnitus, perilymphatic fistulas, cochlear implants, superior canal dehiscence, tympanic membrane perforation repair, stem cell transplants, and otic drug safety testing (Martin, 2012b). More recently, chinchillas have been used as models for pathogenesis, diagnostic test development, and vaccine evaluation for a number of inter-related upper respiratory tract pathogens, including *Haemophilus influenzae, Moraxella catarrhalis*, and respiratory syncytial virus (Brockson *et al.*, 2012; Harrison *et al.*, 2013; Hempel *et al.*, 2013; Das *et al.*, 2014; Shaffer *et al.*, 2013; Gitiban *et al.*, 2005; Wang *et al.*, 2014; Ren *et al.*, 2014). Other areas of research utilizing chinchillas include hypothyroidism model development (Martin *et al.*, 2005), repair of dural tears (Shah *et al.*, 2007), evaluation of pathogenic biofilm mediators of *Pseudomonas aeruginosa* (Byrd *et al.*, 2011), and propagation of *Taenia solium taeniasis* eggs and adults for further study (Maravilla *et al.*, 2011).

C. Availability and Sources

Chinchillas are not inbred or widely available commercially. The AALAS Buyer's Guide lists only one source of chinchillas, the Moulton Chinchilla Ranch in Rochester, Minnesota, which has been breeding and selling chinchillas since 1966 (AALAS, 2013). Other sources include local chinchilla fur farms and pet suppliers.

D. Laboratory Management and Husbandry

Management, husbandry, and caging requirements of research chinchillas are similar to those of rabbits and guinea pigs. Modifications may need to be made to prevent escape, as chinchillas can squeeze through small openings. Solid-bottomed caging is preferred, but suspended metal or plastic caging may be used if the perforations are no larger than ½ in × ½ in (15 mm × 15 mm) to prevent foot and leg injuries (Levin *et al.*, 2012; Harkness *et al.*, 2010; Richardson, 2003). A solid floor area should also be provided. There are no published floor space or height requirements for housing chinchillas, but recommendations from the pet trade suggest approximately 1–2 ft^2 (0.1–0.2 m^2) per animal and 12 in (30 cm) of cage height is adequate (Levin *et al.*, 2012). Chinchillas are very agile and will exhibit jumping and climbing behaviors given the opportunity. Multilevel cages provide enrichment opportunities. Other types of enrichment should include items for gnawing to assist with dental health and items that can be orally manipulated, such as steel chains. A shelter or hide-box should also be provided for privacy. Chinchillas will perch on flat-topped structures.

Several commercially available bedding products are suitable for chinchillas such as wood shavings or paper-based products. Wood products containing aromatic hydrocarbons, such as pine shavings, may affect drug metabolism or predispose to respiratory problems and should be avoided (Levin *et al.*, 2012; Harkness *et al.*, 2010). Dropping pans should be lined with absorbent material.

One unique housing requirement of chinchillas is regular access to a dust bath to prevent their fur from becoming matted and greasy. Various mixtures of silver sand, Fuller's earth, diatomaceous earth, and volcanic ash are available commercially. Dust baths should be provided for 15 min daily, or at least several times a week (Mans and Donnelly, 2012; Quesenberry *et al.*, 2012). The bath should be removed and cleaned between uses and should not be shared between enclosures to prevent transmission of diseases such as ringworm. Overuse of dust baths may cause eye irritation and dry skin. Baths should not be offered to near-term females or mothers with litters as the dust may contribute to mastitis and uterine infection (Harkness *et al.*, 2010).

Chinchillas are social animals and should be housed in same-sex pairs or groups. They do best in a dry, draft-free environment, with a temperature range between 63 and 77°F (17–25°C) and humidity between 30 and 60%. They are very prone to heat stress and can die if temperatures exceed 90°F (32°C), particularly if humidity is also high (>60%). A guideline that has been previously proposed is to combine the units of humidity plus the temperature in Fahrenheit, and the sum should not exceed 150 (Donnelly, 2004). However, if chinchillas are allowed to become cold adapted, they can withstand temperatures of 32°F (0°C) or lower, and this is used to stimulate production of a thick fur coat desirable for the fur trade. Ventilation of 10–15 air changes per hour and a 12:12 h light:dark cycle is generally appropriate; however, alterations may be necessary for manipulating breeding behavior (Levin *et al.*, 2012; Harkness *et al.*, 2010).

Wild chinchillas rarely drink water and maintain their hydration by licking dew drops and eating plants. Captive chinchillas adapt readily to water bottles or automatic watering systems.

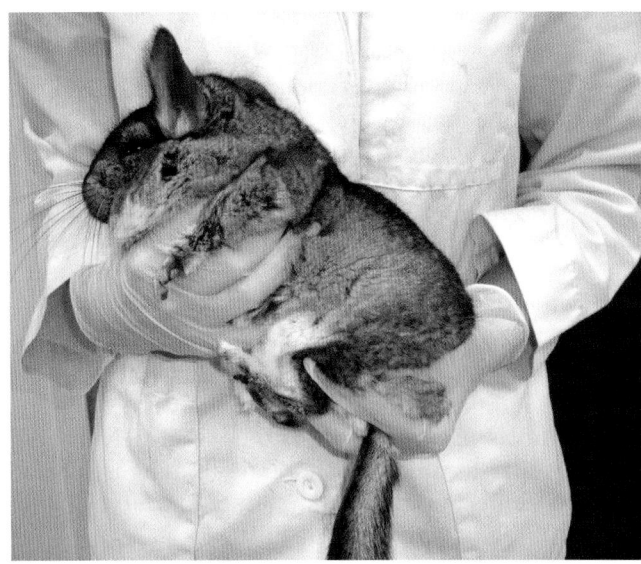

FIGURE 9.4   Proper restraint of a chinchilla by firmly grasping the base of the tail with one hand while the other hand supports the body. *Courtesy of Dr. A. Keffer.*

Chinchillas are not naturally aggressive toward humans and are generally easy to handle. They can be picked up by firmly grasping the base of the tail with one hand while the other hand supports the body (Fig. 9.4). They should never be picked up by the tail alone. Tamer animals can be gently grasped around the thorax while supporting the hind end, similar to guinea pigs. Fur-slip is a protective mechanism employed by chinchillas to evade predators. A patch of hair is simultaneously released from its follicles, leaving a bare area of skin. This phenomenon may occur with improper or rough handling (Harkness *et al.*, 2010).

II. BIOLOGY

A. Unique Physiologic and Anatomic Characteristics

1. The Ear

Chinchillas share similar anatomy and physiology of the inner ear with humans. Like humans, their cochlea has three turns and is readily accessible for microsurgical procedures, and their large, thin-walled tympanic bullae allow easy access to the middle ear. Their range of hearing is also similar to humans. The round window is thinner than in humans, which is useful for ototoxic drug studies. Another similarity shared with humans is a freely mobile conductive apparatus in which the malleus and incus are attached by ligaments and therefore able to move independently. This differs from other rodents such as mice, gerbils, and hamsters where there is bony fusion between the malleus and the tympanic ring. Chinchillas are long-lived, with an average life span of 9–18 years, so their auditory system does not undergo aging as quickly as in mice, making them a more reliable animal model for short-term studies. Their age-related hearing loss is similar to age-related hearing loss in humans, so they are also useful for these types of studies (Alworth and Harvey, 2012; Martin, 2012b; Harkness *et al.*, 2010).

2. Circulatory and Lymphoreticular Systems

The brain of chinchillas is supplied only by a vertebral-basilar artery system, and internal carotid arteries are absent. In addition, the right coronary artery is not present.

Chinchillas have discrete nasal-associated lymphoid tissue similar to other rodents. The thymus is located entirely within the thorax (Alworth and Harvey, 2012; Martin, 2012b; Harkness *et al.*, 2010).

3. Gastrointestinal System

All teeth are open-rooted and grow continuously. The soft palate is continuous with the base of the tongue and contains a palatal ostium, which connects the oropharynx to the rest of the pharynx. The entire gastrointestinal tract can reach 3 m (9.8 ft) in length, with the large intestine being 1.5-times longer than the small intestine. Cecal volume is relatively smaller than in rabbits or guinea pigs. Similar to many rodent species, chinchillas are coprophagic. Cecal pellets are taken directly from the anus with the incisors, masticated, and swallowed. Chinchillas typically ingest only those pellets produced in the daytime, which have higher nitrogen content than night pellets (Bjornhag and Sjoblom, 1977; Hirakawa, 2001). Chinchillas, like rabbits and other rodents, are unable to vomit (Alworth and Harvey, 2012; Harkness *et al.*, 2010).

4. Urinary System

Chinchillas originate from an arid environment and rarely drink water in the wild. The relatively large renal medulla of the chinchilla allows them to conserve water by producing highly concentrated urine (Alworth and Harvey, 2012).

B. Life-Cycle and Physiologic Values

Table 9.1 lists life-cycle information for chinchillas. Table 9.2 outlines physiologic values.

C. Diets, Nutrition, and Feeding Behavior

Chinchillas are monogastric hind-gut fermenters. Exact nutritional requirements of chinchillas have not been determined; however, they do best with a high-fiber, low-energy diet with 16–20% protein, 2.5–5.5%

TABLE 9.1 Life-Cycle Information for Chinchillas[a]

Breeding onset male	7–9 months
Breeding onset female	4–5 months
Cycle length	20–60 days
Gestation period	105–120 days (average 112)
Postpartum estrus	Fertile
Birth weight	30–60 g
Litter size	1–6 (2–3 most common)
Weaning age	6–8 weeks
Breeding life	Up to 10 years

[a]*From Harkness et al. (2010) and Richardson (2003).*

TABLE 9.2 Physiologic Values for Chinchillas[a]

Body weight: adult male	400–500 g
Body weight: adult female	400–600 g
Body temperature	37–38°C (98.6–100.4°F)
Pulse	200–350 bpm
Respirations	45–80/min
Diploid number	64
Life span	9–18 years
Food consumption	30–40 g/day; 5.5 g/100 g/day
Water consumption	10–20 ml/day; 8–9 ml/100 g/day
Gastrointestinal transit time	12–15 h

[a]*From Harkness et al. (2010).*

fat, and 15–23% fiber. A low-protein diet may result in unthriftiness and dry, weak fur (Richardson, 2003). Captive chinchillas are usually provided with a pelleted ration and should be supplemented with free-choice grass hay or other high-fiber substance to ensure gastrointestinal health. Unlike guinea pigs and rabbits, chinchillas tend to sit upright on their haunches and hold food with their forepaws when they eat. Commercial chinchilla pellets are longer than guinea pig pellets to facilitate this behavior. Treats containing high amounts of starch or sugar should be avoided to prevent upsetting the gastrointestinal tract. However, small amounts of well-washed, dark green leafy vegetables can be offered. Mixed feeds containing pellets and seeds should be avoided as chinchillas will pick out and eat only their favorite items. Suspended food hoppers such as hanging J-feeders will prevent waste and contamination of food material. Chinchillas are nocturnal in the wild and feed primarily during the dark (Levin *et al.*, 2012; Harkness *et al.*, 2010; Hirakawa, 2001).

Water intake varies with the amount of moisture present in the feed. Daily intake ranges from 10 to 40 ml/day.

D. Behavior

Chinchillas are quiet, gentle, low-maintenance animals popular in the pet trade. When allowed free-run, they are very agile climbers and jumpers. They will also use running wheels for exercise. Similar to the preference of providing solid-bottom caging, solid running wheels are also available for chinchillas to minimize foot and leg injuries. Chinchillas are social animals and should be housed in same-sex pairs or small groups. Huddling together and mutual grooming are practiced. Similar to other rodents, chinchillas require safe items to chew so they can satisfy their gnawing behavior. They also use their mouths to explore and will manipulate metal chains and other toys with their tongue and lips. Chinchillas are not very vocal but can make a variety of sounds. Normal vocalizations consist of soft, high-pitched grunts, angry barks, and warning whistles. They can become territorial and will stand upright and spray urine at an intruder to defend their territory. Females may become aggressive when in estrus or post-partum, especially toward males. Intact males housed in groups may fight. Like other rodents, chinchillas are fastidious groomers, complete with dust bathing, which should be accommodated in captivity. Chinchillas startle easily and may become stressed by loud noises and activity. Like guinea pigs, they do not adjust very readily to changes in their environment. In the wild, chinchillas are nocturnal but can adapt to a diurnal lifestyle in captivity (Alworth and Harvey, 2012; Harkness et al., 2010).

E. Reproduction

Sexual maturity occurs at about 4–5 months of age in females and 7–9 months of age in males. Female chinchillas are generally larger than males and have a prominent urethral papilla, which can be confused with a penis by inexperienced observers. In addition, the testicles of the male are retractable and are not always obvious on physical exam. The anogenital distance is the most dependable way to determine sex and can be reliably used at any age. In mature males, this distance is approximately 1 cm (2/5 in), which is about twice that of the female (Harkness et al., 2010).

In the northern hemisphere, chinchillas are seasonally polyestrus from November to May. The estrus cycle lasts from 20 to 60 days, with an average of 35 days. Estrus lasts between 12 and 48 h and is characterized by opening of the vaginal closure membrane, accompanied by vaginal reddening and discharge. A wax-like vaginal plug is normally expressed at the onset of estrus. Vaginal cytology can be used to determine stage of estrus with 70% accuracy. Gentle pressure on the urethral papilla will usually open the vagina.

Female chinchillas are monogamous in the wild, but mating systems in captivity typically use a harem scheme with one male for every four to six females. During breeding, each female resides in her own individual cage, which is connected to other cages by a tunnel. Females are fitted with a flat metal disc around their neck, which is slightly larger than the tunnel opening, preventing passage. Males are not fitted with collars and can move freely from cage to cage. This provides males with easy, unrestricted access to females and an area where they can rest and escape. Interested males will make a cooing, chuckling noise, and both sexes may rub their chins on the floor (Richardson, 2003). Receptive females will exhibit lordosis and lateral deviation of the tail and will allow the male to mount. Following mating, the female may become aggressive toward the male. Threats are expressed as growling, chattering teeth, and spraying urine. Severe trauma or death may occur if the male is unable to escape. Mating usually occurs several times during the night. Loss of some fur from the female is normal during this time. The male deposits an ejaculatory plug in the vagina after mating, which remains in place for several hours before falling out (Harkness et al., 2010; Richardson, 2003).

Chinchillas have a notably longer gestation period than other rodents, ranging from 105 to 120 days (Harkness et al., 2010). At about 60 days, the mammary tissue and teats begin to swell and the nipples become reddened. Experienced personnel may be able to palpate fetuses after 60 days' gestation. Monitoring weight gain is more reliable: a gain of 25–30 g/month occurs initially, with a more rapid increase in the last month (Richardson, 2003). Females near parturition become inactive and anorectic. The perineal area, mouth, and nose become wet with amniotic fluid to signal the start of parturition. Parturition generally occurs at night or in the early morning. The strenuous phase of labor usually lasts 1–2 h or less. During that time, the female writhes and stretches, and may vocalize. The interval between kits ranges from a few minutes to several hours, and generally all kits are born within a 4-h period. The female will continually lick her vulva as each fetus emerges and will use her teeth to pull the kits from the birth canal. If the birth is difficult or the young get stuck, the female may cannibalize them. The fetal membranes are normally eaten. A post-partum estrus occurs approximately 12 h after parturition and last for 2 days after which the vaginal closure membrane reforms (Richardson, 2003). Dystocia is uncommon; however, Caesarean section should be considered if more than 4 h of unproductive labor have elapsed. After labor the female should be palpated to ensure no mummified or stillborn fetuses remain, especially if she appears restless and ignores her young (Harkness et al., 2010; Kennedy, 1952; Richardson, 2003). Medical or surgical intervention may be required if mummified or stillborn fetuses are found.

Litter sizes average two to three, although up to six have been reported. Dams do not normally build a nest; however, nest boxes may help reduce mortality (Richardson, 2003). Birth weight ranges from 30 to 60g and kits less than 25g are unlikely to survive. Chinchillas sit on top of their young to nurse them and keep them warm. Newborns are fully furred with a complete set of teeth and are able to walk within 1h. Their eyes open within 24h of birth. Weaning can occur as early as 6 weeks, although lactation can last up to 8 weeks. Newborn kits will begin to eat small amounts of solid food within the first week of life.

Orphans can be fostered onto another female with a small litter of approximately the same age kits, or with a litter ready to be weaned. The orphans can be introduced a few hours after the older pups have been removed (Richardson, 2003).

Assisted breeding techniques such as electroejaculation, artificial insemination, and cryopreservation of spermatozoa have also been extensively studied by researchers at the University of Cordoba in Argentina, who have been facilitating captive breeding programs for this endangered species over the past 10 years (Busso et al., 2005; Busso et al., 2012; Dominchin et al., 2014; Ponzio et al., 2007; Ponzio et al., 2011).

III. DISEASES

A. Infectious Diseases

There are only a handful of reports in the published literature about naturally occurring infectious diseases in chinchillas. Most of these reports describe infections in pet chinchillas or those raised for their pelts in a farm or ranch setting, rather than in laboratory chinchillas. Chinchillas are commonly used as experimental models of otitis media (Bakaletz, 2009; Giebink, 1999), and most of the published literature on infectious diseases in chinchillas describe experimental infections with various infectious agents to which they are susceptible. These agents include experimental infections with respiratory syncytial virus (Brockson et al., 2012; Grieves et al., 2010; Gitiban et al., 2005), adenovirus (Bakaletz and Holmes, 1997; Bakaletz et al., 1993), influenza A virus (Tong et al., 2000b), vesicular stomatitis virus (Kowalczyk and Brandly, 1954), Moraxella catarrhalis (Brockson et al., 2012), Haemophilus influenzae (Novotny et al., 2006), Streptococcus pneumoniae (Tong et al., 2000a; Long et al., 2004; Reid et al., 2009), Pseudomonas aeruginosa (Cotter et al., 1996), and Chlamydia trachomatis (Weber and Koltai, 1991). However, the following sections on infectious diseases in chinchillas will focus primarily on naturally acquired infections. In the laboratory setting, many of these diseases will rarely be encountered if chinchillas are obtained from clean, reputable sources, and if proper facility maintenance, sanitation, and animal husbandry procedures are followed.

1. Bacterial, Mycoplasmal, and Rickettsial Infections

a. Clostridium perfringens

Etiology Clostridium perfringens is a gram-positive, anaerobic, rod-shaped, and spore-forming bacterium that can cause enterotoxemia and necrotizing enteritis. C. perfringens type A, B, and D have been reported in chinchillas (Bartoszcze et al., 1990b; Lucena et al., 2011; Moore and Greenlee, 1975).

Clinical Signs Diarrhea, abdominal pain, prolapsed rectum, lethargy, recumbency, and sudden deaths can be seen in chinchillas naturally infected with C. perfringens. Morbidity and mortality reached as high as 20% in one report (Bartoszcze et al., 1990b).

Epizootiology and Transmission These bacteria are commonly found in the intestines of animals and people, as well as being widespread in the environment (Petit et al., 1999).

Necropsy Findings Gross necropsy findings include extensive hemorrhagic enteritis, mild pulmonary edema, splenomegaly, hepatomegaly, and hepatic lipidosis. Histologically, necrotizing and hemorrhagic enteritis with bacterial aggregates in the epithelium and lamina propria, necrosis of the large intestinal mucosa, centrilobular hepatic necrosis, hepatic lipidosis, splenic white pulp proliferation, and pulmonary edema has been described (Bartoszcze et al., 1990b; Lucena et al., 2011).

Pathogenesis C. perfringens can be classified into five toxinotypes (A through E) based on their production of four major toxins (γ, β, ϵ, and ι), and each toxinotype may cause distinct and specific diseases in animals and people (Petit et al., 1999). Additionally, C. perfringens does not invade healthy cells but rather the toxins and enzymes are responsible for causing disease. C. perfringens from each toxinotype may or may not also produce another toxin, C. perfringens enterotoxin, encoded by the cpe gene. The global distribution of strains carrying the cpe gene is relatively low at only 5%, and C. perfringens type A is considered ubiquitous and the most commonly found strain in the environment (Petit et al., 1999; Marks, 2012). However, the role of C. perfringens in causing disease is complicated by the fact that in other species such as the dog, C. perfringens and its various toxins may be found in both diseased and clinically normal patients (Marks, 2012).

Differential Diagnosis Diagnosis can be made by anaerobic culture and bacterial identification from intestinal contents. Commercially available immunoassays can be used for the detection of enterotoxin from fecal or intestinal contents. Polymerase chain reaction can be used to characterize the toxinotype of

C. perfringens (Lucena *et al.*, 2011; Yoo *et al.*, 1997). Other causes of sudden death may include *Yersinia* sp., *Listeria* sp., *Salmonella*, or *Pseudomonas aeruginosa* infections.

Control and Treatment Treatment of clinically ill animals with antibiotics and supportive care may be attempted but may not be rewarding due to the rapid progression of disease. Sourcing clean animals, proper husbandry, minimizing stress, appropriate antibiotic usage, and providing uncontaminated feed to laboratory chinchillas may minimize chances of infection.

Research Complications Laboratory chinchillas that are clinically ill or die suddenly may complicate research studies. Subclinically infected animals, if present, may be a source of infection for other animals and people.

b. *Pseudomonas aeruginosa*

Etiology *Pseudomonas aeruginosa* is a gram-negative, aerobic, rod-shaped bacterium.

Clinical Signs Most infections are subclinical and only pose a problem in immunodeficient animals. *P. aeruginosa* has been cultured from clinically normal animals (Hirakawa *et al.*, 2010). Clinical signs of infection will depend on the location and extent of infection and may include anorexia, weight loss, enteritis, diarrhea, pneumonia, conjunctivitis with corneal ulceration, inguinal and genital pustules, and otitis with neurologic signs such as facial paralysis, head tilt, ataxia, circling, and rolling (Wideman, 2006; Doerning *et al.*, 1993; Kennedy, 1952). Septicemia and sudden death may also be seen in severe infections.

Epizootiology and Transmission *P. aeruginosa* is ubiquitous and commonly found in soil and water. Infection is acquired from contaminated water sources (Hirakawa *et al.*, 2010; Doerning *et al.*, 1993; Lusis and Soltys, 1971). In a recent study, 47.7% of laboratory chinchillas and 30.4% of pet chinchillas were subclinical carriers of *P. aeruginosa* (Hirakawa *et al.*, 2010).

Necropsy Findings Depending on the site of infection, gross necropsy findings that have been reported include caseous yellow material from the external ear canal, mottled and congested lungs, small pustules filled with thick white exudate in the inguinal and genital skin, enlarged and reddened inguinal lymph nodes, and a yellow and friable liver (Doerning *et al.*, 1993; Wideman, 2006). Histologically, animals with otitis displayed neutrophilic infiltrates with bacterial colonies in the tympanic bulla and inner ear. In animals with inguinal and genital skin pustules, the affected skin had severe hemorrhage, subcutaneous edema, and inflammation extending into the dermis. The mesenteric lymph nodes from these animals contained microabscesses, subcapsular hemorrhages, and neutrophilic inflammation. Histopathologic evidence of septicemia may be seen in the liver and lung (Wideman, 2006).

Pathogenesis *P. aeruginosa* is an opportunistic pathogen. Infection generally does not cause a problem in animals with a normal immune system; however, infection may be problematic in immunocompromised animals.

Differential Diagnosis Bacterial culture and identification from lesions or from the blood in septic animals can be performed to diagnose infection. Swabs of the oral cavity, feces, and water bottles may also be taken for culture (Hirakawa *et al.*, 2010).

Control and Treatment *P. aeruginosa* can be present in many laboratory rodent colonies and is not always considered an excluded agent except in immunodeficient colonies. Therefore, complete elimination or prevention of *P. aeruginosa* infection in conventionally housed laboratory chinchillas may be difficult or impractical. Treatment of the water supply by acidification, autoclaving, reverse osmosis, chlorine treatment, or filtering is required to minimize contamination and should be considered part of any routine animal colony management and husbandry program. However, biofilms may prevent complete sterilization of the water supply. Antibiotic treatment of animals already showing severe signs of clinical illness is unlikely to be successful.

Research Complications Generally, infection in immunocompetent animals is not considered to cause a significant research impact. Animals that become septicemic or show clinical signs of disease may not be suitable research subjects.

c. *Yersinia* Spp.

Etiology Infection with the gram-negative, rod-shaped, facultative anaerobic bacteria *Yersinia pseudotuberculosis* (Langford, 1972; Hubbert, 1972) and *Y. enterocolitica* (Bonke *et al.*, 2011; Raevuori *et al.*, 1979; Wuthe and Aleksic, 1992; Hubbert, 1972) have been reported in the chinchilla.

Clinical Signs Animals may be subclinically infected. Sporadic deaths have been reported with *Y. pseudotuberculosis* and *Y. enterocolitica* infection in chinchillas. Clinical signs include anorexia, weight loss, lethargy, excessive salivation, and diarrhea.

Epizootiology and Transmission Both humans and animals can be infected with *Yersinia* spp. Infection is transmitted by the fecal–oral route. Subclinical carriers may be a source of infection. Vertical transmission including transmission via the milk from mothers to their young may occur.

Necropsy Findings Gray–white, firm, nodular foci containing thick purulent material can be seen in the liver, spleen, intestinal tract, lymph nodes, and less frequently in the lungs. Hepatic and splenic enlargement may also be seen.

Pathogenesis Yersiniosis is an enteric disease that causes mucosal hemorrhage and ulceration of the ileum, cecum, and colon (Mans and Donnelly, 2012). Granulomatous lesions in various organs such as the liver, spleen, and lungs occur after systemic spread of the bacteria.

Differential Diagnosis Diagnosis can be made by bacterial culture and identification from lesioned organs, intestinal tract, or blood. Differential diagnoses include agents capable of causing systemic infections and similar lesions, such as *Listeria* spp. and *Salmonella*.

Control and Treatment Treatment with tetracycline antibiotics given orally or in the drinking water has been reported. Appropriate antibiotics should be selected based on culture and sensitivity as well as suitability for use in chinchillas. Treatment may not be successful in severely ill animals. Sourcing animals from clean colonies, elimination of subclinically infected animals, and environmental decontamination should be performed.

Research Complications Sick animals or animals that die unexpectedly may interfere with research studies. Infected animals may be a source of zoonotic infection.

d. Salmonella

Etiology *Salmonella* are ubiquitous, flagellaed, nonspore forming, facultative anaerobic, gram-negative, rod-shaped bacilli of the family Enterobacteriaceae. The genus *Salmonella* contains two species, although it had previously been considered to contain many more, *S. bongori* which infects mainly poikilotherms and rarely, humans, and *S. enterica* which includes approximately 2500 serovars. The salmonella of historical importance that are now rare include *S. enterica* subsp. *enterica* serovar Typhimurium (aka *S.* Typhimurium) and serovar Enteritidis (*S.* Enteritidis). *Salmonella* sp. (Lucena *et al.*, 2012a), *S.* Dublin (Watson and Watson, 1966), *S.* Enteritidis, *S.* Sofia (Naglic *et al.*, 2003; Misirlioglu *et al.*, 2002), *S.* Pullorum (Jones and Henderson, 1953), *S.* Typhimurium (Misirlioglu *et al.*, 2002), and *S.* Arizona (Mountain, 1989) infection have been reported in chinchillas.

Clinical Signs Infected animals may be subclinical carriers, or they may present with sudden death with no obvious clinical signs. Animals may be emaciated at the time of death. Clinical signs may include those associated with septicemia, anorexia, weight loss, lethargy, diarrhea with or without hemorrhage, tremors, and local paralysis. Mucopurulent or hemorrhagic vaginal secretions and abortions may be seen in females.

Epizootiology and Transmission *Salmonella* infections have been reported in pet chinchillas or those raised for their fur but have not been reported in laboratory chinchillas. All ages are susceptible to infection. In one report, hay fed to chinchillas may have been contaminated with chicken droppings and was suspected as the source of infection (Jones and Henderson, 1953). Transmission occurs by the fecal–oral route.

Necropsy Findings Gastritis, enteritis, extensive cecal ulcerations, enlarged spleens with necrotic foci, hepatitis with focal necrosis, cholecystitis, hemorrhagic and mucopurulent endometritis, and evidence of septicemia can be seen in chinchillas with *Salmonella* infection.

Pathogenesis *Salmonella* organisms are ingested and then colonize the intestines by attaching to the tips of intestinal villi. The host inflammatory response and intestinal injury results in gastroenteritis. *Salmonella* sp. may persist in enterocytes, M cells, or macrophages, and virulent strains may lead to bacteremia.

Differential Diagnosis Diagnosis of *Salmonella* infection can be made by culture and identification. Differential diagnoses for diarrhea or septicemic infections include coliforms, *Pseudomonas aeruginosa*, *Clostridium* spp., *Listeria monocytogenes*, *Yersinia pseudotuberculosis*, parasites, and coccidia and so on.

Control and Treatment Treatment with oxytetracycline, chloramphenicol, and enrofloxacin (Watson and Watson, 1966; Naglic *et al.*, 2003) has been reported. Due to its zoonotic potential and potential for subclinical carrier states, treatment in laboratory chinchillas may not be warranted.

Research Complications Infected chinchillas may show signs of clinical disease or sudden death, interfering with research studies. Subclinical carrier states may be a source of contamination for other experimental animals.

e. *Listeria* Spp.

Etiology Listeriosis is caused by an intracellular, facultative anaerobic, gram-positive, β-hemolytic, rod-shaped bacterial pathogen. Infection with *Listeria monocytogenes* (Cavill, 1967; Finley and Long, 1977; MacDonald *et al.*, 1972; Sabocanec *et al.*, 2000; Shalkop, 1950; Wilkerson *et al.*, 1997; Kirinus *et al.*, 2010; Lucena *et al.*, 2012a) and *L. ivanovii* (Kimpe *et al.*, 2004) has been reported in the chinchilla.

Clinical Signs Listeriosis may be subclinical or cause signs of septicemia, encephalitis, and/or abortions. In chinchillas with listeriosis, it is generally more common to see the septicemic form of the disease causing multiple visceral abscesses. Clinical signs have an acute onset and may include anorexia, lethargy, abdominal discomfort, diarrhea or decreased fecal production, and rectal prolapse. Torticollis and ataxia may be seen when encephalitis is present. Some reports describe a short duration of illness of approximately 1–4 days prior to death (Cavill, 1967; Finley and Long, 1977; Wilkerson *et al.*, 1997). However, sudden death with no previous clinical signs may also be seen. Infection may only affect a few animals, or entire colonies of chinchillas may be severely affected.

Epizootiology and Transmission Listeriosis in chinchillas has been reported worldwide, mainly in farm- or ranch-bred animals raised for their fur (Cavill, 1967; Shalkop, 1950; MacDonald *et al.*, 1972; Sabocanec *et al.*, 2000; Kirinus *et al.*, 2010). Infection of laboratory chinchillas is uncommon. *Listeria* spp. can infect a wide range of host animals (MacDonald *et al.*, 1972) and can be found in soil, water, sewage, decaying vegetation, insects, silage, and even in the intestinal tract of healthy animals (Ramaswamy *et al.*, 2007). Animals of all ages are susceptible to infection. Subclinically infected chinchillas may serve as a source of infection for other animals. Contaminated hay or feed have been suspected as sources of infection (Cavill, 1967; Finley and Long, 1977; Wilkerson *et al.*, 1997).

Necropsy Findings Necropsy findings commonly seen in infected chinchillas are the result of septicemic spread of the bacteria leading to the development of focal necrosis and abscesses in various tissues. Grossly, infected animals have pinpoint to 1–3 mm diameter white to yellow foci in the liver, spleen, cecum and intestines, mesentery, and mesenteric lymph nodes. Splenic and adrenal gland enlargement, impaction of the cecum, hemorrhagic enteritis, intussusception, myocardial abscess, pleuritis, and patchy pneumonia have also been seen. In females, hemorrhagic and necrotic metritis and mucometra have been reported, while fetuses from pregnant females exhibited miliary necrotic foci in the liver (Cavill, 1967). Microscopically, focal areas of necrosis consisting of necrotic debris, polymorphonuclear and mononuclear cell infiltrates, and bacterial colonies are present in the liver, intestines, mesenteric lymph nodes, and spleen. Microabscesses and areas of necrosis can be found in the kidney, cerebrum, brain stem, and adrenal glands. Lungs may reveal a pleuritis, interstitial pneumonia with thickened alveolar walls, foamy alveolar macrophages, and dispersed bacterial colonies (Cavill, 1967; Finley and Long, 1977; Wilkerson *et al.*, 1997).

Pathogenesis After ingestion of the bacteria from contaminated sources, pathogenic *Listeria* spp. disrupt the cecal and intestinal barrier to enter the host then colonize and multiply in the liver. Spread to other organs can occur via the blood and result in abscess formation in the liver, spleen, lymph nodes, brain, lungs, and various other organs (Mans and Donnelly, 2012). The bacteria are able to invade and survive in macrophages as well as a variety of other nonphagocytic cells such as epithelial cells, hepatocytes, and endothelial cells (Ramaswamy *et al.*, 2007). Chinchillas appear to be more susceptible to the septicemic form of the disease rather than the reproductive or encephalitic forms.

Differential Diagnosis A suspected diagnosis of Listeriosis can be made based on clinical signs, gross necropsy findings, and observing the presence of gram-positive organisms morphologically consistent with *L. monocytogenes* or *L. ivanovii* in abscesses. Diagnosis should be confirmed by bacterial culture and identification, and immunohistochemistry. *Yersinia pseudotuberculosis* and *Salmonella* infection may show similar gross lesions at necropsy (Cavill, 1967; Wilkerson *et al.*, 1997).

Control and Treatment Treatment with antibiotics such as oxytetracycline or chloramphenicol have been recommended (Hoefer and Crossley, 2002). However, treatment may not be successful when clinical signs are apparent and may not be warranted due to the pathogen's zoonotic potential. Elimination of the source of contamination and thorough decontamination of the environment should be performed.

Research Complications Infected chinchillas may die unexpectedly or show signs of clinical disease interfering with research studies.

f. *Helicobacter* Spp.

Confirmed disease or pathology caused by *Helicobacter* spp. infection in the chinchilla has not been reported, although an association with a gastric adenocarcinoma has been described (Lucena *et al.*, 2012b). A 5-year-old female chinchilla that died after 5 days of lethargy and anorexia was diagnosed by histopathology with an infiltrative gastric adenocarcinoma. Gross necropsy findings revealed a markedly thickened gastric wall with numerous firm white plaques and nodules in the gastric serosa, a firm white transmural mass obliterating the gastric lumen, and numerous gastric ulcers. Since *Helicobacter* spp. have been associated with the development of gastritis and gastric neoplasms in humans and other animals, the authors employed various diagnostic techniques in search of the organism. Polymerase chain reaction identified *H. pylori* in the gastric mucosa of this chinchilla; however, it is unclear whether this was indeed the causative agent of the adenocarcinoma. The authors report that in unpublished observations from their laboratory, *Helicobacter* spp. infection has been found in 40% of stomachs from approximately 252 routinely necropsied chinchillas in 2010 and 2011. Several of these infected chinchillas had varying degrees of gastritis, lymphoid hyperplasia, intestinal metaplasia, and/or dysplasia.

g. *Campylobacter* Spp.

Only a single meeting presentation abstract describing *Campylobacter lanienae* infection in laboratory chinchillas exists (Turowski *et al.*, 2011). This agent was found by polymerase chain reaction in 12 of 27 juvenile males from a laboratory colony with a history of gastritis, duodenitis, and typhlocolitis. However, further studies are necessary to determine whether or not infection with *C. lanienae* is indeed associated with gastrointestinal pathology in chinchillas.

h. *Klebsiella pneumoniae*

A single report of *Klebsiella pneumoniae* infection in the chinchilla has been described in a colony of breeding animals (Bartoszcze *et al.*, 1990a). Animals were anorexic, depressed, and showed signs of respiratory distress and diarrhea. Death ensued 5 days after onset of clinical signs. *K. pneumoniae* was isolated from visceral organs of animals at necropsy. Gross necropsy findings included congestion and consolidation of the lungs, hydrothorax, cardiomegaly, gastroenteritis, and subcapsular renal petechial hemorrhages. Histologic findings included congestion of alveolar capillaries and venous distention in the lungs, serous to suppurative exudate in the alveoli, and renal tubular necrosis with luminal casts. Treatment with gentamicin was attempted in chinchillas showing clinical signs of illness but only proved effective in half the treated animals.

i. *Escherichia coli*

A recent report of *Escherichia coli* septicemia has been described in an adult male, experimentally naïve chinchilla (Diaz *et al.*, 2013). This chinchilla presented with extreme lethargy and tachypnea and died shortly thereafter. Hematology revealed an overall leukocytosis, neutrophilia with a left-shift, and lymphopenia. Clinical chemistry abnormalities included azotemia, hyperphosphatemia, hyperglycemia, electrolyte imbalances, cholestasis, and hepatocellular damage. Microscopically, this chinchilla had a neutrophilic enterocolitis with surface bacterial colonization by gram-negative rods (Figs. 9.5 and 9.6), as well as lesions suggestive of septicemia such as neutrophilic infiltrates, fibrin thrombi, and edema in the lungs, neutrophilic inflammation in the gastrointestinal tract, and neutrophilic tubulonephritis in the kidneys. Other findings included neutrophilic and erosive gastritis, hepatic lipidosis, cerebral edema and congestion, lymphoid depletion in the spleen and thymus, and testicular degeneration. Cultures of the kidney and spleen revealed infection with an attaching and effacing *E. coli* positive for the intimin virulence factor. The origin of the *E. coli* infection was not found, and none of the remaining chinchillas developed any disease. *E. coli* is not considered part of the normal gastrointestinal flora of captive chinchillas but rather is considered an opportunistic pathogen (Diaz *et al.*, 2013; Mans and Donnelly, 2012). In this case reported by Diaz *et al.* (2013), the authors propose that the findings were consistent with enteric infection with subsequent acute septicemia and disseminated intravascular coagulation.

j. Other Bacteria

Other bacterial agents such as *Bordetella* sp., *Streptococcus* sp., and *Pasteurella* sp. have been suggested as a cause of chronic respiratory disease in chinchillas (Hoefer and Crossley, 2002; Goodman, 2004; Hrapkiewicz *et al.*, 2013). However, it is not clear if these agents are primary pathogens or opportunistic invaders in chinchilla colonies that have other management-related

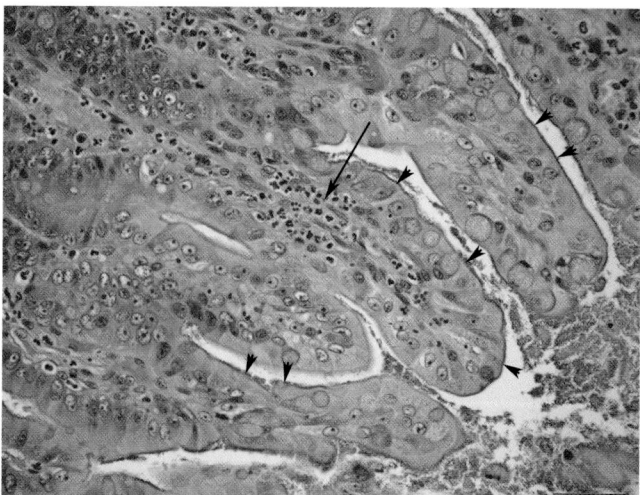

FIGURE 9.5 Neutrophilic enterocolitis in the ileum of an adult male chinchilla that died from an enteric infection and septicemia due to an attaching and effacing *Escherichia coli* infection. The apical surface of the enterocytes of the villi (arrowheads) are lined extensively with rod-shaped bacteria. Moderate numbers of neutrophils are present within the lamina propria of the villi (arrow). Hematoxylin and eosin stain; magnification, 40×; bar, 50 μm. *Image from Diaz et al.* (2013), *reprinted with permission from AALAS.*

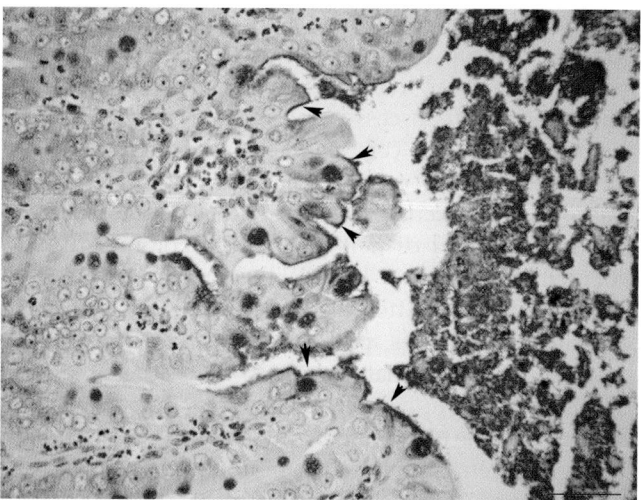

FIGURE 9.6 Gram stain of the ileum of the same chinchilla shown in Figure 9.5 that died from an enteric infection and septicemia due to an attaching and effacing *Escherichia coli* infection. The bacteria lining the apical surface of the enterocytes are gram-negative (arrowheads). Gram stain; magnification, 40×; bar, 50 μm. *Image from Diaz et al.* (2013), *reprinted with permission from AALAS.*

stressors such as inadequate husbandry, overcrowding, poor ventilation, and high humidity. *Proteus* sp. and *E. coli* have been associated with enteritis and diarrhea in chinchillas (Riggs and Mitchell, 2009; Lucena *et al.*, 2012a; Kennedy, 1952).

k. Mycoplasma and Rickettsia

No naturally occurring or experimental infections with mycoplasmal or rickettsial agents have been reported in chinchillas.

2. Chlamydial and Viral Infections

a. Chlamydia

No naturally occurring chlamydial infections have been reported in the chinchilla.

b. Herpes Virus

Etiology Herpes simplex virus 1, also known as human herpes virus 1, is an enveloped DNA virus in the family *Herpesviridae* and genus *Simplexvirus*.

Clinical Signs Chinchillas infected with human herpes virus type 1 may show signs of progressive central neurologic diseases including disorientation, seizures, and atonic lateral recumbency. Other signs may include a conjunctivitis, mydriasis, uveitis, purulent rhinitis, or sudden death.

Epizootiology and Transmission Only two cases of spontaneous herpes virus or herpes-like virus infection in chinchillas have been reported (Goudas and Gilroy, 1970; Wohlsein *et al.*, 2002). One case used histopathology and electron microscopy to visualize herpes-like viral particles in infected tissues (Goudas and Gilroy, 1970), while the other case confirmed infection with human herpes virus 1 using immunohistochemistry, virus isolation, and genomic sequence analysis (Wohlsein *et al.*, 2002). In the latter case, ocular infection was thought to be the primary route of entry, most likely from an infected person.

Necropsy Findings Gross and histologic lesions in the two infected chinchillas included discoloration of the perineal fur, a pale and friable liver, white foci and coagulative necrosis in the adrenal gland, areas of splenic necrosis, polioencephalitis with neuronal necrosis, nonsuppurative meningitis, purulent rhinitis, ulcerative keratitis, uveitis, retinal degeneration and inflammation, optic neuritis, and intranuclear inclusion bodies.

Pathogenesis Ocular infection with transneuronal spread has been suggested. In general, herpes viruses are considered neurotropic and infection is lifelong.

Differential Diagnosis Diagnosis can be confirmed by immunohistochemistry or virus isolation and genetic sequencing. Since infection of chinchillas with human herpes virus 1 is a rare occurrence, other causes of neurologic disease should also be considered.

Control and Treatment Since spread of the virus may occur from infected people, those actively shedding virus should avoid contact with chinchillas. In people within the United States, a seroprevalence of 57.7% has been reported (Xu *et al.*, 2006), indicating infection in people is common. Herpes virus infections are generally considered lifelong, so treatment of affected animals may not be warranted or effective.

Research Complications Infected chinchillas may die unexpectedly or show signs of clinical disease. Although it has not been reported, zoonotic infection may be a potential risk since chinchillas are susceptible to the virus.

c. Lymphocytic Choriomeningitis Virus

Chinchillas have been reported to be susceptible to natural infection with lymphocytic choriomeningitis virus (Maurer, 1964; Wallach and Boever, 1983). Although clinical signs specific to chinchillas after infection have not been described in great detail, it is presumed infection in chinchillas may be subclinical as it is in other rodents. This virus is zoonotic.

3. Parasitic Diseases

a. Protozoa

Toxoplasma and Frenkelia Historically toxoplasmosis was commonly found in fur-ranched chinchillas (Keagy, 1949) but it currently is rare. Necropsy lesions include hemorrhagic lungs, enlarged spleens, and enlarged mesenteric lymph nodes. Turner (1978) reviewed the wide pathological manifestations of toxoplasmosis, with or without necrosis, and tissue cyst formation as it occurs in sheep, cattle, pigs, horses, dogs, cats, chinchillas, and humans. Meingassner and Burtscher (1977) described two chinchillas with focal necrotic meningoencephalitis due to *Toxoplasma gondii*. Independent of and remote from the *Toxoplasma* inflammatory reactions, the authors also found several lobulated cysts up to 0.6 mm diameter in the brains of the two chinchillas. Based on morphology and staining characteristics, these cysts resembled those of the coccidian parasite *Frenkelia* as seen in other rodent species such as *Microtus* (voles) and *Ondatra zibethicus* (muskrat). This was the first report of *Frenkelia* cysts in the chinchilla and the authors suggest that chinchillas, like other rodent species, are likewise susceptible to *Frenkelia* infection. More recently, Dubey *et al.* (2000) described a *Frenkelia microti* cyst found in the brain of a biomedical research chinchilla bred in Minnesota, the first documentation of this organism in a chinchilla in the United States.

Giardia In the past, group-housed chinchillas in fur ranches and research colonies often had a high prevalence of *Giardia* infection (Newberne, 1953; Shelton, 1954a; Shelton, 1954b). Likewise, Eidmann (1992) examined the feces from healthy chinchillas and found that they normally harbor *Giardia* species in large numbers. A case report of *Giardia* infection in chinchillas in Taiwan has been described (Chang *et al.*, 1986), while more recently, *Giardia duodenalis* infection was detected in clinically normal pet and breeding chinchillas at a high prevalence in Belgium (66.3%) and Italy (39.4%)

(Levecke *et al.*, 2011; Veronesi *et al.*, 2012). The two studies by Levecke *et al.* (2011) and Veronesi *et al.* (2012), and another report by Soares *et al.* (2011), provided evidence that chinchillas can be infected with *G. duodenalis* assemblages of zoonotic importance, suggesting chinchillas may serve as a potential reservoir for zoonotic infection. Although infection in chinchillas is typically subclinical, cycles of inappetence and diarrhea leading to weight loss and poor fur condition may be seen (Mans and Donnelly, 2012). Stress and poor husbandry may cause an increased number of *Giardia* organisms and may predispose animals to opportunistic gastroenteric bacterial infections, potentially resulting in severe diarrhea and death. Diagnosis is through microscopic identification of trophozoites or cysts on a fresh fecal smear (Mans and Donnelly, 2012). ELISA on fecal samples has also been used, although results may be difficult to interpret as sensitivity and specificity of the test in chinchillas has not been determined, and clinically normal chinchillas may also shed *G. duodenalis* in their feces (Mans and Donnelly, 2012). Although the pathogenicity of the organism in chinchillas remains unknown, treatment with albendazole (25 mg/kg PO q12h for 2 days), fenbendazole (50 mg/kg PO q24h for 3 days), or metronidazole (10–20 mg/kg PO q12h, with caution) of the affected chinchilla(s), and all those in contact, is indicated. Treatment may inhibit cyst production rather than fully eradicate *Giardia*, so the environment should be thoroughly disinfected to prevent reinfection (Mans and Donnelly, 2012).

Other Protozoa De Vos (1970) and De Vos and Dobson (1970) studied the etiology, pathology, and host range of *Eimeria chinchillae* in chinchillas, guinea pigs, hamsters, mice, rats, and rabbits in South Africa. Individual case reports of hepatic sarcocystosis in a pet female chinchilla that died acutely (Rakich *et al.*, 1992) and gastroenteritis associated with a *Cryptosporidium* sp. in a pet chinchilla (Yamini and Raju, 1986) are described. *Trichomonas muris*, *T. wenyani*, *T. minuta*, and a form resembling *Theileria microta* have been reported in chinchillas (Griffiths, 1971).

b. Nematodes

Sanford (1989, 1991) reported disease outbreaks of cerebral nematodiasis caused by the raccoon ascarid *Baylisascaris procyonis* in chinchillas in western Canada. Affected chinchillas exhibited ataxia, torticollis, paralysis, and tumbling. Exposure was via hay contaminated with raccoon feces (Mans and Donnelly, 2012).

c. Cestodes

Chinchillas can serve as an intermediate host for cestodes, including *Taenia serialis*, *Taenia pisiformis*, *Taenia crassiceps*, *Echinococcus granulosus*, and *Hymenolepis nana*. Exposure can occur via ingestion of hay contaminated

with the feces of an infected dog. Recently, naturally occurring *Echinococcus multilocularis* infection was reported in a pet chinchilla that was euthanized due to abdominal distension (Staebler *et al.*, 2007). Multiple hepatic vesicles and cysts were noted on gross necropsy, and diagnosis of *E. multilocularis* was made on histologic examination. Holmberg *et al.* (2007) described a 4-year-old, intact, male captive-bred pet chinchilla that was examined for unilateral exophthalmos that developed and progressed over a 5-month period. A cyst was removed via ventral transpalpebral orbitotomy and comprised of "multiple invaginated protoscolices, characterized by a prominent scolex with refractile hooklets, suckers, and abundant calcareous corpuscles" which was consistent with *Taenia coenurus*. No recurrence or complications were noted for two years following removal of the cyst.

d. Ectoparasites

Reports of ectoparasitism in chinchillas are quite rare owing to their dense fur. Fur mites (*Cheyletiella*) and fleas (acquired by chinchillas in households including a dog and/or cat) have been reported anecdotally (Hoefer and Crossley, 2002; Richardson, 2003). Chinchillas can be treated with ivermectin (0.2–0.4 mg/kg SC q7–14d), 2.5% lime sulfur dips (q7d), pyrethrin power (q7d), or other appropriate antiparasitic agents (Hoefer and Crossley, 2002; Morrisey and Carpenter, 2012). Potential effects of ectoparasites on research in chinchillas have not been defined.

4. Mycotic Infections

a. Dermatophytes

Etiology Dermatophytosis, also referred to as ringworm, is caused by the dermatophytes *Trichophyton mentagrophytes* (Lucena *et al.*, 2012a; Cabanes *et al.*, 1997; Horvath and Keri, 1980; Hagen and Gorham, 1972), *Microsporum gypseum* (Morganti and Gomez Portugal, 1970), and *M. canis* (Donnelly *et al.*, 2000; Hagen and Gorham, 1972).

Clinical Signs Infections can be subclinical (Chermette *et al.*, 2008; Hagen and Gorham, 1972). When present, clinical signs in chinchillas include well-defined areas of alopecia with variable degrees of scaling, crust formation, and erythema (Chermette *et al.*, 2008; Donnelly *et al.*, 2000). Typically, lesions are non-pruritic and can occur around the eyes, on the nose, head, ears, flanks, tail, and forefeet; however, lesions may be found on any part of the body (Hagen and Gorham, 1972; Morganti and Gomez Portugal, 1970; Chermette *et al.*, 2008).

Epizootiology and Transmission *T. mentagrophytes* is more commonly isolated from chinchillas than *Microsporum* sp. (Donnelly *et al.*, 2000; Hagen and Gorham, 1972; Morganti and Gomez Portugal, 1970). Transmission occurs via direct contact with an infected animal or person, or by contact with infected hair and scale on fomites or in the environment. *T. mentagrophytes* and *M. canis* are zoophilic dermatophytes while *M. gypseum* is a geophilic dermatophyte (Chermette *et al.*, 2008). Wild rodents may be subclinical carriers of *T. mentagrophytes* (Hagen and Gorham, 1972; Chermette *et al.*, 2008).

Necropsy Findings Microscopically, tissue sections stained with periodic acid Schiff (PAS) or methenamine silver stain will stain fungal elements and allow for the detection of arthroconidia and hyphae (Chermette *et al.*, 2008; Donnelly *et al.*, 2000).

Pathogenesis Dermatophytes do not invade living tissue but rather colonize the keratinized layer to utilize keratin as a source of nutrients in tissues such as the skin, hair, and nails (Donnelly *et al.*, 2000). Infection does not occur on healthy, intact skin but rather mild damage is required for infection to take place. An allergic inflammatory response to the fungus or its metabolic products results in clinical disease. The immune status of the host is important in determining susceptibility – young, old, or immunosuppressed animals are predisposed to having clinical infections. Infection in healthy animals is usually self-limiting, and cell-mediated immunity is essential for clinical resolution of disease (Chermette *et al.*, 2008).

Differential Diagnosis Diagnosis can be suspected based on clinical presentation but should be confirmed by fungal culture with dermatophyte test medium (DTM). Microscopic examination of the hair and skin scrapings collected from lesion margins can also be performed to supplement fungal culture. For better visualization of fungal elements, samples should be cleared of keratin with chlorolactophenol or with potassium hydroxide (KOH). A Wood's light can be used to screen for *M. canis* infection, which will produce an apple-green fluorescence. However, this test has a low negative predictive value (Chermette *et al.*, 2008). Therefore, a negative Wood's light examination should not be used to rule out dermatophyte infection, especially since infection with non-fluorescing dermatophytes is more common in chinchillas.

Control and Treatment Infected animals should be isolated or removed to minimize exposure to uninfected animals, and the environment thoroughly disinfected. In healthy animals, the infection may be self-limiting, and lesions may resolve as the immune response successfully controls infection. Treatment may be attempted in non-resolving lesions and should include both topical and system medications. Topical treatments include a 2% chlorhexidine/2% miconazole shampoo or 0.2% enilconazole rinse, while systemic drugs include terbinafine, itraconazole, or ketoconazole (Mans and Donnelly, 2012). However, in the laboratory setting, the benefits of treatment must be weighed against the risk of zoonosis, the long duration of antifungal therapy required to eliminate infection, the potential side-effects of treatment, and the potential to interfere with research studies.

Research Complications Infected animals may not be suitable research subjects if signs of clinical disease are present. Clinically and subclinically infected animals may be a source of zoonotic infection, causing tinea corporis in people (Rosen and Jablon, 2003).

b. *Histoplasma capsulatum*

Histoplasma capsulatum is a fungus that grows in the soil and is most common in the southeastern, mid-Atlantic, and central states of the United States. A naturally occurring infection with *H. capsulatum* has been reported in the chinchilla (Owens *et al.*, 1975). Infection was diagnosed by histopathology in one animal from a colony that had a history of multiple unexpected deaths. Sick animals in this colony had clinical signs of anorexia, weight loss, constipation, and tachypnea with deaths occurring within 2–4 days of the acute respiratory signs. However, besides this single animal diagnosed with histoplasmosis, no other animals evaluated had evidence of this fungal infection. Instead, histopathologic evidence of a bacterial pneumonia was seen. Therefore, this single animal with *H. capsulatum* infection may have been an incidental finding rather than the primary cause of deaths in this chinchilla colony. Even so, *H. capsulatum* was cultured from timothy hay fed to the chinchillas, indicating that this fungus was present in their immediate environment. Gross necropsy findings from the single animal diagnosed with *H. capsulatum* infection included emphysematous lungs with foci of hemorrhage and bronchopneumonia, an enlarged spleen with white nodules, focal necrosis in the liver, and an empty gastrointestinal tract. Histopathology revealed proliferation of septal cells and focal consolidation in the lungs, a fibrinous pleuritis, multiple focal granulomas in the liver, splenic necrosis and abscessation with multiple focal granulomas, glomerular nephritis, and distended lymph node sinuses. *H. capsulatum* organisms were seen in the lungs, liver, spleen, kidneys, and lymph node.

B. Gastrointestinal and Metabolic Diseases

1. *Gastrointestinal Disorders*

In the early 1960s, the Chinchilla Fur-Breeders Association of England showed that approximately half of all deaths in adult chinchillas were due to disorders of the digestive tract, with malocclusion accounting for one-quarter of all deaths (Cousens, 1963; Dall, 1963). Husbandry-related disorders of the digestive tract still remain one of the most frequent problems seen. Cheek tooth crown and root abnormalities are common in chinchillas (Crossley, 1997; Crossley *et al.*, 1997). Crossley *et al.* (1998) used computerized tomographic (CT) scanning to investigate tooth structure in chinchillas and have shown CT to be a useful tool in the early diagnosis of malocclusion. Complications of malocclusion include periodontitis, alveolar periostitis, and alveolar abscessation of maxillary and mandibular cheek teeth (Emily, 1991; Griner, 1983). See Section III, F for additional information on dental disease.

Chinchillas cannot vomit, and esophageal choke has been described in chinchillas of all ages (Cousens, 1963). Affected animals show drooling, retching, dyspnea, and anorexia. Choke is more common in animals that eat their bedding and in postparturient females that eat their placentas. Bloat or gastric tympany is a problem of lactating females and is generally associated with overeating but can also be seen with sudden changes in diet, and in both sexes, with gastrointestinal inflammation (Donnelly, 2004; Kennedy, 1952). Affected animals are distended, laterally recumbent, lethargic, and dyspneic. Treatment to relieve bloat includes decompressing the stomach by passing a gastric tube or inserting a needle or trocar (Donnelly, 2004); however, in some decompensated animals, decompression can result in collapse and death (Mans and Donnelly, 2012). Gastric trichobezoars are often associated with the vice of fur chewing and may be accompanied by anorexia. Papaya tablets and pineapple juice are anecdotal remedies that are at least unlikely to cause harm. Dehydrated and anorexic animals with suspected trichobezoars will benefit from supplemental fluids, gastric motility stimulants, and force-feeding of a high-fiber food supplement such as Critical Care (Oxbow Animal Health, Murdock, NE). Radiographs (Fig. 9.7) to rule out obstruction prior to administering gastric motility medications are recommended.

In the chinchilla, constipation occurs more often than diarrhea (Hartmann, 1993). Chinchillas with constipation strain to defecate, and the few pellets passed are thin, short, hard, and occasionally bloodstained. The usual cause of constipation is insufficient roughage or fiber (Cousens, 1963). Other causes of constipation may include obesity, intestinal obstruction, intestinal compression due to large fetuses (Hartmann, 1993), and intestinal intussusception (Mans and Donnelly, 2012). Increasing fiber in the diet and gradually adding small amounts of foods such as apples, carrots, and dark lettuces, while eliminating grains and raisins, may be sufficient treatment. Otherwise, treatment focuses primarily on rehydration of gut contents by enteral fluid therapy (100 ml/kg PO q24h divided in 4–5 doses); abdominal massage and regular exercise may be beneficial (Mans and Donnelly, 2012). If no intestinal blockage is present, cisapride may be used at 0.5 mg/kg PO q8h to stimulate intestinal motility (Donnelly, 2004). In chronic cases of constipation or gastroenteritis, intestinal torsion and impaction of the cecum or colonic flexure may occur and require surgical intervention (Bowden, 1959; McGreevy and Carn, 1988; Donnelly, 2004). Rectal prolapse may also occur in severe cases of constipation or diarrhea, and may include intussusception of the intestines as well as the descending colon and rectum (Mans and Donnelly, 2012). Among 91 chinchillas necropsied over a 4-year period in a Japanese laboratory, 6% of chinchillas had prolapse of the rectum as the major cause of death, while malocclusion accounted for 10% of deaths (Kuroiwa and Imamichi, 1977). If intussusception is ruled out, and the rectal prolapse is diagnosed and treated promptly, it can be replaced (with the topical application of dextrose or similar solution to reduce edema, if necessary) and fixed with a purse-string suture. A bland, soft diet of baby food and cereals (except rice cereal) should be offered for 10 days post-prolapse, with gradual return to a normal diet after suture removal (Donnelly, 2004). For successful treatment, measures must also be taken to address the underlying cause of the prolapse. In cases involving intestinal intussusception, however, surgical correction of the intussusception, including resection and anastomosis of compromised tissue, is necessary, and the prognosis is usually poor (Mans and Donnelly, 2012).

2. Metabolic Disorders

Marlow (1995) described a case of diabetes mellitus in a 5-year-old overweight female chinchilla. The animal had a 3-week history of poor appetite, lethargy, and weight loss. Diagnostic workup revealed polydipsia, polyuria, and bilateral cataracts. Blood and urine analysis indicated a hyperglycemia greater than 400 mg/dl (22.2 mmol/L), a heavy glucosuria, and ketonuria. Insulin treatment of the animal achieved a decrease of the blood glucose concentration to 210 mg/dl (11.7 mmol/L). However, the condition did not stabilize and the chinchilla was euthanized after 2 weeks of therapy. The pancreatic islets showed prominent vacuolation consistent with diagnosis of diabetes mellitus. Treatment

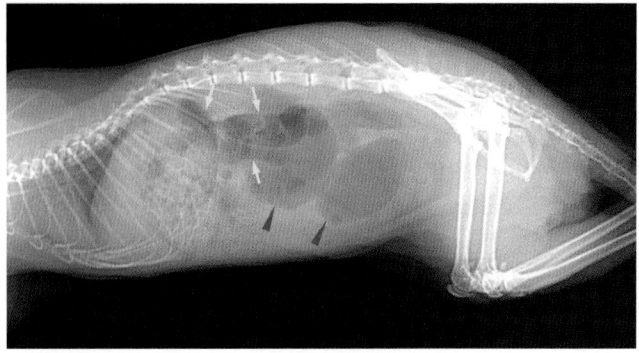

FIGURE 9.7   Right lateral radiograph of a 10-year-old female chinchilla with bloat that presented with inappetence, decreased fecal production, and dental disease. Note the mildly increased gas intermixed with ingesta in the stomach and marked gas dilation of the intestines (yellow arrows) and cecum (red arrowheads). *Courtesy Dr. L. Brazelton.*

of diabetes mellitus in rodents is typically difficult, but adjusting the diet to one that is high in protein and complex carbohydrates, low in fat, and supplemented with 50 μg chromium per kg of diet has been suggested to help regulate the disease (Donnelly, 2004). Fritsche *et al.* (2008) described hyperthyroidism in a pet intact female 6-year-old chinchilla. The chinchilla presented for rapid weight loss and exhibited poor body condition, ptyalism and malodorous breath, multifocal mild alopecia, and unilateral seromucous lacrimation. A diagnosis of suspected diabetes mellitus was initially made based on weight loss and a single high serum glucose. Treatment with glipizide was initiated but then discontinued after a normal serum fructosamine was obtained in conjunction with elevated T4. Treatment with thiamazole ointment applied to the concave aspect of the pinna (initial dose 0.15 ml, then decreased to 0.1 ml), successive dentals to correct overgrown incisors, and nystatin for oral mycosis led to resolution of the hyperglycemia, ptyalism, and unilateral ocular discharge, and to moderate weight gain. The increased weight correlated with a reduction of T_4 to normal levels.

Pathologists often see fatty liver on histology without clinical signs or other histopathology in routine necropsies (Egri *et al.*, 1994). Kruckenberg *et al.* (1975) described clinical toxicities, including adverse effects of alfalfa, in chinchillas (and other rodents and rabbits). Chinchillas with metabolic disease may have altered responses to experimental conditions compared to healthy animals, and the use of animals known or suspected to have a metabolic condition should be avoided in research studies.

C. Traumatic Lesions

1. Fur Slip

Chinchillas possess a predator-avoidance mechanism known as fur slip. When the animal is fighting or roughly handled, it can release a large patch of fur, thus enabling it to escape. A clean, smooth area of skin is left and the hair may take several months to regrow. Fur slip should not be confused with the vice of fur chewing seen when chinchillas chew each other's fur, resulting in a coat with a moth-eaten appearance.

2. Bite Wounds

During breeding, bite wounds that abscess occur frequently in group-housed animals. Culture of the abscesses often yields *Staphylococcus* species (Jenkins, 1992). Often, bite wounds result in the loss of pieces of ears and toes. Female chinchillas are larger than males and more aggressive. They are highly selective in their choice of males for mating and will keep 'unsuitable' males at bay by urinating, kicking, and biting (Bignami and Beach, 1968; Weir,

1970). As previously noted, males may even be killed by the female if unable to escape (Weir, 1970).

3. Fractures

Traumatic fractures of the tibia are commonly seen (Hoefer, 1994) and are associated with the animal catching its hind limb in a cage bar. The tibia is a straight bone longer than the femur and with little overlying soft tissue. The fibula is virtually nonexistent. Tibial fractures are either transverse or short spiral and generally are associated with bony fragments. Simple fractures may be stabilized using a needle as an intramedullary pin (Richardson, 2003), although wire or external fixators (type II Kirscher–Ehmer apparatus) with a stabilizing bandage are more likely to produce satisfactory results. Bandaging alone is seldom successful due to the thin, fragile nature of chinchilla bones and difficulty of stabilization but may be more successful for forelimb fractures of the radius/ulna and distally (Hoefer and Crossley, 2002). Amputation is well tolerated by chinchillas and recommended for comminuted or compound fractures (Richardson, 2003; Mans and Donnelly, 2012). An Elizabethan collar is frequently required to prevent self-mutilation of the affected limb (Richardson, 2003), and strict cage rest for a minimum of 4 weeks is essential for adequate healing and successful recovery (Hoefer and Crossley, 2002; Donnelly, 2004).

4. Other Traumatic Injuries

Other traumatic lesions seen in chinchillas include a report of a diaphragmatic hernia (Dall, 1967) and degloving injuries of the tail (Richardson, 2003).

D. Reproductive, Management-Related, and Iatrogenic Disorders

1. Reproductive Disorders

a. Female Reproductive Disorders and Dystocia

Chinchillas usually give birth in the early morning (before 8:00 a.m.) and rarely late at night (Weir, 1970; Quesenberry *et al.*, 2012). Dystocia is usually associated with the presentation of a single oversized fetus or malpresentation of one or more kits (Cousens, 1963). Uterine inertia (Prior, 1986) and uterine torsion (Hoefer and Crossley, 2002) have also been reported causes of dystocia. Affected females may exhibit restlessness and bleeding as well as frequent crying and attention to the genital region (Mans and Donnelly, 2012). Initial treatment for uterine inertia can be attempted with 0.5–1 IU/kg of oxytocin and 25–50 mg/kg SC of diluted calcium gluconate (Mans and Donnelly, 2012). However, if labor is still unproductive after 4 h, Caesarian section should be considered and is usually well tolerated (Richardson, 2003; Jones, 1990; Prior, 1986; Stephenson, 1990; Caspari, 1990; Sims, 1990;

Hoefer and Crossley, 2002). Pyometras are seldom diagnosed in chinchillas (Hoefer and Crossley, 2002). Acute metritis may be unresponsive to treatment, but the treatment plan should include systemic antibiotics, with or without a dose of oxytocin. Treatment for chronic pyometritis or metritis should consist of ovariohysterectomy and systemic antibiotics (Richardson, 2003).

Gitlin and Adler (1969) described an unusual case report of coexisting intrauterine and intraperitoneal pregnancy due to superfetation in a chinchilla. Kuroiwa and Imamichi (1977) followed birth-to-weaning mortality in a Japanese laboratory colony of chinchillas. Among 91 animals that died, the cause of death in 23 (25.3%) was neonatal-related. Thirty-seven chinchillas gave birth to 71 kits with an average litter size of 1.9, and 59 kits were successfully weaned (1.6 per litter). Of these kits, 50 (1.3 per litter) attained 240 days of age.

In chinchillas, the fine structure of the interhemal membrane of the placental labyrinth is hemomonochorial, consisting of a single layer of syncytial trophoblast. In this respect, the placental labyrinth is similar to that of another caviomorph rodent, the guinea pig (King and Tibbitts, 1976). Tvedten and Langham (1974) described an unusual puerperal disorder of trophoblastic emboli in a chinchilla, resulting in pulmonary embolism. Granson *et al.* (2011) described a 4-year-old nulliparous female chinchilla that presented for a 2-month history of blood being observed intermittently in its cage. There were no other abnormal clinical findings, although of note the chinchilla's littermate had previously been evaluated for similar clinical signs. Ovariohysterectomy of the second presenting chinchilla revealed no gross reproductive lesions, however histology revealed multifocal cystic dilation of the endometrial glands, microhemorrhagic foci, and chronic endometritis. For both animals, ovariohysterectomy resulted in cessation of clinical signs.

b. Fur Ring

Male chinchillas that groom excessively, frequently produce small amounts of urine, strain to urinate, and/ or repeatedly clean their penis may have a fur ring (Mans and Donnelly, 2012). This is a ring of hair around the penis and under the prepuce that eventually stops the penis from retracting into the prepuce. In severe cases, an engorged penis is seen protruding 4–5 cm from the prepuce, resulting in paraphimosis. The condition is painful and may cause urethral constriction and acute urinary retention. Chronic paraphimosis may culminate in infection and severe damage to the penis, affecting the breeding ability of the animal. Getting fur from a female during copulation is the most common cause of fur ring. However, the fur may come from other males or the same animal as the condition is also seen in

group-housed and singly-housed males not exposed to females. Males should be examined for fur rings at least four times a year; active stud males should be examined every few days. In some male chinchillas, the penis will hang out of the prepuce all the time and is not engorged. In these males the cause of this condition is not associated with fur ring but is due to overexcitement brought on by separation from their mates or overexhaustion due to too many females in the same cage. Fur rings can be cut or gently rolled off the penis after applying a sterile lubricant. Occasionally, sedation or anesthesia of the male may be required to remove the fur ring.

2. Management-Related Disorders

a. Heatstroke

Chinchillas exposed to ambient temperatures above the range of 65–80°F (18.3–26.7°C), especially in the presence of high humidity, may succumb to heatstroke. As noted above, a suggested rule of thumb is to add the units of temperature (in Fahrenheit) and humidity, with any value greater than 150 having the potential to induce heatstroke (Donnelly, 2004). Obesity and periods of increased activity (dust bathing) may also predispose to heatstroke (Richardson, 2003). Chinchillas experiencing heatstroke may initially be restless and polydipsic (Richardson, 2003), progressing to recumbency, tachypnea, bright-red mucous membranes and hyperemic pinnae, thickened saliva, and occasionally bloody diarrhea. Rectal temperature often exceeds 103°F (39.4°C). Treatment is aimed at cooling the chinchilla in a tepid water (not ice water) bath and rehydrating with IV or subcutaneous fluids as needed (Donnelly, 2004).

b. Fur-Chewing

Chinchillas will barber and chew their own and cagemates' fur, resulting in an untidy coat with a moth-eaten appearance (Richardson, 2003; Mans and Donnelly, 2012). The dark undercoat may remain in animals that chew their own fur, and the area over the lumbar spine is often affected (Mans and Donnelly, 2012). Eidmann (1992) examined histologic sections of 39 fur-chewing chinchillas and 19 healthy chinchillas of both sexes and various ages. No infectious cause of fur-chewing was identified, and an etiology of nutritional deficiency has been proposed (Richardson, 2003). More recently, the abnormal activity has been considered to be a behavioral disorder in reaction to overcrowding or stress, with up to 20% of animals in some breeding facilities being affected (Mans and Donnelly, 2012). Boredom, small caging, draughts, and high ambient temperature have also been implicated (Richardson, 2003). Correction of social and environmental stressors should be implemented, including removing dominant or aggressive animals, providing multiple sleeping boxes and feeding areas for group-housed animals, and reducing disturbances due to frequent handling or changes in light and noise levels (Mans and Donnelly, 2012). Treatment with fluoxetine (5–10 mg/kg PO q24 h) has been suggested, but not described, based on rabbit and rodent dosages (Mans and Donnelly, 2012).

c. Matted Fur

Chinchillas housed at temperatures exceeding 80°F (26.7°C), at high humidity, or without adequate access to a dust bath may develop matted fur. Recommended dust bath availability is 15 min per day, or at least several times a week (Mans and Donnelly, 2012; Quesenberry *et al.*, 2012).

d. Conjunctivitis

Excessive dust bathing or bathing with dust that has not been changed with sufficient frequency can result in irritation of the eyes and conjunctivitis (Fig. 9.8) in the absence of clinical signs of upper respiratory tract infection. Dirty, poor-quality bedding, inadequate cage ventilation, or underlying nasolacrimal duct obstruction may also contribute to disease. *Pseudomonas aeruginosa* may cause conjunctivitis as a localized infection or as part of systemic infection. Diagnostics should include fluorescein staining to rule out corneal damage, and conjunctival swab for culture and sensitivity. Treatment should include restricting dust bath access and lavaging the conjunctival sac with saline, and use of a broad-spectrum antibiotic ophthalmic ointment. Prompt systemic antibiotic therapy and supportive care are necessary for chinchillas with systemic *Pseudomonas* infection (Mans and Donnelly, 2012) but may not be advisable or justified for animals in a laboratory setting as they may not be suitable research subjects.

3. *Iatrogenic Disorders*
a. Antibiotic-Associated Dysbiosis and Gastroenteritis

Similar to guinea pigs, chinchillas are susceptible to antibiotic-associated dysbiosis and gastroenteritis. Antibiotics that target gram-positive bacteria, such as penicillins, cephalosporins, clindamycin, lincomycin, and erythromycin, may disrupt the normal gut flora and allow overgrowth of opportunistic gastrointestinal bacterial pathogens (Mans and Donnelly, 2012; Hrapkiewicz *et al.*, 2013). Therefore, the use of these antibiotics should be avoided.

b. Metronidazole Toxicity

Rare anecdotal reports of metronidazole administration associated with liver failure in chinchillas exist, although it is unclear if the effect was due to toxicity or to a pre-existing condition, and no reports have arisen in more than a decade (Donnelly, 2004).

E. Neoplastic Diseases

Despite a reported life span of up to 20 years, references on neoplasia in chinchillas are rare. *Post mortem* examinations on 1005 chinchillas before 1949 and another 1000 chinchillas between 1949 and 1952, ranging in age between less than 6 months and 11 years, did not list neoplasia as a cause of death (Brenon, 1955; Brenon, 1953). In contrast, during the 1950s the Annual Reports of the San Diego County Livestock Department listed tumors such as neuroblastoma, carcinoma, lipoma, and hemangioma as occurring in chinchillas. Newberne and Robinson (1957) described a malignant lymphoma in a chinchilla. Schaeffer and Donnelly (1997) reported a uterine leiomyosarcoma in a 1-year-old female chinchilla as an incidental finding at necropsy. Lucena *et al.* (2012b) described gastric adenocarcinoma in a 5-year-old female chinchilla that died after a 5-day period of anorexia and lethargy. Neoplastic cells infiltrated the lamina propria, submucosa, and muscular layers, and were positive for cytokeratin. In addition, similar nodules were noted on the mesentery, visceral surface of the diaphragm, renal capsule, and uterine serosa. Smith *et al.* (2010) reported an undifferentiated salivary gland carcinoma in a 12-year-old female chinchilla; neoplastic cells were positive for vimentin and pan-cytokeratin but negative for alpha-smooth muscle actin, S100, and myosin. Simova-Curd *et al.* (2008) also described a lumbar osteosarcoma in an 11-year-old male chinchilla that presented for anorexia, weight loss, apathy, altered fecal consistency, self-mutilation of the tail tip, and eventual hind limb paralysis.

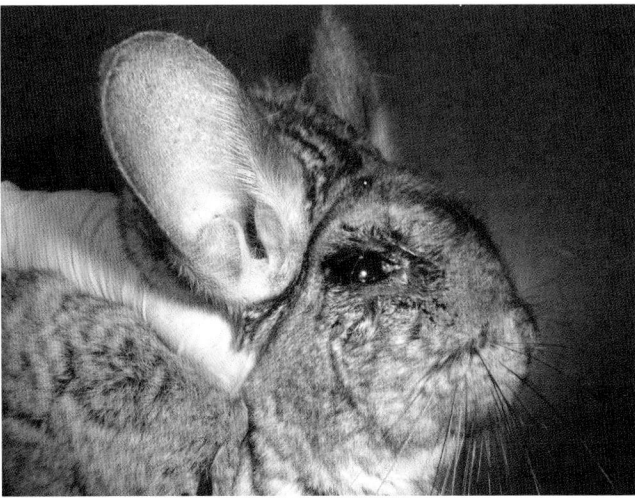

FIGURE 9.8 Gray chinchilla with conjunctivitis and blocked tear ducts, possibly due to a bacterial infection or inflammation created by foreign objects such as dust or hay in the eye. *Courtesy of Dr. A. Keffer.*

F. Miscellaneous Conditions

1. Congenital Disorders

Few congenital abnormalities have been described in chinchillas; however, malocclusion (which may be congenital, traumatic, or of later onset) is an extremely common condition that can have a significant health impact in chinchillas.

a. Embryologic Abnormalities

DeNooij (1985) described a case of abnormal embryological development in a chinchilla, resulting in a schistosomus reflexus fetus.

b. Cardiovascular Disorders

Cardiomyopathy, congenital septal defects, and valvular disease have anecdotally been reported in pet chinchillas (Hoefer and Crossley, 2002; Donnelly, 2004). Cardiomyopathy and valvular disease have been seen at necropsy. Heart murmurs of varying intensity are often detected in chinchillas, including young chinchillas presented for routine examination. While some animals with significant murmurs may have normal echocardiographic findings, one 2-year-old male chinchilla in which a heart murmur was ausculted incidentally during routine exam was found to have a ventricular septal defect and tricuspid regurgitation. The animal died acutely more than a year later (Hoefer and Crossley, 2002). The majority of chinchillas with cardiac disease only present once they have developed advanced clinical signs, including acute dyspnea on exam and pleural effusion, pulmonary edema, and cardiomegaly on radiography. Treatment is empiric, with diuretics and sodium channel blockers such as amlodipine, and fulminant heart failure carries a poor prognosis (Donnelly, 2004; Hoefer and Crossley, 2002; author's experience). There are currently no reports on the prevalence of heart diseases in chinchillas, and the relationship between the occurrence and severity of heart murmurs and underlying cardiovascular pathology is unknown (Donnelly, 2004).

c. Malocclusion

As in guinea pigs, the open-rooted, hypsodont incisors and molars of chinchillas are prone to overgrowth when misaligned, and dental disease is very common in captive chinchillas. A UK study (Crossley, 2001) identified early changes in 35% of apparently healthy chinchillas examined (Hoefer and Crossley, 2002). Continued apical growth of maloccluded teeth results in remodeling of surrounding tissues, facilitating tooth root elongation and producing palpable rounded bony protrusions along the mandible. Tooth root elongation of maxillary premolars and molars can impinge on the lacrimal ducts, causing epiphora (Hoefer and Crossley, 2002; author's experience). Elongation of the second and

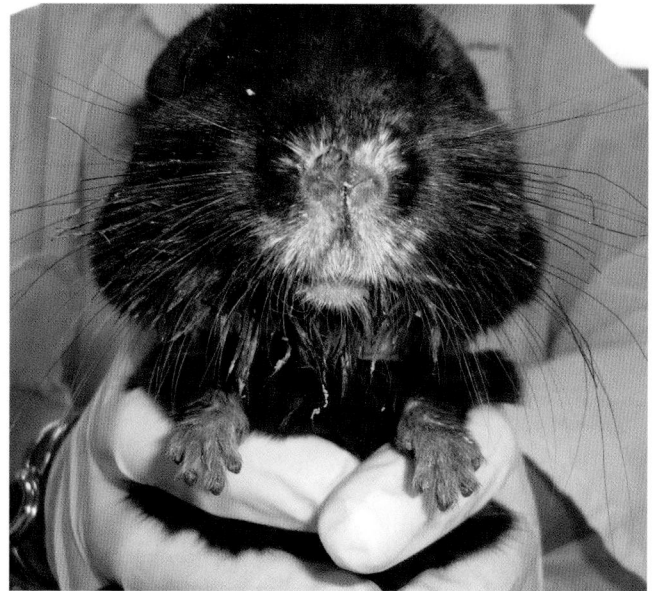

FIGURE 9.9   Ebony chinchilla with malocclusion of the molars causing crown elongation, an inability to close the mouth, and drooling ('slobbers'). *Courtesy of Dr. A. Keffer.*

third maxillary molar roots can interfere with retraction of the eyes into their sockets and can rarely cause proptosis. Altered coordination of tooth eruption and growth rates, which may be affected by extreme nutritional deficiencies, stress, inflammation, trauma, and other disease, also leads to abnormal curvature of the cheek teeth and the formation of spurs or spikes typically on the buccal aspect (Hoefer and Crossley, 2002). In one author's experience (MC), premolar and molar malocclusion and abnormalities appear to be more common and severe than incisor abnormalities in chinchillas, which almost always are secondary to crown elongation of the cheek teeth or absence of the opposing incisors (Crossley, 2001).

Affected animals may present with weight loss, drooling ('slobbers') (Fig. 9.9), unilateral or bilateral epiphora, dysphagia, clear nasal discharge, retained food in the mouth, or, in the early stages, may be subclinical. Examination of the cheek teeth may be difficult in some animals without anesthesia, and a suitable speculum and/or cheek spreaders are essential. Food and hair impaction into periodontal pockets can also lead to lateral and tooth root abscessation (Hoefer and Crossley, 2002). Radiography (Fig. 9.10) or CT of the skull to best assess the extent of tooth root abnormalities is strongly recommended (Donnelly, 2004). Treatment to correct dental overgrowth involves general anesthesia and the use of a fine high-speed dental burr to restore occlusal surfaces to a normal height and remove spurs and spikes. Prevention should consist of ensuring an appropriate diet that includes high fiber grass hays

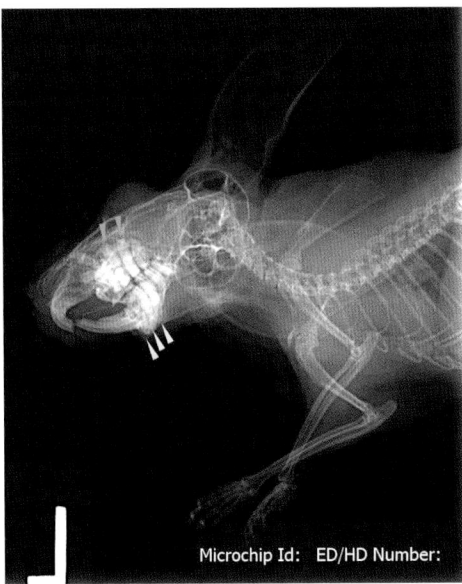

FIGURE 9.10 Left oblique skull radiograph of an adult female chinchilla showing apical elongation and curvature of the upper and particularly lower premolars and molars. Note distortion of the mandible due to elongated roots of lower premolar 1 and first and second molars (yellow arrowheads), and dorsal extension of elongated upper premolar and molar roots into the area of the orbit (green arrowheads). Buccal spur of upper premolar is also visible (red arrow). *Courtesy of Dr. L. Brazelton.*

and monocotyledonous plants, which promote normal chewing patterns. Animals with significant damage to the tongue and buccal surfaces due to spurs or spikes may benefit from administration of NSAIDs such as meloxicam (0.2–0.5 mg/kg q24 h), and antibiotics (enrofloxacin 20 mg/kg q24 h) if abscessation has occurred. When a significant length of the cheek teeth is removed, animals may require supportive feeding for a period as the jaw muscles adapt to the shorter occlusal surfaces (Hoefer and Crossley, 2002). In addition, animals presenting with anorexia, weight loss, and/or decreased fecal output may need supportive feedings, analgesics, parenteral fluid administration, and may benefit from promotility medications. Chinchillas with dental abnormalities, particularly from an early age, should not be used as breeders and may be less desirable as experimental animals due to the periodic stress of inconsistent feed intake and intermittent handling and anesthesia for tooth trimming.

2. Age-Related Disorders

a. Ocular Abnormalities

Peiffer and Johnson (1980) examined the eyes of 14 chinchillas, ages 6–17 years old. They found that the mean intraocular pressure, as measured with a Mackay–Marg applanation tonometer, was 18.5 ± 5.75 mmHg. Using a modern applanation tonometer, Lima *et al.*

(2010) determined a similar intraocular pressure reference range (17.71 ± 4.17 mmHg) for 36 chinchillas, ages 4 ± 2 years and of various color patterns. In contrast, a much lower reference value of 2.9 ± 1.9 mmHg in 61 healthy pet chinchillas of various ages and gender was established by Muller *et al.* (2010) utilizing a different modern tonometer. Peiffer and Johnson (1980) also observed bilateral posterior cortical cataracts and asteroid hyalosis in two animals.

3. Other Disorders

Six spontaneous cases of oxalate nephrosis have been described in adult female chinchillas (Goudas and Lusis, 1970), and urinary calculi and urolithiasis in three male chinchillas have been reported (Jones *et al.*, 1995; Newberne, 1952; Spence and Skae, 1995). A recent study of uroliths from 73 chinchillas showed that calcium carbonate accounted for 90% of the calculi (Mans and Donnelly, 2012; Osborne *et al.*, 2009). Hematuria, dysuria, or stranguria may be seen on presentation. Radiographs may be used to confirm the diagnosis, and treatment consists of surgical removal of the calculi, postoperative antibiotic therapy if bladder culture indicates underlying or concurrent urinary tract infection, and efforts to maintain and encourage hydration (Mans and Donnelly, 2012).

Led and Brandetti (1974) described a case of subcutaneous myiasis by *Cuterebra* larvae in Argentina. Hoefer and Crossley (2002) reported a case of lead poisoning in a pet chinchilla that manifested as acute convulsions and blindness. Increased blood levels of lead were detected, and the animal responded well to chelation therapy with calcium disodium versenate (CaEDTA at 30 mg/kg SC q12 h).

References

AALAS Buyers Guide [Online]. <http://laboratoryanimalsciencebuyersguide.com/>.

Alworth, L.C., Harvey, S.B., 2012. Anatomy, physiology, and behavior. In: Suckow, M.A., Stevens, K.A., Wilson, R.P. (Eds.), The Laboratory Rabbit, Guinea Pig, Hamster, and Other Rodents. Academic Press/Elsevier, London; Waltham, MA, pp. 955–966.

Bakaletz, L.O., 2009. Chinchilla as a robust, reproducible and polymicrobial model of otitis media and its prevention. Expert Rev. Vaccines 8, 1063–1082.

Bakaletz, L.O., Daniels, R.L., Lim, D.J., 1993. Modeling adenovirus type 1-induced otitis media in the chinchilla: effect on ciliary activity and fluid transport function of eustachian tube mucosal epithelium. J. Infect. Dis. 168, 865–872.

Bakaletz, L.O., Holmes, K.A., 1997. Evidence for transudation of specific antibody into the middle ears of parenterally immunized chinchillas after an upper respiratory tract infection with adenovirus. Clin. Diagn. Lab. Immunol. 4, 223–225.

Bartoszcze, M., Matras, J., Palec, S., Roszkowski, J., Wystup, E., 1990a. *Klebsiella pneumoniae* infection in chinchillas. Vet. Rec. 127, 119.

Bartoszcze, M., Nowakowska, M., Roszkowski, J., Matras, J., Palec, S., Wystup, E., 1990b. Chinchilla deaths due to *Clostridium perfringens* A enterotoxin. Vet. Rec. 126, 341–342.

Bignami, G., Beach, F.A., 1968. Mating behaviour in the chinchilla. Anim. Behav. 16, 45–53.

Bjornhag, G., Sjoblom, L., 1977. Demonstration of coprophagy in some rodents. Swed. J. Agric. Res. 7, 105–113.

Bonke, R., Wacheck, S., Stuber, E., Meyer, C., Martlbauer, E., Fredriksson-Ahomaa, M., 2011. Antimicrobial susceptibility and distribution of beta-lactamase A (blaA) and beta-lactamase B (blaB) genes in enteropathogenic yersinia species. Microb. Drug Resist. 17, 575–581.

Bowden, R.S.T., 1959. Diseases of chinchillas. Vet. Rec. 71, 1033–1039.

Brenon, H.C., 1953. Postmortem examinations of chinchillas. J. Am. Vet. Med. Assoc. 123, 310.

Brenon, H.C., 1955. Postmortem examinations of chinchillas. J. Am. Vet. Med. Assoc. 126, 222–223.

Brockson, M.E., Novotny, L.A., Jurcisek, J.A., Mcgillivary, G., Bowers, M.R., Bakaletz, L.O., 2012. Respiratory syncytial virus promotes Moraxella catarrhalis-induced ascending experimental otitis media. PLoS One 7.

Busso, J.M., Ponzio, M.F., Chiaraviglio, M., De Cuneo, M.F., Ruiz, R.D., 2005. Electroejaculation in the chinchilla (Chinchilla lanigera): effects of anesthesia on seminal characteristics. Res. Vet. Sci. 78, 93–97.

Busso, J.M., Ponzio, M.F., Fiol De Cuneo, M., Ruiz, R.D., 2012. Reproduction in chinchilla (Chinchilla lanigera): current status of environmental control of gonadal activity and advances in reproductive techniques. Theriogenology 78, 1–11.

Byrd, M.S., Pang, B., Hong, W., Waligora, E.A., Juneau, R.A., Armbruster, C.E., et al., 2011. Direct evaluation of Pseudomonas aeruginosa biofilm mediators in a chronic infection model. Infect. Immun. 79, 3087–3095.

Cabanes, F.J., Abarca, M.L., Bragulat, M.R., 1997. Dermatophytes isolated from domestic animals in Barcelona, Spain. Mycopathologia 137, 107–113.

Caspari, E.L., 1990. Caesarean section in a chinchilla. Vet. Rec. 126, 490.

Cavill, J.P., 1967. Listeriosis in chinchillas (Chinchilla laniger). Vet. Rec. 80, 592–594.

Chang, W.F., Liu, C.H., Du, S.J., 1986. Giardiasis of chinchilla – a case report. J. Chin. Soc. Vet. Sci. 12, 149–152.

Chermette, R., Ferreiro, L., Guillot, J., 2008. Dermatophytoses in animals. Mycopathologia 166, 385–405.

Cotter, C.S., Avidano, M.A., Stringer, S.P., Schultz, G.S., 1996. Inhibition of proteases in Pseudomonas otitis media in chinchillas. Otolaryngol. Head Neck Surg. 115, 342–351.

Cousens, P.J., 1963. The chinchilla in veterinary practice. J. Small Anim. Pract. 4, 199–205.

Crossley, D.A., 1997. Dental disease in chinchillas. Vet. Rec. 140, 512.

Crossley, D.A., 2001. Dental disease in chinchillas in the UK. J. Small. Anim. Pract. 42, 12–19.

Crossley, D.A., Dubielzig, R.R., Benson, K.G., 1997. Caries and odontoclastic resorptive lesions in a chinchilla (Chinchilla lanigera). Vet. Rec. 141, 337–339.

Crossley, D.A., Jackson, A., Yates, J., Boydell, I.P., 1998. Use of computed tomography to investigate cheek tooth abnormalities in chinchillas (Chinchilla laniger). J. Small Anim. Pract. 39, 385–389.

Dall, J., 1963. Diseases of the chinchilla. J. Small Anim. Pract. 4, 207–212.

Dall, J.A., 1967. Diaphragmatic hernia in a chinchilla. Vet. Rec. 81, 599.

Das, S., Rosas, L.E., Jurcisek, J.A., Novotny, L.A., Green, K.B., Bakaletz, L.O., 2014. Improving patient care via development of a protein-based diagnostic test for microbe-specific detection of chronic rhinosinusitis. Laryngoscope 124, 608–615.

Denooij, P.P., 1985. Schistosomus reflexus in a chinchilla kit. Mod. Vet. Pract. 66, 23–27.

De Vos, A.J., 1970. Studies on the host range of Eimeria chinchillae De Vos & Van der Westhuizen, 1968. Onderstepoort. J. Vet. Res. 37, 29–36.

De Vos, A.J., Dobson, L.D., 1970. Eimeria chinchillae De Vos & Van Der Westhuizen, 1968 and other Eimeria spp. from three South African rodent species. Onderstepoort J. Vet. Res. 37, 185–190.

Diaz, L.L., Lepherd, M., Scott, J., 2013. Enteric infection and subsequent septicemia due to attaching and effacing Escherichia coli in a chinchilla. Comp. Med. 63, 503–507.

Doerning, B.J., Brammer, D.W., Rush, H.G., 1993. Pseudomonas aeruginosa infection in a Chinchilla lanigera. Lab. Anim. 27, 131–133.

Dominchin, M.F., Bianconi, S., Ponzio, M.F., Fiol De Cuneo, M.F., Ruiz, R.D., Busso, J.M., 2014. Seasonal evaluations of urinary androgen metabolites and semen quality in domestic long-tailed chinchilla (Chinchilla lanigera) under natural photoperiod. Anim. Reprod. Sci. 145, 99–104.

Donnelly, T.M., 2004. Disease problems of chinchillas. In: Quesenberry, K.E., Carpenter, J.W. (Eds.), Ferrets, Rabbits, and Rodents: Clinical Medicine and Surgery: Includes Sugar Gliders and Hedgehogs, second ed. W.B. Saunders, St. Louis, MO, pp. 255–265.

Donnelly, T.M., Rush, E.M., Lackner, P.A., 2000. Ringworm in small exotic pets. Semin. Avian Exot. Pet Med. 9, 82–93.

Dubey, J.P., Clark, T.R., Yantis, D., 2000. Frenkelia microti infection in a chinchilla (Chinchilla laniger) in the United States. J. Parasitol. 86, 1149–1150.

Egri, B., Egri, J., Hajnovics, B., 1994. Uber fettinfiltration der leber beim chinchillabockchen (Chinchilla velligera). Tierarztl. Umsch. 49, 42–47.

Eidmann, S. 1992. Studies on etiology and pathogenesis of fur damages in the chinchilla. Doctoral Thesis, Stiftung Tierärztliche Hochschule, Hannover, Germany.

Emily, P., 1991. Problems peculiar to continually erupting teeth. J. Small Exotic. Anim. Med. 1, 56–59.

Finley, G.G., Long, J.R., 1977. Epizootic of listeriosis in chinchillas. Can. Vet. J.–Revue Veterinaire Canadienne 18, 164–167.

Fritsche, R., Simova-Curd, S., Clauss, M., Hatt, J.M., 2008. Hyperthyroidism in connection with suspected diabetes mellitus in a chinchilla (Chinchilla laniger). Vet. Rec. 163, 454–456.

Giebink, G.S., 1999. Otitis media: the chinchilla model. Microb. Drug Resist. – Mech. Epidemiol. Dis. 5, 57–72.

Gitiban, N., Jurcisek, J.A., Harris, R.H., Mertz, S.E., Durbin, R.K., Bakaletz, L.O., et al., 2005. Chinchilla and murine models of upper respiratory tract infections with respiratory syncytial virus. J. Virol. 79, 6035–6042.

Gitlin, G., Adler, J.H., 1969. Coexisting intrauterine and abdominal (intraperitoneal) pregnancy with possible superfoetation (superfecundation) and with adhesion of placenta to foetus in a chinchilla (Chinchilla laniger). Acta. Zool. Pathol. Antverp. 49, 65–76.

Goodman, G., 2004. Infectious respiratory disease in rodents. In Practice 26, 200–205.

Goudas, P., Gilroy, J.S., 1970. Spontaneous herpes-like viral infection in a chinchilla (Chinchilla laniger). Wildl. Dis. 6, 175–179.

Goudas, P., Lusis, P., 1970. Case report. Oxalate nephrosis in chinchilla (Chinchilla laniger). Can. Vet. J. 11, 256–257.

Granson, H.J., Carr, A.P., Parker, D., Davies, J.L., 2011. Cystic endometrial hyperplasia and chronic endometritis in a chinchilla. J. Am. Vet. Med. Assoc. 239, 233–236.

Grieves, J.L., Jurcisek, J.A., Quist, B., Durbin, R.K., Peeples, M.E., Durbin, J.E., et al., 2010. Mapping the anatomy of respiratory syncytial virus infection of the upper airways in chinchillas (Chinchilla lanigera). Comp. Med. 60, 225–232.

Griffiths, H.J., 1971. Some common parasites of small laboratory animals. Lab. Anim. 5, 123–135.

Griner, L.A., 1983. Pathology of Zoo Animals: A Review of Necropsies Conducted over a Fourteen-year Period at the San Diego Zoo and San Diego Wild Animal Park. Zoological Society of San Diego, San Diego, CA.

Hagen, K.W., Gorham, J.R., 1972. Dermatomycoses in fur animals: chinchilla, ferret, mink and rabbit. Vet. Med. Small Anim. Clin. 67, 43–48.

Harkness, J.E., Turner, P.V., Vandewoude, S., Wheler, C.L., 2010. Harkness and 'Wagner's Biology and Medicine of Rabbits and Rodents, fifth ed. Wiley-Blackwell, Ames, IA.

Harrison, A., Santana, E.A., Szelestey, B.R., Newsom, D.E., White, P., Mason, K.M., 2013. Ferric uptake regulator and its role in the pathogenesis of nontypeable Haemophilus influenzae. Infect. Immun. 81, 1221–1233.

Hartmann, K., 1993. Husbandry-related diseases in the chinchilla. Tierarztl. Prax 21, 574–580.

Hempel, R.J., Morton, D.J., Seale, T.W., Whitby, P.W., Stull, T.L., 2013. The role of the RNA chaperone Hfq in Haemophilus influenzae pathogenesis. BMC Microbiol. 13, 134.

Hirakawa, H., 2001. Coprophagy in leporids and other mammalian herbivores. Mammal Rev. 31, 61–80.

Hirakawa, Y., Sasaki, H., Kawamoto, E., Ishikawa, H., Matsumoto, T., Aoyama, N., et al., 2010. Prevalence and analysis of Pseudomonas aeruginosa in chinchillas. BMC Vet. Res. 6: 52.

Hoefer, H.L., 1994. Chinchillas. Vet. Clin. North. Am. Small Anim. Pract. 24, 103–111.

Hoefer, H.L., Crossley, D.A., 2002. Chinchillas. In: Meredith, A., Redrobe, S. (Eds.), BSAVA Manual of Exotic Pets, fourth ed. British Small Animal Veterinary Association, Quedgeley, pp. 65–75.

Holmberg, B.J., Hollingsworth, S.R., Osofsky, A., Tell, L.A., 2007. Taenia coenurus in the orbit of a chinchilla. Vet. Ophthalmol. 10, 53–59.

Horvath, Z., Keri, M., 1980. Dermatomycosis of chinchilla caused by Trichophyton mentagrophytes. Magy. Allatorvosok Lapja 35, 592–601.

Hrapkiewicz, K., Colby, L.A., Denison, P.L., 2013. Chinchillas Clinical Laboratory Animal Medicine: An Introduction, fourth ed. Wiley, Hoboken, NJ, pp. 227–248.

Hubbert, W.T., 1972. Yersiniosis in mammals and birds in the United States: case reports and review. Am. J. Trop. Med. Hyg. 21, 458–463.

Integrated Taxonomic Information System (ITIS) [Online]. <http://www.itis.gov/> (accessed 23.08.13).

IUCN Red List of Endangered Species, 2013. 1 [Online]. <http://www.iucnredlist.org/details/4652/0> (accessed 23.08.13).

Jenkins, J.R., 1992. Husbandry and common diseases of the chinchilla (Chinchilla laniger). J. Small Exot. Anim. Med. 2, 15–17.

Jones, A.K., 1990. Caesarean section in a chinchilla. Vet. Rec. 126, 441.

Jones, R.J., Stephenson, R., Fountain, D., Hooker, R., 1995. Urolithiasis in a chinchilla. Vet. Rec. 136, 400.

Jones, R.K., Henderson, W., 1953. Isolation of Salmonella pullorum from a chinchilla. J. Am. Vet. Med. Assoc. 123, 213.

Keagy, H.F., 1949. Toxoplasma in the chinchilla. J. Am. Vet. Med. Assoc. 114, 15.

Kennedy, A.H., 1952. Chinchilla diseases and ailments. Fur Trade J. Canada, Toronto.

Kimpe, A., Decostere, A., Hermans, K., Baele, M., Haesebrouck, F., 2004. Isolation of Listeria ivanovii from a septicaemic chinchilla (Chinchilla lanigera). Vet. Rec. 154, 791–792.

King, B.F., Tibbitts, F.D., 1976. The fine structure of the chinchilla placenta. Am. J. Anat. 145, 33–56.

Kirinus, J.K., Krewer, C., Zeni, D., Monego, F., Da Silva, M.C., Kommers, G.D., et al., 2010. Outbreak of systemic listeriosis in chinchillas. Ciencia Rural 40, 686–689.

Kowalczyk, T., Brandly, C.A., 1954. Experimental infection of dogs, ferrets, chinchillas and hamsters with vesicular stomatitis virus. Am. J. Vet. Res. 15, 98–101.

Kruckenberg, S.M., Cook, J.E., Feldman, B.F., 1975. Clinical toxicities of pet and caged rodents and rabbits. Vet. Clin. North Am. 5, 675–684.

Kuroiwa, J., Imamichi, T., 1977. Growth and reproduction of the chinchilla–age at vaginal opening, oestrous cycle, gestation period, litter size, sex ratio, and diseases frequently encountered. Jikken Dobutsu. 26, 213–222.

Langford, E.V., 1972. Pasteurella pseudotuberculosis infections in Western Canada. Can. Vet. J. 13, 85–87.

Led, J.E., Brandetti, E., 1974. Miiasis por Cuterebra sp., Clark 1815 (Diptera cuterebridae) en una chinchilla (Chinchilla lanigera). Analecta Vet. 8, 29–33.

Levecke, B., Meulemans, L., Dalemans, T., Casaert, S., Claerebout, E., Geurden, T., 2011. Mixed Giardia duodenalis assemblage A, B, C and E infections in pet chinchillas (Chinchilla lanigera) in Flanders (Belgium). Vet. Parasitol. 177, 166–170.

Levin, S.I., Berger, D.M.P., Gluckman, T.L., 2012. Management, husbandry, and colony health. In: Suckow, M.A., Stevens, K.A., Wilson, R.P. (Eds.), The Laboratory Rabbit, Guinea Pig, Hamster, and Other Rodents. Academic Press/Elsevier, London; Waltham, MA, pp. 967–976.

Lima, L., Montiani-Ferreira, F., Tramontin, M., Dos Santos, L.L., Machado, M., Lange, R.R., et al., 2010. The chinchilla eye: morphologic observations, echobiometric findings and reference values for selected ophthalmic diagnostic tests. Vet. Ophthalmol. 13, 14–25.

Long, J.P., Tong, H.H., Demaria, T.F., 2004. Immunization with native or recombinant Streptococcus pneumoniae neuraminidase affords protection in the chinchilla otitis media model. Infect. Immun. 72, 4309–4313.

Lucena, R.B., Farias, L., Libardoni, F., Vargas, A.C., Giaretta, P.R., Barros, C.S.L., 2011. Necrotizing enteritis associated with Clostridium perfringens Type B in chinchillas (Chinchilla lanigera). Pesquisa Vet. Brasil. 31, 1071–1074.

Lucena, R.B., Giaretta, P.R., Tessele, B., Fighera, R.A., Kommers, G.D., Irigoyen, L.F., et al., 2012a. Diseases of chinchilla (Chinchilla lanigera). Pesquisa Vet. Brasil. 32, 529–535.

Lucena, R.B., Rissi, D.R., Queiroz, D.M.M., Barros, C.S.L., 2012b. Infiltrative gastric adenocarcinoma in a chinchilla (Chinchilla lanigera). J. Vet. Diagn. Invest. 24, 797–800.

Lusis, P.I., Soltys, M.A., 1971. Immunization of mice and chinchillas against Pseudomonas aeruginosa. Can. J. Comp. Med. 35, 60–66.

Macdonald, D.W., Wilton, G.S., Howell, J., Klavano, G.G., 1972. Listeria monocytogenes isolations in Alberta 1951–1970. Can. Vet. J. 13, 69–71.

Mans, C., Donnelly, T.M., 2012. Disease problems of chinchillas. In: Quesenberry, K.E., Carpenter, J.W. (Eds.), Ferrets, Rabbits, and Rodents: Clinical Medicine and Surgery, third ed. Elsevier/Saunders, St. Louis, MO, pp. 311–325.

Maravilla, P., Garza-Rodriguez, A., Gomez-Diaz, B., Jimenez-Gonzalez, D.E., Toral-Bastida, E., Martinez-Ocana, J., et al., 2011. Chinchilla laniger can be used as an experimental model for Taenia solium taeniasis. Parasitol. Int. 60, 364–370.

Marks, S.L., 2012. Enteric bacterial infections. In: Greene, C.E. (Ed.), Infectious Diseases of the Dog and Cat, fourth ed. Elsevier/Saunders, St. Louis, MO, pp. 370–398.

Marlow, C., 1995. Diabetes in a chinchilla. Vet. Rec. 136, 595–596.

Martin, B.J., 2012a. Taxonomy and history. In: Suckow, M.A., Stevens, K.A., Wilson, R.P. (Eds.), The Laboratory Rabbit, Guinea Pig, Hamster, and Other Rodents. Academic Press/Elsevier, London; Waltham, MA, pp. 949–953.

Martin, L., 2012b. Chinchillas as experimental models. In: Suckow, M.A., Stevens, K.A., Wilson, R.P. (Eds.), The Laboratory Rabbit, Guinea Pig, Hamster, and Other Rodents. Academic Press/Elsevier, London; Waltham, MA, pp. 1009–1028.

Martin, L.B., Chidambaram, R.M., Schroeder, K.E., Mcfadden, S.L., 2005. Thyroparathyroidectomy procedures and thyroxine levels in the chinchilla. Contemp. Top. Lab. Anim. Sci. 44, 31–36.

Maurer, F.D., 1964. Lymphocytic Choriomeningitis. Lab. Anim. Care. 14, 415–419.

McGreevy, P.D., Carn, V.M., 1988. Intestinal torsion in a chinchilla. Vet. Rec. 122, 287.

Meingassner, J.G., Burtscher, H., 1977. Double infection of the brain with frenkelia species and Toxoplasma gondii in Chinchilla laniger. Vet. Pathol. 14, 146–153.

Misirlioglu, D., Cetin, C., Kahraman, M.M., Caner, V., Ozyigit, M.O., 2002. Salmonella infection in a chinchilla farm. Turkish J. Vet. Anim. Sci. 26, 151–155.

Moore, R.W., Greenlee, H.H., 1975. Enterotoxaemia in chinchillas. Lab. Anim. 9, 153–154.

Morganti, L., Gomez Portugal, E.A., 1970. *Microsporum gypseum* infection in chinchillas. Sabouraudia 8, 39–40.

Morrisey, J.K., Carpenter, J.W., 2012. Formulary. In: Quesenberry, K.E., Carpenter, J.W. (Eds.), Ferrets, Rabbits, and Rodents: Clinical Medicine and Surgery, third ed. Elsevier/Saunders, St. Louis, MO, pp. 566–575.

Mountain, A., 1989. *Salmonella arizona* in a chinchilla. Vet. Rec. 125 25–25.

Muller, K., Mauler, D.A., Eule, J.C., 2010. Reference values for selected ophthalmic diagnostic tests and clinical characteristics of chinchilla eyes (*Chinchilla lanigera*). Vet. Ophthalmol. 13 (Suppl), 29–34.

Naglic, T., Seol, B., Bedekovic, M., Grabarevic, Z., Listes, E., 2003. Outbreak of *Salmonella enteritidis* and isolation of *Salmonella sofia* in chinchillas (*Chinchilla laniger*). Vet. Rec. 152, 719–720.

Newberne, J.W., Robinson, V.B., 1957. Malignant lymphoma in the South American chinchilla. North Am. Vet. 38, 362–372.

Newberne, P.M., 1952. Urinary calculus in a chinchilla. N. Am. Vet. 33, 334.

Newberne, P.M., 1953. An outbreak of bacterial gastroenteritis in the South American chinchilla. North Am. Vet. 34, 187–188.

Novotny, L.A., Jurcisek, J.A., Godfroid, F., Poolman, J.T., Denoel, P.A., Bakaletz, L.O., 2006. Passive immunization with human anti-protein D antibodies induced by polysaccharide protein D conjugates protects chinchillas against otitis media after intranasal challenge with Haemophilus influenzae. Vaccine 24, 4804–4811.

Osborne, C.A., Albasan, H., Lulich, J.P., Nwaokorie, E., Koehler, L.A., Ulrich, L.K., 2009. Quantitative analysis of 4468 uroliths retrieved from farm animals, exotic species, and wildlife submitted to the Minnesota Urolith Center: 1981 to 2007. Vet. Clin. North Am. Small Anim. Pract. 39, 65–78.

Owens, D.R., Menges, R.W., Sprouse, R.F., Stewart, W., Hooper, B.E., 1975. Naturally occurring histoplasmosis in the chinchilla (*Chinchilla laniger*). J. Clin. Microbiol. 1, 486–488.

Peiffer, R.L., Johnson, P.T., 1980. Clinical ocular findings in a colony of chinchillas (*Chinchilla laniger*). Lab. Anim. 14, 331–335.

Petit, L., Gibert, M., Popoff, M.R., 1999. Clostridium perfringens: toxinotype and genotype. Trends. Microbiol. 7, 104–110.

Ponzio, M.F., Busso, J.M., Ruiz, R.D., De Cuneo, M.F., 2007. Time-related changes in functional activity and capacitation of chinchilla (*Chinchilla lanigera*) spermatozoa during *in vitro* incubation. Anim. Reprod. Sci. 102, 343–349.

Ponzio, M.F., Roussy-Otero, G.N., Ruiz, R.D., Fiol De Cuneo, M., 2011. Seminal quality and neutral alpha-glucosidase activity after sequential electroejaculation of chinchilla (*Ch. laniger*). Anim. Reprod. Sci. 126, 229–233.

Prior, J.E., 1986. Caesarean section in the chinchilla. Vet. Rec. 119, 408.

Quesenberry, K.E., Donnelly, T.M., Mans, C., 2012. Biology, husbandry, and clinical techniques of guinea pigs and chinchillas. In: Quesenberry, K.E., Carpenter, J.W. (Eds.), Ferrets, Rabbits, and Rodents: Clinical Medicine and Surgery, third ed. Elsevier/ Saunders, St. Louis, MO, pp. 279–294.

Raevuori, M., Harvey, S.M., Pickett, M.J., 1979. *Yersinia enterocolitica –* experimental pathogenicity for chinchilla. Acta Vet. Scand. 20, 82–91.

Rakich, P.M., Dubey, J.P., Contarino, J.K., 1992. Acute hepatic sarcocystosis in a chinchilla. J. Vet. Diagn. Invest. 4, 484–486.

Ramaswamy, V., Cresence, V.M., Rejitha, J.S., Lekshmi, M.U., Dharsana, K.S., Prasad, S.P., et al., 2007. Listeria – review of epidemiology and pathogenesis. J. Microbiol. Immunol. Infect. 40, 4–13.

Reid, S.D., Hong, W.Z., Dew, K.E., Winn, D.R., Pang, B., Watt, J., et al., 2009. *Streptococcus pneumoniae* forms surface-attached communities in the middle ear of experimentally infected chinchillas. J. Infect. Dis. 199, 786–794.

Ren, D., Kordis, A.A., Sonenshine, D.E., Daines, D.A., 2014. The ToxAvapA toxin–antitoxin locus contributes to the survival of

nontypeable Haemophilus influenzae during infection. PLoS One 9, e91523.

Richardson, V.C.G., 2003. Chinchillas Diseases of Small Domestic Rodents, second ed. Blackwell Publishing, Oxford, UK, pp. 1–54.

Riggs, S.M., Mitchell, M.A., 2009. Chinchillas. In: Mitchell, M.A., Tully, T.N. (Eds.), Manual of Exotic Pet Practice. Saunders, St. Louis, MO, pp. 474–492.

Rosen, T., Jablon, J., 2003. Infectious threats from exotic pets: dermatological implications. Dermatol. Clin. 21, 229–236.

Sabocanec, R., Culjak, K., Ramadan, K., Naglic, T., Seol, B., Maticic, D., 2000. Incidence of listeriosis in farm chinchillas (*Chinchilla laniger*) in Croatia. Vet. Arh. 70, 159–167.

Sanford, S.E., 1989. Cerebral nematodiasis caused by the raccoon ascarid (*Baylisascaris procyonis*) in chinchillas. Can. Vet. J. 30, 902.

Sanford, S.E., 1991. Cerebrospinal nematodiasis caused by *Baylisascaris procyonis* in chinchillas. J. Vet. Diagn. Invest. 3, 77–79.

Schaeffer, D.O., Donnelly, T.M., 1997. Disease problems of guinea pigs and chinchillas. In: Hillyer, E.V., Quesenberry, K.E. (Eds.), Ferrets, Rabbits, and Rodents: Clinical Medicine and Surgery. W.B. Saunders Co., Philadelphia, PA, pp. 260–283.

Shaffer, T.L., Balder, R., Buskirk, S.W., Hogan, R.J., Lafontaine, E.R., 2013. Use of the Chinchilla model to evaluate the vaccinogenic potential of the Moraxella catarrhalis filamentous hemagglutinin-like proteins MhaB1 and MhaB2. PLoS One 8, e67881.

Shah, A.R., Pearlman, A.N., O'Grady, K.M., Bhattacharyya, T.K., Toriumi, D.M., 2007. Combined use of fibrin tissue adhesive and acellular dermis in dural repair. Am. J. Rhinol. 21, 619–621.

Shalkop, W.T., 1950. *Listeria monocytogenes* isolated from chinchillas. J. Am. Vet. Med. Assoc. 116, 447–448.

Shelton, G.C., 1954a. Giardiasis in the chinchilla. I. Observations on morphology, location in the intestinal tract, and host specificity. Am. J. Vet. Res. 15, 71–74.

Shelton, G.C., 1954b. Giardiasis in the chinchilla. II. Incidence of the disease and results of experimental infections. Am. J. Vet. Res. 15, 75–78.

Simova-Curd, S., Nitzl, D., Pospischil, A., Hatt, J.M., 2008. Lumbar osteosarcoma in a chinchilla (*Chinchilla laniger*). J. Small. Anim. Pract. 49, 483–485.

Sims, E., 1990. Caesarean section in a chinchilla. Vet. Rec. 126, 490.

Smith, J.L., Campbell-Ward, M., Else, R.W., Johnston, P.E., 2010. Undifferentiated carcinoma of the salivary gland in a chinchilla (*Chinchilla lanigera*). J. Vet. Diagn. Invest. 22, 152–155.

Soares, R.M., De Souza, S.L., Silveira, L.H., Funada, M.R., Richtzenhain, L.J., Gennari, S.M., 2011. Genotyping of potentially zoonotic Giardia duodenalis from exotic and wild animals kept in captivity in Brazil. Vet. Parasitol. 180, 344–348.

Spence, S., Skae, K., 1995. Urolithiasis in a chinchilla. Vet. Rec. 136, 524.

Staebler, S., Steinmetz, H., Keller, S., Deplazes, P., 2007. First description of natural *Echinococcus multilocularis* infections in chinchilla (*Chinchilla laniger*) and Prevost's squirrel (*Callosciurus prevostii borneoensis*). Parasitol. Res. 101, 1725–1727.

Stephenson, R.S., 1990. Caesarean section in a chinchilla. Vet. Rec. 126, 370.

Tong, H.H., Blue, L.E., James, M.A., Demaria, T.F., 2000a. Evaluation of the virulence of a *Streptococcus pneumoniae* neuraminidase-deficient mutant in nasopharyngeal colonization and development of otitis media in the chinchilla model. Infect. Immun. 68, 921–924.

Tong, H.H., Fisher, L.M., Kosunick, G.M., Demaria, T.F., 2000b. Effect of adenovirus type 1 and influenza A virus on *Streptococcus pneumoniae* nasopharyngeal colonization and otitis media in the chinchilla. Ann. Otol. Rhinol. Laryngol. 109, 1021–1027.

Turner, G.V.S., 1978. Some aspects of pathogenesis and comparative pathology of toxoplasmosis. J. S. Afr. Vet. Assoc. 49, 3–8.

Turowski, E.E., Shen, Z., Ducore, R.M., Parry, N., Fox, J.G., 2011. Identification of *Campylobacter lanienae* from laboratory chinchillas (*Chinchilla laniger*). J. Am. Assoc. Lab. Anim. Sci. 50 796–796.

Tvedten, H.W., Langham, R.F., 1974. Trophoblastic emboli in a chinchilla. J. Am. Vet. Med. Assoc. 165, 828–829.

Veronesi, F., Piergili Fioretti, D., Morganti, G., Bietta, A., Moretta, I., Moretti, A., et al., 2012. Occurrence of Giardia duodenalis infection in chinchillas (*Chincilla lanigera*) from Italian breeding facilities. Res. Vet. Sci. 93, 807–810.

Wallach, J.D., Boever, W.J., 1983. Rodents and Lagomorphs Diseases of Exotic Animals: Medical and Surgical Management. Saunders, Philadelphia, PA, pp. 135–195.

Wang, W., Joslin, S.N., Pybus, C., Evans, A.S., Lichaa, F., Brautigam, C.A., et al., 2014. Identification of an Outer Membrane Lipoprotein Involved in Nasopharyngeal Colonization by Moraxella catarrhalis in an animal model. Infect. Immun.

Watson, W.A., Watson, F.I., 1966. An outbreak of *Salmonella dublin* infection in chinchillas. Vet. Rec. 78, 15–17.

Weber, P.C., Koltai, P.J., 1991. *Chlamydia trachomatis* in the etiology of acute otitis media. Ann. Otol. Rhinol. Laryngol. 100, 616–619.

Weir, B.J., 1970. Chinchilla. In: Hafez, E.S.E. (Ed.), Reproduction and Breeding Techniques for Laboratory Animals. Lea & Febiger, Philadelphia, PA, pp. 209–223.

Wideman, W.L., 2006. *Pseudomonas aeruginosa* otitis media and interna in a chinchilla ranch. Can. Vet. J.–Revue Vet. Can. 47, 799–800.

Wilkerson, M.J., Melendy, A., Stauber, E., 1997. An outbreak of listeriosis in a breeding colony of chinchillas. J. Vet. Diagn. Invest. 9, 320–323.

Wohlsein, P., Thiele, A., Fehr, M., Haas, L., Henneicke, K., Petzold, D.R., et al., 2002. Spontaneous human herpes virus type 1 infection in a chinchilla (*Chinchilla lanigera f. dom.*). Acta Neuropathol. 104, 674–678.

Wuthe, H.H., Aleksic, S., 1992. *Yersinia enterocolitica* serovar 1,2a,3 biovar 3 in chinchillas. Zentralbl. Fur Bakteriol.–Int. J. Med. Microbiol. Virol. Parasitol. Infect. Dis. 277, 403–405.

Xu, F., Sternberg, M.R., Kottiri, B.J., Mcquillan, G.M., Lee, F.K., Nahmias, A.J., et al., 2006. Trends in herpes simplex virus type 1 and type 2 seroprevalence in the United States. JAMA 296, 964–973.

Yamini, B., Raju, N.R., 1986. Gastroenteritis associated with a *Cryptosporidium* sp. in a chinchilla. J. Am. Vet. Med. Assoc. 189, 1158–1159.

Yoo, H.S., Lee, S.U., Park, K.Y., Park, Y.H., 1997. Molecular typing and epidemiological survey of prevalence of Clostridium perfringens types by multiplex PCR. J. Clin. Microbiol. 35, 228–232.

CHAPTER

10

Biology and Diseases
of Rabbits

Megan H. Nowland DVM, BS, DACLAM[a],
David W. Brammer DVM, DACLAM[b], Alexis Garcia DVM, BS[c]
and Howard G. Rush DVM, MS, DACLAM[d]

[a]University of Michigan, Unit for Laboratory Animal Medicine, Ann Arbor, MI, USA
[b]University of Houston, Animal Care Operations, Houston, TX, USA
[c]Massachusetts Institute of Technology, Division of Comparative Medicine, Cambridge, MA, USA
[d]University of Michigan, Unit for Laboratory Animal Medicine, Ann Arbor, MI, USA

OUTLINE

I. INTRODUCTION

Beginning in 1931, an inbred rabbit colony was developed at the Phipps Institute for the Study, Treatment and Prevention of Tuberculosis at the University of Pennsylvania. This colony was used to study natural resistance to infection with tuberculosis (Robertson *et al.*, 1966). Other inbred colonies or well-defined breeding colonies were also developed at the University of Illinois College of Medicine Center for Genetics, the Laboratories of the International Health Division of The Rockefeller Foundation, the University of Utrecht in the Netherlands, and Jackson Laboratories. These colonies were moved or closed in the years to follow. Since 1973, the U.S. Department of Agriculture (USDA) has reported the total number of certain species of animals used by registered research facilities (1997). In 1973, 447,570 rabbits were used in research. There has been an overall decrease in numbers of rabbits used. This decreasing trend started in the mid-1990s. In 2010, 210,172 rabbits were used in research. Despite the overall drop in the number used in research, the rabbit is still a valuable model and tool for many disciplines.

A. Taxonomy

Rabbits are small mammals in the Lagomorpha order and Leporidae family. There are eight different genera classified as rabbits including *Brachylagus, Bunolagus, Nesolagus, Oryctolagus, Pentalagus, Poelagus, Romerolagus,* and *Sylvilagus*. The nonscientific names for rabbits are often confusing. An *Oryctolagus cuniculus* is commonly called a European rabbit. Several unique breeds of *Oryctolagus cuniculus* have been developed including the New Zealand White rabbit and the Dutch belted rabbit. To further complicate naming issues, the terms 'rabbit' and 'hare' are often misused when referring to

common names or breeds of rabbits (Fox, 1994; Nowak and Paradiso, 1983). Animals classified in the genus *Lepus* are the only true hares. *Oryctolagus cuniculus* is the only domesticated rabbit, and consequently the only species from which unique breeds have been derived.

Many breeds have been developed simply by selectively breeding for different physical characteristics. Currently, there are 127 different breeds of rabbits. Some are recognized by the American Rabbit Breeders Association or the British Rabbit Council, whereas others are not recognized by either organization. There are also several color variations of these breeds. A list of breeds is found in Table 10.1.

The following list shows the complete taxonomic position of animals in the order Lagomorpha:

Class: Mammalia
Order: Lagomorpha
Family: Ochotonidae (pikas)
 Genus: *Ochotona*
 Species: 19 species

TABLE 10.1   Breeds of Rabbits

Alaska	Blue of Sint-Niklaas
Altex	Bourbonnais Grey
American Blue	Brazilian
American White	Britannia Petite
American Fuzzy Lop	British Giant
American Sable	Brown Chestnut of Lorraine
Argente Bleu	Caldes
Argente Brun	Californian
Argente Clair	Carmagnola Grey
Argente Crème	Cashmere Lop
Argente de Champagne	Chaudry
Argente Noir	Checkered Giant
Argente St. Hubert	Chinchilla (American)
Baladi	Chinchilla (Giant)
Bauscat	Chinchilla (Giganta)
Beige	Chinchilla (Standard)
Belgian Hare	Cinnamon
Beveren	Continental Giant
Blanc de Bouscat	Criollo
Blanc de Hotot	Cuban Brown
Blanc de Popielno	Czech Albin
Blanc de Termonde	Czech Red rabbit
Blue of Ham	Czech Spot

(Continued)

TABLE 10.1 (Continued)

Deilenaar	New Zealand
Dutch	New Zealand Red
Dutch (Tricolored)	Orestad
Dwarf Hotot	Palomino
Dwarf lop	Pani
Elfin	Pannon White
Enderby Island	Perlfee
English Angora	Plush Lop (Mini)
English Lop	Plush Lop (Standard)
English Spot	Pointed Beveren
Fauve de Bourgogne	Polish
Fee de Marbourg (Marburger)	Rex (Astrex)
Flemish Giant	Rex (Mini)
Florida White	Rex (Opossum)
French Angora	Rex (Standard)
French Lop	Rhinelander
Gabali	Sachsengold
German Angora	Sallander
German Lop	San Juan
Giant Angora	Satin
Giant Papillon	Satin (Mini)
Giza White	Satin Angora
Golden Glavcot	Siamese Sable
Gotland	Siberian
Grey Pearl of Halle	Silver
Güzelçamlı rabbit	Silver Fox
Harlequin	Silver Marten
Havana	Smoke Pearl
Himalayan	Spanish Giant
Hulstlander	Squirrel
Hungarian Giant	Sussex
Jersey Wooly	Swiss Fox
Kabyle	Tadla
Lilac	Tan
Lionhead	Teddywidder
Liptov Baldspotted Rabbit	Thrianta
Meissner Lop	Thuringer
Mini Lion Lop	Vienna
Miniature Lop (Holland Lop in the United States)	Wheaten
Netherland Dwarf	Wheaten Lynx
	Zemmouri

Despite the different breed names and the use of the word hare for some breeds, all are derived from Oryctolagus cuniculus

Family: Leporidae (rabbits and hares)
  Subfamily: Leporinae
  Genus/Species:
    Bunolagus monticularis (Bushman rabbit)
    Brachylagus idahoensis (Idaho pygmy rabbit)
    Caprolagus hispidus (hispid hare)
    Lepus, 22 species ('true' hares, jackrabbits)
    Nesolagus netscheri (Sumatra short-eared rabbit)
    Oryctolagus cuniculus (European rabbit, Old
    World rabbit)
    Pentalagus furnessi (Amami rabbit)
    Poelagus marjorita (Bunyoro rabbit)
    Pronolagus, three species (rock hare)
    Romerolagus diazzi (volcano rabbit)
    Sylvilagus, 14 species (cottontail rabbits)

B. Use in Research

The rabbit has been utilized in immunology research for many years especially in regard to the structure of immunoglobulins and the genetic control of their formation. In addition, the rabbit is commonly used for the production of polyclonal antibodies for use as immunologic reagents (Mage, 1998; Pinheiro *et al.*, 2011). The relatively large body size and blood volume, easy access to the vascular system, and an existent large body of information on the purification of rabbit immunoglobulins are a few reasons the rabbit is preferred over other common laboratory animal species for polyclonal antibody production (Stills, 1994).

The organization of the lymphoid system of the rabbit is comparable to that of other mammals. However, the rabbit does possess two gut-associated lymphoid tissues (GALT) with specialized functions in the maturation of IgM$^+$ B cells. These are the vermiform appendix at the distal end of the cecum and the sacculus rotundus at the ileocecal junction (Mage, 1998).

For many years, the lack of rabbit-specific immunological reagents has limited the study of inflammation and immunity in the rabbit. The use of real-time polymerase chain reaction (RT-PCR) techniques has overcome this limitation and permitted such studies in many species other than man and mice. A quantitative real-time RT-PCR assay for measuring mRNA for rabbit cytokines IFN-γ, IL-2, IL-4, IL-10, and TNF-α has been described (Godornes *et al.*, 2007). Recently, Schnupf and Sansonetti (2012) reported on RT-PCR primer pairs for analysis of three chemokines (IL-8, CCL-4, and CCL20) and 16 cytokines (IL-1β, IL-2, IL-4, IL-6, IL-10, IL-12p35, IL12p40, IL-17A, IL-17F, IL-18, IL-21, IL-22, IFN-β, IFN-γ, TGF-β, and TNF-α). The profile of cytokines in the rabbit appears similar to other mammals.

In mice and humans, the primary antibody repertoire is created by combinatorial rearrangement of a large number of immunoglobulin gene segments. Other species (chicken, sheep, cattle, and rabbit) that have a limited number of gene segments utilize somatic gene conversion and/or somatic hypermutation (Pinheiro *et al.*, 2011). In the former, a portion of the immunoglobulin gene is replaced with a gene sequence from a nonfunctional pseudogene. In the latter, single-nucleotide changes are made in the immunoglobulin genes (Jenne *et al.*, 2003). In the rabbit, gene diversification occurs initially in the fetus and the neonate in sites such as the bone marrow. Subsequently, between 4 and 8 weeks of age, immature IgM$^+$ B cells undergo further diversification in the GALT (appendix, sacculus rotundus, and Peyer's patches) (Mage *et al.*, 2006; Pinheiro *et al.*, 2011). Furthermore, certain species of intestinal bacteria (*Bacteroides fragilis* and *Bacillus subtilis*) are required for appendix follicle development and antibody diversification to occur (Hanson and Lanning, 2008; Mage *et al.*, 2006).

Most mammals express five classes of immunoglobulins: IgM, IgD, IgG, IgA, and IgE. However, the rabbit lacks IgD (Sun *et al.*, 2013).

The area of cardiovascular research has used the rabbit in a variety of different models. Numerous dietary modifications will induce or exacerbate cholesterol-induced atherosclerosis in the rabbit. A brief overview of some of these dietary modifications can be found elsewhere (Jayo *et al.*, 1994). Research efforts into cholesterol metabolism have used the Watanabe heritable hyperlipidemic (WHHL) (Atkinson *et al.*, 1992; Kita *et al.*, 1981) and the St. Thomas Hospital strain rabbits (Laville *et al.*, 1987). The WHHL rabbit has a marked deficiency of low-density lipoprotein (LDL) receptors in the liver and other tissues. Selective breeding of the WHHL rabbit will increase the incidence of coronary artery atherosclerosis without increasing the incidence of aortic atherosclerosis (Watanabe *et al.*, 1985). In contrast, the St. Thomas Hospital strain has a normal functioning LDL receptor but still maintains a hypercholesterolemic state (Laville *et al.*, 1987).

Genetically modified rabbits have been created via both intracytoplasmic injection (Li *et al.*, 2010) and retroviral vectors (Hiripi *et al.*, 2010). This has resulted in a multitude of new strains to address interesting research questions. Cardiovascular disease (Lombardi *et al.*, 2009; Peng, 2012; Sanbe *et al.*, 2005; Stanley *et al.*, 2011) including models of long QT interval for exploration of treatments (Biermann *et al.*, 2011; Jindal *et al.*, 2012; Liu *et al.*, 2012a; Peng, 2012; Sanbe *et al.*, 2005; Ziv *et al.*, 2009) and atherosclerosis (Araki *et al.*, 2000; Masson *et al.*, 2011; Tjwa *et al.*, 2006) are the main focus of model development. Strains have also been developed that express human recombinant proteins in rabbit milk (Chrenek *et al.*, 2007; Dragin *et al.*, 2005; Hiripi *et al.*, 2010; Houser *et al.*, 2010; Lipinski *et al.*, 2012; Simon *et al.*, 2011; Soler *et al.*, 2005). This ability can be passed down for multiple generations (Chrenek *et al.*, 2007; Dragin *et al.*, 2005).

These human proteins have resulted in antigen production for rotavirus vaccine creation, human factor VIII that could be used to treat hemophilia (Chrenek *et al.*, 2007; Krylov *et al.*, 2008; Simon *et al.*, 2011) and human growth hormone that could supplement a deficiency in that hormone (Lipinski *et al.*, 2012). Rabbits that express enhanced green fluorescent protein (EGFP) in various tissues have been created for the purpose tracking cells, which is important for tissue engineering and regenerative medicine studies (Chrenek *et al.*, 2011; Takahashi *et al.*, 2007; Yin *et al.*, 2013).

II. BIOLOGY

A. Comparative Anatomy and Physiology

1. Digestive System

The mouth of the rabbit is relatively small, and the oral cavity and pharynx are long and narrow. The dental formula is i2/1, c0/0, pm3/2, m2-3/3 × 2 = 26 or 28 teeth.

A small pair of incisors is present directly caudal to the primary maxillary incisors and is referred to as 'peg' teeth. The peg teeth are used along with the primary incisors to bite and shear food. The absence of second incisors has been noted in some rabbit colonies as a dominant trait (I^2/I^2 or I^2/i^2). The teeth of rabbits erupt continuously throughout life and therefore will continue to grow unless normal occlusion and use are sufficient to wear teeth to a normal length. Molars do not have roots and are characterized by deep enamel folds. Rabbits normally masticate with a chewing motion that facilitates grinding of food by movement of the premolars and molars from side to side and front to back.

The rabbit has four pairs of salivary glands, including the parotid, submaxillary, sublingual, and zygomatic. The parotid is the largest and lies laterally just below the base of the ear. The zygomatic salivary gland does not have a counterpart in humans.

The esophagus of the rabbit has three layers of striated muscle that extend the length of the esophagus down to, and including, the cardia of the stomach. This is in contrast to humans and many other species, which have separate portions of striated and smooth muscle along the length of the esophagus. There are no mucous glands in the esophagus of the rabbit.

Although the stomach of the rabbit holds approximately 15% of the volume of the gastrointestinal tract, it is never entirely empty in the healthy rabbit. The gastric contents often include a large amount of hair ingested as the result of normal grooming activity. The stomach is divided into the cardia, fundus, and pylorus.

The liver has four lobes. The gallbladder is located on the right. From the liver, the common bile duct empties into the duodenum posterior to the pylorus. Rabbits produce relatively large amounts of bile compared to other common species. The pancreas is diffuse within the mesentery of the small intestine and enters the duodenum 30–40 mm distal to the common bile duct.

The small intestine of the rabbit is short relative to that of other species and comprises approximately 12% of the total length of the gastrointestinal (GI) tract. Because the GI tract of the rabbit is relatively impermeable to large molecules, kits receive most of their passive immunity via the yolk sac prior to birth rather than by colostrum. Peyer's patches are found along the ileum, particularly near the cecal junction. The sacculus rotundus is a large bulb of lymphoid tissue located at this junction.

The large intestine includes the cecum, the ascending colon, the transverse colon, and the descending colon. The ileocecal valve regulates flow of chyme into the cecum and retards reverse flow back into the ileum. The cecum is very large with a capacity approximately 10-times that of the stomach. The cecum ends in a blind sac, the appendix.

The colon is divided into proximal and distal portions by the fusus coli, which serves to regulate the elimination of hard versus soft fecal pellets. Hard pellets comprise about two-thirds of the fecal output. Soft pellets, or 'cecotrophs,' have a high moisture content and are rich in nitrogen-containing compounds (Ferrando *et al.*, 1970) and the B vitamins niacin, riboflavin, pantothenate, and cyanocobalamin. Rabbits consume cecotrophs directly from the anus to obtain significant nutritional benefit. Soft pellets are sometimes termed 'night feces,' since they are generally produced at night in domestic rabbits. In contrast, the circadian rhythm of cecotrophy is reversed in wild rabbits, occurring during the day when the animals are in their burrows (Hornicke, 1977).

2. Respiratory System

Nostrils of rabbits are well equipped with touch cells, and they have a well-developed sense of smell. Nasal breathing in rabbits is characterized by twitching of the nostrils at rates varying from 20 to 120 times per minute, although twitching may be absent in the relaxed rabbit. It has been speculated that inspiration occurs as the nostril moves up and that this serves to direct the flow of air over the turbinate bones where the olfactory cells are most concentrated.

The musculature of the thoracic wall contributes little to respiratory efforts. Instead, rabbits rely mostly on the activity of the diaphragm. Because of this, artificial respiration is easily performed by alternating the head of the rabbit between the up and down positions, 30–45 times per minute, while holding the animal. Compression and release of the chest wall is an ineffective means of artificial respiration in the rabbit.

The pharynx of the rabbit is long and narrow, and the tongue is relatively large. These features make endotracheal intubation difficult. The procedure is further complicated by the propensity of the rabbit to laryngo-spasm during attempts to intubate the trachea.

The rabbit lungs consist of six lobes. Both right and left sides have cranial, middle, and caudal lobes, with the right caudal being further subdivided into lateral and medial portions. Flow volume of air to the left lung is higher than that to the right due to the lower resistance of the proximal airways per unit volume (Yokoyama, 1979). In rabbits, lung volume increases with age, in contrast to that of humans and dogs, in which it decreases. Bronchial-associated lymphoid tissue (BALT) is present as distinct tissue.

3. Cardiovascular System

A unique feature of the cardiovascular system of the rabbit is that the tricuspid valve of the heart has only two cusps, rather than three as in many other mammals. A small group of pacemaker cells generate the impulse of the sinoatrial (SA) node in the rabbit, a feature that facilitates precise determination of the location of the pacemaker (Bleeker et al., 1980; Hoffman, 1965; West, 1955). The SA and atrioventricular (AV) nodes are slender and elongated, and the AV node is separated from the annulus fibrosus by a layer of fat (Truex and Smythe, 1965).

Additional unique anatomic features of the cardiovascular system of the rabbit have been utilized to advantage. The aortic nerve subserves no known chemoreceptors (Kardon et al., 1974; Stinnett and Sepe, 1979) and responds to baroreceptors only. Because the aortic nerve, which becomes the depressor nerve, runs alongside but separate from the vagosympathetic trunk, it lends itself readily to implantation of electrodes (Karemaker et al., 1980).

The blood supply to the brain is restricted mainly to the internal carotid artery. Blood supplied via the vertebral arteries is limited. The aorta of the rabbit demonstrates rhythmic contractions that arise from neurogenic stimulation in a pattern related to the pulse wave (Mangel et al., 1981).

4. Urogenital System

The kidneys of the rabbit are unipapillate in contrast to those of most other mammals, which are multipapillate. This feature increases the ease with which cannulization is performed. The right kidney lies more cranial than the left.

Glomeruli increase in number after birth in rabbits, whereas all of the glomeruli are present at birth in humans (Smith, 1951). Ectopic glomeruli are normal in the rabbit (Steinhausen et al., 1990). Blood vessels that perfuse the medulla remain open during many conditions under which vasoconstriction of the cortical tissue occurs; thus, the medullary tissue may be perfused, while the cortex is ischemic (Trueta et al., 1947).

The urine of adult rabbits is typically cloudy due to a relatively high concentration of ammonium magnesium phosphate and calcium carbonate monohydrate precipitates (Flatt and Carpenter, 1971). The urine may also take on hues ranging from yellow or reddish to brown. In contrast, the urine of young rabbits is typically clear, although healthy young rabbits may have albuminuria. The urine is normally yellow but can also take on reddish or brown hues once animals begin to eat green feed and cereal grains. Normal rabbits have few cells, bacteria, or casts in their urine. The pH of the urine is typically alkaline at about 8.2 (Williams, 1976). A normal adult rabbit produces approximately 50–75 ml/kg of urine daily (Gillett, 1994), with does urinating more copiously than bucks.

The urethral orifice of the buck is rounded, whereas that of the doe is slit-like. This feature is useful for distinguishing the sexes. The testes of the adult male usually lie within the scrotum; however, the inguinal canals that connect the abdominal cavity to the inguinal pouches do not close in the rabbit. For this reason, the testes can easily pass between the scrotum and the abdominal cavity. This feature necessitates closure of the superficial inguinal ring following orchiectomy by open technique to prevent herniation.

The reproductive tract of the doe is characterized by two uterine horns that are connected to the vagina by separate cervices (bicornuate uterus). A common tube, the urogenital sinus or vestibulum, is present where the urethra enters the vagina. The placenta is hemochorial, and maternal blood flows into sinus-like spaces where the transfer of nutrients and other substances to the fetal circulation occurs (Jones and Hunt, 1983).

Inguinal pouches are located lateral to the genitalia in both sexes. The pouches are blind and contain scent glands that produce white to brown secretions that may accumulate in the pouch.

5. Metabolism

The metabolic rate of endotherms is generally related to the body surface area. Including the ears, the rabbit has a relatively low metabolic rate (MR); however, if the surface area of the ears is discounted, the MR of the rabbit is similar to that of other endotherms.

Neonatal rabbits have an amount of body fat comparable to that of the human infant (16% of body weight) (Cornblath and Schwartz, 1976). The neonatal rabbit is essentially an ectotherm until about day 7 (Gelineo, 1964). The glucose reserves of the neonatal rabbit are quickly depleted, usually within about 6 h after birth (Shelley, 1961). The fasting neonatal rabbit quickly becomes hypoglycemic and ketotic (Callikan and Girard, 1979).

The normal rectal temperature of the adult New Zealand White rabbit at rest is approximately 38.5–39.5°C (Ruckebusch et al., 1991). The ears serve an important thermoregulatory function. Because they have a large surface area and are highly vascular with an extensive arteriovenous anastomotic system, the ears help the rabbit sense and respond to cold *versus* warm temperatures (Kluger *et al.*, 1972). In addition, the ears serve as a countercurrent heat-exchange system to help adjust body temperature.

Early studies found that the body of the adult rabbit (3 kg body weight) consists of greater than 50% water (58%), with a half-time turnover of about 3.9 days and a loss of about 340 ml daily (Richmond *et al.*, 1962). The amount of water ingested varies with the amount and type of feed consumed and the environmental temperature. In general, rabbits will drink more water when consuming dry, pelleted feed than when consuming foodstuffs high in moisture, such as fresh greens. Conversely, rabbits deprived of water will decrease food consumption. After 3 days of complete water deprivation, food intake falls to less than 2% of normal (Cizek, 1961).

B. Normative Physiological Values

Normal values for various systems and parameters are provided as a general indication for these values in the rabbit. It is important to recognize, however, that most of these values have been obtained through the study of adult New Zealand White rabbits. As with any experiment, values can vary significantly between breeds, laboratories, methods of sampling and measurement, and individual rabbits due to age, sex, breed, health, handling, and husbandry (Hewitt *et al.*, 1989; Lidena and Trautschold, 1986; Mitruka and Rawnsley, 1981; Wolford *et al.*, 1986; Yu *et al.*, 1979). For this reason, individual laboratories should strive to establish their own normal values, whenever possible.

1. Hematologic Values

Values for hematologic parameters are shown in Table 10.2. These values represent those typical of adult New Zealand White rabbits. In general, males have slightly greater hematocrit and hemoglobin values than females (Mitruka and Rawnsley, 1981).

Anisocytosis is normal and accounts for variation in reported values for red blood cell diameter (Sanderson and Phillips, 1981). Reticulocyte values are usually between 2% and 4% in healthy rabbits (Corash *et al.*, 1988). The neutrophil of the rabbit is sometimes referred to as a 'pseudoeosinophil' or 'heterophil,' due to the presence of red-staining granules in the cytoplasm. The heterophil (10–15 mm in diameter) is, however, smaller than the eosinophil (12–16 mm in diameter) (Sanderson and Phillips, 1981). In addition, the red granules of the heterophil are smaller than the red granules of the eosinophil. The nucleus of the eosinophil may be either bilobed or horseshoe-shaped.

2. Blood and Serum Chemistry and Enzyme Values

As mentioned earlier, chemistry values can vary because of a number of factors. For this reason, each laboratory should establish its own normal values.

TABLE 10.2 Hematologic Values for the Adult Rabbit[a]

Hematologic parameter	Typical value
Blood volume	55–65 ml/kg
Plasma volume	28–50 ml/kg
Hemoglobin	9.8–14.0 g/dl
Packed cell volume	34–43%
Erythrocytes	5.3–6.8 cells (10^6/µl)
Reticulocytes	1.9–3.8%
Mean corpuscular volume (MCV)	60–69 fl
Mean corpuscular hemoglobin (MCH)	20–23 pg
MCH concentration (MCHC)	31–35%
Sedimentation rate	0.92–3.00 mm/h
White blood cells	5.1–9.7 cells (10^3/µl)
Neutrophils (heterophils)	25–46%
Lymphocytes	39–68%
Eosinophils	0.1–2.0%
Basophils	2.0–5.0%
Monocytes	1.0–9.0%
Platelets	158–650 (10^3/µl)

[a]*Values obtained from the following sources: Burns and DeLannoy (1966), Gillett (1994), Kabata et al. (1991), Mitruka and Rawnsley (1981), and Woolford et al. (1986).*

Aspartate aminotransferase (AST) is present in the liver, heart, skeletal muscle, kidney, and pancreas. Collection of blood samples in rabbits by decapitation, cardiac puncture, or aortic incision, or the use of restraint that causes exertion will elevate AST levels due to muscle damage (Lidena and Trautschold, 1986). Similarly, levels of creatinine kinase are sensitive to muscle damage since that enzyme is present in the skeletal muscle, brain, and heart (Lidena and Trautschold, 1986; Mitruka and Rawnsley, 1981).

Although most mammals have two isoenzymes (intestinal and a liver/kidney/bone form) of alkaline phosphatase (AP), rabbits are unique in having three forms of AP, including an intestinal form and two forms that are both present in the liver and the kidney (Noguchi and Yamashita, 1987).

Values for blood and serum chemistry are shown in Table 10.3.

3. Respiratory, Circulatory, and Miscellaneous Biologic Parameters

Cardiovascular and respiratory functions are often altered with experimental manipulation, anesthesia, or disease. Normal values for these parameters and other miscellaneous biologic characteristics of the rabbit are listed in Table 10.4.

TABLE 10.3 Values of Serum Biochemical and Enzyme Parameters of the Adult Rabbits

Biochemical parameter	Typical value
Total protein	5.0–7.5 g/dl
Globulin	1.5–2.7 g/dl
Albumin	2.7–5.0 g/dl
Glucose	74–148 mg/dl
Sodium	125–150 mEq/l
Chloride	92–120 mEq/l
Potassium	3.5–7.0 mEq/l
Phosphorus	4.0–6.0 mg/dl
Calcium	5.60–12.1 mg/dl
Magnesium	2.0–5.4 mg/dl
Acid phosphatase	0.3–2.7 IU/l
Alkaline phosphatase	10–86 IU/l
Acid phosphatase	0.30–2.70 IU/l
Lactate dehydrogenase	33.5–129 IU/l
γ-Glutamyltransferase	10–98 IU/l
Aspartate aminotransferase *AST*	20–120 IU/l
Creatine kinase	25–120 IU/l
Alanine aminotransferase (SGPT) *ALT*	25–65 IU/l
Sorbitol dehydrogenase	170–177 U
Urea nitrogen	5–25 mg/dl
Creatinine	0.5–2.6 mg/dl
Total bilirubin	0.2–0.5 mg/dl
Uric acid	1.0–4.3 mg/dl
Amylase	200–500 IU/l
Serum lipids	150–400 mg/dl
Phospholipids	40–140 mg/dl
Triglycerides	50–200 mg/dl
Cholesterol	10–100 mg/dl
Corticosterone	1.54 μg/dl

Values obtained from the following sources: Burns and DeLannoy (1966), Fox (1989), Gillett (1994), Kraus et al. (1984), and Loeb and Quimby (1989).

TABLE 10.4 Respiratory, Circulatory, and Miscellaneous Biologic Parameters of the Rabbit[a]

Parameter	Typical value
Life span	5–7 years
Body weight	2–5 kg
GI transit time	4–5 hr
Number of mammary glands	8 or 10
Diploid chromosome number	44
Body temperature	38.5–39.5°C
Respiratory rate	32–60 breaths/min
Lung weight (2.4-kg rabbit)	9.1 g
Total lung capacity	111 ± 14.7 ml
Minute volume	0.6 l/min
Tidal volume	4–6 ml/kg body weight
Mean alveolar diameter	93.97 μm
Heart rate	200–300 beats/min
pO_2	85–102 mmHg
pCO_2	20–46 torr
HCO_3	12–24 mmol/l
Arterial oxygen	12.6–15.8% volume
Arterial systolic pressure	90–130 mmHg
Arterial diastolic pressure	80–90 mmHg
Arterial blood pH	7.2–7.5
Interstitial fluid (IF) colloid osmotic pressure	13.6 mmHg
IF viscosity (water = 1)	1.9
IF protein	2.7
Cerebrospinal fluid (CSF) white blood cells	0–7 cells/mm^3
CSF lymphocytes	40–79%
CSF monocytes	21–60%

[a]Values obtained from the following sources: Barzago et al. (1992), Curiel et al. (1982), Gillett (1994), Kozma et al. (1974), Sanford and Colby (1980), Suckow and Douglas (1997), and Zurovsky et al. (1995).

C. Nutrition

Rabbits are strictly herbivorous with a preferred diet of herbage that is low in fiber and high in protein and soluble carbohydrate (Cheeke, 1987; Cheeke, 1994). Rabbits will generally accept a pelleted feed more readily than one in meal form. When a meal diet is needed, a period of adjustment should be allowed for the rabbits to accommodate to the new diet. Examples of adequate diets are shown in Table 10.5.

The requirement for fiber in the diet of rabbits has been reviewed (Gidenne, 2003). Fiber is especially important in the early postweaning period when low fiber intake is associated with an increase in digestive disorders (Gidenne, 2003).

The exact nutrient requirements for individual rabbits vary with age, reproductive status, and health of the animal. On occasion, the need arises for use of highly purified diets. A suggested purified diet has been described elsewhere (Subcommittee on Rabbit Nutrition, 1977). It should be noted that overfeeding of

TABLE 10.5 Examples of Adequate Diets for Commercial Production[a]

Kind of animal	Ingredients	Percentage of total diet[b]
Growth, 0.5–4 kg	Alfalfa hay	50.00
	Corn, grain	23.50
	Barley, grain	11.00
	Wheat bran	5.00
	Soybean meal	10.00
	Salt	0.50
Maintenance, does and bucks, average 4.5 kg	Clover hay	70.00
	Oats, grain	29.50
	Salt	0.50
Pregnant does, average 4.5 kg	Alfalfa hay	50.00
	Oats, grain	45.50
	Soybean meal	4.00
	Salt	0.50
Lactating does, average 4.5 kg	Alfalfa hay	40.00
	Wheat, grain	25.00
	Sorghum grain	22.50
	Soybean meal	12.00
	Salt	0.50

[a]*From Subcommittee on Rabbit Nutrition (1977). Used with permission.*
[b]*Composition given on an as-fed basis.*

laboratory rabbits resulting in obesity is common, but can be prevented by either reducing the amount of feed or by providing a low-energy, high-fiber maintenance diet (Donnelly, 2004).

As mentioned earlier, rabbits engage in cecotrophy, and by doing so supplement their supply of protein and B vitamins (Carabaño et al., 2010; Gidenne et al., 2010). Rabbits fed a diet high in fiber ingest a greater quantity of cecotropes than those on a lower fiber diet (Fekete and Bokori, 1985).

Unlike most other species, both calcium absorption in the small intestine and serum calcium levels increase in proportion to the amount of calcium in the diet (Cheeke, 1987). Prolonged feeding of diets high in calcium, such as those with a high level of alfalfa meal, can result in renal disease. Consumption of diets containing excessive vitamin D can result in calcification of soft tissues, including the liver, kidney, vasculature, and muscles (Besch-Williford et al., 1985; Lebas, 2000).

Diets that are either too high or too low in vitamin A can result in reproductive dysfunction and congenital hydrocephalus (Cheeke, 1987; DiGiacomo et al., 1992). The exact requirement for vitamin A in the rabbit has not

been determined; however, a level of 6000–10,000 IU/kg of diet is generally adequate (Lebas, 2000).

Vitamin E deficiency has been associated with infertility, muscular dystrophy, fetal death, neonatal death, and colobomatous microphthalmos in rabbits (Lebas, 2000; Nielsen and Carlton, 1995; Ringler and Abrams, 1970; Ringler and Abrams, 1971). McDowell (1989) suggested that serum vitamin E levels of less than 0.5 µg/ml are indicative of hypovitaminosis E.

Relative to other species, rabbits have a high water intake. In general, daily water intake is approximately 120 ml/kg of body weight. Consumption of water is influenced by environmental temperature, disease states, and feed composition and intake (Cizek, 1961; Tschudin et al., 2011). Consumption of diets high in dry matter results in increased water intake (Tschudin et al., 2011). Water consumption also increases with food deprivation.

D. Behavior

Rabbits are social animals and attempts at group housing often meet with success, although mature males will fight and can inflict serious injury on one another (Love, 1994; Podberscek et al., 1991; Whary et al., 1993). Group-penned female rabbits allowed to choose between single or paired housing prefer being in the same cage with other rabbits (Huls et al., 1991). In general, rabbits are timid and nonaggressive. Some animals will display defensive behavior, typically characterized by thumping the cage floor with the rear feet, biting, and charging toward the front of the cage when opened. Laboratory-housed rabbits demonstrate diurnal behavior, in contrast to the nocturnal pattern exhibited by wild rabbits (Jilge, 1991).

The ethogram of the laboratory rabbit has been described (Chu et al., 2004; Gunn and Morton, 1995). The most common behaviors of individually housed rabbits included lie alert, doze, groom, sleep, and eat. Individually housed rabbits were inactive the majority of the time (Gunn and Morton, 1995). Individually housed female rabbits showed an increase in abnormal behaviors compared to pair-housed rabbits (Chu et al., 2004). Rabbits housed in pairs in double-wide cages locomoted more than individually housed rabbits (Chu et al., 2004).

E. Reproduction

1. Sexual Maturity

The age of puberty varies with the breed of rabbit. Puberty generally occurs at 4–5 months of age in small breeds, 4–6 months in medium breeds, and 5–8 months in large breeds (Donnelly, 2004). Female New Zealand White rabbits reach maturity at 5 months of age and males at 6–7 months.

The breeding life of a doe typically lasts approximately 1–3 years, although some remain productive for up to 5 or 6 years. In later years, litter sizes usually diminish. In comparison, most bucks will remain reproductively useful for an average of 5–6 years.

Because does often will engage in reproductive behavior before being able to ovulate, it is advisable not to breed does until they are fully grown.

2. Reproductive Behavior

Does do not have a distinct estrous cycle, but rather demonstrate a rhythm with respect to receptivity to the buck. Receptivity is punctuated by periods (1–2 days every 4–17 days) of anestrus and seasonal variations in reproductive performance (Hafez, 1970). During periods of receptivity, the vulva of the doe usually becomes swollen, moist, and dark pink or red. Receptivity of the doe is usually signaled by lordosis in response to the buck's attempt to mount, vulvar changes as described above, restlessness, and rubbing of the chin on the hutch or cage (Donnelly, 2004). Vaginal cytology is generally not useful for determination of estrus or receptivity in the rabbit.

Typically, the doe is brought to the buck's cage for breeding, since the doe can be very territorial and may attack the male in her own quarters. A period of 15–20 min is usually sufficient to determine compatibility of the doe and buck. If receptive, the doe will lie in the mating position and raise her hindquarters to allow copulation. If fighting or lack of breeding is observed, the doe may be tried with another buck. A single buck is usually sufficient to service 10–15 does.

Ovulation is induced and occurs approximately 10–13 h after copulation (Donnelly, 2004). Up to 25% of does fail to ovulate following copulation. Ovulation can also be induced by administration of luteinizing hormone (Kennelly and Foote, 1965), human chorionic gonadotropin (Williams et al., 1991), or gonadotropic releasing hormone (Foote and Simkin, 1993).

Does may be bred immediately after kindling; however, most breeders delay until after the kits have been weaned. Success at postpartum breeding varies, but one can produce a large number of kits in a relatively short time period by foster nursing the young and rebreeding the doe immediately. While conventional breeding, nursing, and weaning schedules allow for only 4 litters per year, early postpartum breeding allows for up to 11 litters per year.

3. Pregnancy and Gestation

Pregnancy can often be confirmed as early as day 14 of gestation by palpation of the fetuses within the uterus. Radiographic procedures permit pregnancy determination as early as day 11. Conception rates have been observed to have an inverse relationship with ambient temperature but not light cycle. Gestation in rabbits usually lasts for 30–32 days (Donnelly, 2004). Does beyond 2–3 weeks of gestation will usually refuse a buck.

Does begin hair pulling and nest building during the last 3–4 days of gestation (Donnelly, 2004). A nesting box with shredded paper or other soft material such as straw should be provided to the doe several days prior to the expected kindling (parturition) date. The doe will usually line the box with her own hair. The nesting box should not be placed in the corner of the cage where the individual doe has been observed to urinate.

4. Pseudopregnancy

Pseudopregnancy is common in rabbits and can follow a variety of stimuli, including mounting by other does, sterile matings by bucks, administration of luteinizing hormone, or the presence of bucks nearby. In such circumstances, ovulation is followed by a persistent corpus luteum that lasts 15–17 days. The corpus luteum or corpora lutea secretes progesterone during this time, causing the uterus and mammae to enlarge. The doe may have the appearance of a normally pregnant rabbit. Toward the end of pseudopregnancy, many does will begin to pull hair as part of ritual nest-building behavior.

5. Parturition

The process of parturition is referred to as 'kindling' when it relates to rabbits. Kindling normally occurs during the early morning hours and takes approximately 30–60 min. Impending kindling is often signaled by nest building and decreased food consumption during the preceding 2–3 days. Both anterior and breech presentations are normal in the rabbit. Fetuses retained beyond 35 days generally die and may harm future reproductive ability of the doe if not expelled.

The average number of kits born is seven to nine per litter, although smaller litters and litters of up to 10 kits are not uncommon. Breed, parity, nutritional status, and environmental factors influence litter size. Polish rabbits usually have fewer than four kits per litter; Dutch or Flemish Giant, four to five; and New Zealand White, eight to ten.

After the young have been cleaned following parturition, the doe typically consumes the placenta. Cannibalism of the young by the doe sometimes occurs and may be related to environmental or hereditary factors or due to environmental stressors.

6. Lactation

Does usually have either four or five pairs of nipples, whereas bucks have none. During the last week of pregnancy, marked development of the mammary gland occurs. The doe normally nurses the kits once daily for several minutes, usually in the early morning or in the evening, regardless of how many kits are present or how many times they attempt to suckle. Milk yield is normally between 160 and 220 g/day. During the first week of life, kits consume 15–25 g of milk per day. Milk intake increases gradually to a maximum of 30 g/day between 17 and 25 days of age (Gidenne et al., 2010). Maximum output occurs at 2 weeks following kindling and then declines during the fourth week. Rabbit milk contains approximately 12.5% protein, 13% fat, 2% lactose, and 2.5% minerals. Nursing may last 5–10 weeks. Kits may begin consuming solid food by 3 weeks of age, with weaning generally occurring by 5–8 weeks of age.

F. Management and Husbandry

1. Housing

The facilities present in most modern research animal facilities would be suitable for housing rabbits. General construction should include adequate heating, ventilation, and air conditioning to house rabbits at appropriate temperature and humidity. In addition, lighting should be adequate to allow easy visualization of the rabbits. Surfaces, such as the floors, walls, and ceilings, should be easily sanitizable (National Research Council, 2011).

Rabbit cages should provide a safe environment with easy access to food and water. Adults can be caged individually or in compatible groups and should have sufficient floor space to lie down and stretch out. In the United States, minimum cage sizes are determined by the Animal Welfare Act (AWA) and the Guide for the Care and Use of Laboratory Animals (Guide). In both cases, sizes vary with the weight of the animal. Currently, the AWA regulations and the Guide require 3.0 ft² of floor space and 16 in of cage height for rabbits weighing 2–4 kg (National Research Council, 2011).

Cages should be constructed of durable materials that will resist corrosion and harsh detergents and disinfectants used in cleaning. Consequently, in the research environment, rabbit cages are most often constructed of stainless steel or plastics. Rabbits are usually housed in cages with mesh or slatted floors to permit urine and feces to drop through into a catch pan. Mesh floors with catch pans do not prevent rabbits from engaging in the normal practice of coprophagy.

Information on environmental enrichment of laboratory rabbits has been published (Baumans, 2005). The behavior of rabbits in conventional cages was compared to that of rabbits provided with enriched cages that contained shelter, a shelf, and increased vertical space. Rabbits in conventional cages were more restless, groomed excessively, exhibited more bar-gnawing, and were more timid than those housed in enriched cages (Hansen and Berthelsen, 2000). Indeed, fecal glucocorticoid levels in rabbits declined when they were provided with a wooden structure for resting

and gnawing (Buijs et al., 2011). Rabbits will play with objects placed in their cages. Huls et al. (1991) noted that rabbits would use wooden sticks, wooden rings, and brass wire balls as toys. Rabbits provided with objects (toys) spent significantly more time chewing than rabbits without toys (Poggiagliolmi et al., 2011). Female rabbits can also be housed in compatible pairs or groups. Singly housed female rabbits exhibited more abnormal behaviors compared to pair housed rabbits (Chu et al., 2004). Group housing of unfamiliar males is not recommended because of the likelihood of fighting and injury.

2. Environment

Rabbits are optimally housed in cooler room temperatures than most other common species of laboratory animals. The Guide recommends that temperatures in rabbit rooms be maintained between 61 and 72°F.

No specific illumination requirements for rabbits have been described. It is common practice to provide rabbits with 12–14 h of light in the light–dark cycle. In breeding colonies, females should be provided with 14–16 h of light.

Rabbits are easily startled by sudden, loud noises. For this reason, they should not be housed near noisy species such as dogs or monkeys, nor should they be housed near noise-generating operations such as the cage-wash area.

3. Sanitation

Catch pans should be cleaned as often as necessary to prevent the formation of ammonia. Cages are generally sanitized on at least a weekly basis.

Rabbit urine contains large amounts of protein and minerals, and often forms deposits on cages and catch pans. It is common practice to soak equipment having urine deposits in acid washes to remove the scale before washing.

Ammonia production in rabbit rooms can be a significant problem; therefore, rabbit rooms should be ventilated at 10–15 air changes per hour (National Research Council, 2011). It is also important to change excreta pans often to prevent the buildup of ammonia.

III. DISEASES

A. Bacterial Diseases

1. Pasteurellosis

Etiology *Pasteurella multocida* is a Gram-negative nonmotile coccobacillus that causes pasteurellosis, also known as 'snuffles', the primary respiratory disease affecting domestic rabbits (Deeb and DiGiacomo, 2000; Guo et al., 2012). Historically, serogroup A isolates have been associated with pneumonic and septicemic pasteurellosis in laboratory rabbits; however, capsular type A is also isolated from rabbits that appear clinically healthy (Confer *et al.*, 2001; El Tayeb *et al.*, 2004).

Clinical Signs *Pasteurella multocida* infection is often subclinical, but pasteurellosis may cause fever, coughing, dyspnea, rhinitis (nasal discharge (serous to mucopurulent), sneezing, and upper airway stentor), pneumonia, otitis, septicemia, meningitis, abscesses (of viscera and subcutaneous sites), and death (Al-Lebban *et al.*, 1989; Confer *et al.*, 2001; Franco and Cronin, 2008; Guo *et al.*, 2012; Suckow *et al.*, 2002; Wilkie *et al.*, 2012). Pasteurellosis may also be associated with pericarditis, pleuritis, sinusitis, dacryocystitis, conjunctivitis, iritis/uveitis, phlegmon, mastitis, endometritis, pyometra, salpingitis, and orchitis (Deeb and DiGiacomo, 2000; Ferreira *et al.*, 2012; Stahel *et al.*, 2009; Williams, 2012).

Epizootiology *P. multocida* can be endemic in rabbitries and is carried in the rabbit's nasal cavity (Confer *et al.*, 2001; Deeb *et al.*, 1990; DiGiacomo *et al.*, 1991; Suckow *et al.*, 2008). Transmission is by direct contact between rabbits (Wilkie *et al.*, 2012). Coinfection with *Bordetella bronchiseptica* may be observed in clinically affected rabbits (Deeb *et al.*, 1990). Stress-related factors associated with pasteurellosis include crowded or unsanitary conditions, transportation, and high ammonia concentrations in the air (Confer *et al.*, 2001). Previous studies reported a high prevalence of *P. multocida* infection (Jaslow *et al.*, 1981). Colonization in immature rabbits occurs more commonly in the sinuses followed by the trachea, middle ears, and lungs (Glass and Beasley, 1989). Similar to cats and dogs, rabbits may transmit *P. multocida* infection to humans (Per *et al.*, 2010; Silberfein *et al.*, 2006).

A study utilizing repetitive extragenic palindromic PCR (REP-PCR) and sequencing determined that 82% of the isolates were characterized as *P. multocida* subsp. *multocida*, 3% as *P. multocida* subsp. *septica*, 5% as atypical subspecies of *P. multocida*, 5% as *P. canis*, and 5% as an unknown species of the family Pasteurellaceae (Stahel *et al.*, 2009).

The pathogenesis of *P. multocida* has been reviewed (Wilkie *et al.*, 2012). The *ptfA* gene, encoding a type 4 fimbrial subunit and involved in bacterial fixation on the surface of epithelial cells, may be highly prevalent in *P. multocida* isolates from rabbits (Ferreira *et al.*, 2012). The *P. multocida* toxin is a major virulence factor in atrophic rhinitis of rabbits and acts by causing constitutive activation of G proteins (Chrisp and Foged, 1991; Frymus *et al.*, 1991; Orth *et al.*, 2009; Suckow *et al.*, 1991).

Pathology The specific pathologic findings will vary with the site of infection, but the underlying host response is characterized by acute or chronic suppurative inflammation with the infiltration of large numbers of neutrophils.

Rhinitis and sinusitis are accompanied by a mucopurulent nasal exudate. Neutrophil infiltration of the tissues is extensive. The nasal passages are edematous, inflamed, and congested, and there may be mucosal ulcerations. The turbinate bones may atrophy (Chrisp and Foged, 1991; DiGiacomo *et al.*, 1989). Purulent conjunctivitis may be present.

Pneumonia is primarily cranioventral in distribution. The lungs can exhibit consolidation, atelectasis, and abscess formation. A purulent to fibrinopurulent exudate is evident, and there may be areas of hemorrhage and necrosis. In some rabbits, fibrinopurulent pleuritis and pericarditis are prominent features (Glavits and Magyar, 1990). This is probably due to elaboration of a heat-labile toxin in some strains of the bacteria (Chrisp and Foged, 1991). Acute hepatic necrosis and splenic lymphoid atrophy are also seen in association with the pleuritis and pneumonia induced by toxigenic strains.

Otitis media is characterized by a suppurative exudate with goblet cell proliferation and lymphocytic and plasma cell infiltration.

In female rabbits with genital tract infections, the uterus may be enlarged and dilated. In the early stages of infection, the exudate is watery; later it thickens and is cream-colored. The exudate contains numerous neutrophils. Focal endometrial ulceration can be found (Johnson and Wolf, 1993). In the male, the testes are enlarged and may contain abscesses.

Systemic and visceral abscesses are characterized by a necrotic center, an infiltrate made up of polymorphonuclear neutrophils, and a fibrous capsule.

Septicemia may only present as congestion and petechial hemorrhages in many organs.

Severe pleuritis with accumulation of fibrinopurulent exudate in the thoracic cavity, serous rhinitis and tracheitis, acute hepatitis with necrotic foci in the parenchyma, and atrophy of lymphoid organs and tissues have been observed after experimental *P. multocida* infection in rabbits (Glavits and Magyar, 1990).

Diagnosis Sterile swabs can be used to collect samples from the nares or nasal cavity of rabbits for culture (Ferreira *et al.*, 2012; Jaslow *et al.*, 1981). Nasal lavage can also be used as a culture sample to isolate *Pasteurella* (Suckow *et al.*, 2002). *P. multocida* isolates can be classified into five serogroups based on capsular antigens (A, B, D, E, and F) and into 16 serotypes based on somatic LPS antigens (Adler *et al.*, 1999; Liu *et al.*, 2012b; Manning, 1982). Biochemical characterization of isolates may show high heterogeneity; however, REP-PCR and phylogenetic analysis using 16S ribosomal RNA and *rpoB* genes can be used for precise characterization of rabbit isolates (Stahel *et al.*, 2009). Classification of *P. multocida* into subspecies and/or by virulence profiles is useful for epidemiological investigations (Ferreira *et al.*, 2012; Stahel *et al.*, 2009). Random amplified polymorphic

DNA PCR (RAPD-PCR) has also been used to subtype rabbit *P. multocida* isolates (Al-Haddawi *et al.*, 1999; Dabo *et al.*, 2000; Williams *et al.*, 1990). PCR can detect capsule biosynthesis genes cap A, B, D, E, and F as well as virulence-related genes (Ferreira *et al.*, 2012). Serological tests can be used to detect antibodies against *P. multocida* (Deeb *et al.*, 1990; Delong *et al.*, 1992; DiGiacomo *et al.*, 1990; Glass and Beasley, 1989; Lukas *et al.*, 1987).

Differential Diagnoses If radiographs reveal an internal mass associated with *P. multocida* infection, the differential diagnoses should include abscess, granuloma, neoplasia, and parasitic cyst (Franco and Cronin, 2008).

Treatment, Prevention, and Control Previous studies have investigated the use of vaccines to protect rabbits against *P. multocida* infection (Confer *et al.*, 2001). Immunization of rabbits with inactivated heat-labile *P. multocida* toxin or a commercial swine *P. multocida* bacterin-toxoid conferred protective immunity against challenge with the *P. multocida* heat-labile toxin (Suckow, 2000; Suckow *et al.*, 1995). A vaccine administered intranasally stimulated immunity against experimental pneumonic pasteurellosis and significantly reduced nasal bacterial counts (Confer *et al.*, 2001). Oral immunization of rabbits with a *P. multocida* thiocyanate extract (PTE) in microparticles was immunogenic and significantly reduced the colony-forming units of homologous *P. multocida* recovered from the lungs and nasopharynx (Suckow *et al.*, 2002). Protective immunity to a heterologous strain of *P. multocida* can be achieved by vaccinating rabbits with PTE via the subcutaneous route (Suckow *et al.*, 2008). A *P. multocida* bacterin known as BunnyVac is currently licensed by the USDA and is intended to be effective in preventing death and limiting disease due to *Pasteurella* in rabbits. BunnyVac is manufactured by Colorado Serum Company and distributed by Pan American Veterinary Laboratories (http://pavlab.com/). Control of pasteurellosis in rabbitries entails testing and culling animals that are positive for *Pasteurella* spp. (Ferreira *et al.*, 2012). Furthermore, rabbits free of *Pasteurella* and other infectious agents can be obtained by enrofloxacin treatment and through cesarean section or hysterectomy rederivation (Pleasants, 1959; Suckow *et al.*, 1996; Syukuda, 1979). Commercial suppliers of laboratory rabbits tend to exclude *Pasteurella* from their colonies.

Treatment with antibiotics should be based on culture and sensitivity. Antibiotic treatment of affected rabbits can alleviate clinical signs or delay disease progression but may not eradicate the disease (El Tayeb *et al.*, 2004; Ferreira *et al.*, 2012). Antibiotic treatment may suppress virulence gene expression without complete elimination of *P. multocida* (Boyce *et al.*, 2012). Internal abscesses may not be treatable using antibiotics (Franco and Cronin, 2008). Penicillin therapy does not seem to be effective against *Pasteurella* infection and may also lead to diarrhea and *Clostridium difficile* colitis in rabbits (Jaslow *et al.*, 1981; Rehg and Lu, 1981). One study from Brazil determined that all tested strains were sensitive to ceftiofur, florfenicol, norfloxacin, enrofloxacin, ciprofloxacin, tetracycline, and doxycycline (Ferreira *et al.*, 2012). Other studies also indicate that fluoroquinolones are useful for the treatment of *P. multocida* infection in rabbits (Abo-El-Sooud and Goudah, 2010; Broome and Brooks, 1991; Franco and Cronin, 2008; Hanan *et al.*, 2000; Okewole and Olubunmi, 2008). Oral ciprofloxacin (20 mg/kg per day for 5 days) has been used in rabbits (Hanan *et al.*, 2000).

Research Complications Pasteurellosis can cause considerable economic losses (El Tayeb *et al.*, 2004; Ferreira *et al.*, 2012; Stahel *et al.*, 2009) and has the potential to affect different types of research studies using rabbits due to the multisystemic nature of the disease, and the possibility of high morbidity and mortality. Therefore, *Pasteurella* should be excluded from laboratory rabbit colonies.

2. Clostridial Diseases

The class *Clostridia* belongs to the phylum Firmicutes (Yutin and Galperin, 2013). Recent genomic analyses suggest assigning some *Clostridium* species that fall outside the family Clostridiaceae into new genera. The genera *Tyzzerella*, *Erysipelatoclostridium*, and *Peptoclostridium* have been proposed for *C. piliforme*, *C. spiroforme*, and *C. difficile*, respectively (Yutin and Galperin, 2013).

a. Tyzzer's Disease

Etiology *C. piliforme* is a pleomorphic, Gram-negative, spore-forming, motile, obligate intracellular rod-shaped bacterium that causes Tyzzer's disease and infects various animals including mice, nonhuman primates, gerbils, rats, rabbits, and others (Allen *et al.*, 1965; Ganaway *et al.*, 1971; Pritt *et al.*, 2010). Infection has also been reported in a human patient with human immunodeficiency virus-1 (Smith *et al.*, 1996). Phylogenetic analyses determined that microorganisms identified as *C. piliforme* form three clusters within a single clade and that the nearest related distinguishable species is *C. colinum* (Feldman *et al.*, 2006).

Clinical Signs The first reported outbreaks in laboratory rabbits described profuse watery to mucoid diarrhea usually followed by death in 12–48 h in 3- to 8-week old rabbits (Allen *et al.*, 1965). Rabbits in affected litters usually died within a week after the first fatality (Allen *et al.*, 1965). The dams of affected litters occasionally died after a diarrheal disease that was more protracted than that of the offspring (Allen *et al.*, 1965). These outbreaks lasted for 6–8 months and affected multiple rabbit rooms. *C. piliforme* infection may also be subclinical and transient as immunocompetent hosts may clear the infection (Ganaway *et al.*, 1971; Pritt *et al.*, 2010). Weanling rabbits with the acute form of Tyzzer's disease exhibit diarrhea, listlessness, anorexia, and dehydration usually followed by death within 72 h (Cutlip *et al.*, 1971). The mortality rate in clinically affected rabbits was estimated to be 90–95% (Cutlip *et al.*, 1971). Anorexia and stunting were observed in chronic cases associated with intestinal stenosis (Cutlip *et al.*, 1971). Acute and chronic Tyzzer's disease types have been described in rabbits; however, large numbers of 'attaching' *Escherichia coli* were recovered from the cecum of most rabbits (Prescott, 1977).

Epizootiology   The vegetative cell is the active stage responsible for the disease and depends on the intracellular environment (Ganaway, 1980). Therefore, the spore, a resistant stage, appears to be the essential element in the transmission of Tyzzer's disease (Ganaway, 1980; Ganaway *et al.*, 1971). Contact with soiled bedding or diseased rabbits have been used experimentally to transmit the disease to other rabbits (Allen *et al.*, 1965). It is possible that subclinically infected rabbits (carriers) may introduce the organism into a colony (Allen *et al.*, 1965; Pritt *et al.*, 2010). In mice, increased susceptibility to infection has been associated with stress (Allen *et al.*, 1965). Furthermore, treatment with cyclophosphamide, cortisone, and prednisolone has been used experimentally to reproduce the disease in animals, suggesting that immunosuppression plays a role in pathogenesis (Allen *et al.*, 1965; Cutlip *et al.*, 1971; Pritt *et al.*, 2010). Animals stressed by poor environmental conditions including overcrowding and extreme temperatures can develop the disease (Cutlip *et al.*, 1971; Wobeser *et al.*, 2009). Significant modifications of the intestinal flora and an impaired immune system may play a role in pathogenesis (Licois, 1986). *C. piliforme* may be transported from the intestine to the liver through the portal circulation and to the heart through the lymphatics (Allen *et al.*, 1965). Some *C. piliforme* isolates can induce cytopathic effects on cell cultures, and *in vivo*, concomitant infection with other enteric pathogens such as *E. coli* may contribute to the severity of the disease (Prescott, 1977; Riley *et al.*, 1992).

Pathology   Lesions can be found in the distal ileum, cecum, proximal colon, liver, and heart (Allen *et al.*, 1965). Intestinal lesions are common, and histologically are characterized by necrosis of the mucosa and edema of the submucosa and serosa (Allen *et al.*, 1965). Bacilli appear as bundles of parallel rods or as criss crossed sticks in the cytoplasm of epithelial cells distributed from the surface of the mucosa to the base of the glands (Allen *et al.*, 1965). The lesions in the liver are punctate areas of parenchymal necrosis that appear grossly as white spots, usually ≤ 2 mm in diameter. Large numbers of bacilli are found in the cytoplasm of cells in the zone of transition between the necrotic lesion and the healthy parenchyma

(Allen *et al.*, 1965). Myocardial lesions appear as white streaks 0.5–2 mm wide and 4–8 mm long extending from the region of the left interventricular groove laterally across the left ventricle (Allen *et al.*, 1965). In the myocardium, bacilli may be noted in partially degenerated and normal looking cells at the sharply delineated borders of the lesions (Allen *et al.*, 1965).

Diagnosis   *C. piliforme* cannot be cultured in artificial (cell-free) media making its diagnosis difficult (Allen *et al.*, 1965; Cutlip *et al.*, 1971; Ganaway *et al.*, 1971; Niepceron and Licois, 2010). Other bacteria, including *E. coli*, have been isolated from the liver of diseased rabbits and are considered secondary invaders (Allen *et al.*, 1965; Cutlip *et al.*, 1971). The isolation of the Tyzzer's agent using liver extract agar has been described (Kanazawa and Imai, 1959). *C. piliforme* can be grown in primary monolayer cultures of adult mouse hepatocytes, in mouse fibroblasts, in rat hepatocytes, and in embryonated eggs (Craigie, 1966; Duncan *et al.*, 1993; Ganaway *et al.*, 1971; Kawamura *et al.*, 1983; Pritt *et al.*, 2010; Riley *et al.*, 1992).

Serology for *C. piliforme* is commonly used for surveillance of laboratory animals because it is rapid and inexpensive (Pritt *et al.*, 2010). Immunofluorescence assay (IFA) and multiplexed fluorometric immunoassay (MFIA) have been utilized (Pritt *et al.*, 2010). In addition, *C. piliforme* PCR assays have been developed (Feldman *et al.*, 2006; Gao *et al.*, 2012; Niepceron and Licois, 2010; Pritt *et al.*, 2010). *Clostridium piliforme* seropositive rabbits may be negative for the organism by PCR and histopathological evaluation (Pritt *et al.*, 2010). Therefore, positive serological findings are not sufficient for a definitive diagnosis of *C. piliforme* infection and PCR testing and/or histopathology should be used for confirmation (Pritt *et al.*, 2010).

Definitive diagnosis is based on identification of typical gross lesions and histological demonstration of intracellular *C. piliforme* at the periphery of the necrotic foci (Niepceron and Licois, 2010; Pritt *et al.*, 2010). Giemsa solution (pH 4), Warthin–Starry silver method, Levaditi silver method, and the periodic acid–Schiff (PAS) reaction have been used to demonstrate *C. piliforme* (Allen *et al.*, 1965; Cutlip *et al.*, 1971). Different morphologic forms of *C. piliforme* can be observed microscopically (Allen *et al.*, 1965; Ganaway *et al.*, 1971).

Differential Diagnoses   Clinically, other diarrheal diseases of rabbits can be included in the differential diagnoses. Grossly, the multifocal white areas on the liver could be from *Eimeria stiedae* infection (hepatic coccidiosis).

Treatment, Prevention, and Control   For prevention, avoid introduction of rabbits of unknown *C. piliforme* status into a colony. Minimize stress-related factors especially in young animals. Good husbandry practices including regular bedding changes and disinfection should decrease the likelihood of spreading *C. piliforme* in a colony.

In one report, a Tyzzer's disease outbreak was observed 7–10 days after rabbits were weaned and transferred to a facility in which the temperature fluctuated from 6 to 35°C. The outbreak was controlled by transferring weanling rabbits to a building maintained at the same temperature as the breeder house (22–26°C) (Cutlip *et al.*, 1971). Spores treated with heat (70 or 80°C) or with either peracetic acid (1%) in a wetting agent (sodium alkylarylsulfonate) or sodium hypochlorite solution (0.3%) for 5 min lose infectivity (Ganaway, 1980). However, spores do not lose infectivity when treated with a phenolic germicidal agent, ethanol, or quaternary ammonium compounds (containing 9% or 17% benzalkonium chloride) (Ganaway, 1980). Sodium hypochlorite solution (0.3%) has been recommended as a surface disinfectant in animal facilities for prevention and control of Tyzzer's disease (Ganaway, 1980).

The sensitivity of *C. piliforme* to antibiotics has been investigated (Kanazawa and Imai, 1959). In one study, none of the antibacterials tested were completely inhibitory (Ganaway *et al.*, 1971). Group treatment of rabbits with tetracyclines in the drinking water and food was effective in lowering the incidence of diarrhea and death (Prescott, 1977).

Research Complications The high morbidity and mortality associated with Tyzzer's disease can affect the overall population of rabbits in a colony thereby decreasing the number of rabbits suitable or available for experimentation. In addition, research studies involving experimental infection with enteric pathogens in rabbits may be confounded by *C. piliforme*-associated intestinal pathology.

b. Enterotoxemia

Enterotoxemia refers to conditions of the bowel caused by toxigenic clostridia (Carman and Evans, 1984). Diagnosis of enterotoxemia should be based on culture of a toxigenic clostridium and demonstration of the toxin from the intestinal contents of the diseased animal (Carman and Evans, 1984; Songer, 1996).

i. CLOSTRIDIUM SPIROFORME

Etiology *C. spiroforme* is a Gram-positive, spore-bearing, helically coiled, semicircular, anaerobic bacterium that can produce iota toxin (Borriello and Carmen, 1983; Carman and Borriello, 1984; Peeters *et al.*, 1986). The disease caused by *C. spiroforme* is known as 'iota enterotoxemia' (Keel and Songer, 2006; Peeters *et al.*, 1986).

Clinical Signs Diarrhea, fecal soiling of the perineum, and cyanosis may be observed (Carman and Borriello, 1984). Diarrhea may be peracute and may lead to 'spontaneous' death or a moribund state (Carman and Borriello, 1984).

Epizootiology *C. spiroforme* is thought to be acquired from the environment (Carman and Evans, 1984; Songer, 1996). Weaning is associated with spontaneous disease and administration of antibiotics can also induce the disease (Borriello and Carmen, 1983; Carman and Borriello, 1984). A study determined that disease results from exposure of weanling rabbits to *C. spiroforme* and also from exposure of adult rabbits with a disrupted gut flora (due to clindamycin treatment) to *C. spiroforme* suggesting that this bacterium is not a normal component of the rabbit gut flora (Carman and Borriello, 1984). *C. spiroforme*-mediated diarrhea may be favored by maldigestion initiated by infectious agents and/or nutritional factors (Peeters *et al.*, 1986). Other clostridia, *E. coli* (EPEC), viruses, and parasites, may coinfect rabbits (Peeters *et al.*, 1986). The iota toxin of *C. spiroforme* binds the same host cell receptor as the iota toxin of *C. perfringens* and the binary toxin of *C. difficile* (Papatheodorou *et al.*, 2012). Poor hygiene, stress, and diet can influence pathogenesis of the disease (Bain *et al.*, 1998; Songer, 1996).

Pathology Grossly, ceca may be enlarged with gas, may exhibit serosal hemorrhages, and have liquid contents (Carman and Borriello, 1984). Cecal contents may be stained with blood (Peeters *et al.*, 1986). *C. spiroforme* is mainly associated with lesions in the cecum, but may also involve lesions in the proximal colon and distal ileum (Keel and Songer, 2006). Mucosal necrosis can be observed microscopically (Keel and Songer, 2006). The mucosa of the ileum, cecum, and colon may be denuded. Cellular debris, red blood cells, and fibrin may be found in the intestinal lumen. Polymorphonuclear cell infiltration and edema can be found in the lamina propria and submucosa. Epithelial degeneration and dilation were found in the renal tubules of some rabbits (Peeters *et al.*, 1986).

Diagnosis Gram staining of smears prepared from intestinal contents can be used to detect *C. spiroforme* (Bain *et al.*, 1998). Clostridial culture and toxin detection assays have been described (Agnoletti *et al.*, 2009; Bain *et al.*, 1998; Borriello and Carmen, 1983; Peeters *et al.*, 1986). *C. spiroforme* can be isolated from the intestinal contents of rabbits by high-speed centrifugation (Holmes *et al.*, 1988). PCR assays for *C. spiroforme* and the iota toxin (binary toxin) have been developed (Drigo *et al.*, 2008).

Differential Diagnoses The differential diagnoses should include other clostridia, *E. coli*, viruses, and parasites (Peeters *et al.*, 1986).

Treatment, Prevention, and Control The iota toxin from *C. spiroforme* is neutralized by serum prepared against the iota toxin of *C. perfringens* type E (Borriello and Carmen, 1983; Carman and Borriello, 1984; Songer, 1996). Prevention, via reduction of risk factors and prudent use of antibiotics, is probably more important than treatment (Agnoletti *et al.*, 2009). Cholestyramine has been used to prevent experimental enterotoxemia induced by clindamycin in rabbits (Lipman *et al.*, 1992). Fecal flora transplants using nonpathogenic *C. spiroforme* or *C. difficile* have been suggested for competitive inhibition of toxigenic strains (Carman and Evans, 1984). No commercial vaccines are available for rabbits; however, vaccination of weanling rabbits with a toxoid imparted protection to intraperitoneal challenge with iota toxin (Songer, 1996). Administration of antibiotics and change in diet are usually the treatment for *C. spiroforme* infections (Songer, 1996). The antibiotic susceptibility of *C. spiroforme* has been investigated (Agnoletti *et al.*, 2009; Carman and Wilkins, 1991). *C. spiroforme* can have a wide range of resistance to antimicrobial classes used in rabbit therapy (Agnoletti *et al.*, 2009). Feeding fresh meadow hay has been suggested (Bain *et al.*, 1998).

Research Complications The mortality due to enterotoxemia caused by *C. spiroforme* would be disruptive to ongoing studies. No other complications have been reported.

ii. CLOSTRIDIUM DIFFICILE

Etiology *C. difficile* is a Gram-positive, spore-forming, anaerobic bacillus commonly associated with diarrhea and colitis in humans and animals (Keel and Songer, 2006).

Clinical Signs *C. difficile* infection may be associated with anorexia, depression, diarrhea, fecal-staining of the perineum, decreased fecal output, abdominal distention, and death (Perkins *et al.*, 1995; Rehg and Lu, 1981). Peracute death, without clinical signs, is also a common presentation in rabbits (Keel and Songer, 2006; Perkins *et al.*, 1995).

Epizootiology The spread of *C. difficile* involves carrier animals that do not show clinical signs of disease (Keel and Songer, 2006). The carrier state may depend on the age of the individual (Keel and Songer, 2006). *C. difficile* is thought to be acquired from the environment due to persistent contamination with spores (Keel and Songer, 2006).

Disease is associated with antibiotic treatment but can also develop spontaneously (without antibiotic treatment) (Perkins *et al.*, 1995; Rehg and Lu, 1981). The disease may also occur after stressful events such as weaning, sudden dietary changes, lactation, kindling, and illness (Perkins *et al.*, 1995). Rabbits that have been recently weaned are the most susceptible (Perkins *et al.*, 1995). Newborn rabbits are resistant to *C. difficile* disease possibly due to the lack of receptors for the toxins (Keel and Songer, 2006). Similar to *C. spiroforme*, the pathogenesis is associated with disruption of the gut flora and with colonization and proliferation of toxigenic *Clostridium*.

Pathology Grossly, a fluid-filled cecum and colon may be found on necropsy (Rehg and Lu, 1981). Spontaneous disease in rabbits is associated with lesions in the small intestine, most commonly in the ileum (Keel and Songer, 2006). In one study, the small intestine was distended with fluid and the cecum was distended with chyme (Perkins *et al.*, 1995). *C. difficile* is also associated with hemorrhagic typhlitis in hares (Dabard *et al.*, 1979).

C. difficile causes severe jejunal lesions in rabbits, but cecal lesions may occur (Keel and Songer, 2006; Perkins *et al.*, 1995). Mural hemorrhages, mucosal necrosis, and submucosal edema have been observed (Perkins *et al.*, 1995). Toxins A (enterotoxin) and B (cytotoxin) act synergistically and are essential virulence factors of *C. difficile* that enter the cells through receptor-mediated endocytosis (Keel and Songer, 2006). Toxins A and B disrupt the actin cytoskeleton by disrupting Rho-subtype intracellular signaling molecules that affect cellular function (Keel and Songer, 2006). Inflammation and neurogenic stimuli also are involved in the pathogenesis of *C. difficile* disease (Keel and Songer, 2006). In addition to toxins A and B, some *C. difficile* strains produce an actin-specific ADP-ribosyltransferase or binary toxin (Stubbs *et al.*, 2000).

Diagnosis *C. difficile* isolation and toxin assays have been described (Keel and Songer, 2006; Perkins *et al.*, 1995; Rehg and Lu, 1981). *C. difficile* selective agar is commercially available. The tissue culture cytotoxin assay for *C. difficile* toxin B is considered the 'gold standard' (Belanger *et al.*, 2003). *C. difficile* toxin B can be neutralized with *C. sordelli* antiserum, but not with *C. spiroforme* antiserum (Perkins *et al.*, 1995). Commercially available enzyme immunoassays to detect *C. difficile* toxin(s) have been used to diagnose rabbit cases (Garcia *et al.*, 2002; Perkins *et al.*, 1995). PCR assays have been developed (Belanger *et al.*, 2003; Goldenberg *et al.*, 2010; Houser *et al.*, 2010; Pallis *et al.*, 2013).

Differential Diagnoses The differential diagnosis of peracute death in rabbits should include infection with *Clostridium* spp. and/or EHEC infection (Garcia *et al.*, 2002; Perkins *et al.*, 1995).

Treatment, Prevention, and Control As with *C. spiroforme*, the reduction of risk factors and the prudent use of antibiotics are recommended (Agnoletti *et al.*, 2009). Cholestyramine may also be used for prevention (Lipman *et al.*, 1992). Fecal flora transplants have been suggested and commercial probiotic strains are able to inhibit *C. difficile* and *C. perfringens in vitro* (Carman and Evans, 1984; Schoster *et al.*, 2013).

Research Complications The sporadic nature of deaths due to *C. difficile* infection is unlikely to result in significant complications to research.

iii. CLOSTRIDIUM PERFRINGENS
C. perfringens type E produces alpha and iota toxins and is an

uncommon cause of enterotoxemia in rabbits (Redondo *et al.*, 2013; Songer, 1996). Because of the similarity between the iota toxins of *C. spiroforme* and *C. perfringens* type E, detection of toxin alone for diagnostic purposes will not differentiate between the two organisms (Songer, 1996). PCR can be used for typing *C. perfringens* based on amplification of toxin genes (Daube *et al.*, 1994).

3. Colibacillosis

Historically, a disease process associated with *E. coli* infection was known as colibacillosis. Currently, *E. coli* is classified based on the virulence factors that are genetically encoded and expressed in the bacteria. Different virulence factors are associated with different *E. coli* 'pathotypes'. Pathotypes may be associated with three general clinical syndromes: enteric/diarrheal disease, urinary tract infections, and sepsis/meningitis (Kaper *et al.*, 2004). The Centers for Disease Control and Prevention currently recognizes six pathotypes associated with diarrhea in humans: enteropathogenic *E. coli* (EPEC), Shiga toxin (Stx)-producing *E. coli* (STEC; also known as enterohemorrhagic *E. coli* (EHEC) or verocytotoxin-producing *E. coli* (VTEC)), enterotoxigenic *E. coli* (ETEC), enteroaggregative *E. coli* (EAEC), enteroinvasive *E. coli* (EIEC), and diffusely adherent *E. coli* (DAEC) (http://www.cdc.gov/ecoli/general/). Comparative genomic analyses identified genes that were isolate- and pathovar-specific and clustered strains according to pathotypes (Lukjancenko *et al.*, 2010; Rasko *et al.*, 2008). Two more emerging pathotypes have been suggested: adherent invasive *E. coli* (AIEC; associated with Crohn's disease in humans) and Shiga toxin-producing enteroaggregative *E. coli* (STEAEC; associated with a large outbreak of hemolytic uremic syndrome (HUS) in Europe) (Clements *et al.*, 2012). Of these pathotypes, EPEC and STEC are associated with natural disease in rabbits (Cantey and Blake, 1977; Garcia *et al.*, 2002). In addition, necrotoxigenic *E. coli* (NTEC) are associated with disease in rabbits (Blanco *et al.*, 1996). Pathogenic animal and human strains are very closely related and have virulence genes in common (Clermont *et al.*, 2011). Therefore, it is important to determine which *E. coli* pathotype(s) are associated with disease in rabbits in order to characterize new diseases and/or more accurately diagnose, prevent, control, and treat the condition as well as for epidemiological investigations.

a. EPEC and STEC

Etiology EPEC carry the *eae* gene that encodes intimin, a protein involved in induction of attaching and effacing lesions in the intestine. *E. coli* serotype O15, also known as RDEC-1, is the prototype EPEC strain which was isolated from rabbits with diarrhea and has been used experimentally as a model to study EPEC-induced disease (Cantey and Blake, 1977). EPEC is an important

cause of potentially fatal infant diarrhea in developing countries (Kaper *et al.*, 2004; Swennes *et al.*, 2012).

Clinical Signs EHEC O153 was isolated from an outbreak of bloody diarrhea and sudden death in Dutch Belted rabbits (Fig. 10.1) (Garcia *et al.*, 2002). Acute diarrhea following shipment was associated with EPEC O145:H2 infection in laboratory rabbits (Swennes *et al.*, 2012). Laboratory rabbits can be reservoir hosts of pathogenic *E. coli* without exhibiting clinical signs (García and Fox, 2003; Swennes *et al.*, 2013). Patent or occult blood may be detected in the feces of infected rabbits (Camguilhem and Milon, 1989; Garcia *et al.*, 2002).

Epizootiology EPEC and EHEC can be enzootic in rabbit colonies and these bacteria are transmitted by the fecal–oral route (García and Fox, 2003; Swennes *et al.*, 2013; Swennes *et al.*, 2012). EPEC and EHEC coinfections are possible (García and Fox, 2003; Garcia *et al.*, 2002). EHEC are a subset of STEC that carry *stx* gene(s) that encode Stx(s) and also carry the *eae* gene that encodes intimin (Melton-Celsa *et al.*, 2012). Rabbits can harbor STEC strains and are recognized as their vectors and reservoir hosts (Bailey *et al.*, 2002; Blanco *et al.*, 1996; García and Fox, 2003; Kim *et al.*, 1997; Leclercq and Mahillon, 2003; Pohl *et al.*, 1993; Pritchard *et al.*, 2001; Scaife *et al.*, 2006).

Pathology Grossly, paintbrush hemorrhages of the cecal serosa may be observed after experimental infection with EPEC (Camguilhem and Milon, 1989). Also, experimentally, the serosal surface of the cecum and/or proximal colon can develop petechial or echymotic hemorrhages and may become edematous and thickened (García *et al.*, 2006). Histologically and ultrastructurally, attaching and effacing lesions with pedestal formation can be observed with EPEC or EHEC infections

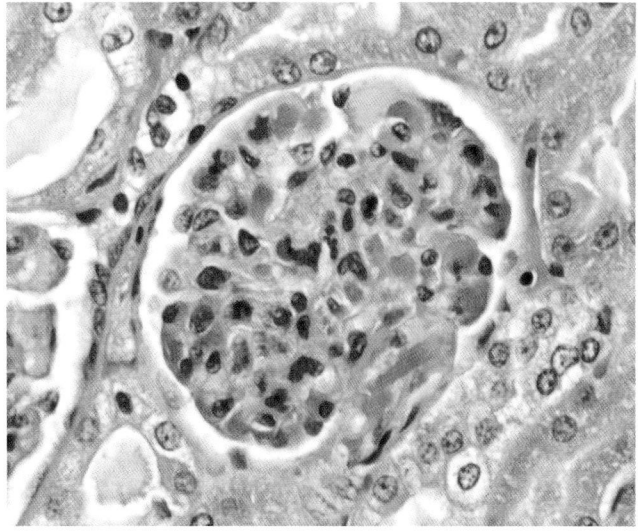

FIGURE 10.1 Glomerulus of a Dutch Belted rabbit naturally infected with EHEC O153. There are heterophils within the glomerulus.

(Kaper *et al.*, 2004; Peeters *et al.*, 1988). Enterocolitis, nephropathy, and thrombotic microangiopathy can be observed in EHEC-infected rabbits (García *et al.*, 2006).

Diagnosis Feces or intestinal contents can be enriched in broth and then cultured using blood agar, MacConkey agar, or EHEC-selective media such as Sorbitol MacConkey agar or Raibow® agar (García and Fox, 2003; Tarr, 2009; Tarr *et al.*, 2005). After isolation of *E. coli* in pure culture, samples can be biotyped using commercial methods such as the API® 20E strips (bioMérieux). Serotyping and molecular characterization of isolates can be performed by the *E. coli* Reference Center (http://ecoli.cas.psu.edu/) at The Pennsylvania State University. PCR assays can be utilized to detect virulence factors characteristic of EPEC, EHEC, or other pathogenic *E. coli* as well as for high-resolution genotyping for epidemiological studies (Blanco *et al.*, 1996; García and Fox, 2003). Molecular characterization of STEC strains can be performed by the STEC Center (http://www.shigatox.net/new/) at Michigan State University.

Differential Diagnoses The differential diagnoses should include other causes of diarrhea in rabbits including the clostridial diseases and intestinal coccidiosis.

Treatment, Prevention, and Control For prevention, avoid introduction of rabbits of unknown pathogenic *E. coli* status into a colony. Rabbits should be screened by culture and *E. coli* isolates characterized for virulence factors by PCR. Also, since it is known that EHEC can contaminate plants and vegetables, laboratory personnel should be aware that rabbit feeds such as hay, alfalfa, and other greens have the potential to introduce enteric pathogens such as EHEC into laboratory rabbits (Berger *et al.*, 2010; García and Fox, 2003). EHEC O157 can survive for 60 days in grass hay feed (Davis *et al.*, 2005).

Cesarean section rederivation and antibiotic treatment have been suggested for eradication of pathogenic *E. coli* in rabbits (Swennes *et al.*, 2012). A 'One Health' approach should be incorporated to control EHEC infections because outbreaks such as with EHEC O157 in humans was linked to consumption of spinach contaminated by feral swine and was additionally isolated from domestic cattle, surface water, sediment, and soil (Garcia *et al.*, 2010) – a good example of integrating human, animal, and environmental health (Monath *et al.*, 2010).

Antibiotic treatment should be based on culture and sensitivity. Importantly, in humans infected with EHEC, treatment with antibiotics is controversial due to the possibility of induction of Stx-encoding bacteriophages and worsening of the clinical condition due to Hemolytic Uremic Syndrome (Tarr *et al.*, 2005); therefore, antibiotic treatment of rabbits infected with EHEC may not be recommended. Clinically affected rabbits can be treated with fluids as this intervention is nephroprotective in humans (Hickey *et al.*, 2011). In addition, rabbit EPEC

strains may carry extended-spectrum beta-lactamases making them resistant to antibiotics (Poeta *et al.*, 2010). Parenteral enrofloxacin administered prior to shipment decreased morbidity and mortality associated with endemic EPEC (Swennes *et al.*, 2012).

Research Complications EPEC infection can cause high morbidity and mortality in laboratory rabbit colonies and can affect studies involving intestinal physiology in rabbits. EPEC and EHEC present a zoonotic risk (Garcia *et al.*, 2010; Poeta *et al.*, 2010; Swennes *et al.*, 2013).

Treponematosis

Etiology *Treponema paraluiscuniculi* is a noncultivable species that infects rabbits and causes venereal spirochetosis or treponematosis (also known as rabbit syphilis, vent disease, or cuniculosis) (Smajs *et al.*, 2011). Although its genome structure is closely related to other pathogenic *Treponema* species including *T. pallidum* subsp. *pallidum*, the etiological agent of human syphilis, *T. paraluiscuniculi* does not infect humans (Smajs *et al.*, 2011). Genome sequencing revealed that *T. paraluiscuniculi* evolved from a *T. pallidum*-like ancestor and adapted to rabbits during loss of infectivity to humans (Smajs *et al.*, 2011). *T. paraluiscuniculi* can also infect hares, and causes seroconversion, but no clinical signs. In contrast, the related organism, *T. paraluisleporis*, can infect and induce disease in rabbits and hares. The close phylogenetic association between *T. paraluiscuniculi* and *T. paraluisleporis* suggests that these organisms could be given a subspecies or ecovar status rather than species status (Lumeij *et al.*, 2013).

Clinical Signs In naturally infected rabbits lesions commonly occur in the vulva or prepuce (Cunliffe-Beamer and Fox, 1981a). Other parts of the body that may be affected, in descending order, include the anal region, nose, eyelid, and lip (Cunliffe-Beamer and Fox, 1981a). Naturally infected rabbits develop lesions of the ear, face, prepuce, and anus (Small and Newman, 1972). In a study involving intratesticular inoculation of *T. paraluiscuniculi*, single lesions were found in the prepuce or scrotum and multiple lesions were found in the nose, mouth, ear, prepuce, foot, and scrotum (Small and Newman, 1972). All lesions had abundant treponemes by dark-field examination (Small and Newman, 1972).

Epizootiology Susceptibility to, and expression of, venereal spirochetosis, may vary with the strain of rabbit (Cunliffe-Beamer and Fox, 1981b). The prevalence of *T. paraluiscuniculi* infection increased with parity in adult females and most adult males seroconverted within 6 months of entering the breeding program. These findings suggested that *T. paraluiscuniculi* spreads by horizontal transmission in adult rabbits (DiGiacomo *et al.*, 1983). In an enzootically infected conventional rabbit colony, the frequency of venereal spirochetosis was lower in rabbits less than 6 months of age than in adult rabbits (Cunliffe-Beamer and Fox, 1981b). Experiments involving cross fostering of newborns indicated that infection occurred at birth (vertical transmission) and during the suckling period (Cunliffe-Beamer and Fox, 1981b). In addition, horizontal transmission by coitus and skin contact occurs (Small and Newman, 1972). Experimental topical or intradermal-subcutaneous genital inoculation of adult rabbits confirmed these routes of transmission (Cunliffe-Beamer and Fox, 1981b).

The *T. pallidum* repeat (*tpr*) genes in *T. pallidum* subsp. *pallidum* are thought to code for potential virulence factors. TprK was the only Tpr homolog found in *T. paraluiscuniculi* that induced antibody and T cell responses after experimental inoculation of rabbits indicating that TprK may be an important virulence factor in venereal spirochetosis (Giacani *et al.*, 2004). Virulence factors and pathogenesis have been recently reviewed (Smajs *et al.*, 2012).

Pathology The lesions include erythemathous macules or papules to erosions, ulcers, and crusts (Cunliffe-Beamer and Fox, 1981a).

Diagnosis Serologic tests that have been used include the nontreponemal antigen tests (Venereal Disease Research Laboratory (VDRL) and rapid plasma reagin), microhemagglutination, and fluorescent treponemal antibody absorption tests (DiGiacomo *et al.*, 1983). Although the nontreponemal antigen tests were not completely satisfactory, the VDRL test was more sensitive and the plasma reagin test was more specific in detecting *T. paraluiscuniculi* infection (DiGiacomo *et al.*, 1983). The sensitivity and specificity of the microhemagglutination test compared favorably with the fluorescent treponemal antibody absorption test and was recommended as the optimal assay to make a diagnosis (DiGiacomo *et al.*, 1983). Detection of *T. paraluiscuniculi* in lesions can be achieved by dark-field microscopic examination of scrapings from lesions and by histological evaluation of silver-stained testicular sections (Cunliffe-Beamer and Fox, 1981a; Faine, 1965). PCR has been used for molecular characterization of treponemes including *T. paraluiscuniculi* (Cejkova *et al.*, 2013).

Differential Diagnoses The skin lesions may be confused with abrasions (trauma), mycotic infections, and lesions of ectoparasites (acariasis) (Small and Newman, 1972).

Treatment, Prevention, and Control There are no vaccines available at this time to prevent treponematosis in rabbits; however, rabbits have been used as experimental models to test vaccines against *T. pallidum* in humans (Ho and Lukehart, 2011). Hysterectomy derivation can eliminate venereal spirochetosis (Cunliffe-Beamer and Fox, 1981b). A study investigating two different doses (42,000 or 84,000 IU/kg body weight/week) of benzathine penicillin G-procaine penicillin G to treat rabbits at 7-day intervals found that both dosages

were effective. Lesions healed within 2 weeks of the first treatment and the plasma reagin titers declined markedly or disappeared by the sixth week after the first treatment (Cunliffe-Beamer and Fox, 1981c).

Research Complications *T. paraluiscuniculi* can affect studies of *T. pallidum* in rabbits (Small and Newman, 1972). Partial immunological cross-protection has been observed between *T. paraluiscuniculi* and *T. pallidum* (Smajs *et al.*, 2011; Turner and Hollander, 1957).

5. Proliferative Enteropathy

Etiology *Lawsonia intracellularis* is a Gram-negative, curved to spiral-shaped, obligate intracellular bacterium that causes proliferative enteropathy in rabbits and other species of animals (Sait *et al.*, 2013; Schauer *et al.*, 1998).

Clinical Signs An intraepithelial 'vibrio' was associated with acute typhlitis in rabbits 1–4 weeks after weaning (Moon *et al.*, 1974). Diarrhea was reported in Japanese White rabbits with presumptive *L. intracellularis* infection and histiocytic enteritis (Umemura *et al.*, 1982). In another report, sucklings and weanlings were affected and the feces of most of the rabbits were characterized as semifluid and mucinous or pasty, and three rabbits had watery diarrhea (Schoeb and Fox, 1990). These affected rabbits were afebrile and lethargic, refused food and water, and most died within a few days after the onset of diarrhea (Schoeb and Fox, 1990). Diarrhea, depression, and dehydration that resolved over the course of 1–2 weeks were reported in 5- to 8-week-old New Zealand White (NZW) rabbits (Hotchkiss *et al.*, 1996). Diarrhea and weight loss were reported in a 3-month-old rabbit (Horiuchi *et al.*, 2008). An outbreak of diarrhea with high (70%) mortality was reported in 2- to 4-month-old NZW rabbits with proliferative enterocolitis associated with *L. intracellularis* and EPEC (Schauer *et al.*, 1998).

Epizootiology Proliferative enteropathy generally occurs as isolated cases or occasional minor outbreaks in species other than the pig, blue fox, and hamster (Lawson and Gebhart, 2000). Infected rabbits can serve as reservoir hosts for *L. intracellularis* infection in other species including foals (Pusterla *et al.*, 2012a, 2013). However, *L. intracellularis* appears to adapt to the specific animal species it infects (Vannucci *et al.*, 2012).

The pathogenesis of *L. intracellularis* infection has been reviewed (Lawson and Gebhart, 2000; Smith and Lawson, 2001). Studies using interferon (IFN)-gamma receptor knockout mice determined that interferon IFN-gamma plays a significant role in limiting intracellular infection and increased cellular proliferation associated with *L. intracellularis* infection (Smith *et al.*, 2000). Lawsonia surface antigen (LsaA) plays a role during *L. intracellularis* attachment to and entry into intestinal epithelial cells (McCluskey *et al.*, 2002). BALB/cA mice are susceptible to rabbit *L. intracellularis* isolates but not to pig *L. intracellularis* isolates suggesting that there are biological differences between the proliferative enteropathy isolates from rabbits and pigs (Murakata *et al.*, 2008).

Pathology   Distention and diffuse mucosal thickening of the jejunum and proximal ileum with enlarged cranial mesenteric lymph nodes was observed in 5- to 6-month-old rabbits (Umemura *et al.*, 1982). Thickening of the mucosa was associated with distention of the lamina propria with macrophages and the enlargement of the lymph nodes was also associated with infiltration of macrophages (Umemura *et al.*, 1982). Minute bacilli were observed in the apical cytoplasm of mucosal epithelial cells using toluidine blue (Umemura *et al.*, 1982). Thickening of the cecum and proximal colon has also been reported (Hotchkiss *et al.*, 1996). In another study, no gross lesions were found in the small intestine, but two suckling rabbits had reddened ceca with congested vessels (Schoeb and Fox, 1990). In this study two types of microscopic lesions were characterized: (1) erosive and suppurative cecitis and colitis, and (2) proliferative lesions in the cecum, sacculated colon, ileum, and distal jejunum, or a combination of these (Schoeb and Fox, 1990). Some animals had both erosive and proliferative lesions. Narrow curved or spiral bacteria were detected in rabbits with erosive and proliferative lesions using Warthin–Starry stain and these bacteria were more abundant in cases with severe lesions (Schoeb and Fox, 1990). Proliferative intestinal lesions contained curved to spiral argyrophilic intracellular bacteria in the apical cytoplasm of crypt enterocytes (Hotchkiss *et al.*, 1996).

Diagnosis   The 16S ribosomal DNA sequences from *L. intracellularis* isolates from different species of animals are highly similar (Cooper *et al.*, 1997a). However, antigenic differences have been found between pig and rabbit isolates (Watarai *et al.*, 2008). The complete genome sequence of a porcine strain has been recently reported (Sait *et al.*, 2013). *L. intracellularis* can be detected in feces from healthy and diarrheic rabbits (Lim *et al.*, 2012).

PCR assays to detect *L. intracellularis* DNA in feces have been evaluated (Pedersen *et al.*, 2010). These assays can be used for *ante mortem* diagnosis of proliferative enteropathy in pigs (Pedersen *et al.*, 2010). PCR primers used to diagnose *Lawsonia* in other animals species have been used in rabbit cases (Cooper *et al.*, 1997b; Duhamel *et al.*, 1998; Fox *et al.*, 1994; Horiuchi *et al.*, 2008; Hotchkiss *et al.*, 1996; Jones *et al.*, 1993). Other diagnostic methods include enzyme-linked immunosorbent assay (ELISA) using synthetic peptides of LsaA and immunomagnetic separation using anti-LsaA antibody to capture *L. intracellularis* in fecal samples followed by detection with ATP bioluminescence (Watarai *et al.*, 2004, 2005). In tissue sections, *L. intracellularis* can be detected using silver stains such as Warthin–Starry stain (Duhamel *et al.*, 1998; Horiuchi *et al.*, 2008; Hotchkiss *et al.*, 1996; Schauer *et al.*, 1998; Schoeb and

Fox, 1990). Indirect immunofluorescence has also been used in deparaffinized intestinal sections from infected rabbits (Schoeb and Fox, 1990). Immunohistochemistry using antiserum against synthetic peptides of LsaA has also been used to detect *L. intracellularis* in the ileum of a naturally infected rabbit (Watarai *et al.*, 2004). Electron microscopy reveals organisms that are ~0.23–0.32 μm wide and ≤ 1.7 μm long in the apical cytoplasm of villous and crypt epithelial cells (Duhamel *et al.*, 1998). *L. intracellularis* can be cultured from homogenized intestinal tissue in cell lines including IEC-18 (rat small intestinal cells) and McCoy cells (mouse fibroblasts) (Lawson and Gebhart, 2000; Watarai *et al.*, 2008). A quantitative PCR (qPCR) assay that is able to assess the growth of *L. intracellularis* in cultured cells has also been used to detect the organisms in pig fecal samples and could be used in other animal species (Drozd *et al.*, 2010).

Differential Diagnoses   Clinically, the differential diagnosis should include other causes of diarrhea in rabbits. *Mycobacterium avium* subsp. *paratuberculosis* can infect rabbits and induce thickening of the intestinal mucosa (Beard *et al.*, 2001; Greig *et al.*, 1997). Therefore, rabbit intestinal sections should be examined for acid-fast organisms using stains such as Ziehl–Neelsen stain (Duhamel *et al.*, 1998; Horiuchi *et al.*, 2008; Schoeb and Fox, 1990; Umemura *et al.*, 1982). Furthermore, other intestinal organisms may colonize the intestine during *L. intracellularis* infection in rabbits (Duhamel *et al.*, 1998; Hotchkiss *et al.*, 1996; Lim *et al.*, 2012; Schauer *et al.*, 1998). Other bacterial diseases have been sporadically reported in rabbits. These are summarized in Table 10.6.

Treatment, Prevention, and Control   Vaccination strategies have been tested and developed for pigs and horses, but not for rabbits (Nogueira *et al.*, 2013; Pusterla *et al.*, 2012b; Weibel *et al.*, 2012). Testing rabbits by PCR prior to introduction to a laboratory colony may be necessary for exclusion of this organism. Oral neomycin (50 mg/rabbit) was used to treat surviving rabbits during an outbreak of presumptive *L. intracellularis* and the diarrhea subsided (Umemura *et al.*, 1982). Because *L. intracellularis* infects the intestine and IFN-gamma appears to be involved in pathogenesis, research involving rabbit gastrointestinal pathology and immune responses may be confounded by infection with this organism.

Research Complications   The mortality associated with *L. intracellularis* infection would be disruptive to ongoing studies.

B. Viral Diseases

1. Poxvirus Infections

a. Myxomatosis

Etiology   Myxomatosis is caused by myxoma virus, a member of the family Poxviridae, genus *Leporipoxvirus* (Kerr and Donnelly, 2013; Spiesschaert *et al.*, 2011).

Clinical Signs The severity of disease varies with the strain of virus and the host species and breed. Rabbits of the genus *Oryctolagus* are particularly susceptible and often develop a fatal disease characterized by mucinous skin lesions and tumors. Affected animals also exhibit edema around the mouth, nose, anus, and genitals as well as progressive conjunctivitis with serous and mucopurulent secretions from the eyes and nose (Brabb and Di Giacomo, 2012; Kerr and Donnelly, 2013; Spiesschaert *et al.*, 2011). Bacterial pneumonia commonly develops and animals die 10–14 days after infection. The virus is spread by arthropod vectors and direct contact.

Epizootiology Myxomatosis has a worldwide distribution. Various species of *Sylvilagus* and *Lepus* are naturally susceptible (Brabb and Di Giacomo, 2012). The myxoma virus genome encodes for a number of immunomodulatory proteins which greatly affect the host immune response by inhibiting apoptosis, interfering with leukocyte chemotaxis, and suppressing leukocyte activation, thereby fostering viral replication and spread (Spiesschaert *et al.*, 2011).

Pathology Histopathology shows these 'myxomas' to be composed of undifferentiated stellate mesenchymal cells embedded in a matrix of mucinous material and interspersed with capillaries and inflammatory cells (Brabb and Di Giacomo, 2012; Kerr and Donnelly, 2013).

Diagnosis Diagnosis can be made by PCR or ELISA. Definitive diagnosis depends on culture of the virus from infected tissues.

Differential Diagnoses Rabbits of the genus *Sylvilagus* develop fibroma-like lesions that may be indistinguishable from those caused by rabbit fibroma virus. The two diseases have been distinguished by inoculation of fibroma material into *Oryctolagus* rabbits. They develop fatal disease if the myxoma virus is the etiologic agent, or fibromas if rabbit fibroma virus is responsible.

Treatment, Prevention, and Control Since the disease is spread by fleas and mosquitoes as well as by direct contact, control measures should include prevention of contact with arthropods and quarantine of infected rabbits. Vaccines have been used in Europe with some success. Most recently, a live recombinant vaccine for both myxomatosis and rabbit hemorrhagic disease has been released in the United Kingdom (Spibey *et al.*, 2012).

Research Complications None have been reported.

b. Rabbit (Shope) Fibroma Virus

Rabbit (Shope) fibroma virus is a *Leporipoxvirus* that is antigenically related to myxoma virus. Fibromatosis is endemic in wild rabbits; however, an outbreak in commercial rabbits caused extensive mortality (Joiner *et al.*, 1971). Usually, less virulent strains cause skin tumors in domestic rabbits (Raflo *et al.*, 1973). The disease is probably spread by arthropods (Brabb and Di Giacomo, 2012; Kerr and Donnelly, 2013). Fibromas are flat, subcutaneous, easily movable tumors, and most often found on the legs and face. Tumors may persist for some time but eventually regress. Metastasis does not occur.

c. Rabbit Pox

Rabbit pox is a rare disease induced by an *Orthopoxvirus* taxonomically similar to vaccina virus that has caused outbreaks of fatal disease in laboratory rabbits in the United States and Holland (Brabb and Di Giacomo, 2012). Rabbits with the disease may or may not present with 'pox' lesions in the skin. The animals have a fever and nasal discharge 2 or 3 days after infection. Most rabbits have eye lesions including blepharitis, conjunctivitis, and keratitis with subsequent corneal ulceration. Skin lesions, when present, are widespread. They begin as a macular rash and progress to papules up to 1 cm in diameter by 5 days postinfection. The lymph nodes are enlarged, the face is often edematous, and there may be lesions in the oral and nasal cavity. At gross necropsy, nodules can be found in the liver, gall bladder, spleen, lung, and reproductive organs. Necrosis is widespread. Characteristic cytoplasmic inclusions seen in many poxvirus infections are rare in this disease. Mortality is high in affected animals. The virus is apparently spread by aerosols and is difficult to control. Rabbit pox is used as a model of smallpox in humans in response to the potential use of smallpox as a bioterrorism agent. It is an effective model for the evaluation of potential therapies against smallpox (Nalca and Nichols, 2011; Rice *et al.*, 2011).

2. Herpesvirus Infections

Four herpesviruses (leporid herpesviruses 1, 2, 3, and 4) have been isolated from rabbits and hares (Davison, 2010). Leporid herpesvirus 1 (LHV-1) was isolated from cottontail rabbits and is also known as cottontail rabbit herpesvirus. It is not pathogenic for domestic rabbits. LHV-2 (*Herpesvirus cuniculi*) was isolated from domestic rabbits (*O. cuniculus*) and causes subclinical infections. LHV-3 (*Herpesvirus sylvilagus*) was isolated from cottontail rabbits. Cottontail rabbits infected with the virus develop a lymphoproliferative disease with lymphoid infiltration of many organs (Hesselton *et al.*, 1988). LHV-3 does not infect domestic rabbits. LHV-1–3 are tentatively classified in the genus *Radinovirus*, subfamily Gammaherpesvirinae. LHV-4 was isolated from domestic rabbits and caused severe disease in preweanlings (Jin *et al.*, 2008a, b). Clinical signs included weakness, anorexia, conjunctivitis, keratitis, and periocular swelling. Some animals also developed skin ulcers. LHV-4 is genus *Simplexvirus*, subfamily Alphaherpesvirinae.

3. Papillomavirus Infections

The cottontail rabbit is the natural host of the cottontail (Shope) papillomavirus, a *Kappapapillomavirus*,

TABLE 10.6 Other Bacterial Infections of Rabbits[a]

GRAM NEGATIVE

Disease [Frequency][b]	Etiologic agent	Presentation[b]	Clinical signs/lesions	Organ and/or system affected	Selected references
Colibacillosis† [*E. coli* infection is common]	Necrotoxigenic *E. coli* 1 or 2 (NTEC-1 or NTEC-2)	Epizootic, sporadic	Diarrhea	Gastrointestinal	Ansuini et al., 1994; Blanco et al., 1996b; Blanco et al., 1994; Caprioli et al., 1989; De Rycke et al., 1999; Falbo et al., 1992
Salmonellosis[c] [Uncommon]	*Salmonella enterica* serotypes Typhimurium or Enteritidis, *S. mbandaka*, other serotypes	Epizootic (can be associated with stress or immunosuppression); no clinical signs (carriers)	Peracute death due to septicemia (with no clinical signs), anorexia, pyrexia, depression, diarrhea, abortion, dyspnea, and cyanosis	Reproductive, respiratory, gastrointestinal	Borrelli et al., 2011; Camarda et al., 2013; de Boer et al., 1983; Habermann and Williams, 1958; Harwood, 1989; Newcomer et al., 1983; Newcomer et al., 1984; Vieira-Pinto et al., 2011
Necrobacillosis[c] (Schmorl's disease) [Uncommon]	*Fusobacterium necrophorum*, *F. nucleatum*	Sporadic	Inflammation, abscessation (*F. nucleatum* associated with mandibular and maxillary abscesses), ulceration, and necrosis. Anorexia and cachexia in chronic disease	Skin and subcutaneous tissue (head and neck more commonly; also plantar surface of feet); bone (mandible or maxilla); other organs (embolic abscesses)	Garibaldi et al., 1990b; Kaur and Falkler, 1992; Seps et al., 1999; Tyrrell et al., 2002; Ward et al., 1981
Tularemia[c] [Common in hares and wild rabbits; rare in domestic rabbits]	*Francisella tularensis* (subsp. *tularensis* and *holartica*)	Enzootic (wild rabbits and hares); no clinical signs (carriers)	Sudden (peracute) death, depression, anorexia, ataxia	Liver, spleen, bone marrow, intestine	Foley and Nieto, 2010; Hoff et al., 1975; Kim et al., 2010; Lepitzki et al., 1990; Morner et al., 1988; Wobeser et al., 2009b
Actinobacillosis[c] [Uncommon in domestic rabbits]	*Actinobacillus capsulatus*, *A. equuli*	Enzootic (in wild lagomorphs) and sporadic (in pet rabbits)	Inflammation around joints of extremities, febrile illness, septicemia	Lungs, liver, soft tissue around joints	Ashhurst-Smith et al., 1998; Meyerholz and Haynes, 2005; Moyaert et al., 2007; Zarnke et al., 1990; Zarnke and Schlater, 1988
Bordetella infection[c] [Common]	*Bordetella bronchiseptica*	Enzootic (no clinical signs)	Respiratory signs (occur when there is coinfection with a respiratory pathogen such as *P. multocida*)	Respiratory, immune system	Broughton et al., 2010; Deeb and DiGiacomo, 2000b; Deeb et al., 1990a; Suzuki et al., 1990; Zeligs et al., 1986
Brucellosis[c] [Rare in domestic rabbits, common in wild lagomorphs (*Lepus*)]	*Brucella suis* (most common), *B. melitensis*, *B. abortus*	Enzootic	Multifocal chronic granulomatous inflammation	Reproductive system, liver, and spleen	Becker, 1964; Gyuranecz et al., 2011; Jacotot and Vallee, 1951; Jacotot and Vallee, 1954; Mykhailova, 1959; Szulowski et al., 1999; Szyfres et al., 1968; Thorpe et al., 1965; Tworek and Serokowa, 1956; Vitovec et al., 1976
Cilia-associated respiratory (CAR) bacillus infection [Common in some colonies]	CAR bacillus	Enzootic (in some colonies)	Slight hypertrophy and hyperplasia of ciliated epithelium and inflammation (bronchi and trachea)	Respiratory	Caniatti et al., 1998; Cundiff et al., 1994; Cundiff et al., 1995; Kurisu et al., 1990; Oros et al., 1997; Schoeb et al., 1993

Disease	Organism	Occurrence	Clinical signs	Organs affected	References
Chlamydiosis[c] [Uncommon in domestic rabbits]	*Chlamydia* or *Chlamydophila* (*Cp.*)	Epizootic (*Cp. psittaci* M56 in *Lepus americanus*)	Congestion and necrosis of liver and spleen (*Cp. psittaci* M56); conjunctivitis, pneumonia	Liver and spleen; eyes, respiratory	Flatt and Dungworth, 1971; Pantchev *et al.*, 2010; Spalatin *et al.*, 1966; Spalatin *et al.*, 1971
Helicobacter infection[c] [Uncommon in laboratory rabbits]	*Helicobacter* spp.	Sporadic	No clinical signs	Stomach (possibly)	Revez *et al.*, 2013; Vaira *et al.*, 1992; Van den Bulck *et al.*, 2005a; Van den Bulck *et al.*, 2005b; Van den Bulck *et al.*, 2006
Campylobacter infection[c] [Common]	*Campylobacter* spp.	Enzootic	No clinical signs	No apparent organs affected	de Boer *et al.*, 1983; Revez *et al.*, 2013; Wahlström *et al.*, 2003
Moraxella infection [Infection is common but disease is rare]	*Moraxella bovis*	Sporadic	Metritis, vaginal discharge, septicemia, pneumonia, hepatic necrosis	Reproductive, lungs, liver	Marini *et al.*, 1996b; Soave *et al.*, 1977
Pasteurella spp. infection (not *P. multocida*) [Uncommon]	*Pasteurella pneumotropica*; *P. aerogenes*	Sporadic	Rhinitis (with *P. pneumotropica*); metritis and abortion (with *P. aerogenes*); or no clinical signs	Respiratory (*P. pneumotropica*); reproductive (*P. aerogenes*)	Kirchner *et al.*, 1983; Okuda and Campbell, 1974; Stahel *et al.*, 2009b; Thigpen *et al.*, 1978
Pseudomoniasis [Uncommon disease]	*Pseudomonas aeruginosa*	Sporadic, enzootic, or epizootic	Exudative, moist dermatitis (of dewlap or other skin areas) with blue-green discoloration; abscesses, septicemia, pneumonia, diarrhea	Skin, respiratory, gastrointestinal	Dominguez *et al.*, 1975; Garibaldi *et al.*, 1990a; McDonald and Pinheiro, 1967; O'Donoghue and Whatley, 1971; Pogany Simonova *et al.*, 2010; Schoenbaum, 1981; Weisner *et al.*, 2005; Williams and Gibson, 1975
Yersiniosis (pseudotuberculosis)[c] [Rare in domestic rabbits]	*Yersinia pseudotuberculosis*; *Y. enterocolitica*	Enzootic and epizootic (in wild lagomorphs-reservoirs)	Caseous necrosis	Mesenteric lymph nodes, spleen, liver, Peyer's patches, intestine, lungs, and kidney	de Boer *et al.*, 1983; Mollaret and Lucas, 1965; Nikolova *et al.*, 2001; Sterba, 1985; Tsubokura *et al.*, 1984; Wobeser *et al.*, 2009b; Wuthe and Aleksic, 1997
Borreliosis[c] (Lyme's disease) [Spirochetemia may be common in wild rabbits]	*Borrelia burgdorferi*	Enzootic in wild lagomorphs	No clinical signs	Blood (spirochetemia)	Anderson *et al.*, 1989; Lane and Burgdorfer, 1988; Magnarelli *et al.*, 2012; Telford and Spielman, 1989a; Telford and Spielman, 1989b
Haemophilosis [Uncommon]	*Haemophilus* spp., *H. paracuniculus*	Sporadic	Conjunctivitis, mucoid enteropathy	Eyes, gastrointestinal tract	Srivastava *et al.*, 1986; Targowski and Targowski, 1979
Leptospirosis[c] [Not described in domestic rabbits]	*Leptospira* spp.	Enzootic (in some populations of wild lagomorphs; rabbits may be an important reservoir)	No clinical signs, focal nephritis	Kidney	Asmera, 1959; Asmera, 1960; Giraudo *et al.*, 1985; Hartman and Broekhuizen, 1980; Shotts *et al.*, 1971

(*Continued*)

TABLE 10.6 (Continued)

GRAM NEGATIVE

Disease [Frequency][b]	Etiologic agent	Presentation[b]	Clinical signs/lesions	Organ and/or system affected	Selected references
GRAM POSITIVE					
Staphylococcosis[c] [Common]	*Staphylococcus aureus*	Sporadic or epizootic (stress can increase disease susceptibility); no clinical signs (carriers)	Death due to septicemia, abscesses (subcutaneous and visceral), pododermatitis, and mastitis. Sometimes pneumonia, rhinitis, conjunctivitis, and otitis media	Skin and subcutaneous tissue more commonly; Also, mammary gland, respiratory system; any organ (with septicemia)	Deeb and DiGiacomo, 2000b; Goni et al., 2004; Millichamp and Collins, 1986; Rodriguez-Calleja et al., 2006; Simonova et al., 2007; Snyder et al., 1976; Sterba, 1985; Vancraeynest et al., 2004, 2006; Viana et al., 2007; Walther et al., 2008
Listeriosis[c] [Uncommon]	*Listeria monocytogenes*	Sporadic or epizootic (can be associated with stress, pregnancy, or immunosuppression); no clinical signs (carriers)	Sudden death due to septicemia (acute cases); anorexia, depression, cachexia (chronic cases); abortion, vaginal discharge	Reproductive system, liver, spleen, adrenals	Briones et al., 1989; Rodriguez-Calleja et al., 2006; Watson and Evans, 1985
Mycobacteriosis[c] [Rare except in pygmy rabbits]	*Mycobacterium bovis, M. avium* (subsp. *paratuberculosis*), *M. tuberculosis*	Sporadic, enzootic, or epizootic	Anorexia, weight loss, pallor, diarrhea (with *M. avium*), swollen joints, ocular lesions, granulomas	Lungs, lymphoid organs, kidney, liver, bone, central nervous system, eyes, intestine	Beard et al., 2001a, c, d; Collins et al., 1983; Greig et al., 1997; Harrenstien et al., 2006; Himes et al., 1989; Judge et al., 2006; McClure, 2012; Reavill and Schmidt, 2012
Actinomycosis [Uncommon]	*Actinomyces israelii*	Sporadic	Osteitis, osteolysis, abscesses (mandibular or maxillary)	Bone and soft tissue	Hong et al., 2009; Sirotek et al., 2006; Tyrrell et al., 2002
Corynebacterium infection [Rare]	*Corynebacterium bovis*	Sporadic	Testicular abscess	Reproductive	Arseculeratne and Navaratnam, 1975
Dermatophilosis[c] [Rare]	*Dermatophilus congolensis*	Sporadic	Skin lesions in foot pads, legs, and perineum	Skin	Shotts and Kistner, 1970; Towersey et al., 1993; Zaria, 1993
Streptococcosis[c] [Uncommon]	*Streptococcus* spp.; *S. agalactiae*	Sporadic	Acute septicemic syndrome; abscess and osteomyelitis; acute respiratory distress syndrome, convulsions, paddling, and fever (*S. agalactiae*)	Subcutaneous tissue; bone; respiratory	Ren et al., 2013; Yanoff, 1983
'Epizootic Rabbit Enteropathy' [Common in rabbit farms in Europe]	The etiology is unknown but bacteria appear to play a role in pathogenesis	Epizootic in rabbit farms (causes high morbidity and mortality)	'Rambling noise', weight loss, abdominal distention (gastrointestinal dilation), diarrhea, mucus excretion	Gastrointestinal	Huybens et al., 2011a, b, 2013; Licois et al., 2005

[a]Some of these bacterial infections have been described in more detail (DeLong, 2012).
[b]Apparent frequency or presentation.
[c]Etiologic agent(s) could be or is/are zoonotic.

which causes horny warts primarily on the neck, shoulders, and abdomen. The disease has a wide geographic distribution with the highest incidence occurring in rabbits in the midwest (Brabb and Di Giacomo, 2012). As many as 25% of infected *Sylvilagus* rabbits develop squamous cell carcinomas. Natural outbreaks in domestic rabbits have been reported (Hagen, 1966). In these natural outbreaks, papillomas were more common on the eyelids and ears. The virus is transmitted by arthropod vectors. This virus is used extensively as a model for the study of oncogenic virus biology and as a model for the treatment and prevention of papillomavirus infections in humans (Christensen, 2005; Salmon *et al.*, 1997; Sundarum *et al.*, 1998).

Oral papillomatosis in domestic rabbits is caused by a *Kappapapillomavirus* that is related to but distinct from the cottontail rabbit papilloma virus. Naturally occurring lesions have been seen in laboratory rabbits and appear as small, white, discrete growths on the ventral surface of the tongue (Kerr and Donnelly, 2013). Lesions may ulcerate. Microscopic examination shows them to be typical papillomas. Most lesions eventually regress spontaneously (Brabb and Di Giacomo, 2012; Kerr and Donnelly, 2013).

4. Rotavirus Infections

Etiology   Rabbit rotavirus is a member of the family Reoviridae. All isolates of rabbit rotavirus have been classified as group A and have been serotype 3 (Brabb and Di Giacomo, 2012; Kerr and Donnelly, 2013).

Clinical Signs   The severity of disease in naturally occurring outbreaks has been variable. In severe outbreaks, affected animals exhibit anorexia, dehydration, and watery to mucoid diarrhea and mortality can be quite high. In other reported outbreaks, mild, transient diarrhea has been reported (Brabb and Di Giacomo, 2012; Kerr and Donnelly, 2013).

Similarly, attempts to experimentally produce clinical disease have had variable results. Mild diarrhea is usually seen, but in some studies there has been significant mortality. It is probable that other factors, such as maternal antibodies, diet, and the presence of pathogenic bacteria, affect the severity of clinical disease in outbreaks. For example, in combined experimental infections with both rotavirus and *E. coli*, the inoculation of both organisms led to more serious clinical signs than when given alone, indicating that rotavirus may have been a more significant determinant in the manifestation of this disease (Thouless *et al.*, 1996). These investigators also showed that older rabbits were naturally more resistant to the combined infection with rotavirus and *E. coli*.

Epizootiology   Rotavirus infections of domestic rabbits are common (Brabb and Di Giacomo, 2012). Many colonies of rabbits are serologically positive, and rotavirus can be isolated readily from rabbit feces. In endemically infected colonies, maternal antibodies to rotaviruses are passed transplacentally and decline at around the time of weaning (Brabb and Di Giacomo, 2012). Rabbits of weaning age are most susceptible.

Very young rabbits appear to be protected from rotavirus infection by passive immunity, when present, but are quite susceptible when there is none (Schoeb *et al.*, 1986). This is also the time when they are most likely to be subjected to diet changes that may contribute to a change in microbial flora.

Pathology   In affected animals, there is villous atrophy and loss of epithelial cells in the small intestines. A lymphocytic infiltrate is present.

Diagnosis   Immunoassays (ELISA and multiplex fluorescent immunoassay) are commercially available for rabbit rotavirus. A commercial immunochromatography kits for detecting human rotavirus infection was used successfully to diagnose rabbit rotavirus infection (Fushuku and Fukuda, 2006).

Differential Diagnoses   *C. piliforme, C. spiroforme, C. difficile, E. coli, Lawsonia intracellularis,* coronavirus, coccidiosis, and intestinal parasites should be considered.

Treatment, Prevention, and Control   Treatment is limited to supportive therapy.

Research Complications   Colony mortality would be disruptive to ongoing studies.

5. Coronavirus Infections

Pleural effusion disease/infectious cardiomyopathy was diagnosed in rabbits inoculated with *T. pallidum*-infected stocks of testicular tissue. Because these treponemes could not be grown *in vitro*, the organism was propagated by passage in rabbits. The stocks were contaminated with a coronavirus, although it is not known whether this virus originated from rabbits or was a virus of human origin that had adapted to rabbits. With continued passage, the virus became more virulent, and significant mortality ensued. Evidence indicated that it was not transmitted by direct contact. Rabbits died due to congestive heart failure, and microscopic examination showed there was widespread necrosis of the heart muscle. It has been suggested that infection with this virus might be a model for the study of virus-induced cardiomyopathy (Brabb and Di Giacomo, 2012; Kerr and Donnelly, 2013).

Rabbit enteric coronavirus has been isolated from tissue cultures from rabbits (Brabb and Di Giacomo, 2012; Kerr and Donnelly, 2013; Lapierre *et al.*, 1980) and has been associated with one naturally occurring outbreak of diarrhea in a barrier-maintained breeding colony (Eaton, 1984). These rabbits developed severe diarrhea, and most died within 48h of onset of clinical signs. Attempts to reproduce the disease led to watery diarrhea, which lasted a short time; however, none of the rabbits died. It is quite probable that other microorganisms or unknown environmental factors contributed to the severity of this outbreak.

6. Calicivirus Infections

Etiology　Rabbit hemorrhagic disease virus is a calicivirus of the genus *Lagovirus* and is the causative agent of rabbit hemorrhagic disease (RHD) (Abrantes *et al.*, 2012; Brabb and Di Giacomo, 2012; Kerr and Donnelly, 2013).

Clinical Signs　Three clinical syndromes are seen (Abrantes *et al.*, 2012). The peracute form is characterized by sudden death without clinical signs. Acutely affected animals demonstrate anorexia and depression. In addition, neurologic signs, respiratory signs, ocular hemorrhage, and epistaxis may be seen. Morbidity and mortality are extremely high. Lymphopenia and abnormalities in coagulation parameters are also seen. In the subacute form, similar signs may occur but are considerably milder and most of these rabbits survive (Abrantes *et al.*, 2012; Kerr and Donnelly, 2013).

Epizootiology　Rabbit hemorrhagic disease was first reported in China in 1984 and is currently endemic in Europe, Asia, Africa, Australia, and New Zealand. In addition, isolated outbreaks have been reported in numerous countries.

The virus is transmitted by the fecal–oral route. The role of fomites and arthropod vectors is also suspected (Brabb and Di Giacomo, 2012; Kerr and Donnelly, 2013). The incubation period may be as short as 1 or 2 days, and sudden death with no previous signs is common.

Pathology　Periportal hepatic necrosis is the only consistent microscopic lesion, and the animals die due to disseminated intravascular coagulopathy and thrombosis (Abrantes *et al.*, 2012; Kerr and Donnelly, 2013).

Diagnosis　The virus has not been successfully grown *in vitro*; however, diagnosis can be confirmed with negative-contrast electron microscopy of liver tissue. Specific antibodies can be detected by ELISA or by hemagglutination inhibition.

Differential Diagnoses　A related calicivirus, European brown hare virus, has caused disease in hares in several countries in Europe (Brabb and Di Giacomo, 2012). Animals present with necrotic hepatitis, hemorrhages in the trachea and lungs, and pulmonary edema. A monoclonal antibody ELISA is available for serodiagnosis, and control measures are similar to those for RHD.

Treatment, Prevention, and Control　The agent resists drying, can be carried on fomites, and may be transmitted via respiratory and intestinal secretions (Mitro and Krauss, 1993). Any rabbit colonies with this disease should be quarantined and depopulated, and the environment thoroughly cleansed and disinfected.

Research Complications　Colony mortality would be disruptive to ongoing studies.

Other Viral Infections　Several other viruses have been isolated from rabbit tissues, but have not been shown to produce disease. These include paramyxoviruses and bunyaviruses. Serologic titers to togaviruses and flaviviruses have also been demonstrated in rabbits (Brabb and Di Giacomo, 2012; Kerr and Donnelly, 2013).

C. Protozoal Diseases

1. Hepatic Coccidiosis

Etiology　Hepatic coccidiosis is caused by the parasite *Eimeria stiedae*, which has also been referred to as *Monocystis stiedae*, *Coccidium oviforme*, and *C. cuniculi* (Hofing and Kraus, 1994).

Clinical Signs　The clinical disease has a wide range of manifestations. Mild infections often result in no apparent disease. Most clinical signs are the result of interruption of normal hepatic function and blockage of the bile ducts. These signs are more common in juvenile rabbits and can include hepatomegaly, icterus, and anorexia (Schoeb et al., 2007). Diarrhea can occur at the terminal stages of the disease (Hofing and Kraus, 1994). Decreased growth rates and weight loss are common. Joyner *et al.* (1987) demonstrated that infected rabbits begin to lose weight within 15 days.

Enlargement of the liver (hepatomegaly) is common. The liver normally is approximately 3.7% of the body weight, but rabbits with severe hepatic coccidiosis may have livers that contribute to greater than 20% of the body weight (Lund, 1954b).

The age of the host strongly affects parasite development and oocyst production. Four-month-old, coccidia-free rabbits experimentally infected with *E. stiedae* produced fewer oocysts than similarly infected 2-month-old rabbits (Gomez-Bautista *et al.*, 1987).

Epizootiology　*E. stiedae* is found worldwide, although rabbits bred for use in research are commonly free of the parasite. Transmission occurs by the fecal–oral route, as for other coccidia. The organism has also been experimentally transmitted by intravenous, intraperitoneal, and intramuscular administration of oocysts (Pellérdy, 1969).

Smetana (1933) demonstrated that infection of the entire liver occurred following ligation of the right bile duct and inoculation of *E. stiedae* oocysts. The study also showed that infection occurred earliest within the small intrahepatic ducts, leading to the theory that infection occurred via blood or lymph. The precise life cycle is still undetermined, although a number of studies have examined it (Horton, 1967; Owen, 1970; Rose, 1959). Sporozoites have been demonstrated in the lymph nodes following experimental inoculation (Horton, 1967; Rose, 1959).

Pathology　Necropsy often shows the liver to be enlarged and discolored, with multifocal yellowish white lesions of varying size (Fig. 10.2). Exudate in the biliary tree is common, along with dilatation of bile ducts. Microscopically, papillomatous hyperplasia of the ducts along with multiple life-cycle stages of the organism can be observed in the biliary epithelium (Fig. 10.3).

Diagnosis Infected rabbits may have decreased fibrinogen when compared to uninfected rabbits (Cam *et al.*, 2006). Serum bilirubin levels can rise to 305 mg/dl, increasing as soon as day 6 of infection and increasing through days 20–24 before moderating (Rose, 1959). Leukocytosis and anemia can be observed and acute phase proteins are notably increased by 7 days post infection (Freitas *et al.*, 2011).

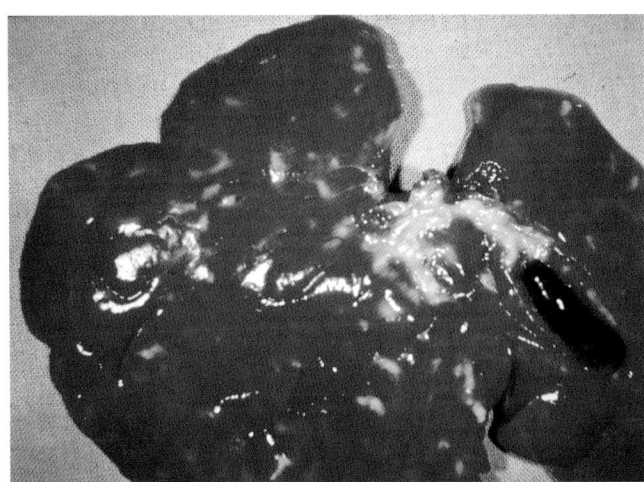

FIGURE 10.2   *Eimeria stiedae* lesions in a rabbit liver. *Photo courtesy of The Rabbit booklet (Copyright 1976, G.L. Van Hoosier, Jr.). Used with permission.*

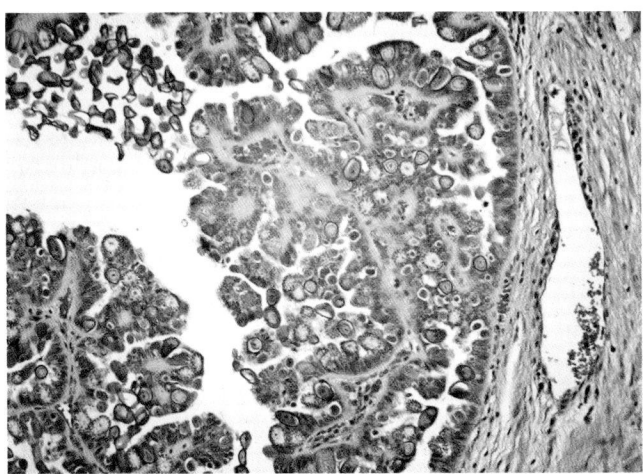

FIGURE 10.3   Histopathology section of a rabbit liver infested with *Eimeria stiedae.* The bile ducts are dilated with hyperplastic epithelium thrown into folds. The epithelial cells contain the various stages of developing coccidia and the lumen contains numerous oocysts. *Photo courtesy of Division of Comparative Medicine, MIT.*

Diagnosis can be made by examination of fecal material, by either flotation or concentration methods. Oocysts can also be detected within the gallbladder exudate (Hofing and Kraus, 1994). Alternatively, oocysts can sometimes be observed by microscopic examination of impression smears of the cut surface of the liver. Ultrasonography may be a useful tool for diagnosis, with dilated vessels and bile ducts and increased echogenicity of the liver parenchyma (Cam *et al.*, 2008).

Differential Diagnoses The hyperplastic biliary ducts can be mistaken grossly for neoplasia. Other types of parasitic hepatitis should be considered as differential diagnoses. Less frequently, hepatitis secondary to bacterial infections can occur.

Treatment, Prevention, and Control Control of the infection until development of natural immunity is one strategy to minimize the severity of disease. Davies *et al.* (1963) demonstrated that immunity occurs following a light infection with *E. stiedae*. In the rabbit, immunity to *Eimeria* may be lifelong (Niilo, 1967; Pellérdy, 1965). Prevention of hepatic coccidiosis with sulfaquinozaline in the feed (250 ppm) was shown to prevent infection when experimental challenged with 100,000 sporulated oocysts (Joyner *et al.*, 1987). Sulfonamides have been shown effective against *Eimeria* spp. (Hagen, 1958; Horton-Smith, 1947; Jankiewicz, 1945; Lund, 1954a; Tsunoda *et al.*, 1968). Treatment with toltrazuril (50 ppm in drinking water for one day) has been shown to effectively treat infected animals (Cam *et al.*, 2008). Thorough sanitation of potentially contaminated surfaces is critical to control of coccidiosis.

Research Complications Potential research complications arising from hepatic coccidiosis are considerable. The resulting liver damage and decreased weight gains can complicate both the supply of rabbits for research as well as adversely affect research protocols.

2. Intestinal Coccidiosis

Etiology There are at least 14 different pathogenic species of intestinal coccidia in rabbits, including *Eimeria coecicola, E. elongate, E exigua, E. intestinalis, E. flavescens, E. irresidua, E. magna, E. matsubayashii, E. media, E. nagnurensis, E. neoleporis, E. piriformis, E. vejdovskyi,* and *E. perforans* (Pakandl, 2009). All of these coccidia are presented here as a group rather than as individual species of intestinal coccidia.

Clinical Signs Although intestinal coccidiosis may be subclinical, clinical signs can range from mild to severe and can result in death of the animal. Postweanling rabbits are the most likely to experience mortality related to intestinal coccidiosis. Suckling rabbits (<20 days old) are generally considered to be resistant to infection (Pakandl and Hlaskova, 2007). Clinical signs also depend on the species of coccidia that are present. Severe diarrhea, weight loss, or mild reduction in growth rate are all possibilities. Fecal occult blood may be detected with *E. perforans* infection (Li and Ooi, 2009). Death is usually associated with severe dehydration subsequent to diarrhea (Frenkel, 1971).

Epizootiology Intestinal coccidiosis is a common rabbit disease worldwide (Varga, 1982). Transmission is by the fecal–oral route through ingestion of sporocysts. Unsporulated oocysts are passed in the feces and are not infective. Such oocysts will, however, sporulate to an infective stage within 3 days after shedding; thus, it is important that sanitation be frequent enough to remove infective stages from the environment. The oocyst burden of feces can be enormous. Gallazzi (Gallazzi, 1977) demonstrated that a subclinical carrier of intestinal coccidia had 408,000 oocysts/gram of feces and that a rabbit with diarrhea could shed in excess of 700,000 oocysts/gram of feces. Environmental contamination with oocysts can be a problem when large numbers of oocysts are being excreted.

The life cycles of *Eimeria* spp. are similar to those of other coccidia. Schizogony, gametogony, and sporogony are the three phases of this life cycle. Other sources can be consulted for greater detail on the life cycle of these protozoans (Davies *et al.*, 1963; Pakandl, 2009; Pakandl and Jelinkova, 2006; Pellérdy, 1965; Rutherford, 1943).

Pathology Lesions are apparent in the small and large intestines. Necrotic areas of the intestinal wall appear as white foci (Pakes, 1974; Pakes and Gerrity, 1994). The location and extent of the lesions depend on the species of coccidia.

Diagnosis Diagnosis of intestinal coccidiosis can be made through identification of the oocysts in the feces (Pakes and Gerrity, 1994). A PCR has been developed (Oliveira *et al.*, 2011) that differentiates between 11 of the different *Eimeria* species that infect the domestic rabbit. This test has excellent sensitivity, with the ability to detect 0.8–1.7 sporulated oocysts per sample. Smaller scale PCR for detection and differentiation between the more pathogenic species (*E. intestinalis*, *E. flavicenens*, and *E. stiedae*) has also been developed (Yan *et al.*, 2013).

Differential Diagnoses Other causes of diarrhea in rabbits should be considered including Tyzzer's disease, the Clostridial diseases, colibacillosis, *L. intracellularis*, enteric coronovairus and rotavirus, protozoons, or intestinal parasites.

Treatment, Prevention, and Control Because intestinal coccidiosis is most common in postweanling rabbits, prevention of the disease should focus on the preweaning period. An oral vaccination has been developed and consists of a nonpathogenic strain of *E. magna*. This vaccine is sprayed into the nest box when rabbits are 25 days of age. The preweanling rabbits develop immunity subsequent to infection with the nonpathogenic strain and are then resistant to wild-type strains of *E. magna* at 35 days of age (Drouet-Viard *et al.*, 1997).

Other oral vaccines developed from various *Eimeria* strains are also in development (Akpo *et al.*, 2012).

Prevention and control of infection can be accomplished by providing 0.02% sulfamerazine or 0.05% sulfaquinoxaline in the drinking water (Kraus *et al.*, 1984). A combination of sulfaquinoxaline, strict sanitation, and elimination of infected animals has been shown to eliminate intestinal coccidiosis from a rabbit breeding colony (Pakes and Gerrity, 1994). As for hepatic coccidiosis, sulfaquinoxaline provided in the feed (250 ppm) is an effective treatment.

Research Complications Intestinal coccidiosis can impact studies of the gastrointestinal tract, or have an impact on survival of postweanling rabbits.

3. Cryptosporidiosis

Etiology The protozoan organism *Cryptosporidium cuniculus* has been found in the intestinal tract of the rabbit (Hadfield and Chalmers, 2012; Inman and Takeuchi, 1979; Kaupke *et al.*, 2014; Rehg *et al.*, 1979; Robinson *et al.*, 2010; Shiibashi *et al.*, 2006; Zhang *et al.*, 2012).

Clinical Signs Clinical signs related to cryptosporidiosis seem to be quite variable in the rabbit. A large farm outbreak (Kaupke *et al.*, 2014) had rabbits that presented with lethargy, anorexia and diarrhea. Animals showing clinical signs died within 5–10 days. The stress of weaning is thought to have exacerbated these signs. Another report describes small intestinal dilatation observed during surgery in a rabbit without other clinical signs (Inman and Takeuchi, 1979).

Epizootiology Transmission is likely via ingestion of thick-walled sporulated oocysts. Experimentally infected juvenile rabbits began shedding oocysts in their feces 4–7 days post infection and continued to shed until 14 days post infection without clinical signs (Robinson *et al.*, 2010).

Pathology Histopathology of the small intestine of the reported rabbit was characterized by shortened, blunted villi and mild edema of the lamina propria. The lacteals of the ileum were also dilated, and an inflammatory response was observed (Inman and Takeuchi, 1979).

Diagnosis *C. cuniculus* is emerging as a potential zoonotic pathogen with several reports in recent years (Chalmers *et al.*, 2009, 2011; Zhang *et al.*, 2012). In response to this, real-time PCR assays are in development (Hadfield and Chalmers, 2012) that detect and differentiate *C. cuniculus* from *C. parvum* and *C. hominis*.

Differential Diagnoses *C. cuniculus* can only be differentiated from *C. hominis* and *C. parvum* via genetic analysis (Robinson *et al.*, 2010). Differential diagnoses would include infection with *Clostridium piliforme*, *C. spiroforme*, *C. difficile*, *E. coli*, *Lawsonia intracellularis*, coronavirus, rotavirus, protozoans, or intestinal parasites.

Treatment, Prevention, and Control Minimizing stress can possibly prevent or reduce clinical signs

(Kaupke *et al.*, 2014). Antibiotics were ineffective in the large farm outbreak. Presumably, supportive care (fluids) would be indicated in animals showing clinical signs (Schoeb *et al.*, 2007). Prevention requires husbandry and sanitation practices that prevent exposure.

Research Complications This organism is emerging as a human pathogen, so appropriate precautions should be made to protect research personnel from rabbits positive for *C. cuniculus*.

4. Encephalitozoonosis

Etiology The etiologic agent responsible for encephalitozoonosis is *Encephalitozoon cuniculi.* This agent is historically known by the name *Nosema cuniculi* (Pakes and Gerrity, 1994) and has been divided into three strains (I – rabbit strain, II – mouse strain, III – dog strain) (Didier *et al.*, 1995). The disease was first described in 1922 as an infectious encephalomyelitis causing motor paralysis in young rabbits (Wright and Craighead, 1922).

Clinical Signs Encephalitozoonosis typically has a delayed onset (weeks to months post infection) prior to the exhibition of clinical signs. Early infection affects the kidney, liver and lung, while alterations later in the infection are most severe in the kidneys and brain (Kunzel and Joachim, 2010). The organism can be found in the tissues without an inflammatory response (Pakes and Gerrity, 1994).

Although named for the motor paralysis in young rabbits, the disease is usually latent. If clinical signs are present, they can include convulsions, tremors, torticollis, paresis, and coma (Pattison *et al.*, 1971) as well as signs of kidney failure. Intrauterine infection can result in phacoclastic uveitis leading to rupture of the lens capsule (Kunzel and Joachim, 2010).

Epizootiology Transmission is likely horizontal via direct contact or environmental contamination (Kunzel and Joachim, 2010), primarily from ingestion of infected urine (Schoeb *et al.*, 2007; Wasson and Peper, 2000). The pathogen can also be transmitted vertically, as evidenced by *in utero* PCR positivity reported by Baneux and Pognan (2003).

Pathology The kidneys commonly have lesions at necropsy. Typically, there are multiple white, pinpoint areas or gray, indented areas on the renal cortical surface (Kraus *et al.*, 1984). Microscopically, these areas are characterized by granulomatous inflammation. Interstitial infiltration of lymphocytes and plasma cells and tubular degeneration may also be present (Flatt and Jackson, 1970). Granulomatous encephalitis is a characteristic lesion (Fig. 10.4) (Pakes and Gerrity, 1994). Lesions of the spinal cord can also occur (Koller, 1969). The organisms are often not observed in histologic sections of the lesions. Organisms may be seen floating free in the tubules of the kidney (Pakes and Gerrity, 1994).

Diagnosis Diagnosis of encephalitozoonosis can be made using several different methods. Histologic examination of tissues and observation of the organism is definitive. Brain and kidney samples yield the best detection rates for histopathological diagnosis (Leipig *et al.*, 2013). The *Encephalitozoon* organism does not stain well with hematoxylin and eosin, and is better demonstrated using Giemsa stain, Gram stain, or Goodpasture's carbol fuchsin stain (Pakes, 1974). Many different serologic tests exist for the organism. Indirect fluorescence antibody technique and ELISA are both available and reliable (Kunzel and Joachim, 2010).

Advances in diagnostic techniques have been made in human medicine due to the susceptibility of immunosuppressed patients to this particular infection. Several PCR tests for diagnosis and species differentiation of encephalitozoonosis have been developed (Croppo *et al.*, 1998; Franzen *et al.*, 1998; Weiss and Vossbrinck, 1998). PCR can be performed on the intestine, brain, heart, liver, lung, or kidney tissue with a good (86%) overall detection rate reported (Leipig *et al.*, 2013).

Differential Diagnoses If the animals are demonstrating motor paralysis, conditions such as splay leg should be considered. For neurological signs, consider bacterial meningitis due to *P. multocida* infection or rabbit hemorrhagic disease.

Treatment, Prevention, and Control Prevention and control of the organism in the colony are done by elimination of the organism from the colony of infected rabbits. Because this is a latent disease in rabbits, serologic methods must be used to identify carriers of the organism. The indirect fluorescence antibody test has

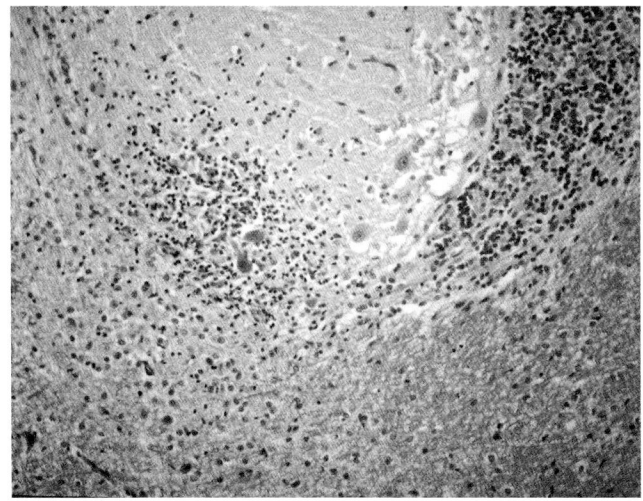

FIGURE 10.4 Histopathology section of a rabbit brain demonstrating small granulomas composed primarily of glial cells present in both the cerebrum and the cerebellum. They are usually observed in association with, or adjacent to, a capillary and are suggestive of *Encephalitozoon* infection. *Photo courtesy of Division of Comparative Medicine, MIT.*

been used successfully to identify infected rabbits (Cox, 1977). The elimination of infected rabbits must be accompanied by disinfection of the environment. Several disinfectants have been effective against this organism. Encephalitozoon was killed by 2% (v/v) Lysol, 10% (v/v) Formalin, and 70% (v/v) ethanol (Shadduck and Polley, 1978) 1% hydrogen peroxide, and 1% sodium hydroxide (Kunzel and Joachim, 2010).

Successful treatment and prevention of *E. cuniculi* in the rabbit has been reported with use of fenbendazole (Suter *et al.*, 2001). For cases of phacoclastic uveitis, removal of the lens is the treatment of choice (Kunzel and Joachim, 2010).

Research Complications Encephalitozoonosis is most commonly subclinical disease, which makes it difficult to determine the effects it may have on research. Granulomatous reactions would complicate renal physiology and neurologic research. Depression of the IgG response and an increase in the IgM response to *Brucella abortus* antigens has been demonstrated in rabbits infected with *Encephalitozoon* organisms (Cox, 1977).

Encephalitozoonosis is also a recognized disease in immunodeficient humans. It is recommended that such individuals seek medical counsel prior to handling rabbits. Isolates from humans have been shown to be infectious for rabbits (Mathis *et al.*, 1997).

D. Arthropod and Helminth Diseases

1. Psoroptes cuniculi *(Rabbit Ear Mite)*

Etiology *Psoroptes cuniculi* is a nonburrowing mite and the causative agent of psoroptic mange, also called ear mange, ear canker, or otoacariasis. The organism is distributed worldwide, but with modern husbandry practices, it is mostly historical in laboratory rabbit colonies (Schoeb *et al.*, 2007).

Clinical Signs Lesions occur primarily in the inner surfaces of the external ear. The lesions are pruritic and can result in scratching, head shaking, pain, and even self-mutilation (Hofing and Kraus, 1994). A tan, crusty exudate accumulates in the ears over the lesions and can become quite extensive and thick (Fig. 10.5). The skin under the crust is moist and reddened. The ears may become malodorous.

Epizootiology All stages of the mite (egg, larva, protonymph, and adult) occur on the host. Early in the infestation, mites feed on sloughed skin cells and lipids. As local inflammation increases, they ingest serum, hemoglobin, and red blood cells (Deloach and Wright, 1981; Hofing and Kraus, 1994). The entire life cycle is complete in 21 days. Mites are relatively resistant to drying and temperature and can survive off the host for 7–20 days in a temperature range of 5–30°C and relative humidity of 20–75%.

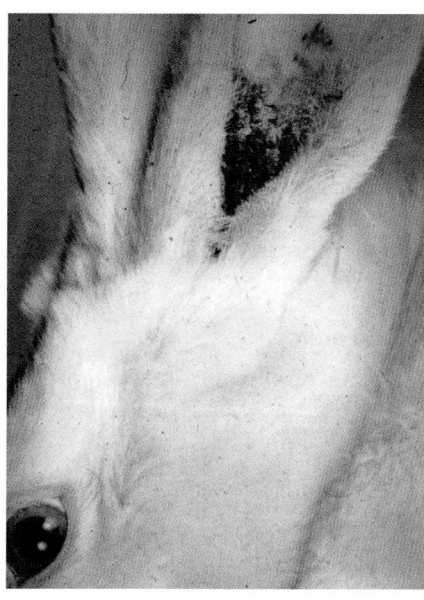

FIGURE 10.5 Dry, brown, crusty exudate on the inner surface of the pinna, consistent with *Psoroptes cuniculi*. *Photo courtesy of The Rabbit booklet (Copyright 1976, G.L. Van Hoosier, Jr.). Used with permission.*

Pathology Lesions are characterized histologically by chronic inflammation, hypertrophy of the Malpighian layer, parakeratosis, and epithelial sloughing. A hypersensitivity response to the mites, mite feces, and saliva likely contributes to lesions (Hofing and Kraus, 1994).

Diagnosis Mites are large enough to be seen with the unaided eye or with an otoscope. Material scraped from the inner surface of the ear can also be examined using a dissecting microscope. Mites are oval-shaped with well-developed legs that project beyond the body margin. Adult males measure 431–547 μm × 322–462 μm, and females measure 403–749 μm × 351–499 μm (Hofing and Kraus, 1994).

Differential Diagnoses Rarely, infection with *Sarcoptes scabiei* or *Cheyletiella parasitovorax* should be considered as differential diagnoses.

Treatment, Prevention, and Control Several successful treatments have been reported. Prior to local treatment, the ears should be cleaned gently to remove accumulated exudate. One treatment involves the application of 3% rotenone in mineral oil (1:3) every 5 days for 30 days. Ivermectin is an effective treatment at dosages of 400–440 μg/kg SC or IM (Curtis *et al.*, 1990; McKellar *et al.*, 1992; Wright and Riner, 1985). One or two doses were utilized for effective treatment. Treatment of moderate to severe infestations with ivermectin alone can fail. Using adjunct vitamin therapy to minimize oxidative tissue damage has been shown to enhance treatment success (Singh *et al.*, 2012). A single dose of topical selamectin at a minimum of 6 mg/kg selamectin (Kurtdede *et al.*, 2007) and a single injection of eprinomectin at 200 or 300 μg/kg (Pan *et al.*, 2006) were found to be effective treatments. Regardless of treatment modality, it is generally recommended that the entire group of rabbits be treated at the same time. Heat (40°C) and desiccation (<20% humidity) will kill parasites that are not on the host (Arlain *et al.*, 1984).

Vaccine targets have been investigated, with gut surface antigen being the primary focus (Rossi *et al.*, 2007).

Research Complications P. *cuniculi* has been associated with immune suppression and a systemic inflammatory reaction (Shang *et al.*, 2014). Ear trauma secondary to *Psoroptes* infestation can limit access to the auricular artery and veins.

2. Cheyletiella *spp.* (C. parasitovorax, C. takahasii, C. ochotonae, C. johnsoni)

Etiology *Cheyletiella* mites are nonburrowing skin mites of rabbits. They are distributed worldwide. Several closely related species have been reported to occur on rabbits, namely, *C. parasitovorax*, *C. takahasii*, *C. ochotonae*, and *C. johnsoni* (Hofing and Kraus, 1994).

Clinical Signs The anatomic site most commonly infested is the area over the scapulae. There may be mild hair loss in the area, and the skin may have a gray–white scale (Cloyd and Moorhead, 1976). Affected rabbits do not scratch, and there is no evidence of pruritus. Skin lesions are mild or nonexistent.

Epizootiology All stages (egg, larva, pupa, and adult) in the life cycle occur on the host. Mites remain in association with the keratin layer of the skin and feed on tissue fluid (Myktowycz, 1957). Transmission is probably by direct contact (Schoeb *et al.*, 2007).

Pathology When present, skin lesions are characterized by mild dermatitis, hyperkeratosis, and an inflammatory cell infiltrate (Hofing and Kraus, 1994).

Diagnosis Mites can be isolated by scraping or brushing fur in the affected areas onto a slide. Clearing samples with 5–10% potassium hydroxide will improve visibility of the mites, which can then be identified using a dissecting microscope. The female measures 450 × 200 μm, and the male is 320 × 160 μm. *Cheyletiella* mites have a large, distinctive curved claw on the palpi (Pegg, 1970).

Differential Diagnoses Other skin mites (such as *Sarcoptes scabei*) or fur mites (*Leporacarus gibbus*) that can affect rabbits should be considered as well as the possibility of dermatophytosis.

Treatment, Prevention, and Control Topical acaricides are often used and are effective at controlling infestation. Ivermectin (subcutaneous or subcutaneous and oral) and selamectin (topical) treatments have been used successfully. Eggs in the environment can reinfest the host, so posttreatment environmental sanitation is important (Mellgren and Bergvall, 2008).

Research Complications Cheyletid mites can cause a transient dermatitis in humans who are in close contact with infested animals (Cohen, 1980; Lee, 1991). For this reason, these mites can be considered a zoonotic pathogen.

3. Sarcoptes scabiei

Etiology *Sarcoptes scabiei* is a burrowing mite and the causative agent of sarcoptic mange. Mites of the genus *Sarcoptes* are generally considered to be one species, *S. scabiei*, but are often further identified by a variety name corresponding to the host species (e.g., *S. scabiei* var. *cuniculi*). The organisms are commonly referred to as itch or scab mites. The disease has a worldwide distribution.

Clinical Signs Affected rabbits will exhibit intense pruritus with hair loss and abrasions as a resulting from scratching. Serous encrustations on the skin and secondary bacterial infections are common. There has been one report of a secondary infection with the yeast *Malassezia* (Radi, 2004). Anemia and leukopenia can also be observed in affected rabbits (Arlain *et al.*, 1988).

Epizootiology Sarcoptic are similar to notoedric mites (*Notoedres cati*) in morphology, life cycle, and public health significance. Mites burrow and produce an intensely pruritic dermatitis. Lesions are most common on the head (Hofing and Kraus, 1994).

All stages of sarcoptic mange mites occur on the host. The females burrow into the skin to lay eggs. Young larvae can also be found in the skin, whereas older larvae, nymphs, and males reside on the skin surface. Mites feed on lymph and epithelial cells (Hofing and Kraus, 1994).

Pathology Amyloidosis of the liver and glomerulus have been reported in rabbits with severe infestation (Arlain *et al.*, 1990). The skin itself is hyperplastic and hyperkeratotic, with inflammatory response evident in the dermis (Schoeb *et al.*, 2007).

Diagnosis Because *Sarcoptes* is a burrowing mite, skin scrapings are necessary to diagnose infestation. Samples may be cleared with 5–10% potassium hydroxide. Female mites measure 303–450 μm × 250–350 μm. The body shape is round, and the legs are very short.

Differential Diagnoses Other causes of dermatitis in rabbits (such as *Cheyletiella* spp., P. *cuniculi* or dermatophytosis) should be considered.

Treatment, Prevention, and Control Ivermectin is effective at eliminating infestation at 100 μg/kg administered subcutaneously. A single topical dose of selamectin at 10–12 mg/kg reduced the number of mites found on skin scrapings of Angora rabbits (Kurtdede *et al.*, 2007) and eliminated clinical signs and parasitic infestation in a group of mixed-breed rabbits at a dose of 30 mg/rabbit (Farmaki *et al.*, 2009). As with *Psoroptes*, more 'natural' treatments are being investigated with good preliminary results from eugenol (Pasay *et al.*, 2010) and *Eupatorium* spp. (Nong *et al.*, 2013).

Research Complications No specific research complications have been reported. *Sarcoptes* can cause a self-limiting dermatitis in humans.

4. Other Arthropod Parasites

A wide variety of arthropod parasites has been reported in wild rabbits but they are extremely rare in laboratory rabbits. For an extensive listing the reader is referred to other sources (Hofing and Kraus, 1994).

5. Oxyuriasis (Pinworm Infestation)

Etiology Historically, the rabbit pinworm was identified as *Oxyuris ambigua*, but is now known as *Passalurus ambiguus* (Hofing and Kraus, 1994).

Clinical Signs Even when rabbits have heavy oxyurid burdens, clinical signs are not usually apparent (Erikson, 1944; Soulsby, 1968). One case report described unsatisfactory breeding performance and poor condition in a rabbit colony infested with the parasite.

Epizootiology *P. ambiguus* has a direct life cycle. Mature pinworms are found in the lumen of the cecum or colon of the rabbit. After ingestion, the eggs hatch in the small intestine, and the larvae molt with maturation in the cecum. The prepatent period is between 56 and 64 days (Taffs, 1976).

Transmission occurs easily via ingestion, given that individual rabbits have been found with over 1000 adult parasites (Hofing and Kraus, 1994) and that embryonated eggs pass out in the feces and are immediately infective (Schoeb *et al.*, 2007; Taffs, 1976).

Pathology Minimal to no lesions are associated with this pinworm (Schoeb *et al.*, 2007).

Diagnosis Eggs can be found in feces, cecum, or colon.

Differential Diagnoses This is the only reported pinworm in rabbits and it is not known to cause lesions or disease.

Treatment, Prevention, and Control Several successful treatment strategies for rabbit oxyuriasis have been reported. Piperazine citrate at 100 mg/100 ml of drinking water for 1 day was successful in eliminating infestation (Hofing and Kraus, 1994). At 25 and 50 ppm, fenbendazole mixed in the food for 5 days eliminated all immature and adult pinworms (Duwell and Brech, 1981). Subcutaneous doses of ivermectin (0.4 mg/kg) were reported to be ineffective in reducing the burden of *Passalurus* organisms in field populations of snowshoe hares (*Lepus americanus*) (Sovell and Holmes, 1996). Due to the direct life cycle, strict husbandry and sanitation practices are required to prevent introduction and spread throughout a rabbit colony (Schoeb *et al.*, 2007).

Research Complications None have been described.

E. Mycotic Diseases

1. Dermatophytosis

Etiology Dermatophytosis, also known as 'ringworm' or 'tinea', refers to a skin infection caused by a dermatophyte, a keratinophilic and keratinolytic fungus (Chermette *et al.*, 2008; Mendez-Tovar, 2010; Robert and Pihet, 2008). Dermatophytes are a group of closely related filamentous fungi that are able to invade the stratum corneum of the epidermis and keratinized tissues including the skin, nail, and hair (Kanbe, 2008). Dermatophytes can infect various animal species, including humans, and the disease is considered contagious and zoonotic (Cafarchia *et al.*, 2012b; Chermette *et al.*, 2008; Kramer *et al.*, 2012). The zoophilic dermatophytes *Trichophyton mentagrophytes* and *Microsporum canis* infect rabbits (Cafarchia *et al.*, 2010, 2012a; Chermette *et al.*, 2008; Kramer *et al.*, 2012).

Clinical Signs The general presentation of dermatophytosis in animals is an area of circular alopecia with erythematous margin and thin desquamation (Chermette *et al.*, 2008). Pruritus is generally absent and lesions can be single or multiple (Chermette *et al.*, 2008). Although lesions can be localized in any region, the anterior part of the body and the head seem to be more frequently involved (Chermette *et al.*, 2008). In rabbits, lesions are often found on the ears and the face (around the eyes and on the nose) and these lesions show scaling and crusting (Chermette *et al.*, 2008; Kramer *et al.*, 2012). Infected rabbits may not exhibit clinical signs and may serve as carriers (Balsari *et al.*, 1981; Cafarchia *et al.*, 2010, 2012a; Chermette *et al.*, 2008; Lopez-Martinez *et al.*, 1984).

Epizootiology Although dermatophytosis is a common cutaneous disease of rabbits and other animals, its incidence is low in well-managed laboratory animal facilities (Chermette *et al.*, 2008; Connole *et al.*, 2000). Contact with infected animals or contaminated environments represent the major risk of infection (Chermette *et al.*, 2008). Young or immunocompromised rabbits are more susceptible (Connole *et al.*, 2000; Kramer *et al.*, 2012). On rabbit farms, the occurrence of lesions, the age of the rabbits, and farm management practices were identified as the most significant risk factors for the occurrence of dermatophytosis (Cafarchia *et al.*, 2010).

Clinically, disease expression varies depending on the host, fungal species, and enzyme production (Cafarchia *et al.*, 2012a; Vermout *et al.*, 2008). The pathogenesis involves contact, adherence, germination, invasion, and penetration (Cafarchia *et al.*, 2012a; Mendez-Tovar, 2010; Vermout *et al.*, 2008). These stages can be associated with the secretion of enzymes that degrade the infected tissue components (Cafarchia *et al.*, 2012a). *T. mentagrophytes* isolates from rabbits with skin lesions showed a significantly higher elastase and gelatinase activity compared to isolates from clinically unaffected rabbits and from the environment (Cafarchia *et al.*, 2012a). Furthermore, *M. canis* isolates from rabbits with skin lesions showed a significantly higher lipase activity compared to isolates from clinically unaffected rabbits and from the environment (Cafarchia *et al.*, 2012a).

Pathology   Histopathologic changes consist of mild to severe dermatitis.

Diagnosis   The Wood's lamp (ultraviolet light) method and direct examination of hairs and scales are fast and affordable tests (Chermette *et al.*, 2008; Robert and Pihet, 2008). The Wood's lamp can be used to screen for infections caused by *M. canis* (Chermette *et al.*, 2008). *M. canis*-infected hairs fluoresce with an apple-green color and can be collected for microscopic examination and culture (Chermette *et al.*, 2008). The results of the Wood's lamp examination should be systematically confirmed by direct examination of hairs and/or fungal culture (Chermette *et al.*, 2008). Deep skin scraping should be performed to obtain hair and scales and confirm the absence of ectoparasites such as mites that can be associated with dermatophytosis (Cafarchia *et al.*, 2010; Chermette *et al.*, 2008). Clearing solutions such as chlorolactophenol or 10% potassium hydroxide (KOH) can then be used to digest keratin prior to microscopic examination (Chermette *et al.*, 2008; Robert and Pihet, 2008). The surface of the hair typically demonstrates clusters or chains of arthroconidia (Chermette *et al.*, 2008). Giemsa-stained skin scrapings allow observation of the arthroconidia along the hair (Chermette *et al.*, 2008).

Fungal culture is the 'gold standard' for the diagnosis of dermatophytosis and the only method for the phenotypic identification of dermatophyte species (Chermette *et al.*, 2008). The fungal culture must be complemented with direct examination of samples for optimal interpretation of the results (Chermette *et al.*, 2008; Robert and Pihet, 2008). Samples for fungal culture may include hairs, scales, crusts, skin scrapes, and tissue biopsies (Chermette *et al.*, 2008). Samples that are obtained from the margin of new skin lesions enhance fungal recovery by culture (Chermette *et al.*, 2008). A brush can also be impressed on the surface of the culture medium after combing the fur and obtaining fungal spores with hair and debris (Robert and Pihet, 2008). Two media that can be used for fungal culture include Sabouraud dextrose agar (supplemented with cycloheximide and antibiotics) and Dermatophyte Test Media (DTM) (Chermette *et al.*, 2008; Robert and Pihet, 2008). If histological examination is performed, periodic acid Schiff (PAS), or methylamine silver stain can be used to detect arthroconidia and hyphae (Chermette *et al.*, 2008). Molecular methods to identify dermatophytes have also been described and include PCR-RFLP and sequencing of the internal transcribed spacer (ITS) region (Chermette *et al.*, 2008; Kanbe, 2008; Robert and Pihet, 2008). Specific identification of the dermatophyte is essential for a better understanding of the epidemiology and prevention of the disease (Chermette *et al.*, 2008).

Differential Diagnoses   The differential diagnoses can include other dermatoses caused by bacteria or ectoparasites (Cafarchia *et al.*, 2010; Chermette *et al.*, 2008).

Treatment, Prevention, and Control   Dermatophytosis is considered a self-limiting disease in immunocompetent animals (Chermette *et al.*, 2008). However, rabbits with dermatophytosis should be culled or separated from a laboratory animal colony due to the contagious and zoonotic nature of the disease (Chermette *et al.*, 2008).

The best method to prevent dermatophyte infection is to prevent contact with infected animals and contaminated environments including fomites (Chermette *et al.*, 2008). An animal that contacts an infected animal or a contaminated environment can be washed with antifungal shampoo (Chermette *et al.*, 2008). Two vaccines incorporating live attenuated cells of *T. mentagrophytes* have been used to prevent disease in rabbits and other animals (Lund and Deboer, 2008). The Mentavak vaccine is from Russia and the Trichopelen vaccine (http://www.bioveta.cz/en/veterinary-division/home/) is from the Czech Republic (Lund and Deboer, 2008). Trichopelen is also indicated for treatment of dermatophytosis (Lund and Deboer, 2008).

Enzootic dermatophytosis may be the result of the high resistance of the arthroconidia in the environment, the number of host species involved, and the close confinement of animals (Chermette *et al.*, 2008). Isolation or culling of infected animals plus environmental and equipment disinfection are required to control this disease (Chermette *et al.*, 2008). A 1:10 dilution of household bleach or a 0.2% enilconazole solution can be used to disinfect the environment (Chermette *et al.*, 2008). Infected animals should be handled with care to avoid zoonotic transmission (Chermette *et al.*, 2008).

If treatment is elected, antifungal treatment shortens the course of the infection and reduces dissemination of arthroconidia to other animals and into the environment (Chermette *et al.*, 2008). Systemic and topical antifungal treatment can be used in combination (Chermette *et al.*, 2008). Systemic drugs include griseofulvin (gold standard) or azole derivatives such as itraconazole (Chermette *et al.*, 2008; Vella, 2013). It is important to know that these drugs can have side effects and be contraindicated due to their teratogenic potential (Chermette *et al.*, 2008). Topical treatment may include 0.2% enilconazole, a combination of 2% miconazole and 2% chlorhexidine, or lime sulfur (Chermette *et al.*, 2008; Vella, 2013). Treatment can be discontinued after two negative fungal culture results (Chermette *et al.*, 2008).

Research Complications Dematophyte lesions could confound histological studies involving the skin (Connole *et al.*, 2000).

2. *Pneumocystosis*

Etiology Pneumocystosis in rabbits is caused by the fungus *Pneumocystis oryctolagi* (Dei-Cas *et al.*, 2006).

Clinical Signs Infected rabbits may not develop clinical signs, but immunocompromised hosts can develop severe interstitial pneumonitis (Dei-Cas *et al.*, 2006; Sheldon, 1959).

Epizootiology Corticosteroid treatment can induce disease in infected rabbits; however, spontaneous disease (not associated with drug treatment) can also occur (Dei-Cas *et al.*, 2006; Sheldon, 1959; Soulez *et al.*, 1989). *P. oryctolagi* is transmitted through the transplacental route (Cere *et al.*, 1997a; Sanchez *et al.*, 2007) and through direct contact and aerosolization (Cere and Polack, 1999; Cere *et al.*, 1997b; Hughes, 1982; Wakefield, 1994, 1996). Spontaneous pneumocystosis can occur at weaning, evolves during 7–10 days, and induces lung lesions and blood biochemical profile changes (Dei-Cas *et al.*, 2006; Soulez *et al.*, 1989). The organisms attach specifically to Type 1 epithelial alveolar cells and proliferate, filling up pulmonary alveoli cavities leading to respiratory failure (Dei-Cas *et al.*, 2006). Changes in surfactant appear to be necessary for *Pneumocystis* proliferation (Prevost *et al.*, 1997). *Pneumocystis* colonization decreases and becomes very low in 60-day-old rabbits (Dei-Cas *et al.*, 2006). Most rabbits recover from pneumocystosis within 3–4 weeks (Dei-Cas *et al.*, 2006). The spontaneous resolution of pneumocystosis in rabbits may be associated with expression of interferon gamma (Allaert *et al.*, 1997). Immunosuppression may be suspected in cases of severe pulmonary disease associated with spontaneous pneumocystosis (Sheldon, 1959).

Pathology Histologically, cystic forms of the organism can be detected in the lungs using toluidine blue O (TBO), GMS, or PAS stains (Dei-Cas *et al.*, 2006). Interstitial thickening of alveolar septa and increased numbers of Type 2 epithelial alveolar cells are characteristic of this infection (Creusy *et al.*, 1996).

Diagnosis For diagnosis, samples from nasal cavity wash, or *post-mortem*, from terminal bronchoalveolar lavage (BAL) or lung homogenates can be used for *Pneumocystis* detection by nested PCR (Dei-Cas *et al.*, 2006; Tamburrini *et al.*, 1999; Wakefield, 1996). Serological diagnosis can also be performed (Tamburrini *et al.*, 1999). Lung impression smears, lung-homogenate smears, and BAL fluid samples can be stained for microscopic detection of *Pneumocystis* (Dei-Cas *et al.*, 2006). Useful stains include TBO, Gomori–Grocott's methenamine silver nitrate (GMS), and methanol–Giemsa or Giemsa-like stains (Dei-Cas *et al.*, 2006). Other useful detection methods include phase-contrast microscopy and the use of *Pneumocystis*-specific fluorescein-labeled antibodies (Dei-Cas *et al.*, 2006).

Differential Diagnoses *P. multocida* can induce respiratory disease in rabbits and can be included in the differential diagnoses.

Treatment, Prevention, and Control For prevention, new rabbits should be negative for *Pneumocystis*. Cotrimoxazole treatment and nested PCR have been used as a screening mechanism to eliminate *Pneumocystis* from colony-maintained rabbits (Cere *et al.*, 1997c). Decontamination practices and air filtration were also important for eradication (Cere *et al.*, 1997c). Confirmation of a *Pneumocystis*-free status in a rabbit colony was demonstrated by negative PCR results and/or failure to induce pneumocystosis after experimental corticosteroid challenge (Dei-Cas *et al.*, 2006).

Research Complications Research studies may be affected if rabbits of unknown *Pneumocystis* status are experimentally treated with corticosteroids or other immunosuppressant drugs (Sheldon, 1959). Pulmonary lesions may be found in infected rabbits and could potentially confound respiratory research studies (Sheldon, 1959).

F. Management-Related Diseases

1. *Gastric Trichobezoar (Hairball)*

Etiology Unknown.

Clinical Signs Trichobezoar is often subclinical. If the trichobezoar causes partial or complete blockage, clinical signs of gastric or intestinal obstruction will result. Death can occur due to prolonged anorexia and metabolic imbalances (Gillett *et al.*, 1983). It appears that obstruction of the pylorus, and not the volume of the gastric mass, is the critical factor in determining the clinical progress of the animal (Leary *et al.*, 1984).

Epizootiology The condition occurs sporadically in rabbit colonies.

Pathology The discovery of a hairball in a rabbit is often an incidental finding during necropsy. Up to 21% of rabbits have been found to have gastric trichobezoars during routine necropsy (Leary *et al.*, 1984). Gastric rupture can also result from an obstructive trichobezoar (Gillett *et al.*, 1983).

Diagnosis Diagnosis is often difficult because the clinical signs are nonspecific and the disease often progresses gradually. Some cases involving acute pyloric obstruction result in sudden clinical disease and rapid clinical decline of the animal. Manual palpation may indicate the presence of a firm mass in the cranial abdomen. Gastric radiographs using contrast media may aid in the diagnosis, but definitive diagnosis is often made during exploratory surgery (Gillett *et al.*, 1983).

Differential Diagnoses Constipation and intestinal foreign body should be considered in the differential list.

Treatment, Prevention, and Control   Treatment of trichobezoar is often unsuccessful. Oral administration of mineral oil at 10 ml/day has been reported (Suckow and Douglas, 1997). Alternatively, oral administration of 5–10 ml of fresh pineapple juice daily has been reported as a possible treatment modality (Harkness and Wagner, 1995). If medical treatment does not resolve the condition, a gastrotomy should be performed. Early surgical intervention is important in such cases, as other, subsequent metabolic abnormalities may quickly increase the surgical risk to the rabbit (Bergdall and Dysko, 1994).

Research Complications   None have been reported.

2. Traumatic Vertebral Fracture (Broken Back)

Etiology   Subluxation or compression fractures of lumbar vertebrae are often secondary to struggling during restraint, particularly when the hindquarters of the rabbit are not supported (Bergdall and Dysko, 1994). The seventh lumbar vertebra (L7) or its caudal articular processes are considered the most frequent sites of fractures, with fracture occurring more commonly than dislocation (Flatt *et al.*, 1974).

Clinical Signs   Clinical signs include posterior paresis or paralysis, loss of sensation in the hindlimbs, urinary and/or fecal incontinence, and perineal staining.

Pathology   Spinal cord hemorrhage and necrosis can be found.

Diagnosis   Diagnosis is based on clinical signs, history of recent restraint, struggling or other trauma, and palpation or radiographic analysis of the vertebral column.

Differential Diagnoses   Spinal cord trauma.

Treatment, Prevention, and Control   Euthanasia of affected animals is usually warranted. Moderate cases (subluxation with spinal edema) may resolve over time. The decision to euthanize should be based on severity of clinical signs. Supportive care includes regular expression of the urinary bladder and prevention and treatment of decubital ulcers. Corticosteroid and diuretic therapy may be effective for cases of subluxation with spinal edema (Bergdall and Dysko, 1994).

Research Complications   Loss of valuable research animals is the primary complication.

3. Ulcerative Pododermatitis

Although the condition is often referred to as 'sore hocks,' the correct name is ulcerative pododermatitis. Despite the name, the condition rarely affects the hocks, but rather occurs most frequently on the plantar surface of the metatarsal and, to a lesser extent, the metacarpal regions. The condition is believed to be initiated by wire-floor housing, foot stomping, or having thin plantar fur pads. Poor sanitation may worsen the condition. Solid resting areas on the cage floors are associated with a decreased incidence of ulcerative pododermatitis,

whereas a high-energy diet and increased body condition scores are associated with an increased incidence (Sanchez *et al.*, 2012).

G. Heritable Diseases

The whole genome sequence from a single female rabbit of the partially inbred Thorbecke rabbit strain was published in 2009 (OryCun2.0; accession AAGW02000000). The annotated assembly is now available at the National Center for Biotechnology Information (NCBI), the University of California Santa Cruz (UCSC), and Ensembl. The rabbit chosen by the Broad Institute for sequencing was obtained from Covance in 2004. The assembly has 2.24 Gbp in 21 autosome and X chromosomes and 489 Mbp in 3219 unplaced scaffolds including mitochondria (Gertz *et al.*, 2013). The nucleotide sequence of the complete mitochondrial DNA (mtDNA) molecule of the *O. cuniculus* has been determined (Gissi *et al.*, 1998). The compositional differences between the two mtDNA strands have also been detailed (Gissi *et al.*, 1998).

The sequencing of the rabbit genome, understanding of rabbit reproduction, and advances in genetic manipulation in the mouse production colonies have led to the ability to produce genetically engineered rabbits. The rabbit offers an alternative model when size or tissue characteristics of a genetically modified mouse are not appropriate. These genetic manipulation techniques were first described by Robl (Robl and Burnside, 1994). Additional methods have been developed and include pronuclear injection of single cell embryos, injection of genetically modified embryonic stem cells into blastocysts, sperm-mediated gene transfer, and genetically modified somatic cell and nuclear transfer (Christensen and Peng, 2012). Commercial companies have been formed to provide genetic modification services with emphasis on production of a unique protein in the milk of rabbits.

This section will outline spontaneous hereditary conditions of the rabbit that have been well characterized. Some conditions represent conditions that have been identified in humans and other conditions offer insight into the mechanism(s) of particular organ or immune function.

1. Hydrocephalus

Hydrocephalus refers to dilatation of the cerebral ventricles and is usually accompanied by accumulation of cerebrospinal fluid within the dilated spaces. Some cases of hydrocephalus in rabbits have been presumed to be related to a single autosomal recessive gene (*hy/hy*); however, occurrence with other abnormalities suggests that inheritance may be more complicated (Lindsey and Fox, 1994). In some cases, the condition appears to be inherited along with various ocular anomalies as an autosomal gene with incomplete dominance. Hydrocephalus may also occur in rabbits as a congenital condition related to hypovitaminosis A in pregnant does (Lindsey and Fox, 1994).

2. Buphthalmia (Glaucoma, Hydrophthalmia, Congenital or Infantile Glaucoma)

Etiology Buphthalmia is inherited as an autosomal recessive trait, although penetrance is presumably incomplete since severity and the age of onset vary greatly and some *bu/bu* individuals do not develop buphthalmia (Hanna *et al.*, 1962).

Clinical Signs Rabbits with hereditary glaucoma develop ocular changes that resemble human congenital glaucoma and buphthalmia. Newborn *bu/bu* rabbits initially have normal intraocular pressure (IOP; 15–23 mmHg) but increased pressures of 26–48 mmHg may develop after 1–3 months of age (Burrows *et al.*, 1995; Knepper *et al.*, 1997). The eyes become progressively buphthalmic (either uni- or bilaterally) but the IOP can return to normal or to sub-normal levels after 6–10 months. Typical clinical changes include increased corneal diameter as the globe enlarges because the sclera is still immature. The cornea may develop a cloudy or bluish tint, corneal edema, increased corneal vascularity, and flattening of the cornea. Structural changes may include widening of the angle, thickening of Descmet's membrane, atrophy of the ciliary process, and excavation of the optic disk. Impaired aqueous outflow may be due to incomplete cleavage of the drainage angle with abnormal insertion of uveal tissue into the cornea (Tesluk *et al.*, 1982). In some cases, the cornea ulcerates and ruptures.

There is also a marked reduction in semen concentration in buphthalmics, with a decrease in libido and decreased spermatogenesis in affected males (Fox *et al.*, 1969).

Epizootiology The condition is common in New Zealand White rabbits.

Pathology By 2 weeks of age, the morphology of the congenital glaucoma trabecular network becomes abnormal with a smaller entrance to the trabecular network at the iris base, smaller intertrabecular openings within and between the trabecular lamellae, and by 6 weeks, iris pillars with extensive lateral extensions in the angle recess can be observed. Most intertrabecular spaces remain open; however, the inner intertrabecular spaces adjacent to the aqueous plexus become compressed.

Diagnosis Diagnosis is based on clinical signs and measurement of intraocular pressure.

Treatment, Prevention, and Control Specific treatment of buphthalmia has not been described for rabbits; however, affected individuals should not be used for breeding purposes.

Research Complications Loss of valuable research animals is the primary complication.

3. Mandibular Prognathism (Malocclusion, Walrus Teeth, Buckteeth)

Etiology Mandibular prognathism is the most common inherited disease of domestic rabbits. The condition is inherited as an autosomal recessive trait (*mp/mp*) with incomplete penetrance (Fox and Crary, 1971; Huang *et al.*, 1981; Lindsey and Fox, 1994).

Clinical Signs Malocclusion related to mandibular prognathia may be clinically apparent as early as 2–3 weeks of age, but is more typically seen in older rabbits post weaning. Clinical signs may include anorexia and weight loss. If severe enough and left untreated, affected animals will starve since they cannot properly prehend and masticate food.

Epizootiology Normally, the lower incisors occlude with the large upper incisors, as well as with a pair of small secondary incisors that are immediately caudal to the primary maxillary incisors. The lower set of incisors typically wear against the upper set during normal biting activity, along an arc formed by biting movements of the lower incisors, whereas the maxillary secondary incisors wear at right angles to the mandibular incisors. The incisors wear more quickly at the posterior aspect in rabbits, partly because the enamel layer is thinner on that side. Affected rabbits have a normal dental formula.

The specific abnormality associated with mandibular prognathism is that the maxilla is short relative to a mandible of normal length. Thus, although the mandible appears abnormally long, the primary defect involves the maxilla. In rabbits, the teeth (including the molars and premolars) grow continuously throughout life. The incisors, for example, grow at the rate of 2.0–2.4 mm/week. When occlusion is normal, the teeth wear against one another and in this way remain a normal length. However, when occlusion is abnormal because of conditions that include mandibular prognathia, the teeth may become greatly elongated because typical attrition of the incisors does not occur. In affected animals the lower incisors often extend anterior to the upper incisors and protrude from the mouth, whereas the upper primary incisors grow past the lower incisors and curl within the mouth. In some instances, the upper incisors curl around dorsally and lacerate the mucosa of the hard palate. Secondary infection and abscessation may occur in such cases.

Diagnosis Diagnosis is based on clinical signs.

Differential Diagnoses Malocclusion secondary to mandibular or maxillary fracture should be considered.

Treatment, Prevention, and Control Overgrown teeth should be trimmed every 2–3 weeks or more frequently if needed. Trimming is preferably performed with a dental bur to avoid cracking the tooth, which may happen more frequently if a bone or wire cutter is used. Care should be taken to avoid exposing the pulp cavity as the result of excessive trimming. Because the condition is hereditary, use of affected animals as breeding stock should be avoided.

Research Complications No specific research complications have been reported.

4. Splay Leg

A number of disorders characterized clinically by complete abduction of one or more legs and the inability to assume a normal standing position are described by the term 'splay leg'. Young kits of 3–4 weeks of age are most commonly affected. Affected rabbits cannot adduct limbs and have difficulty in making normal locomotory movements. Most commonly, animals are affected in the right rear limb, although the condition may be uni- or bilateral and may affect the anterior, posterior, or all four limbs. Rabbits with splay leg may have difficulty in accessing food and water; thus, attention to adequate nutrition is required as part of proper clinical care.

The clinical signs of splay leg may be due to an overall imbalance of development of the neural, muscular, and skeletal systems. Possibly, some animals compensate with torsion and exorotation of the limb at the hip, whereas rabbits that are unable to compensate are clinically affected.

Although the precise pathogenesis of splay leg is not entirely understood, at least some cases are ascribed to inherited disorders. Typical clinical signs are secondary to femoral endotorsion, with a shallow acetabulum but without luxation of the femur at the hip. The semitendinosus muscle of affected animals is abnormal, with smaller fibers and abnormal mitochondria. Some reports suggest that the condition is associated with inherited achondroplasia of the hip and shoulder, whereas others indicate that a recessively inherited anteversion of the femoral head can be involved.

5. Inherited Self-Mutilating Behavior

Self-mutilating behavior in a Checkered cross (cross between English Spot, German Checkered Giant, and Checkered of Rhineland rabbits) was reported to occur as an inherited trait (Iglauer *et al.*, 1995). Autotraumatization of the feet and pads was observed. The abnormal behavior could be interrupted by administration of haloperidol.

6. Atropine Esterase Activity

Although not manifested as a disease, the presence of serum atropine esterase allows rabbits to inactivate atropine when administered for therapeutic purposes (Liebenberg and Linn, 1980; Stormont and Suzuki, 1970).

The enzyme also permits rabbits to consume diets containing belladonna compounds.

The enzyme is produced by a semidominant gene *Est*-2F. Three phenotypes are recognized depending on the number of genes expressed. The enzyme first appears in the serum at 1 month of age, and enzyme levels are greater in females than in males (Lindsey and Fox, 1994). The *Est*-2F gene is linked to genes controlling the black pigment in the coat (Forster and Hannafin, 1979; Fox and van Zutphen, 1977; Sawin and Crary, 1943).

7. Complement 3 Deficiency

Hereditary deficiency of the third component of complement (C3) was found in a strain of rabbits. This same strain also exhibited a hereditary C8 alpha-gamma deficiency. The serum C3 concentration, hemolytic C3 activity, and total complement hemolytic activity of these animals were significantly reduced. The low level of serum C3 in these rabbits was not due to C3 conversion, partial C3 antigenicity, and presence of a C3 inhibitor or hypercatabolism of normal C3. The C3 deficiency was transmitted as a simple autosomal co-dominant trait. Rabbits with this trait have a lower survival at 3 months than normal rabbits (Komatsu *et al.*, 1988).

8. Complement 6 Deficiency

This complement deficiency syndrome in the rabbit has been well characterized. This syndrome was initially reported in 1964 in a strain of rabbits that lacked the sixth component of the hemolytic complement system (Rother *et al.*, 1966). Whole blood clotting time in glass or plastic was prolonged and prothrombin consumption was decreased in blood from the deficient animals. Other parameters of blood coagulation were normal, including prothrombin time, partial thromboplastin time, specific clotting factor activities, platelet factor III function, platelet count, and bleeding time (Zimmerman *et al.*, 1971). Abnormal platelet response is also characteristic of this syndrome in the rabbit (Lee *et al.*, 1974). Complement C6-deficient rabbits are protected against diet-induced atherosclerosis despite having similar profiles in cholesterol levels and plasma lipoprotein. When compared to normal rabbits, differences in atherosclerotic plaque formation were discernible macroscopically, with extensive aortic lesions being visible in all normal rabbits while absent in all C6-deficient animals (Schmiedt *et al.*, 1998). The inheritance pattern for this defect is autosomal recessive (Abe *et al.*, 1979).

A progressive neurological syndrome has also been observed in the C6-deficient rabbits. This syndrome is clinically characterized by subacute motor neuropathy. Pathological studies of affected animals revealed (1) severe axonal degeneration in the sciatic nerve involving mainly motor fibers; (2) occasional peripheral axonal enlargement closely associated with axonal degeneration; (3) presence of structured abnormal material in normal-size myelinated fibers of the central and peripheral nervous systems; and (4) widespread occurrence of dystrophic axons and axonal spheroids in the gray matter of the central nervous system. By ultrastructural examination, dystrophic axons were filled with tubulovesicular material, appearing as stalks of parallel membranes and dense bodies similar to what is described in human neuroaxonal dystrophies (NAD). The disease manifested by C6-deficient rabbits may represent an animal model of primary human NAD (Giannini *et al.*, 1992).

9. Complement 8 Deficiency

Genetic deficiency of the alpha-gamma-subunit of the eighth complement component (C8 alpha-gamma) was found in a substrain of the New Zealand White rabbits. The serum of this deficient rabbit lacked the immunochemical and functional alpha-gamma-subunit of C8 (C8D). This syndrome is transmitted as a simple autosomal recessive trait. The syndrome is characterized by smaller body weight compared to those of heterozygous and normal rabbits. In addition, survival rates for the first 3 months of life of the deficient animals tended to be lower than those of heterozygous and normal littermates (Komatsu *et al.*, 1985). All C8D rabbits (more than 180 animals obtained thus far) were consistently smaller than normal littermates from birth to adulthood, i.e., 86% of normal size at birth, 57% of normal size at 35 days of age, and 68% of normal size at adulthood. The C8α-γ deficiency in rabbits is always associated with dwarfism. Furthermore, there appears to be a discrete recessive dwarf gene (dw-2), whose locus is not linked to C8D. Rabbits double-homozygous for C8D and dw-2 (severe dwarf) were smaller than the C8D or dwarf rabbits and almost all of the severe dwarf rabbits died within 35 days after birth. The actual and relative weights of the thymus in the C8D rabbits were consistently lower than those of normal rabbits, but histological examination of the C8D thymus did not reveal any abnormalities. The C8D and dwarf rabbits were fertile; however, crosses of C8D females with C8D or dwarf males led to a reduced delivery rate and small litter size. The C8D locus is loosely linked to the C3 hypocomplementemic locus (C3-hypo) (map distance 24 cM) but not to the hemoglobin blood group locus (Komatsu *et al.*, 1990).

10. Hypercholesterolemia (Kurosawa and Kusanagi Hypercholesterolemic Rabbit)

The inherited characteristics of the Kurosawa and Kusanagi hypercholesterolemic (KHC) rabbit include persistent hypercholesterolemia. This strain of rabbits was produced by inbreeding mutants discovered in 1985. These KHC rabbits had serum cholesterol, triglyceride, and phospholipid levels 8–10 times greater than clinically normal *O. cuniculus*. The KHC rabbits also had decreased serum high-density lipoprotein cholesterol concentration, about one-third the value in clinically normal rabbits. In addition, the serum lipoprotein electrophoretic patterns were characterized by a strong, broad beta-lipoprotein band and a diminished alpha-lipoprotein band. Fractionation of lipoprotein lipids revealed increased cholesterol, phospholipid, and triglyceride in the LDL fraction; increased cholesterol and phospholipid in the very LDL fraction; and decreased cholesterol and triglyceride in the high-density lipoprotein fraction. The inheritance is thought to be a single autosomal recessive gene mutation, and analysis of the LDL receptor indicated that the KHC rabbit has a 12-base pair deletion in the LDL receptor mRNA. Macroscopic analysis of the aorta revealed the atheromatous lesions at 2 months of age, drastically increased lesional areas in the total aortic surface at 8 months of age, and a high incidence of coronary atheromas and xanthomas (Kurosawa *et al.*, 1995).

11. Hyperlipidemia

A spontaneous phenotype in a rabbit was discovered with an elevation of serous lipid ingredients including cholesterol and beta-lipoprotein (beta-LP). Atherosclerotic lesions were evident in the aorta and renal arteries. Nodular xanthomas were also present on the front and rear feet. The HLR strain was inbred to accentuate these characteristics (Watanabe *et al.*, 1977). The strain was eventually designated the Watanabe-heritable hyperlipidemic rabbit (WHHL-rabbit). An additional report of this strain of rabbits indicated that the WHHL-rabbits spontaneous developed aortic atherosclerosis by 5 months of age and xanthoma of digital joints in 60% of the rabbits aged to 16 months (Watanabe, 1980).

H. Neoplasia

Historically, spontaneous neoplasia in the laboratory rabbit has not been widely reported because neoplasia in the rabbit is very uncommon before 2 years of age and many laboratory rabbits are not maintained beyond this age (Weisbroth, 1994). Endometrial adenocarcinoma is the most common tumor in aged female rabbits, with an incidence of 79% reported in a colony of 5-year-old rabbits (Baba and Von Haam, 1972). Tinkey *et al.* complied an extensive review of the literature dealing with spontaneous neoplasia in the domestic rabbit. This review contained data on case reports, descriptions of biologic aspects of naturally occurring tumors and reports of experimentally induced tumor models. Neoplasia in *Sylvilagus* and *Lepus* were also discussed (Tinkey *et al.*, 2012).

1. Neoplasia of Genitourinary System and Mammary Gland

Uterine adenocarcinoma is by far the most common tumor in rabbits. Typically, the disease is present as multiple tumors and is malignant, often metastasizing to the liver, lungs, and other organs. There is evidence that inheritance plays a role in susceptibility, but parity does not. Uterine leiomyomas and leiomyosarcomas are much less common (Weisbroth, 1994). There are a few reports of vaginal squamous cell carcinomas (Weisbroth, 1994) and an ovarian hemangioma has been described (Greene and Strauss, 1949).

Mammary adenocarcinomas are fairly common in older female rabbits and may occur in animals with uterine adenocarcinoma (Weisbroth, 1994). Papillomas have been described, but mammary adenocarcinomas are much more important. These malignant tumors may metastasize, but the cause of death in affected rabbits is often due to uterine adenocarcinoma. Serial biopsy studies indicate that these tumors are preceded by cystic mastopathy as well as changes in the adrenal and pituitary glands (Greene, 1965). There may also be small prolactin-secreting pituitary adenomas in rabbits with mammary dysplasia (Lipman et al., 1994).

Testicular tumors in the rabbit appear to be relatively uncommon. Interstitial tumors are the most common testicular tumor in the rabbit. Seminomas and teratomas have also been reported (Weisbroth, 1994).

Embryonal nephromas are one of the most common tumors in laboratory rabbits. These tumors are often found incidentally, occur in younger animals, and seldom cause clinical signs (Weisbroth, 1994). There has been one report of a renal carcinoma in the rabbit (Kaufman and Quist, 1970) and one report of a leiomyoma arising in the urinary bladder (Weisbroth, 1974).

2. Neoplasia of Hematopoietic System

Malignant lymphomas (lymphosarcomas) are relatively common in rabbits. They may occur in rabbits that are less than 2 years of age (Weisbroth, 1994), but older rabbits may also be affected. According to (Weisbroth, 1994), a tetrad of lesions is often seen. These lesions include enlarged kidneys, splenomegaly, hepatomegaly, and lymphadenopathy. Older rabbits have presented with skin nodules and eye lesions; however, malignant lymphomas in the rabbit are seldom leukemic. Most cases of malignant lymphoma appear to resemble the lymphoblastic subtype as seen in humans and mice. Malignant lymphoma is more prevalent in some strains of rabbits than in others, and there is some evidence for a retroviral cause of lymphomas in rabbits (Weisbroth, 1994). True thymomas (containing both lymphoid and epithelial components) (Vernau et al., 1995) and plasma cell myelomas (Pascal, 1961)

are rare in rabbits. One case of myeloid leukemia has been reported (Meier et al., 1972).

3. Neoplasia of Skin and Subcutaneous Tissue

Basal cell tumors are reported to be rare (Weisbroth, 1994), but they may be underreported (Li and Schlafer, 1992). Squamous cell carcinomas are also uncommon, and there is no apparent predilection for any particular area of the body (Weisbroth, 1994). Other cited skin-associated tumors include a trichoepithelioma (Altman et al., 1978), a sebaceous gland carcinoma (Port and Sidor, 1978), and two malignant melanomas (Hotchkiss et al., 1994).

4. Neoplasia of Bone, Muscle, and Connective Tissue

Osteosarcomas are extremely rare in rabbits, and most have arisen in the mandible or maxilla, with only one found in a long bone (Weisbroth, 1994). No primary tumors arising in cartilage have been described, although some of the reported osteosarcomas have had cartilaginous elements. One tumor of skeletal muscle, a rhabdomyosarcoma, has been reported. A few fibrosarcomas and one fibrosarcoma involving the foot have been reported (Weisbroth, 1994).

5. Miscellaneous Neoplasia

A number of case reports of single tumors are found in the literature. These include a peritoneal mesothelioma (Lichtensteiger and Leathers, 1987), an intracranial teratoma (Bishop, 1978), an ependymoma (Kinkier and Jepsen, 1979), a neurofibrosarcoma, two hemangiosarcomas (Pletcher and Murphy, 1984), and a malignant fibrous histiocytoma (Yamamoto and Fujishiro, 1989). There are a few very old reports of lung tumors dating to the first part of the 20th century (Weisbroth, 1994).

6. Neoplasia Models Derived from Rabbits

There are several tumor models in which the cells used for inoculation were originally derived from rabbit tumors. These include the vx–2 carcinoma (Kidd and Rous, 1940), the Brown Pearce carcinoma (Brown and Pearce, 1923), and the Greene melanoma (Greene, 1958). The vx–2 carcinoma originated from a squamous cell carcinoma in a rabbit carrying a Shope papilloma. The most common modern use of this transplantable tumor is as a model for the study of various cancer treatment modalities for metastatic tumors (Stetson et al., 1991).

The Brown Pearce carcinoma arose from a tumor in a rabbit testis, but the exact tissue of origin of the tumor was never determined. The tumor was readily transplantable and caused stable metastases. Because some tumors regress, even after widespread metastases, this tumor has been used as a model for the study of tumor immunology (Weisbroth, 1994). The Brown Pearce carcinoma, although extensively characterized and historically used, has been reported in the literature only five times from 1990 to 2009 (Tinkey *et al.*, 2012).

I. Miscellaneous Diseases

1. *Hydrometra*

Hydrometra has been described as a clinical condition of rabbits. All cases were in unmated rabbits that were used experimentally for the production of serum antibodies (Bray *et al.*, 1991; Hobbs and Parker, 1990; Morrell, 1989). Clinical signs included abdominal distension and tachypnea. Cases were characterized by distension of the uterine horns with a transudative fluid. One case was associated with uterine torsion (Hobbs and Parker, 1990). One case had resolved with diuretic therapy, only to return later (Bray *et al.*, 1991).

2. *Liver Lobe Torsion*

Most cases of liver lobe torsion in rabbits involve the caudate lobe (Bergdall and Dysko, 1994), although one case report described torsion of the left hepatic lobe (Wilson *et al.*, 1987). Most reported cases have been incidental findings at necropsy. Incidental hepatic lobe torsions have also been identified in three adult New Zealand white rabbits that died from pasteurellosis (Weisbroth, 1975). Three cases of hepatic torsion in pet rabbits were reported by Wenger in 2009 (Wenger *et al.*, 2009). All rabbits presented with an acute onset of lethargy, anorexia, abdominal pain, pale mucous membranes, and jaundice. One rabbit also had hematuria. Another report of caudate liver lobe torsion also described a rabbit that was jaundiced, anemic, and anorexic, with elevated alanine aminotransferase. Torsion of the caudate liver lobe was seen at necropsy (Fitzgerald and Fitzgerald, 1992). In all reported clinical cases, rabbits were euthanized, or died during postoperative recovery.

3. *Urolithiasis*

Calcium carbonate and triple phosphate crystals are present in the urine of normal rabbits. These crystals contribute to the cloudy consistency of the urine (Williams, 1976). A 9-year retrospective study of hematuria in 14 New Zealand White rabbits was conducted by Garibaldi (Garibaldi *et al.*, 1987). Physical examination, laboratory tests, radiography, and *postmortem* examination were utilized in most cases to verify the presence of hematuria and to determine its etiology. Uterine adenocarcinoma was diagnosed in two rabbits. Three rabbits had uterine polyps with hemorrhage. Renal infarction with hemorrhage was diagnosed in three rabbits. Urolithiasis with secondary urethral obstruction and hemorrhagic cystitis was identified as the cause of hematuria in four rabbits. Other causes of hematuria included chronic cystitis,

disseminated intravascular coagulation, bladder polyps and pyelonephritis. Hematuria of undetermined origin was observed in one rabbit which emphasizes that hyperpigmented urine should be a rule out in all cases of suspected hematuria in rabbits (Garibaldi *et al.*, 1987). One case of urolithiasis with hydronephrosis in a New Zealand White rabbit was also reported (Labranche and Renegar, 1996). This condition must be distinguished from hematuria caused by endometrial venous aneurysm in female rabbits (Bray *et al.*, 1992).

4. *Lumbar Hernia*

Herniation of the kidney along with perinephric fat has been reported (Suckow and Grigdesby, 1993). The affected rabbit was clinically normal except for a subcutaneous mass that had passed through the body wall. The precise etiology is not known, although it was speculated that herniation might have occurred as the result of unreported trauma.

5. *Anomalous Nasolacrimal Duct Apparatus*

Occlusion of the nasolacrimal duct, presumably due to accumulation of fat droplets, has been described as a putative cause of epiphora in some rabbits (Marini *et al.*, 1996). Although the obstruction occurred at the dorsal flexure, it is not clear if this was due to congenital rather than acquired stenosis. In a retrospective study of 28 rabbits it was determined that the mean age of the rabbits presenting with ocular discharge from the nasolacrimal duct was 4.4 years. In 25 rabbits (89%), dacryocystitis was a unilateral finding. No underlying cause could be determined in 10 animals (35%). Dental malocclusion was observed in 14 rabbits (50%) and rhinitis in two animals (7%), with one animal showing both signs (4%). One rabbit (4%) presented with panophthalmitis. Most animals (96%) received topical antibiotic treatment. Regarding the clinical outcome, 12 animals (43%) showed complete recovery, eight rabbits (28%) were euthanized, three (11%) died due to unrelated causes, and three (11%) were lost to follow-up. Two rabbits (7%) continued to display signs of dacryocystitis (Florin *et al.*, 2009).

References

Abe, T., Komatsu, M., Oishi, T., Yamamoto, K., 1979. Development and genetic differences of complement activity in rabbits. Anim. Blood Groups Biochem. Genet. 10, 19–26.

Abo-El-Sooud, K., Goudah, A., 2010. Influence of *Pasteurella multocida* infection on the pharmacokinetic behavior of marbofloxacin after intravenous and intramuscular administrations in rabbits. J. Vet. Pharmacol. Ther. 33, 63–68.

Abrantes, J., Van Der Loo, W., Le Pendu, J., Esteves, P.J., 2012. Rabbit haemorrhagic disease (RHD) and rabbit haemorrhagic disease virus (RHDV): a review. Vet. Res. 43, 12.

Adler, B., Bulach, D., Chung, J., Doughty, S., Hunt, M., Rajakumar, K., et al., 1999. Candidate vaccine antigens and genes in *Pasteurella multocida*. J. Biotechnol. 73, 83–90.

Agnoletti, F., Ferro, T., Guolo, A., Marcon, B., Cocchi, M., Drigo, I., et al., 2009. A survey of *Clostridium spiroforme* antimicrobial susceptibility in rabbit breeding. Vet. Microbiol. 136, 188–191.

Akpo, Y., Kpodekon, M.T., Djago, Y., Licois, D., Youssao, I.A., 2012. Vaccination of rabbits against coccidiosis using precocious lines of *Eimeria magna* and *Eimeria media* in Benin. Vet. Parasitol. 184, 73–76.

Al-Haddawi, M.H., Jasni, S., Son, R., Mutalib, A.R., Bahaman, A.R., Zamri-Saad, M., et al., 1999. Molecular characterization of *Pasteurella multocida* isolates from rabbits. J. Gen. Appl. Microbiol. 45, 269–275.

Allaert, A., Jouault, T., Rajagopalan-Levasseur, P., Odberg-Ferragut, C., Dei-Cas, E., Camus, D., 1997. Detection of cytokine mRNA in the lung during the spontaneous *Pneumocystis carinii* pneumonia of the young rabbit. J. Eukaryot. Microbiol. 44, 45S.

Al-Lebban, Z.S., Kruckenberg, S., Coles, E.H., 1989. Rabbit pasteurellosis: respiratory and renal pathology of control and immunized rabbits after challenge with *Pasteurella multocida*. Histol. Histopathol. 4, 77–84.

Allen, A.M., Ganaway, J.R., Moore, T.D., Kinard, R.F., 1965. Tyzzer's disease syndrome in laboratory rabbits. Am. J. Pathol. 46, 859–882.

Altman, N.H., Damaray, S.Y., Lamborn, P.B., 1978. Trichoepithelioma in a rabbit. Vet. Pathol. 15, 671–672.

Araki, M., Fan, J., Challah, M., Bensadoun, A., Yamada, N., Honda, K., et al., 2000. Transgenic rabbits expressing human lipoprotein lipase. Cytotechnology 33, 93–99.

Arlain, L.G., Ahmed, M., Vyszenski-Moher, D.L., 1988. Effects of *Sarcoptes scabei* var. *canis* (Acari: Sarcoptidae) on blood indexes of parasitized rabbits. J. Med. Entomol. 25, 360–369.

Arlain, L.G., Runyan, B.S., Sorlie, B.S., Estes, S.A., 1984. Host-seeking behavior of *Sarcoptes scabei*. Am. Acad. Dermatol. 11, 594–598.

Arlain, L.G., Bruner, R.H., Stuhlman, R.A., Ahmed, M., Vyszenski-Moher, D.L., 1990. Histopathology in hosts parasitized by *Sarcoptes scabei*. J. Parasitol. 76, 889–894.

Atkinson, J.B., Swift, L.L., Virmani, R., 1992. Watanabe heritable hyperlipidemic rabbits. Familial hypercholesterolemia. Am. J. Pathol. 140, 749–753.

Baba, N., Von Haam, E., 1972. Animal model: spontaneous adenocarcinoma in aged rabbits. Am. J. Pathol. 68, 653–656.

Bailey, J.R., Warner, L., Pritchard, G.C., Williamson, S., Carson, T., Willshaw, G., et al., 2002. Wild rabbits – a novel vector for Vero cytotoxigenic *Escherichia coli* (VTEC) O157. Commun. Dis. Public Health 5, 74–75.

Bain, M.S., Naylor, R.D., Griffiths, N.J., 1998. *Clostridium spiroforme* infection in rabbits. Vet. Rec. 142, 47.

Balsari, A., Bianchi, C., Cocilovo, A., Dragoni, I., Poli, G., Ponti, W., 1981. Dermatophytes in clinically healthy laboratory animals. Lab. Anim. 15, 75–77.

Baneux, P.J., Pognan, F., 2003. In utero transmission of *Encephalitozoon cuniculi* strain type I in rabbits. Lab. Anim. 37, 132–138.

Baumans, V., 2005. Environmental enrichment for laboratory rodents and rabbits: requirements of rodents, rabbits, and research. ILAR J. 46, 162–170.

Beard, P.M., Rhind, S.M., Buxton, D., Daniels, M.J., Henderson, D., Pirie, A., et al., 2001. Natural paratuberculosis infection in rabbits in Scotland. J. Comp. Pathol. 124, 290–299.

Belanger, S.D., Boissinot, M., Clairoux, N., Picard, F.J., Bergeron, M.G., 2003. Rapid detection of *Clostridium difficile* in feces by real-time PCR. J. Clin. Microbiol. 41, 730–734.

Bergdall, V.K., Dysko, R.C., 1994. Metabolic, traumatic, mycotic, and miscellaneous diseases of rabbits. In: Manning, P.J., Ringler, D.H., Newcomer, C.E. (Eds.), Biology of the Laboratory Rabbit, second ed. Academic Press, Orlando, FL, pp. 335–353.

Berger, C.N., Sodha, S.V., Shaw, R.K., Griffin, P.M., Pink, D., Hand, P., et al., 2010. Fresh fruit and vegetables as vehicles for the transmission of human pathogens. Environ. Microbiol. 12, 2385–2397.

Besch-Williford, C., Matherne, C., Wagner, J., 1985. Vitamin D toxicosis in commercially reared rabbits. Lab. Anim. Sci. 35, 528.

Biermann, J., Wu, K., Odening, K.E., Asbach, S., Koren, G., Peng, X., et al., 2011. Nicorandil normalizes prolonged repolarisation in the first transgenic rabbit model with long-QT syndrome 1 both in vitro and in vivo. Eur. J. Pharmacol. 650, 309–316.

Bishop, L., 1978. Intracranial teratoma in a domestic rabbit. Vet. Pathol. 15, 525–530.

Blanco, J.E., Blanco, M., Blanco, J., Mora, A., Balaguer, L., Mourino, M., et al., 1996. O serogroups, biotypes, and eae genes in *Escherichia coli* strains isolated from diarrheic and healthy rabbits. J. Clin. Microbiol. 34, 3101–3107.

Bleeker, W.K., Mackay, A.J., Masson-Pevet, M., Bouman, L.N., Becker, A.E., 1980. Functional and morphological organization of the rabbit sinus node. Circ. Res. 46, 11–22.

Borriello, S.P., Carmen, R.J., 1983. Association of iota-like toxin and *Clostridium spiroforme* with both spontaneous and antibiotic-associated diarrhea and colitis in rabbits. J. Clin. Microbiol. 17, 414–418.

Boyce, J.D., Seemann, T., Adler, B., Harper, M., 2012. Pathogenomics of *Pasteurella multocida*. Curr. Top. Micro. Immuno. 361, 23–38.

Brabb, T., Di Giacomo, R.F., 2012. Viral diseases. In: Suckow, M.A., Stevens, K.A., Wilson, R.P. (Eds.), The Laboratory Rabbit, Guinea Pig, Hamster, and Other Rodents, Elsevier, Amsterdam, pp. 365–413.

Bray, M.V., Gaertner, D.J., Brownstein, D.G., Moody, K.D., 1991. Hydrometra in a New Zealand White rabbit. Lab. Anim. Sci. 41, 628–629.

Bray, M.V., Weir, E.C., Brownstein, D.G., Delano, M.L., 1992. Endometrial venous aneurysms in three New Zealand White Rabbits. Lab. Anim. Sci. 42, 360–362.

Broome, R.L., Brooks, D.L., 1991. Efficacy of enrofloxacin in the treatment of respiratory pasteurellosis in rabbits. Lab. Anim. Sci. 41, 572–576.

Brown, W.H., Pearce, L., 1923. Studies based on a malignant tumor of the rabbit. I. The spontaneous tumor and associated abnormalities. J. Exp. Med. 37, 601–630.

Buijs, S., Keeling, L.J., Rettenbacher, S., Maertens, L., Tuyttens, F.A., 2011. Glucocorticoid metabolites in rabbit faeces – Influence of environmental enrichment and cage size. Physiol. Beh. 104, 469–473.

Burns, K.F., DeLannoy Jr., C.W., 1966. Compendium of normal blood values of laboratory animals with indication of variations. Toxicol. Appl. Pharmacol. 8, 429–437.

Burrows, A.M., Smith, T.D., Atkinson, C.S., Mooney, M.P., Hiles, D., Losken, H.W., 1995. Development of ocular hypertension in congenitally buphthalmic rabbits. Lab. Anim. Sci. 45, 443–444.

Cafarchia, C., Camarda, A., Coccioli, C., Figueredo, L.A., Circella, E., Danesi, P., et al., 2010. Epidemiology and risk factors for dermatophytoses in rabbit farms. Med. Mycol. 48, 975–980.

Cafarchia, C., Figueredo, L.A., Coccioli, C., Camarda, A., Otranto, D., 2012a. Enzymatic activity of *Microsporum canis* and *Trichophyton mentagrophytes* from breeding rabbits with and without skin lesions. Mycoses 55, 45–49.

Cafarchia, C., Weigl, S., Figueredo, L.A., Otranto, D., 2012b. Molecular identification and phylogenesis of dermatophytes isolated from rabbit farms and rabbit farm workers. Vet. Microbiol. 154, 395–402.

Callikan, S., Girard, J., 1979. Perinatal development of glucogenic enzymes in rabbit liver. Biol. Neonate. 1, 78–84.

Cam, Y., Cetin, E., Ica, A., Atalay, O., Cetin, N., 2006. Evaluation of some coagulation parameters in hepatic coccidiosis experimentally induced with *Eimeria stiedai* in rabbits. Zentralbl. Veterinarmed. B 53, 201–202.

Cam, Y., Atasever, A., Eraslan, G., Kibar, M., Atalay, O., Beyaz, L., et al., 2008. *Eimeria stiedae*: experimental infection in rabbits and the effect of treatment with toltrazuril and ivermectin. Exp. Parasitol. 119, 164–172.

Camguilhem, R., Milon, A., 1989. Biotypes and O serogroups of *Escherichia coli* involved in intestinal infections of weaned rabbits: clues to diagnosis of pathogenic strains. J. Clin. Microbiol. 27, 743–747.

Cantey, J.R., Blake, R.K., 1977. Diarrhea due to *Escherichia coli* in the rabbit: a novel mechanism. J. Infect. Dis. 135, 454–462.

Carabaño, R., Piquer, J., Menoyo, D., Badiola, I., 2010. The digestive system of the rabbit. In: De Blas, C., Wiseman, J. (Eds.), Nutrition of the Rabbit, second ed. CABI, Wallingford, pp. 1–18.

Carman, R.J., Borriello, S.P., 1984. Infectious nature of *Clostridium spiroforme*-mediated rabbit enterotoxaemia. Vet. Microbiol. 9, 497–502.

Carman, R.J., Evans, R.H., 1984. Experimental and spontaneous clostridial enteropathies of laboratory and free living lagomorphs. Lab. Anim. Sci. 34, 443–452.

Carman, R.J., Wilkins, T.D., 1991. In vitro susceptibility of rabbit strains of *Clostridium spiroforme* to antimicrobial agents. Vet. Microbiol. 28, 391–397.

Cejkova, D., Zobanikova, M., Pospisilova, P., Strouhal, M., Mikalova, L., Weinstock, G.M., et al., 2013. Structure of rrn operons in pathogenic non-cultivable treponemes: sequence but not genomic position of intergenic spacers correlates with classification of *Treponema pallidum* and *Treponema paraluiscuniculi* strains. J. Med. Microbiol. 62, 196–207.

Cere, N., Polack, B., 1999. Animal pneumocystosis: a model for man. Vet. Res. 30, 1–26.

Cere, N., Drouet-Viard, F., Dei-Cas, E., Chanteloup, N., Coudert, P., 1997a. In utero transmission of *Pneumocystis carinii* sp. *f. oryctolagi*. Parasite 4, 325–330.

Cere, N., Polack, B., Chanteloup, N.K., Coudert, P., 1997b. Natural transmission of *Pneumocystis carinii* in nonimmunosuppressed animals: early contagiousness of experimentally infected rabbits (*Oryctolagus cuniculus*). J. Clin. Microbiol. 35, 2670–2672.

Cere, N., Polack, B., Coudert, P., 1997c. Obtaining a *Pneumocystis*-free rabbit breeding stock (*Oryctolagus cuniculus*). J. Eukaryot. Microbiol. 44, 19S–20S.

Chalmers, R.M., Robinson, G., Elwin, K., Hadfield, S.J., Xiao, L., Ryan, U., et al., 2009. *Cryptosporidium* sp. rabbit genotype, a newly identified human pathogen. Emerg. Infect. Dis. 15, 829–830.

Chalmers, R.M., Elwin, K., Hadfield, S.J., Robinson, G., 2011. Sporadic human cryptosporidiosis caused by *Cryptosporidium cuniculus*, United Kingdom, 2007–2008. Emerg. Infect. Dis. 17, 536–538.

Cheeke, P.R., 1987. Rabbit Feeding and Nutrition. Academic Press, New York.

Cheeke, P.R., 1994. Nutrition and nutritional diseases. In: Manning, P.J., Ringler, D.H., Newcomer, C.E. (Eds.), Biology of the Laboratory Rabbit, second ed. Academic Press, Orlando, FL, pp. 321–333.

Chermette, R., Ferreiro, L., Guillot, J., 2008. Dermatophytoses in animals. Mycopathologia 166, 385–405.

Chrenek, P., Ryban, L., Vetr, H., Makarevich, A.V., Uhrin, P., Paleyanda, R.K., et al., 2007. Expression of recombinant human factor VIII in milk of several generations of transgenic rabbits. Transgenic Res. 16, 353–361.

Chrenek, P., Bauer, M., Makarevich, A.V., 2011. Quality of transgenic rabbit embryos with different EGFP gene constructs. Zygote 19, 85–90.

Chrisp, C.E., Foged, N.T., 1991. Induction of pneumonia in rabbits by use of a purified protein toxin from *Pasteurella multocida*. Am. J. Vet. Res. 52, 56–61.

Christensen, N.D., 2005. Cottontail rabbit papillomavirus (CRPV) model system to test antiviral and immunotherapeutic strategies. Antiviral Chem. Chemother. 16, 355–362.

Christensen, N.D., Peng, X., 2012. Rabbit Genetics and Transgenic Models. In: Suckow, M.A., Stevens, K.A., Wilson, R.P. (Eds.), The Laboratory Rabbit, Guinea Pig, Hamster, and Other Species. Academic Press, Orlando, FL.

Chu, L.-R., Garner, J.P., Mench, J.A., 2004. A behavioral comparison of New Zealand White rabbits (*Oryctolagus cuniculus*) housed individually or in pairs in conventional laboratory cages. Appl. Anim. Behav. Sci. 85, 121–139.

Cizek, L.J., 1961. Relationship between food and water ingestion in the rabbit. Am. J. Physiol. 201, 557–566.

Clements, A., Young, J.C., Constantinou, N., Frankel, G., 2012. Infection strategies of enteric pathogenic *Escherichia coli*. Gut Microbes 3, 71–87.

Clermont, O., Olier, M., Hoede, C., Diancourt, L., Brisse, S., Keroudean, M., et al., 2011. Animal and human pathogenic *Escherichia coli* strains share common genetic backgrounds. Infect. Genet. Evol. 11, 654–662.

Cloyd, G.C., Moorhead, D.P., 1976. Facial alopecia in the rabbit associated with *Cheyletiella parasitovorax*. Lab. Anim. Sci. 26, 801–803.

Cohen, S.R., 1980. Cheyletiella dermatitis: a mite infestation of rabbit, cat, dog, and man. Arch. Dermatol. 116, 435–437.

Confer, A.W., Suckow, M.A., Montelongo, M., Dabo, S.M., Miloscio, L.J., Gillespie, A.J., et al., 2001. Intranasal vaccination of rabbits with *Pasteurella multocida* A:3 outer membranes that express iron-regulated proteins. Am. J. Vet. Res. 62, 697–703.

Connole, M.D., Yamaguchi, H., Elad, D., Hasegawa, A., Segal, E., Torres-Rodriguez, J.M., 2000. Natural pathogens of laboratory animals and their effects on research. Med. Mycol. 38 (Suppl 1), 59–65.

Cooper, D.M., Swanson, D.L., Barns, S.M., Gebhart, C.J., 1997a. Comparison of the 16S ribosomal DNA sequences from the intracellular agents of proliferative enteritis in a hamster, deer, and ostrich with the sequence of a porcine isolate of *Lawsonia intracellularis*. Int. J. Syst. Bacteriol. 47, 635–639.

Cooper, D.M., Swanson, D.L., Gebhart, C.J., 1997b. Diagnosis of proliferative enteritis in frozen and formalin-fixed, paraffin-embedded tissues from a hamster, horse, deer and ostrich using a *Lawsonia intracellularis*-specific multiplex PCR assay. Vet. Microbiol. 54, 47–62.

Corash, L., Rheinschmidt, M., Lieu, S., Meers, P., Brew, E., 1988. Fluorescence-activated flow cytometry in the hematology clinical laboratory. Cytometry Suppl. 3, 60–64.

Cornblath, M., Schwartz, R., 1976. Disorders of Carbohydrate Metabolism in Infancy. Saunders, Philadelphia, PA.

Cox, J.C., 1977. Altered immune responsiveness associated with *Encephalitozoon cuniculi* infection in rabbits. Infect. Immun. 15, 392–395.

Craigie, J. 1966. '*Bacillus piliformis*' (Tyzzer) and Tyzzer's disease of the laboratory mouse. I. Propagation of the organism in embryonated eggs. Proc. R. Soc. Lond., B, Biol. Sci., 165, 35–60.

Creusy, C., Bahon-Le Capon, J., Fleurisse, L., Mullet, C., Dridba, M., Cailliez, J.C., et al., 1996. *Pneumocystis carinii* pneumonia in four mammal species: histopathology and ultrastructure. J. Eukaryot. Microbiol. 43, 47S–48S.

Croppo, G.P., Moura, H., Dasilva, A.J., Leitch, G.J., Moss, D.M., Wallace, S., et al., 1998. Ultrastructure, immunoflourescence, western blot, and PCR analysis of eight isolates of *Encephalitozoon (Septata) intestinalis* established in culture from sputum and urine samples and duodenal aspirates of five patients with AIDS. J. Clin. Microbiol. 36, 1201–1208.

Cunliffe-Beamer, T.L., Fox, R.R., 1981a. Venereal spirochetosis of rabbits: description and diagnosis. Lab. Anim. Sci. 31, 366–371.

Cunliffe-Beamer, T.L., Fox, R.R., 1981b. Venereal spirochetosis of rabbits: epizootiology. Lab. Anim. Sci. 31, 372–378.

Cunliffe-Beamer, T.L., Fox, R.R., 1981c. Venereal spirochetosis of rabbits: eradication. Lab. Anim. Sci. 31, 379–381.

Curtis, S.K., Housley, R., Brooks, D.L., 1990. Use of ivermectin for treatment of ear mite infestation in rabbits. J. Am. Vet. Med. Assoc. 196, 1139–1140.

Cutlip, R.C., Amtower, W.C., Beall, C.W., Matthews, P.J., 1971. An epizootic of Tyzzer's disease in rabbits. Lab. Anim. Sci. 21, 356–361.

Dabard, J., Dubos, F., Martinet, L., Ducluzeau, R., 1979. Experimental reproduction of neonatal diarrhea in young gnotobiotic hares simultaneously associated with *Clostridium difficile* and other *Clostridium* strains. Infect. Immun. 24, 7–11.

Dabo, S.M., Confer, A.W., Lu, Y.S., 2000. Single primer polymerase chain reaction fingerprinting for *Pasteurella multocida* isolates from laboratory rabbits. Am. J. Vet. Res. 61, 305–309.

Daube, G., China, B., Simon, P., Hvala, K., Mainil, J., 1994. Typing of *Clostridium perfringens* by in vitro amplification of toxin genes. J. Appl. Bacteriol. 77, 650–655.

Davies, S.F.M., Joyner, L.P., Kendall, S.B., 1963. Coccidiosis. Oliver & Boyd, Edinburgh.

Davis, M.A., Cloud-Hansen, K.A., Carpenter, J., Hovde, C.J., 2005. *Escherichia coli* O157: H7 in environments of culture-positive cattle. Appl. Environ. Microbiol. 71, 6816–6822.

Davison, A.J., 2010. Herpesvirus systematics. Vet. Microbiol. 143, 52–69.

Deeb, B.J., DiGiacomo, R.F., 2000. Respiratory diseases of rabbits. Vet. Clin. North Am. Exot. Anim. Pract. 3, 465–480. vi–vii.

Deeb, B.J., DiGiacomo, R.F., Bernard, B.L., Silbernagel, S.M., 1990. *Pasteurella multocida* and *Bordetella bronchiseptica* infections in rabbits. J. Clin. Microbiol. 28, 70–75.

Dei-Cas, E., Chabe, M., Moukhlis, R., Durand-Joly, I., Aliouat El, M., Stringer, J.R., et al., 2006. *Pneumocystis oryctolagi* sp. nov., an uncultured fungus causing pneumonia in rabbits at weaning: review of current knowledge, and description of a new taxon on genotypic, phylogenetic and phenotypic bases. FEMS Microbiol. Rev. 30, 853–871.

Deloach, J.R., Wright, P.C., 1981. Ingestion of rabbit erythrocytes containing 51Cr-labeled hemoglobin by *Psoroptes* spp. that originated on cattle, mountain sheep, or rabbits. J. Med. Entomol. 18, 345–348.

Delong, D., Manning, P.J., Gunther, R., Swanson, D.L., 1992. Colonization of rabbits by *Pasteurella multocida*: serum IgG responses following intranasal challenge with serologically distinct isolates. Lab. Anim. Sci. 42, 13–18.

Didier, E.S., Vossbrinck, C.R., Baker, M.D., Rogers, L.B., Bertucci, D.C., Shadduck, J.A., 1995. Identification and characterization of three *Encephalitozoon cuniculi* strains. Parasitol 111 (Pt 4), 411–421.

DiGiacomo, R.F., Talburt, C.D., Lukehart, S.A., Baker-Zander, S.A., Condon, J., 1983. *Treponema paraluis-cuniculi* infection in a commercial rabbitry: epidemiology and serodiagnosis. Lab. Anim. Sci. 33, 562–566.

DiGiacomo, R.F., Deeb, B.J., Giddens, W.E., Bernard, B.L., Chengappa, M.M., 1989. Atrophic rhinitis in New Zealand White rabbits infected with Pasteurella multocida. Am. J. Vet. Res. 50, 1460–1465.

DiGiacomo, R.F., Taylor, F.G., Allen, V., Hinton, M.H., 1990. Naturally acquired *Pasteurella multocida* infection in rabbits: immunological aspects. Lab. Anim. Sci. 40, 289–292.

DiGiacomo, R.F., Xu, Y.M., Allen, V., Hinton, M.H., Pearson, G.R., 1991. Naturally acquired *Pasteurella multocida* infection in rabbits: clinicopathological aspects. Can. J. Vet. Res. 55, 234–238.

DiGiacomo, R.F., Deeb, B.J., Anderson, R.J., 1992. Hypervitaminosis A and reproductive disorders in rabbits. Lab. Anim. Sci. 42, 250–254.

Donnelly, T.M., 2004. Ferrets, Rabbits, and Rodents, Clinical Medicine and Surgery in: Quesenberry, K.E., Carpenter, J.W. (Eds.). Ferrets, Rabbits, and Rodents, Clinical Medicine and Surgery, second ed. WB Saunders, Philadelphia, PA.

Dragin, S., Chrastinova, L., Makarevich, A., Chrenek, P., 2005. Production of recombinant human protein C in the milk of transgenic rabbits from the F3 generation. Foila Biol. 53, 129–132.

Drigo, I., Bacchin, C., Cocchi, M., Bano, L., Agnoletti, F., 2008. Development of PCR protocols for specific identification of *Clostridium spiroforme* and detection of sas and sbs genes. Vet. Microbiol. 131, 414–418.

Drouet-Viard, F., Coudert, P., Licois, D., Boivin, M., 1997. Vaccination against *Eimeria magna* coccidiosis using spray dispersion of precocious line oocysts in the nest box. Vet. Parasitol. 70, 61–66.

Drozd, M., Kassem, II, Gebreyes, W., Rajashekara, G., 2010. A quantitative polymerase chain reaction assay for detection and quantification of *Lawsonia intracellularis*. J. Vet. Diagn. Invest. 22, 265–269.

Duhamel, G.E., Klein, E.C., Elder, R.O., Gebhart, C.J., 1998. Subclinical proliferative enteropathy in sentinel rabbits associated with *Lawsonia intracellularis*. Vet. Pathol. 35, 300–303.

Duncan, A.J., Carman, R.J., Olsen, G.J., Wilson, K.H., 1993. Assignment of the agent of Tyzzer's disease to *Clostridium piliforme* comb. nov. on the basis of 16S rRNA sequence analysis. Int. J. Syst. Bacteriol. 43, 314–318.

Duwell, D., Brech, K., 1981. Control of oxyuriasis in rabbits by fenbendazole. Lab. Anim. 15, 101–105.

Eaton, P., 1984. Preliminary observations on enteritis associated with a coronavirus-like agent in rabbits. Lab. Anim. 18, 71–74.

El Tayeb, A.B., Morishita, T.Y., Angrick, E.J., 2004. Evaluation of *Pasteurella multocida* isolated from rabbits by capsular typing, somatic serotyping, and restriction endonuclease analysis. J. Vet. Diagn. Invest. 16, 121–125.

Erikson, A.B., 1944. Helminth infection in relation to population fluctuations in snowshoe hare. J. Wildl. Manage. 8, 134–153.

Faine, S., 1965. Silver staining of spirochaetes in single tissue sections. J. Clin. Pathol. 18, 381–382.

Farmaki, R., Koutinas, A.F., Papazahariadou, M.G., Kasabalis, D., Day, M.J., 2009. Effectiveness of a selamectin spot-on formulation in rabbits with sarcoptic mange. Vet. Rec. 164, 431–432.

Fekete, S., Bokori, J., 1985. The effect of the fiber and protein level of the ration upon the cecotrophy of rabbits. J. Appl. Rabbit Res. 8, 68–71.

Feldman, S.H., Kiavand, A., Seidelin, M., Reiske, H.R., 2006. Ribosomal RNA sequences of *Clostridium piliforme* isolated from rodent and rabbit: re-examining the phylogeny of the Tyzzer's disease agent and development of a diagnostic polymerase chain reaction assay. J. Am. Assoc. Lab. Anim. Sci. 45, 65–73.

Ferrando, R., Wolter, R., Vilat, J.C., Megard, J.P., 1970. Teneur en acides amines des deux categories de fèces du lapin: caecotrophes et fèces durés. Comptes Rendus 20, 2202–2205.

Ferreira, T.S., Felizardo, M.R., Sena De Gobbi, D.D., Gomes, C.R., Nogueira Filsner, P.H., Moreno, M., et al., 2012. Virulence genes and antimicrobial resistance profiles of *Pasteurella multocida* strains isolated from rabbits in Brazil. Sci. World J. 2012, 685028.

Fitzgerald, A.L., Fitzgerald, S.D., 1992. Hepatic lobe torsion in a New Zealand White rabbit. Canine Pract. 17, 16–19.

Flatt, R.E., Carpenter, A.B., 1971. Identification of crystalline material in urine of rabbits. Am. J. Vet. Res. 32, 655–658.

Flatt, R.E., Jackson, S.J., 1970. Renal nosematosis in young rabbits. Vet. Pathol. 7, 492–497.

Flatt, R.E., Weisbroth, S.H., Kraus, A.L., 1974. Metabolic, traumatic, mycotic, and miscellaneous disease of rabbits. In: Weisbroth, S.H., Flatt, R.E., Kraus, A.L. (Eds.), The Biology of the Laboratory Rabbit, first ed. Academic Press, Orlando, FL, pp. 435–453.

Florin, M., Rusanen, E., Haessig, M., Richter, M., Spiess, B.M., 2009. Clinical presentation, treatment, and outcome of dacryocystitis in rabbits: a retrospective study of 28 cases (2003–2007). Vet. Ophthalmol. 12, 350–356.

Foote, R.H., Simkin, M.E., 1993. Use of gonadotropic releasing hormone for ovulating the rabbit model. Lab. Anim. Sci. 43, 383–385.

Forster, R.P., Hannafin, J.A., 1979. Influence of a genetically determined atropinesterase on atropine inhibition of the "smoke (dive) reflex" in rabbits. Gen. Pharmacol. 10, 41–46.

Fox, J.G., Dewhirst, F.E., Fraser, G.J., Paster, B.J., Shames, B., Murphy, J.C., 1994. Intracellular *Campylobacter*-like organism from ferrets and hamsters with proliferative bowel disease is a *Desulfovibrio* sp. J. Clin. Microbiol. 32, 1229–1237.

Fox, R.R., 1989. The rabbit. In: Loeb, W.F., Quimby, F.W. (Eds.), The Clinical Chemistry of Laboratory Animals. Pergamon, New York, pp. 41–46.

Fox, R.R., 1994. Taxonomy and genetics. In: Manning, P.J., Ringler, D.H., Newcomer, C.E. (Eds.), Biology of the Laboratory Rabbit, second ed. Academic Press, Orlando, FL, pp. 1–26.

Fox, R.R., Crary, D.D., 1971. Mandibular prognathism in the rabbit. Genetic studies. J. Hered. 62, 23–27.

Fox, R.R., van Zutphen, L.F., 1977. Strain differences in the prealbumin serum esterases of JAX rabbits. J. Hered. 68, 227–230.

Fox, R.R., Crary, D.D., Babino, E.J., Sheppard, L.B., 1969. Buphthalmia in the rabbit. Pleiotropic effects of the (bu) gene and a possible explanation of mode of gene action. J. Hered. 60, 206–212.

Franco, K.H., Cronin, K.L., 2008. What is your diagnosis? Respiratory abscess. J. Am. Vet. Med. Assoc. 233, 35–36.

Franzen, C., Muller, A., Hartmann, P., Hegener, P., Schrappe, M., Diehl, V., et al., 1998. Polymerase chain reaction for diagnosis and species differentiation of microsporidia. Folia Parsitol. 45, 140–148.

Freitas, F.L., Yamamoto, B.L., Freitas, W.L., Fagliari, J.J., Almeida Kde, S., Machado, R.Z., et al., 2011. Systemic inflammatory response indicators in rabbits (Oryctolagus cuniculus) experimentally infected with sporulated oocysts of Eimeria stiedai (Apicomplexa: Eimeriidae). Braz. J. Vet. Parasitol. 20, 121–126.

Frenkel, J.K., 1971. Pathology of protozoal and helminthic diseases. In: Marcial-Rojas, R.A. (Ed.), Protozoal Diseases of Laboratory Animals Williams & Wilkins, Baltimore, MD, pp. 318–369.

Frymus, T., Bielecki, W., Jakubowski, T., 1991. Toxigenic Pasteurella multocida in rabbits with naturally occurring atrophic rhinitis. Zentralbl. Veterinarmed. B 38, 265–268.

Fushuku, S., Fukuda, K., 2006. Examination of the applicability of a commercial human rotavirus antigen detection kit for use in laboratory rabbits. Exp. Anim. 55, 71–74.

Gallazzi, D., 1977. Cyclical variations in the excretion of intestinal coccidial oocysts in the rabbit. Folia Vet. Lat. 7, 371–380.

Ganaway, J.R., 1980. Effect of heat and selected chemical disinfectants upon infectivity of spores of Bacillus piliformis (Tyzzer's disease). Lab. Anim. Sci. 30, 192–196.

Ganaway, J.R., Allen, A.M., Moore, T.D., 1971. Tyzzer's disease of rabbits: isolation and propagation of Bacillus piliformis (Tyzzer) in embryonated eggs. Infect. Immun. 3, 429–437.

Gao, Z.Q., Yue, B.F., He, Z.M., 2012. Development and application of TaqMan MGB probe fluorescence quantitative PCR method for rapid detection of Clostridium piliforme. Zhonghua Liu Xing Bing Xue Za Zhi 33, 226–228.

García, A., Fox, J.G., 2003. The rabbit as a new reservoir host of enterohemorrhagic Escherichia coli. Emerg. Infect. Dis. 9, 1592–1597.

Garcia, A., Marini, R.P., Feng, Y., Vitsky, A., Knox, K.A., Taylor, N.S., et al., 2002. A naturally occurring rabbit model of enterohemorrhagic Escherichia coli-induced disease. J. Infect. Dis. 186, 1682–1686.

García, A., Bosques, C.J., Wishnok, J.S., Feng, Y., Karalius, B.J., Butterton, J.R., et al., 2006. Renal injury is a consistent finding in Dutch Belted rabbits experimentally infected with enterohemorrhagic Escherichia coli. J. Infect. Dis. 193, 1125–1134.

Garcia, A., Fox, J.G., Besser, T.E., 2010. Zoonotic enterohemorrhagic Escherichia coli: A One Health perspective. ILAR J. 51, 221–232.

Garibaldi, B.A., Fox, J.G., Otto, G., Murphy, J.C., Pecquet-Goad, M.E., 1987. Hematuria in rabbits. Lab. Anim. Sci. 37, 769–772.

Gelineo, S., 1964. Organ systems in adaptation: the temperature regulating system. In: Dill, D.B., Adolph, E.F., Wilber, C.G. (Eds.), Handbook of Physiology. Am. Physiol. Soc., Washington, DC, pp. 259–282.

Gertz, E.M., Schaffer, A.A., Agarwala, R., Bonnet-Garnier, A., Rogel-Gaillard, C., Hayes, H., et al., 2013. Accuracy and coverage assessment of Oryctolagus cuniculus (rabbit) genes encoding immunoglobulins in the whole genome sequence assembly (OryCun2.0) and localization of the IGH locus to chromosome 20. Immunogenetics 65, 749–762.

Giacani, L., Sun, E.S., Hevner, K., Molini, B.J., Van Voorhis, W.C., Lukehart, S.A., et al., 2004. Tpr homologs in Treponema paraluiscuniculi Cuniculi A strain. Infect. Immun. 72, 6561–6576.

Giannini, C., Monaco, S., Kirschfink, M., Rother, K.O., Lorbacher De Ruiz, H., Nardelli, E., et al., 1992. Inherited neuroaxonal dystrophy in C6 deficient rabbits. J. Neuropathol. Exp. Neurol. 51, 514–522.

Gidenne, T., 2003. Fibres in rabbit feeding for digestive troubles prevention: respective role of low-digested and digestible fibre. Livestock Prod. Sci. 81, 105–117.

Gidenne, T., Lebas, F., Fortun-Lamothe, L., 2010. Feeding behaviour of rabbits. In: De Blas, C., Wiseman, J. (Eds.), Nutrition of the Rabbit, second ed. CABI, Wallingford and Cambridge, MA, pp. 233–252.

Gillett, C.S., 1994. Selected drug dosages and clinical reference data. In: Manning, P.J., Ringler, D.H., Newcomer, C.E. (Eds.), Biology of the Laboratory Rabbit, second ed. Academic Press, Orlando, FL, pp. 467–472.

Gillett, N.A., Brooks, D.L., Tillman, P.C., 1983. Medical and surgical management of gastric obstruction from a hairball in the rabbit. J. Am. Vet. Med. Assoc. 183, 1176–1178.

Gissi, C., Gullberg, A., Arnason, U., 1998. The complete mitochondrial DNA sequence of the rabbit, Oryctolagus cuniculus. Genomics 50, 161–169.

Glass, L.S., Beasley, J.N., 1989. Infection with and antibody response to Pasteurella multocida and Bordetella bronchiseptica in immature rabbits. Lab. Anim. Sci. 39, 406–410.

Glavits, R., Magyar, T., 1990. The pathology of experimental respiratory infection with Pasteurella multocida and Bordetella bronchiseptica in rabbits. Acta. Vet. Acad. Sci. Hung. 38, 211–215.

Godornes, C., Leader, B.T., Molini, B.J., Centurion-Lara, A., Lukehart, S.A., 2007. Quantitation of rabbit cytokine mRNA by real-time RT-PCR. Cytokine 38, 1–7.

Goldenberg, S.D., Dieringer, T., French, G.L., 2010. Detection of toxigenic Clostridium difficile in diarrheal stools by rapid real-time polymerase chain reaction. Diagn. Microbiol. Infect. Dis. 67, 304–307.

Gomez-Bautista, M., Rojo-Vazquez, F., Alunda, J.M., 1987. The effect of host's age on the pathology of Eimeria stiedae infection in rabbits. Vet. Parasitol. 24, 47–57.

Greene, H.S.N., 1958. A spontaneous melanoma in the hamster with a propensity for amelanotic alteration and sarcomatous transformation during transplantation. Cancer Res. 18, 422–425.

Greene, H.S.N., 1965. Diseases of the rabbit. In: Ribelin, W.W., Mccoy, J.R. (Eds.), The Pathology of Laboratory Animals. Thomas, Springfield, IL, pp. 340–348.

Greene, H.S.N., Strauss, J.S., 1949. Multiple primary tumors in the rabbit. Cancer Res. 2, 673–691.

Greig, A., Stevenson, K., Perez, V., Pirie, A.A., Grant, J.M., Sharp, J.M., 1997. Paratuberculosis in wild rabbits (Oryctolagus cuniculus). Vet. Rec. 140, 141–143.

Gunn, D., Morton, D.B., 1995. Inventory of the behaviour of New Zealand White rabbits in laboratory cages. Appl. Anim. Behav. Sci. 45, 277–292.

Guo, D., Lu, Y., Zhang, A., Liu, J., Yuan, D., Jiang, Q., et al., 2012. Identification of genes transcribed by Pasteurella multocida in rabbit livers through the selective capture of transcribed sequences. FEMS Microbiol. Lett. 331, 105–112.

Hadfield, S.J., Chalmers, R.M., 2012. Detection and characterization of Cryptosporidium cuniculus by real-time PCR. Parasitol. Res. 111, 1385–1390.

Hafez, E.S.E.(Ed.), 1970. Rabbits. In: Reproduction and Breeding Techniques for Laboratory Animals. Lea & Febiger, Philadelphia, PA.

Hagen, K.W., 1958. The effects of continuous sulfaquinoxaline feeding on rabbit mortality. Am. J. Vet. Res. 19, 494–496.

Hagen, K.W., 1966. Spontaneous papillomatosis in domestic rabbits. Bull. Wildl. Dis. Assoc. 2, 108–110.

Hanan, M.S., Riad, E.M., El-Khouly, N.A., 2000. Antibacterial efficacy and pharmacokinetic studies of ciprofloxacin on Pasteurella multocida infected rabbits. Dtsch. Tierarztl. Wochenschr. 107, 151–155.

Hanna, B.L., Sawin, P.B., Sheppard, L.B., 1962. Recessive buphthalmos in the rabbit. Genetics 47, 519–529.

Hansen, L., Berthelsen, H., 2000. The effect of environmental enrichment on the behaviour of caged rabbits (Oryctolagus cuniculus). Appl. Anim. Behav. Sci. 68, 163–178.

Hanson, N.B., Lanning, D.K., 2008. Microbial induction of B and T cell areas in rabbit appendix. Dev. Comp. Immunol. 32, 980–991.

Harkness, J.E., Wagner, J.E., 1995. The Biology and Medicine of Rabbits and Rodents. Williams & Wilkins, Baltimore, MD.

Hesselton, R.M., Yang, W.C., Medveczky, P., Sullivan, J.L., 1988. Pathogenesis of Herpesvirus sylvilagus infection in cottontail rabbits. Am. J. Pathol. 133, 639–647.

Hewitt, C.D., Innes, D.J., Savory, J., Willis, M.R., 1989. Normal biochemical and hematological values in New Zealand White rabbits. Clin. Chem. 35, 1777–1779.

Hickey, C.A., Beattie, T.J., Cowieson, J., Miyashita, Y., Strife, C.F., Frem, J.C., et al., 2011. Early volume expansion during diarrhea and relative nephroprotection during subsequent hemolytic uremic syndrome. Arch. Pediatr. Adolesc. Med. 165, 884–889.

Hiripi, L., Negre, D., Cosset, F.L., Kvell, K., Czompoly, T., Baranyi, M., et al., 2010. Transgenic rabbit production with simian immunodeficiency virus-derived lentiviral vector. Transgenic Res. 19, 799–808.

Ho, E.L., Lukehart, S.A., 2011. Syphilis: using modern approaches to understand an old disease. J. Clin. Invest. 121, 4584–4592.

Hobbs, B.A., Parker, R.F., 1990. Uterine torsion associated with either hydrometra or endometritis in two rabbits. Lab. Anim. Sci. 40, 535–536.

Hoffman, B.F., 1965. Atrioventricular conduction in mammalian hearts. Ann. N. Y. Acad. Sci. 127, 105–112.

Hofing, G.L., Kraus, A.L., 1994. Arthropod and helminth parasites. In: Manning, P.J., Ringler, D.H., Newcomer, C.E. (Eds.), Biology of the Laboratory Rabbit, second ed. Academic Press, Orlando, FL, p. 483.

Holmes, H.T., Sonn, R.J., Patton, N.M., 1988. Isolation of Clostridium spiroforme from rabbits. Lab. Anim. Sci. 38, 167–168.

Horiuchi, N., Watarai, M., Kobayashi, Y., Omata, Y., Furuoka, H., 2008. Proliferative enteropathy involving Lawsonia intracellularis infection in rabbits (Oryctlagus cuniculus). J. Vet. Med. Sci. 70, 389–392.

Hornicke, H., 1977. Coecotrophy in rabbits—A circadian function. J. Mammal. 58, 240–242.

Horton, R.J., 1967. The route of migration of Eimeria stiedae (Lindemann, 1865) sporozoites between the duodenum and bile duct of the rabbit. Parasitology 57, 9–17.

Horton-Smith, C., 1947. The treatment of hepatic coccidiosis in rabbits. Br. Vet. J. 103, 207–213.

Hotchkiss, C.E., Norden, H., Collins, B.R., Ginn, P.E., 1994. Malignant melanomas in two rabbits. Lab. Anim. Sci. 44, 377–379.

Hotchkiss, C.E., Shames, B., Perkins, S.E., Fox, J.G., 1996. Proliferative enteropathy of rabbits: the intracellular Campylobacter-like organism is closely related to Lawsonia intracellularis. Lab. Anim. Sci. 46, 623–627.

Houser, B.A., Hattel, A.L., Jayarao, B.M., 2010. Real-time multiplex polymerase chain reaction assay for rapid detection of Clostridium difficile toxin-encoding strains. Foodborne Path. Dis. 7, 719–726.

Huang, C.M., Mi, M.P., Vogt, D.W., 1981. Mandibular prognathism in the rabbit: discrimination between single-locus and multifactorial models of inheritance. J. Hered. 72, 296–298.

Hughes, W.T., 1982. Natural mode of acquisition for de novo infection with Pneumocystis carinii. J. Infect. Dis. 145, 842–848.

Huls, W.L., Brooks, D.L., Bean-Knudsen, D., 1991. Response of adult New Zealand White rabbits to enrichment objects and paired housing. Lab. Anim. Sci. 41, 609–612.

Iglauer, F., Beig, C., Dimigen, J., Gerold, S., Gocht, A., Seeburg, A., et al., 1995. Hereditary compulsive self-mutilating behaviour in laboratory rabbits. Lab. Anim. 29, 385–393.

Inman, L.R., Takeuchi, A., 1979. Spontaneous cryptosporidiosis in an adult female rabbit. Vet. Pathol. 16, 89–95.

Jankiewicz, H.A., 1945. Liver coccidiosis prevented by sulfasuxidine. J. Parasitol. Vol 31, Suppl pg 3.

Jaslow, B.W., Ringler, D.H., Rush, H.G., Glorioso, J.C., 1981. Pasteurella associated rhinitis of rabbits: efficacy of penicillin therapy. Lab. Anim. Sci. 31, 382–385.

Jayo, J.M., Schwenke, D.C., Clarkson, T.B., 1994. Atherosclerotic research. In: Manning, P.J., Ringler, D.H., Newcomer, C.E. (Eds.), Biology of the Laboratory Rabbit, second ed. Academic Press, Orlando, FL, pp. 367–380.

Jenne, C.N., Kennedy, L.J., Mccullagh, P., Reynolds, J.D., 2003. A new model of sheep Ig diversification: shifting the emphasis toward combinatorial mechanisms and away from hypermutation. J. Immunol. 170, 3739–3750.

Jilge, B., 1991. The rabbit: a diurnal or nocturnal animal? J. Exp. Anim. Sci. 34, 170–175.

Jin, L., Lohr, C.V., Vanarsdall, A.L., Baker, R.J., Moerdyk-Schauwecker, M., Levine, C., et al., 2008a. Characterization of a novel alphaherpesvirus associated with fatal infections of domestic rabbits. Virology 378, 13–20.

Jin, L., Valentine, B.A., Baker, R.J., Lohr, C.V., Gerlach, R.F., Bildfell, R.J., et al., 2008b. An outbreak of fatal herpesvirus infection in domestic rabbits in Alaska. Vet. Pathol. 45, 369–374.

Jindal, H.K., Merchant, E., Balschi, J.A., Zhangand, Y., Koren, G., 2012. Proteomic analyses of transgenic LQT1 and LQT2 rabbit hearts elucidate an increase in expression and activity of energy producing enzymes. J. Proteomics 75, 5254–5265.

Johnson, J., Wolf, A.M., 1993. Ovarian abscesses and pyometra in a domestic rabbit. J. Am. Vet. Med. Assoc. 203, 667–669.

Joiner, G.N., Jardine, J.H., Gleiser, C.A., 1971. An epizootic of Shope fibromatosis in a commercial rabbitry. J. Am. Vet. Med. Assoc. 159, 1583–1587.

Jones, G.F., Ward, G.E., Murtaugh, M.P., Lin, G., Gebhart, C.J., 1993. Enhanced detection of intracellular organism of swine proliferative enteritis, ileal symbiont intracellularis, in feces by polymerase chain reaction. J. Clin. Microbiol. 31, 2611–2615.

Jones, T.C., Hunt, R.D., 1983. Veterinary Pathology. Lea & Fibiger, Philadelphia, PA.

Joyner, L.P., Catchpole, J., Berrett, S., 1987. Eimeria stiedae in rabbits: the demonstration of responses to chemotherapy. Res. Vet. Sci. 34, 64–67.

Kanazawa, K., Imai, A., 1959. Pure culture of the pathogenic agent of Tyzzer's disease of mice. Nature 184 (Suppl. 23), 1810–1811.

Kanbe, T., 2008. Molecular approaches in the diagnosis of dermatophytosis. Mycopathologia 166, 307–317.

Kaper, J.B., Nataro, J.P., Mobley, H.L., 2004. Pathogenic Escherichia coli. Nat. Rev. Microbiol. 2, 123–140.

Kardon, M.B., Peterson, D.F., Bishop, V.S., 1974. Beat-to-beat regulation of heart rate by afferent stimulation of the aortic nerve. Am. J. Physiol. 227, 598–600.

Karemaker, J.M., Borst, C., Schreurs, A.W., 1980. Implantable stimulating electrode for baroreceptor afferent nerves in rabbits. Am. J. Physiol. 239, H706–H709.

Kaufman, A.F., Quist, K.D., 1970. Spontaneous renal carcinoma in a New Zealand White rabbit. Lab. Anim. Care 20, 530–532.

Kaupke, A., Kwit, E., Chalmers, R.M., Michalski, M.M., Rzezutka, A., 2014. An outbreak of massive mortality among farm rabbits associated with Cryptosporidium infection. Res. Vet. Sci. 97, 85–87.

Kawamura, S., Taguchi, F., Ishida, T., Nakayama, M., Fujiwara, K., 1983. Growth of Tyzzer's organism in primary monolayer cultures of adult mouse hepatocytes. J. Gen. Microbiol. 129, 277–283.

Keel, M.K., Songer, J.G., 2006. The comparative pathology of Clostridium difficile-associated disease. Vet. Pathol. 43, 225–240.

Kennelly, J.J., Foote, R.H., 1965. Superovulatory response of pre-and post-pubertal rabbits to commercially available gonadotropins. J. Reprod. Fertil. 9, 177–183.

Kerr, P.J., Donnelly, T.M., 2013. Viral infections of rabbits. Vet. Clin. North Am. Exot. Anim. Pract 16, 437–468.

Kidd, J.G., Rous, P., 1940. A transplantable rabbit carcinoma originating in a virus-induced papilloma and containing the virus in masked or altered form. J. Exp. Med. 71, 813–838.

Kim, S.H., Cha, I.H., Kim, K.S., Kim, Y.H., Lee, Y.C., 1997. Cloning and sequence analysis of another Shiga-like toxin IIe variant gene (slt-IIera) from an *Escherichia coli* R107 strain isolated from rabbit. Microbiol. Immunol. 41, 805–808.

Kinkier, R.J., Jepsen, P.L., 1979. Ependymoma in a rabbit. Lab. Anim. Sci. 29, 255–256.

Kita, T., Brown, M.S., Watane, Y., Goldstein, J.L., 1981. Deficiency of low density lipoprotein receptors in liver and adrenal gland of the WHHL rabbit, an animal model of familial hypercholesterolemia. Proc. Natl. Acad. Sci. USA 78, 2268–2272.

Kluger, M.J., Gonzalez, R.R., Hardy, J.D., 1972. Peripheral thermal sensitivity in the rabbit. Am. J. Physiol. 222, 1031–1034.

Knepper, P.A., Goossens, W., Mclone, D.G., 1997. Ultrastructural studies of primary congenital glaucoma in rabbits. J. Pediatr. Ophthalmol. Strabismus. 34, 365–371.

Koller, L.D., 1969. Spontaneous *Nosema cuniculi* infection in laboratory rabbits. J. Am. Vet. Med. Assoc. 155, 1108–1114.

Komatsu, M., Yamamoto, K., Kawashima, T., Migita, S., 1985. Genetic deficiency of the alpha-gamma-subunit of the eighth complement component in the rabbit. J. Immunol. 134, 2607–2609.

Komatsu, M., Yamamoto, K., Nakano, Y., Nakazawa, M., Ozawa, A., Mikami, H., et al., 1988. Hereditary C3 hypocomplementemia in the rabbit. Immunology 64, 363–368.

Komatsu, M., Imaoka, K., Satoh, M., Mikami, H., 1990. Hereditary C8α-γ deficiency associated with dwarfism in the rabbit. J. Hered. 81, 413–417.

Kramer, A., Muller, R.S., Hein, J., 2012. Environmental factors, clinical signs, therapy and zoonotic risk of rabbits with dermatophytosis. Tierarztl Prax Ausg K Kleintiere Heimtiere 40, 425–431.

Kraus, A.L., Weisbroth, S.H., Flatt, R.E., Brewer, N., 1984. Biology and diseases of rabbits. In: Fox, J.G., Cohen, J., Loew, F.M. (Eds.), Laboratory Animal Medicine. Academic Press, Orlando, FL, pp. 207–240.

Krylov, V., Tlapakova, T., Macha, J., Curlej, J., Ryban, L., Chrenek, P., 2008. Localization of human coagulation factor VIII (hFVIII) in transgenic rabbit by FISH-TSA: identification of transgene copy number and transmission to the next generation. Foila Biol. 54, 121–124.

Kunzel, F., Joachim, A., 2010. Encephalitozoonosis in rabbits. Parasitol. Res. 106, 299–309.

Kurosawa, T., Kusanagi, M., Yamasaki, Y., Senga, Y., Yamamoto, T., 1995. New mutant rabbit strain with hypercholesterolemia and atherosclerotic lesions produced by serial inbreeding. Lab. Anim. Sci. 45, 385–392.

Kurtdede, A., Karaer, Z., Acar, A., Guzel, M., Cingi, C.C., Ural, K., et al., 2007. Use of selamectin for the treatment of psoroptic and sarcoptic mite infestation in rabbits. Vet. Dermatol. 18, 18–22.

Labranche, G.S., Renegar, K., 1996. Urinary calculus and hydronephrosis in a New Zealand White rabbit. Contemp. Top. Lab. Anim. Sci. 35, 71–73.

Lapierre, J., Marsolais, G., Pilon, P., Descoteaux, J.P., 1980. Preliminary report on the observation of a coronavirus in the intestine of the laboratory rabbit. Can. J. Microbiol. 26, 1204–1208.

Laville, A., Turner, P.R., Pittilo, R.M., Martini, S., Marenah, C.B., Rowles, P.M., et al., 1987. Hereditary hyperlipidemia in the rabbit due to overproduction of lipoproteins, I. Biochemical studies. Arteriosclerosis 7, 105–112.

Lawson, G.H., Gebhart, C.J., 2000. Proliferative enteropathy. J. Comp. Pathol. 122, 77–100.

Leary, S.J., Manning, P.J., Anderson, L.C., 1984. Experimental and naturally-occuring gastric foreign bodies in laboratory rabbits. Lab. Anim. Sci. 34, 58–61.

Lebas, F., 2000. Vitamins in rabbit nutrition: literature review and recommendations. World Rabbit Sci. 8, 185–192.

Leclercq, A., Mahillon, J., 2003. Farmed rabbits and ducks as vectors for VTEC O157:H7. Vet. Rec. 152, 723–724.

Lee, B.W., 1991. Cheyletiella dermatitis: a report of fourteen cases. Cutis 47, 111–114.

Lee, M.J., Lee, M.Y., Dalmasso, A.P., Swaim, W.R., 1974. Abnormal platelet response to thromboplastin infusion in rabbits deficient in the sixth component of complement. Proc. Soc. Exp. Biol. Med. 146, 732–737.

Leipig, M., Matiasek, K., Rinder, H., Janik, D., Emrich, D., Baiker, K., et al., 2013. Value of histopathology, immunohistochemistry, and real-time polymerase chain reaction in the confirmatory diagnosis of *Encephalitozoon cuniculi* infection in rabbits. J. Vet. Diagn. Invest. 25, 16–26.

Li, M.H., Ooi, H.K., 2009. Fecal occult blood manifestation of intestinal *Eimeria* spp. infection in rabbit. Vet. Parasitol. 161, 327–329.

Li, Q., Hou, J., Wang, S., Chen, Y., An, X.R., 2010. Production of transgenic rabbit embryos through intracytoplasmic sperm injection. Zygote 18, 301–307.

Li, X., Schlafer, D.H., 1992. A spontaneous skin basal cell tumor in a black French minilop rabbit. Lab. Anim. Sci. 42, 94–95.

Lichtensteiger, C., Leathers, C.W., 1987. Peritoneal mesothelioma in the rabbit. Vet. Pathol. 24, 464–466.

Licois, D., 1986. Tyzzer's disease. Ann. Rech. Vet. 17, 363–386.

Lidena, J., Trautschold, I., 1986. Catalytic enzyme activity concentration in plasma of man, sheep, dog, cat, rabbit, guinea pig, rat, and mouse. J. Clin. Chem. Clin. Biochem. 24, 11–18.

Liebenberg, S.P., Linn, J.M., 1980. Seasonal and sexual influence on rabbit atropinesterase. Lab. Anim. 14, 297–300.

Lim, J.J., Kim, D.H., Lee, J.J., Kim, D.G., Kim, S.H., Min, W., et al., 2012. Prevalence of *Lawsonia intracellularis*, *Salmonella* spp. and *Eimeria* spp. in healthy and diarrheic pet rabbits. J. Vet. Med. Sci. 74, 263–265.

Lindsey, J.R., Fox, R.R., 1994. Inherited diseases and variations. In: Manning, P.J., Ringler, D.H., Newcomer, C.E. (Eds.), Biology of the Laboratory Rabbit, second ed. Academic Press, Orlando, Florida, pp. 293–319.

Lipinski, D., Zeyland, J., Szalata, M., Plawski, A., Jarmuz, M., Jura, J., et al., 2012. Expression of human growth hormone in the milk of transgenic rabbits with transgene mapped to the telomere region of chromosome 7q. J. Appl. Genet. 53, 435–442.

Lipman, N.S., Weischedel, A.K., Connors, M.J., Olsen, D., Taylor, N.S., 1992. Utilization of cholestyramine resin as a preventative treatment for antibiotic (clindamycin) induced enterotoxemia in the rabbit. Lab. Anim. 26, 1–8.

Lipman, N.S., Zhao, Z.B., Andrutis, K.A., Hurley, R.J., Fox, J.G., White, H.J., 1994. Prolactin-secreting pituitary adenomas with mammary dysplasia in New Zealand White rabbits. Lab. Anim. Sci. 44, 114–120.

Liu, G.X., Choi, B.R., Ziv, O., Li, W., De Lange, E., Qu, Z., et al., 2012a. Differential conditions for early after-depolarizations and triggered activity in cardiomyocytes derived from transgenic LQT1 and LQT2 rabbits. J. Physiol. 590, 1171–1180.

Liu, W., Yang, M., Xu, Z., Zheng, H., Liang, W., Zhou, R., et al., 2012b. Complete genome sequence of *Pasteurella multocida* HN06, a toxigenic strain of serogroup D. J. Bacteriol. 194, 3292–3293.

Lombardi, R., Rodriguez, G., Chen, S.N., Ripplinger, C.M., Li, W., Chen, J., et al., 2009. Resolution of established cardiac hypertrophy and fibrosis and prevention of systolic dysfunction in a transgenic rabbit model of human cardiomyopathy through thiol-sensitive mechanisms. Circulation 119, 1398–1407.

Lopez-Martinez, R., Mier, T., Quirarte, M., 1984. Dermatophytes isolated from laboratory animals. Mycopathologia 88, 111–113.

Love, J.A., 1994. Group housing: meeting the physical and social needs of the laboratory rabbit. Lab. Anim. Sci. 44, 5–11.

Lukas, V.S., Ringler, D.H., Chrisp, C.E., Rush, H.G., 1987. An enzyme-linked immunosorbent assay to detect serum IgG to *Pasteurella multocida* in naturally and experimentally infected rabbits. Lab. Anim. Sci. 37, 60–64.

Lukjancenko, O., Wassenaar, T.M., Ussery, D.W., 2010. Comparison of 61 sequenced *Escherichia coli* genomes. Microb. Ecol. 60, 708–720.

Lumeij, J.T., Mikalova, L., Smajs, D., 2013. Is there a difference between hare syphilis and rabbit syphilis? Cross infection experiments between rabbits and hares. Vet. Microbiol. 164, 190–194.

Lund, A., Deboer, D.J., 2008. Immunoprophylaxis of dermatophytosis in animals. Mycopathologia 166, 407–424.

Lund, E.E., 1954a. The effect of sulfaquinoxaline on the course of *Eimeria stiedae* infection in the domestic rabbit. Exp. Parasitol. 3, 497–503.

Lund, E.E., 1954b. Estimating relative pollution of the environment with oocysts of *Eimeria stiedae*. J. Parasitol. 40, 663–667.

Mage, R.G., 1998. Immunology of Lagomorphs. In: Pastoret, P.P., Bazin, H., Griebel, H.P., Govaerts, H. (Eds.), Handbook of Vertebrate Immunology. Academic Press, London, pp. 223–260.

Mage, R.G., Lanning, D., Knight, K.L., 2006. B cell and antibody repertoire development in rabbits: the requirement of gut-associated lymphoid tissues. Dev. Comp. Immunol. 30, 137–153.

Mangel, A., Fahim, M., Van Breemen, C., 1981. Rhythmic contractile activity of the in vivo rabbit aorta. Nature 289, 892–894.

Manning, P.J., 1982. Serology of *Pasteurella multocida* in laboratory rabbits: a review. Lab. Anim. Sci. 32, 666–671.

Marini, R.P., Foltz, C.J., Kersten, D., Batchelder, M., Kaser, W., Li, X., 1996. Microbiologic, radiographic, and anatomic study of the nasolacrimal duct apparatus in the rabbit (*Oryctolagus cuniculus*). Lab. Anim. Sci. 46, 656–662.

Masson, D., Deckert, V., Gautier, T., Klein, A., Desrumaux, C., Viglietta, C., et al., 2011. Worsening of diet-induced atherosclerosis in a new model of transgenic rabbit expressing the human plasma phospholipid transfer protein. Arterioscler. Thromb. Vasc. Biol. 31, 766–774.

Mathis, A., Michel, M., Kuster, H., Muller, C., Weber, R., Deplazes, P., 1997. Two *Encephalitozoon cuniculi* strains of human origin are infectious to rabbits. Parasitol 114, 29–35.

McCluskey, J., Hannigan, J., Harris, J.D., Wren, B., Smith, D.G., 2002. LsaA, an antigen involved in cell attachment and invasion, is expressed by *Lawsonia intracellularis* during infection in vitro and in vivo. Infect. Immun. 70, 2899–2907.

McDowell, L.R., 1989. Vitamins in Animal Nutrition. Academic Press, San Diego, CA.

McKellar, Q.A., Midgeley, D.M., Galbraith, E.A., Scott, E.W., Bradley, A., 1992. Clinical and pharmacological properties of ivermectin in rabbits and guinea pigs. Vet. Rec. 25, 71–73.

Meier, H., Fox, R.R., Cary, D.D., 1972. Myeloid leukemia in the rabbit. Cancer Res. 32, 1785–1787.

Mellgren, M., Bergvall, K., 2008. Treatment of rabbit chyletiellosis with selamectin or ivermectin: a retrospective case study. Acta. Vet. Scand., 50.

Melton-Celsa, A., Mohawk, K., Teel, L., O'Brien, A., 2012. Pathogenesis of Shiga-toxin producing *Escherichia coli*. Curr. Top. Micro. Immuno. 357, 67–103.

Mendez-Tovar, L.J., 2010. Pathogenesis of dermatophytosis and *Tinea versicolor*. Clin. Dermatol. 28, 185–189.

Mitro, S., Krauss, H., 1993. Rabbit hemorrhagic disease: a review with special reference to its epizootiology. Eur. J. Epidemiol. 9, 70–78.

Mitruka, B.M., Rawnsley, H.M., 1981. Clinical Biochemical and Hematological Reference Values in Normal Experimental Animals and Normal Humans. Masson, New York.

Monath, T.P., Kahn, L.H., Kaplan, B., 2010. Introduction: one health perspective. ILAR J. 51, 193–198.

Moon, H.W., Cutlip, R.C., Amtower, W.C., Matthews, P.J., 1974. Intraepithelial vibrio associated with acute typhlitis of young rabbits. Vet. Pathol. 11, 313–326.

Morrell, J.M., 1989. Hydrometra in the rabbit. Vet. Rec. 125, 325.

Murakata, K., Sato, A., Yoshiya, M., Kim, S., Watarai, M., Omata, Y., et al., 2008. Infection of different strains of mice with *Lawsonia intracellularis* derived from rabbit or porcine proliferative enteropathy. J. Comp. Pathol. 139, 8–15.

Myktowycz, R., 1957. Ectoparasites of the wild rabbit, *Oryctolagus cuniculus* (L.) in Australia. Wildl. Res. 2, 1–4.

Nalca, A., Nichols, D.K., 2011. Rabbitpox: a model of airborne transmission of smallpox. J. Gen. Virol. 92, 31–35.

National Research Council, 2011. Guide for the Care and Use of Laboratory Animals. National Academies Press, Washington, DC.

Nielsen, J.N., Carlton, W.W., 1995. Colobomatous microphthalmos in a New Zealand White rabbit, arising from a colony with suspected vitamin E deficiency. Lab. Anim. Sci. 45, 320–322.

Niepceron, A., Licois, D., 2010. Development of a high-sensitivity nested PCR assay for the detection of *Clostridium piliforme* in clinical samples. Vet. J. 185, 222–224.

Niilo, L., 1967. Acquired resistance to reinfection of rabbits with *Eimeria magna*. Can. Vet. J. 8, 201–208.

Noguchi, T., Yamashita, Y., 1987. The rabbit differs from other mammalian species in the tissue distribution of alkaline phosphatase isoenzymes. Biochem. Biophys. Res. Commun. 143, 15–19.

Nogueira, M.G., Collins, A.M., Donahoo, M., Emery, D., 2013. Immunological responses to vaccination following experimental *Lawsonia intracellularis* virulent challenge in pigs. Vet. Microbiol. 164, 131–138.

Nong, X., Ren, Y.J., Wang, J.H., Xie, Y., Fang, C.L., Yang, D.Y., et al., 2013. Clinical efficacy of botanical extracts from *Eupatorium adenophorum* against the *Sarcoptes scabiei* (Sarcoptidae: Sarcoptes) in rabbits. Vet. Parasitol. 195, 157–164.

Nowak, R.M., Paradiso, J.L., 1983. Walker's Mammals of the World. Johns Hopkins University Press, Baltimore, MD.

Okewole, E.A., Olubunmi, P.A., 2008. Antibiograms of pathogenic bacteria isolated from laboratory rabbits in Ibadan, Nigeria. Lab. Anim. 42, 511–514.

Oliveira, U.C., Fraga, J.S., Licois, D., Pakandl, M., Gruber, A., 2011. Development of molecular assays for the identification of the 11 *Eimeria* species of the domestic rabbit (*Oryctolagus cuniculus*). Vet. Parasitol. 176, 275–280.

Orth, J.H., Preuss, I., Fester, I., Schlosser, A., Wilson, B.A., Aktories, K., 2009. *Pasteurella multocida* toxin activation of heterotrimeric G proteins by deamidation. Proc. Natl. Acad. Sci. USA 106, 7179–7184.

Owen, D., 1970. Life cycle of *Eimeria stiedae*. Nature 227, 304.

Pakandl, M., 2009. Coccidia of rabbit: a review. Folia Parsitol. 56, 153–166.

Pakandl, M., Hlaskova, L., 2007. The reproduction of *Eimeria flavescens* and *Eimeria intestinalis* in suckling rabbits. Parasitol. Res. 101, 1435–1437.

Pakandl, M., Jelinkova, A., 2006. The rabbit coccidium *Eimeria piriformis*: selection of a precocious line and life-cycle study. Vet. Parasitol. 137, 351–354.

Pakes, S.P., 1974. Protozoal diseases. In: Weisbroth, S.H., Flatt, R.E., Kraus, A.L. (Eds.), The Biology of the Laboratory Rabbit, first ed. Academic Press, Orlando, FL, pp. 263–286.

Pakes, S.P., Gerrity, L.W., 1994. Protozoal diseases. In: Manning, P.J., Ringler, D.H., Newcomer, C.E. (Eds.), Biology of the Laboratory Rabbit, second ed. Academic Press, Orlando, FL, pp. 205–230.

Pallis, A., Jazayeri, J., Ward, P., Dimovski, K., Svobodova, S., 2013. Rapid detection of *Clostridium difficile* toxins from stool samples using real-time multiplex PCR. J. Med. Microbiol. 62, 1350–1356.

Pan, B., Wang, M., Xu, F., Wang, Y., Dong, Y., Pan, Z., 2006. Efficacy of an injectable formulation of eprinomectin against Psoroptes cuniculi, the ear mange mite in rabbits. Vet. Parasitol. 137, 386–390.

Papatheodorou, P., Wilczek, C., Nolke, T., Guttenberg, G., Hornuss, D., Schwan, C., et al., 2012. Identification of the cellular receptor of *Clostridium spiroforme* toxin. Infect. Immun. 80, 1418–1423.

Pasay, C., Mounsey, K., Stevenson, G., Davis, R., Arlian, L., Morgan, M., et al., 2010. Acaricidal activity of eugenol based compounds against scabies mites. PLoS One 5, e12079.

Pascal, R.R., 1961. Plasma cell myeloma in the brain of a rabbit. Cornell Vet. 51, 528–535.

Pattison, M., Clegg, F.G., Duncan, A.L., 1971. An outbreak of encephalomyelitis in broiler rabbits caused by *Nosema cuniculi*. Vet. Rec. 88, 404–405.

Pedersen, K.S., Holyoake, P., Stege, H., Nielsen, J.P., 2010. Diagnostic performance of different fecal *Lawsonia intracellularis*-specific polymerase chain reaction assays as diagnostic tests for proliferative enteropathy in pigs: a review. J. Vet. Diagn. Invest. 22, 487–494.

Peeters, J.E., Geeroms, R., Carman, R.J., Wilkins, T.D., 1986. Significance of *Clostridium spiroforme* in the enteritis-complex of commercial rabbits. Vet. Microbiol. 12, 25–31.

Peeters, J.E., Geeroms, R., Orskov, F., 1988. Biotype, serotype, and pathogenicity of attaching and effacing enteropathogenic *Escherichia coli* strains isolated from diarrheic commercial rabbits. Infect. Immun. 56, 1442–1448.

Pegg, E.J., 1970. Three ectoparasites of veterinary interest communicable to man. Med. Bio. Illus. 20, 106–110.

Pellérdy, L., 1965. Coccidia and Coccidiosis. Hungarian Academy of Science, Budapest, Hungary.

Pellérdy, L., 1969. Parenteral infection experiments with Eimeria stiedae. Acta. Vet. Acad. Sci. Hung. 19, 171–182.

Peng, X., 2012. Transgenic rabbit models for studying human cardiovascular diseases. Comp. Med. 62, 472–479.

Per, H., Kumandas, S., Gumus, H., Ozturk, M.K., Coskun, A., 2010. Meningitis and subgaleal, subdural, epidural empyema due to *Pasteurella multocida*. J. Emerg. Med. 39, 35–38.

Perkins, S.E., Fox, J.G., Taylor, N.S., Green, D.L., Lipman, N.S., 1995. Detection of *Clostridium difficile* toxins from the small intestine and cecum of rabbits with naturally acquired enterotoxemia. Lab. Anim. Sci. 45, 379–384.

Pinheiro, A., Lanning, D., Alves, P.C., Mage, R.G., Knight, K.L., Van Der Loo, W., et al., 2011. Molecular bases of genetic diversity and evolution of the immunoglobulin heavy chain variable region (IGHV) gene locus in leporids. Immunogenetics 63, 397–408.

Pleasants, J.R., 1959. Rearing germfree cesarean-born rats, mice, and rabbits through weaning. Ann. N. Y. Acad. Sci. 78, 116–126.

Pletcher, J.M., Murphy, J.C., 1984. Spontaneous malignant hemangiosarcomas in two rabbits. Vet. Pathol. 21, 542–544.

Podberscek, A.L., Blackshaw, J.K., Beattie, A.W., 1991. The behaviour of group penned and individually caged laboratory rabbits. Appl. Anim. Behav. Sci. 28, 353–359.

Poeta, P., Radhouani, H., Goncalves, A., Figueiredo, N., Carvalho, C., Rodrigues, J., et al., 2010. Genetic characterization of antibiotic resistance in enteropathogenic *Escherichia coli* carrying extended-spectrum beta-lactamases recovered from diarrhoeic rabbits. Zoonoses Public Hlth. 57, 162–170.

Poggiagliolmi, S., Crowell-Davis, S.L., Alworth, L.C., Harvey, S.B., 2011. Environmental enrichment of New Zealand White rabbits living in laboratory cages. J. Vet. Behav. 6, 343–350.

Pohl, P.H., Peeters, J.E., Jacquemin, E.R., Lintermans, P.F., Mainil, J.G., 1993. Identification of *eae* sequences in enteropathogenic *Escherichia coli* strains from rabbits. Infect. Immun. 61, 2203–2206.

Port, C.D., Sidor, M.A., 1978. A sebaceous gland carcinoma in a rabbit. Lab. Anim. Sci. 28, 215–216.

Prescott, J.F., 1977. Tyzzer's disease in rabbits in Britain. Vet. Rec. 100, 285–286.

Prevost, M.C., Aliouat, E.M., Escamilla, R., Dei-Cas, E., 1997. Pneumocystosis in humans or in corticosteroid-untreated animal models: interactions between pulmonary surfactant changes and *Pneumocystis carinii* in vivo or in vitro growth. J. Eukaryot. Microbiol. 44, 58S.

Pritchard, G.C., Williamson, S., Carson, T., Bailey, J.R., Warner, L., Willshaw, G., et al., 2001. Wild rabbits—a novel vector for verocytotoxigenic *Escherichia coli* O157. Vet. Rec. 149, 567.

Pritt, S., Henderson, K.S., Shek, W.R., 2010. Evaluation of available diagnostic methods for *Clostridium piliforme* in laboratory rabbits (*Oryctolagus cuniculus*). Lab. Anim. 44, 14–19.

Pusterla, N., Mapes, S., Gebhart, C., 2012a. Further investigation of exposure to Lawsonia intracellularis in wild and feral animals captured on horse properties with equine proliferative enteropathy. Vet. J. 194, 253–255.

Pusterla, N., Vannucci, F.A., Mapes, S.M., Nogradi, N., Collier, J.R., Hill, J.A., et al., 2012b. Efficacy of an avirulent live vaccine against *Lawsonia intracellularis* in the prevention of proliferative enteropathy in experimentally infected weanling foals. Am. J. Vet. Res. 73, 741–746.

Pusterla, N., Sanchez-Migallon Guzman, D., Vannucci, F.A., Mapes, S., White, A., Difrancesco, M., et al., 2013. Transmission of *Lawsonia intracellularis* to weanling foals using feces from experimentally infected rabbits. Vet. J. 195, 241–243.

Radi, Z.A., 2004. Outbreak of sarcoptic mange and malasseziasis in rabbits (*Oryctolagus cuniculus*). Comp. Med. 54, 434–437.

Raflo, C.P., Olsen, R.G., Pakes, S.P., Webster, W.S., 1973. Characterization of a fibroma virus isolated from naturally-occurring skin tumors in domestic rabbits. Lab. Anim. Sci. 23, 525–532.

Rasko, D.A., Rosovitz, M.J., Myers, G.S., Mongodin, E.F., Fricke, W.F., Gajer, P., et al., 2008. The pangenome structure of *Escherichia coli*: comparative genomic analysis of *E. coli* commensal and pathogenic isolates. J. Bacteriol. 190, 6881–6893.

Redondo, L.M., Farber, M., Venzano, A., Jost, B.H., Parma, Y.R., Fernandez-Miyakawa, M.E., 2013. Sudden death syndrome in adult cows associated with *Clostridium perfringens* type E. Anaerobe 20, 1–4.

Rehg, J.E., Lawton, G.W., Pakes, S.P., 1979. *Cryptosporidium cuniculus* in the rabbit (*Oryctolagus cuniculus*). Lab. Anim. Sci. 29, 656–660.

Rehg, J.E., Lu, Y.S., 1981. *Clostridium difficile* colitis in a rabbit following antibiotic therapy for pasteurellosis. J. Am. Vet. Med. Assoc. 179, 1296–1297.

Rice, A.D., Adams, M.M., Lampert, B., Foster, S., Robertson, A., Painter, G., et al., 2011. Efficacy of CMX001 as a prophylactic and presymptomatic antiviral agent in New Zealand white rabbits infected with rabbitpox virus, a model for orthopoxvirus infections of humans. Viruses 3, 63–82.

Richmond, C.R., Langham, W.H., Trujillo, T.T., 1962. Comparative metabolism of tritiated water by mammals. J. Cell. Comp. Physiol. 59, 45–53.

Riley, L.K., Caffrey, C.J., Musille, V.S., Meyer, J.K., 1992. Cytotoxicity of Bacillus piliformis. J. Med. Microbiol. 37, 77–80.

Ringler, D.H., Abrams, G.D., 1970. Nutritional muscular dystrophy and neonatal mortality in a rabbit breeding colony. J. Am. Vet. Med. Assoc. 157, 1928–1934.

Ringler, D.H., Abrams, G.D., 1971. Laboratory diagnosis of vitamin E deficiency in rabbits fed a faulty commercial ration. Lab. Anim. Sci. 21, 383–388.

Robert, R., Pihet, M., 2008. Conventional methods for the diagnosis of dermatophytosis. Mycopathologia 166, 295–306.

Robertson, J.M., Samankova, L., Ingalls, T.H., 1966. Hydrocephalus and cleft palate in an inbred rabbit colony. J. Hered. 57, 142–148.

Robinson, G., Wright, S., Elwin, K., Hadfield, S.J., Katzer, F., Bartley, P.M., et al., 2010. Re-description of Cryptosporidium cuniculus Inman and Takeuchi, 1979 (Apicomplexa: Cryptosporidiidae): morphology, biology and phylogeny. Int. J. Parsitol. 40, 1539–1548.

Robl, J.M., Burnside, A.S., 1994. Production of transgenic rabbits. In: Pinker, C.A. (Ed.), Transgenic Animal Technology: A Laboratory Handbook. Academic Press, Orlando, FL, pp. 251–260.

Rose, M.E., 1959. A study of the life cycle of Eimeria stiedae (Lindemann, 1865) and the immunological response of the host. Ph.D. thesis, Cambridge University.

Rossi, G., Donadio, E., Perrucci, S., 2007. Immunocytochemistry of Psoroptes cuniculi stained by sera from naive and infested rabbits: preliminary results. Parasitol. Res. 100, 1281–1285.

Rother, K., Rother, U., Muller-Eberhard, H.J., Nilsson, J.R., 1966. Deficiency of the sixth component of complement in rabbits with an inherited complement defect. J. Exp. Med. 124, 773–785.

Ruckebusch, Y., Phaneuf, L.P., Dunlop, R., 1991. Physiology of Small and Large Animals. Dekker, Philadelphia, PA.

Rutherford, R.L., 1943. The life cycle of four intestinal coccidia of the domestic rabbit. J. Parasitol. 29, 10–32.

Sait, M., Aitchison, K., Wheelhouse, N., Wilson, K., Lainson, F.A., Longbottom, D., et al., 2013. Genome Sequence of Lawsonia intracellularis Strain N343, Isolated from a Sow with Hemorrhagic Proliferative Enteropathy. Genome Announc. 1 http://dx.doi.10.1128/genomeA.00027-13. Epub 2013 Feb 28.

Salmon, J., Ramoz, N., Cassonnet, P., Orth, G., Breitburd, F., 1997. A cottontail rabbit papillomavirus strain (CRPVb) with striking divergent E6 and E7 oncoproteins: an insight in the evolution of papillomaviruses. Virology 235, 228–234.

Sanbe, A., James, J., Tuzcu, V., Nas, S., Martin, L., Gulick, J., et al., 2005. Transgenic rabbit model for human troponin I-based hypertrophic cardiomyopathy. Circulation 111, 2330–2338.

Sanchez, C.A., Chabe, M., Aliouat El, M., Durand-Joly, I., Gantois, N., Conseil, V., et al., 2007. Exploring transplacental transmission of Pneumocystis oryctolagi in first-time pregnant and multiparous rabbit does. Med. Mycol. 45, 701–707.

Sanchez, J.P., De La Fuente, L.F., Rosell, J.M., 2012. Health and body condition of lactating females on rabbit farms. J. Anim. Sci. 90, 2353–2361.

Sanderson, J.H., Phillips, C.E., 1981. An Atlas of Laboratory Animal Haematology. Oxford University, Oxford.

Sawin, P.B., Crary, D.D., 1943. Atropinesterase, a genetically determined enzyme in the rabbit. Proc. Natl. Acad. Sci. USA 29, 55–59.

Scaife, H.R., Cowan, D., Finney, J., Kinghorn-Perry, S.F., Crook, B., 2006. Wild rabbits (Oryctolagus cuniculus) as potential carriers of verocytotoxin-producing Escherichia coli. Vet. Rec. 159, 175–178.

Schauer, D.B., Mccathey, S.N., Daft, B.M., Jha, S.S., Tatterson, L.E., Taylor, N.S., et al., 1998. Proliferative enterocolitis associated with dual infection with enteropathogenic Escherichia coli and Lawsonia intracellularis in rabbits. J. Clin. Microbiol. 36, 1700–1703.

Schmiedt, W., Kinscherf, R., Deigner, H.P., Kamencic, H., Nauen, O., Kilo, J., et al., 1998. Complement C6 deficiency protects against diet-induced atherosclerosis in rabbits. Arterioscler. Thromb. Vasc. Biol. 18, 1790–1795.

Schnupf, P., Sansonetti, P.J., 2012. Quantitative RT-PCR profiling of the rabbit immune response: assessment of acute Shigella flexneri infection. PLoS One 7, e36446.

Schoeb, T.R., Fox, J.G., 1990. Enterococecolitis associated with intraepithelial Campylobacter-like bacteria in rabbits (Oryctolagus cuniculus). Vet. Pathol. 27, 73–80.

Schoeb, T.R., Casebolt, D.B., Walker, V.E., Potgieter, L.N.D., Thouless, M.E., DiGiacomo, R.F., 1986. Rotavirus-associated diarrhea in a commercial rabbitry. Lab. Anim. Sci. 36, 149–152.

Schoeb, T.R., Cartner, S.C., Baker, R.A., Gerrity, L.W., Baker, D.G., 2007. Parasites of Rabbits. In: Baker, D.G. (Ed.), Flynn's Parasites of Laboratory Animals, second ed. Wiley-Blackwell, Oxford, UK, pp. 451–499.

Schoster, A., Kokotovic, B., Permin, A., Pedersen, P.D., Dal Bello, F., Guardabassi, L., 2013. In vitro inhibition of Clostridium difficile and Clostridium perfringens by commercial probiotic strains. Anaerobe 20, 36–41.

Shadduck, J., Polley, M.B., 1978. Some factors in the in vitro infectivity and replication of Encephalitozoon cuniculi. J. Protozool. 25, 491–496.

Shang, X., Wang, D., Miao, X., Wang, X., Li, J., Yang, Z., et al., 2014. The oxidative status and inflammatory level of the peripheral blood of rabbits infested with Psoroptes cuniculi. Parasit Vectors 7, 124.

Sheldon, W.H., 1959. Experimental pulmonary Pneumocystis carinii infection in rabbits. J. Exp. Med. 110, 147–160.

Shelley, H.J., 1961. Glycogen reserves and their changes at birth. Br. Med. Bull. 17, 137–143.

Shiibashi, T., Imai, T., Sato, Y., Abe, N., Yukawa, M., Nogami, S., 2006. Cryptosporidium infection in juvenile pet rabbits. J. Vet. Med. Sci. 68, 281–282.

Silberfein, E.J., Lin, P.H., Bush, R.L., Zhou, W., Lumsden, A.B., 2006. Aortic endograft infection due to Pasteurella multocida following a rabbit bite. J. Vasc. Surg. 43, 393–395.

Simon, M., Antalikova, J., Chrenek, P., Horovska, L., Hluchy, S., Michalkova, K., et al., 2011. Analysis of the expression of platelet antigens CD9 and CD41/61 in transgenic rabbits with the integrated human blood clotting factor VIII gene construct. Gen. Physiol. Biophys. 30 (Spec No), S83–S87.

Singh, S.K., Dimri, U., Sharma, M.C., Swarup, D., Kumar, M., Tiwary, R., 2012. Psoroptes cuniculi induced oxidative imbalance in rabbits and its alleviation by using vitamins A, D3, E, and H as adjunctive remedial. Trop. Anim. Health Prod. 44, 43–48.

Smajs, D., Zobanikova, M., Strouhal, M., Cejkova, D., Dugan-Rocha, S., Pospisilova, P., et al., 2011. Complete genome sequence of Treponema paraluiscuniculi, strain Cuniculi A: the loss of infectivity to humans is associated with genome decay. PLoS One 6, e20415.

Smajs, D., Norris, S.J., Weinstock, G.M., 2012. Genetic diversity in Treponema pallidum: implications for pathogenesis, evolution and molecular diagnostics of syphilis and yaws. Infect. Genet. Evol. 12, 191–202.

Small, J.D., Newman, B., 1972. Venereal spirochetosis of rabbits (rabbit syphilis) due to Treponema cuniculi: a clinical, serological, and histopathological study. Lab. Anim. Sci. 22, 77–89.

Smetana, H., 1933. Coccidiosis of the live rabbit II, Experimental study on the mode of infection of the liver by sporozoites of Eimeria stiedae Arch. Pathol. 15, 330–339.

Smith, D.G., Lawson, G.H., 2001. Lawsonia intracellularis: getting inside the pathogenesis of proliferative enteropathy. Vet. Microbiol. 82, 331–345.

Smith, D.G., Mitchell, S.C., Nash, T., Rhind, S., 2000. Gamma interferon influences intestinal epithelial hyperplasia caused by Lawsonia intracellularis infection in mice. Infect. Immun. 68, 6737–6743.

Smith, H.W., 1951. The Kidney. Oxford University Press, New York.

Smith, K.J., Skelton, H.G., Hilyard, E.J., Hadfield, T., Moeller, R.S., Tuur, S., et al., 1996. Bacillus piliformis infection (Tyzzer's disease) in a patient infected with HIV-1: confirmation with 16S ribosomal RNA sequence analysis. J. Am. Acad. Dermatol. 34, 343–348.

Soler, E., Le Saux, A., Guinut, F., Passet, B., Cohen, R., Merle, C., et al., 2005. Production of two vaccinating recombinant rotavirus proteins in the milk of transgenic rabbits. Transgenic Res. 14, 833–844.

Songer, J.G., 1996. Clostridial enteric diseases of domestic animals. Clin. Microbiol. Rev. 9, 216–234.

Soulez, B., Dei-Cas, E., Charet, P., Mougeot, G., Caillaux, M., Camus, D., 1989. The young rabbit: a nonimmunosuppressed model for Pneumocystis carinii pneumonia. J. Infect. Dis. 160, 355–356.

Soulsby, E.J.L., 1968. Helminth, Arthropods, and Protozoa of Domestic Animals. Williams & Wilkins, Baltimore, MD.

Sovell, J.R., Holmes, J.C., 1996. Efficacy of ivermectin against nematodes infecting field populations of snowshoe hares (Lepus americanus) in Yukon, Canada. J. Wildl. Dis. 32, 23–30.

Spibey, N., McCabe, V.J., Greenwood, N.M., Jack, S.C., Sutton, D., Van Der Waart, L., 2012. Novel bivalent vectored vaccine for control of myxomatosis and rabbit haemorrhagic disease. Vet. Rec. 170, 309.

Spiesschaert, B., McFadden, G., Hermans, K., Nauwynck, H., Van De Walle, G.R., 2011. The current status and future directions of myxoma virus, a master in immune evasion. Vet. Res. 42, 76.

Stahel, A.B., Hoop, R.K., Kuhnert, P., Korczak, B.M., 2009. Phenotypic and genetic characterization of *Pasteurella multocida* and related isolates from rabbits in Switzerland. J. Vet. Diagn. Invest. 21, 793–802.

Stanley, B.A., Graham, D.R., James, J., Mitsak, M., Tarwater, P.M., Robbins, J., et al., 2011. Altered myofilament stoichiometry in response to heart failure in a cardioprotective alpha-myosin heavy chain transgenic rabbit model. Proteomics 5, 147–158.

Steinhausen, M., Endlich, K., Wiegman, D.L., 1990. Glomerular blood flow. Kidney Int. 38, 769–784.

Stetson, P.L., Normolle, D.P., Knol, J.A., et al., 1991. Biochemical modulation of 5-bromo-2′-deoxyuridine and 5-iodo-2′-deoxyuridine incorporation into DNA in VX2 tumor-bearing rabbits. J. Natl. Cancer Inst. 83, 1659–1667.

Stills, J.H.F., 1994. Polyclonal antibody production. In: Manning, P.J., Ringler, D.H., Newcomer, C.E. (Eds.), Biology of the Laboratory Rabbit, second ed. Academic Press, Orlando, FL, pp. 435–448.

Stinnett, H.O., Sepe, F.J., 1979. Rabbit cardiovascular responses during PEEP before and after vagotomy. Proc. Soc. Exp. Biol. Med. 162, 485–494.

Stormont, C., Suzuki, Y., 1970. Atropinesterase and cocainesterase of rabbit serum: localization of the enzyme activity in isozymes. Science 167, 200–202.

Stubbs, S., Rupnik, M., Gibert, M., Brazier, J., Duerden, B., Popoff, M., 2000. Production of actin-specific ADP-ribosyltransferase (binary toxin) by strains of *Clostridium difficile*. FEMS Microbiol. Lett. 186, 307–312.

Subcommittee on Rabbit Nutrition, Committee on Animal Nutrition, Board on Agriculture and Renewable Resources & National Research Council, 1977. Nutrient Requirements of Rabbits. National Academy of Sciences, Washington, DC.

Suckow, M., Douglas, F., 1997. The Laboratory Rabbit. CRC Press, Boca Raton, FL.

Suckow, M., Grigdesby, C.F., 1993. Spontaneous lateral abdominal (lumbar) hernia in a New Zealand White rabbit. Lab. Anim. Sci. 43, 106–107.

Suckow, M.A., 2000. Immunization of rabbits against *Pasteurella multocida* using a commercial swine vaccine. Lab. Anim. 34, 403–408.

Suckow, M.A., Chrisp, C.E., Foged, N.T., 1991. Heat-labile toxin-producing isolates of *Pasteurella multocida* from rabbits. Lab. Anim. Sci. 41, 151–156.

Suckow, M.A., Bowersock, T.L., Nielsen, K., Chrisp, C.E., Frandsen, P.L., Janovitz, E.B., 1995. Protective immunity to *Pasteurella multocida* heat-labile toxin by intranasal immunization in rabbits. Lab. Anim. Sci. 45, 526–532.

Suckow, M.A., Martin, B.J., Bowersock, T.L., Douglas, F.A., 1996. Derivation of *Pasteurella multocida*-free rabbit litters by enrofloxacin treatment. Vet. Microbiol. 51, 161–168.

Suckow, M.A., Jarvinen, L.Z., Hogenesch, H., Park, K., Bowersock, T.L., 2002. Immunization of rabbits against a bacterial pathogen with an alginate microparticle vaccine. J. Contr. Release 85, 227–235.

Suckow, M.A., Haab, R.W., Miloscio, L.J., Guillou, N.B., 2008. Field trial of a *Pasteurella multocida* extract vaccine in rabbits. J. Am. Assoc. Lab. Anim. Sci. 47, 18–21.

Sun, Y., Wei, Z., Li, N., Zhao, Y., 2013. A comparative overview of immunoglobulin genes and the generation of their diversity in tetrapods. Dev. Comp. Immunol. 39, 103–109.

Sundarum, P., Tigelaar, R.E., Brandsma, J.L., 1998. Intracutaneous vaccination of rabbits with the cottontail rabbit papillomavirus (CRPV) L1 gene protects against virus challenge. Vaccine 16, 613–623.

Suter, C., Muller-Doblies, U., Hatt, J., Deplazes, P., 2001. Prevention and treatment of Encephalitozoon cuniculi infection in rabbits with fenbendazole. Vet. Rec. 148, 478–480.

Swennes, A.G., Buckley, E.M., Madden, C.M., Byrd, C.P., Donocoff, R.S., Rodriguez, L., et al., 2013. Enteropathogenic Escherichia coli prevalence in laboratory rabbits. Vet. Microbiol. 163, 395–398.

Swennes, A.G., Buckley, E.M., Parry, N.M., Madden, C.M., Garcia, A., Morgan, P.B., et al., 2012. Enzootic enteropathogenic Escherichia coli infection in laboratory rabbits. J. Clin. Microbiol. 50, 2353–2358.

Syukuda, Y., 1979. Rearing of germfree rabbits and establishment of an SPF rabbit colony. Jikken Dobutsu 28, 39–48.

Taffs, L.F., 1976. Pinworm infection in laboratory rodents: a review. Lab. Anim. 10, 1–13.

Takahashi, R., Kuramochi, T., Aoyagi, K., Hashimoto, S., Miyoshi, I., Kasai, N., et al., 2007. Establishment and characterization of CAG/EGFP transgenic rabbit line. Transgenic Res. 16, 115–120.

Tamburrini, E., Ortona, E., Visconti, E., Mencarini, P., Margutti, P., Zolfo, M., et al., 1999. *Pneumocystis carinii* infection in young non-immunosuppressed rabbits. Kinetics of infection and of the primary specific immune response. Med. Microbiol. Immunol. 188, 1–7.

Tarr, P.I., 2009. Shiga toxin-associated hemolytic uremic syndrome and thrombotic thrombocytopenic purpura: distinct mechanisms of pathogenesis. Kidney Int. Suppl., S29–S32.

Tarr, P.I., Gordon, C.A., Chandler, W.L., 2005. Shiga-toxin-producing Escherichia coli and haemolytic uraemic syndrome. Lancet 365, 1073–1086.

Tesluk, G.C., Peiffer, R.L., Brown, D., 1982. A clinical and pathological study of inherited glaucoma in New Zealand White rabbits. Lab. Anim. 16, 234–239.

Thouless, M.E., DiGiacomo, R.F., Deeb, B.J., 1996. The effect of combined rotavirus and Escherichia coli infection in rabbits. Lab. Anim. Sci. 46, 381–385.

Tinkey, P., Uthamanthil, R.K., Weisbroth, S.T., 2012. Rabbit neoplasia. In: Suckow, M.A., Stevens, K.A., Wilson, R.P. (Eds.), The Laboratory Rabbit, Guinea Pig, Hamster, and Other Rodents. Academic Press, Orlando, FL.

Tjwa, M., Carmeliet, P., Moons, L., 2006. Novel transgenic rabbit model sheds light on the puzzling role of matrix metalloproteinase-12 in atherosclerosis. Circulation 113, 1929–1932.

Trueta, J., Barclay, A.E., Daniel, P.M., Franklin, K.J., Prichard, M.M.L., 1947. Studies on the Renal Circulation. Blackwell, Oxford.

Truex, R.C., Smythe, M.Q., 1965. Comparative morphology of the cardiac conduction tissue in animals. Ann. N. Y. Acad. Sci. 127, 19–33.

Tschudin, A., Clauss, M., Codron, D., Liesegang, A., Hatt, J.M., 2011. Water intake in domestic rabbits (Oryctolagus cuniculus) from open dishes and nipple drinkers under different water and feeding regimes. J. Anim. Physiol. Anim. Nutr. (Berl.) 95, 499–511.

Tsunoda, K., Imai, S., Tsutsumi, Y., Inouye, S., 1968. Intermittent medication of sulfadimethoxine and sulfamonomethoxine for the treatment of coccidiosis in domestic rabbits. Natl. Inst. Anim. Health Q. (Tokyo) 8, 74–80.

Turner, T.B., Hollander, D.H., 1957. Biology of the treponematoses based on studies carried out at the International Treponematosis Laboratory Center of the Johns Hopkins University under the auspices of the World Health Organization. Monogr. Ser. World Health Organ., 3–266.

Umemura, T., Tsuchitani, M., Totsuka, M., Narama, I., Yamashiro, S., 1982. Histiocytic enteritis of rabbits. Vet. Pathol. 19, 326–329.

Vannucci, F.A., Pusterla, N., Mapes, S.M., Gebhart, C., 2012. Evidence of host adaptation in Lawsonia intracellularis infections. Vet. Res. 43, 53.

Varga, I., 1982. Large-scale management systems and parasite populations: coccidia in rabbits. Vet. Parasitol. 11, 69–84.

Vella, D., 2013. Rabbits, dermatopathies. In: Donnelly, T.M. (Ed.), Clinical Veterinary Advisor Birds and Exotic Pets. Elsevier Saunders, Philadelphia, pp. 360–364.

Vermout, S., Tabart, J., Baldo, A., Mathy, A., Losson, B., Mignon, B., 2008. Pathogenesis of dermatophytosis. Mycopathologia 166, 267–275.

Vernau, K.M., Grahn, B.H., Clarke-Scott, H., Sullivan, N., 1995. Thymoma in a rabbit with hypercalcemia and periodic exophthalmus. J. Am. Vet. Med. Assoc. 206, 820–822.

Wakefield, A.E., 1994. Detection of DNA sequences identical to *Pneumocystis carinii* in samples of ambient air. J. Eukaryot. Microbiol. 41, 116S.

Wakefield, A.E., 1996. DNA sequences identical to *Pneumocystis carinii* f. sp. *carinii* and *Pneumocystis carinii* f. sp. *hominis* in samples of air spora. J. Clin. Microbiol. 34, 1754–1759.

Wasson, K., Peper, R.L., 2000. Mammalian microsporidiosis. Vet. Pathol. 37, 113–128.

Watanabe, Y., 1980. Serial inbreeding of rabbits with hereditary hyperlipidemia (WHHL-rabbit). Atherosclerosis 36, 261–268.

Watanabe, Y., Ito, T., Kondo, T., 1977. Breeding of a rabbit strain of hyperlipidemia and characteristic of this strain (author's transl). Jikken Dobutsu 26, 35–42.

Watanabe, Y., Ito, T., Shiomi, M., 1985. The effect of selective breeding on the development of coronary atherosclerosis in WHHL rabbits. An animal model for familial hypercholesterolemia. Atherosclerosis 56, 71–79.

Watarai, M., Yamato, Y., Horiuchi, N., Kim, S., Omata, Y., Shirahata, T., et al., 2004. Enzyme-linked immunosorbent assay to detect *Lawsonia intracellularis* in rabbits with proliferative enteropathy. J. Vet. Med. Sci. 66, 735–737.

Watarai, M., Yamato, Y., Murakata, K., Kim, S., Omata, Y., Furuoka, H., 2005. Detection of *Lawsonia intracellularis* using immunomagnetic beads and ATP bioluminescence. J. Vet. Med. Sci. 67, 449–451.

Watarai, M., Yoshiya, M., Sato, A., Furuoka, H., 2008. Cultivation and characterization of *Lawsonia intracellularis* isolated from rabbit and pig. J. Vet. Med. Sci. 70, 731–733.

Weibel, H., Sydler, T., Brugnera, E., Voets, H., Grosse Liesner, B., Sidler, X., 2012. Efficacy of simultaneous vaccination with Enterisol(R) Ileitis and Ingelvac(R) CircoFLEXTM in a Swiss breeding farm. Schweiz. Arch. Tierheilkd. 154, 445–450.

Weisbroth, S.H., 1974. Neoplastic diseases. In: Weisbroth, S.H., Flatt, R.E., Kraus, A.L. (Eds.), The Biology of the Laboratory Rabbit, first ed. Academic Press, San Diego, CA, pp. 331–375.

Weisbroth, S.H., 1975. Torsion of the caudate lobe of the liver in the domestic rabbit (Oryctolagus). Vet. Pathol. 12, 13–15.

Weisbroth, S.H., 1994. Neoplastic diseases. In: Manning, P.J., Ringler, D.H., Newcomer, C.E. (Eds.), Biology of the Laboratory Rabbit, second ed. Academic Press, Orlando, FL, pp. 259–289.

Weiss, L.M., Vossbrinck, C.R., 1998. Microsporidiosis: molecular and diagnostic aspects. Adv. Parasitol. 40, 351–395.

Wenger, S., Barrett, E.L., Pearson, G.R., Sayers, I., Blakey, C., Redrobe, S., 2009. Liver lobe torsion in three adult rabbits. J. Small Anim. Pract. 50, 301–305.

West, T.C., 1955. Ultramicroelectric recording from cardiac pacemaker. J. Pharmacol. Exp. Ther. 115, 283–290.

Whary, M., Peper, R., Borkowski, G., Lawrence, W., Ferguson, F., 1993. The effects of group housing on the research use of the laboratory rabbit. Lab. Anim. 27, 330–336.

Wilkie, I.W., Harper, M., Boyce, J.D., Adler, B., 2012. *Pasteurella multocida*: diseases and pathogenesis. Curr. Top. Micro. Immuno. 361, 1–22.

Williams, C.S.F., 1976. Practical Guide to Laboratory Animals. Mosby, St. Louis, MO.

Williams, D.L., 2012. Ophthalmology of Exotic Pets. Wiley-Blackwell, Chichester, UK.

Williams, J., Gladen, B.C., Turner, T.W., 1991. The effects of ethylene dibromide on semen quality and fertility in the rabbit: evaluation of a model for human seminal characteristics. Fundam. Appl. Toxicol. 16, 687–691.

Williams, J.G., Kubelik, A.R., Livak, K.J., Rafalski, J.A., Tingey, S.V., 1990. DNA polymorphisms amplified by arbitrary primers are useful as genetic markers. Nucleic Acids Res. 18, 6531–6535.

Wilson, R.B., Holscher, M., Sly, D.L., 1987. Liver lobe torsion in a rabbit. Lab. Anim. Sci. 37, 506–507.

Wobeser, G., Campbell, G.D., Dallaire, A., Mcburney, S., 2009. Tularemia, plague, yersiniosis, and Tyzzer's disease in wild rodents and lagomorphs in Canada: a review. Can. Vet. J. 50, 1251–1256.

Wolford, S.T., Schroer, R.A., Gohs, F.X., Gallo, P.P., Brodeck, M., Falk, H., et al., 1986. Reference range data base for serum chemistry and hematology values in laboratory animals. J. Toxicol. Environ. Health 18, 161–188.

Wright, J.H., Craighead, E.M., 1922. Infectious motor paralysis in young rabbits. J. Exp. Med. 36, 135–140.

Wright, P., Riner, J., 1985. Comparative efficacy of injection routes and doses of ivermectin against Psoroptes in rabbits. Am. J. Vet. Res. 46, 752–754.

Yamamoto, H., Fujishiro, K., 1989. Pathology of spontaneous malignant fibrous histiocytoma in a Japanese White rabbit (Oryctolagus cuniculus). Lab. Anim. Sci. 38, 165–169.

Yan, W., Wang, W., Wang, T., Suo, X., Qian, W., Wang, S., et al., 2013. Simultaneous identification of three highly pathogenic Eimeria species in rabbits using a multiplex PCR diagnostic assay based on ITS1-5.8S rRNA-ITS2 fragments. Vet. Parasitol. 193, 284–288.

Yin, M., Fang, Z., Jiang, W., Xing, F., Jiang, M., Kong, P., et al., 2013. The Oct4 promoter-EGFP transgenic rabbit: a new model for monitoring the pluripotency of rabbit stem cells. Int. J. Dev. Bio. 57, 845–852.

Yokoyama, E., 1979. Flow-volume curves of excised right and left rabbit lungs. J. Appl. Physiol. 46, 463–468.

Yu, L., Pragay, D.A., Chang, D., Wicher, K., 1979. Biochemical parameters of normal rabbit serum. Clin. Biochem. 12, 83–87.

Yutin, N., Galperin, M.Y., 2013. A genomic update on clostridial phylogeny: gram-negative spore formers and other misplaced clostridia. Environ. Microbiol. 15, 2631–2641.

Zhang, W., Shen, Y., Wang, R., Liu, A., Ling, H., Li, Y., et al., 2012. Cryptosporidium cuniculus and Giardia duodenalis in rabbits: genetic diversity and possible zoonotic transmission. PLoS One 7, e31262.

Zimmerman, T.S., Arroyove, C.M., Muller-Eberhard, H.J., 1971. A blood coagulation abnormality in rabbits deficient in the sixth component of complement (C6) and its correction by purified C6. J. Exp. Med. 134, 1591–1600.

Ziv, O., Morales, E., Song, Y.K., Peng, X., Odening, K.E., Buxton, A.E., et al., 2009. Origin of complex behaviour of spatially discordant alternans in a transgenic rabbit model of type 2 long QT syndrome. J. Physiol. 587, 4661–4680.

Microbiological Quality Control for Laboratory Rodents and Lagomorphs

William R. Shek, DVM, PhD[a], Abigail L. Smith, MPH, PhD[b]
and Kathleen R. Pritchett-Corning, DVM[c]

[a]Research Animal Diagnostics, Charles River Laboratories, Wilmington, MA, USA [b]Department of
Pathobiology, University of Pennsylvania School of Veterinary Medicine, Philadelphia, PA, USA
[c]Office of Animal Resources, Harvard University, Faculty of Arts and Sciences, and Department of
Comparative Medicine, University of Washington, Cambridge, MA, USA

I. INTRODUCTION

Mice (*Mus musculus*), rats (*Rattus norvegicus*), other rodent species, and domestic rabbits (*Oryctolagus cuniculus*) have been used in research for over 100 years. During the first half of the 20th century, microbiological quality control (QC) of lab animals was at best rudimentary as colonies were conventionally housed and little or no diagnostic testing was done. Hence, animal studies were often curtailed and confounded by infectious disease (Mobraaten and Sharp, 1999; Morse, 2007; Weisbroth, 1999). By the 1950s, it became apparent to

veterinarians in the nascent field of comparative medicine that disease-free animals suitable for research could not be produced by standard veterinary disease control measures (e.g., improved sanitation and nutrition, antimicrobial treatments) in conventional facilities. Henry Foster, the veterinarian who founded Charles River Breeding Laboratories in 1948 and a pioneer in the large-scale production of laboratory rodents, stated in a seminar presented at the 30th anniversary of the American Association for Laboratory Animal Science, "After a variety of frustrating health-related problems, it was decided that a major change in the company's philosophy was required and an entirely different approach was essential." Consequently, he and others developed innovative biosecurity systems to eliminate and exclude pathogens (Allen, 1999). In 1958, Foster reported on the Cesarean-originated barrier-sustained (COBS) process for the large-scale production of specific pathogen-free (SPF) laboratory rodents (Foster, 1958). To eliminate horizontally transmitted pathogens, a hysterectomy was performed on a near-term dam from a contaminated or conventionally housed colony. The gravid uterus was pulled through a disinfectant solution into a sterile flexible film isolator where the pups were removed from the uterus and suckled on axenic (i.e., germ-free) foster dams. After being mated to expand their number and associated with a cocktail of nonpathogenic bacteria to normalize their physiology and prime their immune system, rederived rodents were transferred to so-called barrier rooms for large-scale production. The room-level barrier to adventitious infection entailed disinfection of the room, equipment and supplies, limiting access to trained and properly gowned personnel, and the application of new technologies such as high-efficiency particulate air (HEPA) filtration of incoming air (Dubos and Schaedler, 1960; Foster, 1980; Schaedler and Orcutt, 1983; Trexler and Orcutt, 1999). The axenic and associated rodents mentioned in the COBS process are collectively classified as gnotobiotic to indicate that they have a completely known microflora. By contrast, barrier-reared rodent colonies are not gnotobiotic because they are housed in uncovered cages and thus acquire a complex microflora from the environment, supplies, personnel, and other sources. Instead, they are described as SPF to indicate that according to laboratory testing, they are free from infection with a defined list of infectious agents, commonly known as an 'exclusion' list.

The advances in cell biology, genetics, and analytical methods that coincided with the progress in research animal biosecurity led to discoveries of infections, often by viruses, which although inapparent nonetheless confounded experimental findings by contaminating biological reagents and distorting or modulating *in vivo* and *in vitro* responses dependent on infected host cells (Hartley and Rowe, 1960; Kilham and Olivier, 1959; Riley *et al.*, 1960; Rowe *et al.*, 1962). There are also documented cases of unrecognized infections altering the phenotype of animal models as has been reported for infections with *Helicobacter* spp. (Horowitz *et al.*, 2007; Jurjus *et al.*, 2004; Kuhn *et al.*, 1993; Kullberg *et al.*, 1998; Mombaerts *et al.*, 1993; Powrie and Leach, 1995; Strober and Ehrhardt, 1993). In addition, mice and rats were shown to be the reservoir species for zoonotic viruses responsible for disease outbreaks in laboratory personnel exposed to silently infected cell lines or cell line-inoculated rodents (Baum *et al.*, 1966; Bhatt *et al.*, 1986a; Himan, 1975; Lewis *et al.*, 1965; Lloyd and Jones, 1986). Thus, the absence of overt disease was no longer sufficient evidence that animals were either suitable or safe for research. Rather, routine laboratory screening, commonly referred to as health monitoring (HM), was required to detect inapparent infections capable of interfering with research. The traditional HM methodologies used for over half a century have included direct gross and microscopic examinations of animal specimens for parasites and pathology, microbiology consisting of cultural isolation, and phenotypic identification of primary and opportunistically pathogenic bacteria and fungi, and serology, that is, immunoassays of serum or blood samples for specific antibodies formed in response to infections with viruses and several fastidious and invasive microbial pathogens. The newest methodology, molecular diagnostics by polymerase chain reaction (PCR), was introduced in general and to lab animal diagnostics in the mid-1990s; since then, its use in HM has grown, in recent years dramatically, for reasons that will be discussed later (Compton and Riley, 2001; Compton *et al.*, 1995; Lipman and Homberger, 2003; Livingston and Riley, 2003; Shek and Gaertner, 2002; Weisbroth *et al.*, 1998).

Although rederivation, barrier room production, and HM had become standard practice for commercial rodent breeders by the1970s, a considerable percentage of vendor barrier-reared colonies were reported in the early 1980s still to be infected with a variety of rodent viruses and parasites (Casebolt *et al.*, 1988). Moreover, it was apparent that many research establishments were not prepared to maintain the SPF status of commercial rodents, which often became ill or seropositive shortly after being received. Subsequently, major commercial breeders greatly reduced the incidence of barrier room contaminations by more thorough disinfection of rooms prior to stocking, rigorous adherence to standard operating procedures (SOPs), and validation and routine certification of the procedures and equipment for disinfecting supplies. They also discontinued direct room-to-room transfers based on negative HM results, as this practice surely contributed to the inadvertent dissemination of unrecognized pathogens such as the then-novel rodent parvovirus serotypes (Ball-Goodrich and Johnson, 1994; Ball-Goodrich *et al.*, 1998; Besselsen *et al.*, 1995a, 1996; Jacoby *et al.*, 1995; Mckisic *et al.*, 1993; Smith *et al.*, 1993a) and enterohepatic species of *Helicobacter* (Fox *et al.*, 1994, 1996; Ward *et al.*, 1994b) identified in the 1990s, and murine norovirus (MNV) first reported in 2003 (Henderson, 2008; Hsu *et al.*, 2006; Karst *et al.*, 2003; Ward *et al.*, 2006). At research institutions, the incidence and prevalence of adventitious infections – where incidence indicates the rate of new contaminations, or outbreaks (e.g., 10 mouse parvovirus (MPV) contaminations/1000 racks/year), and prevalence is the % positive within a time period (e.g., 40% of mice in North America were MNV seropositive in 2012) – were greatly reduced by switching from housing rodents in uncovered cages, perhaps in barrier rooms, to static and then individually ventilated microisolation cage-level barrier systems shown to be highly effective at excluding and impeding the transmission of adventitious agents (Bohr *et al.*, 2006; Hessler, 1999; Lipman, 1999; Sedlacek and Mason, 1977).

While these biosecurity improvements have nearly or completely eliminated once-common pathogens such as Sendai virus from production and research colonies, outbreaks with environmentally stable and highly contagious enterotropic pathogens, such as MPV, mouse rotavirus, and hepatitis virus (MHV), continue to occur (Pritchett-Corning *et al.*, 2009). Additionally, transgenic and gene-targeted genetically engineered mouse models for human diseases, which make up a large and rapidly growing proportion of the animals used in research, have been shown often to harbor pathogens such as *Helicobacter* spp., MNV, *Pasteurella pneumotropica*, and parasites largely eliminated from commercial colonies (Carty, 2008; Jacoby and Lindsey, 1998; Pritchett-Corning *et al.*, 2009). Likely reasons for this include the recurrent and expanding exchange of genetically engineered mice among research institutions worldwide where QC practices vary and infected rodents may be housed and the initially inadvertent distribution of mice infected with *Helicobacter* spp. and MNV before these agents were recognized and testing for them was available. Thus, genetically engineered mice represent a significant source of adventitious agents capable of confounding experiments, not least of all in genetically engineered models in which these infections have been shown to alter or obscure the effects of genetic modifications, or cause severe and sometimes atypical disease (Compton *et al.*, 2003; Franklin, 2006).

The continued occurrence of adventitious infections and the discovery of pathogens underscore the importance of HM results that accurately represent the pathogen status of research animals, but also highlight the limitations of HM and the need for all aspects of microbiological QC including biosecurity with rederivation to eliminate and prevent the dissemination of yet-to-be recognized as well as known pathogens. It is worth noting that this is comparable to the complementary approaches of strict control of production processes and comprehensive quality testing, which are the basis of Current Good Manufacturing Practices (CGMPs) for regulated pharmaceuticals (Tolbert and Rupp, 1989). While the degree of rigor engendered in CGMPs of regulated pharmaceuticals may be excessive for laboratory research, applying the essential aspects of CGMPs to microbiological QC of research animals and biological reagents is a prerequisite for meaningful biomedical research. Insufficient microbiological QC during research can lead to inaccurate findings, the need to repeat experiments, and biological product development setbacks and failures.

In addition to depending on an assay's ability to correctly classify positive and negative samples, the accuracy of microbiological surveillance is contingent on testing specimens that are both representative of the pathogen status of the principal animals and suitable for the assay method. The term 'principals' (or principal animals) refers to the animal populations, or groups, being monitored, whether resident or in quarantine. Residents include colony and study animals housed at a facility. Collecting specimens from microisolation caging systems that are representative of the principals' pathogen status and suitable for the test method is challenging because of the often low prevalence of infection and the shortcomings of soiled bedding sentinel monitoring. PCR testing of non-invasive specimens collected directly from resident and quarantined animals, and of environmental samples not suitable for traditional methodologies is helping address these challenges (Bauer and Riley, 2006; Compton *et al.*, 2004c; Henderson *et al.*, 2013; Jensen *et al.*, 2013; Macy *et al.*, 2009, 2011). The process of containing and eradicating adventitious infections is inevitably costly and disruptive to research. Therefore, it is crucial that repeat testing, employing complementary methodologies if possible, be carried out to verify infection of the resident animals before taking remedial measures. Once the occurrence of an adventitious infection has been verified, actions are taken to contain, eradicate, and investigate the contamination with the goal of preventing a recurrence.

In sum, as biomedical research has become more sophisticated, the list of pathogens shown to interfere with research has grown, and hence, research animal SPF specifications have become more rigorous. This chapter reviews the main elements of microbiological QC needed to meet these specifications including biosecurity to eliminate, exclude, and contain pathogens, HM, and the management, eradication, and investigation of contaminations. Although microbiological QC for rodents will be emphasized, the methodologies considered are applicable to laboratory animals in general.

II. MICROBIOLOGICAL QUALITY SPECIFICATIONS

Gnotobiotic animals, whether axenic (i.e., germ-free) or associated with a defined microbiome consisting of a few nonpathogenic bacteria, make up a small fraction of the animals used in research; however, their usage is likely to increase with the growth of research into the profound influences and diverse effects of the microbiome on human health and the experimental responses of research models (Bech-Nielsen *et al.*, 2012; Friswell *et al.*, 2010; Grada and Weinbrecht, 2013). As already mentioned, most lab animals are referred to as SPF to indicate that they have been shown by HM to be free of pathogens on an exclusion list.

Exclusion lists for rodents, rabbits, and other common lab animal species have been substantially harmonized throughout the developed world due to the efforts of lab animal science organizations (Guillen, 2012; Nicklas, 2008; Nicklas et al., 2002), and the globalization of biomedical research. In addition, competition for customers encourages vendors to offer SPF animals free of newly discovered pathogens and diagnostic laboratories to develop tests for those pathogens (Shek, 2000). The exclusion lists for SPF mice and rats are more extensive than those for rabbits and other common lab animal species for a number of reasons. First, as mice and rats account for the vast majority of animals used in research, it stands to reason that more is known about their indigenous pathogens than those of other less used lab animal species. The diversity of inbred, and naturally and genetically engineered immunodeficient mutant rodent strains highly susceptible to infectious disease (Compton et al., 2003; Franklin, 2006), in conjunction with sensitive immunoassay methods (Smith, 1986b) and advances in molecular genetics (Compton and Riley, 2001), has contributed to the discovery and characterization of rodent pathogens (Fox et al., 1994; Ward et al., 1994a) found to be the cause of ubiquitous, inapparent infections of laboratory rodent colonies (Hsu et al., 2006; Shames et al., 1995). In addition, the predominance of murine rodent research models has provided strong incentives for diagnostic laboratories and vendors to develop and offer specific serologic and PCR assays for viral and other fastidious microbial pathogens – not amenable to detection by direct microscopic examination or cultural isolation – soon after their discovery. By contrast, commercial vendors and diagnostic laboratories have had little demand from the research and lab animal medicine communities to provide routine serologic and PCR testing for rabbit viruses recognized decades ago, such as lapine parvovirus (Matsunaga and Matsuno, 1983) (which sequencing has recently shown to be a bocavirus (personal communication, K Henderson)), rabbit enteric coronavirus (Deeb et al., 1993; Descoteaux and Lussier, 1990; Descoteaux et al., 1985), and leporid herpesvirus 2 (Matsunaga and Yamazaki, 1976). Finally, rederivation by hysterectomy or embryo transfer (ET) to eliminate all exogenous pathogens is the standard practice for SPF mice and rats, but not for other species.

SPF exclusion lists for mice and rats have included all known exogenous viruses regardless of virulence because as obligate intracellular parasites, viruses are inherently invasive; furthermore, even noncytopathic viral infections have been shown to alter the metabolism of host cells (Oldstone et al., 1982). Strict adherence to the dogma of excluding all exogenous viruses from SPF mice and rats, however, has become impractical at many research

institutions where asymptomatic MNV infections, primarily in genetically engineered mice, are considered to be too widespread to be eliminated. Leading-edge molecular genetic techniques have recently uncovered a murine astrovirus (Farkas et al., 2012), possibly more common in mice than MNV, and will surely find additional prevalent viruses that have so far eluded detection because they, like MPV, MNV, and murine astrovirus, are highly host-adapted and by and large apathogenic even for immunodeficient hosts. As noted, viral exclusion lists for rabbits and other lab animal species are less comprehensive than for murine rodents.

Ectoparasites, helminths, pathogenic protozoa, bacteria, and fungi are part of the exclusion lists of all SPF animal species. The pathogenic bacteria and fungi excluded for SPF animals are mainly distinguished from commensal and autochthonous (i.e., indigenous) organisms by their ability to cross anatomic and biochemical barriers to establish themselves in niches devoid of other microorganisms such as the lower respiratory and urogenital tracts, internal organs, and intracellularly (Casadevall and Pirofski, 2000; Council, 2009; Merrell and Falkow, 2004). Pathogenicity is not necessarily an immutable characteristic of the microbial species as normally commensal microbes such as Escherichia coli have been transformed into pathogens through the acquisition of virulence genes transferred from other bacteria in mobile genetic elements such as plasmids, phages, and transposons (Dobrindt et al., 2004).

Microbes are classified as primary pathogens if they can cause disease in immunocompetent hosts. Examples include Salmonella, Mycoplasma pulmonis, Helicobacter hepaticus, and Clostridium piliforme (the etiology of Tyzzer's disease). Opportunistic pathogens such as Pseudomonas aeruginosa, β-hemolytic streptococci, Staphylococcus aureus, and Pneumocystis fungi cause disease mainly in immunocompromised hosts, whether (1) immunosuppressed by irradiation or chemotherapy (Bosma et al., 1983; Cryz et al., 1983; Flynn, 1963; Homberger et al., 1993; Rosen and Berk, 1977; Waggie et al., 1988; Walzer et al., 1989; Weir et al., 1986; Weisbroth et al., 1999) or (2) inherently immunodeficient, such as athymic nude and severe combined immunodeficient (SCID) mice (Bosma et al., 1983; Clifford et al., 1995; Dole et al., 2013b; Henderson et al., 2012; Pantelouris, 1968; Ward et al., 1996). For the most part, only primary microbial pathogens are included in SPF exclusion lists for immunocompetent animals. Opportunists are added, chiefly by commercial vendors, to lists for immunodeficient and genetically engineered mutant lines. Because it is not unusual for opportunists such as S. aureus to cause disease in standard (i.e., nongenetically engineered) immunocompetent strains of rodents (Besch-Williford and Franklin, 2007), which are often used in rederivation and breeding schemes for genetically engineered lines, the demand for standard, immunocompetent rodent strains and stocks free of opportunistic as well as primary pathogens has increased. This subset of SPF animals has been referred to as SOPF for specific opportunistic pathogen-free.

To summarize, the infectious agents on SPF exclusions lists are determined by general and institution-specific criteria. In general, the SPF exclusion lists of mice and rats are more comprehensive than those of less popular animal species because more of the indigenous murine viral and host-adapted microbial pathogens have been identified and studied; serologic and PCR assays are made available for murine pathogens soon after their discovery; and rederivation to eliminate all exogenous pathogens from SPF mouse and rat populations is standard practice. The SPF exclusion lists of all species typically contain ectoparasites, endoparasites, and microbes classified as primary pathogens as well as viruses; vendors often add opportunistic pathogens for immunodeficient and genetically engineered mutant murine models.

Complying with consensus SPF standards can be problematic at an institution if the prevalence of infection is high or barrier systems and practices are inadequate to prevent adventitious infections from recurring and spreading. Many research-intensive academic institutions have decided that the benefits of eliminating prevalent infections with recently recognized agents such as MNV and *Helicobacter*, which rarely produce disease and/or have been endemic to their research colonies for many years, are outweighed by the disruption to research and costs of doing so. However, the elimination (and exclusion) of prevalent pathogens and compliance with consensus SPF standards reduces the risk that a pathogen will infect additional colonies and interfere with research, and simplifies the exchange of animal models and collaborative studies with other investigators and institutions.

III. BIOSECURITY

Lab animal biosecurity consists of all measures taken to eliminate, exclude, contain, and eradicate adventitious infections. Containment and eradication will be discussed further in the section on Outbreak Management and Investigation.

A. Elimination

1. *Rederivation*

Rederivation of SPF lab animal stocks from those that are harboring pathogens is widely regarded as the most dependable approach for eliminating infections with unrecognized as well as known pathogens. In association with advances in assisted reproductive technologies, ET into SPF pseudopregnant recipient females has supplanted nursing of Cesarian section-originated pups by gnotobiotic or SPF foster mothers as the gold standard for rederivation (Suzuki *et al.*, 1996; Van Keuren and Saunders, 2004). Cesarean rederivation is considered to be less reliable than ET because vertical transmission of infections to fetuses has been demonstrated for viruses (Barthold *et al.*, 1988; Jacoby *et al.*, 2001; Katami *et al.*, 1978; Lehmann-Grube, 1982) and for bacteria capable of colonizing the uterus (Brown and Steiner, 1996; Matsumiya and Lavoie, 2003; Reyes *et al.*, 2000, 2004; Ward *et al.*, 1978). Vertical transmission by ET is unlikely because the zona pellucida that surrounds embryos and oocytes excludes pathogens (Peters *et al.*, 2006) and the risk of infecting the recipient females is minimized by extensive washing of the embryos. In a recent study, ET from MPV-infected SCID mice eliminated the infection (Besselsen *et al.*, 2008b). Other advantages of ET *vis-à-vis* Cesarean rederivation are that it can be combined with other artificial methods like *in vitro* fertilization (IVF) and intracytoplasmic injection of sperm (ICSI) to overcome the reproductive defects that are common in aged and in naturally and genetically engineered mutant mice (Suzuki *et al.*, 1996). Embryos, ova, and sperm (i.e., germplasm) can be cryopreserved to reduce *per diem* costs, save valuable cage space, and assure that unique genetically engineered strains can be rederived at any time and, hence, are never lost. Finally, ET is more efficient because embryo donors are usually superovulated resulting in more offspring per female than are obtained from natural matings (Mazur *et al.*, 2008).

Cesarean rederivation, however, is still extensively used by commercial vendors for standard rodent strains and stocks, and may be preferable to ET for certain genetically engineered rodent lines with fertility issues or whose embryos exhibit low viability in culture. Although less dependable than ET, Cesarean rederivation is highly effective as supported by the observation at Charles River Laboratories that thousands of isolator-maintained rodent colonies, originated by Cesarean rederivations carried out over many years, were without exception free of murine parvoviruses, *Helicobacter* spp. and MNV when these agents were first recognized (W. Shek, unpublished). Neonatal transfer of mouse pups within several days of parturition to SPF foster mothers, after being immersed in disinfectant, has been reported to successfully eliminate a variety of common mouse pathogens including MPV, MHV, MNV, and *Helicobacter* spp., and has the advantages in comparison with Cesarean section of being less expensive and not requiring that valuable breeders be euthanized (Huerkamp *et al.*, 2005; Lipman *et al.*, 1987; Truett *et al.*, 2000; Watson *et al.*, 2005).

Rederivation with rare exception requires pathogen-free animals of the same species to receive embryos or nurse offspring, and to associate progeny with a normal autochthonous microbiome. For mice and rats, this has been accomplished over many years by overcoming various technical hurdles such as (1) hand rearing and meeting the unique nutritional needs of germfree animals; (2) development of defined cocktails of non-pathogenic bacteria to colonize the intestinal tract of ex-germfree animals in order to resist colonization by pathogenic microbes, to normalize host physiology, and to stimulate the immune system; and (3) maintaining rodents in isolators or microisolation cages on sterile supplies to exclude all exogenous microbes from axenic and defined flora animals (Foster, 1980; Schaedler and Orcutt, 1983; Trexler, 1983; Trexler and Orcutt, 1999). The production of defined flora pathogen-free animals is uncommon for other lab animal species but has been described for rabbits (Boot et al., 1985, 1989b; Yanabe et al., 1999) and guinea pigs (Boot et al., 1989a). Cross-fostering offspring onto SPF animals of a different species has been attempted when SPF animals of the same species are not available. In a successful example, H. hepaticus was eliminated from Mongolian gerbils by Cesarean rederivation with cross-fostering of the offspring onto SPF mice and rats. The percent survival of rederived gerbils was higher for those nursed by mice (Glage et al., 2007).

2. Alternatives to Rederivation

Although not considered to be as dependable as rederivation, chemotherapeutic treatments and test-and-cull procedures (Macy et al., 2011; Smith, 2010) are increasingly employed to eliminate, or eradicate, adventitious infections from the colonies of unique genetically engineered mutant mouse lines that may not be available from commercial sources and hence are difficult to replace. Microisolation caging systems have contributed substantially to the feasibility and efficacy of these alternatives to rederivation by keeping the prevalence of infection low (Bohr et al., 2006), minimizing the level of environmental contamination, and thereby reducing the chance of reinfection. Nevertheless, rederivation and eventual cryopreservation of unique mutant animal models are considered crucial to ensuring their survival, availability, and freedom from known and yet-to-be recognized pathogens.

Chemotherapy is mainly employed to cure or prophylactically treat pinworm and mite infestations of quarantined and resident rodents housed in microisolation cages. The most effective and frequently administered antiparasite medications are the avermectins (e.g., ivermectin and selamectin) and benzimidazoles (e.g., fendbendazole); they are normally added to the diet or drinking water, or applied topically (Pritchett and

Johnston, 2002; Ricart Arbona et al., 2010b). Therapeutic doses of these drugs, however, may cause toxicity as has been demonstrated for ivermectin given to rodents with compromised blood–brain barriers because of young age (Lankas et al., 1989; Skopets et al., 1996), genetic background (Jackson et al., 1998; Lankas et al., 1997), or genetically engineered mutations (Schinkel et al., 1994, 1997). Antibiotic treatments have been shown to eliminate infections with host-adapted bacterial pathogens, such as P. pneumotropica (Goelz et al., 1996; Matsumiya and Lavoie, 2003) and H. hepaticus (Foltz et al., 1996; Kerton and Warden, 2006; Russell et al., 1995), which do not survive for long ex vivo and, therefore, are unlikely to reinfect hosts after treatment is stopped. Even when effective, however, drug therapies may be too expensive or laborious to be practical, particularly when treating large numbers of animals. However, the labor and cost of large-scale chemotherapy have been greatly reduced by using commercially available medicated diets for treating parasite infestations (Ricart Arbona et al., 2010b) and Helicobacter infections (Kerton and Warden, 2006; Whary and Fox, 2006).

Unlike the parasite infestations and bacterial infections just mentioned, viral infections cannot be treated; however, low-prevalence viral infections can be eradicated from rodents housed in microisolation cages by test-and-cull procedures discussed further in Section V. Briefly, breeding and the introduction of naive animals to the infected room(s) and rack(s) are stopped and 100% of microisolation cages are tested at regular intervals by serology, PCR, or both. Positive cages are culled and testing at regular intervals is continued for a limited period until either the remaining cages are repeatedly negative or the rack(s) are depopulated and resident animals euthanized, relocated, and/or rederived. Test-and-cull procedures have been successfully utilized to eradicate outbreaks with Helicobacter spp. (Beckwith et al., 1997; Fermer et al., 2002; Hodzic et al., 2001; Mahler et al., 1998; Shames et al., 1995), murine parvoviruses (Bauer and Riley, 2006; Macy et al., 2009, 2011), MHV (Compton et al., 2004a; Manuel et al., 2008), MNV (Manuel et al., 2008), and murine rotavirus (A.L. Smith, unpublished).

Another alternative to rederivation applied historically to nonpersistent infections of immunocompetent hosts with enveloped viruses (e.g., Sendai virus and sialodacryoadenitis virus (SDAV)) is to break the cycle of infection by instituting a 6- to 8-week moratorium on breeding and the introduction of naive animals (Bhatt and Jacoby, 1985). During this period, it was expected that all animals in the colony would recover from infection and stop shedding virus, and that the excreted virus would quickly become noninfectious due to the environmental lability of these agents. Historical success was enhanced by the small size of the affected population, and contemporary mouse housing rooms are likely to contain 700–800 cages. A time-efficient alternative to a breeding moratorium is to start a new colony with seropositive, noncontagious breeders (Brammer *et al.*, 1993). It is worth emphasizing that breaking the cycle of infection, commonly called 'burnout', is not recommended in contemporary rodent colonies due to the increasing proportion of genetically modified rodents in populations and the frequently unknown immune competence and atypical response to infection of such animals. The relevance of burnout has been further eroded by the virtual disappearance from research colonies of infections with enveloped respiratory viruses to which this approach was applicable. Most of the enteric viruses that continue to be present in research colonies today are nonenveloped and hence environmentally stable, and persist for prolonged or indefinite periods in the tissues of hosts, including those that are immunocompetent and seropositive. MNV, the most prevalent pathogen of mice, is shed indefinitely (Hsu *et al.*, 2006; Manuel *et al.*, 2008). If despite these caveats breaking the cycle of infection is attempted, confirmation of eradication is best achieved by PCR or by serosurveillance of sentinels instead of the colony offspring that will likely have maternal antibodies.

B. Exclusion

To exclude pathogens, research animals are maintained behind sanitized and disinfected room- to cage-level barriers provided with filtered air and disinfected supplies and equipment. Biosecurity procedures pertaining to personnel, animal maintenance, pest control, disinfection, and so forth should be regularly reviewed and revised to further reduce the risks associated with potential sources of adventitious infection.

1. Barrier Systems

Barrier rooms, with animals kept in open cages, continue to be employed by commercial breeders for the efficient, large-scale production of immunocompetent rodents and rabbits. Because opportunistic pathogens are not reliably excluded from barrier room colonies (Blackmore and Francis, 1970; Fallon *et al.*, 1988; Geistfeld *et al.*, 1998), the production of mice and rats that need to be SOPF, in particular known and potentially immunodeficient mice and rats, has been transferred from barrier rooms to flexible-film and semirigid isolators, and filter-covered microisolation cages that provide a higher degree of biosecurity.

Although the effectiveness of filter-covered cages for excluding and controlling the spread of infections had already been demonstrated for mouse rotavirus in1958 (Kraft, 1958), this cage-level barrier strategy did not become popular until the 1980s when commercial microisolation caging systems were introduced. The first

microisolation cages were referred to as 'static' to indicate that they relied on passive ventilation. As the temperatures, humidity levels, and noxious gas concentrations (such as CO_2 and NH_3) in static cages were found to be significantly elevated in comparison with room levels, actively ventilated microisolation caging systems were developed to enhance the cage microenvironment (Les, 1983) and to allow for higher animal densities with fewer cage changes. Moreover, ventilated systems can be exhausted directly into the facility HVAC to improve the room environment and can be run under a negative pressure differential for pathogen containment. To maximize biosecurity, microisolation cages should only be opened in a HEPA-filtered air laminar flow change stations or biological safety cabinets by technicians wearing personal protective equipment (PPE) and following sterile technique when manipulating animals. Microisolation cages are often located in barrier rooms to provide a further obstacle to microbial contamination (Hessler, 1999; Lipman, 1999; Sedlacek and Mason, 1977; Trexler and Orcutt, 1999). Today, microisolation caging systems house the majority of rodents at research-intensive academic, biotechnical, and pharmaceutical institutions. There is little doubt that the effectiveness of these cage-level barrier systems at excluding and impeding the spread of infections, and their tolerance of systemic deficiencies and operator errors, has played a major part in lowering the frequency of microbial contaminations at biomedical research facilities and keeping the prevalence of infection low following an outbreak (Macy *et al.*, 2011; Shek, 2008; Whary *et al.*, 2000a). The challenges that this low prevalence presents to obtaining test results that accurately represent the pathogen status of principal animals (i.e., the resident colony or study animals, or the quarantined animals being monitored) will be discussed in Section IV.

2. Mitigating Risks from Sources of Infection

Irrespective of the barrier system, successful exclusion of pathogens from rodent colonies depends on an understanding of the chain of adventitious infection, which comprises reservoirs, sources, and modes of transmission (Fig. 11.1), and mitigating the risks associated with sources of infection (Table 11.1). The reservoir, or ecological niche, of a microorganism can be an animal species or the environment (Brachman, 1996). For example, the reservoir for lymphocytic choriomeningitis virus (LCMV) is the wild mouse (Lehmann-Grube, 1982), whereas *Listeria monocytogenes* is found in various avian and mammalian species as well as throughout the environment (Broome *et al.*, 1998). The source of an organism for transmission to a susceptible host is not necessarily the same as its reservoir. The source of *L. monocytogenes* for an SPF colony might be food or bedding that was contaminated by carrier animals or the environment. The distinction between reservoir and

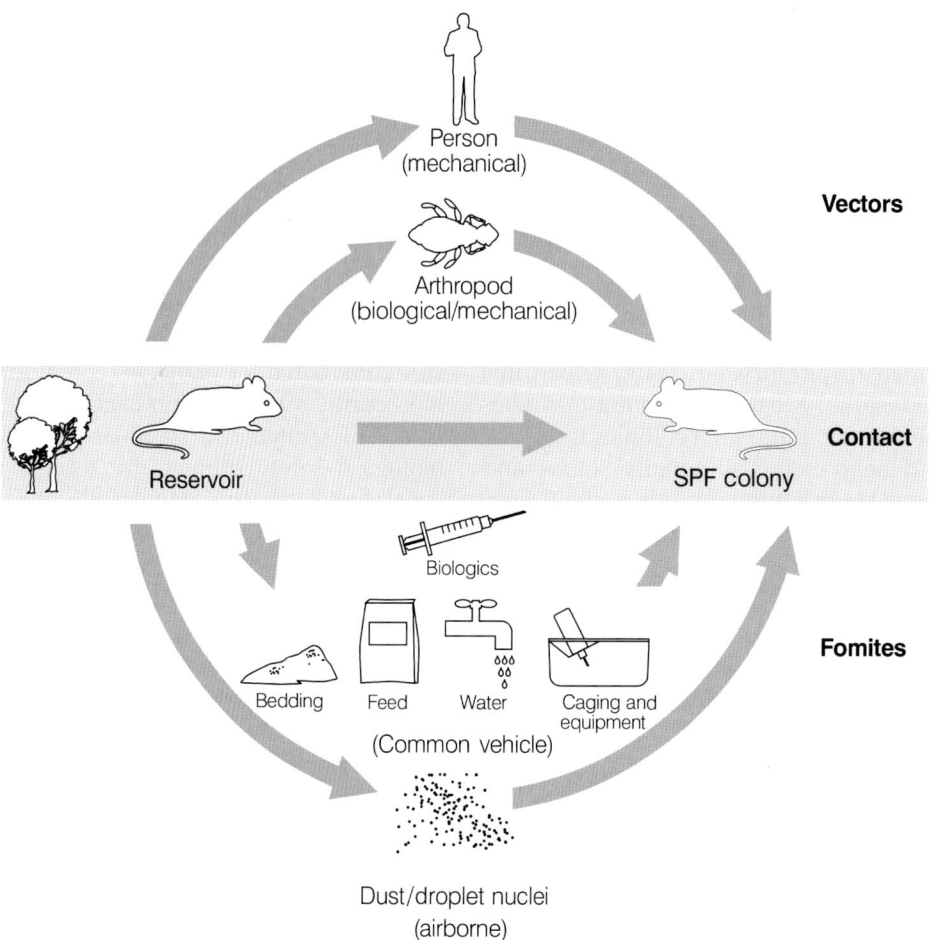

FIGURE 11.1 Chain of adventitious infection for laboratory rodents. The reservoir, or ecological niche, of a microorganism can be an animal species or the environment. The principal reservoirs of adventitious infection for SPF rodents are other rodents of the same or related species. Infection can be transmitted directly from animal to animal or indirectly by an inanimate vehicle, also termed a fomite, or a vector.

source is important in the case of lab animal biosecurity because, in general, it is much more practical to control a pathogen's source than its reservoir.

Given that most pathogens are obligate parasites with a limited host range, it stands to reason that infected animals of the same or related species are the principal reservoirs of adventitious infection for SPF lab animal populations. Infection can be transmitted directly from animal to animal or indirectly by an inanimate vehicle, also termed a fomite, or an animate vector.

Contact transmission is vertical when it takes place *in utero* or at birth, or horizontal if it occurs postpartum through the transfer of droplets or by intimate contact, as exemplified by venereal diseases. Most pathogens of rodents and rabbits are efficiently transmitted by direct contact (Parker and Reynolds, 1968; Shek *et al.*, 1998; Thigpen *et al.*, 1989; Yang *et al.*, 1995). Lactate dehydrogenase-elevating virus (LDV) is a notable exception that is mainly spread by parenteral injection of naive mice with transplantable mouse cell lines (Collins and Parker, 1972;

Nicklas *et al.*, 1993; Riley, 1974). LDV has been recently shown to contaminate a basement membrane matrix used by tumor biologists and the cell line from which it was derived (Carlson Scholz *et al.*, 2011; Liu *et al.*, 2011; Nagaoka *et al.*, 2010). The efficacy of Cesarean rederivation shows that vertical transmission of rodent pathogens is uncommon although it has been demonstrated to occur for various viruses in immunodeficient or acutely infected dams (Barthold *et al.*, 1988; Jacoby *et al.*, 2001; Katami *et al.*, 1978; Lehmann-Grube, 1982), for LCMV in enzootically infected mice (Lehmann-Grube, 1982) and for bacterial pathogens capable of colonizing the uterus (Brown and Steiner, 1996; Matsumiya and Lavoie, 2003; Reyes *et al.*, 2000, 2004; Ward *et al.*, 1978).

Fomite transmission can be airborne, referring to the spread of contaminated droplet nuclei (i.e., the residue of dried droplets) or dust for a distance of more than several feet (Brachman, 1996), or by way of common vehicles such as food, water, bedding, and equipment. Aerosol transmission of enveloped respiratory viruses to

TABLE 11.1 Mitigating Risks for Sources of Infection

Transmission	Source	Risk mitigation
Direct contact	Wild or escaped rodents	Rodent proof construction Pest control program Barrier maintenance
	Imported animals	HM records from source Quarantine with HM Rederivation
	Personnel	Gowned (PPE) Animals manipulated in hood/ isolator Restricted access Pet policy
Fomite	Room/equipment surfaces	Chemical disinfection Manipulate animals in hood
	Food, bedding, supplies	Autoclaving, gamma irradiation
	Airborne	HEPA filtration Air pressure differential
	Waterborne	Filtration, chlorination, UV irradiation
Vector	Insects	As for wild rodents
	Personnel	As above
Inoculation of biologic	All biologics	Testing: PCR for rodent pathogens, sterility/bioburden, mycoplasma
	Cell line	Bank cells
	Other biologics	Physical or chemical disinfection

sentinels has been demonstrated in ventilated microisolation caging systems by housing sentinels in cages with unfiltered exhaust air from infected colony cages (Compton et al., 2004c); however, its overall significance to the spread of disease in laboratory rodents has been diminished based on the eradication of rodent respiratory pathogens and the predominance of covered microisolation cages, which minimize the opportunity for airborne spread. By contrast, common vehicles continue to be highly important for two reasons. First, soiled bedding is usually the primary or only source of infection for microisolation cage sentinels, and studies have shown that infections with host-adapted bacteria, enveloped viruses, and other organisms that are unstable *ex vivo* are not transmitted efficiently or at all in soiled bedding (Artwohl et al., 1994; Compton et al., 2004c; Cundiff et al., 1995; Dillehay et al., 1990; Henderson et al., 2013; Ike et al., 2007; Thigpen et al., 1989). Fortunately, soiled bedding has been reported to transmit many of the

enteric viruses and microbial pathogens that are common today (Compton et al., 2004c; Grove et al., 2012; Livingston et al., 1998; Manuel et al., 2008; Perdue et al., 2007; Smith et al., 2007; Whary et al., 2000b), provided that the sentinels are exposed to a sufficient dose of the pathogen to infect them (Smith et al., 2007). Second, evidence supports food and bedding as important sources of the multi-institutional MPV and mouse rotavirus outbreaks that have repeatedly occurred over the years. For instance, at institutions where some colonies were given gamma-irradiated or autoclaved food and bedding and others were not, outbreaks were by and large restricted to the colonies receiving non-disinfected supplies (Reuter et al., 2011). Furthermore, a noticeable drop in the incidence of MPV and mouse rotavirus outbreaks has been observed at vivaria that have switched to disinfected (typically γ-irradiated) food and bedding. A recent report linked MPV-1 and MPV-2 outbreaks to medicated diet that had not been disinfected by showing that the locations of mice experiencing the outbreaks matched the distribution of the untreated medicated diet (Watson, 2013). In another recent study, concomitant mouse rotavirus outbreaks at five institutions were related to the use of non-disinfected bedding from a common source by showing that the genetic sequences of mouse rotaviruses from the different institutions were identical (Dole et al., 2013a).

Vectors can be biological, i.e., essential to the life cycle of the pathogenic organism, or mechanical (Brachman, 1996; Cohen, 1998; Prince et al., 1991; Waggie et al., 1994). Arthropod vectors play a minor role in the transmission of rodent pathogens. Lice are known biological vectors for the erythrocyte parasites *Eperythrozoon coccoides* and *Mycoplasma haemofelis*, formerly *Haemobartonella muris* (Neimark et al., 2002), of mice and rats, respectively (Hildebrandt, 1982), but these louse vectors and rickettsial parasites are no longer encountered in laboratory mice (Jacoby and Lindsey, 1998), although they still may be common in pet and wild mouse population. Both insects and people have been incriminated as mechanical vectors for adventitious viral infections (Ishii et al., 1974; Tietjen, 1992). To summarize, adventitious infection occurs when an etiologic agent is accidentally transmitted from its reservoir, most often animals of the same species, into an SPF animal colony by direct animal-to-animal contact or indirectly through a fomite or vector.

a. Animals

As mentioned, the most likely animal reservoir of infection for SPF rodent colonies are other rodents, whether wild or feral (i.e., escaped), housed nearby in the same facility, or imported. Wild rodents have been shown to carry a variety of pathogens that contaminate SPF facilities (Behnke, 1975; Bhatt et al., 1986b; Chabe et al., 2010; Childs et al., 1989; Ike et al., 2007; Parker et al., 2009; Singleton et al., 1993; Skinner et al., 1977; Smith et al., 1993b). The risk of their contaminating an SPF colony is expected to increase when a rodent control program is not in place or the structural barriers to entry are inadequate (Lussier et al., 1988). Pest control services are best provided by a reputable and licensed commercial vendor. Animal facilities should be constructed and maintained so that potential nest areas and routes of ingress or egress are not present. All holes and cracks in the facility should be sealed. No matter how careful the oversight of construction projects, there may be unanticipated problems. A relatively new housing facility very suddenly revealed evidence of increased wild/feral mouse activity. Doors that were to be completely sealed were found to have small holes on the bottom surface and mice were breeding in the Styrofoam filler that was used in the doors for noise abatement (A.L. Smith, unpublished). A widespread fur mite outbreak in that vivarium about 1 year later was attributed to the earlier mouse infestation and necessitated treatment of all mice in the facility at a cost of $102,000. Trapping devices should be used to detect and eliminate loose rodents. Those that are captured alive should be identified as to species, handled as if they were infected, anesthetized, bled for serology, and examined for internal and external parasites prior to euthanasia. Whether loose rodents are captured dead or alive, specimens from them (e.g., tissues, feces, and swabs) are suitable for testing by microbial PCR as an adjunct or alternative to traditional diagnostic methodologies. Food, bedding, and garbage attract loose rodents and therefore should be stored off the floor in a secure area in sealed containers (Hoddenbach et al., 1997; Small, 1983). Vivaria that are located in multiuse buildings, frequently including offices and common areas at academic institutions, are at high risk because food is often present and may not be cleared until the next day after late social events. Sealed trash containers should be used in these situations to decrease the likelihood of rodents having access to food.

The risk of introducing pathogens through the transfer or importation of animals from another investigator or institution is affected by a variety of factors that are not mutually exclusive. These include the type of animals being imported, the source institution's microbiological QC program, the prevalence and incidence of infections, and the method of transportation.

It is generally the case that genetically engineered mutant mice produced at academic institutions have a high prevalence of infection with MNV, Helicobacter spp., P. pneumotropica, and parasites (Carty, 2008; Jacoby and Lindsey, 1998; Pritchett-Corning et al., 2009). By contrast, the risk of unexpectedly introducing pathogens with rodents and rabbits from large commercial breeders is minimal. Commercial vendors that have historically low rates of contamination, transportation dedicated to SPF

animals, and a track record of reliability are usually put on an institution's 'approved vendors list', which exempts their animals from quarantine. At large, research-intensive academic institutions, the vast majority of rodents acquired by scientists are likely to be procured from 'approved' commercial vendors. However, while the absolute number of animals is much smaller, these same scientists frequently need to procure unique strains of rodents from colleagues at academic institutions or biotech or pharmaceutical companies. These are so-called nonapproved vendors and most institutions have policies and programs that provide quality control testing of these animals prior to their release into the general resident population. Among the steps taken to mitigate risks associated with importing these rodents are (1) review of health reports from the source colony (often 1 year's worth of data may be requested) to ensure the animals are not likely to carry an agent excluded by the recipient institution; (2) quarantine of the newly arrived rodents in a remote area that provides barriers to transmission of agents to colony animals; and (3) a program to monitor the health of the animals prior to release from the quarantine area. Some quarantine facilities house rodents in static microisolation cages, some on ventilated racks, some in individually ventilated cubicles, and, although more rarely, some in semirigid isolators. Used properly, any of these housing modalities can provide effective isolation. Isolators are labor-intensive to use and service but provide very good isolation.

During the quarantine period, the principal animals being monitored for infection ideally should be cohoused with SPF sentinels for part or all of the quarantine to maximize the chance of sentinel infection. The quarantine typically lasts 4–8 weeks to allow sufficient time for sentinels to get infected and seroconvert. Alternatively, the need for sentinel testing can be bypassed and the time in quarantine reduced to about 2 weeks by PCR testing of noninvasive, ante mortem specimens (e.g., feces and swabs of the fur, perianal region, and oral cavity) collected directly from the principals within a week of their arrival. By reducing the time in quarantine, direct PCR testing of principals makes more efficient use of quarantine space, decreases the chance of cross-infection among imported cohorts, and affords investigators quicker access to their animals. Most importantly, as shown in a recent study, direct PCR testing of principals is more sensitive than indirect sentinel screening (Henderson et al., 2013), which is not unexpected as PCR typically detects pathogen levels well below the infectious dose for animals and cell culture (Bauer et al., 2004; Bauer and Riley, 2006; Blank et al., 2004).

One reason to monitor the health of the imported mice is to ensure that they were not inadvertently exposed to any excluded pathogens during transport. Whereas approved vendors usually employ dedicated trucks that carry animals of known health status, non-approved source rodents are normally transported by commercial carriers and private couriers whose quality control practices cannot be monitored. Also, a proportion of the nonapproved source animals come from laboratories with HM programs of unknown quality, so checking the health status of the imported animals is a good insurance policy and protects the health of the destination colony.

b. Supplies and Equipment as Common Vehicles

The risk of fomite transmission may be reduced by using physical and chemical processes to sterilize or disinfect equipment and supplies. Sterilization is the elimination or inactivation of all microorganisms, whereas disinfection is less complete. For example, a disinfection process might destroy vegetative bacteria but not bacterial spores (Block, 1991). Supplies for gnotobiotic colonies must be sterilized, whereas disinfection, or pasteurization, generally suffices for supplies being transferred into an SPF area (Foster, 1980; Foster et al., 1964; Trexler, 1983). Rational selection of a disinfection or sterilization process is aided by knowledge of the process's mechanism of action and the physicochemical characteristics of the microorganisms to be eliminated. In general, bacterial spores, free-living stages of parasites (e.g., pinworm eggs and protozoan cysts), and hydrophilic nonenveloped viruses (e.g., MPV) are resistant to inactivation (Ganaway, 1980; Hoover et al., 1985; Leland, 1991; Prince et al., 1991; Russell, 1991; Van Der Gulden and Van Erp, 1972). The best method for disinfection is also determined by the process's applicability to a particular medium (e.g., air, food, water, and surfaces), hazards (including corrosive properties), and the toxicity of treatment, ease of application, and cost. The efficacy of disinfection procedures and equipment should be validated and routinely monitored using biological, chemical, and/or physical indicators (Russell, 1992).

Physical Processes of Disinfection Physical processes of disinfection, such as autoclaving and electromagnetic irradiation, are the treatments of choice for food and bedding. By contrast to chemical disinfection, these methods do not leave a residue or by-products that may be toxic for or cause physiologic changes in animals (Hermann et al., 1982). Raw materials used in the preparation of animal feed and bedding frequently have a high bacteria count. The heating of food to 75–80°C during pelleting substantially reduces the bacterial count but is not sufficient to inactivate thermostable pathogens. In addition, food and bedding may become recontaminated after processing (Clarke et al., 1977). Therefore, they should be sterilized or pasteurized for gnotobiotic or SPF rodent colonies, respectively. As mentioned, this has traditionally been accomplished by autoclaving (i.e., saturated steam heat) or gamma irradiation. In comparison

with gamma irradiation, autoclaving is less expensive but causes a greater reduction in the nutritional value of food (Ferrando et al., 1981). Another drawback of autoclaving is the difficulty in achieving uniform steam penetration and temperature throughout a load (Small, 1983). Presterilization vacuum cycles help preserve the nutritional value of food by promoting rapid and uniform steam penetration, which allows autoclave times to be kept short (Foster et al., 1964; Maerki et al., 1989).

Gamma radiation, usually emitted from a cobalt-60 source, is a type of ionizing radiation. Although ionizing irradiation has a variety of physical and biochemical effects, it mainly renders microorganisms nonviable by causing breakage in their nucleic acid (Silverman, 1991). Ultraviolet (UV) radiation (210–328 nm), which does not possess sufficient energy to cause ionization, also inactivates microorganisms by damaging their DNA but does not cause DNA breakage. Instead, UV irradiation produces thymine and other pyrimidine dimers. As one might expect, the bactericidal activity of UV irradiation is maximal near the peak of DNA absorption, which is 260 nm (Russell, 1991). Gamma radiation passes through solid objects; by contrast, UV radiation does not and therefore is effective only for disinfection of surfaces and drinking water. UV inactivation of microbes in drinking water is reduced as the UV light source loses intensity or becomes dirty and by the presence of particles and dissolved organics in the water (Sobsey, 1989). Nonetheless, UV irradiation is an attractive option for water disinfection because it is virucidal and, in contrast to chlorination, does not convert organic precursors into potentially carcinogenic trihalomethanes (Flood, 1995).

The radiosensitivity of organisms has been shown to correlate with genome volume and the ability of the organism to repair DNA damage (Silverman, 1991). This is the reason why comparatively small viruses, such as parvoviruses, are highly resistant to UV and gamma irradiation (Hanson and Wilkinson, 1993), as are bacterial spores, protozoan cysts, and vegetative bacteria with highly efficient DNA repair capabilities (Russell, 1991). Accordingly, irradiation should not be relied on as the sole treatment for sterilization of supplies intended for gnotobiotic rodents.

Filtration is the process most often employed to remove microbes from air and water (Denyer, 1992; Levy and Leahy, 1991). Depth filters entrap and adsorb, whereas membrane filters exclude particles according to pore size. They have high 'dirt-handling' capacity, and therefore they are used for HEPA filtration and for clarification of particle-laden liquids. Because depth filters have no meaningful pore size, they are given nominal ratings to indicate the efficiency with which they retain particles of a particular size. The 99.97% rating given HEPA filters is based on the efficiency with which they retain 0.3-μm particles (Avery, 1996).

A filtration process can be classified according to the minimum size of particles retained as microfiltration (range 0.1–10.0 µm), ultrafiltration (range 1000–1,000,000 molecular weight), or reverse osmosis (low-molecular-weight molecules, including salts). Microfiltration of water retains bacteria, fungi, and their spores, but it cannot be relied upon to exclude viruses (Block, 1991). Removal of virus from water can be achieved, however, by ultrafiltration or reverse osmosis. Although there are no reports implicating water as a source of adventitious viral infections for laboratory rodents, the possibility should be taken seriously because rodents are susceptible to infection with viruses that are taxonomically related to waterborne human viruses. Characteristically, waterborne viruses are of small to medium size, nonenveloped (and hence stable), and shed in the feces (Block and Schwartzbrod, 1989).

Chemical Disinfection   Chemical disinfectants are commonly utilized to decontaminate a room or an isolator before the introduction of SPF animals and to treat the surfaces of materials and containers being brought into an SPF colony or removed from a quarantine colony (Small and New, 1981). Water is often disinfected through chemical processes such as chlorination (Hermann *et al.*, 1982; Homberger *et al.*, 1993) or ozonation (Flood, 1995; Shek *et al.*, 1991). Chemical disinfectants inactivate microorganisms by acting as denaturants that disrupt protein or lipid structures, reactants that form or break covalent bonds, or oxidants (Table 11.2) (Prince *et al.*, 1991). Of these, oxidants such as chlorine dioxide, bleach, vapor-phase H_2O_2, and the peroxygen Virkon® S (from Dupont) are most frequently utilized because they are generally considered more effective than reactants and denaturants for inactivating resistant pathogens such as spore-forming bacteria, nonenveloped viruses and free-living forms of parasites.

The principles of effective chemical disinfection are as follows: (1) starting with a clean surface and freshly prepared disinfectant; (2) applying multiple, or 'layering', chemicals when disinfection requirements are especially strict; (3) allowing adequate contact time as recommended by the disinfectant manufacturer; (4) rinsing if the disinfectant is corrosive to the surface; and (5) selecting disinfectant (s) shown to inactivate the most stable pathogens on your SPF exclusions lists. Various schemes have been developed to link the physicochemical characteristics of microorganisms with susceptibility to chemical inactivation. For example, the Klein–DeForest scheme for viruses, associates sensitivity to disinfectants with viral solubility (Table 11.3). Phenolics and quaternary ammonium compounds, which disrupt lipid membranes, are more potent against lipophilic, enveloped viruses than against hydrophilic, nonenveloped viruses. Oxidants attack all organic compounds and thus inactivate hydrophilic as well as lipophilic viruses (Klein and Deforest, 1983; Prince *et al.*, 1991). A disinfection scale for all microbial taxa likely to be encountered in lab animals, derived from one proposed by Prince *et al.* (1991), is presented in Table 11.4. In brief, this scale recapitulates

TABLE 11.3   Klein–DeForest Scheme for Viral Sensitivity to Disinfectants

Category	Solubility	Structure	Sensitivity	Examples
A	Lipophilic	Lipid envelope + capsid	Marked	Paramyxo (Sendai, PVM) Corona (MHV, SDAV) Arena (LCMV)
B	Hydrophilic	Naked capsid	Slight	Picorna (TMEV) Parvo (MVM, MPV, KRV, RPV)
C	Intermediate	Partially lipophilic capsid	Moderate	Adeno (MAV-1,2) Reo (Reo-3) Rota (EDIM, IDIR)

PVM, pneumonia virus of mice; MHV, mouse hepatitis virus; SDAV, sialodacryoadenitis virus; LCMV, lymphocytic choriomeningitis virus; TMEV, Theiler's mouse encephalomyelitis virus; MVM, minute virus of mice; MPV, mouse parvovirus; KRV, Kilham's rat virus; RPV, rat parvovirus; MAV, mouse adenovirus; EDIM, epizootic diarrhea of infant mouse virus; IDIR, infectious diarrhea of infant rat virus.

TABLE 11.2   Chemical Disinfectant Categories

Category	Examples
Denaturants	Quaternary ammonium compounds (benzalkonium chloride) Phenolics Alcohols
Reactants	Aldehydes (formaldehyde, glutaraldehyde) Ethylene oxide
Oxidants	Halogens (chlorine bleach, chlorine dioxide, povidone-iodine) Peroxygens (vapor-phase H_2O_2, Virkon® S[a])

[a]*Virkon® is a registered trademark of DuPont.*

TABLE 11.4   Approximate Scale for Susceptibility of Laboratory Animal Pathogens to Disinfectants

Susceptibility category[a]	Type of microorganism
A	Enveloped viruses, non-spore-forming bacteria
B	Partially lipophilic, nonenveloped viruses
C	Hydrophilic, nonenveloped viruses
D	Bacterial endospores and parasite ova and cysts

[a]*Susceptibility decreases from A→D.*

the generalization made at the beginning of this section that enveloped viruses and vegetative bacteria are considerably easier to inactivate than are nonenveloped viruses, bacterial endospores, and free-living parasite stages. For the most part, a disinfectant that has been shown to inactivate microorganisms of a particular susceptibility group will inactivate infectious agents in more susceptible groups. For instance, a disinfectant that inactivates parvoviruses (Table 11.3, Category C) will certainly kill non-spore-forming bacteria such as *S. aureus* (Table 11.3, Category A).

The potency of a disinfectant can be enhanced through chemical modification or the addition of synergistic ingredients to the formulation. Conversely, physical factors, including temperature, pH, and the chemical 'demand' of the medium being treated, can diminish potency by reducing the concentration or stability of the active form of the disinfectant. Using chlorine as a case in point, increasing the pH or temperature of water reduces the concentration of hypochlorous acid in favor of the hypochlorite (OCl^-) ion, which is less biocidal. Chlorine is a strong oxidant that reacts not only with living microorganisms but also with inorganic reducing substances such as ferrous iron and organic impurities, including dissolved proteins. These reactions exert a chemical demand that reduces the concentration of free chlorine available for disinfection (Dychadala, 1991; Russell, 1992; Wickramanayake and Sproul, 1991).

Association with dirt and organic matter has been shown to protect microorganisms from disinfectants (Grossgebauer *et al.*, 1975; Russell, 1992; Wickramanayake and Sproul, 1991). Upon colonizing surfaces, bacteria such as *P. aeruginosa* are notorious for forming biofilms, i.e., large clumps of bacteria surrounded in slime, that resist chemical disinfectants (Potera, 1996). It is therefore crucial that soiled surfaces be cleaned before being disinfected in order to reduce chemical demand and to ensure that microorganisms are adequately exposed to disinfectant. Biofilms in water systems can reportedly be removed by treatment with H_2O_2 or alkaline peroxide (Klein and Deforest, 1983; Kramer, 1992).

c. Vectors

Previously in this chapter, it was noted that although biological vectors are rarely involved in the transmission of rodent pathogens, both insects and people have been incriminated as mechanical vectors. People are also carriers of opportunistic bacterial pathogens such as β-hemolytic streptococci and *S. aureus* (Foster, 1996; Patterson, 1996). The keys to controlling insects – mostly flies and cockroaches – are deterrence to entry, sanitation, and the application of control methods, resorting lastly to the use of insecticides that might alter rodent physiology (Small, 1983). Entomologists with a detailed understanding of insect life cycles can often minimize or obviate chemical use. Risk factors for personnel becoming vehicles of infection include (1) exposure to a reservoir, such as an infected colony; (2) access to multiple colonies, especially going from conventional to SPF; and (3) unprotected human–animal contact, as exemplified by a technician handling animals without wearing gloved ideally disinfected or changed between animal groups.

To state the obvious, because people who care for and use research animals do not themselves live in isolators or barrier rooms, contact between people and reservoirs of infection can never be completely avoided. However, practices can be instituted that reduce this risk. Animal care technicians should be prohibited from having pet rodents although enforcement is challenging. There is also a risk associated with procuring rodents from pet stores for feeding snakes or other reptiles kept as pets. In many institutions, visitors are permitted to enter animal facilities only if they have not had recent contact with lab animals. Breeders with large production rooms may have a dedicated staff for each room. Access to smaller colonies, for which a dedicated staff is not practical, should still be restricted, and the flow of people and supplies should always be from 'clean' to 'dirty' areas. Personnel entering a barrier room should gown in a manner that keeps areas of exposed skin to a minimum in order to reduce the potential for transmitting infectious agents. Alternatively, it has become common practice to limit animal–human contact by housing rodents in microisolation cages (Lipman, 1999) or isolators (Trexler, 1983). Contact is limited further by manipulating rodents in a laminar flow hood and by handling them with disinfected gloves or forceps.

d. Cell Lines and Other Biologicals

Inoculation of rodents and other lab animals with untested biologicals, particularly transplantable tumor lines and reagents derived from animal tissues and fluids (Collins and Parker, 1972; Dick *et al.*, 1996; Lipman *et al.*, 2000; Nicklas *et al.*, 1993), has represented a major risk for adventitious viral infections. In fact, many indigenous rodent viruses were discovered as contaminants of animal-derived biologicals that confounded research findings (Bonnard *et al.*, 1976; Hartley and Rowe, 1960; Mckisic *et al.*, 1993; Riley *et al.*, 1960; Rowe and Capps, 1961). Failing to screen biological materials for rodent viruses has also been a public health concern as LCMV has been a relatively prevalent contaminant of cell lines (Bhatt *et al.*, 1986a; Lewis *et al.*, 1965; Simon *et al.*, 1982) and hantaviruses have been isolated from transplantable rat tumors (Lloyd and Jones, 1986; Yamanishi *et al.*, 1983). Traditionally, biologicals were screened for rodent viruses by the mouse and rat antibody production (MAP and RAP) tests (Collins and Parker, 1972; Desousa and Smith, 1989; Lewis and Clayton, 1971; Nicklas *et al.*,

1993; Shek, 1983) as well as other *in vivo* and cultural isolation techniques (Lussier, 1991; Smith, 1986a). Briefly, in an antibody production test, SPF rodents are inoculated with the test article orally and parenterally, held in isolation for a month, and tested by serology for antibodies to rodent viruses; detection of viral antibodies is tantamount to demonstrating infective virus in the test article. MAP and RAP tests continue to be required for cell substrates used in the production of regulated biopharmaceuticals. However, viral PCR tests have replaced antibody production tests of research biologicals because PCR assays are faster, more sensitive, and less costly, and achieve the goal of reduced animal usage espoused in the Three Rs [replacement, reduction, refinement] (3Rs) (Bauer *et al.*, 2004; Blank *et al.*, 2004).

In addition to being tested for viruses, it is of paramount importance that research biologicals for parenteral injection and those used to produce reagents for animal inoculation are cultured for extraneous bacteria and fungi to demonstrate that they are sterile or at least have a low bioburden. Maintaining a low bioburden is especially challenging for transplantable tumors passaged in animals; moreover, microbial contaminants can include prevalent pathogens such as *H. hepaticus* (Goto *et al.*, 2001). A high bioburden is problematic even when free of pathogens because commensal bacteria are more likely to cause disease by circumventing natural host defenses when parenterally injected along with tumor cells into immunodeficient recipients such as nude or SCID mice.

A common contaminant of cells propagated in culture is mycoplasma. Testing cell cultures for mycoplasma infection (usually by culture or PCR) is worthwhile because of the wide range of adverse effects these infections cause such as inhibition of cell growth due to competition for nutrients, cytopathic effects, mutagenesis and interference with viral synthesis, and interferon induction (Hendershot and Levitt, 1985; Mcgarrity *et al.*, 1984). However, 99% of the mycoplasma species found in cell culture are of human, porcine, and bovine origin (Erickson *et al.*, 1989; Mcgarrity *et al.*, 1983; Moore, 1992; Thornton, 1986) and do not infect rodents or rabbits to our knowledge.

A theme of this chapter has been that the complementary approaches of strict control of production processes and comprehensive quality testing, emphasized in CGMPs, are central to microbiological QC of research animals. As neither barrier systems nor the people who maintain rodent colonies are infallible and assays inevitably yield some level of inaccurate results, the complementary approaches of rigorous biosecurity and routine HM are essential to maintaining SPF lab animals. Similarly, QC for biological research reagents should complement testing with procedures to reduce the risk of microbial contamination including (1) obtaining biological reagents from reputable suppliers able to provide material traceability and lot analysis information, i.e., a Certificate of Analysis. Tissues, cells, blood, and so on. should be from animal populations shown to be healthy and SPF according to observations and testing carried out over an extended period. (2) Applying physical or chemical treatments to reagents that are able to withstand them to remove or inactivate infectious agents, e.g., heat inactivation or detergent treatment of serum. (3) Preventing operator-induced contaminations by using PPE, a biological safety hood, and sterile technique. (4) Banking (i.e., cryopreserving vials of) cell lines and microorganisms to ensure that you always have access to starting material that is well characterized and free of extraneous or pathogenic microorganisms, and for which you have documented key information such as designation, lot, species and strain, provenance, preparation method, and QC test results (Shek, 2007).

IV. HEALTH MONITORING

Laboratory testing commonly referred to as 'health monitoring' (HM) is an essential component of a lab animal microbiological QC program. Although the familiar term HM has been used throughout this chapter, specific-pathogen, or microbiological, monitoring (or surveillance) would have been more correct as all but profoundly immunodeficient and disease susceptible research animal strains remain healthy following infections with the highly host-adapted pathogens that are common today. Thus, the main purpose of HM is to detect silent infections of animals and biologicals that nevertheless are capable of confounding research and, if zoonotic, endangering the health of personnel, and to detect those infections early to limit their spread (Lipman and Homberger, 2003).

The traditional HM diagnostic methodologies employed for over half a century are as follows: (1) direct gross and microscopic examinations of animal specimens for pathology, specifically lesions consistent with infectious etiologies, and for parasites; (2) microbiology consisting of cultural isolation of bacteria and fungi and identification of isolates according to their phenotypic characteristics, such as colonial and cellular morphology and biochemical pattern; and (3) serology, i.e., immunoassays of blood or serum samples for antibodies to viruses and several fastidious and invasive microbial pathogens. The newest HM methodology, molecular diagnostics, utilizes molecular genetic techniques to detect and characterize pathogens of all types including viruses, bacteria, fungi, and parasites (Compton and Riley, 2001; Lipman and Homberger, 2003; Livingston and Riley, 2003; Shek and Gaertner, 2002; Weisbroth *et al.*, 1998).

The molecular assay method employed most often in HM is the PCR, in which a targeted microbial genomic DNA sequence is specifically and exponentially amplified (i.e., copied) entirely *in vitro* in a matter of hours. Because of exponential amplification, PCR assays characteristically achieve sensitivity levels that far and away surpass those of other test methods. The role of PCR testing in HM has expanded substantially in recent years because PCR assays have been made available for most or all reportable research animal pathogens, including bacteria, fungi, and parasites as well as viruses; moreover, PCR can specifically detect tiny quantities of targeted microbial genomic sequences in a broad array of complex and heavily pooled specimens, including environmental and *ante mortem* animal specimens that are not likely to contain enough viable bacteria and fungi or intact parasites to be suitable for traditional microbiology or parasitology, respectively.

The resident populations and the imported animal groups in quarantine that are being monitored for adventitious infections are referred to as the 'principal' animals. Resident groups comprise the breeding colony and study animals maintained at a facility. HM of resident animal populations verifies the effectiveness of biosecurity measures to eliminate, exclude, or contain and eradicate infections. Animals imported from unapproved sources, such as other research facilities (as opposed to approved commercial breeding colonies) are placed in quarantine; HM determines whether imported animals meet the institutional SPF standards for release from quarantine.

HM has been referred to as direct when it is performed on specimens from the principals and indirect when testing samples from sentinels (Koszdin and Digiacomo, 2002). Direct HM is common for commercial breeding colonies, but otherwise most surveillance has been indirect because lethal sampling of investigator animals for *postmortem* examinations and microbiologic specimen collections is seldom permitted, and in most situations would be impractical and cost-prohibitive. In addition, the principals might be immunodeficient and hence not suitable for serosurveillance.

Irrespective of the diagnostic methodology, detection of a contamination by indirect sentinel surveillance requires transmission of infection from the principals to the sentinels; this occurs most reliably by contact and by exposing sentinels to a high infectious dose of the adventitious agent (Grove *et al.*, 2012; Henderson *et al.*, 2013; Smith *et al.*, 2007). While contact sentinels are an option for imported rodents in quarantine, they are generally inappropriate for routine surveillance of resident animals in popular microisolation caging systems because to be effective the sentinels would have to be moved among resident cages, which, besides

being unworkable, would defeat the cage-level barrier. Consequently, sentinels are kept in separate cages supplied with regular changes of soiled bedding pooled from resident cages. Reliance on soiled bedding transmission alone, however, is problematic because microisolation cages impede the spread of infection (Compton *et al.*, 2012; Jensen *et al.*, 2013; Whary *et al.*, 2000a). Thus, the percentage of cages containing contagious animals following an outbreak often remains low and can be as low as 2% (Smith, 2010). The lower the prevalence of infection, the greater the risk that the dose of pathogen in pooled bedding will not be sufficient to infect sentinels. Other factors contributing to this risk include the high degree of pooling that is common because it is typical for a rack of more than 50 cages to have just one or two sentinel cages. In addition, certain pathogens, such as respiratory viruses, host-adapted bacteria, and parasites, are transmitted inefficiently or not at all in soiled bedding (Artwohl *et al.*, 1994; Compton *et al.*, 2004c; Cundiff *et al.*, 1995; Dillehay *et al.*, 1990; Henderson *et al.*, 2013; Ike *et al.*, 2007; Lindstrom *et al.*, 2011; Thigpen *et al.*, 1989). Finally, sentinels can be resistant to infection with certain pathogens due to their age (Riepenhoff-Talty *et al.*, 1985) or genetic background (Besselsen *et al.*, 2000; Filipovska-Naumovska *et al.*, 2010b; Henderson *et al.*, 2015; Hirai *et al.*, 2010; Shek *et al.*, 2005; Thomas *et al.*, 2007).

As described earlier in this section, the exquisite sensitivity and high analytical specificity of PCR assays allow them to detect low concentrations of the targeted microbial genomic sequences in complex, heavily pooled and therefore highly representative specimens not suitable for traditional methodologies. These include specimens from the environment, such as swabs of cages and room or individually ventilated cage (IVC) rack, exhaust air dust, and those that can be collected *ante mortem* directly from animals in residence or quarantine, such as feces and swabs of the upper respiratory tract, skin, and fur (Bauer and Riley, 2006; Dole *et al.*, 2011; Henderson *et al.*, 2013; Jensen *et al.*, 2013). PCR surveillance of these nonsentinel specimens is increasingly employed to lessen the risk of missing adventitious agents that is associated with dependence on transmission of infections to sentinels, particularly those exposed by soiled bedding transfer alone. By eliminating the time required for sentinels to get infected and seroconvert, direct PCR HM of imported animals has been able to reduce the time they spend in quarantine from 2 months or longer for sentinel HM to just 2 weeks. In addition, environmental and direct PCR HM can reduce sentinel usage in accordance with the goals of the 3Rs as well as the expense, logistical, and animal welfare issues of shipping live animals to diagnostic laboratories for pathology and traditional parasitology and microbiology.

A. Methodologies

1. Direct Gross and Microscopic Examination of Animal Specimens

Direct examination continues to be a fundamental diagnostic methodology for pathology and parasitology, despite the increasing availability of rapid and specific *in vitro* PCR and serologic assays for pathogens on SPF exclusion lists. As still common pathogens are highly host-adapted and rarely cause disease, direct examinations should be given a high priority when investigating disease outbreaks. This is highlighted by the pivotal contribution made by gross and microscopic pathology to (1) the discovery of hitherto unrecognized pathogens such as *H. hepaticus*, shown to be the agent responsible for hepatitis and hepatocellular carcinoma in mice in a long-term toxicology study (Fox *et al.*, 1994, 1996; Ward *et al.*, 1994b, 1996), and MNV, found to cause of lethal, systemic disease in mice genetically engineered to be deficient in innate and acquired immunity (Henderson, 2008; Hsu *et al.*, 2006; Karst *et al.*, 2003) and (2) the association recognized pathogens with atypical, novel disease manifestations (Compton *et al.*, 2003; Henderson *et al.*, 2012; Livingston *et al.*, 2011). In addition, direct examination has been a necessary or useful approach to monitor for infectious diseases (Albers *et al.*, 2009; Cundiff *et al.*, 1992; Gibson *et al.*, 1987) and parasite infestations (Watson, 2008) when specific assays have not been available. Finally, direct examination can be used in combination with other test methods to arrive at a specific diagnosis (see below), or to corroborate findings obtained by other assays. For example, microscopic examination of Warthin–Starry silver-stained tissue sections for intracellular bacteria from rodents following disease provocation by immunosuppressive treatment with cyclophosphamide or dexamethasone has been used to verify a preliminary diagnosis of *C. piliforme* infection made by serology or PCR (Nakayama *et al.*, 1984; Riley *et al.*, 1994; Waggie *et al.*, 1981).

a. Techniques

Pathology Tissues and organs are inspected for gross abnormalities during routine HM. Selected tissue specimens, including those with gross abnormalities, may then be fixed in buffered formalin, embedded in paraffin blocks, sectioned onto slides, stained with hematoxylin and eosin, and then examined microscopically for histopathological changes (Weisbroth *et al.*, 1998). Special stains can be applied to tissue sections to enhance the visibility of certain pathogens (Clifford *et al.*, 1995; Gibson *et al.*, 1987; Hoover *et al.*, 1985; Thompson *et al.*, 1982; Waggie *et al.*, 1983; Ward *et al.*, 1994b). In diagnostic and experimental lab animal microbiology, microbial antigens or nucleic acid in tissue sections can be specifically stained by immunohistochemistry (Allen *et al.*, 1981; Brownstein and Barthold, 1982; Cera *et al.*,

1994; Hall and Ward, 1984; Jacoby *et al.*, 1975; Sundberg *et al.*, 1989) or *in situ* hybridization (Gaertner *et al.*, 1993; Jacoby *et al.*, 1995; Smith *et al.*, 1993a), respectively. However, these specific staining techniques are rarely if ever used in routine HM. Instead, the presence of pathogens in tissues is demonstrated by PCR of nucleic acid extracted usually from tissue homogenates, but also fixed tissue sections (Henderson *et al.*, 2012).

Parasitology Low-power dissecting microscopy is used to inspect the pelage and skin of lab animal carcasses for mites and lice, and the macerated gastrointestinal tract for adult helminths (Flynn, 1973; Parkinson *et al.*, 2011). The latter method has been considered the gold standard for diagnosing helminth infestations (Huerkamp, 1993; West *et al.*, 1992). Microscopic examination of skin scrapings may be necessary to detect mites, such as *Demodex* and *Notoedres*, which burrow into the epidermis (Weisbroth, 1979b; Wescott, 1982). It has been reported that fur mites can be found in a higher percentage of mice by microscopic examination of adhesive tape applied to the dorsal fur than by checking the skin or skin scrapings (Ricart Arbona *et al.*, 2010a; West *et al.*, 1992). Fur 'plucks' taken from multiple sites on the dorsal surface (e.g., between the scapulae, near base of the tail) and microscopically examined in Petri dishes also yield reasonably accurate results (Rice *et al.*, 2013), but all of these are limited by sampling 'error' compared to pelt digestion (Owen, 1972), which samples the entire, but deceased, host. Fur mite eggs can also be observed on perianal tape tests used to detect pinworm eggs if the mite infestation is very heavy. Infections with enteric protozoa are diagnosed by examining wet mounts of mucosal scrapings of the small and large intestines with a phase-contrast microscope, which makes it possible to see unstained microorganisms (Brock, 1970; Weisbroth *et al.*, 1996); however, histologic examination of the gastrointestinal tract is best for detecting *Cryptosporidium* (Wasson, 2007). Phase-contrast microscopy is also used for more precise morphologic identification of adult helminths and mites, and to examine fecal floats or centrifugation concentrates for helminth ova and protozoan cysts, tape applied perianally for *Syphacia* pinworm eggs, and tape applied to the fur for mites (Rice *et al.*, 2013; Weisbroth, 1979b, 1998; Weiss *et al.*, 2012).

b. Limitations

Gross and microscopic lesions are seldom diagnostic. Furthermore, direct examinations are characterized by low analytical sensitivity, that is, the lesions and organisms in stained tissue sections and the intact parasite stages that these tests target must be present at high concentrations to be observed, particularly when specimens are examined microscopically as is almost always done. As the level of magnification increases, there is a commensurate rise in the minimum target concentration required for detection. As an extreme example, the minimum concentration of virus that can be detected by transmission electron microscopy is 10^5–10^6 particles per milliliter (Miller, 1995). High magnification further limits sensitivity by constraining the amount of sample that is practical to examine.

According to sampling statistics (Anonymous, 1976; Clifford, 2001; Dubin and Zietz, 1991; Selwyn and Shek, 1994), the likelihood of detecting an outbreak is enhanced by increasing the number of animals evaluated, but this also increases the labor of sample collection along with the cost of testing. One way of increasing the sample size, while controlling HM costs, is to test sample pools; however, sample pooling is limited by the low analytical sensitivity of direct examinations. Because principal animals at research institutions are seldom made available to be euthanized for routine HM, the number of animals that can be sampled is further restricted by the need to examine *postmortem* specimens for optimal detection of some types of parasites, such as macerated gastrointestinal tract for adult helminths, intestinal scrapings for protozoan trophozoites, and the pelt for ectoparasites (Parkinson *et al.*, 2011). Therefore, *postmortem* specimen collection and examinations are usually restricted to a small number of sentinels (e.g., one or two sentinels per rack). In addition to limiting sample size, the main shortcoming of sentinel surveillance is the risk that sentinels will not become infected (or infested) with pathogens harbored by the principal animals. This is of greatest concern when monitoring resident rodents housed in microisolation cages using sentinels exposed to pooled soiled bedding because, as discussed, certain pathogens including mites (Grove *et al.*, 2012; Henderson *et al.*, 2013; Lindstrom *et al.*, 2011) are poorly transmitted in bedding and sentinels may be exposed to subinfectious doses of pathogens when the prevalence of infection is low, as commonly occurs in microisolation cages, or when sentinels are resistant to an infection due to their age or genetic background.

2. Microbiology: Cultural Isolation and Identification

This section focuses on testing animal specimens for pathogenic microorganisms. Other routine applications of traditional microbiology not covered here are bioburden and sterility testing to monitor the efficacy of disinfection procedures for facilities, equipment, and supplies (Ednie *et al.*, 2005; Meier *et al.*, 2008; Schondelmeyer *et al.*, 2006; Small, 1983). By demonstrating deficiencies in biosecurity measures, monitoring of disinfection processes can help prevent contaminations.

a. Techniques

Cultural Isolation Animal specimens, artificial cell-free agar and broth media, and incubation conditions are chosen to favor the isolation and cultivation of primary and opportunistic microbial pathogens while limiting the growth of commensal and autochthonous microorganisms (Ganaway, 1976; Orcutt, 1980; Weisbroth, 1979a; Weisbroth *et al.*, 1998). The animal sites most often sampled – the upper respiratory tract and large intestine – possess a complex microbiome that can overgrow cultures and obscure colonies of interest. To lessen this problem, specimens are cultured with selective media that contain additives, such as dyes or antibiotics, to inhibit the growth of certain microorganisms. MacConkey's agar, e.g., contains crystal violet and bile salts that selectively inhibit the growth of gram-positive bacteria, while allowing most gram-negative bacteria to grow (Forbes *et al.*, 1998). Media for the isolation of *Helicobacter* spp. from fecal or intestinal specimens contain a mixture of antibiotics to selectively inhibit the growth of the intestinal microbiome (Fox *et al.*, 1994). Overgrowth can be further reduced by culturing sites that do not possess a normal microbiome to obscure invasive bacteria. Tracheal cultures from *Bordetella bronchiseptica*-infected animals contain few extraneous bacteria, making it easier to view *B. bronchiseptica* colonies (Bemis *et al.*, 2003; Brownstein *et al.*, 1985). *Corynebacterium kutscheri* is most reliably isolated from the submaxillary lymph nodes of infected rats (Brownstein *et al.*, 1985). Enrichment media are used to encourage the growth of particular bacteria, which are at low concentration in a specimen containing many microorganisms. Selenite broth is an enrichment medium that is used to recover salmonella from feces or the intestinal tract (Orcutt, 1980). Media are categorized as differential when they allow colonies to be morphologically differentiated based on metabolic characteristics. On MacConkey's agar, lactose-fermenting bacteria produce pink to red colonies, whereas colonies of non-lactose fermenters remain colorless (Forbes *et al.*, 1998). Cultures are usually incubated aerobically at 35–37°C because the majority of clinically important bacteria are facultative anaerobes that will grow under these conditions, whereas the strict anaerobes that constitute the autochthonous microbiome will not. PCR and/or serology are used instead of culture to screen for fastidious and noncultivable microbial pathogens such as *M. pulmonis* (Davidson *et al.*, 1981; Kraft *et al.*, 1982; Loganbill *et al.*, 2005), *Helicobacter* spp. (Whary *et al.*, 2000b), *C. piliforme* (the etiology of Tyzzer's disease) (Goto and Itoh, 1996; Motzel and Riley, 1991; Pritt *et al.*, 2010), cilia-associated respiratory (CAR) bacillus (Cundiff *et al.*, 1994a; Lukas *et al.*, 1987; Matsushita *et al.*, 1987), and *Pneumocystis* spp. (Henderson *et al.*, 2012; Hong *et al.*, 1995; Livingston *et al.*, 2011).

Phenotypic and Genetic Identification After incubation, isolated colonies on agar media are examined to assess their morphology and number; colonies of interest are characterized further. Cellular morphology, size, and motility are evaluated by examining a wet mount of an isolate with a phase-contrast microscope or a slide of gram-stained cells with a bright-field microscope. Additional tests are performed to determine the identity of isolates suspected to be pathogens. A metabolic profile is established by performing panels of biochemical tests as individual assays (e.g., catalase) and in automated multitest systems (Carroll and Weinstein, 2007; Macfaddin, 1980).

Serotyping may also be necessary or helpful to determine the identity and clinical significance of an isolate. For *Salmonella*, serotypes are based on the somatic O and flagellar H antigens (Ganaway, 1982; Giannella, 1996). β-Hemolytic streptococci usually have group-specific, cell-wall carbohydrate (C) antigens, which are the basis of the Lancefield classification system (Corning *et al.*, 1991; Patterson, 1996; Washington, 1996).

As the identification of microbial isolates according to their phenotypic properties may be imprecise or simply inaccurate, biochemical and serologic tests are being augmented or supplanted by PCR and gene sequencing methods that provide highly accurate, reproducible classifications of microorganisms (Dole *et al.*, 2010, 2013b; Gentsch *et al.*, 1992; Tenover, 1998; Tenover *et al.*, 1994; Ushijima *et al.*, 1992). Related to their characteristically high analytical specificity and sensitivity, PCR assays can be performed directly on microbially complex clinical specimens, bypassing the need for cultural isolation, which is impractical for routine detection of fastidious microbes such as *Helicobacter* spp. (Whary *et al.*, 2000b; Whary and Fox, 2006). So-called next-generation sequencing in which millions of DNA fragments from a single sample are sequenced in unison is already being used to characterize the intestinal microbiome (Friswell *et al.*, 2010), but currently is far too expensive and complicated for routine identification of microbial pathogens in clinical specimens (Grada and Weinbrecht, 2013).

Matrix-assisted laser desorption ionization time-of-flight mass spectrometry (MALDI-TOF MS) is an alternative to conventional phenotypic tests for identification of bacterial isolates that, although proposed over 30 years ago, have only recently been made commercially available. Identifications by the MALDI-TOF MS are performed on actively growing cultures, or extracts made from them, and are based on unique peptidic spectra primarily of ribosomal and other housekeeping proteins that are expressed at high levels. The peak intensity and position of the spectra are compared to those in a database to establish identifications. The principal advantages of MALDI-TOF MS in comparison with biochemical testing are that it is much more rapid (completed in minutes instead of hours to days) and has a lower cost per identification, although the mass spectrometer instrument is very expensive. MALDI-TOF MS is also highly reliable and accurate since it is based on

molecules that are less dependent on growth conditions and not subject to the expression variability seen in phenotypic systems (Seng *et al.*, 2009). Because of the aforementioned advantages, MALDI-TOF MS is increasingly employed, in place of traditional phenotypic techniques, for human and veterinary diagnostic microbiology.

b. Limitations

Microbiology is limited to microorganisms that can be cultivated in cell-free media. Serology and PCR assays have been developed to monitor for noncultivable microbial pathogens such as *C. piliforme*, CAR bacillus, and *Pneumocystis* spp., and have replaced culture when testing for fastidious, slow growing bacteria such as *M. pulmonis* and *Helicobacter* spp. Because the preferred respiratory and intestinal specimens for culture are collected *postmortem*, microbiology of resident animals at research institutions is largely restricted to indirect surveillance of a few sentinels, with the associated risk of missing adventitious infections when the prevalence is low; the pathogen is poorly transmitted in soiled bedding or the sentinels are resistant to infection due to their genetic background or age. The complex microbiome of respiratory and gastrointestinal specimens necessitates that bacteria of interest be viable and present in high numbers in order to obtain isolated colonies for identification.

3. *Serology*

Serology has been the most commonly used methodology to detect rodent infections because it is easily used to monitor viral infections, which are among the most common adventitious agents infecting rodents (Lussier and Descoteaux, 1986; Pritchett-Corning *et al.*, 2009; Schoondermark-Van De Ven *et al.*, 2006; Zenner and Regnault, 2000). They also have high impact due to their effects on research (Bhatt *et al.*, 1986b) and because, unlike parasites, they cannot be treated. Although virus isolation has been used for diagnosis on occasion, that approach can be problematic because (1) many field strains are either difficult to cultivate or noncultivable; (2) virus isolation is time-consuming and expensive (Schmidt, 1979); and (3) live virus may be present in host tissue and shed for relatively short periods of time. By contrast, serum antibody responses are usually detectable by 1–2 weeks post infection and last for long periods (at least months and sometimes for the life of the rodent) and the tests are highly accurate, fast, and relatively inexpensive (Barthold and Smith, 1983; Bhatt and Jacoby, 1985; Homberger *et al.*, 1992; Parker and Reynolds, 1968; Peters and Collins, 1981; Smith *et al.*, 1984).

a. Techniques

As a consequence of serology's central role in HM, substantial resources have been dedicated over the years toward upgrading the immunoassay and related technologies it employs. In the mid-1980s, traditional homogenous serologic techniques (with the term homogeneous indicating that sample and assay reagents are mixed and incubated together in solution) such as hemagglutination inhibition (HAI), complement fixation, and virus neutralization were supplanted by more sensitive and broadly applicable heterogeneous solid-phase immunoassays, notably the indirect enzyme-linked immunosorbent assay (ELISA) and immunofluorescence assay (IFA) schematically depicted in Figs. 11.2 and 11.3b,

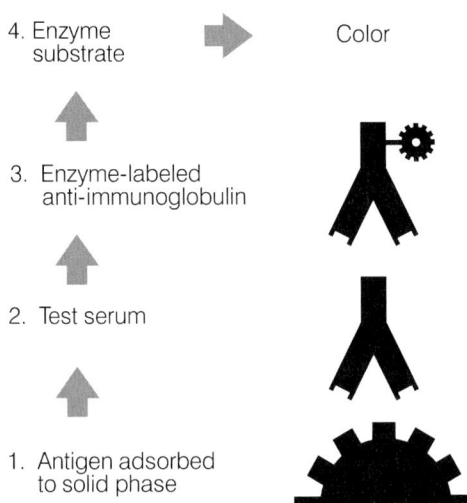

FIGURE 11.2 Indirect ELISA for microbial antibodies. Antigen, such as virus particles or lysates, microbial cell extracts, or recombinant proteins, is adsorbed to wells in microtiter plates. Separate wells may be coated with a 'tissue control', i.e., an extract of uninfected host cells (or of a related microorganism) to detect nonspecific binding of Ig. The numbers denote incubations; incubations 1–3 are followed by washing to remove unbound antibodies and other substances that might interfere with the assay. The rate at which chromogenic substrate is converted to a colored product is proportional to the amount of enzyme-labeled anti-Ig and, hence, serum antibodies bound to the solid phase. The color development can be scored visually, but is more commonly measured as optical density by an ELISA plate reader. *Adapted from Mahony and Chernesky (1999), Fig. 4A, p. 208.*

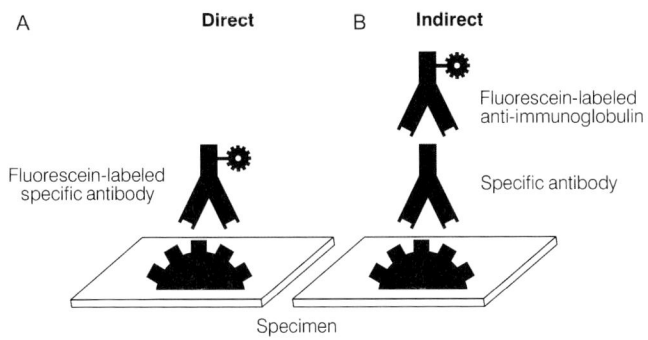

FIGURE 11.3 Direct (A) and indirect (B) immunofluorescence assays. *Adapted from Mahony and Chernesky (1999), Fig. 2, p. 206.*

respectively (Kraft *et al.*, 1982; Mahoney and Chernesky, 1999; Parker *et al.*, 1979; Smith, 1983a, b, 1986b; Takahashi *et al.*, 1986; Voller *et al.*, 1982). The 'solid phase' denotes the surface to which the antigen is attached. For ELISA, antigen, consisting of purified virus particles, microbial cell extracts, or recombinant proteins encoded by microbial genes of interest, is immobilized on the surface of wells in microtiter plates made of specially prepared polystyrene or polyvinyl; separate wells may be coated with an extract of uninfected host cells (or with antigen from other microorganisms), often called a 'tissue control', to detect nonspecific binding of immunoglobulin (Ig). For IFA, infected and uninfected cells are fixed to wells on glass slides. The fixative is usually cold acetone, which permeabilizes the cell membrane, making the intracellular viral antigens accessible to antibodies in the serum samples. 'Heterogeneous' indicates that each incubation period is followed by a wash step to separate antibody bound to the solid phase from unbound antibody. The wash step also removes interfering substances in a specimen that could compromise the sensitivity or specificity of a corresponding traditional homogeneous test. 'Indirect' refers to detection of serum antibodies bound to the solid phase (whether as specific antigen–antibody complexes or nonspecifically) by labeled anti-immunoglobulin (anti-Ig), such as goat IgG anti-mouse IgG, or Ig-binding bacterial proteins including Proteins A and G (Delellis, 1981; Hrapchak, 1980). Common non-radioisotopic labels include the enzymes horseradish peroxidase and alkaline phosphatase for ELISA and the fluorescent dye fluorescein for IFA (Mahoney and Chernesky, 1999; Voller *et al.*, 1982).

A direct solid-phase immunoassay, as shown in Fig. 11.3a, is one in which a label is coupled to the microbial antibodies rather than anti-Ig or Ig-binding bacterial protein for indirect labeling. Although labeled microbial antibodies are incorporated into blocking or competitive assays for serum antibodies (Vonderfecht *et al.*, 1985), they are more commonly used in fluorescence and enzyme immunoassays when doing research on the time course and distribution of infections *in situ*, i.e., in animal tissues and cells (Allen *et al.*, 1981; Brownstein and Barthold, 1982; Cera *et al.*, 1994; Dick *et al.*, 1996; Jacoby *et al.*, 1975; Kimsey *et al.*, 1986; Sundberg *et al.*, 1989; Weir *et al.*, 1988) and in specimens using techniques such as the double-antibody sandwich antigen capture method (Jure *et al.*, 1988; Newsome and Coney, 1985; Vonderfecht *et al.*, 1988). While solid-phase antigen capture immunoassays for pathogens have been popular in domestic and companion animal and human diagnostics, they have seldom been utilized in laboratory HM for a variety of reasons. First, as already discussed, the window of active infection and shedding is often short-lived. Even when an infection is active, the concentration of microbial antigens in animal specimens may be below the assay's detection limit, which is why MPV pathogenesis studies have utilized *in situ* hybridization (Jacoby *et al.*, 1995; Smith *et al.*, 1993a) and PCR (Besselsen *et al.*, 2000, 2007) to detect viral DNA rather than antigens. Also, antigen immunoassay development, particularly obtaining or producing microbial antibodies of the appropriate specificity, can be a long and expensive process with an unpredictable outcome; this helps explain why most of the few evaluations of antigen-capture immunoassays for HM have utilized commercial kits that had been developed for other host species, but recognized a group antigen shared with the related lab animal pathogen. Human group-A rotavirus kits, for instance, have been assessed for detection of mouse rotavirus in fecal specimens (Jure *et al.*, 1988; Newsome and Coney, 1985). Finally, the importance of antigen-capture immunoassays in diagnostics has been substantially diminished by the advent of more sensitive and specific molecular genetic assays – especially PCR assays – that are better suited to direct detection of infectious agents in animal and environmental samples (Wilde *et al.*, 1990).

After the labeled antibody incubation and final wash (Fig. 11.2), ELISA reactions are developed by adding an enzyme substrate to test plate wells; most substrates are chromogenic, that is, they are converted by the enzyme to a colored product at a rate proportional to the quantity of enzyme-labeled anti-Ig and, hence, serum antibodies attached to the solid phase. Color development can be read visually in a qualitative or semiquantitative fashion, but is usually read with a spectrophotometer, or ELISA plate reader, that exports optical density readings to a computer for analysis and reporting (Mahoney and Chernesky, 1999; Voller *et al.*, 1982). By contrast, IFA reactions are examined manually using a fluorescence microscope; analysts classify test serum reactions as negative to strong positive or nonspecific by comparing the pattern, intracellular location, and intensity of fluorescence to those observed with standard immune and nonimmune control sera (Lyerla and Forrester, 1979).

Because ELISA are generally performed in 96-well microtiter plates and reactions can be instrument-read and processed by computer, they are better suited than IFA to high-throughput testing and, hence, have been preferred for primary screening of serum samples. The IFA, however, has proven to be an excellent method for confirmatory testing because the pattern of fluorescence and whether it is located in the host cell nucleus, cytoplasm, or both is useful in distinguishing specific from nonspecific reactions. In addition, IFA are generally as sensitive as corresponding ELISA (Homberger *et al.*, 1995; Kraft *et al.*, 1982; Smith, 1983a) and they can be more 'inclusive', i.e., better able to detect seroconversion to heterologous viral strains and serotypes (OIE, 2013), when the host develops antibodies to highly conserved nonstructural viral protein antigens found in

the infected cells that compose IFA antigen, but not necessarily in ELISA antigen consisting of purified virus particles. The inclusivity of the IFA (specifically, its ability to detect antibodies to the nonstructural proteins conserved among rodent parvoviruses in mouse and rat populations that were largely MVM and rat virus (RV) seronegative by serotype-specific HAI and by ELISA with virus particle antigen) provided the initial evidence for the existence of then-novel rodent parvoviruses later identified as MPV, rat parvovirus, and rat minute virus (Jacoby *et al.*, 1996).

The prior rodent parvovirus example demonstrates that inclusivity is a preferred attribute of primary assays because it can enhance diagnostic sensitivity, i.e., the proportion of infected animals that test positive. Moreover, a single inclusive assay can replace several 'exclusive', i.e., strain-specific tests, thereby reducing the number tests and the cost of surveillance; however, this comes with a risk of false-negative (FN) findings if the antibody response to the conserved antigen (variously called shared or group-specific antigens) is delayed, weak, or absent, as has been demonstrated for the antibody response of rodents to the parvovirus nonstructural protein NS1 (Besselsen *et al.*, 2000; Filipovska-Naumovska *et al.*, 2010a; Henderson *et al.*, 2015; Livingston *et al.*, 2002). Solid-phase immunoassays tend to be more inclusive than corresponding traditional tests because they can detect antibodies to any of the epitopes (i.e., antigenic sites) presented by the microbial antigens attached to the solid phase and at much lower levels (Parker *et al.*, 1979), which improves detection of low-titered 'cross-reacting' antibodies to shared or group-specific antigens. By contrast, virus neutralization and HAI are highly exclusive because by definition they only recognize antibodies to viral surface protein antigens that are unique to the serotype or strain of virus being used in the test. Although this high level of exclusivity is not favored for primary surveillance, it is desirable for confirmatory testing to delineate the strain or serotype specificity and, thus, the etiology of the viral antibody response (Parker *et al.*, 1965). The inclusivity and high analytical sensitivity of solid-phase immunoassays has expanded lab animal serosurveillance to pathogens for which traditional serologic tests had not been developed because they were not sufficiently sensitive or applicable. Examples of agents added to serologic panels after the advent of solid-phase methods are mouse rotavirus (Smith) and invasive microbial pathogens including *M. pulmonis* (Cassell *et al.*, 1983; Minion *et al.*, 1984), *C. piliforme* (Motzel and Riley, 1991; Waggie *et al.*, 1987), *Helicobacter* spp. (Fox *et al.*, 1996; Whary *et al.*, 2000b), and CAR bacillus (Lukas *et al.*, 1987; Matsushita *et al.*, 1987), *Pneumocystis carinii* (Henderson *et al.*, 2012; Hong *et al.*, 1995) and *Encephalitozoon cuniculi* (Digiacomo *et al.*, 1983).

To be performed optimally, ELISA and other solid-phase immunoassays generally require antigen that is more concentrated and pure than was needed for the traditional homogenous tests they replaced. During the 1990s, advances in recombinant DNA technology made it possible to produce large quantities of recombinant protein rapidly from a cloned gene of interest inserted into microbial, mammalian, or baculovirus (an insect virus) expression vector systems. These systems have facilitated the production of pure and potent antigen, particularly for infectious agents that are fastidious, noncultivable, or zoonotic (Ball-Goodrich *et al.*, 2002; Filipovska-Naumovska *et al.*, 2010a; Homberger *et al.*, 1995; Katz *et al.*, 2012; Schmaljohn *et al.*, 1990). Thus, these systems have obviated the need to propagate a pathogen in culture and the recombinant proteins they generate are noninfectious. In addition, microbial genes of interest have been 'fused' to sequences that encode affinity tags, such as 6 × histidine, to permit purification of the recombinant proteins by affinity chromatography (Ball-Goodrich *et al.*, 2002; Riley *et al.*, 1996b; Seletsakia *et al.*, 2004). Recombinant viral capsid proteins, such as the parvovirus VP2, that self-assemble into virus-like particles, or VLPs, can also be purified by gradient centrifugation and other conventional techniques (Kahn *et al.*, 2008; Livingston *et al.*, 2002). Finally, incorporating recombinant protein antigens representing different viral strains and proteins into serosurveillance panels has enhanced diagnostic accuracy by being more inclusive and permitting confirmation and characterization of antibody specificity.

In the 2000s, novel systems became commercially available for assay multiplexing, i.e., for performing an array of tests simultaneously, in a single well, tube, or chip location. Among the most popular of these for lab animal serology has been Luminex's Multi-Analyte Profile (xMAP) platform (Adams and Myles, 2013; Besselsen *et al.*, 2008a; Hsu *et al.*, 2005; Khan *et al.*, 2005; Wunderlich *et al.*, 2011), which is termed a suspension microarray because the solid phase is a color-coded 5.6-μm polystyrene bead available in at least 100 different color sets. At the conclusion of an assay procedure, beads from test wells flow single file through an array reader (which is a modified flow cytometer); each bead is interrogated by two laser beams: one to identify the bead color set (i.e., test) and the other to measure the intensity of fluorescence emitted by the reporter dye phycoerythrin (Fig. 11.4). A predetermined minimum number of beads are read for each assay (i.e., bead set) in a well and the intensity of fluorescence for each test is reported as median fluorescence intensity (MFI) (De Jager *et al.*, 2003; Richens *et al.*, 2010).

The xMAP antibody immunoassays for serosurveillance, abbreviated as MFI or MFIA for multiplexed fluorescence or fluorometric immunoassay, are indirect,

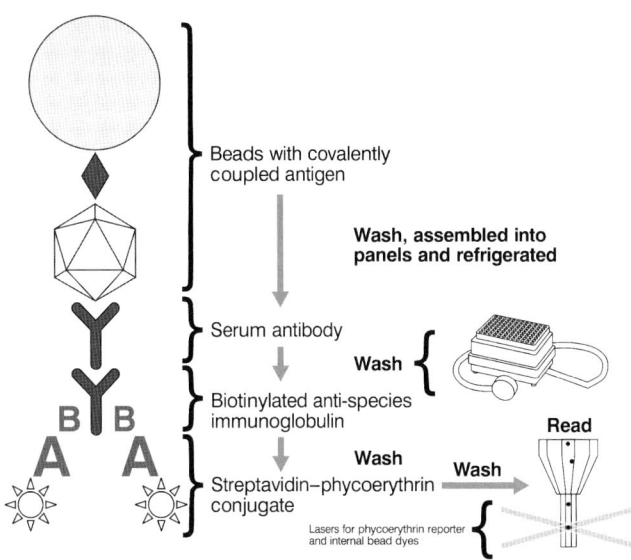

FIGURE 11.4 Multiplexed fluorometric immunoassay. An antigen or control (e.g., tissue control) is covalently coupled to beads of an assigned color set, of which there are 100. Serum antibodies bound to the bead are labeled with the reporter dye phycoerythrin by incubations with biotinylated anti-species Ig (e.g., goat IgG anti-mouse IgG) and phycoerythrin-conjugated streptavidin. An array reader evaluates a predetermined minimum number of beads of each color set in the panel. Each bead is interrogated by two laser beams, one to identify the bead color set, which corresponds to a test, and the other to measure the intensity of fluorescence emitted by the reporter dye phycoerythrin. The array reader reports the phycoerythrin median fluorescence intensity (MFI) for each assay.

heterogeneous solid-phase tests. Hence, the MFIA steps depicted in Fig. 11.4 are essentially the same as those described for the ELISA. Briefly, an antigen or control (e.g., tissue control) is covalently coupled to beads of a specific color. Although up to 100 different tests could be included in an MFIA panel, the largest serologic panels for HM contain fewer than 40. Antigen–antibody complexes that form during the serum incubation (as well as nonspecifically bound antibodies) are detected by phycoerythrin-conjugated anti-Ig or by biotinylated anti-Ig followed by phycoerythrin-conjugated streptavidin (a protein that binds strongly to biotin). The array reader reports the MFI for each assay in a well as described (Wunderlich *et al.*, 2011). Overall, the diagnostic performance of MFIA has been shown to be comparable to that of ELISA (Khan *et al.*, 2005).

Multiplexing has been a very important advance for serosurveillance because an extremely small volume of serum (e.g., 1–2 μl for MFIA) suffices for even the largest surveillance panels. Moreover, multiplexing conserves reagents, reduces the volume of waste fluids, and permits high-throughput testing without complex and expensive automation. These efficiencies have made it practical to add confirmatory antibody assays for common adventitious agents and internal controls to panels to enhance the quality and reliability of serologic findings. In addition to standard tissue control bead sets for detecting nonspecific binding of serum Ig, MFIA panels have incorporated a bead set coated with Ig of the test species to detect procedural errors such as the failure to add labeled anti-Ig to a well and a set coated with anti-test species Ig to identify samples with inadequate levels of Ig; failures of the latter control occur most often because the sample is from an animal that is immunocompromised or different from the test species.

The dried blood spot (DBS) has recently been shown to be a suitable alternative to serum for serology in large part because multiplexing has made it feasible to perform the largest test panels on the single drop of blood used to prepare a DBS. Although new to HM, DBS technology has long been used for human neonatal screening (Mei *et al.*, 2001) and is increasingly employed for serial sampling of rodents in pharmacologic studies (Beaudette and Bateman, 2004). Collecting the drop of blood for preparing a DBS is minimally invasive and therefore can easily be performed on unanesthetized animals. In addition, the use of DBS eliminates the steps, reagents, and equipment required for serum preparation and DBS can be safely shipped in envelopes at ambient temperature in contrast to serum samples. *Ante mortem* blood collection for preparing DBS facilitates direct sampling of colony animals to supplement sentinel monitoring, to verify positive sentinel findings, and to identify infected animals to be culled.

b. Limitations

Despite the rapidity and low cost of serologic tests, they do have some important limitations. They are applicable mainly to viruses and seldom used for bacteria, with the exception of *M. pulmonis*, CAR bacillus, and *E. cuniculi*, or fungi due to poor specificity compared to viruses, which are less complex with their smaller genomes. Bacteria and fungi also induce weak antibody responses unless they are invasive. Poor sensitivity can occur when antigen purified from one bacterial strain does not cross-react with antibodies to others (Manning *et al.*, 1994). Additional limitations of serology include the requirement for an immunocompetent host that is susceptible to infection by virtue of age and genotype. Thus, serology is not suitable for direct testing of known immunodeficient or 'immunovague' genetically engineered principals to confirm or eradicate an adventitious infection. There is also a period of at least a week to 10 days between infection and seroconversion.

4. Molecular Diagnostics – PCR

The revolutionary advances in molecular genetics that have gained pace in recent decades have caused a shift from the just-described traditional diagnostic methodologies, which identify pathogens by their phenotypic characteristics (e.g., morphology, biochemical profile, serotype, or serum antibody specificity) to molecular assays for specific microbial gene sequences. Key among these advances has been the development and general availability of robust, rapid, and inexpensive tools for (1) amplifying, cloning, and sequencing genes; (2) analyzing and comparing gene sequences to identify those that are shared by related pathogens or strain-specific to target for inclusive surveillance or exclusive confirmatory assays, respectively; and (3) selecting and synthesizing DNA (or RNA) fragments with nucleotide sequences complementary to those targeted. This highly engineered process has led to the very rapid development of extremely sensitive molecular assays for newly recognized as well as known infectious agents of all types, with specificities that are generally more predictable and definitive than those of phenotypic tests (Tang and Persing, 1999; Tenover, 1998).

a. Techniques

The annealing of a known fragment (or collection of fragments) of RNA or DNA to complementary RNA or DNA sequences in a sample is fundamental to the principal molecular assay strategies (for infectious agents) of (1) labeled probe hybridization and (2) biochemical amplification. Reporter probes (usually 100–1000 bases long) for hybridization assays are directly or indirectly labeled with a radioisotope, an enzyme that acts on a chromogenic or chemiluminescent substrate, or a fluorescent dye. Assays begin with immobilization of the sample nucleic acid *in situ* or by blotting onto nitrocellulose or nylon membranes. For example, Southern (after the developer E.M. Southern) and Northern (a play on words) refer to blots of DNA and RNA, respectively (Cundiff *et al.*, 1994b; Hsu and Choppin, 1984). Alternatively, target sequences in a specimen can be captured by an unlabeled probe attached to a solid phase, e.g., a chip, bead, or microtiter plate well (Goto and Itoh, 1996). Prior to hybridization, double-stranded sample and probe DNA must be denatured to single-stranded DNA by heating (e.g., 90–100°C) or exposure to alkaline conditions. The reaction mixture is then cooled (to 55–65°C) to permit the formation of stable probe-target hybrids (which can be RNA to RNA, DNA to DNA, or DNA to RNA). Raising the temperature of incubation during hybridization enhances assay specificity by increasing the degree of complementarity necessary for stable probe–target hybrids to form. Free probe can be removed by washing (as is done in heterogeneous solid-phase immunoassays) or digestion with an enzyme that attacks single-stranded nucleic acids. Finally, the degree of hybridization is determined by measuring the signal emitted by the probe label or the enzyme-substrate product (Fig. 11.5) (Tang and Persing, 1999; Tenover, 1998).

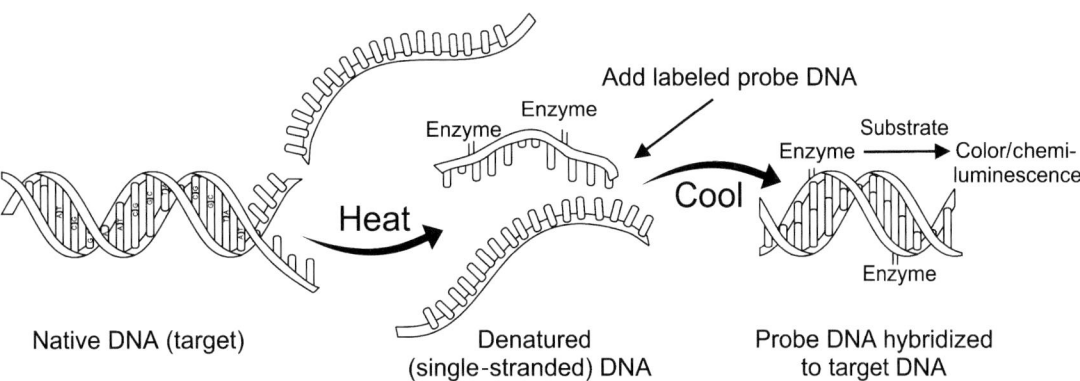

FIGURE 11.5   Hybridization with an enzyme-labeled DNA probe. Native (double-stranded) DNA is denatured by heating (to 90–100°C). The reaction mixture is then cooled (to 55–65°C) to permit the formation of stable probe–target hybrids. Free probe is removed by washing or by digestion with an enzyme that attacks single-stranded nucleic acids. The degree of hybridization corresponds to the amount of color or luminescence from the enzyme-substrate product. *Adapted from Tenover (1998), Fig. 14-1, p. 153.*

The sensitivity of probe hybridization assays for direct detection of pathogens in clinical specimens, like that of immunoassays, is constrained by the quantity of organisms typically found in specimens and background due to nonspecific binding of the labeled probe (Mahoney and Chernesky, 1999; Tang and Persing, 1999). These limitations have been overcome by the development of practical and robust technologies for rapid biochemical amplification, or copying, of target (or probe) nucleic acid sequences entirely *in vitro*. The best developed and most widely used of these, the PCR, was the invention for which Kary Mullis was awarded the Nobel Prize for Medicine in 1993 (Mullis, 1990). Because of its versatility, speed, exquisite sensitivity, and definitive specificity, PCR has become the preeminent diagnostic technique for demonstrating infectious agents (including those of lab animals) in clinical and environmental specimens and biologics.

The PCR consists of repeated cycles of heating and cooling, termed thermal cycling, during which a DNA template is enzymatically replicated, i.e., amplified (Fig. 11.6). The repeated, sequence-specific amplification that occurs in PCR is enabled by (1) synthetic oligonucleotide primers (15–25 bases long) that anneal in opposite directions to complementary strands of the DNA template at sites separated by up to 500 base pairs (for surveillance assays) and (2) a heat-stable DNA polymerase (such as the Taq DNA polymerase originally isolated from the thermophilic bacterium *Thermus aquaticus*) with the unique ability to tolerate the 95°C denaturation step in a PCR cycle (Cooper, 1997; Tang and Persing, 1999; Tenover, 1998).

Primers are designed by analyzing sequence data obtained from published sources (e.g., databases and scientific journals), from colleagues, and by DNA sequencing of laboratory and field strains of the agent of interest (Ball-Goodrich and Johnson, 1994; Battles *et al.*, 1995;

Besselsen *et al.*, 2006; Henderson *et al.*, 2012). To reduce the risk of missing an adventitious infection, primary PCR assays for microbiological surveillance maximize inclusivity by using primers targeting genes that are conserved among strains of a pathogen, such as the nonstructural NS-1 gene of parvoviruses (Besselsen *et al.*, 1995a), or a mixture of primers that account for strain variation. By contrast, the secondary PCR assays for confirming or investigating outbreaks frequently emphasize exclusivity by targeting genes that differentiate among pathogen variants, such as the capsid gene of parvoviruses (Besselsen *et al.*, 1995b). PCR primers for bacteria and parasites chiefly target sequences in the ribosomal genes (Battles *et al.*, 1995; Beckwith *et al.*, 1997; Fox *et al.*, 1994; Goto and Itoh, 1996; Greisen *et al.*, 1994; Grove *et al.*, 2012; Loganbill *et al.*, 2005; Shames *et al.*, 1995), which have been extensively analyzed and contain both conserved and differential regions, but sequences in other well-characterized genes are targeted too, for instance, the RNA polymerase *rpoB* gene of bacteria (Dole *et al.*, 2010, 2013b; Gundi *et al.*, 2009).

Although the PCR can only copy DNA, RNA templates such as the genomes of MHV (Casebolt *et al.*, 1997; Homberger *et al.*, 1991; Matthaei *et al.*, 1998) and MNV (Hsu *et al.*, 2006; Taylor and Copley, 1993) can be detected by PCR provided they are first transcribed by a reverse transcriptase to a complementary DNA template. PCR assays of this type are referred to as reverse transcription (RT) PCR (RT-PCR). Priming options for RT include sequence-specific primers, which are the most efficient, and nonspecific primers such as oligo-dT (which anneal to the polyA sequence appended to RNA transcripts) and random hexaxers. There are advantages and disadvantages of each primer type, but nonspecific priming of RT is preferred when testing for multiple RNA viruses (Compton and Riley, 2001; Henderson *et al.*, 2013; Lifetechnologies, 2014).

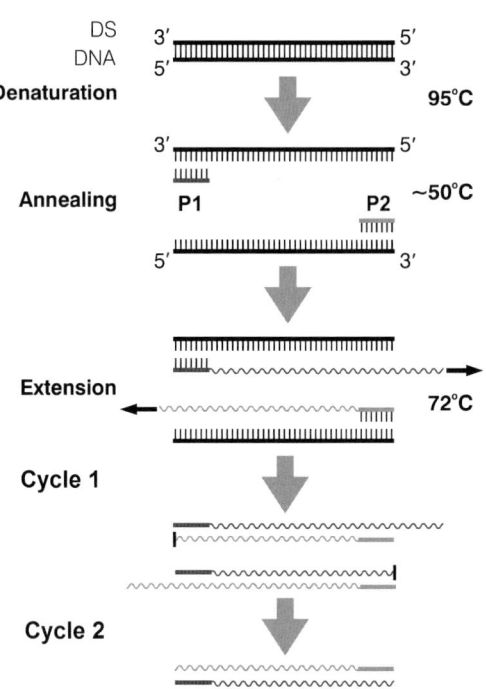

FIGURE 11.6 Steps of PCR. First, nucleic acid isolated from a clinical specimen is denatured at high temperature. Next, the reaction temperature is lowered to allow the oligonucleotide primer pair (P1 and P2) to anneal to complementary target microbial sequences. Last, the heat-stable DNA polymerase synthesizes copies of the target sequences by extending the primers. Copies made in a cycle act as template subsequent cycles, resulting in exponential amplification (Fig. 11.7).

As illustrated in Fig. 11.6, each PCR cycle comprises three steps including denaturation, annealing, and elongation. Following denaturation (at approximately 95°C), reactions are cooled to the annealing temperature, which varies (from 50 to 70°C) according to the melting temperature of the primer–template hybrid, and then reheated (e.g., to 72°C) for the elongation step during which the DNA polymerase synthesizes complementary DNA strands by extending the hybridized primer. Elongation of the forward and reverse primers (which match sequences in the 5′ results in complementary sense and antisense strands of DNA, respectively). A PCR assay consists of 30–50 of these cycles, each lasting no more than several minutes and performed automatically by a programmable heating block called a thermocycler. As the PCR progresses, DNA synthesized in one cycle serves as a template for subsequent cycles, setting in motion a chain reaction (hence, the name polymerase chain reaction) in which the targeted gene sequence is exponentially amplified (Fig. 11.7). For example, after 25 cycles, the PCR can theoretically produce 100,000 copies from a single starting copy of the gene of interest.

In the standard 'gel-based' method, the PCR product, or amplicon, is identified in an ethidium bromide-stained gel electrophoretogram exposed to UV light as a visible fluorescent band of an expected size. To rule out nonspecific amplification, the identity of a PCR product determined by size can be substantiated by sequence-specific methods such as restriction enzyme analysis, DNA sequencing, or labeled probe hybridization (Besselsen *et al.*, 2006; Goto and Itoh, 1996; Goto *et al.*,

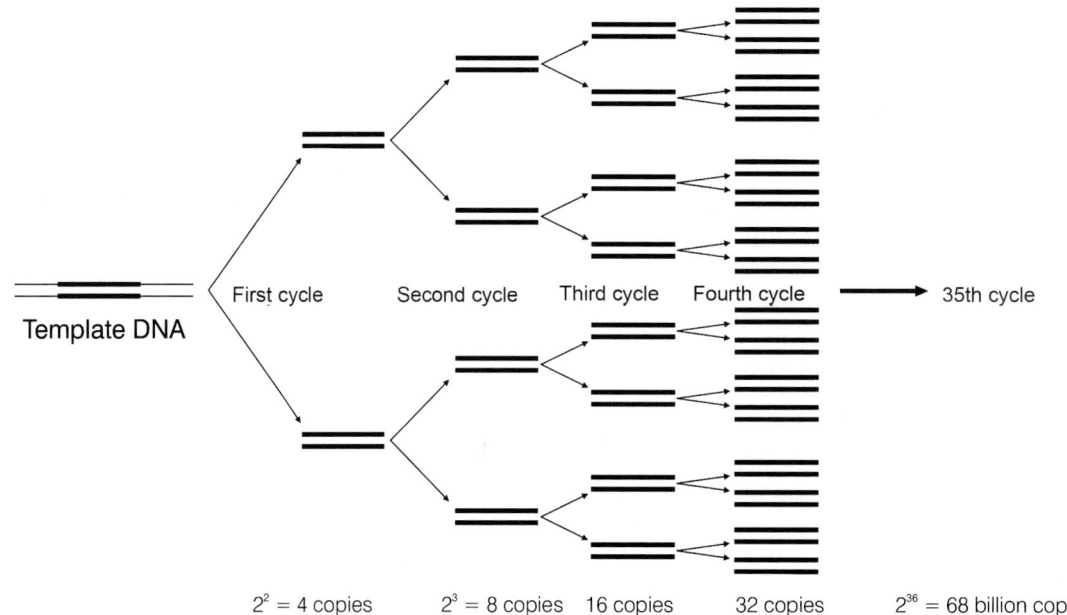

FIGURE 11.7 Exponential amplification by PCR. DNA synthesized in one cycle serves as template for subsequent cycles, setting in motion a chain reaction in which the targeted gene sequence is exponentially amplified.

1998; Riley *et al.*, 1996a; Xiao *et al.*, 1992). The latter is increasingly used as the primary method for identifying PCR product because it is more specific, sensitive, and amenable to automation and computer data processing than the gel-based method (Tang and Persing, 1999).

The most widely used PCR technique that relies on labeled probe hybridization for sequence-specific identification of amplicons is the fluorogenic nuclease, or TaqMan, assay, in which amplification and hybridization occur concurrently (Heid *et al.*, 1996; Holland *et al.*, 1991). The TaqMan probe is an oligonucleotide that anneals to a DNA template sequence between the forward and reverse primers and is tagged on opposite ends with a fluorescent reporter dye and a quencher dye. As long as the probe is intact and the dyes are in close proximity, the reporter signal is quenched. But when extending a primer, the Taq DNA polymerase uses its 5'–3' exonuclease activity to digest annealed probe (Fig. 11.8A). The resultant separation of the reporter from its quencher generates a sequence-specific fluorescent signal that can be read after each amplification cycle, i.e., in 'real time', or once at the end of the PCR assay. In the real-time assay, results are reported as the number of cycles

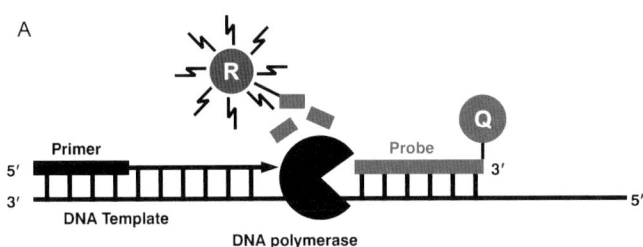
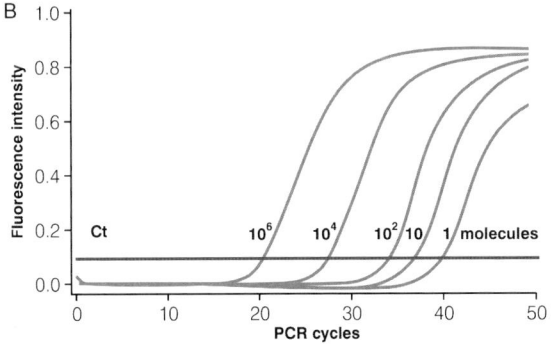

FIGURE 11.8 Real-time fluorogenic nuclease qPCR. The oligonucleotide probe tagged on opposite ends with a fluorescent reporter dye (R) and a quencher dye (Q), anneals to the DNA template between the forward and reverse primers. During the extension phase of the cycle, the DNA polymerase uses its 5'–3'exonuclease activity to digest annealed probe; cleavage of the report dye from the probe (and thus, separation from the quencher) generates a sequence-specific fluorescent signal (A). When the fluorescence intensity is read in 'real time', i.e., after each amplification cycle, the number of cycles required to reach a threshold signal (Ct) is inversely related to the copies of DNA template added to the reaction (B).

required to reach a (low) threshold signal, or Ct (for cycle threshold), which is inversely related to the copies of DNA template added to the reaction (Gibson *et al.*, 1996; Heid *et al.*, 1996; Kendall *et al.*, 2000; Kutyavin *et al.*, 2000; Leutenegger, 2001) (Fig. 11.8B). To avoid the confusion that would arise if both the real-time and reverse transcription PCR used the prefix RT, real-time assays are referred to as quantitative (q) PCR. Particularly for pathogens that are present in very high copy numbers in specimens from infected animals, estimating the copy number is helpful for identifying and discounting low-copy positive results due to contamination with template from other samples, controls, or the environment. Other important advantages of the TaqMan technique in comparison with the gel-based method include better analytical specificity and sensitivity due to the internal probe, less risk of contamination because reaction tubes stay closed post amplification, and higher throughput as there are no post-PCR processing steps and reactions are automatically read by a fluorometer and transferred to a computer for analysis and reporting. Moreover, several systems are available for creating spatial multiplexes of TaqMan PCR, including the OpenArray platform, which has been used in research animal HM (Henderson *et al.*, 2013) and biologics testing. As each test in an OpenArray chip occupies a separate location, the OpenArray avoids the pitfalls of competitive inhibition (Hamilton *et al.*, 2002) and low specificity (Lo *et al.*, 1998) that can affect standard homogenous PCR multiplexes created by mixing of multiple primer sets together in a single well. Because of these advantages, fluorogenic nuclease PCR has been developed for many pathogens of rodents including viruses (Besselsen *et al.*, 2003; Blank *et al.*, 2004; Drazenovich *et al.*, 2002; Ge *et al.*, 2001; Redig and Besselsen, 2001; Uchiyama and Besselsen, 2003; Wagner *et al.*, 2003, 2004), microbes (Dole *et al.*, 2010, 2013b; Drazenovich *et al.*, 2002; Ge *et al.*, 2001; Henderson *et al.*, 2012; Whary *et al.*, 2001), and parasites (Dole *et al.*, 2011; Jensen *et al.*, 2013; Rice *et al.*, 2013; Weiss *et al.*, 2012).

The exponential amplification that accounts for the extreme sensitivity of PCR assays is analogous to culture, with the advantages that PCR is completed in hours instead of days to weeks, avoids the biosecurity and health risks associated with propagating pathogens, is applicable to fastidious and noncultivable agents, and is minimally affected by the complexity of the specimen microbiome because amplification is sequence-specific. PCR can detect low concentrations of infectious agent template in heavily pooled and therefore highly representative samples such as room or ventilated rack exhaust air dust and noninvasive specimens collected *ante mortem* directly from animals in residence or quarantine – samples that are unlikely to contain enough viable bacteria and fungi or intact parasites to be suitable for traditional microbiology or parasitology, respectively.

Thus, by allowing testing of principal and environmental samples, PCR addresses the main shortcomings of sentinel HM, which is that it depends on transmission of adventitious infections of the principal animals to the sentinels. This transmission, however, may not occur when the adventitious agent is inactivated in soiled bedding; the percentage of actively infected animals is low as is common for rodents housed in microisolation caging systems; or sentinels are resistant to infection due to their age or genetic background.

b. Limitations

Detection of microbial nucleic acid template by PCR can occur in the absence of infection. The exquisite sensitivity of the PCR makes it especially vulnerable to false-positive (FP) findings following even minute levels of template contamination from test samples (and is most likely to occur for prevalent organisms that are present in high copy numbers), controls, the environment, and so forth. This risk of contamination, which represents a significant challenge to high-throughput screening, can be reduced by physical separation of pre- and postamplification procedures, decontamination of work surfaces with chemicals or UV irradiation, and enzymatic digestion or chemical inactivation of amplified template. Estimating the copy number by qPCR can be helpful in discounting low-copy positive results not associated with an active infection.

PCR may miss infections with viruses and other pathogenic organisms that are shed transiently, particularly in sentinels tested quarterly, although PCR has been shown to detect MHV and MPV in feces for weeks to months after infected mice are no longer contagious (Besselsen et al., 2007; Compton et al., 2004a). Furthermore, PCR continues to detect template in exhaust air dust swabs even after principal and sentinel animals have stopped shedding a pathogen. PCR results can be FN due to sample-mediated inhibition, but this can be detected by including an internal control assay or by spiking a duplicate reaction with template. Finally, PCR is still relatively labor-intensive and costly, although the cost of PCR testing can be contained by pooling of samples from various animal sites appropriate to the organisms being detected and the environment.

B. Factors Affecting Accuracy of HM

The importance of HM results that correctly represent the current pathogen status of the principal populations being monitored has been accentuated by (1) the continued incidence of outbreaks, particularly with environmentally stable nonenveloped viruses that are resistant to disinfection; (2) the frequent and growing exchange among investigators and institutions of genetically engineered mutant mice harboring pathogens; and

(3) the use of research animal-derived reagents and cell substrates in the development and production of parenterally administered biopharmaceuticals. The key factors determining the likelihood that HM findings correspond to the pathogen status of the principal animal population are the accuracy of the assay results and the degree to which samples are representative and suitable for the diagnostic methodologies by which they are tested. This section will review these factors, with emphasis on the challenges to obtaining accurate HM results for rodents housed in microisolation caging systems, including the typically low prevalence of infection and reliance on soiled bedding sentinel monitoring, and the role that PCR is playing in addressing these challenges by enabling testing of pooled environmental and *ante mortem* animal specimens not suitable for traditional methodologies.

1. Assay Accuracy

The key indicators of accuracy for primary surveillance tests are diagnostic sensitivity (DSe) and specificity (DSp), i.e., the proportions of correctly classified known positive and negative samples, respectively (reviewed in Jacobson, 1998; OIE, 2013; Pepe, 2003; Tyler and Cullor, 1989; Zweig and Robertson, 1987). Estimates of DSe and DSp are obtained by testing known positive and negative samples from pathogen-infected and pathogen-free animals, respectively, and by comparing an assay's results to those of a 'gold-standard' reference test. For serologic and PCR assay methods that yield numeric titers or instrument readings such as optical density or fluorescence intensity, sample results are classified as positive (+), negative (−), or equivocal (+/−) compared to positive and negative cutoff values, as shown in Fig. 11.9. Raw instrument readings may be used as the result values, but a common practice is to calculate values from one or more instrument readings in order to simplify the examination and classification of test results by (1) reducing the number of digits and decimals, (2) subtracting background so that negative result values are near zero, and/or (3) normalizing values, e.g., scoring sample readings in comparison with the positive control for the assay run. In addition, a sample result may be classified as indeterminate when a sample suitability control fails because the sample reacted nonspecifically or was inhibitory, or its quantity or target concentration was insufficient. Examples of the system and sample suitability controls utilized for serology by MFIA and for PCR assays are shown in Table 11.5. Sample results should only be classified (and reported) if the standard positive and negative system suitability control results were satisfactory, thereby demonstrating that assay sensitivity and specificity were acceptable. Thus, including the appropriate system and sample suitability controls in each assay run is essential to diagnostic accuracy.

A **Assay optimization**

B **Adjusting cutoff**

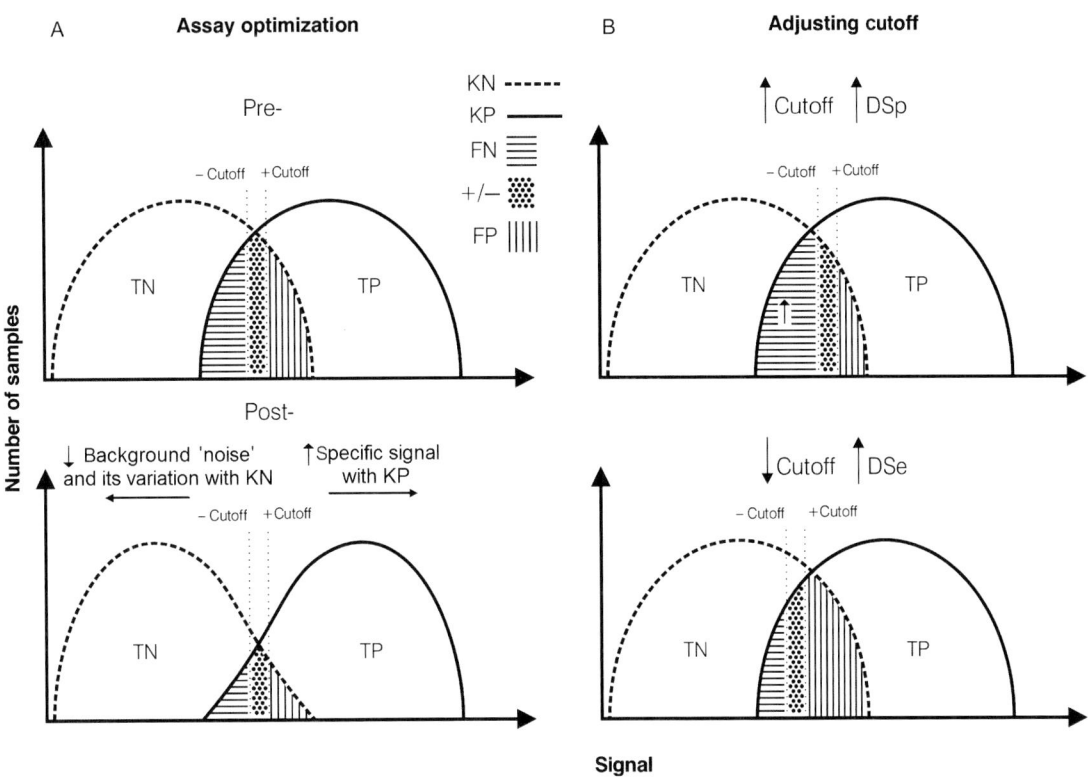

FIGURE 11.9 Classification of assay results. Serologic and PCR assays yield numeric titers or instrument readings such as optical density or fluorescence intensity. These numeric data, or values calculated from them, are classified as positive (+), negative (−), or equivocal (+/−) by comparison to positive and negative cutoff values, which are determined by testing known positive (KP) and known negative (KN) samples from pathogen-free and infected animals. Diagnostic sensitivity (DSe) and specificity (DSp) are the percentages of KP and KN samples correctly classified as true positive (TP) and true negative (TN), respectively. The schematic graphs in panel A depict the distribution of results for KP and KN samples tested by a hypothetical assay 'pre-' and 'post'-optimization. The goal of assay optimization is to reduce the percentages of samples that yield false-negative (FN), false-positive (FP), or +/− results by increasing the specific signal given by KP samples and decreasing the background 'noise' level and variation for KN samples. Following optimization, as shown in panel B, cutoffs can be adjusted to favor DSe or DSp depending on whether FN or FP determinations are more problematic. For example, cutoffs may be increased to favor DSp and avoid FP findings in tests for rare pathogens or decreased to favor DSe and avoid FN when testing for common pathogens.

Cutoff values are chosen initially based on analysis of data from assay development and validation; subsequently, they may be adjusted in accordance with the results of routine quality control and surveillance. Receiver operating characteristic curve analysis, comprising various graphs and statistics to summarize the DSe and DSp for a range of cutoffs values, is a common methodology for empirically evaluating the optimality of cutoffs (Greiner et al., 2000; Pepe, 2003; Zweig and Campbell, 1993). Cutoffs can be adjusted to favor DSe or DSp depending on whether FN or FP determinations are more 'costly'. Assay cutoff values might be increased to favor DSp and avoid FP results in tests for rare pathogens; conversely, they may be decreased to enhance DSe when testing for common agents to reduce the likelihood that adventitious infections will be missed due to FN findings (Fig. 11.9B).

The basic strategy for optimizing the diagnostic accuracy of a primary surveillance test is to decrease the 'noise', i.e., the strength and variation of the background

signals given by known negative samples from pathogen-free animals, and to boost the specific signal or titer given by known positive samples from infected animals, thereby reducing the number of samples with signals or titers near the cutoffs that are most likely to be FN or FP (Fig. 11.9A). The amount of separation between positive and negative signals is dependent on an assay's analytical sensitivity and specificity. The former is measured as the limit of detection (LOD), which is the lowest concentration of a target analyte (e.g., antibody, organism, or genomic sequence) in a specific matrix (e.g., serum, tissue homogenate, or feces) that can consistently yield a positive result. For PCR, samples can be 'spiked' with a known number of template copies to determine LOD; however, as quantifying the actual concentration of polyclonal serum antibodies to multivalent microbial antigens is not feasible, the LOD of serologic immunoassays is usually presented as a comparison of titration endpoints for an antiserum by two or more tests. The analytical sensitivity needed for a surveillance assay

TABLE 11.5   System and Sample Suitability Controls for Serology by the MFIA and for the PCR Assay

Method	Type	Qualification of	Assay for	Sample	Satisfactory
MFIA	System[a]	Analytical sensitivity	Microbial antibodies	Control-positive (C+) standard (std) antiserum	+
		Analytical specificity	Microbial antibodies	Control-negative (C−) std SPF serum	−
			Microbial antibodies	Diluent (Blank)	−
		Assay procedure (process)	Microbial antibodies	Std serum processed with test (i.e., noncontrol) samples	+ or −
			Labeled anti-species IgG probe	BiotinαIgG, phycoerythrin-streptavidin	+
	Sample[b]	Low nonspecific background	Nonspecific antibody binding	Test serum	−
		Adequate antibody quantity	Serum total IgG	Test serum	+
PCR	System[a]	Analytical sensitivity	Microbial template	Positive template control (PTC)	+
		Analytical specificity	Microbial template	Negative template control (NTC)	−
		Procedure: extraction and RT[c]	RNA template spike recovery	Exogenous RNA template	+
		Procedure: sample processing	Mock extraction	None or NTC	−
	Sample[b]	DNA recovery and purity (i.e., lack of PCR inhibitors)	PTC template Internal host cell template	Test specimen + PTC spike added to PCR Test specimen	+
		Recovery: RNA from extraction and cDNA from RT step	RNA template spike recovery	Test specimen + RNA template spike added to sample before extraction	+

[a]*System suitability controls qualify the overall performance of the assay run; the most commonly employed of these controls are the C+ and C−, which are tested to verify that analytical sensitivity and specificity, respectively, are satisfactory; others confirm that the procedure steps are being carried out and are performing properly, i.e., labeled anti-species IgG has been added to test wells or that cross-contamination (of the PCR mock control) did not occur during nucleic acid extraction. All samples in a test run with one or more failed system suitability controls should be retested.*

[b]*Sample suitability controls assess the fitness of the sample for the assay methods. For example, if a test serum gives a high background signal in the tissue control test for detection of nonspecific binding of serum antibodies to the solid phases, a positive signal in a microbial antibody MFIA is classified as indeterminate because it could also be nonspecific; a specimen negative by PCR is reported indeterminate if the PTC spike control reaction is negative, indicating that the sample is inhibiting the PCR.*

[c]*RT = reverse transcription of viral genomic RNA into complementary DNA by a reverse transcriptase enzyme (often originating from a retrovirus). This step is necessary for RNA viruses because the PCR DNA polymerase cannot directly copy RNA templates.*

depends on the expected range of concentrations of target analyte in specimens and the volume of sample tested. For example, a 'moderate' level of sensitivity suffices for the immunoassays used to screen for common viruses because these viruses typically elicit a strong antibody response in immunocompetent sentinels. By contrast, the extreme analytical sensitivity of PCR assays is important to their DSe because it allows detection of the low pathogen concentrations (or more correctly nucleic acid template copy number) expected in heavily pooled (e.g., 10:1) animal and environmental specimens; conversely, extreme analytical sensitivity can negatively impact the DSp of PCR when amplification of small quantities of template not associated with an active infection yields FP findings. As already mentioned and reviewed in the next section, sample selection errors, such as performing serology on acutely infected or PCR on convalescent hosts, can reduce the concentration of the targeted analyte below the test LOD.

Analytical specificity is defined as the ability of an assay to distinguish target from nontarget analytes, including matrix (i.e., specimen) components; it comprises selectivity, inclusivity, and exclusivity, (OIE, 2013). A selective assay is one with the capacity to resist matrix-mediated effects such as those detected by sample suitability controls including sample-mediated inhibition of the PCR, nonspecific binding of the serum antibodies (or labeled anti-Ig) to the solid phase, and target analyte degradation. Inclusivity refers to the ability of a single test to detect related organisms of interest, whereas exclusivity describes a test able to differentiate an infectious agent from others that are closely related. As a general strategy, inclusive assays are preferred for primary testing because they can reduce both the chance of missing an adventitious infection and the number of assays needed for surveillance. For example, lab animals are commonly screened for *Helicobacter* infection by a single inclusive PCR test that detects all species of the *Helicobacter* genus.

Exclusive assays, however, are important for confirmatory testing to corroborate preliminary findings and to determine the species, strain, serotype, or genotype of an adventitious agent when it is relevant to the SPF status of the principals or useful for investigating an outbreak. In the case of *Helicobacter*, additional testing by a number of species-specific PCR tests is carried out to corroborate initial findings and because the *Helicobacter* species can affect the course of action. For instance, certain species, such as *H. hepaticus* and *H. bilis*, are considered to be more pathogenic and likely to interfere with research than others (Drazenovich *et al.*, 2002; Henderson *et al.*, 2013; Whary and Fox, 2004). An additional example of the importance of sequencing is derived from an investigation of murine rotaviruses recovered from concomitant outbreaks at multiple institutions. The agents had identical genotypes, and repeated testing that included genomic sequencing provided convincing evidence that linked the outbreaks to a common source of contaminated bedding (Dole *et al.*, 2013a).

The analytical specificity of serologic and PCR assays is chiefly determined by the antigen bound to the immunoassay solid phase and the genomic sequences to which the primers (and probe for qPCR) anneal, respectively. Antigen for ELISA or MFIA may consist of organisms purified to varying degrees, organism extracts, or recombinant proteins, which have facilitated the development of assays with predictable analytical specificity. For example, ELISA and MFIA for viral antibodies that utilize a recombinant protein antigen conserved among related viruses, such as the nonstructural NS1 protein of parvoviruses (Riley *et al.*, 1996b), the VP6 capsid of group A rotaviruses (Zhu *et al.*, 2013), and the nucleocapsid NP protein of LCMV (Homberger *et al.*, 1995), are inclusive, whereas those employing recombinant envelope or capsid protein antigen that possesses neutralizing epitopes, such as the parvovirus capsid protein VP2 capsid protein (Henderson *et al.*, 2015; Livingston *et al.*, 2002), are exclusive (i.e., primarily detect serotype specific antibodies). IFAs for viral antibodies are intrinsically inclusive because they typically use as antigen-infected cells containing all virally encoded proteins. By detecting antibodies to conserved nonstructural proteins, rodent parvovirus IFA provided the initial evidence in the 1980s for the existence of parvovirus serotypes in addition to those represented by the prototypical strains used at the time in serotype-specific HAI tests (Jacoby *et al.*, 1996). Inclusivity achieved with complex antigen consisting of whole organisms, infected cells, or crude extracts of those, however, can increase the rate of false-positive findings when antibodies bind to nonmicrobial constituents of the antigen preparation or to antigenic determinants shared with commensal microbes; moreover, raising the positive cutoff to compensate for higher background is likely to reduce DSe. Relying on a single conserved recombinant protein antigen can also compromise DSe when the antigen is not consistently immunogenic or elicits an antibody response that is weak or delayed, as has been demonstrated for the rodent parvovirus antibody response to NS1 *vis-à-vis* capsid proteins.

PCR assays are made inclusive or exclusive by designing primers (and probes for qPCR) that anneal to genomic sequences, which are shared by or unique to variants of the agent of interest, respectively. Designing primers that fulfill these criteria and amplify a small product (e.g., under <200 bp) for optimal sensitivity can be demanding when the targeted pathogen species or group is very heterogeneous or there is a paucity of DNA sequence information available for commensal and other extraneous organisms likely to be present in clinical specimens. These challenges have been eased by access to increasingly sophisticated and cost-effective tools, techniques, and services for DNA sequencing and analysis that have expedited the identification of conserved and differential genomic sequences for PCR amplification in a wide variety of infectious agents. PCR (and probe hybridization) targets are generally more plentiful than those that can be distinguished by phenotypic tests because (1) they can be located in regions of the microbial genome that do not encode proteins and (2) the sequence of a gene often varies more than the amino acid sequence of the protein it encodes due to the degeneracy of the genetic code (i.e., multiple codons are translated into the same amino acid). In addition, the analytical specificity of genetic targets are unaffected by environmental and host-related factors that can alter the phenotype of an organism or humoral immune response to infection. Thus, the analytical specificity of PCR assays by and large exceeds that achievable by traditional tests.

The probability that a positive or negative result is correct is referred to as its predictive value. Besides being a function of assay DSe and DSp, predictive values are substantially affected by the prevalence of infection. The positive predictive value (PPV), which is the percentage of all positive results that are true positive, decreases along with the prevalence (Laregina and Lonigro, 1988; OIE, 2013; Zweig and Robertson, 1987). When the prevalence of infection is very low, as has been found for adventitious infections of animals housed in microisolation cages, a substantial percentage of positive results are expected to be FP, even for assays with DSp approaching 100%. The example shown in Fig. 11.10 illustrates that for an assay with DSp and DSe that are 99%, dropping the prevalence of infection from 50% to 2% decreased the PPV from 99% to 67%; to put it another way, one-third of the positive results are expected by FP when the prevalence of infection is 2%. This underscores the need, emphasized throughout this chapter, for repeat testing to corroborate new positive findings.

Number of Samples Tested: 10,000   **DSe:** 99%   **DSp:** 99%

Value		Formula	Prevalence	
			50%	2%
Samples	KP:	# Tested × Prevalence	5000	200
	KN:	# Tested × (1−Prevalence)	5000	9800
Positive results	TP:	KP × DSe	4950	198
	FP:	KN × (1−DSp)	50	98
	Total:	TP + FP	5000	296
			99%	**67%**
	PPV:	TP/(TP+FP)		
			1% FP	**33% FP**

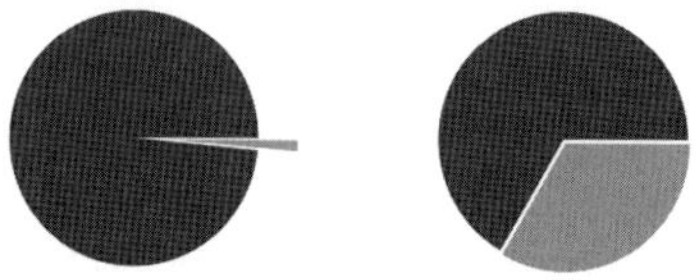

FIGURE 11.10   Effect of prevalence on PPV. The PPV is the percentage of all positive results – including true-positive (TP) and false-positive (FP) results given by known positive (KP) and known negative (KN) samples, respectively – that are TP. For an assay with diagnostic sensitivity (DSe) and specificity (DSp) both equal to 99%, dropping the prevalence of infection from 50% to 2% decreased the PPV from 99% to 67%. That one-third of the positive results for this highly accurate assay are expected to be FP when the prevalence is 2% underscores the critical importance of repeat testing to corroborate new positive findings.

2. Sample Selection

The overall goal of an HM program is to obtain results that are reflective of rodent colony health status. In addition to the influence of test accuracy, the correspondence of HM findings to the actual health status of the population being monitored is affected by the degree to which the samples are representative of the population and specimens are suitable for the tests employed. For commercial barrier rooms, HM is performed directly on colony animals of both sexes and multiple age groups. Commercial breeders may house their animals in open-topped cages to promote rapid and unimpeded spread of infection by all modes. Aerosols are generated that fall into other cages, as do bedding and feces from nearby cages. Animals are transferred among cages for breeding and stocking, and technicians manipulate multiple cages in succession. All of these factors promote transmission and, therefore, early detection of any microbial contamination. In addition, commercial breeders monitor their colonies on an almost continuous basis, in contrast to academic and other institutions that usually monitor on a quarterly schedule.

a. Principal Animals

Using resident colony animals for HM avoids the chance of introducing unwanted infectious agents that might be present in sentinel animals. Additionally, there is no time lag as occurs with exposure of externally sourced sentinels; whenever a sample is needed, one merely selects the desired number of animals directly from the population in question. However, use of resident animals for HM involves certain assumptions. One assumption is that the animals selected for monitoring have been adequately exposed to any infectious agents present. Exposure may be accomplished through husbandry practices, through the use of open-topped cages, or through transfer of potentially contaminated fomites such as soiled bedding. Sampling colony animals that are housed in individually ventilated cages without additional exposure such as through transfer of soiled bedding may be unlikely to test positive for any infectious agents present, as only a very small percentage of cages may be contaminated (Shek and Gaertner, 2002; Shek et al., 2005). Another assumption is that all animals in the population are genetically susceptible to infection with the agents being monitored and the panoply of inbred strains and genetic modifications in contemporary mouse populations militates against that.

Animals selected from the colony for serologic monitoring must be immunocompetent and therefore able to produce antibodies to viral or microbial agents. Immunocompetence may be difficult to determine or unknown in some genetically engineered animals, as there are numerous anecdotal reports of incomplete immune responses in genetically engineered mice previously thought to be immunocompetent. By contrast, intentional use of immunodeficient animals may enhance the sensitivity of surveillance relying on direct detection of infectious agents, such as PCR, bacteriology, or parasitology, because immunodeficient animals may sustain infectious agents for long periods, if not indefinitely (Besselsen *et al.*, 2007; Compton *et al.*, 2004b; Henderson *et al.*, 2012; Macy *et al.*, 2013).

Selecting resident animals of the appropriate age is more problematic than selecting the appropriate age of sentinel animals. In general, the oldest animals in a population are the most likely to have encountered (and seroconverted to) an infectious agent during their tenure. However, immunocompetent animals mount a host response and partially or entirely clear many parasitic, microbial, and viral infections, so that aged animals are less likely to test positive by direct examination and cultural isolation. In enzootically infected colonies in which newborns are protected by maternal antibodies, recently weaned to young adult animals are those most likely to be heavily infested with protozoan and metazoan parasites and actively infected with viruses and microbial pathogens, such as *C. piliforme* and *P. carinii* (An *et al.*, 2003; Henderson *et al.*, 2012; Waggie *et al.*, 1987), that are cleared by the host adoptive immune response.

In theory, the number of animals tested is based on the predicted prevalence of the infectious agent in the colony (Anonymous, 1976; Clifford, 2001; Dubin and Zietz, 1991; Selwyn and Shek, 1994). For barrier room colonies housed in open-topped cages, which are monitored by sampling of colony animals, this means that eight animals are sampled at each testing interval. This gives a 95% probability of detecting a pathogen when it reaches a prevalence of approximately 30% in the population; experience has shown that recently introduced viruses actually reach a prevalence above 50% within a single 4-week monitoring interval (Selwyn and Shek, 1994; Shek *et al.*, 2005). For greater security, this type of facility may (and frequently does) choose to monitor more animals and/or sample more frequently. Today, a majority of research rodents are housed in static or ventilated microisolation cages where the prevalence of an agent is kept low by the very nature of this type of housing. If an agent were present at a 10% prevalence, 30 animals would need to be screened for a 95% chance of detection, and if an agent were present in only 1% of animals, then 300 animals would need to be screened (Clifford, 2001). Prevalence as low as 2% has been considered realistic for MPV infection of mice in IVC (Macy *et al.*, 2009; Smith, 2010). Because sampling of sufficient numbers of mice to detect such low-prevalence infections is not feasible, most facilities use testing of sentinel animals.

b. Sentinel Animals

In reality, principal animals being used in research are rarely made available by scientists for blood draws or euthanasia for conventional HM, and consequently, colonies are monitored indirectly by testing sentinels. Sentinel animals are generally externally sourced

animals that are introduced into a population, exposed to animals or soiled bedding from the population, and sampled in lieu of the principal animals. Sentinels should be immunocompetent so that they are suitable subjects for serology, and should have a mature immune system when sampled. Outbred stocks are recommended because they are generally good serologic responders and are usually less expensive. Conversely, inbred sentinels should be avoided because some inbred strains have been shown to be comparatively resistant to infection with or to mount a delayed antibody response to certain pathogens (Besselsen *et al.*, 2000; Brownstein *et al.*, 1981; Drake *et al.*, 2008; Henderson *et al.*, 2015; Hirai *et al.*, 2010; Shek *et al.*, 2005). Sentinels should be female, which will decrease fighting within the sentinel cage and lessen the chance of genetic contamination of the principal animals from contact sentinels. They should of course be free of all infectious agents, which would be of concern for the principals being monitored. If those agents include opportunistic pathogens, as might be the case for immunodeficient models, then sentinels should be obtained from gnotobiotic or SOPF colonies raised in isolators rather than barrier rooms. As mentioned, sentinels are externally sourced from commercial vendors because this is considered to be simpler and less expensive than attempting to produce clean sentinels internally. If, however, sentinel animals are bred at the facility, they should be monitored at an increased frequency, perhaps monthly, as they are a potential source of infection for the entire facility. However, there is a biosecurity risk associated with the routine receipt of sentinels from commercial vendors that is low but not zero (Pullium *et al.*, 2004; Shek *et al.*, 2005).

The current standard practice for routine surveillance of resident animals is to keep sentinels in separate cages supplied with regular changes of soiled bedding pooled from colony cages. Typically, one or two sentinel cages are set up for a rack of cages (frequently one cage per side of a rack). Contact sentinels are impractical for routine surveillance for several reasons, the most important being their potential to contribute to the spread of infection. Reliance on soiled bedding alone to transmit infections to sentinels, however, is problematic because infections with certain respiratory viruses, host-adapted bacteria, and parasites are transmitted inefficiently or not at all in soiled bedding (Artwohl *et al.*, 1994; Compton *et al.*, 2004c; Cundiff *et al.*, 1995; Dillehay *et al.*, 1990; Henderson *et al.*, 2013; Ike *et al.*, 2007; Lindstrom *et al.*, 2011; Thigpen *et al.*, 1989). In addition, the ability of microisolation cages to control the spread of infection frequently keeps the percentage of cages with actively infected rodents low, thus presenting challenges for detection by the HM program. Irrespective of the test methodology used, detection of transmission to sentinels is dependent on exposure of those animals to an infectious dose of the microbial contaminant. Thus, the lower the prevalence of infection, the greater the risk that the pathogen dose in pooled bedding will not be sufficient to infect sentinels. As cited above, that risk may increase as sentinels become older and less susceptible to infection with certain agents. However, a recent study demonstrated that the transmission of common adventitious viruses (including MPV) and pinworms to sentinels via soiled bedding did not differ according to whether the sentinels were weanlings, young adults, or aged (Grove et al., 2012).

c. General Principles of Sentinel Exposure

Sentinels should be exposed to new soiled bedding at each cage change, keeping in mind that the shedding of many pathogens eventually stops. As much soiled bedding as possible should be placed in the sentinel cage to minimize the diluting of infectious material; most facilities transfer 5–15 ml from each principal cage. Clean bedding should not be placed in a sentinel cage because it further dilutes infectious agents in the soiled bedding, possibly to concentrations below the infectious dose for the sentinels (Besselsen et al., 2008a; Smith et al., 2007). The placement of new nesting material into the sentinel cage is a reasonable compromise and is recommended wherever this enrichment method is in use. Sentinels should be given a period of at least several weeks to become infected and seropositive, but since HM at research facilities is done quarterly or less often, sentinels are exposed for a minimum of 3 months before being tested.

Depending on the required health status of the principal animals and the types of organisms to be excluded as well as the type of husbandry and housing systems used, the composition of the sentinel cage group(s) and the number of sentinel animals per cages may vary. Typical recommendations are that one sentinel cage of two to three sentinels be used for monitoring a 50–80-cage rack or side of a rack, but often additional sentinel cages are used to increase the amount of soiled bedding which can be sampled from each principal cage. Housing more than one sentinel per cage is beneficial when unexpected deaths occur or when a cage mate is required to confirm an unexpected positive result. Risks and costs should be balanced by the institution. For example, finding an unexpected positive might require individual testing of 50–80 colony cages versus the cost of monitoring two sentinel cages and then individually testing 25–40 colony cages, should there be a positive.

An economical alternative to testing all sentinels in a cage for all agents is to test only one per cage (or to test a pool of ante mortem specimens). At the time those samples are submitted, new sentinels can be added to the cage as a 'bridge' for any recent infections or exposures to which the previous sentinels had not yet seroconverted. When the results from the submitted samples are received, the remaining 'old' sentinels can be euthanized, can be used for confirmation of any positive findings, or can be used to sample for agents of particular concern, e.g., any present in the facility, or even for a full panel. It should be noted that occasionally not all animals in a cage will seroconvert to MPV, so testing only a subset of the sentinels slightly decreases the sensitivity of the sentinel program. However, facilities may accept this slight decrease in sensitivity in exchange for the cost savings, or they may choose to test the second sentinel only for parvoviruses. Alternatively, mesenteric lymph nodes can be collected for PCR testing as a supplement to MPV serology.

C. Health Management Program Management

HM programs should be designed by a knowledgeable person, based on the needs of the facility/institution, and subject to frequent review and updates as necessary. It is important to remember that the goal of an HM program is not necessarily to exclude all possible infectious organisms, but rather to monitor for the presence or absence of a select set of organisms that have the potential to affect research conducted in that facility. A positive for an infectious agent on a health report does not necessarily mean that the facility should be depopulated or that the animals are not usable. While recommendations for exclusion lists exist (Guillen, 2012; Nicklas et al., 2002), those recommendations should always be interpreted by someone with knowledge of the needs of the facility or institution. Financial constraints may also play a role in decisions regarding exclusion; for instance, a large institution with rodents housed in multiple facilities, all of which are positive for Helicobacter spp., may decide to eliminate it from a subset of those facilities, depending on the needs of scientists using the animals. Thus, detection of an agent could result in immediate eradication, planned eradication, or acceptance, depending on research goals.

HM programs should be as simple in design as possible and any components that can be computerized, especially for large programs, will help in simplification. Factors to consider at the earliest stages include the host species that will be monitored (including immune function and pathogen status); the source of animals that will be monitored (all from approved commercial breeders or nonapproved sources, such as academic institutions, or a combination of the two); how the animals are used (e.g., breeding and distribution or research); and biosecurity level available at institution (barrier or nonbarrier and/or static or ventilated microisolation cage, isolators, or a combination). If animals will be obtained from nonapproved sources, it is critical to consider the availability of a space in which incoming animals can be quarantined prior to introduction into existing colonies, keeping in mind that these animals are not transported in dedicated vehicles.

1. Design and Implementation

Large and complex academic programs tend to be geographically dispersed and have vivaria that cater to many research needs. These include barrier facilities from which rodents make 'one-way' trips (e.g., breeding colonies), conventional facilities that may permit animals to be transported to laboratory space with subsequent return to the vivarium, and specialized housing for rodents used in behavioral testing, sequential imaging procedures, or metabolic assays.

Designing an HM program for such diverse housing and research modalities can be daunting. As a first step, the program should have universal features that are applied to all vivarial situations. These can be customized to meet the needs of the research performed in the various types of housing modalities; however, customization should probably be minimized so that the simplicity suggested above is retained, resulting in lower likelihood of human error. An animal resource leader knowledgeable about institutional needs and financial constraints must decide on methodologies to be used (e.g., serology, culture, physical and microscopic examinations versus PCR); testing intervals (quarterly, semiannually, annually); test panels (basic versus comprehensive); animals/materials to be tested (soiled bedding or contact sentinels, principals, environment); and samples to be collected (serum or DBS, feces and swabs (from animals or environment), or live animals). In considering methods, one must keep in mind that serology and PCR yield different information, the former simply indicating infection at some prior, undetermined time and the latter indicating the current infection or nucleic acid presence. Based on scientific needs, an exclusion list should be established and a plan devised for actions taken when an excluded agent is detected (immediate versus 'planned' eradication).

Testing is usually performed quarterly, after full exposure of the sentinels to all cages of the sampling area. Sentinels should not be kept more than 6 months as their sensitivity to certain excluded pathogens may decrease as they age (Riepenhoff-Talty et al., 1985). However, sentinels may take months to become infected and seroconvert (Henderson, 2008). Thus, quarterly rotation and testing of sentinels seems to best fit the optimal time window for serologic detection of the most prevalent infectious agents.

For routine HM, most facilities choose to monitor quarterly as the default, with increased frequency of monitoring used to assist disease eradication or containment efforts for particular agents. A frequently used paradigm includes testing three times each year for the most prevalent agents (those that are most likely to be introduced into a vivarium), and annually for a more comprehensive panel of infectious agents. The comprehensive panel is employed to satisfy import requirements of collaborating institutions, to address any inquiries by regulatory bodies, and to detect infections which are rare in contemporary lab animals but still common in wild and pet rodents, and which may also be present in materials archived in freezers from the days when more viral and bacterial infections, including some zoonoses, were prevalent.

Once the details of the program designs have been established, programs are implemented by assigning them to locations and colonies, and by generating a master HM schedule for collecting and submitting samples (Table 11.6). For a campus managing multiple vivaria with each housing variable numbers of rodents, the schedule can be adjusted to even-out the workflow for the HM technicians over the course of a year. Simple modifications, such as PCR testing of feces for MPV in barrier-maintained sentinels, can be easily inserted into the master schedule without too much concern that this

TABLE 11.6 HM Program Design and Implementation

STEPS

DESIGN

Develop specifications, i.e., lists of excluded and other reportable agents, by species, immune status, barrier system, source, use, etc.

Determine frequency of testing for each agent according to risk and cost of contamination

Select/create/customize test panels by species, diagnostic methodology, and frequency of testing for specific agents

For each panel, choose sample and specimens types that are suitable for the HM methodology and determine the sample number.

By program, arrange protocols (i.e., panels + samples) in the appropriate order, separated by intervals corresponding to the frequency of testing.

For results summarization, define diagnoses and the laboratory tests they comprise.

IMPLEMENTATION

List animal locations (typically by facility, building, and room) and colonies (which can be actual colonies or monitoring units such as a cage racks).

Assign HM programs to colonies.

Generate master schedule indicating the location, colony, collection date, protocol, and testing laboratory.

Collect and submit samples according to schedule.

Review and file reports.

Maintain 12–18-month longitudinal summary of results (as positive/tested) by species, location, and colony.

will be forgotten by the HM technicians packing and submitting the animals.

Although we have emphasized serologic and direct sampling monitoring of sentinel animals in this section and in the accompanying table, there is an emerging trend away from sentinel use and toward environmental monitoring as a way to better sample principal animals that are housed in ventilated caging systems. Such non-sentinel monitoring also has the advantage of detecting agents that are difficult or impossible to transmit via soiled bedding (Artwohl et al., 1994; Compton et al., 2004c; Cundiff et al., 1995; Dillehay et al., 1990; Henderson et al., 2013; Ike et al., 2007; Thigpen et al., 1989) and it supports the 3Rs principles.

2. Results Analysis and Summarization

Data generated by an HM program should be reviewed by an individual at the institution who understands the biology of the agents and the scientific goals of the rodent users and is responsible for the overall biosecurity program. This person should examine the data for anomalous or unexpected findings and then initiate appropriate action. Actions might include report filing or data compilation if no actionable results are received, communication with the testing laboratory for all unexpected or actionable results, or notification of other responsible individuals at the institution. Because of the significant consequences of many infections and the equally significant consequences of erroneously taking action in situations where no infection exists, the first step should always be to contact the testing laboratory prior to executing any eradication plan or other research-inhibiting actions. The testing laboratory cannot only give some idea of the level of confidence in the results (i.e., was it a strong positive versus near-threshold result? Does that particular assay often give FP results? Is the positive predictive value of the result low because that particular agent is very rare?), but can also help plan the quickest and most definitive confirmation testing.

Health reports that require the reader, often the import coordinator at a potential recipient institution, to sift through many pages to identify the room or vivarium of interest are not useful and generally end up as reams of wasted paper, even if recycled. The results of HM testing should be summarized into a one- or two-page HM report for areas within institutions (usually for individual vivaria at academic institutions). This allows for easier interpretation for import/export of animals and less confusion by shipping and receiving institutions as to the agents tested and results obtained. A useful health report does not only give results from the most recent and historical (up to 18 months) testing but must also provide additional information about housing and maintenance procedures,

TABLE 11.7 HM Summary Report Information

Results	Diagnosis[a]
	Primary assay
	Most recent # Positive/# Tested
	Longitudinal # Positive/# Tested
	Longitudinal period in months
	Frequency of testing by diagnosis
	Frequency of testing by protocols[b]
Colony	Institution location
	Species, strain
	Specification (e.g., SPF, SOPF)
	Barrier system
	Treatments
	Other colonies in location

[a]An infectious agent, based on assays performed in one or more laboratories.
[b]Protocols include the laboratory, assay panels, and samples (e.g., principals, sentinels, exhaust air dust, etc.).

any treatment provided, and the HM program and exclusion list (Nicklas et al., 2002) (Table 11.7). It is also important to provide contact information for the person responsible for the HM program in the animal facility in case additional information is requested. Not all of these data are easily provided on a health report, and ideally institutions should also provide a one- to two-page HM program description with the HM results. It should be emphasized that a high-quality HM program is of utmost importance to institutions exporting large numbers of rodents. Having a reputation for outsourcing infectious disease outbreaks is not a winning strategy.

V. OUTBREAK MANAGEMENT AND INVESTIGATION

A. Repeat Testing to Corroborate New Positive Findings

As the prevalence of infection decreases, so does the PPV. When the prevalence of infection is very low, as is frequently the case following contamination of rodents in microisolation cages, a substantial percentage of positive results are likely to be FP, even for assays having diagnostic accuracy (i.e., DSp and DSe) near 100% (Fig. 11.10). In addition, irrespective of diagnostic accuracy, no assay is immune to sample selection errors (Table 11.8) and mistakes made in the laboratory including sample mix-ups, noncompliance with SOPs,

TABLE 11.8 HM Animal Sample Selection Errors

Principals/ HM	Methodology	Animals sampled
Infected/ HM-negative	Serology	Acutely infected, prior to seroconversion Immunodeficient, unable to mount antibody response
	PCR/ bacteriology/ parasitology	Older and recovered from infection From sites where organism is not resident or target concentration is below the test LOD

	All	Too few in number for low prevalence of infection
		Uninfected sentinels because
		  Prevalence of infection in principals was low
		  Pathogen not transmitted via soiled bedding
		  Resistant to infection due to age or genetic background
		Unintentionally from the wrong colony or samples mislabeled postcollection

Uninfected/ HM-positive	Serology	Tissue reactive antibodies because of
		  Age or autoimmune disease
		  Inoculated with biologic
		Elevated levels of serum Ig due to age
		Maternal antibodies

	PCR	Were negative, but samples from them were contaminated during collection or processing Low levels of template not associated with active infection (e.g., ingested noninfective template from the environment)
	All	Were sentinels infected from extraneous, i.e., noncolony source, e.g., while in transit Unintentionally from the wrong colony or samples mislabeled postcollection

data calculation and transcription errors, incorrect interpretation of findings, and so forth. Therefore, we cannot overemphasize the importance of confirming new positive findings – even those made by direct examinations that would seem irrefutable – before undertaking disruptive and costly actions to eradicate an infection. When one considers that most programs rely on quarterly testing and an adventitious infection is likely to require at least several weeks to spread to and reach a detectable level or elicit seroconversion in sentinels, it is reasonable to expect that a period of a month or longer has elapsed between the occurrence and detection of an outbreak. Thus, taking few a more days to a week to corroborate initial findings poses little additional risk to other animals in the facility, especially if the animals are maintained in microisolation cages that provide biocontainment.

Confirmatory testing, employing when feasible alternative assay methods and target analytes (i.e., antigens for serology or genomic sequences for PCR) as well as complementary methodologies, is frequently performed concomitantly on samples from the sentinel cage mate(s) and resident animals on the suspect side(s) of the rack monitored by the positive sentinel(s). Confirming infection of resident animals is worthwhile because sentinels may have acquired the infection from an extraneous source prior to placement, e.g., while in transit or quarantine. In addition, environmental specimens such as swabs of cages or the exhaust air dust from ventilated rack plenums or filters can be submitted for molecular testing (Jensen *et al.*, 2013). The rule of thumb at one author's institution is that positive samples detected using commercially available antigen-coated ELISA plates are retested by IFA using cells infected with virus from different sources. Even when both tests are positive, the suspect sample is shipped to a commercial lab that runs MFIA with additional antigens and IFA using further, independently prepared reagents.

Determining the appropriate assay methods and specimens for repeating testing should be based on the knowledge of the adventitious agent's pathobiology including the time course and sites of infection and shedding, and the time to seroconversion. For instance, a murine rotavirus seropositive sentinel might lead to testing its cage mate by fecal PCR. A negative PCR result would not clarify the accuracy of the earlier result. This is because murine rotavirus causes an acute, self-limiting infection with shedding and transmission ceasing at some point after antibody development (Riepenhoff-Talty *et al.*, 1985). More useful follow-up data could result from serologic testing of the cage mate and/or PCR on fecal pools of the relevant colony population or on IVC exhaust. In the case of an MPV seropositive sentinel whose cage mate was subsequently found to be negative by fecal PCR, additional testing would be required. MPV shedding and transmission wane after seroconversion, but viral DNA persists in selected tissues, notably mesenteric lymph node (Besselsen *et al.*, 2007; Henderson *et al.*, 2015; Jacoby *et al.*, 1995; Shek *et al.*, 1998; Smith *et al.*, 1993a). If PCR on mesenteric lymph node yielded a negative result, one could infer that the serologic finding represented a false positive. Because MNV continues be shed at high levels in the feces of seropositive mice, negative PCR results for feces from a seropositive sentinel and/or its cage mate(s) provide significant support for the serology being FP. The patterns of infection and shedding in relation to seroconversion

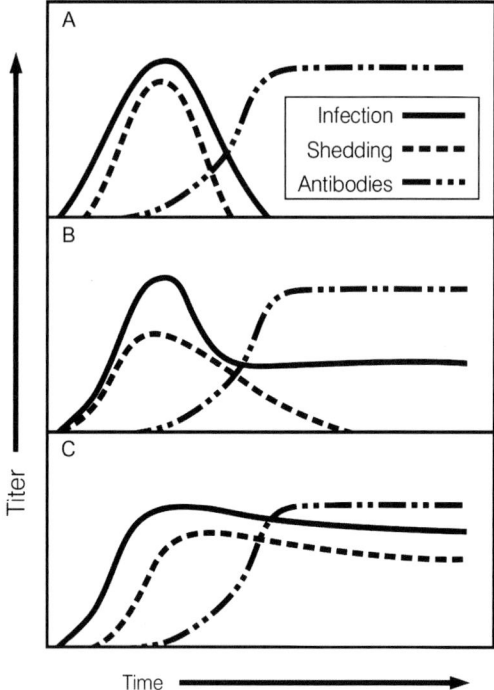

FIGURE 11.11   Basic patterns of infection and shedding in relation to seroconversion. Following seroconversion, an infectious agent may be cleared from (A) or persist in (B, C) host tissues; for a persistent infection, shedding of the organism may wane rapidly (B) or continue for a prolonged or indefinite period (C). As discussed at the beginning of Section V, knowing the pattern that an infectious agent follows is crucial when carrying out repeat testing to substantiate new positive findings.

by immunocompetent hosts just described for murine rotavirus, MPV, and MNV are schematically depicted in Fig. 11.11A, B, and C, respectively.

B. Containment and Eradication

Once the presence of an excluded agent has been confirmed, the outbreak must be contained and managed. At academic institutions that generally provide scientists with 24/7 vivarial access, containment can be a challenge. Although investigators may view the approach as draconian, one solution is to change locks on housing rooms prior to announcing quarantine. A meeting with personnel affected by the quarantine should be scheduled as quickly as possible. During that meeting, investigators and their staffs should be informed of the facts as known at the time and the proposed management plan. Access to rooms operating under quarantine conditions should be limited to the extent possible, preferably to a single individual from each lab (often the lab manager). Breeder cages should be broken down so pups will not be delivered after a certain point in the quarantine process. Litters that are within a few days of weaning may be

retained. New animals, either from approved vendors or from other locations on the campus, should never enter a room quarantined for a virus infection, thus limiting the population of susceptible animals. If investigators housing mice in the affected room(s) have standing orders with approved vendors, those orders should be cancelled for at least 90 days, allowing time for an initial 100% screen of the room plus two additional screens at 21- to 28-day intervals. A critical early step is tracking any relocations or exports that have occurred within the last 90 days prior to detection of the excluded agent. If either has occurred, the destination room(s) must be tested for 'collateral damage' and/or recipient institutions must be notified that the animals received may have been infected. The scientist(s) having mice in the affected room might also house mice in other rooms and/or vivaria on the campus. Rodents in those areas should also be screened since traffic patterns of laboratory staff usually cannot be easily monitored. Supplies exiting a room operating under quarantine conditions should be bagged and autoclaved to reduce chances of further spread within the vivarium. This, of course, adds substantially to the workload of husbandry staff and may necessitate overtime and, thus, increased financial burden to the animal resource. Each cage in a quarantined room is sampled (e.g., serum for serology provided the principals are immunocompetent or feces for PCR to detect enterotropic pathogens) at 3- to 4-week intervals. Two consecutive negative screens of 100% of cages in the room are required to lift quarantine. Depending on the prevalence of infection at the baseline interval – and the nature of the mice – the management approach may be test-and-cull or the room may be depopulated by a combination of culling and rederivation (Smith, 2010). As discussed earlier, rederivation can be accomplished by a variety of means and the choice may hinge on the age and fecundity of the available animals. If the infecting agent is zoonotic, the institution may very well opt for depopulation via euthanasia, decontamination, and safe disposal.

Because pathogens often cause immunological perturbations, and because these disturbances can persist even in recovered animals (Compton et al., 1993), the use of infected animals in immunological research should be avoided. Tissues, organs, fluids, or tumors from mice in a room quarantined for a virus infection should never be collected for transplant into other animals. A virus might contaminate these materials, especially if it causes a persistent infection (Compton et al., 2004d; Riley et al., 1960), has a broad host range (Bhatt et al., 1986a), or has a predilection for replicating in rapidly dividing cells (Bonnard et al., 1976; Mckisic et al., 1993).

Control and eradication are most reliably achieved by depopulation, disinfection, and repopulation with SPF replacements or rederived descendants of the infected colony. Proper chemical disinfection following depopulation is critical to preventing the recurrence and spread of an outbreak. Consequently, the principles of effective chemical disinfection, reviewed in Section III, will be restated here. Thorough sanitization and disinfection of the affected area are necessary to prevent recurrence or spread throughout a facility. Animal areas (including shared equipment, such as anesthesia equipment or behavioral testing apparatus) should be cleaned with detergent, then, at a minimum, disinfected with compounds known to inactivate the contaminating infectious agent. General cleaning should be undertaken before disinfection or sterilization, because chemical disinfectants are inactivated by the presence of organic matter (animal room soil). Detergents are best for removing soil, whereas disinfectants and sterilants work best on clean surfaces. Sterilants will, by default, kill a broader range of organisms, and therefore are usually the best choice for general decontamination purposes. Such sterilization agents include, but are not limited to, vapor-phase hydrogen peroxide, chlorine dioxide gas, and formaldehyde. A general plan, if a room has been contaminated, might consist of the following:

- Depopulate the room.
- Discard any nonessential or easily replaceable equipment.
- Place any materials leaving the room in a bag; spray the outer surface of the bag with a disinfectant and then place it into a second bag outside the room. The bagged caging may then be autoclaved, cleaned, and then autoclaved again before reentering a clean room.
- Clean the floors, walls, and room surfaces thoroughly with a detergent solution and then rinse.
- After rinsing, apply an aqueous-based disinfectant as per the manufacturer's recommendations (concentration, time, temperature, humidity, etc.).
- Rinse again.
- Apply at least one other aqueous-based disinfectant (with a different mode of action than the first). Many facilities will go further and use a sterilant such as vapor-phase hydrogen peroxide or chlorine dioxide.

When this approach is not feasible for scientific or financial reasons, a test-and-cull protocol can be implemented with recognition that this may be a protracted process. In all cases, steps should be taken to ensure that the likely sources of infection are adequately disinfected or eliminated. The postquarantine process should include encouraging investigators to cryopreserve unique genotypes. This ensures that unique strains will not be lost in future outbreaks or disasters such as floods or prolonged power outages. This strategy can have the added benefit of reducing per diems for on-the-shelf animals that are less frequently needed for experiments. It also conserves cage space, which is an advantage for the animal resource and colleagues who may need additional space.

C. Investigation

One of the first questions an animal resource representative may hear at the first user meeting scheduled after imposition of quarantine is: how did this happen? In many cases, that question remains unanswered. Nevertheless, systematically investigating the potential direct and indirect sources of contamination discussed in Section III often reveals procedural or engineering gaps that can be easily closed to reduce the chance that outbreaks will recur. A few of the possibilities are noncompliance with SOPs for animal importation and on-campus relocations; noncompliance with human traffic flow SOPs; improper disinfection of supplies; failure by animal resource to calibrate and maintain equipment; improper use of PPE; improper storage of diet or other supplies used by investigators; improper handling of cages by lab staff (opening cages outside a laminar flow hood); home maintenance of reptiles or rodents by staff members; and injection of biological products that have not been tested for adventitious agents. The advent of bar-coded cage cards has permitted much improved on-campus tracking of cages that have relocated. Vivaria should also have the capacity to store experimental diets so that investigators do not keep these in the lab which may have less rigorous pest control practices than the vivarial space.

In order to detect outbreaks earlier, institutions with ventilated racks might consider the use of PCR testing of swabs taken of exhaust air dust and of noninvasive fecal and swab specimens collected directly from resident and quarantined animals, and further mitigation of risks associated with possible sources of infection include autoclaving or gamma irradiation of feed and bedding. If significant noncompliance is shown to be responsible for an outbreak, mandatory retraining and/or Institutional Animal Care and Use Committee intervention may be imposed.

References

Adams, V., Myles, M.H., 2013. Multiplex fluorescent immunoassay for detection of mice infected with lactate dehydrogenase elevating virus. J. Am. Assoc. Lab. Anim. Sci. 52, 253–258.

Albers, T.M., Simon, M.A., Clifford, C.B., 2009. Histopathology of naturally transmitted "rat respiratory virus": progression of lesions and proposed diagnostic criteria. Vet. Pathol. 46, 992–999.

Allen, A.M., 1999. Evolution of disease monitoring in laboratory rodents. In: Mcpherson, C.W., Mattingly, S. (Eds.), Fifty Years of Laboratory Animal Science American Association of Laboratory Animal Science, Memphis, TN. Chapter 18.

Allen, M.A., Clarke, G.L., Ganaway, J.R., Lock, A., Werner, R.M., 1981. Pathology and diagnosis of mousepox. Lab. Anim. Sci. 31, 599–608.

An, C.L., Gigliotti, F., Harmsen, A.G., 2003. Exposure of immunocompetent adult mice to *Pneumocystis carinii* f. sp. *muris* by cohousing: growth of *P. carinii* f. sp. *muris* and host immune response. Infect. Immun. 71, 2065–2070.

Anonymous, 1976. Long-term holding of laboratory rodents. Ilar. News. 19, L1–L25.

Artwohl, J.E., Cera, L.M., Wright, M.F., Medina, L.V., Kim, L.J., 1994. The efficacy of a dirty bedding sentinel system for detecting Sendai virus infection in mice: a comparison of clinical signs and seroconversion. Lab. Anim. Sci. 44, 73–75.

Avery, R.H., 1996. HEPA and ULPA filter testing. In: Sufka, A., Harden, R., Mckenna, S.M. (Eds.), NAFA Guide to Air Filtration National Air Filtration Association, Washington, DC.

Ball-Goodrich, L.J., Johnson, E., 1994. Molecular characterization of a newly recognized mouse parvovirus. J. Virol. 68, 6476–6486.

Ball-Goodrich, L.J., Leland, S.E., Johnson, E.A., Paturzo, F.X., Jacoby, R.O., 1998. Rat parvovirus type 1: the prototype for a new rodent parvovirus serogroup. J. Virol. 72, 3289–3299.

Ball-Goodrich, L.J., Hansen, G., Dhawan, R., Paturzo, F.X., Vivas-Gonzalez, B.E., 2002. Validation of an enzyme-linked immunosorbent assay for detection of mouse parvovirus infection in laboratory mice. Comp. Med. 52, 160–166.

Barthold, S.W., Smith, A.L., 1983. Mouse hepatitis virus S in weanling Swiss mice following intranasal inoculation. Lab. Anim. Sci. 33, 355–360.

Barthold, S.W., Beck, D.S., Smith, A.L., 1988. Mouse hepatitis virus and host determinants of vertical transmission and maternally-derived passive immunity in mice. Arch. Virol. 100, 171–183.

Battles, J.K., Williamson, J.C., Pike, K.M., Gorelick, P.L., Ward, J.M., Gonda, M.A., 1995. Diagnostic assay for *Helicobacter hepaticus* based on nucleotide sequence of Its 16S rRNA gene. J. Clin. Microbiol. 33, 1344–1347.

Bauer, B.A., Riley, L.K., 2006. Antemortem detection of mouse parvovirus and mice minute virus by polymerase chain reaction (PCR) of faecal samples. Lab. Anim. 40, 144–152.

Bauer, B.A., Besch-Williford, C.L., Riley, L.K., 2004. Comparison of the mouse antibody production (MAP) assay and polymerase chain reaction (PCR) assays for the detection of viral contaminants. Biologicals 32, 177–182.

Baum, S.G., Lewis Jr., A.M., Rowe, W.P., Huebner, R.J., 1966. Epidemic nonmeningitic lymphocytic-choriomeningitis-virus infection. An outbreak in a population of laboratory personnel. N. Engl. J. Med. 274, 934–936.

Beaudette, P., Bateman, K.P., 2004. Discovery stage pharmacokinetics using dried blood spots. J. Chromatogr. B. Analyt. Technol. Biomed. Life. Sci. 809, 153–158.

Bech-Nielsen, G.V., Hansen, C.H., Hufeldt, M.R., Nielsen, D.S., Aasted, B., Vogensen, F.K., et al., 2012. Manipulation of the gut microbiota in C57BL/6 mice changes glucose tolerance without affecting weight development and gut mucosal immunity. Res. Vet. Sci. 92, 501–508.

Beckwith, C.S., Franklin, C.L., Hook Jr., R.R., Besch-Williford, C.L., Riley, L.K., 1997. Fecal PCR assay for diagnosis of *Helicobacter* infection in laboratory rodents. J. Clin. Microbiol. 35, 1620–1623.

Behnke, J.M., 1975. *Aspiculuris tetraptera* in wild *Mus musculus*. The prevalence of infection in male and female mice. J. Helminthol. 49, 85–90.

Bemis, D.A., Shek, W.R., Clifford, C.B., 2003. *Bordetella bronchiseptica* infection of rats and mice. Comp. Med. 53, 11–20.

Besch-Williford, C., Franklin, C.L., 2007. Aerobic Gram-positive bacteria. In: Fox, J.G., Barthold, S.W., Davisson, M.T., Newcomer, C.E., Quimby, F.W., Smith, A.L. (Eds.), The Mouse in Biomedical Research, second ed. Academic Press, Burlington, MA.

Besselsen, D.G., Becker, M.D., Henderson, K.S., Wagner, A.M., Banu, L.A., Shek, W.R., 2007. Temporal transmission studies of mouse parvovirus 1 in BALB/c and C.B-17/Icr-Prkdc(scid) mice. Comp. Med. 57, 66–73.

Besselsen, D.G., Besch-Williford, C., Pintel, D.J., Franklin, C.L., Hook, R.R., Riley, L.K., 1995a. Detection of newly recognized rodent parvoviruses by PCR. J. Clin. Microbiol., 2859–2863.

Besselsen, D.G., Besch-Williford, C.L., Pintel, D.J., Franklin, C.L., Hook Jr., R.R., Riley, L.K., 1995b. Detection of H-1 parvovirus and Kilham rat virus by PCR. J. Clin. Microbiol. 33, 1699–1703.

Besselsen, D.G., Pintel, D.J., Purdy, G.A., Besch-Williford, C.L., Franklin, C.L., Hook Jr., R.R., et al., 1996. Molecular characterization of newly recognized rodent parvoviruses. J. Gen. Virol. 77 (Pt 5), 899–911.

Besselsen, D.G., Wagner, A.M., Loganbill, J.K., 2000. Effect of mouse strain and age on detection of mouse parvovirus 1 by use of serologic testing and polymerase chain reaction analysis. Comp. Med. 50, 498–502.

Besselsen, D.G., Wagner, A.M., Loganbill, J.K., 2003. Detection of lymphocytic choriomeningitis virus by use of fluorogenic nuclease reverse transcriptase-polymerase chain reaction analysis. Comp. Med. 53, 65–69.

Besselsen, D.G., Romero, M.J., Wagner, A.M., Henderson, K.S., Livingston, R.S., 2006. Identification of novel murine parvovirus strains by epidemiological analysis of naturally infected mice. J. Gen. Virol. 87, 1543–1556.

Besselsen, D.G., Myers, E.L., Franklin, C.L., Korte, S.W., Wagner, A.M., Henderson, K.S., et al., 2008a. Transmission probabilities of mouse parvovirus 1 to sentinel mice chronically exposed to serial dilutions of contaminated bedding. Comp. Med. 58, 140–144.

Besselsen, D.G., Romero-Aleshire, M.J., Munger, S.J., Marcus, E.C., Henderson, K.S., Wagner, A.M., 2008b. Embryo transfer rederivation of C.B-17/Icr-Prkdc(scid) mice experimentally infected with mouse parvovirus 1. Comp. Med. 58, 353–359.

Bhatt, P.N., Jacoby, R.O., 1985. Epizootiological observations of natural and experimental infection with sialodacryoadentitis virus. Lab. Anim. Sci. 35, 129–134.

Bhatt, P.N., Jacoby, R.O., Barthold, S.W., 1986a. Contamination of transplantable murine tumors with lymphocytic choriomeningitis virus. Lab. Anim. Sci. 36, 136–139.

Bhatt, P.N., Jacoby, R.O., Morse, H.C., New, A.E., 1986b. Viral and Mycoplasmal Infections of Laboratory Rodents: Effects on Biomedical Research. Academic Prss, Orlando.

Blackmore, D.K., Francis, R.A., 1970. The apparent transmission of staphylococci of human origin to laboratory animals. J. Comp. Pathol. 80, 645–651.

Blank, W.A., Henderson, K.S., White, L.A., 2004. Virus PCR assay panels: an alternative to the mouse antibody production test. Lab. Anim. (NY) 33, 26–32.

Block, J.C., Schwartzbrod, L., 1989. Waterborne Viruses. Detection and Identification Viruses in Water Systems. VCH Publishers, New York.

Block, S.S., 1991. Definition of terms. In: Block, S.S. (Ed.), Disinfection, Sterilization, and Preservation. Lea & Febiger, Gainesville, FL.

Bohr, U.R., Selgrad, M., Ochmann, C., Backert, S., Konig, W., Fenske, A., et al., 2006. Prevalence and spread of enterohepatic *Helicobacter* species in mice reared in a specific-pathogen-free animal facility. J. Clin. Microbiol. 44, 738–742.

Bonnard, G.D., Manders, E.K., Campbell Jr., D.A., Herberman, R.B., Collins Jr., M.J., 1976. Immunosuppressive activity of a subline of the mouse EL-4 lymphoma. Evidence for minute virus of mice causing the inhibition. J. Exp. Med. 143, 187–205.

Boot, R., Koopman, J.P., Kruijt, B.C., Lammers, R.M., Kennis, H.M., Lankhorst, A., et al., 1985. The "normalization" of germ-free rabbits with host-specific caecal microflora. Lab. Anim. 19, 344–352.

Boot, R., Koopman, J.P., Kruijt, B.C., Lammers, R.M., Kennis, H.M., Lankhorst, A., et al., 1989a. The 'normalization' of germ-free guineapigs with host-specific caecal microflora. Lab. Anim. 23, 48–52.

Boot, R., Koopman, J.P., Lankhorst, A., Stadhouders, A.M., Welling, G.W., Hectors, M.P., 1989b. Intestinal "normalization" of germ-free rabbits with rabbit caecal microflora: effect of dosing regimens. Z. Versuchstierkd. 32, 83–86.

Bosma, G.C., Custer, R.P., Bosma, M.J., 1983. A severe combined immunodeficiency mutation in the mouse. Nature 301, 527–530.

Brachman, P.S., 1996. Epidemiology. In: Baron, S. (Ed.), Medical Microbiology. The University of Texas Medical Branch at Galveston, Galveston, TX.

Brammer, D.W., Dysko, R.C., Spilman, S.C., Oskar, P.A., 1993. Elimination of sialodacryoadenitis virus from the rat production colony by using seropositive breeding animals. Lab. Anim. Sci. 43, 633–634.

Brock, T.D., 1970. The procaryotic cell: microscopical methods. In: Brock, T.D. (Ed.), Biology of Microorganisms. Prentice-Hall, Englewood Cliffs, NJ.

Broome, C., Pinner, R., Schuchat, A., 1998. Listeria monocytogenes. In: Gorbach, S.L., Bartlett, J.G., Blacklow, N.R. (Eds.), Infectious Diseases. W.B. Saunders Company, Philadelphia, PA.

Brown, M.B., Steiner, D.A., 1996. Experimental genital mycoplasmosis: time of infection influences pregnancy outcome. Infect. Immun. 64, 2315–2321.

Brownstein, D.G., Barthold, S.W., 1982. Mouse hepatitis virus immunofluorescence in formalin or Bouin's-fixed tissues using trypsin digestion. Lab. Anim. Sci. 32, 37–39.

Brownstein, D.G., Smith, A.L., Johnson, E.A., 1981. Sendai virus infection in genetically resistant and susceptible mice. Am. J. Pathol. 105, 156–163.

Brownstein, D.G., Barthold, S.W., Adams, R.L., Terwilliger, G.A., Aftosmis, J.G., 1985. Experimental Corynebacterium kutscheri infection in rats: bacteriology and serology. Lab. Anim. Sci. 35, 135–138.

Carlson Scholz, J.A., Garg, R., Compton, S.R., Allore, H.G., Zeiss, C.J., Uchio, E.M., 2011. Poliomyelitis in MuLV-infected ICR-SCID mice after injection of basement membrane matrix contaminated with lactate dehydrogenase-elevating virus. Comp. Med. 61, 404–411.

Carroll, K.C., Weinstein, M.P., 2007. Manual and automated systems for detection and identification of microorganisms. In: Murray, P.R., Baron, E.J., Jorgensen, J.H., Landry, M.L., Pfaller, M.A. (Eds.), Manual of Clinical Micro Biology, nineth ed. American Society for Microbiology, Washington, DC.

Carty, A.J., 2008. Opportunistic infections of mice and rats: Jacoby and Lindsey revisited. ILAR. J. 49, 272–276.

Casadevall, A., Pirofski, L.A., 2000. Host–pathogen interactions: basic concepts of microbial commensalism, colonization, infection, and disease. Infect. Immun. 68, 6511–6518.

Casebolt, D.B., Lindsey, J.R., Cassell, G.H., 1988. Prevalence rates of infectious agents among commercial breeding populations of rats and mice. Lab. Anim. Sci. 38, 327–329.

Casebolt, D.B., Qian, B., Stephensen, C.B., 1997. Detection of enterotropic mouse hepatitis virus fecal excretion by polymerase chain reaction. Lab. Anim. Sci. 47, 6–10.

Cassell, G.H., Davis, J.K., Lindsey, J.R., Davidson, M.K., Brown, M.B., Baker, J.K., 1983. Detection of Mycoplasma pulmonis infections by ELISA. Lab. Anim. 12, 27–38.

Cera, L.M., Artwohl, J.E., Wright, M., Kim, L.J., 1994. Immunohistochemical detection of localized sendai virus antigen in preserved mouse tissue. Lab. Anim. Sci. 44, 88–90.

Chabe, M., Herbreteau, V., Hugot, J.P., Bouzard, N., Deruyter, L., Morand, S., et al., 2010. Pneumocystis carinii and Pneumocystis wakefieldiae in wild Rattus norvegicus trapped in Thailand. J. Eukaryot. Microbiol. 57, 213–217.

Childs, J.E., Glass, G.E., Korch, G.W., Leduc, J.W., 1989. Effects of hantaviral infection on survival, growth and fertility in wild rat (Rattus norvegicus) populations of Baltimore, Maryland. J. Wildl. Dis. 25, 469–476.

Clarke, G.L., Coates, M.E., Eva, J.K., Ford, D., Milner, C.K., O'Donoghue, P.N., et al., 1977. Dietary standards for laboratory animals. Lab. Anim. 11, 1–28.

Clifford, C.B., 2001. Samples, sample selection, and statistics: living with uncertainty. Lab. Anim. (NY) 30, 26–31.

Clifford, C.B., Walton, B.J., Reed, T., Coyle, M.B., White, W.J., Amyx, H.L., 1995. Hyperkeratosis in athymic nude mice caused by a coryneform bacterium: microbiology, transmission, clinical cigns, and pathology. Lab. Anim. Sci. 45, 131–139.

Cohen, M.L., 1998. Epidemiology of community-acquired infections. In: Gorbach, S.L., Bartlett, J.G., Blacklow, N.R. (Eds.), Infectious Diseases. W.B. Saunders Company, Philadelphia, PA.

Collins Jr., M.J., Parker, J.C., 1972. Murine virus contaminants of leukemia viruses and transplantable tumors. J. Natl. Cancer. Inst. 49, 1139–1143.

Compton, S.R., Barthold, S.W., Smith, A.L., 1993. The cellular and molecular pathogenesis of coronaviruses. Lab. Anim. Sci. 43, 15.

Compton, S.R., Winograd, D.F., Gaertner, D.J., 1995. Optimization of in vitro growth conditions for enterotropic murine coronavirus strains. J. Virol. Methods 52, 301–307.

Compton, S.R., Riley, L.K., 2001. Detection of infectious agents in laboratory rodents: traditional and molecular techniques. Comp. Med. 51, 113–119.

Compton, S.R., Ball-Goodrich, L.J., Zeiss, C.J., Johnson, L.K., Johnson, E.A., Macy, J.D., 2003. Pathogenesis of mouse hepatitis virus infection in gamma interferon-deficient mice is modulated by co-infection with Helicobacter hepaticus. Comp. Med. 53, 197–206.

Compton, S.R., Ball-Goodrich, L.J., Johnson, L.K., Johnson, E.A., Paturzo, F.X., Macy, J.D., 2004a. Pathogenesis of enterotropic mouse hepatitis virus in immunocompetent and immunodeficient mice. Comp. Med. 54, 681–689.

Compton, S.R., Ball-Goodrich, L.J., Paturzo, F.X., Macy, J.D., 2004b. Transmission of enterotropic mouse hepatitis virus from immunocompetent and immunodeficient mice. Comp. Med. 54, 29–35.

Compton, S.R., Homberger, F.R., Paturzo, F.X., Clark, J.M., 2004c. Efficacy of three microbiological monitoring methods in a ventilated cage rack. Comp. Med. 54, 382–392.

Compton, S.R., Jacoby, R.O., Paturzo, F.X., Smith, A.L., 2004d. Persistent Seoul virus infection in Lewis rats. Arch. Virol. 149, 1325–1339.

Compton, S.R., Paturzo, F.X., Smith, P.C., Macy, J.D., 2012. Transmission of mouse parvovirus by fomites. J. Am. Assoc. Lab. Anim. Sci. 51, 775–780.

Cooper, G.M., 1997. Fundamentals of molecular biology The Cell. ASM Press, Washington, DC.

Corning, B.F., Murphy, J.C., Fox, J.G., 1991. Group G streptococcal lymphadenitis in rats. J. Clin. Microbiol. 29, 2720–2723.

Council, N.R., 2009. Microbial Evolution and Co-Adaptation: A Tribute to the Life and Scientific Legacies of Joshua Lederberg. The National Academies Press, Washington, DC.

Cryz Jr., S.J., Furer, E., Germanier, R., 1983. Simple model for the study of Pseudomonas aeruginosa infections in leukopenic mice. Infect. Immun. 39, 1067–1071.

Cundiff, D.C., Besch-Williford, C., Riley, L.K., 1992. A review of the cilia-associated respiratory bacillus. CRL Reference Paper Fall, 1–4.

Cundiff, D.C., Besch-Williford, C., Hook, R.R., Franklin, C.L., Riley, L.K., 1994a. Detection of cilia-associated respiratory bacillus by PCR. J. Clin. Microbiol. 32, 1930–1934.

Cundiff, D.C., Besch-Williford, C.L., Hook, R.R., Franklin, C.L., Riley, L.K., 1994b. Characterization of cilia-associated respiratory bacillus isolates from rats and rabbits. Lab. Anim. Sci. 44, 305–312.

Cundiff, D.D., Riley, L.K., Franklin, C.L., Hook Jr., R.R., Besch-Williford, C., 1995. Failure of a soiled bedding sentinel system to detect cilia-associated respiratory bacillus infection in rats. Lab. Anim. Sci. 45, 219–221.

De Jager, W., Te Velthuis, H., Prakken, B.J., Kuis, W., Rijkers, G.T., 2003. Simultaneous detection of 15 human cytokines in a single sample of stimulated peripheral blood mononuclear cells. Clin. Diagn. Lab. Immunol. 10, 133–139.

Davidson, M.K., Lindsey, J.R., Brown, M.B., Schoeb, T.R., Cassell, G.H., 1981. Comparison of methods for detection of *Mycoplasma pulmonis* in experimentally and naturally infected rats. J. Clin. Microbiol. 14, 646–655.

Deeb, B.J., Digiacomo, R.F., Evermann, J.F., Thouless, M.E., 1993. Prevalence of coronavirus antibodies in rabbits. Lab. Anim. Sci. 43, 431–433.

Delellis, R.A., 1981. Basic techniques of immunohistochemistry. In: Delellis, R.A. (Ed.), Diagnostic Immunohistochemistry Masson Publishing.

Denyer, S.P., 1992. Filtration sterilization. In: Russell, A.D., Hugo, W.B., Ayliffe, G.A.J. (Eds.), Principles and Practice of Disinfection, Preservation and Sterilization. Blackwell Science, Oxford.

Descoteaux, J.P., Lussier, G., 1990. Experimental infection of young rabbits with a rabbit enteric coronavirus. Can. J. Vet. Res. 54, 473–476.

Descoteaux, J.P., Lussier, G., Berthiaume, L., Alain, R., Seguin, C., Trudel, M., 1985. An enteric coronavirus of the rabbit: detection by immunoelectron microscopy and identification of structural polypeptides. Arch. Virol. 84, 241–250.

Desousa, M., Smith, A., 1989. Comparison of isolation in cell culture with conventional and modified mouse antibody production tests for detection of murine viruses. J. Clin. Microbiol. 27, 185–187.

Dick, E.J., Kittell, C., Meyer, H., Farrar, P.L., Ropp, S.L., Esposito, J.J., et al., 1996. Mousepox outbreak in a laboratory mouse colony. Lab. Anim. Sci. 46, 602–611.

Digiacomo, R.F., Talburt, C.D., Lukehart, S.A., Baker-Zander, S., Condon, J., 1983. *Treponema paraluis-cuniculi* infection in a commercial rabbitry: epidemiology and serodiagnosis. Lab. Anim. Sci. 33, 562–566.

Dillehay, D.L., Lehner, N.D., Huerkamp, M.J., 1990. The effectiveness of a microisolator cage system and sentinel mice for controlling and detecting MHV and Sendai virus infections. Lab. Anim. Sci. 40, 367–370.

Dobrindt, U., Hochhut, B., Hentschel, U., Hacker, J., 2004. Genomic islands in pathogenic and environmental microorganisms. Nat. Rev. Microbiol. 2, 414–424.

Dole, V.S., Banu, L.A., Fister, R.D., Nicklas, W., Henderson, K.S., 2010. Assessment of rpoB and 16S rRNA genes as targets for PCR-based identification of *Pasteurella pneumotropica*. Comp. Med. 60, 427–435.

Dole, V.S., Zaias, J., Kyricopoulos-Cleasby, D.M., Banu, L.A., Waterman, L.L., Sanders, K., et al., 2011. Comparison of traditional and PCR methods during screening for and confirmation of *Aspiculuris tetraptera* in a mouse facility. J. Am. Assoc. Lab. Anim. Sci. 50, 904–909.

Dole, V.S., Boyd, K., Jackson, K., Wallace, J., Asher, J., Cohen, J., et al., 2013a. Investigation of commonalities among laboratory animal facilities associated with the group a rotavirus outbreaks in spring 2013. J. Am. Assoc. Lab. Anim. Sci. 52, 619–620.

Dole, V.S., Henderson, K.S., Fister, R.D., Pietrowski, M.T., Maldonado, G., Clifford, C.B., 2013b. Pathogenicity and genetic variation of 3 strains of *Corynebacterium bovis* in immunodeficient mice. J. Am. Assoc. Lab. Anim. Sci. 52, 458–466.

Drake, M.T., Riley, L.K., Livingston, R.S., 2008. Differential susceptibility of SD and CD rats to a novel rat theilovirus. Comp. Med. 58, 458–464.

Drazenovich, N.L., Franklin, C.L., Livingston, R.S., Besselsen, D.G., 2002. Detection of rodent *Helicobacter* spp. by use of fluorogenic nuclease polymerase chain reaction assays. Comp. Med. 52, 347–353.

Dubin, S., Zietz, S., 1991. Sample size for animal health surveillance. Lab. Anim. (NY) 20, 29–33.

Dubos, R.J., Schaedler, R.W., 1960. The effect of the intestinal flora on the growth rate of mice, and on their susceptibility to experimental infections. J. Exp. Med. 111, 407–417.

Dychadala, G.R., 1991. Chlorine and chlorine compounds. In: Block, S.S. (Ed.), Disinfection, Sterilization, and Preservation. Lea & Febiger, Gainesville, FL.

Ednie, D.L., Wilson, R.P., Lang, C.M., 2005. Comparison of two sanitation monitoring methods in an animal research facility. Contemp. Top. Lab. Anim. Sci. 37, 71–74.

Erickson, G.A., Landgraf, J.G., Wessman, S.J., Koski, T.A., Moss, L.M., 1989. Detection and elimination of adventitious agents in continuous cell lines. Dev. Biol. Stand. 70, 59–66.

Fallon, M.T., Reinhard, M.K., Gray, B.M., Davis, T.W., Lindsey, J.R., 1988. Inapparent *Streptococcus pneumoniae* type 35 infections in commercial rats and mice. Lab. Anim. Sci. 38, 129–132.

Farkas, T., Fey, B., Keller, G., Martella, V., Egyed, L., 2012. Molecular detection of novel astroviruses in wild and laboratory mice. Virus. Genes. 45, 518–525.

Fermer, C., Lindberg, A.V., Feinstein, R.E., 2002. Development and use of a simple polymerase chain reaction assay to screen for *Helicobacter* spp. and *H. hepaticus* in intestinal and fecal samples from laboratory mice. Comp. Med. 52, 518–522.

Ferrando, R., Vallette, J.P., Sain-Lebe, L., Bonnod, J., Huard, M., 1981. Influence of autoclaving on gamma irradiation on the main constituents of a complete composed diet for laboratory rats and mice. Sciences et Technique de l'Animal de Laboratoire 6, 5–13.

Filipovska-Naumovska, E., Abubakar, S.M., Thompson, M.J., Hopwood, D., Pass, D.A., Wilcox, G.E., 2010a. Serologic prevalence of MPV1 in mouse strains in a commercial laboratory mouse colony determined by using VP1 antigen. J. Am. Assoc. Lab. Anim. Sci. 49, 437–442.

Filipovska-Naumovska, E., Thompson, M.J., Hopwood, D., Pass, D.A., Wilcox, G.E., 2010b. Strain- and age-associated variation in viral persistence and antibody response to mouse parvovirus 1 in experimentally infected mice. J. Am. Assoc. Lab. Anim. Sci. 49, 443–447.

Flood, K.M., 1995. Efficacy of Alternative Disinfectants in the Inactivation of Kilham Rat Virus. The University of Connecticut, MSc.

Flynn, R.J., 1963. *Pseudomonas aeruginosa* infection and radiobiological research at Argonne National Laboratory: effects, diagnosis, epizootiology, control. Lab. Anim. Care 13, 25–35.

Flynn, R.J., 1973. Parasites of Laboratory Animals. Iowa State University Press, Ames, IA.

Foltz, C.J., Fox, J.G., Yan, L., Shames, B., 1996. Evaluation of various oral antimicrobial formulations for eradication of *Helicobacter hepaticus*. Lab. Anim. Sci. 46, 193–197.

Forbes, B.A., Sahm, D.F., Weissfeld, A.S., 1998. Laboratory cultivation and isolation of bacteria. In: Forbes, B.A., Sahm, D.F., Weissfeld, A.S. (Eds.), Bailey & Scott's Diagnostic Microbiology Mosby, St. Louis, MO.

Foster, H.L., 1958. Large scale production of rats free of commonly occurring pathogens and parasites. Proc. Anim. Care. Panel. 8, 92–100.

Foster, H.L., 1980. Gnotobiology. In: Baker, H.J., Lindsey, J.R., Weisbroth, S.P. (Eds.), The Laboratory Rat Volume 1: Biology and Disease. Academic Press, Inc., San Diego, CA.

Foster, H.L., Black, C., Pfau, E., 1964. A pasteurization process for pelleted diets. Lab. Anim. Sci. 14, 373–381.

Foster, T., 1996. *Staphylococcus*. In: Baron, S. (Ed.), Medical Microbiology. The University of Texas Medical Branch at Galveston, Galveston, TX.

Fox, J.G., Dewhirst, F.E., Tully, J.G., Paster, B.J., Yan, L., Taylor, N.S., et al., 1994. *Helicobacter hepaticus* sp. nov., a microaerophilic bacterium isolated from livers and intestinal mucosal scrapings from mice. J. Clin. Microbiol. 32, 1238–1245.

Fox, J.G., Li, X., Yan, L., Cahill, R.J., Hurley, R., Lewis, R., et al., 1996. Chronic proliferative hepatitis in A/JCr mice associated with persistent *Helicobacter hepaticus* infection: a model of helicobacter-induced carcinogenesis. Infect. Immun. 64, 1548–1558.

Franklin, C.L., 2006. Microbial considerations in genetically engineered mouse research. ILAR. J. 47, 141–155.

Friswell, M.K., Gika, H., Stratford, I.J., Theodoridis, G., Telfer, B., Wilson, I.D., et al., 2010. Site and strain-specific variation in gut microbiota profiles and metabolism in experimental mice. PLoS One 5, e8584.

Gaertner, D.J., Jacoby, R.O., Johnson, E.A., Paturzo, F.X., Smith, A.L., 1993. Characterization of acute rat parvovirus infection by in situ hybridization. Virus. Res. 28, 1–18.

Ganaway, J.R., 1976. Bacteria, mycoplasma and rickettsial diseases. In: Wagner, J.E., Manning, P.J. (Eds.), The Biology of the Guinea Pig. Academic Press, New York.

Ganaway, J.R., 1980. Effect of heat and selected chemical disinfectants upon infectivity of spores of *Bacillus piliformis* (Tyzzer's disease). Lab. Anim. Sci. 30, 192–196.

Ganaway, J.R., 1982. Bacterial and mycotic diseases of the digestive system. In: Foster, H.L., Small, J.D., Fox, J.G. (Eds.), The Mouse in Biomedical Research: Diseases. Academic Press, New York.

Ge, Z., White, D.A., Whary, M.T., Fox, J.G., 2001. Fluorogenic PCR-based quantitative detection of a murine pathogen, *Helicobacter hepaticus*. J. Clin. Microbiol. 39, 2598–2602.

Geistfeld, J.G., Weisbroth, S.H., Jansen, E.A., Kumpfmiller, D., 1998. Epizootic of group B *Streptococcus agalactiae* serotype V in DBA/2 mice. Lab. Anim. Sci. 48, 29–33.

Gentsch, J.R., Glass, R.I., Woods, P., Gouvea, V., Gorziglia, M., Flores, J., et al., 1992. Identification of group A rotavirus gene 4 types by polymerase chain reaction. J. Clin. Microbiol. 30, 1365–1373.

Giannella, R.A., 1996. *Salmonella*. In: Baron, S. (Ed.), Medical Microbiology. The University of Texas Medical Branch at Galveston, Galveston, TX.

Gibson, S.V., Waggie, K.S., Wagner, J.E., Ganaway, J.R., 1987. Diagnosis of subclinical *Bacillus piliformis* infection in a barrier-maintained mouse production colony. Lab. Anim. Sci. 37, 786–788.

Gibson, U.E.M., Heid, C.A., Willams, P.M., 1996. A novel method for real time quantitative RT-PCR. Genome Res. 6, 995–1001.

Glage, S., Dorsch, M., Hedrich, H.J., Bleich, A., 2007. Rederivation of *Helicobacter hepaticus*-infected Mongolian gerbils by Caesarean section and cross-fostering to rats and mice. Lab. Anim., 103–110.

Goelz, M.F., Thigpen, J.E., Mahler, J., Rogers, W.P., Locklear, J., Weigler, B.J., et al., 1996. Efficacy of various therapeutic regimens in eliminating *Pasteurella pneumotropica* from the mouse. Lab. Anim. Sci. 46, 280–285.

Goto, K., Ishihara, K.I., Kuzuoka, A., Ohnishi, Y., Itoh, T., 2001. Contamination of transplantable human tumor-bearing lines by *Helicobacter hepaticus* and its elimination. J. Clin. Microbiol. 39, 3703–3704.

Goto, K., Itoh, T., 1996. Detection of *Clostridium piliforme* by enzymatic assay of amplified cDNA segment in microtitration plates. Lab. Anim. Sci. 46, 493–496.

Goto, K., Takakura, A., Yoshimura, M., Ohnishi, Y., Itoh, T., 1998. Detection and typing of lactate dehydrogenase-elevating virus RNA from transplantable tumors, mouse liver tissues, and cell lines, using polymerase chain reaction. Lab. Anim. Sci. 48, 99–102.

Grada, A., Weinbrecht, K., 2013. Next-generation sequencing: methodology and application. J Invest. Dermatol. 133, e11.

Greiner, M., Pfeiffer, D., Smith, R.D., 2000. Principles and practical application of the receiver-operating characteristic analysis for diagnostic tests. Prev. Vet. Med. 45, 23–41.

Greisen, K., Loeffelholz, M., Purohit, A., Leong, D., 1994. PCR primers and probes for the 16S rRNA gene of most species of pathogenic bacteria, including bacteria found in the cerebrospinal fluid. J. Clin. Microbiol. 32, 335–351.

Grossgebauer, K., Spicker, G., Peter, J., 1975. Experiments on terminal disinfection by formaldehyde vapor in the case of smallpox. J. Clin. Microbiol. 2, 519.

Grove, K.A., Smith, P.C., Booth, C.J., Compton, S.R., 2012. Age-associated variability in susceptibility of Swiss Webster mice to MPV and other excluded murine pathogens. J. Am. Assoc. Lab. Anim. Sci. 51, 789–796.

Guillen, J., 2012. FELASA guidelines and recommendations. J. Am. Assoc. Lab. Anim. Sci. 51, 311–321.

Gundi, V.A., Dijkshoorn, L., Burignat, S., Raoult, D., La Scola, B., 2009. Validation of partial rpoB gene sequence analysis for the identification of clinically important and emerging *Acinetobacter species*. Microbiology 155, 2333–2341.

Hall, W.C., Ward, J.M., 1984. A comparison of the avidin–biotin–peroxidase complex (ABC) and peroxidase–anti-peroxidase (PAP) immunocytochemical techniques for demonstrating Sendai virus infection in fixed tissue specimens. Lab. Anim. Sci. 34, 261–263.

Hamilton, M.S., Otto, M., Nickell, A., Abel, D., Ballam, Y., Schremmer, R., 2002. High frequency of competitive inhibition in the Roche Cobas AMPLICOR multiplex PCR for *Chlamydia trachomatis* and *Neisseria gonorrhoeae*. J. Clin. Microbiol. 40, 4393.

Hanson, G., Wilkinson, R., 1993. Gamma radiation and virus inactivation. Art Sci. 12, 1–5.

Hartley, J.W., Rowe, W.P., 1960. A new mouse virus apparently related to the adenovirus group. Virology 11, 645–647.

Heid, C.A., Stevens, J., Livak, K.J., Williams, P.M., 1996. Real time quantitative PCR. Genome Res. 6, 986–994.

Hendershot, L., Levitt, D., 1985. Effects of mycoplasma contamination on immunoglobulin biosynthesis by human B lymphoblastoid cell lines. Infect. Immun. 49, 36–39.

Henderson, K.S., 2008. Murine norovirus, a recently discovered and highly prevalent viral agent of mice. Lab. Anim. (NY) 37, 314–320.

Henderson, K.S., Dole, V., Parker, N.J., Momtsios, P., Banu, L., Brouillette, R., et al., 2012. *Pneumocystis carinii* causes a distinctive interstitial pneumonia in immunocompetent laboratory rats that had been attributed to "rat respiratory virus". Vet. Pathol. 49, 440–452.

Henderson, K.S., Perkins, C.L., Havens, R.B., Kelly, M.J., Francis, B.C., Dole, V.S., et al., 2013. Efficacy of direct detection of pathogens in naturally infected mice by using a high-density PCR array. J. Am. Assoc. Lab. Anim. Sci. 52, 763–772.

Henderson, K.S., Pritchett-Corning, K.R., Perkins, C.L., Banu, L.A., Jennings, S.M., Francis, B.C., et al., 2015. A comparison of mouse parvovirus 1 infection in BALB/c and C57BL/6 mice: Susceptibility, replication, shedding, and seroconversion. *Comp. Med.* 65(1), 5–14.

Hermann, L.M., White, W.J., Lang, C.M., 1982. Prolonged exposure to acid, chlorine, or tetracycline in the drinking water: effects on delayed-type hypersensitivity, hemagglutination titers, and reticuloendothelial clearance rates in mice. Lab. Anim. Sci. 32, 603–608.

Hessler, J.R., 1999. The history of environmental improvements in laboratory animal science: caging systems, equipment and facility design. In: Mcpherson, C.W., Mattingly, S. (Eds.), Fifty Years of Laboratory Animal Science. American Association of Laboratory Animal Science Memphis, TN. Chapter 15.

Hildebrandt, P.K., 1982. Rickettsial and chlamydial diseases. In: Foster, H.L., Small, J.D., Fox, J.G. (Eds.), The Mouse in Biomedical Research: Diseases. Academic Press, New York.

Himan, M.E., 1975. Death of a neighbor (author's transl). Hu. Li. Za. Zhi. 22, 15–17.

Hirai, A., Ohtsuka, N., Ikeda, T., Taniguchi, R., Blau, D., Nakagaki, K., et al., 2010. Role of mouse hepatitis virus (MHV) receptor murine CEACAM1 in the resistance of mice to MHV infection: studies of mice with chimeric mCEACAM1a and mCEACAM1b. J. Virol. 84, 6654–6666.

Hodzic, E., Mckisic, M., Feng, S., Barthold, S.W., 2001. Evaluation of diagnostic methods for *Helicobacter bilis* infection in laboratory mice. Comp. Med. 51, 406–412.

Hoddenbach, G., Johnson, J., Disalvo, C., 1997. Rodent Exclusion Techniques. National Park Service Public Health Program, Washington, DC, pp. 1–55.

Holland, P.M., Abramson, R.D., Watson, R., Gelfand, D.H., 1991. Detection of specific polymerase chain reaction product by utilizing the 5′–3′ exonuclease activity of *Thermus aquaticus* DNA polymerase. Proc. Natl. Acad. Sci. USA 88, 7276–7280.

Homberger, F.R., Smith, A.L., Barthold, S.W., 1991. Detection of rodent coronaviruses in tissues and cell cultures by using polymerase chain reaction. J. Clin. Microbiol. 29, 2789–2793.

Homberger, F.R., Barthold, S.W., Smith, A.L., 1992. Duration and strain-specificity of immunity to enterotropic mouse hepatitis virus. Lab. Anim. Sci. 42, 347–351.

Homberger, F.R., Pataki, Z., Thomann, P.E., 1993. Control of *Pseudomonas aeruginosa* infection in mice by chlorine treatment of drinking water. Lab. Anim. Sci. 43, 635–637.

Homberger, F.R., Romano, T.P., Seiler, P., Hansen, G.M., Smith, A.L., 1995. Enzyme-linked immunosorbent assay for detection of antibody to lymphocytic choriomeningitis virus in mouse sera, with recombinant nucleoprotein as antigen. Lab. Anim. Sci. 45, 493–496.

Hong, S.T., Lee, M., Seo, M., Choo, D.H., Moon, H.R., Lee, S.H., 1995. Immunoblot analysis for serum antibodies to *Pneumocystis carinii* by age and intensity of infection in rats. Korean. J. Parasitol. 33, 187–194.

Hoover, D., Bendele, S.A., Wightman, S.R., Thompson, C.Z., Hoyt, J.A., 1985. Streptococcal enteropathy in infant rats. Lab. Anim. Sci. 35, 635–641.

Horowitz, S., Binion, D.G., Nelson, V.M., Kanaa, Y., Javadi, P., Lazarova, Z., et al., 2007. Increased arginase activity and endothelial dysfunction in human inflammatory bowel disease. Am. J. Physiol. Gastrointest. Liver. Physiol. 292, G1323–G1336.

Hrapchak, B.B., 1980. Immunohistochemistry. In: Sheehan, D.C., Hrapchak, B.B. (Eds.), Theory and Practice of Histotechnology. Battelle Press, Columbus, OH.

Hsu, C.C., Wobus, C.E., Steffen, E.K., Riley, L.K., Livingston, R.S., 2005. Development of a microsphere-based serologic multiplexed fluorescent immunoassay and a reverse transcriptase PCR assay to detect murine norovirus 1 infection in mice. Clin. Diagn. Lab. Immunol. 12, 1145–1151.

Hsu, C.C., Riley, L.K., Wills, H.M., Livingston, R.S., 2006. Persistent Infection with and serologic crossreactivity of three novel murine noroviruses. Comp. Med. 56, 247–251.

Hsu, M., Choppin, P.W., 1984. Analysis of Sendai virus mRNAs with cDNA clones of viral genes and sequences of biologically important regions of the fusion protein. Proc. Natl. Acad. Sci. 81, 7732–7736.

Huerkamp, M.J., 1993. Ivermectin eradication of pinworms from rats kept in ventilated cages. Lab. Anim. Sci. 43, 86–90.

Huerkamp, M.J., Zitzow, L.A., Webb, S., Pullium, J.K., 2005. Cross-fostering in combination with ivermectin therapy: a method to eradicate murine fur mites. Contemp. Top. Lab. Anim. Sci. 44, 12–16.

Ike, F., Bourgade, F., Ohsawa, K., Sato, H., Morikawa, S., Saijo, M., et al., 2007. Lymphocytic choriomeningitis infection undetected by dirty-bedding sentinel monitoring and revealed after embryo transfer of an inbred strain derived from wild mice. Comp. Med. 57, 272–281.

Ishii, A., Yago, A., Nariuchi, H., Shirasaka, A., Wada, Y., Matubashi, T., 1974. Some aspects on the transmission of hepatitis B antigen: model experiments by mosquitoes with murine hepatitis virus. Jpn. J. Exp. Med. 44, 495–501.

Jackson, T.A., Hall, J.E., Boivin, G.P., 1998. Ivermectin toxicity in young mice. Lab. Anim. Pract. 31, 37–41.

Jacobson, R.H., 1998. Validation of serological assays for diagnosis of infectious diseases. Rev. Sci. Tech. 17, 469–526.

Jacoby, R.O., Lindsey, J.R., 1998. Risks of infection among laboratory rats and mice at major biomedical research institutions. ILAR. J. 39, 266–271.

Jacoby, R.O., Bhatt, P.N., Jonas, A.M., 1975. Pathogenesis of sialodacryoadenitis in gnotobiotic rats. Vet. Pathol. 12, 196–209.

Jacoby, R.O., Johnson, E.A., Ball-Goodrich, L., Smith, A.L., Mckisic, M.D., 1995. Characterization of mouse parvovirus infection by in situ hybridization. J. Virol. 69, 3915–3919.

Jacoby, R.O., Ball-Goodrich, L.J., Besselsen, D.G., Mckisic, M.D., Riley, L.K., Smith, A.L., 1996. Rodent parvovirus infections. Lab. Anim. Sci. 46, 370–380.

Jacoby, R.O., Ball-Goodrich, L., Paturzo, F.X., Johnson, E.A., 2001. Prevalence of rat virus infection in progeny of acutely or persistently infected pregnant rats. Comp. Med. 51, 38–42.

Jensen, E.S., Allen, K.P., Henderson, K.S., Szabo, A., Thulin, J.D., 2013. PCR testing of a ventilated caging system to detect murine fur mites. J. Am. Assoc. Lab. Anim. Sci. 52, 28–33.

Jure, M.N., Morse, S.S., Stark, D.M., 1988. Identification of nonspecific reactions in laboratory rodent specimens tested by Rotazyme rotavirus ELISA. Lab. Anim. Sci. 38, 273–278.

Jurjus, A.R., Khoury, N.N., Reimund, J.M., 2004. Animal models of inflammatory bowel disease. J. Pharmacol. Toxicol. Methods. 50, 81–92.

Kahn, J.S., Kesebir, D., Cotmore, S.F., D'abramo Jr., A., Cosby, C., Weibel, C., et al., 2008. Seroepidemiology of human bocavirus defined using recombinant virus-like particles. J. Infect. Dis. 198, 41–50.

Karst, S.M., Wobus, C.E., Lay, M., Davidson, J., Virgin, H.W.T., 2003. STAT1-dependent innate immunity to a Norwalk-like virus. Science 299, 1575–1578.

Katami, K., Taguchi, F., Nakayama, M., Goto, N., Fujiwara, K., 1978. Vertical transmission of mouse hepatitis virus infection in mice. Jpn. J. Exp. Med. 48, 481–490.

Katz, D., Shi, W., Patrusheva, I., Perelygina, L., Gowda, M.S., Krug, P.W., et al., 2012. An automated ELISA using recombinant antigens for serologic diagnosis of B virus infections in macaques. Comp. Med. 62, 527–534.

Kendall, L.V., Besselsen, D.G., Riley, L.K., 2000. Fluorogenic 5′ nuclease PCR (real time PCR). Contemp. Top. Lab. Anim. Sci. 39, 41.

Kerton, A., Warden, P., 2006. Review of successful treatment for Helicobacter species in laboratory mice. Lab. Anim. 40, 115–122.

Khan, I.H., Kendall, L.V., Ziman, M., Wong, S., Mendoza, S., Fahey, J., et al., 2005. Simultaneous serodetection of 10 highly prevalent mouse infectious pathogens in a single reaction by multiplex analysis. Clin. Diagn. Lab. Immunol. 12, 513–519.

Kilham, L., Olivier, L.J., 1959. A latent virus of rats isolated in tissue culture. Virology 7, 428–437.

Kimsey, P.B., Engers, H.D., Hirt, B., Jongeneel, C.V., 1986. Pathogenicity of fibroblast- and lymphocyte-specific variants of minute virus of mice. J. Virol. 59, 8–13.

Klein, M., Deforest, A., 1983. Principals of virus inactivation. In: Block, S.S. (Ed.), Disinfection, Sterilization and Preservation. Lea & Febiger, Philadelphia, PA.

Koszdin, K.I., Digiacomo, R.F., 2002. Outbreak: Detection and Investigation. Contemp. Top. Lab. Anim. Sci. 41, 18–27.

Kraft, L.M., 1958. Observations on the control and natural history of epidemic diarrhea of infant mice (EDIM). Yale. J. Biol. Med. 31, 121–137.

Kraft, V., Meyer, B., Thunert, A., Deerberg, F., Rehm, S., 1982. Diagnosis of *Mycoplasma pulmonis* infection of rats by an indirect immunofluorescence test compared with 4 other diagnostic methods. Lab. Anim. 16, 369–373.

Kramer, D.N., 1992. Myths: cleaning, sanitation and disinfection. Dairy Food Environ. Sanit. 12, 507–509.

Kuhn, R., Lohler, J., Rennick, D., Rajewsky, K., Muller, W., 1993. Interleukin-10-deficient mice develop chronic enterocolitis. Cell 75, 263–274.

Kullberg, M.C., Ward, J.M., Gorelick, P.L., Caspar, P., Hieny, S., Cheever, A., et al., 1998. *Helicobacter hepaticus* triggers colitis in specific-pathogen-free interleukin-10 (IL-10)-deficient mice through an IL-12- and gamma interferon-dependent mechanism. Infect. Immun. 66, 5157–5166.

Kutyavin, I.V., Afonina, I.A., Mills, A., Gorn, V.V., Lukhtanov, E.A., Belousov, E.S., et al., 2000. 3'-Minor groove binder-DNA probes increase sequence specificity at PCR extension temperatures. Nucleic. Acids. Res. 28, 655–661.

Lankas, G.R., Cartwright, M.E., Umbenhauer, D., 1997. P-glycoprotein deficiency in a subpopulation of CF-1 mice enhances avermectin-induced neurotoxicity. Toxicol. Appl. Pharmacol. 143, 357–365.

Lankas, G.R., Minsker, D.H., Robertson, R.T., 1989. Effects of ivermectin on reproduction and neonatal toxicity in rats. Food. Chem. Toxicol. 27, 523–529.

Laregina, M.C., Lonigro, J., 1988. Serologic screening for murine pathogens: basic concepts and guidelines. Lab. Anim., 40–47.

Lehmann-Grube, F., 1982. Lymphocytic choriomeningitis virus. In: Foster, H.L., Small, J.D., Fox, J. (Eds.), The Mouse in Biomedical Research. Academic Press, Inc, New York, New York. ed.

Leland, S.E., 1991. Antiprotozoan, antihelmintic, and other pest management compounds. In: Block, S.S. (Ed.), Disinfection, Sterilization, and Preservation. Lea & Febiger, Gainesville, FL.

Les, E.P., 1983. Pressurized, individually ventilated (PVI) and individually exhausted caging for laboratory mice [abstract]. Lab. Anim. Sci. 33, 495.

Leutenegger, C.M., 2001. The real-time TaqMan PCR and applications in veterinary medicine. Vet. Sci. Tomorrow, 1–15.

Levy, R.V., Leahy, T.J., 1991. Sterilization filtration. In: Block, S.S. (Ed.), Disinfection, Sterilization, and Preservation. Lea & Febiger, Gainesville, FL.

Lewis Jr., A.M., Rowe, W.P., Turner, H.C., Huebner, R.J., 1965. Lymphocytic-choriomeningitis virus in hamster tumor: spread to hamsters and humans. Science 150, 363–364.

Lewis, V.J., Clayton, D.M., 1971. An evaluation of the mouse antibody production test for detecting three murine viruses. Lab. Anim. Sci. 21, 203–205.

Lifetechnologies., 2014. RNA Priming Strategy. Available from: <http://www.lifetechnologies.com/us/en/home/life-science/pcr/reverse-transcription/rna-priming-strategies.html>.

Lindstrom, K.E., Carbone, L.G., Kellar, D.E., Mayorga, M.S., Wilkerson, J.D., 2011. Soiled bedding sentinels for the detection of fur mites in mice. J. Am. Assoc. Lab. Anim. Sci. 50, 54–60.

Lipman, N.S., 1999. Isolator rodent caging systems (state of the art): a critical view. Contemp. Top. Lab. Anim. Sci. 38, 9–17.

Lipman, N.S., Homberger, F.R., 2003. Rodent quality assurance testing: use of sentinel animal systems. Lab. Anim. 32, 36–43.

Lipman, N.S., Newcomer, C.E., Fox, J.G., 1987. Rederivation of MHV and MEV antibody positive mice by cross-fostering and use of the microisolator caging system. Lab. Anim. Sci. 37, 195–199.

Lipman, N.S., Perkins, S., Nguyen, H., Pfeffer, M., Meyer, H., 2000. Mousepox resulting from use of ectromelia virus-contaminated, imported mouse serum. Comp. Med. 50, 426–435.

Liu, H., Bockhorn, J., Dalton, R., Chang, Y.F., Qian, D., Zitzow, L.A., et al., 2011. Removal of lactate dehydrogenase-elevating virus from human-in-mouse breast tumor xenografts by cell-sorting. J. Virol. Methods. 173, 266–270.

Livingston, R.S., Besch-Williford, C.L., Myles, M.H., Franklin, C.L., Crim, M.J., Riley, L.K., 2011. *Pneumocystis carinii* infection causes lung lesions historically attributed to rat respiratory virus. Comp. Med. 61, 45–59.

Livingston, R.S., Besselsen, D.G., Steffen, E.K., Besch-Williford, C.L., Franklin, C.L., Riley, L.K., 2002. Serodiagnosis of mice minute virus and mouse parvovirus infections in mice by enzyme-linked immunosorbent assay with baculovirus-expressed recombinant VP2 proteins. Clin. Diagn. Lab. Immunol. 9, 1025–1031.

Livingston, R.S., Riley, L.K., 2003. Diagnostic testing of mouse and rat colonies for infectious agents. Lab. Anim. (NY) 32, 44–51.

Livingston, R.S., Riley, L.K., Besch-Williford, C.L., Hook Jr., R.R., Franklin, C.L., 1998. Transmission of *Helicobacter hepaticus* infection to sentinel mice by contaminated bedding. Lab. Anim. Sci. 48, 291–293.

Lloyd, G., Jones, N., 1986. Infection of laboratory workers with hantavirus acquired from immunocytomas propagated in laboratory rats. J. Infect. 12, 117–125.

Lo, T.M., Ward, C.K., Inzana, T.J., 1998. Detection and identification of *Actinobacillus pleuropneumoniae* serotype 5 by multiplex PCR. J. Clin. Microbiol. 36, 1704–1710.

Loganbill, J.K., Wagner, A.M., Besselsen, D.G., 2005. Detection of *Mycoplasma pulmonis* by fluorogenic nuclease polymerase chain reaction analysis. Comp. Med. 55, 419–424.

Lukas, V.S., Ruehl, W.W., Hamm, T.E., 1987. An enzyme-linked immunosorbent assay to detect serum IgG in rabbits naturally exposed to cilia-associated respiratory bacillus. Lab. Anim. Sci. 37, 533.

Lussier, G., 1991. Detection methods for the identification of rodent viral and mycoplasmal infections. Lab. Anim. Sci. 41, 199–225.

Lussier, G., Descoteaux, J.P., 1986. Prevalence of natural virus infections in laboratory mice and rats used in Canada. Lab. Anim. Sci. 36, 145–148.

Lussier, G., Guenette, D., Descoteaux, J.P., 1988. Detection of antibodies to mouse thymic virus by enzyme-linked immunosorbent assay. Can. J. Vet. Res. 52, 236–238.

Lyerla, H.C., Forrester, F.T., 1979. Immunofluorescence Methods in Virology, Course No. CDC, Atlanta, 8231-C.

Macfaddin, J.F., 1980. Biochemical Tests for Identification of Medical Bacteria. Williams & Wilkins, Baltimore, MD.

Macy, J.D., Cameron, G.A., Smith, P.C., Ferguson, T.A., Compton, S.R., 2011. Detection and control of mouse parvovirus. J. Am. Assoc. Lab. Anim. Sci. 50, 516–522.

Macy, J.D., Paturzo, F.X., Ball-Goodrich, L.J., Compton, S.R., 2009. A PCR-based strategy for detection of mouse parvovirus. J. Am. Assoc. Lab. Anim. Sci. 48, 263–267.

Macy, J.D., Paturzo, F.X., Compton, S.R., 2013. Effect of immunodeficiency on MPV shedding and transmission. J. Am. Assoc. Lab. Anim. Sci. 52, 467–474.

Maerki, U., Rossbach, W., Leuenberger, J., 1989. Consistency of laboratory animal food following incubation prior to autoclaving. Lab. Anim. 23, 319–323.

Mahler, M., Bedigian, H.G., Burgett, B.L., Bates, R.J., Hogan, M.E., Sundberg, J.P., 1998. Comparison of four diagnostic methods for detection of *Helicobacter* species in laboratory mice. Lab. Anim. Sci. 48, 85–91.

Mahoney, J.B., Chernesky, M.A., 1999. Immunoassays for the diagnosis of infectious diseases. In: Murray, P.R., Baron, E.J., Pfaller, M.A., Tenover, F.C., Yolken, R.H. (Eds.), Manual of Clinical Microbiology. ASM Press, Washington, DC.

Manning, P.J., Delong, D., Swanson, D., Shek, W.R., 1994. Rodent isolates of *Pasteurella pneumotropica*: demonstration of O polysaccharide chains and serologically specific lipopolysaccharide antigens. Lab. Anim. Sci. 44, 399.

Manuel, C.A., Hsu, C.C., Riley, L.K., Livingston, R.S., 2008. Soiled-bedding sentinel detection of murine norovirus 4. J. Am. Assoc. Lab. Anim. Sci. 47, 31–36.

Matsumiya, L.C., Lavoie, C., 2003. An outbreak of *Pasteurella pneumotropica* in genetically modified mice: treatment and elimination. Contemp. Top. Lab. Anim. Sci. 42, 26–28.

Matsunaga, Y., Matsuno, S., 1983. Structural and nonstructural proteins of a rabbit parvovirus. J. Virol. 45, 627–633.

Matsunaga, Y., Yamazaki, S., 1976. Studies on herpesvirus cuniculi. I. Virus isolation and antibody response in rabbits with experimental infection (author's transl). Uirusu 26, 11–19.

Matsushita, S., Kashima, M., Joshima, H., 1987. Serodiagnosis of cilia-associated respiratory bacillus infection by the indirect immunofluorescence assay technique. Lab. Anim. 21, 356–359.

Matthaei, K.I., Berry, J.R., France, M.P., Yeo, C., Garcia-Aragon, J., Russell, P.J., 1998. Use of polymerase chain reaction to diagnose a natural outbreak of mouse hepatitis virus infection in nude mice. Lab. Anim. Sci. 48, 137–144.

Mazur, P., Leibo, S.P., Seidel Jr., G.E., 2008. Cryopreservation of the germplasm of animals used in biological and medical research: importance, impact, status, and future directions. Biol. Reprod. 78, 2–12.

Mcgarrity, G.J., Lindsay, G., Sarama, J., 1983. Prevention and control of mycoplasma infection. In: Tully, J.G., Razin, S. (Eds.), Methods in Mycoplasmology. Volume II. Diagnostic Mycoplasmology. Academic Press, New York.

Mcgarrity, G.J., Vanaman, V., Sarama, J., 1984. Cytogenetic effects of mycoplasmal infection of cell cultures: a review. In Vitro 20, 1–18.

Mckisic, M.D., Lancki, D.W., Otto, G., Padrid, P., Snook, S., Cronin, D.C., et al., 1993. Identification and propagation of a putative immunosuppressive orphan parvovirus in cloned T cells. J. Immunol. 150, 419–428.

Mei, J.V., Alexander, J.R., Adam, B.W., Hannon, W.H., 2001. Use of filter paper for the collection and analysis of human whole blood specimens. J. Nutr. 131, 1631S–1636S.

Meier, T.R., Maute, C.J., Cadillac, J.M., Lee, J.Y., Righter, D.J., Hugunin, K.M., et al., 2008. Quantification, distribution, and possible source of bacterial biofilm in mouse automated watering systems. J. Am. Assoc. Lab. Anim. Sci. 47, 63–70.

Merrell, D.S., Falkow, S., 2004. Frontal and stealth attack strategies in microbial pathogenesis. Nature 430, 250–256.

Miller, S.E., 1995. Diagnosis of viral infection by electron microscopy. In: Edwin, P., Lennette, H., David, A., Lennette, P., Evelyne, T., Lennette, P. (Eds.), Diagnostic Procedures for Viral, Rickettsial, and Chlamydial Infections, seventh ed. American Public Health Association, Washington, DC.

Minion, F.C., Brown, M.B., Cassell, G.H., 1984. Identification of cross-reactive antigens between Mycoplasma pulmonis and Mycoplasma arthritidis. Infect. Immun. 43, 115–121.

Mobraaten, L.E., Sharp, J.J., 1999. Evolution of genetic manipulation of laboratory animals. In: Charles, W.M., Steele, F.M. (Eds.),. Fifty Years of Laboratory Animal Science. American Association of Laboratory Animal Science, Memphis, TN, Chapter 17.

Mombaerts, P., Mizoguchi, E., Grusby, M.J., Glimcher, L.H., Bhan, A.K., Tonegawa, S., 1993. Spontaneous development of inflammatory bowel disease in T cell receptor mutant mice. Cell 75, 274–282.

Moore, W.A., 1992. Experience in cell line testing. Dev. Biol. Stand. 76, 51–56.

Morse, H.C., 2007. Building a better mouse: one hundred years of genetics and biology. In: Fox, J.G., Barthold, S.W., Davisson, M.T., Newcomer, C.E., Quimby, F.W., Smith, A.L. (Eds.), The Mouse in Biomedical Research: Volume I History, Wild Mice, Genetics, second ed. Academic Press, Inc., Burlington, MA.

Motzel, S.L., Riley, L.K., 1991. Bacillus piliformis flagellar antigens for serodiagnosis of Tyzzer's disease. J. Clin. Microbiol. 29, 2566–2570.

Mullis, K.B., 1990. The unusual origin of the polymerase chain reaction. Sci. Am. 262, 56–61, 64–65.

Nagaoka, M., Si-Tayeb, K., Akaike, T., Duncan, S.A., 2010. Culture of human pluripotent stem cells using completely defined conditions on a recombinant E-cadherin substratum. BMC. Dev. Biol. 10, 60.

Nakayama, H., Oguihara, S., Osaki, Toriumi, W., 1984. Effect of cyclophosphamide on Tyzzer's disease of mice. Unknown, pp. 82–88.

Neimark, H., Johansson, K.E., Rikihisa, Y., Tully, J.G., 2002. Revision of haemotrophic Mycoplasma species names. Int. J. Syst. Evol. Microbiol. 52, 683.

Newsome, P.M., Coney, K.A., 1985. Synergistic rotavirus and Escherichia coli diarrheal infection of mice. Infect. Immun. 47, 573–574.

Nicklas, W., 2008. International harmonization of health monitoring. ILAR. J. 49, 338–346.

Nicklas, W., Kraft, V., Meyer, B., 1993. Contamination of transplantable tumors, cell lines, and monoclonal antibodies with rodent viruses. Lab. Anim. Sci. 43, 296–300.

Nicklas, W., Baneux, P., Boot, R., Decelle, T., Deeny, A.A., Fumanelli, M., et al., 2002. Recommendations for the health monitoring of rodent and rabbit colonies in breeding and experimental units. Lab. Anim. 36, 20–42.

OIE, 2013. Principles and methods of validation of diagnostic assays for infectious diseases OIE Terrestrial Manual. World Organisation for Animal Health, Paris, France, (OIE).

Oldstone, M.B., Sinha, Y.N., Blount, P., Tishon, A., Rodriguez, M., Von Wedel, R., et al., 1982. Virus-induced alterations in homeostasis: alteration in differentiated functions of infected cells in vivo. Science 218, 1125–1127.

Orcutt, R.P., 1980. Bacterial diseases: agents, pathology, diagnosis & effects on research. Lab. Anim. 9, 28–43.

Owen, D., 1972. Preparation and identification of common parasites of laboratory rodents. In: "Medical Research Council, Laboratory Animal Centre Handbook No. 1. Her Majesty's Stationery Office, London.

Pantelouris, E.M., 1968. Absence of thymus in a mouse mutant. Nature 217, 370–371.

Parker, J.C., Reynolds, R.K., 1968. Natural history of Sendai virus infection in mice. Am. J. Epidemiol. 88, 112–125.

Parker, J.C., O'Beirne, A.J., Collins Jr., M.J., 1979. Sensitivity of enzyme-linked immunosorbent assay, complement fixation, and hemagglutination inhibition serological tests for detection of Sendai virus antibody in laboratory mice. J. Clin. Microbiol. 9, 444–447.

Parker, S.E., Malone, S., Bunte, R.M., Smith, A.L., 2009. Infectious diseases in wild mice (Mus musculus) collected on and around the University of Pennsylvania (Philadelphia) Campus. Comp. Med. 59, 424–430.

Parker, J.C., Tennant, R.W., Ward, T.G., 1965. Virus studies with germ-free mice. I. Preparation of serologic diagnostic reagents and survey of germfree and monocontaminated mice for indigenous murine viruses. J. Natl. Cancer Inst. 34, 371–380.

Parkinson, C.M., O'Brien, A., Albers, T.M., Simon, M.A., Clifford, C.B., Pritchett-Corning, K.R., 2011. Diagnosis of ecto- and endoparasites in laboratory rats and mice. J. Vis. Exp. (55), e2767. http://dx.doi.org/doi:10.3791/2767

Patterson, M.J., 1996. Streptococcus. In: Baron, S. (Ed.), Medical Microbiology. The University of Texas Medical Branch at Galveston, Galveston, TX.

Pepe, S., 2003. The Statistical Evaluation of Medical Tests for Classification and Prediction. Oxford University Press, New York.

Perdue, K.A., Green, K.Y., Copeland, M., Barron, E., Mandel, M., Faucette, L.J., et al., 2007. Naturally occurring murine norovirus infection in a large research institution. J. Am. Assoc. Lab. Anim. Sci. 46, 39–45.

Peters, D.D., Marschall, S., Mahabir, E., Boersma, A., Heinzmann, U., Schmidt, J., et al., 2006. Risk assessment of mouse hepatitis virus infection via in vitro fertilization and embryo transfer by the use of zona-intact and laser-microdissected oocytes. Biol. Reprod. 74, 246–252.

Peters, R.L., Collins Jr., M.J., 1981. Use of mouse hepatitis virus antigen in an enzyme-linked immunosorbent assay for rat coronaviruses. Lab. Anim. Sci. 31, 472–475.

Potera, C., 1996. Biofilms invade microbiology [news]. Science 273, 1795–1797.

Powrie, F., Leach, M.W., 1995. Genetic and spontaneous models of inflammatory bowel disease in rodents: evidence for abnormalities in mucosal immune regulation. Ther. Immunol. 2, 115–123.

Prince, H.N., Prince, D., Prince, R., 1991. Principles of viral control and transmission. In: Block, S.S. (Ed.), Disinfection, Sterilization, and Preservation. Lea & Febiger, Gainesville, FL.

Pritchett-Corning, K.R., Cosentino, J., Clifford, C.B., 2009. Contemporary prevalence of infectious agents in laboratory mice and rats. Lab. Anim. 43, 165–173.

Pritchett, K.R., Johnston, N.A., 2002. A review of treatments for the eradication of pinworm infections from laboratory rodent colonies. Contemp. Top. Lab. Anim. Sci. 41, 36–46.

Pritt, S., Henderson, K.S., Shek, W.R., 2010. Evaluation of available diagnostic methods for Clostridium piliforme in laboratory rabbits (Oryctolagus cuniculus). Lab. Anim. 44, 14–19.

Pullium, J.K., Benjamin, K.A., Huerkamp, M.J., 2004. Rodent vendor apparent source of mouse parvovirus in sentinel mice. Contemp. Top. Lab. Anim. Sci. 43, 8–11.

Redig, A.J., Besselsen, D.G., 2001. Detection of rodent parvoviruses by use of fluorogenic nuclease polymerase chain reaction assays. Comp. Med. 51, 326–331.

Reuter, J.D., Livingston, R., Leblanc, M., 2011. Management strategies for controlling endemic and seasonal mouse parvovirus infection in a barrier facility. Lab. Anim. (NY) 40, 145–152.

Reyes, L., Shelton, M., Riggs, M., Brown, M.B., 2004. Rat strains differ in susceptibility to maternal and fetal infection with Mycoplasma pulmonis. Am. J. Reprod. Immunol. 51, 211–219.

Reyes, L., Steiner, D.A., Hutchison, J., Crenshaw, B., Brown, M.B., 2000. Mycoplasma pulmonis genital disease: effect of rat strain on pregnancy outcome. Comp. Med. 50, 622–627.

Ricart Arbona, R.J., Lipman, N.S., Wolf, F.R., 2010a. Treatment and eradication of murine fur mites: II. Diagnostic considerations. J. Am. Assoc. Lab. Anim. Sci. 49, 583–587.

Ricart Arbona, R.J., Lipman, N.S., Wolf, F.R., 2010b. Treatment and eradication of murine fur mites: III. Treatment of a large mouse colony with ivermectin-compounded feed. J. Am. Assoc. Lab. Anim. Sci. 49, 633–637.

Rice, K.A., Albacarys, L.K., Metcalf Pate, K.A., Perkins, C., Henderson, K.S., Watson, J., 2013. Evaluation of diagnostic methods for Myocoptes musculinus according to age and treatment status of mice (Mus musculus). J. Am. Assoc. Lab. Anim. Sci. 52, 773–781.

Richens, J.L., Urbanowicz, R.A., Metcalf, R., Corne, J., O'Shea, P., Fairclough, L., 2010. Quantitative validation and comparison of multiplex cytokine kits. J. Biomol. Screen. 15, 562–568.

Riepenhoff-Talty, M., Offor, E., Klossner, K., Kowalski, E., Carmody, P.J., Ogra, P.L., 1985. Effect of age and malnutrition on rotavirus infection in mice. Pediatr. Res. 19, 1250–1253.

Riley, L.K., Franklin, C.L., Hook, R.R., Besch-Williford, C., 1994. Tyzzer's disease: an update of current information. Charles River Lab. Tech. Bull. Fall, 1–6.

Riley, L.K., Franklin, C.L., Hook, R.R., Besch-Williford, C., 1996a. Identification of murine helicobacters by PCR and restriction enzyme analyses. J. Clin. Microbiol. 34, 942–946.

Riley, L.K., Knowles, R., Purdy, G., Salome, N., Pintel, D., Hook, R.R., et al., 1996b. Expression of recombinant parvovirus NS1 protein by a baculovirus and application to serologic testing of rodents. J. Clin. Microbiol. 34, 440–444.

Riley, V., 1974. Persistence and other characteristics of the lactate dehydrogenase-elevating virus (LDH-Virus). Prog. Med. Virol. 18, 198–213.

Riley, V., Lilly, F., Huerto, E., Bardell, D., 1960. Transmissible agent associated with 26 types of experimental mouse neoplasms. Science 132, 545–547.

Rosen, D.D., Berk, R.S., 1977. Pseudomonas eye infections in cyclophosphamide-treated mice. Invest. Ophthalmol. 16, 649–652.

Rowe, W.P., Capps, W.I., 1961. A new mouse virus causing necrosis of the thymus in newborn mice. J. Exp. Med. 113, 831–844.

Rowe, W.P., Hartley, J.W., Huebner, R.J., 1962. Polyoma and other indigenous mouse viruses. In: Harris, R.J.C. (Ed.), The Problems of Laboratory Animal Disease. Academic Press, New York.

Russell, A.D., 1991. Principles of antimicrobial activity. In: Block, S.S. (Ed.), Disinfection, Sterilization, and Preservation. Lea & Febriger, Gainesville, FL.

Russell, A.D., 1992. Factors influencing the efficacy of antimicrobial agents. In: Russell, A.D., Hugo, W.B., Ayliffe, G.A.J. (Eds.), Principles and Practice of Disinfection, Preservation and Sterilization. Blackwell Science, Oxford.

Russell, R., Haines, D.C., Anver, M.R., Battles, J.K., Gorelick, P.L., Blumenauer, L.L., et al., 1995. Use of antibiotics to prevent hepatitis and typhlitis in male SCID mice spontaneously infected with Helicobacter hepaticus. Lab. Anim. Sci. 45, 373–378.

Schaedler, R.W., Orcutt, R.P., 1983. Gastrointestinal microflora. In: Foster, H.L., Small, J.D., Fox, J.G. (Eds.), The Mouse in Biomedical Research. Academic Press, Inc., New York. New York.

Schinkel, A.H., Smit, J.J., Van Tellingen, O., Beijnen, J.H., Wagenaar, E., Van Deemter, L., et al., 1994. Disruption of the mouse mdr1a P-glycoprotein gene leads to a deficiency in the blood–brain barrier and to increased sensitivity to drugs. Cell 77, 491–502.

Schinkel, A.H., Mayer, U., Wagenaar, E., Mol, C.A., Van Deemter, L., Smit, J.J., et al., 1997. Normal viability and altered pharmacokinetics in mice lacking mdr1-type (drug-transporting) P-glycoproteins. Proc. Natl. Acad. Sci. USA 94, 4028–4033.

Schmaljohn, C.S., Chu, Y.K., Schmaljohn, A.L., Dalrymple, J.M., 1990. Antigenic subunits of Hantaan virus expressed by baculovirus and vaccinia virus recombinants. J. Virol. 64, 3162–3170.

Schmidt, N.J., 1979. Cell culture techniques for diagnostic virology. In: Lennette, E.H., Schmidt, N.J. (Eds.), Diagnostic Procedures for Viral, Rickettsial and Chlamydial Infections. American Public Health Association, Washington, DC.

Schondelmeyer, C.W., Dillehay, D.L., Webb, S.K., Huerkamp, M.J., Mook, D.M., Pullium, J.K., 2006. Investigation of appropriate sanitization frequency for rodent caging accessories: evidence supporting less-frequent cleaning. J. Am. Assoc. Lab. Anim. Sci. 45, 40–43.

Schoondermark-Van De Ven, E.M., Philipse-Bergmann, I.M., Van Der Logt, J.T., 2006. Prevalence of naturally occurring viral infections, Mycoplasma pulmonis and Clostridium piliforme in laboratory rodents in Western Europe screened from 2000 to 2003. Lab. Anim. 40, 137–143.

Sedlacek, R.S., Mason, K.A., 1977. A simple and inexpensive method for maintaining a defined flora mouse colony. Lab. Anim. Sci. 27, 667–670.

Seletsakia, E.M., Cowley, J.P., Wunderlich, M.L., Jennings, S.J., Henderson, K.S., Shek, W.R., et al., 2004. Development of a parvovirus assay using rNS-1 his-tagged antigen. Bioprocess. J., 35–39.

Selwyn, M.R., Shek, W.R., 1994. Sample sizes and frequency of testing for health monitoring in barrier rooms and isolators. Contemp. Top. Lab. Anim. Sci. 33, 56–60.

Seng, P., Drancourt, M., Gouriet, F., La Scola, B., Fournier, P.E., Rolain, J.M., et al., 2009. Ongoing revolution in bacteriology: routine identification of bacteria by matrix-assisted laser desorption ionization time-of-flight mass spectrometry. Clin. Infect. Dis. 49, 543–551.

Shames, B., Fox, J.G., Dewhirst, F., Yan, L., Shen, Z., Taylor, N.S., 1995. Identification of widespread Helicobacter hepaticus infection in feces in commercial mouse colonies by culture and PCR assay. J. Clin. Microbiol. 33, 2968–2972.

Shek, W., 2000. Standardization of rodent health surveillance: regulation versus competition. Microbial Status and Genetic Evaluation of Mice and Rats, Proceedings of the 1999 US/Japan Conference. Washington, DC: The National Academies Press.

Shek, W.R., 1983. Detection of murine viruses in biological materials by the mouse antibody production test. In: Seaver, S.S. (Ed.), Commercial Production of Monoclonal Antibodies: A Guide for Scale-Up. Marcel Dekker, Inc., New York.

Shek, W.R., 2007. Quality control testing of biologics. In: Fox, J.G., Barthold, S.W., Davisson, M.T., Newcomer, C.E., Quimby, F.W., Smith, A.L. (Eds.), The Mouse in Biomedical Research, second ed. Academic Press, Burlington, MA.

Shek, W.R., 2008. Role of housing modalities on management and surveillance strategies for adventitious agents of rodents. ILAR. J. 49, 316–325.

Shek, W.R., Gaertner, D.J., 2002. Microbiological quality control for rodents and lagomorphs. In: Fox, J., Anderson, L., Loew, M., Quimby, F. (Eds.), Lab Animal Medicine, second ed. Academic Press, New York.

Shek, W.R., Flood, K.M., Green, D., Jennings, S.M., 1991. Inactivation of Kilham's rat virus (KRV) by ozonation. Annual Meeting, AALASA, Buffalo, NY.

Shek, W.R., Paturzo, F.X., Johnson, E.A., Hansen, G.M., Smith, A.L., 1998. Characterization of mouse parvovirus infection among BALB/c mice from an enzootically infected colony. Lab. Anim. Sci. 48, 294–297.

Shek, W.R., Pritchett, K.R., Clifford, C.B., White, W.J., 2005. Large-scale rodent production methods make vendor barrier rooms unlikely to have persistent low-prevalence parvoviral infections. Contemp. Top. Lab. Anim. Sci. 44, 37–42.

Silverman, G.J., 1991. Sterilization and preservation by ionizing irradiation. In: Block, S.S. (Ed.), Disinfection, Sterilization, and Preservation. Lea & Febiger, Gainesville, FL.

Simon, M., Domok, I., Pinter, A., 1982. Lymphocytic choriomeningitis (LCM) virus carrier cell cultures in Hungarian laboratories. Acta. Microbiol. Acad. Sci. Hung. 29, 201–208.

Singleton, G.R., Smith, A.L., Shellam, G.R., Fitzgerald, N., Muller, W.J., 1993. Prevalence of viral antibodies and helminths in field populations of house mice (Mus domesticus) in southeastern Australia. Epidemiol. Infect. 110, 399–417.

Skinner, H.H., Knight, E.H., Grove, R., 1977. Murine lymphocytic choriomeningitis: the history of a natural cross-infections from wild to laboratory mice. Lab. Anim. 11, 219–222.

Skopets, B., Wilson, R.P., Griffith, J.W., Lang, C.M., 1996. Ivermectin toxicity in young mice. Lab. Anim. Sci. 46, 111–112.

Small, J.D., 1983. Environmental and equipment monitoring. In: Foster, H.L., Small, J.D., Fox, J.G. (Eds.), The Mouse in Biomedical Research: Normative Biology, Immunology and Husbandry. Academic Press, San Diego, CA.

Small, J.D., New, A., 1981. Prevention and control of mousepox. Lab. Anim. Sci. 31, 616–621.

Smith, A.L., 1983a. An immunofluorescence test for detection of serum antibody to rodent coronaviruses. Lab. Anim. Sci. 33, 157–160.

Smith, A.L., 1983b. Response of weanling random-bred mice to inoculation with minute virus of mice. Lab. Anim. Sci. 33, 37–39.

Smith, A.L., 1986a. Methods for potential application to rodent virus isolation and identification. In: Bhatt, P.N., Jacoby, R.O., Morse, H.C., New, A.E. (Eds.), Viral and Mycoplasmal Infections of Laboratory Rodents: Effects on Biomedical Research. Academic Press, Orlando.

Smith, A.L., 1986b. Serologic tests for detection of antibody to rodent viruses. In: Bhatt, P.N., Jacoby, R.O., Morse, S.S., New, A. (Eds.), Viral and Mycoplasmal Infections of Laboratory Rodents: Effects on Biomedical Research. Academic Press, Orlando, FL.

Smith, A.L., 2010. Management of rodent viral disease outbreaks: one institutions (r)evolution. ILAR. J. 51, 127–137.

Smith, A.L., Carrano, V.A., Brownstein, D., 1984. Response of weanling random-bred mice to infection with pneumonia virus of mice (PVM). Lab. Anim. Sci. 34, 35–37.

Smith, A.L., Jacoby, R.O., Johnson, E.A., Paturzo, F., Bhatt, P.N., 1993a. In vivo studies with an "orphan" parvovirus of mice. Lab. Anim. Sci. 43, 175–182.

Smith, A.L., Singleton, G.R., Hansen, G.M., Shellam, G., 1993b. A serologic survey for viruses and Mycoplasma pulmonis among wild house mice (Mus domesticus) in southeastern Australia. J. Wildl. Dis. 29, 219–229.

Smith, P.C., Nucifora, M., Reuter, J.D., Compton, S.R., 2007. Reliability of soiled bedding transfer for detection of mouse parvovirus and mouse hepatitis virus. Comp. Med. 57, 90–96.

Sobsey, M.D., 1989. Inactivation of health-related microorganisms in water by disinfection processes. Water Sci. Tech. 21, 179–195.

Strober, W., Ehrhardt, R.O., 1993. Chronic intestinal inflammation: an unexpected outcome in cytokine or T cell receptor mutant mice. Cell 75, 203–205.

Sundberg, J.P., Burnstein, T., Shultz, L.D., Bedigian, H., 1989. Identification of Pneumocystis carinii in immunodeficient mice. Lab. Anim. Sci. 39, 213–218.

Suzuki, H., Yorozu, K., Watanabe, T., Nakura, M., Adachi, J., 1996. Rederivation of mice by means of in vitro fertilization and embryo transfer. Exp. Anim. 45, 33–38.

Takahashi, Y., Okuno, Y., Yamanouchi, T., Takada, N., Yamanishi, K., 1986. Comparison of Immunofluorescence and hemagglutination inhibition tests and enzyme-linked immunosorbent assay for detection of serum antibody in rats infected with hemorrhagic fever with renal syndrome virus. J. Clin. Microbiol. 24, 712–715.

Tang, Y.W., Persing, D.H., 1999. Molecular detection and identification of microorganisms. In: Murray, P.R., Baron, E.J., Pfaller, M.A., Tenover, F.C., Yolken, R.H. (Eds.), Manual of Clinical Microbiology. ASM Press, Washington, DC.

Taylor, K., Copley, C.G., 1993. Detection of rodent RNA viruses by polymerase chain reaction. Lab. Anim. 28, 31–34.

Tenover, F.C., 1998. Molecular techniques for the detection and identification of infectious agents. In: Gorbach, S.L., Bartlett, J.G., Blacklow, N.R. (Eds.), Infectious Diseases. W.B. Saunders Company, Philadelphia, PA.

Tenover, F.C., Arbeit, R., Archer, G., Biddle, J., Byrne, S., Goering, R., et al., 1994. Comparison of traditional and molecular methods of typing of Staphylococcus aureus. J. Clin. Microbiol. 32, 407–415.

Thigpen, J.E., Lebetkin, E.H., Dawes, M.L., Amyx, H.L., Caviness, G.F., Sawyer, B.A., et al., 1989. The use of dirty bedding for detection of murine pathogens in sentinel mice. Lab. Anim. Sci. 39, 324–327.

Thomas III, M.L., Morse, B.C., O'Malley, J., Davis, J.A., St Claire, M.B., Cole, M.N., 2007. Gender influences infectivity in C57BL/6 mice exposed to mouse minute virus. Comp. Med. 57, 74–81.

Thompson, R.E., Smith, T.F., Wilson, W.R., 1982. Comparison of two methods used to prepare smears of mouse lung tissue for detection of Pneumocystis carinii. J. Clin. Microbiol. 16, 303–306.

Thornton, D.H., 1986. A survey of mycoplasma detection in veterinary vaccines. Vaccine 4, 237–240.

Tietjen, R.M., 1992. Transmission of minute virus of mice into a rodent colony by a research technician. Lab. Anim. Sci. 42, 422.

Tolbert, W.R., Rupp, R.G., 1989. Manufacture of pharmaceutical proteins from hybridomas and other cell substrates. Dev. Biol. Stand. 70, 49–56.

Trexler, P.C., 1983. Gnotobiotics. In: Foster, H.L., Small, J.D., Fox, J.G. (Eds.), The Mouse in Biomedical Research: Normative Biology, Immunology and Husbandry. Academic Press, San Diego, CA.

Trexler, P.C., Orcutt, R.P., 1999. Development of gnotobiotics and contamination control in laboratory animal science. In: Mcpherson, C.W., Mattingly, S. (Eds.), Fifty Years of Laboratory Animal Science American Association of Laboratory Animal Science, Memphis, TN. Chapter 16.

Truett, G.E., Walker, J.A., Baker, D.G., 2000. Eradication of infection with Helicobacter spp. by use of neonatal transfer. Comp. Med. 50, 444–451.

Tyler, J.W., Cullor, J.S., 1989. Titers, test, and truisms: rational interpretation of diagnostic serologic testing. JAVMA 194, 1550–1558.

Uchiyama, A., Besselsen, D.G., 2003. Detection of Reovirus type 3 by use of fluorogenic nuclease reverse transcriptase polymerase chain reaction. Lab. Anim. 37, 352–359.

Ushijima, H., Koike, H., Mukoyama, Hasegawa, A., Nishimura, S., Gentsch, J., 1992. Detection and serotyping of rotaviruses in stool specimens by using reverse transcriptionand polymerase chain reaction amplification. J. Med. Virol. 38, 292–297.

Van Der Gulden, W.J.I., Van Erp, A.J.M., 1972. The effect of parace-tic acid as a disinfectant on worm eggs. Lab. Anim. Sci. 22, 225–226.

Van Keuren, M.L., Saunders, T.L., 2004. Rederivation of transgenic and gene-targeted mice by embryo transfer. Transgenic. Res. 13, 363–371.

Voller, A., Bidwell, D.E., Bartlett, A., 1982. ELISA techniques in virol-ogy. In: Howard, C.R. (Ed.), New Developments in Practical Virology Alan R. Liss, New York.

Vonderfecht, S.L., Miskuff, R.L., Eiden, J.J., Yolken, R.H., 1985. Enzyme immunoassay inhibition assay for the detection of rat rotavirus-like agent in intestinal and fecal specimens obtained from diar-rheic rats and humans. J. Clin. Microbiol. 22, 726–730.

Vonderfecht, S.L., Eiden, J.J., Miskuff, R.L., Yolken, R.H., 1988. Kinetics of intestinal replication of group B rotavirus and relevance to diagnostic methods. J. Clin. Microbiol. 26, 216–221.

Waggie, K., Kagiyama, N., Allen, A.M., Nomura, T., 1994. Manual of Microbiologic Monitoring of Laboratory Animals. National Institutes of Health, Bethesda, (NIH publication no. 94-2498).

Waggie, K.S., Hansen, G., Ganaway, J., Spencer, T.H., 1981. A study of mouse strain susceptibility to Bacillus piliformis (Tyzzer's Disease): the association of B-cell function and resistance. Lab. Anim. Sci. 31, 139–142.

Waggie, K.S., Wagner, J.E., Lentsch, R.H., 1983. A naturally occur-ring outbreak of Mycobacterium avium intracellular infections in C57BL/6N mice. Lab. Anim. Sci. 33, 249–250.

Waggie, K.S., Hansen, G., Moore, T.D., Bukowski, M.A., Allen, A.M., 1988. Cecocolitis in immunodeficient mice associated with an enteroinvasive lactose-negative E. coli. Lab. Anim. Sci. 38, 389–393.

Waggie, K.S., Spencer, T.H., Ganaway, J., 1987. An enzyme-linked immunosorbent assay for detection of anti-Bacillus piliformis serum antibody in rabbits. Lab. Anim. Sci. 37, 176–179.

Wagner, A.M., Loganbill, J.K., Besselsen, D.G., 2003. Detection of Sendai virus and pneumonia virus of mice by use of fluorogenic nuclease reverse transcriptase polymerase chain reaction analysis. Comp. Med. 53, 173–177.

Wagner, A.M., Loganbill, J.K., Besselsen, D.G., 2004. Detection of lac-tate dehydrogenase-elevating virus by use of a fluorogenic nucle-ase reverse transcriptase-polymerase chain reaction assay. Comp. Med. 54, 288–292.

Walzer, P.D., Kim, C.K., Linke, M.J., Pogue, C.L., Heurkamp, M.J., Chrisp, C.E., et al., 1989. Outbreaks of Pneumocysitis carinii pneumo-nia in colonies of immunodefiient mice. Infect. Immun. 57, 62–70.

Ward, G.E., Moffatt, R., Olfert, E., 1978. Abortion in mice associated with Pasteurella pneumotropica. J. Clin. Microbiol. 8, 177–180.

Ward, J.M., Anver, M.R., Haines, D.C., Benveniste, R.E., 1994a. Chronic active hepatitis in mice caused by Helicobacter hepaticus. Am. J. Pathol. 145, 959–968.

Ward, J.M., Fox, J.G., Anver, M.R., Haines, D.C., George, C.V., Collins, M.J., et al., 1994b. Chronic active hepatitis and associated liver tumors in mice caused by a persistent bacterial infection with a novel Helicobacter species. J. Natl. Cancer. Inst. 86, 1222–1227.

Ward, J.M., Anver, M.R., Haines, D.C., Melhorn, J.M., Gorelick, P., Yan, L., et al., 1996. Inflammatory large bowel disease in immuno-deficient mice naturally infected with Helicobacter hepaticus. Lab. Anim. Sci. 46, 15–20.

Ward, J.M., Wobus, C.E., Thackray, L.B., Erexson, C.R., Faucette, L.J., Belliot, G., et al., 2006. Pathology of immunodeficient mice with naturally occurring murine norovirus infection. Toxicol. Pathol. 34, 708–715.

Washington, J.A., 1996. Principles of diagnosis. In: Baron, S. (Ed.), Medical Microbiology. The University of Texas Medical Branch at Galveston, Galveston, TX.

Wasson, K., 2007. Protozoa. In: Fox, J.G., Barthold, S.W., Davisson, M.T., Newcomer, C.E., Quimby, F.W., Smith, A.L. (Eds.), The Mouse in Biomedical Research, second ed. Academic Press, Burlington, MA.

Watson, J., 2008. New building, old parasite: mesostigmatid mites—an ever-present threat to barrier facilities. ILAR. J. 49, 303–309.

Watson, J., 2013. Unsterilized feed as the apparent cause of a mouse parvovirus outbreak. J. Am. Assoc. Lab. Anim. Sci. 52, 83–88.

Watson, J., Thompson, K.N., Feldman, S.H., 2005. Successful rederi-vation of contaminated immunocompetent mice using neonatal transfer with iodine immersion. Comp. Med. 55, 465–469.

Weir, E.C., Brownstein, D.G., Barthold, S.W., 1986. Spontaneous wast-ing disease in nude mice associated with Pneumocystis carinii infec-tion. Lab. Anim. Sci. 36, 140–144.

Weir, E.C., Brownstein, D., Smith, A., Johnson, E.A., 1988. Respiratory disease and wasting in athymic mice infected with pneumonia virus of mice. Lab. Anim. Sci. 38, 133–137.

Weisbroth, S.H., 1979a. Bacterial and mycotic diseases. In: Baker, H.J., Lindsey, J.R., Weisbroth, S.H. (Eds.), The Laboratory Rat: Biology and Diseases. Academic Press, Orlando, FL.

Weisbroth, S.H., 1979b. Parasitic diseases. In: Baker, H.J., Lindsey, J.R., Weisbroth, S.H. (Eds.), The Laboratory Rat: Biology and Diseases. Academic Press, Orlando, FL.

Weisbroth, S.H., 1999. Evolution of disease patterns in laboratory rodent: the post indigenous condition. In: Mcpherson, C.W., Mattingly, S. (Eds.), Fifty Years of Laboratory Animal Science American Association of Laboratory Animal Science, Memphis, TN. Chapter 19.

Weisbroth, S.H., Brobst, R.C., Smiley, D.P., 1996. Diagnosis of low level coccidiosis (Eimeria) infection in laboratory rabbits: evaluation of detection methods. Lab. Anim. Sci. 35, 87–89.

Weisbroth, S.H., Peters, R., Riley, L.K., Shek, W., 1998. Microbiological assessment of laboratory rats and mice. ILAR. J. 39, 272–290.

Weisbroth, S.H., Geistfeld, J., Weisbroth, S.P., Williams, B., Feldman, S.H., Linke, M.J., et al., 1999. Latent Pneumocystis carinii infection in commercial rat colonies: comparison of inductive immunosup-pressants plus histopathology, PCR, and serology as detection methods. J. Clin. Microbiol. 37, 1441–1446.

Weiss, E.E., Evans, K.D., Griffey, S.M., 2012. Comparison of a fur mite PCR assay and the tape test for initial and posttreatment diagno-sis during a natural infection. J. Am. Assoc. Lab. Anim. Sci. 51, 574–578.

Wescott, R.B., 1982. Helminths. In: Foster, H.L., Small, J.D., Fox, J.G. (Eds.), The Mouse in Biomedical Research: Diseases. Academic Press, New York.

West, W.L., Schofield, J.C., Bennett, B.T., 1992. Efficacy of the "micro-dot" technique for administering topical 1% ivermectin for the control of pinworms and fur mites in mice. Contemp. Top. Lab. Anim. Sci. 31, 7–10.

Whary, M.T., Fox, J.G., 2004. Natural and experimental Helicobacter infections. Comp. Med. 54, 128–158.

Whary, M.T., Fox, J.G., 2006. Detection, eradication, and research impli-cations of Helicobacter infections in laboratory rodents. Lab. Anim. (NY) 35, 25–27, 30–36.

Whary, M.T., Cline, J.H., King, A.E., Corcoran, C.A., Xu, S., Fox, J.G., 2000a. Containment of Helicobacter hepaticus by use of husbandry practices. Comp. Med. 50, 78–81.

Whary, M.T., Cline, J.H., King, A.E., Hewes, K.M., Chojnacky, D., Salvarrey, A., et al., 2000b. Monitoring sentinel mice for Helicobacter hepaticus, H. rodentium, and H. bilis infection by use of polymerase chain reaction analysis and serologic testing. Comp. Med. 50, 436–443.

Whary, M.T., Cline, J., King, A., Ge, Z., Shen, Z., Sheppard, B., et al., 2001. Long-term colonization levels of Helicobacter hepaticus in the cecum of hepatitis-prone A/JCr mice are significantly lower than those in hepatitis-resistant C57BL/6 mice. Comp. Med. 51, 413–417.

Wickramanayake, G.B., Sproul, O., 1991. Kinetics of the inactivation of microorganisms. In: Block, S.S. (Ed.), Disinfection, Sterilization, and Preservation. Lea & Febiger, Gainesville, FL.

Wilde, J., Eiden, J., Yolken, R., 1990. Removal of inhibitory sustances from human fecal specimens for detection of group A rotaviruses by reverse transcriptase and polymerase chain reaction. J. Clin. Microbiol. 28, 1300–1307.

Wunderlich, M.L., Dodge, M.E., Dhawan, R.K., Shek, W.R., 2011. Multiplexed fluorometric immunoassay testing methodology and troubleshooting. *J. Vis. Exp.* (58). http://dx.doi.org/doi:10.3791/3715

Xiao, S.Y., Chu, Y.K., Knauert, F., Lofts, R., Dalrymple, J.M., Leduc, J.W., 1992. Comparison of Hantavirus isolates using a genus-reactive primer pair polymerase chain reaction. J. Gen. Virol. 73, 567–573.

Yamanishi, K., Dantas, J.R., Takahashi, M., Yamanouchi, T., Domae, K., Kawamata, J., et al., 1983. Isolation of hemorrhagic fever with renal syndrome (HFRS) virus from a tumor specimen in a rat. Biken. J. 26, 155–160.

Yanabe, M., Shibuya, M., Gonda, T., Asai, H., Tanaka, T., Narita, T., et al., 1999. Production of ex-germfree rabbits for establishment of specific pathogen-free (SPF) colonies. Exp. Anim. 48, 79–86.

Yang, F.C., Paturzo, F.X., Jacoby, R.O., 1995. Environmental stability and transmission of rat virus. Lab. Anim. Sci. 45, 140–144.

Zenner, L., Regnault, J.P., 2000. Ten-year long monitoring of laboratory mouse and rat colonies in French facilities: a retrospective study. Lab. Anim. 34, 76–83.

Zhu, J., Yang, Q., Cao, L., Dou, X., Zhao, J., Zhu, W., et al., 2013. Development of porcine rotavirus vp6 protein based ELISA for differentiation of this virus and other viruses. Virol. J. 10, 91.

Zweig, M.H., Campbell, G., 1993. Receiver-operating characteristic (ROC) plots: a fundamental evaluation tool in clinical medicine. Clin. Chem. 39, 561–577.

Zweig, M.H., Robertson, E.A., 1987. Clinical validation of immunoassays: a well-designed approach to a clinical study. In: Chan, D.W., Perlstein, M.T. (Eds.), Immunoassay: A Practical Guide. Academic Press, Orlando, FL.

CHAPTER

12

Biology and Diseases of Dogs

Jean A. Nemzek, DVM, MS, DACVS[a], Patrick A. Lester, DVM,
MS, DACLAM[a], A. Marissa Wolfe, DVM[b], Robert C. Dysko, DVM,
DACLAM[a] and Daniel D. Myers, Jr., DVM, MPH, DACLAM[a]

[a]Unit for Laboratory Animal Surgery, University of Michigan, Ann Arbor, MI, USA
[b]Department of Comparative Medicine, Medical University of South Carolina, Charleston, SC, USA

OUTLINE

I. INTRODUCTION

A. Taxonomic Considerations

Dogs are mammals in the order Carnivora, suborder Caniformia (or superfamily Canoidea), and family Canidae. The domesticated dog has been designated as a subspecies of the gray wolf: *Canis lupus familiaris* (Wilson and Reeder, 2005). Other members of the genus *Canis* include four species of jackal and the coyote (*C. latrans*). *Canis lupus familiaris* is subdivided into approximately 400 breeds, ranging in size and shape from the teacup chihuahua to the large Irish wolfhound. The domesticated dog may have descended from prehistoric canids in Europe roughly 18,000–32,000 years ago (Thalmann *et al.*, 2013), although an East Asian origin is also possible (Savolainen *et al.*, 2002).

B. Use in Research

1. Historical Use of Dogs in Research

The dog played an important role as a laboratory animal in the early history of biomedical research, primarily because of its status as a cooperative companion animal of reasonable size. Dogs were used in the mid-1600s by William Harvey to study cardiac movement, by Marcello Malpighi to understand the basic lung anatomy and function, and by Sir Christopher Wren to demonstrate the feasibility of intravenous delivery of medications (Gay, 1984). The use of dogs continued as biomedical research advanced, and they were featured in many noteworthy studies, including those by Pavlov to observe and document the conditioned reflex response and by Banting and Best to identify the role of insulin in diabetes

Laboratory Animal Medicine, Third Edition
DOI: http://dx.doi.org/10.1016/B978-0-12-409527-4.00012-2

mellitus. A comprehensive but concise review of the use of the dog as a research subject is available in Gay (1984).

2. Current Use of Dogs in Research

The breed of dog most commonly bred for use in biomedical research is the beagle. Some commercial facilities also breed foxhounds or other larger dog breeds for use in surgical research studies. Some specific breeds with congenital or spontaneous disorders have also been maintained by research institutions (see examples below). Random-source dogs used in research are most frequently mongrels or larger dog breeds (e.g., German shepherd, Doberman pinscher, Labrador and golden retrievers) that are used for surgical research and/or training.

According to a computerized literature search for "beagle" for the years 2012–2013, a significant portion of the biomedical scientific publications identified were in the fields of pharmacology or toxicology. Especially common were studies focusing on pharmacokinetics, alternative drug delivery systems, and cardiovascular pharmacology. Other common areas of research using beagles were dental and periodontal disease and surgery, orthopedic surgery, skeletal physiology, and imaging studies. Other research areas that utilized beagles included canine infectious disease, prostatic urology, and ophthalmology.

Most large-sized dogs (either purpose-bred or random-source) are used in biomedical research because of their suitability for surgical procedures. Anesthetic protocols and systems for dogs are well established and the organs of larger dog breeds are often an appropriate size for trials of potential pediatric surgical procedures. Surgical canine models have been used extensively in cardiovascular, orthopedic, and transplantation research.

There are also some unique spontaneous conditions for which dogs have proven to be valuable animal models. A colony of gray collies had been maintained at the University of Washington (Seattle) for the study of cyclic hematopoiesis. This condition is manifested by periodic fluctuations of the cellular components of the blood, most notably the neutrophil population. These dogs can be used to study the basic regulatory mechanisms involved with hematopoiesis, as well as possible treatments for both the human and the canine conditions (Brabb et al., 1995). Golden retrievers affected with muscular dystrophy have been used as models of Duchenne muscular dystrophy in human children. Duchenne muscular dystrophy is caused by an absence of the muscle protein dystrophin, inherited in an X-linked recessive manner. The dystrophy in golden retrievers is caused by the absence of the same protein and is inherited in the same way. The clinical signs (such as debilitating limb contracture) are also similar between the canine and human conditions (Kornegay et al., 1994). Other genetic disorders studied in dog colonies include hereditary canine spinal muscle atrophy (Cork, 1991) and narcoplexy in

Doberman pinschers (Ripley et al., 2001). Bedlington terriers have been used to study copper storage diseases (such as Wilson's disease) and the development of spontaneous diabetes mellitus and hypothyroidism has been studied in several breeds of dogs for comparisons with the human conditions.

3. Decline in Numbers Used

Although historically the dog has been a common laboratory animal, their use in research has waned over the past 30 years. According to the U.S. Department of Agriculture (USDA), Animal and Plant Health Inspection Service (1998, 2011), the number of dogs used in research has declined from 211,104 in 1979 to 75,429 in 1997 (prior to the previous edition of this text) and 64,930 in 2010. This decrease was caused by a variety of factors, including (but not limited to) decreased availability, local restrictive regulations, conversion to other animal models (such as livestock or rodents), increased cost, and shift in scientific interest from pathophysiology to molecular biology and genetics.

C. Availability and Sources

Dogs used for research are generally segregated into two classes: purpose-bred and random-source. Purpose-bred dogs are those produced specifically for use in biomedical research; they are intended for use in long-term research projects and/or pharmacologic studies in which illness or medication would require removal from the study. Usually these dogs are either beagles or mongrel foxhounds, although other breeds may be available. Purpose-bred dogs typically receive veterinary care throughout their stay at the breeding facility. They are usually vaccinated against rabies virus, canine distemper virus, parvovirus, adenovirus type 2, parainfluenza virus, Leptospira serovars Canicola, Icterohaemorrhagiae, Grippotyphosa, and Pomona, and Bordetella bronchiseptica (Jasmin, personal communication). Purpose-bred dogs are also usually treated prophylactically for intestinal helminths and ectoparasites, and possibly given a heartworm preventative.

Random-source dogs are not bred specifically for use in research. They may be dogs bred for another purpose (e.g., hunting and racing) or stray dogs collected at pounds or shelters. The health status of these dogs can be the same quality as purpose-bred dogs, or it can be an unknown entity. Random-source dogs that have been treated and vaccinated in preparation for use in research are termed conditioned dogs. These dogs are then suitable for long-term studies or terminal preparations that require unperturbed physiologic parameters. Conditioned dogs are often tested for heartworm antigen because of the implications that infestations can have on cardiovascular status and surgical risk. Nonconditioned random-source dogs are useful only in a limited number of research studies, such as nonsurvival surgical training preparations and tissue/organ harvest.

Options for procurement of dogs for biomedical research typically include purchase from a USDA-designated Class A or Class B licensed dealer or directly from a municipal pound. The requirements for USDA licensure are detailed in Code of Federal Regulations (CFR), Title 9, Chapter 1 (1-1-92 edition), Subchapter A, Animal Welfare, 1.1 Definitions, and 2.1 Requirements and Application (Office of the Federal Register, 2002). Briefly, Class A licensees are breeders who raise all animals on their premises from a closed colony. Class B licensees purchase the dogs from other individuals (including unadopted animals from municipal pounds) and resell them to research facilities. There are additional regulations that apply to Class B dealers (such as holding periods and record-keeping documentation) because of the public concern that stolen pets could enter biomedical research facilities in this manner. In December 2013, the National Institutes of Health (NIH) issued notice NOT-OD-14-034 entitled *Notice regarding NIH plan to transition from use of USDA Class B dogs to other legal sources* (National Institutes of Health, 2013). This NIH policy begins in the fiscal year 2015 and prohibits the procurement of dogs from Class B dealers using NIH grant funds. From that point forward, dogs on NIH-funded studies will have to be obtained from Class A vendors, privately owned colonies (such as institutional breeding colonies), or client-owned animals (e.g., animals participating in veterinary clinical trials).

The best resource for identification of possible vendors are online 'Buyer's Guide' sites or 'Buyer's Guide' issues of trade periodicals. Online sites include the Buyer's Guide of the American Association of Laboratory Animal Science (http://laboratoryanimalbuyersguide.com), and the trade journals *Lab Animal* (http://guide.labanimal.com) and *Animal Lab News* (http://www.alnmag.com/content/buyers-guide). A 'Buyer's Guide' typically lists sources for both purpose-bred and random-source dogs, and denotes such features as pathogen-free status, health status, and availability of specific breeds and timed pregnant females. Some suppliers also have separate advertisements within issues of the journals.

D. Laboratory Management and Husbandry

Federal regulations promulgated by the Animal and Plant Health Inspection Service, USDA, in response to the Animal Welfare Act (7 CFR 2.17, 2.51, and 371.2[g]) are described in 9 CFR Chapter 1 (1-1-92 edition), Subchapter A, Animal Welfare (Office of the Federal Register, 2002). Regulations pertaining specifically to the care of dogs used in research are found in Subpart A, Specifications for the Humane Handling, Care,

Treatment, and Transportation of Dogs and Cats of Part 3 (Standards) of Subchapter A. Particular attention should be paid to Section 3.6c (*Primary Enclosures—Additional Requirements for Dogs*) because the space required for housing dogs is calculated using body length rather than weight (a parameter used for other species and also for dogs in the National Research Council (NRC) guidelines). Section 3.8 (Exercise for Dogs) describes the requirements that dealers, exhibitors, and facilities must follow in order to provide dogs with sufficient exercise.

The Institute for Laboratory Animal Research (ILAR) has written the *Guide for the Care and Use of Laboratory Animals* (National Research Council, 2011). The 'Guide' is the primary document used by institutional animal research units to develop their programs and by animal care evaluation groups, such as the Association for Assessment and Accreditation of Laboratory Animal Care International (AAALAC International), to facilitate site visits and inspections. The primary difference between the 7th and 8th editions of the 'Guide' (National Research Council, 1996, 2011) regarding the care of dogs is the notation that "Enclosures that allow greater freedom of movement and unrestricted height (i.e., pens, runs, or kennels) are preferable." The ILAR Committee on Dogs authored *Dogs: Laboratory Animal Management* (National Research Council, 1994). This publication describes "features of housing, management, and care that are related to the expanded use of dogs as models of human diseases" and includes "an interpretive summary of the Animal Welfare Regulations and the requirements of the Public Health Service Policy on Humane Care and Use of Laboratory Animals." The reader is encouraged to use these publications to obtain further information on care and husbandry of dogs in the biomedical research setting.

II. BIOLOGY

A. Normal Values

The information presented in the tables represents a range of normal values that can vary depending on the analytical method, as well as the age, breed, and sex of the animal. Table 12.1 shows representative normal

TABLE 12.1 Normal Vital Signs

Physiologic parameters[a]	Reference ranges
Temperature	37.9–39.9°C, 100.2–103.8°F
Heart rate (beats/min)	70–120
Respiratory rate (breaths/min)	18–34
Capillary refill time (seconds)	<2

[a]*Modified from Detweiler D.K. and Erickson H.H., Regulation of the Heart, in Dukes' Physiology of Domestic Animals, 12th edn., Reece W.O., Ed. Copyright 2004 by Cornell University.*

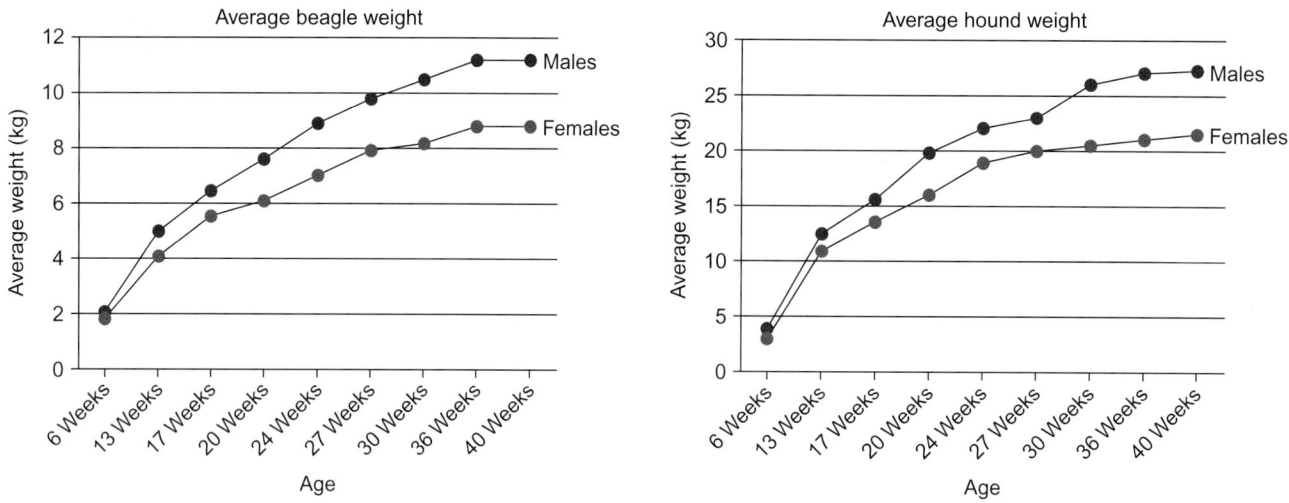

FIGURE 12.1   Average weight in kilograms by age in weeks for male and female beagle and hound dogs. *Data courtesy of Dr. Asheley Wathen, Covance Laboratories, Inc., Madison, WI, and Dr. Kimberley Cohen, Covance Laboratories, Inc., Cumberland, VA (2013).*

TABLE 12.2   Hematology Data from Purpose-Bred Beagles at Covance Laboratories, Inc.

Complete blood count[a]	Reference range	Units	4-Month male beagle	4-Month female beagle	6-Month male beagle	6-Month female beagle	8-Month male beagle	8-Month female beagle
HGB	12.1–20.3	g/dl	12.1	11.8	14.2	14.4	15.2	15.7
HCT	36–60	%	40.8	38.8	47.9	47.6	49.7	51.6
WBC	4.0–15.5	thousand/µl	18.6	20.3	14.4	11.5	11.6	11.8
RBC	4.8–9.3	million/µl	5.61	5.7	6.5	6.5	6.8	7
MCV	58–79	fl	73	68	74	73	73	74
MCH	19–28	pg	21.6	20.8	21.8	22.7	22.4	22.3
MCHC	30–38	g/dl	29.7	30.5	29.6	30.2	30.6	30.4
PLT	17–400	thousand/µl	512	438	436	345	329	344
DIFFERENTIAL								
Neutrophils	3000–13000	µ/l	12211	13172	9265	5202	8844	7074
Bands	0–300	µ/l	0	0	0	0	0	0
Lymphocytes	530–4800	µ/l	4648	5697	3916	3216	3036	3812
Monocytes	100–1800	µ/l	1325	1011	840	717	792	679
Eosinophils	0–1900	µ/l	446	369	310	253	528	187
Basophils	0–150	µ/l	0	0	19	20	0	71
OTHER TESTS								
T4	1.0–4.0	ng/dl	2.1	2.1	2	1.6	2.8	2.3

HGB, hemoglobin; HCT, hematocrit; WBC, white blood cells; RBC, red blood cells; MCV, mean corpuscular volume; MCH, mean corpuscular hemoglobin; MCHC, mean corpuscular hemoglobin concentration; PLT, platelets; T4, thyroxine.

[a]*Beagle baseline data averaged from blood testing performed in December 2011. From Dr. Asheley Wathen, Covance Laboratories, Inc., Madison, WI, and Dr. Kimberley Cohen, Covance Laboratories, Inc., Cumberland, VA (2013).*

physiological data for a mixed population of dogs of both sexes. Fig. 12.1 demonstrates the normal weights and corresponding ages for both male and female beagle and hound dogs. Tables 12.2 and 12.3 feature hematology data from beagles of both sexes from two commercial facilities. Tables 12.4 and 12.5 list serum chemical data for beagles of both sexes from two commercial facilities. Representative blood gas, coagulation

TABLE 12.3 Hematology Data from Purpose-Bred Beagles at Marshall BioResources

Complete blood count[a]	Units	6-Month male beagle (n =>1000)	6-Month female beagle (n =>1000)
HGB	g/dl	14.7 ± 1.3	15.2 ± 1.3
HCT	%	45.6 ± 3.6	47.0 ± 3.7
WBC	Thousand/μl	15.2 ± 3.9	14.7 ± 3.8
RBC	Million/μl	6.5 ± 0.5	6.7 ± 0.5
MCV	fl	70.3 ± 2.7	70.1 ± 3.0
MCH	pg	22.7 ± 0.9	22.7 ± 1.0
MCHC	g/dl	32.3 ± 1.2	32.4 ± 1.3
MPV	fl	11.2 ± 2.1	10.8 ± 1.9
RDW	%	13.6 ± 0.8	13.6 ± 0.9
HDW	g/dl	1.8 ± 0.2	1.8 ± 0.2
PLT	×10³/μl	410.1 ± 112.2	397.0 ± 115.7
DIFFERENTIAL			
Neutrophils	×10³/μl	8.6 ± 3.1	8.3 ± 2.8
Lymphocytes	×10³/μl	5.1 ± 1.1	5.1 ± 1.1
Monocytes	×10³/μl	1.0 ± 0.4	0.9 ± 0.4
Eosinophils	×10³/μl	0.3 ± 0.2	0.2 ± 0.1
Basophils	×10³/μl	0.2 ± 0.1	0.2 ± 0.1
PERCENTAGE			
Neutrophils	%	55.6 ± 6.6	55.7 ± 6.1
Lymphocytes	%	34.4 ± 6.4	35.2 ± 6.1
Monocytes	%	6.3 ± 1.7	5.8 ± 1.4
Eosinophils	%	2.0 ± 1.1	1.6 ± 0.9
Basophils	%	1.2 ± 0.5	1.3 ± 0.5

HGB, hemoglobin; HCT, hematocrit; WBC, white blood cells; RBC, red blood cells; MCV, mean corpuscular volume; MCH, mean corpuscular hemoglobin; MCHC, mean corpuscular hemoglobin concentration; MPV, mean platelet volume; RDW, red cell distribution width; HDW, hemoglobin distribution width; PLT, platelets.
[a]Data generated by the Marshall Farms USA Bayer Advia 120 Hematology Analyzer. From Dr. Bambi Jasmin, Marshall BioResources, North Rose, NY (2013).

data, and normal urinalysis parameters can be found in Tables 12.6–12.8, respectively. Finally, the reviews in *Arterial and Venous Blood Gas Anaylses* (Rieser, 2013) and the *Manual of Canine and Feline Cardiology* (Tilley et al., 2007) are excellent resources.

B. Nutrition

Good nutrition and a balanced diet are essential to the health, performance, and well-being of the animal. The NRC of the United States National Academy of Sciences is the leading provider of nutrient recommendations for dogs and provides average requirements needed to maintain growth and prevent deficiencies (Subcommittee on Dog and Cat Nutrition, 2006). The NRC publications form the basis for the Association of American Feed Control Officials (AAFCO) nutrient profiles, which are updated periodically (Baldwin et al., 2010). The AAFCO is an advisory body comprising state representatives from across the United States. It provides a mechanism for developing and implementing uniform and equitable laws, regulations, standards, and enforcement policies, and establishes nutrient profiles for cat and dog foods (Dzanis, 1994; Thatcher et al., 2010). Additional resources should be consulted for details on the nutritional requirements for dogs of all ages (Dzanis, 1994; Subcommittee on Dog and Cat Nutrition, 2006; Baldwin et al., 2010; Thatcher et al., 2010; Hand et al., 2010).

Recommendations for feeding the appropriate amount of diet are determined by the dog's metabolic requirements. The maintenance energy requirement (MER) is the amount of energy used by a moderately active adult animal in a thermoneutral environment. The MER for most breeds may be calculated using the following equation: MER (metabolizable kcal/day) = BW × 0.75 × 550 kJ DE, where BW = body weight (kg), kJ = kilojoules, DE = digestable energy (Kienzle and Rainbird, 1991).

In-depth overviews of diets used in biomedical research are available in diet-specific literature. *Open-Formula Diets* have defined concentrations of all ingredients and the information is publicly available. This allows researchers to control for this important environmental variable and enables retrospective analysis of possible diet composition effects on research results (Barnard et al., 2009). Open-formula diets occasionally may require changes in formulation to maintain nutrient composition or meet changing nutrient requirements. These changes in quantitative ingredient formulation are made public when open-formula diets are modified. In contrast, *closed-formula diets* are commercially available, balanced diets that meet and label the minimum requirements for protein and fat and the maximum values for ash and fiber; however, the exact composition of ingredients may vary from batch to batch. Ingredient composition varies as the manufacturer applies a least-cost strategy, referring to formulating diets to maximize profit by using the least-expensive ingredients. Although the ingredients are listed, the quantitative ingredient formulation is not publicly available and can vary without public disclosure, due to proprietary nature of commercial diets produced and marketed under vendor trade names. Closed-formula diets have also been referred to as 'fixed formula' or 'constant nutrition' (LabDiets, PMI Nutrition International, St. Louis, Missouri) by manufacturers (Barnard et al., 2009). In *fixed-formula diets*, the quantitative ingredient formulation does not change; however, this information is proprietary and therefore

TABLE 12.4   Clinical Chemistry Data from Beagles at Covance Laboratories, Inc.[a]

Blood chemistry	Reference range	Units	4-Month male beagle	4-Month female beagle	6-Month male beagle	6-Month female beagle	8-Month male beagle	8-Month female beagle
Total protein	5.0–7.4	g/dl	5.4	5.3	5.9	5.5	5.8	5.8
Albumin	2.7–4.4	g/dl	2.9	2.8	3.2	3.2	3.2	3.4
Globulin	1.6–3.6	g/dl	2.5	3.5	2.6	2.4	2.6	2.3
Albumin/globulin ratio	0.8–2.0	ratio	1.2	1.2	1.2	1.4	1.3	1.5
AST (SGOT)	15–66	U/l	51	48	50	36	40	63
ALT (SGPT)	12–118	U/l	41	39	42	47	44	57
ALP	5–131	U/l	124	122	97	98	99	72
GGTP	1–12	U/l	6	5	5	5	6	5
Total bilirubin	0.1–.03	mg/dl	0.1	0.1	0.2	0.2	0.1	0.2
BUN	6–25	mg/dl	20	22	25	24	18	21
Creatinine	0.5–1.6	mg/dl	0.4	0.4	0.4	0.4	0.5	0.5
Phosphorus	2.5–6.0	mg/dl	8.6	9.2	8.2	7.5	6.5	6.3
Glucose	70–138	mg/dl	87	76	65	90	82	80
Calcium	8.9–11.4	mg/dl	11	11	7.9	9.2	10.5	10.4
Magnesium	1.5–2.5	mEq/dl	1.7	1.7	1.8	1.7	1.6	1.9
Sodium (Na)	139–154	mEq/dl	144	147	147	145	145	148
Potassium (K)	3.6–5.5	mEq/dl	5.6	5.5	6.4	5.6	5	5.1
Na/K ratio		ratio	26	27	23	26	28	29
Chloride	102–120	mEq/dl	98	108	105	105	108	109
Cholesterol	92–324	mg/dl	159	152	136	127	151	141
Triglycerides	29–291	mg/dl	91	96	72	64	62	44
Amylase	290–1125	U/l	614	604	713	543	671	597
Lipase	77–695	U/l	160	189	200	224	147	280
CPK	59–895	U/l	945	829	606	318	624	741

AST, aspartate aminotransferase; ALT, alanine aminotransferase; ALP, alkaline phosphatase; GGTP, gamma-glutamyl transpeptidase; BUN, blood urea nitrogen; CPK, creatine phosphokinase.

[a]Beagle baseline data averaged from blood testing performed in December 2011. From Dr. Asheley Wathen, Covance Laboratories, Inc., Madison, WI, and Dr. Kimberley Cohen, Covance Laboratories, Inc., Cumberland, VA (2013).

not disclosed publically (Barnard *et al.*, 2009). *Semi-purified and purified* diets provide the strictest control of ingredients and are formulated from purified components: amino acids, lipids, carbohydrates, vitamins, and minerals. Although purified and semipurified diets do differ in the types of ingredients used, the terms are generally used to mean the same thing. Purified-ingredient diets are generally 'open' formulas, meaning that they are published and available to the scientific community.

The animal care provider should be aware of the manufacture date of the diet, which should be clearly visible on the bag. As a general rule, diets are safe for consumption up to 6 months following the manufacture date when stored at room temperature. Refrigeration may prolong

the shelf-life, but the best strategy is to feed only fresh diets and use each lot based on the date of manufacture. Specifications for feeding and watering of dogs are provided in the regulations of the Animal Welfare Act.

C. Reproduction

Management of a breeding colony requires broad knowledge of the dog's anatomy, reproductive physiology, and behavioral needs during breeding, gestation, and parturition. Although a comprehensive discussion of the biology of canine reproduction is beyond the scope of this chapter, essential features of the broad topics noted above are presented.

TABLE 12.5 Clinical Chemistry Data from Beagles at Marshall BioResources

Blood chemistry[a]	Units	6-Month male beagle (n = 50)	6-Month female beagle (n = 50)
Total protein	g/dl	5.1 ± 0.3	5.2 ± 0.4
Albumin	g/dl	2.7 ± 0.3	2.7 ± 0.3
Globulin	g/dl	2.5 ± 0.1	2.4 ± 0.2
AST (SGOT)	U/l	43.7 ± 7.1	46.3 ± 7.0
ALT (SGPT)	U/l	33.7 ± 5.6	37.5 ± 7.2
ALP	U/l	154.4 ± 36.4	113.3 ± 24.8
GGTP	U/l	6.8 ± 1.0	7.7 ± 2.9
Total bilirubin	mg/dl	0.2 ± 0.1	0.3 ± 0.1
BUN	mg/dl	19.0 ± 4.8	17.7 ± 3.5
Creatinine	mg/dl	0.9 ± 0.2	0.8 ± 0.2
Phosphorus	mg/dl	7.8 ± 0.6	7.8 ± 0.8
Glucose	mg/dl	87.8 ± 10.0	88.7 ± 8.8
Calcium	mg/dl	11.5 ± 0.4	11.1 ± 0.3
Magnesium	mEq/dl	1.9 ± 0.1	1.9 ± 0.1
Sodium (Na)	mEq/dl	146.6 ± 2.5	145.5 ± 1.6
Potassium (K)	mEq/dl	5.2 ± 0.4	5.1 ± 0.4
Na/K ratio	ratio	28.1 ± 2.0	28.7 ± 2.0
Chloride	mEq/dl	114.6 ± 1.8	111.9 ± 1.6
Cholesterol	mg/dl	202.2 ± 32.0	181.8 ± 26.0
Amylase	U/l	688.5 ± 99.2	687.9 ± 84.6
CPK	U/l	243.7 ± 64.1	230.2 ± 52.5

AST, aspartate aminotransferase; ALT, alanine aminotransferase; ALP, alkaline phosphatase; GGTP, gamma-glutamyl transpeptidase; BUN, blood urea nitrogen; CPK, creatine phosphokinase.
[a]Data generated by the Marshall BioResources Vitros 250. From Dr. Bambi Jasmin, Marshall BioResources, North Rose, NY (2013).

TABLE 12.6 Normal Physiologic Data for Dogs

Arterial blood gas[a]	Reference range
pH	7.3–7.5
PCO_2 (mmHg)	30.8–42.8
PO_2 (mmHg)	80.9–103.3
HCO_3 (mEq/l)	18.8–25.6

[a]From Tieser T.M., Arterial and Venous Blood Gas Analysis, Topics in Companion Animal Medicine **28** (2013) 86–90.

1. Anatomy and Reproductive Physiology of the Bitch

Overall health, body condition, nutrition, and age greatly influence reproductive efficiency (Gavrilovic et al., 2008; Johnson, 2008). Therefore, only normal,

TABLE 12.7 Normal Coagulation Data in Dogs

Coagulation tests[a,b]	Time (seconds)
Prothrombin time (OSPT)	6–10
Activated partial thromboplastin time	11–19
Thrombin clotting time	3–8
Activated clotting time	55–80

[a]Modified from The Laboratory Canine, Taylor & Francis, New York, Garrett Field, Todd A. Jackson (2007).
[b]Values from coagulation tests may have wide variability due to collection method, anticoagulant used, analyte (whole blood, serum, plasma, platelet poor plasma), temperature, and method of analysis.

TABLE 12.8 Normal Chemistry-Urinalysis in Dogs

Urine volume and specific gravity[a]	
Volume (ml/kg body weight/day)	24–41
Specific gravity (g/l)	1.016–1.060
pH	5.5–7.5
Glucose/ketones	0

[a]Modified from Reece W.O., Kidney Function in Mammals, in Dukes' Physiology of Domestic Animals, 12th edn., Reece W.O., Ed. Copyright 2004 by Cornell University.

healthy animals in excellent body condition should be used in breeding programs. Beagles between 2 and 3.5 years of age have the best conception rates and litter size with the lowest neonatal mortality. After 5 years of age, conception rates and litter size decline and neonatal mortality increases (Johnson, 2008).

The vagina is a long, musculomembranous canal that extends from the uterus to the vulva. During physical examination, the gloved finger or examination instrument should be introduced through the dorsal commissure of the vulva, avoiding the deep ventral clitoral fossa. Examination should proceed at an angle of approximately 60° until the instrument or fingertip has passed over the ischial arch, after which it can be directed further craniad toward the cervix. The uterus consists of the cervix, uterine body, and uterine horns. The cervix is an abdominal organ, located approximately halfway between the ovaries and the vulva. When the bitch is in proestrus and estrus, the cervix can be distinguished during abdominal palpation as an enlarged, turgid, walnut-shaped structure.

Female dogs are monoestrous, typically nonseasonal, spontaneous ovulators that have a spontaneous luteal phase approximately 5 days longer than the 65 ± 1 days of pregnancy followed by obligate anestrus. Puberty (beginning of the first estrus) occurs between 6 and 14 months in most breeds. The time of onset positively correlates with the body size (Concannon, 2011).

The canine cycle is divided into four phases: proestrus, estrus, diestrus, and anestrus. The duration of proestrus is 5–20 days with an average of 9 days and reflects the follicular phase rise in estrogen. During this stage, the vulva is enlarged and turgid, and a serosanguinous vaginal discharge is present (Concannon, 2011). Estrus may be from 5 to 15 days in duration but generally lasts 9 days. The endocrine feature of estrus is the first abrupt increase in progesterone (>5ng/ml), which occurs concomitantly with the luteinizing hormone (LH) surge 95% of the time, followed by ovulation within 24–72 h. The vulva is softer and smaller than in proestrus. The vaginal discharge persists and may remain serosanquinous or become straw colored.

Diestrus begins approximately 9 days after the onset of standing heat. The end of this stage is 60 days later, which would be coincident with whelping if the bitch had become pregnant. Defined behaviorally as starting when estrous behavior ceases (Concannon, 2011), diestrus represents the peak of serum progesterone. Anestrous may last from 80 to 240 days and is the stage of reproductive quiescence. It is characterized by an absence of ovarian activity and serum progesterone levels of less than 1ng/ml.

2. Anatomy and Reproductive Physiology of the Male Dog

The onset of puberty in the male ranges from 5 to 12 months of age and is affected by breed, season, nutrition, and disease status. This process is initiated by the secretion of LH from the anterior pituitary, which stimulates the production of testosterone by the interstitial or Leydig's cells. At this time, the testicular growth is rapid, the seminiferous tubules begin to differentiate, and Sertoli cells form the blood–testis barrier. Secretion of follicle-stimulating hormone (FSH) by the anterior pituitary stimulates the production of other key hormones by the Sertoli cells, including, inhibin, androgen binding protein, and estrogen. FSH stimulates spermatogenesis in the presence of testosterone, whereas inhibin and estrogen provide negative feedback to the pituitary gland to decrease FSH production. Spermatogenesis in the dog is completed in 45 days, with subsequent maturation of sperm occurring in the epididymis for approximately 15 days. Thus, the entire process from the initiation of spermatogonial mitosis to the delivery of mature sperm to the ejaculate is 60 days.

A breeding soundness exam should be conducted to assess the probability of a male dog's successful production of offspring. Factors affecting male fertility include libido, ability to copulate, testicular size, and quality semen production. Supression of sexual behavior and problems with libido may occur in dogs due to early weaning, isolation, or inherited abnormalities. Animals with poor hind limb conformation or trauma to the back may be unable to properly mount the female. There is a positive correlation between scrotal circumference and

the number of sperm produced. Finally, the quality of sperm is assessed by motility, morphology, volume, and concentration. An ejaculate (5ml) that contains approximately 500 million progressively motile sperm without significant morphological abnormalities is a good indicator of normal male fertility. Complete anatomy of the bitch and dog can be found in *Miller's Anatomy of the Dog* (Evans and de Lahunta, 2012).

3. Detection of Estrus and Pregnancy

Cells of the vaginal epithelium mature to keratinized squamous epithelium under the influence of estrogen. Because of the rise in estrogen throughout proestrus, with peak levels occurring just prior to the onset of standing heat, the vaginal smear can be used as an indicator of the bitch's readiness for breeding. The smear will not confirm the presence of ovulation nor is it of prognostic value in normal bitches during anestrus.

The percentage of vaginal epithelial cell cornification is an index of estrogen secretion by the ovarian follicles. Cornification occurs approximately 2 days prior to the estrogen peak and 4 days prior to standing heat. As cornification of vaginal epithelial cells proceeds, the cells become larger, with more angular borders. The nuclear/cytoplasmic ratio decreases until the nuclei reach a point where they no longer take up stain (coincident with the onset of estrus). The cells appear 'anuclear' and are classified as 'cornified' or 'anuclear squames.' The vaginal cytology smear of the bitch changes from predominantly cornified to noncornified 6 days after ovulation. The day of this change is the first day of diestrus. Other epithelial cell types noted on vaginal cytology include superficial cells (large, angular cells with small nuclei); intermediate cells (round or oval cells with abundant cytoplasm and large, vesicular nuclei); and parabasal cells (small round or elongated cells with large, well-stained nuclei, and a high nuclear/cytoplasmic ratio). Based on vaginal cytology, the estrous cycle is classified as follows:

Proestrus, early: intermediate and superficial cells, red blood cells, and neutrophils
Proestrus, late: superficial cells, anuclear squames, and red blood cells
Estrus: more than 50% anuclear squames, superficial cells, ± red blood cells
Diestrus: more than 50% intermediate cells, superficial cells, and squames early, but becoming completely noncornified with neutrophils present as diestrus proceeds
Anestrus: small numbers of parabasal cells and intermediate cells, ± neutrophils

Although vaginal cytology is a useful tool, observation of behavioral estrus is the best criterion to use in breeding management. During proestrus, the male is attracted to the bitch and will investigate her hindquarters, but she will not accept breeding. Estrus is characterized by proactive receptivity to mounting by males and increased male-seeking behavior (Concannon, 2011). During this stage, the bitch will exhibit 'flagging,' or elevation of her tail with muscular elevation of the vulva to facilitate penetration by the male. In order to maximize the conception rate and litter size, it is recommended to breed the bitch on days 1, 3, and 5 of the standing heat. Due to the long life span of canine sperm, fertilization occurs in the oviduct up to 8 days after coitus. The ovulated oocyte is a primary oocyte that must undergo two meiotic divisions before fertilization can occur. This overall maturation process takes approximately 2 days. After maturation, the oocyte remains viable for 4–5 days. Optimal conception rates tend to occur when the bitch is bred from 4 days before to 3 days after ovulation; best litter size is achieved when the bitch is bred 2 days after ovulation.

4. Pregnancy

Implantation is evident by areas of local endometrial edema 17–18 days after breeding. There is no correlation between the number of corpora lutea and the number of fetuses in the corresponding uterine horn, suggesting transuterine migration of embryos.

The dog has endotheliochorial placentation. The endothelium of uterine vessels lies adjacent to the fetal chorion, mesenchymal, and endothelial tissues, so that maternal and fetal blood are separated by four layers. The canine placenta is also classified as zonary, indicating the placental villi are arranged in a belt, and deciduate, reflecting that maternal decidual cells are shed with fetal placentas at parturition.

The length of gestation is 59–63 days. Luteal progesterone is responsible for maintaining pregnancy and canine corpora lutea retain their structural development throughout gestation. Serum progesterone rises from less than 1 ng/ml in late proestrus to a peak of 30–60 ng/ml during gestation, and then declines to 4–5 ng/ml just prior to parturition. Progesterone is essential for endometrial gland growth, secretion of uterine milk, attachment of the placentas, and inhibition of uterine motility (Johnson, 2008; Verstegen-Onclin and Verstegen, 2008).

Pregnancy detection can be performed by several methods. Abdominal palpation of the uterus may be most informative at approximately 28 days after breeding. The embryos and chorioallantoic vesicles form a series of ovoid swellings and are approximately 2 inches in length at 28–30 days. By day 35, the uterus begins to enlarge diffusely and the vesicles become difficult to identify by palpation. Radiology can be used to confirm pregnancy and facilitate determination of gestational age, beginning 45 days after the LH surge (Lopate, 2008). Bitches in which a difficult whelping is anticipated should be radiographed in late pregnancy to determine

the litter size and to evaluate the size of the fetal skulls in relation to the bony maternal birth canal.

Ultrasonography can be used to confirm pregnancy beginning on days 18–22, at which point the gestational sacs will be approximately 1 cm in diameter, and until parturition (Shille and Gontarek, 1985; Lopate, 2008). Ultrasonography can assess fetal viability by visualizing fetal heartbeats and fetal movement beginning on gestational days 23–25 and 35, respectively (Lopate, 2008). It can also predict gestational age using the inner diameter of the chorionic cavity in early pregnancy and the biparietal diameter in late pregnancy (Beccaglia and Luvoni, 2006; Luvoni and Beccaglia, 2006). However, ultrasonography for determination of gestational age is most accurate at day 30 of pregnancy when using correction factors for small (<9 kg) and large (>40 kg) body weight dogs (Kutzler et al., 2003).

5. Parturition and the Neonate

Thermal support should be provided prior to parturition. Dogs housed on grated flooring should be provided with mats and those on solid floors would benefit from blankets placed in a corner of the primary enclosure. Shavings are discouraged because they may adhere to the umbilical cord and predispose to ascending infections. Heat lamps may be placed 24 h prior to parturition and remain until all neonates demonstrate vigorous suckling behavior. However, the use of heat lamps necessitates strict supervision in order to prevent thermal burns. If possible, whelping bitches should be housed in a quiet corridor in order to decrease periparturient stress, especially in primiparous or young mothers. Monitoring of parturition is important, but human intervention should be minimal in order to prevent stress-induced cannibalism.

An abrupt drop in body temperature to less than 100°F indicates impending parturition within 18–24 h. The process of parturition has been divided into three stages. Stage 1 of labor lasts 6–12 h and is characterized by uterine contractions and cervical dilation. During this stage, the bitch may appear restless, nervous, and anorexic. Other common clinical signs include panting and increased pulse rate (Johnson, 2008).

Fetal expulsion occurs during stage 2, which lasts approximately 3–6 h. As the fetus engages the cervix, there is release of oxytocin, referred to as the Ferguson reflex, which strengthens the uterine contractions and may elicit abdominal contractions as well. The bitch is able to inhibit this stage of labor if disturbed. The chorioallantois ruptures either during passage of each neonate through the birth canal or by the bitch's teeth at birth. Interestingly, posterior presentation is common in dogs but does not predispose to dystocia. The time interval between deliveries of each pup is irregular, but the average is less than 1 h between pups. Veterinary assistance is necessary if the bitch remains in stage 2 for more than 5h without delivering the first pup, or for more than 2h before delivering subsequent pups.

During stage 3 of labor, the placentas are expelled either immediately or within 15min of delivery of each pup. If two pups are delivered from alternate uterine horns, then the birth of both puppies may precede expulsion of the respective placentas. The bitch will lick the newborn vigorously to remove the membranes from its head and to promote respiration. She will also sever the umbilical cord. The bitch may ingest the placentas, although they confer no known nutritional benefit and may induce a transient diarrhea.

The peripartum use of oxytocin is required only in the event of uterine inertia, stillbirths, or agalactia. Oxytocin should not be used in the event of systemic illness or abnormalities precluding vaginal delivery. Indications for its use include lack of delivery 24h after onset of stage 1 labor, greater than 1h of unproductive stage 2 labor, inadequate contractions, or abnormal vaginal discharge. In these cases, radiographs are recommended to assess fetal size in relation to the birth canal and any possible obstructions, followed by 0.25–2.00 IU of oxytocin intramuscularly or subcutaneously. The oxytocin can be repeated 30–60min after the first dose for a total of two doses (Plunkett, 1993). In some cases, treatment with 0.5–1.5ml/kg of 10% calcium gluconate, delivered slowly IV while monitoring closely for bradycardia, and 25% dextrose IV may be indicated.

Uterine involution occurs during anestrus within 4–5 weeks of parturition. During this time, a greenish to red–brown vaginal discharge, or lochia, is considered normal. The presence of an odiferous, purulent discharge, accompanied by systemic signs of illness, indicates metritis or pyometra. Desquamation of the endometrium begins by the 6th postpartum week, with complete repair by 3 months.

Newborn puppies are easily sexed by examination of the anogenital distance. In female puppies, the vulva is evident a short distance from the anus, whereas the prepuce of male puppies is nearly adjacent to the umbilicus. Eyes are open at approximately 12 days, and ears are patent at approximately 12–20 days. Solid food can be introduced between 4.5 and 6 weeks of age, and puppies can be weaned at 6–8 weeks.

6. Artificial Insemination

Artificial insemination (AI) is indicated when the male is physically incapable of mounting or penetrating the bitch, when there are vaginal abnormalities such as a vaginal–vestibular stricture, narrow vagina, vaginal septum, and vaginal hyperplasia, or if there is a behavioral incompatibility between the male and female dogs (Kutzler, 2005).

Semen is collected using a plastic centrifuge tube and rubber latex artificial vagina. The male is introduced to the scent of an estrous bitch and manually stimulated. The first two fractions are collected followed by a sufficient amount of the third fraction (predominantly of prostatic fluid) to bring the total semen volume to 4–6ml.

The semen can be introduced into the cranial vagina or directly into the uterus either through trans-cervical catheterization with a Norwegian AI catheter or utilizing fiberoptic endoscopy. Use of the Norwegian AI catheter for intrauterine insemination of frozen-thawed, fresh, and chilled-extended semen results in significantly higher whelping rates than intravaginal insemination (Linde-Forsberg et al., 1999; Thomassen and Farstad, 2009). For trans-cervical insemination, the bitch is either standing on all four legs or standing with hindquarters raised. The AI catheter and guiding tube are inserted into the vestibulum as far as the pseudocervix. Firm abdominal palpation is then used to locate and fix the cervix in the other hand, at which point the catheter is further inserted along the dorsal vaginal fold until the cervical opening is located and semen is deposited into the uterus lumen (Thomassen and Farstad, 2009).

Surgical and laparoscopic AI has been used successfully for intrauterine and intratubal insemination; however, these techniques are invasive and require anesthesia. Therefore, the nonsurgical techniques mentioned above are recommended, as these approaches are less invasive and can be completed without anesthesia in nonsedated or sedated dogs depending on the experience of the personnel and personality of the dogs.

AI with freshly collected sperm can be done on days 1, 3, and 5 of standing heat or on days of maximal vaginal cornification. The viability of frozen-thawed sperm is significantly reduced compared to fresh or chilled sperm that may live up to 5 or 6 days in the reproductive tract of the bitch; frozen-thawed sperm live only a few hours. Therefore, the ova must be mature and insemination with frozen-thawed semen must be done 2–3 days after ovulation in the bitch as determined by serum progesterone concentrations (Thomassen et al., 2006).

7. False Pregnancy

False pregnancy (pseudocyesis), a stage of mammary gland development and lactation associated with nesting or mothering behavior, is common in the bitch. The condition occurs after the decline in serum progesterone toward the end of diestrus. There is no age or breed predisposition. Pseudopregnancy does not predispose the bitch to reproductive disease or infertility. A comprehensive review of canine pseudocyesis exploring its cause, clinical features, and treatments is covered by C. Gobello (Gobello et al., 2001).

8. Reproductive Life Span

Reproductive performance in the bitch is optimal prior to 4 years of age. Cycling does not completely cease; however, after 5–8 years of age, bitches demonstrate significant decreases in conception rate and the number of live pups whelped. By 8–9 years of age, pathologic conditions of the uterus, such as cysts, hyperplasia, atrophy, and neoplasia, are extremely common.

D. Behavior

Dogs prefer living in a social environment. Dogs have well developed olfactory glands, vision, and auditory and tactile senses that allow them to gain environmental cues and information from other dogs and humans (Field and Jackson, 2006; Joint Working Group on Refinement, 2004). Much of their instinctive behavior is dependent on learning to interact with other members of their species. Beagles have been a popular animal model because of their docile nature. They are easily handled and, for the most part, respond favorably to repetitive manipulations such as body weight measurements, physical examination, electrocardiograms (ECGs), oral gavage, and venipuncture.

Although sexually mature by 6–9 months of age, dogs are not socially mature until 18–36 months of age. The socialization process should begin early during development, when puppies are receptive to conspecific and human contact. For example, from 3 to 8 weeks of age, puppies are most capable of learning about how to interact with other dogs. Between weeks 5 and 12, puppies are most capable of learning how to interact with people. By 10–12 weeks of age, dogs voluntarily wander and explore new environments. Thus, early handling and mild stress (such as vaccination) appear to be extremely beneficial components of a dog's social exposure.

Canid social systems use signals and displays that minimize the probability of outright aggression. These behavior patterns are most likely elicited during distressful situations, such as strange environments, being handled by strange people, or encountering new animals. An excellent, illustrated discussion of normal canine behavior patterns can be found in the canine behavior section of the *Manual of Clinical Behavioral Medicine for Dogs and Cats* (Overall, 2013).

III. DISEASES

By virtue of the dog's status as a companion animal, there are many veterinary publications and reference texts on the diagnosis, medical management, pathology, and epidemiology of its disorders. The authors of this chapter have chosen to emphasize those diseases that are more frequently encountered in the research setting, especially infectious diseases associated with the use of random-source dogs and conditions seen frequently in the beagle. For more thorough and detailed discussion of these diseases, as well as those not discussed in this chapter, the reader should consult standard veterinary textbooks.

A. Infectious Diseases

1. Bacterial and Mycoplasmal Diseases

a. Canine Infectious Respiratory Disease (Kennel Cough Complex and Infectious Tracheobronchitis)

Etiology Canine infectious respiratory disease (CIRD) is a highly contagious illness and several organisms have been incriminated including *Bordetella bronchiseptica*; *Streptococcus equi* subsp. *zooepidemicus*; canine parainfluenza virus (CPIV); canine influenza virus (CIV); canine respiratory coronavirus; canine adenovirus type 2 (CAV-2); canine herpesvirus; canine reovirus types 1, 2, and 3; and mycoplasma and ureaplasma. Naturally occuring infection can result in coinfection by two or more organisms (Garnett *et al.*, 1982; Ford, 2012).

Clinical Signs CIRD can be subdivided into mild or severe forms. The mild form is more common and is characterized by an acute onset of a loud, dry, hacking cough. Increased formation of mucus sometimes results in a productive cough, followed by gagging or retching motions. Cough may be elicited by tracheal palpation and may be more frequent with excitement or exercise. Otherwise, dogs are typically asymptomatic. Mild tracheobronchitis usually lasts 7–14 days, even when untreated.

The severe form results from poor general health, immunosuppression, or lack of vaccination. Secondary bronchopneumonia can occur and can be the determinant of severity (Sherding, 1994). Animals are clinically ill and may be febrile, anorexic, and depressed. Productive cough and mucopurulent naso-ocular discharge are more common than in the mild form.

Epizootiology and Transmission The natural reservoir for *B. bronchiseptica* is the respiratory tract (Bemis, 1992), and it is very easily spread by aerosol and direct contact. Transmission is heightened by confined housing of multiple animals. *Bordetella bronchiseptica* is highly infectious with an incubation period of 3–10 days.

Pathogenesis The most common clinical isolates are CPIV and *B. bronchiseptica* (Mochizuki *et al.*, 2008). However, *B. bronchiseptica* is often recovered from clinically healthy animals (Chalker *et al.*, 2003). During clinical infection, *B. bronchiseptica* attaches to the cilia of the upper airway epithelium, causing suppurative tracheobronchitis and bronchiolitis. Infections with CPIV or CAV-2 alone are usually subclinical but can cause necrotizing tracheobronchiolitis (Dungworth, 1985).

Diagnosis and Differential Diagnosis Diagnosis is often based on clinical signs and known history; however, cough elicited by tracheal palpation may be inconsistent and should not be used for definitive diagnosis. Presumptive diagnosis can be made by isolation of *B. bronchiseptica* or mycoplasma by nasal swabs. Viral isolation or paired serology is often impractical and expensive. If cough persists for more than 14 days, other disease conditions should be considered. Differential diagnoses include CIV, canine distemper virus, pneumonia, heartworm disease, tracheal collapse, mycotic infections, and diseases resulting in tracheal compression (Johnson, 2000).

Prevention Prevention is best achieved by avoiding exposure to infected animals. Dogs should be vaccinated prior to or upon admission to the animal facility. Intranasal vaccines protect against infection and disease and can be given to dogs as young as 3 weeks of age (Greene and Levy, 2012). Combination vaccines for *B. bronchiseptica*, CAV-2, and CPIV are preferred. Vaccinations should be boostered every 6 months when multiple animals are housed in a confined area.

Control Staff must practice proper hygiene to prevent transmission by fomites. Sanitation, proper ventilation, and proper humidity are critical for control. Symptomatic animals should be isolated and kennels should be disinfected with agents such as bleach, chlorhexidine, or quaternary ammonium chloride.

Treatment Bordetella bronchiseptica is sensitive to potentiated sulfas, chloramphenicol, quinolones, tetracyclines, gentamicin, and kanamycin. Use of antibiotics is indicated when severe or persistent clinical signs occur and should be continued for 14 days. For severe or unresponsive infection, treatment should be based on bacterial culture/sensitivity patterns. Nebulized gentamicin or kanamycin may be helpful in severe cases. Antitussives should be avoided if the cough is productive; however, their use is indicated if coughing is causing discomfort or interfering with sleep. Bronchodilators such as aminophylline, theophylline, or terbutaline can be helpful in reducing reflex bronchoconstriction.

Research Complications Due to the altered respiratory tract physiology, infected animals should not be used for pulmonary studies.

b. Group C Streptococcus Infections

Etiology β-Hemolytic Lancefield's group C streptococcus (*S. equi* ssp. *zooepidemicus*) is a gram-positive, non-spore-forming coccus that causes pneumonia and sepsis in dogs.

Clinical Signs Clinical signs vary based on the organ system affected. Pneumonic disease is typically associated with sudden onset of clinical signs including

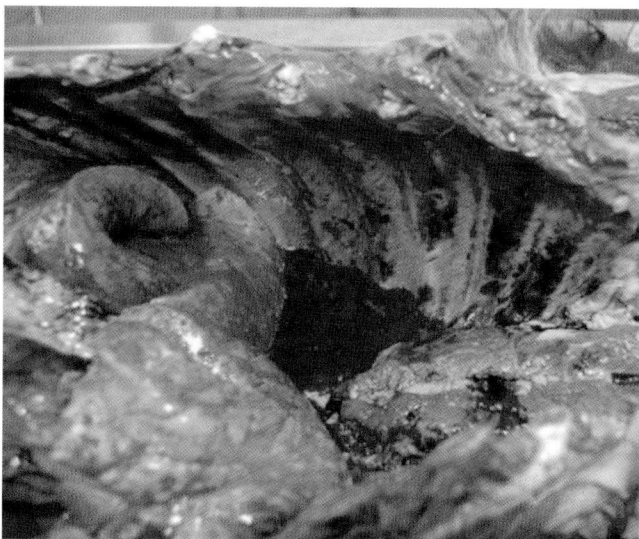

FIGURE 12.2 Open view within the thoracic cavity of a dog after acute death from *Streptococcus equi* subsp. *zooepidemicus*. Petechial and eccymotic hemorrhages evident on the parietal pleura and hemorrhagic fluid within the thoracic cavity. *Reprinted from The Veterinary Journal, vol. 188, Priestnall, S. and Erles, K., Streptococcus zooepidemicus: an emerging canine pathogen, pp. 142–148, 2011, with permission from Elsevier.*

coughing, weakness, fever, dyspnea, and hematemesis. The rapid progression of disease is similar to that seen in humans with toxic shock syndrome (TSS) caused by *Streptococcus pyogenes*. Peracute death has been reported in research and shelter dogs (Bergdall *et al.*, 1996; Pesavento *et al.*, 2008).

Epizootiology and Transmission Streptococcus *equi* ssp. *zooepidemicus* is not considered a commensal of healthy dogs as most of the β-hemolytic commensal organisms belong to group G, specifically *Streptococcus canis*. Asymptomatic carriers are suspected to be the route by which infection enters populations. *Streptococcus equi* ssp. *zooepidemicus* is considered an opportunistic pathogen and stressful factors such as transport can predispose to disease (Priestnall *et al.*, 2010).

Pathologic Findings In peracute cases, hemorrhage from the mouth and nose and within the pleural cavity can be the most striking lesion. Ecchymotic and petechial hemorrhages can be noted on several organs (Fig. 12.2). 'Bull's-eye' lesions may be observed on the pleural surface of affected lung lobes. Histologic lesions can include fibrino-suppurative, necrotizing, and hemorrhagic pneumonia. Gram-positive cocci can be found in intracellular clusters throughout the lung (Fig. 12.3), tonsils, and spleen of affected animals (Bergdall *et al.*, 1996; Priestnall and Erles, 2011).

Pathogenesis Predisposing factors such as transport stress and viral coinfection have been shown to contribute to the virulence of *S. zooepidemicus* (Priestnall and Erles, 2011). Due to the similarities with the clinical

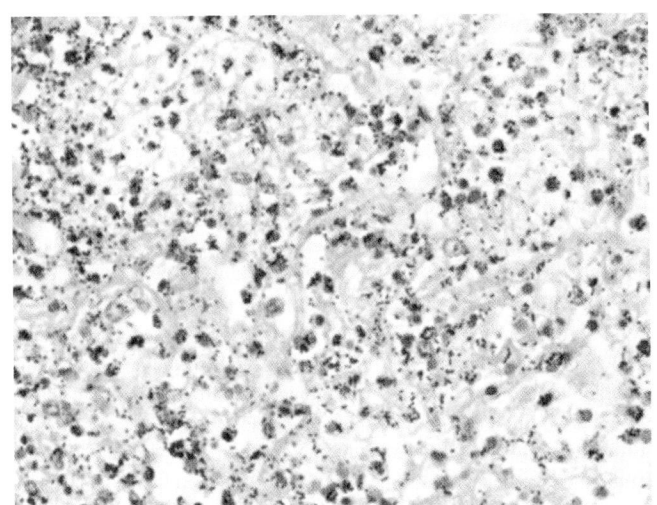

FIGURE 12.3 Gram stain of *Streptococcus zooepidemicus*-positive canine lungs. Numerous gram-positive coccoid bacteria within the alveolar spaces. Some bacteria evident within neutrophil cytoplasm. Magnification ×400. *Reprinted from The Veterinary Journal, vol. 188, Priestnall, S. and Erles, K., Streptococcus zooepidemicus: an emerging canine pathogen, pp. 142–148, 2011, with permission from Elsevier.*

signs seen in human cases of TSS, superantigens are thought to contribute to the virulence of *S. zooepidemicus* in cases of acute hemorrhagic pneumonia. These superantigens work by bypassing the conventional mechanisms of antigen presentation and binding to major histocompatibility complex class II receptors. As a result, there is a hyperactive proinflammatory response and an 'avalanche' of cytokines including interleukin 1β (IL-1β), interleukin 6 (IL-6), and tumor necrosis factor alpha (TNF-α). Three novel superantigen-encoding genes have been identified from a case of acute fatal hemorrhagic pneumonia, *szeF*, *szeN*, and *szeP*. However, it is currently unclear what effect these superantigens have *in vivo* (Paillot *et al.*, 2010; Priestnall *et al.*, 2010). While superantigens have been detected in some isolates, there is not enough data to determine if superantigens play a role in the pathogenesis (Byun *et al.*, 2009; Kim *et al.*, 2007).

Diagnosis and Differential Diagnosis Definitive diagnosis is based on bacterial culture of nasal swabs or transtracheal lavage. Polymerase chain reaction (PCR) can be done on post-mortem lung tissue. Bacterial pneumonias or bacteremias can be caused by other pathogenic *Streptococcus* spp., *Staphylococcus* spp., *Escherichia coli*, *Pasteurella multocida*, *Pseudomonas* spp., *Klebsiella pneumoniae*, and *B. bronchiseptica*. Nonbacterial causes of respiratory disease include rodenticide intoxication, coagulopathies, heartworm disease, pulmonary thromboembolism, ruptured aneurysm, and left-sided congestive heart failure.

Prevention and Control There is no vaccine for prevention of *S. zooepidemicus*. The organism has been

isolated from the environment during active outbreaks (Pesavento *et al.*, 2008), so dogs diagnosed with *S. zooepidemicus* should be quarantined and any potential fomites (e.g. food bowls, enrichment) should be properly disinfected.

Treatment Antibiotic therapy should be based on culture and sensitivity. Resistance to doxycycline and tetracycline has been demonstrated (Garnett *et al.*, 1982; Pesavento *et al.*, 2008).

Research Complications Dogs with severe hemorrhagic pneumonia or systemic disease are not appropriate for research study. The association between epizootics of this disease and transportation supports operational policies that require adequate acclimation periods for animals upon arrival.

c. Leptospirosis

Etiology Serovars Canicola, Bratislava, and Grippotyphosa result in renal or hepatic disease, whereas serovars Icterohaemorrhagiae and Pomona predominantly result in hepatic disease (Greene *et al.*, 2012).

Clinical Signs Canine leptospirosis can present as subclinical, acute, or chronic disease. Clinical signs in acute infection can be nonspecific and include lethargy, depression, abdominal discomfort, stiffness, anorexia, vomiting, muscle tenderness, and pyrexia. Clinical signs can be related to renal failure including polyuria and polydipsia, with or without azotemia, oliguria, or anuria. Leptospirosis can also lead to hepatic failure with signs such as icterus or bleeding abnormalities. Peracute leptospirosis is characterized by shock, vascular collapse, and rapid death. Uveitis, abortions, stillbirths, and pulmonary hemorrhage have also been associated with leptospirosis (Klopfleisch *et al.*, 2010; van de Maele *et al.*, 2008).

Epizootiology and Transmission Bivalent vaccines against the most common canine serovars, Icterohaemorrhagiae and Canicola, have resulted in the increased prevalence of other serovars including Grippotyphosa, Pomona, Bratislava, and Autumnalis. Increased movement of wild animal reservoirs (rats, raccoons, skunks, opossums) into urban/suburban areas have also contributed to the greater prevalence of previously uncommon serovars (Sykes *et al.*, 2011). Transmission occurs primarily through environmental contact, although direct transmisson between hosts may also occur. Leptospires passing from urine into water is the most common route of contamination (Goldstein, 2010). Leptospirosis is a zoonotic disease.

Pathologic Findings The kidneys consistently have gross and microscopic lesions. In the acute phase, the kidneys are swollen with subcapsular and cortical ecchymotic hemorrhages. Petechial or ecchymotic hemorrhages and swelling of the lungs may also be noted. Hepatic lesions during the acute phase consist of diffuse hemorrhage and necrotic foci (Searcy, 1995). In chronic stages of leptospirosis, the kidneys become small and fibrotic. Endothelial cell degeneration and focal to diffuse lymphocytic–plasmacytic interstitial nephritis are the characteristic histopathological findings.

Pathogenesis The severity and course of leptospirosis depend on the causative serovar as well as the age and immune status of the dog. Infection occurs after the leptospires penetrate a mucous membrane or abraded skin. The organisms then invade the vascular space and multiply rapidly, reaching the renal tubular epithelium several days postinfection. Acute or progressive renal failure leading to oliguria or anuria may occur. Nephritis may or may not be accompanied by hepatitis, uveitis, pulmonary hemorrhage, and meningitis. Disseminated intravascular coagulation is often a secondary complication.

Diagnosis and Differential Diagnosis Paired serology for the microscopic agglutination test is the most reliable means of definitive diagnosis, and successive serum sampling should be done 7–14 days after the first sample. PCR can be used to identify active infection early in the disease when serologic testing is negative or in previously vaccinated animals (Sykes *et al.*, 2011). Differential diagnoses include other causes of acute renal failure and hepatitis.

Prevention and Control According to the American Animal Hospital Association's 2011 vaccination guidelines, vaccination for leptospirosis is recommended based on geographic location and exposure risk (Welborn *et al.*, 2011). Both quadrivalent and bivalent inactivated bacterins are available. Quadrivalent bacterins protect against Canicola, Icterohaemorrhagiae, Grippotyphosa, and Pomona serovars, whereas bivalent bacterins cover only Canicola and Icterohaemorrhagiae. Immunization does not prevent the development of the carrier state or protect against other serovars. Control requires preventing contact with wildlife reservoirs as well as identification of carrier animals.

Treatment Doxycycline is the drug of choice as it can eliminate renal colonization. If vomiting or allergic reactions prohibit treatment with doxycycline, ampicillin or other penicillins should be utilized. Aggressive fluid therapy and supportive care may also be needed.

Research Complications Due to the zoonotic potential, dogs with clinical leptospirosis should not be used in research studies.

d. Campylobacteriosis

Etiology *Campylobacter* spp. are thin, curved or spiral, microaerophilic, thermophilic motile gram-negative rods. Many species of *Campylobacter* have been isolated from normal and diarrheic animals; however, the most common pathogenic species include *Campylobacter jejuni* ssp. *jejuni* and *C. coli* (Marks *et al.*, 2011).

Clinical Signs Most adult animals infected with *C. jejuni* are asymptomatic carriers; clinical signs are most commonly noted in dogs that are less than 6 months of age (Greene, 2000; Burnens *et al.*, 1992). In cases of clinical illness, mild and intermittent mucoid or watery diarrhea, with or without frank blood, is most commonly noted. Signs typically last 5–21 days but can persist for several months. Tenesmus, inappetance, vomiting, and a mild fever may accompany the diarrhea (Marks *et al.*, 2011). Bacteremia and cholecystitis secondary to *C. jejuni* have also been documented in dogs (Fox, 2012).

Epizootiology and Transmission The role of *Campylobacter* spp. as a primary pathogen has been questioned; it may require a coenteropathy to produce disease (Sherding and Johnson, 1994). Stress or immunosuppression may make animals more susceptible. Transmission is via the fecal–oral route, mostly through contaminated food or water. *Campylobacter jejuni* can be zoonotic with immunocompromised individuals at greatest risk.

Pathologic Findings Lesions depend on the mechanism of the enteropathy (Van Kruiningen, 1995). Enterotoxin production results in dilated, fluid-filled bowel loops, with little or no histopathologic alteration. Cytotoxin-mediated disease results in a friable, hemorrhagic mucosal surface. Histologically, the mucosa is ulcerated with lymphoplasmacytic infiltration. Translocation can result in edema and congestion of the lamina propria with focal accumulation of granulocytes. Epithelial hyperplasia and decreased goblet cell numbers are also noted. *Campylobacter jejuni* may be visualized between enterocytes with Warthin–Starry silver-stained sections.

Pathogenesis Clinical disease may be produced by several different mechanisms as *Campylobacter* spp. have a variety of virulence factors including enterotoxins, cytotoxins, and adherence or invasion properties. *Campylobacter jejuni* can cause an erosive enterocolitis by invasion of epithelium and production of the cytolethal distending toxin (cdt) (Fox, 2012; Van Kruiningen, 1995). In addition, *C. jejuni* can produce illness via translocation to regional lymph nodes causing a mesenteric lymphadenitis.

Diagnosis and Differential Diagnosis Fresh feces (per rectum) can be used for presumptive diagnosis by demonstration of highly motile, curved or spiral organisms with dark-field or phase-contrast microscopy. Gram-stained *C. jejuni* appear as gull-winged rods. Definitive diagnosis requires isolation of the organism (Sherding and Johnson, 1994). Culture requires selective isolation media, and growth is favored by reduced oxygen tension and a temperature of 37°C. A PCR multiplex assay for differentiation of *C. jejuni*, *C. coli*, *C. lari*, *C. upsaliensis*, and *C. fetus* ssp. *fetus* has been developed (Wang *et al.*, 2002). Any disorder that can cause diarrhea in dogs should be considered as a differential diagnosis.

Prevention and Control Proper environmental sanitation, waste disposal, and food storage can prevent campylobacteriosis. In enzootic situations, group housing should be avoided. Outbreaks are controlled by isolation and treatment of affected individuals.

Treatment Antibacterial treatment should be considered in severely ill dogs. Erythromycin, neomycin, enrofloxacin, clindamycin, and doxycycline are all effective. Resistance to quinolones and ciprofloxacin has been documented (Acke *et al.*, 2009). Treatment should be a minimum of 10–14 days with bacterial cultures repeating 1 and 4 weeks after treatment.

Research Complications Dogs with clinical campylobacteriosis have temporary derangements to digestive and absorptive functions.

e. Helicobacteriosis

Etiology Helicobacters are gram-negative, microaerophilic, spiral bacteria that infect the gastrointestinal tract. *Helicobacter* spp. can be separated into gastric and enterohepatic groups. The gastric helicobacters commonly identified in dogs are referred to as non-*Helicobacter pylori* helicobacters or *H. heilmannii sensu lato* and include *H. felis*, *H. bizzozeronii*, *H. salomonis*, *H. cynogastricus*, and *H. heilmannii sensu stricto*, formerly *Candidatus H. heilmanni* (Haesebrouck *et al.*, 2011; Joosten *et al.*, 2013). The most common enterohepatic species found in dogs include *H. bilis*, *H. canis*, and *H. cinaedi* (Castiglioni *et al.*, 2012; Dewhirst *et al.*, 2005; Fox, 2012). Canine *Helicobacter* spp. isolated from human tissues, suggesting zoonotic transmission, include *H. bizzozeronii*, *H. salomonis*, *H. bilis*, *H. canis*, and *H. heilmannii s.s.* (Haesebrouck *et al.*, 2009; Fox, 2012).

Clinical Signs Most infections are subclinical in the dog. Gastric infections may present with vomiting, diarrhea, and fever, accompanied by anorexia, pica, or polyphagia. Enterohepatic helicobacters have been linked with inflammatory bowel disease in experimental animal models. Heavy infections in dogs have been associated with inflammatory lesions of the large intestine (Castiglioni *et al.*, 2012; Nguyen *et al.*, 2013).

Epizootiology and Transmission The epizootiology and transmission of *Helicobacter* spp. in the dog remain unknown. Both oral–oral and fecal–oral routes for transmission have been suggested in humans, but transmission via canine saliva is a less reliable source of infection (Craven *et al.*, 2011). Enterohepatic infections of pet dogs are as high as 52% (Castiglioni *et al.*, 2012). Prevalence of gastric *Helicobacter* infections in colony or shelter dogs can be as high as 82–100% (Fox, 1995; Hermanns *et al.*, 1995).

Pathologic Findings Gastritis is usually mild and characterized by reduced mucus content of the surface epithelium with vacuolation, swelling, karyolysis, and karyorrhexis of parietal cells. Multifocal infiltrates of plasma cells and neutrophils occur around blood vessels and between gastric pits (Hermanns *et al.*, 1995). Intestinal lesions include mild to moderate lymphoplasmacytic infiltration as well as crypt dilation and crypt hyperplasia (Castiglioni *et al.*, 2012).

Pathogenesis Gastric helicobacters are urease positive, which assists with survival in the acidic environment of the stomach (Kusters *et al.*, 2006; Uberti *et al.*, 2013). Enterohepatic helicobacters are urease negative and typically reside in the lower intestine. The mechanism by which enterohepatic helicobacters colonize the liver is thought to be through portal circulation after uptake by enterocytes or through retrograde movement from the intestine into the bile duct (Fox, 2012).

Diagnosis and Differential Diagnosis Organisms may be demonstrated with histopathology on endoscopic or surgical biopsy tissue samples. Warthin–Starry silver stain may increase the sensitivity for histopathologic diagnosis. Culture may be difficult depending on the *Helicobacter* spp. For species that produce urease, a positive urease test on a gastric biopsy specimen may give a presumptive diagnosis. The urea breath test has been successfully used to diagnose *Helicobacter* spp. in laboratory beagles with a sensitivity and specificity of 89% (Kubota *et al.*, 2013). Western blot has been used to detect serum antibodies to enterohepatic species and PCR can be used to detect *Helicobacter* spp. in fecal samples (Oyama *et al.*, 2012; Wadström *et al.*, 2009). Any causes of acute or chronic vomiting and diarrhea in the dog are differential diagnoses.

Prevention and Control Until more is known about the epizootiology and transmission of *Helicobacter* spp., specific recommendations cannot be made for prevention and control.

Treatment For gastric species, combination therapy of amoxicillin (10 mg/kg q12h), metronidazole (30 mg/kg q24h), and sucralfate (0.25–0.5 mg/kg q8h) has proven to be most effective (Hall and Simpson, 2000). Replacing sucralfate with famotidine, omeprazole, or bismuth subsalicylate may also be effective (Marks, 1997; Jenkins and Bassett, 1997; DeNovo and Magne, 1995). Recurrence rates within 60 days of treatment can be as high as 80% (Anacleto *et al.*, 2011). Treatment of enterohepatic helicobacters may depend on species susceptibility. Aminoglycosides have been successful in treating *H. cinaedi*, but resistance to fluoroquinolones has been documented (Tomida *et al.*, 2013). Combination therapy of amoxicillin, clarithromycin, metronidazole, and omeprazole in medicated chow has been successful in eliminating various enterohepatic helicobacters from mice (del Carmen Martino-Cardona *et al.*, 2010). Long-term antibiotic treatment at a minimum of 21 days is suggested for enterohepatic and gastric helicobacters.

Research Complication Dogs used in gastrointestinal physiology or oral pharmacology studies should be free from helicobacteriosis.

2. Viral and Chlamydial Diseases

a. Canine Parvovirus Enteritis

Etiology Parvoviral enteritis in dogs is caused by canine parvovirus strain 2 (CPV-2) of the family Parvoviridae, genus *Protoparvovirus*, species *Carnivore protoparvovirus 1*. Currently, there are three antigenic variants, 2a, 2b, and 2c. Parvoviruses are nonenveloped, single-stranded DNA viruses.

Clinical Signs While parvoviral infection can affect the gastrointestinal tract, bone marrow, myocardium, and nervous tissues, the most common manifestation of disease is acute enteritis. Clinical signs usually appear 5 days after fecal–oral inoculation and include anorexia, fever, depression, vomiting, and profuse intractable diarrhea which may become hemorrhagic. Excessive fluid and protein losses through the gastrointestinal tract result in rapid and severe dehydration. Dogs can develop severe leukopenia with a total leukocyte count of 1000 cells/μl or less. Repeated hemograms may provide prognostic value, as rebounds in leukocyte counts are indicative of impending recovery. Terminally ill dogs may develop hypothermia, icterus, or disseminated intravascular coagulation due to endotoxemia.

Epizootiology and Transmission Parvovirus can infect dogs of any age, but puppies between 6 and 20 weeks of age are particularly susceptible. Puppies less than 6 weeks of age are protected by passive maternal antibody. Strain CPV-2c has been associated with severe disease in adult vaccinated dogs (Calderon *et al.*, 2009).

Pathogenesis Canine parvovirus has an affinity for rapidly dividing cells of the intestine and causes acute enteritis with intestinal crypt necrosis and villus atrophy. The virus also has tropism for the bone marrow and lymphoid tissues; thus, leukopenia and lymphoid depletion accompany the intestinal destruction.

Diagnosis and Differential Diagnosis Parvovirus can be detected with a commercially available fecal enzyme-linked immunosorbent assay (ELISA). Due to intermittent and brief shedding of the virus, fecal ELISAs can have false-negative results. PCR can be used to confirm an ELISA result and to differentiate the viral strain. At necropsy, diagnosis is based on gross and histopathologic evidence of necrosis and dilatation of intestinal crypt cells with secondary villous collapse.

Prevention and Control Parvoviral-positive animals should be quarantined for at least 10 days as the infectious virus is shed for several days after onset of clinical signs. Although PCR has been used to detect viral DNA in feces for up to 6 weeks (Decaro *et al.*, 2005), it is currently unknown if the material being shed at this time is still infectious. Disinfection of exposed areas with dilute bleach (1:30) or a commercial disinfectant is essential for elimination of the virus. Six-week-old puppies should be vaccinated every 2–4 weeks with a modified live vaccine until at least 16 weeks of age.

Treatment Treatment is largely supportive and aimed at restoring fluid and electrolyte balance. Antimicrobial therapy is recommended due to intestinal compromise and risk of sepsis. Early nutritional support continued throughout the disease has been shown to decrease recovery times (Mohr *et al.*, 2003).

Research Complications Infection with parvovirus precludes the use of a particular dog in an experimental protocol. Due to the significant discomfort of the animal, as well as the intensive therapy required, humane euthanasia is usually chosen in a research setting.

b. Rabies

Etiology Rabies virus is a *Lyssavirus* belonging to the family Rhabdoviridae.

Clinical Signs Clinical progression of neurologic disease occurs in three stages. The first, prodromal, stage is characterized by a change in species-typical behavior. The loss of the instinctive fear of humans by a wild animal is a classic sign of impending rabies. In the second, furious, stage, animals are easily excited or hyperreactive to external stimuli and will readily bite at inanimate objects. The third, paralytic, stage is characterized by incoordination and ascending ataxia of the hindlimbs due to viral-induced damage of motor neurons. Death due to respiratory failure usually occurs after onset of the third stage.

Epizootiology and Transmission Wild animals such as raccoons, skunks, and bats are common reservoirs of infection for domestic animals, which in turn are the principal source of infection for humans. Transmission occurs primarily by contact with infected saliva, usually via bite wounds.

Pathogenesis The incubation period for rabies is 3–8 weeks to the onset of clinical signs but can range from 1 week to 1 year. Bites to the head and neck result in shorter incubation periods due to the close proximity to the brain. Following infection, the virus migrates centripetally via peripheral nerve fibers to neurons within the brain, resulting in neurologic dysfunction. On reaching the brain, the virus migrates centrifugally to the salivary glands, thus enabling shedding and subsequent transmission.

Diagnosis and Differential Diagnosis Definitive diagnosis is based on immunofluorescence of the virus in Negri bodies of hippocampal cells. Submission of the whole, unfixed brain, including the cerebellum and proximal brain stem, should be done within 48 h of collection. The tissue should be kept refrigerated as freezing can cause delays in testing. Differential diagnoses include pseudorabies, canine distemper, bacterial meningitis, and toxicants that affect neurologic function.

Prevention and Treatment Puppies should be vaccinated by 16 weeks of age, again at 1 year, and then annually or triennially, depending on state and local laws.

Research Complications Immuno-prophylaxis is recommended for animal care and research personnel who may have work-related risks of exposure. Due to risk of human exposure, animals with suspected infection should be humanely euthanized and brain tissue should be submitted for confirmation.

3. Parasitic Diseases

a. Protozoa

Giardiasis Giardia lamblia, also known as *G. duodenalis* and *G. intestinalis*, is a binucleate flagellate protozoan that usually causes subclinical infestation of the small intestine. Clinical disease is usually seen in young dogs and the characteristic sign is voluminous, light-colored, foul-smelling, soft to watery diarrhea, which is the result of malabsorption and hypersecretion. *Giardia* has a direct life cycle with infection resulting after consuming cyst-contaminated food or water. The change in pH between the stomach and duodenum activates excystation and trophozoites then attach to the enterocytes. For diagnosis, direct fecal smears are considered best for observing trophozoites and zinc sulfate centrifugation is preferred for detection of cysts. A commercial ELISA kit is licensed for use in dogs, but the positive predictive value is poor and zinc sulfate centrifugation techniques should be used in conjunction with ELISA (Rishniw *et al.*, 2010). PCR assays are also available for diagnosing giardiasis. Differential diagnoses for giardiasis include bacterial and protozoal enteritis, coccidiosis, and whipworm infestation. Metronidazole at 25–30 mg/kg PO q12 h for 5–10 days is effective at treating giardiasis as well as other enteric protozoans, which may be potential differential diagnoses or coinfections. Albendazole, fenbendazole, pyrantel, and praziquantel are also effective.

Coccidiosis Intestinal coccidia associated with enteropathy in dogs include *Isospora canis, I. ohioensis, I. neorivolta, I. burrowsi*, and *Hammondia heydorni* (Dubey and Greene, 2012). Coccidian oocysts can be found in feces of clinically healthy dogs, as well as animals with diarrhea. Clinically affected animals are young or immunosuppressed and develop diarrhea, which can vary from soft to watery and may contain blood or mucus. Vomiting, dehydration, lethargy, and weight loss can also be seen. Coccidia oocysts are typically spread by fecal–oral transmission, but dogs can ingest monozoic cysts in intermediate host tissues. The coccidian life cycle is both sexual and asexual, and results in the release of unsporulated eggs, which sporulate under appropriate environmental conditions. Other causes for diarrhea should be excluded before a coccidial etiology is implicated. Treatment may not be necessary, as infections are typically self-limiting and clinically insignificant. Treatment may help to limit the number of oocysts shed in a kennel-housing situation and may be necessary in cases of protracted clinical illness. Possible choices for treatment include daily administration of sulfadimethoxine (50–60 mg/kg PO q24 h for 10–20 days) or trimethoprim sulfa (30 mg/kg PO q8 h for 10 days).

b. Nematodes

Ascarids Roundworms of dogs are most often *Toxocara canis*; however, *Toxascaris leonina* can also affect dogs. Clinical illness is usually only seen in young animals with large worm burdens. Diarrhea, vomiting, dehydration, and abdominal discomfort with vocalization can be seen. Puppies may have a classical 'potbellied' appearance. Heavy infestations can cause intussusception and/or intestinal obstruction. Puppies that experience lung migrations of larval worms can develop fatal pneumonia. *Toxascaris canis* can infect dogs by transplacental migration, transmammary migration, or ingestion of infective eggs. The infective stage of *T. canis* is the third-stage larva (L3). In transplacental infections, puppies may be born with L3 larvae in their lungs (Sherding, 1989). For diagnosis, large (70–85 μm in diameter) and relatively round ascarid eggs can be seen by standard fecal flotation methods. Monthly administration of milbemycin or ivermectin plus pyrantel pamoate is recommended for prevention (Hall and Simpson, 2000). Most anthelmintics are effective for treatment. Puppies should be treated early and often (every other week until 16 weeks of age) because of the possibility of prenatal or neonatal infection. Pregnant bitches can be treated with extended fenbendazole therapy (50 mg/kg PO once a day from day 40 of gestation through day 14 of lactation).

Hookworms The most common and most pathogenic hookworm of dogs is *Ancylostoma caninum*. *Ancylostoma braziliense* can also be found in dogs, but only *A. caninum* infestation typically results in clinical illness. Puppies with hookworm infections can present as anemic with bloody diarrhea or melena. Other clinical signs include lethargy, anorexia, dehydration, vomiting, and poor weight gain. These signs are a direct result of the worms' consumption of blood and body fluids. Infective larvae (L3) are ingested from the environment and develop directly in the intestinal tract. Infestation can also be transmammary, from ingestion of a paratenic host, and, less often, by transplacental migration. On histological sections, embedded worms with mouthparts may be identified. Diagnosis is made by identification of eggs or larvae by either fecal flotation or direct smear.

A differential diagnosis of parvovirus should be considered for puppies with bloody diarrhea, and autoimmune hemolytic anemia should be considered in young dogs with anemia. Pyrantel pamoate is the anthelmintic of choice because it is safest in young ill animals. Monthly administration of milbemycin or ivermectin plus pyrantel pamoate is recommended for prevention and control (Hall and Simpson, 2000). Due to transplacental or milk-borne infection, puppies should be treated q2 weeks from 2 to 16 weeks of age.

Whipworms *Trichuris vulpis*, the canine whipworm, can cause acute or chronic large intestinal diarrhea. The adult worm resides in the cecum or ascending colon. Most infections are subclinical, but in symptomatic cases, the typical clinical sign is diarrhea with blood and/or mucus. Abdominal pain, anorexia, and weight loss may also be seen. Dogs may have eosinophilia, anemia, and/or hypoproteinemia on clinical hematology. *Trichuris vulpis* has a direct life cycle with eggs passed in the feces. The penetration of the adult worm into the enteric mucosa, and the associated inflammation, can lead to diarrhea. Factors that influence development of clinical symptoms are the number and location of adult whipworms; the severity of inflammation, anemia, or hypoproteinemia in the host; and the overall condition of the host. Whipworm infestation is diagnosed by the presence of barrel-shaped, thick-walled eggs with bipolar plugs on fecal flotation. Adult worms intermittently release eggs; therefore, negative results do not exclude infection. Differential diagnoses for whipworm infestation include giardiasis, coccidiosis, and bacterial enteritis. Fenbendazole, oxibendazole, and milbemycin have all been recommended for treatment of whipworms. Treatment for whipworm infestation should be at monthly intervals for 3 months (Jergens and Willard, 2000).

c. Cestodes (Tapeworms)

Several species of cestodes parasitize the small intestine of dogs. The most common is *Dipylidium caninum*. Other species include *Taenia pisiformis* and, more rarely, *Echinococcus granulosus*, *Multiceps* spp., *Mesocestoides* spp., and *Spirometra* spp. Most cestode infestations are subclinical, but severe infestations with *Dipylidium* can cause diarrhea, weight loss, and poor growth. The cestode requires an intermediate host, which for *D. caninum* are fleas and lice. Ingestion of these arthropods results in transmission of the tapeworm. Definitive diagnosis is usually made by the identification of egg capsules or proglottids (tapeworm segments) on the surface of the feces or around the anus. The most significant means to limit cestode infestation is to control flea and/or louse exposure. Praziquantel at 5–12.5 mg/kg orally or subcutaneously is the standard treatment for cestodiasis, especially *Taenia* or *Echinococcus* species. Fenbendazole,

mebendazole, or oxfendazole may also be effective against *D. caninum* (Hall and Simpson, 2000).

d. Mites

Demodicosis Canine demodicosis is caused by *Demodex canis*, a commensal mite that lives in the hair follicles and is passed from dams to nursing pups. Localized demodicosis is typically asymptomatic, but disease can present with variable and nonspecific clinical signs, such as alopecia, erythema, pruritus, crusts, and hyperpigmentation. It can occur anywhere on the body but is often seen on the feet and face, and around the ears (DeManuelle, 2000a). Generalized demodicosis can develop in juvenile or adult populations and is indicative of an underlying immunosuppressive disorder. *Demodex* has a characteristic 'cigar shape' and can be identified from deep skin scrapings mounted on mineral oil (Campbell, 2000; Noli, 2000). Differential diagnoses include dermatophytosis, allergic contact dermatitis, and seborrheic dermatitis. The primary differential diagnosis for generalized demodicosis is primary bacterial pyoderma, which is also a common secondary complication of generalized demodicosis. Ivermectin at 200–600 µg/kg and oral milbemycin at 1–2 mg/kg/day are effective treatments. Treatment duration can be extensive and must be accompanied by repeated skin scrapings.

Sarcoptic Mange Canine sarcoptic mange is caused by *Sarcoptes scabiei* var. *canis*, which is zoonotic. The most common clinical sign is an intense pruritus, usually beginning at sparsely furred areas of the ear pinnae, elbows, ventral thorax, and abdomen. Lesions are characterized by alopecia and yellowish dry crusts with a macular papular eruption. These lesions may be exacerbated by excoriation due to the pruritic nature of the condition. Adult mites, mite eggs, or mite feces may be observed on superficial skin scrapings, but diagnosis may be difficult because multiple skin scrapings may yield negative results. Even if scrapings are negative, a therapeutic trial should be initiated if the clinical signs and history suggest a *Sarcoptes* etiology. Demonstration of anti-mite IgE either in the serum or via an intradermal antigen test can be used as a diagnostic aid (Campbell, 2000). Histologic examination is nondiagnostic; however, suggestive lesions include small foci of edema, exocytosis, degeneration, and necrosis (Scott *et al.*, 1995). An important differential diagnosis is flea allergy dermatitis (FAD). Unless antiparasitic therapy would interfere with research objectives, all dogs with sarcoptic mange should be treated. In addition, their kennel mates should also be treated due to the contagious nature of the disease and its zoonotic potential. The usual means of treatment is either ivermectin at 200–400 µg/kg q14 days or milbemycin at 2 mg/kg q7 days for three oral doses (Scott *et al.*, 1995).

e. Ticks and Fleas

Ticks Ticks are obligate arachnid parasites that require vertebrate blood as their sole food source. Genera that more commonly infest dogs in the United States include species of *Rhipicephalus, Dermacentor, Amblyomma,* and *Ixodes.* The primary significance of tick infestation is vector-borne infectious diseases, including Rocky Mountain spotted fever (*Rickettsia rickettsii*), Lyme disease (*Borrelia burgdorferi sensu stricto*), thrombocytic anaplasmosis (*Anaplasma platys*), and canine monocytic ehrlichiosis (*Ehrlichia canis*). Ticks alone cause minimal signs unless the dog develops a hypersensitivity reaction leading to a more granulomatous response at the bite location (Merchant and Taboada, 1991). Some species (primarily *Dermacentor andersoni* and *D. variabilis*) produce a salivary neurotoxin that causes an ascending flaccid paralysis (Malik and Farrow, 1991). Uncomplicated tick bites and tick-bite paralysis are diagnosed by identification of the tick and clinical signs of paralysis. Dogs with tick-bite paralysis usually show improvement within 24h of tick removal, with complete recovery within 72h (Malik and Farrow, 1991). Formamidines (amitraz), pyrethroids, and phenylpyrazoles (fipronil) are available as spot-ons, collars, sprays, and foggers to treat tick infestations in both the animal and the environment (Halos *et al.*, 2014; Beugnet and Franc, 2012). Differential diagnoses for tick-bite paralysis include botulism, snakebite, polyradiculoneuritis, and idiopathic polyneuropathy (Malik and Farrow, 1991).

Fleas The most common flea to infest dogs is *Ctenocephalides felis felis*, the cat flea (Sousa, 2010). Flea infestations usually cause foci of alopecia and pruritus. Dogs that are hypersensitive to antigenic proteins in flea saliva develop severe FAD, which features papules, crusting, and excoriations over the lumbosacral region, flanks, thighs and abdomen. These animals may require oral corticosteroids to relieve clinical signs (Muller *et al.*, 1983). Secondary bacterial and fungal infections can also develop. Fleas can also transmit other parasitic diseases, such as *Dipylidium* tapeworms. Flea infestations and FAD are definitively diagnosed by observing the fleas on the host's skin; however, the presence of flea excrement can support a presumptive diagnosis (DeManuelle, 2000b). Treatment of flea infestations should use an integrated pest management (IPM) approach that targets adult fleas, immature stages, and environmental contamination in order to limit the risk of chemoresistance. Combining ovicidal treatments, such as lufenuron and selamectin, with adulticidal treatments, such as fipronil, spinosad, selamectin, and imidacloprid, is recommended (Halos *et al.*, 2014; Beugnet and Franc, 2012; Dryden *et al.*, 2012). Certain chemicals (i.e., imidacloprid and selamectin) have both adulticidal and larvacidal abilities, but the principles of IPM preclude the use of one product solely for both adulticidal and larvacidal properties (Schwassman and Logas, 2009). Differential diagnoses include mite and louse infestations, bacterial folliculitis, and allergic or atopic conditions that present with skin lesions in dogs.

4. Fungal Diseases
a. Superficial Dermatophytoses (Ringworm)

Canine dermatophytoses are commonly caused by *Microsporum* spp., *Trichophyton* spp., and *Epidermophyton* spp. (Moriello and DeBoer, 2012). Uncomplicated infections are characterized by circular areas of alopecia and crusting with or without follicular papules, usually around the face, neck, and forelimbs. Dermatophytes infect the hair shaft and follicle, as well as the surrounding skin. Infected hairs become brittle and broken shafts remain infective in the environment for months. Dermatophytoses are zoonotic and easily transmitted to other animals through the environment or by direct contact. Definitive diagnosis is made using dermatophyte test medium for culture. Hair and crust material from infected sites can be plucked and placed on culture; however, the 'toothbrush' method is more effective for sampling multiple sites. The brush is used to comb hairs and scales from several infected sites and then pressed into the culture media. Media plates should be visually inspected daily for 14 days. Positive cultures will become red at the same time as growth of a fluffy white colony. Microscopic examination of hairs and scales to visualize fungal elements can be done using skin scrapings in 20% KOH or mineral oil; however, this method is not very sensitive. Topical and systemic therapy should be initiated together after all suspected areas are clipped to reduce spreading of contaminated fragile hairs. Whole-body topical therapies with antifungal shampoos, rinses, and creams are recommended rather than spot treatment. Systemic therapy can be achieved with griseofulvin, ketoconazole, itraconazole, or fluconazole. Due to the highly infective nature of this disease, animals should be isolated and the environment thoroughly disinfected. Chlorhexidine and Virkon® S are ineffective at clearing environmental spores, but lime sulfur (1:33), enilconazole (0.2%), and bleach (1:10) are effective across many strains of *Microsporum canis* (Moriello and DeBoer, 2002).

B. Metabolic and Nutritional Diseases
1. Endocrine Disorders
a. Hypothyroidism

Although the incidence of hypothyroidism in the canine population is not high (Kemppainen and Clark, 1994), deficiency in thyroid hormone can significantly affect basal metabolism and immune function. Because these factors are important in many biomedical research studies, it is imperative that laboratory animal veterinarians be able to recognize, diagnose, and treat this problem.

Etiology   Primary hypothyroidism affects the thyroid gland directly, whereas secondary hypothyroidism has indirect effects through dysfunction of the pituitary gland (Seguin and Brownlee 2012). Both of these causes result in a gradual loss of functional thyroid tissue (Avgeris *et al.*, 1990; Kemppainen and Clark, 1994). The majority of cases of canine hypothyroidism are due to lymphocytic thyroiditis, an autoimmune disorder, or idiopathic atrophy of the thyroid gland. Lymphocytic thyroiditis is the major cause of hypothyroidism in laboratory beagles and appears to be familial in that breed (Tucker, 1962; Beierwaltes and Nishiyama, 1968; Manning 1979). Rarely, congenital defects or nonfunctional tumors may cause hypothyroidism (Peterson and Ferguson, 1989; Kemppainen and Clark, 1994).

Clinical Signs   Because it affects metabolism in general, hypothyroidism can produce a large number of clinical signs referable to many organ systems. An individual dog with hypothyroidism may have one or any combination of clinical signs. Hypothyroidism reduces the dog's metabolic rate, which then produces such signs as obesity, lethargy, cold intolerance, and constipation. Additionally, hypothyroidism can produce several dermatologic abnormalities, including nonpruritic, bilaterally symmetrical alopecia, hyperpigmentation, seborrhea, and pyoderma (Avgeris *et al.*, 1990; Peterson and Ferguson, 1989; Panciera, 1994). Several clinicopathologic abnormalities have also been reported in a large percentage of hypothyroid dogs. These aberrations include increased serum cholesterol and triglycerides due to a decrease in lipolysis and decreased numbers of low-density lipopolysaccharide receptors (Peterson and Ferguson, 1989; Panciera, 1994). Normocytic, normochromic, nonregenerative anemia may be seen in approximately one-half of the cases (Avgeris *et al.*, 1990). Increased serum alkaline phosphatase and creatine kinase have also been reported in a significant number of hypothyroid dogs (Peterson and Ferguson, 1989; Panciera 1994). Neurologic signs of hypothyroidism, which include lameness, foot dragging, and paresis, may be caused by several mechanisms such as segmental nerve demyelination or nerve entrapment secondary to myxedema (Peterson and Ferguson, 1989). Mental impairment and dullness have also been reported in hypothyroid dogs, secondary to atherosclerosis and cerebral myxedema (Peterson and Ferguson, 1989). Hypothyroidism has been implicated in other neurological abnormalities such as Horner's syndrome, facial nerve paralysis, megaesophagus, and laryngeal paralysis; however, these conditions do not always resolve

with treatment (Bichsel *et al.*, 1988; Panciera, 1994), and a true causal relationship with hypothyroidism has not been completely defined (Panciera, 1994). Myopathies associated with hypothyroidism are caused by metabolic dysfunction and atrophy of type II muscle fibers and can present with signs similar to neurological disease (Peterson and Ferguson, 1989). Hypothyroidism can also cause abnormalities of the cardiovascular system including bradycardia, hypocontractility, increased vascular volume, and atherosclerosis (Seguin and Brownlee 2012). Abnormalities that may be detected by ECG include a decrease in P- and R-wave amplitude (Peterson and Ferguson, 1989) and inverted T waves (Panciera, 1994). These ECG abnormalities are caused by lowered activity of ATPases and calcium channel function.

An association between hypothyroidism and von Willebrand disease has been suggested. However, the relationship is probably one of shared breed predilection and not a true correlation. Contradictory studies have shown either deficient (Avgeris *et al.*, 1990) or normal (Panciera and Johnson 1994, 1996; Avgeris *et al.*, 1990) von Willebrand factor antigen and bleeding times in hypothyroid dogs. Most importantly, hypothyroidism does not appear to cause overt, clinical von Willebrand disease. However, it may exacerbate existing subclinical von Willebrand disease (Seguin and Brownlee, 2012).

Epizootiology   The prevalence of hypothyroidism in the general canine population is reportedly less than 1% (Panciera, 1994). The disorder occurs most often in middle-aged, larger breed dogs (Avgeris *et al.*, 1990), and reports suggest a higher incidence of hypothyroidism in spayed, female dogs (Panciera, 1994; Peterson and Ferguson, 1989). Doberman pinschers and golden retrievers appear to have a higher incidence of hypothyroidism compared with other breeds (Panciera, 1994; Peterson and Ferguson, 1989; Scarlett, 1994). There have been several reports about hypothyroidism in laboratory colonies of beagles (Manning, 1979; Tucker, 1962; Beierwaltes and Nishiyama, 1968).

Diagnosis and Differential Diagnosis   Because of the large number of clinical manifestations in dogs, the recognition of hypothyroidism is not always straightforward. Likewise, the diagnosis of hypothyroidism can be difficult because of the lack of definitive diagnostic tests available for the dog. A complete understanding of the diagnosis of hypothyroidism requires a familiarity with thyroid hormone metabolism and function that is beyond the scope of this writing. For additional information, the reader is referred to one of several manuscripts available (Peterson and Ferguson, 1989; Ferguson, 1994).

Currently, the ability to diagnose hypothyroidism relies heavily on the measurement of serum total T_4 (thyroxine) and free T_4 (Peterson and Ferguson, 1989; Ferguson, 1994). T_4 serves primarily as a precursor for T_3 and is heavily protein bound. Free T_4 represents the unbound fraction that is available to the tissues (Peterson and Ferguson, 1989). The measurement of total T_4 carries a sensitivity of around 95% and can be used as a good screening tool. With the measurement of both serum total T_4 and free T_4, hypothyroidism can usually be ruled out if the values are within the normal range or higher. If both hormone concentrations are low, it is highly likely that the patient has hypothyroidism, and a therapeutic trial may be in order (Peterson and Ferguson, 1989). However, nonthyroidal illnesses and some drugs (e.g., glucocorticoids, anticonvulsants, phenylbutazone, salicylates) can falsely lower these values (Peterson and Ferguson, 1989; Ferguson, 1994). Therefore, low values do not always indicate that hypothyroidism is present and animals should not be treated solely on the basis of serum hormone levels if clinical signs are not present. If the clinical signs are equivocal or only total T_4 or free T_4 is decreased, further diagnostic testing is warranted (Peterson and Ferguson, 1989). Although T_3 is the most biologically active form of thyroid hormone, the measurement of serum T_3 levels is an unreliable indicator of hypothyroidism (Peterson and Ferguson, 1989; Ferguson, 1994). Serum T_3 can be falsely lowered by many nonthyroidal illnesses and many drugs (see above). In addition, T_3 may be preferentially released and conversion of T_4 to T_3 may be enhanced by the failing thyroid (Peterson and Ferguson, 1989; Ferguson, 1994), particularly early in the disease. In one study, T_3 was within normal limits in 15% of the hypothyroid dogs (Panciera, 1994). Autoantibodies can be responsible for false elevations in the concentrations of T_3 and T_4 found in these respective assays. It has been recommended that free T_4, measured by equilibrium dialysis, be assayed in dogs that are suspected of hypothyroidism and have autoantibodies with normal or high T_3 and T_4. Autoantibodies have been found in less than 1% of the samples submitted to one laboratory (Kemppainen and Behrend, 2000).

Other means of diagnosing hypothyroidism have been described. In humans, endogenous thyroid-stimulating hormone (TSH) levels provide reliable information on thyroid status, and an assay is available for dogs. However, endogenous TSH levels can be normal in some dogs with hypothyroidism and high TSH levels have been noted in normal dogs and sick animals that are actually euthyroid. It is therefore recommended that TSH levels be considered along with other information (clinical signs, T_4) prior to diagnosis and treatment (Kemppainen and Behrend, 2000). TSH stimulation testing using exogenous bovine TSH provides a good and reliable method for establishing a diagnosis. Unfortunately, the availability and expense of TSH limit the use of this diagnostic tool (Peterson and Ferguson, 1989; Ferguson, 1994). Another drawback of TSH testing is that the test must be postponed for 4 weeks if thyroid supplementation has been given (Peterson and Ferguson, 1989). When TSH is available for testing, there are several recommendations for dosage, routes of administration, and sampling times. One recommendation is 0.045 U of TSH per pound of body weight (up to a maximum of 5 U) to be administered IV. For this protocol, blood samples are taken prior to administration of TSH and 6 h after. A normal response to the administration of TSH should create an increase of T_4 levels at least 2 µg/dl above the baseline levels or an absolute level that exceeds 3 µg/dl (Peterson and Ferguson, 1989; Wheeler et al., 1985).

Treatment The treatment of choice for hypothyroidism in the dog is L-thyroxine (sodium levothyroxine). A recommended dosing regimen is 0.01–0.02 mg/kg once a day (Avgeris et al. 1990). If drugs that decrease thyroxine levels are being administered concurrently, it may be necessary to divide the thyroxine dose for twice daily administration. After the supplementation has begun, the thyroid hormone level should be rechecked in 6–8 weeks, and blood samples should be drawn 4–8 h after the morning pill. A clinical response is usually seen in 6–8 weeks and would include weight loss, hair regrowth, and resolution of other signs (Panciera, 1994). ECG abnormalities also return to normal (Peterson and Ferguson, 1989). For dogs with neurologic signs, the prognosis is guarded, because the signs do not always resolve with supplementation (Panciera, 1994).

2. Management-Related Issues

a. Obesity

Weight gain and eventual obesity are frequent findings in dogs in the research environment. Because obesity can adversely affect several body systems as well as general metabolism, the laboratory animal veterinarian must address obesity and its potential effects on animal welfare and research results.

Etiology Obesity is defined as a body weight 20–25% over the ideal. In general, obesity occurs when the intake of calories exceeds the expenditure of energy, the result of overeating or eating an unbalanced diet. Overeating is a common cause of obesity in pet dogs and may be triggered by boredom, nervousness, or conditioning (MacEwen, 1992). In addition, pet animals are often subjected to unbalanced diets supplemented with high-fat treats. In the laboratory animal setting, overeating is less likely than in a household because access to food is more restricted, and diets are usually a commercially prepared balanced ration. However, obesity can still be a problem if specific guidelines for energy requirements are not followed. In addition, the necessary caging of dogs in the research environment and limitation to exercise reduces energy expenditure. It is also important to realize that other factors may predispose dogs to obesity, even when guidelines for caloric intake and energy expenditure are followed (Butterwick and Hawthorne, 1998). As in humans, genetics plays an important role in the development of obesity in dogs, and certain breeds are more predisposed toward obesity. In a study of dogs visiting veterinary clinics in the United Kingdom, Labrador retrievers were most likely to be obese. Other breeds affected included Cairn terriers, dachshunds, basset hounds, golden retrievers, and cocker spaniels. The beagle was also listed as a breed predisposed to obesity in the household environment (Edney and Smith, 1986).

Several metabolic or hormonal changes are also associated with obesity. It has been well established that neutering promotes weight gain. In one study, spayed female dogs were twice as likely to be obese compared with intact females (MacEwen, 1992). The authors proposed that the absence of estrogen promotes an increase in food consumption. A similar trend toward obesity was found in castrated male dogs (Edney and Smith, 1986). In addition, hypothyroidism and hyperadrenocorticism may present with obesity as one of the clinical signs (MacEwen, 1992).

Differential Diagnosis The diagnosis of obesity is somewhat subjective and relies on an estimate of ideal body weight. The ideal body condition for dogs is considered to be achieved when the ribs are barely visible but easily palpated beneath the skin surface. When the ribs are not easily palpated and/or the dog's normal function is impaired by its weight, the animal is considered obese. There are few objective, quantifiable methods for establishing this diagnosis. Ultrasound has been evaluated for measurement of subcutaneous fat in dogs, and measurements taken from the lumbar area can be used to reliably predict the total body fat (Wilkinson and McEwan, 1991). After a diagnosis of obesity has been made, additional diagnostic tests should be performed to determine if there is an underlying cause for the problem. A complete physical exam should be performed to look for signs of concurrent disease and to establish if obesity has adversely affected the individual. Serum thyroid hormones should be evaluated (see above), and serum chemistry may reveal an increased alkaline phosphatase associated with hyperadrenocorticism.

Treatment Restricting food intake readily treats obesity, and this is easily done in the research setting. It has been suggested that a good weight loss program involves restriction of intake to 60% of the calculated energy requirement to maintain ideal body weight. It has been shown that restriction of calories down to 50% produces no adverse health effects. However, T_3 levels will decrease in direct proportion with caloric intake. Ideally, weight loss will occur at a rate of 1–2% of body weight per week (Laflamme et al., 1997). With more severe calorie restriction and more rapid weight loss, the individual is more likely to have rebound weight gain after restrictions are relaxed.

There has been a great deal of attention in humans as to the correct diet to encourage weight loss. Likewise, the type of diet fed to dogs has been examined. As mentioned above, the restriction of calories is most important, and feeding less of an existing diet can do this. Alternatively, several diet dog foods are available, and there is some evidence that these diets are superior to simple volume restriction (MacEwen, 1992). There has been much concern about the addition of fiber to the diet as a method for reducing caloric intake while maintaining the volume fed. Studies in dogs have examined the addition of both soluble and insoluble fibers to calorie-restricted diets. These studies have shown that the addition of fiber does not have an effect on satiety in dogs and therefore does not have a beneficial effect in weight loss protocols (Butterwick et al., 1994; Butterwick and Markwell, 1997).

Research Complications It is important to control weight gain in research animals because of the association of obesity with metabolism. Although an association between obesity and reproductive, dermatologic, and neoplastic problems has been reported (MacEwen, 1992), this relationship is not consistently apparent (Edney and Smith, 1986). Joint problems including osteoarthritis and hip dysplasia have also been related to obesity (MacEwen, 1992; Kealy et al., 1997). In addition, diabetes mellitus has been linked to obesity and obesity-induced hyperinsulinism in several experimental models (MacEwen, 1992). A recent study demonstrated metabolic disease, typified by hyperinsulinemia and hypoadiponectinemia, in approximately 20% of obese dogs (Tvarijonaviciute et al., 2012). Research that requires anesthesia may be complicated by a greater risk of cardiovascular diseases (Edney and Smith, 1986) including hypertension and compromise to the respiratory tract.

C. Traumatic Disorders

1. Traumatic Wounds

Etiology In the laboratory setting, the majority of traumatic wounds will be small in size and quickly observed. Occasionally, dogs may sustain minor trauma during transport or have a small, previously undetected, chronic wound upon arrival at the facility. When dogs are group housed, they may sustain bite wounds during early socialization periods. Under these conditions, proper initial treatment will lead to uncomplicated wound healing. Complications such as infection and delayed healing arise when wounds are not noticed immediately or when the basic principles of wound management are not followed.

Clinical Signs The signs and appearance of a traumatic wound will vary with the cause and the duration of time since wounding. Abrasions, sustained by shear forces, are partial thickness skin wounds characterized by minimal bleeding or tissue disruption. Puncture wounds have a small surface opening but penetrate into deep tissues with the potential for contamination. Lacerations are wounds caused by sharp separation of skin that may extend to deeper tissues. Acute wounds are characterized by bleeding tissue, sharp edges and no obvious devitalization. They have variable degrees of contamination. Chronic wounds generally do not exhibit active bleeding and will have curled or rounded edges. These wounds often have necrotic tissue and are considered contaminated.

Treatment To aid decision making about wound therapy, several classification systems have been developed for traumatic injuries. At one time, decisions about wound therapy were largely based upon the length of time since wounding, or the concept of a 'golden period.' It is now recognized that several factors must be considered prior to initiating wound care, including (but not limited to) the type and size of the wound, the degree of wound contamination, and the competence of the host's defense systems (Swaim, 1980; Waldron and Trevor, 1993). One of the most widely used classification systems is based upon wound contamination and categorizes wounds as clean, clean-contaminated, contaminated, or dirty (see Table 12.9).

The vast majority of the wounds seen in the laboratory setting will fall into the clean and clean-contaminated categories. These wounds may be treated with the basic wound care described below and primary closure of the wound. Contaminated and dirty wounds require more aggressive therapy. Postsurgical infections or complications of initial therapy would be considered dirty wounds. When in doubt as to the classification of a wound, the worst category should be presumed in order to provide optimal therapy and reduce the chance for complications.

The initial treatment of a wound is the same regardless of its classification. When first recognized, the wound should be covered with a sterile dressing until definitive treatment can be rendered. Bleeding should be controlled with direct pressure; tourniquets are discouraged because of the complications that may arise with inappropriate placement (Swaim, 1980). It is best to avoid using topical disinfectants in the wound until further wound treatment (culture, debridement, lavage) has been performed (Swaim, 1980). Anesthesia or analgesia may be necessary and the choice of agent will depend on the size and location of the wound as well as the preference of the clinician. If the wound is contaminated or dirty, bacterial cultures, both aerobic and anaerobic, should be performed. Then a water-soluble lubricant gel may be applied directly to the wound to prevent it from further contamination during the hair removal process. A wide margin of hair should be clipped and a surgical scrub performed around the edges of the wound. Povidone-iodine alternating with alcohol or chlorhexidine gluconate scrub alternating with water is most often recommended for surgical preparation of the skin surface (Osuna *et al.*, 1990a, b). Simple abrasions that involve only a partial thickness of the skin do not generally require further treatment. Full-thickness wounds require further attention, including irrigation with large quantities of a solution delivered under pressure. Several irrigation solutions have been recommended (Lozier *et al.*, 1992; Waldron and Trevor, 1993; Sanchez *et al.*, 1988), but type may not be as important as the volume and pressure of delivery. It has been suggested that 8 psi is required to obtain adequate tissue irrigation, and this may be achieved by using a 35-ml syringe with an 18- or 19-gauge needle (Waldron and Trevor, 1993).

For wounds that are contaminated or dirty, debridement is an important part of initial therapy. Debridement usually proceeds from superficial to deeper layers. Skin that is obviously necrotic should be removed. Although it is often recommended to remove skin back to the point at which it bleeds, this may not be feasible with large wounds on the limbs. In addition, other factors such as edema or hypovolemia may reduce bleeding in otherwise viable skin (Waldron and Trevor, 1993). If one is unsure about tissue viability in areas that are devoid of

TABLE 12.9 Classification and Treatment of Traumatic Wounds[a]

Classification	Description	Examples	Treatment options
Clean	Aseptic wound	Surgical incision	Aseptic, immediate closure
Clean-contaminated	Recent wound with minimal, easily removed contamination	Simple laceration, broken toenail	Wound lavage, debridement, ± immediate closure
Contaminated	Several hours since wounding; grossly contaminated	Bite wounds, old lacerations, fecal contamination	Wound lavage, debridement, ± drain placement, ± delayed closure
Dirty	Purulent exudate and infection already present	Infected bite wound, anal sac abscess, postsurgical infection	Wound lavage, debridement, drain placement, delayed or no closure

[a]*Modified from Waldron and Trevor (1993).*

extra skin, the tissue may be left (Swaim, 1980; Waldron and Trevor, 1993), and nonviable areas will demarcate within 2–3 days (Waldron and Trevor, 1993). Necrotic fat should be resected liberally, because it does not have a large blood supply and will provide an environment for infection. Often, resection of subcutaneous fat is necessary to remove debris and hair that could not be removed during wound irrigation. Damaged muscle should also be liberally resected (Swaim, 1980). The wound should be irrigated several times during debridement and again after completion.

After initial wound treatment, the options concerning wound closure must be weighed. The principles of basic surgery are discussed in several good texts, and readers are encouraged to pursue additional information. Primary wound closure is defined as closure at the time of initial wound therapy and is the treatment of choice for clean and clean-contaminated wounds. Closure is performed in two or more layers, carefully apposing tissues and obliterating dead space. If dead space will remain in the wound, a drain should be placed. Subcutaneous closure should be performed with absorbable suture such as polydioxanone, polyglactin 910, or polyglycolic acid. It is best to use interrupted sutures and avoid leaving excess suture material in the wound. It may be necessary to choose tension-relieving suture patterns, such as horizontal mattress. Skin closure is generally performed with nylon (3-0 or 4-0).

In situations where gross contamination cannot be completely removed, closure of the wound should be delayed or avoided. After debridement and irrigation, the wound should be bandaged. The wound may be covered by a nonadherent dressing such as vaseline-impregnated gauze (Swaim, 1980). The contact layer is covered by cotton padding, and the entire bandage is covered by a supportive and protective layer. The bandages should be changed once or twice daily, depending upon the amount of discharge coming from the wound. Wound closure within 3–5 days of wounding (prior to the formation of granulation tissue) is considered delayed primary closure. When the wound is closed after 5 days, this is considered secondary closure (Waldron and Trevor, 1993). Second-intention healing involves allowing the wound to heal without surgical intervention. This type of healing is often used on limbs when there is an insufficient amount of skin to allow complete closure (Swaim, 1980). It is important to note that second-intention healing will take longer than with surgical repair, and, in the case of large wounds, it will be more expensive because of the cost of bandaging materials.

Several factors must be weighed when considering the use of antibiotics in traumatic wound care, including the classification and site of the wound, host defenses, and concurrent research use of the animal. When wounds are clean or clean-contaminated, antibiotics are seldom necessary unless the individual is at high risk for infection. When wounds have been severely contaminated or are dirty, antibiotics are indicated and the type of antibiotic will ultimately depend on culture and sensitivity results. Until such results are available, the choice of antibiotic is based on the most likely organism to be encountered. Topical application of bacitracin, neomycin sulfate, and polymixin B combinations may be used in wounds with minor contamination. In skin wounds with more extensive contamination, *Staphylococcus* spp. are generally of concern, whereas *Pasteurella multocida* should be considered in bite wounds. When systemic antibiotics are necessary, cephalosporins, amoxicillin-clavulanate, and trimethoprim sulfas are often recommended for initial antibiotic therapy (Waldron and Trevor, 1993).

Prevention In facilities with good husbandry practices and a diligent staff, potentially injurious equipment or surfaces are identified quickly. Appropriate attention to surgical technique and to initial wound care will generally reduce the occurrence of postprocedure wound infection.

2. Pressure Sores (Decubital Ulcers)

Etiology Pressure sores (decubital ulcers) can be a problem in long-term studies and housing situations that require chronic skin contact with hard surfaces. Decubital ulcers often develop over a bony prominence such as the elbow, tuber ischii, tarsus, or carpus. The compression of soft tissues between hard surfaces results in vascular occlusion, ischemia, and ultimately tissue death (Swaim and Angarano, 1990). Several factors that increase pressure at the site and/or affect the integrity of the skin will predispose an individual to develop pressure sores, including poor hygiene, self-trauma, low-protein diet, preexisting tissue damage, muscle wasting, inadequate bedding, and ill-fitting coaptation devices (Swaim and Angarano, 1990).

Clinical Signs Initially, the skin will appear red and irritated. Over time, constant trauma can result in full-thickness skin defects and can progress to necrosis of underlying tissues. The severity of the sores may be graded from I to IV according to the depth of the wound and the tissues involved, from superficial skin irritation to involvement of underlying bone (Waldron and Trevor, 1993).

Epizootiology The problem usually occurs in large dog breeds, but any type of dog can be affected.

Prevention and Control Minimizing or eliminating predisposing factors is important to both the prevention and treatment of this condition. If a dog will experience long periods of recumbency, adequate bedding or padding must be provided. Recumbent animals should be moved frequently, ideally every 2 h, to prevent continuous compression on a specific area (Waldron and Trevor, 1993). Skin hygiene is of the utmost importance when trying to prevent or treat pressure sores. The skin should be kept clean and dry at all times. If urine scalding is a problem, the affected area should be clipped, bathed, and dried thoroughly at least once or twice daily. Finally, an appropriate diet to maintain body weight will minimize compressive forces experienced over areas susceptible to ulceration (Swaim and Angarano, 1990).

Treatment The treatment of pressure sores must involve care of the wound and attention to the factors causing the wound. The extent of initial wound management will largely depend on the depth of the wound. For simple abrasions and small wounds involving the skin only, simple wound cleansing and open-wound management provide adequate treatment. When wounds involve deeper tissues, including fat, fascia, or bone, more aggressive diagnostics and therapy must be performed. The affected area should be radiographed to assess bone involvement and the wound should be cultured. All of the damaged tissue should be debrided and basic wound management guidelines should be followed (see above). When a healthy granulation bed has formed over the entire wound, a delayed closure over a drain may be performed (Swaim and Angarano, 1990). With extensive lesions, reconstruction with skin flaps may be necessary (Waldron and Trevor 1993).

Bandaging should be performed on all full-thickness wounds; however, it is important to remember that ill-fitting or inadequately padded bandages or casts may worsen the problem. The area over the wound itself should not be heavily padded. The wounded area should be lightly covered and then a doughnut, created from rolled gauze or towel, should be fitted around the wound, in order to displace pressure over a larger area and onto healthier tissue. The doughnut is then incorporated into a padded bandage. If a cast has been applied to the area for treatment or research purposes, a hole can be cut over the wound to reduce pressure in that area and allow treatment of the wound (Swaim and Angarano, 1990). Bandages should be removed at least once or twice a day to allow wound care.

3. Acral Lick Granuloma

Etiology An acral lick granuloma is a skin lesion caused by self-trauma. In a few cases, the self-trauma is due to initial irritation caused by an identifiable neurologic or orthopedic condition (Tarvin and Prata, 1980). Allergy may also be a source of irritation that leads to self-trauma. However, the majority of cases begin because of repetitive licking by dogs that are confined and lack external stimuli (Swaim and Angarano, 1990). It has been theorized that the self-trauma promotes the release of endogenous endorphins, which act as a reward for the abnormal behavior (Dodman *et al.*, 1988).

The laboratory environment could promote the abnormal behavior and lead to acral lick granuloma.

Epizootiology The lesions associated with acral lick granuloma are seen most often in large dog breeds, particularly Dobermans. However, any type of dog can be affected (Walton, 1986).

Clinical Signs Early lesions appear as irritated, hairless areas usually found on the distal extremities (Swaim and Angarano, 1990). The predilection for the limbs may be due to accessibility or possibly a lower threshold for pruritus in these areas. As the lesions progress, the skin becomes ulcerated and the wound develops a hyperpigmented edge. The wounds may partially heal and then be aggravated again when licking resumes.

Diagnosis and Differential Diagnosis Acral lick granulomas must be differentiated from several other conditions, including bacterial or fungal infection, foreign bodies, and pressure sores. In addition, mast cell tumors and other forms of neoplasia can mimic the appearance of acral lick granuloma. Many of the aforementioned problems can be ruled out by the history of the animal. However, a complete history may be unavailable in the laboratory setting. Fungal cultures and allergy testing may aid in diagnosis. Biopsy of the affected area would rule out neoplasia. An uncomplicated acral lick granuloma would feature hyperplasia, ulceration, and fibrosis without evidence of infection or neoplasia (Walton, 1986).

Prevention and Control Behavior modification and relief of boredom are important aspects of preventing (and treating) acral lick granuloma. Environmental enrichment including exercise, co-housing and various toys is already a basic requirement and may be increased to combat self injurious behaviors.

Treatment Several treatments have been reported for acral lick granuloma and the selection of a treatment should be based on the underlying cause. One of the most important aspects of treatment is to break the cycle of self-trauma. Mechanical restraint with an Elizabethan collar is one of the easiest methods to accomplish this goal. Several direct treatments have been examined, including intralesional and topical steroids, perilesional cobra venom, acupuncture, radiation, and surgery (Swaim and Angarano, 1990; Walton, 1986). Opioid antagonists have been applied as treatments for acral lick granulomas and self-injurious behaviors with the theory that this will block the effects of endogenous opioids. Naltrexone and nalmefene have been used successfully to reduce excessive licking behaviors and resolve associated lesions. However, lesions did recur after the drugs were discontinued (Dodman *et al.*, 1988; White, 1990). The topical administration of a mixture of flunixin meglumine, steroid, and dimethyl sulfoxide has also been shown to be effective (Walton, 1986). In addition, psychoactive drugs have been suggested to relief of boredom or anxiety. These have included phenobarbital, megestrol acetate, and progestins. However, side effects have been reported (Swaim and Angarano, 1990). Other behavior-modifying medications such as clomipramine may be effective in the treatment of compulsive anxiety disorder. The potential for effects that could interfere with experimental results must be determined prior to initiation of treatment. It is important to note that none of the above-mentioned treatments have been successful in all cases. The overall prognosis for acral lick granuloma should be considered guarded since the lesions often recur when treatment is discontinued.

4. Elbow Hygroma

Etiology Hygromas are fluid-filled sacs that develop as a result of repeated trauma or pressure over a bony prominence. The area over the olecranon is most frequently affected, but hygromas have been reported in association with the tuber calcis, greater trochanter, and stifle (Newton *et al.*, 1974).

Epizootiology Elbow hygromas are most frequently reported in large and giant breeds of dogs, less than 2 years of age (Johnston, 1975; White, 2003; Cannap *et al.*, 2012). Elbow hygromas are seen infrequently in the laboratory animal setting because the commonly affected breeds are seldom used in research. However, the housing environment of research dogs, especially cage bottoms and cement runs, may predispose them to hygromas. For this reason, laboratory animal veterinary and husbandry staff should be familiar with this condition.

Clinical Signs The clinical presentation will depend upon the chronicity of the problem. A dog with an elbow hygroma usually presents with a painless, fluctuant swelling over the point of the elbow without signs of lameness. The condition may be unilateral or bilateral. Over a long period of time, elbow hygromas may become inflamed and ulcerated. If the hygroma becomes secondarily infected, the animal may exhibit pain and fever (Johnston, 1975; White, 2003).

Pathology The fluid-filled cavity in the hygroma is lined by granulation and fibrous tissue. Hygromas lack an epithelial lining and therefore are not true cysts. The fluid within the cavity is a yellow or red serous transudate. This fluid is less viscous than joint fluid and elbow hygromas do not communicate with the joint (Johnston, 1975).

Treatment The treatment of elbow hygromas should be conservative whenever possible. Conservative management of the elbow hygroma is aimed at relieving the source of pressure at the point of the elbow. In early and mild cases, simply providing padding to cover hard surfaces will result in resolution of the hygroma. A soft padded bandage or doughnut bandage around the affected site may also be of benefit. Neoprene/polyester sleeves that cover the elbows and fit over the shoulders are also available as an option for either prevention or treatment of hygromas (Cannap *et al.*, 2012). More aggressive therapies, including needle drainage and injection of corticosteroids into the hygroma, have been described but are not recommended due to the risk of infection (Johnston, 1975). Surgical options should be reserved for complicated or refractory cases. Even simple excision can be associated with complications such as wound dehiscence and ulceration (Johnston, 1975) due to the location of the bony prominence at the surgical site. This issue may be avoided by using a skin advancement flap (White, 2003) that allows intact, healthy skin to cover the boney prominence. A muscle advancement flap has also been described (Green *et al.*, 2008). Regardless of the method used to treat an elbow hygroma, recurrence of the problem is likely unless the predisposing factors are identified and relieved.

5. Corneal Ulcers

Etiology In the research environment, corneal ulcers are most often associated with direct trauma, contact with irritating chemicals, or exposure to the drying effects of air during long periods of anesthesia. Chronic or recurrent corneal ulcers may also be associated with infection or hereditary causes in some breeds of dogs; however, these would be rare in the laboratory setting.

Clinical Signs The signs of corneal ulceration are blepharospasm, epiphora, and photophobia. The eye may appear irritated and inflamed. In minor cases, the cornea may appear normal however, in cases of deeper ulceration, the cornea may appear roughened or have an obvious defect. In addition, the periocular tissues may be swollen and inflamed because of self-inflicted trauma from rubbing at the eye.

Diagnosis A tentative diagnosis of corneal ulcer or abrasion may be based on the clinical signs. A definitive diagnosis of corneal ulcers is made by the green appearance of the cornea when stained with fluorescein dye. When a corneal ulcer has been diagnosed, the eye should be inspected for underlying causes such as foreign bodies, abnormal eyelids, or abberant cilia.

Treatment The treatment of corneal ulcers will depend on the depth and size of the affected area, as well as the underlying cause. Superficial abrasions are generally treated with topical application of antibiotics. A triple antibiotic ointment that does not contain steroids given three times a day for 2–3 days usually provides adequate treatment. Simple corneal ulcers are restained with fluorescein after 3 days and should show complete healing at that time. If the ulcer is not healed, this may indicate that the ulcer has an undermined edge impeding proper healing. Topical anesthetic should be applied to the eye, and a cotton-tipped applicator can be rolled over the surface of the ulcer toward its edge.

This will remove the unattached edge of the cornea and healing should progress normally after debridement. Deep ulcers may require further debridement and primary repair. In such cases, a third eyelid or conjunctival flap may be applied to the eye until experienced help can be obtained. In all cases, an Elizabethan collar or other restraint may be necessary to prevent additional trauma to the eye. Ulcers caused by entropion, ectropion, or dystichiasis will not resolve until the condition is repaired, and descriptions for this can be found elsewhere.

Prevention The proper application of lubricant eye ointment at the time of anesthesia will prevent drying due to exposure and may also protect the eye from scrub solutions applied near the eye. Early treatment of superficial ulcers should prevent self-trauma and progression of the wound.

D. Iatrogenic Diseases

1. Implant and Catheter Infections

Etiology Research protocols often require the placement of chronic implants. Implants such as cardiac or other biomedical devices may be the primary focus of the research study. Implants may also be used as chronic monitoring devices, for delivery of compounds, or to collect serial samples. Infection may occur at the time of implant. Alternatively, the implant may serve as a nidus after hematogenous spread from other sources. One of the most common sources of infection is from colonization of the device from an external component, which is a frequent complication with indwelling catheters.

The actual incidence of complications associated with indwelling vascular catheters in dogs is unknown. One study (Hysell and Abrams, 1967) examined the lesions found at necropsy in animals with chronic indwelling catheters, which included traumatic cardiac lesions, visceral infarcts, and fatal hemorrhages. These lesions were primarily associated with catheter-induced trauma or secondary to embolization of fibrin. In a veterinary clinical setting, infections in peripheral catheters were more likely when the catheters were used for blood collection immediately after placement and when a 'T' connector rather than a 'Y' connector was used. (Jones *et al.*, 2009).

Intestinal access ports have been used to study the pharmacokinetics of drugs at various levels in the intestinal tract. These catheters are usually vascular access ports with several modifications to allow secure placement in bowel (Meunier *et al.*, 1993). The most frequently reported complication associated with these catheters is infection around the port site (Meunier *et al.*, 1993; Kwei *et al.*, 1995).

Clinical Signs Dogs with implant infections may not exhibit signs initially (Jones *et al.*, 2009). Localized swelling around the implant may occur. In the case of indwelling catheters, signs may include redness and swelling of the skin around the external port or discharge from the skin wound. Vascular access ports may develop fluctuant subcutaneous abscesses. In more severe cases, systemic signs may be noted (Bach *et al.*, 1998; Hysell and Abrams, 1967). The systemic signs of infection are covered elsewhere in this chapter.

Treatment The treatment of catheter infections almost invariably requires removal of the catheter, as demonstrated in both dogs and monkeys (Ringler and Peter, 1984; DaRif and Rush, 1983). Superficial wound irritation or infection may be treated locally with antibiotic ointment, sterile dressing changes, and efforts to minimize catheter movement; however, more extensive problems require aggressive therapy. Localized abscesses or sinus tracts may be managed by establishing drainage and copious flushing. Aerobic and anaerobic cultures of blood and locally infected sites should be performed prior to initial treatment (Ringler and Peter, 1984). Systemic antibiotic therapy should be initiated for a 10-day period. The choice of drug will ultimately be based on previous experience and culture results. If retention of a catheter is important, the catheter lumen may be safely disinfected with chlorine dioxide solution (Dennis *et al.*, 1989). The solution is removed after 15 min and replaced with heparinized saline. All of the extension lines and fluids used with an infected catheter should be discarded. The blood cultures should be repeated 3 days after the antibiotic therapy has ceased. If bacteria are still cultured, the catheter must be removed.

Prevention It is highly desirable to prevent complications that may result in loss of an implanted device. Catheters and other implants should be made of nonthrombogenic material and be as simple as possible. A catheter with extra ports or multiple lumens requires additional management and supplies more routes for infection. The initial placement of an indwelling catheter must be done under aseptic conditions by individuals who are familiar with the procedure. Intravenous catheters that are used for delivery of drugs or blood sampling should be positioned in the vena cava and not in the right atrium, thereby minimizing trauma to the tricuspid valve. Ideally, catheters are secured to reduce movement and irritation of the skin, which may predispose to infection around external ports. The use of vascular access ports that lie entirely under the skin eliminates many problems with infection. It has also been found that long extension tubing connected to the port may actually reduce the potential for infection of the catheter (Ringler and Peter, 1984). For intestinal access ports, catheter security may be improved with a synthetic cuff added to the end of the catheter allowing better attachment to the intestine (Meunier *et al.*, 1993). After any catheter placement, animals should be observed daily for signs of either local or systemic infection. The catheter entry site should be disinfected, coated with antibiotic ointment, and rebandaged every other day. Once a month, the catheter line may be disinfected with chlorine dioxide. In addition, a solution of the antibiotic ceftazidime used on alternate days with the heparin locking solution has been shown to effectively reduce infections in indwelling vascular catheters (Bach *et al.*, 1998).

Throughout the life of the catheter, injections into and withdrawals from the catheter should be done in a sterile manner, and the number of breaks in the line should be kept to a minimum. Periodically, the placement of an indwelling catheter may be verified by radiography. When placed and managed correctly, catheters and ports of any kind may remain in place for months without complications.

2. Sepsis

Etiology   Sepsis is defined as the systemic response to infection caused by bacteria (gram negative and/or gram positive), fungi, or viruses. In laboratory animals, sepsis is most often seen as a complication of surgical procedures or associated with chronic implants. Sepsis may also be seen as a complication of infectious diseases such as parvovirus.

Clinical Signs   The signs of sepsis can vary, depending on the source of the infection and the stage of the disease. Early in the course, dogs may present with signs of a hyperdynamic sepsis, including increased heart rate, increased respiratory rate, red mucous membranes, and a normal-to-increased capillary refill time. Systemic blood pressure and cardiac output will be increased or within the normal range. The animals will often be febrile. Later in the course of the syndrome, the animals may show classic signs of septic shock including decreased temperature, pale mucous membranes, and a prolonged capillary refill time. Cardiac output and blood pressure are decreased as shock progresses. Peripheral edema and mental confusion have also been reported (Hauptman and Chaudry, 1993).

Pathogenesis   The pathophysiology of sepsis is complex and is mediated by immune responses involving mediators such as cytokines, eicosinoids, complement, superoxide radicals, and nitric oxide. The body responds to overwhelming infection with an attempt to optimize metabolic processes and maximize oxygen delivery to tissues. However, if inflammation is left unchecked, the system may be unable to compensate, and the result is cardiovascular collapse.

Diagnosis   In general, a presumptive diagnosis of sepsis is made based on the occurrence of several in a group of signs, including altered body temperature, increased respiratory and/or heart rate, increased or decreased white blood cell (WBC) count, increased number of immature neutrophils, decreased platelet count,

decreased blood pressure, hypoxemia, and altered cardiac output. However, extreme inflammation without infection (e.g., pancreatitis, trauma) may create similar signs. One study examined the diagnosis of sepsis in canine patients at a veterinary hospital based on easily obtainable physical and laboratory findings. That study found that septic individuals had higher temperatures, WBC counts, and percentage of band neutrophils than nonseptic individuals, whereas platelet counts were lower in the septic dogs. There were no differences in respiratory rate or glucose levels between the groups. Using these criteria, the results had a high sensitivity and a tendency to overdiagnose sepsis (Hauptman *et al.*, 1997). Ultimately, the presence of a septic focus simplifies diagnosis greatly; however, the focus may not be obvious. If the signs of sepsis are evident but the focus is not, several areas should be evaluated for infection, including the urinary, reproductive, respiratory, alimentary, and cardiovascular systems, as well as the abdominal cavity (Kirby, 1995).

Treatment   The treatment of sepsis has three aims. The first aim is to support the cardiovascular system. All septic animals should be treated with fluids to replace deficits and to maximize cardiac output. Crystalloids are most frequently used to maintain vascular volume, primarily because of their low cost. Colloids offer the advantage of maintaining volume without fluid overload and may have other positive effects on the cardiovascular system. Acid–base and electrolyte imbalances should also be addressed.

After the animal has stabilized, the treatment of sepsis should be aimed at removing the septic focus. Obvious sources of infection should be drained or surgically removed. If an implant is infected, it should be removed. Antibiotic therapy should also be instituted. The choice of antibiotic will ultimately depend upon the results of culture; however, the initial choice of antibiotics is based on previous experience, source of infection, and gram stains. The organisms associated with sepsis are often gram-negative bacteria of gastrointestinal origin or are previously encountered nosocomial infections. Ideally, the antibiotic chosen for initial therapy should be a broad-spectrum, bactericidal drug that can be administered intravenously. Second- or third-generation cephalosporins provide good coverage, as does combination therapy with enrofloxacin plus metronidazole or penicillin.

Finally, the treatment of sepsis is aimed at blocking the mediators of the systemic response. This category of sepsis treatment is the focus of much research. Several studies have examined the effects of steroids, nonsteroidal anti-inflammatory drugs, and antibodies directed against endotoxin, cytokines, or other mediators of the inflammatory response; however, none of these treatments have proven greatly effective in clinical trials.

Consequently, there is no 'magic bullet' for the treatment of sepsis at this time. Successful therapy remains dependent on aggressive supportive care coupled with identification and elimination of the inciting infection.

3. Aspiration Lung Injury

Etiology In research animals, aspiration may occur accidentally during the oral administration of various substances or by the misplacement of gastric tubes. Aspiration of gastric contents may also occur as a complication of anesthesia. In pet animals, aspiration is often seen as a result of metabolic and anatomical abnormalities; however, such occurrence would be rare in the research setting.

Pathogenesis Aspirated compounds can produce direct injury to lung tissue, but more importantly, the aspiration provokes an inflammatory response, probably mediated by cytokines. The result is a rapid influx of neutrophils into the lung parenchyma and alveolar spaces. The inflammation leads to increased vascular permeability with leakage of fluid into the alveolar spaces and can eventually lead to alveolar collapse. If the condition is severe, it may result in adult respiratory distress syndrome and respiratory failure. It should be noted that infection is not present in the early stages of this condition but may complicate the problem after 24–48 h.

Clinical Signs The severity and clinical manifestation of aspiration lung injury are dependent upon the pH, osmolality, and volume of the aspirate. The signs of aspiration lung injury may include cough, increased respiratory rate, pronounced respiratory effort, and fever. When respiration is severely affected, the oxygen saturation of blood will be decreased. The diagnosis of this problem is based on witness of aspiration, history consistent with aspiration, and/or the physical findings. Classically, radiographs of the thorax demonstrate a bronchoalveolar pattern in the cranioventral lung fields. However, these lesions may not appear for several hours after the incident of aspiration. In addition, the location of the lesions may be variable, depending on the orientation of the animal at the time of aspiration.

Treatment The treatment of aspiration lung injury is largely supportive and depends upon the severity of the inflammation and the clinical signs. If the aspiration is witnessed, the mouth and, ideally, the upper airway should be cleared of residual material. When small amounts of a relatively innocuous substance (e.g., barium) have been aspirated, treatment may not be necessary. When severe inflammation is present, systemic as well as localized therapy may be necessary. Oxygen therapy may be instituted; however, the concentration and time frame are controversial, because lung injury may be exacerbated by long-term administration of oxygen at high concentrations (Nader-Djahal *et al.*, 1997).

Fluid therapy may also be necessary in severe cases; however, cardiovascular support should be performed judiciously as fluid overload could lead to an increase in pulmonary edema. The use of colloids is also controversial because of the increase in vascular permeability that occurs in the lungs. Several studies have addressed the use of anti-inflammatory agents to reduce lung injury associated with aspiration; however, none are used clinically in human or veterinary medicine at this time. Corticosteroids are contraindicated (Raghavendran *et al.*, 2011).

In humans, antibiotics are reserved for cases with confirmed infection, in order to prevent the development of antibiotic-resistant pneumonia. It has been suggested that dogs should be immediately treated with antibiotics when the aspirated material is not acidic or has potentially been contaminated by oral bacteria associated with severe dental disease. Amoxicillin-clavulanate has been recommended as a first line of defense, reserving enrofloxacin for resistant cases (Hawkins, 2000). The presence of pneumonia should be verified by tracheal wash and cultures.

Prevention Aspiration of drugs and other compounds may be avoided through careful administration of oral medications by experienced individuals. Likewise, gavage or orogastric administration of liquids should be performed by experienced individuals, and the procedure should be aborted if coughing or other respiratory signs occur. The aspiration of stomach contents can largely be avoided by appropriate fasting prior to anesthesia for at least 12 h for food and 2 h for water. If appropriate fasting times are not observed, anesthesia should be postponed whenever possible, particularly if intended procedures require manipulation of the viscera or head-down positioning of the dog. If anesthesia cannot be avoided, it should be rapidly induced and the dog should be intubated. During recovery from anesthesia, the endotracheal tube should be removed with the cuff partially inflated and with the dog in a head-up position (Haskins, 1993).

4. Burn Wounds

Based on the source of energy, burn wounds may be categorized into four groups: thermal, chemical, radiation, and electrical. In laboratory animals, accidental burns are usually the result of thermal injury (heating pads, water bottles), chemicals (strong alkalis, acids, disinfectants, drugs), or experimental irradiation protocols.

a. Thermal Injury

Etiology Inappropriate use of external heating devices is the most common cause of burns in laboratory animal medicine. The insult to the skin results in desiccation of the tissue and coagulation of proteins.

In addition, the severely injured area is surrounded by a zone of vascular stasis, which promotes additional tissue damage. Even small burns can result in significant inflammation that could affect the outcome of some research investigations and cause considerable discomfort to the animal. The proper and immediate treatment of burn wounds can reduce the effects of the injury on both the individual and the research.

Clinical Signs   The clinical signs vary with the depth, location, and surface area of burn injury. Classification systems for thermal burns are generally based on the depth of the injury, varying from superficial involvement of only epidermis to complete destruction of skin and subcutaneous tissues (Bohling, 2012). Superficial burns appear erythematous and inflamed. In some cases, matting of the overlaying hair with exudate may be the first sign of a previously undetected skin lesion. Progressive hair and skin loss may be evident over the first few days after injury (Johnston, 1993). Although blistering is a characteristic of partial thickness burns in humans, this is rarely seen in dogs (Bohling, 2012). Uncomplicated, superficial burn wounds heal by reepithelialization within 3–5 days. Deeper burn wounds are characterized by a central area of nonviable tissue surrounded by edematous, inflamed tissues. A thick eschar, composed of the coagulated proteins and desiccated tissue fluid, develops over deep burn wounds. These wounds heal by granulation under the eschar, which will eventually slough.

The amount of pain associated with burns depends upon several factors including the depth and area of the wound, procedural manipulations, and movement at the affected site (Bohling, 2012). Pain associated with superficial burn wounds usually subsides in 2–3 days. Theoretically, deep burns destroy nerve endings and result in less pain than superficial burns. However, inflammatory pain may still be present due to the tissue reaction around the necrotic site. In addition, sharp procedural pain and breakthrough pain have been described in humans during the healing phases of burn injuries and should be considered as potential complications in dogs as well (Bohling, 2012).

Severe and widespread accidental burn injury can result in clinical signs associated with multiple organs including the pulmonary, gastrointestinal, hematopoietic, and immune systems. In addition, extensive burn injury can predispose to infection and even sepsis. This type of injury with the associated complications would be extremely rare in the laboratory setting.

Treatment   Appropriate and timely treatment of a burn wound will reduce the extent of tissue damage and associated pain. Thermal injuries should be immediately exposed to cool water (15°C) to reduce edema and pain. Exposure to very cold water and ice does not improve outcomes (Bohling, 2012). Topical wound dressings are recommended in the early stages of treatment for both partial- and full-thickness burns that are of small size.

Systemic antibiotics are unable to penetrate eschar and are not adequately distributed through the abnormal blood supply of burned tissues. Therefore, a thin film of a water-soluble, broad-spectrum antibiotic ointment should be applied to the wound surface. Silver sulfadiazine has a broad spectrum, penetrates eschar, and is often the preparation of choice for burn wound therapy. Povidone-iodine ointment will also penetrate thin eschar and provides a broad spectrum. Mafenide has a good spectrum that covers gram-negative organisms well and is often used to treat infected wounds, although it has been associated with pain upon application (Demling and Lalonde, 1989). Once a topical antibiotic has been applied, a nonadherent dressing should be placed on the wound. Burn wounds covered in such a manner tend to epithelialize more rapidly and are less painful than uncovered wounds (Demling and Lalonde, 1989; Bohling, 2012). After the initial treatment, burn wounds should be gently cleansed two to three times a day, followed by reapplication of the topical antibiotic and rebandaging (Demling and Lalonde, 1989). Systemic antibiotics are indicated in cases where local or systemic infection is present and their ultimate selection should be based on culture results. Burn wounds can be extremely painful, and analgesia should be instituted immediately and adjusted accordingly throughout the treatment period.

Surgical intervention may be necessary in some cases. With small or moderately sized wounds, the eschar over the burn wound may actually impede wound contraction and reepithelialization. In such cases, once the eschar has become fully defined, a complete resection may improve wound healing. With large and severe burn wounds, repeated debridement by surgery or other means might be necessary. In the laboratory setting, a decision to pursue extensive surgical intervention would be dependent upon full consideration of the effects on animal welfare and research results.

Prevention   Thermal burns can be prevented in the research setting. Electric heating pads and heat lamps should be avoided if possible. Only heated water blankets or circulating warm air devices should be used to provide warmth to the animals. In rare instances, heated water blankets have also caused burns; therefore, these devices should be carefully monitored. As a precaution, a thin towel may be placed between the animal and the water blanket. Basic fire prevention precautions should be taken particularly around oxygen sources and flammable agents

b. Chemical Injury

Etiology   Chemical injury may be due to skin contact with concentrated solutions such as disinfectants or inadvertent exposure to laboratory chemicals. In addition, perivascular injection of certain drugs (pentobarbital, thiamylal, thiopental, thiacetarsemide, vincristine, vinblastine, and doxorubicin) have been associated with extensive tissue damage (Swaim and Angarano, 1990; Waldron and Trevor, 1993). The mechanism of action will vary depending upon the pH, osmolality, and chemical composition of the agent and may include oxidation, reduction, disruption of lipid membranes, or other reactions (Bohling, 2012; Swaim, 1990; Waldron and Trevor, 1993).

Clinical Signs Surface contact with chemicals may result in mild irritation and redness of superficial layers of the skin. However, many agents may cause progressive injury until the chemical reaction has been neutralized. This may result in tissue necrosis and secondary infection. The immediate signs of perivascular injection are withdrawal of the limb or other signs of discomfort and swelling at the injection site. The area may appear red, swollen, and painful as inflammation progresses. There may eventually be necrosis of the skin around the injection site. In cases of doxorubicin extravasation, signs may develop up to a week after the injection, and the affected area may progressively enlarge over a 1- to 4-month period. This is because the drug is released over time from the dying cells (Swaim and Angarano, 1990).

Treatment In cases of skin contact with chemical agents, the affected area should be thoroughly and repeatedly lavaged with warm water to dilute or remove the substance. The material safety data sheet for the substance should be consulted for any possible neutralization protocol. Additional treatment will depend upon the severity of the tissue damage and will follow the same guidelines as for the thermal injury described earlier. For the treatment of perivascular injections, dilution of the drug with subcutaneous injections of saline is recommended. In addition, steroids may be infiltrated locally to reduce inflammation. Topical application of dimethyl sulfoxide (DMSO) may also be helpful in reducing the immediate inflammation and avoiding the development of chronic lesions. The addition of lidocaine to subcutaneous injections of saline has been used in cases of thiacetarsemide injection (Hoskins, 1989). The local infiltration of hyaluronidase accompanied by warm compresses has been suggested for perivascular vinblastine (Waldron and Trevor, 1993) and for doxirubicin. The use of DMSO or another free radical scavenger, dexrazoxane, infused at the site has also been suggested for doxorubicin toxicities. Despite these treatments, necrosis of skin may be observed and would require serial debridement of tissues with secondary wound closure or skin grafting. In cases of doxorubicin extravasation, early excision of affected tissues is advocated to prevent the progressive sloughing caused by sustained release of the drug from dying tissues (Swaim and Angarano, 1990). In all cases, the condition can be painful and analgesia should be addressed.

Prevention Prior to the use of any substance, the investigator should be aware of its chemical composition and the potential for problems. The material safety data sheets should be available for all compounds and storage recommendations followed closely. For intravenous administration of toxic compounds, insertion of an indwelling catheter is extremely important. Prior to the injection, the catheter should be checked repeatedly for patency by withdrawal of blood and injection of saline. Any swelling at the catheter site or discomfort by the subject indicates that the catheter should not be used. Access to a central vessel such as the cranial or caudal vena cava is preferred over the use of peripheral vessels. When peripheral catheters are used, the injection should be followed by a vigorous amount of flushing with saline or other physiological solution and removal of the catheter. Additional injections are best given through newly placed catheters in previously unused vessels. The repeated use of an indwelling peripheral catheter should be approached cautiously and done only out of necessity.

c. Radiation Injury

Etiology Radiation burns are generally a complication of therapeutic administration and are a result of free oxygen radical formation (Waldron, 1993). The severity of radiation burns and their treatment will depend upon the dose, frequency, total surface area, and location of the radiation. Damage to epithelial layers of the skin can lead to desquamation. Direct injury to fibroblasts results in decreased collagen production and poor wound healing. In addition, there may be fibrosis of blood vessels (Pavletic, 2010) and subsequent hypoxia causing necrosis of deeper tissues.

Clinical Signs The tissues most often affected are the skin and mucus membranes. With superficial injury, affected skin may exhibit hair loss and erythema, and produce a clear exudate. The intensity of the inflammation may increase for 1–2 weeks after the completion of radiation treatment. Deeper and more serious injury manifests with subcutaneous fibrosis and can lead to disfigurement (Johnston *et al.*, 1993). The skin and underlying deep structures including the bone may become necrotic over several weeks (Pavletic, 2010). These deeper injuries are prone to infection due to their lack of blood supply. Systemic signs such as vomiting are rare in dogs unless there has been direct radiation treatment to organs (Johnston *et al.*, 1993).

Treatment With superficial skin burns, the wound should be kept clean and should be covered if possible. In cases of oral mucous membrane damage, there may be special feeding requirements. When wounds are ulcerated, avascular tissues should be excised. Treatments with silver sulfadiazine, mafenide acetate, or other topical agents are recommended to control infection. In addition, infection is avoided by closure of the wound as soon as possible. The goal of surgery is to cover the wound with healthy tissue to promote vascularization of the area. In some cases, this may require muscle and/ or skin grafts.

Prevention Radiation burns can be limited by selection of appropriate, fractionated therapy and application of shielding to reduce exposure. Prompt treatment of the injuries can reduce the occurrence of infection. Since radiation is associated with poor wound healing, complications may arise when additional procedures are required. It is recommended to wait at least 1 week (Pavletic, 2010) or even longer (Laing, 1990) prior to administering radiation to a surgical site. After radiation, routine surgeries should be avoided for 1–2 months (Pavletic, 2010).

E. Neoplastic Diseases

1. Introduction

The prevalence of cancer in the general canine population has increased over the years (Dorn, 1976). This can be attributed to the longer life spans resulting from improvements in nutrition, disease control, and therapeutic medicine. Because of these changes, cancer has become a major cause of death in dogs (Bronson, 1982).

In a lifetime cancer mortality study of intact beagles of both sexes, Albert *et al.* (1994) found death rates similar to the death rate of the at-large dog population (Bronson, 1982). Approximately 22% of the male beagles died of cancer. The majority of the tumors were lymphomas (32%) and sarcomas (29%), including hemangiosarcomas of the skin and fibrosarcomas. Of the female beagles dying of cancer (26% of the population studied), three-quarters had mammary cancer (40%), lymphomas (18%), or sarcomas (15%). Of the sarcomas in females, one-third were mast cell tumors. In addition to these tumors that cause mortality, the beagle is also at risk for thyroid neoplasia (Hayes and Fraumeni, 1975; Benjamin *et al.*, 1996).

Because of the popularity of the beagle as a laboratory animal, discussion of specific neoplasms will focus on the tumors for which this breed is at risk, as well as tumors that are common in the general canine population. A complete review of clinical oncology in the dog is beyond the scope of this chapter but can be found elsewhere (Withrow *et al.*, 2013).

2. Biopsy Techniques

Fine-needle aspirates are generally the first diagnostic option for palpable masses, because they can easily be performed in awake, cooperative patients. This technique allows for rapid differentiation of benign and neoplastic processes. In cases where cytologic results from fine-needle aspirates are not definitive, more invasive techniques must be used.

Needle-punch or core biopsies can also be performed in awake patients with local anesthesia. An instrument such as a Tru-Cut® needle (Travenol Laboratories, Inc., Deerfield, Illinois) is used to obtain a 1-mm × 1–1.5-cm biopsy of a solid mass. A definitive diagnosis may be limited by the size of the sample acquired using this technique.

Incisional and excisional biopsies are utilized when less invasive techniques fail to yield diagnostic results. Excisional biopsies aid in histopathological examination and are the treatment of choice when surgery is necessary, because the entire mass is removed. Surgical margins should extend at least 1 cm around the tumor and 3 cm if mast cell tumors are suspected (Morrison *et al.*, 1993). Incisional biopsies are performed when large soft-tissue tumors are encountered and/or when complete excision would be surgically difficult or life-threatening. When performing an incisional biopsy, always select tissue from the margin of the lesion and include normal tissue in the submission.

3. Neoplastic Disease

a. Lymphomas

Etiology Lymphomas are a diverse group of neoplasms that originate from lymphoreticular cells. Canine lymphoma represents 5–7% of canine tumors and a majority (85%) of canine hematopoetic disease (Ettinger, 2003; Vail and Young, 2013). Whereas retroviral etiologies have been demonstrated in a number of species (e.g., cat, mouse, chicken), conclusive evidence of a viral etiology has not been established in the dog. In humans, data implicate the herbicide 2,4-dichlorophenoxyacetic acid as a cause of non-Hodgkin's lymphoma, but studies in dogs with similar conclusions have come under scrutiny (MacEwen and Young, 1991). In addition, tobacco smoke, environmental chemicals, and waste emissions are considered possible risk factors (Marconato *et al.*, 2009; Gavazza *et al.*, 2001)

Clinical Signs Multicentric high-grade lymphoma (MHGL) accounts for the majority of reported cases of canine lymphoma. Depending upon grade, immunophenotype, and location involved, dogs with MHGL usually present with painless, enlarged lymph nodes and nonspecific signs such as anorexia, weight loss, polyuria, polydypsia, fever, and lethargy. When the liver and spleen are involved, generalized organomegaly may be felt on abdominal palpation.

Less commonly, dogs develop alimentary, mediastinal, cutaneous, and extranodal lymphomas. Alimentary lymphoma is associated with vomiting and diarrhea, in addition to clinical signs associated with MHGL. Dogs with mediastinal lymphoma often present with respiratory signs (dyspnea and exercise intolerance) secondary to pleural effusion or cranial vena caval syndrome.

Hypercalcemia is most frequently associated with this form of lymphoma and may result in polyuria, polydypsia, and weakness. Cutaneous lymphoma is an uncommon epitheliotrophic form of lymphoma. It is often referred to as mycosis fungoides and is typically of a CD8+ T-cell immunophenotype. It varies in presentation from solitary to generalized and may mimic any of a number of other inflammatory skin disorders including oral mucosal lesions. The lesions may occur as erythema, plaques, erosions, scales, nodules, crusts, hypopigmentation, and alopecia (Fontaine *et al.*, 2009). Approximately half of the cases are pruritic. A number of extranodal forms of lymphoma have been reported, including tumors affecting the eyes, central nervous system, kidneys, or nasal cavity. Clinical presentation varies, depending on the site of involvement (e.g., nervous system: seizures, paresis, paralysis).

Epizootiology   The incidence of lymphoma is highest in dogs 5–11 years old, accounting for 80% of cases. Although the neoplasm generally affects dogs older than 1 year, cases in puppies as young as 4 months have been reported (Dorn *et al.*, 1967). No gender predilection has been reported.

Diagnosis and Pathologic Findings   A fine-needle aspirate is initially performed on accessible lymph nodes. Thoracic radiographs and abdominal ultrasound ± fine needle aspiration of the liver or spleen can be used if mediastinal or abdominal involvement is suspected. Additional staging can be determined through complete blood counts, serum biochemistry, flow cytometry for immunotyping, bone marrow aspiration, or surgical lymphadenectomy and histology. Enlarged neoplastic lymph nodes vary in diameter from 1 to 9cm and are moderately firm. Some may have areas of central necrosis and are soft to partially liquefied. The demarcation between cortex and medulla is generally lost, and on cut section, the surface is homogenous. The spleen may have multiple small nodular masses or diffuse involvement with generalized enlargement. The enlarged liver may have disseminated pale foci or multiple large, pale nodules. In the gastrointestinal tract, both nodular and diffuse growths are observed. These masses may invade through the stomach and intestinal walls.

Flow cytometry and lymphoblastic markers (CD34) can aid in diagnosis and subtyping of tumors. In addition, positron emission tomography is being explored for detection of extranodal and metastatic lymphoma (LeBlanc *et al.*, 2009; Marconato, 2011; Elstrom *et al.*, 2003).

Classification of lymphoma types is based upon cytological, morphological, and immunological characteristics using the Kiel classification criteria (Vail and Young, 2013). Histologically, the most common lymphomas are classified as intermediate to high grade and of large-cell (histiocytic) origin. The neoplastic lymphocytes typically obliterate the normal architecture of the lymph nodes and may involve the capsule and perinodal areas. Lymphoma subtypes can be further characterized based upon genetic, molecular, and immunological criteria (Ponce *et al.*, 2004).

Pathogenesis   All lymphomas regardless of location should be considered malignant. A system for staging lymphoma has been established by the World Health Organization. The average survival time for dogs without treatment is 4–6 weeks. Survival of animals undergoing chemotherapy is dependent on the treatment regimen as well as the form and stage of lymphoma (MacEwen and Young, 1991). Median survival time with aggressive therapy is generally less than 12 months.

Hypercalcemia is a paraneoplastic syndrome frequently associated with lymphoma. The pathogenesis of this phenomenon is not fully understood but may be a result of a parathormone-like substance produced by the neoplastic lymphocytes.

Differential Diagnosis   Differential diagnoses for multicentric lymphoma include systemic mycosis; salmon-poisoning and other rickettsial infections; lymph node hyperplasia from viral, bacterial, and/or immunologic causes; and dermatopathic lymphadenopathy. Alimentary lymphoma must be distinguished from other gastrointestinal tumors, foreign bodies, and lymphocytic–plasmacytic enteritis. In order to make a definitive diagnosis, whole lymph node biopsies and full-thickness intestinal sections for histopathologic examination may be needed.

Treatment   Therapy for lymphoma primarily consists of one or a combination of several chemotherapeutic agents. In addition, radiation therapy and bone marrow transplantation have been utilized. The treatment regimen is based on the staging of the disease, the presence of paraneoplastic syndromes, and the overall condition of the patient. Although treatment may induce clinical remission and prolong short-term survival, most treatment is palliative and aimed at improving quality of life. A thorough discussion of therapeutic options for the treatment of lymphomas in the dog can be found elsewhere (Chun, 2009; Marconato, 2011). Future directions include development of molecular and cellular targeted therapies to enhance traditional chemotherapy treatment, prolong remission, and treat immunologic subtypes of lymphoma (e.g., T-cell lymphoma).

Research Complications   Given the grave prognosis for lymphoma with or without treatment, euthanasia should be considered for research animals with significant clinical illness.

b. Mast Cell Tumors

Etiology   Mast cells are derived from CD34+ bone marrow progenitor cells. Neoplastic proliferations of mast cells are the most commonly observed skin tumor of the dog and may account for up to 21% of canine skin tumors (Bostock, 1986; Welle *et al.*, 2008). Mast cells are normally found in the connective tissue beneath serous surfaces and mucous membranes, and within the skin, lung, liver, and gastrointestinal tract. Current research has linked mast cell tumor development to multifactorial causes including breed predisposition and a genetic component, chronic inflammation, and mutations in the surface growth factor, *c-kit* (Ma *et al.*, 1999; Reguera *et al.*, 2000; Webster *et al.*, 2006).

Clinical Signs   Well-differentiated mast cell tumors are typically solitary, well-circumscribed, slow-growing, 1- to 10-cm nodules in the dermis and subcutaneous tissue. Alopecia may be observed, but ulceration is not usual. Poorly differentiated tumors grow rapidly, may ulcerate, and may cause irritation, inflammation, and edema to surrounding tissues. Mast cell tumors can be found on any portion of the dog's skin but frequently affect the trunk and hind limb extremeties along with perineal and preputial areas. The tumors usually appear to be discrete masses, but they frequently extend deep into surrounding tissues. Abdominal organs are rarely involved but may be associated with anorexia, vomiting, melena, abdominal pain, and gastrointestinal ulceration. Mast cell tumors have also been reported in extracutaneous areas such as the salivary glands, larynx, nasopharynx (London and Thamm, 2013) and conjunctiva (Fife *et al.*, 2011). Mast cell tumors within the perineal, preputial, or inguinal areas are associated with a greater predilection for recurrence or metastasis (Misdorp, 2004).

Epizootiology   These tumors tend to affect middle-aged dogs but have been observed in dogs ranging from 4 months to 18 years (Pulley and Stannard, 1990).

Pathologic Findings   Because of the substantial variation in histologic appearance of mast cell tumors, a classification and grading system described by Patnaik *et al.* (1986) has become widely accepted. In this system, grade I has the best prognosis and are well differentiated, with round to ovoid, uniform cells with distinct cell borders. The nuclei are round and regular, the cytoplasm is packed with large granules that stain deeply, and mitotic figures are rare to absent. Grade II (intermediately differentiated) mast cell tumors have indistinct cytoplasmic boundaries with higher nuclear–cytoplasmic ratios, fewer granules, and occasional mitotic figures. Grade III (anaplastic or undifferentiated) mast cell tumors have the worst prognosis. The cells contain large, irregular nuclei with multiple prominent nucleoli and few cytoplasmic granules. Mitotic figures are much more frequent. Cells are pleomorphic with indistinct borders. In addition to associated skin lesions (e.g., ulceration, collagenolysis, necrosis, and infection), mast cell tumors have been associated with gastric ulcers in the fundus, pylorus, and/or proximal duodenum, most likely secondary to tumor production of histamine. Histamine stimulates the H_2 receptors of the gastric parietal cells,

causing increased acid secretion. Gastric ulcers have been observed in large numbers (>75%) of dogs with mast cell tumors (Howard *et al.*, 1969).

Pathogenesis   Although all mast cell tumors should be considered potentially malignant, the outcome in individual cases can be correlated with the histologic grading of the tumor. Grade III tumors are most likely to disseminate internally. This spread is usually to regional lymph nodes, spleen, and liver, and less frequently to the kidneys, lungs, and heart.

Diagnosis and Differential Diagnosis   Using fine-needle aspiration, mast cell tumors can be distinguished cytologically from other round cell tumors (such as histiocytomas and cutaneous lymphomas) by using toluidine blue to metachromatically stain the cytoplasmic granules red or purple. Mast cell granules can also be stained with Wright's, Giemsa, and Romanowsky stains. In addition, mast cells may contain tryptase, chymase, or both (Fernandez *et al.*, 2005). Histological evaluation is generally required for grading. Examination of regional lymph nodes may be warranted if metastatic or systemic disease is suspected. In addition, radiographs and ultrasound with guided aspirates of the liver, spleen, or sublumbar lymph nodes can be used to determine metastatic disease.

Treatment   Depending upon the grade, initial treatment for mast cell tumors is generally wide surgical excision (3-cm margins), which may be followed by radiation, chemotherapy, or glucocorticoid therapy. Aspiration or surgical removal of regional lymph nodes is recommended if lymphatic tumor drainage is suspected. If the tumor is not completely resectable or is grade II or III (moderately to undifferentiated), then debulking surgery and adjunct therapy may be used. Treatment algorithms are outlined elsewhere (Withrow *et al.*, 2013)

Research Complications   Because of the potential for systemic release of substances such as histamine, vasoactive substances, heparin, eosiniphilic chemotactic factor, and proteolytic enzymes, along with the possibility of delayed wound healing and tumor recurrence, dogs with mast cell tumors are not good candidates for research studies. Grade I mast cell tumors may be excised, allowing dogs to continue on study; however, monitoring for local recurrence should be performed monthly. Grade II tumors are variable; animals that undergo treatment should be monitored for recurrence monthly, and evaluation of the buffy coat should be performed every 3–6 months for detection of systemic mastocytosis. Because of the poor prognosis for grade III tumors, treatment is unwarranted in the research setting.

c. Canine Transmissible Venereal Tumors

Etiology   Also known as infectious or venereal granuloma, Sticker tumor, transmissible sarcoma, and contagious venereal tumor, the canine transmissible venereal tumor (CTVT) is transmitted horizontally to the genitals by coitus (Nielsen and Kennedy, 1990). CTVT is a 'parasitic-like' tumor that appears to have originated from dogs or wolves thousands of years ago and despite immense mutation, CTVT adapted, survived, and spread across multiple continents making it the oldest known continuously passaged somatic cell line (Rebbeck *et al.*, 2009; Murchison *et al.*, 2014; Murgia *et al.*, 2006). It has been described as a round cell tumor of histiocytic origin. Although this tumor has been reported in most parts of the world, it is most prevalent in tropical or temperate climates (MacEwen, 1991).

Clinical Signs The tumors are usually cauliflower-like masses on the external genitalia, but they can also be pedunculated, nodular, papillary, or multilobulated. These friable masses vary in size up to 10 cm, and hemorrhage is frequently observed. In male dogs, the lesions are found on the caudal part of the penis from the crura to the bulbus glandis or on the glans penis. Less frequently, the tumor is found on the prepuce. Females typically have lesions in the posterior vagina at the junction of the vestibule and vagina. When located around the urethral orifice, the mass may protrude from the vulva. These tumors have also been reported in the oral cavity, skin, and eyes.

Epizootiology and Transmission CTVTs are most commonly observed in young, sexually active dogs. Transmission takes place during coitus when injury to the genitalia allows for exfoliation and transplantation of the tumor. Genital to oral to genital transmission has also been documented (Nielsen and Kennedy, 1990). Extragenital lesions may be the result of oral contact with previously traumatized areas.

Pathologic Findings Histologically, cells are arranged in compact masses or sheets. The cells are round, ovoid, or polyhedral, and have large, round nuclei with coarse chromatin. The cytoplasm is eosinophilic with small vacuoles arranged in a 'string of pearls' pattern.

Pathogenesis Tumor growth occurs within 2–6 months after mating or implantation, and then growth generally slows. Metastasis is rare (<5–17% of cases) but may involve the superficial inguinal and external iliac lymph nodes as well as distant sites. Spontaneous regression may occur within 6–9 months of tumor development.

Diagnosis and Differential Diagnosis Transmissible venereal tumors have been confused with lymphomas, histiocytomas, mast cell tumors, and amelanotic melanomas. However, cytological examination of impression smears, swabs, and fine-needle aspirates generally provide a definitive diagnosis. Although not usually required, histopathology of a biopsy from the mass can aid in diagnosis.

Prevention Thorough physical examinations prior to bringing new animals into a breeding program should prevent introduction of this tumor into a colony.

Control Removing affected individuals from a breeding program should stop further spread through the colony.

Treatment Surgery and radiation can be used for treatment, but chemotherapy is the most effective. Vincristine (0.5–0.7 mg/m^2) IV once weekly for four to six treatments will induce remission and cure in greater than 90% of the cases (MacEwen, 1991).

Research Complications Experimental implantation of CTVTs has been shown to elicit formation of tumor-specific IgG (Cohen, 1972). This response may occur in natural infections and could possibly interfere with immunologic studies.

d. Mammary Gland Tumors

Etiology Dogs are susceptible to a wide variety of mammary gland neoplasms, most of which are influenced by circulating reproductive steroidal hormones.

Clinical Signs Single nodules are found in approximately 75% of the cases of canine mammary tumors. The nodules can be found in the glandular tissue or associated with the nipple. Masses in the two most caudal glands (fourth and fifth) account for a majority of the tumors. Benign tumors tend to be small, well circumscribed, and firm, whereas malignant tumors are larger, invasive, and coalescent with adjacent tissues. Inflammatory mammary carcinomas may mimic mastitis or severe dermatitis and must be ruled out to prevent misdiagnosis.

Epizootiology Mammary tumors are uncommon in dogs under 5 years of age with the incidence rising sharply after that. The median age at diagnosis is 10–11 years. A longitudinal study of a large beagle colony showed that significant risk for development of mammary tumors begins at approximately 8 years of age (Taylor *et al.*, 1976). Mammary tumors occur almost exclusively in female dogs, with most reports in male dogs being associated with endocrine abnormalities, such as estrogen-secreting Sertoli cell tumors.

Pathologic Findings The T (tumor size), N (lymph node involvement), and M (metastasis) system is commonly used to stage mammary tumors. Based on histologic classification of mammary gland tumors, approximately half of the reported tumors are benign (fibroadenomas, simple adenomas, and benign mesenchymal tumors), and half are malignant (solid carcinomas, tubular adenocarcinomas, papillary adenocarcinomas, anaplastic carcinomas, sarcomas, and carcinosarcomas) (Bostock, 1977). Histopathologic grades are scored based upon tubule formation, nuclear pleomorphism, and mitosis (Elston and Ellis, 2002). Extensive discussions of classification, staging, and histopathologic correlations can be found elsewhere (Moulton, 1990; Sorenmo *et al.*, 2011).

Pathogenesis Mammary tumors of the dog develop under the influence of hormones. Receptors for both estrogen and progesterone can be found in 60–70% of tumors. Malignant mammary tumors typically spread through the lymphatic vessels. Metastasis from the first, second, and third mammary glands is to the ipsilateral axillary or anterior sternal lymph nodes. The fourth and fifth mammary glands drain to the superficial inguinal lymph nodes where metastasis can be found. Many mammary carcinomas will eventually metastasize to the lungs and extraskeleton.

Diagnosis and Differential Diagnosis   Both benign and malignant mammary tumors must be distinguished from mammary hyperplasia, mastitis, and severe dermatitis. Cytological evaluation from fine-needle aspirates correlates well with histological examination of benign and malignant tumors (Simon *et al.*, 2009). Radiographs and possibly ultrasound should be performed to rule out metastatic disease prior to surgery.

Prevention   The lifetime risk of developing mammary tumors can effectively be reduced to 0.5% by spaying bitches prior to the first estrus (Schneider *et al.*, 1969). This is commonly done in the general pet population at 6 months of age. The protective effects of early spay rapidly decrease after several estrus cycles. Dogs spayed prior to the first estrus had a risk of 0.8%, whereas dogs spayed after the first and second estrus had risks of 8% and 26%, respectively.

Treatment   Surgery is the treatment of choice for mammary tumors, because chemotherapy and radiation therapy have not been reported to be effective. The extent of the surgery is dependent on the area involved. Single mammary tumors should be surgically removed with 2-cm lateral margins or margins wide enough for complete resection. Deep margins may include removing sections of abdominal fascia or musculature *en bloc* with mammary tumor. Multiple mammary tumors should be removed via regional or unilateral chain mastectomies. Bilateral, staged mastectomies are reserved for more aggressive tumors. There is insufficient evidence at this time to recommend routine complete unilateral or bilateral chain mastectomies. At the time of surgery, axillary lymph nodes are removed only if enlarged or positive on cytology for metastasis. Sorenmo *et al.* (2013) provide a thorough review of canine mammary gland neoplasia.

Research Complications   Treatment of early-stage or low-grade mammary tumors may be rewarding, allowing dogs to continue on study. If removed early enough, malignant masses could yield the same results. All dogs should be monitored regularly for recurrence and new mammary tumors.

F. Miscellaneous Diseases

1. Congenital Disorders

Beagles are subject to many of the inherited and/or congenital disorders that affect dogs in general. In a reference table on the congenital defects of dogs (Hoskins, 2000), disorders for which beagles are specifically mentioned include brachyury (short tail), spina bifida, pulmonic stenosis, cleft palate–cleft lip complex, deafness, cataracts, glaucoma, microphthalmos, optic nerve hypoplasia, retinal dysplasia, tapetal hypoplasia, factor VII deficiency, pyruvate kinase deficiency, pancreatic hypoplasia, epilepsy, GM_1 gangliosidosis, globoid cell leukodystrophy, XX sex reversal, and cutaneous asthenia (Ehlers–Danlos syndrome). Other defects observed include cryptorchidism, monorchidism, limb deformity, inguinal hernia, diaphragmatic hernia, hydrocephaly, and fetal anasarca. Each of these other congenital defects occurred at less than 1.0% incidence.

2. Age-Related Diseases

a. Benign Prostatic Hyperplasia

Etiology   Benign prostatic hyperplasia (BPH) is an age-related condition in intact male dogs. The hyperplasia of prostatic glandular tissue is a response to the presence of both testosterone and estrogen.

Clinical Signs   BPH is often subclinical. Straining to defecate (tenesmus) may be seen because the enlarged gland impinges on the rectum. Urethral discharge (yellow to red) and hematuria can also be presenting clinical signs.

Epizootiology and Transmission   BPH typically affects older dogs (>4 years), although glandular hyperplasia begins as early as 3 years of age. Approximately 95% of inact male dogs will develop BPH by 9 years of age (Smith, 2008).

Pathologic Findings   In the early stages of BPH, there is hyperplasia of the prostatic glandular tissue. This is in contrast to human BPH, which is primarily stromal in origin. Eventually, the hyperplasia tends to be cystic, with the cysts containing a clear to yellow fluid. The prostate becomes more vascular with a honeycomb appearance (resulting in hematuria or hemorrhagic urethral discharge), and BPH may be accompanied by mild chronic inflammation.

Pathogenesis   BPH occurs in older intact male dogs because increased production of estrogens (estrone and estradiol), combined with decreased secretion of androgens, sensitizes prostatic androgen receptors to dihydrotestosterone. The presence of estrogens may also increase the number of androgen receptors, and hyperplastic prostate glands also have an increased ability to metabolize testosterone to 5α-dihydrotestosterone (Kustritz and Klausner, 2000) mediating BPH.

Diagnosis and Differential Diagnosis   BPH is diagnosed in cases of nonpainful symmetrical swelling of the prostate gland in intact male dogs, with normal hematologic profiles and urinalysis that may be characterized by hemorrhage. A prostatic biopsy can be performed to confirm diagnosis. Differential diagnoses include squamous metaplasia of the prostate, para-prostatic cysts, bacterial prostatitis, prostatic abscessation, and prostatic neoplasia (primarily adenocarcinoma). These differential diagnoses also increase in frequency with age and, except for squamous metaplasia, can also occur in castrated dogs. As such, these conditions do not necessarily abate or resolve with castration.

Prevention Castration is the primary means for prevention of benign prostatic hyperplasia.

Treatment The first and foremost treatment for BPH is castration. In pure cases of BPH, castration results in involution of the prostate gland detectable by rectal palpation within 7–10 days. For most dogs in research studies, this is a viable option to rapidly improve the animal's condition. The alternative to castration is hormonal therapy, primarily with estrogens. This may be applicable in cases where semen collection is necessary from a valuable breeding male (e.g., genetic diseases). If the research study concerns steroidal hormone functions, then neither the condition nor the treatment is compatible. Finasteride, a synthetic 5α-reductase inhibitor, has been used in dogs to limit the metabolism of testosterone to 5α-dihydrotestosterone. Treatment at daily doses of 0.1–0.5 mg/kg orally for 16 weeks was shown to reduce prostatic diameter and volume without affecting testicular spermatogenesis (Sirinarumitr *et al.*, 2001). Upon discontinuation of finasteride, the prostate generally returns to its pretreatment size within several months (Smith, 2008). Gonadotropin-releasing hormone analogs such as desorelin inhibit production of testosterone and estrogen via negative feedback on the hypothalamus–pituitary axis. This is available in a sustained release subcutaneous implant, which has demonstrated efficacy in reducing prostatic size in dogs (Junaidi *et al.*, 2009). However, medical therapy has not shown to be as advantageous as castration.

Research Complications BPH can cause complications to steroidal hormone studies, in that the condition may be indicative of abnormal steroidal hormone metabolism, and neither castration nor estrogen therapy is compatible with study continuation. The development of tenesmus as a clinical sign may also affect studies of colorectal or anal function.

Research Model Older dogs with benign protastic hypertrophy are used in research to evaluate the use of ultrasonic histotripsy as a precise nonsurgical urethral-sparing alternative to prostate surgery (Lake *et al.*, 2008; Hall *et al.*, 2009; Schade *et al.*, 2012).

b. Juvenile Polyarteritis Syndrome

Etiology Juvenile polyarteritis syndrome (JPS), also known as steroid-responsive meningitis-arteritis, is a painful disorder seen in young beagles (occasionally reported in other breeds) caused by a systemic necrotizing vasculitis. The cause of the vasculitis has not been established but appears to have an autoimmune-mediated component and may have a hereditary predisposition.

Clinical Signs Clinical signs of JPS include fever, anorexia, lethargy, and reluctance to move the head and neck. The dogs tend to have a hunched posture and/or an extended head and neck. Most dogs seem to be in pain when touched, especially in the neck region. Neurological examination may reveal proprioceptive deficits, paresis, or paralysis. The syndrome typically has a course of remissions and relapses characterized by 3–7 days of illness and 2–4 weeks of remission (Scott-Moncrieff *et al.*, 1992). There may be a component of this condition that is subclinical, given that vasculitis has been diagnosed postmortem in beagles that had no presenting signs.

Epizootiology and Transmission JPS typically affects young beagles (6–40 months), with no sex predilection. JPS has been reported in other breeds including sibling Welsh Springer Spaniels (Caswell and Nykamp, 2003).

Pathologic Findings On gross necropsy, foci of hemorrhage can be seen in the coronary grooves of the heart, cranial mediastinum, and cervical spinal cord meninges (Snyder *et al.*, 1995). Local lymph nodes may be enlarged and hemorrhagic. Histologically, necrotizing vasculitis and perivasculitis of small to medium-sized arteries are seen. These lesions are most noticeable where gross lesions are observed, but they may be seen in other visceral locations. Arterial fibrinoid necrosis leading to thyroid gland hemorrhage and inflammation was also reported (Peace *et al.*, 2001). The perivasculitis often results in nodules of inflammatory cells that eccentrically surround the arteries. The cellular composition of these nodules is predominantly neutrophils, but it can also consist of lymphocytes, plasma cells, or macrophages (Snyder *et al.*, 1995). Fibrinous thrombosis of the affected arteries is also seen. A subclinical vasculitis has also been diagnosed in beagles post mortem; it is not known whether this subclinical condition is a different disorder or part of a JPS continuum. This subclinical vasculitis often affects the coronary arteries (with or without other sites).

Pathogenesis The initiating factors for JPS are unknown. It was once presumed to be a reaction to test compounds by laboratory beagles, but this may have been coincident to the fact that the beagle is the breed most often affected with JPS. Immune mediation of JPS is strongly suspected, because the clinical signs have a cyclic nature and respond to treatment with corticosteroids, and the affected dogs have elevated α$_2$-globulin fractions and abnormal immunologic responses. There may be hereditary predisposition, given that pedigree analysis has indicated that the offspring of certain sires are more likely to be affected, and breeding of two affected dogs resulted in one in seven affected pups (Scott-Moncrieff *et al.*, 1992).

Diagnosis and Differential Diagnosis Differential diagnoses include encephalitis, meningitis, injury or degeneration of the cervical vertebrae or disks, and arthritis. In the research facility, the disorder may be readily confused with complications secondary to the experimental procedure, or with postsurgical pain. Beagles with JPS that were in an orthopedic research study were evaluated for postsurgical complications and skeletal abnormalities prior to the postmortem diagnosis of systemic vasculitis (authors' personal experience).

Prevention and Control No prevention and control measures are known at this time.

Treatment Clinical signs can be abated by administration of corticosteroids. Prednisone administered orally at 1.1 mg/kg, q12h, was associated with rapid relief of clinical symptoms. Maintenance of treatment at an alternate-day regimen of 0.25–0.5 mg/kg was shown to relieve symptoms for several months. However, withdrawal of corticosteroid therapy led to the return of clinical illness within weeks.

Research Complications Because of the potentially severe clinical signs and the need for immunosuppressive treatment, JPS is often incompatible with use of the animal as a research subject. It is unknown whether subclinical necrotizing vasculitis causes sufficient aberrations to measurably alter immunologic responses.

3. Other Miscellaneous Diseases

a. Interdigital Cysts

Etiology Interdigital cysts are chronic inflammatory lesions (not true cysts) that develop in the webbing between the toes. The cause for most interdigital cysts is usually not identified unless a foreign body is present. Bacteria may be isolated from the site, but the lesions may also be sterile (hence the synonym 'sterile pyogranuloma complex').

Clinical Signs Dogs with interdigital cysts are usually lame on the affected foot, with licking and chewing at the interdigital space. Exudation may be noticed at the site of the lesion. The lesion appears as a cutaneous ulcer, usually beneath matted hair, with possible development of sinus tracts and purulent exudate.

Epizootiology and Transmission Interdigital cysts are common in a variety of canine breeds, including German shepherds. Beagles have been affected in the research setting. Interdigital cysts usually occur in the third and fourth interdigital spaces (Bellah, 1993). A retrospective study of beagles housed in a research industry setting, linked development of interdigital cysts to body codition score, age, location of cyst, and type of caging, and may result from chronic interdigital dermatitis (Kovacs *et al.*, 2005).

Pathologic Findings Histopathologically, interdigital cysts are sites of chronic inflammation, typically described as pyogranulomatous.

Pathogenesis Initial development of the cysts is unknown, except for those cases in which a foreign body can be identified.

Diagnosis and Differential Diagnosis Bacterial culture swabs and radiographs should be taken of the cysts to rule out bacterial infection and radiopaque foreign bodies or bony lesions, respectively. A biopsy should be taken if neoplasia is suspected.

Treatment If a foreign body is associated with the lesion, then removal is the first order of treatment. If biopsy of the site provides a diagnosis of sterile pyogranuloma complex, then systemic corticosteroid therapy (e.g., prednisolone at 1 mg/kg q12h) can be initiated and then tapered once the lesion heals. Interdigital cysts that are refractory to medical therapy require surgical removal. Excision includes the removal of the lesion and the interdigital web, and a two-layer closure of the adjacent skin and soft tissues is recommended (Bellah, 1993). The foot should be put in a padded bandage and a tape hobble placed around the toes to reduce tension when the foot is weight-bearing. The prognosis for idiopathic interdigital cysts is guarded, because the cysts tend to recur (Bellah, 1993).

Research Complications Research complications from the cysts are minimal, unless the dogs need to be weight-bearing for biomechanic or orthopedic studies. Treatment with systemic steroids could be contraindicated with some experimental designs.

b. Hyperplasia of the Gland of the Nictitating Membrane

Etiology 'Cherry eye' is a commonly used slang term for hyperplasia and/or prolapse of the gland of the nictitating membrane (third eyelid). This is not considered a congenital anomaly, but there is breed disposition for this condition, including beagles. A specific etiology is not known.

Clinical Signs The glandular tissue of the nictitating membrane protrudes beyond the membrane's edge and appears as a reddish mass in the ventromedial aspect of the orbit. Excessive tearing to mucoid discharge can result, and severe cases can be associated with corneal erosion.

Pathologic Findings Typically, the glandular tissue is hyperplastic, possibly with inflammation. Rarely is the tissue neoplastic.

Pathogenesis Prolapse of the gland may be a result of a congenital weakness of the connective tissue band between the gland and the cartilage of the third eyelid (Helper, 1989).

Prevention Hyperplasia of the third eyelid cannot be prevented, but dogs that develop this condition unilaterally should have the other eye evaluated for potential glandular prolapse. Preventative surgical measures might be warranted.

Treatment Corticosteroid treatment (topical or systemic) can be used to try to reduce the glandular swelling. However, surgical reduction or excision of the affected gland is typically required to resolve the condition. In the reduction procedure, the prolapsed gland is sutured to fibrous tissue deep to the fornix of the conjunctiva (Helper, 1989). If reduction is not possible (as with deformed nictitating cartilage) or is unsuccessful, removal of the gland can be performed. Such excision is fairly straightforward and can be done without removal of the nictitating membrane itself. The gland of the third eyelid is important in tear production; although the rest of the lacrimal glands should be sufficient for adequate tear production, keratoconjunctivitis sicca is a possible consequence after removal of the gland of the nictitating membrane.

Research Complications In most cases, research complications would be minimal, especially if treated adequately. Either the presence of the hyperplastic gland or its removal might compromise ophthalmologic studies.

Acknowledgments

The authors thank Dr. Bambi Jasmin of Marshall Farms for contributions on preventive health practices for Class A dogs.

References

Acke, E., Mcgill, K., Quinn, T., Jones, B.R., Fanning, S., Whyte, P., 2009. Antimicrobial resistance profiles and mechanisms of resistance in *Campylobacter jejuni* isolates from pets. Foodborne Pathog. Dis. 6 (6), 705–710.

Albert, R.E., Benjamin, S.A., Shukla, R., 1994. Life span and cancer mortality in the beagle dog and human. Mech. Ageing Dev. 74 (3), 149–159.

Anacleto, T.P., Lopes, L.R., Andreollo, N.A., Bernis Filho, W.O., Resck, M.C.C., Macedo, A., 2011. Studies of distribution and recurrence of Helicobacter spp. gastric mucosa of dogs after triple therapy. Acta Cir. Bras. 26 (2), 82–87.

Avgeris, S., Lothrop Jr., C.D., McDonald, T.P., 1990. Plasma von Willebrand factor concentration and thyroid function in dogs. J. Am. Vet. Med. Assoc. 196 (6), 921–924.

Bach, A., Just, A., Berthold, H., Ehmke, H., Kirchheim, H., Borneff-Lipp, M., et al., 1998. Catheter–related infections in long-term catheterized dogs. Observations on pathogenesis, diagnostic methods, and antibiotic lock technique. Zentralbl. Bakteriol. 288 (4), 541–552.

Baldwin, K., Bartges, J., Buffington, T., Freeman, L.M., Grabow, M., Legred, J., et al., 2010. AAHA nutritional assessment guidelines for dogs and cats. J. Am. Anim. Hosp. Assoc. 46 (4), 285–296.

Barnard, D.E., Lewis, S.M., Teter, B.B., Thigpen, J.E., 2009. Open- and closed-formula laboratory animal diets and their importance to research. J. Am. Assoc. Lab. Anim. Sci. 48 (6), 709–713.

Beccaglia, M., Luvoni, G.C., 2006. Comparison of the accuracy of two ultrasonographic measurements in predicting the parturition date in the bitch. J. Small Anim. Pract. 47 (11), 670–673.

Beierwaltes, W.H., Nishiyama, R.H., 1968. Dog thyroiditis: occurrence and similarity to Hashimoto's struma. Endocrinology 83 (3), 501–508.

Bellah, J.R., 1993. Surgical management of specific skin disorders. In: Slatter, D. (Ed.), Textbook of Small Animal Surgery, second ed. Saunders, Philadelphia, PA, pp. 341–354.

Bemis, D.A., 1992. Bordetella and mycoplasma respiratory infections in dogs and cats. Vet. Clin. North Am. Small Anim. Pract. 22 (5), 1173–1186.

Benjamin, S.A., Stephens, L.C., Hamilton, B.F., Saunders, W.J., Lee, A.C., Angleton, G.M., et al., 1996. Associations between lymphocytic thyroiditis, hypothyroidism, and thyroid neoplasia in beagles. Vet. Pathol. 33 (5), 486–494.

Bergdall, V.K., Eng, V., Rush, H.G., 1996. Diagnostic exercise: peracute death in a research dog. Lab. Anim. Sci. 46 (2), 226–227.

Beugnet, F., Franc, M., 2012. Insecticide and acaricide molecules and/or combinations to prevent pet infestation by ectoparasites. Trends Parasitol. 28 (7), 267–279.

Bichsel, P., Jacobs, G., Oliver Jr., J.E., 1988. Neurologic manifestations associated with hypothyroidism in four dogs. J. Am. Vet. Med. Assoc. 192 (12) 1745–1417.

Bohling, M.W., 2012. Burns. In: Tobias, K.M., Johnston, S.A. (Eds.), Veterinary Surgery: Small Animal, first ed. Saunders, St. Louis, MO, pp. 1291–1302.

Bostock, D.E., 1986. Neoplasms of the skin and subcutaneous tissues in dogs and cats. Br. Vet. J. 142 (1), 1–19.

Bostock, R., 1977. Neoplasia of the skin and mammary glands of dogs and cats. In: Kirk, R.W. (Ed.), Current Veterinary Therapy VI: Small Animal Practice. Saunders, Philadelphia, PA, pp. 493–496.

Brabb, T., Maggio-Price, L., Dale, D., Deeb, B., Liggitt, D., 1995. Pancreatic adenocarcinoma in two grey collie dogs with cyclic hematopoiesis. Lab. Anim. Sci. 45 (4), 357–362.

Bronson, R.T., 1982. Variation in age at death of dogs of different sexes and breeds. Am. J. Vet. Res. 43 (11), 2057–2059.

Burnens, A.P., Angeloz-Wick, B., Nicolet, J., 1992. Comparison of *Campylobacter* carriage rates in diarrheic and healthy pet animals. Zentralbl. Veterinarmed. B. 39 (3), 175–180.

Butterwick, R.F., Hawthorne, A.J., 1998. Advances in dietary management of obesity in dogs and cats. J. Nutr. 128 (12 Suppl.), 2771S–2775S.

Butterwick, R.F., Markwell, P.J., 1997. Effect of amount and type of dietary fiber on food intake in energy-restricted dogs. Am. J. Vet. Res. 58 (3), 272–276.

Butterwick, R.F., Markwell, P.J., Thorne, C.J., 1994. Effect of level and source of dietary fiber on food intake in the dog. J. Nutr. 124 (12 Suppl.), 2695S–2700S.

Byun, J.W., Yoon, S.S., Woo, G.H., Jung, B.Y., Joo, Y.S., 2009. An outbreak of fatal hemorrhagic pneumonia caused by Streptococcus equi subsp. zooepidemicus in shelter dogs. J. Vet. Sci. 10 (3), 269–271.

Calderon, M.G., Mattion, N., Bucafusco, D., Fogel, F., Remorini, P., La Torre, J., 2009. Molecular characterization of canine parvovirus strains in Argentina: Detection of the pathogenic variant CPV2c in vaccinated dogs. J. Virol. Methods 159 (2), 141–145.

Campbell, K.L., 2000. External parasites: identification and control. In: Ettinger, S.J., Feldman, E.C. (Eds.), Textbook of Veterinary Internal Medicine, fifth ed. Saunders, Philadelphia, PA, pp. 58–62.

Canapp, S.O., Campana, D.M., Fair, L.M., 2012. Orthopedic coaptation devices and small-animal prosthetics. In: Tobias, K.M., Johnston, S.A. (Eds.), Veterinary Surgery, first ed. Saunders, Philadelphia, PA, pp. 638–639.

Castiglioni, V., Vailati Facchini, R., Mattiello, S., Luini, M., Gualdi, V., Scanziani, E., et al., 2012. Enterohepatic Helicobacter spp. in colonic biopsies of dogs: molecular, histopathological and immunohistochemical investigations. Vet. Microbiol. 159 (1–2), 107–114.

Caswell, J.L., Nykamp, S.G., 2003. Intradural vasculitis and hemorrhage in full sibling Welsh springer spaniels. Can. Vet. J. 44 (2), 137–139.

Chalker, V.J., Toomey, C., Opperman, S., Brooks, H.W., Ibuoye, M.A., Brownlie, J., et al., 2003. Respiratory disease in kennelled dogs: serological responses to *Bordetella bronchiseptica* lipopolysaccharide do not correlate with bacterial isolation or clinical respiratory symptoms. Clin. Diagn. Lab. Immunol. 10 (3), 352–356.

Chun, R., 2009. Lymphoma: which chemotherapy protocol and why? Top. Companion Anim. Med. 24 (3), 157–162.

Cohen, D., 1972. Detection of humoral antibody to the transmissible venereal tumor of the dog. Int. J. Cancer 10 (1), 207–212.

Committee on Dogs, Institute of Laboratory Animal Research, Commission on Life Sciences, National Research Council, 1994. Laboratory Animal Management: Dogs. National Academies Press, Washington, DC.

Concannon, P.W., 2011. Reproductive cycles of the domestic bitch. Anim. Reprod. Sci. 124 (3–4), 200–210.

Cork, L.C., 1991. Hereditary canine spinal muscular atrophy: an animal model of motor neuron disease. Can. J. Neurol. Sci. 18 (3 Suppl.), 432–434.

Craven, M., Recordati, C., Gualdi, V., Pengo, G., Luini, M., Scanziani, E., et al., 2011. Evaluation of the Helicobacteraceae in the oral cavity of dogs. Am. J. Vet. Res. 72 (11), 1476–1481.

DaRif, C.A., Rush, H.G., 1983. Management of septicemia in rhesus monkeys with chronic indwelling catheters. Lab. Anim. Sci. 33 (1), 90–94.

Decaro, N., Desario, C., Campolo, M., Elia, G., Martella, V., Ricci, D., et al., 2005. Clinical and virological findings in pups naturally infected by canine parvovirus type 2 Glu-426 mutant. J. Vet. Diagn. Invest. 17 (2), 133–138.

Del Carmen Martino-Cardona, M., Beck, S.E., Brayton, C., Watson, J., 2010. Eradication of Helicobacter spp. by using medicated diet in mice deficient in functional natural killer cells and complement factor D. J. Am. Assoc. Lab. Anim. Sci. 49 (3), 294–299.

DeManuelle, T.C., 2000a. Client information series: canine demodicosis. In: Ettinger, S.J., Feldman, E.C. (Eds.), Textbook of Veterinary Internal Medicine, fifth ed. Saunders, Philadelphia, PA, p. 1970.

DeManuelle, T.C., 2000b. Client information series: fleas and flea allergy dermatitis. In: Ettinger, S.J., Feldman, E.C. (Eds.), Textbook of Veterinary Internal Medicine, fifth ed. Saunders, Philadelphia, PA, p. 1971.

Demling, R.H., Lalonde, C., 1989. Management of the burn wound Burn Trauma. Thieme Medical Publ., Philadelphia, PA, pp. 42–65.

Dennis Jr., M.B., Jones, D.R., Tenover, F.C., 1989. Chlorine dioxide sterilization of implanted right atrial catheters in rabbits. Lab. Anim. Sci. 39 (1), 51–55.

DeNovo, R.C., Magne, M.L., 1995. Current concepts in the management of Helicobacter associated gastritis. Proceedings of the 13th Annual ACVIM Forum. Lake Buena Vista, FL, pp. 57–61.

Dewhirst, F.E., Shen, Z., Scimeca, M.S., Stokes, L.N., Boumenna, T., Chen, T., et al., 2005. Discordant 16S and 23S rRNA gene phylogenies for the genus Helicobacter: implications for phylogenetic inference and systematics. J. Bacteriol. 187 (17), 6106–6118.

Dodman, N.H., Shuster, L., White, S.D., Court, M.H., Parker, D., Dixon, R., 1988. Use of narcotic antagonists to modify stereotypic self-licking, self-chewing, and scratching behavior in dogs. J. Am. Vet. Med. Assoc. 193 (7), 815–819.

Dorn, C.R., 1976. Epidemiology of canine and feline tumors. J. Am. Anim. Hosp. Assoc. 12, 307–312.

Dorn, C.R., Taylor, D.O., Hibbard, H.H., 1967. Epizootiologic characteristics of canine and feline leukemia and lymphoma. Am. J. Vet. Res. 28 (125), 993–1001.

Dryden, M.W., Payne, P.A., Smith, V., Ritchie, D.L., Allen, L., 2012. Evaluation of the ovicidal cctivity of lufenuron and spinosad on fleas' eggs from treated dogs. Int. J. Appl. Res. Vet. Med. 10 (3), 198–204.

Dubey, J.P., Greene, C.E., 2012. Enteric coccidiosis. In: Greene, C.E. (Ed.), Infectious Diseases of the Dog and Cat, fourth ed. Elsevier Saunders, St. Louis, MO, pp. 828.

Dungworth, D.L., 1985. The respiratory system. In: Jubb, K.V., Kennedy, P.C., Palmer, N. (Eds.), Pathology of Domestic Animals, third ed. Academic Press, London, pp. 413–556.

Dzanis, D.A., 1994. The Association of American Feed Control Officials Dog and Cat Food Nutrient Profiles: substantiation of nutritional adequacy of complete and balanced pet foods in the United States. J. Nutr. 124 (12 Suppl.), 2535S–2539S.

Edney, A.T., Smith, P.M., 1986. Study of obesity in dogs visiting veterinary practices in the United Kingdom. Vet. Rec. 118 (14), 391–396.

Elston, C.W., Ellis, I.O., 2002. Pathological prognostic factors in breast cancer. I. The value of histological grade in breast cancer: experience from a large study with long-term follow-up. Histopathology 41 (3A), 154–161.

Elstrom, R., Guan, L., Baker, G., Nakhoda, K., Vergilio, J.A., Zhuang, H., et al., 2003. Utility of FDG-PET scanning in lymphoma by WHO classification. Blood 101 (10), 3875–3876.

Ettinger, S.N., 2003. Principles of treatment for canine lymphoma. Clin. Tech. Small Anim. Pract. 18 (2), 92–97.

Evans, H.E., de Lahunta, A., 2012. Miller's Anatomy of the Dog, fourth ed. Saunders, St. Louis, MO.

Ferguson, D.C., 1994. Update on diagnosis of canine hypothyroidism. Vet. Clin. North Am. Small Anim. Pract. 24 (3), 515–539.

Fernandez, N.J., West, K.H., Jackson, M.L., Kidney, B.A., 2005. Immunohistochemical and histochemical stains for differentiating canine cutaneous round cell tumors. Vet. Pathol. 42 (4), 437–445.

Field, G., Jackson, T.A., 2006. The Laboratory Canine. CRC Press, New York.

Fife, M., Blocker, T., Fife, T., Dubielzig, R.R., Dunn, K., 2011. Canine conjunctival mast cell tumors: a retrospective study. Vet. Ophthalmol. 14, 153–160.

Fontaine, J., Bovens, C., Bettenay, S., Mueller, R.S., 2009. Canine cutaneous epitheliotropic T-cell lymphoma: a review. Vet. Comp. Oncol. 7 (1), 1–14.

Ford, R.B., 2012. Canine infectious respiratory disease. In: Greene, C.E. (Ed.), Infectious Diseases of the Dog and Cat, fourth ed. Elsevier Saunders, St. Louis, MO, pp. 55–57.

Fox, J.G., 1995. Helicobacter-associated gastric disease in ferrets, dogs, and cats. In: Bonagura, J.D. (Ed.), Kirk's Current Veterinary Therapy XII: Small Animal Practice. Saunders, Philadelphia, PA, pp. 720–723.

Fox, J.G., 2012. Enteric bacterial infections. In: Greene, C.E. (Ed.), Infectious Diseases of the Dog and Cat, fourth ed. Elsevier Saunders, St. Louis, MO, pp. 370–380.

Garnett, N.L., Eydelloth, R.S., Swindle, M.M., Vonderfecht, S.L., Strandberg, J.D., Luzarraga, M.B., 1982. Hemorrhagic streptococcal pneumonia in newly procured research dogs. J. Am. Vet. Med. Assoc. 181 (11), 1371–1374.

Gavazza, A., Presciuttini, S., Barale, R., Lubas, G., Gugliucci, B., 2001. Association between canine malignant lymphoma, living in industrial areas, and use of chemicals by dog owners. J. Vet. Intern. Med. 15 (3), 190–195.

Gavrilovic, B.B., Andersson, K., Linde Forsberg, C., 2008. Reproductive patterns in the domestic dog—a retrospective study of the Drever breed. Theriogenology 70 (5), 783–794.

Gay, W.I., 1984. The dog as a research subject. Physiologist 27 (3), 133–141.

Gobello, C., de la Sota, R.L., Goya, R.G., 2001. A review of canine pseudocyesis. Reprod. Domest. Anim. 36 (6), 283–288.

Goldstein, R.E., 2010. Leptospirosis. In: Ettinger, S.J., Feldman, E.C. (Eds.), Textbook of Veterinary Internal Medicine, seventh ed. Elsevier Saunders, St. Louis, MO, pp. 863–868.

Green, M.L., Miller, J.M., Lanz, O.I., 2008. Surgical treatment of an elbow hygroma utilizing microvascular free muscle transfer in a newfoundland. J. Am. Animal Hosp. Assoc. 44 (4), 218–223.

Greene, C.E., 2000. Bacterial diseases. In: Ettinger, S.J., Felman, E.C. (Eds.), Textbook of Veterinary Internal Medicine, fifth ed. Saunders, Philadelphia, PA, pp. 390–400.

Greene, C.E., Levy, J.K., 2012. Immunoprophylaxis. In: Greene, C.E. (Ed.), Infectious Diseases of the Dog and Cat, fourth ed. Elsevier Saunders, St. Louis, MO, pp. 1196–1197.

Greene, C.E., Sykes, J.E., Moore, G.E., Goldstein, R.E., Schultz, R.D., 2012. Leptospirosis. In: Greene, C.E. (Ed.), Infectious Diseases of the Dog and Cat, fourth ed. Elsevier Saunders, St. Louis, MO, pp. 863–868.

Haesebrouck, F., Pasmans, F., Flahou, B., Chiers, K., Baele, M., Meyns, T., et al., 2009. Gastric helicobacters in domestic animals and non-human primates and their significance for human health. Clin. Microbiol. Rev. 22 (2), 202–223.

Haesebrouck, F., Pasmans, F., Flahou, B., Smet, A., Vandamme, P., Ducatelle, R., 2011. Non-*Helicobacter pylori* Helicobacter species in the human gastric mucosa: a proposal to introduce the terms *H. heilmannii sensu lato* and *sensu stricto*. Helicobacter 16 (4), 339–340.

Hall, E.J., Simpson, K.W., 2000. Diseases of the small intestine. In: Ettinger, S.J., Feldman, E.C. (Eds.), Textbook of Veterinary Internal Medicine, fifth ed. Saunders, Philadelphia, PA, pp. 1182–1237.

Hall, T.L., Hempel, C.R., Wojno, K., Xu, Z., Cain, C.A., Roberts, W.W., 2009. Histotripsy of the prostate: dose effects in a chronic canine model. Urology 74 (4), 932–937.

Halos, L., Beugnet, F., Cardoso, L., Farkas, R., Franc, M., Guillot, J., et al., 2014. Flea control failure? Myths and realities. Trends Parasitol. 30 (5), 228–233.

Hand, M.S., Thatcher, C.D., Remillard, R.L., Roudebush, P., Novotny, B.J., 2010. Small Animal Clinical Nutrition, fifth ed. Mark Morris Institute, Topeka, KS.

Haskins, S., 1993. Operating room emergencies. In: Slatter, D. (Ed.), Textbook of Small Animal Surgery, second ed. WB Saunders, Philadelphia, PA, p. 247.

Hauptman, J.G., Chaudry, I.H., 1993. Shock. In: Bojrab, M.J. (Ed.), Disease Mechanisms in Small Animal Surgery. Lea and Febiger, Philadelphia, PA, pp. 17–20.

Hauptman, J.G., Walshaw, R., Olivier, N.B., 1997. Evaluation of the sensitivity and specificity of diagnostic criteria for sepsis in dogs. Vet. Surg. 26 (5), 393–397.

Hawkins, E.C., 2000. Pulmonary parenchymal disease. In: Ettinger, S.J., Feldman, E.C. (Eds.), Textbook of Veterinary Internal Medicine, fifth ed. Saunders, Philadelphia, PA, pp. 1061–1091.

Hayes Jr., H.M., Fraumeni, J.F., 1975. Canine thyroid neoplasms: epidemiologic features. J. Natl. Cancer Inst. 55 (4), 931–934.

Helper, L.C., 1989. Magrane's Canine Ophthalmology, fourth ed. Lea and Febiger, Philadelphia, PA.

Hermanns, W., Kregel, K., Breuer, W., Lechner, J., 1995. *Helicobacter*-like organisms: histopathological examination of gastric biopsies from dogs and cats. J. Comp. Pathol. 112 (3), 307–318.

Hoskins, J.D., 1989. Thiacetarsamide and its adverse effects. In: Kirk, R.W. (Ed.), Current Veterinary Therapy X: Small Animal Practice. Saunders, Philadelphia, PA, pp. 131–134.

Hoskins, J.D., 2000. Congenital defects of the dog. In: Ettinger, S.J., Feldman, E.C. (Eds.), Textbook of Veterinary Internal Medicine, fifth ed. Saunders, Philadelphia, PA, pp. 1983–1996.

Howard, E.B., Sawa, T.R., Nielson, S.W., Kenyon, A.J., 1969. Mastocytoma and gastroduodenal ulceration. Gastric and duodenal ulcers in dogs with mastocytoma. Pathol. Vet. 6 (2), 146–158.

Hysell, D.K., Abrams, G.D., 1967. Complications in the use of indwelling vascular catheters in laboratory animals. Lab. Anim. Care 17 (3), 273–280.

Jenkins, C.C., Bassett, J.R., 1997. *Helicobacter* infection. Compend. Contin. Educ. Pract. Vet. 19 (3), 267–279.

Jergens, A.E., Willard, M.D., 2000. Diseases of the large intestine. In: Ettinger, S.J., Feldman, E.C. (Eds.), Textbook of Veterinary Internal Medicine, fifth ed. Saunders, Philadelphia, PA, pp. 1238–1256.

Johnson, C.A., 2008. Pregnancy management in the bitch. Theriogenology 70 (9), 1412–1417.

Johnson, L., 2000. Tracheal collapse. Diagnosis and medical and surgical treatment. Vet. Clin. North Am. Small Anim. Pract. 30 (6), 1253–1266. vi.

Johnston, D.E., 1975. Hygroma of the elbow in dogs. J. Am. Vet. Med. Assoc. 167 (3), 213–219.

Johnston, D.E., 1993. Thermal injuries. In: Bojrab, M.J. (Ed.), Disease Mechanisms in Small Animal Surgery, second ed. Lea and Febiger, Philadelphia, PA, pp. 170–177.

Johnston, G., Whiteley, M.A., Kestenman, D.B., Feeney, D., 1993. Radiation Therapy. In: Slatter, D. (Ed.), Textbook of Small Animal Surgery, second ed. WB Saunders, Philadephia, PA, p. 2060.

Joint Working Group on Refinement, 2004. Refining dog husbandry and care. Eighth report of the BVAAWF/FRAME/RSPCA/UFAW Joint Working Group on Refinement. Lab. Anim. 38 (Suppl. 1), 1–94.

Jones, I.D., Case, A.M., Stevens, K.B., Boag, A., Rycroft, A.N., 2009. Factors contributing to the contamination of peripheral intravenous catheters in dogs and cats. Vet. Rec. 164 (20), 616–618.

Joosten, M., Blaecher, C., Flahou, B., Ducatelle, R., Haesebrouck, F., Smet, A., 2013. Diversity in bacterium–host interactions within the species Helicobacter heilmannii sensu stricto. Vet. Res. 44 (1), 65.

Junaidi, A., Williamson, P.E., Trigg, T.E., Cummins, J.M., Martin, G.B., 2009. Morphological study of the effects of the GnRH superagonist deslorelin on the canine testis and prostate gland. Reprod. Domest. Anim. 44 (5), 757–763.

Kealy, R.D., Lawler, D.F., Ballam, J.M., Lust, G., Smith, G.K., Biery, D.N., et al., 1997. Five-year longitudinal study on limited food consumption and development of osteoarthritis in coxofemoral joints of dogs. J. Am. Vet. Med. Assoc. 210 (2), 222–225.

Kemppainen, R.J., Behrend, E.N., 2000. CVT update: interpretation of endocrine diagnostic test results for adrenal and thyroid disease. In: Bonagura, J.D. (Ed.), Kirk's Current Veterinary Therapy XIII: Small Animal Practice. Saunders, Philadelphia, PA, pp. 321–324.

Kemppainen, R.J., Clark, T.P., 1994. Etiopathogenesis of canine hypothyroidism. Vet. Clin. North Am. Small Anim. Pract. 24 (3), 467–476.

Kienzle, E., Rainbird, A., 1991. Maintenance energy requirement of dogs: what is the correct value for the calculation of metabolic body weight in dogs? J. Nutr. 121 (11 Suppl.), S39–S40.

Kim, M.K., Jee, H., Shin, S.W., Lee, B.C., Pakhrin, B., Yoo, H.S., et al., 2007. Outbreak and control of haemorrhagic pneumonia due to Streptococcus equi subspecies zooepidemicus in dogs. Vet. Rec. 161 (15), 528–530.

Kirby, R., 1995. Septic shock. In: Bonagura, J.D. (Ed.), Kirk's Current Veterinary Therapy XII: Small Animal Practice. Saunders, Philadelphia, PA, pp. 139–146.

Klopfleisch, R., Kohn, B., Plog, S., Weingart, C., Nöckler, K., Mayer-Scholl, A., et al., 2010. An emerging pulmonary haemorrhagic syndrome in dogs: similar to the human leptospiral pulmonary haemorrhagic syndrome? Vet. Med. Int. 2010, 1–7.

Kornegay, J.N., Sharp, N.J., Scheuler, R.O., Betts, C.W., 1994. Tarsal joint contracture in dogs with golden retriever muscular dystrophy. Lab. Anim. Sci. 44 (4), 331–333.

Kovacs, M.S., McKiernan, S., Potter, D.M., Chilappagari, S., 2005. An epidemiological study of interdigital cysts in a research beagle colony. Contemp. Top. Lab. Anim. Sci. 44 (4), 17–21.

Kubota, S., Ohno, K., Tsukamoto, A., Maeda, S., Murata, Y., Nakashima, K., et al., 2013. Value of the (13)C-urea breath test for detection of gastric helicobacter spp. infection in dogs undergoing endoscopic examination. J. Vet. Med. Sci. 75 (8), 1049–1054.

Kusters, J.G., van Vliet, A.H., Kuipers, E.J., 2006. Pathogenesis of Helicobacter pylori infection. Clin. Microbiol. Rev. 19 (3), 449–490.

Kustritz, M.V.R., Klausner, J.S., 2000. Prostatic diseases. In: Ettinger, S.J., Feldman, E.C. (Eds.), Textbook of Veterinary Internal Medicine, fifth ed. Saunders, Philadelphia, PA, pp. 1687–1698.

Kutzler, M.A., 2005. Semen collection in the dog. Theriogenology 64 (3), 747–754.

Kutzler, M.A., Yeager, A.E., Mohammed, H.O., Meyers-Wallen, V.N., 2003. Accuracy of canine parturition date prediction using fetal measurements obtained by ultrasonography. Theriogenology 60 (7), 1309–1317.

Kwei, G.Y., Gehret, J.R., Novak, L.B., Drag, M.D., Goodwin, T., 1995. Chronic catheterization of the intestines and portal vein for absorption experimentation in beagle dogs. Lab. Anim. Sci. 45 (6), 683–685.

Laflamme, D.P., Kuhlman, G., Lawler, D.F., 1997. Evaluation of weight loss protocols for dogs. J. Am. Anim. Hosp. Assoc. 33 (3), 253–259.

Laing, E.J., 1990. Problems in wound healing associated with chemotherapy and radiation therapy. Probl. Vet. Med. 2 (3), 433–441.

Lake, A.M., Hall, T.L., Kieran, K., Fowlkes, J.B., Cain, C.A., Roberts, W.W., 2008. Histotripsy: minimally invasive technology for prostatic tissue ablation in an in vivo canine model. Urology 72 (3), 682–686.

Leblanc, A.K., Jakoby, B.W., Townsend, D.W., Daniel, G.B., 2009. 18FDG-PET imaging in canine lymphoma and cutaneous mast cell tumor. Vet. Radiol. Ultrasound 50 (2), 215–223.

Linde-Forsberg, C., Ström Holst, B., Govette, G., 1999. Comparison of fertility data from vaginal vs intrauterine insemination of frozen-thawed dog semen: a retrospective study. Theriogenology 52 (1), 11–23.

London, C.A., Thamm, D.H., 2013. Mast cell tumors. In: Withrow, S.J., Vail, D.M., Page, R.L. (Eds.), Withrow & MacEwen's Small Animal Clinical Oncology. Saunders, Philadelphia, PA, pp. 335–336.

Lopate, C., 2008. Estimation of gestational age and assessment of canine fetal maturation using radiology and ultrasonography: a review. Theriogenology 70 (3), 397–402.

Lozier, S., Pope, E., Berg, J., 1992. Effects of four preparations of .05% chlorhexidine diacetate on wound healing in dogs. Vet. Surg. 21 (2), 107–112.

Luvoni, G.C., Beccaglia, M., 2006. The prediction of parturition date in canine pregnancy. Reprod. Domest. Anim. 41 (1), 27–32.

Ma, Y., Longley, B.J., Wang, X., Blount, J.L., Langley, K., Caughey, G.H., 1999. Clustering of activating mutations in c-kit's juxtamembrane coding region in canine mast cell neoplasms. J. Invest. Dermatol. 112, 165–170.

MacEwen, E.G., 1991. Transmissible venereal tumors. In: Withrow, S.J., MacEwen, E.G. (Eds.), Small Animal Clinical Oncology, second ed. Saunders, Philadelphia, PA, pp. 533–538.

MacEwen, E.G., 1992. Obesity. In: Kirk, R.W., Bonagura, J.D. (Eds.), Kirk's Current Veterinary Therapy 11: Small Animal Practice. Saunders, Philadelphia, PA, pp. 313–318.

MacEwen, E.G., Young, K.M., 1991. Canine lymphoma and lymphoid leukemias. In: Withrow, S.J., MacEwan, E.G. (Eds.), Small Animal Clinical Oncology, second ed. Saunders, Philadelphia, PA, pp. 451–479.

Marconato, L., 2011. The staging and treatment of multicentric high-grade lymphoma in dogs: a review of recent developments and future prospects. Vet. J. 188, 34–38.

Marconato, L., Leo, C., Girelli, R., Salvi, S., Abramo, F., Bettini, G., et al., 2009. Association between waste management and cancer in companion animals. J. Vet. Intern. Med. 23, 564–569.

Malik, R., Farrow, B.R.H., 1991. Tick paralysis in North America and Australia. Vet. Clin. North Am. Small Anim. Pract. 21, 157–171.

Manning, P.J., 1979. Thyroid gland and arterial lesions of beagles with familial hypothyroidism and hyperlipoproteinemia. Am. J. Vet. Res. 40, 820–828.

Marks, S.L., 1997. Bacterial gastroenteritis in dogs and cats: more common than you think. In: Proceedings of the 15th Annual ACVIM Forum, May 22–25, Lake Buena Vista, FL, pp. 237–239.

Marks, S.L., Rankin, S.C., Byrne, B.A., Weese, J.S., 2011. Enteropathogenic bacteria in dogs and cats: diagnosis, epidemiology, treatment, and control. J. Vet. Intern. Med. 25, 1195–1208.

Merchant, S.R., Taboada, J., 1991. Dermatologic aspects of tick bites and tick-transmitted diseases. Vet. Clin. North Am. Small Anim. Pract. 21, 145–155.

Meunier, L.D., Kissinger, J.T., Marcello, J., Nichols, A.J., Smith, P.L., 1993. A chronic access port model for direct delivery of drugs into the intestine of conscious dogs. Lab. Anim. Sci. 43, 466–470.

Misdorp, W., 2004. Mast cells and canine mast cell tumours: a review. Vet. Q. 26, 156–169.

Mochizuki, M., Yachi, A., Ohshima, T., Ohuchi, A., Ishida, T., 2008. Etiologic study of upper respiratory infections of household dogs. J. Vet. Med. Sci. 70, 563–569.

Mohr, A.J., Leisewitz, A.L., Jacobson, L.S., Steiner, J.M., Ruaux, C.G., Williams, D.A., 2003. Effect of early enteral nutrition on intestinal permeability, intestinal protein loss, and outcome in dogs with severe parvoviral enteritis. J. Vet. Intern. Med. 17, 791–798.

Moriello, K.A., DeBoer, D.J., 2002. Determination of strain variability of Microsporum canis to disinfectants. Vet. Dermatol. 13, 211–229.

Moriello, K.A., Deboer, D.J., 2012. Cutaneous fungal infections. In: Greene, C.E. (Ed.), Infectious Diseases of the Dog and Cat, fourth ed. Elsevier Saunders, St. Louis, MO.

Morrison, W.B., Hamilton, T.A., Hahn, K.A., Richardson, R.C., Janas, W., 1993. Diagnosis of neoplasia. In: Slatter, D. (Ed.), Textbook of Small Animal Surgery, second ed. Saunders, Philadelphia, PA, pp. 2036–2048.

Moulton, J., 1990. Tumors of the mammary gland. In: Moulton, J.E. (Ed.), Tumors in Domestic Animals, third ed. Saunders, Philadelphia, PA, pp. 518–552.

Muller, G.H., Kirk, R.W., Scott, D.W., 1983. Small Animal Dermatology, third ed. Saunders, Philadelphia, PA.

Murchison, E.P., Wedge, D.C., Alexandrov, L.B., Fu, B., et al., 2014. Transmissible dog cancer genome reveals the origin and history of an ancient cell lineage. Science 343, 437–440.

Murgia, C., Pritchard, J.K., Kim, S.Y., Fassati, A., Weiss, R.A., 2006. Clonal origin and evolution of a transmissible cancer. Cell 126, 477–487.

Nader-Djahal, N., Knight, P.R., Davidson, B.A., Johnson, K., 1997. Hyperoxia exacerbates microvascular injury following acid aspiration. Chest 112, 1607–1614.

National Institutes of Health, 2013. Notice regarding NIH plan to transition from use of USDA Class B dogs to other legal sources (NOT-OD-14-034). Available from: <http://grants.nih.gov/grants/guide/notice-files/NOT-OD-14-034.html> (accessed 06.27.14).

National Research Council, 1994. Dogs: Laboratory Animal Management. National Academy Press, Washington, DC.

National Research Council, 1996. Guide for the Care and Use of Laboratory Animals, seventh ed. National Academy Press, Washington, DC.

National Research Council, 2011. Guide for the Care and Use of Laboratory Animals, eighth ed. National Academy Press, Washington, DC.

Newton, C.D., Wilson, G.P., Allen, H.L., Swenberg, J.A., 1974. Surgical closure of elbow hygroma in the dog. J. Am. Vet. Med. Assoc. 164 (2), 147–149.

Nguyen, D.D., Muthupalani, S., Goettel, J.A., Eston, M.A., Mobley, M., Taylor, N.S., et al., 2013. Colitis and colon cancer in WASP-deficient mice require helicobacter species. Inflamm. Bowel Dis. 19 (10), 2041–2050.

Nielsen, S.W., Kennedy, P.C., 1990. Tumors of the genital system. In: Moulton, J.E. (Ed.), Tumors in Domestic Animals, third ed. Saunders, Philadelphia, PA, pp. 479–517.

Noli, C., 2000. Practical laboratory methods for the diagnosis of dermatologic diseases. In: Bongura, J.D. (Ed.), Kirk's Current Veterinary Therapy 13: Small Animal Practice. Saunders, Philadelphia, PA, pp. 526–536.

Office of the Federal Register, 2002. Code of Federal Regulations, Title 9, Animals and Animal Products, subchapter A, parts 1, 2, and 3. Animal Welfare, Washington, DC.

Osuna, D.J., DeYoung, D.J., Walker, R.L., 1990a. Comparison of three skin preparation techniques in the dog. Part 1: Experimental trial. Vet. Surg. 19 (1), 14–19.

Osuna, D.J., DeYoung, D.J., Walker, R.L., 1900b. Comparison of three skin preparation techniques in the dog. Part 2: Clinical trial in 100 dogs. Vet. Surg. 19 (1), 20–23.

Overall, K.L., 2013. Manual of Clinical Behavioral Medicine for Dogs and Cats. Mosby-Year Book, St. Louis, MO.

Oyama, K., Khan, S., Okamoto, T., Fujii, S., Ono, K., Matsunaga, T., et al., 2012. Identification of and screening for human Helicobacter cinaedi infections and carriers via nested PCR. J. Clin. Microbiol. 50, 3893–3900.

Paillot, R., Darby, A.C., Robinson, C., Wright, N.L., Steward, K.F., Anderson, E., et al., 2010. Identification of three novel superantigen-encoding genes in Streptococcus equi subsp. zooepidemicus, szeF, szeN, and szeP. Infect. Immun. 78, 4817–4827.

Panciera, D.L., 1994. Hypothyroidism in dogs: 66 cases (1987–1992). J. Am. Vet. Med. Assoc. 204 (5), 761–767.

Panciera, D.L., Johnson, G.S., 1994. Plasma von Willebrand factor antigen concentration in dogs with hypothyroidism. J. Am. Vet. Med. Assoc. 206 (5), 594–596.

Panciera, D.L., Johnson, G.S., 1996. Plasma von Willebrand factor antigen concentration and buccal bleeding time in dogs with experimental hypothyroidism. J. Vet. Intern. Med. 10 (2), 60–64.

Patnaik, A.K., Ehler, W.J., MacEwen, E.G., 1986. Canine cutaneous mast cell tumor: morphologic grading and survival time in 83 dogs. Vet. Pathol. 21, 469–474.

Pavletic, M.M., 2010. Atlas of Small Animal Wound Management and Reconstructive Surgery, third ed. Wiley-Blackwell, Ames, IA, pp. 189–190.

Peace, T.A., Goodchild, L.R., Vasconcelos, D.Y., 2001. What's your diagnosis? Fever and leukocytosis in a young beagle. Canine juvenile polyarteritis syndrome (beagle pain syndrome). Lab. Anim. (NY) 30, 23–26.

Pesavento, P.A., Hurley, K.F., Bannasch, M.J., Artiushin, S., Timoney, J.F., 2008. A clonal outbreak of acute fatal hemorrhagic pneumonia in intensively housed (shelter) dogs caused by Streptococcus equi subsp. zooepidemicus. Vet. Pathol. 45, 51–53.

Peterson, M.E., Ferguson, D.C., 1989. Thyroid diseases. In: Ettinger, S.J. (Ed.), Textbook of Veterinary Internal Medicine, third ed. Saunders, Philadelphia, PA, pp. 1632–1675.

Plunkett, S., 1993. Urogenital emergencies Emergency Procedures for the Small Animal Veterinarian. WB Saunders, Philadelphia, PA.

Ponce, F., Magnol, J.P., Ledieu, D., Marchal, T., Turinelli, V., Chalvet-Monfray, K., et al., 2004. Prognostic significance of morphological subtypes in canine malignant lymphomas during chemotherapy. Vet. J. 167, 158–166.

Priestnall, S., Erles, K., 2011. Streptococcus zooepidemicus: an emerging canine pathogen. Vet. J. 188, 142–148.

Priestnall, S.L., Erles, K., Brooks, H.W., Cardwell, J.M., Waller, A.S., Paillot, R., et al., 2010. Characterization of pneumonia due to Streptococcus equi subsp. zooepidemicus in dogs. Clin. Vaccine Immunol. 17, 1790–1796.

Pulley, L.T., Stannard, A.A., 1990. Tumors of the skin and soft tissue. In: Moulton, J.E. (Ed.), Tumors in Domestic Animals, third ed. Saunders, Philadelphia, PA, pp. 23–87.

Raghavendran, K., Nemzek, J., Napolitano, L.M., Knight, P.R., 2011. Aspiration-induced lung injury. Crit. Care Med. 39 (4), 818–826.

Rebbeck, C.A., Thomas, R., Breen, M., Leroi, A.M., Burt, A., 2009. Origins and evolution of a transmissible cancer. Evolution 63, 2340–2349.

Reguera, M.J., Rabanal, R.M., Puigdemont, A., Ferrer, L., 2000. Canine mast cell tumors express stem cell factor receptor. Am. J. Dermatopathol. 22, 49–54.

Rieser, T.M., 2013. Arterial and venous blood gas analyses. Top. Companion Anim. Med. 28, 86–90.

Ringler, D.H., Peter, G.K., 1984. Dogs and cats as laboratory animals. In: Fox, J.G., Cohen, B.J., Loew, F.M. (Eds.), Laboratory Animal Medicine. Academic Press, Orlando, FL, pp. 241–271.

Ripley, B., Fujiki, N., Okura, M., Mignot, E., Nishino, S., 2001. Hypocretin levels in sporadic and familial cases of canine narcolepsy. Neurobiol. Dis. 8 (3), 525–534.

Rishniw, M., Liotta, J., Bellosa, M., Bowman, D., Simpson, K.W., 2010. Comparison of 4 Giardia diagnostic tests in diagnosis of naturally acquired canine chronic subclinical giardiasis. J. Vet. Intern. Med. 24, 293–297.

Sanchez, I.R., Swaim, S.F., Nusbaum, K.E., Hale, A.S., Henderson, R.A., McGuire, J.A., 1988. Effects of chlorhexidine diacetate and povidone-iodine on wound healing in dogs. Vet. Surg. 17 (6), 291–295.

Savolainen, P., Zhang, Y., Luo, J., Lundeberg, J., Leitner, T., 2002. Genetic evidence for an East Asian origin of domestic dogs. Science 298, 1610–1613.

Schade, G.R., Hall, T.L., Roberts, W.W., 2012. Urethral-sparing histotripsy of the prostate in a canine model. Urology 80, 730–735.

Schneider, R., Dorn, C.R., Taylor, D.O.N., 1969. Factors influencing canine mammary cancer development and postsurgical survival. J. Natl. Cancer Inst. 43, 1249–1261.

Schwassman, M., Logas, D., 2009. How to treat common parasites safely. In: August, J.R. (Ed.), Consultations in Feline Internal Medicine. Elsevier Saunders, Philadelphia, PA.

Scott, D.W., Miller Jr., W.H., Griffin, C.E., 1995. Muller and Kirk's Small Animal Dermatology, fifth ed. Saunders, Philadelphia, PA.

Scott-Moncrieff, J.C.R., Snyder, P.W., Glickman, L.T., Davis, E.L., Felsburg, P.J., 1992. Systemic necrotizing vasculitis in nine young beagles. J. Am. Vet. Med. Assoc. 201 (10), 1553–1558.

Searcy, G.P., 1995. Hemopoietic system. In: Carlton, W.W, McGavin, D.M. (Eds.), Thomson's Special Veterinary Pathology, second ed. Mosby-Year Book, St. Louis, MO, pp. 285–331.

Seguin, B., Brownlee, L., 2012. Thyroid and parathyroid glands. In: Tobias, K., Johnston, S. (Eds.), Veterinary Surgery. Saunders, Philadelphia, PA, pp. 2053–2054.

Sherding, R.G., 1989. Diseases of the small bowel. In: Ettinger, S.J. (Ed.), Textbook of Veterinary Internal Medicine, third ed. Saunders, Philadelphia, PA, pp. 1344–1350.

Sherding, R.G., 1994. Canine infectious tracheobronchitis (kennel cough complex). In: Birchard, S.J., Sherding, R.G. (Eds.), Saunders Manual of Small Animal Practice, first ed. Saunders, Philadelphia, PA, p. 104.

Sherding, R.G., Johnson, S.E., 1994. Diseases of the intestines. In: Birchard, S.J., Sherding, R.G. (Eds.), Saunders Manual of Small Animal Practice, first ed. Saunders, Philadelphia, PA, p. 702.

Shille, V.M., Gontarek, J., 1985. The use of ultrasonography for pregnancy diagnosis in the bitch. J. Am. Vet. Med. Assoc. 187, 1021–1025.

Simon, D., Schoenrock, D., Nolte, I., Baumgartner, W., Barron, R., Mischke, R., 2009. Cytologic examination of fine-needle aspirates from mammary gland tumors in the dog: diagnostic accuracy with comparison to histopathology and association with postoperative outcome. Vet. Clin. Pathol. 38, 521–528.

Sirinarumitr, K., Johnston, S.D., Kustritz, M.V., Johnston, G.R., Sarkar, D.K., Memon, M.A., 2001. Effects of finasteride on size of the prostate gland and semen quality in dogs with benign prostatic hypertrophy. J. Am. Vet. Med. Assoc. 218, 1275–1280.

Smith, J., 2008. Canine prostatic disease: a review of anatomy, pathology, diagnosis, and treatment. Theriogenology 70, 375–383.

Snyder, P.W., Kazacos, E.A., Scott-Moncrieff, J.C., HogenEsch, H., Carlton, W.W., Glickman, L.T., et al., 1995. Pathologic features of naturally occurring juvenile polyarteritis in beagle dogs. Vet. Pathol. 32, 337–345.

Sorenmo, K.U., Rasotto, R., Zappulli, V., Goldschmidt, M.H., 2011. Development, anatomy, histology, lymphatic drainage, clinical features, and cell differentiation markers of canine mammary gland neoplasms. Vet. Pathol. 48, 85–97.

Sorenmo, K.U., Worley, D.R., Goldschmidt, M.H., 2013. Tumors of the mammary gland. In: Withrow, S.J., Vail, D.M., Page, R.L. (Eds.), Withrow & Macewen's Small Animal Clinical Oncology. Saunders, Philadelphia, PA.

Sousa, C.A., 2010. Fleas, flea allergy, and flea control. In: Ettinger, S.J., Feldman, E.C. (Eds.), Textbook of Veterinary Internal Medicine, seventh ed. Elsevier Saunders, St. Louis, MO.

Subcommittee on Dog and Cat Nutrition, C.O.A.N., Board on Agriculture and Natural Resources, Division on Earth and Life Studies, National Research Council, 2006. Nutrient Requirements of Dogs and Cats (Nutrient Requirements of Domestic Animals). National Academies Press, Washington, DC.

Swaim, S.F., 1980. Trauma to the skin and subcutaneous tissues of dogs and cats. Vet. Clin. North Am. Small Anim. Pract. 10 (3), 599–618.

Swaim, S.F., Angarano, D.W., 1990. Chronic problem wounds of dog limbs. Clin. Dermatol. 8 (3–4), 175–186.

Sykes, J.E., Hartmann, K., Lunn, K.F., Moore, G.E., Stoddard, R.A., Goldstein, R.E., 2011. 2010 ACVIM small animal consensus statement on leptospirosis: diagnosis, epidemiology, treatment, and prevention. J. Vet. Intern. Med. 25, 1–13.

Tarvin, G., Prata, R.G., 1980. Lumbosacral stenosis in dogs. J. Am. Vet. Med. Assoc. 177, 154–159.

Taylor, G.N., Shabestari, L., Williams, J., Mays, C.W., Angus, W., Mcfarland, S., 1976. Mammary neoplasia in a closed beagle colony. Cancer Res. 36, 2740–2743.

Thalmann, O., Shapiro, B., Cui, P., Schuenemann, V.J., Sawyer, S.K., Greenfield, D.L., et al., 2013. Complete mitochondrial genomes of ancient canids suggest a European origin of deomestic dogs. Science 342 (6160), 871–874.

Thatcher, C.D, Hand, M.S., Remillard, R.L., 2010. Small animal clinical nutrition: an iterative process. In: Hand, M.S., Thatcher, C.D., Remillard, R.L., Roudebush, P., Novotny, B.J. (Eds.), Small Animal Clinical Nutrition, fifth ed. Mark Morris Institute, Topeka, KS.

Thomassen, R., Farstad, W., 2009. Artificial insemination in canids: a useful tool in breeding and conservation. Theriogenology 71, 190–199.

Thomassen, R., Sanson, G., Krogenaes, A., Fougner, J.A., Berg, K.A., Farstad, W., 2006. Artificial insemination with frozen semen in dogs: a retrospective study of 10 years using a non-surgical approach. Theriogenology 66, 1645–1650.

Tilley Jr., L.P., Smith, F.W.K., Oyama, M., 2007. Manual of Canine and Feline Cardiology, fourth ed. Saunders, Philadelphia, PA.

Tomida, J., Oumi, A., Okamoto, T., Morita, Y., Okayama, A., Misawa, N., et al., 2013. Comparative evaluation of agar dilution and broth microdilution methods for antibiotic susceptibility testing of Helicobacter cinaedi. Microbiol. Immunol. 57, 353–358.

Tucker, W.E., 1962. Thyroiditis in a group of laboratory dogs: a study of 167 beagles. Am. J. Clin. Pathol. 38 (1), 70–74.

Tvarijonaviciute, A., Ceron, J.J., Holden, S.L., Cuthbertson, D.J., Biourge, V., Morris, P.J., et al., 2012. Obesity-related metabolic dysfunction in dogs: a comparison with human metabolic syndrome. BMC Vet. Res. 8, 147.

Uberti, A.F., Olivera-Severo, D., Wassermann, G.E., Scopel-Guerra, A., Moraes, J.A., Barcellos-De-Souza, P., et al., 2013. Pro-inflammatory properties and neutrophil activation by Helicobacter pylori urease. Toxicon 69, 240–249.

U.S. Dept. of Agriculture, Animal and Plant Health Inspection Service, (1998). Animal Welfare Report: Fiscal Year 1997, Table 6, p. 36.

U.S. Dept. of Agriculture, Animal and Plant Health Inspection Service, (2011). Annual Report Animal Usage by Fiscal Year. Available from: <www.aphis.usda.gov/animal_welfare/efoia/downloads/2010_Animals_Used_In_Research.pdf> (Accessed 11.15.13).

Vail, D.M., Young, K.M., 2013. Hematopoietic Tumors. In: Withrow, S.J., Vail, D.M., Page, R.L. (Eds.), Withrow & Macewen's Small Animal Clinical Oncology. Saunders, Philadelphia, PA.

van de Maele, I., Claus, A., Haesebrouck, F., Daminet, S., 2008. Leptospirosis in dogs: a review with emphasis on clinical aspects. Vet. Rec. 163, 409–413.

Van Kruiningen, H.J., 1995. Gastrointestinal system. In: Carlton, W.W., McGavin, D.M. (Eds.), Thomson's Special Veterinary Pathology, second ed. Mosby-Year Book, St. Louis, MO, pp. 1–80.

Verstegen-Onclin, K., Verstegen, J., 2008. Endocrinology of pregnancy in the dog: a review. Theriogenology 70, 291–299.

Wadström, T., Hau, J., Nilsson, I., Ljungh, Å., 2009. Immunoblot analysis as an alternative method to diagnose enterohepatic helicobacter infections. Helicobacter 14, 172–176.

Waldron, D.R., Trevor, P., 1993. Management of superficial skin wounds. In: Slatter, D. (Ed.), Textbook of Small Animal Surgery, second ed. Saunders, Philadelphia, PA, pp. 269–280.

Walton, D.K., 1986. Psychodermatosis. In: Kirk, R.W. (Ed.), Current Veterinary Therapy 9: Small Animal Practice. Saunders, Philadelphia, PA, pp. 557–559.

Wang, G., Clark, C.G., Taylor, T.M., Pucknell, C., Barton, C., Price, L., et al., 2002. Colony multiplex PCR assay for identification and differentiation of Campylobacter jejuni, C. coli, C. lari, C. upsaliensis, and C. fetus subsp. fetus. J. Clin. Microbiol. 40, 4744–4747.

Webster, J.D., Yuzbasiyan-Gurkan, V., Kaneene, J.B., Miller, R., Resau, J.H., Kiupel, M., 2006. The role of c-kit in tumorigenesis: evaluation in canine cutaneous mast cell tumors. Neoplasia 8, 104–111.

Welborn, L.V., Devries, J.G., Ford, R., Franklin, R.T., Hurley, K.F., Mcclure, K.D., et al., 2011. 2011 AAHA Canine Vaccination Guidelines [Online]. Available: <https://www.aahanet.org/publicdocuments/caninevaccineguidelines.pdf>.

Welle, M.M., Bley, C.R., Howard, J., Rufenacht, S., 2008. Canine mast cell tumours: a review of the pathogenesis, clinical features, pathology and treatment. Vet. Dermatol. 19, 321–339.

Wheeler, S.L., Husted, P.W., Roscychuk, R.A. W., Allen, T.A., Nett, T.M., Olson, P.N., 1985. Serum concentrations of thyroxine and 3,5,3'-triiodothyronine before and after intravenous or intramuscular thyrotropin administration in dogs. Am. J. Vet. Res. 26 (12), 2605–2608.

White, R.A.S., 2003. Surgical treatment of specific skin disorders. In: Slatter, D.H. (Ed.), Textbook of Small Animal Surgery. WB Saunders, Philadelphia, PA, pp. 339–355.

White, S.D., 1990. Naltrexone for treatment of acral lick dermatitits in dogs. J. Am. Vet. Med. Assoc. 196 (7), 1073–1076.

Wilkinson, M.J.A., McEwan, N.A., 1991. Use of ultrasound in the measurement of subcutaneous fat and prediction of total body fat in dogs. J. Nutr. 121, S47–S50.

Wilson, D.E., Reeder, D.M. (Eds.), 2005. Mammal Species of the World: A Taxonomic and Geographic Reference, third ed. Johns Hopkins University Press, Baltimore, MD. Available online at: <www.departments.bucknell.edu/biology/resources/msw3>.

Withrow, S.J., Vail, D.M., Page, R.L., 2013. Withrow & MacEwen's Small Animal Clinical Oncology. Saunders, Philadelphia, PA.

13

Biology and Diseases of Cats

Tanya Burkholder, DVM, DACLAM[a], Carmen Ledesma Feliciano, DVM[b], Sue VandeWoude, DVM, DACLAM[c] and Henry J. Baker, DVM, DACLAM[d]

[a]Veterinary Medicine Branch, ORS/DVR, National Institutes of Health, Bethesda, MD, USA
[b]Comparative Medicine Resident, Laboratory Animal Medicine, Colorado State University, Fort Collins, CO, USA [c]Department of Micro-, Immuno- and Pathology, College of Veterinary Medicine and Biomedical Sciences, Colorado State University, Fort Collins, CO, USA [d]Scott-Ritchey Research Center, College of Veterinary Medicine, Auburn University, AL

I. INTRODUCTION

A. Unique Contributions of Cats to Biomedical Research

Domestic cats *(Felis cattus)* comprise a small (2%) percentage of the nonrodent animals used in biomedical research. In 2011, 21,700 cats of a total 1,134,693 nonrodent animals were used in research (APHIS, 2011). According to the National Research Council Committee on Scientific and Humane Issues in the Use of Random Source Dogs and Cats in Research (National Research Council, 2009), peak use of cats occurred in 1974. Since that time, the number of cats used in research has fallen

Laboratory Animal Medicine, Third Edition
DOI: http://dx.doi.org/10.1016/B978-0-12-409527-4.00013-4

by 71%, with more than 98% of those cats being purpose bred for research. Cats are a U.S. Department of Agriculture (USDA) covered species with special housing requirements defined in the Animal Welfare Act and the *Guide for the Care and Use of Laboratory Animals* (NRC, 2011). At the request of congress, a committee of experts formed by the National Research Council examined the use of random source dogs and cats and concluded that obtaining dogs and cats from Class B dealers is not necessary for NIH funded research (National Research Council, 2009). While the number of cats used in biomedical research has declined, cats continue to contribute uniquely to biomedical science and are valuable research model for several disciplines, including aspects of neurology involved in locomotion and spinal trauma, retrovirus and zoonotic disease research, and for developing therapeutic strategies for inherited diseases.

B. Infectious Disease Models

Domestic cats are susceptible to a wide variety of infectious diseases and thus are used for studies that relate to basic pathogenesis to therapeutic trials for testing interventions to aid studies of both human and domestic cat therapies. Several of these infections are zoonotic and, as domestic cats play a critical role in transmission to humans, are studied to understand pathogenesis

and mechanisms of transmission to humans. Examples of infections that have been studied in laboratory settings are listed in Table 13.1. While SPF colonies are typically tested for presence of some viral diseases and toxoplasmosis, not all infections are excluded in laboratory SPF colonies. This is particularly true for colonies that originate for the purposes of establishing models of inherited diseases, as founder animals are typically not SPF derived.

1. Feline Retroviruses: Models of Human AIDS and Potential Viral Vectors for Vaccine Delivery

Domestic cats are susceptible to three retroviruses: feline immunodeficiency virus (FIV), genus *Lentivirus*; feline leukemia virus (FeLV), genus *Gammaretrovirus*; and feline foamy virus (FFV), genus *Spumavirus*. Each of these infections results in a typical retroviral infection – i.e., a DNA copy of the retroviral genome is incorporated into the host genome. However, each of these infections has a different clinical outcome in its host. FFV is generally considered asymptomatic, and thus has been considered to be a potential vehicle for gene therapy delivery (Liu *et al.*, 2013). FeLV can cause either fulminant disease resulting in immunodeficiency and death, or may be controlled and all but eliminated. Effective vaccines are commercially available for FeLV; this, along with testing and isolation or euthanasia

TABLE 13.1   Infectious Diseases Studied in Cats

Agent	Aspects studied	References
VIRUSES		
Feline foamy virus (FFV)	Use as viral vectors	Liu *et al.* (2013)
Feline immunodeficiency virus (FIV)	Animal model for HIV/AIDS	Hartmann (2012), Magden *et al.* (2011), Elder *et al.* (2010)
Feline Leukemia Virus (FeLV)	Animal model for HIV/AIDS and retroviral disease	Hartmann (2012), Willett and Hosie (2013)
Feline calicivirus	Development of vaccines; model for human norovirus infection	Shimizu-Onda *et al.* (2013), Horzinek *et al.* (2013), Scipioni *et al.* (2008), Patel and Heldens (2009), Poulet *et al.* (2008), Huang *et al.* (2010)
Feline coronavirus	SARS vaccine research	Roper and Rehm (2009)
Feline parvovirus	*Parvoviridae* Cross-species transmission; vaccine development	Allison *et al.* (2012, 2013), Hoelzer and Parrish (2010), Truyen and Parrish (2013)
BACTERIA		
Helicobacter pylori, H. felis	Pathogenesis and zoonotic aspects	Perkins *et al.* (1996), Lee *et al.* (1988)
Yersinia pestis	Pathogenesis and zoonotic aspects	Gerhold and Jessup (2013), Watson *et al.* (2001), Carlson (1996)
Bartonella henselae	Pathogenesis and zoonotic aspects	Stutzer and Hartmann (2012), Athanasiou *et al.* (2012)
PROTOZOA		
Toxoplasma gondii	Vaccine development; zoonotic aspects	Gerhold and Jessup, 2013, Esch and Petersen, 2013, Lappin, 2010a

of FeLV positive individuals, has decreased the FeLV incidence in feral and companion cats. FeLV has been studied to understand retroviral-induced immunodeficiency, particularly hematopoietic tumors such as acute lymphoblastic leukemia and lymphoma. After infection with FeLV, a fraction of cats become persistently viremic and virus is excreted, particularly through saliva and nasal secretions. Serological tests are based on detection of the major viral core protein of FeLV (p27 gag) in serum or plasma by enzyme-linked immunosorbent assay (ELISA). Strengths of this model include substantial information on FeLV, pathogenesis of the disease, responses of the immune system, availability of FeLV strains of known virulence, and the ease of inducing infection and disease in cats (Hartmann, 2012; Willett and Hosie, 2013).

Immunodeficiency disease of cats caused by the lentivirus FIV is considered by many to be one of the most relevant naturally occurring models of human acquired immune deficiency syndrome (AIDS) (Hartmann, 2012; Magden et al., 2011; Elder et al., 2010). The advantages of the feline disease model include the similarities with human immunodeficiency virus (HIV, the human lentivirus), similarities in pathogenesis and clinical signs, ease of experimental infection, and predictable disease progression. A weakness of the model relates to the limited variety of reagents available for identifying cells of the cat immune system. FIV has been molecularly cloned and resembles HIV in tissue and cell tropism but is antigenically distinct. Experimental transmission is achieved readily with infected blood or cultured cells. Cell-associated viremia occurs within 1–2 weeks and remains persistent, even after development of antibodies and T cell immunity. Characteristic changes in the immune system include lymphadenopathy, neutropenia, decreased lymphocyte proliferative response, and increased susceptibility to opportunistic infections (Elder et al., 2010). B-cell lymphomas and myeloproliferative disease are seen in some infected cats (Magden et al., 2011). Interestingly, a commercially available vaccine provides reasonable protection against challenge with heterologous viral strains (Yamamoto et al., 2010).

Helicobacter pylori is the etiologic agent responsible for a sequence of degenerative changes in the human gastric mucosa, starting with gastritis, progressing to peptic ulcers, and ending in gastric carcinoma. *Helicobacter felis* is a naturally occurring pathogen in cats that appears to be prevalent in some colonies, but its prevalence or significance as an agent of clinical diseases in the general cat population is not clear (Lee et al., 1988; Perkins et al., 1996). *H. felis* is one of the most interesting *Helicobacter* species infecting animals because of its wide host range, and its ability to induce many of the lesions found in human *Helicobacter* disease, particularly those associated with the chronic infection (Enno et al., 1995; Wang et al.,

2000). In addition to *H. felis* infection, cats appear also to be naturally infected with *H. pylori*, raising the possibility that domestic cats could serve as a reservoir for this human pathogen (Perkins et al., 1996).

C. Spinal Cord Injury

Traumatic spinal cord injury (SCI) affects more than 10,000 people in the United States (Majczynski and Slawinska, 2007) and many veterinary patients annually due to accidents and intervertebral disk diseases among other causes (Webb et al., 2010). Cats have been the preferred species for investigating SCI since the early part of the 20th century (Hultborn and Nielson, 2007) because, despite their small body size, the spinal cord of cats is similar in length (34 cm) and anatomy to the human spinal cord which is 40–45 cm (Perese and Fracasso, 1959). In the SCI model, cats are taught to walk on a treadmill for a period of 3–4 weeks followed by surgery to implant electrodes in the brain and muscles of the rear legs and to create a lesion in the spinal cord, generally at the last thoracic segment (T13) (Rossignol et al., 2002). After a period of recovery, cats are able to regain a normal locomotor pattern using a combination of training, electrical stimulation, and pharmacologic agents which demonstrates that the spinal cord has intrinsic circuitry that generates locomotion (Martinez and Rossignol, 2013). Cats were favored for this research because their size allowed electrophysiological studies to be conducted with ease. The research focus during the last few decades has shifted to transplantation of embryonic stem cells, evaluation of the neurotransmitters and the molecular genetics of the circuitry controlling locomotion in the spinal cord (Hultborn and Nielson, 2007) For these types of studies, mice and rats are more commonly used. However, preclinical translational work for SCI will likely continue to be conducted in large animals, including cats (Kwon et al., 2010). A recent study in cats demonstrated successful grafting of peripheral nerves onto the spinal cord (Hanna et al., 2011) which offers a promising potential therapy for patients with SCI.

D. Sleep Research

Adult cats spend up to two-thirds of their time sleeping which, together with their small size and gentle dispositions, has made them popular models of sleep research. Neuzeret et al. described a new cat model of obstructive sleep apnea (OSA) in which cats are habituated to sleeping in a hammock in one of four positions: supine neck extended, supine neck flexed, prone neck extended, and prone neck flexed. The cats are also habituated to wearing a contiguous positive airway pressure (CPAP), which is the gold standard treatment for OSA in humans. In the cats, OSA occurs when the cats sleep in the supine position with their neck flexed. CPAP treatment results in fewer arousals, a reduced number of sleep shifts and an increase in REM sleep, both of which are analogous to the situation in humans (Neuzeret et al., 2011).

Parkinson's disease can be induced in cats and many other species using 1-methyl-4-phenul-1,2,3,6-tetrahydropyridine (MPTP) (Aznavour et al., 2012). However, unlike the disease in humans, cats are able to recover from the syndrome. During the acute phase cats experience interruptions in their sleep patterns (Aznavour et al., 2012). Humans with with Parkinson's disease also experience prominent difficulties in maintaining sleep due to painful night-time abnormal movements, and subsequent daytime sleepiness, sometimes culminating in sleep attacks (Arnulf, 2006). While not yet fully explored, the cat MPTP model has been proposed as a model of sleep disorders in Parkinson's disease (Arnulf et al., 2005).

E. Feline Genomics and Inherited Feline Diseases as Models of Human Diseases

The domestic cat is one of only a few mammals (human, chimpanzee, mouse, rat, dog, and cow) for which extensive information has been generated on its genome. The cat was selected for genetic sequencing by the National Human Genome Research Institute due to the substantial number of naturally occurring inherited diseases that are homologous to human disease (Pontius et al., 2007; Mullikin et al., 2010). Table 13.2 lists some of the genetic disorders of cats which share similar clinical and pathologic characteristics to those of its human counterpart. Cat colonies with homologous diseases make excellent models for the evaluation of human directed preclinical gene therapy trials because of their large size (compared to rodents), outbred genetic diversity, and longevity, which allows for long-term evaluation of the stability of the treatment. Cats have been used extensively to study the central nervous system and the brain of the cat is well characterized and has similar anatomy to the human brain, making cats a good model for gene therapy trials for neurological disorders such as lysosomal storage disease (Blagbrough and Zara, 2009; Vite et al., 2005).

Given the importance of the cat as a genetic model of human disease, several centers for feline inherited diseases have been established, including the Center for Comparative Medical Genetics (CCMG) and the Cat Phenotype and Health Information Registry (CAT PHIR). CCMG characterizes, utilizes and makes available cat models of human diseases and performs collaborative as well as fee-for-service studies. In addition, CCMG has cryopreserved resources as well as colonies of animals maintained for study of α-mannosidosis, mucolipidosis II, Neimanpick-C, glycogen storage IV, pyruvate kinase

deficiency, porphyria, and hypothyroidism. Cat PHIUR defines feline genetic models and characterizes the specific mutations. Important models characterized by this resource include polycystic kidney disease and progressive retinal atrophy in Persian cats, and hypotrichinosis in Cornish Rex cats (Gandolfi et al., 2010).

The National Cancer Institute's Laboratory of Genomic Diversity also maintains a frozen repository. The models preserved in this resource include: Spinal muscular atrophy (gene: *LIX1*); rdAc – retinal degeneration in Abyssinian cats (gene: *CEP290*); cone-rod dystrophy – gene: *CRX*; white, deaf cat aganglionic colon; polycystic kidney disease (PKD1).

II. SOURCES OF CATS

A. Directories of Sources

The Laboratory Animal Science Buyers Guide, (http:// laboratoryanimalsciencebuyersguide.com), is a reliable and easy method for locating information on sources of purpose-bred cats. The Office of Research Infrastructure Programs, Division of Comparative Medicine provides information on cat genetic resources that are supported by that organization. The *Lab Animal Buyers Guide* provides information on both purpose-bred sources and random sources for cats.

B. Random Sources

Random-source cats derived from animal control agencies and dealers make up less than 2% of cats used in research most likely due to the risk these cats carry of unknown morbidity and mortality from infectious diseases (including zoonoses), unknown reproductive status, and variable tractability. The addition of random-source cats into facilities with stable research colonies of cats introduces unacceptable risks because, even after long periods of quarantine, inapparent or latent diseases such as feline immunodeficiency disease and feline infectious peritonitis (FIP) may be transmitted to healthy cats. Random-source cats continue to be valuable for training veterinary students and for the establishment of genetic models of human diseases that have been identified in a pet population. In the latter case, a prolonged (8- to 12-week) isolation and observation period is needed to identify diseases, eliminate parasites and vaccinate in order to minimize pathogen transmission. When feasible, assisted reproductive techniques such as artificial insemination can be used to establish genetically valuable colonies. The National Research Council report on use of random-source cats states that for the reasons stated above, Institutional Animal Care and Use Committees must give rigorous consideration

TABLE 13.2   Inherited Diseases Common to Cats and Humans

Disease	Protein affected	Reference(s)
Amyloidosis	AA amyloid	Niewold *et al.* (1999), Boyce *et al.* (1984)
Cerebellar degeneration	Unknown	Inada *et al.* (1996)
Chediak–Higashi syndrome	Nidogen?	Narfstrom (1999), Kramer *et al.* (1977)
Chylomicronemia	Lipoprotein lipase	Ginzinger *et al.* (1996)
Ehlers–Danlos syndrome, type II	Procollagen peptidase	Freeman *et al.* (1989)
Endocardial fibroelastosis	Unknown	Rozengurt (1994), Paasch and Zook (1980)
Globoid cell leukodystrophy	Galactocerebroside	Alroy *et al.* (1986), Salvadori *et al.* (2005)
Glycogenosis II	α-1,4-Glucosidase	Vite *et al.* (2005)
Glycogenosis IV	Glycogen branching enzyme	Gaschen *et al.* (2004)
GM$_2$ gangliosidosis	Hexosaminidase B	Muldoon *et al.* (1994), Bradbury *et al.* (2013)
Gyrate atrophy of choroid and retina	Ornithine δ-Aminotransferase	Valle *et al.* (1981)
Hageman trait bleeding disorder	Factor XII	Kier *et al.* (1980, 1990)
Hemophilia A	Factor VIII	Barr and McMichael (2012)
Hemophilia B	Factor IX	Barr and McMichael (2012), Xu *et al.* (2007), Maggo-Price and Dodds (1993)
Hypokalaemic periodic polymyopathy	WNK4	Gandolfi *et al.* (2012)
Hypertrophic cardiomyopathy	MYPBC3 and others	Trehiou-Sechi *et al.* (2012), Meurs *et al.* (2009)
Klinefelter's syndrome	X chromosome chimerism	Centerwall and Benirschke (1975)
α-Mannosidosis	α-Mannosidase	Vite *et al.* (2005), Berg *et al.* (1997)
Methemoglobinemia	NADH-methemoglobin reductase	Harvey *et al.* (1994), Harvey (2006)
Mucolipidosis type II	Mannose 6 Phosphotransferase	Hubler *et al.* (1996)
MPS I, VI, VII	IDUA, ASB, GUSB	Sands and Haskins (2008), Ferla *et al.* (2013)
Muscular dystrophy	Dystrophin	Smith (2011)
Polycystic kidney disease	PKD1	Young *et al.* (2005), Lyons (2010)
Porphyria	Porphyrin	Clavero *et al.* (2010), Glenn *et al.* (1968)
Progressive retinal atrophy	Unknown	Glaze (2005)
Pyruvate kinase deficiency	Erythrocytic R-type phyruvate kinase	Young *et al.* (2005)
Retinal degeneration	CEP290 peptide	Menotti-Raymond *et al.* (2010), Narfstrom *et al.* (2011), Seiler *et al.* (2009)
Sphingomyelin lipidosis, or Niemann–Pick disease, type C	Sphingomyelinase	Stein *et al.* (2012)
Spinal muscular atrophy	LIX1	Fyfe *et al.* (2006)
Waardenburg's syndrome	Homeobox?	Klein (1983)

to the scientific justification for the use of random-source rather than purpose-bred cats (National Research Council, 2009). In fact, the report concludes that "random source dogs and cats used for research probably endure greater degrees of stress and distress compared to purpose-bred animals. This conclusion has implications both for the welfare of random source animals and for their reliability as research models."

C. Commercial Purpose-Bred Colonies

Very few purpose-bred cat vendors are available; several universities maintain SPF breeding colonies (see below). Factors to be considered in selecting purpose-bred cats are how the colony was established (e.g., cesarean-derived), is the colony maintained under barrier conditions, is the disease status SPF, are non-vaccinated animals available, and importantly, are the animals well socialized with a good temperament? Referrals from previous customers will provide an indication of the health and behavioral characteristics of cats from a particular source. Vendors should be able to provide reports of health examinations, vaccine protocols, and serology results.

D. Institutional Breeding Colonies

Projects that require a regular source of substantial numbers of normal cats or that depend on special characteristics such as perpetuation of an inherited trait can best be satisfied by establishment of an institutional breeding colony. Careful analysis of cost and complexity should be undertaken to determine if this approach is justified. In this chapter, we provide basic information on housing and reproduction useful for establishing an institutional breeding program. When possible, breeders should be derived from minimal-disease stock, and a rigorous program of vaccination and health testing must be followed to ensure continued good health. Periodic assessment of reproductive success, ability to meet the needs of research projects, and colony health status is useful in making corrective adjustments and ensuring that the breeding colony effort is economical and serves its intended purpose.

III. HOUSING

A. Caging Design and Operating Procedures

Although cats adapt well to high-density housing, such conditions can introduce a number of management issues, including abnormal behavior, infectious disease transmission, and reproductive failure. Careful planning of facility design, adoption of strict management protocols, thorough training and supervision of personnel, and oversight by a knowledgeable professional will facilitate successful laboratory cat management.

Primary enclosures should allow enough space and complexity for cats to rest comfortably and express species-specific behaviors. Enclosure requirements have been published in the USDA's Animal Welfare Act (AWA, 2008) and the Institute for Laboratory Animal Research (ILAR) *Guide for the Care and Use of Laboratory Animals* (NRC, 2011). Facilities housing cats have the following requirements: primary enclosures having a height of at least 24 in and floor space of 3 ft^2 for cats weighing less than 8.8 lb (4 kg) or 4 ft^2 for cats weighing more. Queens (intact females) with nursing kittens require additional space (AWA, 2008).

Cats are commonly housed in three basic arrangements: single cages, multiple runs within a room, and free ranging in a room. Domestic cats develop highly structured interactive social groups, and most cats do not thrive in isolation. Therefore, individual housing should be avoided unless particular experimental objectives dictate the use of single-cage housing or if caging is needed for short periods of time to permit collection of specimens, administer material individually, or accomplish treatments and/or observations. Cats that are vicious or aggressive towards other cats should also be singly housed. If caged, cats should be allowed out of their cages daily to exercise, unless activity is contraindicated due to medical concerns. Cats should be housed in compatible pairs or, preferably, in small groups of the same sex. Females in heat should not be placed in the same primary enclosure as toms (inact males), unless for breeding purposes (AWA, 2008). Breeding colonies are typically organized in harem groupings; this may consist of approximately four to six queens per tom. Twenty to twenty-five animals is typically the maximal number of cats successfully housed in a single breeding room, as long as enough floor, perch, feeding, and litter space is provided (Rochlitz, 2000) (Fig. 13.1). Housing compatible pregnant queens together before they deliver may lead to shared nursing and neonatal care. After delivery, pairing becomes more problematic. Queens nursing litters and kittens that are under 4 months of age should not be housed with other adult

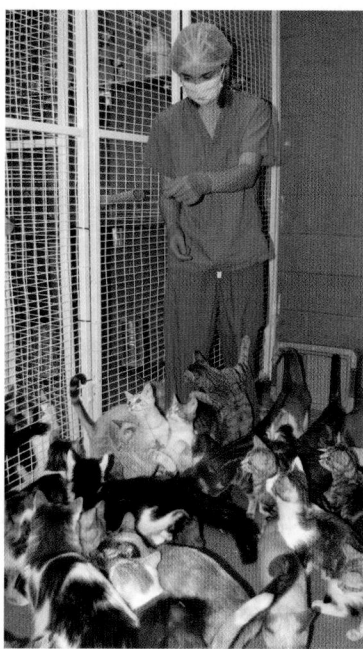

FIGURE 13.1   Social housing for cats using a room as a primary enclosure.

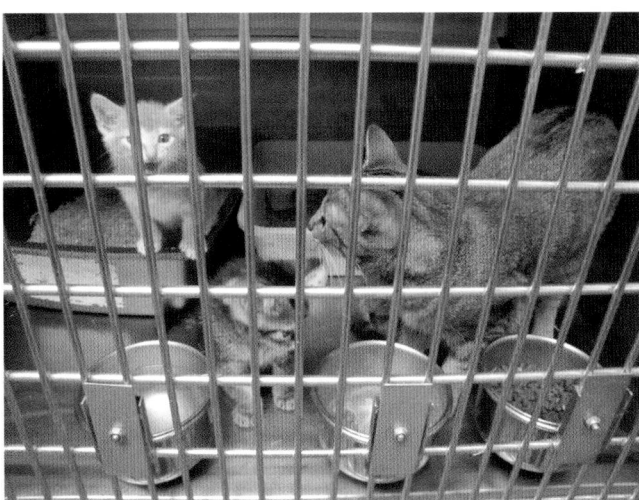

FIGURE 13.2 Nursing mothers and their kittens should be housed separately from the main cat colony to prevent.

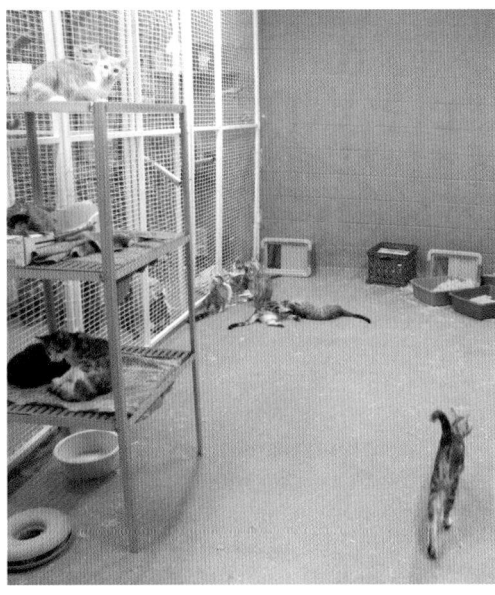

FIGURE 13.3 Social housing for cats using a run with shelving units to provide opportunities for the cats to climb.

cats to decrease interspecific aggression and to promote maternal care (Fig. 13.2).

Installation of multiple runs within a room is often the most economical use of floor space (Fig. 13.3). Depending on the dimensions of the room, runs can be 3–4 ft wide, 4–6 ft long, and 6 ft high (12–24 ft^2 of floor area). The smaller runs are adequate for pregnant or lactating queens and their litters or two to three juveniles. Larger runs are best for breeding groups of toms and queens, postweaning family groups, and single-sex adult groups. Galvanized wire panels with 1–inch mesh fence wire and a top panel are inexpensive, durable materials for run construction. Primary enclosures must

be free of sharp edges, protrusions, or open spaces that would cause injury to its feline occupants. When a free-ranging room arrangement is used, a chain-link fence 'foyer' is usually constructed at the door inside the room to allow personnel entry into the room without giving any opportunity for a cat to escape into the hallway.

Cats commonly make use of vertical space in their primary enclosures (Rochlitz, 2000); as such, enclosures must contain elevated resting surfaces. USDA regulations require that enough perch space is available for all of the cats to rest comfortably on a perch surface simultaneously. If the resting areas are placed so low to the ground that a cat cannot comfortably rest underneath it, the resting surface will be considered floor space (AWA, 2008). Perches also provide environmental enrichment and opportunities to escape from socially dominant members of the group (Fig. 13.3).

Enclosed nesting boxes (e.g., 24 in^2 with a doorway cut into one side) are useful for pregnant and lactating queens and their litters. Open boxes of the same size with walls 12 in high are preferred for juveniles and adults. Boxes also serve to enhance the comfort of housed cats by providing places to hide and substrates for scratching, behaviors that are both fundamental needs of cats.

Regardless of the cage arrangement used, wall, floor, and ceiling surfaces must be easily sanitized to achieve pathogen control measures. Litter pans and utensils for food and water may be durable plastic or stainless steel and should be able to withstand 180°F wash water. Litter can be any clean, dust-free, absorbent material, including extruded corncob pellets. One box per two cats is recommended (Rochlitz, 2000), and is dependent upon the total number of cats in the enclosure. Soiled litter must be removed and replaced daily to minimize cat-to-cat transmission of enteric pathogens, and to control odors. While most captive colony cats will not likely be excreting *Toxoplasma gondii* oocysts, daily litter box cleaning would also serve to diminish personnel risk of exposure to infective oocyst, as they require 1–5 days to sporulate and become infective (Esch and Petersen, 2013). Room illumination must be controlled to provide duration, intensity, and spectrum of light that is optimal for specific needs of an experiment. In general, daylight-spectrum fluorescent tubes and daylight–dark cycles of 12:12 or 14:10 h are useful and are required for successful breeding. The *Guide* also suggests housing cats within a temperature range of 64–84°F and 30–70% environmental humidity (NRC, 2011).

B. Animal Care Staff

Animal care staff must be knowledgable about and enjoy working with cats. Staff must be willing to interact daily with animals to ensure socialization and tractability, which becomes even more important when cats are singly housed. The staff members become aware of the personalities of individual animals and assist with detection of estrous cycling, potential health problems, or incompatibility of runmates caused by social dominance. Animal care staff should also adopt gentle and predictable practices with cats; any rough handling or erratic management practices could produce undesirable and aggressive behaviors (Rodan et al., 2011). If followed consistently, gentle handling practices could lead to cats becoming accustomed to procedures such as venipuncture that would otherwise require sedation. The staff must be trained to follow prescribed sanitation procedures, complete and record husbandry activities on a daily basis, follow proper room flow, and adhere to personal protective equipment protocols (e.g., facility scrubs, shoes or shoecovers, and face-masks).

C. Feline Social Behavior

As natural predators, cats possess keen senses and heightened fight-or-flight responses, making them particularly susceptible to environmental stress (Greco, 1991). In a laboratory setting, cats become readily entrained to daily activity patterns and respond strongly to their surroundings as well as to their human caretakers. Unpredictable caretaking and handling are potent stressors in cats (Carlstead et al., 1993). Behaviors typically observed in cats suffering from stress include: decreased activity, such as grooming and social interactions, withdrawal behavior, increased time spent awake with vigilant behavior, and altered appetite (Overall et al., 2004). Overcrowding and insufficient resting and hiding places also increase stress (Carlstead et al., 1993). The ability to control aversive stimuli through hiding profoundly decreases cortisol concentrations in cats when measured over time or in response to adrenocorticotropic hormone (ACTH) (Carlstead et al., 1993). As in many species, persistence of stress may compromise both immune and reproductive function as well as alter normal behavior (Griffin, 1989). In our experience, provision of proper social housing, exercise, environmental enrichment, and a predictable routine dramatically reduces the incidence of behavioral problems, including urine spraying, fighting, hiding, and silent heat.

With the exception of being solitary hunters, free-roaming cats are social creatures (Crowell-Davis et al., 1997). Communication between cats takes place through a variety of visual, auditory, olfactory, and tactile cues. Expressions of the face and posturing of the body are visual cues; a cat with ears facing another cat and a relaxed tail would indicate a more curious approach, whereas ears flattened against the head and a crouched body position indicate a defensive attitude. Auditory cues can range from casual meowing and chirps that indicate curiosity versus hissing and shrieking, which point to a more defensive or scared attitude. Tactile cues such as body and nose rubbing are more indicative of positive interactions. Olfactory cues are those that result from urine spraying or by rubbing scent glands onto other cats, humans, or surfaces (Overall et al., 2004).

The majority of feline activities are performed within stable social groups in which cooperative defense, cooperative care of young, and a variety of affiliative behaviors are practiced. Affiliative behaviors are those that facilitate proximity or contact. Cats within groups commonly practice mutual grooming and allorubbing, in which cats rub their heads and faces against one another. This may serve as a greeting or as an exchange of odor for recognition, familiarization, marking, or development of a communal scent. Although both males and females exhibit affiliative behavior, these behaviors are more common in females. Play behavior and food sharing are common in kittens and adolescent cats.

The formation of social hierarchy occurs within groups of cats. Establishment of ranking order is a social adaptation that minimizes agonistic behavior between individuals within a group. Signals of dominance and submission may be subtle or obvious and include vocalization (growling, hissing), visual cues (facial expression, posturing of the body, ears, and tail), and scent marking (urine, feces, various glands of the skin). Cats that are high ranking in a colony may try to control resources such as food, water, resting surfaces, or preferred litter boxes; providing multiple of these helps to reduce antagonistic behavior between dominant and submissive cats.

Maternal behavior is the primary social pattern of the female cat. Queens exhibit strong maternal instincts. Adult queens form social groups along with their kittens and juvenile offspring (Crowell-Davis et al., 1997). They nest communally and care for each other's kittens. Cooperative nursing is common. Kittens raised in communal nests develop faster and leave the nest sooner than kittens raised by solitary mothers. Between 3 and 8 weeks of age, kittens undergo a critical socialization period that can affect their behavior later in life towards other cats and humans. It is especially important that kittens in breeding colonies are handled during this period to ensure tractability (Overall et al., 2004).

Adult toms reside within one group or roam between a few established groups. Although they are social animals also, tomcats commonly exhibit aggressive behavior toward one another during the establishment of dominance in relationships and during competition for territory, breeding, food, and other resources (Crowell-Davis et al., 1997). Urine spraying and fighting are the most common undesirable male behaviors. In contrast to their interaction with other males, tomcats commonly display affiliative or 'friendly' behavior with females regardless of their reproductive status. For these reasons, tomcats should be housed with spayed females when not breeding. If not used for breeding, toms should be castrated. Neutering before puberty is best for prevention of undesirable male behaviors such as urine spraying and fighting. If the sexually mature tomcat is neutered, these behaviors will usually subside within a few weeks, facilitating intersex group housing. Neutered males display less agonistic behaviors towards other cats (Finkler et al., 2011).

Once social order is established in group housed animals, particularly those in a free-ranging room group, introduction or removal of individuals requires a period of adjustment that is usually stressful, induces fighting, and may disrupt breeding until a new social hierarchy and territorial limits are established (Rochlitz, 2000; Overall et al., 2004; Ellis et al., 2013). Introducing a new animal is ideally gradual and supervised, such as by placing the newcomer in a transport cage in the larger multicat enclosure for a period of time (possibly up to 2 weeks) before allowing the cat to roam freely in the group (Rochlitz, 2000). Even in multiple-run housing in a single room, rearrangement of run groups or even relocation of an entire group within the room may induce imbalance of the social order and anxiety. Therefore, every effort should be made to minimize reorganization of groups once they are established, and if restructuring is necessary, ample time should be allowed for restabilization of social order before experimental interventions are attempted to avoid social and stress-induced variables that may affect physiological and immunological parameters.

D. Housing to Exclude Pathogens

As with other laboratory species, infectious disease control for cats is based on exclusion. This requires that members of the colony are free from specific pathogens when the group is established, that any incoming animals are accepted into the colony only after rigorous health standards of the group are met, that proper preventive medicine protocols are followed rigorously, that barrier procedures (such as room order) and sanitization protocols are followed, and that staff is properly trained on feline biology, barrier procedures, and sanitization protocols.

To adequately reduce disease transmission, a facility should have various areas that segregate cats into life stage, health status, quarantine status, and research use. Traffic patterns should start with rooms housing pathogen-free and healthy animals, then quarantine animals whose health status has not been verified, and finally diseased animals in isolation (Hurley, 2005; Mostl et al., 2013). Animals in isolation rooms should ideally also be subdivided based on whether they have respiratory, dermatologic, or gastrointestinal disease (Hurley, 2005). Cats that have had exposure to infectious diseses (i.e., non-SPF cats) should ideally remain in quarantine for at least 6 weeks, which is the time it takes cats to seroconvert against FIV or become antigen-positive to FeLV (Mostl et al., 2013). Cats from SPF sources should ideally be quarantined for at least a week after receipt to monitor for signs of shipment-related diseases, and serologic evaluation is recommended prior to mixing cats from different sources (Mostl et al., 2013). The youngest and most immunocompromised animals should be handled before older animals that could transmit disease. In addition, queens with litters should be housed separately and handled prior to handling the rest of the colony to prevent disease spread from adults to kittens that are not yet immunocompetent (Mostl et al., 2013). Finally, the entry order of the rooms depends on the research being conducted at the animal facility, e.g., animal rooms housing infectious disease studies need to be entered after rooms housing cats used in non-infectious research. If rooms must be entered out of order, it is imperative that proper barrier protocol is followed, such as showering between rooms or changing scrubs/shoes.

Equipment used in separate rooms should be room-specific. This includes scrubs and shoes worn by animal care staff (street-wear should be avoided to decrease outside pathogens accessing the colony), cleaning utensils and disinfectants, and cat-related items such as food bowls, litterboxes, and enrichment items. Enough litter boxes should be provided to decrease waste material accumulation and disease spread (Mostl et al., 2013). All of these items should be sanitizable or disposable to prevent fomite transmission of disease.

Attention to air quality in individual rooms is very important. Poor ventilation can lead to disease spread through aerosolization of infectious particles or irritation of a cat's respiratory mucosa by cleaning agents (Hurley, 2005; Mostl et al., 2013). Air exchanges of 10–12 per hour help reduce air contaminants, as do cleaning litter boxes regularly, diluting cleaning agents correctly, and using filtration in the air-supply system (Hurley, 2005).

Facility design that encourages a high level of sanitation and operational policies that ensure cleanliness are essential to minimize infectious disease transmission. Daily operations should include vacuuming and mopping floors, disposal of soiled litter, replacing soiled cardboard nesting boxes, and washing utensils for water and food as needed. Weekly procedures should include washing litter boxes and food/water utensils in 180°F water, scrubbing soiled areas, and replacing nesting boxes. Individual cages should be accorded the same level of sanitation and processed through a mechanical cage washer weekly, because soiling in these closely confined cages is unavoidable, and daily hand washing is usually inadequate to maintain sanitation. Food and water should be separated from litter as much as possible.

Selection of disinfectants is very important because different pathogens are susceptible to different disinfectants; attention must also be paid to proper dilution and surface contact time to ensure efficacy. For example, disinfectants used against nonenveloped viruses like feline panleukopenia virus and feline calicivirus (FCV) have aldehydes, hypochlorite, or peracetic acid as active ingredients, among others (Mostl et al., 2013). On the other hand, dermatophytes are eliminated with hypochlorite at much higher concentrations and repeated applications than nonenveloped viruses (Hurley, 2005). Disinfection where coccidial infection has taken place would require steam cleaning and disinfectants specifically tested against coccidia (Mostl et al., 2013). As is true for all species, staff must ensure that chemical disinfectant residues are thoroughly rinsed from all surfaces to prevent cats from ingesting chemicals and suffering toxicity.

E. Environmental Enrichment

Environmental enrichment is essential for behavioral health of closely confined cats and should allow them to express natural behaviors. Cats are hunters, and typically eat up to 20 small prey in a day (Ellis, 2009); providing toys and play that appeal to a cat's predatory instincts is beneficial to its well-being. Examples of these include hiding food kibble or treats for them to 'hunt' and find, using feathered toys they can catch and 'capture', and soft toys that can be bitten and moved around like prey. Items should also be provided for scent marking (Fig. 13.3). Whatever play items are provided, they should be easily sanitizable or disposable in the event they become soiled. Interspecies enrichment takes place with cats that are housed in groups. Cats that are group housed should be provided multiple environmental enrichment items so dominant cats do not manipulate all available resources. Hiding areas should also be provided for more timid cats to rest comfortably and avoid stressful encounters with dominant run-mates. Cats that are singly housed should be given extra attention by care staff to ensure socialization. The most effective environmental enrichment is a staff that enjoys interacting with cats and is willing to spend adequate time to ensure their socialization; this can include daily gentle interactions to playing with laser pointers and 'wand'-type toys. Rest boards are required for comfort and contentment of cats because cats instinctively feel more secure when they can perch at a high point. These also provide an opportunity for lactating females to have rest periods away from their young. Boards should be constructed of dense plastic and anchored in such a way that crevices that accumulate hair and debris are avoided. Primahedrons can be attached to the ceiling to provide cats with the opportunity to climb and perch (Fig. 13.4).

IV. BREEDING COLONY MANAGEMENT

Because optimal conditions for exclusion of infectious diseases depend on use of purpose-bred cats, breeding colony management becomes exceedingly important for the use of cats in research. Fortunately, domestic cats are very prolific and high rates of production can be achieved in a laboratory environment with minimal complications. However, certain characteristics of feline reproduction are unique and must be recognized to achieve optimal breeding performance.

A. Reproductive Biology

On average, queens reach puberty or experience their first estrous cycle between 5 and 9 months of age, although the onset may range from 3.5 to 18 months of age. In addition to age, factors that affect the onset of puberty include breed, time of year or photoperiod, social environment, health, physical condition, and nutritional status. With proper health maintenance, nutrition, and control of light cycles, adolescent queens begin to cycle after attaining a body weight of 2 kg or more. Group housing, especially the introduction of a tomcat or estral queen, provides social stimuli that hasten the onset of estrus (Michel, 1993).

Free-roaming queens are seasonally polyestrous. In the Northern Hemisphere, the season begins in January or February after the winter solstice, as the days get longer, and lasts until fall. Anestrus persists from October through December until the next breeding season begins in January or February. Cats are extremely sensitive to photoperiod. In an environmentally controlled laboratory setting, 10 or more hours of light in a 24-h period is required for reproductive cycling (Shille and Sojka, 1995). Maintaining a 14-h light photoperiod and the use of natural daylight spectrum fluorescent bulbs ensures the maximum fertility period and estrous cycling (H. J. Baker, unpublished observations, 1999). Estrous cycling typically occurs within 7–10 weeks of instituting such a light cycle (Dawson, 1941; Scott and Lloyd-Jacob, 1959); however, this period can be shortened if preceded by a nonstimulatory light cycle of 8 or fewer hours of light (Hurni, 1981), or if a tomcat or queen in estrus is introduced at the time of increasing the duration of light (Michel, 1993).

Peak sexual activity occurs between 1.5 and 7 years of age, with an average of two to three litters per year, with three to four kittens per litter (range 1–15 kittens per litter). Queens can bear 50–150 kittens in a breeding life of approximately 10 years if allowed to mate naturally. Like tomcats, queens are polygamous and rarely form long-term bonds with a mate, although they often display preferences for particular mates. If allowed, a female may accept a number of males, and therefore litters may have

High-quality commercial feline diets formulated for laboratory cats are available in both wet (canned) and dry formulations. Consideration should be given to using diets from manufacturers of research formulas that have undergone additional testing to ensure nutritional adequacy and safety when maintenance of specific pathogen-free status of a colony is required or if diets must be irradiated or sterilized for specific protocols. Laboratory-housed cats are often provided continuous access to dry food which can be left out overnight without spoiling. Continuous access to food allows cats to mimic the feeding pattern of free-ranging cats that consume multiple small meals over the course of 24 h (MacDonald et al., 1984; Ellis, 2009), but can lead to excess weight and obesity if body weight and condition are not closely monitored and assessed. Canned foods tend to be highly palatable, although they are more expensive, more labor-intensive to use, and may spoil if left for more than 8–12 h.

B. Energy Requirements

Age, life stage, activity level, reproductive status, and environment all affect energy requirements. The estimated energy need of adult lean cats at maintenance is $100 \, \text{kcal}/(\text{kg body weight})^{0.67}$ per day (NRC, 2006), which can be used as an initial estimate for the amount of food that should be offered daily. An individual cat's energy requirements for maintenance of optimal weight and body condition can vary widely, exceeding more than 50% under or over the estimated amount and is best determined by weighing all colony cats monthly and assessing their body (Laflamme, 1997) and muscle condition (Michel et al., 2011) by palpation using established scoring criteria. Properly fed adult cats should be well muscled and the ribs should be readily palpable beneath a slight layer of fat. Viewing the cat from the side, the waist should be moderately tucked up behind the last rib, and the inguinal fat pad should be minimal (Laflamme, 1997). Assessing muscle condition is important because cats tend to catabolize lean body tissue under conditions of acute stress either due to environmental factors or disease, and loss of muscle tissue may not be readily appreciated with traditional body condition scores that focus on body silhouette and fat stores (Baldwin et al., 2010; Michel et al., 2011).

A significant risk for group-housed, ad libitum-fed cats is the development of obesity. Obesity is the most common nutritional disease in pet cats in the Western hemisphere (Laflamme, 2012), and is common in laboratory-raised cats, particularly those on long-term studies. Obesity leads to increased health risks including the development of diabetes mellitus, hepatic lipidosis, and urinary tract diseases (Laflamme, 2012). White adipose tissue is now recognized to be an important endocrine organ that secretes a variety of substances that are active in energy metabolism and appetite control such as steroid hormones, growth factors and various cytokines such as leptin, adiponectin, resistin, and visfatin, which are collectively known as adipokines (Zoran, 2010). Leptin is several-fold higher in obese cats compared to lean cats without leading to the appropriate physiological response of appetite suppression (Hoenig, 2012). Obesity in cats also leads to upregulation of mRNA expression of the pro-inflammatory cytokines tumor necrosis factor-α and interferon-γ in adiposites (Van de Velde et al., 2013). While an initial, small study in cats did not demonstrate an adverse impact of obesity on white blood cell counts or lymphocyte function (Jaso-Friedmann et al., 2008) the potential impacts of inflammation during obesity on the immune system continue to be investigated. Obesity in cats is more easily prevented than treated. Cats becoming overconditioned with ad libitum access to food should be fed a fixed amount of food twice daily. This can be problematic in colonies maintained in group-housed situations over long periods of time, and may require specialized exercise or feeding plans.

Reproductively active cats and growing kittens need to be fed a high-quality feline diet designed for reproduction and growth. Queens gain weight throughout gestation in a linear fashion, with their energy requirements increasing by 25–30% by mid-gestation (Buffington, 1991). After parturition, energy requirements continue to rise to three- to four-times those of maintenance, as queens nurse their kittens (Lawler and Bebiak, 1986). Peak lactation occurs at 2–3 weeks postpartum. Maintaining adequate nutrition during this time is extremely important to ensure production of sufficient quantities of milk, particularly in queens with large litters. After weaning, milk production and mammary congestion can be decreased by fasting queens for 24 h before returning to maintenance feeding. As is true for most species, a continuous supply of fresh, clean drinking water must be available.

VI. INFECTIOUS DISEASE EXCLUSION AND CONTROL

Veterinary graduates are well versed in the breadth of infectious diseases affecting cats, including pathogenesis, diagnosis, and therapy. Additionally, abundant texts and journal references are available on practice management of these diseases. Therefore, this chapter will emphasize infectious disease issues that apply uniquely to colonies of cats and that are critically important to health management of cats used in research.

A. Preventive Medicine

Preventive health care involves recognizing and managing factors that affect disease transmission, including genetics, environmental stress, immunization, disease surveillance, nutrition, housing design, maintenance, and sanitation (Mostl et al., 2013; Hurley, 2005; AAHA-AVMA, 2011). Selection for disease resistance and docile temperaments should be considered. For example, queens repeatedly producing kittens with congenital abnormalities, or dams that are not able to successfully raise the majority of their kittens to weaning should be removed from breeding stock. Small colonies will rapidly lose genetic heterozygosity, and formerly recessive traits may become more commonly expressed. It may be necessary to include periodic expansion from other colonies with similar disease background to avoid inbreeding depression. This is problematic in colonies maintained to preserve a genetic disorder.

Yearly physical examinations conducted by a veterinarian and regular diagnostics to monitor for common feline pathogens are recommended (Overall et al., 2004). Immunization protocols will vary for each feline colony based on risk–benefit assessments depending on the individual animal and research use. Cats used in infectious disease research may not be vaccinated, or may be vaccinated only with killed vaccines to avoid perturbations to the immune response. Cats used in vaccine studies will also not typically be routinely vaccinated with commercial vaccines, as these may interfere with candidate vaccine study outcomes. Cats maintained for preservation of genetic traits may undergo preventative health maintenance more akin to cats kept as pets. Scherk et al. (2013) lists specific immunization recommendations for cats maintained as companion animals. These recommendations can be modified for laboratory housed cats based on the research use of the animals. Early cessation of immunization protocols is the most common form of immunization failure (Scherk et al., 2013).

Young kittens (less than 6 months old) represent one of the main target populations for immunization due to their increased susceptibility to infection compared to older cats (Scherk et al., 2013). Maternal antibodies acquired through colostrum can also interfere with immunization as late as 16 weeks of age in kittens and will vary depending on the pathogen. The health status of the individual cat will also affect immune response to immunization as immunocompromised animals will likely not mount an appropriately robust response to afford protection (Day, 2006; Scherk et al., 2013). The closed/open status of a colony, animal density, research use of animals, and potential exposure (either through fomites carried into the facility or geographical presence of pathogens) should be considered when develoing immunization protocols (Scherk et al., 2013). The type of vaccine administered can vary depending on the reproductive status of the individual animal. Vaccinating pregnant queens is generally not recommended due to the possibility of infecting the fetus during pregnancy or lactation. For example,

administering a modified-live feline panleukopenia virus vaccine to a pregnant queen could cause cerebellar hypoplasia in her kittens; in cases like these, inactivated vaccines should be used instead (Scherk et al., 2013).

Vaccine-related adverse reactions are a possibility whenever immunizations are administered. A retrospective study of over 400,000 cats in 329 hospitals performed by Moore et al. found the most common reactions to be nonspecific: pyrexia, lethargy, anorexia, and pain and swelling at the injection site. Multivalent panleukopenia vaccines were found to induce more lethargy postvaccination (Moore et al., 2007).

Stress has a profound influence on disease transmission, and commonly reactivates latent viral respiratory infections, leading to increased virus shedding and even recurrence of clinical disease (Mostl et al., 2013; Thiry et al., 2009). Overcrowding is one of the most potent stressors recognized in cats; as it increases the number of pathogens, susceptible animals, and the number of asymptomatic carriers in a given group, while increasing the likelihood of disease transmission between group members through both direct contact and exposure to contaminated fomites (Carlstead et al., 1993; Mostl et al., 2013; Hurley, 2005). While there is no specific number of animals that constitute overcrowding, it is recommended that groups be kept as small and stable as possible. For example, to reduce risk of coronavirus spread, keeping animals in groups of up to three cats can reduce risk of spread, while groups consisting of more than six animals were found to consistently have coronavirus infections (Pedersen, 2009; Addie et al., 2009). Kittens should remain only with their queens and littermates until weaning (Mostl et al., 2013). Other stressors that should be avoided include irregular feeding and husbandry schedules, unpredictable daily manipulations, and infrequent or indifferent human contacts (Carlstead et al., 1993; Mostl et al., 2013; Hurley, 2005; Overall et al., 2004).

Synthetic feline facial pheromones (FFP) have been recommended in the treatment of stress-related behaviors due to their apparent anxiolytic effect on cats. A meta-analysis conducted by Mills et al. found that the use of FFP decreased urine-spraying incidence in a group of cats just 4 weeks after initiating pheromone treatment (Mills et al., 2011). Analysis of FFP study data, however, found insufficient evidence in Mills' and similar studies to conclude that FFP is beneficial in treating stress-related behaviors and reducing stress in unfamiliar environments (Frank et al., 2010). Despite this, FFP use, continues to be recommended by veterinarians based on subjective experience, and may have application in colony settings (Beck, 2013).

B. Pathogen Control

Although domestic cats are susceptible to a large number of viral diseases, only a few are significant for colony-reared cats. FeLV and FIV diseases can be excluded from research colonies by preventive measures described in Section VI, A. With care, other viruses listed below can also be excluded from SPF colonies.

1. Upper Respiratory Infection

Etiology Upper respiratory tract infections (URI) are common in non-SPF cats and result in oculonasal discharge and sneezing (Dinnage *et al.*, 2009). Respiratory disease spreads rapidly in a research colony, negatively impacting the cat's welfare and is an adverse confounder for many research studies. As a result, URI should be excluded from SPF research colonies. Feline herpesvirus-1 (FHV-1) and FCV are the primary etiologic agents in 80% of all URI in cats (Knowles and Gaskell, 1991; Lawler and Evans, 1997). Other agents, including *Chlamydia*, *Mycoplasma*, reovirus, and *Bordetella* may cause infections that are primary, concurrent, or secondary to the viral diseases (Dinnage *et al.*, 2009; Bannasch and Foley, 2005). The severity of clinical signs is dependent on population density, the duration of exposure, the challenge dose of the virus, and the cat's age at time of infection, the quality and duration of its acquired maternal immunity, nutritional plane, stress level, and general health (Hurley, 2005; Mostl *et al.*, 2013; Dinnage *et al.*, 2009; Overall *et al.*, 2004). Once enzootic in a population of cats, upper respiratory viruses manifest primarily as acute disease in young kittens as passive immunity is lost and, at that point, may be difficult to control.

Chlamydophila felis is normally associated with serous conjunctivitis but can also cause mild upper respiratory infections that self-resolve and are easily eliminated with use of antibiotics. A multivalent vaccine is available that can be used if there is a history of *C. felis* infection in the colony (Scherk *et al.*, 2013). *Mycoplasma felis*, more commonly associated with primary conjunctivitis and anemia, has also been associated with upper respiratory infections and can be treated with antimycoplasmal drugs (Burns *et al.*, 2011; Bannasch and Foley, 2005). *Bordetella bronchiseptica* has been implicated as a cause of acute bronchitis and pneumonia, ocular discharge, and even death (Egberink *et al.*, 2009). While the significance of *Bordetella* in the pet population is not known, it can result in significant morbidity in feline colonies. Vaccination may be warranted in colonies with a history of *Bordetella* infection (Scherk *et al.*, 2013).

Feline viral rhinotracheitis, caused by FHV-1 subfamily *Alphaherpesvirinae*, is characterized by acute rhinitis, conjunctivitis and corneal ulcers (dendritic ulcers particularly), as well as sneezing, conjunctival hyperemia, and coughing. The virus is shed in oculonasal discharge and transmission is through direct contact (Gaskell *et al.*, 2007). Acute disease tends to resolve in 10–14 days while

viral shedding begins 24 h after infection and can last up to 3 weeks (Thiry *et al.*, 2009). FCV infections typically cause acute URI and acute stomatitis characterized by oral musocal and lingual ulceration. Chronic stomatitis (possibly immune-mediated) and a limping syndrome due to an idiopathic acute synovitis are also described (Thiry *et al.*, 2009). Cats are infected with FCV through oronasal routes with a transient viremia in the following 3–4 days that can be detected in a variety of tissues. Healing takes place within 3–4 weeks following infection (Thiry *et al.*, 2009). A recent virulent systemic disease associated with FCV has been reported in the United States and Europe. It is characterized by systemic inflammatory disease, disseminated intravascular coagulation, organ failure, and ultimately, death. Mortality rates of up to 67% have been reported (Thiry *et al.*, 2009).

Following entry through oral mucosa or conjunctiva and resolution of clinical disease, FHV-1 spreads to the trigeminal nerve to establish latency (Thiry *et al.*, 2009). Over 80% of cats that recover from FHV-1 become carriers and intermittently shed virus in oronasal and conjunctival secretions for life (Knowles and Gaskell, 1991; Lawler and Evans, 1997). Under natural conditions, approximately 45% of latently infected cats shed virus following stress. The most common stressors include glucocorticoid administration, followed by parturition and relocalization of cats (Gaskell and Povey, 1977). Virus shedding usually begins within 1 week after a stressful episode and continues for approximately 2 weeks (Gaskell *et al.*, 2007). Cats infected with FCV shed virus for 30 days. Even though many cats clear FCV, others can continually shed virus, potentially for the rest of their lives (Radford *et al.*, 2009). Studies on colonies with endemic FCV have showed that long-term shedding is rare, and that most cats that continue to shed FCV through their lives tend to do so after re-infection with FCV variants of the same strain or new strains (Radford *et al.*, 2009). FCV may also undergo mutations that cause changes to its capsid protein, possibly avoiding the host's immune response (Radford *et al.*, 2009).

Prevention and Control Treatment for URI is largely supportive. Eyes and noses should be kept clean of discharge with the use of saline. Mucolytic agents can be administered if there is excessive mucoid nasal discharge. Nebulization with saline can also help hydrate respiratory mucosa (Thiry *et al.*, 2009). Hydration status, electrolyte levels, and pH balance must be maintained through intravenous fluid administration. Nutrition maintenance is also important as cats often become anorexic due to feeling ill and suffer decreased interest in food due to congested nares. In cases where cats have not eaten, parenteral nutrition must be administered (Thiry *et al.*, 2009). Strong-smelling and highly palatable moist canned foods stimulate the appetite, aid in maintenance of hydration and are gentler on sore throats than dry products. If secondary bacterial infection develops, administration of antibiotics may be necessary. It is important to use antibiotics that have penetrance of respiratory and oral mucosa (Thiry *et al.*, 2009). Antiviral drugs, such as acyclovir and famcyclovir can have beneficial effects on cats suffering from FHV-1 (Thiry *et al.*, 2009; Malik *et al.*, 2009).

Both parenteral and intranasal vaccines are available for FHV-1 and FCV. Multivalent vaccines, coupled with FPV are commonly used and follow a similar vaccination protocol (Scherk *et al.*, 2013). It must be noted that vaccination against FCV will not prevent shedding or clinical disease, and it does not protect against all FCV strains (Radford *et al.*, 2009). FHV-1 is very labile in the environment, tending to persist in the environment for only 24 h, and can be eliminated with most disinfectants (Thiry *et al.*, 2009). FCV persists in the environment for up to 2 weeks and can be transmitted by fomites. It can be eliminated from the environment with household bleach under proper dilution and contact time (Radford *et al.*, 2009).

2. Feline Parvovirus

Etiology, Clinical Signs, Epizootiology, Pathology, Diagnosis, Prevention, and Control   Feline panleukopenia, caused by a parvovirus, is highly contagious and causes serious clinical disease but fortunately can be easily controlled by vaccination. Transmission is usually indirect through the fecal–oral route. Clinical signs include diarrhea, lymphopenia, neutropenia, thrombocytopenia, anemia, cerebellar hypoplasia in kittens, and abortion. While both adults and young are affected, kittens are the most vulnerable population and suffer mortality rates as high as 90% (Truyen *et al.*, 2009). Treatment is largely supportive. This nonenveloped virus is very resistant to environmental conditions and many disinfectants, is highly contagious, and rapidly accumulates in the environment due to high shedding of virions from affected animals. Passive immunity from maternally acquired antibodies tends to last 6–8 weeks before levels of antibody begin to decline. At this point, an immunity gap can take place, where levels of antibody are too low to protect the kitten but high enough to interfere with vaccination (Truyen *et al.*, 2009). Therefore, it is recommended that kittens at risk of exposure receive vaccines for panleukopenia as early as 6 weeks of age, repeated every 3–4 weeks until 16–20 weeks of age. Revaccination should occur 1 year later, and then every 3 years (Scherk *et al.*, 2013).

3. Feline Infectious Peritonitis

Etiology   FIP is a potentially important infection of colony cats because it may arise in otherwise healthy cats, cannot be distinguished serologically from other coronaviruses, and because it causes recurring appearance of disease that tends to be fatal. Two types of coronaviruses infect cats: feline enteric coronavirus (FECV) and FIP virus (FIPV), both members of the genus *Alphacoronavirus*. FECV is ubiquitous and avirulent while FIPV frequently coexists with FECV and is virulent. FECV and FIPV are antigenically and morphologically indistinguishable from each other (Pedersen, 2009).

Epizootiology   FECV is endemic in nearly all environments where a large number of cats share close quarters (Addie *et al.*, 2009). It is spread by the fecal–oral route and associated with subclinical or self-limiting gastrointestinal signs, especially diarrhea (Pedersen, 2009). Viral shedding from small and large intestine is typically seen 1 week after infection and can persist for 18 months or more. Immunity is not life-long, as recovered cats can become re-infected with typically the same strain. Immunity between FECV and FIPV is not cross-protective (Pedersen, 2009).

Up to 12% of cats infected with feline coronavirus may succumb to FIP (Addie *et al.*, 2009). A mutation in FECV is believed to lead to the virulent FIPV. Several previous studies have implicated a variety of mutations in FECV genes that correlate with development of virulence (Pedersen, 2009; Brown *et al.*, 2009). Licitra *et al.* recently identified a mutation at a spike protein cleavage site in a high percentage of cats that developed FIP. This mutation was theorized to lead to altered fusion properties that would provide for macrophage cell tropism, systemic spread, and development of FIP and was observed in cats that were still asymptomatic for FIP as well (Licitra *et al.*, 2013).

FECV mutations differ between littermates and even within different tissues in the same animal, which supports a mode of internal mutation and consequent disease instead of spread of virulent mutated forms between cats (Licitra *et al.*, 2013; Pedersen, 2009). Kittens are most susceptible to this mutation during primary infection due to production of high levels of FECV and a decreased resistance to mutation early in life (Pedersen, 2009). Coinfections with other viruses (such as FPV) and stress also increase incidence of FIP (Addie *et al.*, 2009). Clinical disease is seen more commonly in young animals ranging from 5–6 weeks up to 16 months of age (Addie *et al.*, 2009; Radford *et al.*, 2009). Other risk factors for development of FIP include genetic susceptibility, coronavirus titer, proportion of FECV shedding, and prevalence of chronic shredders in the colony (Pedersen, 2009).

Clinical Signs and Pathology   Two forms of clinical FIP exist: an effusive 'wet' form and a dry form. The effusive form is more common and has a shorter incubation period (2–14 days) than the dry form. The effusive form may be subclinical for weeks, with affected young animals appearing unthrifty, before clinical disease is manifested (Pedersen, 2009). The onset of the effusive form includes fever, anorexia, malaise, and weight loss. Painless abdominal distention due to ascites is the most common clinical sign observed in affected animals; the effusion tends to be yellow-tinged and mucinous and amounts can reach up to a liter in severe cases. Other clinical signs include dyspnea from pleural involvement or thoracic effusion, ocular and neurologic signs, scrotal edema in intact males, and synovitis due to immune-complex formation and deposition (Pedersen, 2009). The 'dry' form of FIP is less common and is characterized by granulomatous lesions in various organs as well as central nervous system involvement and ocular disease. Granulomatous lesions are commonly found in the kidneys, mesenteric lymph nodes, and liver, and tend to be painful on palpation; smaller granulomas can also be found in the lungs (Pedersen, 2009).

Diagnosis Serological testing does not differentiate FECV from FIPV and therefore is not an effective diagnostic tool. A high percentage of cats are FECV positive and will yield a false-positive for FIPV when tested (Addie *et al.*, 2009). Effusions should be aspirated and analyzed, as they provide a higher diagnostic value than blood analyses (Addie *et al.*, 2009). Protein content of the effusion is typically very high (>35 g/l) and is consistent with exudative effusion. Cytologic evaluation will show an abundance of neutrophils and macrophages (Addie, *et al.*, 2009). The recent finding from Licitra *et al.* implies that, due to the specific mutation at the S1/S2 site, diagnosis of FIP is a possibility prior to development of disease; this would also carry preventive and treatment implications as well (Licitra *et al.*, 2013).

Prevention and Control FIPV infection is usually fatal and has no current effective treatment. In addition, a reliable vaccine against FIPV has not been developed (Pedersen, 2009). The virus may persist up to 2 months in the environment. Effective prevention depends on minimizing fecal–oral spread, such as diligently cleaning litterboxes (Addie *et al.*, 2009).

C. Eliminating Parasites

Although cats are susceptible to a wide range of parasites, effective antiparasitic drugs are available, and the high level of sanitation that should be practiced in research colonies makes them easily eliminated. The most common parasites include fleas, ear mites, cestodes, ascarids, hookworms, and coccidia.

Fleas cause marked allergic dermatitis in many adults and serve as vectors for transmission of infectious diseases and tapeworms (*Dipylidium caninum*). Several very effective commercial products are available for flea control. Because both cats and kittens are extremely sensitive to toxic effects from insecticides, products should be selected carefully and used only on animals of the age for which they are intended. After eliminating fleas on adult cats, eradication can be achieved because sanitation eliminates opportunities for larval development.

Ear mites (*Otodectes cynotis*) are the most common cause of otitis externa in the cat. They live in the external ear canal, feeding on tissue fluids and producing irritation. Their presence results in the formation of a thick, dark-brown exudate consisting of cerumen and exfoliated debris. Infested cats shake their heads, scratch their ears, and often excoriate their pinnae. Untreated infestations may result in permanent damage to the ear. Diagnosis is made on close visual inspection of aural exudate where the mites are barely visible with the naked eye or by microscopic examination of exudate in mineral oil at ×10 magnification with a light microscope. If ear mites are diagnosed in a colony, all cats, whether infected or not, should be treated. Although not labeled for this use, ivermectin (200–300 μg/kg SQ q2 weeks × 2 treatments) is safe, practical, inexpensive, and extremely effective.

Endoparasites include ascarids or roundworms (*Toxocara cati* and *Toxascaris leonina*), hookworms (*Ancylostoma* and *Uncinaria*), and coccidia. Transmammary transmission is the most common route of transmission for both roundworms and hookworms, although cats may become infested by ingesting contaminated soil. Larvae ingested by adult cats migrate to body tissues and persist for years. During pregnancy, these larvae are reactivated and travel to the mammary glands, where they are shed into the milk and ingested by nursing neonates. Infested kittens may develop diarrhea as early as 2–3 weeks of age. Hookworms cause blood loss and anemia. Female worms produce eggs that pass in the feces and may persist in the soil for years. Control is readily achieved through proper sanitation and routine deworming of kittens. Pyrantel pamoate (8–10 mg/kg PO q3 weeks × 3 treatments) is highly effective against both roundworms and hookworms and is cost-effective and easy to administer. Adult cats acquire immunity and rarely experience reinfestation. In humans, hookworms and ascarids are associated with cutaneous larval migrans and visceral larval migrans, respectively.

Protozoal parasites (coccidia and, less commonly, giardia) may occur in conditions of poor sanitation, particularly in kittens. Parasitization of the small intestine may result in diarrhea. Although uncommon, giardiasis is potentially zoonotic. Eradication consists of treatment of all cats with giardiacidal drugs (metronidazole at 50 mg/kg PO daily for 5 days or fenbendazole at 50 mg/kg PO daily for 5 days) and proper sanitation. Cats are definitive hosts for *Isospora felis* and *Isospora rivolta*. Young kittens, and weak and immunocompromised animals are usually affected. Eggs are passed in the feces and can sporulate in as little as 12 h. Adult forms replicate in the small intestine and cause villous atrophy, dilated lacteals, and lymphoid proliferation of Peyer's Patches (Lappin, 2010b). Clinical signs include watery diarrhea that may contain blood, vomiting, abdominal discomfort, and anorexia. Sulfadimethoxine (50–60 mg/kg daily for 5–20 days) and supportive treatment speed recovery. Eggs can easily be identified on fecal flotation and are resistant to many disinfectants. Prompt removal of feces and steam cleaning surfaces help decrease coccidial egg load in the environment (Lappin, 2010b).

D. Personnel Health Risks

Complete lists of infectious diseases of cats with zoonotic potential are available in the literature (Gerhold and Jessup, 2013; Guptill, 2010; Bond, 2010). Although no potential human health risk should be underestimated, in fact there are only a few of these infections that should be of any concern for a minimal-disease, closed cat colony. Infections of primary concern include cat scratch disease, dermatophytosis, and toxoplasmosis. 'Cat Scratch Disease' is caused by infection by *Bartonella henselae* that may be carried inapparently by cats and are transmitted to humans by bite or scratch wounds or fleas. Personell handling cats should be aware of the potential for this infection and should thoroughly wash bite or scratch wounds and seek medical attention, particularly for a wound that does not respond to the usual treatment (Guptill, 2010). Dermatophytosis usually results from *Microsporum canis* and can be diagnosed by culture of the organism. It can be a difficult disease to treat in large groups of cats, and if treatment is attempted, the risk of human exposure must be considered (DeBoer and Moriello, 1995; Moriello and DeBoer, 1995; Bond, 2010). Toxoplasmosis is an obligate intracellular protozoan parasite that can be transmitted to cats and humans by ingestion of infected feces/soil or undercooked meat. Diagnosis is difficult, but the simple expedient of changing litter daily, using gloves when handling litter and litter pans, and washing hands will eliminate risk (Gerhold and Jessup, 2013). Rabies vaccination of cats should be considered because of legal obligations and interstate shipping regulations; otherwise, while contact with feral or 'barn cats' poses a potential risk, there is little or no risk to cats maintained in a closed colony derived from disease-free stock (Gerhold and Jessup, 2013).

Cat salivary and urine proteins are potent allergens, and many people experience severe allergic reactions when exposed to cats. Five cat allergens have been characterized (Acedoyin, 2007). Cats are more commonly implicated in asthma and allergic disease than other pet species (Dharmage *et al.*, 2012). Personnel with known allergy to cats should not work with them unless they take special precautions such as using face masks and gloves, and exposure to cats should be considered as an occupational health risk factor.

Acknowledgments

The authors thank Dr. Charmaine Foltz and Dr. William Burkholder for editorial assistance with the first draft of this manuscript. The preparation of this manuscript was partially funded by the Office of Research Services, National Institutes of Health (Burkholder).

References

AAHA-AVMA, 2011. Development of new canine and feline preventive healthcare guidelines designed to improve pet health. J. Am. Anim. Hosp. Assoc. 47, 306–311.

Acedoyin, J.L., 2007. Cat IgA, representative of new carbohydrate cross-reactive allergens. J. Allergy Clin. Immunol. 119, 640–645.

Addie, D., Belák, S., Boucraut-Baralon, C., Egberink, H., Frymus, T., Gruffydd-Jones, T., et al., 2009. Feline infectious peritonitis. ABCD guidelines on prevention and management. J. Feline. Med. Surg. 11, 594–604.

Allison, A.B., Harbison, C.E., Pagan, I., Stucker, K.M., Kaelber, J.T., Brown, J.D., et al., 2012. Role of multiple hosts in the cross-species transmission and emergence of a pandemic parvovirus. J. Virol. 86, 865–872.

Allison, A.B., Kohler, D.J., Fox, K.A., Brown, J.D., Gerhold, R.W., Shearn-Bochsler, V.I., et al., 2013. Frequent cross-species transmission of parvoviruses among diverse carnivore hosts. J. Virol. 87, 2342–2347.

Alroy, J., Ucci, A.A., Goyal, V., Aurilio, A., 1986. Histochemical similarities between human and animal globoid cells in Krabbe's disease: a lectin study. Acta Neuropathol. 71, 26–31.

APHIS, 2011. *Annual Report Animal Usage by Fiscal Year [Online]*. United States Department of Agriculture Animal and Plant Inspection Service. Available from: <http://www.aphis.usda.gov/animal_welfare/efoia/downloads/2010_Animals_Used_In_Research.pdf> (Accessed 09.12.13).

Arnulf, I., 2006. Sleep and wakefulness disturbances in Parkinson's disease. J. Neural. Transm. Suppl., 357–360.

Arnulf, I., Crochet, S., Buda, C., 2005. Sleep–wake changes in MPTP-treated cats: an experimental model for studying sleep–wake disorders in Parkinson's disease? Sleep (Suppl.) 28, A17–A18.

Athanasiou, L.V., Chatzis, M.K., Kontou, I.V., Kontos, V.I., Spyrou, V., 2012. Feline bartonellosis. A review. J. Hell. Vet. Med. Soc. 63, 63–73.

AWA [Animal Welfare Act]. 2008. PL (Public Law) 89–544. Available from: <www.nal.usda.gov/awic/legislat/awa.htm/> (Accessed 04.17.14).

Aznavour, N., Cendres-Bozzi, C., Lemoine, L., Buda, C., Sastre, J.P., Mincheva, Z., et al., 2012. MPTP animal model of Parkinsonism: dopamine cell death or only tyrosine hydroxylase impairment? A study using PET imaging, autoradiography, and immunohistochemistry in the cat. CNS Neurosci. Ther. 18, 934–941.

Baldwin, K., Bartges, J., Buffington, T., Freeman, L.M., Grabow, M., Legred, J., et al., 2010. AAHA Nutritional assessment guidelines for dogs and cats. J. Am. Anim. Hosp. Assoc. 46, 285–296.

Bannasch, M.J., Foley, J., 2005. Epidemiologic evaluation of multiple respiratory pathogens in cats in animal shelters. J. Feline. Med. Surg. 7, 109–119.

Barr, J.W., McMichael, M., 2012. Inherited disorders of hemostasis in dogs and cats. Top. Companion. Anim. Med. 27, 53–58.

Beck, A., 2013. Use of pheromones to reduce stress in sheltered cats. J. Feline. Med. Surg. 15, 829–830.

Berg, T., Tollersrud, O.K., Walkley, S.U., Siegel, D., Nilssen, O., 1997. Purification of feline lysosomal α-mannosidase, determination of its cDNA sequence, and identification of a mutation causing α-mannosidosis in Persian cats. Biochem. J. 328, 863–870.

Blagbrough, I.S., Zara, C., 2009. Animal models for target diseases in gene therapy – using DNA and siRNA delivery strategies. Pharm. Res. 26, 1–18.

Bond, R., 2010. Superficial veterinary mycoses. Clin. Dermatol. 28, 226–236.

Boyce, J.T., DiBartola, S.P., Chen, D.J., Gasper, P.W., 1984. Familial renal amyloidosis in Abyssinian cats. Vet. Pathol., 21.

Bradbury, A.M., Cochran, J.N., McCurdy, V.J., Johnson, A.K., Brunson, B.L., Gray-Edwards, H., et al., 2013. Therapeutic response in feline sandhoff disease despite immunity to intracranial gene therapy. Mol. Ther. 21, 1306–1315.

Brown, M.A., Troyer, J.L., Pecon-Slattery, J., Roelke, M.E., O'Brien, S.J., 2009. Genetics and pathogenesis of feline infectious peritonitis virus. Emerg. Infect. Dis. [Online] Available from: <http://www.nc.cdc.gov/eid/article/15/9/08-1573.htm> (accessed 17.09.13).

Buffington, T., 1991. Meeting the nutritional needs of your feline patients. Vet. Med. 86, 720–727.

Burns, R.E., Wagner, D.C., Leutenegger, C.M., Pesavento, P.A., 2011. Histologic and molecular correlation in shelter cats with acute upper respiratory infection. J. Clin. Microbiol. 49, 2454–2460.

Carlson, M.E., 1996. Yersinia pestis infection in cats. J. Fel. Prac. 24, 22–24.

Carlstead, K., Brown, J.L., Strawn, W., 1993. Behavioral and physiological correlates of stress in laboratory cats. Appl. Animl. Behav. Sci. 38, 143–158.

Casal, M.L., Jezyk, P.F., Giger, U., 1996. Transfer of colostral antibodies from queens to their kittens. Am. J. Vet. Res. 57, 1653–1658.

Cassidy, J.P., Caulfield, C., Jones, B.R., Worrall, S., Conlon, L., Palmer, A.C., et al., 2007. Leukoencephalomyelopathy in specific pathogen-free cats. Vet. Pathol. 44, 912–916.

Caulfield, C.D., Cassidy, J.P., Kelly, J.P., 2008. Effects of gamma irradiation and pasteurization on the nutritive composition of commercially available animal diets. J. Am. Assoc. Lab. Anim. Sci. 47, 61–66.

Centerwall, W.R., Benirschke, K., 1975. An animal model for the XXY Klinefelter's syndrome in man: tortoiseshell and calico male cats. Am. J. Vet. Res. 36, 1275–1280.

Clavero, S., Bishop, D.F., Giger, U., Haskins, M.E., Desnick, R.J., 2010. Feline congenital erythropoietic porphyria: two homozygous UROS missense mutations cause the enzyme deficiency and porphyrin accumulation. Mol. Med. 16, 381–388.

Crowell-Davis, S.L., Barry, K., Wolfe, R., 1997. Social behavior and aggressive problems of cats. Vet. Clin. North Am. Small Anim. Pract. 27, 549–568.

Dawson, A.B., 1941. Early estrus in the cat following increased illumination. Endocrinology 28, 907–910.

Day, M.J., 2006. Vaccine side effects: fact and fiction. Vet. Microbiol. 117, 51–58.

DeBoer, D.J., Moriello, K.A., 1995. Inability of two topical treatments to influence the course of experimentally induced dermatophytosis in cats. J. Am. Vet. Med. Assoc. 207, 52–57.

Dharmage, S.C., Lodge, C.L., Matheson, M.C., Campbell, B., Lowe, A.J., 2012. Exposure to cats: update on risks for sensitization and allergic diseases. Curr. Allergy. Asthma. Rep. 12, 413–423.

Dinnage, J.D., Scarlett, J.M., Richards, J., 2009. Descriptive epidemiology of feline upper respiratory tract disease in an animal shelter. J. Feline. Med. Surg. 11, 538–546.

Egberink, H., Addie, D., Belák, S., Boucraut-Baralon, C., Frymus, T., Gruffydd-Jones, T., et al., 2009. Bordetella bronchiseptica infection in cats. ABCD guidelines on prevention and management. J. Feline. Med. Surg. 11, 610–614.

Elder, J.H., Lin, Y.C., Fink, E., Grant, C.K., 2010. Feline immunodeficiency virus (FIV) as a model for study of lentivirus infections: parallels with HIV. Curr. HIV. Res. 8, 73–80.

Ellis, S.L., 2009. Environmental enrichment: practical strategies for improving feline welfare. J. Feline. Med. Surg. 11, 901–912.

Ellis, S.L., Rodan, I., Carney, H.C., Heath, S., Rochlitz, I., Shearburn, L.D., et al., 2013. AAFP and ISFM feline environmental needs guidelines. J. Feline. Med. Surg. 15, 219–230.

Enno, A., O'Rourke, J.L., Howlett, C.R., Jack, A., Dixon, M.F., Lee, A., 1995. MALToma-like lesions in the murine gastric mucosa after long-term infection with Helicobacter felis. A mouse model of Helicobacter pylori-induced gastric lymphoma. Am. J. Pathol. 147, 217–222.

Esch, K.J., Petersen, C.A., 2013. Transmission and epidemiology of zoonotic protozoal diseases of companion animals. Clin. Microbiol. Rev. 26, 58–85.

Feldman, E.C., Nelson, R.W., 1996. Feline reproduction. Canine and Feline Endocrinology and Reproduction, second ed. Saunders, Philadelphia, PA.

Ferla, R., O'Malley, T., Calcedo, R., O'Donnell, P., Wang, P., Cotugno, G., et al., 2013. Gene therapy for mucopolysaccharidosis type VI is effective in cats without pre-existing immunity to AAV8. Hum. Gene. Ther. 24, 163–169.

Finkler, H., Gunther, I., Terkel, J., 2011. Behavioral differences between urban feeding groups of neutered and sexually intact free-roaming cats following a trap-neuter-return procedure. J. Am. Vet. Med. Assoc. 238, 1141–1149.

Frank, D., Beauchamp, G., Palestrini, C., 2010. Systematic review of the use of pheromones for treatment of undesirable behavior in cats and dogs. J. Am. Vet. Med. Assoc. 236 (12): 1308–1316.

Freeman, L.J., Hegreberg, G.A., Robinette, J.D., Kimbrell, J.T., 1989. Biomechanical properties of skin and wounds in Ehlers–Danlos syndrome. Vet. Surg. 18, 97–102.

Food and Drug Administration, (2014). Animal and Veterinary Recalls and Withdrawls. Available from: <http://www.fda.gov/AnimalVeterinary/SafetyHealth/RecallsWithdrawals/default.htm> (accessed 6.31.14).

Fyfe, J.C., Menotti-Raymond, M., David, V.A., Brichta, L., Schaffer, A.A., Agarwala, R., et al., 2006. An approximately 140-kb deletion associated with feline spinal muscular atrophy implies an essential LIX1 function for motor neuron survival. Genome Res. 16, 1084–1090.

Gandolfi, B., Outerbridge, C.A., Beresford, L.G., Myers, J.A., Pimentel, M., Alhaddad, H., et al., 2010. The naked truth: Sphynx and Devon Rex cat breed mutations in KRT71. Mamm. Genome 21, 509–515.

Gandolfi, B., Gruffydd-Jones, T.J., Malik, R., Cortes, A., Jones, B.R., Helps, C.R., et al., 2012. First WNK4-hypokalemia animal model identified by genome-wide association in Burmese cats. PLoS One 7, e53173.

Gaschen, F., Jaggy, A., Jones, B., 2004. Congenital diseases of feline muscle and neuromuscular junction. J. Feline. Med. Surg. 6, 355–366.

Gaskell, R.M., Povey, R.C., 1977. Experimental induction of feline viral rhinotracheitis virus re-excretion in FVR-recovered cats. Vet. Rec. 12, 128–133.

Gaskell, R.M., Dawson, S., Radford, A.D., Thiry, E., 2007. Feline herpesvirus. Vet. Res. 38, 337–354.

Gerhold, R.W., Jessup, D.A., 2013. Zoonotic diseases associated with free-roaming cats. Zoonoses Public Health 60, 189–195.

Ginzinger, D.G., Lewis, M.E., Ma, Y., Jones, B.R., Liu, G., Jones, S.D., 1996. A mutation in the lipoprotein lipase gene is the molecular basis of chylomicronemia in a colony of domestic cats. J. Clin. Invest. 97, 1257–1266.

Glaze, M.B., 2005. Congenital and hereditary ocular abnormalities in cats. Clin. Tech. Small. Anim. Pract. 20, 74–82.

Glenn, B.L., Glenn, H.G., Omtvedt, I.T., 1968. Congenital porphyria in the domestic cat: preliminary investigations on inheritance pattern. Am. J. Vet. Res. 29, 1653.

Greco, D.S., 1991. The effect of stress on the evaluation of feline patients. In: August, J.R. (Ed.), Consultations in Feline Internal Medicine. Saunders, Philadelphia, PA.

Griffin, J.F.T., 1989. Stress and immunity: a unifying concept Veterinary Immunology and Immunopathology. Elsevier Science Publ., Amsterdam.

Guptill, L., 2010. Bartonellosis. Vet. Microbiol. 140, 347–359.

Hanna, A.S., Cote, M.P., Houle, J., Dempsey, R., 2011. Nerve grafting for spinal cord injury in cats: are we close to translational research? Neurosurgery 68, N14–N15.

Hartmann, K., 2012. Clinical aspects of feline retroviruses: a review. Viruses 4, 2684–2710.

Harvey, J.W., 2006. Pathogenesis, laboratory diagnosis, and clinical implications of erythrocyte enzyme deficiencies in dogs, cats, and horses. Vet. Clin. Pathol. 35, 144–156.

Harvey, J.W., Dahl, M., High, M.E., 1994. Methemoglobin reductase deficiency in a cat. J. Am. Vet. Med. Assoc. 205, 1290–1291.

Hayes, K., Carey, R., 1975. Retinal degeneration associated with taurine deficiency in the cat. Science 188, 949–951.

Hoelzer, K., Parrish, C.R., 2010. The emergence of parvoviruses of carnivores. Vet. Res. 41, 39.

Hoenig, M., 2012. The cat as a model for human obesity and diabetes. J. Diabetes Sci. Technol. 6, 525–533.

Horzinek, M.C., Addie, D., Belak, S., Boucraut-Baralon, C., Egberink, H., Frymus, T., et al., 2013. ABCD: update of the 2009 guidelines on prevention and management of feline infectious diseases. J. Feline. Med. Surg. 15, 530–539.

Huang, C., Hess, J., Gill, M., Hustead, D., 2010. A dual-strain feline calicivirus vaccine stimulates broader cross-neutralization antibodies than a single-strain vaccine and lessens clinical signs in vaccinated cats when challenged with a homologous feline calicivirus strain associated with virulent systemic disease. J. Feline. Med. Surg. 12, 129–137.

Hubler, M., Haskins, M.E., Arnold, S., Kaser-Hotz, B., Bosshard, N.U., Briner, J., et al., 1996. Mucolipidosis type II in a domestic shorthair cat. J. Small Anim. Pract. 37, 435–441.

Hultborn, H., Nielson, J.B., 2007. Spinal control of locomotion – from cat to man. Acta Physiol. 189, 111–121.

Hurley, K.F., 2005. Feline infectious disease control in shelters. Vet. Clin. North Am. Small Anim. Pract. 35, 21–37.

Hurni, H., 1981. Day length and breeding in the domestic cat. Lab. Anim. 15, 229–233.

Inada, S., Mochizuki, M., Izumo, S., Kuriyama, M., Sakamoto, H., Kawasaki, Y., et al., 1996. Study of hereditary cerebellar degeneration in cats. Am. J. Vet. Res. 57, 296–301.

Jaso–Friedmann, L., Leary III, J.H., Praveen, K., Waldron, M., Hoenig, M., 2008. The effects of obesity and fatty acids on the feline immune system. Vet. Immunol. Immunopathol. 122, 146–152.

Kier, A.B., Bresnahan, J.F., White, F.J., Wagner, J.E., 1980. The inheritance pattern of factor XII (Hageman deficiency) in domestic cats. Can. J. Comp. Med. 44, 309–314.

Kier, A.B., McDonnell, J.J., Stern, A., Ratnoff, O.D., 1990. The Arthus reaction in cats deficient in Hageman factor (factor XII). J. Comp. Pathol. 102, 33–47.

Klein, D., 1983. Historical background and evidence for dominant inheritance of the Klein–Waardenburg syndrome (type III). Am. J. Med. Genet. 14, 231–239.

Knowles, J.O., Gaskell, R.M., 1991. Control of upper respiratory diseases in multiple cat households and catteries. In: August, J.R. (Ed.), Consultations in Feline Internal Medicine 2. Saunders, Philadelphia, PA.

Kramer, J.W., Davis, W.C., Prieur, D.J., 1977. The Chediak–Higashi syndrome of cats. Lab. Invest. 36, 554–562.

Kwon, B.K., Hillyer, J., Tetzlaff, W., 2010. Translational research in spinal cord injury: a survey opinion from the SCI community. J. Neurotrauma 27, 21–33.

Laflamme, D., 1997. Development and validation of a body condition score system for cats: A clinical tool. Fel. Pract. 25, 13–18.

Laflamme, D.P., 2012. Companion Animal Symposium: obesity in dogs and cats: what is wrong with being fat? J. Anim. Sci. 90, 1653–1662.

Lambo, C.A., Grahn, R.A., Lyons, L.A., Bateman, H., Newsom, J., Swanson, W.F., 2012. Comparative fertility of freshly collected vs frozen-thawed semen with laparoscopic oviductal artificial insemination in domestic cats. Reprod. Domest. Anim. 47 (Suppl. 6), 284–288.

Lappin, M.R., 2010a. Undate on the diagnosis and management of Toxoplasma gondii infection in cats. Top. Companion. Anim. Med. 2, 136–141.

Lappin, M.R., 2010b. Update on the diagnosis and management of Isospora spp infections in dogs and cats. Top. Companion. Anim. Med. 25, 133–135.

Lawler, D.F., Bebiak, D.M., 1986. Nutrition and management of reproduction in the cat. Vet. Clin. North Am. Small Anim. Pract. 16, 495–519.

Lawler, D.F., Evans, R.H., 1997. Strategies for controlling viral infections in feline populations. In: August, J.R. (Ed.), Consultations in Feline Internal Medicine 3. Saunders, Philadelphia, PA.

Lee, A., Hazell, S.L., O'Rourke, J., Kouprach, S., 1988. Isolation of a spiral-shaped bacterium from the cat stomach. Infect. Immun. 56, 2843–2850.

Licitra, B.N., Millet, J.K., Regan, A.D., Hamilton, B.S., Rinaldi, V.D., Duhamel, G.E., et al., 2013. Mutation in spike protein cleavage site and pathogenesis of feline coronavirus. Emerg. Infect. Dis. 19, 1066–1073.

Liu, W., Lei, J., Liu, Y., Lukic, D.S., Rathe, A.M., Bao, Q., et al., 2013. Feline foamy virus-based vectors: advantages of an authentic animal model. Viruses 5, 1702–1718.

Löfstedt, R.M., 1982. The estrous cycle of the domestic cat. Compend. Contin. Educ. 4, 52–58.

Lyons, L.A., 2010. Feline genetics: clinical applications and genetic testing. Top. Companion. Anim. Med. 25, 203–212.

MacDonald, M.L., Rogers, Q.R., Morris, J.G., 1984. Nutrition of the domestic cat, a mammalian carnivore. Annu. Rev. Nutr. 4, 521–562.

Magden, E., Quackenbush, S.L., VandeWoude, S., 2011. FIV associated neoplasms – a mini-review. Vet. Immunol. Immunopathol. 143, 227–234.

Maggo-Price, L., Dodds, W.J., 1993. Factor IX deficiency (hemophilia B) in a family of British shorthair cats. J. Am. Vet. Med. Assoc. 203, 1702–1704.

Majczynski, H., Slawinska, U., 2007. Locomotor recovery after thoracic spinal cord lesions in cats, rats and humans. Acta Neurobiol. Exp. 67, 235–257.

Malik, R., Lessels, N.S., Webb, S., Meek, M., Graham, P., Vitale, C., et al., 2009. Treatment of feline herpesvirus-1 associated disease in cats with famciclovir and related drugs. J. Fel. Med. Surg. 11, 40–48.

Martinez, M., Rossignol, S., 2013. A dual spinal cord lesion paradigm to study spinal locomotor plasticity in the cat. Ann. N.Y. Acad. Sci. 1279, 127–134.

Menotti-Raymond, M., David, V.A., Pflueger, S., Roelke, M.E., Kehler, J., O'Brien, S.J., et al., 2010. Widespread retinal degenerative disease mutation (rdAc) discovered among a large number of popular cat breeds. Vet. J. 186, 32–38.

Meurs, K.M., Norgard, M.M., Kuan, M., Haggstrom, J., Kittleson, M., 2009. Analysis of 8 sarcomeric candidate genes for feline hypertrophic cardiomyopathy mutations in cats with hypertrophic cardiomyopathy. J. Vet. Intern. Med. 23, 840–843.

Michel, C., 1993. Induction of oestrus in cats by photoperiodic manipulations and social stimuli. Lab. Anim. 27, 278–280.

Michel, K.E., Andeson, W., Cupp, C.J., Laflamme, D.P., 2011. Correlation of a feline muscle mass score with body composition determined by dual-energy X-ray absorptiometry. Br. J. Nutr. 106, S57–S59.

Mills, D.S., Redgate, S.E., Landsberg, G.M., 2011. A meta-analysis of studies of treatments for feline urine spraying. PLoS ONE 6, e18448.

Moore, G.E., DeSantin-Kerr, A.C., Guptil, L.F., Glickman, N.W., Lewis, H.B., Glickman, L.T., 2007. Adverse events in cats after vaccine administation in cats: 2,560 cases (2002–2005). J. Feline. Med. Surg. 231, 94–100.

Moriello, K.A., DeBoer, D.J., 1995. Efficacy of griseofulvin and itraconazole in the treatment of experimentally induced dermatophytosis in cats. J. Am. Vet. Med. Assoc., 439–444.

Mostl, K., Egberink, H., Addie, D., Frymus, T., Boucraut-Baralon, C., Truyen, U., et al., 2013. Prevention of infectious diseases in cat shelters: ABCD guidelines. J. Feline. Med. Surg. 15, 546–554.

Muldoon, L.L., Pagel, M.A., Neuwelt, E.A., Weiss, D.L., 1994. Characterization of the molecular defect in a feline model for type II GM2 gangliosidosis. Am. J. Pathol. 144, 109.

Mullikin, J.C., Hansen, N.F., Shen, L., Ebling, H., Donahue, W.F., Tao, W., et al., 2010. Light whole genome sequence for SNP discovery across domestic cat breeds. BMC Genomics 11, 406.

Narfstrom, K., 1999. Hereditary and congenital ocular disease in the cat. J. Feline. Med. Surg. 1, 135–141.

Narfstrom, K., Deckman, K.H., Menotti-Raymond, M., 2011. The domestic cat as a large animal model for characterization of disease and therapeutic intervention in heriditary retinal blindness. J. Opthalmol. 1–8.

National Research Council (NRC), 2006. Nutrient Requirements of Dogs and Cats. The National Academies Press, Washington, DC.

National Research Council, 2009. Scientific and Humane Issues in the Use of Random Source Dogs and Cats in Research. The National Academies Press, Washington, DC.

National Research Council, 2011. Guide for the Care and Use of Laboratory Animals, eighth ed. The National Academies Press, Washington, DC.

Neuzeret, P.C., Gormand, F., Reix, P., Parrot, S., Sastre, J.P., Buda, C., et al., 2011. A new animal model of obstructive sleep apnea responding to continuous positive airway pressure. Sleep 34, 541–548.

Niewold, T.A., van der Linde-Sipman, J.S., Murphy, C., Tooten, P.C., Gruys, E., 1999. Familial amyloidosis in cats: Siamese and Abyssinian AA proteins differ in primary sequence and pattern of deposition. Amyloid 6, 205–209.

Overall, K.L., Rodan, I., Beaver, B.V., Carney, H., Crowell-Davis, S., Hird, N., et al. (2004). Feline behavior guidelines from the American Association of Feline Practitioners [Online]. Available from: <http://www.catvets.com/public/PDFs/PracticeGuidelines/FelineBehaviorGLS.pdf>.

Paasch, L.H., Zook, B.C., 1980. The pathogenesis of endocardial fibroelastosis in Burmese cats. Lab. Invest. 42, 197–204.

Patel, J., Heldens, J., 2009. Review of companion animal viral diseases and immunoprophylaxis. Reply to Day et al. Vaccine 27, 3689.

Pedersen, N.C., 2009. A review of feline infectious peritonitis virus infection: 1963–2008. J. Feline. Med. Surg. 11, 225–258.

Perese, D.M., Fracasso, J.E., 1959. Anatomical considerations in surgery of the spinal cord: a study of vessels and measurements of the cord. J. Neurosurg. 16, 314–325.

Perkins, S.E., Yan, L.L., Shen, Z., Hayward, A., Murphy, J.C., Fox, J.G., 1996. Use of PCR and culture to detect Helicobacter pylori in naturally infected cats following triple antimicrobial therapy. Antimicrob. Agents. Chemother. 40, 1486–1490.

Pion, P.D., Kittleson, M.D., Rogers, Q.R., Morris, J.G., 1987. Myocardial failure in cats associated with low plasma taurine: a reversible cardiomyopathy. Science 237, 764–768.

Plantinga, E.A., Bosch, G., Hendriks, W.H., 2011. Estimation of the dietary nutrient profile of free-roaming feral cats: possible implications for nutrition of domestic cats. Br. J. Nutr. 106, S35–S48.

Pontius, J.U., Mullikin, J.C., Smith, D.R., Agencourt Sequencing, T., Lindblad-Toh, K., Gnerre, S., et al., 2007. Initial sequence and comparative analysis of the cat genome. Genome Res. 17, 1675–1689.

Poulet, H., Jas, D., Lemeter, C., Coupier, C., Brunet, S., 2008. Efficacy of a bivalent inactivated non-adjuvanted feline calicivirus vaccine: relation between in vitro cross-neutralization and heterologous protection in vivo. Vaccine 26, 3647–3654.

Radford, A.D., Addie, D., Belák, S., Boucraut-Baralon, C., Egberink, H., Frymus, T., et al., 2009. Feline calicivirus infection. ABCD guidelines on prevention and management. J. Feline. Med. Surg. 11, 556–648.

Reisner, I.R., Houpt, K.A., Erb, H.N., Quimby, F.W., 1994. Friendliness to humans and defensive aggression in cats: the influence of handling and paternity. Physiol. Behav. 55, 1119–1124.

Rochlitz, I., 2000. Recommendations for the housing and care of domestic cats in laboratories. Lab. Anim. 34, 1–9.

Rodan, I., Sundahl, E., Carney, H., Gagnon, A.C., Heath, S., Landsberg, G., et al., 2011. American Animal Hospital Association. AAFP and ISFM feline-friendly handling guidelines. J. Feline. Med. Surg. 13, 364–375.

Roper, R.L., Rehm, K.E., 2009. SARS vaccines: where are we? Expert Rev. Vaccines 8, 887–898.

Rossignol, S., Chau, C., Giroux, N., Brustein, E., Bouyer, L., Marcoux, J., et al., 2002. The cat model of spinal injury. Prog. Brain. Res. 137, 151–168.

Rozengurt, N., 1994. Endocardial fibroelastosis in common domestic cats in the UK. J. Comp. Pathol. 110, 295–301.

Salvadori, C., Modenato, M., Corlazzoli, D.S., Arispici, M., Cantile, C., 2005. Clinicopathological features of globoid cell leucodystrophy in cats. J. Comp. Pathol. 132, 350–356.

Sands, M.S., Haskins, M.E., 2008. CNS-directed gene therapy for lysosomal storage diseases. Acta Paediatr. Suppl. 97, 22–27.

Scherk, M.A., Ford, R.B., Gaskell, R.M., Hartmann, K., Hurley, K.F., Lappin, M.R., et al., 2013. AAFP Feline Vaccination Advisory Panel Report. J. Feline. Med. Surg. 15, 785–808.

Scipioni, A., Mauroy, A., Vinje, J., Thiry, E., 2008. Animal noroviruses. Vet. J. 178, 32–45.

Scott, P.P., Lloyd-Jacob, M.A., 1959. Reduction in the anoestrus period of laboratory cats by increased illumination. Nature 184, 2022.

Seiler, M.J., Aramant, R.B., Seeliger, M.W., Bragadottir, R., Mahoney, M., Narfstrom, K., 2009. Functional and structural assessment of retinal sheet allograft transplantation in feline hereditary retinal degeneration. Vet. Ophthalmol. 12, 158–169.

Shille, V.M., Sojka, N.J., 1995. Feline reproduction. In: Ettinger, S.J., Feldman, E.C. (Eds.), Textbook of Veterinary Internal Medicine. Saunders, Philadelphia, PA.

Shimizu-Onda, Y., Akasaka, T., Yagyu, F., Komine-Aizawa, S., Tohya, Y., Hayakawa, S., et al., 2013. The virucidal effect against murine norovirus and feline calicivirus as surrogates for human norovirus by ethanol-based sanitizers. J. Infect. Chemother. 19, 779–781.

Smith, K., 2011. Feline muscular dystrophy: parallels between cats and people. Vet. Rec. 168, 507–508.

Stein, V.M., Crooks, A., Ding, W., Prociuk, M., O'Donnell, P., Bryan, C., et al., 2012. Miglustat improves purkinje cell survival and alters microglial phenotype in feline Niemann–Pick disease type C. J. Neuropathol. Exp. Neurol. 71, 434–448.

Stutzer, B., Hartmann, K., 2012. Chronic Bartonellosis in cats: what are the potential implications? J. Feline. Med. Surg. 14, 612–621.

Swanson, W., 2012. Laparoscopic oviductal embryo transfer and artificial insemination in felids – challenges, strategies and successes. Reprod. Domest. Anim. 47 (Suppl. 6), 136–140.

Thiry, E., Addie, D., Belák, S., Boucraut-Baralon, C., Egberink, H., Frymus, T., et al., 2009. Feline herpesvirus infection. ABCD guidelines on prevention and management. J. Feline. Med. Surg. 11, 547–555.

Trehiou-Sechi, E., Tissier, R., Gouni, V., Misbach, C., Petit, A.M., Balouka, D., et al., 2012. Comparative echocardiographic and clinical features of hypertrophic cardiomyopathy in 5 breeds of cats: a retrospective analysis of 344 cases (2001–2011). J. Vet. Intern. Med. 26, 532–541.

Truyen, U., Parrish, C.R., 2013. Feline panleukopenia virus: its interesting evolution and current problems in immunoprophylaxis against a serious pathogen. Vet. Microbiol. 165, 29–32.

Truyen, U., Addie, D., Belák, S., Boucraut-Baralon, C., Egberink, H.F.T., Gruffydd-Jones, T., et al., 2009. Feline panleukopenia. ABCD guidelines on prevention and management. J. Feline. Med. Surg. 11, 538–546.

Turner, D.C., Feaver, J., Mendl, M., Bateson, P., 1986. Variation in domestic cat behavior towards humans: a paternal effect. Anim. Behav. 34, 1890–1892.

Valle, D.L., Boison, A.P., Jezyk, P., Aguirre, G., 1981. Gyrate atrophy of the choroid and retina in a cat. Invest. Ophthalmol. Vis. Sci. 20, 251–255.

Van de Velde, H., Janssens, G.P., de Rooster, H., Polis, I., Peters, I., Ducatelle, R., et al., 2013. The cat as a model for human obesity: insights into spot-specific inflammation associated with feline obesity. Br. J. Nutr. 110, 1326–1335.

Villaverde, B., Fioratti, E.G., Penitenti, M., Ikoma, M.R., Tsunemi, M.H., Papa, F.O., et al., 2013. Cryoprotective effect of different glycerol concentrations on domestic cat spermatozoa. Theriogenology 80, 730–737.

Vite, C.H., McGowan, J.C., Niogi, S.N., Passini, M.A., Drobatz, K.J., Haskins, M.E., et al., 2005. Effective gene therapy for an inherited CNS disease in a large animal model. Ann. Neurol. 57, 355–364.

Wang, T.C., Dangler, C.A., Chen, D., Goldenring, J.R., Koh, T., Raychowdhury, R., et al., 2000. Synergistic interaction between hypergastrinemia and Helicobacter infection in a mouse model of gastric cancer. Gastroenterology 118, 36–47.

Watson, R.P., Blanchard, T.W., Mense, M.G., Gasper, P.W., 2001. Histopathology of experimental plague in cats. Vet. Pathol. 38, 165–172.

Webb, A.A., Ngan, S., Fowler, J.D., 2010. Spinal cord injury I: a synopsis of the basic science. Can. Vet. J. 51, 485–492.

Willett, B.J., Hosie, M.J., 2013. Feline leukaemia virus: half a century since its discovery. Vet. J. 195, 16–23.

Wongsrikeao, P., Saenz, D., Rinkoski, T., Otoi, T., Poeschla, E., 2011. Antiviral restriction factor transgenesis in the domestic cat. Nat. Methods 8, 853–859.

Xu, L., Mei, M., Haskins, M.E., Nichols, T.C., O'Donnell, P., Cullen, K., et al., 2007. Immune response after neonatal transfer of a human factor IX-expressing retroviral vector in dogs, cats, and mice. Thromb. Res. 120, 269–280.

Yamamoto, J.K., Sanou, M.P., Abbott, J.R., Coleman, J.K., 2010. Feline immunodeficiency virus model for designing HIV/AIDS vaccines. Curr. HIV. Res. 8, 14–25.

Young, A.E., Biller, D.S., Herrgesell, E.J., Roberts, H.R., Lyons, L.A., 2005. Feline polycystic kidney disease is linked to the PKD1 region. Mamm. Genome 16, 59–65.

Zoran, D.L., 2010. Obesity in dogs and cats: A metabolic and endocrine disorder. Vet. Clin. Small Anim. 40, 221–239.

Zoran, D.L., Buffington, C.A.T., 2011. Effects of nutrition choices and lifestyle changes on the well-being of cats, a carnivore that has moved indoors. JAVMA 239, 596–606.

14

Biology and Diseases of Ferrets

Joerg Mayer, Dr. med.vet., MSc, Dipl. ACZM, Dipl. ECZM (small mammal), Dipl. ABVP (ECM)[a], Robert P. Marini, DVM[b] and James G. Fox, DVM, MS, DACLAM[b]

[a]College of Veterinary Medicine, University of Georgia Athens, Georgia [b]Division of Comparative Medicine, Massachusetts Institute of Technology, Cambridge, Massachusetts, MA, USA

I. INTRODUCTION

A. Taxonomic Considerations

Ferrets (*Mustela putorius furo*) belong to the ancient family Mustelidae, which is believed to date back to the Eocene period, some 40 million years ago. The taxonomic groups in the family Mustelidae, as recognized by Nowak (1999), include 67 species in 25 genera from North, Central, and South America; Eurasia; and Africa. No other carnivore shows such diversity of adaptation, being found in a wide variety of ecosystems ranging from arctic tundra to tropical rainforests. Mustelids have retained many primitive characteristics, which include relatively small size, short stocky legs, five toes per foot, elongated braincase, and short rostrum (Anderson, 1989). The Mustelinae is the central subfamily of the Mustelidae. The best-known members of the Mustelinae are the weasels, mink, ferrets (genus *Mustela*), and the martens (genus *Martes*) (Anderson, 1989). The genus *Mustela* is divided into five subgenera: *Mustela* (weasels), *Lutreola* (European mink), *Vison* (American mink), *Putorius* (ferrets), and *Grammogale* (South American weasels). The smallest member of the Mustelidae family is the least weasel (*Mustela nivalis*), which weighs as little as 25 g, and the largest member is the sea otter (*Enhydra lutris*), which can weigh as much as 45 kg (Nowak, 1999).

Laboratory Animal Medicine, Third Edition
DOI: http://dx.doi.org/10.1016/B978-0-12-409527-4.00014-6

According to one author, ferrets (*Mustela putorius furo*) have been domesticated for more than 2000 years (Davidson *et al.*, 1999). Earlier references to ferrets are probably the basis of the belief that ferrets originated in North Africa (Thomson, 1951). Evidently they were bred specifically for rabbiting (rabbit hunting) and were muzzled before being sent into rabbit burrows. This practice was later introduced into Europe, Asia, and the British Isles, where the sport is still practiced today.

Although the ferret has been historically used for hunting, more recently it has been increasingly used in biomedical research and is popular in North America as a pet. It is most likely a domesticated version of the wild European ferret or polecat (*M. putorius* or *M. furo*) (Thomson, 1951). Alternatively, several authors have at least considered whether *M. putorius*, *M. eversmannii*, and the endangered *M. nigripes* from North America (black-footed ferret) could be viewed as one Holarctic species (Davidson *et al.*, 1999).

The domesticated ferret, although introduced to North America by the early English settlers some 300 years ago, has not unequivocally established feral colonies on this continent. Feral populations have established themselves in New Zealand, however, where they have contributed to the decline of vulnerable native species. A large bibliography emphasizing predatory behavior, environmental impact, and the potential of ferrets to establish feral colonies has been published by the California Department of Fish and Game (Whisson and Moore, 1997).

B. Use in Research

The ferret was not recognized as having potential as an animal model for biomedical research until the 1900s. Early studies utilized the ferret in classic experiments with influenza virus pathogenesis (Pyle, 1940). Its use was cited infrequently; an article published in 1940, detailing the use of ferrets in research, cited only 26 publications (Pyle, 1940). Literature reviews undertaken in 1967, 1969, 1973, and 1985, however, revealed an increasing appreciation for the ferret's usefulness and versatility in the study of human physiologic, anatomic, and disease mechanisms (Hahn and Wester, 1969; Marshall and Marshall, 1973; Shump *et al.*, 1974; Frederick and Babish, 1985). In 1991, a bibliography containing 'selected' literature citations on the ferret and its use in biomedical research was published (Clingerman *et al.*, 1991). The document was designed to serve as a reference tool for individuals involved in the care or use of ferrets in the laboratory setting. Although not comprehensive, the document provides extensive coverage of ferret biology, diseases, and use as an animal model. The domesticated ferret has been and continues to be used extensively in studies involving virology, neuroscience, carcinogenesis, cardiovascular physiology, and emesis (Morgan and Travers, 1998).

An extensive overview of different uses of the ferret as an animal model has been compiled by the USDA. It contains more than 30 publications and was last updated in 2006. It can be accessed online at: http://www.nal.usda.gov/awic/pubs/Ferrets06/animal_models.htm.

C. Availability and Sources

The ferret's increasing popularity in research and as a pet is mainly a result of large-scale commercial production. Commercial farms have been raising ferrets for almost 50 years. Biomedical researchers in the United States can request animals of a specific sex, weight, and age for individual experiments. Investigators in other countries may acquire ferrets from fur operations or may make arrangements with commercial vendors in the United States. Even though the ferret is nonstandardized with regard to exact genotype and pedigree, its routine availability in a clinically healthy state has aided immeasurably its acceptance as a research animal. Readily available commercial stocks, based on coat color, are albino, sable (or fitch), Siamese, silver mitt, and Siamese-silver mitt (Siamese with white chest and feet) (McLain *et al.*, 1985). The fitch or so-called wild coat color is the most common, recognized by yellow–buff fur with patches of black or dark brown, particularly on the tail and limbs (Andrews and Illman, 1987). The production of ferrets by large commercial operations has raised concern by some that inbreeding of these animals has made the ferret more susceptible to diseases, e.g., endocrine-related disorders. Anecdodally, it has been suggested that 75% of US ferrets with a blaze or white head can suffer from the Waardenburg syndrome and are deaf (J. Mayer, personal observation). The only study providing a physiologic basis for auditory impairment describes a reduction in the ipsilateral projections of the cochlear nucleus to the auditory midbrain in albino ferrets (Moore and Kowalchuk, 1988). Albino ferrets also have impaired motion perception and contrast sensitivity (Hoffmann *et al.*, 2004; Price and Morgan, 1987; Akerman *et al.*, 2003; Hupfeld *et al.*, 2006).

D. Laboratory Management and Husbandry

1. Housing and Husbandry

Housing of ferrets in a research facility is similar to that of other small carnivores such as cats (Fox, 1998c). Ferrets tolerate low temperatures well and high temperatures poorly; the recommended temperature range for juvenile and adult animals is 4–18°C (39.2–64.4°F) (Hammond and Chesterman, 1972). Ferrets less than 6 weeks of age should be housed at >15°C. Kits under this age require a heat source if separated from the dam; older kits that are group-housed do not. Elevated temperatures (>30°C; 86°F) cannot be tolerated by ferrets, because they have poorly developed sweat glands and are susceptible to heat prostration. Signs of hyperthermia include panting, flaccidity, and vomiting. The preferred humidity is 40–65%.

For non-breeding animals that will remain in the facility for a short time, a conventional dark–light cycle at 12:12 h is adequate. Lighting may be altered to control breeding cycles. Breeding and lactating jills should be exposed to 16 h of light daily. Ferrets that are maintained for breeding or for use beyond 6 months should be exposed to 'winter' light – 6 weeks per year of 14 h of dark daily – to maintain physiologic normalcy. It is also essential that researchers receiving time-pregnant jills preserve the photoperiod to which jills were exposed prior to shipment. Failure to do so may cause inappetence, with subsequent negative energy balance and pregnancy toxemia.

Similar to other laboratory animal species, ferrets should be housed with 10–15 air changes per hour (USDHHS, 1996). It is important to use nonrecirculated air because of the strong odor of ferrets and the susceptibility of ferrets to human respiratory tract infections such as influenza. The ferret odor should not overlap into any rodent housing areas, because rodents have an instinctive fear of ferrets, and the ferret scent can disrupt rodent breeding and physiology (Fox, 1998c).

2. Caging

Female ferrets can be housed singly or in groups, but estrous females that are cohoused may become pseudopregnant (Beck et al., 1976). Intact males in breeding condition should be housed individually after 12 weeks of age.

Molded plastic caging used to house rabbits works very well for ferrets. The solid bottom is perforated with holes and is readily sanitizable. An absorbable paper liner may be used in the pan beneath the cage to facilitate daily disposal of urine and feces. In a research setting, the plastic caging should be washed weekly to avoid excessive soiling. Use of one or two additional pieces of cage board or similar substance within the cage also helps maintain cleanliness, and ferrets enjoy burrowing beneath and between the sheets of paper. The spacing of grid walls should be 1.0 × 0.5 inches apart, or 0.25 inch if using wire mesh. Ferrets like to lick and bite at their enclosures, so sharp edges and galvanized metal should be avoided. Fractured teeth are often a consequence if this behavior is not corrected. Zinc toxicosis has been reported from licking galvanized bars from which metals had leached during steam sterilization (Straube and Walden, 1981) (Table 14.1) Ferrets can be trained to use a litter box because they repeatedly urinate or defecate in one corner of the cage. Clay litters have been reported to cause chronic upper respiratory irritation from inhaled dust (Jenkins and Brown, 1993). Ferrets prefer sleeping in a soft isolated area, and in a research facility this can

TABLE 14.1   Housing Ferrets in Research

Parameter	Comment
Cage size	24 × 24 × 18 inches (adequate for two adult ferrets)
Grid size	1 × 0.5 inches (0.25 inch if wire mesh or slatted flooring)
Temperature range	4–18°C (40–64.5°F); animals less than 6 weeks (>15°C; 60°F)
Humidity range	40–65%
Air handling	10–15 complete air changes/h (nonrecirculated)
Animals amenable to group/pair housing	Female ferrets
	Anestrous
	Nonlactating
	Weanling ferrets (4–12 weeks old)
	Males separated at 12 weeks
Photoperiod (hours light:hours dark)	Breeding; lactation (16:8)
	Winter cycle (10:14)
	Nonbreeders housed for <6 months (12:12)
Diet (protein source: meat)	Nonbreeding adult males and females: 18–20% fat, 30–40% protein
	Breeding males and females: minimum 25% fat, minimum 35% protein
	Peak lactation: 30% fat minimum, 35% protein
Feeding schedule	Ad libitum
Quantity consumed (dry-weight basis)	43 g/kg body weight
Water consumption (adults)	75–100 ml daily

be accomplished by providing a washable 'snooze tube' or hammock (Fox, 1998c). Environmental enrichment is now commonly used in order to prevent boredom or misplaced reactions towards cagemates. Some studies suggest that the lack of environmental stumuli has potentially wide-ranging effects on the overall well-being of ferrets. Chivers and Einon (1982) found that some of the isolation-induced effects on behavior seen in rats also occurred in ferrets, with deprivation of rough and tumble social play causing hyperactivity that persisted into adulthood. Socially reared ferrets whose environment was enriched with a series of changing tube systems (Weiss-Buerger, 1981) were superior in maze learning and reversal. Korhonen (1995) demonstrated that optimal health occurred when ferrets were provided with increased floor space and compatible cagemates and when offered balls and bite cups with which to play. Russell (1990) found that ferrets raised in enriched conditions would choose the arm of a maze leading to the more prey-like of two play objects and were superior in capturing prey-models. These forms of enrichment are easy to implement and carry a minimal risk of injury to the animal. Examples of enrichment ideas include making tunnels from PCV pipe or dryer hose, and filling a box with rice, plastic balls, or crumpled paper balls, in order to let the ferrets fulfill their instinctive digging behaviors. All these items can easily be sterilized or exchanged between uses. Care must be taken that the enrichment items are not ingested by the ferret. Foreign body ingestion in ferrets is usually a true medical emergency.

Research with the black-footed ferret has demonstrated that enrichment lowers fecal glucocorticoid metabolites (FGM) in juvenile males (Poessel et al., 2011). Enrichment had no effect on FGM in juvenile females and adult males. The study also showed that juvenile males interacted more with enrichment items than adult females. The authors concluded that an environmental enrichment program could benefit captive juvenile male ferrets by reducing adrenocortical activity.

II. BIOLOGY

A. Unique Anatomic and Physiologic Characteristics

The thorax of the ferret is narrow and elongated, and as a result the trachea is proportionally long. This makes the ferret an ideal species for studies of tracheal physiology. The tracheal size and laryngeal anatomy make endotracheal intubation somewhat challenging, and as a result the ferret has been advocated as a species suitable for use in pediatric intubation training (Powell et al., 1991). The lungs are relatively large, and the total lung capacity is nearly three-times that which would be predicted based on body size, as compared with other mammals. This characteristic, together with a higher degree of bronchiolar branching and more extensive bronchial submucosal glands (as compared with the dog), makes the ferret an attractive model for pulmonary research studies (Vinegar et al., 1985). Although a previous report (Willis and Barrow, 1971) commented that the carotid arterial branching pattern in the ferret is unusual, it is actually typical for a carnivore. As is the case in the dog and the cat, the paired common carotid arteries arise from the brachiocephalic trunk (sometimes called the innominate artery) at the level of the thoracic inlet (Andrews et al., 1979b).

The ferret's gastrointestinal tract is specialized to fit its carnivorous nature. The simple monogastric stomach is similar to that of the dog. There is no cecum present, and the indistinct ileocecal transition makes it difficult to identify the junction of the small and large intestines during a gross examination. The overall length of the alimentary tract is very short relative to the body size, resulting in a gastrointestinal transit time as short as 3 h (Bleavins and Aulerich, 1981).

As in other mustelids, the paired anal scent glands of the ferret are well developed. Although not as potent as those of the skunk, the secretions of the ferret are sufficiently odoriferous that many pet or research ferrets are descented. Surgical techniques for this procedure have been described (Creed and Kainer, 1981; Mullen, 1997). Ferrets, especially intact males and estrous jills, may possess a distinctive musky odor even after a successful descenting, because of normal sebaceous secretions. Ferrets lack well-developed sweat glands for use in thermal regulation, and as a result they are predisposed to heat prostration when ambient temperatures reach 32°C (90°F) (Ryland et al., 1983).

Extramedullary hematopoiesis is commonly found during histological examination of the spleen, and in some cases it may result in a grossly evident splenomegaly (Erdman et al., 1998). This must be differentiated from splenomegaly that can arise from a variety of pathologic conditions or from isoflurane administration (see Section III, E). Experimental evidence suggests that ferrets have no naturally occurring antibodies against unmatched erythrocyte antigens, and that none develop even in the face of repeated transfusions (Manning and Bell, 1990b). One of the authors (JM) has transfused multiple ferrets with multiple sessions and not seen an anaphylactic reaction to date.

Ferrets are seasonal breeders, and the resulting pronounced physiological variations in body weight, behavior, and gametogenesis are utilized in scientific studies of photoperiod responses and neuroendocrine control. Prolonged estrus in unbred females can cause an aplastic anemia, an effect that can be reproduced with exogenous estrogen administration (Bernard et al., 1983). The male has a radiographically evident os penis, and, contrary to some earlier reports, a prostate gland is present in males (Evans and An, 1998).

B. Normal Values

Newborn ferret kits weigh 6–12 g at birth and will grow to 400 g by the time they are weaned at 6–8 weeks (Shump and Shump, 1978). In sexually intact populations, males (1.0–2.0 kg) can be twice the size of females (0.5–1.0 kg). The adult weight of nonobese male and female ferrets that have been gonadectomized prior to weaning and raised in captivity will generally fall between 0.8 and 1.2 kg (Brown, 1997a). Adult animals (especially those that are sexually intact) may be subject to seasonal fluctuations in body fat percentage, which can cause body weight to fluctuate by 30–40% (Fox and Bell, 1998). The approximate life span for the ferret is 6–8 years, but on rare occasions they may live as long as 11 years (Table 14.2).

TABLE 14.2 Selected Normative Data for the Ferret[a]

Parameter	Value
Life span (average)	5–11 years
Body temperature	38.8°C (37.8–40°C)
Chromosome number (diploid)	40
Dental formula	2 (I 3/3, C 1/1, P 4/3, M 1/2)
Vertebral formula	$C_7T_{15}L_5S_3C_{14}$
Age of sexual maturity	4–12 months[b]
Length of breeding life	2–5 years
Gestation	42 ± 2 days
Litter size	8, average (range, 1–18)
Birth weight	6–12 g
Eyes open	34 days
Onset of hearing	32 days
Weaning	6–8 weeks
Water intake	75–100 ml/24 h
Urine volume	26–28 ml/24 h
Urine pH	6.5–7.5
Cardiovascular/respiratory	
Arterial blood pressure	
Mean systolic	Female 133, male 161 mmHg (conscious)
Mean diastolic	110–125 mmHg (anesthetized)
Heart rate	200–400 beats/min
Cardiac output	139 ml/min
Circulation time	4.5–6.8 s
Respirations	33–36/min

[a]Adapted from Fox (1998e).
[b]Dependent on photoperiod.

TABLE 14.3 Hematology Values of Normal Ferrets[a]

Parameter (unit)	Observed range
WBC (10^3/mm^3)	1.7–13.4
RBC (10^3/mm^3)	9.7–13.2
Hematocrit (%)	47–59
Hemoglobin (gm/dl)	14.5–18.5
Total protein (gm/dl)	6.2–7.7
Neutrophils (%)	22–75
Bands (%)	0–2
Lymphocytes (%)	20–73
Monocytes (%)	0–4
Eosinophils (%)	0–3
Basophils (%)	0–1

[a]Combined ranges from orbital and cardiac venipuncture of anesthetized male ferrets (Fox et al., 1986b).

TABLE 14.4 Serum Chemistry Values of Normal Ferrets

Serum analyte (unit)	Observed range[a]	Mean ± SEM Female[b]	Male[b]
Glucose (mg/dl)	99–135	104.9 ± 16.4	104.0 ± 15.0
Urea nitrogen (mg/dl)	11–25	33.3 ± 7.6	22.0 ± 6.3
Creatinine (mg/dl)	0.3–0.8	0.40 ± 0.10	0.40 ± 0.10
Sodium (mEq/l)	152–164	150.4 ± 1.50	154.4 ± 3.60
Potassium (mEq/l)	4.1–5.2	4.90 ± 0.30	4.90 ± 0.20
Chloride (mEq/l)	118–126	117.1 ± 1.90	112.5 ± 9.10
Calcium (mg/dl)	7.5–9.9	9.0 ± 0.30	9.5 ± 0.60
Phosphorus (mg/dl)	4.8–7.6	6.70 ± 0.60	6.70 ± 1.20
Alanine aminotransferase (IU/l)	78–149	150.3 ± 49.3	157.6 ± 79.9
Aspartate aminotransferase (IU/l)	57–248	ND[c]	101.0 ± 35.25
Alkaline phosphatase (IU/l)	31–66	44.3 ± 11.3	52.4 ± 11.6
Lactate dehydrogenase (IU/l)	221–752	ND	434 ± 113.5
Sorbitol dehydrogenase (IU/l)	ND	2.6 ± 2.2	5.4 ± 4.5
Protein, total (gm/dl)	5.0–6.8	6.0 ± 0.5	5.9 ± 0.3
Albumin (gm/dl)	3.3–4.2	3.8 ± 0.2	3.7 ± 0.1
Cholesterol (mg/dl)	119–209	174.0 ± 43.5	156.0 ± 37.0
Triglycerides (mg/dl)	10–32	ND	18.5 ± 5.1
Bilirubin, total (mg/dl)	0–0.1	ND	0.55 ± 0.225
Uric acid (mg/dl)	0.7–2.7	ND	ND
Globulin (mg/dl)	1.8–3.1	ND	ND
Carbon dioxide (mmol/l)	16–28	ND	ND

[a]Combined ranges (Fox et al., 1986b).
[b]Four- to 8-month-old ferrets (Loeb and Quimby, 1999).
[c]ND, Not done.

Normal hematology and serum chemistry values have been reported for the ferret (Tables 14.3, 14.4) (Thornton et al., 1979; Lee et al., 1982; Fox, 1998e). These values are not greatly dissimilar from those of other domestic carnivores. One distinctive hematological characteristic of the ferret is the presence of a relatively robust erythron, characterized by hematocrit, hemoglobin, and total erythrocyte and reticulocyte counts that are generally higher than those of the dog or cat. Reported neutrophil–lymphocyte ratios range from 1.7:1 to 0.7:1. Representative hematology and chemistry ranges of pet ferrets have recently been published and are listed in Table 14.5 (Hein et al., 2012). While these values are reliable and complete for diagnostic purposes, any laboratory that evaluates ferret samples should develop its

TABLE 14.5   Reference ranges for laboratory parameters in ferrets

Parameter	Unit	Median	Reference interval	90% CI for lower limit	90% CI for upper limit
HAEMATOLOGY*					
Red blood cells	$10^{12}/l$	10.5	7.4–13.0	6.8–7.9	12.7–13.3
Packed cell volume	l/l	0.6	0.4–0.7	0.4–0.5 0.7	0.7–0.7
Hemoglobin	mmol/l	11.1	8.6–13.6	8.2–9.0	13.2–13.9
Mean corpuscular volume	fl	54.3	49.6–60.6	49.0–50.2	59.6–61.5
Mean corpuscular hemoglobin concentration	mmol/l	19.3	17.8–20.9	17.5–18.0	20.7–21.2
Mean corpuscular hemoglobin	fmol/l	1.1	1.0–1.2	0.9–1.0	1.2–1.2
Platlets	$10^9/l$	807.0	171.7–1280.6	21.0–304.8	1219.7–1338.1
White blood cells	$10^9/l$	7.2	3.0–16.7	2.7–3.4	14.9–18.8
DIFFERENTIAL BLOOD COUNT (ABSOLUTE VALUES)					
Monocytes	$10^9/l$	0.2	0.0–0.5	0.0–0.0	0.5–0.6
Lymphocytes	$10^9/l$	3.4	0.6–10.5	0.3–0.8	9.3–12.0
Band neutrophilic granulocytes	$10^9/l$	0.0	0.0–0.1	0.0–0.0	0.1–0.2
Segmented neutrophilic granulocytes	$10^9/l$	3.0	0.9–7.4	0.7–1.1	6.6–8.2
Eosinophilic granulocytes	$10^9/l$	0.1	0.0–0.7	0.0–0.0	0.6–0.8
Basophile granulocytes	$10^9/l$	0.0	0.0–0.2	0.0–0.0	0.1–0.2
DIFFERENTIAL BLOOD COUNT (RELATIVE VALUES)					
Monocytes	%	2.0	0.0–6.5	0.0–0.0	5.7–7.1
Lymphocytes	%	53.0	12.6–80.6	5.3–19.8	77.0–83.8
Band neutrophilic granulocytes	%	0.0	0.0–1.2	0.0–0.0	0.9–1.5
Segmented neutrophilic granulocytes	%	43.0	17.2–81.9	15.5–19.5	75.9–87.7
Eosinophilic granulocytes	%	2.0	0.0–5.7	0.0–0.0	5.1–6.3
Basophile granulocytes	%	0.0	0.0–1.4	0.0–0.0	1.1–1.7
ENZYMES**					
ALT	IU/l	110.0	49.0–242.8	45.7–53.9	217.6–271.3
AST	IU/l	74.0	40.1–142.7	37.8–43.3	129.8–152.8
AP	IU/l	34.0	13.3–141.6	13.0–14.2	113.4–175.7
GLDH	IU/l	1.0	0.0–2.5	0.0–0.0	2.1–2.8
γ-GT	IU/l	4.0	0.2–14.0	0.0–0.5	11.9–16.3
LDH	IU/l	325.0	154.4–1780.6	149.8–162.3	1401.8–2236.4
CK	IU/l	203.0	94.0–730.9	86.3–102.5	580.2–907.3
α-Amylase	IU/l	38.0	19.4–61.9	17.4–22.0	58.3–65.4
Lipase	IU/l	204.0	73.2–351.1	62.0–91.0	326.2–372.8
CHE	IU/l	526.0	262.1–1017.5	235.6–295.5	933.0–1108.4

(*Continued*)

TABLE 14.5 (Continued)

Parameter	Unit	Median	Reference interval	90% CI for lower limit	90% CI for upper limit
SUBSTRATES*					
Glucose	mmol/l	6.0	3.0–8.5	2.5–3.5	8.2–8.8
Fructosamine	μmol/l	163.0	121.1–201.6	114.8–127.4	195.9–206.9
Cholesterol	mmol/l	4.9	2.4–7.1	2.1–2.8	6.8–7.4
Triglycerides	mmol/l	1.0	0.5–2.8	0.4–0.5	2.3–3.6
Serum bile acids	μmol/l	5.7	0.0–28.9	0.0–0.0	23.7–34.8
Bilirubin	μmol/l	1.1	0.0–3.3	0.0–0.0	2.8–3.8
Urea	mmol/l	9.8	4.8–16.9	4.2–5.4	15.8–18.1
Creatinine	μmol/l	44.0	23.0–76.7	20.7–25.4	71.0–82.8
Total protein	g/l	67.8	54.7–77.9	52.4–57.0	76.3–79.4
Albumin	g/l	36.1	28.0–43.9	26.7–29.1	43.0–44.9
ELECTROLYTES[†]					
Calcium	mmol/l	2.3	2.0–2.6	1.9–2.0	2.5–2.6
Phosphate	mmol/l	1.8	1.0–3.1	1.0–1.1	2.9–3.4
Magnesium	mmol/l	1.2	0.9–1.6	0.9–1.0	1.5–1.7
Sodium	mmol/l	154.0	140.1–169.7	138.0–142.5	166.7–172.5
Potassium	mmol/l	5.0	3.9–5.9	3.7–4.1	5.8–6.0
Chloride	mmol/l	114.0	108.0–119.9	107.1–108.7	118.9–120.8
Iron	μmol/l	33.8	11.7–56.3	8.4–14.5	53.1–59.6
HORMONES[††]					
Cortisol	nmol/l	6.6	0.0–101.5	0.0–0.0	80.5–122.8
Thyroxine	nmol/l	27.0	15.9–42.0	14.3–17.8	39.6–44.7
Progesterone	ng/ml	0.0	0.0–0.4	0.0–0.0	0.3–0.5
Oestradiol	pg/ml	5.0	0.0–12.2	0.0–3.0	7.7–16.3

Hein et al. (2012).
Number of ferrets = 105–106.
**Number of ferrets = 102–106; γ-GT = 94.*
***Number of ferrets = 100–109; serum bile acids = 95.*
[†]*Number of ferrets = 102–109.*
[††]*Number of ferrets = 70–94.*

own set of specific normal ranges. A low-grade proteinuria may be identified by urinalysis in normal, healthy ferrets (Thornton *et al.*, 1979) (Table 14.6). The specifics of the urinalysis have been published and mean urine specific gravity reported was 1051 for intact males and 1042 for intact females (Eshar *et al.*, 2012).

C. Nutrition

Ferret diets have been formulated both empirically and based upon the nutrient requirements of other mustelids (Fox and McLain, 1998). Specific requirements for various life-cycle stages have not been determined experimentally. Available commercial diets are certainly capable of supporting growth, reproduction, and maintenance

TABLE 14.6 Urine Analytes of Normal Ferrets

Urine analyte	Units	Female[a]	Male[a]
Volume	ml/24h	8–140	8–48
pH		6.5–7.5	6.5–7.5
Protein	mg/100ml	0–32	7–33
Sodium	mmol/24h	0.2–5.6	0.4–6.7
Potassium	mmol/24h	0.9–5.4	1.0–9.6
Chloride	mmol/24h	0.3–7.5	0.7–8.5

[a]*Four- to 8-month-old ferrets (Loeb and Quimby, 1999).*

in conventional settings. In recent years speciality diets designed for ferrets have entered the commercial market. Some of these diets contain extremely high crude protein contents (up to ~50%) and low charbohydrate values (<10%) in order to try to mimic a more natural composition of a whole-prey diet. Other speciality foods are considered hypoallergenic as they are made with turkey, venison, and lamb, and contain no chicken. In the absence of careful analysis, however, it is uncertain whether the proportion and quantity of ingredients in these diets is optimal or even beneficial.

Ferrets are strict carnivores with a high requirement for dietary fat and protein. Their short digestive tract and rapid gastrointestinal transit time require protein to be readily digestible. There is general agreement that ferrets should not be given diets high in complex carbohydrates or fiber. Diets that are high in fish products are also not recommended for ferrets (Fox and McLain, 1998). The use of any raw chicken, beef, or other meats is strongly discouraged because of the potential contamination by *Campylobacter, Salmonella, Listeria, Mycobacterium,* and *Streptococcus* (Fox, 1998a). The daily maintenance energy requirement of the ferret is estimated to be 0.5 MJ metabolizable energy (ME)/kg metabolic body weight (BW$^{0.75}$; Kamphues *et al.*, 1999). The requirement may reach multiples of the above value during growth, pregnancy and lactation (Bell, 1996).

Calorie–percent protein ratios have been determined for mink (*Mustela vison*) kits up to and after 16 weeks of age (Sinclair *et al.*, 1962; Allen *et al.*, 1964). A ratio of 13 and a caloric density of 550 kcal/100 g of feed, corresponding to 42% protein, provided optimum growth for male kits up to 16 weeks. After 16 weeks, ratios of 17 and 21, corresponding to 36% and 26% protein, respectively, were recommended. Diets containing 9–28% fat and 22–42% carbohydrate have been used successfully to maintain ferrets. One author recommends 30–40% protein and 18–20% fat for adult, nonbreeding animals and a minimum of 35% protein and 25% fat for reproductively active animals and those that have not reached sexual maturity (Brown, 1997a). The long-term impact of diets containing high levels of fat and protein are unknown. A recent study demonstrates that the digestibility of crude protein in ferrets is significantly lower than in cats while the digestibility of crude fat is significantly higher (Fekete *et al.*, 2005). The study concludes that the ferret cannot be used as a model animal for cats with respect to either feed preference or nutrient digestibility and care must be taken when extrapolating data obtained from feline research to the ferret.

The quality and origin of the protein also appear to be a significant factor as it has been shown that very high levels of plant proteins in the diet can lead to urolithiasis (Bell, 1999).

Another controversial topic is the carbohydrate content of the diet. While in the wild, the ferret would have an extremely limited intake of carbohydrates, most commercial pellets contain a significant amount of carbohydrates. It has been suggested that the starch content of the diet should not exceed 30–36% (Naismith and Cursiter, 1972). As a general rule it has been accepted that a diet low in carbohyrates appears to be preferred for the maintenance of ferrets. However, it has been observed that pups of ferret bitches fed a high-fat and high-protein but carbohydrate-free diet had poorer viability, probably as a result of hypoglycaemia (Hebeler and Wolf, 2001).

Ferrets have been used to investigate the absorption, metabolism, and interaction of the dietary micronutrients β-carotene and vitamin E. Ferrets, like humans, convert β-carotene to vitamin A in the gut and absorb β-carotene intact (Fox and McLain, 1998). In intestinal perfusion experiments in ferrets, it was demonstrated that β-carotene, retinol, and retinyl esters are absorbed intact into lymph and that cleavage products, including β-apo-12′-carotenal, β-apo-10′-carotenal, and retinoids, accumulate in the intestinal mucosa (Wang *et al.*, 1992). The intestinal mucosa is capable of converting β-carotene into retinoic acid and other polar metabolites, which are then transported via the portal vein to the liver (Wang *et al.*, 1993). β-Carotene absorption is enhanced by co-perfusion with α-tocopherol, and the perfusion of the latter is unaltered by the presence of β-carotene. The conversion of β-carotene into retinol is also enhanced by the presence of α-tocopherol (Wang *et al.*, 1995). Studies have shown that ferrets have the capacity to excrete retinol and retinyl esters in the urine. This response seems dependent on oral vitamin A supplementation (Raila *et al.*, 2002). Based on the various studies available, it can be concluded that the ferret can be used as a model to investigate aspects of beta-carotene metabolism as well as aspects of the metabolism of vitamin A such as absorption in the gut, regulation of incorporation of retinyl esters into lipoproteins in the liver, and renal uptake and regulated urinary excretion of vitamin A.

A lung cancer model of ferrets exposed to tobacco smoke has been used to evaluate the cancer-modulating properties of these micronutrients (Kim *et al.*, 2006a, b, 2012).

Adult ferrets drink 75–100 ml of water daily, depending on the dry-matter content of the feed (Andrews and Illman, 1987). Fresh water can be provided *ad libitum* in stainless steel bowls or water bottles with sipper tubes. Ferrets are playful and will overturn bowls or water bottles that are not well secured.

D. Reproduction

1. Reproductive Physiology

Features of ferret reproduction may be found in Table 14.7. Female ferrets are seasonal breeders and induced ovulators. The season under natural illumination in the Northern Hemisphere is from March to August for females and from December to July for

TABLE 14.7   Ferret Reproductive Data[a]

Parameter	Value
Age at puberty	
Female (adult, range 750–1500 g)	6–12 months
Male (adult, range 1500–2500 g)	6–12 months
Minimum breeding age	8–12 months (male); 4–5 months (female)
Estrous cycle[b]	Monestrus, March through August[c]
Duration of estrous cycle	Continuous until intromission
Type of ovulation	Induced by copulation
Ovulation time	30–40 h after mating
Number of ova	12 (range, 5–13)
Copulation time	Up to 3 h
Sperm deposition site	Posterior os cervix
Ovum transit time	5–6 days
Viability of sperm in female tract	36–48 h
Cleavage to formation of blastocoele	Uniform rate
Implantation	12–13 days
Gestation period	42 ± 1 days
Implantation–parturition	30 ± 1 days
Litter size	8 average (range, 1–18)
Size at birth	6–12 g
Return to estrus	Next March[b], occasionally postpartum estrus
Solid food eaten	3 weeks, before eyes are open
Breeding life of female	2–5 years
Breeding life of male	5 + years
Breeding habits	One male to several females; in colony production

[a]Adapted from Fox and Bell (1998).
[b]Dependent on photoperiod.
[c]Polyestrous in this period if a litter is produced.

males, corresponding temporally to increasing day length. Ferrets born in the late spring or early summer and maintained under natural lighting will not assume an adult pattern of gonadal activity (i.e., puberty) until the following season (Baum, 1998). Under artificial illumination, jills that are maintained at 8 h light–16 h dark reach puberty at 10–12 months. Stimulatory photoperiods may be used, however, in the laboratory or intensive production setting, as a method of breeding ferrets out of the natural season. However, the transfer from short to long photoperiods should not occur prior to 90 days of age, because jills that are prematurely transferred will remain anestrous (Hammond and Chesterman, 1972). Management practices in one breeding facility are such that jills commence breeding at 7–10 months, average 3.7 litters a year, and are cycled out of reproduction after six litters. In another strategy, ferrets are exposed to a 16:8 h photoperiod at 12 weeks of age, are bred at 16 weeks during their first estrus, and whelp at 5½ months.

Vulvar swelling is the hallmark of estrus in jills. The ease with which estrus is detected in the ferret, as well as the size of the ferret and ease of its maintenance in captivity have made the ferret a model for study of neuroendocrine events and their gonadal correlates. Along with the hamster, the ferret has contributed extensively to an understanding of the photoperiodic influences on the hypothalamic–pituitary–gonadal axis (Baum, 1998). As in females of other species, estradiol concentrations are responsible for controlling the development of the female reproductive tract and secondary sexual characteristics, and the tonic inhibition of luteinizing hormone (LH) secretion by the anterior pituitary during both prepubertal life and anestrus. The sensitivity of the hypothalamic gonadostat to negative feedback inhibition by estradiol changes at the time of puberty, and under the influence of increasing light exposure, LH levels rise despite estradiol (Ryan, 1984). Similarly, age differences in the sensitivity of negative feedback inhibition of the hypothalamic secretion of gonadotropin-releasing hormone (GnRH) by testosterone, or to estrogenic compounds derived from the aromatization of testosterone, appear to be essential in determining puberty and seasonality of reproduction in the male (Baum, 1998).

2. Detection of Estrus and Pregnancy

Estrus in jills is characterized by dramatic vulvar swelling from an anestrous diameter of 5–16 mm to an estrous diameter of 17–33 mm. Changes in vaginal cytology have also been described for the ferret and other mustelid species, but these changes are seldom used to determine onset of estrus or to schedule breeding (Williams et al., 1992). After a 2- to 3-week proestrus, estrus occurs. Estrus onset is not associated with elevated serum FSH in the ferret, as it is in the rodent. Once estrus has occurred, it may terminate in coitus-induced ovulation and pregnancy, pseudopregnancy after infertile mating, pharmacologic termination (by injection of human chorionic gonadotropin [hCG], GnRH or GnRH analogs), death due to estrogen-induced aplastic anemia, or spontaneous remission and anestrus due to reduced photoperiod. Waves of follicular development occur in estrus, and five to 13 ova are ovulated approximately 30–40 h after coitus. Female ferrets are brought to the male approximately 14 days after vulvar enlargement. Females and males copulate many times and for prolonged periods of time; they are typically left together for 2 days. Both intromission and neck restraint by the male are apparently required for induction of ovulation (Baum, 1998). An LH surge accompanies coitus in females, but the same is not true of males (Carroll *et al.*, 1987). Implantation occurs 12 days after mating; both a functional corpus luteum and the anterior pituitary are required for implantation and maintenance of pregnancy. Placentation is typical of carnivores and is zonary and endotheliochorial (Morrow, 1980). Pregnancy may be detected by ultrasonographic demonstration of 3- to 5-mm discrete nonechogenic structures as early as day 12 (Peter *et al.*, 1990), by palpation as early as day 14, or by radiographic demonstration of calcified fetal skeletons at approximately 30 days of gestation.

3. Husbandry Needs

Jills within 2 weeks of parturition should be singly housed and provided with a secluded place in which to deliver their kits. When rabbit cages are used for housing, nest boxes may take the form of polypropylene rat cages or other plastic boxes (cat litter box or dish pan). Nest boxes should have bedding provided for warmth and comfort. Materials suitable for bedding include pieces of fabric (towels), ripped cageboard, shredded paper, or cotton batting. The nest box should be at least 6 inches deep and should prevent the kits from wandering from the jill. Entrance to the nest box should be smooth, to avoid injury to the teats and mammary gland. At our institution, jills are provided a stainless steel rectangular box with a smooth-surfaced plastic entrance (Fig. 14.1). A retractable steel roof panel and a guillotine side panel exposing a Plexiglas sidewall allow access to the jill and permit observation with minimal disturbance. One major supplier of ferrets uses sunken tubs filled with bedding to promote a sense of security and isolation of the jill. Most jills will leave the nest box to eat and drink. If the jill will not leave, however, low-sided food bowls should be placed within the nest box. Adequate nutritional care for the pregnant jill is of utmost importance, as during pregnancy the ferret fetuses have a large

glucose demand that must be satisfied by the mother. If the fetal demand and the maternal supply become imbalanced due to fasting of the mother or increased nutritional demands of the rapidly developing fetal placental unit, females suffer from negative energy balance and succumb to severe hypoglycemia (Batchelder *et al.*, 1999; Dalrymple, 2004). Prohaczik *et al.* (2009) describe in detail the metabolic changes which occur during pregnancy toxemia and how to monitor for them. Their findings showed that in contrast to healthy animals, hypoglycemia, hyperketonemia, hypoinsulinemia, and decreased T4 and T3 levels were detected in females with pregnancy toxemia. Necropsy showed excessive hepatic lipidosis (Batchelder *et al.*, 1999; Dalrymple, 2004; Prohaczik *et al.*, 2009).

4. Parturition

Parturition occurs rapidly in ferrets and may last as little as 2–3 h. Primiparous jills typically deliver on day 41 of gestation whereas multiparous jills deliver on day 42. There are few signs of impending parturition, although abdominal enlargement and mammary development do occur in the last week or two. Small litters (fewer than three) may result in inadequate stimulus for parturition. Jills that pass their due date without delivery should be palpated for fetuses. Kits remaining *in utero* beyond the 43rd day typically die; kits with congenital malformations such as cyclopia and exencephaly may also delay the initiation of labor. Dystocia is common in ferrets because of positional abnormalities and fetal oversize and should be treated by cesarean section. Jills tolerate cesareans well and will nurse kits delivered in this way. If small litter size is responsible for delayed parturition, prostaglandins (0.5–1.0 mg Lutalyse) may be used, followed by 0.3 ml oxytocin (6 U) after 3 h (Fox and Bell, 1998). Failure to deliver within 8 h of administration of prostaglandin is an indication for cesarean section. Jills should be provided heat, energy, hydration, and analgesia following cesarean.

Kits will attempt to nurse soon after parturition, but jills experiencing difficult labor may not allow them to nurse until all kits are delivered. Jills that are not attentive to their kits should be palpated for the presence of additional, undelivered kits. Oxytocin may be used to facilitate delivery of remaining kits. Offering the jill regular chow mixed with warm water may promote maternal acceptance. Kits should be kept warm pending acceptance by the jill. Jills should be left undisturbed for the first several days postpartum to minimize as much as possible provoking litter cannibalization. Cross-fostering to other jills may be successfully accomplished, provided that the kits are warm and that the foster jill has kits of similar age. Kits to be fostered should be allowed to mingle with the foster jill's own kits while their dam is absent so that rejection due to olfactory stimuli will not occur.

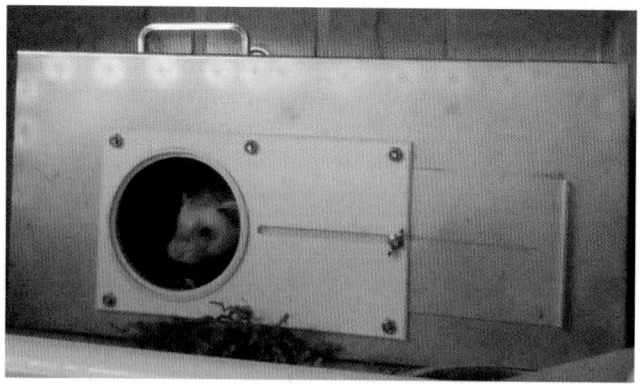

FIGURE 14.1   Ferret nesting box. Top and side panels allow inspection without disturbing the jill.

5. Early Development of the Newborn

Kits are born in an altricial state, covered by lanugo hair and with their eyes closed. By 3 days of age, albino ferrets retain their white hair whereas pigmented ferrets acquire a gray coat. They are completely dependent on the jill for the first 3 weeks of life. Defecation and urination are stimulated by jills through anogenital licking of the kits. Kits are born weighing 6–12 g, double their weight in 5 days, and triple it in 10 days to a weight of 30 g. The 3-week-old male kit should weigh at least 100 g. Sexual dimorphism in size is apparent by week 7 and persists into adulthood.

Developmental landmarks include ability to hear at 32 days, opening of the eyes at 34 days, eruption of deciduous teeth at 14 days, eruption of permanent canines at 47–52 days, and displacement of deciduous canines by 56–70 days (Fox and Bell, 1998). The ear canals of a ferret do not open until approximately 32 days postnatally (as compared with 6 days in a cat), which coincides with the appearance of a startle response to loud hand claps and the recording of acoustically activated neurons in the midbrain (Moore, 1982). This late onset of hearing may explain why kits produce exceptionally loud, piercing sounds during the first 4 weeks of life. Lactating jills are tuned in to kit vocalizations and will respond to high-frequency (greater than 16 kHz) sounds in a maze test, whereas males and nonlactating females will ignore these sounds (Shimbo, 1992). Kits of wild polecats have a critical period of learning the scent of prey which, according to Apfelbach (1986), is between 60 and 90 days of age.

6. Sexing

Gender may be distinguished in neonatal ferrets, as in other species, by anogenital distance, with the distance being much shorter in females than in males. In males, the urogenital opening is seen just caudal to the umbilicus. The prominent midline raphe penis overlying the palpable os penis is also a distinctive feature in the male.

7. Weaning

Ferrets are typically weaned at 6 weeks of age. Early weaning may be encouraged by making a slurry of the jill's chow available at 3–4 weeks; fat may be added to achieve a fat content of 30%. The fatty acid supplement Linatone (Lambert Kay, Cranberry, New Jersey) is recommended by one author (Brown, 1997a). The diet should contain approximately 30% fat and 40% protein. The slurry should be fed twice daily for a restricted time and then removed to avoid having kits walking through and defecating in the diet. Unthrifty kits over 14 days of age may be supplemented with canine or feline milk replacers administered per os by Tygon-tipped Pasteur pipette (Manning and Bell, 1990a). Weaned ferrets are best housed in groups until sexually mature. Males over

12 weeks old may begin to fight if exposed to greater than 12 h light per day.

Jills may return to estrus during the second or third week of lactation if they have fewer than five kits or 2 weeks after weaning if the litter is of normal size. Jills should be rebred or administered hCG to terminate estrus, even if still lactating. A high-quality, calorie-dense diet is required for lactation and to maintain pregnancy. If maintained on a stimulatory photoperiod and adequate nutrition, jills may have two to three litters of six or more kits yearly until they are 5 years old (Fox and Bell, 1998). A nonstimulatory photoperiod should be used 6 weeks per year to rest the ferret and preserve maximum fertility; a maintenance diet can be given at this time. Jills return to estrus approximately 3 weeks after reinstitution of the longer photoperiod.

8. Artificial Insemination

A visual transcervical artificial insemination technique with the aid of an endoscope has been described in the domestic ferret (Kidder et al., 1998). However, artificial insemination is not commonly performed in ferrets but has been studied in the context of providing strategies for species perpetuation of the endangered black-footed ferret (Wildt et al., 1989; Howard et al., 2003).

9. Synchronization

Synchronization of estrus as practiced in rodent production is not used as a tool of reproductive management in the ferret. Synchronization of jills may be approximated, however, by manipulation of photoperiod. If exposed only to natural lighting, the hob will become reproductively active a full 1 to 2 months before the jill. With natural illumination in outdoor housing, jills all come into estrus within a 1- to 2-week period (Baum, 1998). In the laboratory setting, when jills are maintained in a nonstimulatory photoperiod (8 h light–16 h dark) for 6–8 weeks, followed by reversal of the cycle (16 h light–8 h dark), estrus will follow in 4 weeks (immature jills) or 3 weeks (mature jills) after the change (Carroll et al., 1985). This correlates with follicular development and increased plasma estradiol.

III. DISEASES

A. Infectious Diseases

1. Bacterial Infections

The occurrence of infectious disease affects animal health and well-being and may complicate research efforts. A program combining good animal husbandry, optimal nutrition, health monitoring practices, and clinical care is essential to maintaining a healthy ferret colony.

a. *Clostridium perfringens* Type A

Etiology   The etiologic agent is *Clostridium perfringens* type A (*Clostridium welchii*).

Epizootiology and Transmission   *Clostridium perfringens* is ubiquitous and is present in the intestinal contents of humans and animals. *Clostridium perfringens* type A has been associated with the occurrence of acute abdominal distension, dyspnea, and cyanosis in weanling ferrets (Field and Laboratory Service Veterinary Staff, 1984) and an outbreak of gastroenteritis in weanling black-footed ferrets (Schulman *et al.*, 1993). The exact cause of these conditions is uncertain, but predisposing factors such as overeating, sudden changes in diet, the proliferation of *C. perfringens* type A, and the production of overwhelming amounts of toxins are suspected (Field and Laboratory Service Veterinary Staff, 1984; Schulman *et al.*, 1993). The alpha toxin is the principal lethal toxin. It is hemolytic and necrotizing and possesses the ability to split lecithin or lecithin–protein complexes, leading to destruction of cell membranes and subsequent necrosis. Reported cases have involved weanling animals exclusively.

Clinical Signs   Ferrets may present with acute abdominal distension, dyspnea, and cyanosis, or may be found dead and bloated (Field and Laboratory Service Veterinary Staff, 1984; Schulman *et al.*, 1993).

Diagnosis   Isolation of *C. perfringens* type A from gastric and small-intestinal contents is required. Toxin identification may be performed by the use of a mouse protection assay (Smith, 1975).

Necropsy Findings   Gross findings include markedly distended stomachs and intestines containing a large amount of gas and a moderate amount of brown, semiliquid ingesta, and subcutaneous emphysema with minimal or no putrefaction (Field and Laboratory Service Veterinary Staff, 1984; Schulman *et al.*, 1993). Histologic findings observed in weanling black-footed ferret cases included the observation of abundant gram-positive bacilli in smears of gastric and intestinal contents. Other findings included varying degrees of gastrointestinal mucosal necrosis, numerous gram-positive bacilli lining the denuded mucosal surface and extending into the gastric glands and intestinal crypts; lymphoid necrosis of lymph nodes, spleen, and thymus; mild to moderate dilatation of central hepatic sinusoids with mild, acute, centrilobular hepatocellular dissociation and multifocal aggregates of small numbers of necrotic neutrophils within portal areas (Schulman *et al.*, 1993).

Treatment and Control   Prevention through good management and feeding practices is the primary means of control. In the reported cases of *C. perfringens* type A-associated gastroenteritis in black-footed ferret weanlings, supportive care and gastric trocharization were unrewarding. The occurrence of the condition was eliminated by restricting feeding of weanlings to twice a day instead of three times daily.

b. Campylobacteriosis

Etiology   Campylobacteriosis is caused by infection with *Campylobacter jejuni*.

Epizootiology and Transmission   *Campylobacter jejuni* is a gram-negative, spirally curved microaerophilic bacterium that is recognized as a significant cause of human enteritis and is associated with diarrheic illness in several animal species, including dogs, cats, cows, goats, pigs, mink, ferrets, and sheep (Carter *et al.*, 1995). It also known to cause mastitis in cows, infectious hepatitis of chickens, and abortion in cattle, sheep, goats, dogs, and mink (Carter *et al.*, 1995). The organism may also be cultured from the feces of normal asymptomatic dogs, cats, and ferrets (Fox *et al.*, 1983; Carter *et al.*, 1995).

Transmission occurs by ingestion of organisms through direct contact with feces or contaminated food and water (Carter *et al.*, 1995). There have been reports linking the disease in humans to pets. Many of these outbreaks were associated with dogs, puppies, and kittens recently obtained from animal shelters or pounds and displaying diarrhea before the human illness occurred (Fox *et al.*, 1983). Isolation of *Campylobacter jejuni* from asymptomatic ferrets also implies a potential for zoonotic transmission (Fox *et al.*, 1982, 1983).

Clinical Signs   Experimental oral inoculation of ferret kits with various strains of *C. jejuni* produced a self-limiting diarrhea that ranged in character from very mild to watery (Fox *et al.*, 1987; Bell and Manning, 1990a, 1991). The presence of mucus and/or blood was also noted in the feces of affected animals. Anorexia, dehydration, and tenesmus with watery diarrhea were also observed. Intravenous inoculation of four pregnant mink and seven pregnant ferrets resulted in reproductive failure, ranging from fetal resorption to expulsion of dead or premature living kits (Bell and Manning, 1990b). Oral inoculation resulted in abortion in a majority of the infected animals (Bell and Manning, 1990b). In one study, 86.7% of the animals infected orally with *C. jejuni* developed diarrhea and inflammatory responses that were similar to those seen in human infection (Nemelka *et al.*, 2009). During the acute clinical phase in this study, *C. jejuni* was isolated from the livers of 7 of 9 (78%) animals, and bacteria were visualized immunohistochemically in the livers from five of the seven animals (71%) from which *C. jejuni* was isolated.

Diagnosis   Diagnosis is based on history, clinical signs, and culture of affected animals. Reports of spontaneous cases in ferrets require diagnostic confirmation and differentiation from cases of proliferative bowel disease and other infectious and noninfectious causes of diarrhea. *Campylobacter jejuni* grows slowly and has specific culture requirements that involve the use of selective media or filtration techniques, and a requirement for thermophilic (42–43°C) and microaerophilic conditions (Fox, 1998a). Cultures should be examined every 48h for round, raised, translucent, and sometimes mucoid colonies (Fox, 1998a).

Necropsy Findings　Studies involving oral inoculation of ferrets with *Campylobacter jejuni* revealed small focal neutrophilic infiltrates in the lamina propria of the colon of relatively few infected animals (Fox *et al.*, 1987). Bell and Manning (1991) noted mild to moderate enterocolitis with neutrophilic infiltration of the lamina propria, which was most severe in kits with concurrent cryptosporidiosis. Placentitis was the most notable histologic finding in pregnant ferrets and mink after experimental inoculation of a strain of an abortion storm-associated isolate of *C. jejuni* (Bell and Manning, 1990b).

Treatment and Control　In a study to eliminate the carrier state in ferrets, erythromycin was ineffective even though *in vitro* isolates of *C. jejuni* were sensitive to the antibiotic (Fox *et al.*, 1983). According to the author, reasons for therapeutic failure included dose selection, interspecies differences in pharmacokinetics and possible reinfection. Supportive care should be instituted, and choice of antibiotic therapy in confirmed diarrheic cases should be based on culture and sensitivity. In addition, because of its zoonotic potential, isolation of affected animals and good hygiene practices are recommended. Reculture of animals after treatment to ensure elimination of the organism is recommended. Azithromycin and fluoroquinolones are common agents used in humans.

In one study investigating a vaccine against *C. jejuni* infections, ferrets were used to demonstrate the potential of a killed whole cell vaccine prepared from *Campylobacter jejuni* to protect against disease (Burr *et al.*, 2005). The results of the study showed that the vaccine can be used to protect against disease caused by *Campylobacter*. After four doses of the vaccine were given 48h apart, 80% of the animals were free of diarrhea after subsequent challenge (Burr *et al.*, 2005).

c. *Helicobacter mustelae*

Epizootiology and Transmission　In 1985, a gastric helicobacter like organism was isolated from the margins of a duodenal ulcer of a ferret and named *Helicobacter mustelae* (Fox *et al.*, 1986a, 1989a). Subsequently, in the United States, gastritis and peptic ulcers have been routinely reported in ferrets colonized with *H. mustelae* (Fox *et al.*, 1988b, 1991a). Every ferret with chronic gastritis is infected with *H. mustelae*, whereas specific pathogen-free (SPF) ferrets not infected with *H. mustelae* do not have gastritis, gastric ulcers, or detectable IgG antibody to the organism (Fox *et al.*, 1990, 1991a). *Helicobacter mustelae* has also been isolated from the stomachs of ferrets living in England, Canada, Australia and, most recently, from

ferrets in New Zealand (Forester *et al.*, 2000; Tompkins *et al.*, 1988).

Koch's postulates have been fulfilled: by oral inoculation of *H. mustelae* into naive ferrets uninfected with *H. mustelae*, the infection induced a chronic, persistent gastritis similar to that observed in ferrets naturally infected with *H. mustelae* (Fox *et al.*, 1991b). Experimental inoculation and other studies have also established *Helicobacter gastritis* in the ferret as a robust model for *H. pylori* gastritis in humans. The *H. mustelae* genome has been sequenced (O'Toole *et al.*, 2010).

It is now known that *H. mustelae* colonizes nearly 100% of ferrets shortly after weaning. Feces from weanling and adult ferrets have been screened for the presence of *H. mustelae* to determine whether fecal transmission could explain the 100% prevalence observed in weanling and older ferrets (Fox *et al.*, 1988b, 1992b). *Helicobacter mustelae* was isolated from the feces of eight of 74 9-week-old and three of eight 8-month-old ferrets. Ferrets placed on proton pump inhibitors, which raise gastric pH, have a statistically higher recovery of *H. mustelae* from feces when compared with age-matched untreated control ferrets (Fox *et al.*, 1993).

Clinial Signs and Pathology　*Helicobacter mustelae*-infected ferrets examined in our laboratory are usually asymptomatic. Ferrets with gastric or duodenal ulcers can be recognized clinically by vomiting, melena, chronic weight loss, and lowered hematocrit. Clinical signs in ferrets with *H. mustelae*-associated gastric adenocarcinoma have consisted of vomiting, anorexia, and weight loss, signs that may be confused with gastric foreign body.

Diagnosis　Gastric and duodenal ulcers are observable endoscopically. It is interesting that the ferret is the only domesticated animal to date that has naturally occurring helicobacter associated ulcer disease. The *H. mustelae* isolated from ferrets has similar but not identical biochemical features to those of *H. pylori*, particularly in regard to the production of large amounts of urease. Gastric samples collected by endoscopy or necropsy are minced with sterile scalpel blades and inoculated onto blood agar plates supplemented with trimethoprim, vancomycin, and polymixin B (Remel, Lenexa, Kansas). The plates are incubated at 37 or 42°C in a microaerobic atmosphere (80% N_2, 10% H_2, and 10% CO_2) in vented jars for 3–7 days. Bacteria are identified as *H. mustelae* on the basis of gram-stain morphology; production of urease, catalase, and oxidase; resistance to cephalothin; and sensitivity to nalidixic acid.

Necropsy and Histopathologic Findings　The histopathological changes occurring in the stomach closely coincided in topography with the presence of *H. mustelae* (Fox *et al.*, 1990). A superficial gastritis present in the body of the stomach showed that *H. mustelae* was located on the surface of the mucosa but not in the crypts. Inflammation occupied the full thickness of the distal antral mucosa, the so-called diffuse antral gastritis described in humans (Fig. 14.2a, b). In this location, *H. mustelae* was seen at the surface, in the pits, and on the superficial portion of the glands. In the proximal antrum and the transitional mucosa, focal glandular atrophy, a precancerous lesion, and regeneration were present, in addition to those lesions seen in the distal antrum. Also, deep colonization of *H. mustelae* was observed focally in the affected antral glands. Argyrophilic bacteria have also been demonstrated in the liver and biliary tract of ferrets with chronic cholangiohepatitis, bile duct hyperplasia, and cholangiocellular carcinoma. Organisms shared sequence homology with *H. cholecystus* (Garcia *et al.*, 2002).

Animals infected with *Helicobacter* spp. may also be susceptible to gastric cancer (Fox *et al.*, 1994; Yu *et al.*, 1995). There is documentation of the presence of argyrophilic bacteria, compatible in location and morphology to *H. mustelae*, within the pyloric mucosa of two male ferrets with pyloric adenocarcinoma (Fox *et al.*, 1997). In humans, epidemiologic data strongly support the association between *H. pylori* and development of gastric adenocarcinoma. Similarly, we have recently documented a series of *H. mustelae*-infected ferrets with gastric mucosa-associated lymphoid tissue (MALT) lymphoma that parallels the same syndrome found in humans. Lymphoma was diagnosed in the wall of the lesser curvature of the pyloric antrum, corresponding to the predominant focus of *H. mustelae*-induced gastritis in ferrets. Gastric lymphomas demonstrated characteristic lymphoepithelial lesions, and the lymphoid cells were IgG positive in all ferrets (Erdman *et al.*, 1997). These findings and their parallels in *H. pylori*-infected humans implicate the involvement of *H. mustelae* in the pathogenesis of gastric cancer in ferrets.

Treatment Studies in ferrets indicate that triple therapy consisting of oral amoxicillin (30 mg/kg), metronidazole (20 mg/kg), and bismuth subsalicylate (17.5 mg/kg) (Pepto-Bismol original formula, Procter and Gamble) three times a day for 3–4 weeks has successfully eradicated *H. mustelae* (Otto *et al.*, 1990). Clinical improvement, including increased appetite and resolution of melena, may occur within 48 h of initiation of triple therapy. A new treatment regimen being used to eradicate *H. pylori* in humans has also been used successfully for eradication of *H. mustelae* from ferrets (Marini *et al.*, 1999). Ferrets received 24 mg/kg ranitidine bismuth and 12.5 mg/kg clarithromycin *per os* three times daily for 2 weeks. Culture of tissue collected by gastric endoscopic biopsy at 16, 32, and 43 weeks after termination of treatment indicated that long-term eradication was achieved in all six ferrets. Eradication was associated with decrease in anti-*H. mustelae* IgG antibody titers, results that are consistent with findings in humans after *H. pylori* eradication.

Omeprazole in ferrets at an oral dose of 0.7 mg/kg once daily effectively induces hypochlorhydria and may be used in conjunction with antibiotics to treat *H. mustelae*-associated duodenal or gastric ulcers. Cimetidine at 10 mg/kg TID *per os* can also be used to suppress acid secretion. Sucralfate given at 100 mg/animal three times a day also provides quick relief of clinical signs due to stomach ulcers. Acute bleeding ulcers must be treated as emergencies, and fluid and blood transfusions are essential.

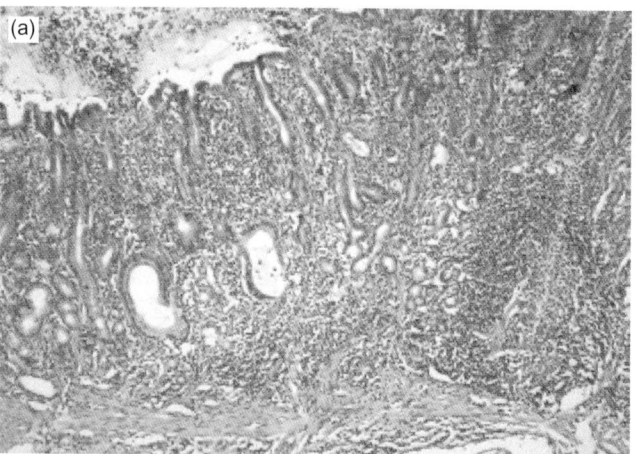

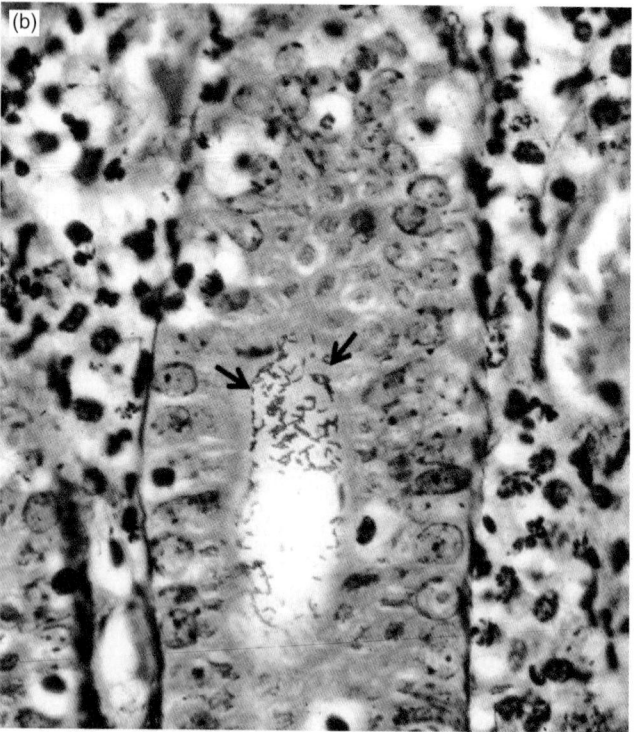

FIGURE 14.2   (a) Diffuse antral gastritis of the *Helicobacter mustelae*-infected ferret stomach; (b) *Helicobacter mustelae* organisms colonizing the gastric mucosa (arrowheads, Warthin–Starry stain). *Courtesy of J.G. Fox.*

d. Proliferative Bowel Disease

Etiology Proliferative bowel disease is caused by intracellular *Campylobacter*-like organisms, closely related to *Desulfovibrio* spp., that are now classified as *Lawsonia intracellularis* in proliferative enteropathy of swine (Fox, 1998a). The organisms are gram-negative, comma- to spiral-shaped bacteria.

Epizootiology and Transmission Proliferative bowel disease is a disease observed in young ferrets. Fecal–oral spread is suspected. The disease typically involves the large bowel, although it has been observed to affect the small bowel (Rosenthal, 1994). *Campylobacter* spp., coccidia, and chlamydia have been isolated from some cases of proliferative bowel disease in ferrets (Li *et al.*, 1996b). The role, if any, of co-pathogens in this disease is unclear.

Clinical Signs Clinical signs include chronic diarrhea, lethargy, anorexia, weight loss (which is often marked), and dehydration. Diarrhea may be blood-tinged, may contain mucus, and is often green in color. Rectal prolapse may be observed in affected animals. Ataxia and muscle tremors have also been observed (Fox *et al.*, 1982).

Diagnosis Diagnosis is based on clinical signs, a palpably thickened colon, and colonic biopsy. It is important to rule out other causes of diarrhea and weight loss through diagnostic tests that include but are not limited to a complete blood count, chemistry profile, radiographs, and fecal analysis and culture.

Necropsy Findings Gross findings include a segmented, thickened lower bowel, usually the terminal colon but occasionally including the ileum and rectum (Fox *et al.*, 1982; Fox, 1998a). Histologic examination consistently reveals marked mucosal proliferation and intracytoplasmic *L. intracellularis* demonstrated with silver stain within the apical portion of epithelial cells in the hyperplastic epithelial cells (Fox *et al.*, 1982; Fox, 1998a) (Fig. 14.3a, b). Other common histologic changes observed include the presence of a mixed inflammatory infiltrate that is variable in severity, reduced goblet cell production, hyperplasia of the glandular epithelium, glandular irregularity with penetration of the mucosal glands through the muscularis mucosa, and an increase in thickness of the tunica muscularis (Fox *et al.*, 1982; Fox, 1998a). Translocation of proliferating glandular tissue to extraintestinal sites, including regional lymph nodes and liver, has been described in two ferrets (Fox *et al.*, 1989b).

Differential Diagnosis Proliferative bowel disease should be differentiated from other diseases that may cause diarrhea and wasting, including dietary changes, eosinophilic gastroenteritis, gastric foreign bodies, lymphoma, Aleutian disease (AD), and gastric ulcers (Bell, 1997b). A complete physical exam that includes palpation of the abdomen should reveal a palpably thickened intestine in cases of proliferative bowel disease. It appears that true, confirmed Lawsonia cases are not frequently reported by pathologists and the incidence of clinical cases appears rare (J. Mayer, personal observation).

Treatment and Control Supportive care, including fluid therapy and nutritional support, should be provided. Treatment with chloramphenicol (50 mg/kg BID PO, SQ, IM) or metronidazole (20 mg/kg BID PO) for 2 weeks is reported to be effective (Krueger *et al.*, 1989; Bell, 1997b). Clinical improvement may be apparent within 48 h.

e. Tuberculosis

Etiology Tuberculosis can be caused by a variety of Mycobacteria, including *Mycobacterium bovis*, *M. avium*, and *M. tuberculosis*.

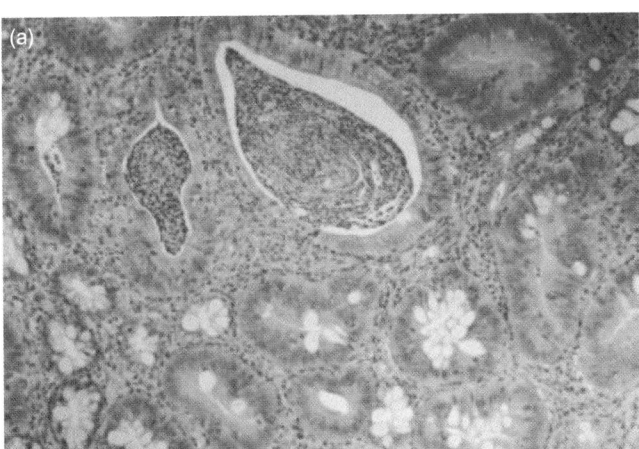 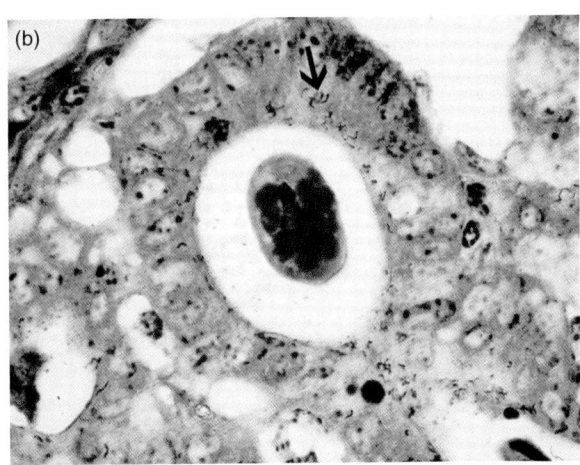

FIGURE 14.3 (a) Proliferative colitis of the ferret with marked epithelial hyperplasia, mixed inflammatory cell infiltrate, and reduction of goblet cells; (b) intracytoplasmic microorganisms in hyperplastic colonic tissue (arrow, Warthin–Starry stain). *Courtesy of J.G. Fox.*

Epizootiology and Transmission Mycobacteria are aerobic, gram-positive, non-branching, non-spore-forming, acid-fast rods. Ferrets might be more susceptible to mycobacterial infections than other species. Natural infections with *Mycobacterium bovis* and *M. avium* have been reported in the ferret (de Lisle *et al.*, 2008; Saunders and Thomsen, 2006). Ferrets are also susceptible to experimental infection with human tubercle bacillus. Most reports of tuberculosis in ferrets are in animals that were used for research in England and the rest of Europe between the years of 1929 to 1953 and were likely related to the feeding of raw poultry, raw meat, and unpasteurized milk to ferrets during this time (Fox, 1998a). In New Zealand the prevalence rate in the endemic area for *M. bovis* was 17.9% for feral ferrets (*n* = 548) (Ragg *et al.*, 1995a) The feeding of commercially prepared diets and widespread tuberculosis testing and elimination in livestock and poultry have resulted in the reduced incidence of the disease in ferrets. *Mycobacterium avium*-infected wild birds shed the organism in feces; prevention of contamination of food and outdoor housing areas of ferrets is warranted. Horizontal transmission of *M. bovis* infection was demonstrated in ferrets under experimental housing conditions. Several behavioral interactions were observed that could result in *M. bovis* transmission, including den sharing, playing, fighting, sniffing of orifices and faeces, cannibalism, and aggressive breeding behavior (Qureshi *et al.*, 2000).

Clinical Signs and Necropsy Findings Clinical signs and lesions are dependent on the infective strain. Ferrets experimentally infected with *M. bovis* invariably had microscopic foci of infection or tissue necrosis typical of tuberculosis, whereas ferrets experimentally infected with *M. avium* did so in only one of nine animals (Cross *et al.*, 2000). Based on these findings, the authors suggested that ferrets ingesting *M. avium*-infected tissue in the field are unlikely to develop mycobacterial disease, although they may harbor low numbers of viable *M. avium* organisms without stimulating the immune system.

Systemic infection with the bovine strain in ferrets results in disseminated disease with weight loss, anorexia, lethargy, death, and miliary lesions involving the lungs and other viscera (Fox, 1998a). In *M. bovis*-infected ferrets, only 2.9% of the pathologic changes were localized to the respiratory tract, whereas 34.5% of the mesenteric lymph nodes had tuberculous lesions, suggesting the importance of oral infection (Ragg *et al.*, 1995b).

Progressive paralysis has also been reported in a case of spontaneously occurring bovine tuberculosis in a ferret (Symmers and Thomson, 1953). A 3-year-old, neutered male, domestic ferret infected with *Mycobacterium celatum* was examined for a 5-month history of coughing, recent weight loss, reduced general condition, vomiting, and mild diarrhea. A chest radiograph showed multiple nodular densities in the lungs. At necropsy, the lungs

contained multifocal firm, light brown nodules, 6–10 mm in diameter). Spleen and lymph nodes (cervical, retropharyngeal, bronchial, gastric, mesenteric, popliteal) were enlarged. Histologic examination of lung, lymph nodes, spleen, liver, and brain showed granulomatous inflammation with predominantly macrophages, epithelioid cells (in the lung, including the bronchioles), and some multinucleated giant cells (Ludwig *et al.*, 2011).

Mycobacterium bovis lesions contain numerous acid-fast bacilli within macrophages with little cellular reaction (Fox, 1998a). In contrast, infection of ferrets with the human tubercle bacilli results in localized infection, often confined to the site of injection and adjacent lymph nodes; microscopically few organisms are observed. An impaired cell-mediated response may account for the large number of organisms observed in *M. bovis* lesions. It is interesting to note that nearly one-third of infected ferrets may have no gross lesions at necropsy (Lugton *et al.*, 1997). Primary infection of the lungs appears to be rare (Lugton *et al.*, 1997). These findings corroborate those of Ragg *et al.* (1995b).

Vomiting, diarrhea, anorexia, and weight loss were observed in a pet ferret with granulomatous enteritis caused by *M. avium* (Schultheiss and Dolginow, 1994). Granulomatous inflammation characterized by large numbers of epithelioid macrophages containing numerous acid-fast bacilli were present in the lamina propria and submucosa of the jejunum and pylorus. Other sites of granulomatous inflammation included peripancreatic adipose tissue, mesenteric lymph nodes, spleen, and liver. A source of infection was not identified in this report. Pulmonary infection with *M. avium* has also been reported in three ferrets in a zoo in France (Viallier *et al.*, 1983).

Diagnosis Definitive diagnosis of tuberculosis requires isolation and identification of the organism from suspect tissue specimens. Lesions are most frequently described in the retropharyngeal and mesenteric nodes (Ragg *et al.*, 1995b; Lugton *et al.*, 1997). Great care should be exercised in handling suspect clinical specimens, and an appropriately equipped laboratory should be identified for culture and identification of the organism.

Although there has been some experimental work in the area of the intradermal tuberculin skin-test response in ferrets and its apparent use in controlling tuberculosis in a breeding colony of ferrets, a tuberculin skin-testing regimen, including dose and type, has not been definitively characterized for clinical use in ferrets (Kauffman, 1981).

Treatment and Control Because of the zoonotic risk, ferrets infected with *M. bovis* and *M. tuberculosis* should be euthanized (Fox, 1998a). Recurrent *M. bovis* infection involving the palmar aspect of the wrist of a 63-year-old man, which developed after he was bitten by a ferret at the age of 12, was reported and demonstrates the zoonotic potential (Jones *et al.*, 1993). *Mycobacterium avium* infection is not reportable but may pose a risk to immunocompromised patients (Fox, 1998a). Personnel at risk should be followed up by a physician for appropriate diagnostic testing (Fox, 1998a). While treatment is usually not recommended, in cases where survival of the animal is desired, management with clarithromycin (8–10 mg/kg PO, BID for 3 months) has been reported (Lunn *et al.*, 2005) Therapy with rifampicin, clofazimine, and clarithromycin was reported in one publication to have potentially cured the infection in two affected animals (Lucas *et al.*, 2000).

Mycobacterium celatum, is a slowly growing, potentially pathogenic mycobacterium and a case of a disseminated *Mycobacterium celatum* (type 3) infection has been described in a domestic ferret (Valheim *et al.*, 2001). Dyspnea, dehydration, depression, emaciation, and poor coat quality were noted during clinical examination. Accurate diagnosis of these cases is difficult as *M. celatum* reacted positively with polyclonal antibodies against *M. paratuberculosis* and *M. bovis*. The isolated mycobacterium in this case was identified as *M. celatum* type 3 using 16S rRNA sequence analysis.

f. Salmonellosis

Etiology Salmonellosis is caused by infection with organisms of the genus *Salmonella*.

Epizootiology and Transmission Salmonella are gram-negative, non-spore-forming, facultative anaerobic rods in the family Enterobacteriaceae (Carter *et al.*, 1995). The genus *Salmonella* contains two species, *S. bongori* which infects mainly poikilotherms and rarely, humans, and *S. enterica* which includes approximately 2500 serovars, and is major cause of food-borne illness in humans. Salmonella are properly designated using their serovar (which was often a species name formerly), so, for example, *S. enterica* subsp. *enterica* serovar Typhimurium (aka *S.* Typhimurium) and serovar Enteritidis (*S.* Enteritidis). Infection is by the oral route. Transmission may be direct from infected carrier animals or humans or through contaminated food products or water (Carter *et al.*, 1995). Several *Salmonella* serovars have been isolated from mink with gastroenteritis and abortion (Gorham *et al.*, 1949). Contaminated raw meat products were suspected as the source in one outbreak. *S.* Typhimurium was isolated in ferrets in an outbreak of clinical disease (Coburn and Morris, 1949) and several serotypes including *S.* Hadar, *S.* Enteritidis, *S.* Kentucky, and *S.* Typhimurium were isolated from the feces of ferrets surveyed in a research colony (Fox *et al.*, 1988a).

Clinical Signs and Necropsy Findings Clinical signs of an outbreak of *S.* Typhimurium in ferrets included conjunctivitis, rapid weight loss, tarry stools, and febrile temperature fluctuations (Coburn and Morris, 1949). Gross findings in two ferrets 10 days after inoculation with *S.* Typhimurium of ferret origin included marked tissue pallor, petechiae in the gastric mucosa, and the presence of melena in one and a dark-colored fibrinous exudate in the large intestine of the other ferret (Coburn and Morris, 1949). Studies involving experimental inoculation with *S.* Enteritidis, *S.* Newport, and *S.* Choleraesuis via the oral route to healthy, distemper-infected, and feed-depleted ferrets and mink showed a fairly high resistance to infection (Gorham *et al.*, 1949). Only two animals of 29 in the diet-restricted group – 1 ferret and 1 mink – showed clinical signs of infection after feeding *S.* Newport culture. Signs included lethargy, anorexia, trembling, and fecal blood. The gastrointestinal tract showed a large amount of mucus containing red blood cells; bits of desquamated epithelium and few mononuclear cells overlying the gastric mucosa; an exudate in the small intestine consisting of mucoid material, red blood cells, and desquamated small intestinal villi; edematous villi in the ileum; and a diffuse infiltrate of the small intestinal mucosa with lymphocytes and macrophages. Necrotic foci in the liver, spleen, and, less commonly, the kidney, as well as splenomegaly and visceral lymphadenopathy, were observed in chronic fatal infections (Coburn and Morris, 1949). Abortion and gastroenteritis have been reported in mink (Gorham *et al.*, 1949). A recent outbreak of *Salmonella* Dublin infection was recorded in a large number of Danish mink farms (Dietz *et al.*, 2006). All of the affected farms suffered extensive disease problems; clinical and pathological observations included abortion, stillbirths, necrotizing endometritis, and increased mortality. The outbreaks took place mainly during April and May, around the time of whelping when the animals are very susceptible to *Salmonella* infections. The most common lesion at necropsy was a characteristic dark-red, very fragile uterus which correlated histologically with severe, necrotizing endometritis, often complicated with endometrial rupture and concurrent, diffuse, purulent peritonitis. The strain was identified as *S.* Dublin.

Diagnosis Diagnosis is based on history, clinical signs, and isolation of the organism. The organism can be cultured on enrichment and selective media and then characterized serologically. Samples of blood, feces, exudates, tissues, and intestinal material may be cultured.

Treatment and Control Coburn and Morris (1949) treated six of 12 ferrets experimentally infected with *S.* Typhimurium with sulfathalidine in the feed (Coburn and Morris, 1949). *Salmonella* Typhimurium was isolated in four of six control animals and none of the treated animals 3 days after the administration of the last dose. Sulfathalidine was administered by the same authors to a colony of 77 ferrets in which an outbreak of salmonellosis occurred. The group was surveyed 2 days after sulfathalidine treatment and showed weight gain, improvement in condition, and a reduction in the number of salmonella-infected ferrets (Coburn and Morris, 1949). *Salmonella* serovars isolated from ferrets may show resistance to a number of antibiotics (Fox, 1998a). Treatment includes appropriate use of antimicrobials and supportive care, which may include fluid therapy, nutritional support, maintenance of electrolyte balance, treatment of concurrent diseases, recognition of and attention to shock, and reduction of stress (Fox, 1998a).

g. Pneumonia

Etiology *Streptococcus zooepidemicus* and other group C and G streptococci, *Escherichia coli, Klebsiella pneumoniae, Pseudomonas aeruginosa*, and *Bordetella bronchiseptica* have been reported as primary and secondary bacterial pathogens in pneumonia in ferrets (Fox, 1998a).

Epizootiology and Transmission From a clinical point of view, primary pneumonia is not very common and if bacterial pneumonia is diagnosed, the clinician should continue to try to rule out another primary pathology. A good example is bacterial pneumonia which occurs secondary to megaesophagus in the ferret. An influenza virus–bacteria synergism has been the subject of several studies in ferrets (Fox, 1998a; McCullers *et al.*, 2010). Debilitated and immunosuppressed animals and animals with concurrent diseases such as influenza may be more susceptible to bacterial pneumonias (Fox, 1998a; Martínez *et al.*, 2012; Kendrick, 2000; Peltola *et al.*, 2006). One exception to this commonly seen secondary pneumonia is the description of an outbreak of severe respiratory disease associated with a novel *Mycoplasma* species in ferrets (Kiupel *et al.*, 2012). This report describes an outbreak of respiratory disease characterized by a dry, nonproductive cough which was observed in 6- to 8-week-old ferrets. While almost 95% of the ferrets were affected, almost none died.

Clinical Signs Clinical signs may include nasal discharge, dyspnea, lethargy, anorexia, increased lung sounds, cyanosis, and fever (Rosenthal, 1997). Fulminant pneumonia may progress to sepsis and death (Fox, 1998a).

Diagnosis Diagnosis is based on history, clinical findings, a complete blood count, culture and cytology of a tracheal wash or lung wash, and radiographs (Rosenthal, 1997).

Differential Diagnosis Diagnostic rule-outs include dilatative cardiomyopathy, heartworm disease, mycotic pneumonia, pneumocystis pneumonia in immunosuppressed animals, neoplasia, and influenza.

Treatment and Control Treatment should consist of appropriate antimicrobial therapy and supportive care, which may include the administration of oxygen, fluid therapy, and force feeding (Rosenthal, 1997). In the Mycoplasma outbreak, affected ferrets received broad-spectrum antimicrobial drugs, bronchodilators, expectorants, nonsteroidal anti-inflammatory drugs, and nebulization; all clinical signs except the dry cough temporarily decreased. However, numerous affected ferrets have been observed for a longer period of time and have had their cough persist for as long as 4 years (Kiupel *et al.*, 2012).

h. Abscesses

Etiology A variety of bacteria have been associated with abscesses and localized infection of the lung, liver, uterus, vulva, skin, mammary glands, and oral cavity. These include *Staphylococcus* spp., *Streptococcus* spp., *Corynebacterium* spp., *Pasteurella, Actinomyces*, hemolytic *Escherichia coli*, and *Aeromonas* spp. (Fox, 1998a).

Epizootiology and Transmission Abscesses in ferrets may result from wounds that are inflicted secondary to biting during fighting, playing, mating, or chewing sharp objects.

Clinical Signs Localized or subcutaneous abscesses present as swellings with or without draining tracts. The swelling may be fluctuant. In most cases, the abscess is walled off and does not result in systemic signs (Fox, 1998a). Abscesses or infection involving visceral organs may give rise to organ-specific and/or systemic signs. Dental abscesses can occur due to infected teeth. A thorough oral exam is always indicated to check for gingivitis or fractured canine teeth. The canine teeth often fracture due to the animal's inquisitive behavior, which is often manifested in repeated bar biting of the cages. Stranguria in males is often related to prostatic abscessation, which is most often secondary to hyperadrenocortism.

Diagnosis Cytologic and gram staining of an aspirate of a suspect subcutaneous swelling will aid in the definitive diagnosis. Culture and sensitivity of the aspirate should also be performed to identify the causative organism and guide appropriate antibiotic therapy.

Differential Diagnosis Differential diagnosis of a subcutaneous swelling in a ferret should include myiasis, granuloma, hematoma, and neoplasia. Clinicians should search for potential primary causes as mentioned with the dental abscessation or hyperadrenocortism.

Treatment and Control Prevention of ferrets from exposure to sharp objects in the cage and feed, and limiting the exposure of male and female during breeding, can minimize the occurrence of abscesses. Treatment of localized abscesses should include appropriate antibiotic therapy and establishment of drainage and debridement if necessary. Bacterial culture and sensitivity of the exudate should be performed. A broad-spectrum antimicrobial may be used pending results of culture and sensitivity (Orcutt, 1997).

i. Mastitis

Etiology Gram-positive cocci such as *Streptococcus* spp., *Staphylococcus aureus*, and coliforms such as hemolytic *E. coli* are the most frequently associated organisms (Bernard *et al.*, 1984; Bell, 1997a).

Epizootiology and Transmission Although the exact pathogenesis of mastitis in ferrets is not clear, a number of factors may play a role and include the stress of lactation, injury to mammary glands by the kits' teeth, environmental contamination, and the virulence of the organism. In one report, the causative organism, hemolytic *E. coli*, was cultured from the feces of mastitic and healthy ferrets and the oral cavity of suckling kits (Liberson *et al.*, 1983). The high level of perineal contamination and the presence of the organism in the oral cavity of suckling kits may enhance transmission and introduction of this organism into mammary tissue. In another outbreak, the causative organisms were cultured from bovine meat fed prior to the outbreak, and the meat was suspected as a possible source.

Clinical Signs Mastitis occurs in nursing jills and has been characterized as acute or chronic (Bell, 1997a). The acute form is reported to occur soon after parturition or after the third week of lactation. Examination of affected jills reveals swollen, firm, red or purple, and painful glands. Affected glands may quickly become gangrenous. The chronic form, which may occur when kits are 3 weeks old or as a sequela to the acute form, is characterized by glands that are firm but not painful or discolored.

Diagnosis Diagnosis is based on history, clinical signs, physical examination findings, and isolation of the causative organism. Clinical isolates of *E .coli* from a number of conditions including mastitis have been shown to be positive for cytotoxic necrotizing factor 1 (cnf1). Isolates containing cnf1 tend to produce extraintestinal disease and are referred to as necrotoxigenic *E. coli* (NTEC) (Marini *et al.*, 2004).

Necropsy Findings In acute mastitis, grossly affected glands are swollen, and the skin overlying the gland may be discolored. Surgical biopsies and necropsies of eight ferrets with mastitis caused by hemolytic *E. coli* (Liberson *et al.*, 1983) revealed extensive edema, hemorrhage, and coagulative and liquefactive necrosis involving the glandular tissue as well as surrounding subcutaneous tissue. Other findings included the presence of a mixed leukocytic infiltrate composed primarily of polymorphonuclear leukocytes; large numbers of bacteria; and thrombosis and necrosis of vessels within and immediately adjacent to areas of inflammation (Liberson *et al.*, 1983).

In an outbreak of mastitis in mink due to *Staphylococcus aureus* and *Escherichia coli*, histologic examination of affected glands revealed an acute suppurative mastitis with desquamation of alveolar epithelium, edema of the connective tissue stroma, alveoli filled with neutrophils and cellular debris, and lactiferous ducts filled with purulent exudate and mats of bacteria within lobules (Trautwein and Helmboldt, 1966).

Treatment Broad-spectrum antibiotic therapy may be instituted pending culture and sensitivity results of the milk. Enrofloxacin (10mg/kg BID PO) is often effective. Jills may require aggressive care, because acute mastitis may progress rapidly and animals may become septicemic and moribund (Liberson *et al.*, 1983). Oral antibiotic administration to kits nursing on affected jills is recommended (Bell, 1997a). Supplementation of kits with milk replacer may also be necessary, because jills with acute mastitis are reluctant to nurse, and jills with the chronic form have diminished lactation as milk-producing tissue is replaced by scar tissue (Bell, 1997a). Surgical resection and debridement of affected glands and supportive care may be necessary for jills with acute mastitis. In the laboratory setting, in which foster mothers are often available, it is far more common to remove and foster the kits, after which jills are treated medically. When cross-fostering kits is required, kits may spread infection to healthy jills. Maintaining thorough personal hygiene practices when handling affected jills is important in minimizing spread to other lactating jills. Jills with the chronic form of mastitis should be culled (Bell, 1997a).

2. Viral Infections

a. Canine Distemper

Etiology Canine distemper (CD) is caused by a paramyxovirus of genus *Morbillivirus* that is related to measles and rinderpest (Budd, 1981). There are several strains, including a ferret-adapted strain of canine distemper virus (CDV), that differ in incubation, clinical signs, and duration (Fox *et al.*, 1998b). The virus can be inactivated by heat, light, and various chemicals, including phenol, Roccal, sodium hydroxide, and formalin (Shen and Gorham, 1980; Budd, 1981). Infectious virions have been recovered from fomites after 20min at room temperature. CD is the most serious viral infection of ferrets. Mortality approaches 100%, making appropriate husbandry and vaccination imperative (Perpiñán *et al.*, 2008).

The disease has a catarrhal phase and a neurological, or central nervous system (CNS), phase. The catarrhal phase is 7–10 days postinfection and is characterized by anorexia, pyrexia, photosensitivity, and serous nasal discharge. An erythematous pruritic rash spreads from the chin to the inguinal region. It is suspected that the rash results from cell-mediated immunity to infected endothelial cells, similar to the response seen in humans with measles (Norrby and Oxman, 1990). Hyperkeratosis of footpads, called hard pad, is an inconsistent feature. Secondary bacterial infections result in mucopurulent ocular and nasal discharge and possibly bacterial pneumonia. The CNS phase, with ataxia, tremors, and paralysis, may or may not be preceded by the catarrhal phase. Death occurs in 12–16 days from ferret strains of CDV and up to 35 days with canine strains. Infection is uniformly fatal.

Epizootiology and Transmission Virus is shed from infected hosts from conjunctival, nasal, and oral exudates, urine, feces, and sloughed skin (Gorham and Brandly, 1953). Transplacental infection is not reported in ferrets. It is important to remember that ferrets are very susceptible to distemper when infected by the respiratory route (Ludlow *et al.*, 2012). Attenuated CDV vaccine strains have not been recovered from the body secretions of ferrets following vaccination (Shen *et al.*, 1981). Unvaccinated dogs and other canids, mustelids, and procyonids may serve as reservoirs of infection.

Viremia is detectable 2 days postinfection and persists until the ferret dies or mounts a neutralizing antibody response (Liu and Coffin, 1957). The primary site of replication is the respiratory and lymphatic systems, and CDV has been recovered from the nasal secretions of ferrets 5–13 days postinfection. A decrease in lymphocyte subsets is detectable 5–30 days postinfection. While the spread of the virus beyond the blood–brain barrier is still under investigation, it was recently shown that hematogenous infection of the choroid plexus is not a significant route of virus spread into the CSF (Ludlow *et al.*, 2012). Instead, viral spread into the subarachnoid space in infected animals was triggered by infection of vascular endothelial cells and the hematogenous spread of virus-infected leukocytes from meningeal blood vessels into the subarachnoid space. This resulted in widespread infection of cells of the pia and arachnoid mater of the leptomeninges over large areas of the cerebral hemispheres (Ludlow *et al.*, 2012).

Clinical Signs and Necropsy Findings Histologically, intracytoplasmic and intranuclear inclusion bodies may be observed in tracheal, bronchial, epithelia, and bile duct as well as transitional epithelium in the bladder (Liu and Coffin, 1957) (Fig. 14.4). The eosinophilic (hematoxylin–eosin) inclusions appear orange using Pollack's trichrome stain.

Diagnosis and Differential Diagnoses Presumptive diagnosis is based on clinical observation, questionable vaccination history, and exposure. A fluorescent antibody test can be used on peripheral blood and conjunctival mononuclear cells to detect infection. Reverse transcriptase–polymerase chain reaction (RT-PCR) has also been used to detect experimental infection (Stephensen *et al.*, 1997). Differential diagnoses should include infection with influenza virus or *Bordetella bronchiseptica*. Influenza does not rapidly progress to mucopurulent ocular and nasal discharge as CD does. Cytologic examination of a conjunctival scraping is a useful and quick clinical test. If inclusions are detected in the epithelial cells, influenza should be ruled out as influenza is more likely.

Treatment and Control During an outbreak, clinically affected ferrets should be isolated and the remainder

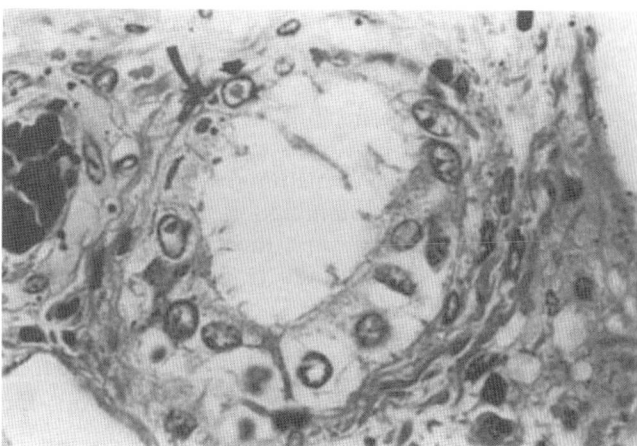

FIGURE 14.4 Intracytoplasmic (curved arrow) and intranuclear (arrowhead) inclusion bodies of canine distemper virus in the bile duct epithelium of a ferret.

of the colony vaccinated. Humane euthanasia of affected animals is recommended due to the absence of any literature reports of an animal surviving active infection. Distemper infection can be prevented by vaccination with modified live vaccine (MLV) of chicken embryo tissue culture origin (CETCO) administered subcutaneously or intramuscularly. Kits should be vaccinated every 2–3 weeks, starting at age 6 weeks, until 14 weeks and annually thereafter (Fox *et al.*, 1998b). It is important to adhere to the prescribed vaccination protocol, because ferret deaths have been reported following double-dose vaccination (Carpenter *et al.*, 1976). Vaccine reactions manifest as vomiting, diarrhea, fever, and collapse. A report evaluating a large number of such reactions found an event rate of 1% for distemper administered as a sole vaccine. This incidence was associated with the cumulative number of distemper vaccines received (Moore *et al.*, 2005). Diphendramine (0.5–2 mg/kg IV, IM) or epinephrine (20 μg/kg SQ, IV, IM, intratracheally) with standard supportive care should be initiated. Inactivated distemper vaccines do not elicit consistent, effective immunity and are not recommended. It is important to know the vaccination schedule of your ferret supplier and to vaccinate supplementally as appropriate. New ferrets should be held in quarantine for 2 weeks prior to introduction into the resident colony.

CD is used experimentally to study morbillivirus infection and vaccine strategies in humans (von Messling *et al.*, 2003).

Ferrets have been experimentally infected with feline panleukopenia, canine parvovirus, canine parainfluenza virus, mink enteritis virus, respiratory syncytial virus, transmissible mink encephalopathy, and pseudorabies, but natural infection with these viruses has not been reported (Fox *et al.*, 1998b).

b. Aleutian Disease

Etiology Aleutian mink disease virus (ADV) is a parvovirus (genus *Amdoparvovirus*, species *Carnivore amdoparvovirus 1*) with strains of varying virulence and immunogenicity. Mink-derived strains are more virulent to mink than are ferret-derived strains (Fox *et al.*, 1998b). Although the mink virus can infect ferrets, at least three separate viral strains that are distinct from the mink ADV have been documented in ferrets. The most common strain is called ADV-F (Morrisey and Kraus, 2011).

Epizootiology and Transmission AD is a chronic progressive illness that was first described in mink (Oxenham, 1990). It was originally named hypergammaglobulinemia (HGG) because of this remarkable finding. Infection may be subclinical for years. Because the immunomodulation associated with ADV infection is disruptive to biomedical research, it is important to seek sources of ADV-free ferrets (Fox *et al.*, 1998b).

Transmission between ferrets may be direct or via aerosol of urine, saliva, blood, feces, and fomites (Kenyon *et al.*, 1963; Gorham *et al.*, 1964; Pennick *et al.*, 2005). Vertical transmission is established in mink but is unproven in ferrets.

Clinical Signs Ferrets infected with ADV as adults develop persistent infection but rarely disease, although chronic progressive weight loss, cachexia, malaise, and melena have been described (Porter *et al.*, 1982). AD may also cause ataxia, paralysis, tremors, and convulsions (Oxenham, 1990; Welchman *et al.*, 1993). The lesions are typically immune-mediated, and there is elevation of the gammaglobulins to generally greater than 20% of the total proteins (Porter *et al.*, 1982; Fig. 14.5). The precise mechanism of immunomodulation is unknown, but in mink there is depression of B- and T-cell responses.

Diagnosis and Differential Diagnoses Presumptive diagnosis is based on HGG and chronic weight loss. Diagnosis is confirmed by immunofluorescent antibody (IFA) or counter-immunoelectrophoresis (CIEP) for antibody to ADV antigen (Palley *et al.*, 1992). ELISA and PCR-based assays have also been used and are now readily available from several commercial laboratories (Erdman *et al.*, 1996b; Saifuddin and Fox, 1996; Erdman *et al.*, 1997, Morrisey and Kraus, 2011). However, it is important to remember that the presence of ADV antibody in a ferret is not necessarily diagnostic of the disease in an animal. In serologic surveys of ferret populations, up to 10% of ferrets surveyed were antibody positive without clinical signs of disease (Welchman *et al.*, 1993).

Differential diagnoses include the neurotropic form of CD, as well as chronic wasting diseases such as neoplasia, malabsorption, maldigestion, and bacterial enteritis (Fox *et al.*, 1998b).

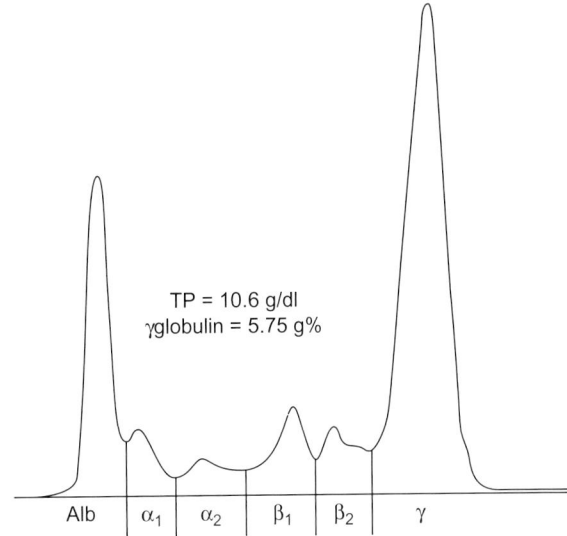

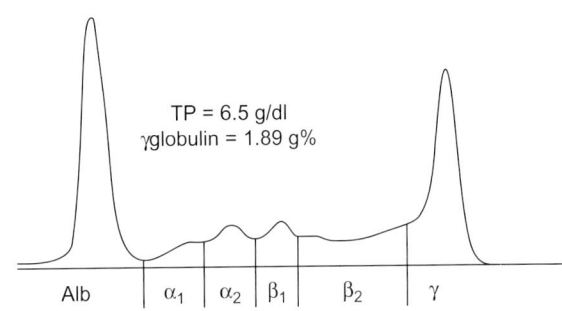

FIGURE 14.5 Serum protein electrophoretograms of two ferrets with Aleutian mink disease-associated syndromes. Note that gammaglobulin concentrations exceed 20% of the total serum protein. *Reprinted from Palley et al. (1992).*

Treatment and Control Vaccination against ADV would be contraindicated because of the immune-mediated reaction, and a vaccine is not available.

Chemical disinfection may be achieved with formalin, sodium hydroxide, and phenolics (Shen *et al.*, 1981). There is no general treatment for AD, and infected ferrets should be culled from the colony. However, treatment of infected mink kits with gamma globulin-containing ADV antibody has decreased mortality rates (Aasted *et al.*, 1988).

Necropsy Ferrets may have no lesions upon necropsy, or infrequently they may have hepatosplenomegaly and lymphadenopathy. The most consistent histological finding is periportal lymphocytic infiltrates (Fig. 14.6). Bile duct hyperplasia and periportal fibrosis have also been reported. Membranous glomerulonephritis has been described (Ohshima *et al.*, 1978). Although lesions are subtle, use of ADV-infected ferrets in biomedical research is contraindicated because histological lesions interfere with the interpretation of study results (Fox *et al.*, 1998b). The DNA of ADV can be detected by *in situ* hybridization, confirming infection

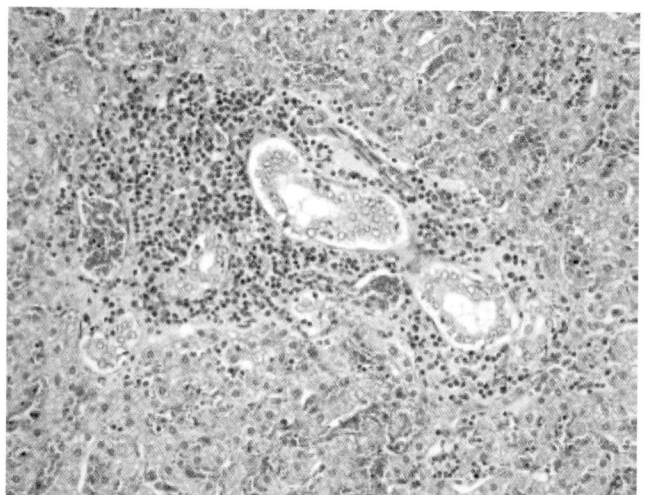

FIGURE 14.6   Lymphocytic infiltrate of portal triad associated with Aleutian mink disease virus.

and identifying infected cells. This technique can also be used on formalin-fixed, paraffin-embedded biopsy samples (Haas *et al.*, 1988).

c. Influenza

Etiology   Influenza is caused by an orthomyxovirus that is transmissible from humans to ferrets and ferrets to humans (Smith and Stuart-Harris, 1936). Human influenza viruses A and B are pathogenic to ferrets (Fox *et al.*, 1998b). However, the pathogenicity of type B influenza virus in ferrets appears to be low (Barron and Rosenthal, 2011).

Ferrets are also susceptible to avian, phocine, equine, and swine influenza, although only porcine influenza causes clinical signs. Because the viruses can be readily transmitted from humans to ferrets, precautions such as requiring handlers to have been vaccinated against currently circulating strains, avoiding contact with ferrets when there are any signs of respiratory/influenza illness in the handler or family members, and use of PPE such as masks and gloves should be in place to minimize transmission. Use of microisolator style caging and biosafety cabinets/ventilated cage change stations may also be useful to prevent cross contamination when conducting influenza research work in ferrets.

Epizootiology, Transmission, and Clinical Signs   Influenza virus generally remains localized in nasal epithelium in ferrets but may cause pneumonia. Clinical signs appear 48 h postinfection and include anorexia, fever, sneezing, and serous nasal discharge. Conjunctivitis, photosensitivity, and otitis are also sometimes seen (Fox *et al.*, 1998b). Secondary bacterial infection by *Streptococcus* spp. and occasionally *Bordetella bronchiseptica* may prolong recovery. Transmission occurs via aerosol and direct contact.

Diagnosis   Diagnosis is based on typical clinical presentation and recovery within 4 days, unlike with CDV, which progresses to more severe disease and death. Hemagglutination inhibition antibody titers on acute and convalescent sera are rarely needed.

Treatment and Control   Antibiotic therapy may be instituted to preclude secondary bacterial infection. Amantadine (6 mg/kg PO q12h) has been experimentally effective in treating ferrets with influenza (Barron and Rosenthal, 2011). Other antiviral medications include neuraminidase inhibitors like zanamivir (12.5 mg/kg as a one-time intranasal dose) and oseltamivir (5 mg/kg PO q12 h × 10 days). These have been shown to prevent and treat influenza infection and either agent may be used to greater effect in combination with amantadine (Barron and Rosenthal, 2011). Animal technicians and investigators suffering from influenza should avoid contact with ferrets.

Ferrets have been used extensively as a model for influenza research because the biological response to infection is similar to that in humans (Fox *et al.*, 1998b; O'Donnell and Subbarao, 2011). Ferrets have been used in influenza A research to study pathogenesis, to investigate Reye's syndrome, and to evaluate vaccine trials (Desmukh, 1987; Sweet *et al.*, 1987; Belser *et al.*, 2011).

d. Rabies

Etiology   Rabies is caused by a rhabdovirus in the genus *Lyssavirus*. Rabies infection is infrequently reported in ferrets, and until recently, research on rabies in ferrets was lacking (Fox *et al.*, 1998b). Ferrets in a well-managed facility would have low risk of exposure to rabies virus. In experimentally induced rabies in ferrets, the mean incubation period was between 28 and 33 days; the mean morbidity was 4–5 days (Niezgoda *et al.*, 1998).

Treatment and Control   A USDA-approved, killed rabies vaccine given subcutaneously at ages 3 months and 1 year and annually thereafter is recommended to protect ferrets against rabies (Rupprecht *et al.*, 1990). MLV is not recommended, because there is at least one case of rabies in a ferret that was vaccinated with MLV rabies vaccine (Fox *et al.*, 1998b). There is no treatment for rabies.

Clinical Signs and Pathogenesis   Clinical signs of rabies infection in ferrets may include anxiety, lethargy, and posterior paresis. In one experimental infection, 11 of 40 ferrets died, and Negri bodies were seen in the brain of only two of the 11 (Blancou *et al.*, 1982). There is conflicting data on the isolation of rabies virus from the salivary glands following experimental infection. In one study using the raccoon variant of rabies for infection, more than half of the ferrets had rabies isolated from the salivary glands (Fox *et al.*, 1998b). In a more recent study the virus was detected in the salivary glands of 63% and in saliva of 47% of the rabid ferrets (Niezgoda et al., 1998).

Ferrets at risk for exposure to rabies virus that bite or scratch a human should be placed under quarantine for not less than 10 days of observation. Veterinarians and facility managers should seek assistance from state public health officials. A recent case report documented the recovery and clearance of rabies virus in a domestic ferret (Hamir et al., 2011). The ferret remained healthy for 80 days after inoculation of rabies virus at a dose of $10^{2.5}$ MICLD$_{50}$ as a single 100-μl injection in the right gastrocnemius muscle. On day 81 after inoculation, the ferret presented with hindlimb paresis and paralysis that progressed to paralysis of the hindquarters within 24 h. The ferret survived for 100 days after onset of clinical signs, with continued paraplegia.

Diagnosis and Differential Diagnoses Differential diagnosis includes the neurotropic form of CD. Diagnosis is based on direct IFA of brain tissue. Because rabies in ferrets is poorly understood, the head from ferrets that exhibit signs compatible with rabies and that have exposure histories that raise concerns about rabies should be shipped to the state public health authority for confirmation.

e. Rotavirus

Etiology Rotaviruses cause diarrhea in young of many species, including humans, calves, pigs, sheep, and rats. Diarrhea in ferret kits is thought to be caused by a poorly characterized, atypical rotavirus that has not been cultivated *in vitro* (Torres-Medina, 1987). Atypical rotaviruses lack the rotavirus common antigen. Definitive identification of a group C rotavirus in ferrets has recently been published (Wise et al., 2009).

Epizootiology, Transmission, and Clinical Signs Clinical disease may occur in kits as young as 1–4 days old or in older animals up to 6 weeks of age. Diarrhea soils the perineum and possibly the fur and nest material. Mortality rates are age-dependent, with high mortality occurring in young kits and lower mortality occurring in kits over 10 days of age (Bell, 1997a; Fox et al., 1998b). Secondary bacterial infection may influence the severity of diarrhea.

Necropsy and Pathogenesis Lesions are restricted to the gastrointestinal tract. Yellow–green liquid or mucous feces may be seen in the terminal colon on necropsy. Subtle small-intestinal villous atrophy and epithelial cell vacuolation are detectable histologically.

Diagnosis and Differential Diagnoses Clinical diagnosis can be confirmed by using clarified and ultra-centrifuged fecal pellets for electron microscopy. The ferret rotavirus does not cross-react with commercially available enzyme immunoassays (Torres-Medina, 1987).

Treatment and Control It is desirable to avoid sources that are known to be infected with ferret rotavirus. Affected kits may be supplemented with kitten milk replacer, using a medicine dropper. Mortality is reduced if the kits continue nursing. Treatment of secondary bacterial infections may reduce severity of the diarrhea, and supportive care, including subcutaneous fluid administration for young kits, may be required (Fox et al., 1998b). Jills develop immunity to rotavirus infection, and subsequent litters are protected.

f. Coronavirus Diseases: Epizootic Catarrhal Enteritis

Etiology A transmissible diarrhea, first referred to as 'green slime disease' and eventually, epizootic catarrhal enteritis (ECE) emerged in early 1993 (Fox et al., 1998b; Murray et al., 2010). Williams et al., (2000) first implicated a coronavirus as the cause of this disease.and the novel *Alphacoronavirus*, ferret enteric coronavirus (FRECV), was subsequently identified in ferrets with ECE (Wise et al., 2006).

Epizootiology and Transmission This highly infectious disease commonly occurs in the setting of a young animal being introduced into a colony of adults, though a susceptible animal of any age can be infected and experience disease. Virions are shed into feces and saliva, rapidly infecting other ferrets by the oral route. Intermittent shedding can occur long after clinical signs have resolved. ECE is a disease of high morbidity and low mortality and is now considered enzootic (Murray et al., 2010).

Clinical Signs Ferrets present with decreased appetite, weight loss, lethargy, diarrhea and vomiting. Diarrhea is green and mucoid, and ferrets can become rapidly dehydrated. With chronicity, malabsorption can occur and feces may be characterized by small, ovoid stools resembling bird seed. Some ferrets develop elevated liver enzymes and non-specific hematologic abnormalities (Murray et al., 2010). Younger ferrets may have milder disease than older animals.

Diagnosis Characteristic history and clinical signs are typically used for diagnosis, but these are not exclusive to ECE. Definitive diagnosis requires intestinal biopsy and histopathology with demonstration of viral antigen or nucleic acid by immunohistochemistry or *in situ* hybridization. RT-PCR and electron microscopy can be used on ferret feces. A serologic test exists but should be evaluated in the context of clinical signs (Murray et al., 2010).

Necropsy Findings and Histopathology Gross necropsy findings include enteritis with watery intestinal contents and enlarged mesenteric lymph nodes. The histologic hallmark is lymphocytic enteritis with villous atrophy and necrosis and vacuolization of enterocytes on the tips. Villous blunting and fusion occur with chronicity. Lesions are predominantly found in the jejeunum and ileum.

Treatment and Control Treatment involves aggressive oral and systemic fluid therapy. Antibiotics may be used for prophylaxis or treatment of secondary bacterial infection. Drugs which have anti-inflammatory as well as antibacterial properties such as metronidazole (20 mg/kg PO bid) have been recommended. Control depends on avoidance of ferrets showing clinical signs and adequate sanitation of ferret housing areas. Most available detergents and disinfectants will kill environmental coronavirus.

g. Coronavirus Diseases: Ferret Systemic Coronaviral Disease

Etiology A systemic granulomatous disease has recently emerged in ferrets and is due to a coronavirus, ferret systemic coronavirus (FRSCV), also of the genus *Alphacoronavirus*, which behaves in a manner analogous to feline infectious peritonitis (FIP) in cats (Perpiñán and López, 2008; Garner *et al.*, 2008). In cats, virulent mutants of feline enteric coronavirus can cause FIP in one of two classic forms, the 'wet' form characterized by effusion, or the 'dry' granulomatous form. The ferret disease, ferret systemic coronaviral disease (FSCD), has associated signs and lesions typical of the dry form of FIP. These similarities have led to speculation that FRSCV and FIP have a common pathogenesis. While FRSCV is more closely related to FRECV than it is to other coronaviruses, experimental confirmation has not yet been achieved (Wise *et al.*, 2006, 2010).

Epizootiology and Transmission FSCD first appeared in Spain in 2004 but has now been diagnosed in the United States (Martinez *et al.*, 2006). It typically affects animals under 1 year of age. The mechanism of transmission is unkown but is most likely ingestion.

Clinical Signs Signs are non-specific and dependent on the organ system(s) affected. Lethargy, decreased appetite, diarrhea, vomiting, and weight loss are commonly seen. Some animals will present with neurologic lesions such as ataxia, paresis, tremor, head tilt, and seizure.

Diagnosis Histologic evaluation of tissues submitted for biopsy and demonstration of intralesional coronaviral nucleic acid provides the definitive diagnosis. Immunohistochemistry using a monoclonal antibody (FIPV3-70) will localize viral nucleic acid (Garner *et al.*, 2008) and an RT-PCR assay has been used to identify virus in tissues and is capable of differentiating FRSCV from FRECV (Garner *et al.*, 2008; Murray *et al.*, 2010). Clinical signs and characteristic hematology are strongly suggestive. Typical hematology findings include nonregenerative anemia, hyperglobulinemia, hypoalbuminemia, and thrombocytopenia. A polyclonal gammopathy exists and requires clinicans to rule out AD and other conditions in which hypergammablobulinemia can occur. Serum chemistry values will reflect specific organ involvement. Radiography and endoscopy can be useful in characterizing palpated masses (Garner *et al.*, 2008; Perpiñán and López, 2008; Murray *et al.*, 2010).

Necropsy and Pathogenesis The predominant necropsy findings are enlarged mesenteric lymph nodes and multiple, coalescing, tan nodules of various sizes that course along serosal surfaces and mesenteric vessels. These nodules can encompass the intestines and project onto the surface of and into the parenchyma of various organs. Lesions are most commonly seen in liver, kidney, spleen, and lung. The characteristic histopathologic finding is severe pyogranulomatous inflammation, often surrounding vessels, that infiltrates, destroys, and replaces affected parenchyma. All parenchymatous organs can be affected, with subsequent organ-specific clinical manifestations. In the brain, the lesions are pyogranulomatous meningoecephalomyelitis, with a distribution centered on blood vessels, and parenchymal involvement which is most severe periventricularly (Garner *et al.*, 2008).

Treatment Supportive care including nutritional supplements, vitamins, iron in anemic animals, gastroprotectants, and immunostimulatory antibiotics like doxycycline can be instituted. Treatment regimens used in cats with the granulomatous form of FIP, including steroids and other immunomodulatory agents, have not as yet been critically evaluated in ferrets. Most animals die or are euthanized within weeks of diagnosis (Murray *et al.*, 2010; Perpiñán and López, 2008)

h. Other Viruses

Bovine herpesvirus 1 (Infectious bovine rhinotracheitis; IBR) was isolated from the liver, spleen, and lung of clinically normal ferrets (Porter *et al.*, 1975). Raw beef was suspected as the source of infection, reinforcing the need to exclude raw meat products from the diet of ferrets used for research. In experimental inoculation studies, IBR either caused no significant respiratory pathology (Porter *et al.*, 1975) or caused acute suppurative pharyngitis (Smith, 1978).

Hepatitis E virus was detected by nested PCR from four of 43 (9.3%) fecal samples of ferrets from four different locations in the Netherlands. These ferrets showed no overt sign of disease and had been sampled for the purpose of attempting to define potential reservoirs of the virus. The ferret virus grouped with rat virus isolates. The relevance of these findings to ferret health or zoonotic risk is unknown (Raj *et al.*, 2012).

Suid herpesvirus 1 (pseudorabies virus [PRV], Aujeszky's disease) has been listed as an infectious agent in the ferret (USDA Aphis, 2013; Williams and Barker, 2001). The consumption of raw pig meat by ferrets should therefore be avoided. The outcome in most species infected with the virus is usually fatal.

3. Parasitic Infections

a. Protozoa

i. ENTERIC COCCIDIOSIS

Etiology Three species of the genera *Isospora* and *Eimeria* have been reported to infect the ferret: *Isospora laidlawi*, *Eimeria furonis*, and *E. ictidea* (Blankenship-Paris et al., 1993).

Epizootiology and Transmission Infection occurs from ingestion of sporulated oocysts.

Clinical Signs Coccidiosis in ferrets is usually subclinical but has been reported to be associated with diarrhea, lethargy, and dehydration in one ferret (Blankenship-Paris *et al.*, 1993). Clinical signs are often seen in young, newly acquired ferrets and are more common after a stressful event (Rosenthal, 1994). Rectal prolapse can also develop in association with coccidial infection (Rosenthal, 1994). Severe clinical signs were reported in a recent outbreak in which morbidity rate was high, including an appreciable number of deaths, and ferrets of all ages were affected (Sledge *et al.*, 2011). One case of biliary infestation with *Eimeria furonis* has been reported in the scientific literature (Williams *et al.*, 1996).

Diagnosis Diagnosis is generally made by any of the fecal flotation methods commonly used in veterinary practice or by direct wet mount of feces and microscopic examination for sporulated or unsporulated oocysts. Because coccidial oocysts are small, slides should be examined under higher magnification. The case in which the biliary tract was involved had significant change in multiple analytes of the serum chemistry profile.

Necropsy Findings Diagnosis is usually made *ante mortem*. Pathologic lesions associated with enteric coccidiosis in a laboratory-reared ferret that was euthanized were described in one published report (Blankenship-Paris *et al.*, 1993). Microscopic lesions were confined to the jejunum and ileum and consisted of villous and epithelial thickening. Parasitic cysts and microorganisms within epithelium, and a mild granulomatous inflammation in the villar lamina propria, were also observed. A recent report documents clinical and anatomic pathology associated with biliary coccidiosis in a weanling ferret (Williams *et al.*, 1996).

Differential Diagnosis Diarrhea may be observed in ferrets that present with gastroenteritis secondary to gastrointestinal foreign bodies and dietary indiscretion, as well as other nutritional, inflammatory, infectious, or other systemic diseases. Infectious causes such as proliferative colitis, salmonellosis, giardiasis, rotavirus, and campylobacteriosis should be considered. Diarrhea may also be seen in eosinophilic gastroenteritis, an uncommonly reported condition in ferrets. At necropsy of the biliary case, the liver was grossly enlarged and pale with enlarged, firm bile ducts, and the gallbladder wall was notably thickened (Williams *et al.*, 1996).

Treatment and Control Good husbandry practices that include sanitation and frequent disposal of feces reduce the number of oocysts in the environment. Cleaning cages with a strong ammonium hydroxide solution is reported to be effective (Kirkpatrick and Dubey, 1987). Heat treatment of surfaces and utensils may also be effective (Kirkpatrick and Dubey, 1987). Treatment of ferrets with sulfadimethoxine at 50 mg/kg orally once and then 25 mg/kg orally every 24 h for 9 days is recommended (Rosenthal, 1994). As in dogs and cats, the complete elimination of a coccidial infection requires an immunocompetent host. Ponazuril (Marquis™) is a triazine coccidiocidal drug that is related to toltrazuril. This newer drug has been used in a variety of small mammals at a dose of 10–50 mg/kg once daily for 10 days (Mitchell, 2008). The coccidiocidal classification of the drug will help to eliminate an infestation with coccidia faster then treatments with coccidiostatic drugs.

ii. CRYPTOSPORIDIOSIS

Etiology Cryptosporidiosis is caused by infection with *Cryptosporidium* spp.

Epizootiology and Transmission *Cryptosporidium* is a protozoan in the class Sporozoa, subclass Coccidia, which inhabits the respiratory and intestinal epithelium of birds, reptiles, mammals, and fish (Regh *et al.*, 1988). It is known to cause gastrointestinal tract disease in many species, including rodents, dogs, cats, calves, and people (Hill and Lappin, 1995). It has a life cycle similar to other coccidian parasites and is transmitted by ingestion of sporulated oocysts. Autoinfection is also a characteristic of the life cycle.

Transmission may occur through consumption of contaminated food or water. Cattle, dogs, and cats, shedding oocysts, are reported to be potential sources of human infection (Hill and Lappin, 1995; Fox, 1998g). Immunosuppressed people are at greatest risk of developing severe fulminating gastrointestinal disease (Hill and Lappin, 1995). The finding of cryptosporidiosis in two ferrets that died from unrelated causes in one animal facility resulted in a survey of the existing ferret population and new arrivals into the facility to determine the prevalence and incidence of infection (Regh *et al.*, 1988). Findings indicated that 40% of the resident population and 38–100% of new arrivals had oocysts in their feces but showed no clinical signs.

Clinical Signs Subclinical infection has been reported in both immunocompetent and immunosuppressed ferrets (Regh *et al.*, 1988). Another publication reports vague and non-specific clinical signs in adult animals, which ended in death 48–72 h after the onset of clinical signs (Gómez-Villamandos *et al.*, 1995).

Diagnosis Diagnosis is based on the identification of the organism in feces. The oocysts are small when compared with other coccidia and may be overlooked or mistaken for yeasts (Kirkpatrick and Dubey, 1987). Yeasts are oval, whereas cryptosporidium oocysts are spherical or ellipsoidal. Additionally, yeasts will stain with iodine and are not acid-fast, whereas Cryptosporidium has the opposite staining characteristics. The oocyst residuum is seen as a refractive dot under phase-contrast microscopy, a structure lacking in yeast (Kirkpatrick and Dubey, 1987). Sugar-solution centrifugation and fecal sedimentation using formalin-ether or formalin-ethyl acetate are effective diagnostic concentration techniques (Hill and Lappin, 1995). Oocysts may then be viewed with phase-contrast or bright-field microscopy of specimens stained with an acid-fast method. A direct fecal smear may be methanol- or heat-fixed and stained with an acid-fast method (Hill and Lappin, 1995).

Necropsy Findings Histologic evaluation reveals the presence of organisms, spherical to ovoid in shape and from 2 to 5 μm in diameter, associated with the brush border of the villi. A mild eosinophilic infiltrate was observed in the lamina propria of the small intestine in most animals. The ileum was the most common and heavily infected section of small intestine (Regh *et al.*, 1988).

Treatment and Control There is no known definitive treatment for cryptosporidiosis (Fox, 1998g). Supportive and symptomatic care should be provided in clinical cryptosporidiosis. Infections are self-limiting in immunocompetent patients (Fox, 1998g). Control is aimed at eliminating or reducing infective oocysts in the environment and avoidance of contact with known sources. Because of the potential for zoonotic transmission, restricting contact of children and immunosuppressed individuals with infected ferrets and practicing good hygiene may help reduce the potential for infection. Drying, freeze-thawing, and steam cleaning inactivate the organism (Hill and Lappin, 1995). There are few effective commercial disinfectants.

b. Ectoparasites and Mites

i. SARCOPTIC MANGE

Etiology Sarcoptic mange is caused by infection with *Sarcoptes scabiei*.

Epizootiology and Transmission Transmission occurs through direct contact with infected hosts or contact with fomites. This parasitic infection is rare under research conditions.

Clinical Signs Infection of ferrets with *S. scabiei* may occur in a generalized or a pedal form (Bernard *et al.*, 1984). In the generalized form, lesions consist of focal or generalized alopecia with intense pruritus. In the pedal form, lesions are confined to the toes and feet, which become swollen and encrusted with scabs. Nails may be deformed or lost if the condition is left untreated.

Diagnosis Diagnosis is made by finding the mites in skin scrapings or removing crusts, breaking them up,

and clearing with 10% KOH for microscopic examination (Phillips *et al.*, 1987). False-negative results are possible; multiple scrapings may be necessary.

Differential Diagnosis Differential diagnosis should include other pruritic external parasitic conditions, including flea infestation. Demodicosis has been reported to cause mild pruritus and alopecia in ferrets (Noli *et al.*, 1996).

Treatment and Control In the pedal form, treatment consists of trimming the claws and removing the scabs after softening them in warm water (Bernard *et al.*, 1984). Treatments that have been used include ivermectin, 0.2–0.4 mg/kg, administered subcutaneously and repeated every 7–14 days until mites are gone; shampoos or soaks to reduce the pruritus; and topical or systemic antibiotic administration for treatment of secondary bacterial dermatitis (Hillyer and Quesenberry, 1997b). Selamectin appears to be a very safe alternative and can be used once monthly at 18 mg/kg (Fisher *et al.*, 2007). Alternatively, weekly dips in 2% lime sulfur until 2 weeks after clinical cure have been shown to be effective (Fox, 1998a). Decontamination of enclosures and bedding, as well as treatment of all affected and contact animals are recommended.

ii. DEMODICOSIS

Etiology Demodicosis is caused by infection by *Demodex* spp.

Epizootiology and Transmission The parasite is found in normal skin of and is not considered contagious. Predisposing factors such as immunologic or genetic conditions have been suggested (Kwochka, 1986). One clinical report describes demodicosis in two adult ferrets that had been treated with an ear ointment containing triamcinolone acetonide for recurrent ear infections daily for three periods of 3 months each during the course of a year (Noli *et al.*, 1996).

Clinical Signs In the report mentioned above, the ferrets presented with alopecia, pruritus, and orange discoloration of the skin behind the ears and on the ventral surface of the abdomen and an accompanying seborrhea (Noli *et al.*, 1996).

Diagnosis Deep skin scrapings should be performed to demonstrate mites. Finding a large number of live adult mites or immature forms and eggs is necessary to confirm the diagnosis. In very chronic cases, the skin may be so thickened that scrapings may be unrewarding. In these cases, a skin biopsy may be diagnostic (Kwochka, 1986).

Necropsy Findings Histologic evaluation of skin biopsies obtained in the case report described above revealed mites with a short, blunted abdomen similar to that of *Demodex criceti* and located in the infundibulum of hairs. The epidermis was slightly hypertrophic, and there was a mild superficial orthokeratotic hyperkeratosis. A very mild superficial and perivascular mixed cellular infiltrate was also observed in the dermis.

Differential Diagnosis Generalized demodicosis should be differentiated from sarcoptic mange and flea infestation. Primary or secondary bacterial dermatitis or pyoderma should also be considered.

Treatment and Control The ferrets in the above-mentioned clinical report were treated initially with a suspension of 0.0125% amitraz applied as a dip three times at 7-day intervals for three treatments. Two drops of the same solution were applied in each ear every other day. After the initial treatment, the ferrets were re-examined, and treatment was continued with the same concentration of solution applied once every 5 days, while the tail was washed with a higher concentration of amitraz (0.025%) once every other day. Thereafter, three final treatments with 0.0375% amitraz every 5 days for the body, and every other day for the ears and tail, were administered. The ferrets were evaluated and skin scrapings were performed regularly during treatment and post-treatment to monitor response to therapy. Various treatments have been used in the clinical settings in ferrets without any side-effects. Commonly used safe drugs include imidacloprid-moxidectin (Advocate® spot-on for small cats and ferrets; once monthly for several months), ivermectin administered orally or topically (up to 0.5 μg/kg q 24 h), and selamectin (20 mg/kg q 30 d). Treatment of any associated pyodermas, systemic illnesses, or management problems should also be included as part of the therapeutic regimen.

iii. EAR MITES

Etiology The ear mite, *Otodectes cynotis*, which commonly infects dogs and cats, is also a common clinical problem in ferrets (Fox, 1998g).

Epizootiology and Transmission Ear mites are transmitted through direct contact with infested ferrets, dogs, or cats (Fox, 1998g). The entire life cycle is completed in 3 weeks.

Clinical Signs Ear mite infestation in the ferret is usually asymptomatic (Orcutt, 1997). However, clinical signs may include head shaking; mild to severe pruritus with inflammation and excoriation; secondary otitis interna with ataxia; circling; torticollis; and Horner's syndrome (Orcutt, 1997; Fox, 1998g). A brownish-black waxy discharge is often present.

Diagnosis Diagnosis is based on direct observation of mites via otoscopic examination or microscopic identification of the ear mite or any of the life-cycle stages of the mite in exudate from the ear canal.

Treatment and Control A study using three treatment regimens – two topical and one injectable – revealed that topical treatments were more efficacious than the injectable in reducing or eradicating ear mites (Patterson *et al.*, 1999). Efficacy was evaluated by

microscopic evidence of ear mites in debris from aural swabs taken weekly for an 8-week period. Topical 1% ivermectin (Ivomec, Merck AgVet Division, Rahway, New Jersey), diluted 1:10 in propylene glycol at a dosage of 400 μg/kg body weight divided equally between the two ear canals and administered on days 1 and 14 of the study, was the most effective treatment. However, more recent publications suggest that because of the anatomical characteristics of the ear of the ferret, conventional treatment involving instillation of drops into the ear canal is of very limited efficacy (Fisher *et al.*, 2007). A single topical application of approximately 15 mg/kg selamectin per ferret has been reported to be highly effective in the treatment of this irritant infestation. Another study showed that the combination of imidacloprid 10% + moxidectin 1% (Advocate® spot-on for small cats and ferrets) applied to ferrets naturally infested with *O. cynotis* achieved 100% cure after two or three treatments at 2-week intervals (Le Sueur *et al.*, 2011). These medications can be partially given into the ear canal with the rest applied directly to the skin of the interscapular region.

Other ferrets diagnosed with an *O. cynotis* infestation were treated with 45 mg selamectin in the form of a complete 0.75-ml single-dose tube (Stronghold Cat; Pfizer), administered topically between the shoulder blades and without cleaning the external ear canal. These infestations were successfully resolved after one treatment, based on resolution of clinical signs, otoscopic examinations and repeat ear swabs conducted 30 days later (Miller *et al.*, 2006).

High doses of injectable ivermectin (0.2 ml of 1% ivermectin) administered to jills at 2–4 weeks of gestation resulted in high rates of congenital defects (Orcutt, 1997).

iv. FLEAS

Etiology *Ctenocephalides* species can infest ferrets (Hutchinson *et al.*, 2001).

Epizootiology and Transmission Transmission requires direct contact with another infested animal or a flea-infested environment.

Clinical Signs Flea infestation may be asymptomatic or may cause mild to intense pruritus and alopecia of the dorsal thorax and neck (Timm, 1988).

Diagnosis Diagnosis is based on clinical signs and identification of fleas or flea excrement.

Differential Diagnosis Sarcoptic and demodectic mange should be included in the differential diagnosis of pruritic skin disease in the ferret. Close examination of the pelage for fleas or flea excrement should be performed. Skin scrapings may be indicated.

Treatment and Control As with flea infestation in dogs and cats, concurrent treatment of the environment, as well as all animals in the household, is essential for effective flea control. Compounds approved for flea control in cats such as rotenone or pyrethrin powders or sprays may be used in ferrets (Hillyer and Quesenberry, 1997a). Selamectin topically (20 mg/kg q 30 d) can be used as a preventative or as a treatment. Ferrets treated topically with an imidacloprid spot-on formulation at a dose rate of 10 mg/kg body weight showed reduced flea burdens by 95.3% within 8 h of treatment and 100% efficacy was recorded at 24 h (Hutchinson et al., 2001).

4. Fungal Diseases

Ferrets may develop systemic disease from *Blastomyces, Coccidioides, Cryptococcus,* and *Histoplasma.* The reservoir of most of these fungi is the soil, however, making infection unlikely in a research facility. In production facilities, exposure can be minimized through careful selection of source animals, appropriate sanitation, and control of pests, particularly birds.

a. Pneumocystis carinii

Pneumocystis carinii has been recently reclassified as a fungus. Although *P. carinii* inhabits the lungs of many different species, recent transmission studies suggest that these fungi are highly species-specific (Gigliotti et al., 1993; Fox et al., 1998b). Clinical disease is evident only in immunocompromised ferrets and can be induced using high doses of exogenous steroids (Stokes et al., 1987). Lesions include interstitial pneumonitis with mononuclear cell infiltrates; cysts and trophozooites are evident with Gomori methanamine-silver nitrate and Giemsa on bronchoalveolar lavage. Treatment with trimethoprim sulfamethoxazole probably controls but does not eliminate infection (Fox et al., 1998b).

b. Mucormycosis

Ferrets are susceptible to secondary fungal infection of the outer ear canal with *Absidia corymbifera* or *Malassezia* spp. (Dinsdale and Rest, 1995; Fox, 1998d). The fungi are widespread in the environment and will cause a secondary fungal infection in the ears of ferrets infested with *Otodectes cynotis.* The yeasts can be visualized by impressions of ear exudates. Treatment involves eradication of the underlying mite infestation followed by oral and topical ketoconazole, miconazole, and polymyxin B.

c. Dermatomycosis

Dermatomycoses in ferrets are caused by *Microsporum canis* and *Trichophyton mentagrophytes.* Dermatophytes are transmissible to humans and are a zoonosis; thus affected animals should be quarantined and removed from the facility to minimize risk (Dinsdale and Rest, 1995; Scott et al., 1995; Fox et al., 1998b). Control of infection includes general disinfection and destruction of

contaminated bedding. Lesions are circumscribed areas of alopecia and inflammation, which begin as small papules that spread peripherally in a scaly inflamed ring. The yellow–green fluorescence of *M. canis* under ultraviolet light helps distinguish it from *T. mentagrophytes.* Skin scrapings digested with 10% potassium hydroxide reveal characteristic arthrospores. Treatment with griseofulvin (at 25 mg/kg per os every 24 h for at least 21–30 days) causes clinical remission but may not clear infection (Hoppmann and Barron, 2007).

d. Cryptococcosis

In recent years, publications concerning cryptococcosis in ferrets have increased significantly. As of 2013, there are 16 publications on this emerging disease (Wyre et al., 2013). Of 13 published cases, six ferrets were infected with *C. neoformans* and six were infected with *C. gatti.* In many of the reported cases, it appears that immunosuppression might have been a contributing factor. The risk for indoor-housed ferrets appears low as cryptococcus is found in soil, bird droppings, and trees, which puts ferrets with outdoor access at an increased risk. The prognosis for this condition is guarded and treatment is usually difficult, but mimics current treatment suggested in dogs and cats. A case treated with itraconazole at 15 mg/kg PO q24 h for 10 months resulted in a successful outcome after the diagnosis of *Cryptococcus neoformans* variety *grubii* from an enlarged submandibular lymph node (Hanley et al., 2006).

5. Other

Other ectoparasitic infections observed to occur in ferrets include cutaneous myiasis and tick infestation. Granulomatous masses in the cervical region caused by the larval stage of *Hypoderma bovis* have been reported in ferrets (Fox, 1998g). *Cuterebra* larvae, although uncommonly observed in ferrets, may cause subdermal cysts found in the subcutis of the neck (Orcutt, 1997). Infestation with the flesh fly has been reported as a problem in commercially reared mink and ferrets housed outdoors (Fox, 1998g).

Ticks may be found on ferrets housed outdoors or on those used for hunting rabbits (Fox, 1998g). Ticks should be removed carefully with hemostats or tweezers, ensuring that the entire head and mouthparts are removed from the skin. Appropriate caution should be exercised in tick removal, because ticks are responsible for transmission of various zoonotic pathogens; gloves should be worn.

6. Nematodes
a. Heartworm

Etiology The ferret is susceptible to natural and experimental infection with *Dirofilaria immitis.*

Epizootiology and transmission *Dirofilaria immitis* is a filarial parasite that is transmitted by mosquitoes, which serve as the intermediate host and vector. Microfilaria are ingested by mosquitoes and, after two molts, become infective third-stage larvae. Infective larvae are deposited onto the skin when mosquitoes feed, and larvae find their way into the body of the final host through the bite wound and migrate subcutaneously to the thorax and eventually to the heart (Knight, 1987). The primary reservoir of infection is dogs, but heartworm may be found in a variety of mammals, including humans. All species except wild and domestic canids, domestic felines, ferrets, and the California sea lion are considered aberrant hosts (Knight, 1987).

Clinical Signs The following clinical signs have been reported in clinical reports describing cases of *D. immitis* in the ferret: weakness, lethargy, depression, dyspnea, cyanosis, anorexia, dehydration, cough, and pale mucous membranes (Miller and Merton, 1982; Parrott *et al.*, 1984; Moreland *et al.*, 1986; Wagner, 2009). Moist lung sounds and/or muffled heart sounds were revealed by thoracic auscultation in many of these cases. Pleural or abdominal effusion may be observed radiologically. The ferrets described in these cases were housed outdoors and either died or were euthanized. In one case the key clinical signs included the caval syndrome, mild anemia and biliverdinuria (Sasai *et al.*, 2000). One of the authors (JM) has also observed biliverdinuria in a confirmed case of dirofilariasis, suggesting that biliverdinuria development in heartworm-infected ferrets may be of increase diagnostic value for this condition.

Diagnosis Diagnosis of heartworm is based on clinical signs, radiographic findings, and testing for circulating microfilariae and heartworm antigen. Ultrasound was used successfully to diagnose a ferret which was affected by one four *Dirofilaria immitis* parasites (Sasai *et al.*, 2000). Microfilaremia is not consistently observed in naturally occurring and experimental cases of heartworm infection in ferrets (Fox, 1998g). Testing for heartworm antigen appears to be more diagnostically useful (Stamoulis *et al.*, 1997). In a study to determine the minimum oral dose of ivermectin needed for monthly heartworm prophylaxis in ferrets, the use of an antigen test (Uni-Tec Canine Heartworm test, Pitman-Moore Co., Mundelein, Illinois) detected infection in more untreated control animals than did the modified Knott's test for detection of circulating microfilaria in the same ferrets (Supakorndej *et al.*, 1992).

Necropsy Findings Cardiomegaly, pleural and/or abdominal fluid, and pulmonary congestion are common findings at necropsy. Grossly, adult worms have been observed in the right atrium, right ventricle, pulmonary artery, and cranial and caudal vena cava. Microscopically, microfilaria may be seen in small and large vessels of the lung.

Differential Diagnosis Differential diagnosis should include primary cardiac diseases, such as dilatative cardiomyopathy, and other systemic or pulmonary diseases.

Treatment and Control Control is best directed at prevention through the administration of heartworm preventative and it is recommended that ferrets in heartworm-endemic areas receive monthly oral ivermectin or topical selamectin throughout the year (Stamoulis *et al.*, 1997; Fox, 1998g). The dosage recommended for ferrets by the American Heartworm Society is 0.006 mg ivermectin per kg body weight monthly (Fox, 1998g). Housing ferrets indoors, particularly during the mosquito season, would help minimize exposure. Successful adulticide treatment in ferrets has been described and includes the administration of thiacetarsemide, with the same precautions used in dogs: antithrombotic therapy, treatment for heart failure, and strict cage confinement (Stamoulis *et al.*, 1997). The current recommended treatment protocol for affected ferrets is ivermectin (50 µg/kg SC q30d) given until clinical signs resolve and microfilaremia is absent. Previous treatment protocols using adulticide therapy with melarsomine have fallen out of favor because of adverse reactions (Morrisey and Kraus, 2011). One should follow up with heartworm antigen tests until negative and resume heartworm prevention 1 month after adulticide treatment (Stamoulis *et al.*, 1997). A ferret with clinically-apparent dirofilariasis was successfully treated via transvenous heartworm extraction (Bradbury *et al.*, 2010).

Ferrets are also susceptible to infection with the following nematodes: *Toxascaris leonina; Toxocara cati; Ancylostoma* spp.; *Dipylidium caninum; Mesocestoides* spp.; *Atriotaenia procyonis; Trichinella spiralis; Filaroides martis;* and *Spiroptera nasicola* (Rosenthal, 1994; Fox, 1998g).

B. Metabolic and Nutritional Diseases

1. Pregnancy Toxemia

Pregnancy toxemia in the ferret occurs predominantly in primiparous jills carrying large litters. An inadvertent fast in late gestation is sometimes implicated. At least 75% of jills carrying more than eight kits will develop pregnancy toxemia if subjected to 24h of food withdrawal in late gestation (Bell, 1997a; Batchelder *et al.*, 1999). Any jill with 15 or more kits may develop pregnancy toxemia because abdominal space is not adequate for both the gravid uterus and the volume of food required to support it. Pregnancy toxemia of the ferret is of the metabolic type and shares features with similar conditions in pregnant sheep, obese cattle, pregnant camelids, obese guinea pigs, and starved pregnant rats, as well as with the condition feline idiopathic hepatic lipidosis. It is characterized by abnormal energy metabolism with consequent hyperlipidemia, hypoglycemia, ketosis, and hepatic lipidosis. In this condition, energy demand exceeds intake, leading to excessive mobilization of free fatty acids and a chain of metabolic events that culminates in a shift from fatty acid metabolism and export to ketosis and hepatic lipidosis. A study evaluating the metabolic and endocrine characteristics of pregnancy toxemia in ferrets showed that in contrast to healthy animals, hypoglycemia, hyperketonemia, hypoinsulinemia, and decreased T4 and T3 levels were detected in females with pregnancy toxemia. Necropsy showed excessive hepatic lipidosis (Prohaczik *et al.*, 2009).

Clinical signs of affected animals usually include anorexia, lethargy, melena, dehydration, and easily epilated hair. Differentials include dystocia, metritis, pyometra, septicemia, renal failure, and *Helicobacter mustelae*-induced gastric ulcer. In a study of ferrets with pregnancy toxemia, consistent clinical chemistry abnormalities included azotemia (100%), hypocalcemia (83%), hypoproteinemia (70%), and elevated liver enzymes (100%) (Batchelder *et al.*, 1999). Anemia was found in 50% of ferrets tested. Necropsy findings included tan or yellow discolored liver, gastric hemorrhage, and gravid uterus. Treatment for jills within a day of their due date should include cesarean section and intensive postoperative support, including force-feeding a gruel of high-quality cat food and ferret chow, nutritive pastes, intravenous fluids containing glucose, and supplemental heat. Ceasarean section should be performed under isoflurane or sevoflurane anesthesia because hepatic dysfunction prolongs the metabolism of injectable agents. Agalactia is common after cesarean section, and kits may require hand feeding with kitten or puppy milk replacers, administered *per os* by fine-tipped syringe six times daily for the first 24 h. Cross-fostering is an effective method of enhancing kit survival; hand rearing of kits if the jill fails to nurse within a day postoperatively is energy-consuming and generally unrewarding. For jills that develop pregnancy toxemia before day 40 of gestation, fluids and nutritional support must be provided until viable kits can be delivered by cesarean.

Pregnancy toxemia may be avoided by close monitoring of the appetite of jills in late gestation, provision of a highly palatable diet with >20% fat and >35% crude protein, and avoidance of stress and dietary change. Water should be made available in both bowls and water bottles, and food should be provided *ad libitum* in several bowls.

2. Hyperestrogenism

Ferrets are induced ovulators and may remain in persistent estrus if they are not bred or if estrus is not terminated chemically or via ovariohysterectomy (Bell, 1997a). Jills that remain in estrus for more than 1 month are at risk for developing estrogen-induced anemia. Hyperestrogenism from persistent estrus causes bone marrow hypoplasia of all cell lines in approximately half of ferrets in prolonged estrus (Ryland *et al.*, 1983).

Clinical signs include vulvar enlargement, bilaterally symmetric alopecia of the tail and abdomen, weakness, anorexia, depression, lethargy, weight loss, bacterial infection, and mucopurulent vaginal discharge. Hematology findings may vary from an initial neutrophilia and thrombocytosis early in the disease course to lymphopenia, thrombocytopenia, neutropenia, and anemia. The anemia begins as normocytic normochromic but progresses to macrocytic hypochromic (Sherrill and Gorham, 1985). Coagulopathy associated with hepatic dysfunction and thrombocytopenia combine to produce extensive manifestations of bleeding, pallor, melena, petechiation or ecchymosis, subdural hematoma, and hematomyelia (Hart, 1985; Fox and Bell, 1998). At necropsy, tissue pallor, light tan to pale pink bone marrow, hemorrhage, bronchopneumonia, hydrometra, pyometra, and mucopurulent vaginitis may be seen. Histopathology may reveal cystic endometrial hypoplasia, hemosiderosis, diminished splenic extramedullary hematopoiesis, and mild to moderate hepatic lipidosis (Sherrill and Gorham, 1985; Bell, 1997a). Treatment consists of terminating estrus while supporting the animal with antibiotics, blood transfusion, B vitamins, and nutritional supplementation. Estrus may be terminated by injection with 50–100 IU of human chorionic gonadotropin (hCG) or 20 μg of gonadotropin-releasing hormone (GnRH), repeated 1 week after initial injection if required. Ovariohysterectomy may be considered for ferrets that are stable and have adequate numbers of platelets and red cells. Ferrets with a packed cell volume (PCV) of 25% or greater have a good prognosis and require only termination of estrus for resolution of aplastic anemia. Jills with a PCV of 15–25% may require blood transfusions and have a guarded prognosis. Ferrets with a PCV of less than 15% have a poor prognosis and require aggressive therapy with multiple transfusions. The lack of identifiable blood groups in ferrets makes multiple transfusions uncomplicated by potential transfusion reactions (Manning and Bell, 1990b).

Estrogen-induced anemia may be avoided by ovariohysterectomy of nonbreeding females, use of vasectomized hobs, or pharmacologic termination of estrus initiated 10 days after estrus onset. A 40- to 45-day pseudopregnancy then follows, except in the case of ovariohysterectomy. Repeated administration of hCG may result in sensitization and anaphylaxis. After several administrations, hCG is unlikely to be effective in termination of estrus. Anaphylaxis is manifest as incoordination, tremor, vomiting, and diarrhea and may be reversed by prompt administration of diphenhydramine. In order to avoid the risk of anaphylaxis, GnRH can be injected, as it is a smaller molecule and anaphylaxis to it is extremely rare. A GnRH analog (Deslorelin)-releasing implant has recently been approved in ferrets for the treatment of hyperadrenocortisism in the United States. This implant could also be used to 'chemically' sterilize the female. The 4.7-mg implant has been shown to suppress clinical signs of hyperadrenocorticism for up to 30 months with an average of 17.5 months (Wagner et al., 2005).

3. Hyperammonemia

Arginine-free diets are unlikely to be fed in the laboratory setting, but administration of such a diet to young ferrets fasted for 16h leads to hyperammonemia and encephalopathy within 2–3h (Thomas and Desmukh, 1986). Exacerbation of signs may be achieved by challenging young ferrets with influenza virus and aspirin (Desmukh et al., 1985) and constitutes a model of Reye's syndrome in children. Lethargy and aggressiveness yield to prostration, coma, and death in affected ferrets. Hyperammonemia presumably occurs because of the inability of ferrets to produce adequate amounts of ornithine from non-arginine precursors. Detoxification of ammonia is thereby compromised. Ferrets more than 18 months old are unaffected by arginine-free diets.

4. Zinc Toxicosis

Ferrets of all ages are susceptible to zinc toxicosis, and the condition has been documented in two ferret farms in New Zealand (Straube and Walden, 1981). Leaching of zinc from steam-sterilized galvanized food and water bowls was implicated. Clinical signs included pallor, posterior weakness, and lethargy. Definitive diagnosis requires demonstration of elevated concentrations of zinc in kidney and liver. At necropsy, kidneys are enlarged, pale, and soft; livers are orange, and gastric hemorrhage may be seen. Histopathology reveals glomerular collapse, tubular dilation, tubular proteinaceous debris, focal cortical fibrosis, hepatic periacinar infiltration, and depression of the erythroid series. Avoidance of galvanized materials precludes the development of zinc toxicosis.

5. Hypothyroidism

Hypothyroidism appears to be an emerging disease as clinical reports have increased recently (J. Mayer, personal observation). Anecdotal reports suggest that the clinical presentation is very much similar to the classical signs in domesticated animals, which are most consistently obesity, lethargy, decreased activity, and excessive sleeping. Ante mortem diagnosis can be challenging but a recent publication reports T4 levels using human recombinant TSH (Thyrogen) in 11 neutered ferrets, and successful stimulation of the thyroid axis was achieved by this method. Prestimulation values for T4 in neutered male and female ferrets were determined to be 29.9 ± 5.8ng/ml and 21.8 ± 3.3ng/ml, respectively. Ferrets were stimulated using 100mg Thyrogen intramuscularly, and euthyroid ferrets were found to have an increase of 1.4-times basal levels after 4h (Wagner, 2012). Another study involving 25 laboratory and pet neutered ferrets using the same protocol noted a median poststimulation T4 level at 34.8% above prestimulatory levels, and found the mean plasma T4 of euthyroid ferrets to be 21.3nmol/l (Mayer et al., 2013). The prognosis for confirmed cases is good as oral levothyroxine at 50–100mg every 12h has been shown to be effective (Wagner, 2012).

C. Traumatic Disorders

Hobs are typically separated at 12 weeks of age. Fighting can occur, especially in the intact male during the breeding season. Clinicians will notice aggressive sexual play between hobs. Puncture wounds, scratches and subsequent scabs and cellulitis are evident between the scapulae and on the dorsal surface of the neck.

Traumatic elbow luxation is common in ferrets. It typically occurs when the animal changes directions after getting a leg caught on cage flooring. Open reduction should be used because closed reduction is seldom successful in ferrets. A transarticular pin applied for 4 weeks in the reduced limb has been successful. The leg should be splinted throughout this time and for 4 weeks after pin removal.

D. Iatrogenic Diseases

Hydronephrosis may occasionally occur in the ferret and is most commonly associated with inadvertent ligation of the ureter during ovariohysterectomy. Ovarian remnants are another potential sequela to ovariohysterectomy. Ovarian remnants in ferrets may be associated with estrus, vulvar enlargement, and alopecia. Appropriate diagnostic procedures include ultrasonography and plain and contrast radiography for hydronephrosis and ultrasonography and serum hormone concentrations for ovarian remnants. Exploratory celiotomy confirms the diagnosis, and unilateral nephrectomy or ovariectomy is indicated if the remaining kidney is normal and the ferret is otherwise healthy.

E. Neoplastic Diseases

Ferrets are subject to a wide variety of neoplastic conditions (Li et al., 1998). However, four categories of cancer account for the majority of ferret neoplasms: pancreatic islet cell tumors, adrenocortical cell tumors, lymphoma, and skin cancers.

1. Insulinoma

Functional pancreatic islet cell tumors (insulinomas) are the most common neoplasm diagnosed in ferrets (Li et al., 1998). Disease may be evident in ferrets as young as 2 years old, but later onset (at 4–5 years of age) is typical

(Caplan *et al.*, 1996; Ehrhart *et al.*, 1996). Nonspecific presenting signs include weight loss, vomiting, and ataxia. Weakness is often evident, ranging from lethargy to posterior paresis or outright collapse (Caplan *et al.*, 1996). Hypoglycemia caused by excess production of insulin by neoplastic β-cells may cause tremors, disorientation, or seizures (Fox and Marini, 1998). Excessive salivation (ptyalism) or pawing at the mouth is a frequent finding. Clinical signs are often intermittent or episodic. Other common findings include hindlimb weakness, splenomegaly, and lymphocytosis. Presumptive diagnosis is made based on clinical signs in conjunction with the demonstration of hypoglycemia. Blood glucose determinations for the diagnosis of insulinoma are most useful when taken after a 4-h fasting period. Fasting glucose concentrations below 60 mg/dl (3.33 mmol/l) are considered diagnostic for the condition (Quesenberry and Carpenter, 2012), whereas values between 60 and 85 mg/dl (3.33–4.72 mmol/l) are suspect and the test should be repeated (Fox and Marini, 1998). The repeat test should be standardized by force feeding the ferret some amount of food with subsequent fasting for 4 h prior to the repeat blood collection. Other potential causes for hypoglycemia should be ruled out, including anorexia, starvation, hepatic disease, sepsis, and nonpancreatic neoplasia (Antinoff, 1997). Demonstration of concurrent hyperinsulinemia aids the diagnosis (Caplan *et al.*, 1996) but secretion of insulin from the pancreas can be erratic in ferrets with insulinoma, resulting in non-diagnostic baseline insulin levels. Normal insulin concentrations have been reported to be between 4.88 and 34.84 mU/ml (35–250 pmol/l) (Jenkins, 2000). Medical management using prednisone and/or diazoxide along with dietary modification such as frequent feeding of high-protein meals can minimize or control clinical signs but will not affect the underlying tumor (Quesenberry and Rosenthal, 1997). Surgical exploration of the pancreas and tumor excision are recommended for animals that are healthy enough to be subjected to anesthesia and surgery. In a comparison of medical *versus* surgical treatment, Weiss *et al.*, (1998) found that surgery improved disease-free interval and survival time. Histological examination of the tissue removed can provide a definitive diagnosis, and although the effect may be transient, clinical signs are often reduced or eliminated after surgical debulking (Figs. 14.7 and 14.8) (Ehrhart *et al.*, 1996). Histologically, these tumors reveal malignant proliferation of pancreatic β-cells, and local recurrence or metastasis to lymph nodes, mesentery, spleen, or liver may occur (Caplan *et al.*, 1996) but it is considered uncommon.

2. Adrenal Tumors

Adrenocortical cell tumor is the second most common type of neoplasia in ferrets (Li *et al.*, 1998) and is generally diagnosed between 3 and 6 years of age. If

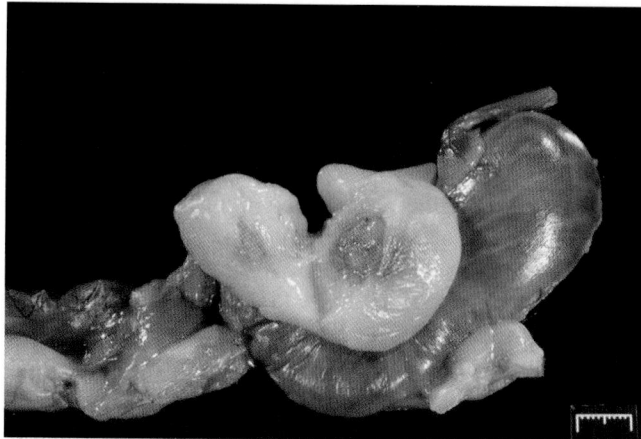

FIGURE 14.7   Gross appearance of islet cell tumors in the ferret. Note the isoflurane-induced splenomegaly.

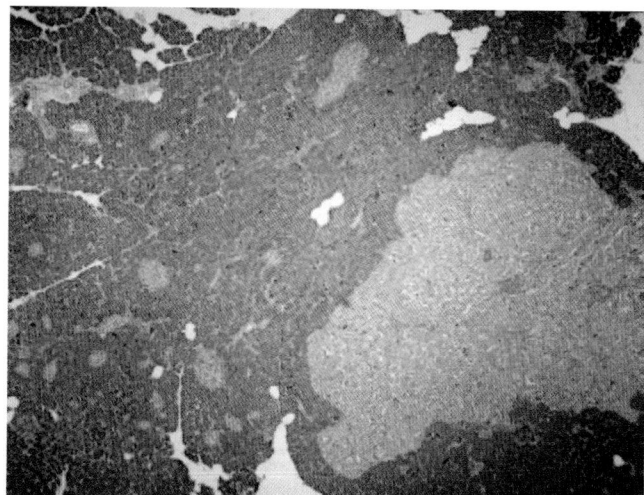

FIGURE 14.8   Histologic appearance of an islet cell tumor.

clinical signs are present, they often include weight loss and a bilateral, symmetric alopecia. Pruritus is a variable finding (Quesenberry and Rosenthal, 1997). These primary clinical signs in ferrets are directly related to the increase of sex steroids in the blood resulting in estrogen toxicity. Although ferrets with this syndrome have been called 'cushingoid,' it is rare to diagnose elevated resting levels of glucocorticoids or an abnormal response to adrenocorticotropic hormone (ACTH) stimulation or dexamethasone suppression testing. The pathophysiologic difference between the ferret adrenal disease and the typical Cushing presentation is the production in affected ferrets of a significant increase of the sex steroids by the zona reticularis and not significant levels of cortisol from the zona fasciculata. The sex steroids that are usually elevated are estradiol, 17-hydroxyprogesterone, testosterone, and androstenedione. The elevation of the adrenal sex hormones leads to characteristic changes such as estrus-like vulvar swelling in spayed females and prostatic changes and cystitis in males (Rosenthal and Peterson, 1996; Coleman *et al.*, 1998). Rule-outs for enlarged vulva include estrus in an intact female or functional ovarian remnants in a spayed female (Patterson *et al.*, 2003). Abdominal palpation may reveal cranial abdominal masses, and ultrasound is extremly useful in documenting a potential increase in size of the adrenal glands. However, with an endocrine disease, the size of the organ does not always correlate with the clinical signs. It is not uncommon for a ferret to have severe clinical signs without having a truly enlarged adrenal gland (J. Mayer, personal observation). In these cases, a serum assay for abnormal levels of the sex hormones listed above should be considered (Lipman *et al.*, 1993; Wagner and Dorn, 1994; Rosenthal and Peterson, 1996). Adrenal panels are available from the endocrinology Laboratory, School of Veterinary Medicine.

In many cases the alopecia begins as a seasonally intermittent partial hair loss that becomes more severe in successive seasons (Fig. 14.9). Even severe manifestations of this endocrine alopecia can spontaneously reverse in the absence of specific therapy, as demonstrated in a group of five ferrets referred to our facility (JGF, RPM) for diagnostic workup. In each of these five ferrets, near total alopecia resolved within a few months of being housed in a research environment. Despite being asymptomatic at the end of the study, all five were shown to have histologic evidence of adrenocortical neoplasia.

In our experience, adrenal cortical hyperplasia with or without neoplasia is an extremely common finding in aging ferrets, even in those not showing clinical signs. In one retrospective survey of our necropsy records it was found that more than 90% of ferrets greater than 4 years

of age had hyperplastic or neoplastic adrenal changes when examined (data not shown). For this reason, careful considerations of other possible disease processes should be made before attributing clinical signs solely to adrenal enlargement.

Medical treatment of the condition can be achieved with monthly injections of Lupron® (leuprolide acetate) at 0.1 mg/animal if less than 1 kg, and 0.2 mg/animal if over 1 kg of bodyweight. The drug is considered a GnRH superagonist and will stop the production of LH and FSH due to negative feedback inhibition from persistent stimulation of the hypophysis. This process is call 'desensitization.' It is important to remember that this treatment only affects response to the hormones and does not interfere at all with tumor growth. It has also been noted that a 'resistance' seems to develop over time and higher doses are needed to control the clinical signs. In rare cases the adrenal gland will produce hormones independent of LH and FSH regulation. In these cases Lupron treatment is completely ineffective.

Deslorelin implants have been approved in the USA for ferrets with adrenal gland disease and these are now considered the medical treatment of choice. The response to a single 4.7-mg implant of deslorelin acetate in a cohort of ferrets lasted between 8 and 30 months with a mean time to recurrence of clinical signs of 13 months (Wagner *et al.*, 2009). It could also be argued that the medication might be able to prevent the onset of adrenal disease if used prior to the onset of clinical disease. Some evidence to this theory was provided in the form of the use of a GnRH vaccine (GonaCon™) in the ferret. Miller *et al.*, (2013) showed that vaccinated ferrets with similar status to deslorelin-treated animals had a significantly lower rate of adrenal disease than control ferrets over the course of 9 years.

Another option for medical treatment is the use of melatonin to suppress hormone release. Melatonin is normally released during the dark phase of the day by the pineal gland. It directly inhibits GnRH release and therefore suppresses LH and FSH production. The importance of the pineal gland and its influence on gonadal activity has been validated as long as 30 years ago in the ferret (Baum *et al.*, 1986). Melatonin treatment is achieved by using a commercially available melatonin implant (Ferretonin™) which can be injected under the skin and releases a steady amount of melatonin for three months. Adrenolytic agents such as mitotane should not be used due to their limited success.

Surgical exploration and removal of enlarged adrenals are commonly performed to establish the diagnosis and to remove hyperfunctional tissue. Unilateral adrenalectomy early in the disease may be curative, but because bilateral neoplastic involvement is not uncommon, full or partial removal of both glands may be required. Bilateral gland involvement has been reported in 16–68%

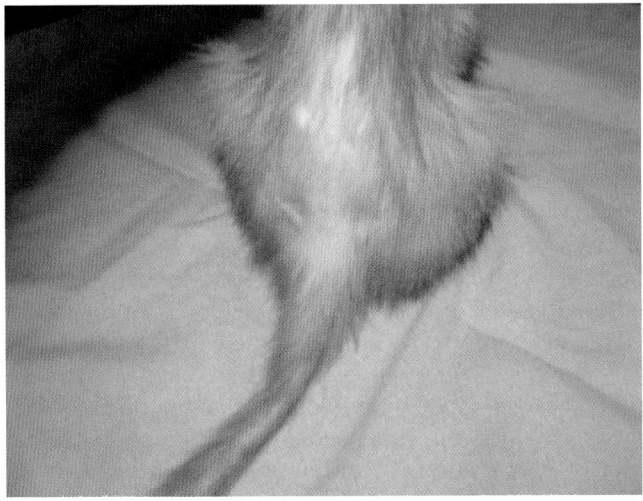

FIGURE 14.9   Adrenal-associated endocrine alopecia in the ferret.

of ferrets with adrenocortical disease (Rosenthal et al., 1993; Weiss et al., 1999). Contrary to popular belief it is possible to remove both adrenal glands at the same time without creating significant hormonal issues. It is best to medicate these animals with dexamethsone (1™ mg/kg IM) during post-op recovery, and then to continue medication with oral prednisone (1 mg/kg SID PO) for a few weeks after surgery before the animal can be weaned off the drugs. Supplementation with glucocorticoids can sometimes be needed if the gland remaining after unilateral adrenalectomy has been suppressed by the hyperactive one.

One of the authors has also achieved acceptable results after alcohol injection into the diseased gland via ultrasound guidance. The injection of alcohol into the adrenal and other tumor sites has been used in human medicine and is well documented. The treated gland appears to shrink, and this has been documented with abdominal ultrasound examinations. This localized treatment option may provide a solution to cases where complete excision or medical management is not possible. Frequently a tumor of the right adrenal will have invaded significantly into the vena cava, making partial resection or a complete removal of the vena cava the only surgical option. In cases where the vena cava has been slowly invaded or occluded by the tumor, a network of collateral vessels into which blood will be diverted to the vertebral sinuses has been established. Survivors must be treated with aggressive fluid therapy for 2–3 days postoperatively, and renal values should be closely monitored for signs of renal failure due to impaired perfusion.

Excised tissues should always be submitted for histological analysis in order to differentiate between hyperplasia, adenoma and adenocarcinoma. Histologically, adrenocortical adenomas are generally 1 cm or less in diameter and are composed of well-differentiated cells with a granular or vacuolated cytoplasm. Adrenal cell carcinomas are less commonly found and are larger, with a more pleomorphic and invasive character (Li et al., 1998). Metastasis to nearby tissues can occur but is rare.

3. Lymphoma

Lymphoma is a complex disease process and the authors suggest that readers consult The Biology of the Ferret, 3rd edition, for a detailed discussion of this common disease in the ferret.

Lymphoma is seen at all ages; however, in the juvenile ferret (younger than 2 years of age), an aggressive form of lymphoma is often found. A mediastinal mass is often part of the initial finding. Older ferrets (older than 2 years of age) are more likely to develop a more indolent form of lymphoma. Common forms are multicentric or gastrointestinal lymphoma. The early age

of onset in some ferrets and reports of case clustering have led to investigation into potential infectious etiologies for lymphoma in the ferret (Erdman et al., 1996b). Earlier reports of feline leukemia virus (FeLV) seroconversion in affected animals have not been substantiated. However, experimental and epidemiological evidence suggests that a retrovirus that is distinct from FeLV may be involved (Erdman et al., 1995). In one study, whole or filtered lymphoma cells from a 3-year-old ferret with spontaneous lymphoma were injected IP into 6 recipient ferrets (Erdman et al., 1995). Two of the six ferrets were euthanized after 14 months, but the remaining four developed splenomegaly, lymphocytosis, and lymphoma. One ferret that received cell-free materials developed multicentric lymphoma with prominent cutaneous lymphoma nodules. Elevated reverse transcriptase activity and retrovirus-like particles evident by electron microscopy were seen in the donor and all of the affected recipient ferrets.

Other potential etiologies that have been considered include two infectious agents that are known to cause chronic immune stimulation in affected ferrets, the ADV and Helicobacter mustelae. A link with ADV has not been proven, but H. mustelae seems to be responsible for the development of a very specific type of gastric B-cell lymphoma (Erdman et al., 1997).

Unfortunately, in spite of the frequency of occurance, lymphoma is one of the more difficult diseases to accurately diagnose. Affected ferrets may exhibit localizing signs (e.g., dyspnea in a ferret with mediastinal involvement or peripheral lymphadenopathy in an animal with a multicentric distribution) but as is the case in many species, lymphoma is a 'masquerader,' and affected ferrets often present with chronic, nonspecific signs. Weight loss, anorexia, and lethargy are often reported. Splenic and/or hepatic enlargement may be evident. Cutaneous involvement has been documented (Li et al., 1995; Rosenbaum et al., 1996). Blood work should not be used as a primary diagnostic tool but it should be performed in every patient with lymphoma to evaluate overall health. Although hematological examination typically reveals anemia, which is usually mild and nonregenerative, and lymphopenia, lymphocytosis may be found, especially in younger ferrets. Lymphocytosis should not be immediately interpreted as leukemia. Ferrets with chronic inflammatory/infectious disease will often present with persistent lymphocytosis. Atypical lymphocytes are identified in the circulation in some cases. Ante mortem definitive diagnosis of lymphoma can be made by cytological examination of specimens obtained via fine-needle aspiration or excisional biopsy. Hypercalcemia can be observed in ferrets with T-cell lymphoma, but in general serum chemistry findings are usually non-pathognomonic. Ferrets with liver involvement may have elevated liver values; patients with renal lymphoma will often present with azotemia. Radiographs are useful in detecting mediastinal forms of lymphoma (Fig. 14.10a); ultrasonography is the imaging modality of choice for abdominal forms of lymphoma (Fig. 14.10b).

To determine cell immunophenotype, routine immunohistochemistry should be performed on affected tissue(s). The use of anti-CD3 and anti-CD79a antibodies is recommended to differentiate between B- and T-cell lymphoma in the ferret. Although there is a paucity of information in the veterinary literature that correlates immunophenotype with disease prognosis in ferrets, one small study found that ferrets treated with chemotherapy survived an average of 4.3 months (T-cell lymphoma) or 8.8 months (B-cell lymphoma). A proposal for a standardized classification of ferret lymphoma has been suggested in order to be able to compare cases for future evaluation and to standardize communication about cases (Table 14.8) (Mayer and Burgess, 2012). The staging process should include the detailed anatomical description based on the following categories: anatomical site, number of lesions, location of the lesions relative to the diaphragm, nodal *versus* extranodal lesions, and involvement of the blood or bone marrow.

Tan-colored masses involving lymph nodes, spleen, liver, or other organs are commonly found at necropsy (Fig. 14.11). Diffuse involvement may lead to uniform enlargement of these organs or to a thickening of the wall of the stomach or intestines. As in other species, histological evaluation reveals neoplastic lymphocytes in affected tissues, generally evident as a monomorphic population (Fig. 14.12) (Erdman et al., 1996a). Although surgery and radiation therapy may be useful in certain cases, most attempts to treat ferret lymphoma

have utilized chemotherapeutic regimens with dosages extrapolated from other domestic animals or humans. Treatment generally results in a remission that may last from 3 months to 5 years (Brown, 1997b; Erdman *et al.*, 1998). Different treatment protocols have been published in the past. Unfortunately, the paucity of information regarding remission durations and survival make comparison between the different protocols impossible. The simplest form of chemotherapy for lymphoma is oral prednisolone/prednisone given at 1–2 mg/kg PO q 12–24 h. This treatment will achieve partial or complete, short-lived remission. It is important that the animal should not be exposed to steriods prior to the diagnostic biopsy as the remission can occur very quickly and a false negative biopsy report would follow if the animal has been medicated for longer than 48 h. In addition, chemotherapy may be less effective in ferrets receiving chronic immunosuppressive doses of prednisolone at the start of therapy (e.g., as part of a medical insulinoma management). Most of the commonly used protocols are modified feline lymphoma protocols, which include commonly used drugs for which repeated IV access is needed. Several multidrug chemotherapy protocols have been described, using L-asparaginase, vincristine, cyclophosphamide, doxorubicin, methotrexate, and prednisone. Due to the possible complication of extravasation of these drugs and the perceived invasive charater of these protocols, one of the authors (JM) was part of a team who developed and successfully implemented a non-invasive protocol (Tables 14.9, 14.10). This protocol involves only oral and SC drugs, which allow for a relatively easy implementation of the protocol without much risk or the need to hospitalize the patient. In general, chemotherapy can be considered chronic treatment because the treatment usually lasts for weeks to months.

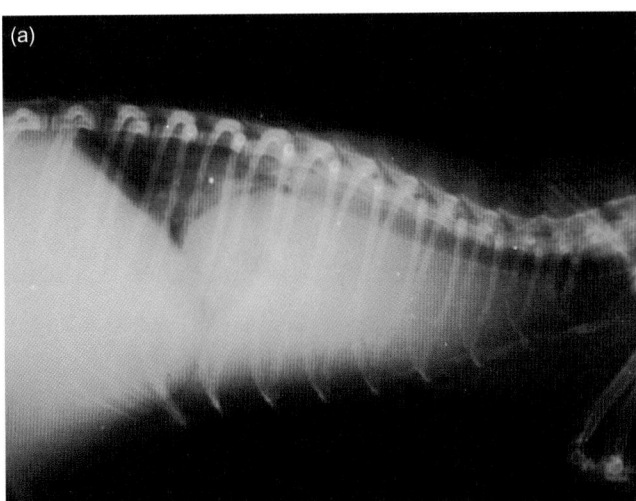
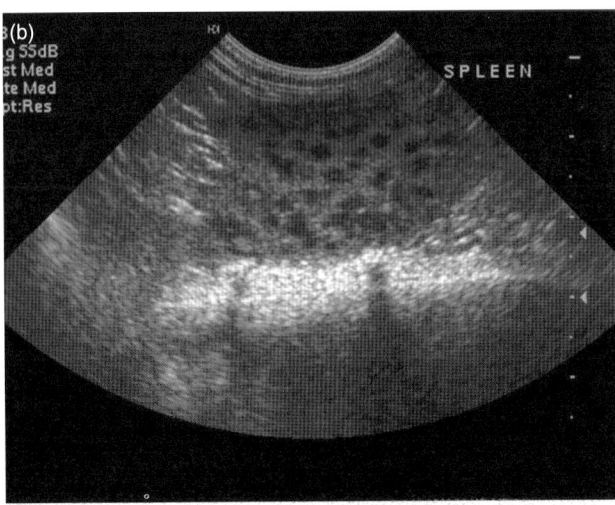

FIGURE 14.10   Radiographic (a) and ultrasonic (b) appearance of lymphoma in a ferret: (a) shows a mediastinal mass cranial to the heart; (b) shows typical 'leopard spots' in the spleen.

TABLE 14.8   Suggested Criteria to Uniformly Describe a Lymphoma

Anatomical site	Stage	Immunophenotyping
A: generalized	Stage 1: Single anatomic lesion (nodal or extranodal)	B-cell lymphoma (e.g., positive for CD79a)
	a: without clinical signs	
	b: with systemic signs	
B: alimentary	Stage 2: Single lesion with regional lymph node involvement limited to one side of the diaphragm	T-cell lymphoma (e.g., positive for CD3)
	a: without clinical signs	
	b: with systemic signs	
C: thymic	Stage 3: Lesions on both sides of the diaphragm including intra-abdominal or GI locations	
	a: without clinical signs	
	b: with systemic signs	
D: skin	Stage 4: Multiple sites on both sides of the diaphragm are affected ± visceral organs	
	a: without clinical signs	
	b: with systemic signs	
E: leukemia (true)	Stage 5: Manifestation in the blood and involvement of bone marrow and/or other organ systems	
	a: without clinical signs	
	b: with systemic signs	
F: others (including solitary renal tumors)		

(Mayer and Burgess, 2012).

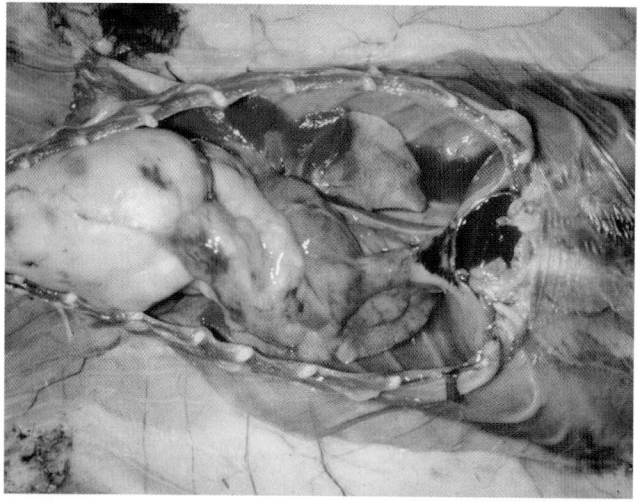

FIGURE 14.11   Cranial mediastinal mass consistent with lymphoma in a ferret.

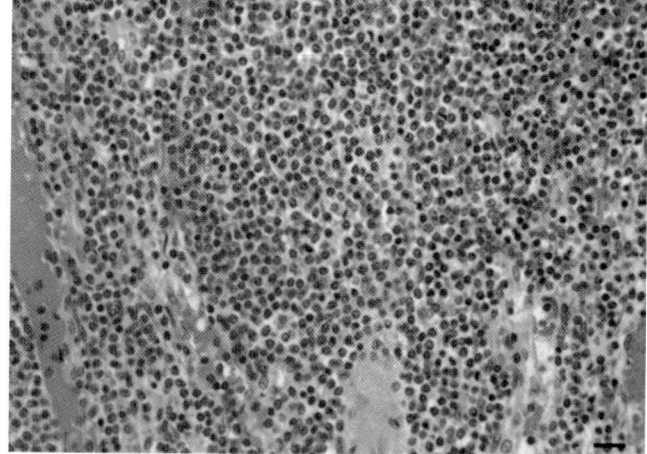

FIGURE 14.12   Monomorphic population of lymphocytes in a case of lymphoma in a ferret.

When choosing a chemoprotocol, different factors should be included in order to provide the best and most practical care. The more rapidly progressive disease encountered in young animals should likely be treated more aggressively than the indolent form commonly seen in adult animals. IV drugs should be administered with great caution through a perfectly placed catheter. Doxorubicin, and to a lesser extent, vincristine extravasation can result in severe tissue sloughing. Oral

TABLE 14.9 Non-Invasive Chemotherapy Protocol for Lymphoma in Ferrets

Week 1	L-asparaginase	10,000 IU/m² SQ
	Cyclophospamide	250 mg/m² PO
	Prednisone	2 mg/kg PO daily for 7 days
Week 2	L-asparaginase	10,000 IU/m² SQ
	CBC	
Week 3	L-asparaginase	10,000 IU/m² SQ
	Cytosar	300 mg/m² SQ × 2 days
Week 4	CBC	
Week 5	Cyclophospamide	250 mg/m² PO
Week 7	Methotrexate	0.8 mg/kg IM
Week 8	CBC	
Week 9	Cyclophospamide	250 mg/m² PO
Week 11	Cytosar	300 mg/m² SQ × 2 days
	Chlorambucil	1 tab/head PO or ½ tab daily for 2 days
Week 12	CBC	
Week 13	Cyclophospamide	250 mg/m² PO
Week 15	Procarbazine	50 mg/m² PO daily for 14 days
Week 16	CBC	
Week 17	CBC	
Week 18	Cyclophospamide	250 mg/m² PO
Week 20	Cytosar	300 mg/m² SQ × 2 days
	Chlorambucil ×2 days	1 tab/head PO or ½ tab daily for 2 days
Week 23	Cyclophospamide	250 mg/m² PO
Week 26	Procarbazine	50 mg/m² PO daily for 14 days
Week 27	CBC, chem.	

If not in remission, continue weeks 20–27 for three cycles

Mayer et al. (2014).
PRED = Prednisone(non) – 2 mg/kg PO daily × 1 week then QOD. L-ASP = L-asparaginase – (non) 10,000 IU/m² SQ. CTX = Cytoxan (mod) – 250 mg/m² PO GIVE WITH 50 ml/kg of LRS once. CYTOSAR = Cytosar (mod) – 300 mg/m² SQ × 2 days (dilute 100 mg with 1 ml saline). MTX = Methotrexate (mild) – 0.8 mg/kg IM. LEUK = Leukeran (mild) – 1 tab/ferret PO (or ½ tablet daily for 2 days). PCB = Procarbazine (mild) – 50 mg/m² PO daily for 14 days. Dose Reductions: if CBC indicates severe myelosuppression, reduce dosage by 25% for next treatment. mod. = moderately myelo-suppressive; mild = mildly myelo-suppressive; non = nonmyelo-suppressive.

TABLE 14.10 Conversion of Bodyweight in kg to Bodysurface in m²

kg	BSA
0.2	0.034
0.3	0.045
0.4	0.054
0.5	0.063
0.6	0.071
0.7	0.079
0.8	0.086
0.9	0.093
1	0.100
1.1	0.107
1.2	0.113
1.3	0.119
1.4	0.125
1.5	0.131
1.6	0.137
1.7	0.142
1.8	0.148
1.9	0.153
2	0.159
2.1	0.164
2.2	0.169
2.3	0.174
2.4	0.179
2.5	0.184
2.6	0.189
2.7	0.194
2.8	0.199
2.9	0.203
3	0.208

(Mayer and Burgess, 2012).

drugs can be compounded by specialty pharmacies for accurate dosing. Remember that chemotherapy administration should always be performed observing rules of maximum safety (e.g., gloves, mask, gown, goggles, dedicated area, closed administration systems, surface decontamination with bleach, etc.). To avoid the risk of extravasation and the need for repeated placement of intravenous catheters, use of a subcutaneous vascular access port (VAP) has been described (Rassnick et al., 1995). However, a surgical procedure is needed for placement of the VAP. One of the authors (JM) has also used radiation to treat lymphoma where chemotherapy was not successful or possible. Different options for radiation include targeted areas such as the lumbar spine for spinal lymphoma, half-body radiation in case of a more disseminated form (e.g., Stage 2 form), or full-body radiation for advanced forms of the disease.

4. Skin Tumors

Mast cell tumors are among the most commonly reported integumentary tumors in ferrets (Parker and Picut, 1993; Li and Fox, 1998). Cutaneous mastocytomas may occur anywhere on the body and present as firm, nodular skin lesions 2–10 mm in size that are often associated with alopecia or crusty ulceration of the overlying skin. Pruritis is common (Stauber et al., 1990). Histologically, they are composed of well-differentiated mast cells with metachromatic cytoplasmic granules that may be difficult to detect in sections stained with hematoxylin–eosin, but are more evident in toluidine blue-stained sections.

A variety of tumors of epithelial origin occur in ferrets, and they can appear at any site on the body. The most common are the basal cell tumors, which present as firm plaques or pedunculated nodules that are white or pink (Parker and Picut, 1993). They may grow rapidly and become ulcerated. The percentage of basiloid cells present in these tumors, and the degree of associated squamous or sebaceous differentiation can vary, resulting in a spectrum of tumor subtypes and associated histological diagnoses (Orcutt, 1997). However, as is the case with mastocytomas, most are benign and will not recur after excision. Resected tumors should be examined histologically to rule out less common tumors that might have a more guarded prognosis, such as squamous cell carcinoma or apocrine gland adenocarcinoma.

Chordomas are not epithelial tumors, but they often present as readily evident firm masses on the tail that may cause ulceration of the overlying skin. These neoplasms arise along the axial skeleton from notochord remnants and are typically slow-growing (Dunn et al., 1991). Tumors involving the tail generally do not recur after amputation of the affected region, but a wide surgical margin should be maintained by removing several vertebrae proximal to the tumor. The prognosis is guarded for those rare chordomas that arise in the cervical region, and metastasis has been documented (Williams et al., 1993). Because of their aggressive nature, extirpation of a chordoma from affected vertebrae is usually not feasible and eventual loss of function and pathologic fracture will result (Antinoff and Williams, 2011).

F. Miscellaneous Diseases

1. Placental–Umbilical Entanglement

Placental–umbilical entanglement may occur in ferrets on the day of parturition and has been associated with fine-particle bedding, large litters, and short kit-birth intervals (Bell, 1997a; Fox et al., 1998a). Jills may neglect to clean placentas from their kits, or kits may be born so rapidly that there is not adequate time for the jill to clean the kits of placental membranes, thereby predisposing to entanglement. Entangled kits may succumb to dehydration, hypothermia, and hypoglycemia because they are unable to nurse and the jill cannot curl around them. Detailed dissection with fine scissors and forceps under a heat lamp or on a heated surface can free the kits. Occasionally, kits may need to be rotated on their umbilical pedicle to achieve adequate clearance to cut the cord; cords should be cut as far from the umbilicus as possible. The use of warm saline or water may help soften the mass. Some kits in the tangle may present with dark, swollen extremities or prolapsed umbilical cords and may require euthanasia. Parturition should be supervised, if possible, to avoid umbilical entanglement.

2. Congenital Lesions

Congenital defects identified in ferrets include a variety of neural tube defects, gastroschisis, cleft palate, amelia, corneal dermoids, cataracts, and supernumerary incisors (Willis and Barrow, 1971; Ryland and Gorham, 1978; McLain et al., 1985; Besch-Williford, 1987). Cystic or polycystic kidneys have been observed (Andrews et al., 1979a; Dillberger, 1985). This has to be differentiated from the common renal cysts that can be seen during an abdominal ultrasound exam in healthy animals (Jackson et al., 2008). Cystic genitourinary anomalies associated with the prostate, bladder, and/or proximal urethra most likely develop secondary to aberrant hormone secretion by adrenocortical tumors (Li et al., 1996a; Coleman et al., 1998). Newborn ferrets are normally born with a closed orbital fissure and are prone to developing subpalpebral conjunctival abscesses. Treatment involves surgically opening the lids (a minor procedure) to establish drainage and to allow topical antibiotics to be administered (Bell, 1997a).

3. Aging and Degenerative Disease

Cardiomyopathy is a common cause of disease in aging ferrets. The dilatative form of the disease is most commonly diagnosed. Affected animals commonly present with lethargy, weight loss, and anorexia. Physical examination may reveal signs of congestive heart failure such as hypothermia, tachycardia, cyanosis, jugular distension, and respiratory distress (Lipman et al., 1987; Heatley, 2011). Auscultation may reveal a heart murmur and/or muffled cardiac sounds. Hepatomegaly and splenomegaly are often identified. Radiographs may reveal an enlarged cardiac silhouette and evidence of pulmonary edema or pleural effusion (Greenlee and Stephens, 1984). Electrocardiography and echocardiography can help make the definitive diagnosis (Malakoff et al., 2012; Wagner, 2009). Medical therapy (supportive care, diuretics, and inotropic drugs) may relieve clinical signs and improve the quality of life for a period of months (Stamoulis et al., 1997). The long-term prognosis for survival is guarded to poor.

Splenomegaly is a common finding in ferrets. In many cases the enlarged spleen appears to be a secondary manifestation of another disease (e.g., insulinoma, cardiomyopathy, or adrenal tumor) and is of unknown significance (Stamoulis *et al.*, 1997). Histologic examination of affected organs has revealed that the most common cause for splenic enlargement (in the absence of a neoplastic infiltrate) is extramedullary hematopoiesis (EMH) (Erdman *et al.*, 1998). This may be an incidental finding, but it has been suggested that in some cases a pathologically enlarged spleen may play a role in chronic anemia that may respond to splenectomy, a syndrome known as hypersplenism (Ferguson, 1985). Splenomegaly can also be commonly found in conjunction with lymphoma, with or without intrasplenic neoplastic lymphoid accumulations. In anesthetized ferrets, splenomegaly may be caused by splenic sequestration of erythrocytes (Marini *et al.*, 1994, 1997). Because this is a transient effect, the normalization of splenic size upon recovery from anesthesia can help in the differentiation of anesthetic-induced splenomegaly from that due to other causes.

Eosinophilic gastroenteritis is an idiopathic disorder characterized by peripheral eosinophilia (sometimes 10–35% of circulating leukocytes), hypoalbuminemia, and diffuse infiltration of the gastrointestinal tract with eosinophils (Fox *et al.*, 1992a). The incidence of the peripherial eosinophilia appears to be variable. Publications include numerous cases of eosinophilic gastroenteritis in which there were no changes in eosinophil concentration in peripheral blood. Presenting signs for this syndrome generally include chronic weight loss, anorexia, diarrhea, and occasionally, vomiting. Eosinophilic granulomas have been found in the mesenteric lymph nodes of most affected ferrets, and in some cases other organs (e.g., lung or liver) may be involved. An interesting finding in many ferrets is the presence in inflamed lymph nodes of Splendore–Hoeppli material, a histological phenomenon that has been associated in other species with helminths, bacteria, fungi, and foreign bodies (Fig. 14.13). An etiological agent has not been identified; consequently, therapy consists largely of supportive care to treat the chronic enteritis (Fox, 1998b). Based on the biology of eosinophils, however, the use of corticosteroids or ivermectin has been attempted and may be beneficial (Bell, 1997b).

Megaesophagus has been diagnosed in ferrets presenting with a variety of signs, including weight loss, anorexia, difficulty in eating, or repeated regurgitation. The cause is generally unknown, and the prognosis is poor, despite efforts at supportive care (Blanco *et al.*, 1994).

Disseminated idiopathic myofasciitis is an emerging ferret disease first described in 2003. It is characterized by inflammation of muscle and surrounding tissue.

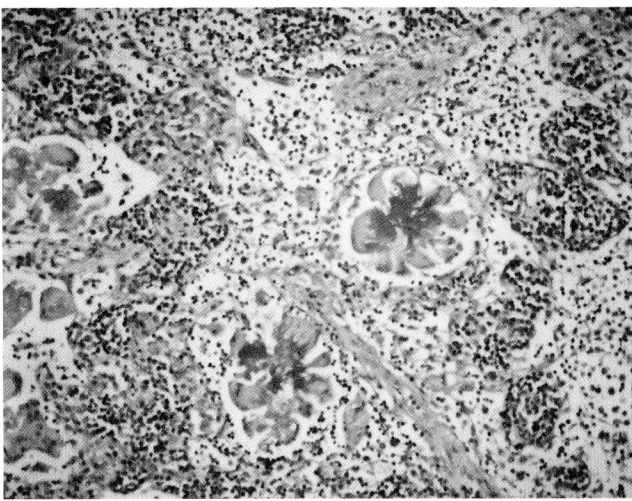

FIGURE 14.13 Splendore–Hoeppli phenomenon in the lymph node of a ferret with eosinophilic gastroenteritis (Giemsa stain).

Ferrets under 18 months are most commonly but not exclusively afftected. Clinical signs include fever, lethargy, depression, paresis, and inappetance. Some animals have lumbosacral or hind limb pain. The clinical course may extend from weeks to months, and progressive disability leads to euthanasia in most cases. Physical examination findings include wasting, muscle atrophy, and sometimes lymphadenopathy and splenomegaly. Hematologic findings can be normal but a mild to marked absolute neuthrophilia can be seen. ALT may be moderately elevated but creatine kinase is not; hypoproteinemia and hypoglobulinemia are somethimes observed. Muscle biopsy from several muscle groups is required for diagnosis.

Necropsy findings depend upon chronicity but can include areas of pallor or white streaks in various muscle groups including the esophagus, diapraghm and both axial and appendicular skeletal muscle. Histologic features are those of muscle fiber atrophy and neutrophilic to pyogranulomatous infiltrate within and around muscle fibers of smooth, cardiac, and skeletal muscle. Necrosis is rare. Transmural and circumferential esophageal infiltrate along the length of the organ is a characteristic lesion. Treatment is supportive; a combination of prednisone, cyclophosphamide, and chloramphenicol may be successful (Ramsell and Garner, 2010).

Gray, yellow, or white small raised lesions may be found on the surface of ferret lungs at gross examination. Histologically, these lesions are composed of a superficial thickening of the lung tissue with mononuclear cell infiltration and varying degrees of fibrosis, with or without cholesterol-like clefts. The etiology of this condition (known as subpleural histiocytosis, pleural lipidosis, or lipid pneumonia) is unknown, and it appears to be an incidental lesion (Fox, 1998f).

Acknowledgment

The authors acknowledge the contributions of the 2nd Edition authors: Glen Otto, Susan Erdman, and Lori Palley.

References

Aasted, B., Alexandersen, S., Hansen, M., 1988. Treatment of neonatally Aleutian disease virus (ADV) infected mink kits with gamma-globulin containing antibodies to ADV reduces the death rate of mink kits. Acta. Vet. Scand. 29 (3–4), 323–330.

Akerman, C.J., Tolhurst, D.J., Morgan, J.E., Baker, G.E., Thompson, I.D., 2003. The relay of visual information to the lateral geniculate nucleus and the visual cortex in albino ferrets. J. Comp. Neurol. 461, 217–235.

Allen, R.P., Evans, E.V., Sibbald, I.R., 1964. Energy: protein relationships in the diets of growing mink. Can. J. Physiol. Pharmacol. 47, 733.

Anderson, E., 1989. The phylogeny of mustelids and the systematics of ferrets. In: Seal, U.S., Thorne, E.T., Bogan, M.A., Anderson, S.H. (Eds.), Conservation Biology and the Black-footed Ferret. Yale Univ. Press, New Haven, CT.

Andrews, P., Illman, O., Mellersh, A., 1979a. Some observations of anatomical abnormalities and disease states in a population of 350 ferrets (Mustela furo). Z. Versuchstierkd. 21, 346–353.

Andrews, P.L., Bower, A.J., Illman, O., 1979b. Some aspects of the physiology and anatomy of the cardiovascular system of the ferret. Mustela Putorius Furo. Lab. Anim. 13, 215–220.

Andrews, P.L.R., Illman, O., 1987. The ferret. In: Poole, T. (Ed.), UFAW Handbook on the Care and Management of Laboratory Animals, sixth ed. Longmans, London.

Antinoff, N., 1997. Musculoskeletal and neurological diseases. In: Hillyer, E.V., Quesenberry, K.E. (Eds.), Ferrets, Rabbits, and Rodents: Clinical Medicine and Surgery. Saunders, Philadelphia, PA, pp. 126–130.

Antinoff, N., Williams, B.H., 2011. Neoplasia. Chapter 8. In: Quesenberry, K., Carpenter, J. (Eds.), Ferrets, Rabbits, and Rodents, third ed. Saunders, St. Louis. MO, pp. 118–119.

Apfelbach, R., 1986. Imprinting on prey odours in ferrets (Mustela putorius F. furo L.) and its neural correlates. Behav. Process. 12 (4), 363–381.

Barron, H.W., Rosenthal, K.L., 2011. Respiratory diseases Chapter 6. In: Quesenberry, K., Carpenter, J. (Eds.), Ferrets, Rabbits, and Rodents, third ed. Saunders, St. Louis. MO, pp. 80–81.

Batchelder, M.A., Bell, J.A., Erdman, S.E., Marini, R.P., Murphy, J.C., Fox, J.G., 1999. Pregnancy toxemia in the European ferret (Mustela putorius furo). Lab. Anim. Sci. 49, 372–379.

Baum, M.J., 1998. Use of the ferret in reproductive neuroendocrinology. In: Fox, J.G. (Ed.), Biology and Diseases of the Ferret. Williams & Wilkins, Baltimore, MD, pp. 521–536.

Baum, M.J., Lynch, H.J., Gallagher, C.A., Deng, M.H., 1986. Plasma and pineal melatonin levels in female ferrets housed under long or short photoperiods. Biol. Reprod. 34 (1), 96–100.

Beck, F., Schion, H., Mould, G., Swidzinska, P., Curry, S., Grauwiler, J., 1976. Comparison of the teratogenic effects of mustine hydrochloride in rats and ferrets. The value of the ferret as an experimental animal in teratology. Teratology 13, 151.

Bell, J.A., 1999. Ferret nutrition. Vet. Clin. North Am. Exot. Anim. Pract. 2, 169–192.

Bell, J.A., 1996. Ensuring proper nutrition in ferrets. Vet. Med. 91, 1098.

Bell, J., 1997a. Periparturient and neonatal diseases. In: Hillyer, E.V., Quesenberry, K.E. (Eds.), Ferrets, Rabbits, and Rodents: Clinical Medicine and Surgery. Saunders, Philadelphia, PA, pp. 58–60.

Bell, J.A., 1997b. Helicobacter mustelae gastritis, proliferative bowel disease, and eosinophilic gastroenteritis. In: Hillyer, E.V., Quesenberry, K.E. (Eds.), Ferrets, Rabbits, and Rodents: Clinical Medicine and Surgery. Saunders, Philadelphia, PA, pp. 37–43.

Bell, J.A., Manning, D.D., 1990a. A domestic ferret model of immunity to Campylobacter jejuni-induced enteric disease. Infect. Immun. 58, 1848–1852.

Bell, J.A., Manning, D.D., 1990b. Reproductive failure in mink and ferrets after intravenous or oral inoculation of Campylobacter jejuni. Can. J. Vet. Res. 54, 432–437.

Bell, J.A., Manning, D.D., 1991. Evaluation of Campylobacter jejuni colonization of the domestic ferret intestine as a model of proliferative colitis. Am. J. Vet. Res. 52, 826–832.

Belser, J.A., Katz, J.M., Tumpey, T.M., 2011. The ferret as a model organism to study influenza A virus infection. Dis. Model Mech. 4, 575–579.

Bernard, S.L., Leathers, C.W., Brobst, D.F., Gorham, J.R., 1983. Estrogen-induced bone marrow depression in ferrets. Am. J. Vet. Res. 44, 657–661.

Bernard, S.L., Gorham, J.R., Ryland, L.M., 1984. Biology and diseases of ferrets. In: Fox, J.G., Cohen, B.J., Loew, F.M. (Eds.), Laboratory Animal Medicine. Academic Press, Orlando, FL, p. 394.

Besch-Williford, C.L., 1987. Biology and medicine of the ferret. Vet. Clin. North Am. Small Anim. Pract. 17, 1155–1183.

Blanco, M.C., Fox, J.G., Rosenthal, K., Hillyer, E.V., Quesenberry, K.E., Murphy, J.C., 1994. Megaesophagus in nine ferrets. J. Am. Vet. Med. Assoc. 205, 444–447.

Blancou, J., Aubert, J.F.A., Artois, M., 1982. Rage experimetale du furet (Mustela putorius furo). Rev. Med. Vet. 133, 553.

Blankenship-Paris, T.L., Chang, J., Bagnell, C.R., 1993. Enteric coccidiosis in a ferret. Lab. Anim. Sci. 43, 361–363.

Bleavins, M.R., Aulerich, R.J., 1981. Feed consumption and food passage time in mink (Mustela vison) and European ferrets (Mustela putorius furo). Lab. Anim. Sci. 31, 268–269.

Bradbury, C., Saunders, A.B., Heatley, J.J., Gregory, C.R., Wilcox, A.L., Russell, K.E., 2010. Transvenous heartworm extraction in a ferret with caval syndrome. J. Am. Anim. Hosp. Assoc. 46 (1), 31–35.

Brown, S.A., 1997a. Basic anatomy, physiology, and husbandry. In: Hillyer, E.V., Quesenberry, K.E. (Eds.), Ferrets, Rabbits, and Rodents: Clinical Medicine and Surgery. Saunders, Philadelphia, PA, pp. 3–13.

Brown, S.A., 1997b. Neoplasia. In: Hillyer, E.V., Quesenberry, K.E. (Eds.), Ferrets, Rabbits, and Rodents: Clinical Medicine and Surgery. Saunders, Philadelphia, PA, pp. 99–114.

Budd, J., 1981. Distemper. In: Davis, J.W., Karstad, L.H., Trainer, D.O. (Eds.), Infectious Diseases of Wild Mammals. Iowa State University Press, Ames, IA.

Burr, D.H., Rollins, D., Lee, L.H., Pattarini, D.L., Walz, S.S., Tian, J.H., et al., 2005. Prevention of disease in ferrets fed an inactivated whole cell Campylobacter jejuni vaccine. Vaccine 23 (34), 4315–4321.

Caplan, E.R., Peterson, M.E., Mullen, H.S., Quesenberry, K.E., Rosenthal, K.L., Hoefer, H.L., et al., 1996. Diagnosis and treatment of insulin-secreting pancreatic islet cell tumors in ferrets: 57 cases (1986–1994). J. Am. Vet. Med. Assoc. 209, 1741–1745.

Carpenter, J.W., Appel, M.J.G., Erickson, R.C., 1976. Fatal vaccine-induced canine distemper virus infection in black-footed ferrets. J. Am. Vet. Med. Assoc. 169, 961–964.

Carroll, R.S., Erskine, M.S., Doherty, P.C., Lundell, L.A., Baum, M.J., 1985. Coital stimuli controlling luteinizing hormone secretion and ovulation in the female ferret. Biol. Reprod. 32, 925–933.

Carroll, R.S., Erskine, M.S., Baum, M.J., 1987. Sex difference in the effect of mating on the pulsatile secretion of luteinizing hormone in a reflex ovulator, the ferret. Endocrinology 121, 1349–1359.

Carter, G.R., Chengapa, M.M., Roberts, A.W., 1995. Campylobacter and Helicobacter Essentials of Veterinary Microbiology, fifth ed. Williams & Wilkins, Baltimore, MD, pp. 214–215.

Chivers, S.M., Einon, D.F., 1982. Effects of early social experience on activity and object investigation in the ferret. Dev. Psychobiol. 15 (1), 75–80.

Clingerman, K.J., Fox, J.G., Walke, M., 1991. Ferrets as Laboratory Animals: A Bibliography. National Agricultural Library, Beltsville, MD.

Coburn, D.R., Morris, J.A., 1949. The treatment of *Salmonella typhimurium* infection in ferrets. Cornell Vet. 39, 183–192.

Coleman, G.D., Chavez, M.A., Williams, B.H., 1998. Cystic prostatic disease associated with adrenocortical lesions in the ferret (*Mustela putorius furo*). Vet. Pathol. 35, 547–549.

Creed, J.E., Kainer, R.A., 1981. Surgical extirpation and related anatomy of anal sacs of the ferret. J. Am. Vet. Med. Assoc. 179, 575–577.

Cross, M.L., Labes, R.E., Mackintosh, C.G., 2000. Oral infection of ferrets with virulent Mycobacterium bovis or *Mycobacterium avium*: susceptibility, pathogenesis and immune response. J. Comp. Pathol. 123 (1), 15–21.

Dalrymple, E.F., 2004. Pregnancy toxemia in a ferret. Can. Vet. J. 45, 150–152.

Davidson, A., Birks, J., Griffiths, H., Kitchener, A., Biggens, D., 1999. Hybridization and the phylogenetic relationship between polecats and the domestic ferret in Britain. Biol. Conserv. 87, 155–161.

de Lisle, G.W., Kawakami, R.P., Yates, G.F., Collins, D.M., 2008. Isolation of *Mycobacterium bovis* and other mycobacterial species from ferrets and stoats. Vet. Microbiol. 132, 402–407.

Desmukh, D.R., 1987. Reye's syndrome. Comp. Pathol. Bull. 19, 2.

Desmukh, D.R., Thomas, P.E., McArthur, M.B., 1985. Serum glutamate-dehydrogenase and ornithine carbamyl transferase in Reye's syndrome. Enzyme 33, 171–174.

Dietz, H.H., Chriél, M., Andersen, T.H., Jørgensen, J.C., Torpdahl, M., Pedersen, H., et al., 2006. Outbreak of *Salmonella* Dublin-associated abortion in Danish fur farms. Can. Vet. J. 47 (12), 1201–1205.

Dillberger, J.E., 1985. Polycystic kidneys in a ferret. J. Am. Vet. Med. Assoc. 186, 74–75.

Dinsdale, J.R., Rest, J.R., 1995. Yeast infection in ferrets [letter]. Vet. Rec. 16, 647.

Dunn, D.G., Harris, R.K., Meis, J.M., Sweet, D.E., 1991. A histomorphologic and immunohistochemical study of chordoma in 20 ferrets (*Mustela putorius furo*). Vet. Pathol. 28, 467–473.

Ehrhart, N., Withrow, S.J., Ehrhart, E.J., Wimsatt, J.H., 1996. Pancreatic beta cell tumor in ferrets: 20 cases (1986–1994). J. Am. Vet. Med. Assoc. 209, 1737–1740.

Erdman, S.E., Reimann, K.A., Moore, F.M., Kanki, P.J., Yu, Q.C., Fox, J.G., 1995. Transmission of a chronic lymphoproliferative syndrome in ferrets. Lab. Invest. 72, 539–546.

Erdman, S.E., Brown, S.A., Kawasaki, T.A., Moore, F.M., Li, X., Fox, J.G., 1996a. Clinical and pathogic findings in ferrets with lymphoma: 60 cases (1982–1994). J. Am. Vet. Med. Assoc. 208, 1285–1289.

Erdman, S.E., Kanki, P.J., Moore, F.M., Brown, S.A., Kawasaki, T.A., Mikule, K.W., et al., 1996b. Clusters of malignant lymphoma in ferrets. Cancer Invest. 14, 225–230.

Erdman, S.E., Correa, P., Li, X., Coleman, L.A., Fox, J.G., 1997. *Helicobacter mustelae*-associated gastric mucosa associated lymphoid tissue (MALT) lymphoma in ferrets. Am. J. Pathol. 151, 273–280.

Erdman, S.E., Li, X., Fox, J.G., 1998. Hematopoietic diseases. In: Fox, J.G. (Ed.), Biology and Diseases of the Ferret, second ed. Williams & Wilkins, Baltimore, MD, pp. 231–246.

Eshar, D., Wyre, N.R., Brown, D.C., 2012. Urine specific gravity values in clinically healthy young pet ferrets (*Mustela furo*). J. Small Anim. Pract. 53 (2), 115–119.

Evans, H.E., An, N.Q., 1998. Anatomy of the ferret. In: Fox, J.G. (Ed.), Biology and Diseases of the Ferret. Williams & Wilkins, Baltimore, MD, pp. 19–69.

Fekete, S. Gy., Fodor, K., Proháczik, A., Andrásofszky, E., 2005. Comparison of feed preference and digestion of three different commercial diets for cats and ferrets. J. Anim. Physiol. Anim. Nutr. 89, 199–202.

Ferguson, D.C., 1985. Idiopathic hypersplenism in a ferret. J. Am. Vet. Med. Assoc. 186, 693–695.

Field and Laboratory Service Veterinary Staff, 1984. Diseases of the fitch. Surveillance 11, 18.

Fisher, M., Beck, W., Hutchinson, M.J., 2007. Efficacy and safety of selamectin (Stronghold®/Revolution™) used off-label in exotic pets. Intern. J. Appl. Res. Vet. Med. 5 (3)., 87–96.

Forester, N.T., Parton, K., Lumsden, J.S., O'Toole, P.W., 2000. Isolation of *Helicobacter mustelae* from ferrets in New Zealand. N. Z. Vet. J. 48, 65–69.

Fox, J.G., 1998a. Bacterial and mycoplasma diseases. In: Fox, J.G. (Ed.), Biology and Diseases of the Ferret, second ed. Williams & Wilkins, Baltimore, MD, pp. 321–354.

Fox, J.G., 1998b. Diseases of the gastrointestinal system. In: Fox, J.G. (Ed.), Biology and Diseases of the Ferret, second ed. Williams & Wilkins, Baltimore, MD, pp. 273–290.

Fox, J.G., 1998c. Housing and management. In: Fox, J.G. (Ed.), Biology and Diseases of the Ferret, second ed. Williams & Wilkins, Baltimore, MD, pp. 173–182.

Fox, J.G., 1998d. Mycotic diseases. In: Fox, J.G. (Ed.), Biology and Diseases of the Ferret, second ed. Williams & Wilkins, Baltimore, MD, pp. 393–404.

Fox, J.G., 1998e. Normal clinical and biologic parameters. In: Fox, J.G. (Ed.), Biology and Diseases of the Ferret, second ed. Williams & Wilkins, Baltimore, MD, pp. 183–210.

Fox, J.G., 1998f. Other systemic diseases. In: Fox, J.G. (Ed.), Biology and Diseases of the Ferret, second ed. Williams & Wilkins, Baltimore, MD, pp. 307–320.

Fox, J.G., 1998g. Parasitic diseases. In: Fox, J.G. (Ed.), Biology and Diseases of the Ferret, second ed. Williams & Wilkins, Baltimore, MD, pp. 375–392.

Fox, J.G., Bell, J.A., 1998. Growth, reproduction, and breeding. In: Fox, J.G. (Ed.), Biology and Diseases of the Ferret, second ed. Williams & Wilkins, Baltimore, MD, pp. 211–227.

Fox, J.G., Marini, R.P., 1998. Diseases of the endocrine system. In: Fox, J.G. (Ed.), Biology and Diseases of the Ferret, second ed. Williams & Wilkins, Baltimore, MD, pp. 291–305.

Fox, J.G., McLain, D.E., 1998. Nutrition. In: Fox, J.G. (Ed.), Biology and Diseases of the Ferret, second ed. Williams & Wilkins, Baltimore, MD, pp. 149–172.

Fox, J.G., Murphy, J.C., Ackerman, J.I., Prostak, K.S., Gallagher, C.A., Rambow, V.J., 1982. Proliferative colitis in ferrets. Am. J. Vet. Res. 43, 858–864.

Fox, J.G., Ackerman, J., Newcomer, C.E., 1983. Ferret as a potential reservoir for human campylobacteriosis. Am. J. Vet. Res. 44, 1049–1052.

Fox, J.G., Edrise, B.M., Cabot, E., Beaucage, C., Murphy, J.C., Prostak, K.S., 1986a. *Campylobacter*-like organisms isolated from gastric mucosa of ferrets. Am. J. Vet. Res. 47, 236–239.

Fox, J.G., Hotaling, L., Ackerman, J.B., Hewes, K., 1986b. Serum chemistry and hematology reference values in the ferret (*Mustela putorius furo*). Lab. Anim. Sci. 36, 583.

Fox, J.G., Ackerman, J.I., Taylor, N., Claps, M., Murphy, J.C., 1987. *Campylobacter jejuni* infection in the ferret: an animal model of human campylobacteriosis. Am. J. Vet. Res. 48, 85–90.

Fox, J.G., Adkins, J.A., Maxwell, K.O., 1988a. Zoonoses in ferrets. Lab. Anim. Sci. 38, 500. (Abstract).

Fox, J.G., Cabot, E.B., Taylor, N.S., Laraway, R., 1988b. Gastric colonization of *Campylobacter pylori* subsp. *mustelae* in ferrets. Infect. Immun. 56, 2994–2996.

Fox, J.G., Chilvers, T., Goodwin, C.S., Taylor, N.S., Edmonds, P., Sly, L.I., et al., 1989a. *Campylobacter mustelae*, a new species resulting from the elevation of *Campylobacter pylori* subsp. *mustelae* to species status. Int. J. Syst. Bacteriol. 39, 301–303.

Fox, J.G., Murphy, J.C., Otto, G., Pecquet-Goad, M.E., Lawson, G.H.K., Scott, J.A., 1989b. Proliferative colitis in ferrets: epithelial dysplasia and translocation. Vet. Pathol. 26, 515–517.

Fox, J.G., Correa, P., Taylor, N.S., Lee, A., Otto, G., Murphy, J.C., et al., 1990. *Helicobacter mustelae*-associated gastritis in ferrets: an animal model of *Helicobacter pylori* gastritis in humans. Gastroenterology 99, 352–361.

Fox, J.G., Otto, G., Murphy, J.C., Taylor, N.S., Lee, A., 1991a. Gastric colonization of the ferret with *Helicobacter* species: natural and experimental infections. Rev. Infect. Dis. 13, S671–S680.

Fox, J.G., Otto, G., Taylor, N.S., Rosenblad, W., Murphy, J.C., 1991b. *Helicobacter mustelae*-induced gastritis and elevated gastric pH in the ferret (*Mustela putorius furo*). Infect. Immun. 59, 1875–1880.

Fox, J.G., Palley, L.S., Rose, R., 1992a. Eosinophilic gastroenteritis with Splendore–Hoeppli material in the ferret (*Mustela putorius furo*). Vet. Pathol. 29, 21–26.

Fox, J.G., Paster, B.J., Dewhirst, F.E., Taylor, N.S., Yan, L.-L., Macuch, P.J., et al., 1992b. *Helicobacter mustelae* isolation from feces of ferrets: evidence to support fecal–oral transmission of a gastric *Helicobacter*. Infect. Immun. 60, 606–611.

Fox, J.G., Blanco, M., Yan, L., Shames, B., Polidoro, D., Dewhirst, F.E., et al., 1993. Role of gastric pH in isolation of *Helicobacter mustelae* from the feces of ferrets. Gastroenterology 104, 86–92.

Fox, J.G., Andrutis, K., Yu, J., 1994. Animal models for *Helicobacter*-induced gastric and hepatic cancer. In: Hunt, R.H., Tytgat, G.N.J. (Eds.), Helicobacter Pylori: Basic Mechanisms to Clinical Cure. Kluwer Academic Publ., Dordrecht, Holland, pp. 504–522.

Fox, J.G., Dangler, C.A., Sager, W., Borkowski, R., Gliatto, J.M., 1997. *Helicobacter mustelae*-associated gastric adenocarcinoma in ferrets (*Mustela putorius furo*). Vet. Pathol. 34, 225–229.

Fox, J.G., Pearson, R.C., Bell, J.A., 1998a. Diseases of the genitourinary system. In: Fox, J.G. (Ed.), Biology and Diseases of the Ferret, second ed. Williams & Wilkins, Baltimore, MD, pp. 247–272.

Fox, J.G., Pearson, R.C., Gorham, J.R., 1998b. Viral diseases. In: Fox, J.G. (Ed.), Biology and Diseases of the Ferret, second ed. Williams & Wilkins, Baltimore, MD, pp. 355–374.

Frederick, K.A., Babish, J.G., 1985. Compendium of recent literature on the ferret. Lab. Anim. Sci. 35, 298–318.

Garcia, A., Erdman, S.E., Xu, S., Feng, Y., Rogers, A.B., et al., 2002. Hepatobiliary inflammation, neoplasia, and argyrophilic bacteria in a ferret colony. Vet. Pathol. 39, 173–179.

Garner, M.M., Ramsell, K., Morera, N., Juan-Salles, C., Jimenez, J., Ardiaca, M., et al., 2008. Clinicopathologic features of a systemic coronavirus-associated disease resembling feline infectious peritonitis in the domestic ferret (*Mustela putorius*). Vet. Pathol. 45, 236–246.

Gigliotti, F., Harmsen, A.G., Haidaris, C.G., Haidaris, P.J., 1993. *Pneumocystis carinii* is not universally transmissible between mammalian species. Infect. Immun. 61, 2886–2890.

Gómez-Villamandos, J.C., et al., 1995. Fatal cryptosporidiosis in ferrets (*Mustela putorius furo*): a morphopathologic study. J. Zoo. Wildl. Med. 26 (4), 539.

Gorham, H.R. and Brandly, C.A., 1953. The transmission of distemper among ferrets and mink. Paper presented at the 90th Meeting of the American Veterinary Medical Association.

Gorham, J.R., Gordy, D.R., Quortrup, E.R., 1949. *Salmonella* infections in mink and ferrets. Am. J. Vet. Res. 10, 183–192.

Gorham, J.R., Leader, R.W., Henson, K.B., 1964. The experimental transmission of a virus causing hypergammagloblinemia in mink: sources and modes in infection. J. Infect. Dis. 114, 341.

Greenlee, P.G., Stephens, E., 1984. Meningeal cryptococcosis and congestive cardiomyopathy in a ferret. J. Am. Vet. Med. Assoc. 184, 840–841.

Haas, L., Lochelt, M., Kaaden, O.R., 1988. Detection of Aleutian disease virus DNA in tissues of naturally infected mink. J. Gen. Virol. 69, 705–710.

Hahn, E.W., Wester, R.C., 1969. The Biomedical Use of Ferrets in Research. Marshall Farms Animals, North Rose, New York.

Hamir, A.N., Niezgoda, M., Rupprecht, C.E., 2011. Recovery from and clearance of rabies virus in a domestic ferret. J. Am. Assoc. Lab. Anim. Sci. 50 (2), 248–251.

Hammond, J., Chesterman, F.C., 1972. The ferret. In: UFAW, The Universities Federation for Animal Welfare Handbook on the Care and Management of Laboratory Animals, fifth ed. Churchill Livingstone, London.

Hanley, C.S., MacWilliams, P., Giles, S., Paré, J., 2006. Diagnosis and successful treatment of *Cryptococcus neoformans* variety *grubii* in a domestic ferret. Can. Vet. J. 47 (10), 1015–1017.

Hart, J.E., 1985. Endocrine factors in hematological changes seen in dogs and ferrets given estrogens. Med. Hypotheses 16, 159–163.

Heatley, J.J., 2011. Ferret cardiomyopathy. Compen. Stand. Care Emerg. Crit. Care Med. 8, 7–11.

Hebeler, D., Wolf, P., 2001. Fütterung von Frettchen in der Heimtierhaltung. Kleintierpraxis 46, 225.

Hein J., Spreyer F., Sauter-Louis C., Hartmann K., 2012. Veterinary Record 10.1136/vr.100628

Hill, S.L., Lappin, M.R., 1995. Cryptosporidiosis in the dog and cat. In: Bonagura, J.D., Kirk, R.W. (Eds.), Kirk's Current Veterinary Therapy. Saunders, Philadelphia, PA, pp. 728–731.

Hillyer, E.V., Quesenberry, K.E., 1997a. Dematologic diseases. In: Hillyer, E.V., Quesenberry, K.E. (Eds.), Ferrets, Rabbits, and Rodents: Clinical Medicine and Surgery. Saunders, Philadelphia, PA, pp. 119–120.

Hillyer, E.V., Quesenberry, K.E. (Eds.), 1997b. Ferrets, Rabbits, and Rodents: Clinical Medicine and Surgery. Saunders, Philadelphia, PA.

Hoffmann, K.-P., Garipis, N., Distler, C., 2004. Optokinetic deficits in albino ferrets (Mustela putorius furo): a behavioural and electrophysiological study. J. Neurosci. 24, 4061–4069.

Hoppmann, E., Barron, H.W., 2007. Ferret and rabbit dermatology. J. Exot. Pet. Med. 16 (4), 225–237.

Howard, J., Marinari, P.E., Wildt, D.E., 2003. Black-footed ferret: model for assisted reproductive technologies contributing to in situ conservation. In: Holt, W.V., Pickard, A., Rodger, J.C., Wildt, D.E. (Eds.), Reproductive Sciences and Integrated Conservation. Cambridge University Press, Cambridge, pp. 249–266.

Hupfeld, D., Distler, C., Hoffmann, K.-P., 2006. Motion perception deficits in albino ferrets (Mustela putorius furo). Vision Res. 46 (18), 2941–2948.

Hutchinson, M.J., Jacobs, D.E., Mencke, N., 2001. Establishment of the cat flea (*Ctenocephalides felis felis*) on the ferret (*Mustela putorius furo*) and its control with imidacloprid. Med. Vet. Entomol. 15 (2), 212–214.

Jackson, C.N., Rogers, A.B., Maurer, K.J., Lofgren, J.L.S., Fox, J.G., Marini, R.P., 2008. Cystic renal disease in the domestic ferret. Comp. Med. 58, 161–167.

Jenkins, J.R., 2000. Ferret metabolic testing. In: Fudge, A.M. (Ed.), Laboratory Medicine: Avian and Exotic Pets. WB Saunders, Philadelphia, PA, pp. 305–309.

Jenkins, J.R., Brown, S.A., 1993. A Practitioner's Guide to Rabbits and Ferrets. American Animal Hospital Association, Lakewood, CO.

Jones, J.W., Pether, J.V.S., Rainey, H.A., Swinburn, C.R., 1993. Recurrent *Mycobacterium bovis* infection following a ferret bite [letter]. J. Infect. 26, 225–226.

Kamphues, J., Schneider, D., Leibetseder, J., 1999. Frettchen Supplemente zu Vorlesungen und Übungen in der Tierernährung. M & H Schaper, Alfeld-Hannover, 262 pp.

Kauffman, C.A., 1981. Cell mediated immunity in ferrets: delayed dermal hypersensitivity, lymphocyte transformation, and macrophage migration inhibitory factor production. Dev. Comp. Immunol. 5, 125–134.

Kendrick, R.E., 2000. Ferret respiratory diseases. Vet. Clin. North Am. Exot. Anim. Pract. 2, 453–464.

Kenyon, A.J., Helmboldt, C.F., Nielson, S.W., 1963. Experimental transmission of Aleutian disease with urine. Am. J. Vet. Res. 24, 1066.

Kidder, J.D., Foote, R.H., Richmond, M.E., 1998. Transcervical artificial insemination in the domestic ferret (Mustela putorius furo). Zoo Biol. 17, 393–404.

Kim, Y., Chongviriyaphan, N., Liu, C., Russell, R.M., Wang, X.D., 2006a. Combined antioxidant (beta-carotene, alpha-tocopherol and ascorbic acid) supplementation increases the levels of lung retinoic acid and inhibits the activation of mitogen-activated protein kinase in the ferret lung cancer model. Carcinogenesis 27 (7), 1410–1419.

Kim, Y., Liu, X.S., Liu, C., Smith, D.E., Russell, R.M., Wang, X.D., 2006b. Induction of pulmonary neoplasia in the smoke-exposed ferret by 4-(methylnitrosamino)-1-(3-pyridyl)-1-butanone (NNK): a model for human lung cancer. Cancer Lett., 209–219.

Kim, Y., Chongviriyaphan, N., Liu, C., Russell, R.M., Wang, X.D., 2012. Combined alpha-tocopherol and ascorbic acid protects against smoke-induced lung squamous metaplasia in ferrets. Lung Cancer 75 (1), 15–23.

Kirkpatrick, C.E., Dubey, J.P., 1987. Enteric coccidial infections. Vet. Clin. North Am. Small Anim. Pract. 17, 1414–1416.

Kiupel, M., Desjardins, D.R., Lim, A., Bolin, C., Johnson-Delaney, C.A., Resau, J.H., et al., 2012. Mycoplasmosis in Ferrets. Emerg. Infect. Dis. 18 (11), 1763–1770.

Knight, D., 1987. Heartworm infections. Vet. Clin. North Am. Small Anim. Pract. 17, 1463–1518.

Korhonen, H., 1995 1995. The effects of environmental enrichment in ferrets. In: Smith, C.P., Taylor, V. (Eds.), Environmental Enrichment Information Resources for Laboratory Animals: 1965–1995: Birds, Cats, Dogs, Farm Animals, Ferrets, Rabbits, and Rodents. U.S. Department of Agriculture, Beltsville, MD. AWIV Resource Series No. 2. In: Smith, C.P., Taylor, V. (Eds.), Environmental Enrichment Information Resources for Laboratory Animals: 1965–1995: Birds, Cats, Dogs, Farm Animals, Ferrets, Rabbits, and Rodents. U.S. Department of Agriculture, Beltsville, MD.

Krueger, K.L., Murphy, J.C., Fox, J.G., 1989. Treatment of proliferative colitis in ferrets. J. Am. Vet. Med. Assoc. 194, 1435–1436.

Kwochka, K.W., 1986. Canine demodicosis. In: Kirk, R. (Ed.), Current Veterinary Therapy 11. Saunders, Philadelphia, PA, pp. 531–537.

Lee, E.J., Moore, W.E., Fryer, H.C., Minocha, H.C., 1982. Haematological and serum chemistry profiles of ferrets (Mustela putorius furo). Lab. Anim. 16, 133–137.

Le Sueur, C., Bour, S., Schaper, R., 2011. Efficacy and Safety of the Combination Imidacloprid 10 % / moxidectin 1.0 % Spot-on (Advocate® Spot-on for Small Cats and Ferrets) in the Treatment of Ear Mite Infection (Otodectes cynotis) in Ferrets. Parasitol. Res. 109 (1 Suppl), 149–156.

Li, X., Fox, J.G., 1998. Neoplastic diseases. In: Fox, J.G. (Ed.), Biology and Diseases of the Ferret, second ed. Williams & Wilkins, Baltimore, MD, pp. 405–448.

Li, X., Fox, J.G., Erdman, S.E., Aspros, D.G., 1995. Cutaneous lymphoma in a ferret (Mustela putorius furo). Vet. Pathol. 32, 55–56.

Li, X., Fox, J.G., Erdman, S.E., Lipman, N.S., Murphy, J.C., 1996a. Cystic urogenital anomalies in the ferret (Mustela putorius furo). Vet. Pathol. 33, 150–158.

Li, X., Pang, J., Fox, J.G., 1996b. Coinfection with intracellular Desulfovibrio species and coccidia in ferrets with proliferative bowel disease. Lab. Anim. Sci. 46, 569–571.

Li, X., Fox, J.G., Padrid, P.A., 1998. Neoplastic diseases in ferrets: 574 cases (1968–1997). J. Am. Vet. Med. Assoc. 212, 1402–1406.

Liberson, A.J., Newcomer, C.E., Ackerman, J.I., Murphy, J.C., Fox, J.G., 1983. Mastitis caused by hemolytic Escherichia coli in the ferret. J. Am. Vet. Med. Assoc. 183, 1179–1181.

Lipman, N.S., Murphy, J.C., Fox, J.G., 1987. Clinical, functional, and pathologic changes associated with a case of dilatative cardiomyopathy in a ferret. Lab. Anim. Sci. 37, 210–212.

Lipman, N.S., Marini, R.P., Murphy, J.C., Zhibo, Z., Fox, J.G., 1993. Estradiol-17β-secreting adrenocortical tumor in a ferret. J. Am. Vet. Med. Assoc. 203, 1552–1555.

Liu, C., Coffin, D.L., 1957. Studies on canine distemper infection by means of fluorescein-labeled antibody. 1. The pathogenesis, pathology, and diagnosis of the disease in experimentally infected ferrets. Virology 3, 115.

Loeb, W., Quimby, F. (Eds.), 1999. The Clinical Chemistry of Laboratory Animals. Taylor and Francis, Philadelphia, PA.

Lucas, J., Lucas, A., Furber, H., et al., 2000. Mycobacterium genavense infection in two aged ferrets with conjunctival lesions. Aust. Vet. J. 78, 685–689.

Ludlow, M., Nguyen, D.T., Silin, D., Lyubomska, O., de Vries, R.D., von Messling, V., et al., 2012. Recombinant canine distemper virus strain snyder hill expressing green or red fluorescent proteins causes meningoencephalitis in the ferret. J. Virol. 86 (14), 7508–7519.

Ludwig, E., Reischl, U., Holzmann, T., Melzl, H., Janik, D., Gilch, C., et al., 2011. Risk for Mycobacterium celatum infection from ferret. Emerg. Infect. Dis. 17 (3), 553–555.

Lugton, I.W., Wobeser, G., Morris, R.S., Caley, P., 1997. Epidemiology of Mycobacterium bovis infection in feral ferrets (Mustela furo) in New Zealand: II. Routes of infection and excretion. N. Z. Vet. J. 45 (4), 151–157.

Lunn, J.A., Martin, P., Zaki, S., et al., 2005. Pneumonia due to Mycobacterium abscessus in two domestic ferrets (Mustela putorius furo). Aust. Vet. J. 83, 542–546.

Malakoff, R.L., Laste, N.J., Orcutt, C.J., 2012. Echocardiographic and electrocardiographic findings in client-owned ferrets: 95 cases (1994–2009). J. Am. Vet. Med. Assoc. 241, 1484–1489.

Manning, D., Bell, J.A., 1990a. Derivation of gnotobiotic ferrets: perinatal diet and hand-rearing requirements. Lab. Anim. Sci. 40, 51–55.

Manning, D.D., Bell, J.A., 1990b. Lack of detectable blood groups in domestic ferrets: implications for transfusion. J. Am. Vet. Med. Assoc. 197, 84–86.

Marini, R.P., Jackson, L.R., Esteves, M.I., Andrutis, K.A., Goslant, G.M., Fox, J.G., 1994. The effect of isoflurane on hematologic variables in ferrets. Am. J. Vet. Res. 55, 1479–1483.

Marini, R.P., Callahan, R.J., Jackson, L.R., Jyawook, S., Esteves, M.I., Fox, J.G., et al., 1997. Distribution of technetium 99m-labeled red blood cells during isoflurane anesthesia in ferrets. Am. J. Vet. Res. 58, 781–785.

Marini, R.P., Fox, J.G., Taylor, N.S., Yan, L., McColm, A., Williamson, R., 1999. Ranitidine-bismuth citrate and clarithromycin, alone or in combination, for eradication of Helicobacter mustelae infection in ferrets. Am. J. Vet. Res. 60, 1280–1286.

Marini, R.P., Taylor, N.S., Liang, A.Y., Knox, K.A., Pena, J.A., et al., 2004. Characterization of hemolytic Escherichia coli strains in ferrets: recognition of candidate virulence factor CNF1. J. Clin. Microbiol. 42, 5904–5908.

Marshall, K.R., Marshall, G.W., 1973. The Biomedical Use of Ferrets in Research. Marshall Farms Animals, North Rose, New York.

Martinez, J., Ramis, A.J., Reinacher, M., Perpiñán, D., 2006. Detection of feline infectious peritonitis virus-like antigen in ferrets. Vet. Rec. 158, 523.

Martínez, J., Martorell, J., Abarca, M.L., Olvera, A., Ramis, A., Woods, L., et al., 2012. Pyogranulomatous pleuropneumonia and mediastinitis in ferrets (Mustela putorius furo) associated with Pseudomonas luteola infection. J. Comp. Pathol. 146, 4–10.

Mayer, J., Burgess, K., 2012. An update on ferret lymphoma: a proposal for a standardized classification of ferret lymphoma. J. Exot. Pet. Med. 21, 123–125.

Mayer, J., Wagner, R., Mitchell, M.A., Fecteau, K., 2013. Use of recombinant human thyroid-stimulating hormone for thyrotropin stimulation test in euthyroid ferrets. J. Am. Vet. Med. Assoc. 243 (10).

McCullers, J.A., McAuley, J.L., Browall, S., Iverson, A.R., Boyd, K.L., et al., 2010. Influenza enhances susceptibility to natural acquisition of and disease due to *Streptococcus pneumoniae* in ferrets. J. Infect. Dis. 202, 1287–1295.

McLain, D.E., Harper, S.M., Roe, D.A., Babish, J.G., Wilkinson, C., 1985. Congenital malformations and variations in reproductive performance in the ferret: effects of maternal age, color, and parity. Lab. Anim. Sci. 35, 251–255.

Miller, W.R., Merton, D.A., 1982. Dirofilariasis in a ferret. J. Am. Vet. Med. Assoc. 180, 1103–1104.

Miller, D.S., Eagle, R.P., Zabel, S., Rosychuk, R., Campbell, T.W., 2006. Efficacy and safety of selamectin in the treatment of *Otodectes cynotis* infestation in domestic ferrets. Vet. Rec. 159, 748. http://dx.doi.org/10.1136/vr.159.22.748

Miller, L.A., Fagerstone, K.A., Wagner, R.A., Finkler, M., 2013. Use of a GnRH vaccine, GonaConTM, for prevention and treatment of adrenocortical disease (ACD) in domestic ferrets. Vaccine 31 (41), 4619–4623.

Mitchell, M., 2008. Ponazuril. J. Exot. Pet Med. 17 (3), 228–229.

Moore, D.R., 1982. Late onset of hearing in the ferret. Brain Res. 235 (1–2), 309–311.

Moore, G.E., Glickman, N.W., Ward, M.P., Engler, K.S., Lewis, H.B., et al., 2005. Incidence of and risk factors for adverse events associated with distemper and rabies vaccine administration in ferrets. J. Am. Vet. Med. Assoc. 226, 909–912.

Moore, D.R., Kowalchuk, N.E., 1988. Auditory brainstem of the ferret: Effects of unilateral cochlear lesions on cochlear nucleus volume and projections to the inferior colliculus. J. Comp. Neurol. 272, 503–515.

Moreland, A.F., Battles, A.H., Nease, J.H., 1986. Dirofilariasis in a ferret. J. Am. Vet. Med. Assoc. 188, 864.

Morgan, J.P., Travers, K.E., 1998. Use of the ferret in cardiovascular research. In: Fox, J.G. (Ed.), Biology and Diseases of the Ferret, second ed. Williams & Wilkins, Baltimore, MD, pp. 499–510.

Morrisey, J.K., Kraus, M.S., 2011. Cardiovascular and other diseases Chapter 5. In: Quesenberry, K., Carpenter, J. (Eds.), Ferrets, Rabbits, and Rodents, third ed. Saunders, St. Louis. MO, pp. 71–73.

Morrow, D.A., 1980. Current Therapy in Theriogenology. Saunders, Philadelphia, PA.

Mullen, H., 1997. Soft tissue surgery. In: Hillyer, E.V., Quesenberry, K.E. (Eds.), Ferrets, Rabbits, and Rodents: Clinical Medicine and Surgery. Saunders, Philadelphia, PA, pp. 131–144.

Murray, J., Kiupel, M., Maes, R.K., 2010. Ferret coronavirus-associated diseases. Vet. Clin. North Am. Exot. Anim. Pract. 13, 543–560.

Naismith, D.J., Cursiter, M.C., 1972. Is there a specific requirement for carbohydrate in the diet? In: Proceedings of the Nutrition Society 31, 94A.

Nemelka, K.W., Brown, A.W., Wallace, S.M., Jones, E., Asher, L.V., Pattarini, D., et al., 2009. Immune response to and histopathology of Campylobacter jejuni infection in ferrets (*Mustela putorius furo*). Comp. Med. 59 (4), 363–371.

Niezgoda, M., Briggs, D.J., Shadduck, J., et al., 1998. Viral excretion in domestic ferrets (*Mustela putorius furo*) inoculated with a raccoon rabies isolate. Am. J. Vet. Res. 59, 1629–1632.

Noli, C., van der Horst, H., Wjillemse, T., 1996. Demodiciasis in ferrets (*Mustela putorius furo*). Vet. Q. 18, 28–31.

Norrby, E., Oxman, M.N., 1990. Measles virus. In: Fields, B.N., Knipe, D.M., Chanock, R.M. (Eds.), Fields Virology. Raven Press, New York, pp. 1013–1044.

Nowak, R.M., 1999. Walker's Mammals of the World, sixth ed. Johns Hopkins Univ. Press, Baltimore.

O'Donnell, C.D., Subbarao, K., 2011. The contribution of animal models to the understanding of the host range and virulence of influenza A viruses. Microbes Infect. 13 (5), 502–515.

Ohshima, K., Shen, D.T., Henson, J.B., Gorham, J.R., 1978. Comparison of the lesions of Aleutian disease in mink and hypergammaglobulinemia in ferrets. Am. J. Vet. Res. 39, 653–657.

Orcutt, C., 1997. Dermatologic diseases. In: Hillyer, E.V., Quesenberry, K.E. (Eds.), Ferrets, Rabbits, and Rodents: Clinical Medicine and Surgery. Saunders, Philadelphia, PA, pp. 115–125.

O'Toole, P.W., Snelling, W.J., Canchaya, C., Forde, B.M., Hardie, K.R., et al., 2010. Comparative genomics and proteomics of *Helicobacter mustelae*, an ulcerogenic and carcinogenic gastric pathogen. BMC Genomics 11, 164.

Otto, G., Fox, J.G., Wu, P.-Y., Taylor, N.S., 1990. Eradication of *Helicobacter mustelae* from the ferret stomach: an animal model of *Helicobacter* (*Campylobacter*) *pylori* chemotherapy. Antimicrob. Agents Chemother. 34, 1232–1236.

Oxenham, M., 1990. Aleutian disease in the ferret. Vet. Rec. 126, 585.

Palley, L.S., Corning, B.F., Fox, J.G., Murphy, J.C., Gould, D.H., 1992. Parvovirus-associated syndrome (Aleutian disease) in two ferrets. J. Am. Vet. Med. Assoc. 201, 100–106.

Parker, G.A., Picut, C.A., 1993. Histopathologic features and postsurgical sequelae of 57 cutaneous neoplasms in ferrets (*Mustela putorius furo* L.). Vet. Pathol. 30, 499–504.

Parrott, T.Y., Greiner, E.C., Parrott, J.D., 1984. *Dirofilaria immitis* in three ferrets. J. Am. Vet. Med. Assoc. 184, 582–583.

Patterson, M.M., Kirchain, S.M., Whary, M.T., 1999. Clinical trial to control ear mites in a ferret colony. Lab. Anim. Sci. 49, 437.

Patterson, M.M., Rogers, A.B., Schrenzel, M.D., Marini, R.P., Fox, J.G., 2003. Alopecia attributed to neoplastic ovarian tissue in two ferrets. Comp. Med. 53, 213–217.

Peltola, V.T., Boyd, K.L., McAuley, J.L., Rehg, J.E., McCullers, J.A., 2006. Bacterial sinusitis and otitis media following influenza virus infection in ferrets. Infect. Immun. 74, 2562–2567.

Pennick, K.E., Stevenson, M.A.M., Latimer, K.S., Ritchie, B.W., Gregory, C.R., 2005. Persistent viral shedding during asymptomatic Aleutian mink disease parvoviral infection in a ferret. J. Vet. Diagn. Invest. 17, 594–597.

Perpiñán, D., López, C., 2008. Clinical aspects of systemic granulomatous inflammatory syndrome in ferrets (*Mustela putorius furo*). Vet. Rec. 162, 180–184.

Perpiñán, D., Ramis, A., Tomás, A., Carpintero, E., Bargalló, F., 2008. Outbreak of canine distemper in domestic ferrets (*Mustela putorius furo*). Vet. Rec. 163, 248–252.

Peter, A.T., Bell, J.A., Manning, D.D., Bosu, W.T., 1990. Real-time ultrasonography determination of pregnancy and gestational age in ferrets. Lab. Anim. Sci. 40, 91–92.

Phillips, P.H., O'Callaghan, M.G., Moore, E., Baird, R.M., 1987. Pedal *Sarcoptes scabiei* infestation in ferrets (*Mustela putorius furo*). Aust. Vet. J. 64, 289–290.

Poessel, S.A., Biggins, D.E., Santymire, R.M., Livieri, T.M., Crooks, K.R., Angeloni, L., 2011. Environmental enrichment affects adrenocortical stress responses in the endangered black-footed ferret. Gen. Comp. Endocrinol. 172 (3), 526–533.

Porter, D.D., Larsen, A.E., Cox, N.A., 1975. Isolation of infectious bovine rhinotracheitis virus from Mustelidae. J. Clin. Microbiol. 1, 112–113.

Porter, H.G., Porter, D.D., Larsen, A.E., 1982. Aleutian disease in ferrets. Infect. Immun. 36, 379–386.

Powell, D.A., Gonzales, C., Gunnels, R.D., 1991. Use of the ferret as a model for pediatric endotrocheal intubation training. Lab. Anim. Sci. 41, 86–89.

Prohaczik, A., Kulcsar, M., Huszenicza, G., 2009. Metabolic and endocrine characteristics of pregnancy toxemia in the ferret. Vet. Med. 54 (2), 75–80.

Price, D.J., Morgan, J.E., 1987. Spatial properties of neurons in the lateral geniculate nucleus of the pigmented ferret. Exp. Brain Res. 68 (1), 28–36.

Pyle, N.J., 1940. Use of ferrets in laboratory work and research investigators. Am. J. Public Health 30, 787.

Quesenberry, E., Carpenter, J. (Eds.), 2012. Ferrets, Rabbits, and Rodents, Clinical Medicine and Surgery, third ed. Saunders, Philadelphia, PA.

Quesenberry, K.E., Rosenthal, K.L., 1997. Endocrine diseases. In: Hillyer, E.V., Quesenberry, K.E. (Eds.), Ferrets, Rabbits, and Rodents: Clinical Medicine and Surgery. Saunders, Philadelphia, PA, pp. 85–98.

Qureshi, T., Labes, R.E., Lambeth, M., Montgomery, H., Griffin, J.F.T., Mackintosh, C.G., 2000. Transmission of *Mycobacterium bovis* from experimentally infected ferrets to non-infected ferrets (*Mustela furo*). N. Z. Vet. J. 48 (4)., 99–104.

Ragg, J.R., Moller, H., Waldrup, K.A., 1995a. The prevalence of bovine tuberculosis (*Mycobacterium bovis*) infections in feral populations of cats (*Felis catus*), ferrets (*Mustela furo*) and stoats (*Mustela erminea*) in Otago and Southland, New Zealand. N. Z. Vet. J. 43 (7), 333–337.

Ragg, J.R., Walderup, K.A., Moller, H., 1995b. The distribution of gross lesions of tuberculosis caused by *Mycobacterium bovis* in feral ferrets (*Mustela furo*) from Otago, New Zealand. N. Z. Vet. J. 43, 338–341.

Raila, J., Gomez, C., Schweigert, F.J., 2002. The ferret as a model for vitamin A metabolism in carnivores. J. Nutr. 132 (6 Suppl 2), 1787S–1789SS.

Raj, V.S., Smits, S.L., Pas, S.D., Provacia, L.B., Moorman-Roest, H., Osterhaus, A.D., et al., 2012. Novel hepatitis E virus in ferrets, the Netherlands. Emerg. Infect. Dis. 18, 1369–1370.

Ramsell, K.A., Garner, M.M., 2010. Disseminated idiopathic myofasciitis in ferrets. VCNA 13, 561–575.

Rassnick, K.M., et al., 1995. Use of a vascular access system for administration of chemotherapeutic agents to a ferret with lymphoma. J. Am. Vet. Med. Assoc. 206, 500–504.

Regh, J.E., Gigliotti, F., Stokes, D., 1988. Cryptosporidiosis in ferrets. Lab. Anim. Sci. 38, 155–158.

Rosenbaum, M.R., Affolter, V.K., Usborne, A.L., Beeber, N.L., 1996. Cutaneous epitheliotropic lymphoma in a ferret. J. Am. Vet. Med. Assoc. 209, 1441–1444.

Rosenthal, K., 1994. Ferrets. Vet. Clin. North Am. 24 (1), 1–23.

Rosenthal, K.L., 1997. Respiratory diseases. In: Hillyer, E.V., Quesenberry, K.E. (Eds.), Ferrets, Rabbits, and Rodents: Clinical Medicine and Surgery. Saunders, Philadelphia, PA, pp. 77–84.

Rosenthal, K.L., Peterson, M.E., 1996. Evaluation of plasma androgen and estrogen concentrations in ferrets with hyperadrenocorticism. J. Am. Vet. Med. Assoc. 209, 1097–1102.

Rosenthal, K.L., Peterson, M.E., Quesenberry, K.E., et al., 1993. Hyperadrenocorticism associated with adrenocortical tumor or nodular hyperplasia of the adrenal gland in ferrets: 50 cases (1987–1991). J. Am. Vet. Med. Assoc. 203, 271–275.

Rupprecht, C.E., Gilbert, J., Pitts, R., Marshall, K.R., Koprowski, H., 1990. Evaluation of an inactivated rabies virus vaccine in domestic ferrets. J. Am. Vet. Med. Assoc. 196, 1614–1616.

Russell, J., 1990. Predatory object play in the ferret. University of London, PhD Thesis, University of London. Accessed at <http://www.nal.usda.gov/awic/pubs/enrich/ferrets.htm>.

Ryan, K.D., 1984. Hormonal correlates of photoperiod-induced puberty in a reflux ovulator, the female ferret. Biol. Reprod. 31, 925.

Ryland, L.M., Gorham, J.R., 1978. The ferret and its diseases. J. Am. Vet. Med. Assoc. 173, 1154–1158.

Ryland, L.M., Bernard, S.L., Gorham, J.R., 1983. A clinical guide to the pet ferret. Compend. Contin. Educ. Pract. Vet. 5, 25.

Saifuddin, M., Fox, J.G., 1996. Identification of a DNA segment in ferret aleutian disease virus similar to hypervariable capsid region of mink Aleutian disease parvovirus. Arch. Virol. 141, 1329–1336.

Sasai, H., Kato, K., Sasaki, T., Koyama, S., Kotani, T., Fukata, T.J., 2000. Echocardiographic diagnosis of dirofilariasis in a ferret. Small Anim. Pract. 41 (4), 172–174.

Saunders, G.K., Thomsen, B.V., 2006. Lymphoma and *Mycobacterium avium* infection in a ferret (Mustela putorius furo). J. Vet. Diagn. Invest. 18, 513–515.

Schulman, F.Y., Montall, R.J., Hauer, P.J., 1993. Gastroenteritis associated with *Clostridium perfringens* type A in black-footed ferrets (*Mustela nigripes*). Vet. Pathol. 30, 308–310.

Schultheiss, P.C., Dolginow, S.Z., 1994. Granulomatous enteritis caused by *Mycobacterium avium* in a ferret. J. Am. Vet. Med. Assoc. 204, 1217–1218.

Scott, D.W., Miller, W.H., Griffin, C.E., 1995. Small Animal Dermatology. Saunders, Philadelphia, PA.

Shen, D.T., Gorham, J.R., 1980. Survival of pathogenic distemper virus at 5°C and 25°C. Vet. Med. Small Anim. Clin. 75, 69–72.

Shen, D.T., Gorham, J.R., Ryland, L.M., Strating, A., 1981. Using jet injection to vaccinate mink and ferrets against canine distemper, mink viral enteritis, and botulism, type C. Vet. Med. Small Anim. Clin. 76, 856–859.

Sherrill, A., Gorham, J.R., 1985. Bone marow hypoplasia associated with estrus in ferrets. Lab. Anim. Sci. 35, 280–286.

Shimbo, F.M., 1992. A Tao Full of Detours, the Behavior of the Domestic Ferret. Ministry of Publications, Elon College, NC.

Shump, A., et al., 1974. A Bibliography of Mustelids. Part 1: Ferrets and Polecats. Michigan Agricultural Experiment Station 6977, East Lansing, MI.

Shump, A.U., Shump Jr., K.A., 1978. Growth and development of the European ferret (*Mustela putorius*). Lab. Anim. Sci. 28, 89–91.

Sinclair, D.G., Evans, E.V., Sibbald, I.R., 1962. The influence of apparent digestible energy and apparent digestible nitrogen in the diet on weight gain, feed consumption, and nitrogen retention of growing mink. Can. J. Biochem. Physiol. 40, 1375–89.

Sledge, D.G., Bolin, S.R., Lim, A., Kaloustian, L.L., Heller, R.L., Carmona, F.M., et al., 2011. Outbreaks of severe enteric disease associated with *Eimeria furonis* infection in ferrets (*Mustela putorius furo*) of 3 densely populated groups. J. Am. Vet. Med. Assoc. 239 (12), 1584–1588.http://dx.doi.org/10.2460/javma.239.12.1584

Smith, L., 1975. The Pathogenic Anaerobic Bacteria. Charles C. Thomas, Springfield, IL.

Smith, P.C., 1978. Experimental infectious bovine rhinotracheitis virus infection of English ferrets. Am. J. Vet. Res. 39, 1369–1372.

Smith, W., Stuart-Harris, C.H., 1936. Influenza infection of man from the ferret. Lancet 2, 21.

Stamoulis, M.E., Miller, M.S., Hillyer, E.V., 1997. Cardiovascular diseases. In: Hillyer, E.V., Quesenberry, K.E. (Eds.), Ferrets, Rabbits, and Rodents: Clinical Medicine and Surgery. Saunders, Philadelphia, PA, pp. 63–70.

Stauber, E., Robinette, J., Basaraba, R., 1990. Mast cell tumors in three ferrets. J. Am. Vet. Med. Assoc. 196, 766–767.

Stephensen, C.B., Welter, J., Thaker, S.R., Taylor, J., Tartaglia, J., Paoletti, E., 1997. Canine distemper virus (CDV) infection of ferrets as a model for testing *Morbillivirus* vaccine strategies: NYVAC- and ALVAC-based CDV recombinants protect against symptomatic infection. J. Virol. 71, 1506–1513.

Stokes, D.C., Gigliotti, F., Rehg, J.E., Snellgrove, R.L., Hughes, W.T., 1987. Experimental *Pneumocystis carinii* pneumonia in the ferret. Br. J. Exp. Pathol. 68, 267–276.

Straube, E.F., Walden, N.B., 1981. Zinc poisoning in ferrets (*Mustela putorius furo*). Lab. Anim. 15, 45–47.

Supakorndej, P., McCall, J.W., Lewis, R.E., 1992. Biology, Diagnosis, and Prevention of Heartworm Infection in Ferrets. American Heartworm Society, Batavia, IL, pp. 59–69.

Sweet, C., Bird, R.A., Jakeman, K., Coates, D.M., Smith, H., 1987. Production of passive immunity of neonatal ferrets following maternal vaccination with killed influenza A virus vaccines. Immunology 60, 83–89.

Symmers, W., Thomson, A., 1953. Observations on tuberculosis in the ferret (*Mustela furo* L.). J. Comp. Pathol. 63, 20–29.

Thomas, P.E., Desmukh, D.R., 1986. Effect of arginine-free diet on ammonia metabolism in young and adult ferrets. J. Nutr. 116, 545–551.

Thomson, A., 1951. A history of the ferret. J. Hist. Med. Allied Sci. 6, 471.

Thornton, P.C., Wright, P.A., Sacra, P.J., Goodier, T.E., 1979. The ferret, *Mustela putorius furo*, as a new species in toxicology. Lab. Anim. 13, 119–124.

Timm, K.I., 1988. Pruritis in rabbits, rodents, and ferrets. Vet. Clin. North Am. 18, 1088–1089.

Tompkins, D.S., Watt, J.I., Rathbone, B.J., West, A.P., 1988. The characterization and pathological significance of gastric *Campylobacter*-like organisms in the ferret: a model of chronic gastritis? Epidemiol. Infect. 101, 269–278.

Torres-Medina, A., 1987. Isolation of atypical rotavirus causing diarrhea in neonatal ferrets. Lab. Anim. Sci. 37, 167.

Trautwein, G.W., Helmboldt, C.F., 1966. Mastitis in mink due to *Staphylococcus aureus* and *Escherichia coli*. J. Am. Vet. Med. Assoc. 149, 924–928.

USDA Aphis., 2013. Pseudorabies (Aujeszky's Disease) and Its Eradication <http://www.aphis.usda.gov/publications/animal_health/content/printable_version/pseudo_rabies_report.pdf> (accessed Dec 2013.).

USDHHS, 1996. Guide for the Care and Use of Laboratory Animals. National Academy Press, Washington, DC, p. 32.

Valheim, M., Djønne, B., Heiene, R., Caugant, D.A., 2001. Disseminated *Mycobacterium celatum* (type 3) infection in a domestic ferret (*Mustela putorius furo*). Vet. Pathol. 38 (4), 460–463.

Viallier, J., Viallier, G., Prave, M., 1983. Place de *Mycobacterium avium* dans l'epidemiologies mycobacterienne actuelle chez les animaux domestiques et savages. Sci. Vet. Med. Comp. 85, 103–109.

Vinegar, A., Sinnett, E.E., Kosch, P.C., Miller, M.L., 1985. Pulmonary physiology as a model for inhalation toxicology. Lab. Anim. Sci. 35, 246–250.

von Messling, V., Springfeld, C., Devaux, P., Cattaneo, R., 2003. A ferret model of canine distemper virus virulence and immunosuppression. J. Virol. 77, 12579–12591.

Wagner R., 2012. Hypothyroidism in ferrets. Association of Exotic Mammal Veterinarians 11th Annual Conference. Oakland (CA), October 25, pp. 29–31.

Wagner, R.A., 2009. Ferret cardiology. Vet. Clin. North Am. Exot. Anim. Pract. 12, 115–134.

Wagner, R.A., Dorn, D.P., 1994. Evaluation of serum estradiol concentrations in alopecic ferrets with adrenal gland tumors. J. Am. Vet. Med. Assoc. 205, 703–707.

Wagner, R.A., Piché, C.A., Jöchle, W., et al., 2005. Clinical and endocrine responses to treatment with deslorelin acetate implants in ferrets with adrenocortical disease. Am. J. Vet. Res. 66, 910–914.

Wagner, R.A., et al., The treatment of adrenal cortical disease in ferrets with 4.7-mg deslorelin acetate implants. J. Exotic. Pet. Med. 18(2), 146–152.

Wang, X.-D., Krinksy, N.L., Marini, R.P., Tang, G., Yu, J., Hurley, R., et al., 1992. Intestinal uptake and lymphatic absorption of β-carotene in ferrets: a model for human β-carotene metabolism. Am. Physiol. Soc. 263, G480–G486.

Wang, X.-D., Russel, R.M., Marini, R.P., Tang, G., Dolnikowski, G., Fox, J.G., et al., 1993. Intestinal perfusion of β-carotene in the ferret raised retinolc acid level in portal blood. Biochim. Biophys. Acta. 1167, 159–164.

Wang, X.-D., Marini, R.P., Hebuterne, X., Fox, J.G., Krinksy, N.I., Russell, R.M., 1995. Vitamin E enhances the lymphatic transport of β-carotene and its conversion to vitamin A in the ferret. Gastroenterology 108, 719–726.

Weiss, C.A., Williams, B.H., Scott, J.B., et al., 1999. Surgical treatment and long-term outcome of ferrets with bilateral adrenal tumors or adrenal hyperplasia: 56 cases (1994–1997). J. Am. Vet. Med. Assoc. 215, 820–823.

Weiss, C.A., Williams, B.H., Scott, M.V., 1998. Insulinoma in the ferret: clinical findings and treatment comparison of 66 cases. J. Am. Anim. Hosp. Assoc. 34, 471–475.

Weiss-Buerger, M., 1981. An investigation of the influence of exploration and playing on learning by polecats, *mustela-putorius-x-mustela-furo*. Zeitschrift für Tierpsychologie 551, 33–62.

Welchman, Dd.B., Oxenham, M., Done, S.H., 1993. Aleutian disease in domestic ferrets: diagnostic findings and survey results. Vet. Rec. 132, 479–484.

Whisson, D., Moore, T., 1997. An annotated bibliography on the ferret (Mustela putorius furo). Calif. Dep. Fish and Game, Wildl. Manage. Div., Bird and Mammal Conservation Program Rep. 97-3, Sacramento, CA, pp. 37.

Wildt, D.E., Bush, M., Morton, C., 1989. Semen characteristics and testosterone profiles in ferrets kept in a long-day photoperiod, and the influence of hCG timing and sperm dilution medium on pregnancy rate after laporoscopic insemination. J. Reprod. Fertil. 86, 349–358.

Williams, E.S., Barker, I.K. (Eds.), 2001. Print Infectious Diseases of Wild Mammals, third ed. Iowa State University Press, ISBN: 9780813825564.

Williams, E.S., Thorne, E.T., Kwiatkowski, D.R., 1992. Comparative vaginal cytology of the estrous cycle of black-footed ferrets (*Mustela nigripes*), Siberian polecats (*M. eversmanni*), and domestic ferrets (*M. putorius furo*). J. Vet. Diagn. Invest. 4, 38–44.

Williams, B.H., Eighmy, J.J., Berbert, M.H., Dunn, D.G., 1993. Cervical chordoma in two ferrets (*Mustela putorius furo*). Vet. Pathol. 30, 204–206.

Williams, B.H., Chimes, M.J., Gardiner, C.H., 1996. Biliary coccidiosis in a ferret (*Mustela putorius furo*). Vet. Pathol. 33, 437–439.

Williams, B.H., Kiupel, M., West, K.H., Raymond, J.T., Grant, C.K., Glickman, L.T., 2000. Coronavirus-associated epizootic catarrhal enteritis in ferrets. J. Am. Vet. Med. Assoc. 217, 526–530.

Willis, L.S., Barrow, M.V., 1971. The ferret (*Mustela putorius furo*) as a laboratory animal. Lab. Anim. Sci. 21, 712–716.

Wise, A.G., Kiupel, M., Maes, R.K., 2006. Molecular characterization of a novel coronavirus associated with epizootic catarrhal enteritis (ECE) in ferrets. Virology 349, 164–174.

Wise, A.G., Smedley, R.C., Kiupel, M., Maes, R.K., 2009. Detection of group C rotavirus in juvenile ferrets (*Mustela putorius furo*) with diarrhea by reverse transcription polymerase chain reaction: sequencing and analysis of the complete coding region of the VP6 gene. Vet. Pathol. 46 (5), 985–991.

Wise, A.G., Kiupel, M., Garner, M.M., Clark, A.K., Maes, R.K., 2010. Comparative sequence analysis of the distal one-third of the genomes of a systemic and an enteric ferret coronavirus. Virus Res. 149, 42–50.

Wyre, N.R., Michels, D., Chen, S., 2013. Selected emerging diseases in ferrets. Vet. Clin. North Am. Exot. Anim. Pract. 16 (2), 469–493.

Yu, J., Russell, R.M., Salomon, R.N., Murphy, J.C., Palley, L.S., Fox, J.G., 1995. Effect of *Helicobacter mustelae* infection on epithelial cell proliferation in ferret gastric tissues. Carcinogenesis 16, 1927–1931.

ALPACAS –
3 CHAMBERED OR STEM
STOMACH
OF 4
ARE PSEUDO RUMINANTS

Biology and Diseases of Ruminants (Sheep, Goats, and Cattle)

Wendy J. Underwood, DVM, MS, DACVIM[a],
Ruth Blauwiekel, DVM, PhD, DACLAM[b], Margaret L. Delano,
MS, DVM, Rose Gillesby, DVM[c], Scott A. Mischler, DVM,
PhD, DACLAM[d] and Adam Schoell, DVM, DACLAM[e]

[a]Eli Lilly and Company, Indianapolis, Indiana, USA [b]University of Vermont, Hills Building, Carrigan Drive, Burlington, VT, USA [c]Veterinary Services and Biocontainment Research, Animal Research Support, Zoetis, Richland, MI, USA [d]Worldwide Comparative Medicine, Pfizer Inc., Middletown Rd., Pearl River, NY, USA [e]Zoetis, Portage St, Kalamazoo, MI, USA

I. INTRODUCTION

Since the first edition of this book, the use of ruminants as research subjects has changed dramatically. Formerly large animals were used primarily for agricultural research or as models of human diseases. Although ruminants have continued in their traditional agricultural research role, they are now extensively used for studies in molecular biology, genetic engineering and biotechnology for basic science, agricultural, and clinical applications. Concern and interest for the welfare for these species and improved understanding of their biology

TABLE 15.1   Terminology

Species	Female	Male	Young animals	Castrated male	Parturition
Cattle	Cow	Bull	Calf (heifer calf, bull calf)	Steer	Calving
			Heifer (nulliparous female)		
Sheep	Ewe	Ram	Lamb (ewe lamb, ram lamb)	Wether	Calving
Goat	Doe or nanny	Buck or billy	Kid or goatling	Wether	Kidding

and behavior have continued and are reflected in changing husbandry and management systems. This chapter addresses basic biology, husbandry, and the more common or important diseases of the three ruminant species used most commonly in the laboratory, namely sheep, goats, and cattle. One chapter is simply not adequate, however, to address the many details and complexities of biology, management, and diseases of these species. References provided at the end of this chapter and noted in the text offer more information to the interested reader.

A. Taxonomy

Sheep, goats, and cattle are ungulates, 'hooved' animals that are members of the Order Artiodactyla (animals with cloven hooves), suborder Ruminatia (ruminants or cud-chewing animals) and Family Bovidae. Members of the Bovidae group of mammals are distinguished by characteristics such as even number of toes, a compartmentalized forestomach, and horns. These animals are herbivores, and as adults, derive all their glucose from gluconeogenesis. The subfamily Capra includes sheep and goats. The genus and subgenus *Ovis* includes domestic sheep as well as wild Asian and European sheep species. Domestic sheep are *Ovis aries*. *Capra hircus* is the domestic goat which originated from western Asian goats. The subfamily Bovinae and genus *Bos* include all domestic and wild cattle, including the yak and Banteng (Bali cattle). The subgenus *Taurus* contains all of today's domestic cattle. *Bos taurus* (domestic cattle) originate from the European continent, and have no hump over the withers. *Bos indicus*, known as Zebu cattle, have a hump over the withers and drooping ears.

There are many breeds of sheep worldwide that are distinguished as either 'meat,' 'wool,' or 'dual' purpose breeds. Some wool or hair breeds have varying coat colors. Some breeds are raised for milk (cheese) production. Common breeds raised for meat in the United States include the Dorset, Columbia, Suffolk, and Hampshire. Slightly smaller meat breeds include the Southdown and Border Cheviot. Wool breeds include the Merino, Rambouillet, Lincoln, and Romney and are subclassified according to properties of the wool.

Goat breeds are numerous and are usually classified according to use as dairy-, meat-, fiber-, or skin-type breeds. The major dairy breeds are the Alpine, Nubian, Toggenburg, La Mancha, and Saanen, all of which have origins on the European continent. The Nubian breed was developed from crossbreeding British stock with Egyptian and Indian goats. Fiber breeds include the Angora and the Cashmere. The La Mancha has rudimentary ears that are a genetically dominant distinguishing characteristic of the breed. Meat breeds include the Boer, Kiko, and Pygmy.

Most breeds of cattle are classified as 'dairy' or 'beef,' while a few breeds are considered 'dual-purpose.' Common dairy breeds in the United States include Holstein (also known as 'Holstein–Friesian'), Brown Swiss, Jersey, Ayrshire, and Guernsey. Holsteins and Brown Swiss have the largest body size, while Jerseys have the smallest. Of the many beef breeds, the more common in the United States include Angus, Hereford, and Simmental.

More detailed information regarding these and other ruminant breeds is available (Integrated Taxonomic Information System: http://www.itis.gov). Minor breeds of sheep, goats, and cattle are studied for their genetic and production characteristics. Discussions of these and efforts at conservation are described in detail elsewhere (American Livestock Breeds Conservancy, http://www.albc-usa.org; Gibbs *et al.*, 2009).

Some of the terminology used with respect to ruminants is given in Table 15.1.

B. Comments About and Examples of Use in Research

Ruminants have been used as research models since the inception of the Land Grant College System, first in production agriculture, and now also in anatomic and physiologic sciences and in biomedical research. Healthy, normal young ruminants serve as models of cardiac transplantation and as pre-clinical models for evaluation of cardiac assist or prosthetic devices such as vascular stents or cardiac valves (Salerno *et al.*, 1998). Ruminants have been useful research subjects for reproductive research such as embryo transfer, artificial insemination (AI), and control of the reproductive cycle (Wall *et al.*, 1997). Several important milestones in gene transfer, cloning, and genetic engineering techniques have been developed or demonstrated using these species (Cibelli *et al.*, 1998a, b). One of many proposed uses of genetically engineered ruminants is the production of proteins to be secreted in the milk and later isolated. Healthy sheep and goats are also often used for antibody production.

Genome mapping has developed rapidly since 1998. The *Genome Sequence of Taurine Cattle: A Window to Ruminant Biology and Evolution* is available for ruminants and other domestic species (Elsik *et al.*, 2009). Other references for genome mapping exist (Broad *et al.*, 1998; Womack, 1998; http://www.marc.usda.gov/genome/sheep/sheep.html; http://www.marc.usda.gov/genome/cattle/cattle.html).

Sheep provide obvious benefits over the use of cattle in research from the standpoint of size, ease of handling, and cost of maintenance. Sheep are widely used models for basic and applied fetal and reproductive research. The species is used for investigating circadian rhythms and the interaction between olfactory cues and behavior. Natural disease models include congenital hyperbilirubinemia/hepatic organic anion excretory defect (Dubin–Johnson Syndrome) in the Corriedale breed, congenital hyperbilirubinemia/hepatic organic anion uptake defect (Gilbert's syndrome) in the Southdown breed, gamma-glutamyl carboxylase deficiency in Rambouillets, lysosomal storage diseases, and pulmonary adenomatosis (Jaagsiekte) in several breeds. Induced models include arteriosclerosis, hemorrhagic shock, copper poisoning (Wilson's disease), and metabolic toxicosis. Sheep have been utilized as research models for orthopedic procedures, airway disease/asthma and in the areas of human device, drug discovery, and implantation research (Easley *et al.*, 2008; Griffiths *et al.*, 2010; Herfat, 2005; Scheerlinck *et al.*, 2008).

Goats are used in a wide variety of disciplines such as immunology, mastitis, and nutrition and parasitology. Vascular researchers select the goat because of the large, readily accessible jugular veins. Goats with inherited caprine myotonia congenita ('fainting goats') have been used as a model for human myotonia congenita, or Thomson's disease (Kuhn, 1993). A line of inbred Nubians serve as models for beta-mannosidosis and prenatal therapeutic cell transplantation strategies (Lovell *et al.*, 1997). These disorders are discussed in more detail later under genetic diseases. Goats are also used as a model for osteoporosis research (Welch *et al.*, 1996).

Cattle are often used as a source of ruminal fluid for research, teaching, or treatment of other cattle, by placing a permanent fistula in the left abdominal wall to allow sampling of ruminal fluid (Dougherty, 1981). Cattle also serve as models of many infectious diseases and several inherited metabolic diseases. Bovine trichomoniasis, caused by *Tritrichomonas (Trichomonas) fetus* has been identified as a useful model for the human infection by *Trichomonas vaginalis* (Corbeil, 1995). Inherited

cardiomyopathies have been found in the Holstein and other breeds (Weil *et al.*, 1997). Lipofuscinosis has been identified in Ayrshires, glycogenosis in Shorthorn and Brahman cattle, and hemochromatosis in Salers. Holstein cattle serve as a model for leucocyte adhesion deficiency syndrome (AFIP, 1995) and achrondroplasia occurs in several breeds.

C. Availability and Sources

Common breeds of normal healthy ruminants are usually readily available, although seasonality may play a role as noted below. Agricultural sources may be located through agricultural schools, cooperative extension, and regional breeders' associations. Commercial sources of purpose-bred animals are found in technical publications and research animal vendor listings.

Purpose-bred research sheep and goats are available from commercial vendors and are usually maintained in registered facilities under federal standards that are also acceptable to research animal accrediting agencies. These animals are frequently described as 'specific pathogen free' (SPF) and are housed as biosecure or closed flocks. Animal health programs are in place and health reports usually are available on request. Agricultural sources of sheep or goats may be acceptable depending on specific research needs. Lambs and kids may be difficult to locate in fall and winter months because most breeds of sheep and goats are seasonal breeders.

Most cattle used as animal models in research in the United States are Holstein, because this dairy breed is now the most common. Purpose-bred, SPF research cattle are not typically available. Due to selection and the management of dairy production units, calves and young stock are available year round. Availability of young beef cattle is more seasonal according to typical production cycles.

Auction or sale barns are not appropriate sources for research ruminants. Many of these animals are culls of unknown genetics and poor health status. Selection of animal suppliers should be made only after research needs have been carefully considered. It is best to buy directly from as few sources as possible. Certain types of research (e.g., agricultural nutrition studies) may better be served by selecting animals from local agricultural suppliers rather than commercial vendors located in a different geographical area. Selection considerations for sources for research ruminants include flock or herd record keeping; health monitoring, vaccination, biosecurity, and preventative medicine programs; production standards and management practices consistent with the industry; vermin and insect control measures (especially flies and other flying insects); rearing programs and condition of young stock; and animal housing facilities.

Cattle used for research should be prepared with an appropriate transitional diet and vaccination program ('backgrounding'). Preliminary and periodic visits to the source farms should be conducted. It is important to establish a good relationship with local attending large animal veterinarians who will be valuable resources for current approved therapies and practices. Creative ways can be used to initiate and foster a good working relationship between the agricultural supplier and the research facility. Supplying vaccines or dewormers required for flock health programs, providing services such as quarterly serological testing or fecal examinations for the herd or flock, and paying a premium (above market price) for animals that meet desired quality research criteria are often helpful ways to manage this relationship.

A set of testing standards can be developed based on one high-quality supplier. Then flocks or herds can be 'qualified' by testing either a percentage of the herd or flock, or the entire flock or herd, for relevant infectious agents. The testing regimen itself should be carefully developed and evaluated for each source and research program need. Once qualified, each source farm should be re-evaluated periodically to maintain its status. Slaughter checks, necropsy of sentinel animals, or other screening tests may be required. Vaccination and deworming regimens should be instituted. Quarantine is advisable when animals arrive at the research facility. The animal screening process also depends on the origin of the animal (state, country) and the scientific program. Federal and State regulations must be followed.

Several texts on industry standards for flock or herd management provide a helpful orientation to those unfamiliar with ruminant husbandry and health care. These references also provide information regarding vaccination products licensed for use in ruminants as well as typical herd and flock vaccination and/or parasite control schedules. These texts are listed under 'Major references' at the end of this chapter (Anderson and Rings, 2009; Smith, 2009; Smith and Sherman, 2009).

When designing a vaccination program during qualification either at the source or at the research facility, it is important to evaluate the local disease incidence, the potential for exposure, and the cost effectiveness of vaccination. Labor and vaccine expenses may be much higher than the potential animal morbidity or mortality for diseases in a particular locality. Not all of the vaccines mentioned below will be necessary in all herds or flocks.

Typical health screening programs for sheep may include testing for Q Fever (*Coxiella burnetii*); contagious ecthyma; caseous lymphadenitis (*Corynebacterium pseudotuberculosis*); Johne's Disease (*Mycobacterium paratuberculosis*); ovine progressive pneumonia; and internal and external parasitism. For goats, screening might include Q Fever (*Coxiella burnetii*), caprine arthritis and encephalomyelitis (CAE), brucellosis, tuberculosis, and Johne's Disease (*Mycobacteria paratuberculosis*). Goats may also be tested for caseous lymphadenitis, contagious ecthyma,

or mycoplasma as needed. The supplier should be queried about the vaccination program; at a minimum, vaccinations should include tetanus toxoid and other clostridial diseases. Because of the limited number of biologics approved for small ruminants, products licensed for cattle have been used with success in sheep, and some licensed for sheep are used in goats (American Association of Small Ruminant Practitioners, AASRP, 1994; Council Report, 1994). In some cases, approved feed additives, such as coccidiostats, are fed to sheep.

Depending on source, cattle may be screened for Johne's disease, brucellosis, tuberculosis, persistent infection with bovine viral diarrhea virus (BVDV), respiratory diseases, internal and external parasitism, and foot conditions such as hairy heel warts or foot rot. Determination of herd status with bovine leukosis virus (BLV) may be critical to some research endeavors. Vaccination programs should include BVDV, infectious bovine rhinotracheitis virus (IBR), bovine respiratory syncytial virus (BRSV), bovine parainfluenza-3 (PI-3), and *Leptospira* spp. Other vaccination programs, dependent on herd status, endemic diseases, or geographic location, may include immunizations against venereal diseases, clostridial diseases, pathogens causing neonatal diarrhea or respiratory disease, *Moraxella bovis* (pinkeye), *Fusobacterium necrophorum* (footrot), *Staphylococcus aureus* (mastitis), *Histophilus somni*, or rabies.

Transportation of animals from the source to the research facility must be carefully planned and coordinated, and all applicable livestock travel regulations must be followed. If commercial haulers are used, disinfection of trucks, trailers, and associated equipment (i.e., ramps and chutes) beforehand is particularly important. The loading, footing, distribution of animals within the trailers or trucks, and environmental conditions during shipping are important areas to evaluate so that stress or injury to animals is minimized or eliminated. Sufficient time for acclimation to the new facility, pen, handler, feed, and water must be allowed post arrival at the destination (Grandin, 2007).

D. Summary of Laboratory Management and Husbandry

Many recent publications address facility, husbandry and space requirements and standard husbandry practices for research and production ruminants. The United States Department of Agriculture (USDA) regulates the use of farm animal species used in biomedical and other nonagricultural research Code of Federal Regulations (CFR), 1985. The *Guide for the Care and Use of Agricultural Animals in Agricultural Research and Teaching* (i.e., the FASS 'Guide') and the *Guide for the Care and Use of Laboratory Animals* (i.e., the ILAR 'Guide') provide additional information to supplement the existing Animal Welfare Act regulations (FASS, 2010; Hays *et al.*, 1998; NRC, 2011; USDA, 2011).

Handler training and facility modification should be considered when appropriate to minimize stress in the husbandry and handling of ruminants. Stress decreases feed intake and affects growth and development in younger animals and reproductive performance in adults. Standard husbandry practices such as weaning, castration, dehorning, vaccinations, deworming or treatments for external parasites, shipping with the associated feed and water deprivation, introduction to new housing environments and novel personnel, and intercurrent disease are all stressors (Houpt, 2010). Animals should be acclimated to the use of halters, and other handling equipment (i.e., chutes and head gates) associated with the research program and personnel must be trained in appropriate handling techniques. Appreciation for ruminant behavior has grown in recent years resulting in refinement of ruminant handling techniques (Houpt, 2010; Grandin, 2007).

When ruminants are confinement housed, proper ventilation is critical. Ammonia buildup and other waste gases may induce respiratory problems. In cold weather, if the ceiling, walls or water pipes condense water vapor, the ventilation should be increased at the expense of lower temperatures. Adult goats and younger cattle are quite comfortable in colder temperatures if provided adequate amounts of dry dust-free bedding and draft protection. Sheep, because of their wool, are remarkably tolerant to both hot and cold extremes. Newborn lambs and recently shorn adults are susceptible to hypothermia, hyperthermia, and sunburn. Therefore, in outside housing areas, sheep should be provided with shelters to minimize exposure to sun and inclement weather.

Animals housed under intensive confinement conditions must be kept clean by daily removal of excreta from pens or enclosures. Feed and water equipment should be maintained in sound, clean condition and should be constructed to prevent fecal contamination. Waterers should not create a muddy environment in paddocks or pens and sufficient access to waterers provided to prevent competition or fighting. Feeders should be constructed according to species size and feeding characteristics and should prevent entrapment of head and limbs. Pens, passageways, chutes, and floors must be sturdy to withstand factors such as frequent cleaning as well as the strength, weight and curiosity of all ages of animals, especially the investigative and climbing behaviors of goats. Chain-link fences are dangerous because goats (as well as some breeds and ages of sheep) are curious and tend to stand on their hind legs against fencing or walls. Forelimbs may be caught easily in the mesh. Floors in any area where animals will be housed, led or herded must ensure secure footing to prevent slipping injuries. Ruminants are social herding animals and should be housed in groups, or minimally within eyesight and hearing of other animals. Singly housed animals must have regular human contact. Durable environmental enrichment items should be supplied to those animals that are housed in confinement. Singly housed or recently weaned calves, in particular, need play objects (FASS, 2010; Morrow-Tesch, 1997).

Photoperiod must be considered because sheep and goats are sensitive to changes in light cycle (especially reproductive parameters). Normally, sheep and goats should be maintained on a cycle comparable to natural conditions. Light intensity should be maintained at about 220 lux (ILAR, 1996; FASS, 2010). Light cycles can be manipulated for experimental reasons.

II. BIOLOGY

A. Unique Physiological Characteristics and Attributes, with Emphasis on Comparative Physiology

The development of the digestive system, including the unique function of the rumen, is among the most notable comparative anatomic and physiologic characteristic of ruminants. These species have a three-compartment forestomach (rumen, reticulum, and omasum) and a true stomach (abomasum). The mature rumen functions as an anaerobic fermentation chamber in which the enzymes, such as cellulase, of the resident bacteria (10^9–10^{10}/ml), allow the animal to prosper as an herbivore. Digestion is also aided by other microorganisms, such as protozoa (10^5–10^6/ml) and fungi, which contribute to the rumen ecosystem. The result is the production of volatile fatty acids (VFA: acetic, propionic, and butyric). Unlike the monogastrics, fermentative digestion and VFA absorption also occur in the large intestines. These VFA serve as the main sources of energy for ruminants rather than glucose. Glucose is formed from propionic acid (or from amino acids) for metabolism in the central nervous system, uterus, and mammary gland. Plasma glucose is much lower and regulated differently in ruminants than in nonruminants. Rumen microorganisms also synthesize B-complex vitamins and vitamin K, and provide protein utilized by the animals' systems. Large amounts of fermentation gases such as carbon dioxide and methane are naturally eructated (Jurgens *et al.*, 2013; Reece 2004). Sheep and goats have tidy 'pelleted' dark-green feces. Cattle have pasty, moist, dark-green–brown feces.

Intestinal immunoglobulin absorption in neonates is crucial to the success of passive transfer. This transfer mechanism is functional for approximately the first 36 h after birth. Neonatal ruminants are immunocompetent, and this advantage is utilized when vaccinating calves

TABLE 15.2   Normal Values for Sheep, Goats, and Ruminants: Vital Signs, Life Spans, and Weights

Parameter/species	Sheep	Goats	Cattle
Chromosome number	54	60	60
Body temperature (°C) young	39.5–40.5	39–40.5	39–40.5
Body temperature (°C) adult	39–40	38.5–39.5	38–39
Heart rate (beats/min) young	140 (120–160)	140 (120–160)	120 (100–140)
Heart rate (beats/min) adult	75 (60–120)	85 (70–110)	60 (40–80)
Respiration rate young (breaths/min)	50 (30–70)	50 (40–65)	48 (30–60)
Respiration rate adult (breaths/min)	36 (12–72)	28 (15–40)	24 (12–36)
Life span (years)	10–15	8–12 years	20–25
Body weights (lbs)			
Birth	3–25		
1 month		25	
3 months		55	400
6 months	110	85	
9 months		110	
12 months		130	720
18 months		155	
24 months	300 (ram)	170	1100
	200 (ewe)		
36 months		205	
Deciduous dental formula	(for sheep, goats, and cattle)	2 (Di 0/3 Dc 0/1 Dp3/3)	=20
Permanent dental formula	(for sheep, goats, and cattle)	2 (I 0/3 C0/1 P 3/3 M 3/3)	=32

Vital sign data for goats is from (Smith and Sherman, 2009). Sheep weight data represent weights of feeder lamb and adult dry ewe (FASS, 2010). Goat weight data is for a large breed male goat. Cattle weight data represent weights of female Holstein or Guernsey dairy cattle (FASS, 2010). Life span data for sheep and cattle is from Brooks *et al.*, 1984.

against some common neonatal or juvenile diseases when the dams' colostrum is lacking antibody against those pathogens.

Three major ovine histocompatibility classes have been identified and are designated as OVAR (Ovis aries) Class I, II, and III (Franz-Werner *et al.*, 1996; Gao *et al.*, 2010). Bovines have several unique aspects of their immune systems. The bovine lymphocyte antigen system (BoLA) ranks after the human (HLA) and murine (H-2) systems in terms of depth of knowledge (Lewin, 1996). The complexity of the immunobiology of the bovine mammary gland is being studied extensively because mastitis is the most prevalent disease in the dairy industry. Several innate immune mechanisms and cellular defenses, and their variation throughout lactation, have been described (Sordillo and Streicher, 2002).

Bovine corneal epithelium is distinguished from other species because of its ability to heal without treatment, even when severely infected. Corneal ulcers are uncommon in sheep or goats.

B. Normal Values: Growth, Longevity, Hematology, Clinical Chemistry

Hematology and clinical reference texts are available for the ruminant species and include overviews of normal values, ranges, and discussions of the influence on the hemogram of many metabolic, nutritional, and other variables (Kaneko *et al.*, 1997; Weiss and Wardrop, 2010). These references should be consulted when preparing to include blood collection data in research protocols and when reviewing hematologic findings. Most veterinary diagnostic laboratories have also developed databases for normal ranges for hematologic and clinical chemistry values based on subjects from their service areas. Appropriate control groups must be incorporated into each research plan to establish the normal values for the particular locale, diagnostic facilities, breed, and so on.

Normal vital sign, life span, and weight values for sheep, goats, and ruminants are presented in Table 15.2.

TABLE 15.3 Normal Values, Hematology

Parameter	Sheep	Goat	Cattle
PCV (%)	27–45	22–38	24–46
Hgb (g/dl)	9–15	8–12	8–15
RBC (×10⁶/μl)	9–15	8–18	5–10
WBC (×10³)	4–12	4–13	4–12
Total Protein (g/dl)	6.0–7.5	6–7.5	7–8.5
MCV (fl)	28–40	16–25	40–60
MCH (pg)	8–12	5.2–8	11–17
MCHC (g/dl)	31–34	30–36	30–36
Reticulocytes (%)	0	0	0
RBC diameter (μm)	3.2–6	2.5–3.9	4.8
RBC life (days)	140–150	125	160
M:E ratio	0.77–1.68:10	0.69:10	0.31–1.85:10
Platelets (×10³/μl)	250–750	300–600	100–800
Fibrinogen (mg/dl)	100–500	100–400	300–700
WBC Diff	Absolute count/μl (% of total)		
Stabs, Bands	Rare	Rare	0–250 (0–2)
Segs	400–6000 (10–50)	1200–6250 (30–48)	600–5400 (15–45)
Lymphs	1600–9000 (40–75)	2000–9100 (50–70)	1800–9000 (45–75)
Monos	0–750 (0–6)	0–550 (0–4)	80–850 (2–7)
Eos	0–1200 (0–10)	50–1050 (1–8)	80–2400 (2–20)
Basos	0–350 (0–3)	0–150 (0–1)	0–250 (0–2)
Coagulation tests (s)			
PT	13.5–15.9	9.0–14.0	6.8–8.4
PTT	27.9–40.7		11.0–17.4
TT	4.8–8.0	20.9–33.4	4.3–7.1

Normal hematologic and clinical biochemistry data is presented in Tables 15.3 and 15.4.

Ruminants generally have fewer neutrophils than lymphocytes. Blood urea nitrogen (BUN) values cannot be used as an indicator of renal function due to the metabolism of urea nitrogen by rumen microflora. Because of the large volume of rumen water, adult ruminants can generally go several days without drinking before significant dehydration occurs. Erythrocytes may become more fragile during rehydration, resulting in some degree of hemolysis and hemoglobinuria. However, severe dehydration can occur quickly in animals that are ill, particularly in pre-ruminant neonates. Urine pH is generally alkaline in adult ruminants.

Ruminant erythrocytes are smaller and more fragile than those of most other mammals; hematocrits tend to be overestimated unless blood samples are centrifuged for extended periods of time. Rouleaux formation does not occur in cattle, but does occur to a limited extent in sheep and goats. Normal caprine erythrocytes lack central pallor because they are flat and lack biconcavity, but they may exhibit poikilocytosis. In addition to fetal hemoglobin, sheep are reported to have at least six different hemoglobins. Sheep blood coagulation is similar to that of humans. At least seven blood group systems have been identified in sheep (A, B, C, D, M, R, and X) and at least five in goats (B, C, M, R-O, and X) (Rychlik and Krawczyk, 2009; Cornell Animal Health Diagnostic Center http://ahdc.vet.cornell.edu/clinpath/modules/coags/typeoth.htm). Because transfusion reaction rates may be as high as 2–3%, cross-matching is advisable, although not always practical (Smith, 2009). Blood may safely be obtained in volumes of 10 ml/kg body weight, and given in volumes of 10–20 ml/kg.

TABLE 15.4   Normal Values, Clinical Biochemistry

Parameter/species	Sheep	Goat	Cattle
Alanine aminotransferase (ALT, GPT; U/l) s, hp	30 ± 4	6–19	11–40
			(27 ± 14)
Albumin (g/l)	24–3.0	27.0–39.0	30.3–35.5
	(27 ± 1.9)	33.0 ± 3.3)	(32.9 ± 1.3)
Alk. phosphatase (AlkP, U/l)	68–387	93–387	0–488
	(178 ± 102)	(219 ± 76)	(194 ± 126)
Aspartate Aminotransferase (AST, GOT; U/l) s, hp	60–280	167–513	78–132
	(307 ± 43)		(105 ± 27)
Bicarbonate (HCO$_3$, mmol/l)	20–25		17–29
Bilirubin, conjugated (mg/dl) s, p, hp	0–0.27		0.04–0.44 (0.18)
	(0.12)		
Bilirubin, unconjugated (mg/dl)	0–0.12		0.03
Bilirubin, Total (Tbili, mg/dl)	0.1–0.5	0.01	0.01–0.5
	(0.23 ± 0.1)		(0.2)
Blood urea nitrogen (BUN; mg/dl) s, p, hp	8–20	10–20	20–30
		(15 ± 2.0)	
Calcium, total (mg/dl) s, hp	11.5–12.8	8.9–11.7	9.7–12.4
Carbon dioxide, Total (mmol/L) s, hp	21–28	25.6–29.6	21.2–32.2
	(26.2)	(27.4 ± 1.4)	(26.5)
Chloride (Cl; mmol/L) s, hp	95–103	99–110.3	97–111
		(105.1 ± 2.9)	(104)
Creatine kinase (CK) U/l s, hp	8.1–12.9	0.8–8.9	4.8–12.1
	(10.3 ± 1.6)	(4.5 ± 2.8)	(7.4 ± 2.4)
Creatinine (mg/dl) s, p, hp	1.2–1.9	1.0–1.8	1.0–2.0
Gamma glutamyltransferase (GGT; U/l) s, p	20–52	20–56	6.1–17.4
	(33.5 ± 4.3)	(38 ± 13)	(15.7 ± 4.0)
Globulin (g/l) s	35.0–57.0	27.0–41.0	30.0–34.8
	(44.0 ± 5.3)	(36.0 ± 5.0)	(32.4 ± 2.4)
Glucose (mg/dl) s, p, hp	50–80	50–75	45–75
	(68.4 ± 6.0)	(62.8 ± 7.1)	(57.4 ± 6.8)
Lactate dehydrogenase (U/l) s, hp	238–440		692–1445
	(352 ± 59)		(1061 ± 222)
Magnesium (mg/dl) s	2.2–2.8	2.8–3.6	1.8–2.3
Phosphorus (P; mg/dl) hp	5.0–7.3	4.2–9.1	5.6–6.5
	(6.4 ± 0.2)	(6.5)	
Potassium (K; mmol/l) hp	3.9–5.4	3.5–6.7	3.9–5.8
	(4.8)	(4.3 ± 0.5)	(4.8)
Sorbitol dehydrogenase (SDH; U/L) hp	5.8–27.9	14.0–23.6	4.3–15.3
	(15.7 ± 7.5)	(19.4 ± 3.6)	(9.2 ± 3.1)
Sodium (Na; mmol/l) hp	139–152	142–155	132–152
		(150 ± 3.1)	(142)
Total protein (TP, g/l) s	60.0–79.0	64.0–70.0	67.4–74.6
	(72.0 ± 5.2)	(69.0 ± 4.8)	(71.0 ± 1.8)

Clinical biochemistry data from Kaneko et al. (1997).
Data presented as ranges with mean and standard bieviation in parentheses. S = serum; p = plasma; hp = heparinized plasma.

In general, aspartate amino transferase (AST) and lactate dehydrogenase (LDH) are not liver specific in ruminants, and alanine amino transferase (ALT) cannot be used to evaluate hepatic disease in goats. Gamma glutamyl transferase (GGT) and alkaline phosphatase (AP) are associated with biliary stasis, and elevations in GGT are generally associated with hepatic damage.

C. Nutrition

The nutritional needs of ruminants vary considerably according to the species, breed type, age, physiologic state, and environment. For example, mineral and other nutritional requirements vary even among breeds of cattle. Several references are available that describe the varying requirements and nutrient content of common feedstuffs (National Research Council (NRC), 2000, 2001, 2007; Smith, 2009). Computer programs are readily available for those who may need to formulate and balance rations.

Pre-formulated commercial feeds, concentrates, and supplements are available for the different species and production classes of ruminants. Often these are used as supplements for pasture, hay, and/or other forages. Concentrate mixtures typically contain a protein source such as soybean meal; salt and other required macro- and microminerals; and vitamins A, D, and E. Palatability of feeds should be taken into account. Mineral deficiencies and supplementation can influence several physiologic parameters such as reproduction and immune function. Whenever possible, introduction of new stock to a research facility should include continuation of the source feeding program followed by gradual transition to appropriate local feedstuffs (NRC, 2000, 2001, 2007).

Good-quality pasture meets the nutritional requirements for maintenance and growth of ruminants under many circumstances. However, lush spring pastures, especially pastures containing alfalfa, can induce bloat, diarrhea, grass tetany, or nitrate poisoning. Ruminants not acclimated to lush pasture should be fed good-quality hay and slowly introduced to those pasture environments.

When ruminants have access to pasture, it is important to be aware of different eating habits. Sheep and cattle are grazers. Goats are browsers and will readily eat not only grasses, but also seeds, nuts, fruits, and woody-stemmed plants. Since goats are selective eaters, they tend to consume the leafy or more nutritious parts of the plant and often require no grain supplementation (Bretzlaff et al., 1991). If needed, pelleted concentrates are preferred because the goat will pick out large particles in mixes. When given access to a salt block, ruminants will generally self-regulate intake. Horse and sheep feeds may be fed to goats; sheep are susceptible to copper toxicity and should not be fed supplements formulated

for horses. Goats will consume 5–8% of body weight in dry matter intake (whereas cattle will usually consume only 4% of body weight).

Rations that contain excessive phosphorus, a low calcium–phosphorus ratio, or elevated magnesium levels may induce urinary calculi in male ruminants. Calculi may also develop when forage grasses are high in silicates and oxalates. Ideally, roughage sources should be analyzed for nutrient content and supplements formulated which provide a nutrient profile complementary to available forage.

To increase ovulation rate in does and ewes, some producers 'flush' females by feeding 200–400g of concentrate per head per day for several weeks before and after the initiation of the breeding season. Thin pregnant does and ewes should receive supplemental grain and ad libitum forage during the last 6 weeks of gestation.

All newborn ruminants must receive passive immunity from colostrum, the first postpartum milk of a dam. Colostrum contains concentrated maternal antibodies (mostly as IgG1), functional leukocytes, and cytokines. The quality of the colostrum is affected by vaccination programs and the dam's overall condition and nutrition throughout gestation and at the time of parturition. Ensuring effective passive immune transfer primarily is dependent on the timing and volume of colostrum ingested by the neonate. Reliance on suckling in dairy calves has been associated with failure of passive immune transfer (NAHMS Dairy Studies, 2007). Frozen or 'banked' colostrum may be used for animals whose dams have poor quality or inadequate volume of colostrum. Colostrum immunoglobulin content can be estimated by specific gravity, by a Brix refractometer, or by commercial test kits designed for on-farm use (Brujeni et al., 2010). Commercial colostrum replacers or supplements also are available. A Holstein calf should receive its first 2-l meal of colostrum within 4h of birth and should consume at least 100g of IgG within the first 24h of life. In general, this IgG requirement can be met with 4l of good-quality colostrum. After 2–3 days, dairy calves are fed milk replacer or whole milk. Due to infectious disease concerns, waste milk should not be fed to calves unless it has been pasteurized.

Commercially available milk replacers that provide complete nutrition for the neonate are available for the common livestock species and should be prepared and fed according to the manufacturer's recommendations. Containers used to prepare and feed these replacers should be sanitized after each feeding. In agricultural settings, calves housed either outside or in cold housing must receive additional calories (milk or milk replacer) when ambient temperatures fall below the thermo-neutral zone.

Young ruminants can be offered good-quality hay to nibble on by 1 week of age. Rumen development in calves has been shown to be enhanced by supplementation with

TABLE 15.5   Reproductive Parameters for Ruminants

Species	Age at puberty (months)	Cycle type	Duration of cycle (days)	Length of estrus (hours)	Gestation (days)
Cattle	4–18 (mean 12)	Polyestrus	18–24 (21)	10–24 (mean 18)	270–292
Sheep	7–8	Seasonally polyestrus	14–19 (mean 17)	24–30	147–150
Goat	4–8	Seasonally polyestrus	18–24	24–96 (mean 40)	144–155

a concentrate feed (Davis and Drackley, 1998). Commercial 'starter' feeds with appropriate levels of energy and protein should be fed according to the manufacturer's recommendations by 2–3 weeks of age. Young animals should have access to fresh water, if not continually, then offered at least twice daily. Lambs and beef calves typically are fed a 'creep' supplement to provide additional nutrients and accustom them to solid feed prior to weaning.

D. Biology of Reproduction

Several useful references addressing ruminant reproduction in detail are available. These references are available in the back of this chapter under 'Major references' (Anderson and Rings, 2009; Smith, 2009; Youngquist and Threlfall, 2007; Hafez and Hafez, 2000).

1. Reproductive Physiology

Sheep and goats are seasonally polyestrus with estrus (heat) brought about by decreasing day length. Some breeds of sheep may cycle both in the fall and spring. In a research environment, ewes can be artificially stimulated to progress from anestrus to estrus cyclicity by maintaining the females in 8h of light and 16h of dark for 8–10 weeks. Older ewes tend to have multiple lambs, and Finn and Dorset breeds are especially prolific. Does also can bear singles, twins, or triplets.

The reproductive physiology and management of cattle are addressed in detail in texts and references oriented toward herd and production management (Anderson and Rings, 2009). Cows usually bear single calves, although twin births do occur. When twins are combinations of male and female calves, the female should be evaluated for freemartinism (see below under 'sexing'). Reproductive parameters for ruminants are given in Table 15.5.

2. Detection of Estrus and Pregnancy

Typically, ewes in heat will show a mild enlargement of the vulva with slight increases of mucus secretion. Ewes may isolate from the flock and appear anxious. It is most reliable to employ the help of a sterile ram to mark females when they are in standing heat. Ewes may be 'hand mated,' in which they are placed either singly or in small groups with the ram of choice and removed as serviced, or 'group mated' in which a mature ram is placed with 50–60 ewes for the entire 6-week breeding season. In either mating system, it is best to attach a marking harness to the male so that individual ewes can be identified as serviced.

Transabdominal ultrasound or interrectal Doppler probes are used for pregnancy detection: accuracy is generally best beyond 60 days of gestation. Commercial tests for serum pregnancy-specific protein B can confirm pregnancy beyond approximately day 30 in sheep and goats.

Signs of estrus in goats include uneasiness, tail switching or 'flagging,' redness and swelling of the vulva, clear vaginal discharge that becomes white by the end of estrus, and vocalization. Does can be induced to show signs of heat by buck exposure, and will ovulate within 7 to 10 days after introduction of the buck. Most goats ovulate between 24 and 36h after the onset of estrus and should be mated once signs of estrus are recognized and every 12h until the end of estrus. Once bred successfully, a goat will only rarely show signs of heat again. Pregnancy can be confirmed similarly to sheep. Dairy goats should have at least a 6- to 8-week dry period for the udder to fully involute and prepare for the next milking period.

The hallmark of estrus in the bovine is standing to be mounted by another animal, a behavioral sign of estrus which lasts approximately 12–16h with a range of 6–24h (Smith, 2009). A clear vaginal mucous discharge is a secondary sign of estrus. Ovulation occurs 12–18h after the onset of estrus. Detection of estrus is usually accomplished by visual observation of mounting behavior by other females (i.e., the cow standing to be mounted is the individual in estrus) or receptivity to a bull (willingness to stand). Teaser animals outfitted with marking devices are also used. Other methods of detecting estrus include monitoring blood progesterone levels, change in conductivity of cervical mucus, change in vaginal pH and body temperature, and evaluating activity levels by the use of pedometry (Hafez and Hafez, 2000).

In the cow, as in small ruminants, presumptive diagnosis of pregnancy can be inferred by failure to return to estrus. Real-time ultrasonography can be used to determine pregnancy as early as 28–32 days after insemination. Fetal gender can also be determined by experienced personnel using this method by about day 55. Pregnancy also can be diagnosed by 30–40 days post conception by palpation per rectum. Levels of bovine pregnancy-specific protein B may also be measured using one of several commercial tests for serum or milk.

Placentation in sheep, goats, and cattle is epitheliochorial and cotyledonary. The placentomes, the infolded functional units of the placenta, are formed as the result of fusion of the villi of the fetal cotyledons projecting into the crypts of the maternal caruncles (specialized projections of uterine mucosa). Caruncles of sheep and goats are concave in shape while those of cows are convex. In all three species, placentomes are distributed between the pregnant and nonpregnant horns of the uterus, athough the placentomes in the nongravid horn will be smaller than in the gravid horn.

3. Husbandry Needs

Pregnant dams must have a proper plane of nutrition (not overnutrition) and adequate exercise. The dam should be confined to a small pasture or sanitized maternity pen a few days to hours prior to parturition. The birthing environment will be very important in the overall health of the dam and offspring. Outdoor parturition in a small birthing pasture has advantages. There is less stress and intensity of pathogens. Indoor maternity pens should be clean, dry, well bedded, well ventilated and well lit. Management of these pens is important to minimize pathogens to which dam and young are exposed. Water troughs or buckets should be elevated or placed outside the pen because lambs and kids have a tendency to fall or be pushed into them. Between dams, the area should be cleaned, sanitized and allowed to dry, and fresh bedding installed for the next occupant. Moving the female immediately before or during parturition may delay the birthing process. Dams should be monitored closely during parturition for dystocia which may result in dead or severely weakened offspring from the prolonged birthing process.

Prior to parturition, the tail and perineal area of ewes and does should be clipped and cleaned. The pregnant doe or ewe needs approximately 1.4–1.5 m^2 of area for the birthing process. Each cow should have a minimum pen area of 9 m^2. Evaluation of a cow's udder as parturition approaches is important in order to ensure adequate passive transfer to the neonate. In the case of dairy cows, young calves are often hand-fed colostrum rather than being allowed to nurse from the dam. Inexperienced heifers may react indifferently or aggressively to their offspring and should be monitored more closely than older, multiparous cows with uneventful calving histories.

4. Parturition

Ewes approaching parturition generally isolate themselves from the flock, become restless, stamp their feet, blat, and periodically turn and look at their abdomen. The pelvic region will appear relaxed and milk will be present in the udder. Once hard labor contractions begin, lambs will usually be born quickly. Animals that don't appear to be progressing in labor should be examined for dystocia. Most cases of fetal malpresentation can be corrected via vaginouterine manipulation. Occasionally caesarean sections will be necessary. Sanitation, cleanliness, and adequate lubrication are of utmost importance when performing obstetrical procedures in all ruminant animals.

Does nearing parturition have an obviously swollen udder and red swollen vulva. Pelvic ligaments at the base of tail relax. Approximately 24 h prior to birth, rectal temperature will drop slightly below normal. Signs of impending parturition include restlessness; vocalization (bleating softly); uneasiness including getting up and down, pawing and bedding; and, a mucous discharge leading to a moist tail. Most goats prefer to kid alone and do so unaided. However, if labor is prolonged for more than 1 h, a vaginal exam is indicated. Many large dairy goat facilities attempt to control the onset of parturition in order to assist birthing. The drug of choice to induce parturition in the goat is prostaglandin F$_{2\alpha}$ (PGF2α) (Ott, 1982). On day 144 of gestation, goats given PGF2α (2.5–5 mg) will deliver kids within 28–57 h. Prostaglandins and glucocorticoids also can be used to induce parturition in the bovine.

The goat is one of the few ungulate species that commonly exhibit 'false pregnancy,' or pseudopregnancy. Does may have characteristically distended abdomens, may develop hydrometra and 'deliver' large volumes of cloudy fluid at expected due dates. Subsequent pregnancies can be normal. Prostaglandin use has been successful in treating false pregnancy.

At the time of calving, cows will separate themselves from the rest of the herd. A cow will lift her tail and arch her back when she is within a few hours of delivering the calf, and most are recumbent during delivery. Typically, the whole birthing process takes about 100 min. The length of labor of cows carrying larger calves or in primiparous animals will be longer. If animals are disturbed, labor may be delayed.

All postparturient animals should be monitored for successful delivery of the fetal membranes within 12 h of birth. If fetal membranes are not expelled, the dam should be monitored daily for temperature, attitude, and appetite. It is not recommended that the placenta be manually removed or that intrauterine boluses be placed in the uterus. Cows and sheep occasionally eat placentas which may subsequently obstruct rumen outflow and require surgical correction. Remove membranes that have been passed to prevent ingestion.

5. Early Development of the Newborn

Many neonatal ruminants will not need much assistance following birth. Dams are usually attentive to their young and will clean their offspring by licking, stimulating them to breath and to rise. When human assistance is given, the newborn's nose and mouth should be wiped free of secretions; gently swinging the animal, head down, aids in removal of these fluids. The neonate should be dried off and stimulated through rubbing to aid its breathing and the navel should be dipped in an iodine solution to prevent subsequent navel infections. Young may be identified by the application of an ear tag or ear notch. It is extremely important that all neonatal ruminants be supplied with high-quality colostrum within the first 12–24 h of birth. Young that are not nursing on their own should be tube fed with colostrum that has been collected and saved previously (i.e., frozen), or collected from the mother after parturition. Kids and lambs may require supplemental heat (as from a heat lamp) during cold weather.

To control transmission of infectious diseases such as CAE or Johnes' disease, young ruminants may be removed immediately from the dam and hand-fed heat-treated colostrum. The first feeding can be up to 125 ml of colostrum (lambs and kids) or up to 4 l (calves). Milk fed can be reduced by 4 weeks by decreasing either the volume fed or the number of feedings.

Kids should be dehorned and castrated within the first few days of life. Due to the thin calvarium and relatively small frontal sinus in goat kids, electric or butane dehorners should be used with great caution to avoid heat damage to the cerebral cortex. Dehorning of calves is performed when hornbuds appear (3–6 weeks) and castration is performed between 2 and 9 weeks of age or later. Sedation, local anesthesia, and post-procedural analgesia (generally NSAIDs) are appropriate for dehorning and castration procedures.

6. Sexing

Sexing the young in any of the ruminant species is straightforward. The vulva of the female young is located just ventral to the anus. The genitalia of the male include a penis located along the ventral midline and a scrotum located in the inguinal region. The phenomenon of 'freemartin,' a genetic female born as a twin to a male, is the result of anastomoses between placental circulations of the twin fetuses, with mixing of blood-forming cells and germ cells, resulting in XX/XY chimeras. This occurs in 85–90% of phenotypic bovine females born twin to males. The female will often have an abnormal vulva and clitoris and the vagina will be a blind end due a lack of a cervix. Sometimes singleton freemartins

are born if the male fetus is lost after 30 days gestation. Multiple births are selected for and are common in sheep; but the freemartin phenomenon is regarded as rare in this species. Twinning is common in goats and freemartinism occurs in about 6% of male–female pairs of twins. Intersexes are seen in some goat breeds, and when polled goats are mated (see Section III, B, 1).

7. Weaning

Grain, and later roughage, should be offered to lambs well in advance of weaning so that they can adjust to the feedstuffs. To prevent the ewe from ingesting the lamb ration, a 'creep' can be set up in an area adjacent to the ewe/lamb pen by devising a slatted entry for the lambs to enter but not the ewes.

Lambs that are consuming 0.6–0.8 kg of creep feed per day may be weaned. Depending on the individual program, lambs may be weaned as early as 4 weeks of age; although, 6–8 weeks of age is more common. The lambs should be monitored after weaning to ensure that they continue to gain weight and are eating the new ration. Kids should be introduced to forages within the first week of life because the natural curiosity of these animals will cause them to investigate sources of feed. Hand-fed milk should be reduced by 4 weeks of age and kids can be weaned by 6–10 weeks or 18–25 pounds. Dairy calves are usually removed from their dams immediately after birth and fed milk replacer or whole milk until weaning at 4–7 weeks. Stressful procedures, such as castration, dehorning, and vaccinations should be avoided in the week prior to and following weaning.

Passive immunity provided by dams' colostrum decreases gradually until the young are about 6 months old. In calves, the duration of passive immunity varies considerably. Although vaccinations are not necessary during this time, calves have been shown to mount memory B and T cell responses to vaccination even in the presence of colostral antibody so it is not uncommon for calves to receive vaccinations at 4 months of age (Endsley et al., 2003). Some producers choose to begin vaccinating calves at 1–2 months of age, and continue with monthly booster immunizations until the animals are 7 months old and passive immunity is no longer a possibility.

8. Artificial Insemination

AI is now an integral part of dairy herd management; natural insemination in dairy cattle is relatively rare. Technicians performing the AI technique are available through commercial enterprises, although on many dairy farms employees are trained to perform AI. Information regarding the storage and handling of the semen; and the skills and record-keeping is covered extensively elsewhere Youngquist and Threlfall, 2007). In sheep, AI is more difficult than in cattle. Laparoscopic AI involves the surgical instillation of semen into the uterus through a small abdominal opening. The procedure has achieved as high as a 70% pregnancy rate with frozen semen (McCappin and Murray, 2011), but is technically involved and costly. Cervical AI involves the transvaginal introduction of semen into the cervix. A modification of this technique (Transcervical AI) allows for penetration through the cervix, into the uterus. This method (called the Guelph System for Transcervical AI) leads to successful penetration into the uterus in up to 75% of ewes when performed by an experienced inseminator.

9. Synchronization

Control of breeding in the goat has been studied mostly in dairy breeds in order to produce milk throughout the year and to reduce kidding labor. Goats in the luteal phase of the estrus cycle, days 4–16, are sensitive to $PGF_{2\alpha}$ (2.5–5 mg IM) and will show estrus in 36–60 h post injection (Youngquist and Threlfall, 2007). Pheromones may be utilized by introduction of the buck to a group of does, which will induce ovulation and may even synchronize does. Does that are kept separate from the buck will show signs of estrus, and ovulate within 6–10 days when introduced to a buck. Vaginal pessaries of fluorogestone acetate left in place for 21 days in the doe followed by an injection of pregnant mare serum gonadotrophin (PMSG) at the time of pessary removal also has proven successful.

Synchronization of cattle estrous cycles and superovulation are used in many dairy production settings where estrus synchronization and/or embryo transfer are advantageous to production and management. The options and dosing regimens are described in detail in veterinary clinical texts (Hafez and Hafez, 2000; Youngquist and Threlfall, 2007). One of the more common practices involves the use of products approved for use in cattle such as PGF2α or one of its analogs to induce luteolysis. Progestogens are also used in the form of vaginal suppositories. Another approach is to synchronize ovulation (OvSynch®) with scheduled delivery of PGF2α followed by gonadotropin-releasing hormone. Estrus may be suppressed in beef heifers in a feedlot setting by the feeding of melengestrol acetate, a synthetic progestogen.

Because sheep are hormonally similar to other ruminants, estrus synchronization techniques are comparable. Ewes may be exposed to vasectomized rams prior to the beginning of the normal fall mating period. Pheromones released from males naturally stimulate the females to cycle and to synchronize their heats. Artificial or natural progesterones can be administered in the feed, through parenteral injection, subcuticular implants and vaginal pessaries. Other synchronization methods using gonadotropins and prostaglandins have also been shown to be effective (Titi *et al.*, 2010).

10. Embryo Transfer

Embryo transfer involves the removal of multiple embryos from a superovulated embryo donor and transferring them to synchronized recipients. This method maximizes the genetic potential of the donor animal. The donor animal is superovulated with gonadotropins and inseminated. In sheep, embryos are surgically removed from the donor's uterus about 1 week after breeding. In cattle, the procedure is a nonsurgical transcervical flush of the uterus. About 75% of expected embryos (determined by counting corpora lutea) can be recovered; successful recovery is affected by factors such as age of the donor, reproductive health, and surgeon or technician expertise. Recipients are hormonally synchronized with the donor animals. On the day of embryo collection, transferable embryos are implanted into the uterus of the recipient using methods similar to AI. Pregnancy rates average about 70%. If recipients are not available, embryos, like sperm, can be frozen and kept for later transfer. Disease screening for all animals involved is important because several pathogens can be transmitted directly or indirectly, such as BVDV, bluetongue virus, infectious bovine rhinotracheitis virus, and mycoplasmal species.

11. Miscellaneous Management Considerations

a. Management of Male Animals

In sheep flocks and goat herds, as noted, male young are usually castrated by 1 month of age. The elastrator method is the more popular for animals less than 1 week of age. Other methods include crushing the spermatic cord with an emasculatome and surgical castration. The distress associated with castration and tail docking in lambs is the subject of debate and has been researched recently. The reader is referred to journal articles and the AVMA website regarding welfare implications (Stafford, 2007; AVMA, 2012). Bull calves should be castrated as early as possible, but no later than 3 month of age. In some production situations, however, where maximum hormone responsive muscle development and grouping animals together for procedures dictate scheduling, the procedure may be performed on older males with appropriate sedation and analgesia.

Breeding and vasectomized rams and bucks are usually maintained by medium to large production farms. Smaller farms often borrow breeding males. Vasectomized males are often retired breeders and should be tattooed or identified clearly. The vasectomy technique for both species is comparable (Smith and Sherman, 2009). Rams may be housed together for most of the year while bucks are penned separately.

Because ewes will only exhibit a limited number of estrous cycles before becoming reproductively quiescent, it is critical that the male be capable of successfully breeding the female in an expeditious manner. Any defects in the external genitalia, reproductive diseases or musculoskeletal abnormalities may prevent successful copulatory behaviors. Furthermore, it is important to know the semen quality of the ram as one indicator of fertility. Semen can be collected via electroejaculation or by use of a teaser mount. Once semen is collected, it should be handled carefully and kept warm to prevent sperm death leading to improper conclusions about the male. Determination of sperm quality is based on volume, motility, sperm cell concentration, and morphology.

The extensive use of AI in the dairy cattle industry has minimized the use of bulls on many farms. Breeding bulls used in dairy operations should be monitored for excessive weight gain and for lameness due to laminitis, often a result of feeding bulls the relatively energy-dense diets used for dairy cows. The use of natural service is much more common in beef production systems. Breeding bulls must be part of the herd vaccination program, with special attention to appropriate timing of immunizations for the commonly transmitted venereal diseases, campylobacteriosis and trichomoniasis. During an intensive breeding season, providing an adequate number of bulls to service eligible cows is critical to breeding success.

Cattle tail docking is a relatively recent development in dairy herd management and practiced in the belief that it will minimize bacterial contamination of the udder and therefore the milk. Tails are typically docked to about 10 inches in length. To date, published research does not support this practice as a means of improving milk quality or cow cleanliness. Tail docking is a common husbandry practice in sheep. The reader is referred to the AVMA website regarding welfare implications (AVMA, 2012).

E. Behavior

Healthy ruminants have good appetites, are alert and curious, and move without hindrance. Even adult animals will play when provided sufficient space. Ruminants normally vocalize, and handlers will learn to recognize normal communication among the group in contrast to excessive, strained vocalizations which may be a sign of fear, anxiety or stress. 'Bruxism' or grinding of the teeth by a ruminant is usually associated with discomfort or pain. Other signs of discomfort, stress, or illness include decreased time spent eating and cud chewing, restlessness, prolonged recumbency with outstretched neck and head, and hunched back when standing. Unhealthy ruminants may be thin, may have external lumps or swollen joints, an unusual abdominal profile, or rough or dull coats.

All ruminants are herd animals and exhibit social behavior, therefore, every effort should be made to allow contact among individuals in terms of either direct contact, sound, smell, or sight. Sheep in particular are gregarious and should be handled as a group. Human contact and handling should be initiated promptly and maintained regularly throughout the animal's stay in the research facilities. Animals should be provided sufficient time to acclimate to handlers and research staff. Cattle and sheep can hear at higher frequencies than humans can and may react to sounds not perceived by handlers.

Movement of animals is simplified by proper facility design. Chutes should have solid walls and allow animals to follow a lead animal. Ruminants have a wide-angle visual field but are easily startled by activities taking place behind them. Animal movement often is disrupted by contrasts such as light and shadows impinging on a chute or corral. Livestock always should be moved slowly and calmly; handlers should avoid the use of prods, loud noises, or sudden movements. Ruminant animals have a flight zone (minimum zone of comfort) which when penetrated, will result in scattering of the herd or flock. This minimal flight distance can be modified by increasing handling of the animals and by working at the edge of the zone. Minimal flight distances should always be considered when working with animals in chutes, pens, or other confined areas.

Goats exhibit behavioral characteristics that make them quite distinct from other ruminants. Their browsing activity makes them quite orally investigative. Goats will readily nibble or chew just about anything they come in contact with so researchers should keep all paperwork and equipment out of reach. Goats are inquisitive, restless, agile jumpers and climbers, and quite mischievous. If maintained in paddocks, strong high fences are essential as are adequate spaces for exercise or boulders or rock piles for hoof maintenance and recreational climbing. Goats are more tolerant of isolation and are more easily acclimated to human contact than sheep and cattle. Goats with horns will use them to their advantage and horns may also become entangled in fencing. Although less strongly affected by flock behavior, goats are social animals. Most goats raised in close human contact are personable and cooperative and can easily be taught to stand for various procedures including blood collection.

Ruminants of all ages, especially cattle, should be handled with an appreciation of the potential for serious injury to human handlers that may result (Houpt, 2010). While dairy cattle have been bred and selected over centuries for docility, beef breeds are generally more difficult to handle and restrain. All cattle respond well to feed as a reward for desired behavior. Healthy cattle typically are very curious and watchful and are alert to sounds and smells. Because of ruminant digestive and metabolic needs, much of the day is spent eating or cud chewing. Isolation from other cattle, rough handling by attendants, and unfamiliar visual patterns, routines, or environments are all sources of stress to cattle. These stressors increase the difficulty of handling and may exacerbate signs of systemic illnesses.

Estrous behavior in dairy cattle can be easily identified and a number of tools exist (pedometers, pressure sensitive transponders, dyes placed on cows' backs) to facilitate identification of this behavior. In addition to mounting or standing to be mounted, common estrous behaviors include decreased feed consumption, hyperactivity, flehmen, standing behind other cows resting their chins on their backs, licking, and sniffing.

Calves are known for non-nutritive suckling, bar licking, and tongue rolling. Non-nutritive suckling behavior is greater in hungry calves and also immediately after a milk meal. It is best to provide nipples and other clean noninjurious materials for the animals to suck. Non-nutritive suckling can be detrimental in group-housed calves since it can result in disease transmission particularly mastitis, and hairball formation. Environmental enrichment devices have been developed to cope with this behavior. The behavior diminishes as the animals are weaned on to solid food (Morrow-Tesch, 1997; Houpt, 2010).

Play activity and vocalizations of calves mimic adult dominance behaviors. Play activity by young adult cattle is more common in males, can be quite rough, and is often triggered by a change in the environment. Social hierarchies are established within a herd by dominance behavior; the presence of horns, increasing age and body size are important determinants of dominance. Aggression is most common among intact adult males.

III. DISEASES

This section focuses primarily on the more common diseases affecting sheep, goats, and cattle in the United States and North America and those that are reportable. For detailed information not included in this limited overview and for diseases of importance internationally, the authors recommend several excellent comprehensive and focused veterinary clinical texts and periodicals: these are listed under 'Major references' at the end of this chapter.

Several of the infectious diseases described herein are reportable to the USDA. The status of these diseases can change from month-to-month and vary by regions across the United States and the world. For up-to-date information on reportable livestock diseases and reporting procedures, veterinarians are encouraged to make use of online resources from both State and Federal animal health authorities, as reportable diseases may differ from state to state. The USDA/APHIS website (http://www.aphis.usda.gov/wps/portal/aphis/home) has abundant materials on program diseases (such as brucellosis

and bovine tuberculosis), foreign animal diseases, and other diseases of interest, and also a directory of Area Veterinarians in Charge (AVICs).

Recommendations for current drug therapies, both approved and off-label use in ruminants, including withholding times prior to slaughter, formularies, and related information also can be found in the references noted above and formularies (Hawk and Leary, 2005; Plumb, 2011). In addition, the Food Animal Residue Avoidance Databank (FARAD), accessible on the Internet, should be used as a resource. FARAD is a food safety project of the USDA, and is an information resource to prevent drug and pesticide residues in food animals and animal products.

Extra-label drug use is defined by the Animal Medicinal Drug Use Clarification Act of 1994 (AMDUCA, 1994) as "Actual use or intended use of a drug in an animal in a manner that is not in accordance with the approved labeling. This includes, but is not limited to, use in species not listed in the labeling, use for indications (diseases and other conditions) not listed in the labeling, use at dosage levels, frequencies, or routes of administration other than those stated in the labeling, and deviation from labeled withdrawal time based on these different uses" (21 CFR 530, 1994). The FDA under the provisions of AMDUCA recognizes the professional judgment of veterinarians and allows the use of extra-label drugs *by veterinarians* within the context of a valid veterinarian–client relationship under certain conditions:

i. There is no approved new animal drug that is labeled for the intended use that contains the same active ingredient in the required dosage form and concentration.
ii. A veterinarian has made a careful diagnosis and evaluation of the condition.
iii. The veterinarian has established an extended withdrawal period prior to marketing.
iv. The identity of the treated animal is assured and maintained.
v. Ensure that no illegal drug residues occur in any food-producing animal subjected to extra-label treatment.
vi. The prescribed or dispensed extra-label drug must bear labeling information which is adequate to assure the safe and proper use of the product.

Note: Extra-label use is limited to circumstances when the health of an animal is threatened or suffering or death may result from failure to treat. Use of extra-label drugs for the purpose of enhancing production is prohibited. Additionally, the FDA can prohibit the extra-label use of a new animal drug if no sufficient analytical method exists for detection of residues and/or if the drug poses a risk to human health. The extra-label use of the following drugs is prohibited *even if the criteria for extra label drug use has been met.*

1. Chloramphenicol;
2. Clenbuterol;
3. Diethylstilbestrol (DES);
4. Dimetridazole;
5. Ipronidazole;
6. Other nitroimidazoles;
7. Furazolidone;
8. Nitrofurazone;
9. Sulfonamide drugs in lactating dairy cattle (except approved use of sulfadimethoxine, sulfabromomethazine, and sulfaethoxypyridazine);
10. Fluoroquinolones;
11. Glycopeptides;
12. Phenylbutazone in female dairy cattle 20 months of age or older;
13. Cephalosporin (excluding cephapirin) use in cattle, swine, chickens, and turkeys:
    Using cephalosporin drugs at unapproved dose levels, frequencies, durations, or routes of administration is prohibited;
    Using cephalosporin drugs in cattle, swine, chickens, or turkeys that are not approved for use in that species (e.g., cephalosporin drugs intended for humans or companion animals);
    Using cephalosporin drugs for disease prevention.

The following drugs, or classes of drugs, approved for treating or preventing influenza A in humans, are prohibited from extra-label drug use in chickens, turkeys, and ducks:

1. Adamantanes;
2. Neuraminidase inhibitors.

A. Infectious Diseases

1. *Bacterial/Mycoplasmal/Rickettsial*

a. Actinobacillosis ('Wooden Tongue')

Etiology *Actinobacillus lignieresii* is an aerobic, nonmotile, nonspore forming, gram-negative coccobacilli that is widespread in soil and manure and is found as normal flora of the respiratory and upper gastrointestinal tract of ruminants. In sheep and cattle, *A. lignieresii* causes sporadic, noncontagious, and potentially chronic disease characterized by diffuse abscess and granuloma formation in tissues of the head and occasionally other body organs. This disease has not been documented in goats.

Clinical Signs Skin lesions are common, with tumorous abscesses of the tongue (cattle) and lip lesions (sheep). Soft-tissue or lymph node swelling accompanied by draining tracts are observed also in the head and neck regions, as well as other areas. The swollen tongue may protrude from the mouth causing difficulty prehending food, anorexia, and excessive salivation.

Epizootiology and Transmission The organism penetrates wounds of the skin, mouth, nose, gastrointestinal tract, testicles, and mammary gland causing chronic inflammation and abscess formation. Rough feed material and foreign bodies may play a role in causing abrasions.

Necropsy Findings Purulent discharges of white–green exudate containing small white–gray granules drain from the tracts that often extend from the area of colonization to the skin surface.

Differential Diagnosis Contagious ecthyma, caseous lymphadenitis and *Actinomyces bovis* (lumpy jaw) are the primary differentials, but rabies should also be considered. Diagnosis can be confirmed by microscopic examination of smears made from pus or by biopsy and culturing of the lesion.

Treatment IV administration of sodium iodide is the treatment of choice; oral potassium iodide also may be used. Clinical response is generally seen within 48 h of starting IV treatment. Systemic antibiotics such as ceftiofur, ampicillin, or florfenicol may be effective. Treatment can include surgical debridement and flushing with iodine.

Prevention and Control Avoid poor quality, coarse feed. Isolation or disposal of animals with disease is recommended. No vaccine is available.

b. Actinomycosis ('Lumpy Jaw') ARCANOBACTERIUM

Etiology *Actinomyces bovis* are anaerobic, nonmotile, nonspore forming, gram-positive, nonacid fast pleomorphic rods to coccobacilli associated with 'Lumpy Jaw' in cattle; rarely seen in sheep and goats.

Clinical Signs and Diagnosis *A. bovis* causes chronic, progressive, pyogranulomatous osteomyelitis of the mandible, maxillae, or other bony tissues of the head. The mass will be slow growing, firm, nonpainful and is attached to the mandible. Ulceration occurs with or without tracts draining purulent material. The alveoli of the roots of the cheek teeth are frequently involved causing loose teeth making chewing difficult. Painful eating and weight loss are evident.

Epizootiology and Transmission These organisms are normal flora of the gastrointestinal tract of ruminants and gain entrance into tissues through abrasions and penetrating wounds from wire or coarse hay or sticks. It is important to note that *Actinomyces bovis* is a zoonotic organism causing granulomas, abscesses, skin lesions, and bronchopneumonia in humans.

Necropsy Draining lesions with sulfur-like granules (as with Actinobacillosis) are frequently observed.

Differential Diagnosis *Actinobacillus lignieresii* and caseous lymphadenitis are important differentials for draining tracts. Tumors, trauma to the affected area, such as the mandible, and dental disease or oral foreign body should also be considered.

Prevention and Control   Avoid feeds with coarse or sharp ingredients.

Treatment   Sodium iodide IV is the treatment of choice and is repeated several times at 7- to 10-day intervals. Concurrent antibiotic treatment may also be used, most often penicillin or oxytetracycline. Prognosis is poor in the presence of bone involvement; surgical excision is an option and may be helpful.

c. Trueperella Associated with Omphalophlebitis (See Navel Ill Below)

Omphalophlebitis, omphaloarteritis, omphalitis, and Navel Ill are terms referring to infection of the umbilicus in young animals.

Etiology   *Trueperella pyogenes*, frequently combined with *E. coli*, is the most common organism causing omphalophlebitis, an acute localized inflammation and infection of the external umbilicus.

Clinical Signs   Most cases occur within the first 3 months of age and animals are presented with a painful enlargement of the umbilicus. Animals may exhibit various degrees of depression and anorexia, and purulent discharges may be seen draining from the umbilicus. Involvement of the urachus is usually followed by cystitis and associated signs of dysuria, hematuria, and so on. Severe sequelae may include septicemia, peritonitis, septic arthritis ('joint ill'), meningitis, patent urachus, urachal abscesses, umbilical hernias, osteomyelitis, and endocarditis.

Diagnosis   Diagnosis is by bacteriologic culture and identification of the organism.

Treatment   Debridement, drainage, and antimicrobials may be useful in treatment. In addition to treatment, husbandry deficiencies resulting in poor hygine must be addressed. Animal caretakers should be trained to ensure appropriate naval dipping is occurring.

Research Complications   Omphalophlebitis is a potential source for recurrent septicemia.

d. Anthrax

Etiology   *Bacillus anthracis* is a zoonotic nonmotile, capsulated, spore-forming, aerobic, gram-positive bacillus that is found in alkaline soil, contaminated feeds (such as bone meal), and water. The common names for the disease are woolsorter's disease, splenic fever, charbon, and milzbrand. Cases of anthrax must be reported to animal health authorities.

Clinical Signs   Anthrax is a sporadic but very serious infectious disease of cattle, sheep, and goats characterized by septicemia, hyperthermia, anorexia, depression, listlessness, and tremors. The incubation period is generally 3–7 days and ranges from peracute to chronic. The peracute form is most common in cattle and sheep and is characterized by sudden onset of staggering, dyspnea, trembling, collapse, and convulsions leading to death. Often the onset is so rapid that illness is not observed and the animal is found dead. Hematuria and bloody diarrhea often occur. The disease is usually fatal, especially in sheep and goats, after 1–3 days. Death is the result of shock, renal failure and anoxia.

Diagnosis   Diagnosis based on clinical signs alone is difficult. Laboratory confirmation should be attempted: the ideal sample is a cotton swab soaked in the blood and allowed to dry. Specific tests include bacterial culture, PCR tests, and fluorescent antibody stains to demonstrate the presence of the organism. Stained blood smears may show short, single to chained bacilli. Blood may be collected from a superficial vein and submitted for culture. Western blot and ELISA blood tests for antibodies are available.

Epizootiology and Transmission   Anthrax has been reported from nearly every continent; most cases in the United States occur in the central and western states. Epizootics occur in agricultural regions associated with drought, flooding, or other types of soil disturbance. Spores remain infective in the soil for many years during which time they are a potential source of infection for grazing livestock. The anthrax organisms (primarily spores) are generally ingested, sporulate, and replicate in the local tissues. Anthrax is zoonotic and may be seen in humans exposed to tissue from infected animals, contaminated animal products or directly to spores under certain conditions. Cattle and sheep tend to be affected more commonly than goats due to grazing habits.

Necropsy   Necropsies should not be performed as the spores contaminate the environment. Definitive diagnoses may be made without opening the animals. Incomplete *rigor mortis*, rapid putrefaction, and dark uncoagulated blood exuding from all body orifices are common findings. Splenomegaly, cyanosis, epicardial and subcutaneous hemorrhages, and lymphadenopathy are characteristic of the disease.

Differential Diagnosis   Although anthrax should always be considered when an animal that was healthy on the previous day dies acutely, other causes of acute death in ruminants should be considered, e.g., bloat, enterotoxemia, malignant edema, blackleg, and black disease.

Prevention and Control   Anthrax is of particular concern as a bioterrorism agent. Control is achieved through vaccination programs and rapid detection and reporting with treatment of asymptomatic animals and burning or burial of suspect and confirmed cases. Herds in endemic areas and along waterways are routinely vaccinated with the Sterne-strain spore vaccine (virulent, nonencapsulated). The disease is a serious public health risk; a vaccine is available for personnel working with the agent.

Treatment Treatment of animals in early stages with penicillin or other long-acting antibiotics may be helpful. Vaccination should follow 7–10 days after the conclusion of antibiotic therapy. During epidemics, animals should be vaccinated with the Sterne vaccine.

Research Complications Natural and experimental anthrax infections are a risk to research personnel. The organism sporulates when exposed to air and spores may be inhaled during post mortem examinations. *B. anthracis* is considered a select agent. Readers are referred to the Center for Disease Control (CDC) National Select Agent Registry (http://www.selectagents.gov) for additional information.

e. Brucellosis

Etiology *Brucella* are nonmotile, nonspore forming, nonencapsulated, gram-negative coccobacilli. *B. abortus* (*B. melitensis biovar Abortus*) is one of several *Brucella* species that infects domestic animals but cross species infections occur rarely. *B. abortus* or *B. melitensis* may cause brucellosis in sheep, cattle and goats. *B. melitensis* (biovar 1, 2, or 3) is the primary cause of the disease in sheep but does not occur in the U.S. *B. abortus* is almost exclusively the cause of disease in cattle but has been largely eliminated in developed countries. Both *B. abortus* and *B. melitensis* are significant human pathogens. *B. ovis* causes pyogranulomatous epididymitis and orchitis, but is not zoonotic. Because brucellosis is unlikely to be encountered in research settings in developed countries, the reader is referred to the 'Major References' at the end of this chapter, and to websites such as http://www.aphis.usda.gov.

f. Campylobacteriosis (Vibriosis): *Campylobacter Fetus* Subsp. *Intestinalis; C. Jejuni*

Etiology *Campylobacter (Vibrio) fetus* subsp. *intestinalis*, a pleomorphic curved to coccoid, motile, nonspore forming, gram-negative bacterium, causes campylobacteriosis, the most important cause of ovine abortion in the United States Vibriosis is derived from the name formerly given to the genus; the term is still frequently used.

Clinical Signs and Diagnosis Ovine vibriosis is a contagious disease that causes abortion, stillbirths and weak lambs. The organism inhabits the intestines and gallbladder in subclinical carriers. Abortion generally occurs in the last trimester and abortion storms may occur as more susceptible animals, such as maiden ewes, become exposed to the infectious tissues. Some lambs may be born alive but will be weak; dams will be agalactic.

Diagnosis is achieved by microscopic identification or isolation of the organism from placenta, fetal abomasal contents, and maternal vaginal discharges using Giemsa or Ziehl–Neelsen stained smears.

Epizootiology and Transmission Campylobacteriosis occurs worldwide. *Campylobacter* spp., such as *C. jejuni*, normally inhabits ovine gastrointestinal tracts and is shed in the feces. In abortion storms, considerable contamination of the environment will occur due to shedding in placenta, fetuses, and uterine fluids. Ewes may have active *Campylobacter* organisms in uterine discharges for several months after abortion. There is no venereal transmission in the ovine.

Necropsy Aborted fetuses will be edematous with accumulation of serosanguinous fluids within the subcutis and muscle tissue fascia. The liver may contain 2- to 3-cm pale foci. Placental tissues will be thickened and edematous, and will contain serous fluids similar to the fetus. The placental cotyledons may appear gray.

Differential Diagnosis *Toxoplasma gondii, Chlamydophila abortus*, and *Listeria monocytogenes* should be considered in late gestation ovine abortions.

Prevention and Control A bacterin is available to prevent the disease. Carrier states have been cleared by treating with a combination of antibiotics including penicillin and oral chlortetracycline. Aborting ewes should be isolated immediately from the rest of the flock. After an outbreak, ewes will develop immunity lasting 2 or 3 years.

Treatment Infected animals should be isolated and provided with supportive therapy. Prompt decontamination of the area and disposal of the aborted tissues and discharges is important.

Research Complications Losses from abortion may be considerable. *Campylobacter* ssp. are zoonotic agents and *C. fetus* ssp. *intestinalis* may be the cause of 'shepherd's scours.'

g. Campylobacteriosis (Bovine *Vibriosis*): *Campylobacter Fetus* Subsp. *Venerealis*

Etiology *Campylobacter fetus* subsp. *venerealis* is the main cause of bovine Campylobacteriosis abortions. It does not cause disease in other ruminant species.

Clinical Signs and Diagnosis Preliminary signs of a problem in the herd will be a high percentage of cows returning to estrus after breeding and temporary infertility. This will be particularly apparent in virgin heifers that may return to estrus by 40 days after breeding. Spontaneous abortions may occur, typically during the 5th to 8th months of gestation. The aborted fetus may be fresh or severely autolyzed. Severe endometritis may lead to salpingitis and permanent infertility.

Demonstration or isolation of the organism, a curved rod with corkscrew motility, is the basis for diagnosis. Campylobacter can be identified by darkfield examination of abomasal contents or from culture of the placenta or abomasal contents. A fluorescent antibody test on genital discharge from the bull or cow can also be diagnostic; a PCR test is available for detection of *Campylobacter* in semen.

Epizootiology and Transmission The bacterium is an obligate, ubiquitous organism of the genital tract. Transmission is from infected bulls to heifers. Bulls are carriers of the disease but show no clinical signs. Older cows develop effective immunity.

Necropsy Findings Necrotizing placentitis with hemorrhagic cotyledons, dehydration, and fibrinous serositis will be found grossly. In addition, broncho-pneumonia and hepatitis will be seen histologically.

Differential Diagnosis The primary differential for campylobacteriosis in cattle is trichomoniasis. Other differentials include brucellosis, mycoplasmosis, infectious bovine rhinotracheitis–pustular vulvovaginitis (IBR–IPV), bovine viral diarrhea (BVD), and leptospirosis.

Prevention and Control Killed bacterin vaccines are available; annual boosters should be given after the initial immunization and as part of the regular prebreeding regimen. AI is particularly useful at controlling the disease.

Treatment Cows will usually recover from the infection. Treatment with antibiotics, such as penicillin, administered as an intrauterine infusion improves the chances of returning to breeding condition.

h. Caprine Staphylococcal Dermatitis

Etiology The most common caprine bacterial skin infection is caused by *Staphylococcus intermedius* or *S. aureus* and is known as staphylococcal dermatitis (Smith and Sherman, 2009). The *Staphylococcus* organisms are cocci and are categorized as primary pathogens or ubiquitous skin commensals of humans and animals.

Clinical Signs and Diagnosis Small pustular lesions, caused by bacterial infection and inflammation of the hair follicle, occur around the teats and perineum. Occasionally, the infection may involve the flanks, underbelly, axilla, inner thigh, and neck. Diagnosis is based on lesions and positive culture.

Differential Diagnosis Contagious ecthyma is a differential diagnosis along with fungal skin infections and nutritional causes of skin disease.

Treatment Severe infections should be treated with antibiotics based on culture and sensitivity. Lesions may benefit from periodic cleaning with an iodophor shampoo and spraying with an antibiotic and an astringent (Smith and Sherman, 2009).

i. Clostridial Diseases

i. C. PERFRINGENS, TYPE C (ENTEROTOXEMIA AND STRUCK)

Etiology C. *perfringens* is an anaerobic, gram-positive, non-motile, spore-forming bacterium that lives in the soil, contaminated feed and gastrointestinal tracts of ruminants. The bacterium is categorized by toxin production. Toxins include alpha (hemolytic), beta (necrotizing), delta (cytotoxic and hemolytic), epsilon, and iota. Types of *C. perfringens* are A, B, C, D, and E. Infection is a common and economically significant disease of sheep, goats, and cattle.

Clinical Signs and Diagnosis The lethal beta toxin associated with overgrowth of this bacterium results in a hemorrhagic enterocolitis within the first 72 h of a well-fed young ruminant's life. Animals may simply be found dead with no clinical presentation. Affected animals are acutely anemic, dehydrated, anorexic, depressed, and may display tremors or convulsions as well as abdominal pain. Calves experience an acute diarrhea, dysentery, abdominal pain, convulsions, and opisthotonos with death occurring in a few hours. Less severe cases can survive for a few days and recovery is possible. Feces may range from loose gray–brown to dark red and malodorous. Morbidity and mortality may be nearly 100%.

A similar noncontagious but acutely fatal form of enterotoxemia in adult sheep, called 'Struck,' occurs in yearlings and adults. Struck is rare in the United States. The disease is also caused by the beta toxin of *C. perfringens* type C and is often associated with rapid dietary changes or shearing stresses in sheep. Although affected animals are usually found dead, clinical signs include uneasiness, depression, and convulsions. Mortality is usually less than 15%.

Diagnosis is usually based on necropsy findings. Identification of the beta toxin in intestinal contents may be difficult due to instability of the toxin, but filtrates made for detection of toxin and future identification by neutralization with specific antisera is possible.

Epizootiology and Transmission Clostridial organisms are ubiquitous in the environment as well as in the gastrointestinal tract and contaminated feeds. Transmission is by ingestion of contaminated material.

Necropsy Findings Necropsy findings include a milk-filled abomasum as well as hemorrhage in the distal small and large intestines. The affected portion of the intestine may be deep blue to purple in color and resemble a mesenteric torsion. Petechial hemorrhages of the serosal surfaces of many organs, especially the thymus, heart, and gastrointestinal tract will be visible. Hydropericardium, hydroperitoneum, and hemorrhagic mesenteric lymph nodes will also be present. Pulmonary and brain edema may also be seen (Blackwell and Butler, 1992).

Differential Diagnoses Other Clostridial diseases such as blackleg and black disease as well as coccidiosis, salmonellosis, anthrax, and acute poisoning.

Prevention and Control A commercial toxoid is available and should be administered to the pregnant animals during the last third of preganancy. Initial vaccination of young animals should consist of two vaccinations, 1 month apart, and then annually.

Treatment   Treatment is difficult and usually unsuccessful due to the severity of the disease. Antitoxin may be useful in milder cases, and antiserum may be administered immediately after birth in the face of an outbreak.

ii. C. PERFRINGENS, *TYPE D (PULPY KIDNEY DISEASE)*

Etiology   *C. perfringens* type D releases epsilon toxin that is proteolytically activated by trypsin. This disease caused by *C. perfringens* tends to be associated with sheep and is of less importance in goats and cattle.

Clinical Signs   The peracute condition in younger animals is characterized by sudden deaths, which are occasionally preceded by neurological signs such as incoordination, opisthotonus, and convulsions. Because the disease progresses so rapidly to death (within 1–2 h) clinical signs are rarely observed. The largest, fastest-growing animals generally are predisposed to this condition.

Necropsy Findings   These are similar to those seen with *C. perfringens* type C. Additionally, extremely necrotic, soft kidneys ('pulpy kidneys') are usually observed immediately following death. Focal encephalomalacia, and petechial hemorrhages on serosal surfaces of the brain, diaphragm, gastrointestinal tract and heart are common findings. See Uzal and Songer (2008) for further information.

Differential Diagnosis   Tetanus, enterotoxigenic *E. coli*, botulism, polioencephalomalacia, grain overload, and listeriosis are differentials.

Prevention and Control   Vaccination prevents the disease. Maternal antibodies last approximately 5 weeks postpartum; thus, young animals should be vaccinated at about this time. Feeding regimens to young or fast-growing animals and feeding of concentrates to adults should be evaluated carefully.

Treatment   Treatment consists of support (fluids, warmth), antitoxin administration, oral antibiotics, and diet adjustment.

iii. C. TETANI *(TETANUS, LOCKJAW)*

Etiology   *Clostridium tetani* is a strictly anaerobic, motile, spore forming, gram-positive rod that persists in soils, manure, and within the gastrointestinal tract. Tetanus toxemia is caused by a specific neurotoxin produced by *Clostridium tetani* in necrotic tissue. It is introduced into the tissue through wounds, specifically deep punctures which provide the necessary anaerobic environment. The uterus is the most common site of infection in post parturient dairy cattle with retained placentas. Banding castrations are another common etiology of the condition.

Clinical Signs   Infection by *C. tetani* is characterized by a sporadic, acute, and fatal neuropathy. After an incubation period of 4 days to 3 weeks, the animal exhibits bloat, muscular spasticity, prolapse of the third eyelid, rigidity and extension of the limbs leading to a stiff gait, an inability to chew, and hyperthermia. Retracted lips, drooling, hypersensitivity to external stimuli, and a 'saw-horse' stance are frequent signs. The animal may convulse. Death occurs within 3–10 days and mortality is nearly 100%, primarily from respiratory failure. Diagnosis is based on clinical signs.

Epizootiology and Transmission   *C. tetani* is a soil contaminant and is often found as part of the gut microflora of herbivores. The organisms sporulate and persist in the environment. All species of livestock are susceptible, but sheep and goats are more susceptible than cattle, with horses being the most susceptible. Individual cases may occur or herd outbreaks may follow castration, tail docking, ear tagging, or dehorning.

Differential Diagnoses   Differentials include bloat, rabies, hypomagnesemic tetany, polioencephalomalacia, white muscle disease, enterotoxemia in lambs, and lead poisoning.

Necropsy Findings   Findings are nonspecific except for the inflammatory reaction associated with the wound.

Treatment   Treatment consists of cleaning and aggressively debriding the infected wound, administration of tetanus antitoxin, vaccination with tetanus toxoid, administration of antibiotics both parenterally and flushed into the cleaned wound, a sedative or tranquilizer and a muscle relaxant, and keeping the animal in a dark, quiet environment. Supportive fluids and glucose must be administered until the animal is capable of feeding.

Prevention and Control   The disease can be controlled and prevented by following good sanitation measures, aseptic surgical procedures, and vaccination programs. Tetanus toxoid vaccine is available and very effective for stimulating long-term immunity. Animals should be vaccinated two to three times during the first year of life. Does and ewes should receive booster vaccinations within 2 months of parturition to ensure colostral antibodies. For sheep, goats, and cattle, the tetanus toxoid vaccine is available in combination with other clostridial diseases. Tetanus antitoxin can be administered as a preventative or in the face of disease as an adjunct to therapy.

Research Complications   Unprotected, younger ruminants may be affected following routine flock or herd management procedures.

iv. C. NOVYI *(BIGHEAD; BLACK DISEASE; BACILLARY HEMOGLOBINURIA [RED WATER]);* C. CHAUVOEI *(BLACKLEG)*

Etiology   *Clostridium novyi*, an anaerobic, motile, spore-forming, gram-positive bacteria, is the agent of bighead and black disease. *C. novyi* Type D (*C. hemolyticum*) is the cause of bacillary hemoglobinuria. *C. chauvoei* is the causative agent of blackleg.

Clinical Signs Bighead is a disease of rams characterized by a nongaseous, nonhemorrhagic edema of the head and neck. The edema may migrate to ventral regions such as the throat. Additional clinical signs include swelling of the eyelids, and nostrils. Most animals will die within 48–72 h. Black disease or infectious necrotic hepatitis is a peracute, fatal disease associated with *C. novyi*. It is more common in cattle and sheep, but may be seen in goats. The clinical course is 1–2 days in cattle, and slightly shorter in sheep. Otherwise healthy-appearing 2- to 4-year-old animals are often affected. Clinical signs are rarely seen because of the peracute nature of the disease. Occasionally, hyperthermia, tachypnea, inability to keep up with other animals, and recumbency are observed prior to death. Bacillary hemoglobinuria is an acute disease seen primarily in cattle, characterized by fever and anorexia in addition to the hemoglobinemia and hemoglobinuria indicated by the name. Animals that survive a few days will develop icterus. Mortality may be high.

Blackleg, a disease similar to bighead, causes necrosis and emphysema of muscle masses (clostridial myositis), serohemorrhagic fluid accumulation around the infected area, and edema. Blackleg is more common in cattle than sheep. The clinical course is short, 24–48 h, and animals die regardless of treatment. Blackleg in cattle can be associated with subcutaneous edema or crepitation; these lesions do not usually occur in sheep. Most lesions are associated with muscles of the face, neck perineum, thigh, and back.

Epizootiology and Transmission Bighead is caused by the toxins of *C. novyi* which enters through wounds often associated with horn injuries during fighting. *C. novyi* Type D is endemic in western USA *C. chauvoei* spores remain viable in the soil for years and are the potential source of infection. Outbreaks are often seen after excavation or flooding and are more common in summer and fall. It is suspected the organism is ingested, gains access to the bloodstream via the gastrointestinal tract and enters the muscles. Black disease and bacillary hemoglobinuria are associated with concurrent liver disease often associated with *Fasciola* infections (liver flukes); it is sometimes seen as sequelae to liver biopsies. Ingested spores are believed to develop in hepatic tissue damaged and anoxic from the fluke migrations.

Necropsy Diagnosis of black disease is usually based on *post mortem* lesions. Subcutaneous vessels will be engorged with blood resulting in dried skin having a dark appearance. Carcasses putrefy quickly. In addition, hepatomegaly and endocardial hemorrhages are common, and hepatic damage from flukes may be so severe that diagnosis is difficult.

Differential Diagnosis Differentials include other clostridial diseases; hemolytic diseases such as babesiosis, leptospirosis, and hemobartonellosis; and photosensitization.

Treatment For *C. chauvoei* and bighead, early aggressive treatment including aggressive wound debridement, oxygenation, and penicillin or tetracycline may be helpful. Treatment for black disease is not rewarding. For *C. novyi* (*C. haemolyticum*) early treatment with penicillin or tetracycline in high doses along with a blood transfusion and fluids may be helpful.

Prevention and Control Vaccinating animals with multivalent clostridial vaccines will prevent these diseases and may be useful in an outbreak. Control of fascioliasis is very important in prevention and control of black disease.

v. C. SEPTICUM (MALIGNANT EDEMA)

Etiology *Clostridium septicum* is the species usually associated with malignant edema, but mixed infections involving other clostridial species such as *C. chauvoei*, *C. novyi*, *C. sordelli*, and *C. perfringens* may occur.

Clinical Signs Malignant edema or gas gangrene is an acute and often fatal bacterial disease caused by clostridium spp. The affected area will be warm and will contain gaseous accumulations that can be palpated as crepitation of the subcutaneous tissue around the infected area. The skin over the infected area generally has a blue color characteristic of gangrene. Regional lymphadenopathy and fever may occur. The animal becomes anorexic, severely depressed and possibly hyperthermic. Pitting edema and crepitation may be noted around the wound; death occurs within 12 h to 2 days.

Epizootiology and Transmission The organisms are ubiquitous in the environment worldwide, are found in the intestinal contents of animals, and may survive in the soil for years. The disease is especially prevalent in animals that have had recent wounds containing devitalized tissue such as those that have undergone castration, docking, ear notching, shearing, or dystocia.

Necropsy Findings The tissue necrosis and hemorrhagic serous fluid accumulations resemble those of other clostridial diseases. Spreading, crepitant lesions around wounds are suggestive of malignant edema. Gas and serosanguineous fluids with foul odors infiltrate the tissue planes.

Treatment Infected animals can be treated with large doses of penicillin, anti-inflammatories and fenestration of the wound is recommended. Affected tissues usually slough.

Prevention and Control Proper preparation of surgical sites, sanitation of instruments and the housing environment and attention to post-operative wounds will help prevent this disease. Multivalent clostridial vaccines are available.

j. Colibacillosis

Etiology *Escherichia coli* is a motile, aerobic, gram-negative, nonspore-forming coccobacillus commonly found in the environment and gastrointestinal tracts of ruminants. *E. coli* organisms have three areas of surface antigenic complexes ('O' – somatic, 'K' – envelope or pili, and 'H' – flagellar) that are used to 'group' or classify serotypes. Colibacillosis is the common term for infections in younger animals caused by this bacterium.

Clinical Signs Presentation of *E. coli* infections vary with the animal's age and the type of *E. coli* involved. Exposure is primarily fecal–oral but can also occur through the umbilicus. Entertoxigenic *E. coli* infection causes gastroenteritis and/or septicemia in neonates. Colibacillosis generally develops within the first 72 h of life when newborn animals are exposed to the organism. The enteric infection causes a semifluid, yellow to gray diarrhea. Occasionally blood streaking of the feces may be observed. Listlessness along with a loss of suckling interest is followed by abdominal pain, evidenced by arching of the back and extension of the tail. Hyperthermia is rare and temperature may be subnormal. Severe acidosis, depression, recumbancy, and lack of response to external stimuli ensue. Mortality may be as high as 75%. This form of the disease is very acute with the clinical course lasting only 3–8 h. The septicemic form generally occurs between 2 and 6 weeks of age. Animals display an elevated body temperature and show signs suggestive of nervous system involvement such as incoordination, head pressing, circling and the appearance of blindness. Opisthotonos, depression and death follow due to endotoxemic shock. Occasionally, swollen, painful joints may be observed with septicemic colibacillosis. Blood cultures may be helpful in identifying the septicemic form.

In ruminants, *E. coli* also may cause cystitis and pyelonephritis. Cystitis is characterized by dysuria and pollakiuria, although gross hematuria and pyuria may be present. In cases of pyelonephritis, a cow will be acutely depressed, have a fever, ruminal stasis, and be anorectic.

Epizootiology and Transmission *E. coli* is one of the most common gram-negative pathogens isolated from ruminant neonates affecting calves and lambs. Overcrowding, poor sanitation, and failure of passive immune transfer contribute significantly to the development of this disease in young animals. The organism will be endemic in a contaminated environment and present on dams' udders. The bacteria rapidly proliferate in the neonates' small intestines. The bacteria and associated toxins cause a secretory diarrhea resulting in the loss of water and electrolytes. If the bacteria infiltrate the intestinal barrier and enter the blood, septicemia results. Immunoglobulin-deficient calves are far more susceptible to both enteritis and septicemia.

Diagnosis Diagnosis of the enteric form can be made by observation of clinical signs including diarrhea, staining of the tail and wool and demonstration of

a deficiency of circulating IgG. ELISA and latex agglutination tests are available diagnostic tools.

Necropsy Findings Swollen, yellow to gray, fluid-filled small and large intestines, swollen and hemorrhagic mesenteric lymph nodes, and generalized tissue dehydration are common. Septicemic animals may have serofibrinous fluid in the peritoneal, thoracic and pericardial cavities, enlarged joints containing fibrinopurulent exudates, and congested and inflamed meninges.

Differential Diagnosis These include the enterotoxemias caused by *C. perfringens* A, B, or C; *Campylobacter jejuni*; *Coccidia* spp., rotavirus, coronavirus, *Salmonella*, *Streptococcus* spp., *Pasteurella* spp., and *Cryptosporidia*.

Prevention and Control The best preventative measures include scrupulous attention to colostrum quality and delivery, prevention of overcrowding and frequent sanitization of maternity areas.

Treatment Antibiotics with known efficacy against gram-negative organisms such as trimethoprim/sulfadiazine, enrofloxacin, cephalothin, and ceftiofur may be helpful. Oral antibiotics are not recommended. Aggressive use of Ringers solution supplemented with dextrose and electrolytes is critical, including bicarbonate for metabolic acidosis, and nonsteroidal anti-inflammatories help with pain relief. High mortalities should be expected even with quick and aggressive intervention. Vaccines may be given to the dam prior to calving to boost colostral immunity.

k. *Corynebacterium pseudotuberculosis* (Caseous Lymphadenitis)

Etiology *Corynebacterium pseudotuberculosis* (previously *C. ovis*) is a nonmotile, nonspore forming, aerobic, short and curved, gram-positive coccobacilli. Caseous lymphadenitis (CLA) is such a common, chronic contagious disease of sheep and goats that any presentation of abscessing and draining lymph nodes should be presumed to be this disease until proven otherwise. The disease has been reported occasionally in cattle.

Clinical Signs and Diagnosis Abscessation of both superficial and deep lymph nodes is typical. Radiographs may be helpful in identifying affected central nodes. Peripheral lymph nodes may erode and drain caseous, 'cheesy,' yellow–green–tan secretions. The incubation period may be weeks to months. Over time, an infected animal may become exercise-intolerant, anorectic, and debilitated. Fever, increased respiratory rates, and pneumonia may also be common signs. Morbidity up to 15% is common, and morbid animals will often eventually succumb to the disease. See Dorella *et al.* (2006) for additional discussion.

Diagnosis is based on clinical lesions, and culturing or gram-staining of lymph node aspirates. ELISA serological testing is also available.

Epizootiology and Transmission The organism can survive for 6 months or more in the environment and enters via skin wounds such as shearing, castration, or docking. Ingestion and aerosolization (leading to pulmonary abscesses) have been reported as alternative routes of entry.

Necropsy Findings Disseminated superficial abscesses as well as lesions of the mediastinal and mesenteric lymph nodes will be identified. Cut surfaces of the affected lymph nodes may appear lamellated. Lungs, liver, spleen, and kidneys may also be affected. Cranioventral lung consolidation with hemorrhage, fibrin, and edema are seen histologically.

Differential Diagnosis Differentials include pathogens causing lymphadenopathy and abscessation as well as injection site reactions from clostridial vaccines.

Treatment Antibiotic therapy is not usually helpful. Abscesses can be surgically lanced and flushed with iodine-containing and/or hydrogen peroxide solutions, or removed entirely from valuable animals. Because of the contagious nature of the disease, animals with draining and lanced lesions should be isolated from CLA-negative animals at least until healed. Commercial vaccines are available (Piontkowski and Shivvers, 1998).

Prevention and Control Minimizing contamination of the environment, proper sanitation methods for facilities and instruments, segregation of affected animals, and precautions to prevent injuries are all important.

Research Complications This pathogen is a risk for animals undergoing routine management procedures, or invasive research procedures, due to the persistence in the environment, a long clinical incubation period, and poor response to antibiotics.

l. *Corynebacterium renale, C. cystitidis,* and *C. pilosum* (Pyelonephritis, Posthitis, and Ulcerative Vulvovaginitis)

Etiology *Corynebacterium renale, C. cystitidis,* and *C. pilosum* are sometimes referred to as the 'C. renale group.' These are piliated and non-motile gram-positive rods and are distinguished biochemically. *C. renale* causes pyelonephritis in cattle, and *C. pilosum* and *C. cystitis* cause posthitis, also known as pizzle rot or sheath rot, in sheep and goats. The bacteria are ubiquitous in the environment and inhabit the vagina and prepuce. High-protein diets, resulting in higher urea excretion, more basic urine, and irritation of the preputial and vaginal mucous membranes are contributing factors.

Clinical Signs and Diagnosis Acute pyelonephritis is characterized by fever, anorexia, polyuria, hematuria, pyuria, and arched-back posture. First signs may be blood-tinged urine in a seemingly normal cow. Untreated infections usually become chronic with

discomfort, frequent urination, weight loss, anorexia, hematuria or pyuria and loss of production in dairy animals. Chronic cases are characterized by diarrhea, polyuria, polydipsia, stranguria, and anemia. Relapses are common, and some infections are severe and fatal. Diagnosis of pyelonephritis is based on clinical signs and urinalysis (proteinuria and hematuria) and rectal or vaginal palpation (assessing ureteral enlargement).

Posthitis and vulvovaginitis are characterized by ulcers, crusting, swelling, and pain. The area may have a distinct malodor. Necrosis and scarring may be sequelae of more severe infections. Fly strike may also be a complication. Diagnosis is based on clinical signs.

Epizootiology and Transmission Although ascending urinary tract infections with cystitis, ureteritis, and pyelonephritis are widespread problems, the incidence is relatively low. The vaginitis and posthitis contribute to venereal transmission. Indirect transmission is possible because organisms are present on wool or scabs shed from affected animals. Posthitis occurs in intact and castrated sheep and goats.

Necropsy Findings Pyelonephritis, multifocal kidney abscessation, dilated and thickened ureters, cystitis, and purulent exudate in many sections of the urinary tract are common findings at gross necropsy.

Differential Diagnosis Urolithiasis is a primary consideration for these diseases. Contagious ecthyma should be considered although the lesions of contagious ecthyma are more likely to develop around the mouth.

Prevention Feeding practices must be reconsidered. Clipping long wool and hair also is helpful. Affected animals should be isolated to control build-up of the organisms.

Treatment Long term (3 weeks) penicillin administration is effective for pyelonephritis as is trimethoprim-sulfadioxine for 3 weeks. Reduction of dietary protein, clipping and cleaning skin lesions, treating for or preventing fly strike, and topical antibacterial treatments are effective for posthitis/vulvovaginitis; systemic therapy may be necessary for severe cases.

m. Dermatophilosis (Cutaneous Streptothricosis, Lumpy Wool, Strawberry Footrot)

Etiology *Dermatophilus congolensis* is a gram-positive, nonacid-fast, facultative anaerobic actinomycete. Dermatophilosis is a chronic bacterial skin disease characterized by crustiness and exudates accumulating at the base of the hair or wool fibers. Various strains can be present within a group of animals experiencing an outbreak. The natural habitat of the organism is unknown as it has not been successfully isolated from soil.

Clinical Signs Animals will be painful but not pruritic. Two forms exist in sheep, mycotic dermatitis (also known as lumpy wool) and strawberry footrot. Mycotic dermatitis is characterized by crusts and wool matting with exudates over the back and sides of adult animals and about the face of lambs. Strawberry footrot is rare in the United States but is characterized by crusts and inflammation between the carpi and/or tarsi and the coronary bands. Animals will be lame. In goats and cattle, similar clinical signs of crusty, suppurative dermatitis are seen; the disease is often referred to as cutaneous streptothricosis in these species. In cattle, most lesions are raised, matted tufts of hair and are distributed over the head, dorsal surfaces of the neck and body. Lesions in younger goats are seen along the tips of the ears and under the tail. Most affected animals will recover within 3–4 weeks and lesions have little effect on overall health. Animals that develop severe generalized infections often lose condition. Movement and eating become difficult if the feet, lips and muzzle are involved. Cattle with lesions over 50% of their bodies are likely to become seriously ill. Rare human infections have occurred from handling diseased animals.

Diagnosis　Diagnosis is based on clinical signs as well as the typical microscopic appearance on stained skin scrapings and crusts, cultures and serology. The organism can be isolated via culture and/or skin biopsy.

Epizootiology and Transmission　The disease occurs worldwide and the *Dermatophilus* organism is believed to be a saprophyte. Transmission occurs by direct contact with infected animals, although contaminated environments and biting insects are also suspected indirect methods of transmission. Development of disease may be influenced by factors such as prolonged wetness, high humidity, high temperatures, and ectoparasites such as ticks and lice which serve to reduce the natural barriers of the skin.

Necropsy Findings　Death is unusual so necropsy is not often performed.

Prevention and Control　Potash alum and aluminum sulfate have been used as wool dusts in sheep to prevent dermatophilosis. Minimizing moist conditions is helpful in controlling and preventing the disease. In addition, controlling external parasites or other factors that cause skin lesions is important. Lesions will resolve during dry periods.

Treatment　Animals can be treated with antibiotics such as penicillin and oxytetracycline as the organism is susceptible to a wide range of antibiotics. Antimicrobial therapy is augmented by topical applications of lime sulfur as well as control of ectoparasites and biting flies. Treating the animals with povidone iodine shampoos or chlorhexidine solutions also is useful in clearing the disease.

Research Complications　*D. congolensis* is a zoonotic organism. Research personnel must be trained in zoonosis and should fully understand the risks of working with infected animals.

n. *Dichelobacter* (*Bacteroides*) *nodosus* and *Fusobacterium necrophorum* (Virulent Foot Rot; Contagious Foot Rot of Sheep and Goats; Footscald)

Etiology　Two bacteria, *Dichelobacter* (*Bacteroides*) *nodosus* and *Fusobacterium necrophorum*, work synergistically in causing contagious foot rot in sheep and goats. Both are nonmotile, nonspore forming, anaerobic, gram-negative bacilli. Foot rot is a contagious, acute or chronic dermatitis involving the hoof and underlying tissues (Bulgin, 1986). It is the leading cause of lameness in sheep. Footscald, an interdigital dermatitis is caused primarily by *D. nodosus* alone.

Clinical Signs　Varying degrees of lameness are observed in all ages of animals within 2–3 weeks of exposure to the organisms. Severely infected animals will show generalized signs of weight loss, decreased productivity, and anorexia associated with an inability to move. The interdigital skin and hooves will be moist with a very distinct necrotic odor. Diagnosis is based on clinical signs. Smears and cultures confirm the definitive agents. Clinical signs of the milder disease, footscald, include mild lameness, redness and swelling, and little to no odor.

Epizootiology and Transmission　*F. necrophorum* is ubiquitous in soil and manure, in the gastrointestinal tract, and on the skin and hooves of domestic animals. In contrast, *Dichelobacter* is an obligate pathogen of the ovine foot; the organism contaminates the soil and manure but rarely remains in the environment for over about 2 weeks. Some animals may be chronic carriers. Overcrowded, warm and moist environments are key elements in transmission.

Differential Diagnoses　Foot abscesses, selenium/vitamin E deficiencies, strawberry footrot, bluetongue virus infection (manifested with myopathy and coronitis), and trauma are among the many differentials that must be considered.

Treatment　Affected animals are best treated by manually trimming the necrotic debris from the hooves, followed by application of local antibiotics and foot wraps. Systemic antibiotics such as penicillin, oxytetracycline, and erythromycin may be used. Footbaths containing 10% zinc or copper sulfate or 10% formalin (not legal in all states) can be used for treatment as well as prevention of the disease. Affected animals should be separated from the flock See Kimberling and Ellis (1990) for more information. Vaccination has been shown to be effective as part of the treatment regimen.

Prevention and Control　These programs involve scrutiny of herd and flock management; quarantine of incoming animals; vaccination; segregation of affected animals; careful and regular hoof trimming; avoiding muddy pens and holding areas; and culling individuals with chronic and nonresponsive infections. *D. nodosus* bacterins are commercially available, but cross protection between serotypes varies. Footbaths are also considered effective preventative measures. Due to the potential for toxicity, copper sulfate footbaths should be employed with great caution in sheep.

Research Complications Treating and controlling footrot is very costly in terms of time, treatment and follow-up, and extra housing space requirements.

o. *Fusobacterium necrophorum* and *Prevotella melaninogenic* (Formerly *Bacteroides melaninogenicus*) (Footrot of Cattle, Interdigital Necrobacillosis, Interdigital Phlegmon of Cattle, Foot Abscesses of Sheep)

Etiology Interdigital necrobacillosis of cattle is caused by *F. necrophorum* and several other organisms. Incidence in cattle has decreased as dairy cows spend less time on pasture, however foot rot still causes up to 15% of claw diseases. *F. necrophorum* is also associated with foot abscesses or infection of the deeper structures of the foot in sheep and goats. One or both claws of the affected hoof may be involved. Animals will be 'three-legged lame' and the affected hoof will be hot. Pockets of purulent material may be in the heel or toe.

Clinical Signs and Diagnosis Clinical signs include mild-to-moderate lameness of sudden onset. Hindlimbs are more commonly affected. The interdigital space will be swollen, as will be the coronet and bulb areas. The claws will be markedly separated and inflammation may extend to the pastern and fetlock. Characteristic malodors will be noted, but there will be little purulent discharge. In more severe cases, animals will have elevated body temperatures and loss of appetite. Lesions progress to fissures with necrosis until sloughing and healing occurs. The diagnosis is by the odor and appearance. If the condition is not treated and allowed to progress, weight loss and decrease in milk production will occur. Diagnosis is based on clinical signs, assessment of the environmental and housing conditions of the animal and anaerobic culture confirms the organisms involved.

Epizootiology and Transmission Cases may be sporadic or epizootics may occur. Dairy cattle breeds are more commonly affected.

Necropsy Findings These include dermatitis and necrosis of the skin and subcutaneous tissues. Although necropsy would rarely be performed, secondary osteomyelitis may be noted in severe cases.

Differential Diagnoses The most common differentials for sudden lameness include hairy heel warts, laminitis, and subsolar abscesses. Bluetongue virus should also be considered.

Prevention and Control As with footrot in smaller ruminants, management of the area and herd are important. Paddocks and pens should be kept dry and well drained and free of material that will damage feet. Footbaths have been shown to control incidence. Affected animals should be segregated during treatment. Chronically affected or severely lame animals should be culled. New cattle should be quarantined and evaluated.

Treatment Successful treatment includes cleaning the feet; trimming necrotic tissue; and use of parenteral antimicrobials such as ceftiofur, oxytetracycline, or procaine penicillin. Twice-a-day footbaths (such as 10% zinc sulfate, 2.5 % formalin when allowed, or 5% copper sulfate) can be effective. In severe cases, more aggressive therapy such as bandaging the feet may be needed. Animals can recover without treatment but may be lame for several weeks.

Research Complications These are comparable to those noted for footrot in smaller ruminants.

p. Heel Warts (Bovine Digital Dermatitis, Papillomatous Digital Dermatitis [PDD], Hairy Foot Warts)

Etiology Digital dermatitis is highly contagious and can cause morbidity of up to 90% in a herd. The causative agent of digital dermatitis is uncertain and may be caused by more than one bacterium. Bacteria such as *Fusobacteria* spp., *Prevotella* spp. (*Bacteroides* spp, *Treponema*), and *Dichelobacter nodosus* have been isolated from bovine heel lesions. Several species of *Treponema* have also been confirmed in the lesions of cows with papillomatous digital dermatitis (PDD) in the United States and Europe.

Clinical Signs All lesions occur on the haired digital skin. One or more feet may be affected. Most lesions occur on the plantar surface of the hind foot (near the heel bulbs and/or extending from the interdigital space), but the palmer and dorsal aspect of the interdigital spaces may also be involved. Moist plaques begin as red, granular areas; plaques enlarge, turn gray or black, and 'hairs' protrude from the roughened surface. Lesioned areas are very painful. Heel warts differentiate from foot rot as swelling and fever are absent.

Epizootiology and Transmission Poorly drained loafing areas, damp and dirty bedding areas, and overcrowding have been implicated as contributing factors. Interdigital lesions occur commonly in young stock and dairy facilities throughout the world. Introduction of new cattle into a herd that has not previously been affected can cause a large outbreak. The disease is seen only in cattle.

Differential Diagnoses Differentials for lameness will include foot rot, sole abscesses, laminitis, and trauma.

Prevention and Control Biosecurity is a key component for control. Purchasing replacement heifers should be avoided in uninfected herds. Equipment used for hoof trimming should be sterilized. Trucks and trailers should be sanitized between groups. Routine use of footbaths that contain copper sulfate, zinc sulfate, formalin, or antibiotics such as tetracycline or lincomycin have been useful in reducing incidence. The footbaths must be well maintained, minimizing contamination by feces and other materials. Tandem arrangements, such as use of cleaning footbaths followed by medicated footbaths or sprays are useful.

Treatment   Lesions should be debrided or removed followed by topical antibiotic and antiseptic regimens.

Research Complications   PPD is one of the major causes of lameness among heifers and dairy cattle and is a costly problem to treat.

q. *Histophilus somni* (Formerly *Haemophilus somnus*) (Thromboembolic Meningoencephalitis [Teme])

Etiology   *Histophilus somni* is a pleomorphic, n on (Kirk and Glenn, 1996)bencapsulated, nonsporeforming gram-negative coccobacillus. Diseases caused by this organism include thromboembolic meningoencephalitis, septicemia, arthritis, and reproductive failures due to genital tract infections in males and females. *H. somni* is a commensal of the bovine mucous membranes; pathogenic and non-pathogenic strains have been found. The nasal and urogenital secretions are believed to be the source of the organism and a major contributor to the bovine respiratory disease complex (BRDC). *Histophilus* spp. also have been associated with respiratory disease in sheep and goats.

Clinical Signs   Sudden death is often the first sign noted of *H. somni* pneumonia in a group of animals. If animals are found prior to death, marked dyspnea is present. Depression is often the first notable sign of the neurologic presentation. Other clinical signs include ataxia, falling, and conscious proprioceptive deficits. Clinical signs such as head tilt from otitis interna-media, opisthotonus and convulsions may be seen when the brainstem is affected. High fever, extreme morbidity and death within 36 h may occur. Respiratory infections with *H. somni* contribute to BRDC in conjunction with one of the respiratory viruses. In acute neurologic as well as chronic pneumonic infections, polyarthritis may develop. *H. somni* may cause abortion, vulvo-vaginitis, endometritis, placentitis and infertility.

Diagnosis is achieved by examination of tissues collected at necropsy. Isolation of the organism from CSF, brain, blood, urine, joint fluid or other internal organs is confirmatory. Paired serum samples are recommended.

Epizootiology and Transmission   Because the organism is considered part of the normal flora of cattle and can be isolated from numerous tissues, the distinction between the normal flora and the status of chronic carrier is not clear. After inhalation, the organism colonizes the respiratory tract and gains access to the bloodstream. Colonization of the male and female reproductive tracts may lead to venereal spread. Stresses of travel and co-infection with other respiratory pathogens may be involved. Transmission is by respiratory and genital tract secretions. The organism does not persist in the environment.

Necropsy Findings   Pathognomonic central nervous system lesions include multifocal red–brown foci of necrosis and inflammation on and within the brain and the meninges. Many thrombi with bacterial colonies will be seen in these affected areas. Ocular lesions may also be seen including conjunctivitis, retinal hemorrhages and edema. The respiratory tract lesions include bronchopneumonia and fibrinous pleuritis. A focal myocardial lesion (in the papillary muscle of the left ventricle) along with fibrinous pericarditis, bronchopneumonia, polyarthritis, and fibrinous laryngitis may also be seen. Aborted fetuses will not show lesions, but necrotizing placentitis will be evident histologically. Pure cultures of *H. somni* may be possible from these tissues.

Differential Diagnoses   Differentials in all ruminants include other pathogens associated with neurological disease and respiratory disease such as *M. hemolytica* and *P. multocida*. In smaller ruminants, *C. pseudotuberculosis* should be considered.

Prevention and Control   The organism is susceptible in vitro to many antimicrobials. However, the use of antibiotics metaphylactically has not shown great success. Late-stage polyarthritis is resistant to antibiotic therapy due to failure to reach the site of infection. Planning vaccination programs carefully will decrease chances of outbreaks; for example; vaccinations for respiratory pathogens should be avoided during times of acute stress. Killed whole-cell bacterins are commercially available that produce a humoral response. Calves should be immunized prior to entering a confinement housing situation (feedlot) with a second vaccination upon arrival to the feedlot.

Treatment   Rapid treatment at the first signs of neurologic disease is important in an outbreak but effective treatment is difficult due to the rapid course of the disease.

r. Leptospirosis

Etiology   Fourteen different species of the spirochete genus *Leptospira* are now recognized, and pathogenic serovars exist within each species. *Leptospira interrogans* serovars *pomona*, *icterohaemorrhagiae*, *grippotyphosa*, *interrogans*, and *hardjo* are recognized pathogens. *L. hardjo* and *L. pomona* are the serovars most commonly diagnosed in cattle, with *L. hardjo* the major serovar in sheep. Goats are susceptible to several serovars.

Clinical Signs   Acute and chronic infections in cattle are more common than in sheep and goats. Infections in cattle often are subclinical, especially in non-pregnant and non-lactating animals. Acute infection in calves can be severe and present with high fever, hemolytic anemia, hemoglobinuria, jaundice, and pulmonary congestion; meningitis and death may result. Lactating cows will have severe drops in production. Chronic cases may lead to abortion, with retained placenta, weakened calves or chronic carrier state. Infertility may also be a sequela. Leptospirosis causes similar symptoms in sheep and goats but is relatively uncommon in these species; however, mortality rates of above 50% have been reported in infected ewes and lambs.

Epizootiology and Transmission Leptospires are a large genus making the disease difficult to prevent, treat and control. The organism survives well in the environment, especially in moist, warm, stagnant water. Wild animals often serve as maintenance hosts, but domestic livestock may be reservoirs also. Organisms are shed in the urine, uterine discharges and through the milk. Infection occurs via ingestion of contaminated feed, water, placental fluids, or through the mucous membranes of the susceptible animal. Chronically infected animals may shed the organism in the urine for 60 days or longer.

Necropsy Diagnosis is confirmed by identification of leptospires in fetal tissues. The leptospires are visible in silver- or fluorescent antibody-stained sections of liver or kidney. Leptospires may also be seen under dark-field or phase-contrast microscopy of fetal stomach contents. Serologic testing coupled with immunofluorescence or PCR of urine from a representative sample of cattle aids in diagnosis.

Differential Diagnoses Because of the associated anemia, differential diagnoses should include copper toxicity and parasites in addition to other abortifacient diseases.

Prevention and Control Polyvalent vaccines, tailored to common serovars regionally, are available and effective for preventing leptospirosis in cattle. Immunity is serovar specific. Because serological titers tend to diminish rapidly (within 40–50 days in sheep), frequent vaccination may be necessary.

Treatment Antibiotic treatment is aimed at treating ill animals and trying to clear the carrier state. Vaccination and antibiotic therapy can be combined in an outbreak.

Research Complications Leptospirosis is zoonotic and may be associated with flu-like signs, meningitis or hepatorenal failure in humans.

s. Listeriosis (Circling Disease, Silage Disease)

Etiology *Listeria monocytogenes* is a gram-positive, pleomorphic, motile, non-spore-forming, beta-hemolytic coccobacillus that survives in soil, feeds and other organic materials for long periods of time. The organism is often found in fermented feedstuffs such as spoiled silage. Listeria is a saprophyte and a psychrophile that prefers microaerophilic conditions. See Liu (2009) for information on Listeria.

Clinical Signs Listeriosis is an acute, sporadic, non-contagious disease associated with neurological signs, mastitis or abortions in sheep and other ruminants. The overall case rate is low. Three forms of disease are described: encephalitis, placentitis with abortion, and septicemia with hepatitis and pneumonia. The encephalitic form is most common in ruminants; the symptoms attributable to encephalitis are responsible for the 'circling disease.' The placental form usually results in third-trimester abortions in adult females who typically survive this form of the disease.

Epizootiology and Transmission The organism most commonly is transmitted by ingestion of contaminated feeds and water. When severe outbreaks occur, feedstuffs should be assessed for spoilage. *Listeria* organisms can be shed by asymptomatic carriers, especially at the end of pregnancy and at parturition.

Diagnosis and Necropsy Findings Diagnosis is usually made from clinical signs, confirmed by culture (cold enrichment at 20°C improve success), impression smears of brain or reproductive tissue or tissue fluorescent antibody techniques. Microabscesses of the midbrain with gram-positive bacilli are characteristic of encephalitis.

Differential Diagnoses Rabies, bacterial meningitis, brain abscess, lead toxicity, PEM, and otitis media must be considered as differentials; in sheep, organisms causing abortion, pregnancy toxemia, and enterotoxemia due to *C. perfringens* Type D and in goats, CAE viral infection.

Prevention and Control Affected dams should be segregated and treated. Other animals in the group may be treated with oxytetracycline as needed. Aborted tissues should be removed immediately. Proper storage of fermented feeds minimizes this source of contamination.

Treatment Affected animals should be treated early and aggressively with penicillin (drug of choice) or other antibiotics. Severely affected animals should receive appropriate fluid support and nursing care.

Research Complications *Listeria* can cause mild to severe flu-like signs in humans, and may be a particular risk for pregnant women and older or immune compromised individuals. Listeriosis in humans is a reportable disease.

t. Mastitis

Mastitis in Sheep and Goats Mastitis in ewes and does may be acute, subclinical, or chronic (Kirk and Glenn, 1996). Acute mastitis usually results in abnormal appearance and composition of milk, heat, pain, and swelling in the mammary gland and systemic signs (fever, anorexia). In sheep, *Mannheimia hemolytica* is the most common cause of acute mastitis. In goats, the primary causative organisms are *Staphylococcus epidermidis* and other coagulase-negative *Staphylococcus* species. Subclinical mastitis is diagnosed by determining somatic cell count in milk, performing a California Mastitis Test or culturing the affected glands. An indication of subclinical mastitis in ewes or does may be thin, poorly growing offspring. Diffuse chronic mastitis or 'hardbag' results from interstitial accumulations of lymphocytes in the udder, usually bilaterally. Redness and swelling are absent. Serological evidence suggests that diffuse chronic mastitis is caused by the retrovirus that causes ovine progressive pneumonia (OPP, Visna/maedi virus) in sheep and the related CAE virus (CAEV) in goats.

Treatment for acute bacterial mastitis should include aggressive application of broad-spectrum antibiotics (intramammary and systemic) and supportive therapy such as fluids and anti-inflammatory drugs. It is necessary to frequently milk out the infected gland; oxytocin injections preceding milking will improve gland evacuation. There is currently no treatment available for diffuse chronic mastitis.

Bovine Mastitis Mastitis is the disease of greatest economic importance for the dairy cattle industry, and a thorough discussion is beyond the scope of this reference. The most common bovine mastitis pathogens include *Staphylococcus aureus*, *Streptococcus agalactiae*, *Strep.* spp., *Corynebacterium bovis* (summer mastitis of heifers, dry cows, and beef breeds), coliform agents (*E. coli* and *Klebsiella pneumonia*), and *Mycoplasma* spp. including *M. bovis* (California mastitis). Many of these agents can cause acute as well as chronic mastitis and severe systemic dysfunction including fever and anorexia. Symptoms and treatment of mastitis in cattle are similar to those in small ruminants.

There are many interrelated factors associated with prevention and control of mastitis in a herd including herd health and dry cow management, milking procedures and equipment, and the condition of the environment. Teat and udder cleaning practices include washing and drying with single service paper or cloth towels and pre- and post-milking dipping with disinfecting agents. Milking equipment must be maintained to provide proper vacuum levels and pulsation rates. Management of the overall herd includes aspects such as vaccination programs; nutrition; isolation of incoming animals; and quarantine, treatment, or culling of diseased individuals. Culturing or testing newly freshened cows and periodic bulk tank milk cultures help to monitor subclinical mastitis. At the time of dry off, all cows should be treated with intramammary antibiotics. Some chronic infections can be successfully cleared during this time. Younger, disease-free animals should be milked first; any animals with diagnosed problems should be milked after the rest of the herd and/or segregated during treatment.

Facilities that provide clean and dry areas for the animals to rest and feed as well as control insect burden will reduce exposures to mastitis pathogens.

u. *Moraxella bovis* (Infectious Bovine Keratoconjunctivitis [IBK] or 'Pinkeye' in Cattle)

Etiology *Moraxella bovis*, a gram-negative coccobacillus causes infectious bovine keratoconjunctivitis (IBK) in cattle. This organism is not a cause of keratoconjunctivitis in sheep and goats. The disease includes conjunctivitis and ulcerative keratitis.

Clinical Signs IBK is characterized by acute onset and rapid course characterized initially by lacrimation, photophobia, and blepharospasm. Conjunctival injection and chemosis develop within a day of exposure, and then keratitis with corneal edema and ulcers. Anterior uveitis may be a sequel within a few days, and thicker mucopurulent ocular discharge may be seen. Corneal vascularization begins by 10 days after onset. Re-epithelialization of the corneal ulcers occurs by 2–3 weeks after onset. Most ulcers will heal without loss of vision, but corneal rupture and blindness can occur in severe cases. Diagnosis is usually based on clinical signs, but culturing is helpful and fluorescein staining is useful for demonstrating corneal ulceration.

Epizootiology and Transmission The disease is more severe in younger cattle. The bacteria are shed in nasal secretions, and cattle may be subclinical carriers. Transmission is by fomites, flies, aerosols, and direct contact. Other factors contributing to infection include ultraviolet light and trauma from dust or plant materials. Incidence is higher in warm weather.

Necropsy Findings Necropsy is not typically performed on these cases.

Differential Diagnoses With *M. bovis* it is important to first determine that the lesions are not due to foreign bodies or parasites. Infectious bovine rhinotracheitis virus causes conjunctivitis but the central corneal ulceration characteristic of IBK is not seen with *M. bovis* infections.

Prevention and Control Available vaccines help to decrease incidence and severity. Other preventative measures include control of insect pests; mowing high pasture grass to minimize ocular trauma; provision of shade; controlling dust and sources of other mechanical trauma; and segregation of animals by age.

Treatment Cattle can recover without treatment, but younger animals should be treated as soon as the infection is detected. Antibiotic treatments include topical and subconjunctival administration. Third-eyelid flaps, temporary tarsorrhaphy, or eye patches often are beneficial.

Research Complications This pathogen presents a research complication due to the carrier status of some animals, the severity of disease in younger animals and treatment and labor costs associated with infections. The overall condition of the cattle will be affected for several weeks, and permanent visual impairment or loss and ocular disfigurement may occur.

v. Mycobacterial Diseases

i. MYCOBACTERIUM BOVIS (TUBERCULOSIS)

Etiology Mycobacteria are aerobic, nonmotile, nonspore forming, acid-fast pleomorphic bacilli. Most cases of tuberculosis in sheep are related to *M. bovis* or *M. avium*. Cases in goats have been attributed to *M. bovis*, *M. avium*, or *M. tuberculosis*. *M. bovis* causes tuberculosis in cattle, but also has a wide host range.

Clinical Signs and Diagnosis Tuberculosis is a sporadic, chronic, granulomatous contagious disease of practically all vertebrates including humans. The infection is often asymptomatic and may be diagnosed only at necropsy. The primary sites of infection are the respiratory system (*M. bovis*) and the digestive system (*M. avium*). Other tissues such as mammary tissue and reproductive tract may be involved. Locations of the characteristic tubercles will determine whether clinical signs are seen. Respiratory signs may include dyspnea, coughing, and pneumonia. Digestive tract signs include diarrhea (most commonly), bloat, or constipation. The most important diagnostic test for TB is the intradermal tuberculin test using purified protein derivatives (PPD). Confirmation of diagnosis is achieved by culture or by PCR.

Epizootiology and Transmission *M. bovis* survives for months in the environment, especially in cattle feces. Animals acquire the infection from the environment or from other animals via aerosols, contaminated feed and water, and in secretions such as milk, semen, genital discharges, urine and feces. Subclinically infected animals serve as carriers.

Necropsy Findings Yellow primary tubercles (granulomas) with central areas of caseous necrosis and calcification are present in the lungs. Touch impressions of lesions will have acid-fast bacteria (AFB). Caseous nodules are also associated with gastrointestinal organs and mesenteric lymph nodes.

Prevention and Control The main reservoirs of infection are humans and cattle. Significant progress has been made in eradication programs in the United States during the past several decades but infected animals continue to be found, particularly in captive deer herds and along the southern border with Mexico. Notification of state officials is required following identification of intradermal-positive animals. Great care must be exercised in any tissue handling or necropsies of reactors, and state animal health officials should be consulted regarding disposal of materials and cleaning of premises following depopulation of positive animals.

Treatment Treatment is usually not allowed due to the zoonotic potential, chronicity of the disease, and the treatment costs. Slaughter is required to prevent potential transmission to humans.

Research Complications The pathogen is zoonotic. Identification will result in quarantine of facilities.

ii. PARATUBERCULOSIS (M. AVIUM SUBSPECIES PARATUBERCULOSIS; JOHNE'S DISEASE)

Etiology Mycobacterium avium subspecies paratuberculosis, the causative agent of Johne's disease, is a fastidious, nonspore forming, acid-fast, gram-positive rod. The organism is a subspecies of *M. avium*.

Clinical Signs and Diagnosis Johne's disease is a chronic, contagious, granulomatous disease of adult ruminants characterized by unthriftiness, weight loss, and intermittent diarrhea. The incubation period is long and infected cattle can appear healthy for months to years. Milk production may fall or fail to reach expected levels. In sheep and goats, chronic wasting is usually observed with only occasional pasty (cow-pat) feces or diarrhea, usually only in advanced disease. Although clinical signs are nonspecific, Johne's should be considered if the diarrheic animals have a good appetite and are on a good anthelmintic program.

The three main areas of focus for testing are (1) detection of the organism in feces or tissue by culture or PCR; (2) evidence of cellular immune response to infection by skin or interferon-γ testing; and (3) detection of antibody to *M. paratuberculosis* by ELISA or AGID (Sergeant et al., 2003). *Post-mortem* testing at necropsy with culture and histopathology on multiple tissues remains the gold standard for definitive diagnosis. The ELISA tests are the most sensitive and specific and should be used to determine the prevalence of infection within a herd of cattle. See the Johne's information center (http://www.johnes.org; Robbe-Austerman (2011)) for additional information on Johne's disease in various species.

Epizootiology and Transmission The organism is prevalent in the environment and most commonly is transmitted to young animals by ingestion of milk or by direct or indirect contact. Cattle exposed as adults are less likely to become infected. It is important to note that fecal shedding occurs before exhibiting clinical signs, therefore making the 'silent' stage of infection an important source of transmission.

Necropsy and Diagnosis The ileum from infected cattle is grossly thickened; but this is not seen in sheep or goats. Ileal and ileocecal lymph nodes provide the best samples for histology and acid fast staining.

Differential Diagnoses Other diseases causing chronic wasting and poor body condition include chronic salmonellosis, severe parasitism, lentiviruses in small ruminants, and pyelonephritis.

Treatment Treatment is not worthwhile.

Prevention and Control Prevention is the most effective method to manage this pathogen. Efforts should be focused on eliminating the disease through test and slaughter, and on breaking the chain of transmission to neonates. Calves should be removed from the dam immediately, fed pasteurized colostrum from a bottle and then raised separate from adult cattle until 1 year of age. Prolonged survival in the soil (up to 1 year) and wildlife reservoirs (hares) can make control of established infections challenging.

Other Considerations   *Mycobacterium avium* subspecies *paratuberculosis* is being investigated as a factor in the development of Crohn's disease in humans. However, there remains no evidence of zoonotic potential.

w. Navel Ill (Omphalitis, Omphalophlebitis, Omphaloarteritis, Joint Ill)

Etiology   The most common organism causing infection of the umbilicus is *Trueperella* (formerly *Actinomyces, Corynebacterium*) *pyogenes*; other bacteria may be present. *Arcanobacterium* are anaerobic, non-motile, nonspore forming, gram-positive, pleomorphic rods to coccobacilli. Other environmental contaminants associated with this disease include *E. coli, Enterococcus* spp., *Proteus, Streptococcus* spp., and *Staphylococcus* spp.

Clinical Signs and Diagnosis   Navel ill is an acute localized inflammation and infection of the external umbilicus. Animals present with fever, painful enlargement of the umbilicus, varying degrees of depression and anorexia. Purulent discharges may be seen draining from the umbilicus. Involvement of the urachus is usually followed by cystitis and associated signs of dysuria, stranguria, and hematuria. Other common severe sequelae include septicemia, pneumonia, peritonitis, septic arthritis (joint ill), patent urachus and urachal abscesses, umbilical hernias, meningitis, osteomyelitis, uveitis, endocarditis, and diarrhea.

Epizootiology and Transmission   Many cases occur in neonates and most cases occur within the first 3 months of age. Cleanliness of the birthing or housing environment and successful transfer of passive immunity are important factors in the occurrence of the disease.

Diagnosis   Navel ill is diagnosed by typical clinical signs and should always be considered for young ruminants during the first week of life with fever of unknown origin and for slightly older lambs, kids, or calves that are not thriving.

Differential Diagnosis   The major differential is an umbilical hernia which will typically not be painful and infected and can often be reduced.

Treatment   Omphalitis can be treated with a 10- to 14-day course of broad-spectrum antibiotics such as ampicillin, ceftiofur, florfenicol, or erythromycin. If an isolated abscess is palpable, it should be surgically opened and repeatedly flushed with iodine solutions. The prognosis for recovery is good if systemic involvement has not occurred.

Prevention and Control   The disease is best prevented and controlled by providing clean birthing environments, ensuring adequate colostral immunity, and dipping the umbilicus of newborns with tincture of iodine or strong iodine solution.

Research Complications   The disease can be costly to treat and the toll taken on the young animals due to the consequences of systemic infection may detract from their research value.

x. Pasteurellosis (Shipping Fever, Hemorrhagic Septicemia, Enzootic Pneumonia)

i. MANNHEIMIA HAEMOLYTICA, PASTEURELLA MULTOCIDA, HISTOPHILUS SOMNI

Etiology   *Mannheimia haemolytica* and *Pasteurella multocida* are aerobic, nonmotile, nonspore-forming, bipolar, gram-negative rods, associated with pneumonia and septicemia in all ruminants.

Clinical Signs   Pasteurellosis is an acute bacterial disease characterized by bronchopneumonia, septicemia, and sudden death. The organism invades the mucosa of the gastrointestinal or respiratory tract and causes localized areas of necrosis, hemorrhage, and thrombosis. The lungs and liver are frequent locations for formation of microabscesses. Acute rhinitis or pharyngitis often precedes the respiratory form. The organism also may invade the bloodstream causing disseminated septicemia. Animals may exhibit nasal discharge of mucopurulent to hemorrhagic exudate, hyperthermia, coughing, dyspnea, anorexia, and depression. With the respiratory form, auscultation of the thorax suggests dullness and consolidation of anteroventral lobes that will be confirmed by radiographs. The disease is diagnosed by clinical signs, blood cultures from septicemic animals, blood smears showing bipolar organisms, and history of predisposing stressors.

Epizootiology and Transmission   The organism is ubiquitous in the environment and in the respiratory tract. Younger ruminants, between 2 and 12 months of age, are especially prone to infection during times of stress such as weaning, transportation, dietary changes, weather changes, and overcrowding. The pneumonic form appears as a component of BRDC associated with concurrent infections such as parainfluenza-3, BRSV, and in cattle, bovine herpes virus 1 or BVDV. The organism is transmitted between animals by direct and indirect contact through inhalation or ingestion.

Necropsy Findings   With the pneumonic form, serofibrinous exudates fill the alveoli and ventral lung lobes are consolidated, congested and purple–gray in color. Degenerate streaming leukocytes (oat cells) are pathognomonic for *M. haemolytica*. Fibrinous pleuritis, pericarditis, and hematogenously induced arthritis also may be evident as well as areas of necrosis and hemorrhage in the small intestines and multifocal lesions on the surface of the liver.

Pathogenesis Stress and concurrent viral infection are considered to be key factors in the pathogenesis of *M. haemolytica* and *Pasteurella* infections. Macrophages and neutrophils are lysed by bacterial leukocidin as they arrive at the lung, and enzymes released by phagocytes cause additional damage to lung tissue.

Differential Diagnosis *Mycoplasma bovis* pneumonia.

Treatment Treatment includes the use of antibiotics and anti-inflammatories. In outbreaks, cultures from fresh necropsies are helpful for determining sensitivities useful for the remaining group.

Prevention and Control The incidence of disease can be decreased by minimizing sources of stress and by vaccinating for viral respiratory pathogens. *M. haemolytica-P. multocida* bacterins labeled for cattle, sheep, and goats are available. Passive immunity is protective in young animals. Preventative measures include maintaining good ventilation in enclosures and barns and metaphylaxis of at-risk animals with approved drugs.

y. Salmonellosis

Etiology *Salmonella enterica* is a motile, aerobic to facultatively anaerobic, nonspore-forming, gram-negative bacillus and is a common inhabitant of the gastrointestinal tract of ruminants. The genus *Salmonella* contains two species, *S. bongori* which infects mainly poikilotherms and rarely, humans, and *S. enterica* which includes approximately 2500 serovars and are a major cause of food-borne illness in humans. *Salmonella* are properly designated using their serovar (which was often formerly a species name), so, for example, *S. enterica* subsp. *enterica* serovar Typhimurium (aka *S.* Typhimurium) and serovar Enteritidis (*S.* Enteritidis). The organism is associated with enteric disease and abortions. The most common serovars in animals (as reported to the CDC) are *S.* Typhimurium, *S.* Newport, *S.* Agona, *S.* Heidelberg; *S.* Dublin and *S.* Abortusovis have been implicated with bovine and ovine abortions (Center for Food Security and Public Safety, 2005).

Clinical Signs and Diagnosis Salmonellosis causes acute gastroenteritis, dysentery, and septicemia in all domestic ruminants; feces may contain mucous and/or blood and have a distinctive, 'septic tank' odor. The animals are anorexic and hyperthermic and become severely depressed and weak, losing a high percentage of their body weight. Animals may die in 1–5 days due to dehydration associated with dysenteric fluid loss, septicemia, shock, and acidosis. Morbidity may be 25%, and mortality may reach 100%. Morbidity and mortality will be highest in neonates and some may simply be found dead. Septicemia may result in subsequent meningitis, polyarthritis, and pneumonia. Chronically infected animals may have intermittent diarrhea.

Salmonella may cause abortions in sheep, goats, and cattle throughout gestation. Hemorrhage, placental necrosis, and edema will be present. Metritis and placental retention may occur. Some mortality of dams may occur.

Diagnosis is based on clinical signs, and can be confirmed by culturing fresh feces or at necropsy. Because shedding of organisms is intermittent, repeated cultures are recommended. Leukopenia and a degenerative left shift are common hematological findings.

Epizootiology and Transmission Stresses associated with recent shipping, overcrowding, and inclement weather may predispose the animal to enteric infection. Birds and rodents may be natural reservoirs of *Salmonella* in external housing environments. Transmission is fecal–oral. Animals that survive may become chronic carriers and shedders of the organisms and this has been demonstrated experimentally.

Necropsy Findings and Diagnosis Animals will have noticeable perineal staining. Intestines (particularly the ileum, cecum, and colon) contain mucoid feces with or without hemorrhages. Petechial hemorrhages and areas of necrosis may be noticed on the surface of the liver, heart, and mesenteric lymph nodes. The wall of the intestines, gall bladder, and mesenteric lymph nodes will be edematous; and a pseudodiphtheritic membrane lining the distal small intestines and colon may be observed in cattle and sheep. Splenomegaly may be present. Necrosuppurative inflammation of the Peyer's patches is characteristic. Fibrinous cholecystitis is considered pathognomonic.

Pathogenesis After ingestion, the organism proliferates in the intestine. Bacteria are selectively taken up by the M cells of the Peyer's patches and gut-associated lymphoid tissue. Damage to the intestines and the resulting diarrhea are due to the bacterial production of cytoxin and endotoxin. Although the *Salmonella* organisms will be taken up by phagocytic cells involved in the inflammatory response, they survive and multiply further. Septicemia is a common sequel with the bacteria localizing throughout the body.

Differential Diagnoses In young animals, differentials include other enteropathogens such as *E. coli*, rotavirus and coronavirus, clostridial infections, cryptosporidiosis, and coccidiosis. These pathogens may also be present in the affected animals. Differentials in adults include bovine viral diarrhea and winter dysentery in cattle, and parasitemia and enterotoxemia in all ruminants.

Prevention and Control Affected animals should be isolated during herd outbreaks. Samples for culture should include herdmates, water and feed sources, recently arrived livestock (including other species), and area wildlife including birds and rodents. Culling carrier animals, pest control, and intensive cleaning and disinfection of facilities are all important during outbreaks.

Treatment Nursing care includes rehydration and correction of acid–base abnormalities. Antibiotic therapy may be useful in cases with septicemia, but the use of oral antibiotics is controversial because it may induce carrier animals.

Research Complications Salmonellosis is zoonotic, and some serotypes of the organism have caused fatalities even in immunocompetent humans.

z. Tularemia

Etiology Tularemia is caused by *Francisella tularensis*, a nonmotile, nonspore-forming, aerobic, gram-negative, rod-shaped bacterium.

Clinical Signs and Diagnosis Sheep are most commonly affected. The disease is characterized by hyperthermia, muscular stiffness, and lymphadenopathy. Anemia and diarrhea may develop, and infected lymph nodes enlarge and may ulcerate. Mortality may reach 40%. Diagnosis is confirmed by prompt culturing of the organism from lymph nodes, spleen, or liver where granulomatous lesions form; serological findings may also be helpful.

Epizootiology and Transmission The disease is most commonly transmitted by ticks or biting flies. The wood tick, *Dermacenter andersoni*, is an important vector in transmitting the disease in western states; wild rodents and rabbits serve as natural reservoirs. The organism can also be transmitted orally through contaminated water.

Necropsy Findings Suppurative, necrotic lymph nodes are typical. Lungs will be congested and edematous. Necrosuppurative splenitis.

Treatment Infected animals can be treated with oxytetracycline, aminoglycosides, or cephalosporins.

Differential Diagnoses When tick infestations are heavy, *F. tularensis* should be suspected. *Mannheimia hemolytica* (sheep), *Histophilus somni* (cattle), and *Mycoplasma mycoides* (goats), and anthrax (all ruminant species) should be considered as differentials.

Prevention and Control Eliminating the tick vectors and deer flies can prevent tularemia.

Research Complications The disease is zoonotic and transmission to people may result from tick or fly bites or from handling contaminated tissues. This is a USDA reportable disease.

aa. Mycoplasmal Diseases

i. MYCOPLASMA BOVIGENITALIUM, MYCOPLASMA BOVIS

Etiology *M. bovigenitalium* and *M. bovis* are associated sporadically with bovine infertility and abortions. Mycoplasma bovis is a significant respiratory pathogen. This pathogen has also been reported associated with similar clinical signs in sheep and goats.

Clinical Signs and Diagnosis Infertility is more commonly caused by *M. bovigenitalium* infections and

granular vulvovaginitis and endometritis will be present. Granular vulvovaginitis is characterized by raised papules on the mucous membranes and mucopurulent exudate. Abortions and mastitis are associated with *M. bovis* infections. Calves that are born may be weak. *M. bovis* is a big economic concern in beef and dairy and has been called an 'all purpose pathogen' causing acute and chronic arthritis, middle and inner ear infections, acute and chronic pneumonia, and mastitis.

Epidemiology and Transmission Mycoplasmal species are considered ubiquitous, are carried in the genital tracts of males and females, and are transmitted during natural breeding or through contaminated insemination materials. Transmission occurs by aerosol, by passage through the birth canal, by direct contact, and by contamination from urine of infected animals. Feeding unpasteurized milk (particularly waste milk) to dairy calves is a major risk factor.

Treatment Fluoroquinolone, oxytetracycline, tilmicosin, and tulathromycin antibiotics may be useful for treating *Mycoplasma*-induced reproductive diseases. Prevention is far more rewarding than treatment.

ii. MYCOPLASMA OVIPNEUMONIAE (OVINE MYCOPLASMAL PNEUMONIA)

Etiology *Mycoplasma ovipneumoniae* causes acute or chronic pneumonia in lambs.

Clinical Signs *Mycoplasma* induces serious diseases in sheep causing acute and chronic pneumonia, conjunctivitis, and genitourinary disease. The disease may be coincidental with pasteurellosis. Respiratory distress, coughing and nasal discharge are observed in infected animals. Bronchoalveolar lavage followed by culture is the best method for diagnosis; however, Mycoplasmas are fastidious organisms requiring special handling techniques. Mycoplasmas are isolated from the genitourinary tract of sheep. Vulvovaginitis and reproductive problems are associated conditions.

Treatment Tylosin, quinolones, oxytetracycline, and gentamicin are good choices for therapy.

iii. M. MYCOIDES BIOTYPE F38 (CONTAGIOUS CAPRINE PLEUROPNEUMONIA, CAPRINE PNEUMONIA, PLEURITIS, AND PLEUROPNEUMONIA)

Etiology *M. mycoides* biotype F38 is the agent of contagious caprine pleuropneumonia and is found worldwide. In the United States, caprine pneumonia is also caused by *M. ovipneumoniae*, *M. mycoides* subspecies *capri*, and *M. mycoides* subspecies *mycoides* (Large Colony Type).

Clinical Signs Contagious Caprine Pleuropneumonia is characterized by severe dyspnea, nasal discharge, cough, and fever. Infections with other *Mycoplasma* species also have similar clinical signs.

Epizootiology and Transmission This disease is highly contagious, with high morbidity and mortality. Transmission is by aerosols. *M. mycoides* subspecies *mycoides* has become a serious cause of morbidity and mortality of goat kids in the United States.

Necropsy Large amounts of pale straw-colored fluid and fibrinous pneumonia and pleurisy are typical. Some lung consolidation may be present. Meningitis, fibrinous pericarditis, and fibrinopurulent arthritis may also be found. Organisms may be cultured from lungs and other internal organs.

Differential Diagnosis In the United States, the principal differential for *M. mycoides* subspecies *mycoides* is CAE.

Treatment Tylosin and oxytetracycline are effective. Some infections are slow to resolve.

Prevention and Control Vaccines are available in some areas. Infected herds are quarantined. New goats should be quarantined before introduction to the herd.

Research Complications The worldwide distribution of the F38 biotype, potential for aerosol transmission and high morbidity and mortality of Mycoplasmal infections make them economically important diseases in goats. Chronic subclinical infections can result in anesthetic complications in sheep.

iv. MYCOPLASMA CONJUNCTIVAE (MYCO-PLASMAL KERATOCONJUNCTIVITIS)

Etiology *M. conjunctivae* and other species cause infectious conjunctivitis or pinkeye in sheep and goats with associated hyperemia, edema, lacrimation, and corneal lesions. Respiratory disease and other infections, such as mastitis, may also be observed.

Clinical Signs and Diagnosis All ages of animals may be affected. Initially, lacrimation, conjunctival vessel injection, then keratitis and neovascularization are seen. Sometimes uveitis is evident. The presentation is usually unilateral, and recurring infections are common.

Epizootiology and Transmission The infection is passed easily between animals by direct contact. Animals can become reinfected and carrier animals may be a factor in outbreaks.

Necropsy It is unlikely animals would undergo necropsy for this problem.

Differential Diagnoses The primary differential in sheep and goats is *Chlamydophila*, as well as *Branhamella*, *Rickettsia (Colesiota) conjunctivae*, and IBR in goats only.

Treatment Animals recover spontaneously within about 10 weeks. Tetracycline ointments and powders are also used. Third eyelid flaps may be necessary if corneal ulceration develops.

Prevention and Control New animals should be quarantined, and if necessary treated, before introduction to the flock or herd.

v. MYCOPLASMA MASTITIS

Etiology and Transmission *Mycoplama* spp. can spread from cow to cow via aerosol transmission. Prior to bacteremia, the pathogen is spread during milking by milker's hands or the milking unit. The bacteria are spread in the milk in large numbers before clinical signs appear and very few organisms are required to infect a quarter. Infected cows may have normal somatic cell counts (SCCs), therefore a cow may be asymptomatic with a normal SCC and serve as a source of infection for other cows.

Clinical Signs and Diagnosis Initial presentation is a swollen quarter that is sensitive to the touch and has decreased milk production. Abnormal milk generally develops 1–3 days later. The milk initially will have visible particles that progress to puss and eventually become watery. Affected cows do not appear sick and maintain good appetites. Generally more than one quarter is infected and it will often invade quarters that are already infected with another organism. Cows that have recovered from the clinical presentation generally always have a subclinical infection.

Necropsy This disease does not generally result in death.

Diagnosis Mycoplasma should be suspected if there are an increase number of clinical cases of mastitis that are nonresponsive to therapy. Diagnosis is made by culturing the organism from the milk. Normal milk culture media will not grow the bacteria from the milk, so *Mycoplasma* must be specifically requested. Considering cows are generally infected with other pathogens as well, this can complicate and delay diagnosis.

Treatment There is no effective treatment for *Mycoplasma mastitis*. If other organisms are cultured from the milk, those should be treated. If the cow has a good immune health status, she may eventually eliminate the infection. Cows may develop normal milk, but still be subclinically infected and therefore shedding the bacteria into the next lactation.

Prevention and Control Screen new animals before they enter the milking herd. Three to five negative individual cow or bulk tank cultures is highly recommended.

ab. Rickettsial Diseases

i. Q OR QUERY FEVER (COXIELLA BURNETII)

Etiology *C. burnetii* is a small, gram-negative, obligate intracellular organism. It is the etiologic agent of Query Fever, or Q Fever (Queensland fever, nine-mile agent), and is regarded as a major cause of late abortion in sheep. Historically considered a Rickettsial organism, it now is thought to be more closely related to *Legionella* and *Francisella* than to *Rickettsia* (Merck Veterinary Manual Online, 2011).

Clinical Signs Infection of ruminants with *C. burnetii* is usually asymptomatic. Experimental inoculation in other mammals has resulted in transient hyperthermia, mild respiratory disease, and mastitis. Abortions, stillbirths, and births of weak lambs are also seen.

Epizootiology and Transmission *C. burnetii* is extremely resistant to environmental changes as well as disinfectants; persistence in the environment for a year or longer is possible. The organism is associated with either a free-living or an arthropod-borne cycle. Although several tick species may serve as vectors, *Coxiella* may be maintained without a tick intermediate. The organism is especially concentrated in placental tissues, and reproductive fluids. The organism also is shed in milk, urine, feces, and oronasal secretions. Placenta can contain up to 10^9 human ID_{50} per gram. The infectious dose for humans can be as low as a single organism, and bacteria can spread up to 11 miles in the wind. The organism can persist in the environment for months.

Necropsy Findings No specific lesion will be seen in aborted or stillborn fetuses but necrotizing placentitis will be a finding in cases of abortion. The placenta will contain white chalky plaques and a red–brown exudate. Intracytoplasmic organisms within trophoblasts are characteristic. The organism stains red with modified Ziehl–Neelsen and Macchiavello stains and purple with Giemsa stain.

Differential Diagnoses Specific diagnosis of Q fever is based upon detection of antibodies. Within 2–3 weeks post-infection, immunoglobulin M (IgM) and IgG antiphase II antibodies against *C. burnetii* are detected. The presence of IgG antiphase I *C. burnetii* antibodies at titers of $\geq$1:800 by microimmunofluorescence is indicative of chronic Q fever (Maurin and Raoult, 1999). PCR of genital swabs, milk, and fecal samples also has been used (Maurin and Raoult, 1999; Merck Veterinary Manual Online, 2011; Van Metre, 1996). Because of the risk of laboratory acquired infection, culture is not recommended.

Treatment *Coxiella* can be treated with oxytetracyclines. Vaccines for ruminants are not commercially available in the United States.

Prevention and Control Any aborting animals should be segregated from other animals, and other pregnant animals treated prophylactically with tetracycline. Serologic screening of ruminant sources should be performed routinely. Barrier housing, a review of ventilation exhaust, and defined handling procedures are often required. All placentas and all aborted tissues should be handled and disposed carefully. Q Fever has been reported in many mammalian species, including cats.

Research Complications *C. burnetii*-free animals are particularly important in studies involving fetuses and placentation. Because of its zoonotic potential, *C. burnetii* presents a unique problem in the animal research facility environment. Of greatest concern are risks to immunocompromised individuals, pregnant women, other animals, and the presence of carrier animals that may shed the organism in the placenta. *C. burnetii* is considered a select agent. Readers are referred to the Center for Disease Control (CDC) and Animal and Plant Inspection Services (APHIS) National Select Agent Registry (http://www.selectagents.gov) for additional information as well as an excellent review on Q Fever (Maurin and Raoult, 1999; Van Metre, 1996).

2. Viral/Chlamydophilal

a. Viral Diseases

i. BLUETONGUE (REOVIRIDAE)

Etiology The bluetongue virus is an RNA virus in the genus *Orbivirus*, and family Reoviridae. Twenty-six serotypes have been identified, with 15 from the United States. Bluetongue is an acute arthropod-borne viral disease of ruminants characterized by stomatitis, depression, coronary band lesions and congenital abnormalities (Bulgin, 1986). It is mostly found in western states.

Clinical Signs and Diagnosis Sheep are the most likely to show clinical signs. Clinical disease is less common in goats and cattle. Early in the infection, animals will spike a fever, and will develop hyperemia and congestion of tissues of the mouth, lips, and ears. The virus name, bluetongue, is associated with the typical cyanotic membranes. The fever may subside; but tissue lesions erode causing ulcers. Increased salivary discharges and anorexia are often related to ulcers of the dental pad, lips, gums, and tongue, although salivation and lacrimation may precede apparent ulceration. Chorioretinitis and conjunctivitis are also common signs in cattle and sheep; lameness, skin lesions such as drying and cracking of the nose and mammary gland, and alopecia are also observed. Secondary bacterial pneumonia may occur, and animals may develop severe diarrhea. Sudden deaths may occur due to cardiomyopathy at any time during the disease. Hematologically, animals will be leukopenic. The course of the disease is about 2 weeks and mortality may reach 80%.

If animals are pregnant, the virus crosses the placenta and causes central nervous system lesions. Abortions may occur at any stage of gestation in cattle. Prolonged gestation may result from cerebellar hypoplasia and lack of normal sequence to induce parturition. Cerebellar hypoplasia will also be present in young born of infected dams as well as hydrocephalus, cataracts, gingival hyperplasia, or arthrogryposis.

Diagnosis is based on characteristic clinical signs and confirmed by virus isolation on blood collected during the febrile stage of the disease or brain tissue is collected from aborted fetuses. Fluorescent antibody tests, ELISA, virus neutralization tests, PCR, and Agar gel immunodiffusion (AGID) tests may be used to confirm the diagnosis.

Epizootiology and Transmission The disease is most common in outdoor-housed animals in the western United States. The virus is primarily transmitted by biting midges, *Culicoides*. A combination of factors associated with viral strain, available and susceptible hosts, environmental conditions (such as damp areas where flies breed), and vector presence are factors in the severity of outbreaks. Some sheep breeds such as Charolais and Merino may be more susceptible. Direct contact, virus-contaminated semen or other animal products, or transplacental transfer are other possible but not common means of transmission.

Necropsy Findings At necropsy, erosive lesions may be observed around the mouth, tongue, palate, esophagus, and pillars of the rumen. Ulceration or hyperemia of the coronary bands may also be seen. Many of the internal organs will contain surface petechial and ecchymotic hemorrhages. Subintimal hemorrhages of the large pulmonary arteries are nearly pathognomonic.

Pathogenesis After entering the host, the virus causes prolonged viremia. The incubation period is 6–14 days. The virus migrates to and attacks the vascular endothelium. The resulting vasculitis accounts for the lesions of the skin, mouth, tongue, esophagus and rumen, and the edema often found in many tissues.

Differential Diagnoses Differentials include other infectious vesicular diseases such as foot-and-mouth disease, contagious ecthyma, bovine virus diarrhea, mucosal disease, infectious bovine rhinotracheitis virus, bovine papular stomatitis, and malignant catarrhal fever.

Prevention and Control Modified live vaccines are available in some parts of the United States but should not be used in pregnant animals. Congenital defects are more common from vaccine use than from naturally occurring infection. Vaccinating lambs and rams in an outbreak is worthwhile. Minimizing exposure to the vector in endemic areas will decrease the incidence of the disease.

Treatment Supportive and nursing care is helpful including gruels or softer feeds, easily accessed water and shaded resting places. Nonsteroidal anti-inflammatory drugs are often administered.

Research Complications This is a reportable disease because clinical signs resemble foot and mouth disease and other exotic vesicular diseases.

ii. ENZOOTIC BOVINE LYMPHOMA (BOVINE LEUKEMIA VIRUS, BOVINE LEUKOSIS)

Etiology The term 'bovine lymphosarcoma' may refer to either sporadic lymphoproliferative disease affecting young cattle (juvenile, thymic, or cutaneous) as well as diseases of older cattle which are associated with bovine leukemia virus infection. BLV is a B lymphocyte-associated member of the genus *Deltaretrovirus* (Johnson and Kaneene, 1993a,b,c,d; Rodriguez *et al.*, 2011) which integrates into host target cell DNA by means of the reverse transcriptase enzyme, creating a provirus.

Clinical Signs Only the adult or enzootic form of bovine lymphoma is associated with BLV infection. The majority of animals will not develop any malignancies or clinical signs of infection, and will simply remain permanently infected; approximately 30% will have an elevated peripheral lymphocyte count and subtle immune defects (persistent lymphocytosis). Less than 5% of infected animals develop B cell lymphoma. Clinical signs are loss of condition and a drop in production of dairy cattle, anorexia, diarrhea, ataxia, melena due to bleeding abomasal ulcer, paresis, and other signs dependent on the location of the neoplastic lesions. Tumors will be associated with lymphoid tissues. Common sites include the abomasum, extradural spinal canal, and uterus. Cardiac tumors develop at the right atrial or left ventricular myocardium, and associated beat and rate abnormalities may be ausculted. The common ocular manifestation of the disease is exophthalmus due to retrobulbar masses.

Diagnosis is based on the animal's age, clinical signs, serology, aspirates or biopsies of masses, and necropsy findings. Kits are available for running AGID for which the BLV antigens gp-51 and gp-24 are used; antibodies may be detected within weeks after exposure and may also help in predicting disease in clinically normal cattle. Serology is the most reliable method for diagnosis of BLV although PCR is also used. Most countries recognize AGID as the official import/export test, and ELISA is the most common test for routine diagnostic use. However, serology is unreliable in calves that have ingested colostrum from BLV-positive cows due to passive transfer of antibodies. In addition, the majority of seropositive animals never develop clinical signs.

Epizootiology and Transmission This disease is present worldwide. It is estimated that at least 50% of the cattle in the United States are infected with BLV (USDA, 2007). As few as 1% of these develop lymphoma, but the adult form of the disease described here is the most common bovine neoplastic disease in the United States. In addition to the presence of BLV, the individual's BoLA genotype confers resistance or susceptibility and affects the course of the disease. Transmission is believed to be by inhalation of BLV in secretions; *in utero* or by colostrum; horizontally by contaminated equipment; by rectum during rectal exams or procedures and by breeding bulls during natural service.

Necropsy Findings Tumors may be local or widely distributed; definitive diagnosis of neoplastic tissue specimens is by histology.

Prevention and Control Development and maintenance of a BLV-free herd, or controlling infection within a herd, requires financial and programmatic commitments: BLV-positive and BLV-negative animals maintained separately; repeated serologic testing; single-use needles; washing and disinfecting instruments (including tattoo devices), needles, and other equipment between animals. A fresh rectal exam sleeve and lubricant should be used for each animal examined. Calves should be fed colostrum from serologically negative cows; however, the protective effect of colostral antibody outweighs the risk of infections. Replacing colostrum with a high-quality colostrum replacer can also be considered.

Treatment Treatment regimens of corticosteroids or cancer chemotherapeutic agents provide only short-term improvement.

Research Complications Many U.S. states and several countries, including Australia, New Zealand, and some countries in Europe have official programs for eradication of enzootic bovine leukosis. BLV is closely related to human T-lymphotropic virus type I (HTLV-1), and aspects of the biology and epidemiology of BLV may be relevant in the study of the human virus.

iii. BOVINE HERPES MAMMILLITIS (BOVINE HERPES 2 VIRUS, BOVINE ULCERATIVE MAMMILLITIS)

Etiology Bovine herpes 2 virus causes bovine herpes mammillitis, a widespread disease characterized by acute ulcerative teat and udder lesions as well as oral and skin lesions.

Clinical Signs and Diagnosis Lesions begin suddenly with teat swelling, tenderness and edema. Lesions progress to vesicles then ulcers; these may take 10 weeks to heal. Lesions may extend to the skin of the udder. Affected cows often resist milking, leading to development of mastitis. Secondary mastitis may also occur due to bacteria associated with the scabs. Diagnosis is by clinical signs and confirmed by histopathology or by virus isolation.

Epizootiology and Transmission The virus is reported to be widespread. Occurrence is often seasonal and biting insects may be vectors. Transmission with successful infection requires deep penetration of the skin. Transmission may be by contaminated milker hands, contaminated equipment, and other fomites.

Differential Diagnoses These include other diseases that cause lesions on teats such as pseudocowpox, papillomatosis, vesicular stomatitis and foot-and-mouth disease virus (FMDV).

Prevention and Control Established milking hygiene practices are important control measures: milkers' handwashing with germicidal solutions or wearing gloves, cleaning equipment between animals, and separating affected animals.

Treatment There is no treatment, and affected animals should be separated from the herd and milked last. Lesions can be cleaned and treated with topical antibacterials.

iv. BOVINE VIRUS DIARRHEA AND MUCOSAL DISEASE COMPLEX

Etiology BVDV is a pestivirus of the Flaviviridae family. A broad range of disease and immune effects is produced by BVDV in cattle but recent reports suggest that other ungulates (including pigs, sheep, and goats) also are susceptible. In addition, this virus is important in the etiology of BRDC, one of the most economically important and complex diseases of cattle. Strains of the BVDV are characterized as cytopathic (CP) and noncytopathic (NCP) based on cell culture growth characteristics. The virus has also been categorized as type 1 and type 2 isolates (along with subgenotypes 1a, 1b, etc.). Heterologous strains exist that may confound even sound vaccination programs.

Clinical Signs and Diagnosis Clinical signs of BVDV infections include abortions, congenital abnormalities, reduced fertility, immunosuppression, and acute and fatal disease. The presence of antibodies, whether from passive transfer or immunizations, does not necessarily guarantee protection from the various forms of the disease.

An acute form of the disease, caused by type 2 BVDV, occurs in cattle without sufficient immunity. After an incubation period of 5–7 days, clinical signs include fever, anorexia, oculonasal discharge, oral erosions, and diarrhea. The disease course may be shorter with hemorrhagic syndrome and death can occur within 2 days. Clinical signs of BVDV in calves also include severe enteritis and pneumonia.

When susceptible cows are infected *in utero* from gestational days 50–100, abortion or stillbirth result. Congenital defects caused by BVDV during gestational days 90–170 include thymic atrophy, cerebellar hypoplasia, ocular defects, alopecia or hypothrichosis, and hydrocephalus. Typical signs of cerebellar dysfunction in calves include wide-based stance, weakness, opisthotonus, hyperreflexia, hypermetria, nystagmus, or strabismus. Some severely affected calves will not be able to stand.

Fetuses infected *in utero* also may be normal at birth, or be immunotolerant to the virus and persistently infected (PI). Many PI animals do not survive to maturity, and those that do may have weakened immune systems. The PI animals are important because these animals shed virus throughout their lives, serving as a major source of new infections within the herd, and may develop mucosal disease (MD) caused by a CP BVDV strain. These MD clinical signs include fever, anorexia, and profuse diarrhea that may include blood and fibrin casts, oral and pharyngeal erosions, as well as erosion at the interdigital spaces and on the teats and vulva. Associated clinical signs include anemia, thrombocytopenia, and leucopenia. Secondary effects of hemorrhage and dehydration also contribute to the morbidity and mortality. Animals that do not succumb to the disease will be chronically unthrifty, debilitated, and infection prone.

Diagnosis is based on herd health history, clinical signs, viral culturing, PCR, or serology. Serology must be interpreted with the awareness of the possibility of persistently infected immunotolerant animals. Identifying PI calves is most commonly done by IHC of skin biopsies (ear notching) or blood.

Epizootiology and Transmission BVDV is present throughout the world. Transmission occurs easily by direct contact between cattle, from feed contaminated by secretions, feces, or aborted fetuses and placentas, and fomites such as contaminated boots, clothing, and equipment. Persistently infected females transmit the virus to their fetuses. Semen can also be a source of virus.

Necropsy Findings *In utero* affected calves may have cerebellar hypoplasia. Older animals may have areas of intestinal necrosis and erosions found from the oral cavity throughout the gastrointestinal tract to the cecum. Respiratory tract lesions will often be complicated by secondary bacterial pneumonia. When the hemorrhagic syndrome develops, petechiation and mucosal bleeding will be present.

Differential Diagnoses Differentials for enteritis of calves include viral infections, *Cryptosporidia*, *E. coli*, *Salmonella*, and *Coccidia*. *Salmonella*, winter dysentery, Johne's disease, intestinal parasites, and malignant catarrhal fever (MCF) are differentials for the diarrhea seen in the disease in adult animals. Respiratory tract pathogens such as BRSV, *Mannheimia*, *Pasteurella*, *Histophilus*, and *Mycoplasma* must be considered for the respiratory tract manifestations. Oral lesions are also produced by MCF, FMDV, vesicular stomatitis, bluetongue and papular stomatitis. Infectious bovine herpesvirus 1, leptospirosis, brucellosis, trichomoniasis, and mycosis should be considered in cases of abortion.

Prevention and Control Biosecurity and vaccination are the best ways to prevent BVDV and should be integrated into the herd health program. Vaccine preparations for BVDV are modified live (MLV) or inactivated virus. Each has advantages and disadvantages. The former induces rapid immunity (within 1 week) after a single dose, provides longer duration of immunity against several strains, and induces serum-neutralizing antibodies. However, MLV vaccines are not recommended for use in pregnant cattle, may induce mucosal disease, and may be immunosuppressive at the time of vaccination. Inactivated vaccines require booster doses after the initial immunization and do not induce cell-mediated immunity. Passive immunity may protect most calves up to 6–8 months of age. Subsequent vaccination with MLV may provide lifelong immunity but this is not guaranteed. Annual boosters are recommended to protect against vaccine breaks.

The virus persists in the environment for 2 weeks, and is susceptible to the disinfectants chlorhexidine, hypochlorite, iodophors, and aldehydes. Isolation and testing of new additions to the herd is critical, as is testing and culling PI cattle.

Treatment No specific treatment is available. Supportive care and treatment with antibiotics to prevent secondary infection are recommended.

v. CAE VIRUS

Etiology CAEV occurs worldwide with a high prevalence in the United States. CAE is considered the most important viral diseases of goats. The CAEV is in the genus *Lentivirus* of the family *Retroviridae*. It causes chronic arthritis and mastitis in adults and encephalitis in young. CAEV is in the same viral genus as the ovine progressive pneumonia virus (OPPV).

Clinical Signs and Diagnosis The most common presentation in goats is an insidious, progressive arthritis in animals 6 months of age and older. Animals become stiff, have difficulty getting up, and may be clinically lame in one or both forelimbs. Carpal joints are so swollen and painful that the animal prefers to eat, drink, and walk on its 'knees.' In dairy goats, milk production decreases and udders may become firmer. This retrovirus also causes neurological clinical signs in kids 2–6 months old. Kids may be bright and alert, afebrile, and able to eat normally even when recumbent. Some kids may initially show unilateral weakness in a rear limb which progresses to hemiplegia or tetraplegia. Mild to severe lower motor neuron deficits may be noted, but spinal reflexes are intact. Clinical signs may also include head tilt, blindness, ataxia and facial nerve paralysis.

Older animals in the group may experience interstitial pneumonia or chronic arthritis. The pneumonia is similar to the pneumonia in sheep caused by OPPV. The course of disease is gradual but progressive, and animals will eventually lose weight and have respiratory distress. Some animals in a herd may not develop any clinical signs.

Diagnosis is based on clinical signs, *post mortem* lesions, and positive serology for viral antibodies to CAEV. An AGID test identifies antibodies to the virus and is used for diagnosis. Kids acquire an anti-CAEV antibody in colostrum and this passive immunity may be interpreted as indicative of infection with the virus. The antibody does not prevent viral transmission.

Epizootiology and Transmission The virus is prevalent in most industrialized countries. The most common means of transmission is oral. Adults transfer virus to kids in colostrum and milk in spite of the presence of anti-CAEV antibody in the colostrum. Transmission may occur among adult goats by contact. Intrauterine transmission is believed to be rare.

Necropsy Findings Necropsy and histopathology reveal a striking synovial hyperplasia associated with the joints with infiltrates of lymphocytes, macrophages, and plasma cells. Other histologic lesions include demyelination in the brain and spinal cord with multifocal invasion of lymphocytes, macrophages, and plasma cells. Lung pathology is characteristic. In severe cases of mastitis, the udder may appear to be composed entirely of lymphoid tissue.

Differential Diagnoses The differential diagnosis for the neurologic form of CAEV should include copper deficiency, enzootic pneumonia, white muscle disease, rabies, listeriosis, thiamine deficiency, and spinal cord disease or injury. The differential diagnosis for CAEV arthritis and pneumonia should include *Chlamydophila* and *Mycoplasma*.

Prevention and Control Herds can be screened for CAE by testing serologically using AGID, ELISA, immunoprecipitation, or PCR. Since CAE is highly prevalent in the United States and since seronegative animals can shed organisms in the milk, retesting herds at least annually may be necessary. Control measures include test and culling, prevention of milk transmission, and isolation of affected animals. Parturition must be monitored and kids must be removed immediately and fed heat-treated colostrum (56°C for 1h). CAEV-negative goats should be separated from -positive goats.

Treatment There is no treatment for CAEV.

vi. INFECTIOUS BOVINE RHINOTRACHEITIS VIRUS (IBRV) (INFECTIOUS PUSTULAR VULVOVAGINITIS (IBR-IPV), BOVINE HERPESVIRUS I)

Etiology The infectious bovine rhinotracheitis virus (IBPR) causes or contributes to several bovine syndromes including respiratory and reproductive tract diseases. It is one of the primary pathogens in the BRDC.

Clinical Signs and Diagnosis Diseases caused by the virus include conjunctivitis, rhinotracheitis, pustular vulvovaginitis, balanoposthitis, abortion, encephalomyelitis, and mastitis. The respiratory form is known as IBR or 'red nose.' Clinical signs may range from mild to severe with severity associated with the presence of additional respiratory viral infections or secondary bacterial infections. The mortality rate in more mature cattle is low, however, unless there is secondary bacterial pneumonia. Fever, anorexia, restlessness, hyperemia of the muzzle and nares, gray pustules on the muzzle (that later form plaques), nasal discharge progressing from serous to mucopurulent, hyperpnea, coughing, salivation, conjunctivitis with excessive epiphora, and decreased production in dairy animals are typical signs. Recovery generally occurs 4–5 days after the onset of clinical signs as long as there is no complication with bacterial pneumonia. Neonatal calves may develop respiratory as well as general systemic disease. Young

calves are most susceptible to the encephalitic form; signs include dull attitude, head pressing, vocalizations, nystagmus, head tilt, blindness, convulsions, and coma. This form is usually fatal within 5 days. Abortion may occur simultaneously with as a sequel to the conjunctival or respiratory tract diseases regardless of the severity of the disease in the dam. Abortions are usually seen in the second half of pregnancy, but early embryonic death is possible. Infectious pustular vulvovaginitis (IPV) is most commonly seen in dairy cows; signs include fever, depression, anorexia, vulvar labia swelling, vulvar discharge, and reddened vaginal mucosa due to pustule development. If uncomplicated, the infection lasts about 4–5 days, and lesions heal in 2 weeks. Younger infected bulls may develop balanoposthitis with edema, swelling, and pain such that the animals will not service cows.

Diagnosis is based on clinical signs, virus isolation, or paired serum samples. Diagnosis can be made from aborted fetal tissues by virus isolation or fluorescent antibody staining.

Epizootiology and Transmission IBRV is widely distributed throughout the world, and adult animals are reservoirs of infection. Transmission is primarily by nasal secretions during and after clinical signs of disease.

Necropsy Findings Fibrinonecrotic rhinotracheitis is considered pathognomonic for IBRV respiratory tract infections. When there are secondary bacterial infections, such as *Pasteurella/Mannheimia* bronchopneumonia, findings will include congested tracheal mucosa and petechial and ecchymotic hemorrhages in that tissue. Lesions from the encephalitic form include lymphocytic meningoencephalitis, and will be found throughout the gray matter (neuronal degeneration, perivascular cuffing) and white matter (myelitis, demyelination). In younger animals, erosions and ulcers are coated with debris and may be found in the nose, esophagus, and forestomachs. White foci may be found in the liver, kidney, spleen, and lymph nodes. In the aborted fetus, pale, focal, necrotic lesions in all tissues may be found but are especially prevalent in the liver.

Differential Diagnoses The conjunctivitis of IBR may initially be mistaken for that of a *Moraxella bovis* (Pinkeye) infection; the IBR will be peripheral and there will not be corneal ulceration.

Prevention and Control Vaccination options include inactivated, attenuated, modified live, and genetically altered temperature-sensitive intranasal (IN) and parenteral preparations. Some are in combination with Parainfluenza Virus-3 (PI-3). The MLV preparations are administered intranasally; these are advantageous in calves for inducing mucosal immunity even when serologic passive immunity is already present and adequate. Parenteral MLV may cause abortion in pregnant cattle. Some newer vaccines, with gene deletion, allow for serologic differentiation between antibody responses from infection or immunization. Bulls and breeding and replacement heifers should be immunized when 6–8 months old, prior to breeding and annually afterwards.

Treatment Uncomplicated mild infections will resolve over a few weeks; palliative treatments, such as cleaning ocular discharges and supplying softened food are helpful in recovery. Antibiotics are usually administered because of the high likelihood of secondary bacterial pneumonia. Treatment of encephalitic animals is unrewarding.

vii. PARAINFLUENZA-3 (PI-3)

Etiology Bovine parainfluenza 3 (BPI 3) is an RNA virus of the family *Paramyxoviridae* that causes mild respiratory disease of ruminants when it is the sole pathogen. Viral infection often predisposes the respiratory system to severe disease associated with concurrent viral or bacterial pathogens. Serotypes seen in the smaller ruminants are distinct from those isolated from cattle.

Clinical Signs Uncomplicated viral infections ranging from asymptomatic to mild signs of upper respiratory tract disease are almost never fatal. Clinical signs include ocular and nasal discharges, cough, fever, and increased respiratory rate and breath sounds. In pregnant animals exposure to BPI-3 can result in abortions. Clinical signs become apparent or more severe when additional viral pathogens, such as BVDV, or a secondary bacterial infection, such as *Mannheimia haemolytica*, are involved.

Diagnosis Viral isolation, direct IFA from nasal swabs, or paired serum samples can be useful.

Epizootiology and Transmission The virus is considered ubiquitous in cattle and a common infection in sheep. Presently it is assumed that the virus is widespread in goats but firm evidence is lacking.

Necropsy Findings For an infection of PI-3 only, findings will be negligible. Some congestion of respiratory mucosa, swelling of respiratory tract-associated lymph nodes, and mild pneumonitis may be noted grossly and histologically.

Differential Diagnoses Differentials, particularly in cattle, include infections with other respiratory tract viruses of ruminants: IBRV, BVDV, and BRSV.

Prevention and Control Immunization, management, and nutrition are important for this respiratory pathogen. In cattle, modified live vaccines for parenteral or IN administration are available. The IN vaccine immunizes in the presence of passively acquired antibodies, provides immunity within 3 days of administration, and stimulates the production of interferon. Booster vaccinations are recommended for all preparations within 2–6 months after the initial immunization. All presently marketed vaccine products come in combination with other bovine respiratory viruses (usually IBR). There is no approved PI-3 vaccine for sheep and goats. The use of the cattle formulation has been used.

Treatment Uncomplicated disease is not treated.

viii. RESPIRATORY SYNCYTIAL VIRUSES OF RUMINANTS (RSV)

Etiology The respiratory syncytial viruses are in the genus *Pneumovirus* in the *Paramyxoviridae* family and are common causes of severe disease in ruminants, especially calves and yearling cattle. Two serotypes of the BRSV have been described for cattle; these may be similar or identical to the virus seen in sheep and goats.

Clinical Findings and Diagnosis Infections may be subclinical or may develop into severe illness. Severe respiratory disease occurs upon initial exposure to the virus and subsequent exposures tend to result in mild to subclinical disease. Clinical signs include high fever, hyperpnea, spontaneous or easily induced cough, nasal discharge, and conjunctivitis. Interstitial pneumonia usually develops and harsh respiratory sounds are evident on auscultation. Open-mouthed breathing may be present in later stages of the disease. Emphysema of the dorsal subcutis from ruptured bullae is characteristic when present. Development of emphysema indicates a poor prognosis and death may occur in the severe cases of the viral infection. Secondary bacterial pneumonia, especially with *Mannheimia haemolytica*, with morbidity and mortality, are also common sequelae. Abortions have been associated with BRSV outbreaks.

Diagnosis is based on virus isolation and serology (acute and convalescent). Nasal swabs for virus isolation should be taken when animals have fevers and before onset of respiratory disease.

Epizootiology and Transmission These viruses are considered ubiquitous in domestic cattle and are transmitted by aerosols.

Necropsy Findings Gross lesions include consolidation of anteroventral lung lobes. Edema and emphysema are present. As the name indicates, syncytia, that may have small eosinophilic intracytoplasmic and rarely intranuclear inclusions, form in areas of the lungs infected with the virus. Necrotizing bronchiolitis, bronchiolitis obliterans, and hyaline membrane formation will be evident microscopically.

Differential Diagnoses Differentials should include other ruminant respiratory tract viruses such as BPI3, BVDV and bovine herpesvirus 1.

Prevention and Control Routine vaccination should be part of the standard health program. Passive immunity from colostrum does not appear to prevent BRSV infection, but does reduce the severity of the disease. The virus is easily inactivated in the environment.

Treatment Recovery can be spontaneous, however, antibiotics and supportive therapy are useful to prevent or control secondary bacterial pneumonia. In severe cases, antihistamines and corticosteroids may also be necessary.

ix. BORDER DISEASE (HAIRY SHAKER DISEASE)

Etiology   Border disease, also known as hairy shaker disease, is a disease of sheep caused by a virus closely related to BVDV, a *Pestivirus* of the ~~Togaviridae~~ family. Goats are also affected.   FLAVIVRIDAE

Clinical Signs and Diagnosis   Border disease in ewes causes early embryonic death, abortion of macerated or mummified fetuses, or birth of lambs with developmental abnormalities. Lambs infected *in utero* may be born weak and exhibit a number of congenital defects such as tremor or hirsutism (darkly pigmented over the shoulders and head), hypothyroidism, joint abnormalities including arthrogryposis, and central nervous system defects. Infection produces similar clinical manifestations in goats except that hirsutism is not seen.

Diagnosis includes the typical signs described above, as well as serological evidence of viral infection. Virus isolation, ELISA, or PCR confirms the diagnosis.

Epizootiology and Transmission   The virus is present worldwide and reports of disease are sporadic. Persistently infected animals shed virus in urine, feces, and saliva throughout their lives.

Necropsy Findings   Lesions include placentitis, and characteristic joint and haircoat changes in the fetus.

Prevention and Control   Congenitally affected lambs should be humanely euthanized as soon as possible. Animals new to the flock should be screened serologically. Cattle housed near sheep should be regularly vaccinated for BVDV. Because border disease viruses of sheep have been proven antigenically distinct from BVD of cattle, the BVD vaccines for cattle cannot be recommended for control of border disease in sheep (Merck Veterinary Manual Online, 2011).

Treatment   There is no treatment other than supportive care for affected animals.

x. ORF VIRUS DISEASE (CONTAGIOUS ECTHYMA, CONTAGIOUS PUSTULAR DERMATITIS, SORE MOUTH)

Etiology   Contagious ecthyma, also known as contagious pustular dermatitis, sore mouth, or orf, is an acute dermatitis of sheep and goats caused by a member of the *Parapoxvirus* genus. This disease occurs worldwide and is zoonotic. Naturally occurring disease has also been reported in other species such as musk ox and reindeer.

Clinical Signs and Diagnosis   The disease is characterized by the presence of papules, vesicles or pustules and subsequently scabs of the skin of the face, genitals of both sexes, and coronary bands of the feet. Lesions develop most frequently at mucocutaneous junctions and are found most commonly at the comissures of the mouth. Orf is usually identified in animals less than a year of age. Younger lambs and kids will have difficulty nursing and become weak. Lesions may also develop on udders of nursing dams. Morbidity in a susceptible group of animals may exceed 90%. Mortality is low but the course of the disease may last up to 6 weeks.

Diagnosis is based on characteristic lesions. Disease is confirmed by virus isolation.

Epizootiology and Transmission   All ages of sheep and goats are susceptible. Seasonal occurrences immediately after lambing and after entry into a feedlot are common because stress plays a role in susceptibility to this viral disease. The virus is extremely resistant to environmental conditions and can contaminate small ruminant facilities for many years.

Necropsy Findings   Except in the case of debilitated lambs, this disease does not usually result in necropsy.

Differential Diagnoses   Ulcerative dermatosis and bluetongue virus should be considered in both sheep and goats as differentials. Another important differential in goats is staphylococcal dermatitis.

Prevention and Control   Individuals handling infected animals should be advised of precautions beforehand, wear gloves, and separate work clothing and other personal protective equipment. Clippers, ear tagging devices, and other similar equipment should always be cleaned and disinfected after each use. Vaccinating lambs and kids with commercial vaccine best prevents the disease. Animals that must be introduced to an infected environment should be vaccinated upon arrival. Precautions must be taken when vaccinating animals because the vaccine may induce orf in animal handlers. It is not recommended to vaccinate animals in flocks already free of the disease.

Treatment   Affected animals should be isolated and provided supportive care. Young animals may require tube feeding because mouths are too sore to nurse.

Research Complications   Carrier animals may be a factor in flock or herd outbreaks. Contagious ecthyma is a zoonotic disease, and human-to-human transmission can also occur. Lesions in humans are extremely painful and may last as long as 6 weeks.

xi. FOOT AND MOUTH DISEASE (AFTOSA, FMDV)

Etiology   The FMDV is a picornavirus in the *Aphthovirus* genus. Although epidemics of the disease have occurred worldwide, North and Central America have been free of the virus since the mid-1950s. This is a reportable disease in the United States, and clinical signs are very similar to other vesicular diseases. Cattle are the most susceptible species with swine being important hosts and propagators of the disease. Disease can occur in sheep and is usually subclinical in goats.

Clinical Signs and Diagnosis   In addition to vesicle formation around and in the mouth, hooves and teats, fever, anorexia, weakness, and salivation occur.

Diagnosis must be based on ELISA, virus neutralization, fluorescent antibody tests, and complement fixation. Samples of vesicular fluid or epithelium can be sent to the national laboratory responsible for diagnosis of FMD.

Epizootiology and Transmission   FMDV is the most highly infectious agent described to date. Domestic and wild ruminants and several other species, such as swine, rats, bears, and llamas are hosts. The United States, Canada, Japan, New Zealand, and Australia are FMD-free, but the disease is endemic in most of South America, parts of Europe, and throughout Asia and Africa. The virus is very contagious and is spread primarily by inhaled aerosols which can be carried over long distances (up to 70 miles) or by fomites, such as shoes, clothing and equipment.

Necropsy Findings   Vesicles, erosions and ulcers are present in the oral cavity as well as on rumen pillars and mammary alveolar epithelium.

Differential Diagnoses   Vesicular stomatitis is the principal differential. Other differentials include mucosal disease, contagious ecthyma (orf), bluetongue, malignant catarrhal fever, bovine papular stomatitis, bovine herpes mammillitis, and IBR virus infection.

Prevention and Control   Movement of animals and animal products from endemic areas is regulated. Vaccination, quarantine and slaughter are practiced in outbreaks in endemic areas.

Treatment   Any suspicion of FMD infection should trigger notification of regulatory authorities; infected animals will be destroyed in FMDV-free countries.

Research Complications   Importation into the United States of animals or animal products from endemic areas is prohibited.

xii. MALIGNANT CATARRHAL FEVER

Etiology   Malignant catarrhal fever (MCF) is a severe disease primarily of cattle caused by bovine herpesvirus 6. The agents of MCF are viruses in the subfamily Gammaherpesvirinae and genus *Macavirus*. Disease may occur sporadically or as outbreaks. The sheep-associated form is due to OvHV-2.

Clinical Signs and Diagnosis   Signs range from subclinical to recrudescing latent infections to the lethal disease seen in susceptible species, such as cattle. Sudden death may also occur in cattle. Presentations of the disease may be categorized as alimentary, encephalitis, or skin forms; all three may occur in an animal. Corneal edema starting at the limbus and progressing centripetally is a nearly pathognomonic sign; photophobia, severe keratoconjunctivitis and ocular involvement may follow. Other signs include prolonged fever, oral mucosal erosions, salivation, lacrimation, ropey catarrhal nasal discharge, encephalitis, and pronounced lymphadenopathy. Cattle may also have severe diarrhea. Recovery is usually prolonged and some permanent debilitation may occur. The disease is fatal in severely affected individuals.

Diagnosis is based on history of exposure as well as clinical signs and characteristic lesions Serology,

PCR-based assays, viral isolation and cell culture assays are also used.

Epizootiology and Transmission   Most ruminant species are susceptible to MCF. Sheep are asymptomatic sources of infection for cattle, which are dead-end hosts. Cattle should not be mixed with sheep for this reason. Other ruminants, including goats, may harbor the virus. Infection is spread by aerosol, direct contact and fomites such as water troughs, placental tissues, contaminated fomites, birds, and caretakers. The incubation period may be up to 3 months.

Necropsy   This disease is systemic and lesions can be found in any organ. Gross findings at necropsy include necrotic and ulcerated nasal and oral mucosa; thickened, edematous, ulcerated and hemorrhagic areas of the intestinal tract; swollen, friable and hemorrhagic lymph nodes and other lymphatic tissues; and erosion of affected mucosal surfaces.

Differential Diagnoses   The differentials for this disease are BVDV and mucosal disease, IBR, bluetongue, vesicular stomatitis, and FMD.

Prevention and Control   There is no vaccine available at this time. In North America, sheep, and cattle that have been either exposed or that have survived the disease are reservoirs for outbreaks in other cattle. The virus is very fragile outside of host's cells and will not survive in the environment for more than a few hours.

Treatment   Prognosis is grave. There is no specific treatment for MCF; supportive treatment may improve recovery rates.

xiii. OVINE PROGRESSIVE PNEUMONIA (OPP, VISNA/MAEDI)

Etiology   An RNA virus in the genus *Lentivirus* of the family Retroviridae causes ovine progressive pneumonia (OPP). The 'Maedi' refers to the progressive pneumonia presentation of the disease. The 'Visna' refers to the central nervous system disease which is reported predominantly in Iceland. Genetic susceptibility to OPP has been implicated (Heaton and Leymaster, 2012).

Clinical Signs and Diagnosis   OPP is characterized by weakness, unthriftiness, weight loss, and pneumonia in adult sheep (Pepin *et al.*, 1998; de la Concha Bermejillo, 1997). Clinically, animals exhibit signs of progressive pulmonary disease after an extremely long incubation period of up to 2 years. Respiratory rate and dyspnea gradually increase as the disease progresses; animals progressively lose weight and become weak. Mastitis is a common clinical feature. Thoracic auscultation reveals consolidation of ventral lung lobes, and hematological findings indicate anemia and leukocytosis. Rare neurological signs include flexion of fetlock and pastern joints, tremors of facial muscles, progressive paresis and paralysis, and depression and prostration.

Death occurs in weeks to months; secondary bacterial pneumonia may contribute to the animal's death.

The disease can be serologically diagnosed with AGID tests, virus isolation, serum neutralization, complement fixation and ELISA tests. A quantitative PCR is also available.

Epizootiology and Transmission   Prevalence in some states in the United States is estimated at 60–80% (Herrmann-Hoesing *et al.*, 2007). It is transmitted horizontally via inhalation of aerosolized virus particles and vertically between the infected dam and fetus. Transmission through the milk or colostrum is considered common (Knowles, 1997).

Necropsy Findings   Lesions are observed in lungs, mammary glands, joints, and the brain. Pulmonary adhesions, ventral lung lobe consolidation and bronchial lymph node enlargement, mastitis and degenerative arthritis are visualized grossly. Meningeal edema, thickening of the choroid plexus and foci of leukoencephalomalacia are seen in the central nervous system.

Differential Diagnoses   Differential diagnoses are pulmonary adenomatosis and mycoplasmosis.

Prevention and Control   Isolating or removing infected animals can prevent the disease. Facilities and equipment should also be disinfected. Some states have initiated control programs.

Treatment   Treatment is unsuccessful.

xiv. POXVIRUSES OF RUMINANTS

Ovine Viral Dermatosis   This is a venereal disease of sheep caused by a parapoxvirus distinct from contagious ecthyma (orf). The disease resolves within two weeks in healthy animals but lesions are painful, and resemble those of *C. renale* posthitis/vulvovaginitis. Symptomatic treatment may be necessary in some cases. There is no vaccine. Animals should not be used for breeding while clinical signs are present.

Proliferative Stomatitis (Bovine Papular Stomatitis)

Etiology   A parapoxvirus is the causative agent of bovine papular stomatitis. This virus is considered to be closely related to the parapoxvirus causing contagious ecthyma and pseudocowpox. It is also a zoonotic disease. The disease is not considered of major consequence but high morbidity may be seen in severe outbreaks. In addition, lesions are comparable in appearance to those seen with vesicular stomatitis, BVDV, and FMDV. The disease occurs worldwide.

Clinical Signs and Diagnosis   Raised red papules or erosions and shallow ulcers on the muzzle, nose, oral mucosa (including the hard palate), esophagus and rumen of cattle from 1 month to 2 years old are the most common findings. Morbidity among herds may be 100% but mortalities are rare. The infection may also be asymptomatic. Diagnosis is based on clinical signs and viral isolation. Handlers may develop lesions on their hands at sites of contact with lesions of cattle.

Pseudocowpox (Milker's nodes, Paravaccinia)

Etiology   Pseudocowpox is a worldwide cattle disease caused by a parapox virus related to the causative agents of bovine papular stomatitis and orf (see above). Lesions are confined to the teats. This is also a zoonotic disease.

Clinical Signs and Diagnosis   Minor lesions are usually confined to the teats. Lesions start as small red papules that proceed quickly to small vesicles or pustules and to scabs. These are distinctive due to the ring or horseshoe shape of the scab; some lesions may persist for months causing the teats to have a rough appearance and feel. Removal of scabs is painful. The teat lesions may predispose to mastitis due to the cows' resistance to milking.

Differential Diagnoses   Differentials include bovine herpes mammillitis and papillomatosis.

Prevention and Control   The virus is spread by contaminated hands and equipment, therefore milking hygiene is crucial.

Treatment   Lesions should be treated symptomatically, and affected animals milked last.

Research Complications   Like other related poxviruses, this virus causes nodular lesions on humans.

xv. PULMONARY ADENOMATOSIS (JAAGSIEKTE SHEEP RETROVIRUS)

Etiology   Pulmonary adenomatosis is a rare but progressive wasting disease of sheep with worldwide distribution. Pulmonary adenomatosis is caused by a retrovirus in the genus *Betaretrovirus* antigenically related to the Mason–Pfizer monkey virus and is reportable in some states. Typical clinical signs include progressive respiratory signs such as dyspnea, rapid respiration and wasting. The disease is diagnosed by chronic clinical signs, viral antigen RNA, IHC, immunoblot, and PCR on tissues.

Research Impact   Pulmonary adenomatosis is a common model used for research of retrovirus development, pulmonary neoplasia, and transmissible pulmonary neoplastic diseases.

xvi. PAPILLOMATOSIS (WARTS, VERRUCAE)

Etiology   Cutaneous papillomatosis is a very common disease in cattle but is much less common among sheep and goats. The disease is a viral-induced proliferation of the epithelium of the neck, face, back, and legs. These tumors are caused by a papilloma (DNA) virus in the family Papillomaviridae. Viruses are host specific and often body-site specific. In cattle, the site specificity of papilloma virus strains around the head and neck is particularly well recognized.

Clinical Signs and Diagnosis Papillomas may last for up to 12 months and are seen more frequently in younger animals. Lesions will have typical wart appearances and be single or multiple, small (1 mm) to very large (500 mm). The infections will generally be benign although when infections are severe, weight loss may occur. When warts occur on teats, secondary mastitis may develop. Prognosis in cattle is poor only when papillomatosis involves more than 20% of the body surface.

In sheep and goat, warts are the verrucous type. The disease is of little consequence unless warts develop in an area that causes discomfort or incapacitation such as between the digits, on the lips, or over the joints. Warts on goat udders tend to be persistent.

Diagnosis is made by observing the typical proliferative lesions.

Epizootiology and Transmission The virus is transmitted by direct and indirect (fomites) contact, entering through surface wounds and sites such as tattoos. DNA from papillomavirus has been found in blood, milk, urine, and other fluids obtained from infected animals. The incubation period ranges from 1 to 6 months. The disease is generally self-limiting.

Prevention and Control Commercial (available only for cattle) or autogenous vaccines must be used with a recognition that a host specificity of papillomavirus strains exists and that immunity from infection or vaccination is viral-type specific. Autogenous vaccines are generally considered more effective Virucidal products are recommended for disinfection of contaminated environments. Minimizing cutaneous injuries and sanitizing equipment (tattoo devices, dehorners, ear taggers, etc.) in a virucidal solution between uses are recommended preventative measures.

Treatment Warts will often spontaneously resolve as immunity develops. Warts can be amputated with scissors and autogenous vaccines can be made and administered to help prevent disease spread. Cryosurgery with liquid nitrogen or dry ice has also proven to be successful.

xvii. PSEUDORABIES (MAD ITCH, AUJESZKY'S DISEASE)

Etiology Pseudorabies is an acute encephalitic disease caused by a neurotropic member of the subfamily *Alphaherpesvirinae*, the Suid herpesvirus 1. One serotype is recognized but strain differences exist. The virus has worldwide distribution; it has been eradicated from domestic livestock in the United States but is prevalent in feral swine. It is a primarily a clinical disease of swine and cattle with less frequent reports in sheep and goats.

Clinical Signs and Diagnosis A range of clinical signs is seen during the rapid course of this usually fatal disease. At the site of virus inoculation or in other locations, abrasions, swelling, intense pruritus and alopecia are seen. Animals are hyperthermic and vocalize frantically. Other neurological signs range from hoof stamping, kicking at the pruritic area, salivation, tongue chewing, head pressing and circling, nystagmus and strabismus to paresthesia or hyperesthesia, ataxia, and conscious proprioceptive deficits. Animals may be fearful or depressed, or aggressive. Recumbency and coma precede death.

Diagnosis is by virus isolation and fluorescent antibody testing from nasal or pharyngeal secretions or *post mortem* tissues, and histological findings at necropsy.

Epizootiology and Transmission Swine are the primary hosts for pseudorabies virus, but they are usually asymptomatic and serve as reservoirs for the virus. Other animals are dead-end hosts. The unprotected virus will survive only a few weeks in the environment but may remain viable in meat (including carcasses) for weeks to months. Transmission is by direct contact or fomites, fecal–oral, or aerosol. Pets or wildlife are a risk as they can carry the organism between farms, although they live only 2–3 days after becoming infected. Transmission can also be by inadvertent exposure (e.g., contaminated syringes) of ruminants to the modified live vaccines developed for use in swine.

Necropsy Findings There is no pathognomonic gross lesion. Definitive histologic findings include severe, focal, nonsuppurative encephalitis and myelitis.

Differential Diagnoses Differentials for the neurologic signs of pseudorabies infection include rabies, polioencephalomalacia, salt poisoning, meningitis, lead poisoning, hypomagnesemia, and enterotoxemia. Those for the intense pruritus include psoroptic mange and scrapie in sheep, sarcoptic mange, and pediculosis.

Prevention and Control Pseudorabies is a reportable disease in the United States where a nationwide eradication program exists.

Treatment There is no treatment and most affected animals die.

Research Complications Any suspicion of pseudorabies virus infection should be promptly reported to animal health authorities.

xviii. RABIES (HYDROPHOBIA)

Etiology Rabies is a sporadic but highly fatal acute viral disease affecting the central nervous system. The rabies virus is a neurotropic RNA virus of the genus *Lyssavirus* and the family Rhabdoviridae that can affect any mammal. Sheep, goats, and cattle are susceptible. The zoonotic potential of this virus must be kept in mind at all times when handling moribund animals with neurological signs characteristic of the disease. Rabies is endemic in many areas of the world and within areas of the Unites States. This is a reportable disease in North America.

Clinical Findings and Diagnosis The most reliable signs in all species are acute behavioral changes and unexplained progressive paralysis. Animals generally progress through three phases: prodromal, excitatory, and paralytic. Many signs during these stages are non-specific. During the short prodromal phase, animals are hyperthermic and apprehensive. In the excitatory phase, they refuse to eat and drink, are active and aggressive. Repeated vocalizations, tenesmus, sexual excitement, and salivation occur during this phase. The final paralytic stage, with recumbency and death, occurs over several hours to days. The clinical course is usually 1–4 days.

Diagnosis is based on clinical signs with a progressive and fatal course. Confirmation presently is made with the fluorescent antibody technique on brain tissue.

Epizootiology and Transmission   The rabies virus is transmitted via a bite-wound inflicted by a rabid animal. Cats, dogs, raccoons, skunks, foxes, wild canids, and bats are the common disease vectors in North America.

Necropsy Findings   Few lesions are seen at necropsy. Negri bodies in the cytoplasm of neurons of the hippocampus and in Purkinje cells are pathognomonic histologic findings.

Differential Diagnoses   Rabies should be included on the differential list when clinical signs of neurologic disease are evident. Other differentials for ruminants include herpesvirus encephalitis, thromboembolic meningoencephalitis, nervous ketosis, grass tetany, and nervous coccidiosis.

Control   Vaccines approved for use cattle and sheep are commercially available and contain inactivated virus; no vaccine is currently approved for goats in the United States. Ruminants in endemic areas, such as the East Coast of the United States, should be routinely vaccinated. Monitoring for and exclusion of wildlife from large animal facilities are worthwhile preventative measures.

Research Complications   Personal protective equipment must be worn by individuals handling animals manifesting neurological disease signs, including gloves, face mask, and eye shields.

xix. SCHMALLENBERG VIRUS

Etiology   Schmallenberg virus is an orthobunyavirus named for the city in Germany where it was discovered in late 2011. Sheep, goats, and cattle are susceptible. It is thought to be found only in Europe at present.

Clinical Findings and Diagnosis   Affected animals including sheep, cattle, and goats, present with fever, diarrhea, and decreased milk production in milking animals. Still births are seen in all three species, as well as congenital malformations. No illness has been seen in the dams prior to the reproductive effects. Congenital malformations include scoliosis, hydrocephalus, arthrogryposis, and hypoplasia of the cerebellum. Diagnosis can be accomplished through RT-PCR via a blood sample or brain and spleen tissue.

Differential Diagnoses   Clinical signs and reproductive issues mimic several other pathogens described in this chapter.

Prevention and Control   The virus is thought to be transmitted by midges therefore is primarily seen in warm weather months. Some early information on affected herds has shown some tendency towards naturally acquired immunity. Currently, there are import bans in different countries around Europe and the world involving areas where this virus has been diagnosed (Garrigliany *et al.*, 2012).

xx. TRANSMISSIBLE SPONGIFORM ENCEPHALOPATHIES

Bovine Spongiform Ecephalopathie (BSE or 'Mad Cow Disease')

Subsequent to the BSE outbreak in Great Britain in the 1980s, the USDA restricted importation of live cattle and certain ruminant products from countries affected with BSE. The USDA also has an ongoing BSE surveillance program, designed to detect the disease at the level of 1 case per 1,000,000 cattle. Because the probability of encountering BSE in the research environment is very low, readers are directed to the USDA/APHIS website for current information. Also, investigators should be cognizant of measures taken by suppliers of biological reagents to mitigate the risk of contamination with the BSE agent.

Scrapie

Etiology   Scrapie is the TSE of sheep and goats, and like BSE is a reportable disease. It is enzootic in many countries and is much more common in sheep than goats.

Clinical Signs and Diagnosis   During early clinical stages, animals are excitable and hard to control. Tremors of head and neck muscles, as well as uncoordinated movements and unusual 'bunny hopping' gaits are observed. Lip smacking may also be seen. Animals experience severe pruritus and will self-mutilate while rubbing on fences, trees, and other objects. Blindness and abortion may also be seen. Morbidity may reach 50% within flock. Most animals die within a 4- to 6-week period, although some animals may survive 6 months. In goats, pruritus is generally less severe. Other clinical signs noted in goats include listlessness, stiffness or restlessness, or behavioral changes such as irritability, hunched posture, twitching, and erect tail and ears. As with sheep, the disease gradually progresses to anorexia, debilitation, and death.

Diagnosis is based on clinical signs and histopathological lesions. A newer diagnostic test in live animals is based on a biopsy from the third eyelid (nictitating membrane) by regulatory veterinarians. Blood tests are available for genetic susceptibility.

Epizootiology and Transmission   The Suffolk breed tends to be especially susceptible, although scrapie has also been reported in several other breeds. Genomic research indicates there are three nonsynonymous genetic polymorphisms in the *PRP* gene governing susceptibility at codons 136, 154, and 171. VRQ/VRQ animals are most susceptible; ARR/ARR animals are resistant. Scrapie is transmitted horizontally to neonates or juveniles by direct or indirect contact; nasal secretions or placentas serve as sources of the infectious agent. Transplacental transmission is considered unlikely. Because of the long incubation period (from 2 to 5 years), only adult animals display signs of the disease. State and federal eradication programs exist. See *A Guide to the National Scrapie Eradication Program for Veterinarians* (2009) for additional information.

Necropsy Findings At necropsy, no gross lesion is observed. Histopathologically, neuronal cytoplasmic vacuolization, astrogliosis, and spongiform degeneration are visualized in the brainstem, spinal cord, and especially thalamus.

Differential Diagnoses In sheep and goats, depending on the speed of onset, differentials for the pruritus include ectoparasites, pseudorabies, and photosensitization.

Prevention and Control If diagnosed in a flock, quarantine and slaughter, followed by strict sanitation are required. The USDA is currently leading a National Scrapie Eradication Program. Scrapie-positive animals are identified, reported, and culled. Genetic selection for shipping, breeding and purchasing is then used to eradicate the disease. Scrapie-free flocks are given identification tags and sheep purchases should be done after confirming the status of a flock (USDA/APHIS, 2012).

Treatment No vaccine or treatment is available.

Research Complications As noted, this is a reportable disease. Stringent regulations exist in the United States regarding importation of small ruminants from scrapie-infected countries.

xxi. VESICULAR STOMATITIS VIRUS

Etiology Vesicular stomatitis (VS) is caused by the vesicular stomatitis virus (VSV), a member of the family Rhabdoviridae. It is a reportable disease in the United States and is zoonotic. The New Jersey and Indiana strains cause sporadic disease in cattle in the United States.

Clinical Signs and Diagnosis Adult cattle are most likely to develop VS. Fever and development of vesicles on the oral mucous membranes are the initial clinical signs. Lesions on the teats and interdigital spaces also develop. The vesicles progress quickly to ulcers and erosions. The animal's tongue may be severely involved. Anorexia and salivation are common. Weight loss and decreased milk production are noticeable. Morbidity will be high in an outbreak but mortality will be low to nonexistent.

Due to its similarity to FMDV, regulatory agencies should be involved in diagnostic work-up. Diagnosis is based on analysis of fluid, serum, or membranes associated with the vesicles. Virus isolation, ELISA, CELISA, CF, serum neutralization, and RT-PCR are used for diagnosis.

Epizootiology and Transmission This disease occurs in several other mammalian species, including swine, horses, and wild ruminants. VSV survives well in different environmental conditions, including in soil, extremes of pH, and low temperatures. Equipment, such as milking machines or human hands can serve as mechanical vectors. Transmission may also be from contaminated water, feed, and insects. Incubation period is 2–8 days. It is believed that carrier animals do not occur in this disease.

Necropsy It is rare for animals to be necropsied as the result of this disease.

Differential Diagnoses VSV lesions are identical to FMDV lesions. Other differentials in cattle include bovine viral diarrhea, malignant catarrhal fever, contagious ecthyma, photosensitization, trauma, and caustic agents.

Prevention and Control Quarantine and restrictions on shipping infected animals or animals from the premises housing affected animals are required in an outbreak. Vaccines are available for use in outbreaks. Phenolics, quaternaries, and halogens are effective for inactivating and disinfecting equipment and facilities.

Treatment Affected animals should be segregated from the rest of the herd, provided with separate water and softened feed. Topical or systemic antibiotics control secondary bacterial infections. Cases of mastitis secondary to teat lesions must be treated as necessary.

Research Complications Animals developing vesicular lesions must be reported promptly to eliminate the possibility of FMDV. VSV causes a flu-like illness in humans.

xxii. VIRAL DIARRHEA DISEASES

Rotavirus Rotavirus, a virus in the family *Reoviridae*, induces an acute, transient diarrhea in calves and lambs within the first few weeks of life. The disease is characterized by yellow, semifluid to watery malabsorptive diarrhea occurring 1–4 days after infection. The disease can progress to dehydration, anorexia and weight loss, acidosis, depression, and occasionally death. Transmission is fecal–oral. Virus may remain in the environment for several months. The disease is diagnosed by virus isolation, electron microscopy of feces, fecal fluorescent antibody, fecal ELISA tests (marketed tests generally detect group A rotavirus), and by fecal latex agglutination tests. Rotavirus diarrhea is treated by supportive therapy, including maintaining hydration, electrolyte, and acid–base balance. A rotavirus vaccine is available for cattle; because of cross-species immunity, oral administration of high-quality bovine colostrum from vaccinated cows to lambs at risk may be helpful (Youngquist and Threlfall, 2007).

Coronavirus Bovine coronavirus, of the family *Coronaviridae*, produces a more severe, long-lasting disease compared to rotavirus. Clinical signs in lambs and calves are similar to above, although the incubation period tends to be shorter (20–36h). In addition, mild respiratory disease may be noted (Janke, 1989). Coronavirus infections may be complicated by parasite infestation (e.g., *Cryptosporidia*, *Eimeria*) or bacterial infections (e.g., *E. coli*, *Salmonella*). Treatment is aimed at correcting dehydration, electrolyte imbalances, and acidosis. Strict hygiene and effective passive transfer by developing good colostrum-management protocols are critical. Bovine vaccines are available both for delivery to pre-partum dams and for the neonate.

Rotaviruses, coronavirus, and adenoviruses affect neonatal goats; however, little has been documented on the pathology and significance of these agents in this age group. Unlike calves, it appears that bacteria play a more important role in neonatal kid diarrheal diseases than in neonatal calf diarrheas. Parvovirus and BVDV also may cause diarrhea in neonatal calves.

Winter Dysentery Winter dysentery is an acute epizootic diarrheal disease of housed adult cattle in winter months although it has been reported in 4-month-old calves. The etiology has not yet been defined but coronavirus-like viral particles have been isolated from cattle feces, either the same as or similar to the coronavirus of calf diarrhea. Outbreaks typically last a few weeks, and first lactation or younger cattle are affected first with waves of illness moving through a herd. Individual cows are ill for only a few days. The incubation period is estimated at 2–8 days. Clinical signs include explosive diarrhea, anorexia, depression, and a profound decrease in production. The diarrhea has a distinctive musty, sweet odor, and is light brown and bubbly, but some blood streaks or clots may be mixed in with the feces. Animals will become dehydrated quickly but are thirsty. Respiratory signs such as nasolacrimal discharges and coughing may develop. Recovery is generally spontaneous within a few days. Mortalities are rare. Diagnosis is based on characteristic patterns of clinical signs, and elimination of diarrheas caused by parasites such as coccidia, bacterial organisms such as *Salmonella* or *Mycobacterium paratuberculosis*, and viruses such as BVDV. Pathology is present in the colonic mucosa and necrosis is present in the crypts.

b. Chlamydophilal Diseases

i. ENZOOTIC ABORTION OF EWES (EAE), CHLAMYDOPHILAL ABORTION
Etiology The etiologic agent of Enzootic Abortion of Ewes is now known as *Chlamydophila abortus* (*Chlamydophila psittaci serotype 1*), a nonmotile, obligate intracytoplasmic, gram-negative bacterium.

Clinical Signs Enzootic abortion in sheep and goats is a contagious disease characterized by hyperthermia and late abortion, or birth of stillborn or weak lambs or kids (Rodolakis *et al.*, 1998). The only presenting clinical sign may be serosanguineous vulvar discharges. Other animals may present with arthritis or pneumonia. Infection of animals prior to 120 days of gestation results in abortion, stillbirths, or birth of weak lambs. Infection after 120 days results in potentially normal births, but the dams or offspring may remain latently infected. Ewes or does generally abort only once. Recovered animals will be immune to future infections.

Epizootiology and Transmission The disease is transmitted by direct contact with infectious secretions such as placental, fetal, and uterine fluids; or by indirect contact with contaminated feed and water.

Necropsy Placental lesions include intercotyledonary plaques and necrosis and cotyledonary hemorrhages. Histopathological evidence of leukocytic infiltration, edema, and necrosis is found throughout the placentome. Fetal lesions include giant cell accumulation in mesenteric lymph nodes and lymphohistiocytic proliferations around the blood vessels within the liver.

Diagnosis Diagnosis is based on clinical signs and immunofluorescence, ELISA, cell culture isolation, and RT-PCR methods (Stuen and Longbottom, 2011) Impression smears in placental tissues stained with Giemsa, Gimenez, or modified Ziehl–Neelsen can provide preliminary indications of the causative agent.

Differential Diagnoses Q fever will be the major differential for late-term abortion and necrotizing placentitis. *Campylobacter* and *Toxoplasma* should also be considered for late-term abortion.

Treatment Animals may respond to treatment with oxytetracycline. Vaccination will prevent abortions but not eliminate infections. The vaccine should be administered before breeding and annually to at least the young females entering the breeding herd or flock.

Research Complications In addition to losses or compromise of research animals, pregnant women should not handle aborted tissues.

ii. CHLAMYDOPHILAL POLYARTHRITIS OF SHEEP
Etiology *Chlamydophila pecorum* is a nonmotile, obligate intracellular, gram-negative bacterium causing acute polyarthritis and conjunctivitis in growing and nursing lambs.

Clinical Signs Clinically, animals will appear lame on one or all legs and in major joints including the scapulohumeral, humeroradioulnar, coxofemoral, femorotibial, and tibiotarsal joints. Lambs may be anorexic and febrile. Animals frequently also exhibit concurrent conjunctivitis. The disease usually resolves in approximately four weeks. Joint inflammation usually resolves without chronic articular changes.

Epizootiology and Transmission The disease is transmitted to susceptible animals by direct contact as well as by contaminated feed and water. The organism penetrates the gastrointestinal tract and migrates to joints and synovial membranes as well as the conjunctiva.

Necropsy Findings Lesions are found in joints, tendon sheaths, conjunctiva, and lungs. Pathological sites will be edematous and hyperemic with fibrinous exudates, but without articular changes. Lesions will be infiltrated with mononuclear cells. Lung lesions include atelectasis and alveolar inspissation.

Diagnosis Diagnosis is based on clinical signs. Synovial taps and subsequent smears may allow the identification of chlamydophilal inclusion bodies.

Treatment Animals respond to treatment with parenteral oxytetracycline.

iii. CHLAMYDOPHILAL CONJUNCTIVITIS (INFECTIOUS KERATOCONJUNCTIVITIS; 'PINKEYE')

Etiology *Chlamydophila psittaci* and *Chlamydophila pecorum* are the most common causes of infectious keratoconjunctivitis in sheep. *Chlamydophila* and *Mycoplasma* are considered to be the most common causes of this disease in goats.

Clinical Signs Infectious keratoconjunctivitis is an acute, contagious disease characterized in earlier stages by photophobia, conjunctival hyperemia, epiphora, and edema, and in later stages by ulceration and opacity. Perforation may result from the ulceration. In less severe cases, corneal healing associated with fibrosis and neovascularization occurs in 3–4 days. Lymphoid tissues associated with the conjunctiva and nictitans membrane may enlarge and prolapse the eyelids. Morbidity may reach 80–90%. Bilateral and symmetrical infections characterize most outbreaks. Relapses may occur. Other concurrent systemic infections may be seen such as polyarthritis or abortion in sheep, and polyarthritis, mastitis, and uterine infections in goats.

Epizootiology and Transmission Direct contact as well as mechanical vectors such as flies easily spread the organism.

Necropsy This disease does not usually result in mortality.

Differential Diagnoses Nonchlamydophilal keratoconjunctivitis also occurs in sheep and goats. The primary agents involved include *Mycoplasma conjunctiva*, *Mycoplasma agalactiae* in goats, *Moraxella* (*Branhamella, Neisseria*) *ovis*, and *Colesiota conjunctivae* (a rickettsia-like organism). Other differentials include eyeworms,

trauma, and foreign bodies such as windblown materials (pollen, dust) and poor-quality hay.

Prevention and Control Source of mechanical irritation should be minimized and shade provided. Quarantine of new animals and treatment before introduction into the flock or herd are important measures.

Treatment Infections are self-limiting in 2–3 weeks without treatment. Treatment consists of topical application of tetracycline ophthalmic ointments. Systemic or oral oxytetracycline treatments have been used with the topical treatment. Atropine may be added to the treatment regimen when uveitis is present.

3. Parasitic

a. Protozoan

i. ANAPLASMA

Etiology Anaplasmosis is a transmissible hemolytic disease of cattle caused by the protozoan *Anaplasma marginale*. In sheep and goats, the disease is caused by *A. ovis* and is a relatively rare cause of hemolytic disease. This summary addresses the disease in cattle with limited reference to *A. ovis* infections, but there are many similarities to the disease in cattle.

Clinical Signs and Diagnosis Acute anemia is the predominant sign in anaplasmosis, and fever coincides with parasitemia. Weakness, pallor, lethargy, dehydration, and anorexia are the result of the anemia. The incubation stage may be long, 3–8 weeks, and is characterized by a rise in body temperature as the infection moves to the next stage. Most clinical signs occur during the 4- to 9-day developmental stage, with hemolytic anemia being common. Death is most likely to occur at this stage or at the beginning of the convalescent stage. Death may also occur from anoxia due to the animal's inability to handle any exertion or stress, especially if treatment is initiated when severe anemia exists. Reticulocytosis characterizes the convalescent stage which may continue for many weeks. Morbidity is high and mortality low. The carrier stage is defined as the time in the convalescent stage when the animal host becomes a reservoir of the disease and parasitemia is not discernible.

Diagnosis is made by clinical and necropsy findings. Common serologic tests include the complement fixation and rapid card tests. These become positive after the incubation phase. Staining of thin blood smears with Wright's or Giemsa stains allows detection of basophilic, spherical *A. marginale* bodies near the red blood cell (RBC) peripheries. A negative finding should not eliminate the pathogen from consideration.

Epizootiology and Transmission The disease is common in cattle in the southern and western United States and other tropical and subtropical regions. *Anaplasma* organisms are spread biologically or mechanically. Mechanical transmission occurs when infected

RBC are passed from one host to another on the mouth parts of seasonal biting flies, mosquitos, or instruments such as dehorners or hypodermic needles. Biological transmission occurs when the organism is passed by carrier *Dermacentor andersoni* and *D. occidentalis* ticks. Recovered animals serve as disease reservoirs.

Necropsy Pale tissues and watery, thin blood are typical findings. Splenomegaly, hepatomegaly, and gall bladder distension are common findings.

Pathogenesis The parasites infect the host's RBCs, and acute hemolysis occurs during the parasites' developmental stage.

Differential Diagnosis The clinical disease closely resembles the protozoal disease babesiosis.

Prevention and Control Offspring of immune carriers resist infection up to 6 months of age due to passive immunity. Vector control and attention to hygiene are essential, such as between-animal disinfection of equipment such as dehorners. Vaccination (killed whole organism) is not entirely effective as vaccinated animals can still become infected and become carriers. Vaccine should not be administered to pregnant cows due to the potential for neonatal isoerythrolysis. There is no *A. ovis* vaccine. Identifying carriers serologically and treating with tetracycline during and/or after vector seasons may be an option. Interstate movement of infected animals is regulated.

Treatment A single dose of long-acting tetracycline reduces the severity of the infection during the developmental stage. Other tetracycline treatment programs have been described to help control carriers.

ii. BABESIOSIS (RED WATER, TEXAS CATTLE FEVER, CATTLE TICK FEVER)

Etiology *Babesia bovis* and *Babesia bigeminia* are intraerythrocytic protozoans that cause subclinical infections or disease in cattle. Babesiosis is one of the most important arthropod-borne diseases of cattle and is very prevalent in tropical and subtropical areas worldwide. This disease is not seen in the smaller ruminants in the United States. See Center for Food Security and Public Health (2008) for more information on Babesiosis.

Clinical Signs and Diagnosis The more common presentation is liver and kidney failure due to hemolysis with icterus, hemoglobinuria, and fever. Acute encephalitis is a less common presentation and begins acutely with fever, ataxia, depression, deficits in conscious proprioception, mania and convulsions, and coma. The encephalitic form generally also has a poor prognosis. Sudden death may also occur.

Diagnosis Thin blood smears stained with Giemsa will show *Babesia* trophozoites at some stages of the disease. Complement fixation, immunofluorescent antibody and ELISA are the most favored of the available serologic tests.

Epizootiology and Transmission The primary vectors for Babesia are ticks of the *Boophilus* genus. In addition to domestic cattle, some wild ruminants such as white-tailed deer and American buffalo are also susceptible. *Bos indicus* breeds have resistance to the disease and the tick vectors. Stress can cause disease development.

Necropsy Findings Signs of acute hemolytic crisis are the most common findings and include hepatomegaly, splenomegaly, dark and distended gallbladder, pale tissues, thin blood, scattered hemorrhages, and petechiation. Animals dying after longer course of disease will be emaciated and icteric with thin blood, pale kidneys, and enlarged liver.

Differential Diagnoses In addition to anaplasmosis, leptospirosis, copper toxicity and bacillary hemoglobinuria are differentials for the hemolytic form of the disease. Several differentials in the United States for the encephalitic presentation include rabies, nervous system coccidiosis, polioencephalomalacia, lead poisoning, IBR, and salt poisoning.

Prevention and Control Control or eradication of ticks and cleaning of equipment to prevent mechanical transmission are important preventative measures. Vaccination approaches have been effective in South American and Australia but a commercial product is not available in the United States.

Treatment Supportive care is indicated including blood transfusions, fluids, and antibiotics. Medications such as diminazene diaceturate, diisethionate, and imidocarb dipropionte are most commonly used.

Research Complications Babesiosis is a reportable disease in the Unites States.

iii. COCCIDIOSIS

Etiology Coccidia are protozoal organisms of the phylum Apicomplexa, members of which are obligatory intracellular parasites. Coccidia spp. have a complex lifecycle in which sexual and asexual reproduction occurs in gastrointestinal enterocytes. Sheep, goats, and cattle are all affected by multiple species of the genus *Eimeria*, however, the species of parasite are host-specific as well as host-cell specific.

Clinical Signs and Diagnosis Coccidiosis is an important protozoal disease of young ruminants characterized primarily by hemorrhagic diarrhea. Diarrhea develops 10 days to 3 weeks after infection. Fecal staining of the tail and perineum will be present. Animals will frequently display tenesmus and rectal prolapses may develop. Anorexia, weight loss, dehydration, anemia, fever (infrequently), depression, and weakness may also be seen in all ruminants. The diarrhea is watery and malodorous and will contain variable amounts of blood and fibrinous, necrotic tissues. The intestinal hemorrhage may subsequently lead to anemia and hypoproteinemia.

Concurrent disease with other enteropathogens may also be part of the clinical picture.

The disease is usually diagnosed by history and clinical signs. Numerous oocysts will be observed in fresh fecal flotation (salt or sugar solution) samples as the diarrhea begins. The pre-patent period for *Eimeria* is from 2 to 3 weeks and usually coincides with the development of clinical signs.

Epizootiology and Transmission Subclinically infected adults are the reservoir for the parasites. The disease is transmitted to young animals via ingestion of sporulated oocysts; severity of the disease is correlated primarily with the number of ingested oocysts. Coccidial oocysts remain viable for long periods of time when in moist, shady conditions. Isolated outbreaks in adults may occur after stressful conditions such as transportation or diet changes.

Necropsy Necropsies provide information on specific locations and severity of lesions that correlate with the species involved. Ileitis, typhlitis, and colitis with associated necrosis and hemorrhage will be observed. Mucosal scrapings will frequently yield oocysts.

Differential Diagnoses These include the many enteropathogens associated with acute diarrhea in young ruminants: cryptosporidiosis, colibacillosis, salmonellosis, enterotoxemia, viral diarrheas, and other intestinal parasites such as helminths.

Prevention and Control Proper sanitation of maternity pens and young stock housing and minimizing overcrowding are essential. Coccidiostats added to the feed, water, or milk replacer are helpful in preventing the disease in areas of high exposure.

Treatment Affected animals should be isolated. Treatment should include provision of a dry, warm environment, fluids, electrolytes (orally or intravenously), antibiotics (to prevent bacterial invasion and septicemia), and administration of coccidiostats. Coccidiostats are preferred to coccidiocidals because the former allow immunity to develop. Sulfonamides and amprolium may be used to aid in the treatment of disease, as well as decoquinate, lasalocid and monensin. Labels should be checked for specific approval in a species or indications. Penmates of affected animals should be considered exposed and treated to control early stages of infection.

iv. CRYPTOSPORIDIOSIS

Etiology *Cryptosporidium* organisms are a very common cause of diarrhea in young ruminants. There are at least 16 species and more than 40 genotypes of species, some of which affect multiple host species. Cryptosporidiosis is a zoonotic disease.

Clinical Signs and Diagnosis Cryptosporidiosis is characterized by protracted, malabsorptive diarrhea and debilitation. The diarrhea may last only 6–10 days, or may be persistent and fatal. Infected animals will display tenesmus, anorexia and weight loss, dehydration, and depression. In relapsing cases, animals become cachectic. Overall, morbidity will be high, and mortality variable.

Mucosal scrapings or fixed stained tissue sections may be useful in diagnosis. The disease is also diagnosed by detecting the oocysts on fecal flotation, in iodine-stained feces, or periodic acid Schiff (PAS) or methenamine silver-stained tissues. *Cryptosporidium* also stains red on acid-fast stains such as Kinyoun or Ziehl–Neelsen. Fecal IFA techniques have also been described.

Epizootiology and Transmission Younger ruminants are commonly affected including lambs, kids between the ages of 5–10 days of age, and calves less than 30 days old. *Cryptosporidium* is transmitted via the fecal–oral route. The oocysts are shed sporulated and are immediately infective. Within 2–7 days of exposure, diarrhea and oocyst shedding occurs. The oocysts are extremely resistant to desiccation in the environment and may survive in the soil and manure for many months. Autoinfection within the lumen of the intestines may also occur and result in persistent infections. Cattle are frequently subclinical or asymptomatic carriers. All cattle should be assumed to be *Cryptosporidium* positive and appropriate precautions to prevent zoonotic spread should be instituted.

Necropsy Findings Gross lesions caused by *Cryptosporidium* are nonspecific. Animals will be emaciated. Moderate enteritis, hyperplasia of the crypt epithelial cells with villous atrophy as well as villous fusion, primarily in the lower small intestines, will be present. Organisms are located at the apical margin of the enterocytes in a characteristic intracellular, extracytoplasmic parasitophorous vacuole. Identification of organisms in tissue section is diagnostic.

Differential Diagnoses Other causes of diarrhea in younger ruminants include rota- and coronavirus, other enteric viral infections, enterotoxigenic *E. coli*, *Clostridia*, and other coccidial pathogens. These other agents may be contributing to illness in the affected animals and may complicate the diagnosis and treatment picture.

Prevention and Control Affected animals must be removed and isolated as soon as possible. Animal housing areas should be disinfected with undiluted commercial bleach or 5% ammonia. After cleaning, areas should be allowed to dry thoroughly, and remain unpopulated for a period of time. Use of powerwashers is not recommended, as this will facilitate spread of oocysts. Management and husbandry should be examined. Clinical cryptosporidiosis is often associated with failure of passive immune transfer or inadequate nutrition, so these factors should be scrutinized.

Treatment Halofuginone lactate has been approved in Europe for treatment of cryptosporidiosis in cattle. Nitazoxanide and paromomycin has been approved for treatment of immunocompetent humans but are not approved for veterinary use. The disease is generally self-limiting so symptomatic, supportive therapy aimed at rehydrating, correcting electrolyte and acid–base balance, and providing energy is often effective.

Research Complications Cryptosporidiosis is a zoonotic disease. This disease is easily spread from calves to humans as the result of simply handling clothing soiled by calf diarrhea. The disease can be life threatening in immunocompromised individuals.

v. GIARDIASIS

Etiology Giardia lamblia (also called *G. intestinalis* and *G. duodenalis*) is a flagellate protozoa. Giardiasis is a worldwide diarrheal disease of mammals and some birds.

Clinical Signs and Diagnosis Diarrhea may be continuous or intermittent, is pasty to watery, yellow and may contain blood. Animals exhibit fever, dehydration, and depression. Chronic cases may result in a 'poor doer' syndrome with weight loss and unthriftiness.

Diagnosis is by identifying the motile trophozoites in fresh fecal mounts. Oval cysts can be floated with zinc sulfate solution (33%). Standard solutions tend to be too hyperosmotic and distort the cysts. Newer ELISA, and IFA tests are sensitive and specific.

Epizootiology and Transmission Giardia infection may occur at any age, but young animals are more susceptible. Giardia is quite prevalent in both beef and dairy calves in North America. Calves do not typically develop diarrhea due to giardiaisis until after 4 weeks of age. Chronic oocyst shedding is common. Transmission of the cyst stage is fecal–orally. Wild animals may serve as reservoirs.

Necropsy Findings This disease does not generally result in necropsy.

Prevention and Control Intensive housing and warm environments should be minimized. Cysts can survive in the environment for long periods of time but are susceptible to desiccation. Effective disinfectants include quaternary ammonium compounds, bleach (1:16 or 1:32), steam, or boiling water.

Treatment Giardia has been successfully treated with oral metronidazole. Benzimidazole anthelmintics are also effective but these are not approved for use in animals for this purpose.

Research Complications Giardia is zoonotic. Precautions should be taken when handling infected animals.

vi. NEOSPOROSIS

Etiology Neosporosis is a common, worldwide cause of bovine abortion caused by the protozoal species, *Neospora caninum*. Abortions have also been reported in sheep and goats. Neonatal disease is seen in lambs, kids, and calves.

Clinical Signs and Diagnosis Abortion is the only clinical sign seen in adult cattle, and occurs either sporadically, endemically, or as abortion storms. Bovine abortions occur between the 3rd and 7th month of gestation. Although infections in adults are asymptomatic, decreased milk production has been noted in congenitally infected cows in addition to abortion. *Neospora*-infected calves can be born asymptomatic. Weakness may be evident but this resolves. Rare clinical signs include exophthalmus or asymmetric eyes, weight loss, ataxia, hyperflexion or hyperextension of all limbs, decreased patellar reflexes, and loss of conscious proprioception, opisthotonus, and seizures.

Immunohistochemistry and histopathology of fetal tissue are the most efficient and reliable means of establishing a *post mortem* diagnosis. Serology (IFA and ELISA) is useful, including pre-colostral levels in weak neonates, but this indicates only exposure. Titers of dams will not be elevated at the time of abortion; fetal serology is influenced by the stage of gestation and course of infection. None of the currently available tests is predictive of disease.

Epizootiology and Transmission The parasite is now acknowledged to be widespread in dairy and beef cattle herds, and is considered a common cause of abortion in cattle. The life-cycle of *N. caninum* is complex and many aspects remain to be clarified. The definitive host is the dog (McAllister *et al.*, 1998); infective oocysts are shed in canine feces. Placental or aborted tissues are the most likely sources of infection for the definitive host and may also play a minor role in transmission to the intermediate hosts. The many intermediate hosts include ruminants, deer, and horses. The transplacental route is the major mode of transmission in dairy cattle and is responsible for perpetuated infection; infection is latent and life-long. Seropositive immunity does not protect a cow from future abortions. Many seropositive cows and calves will never abort or show clinical signs, respectively.

Necropsy Findings Aborted fetuses will usually be autolyzed. In those from which tissue can be recovered, tissue cysts are most commonly found in the brain. Cysts and tachyzoites of *N. caninum* cannot reliably be distinguished from those of *Toxoplasma gondii* at the light-microscopic level, and require ultrastructure or molecular techniques (IHC, PCR, etc.) for differentiation.

Differential Diagnoses Even when there is a herd history of confirmed *Neospora* abortions, leptospirosis, BVDV, IBRV, salmonellosis, and campylobacteriosis should be considered. BVDV in particular should be considered for abortion storms. Differentials for weak calves are BVDV, perinatal hypoxia following dystocia, bluetongue virus, *Toxoplasma*, exposure to teratogens, or congenital defects.

Prevention and Control The primary preventative measure is eliminating contact with contaminated dog feces. Dog populations should be controlled, and dogs and other canids should not have access to placentas or aborted fetuses, or to feed bunks and other feed storage areas. Preventative culling is not economically practical for most producers. A vaccine recently became available, although its efficacy is not well-established.

Treatment There is no known treatment or immunoprophylaxis.

vii. SARCOCYSTOSIS

Etiology Sarcocystosis is the disease caused by the cyst-forming sporozoan, *Sarcocystis*. Separate species of *Sarcocystis* infect sheep, goats, and cattle. Definitive hosts are carnivores and all ruminant species are intermediate hosts.

Clinical Signs and Diagnosis Clinical signs of sarcocystosis infection are seen in cattle during the stage when the parasite encysts in soft tissues. Most infections are asymptomatic. Fever, ataxia, symmetric lameness, tremors, tail switch hair-loss ('rat-tail'), excessive salivation, diarrhea, and weight loss occur. Abortions in cattle occur during the second trimester; small ruminants abort approximately 28 days after ingestion of the sporulated oocysts. Sarcocystis in sheep has been known to cause encephalomyelitis. Some sheep may lose wool after recovery from acute infection.

Definitive diagnosis is based on finding merozoites and meronts in fetal neural tissue lesions.

Epizootiology and Transmission Infection rates among cattle in the United States are estimated to be very high (Barr *et al.*, 1998; Dubey, 2005). Transmission is by ingestion of feed and water contaminated by feces of the definitive hosts. Dogs are the definitive hosts for the species infecting the smaller ruminants. Cats, dogs, and primates (including humans when *S. hominis* is involved) are the definitive hosts for the species infecting cattle.

Necropsy Aborted fetuses may be autolyzed. Lesions in neural tissues, including meningoencephalomyelitis, focal malacia, perivascular cuffing, neuronal degeneration, and gliosis, are most marked in the cerebellum and midbrain. Grossly, sarcocysts encysted in skeletal or cardiac muscle may resemble grains of rice. The histologic appearance of the sarcocysts is characteristic.

Pathogenesis Ingestion of muscle flesh from an infected ruminant results in intestinal infection and sarcocystis shedding in feces as sporocysts by the definitive hosts. The sporocysts are eaten by the ruminant, and several stages of development occur in endothelial cell of arteries, culminating in merozoites which enter soft tissues and subsequently encyst.

Prevention and Control Feed supplies of ruminants must be protected from fecal contamination by domestic and wild carnivores. These animals should be controlled and must not have access to carcasses.

Treatment Monensin fed during incubation is prophylactic but the efficacy in clinically affected cattle is not known. Amprolium (100 mg/kg, SID for 30 days) fed prophylactically in cattle and sheep has been shown to reduce illness and even protect experimentally infected animals (Merck Veterinary Manual Online, 2011).

viii. TOXOPLASMOSIS

Etiology Toxoplasmosis is caused by the obligate intracellular protozoan, *Toxoplasma gondii*, a coccidian parasite. Cats are the only definitive hosts and several warm-blooded animals, including ruminants, have been shown to be intermediate hosts. It is a major cause of abortion in sheep and goats and less common in cattle.

Clinical Signs and Diagnosis Toxoplasmosis is typically associated with placentitis, abortion, stillbirths, or birth of weak young (Underwood and Rook, 1992). It has also been shown to cause pneumonia and non-suppurative encephalitis. Infection of the ewe during the first trimester usually leads to fetal resorption, during the second trimester leads to abortion, and during the third trimester leads to birth of weak or normal lambs with subsequent high perinatal mortality. Congenitally infected lambs may display encephalitic signs of circling, incoordination, muscular paresis, and prostration. Although infected adult sheep show no systemic illness, infected adult goats may die of toxoplasmosis.

Diagnosis may be difficult, but biological, serological, and histological diagnostic methods are helpful. Serological tests are the most readily available. Fetal thoracic fluid is especially useful in demonstrating serological evidence of exposure. *In vivo* tests for Toxoplasmosis include IHA, IFA, latex agglutination, or ELISA. Characteristic crescentic tachyzoites in impression smears of tissue can be utilized for diagnosis *post mortem*.

Epizootiology and Transmission This protozoan is considered ubiquitous. Fifty percent of adult western sheep and 20% of feedlot lambs have positive hemagglutination titers of 1:64 or higher (Kimberling, 1988). Transmission among the definitive host is by ingestion of tissue cysts. Transmission to ruminants is through ingestion of cat feces.

Necropsy Findings At necropsy, placental cotyledons contain multiple small white areas that are sites of necrosis, edema and calcification. Fetal brains may show non-specific lesions such as coagulative necrosis, non-suppurative encephalomyelitis, pneumonia, myocarditis, and hepatitis. Giemsa-stained impression smears of retina, myocardium, liver, kidney, or brain provide a rapid means of diagnosis. Identification of the organism in tissue sections (especially the heart and the brain) also confirms the findings.

Pathogenesis The definitive hosts, felids, become infected by ingesting cyst stages in mammalian tissues, by ingesting oocysts in feces, and by transplacental transfer. Infected cats shed millions of oocysts in the feces but only for a few weeks in its life. Ruminants become infected by ingesting sporulated oocyst-contaminated water or feed. The ingested sporozoite invades invades the bloodstream and migrates to tissues such as the brain, liver, muscles, and placenta. Placental infection develops about 14 days after ingestion of the oocysts.

Differential Diagnoses Differentials for abortion include *Neospora caninum*, *Campylobacter*, *Chlamydophila*, and Query Fever.

Prevention and Control Feline populations on source farms must be controlled. Eliminating contamination of feed and water with cat feces is the best preventative measure. Sporulated oocysts can survive in soil and other places for long periods of time and are resistant to desiccation and freezing. Vaccines for abortion prevention in sheep are available in New Zealand and Europe.

Treatment Toxoplasmosis treatment is ineffective, although feeding monensin during pregnancy may be helpful (Underwood and Rook, 1992). However, monensin is not approved for this use in the United States.

Research Complications Because toxoplasmosis is zoonotic, precautions must be taken when handling tissues from any abortions or neurological cases. Infections in immunocompromised humans have been fatal.

ix. TRICHOMONIASIS

Etiology Trichomoniasis is a venereal disease of cattle caused by *Tritrichomonas* (also referred to as *Trichomonas*) *fetus*, a large, pear-shaped, flagellated protozoan which is an obligate parasite of the bovine reproductive tract. In the United States, trichomoniasis is a disease seen primarily in western beef herds.

Clinical Signs and Diagnosis Clinical signs include infertility manifested by low pregnancy rates as well as periodic pyometras and abortions during the first half of gestation. The abortion rate varies from 5% to 30%, and placentas will be expelled or retained. Infection with *T. fetus* causes no systemic signs. Affected cows will clear the infection over a span of months and maintain immunity for about 6 months but bulls may become chronic carriers.

Diagnosis is based on patterns of infertility and pyometras. Trichomonads may be identified or cultured from preputial smegma, cervicovaginal mucus, uterine exudates, placental fluids, or abomasal contents of aborted fetuses. Culturing must be done on specific media, such as Diamond's or modified Pastridge.

Epizootiology and Transmission All transmission is by venereal exposure from either breeding bulls or cows, or in some cases, contaminated breeding equipment.

Necropsy Findings Nonspecific lesions, such as pyogranulomatous bronchopneumonia of fetuses and placentitis, may be seen in aborted material; fetal lung and placenta are the most useful for culturing.

Differential Diagnosis Campylobacteriosis is the other primary differential for reduced reproductive efficiency of a herd.

Prevention and Control A bacterin vaccine is available. AI reduces but does not eliminate the disease. The use of younger vaccinated bulls is recommended in all circumstances. Culling chronically infected bulls is strongly recommended.

Treatment Imidazole compounds have been effective, but the use of these substances is not permitted in food animals in the United States. Therapeutic immunizations are worthwhile when a positive diagnosis has been made.

Research Complications Trichomonas should be considered whenever natural service is used and fertility problems are encountered.

b. Gastrointestinal Nematodiasis

Nematodes are important ruminant pathogens and result in acute, chronic, subclinical, and clinical disease in adults and adolescents. The major helminths may result in gastroenteritis associated with intestinal hemorrhage and malnutrition. The disease is associated with grazing exposure to infective larvae. Animals procured for research may have had exposure to these helminths. Mixed infections of these parasites are common. Generally, older animals develop resistance to some of the species; thus, animals between about 2 months and 2 years of age are most susceptible to infection. Because of the parasites' effects on the animals' physiology, infection in these younger animals is a major contributor to a cycle of poor nutrition and digestion, compromised immune responses, and impaired growth and development. Diagnosis is primarily based on fecal flotation techniques; however, because many of these nematodes have similarly appearing ova, hatching the ova and identifying the larvae is often required (Baermann technique). The pre-patent period for most nematode parasites is 2–3 weeks. A number of anthelmintics can be used to interrupt nematode life-cycles. (See McKellar and Jackson, 2004, and/or Sargison, 2012; Quinton *et al.*, 2004, for comprehensive reviews of treatment and control of nematodiasis.) Those nematodes with the highest potential for pathogenicity in sheep and goats include *Haemonchus contortus* (Barber-pole worm), *Teladorsagia* (formerly *Ostertagia*) *circumcincta* (Medium stomach worm), *Cooperia* (Small intestinal worms), *Trichostrongylus* spp. (Hair worms), *Oesophagostomum columbianum* (Nodule worm disease, pimply gut), *Cooperia curticei*, and *Strongyloides pappilosus*. In cattle, clinical parasitism is often associated with *Haemonchus placei*, *Ostertagia ostertagi*, *Trichostrongylus axei*, *Cooperia* spp., *Strongyloides* spp., and *Oesophagostomum* spp. Trichostrongyles such as *Ostertagia*, *Haemonchus*, *Trichostrongylus*, *Cooperia*, *Dictyocaulus*, and *Oesophagostomum* may undergo seasonal hypobiosis or arrested development of the lifecycle. In the northern hemisphere larvae arrest and accumulate inside grazing animals in the fall, allowing the parasite to overwinter in the animal protected from winter pasture conditions.

Rotation of anthelmintics due to inherent resistance development and appropriate pasture management are key principles in parasite control.

i. DICTYOCAULOSIS (LUNGWORMS) Dictyocaulosis, or lungworm infestation, causes clinical respiratory signs in ruminants. In sheep, *Dictyocaulus filaria*, *Protostrongylus rufescens*, and *Muellerius capillaris* cause disease; *Dictyocaulus* is the most pathogenic. Infections in goats are uncommon. *Dictyocaulus viviparus* is the only lungworm found in cattle. Infections with these parasites in the United States tend to be associated with cool, moist climates. Lungworms induce a severe parasitic bronchitis (known as 'husk,' or verminous pneumonia) in sheep between approximately 2 months and 18 months of age. Sheep and cattle infected with any of the species of lungworms may display coughing, dyspnea, nasal discharge, weight loss, unthriftiness, and occasionally fever. Diagnosis is suggested by clinical signs and is confirmed by identifying larvae in the feces using the Baermann technique or adults in lung tissue samples.

Dictyocaulus has a direct life-cycle. The adult worms reside in the large bronchi, produce embryonated eggs that are coughed up and swallowed; the eggs then hatch in the intestines and larvae are expelled in the feces. The expelled larvae are infectious in about 7–10 days, and after ingestion, penetrate the intestinal mucosa and move through the lymphatics and blood into the lungs where they develop into adults in about 5 weeks. *Protostrongylus* and *Muellerius* require a snail or slug as an intermediate host.

Necropsy lesions include bronchiolitis and bronchitis, atelectasis, and hyperplasia of peribronchiolar lymphoid tissue.

Prevention and control of the disease involves appropriate pasture management to minimize exposure of young, susceptible animals. Elimination of intermediate hosts is important in sheep and goat pastures. Infected animals can be treated with anthelmintics such as ivermectins, milbemycins, or levamisole. An effective irradiated larval vaccine is marketed in the United Kingdom and Western Europe.

ii. PARELAPHOSTRONGYLUS TENUIS (MENINGEAL WORM, BRAIN WORM) *Parelaphostrongylus tenuis* is a nematode parasite common to white tail deer. Sheep and goats, camelids, elk, caribou, and moose may be aberrant hosts. Adult worms in meningeal tissue lay eggs that develop into first stage larvae that migrate through the bloodstream to the lungs. Larvae are coughed up, swallowed, and are expelled in the feces where they are ingested by snails and slugs and develop into second- and third-stage larva. Following accidental ingestion of the gastropods, the larvae migrate to the brain. Neurological and behavioral signs are rare and relatively mild in white tail deer but can be severe in aberrant hosts, sometimes resulting in paraplegia. Goats have been reported to develop vertically oriented pruritic skin lesions on the neck, shoulders, and back (Smith and Sherman, 2009).

c. Cestodiasis (Tapeworms)

i. MONIEZIA EXPANSA, THYSANOSOMA ACTINOIDES Tapeworms are rarely of clinical or economic importance. In younger animals, heavy infections result in pot bellies, constipation or mild diarrhea, poor growth, rough coat, and anemia. *Moniezia expansa*, and less commonly *Moniezia benedini*, inhabit the small intestines of grazing ruminants. *Thysanosoma actinoides* or the fringed tapeworm resides in the duodenum, bile duct, and pancreatic duct of sheep and cattle raised primarily west of the Mississippi River. All have indirect life-cycles. No clinical or pathological sign is usually observed with tapeworm infection, however, *Thysanosoma* infections may result in liver condemnation at slaughter. Diagnosis is made by observing segments in manure or the characteristic triangular-shaped eggs in fecal flotation examinations. Albendazole is an effective cestocide.

ii. ABDOMINAL OR VISCERAL CYSTICERCOSIS AND ECHINOCOCCOSIS (HYDATID CYST DISEASE) Tapeworm eggs from the primary host contain an oncosphere, which hatches and penetrates the intestinal wall when ingested by the intermediate host. The second-stage larva develops in the intermediate host and is called a metacestode which is a space occupying cystic structure. Metacestode forms are tapeworm specific and include the cysticercoid (microscopic and in small intermediate hosts such as insects of mites); cysticercus (small blister to ping-pong ball sized structures); coenurus (usually intracranial in the host) and hydatid cysts (usually intraabdominal in the host). The coenurus and hydatid cysts can become quite large, contain multiple larvae, and can locally bud and spread. When the metacestode form is ingested by the primary host, the larval brood capsules containing protoscolices evaginate to form the tapeworm head called the scolex.

Abdominal or visceral cysticercosis is an occasional finding in ruminants at slaughter. The 'bladder worms' typically affect the liver or peritoneal cavity and are caused by the larval form (metacestode) of *Taenia hydatigena*, the common tapeworm of the dog family. The larval intermediate of another tapeworm of canids, *Echinococcus granulosus*, also may form hydatid cysts, particularly in liver and lungs. Ruminants are intermediate hosts of both parasites, and are infected by feed or water contaminated with gravid segments or ova. Although larval migration may cause nonspecific signs such as anorexia, hyperthermia, and weight loss, affected animals are usually asymptomatic. Infestation is usually diagnosed at necropsy or slaughter, and may result in condemnation of carcasses. Minimizing exposure to canine feces-contaminated feeds and water effectively interrupts the life-cycle. Research animals may have been exposed prior to purchase.

iii. COENUROSIS (GID) *Coenurus cerebralis*, the larval form of the tapeworm of domestic dogs, humans, and some wild carnivores, *Taenia (Multiceps) multiceps* is the causative agent of the rare condition called Gid. The disease occurs in ruminants as well as many other mammalian species. The larval parasite, ingested from fecal-contaminated food and water, invades the brain and spinal cord and develops as a bladderworm that causes pressure necrosis of the nervous tissues. The resultant signs of hyperesthesia, meningitis, paresis, paralysis, ataxia, and convulsions are observed. Diagnosis is usually made at necropsy. Eliminating transfer from the canid hosts prevents the disease.

d. Trematodes

i. FASCIOLIASIS (LIVER FLUKE DISEASE)

Etiology   Liver flukes are an important cause of acute and chronic disease in grazing sheep and cattle. In the continental U.S., *Fasciola hepatica* infections are primarily seen in southeastern and western states. *Fascioloides magna* infections are typically seen in the Texas; Gulf coast; Great Lakes; and northwestern states where ruminants share pasture with deer, elk, and moose. *Dicrocoelium dendriticum* infections occur primarily in the eastern U.S. and Atlantic provinces of Canada, however *Dicrocelium* also occurs in areas of Europe and Asia. Liver fluke eggs are passed in the bile and feces and hatch in 2–3 weeks to form the free-swimming miracidia. It is important to note that each fluke egg represents the source of eventually thousands of cercariae or metacercariae. The miracidia penetrate the body of an intermediate host (usually freshwater snails) and develop through sporocysts and rediae stages, finally forming cercariae. The cercariae leave the intermediate host, swim to grassy vegetation, and become cyst-like metacercariae, which may remain in a dormant stage on the grass for 6 months or longer until ingested by a ruminant. The ingested metacercariae penetrate the small-intestinal wall, migrate through the abdominal cavity to the liver where they locate in a bile duct, mature and remain for up to 4 years.

Clinical Signs   Acute liver fluke disease is related to the damage caused by the migration of immature flukes which leads to liver inflammation, hemorrhage, necrosis, and fibrosis. *F. magna* infections in sheep and goats can be fatal as the result of just one fluke tunneling through hepatic tissue. In cattle, infections are often asymptomatic due to the host's encapsulation of the parasite. Liver fluke damage may predispose to invasion by anaerobic *Clostridium* species such as *C. novyi* that could lead to fatal Black Disease or bacillary hemoglobinuria. Chronic disease may result from fluke-induced physical damage to the bile ducts and cholangiohepatitis. Blood loss into the bile may lead to anemia and hypoproteinemia. Liver damage also is evidenced by increases in liver enzymes such as gamma glutamyl transferase (GGT). Persistent eosinophilia is also seen with liver fluke disease. Other clinical signs of liver fluke disease include anorexia, weight loss, unthriftiness, edema, and ascites. At necropsy, livers will be pale, friable and may have distinct migration tunnels along the serosal surfaces. Bile ducts will be enlarged and areas of fibrosis will be evident.

Diagnosis can be made from clinical signs and *post mortem* analyses. Blood chemistries suggestive of liver disease and eosinophilia support the diagnosis. Liver fluke control involves treatment of infected animals, reduction of the intermediate host population and/or restriction of animal access to snail-infested pastures. In a laboratory setting, liver fluke infection is unlikely. Nonetheless, incoming animals from pasture environments may be infected. Liver flukes can be treated with the anthelmintic clorsulon or albendazole.

e. Mites

i. MANGE   Mites infesting ruminants include those of the genera *Sarcoptes*, *Psoroptes*, *Chorioptes*, and *Demodex*. Depending on the species of mite, signs range from relatively mild flaking and itching to intense pruritus, extensive skin damage, and self-mutilation. Papules, crusts, alopecia, and secondary dermatitis are seen. In more severe cases, anemia, disruption of reproductive cycles, and increased susceptibility to other diseases may also develop.

In the United States, infections of *Sarcoptes* and *Psorergates* must be reported to animal health officials. These mites cause severe signs in cattle, sheep, and goats, but fortunately are rare in North America. Diagnosis is based on clinical signs, examination of skin scrapings, and response to therapy.

Chorioptic mange ('barn itch' or 'leg mange') is common in ruminants, particularly in winter months when animals are housed. Chorioptes species (*C. bovis*, *C. ovis*, *C. caprae*) are relatively specific to their hosts and do not invade the epidermal tissue but rather feed off dead skin. The lower limbs, tail, perineum, and scrotum are most often affected. Pruritis is variable and may be accompanied by papules, crustiness, and alopecia.

Historically, insecticides such as coumaphos, diazinon, and lime sulfur have been used to treat mange in ruminants. These treatments have been largely replaced by the use of macrocyclic lactone anthelmintics (ivermectin), either by injection or topically.

Although relatively uncommon, demodectic mange occurs in cattle, sheep, and goats. Animals develop nodular lesions, typically around the face, head, and shoulders. No effective treatment for demodectic mange in large animals has been found. The differential for mite infestations is pediculosis. In goats, the psoroptic mite, *Psoroptes cuniculi*, commonly occurs in the ear canal and causes head shaking and scratching.

f. Lice/Ticks

i. PEDICULOSIS (LICE) Lice infecting ruminants are of the order *Mallophaga*, the biting or chewing lice (genus *Damalina*), and *Anoplura*, the sucking lice (genus *Linognathus*). These are wingless insects. Lice produce a seasonal (winter to spring) chronic dermatitis.

Pruritus is the most common sign and often results in alopecia and excoriation. The host's rubbing and grooming may not correlate with the extent of infestation. Hairballs can result from overgrooming in cattle. In severe cases, the organisms can lead to anemia, weight loss, damaged wool in sheep, and damaged pelts in other ruminants. Young animals with severe infestations of sucking lice may become anemic or even die. Pregnant animals with heavy infestations may abort. In sheep infected with the foot louse, lameness may result.

Lice are generally species specific, and those infecting ruminants are usually smaller than 5 mm. Transmission is primarily by direct contact between animals or by attachment to flies or fomites.

Biting or chewing lice inhabit the host's face, lower legs, and flanks and feed on epidermal debris and sebaceous secretions. Sucking lice inhabit the host's neck, back, and body region and feed on blood. Lice eggs or nits are attached to hairs near the skin. Three nymphal stages, or instars, occur between egg and adult, and the growth cycle takes about 1 month for all species. Lice cannot survive for more than a few days off the host. All ruminant mite infestations are differentials for the clinical signs seen with pediculosis.

Lice are effectively treated with a variety of insecticides including coumaphos, dichlorvos, crotoxyphos, avermectin, and pyrethroids. Label directions should be read and adhered to including withdrawal times. Only products approved for lactating or dry dairy cattle should be used on female dairy animals >20 months of age. Treatments must be repeated at least twice at intervals appropriate for nit hatches (about every 16 days) because nits will not be killed. Fall treatments are useful in managing the infections. Systemic treatments in cattle are contraindicated when there may be concurrent larvae of cattle grubs (*Hypoderma lineatum* and *H. bovis*). Back rubbers with insecticides, capitalizing on self-treatment, are useful for cattle. Sustained release insecticide-containing ear tags are approved for use in cattle.

ii. TICKS (ARACHNIDS)
Etiology Ruminants are susceptible to many species of Ixodidae (hard shell ticks) and Argasidae (soft-shell ticks). Several diseases, including anaplasmosis, babesiosis, and Q fever are transmitted by ticks.

Clinical Signs and Diagnosis Tick infestations are associated with decreased productivity, loss of blood and blood proteins, transmission of diseases, debilitation, and even death. Feeding sites on the host vary with the tick species. Ticks are associated with an acute paralytic syndrome called Tick Paralysis. This disease is characterized by ascending paralysis and may lead to death if the tick is not removed before the paralysis reaches the respiratory muscles. Diagnosis is based on identification of the species.

Epizootiology and Transmission Ticks are not as host specific as lice. Ticks are classified as one-host, two-host, or three-host ticks which refers to whether they drop off the host between larval and nymphal stages to molt.

Treatment Ticks can be treated using systemic or topical insecticides.

g. Other

i. NEW WORLD SCREWWORM The New World Screw Worm, *Cochliomyia hominivorax*, is a parasitic fly whose larvae are known to eat the living tissue of warm-blooded animals. Although eradicated from the United States, it is present in the New World tropics particularly Mexico and Central America. Screwworms are a reportable species to the state veterinarian in the United States if discovered on livestock.

ii. NASAL BOTS (NASAL MYIASIS, HEAD GRUBS) Nasal myiasis is a chronic rhinitis and sinusitis caused by the larval forms of the botfly, *Oestrus ovis*. The botfly deposits eggs around the nostrils of sheep. The ova hatch and the larvae migrate throughout the nasal cavity and sinuses, feeding on mucus and debris. In 2–10 months, the larvae complete their growing phase, migrate back to the nasal cavity, and are sneezed out. The mature larvae penetrate the soil and pupate for 1–1.5 months and emerge as botflies. Clinically, early in the disease course, animals display unique behaviors such as stamping, snorting, sneezing, and rubbing their noses against each other or objects.

Hypersensitivity to the larvae occurs (Dorchies *et al.*, 1998). Later, mucopurulent nasal discharges will be observed associated with the larval-induced inflammation of mucosal linings. At necropsy, larvae will be observed in the nasal cavity or sinuses. Mild inflammatory reactions, mucosal thickening and exudates will accompany the larvae. The disease is diagnosed by observing the behaviors or identifying organisms at necropsy. Up to 80% of a flock will potentially be infected; treatment should be employed on the rest of the flock. Ivermectins and other insecticides will eliminate the larvae; but treatment should be done in the early fall, when larvae are small. Fly repellents may be helpful at preventing additional infections.

iii. SHEEP KEDS ('SHEEP TICK') In sheep and goats, sheep keds produce a chronic irritation and dermatitis with associated pruritus. The disease is caused by *Melophagus ovinus*, which is a flat, brown bloodsucking, wingless fly; the term 'sheep tick' is incorrectly used. The adult fly lives entirely on the skin of sheep. Females mate and produce 10–15 larvae following a gestation of about 10–12 days. The larvae attach to the wool or hair, and pupate for about 3 weeks. The adult female feeds on blood and lives for 4–5 months, and the life-cycle is completed in about 5–6 weeks. Infection is highest in fall and winter. Pruritus develops around the neck, sides, abdomen, and rump. In severe cases, anemia may occur. Keds can transmit Bluetongue Virus. Keds are diagnosed by gross or microscopic identification. Ivermectin or other insecticides are useful treatment agents.

4. Fungal

a. Dermatophytes (Ringworm)

Etiology Dermatophytosis, infections of the keratinized layers of skin, are caused mostly by species of the genuses *Trichophyton* and *Microsporum*. The primary causes in sheep are *Trichophyton mentagrophytes* and *T. verrucosum*. In goats, the agents are *T. mentagrophytes*, *Microsporum canis*, *M. gypseum*, and *T. verrucosum*. In cattle, *T. verrucosum* is the primary causative agent. Dermatophytosis is a common fungal infection of the epidermis of cattle and less common in sheep and goats.

Clinical Signs and Diagnosis Multiple, gray, crusty, circumscribed, hyperkeratotic lesions are characteristic of infection. Lesions will vary in size. In all ruminants, lesions will be around the head, neck, and ears. In goats and cattle, lesions will extend down the neck, and in cattle, lesions develop particularly around the eyes, and on the thorax. Cattle lesions are unique in the marked crustiness; hair shafts will become brittle and break off. Intense pruritus is often associated with the alopecic lesions.

The disease can be diagnosed by microscopic identification of hyphae and conidia on the hairs following skin scraping and 20% potassium hydroxide digestion.

Dermatophyte Test Media (DTM) culture are the most reliable means to diagnose the fungus. Broken hairs from the periphery of the lesion are the best sources of the fungus.

Epizootiology and Transmission Younger animals are more susceptible, and factors such as crowding, indoor housing, warm and humid conditions, and poor nutrition are also important. Transmission is by direct contact or by contact with contaminated fomites, such as equipment, fencing, or feed bunks.

Treatment Spontaneous recovery occurs in all species in 1–4 months. Immune mechanisms are not well understood and immunity may not be of long duration. Recovery is enhanced by exposure to sunlight, correcting nutritional deficiencies and improving housing and ventilation problems. A number of topical treatments, such as 2–5% lime–sulfur solution, 3% Captan, iodophores, thiabendazole, and 0.5% sodium hypochlorite can be used. In severe cases, systemic therapy with griseofulvin may be successful.

Prevention and Control The animals' environment and overall physical condition should be reassessed with particular attention to ventilation, crowding, sanitation, and nutrition. Pens should be thoroughly cleaned and disinfected.

Research Complications Ringworm is a zoonotic disease.

B. Genetic/Metabolic/Nutritional/Management-Related Diseases

1. Genetic Diseases

a. Entropion

Inverted eyelids are a common inherited disorder of lambs and kids of most breeds. Generally, the lower eyelid is affected and turns inward causing various degrees of trauma to the conjunctiva and cornea. Young animals will display tearing, blepharospasm, and photophobia initially. If left uncorrected, corneal ulcers, perforating ulcers, uveitis and blindness may occur. Placing a suture or surgical staple in the lower eyelid and the cheek, effectively anchoring the lid in an everted position successfully treats the condition.

b. Beta Mannosidosis of Goats

Beta mannosidosis is an autosomal recessive lysosomal storage disease of goats. The disease affects kids of the Nubian breed and is identified by intention tremors and difficulty or inability of newborns to stand. Newborn kids are unable to rise and have characteristic flexion of the carpal joint and hyperextension of the pastern joint. Kids are born deaf with other musculoskeletal deformities such as a domed skull, small narrow muzzle, enophthalmus, and a depressed nasal bridge (Smith and Sherman, 2009). Carrier adults can be identified by plasma measurements of beta mannosidase activity.

c. Congenital Myotonia of Goats

Caprine congenital myotonia is an inherited autosomal dominant disease that affects voluntary striated skeletal muscles. Goats with this disease are commonly known as 'fainting' goats. Fainting is actually transient spasms of skeletal musculature brought about by visual, tactile, or auditory stimuli (Smith and Sherman, 2009). Contractions of skeletal muscle are sustained for up to 1 min. Kids exhibit the condition by 6 weeks of age, and males appear to exhibit more severe clinical signs than females.

d. Polled Intersex Goats

Several western European goat breeds (Saanen, Alpine, Toggenburg) exhibit a well-described genetic relationship between the polled (hornless) phenotype and intersex (or hermaphrodite) characteristics. A gene deletion on chromosome 1 affects the regulation of both horn bud and fetal ovarian development, resulting in genetically female animals who exhibit masculine characteristics such as enlarged clitoris, decreased anogenital distance, and muscular neck development. These animals are not fertile, and testosterone production often results in characteristic male odor and aggressive behavior (Smith and Sherman, 2009).

e. Inherited Conditions of Cattle

i. CONGENITAL ERTHYROPOIETIC PORPHYRIA

Congenital Erthyropoietic Porphyria (CEP) is a rare autosomal recessive disease of cattle seen primarily in Holsteins, Herefords, and Shorthorns. In the homozygous recessive animal, reddish-brown discoloration of teeth and bones is a characteristic as are discolored urine, general weakness and failure to thrive, photosensitization and photophobia. Porphyrins are excreted in varying amounts in the urine and the discoloration fluoresces under a Woods lamp. Bones are fragile compared to those of normal animals. A regenerative anemia occurs as the result of the shortened life span of erythrocytes due to accumulations of porphyrins. The genetic defect is associated with low activity of an essential enzyme, uroporphyrinogen III synthase, in the porphyrin–heme synthesis pathway in erythrocytic tissue. Heterozygotes may have milder clinical signs.

ii. OTHER INHERITED CONDITIONS OF CATTLE

Many other genetic defects, in all major organ systems, have been described in numerous breeds of cattle and are described in detail elsewhere (Smith, 2009). The bovine genome continues to be further characterized and more linkage maps and gene locations will be forthcoming (Womack, 1998). Some bovine genetic defects are also regarded as models of genetic disease, such as leukocyte adhesion deficiency and citrullinemia of Holstein cattle.

Some of the more commonly reported defects include syndactyly and complex vertebral malformation in Holstein and other breeds, arthrogryposis multiplex in Angus, lysosomal storage diseases such as alpha-mannosidosis in some beef breeds, and progressive degenerative myeloencephalopathy ('weaver') in Brown Swiss.

Inherited periodic spasticity ('crampy syndrome') is a relatively common inherited trait in dairy cattle breeds, particularly Holsteins. Affected cattle develop muscle spasms in the hip and upper leg between 3 and 8 years of age. During a spasm, animals will typically extend or flex one rear leg and shake the leg for 15–30 s. The disease is progressive over the course of 1–2 years, and is thought to be transmitted by a single recessive gene.

f. Congenital Dyshormonogenetic Goiter of Sheep

A defect in the synthesis of thyroid hormone has been identified in Merino sheep (Radostits et al., 2007). It has also been identified as an autosomal recessive disease in Corriedale, Dorset Horn, Merino, and Romney sheep and Saanen dwarf goats. Lambs and goats born with the defect have enlargement of the thyroid gland, a silky appearance to the wool and a high degree of mortality. Edema, bowing of the legs, and facial abnormalities have also been noted in animals with this disorder. Immaturity of the lungs at birth causes neonatal respiratory distress and results in dyspnea and respiratory failure.

g. Spider Lamb Syndrome (Hereditary Chondrodysplasia)

Spider lamb syndrome is an inherited, often lethal, musculoskeletal disorder primarily occurring in Suffolk and Hampshire breeds. Severely affected lambs die shortly after birth. Animals that survive the perinatal period develop angular limb deformities, scoliosis, and facial deformities. Muscle atrophy is common. Diagnosis can be based on typical clinical signs, which are similar to those seen with Marfan syndrome in humans (Rook et al., 1986). Long-term survival is rare, and treatment is unsuccessful.

h. Other Inherited Conditions of Sheep

Gangliosidosis (β-galactosidase deficiency) has been documented in Suffolk and Coopworth–Romney sheep; gamma-glutamyl carboxylase deficiency in the Rambouillet breed; globoid cell leukodystrophy (Krabbe's disease or galactocerebroside beta-galactosidase deficiency) in polled Dorset sheep; ceroid lipofuscinosis in South Hampshire, Swedish Landrace, and Rambouillet sheep; neuraxonal dystrophy of the Suffolk breed; and primary cerebellar degeneration of Merino and Charollais sheep.

2. Metabolic Diseases

a. Abomasal Disorders

i. ABOMASAL, DUODENAL ULCERS Abomasal and duodenal ulcers occur more frequently in pre-weaned beef calves and adult dairy cattle than in sheep and goats. Ulcers may be associated with abrupt dietary changes, or stress due to over-crowding, recent transport or recent parturition. Concurrent disease, such as Salmonellosis, Bluetongue or *Clostridium perfringens* abomasitis or overuse of anti-inflammatory drugs also may lead to ulcer formation. In older adult cattle, abomasal lymphoma may be the underlying condition. Ulcers are classified as perforating or non-perforating, and non-perforating ulcers are further classified as non-bleeding or bleeding.

Clinical signs vary with the type of ulcer. Non-perforating ulcers may simply result in reduced feed intake and reduced milk production, or chronic hemorrhage may lead to anemia. Dark feces or melena and abdominal pain may be observed. Arched back, restlessness, kicking at the abdomen, bruxism and anorexia are common signs of abdominal pain (Fecteau and Whitlock, 2009). Fecal occult blood is one of the more reliable diagnostic tests. Marked elevation of BUN with a normal serum creatinine is supportive of a bleeding ulcer. Ulcers often are asymptomatic in calves, but perforation with peritonitis is more common than hemorrhage.

Treatment for ulcers include gastrointestinal protectants and antihistamines. Anemia may be symptomatically treated with parenteral iron injections and anabolic steroids. Preventative measures in cattle herds include minimizing stress to calves, and striving for a herd free of BLV.

ii. ABOMASAL EMPTYING DEFECT Abomasal emptying defect of sheep is a sporadic syndrome associated with abomasal distention and weight loss. Suffolks tend to be especially predisposed, although the disease has been diagnosed in Hampshires, Columbia, and Corriedales. The mechanism of the disease is unknown. Research has shown a link to a defect in the autonomic nervous system, dyautonomia and possible neurotoxicosis (Pugh and Baird, 2012). Affected animals will exhibit a gradual weight loss with a history of normal appetites and normal feces. Ventral abdominal distension associated with abomasal accumulation of feedstuffs will be apparent. Diagnosis is primarily based on history and clinical signs. Elevations in rumen chloride concentrations (>15 mEq/l) are commonly found. Radiography or ultrasonography may be helpful in identifying the distended abomasum. Abomasal emptying defect is eventually fatal. Treatment with metoclopramide and mineral oil may be helpful in early disease.

iii. ABOMASAL DISPLACEMENT Displaced abomasum (DA) is a sporadic disorder usually associated with dairy cows in early lactation but the condition can occur in any stage of lactation, in young calves and in bulls. Left displacement (LDA) is the most common presentation (about 90%). Displacement to the right (RDA) may be further complicated by abomasal volvulus (RAV), a surgical emergency. The DA occurs because of gas accumulation within the abomasum, often associated with periparturient hypocalcemia, allowing the abomasum to migrate up from its normal ventral location to either the right or left lateral abdomen.

Clinical signs include anorexia, lack of cud chewing, decreased frequency of ruminal contractions, shallow respirations, increased heart rate, evidence of abdominal pain, and decreased milk production. Diagnosis is based on characteristic areas of tympanic resonance during auscultation-percussion of the lateral to ventro-lateral abdomen ('pings'), ruminal displacement palpated per rectum, and clinical signs. Clinical chemistry findings include hypoglycemia and ketonuria and moderate to severe electrolyte and acid–base abnormalities.

Risk factors for DA include parity (multiparous cows having higher incidence), twinning, breed, season (higher incidence in winter), the practice of 'lead feeding' concentrate feeds, and many disorders including hypocalcemia, retained placenta, metritis, and mastitis. Body size and conformation may be factors, indicating the possibility of genetic predisposition.

Treatments include surgical and nonsurgical correction of LDA with the former having a better chance of permanent correction. Emergency surgery is necessary for RAV because the disorder can be fatal within 72 h. Reoccurrence is rare after surgical correction. Electrolyte and acid–base imbalances are likely in severe cases and especially RAV. Prevention includes reducing stress in the periparturient period, greater care in the introduction and feeding of concentrates, and reducing incidence of predisposing diseases noted above (Geishauser *et al.*, 2000).

b. Rumen and Reticulum Disorders

i. BLOAT Bloat or rumen tympany refers to an excessive accumulation of gas in the rumen. The condition most frequently occurs in animals that recently have been fed abundant quantities of succulent forages or grains. Bloat is classified into two broad categories: frothy bloat and free-gas bloat. Frothy bloat is associated with ingestion of feeds that produce a stable froth that is not easily expelled from the rumen. Fermentation gases such as CO_2 and methane incorporate into the froth and over-distend the rumen, eventually compromising respiration by limiting diaphragm movement. Typical feedstuffs that cause frothy bloat include fresh or dried legumes (alfalfa or clover) or cereal grains (especially finely ground corn and barley). Free-gas bloat is more often related to rumen atony or physical/pathological problems preventing normal gas eructation. Some causes of free-gas bloat include esophageal obstructions (foreign bodies such as boluses, apples, etc.), positional (e.g., being trapped in a position that precludes eructation), tumors, abscesses, enlarged cervical or thoracic lymph nodes, vagal nerve paralysis or injury, traumatic reticulitis, hypocalcemia, and central nervous system conditions affecting eructation reflexes.

Clinically, rumen distension will be observed in the left paralumbar fossa. Additional signs may include colic-like pain of the abdomen and dyspnea. Passage of a stomach tube helps to differentiate between free-gas bloat and frothy bloat. Obstructions may require manual removal prior to the use of a stomach tube; be sure to consider rabies prior to manual extraction. With free-gas bloat, expulsion of gas through the stomach tube aids in treatment of the disorder. Once rumen distension is alleviated with free-gas bloat, the underlying cause must be investigated to prevent reoccurrence. Frothy bloat is more difficult to treat as the foam blocks the stomach tube. Addition of mineral oil, surfactants or antifermentative compounds via stomach tube may help break down surface tension, allowing gas to be expelled. In acute, life-threatening cases of bloat, treatment should be aimed at alleviating rumen distension by placing a trocar or surgical rumenotomy into the rumen via the left paralumbar fossa. Feeding management is critical in controlling the incidence of bloat; limiting the consumption of feedstuffs known to induce bloat can prevent the disease. In addition, feeding poloxalene will decrease the incidence of legume bloat. Ionophores such as monensin or lasalocid can reduce the incidence of frothy bloat from either legume or concentrate feeds (Streeter, 2009).

ii. LACTIC ACIDOSIS: ACUTE AND SUBACUTE

Lactic acidosis or rumen acidosis may be acute or subacute and typically affects cattle or sheep consuming relatively energy-dense diets such as feedlot animals or dairy cows. Acute metabolic disease usually is caused by sudden engorgement on grains or other highly fermentable carbohydrate sources or by a rapid change from a diet containing high roughage content to one containing a relatively high proportion of grain. Common cereal grains and feedstuffs such as sugar beets, molasses, and potatoes predispose to acidosis. Ingestion of large amounts of these carbohydrate-rich feeds causes proliferation of gram-positive bacteria leading to rapid fermentation with an increase in lactic acid production and reduction of rumen pH. Subsequently gram-negative bacteria die in large numbers and release endotoxin. The high osmolarity of rumen contents results in accumulation of fluid, and the low pH and perturbed rumen microflora cause rumen mucosal inflammation.

Sequelae of acidosis include rumenitis, abomasal ulcers, liver abscesses, lung abscesses leading to episodes of epistaxis, laminitis from absorbed toxins, and polioencephalomalacia from the inability of the altered rumen bacterial populations to produce sufficient B-complex vitamins.

Clinical Signs and Diagnosis In the case of acute ruminal acidosis, animals will become anorexic, depressed, and weak within 1–3 days after the initial insult. Incoordination, ataxia, dehydration and hemoconcentration (hypovolemic and endotoxic shock), rapid pulse and respiration, diarrhea, abdominal pain, and lameness may be noted. Rumen distension (bloat) may also be observed. Rumen pH, which is normally above 6.0 will drop to less than 5.0 and in severe cases may achieve levels as low as 3.8. Similarly, urine pH will become acidic, blood pH will drop below 7.4 and hematocrit will appear to increase due to the relative hemoconcentration. Subacute ruminal acidosis (SARA syndrome) has more subtle signs, but may include intermittent bouts of anorexia and diarrhea, depressed milk fat percentage in dairy cows, sporadic cases of epistaxis and an increased incidence of laminitis. Subacute acidosis is best diagnosed by performing rumenocentesis in a sample of affected cows (Krause and Oetzel, 2006).

Necropsy Findings Necropsy findings will be determined by severity and time-course of the incident. Acute lactic acidosis will cause inflammation, swelling and necrosis of rumen papillae and abomasal hemorrhages and ulcers. More chronic or subacute acidosis will result in parakeratosis of ruminal papillae. Papillae will be short (blunted), thickened, and rough. They will frequently be dark in color, and multiple papillae will clump together. Abscesses may be present in lung and liver. Stellate ruminal scars are telltale signs of previous episodes of acute acidosis.

Treatment Treatment must be applied early in the case of acute acidosis. In early hours of severe carbohydrate engorgement, rumenotomy and evacuation of the contents is appropriate. The patient should be given mineral oil and antifermentatives to prevent the continued conversion of starches to acids and the absorption of the metabolic products; animals in hypovolemic shock should be given hypertonic saline. Bicarbonate or other antacids such as magnesium carbonate or magnesium oxide introduced into the rumen will aid in adjusting rumen pH. Furthermore, animals can be given oral tetracycline or penicillin that will decrease the gram-positive bacterial population. In the case of subacute acidosis, correction of ration formulation and delivery to provide a higher proportion of effective fiber is critical. In the case of animals receiving chopped or processed forages, provision of long hay may be beneficial. Buffers such as sodium bicarbonate or sodium sesquicarbonate also can be incorporated into the rations or provided free-choice.

iii. TRAUMATIC RETICULITIS-RETICULOPERITONITIS (HARDWARE DISEASE)

Etiology   This is a disease primarily of cattle related to their relatively indiscriminant feeding behavior. The disease is rarely seen in smaller ruminants.

Clinical Signs   Clinical signs range from asymptomatic to severe, depending on the penetration and damage by the foreign object after settling in the animal's reticulum. Many signs during the early, acute stages will be attributable to pain and rumen stasis and range from anorexia, listlessness and an arched back, grunting forced to move, a painful response to pressure on the xyphoid or pinching of the withers, fever, abrupt decrease in production, decrease or cessation of ruminal contractions, bloat, regurgitation, tachypnea, and tachycardia. The prognosis is poor when peritonitis becomes diffuse. Sudden death can occur if the heart, coronary vessels, or other large vessels are punctured by the migrating object.

Epizootiology and Transmission   This is a non-contagious disease. The occurrence is directly related to sharp or metallic indigestible linear items in the feed or environment that the cattle can swallow. Multiple cases may present if dairy or feedlot cattle consuming chopped feeds such as silage are presented with shards of metal (e.g., fencing material) which has been processed along with the feedstuffs.

Necropsy Findings   In severe cases, these include extensive inflammation throughout the cranial abdomen, malodorous peritoneal fluid accumulations, and lesions at the reticular sites of migration of the foreign objects. Pericarditis and/or cardiac puncture may be present in those animals succumbing to sudden death.

Pathogenesis   Consumed objects initially settle in the rumen, but are deposited in the reticulum during the digestive process and normal contraction may eventually lead to puncture of the reticular wall. This sets off a localized inflammation, or a more generalized peritonitis. Further damage may result from migration and penetration of the diaphragm, pericardium, and heart. Diagnosis is based on clinical signs and reflection of acute or chronic infection on the hemogram. Ultrasound and abdominocentesis may be useful.

Differential Diagnoses   These include abomasal ulcers, hepatic ulcers, neoplasia (such as lymphoma in older animals or intestinal carcinoma), and cor pulmonale. Infectious diseases that are differentials include systemic leptospirosis and internal parasitism. Diseases causing sudden death may need to be considered.

Prevention and Control   This problem can be prevented entirely by elimination of sharp objects in cattle feed and pasture environments. Adequately sized magnets placed in feed-handling equipment and forestomach magnets (placed *per os* with a balling gun in youngstock at 6–8 months of age) are also significant prevention measures. However, only a single magnet should ever be placed in an animal. The magnets are very strong, and can trap forestomach wall between them resulting in tissue necrosis and perforation. A compass placed near the xiphoid can be used to check for the presence of a magnet.

Treatment   Providing a forestomach magnet, confinement and nursing care, including antibiotics, are the initial treatments. In severe cases, rumenotomy may be considered.

c. Hypocalcemia (Parturient Paresis, Milk Fever)

Etiology   Hypocalcemia is an acute metabolic disease of ruminants that requires emergency treatment; the presentation is slightly different in ewes, does, and cows. High-producing, multiparous dairy cows are the most susceptible, and the Jersey breed is particularly susceptible. Cows that have survived one episode are prone to recurrence. In sheep, hypocalcemia occurs primarily in overweight ewes during the last 6 weeks of pregnancy or during the first few weeks of lactation. The disease is not as common in the dairy goat as in the dairy cow. The disease is not common in beef cattle unless there is an overall poor nutrition program.

Clinical Signs and Diagnosis   In sheep, the disease is seen in ewes during the last 6 weeks of pregnancy, and is characterized by muscle tetany, incoordination, paralysis, and finally coma. Early signs in ewes include stiffness and incoordination of movements, especially in the hind limbs. Later, muscular tremors, muscular weakness, and recumbency will ensue. Morbidity may approach 30% while mortality may reach as high as 90% in untreated animals. Affected does become bloated, weak, unsteady and eventually recumbent. Cows typically are affected within 24–48h before or after parturition. Cows initially are weak and show evidence of muscle tremors, then deteriorate to sternal recumbency, with head usually tucked to the abdomen, and an inability to stand. Muscle weakness predisposes to traumatic injuries such as splayleg or hip fractures. Tachycardia, dilated pupils, anorexia, hypothermia, depression, ruminal stasis, bloat, uterine inertia, and loss of anal tone are also seen at this stage. The terminal stage of disease is a rapid progression from coma to death. Heart rates will be high but pulse may not be detectable.

Hypocalcemia is diagnosed based on the pregnancy stage of the female and on clinical signs. It may later be confirmed by laboratory findings of low serum calcium. With hypocalcemia in ewes, the plasma concentrations of calcium drop from normal values of 8–12 mg/dl to values of 3–6 mg/dl. In cattle, plasma levels below 7.5 mg/dl are hypocalcemic.

Necropsy Findings   There is no pathognomonic or typical finding at necropsy. Dairy cows which have been recumbent for more than 12h may have severe muscle damage due to 'crush syndrome.'

Prevention and Control In sheep, maintaining appropriate body condition during the last trimester is helpful in preventing the disease. Recent information suggests that dry cow diets which rely on legume and grass forages, which are relatively high in potassium, create a slight physiological alkalosis that decreases tissue responsiveness to parathyroid hormone (Goff, 2009). Limiting sodium and potassium in the diet of prepartum cows to levels that will just meet maintenance requirements is critical. In herds with a high incidence or genetic predisposition to hypocalcemia, such as Jersey cows, increasing dietary chlorides is often helpful. Oral calcium supplements (gels or boluses) given to multiparous cows at the time of calving can be effective in preventing hypocalcemia.

Treatment Hypocalcemia must be treated quickly based on clinical signs. Pretreatment blood samples can be saved for later confirmation. Twenty percent calcium borogluconate solution should be administered by slow intravenous infusion. Solutions containing magnesium and phosphorus are also used, particularly in animals prone to relapse. Response will often be rapid with the resolution of the animal's dull mentation. Less severely affected animals will often try to stand in a short time. Relapses are common, however, in sheep and cattle. Heart rate should be monitored closely throughout calcium administration, most conveniently by palpation of the pulse in the facial artery. If an irregular (ventricular premature contractions) or rapid (ventricular tachycardia) heart rate is detected, then calcium treatment should be slowed or discontinued. Care must be taken to avoid extravascular leakage of the highly irritant calcium solution. Calcium gels and boluses available for treatment may be used as an adjunct but are not adequate for animals which have reached the stage of recumbancy.

d. Hypomagnesemic Tetany (Grass Tetany, Grass Staggers)

Unlike calcium, magnesium (Mg) is not under hormonal control, and Mg stores in bone are not readily mobilized. Maintenance of blood magnesium levels relies on the presence of adequate levels of magnesium in the diet. Hypomagnesemic tetany occurs most frequently in early lactation beef cows grazing lush pastures which are high in potassium and nitrogen. Dairy cattle, calves, ewes, and goats also may develop hypomagnesemia.

Clinical Signs Early signs include twitching of muscles and apprehension or hyperexcitability. Muscular spasms become more frequent until the cow becomes ataxic and falls to the ground. Clonic convulsions follow with bruxism and hypersalivation. Heart and respiratory rates are extremely elevated and the animal becomes hyperthermic due to muscular activity. Blood Mg levels below 1.1 mg/dl coincide with clinical signs, but CSF and vitreous humor are more reliable necropsy specimens.

Epizootiology Low magnesium concentrations in rapidly growing forages along with inadequate Mg supplementation are the primary cause. Higher concentration of potassium in these lush, immature forages interferes with absorption of Mg in the rumen. Hypocalcemia often accompanies hypomagnesemia as the lack of Mg impairs PTH secretion and activity at the target tissue (Martens and Schweigel, 2000).

Treatment and Control Treatment of hypomagnesemic convulsions is a medical emergency. Magnesium must be administered intravenously. Many solutions marketed for the treatment of hypocalcemia in dairy cows contain Mg and can be used effectively as treatment. To prevent relapse, oral drenching with Mg salts should be performed as soon as the animal has recovered enough to swallow. To prevent other cases, all other animals in the group should begin to receive Mg supplementation in the diet.

e. Ketosis (Acetonemia), Fat Cow Syndrome, Hepatic Lipidosis, Pregnancy Toxemia, Protein Energy Malnutrition

Etiology Ketosis and hepatic lipidosis are diseases of high-producing dairy cows. Pregnancy toxemia primarily is a metabolic disease of ewes and does in advanced pregnancy, particularly with twins or triplets. Beef heifers are susceptible to protein-energy malnutrition (PEM) syndrome that is also referred to as pregnancy toxemia. These metabolic disease syndromes have slightly different clinical syndromes but are all related to a negative energy balance.

Clinical Signs Clinical signs include anorexia, weakness, and lethargy. In dairy cattle, ketosis occurs in the first 6 weeks of lactation. Weight loss and thin body condition may be seen, and hypoglycemia, ketonemia, and ketonuria are evident. Some caretakers may be able to smell fruity ketones on the animal's breath. Animals with severe ketosis can exhibit neurologic signs, including circling, head-pressing, and apparent blindness. In sheep and goats, pregnancy toxemia generally occurs in the last six weeks of gestation and in ewes and does with multiple fetuses. Lactational ketosis and/or fatty liver disease can also occur during the early postpartum period in small ruminants and manifest similarly to that described for dairy cows. Hypoglycemic and/or ketotic ewes and does may begin to wander aimlessly and move away from the flock. They become anorexic and uncoordinated, frequently leaning against objects, and may display, muscle tremors, teeth grinding, convulsions, and coma. Often the animal is found unable or unwilling to rise, and up to 80% of infected ewes may die from the disease. If fetal death occurs, acute toxemia and death may result.

Pathogenesis Dairy cows normally experience a decrease in dry matter intake in the 2–3 weeks before calving. In obese cows, this drop in intake is exaggerated. Negative energy balance is a result of lower intake in conjunction with increasing nutrient demands of the growing fetus and colostrogenesis. In addition, dairy cows typically mobilize body adipose stores to support the energy demands of milk production for the first 7–8 weeks of lactation. When adipose reserves are mobilized, ketone bodies (acetone, acetoacetate, and beta-hydroxybutyrate) are produced in the liver. Although ketones are utilized by many body tissues as a source of energy, excessive levels in blood lead to ketonemia and ketoacidosis. In addition, mobilization of stored triglycerides in adipose results in increased blood nonesterified fatty acids (NEFAs). A disproportionate amount of NEFA is extracted by the liver, resulting in an accumulation of liver triglycerides which can exceed 20% of tissue dry weight.

In small ruminants and beef cattle, rapid fetal growth and/or lactational demands, a decline in maternal nutrition, or a voluntary decrease in food intake in over-fat animals result in an inadequate supply of glucose needed for both maternal and fetal tissues. The animal develops a severe hypoglycemia in early stages of the disease. The oxidation of fatty acids results in the formation of ketone bodies resulting in ketoacidosis.

PEM in beef cattle occurs in late gestation or the early post-partum period, and also has a higher incidence in cows with twins, and first calf heifers. Heifer cattle have high energy requirements for completing normal body growth and supporting a pregnancy. Additional energy requirements are imposed during pregnancy, cold weather and during concurrent diseases. Marginal diets and poor-quality forage will place the cows in a negative energy balance.

Diagnosis Ketosis is diagnosed by clinical signs; sodium nitroprusside tablets or ketosis dipsticks may be used to identify ketones in the urine or plasma. In dairy cattle, blood glucose is typically less than 40 mg/dl, total blood ketones >30 mg/dl, and milk ketones >10 mg/dl. In small ruminants, blood glucose levels found to be below 25 mg/dl and ketonuria are good diagnostic indicators. Often ketones can be smelled in the cow's breath and milk. In prepartum cattle and in lactating cows, blood levels of NEFA greater than 1000 uEq/l and 325–400 uEq/l are abnormal (Gerloff and Herdt, 2009). Triglyceride analysis of liver biopsy specimens is useful.

Treatment Management of ketosis must be accompanied by a thorough physical exam to determine if concurrent disease (such as metritis or displaced abomasum) is present. Intravenous treatment with 50% glucose followed by oral supplementation with propylene glycol often produces significant clinical improvement. Glucocorticoids and/or long-acting insulin may be used

as adjunct therapy (Smith, 2009). In sheep and goats, reducing glucose demand by inducing abortion or surgical removal of the offspring may be helpful. Because the morbidity in sheep may be as high as 20%, treatment should be directed at the flock rather than the individual. Treating the individual ewe often is unsuccessful.

Necropsy Findings At necropsy, small ruminants often will have multiple fetuses which may have died and decomposed. The liver will be enlarged, yellow, greasy, and friable with fatty degeneration. If severe, the liver will float in formalin or water. Beef heifers will be very thin, and in dairy cattle in addition to a fatty liver, signs of concurrent diseases may be present.

Differential Diagnoses Hypocalcemia is a common differential diagnosis. Toxemia associated with mastitis, enterotoxemia, and peritonitis should be considered. In cattle, differentials include chronic or untreated diseases such as Johne's, lymphoma, parasitism, abomasal disease, vagal indigestion, and chronic respiratory diseases.

Prevention Providing adequate nutrition and managing body weight gain in late lactation, particularly in dairy cattle with prolonged lactation or delayed breeding, helps in prevention. Dry and lactating cows should be maintained and fed separately; their energy, protein, and dry matter requirements are very different. Management of cows in the pre-partum period should focus on reducing stress and maintaining feed intakes. Providing monensin and/or rumen-protected choline in the pre-partum diet may reduce fatty infiltration of the liver. In sheep and does in late pregnancy, the dietary energy and protein should be increased 1.5- to 2-times the maintenance level.

Research Complications In research requiring pregnant animals in late stages of gestation, for example, this disease should be considered if the animals are likely to bear twins and will be transported or stressed in other ways during that time.

f. Urinary Calculi (Obstructive Urolithiasis, Water Belly)

Etiology Urolithiasis is a metabolic disease of intact and castrated male sheep, goats, and cattle characterized by the formation of bladder and urethral crystals, urethral blockage and anuria (Anderson and Rings, 2009). Male sheep and goats have a urethral process that predisposes them to entrapment of calculi. In cattle, the urethra narrows at the sigmoid flexure, and calculi lodge in the distal flexure most frequently. Additionally, the removal of testosterone by early castration is thought to result in hypoplasia of the urethra and penis. The disease is rare in female ruminants.

Clinical Signs and Diagnosis Affected animals will vocalize and begin to show signs of uneasiness, such as treading, straining postures, arched backs, raised tails, and squatting while attempting to urinate. Male cattle may develop swelling along the ventral perineal area. Small amounts of urine may be discharged and crystal deposits may be visible attached to the preputial hairs.

In smaller ruminants, the vermiform urethral appendage (pizzle) often becomes dark purple to black in color. The pulsing pelvic urethra may be detected by manual or digital rectal palpation, and bladder distention may be noticeable in cattle by the same means. As the disease progresses to complete urethral blockage, the animal will become anorexic and show signs of abdominal pain such as kicking at the belly. The abdomen will swell as the bladder enlarges and rupture can occur within 36 h after development of clinical signs; subsequent development of uremia and hyperkalemia will eventually lead to death.

Diagnosis is made by the typical clinical signs. Abdominocentesis may yield urine. Creatinine concentration in abdominal fluid that is 1.5- to 2-fold greater than serum creatinine is diagnostic for uroperitoneum. Calculi are usually composed of calcium phosphate or ammonium phosphate matrices.

Epizootiology and Transmission Clinical disease is usually seen in growing intact or castrated males. The disease may be sporadic or there may be clusters of cases in the flock or herd.

Necropsy Findings Necropsy findings include severe hemorrhage and inflammation of the bladder wall. There may be urine in the abdomen with bladder or urethral rupture. Calculi or struvite crystal sediment will be observed in the bladder and urethra.

Differential Diagnoses Grain engorgement, colic, gastrointestinal blockage, and causes of tenemus, such as enteritis or trauma are differentials. Trauma to the urethral process should be considered.

Prevention and Control One case often is indicative of a potential problem in the group. Urolithiasis can be minimized by maintaining the calcium:phosphorus ratio in the diet at 2–2.5:1 with phosphorus levels at no more than 0.6% of diet dry matter. Increasing the amount of dietary roughage will help balance the mineral intake and increase the amount of phosphorus excreted via feces rather than urine. Increasing the amount of salt (sodium chloride, 2–4%) in the diet to increase water consumption, or adding ammonium chloride to the diet (10 g/head/day or 2% of the ration) to acidify the urine, will aid in the prevention of this disease (Anderson and Rings, 2009). Palatability of and accessibility to water should be assessed as well as functioning of automatic watering equipment.

Treatment Treatment is primarily surgical (Smith and Sherman, 2009). A lumbosacral epidural will relieve pain and facilitate examination of the penis, as will the use of acepromazine as a sedative. Initially, amputation of vermiform urethral appendage may alleviate the disease in small ruminants since urethral blockage often begins here. In more advanced stages, perineal urethrostomy may yield good results. The prognosis is poor when the condition becomes chronic, reoccurs, or surgery is required.

Research Complications Young castrated and intact male ruminants used in the lab setting will be the susceptible age group for this disorder.

3. NUTRITIONAL DISEASES
a. Copper Deficiency (Enzootic Ataxia, Swayback)

Etiology Chronic copper deficiency in pregnant ewes and does may produce a metabolic disorder in their lambs and kids called enzootic ataxia. In goats, this deficiency also causes 'swayback' in the fetuses. Enzootic ataxia is rarely seen as most North American diets have sufficient copper levels to prevent this disease. However, copper antagonists in the feed or forage may predispose to copper deficiencies. The most important of these reactions are the interaction between copper, molybdenum and sulfates.

Clinical Signs and Diagnosis This results in a progressive hind limb ataxia and apparent blindness in lambs up to about 3 months of age. Ewes may appear unthrifty, anemic and have poor quality, depigmented wool with a decrease in wool crimp. Affected kids are born weak, tremble and have the characteristic concavity to the spinal cord giving the name 'swayback.' Copper deficiency in cattle is associated with chronic diarrhea, weight loss, unthriftiness, and changes in coat color. Rarely there will be aortic aneurysms or dissections. Pathologic fractures may occur in young animals. Diagnosis is based on low copper levels found in feedstuffs and tissues at necropsy.

b. Copper Toxicosis

Etiology Acute or chronic copper ingestion or liver injury often causes a severe acute hemolytic anemia in weanling to adult sheep, and in calves and adult dairy cattle. Growing lambs may be the most susceptible. Copper toxicosis is rare in goats.

Clinical Signs and Diagnosis The clinical course in sheep can be as short as 1–4 days and mortality may reach 75%. Intravascular hemolysis, anemia, hemoglobinuria, and icterus characterize the acute hemolytic crisis, associated with copper released from the overloaded liver. Some clinical signs are related to direct irritation to the gastrointestinal tract mucosa. Weakness, vomiting, abdominal pain, bruxism, diarrhea, respiratory difficulty, and circulatory collapse are followed by recumbency and death.

Hepatic biopsy is currently considered the best diagnostic approach. Serum or plasma levels of copper and hepatic enzymes such as AST and GGT may provide some information, but it is generally believed that these will not accurately reflect total copper load or hepatic damage.

Epizootiology and Transmission A single toxic dose for sheep is in the range of 20–100 mg/kg, and for cattle is 220–880 mg/kg. Chronic poisoning in sheep may occur when 3.5 mg/kg is ingested. Copper-containing pesticides, soil additives, therapeutics, and improperly formulated feeds may potentially lead to copper toxicity. The feeding of poultry litter or forages fertilized with poultry or swine manure may also result in toxicity. A common cause of the disease in sheep is feeding concentrates balanced for cattle. Cattle feed and mineral blocks contain higher quantities of copper than are required for sheep. Chronic ingestion of these feedstuffs leads to copper accumulation and toxicity. Copper toxicosis has been reported in calves given regular oral or parenteral copper supplements, and in adult dairy cattle given copper supplements to compensate for copper deficient pasture. Pregnant dairy cattle and Jersey cattle may be more susceptible to copper toxicity. Sources of copper ingestion may include copper sulfate footbaths.

Necropsy Findings Icterus; a soft, dark, friable, enlarged spleen; an enlarged, yellow–brown friable liver; and, 'gun-barrel' black kidneys are common findings. Hemoglobin-stained urine will be visible in the bladder. Copper accumulations in the liver reaching 1000–3000 ppm are toxic.

Differential Diagnoses Other causes of hemolytic disease include babesiosis, trypanosomiasis, anaplasmosis, and plant poisonings such as kale. Arsenic ingestion, organophosphate toxicity, cyanide and nitrate poisoning should also be considered as a cause of poisoning. Urethral obstruction and gastrointestinal emergencies should be considered for the abdominal pain.

Prevention and Control The disease is prevented by carefully monitoring copper access in sheep and copper supplementation in cattle. Sheep and goats should not be fed feedstuffs formulated for cattle, and dairy calf milk replacer should not be used for lambs and kids.

Treatment Oral treatment for sheep or cattle consists of sodium molybdenate (and sodium thiosulfate orally for 3 weeks to aid in excretion of copper. Oral D-penicillamine daily for 6 days (50 mg/kg) has also been shown to increase copper excretion in sheep. Treatment for anemia and nephrosis may be necessary in severe cases.

Research Complications Breeds of sheep, such as the Merino and Merino crosses as well as British breeds, may be more susceptible to copper toxicosis caused by phytogenous sources.

c. Selenium/Vitamin E Deficiency (Nutritional Muscular Dystrophy or NMD Nutritional Myodegeneration, White Muscle Disease)

Etiology Nutritional muscular dystrophy (NMD), or stiff lamb disease, is a muscular dystrophy caused by a deficiency of selenium (Se) or vitamin E or both in young ruminants. Selenium and vitamin E function together as antioxidants that protect cell membranes from oxidative damage. Selenium is a cofactor for glutathione peroxidase which converts hydrogen peroxide to water and other nontoxic compounds. Lack of one or both nutrients results in loss of membrane integrity.

Clinical Signs and Diagnosis Clinically two forms of the disease have been identified: cardiac and skeletal. The cardiac form occurs most commonly in neonates and typically has a rapid onset; animals may be found severely debilitated or dead. Respiratory difficulty will be a manifestation of damage to cardiac, diaphragmatic, and intercostal muscles. In older animals, locomotor disturbances and/or circulatory failure may accompany respiratory signs. Clinically, animals may display paresis, stiffness or inability to stand, rapid but weak pulse, and acute death. Mortality may reach 70% (Hefnawy and Totura-Perez, 2010). Paresis and sudden deaths in neonates with associated pathological signs are frequently diagnostic. With the skeletal form, affected animals are stiff and reluctant to move and muscles of affected animals are painful. Young will be reluctant to get up, and may have difficulty nursing (dysphagia). Subclinical disease results in subtle immune defects.

Diagnosis Definitive diagnosis is based on determination of whole blood levels of Se (>0.07 ppm Se is normal) and plasma levels of vitamin E (<1.1 ppm). Glutathione peroxidase levels in red blood cells can be measured as an indirect test.

Epizootiology and Transmission Se deficiency and NMD occurs in young, rapidly growing calves, lambs, and kids. Se-deficient soils are common in many areas of the United States (including the Northeast, Northwest, and Great Lakes regions) and throughout the world. Diets based on feeds grown in these areas will result in Se deficiency if the mineral is not supplemented. The U.S. Food and Drug Administration limits supplemental Se in complete ruminant diets to 0.3 ppm (no more than 0.7 mg/day for adult sheep and 3 mg/day for adult cattle). This level of supplementation often is not adequate in deficient areas and the use of injectable sources is necessary to prevent clinical deficiencies.

Necropsy Findings Necropsy lesions include petechial hemorrhages and muscle edema. Hallmarks are pale-white streaking of affected skeletal and cardiac muscle, diaphragm, and tongue. However, muscles of young ruminants are normally very pale, and lesions may not be readily visible without histologic examination.

Differential Diagnoses In neonatal ruminants presenting with respiratory and cardiac dysfunction, differentials include congenital cardiac anomalies and pneumonia.

Prevention and Control Awareness of regional selenium deficiencies is important as disease is frequently subclinical. Control involves vitamin E and selenium supplementation, particularly to pregnant dams and/or young animals in deficient areas. Injectable selenium supplements are required to prevent clinical disease in severely deficient regions.

Treatment Affected animals may be treated by administering vitamin E and selenium injections.

d. Selenium Toxicity

Selenium toxicity occurs most frequently as the result of excessive dosing to prevent or correct selenium deficiency, feed manufacturing errors, or following ingestion of Se-concentrating plants. The main preventative measure for the former is the use of the appropriate supplement or injectable product for the species being treated. In the United States, ruminants on arid alkaline soils (found primarily in the western states) may be subject to selenium toxicity especially when pastured in areas containing Se-accumulating plants. Signs of selenosis include weakness, dyspnea, bloating, and diarrhea. Shock, paresis, and death may occur. Initial clinical signs of excessive selenium intake from plants are observed in the distal limb with cracked hoof walls and subsequent infection and irregular hoof growth.

e. Thiamine Deficiency/Polioencephalomalacia

Etiology Polioencephalomalacia (PEM) is a non-infectious, nutritional disease characterized by neurological signs. PEM is caused by thiamine deficiency due to inadequate ruminal thiamine production or bacterial thiaminase production in cattle and sheep consuming diets high in fermentable carbohydrates. Animals exposed to toxic plants (bracken fern or equisetum), moldy feed containing thiaminases, or to feed or water high in sulfates also are at risk. The condition occurs throughout the world and affects cattle, sheep, goats, deer, and camelids.

Clinical Signs and Diagnosis Early clinical signs include anorexia, ataxia and/or hypermetria, bruxism, hypersalivation, hyperesthesia, and muscle tremors. As the disease progresses, cortical blindness, head-pressing, head tilt, opisthotonus, nystagmus, dorsalmedial strabismus, seizures, and death ensue. Body temperatures are normal unless excessive muscle activity has resulted in hyperthermia and ocular reflexes are normal. Morbidity and mortality may be high especially in younger animals. Diagnosis is suggestive from clinical signs, and response to intensive parental thiamine hydrochloride.

Necropsy Signs Cerebral lesions characterized by softening and discoloration are grossly observed in the gray matter. Microscopically, neurons will exhibit edema, chromatolysis, and shrinkage.

Differential Diagnoses Several important differentials include acute lead poisoning, hypomagnesemia, listeriosis, rabies, pregnancy toxemia, infectious thromboembolic meningoencephalitis, and type D clostridial enterotoxemia.

Prevention and Control The disease can be prevented by monitoring the diet and by providing adequate roughage necessary to support ruminal production of B vitamins. If excess sulfates are the primary factor, then immediate removal of the source is critical.

Treatment Early aggressive treatment is essential to save animals. The disease is treated by frequent parenteral administration of thiamine hydrochloride, the first dose being administered intravenously. Dexamethasone, B vitamins, and diazepam may also be required.

Research Complications This is a preventable disease. Although less likely to occur in smaller groups of confined ruminants, the risks of feeding concentrates or moldy feed, for example, with minimal good quality roughage, should be kept in mind.

f. Salt Toxicity

Salt poisoning may result from the practice of feeding high-salt supplements to restrict intake, from consuming water that is high in sodium, from mistakes in formulation or preparation of feedstuffs or electrolyte solutions, and from the feeding of high-sodium byproducts (whey, waste food products). Restriction of water also may result in sodium toxicity.

Clinical Signs Clinical signs of sodium toxicity include colic and diarrhea, blindnesss or 'star-gazing,' hyperexcitability, head-pressing, ataxia, incessant chewing, nystagmus, and seizures progressing to coma and death. Sodium levels will be elevated in serum and CSF. Animals allowed to rehydrate rapidly may develop intravascular hemolysis and hemoglobinuria. Cerebral edema may be present on necropsy (Fecteau and George, 2009).

Treatment and Control Affected animals should receive normal or hypertonic saline intravenously followed by oral fluid replacement. Mannitol (0.5–1 g/kg) may be useful in the treatment of calves and small ruminants. Prognosis is poor for animals with severe neurologic clinical signs. Control relies on providing adequate amounts of fresh water (<7000 ppm sodium), and in particular avoiding water restriction if high-sodium feeds are used. Oral electrolyte solutions for young ruminants must always be prepared according to manufacturers' instructions.

4. MANAGEMENT-RELATED
a. Failure of Passive Transfer

Because of their epitheliochorial placentation, neonatal ruminants are born without immunoglobulins and must receive colostrum as soon as possible after birth. The morbidity and mortality associated with inadequate passive transfer of antibodies in colostrum can be severe.

Measures to ensure passive immunity for neonatal ruminants are covered under management, and clinical signs of illness associated with lack of immunity are addressed under bacterial diseases, such as *E. coli*, and viral diseases, such as diarrheas. Generally, failure of passive transfer is defined by serum concentration of less than 10 mg/ml IgG1 at 48 h after birth. Methods to determine success of transfer should be performed within a week of birth and include: single radial immunodiffusion (quantitates immunogloblin classes), ELISA test kits (available commercially), zinc sulfate turbidity (semiquantitative), sodium sulfite precipitation (semiquantitative), glutaraldehyde coagulation (coagulates above specific level), and serum gamma-glutamyltransferase activity (assays enzyme in high concentration in colostrum and absorbed simultaneously with colostrum). Total serum protein of greater than 5 g/dl measured by refractometer has been associated with adequate immunoglobulin concentrations in hydrated animals.

b. Laminitis (Subsolar Abscesses, White Line Disease)

Laminitis is common in ruminants, particularly in dairy cattle. Laminitis is often a sequel of acute or subacute ruminal acidosis (covered above) caused by sudden changes in diet or by diets containing excessive amounts of nonstructural carbohydrate (starch and sugars) and inadequate fiber. Laminitis also may be associated with febrile episodes such as mastitis, metritis, or respiratory disease. Facility conditions, such as concrete flooring and inadequate resting areas, may also contribute to the pathogenesis of laminitis. Abrupt changes in diet cause changes in rumen microbial populations resulting in acute or subacute ruminal acidosis and endotoxemia. Alterations in the vascular endothelium result in chronic inflammation of the sensitive laminae of the hoof, separation of corium and hoof wall, and rotation of the third phalanx.

Rotation of the third phalanx associated with laminitis frequently leads to subsolar abscesses. These abscesses commonly occur in toe or heel region of the sole due to pressure on the solar corium. Solar abscesses may progress to full-thickness defects in the sole with attendant infection. These animals are severely lame, reluctant to move, and subsequently lose body weight and production.

Diagnosis Affected animals may be reluctant to get up or walk, will shift their weight frequently, and will grind teeth or walk on carpi. Rotation of the third phalanx can result in paint-brush hemorrhages in the hoof sole and eventually sole abscesses. Chronically, the hoof wall takes on a 'slipper' appearance. Treatment consists of identifying and correcting the underlying cause, administering anti-inflammatories (flunixin meglumine) and regular foot trimming. Proper diet formulation, preparation, and delivery are crucial. Sole abscesses can be treated with trimming and bandaging. The cow's comfort and mobility can often be restored by gluing a wooden block or slipper onto the healthy claw in order to remove the weight burden from the claw with the abscess (Van Amstel, 2009).

c. Hemorrhagic Bowel Syndrome (Jejunal Hemorrhage Syndrome)

Hemorrhagic bowel syndrome (HBS) is an acute enteric disease, primarily affecting dairy cows in the first three to 3–4 four months of lactation. HBS was first reported in the 1990s but appears to be increasing in prevalence (NAHMS Dairy Studies, 2007). The disease can strike very rapidly and, at times, previously healthy cows are simply found dead. The notable lesion is hemorrhage into a segment of the small intestine, resulting in a blood clot which produces a functional obstruction. Depending on the rate and volume of the hemorrhage, some cattle may present in hypovolemic shock, with elevated heart rate, weak pulse, pale mucous membranes, and cold extremities. Cases with slower progression may present with abdominal distension, anorexia, fluid splashing sounds, or localized 'pings' in the lower right abdomen. Feces may be normal or tarry-colored or contain clotted blood. Most cases develop fatal septic shock within 24–48 h due to necrosis of the intestinal wall. The case fatality rate is reported to be 80–100%.

The etiology of HBS is not well-understood and is likely to be multifactorial. Many authors implicate *Clostridium perfringens* type A, but *Aspergillus fumigatus* also may play a role in the pathogenesis. The disease is associated with larger and higher-producing dairy herds and with energy-dense diets which have relatively low fiber levels.

On necropsy, purple or red discolored segments of small intestine will be identified. The intestinal contents may be mixed with unclotted blood, or firm blood clots may be tightly adhered to the mucosa (Van Metre, 2009).

Treatment for HBS usually is unsuccessful. Medical treatment with fluids, laxatives, anti-inflammatory agents, and antibiotics typically only prolongs the course of the disease. If the affected area(s) of bowel can be identified by laparotomy, the obstructed area may be relieved by gentle massage or the area of bowel may be resected.

d. Nutritional Diarrhea

In a laboratory setting, young ruminants should consume high-quality milk replacers which rely primarily on dairy products for their protein sources. Milk replacers should be mixed according to directions and fed at a consistent time and temperature. Although 'overfeeding' is often blamed for diarrhea in calves, there is no research to support this. Calves with *ad libitum* access to milk may consume up to 20% of their body weight in milk daily without developing diarrhea. However, poor-quality milk replacers and inconsistent preparation and presentation of milk replacers may exacerbate diarrhea due to enteric pathogens.

e. Photosensitization (Bighead)

Photosensitization is an acute dermatitis associated with an interaction between photosensitive chemicals and sunlight. Photosensitive chemicals are usually ingested but in some cases exposure may be by contact. Animals with a lack of pigment are more susceptible to the disease. Three types of photosensitization occur: primary, secondary or hepatogenous, and aberrant. Primary photosensitization is related to plant pigments or drugs such as phenothiazine, sulfonamides, or tetracyclines. Secondary photosensitization is more common in large animals, and is specifically related to the plant pigment phylloerythrin. Phylloerythrin, a porphyrin compound, is a degradation product of chlorophyll released by rumen microbial digestion. Liver disease or injury, which prevents normal conjugation of phylloerythrin and excretion through the biliary system, predisposes to photosensitization. The only example of aberrant photosensitization is congenital porphyria of cattle (see Section III, B, 1).

Pathologically, the photosensitive chemical is deposited in the skin and is activated by absorbed sunlight. The activated pigments convert local amino acids and proteins to vasoactive substances which increase the permeability of capillaries leading to fluid and plasma protein losses and eventually local tissue necrosis. Photosensitization can occur within hours to days after sun exposure and produces lesions of the face, vulva, and coronary bands. Lesions are most likely to occur on white-haired or thinly haired areas. Initially, edema of the lips, corneas, eyelids, nasal planum, face, vulva, or coronary bands occurs. Facial edema, nostril constriction, and swollen lips potentially lead to difficulty breathing. With secondary photosensitization, icterus is also common. Necrosis and gangrene may occur. Diagnosis is based on clinical lesions and exposure to the photosensitive chemicals and sunlight. Treatment is symptomatic.

f. Reproductive (Vaginal, Uterine) Prolapses

Vaginal and uterine prolapses occur in ewes and cows and less commonly in does. Vaginal prolapses usually occur during late gestation and may be related to relaxation of the pelvic ligaments in response to hormone levels. In sheep, these are most common in overconditioned ewes that are also carrying twins or triplets.

The condition may result from excessive straining associated with dysuria from the pressure of the fetuses and/or abdominal contents on the bladder. If the prolapse obstructs subsequent urination, rupture of the bladder may occur. The vaginal prolapse can be reduced and repaired if discovered early. Techniques for replacement in small and large ruminants are comparable. The animal should be restrained and the prolapsed tissue should be cleansed with disinfectants. Best done under epidural anesthesia, the vagina is replaced into the pelvic canal and the vulvar or vestibular opening is sutured closed (Buhner suture). Alternatively, a commercial device called a bearing retainer (or truss) can be placed into the reduced vagina and tied to the wool, thereby holding the vagina in proper orientation without interfering with subsequent lambing.

Vaginal prolapses may have a hereditary basis in ewes and cows and may recur the following year. These animals should be culled. Vaginal prolapses may occur in nonpregnant animals grazing estrogenic plants or as sequelae to docking the tail too close to the body (Ross, 1989).

Uterine prolapses occur sporadically in postpartum ewes and cattle. The gravid horn invaginates after delivery and protrudes from the vulva. The cause is unknown, but excessive traction utilized to correct dystocia or retained placenta, uterine atony, hypocalcemia and over-conditioning or lack of exercise have been implicated. In cattle, the uterine prolapses usually develop within 24 h of calving, are more common in dairy than beef cows, and are often associated with dystocia or hypocalcemia. Cows may also have concurrent parturient paresis. Initially, the tissue will appear normal, but edema and environmental contamination or injuries of the tissue develop quickly. The weight of the prolapsed uterus can potentially tear the mesometrial arteries resulting in fatal hemorrhage.

Clinical signs will include increased pulse and respiratory rates, straining, restlessness, and anorexia. If identified early, the uterus can be replaced as for vaginal prolapses, taking care to avoid trauma to the exposed endometrium. Electrolyte imbalances (particularly hypocalcemia) should be corrected if present. Passively infusing several gallons of warm fluid into the uterus following reduction will aid in completely inverting the uterine horns. Additional supportive therapy including the use of antibiotics should always be considered. Tetanus prophylaxis should be included. Oxytocin should be administered to induce uterine involution, but only after the uterus has been replaced. Vaginal closures are less successful at retaining uterine prolapses. Preventative and control measures include regular exercise for breeding animals, prevention of hypocalcemia and management of body condition in cows and ewes.

g. Rectal Prolapse

Rectal prolapses are common in growing, weaned lambs and cattle from 6 months to 2 years old. The physical eversion of the rectum through the anal sphincter is usually secondary to other diseases or management-related circumstances. Rectal prolapses may occur secondary to gastrointestinal infection or inflammation, especially when the colon is involved. Diseases such as coccidiosis, salmonellosis, and intestinal parasites that cause tenesmus may result in prolapse. Urolithiasis may result in rectal prolapses as the animal strains to urinate. Any form of cystitis or urethritis, vaginal irritation or vaginal prolapse, and some forms of hepatic disease may lead to rectal prolapses. Abdominal enlargement related to advanced stages of pregnancy, excessive rumen filling or bloat, and overconditioning may cause prolapses as can coughing during respiratory tract infections, or improper tail docking (too short).

Diagnosis is based on clinical signs. Early prolapses may be corrected by holding the animal with the head down, while a colleague places a purse-string suture around the anus. The mucosa and underlying tissue of prolapses that have been present for longer periods of time will often become necrotic, dry, friable, and devitalized and will require surgical amputation or the placement of prolapse rings to remove the tissue. Rectal prolapses may also be accompanied by intestinal intussusceptions that will further complicate the treatment and increase mortality. Occasionally, acute rectal prolapses with evisceration will result in shock and prompt death of the animal. Prognosis depends on the cause, extent of the prolapse as well as timeliness of intervention. In all cases, determination and elimination of the underlying cause is essential.

h. Trichobezoars, Phytobezoars, and Enteroliths

Gastrointestinal accumulations or obstructions of hair, indigestible plant material or other foreign material can occur in cattle and sheep. Cattle that are maintained on a low-roughage diet, that lick their coats frequently, that have long hair coats from outdoor housing, or that have heavy lice or mite infestations, will often develop trichobezoars. In addition, younger calves with abomasal ulcers have been found to more likely to also have abomasal trichobezoars. Enteroliths also can form from indigestible material that the animals have consumed (e.g., plastic bale twine or sheeting).

Clinical signs may be mild or severe according to size, number, and location. Ruminal trichobezoars rarely result in clinical signs. Obstruction will be accompanied by signs of pain, development of bloat, and decreased appetite and fecal production. Diagnosis is based on abdominal auscultation, rectal palpation, and ultrasound (useful in calves and smaller ruminants). Treatment is surgical, such as paracostal laparotomy (for abomasal), rumenotomy, or right paralumbar celiotomy (for obstruction of the duodenum, jejunum, or spiral colon). Supportive care should be administered as necessary to correct electrolyte imbalances and prevent inflammation and sepsis. Prognosis is generally good if the condition is diagnosed and treated before dehydration and imbalances become severe and peritonitis develops. Prevention includes good-quality roughage, treating lice and mange infestations, and avoiding incorporation of plastic materials into mixed rations.

C. Traumatic

1. Wounds, Bites, Entrapped Foreign Bodies

Wounds may be sustained from poorly constructed facilities or from skirmishes among animals. Predators will usually be sources of bite wounds, and the potential for rabies exposure should be considered. Frontal sinusitis is a potential complication of dehorning older ruminants. Standard veterinary wound assessment and care are essential for wounds or bites. Tetanus antitoxin may be indicated. Use of approved antibiotics may be appropriate. Wounds should be cleaned with disinfectants and repaired with primary closure if clean and uncontaminated. Thorough cleaning and regular monitoring and healing by second intention are recommended for older wounds. Abscesses may also occur in the soft tissues of the hooves due to entrapped foreign bodies or hoof cracks filling with dirt. Paraphimosis may be seen in male ruminants associated with hair rings around the penis. Preventative measures include improvement of housing facilities, pens, and pastures; monitoring hierarchies among animals penned together; and implementing predator control measures, such as sound fencing or flock guard dogs or donkeys in pasture situations. Seasonal fly control to avoid maggot infestation of wounds must be considered.

D. Iatrogenic

1. Anaphylactic Reactions

Acute anaphylactic reactions in sheep, goats and cattle are often clinically referable to the respiratory system. The lung is the major target organ in cattle for Type 1 hypersensitivity. Anaphylactic vaccine reactions cause acute lung edema; lungs are the primary site of lesions if collapse and death are sequelae. The animals will also be anxious, shivering and become hyperthermic. Salivation, diarrhea, and bloat also occur. Immediate therapy must include epinephrine (1 ml of 1:1000 per 50 kg body weight for goats; 1:10,000 [0.1 mg/ml], 0.01 mg/kg [about 5 ml], for adult cow) by intravenous infusion. Treatment should also include anti-inflammatories such as corticosteroids (dexamethasone, 5–20 mg IV) or NSAID's. Furosemide (5 mg/kg) may be beneficial to reduce edema. Tracheostomy may be indicated if pharyngeal or laryngeal edema is present. Prognosis is usually guarded. Recovery can occur within 2 h.

2. Catheter Sites, Experimental Surgeries

In a research environment, catheter sites or experimental surgeries may be sources of iatrogenic infection. Traumatic injuries to peripheral nerves or improper injection of pharmaceuticals can cause acute lameness. Contraction of the quadriceps results in the limb being pulled forward. Traumatic injury to the radial nerve can result in a 'dropped elbow.' Husbandry procedures such as tail docking, castration, dehorning, dosing with a balling gun, and shearing may result in superficial lesions, dermal infections, or cases of tetanus. Balling gun injuries to the pharynx may lead to cellulitis with coughing, decreased appetite and sensitivity to palpation.

Standard veterinary assessment and care are essential for these cases. Local and systemic antibiotics with supportive care may be indicated. Swelling around peripheral nerves caused by inoculations may be reduced by diuretics and anti-inflammatories. Mild cases of peripheral nerve damage may recover in 7–14 days. Personnel training, including review of relevant anatomy, pre-procedure preparation, appropriate technique, careful surgical site preparation, rigorous instrument sanitation, and sterile technique will minimize the incidence of potential complications from surgical procedures. Lastly, appropriate facilities and equipment kept in good repair will facilitate safe and effective restraint of large animals and help reduce incidence of these types of iatrogenic conditions.

E. Neoplastic

Neoplasia and tumors are relatively rare in ruminants. Lymphoma/leukemia in sheep has been shown to result from infection by a virus related (or identical) to the bovine leukemia virus. Pulmonary carcinoma (pulmonary adenomatosis) and hepatic tumors are found in sheep. Pulmonary adenosarcoma in sheep, described previously, is a transmissible viral disease. Also, virus-induced papillomatosis as discussed earlier, and squamous cell carcinomas have also been reported in sheep.

In goats, thymoma is one of the two most common neoplasias reported, although no distinct clinical syndrome has been described. Cutaneous papillomas are the most common skin and udder tumor of goats, and although outbreaks involve multiple animals, no wart virus has been identified. Persistent udder papillomas may progress to squamous cell carcinoma. Lymphoma is reported rarely in goats.

Lymphoma of various organ systems and 'cancer eye' (bovine ocular squamous cell carcinoma, BSCC) are the most commonly reported cancers in cattle. Lymphoma is described above under Bovine Leukemia Virus (Section III, B, 2, a, ii). Lack of periocular pigmentation, amount and intensity of exposure to solar ultraviolet light, and age are considered important factors in BSCC. Genetic factors may also play a role as many cases occur in Herefords. The cancer metastasizes through the lymph system to major organs. Treatment in either lymphoma or BSCC is recommended only as a palliative measure, although enucleation may be successful if the disease is still localized. The extent of ocular neoplastic involvement is a significant criterion for carcass condemnation. Papillomatosis (warts) is common in cattle, and the disease is described under viruses.

Forms of bovine lymphoma that are not associated with BLV infection are calf or juvenile; thymic or adolescent (animals 6 month to 2 years); and cutaneous (any age). The calf form is rare and characterized by generalized lymphadenopathy. Onset may be sudden, and the disease is usually fatal within a few weeks. Signs include lymphadenopathy, anemia, weight loss, and weakness. Some animals may be paralyzed due to spinal cord compression from subperiosteal infiltration of neoplastic cells. The adolescent form is also rare, the course rapid, and the prognosis poor. The disease is seen most often in beef breeds such as Hereford cattle and is characterized by space occupying masses in the neck or thorax. Secondary effects of the masses are loss of condition, dysphagia, and rumen tympany. The cutaneous presentation has a longer course that may wax and wane. Masses will be found at the anus, vulva, escutcheon, shoulder, and flank; they will be painful when palpated, will be raised and often ulcerated. The animals will be anemic, and neoplastic involvement may affect cardiac function. Generalized or limited lymphadenopathy may be apparent.

F. Miscellaneous

1. Amyloidosis

Amyloidosis in adult cattle is due to accumulations of amyloid protein in the kidney, liver, adrenal glands, and gastrointestinal tract. The disease is associated with chronic inflammatory disease, although other unknown factors are believed to be involved in some cases. Clinical signs include chronic diarrhea, weight loss, and nonpainful renomegaly and generalized edema. The loss of protein in the urine contributes to abnormal plasma albumin values and foaming urine. The proteinuria also distinguishes amyloidosis (and glomerulonephritis) from other causes of weight loss and diarrhea in cattle such as Johne's disease or parasitism. The diffuse nature and insidious onset make amyloidosis difficult to diagnose. Prognosis is poor and no treatment is reported.

2. Dental Wear

Ruminants have an intermandibular space that is narrower than the intermaxillary space. Dental wear is seen most commonly in sheep. As sheep age, excessive dental wear may lead to an inability to properly masticate feed, manifesting as weight loss and unthriftiness. Dietary contamination with silica (i.e., hays, grains harvested in sandy regions) will lead to mechanical wear on the teeth. Likewise, animals grazing or being fed in sandy environments will have excessive teeth wear. Sheep older than about 5 years of age are especially prone to teeth wear and should be checked frequently; especially if signs of weight loss or malnutrition are evident. Managing the content and consistency of the diets can best prevent the disease.

References

Major References Cited Addressing Husbandry, Management, and Clinical Medicine

American Veterinary Medical Association. <https://www.avma.org/KB/Resources/FAQs/Pages/ELDU-and-AMDUCA-FAQs.aspx>.

Anderson, D.E., Rings, M., 2009. Current Veterinary Therapy: Food Animal Practice, fifth ed. Saunders Elsevier, St. Louis, MO.

Code of Federal Regulations (CFR), 1985. Title 9 (Animals and Animal Products), Subchapter A (Animal Welfare). Office of the Federal Register, Washington, DC, Public Law, 89–544.

Davis, C.L., Drackley, J.M., 1998. The Development, Nutrition and Management of the Young Calf. Iowa State University Press, Ames, IA.

Federation of Animal Science Societies (FASS), 2010. Guide for the Care and Use of Agricultural Animals in Agricultural Research and Teaching, third ed. FASS, Savoy. Champaign, IL.

Grandin, T., 2007. Livestock Handling and Transport, third ed. CAB International, United Kingdom.

Hafez, E.S.E., Hafez, B., 2000. Reproduction in Farm Animals, seventh ed. Lippincott, Williams & Wilkins, Philadelphia, PA.

Hawk, C.T., Leary, S.L., 2005. Formulary for Laboratory Animals, third ed. Iowa State University Press, Ames, IA.

Houpt, K.A., 2010. Domestic Animal Behavior for Veterinarians and Animal Scientists, fifth ed. Wiley-Blackwell, Ames, IA.

Jurgens, M.H., Bregendahl, K., Coverdale, J., Hansen, S., 2013. Animal Feeding and Nutrition, eleventh ed. Kendall/Hunt Publishing Co., Iowa.

Kaneko, J.J., Harvey, J.W., Bruss, M.L., 1997. Clinical Biochemistry of Domestic Animals. Academic Press, San Diego, CA.

Kimberling, C.V., 1988. Jenson and Swift's Diseases of Sheep. Lea & Febiger.

Merck Veterinary Manual Online, 2011. Merk and Co. <www.merck-vetmanual.com>.

National Research Council, 2000. Nutrient Requirements of Beef Cattle, seventh Revised ed. National Academy Press, Washington, DC, Update 2000.

National Research Council, 2001. Nutrient Requirements of Dairy Cattle, seventh Revised ed. National Academy Press, Washington, DC, Update.

National Research Council, 2007. Nutrient Requirements of Small Ruminants: Sheep, Goats, Cervids, and New World Camelids. National Academy Press, Washington, DC.

National Research Council, 2011. Guide for the Care and Use of Laboratory Animals, eighth ed. National Academy Press, Washington, DC.

Plumb, D.C., 2011. Veterinary Drug Handbook, seventh ed. Iowa State University Press, Ames, IA.

Pugh, D.G., Baird, A.N., 2012. Sheep and Goat Medicine, second ed. Elsevier Saunders, Maryland Heights, MO.

Radostits, O.M., Gay, C.C., Hinchliff, K.W., Constable, P.D., 2007. Veterinary Medicine: A Textbook of the Diseases of Cattle, Horses, Sheep, Pigs and Goats, tenth ed. WB Saunders, NY, ISBN 978-0702-07772.

Reece, W.O., 2004. Duke's Physiology of Domestic Animals, twelvth ed. Cornell University Press, Ithaca, NY.

Ross, C.V., 1989. Sheep Production and Management. Prentice-Hall, Inc., Englewood Cliffs, NJ.

Smith, B.P., 2009. Large Animal Internal Medicine, fourth ed. Mosby Elsevier, St. Louis, MO, ISBN 978-0-323-04297-0.

Smith, M.C., Sherman, D.M., 2009. Goat Medicine, second ed. Wiley-Blackwell, Ames, IA.

United States Department of Agriculture (USDA). March 25, 2011. Animal and Plant Health Inspection Service (APHIS), Policy #Farm17, Regulation of Agricultural Animals. Available at: <http://www.aphis.usda.gov/animal_welfare/policy.php?policy=17>.

Weiss, D.J., Wardrop, K.J., 2010. Schalm's Veterinarinay Hematology. Wiley-Blackwell, Hoboken, NJ.

Youngquist, R.S., Threlfall, W.R., 2007. Current Therapy in Large Animal Theriogenology, second ed. Saunders Elsevier, St. Louis, MO.

Additional References Cited or Used in the Preparation of this Chapter

21 CFR 530 1994. Animal Medicinal Drug Use Clarification Act (AMDUCA) <http://www.fda.gov/AnimalVeterinary/GuidanceComplianceEnforcement/ActsRulesRegulations/ucm085377.htm> (accessed 4.23.15).

A Guide to the National Scrapie Eradication Program for Veterinarians, 2009. <http://www.eradicatescrapie.org/Educational%20Resources/Vet%20Guide.html> (accessed 3.08.13).

American Veterinary Medical Association (AVMA) Backgrounders, 2012. <https://www.avma.org/kb/resources/backgrounders/pages/default.aspx> (accessed 3.08.13).

Armed Forces Institute of Pathology (AFIP), 1995. Animal Models of Human Disease. Registry of Comparative Pathology, Washington, DC.

Barr, B.C., Dubey, J.P., Lindsay, D.S., Reynolds, J.P., Wells, S.J., 1998. Neosporosis: its prevalence and economic impact. Suppl. Comp. Cont. Ed. Prac. Vet. 20 11(D).

Blackwell, T.E., Butler, D.G., 1992. Clinical signs, treatment, and postmortem lesions in dairy goats with enterotoxemia: 13 cases (1979–1982). J. Amer. Vet. Med. Assoc. 200 (2), 214–217.

Bretzlaff, K., Haenlein, G., Huston, E., 1991. The goat industry: feeding for optimal production. In: Naylor, J.M., Ralston, S.L. (Eds.), Large Animal Clinical Nutrition Mosby, St. Louis, MO.

Broad, T.E., Hill, D.F., Maddox, J.F., Montgomery, G.W., Nicholas, F.W., 1998. The sheep gene map. In comparative gene mapping. ILAR J. 39, 160–170.

Brujeni, G.N., Jani, S.S., Alidadi, N., Tabatabaei, S., Sharif, H., Mohri, M., 2010. Passive immune transfer in fat-tailed sheep: evaluation with different methods. Small Ruminant Res. 90, 146–149.

Bulgin, M.S., 1986. Diagnosis of lameness in sheep. Comp. Cont. Educ. Pract. Vet. 8, F122–F128.

Center for Food Security and Public Safety, 2005. <www.cfsph.iastate.edu/Factsheets/.../nontyphoidal_salmonellosis.pdf> (accessed 3.08.13).

Center for Food Security and Public Health, 2008. Bovine Babesiosis. Iowa State University, Ames, IA, http://www.cfsph.iastate.edu/Factsheets/pdfs/bovine_babesiosis.pdf.

Cibelli, J.B., Stice, S.L., Golueke, P.J., et al., 1998a. Cloned transgenic calves produced from nonquiescent fibroblasts. Science 280, 1256–1258.

Cibelli, J.B., Stice, S.L., Golueke, P.J., et al., 1998b. Transgenic bovine chimeric offspring produced from somatic cell-derived stem-like cells. Nat. Biotechnol. 16, 642–646.

Corbeil, L.B., 1995. Use of an animal model of trichomoniasis as a basis for understanding this disease in women. Clin. Infect. Dis. 21 (Suppl. 2), S158–S161.

Cornell Animal Health Diagnostic Center. <http://ahdc.vet.cornell.edu/clinpath/modules/coags/typeoth.htm> (accessed 3.08.13).

Council Report: Vaccination guidelines for small ruminants (sheep, goats, llamas, domestic deer, and wapiti), 1994. J. Am. Vet. Med. Assoc. 205, 1539–1544.

de la Concha Bermejillo, A., 1997. Maedi-Visna and ovine progressive pneumonia. Vet. Cin. North Am. Food Anim. Pract. 13, 13–33. (Abstract).

Dorella, F.A., Pacheco, L.G., Oliviera, S.C., Miyoshi, A., Azevedo, V., 2006. Corynebacterium pseudotuberculosis: microbiology, biochemical properties, pathogenesis and molecular studies of virulence. Vet. Res. 37 (2), 201–218. review.

Dorchies, P., Duranton, C., Jacquiet, P., 1998. Pathophysiology of oestrous ovis infection in sheep and goats: a review. Vet. Rec 142 (18), 487–489. Review.

Dougherty, R.W., 1981. Experimental Surgery in Farm Animals. Iowa State University Press, Ames, IA.

Dubey, J.P., 2005. Neosporosis in cattle. Vet. Clin. North Am. Food Anim. Pract. 21, 473–483.

Easley, N.E., Wang, M., McGrady, L.M., Toth, J.M., 2008. Biomechanical and radiographic evaluation of an ovine model for the human lumbar spine. Proc. Inst. Mech. Eng. Part H J. Eng. Med. 22 (6), 915–922.

Elsik, C.G., Tellam, R.L., Worley, K.C., 2009. The genome sequence of taurine cattle: a windo to ruminant biology and evolution. The bovine genome sequencing and analysis consortium. Science 324 (5926), 522–528.

Endsley, J.J., Roth, J.A., Ridpath, J., Neill, J., 2003. Maternal antibody blocks humoral but not T cell responses to BVDV. Biologicals 31 (2), 123–125.

Fecteau, G., George, L.W., 2009. Mentation abnormality, depression, and cortical blindness. In: Anderson, D.E., Rings, M. (Eds.), Current Veterinary Therapy: Food Animal Practice, fifth ed. Saunders-Elsevier, St. Louis, MO, pp. 301–311.

Fecteau, M.E., Whitlock, R.H., 2009. Abomasal ulcers. In: Anderson, D.E., Rings, M. (Eds.), Current Veterinary Therapy: Food Animal Practice, fifth ed. Saunders-Elsevier, St. Louis, MO.

Franz-Werner, S., Maddox, J., Ballingall, K., et al., 1996. The ovine major histocompatibility complex. In: Schook, L.B., Lamont, S.J. (Eds.), The Major Histocompatibility Complex Region of Domestic Animal Species CRC Press, Inc., Taylor and Francis Group, Boca Raton, FL.

Gao, J., Liu, K., Liu, H., et al., 2010. A complete DNA sequence map of the ovine Major histocompatibility complex. BMC Genomics 11, 466.

Garrigliany, M.M., Bayrou, C., Kleijnen, D., et al., 2012. Schmallenberg virus: a new shamonda/sathuperi-like virus on the rise in Europe. Antiviral Res. 95 (2), 82–87.

Geishauser, T., Leslie, K., Duffield, T., 2000. Metabolic aspects in the etiology of displaced abomasum. Metabolic disorders of ruminants. Vet. Clin. North Am. Food Anim. Pract. 16 (2), 255–265. WB Saunders, Philadelphia, PA.

Gerloff, B.J., Herdt, T.H., 2009. Fatty liver in dairy cattle. In: Anderson, D.E., Rings, M. (Eds.), Current Veterinary Therapy: Food Animal Practice, fifth ed. Saunders Elsevier, St. Louis, MO, pp. 146–149.

Gibbs, R.A., Taylor, J.F., Van Tassell, C.P., et al., 2009. Genome-wide survey of SNP variation uncovers the genetic structure of cattle breeds. Science (New York, NY) 324 (5926), 528–532.

Goff, J.P., 2006. Major advances in our understanding of nutritional influences of bovine health. J. Dairy Sci. 89 (4), 1292–1301.

Griffiths, D.J., Martineau, H.M., Cousens, C., 2010. Pathology and pathogenesis of ovine pulmonary adenosarcoma. J. Comp. Path. 142 (4), 260–283.

Hays, J.T., Suckow, M.A., Jackson, G.E., Douglas, F.E., 1998. Considerations in the design and construction of facilities for farm species. Lab. Anim. 27 (6), 22–25.

Heaton, M., Leymaster, K., 2012. Research on Genetic Susceptibility to Ovine Progressive Pneumonia at the USDA Meat Animal Research Center (USMARC). Clay Center, Nebraska, OPP Handout. www.ars.usda.gov.

Hefnawy, A.E.G., Totura-Perez, J.L., 2010. The importance of selenium and the effects of its deficiency in animal health. Small Rum. Res. 89, 185–192.

Herfat, M.T., 2005. Characterizing the Ovine Stifle Model as a Preclinical Biomechanical Surrogate for the Human Knee. PhD Dissertation, University of Cincinnati, OH.

Herrmann-Hoesing, L.M., White, S.N., Lewis, G.S., Mousel, M.R., Knowles, D.P., 2007. Development and validation of an ovine progressive pneumonia virus quantitative PCR. Clin. Vacc. Immun. 14 (10), 1274–1278.

Janke, B.H., 1989. Protecting calves from viral diarrhea. Vet. Med. 803–810.

Johnson, R., Kaneene, J.B., 1993a. Bovine leukemia virus. Part II: risk factors of transmission "Infectious Disease in Food Animal Practice." The Compendium Collection. Veterinary Learning Systems, Trenton, NJ.

Johnson, R., Kaneene, J.B., 1993b. Bovine leukemia virus. Part III: zoonotic potential, molecular epidemiology and an animal model "Infectious Disease in Food Animal Practice." The Compendium Collection. Veterinary Learning Systems, Trenton, NJ.

Johnson, R., Kaneene, J.B., 1993c. Bovine leukemia virus. Part IV: economic impact and control measures "Infectious Disease in Food Animal Practice." The Compendium Collection. Veterinary Learning Systems, Trenton, NJ.

Johnson, R., Kaneene, J.B., 1993d. Bovine leukemia virus. Part I: descriptive epidemiology, clinical manifestations, and diagnostic tests Infectious Disease in Food Animal Practice. The Compendium Collection. Veterinary Learning Systems, Trenton, NJ.

Jones, M.L., Meisner, M.D., 2008. Urolithiasis. In: Anderson, D.E., Rings, M. (Eds.), Current Veterinary Therapy: Food Animal Practice, fifth ed. Saunders Elsevier, St. Louis, MO, pp. 322–325.

Kimberling, C.V., Ellis, R.P., 1990. Advances in the control of foot rot in sheep. Vet. Clin. North Am. Food Anim. Pract. 6 (3), 671–681.

Kirk, J.H., Glenn, J.S., 1996. Mastitis in ewes. Comp. Cont. Educ. Pract. Vet. 18, 582.

Knowles Jr., D.P., 1997. Laboratory diagnostic tests for retrovirus infections of small ruminants. Vet. Clin. North Am. Food Anim. Pract. 13, 1–11. (Abstract).

Krause, K.M., Oetzel, G., 2006. Understanding and preventing subacute ruminal acidosis in dairy herds: a review. Anim. Feed Sci. Tech. 126 (3), 215–236.

Kuhn, E., 1993. Myotonia congenita (Thomsen) and recessive myotonia (Becker). Nervenarzt 64, 766–769.

Lewin, H.A., 1996. Genetic organization, poymorphism, and function of the bovine major histocampaticility complex. In: Schook, L.B., Lamont, S.J. (Eds.), The Major Histocompatibility Complex Region of Domestic Animal Species CRC Press, New York, pp. 65–98.

Liu, D., 2009. Handbook of Listeria Monocytogenes. CRC Press, Taylor & Francis Group, Boca Raton, FL.

Lovell, K.L., Matsuura, F., Patterson, J., Baeverfjord, G., Ames, N.K., Jones, M.Z., 1997. Biochemical and morphological expression of early prenatal caprine beta-mannosidosis. Prenatal Diag. 17, 551–557.

Martens, H., Schweigel, M., 2000. Pathophysiology of grass tetany and other hypomagnesemias: implications for clinical management. Vet. Clin. North Am. Food Anim. Pract. 16 (2), 339–368. WB Saunders, Philadelphia, PA.

Maurin, M., Raoult, D., 1999. Q fever. Clin. Microbiol. Rev. 12 (4), 518–553.

McAllister, M.M., Dubey, J.P., Lindsay, D.S., Jolley, W.R., Wills, R.A., McGuire, A.M., 1998. Dogs are the definitive hosts of Neospora caninum. Int. J. Parasitol. 28, 1473–1478.

McCappin, N., Murray, R.D., 2011. Some factors affecting pregnancy rate in ewes following laparoscopic artificial insemination. Vet. Rec. 168 (4), 99.

McKellar, Q.A., Jackson, F., 2004. Veterinary anthelmintics: old and new. Trends Parasitol. Oct 20 (10), 456–461.

Morrow-Tesch, J., 1997. Environmental enrichment for dairy calves and pigs. Animal welfare information center. Newsletter 7, 3–8.

NAHMS Dairy Studies, 2007. United States Department of Agriculture, Animal and Plant Health Inspection Service. <http://www.aphis.usda.gov/animal_health/nahms/dairy/#dairy2007>.

Ott, R.S., 1982. Dairy goat reproduction comp. Cont. Ed. Pract. Vet 4, s164–s172.

Pepin, M., Vitu, C., Russo, P., Mornex, J.F., Peterhans, E., 1998. Maedi-visna virus in sheep: a review. Vet. Res. 29, 341–367. (Abstract).

Piontkowski, M.D., Shivvers, D.W., 1998. Evaluation of a commercially available vaccine against Corynebacterium pseudotuberculosis for use in sheep. J. Am. Vet. Med. Assoc. 212, 1765–1768. (Abstract).

Quintin, A., McKellar, L., Jackson, F., 2004. Veterinary anthelmintics: old and new. Trends Parasit. 20 (10), 456–461.

Robbe-Austerman, S., 2011. Control of paratuberculosis in small ruminants. Vet. Clin. North Am. Food Anim. Pract. 27 (3), 609–620.

Rodolakis, A., Salinas, J., Papp, J., 1998. Recent advances on ovine chlamydophilal abortion. Vet. Res. 29, 275–288. (Abstract).

Rodriguez, S.M., Florins, A., Gillet, N., et al., 2011. Preventive and therapeutic strategies for bovine leukemia virus: lessons for HTLV. Viruses 3 (7), 1210–1248.

Rook, J.S., Kopcha, M., Spaulding, K., et al., 1986. The spider syndrome: a report on one purebred flock. Comp. Cont. Educ. Pract. Vet. 8, S402–S405.

Rychlik, T., Krawczyk, A., 2009. Class I marker polymorphism in polish mountain sheep of coloured and white varieties. Ann. Anim. Sci. 9 (4), 385–393.

Salerno, C.T., Droel, J., Bianco, R.W., 1998. Current state of in vivo preclinical heart valve evaluation. J. Heart Dis. 7, 158–162.

Sargison, N.D., 2012. Pharmaceutical treatments of gastrointestinal nematode infections of sheep – Future of anthelmintic drugs. Vet. Parasitol. 189 (1), 79–84.

Scheerlinck, J.P., Snibson, K.J., Bowles, V.M., Sutton, P., 2008. Biomechanical applications of sheep models: from asthma to vaccines. Trends Biotechnol. 26 (5), 259–266.

Sergeant, E.S.G., Marshall, D.J., Eamens, G.J., Kearns, C., Whittington, R.J., 2003. Evaluation of an agar gel immunodiffusion test kit for detection of antibodies to mycobacterium paratuberculosis in sheep. J. Am. Vet. Med. Assoc. 208, 401–403.

Sordillo, L.M., Streicher, K.L., 2002. Mammary gland immunity and mastitis susceptibility. J. Mamm. Gland Biol. Neoplasia. 7 (2), 135–146.

Stafford, K.J., 2007. Alleviating the pain caused by the castration of cattle. Vet. J. 173, 333–342.

Streeter, R.N., 2009. Bloat or ruminal tympany. In: Anderson, D.E., Rings, M. (Eds.), Current Veterinary Therapy: Food Animal Practice, fifth ed. Saunders-Elsevier, St. Louis, MO, pp. 9–11.

Stuen, S., Longbottom, D., 2011. Treatment and control of chlamydophilal and ricketsial infections in sheep and goats. Vet. Clin. North Am. Food Anim. Pract. 27 (1), 213–233.

Titi, H.H., Kridli, R.T., Alnimer, M.A., 2010. Estrus synchronization in sheep and goats using combinations of GnRH, progestagen and prostaglandin F2alpha. Reprod. Domest. Anim. 45 (4), 594–599.

Underwood, W.J., Rook, J.S., 1992. Toxoplasmosis infection in sheep. Compend. Contin. Educ. Pract. Vet. 14, 1543–1548.

United States Department of Agriculture, Animal and Plant Health Inspection Service (USDA/APHIS), Animal Health. <http://www.aphis.usda.gov/wps/portal/aphis/ourfocus/animalhealth>.

United States Department of Agriculture, Animal and Plant Health Inspection Service (USDA/APHIS), 2012. Animal Health – Animal Diseases – Scrapie Disease Information – Eradication Program. <www.aphis.usda.gov/animal_health/animal_diseases/scrapie>.

United States Food and Drug Administration; Animal Medicinal Drug Use Clarification Act of 1994 (AMDUCA). <http://www.fda.gov/AnimalVeterinary/GuidanceComplianceEnforcement/ActsRulesRegulations/ucm085377.htm>.

Uzal, F.A., Songer, J.G., 2008. Diagnosis of clostridium perfringens intestinal infections in sheep and goats. J. Vet. Diagn. Invest. 20 (3), 253–265.

Van Amstel, S.R., 2009. Noninfectious disorders of the foot. In: Anderson, D.E., Rings, M. (Eds.), Current Veterinary Therapy: Food Animal Practice, fifth ed. Saunders-Elsevier, St. Louis, MO, pp. 222–234.

Van Metre, D.C., 2009. Hemorrhagic bowel syndrome. In: Anderson, D.E., Rings, M. (Eds.), Current Veterinary Therapy: Food Animal Practice, fifth ed. Saunders-Elsevier, St. Louis, MO, pp. 55–57.

Wall, R.J., Kerr, D.E., Bondoli, K.R., 1997. Transgenic dairy cattle. Genetic engineering on a large scale. J. Dairy Sci. 80, 2213–2224.

Weil, J., Eschenhagen, T., Magnussen, O., et al., 1997. Reduction of myocardial myoglobin in bovine dilated cardiomyopathy. J. Mol. Cell. Cardiol. 29, 743–751.

Welch, R.D., Ashman, R.B., Baker, K.J., Browne, R.H., 1996. Intraosseus infusion of prostaglandin E2 prevents disuse-induced bone loss in the tibia. J. Orthop. Res. 14, 303–310.

Womack, J.E., 1998. The cattle gene map. Comparative gene mapping. Inst. Lab. Anim. Res. J. 39, 153–159.

16

Biology and Diseases of Swine

Kristi L. Helke, DVM, PhD, DACVP[a], Paula C. Ezell, DVM, DACLAM[b], Raimon Duran-Struuck, DVM, PhD, DACLAM[c] and M. Michael Swindle, DVM, DACLAM, DECLAM[d]

[a]Departments of Comparative Medicine and Pathology and Laboratory Medicine, Medical University of South Carolina, Charleston, SC, USA [b]Intuitive Surgical, Inc., Norcross, GA, USA [c]Columbia Center of Translational Immunology, Department of Surgery; Institute of Comparative Medicine; Columbia University Medical Center, New York, NY, USA [d]Medical University of South Carolina, Department of Comparative Medicine and Department of Surgery, Charleston, SC, USA

OUTLINE

I. INTRODUCTION

Swine are used in biomedical research both as general large-animal biological models in teaching and research, and for the study of specific disease conditions due to their anatomic and physiological similarities to humans (Swindle, 2007; Helke and Swindle, 2013; McAnulty, 2012; Swindle *et al.*, 2012; Kobayashi *et al.*, 2012; Matsunari and Nagashima, 2009; Critser *et al.*, 2009). Over the last decade, swine have become the default model for surgery models as well as translational research, which bridges the gaps between basic science research and clinical applications. The Swine Genome Sequencing Consortium has completed the sequencing of the pig genome, which will help researchers find the putative genes needed to facilitate model development in areas such as cardiovascular disease, xenotransplantation, and neurodegeneration. Textbooks specific to the use of swine as laboratory

Laboratory Animal Medicine, Third Edition
DOI: http://dx.doi.org/10.1016/B978-0-12-409527-4.00016-X

animals are available as are websites and proceedings from symposia on the use of swine in research (McAnulty, 2012; Swindle, 2007; Bollen *et al.*, 2010; Minipigs, 2010; Forum, 2013; Tumbleson, 1986; Swindle *et al.*, 1992). Images of all disease entities are available online on several websites (Cornell Veterinary Medicine, 2012; Iowa State University, 2014; Veterinarians, 2013).

While this chapter covers many porcine diseases, many are included for completeness. Some of the diseases have been eradicated from the United States (US) and European Union (EU) and are mentioned here because they are reportable. Also, most readers of this chapter will purchase research animals from a vendor providing specific pathogen-free (SPF) swine. This suggests that there is some essence of biosecurity in place and that many of the diseases are rarely, if ever, seen in the research population. The most important factors to consider when encountering disease in research pigs are as follows: (1) research and husbandry personnel – in this era of global travel, we need to consider reverse zoonosis (especially with swine influenza virus (SIV)), and also protecting people in contact with the animals which may be harboring these diseases, and (2) emerging diseases – since the last iteration of this chapter, we have added porcine circovirus-2 (PCV2), Nipah virus, porcine lymphotrophic herpes virus, Ebola virus, and others, some of which were discovered only after human infection.

A. Taxonomy

Order: Artiodactyla (even-toed ungulates)
Family: Suidae
Species: *Sus scrofa domestica*

B. Availability and Sources

Commercial breeds of domestic swine raised for meat production are available worldwide. There is extensive variability in the health status of the various herds. In the US, the designation SPF has a proprietary connotation. It is a program based on management procedures that reduce or eliminate diseases that stunt growth. Pigs designated SPF are a good source for biomedical research; however, the designation does not mean that the animals are completely free of diseases that may interfere with research. It is best to purchase animals from a herd in which the institutional veterinarian has screened for research-complicating diseases. Commercial breeds have limited availability from commercial suppliers of laboratory animals (Safron and Gonder, 1997; Swindle *et al.*, 1994).

When using domestic breeds of swine, the growth rate is a major consideration. Swine reach sexual maturity and a commercial slaughter weight of approximately 115–130 kg at 5–6 months of age. At birth, they weigh approximately 1.4 kg (average); consequently, there is an

exponential growth phase during the adolescent period. Most swine used in research programs are 15–30 kg and are 8–12 weeks of age. Weight gain during this period may be 2–5 kg per week. When selecting a model, age and maturity factors must also be considered. Consequently, domestic swine are rarely used for long-term projects unless the study includes the effect of growth and maturity factors or the animals are involved in agricultural research. Generally, most projects involving a length of >3 weeks would best be performed in miniature swine (Swindle, 2007; Fisher, 1993; Swindle *et al.*, 1994).

Miniature swine are available from commercial breeders of laboratory animals. Commonly used breeds include Yucatan, Hanford, Sinclair, Hormel, and Göttingen. Other breeds of miniature pigs are available in limited quantities from some market areas and include the Panepinto, Vietnamese potbellied, Ohmini, Pitman–Moore, and Chinese dwarf. Generally, the health status of these animals is higher than that of SPF animals, and they are suitable for most biomedical research projects. These animals range from 30 to 50 kg in body weight at sexual maturity and, consequently, are more amenable than larger commercial breeds to long-term projects (Fisher, 1993; Swindle, 1998, 2007; Panepinto, 1986).

C. Laboratory Management and Husbandry

Individual shipments of swine are best separated by time and distance and, in particular, mixing animals from multiple vendors is poor practice. Swine should be purchased from vendor herds that are validated brucellosis-free and qualified pseudorabies-negative by the U.S. Department of Agriculture (USDA). Commercial sources typically implement a vaccination and parasite-control program beginning at weaning age and dependent on the intended experimental use of the animal, such efforts may or may not need additional attention at the research facility. Quality source suppliers will deworm piglets at 4- to 6-week intervals and administer preventive treatments for ectoparasites. Weanling animals are commonly vaccinated against erysipelas and leptospirosis, and breeding animals should be vaccinated in addition against porcine parvovirus, *Bordetella bronchiseptica, Pasteurella multocida*, and *Escherichia coli*. Newly received animals should be given a minimum of 72 h to adjust to the new environment during which time physical exams and screening tests for parasites can be performed (Smith and Swindle, 2006). Ideally, diet changes should be gradual over several days, with increased fiber if stress-induced diarrhea develops. Adult swine that are housed long term should have, at a minimum, periodic physical exams that include weight and parasite checks. Vaccination programs for adult swine should be implemented based on risk assessment that considers how the animal will be used in research, what the housing conditions are, and how close the research herd is to incoming animals of uncertain health status. Ideally, pigs should be purchased from one source with established health status to take advantage of natural herd immunity. The value of good herd health management is illustrated by the observation that swine herds that maintain SPF status have an odds ratio of 0.2 relative to that of conventional herds for the development of diarrhea (Moller *et al.*, 1998).

Swine are best housed in pens rather than in cages. Pens may be constructed of either chain-link fencing or stainless steel or aluminum bars. Wood is best avoided because of pigs' ability to chew it and the difficulty of sanitation. The chosen material should be of sturdy construction because swine can be very destructive. It is best to provide them with indestructible toys or balls to preoccupy them and to satisfy their rooting instincts (Swindle, 2007).

Flooring for swine deserves special consideration. Smooth flooring, such as seamless epoxy, is best avoided. Swine have difficulty with firm footing on these floors, especially when the floors are wet. If contact flooring is used, it should have a rough surface to provide traction and provide wear on the hooves or it should be covered with deep wood-chip bedding. Wood-chip bedding keeps swine clean and satisfies their rooting instinct. However, wood-chip bedding is eaten by swine, especially when they are fasted. Raised flooring has been found to be satisfactory in many laboratory situations. Plastic-coated metal grids are sturdy and easy to sanitize. However, if a cut becomes apparent in the plastic, swine will strip the flooring and eat the plastic. Slatted fiberglass floors with grit to provide hoof wear are generally ideal in most situations. They are lightweight and easy to remove from pens for sanitation (Swindle, 2007).

Swine readily use automatic watering systems. The system should be checked daily to ensure that the water supply is functional because swine are susceptible to 'salt poisoning,' which results in a neurologic syndrome when they are deprived of water. Individual feeding bowls will reduce food aggressive behavior. Food dishes should be secured to the cage or flooring. Swine will tip movable dishes and lose their feed, especially on raised flooring. They will also chew their feeders, which are best made of an indestructible material such as stainless steel (Swindle, 2007).

Swine prefer to have contact with other members of their species. They may be housed together in groups, but dominance fighting will occur unless animals are socialized. Providing cage walls that allow visual and snout contact between animals (Swindle, 2007; Fisher, 1993; Panepinto, 1986) may also satisfy this social instinct. New guidelines require attempts to be made to house social animals in stable pairs or compatible groups unless single housing is scientifically justified

or behavioral issues prohibit cohabitation (Institute of Laboratory Animal Resources (U.S.), Committee on Care and Use of Laboratory Animals, 2011).

Swine can be restrained in slings, such as the Panepinto sling (Panepinto *et al.*, 1983). This method is more humane than agricultural methods such as snout tying and is therefore preferable. Small swine can also be restrained manually in a manner similar to that of dogs. Swine may be trained to walk on a leash and can also be restrained against the side of the cage with portable handheld panels (typical size 60 × 80 cm) (Swindle, 2007).

Intramuscular injections may be administered in the neck or hind limb. Venous access sites include the following veins: auricular, cephalic, external and internal jugular, anterior vena cava, lateral saphenous, cranial abdominal (mammary), and femoral (Figs 16.1–16.8).

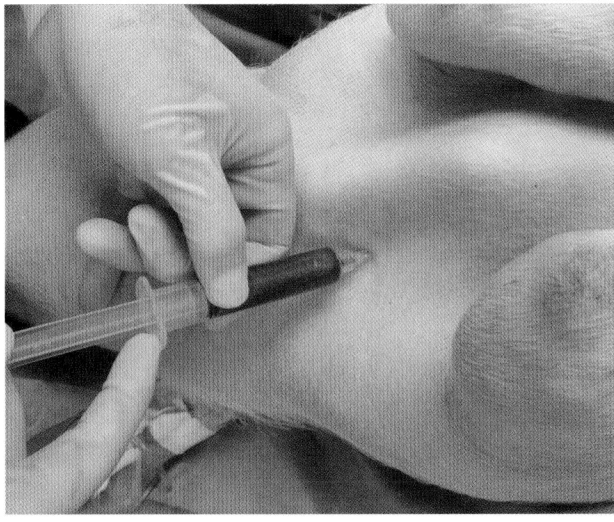

FIGURE 16.1 Blood collection from the cranial vena cava. To prevent damage to the recurrent laryngeal nerve, samples should only be collected from the right side.

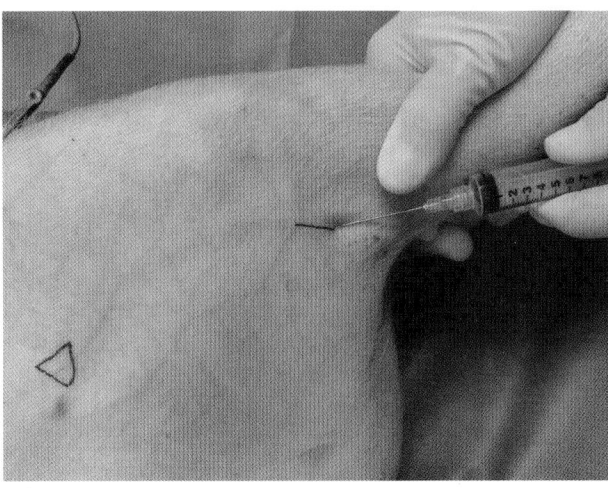

FIGURE 16.2 Venipuncture site of the left saphenous vein.

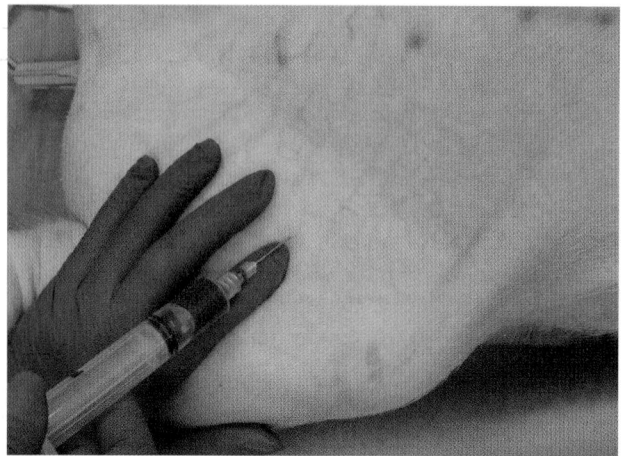

FIGURE 16.3   Venipuncture of femoral vein. Palpate the pulse with a finger and then guide needle into vessel. The vessel is not visualized on the surface.

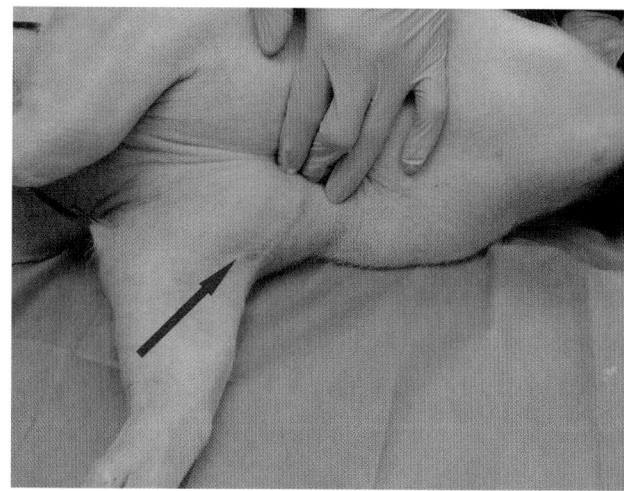

FIGURE 16.6   Venipuncture site of the cephalic vein. The vessel courses from the forelimb into the thoracic inlet. Two branches of the vessel are visible.

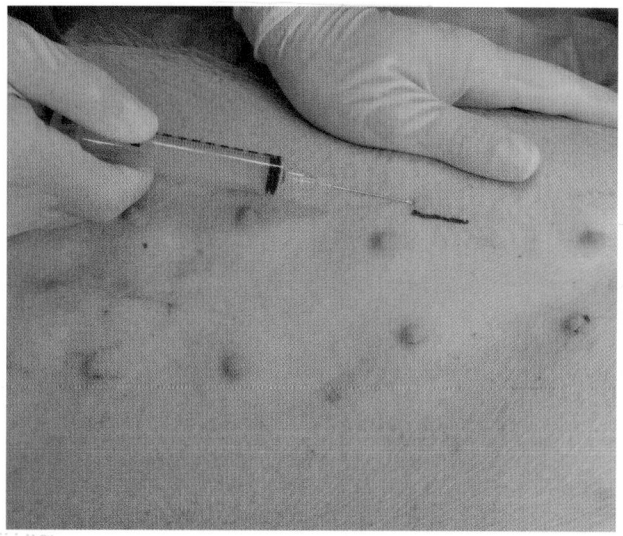

FIGURE 16.4   Venipuncture site of the mammary vein.

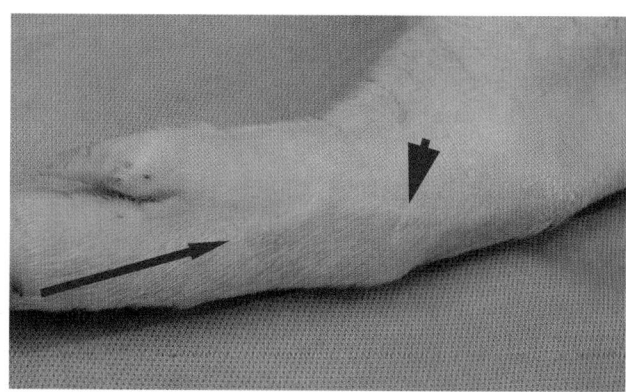

FIGURE 16.7   Venipuncture sites for accessory cephalic vein (arrowhead) and common dorsal digital vein (arrow).

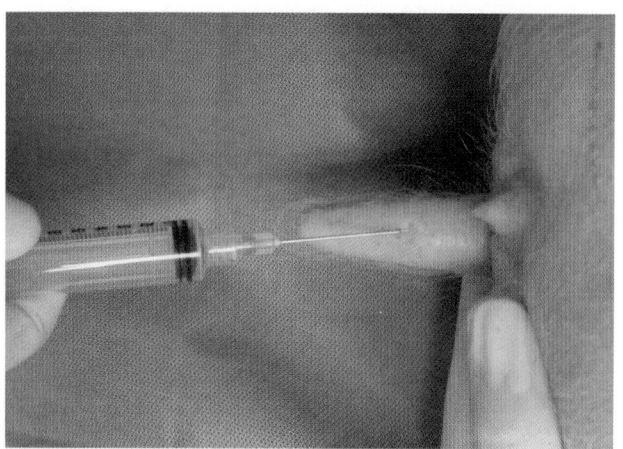

FIGURE 16.5   Venipuncture site of the tail vein.

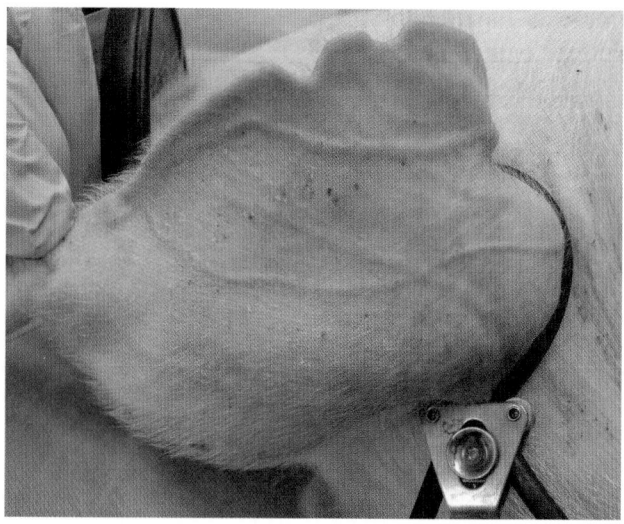

FIGURE 16.8   Dilation of auricular veins using a tourniquet.

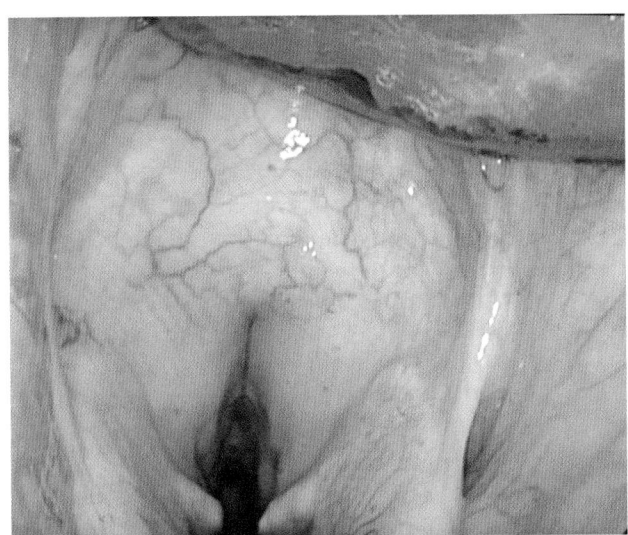

FIGURE 16.9 Visualization of vocal folds using a laryngoscope with animal in dorsal recumbency.

Most of the peripheral vessels are deep and not visible; consequently, knowledge of their anatomic location is essential. Most of the vessels can be accessed with standard-sized needles and a 20-gauge 1.5-inch needle is the largest size that will be required in swine up to 50 kg (Swindle, 1998; Bobbie and Swindle, 1986).

Surgical procedures, anesthesia, and anatomy, including surgical approaches for vascular access and fistulation procedures, are described in detail in other references (Swindle, 2007). A common problem is intubation of the pig. Intubation can easily be performed with the pig in dorsal recumbency using a laryngoscope to lift the tongue and mandible to visualize the vocal cords (Fig. 16.9).

D. Use in Research

Swine have been used mainly for research involving the cardiovascular system because of their unique anatomy and physiology, which makes them similar to humans (Swindle, 2007; Stanton and Mersmann, 1986). Cardiovascular diseases in which the pig is a useful model include atherosclerosis, coronary arterial stenosis and infarction, congenital heart disease, volume- and pressure-overload heart failure, electrophysiology, and testing of grafts, stents, and interventional devices. Swine are also susceptible to atherosclerosis. There are several models, the Rapacz familial hypercholesterol-emia model, and induced models where feeding of high-cholesterol and fat-enhanced diets to standard breeds induces the disease (Bahls et al., 2011, 2013). Some breeds are much more susceptible to diet-induced atherosclerosis than others. A more rapid form of atherosclerosis may be induced by damaging the endothelium with a balloon catheter (balloon endarterectomy). The induced

form has the advantage of producing a lesion in a specific anatomic area. Genetic models of high-membranous ventricular septal defect (VSD) and von Willebrand's disease are also available (Swindle et al., 1990).

Nutritional and gastrointestinal models in swine are studied because of the physiology of their digestion, which is similar to that of humans, and their omnivorous diet. Areas of study include nutrient absorption and growth, gastrointestinal transport, hepatic metabolism, total parenteral nutrition, and necrotizing enterocolitis.

Renal diseases are another area of interest in research. Swine have been used in studies of renal hypertension, vesicoureteral reflux, intrarenal reflux, and urinary obstruction.

Swine have been increasingly used in research and teaching studies that involve surgery, both as a substitute for dogs and as a model based on physiologic characteristics (Swindle, 1986). Swine are the model of choice for most of the laparoscopic and endoscopic procedures because of their size and anatomy. Catheter delivery of interventional devices has also been studied extensively in swine. Transplantation research has been performed on the heart, lung, liver, kidney, and viscera. The size of the organs, the surgical anatomy, and the response to immunosuppressive therapy make them ideal for many of these studies. Swine are being developed as models and donors for xenotransplantation, which has included the development of transgenic strains (Swindle, 1998). The anatomic and physiologic characteristics of the skin have made swine a definitive plastic surgery model. Swine have also been developed as models in a wide variety of other surgical procedures, including fetal surgery and procedures in the musculoskeletal, central nervous, gastrointestinal, urogenital, and cardiopulmonary systems.

Many other biological models have been developed in swine, including the areas of systemic and dermal toxicology, septic and hemorrhagic shock, immunology, diabetes, malignant melanoma, malignant hyperthermia, and gastric ulceration. An exhaustive list of all the developed and potential models in swine is beyond the scope of this chapter. Extensive reviews of that information may be found in general reference and proceedings books.

II. BIOLOGY

A. Unique Physiologic Characteristics and Attributes

References with complete descriptions of swine anatomy and physiology are available (Swindle and Swindle, 2007). However, some of the unique characteristics of swine will be covered in this section.

The cardiovascular system is similar to that of humans, especially the coronary anatomy (Swindle and

Swindle, 2007). The blood supply from the coronary artery is right-side dominant and does not have pre-existing collateral circulation. This makes the coronary blood flow situation similar to 90% of that of the human population, unlike that in other species such as the dog. The electrophysiological system is more neurogenic than myogenic, and there are prominent Purkinje fibers. The left azygous (hemiazygous) vein drains the intercostal vessels into the coronary sinus unlike in most other species. This vessel may be ligated or blocked with a balloon catheter to provide total coronary venous drainage into the coronary sinus. The aorta has a true vaso vasorum like that of humans. Normal values for hematology and serum chemistry and urine physiology for swine are listed in Table 16.1.

The gastrointestinal tract has unique anatomic characteristics (Swindle and Swindle, 2007). The stomach has a muscular outpouching, the torus pyloricus near the pylorus. The bile duct and pancreatic duct enter the duodenum separately in the proximal portion. The anatomic divisions between the duodenum, ileum, and jejunum are indistinct. The mesentery is thin and friable. The mesenteric vessel branches form their vascular arcades in the sub-serosa of the intestine rather than in the mesentery as in other species. The majority of the large intestine is arranged in a spiral colon in the left upper quadrant of the abdomen. This series of centrifugal and centripetal coils includes the cecum and ascending, transverse, and majority of the descending colon. Tenia and haustra are present on the cecum and large intestine. In spite of the anatomic differences from humans, the physiology of digestion and intestinal transport are very similar.

Other unique anatomic features need to be considered (Swindle and Swindle, 2007). The lymph nodes are inverted with the germinal centers being located in the internal portion of the node. The thymus is located on the ventral midline of the trachea near the thoracic inlet rather than proximal to the larynx, and has fused lobes and appears as a single organ. A major portion of the thymus is located in the neck, and the single pair of parathyroid glands is located in the medial aspect of this gland near the larynx. The penis is fibromuscular with a corkscrew-shaped tip located in a preputial diverticulum near the umbilicus. The penis has a sigmoid flexure as it exits the pelvic canal. The male accessory glands include the prostate, vesicular gland, and bulbourethral glands. The female reproductive system is composed of a bicornuate uterus with lengthy tortuous fallopian tubes. The pancreas is bilobed and surrounds and encompasses the superior mesenteric vein. The liver is organized into lobules by microscopic fibrous septae. The cytochrome P450 system is similar to that in humans, but many subtle differences exist which may impact toxicity studies (Helke and Swindle, 2013).

B. Nutrition

A comprehensive text on swine nutrition has been published (Lewis and Southern, 2001). There is considerable variation of the genetic capacity for accretion of lean body mass among the various breeds of swine utilized in biomedical research. The 'farm swine' include breeds developed for meat production and at 6 months of age may have a lean body weight five- to sixfold greater than that of a micropig breed. The published research on swine nutrition is focused on farm swine and maximization of lean growth (Table 16.2). The majority of mini- and microswine nutritional research is proprietary and is reflected in the commercially available formulations offered by feed companies. In general, the nutrient requirements of these breeds are similar; however, the small breeds often require fixed-quantity feeding to control obesity, especially for long-term research studies. This in turn necessitates a higher margin of safety for many nutrient concentrations to prevent deficiencies, since most commercially available diets are designed for free-choice feeding. Diets formulated for the mini- and microbreeds generally have lower energy and higher fiber concentrations. The daily energy and quantity of feed required by farm pigs is quite different from that which is required by mini- and microbreeds.

Swine, unlike ruminants, do not require elemental sulfur in their diets when adequate sulfur-containing amino acids (methionine and cysteine) are available. Sulfur is essential for synthesis of various body compounds such as taurocholic acid, chondroitin sulfate, glutathione, and lipoic acid. Methionine alone can meet the total sulfur-containing amino acid requirement in swine because cysteine can be synthesized from methionine. The amino acid requirements (Table 16.2) refer to the L-isomer, which is the most biologically active form in swine and most common form found in plants and animals (National Research Council (U.S.), Committee on Nutrient Requirements of Swine, 2012).

C. Reproduction

1. Reproductive Physiology

Swine reach sexual maturity at 3–7 months of age, with most miniature breeds becoming sexually mature at 4–6 months of age. Litter size varies among breeds, with domestic swine usually having an average of eight to 12 pigs per litter and miniature breeds, four to six pigs. Litter size also varies with parity, being smallest at the first parity, increasing to a maximum between the third and seventh parities, and then remaining stable or decreasing (Kirkwood et al., 2012).

The pig is polyestrous with an average estrous cycle of 21 days with a range of 17–25 days. Estrus typically lasts 48h (range 1–3 days). Prior to the onset of estrus,

TABLE 16.1 Porcine Hematology and Clinical Chemistry Values

	Farm pigs[a,b,c]	Hanford[a] Male	Female	Yucatan[a,e] micropigs	Gottingen[d,e] Male	Female
RBC	5–8	6.6–9.3	6.4–8.3	5.6–8.8	7.1–8.5	7.2–8.4
Hemoglobin	10–16	11.4–12.8	11.4–13.5	13.1–17.0	11.2–12.8	10.9–12.9
Hematocrit	32–50	35–55	38–56	36.3–53.7	36.7–41.5	36.3–41.7
MCV	50–68	48.1–63.1	54.1–63.9	58.2–72.5	46.1–54.7	46.0–53.6
MCH	17–21	13.7–18.6	15.9–18.8	18.9–24.3	13.9–16.9	13.8–16.6
MCHC	30–34	30.8–33.7	31.7–33.1	31.1–34.5	29.8–31.2	29.6–31.4
Platelets	320–520	172–845	152–751	217–770	406.1–628.1	460.8–666.4
Reticulocytes	0–1	18.9–235.0	18.4–251.0		0.8–2.6	0.6–1.6
Plasma proteins	6–8					
Fibrinogen	100–500				5.6–8.2	4.2–5.4
WBC	11,000–22,000	21,300–32,400	16,800–26,700	6900–21,200	8800–13,600	9200–13,000

NEUTROPHILS

	Farm pigs[a,b,c]	Hanford[a] Male	Female	Yucatan[a,e] micropigs	Gottingen[d,e] Male	Female
Band	0–880	10,800–24,600	7600–19,500	0.0–200		
Segs	3080–10,450			1800–6400	2500–5600	1900–4900
Lymphocytes	4300–13,600	7190–17,980	5590–17,330	2100–7100	5100–8500	5600–8600
Monocytes	200–2200	240–1320	140–1470	200–1500	200–300	300–500
Basophils	0–440	50–210	50–500	0–500	0–100	0–100
Eosinophils	55–2400	10–1490	10–1190	0–1300	0–200	0–200
Glucose (mg/dl)	65–95	94–118	91–123	56–153	85.5–115.1	84.1–116.1
BUN (mg/dl)	8–24	12–17	10–16	10–29	7.4–11.2	5.7–9.9
Creatinine (mg/dl)	1.0–2.7	0.5–1.1	0.6–0.8	1.2–2.0	1.0–1.2	1.0–1.1
Phosphorus	4.0–11.0	5.6–7.3	7.7–10.7	5.0–8.3	7.9–9.9	7.2–10.0
Calcium (mg/dl)	11.0–11.3	10.4–11.4	10.0–11.4	9.3–11.6	10.9–11.9	10.9–11.7
Total protein	7.9–8.9	6.1–7	5.8–6.6	6.3–9.4	4.9–5.7	5.0–5.8
Albumin	1.8–3.3	3.3–4	3.1–4.3	4.1–5.6	2.9–3.5	2.9–3.5
Globulin	5.3–6.4	2.4–3.7	2.1–3.5	1.4–3.6	1.9–2.3	2.0–2.4
A/G		0.9–1.7	0.9–1.9	1.11–3.49		
Sodium (mEq/l)	139–152	140–146	139–144	142–153	142.7–149.3	139–147
Chloride (mEq/l)	100–105	99–102	98–102	95–114	102.1–106.3	99.6–105.4
Potassium (mEq/l)	4.9–7.1	4.7–6.8	4.6–6.3	3.9–5.2	6.3–7.7	5.9–7.3
CO_2	18–26	24–28	20–29			
AGAP		12–17	14–20			
Total bilirubin	0.1–0.2	0.11–0.41	0.09–0.16		0.2–0.4	0.1–0.3
Indirect bilirubin	—	0.09–0.41	0.07–0.15			
Alkaline phosphate	26–362	166–484	206–576		189.1–345.9	199.7–303.3
GGT(IU/l)	10–52	31–75	29–49	20.4–46.8	68.8–93.2	68.9–96.4
AST (U/l)	9–113	42–90	33–59	15–53	21.7–43.9	23.0–36.8
LDH (U/l)	380–630	510–758	490–593			
CK (U/l)	0–500	270–735	221–628		13.6–591.8	107.2–470.6
Na/K	—	21–30	23–31			

[a]From Fox (2002).
[b]Studdert et al. (2012).
[c]Jackson and Cockcroft (2007).
[d]Minipigs (2010).
[e]Swindle (2007).

TABLE 16.2   Daily Nutrient Requirements of Growing Swine[a]

Parameters (body weight in kg)	10–20	20–50	50–80
Digestible energy of diet (kcal/kg)	3400	3400	3400
Estimated digestible energy intake (kcal/day)	3400	6305	8760
Metabolizable energy of diet (kcal/kg)	3265	3265	3265
Estimated metabolizable energy intake (kcal/day)	3265	6050	8410
Estimated feed intake (gm/day)	1000	1855	2575
Crude protein (%)	20.9	18.0	15.5
Water (l) (2.5 l/kg feed consumed)	2.5	4.6	6.4
Fatty acid requirements – linoleic acid (g)	1.0	1.86	2.58

AMINO ACID REQUIREMENTS (G/DAY) (TOTAL BASIS)

Arginine	4.6	6.8	7.1
Histidine	3.7	5.6	6.3
Isoleucine	6.3	9.5	10.7
Leucine	11.2	16.8	18.4
Lysine	11.5	17.5	19.7
Methionine	3.0	4.6	5.1
Methionine + cystine	6.5	9.9	11.3
Phenylalanine	6.8	10.2	11.3
Phenylalanine + tyrosine	10.6	16.1	18.0
Threonine	7.4	11.3	13.0
Tryptophan	2.1	3.2	3.6
Valine	7.9	11.9	13.3

MINERAL ELEMENTS

Calcium (g)	7.0	11.13	12.88
Phosphorus, total (g)	6.0	9.28	11.59
Phosphorus, available (g)	3.2	4.27	4.89
Sodium (g)	1.5	1.86	2.58
Chlorine (g)	1.5	1.48	2.06
Magnesium (g)	0.4	0.74	1.03
Potassium (g)	2.6	4.27	4.89
Copper (mg)	5.0	7.42	9.01
Iodine (mg)	0.14	0.26	0.36
Iron (mg)	80.0	111.3	129.75
Manganese (mg)	3.0	3.71	5.15
Selenium (mg)	0.25	0.28	0.39
Zinc (mg)	80.0	111.3	129.75
Vitamins			
Vitamin A (IU)	1750	2412	3348
Vitamin D$_3$ (IU)	200	278	386

(Continued)

TABLE 16.2   (Continued)

Vitamin E (IU)	11	20	28
Vitamin K (menadione) (mg)	0.5	0.93	1.29
Biotin (mg)	0.05	0.09	0.13
Choline (g)	0.4	0.56	0.77
Folacin (mg)	0.3	0.56	0.77
Niacin, available (mg)	12.50	18.55	18.03
Pantothenic acid (mg)	9.0	14.84	18.03
Riboflavin (mg)	3.0	4.64	5.15
Thiamin (mg)	1.0	1.86	2.58
Vitamin B$_6$ (mg)	1.5	1.86	2.58
Vitamin B$_{12}$ (ng)	15.00	18.55	12.88

[a]Fox (2002).

sows will exhibit signs of vulvar reddening and swelling, mucous discharge, nervousness, and increased activity. During estrus, sows will stand immobile when pressure is applied to the rump (Braun, 1993). Silent estrus is common in swine, but the presence of a boar can facilitate estrus detection (Kirkwood et al., 2012).

Optimal fertilization rates occur when insemination takes place 12 h prior to ovulation. However, the variability in the interval between onset of estrus and ovulation makes it difficult to determine when females ovulate. As a result, commercial producers usually breed sows twice during estrus to maximize conception rates. Litter size also tends to increase with multiple matings per estrus. In pen mating, the sow and boar are left together during estrus. Hand mating involves placing the sow and boar in the same pen at 12- to 24-h intervals during estrus until the female is no longer receptive (Kirkwood et al., 2012). Swine may also be bred by artificial insemination; however, conception rates are typically 10–15% lower compared to natural service. Satisfactory results are obtained if sows are inseminated 10–30 h after the beginning of estrus (Einarsson, 1980).

2. Pregnancy

Failure to return to estrus 18–24 days following mating is the first sign of pregnancy. Non-estrous sows are most easily detected by daily exposure to a boar during this time. In pregnant sows, rooting, walking, standing, and general activity decrease with increases in inactivity and time spent sleeping (Marchant-Forde and Marchant-Forde, 2004). These changes may be subtle and determination of pregnancy can also be based on whether or not the physical and behavioral changes of estrus are observed approximately 21 days post assumed mating date (Braun, 1993). Estrus detection has been reported to be 98% accurate and can be used to determine pregnancy status soon after failure of conception or death of a litter (Kirkwood et al., 2012).

Other pregnancy detection procedures include the use of ultrasound and hormone assays. Ultrasound is <90% accurate and cannot be performed prior to the fourth week of gestation. Amplitude-depth ultrasound units can be used to detect pregnancy reliably between 30 and 90 days and as early as 18 days with some equipment. They are handheld devices that detect interfaces between fluid and tissues, which is the reason why they lose sensitivity at either early or late gestation. Doppler ultrasonography can be used from 4 weeks until farrowing and can also be used to determine litter size as well as fetal viability in late gestation (Kirkwood et al., 2012; Braun, 1993).

Activity of the corpora lutea can be measured by progesterone assays. Progesterone concentrations of <1 ng/ml on days 17–19 of the estrous cycle are typical of non-pregnant females. An elevated progesterone concentration on day 18 after breeding is indicative of pregnancy. Estrone sulfate assays are more accurate for determining pregnancy status than progesterone assays. Estrone sulfate, produced by the fetus, reaches peak blood levels at 23–30 days gestation (Braun, 1993).

3. Parturition and Neonatal Care ~~GESTATION 114-15~~

Swine have a diffuse epitheliochorial placenta necessitating colostrum for maternal antibody protection of the piglets from infectious agents. The gestation period of miniature pigs and commercial pigs is typically 114–115 days. Signs of impending parturition are usually evident during the last week of gestation. The vulva becomes swollen and more reddened during the last 3–4 days. Development and distension of individual mammary glands occur during the last 2–3 days of gestation, and drops of clear or straw-colored fluid can be expressed. This is followed by the initiation of milk secretion. Characteristically, abundant milk can be expressed at the onset of farrowing. The interval between the initiation of milk flow to parturition is typically 6–12 h and provides a somewhat reliable sign of farrowing. Increased respiratory rate is most reliable. Behavioral changes occur during the 24 h preceding farrowing and include restlessness and nesting. Frequent urination, defecation, and chewing or biting on surrounding objects may also be noted. However, just prior to birth, this activity diminishes and the sow becomes recumbent (Braun, 1993; Day, 1980).

Use of a farrowing crate is seldom necessary. The week prior to the anticipated farrowing date, sows should be placed in a quiet room in a stall with abundant bedding material for nest building. Wood chips are ideal for farrowing stalls since they allow the sow to engage in nesting behavior. They also help maintain the neonates' body temperature since newborn piglets lack the ability to effectively thermoregulate. Environmental temperature should be 85–95°F with a supplemental heat source

in the stall that results in a temperature of approximately 90°F at pig level (Fisher, 1993). Hanging heat lamps are commonly used and should be positioned to be effective without causing burns. The sow's comfort level is approximately 68–70°F, which is the reason for having a supplemental heat source just for the neonates. Newborns should not be exposed to drafts or moisture.

The duration of farrowing ranges from less than 1 h up to 8 h, but typically lasts 3–4 h; larger litters may have a longer farrowing duration. The sow displays little physical exertion during the birth process. Sows generally remain laterally recumbent while giving birth but will occasionally change to a standing or ventrally recumbent position. The interval between the birth of piglets is typically 15 min. Assistance should be provided if more than 30–60 min elapse between the delivery of piglets (Day, 1980; Braun, 1993).

The most important factors that contribute to neonatal survival are the ability of the piglets to receive colostrum within the first 12 h of birth, adequate nutrition, and appropriate environmental conditions (Reeves, 1993). Competition is normal among littermates during nursing and can result in inadequate colostrum and milk intake in less dominant animals. Neonates must consume colostrum with in the first 12–24 h before their gut loses the ability to absorb immunoglobulins. Neonates will compete for, and establish, teat order on their day of birth. This hierarchy remains until weaning (Sawatsky, 1993). If necessary, the technique of split suckling can be used to ensure that all animals can nurse. This involves removing half of the litter comprising the largest piglets three to four times a day to allow the smaller animals to nurse adequately (Kirkwood et al., 2012; Reeves, 1993). The sow's milk supply should be checked daily to prevent piglet deaths from dysgalactia. Commercial pig milk replacers are available and should be provided to piglets by bottle or pan feeding if the sow is unable to produce an adequate milk supply.

One nutrient requirement that is particularly important for newborn piglets is iron. Nursing piglets require 21 mg of iron for each kilogram of growth and sow's milk contains approximately 1 mg of iron per liter (National Research Council (U.S.), Committee on Nutrient Requirements of Swine, 2012; Brady et al., 1978). Therefore, a microcytic, hypochromic anemia can develop. Nursing piglets can obtain some additional iron if allowed access to the feces of the sow; however, deficiency is still a common clinical problem. Consequently, it is routine practice in most swine herds to give 100–200 mg of iron dextran IM within 48 h of farrowing to prevent iron deficiency anemia.

Preweaning mortality is enzootic in most herds, but mortality varies depending on the prevalence of the various causes, which include poor viability at birth, chilling, starvation, trauma, diarrhea, and other diseases

(Kirkwood *et al.*, 2012). Trauma includes incidences of piglets that are stepped on, suffocated when lain on, and savaged by the female. Savaging is a behavior observed occasionally in individual animals, resulting in injury to and/or death of the piglets. The only recourse is to remove the piglets from the sow and to cull her from the breeding herd.

Day 1 care for piglets includes disinfection of the navel, clipping of the canine or 'needle' teeth, injection of an iron supplement, identification of individual animals, weighing, and clinical exam (Reeves, 1993; Fisher, 1993). The environmental temperature should remain at 85–90°F for animals up to 3–4 weeks of age. Animals 4–8 weeks old can be housed in rooms with temperatures at 75–80°F. Swine are generally weaned at 3–5 weeks by allowing them access to a solid ration.

D. Behavior

Swine are highly social and intelligent animals. They have a highly developed sense of smell, but poor eyesight. Group-housed swine are frequently observed vocalizing to each other. Pigs have an innate need to root, which can become destructive if they are not provided with an adequate outlet for expression. Housing strategies should accommodate swine behavioral needs as much as possible within the constraints of experimental design. Group housing or housing two animals per cage can be used to allow social interactions among animals. If individual housing is necessary, cages should be close together, and their design should include openings at the bottom to facilitate contact. Providing bedding material such as wood shavings is an excellent way to satisfy pigs' rooting behavior. Bedding material has the additional advantage of absorbing excreta but can be more labor-intensive for the husbandry staff than slatted or mesh flooring. Alternatively, a variety of toys, such as balls, chains, or hoses, can be supplied to help provide cage enrichment (Fisher, 1993; Sawatsky, 1993). Rotation of toys can keep the enrichment experience novel. Providing environmental enrichment that promotes species-specific behavior can enhance the well-being of swine and reduce fighting. Minipigs and farm pigs prefer toys that are chewable and can be easily misshapen. A recent environmental enrichment study indicated that minipigs prefer soft, pliable toys over hard, nonpliable toys (Smith *et al.*, 2009).

Swine are readily trained and respond well to positive reinforcement in contrast to conventional agricultural handling practices. This characteristic can be used to advantage in the research setting when animals must be handled or restrained for research manipulations. Acclimating and training swine to tolerate research equipment that will be used on them should be a standard procedure and can include the use of various types of food rewards given for reinforcing wanted behaviors. Gentle handling and the use of a humane restraint sling are warranted whenever swine need to be transported from their home cages or when restraint is necessary during noninvasive procedures. Many pigs respond to gentle rubbing of the ventral abdomen by rolling over onto their sides, enabling caregivers to perform such minor procedures as wound cleansing or suture removal without restraining the animals. This type of handling is very effective for positively reinforcing contact between pigs and their caretakers and has a calming effect on most animals.

E. Immunology and Use of Swine in Xenotransplantation

1. Immunology

Normative data for the swine immune system, such as lymphoid tissue weights and percentages of cell subsets represented in different tissues, are influenced by the animal health status, as data derived from animals of conventional health status (i.e., farm environments) differ significantly from data derived from those housed under SPF, gnotobiotic, or axenic conditions.

The pig has a large population of what were initially considered 'null' cells, which lack expression of CD2, CD4, or CD8, but are known to express CD3, classifying them as T cells. The lymphoid population is largely comprised of γδ T cells and is found in large numbers in various tissues, especially mucosal sites (such as the uterus). These are also highly prominent in the newborn. γδ T cells from swine are similar to the ones described from ruminants (Davis *et al.*, 1998). Expression of CD4 (T-helper) and CD8 (T-cytotoxic) is mutually exclusive in most species, but swine (similar to human and monkey) have a unique lymphocyte subset that expresses both CD4 and CD8 (Thome *et al.*, 1994). The CD8 marker that is expressed is part of α (and not β) chain. CD4+ CD8+ (αα) upregulation is commonly present in activated T cells. This subset may represent a type of memory cell or a lineage that differentiates from CD4+ CD8– to CD8+. In combination with CD45 and CD62L markers, central versus peripheral and naive versus activated T cells can now be identified in swine. There has been an increase in the identification of cluster of differentiation (CD) markers to phenotype lymphocyte subsets. Many homologous CD markers have now been identified, and a limited number are available commercially from the American Type Culture Collection (Manassas, Virginia) and Pharmingen, Inc. (San Diego, California).

Many hybridomas are available for the research community at the Massachusetts General Hospital Transplantation Biology Research Center. A monoclonal antiporcine CD3 antibody has been identified that is capable of activating or depleting T cells *in vitro* and inducing an immunosuppressive state *in vivo*, which will greatly facilitate studies of the swine immune system, in particular, induction of tolerance in xenotransplantation research (Huang *et al.*, 1999). These have the CD3 antibody linked with diphtheria toxin. Other swine-specific T-cell-depleting antibodies such as CD4 and CD8 have also been used (Pennington *et al.*, 1988). Bone marrow (BM) of swine is more similar to that of humans than of rodents, especially when dealing with toxicity in response to lethal irradiation. This has allowed studies that have demonstrated the benefit of T-cell depletion of donor tissues in preventing graft-versus-host disease (Sakamoto *et al.*, 1987). Immunological rejection is the major barrier to advancement in several areas of swine research. Therefore, thorough understanding of the complex intricacies of the swine immunological system is paramount to facilitating research in disciplines such as cancer, allotransplantation, and xenotransplantation research. A greater understanding of the swine immune system will help researchers develop translational models.

Immunoglobulins (Igs) of the pig are the most studied of those in farm species (Ober *et al.*, 1998). Neonates are colostrum dependent because maternal immunity is not conferred through the placenta. Access to IgG-rich colostrum within the first 6 h postpartum is most critical for 3-week survival rate and weight gain. Colostral leukocytes, largely neutrophils and T cells, are also absorbed by intercellular migration. Intestinal closure for absorption of colostrum is complete by 24–48 h of age. In contrast to most other species, the pig lacks the gene for IgD, which is a precursor immunoglobulin in the differentiation pathway to IgM. The pig does have a large number of IgG subclasses: IgG$_1$, IgG$_{2a}$, IgG$_{2b}$, IgG$_3$, and IgG$_4$. IgA circulates as a dimer in blood and tissues and as a monomer in mucosal secretions; IgE is found in serum and mucosal tissues. High endothelial venules of transplanted swine tissues express adhesion molecules, but information on the relative homology of these 'addressins' is limited in scope due to lack of reagents.

Cytokines and lymphokines in the pig have been studied in models associated with inflammation, such as sepsis, atrophic rhinitis, erysipelas, arthritis, and viral infections (Murtaugh, 1994; Ober *et al.*, 1998). Reports on swine cytokine regulation and function suggest that the biology is similar to that of humans and mice and that there is some limited homology; swine lymphocytes will respond to recombinant human interleukin (IL)-2 *in vitro* and also *in vivo* (Whary *et al.*, 1995). When injected into pigs, upregulation of regulatory T cells for the induction of tolerance has been attempted as a bridge to preclinical human transplantation. Rejection is observed when injected at high concentration. For cancer studies, the use of IL-2 has been controversial as depending on the dose, it may enhance antitumor responses, or if T regulatory cells are unevenly upregulated, then relapse may occur. The swine leukocyte antigens (SLAs), the equivalent of the human major histocompatibility complex (MHC), have been cloned and sequenced and are located in chromosome 7 in swine. Like all other MHC-I molecules, the SLAs are expressed by all nucleated cells and function to restrict CD8+ T-cell activation, particularly antiviral immune responses. The SLA class II (MHC-II) genes have been cloned and are restricted to professional antigen presenting cells such as B cells, macrophages, and dendritic cells. Contrary to mice and similar to humans, SLAs class II genes are also expressed in lymphocytes and vascular endothelium. Upregulation of MHC-II does occur during inflammatory processes. The number of SLA class III genes that have been cloned is lower than that found in other species. Member genes of the SLA class III complex function in the complement system, which in the pig is closely aligned with the human systems of classical and alternate pathways of complement activation. One difference between swine and humans is that elimination of antigen–antibody immune complexes occurs through the lung in the pig, in contrast to the target organs of the liver and spleen in humans (Davies *et al.*, 1995).

Red blood cell (RBC) antigen classification is very complex in the pig, with 16 genetic systems having been developed that consist of 78 blood factors, which are either antigens of the RBC itself or become cell-associated from other tissues when serum concentrations are high (Pescovitz, 1998). Knowledge of red cell surface expression is important during transplantation as disparities between donor and recipient can induce antibody-mediated hyperacute rejection, and thus, it is important to match blood types when working with MHC-characterized miniature swine.

Swine have been used as a model of allotransplantation including pancreatic islet, kidney, intestine, liver, composite tissue antigen, lung, heart, and bone marrow (Huang *et al.*, 2001). Currently, a new method has demonstrated that combining donor bone marrow with skin or solid organ transplant may contribute to tolerance induction (Horner *et al.*, 2008).

Immunodeficient swine are available in which human xenografts are not rejected. Acquired immunodeficient states can also be surgically induced by thymectomy, splenectomy and use of strong pan-immunosuppressants. Management-related or spontaneous cases of immunodeficiency have been attributed to inadequate colostrum, stress, or poor nutrition (Pescovitz, 1998). Autoimmune disease in swine is largely undocumented except for hemolytic disease in neonates related to postnatal absorption of maternal Igs (erythroblastosis fetalis) and two forms of glomerulonephritis. One form appears to be inherited in Norwegian Yorkshire swine, and a second involves spontaneous IgA nephropathy reported in Japanese slaughter pigs (Ober *et al.*, 1998).

2. Use of Swine in Xenotransplantation

About 120,000 people are currently waiting on the organ transplant list in the US. In 2012 a total of 6115 patients died while waiting for a compatible transplant (Sharing, 2013). There are several major concerns regarding the use of swine for xenotransplantation particularly zoonotic risks and ethical issues. First is the risk for acquired zoonoses, particularly in recipients already immunosuppressed by illness and chemotherapy. Second are the anticipated risks associated with normal flora, environmental contaminants, and true pathogens. And third is the concern regarding the unknown risks of viral latency, viral recombination, and endogenous retroviruses (Levy et al., 2000). Risks can be minimized by ensuring that donor animals must be free of potential zoonoses and other complicating diseases (Ye et al., 1994). The term 'xenograft-defined flora' rather than SPF should be used to designate the appropriate health status of donor animals in order to avoid confusion with existing standards (Swindle, 1998).

Although swine have fewer endogenous retroviruses than other vertebrates, and porcine endogenous retrovirus (PERVs) infections have not been documented, vigilant screening is paramount to minimize the risk of zoonotic infection. Despite these concerns, the transplantation community continues to grow, driven by the increasing demand for donor cells, tissues, and organs. There are ethical concerns, however, including public acceptance of these alternatives and regulatory issues. A plethora of organizations throughout the world have been established to address these issues. The World Health Organization has stressed the importance of developing checks and balances for future clinical trials. The Ethics Committee of the International Xenotransplantation Association was founded to promote xenotransplantation as a safe, ethical, and effective therapeutic modality (Anderson, 2006; Yang and Sykes, 2007; Schuurman et al., 2012). As this field develops, guidelines and regulations expand; the European Parliament and Council, the Food and Drug Administration, and the Public Health Service have all published guidelines. Significant steps forward in the process have been accomplished with the completion of swine genome mapping and the creation of transgenic pigs. Further research to understand the intricacies of swine immunology are instrumental in developing tools for xenotransplantation research. The comparable anatomy and physiology of the pig and human, defined herd health status, and the recent finding that over 100 porcine protein sequences share the same amino acids as their human orthologs, have indicated that with targeted genetic modification, the pig may be an ideal model for xenotransplantation. The experimental use of swine organs or tissues for humans faces significant scientific challenges however. These include, but are not restricted to, overcoming hyperacute, acute

and chronic rejection by the host. Nonetheless, despite all of these factors the pig, specifically the miniature pig, continues to be considered the prime candidate for xenotransplantation.

Optimization of miniature swine has been attempted in the last several decades. Development of disease-resistant swine organs has been promoted as a strategy to circumvent failure of transplanted organs resulting from human centric infectious agents such as hepatitis B virus (Mueller et al., 1999).

One important resource has been the cross-breeding of outbred miniature swine from the Andes and the Rockies to develop three lines of miniature swine which are homozygous for different SLA alleles. Once the alleles were identified, the swine were designated as SLA^{aa}, SLA^{cc}, and SLA^{dd}. The 'B' allele was either lost through the breeding process or was never present in the founder animals. These three lines are fixed at the SLA loci and are heterozygous at minor histocompatibility loci. Thus, MHCs matched with minor mismatches or full mismatch transplants are now possible which can reliably emulate clinical paradigms. Pairing donor and recipient within a line is used to model for transplants between MHC identical human siblings, between swine lines as a model for MHC full mismatches, and between F_1 hybrids for haplo-identical transplants, also known as parent-to-offspring transplants. Several recombinant strains have been bred where different SLA MHC-I or MHC-II recombinants exist. These intra-SLA recombinant strains have permitted the study of SLA class I and II differences and demonstrated the relevance of different SLA specific mismatches on graft survival of various tissues. As an example, it is easier to develop tolerance to a full MHC-I mismatched kidney than a full MHC-II. MHC-II is thought to permit optimal function of regulatory T cells, which are dependent on MHC-II matching (Griesemer et al., 2008). Matching of SLA skin grafts without immunosuppression typically has a survival of 7–12 days. The SLA^{dd} line was further inbred (brother sister matings) and currently has >95% consanguinity (Mezrich et al., 2003). Skin grafts between these swine survived more than 340 days before rejection occurred. These animals are several generations away from being fully inbred and the presence of developmental abnormalities has slowed the development of the line.

Pig studies have also been pivotal in the identification of the tolerogenic (or resistance to rejection) properties different organs may have. Some can now be ranked for their 'tolerogenicity'. Though the specifics are beyond the scope of this review, the transplant hierarchy of tolerance (from greater to lesser) is as follows: liver > kidney > heart > lung > skin.

The swine-to-baboon xenotransplantation model holds the promise of future technology transfer to enable swine-to-human solid organ and tissue/cell transplantation. Lack of long-term graft acceptance due to the potent immunological barriers encountered between disparate species has forced the field to generate multiple strategies to minimize rejection. Understanding of the different rejection processes of xenotransplantation is needed. The most immediate and serious causes of graft loss are now better understood and some can be prevented. The mechanisms responsible for hyperacute rejection (seconds to minutes) are no longer a problem. Thus, in some instances the swine grafts have lived in nonhuman primates (NHPs) for several months before being rejected (Yamada *et al.*, 2005), and in some cases, even without evidence of rejection at the time of death (by other causes). When discussing xenogeneic rejection, one must differentiate between humoral and cellular driven processes. Of the two, humoral rejection has been the cause of immediate graft loss known as hyperacute rejection (HAR). HAR is driven by natural antibodies that recognize the sugar moiety Galα1-3Galβ1-4GlcNAc (α1,3Gal) which is present in porcine endothelium. This sugar is produced by the enzyme α-1,3-galactosyltransferase which is present in most mammals but not in humans and old world monkeys. The enzyme was lost through evolution, possibly through the selective advantage of preventing infections by many bacterial pathogens that express α-1,3-Gal. Antibody-mediated recognition of this epitope on the swine vascular epithelium after transplantation triggers the complement cascade (Saadi and Platt, 1999). If HAR is avoided by either absorbing natural anti-Gal antibodies or using grafts deficient of the Gal antigen, a second potent antibody mediated response, inducing acute humoral xenograft rejection (AHXR) is observed. This is generally caused by non-Gal xenoreactive antibodies. The graft is eventually lost over several days/weeks by complement activation. However, other non-complement-mediated mechanisms are also capable of inducing graft loss. This was demonstrated by transplantation of decay accelerating factor DAF−/−(CD55−/−) donor mice into Gal-T KO mice (Shimizu *et al.*, 2006).

Resolution of humoral responses hindering induction of immunological tolerance is paramount; however, other factors of the innate and adaptive immune system elicit slower rejection of xenografts such as T-cell-mediated rejection and rejection caused by natural killer (NK) cells, macrophages, and neutrophils. Delayed rejection of xenografts through cell-mediated responses develops over 3–4 days, involving activation of endothelial cells of the graft as in the acute rejection response (Brouard *et al.*, 1999). Activation leads to loss of thrombomodulin and adenosine triphosphate diphosphohydrolase, which leads to prothrombosis, proinflammatory gene activation increasing the expression of adhesion molecules, prothrombotic factors, and cytokines. Adoptive cell transfer experiments in immunodeficient rodents have demonstrated that engrafted human CD4+ T cells mediate rejection of porcine xenografts as do NK cells and monocytes (Friedman *et al.*, 1999). T-cell-mediated rejection has not been as well characterized as humoral responses because of the difficulty avoiding HAR and AHXR. However, the development of Gal-knockout (KO) pigs has permitted the study in large animals of other non-humoral xenograft rejection mechanisms. Control of CD4+ T-helper cells is not only an important part of a T-cell-mediated response, but will provide control of AHXR (Sachs, 2005). CD8+ T-cell-mediated cytolysis continues to be a potent method of xenograft rejection. Pharmacological and nonpharmacological approaches to minimize their lytic function are crucial.

Activation of cells of the innate immune system via pathogen-associated molecular patterns potentiates NK cell and macrophage xenograft rejection. NK cells function by sensing inhibitory signals through MHC ligation. Because xenogeneic MHC cannot provide the necessary 'inhibitory' signals to the NK cells (when compared to allogeneic responses) NK-cell-mediated xenograft rejection is more potent in this context. (Sachs, 2005). Addition of human MHC expression on Gal-KO pigs will be able to better avoid NK-cell-mediated rejection. Another common NK-cell-mediated kill mechanism is via antibody-dependent cell cytotoxicity (ADCC). Both natural and IgG-specific antibody responses can induce ADCC-mediated xenogeneic rejection (Gourlay *et al.*, 1998). Macrophages are also involved in xenograft rejection, and they phagocytose the target tissues if they do not receive a negative signal through the interaction of CD172 (SIRPα) on the macrophage and CD47 on the cell surface molecule. This provides a common 'do not eat me' signal. Interspecies incompatibilities induce macrophage-mediated xenograft rejection (Wang *et al.*, 2007).

a. Methods to Prevent Rejection of a Xenograft

Removal of natural anti-Gal xenoantibodies can be performed by immunoabsorption. This method is efficient, but incomplete, and often xenoreactive natural antibodies rebound relatively quickly (Kozlowski *et al.*, 1998). There are two approaches for the elimination of natural antibodies: *in vitro*, using α-Gal immunoaffinity columns, or *in vivo*, by extracorporeal perfusion of a donor organ (often the liver is chosen based on its size and vascularity). There is no swine breed available with inherently low α-Gal or animals which have spontaneously lost the α-Gal gene (Chae *et al.*, 1999). Identification of such animals would have been crucial to starting a low α-Gal or α-Gal-deficient herd. In another approach, Brenner *et al.* reported that nonspecific depletion of the majority of recipient immunoglobulins of all isotypes by column immunoapheresis significantly improved graft survival of pig hearts in baboons (Brenner *et al.*, 2000). This strategy is clearly not clinically applicable as patients would not be able to survive long term without antibody-mediated protection.

Based on these facts, Sachs and colleagues knocked out the gene in the most inbred of the MGH miniature swine (the 'D' haplotype) (Kolber-Simonds *et al.*, 2004). These pigs were devoid of α-Gal from the SLA^dd pigs. Thus, these KOs have become the most likely donors to be used in clinical xenotransplantation.

Though beyond the scope of this chapter, there are currently several additional approaches to eliminating xenoantibodies. Anti-CD20 monoclonal antibodies which kill B cells have been used (McGregor *et al.*, 2005), but there are B cells that do not express CD20, and thus are not eliminated. The use of cobra venom factor has been a common (yet toxic) method for preventing activation of complement (Dwyer *et al.*, 2002). The use of pigs expressing human complement inhibitory molecules such as CD46, CD55, and CD59 has also been tried (Dwyer *et al.*, 2002). Transgenic expression of CD59, a human complement regulatory protein, has promoted survival of swine lungs in a pig-to-primate model (Kulick *et al.*, 2000; Yeatman *et al.*, 1999).

The development of immunological tolerance is theorized to be the most effective method to circumvent xenograft rejection (Li and Sykes, 2012). This approach addresses humoral and T-cell-mediated responses and has shown promise in the induction of donor-specific tolerance using bone marrow transplantation to create hematological chimeras. Tolerance to fully MHC-mismatched allografts has been demonstrated in mice and primates after first creating a mixed allogeneic hematopoietic chimerism by engrafting donor bone marrow cells into the recipient. However, this hematopoietic chimerism has been difficult to achieve in the discordant pig-to-primate xenogeneic model, most likely due to species-specific differences in regulatory cytokines and elements of the stromal microenvironment (Sablinski *et al.*, 1999; Emery *et al.*, 1999).

Representative of a typical experimental protocol and illustrative of the complexities involved, recipient primates undergo whole-body irradiation prior to infusion of pig bone marrow. This method was modified to minimize irradiation-induced inflammatory responses. Primate anti-pig xenoantibodies were immuno-adsorbed by extracorporeal perfusion of recipient blood through a pig liver immediately before the intravenous infusion of porcine marrow. In addition to cyclosporine and 15-deoxyspergualin, recombinant pig stem-cell factor and IL-3 were given. Other calcineurin inhibitors such as FK506 (Tacrolimus) are now being used instead. Anti-thymocyte globulin and/or anti-CD2 monoclonal antibodies to target T cells have also been

used. This permits, in part, the decrease of irradiation dosage. Thymic specific irradiation to prevent host resident thymic T cells from rejecting new bone marrow donor-derived thymic emigrants has been performed. Recipient primates required 4 weeks to recover from pancytopenia from whole body irradiation, and anti-pig IgM and IgG antibodies were temporarily depleted by the liver perfusion for 12–14 days. About 2% of the myeloid progenitors in the bone marrow of the recipient were of pig origin, and chimeras were unresponsive (or hyporesponsive) by mixed lymphocyte reaction when challenged with pig-specific stimulators. The first report of long-term survival of discordant xenogeneic bone marrow is in a primate recipient (Sablinski *et al.*, 1999). Others have reported on the poor function of porcine hematopoietic cells in primate marrow microenvironments. Warrens *et al.* found differences between swine and human bone marrow cultures in function of two well-characterized ligands known to be important in hematopoiesis, CD44 and very late antigen-4 (VLA-4), but they concluded that the differences were not significant enough to explain lack of effective porcine hematopoiesis in the primate marrow, suggesting that other unknown interactions may be important (Warrens *et al.*, 1998).

Gene therapy to express swine SLA class II antigens on baboon autologous bone marrow cells has had limited success (Ierino *et al.*, 1999). Transcription of the transgene was transient, and xenografts were rejected after 8–22 days. This experiment was important because it demonstrated that transfer and expression of xenogeneic class II transgenes can be achieved in baboons, and this therapy may prevent late T-cell-dependent responses to porcine xenografts, which include induced non-α-Gal IgG antibody responses. The use of porcine thymic grafts in immunodeficient mice has been found to support normal development of polyclonal, functional human T cells, and these T cells were specifically tolerant to SLA antigens of the porcine thymus donor, suggesting thymic transplantation may be an approach to achieve tolerance in pig-to-human xenotransplantation (Nikolic *et al.*, 1999). Indeed, this approach, by providing a thymokidney graft by Yamada *et al.*, demonstrated that baboon thymic precursors were developing in the pig thymus posttransplant (Yamada *et al.*, 2005).

The bone marrow chimerism tolerance approach is the one which has provided the longest survival and donor-specific tolerance. Refinement of this protocol will likely be the pathway that will lead swine xenotransplantation to the hospital floors. Before swine organs can be utilized as a successful alternative to human organ transplant, further research will be required to determine mechanisms to facilitate xenograft compatibility.

III. DISEASES

A. Infectious Diseases

Incidence of infectious disease in the research laboratory is greatly reduced when pigs are purchased from herds with defined health status, newly introduced animals are adequately quarantined and conditioned, and husbandry conditions are optimum. Veterinarians responsible for swine herd health should be familiar with both classical swine diseases and, more importantly, health problems that can emerge from opportunistic agents in animals stressed by experimental manipulation. Many of the diseases discussed below are in fact rare in the majority of modern, commercially reared pigs and will not be found in the commercially supplied miniature swine herds of high health status. However, new diseases continue to emerge and diseases that were once thought to be geographically isolated can spread.

Implementing treatment of infectious problems should be considered cautiously and is best reserved for those problems with minimal impact on the research use or health status of the research herd as a whole. In the following discussion of infectious diseases, classes of drugs are listed and culture and sensitivity is recommended before selecting and starting treatment. Likewise, the reader is referred to veterinary formularies (Plumb, 2011) for specific doses. Many of the drugs listed are extra-label use in swine; hence, veterinarians must determine a dose from experience with other species.

1. Polysystemic Diseases

a. Porcine Circovirus-2

A relatively new agent has emerged within recent years to cause a multitude of disease manifestations within the porcine world. The virus is often associated with other infectious agents. The disease syndromes are widely varied and affect all organ systems.

In 1998 the first report described porcine circovirus-2 (PCV2) as a causative (or cofactor) agent in porcine multisystemic wasting disease (PMWS) (Ellis et al., 1998; Allan et al., 1999). Many poly-systemic diseases have since been described which were determined to be multifactorial, the common denominator being that animals were nearly always co-infected with PCV2. Since then, PCV2 has been identified as causing or being associated with disease pathogenesis of many porcine syndromes including PMWS, porcine dermatitis and nephropathy syndrome (PDNS), PCV-associated disease (PCVAD), porcine respiratory disease complex (PRDC), acute pulmonary edema (APE), PCV2-associated neuropathy (PAN), reproductive failure, granulomatous enteritis, necrotizing lymphadenitis, and exudative epidermitis.

Etiology Porcine circovirus (family Circoviridae, genus *Circovirus*) is a nonenveloped RNA virus, the smallest virus to infect mammals. Since its initial discovery in cell culture in 1974, another serotype has been discovered (PCV2) which causes disease *in vivo*, and has been further divided into PCV2a and 2b (Tischer et al., 1986). PCV2a and 2b often result in coinfection (Opriessnig and Langohr, 2013). PCV2c, 2d, and 2e have also been identified in various countries and further studies are ongoing on these subtypes (Wang et al., 2009; Opriessnig and Langohr, 2013).

The differences between PCV2a and 2b are only two nucleotides, which have been proposed to lead to differences in pathogenesis. Disease severity has been shown to differ between PCV2a and 2b with 2b infection being associated with pulmonary edema, granulomatous enteritis, as well as lymphoid necrosis and depletion yet it remains unknown whether these differences are due to viral or host factors (Gillespie et al., 2009). However, some studies have found no difference in pathogenicity (Trible and Rowland, 2012).

Epizootiology and Transmission PCV is highly prevalent in the worldwide pig population, and greater than 50% of feral swine are positive for PCV2 antibodies (Rose et al., 2012; Sandfoss et al., 2012). PCV has prolonged shedding in respiratory and oral secretions and is highly resistant within the environment. Complete inactivation is difficult and extended exposure times to disinfectant agents are required (Kim et al., 2009b; Rose et al., 2012). PCV is transmitted via feces, urine, and direct transmission as well as transplacentally, through the colostrum, and via seminal fluid (Gillespie et al., 2009; Rose et al., 2012). After the virus gains access, tonsils and lymph nodes of the head are infected. Initially, type B lymphocytes are infected followed by T cells and peripheral blood mononuclear cells (Gillespie et al., 2009). Animals are typically 4 weeks old before clinical signs appear, suggesting that maternal antibodies are protective (Gillespie et al., 2009). There is evidence of a global shift from PCV2a to PCV2b, which is reported to be associated with more severe disease, and for which the current vaccines are not protective (Rose et al., 2012).

Pathogenesis The pathogenesis of PCV2-associated syndromes remains unclear and has not been fully elucidated (Darwich and Mateu, 2012; Gillespie et al., 2009). Many factors are involved, most of which have been investigated, yet no clear unifying mechanism has yet been discovered (Darwich and Mateu, 2012). Many multisystemic diseases have been attributed to PCV2. Lesions are often only seen when animals are coinfected with other agents such as porcine parvovirus (PPV), porcine reproductive and respiratory syndrome virus (PRRSV), or *Mycoplasma hyopneumoniae*, which prime or activate the immune system. Studies in caesarian-derived, colostrum-deficient pigs inoculated with PCV2 alone can cause lesions, albeit only with immunostimulation via adjuvants.

Current thought is that PCV2 infects macrophages, or endothelial cells directly. PCV2 has been shown to infect endothelial cells resulting in activated phenotype, degeneration of endothelial cells, perivascular and intramural edema, fibrinoid necrosis, and vascular thrombi (Opriessnig and Langohr, 2013). In conventional pigs infected with PCV2a or 2b alone, clinical disease is not observed, nor is there any difference between animals infected with a single serovar. When archival tissue collected from pigs before the advent of PMWS was examined and tested, PCV2 was present, albeit avirulent (Krakowka et al., 2012). Mutational events within a specific epitope led to the increased virulence of PCV2 (Krakowka et al., 2012).

Macrophages in bone marrow, thymus, and thymic lymphocytes label positive for PCV2 in infected animals (Hansen et al., 2013; Nauwynck et al., 2012). Viral replication is present in both thymus and bone marrow (Hansen et al., 2013). Lymphoblasts support active viral replication and while PCV2 is found within macrophages, this is suspected to be due to phagocytosis and not active infection of the cell (Nauwynck et al., 2012). Heparin sulfate and chondroitin sulfate B are PCV2 attachment receptors (Misinzo et al., 2006). The molecule or pathway triggered has not yet been identified (Mankertz, 2012). However, cytoskeleton maintenance, intracellular signaling, and RNA processing have all been implicated in pathogenesis (Mankertz, 2012). PCV2 targets fetal myocardiocytes and hepatocytes (Nauwynck et al., 2012). The virus requires cells in S-phase for DNA replication as the virus replicates faster in active cells (Gillespie et al., 2009). Lymphocytes are most active postvaccination and when infected with another pathogen, thus leading to increased pathology (Gillespie et al., 2009; Nauwynck et al., 2012).

Genetic (Breed Factors) All breeds are susceptible, yet differences exist in degree of susceptibility. Landrace are more susceptible to lesions and disease compared to Durocs and Large Whites (Meerts et al., 2005; Opriessnig et al., 2006).

Other Infections/Immunomodulation Most (98%) pigs with PCVAD have coinfections (Pallares et al., 2002). The most common agents in coinfections are PRRSV, *M. hyopneumoniae*, PPV, and septicemia (Pallares et al., 2002). Other coinfective agents which have been shown to lead to PCVAD are Torque teno virus (TTV), porcine epidemic diarrhea virus (PEDV), SIV, porcine endogenous retrovirus, PCV1, pseudorabies virus (PRV), *Lawsonia intracellularis*, *Salmonella*, and bovine viral diarrhea virus (BVDV) (Opriessnig and Halbur, 2012; Langohr et al., 2012).

PRRSV has been shown to be present in cells containing PCV2 kidney, lymph node, and tonsil using double labeling techniques (Choi and Chae, 2001).

Clinical Signs and Necropsy Findings differ with each syndrome and will be discussed in sections below.

Diagnosis To diagnose PCV2-related diseases or syndromes, a complete tissue set needs to be examined. This includes lymphoid organs, lung, digestive system, kidney, reproductive system, skin, cardiovascular and central nervous systems. Viral detection is typically via immunohistochemistry, *in situ* hybridization, or polymerase chain reaction (PCR) (Opriessnig and Langohr, 2013). Diagnosis is not as straightforward as with other agents, not only because PCV2 is associated with so many syndromes, but also since animals may be infected without showing clinical signs. Diagnosis of a PCV-related syndrome requires presence of three criteria: (1) compatible clinical signs, (2) characteristic microscopic lesions, and (3) PCV2 within lesions (Chae, 2004; Rosell et al., 2000).

Differential Diagnosis Differentials for vasculitis in pigs include PRV, African swine fever (ASFV), classic swine fever (CSF), ovine herpes virus, PRRSV, *Actinobacillus pleuropneumoniae* (APP), *Actinobacillus suis*, *E. coli*, *Pasteurella multocida*, *Salmonella*, and *Streptococcus* spp. (Szeredi et al., 2012).

Prevention/Control Several inactivated subunit vaccines based on PCV2a are commercially available and are effective in controlling and preventing disease, but continued evolution of the virus may evade current vaccines (Opriessnig and Langohr, 2013; Beach and Meng, 2012). Vaccine failure has been reported recently, which prompted examination of the cause which was found to be the presence of PCV2b (Xiao et al., 2012). Since PCV2b has been growing in prevalence over the past few years, vaccines for this serovar are under development (Beach and Meng, 2012). Also, since most cases of clinical PCV2 have coinfections, the vaccine mitigates only the contribution of PCV2, not the coinfection agent.

Research Complications PCV2 also manifests as subclinical disease which results in decreased average weight gain without overt clinical signs (Segales, 2012). More importantly, since overt disease is often seen only with immunomodulation in conjunction with PCV2, research manipulations may result in immunomodulation, thus precipitating overt disease. Many organ systems are potentially susceptible and studies may be compromised due to the presence of PCV2.

Syndromes Postweaning Multisystemic Wasting Syndrome (PMWS).

Pathogenesis An increased number of actively replicating cells within the lymph node correlates with upregulation of virus production (Krakowka et al., 2001). Severe alterations of hematological parameters are seen with PMWS such as anemia, lymphopenia with decrease of CD8+ and IgM-producing cells, monocytosis, and neutrophilia (Darwich et al., 2003). There is cytokine dysregulation with overexpression of IL-10 in the thymus, which is associated with thymic depletion and atrophy, and overexpression of interferon (IFN)-γ in the tonsils (Darwich *et al.*, 2003). The following cytokines are decreased: IL-2 and IL-12p40 in the spleen, IL-4 in tonsils, and IFN-γ, IL10, IL-12p40, and IL-4 in peripheral lymph nodes (Darwich *et al.*, 2003).

These cytokine changes are indicative of T-cell immunosuppression (Darwich *et al.*, 2003).

Clinical Signs/Diagnosis Age at onset of disease differs between the US (7–16 weeks) and EU (5–12 weeks), which is hypothesized to be due to differences in vaccination regimens (Gillespie *et al.*, 2009). First described in 1991, clinical disease includes progressive weight loss, lethargy, jaundice, respiratory disease, diarrhea, lymphadenitis, and anemia (Segales, 2012; Gillespie *et al.*, 2009; Krakowka *et al.*, 2001).

In gnotobiotic piglets, PCV2 alone causes asymptomatic infection without overt evidence of PMWS; however, after activation of the immune system using incomplete Freund's and an immunogen, piglets develop moderate to severe PMWS (Krakowka *et al.*, 2001). PMWS is an acquired immunodeficiency (Darwich and Mateu, 2012).

Necropsy Macroscopic lesions consist of generalized lymphadenopathy, hepatitis with icterus, edema, nephritis, and pneumonia (Krakowka *et al.*, 2001). Lungs fail to collapse and are mottled white to tan (Gillespie *et al.*, 2009). Enlarged lymph nodes have lymphoid depletion with histiocytic replacement (Gillespie *et al.*, 2009; Rosell *et al.*, 2000). Other common lesions include interstitial pneumonia (Figs 16.10, 16.11) and interstitial nephritis, granulomatous inflammation in the liver, spleen, tonsil, thymus, and Peyer's patches (Chae, 2004). Intracytoplasmic botryoid inclusion bodies (Fig. 16.12) are common in epithelial cells of the bronchi, renal tubules, and bronchial glands as well as within macrophages (Huang *et al.*, 2008).

Lesions are typically angiocentric with lymphoplasmacytic and histiocytic to granulomatous inflammation, and multinucleate giant cells (Chae, 2004; Krakowka *et al.*, 2001). In the liver, PCV2 antigen is found in Kupffer cells, hepatocytes, and inflammatory cell infiltrates (Rosell *et al.*, 2000). Renal lesions may consist of tubulointerstitial, lymphoplasmacytic nephritis, interstitial granulomatous nephritis, or mixed patterns (Sarli *et al.*, 2008). Viral load is related to the amount of lymphoplasmacytic inflammation (Sarli *et al.*, 2008).

Porcine Dermatitis and Nephropathy Syndrome
Porcine dermatitis and nephropathy syndrome (PDNS) associated with PCV2 has been reported in a purpose-bred research pig (Phaneuf *et al.*, 2007).

Pathogenesis The current hypothesis is that immune complex deposition is involved in pathogenesis (Wellenberg *et al.*, 2004). This disease is not always

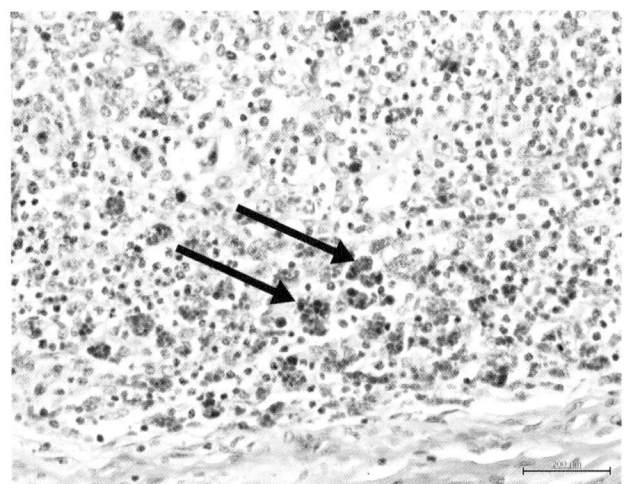

FIGURE 16.11 Porcine circovirus. Macrophages containing botryoid inclusions within the cytoplasm (arrows). *Courtesy of J. Haruna.*

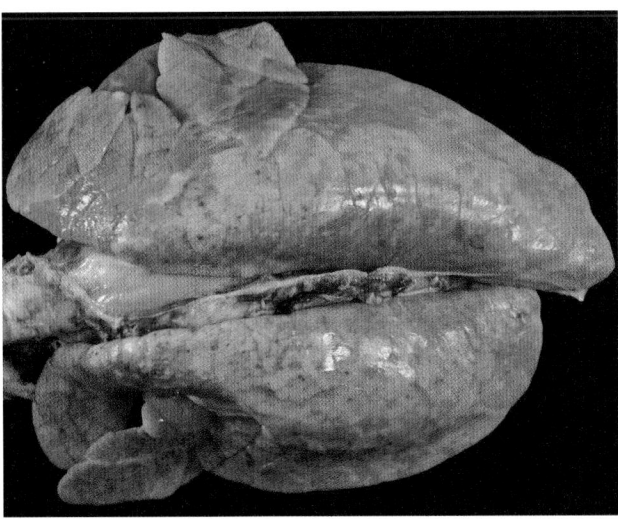

FIGURE 16.10 Porcine circovirus. Lungs with interstitial pneumonia. Lungs are rubbery and fail to collapse. *Courtesy of T. Cecere.*

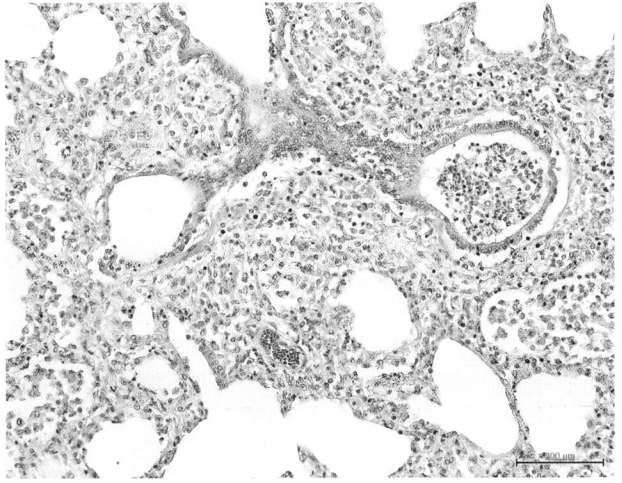

FIGURE 16.12 Porcine circovirus. Lung, broncho-interstitial pneumonia. Bronchi contain inflammatory cells and the interstitium is expanded by inflammatory infiltrates. *Courtesy of J. Haruna.*

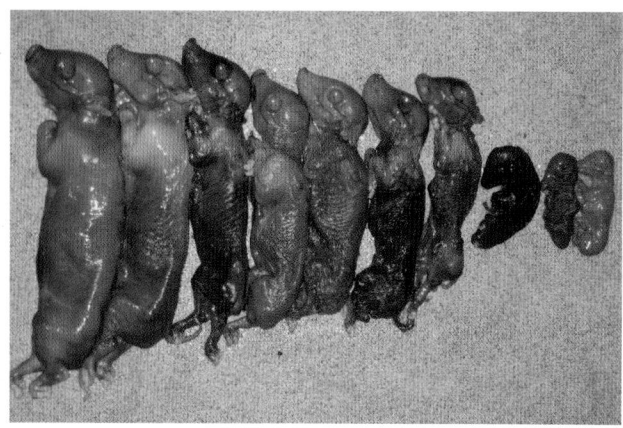

FIGURE 16.13 Porcine circovirus. Reproductive failure with mummification at different gestational ages. *Courtesy of ISU Veterinary Diagnostic Laboratory.*

associated with PCV2, but may also be caused by co-infection of PRRSV and TTV (Krakowka *et al.*, 2008).

Clinical Signs/Diagnosis PDNS is characterized by fever, lethargy, and raised purple lesions on the skin, especially the rear legs (Gillespie *et al.*, 2009) (Fig. 16.13). Skin lesions consist of dark red papules/macules multifocally, primarily on the hind limbs and peri-anal areas (Segales, 2012).

Necropsy The kidneys are enlarged, tan, and waxy with petechial hemorrhages (Segales, 2012; Choi and Chae, 2001; Gillespie *et al.*, 2009). Gross and histological lesions are present in the skin and kidney, but there may also be pulmonary congestion, and multiorgan fibrinoid necrotizing vasculitis with prominent lesions in the dermis, subcutis, stomach, kidneys, lung, spleen, and liver (Phaneuf *et al.*, 2007; Chae, 2005; Choi and Chae, 2001). Cutaneous lesions consist of severe necrotizing vasculitis in dermis and subcutis with leukocytoclastic inflammation of capillaries, small- and medium-sized venules, and arterioles with associated epidermal necrosis, ulceration, and dermal hemorrhage (Choi and Chae, 2001). Renal lesions consist of exudative to fibrinonecrotic glomerulonephritis, interstitial nephritis, and necrotizing arteritis (Segales, 2012; Chae, 2005). Renal and inguinal lymph nodes are also typically enlarged and reddened with necrosis of lymphocytes in the cortex and paracortex with infiltration of multinucleated giant cells (Choi and Chae, 2001; Chae, 2005). Systemic vasculitis is a hallmark lesion of PDNS. Histologically, the vasculitis is similar to type III hypersensitivity.

Porcine Respiratory Disease Complex PCV2 was the most commonly identified pathogen in a study that examined porcine pneumonia, and detection of PCV2 positively correlated with vascular lesions, with PCV2b being the dominant subtype (Szeredi *et al.*, 2012).

Pathogenesis Damage to the lymphoid system after infection is important in the pathogenesis of porcine respiratory disease complex (PRDC) (Szeredi *et al.*, 2012). *In vitro*, activation of endothelial cells has been shown along with diminished coagulation time *in vivo* (Szeredi *et al.*, 2012). Co-infection of animals with PCV2 and another pathogen occurs in most cases, and pathogenesis is thought to occur from virus-induced damage to the immune system (Szeredi *et al.*, 2012). It is suspected that blood vessels play a role in PCV2 pathogenesis, but exact mechanism is not yet known (Szeredi *et al.*, 2012).

Clinical Signs/Diagnosis Animals with PRDC have a decreased growth rate, decreased feed efficiency, lethargy, anorexia, fever, cough, and dyspnea (Chae, 2005; Gillespie *et al.*, 2009). Disease may be due to coinfections with PCV2, PRRSV, SIV, *Mycoplasma hyopneumoniae*, APP, or *Pasteurella multocida* (Chae, 2005).

Necropsy The hallmark lesion is granulomatous bronchointerstitial pneumonia with peribronchial and peribronchiolar fibrosis (Chae, 2005). Mild to severe necrotizing ulcerative bronchiolitis is also seen (Gillespie *et al.*, 2009). Vascular lesions include lymphohistiocytic vasculitis, necrotizing vasculitis, vasculitis with fibrinoid necrosis, intravascular thrombi, along with acute edema, hyaline membranes and acute hemorrhage in the lung (Szeredi *et al.*, 2012). PCV2 antigen is present in endothelial cells, smooth muscle cells of the tunica media, within infiltrating white blood cells (WBCs), intravascular and perivascular macrophages, and intravascular monocytes (Szeredi *et al.*, 2012).

Reproductive Failure

Pathogenesis Infection of piglets is transplacental from PCV2-infected sows (Mateusen *et al.*, 2007). Target cells depend on age. Myocardiocytes are the target cell of fetuses, whereas lymphoid tissues are targeted in neonates (Mateusen *et al.*, 2007). As the fetus develops, replication of virus decreases (Nauwynck *et al.*, 2012).

Clinical Signs/Diagnosis The time of gestation at which the sow is infected determines the course of disease. If the sow is infected at 57 days of gestation, there is increased viral replication with edema, hepatomegaly, and congestion of the fetus, whereas if infected around 90 days of gestation, there are increased reproductive abnormalities (Gillespie *et al.*, 2009). PVC2 infection of pregnant sows can cause fetal death leading to mummification or late-term abortion, stillbirths, mummification (often in the same litter), and preweaning mortality (Fig. 16.14) (Mateusen *et al.*, 2007; Gillespie *et al.*, 2009; Segales, 2012).

Necropsy Dams with reproductive failure show no pathological changes or histological lesions (Opriessnig and Langohr, 2013; Chae, 2005). In piglets, the heart is the most common organ affected and superficial lymph nodes may be enlarged (Mikami *et al.*, 2005; Opriessnig and Langohr, 2013). Histological examination reveals myocardiocyte degeneration, necrosis, fibrosis and

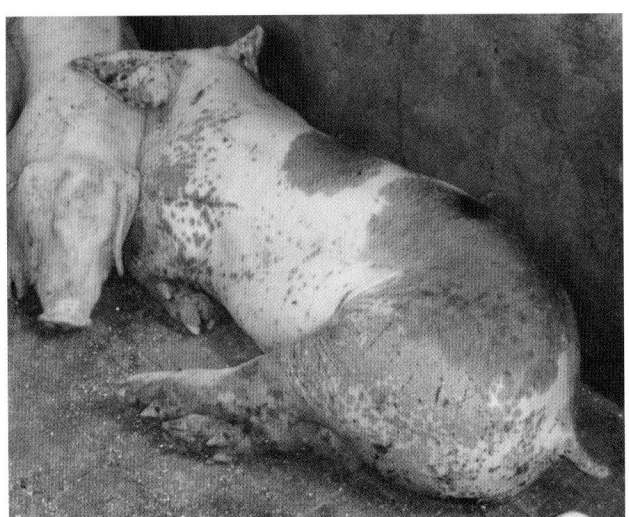

FIGURE 16.14   Porcine circovirus. Porcine dermatitis and nephropathy syndrome (PDNS). Multifocal raised red to purple areas covering hind limbs, forelimbs, and ears. *Courtesy of ISU Veterinary Diagnostic Laboratory.*

mineralization with surrounding lymphocytes, plasma cells, and macrophages (Mikami *et al.*, 2005; O'Connor *et al.*, 2001; Gillespie *et al.*, 2009; Segales, 2012). Intranuclear botryoid inclusion bodies, positive for PCV2 antigen, may be found within the cardiomyocytes (O'Connor *et al.*, 2001). Lymphoid organs often display depletion of lymphocytes with infiltration of multinucleated giant cells containing PCV2 antigen (Mikami *et al.*, 2005).

Granulomatous Enteritis
Pathogenesis   The pathogenesis is currently unknown. When samples were submitted with clinical history suggestive of *Lawsonia intracellulare*, some had dual infection with PCV2, whereas others were infected with *L. intracellulare* only or were infected with PCV2 only (Jensen *et al.*, 2006).

Clinical   Signs/Diagnosis   Clinically,   PCV2-associated granulomatous enteritis affects 2- to 4-month-old pigs and resembles chronic ileitis with diarrhea, unthriftiness, decreased growth, and increased mortality (Chae, 2005; Gillespie *et al.*, 2009). Differentials are *L. intracellulare*, *Brachyspira hyodysenteriae*, *B. pilosicoli*, *Salmonella*, and *E. coli* infection (Jensen *et al.*, 2006).

Necropsy   Lesions are of a necrotizing ileitis and colitis indistinguishable grossly from proliferative ileitis caused by *L. intracellularis* (Jensen *et al.*, 2006). Mesenteric lymph nodes are enlarged and the intestinal mucosa is diffusely thickened (Gillespie *et al.*, 2009). Histologically, there is granulomatous enteritis, composed of epithelioid cells and multinucleated giant cells along with PCV2-type lesions in Peyer's patches but not in other lymphoid tissues (Gillespie *et al.*, 2009; Chae, 2005). Inflammation is primarily in the ileum, but occasionally also found in the colon and cecum (Opriessnig and

Langohr, 2013). There is occasional gastric ulceration (Opriessnig and Langohr, 2013). Other lesions include cytoplasmic inclusion bodies, proliferation of immature enterocytes, and edema in the mesocolon (Jensen *et al.*, 2006).

Acute Pulmonary Edema   With this syndrome, all animals were seropositive for PCV2, with PCV2b being most prevalent (Cino-Ozuna *et al.*, 2011).

Clinical Signs   Animals display a rapid onset of respiratory distress followed nearly immediately by death with no indications of previous disease (Cino-Ozuna *et al.*, 2011). Peracute death in PCV2-vaccinated herds has been associated with PCV2 infection (Cino-Ozuna *et al.*, 2011). Nursery and young finisher pigs are most commonly affected (Cino-Ozuna *et al.*, 2011; Segales, 2012).

Necropsy   Clear fluid accumulates within the thorax with wet, heavy lungs and expansion of interlobular septae with edema (Cino-Ozuna *et al.*, 2011). Cranioventral lobes are consolidated (Cino-Ozuna *et al.*, 2011). Histological changes include diffuse interstitial macrophages and lymphocytes, fibrinoid necrosis of blood vessel walls, and surrounding edema (Cino-Ozuna *et al.*, 2011). Most affected animals display diffuse lymphoid depletion (Cino-Ozuna *et al.*, 2011).

PCV2-Associated Neuropathy   PAN is currently under investigation (Gillespie *et al.*, 2009).

Clinical Signs   Animals display wasting and neurologic deficits which may be associated with congenital tremors, but this has not been confirmed (Seeliger *et al.*, 2007; Gillespie *et al.*, 2009; Opriessnig and Langohr, 2013).

Necropsy   Lesions consist of acute hemorrhages and edema of cerebellar meninges and parenchyma due to necrotizing vasculitis resulting in degeneration and necrosis of the gray and white matter (Seeliger *et al.*, 2007; Gillespie *et al.*, 2009).

Other syndromes which may be associated with PCV2 include exudative dermatitis and necrotizing lymphadenitis (Chae, 2005). Animals with PCV2-associated exudative dermatitis may have concurrent PPV or *Staphylococcus hyicus* (Opriessnig and Halbur, 2012; Opriessnig and Langohr, 2013). Necrotizing lymphadenitis differs from other PCV2-associated diseases in that there is no granulomatous inflammation (Chae, 2005).

b. Salmonellosis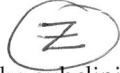
Salmonellosis can be subclinical or present with multiorgan involvement, including septicemia, pneumonia, meningitis, lymphadenitis, abortion, and enterocolitis which can be acute or chronic (Carlson *et al.*, 2012).

Etiology   There are over 2400 serotypes in the genus *Salmonella*, although there are only two species, *Salmonella enterica* and *S. bangori*. Salmonella nomenclature is constantly being updated and this chapter uses the current CDC guidelines.

All members of this genus are motile, non-spore-forming, facultative anaerobic, gram-negative bacilli possessing peritrichous flagella. There are three serotypes that are typically etiologic agents of clinical disease in swine and numerous others that are occasionally associated with disease.

S. enterica ser. Choleraesuis var. *kunzendorf* contains large drug-resistance plasmids and is the most frequent serotype in some parts of the world causing disease in swine, and infection is usually manifested as septicemia and/or pneumonia. *S. enterica* ser. Typhimurium is the most frequently isolated serotype in North America and typically causes enterocolitis. *S. enterica* ser. Typhisuis is associated with localized epizootics characterized by chronic wasting, caseous lymphadenitis, diarrhea, and pneumonia. It is very common to isolate more than one serotype from an individual pig; however, it is unusual that primary disease would be caused by a serotype other than *S. enterica* ser. Choleraesuis or *S. enterica* ser. Typhimurium. *Salmonella* enterocolitis is usually attributed to *S. enterica* ser. Typhimurium and less frequently, *S. enterica* ser. Choleraesuis.

Epizootiology and Transmission   The source of *S. enterica* ser. Choleraesuis for swine is typically other swine and environments contaminated by swine (or other animals). Feed and feed ingredients have also been shown to be a source of serotypes that can cause disease in swine (Harris *et al.*, 1997). Transmission is both vertical and horizontal by fecal–oral spread or nasal secretions. The incubation period ranges from 2 days to several weeks, and survivors become carriers that shed the bacteria in feces for several months. Some form of stress, including shipping, food deprivation, concurrent diseases, research protocols, and mixing pigs from different sources, usually precedes clinical disease. Stress also increases shedding by inapparent carriers. *S. enterica* ser. Choleraesuis is fairly host-specific for swine, but *S. enterica* ser. Typhimurium is not host-specific (Carlson *et al.*, 2012). *S. enterica* ser. Typhimurium is also transmitted via the oronasal route following which organisms have been found in the cecum, colon, and ileal Peyer's patches within 3 h (Fedorka-Cray *et al.*, 1995).

Pathogenesis   Salmonellae have over 200 virulence factors including those involved in adhesion, invasion, cytotoxicity, and resistance to killing (Carlson *et al.*, 2012). They synthesize over 30 proteins that are specific to evading intracellular killing by macrophages. Invasive ability of the organism along with neutrophil recruitment and transmigration are important in pathogenesis. *S. enterica* ser. Typhimurium-secreted proteins activate pathogen elicited epithelial chemotractant and protein kinase C which promotes secretion of IL-8, as well as many other pathways (Lee *et al.*, 2000; Vitiello *et al.*, 2008; Galdiero *et al.*, 2003). Outer membrane proteins such as lipid A and lipopolysaccharide are important mediators of cell damage and microvascular thrombosis and endothelial necrosis which often lead to mucosal ischemia.

S. enterica ser. Typhimurium infection downregulates host local inflammatory response, specifically, TH1 response genes, genes involved in cytoskeletal reorganization, and chaperone proteins (Uthe *et al.*, 2007). Different serovars of salmonella result in different cytokine activation within the host (Skjolaas *et al.*, 2006; Paulin *et al.*, 2007).

The lungs are the site of initial *S. choleraesuis* infection in oronasally exposed pigs (Gray *et al.*, 1996). In pigs exposed via the oral route, *S. enterica* ser. Choleraesuis also can invade the mucosa of the ileum where it is taken up by macrophages. The predominant portal of entry is within the Peyer's patches, specifically through M cells (Meyerholz and Stabel, 2003; Meyerholz *et al.*, 2002). This invasion is followed by dissemination to the spleen and liver via CD18(+) macrophages (Vazquez-Torres *et al.*, 1999). It produces both Shiga-like and cholera-like endotoxins that are responsible for the microthrombosis and ischemia of vessels in the lamina propria and resulting necrosis of the enterocytes. Rectal strictures, particularly of the cranial hemorrhoidal artery, are an outcome of porcine anatomy since pigs have poor to no collateral circulation to the rectum (McGavin and Zachary, 2007). Diarrhea is malabsorptive with extensive fluid loss from the necrotic lesions (Carlson *et al.*, 2012).

Clinical Signs/Diagnosis   Signs characteristic of *Salmonella* septicemia in pigs less than 5 months old include respiratory signs of cough, dyspnea, pneumonia, and cyanosis of the ears and ventral abdomen. Lethargy, anorexia, pyrexia of 40.5–41.6°C, and sometimes jaundice followed by watery yellow diarrhea is also evident. Cyanosis of the extremities and abdomen may also be seen. Diarrhea may be seen, but not until 3–4 days after the other signs are manifest. It can cause abortion in breeding sows.

In *S. enterica* ser. Typhimurium infections, the initial diarrhea is usually watery, yellow and sporadically hemorrhagic and lasts less than a week but may recur. Diarrhea containing blood or mucus is not a prominent feature as it is in diseases such as swine dysentery. Anorexia, pyrexia, and dehydration are seen concurrently with diarrhea. A distended abdomen due to rectal strictures can be a sequela to septicemia. The majority of affected pigs recover; however, some will be carriers and shed the organism for several months. Death may occur in severely affected animals.

Enzyme-linked immunosorbent assays (ELISAs) are available for detection, but definitive diagnosis is achieved via bacterial isolation in conjunction with pathological lesions consistent with *Salmonella* sp. infection (Carlson *et al.*, 2012).

Differential diagnoses for septicemic form include erysipelas and *Streptococcus enterica* ser. Suis as well as other causes of septicemia. A differential list for diarrhea includes other causes of gastroenteritis in recently weaned swine, including colibacillosis, *Lawsonia intracellularis, Serpulina hyodysenteriae,* transmissible gastroenteritis (TGE), PCV2, rotavirus, *Trichuris suis* and coccidiosis.

Treatment Clinical salmonellosis should not be treated because recovered pigs remain carriers and some isolates may be pathogenic for humans. If absolutely necessary, treatments should be based on susceptibility testing.

Prevention/Control Swine may shed *Salmonella* for 5 months or more. Clinically affected swine should be euthanized and the facility sanitized. Removing stressors to minimize fecal shedding by carriers and practicing good sanitation to minimize exposure to the bacteria may help reduce clinical disease. Common surface disinfectants that are efficacious for this bacterium include chlorine, iodine, and phenols. Modified live attenuated vaccines for *S. enterica* ser. Choleraesuis are protective and are thought to be effective because they stimulate cell-mediated immunity. For *S. enterica* ser. Typhimurium, killed bacterins are available and may provide protection. Medication of feed or water with appropriate antibiotics (e.g., carbadox, neomycin) in conjunction with improvements in husbandry, management, and environment may have a prophylactic benefit.

Necropsy *S. enterica* ser. Choleraesuis infection leads to severe pleuropneumonia; cyanosis of the ears, feet, tail, and abdomen; splenomegaly and hepatomegaly; edematous enlarged mesenteric lymph nodes; erosion of the fundic mucosa in the stomach; and a focal to diffuse necrotic typhlocolitis with or without a necrotic ileitis (Turk *et al.*, 1992). Microscopic lesions include paratyphoid nodules in the liver; necrotic lesions involving the intestinal mucosa, submucosa, and lymphoid follicles; and a bronchopneumonia or hemorrhagic pleuropneumonia (Turk *et al.*, 1992; Carlson *et al.*, 2012).

With *S. enterica* ser. Typhimurium, lesions include enterotyphlocolitis involving the ileum, cecum, spiral colon with thickened edematous walls, red roughened mucosa, and multifocal to coalescing erosions and ulcers covered with pseudomembranous gray–yellow fibrinonecrotic debris, with or without button ulcers. Rectal strictures with mural fibrosis and resultant distention of the colon with fecal matter are also seen. Acute lesions include necrosis of Peyer's patches, but later in disease they may be hyperplastic.

Research Complications Pigs proven to be clinically ill or shedding *Salmonella* should not be maintained in a research facility because of chronic fecal shedding and zoonotic risks. *Salmonella* are present at a low subclinical level in the majority of conventional swine herds. Outbreaks of clinical disease are associated with immunosuppression or stress, including experimental stress. Clinical disease caused by *S. enterica* ser. Choleraesuis

has up to 60% morbidity and up to 30% mortality, which would seriously impact any research project (Schwartz, 1991).

c. Glasser's Disease (Haemophilus, Porcine Polyserositis, Infectious Polyarthritis, Fibrinous Polyserositis, and Arthritis)

Etiology *Haemophilus parasuis*, a member of the Pasteurellaceae family, are a small gram-negative pleomorphic coccobacilli. There are currently 15 recognized serovars. Both pathogenic and nonpathogenic strains of the organism exist. Exposure to nonpathogenic strains can induce protective immunity.

Epizootiology and Transmission *H. parasuis* is one of the earliest isolates to be cultured from the nasal cavities of swine in conventional herds. In endemic herds it can be cultured when animals are 1 week of age and is commonly cultured from the upper respiratory tracts of healthy pigs and may be part of normal flora (Macinnes and Desrosiers, 1999). Experimental evidence suggests that the first site of colonization in piglets is the nasal mucosa (Vahle *et al.*, 1995). It is only known to infect swine, suggesting that introduction by other carrier species is unlikely. The role of *H. parasuis* as a respiratory pathogen is not well established; however, some report that it may be a primary etiologic agent in fibrinosuppurative bronchopneumonia (Aragon *et al.*, 2012).

Pathogenesis This organism is an opportunistic pathogen with PRRSV, PCV2, and *B. bronchiseptica*. Organisms adhere to epithelial cells of the upper respiratory tract, which induces apoptosis and cytokine release (Bouchet *et al.*, 2009). Resistance to phagocytosis is likely associated with the capsule and enhances virulence (Aragon *et al.*, 2012). The severity of disease is dependent on *H. parasuis* strain.

Clinical Signs/Diagnoses In conventional herds where *H. parasuis* is enzootic, the clinical signs will be mild with low morbidity. In susceptible herds, the clinical signs occur within a week after exposure and consist of some or all of the following: pyrexia 40–41.7°C, anorexia, coughing, depression, swollen joints with lameness, neurological signs, dyspnea, and sudden death. A markedly increased WBC and decreased packed cell volume (PCV) have been reported in experimentally infected SPF piglets (Wiegand *et al.*, 1997). Long-term sequelae include abortion and chronic arthritis. An oligonucleotide-specific capture plate hybridization assay has been developed and is reported to be specific and more sensitive than culturing for *H. parasuis* from lesions and nasal swabs (Calsamiglia *et al.*, 1999). Differentials include *Mycoplasma hyorhinis* and other bacterial septicemic conditions that affect swine including *Erysipelothrix rhusiopathiae, Salmonella choleraesuis,* and *Streptococcus suis*.

Treatment Parenteral antibiotics should be started as soon as clinical signs become evident. Oral antibiotics are less effective. High doses of penicillin should be given to those with and without clinical signs. Several other antibiotics (cephalosporins, fluoroquinolones, potentiated sulfas, tetracyclines, tylosin) are also effective. Resistance to tetracycline, erythromycin, and penicillin in some strains is increasing.

Prevention/Control   Practices to increase immunity by the use of bacterins and reduction of experimental, environmental, and shipping stress are helpful in prevention and control of disease. Herd-specific autogenous vaccines should be considered, as it is unlikely that any one commercial bacterin will induce immunity to all pathogenic strains in the population (Aragon *et al.*, 2012). Medicated early weaning can be successful if high doses of both parenteral and oral antibiotics are utilized (Aragon *et al.*, 2012). Antimicrobial medication of feed or water of groups of swine at risk may be beneficial.

Necropsy   Gross lesions may include cyanosis of the ears and tail, polyarthritis of one or more joints, fibrinous pleuritis, pericarditis, peritonitis, and leptomeningitis (Fig. 16.15) (Little and Harding, 1971; Aragon *et al.*, 2012). Histopathologic lesions in peracute disease consist of fibrin thickening of alveolar walls and capillary thrombosis of glomerular tufts. Acute disease lesions consist of fibrinopurulent arthritis and synovitis, fibrinous to fibrinopurulent serositis, and fibrinopurulent leptomeningitis (McGavin and Zachary, 2007; Aragon *et al.*, 2012).

Research Complications   This disease will confound cardiovascular studies because the chronic form can produce congestive heart failure and fibrinous pericarditis.

d. Erysipelas (Swine Erysipelas) DIAMOND SKIN DZ

Etiology   Swine erysipelas (SE) is caused by *Erysipelothrix rhusiopathiae* is a gram-positive bacillus

that has 28 serotypes. The majority of isolates from swine are serotypes 1 and 2.

Epizootiology and Transmission   The domestic pig is the primary reservoir of *E. rhusiopathiae*, and probably 30–50% of conventional swine are carriers (Opriessnig and Wood, 2012; Cowart, 1995). These pigs harbor the bacteria in lymphoid tissues (tonsils, Peyer's patches) and shed it in nasal secretions, saliva, and feces. Individuals with acute SE will shed large quantities into the environment, and those with the chronic form are a long-term source of contamination. Additionally, contact with infected sheep, turkeys, chickens, ducks, and emus is a potential source of infection for swine. Swine older than 3 months and younger than 3 years of age are most likely to develop clinical disease. Passive antibodies obtained from the sow protect the young, and acquired immunity from subclinical infections protects the mature animals. This bacterium typically gains entry into the body through contaminated food and water (oral route) and skin wounds.

Pathogenesis   The organisms gain entry to the body via the palatine tonsils or gut-associated lymphoid tissue, and through skin wounds via direct contact or arthropod bites (Chirico *et al.*, 2003). The pathogenesis of the lesions is not completely understood, but virulence factors are currently only partially characterized, but the most important factors include neuraminidase, capsular polysaccharides, and surface proteins (Wang *et al.*, 2010).

Clinical Signs/Diagnosis   Animals with acute SE may have no clinical signs or have a combination of classical rhomboid or diamond-shaped urticarial (pink to purple) skin lesions on the snout, ears, abdomen, and thighs; fever of 40–42°C; anorexia; depression; stiff, stilted gait; sitting posture; abortion; and sudden death. Skin lesions appear 2–3 days post exposure and are erythematous, raised, and palpable, measure 1–8 cm across, and vary in number from few to many (Fig. 16.16)

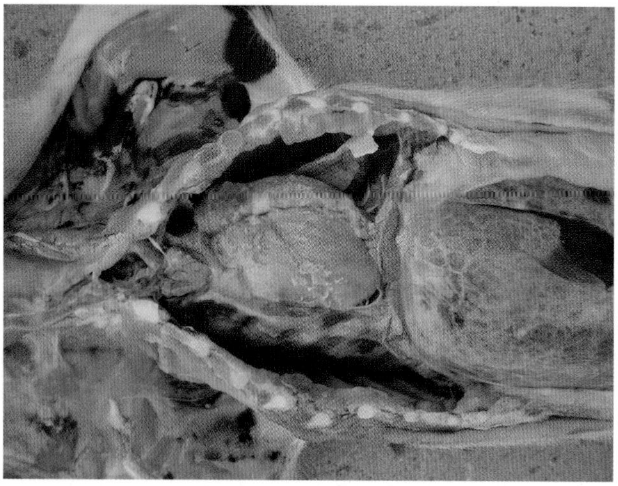

FIGURE 16.15   *H. parasuis* (Glasser's disease). Thoracic and peritoneal fibrinoserositis. *Courtesy of ISU Veterinary Diagnostic Laboratory.*

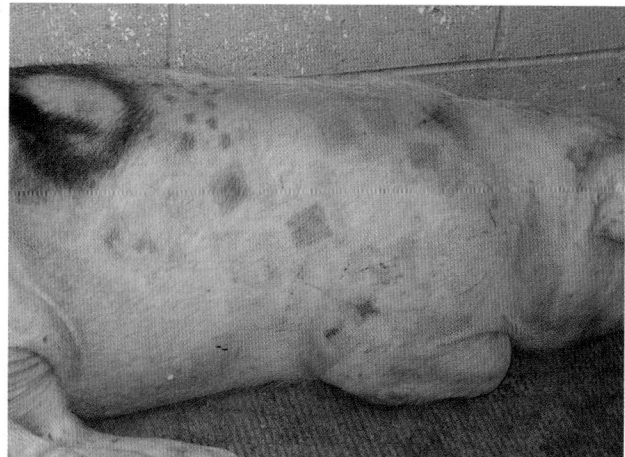

FIGURE 16.16   *E. rhusiopathiae* (diamond skin disease). Multifocal red to purple rhomboid lesions in the skin. *Courtesy of ISU Veterinary Diagnostic Laboratory.*

(Amass and Scholz, 1998). The fever and skin lesions will usually resolve within 1 week.

Enlarged, stiff joints resulting in slight to non-weight-bearing lameness characterize the chronic form of SE. The hock and carpal joints are usually the most visibly affected in those with chronic arthritis. In some cases cardiac insufficiency manifested by exercise intolerance and sudden death may result. Chronic SE may follow subclinical, subacute, and acute forms, sometimes within 3 weeks.

PCR assays can be used, as can formic acid and immunohistochemistry (IHC) to diagnose SE (Brooke and Riley, 1999).

Differentials for the acute form include any bacterial septicemia and PDNS caused by PCV2. The diamond-shaped skin lesions are characteristic. Differentials for chronic SE include other causes of lameness in swine, including *Haemophilus* polyserositis, mycoplasmal polyserositis, and trauma and other bacterial septicemias such as *Actinobacillus suis*.

Treatment Penicillin is the treatment of choice for the acute form of SE. Most strains are susceptible to several classes of antibiotics such as beta lactams, fluoroquinolones and cephalosporins (Yamamoto *et al.*, 2001). Hyperimmune serum has been used historically and can be effective if given early in the course of the disease, especially in suckling piglets. This will provide about 2 weeks of passive immunity. Anti-inflammatory drugs can be used to treat the arthritis associated with chronic SE (Opriessnig and Wood, 2012; Cowart, 1995).

Prevention/Control Vaccination is worthwhile, although neither attenuated vaccines nor bacterins are successful at preventing chronic SE (Cowart, 1995). Immunization with purified protein antigen P64 is protective against experimental challenge (Yamazaki *et al.*, 1999). The surface protein SpaA has potential as an antigen for new vaccines (Makino *et al.*, 1998; Imada *et al.*, 1999; Shimoji *et al.*, 1999). Attenuated vaccines can be injected, given orally in drinking water, or delivered by aerosol with special equipment. Antibiotic treatment should be stopped 10 days prior to giving attenuated live vaccines. Due to the ubiquitous nature of *E. rhusiopathiae*, the ultimate prevention plan is to obtain SPF animals via cesarean derivation or preweaning medication and to maintain them in a barrier facility (Opriessnig and Wood, 2012).

Chronically infected animals should be eliminated from the facility. Routine use of common disinfectants, including hypochlorite, quaternary ammonium, phenolic, and alkali, is important as these bacteria can survive in the environment for long periods.

Necropsy Acute-phase gross lesions are those of a bacteremia and generalized coagulopathy (Wood, 1984). Characteristic rhomboid or rectangular-shaped, slightly raised, firm skin lesions are most commonly found on the skin of the abdomen but also on the thighs, ears, snout, throat, and jowls. There is congestion of the

spleen, lungs, and liver, and there may be petechial to ecchymotic hemorrhages in the cortex of the kidneys, on the atrial epi- and myocardium, and within lymph nodes (Wood, 1984; Opriessnig and Wood, 2012). Microscopic lesions in the acute phase are the result of damage done to endothelial cells in capillaries and venules. In the dermal papillae these lead to fibrin deposition, microthrombi, lymphocytic and plasmacytic perivascular infiltrates, and focal necrosis. Chronic lesions are manifested as a proliferative, nonsuppurative synovitis and arthritis that results in enlarged joints, most commonly involving the stifle, hock, and carpal joints (Wood, 1984; Opriessnig and Wood, 2012).

Research Complications Acute SE can potentially complicate research protocols involving small numbers of swine by causing losses due to sudden death. The chronic form will affect orthopedic and cardiovascular studies since proliferative, nonsuppurative arthritis and vegetative proliferation on the heart valves can result. *E. rhusiopathiae* is a zoonotic disease which in most cases is self-limiting; however, care must be taken to protect personnel when working with infected pigs.

e. Streptococcosis (Streptococcal Meningitis)

Etiology *Streptococcus suis* (Lancefield's group D) is a gram-positive oval cocci found as diplococci or short chains. Capsular types 1–9 are most often associated with clinical disease in swine, with type 2 being the most common (Aarestrup *et al.*, 1998a; Gottschalk, 2012b).

Another streptococcus species, *S. equisimilis*, may be recovered from cases of septicemia associated with subsequent development of swollen joints (Gottschalk, 2012b).

Epizootiology and Transmission Transmission between herds is via flies and carrier animals (Enright *et al.*, 1987). Newborns are infected during parturition and suckling by direct contact, aerosols, and fomites (Berthelot-Herault *et al.*, 2001). Most piglets of carrier sows are colonized before weaning age (Torremorell *et al.*, 1998).

Subclinical carriers harbor the organism in their tonsilar crypts, nasal cavity, and reproductive and gastrointestinal tracts. When a carrier is introduced to a susceptible herd, the signs are usually first evident in recently weaned young between 5 and 12 weeks of age. This bacterium has been cultured from a variety of other animals, including birds, and wild boars (Baums *et al.*, 2007; Devriese *et al.*, 1994). Simultaneous infection with other pathogens, including PRRSV and PRV, can increase the severity of clinical signs (Cowart, 1995; Gottschalk, 2012b).

Pathogenesis The pathogenesis of *S. suis* is believed to begin via colonization of the palatine and pharyngeal tonsils. It is then spread extracellularly or attached to monocytes via the blood or lymph (Gottschalk, 2012b;

Madsen *et al.*, 2002). Pathogenesis is still not fully understood. Most studies are done on serotype 2, but use different animal models. There are different virulence factors between serotypes, but these are not always consistently involved in disease. Hemolysin (suilysin) is one of the best-characterized virulence factors and is toxic to epithelial, endothelial, and phagocytic cells (Gottschalk and Segura, 2000). Bacteria and suilysin colocalize within neutrophils and macrophages localized to meningeal lesions (Zheng *et al.*, 2009).

Clinical Signs/Diagnosis Manifestations of meningitis are the most characteristic signs of *S. suis* type 2 infections in swine, and swine aged 5–16 weeks are most commonly affected. Pyrexia to 42.5°C is usually the initial sign, followed by anorexia, depression, ataxia, paddling, opisthotonus, convulsions, and death. Additional signs of *S. suis* infection include pneumonia, rhinitis, polyarthritis, and less commonly, stillbirths, abscesses, vaginitis, and myocarditis (Gottschalk, 2012b; Staats *et al.*, 1997). Otitis interna has been reported as a sequela to *S. suis* meningitis with involvement of perilymphatic ducts (Madsen *et al.*, 2001).

A PCR assay developed for the detection of strains of serotypes 1 and 2 in tonsilar specimens and an ELISA based on a purified polysaccharide antigen are specific and sensitive to diagnose presence of *Streptococcus* sp. (Wisselink *et al.*, 1999; Kataoka *et al.*, 1996). Isolation of the organism from an area other than the nasal or oral cavity (where organism is part of normal flora) is required, with serotyping being an important part. Isolates from different geographical areas may be genotypically different and make diagnosis more difficult (Rehm *et al.*, 2007). Differentials include other streptococcal infections, *H. parasuis*, *E. rhusiopathiae*, *S. enterica* ser. Choleraesuis, and salt poisoning or water deprivation.

Treatment Treatment should be with a parenteral antibiotic to which the particular herd strain has been shown to be susceptible by testing. Resistance to several antibiotics, including tetracycline, tylosin, and sulfonamides, is a developing concern (Aarestrup *et al.*, 1998b; Rasmussen *et al.*, 1999; Gottschalk, 2012b).

Prevention/Control Rederivation by hysterectomy or hysterotomy and maintenance in a barrier facility will eliminate *S. suis* from an infected herd (Gottschalk, 2012b). The natural history and epizootiology of the disease is such that depopulation with subsequent repopulation with clean animals is a feasible method of control and prevention within a research facility. Antimicrobial therapy and early weaning did not eliminate the tonsilar carrier state (Amass *et al.*, 1996; Macinnes and Desrosiers, 1999).

Minimization of environmental and experimental stress, good sanitation, prophylactic antibiotics, and use of bacterins will help control clinical disease. *S. suis* is susceptible to common disinfectants. Mixing swine

from different sources and of different ages should not occur. Oral medication of feed or water has been shown to be beneficial in controlling streptococcal meningitis. Penicillin, amoxicillin, florfenicol, and gentamicin antimicrobials are often effective, however culture and sensitivity should be performed on isolates (Marie *et al.*, 2002). Bacterin vaccines, including autogenous and whole-cell, have had variable success. Live avirulent strains and vaccines against cell-wall proteins or extracellular proteins, particularly suilysin, have produced protective immunity in swine, yet are inconsistent (Busque *et al.*, 1997; Jacobs *et al.*, 1996; Gottschalk, 2012b).

Necropsy Necropsy findings may include evidence of encephalitis, cerebral edema, and fibrinous pleuritis/pericarditis. Histopathologic findings include suppurative meningitis, choroiditis with hyperemic blood vessels, and fibrinopurulent to suppurative epicarditis (Gottschalk, 2012b).

Research Complications Direct losses from fatal meningitis will certainly affect all types of research. Cardiovascular studies will be confounded by the development of endocarditis and myocarditis. *S. suis* type 2 is zoonotic to humans (Erickson, 1987).

f. Pseudorabies

PRV, also known as Aujeszky's disease, was not considered important in the US prior to 1960. However, since that time new and more virulent strains have emerged. PRV is a reportable disease. In January 1989, the US implemented a national PRV eradication program and in 2005 was declared to be free of the disease (Agriculture, 2008). This program included test and removal, offspring segregation, and depopulation and repopulation. The majority of industrialized nations also have eradication programs.

Etiology The disease is caused by suid herpesvirus 1 in the genus *Varicellovirus*, subfamily Alphaherpesvirinae, family Herpesviridae (Davison *et al.*, 2009). Herpesviridae are known for the ability to establish latent infections, particularly in the sensory ganglia of the nervous system.

Suid herpesvirus 1 can affect a variety of animals, including pigs, cattle, sheep, goats, dogs, cats, rodents, macaques, and marmosets. Reports of human infection are limited and poorly documented (Mettenleiter *et al.*, 2012). Pigs may host subclinical and latent infections whereas infection of all other animals results in death.

Epizootiology and Transmission The single most important mechanism contributing to disease spread is the movement of swine which are shedding the viral particles. Transmission can occur via direct contact, fomites, insemination, inhalation of aerosolized particles, or transplacental transmission. Infective levels of virus can persist for up to 7h in air with relative humidity of 55% (Schoenbaum *et al.*, 1990). Infective levels of viral particles can also be present in tissues of animals that have died from the disease. Consuming infected carcasses or feed that has been contaminated with the virus is another means of transmission. Evidence indicates that avian species are not a significant contributor to the spread of the virus, and the role of insects in the transmission process has not been adequately evaluated (Zimmerman *et al.*, 1989). Animals other than pigs, which are considered dead-end hosts, typically die within 3 days of being infected.

Pathogenesis In natural infections, the virus enters via the mucosal epithelium in the nasopharynx and tonsils and replicates in the epithelium. The virus gains access to neurons of the facial region (olfactory, trigeminal, glossopharyngeal nerves), and reaches neuronal cell bodies via axonal retrograde transport, and then spreads to the medulla and pons where it replicates in neurons and spreads to other parts of the brain resulting in latent infection of the trigeminal ganglia (Mettenleiter *et al.*, 2012). Viremia disseminates virus to many other organs (Kritas *et al.*, 1999; Mettenleiter, 2000).

Clinical Signs/Diagnosis The clinical signs associated with PRV are related to the age of the swine affected, although the strain of virus and infectious dose also play a role. The virus predominantly impacts the respiratory and nervous systems. Neonatal pigs typically respond to exposure with acute signs related to the central nervous system (CNS). Affected pigs will tremble, hypersalivate, stumble, and exhibit nystagmus and opisthotonus, often with epileptiform-like seizures. Because of posterior paresis, the animals may be observed sitting like a dog. Other signs include circling and paddling, vomiting, and diarrhea. Once CNS signs start, death usually follows within 24–36 h, and mortality approaches 100% in neonates and young piglets; mortality may decrease to 50% by 4 weeks of age. As the pigs age, the clinical signs become less severe, fewer pigs develop CNS involvement, and mortality declines. Respiratory signs characterized by sneezing, nasal discharge, and cough become the hallmark of pigs that are infected at greater than 9 weeks of age. Morbidity rate is high, but mortality is low with uncomplicated CNS signs such as muscle tremors that occur only sporadically. The duration of clinical signs is usually 6–10 days, with rapid recovery unless the disease has progressed to pneumonia or a secondary bacterial pneumonia has been initiated. Coinfection with other viruses (PRRSV, PCV2, SIV) may result in severe proliferative and necrotizing pneumonia in weanling and postweanling pigs (Morandi *et al.*, 2010). When CNS signs are exhibited, the clinical diagnosis of PRV becomes much more facile. Sows and boars also develop primarily respiratory signs, although pregnant animals in the first trimester resorb the fetus, and in the second to third trimester, abort.

Serum neutralization is the standard test, but ELISA and latex agglutinations are also commonly used to diagnose. Virus isolation allows for a definitive diagnosis, with the brain, tonsils, and lung being the organs of choice. Trigeminal ganglia, olfactory ganglia, and tonsils are the preferred tissues for isolation/detection of virus using IFA, IHC, or *in situ* hybridization. The main differential diagnoses are SIV, rabies, CSF, ASFV, porcine teschovirus (PTV), Nipah virus, and many others.

Prevention/Control Modified live, killed, and gene-deleted vaccines with foreign-gene insertions are available to aid in the control of PRV (Mulder *et al.*, 1997). The vaccines protect pigs against clinical signs and mortality but do nothing toward eradicating the disease; the vaccine does not eliminate the virus in infected animals, nor does it prevent animals from becoming infected with the virus. Animals that are vaccinated, however, do shed lesser amounts of virus and have limited tissue invasion by the organism. The gene-deleted vaccinations offer the advantage of producing vaccinated animals that lack antibody against the specific protein coded for by the deleted gene to allow the vaccinated pigs to be differentiated serologically from infected pigs.

Necropsy Gross lesions may be minimal or may include a fibrinonecrotic rhinitis; necrotic foci in the tonsils, liver, spleen, lungs, intestines, and adrenals; occasional leptomeningeal hyperemia; endometritis; and necrotizing placentitis (Thomson, 1988). Microscopic lesions include a nonsuppurative meningoencephalitis and ganglioneuritis involving both gray and white matter. Eosinophilic intranuclear inclusions may be found in neurons, astrocytes, oligodendroglia, and endothelial cells (Thomson, 1988). There is a necrotizing bronchitis and alveolitis, necrotizing tonsillitis, lymphohistiocytic endometritis, and necrotizing placentitis with inclusion bodies in necrotic and epithelial cells around the foci of necrosis (Mettenleiter *et al.*, 2012).

Research Complications This is a reportable disease, and as such affected animals need to be euthanized.

g. Encephalomyocarditis Virus

Etiology Encephalomyocarditis virus (EMCV) is found in the genus *Cardiovirus*, family Picornaviridae.

Epizootiology/Transmission Outbreaks of the acute myocarditis form have been reported most frequently in Europe and are often clustered in endemic areas (Koenen *et al.*, 1999; Maurice *et al.*, 2007). Rodents are thought to be a reservoir and can infect food and water that pigs ingest (Alexanersen *et al.*, 2012). Infection of pigs is not uncommon, but clinical disease is infrequent. Infected pigs can excrete virus, and dead pigs are also potential sources of infection.

Pathogenesis Oral exposure is most likely, with virus subsequently found in myocardiocytes, tonsils, intestinal tract and macrophages.

Clinical Signs/Diagnosis There are two forms of disease caused by EMCV, an acute myocarditis and reproductive failure in sows. In young pigs the only clinical sign may be sudden death. Other signs in young animals may include anorexia, listlessness, trembling, staggering, paralysis, or dyspnea. Infected sows may abort or have mummified or stillborn fetuses.

EMCV is diagnosed via virus isolation, virus neutralization, and ELISA. There is currently no treatment for EMCV.

Prevention/Control Vaccines are available to prevent disease caused by EMCV. Minimizing stress will help control disease.

Necropsy In acute infections, heart lesions are prominent. Epicardial hemorrhage may be the only lesion noted, although hydropericardium, hydrothorax, and pulmonary edema are often noted (Alexanersen *et al.*, 2012). Myocardial lesions are most prominent in the right ventricle and are grayish-white in color. Histological lesions of nonsuppurative myocarditis or encephalitis are indicative of EMCV disease (Alexanersen *et al.*, 2012).

Research Complications The virus has only recently been associated with human disease, and it is known to infect and cause disease in nonhuman primates (Czechowicz *et al.*, 2011). The risk of human infection may increase if porcine-to-human xenografts are performed.

h. Porcine Teschovirus

Etiology Teschen disease is caused by porcine teschovirus, a member of the family Picornaviridae, genus *Teschovirus*. There are several PTV serotypes which present with different disease manifestations.

Epizootiology/Transmission The only known host of PTV is the pig. The virus is ubiquitous worldwide, with no herd shown to be free of virus. Disease occurs sporadically. Transmission is primarily fecal–oral, although fomite transmission also occurs. Virus particles remain active in the environment and are highly resistant to inactivation (Derbyshire and Arkell, 1971).

Pathogenesis The virus replicates in the tonsil and intestinal tract. In some animals, there is a viremia, which allows spread to the CNS.

Clinical Signs/Diagnosis Polioencephalomyelitis, reproductive disease, enteric disease, pericarditis, myocarditis, and pneumonia are all signs of PTV, depending on serotype.

Teschen disease is caused by a highly virulent PTV-1 strain: All ages are affected and the main presentation is polioencephalomyelitis although other signs include fever, anorexia, ataxia, opisthotonus, coma, and paralysis. Death is common 3–4 days post initial clinical signs.

Talfan disease is caused by a less virulent PTV-1 strain. Signs are milder than in Teschen disease and typically consist of benign enzootic paresis.

PTV also may cause abortion in swine (Bielaaski and Raeside, 1977). Although there have been reports of enteric disease, pericarditis, myocarditis, and pneumonia associated with PTV, studies have been inconsistent in reproduction of these lesions (Alexanersen *et al.*, 2012).

Reverse transcriptase PCR (RT-PCR) is used to detect viral RNA. The virus can be found in the spinal cord, brainstem, or cerebellum of animals with Teschen disease. Other disease manifestations may be more complicated to isolate virus from.

Treatment Animals with mild disease may recover, but there is no effective treatment.

Prevention/Control Prevention of import of animals from enzootic areas helps control spread of Teschen disease. Elimination of PTV proves difficult, as the viruses have been isolated from SPF herds, and gnotobiotic pigs may be infected due to transplacental transmission (Alexanersen *et al.*, 2012).

Necropsy No specific lesions have been associated with PTV. Histological lesions consist of diffuse chromatolysis and are present throughout the CNS, but especially in the ventral columns of the spinal cord, cerebellar cortex, and brain stem (Alexanersen *et al.*, 2012; Koestner *et al.*, 1966; Holman *et al.*, 1966).

Research Complications Teschen disease is a reportable disease (Health, 2013b).

2. Respiratory Diseases

a. Atrophic Rhinitis

Etiology Toxigenic strains of *P. multocida*, *B. bronchiseptica*, and *H. parasuis* are the bacterial agents of the multifactorial disease atrophic rhinitis (AR). Porcine cytomegalovirus (CMV), which is the cause of inclusion body rhinitis, does not cause nasal turbinate atrophy; however, it may damage the nasal mucosa, predisposing it to colonization with one of these bacterial agents. Environmental air pollutants, namely, high ammonia levels (50–100 ppm) and dust (Hamilton *et al.*, 1999), and genetic factors also play a role. *P. multocida* strains A and D produce *Pasteurella multocida* toxin (PMT), which causes progressive nasal turbinate atrophy. *B. bronchiseptica* produces a heat-labile dermonecrotic toxin (DNT) which alone will produce a moderate self-limiting form of the disease in which damaged tissues may regenerate in time (Roop *et al.*, 1987). *H. parasuis* reportedly causes a mild turbinate atrophy (Cowart, 1995). Combined infections of toxigenic *P. multocida* and *B. bronchiseptica* produce the most severe form of AR. Typically, two or more infectious organisms are required to produce clinical disease with permanent nasal distortion and turbinate atrophy. Recently, the term 'nonprogressive atrophic rhinitis' (NPAR) has been applied to the form caused by *B. bronchiseptica* alone, and the term 'progressive atrophic rhinitis' (PAR) to *P. multocida* alone and combined infections with *B. bronchiseptica* (Register *et al.*, 2012; Brockmeier *et al.*, 2012).

Epizootiology and Transmission The majority of conventional swine herds are infected with *B. bronchiseptica*, and a smaller proportion also have strains A and D of *P. multocida*, the bacterial etiologic agents of atrophic rhinitis.

B. bronchiseptica is spread from pig to pig by aerosol droplets, which probably first occurs with snout-to-snout contact between a sow and a newborn piglet, followed by horizontal spread among littermates; however, transmission can occur at any age. Piglets infected in the first week of life will generally develop more severe lesions than those infected at 4 weeks or later. Those infected at 9 weeks show almost no lesions (Brockmeier *et al.*, 2012). The quantity and quality of passive antibody obtained from the sow also affects the severity of lesions. In SPF herds, the mode of transmission is often the introduction of new carrier animals to the herd. *B. bronchiseptica* can be isolated from many domestic and wild species; however, these strains are usually less pathogenic for swine. This bacterium is commonly cultured from most swine herds and is not always associated with disease.

P. multocida infection in SPF herds typically occurs by the introduction of carrier pigs. Once introduced into a seronegative herd, these bacteria spread quickly by direct contact and aerosols. The pharynx, especially tonsils, and vagina of sows are sources of infection for piglets. Age of first infection inversely affects the severity of lesions; however, older pigs (3–4 months) will still develop lesions, which is in contrast to infection with *B. bronchiseptica* (Brockmeier *et al.*, 2012; Register *et al.*, 2012).

Pathogenesis *B. bronchiseptica* colonizes the ciliated epithelial cells in the nasal epithelium, where it results in loss of cilia. Sequential virulence factors are expressed only at temperatures greater than 77°F (Beier and Gross, 2008). These toxins include DNT, which impairs bone formation; adenylate cyclase toxin (ACT), which is responsible for disruption of innate immune function; tracheal cytotoxin (TCT), which interacts with LPS and is responsible for impaired ciliary function; and others (Horiguchi *et al.*, 1995; Brockmeier *et al.*, 2012). It also produces a toxin that is believed to penetrate the lamina propria and initiate an inflammatory infiltrate and atrophy of the osseous cores (Brockmeier *et al.*, 2012). *B bronchiseptica* is cytotoxic for alveolar macrophages (Brockmeier and Register, 2000). IgG and IgA are both required for complete clearance of the respiratory tract of *B. bronchiseptica*.

P. multocida has been shown to produce a toxin that results in necrosis of osteoblasts and stimulation of osteoclastic bone resorption in the nasal turbinates, leading to turbinate atrophy (Dominick and Rimler, 1988).

In order for *P. multocida* to colonize, decreased ciliary function or increased mucous is typically required. These changes are commonly caused by increased ammonia or infection with other agents such as *B. bronchiseptica* and CMV (Register *et al.*, 2012). Experimental evidence has shown that continuous exposure of piglets to 20 ppm ammonia for 2 weeks will markedly exacerbate *P. multocida* colonization in the upper respiratory tract (Hamilton *et al.*, 1998). Once *P. multocida* colonizes, it produces toxins including PMT, which disrupts G-protein and rho-dependent pathways and stimulates mitogenesis resulting in degenerative and hyperplastic changes, especially within the bony turbinates of the nasal cavity (Register *et al.*, 2012). These toxins incite inflammatory cell infiltrates in the lamina propria and cause atrophy of mucosal glands, osteolysis, and replacement of turbinate bones by fibrous connective tissue. PMT may induce turbinate atrophy via alterations in cytokines and soluble factors affecting osteoclast number and or inhibition of osteoblastic bone formation (Gwaltney *et al.*, 1997).

Clinical Signs/Diagnosis The clinical signs of pure *B. bronchiseptica* infection (NPAR) generally appear in nursery pigs less than 4 weeks of age and consist of sneezing, snuffling, and a mucopurulent nasal discharge. In older pigs, these signs are mild or nonexistent. In very young pigs (3–4 days old), a severe bronchopneumonia can result. This form is much more rare than the nasal infections. Infected animals display a mild fever (39.5–40°C), marked 'whooping' cough, and dyspnea, with high morbidity and mortality possible if untreated. The organism is frequently isolated from pneumonic lesions of older pigs; however, its role as a pathogen in this setting is questionable (Brockmeier *et al.*, 2012).

The clinical signs of *P. multocida* (PAR) typically begin at 1–3 months of age and consist of sneezing and snuffling, which progresses to more violent sneezing with mucopurulent nasal discharge. In some cases epistaxis is seen. Inflammation of the nasolacrimal duct, which causes occlusion of the duct and subsequent tear staining visible at the medial canthus, frequently occurs. The most characteristic clinical sign is the dorsal and/or lateral deviation of the snout as the pig grows. This is caused by abnormal bone growth due to unequal nasal turbinate atrophy. Brachygnathia superior is the most common form seen and is due to slower bone growth in the upper jaw which gives it an upturned appearance. Significant turbinate atrophy can be present without visible snout abnormalities. In the more severe cases, whole-body growth rate will be decreased, which may be due in part to the possibility that PMT affects the growth of the skeletal system (Brockmeier *et al.*, 2012; Ackermann *et al.*, 1996). Coinfection with *B. bronchiseptica* and *P. multocida* can lead to severe upper respiratory signs including epistaxis, brachygnathia, and lateral deformity of the snout.

PCR assays directed at the gene that encodes for the PMT produced by toxigenic strains of *P. multocida* are reportedly specific and sensitive when used on nasal and tonsilar swabs and colostrum (Kamp *et al.*, 1996; Lichtensteiger *et al.*, 1996; Levonen *et al.*, 1996). PCR and ELISAs may be used for herd-health monitoring, facility biosecurity, and clinical diagnosis.

Differentials for PAR include other causes of facial deformities, including paranasal abscesses and breed variations. Other diagnoses to rule out for *B. bronchiseptica* include CMV and other causes of sneezing and rhinitis.

Treatment   Once lesions are present, there is no cure. AR is a disease best prevented.

Prevention/Control   A treatment plan for NPAR and PAR should include a combination of environmental and husbandry improvements followed by a vaccination and antibiotic program tailored to the facility. One approach is to medicate the feed of sows during the last month of gestation to reduce the bacterial load and source of initial exposure for suckling piglets. The oral antibiotics of choice include tilmicosin, sulfonamides, and tetracyclines (Olson and Backstrom, 2000). Piglets can be given weekly or biweekly parenteral injections of oxytetracycline, potentiated sulfonamides, ceftiofur, or penicillin/streptomycin, preferably based on culture and susceptibility, for the first month of life. Medication of feed or water in older weaned pigs at risk for PAR for periods of at least 4–5 weeks will help control clinical signs (Register *et al.*, 2012; Brockmeier *et al.*, 2012).

Vaccines for both *P. multocida* and *B. bronchiseptica* are available as bacterins and toxoids and are considered effective against atrophic rhinitis (Sakano *et al.*, 1997). PMT is an important component of the vaccine to prevent disease. Vaccines are generally given to the sow prefarrowing, as improved colostral immunity is considered more important than piglet vaccination.

Practices such as disinfection between groups of animals housed in a facility, adequate air changes to reduce ammonia levels, good temperature control, adequate nutrition and pen space, and control of concurrent diseases and experimental stress will help. *P. multocida* and *B. bronchiseptica* are sensitive to most common disinfectants.

Development and maintenance of an SPF swine facility using cesarian section, medicated early weaning, and segregated early weaning are the most satisfactory methods of prevention. The focus should be on ensuring freedom from toxigenic *P. multocida* since this is the most pathogenic etiologic agent of this multifactorial disease.

It is possible to keep herds free of significant clinical disease through good sanitation, husbandry, and management.

Necropsy   *B. bronchiseptica* – lesions in young pigs are catarrhal rhinitis, varying degrees of atrophy of the turbinates (most severe in the ventral scroll of the ventral turbinate) (Fig. 16.17), and a bilateral suppurative

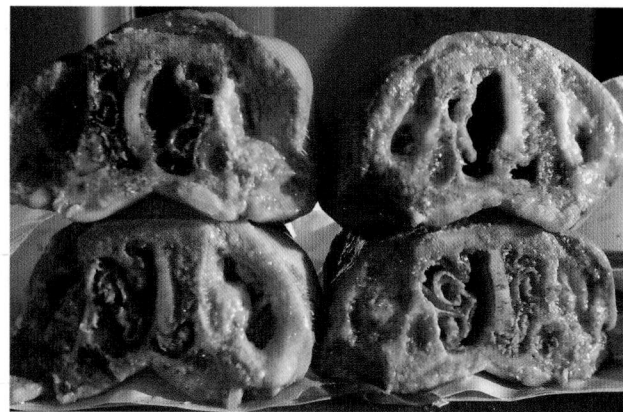

FIGURE 16.17   Atrophic rhinitis. Cross sections of nasal turbinates with loss of turbinate scrolls and deviation of septum. *Courtesy of ISU Veterinary Diagnostic Laboratory.*

bronchopneumonia involving the apical and cardiac lobes (Brockmeier *et al.*, 2012; Duncan *et al.*, 1966b). Commonly, the turbinate atrophy is subjectively measured at necropsy by visual scoring of a section at the level of the second premolar. Techniques for objective quantification of this atrophy by digital image analysis or digitization and computed tomography have been published (Shryock *et al.*, 1998; Gatlin *et al.*, 1996). In the lungs, there is a severe vasculitis, endothelial cell hyperplasia, hemorrhage, and alveolar and perivascular fibrosis (Duncan *et al.*, 1966a).

P. multocida – there are varying degrees of deformity of the snout and the nasal septum. Distortion and atrophy of the turbinates are most severe in the ventral scroll of the ventral turbinates but can also involve the dorsal scroll of the ventral turbinates, dorsal turbinates, and ethmoid turbinates. Microscopic changes include atrophy of the osseous cores of the turbinates and replacement by fibrous connective tissue, metaplasia of respiratory epithelium to stratified squamous, and inflammatory cell infiltrates in the lamina propria (Register *et al.*, 2012).

Research Complications   The toxin produced by severe infections of toxigenic strains of *P. multocida* will induce liver and kidney lesions as well as damage nasal turbinates. *B. bronchiseptica* can induce pneumonic lesions in very young piglets. Therefore, PAR has the potential to affect most chronic research studies.

b. Pasteurellosis

Etiology   *P. multocida* is a gram-negative coccobacillus and a facultative anaerobe. Capsular serotypes A, B, and D have been reported in swine, with A being the most common in pneumonic lungs and B causing the most severe disease (septicemic). The role of toxin production by *P. multocida* as a virulence factor in pneumonic pasteurellosis is not clear; however, it has a defined role in causing atrophic rhinitis.

Epizootiology and Transmission P. *multocida* is a common inhabitant of the upper respiratory tract of swine. It can be cultured from the nose and tonsils of healthy pigs from most herds, including SPF herds (Register *et al.*, 2012). Transmission is by direct contact and aerosols.

Pathogenesis P. *multocida* is not usually a primary agent but results in disease when adherence is facilitated by the presence of other agents such as *M. hyopneumoniae*, PRV, hog cholera, PRRSV, parasites, or *B. bronchiseptica*. P. *multocida* is poorly phagocytized by swine alveolar macrophages and the capsule of the organism interferes with uptake by neutrophils (Register *et al.*, 2012).

Clinical Signs/Diagnosis The predominant signs of the acute form of the disease are dyspnea, cough, anorexia, and fever to 41.7°C. Sudden death is not typical. Morbidity and mortality are variable, and typically pigs will lose weight and have a decreased rate of growth. The chronic form of the disease is characterized by intermittent cough and low fever of 39.5–40°C.

The acute form is clinically similar to pleuropneumonia (APP) without the frequency of sudden death; the chronic form is similar to mycoplasmal pneumonia of swine (MPS). *S. enterica* ser. Choleraesuis should also be considered. *Metastrongylus elongatus* and *Ascaris suum* are additional differentials for the chronic form (Cowart, 1995; Register *et al.*, 2012).

Treatment Animals showing clinical signs should be treated with a parenteral antibiotic based on susceptibility testing. Alternatively, oxytetracycline, ceftiofur, penicillin, florfenicol, enrofloxacin, or doxycycline dosed in the feed has been shown to be effective at controlling pneumonia caused by P. *multocida* and *M. hyopneumoniae*; however, development of resistance to antibiotics is a concern (Burton *et al.*, 1996; Bousquet *et al.*, 1998; Hormansdorfer and Bauer, 1998).

Prevention/Control It is essential to identify and treat or manage any concurrent pathogens since P. *multocida* is usually the secondary agent. Typically, pasteurellosis is a complication of *M. hyopneumoniae* infection. High-quality control of environmental air temperature, humidity, and ammonia levels is critical. Vaccination and medicated feed (tetracyclines, tylosin) and water may be beneficial.

Necropsy Gross findings in the lungs are usually confined to the cranioventral aspects of the lobes and include red to gray areas of consolidation, frothy exudate in the trachea, suppurative pleuritis and pericarditis, pleural adhesions, and pulmonary abscesses (Pijoan and Fuentes, 1987; Register *et al.*, 2012). The histopathologic lesions in the lungs are a severe suppurative bronchopneumonia, with interstitial thickening, fibrinosuppurative pleuritis, and well-defined abscesses.

Research Complications Bronchopneumonia-associated accumulation of purulent fluid in airways will complicate general anesthesia. Severe infections produce fibrinous pleuritis and pericarditis, which will confound most cardiovascular and respiratory system research studies.

c. Pleuropneumonia

Etiology *Actinobacillus pleuropneumoniae* (APP), previously designated as *Haemophilus pleuropneumoniae* or *H. parahaemolyticus*, is the cause of pleuropneumonia of swine. This bacterium is a gram-negative encapsulated coccobacillary rod, which requires nicotinamide adenine dinucleotide (NAD or factor V) for growth. There are currently 15 recognized serotypes (1–15) (Gottschalk, 2012a). Extracellular hemolytic toxins ApxI, ApxII, and ApxIII are some of the more important virulence factors of the *A. pleuropneumoniae* strains that produce them (Reimer *et al.*, 1995; Kamp *et al.*, 1997). All serotypes secrete more than one Apx toxin. There are differences between serotypes as well as differences in geographical prevalence of serotypes (Gottschalk, 2012a).

Epizootiology and Transmission The disease is prevalent worldwide, different countries tend to have a different set of serovars, and multiple serovars can be found in one facility. Transmission is primarily by snout to snout and by aerosol. Recovered swine may become chronic carriers and are a source of transmission within and between herds. Some exposed animals may become subclinical carriers. The spread is likely related to the movement of animals since artificial insemination and embryo transfer are unlikely sources of introduction (Gottschalk, 2012a). Pleuropneumonia is more prevalent in facilities that bring in swine from multiple sources on a regular basis. Typically, in herds where APP is endemic, the piglets are infected in the farrowing pen and a carrier sow is the source. All age groups are affected, and morbidity and mortality are linked to environmental quality, stress, and concurrent infection with other pathogens.

Pathogenesis Inoculation of pigs may result in death in as little as 3 h (Gottschalk, 2012a). Infection with other agents may enhance disease progression of APP. Virulence is also dependent upon serotype specific Apx toxins, LPS, etc. APP binds squamous cells of the tonsil followed by type I pneumocytes of the lower respiratory tract (Chiers *et al.*, 1999; Bosse *et al.*, 2002). Interactions between virulence factors and host immune system, especially macrophages, and neutrophils, along with released cytokines determine pathologic outcome (Cho *et al.*, 2005). Primary damage to the capillary endothelium in alveoli may be the result of endotoxin produced by APP in acute and peracute infections. This results in severe edema and fibrin deposition as well as in thrombosis of capillaries and ischemic necrosis of pulmonary parenchyma (Bertram, 1985). Tissue damage is primarily caused by the host immune response and from lytic factors released from these cells when they are killed by Apx toxins released from APP, whereas death is primarily due to endotoxic shock from APP LPS (Gottschalk, 2012a).

Clinical Signs/Diagnosis The clinical signs of APP can be categorized into peracute, acute, and chronic forms. The peracute form is characterized by rapid development of fever to 41.7°C, anorexia, and depression. There is increased heart rate and the skin becomes cyanotic beginning at the extremities with terminal open-mouth breathing. Near death, there is foamy blood tinged nasal/oral discharge (Gottschalk, 2012a). Animals may be found dead with no prior signs. In the acute form, pigs have fevers of 40.5–41.1°F, depression, anorexia, reddening or congestion of the skin, severe dyspnea with a marked abdominal component, and sometimes death within 36 h The chronic form is characterized by variable cough, decreased rate of body-weight gain, and other complications (pleuritis, abortion, endocarditis, arthritis, abscesses). Serotype 2 has been connected with lameness due to necrotizing osteomyelitis and fibrinopurulent arthritis in 8- to 12-week-old pigs (Jensen *et al.*, 1999). All three forms may be found in the same group of animals. A list of diagnoses to rule out includes *A. suis*, MPS, pasteurellosis, PRRS, *S. enterica* ser. Choleraesuis, and combinations of these agents.

Treatment Parenteral antimicrobials, including ceftiofur, penicillin, tetracyclines, and enrofloxacin, can reduce mortality in the acute stage of the disease (Burton *et al.*, 1996). Marked resistance to amoxicillin, oxytetracycline, and metronidazole and others have increased in recent years (Gottschalk, 2012a). Medicating feed and water with an antimicrobial at a low minimum inhibitory concentration (MIC) for members of an affected group that are still eating and drinking may be successful. A combination of parenteral and oral medication often yields the best results, as many affected animals do not eat. If treating via medicated feed, intake needs to be monitored closely for this reason. Injectable antibiotics may be more reliable. Antimicrobial therapy will not eliminate the chronic form or carrier animals from the herd (Gottschalk, 2012a).

Prevention/Control The most satisfactory prevention program is to maintain a closed, APP-free herd through strict isolation. Artificial insemination and embryo transfer can be utilized when introduction of new genetics is required. Alternatively, only known SPF animals that have been validated by serologic testing (ELISA, CF, or PCR) are added. An ELISA utilizing the *A. pleuropneumoniae* ApxII antigen is useful for this purpose (Leiner *et al.*, 1999). In addition, PCR on mixed bacterial cultures from swine tonsils may be more sensitive than culture for detection and is useful in determining serotype (Gram *et al.*, 1996). Segregated early-weaning practices can potentially eliminate APP; however, this

is difficult because this bacterium is an early colonizer (Macinnes and Desrosiers, 1999). Depopulation and restocking with hysterectomy-derived SPF animals is the most satisfactory means of prevention.

Vaccination of seronegative animals prior to introduction with killed whole-cell, cell-free antigens, or subunit type along with maintaining optimal ambient temperature, ventilation, and humidity may reduce morbidity and mortality (Gottschalk, 2012a; Buettner *et al.*, 2011; Oishi *et al.*, 1995). Oral immunization with live or inactivated *A. pleuropneumoniae* serotype 9 has been shown to provide partial clinical protection from aerosol challenge (Hensel *et al.*, 1995). A vaccine strain of *A. pleuropneumoniae* produced by insertional inactivation of the ApxII operon can be delivered live intranasally and provide cross-serovar protection (Prideaux *et al.*, 1999). Subunit vaccines against Apx1/ApxII/ApxIII have been developed and provide protection against all major serotypes (Ramjeet *et al.*, 2008). Additional control measures include good husbandry practices, including use of disinfectants and minimization of stress.

Necropsy The gross findings in pigs with APP are dependent upon time course and include fibrinous pleuritis, pulmonary edema, and the presence of bloody froth or clotted fibrin plugs in the trachea and bronchi. The lungs contain bilateral lesions that are dark red and firm with a predominance of lesions in the dorsal aspects of the caudal lobes, and there may be a bloody nasal discharge (Didier *et al.*, 1984; Bertram, 1985; Nielsen, 1973). Lung lesions are well-defined abscesses and necrotic areas in the lung. Histopathologic lesions are a necrotizing, fibrinous, and hemorrhagic pneumonia that is predominantly lymphocytic and histiocytic, as well as a vasculitis with thrombosis of vessels and lymphatics (Didier *et al.*, 1984; Nielsen, 1973). Cases of bone necrosis with lysis of growth plates and suppurative osteomyelitis have also been associated with APP serotype 2 (Jensen *et al.*, 1999).

Research Complications APP will affect any research involving the respiratory or cardiovascular systems since pleurisy, pneumonia, and pericarditis may result. If animals survive illness, lungs often contain bacterial sequestrae. The mortality associated with the acute form may terminate most studies.

d. *Actinobacillus Suis*

Etiology *Actinobacillus suis* is a gram-negative bacterium in the Pasteurellaceae family.

Epizootiology/Transmission *A. suis* colonizes the upper respiratory tract with many herds infected, all of which do not always show clinical signs.

Pathogenesis *A. suis* produces toxins similar to APP, but less virulent.

Clinical Signs/Diagnosis Animals may present with septicemia, sudden death, dyspnea, cough, lameness, fever, weakness, wasting, abscesses, neurological signs, abortion, cyanosis, or diffuse hyperemia. There are three forms of disease dependent on the age of animals affected (Yaeger, 1995). The first form is a septicemia affecting suckling and recently weaned piglets where the only signs may be that animals are found dead. The second form is respiratory disease seen in growers and finishers with clinical signs including cough and fever, but they may also be found dead. The third form is an acute septicemia that affects adults with lethargy, anorexia, fever, rhomboid skin lesions, and abortion in pregnant sows.

Diagnosis is based on clinical signs and gross lesions, and confirmed by bacterial culture. Differentials include APP, causes of septicemia, and erysipelas.

Treatment Antibiotics are the treatment of choice and there are no reports of resistance in the literature (Gottschalk, 2012a).

Prevention/Control Vaccines have variable results.

Necropsy Lesions include erysipelas-like lesions, petechiae to ecchymoses in the lung, kidney, heart, liver, spleen, skin, gastrointestinal tract, and petechiae on the ears, abdomen, skin. In acute disease, hemorrhages in multiple organs and serofibrinous exudates in thoracic and abdominal cavities are common. Histological changes include necrotic foci in numerous organs with bacterial thromboemboli. In the form affecting growers and finishers, necrohemorrhagic pneumonia with petechiae in serosal surfaces of abdominal and thoracic organs are seen. Multifocal petechiae and serofibrinous exudates in the thorax and abdomen are seen in the septicemic form that affects adults.

e. Mycoplasmal Pneumonia: Enzootic Pneumonia, Mycoplasmal Pneumonia of Swine

Etiology M. hyopneumoniae is a common pathogen that colonizes the ciliated epithelium of the porcine respiratory tract. Mycoplasmas are small (0.2–0.3 μm), lack a cell wall, and are nonmotile, fastidious, gram-negative facultative anaerobes. They belong to the class Mollicutes and are the smallest free-living cells.

Epizootiology and Transmission Enzootic disease is what is most commonly seen. Epizootic infection is uncommon as it affects naive herds. The spread of MPS is primarily by direct contact with respiratory secretions and aerosols from carrier swine. Generally, it is transmitted from infected sows to suckling piglets prior to weaning; however, pigs of all ages are susceptible. It is probably the most common cause of chronic pneumonia in swine, and most conventional herds are affected.

Pathogenesis M. hyopneumoniae is not a significant sole cause of disease. M. hyopneumoniae adhere to the cilia and apical plasma membrane of the respiratory epithelium in the trachea, bronchi, and bronchioles which results in loss of cilia, ciliostasis, and filling of alveoli with cell debris and exudate and prevent airway clearance of other pathogens (Ackermann *et al.*, 1991). Organisms further suppress innate and acquired pulmonary immunity allowing other bacteria to proliferate, or they can potentiate disease from some viruses (Thacker and Minion, 2012; Thacker *et al.*, 2001). Humoral immunity has an important role in infection and macrophage activity is altered by *M. hyopneumoniae* (Sarradell *et al.*, 2003). IL-10, IL-12 and IL-18 are increased, but IFN-γ is decreased (Thanawongnuwech *et al.*, 2001; Muneta *et al.*, 2006). Tissue damage is due to inflammatory cell factors, not direct damage from the *M. hyopneumoniae* organism (Thacker and Minion, 2012).

Clinical Signs/Diagnosis There are two disease presentations, epizootic and enzootic. Epizootic disease is characterized by coughing, respiratory distress, pyrexia, and death. Enzootic disease manifests via a dry cough, typically when animals are aroused. They also have decreased appetite and fever with endemic disease (Thacker and Minion, 2012). Although younger pigs may be affected, generally clinical signs are not obvious until pigs are 3–6 months of age. Uncomplicated MPS is generally characterized by a reduced growth rate and a chronic cough precipitated by exercise. In some affected animals, the cough may not be readily evident. Morbidity is typically high and mortality low unless complicated by concurrent viral or bacterial infections, or stress of any form. It plays an important role in PRDC when concurrent infection with PRRSV or PCV2 occurs (Thacker *et al.*, 1999; Thacker and Minion, 2012). In these complicated infections, malaise, anorexia, fever, labored respirations, and possibly death may result (Thacker and Minion, 2012). Bacteria that frequently complicate MPS leading to enzootic pneumonia are clinical differentials and include *P. multocida*, *B. bronchiseptica*, *A. pleuropneumoniae*, *S. enterica* ser. Choleraesuis, and *S. suis* (Bousquet *et al.*, 1998; Cowart, 1995).

Culture is not usually feasible since mycoplasmas and *M. hyopneumoniae*, in particular, are difficult to isolate and grow. IFA or IHC and PCR have all been used in diagnosis (Opriessnig *et al.*, 2004). ELISAs are also currently in use to diagnose *M. hyopneumoniae* (Okada *et al.*, 2005).

Treatment Antimicrobials, including lincomycin, tetracyclines, doxycycline in feed, tiamulin, and several quinolone antibiotics, have been shown to be efficacious in reducing the severity of pneumonia and weight reduction due to MPS (Bousquet *et al.*, 1998). This beneficial effect is generally attributed to controlling complicating bacterial infections. Experimental evidence has shown that doxycycline has greater *in vitro* activity than oxytetracycline against *M. hyopneumoniae*, *A. pleuropneumoniae*, and *P. multocida* (Bousquet *et al.*, 1997).

Prevention/Control The most satisfactory form of prevention is to allow only SPF swine into the facility.

M. hyopneumoniae-free herds may be derived by hysterotomy or hysterectomy, medicated early weaning, or segregated early weaning (Dritz *et al.*, 1996). The success of these techniques should be monitored by a combination of ELISA testing of serum or milk, PCR assay of bronchoalveolar lavage fluids or lung tissue, and examination of lungs at necropsy (Baumeister *et al.*, 1998; Stemke, 1997).

Control of clinical disease in infected animals is best accomplished by providing optimal environmental conditions with respect to ammonia levels, humidity, temperature control, air changes, overcrowding, and reduction of stress. Protective immunity will develop in swine recovered from MPS, and vaccines may help alleviate disease, but not colonization (Thacker *et al.*, 2000; Thacker and Minion, 2012). Maternally derived antibodies have been found to inhibit response to *M. hyopneumoniae* vaccination, and the timing of the dosing to avoid this interference varies from herd to herd (Hodgins *et al.*, 2004).

Necropsy In acute disease, the lungs fail to collapse and there is edema of the lungs. The lungs contain pale gray or dark-red foci of consolidation that are most commonly found in the apical lobes and the cranioventral aspects of the middle, accessory, and caudal lobes (Fig. 16.18). Additionally, there may be catarrhal exudate in the bronchi. In enzootic pneumonia, in which secondary bacteria are present, the lungs are mottled by exudate-distended alveoli and the exudate is mucopurulent (Thacker and Minion, 2012). Microscopic lesions consist of perivascular, peribronchial, and peribronchiolar infiltrations of large numbers of lymphoreticular cells, which in chronic lesions may include lymphoid nodules (Piffer and Ross, 1984; Thacker and Minion, 2012). Additionally, differentiation of cuboidal epithelium to pseudostratified epithelium in bronchioles occurs (Ackermann *et al.*, 1991).

Research Complications Uncomplicated infection with *M. hyopneumoniae* will directly interfere with research involving the respiratory system, and complicated infections may also interfere with cardiovascular studies since pericarditis may result. This agent has been found in purpose-bred animals.

f. Mycoplasmal Polyserositis and arthritis

Etiology *Mycoplasma hyorhinis* is probably the easiest of the porcine mycoplasmas to isolate, is a common contaminant of cell culture lines, and is ubiquitous in the swine population. This pathogen has been diagnosed in research swine via PCR.

Epizootiology and Transmission This organism is harbored in the respiratory tract of carrier swine, often without clinical disease. The most likely first exposure for baby pigs is from aerosolization or direct contact with nasal secretions from the sow prior to weaning. The

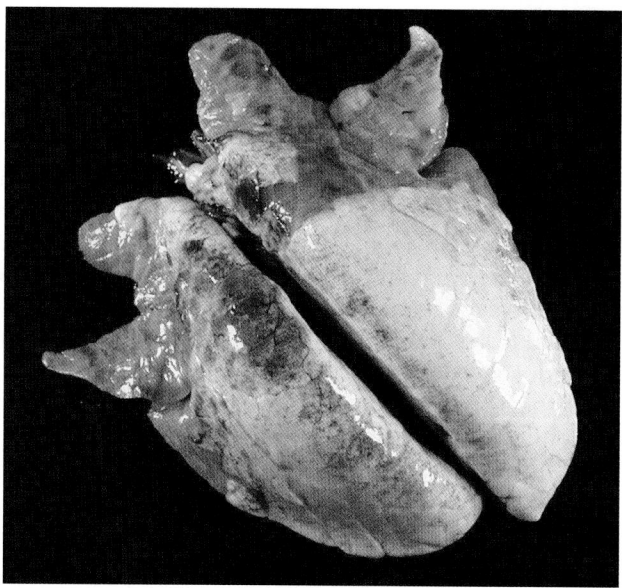

FIGURE 16.18 *M. hyopneumoniae.* Consolidated and red apical lung lobes. *Courtesy of ISU Veterinary Diagnostic Laboratory.*

organism will spread rapidly through group-housed pigs and typically will not cause clinical disease unless the animals are stressed. Stress will induce septicemia and its subsequent lesions (Thacker and Minion, 2012).

Pathogenesis The organism adheres to cilia similar to *M. hyopneumoniae* and is considered normal flora of the respiratory tract. The mechanisms that the organism uses to induce systemic disease is still not known, but once the organism gains entry to other sites, it causes polyserositis and polyarthritis in pigs less than 8 weeks old. In older pigs (3–6 months old), only arthritis is caused (Potgieter *et al.*, 1972; Potgieter and Ross, 1972).

Clinical Signs/Diagnosis The age group most commonly affected is 3–10 weeks of age. Clinical signs typically begin about 1 week after some form of stress or initial exposure to the etiologic agent. The acute signs are lethargy, anorexia, labored respirations, arched back with tucked-up abdomen, lameness, and slight fever and swollen joints. These signs abate in about 2 weeks except that the lameness with swollen joints may persist for several months. Experimental *M. hyorhinis* intranasal inoculation has been shown to cause eustachitis and occasionally otitis media (Morita *et al.*, 1998, 1999). *H. parasuis*, *S. suis*, and *M. hyosynoviae* should be ruled out for this clinical presentation.

Treatment Prophylactic treatment of the entire herd by medicating food or water with lincomycin or tylosin may be beneficial. Antimicrobial treatment of clinically affected swine is unrewarding (Thacker and Minion, 2012; Cowart, 1995).

Prevention/Control Eliminating stress of any type can best prevent clinical outbreaks of disease.

This includes eliminating other diseases, controlling temperature and humidity fluctuations, and avoiding shipping and invasive research protocols. Concurrent infection with *M. hyorhinis* and PRRSV has been found to cause severe pulmonary lesions with respiratory distress (Kawashima *et al.*, 1996) and underscores the need to eliminate other pathogens.

Necropsy Acute lesions include serofibrinous or fibrinopurulent pleuritis, pericarditis, and peritonitis, as well as serofibrinous arthritis with increased synovial fluid and swollen reddish yellow synovial membranes (Ross *et al.*, 1971). The joints most frequently involved are the stifle joints, but the tibiotarsal, cubital, coxofemoral, and shoulder joints may also be involved (Ross *et al.*, 1971). In chronic cases, pannus, erosions of articular cartilage, and fibrous adhesions may be present (Thacker and Minion, 2012).

Research Complications Although mortality is low and morbidity typically less than 25%, clinical disease will confound cardiovascular studies and surgical models because it causes pericarditis, pleuritis, and peritonitis. Orthopedic studies may be compromised by arthritis.

g. Inclusion Body Rhinitis

Etiology Inclusion body rhinitis (IBR) is caused by porcine cytomegalovirus (PCMV) and is found throughout the world. The causative agent is a member of the subfamily Betaherpesvirinae, genus *Proboscivirus* that produces cytomegaly with hallmark basophilic intranuclear inclusions in cytomegalic cells of nasal mucosa. The agent is species-specific and is able to induce latent infection, with shedding of virus occurring even in the presence of circulating antibodies.

Epizootiology and Transmission The virus can be recovered from nasal and ocular secretions, urine, fluids associated with pregnancy, and male reproductive organs. The virus can also be transmitted transplacentally. Dissemination of the agent most commonly occurs via nasal secretions and urine. Viral excretion is highest at 3–8 weeks of age; however, reactivation of excretion can occur when animals are stressed. Lung macrophages are the reservoir of infection.

Pathogenesis The virus enters the body through the mucosa, where it replicates inside the epithelial cells of the mucosal, Harderian, and lacrimal glands. Subsequent viremia results in seeding of mucosal glands, renal tubular epithelium, hepatocytes, and duodenal epithelium, and in neonates or fetal pigs, the reticuloendothelial cells and capillary endothelium (Mettenleiter *et al.*, 2012; Edington *et al.*, 1976). The virus inhibits T-cell function and thus modifies the host defense mechanisms (Kelsey *et al.*, 1977).

Clinical Signs/Diagnosis This disease is usually subclinical in pigs more than 3 weeks of age and may even be totally inapparent in young animals if good management practices are being followed. The clinical sequelae typically associated with this disease include unexpected fetal and piglet death, runting, rhinitis, conjunctival discharge, pneumonia, sometimes neurological signs, and poor weight gain in young pigs (Edington *et al.*, 1977). Some piglets may be born anemic, with edema noted around the jaw and tarsal joints. Adult animals that are exposed to this agent for the first time may develop mild anorexia and lethargy. Coinfection with PCMV and PCV2 exacerbates PRDC (Hansen *et al.*, 2010).

The presence of this disease can be confirmed using a serum ELISA. Virus isolation or PCR can be done on nasal secretions or scrapings, or on whole blood. The virus can be isolated from the nasal mucosa, lung, and kidney. Differential diagnoses include PPV, PCV2, PRRSV, CSF, PRV, and enterovirus.

Prevention/Control Supportive therapy to prevent secondary bacterial infections is important in the face of a viral disease outbreak. Caution should always be taken when introducing new animals into an established grouping as new animals may expose susceptible animals or may stress existing groupings to stimulate resurgence of a latent infection.

Necropsy Gross lesions in piglets are found in the nasal passages, where there is serous rhinitis in early stages of the disease and purulent exudate in older lesions (Thomson, 1988). There may also be sinusitis, and if the disease becomes systemic, there are petechial hemorrhages and edema in the lungs, lymph nodes, subcutaneous tissues, along with pericardial and pleural effusions. The kidneys may contain petechiae, or may be dark purple (Mettenleiter *et al.*, 2012). Histologic findings characteristic for this disease are the presence of large basophilic intranuclear inclusions in the epithelial cells in both the mucosa and the mucosal glands (Thomson, 1988; Edington *et al.*, 1976). If disease is systemic, there may be pneumonia and foci of necrosis in the liver, kidney, CNS, and adrenals, with inclusions in capillary endothelium and sinusoidal cells throughout the body (Thomson, 1988).

Research Complications The virus may be passed to humans in porcine to human xenotransplantation, the consequences of which are currently unknown (Mueller *et al.*, 2004).

h. Swine Influenza

Etiology Swine influenza, first identified in 1918, is caused by a type A influenza virus. The agent is distributed worldwide, and antibodies to the virus are found in about 45% of the sampled pig populations. Influenza A viruses belong to the family of RNA viruses, *Orthomyxoviridae*. The type A viruses are further classified based on the glycoprotein spikes that extend from the viral particle (hemagglutinin [H] and neuraminidase [N]). The antigenic characteristics of these spikes provide the basis for dividing these viruses into subtypes. Antigenic comparison of the H1N1 swine viruses has shown, in contrast to human strains, that there has been little antigenic variation over the last 50 years (Sheerar et al., 1989). This could be attributed to the fact that the virus is able to propagate in an ever-present population of nonimmune pigs. Strains H3N2 and H1N2 are also prevalent in swine and they may also be infected by H3N3, H4N6, H5N1, H5N2, and H9N2 (Van Reeth et al., 2012).

Epizootiology and Transmission   Swine influenza typically appears as a result of new animals entering the herd. Outbreaks rapidly spread through all animals within a group. Once the virus gains purchase within a population of swine, the disease is likely to recur unless the grouping is totally depopulated. Distribution of different subtypes/genotypes varies widely and is dependent on geographical location.

The primary route of transmission is via direct contact with the viral particles present within nasal secretions. There is no evidence that supports a carrier state, and the widespread occurrence and persistence of the virus is attributed to its continued passage to young susceptible animals or animals that have lost protective antibody titers.

The swine influenza viruses (SIVs) have a very wide host range, including humans and birds, and interspecies transmission readily occurs. It can cause acute respiratory disease in humans. It also infects wild boar, domestic turkeys, and free-ranging waterfowl (Van Reeth et al., 2012).

Pathogenesis   The virus enters via the respiratory epithelium. The viral hemagglutinin attaches to host cells via sialic acid containing receptors. Viral replication occurs in both upper and lower respiratory tracts. Virus positive cells are only within the respiratory tract and consist of bronchial and bronchiolar epithelial cells (Jung et al., 2002; De Vleeschauwer et al., 2009). Neutrophils subsequently infiltrate the lungs. Subclinical infection versus disease is determined by viral load and cytokines released. Disease and inflammation are precipitated by increased IFN-α, IFN-γ, tumor necrosis factor (TNF)-α, and IL-1, IL-6, and IL-12 (Van Reeth et al., 1998, 2002; Kim et al., 2009a; Barbe et al., 2011). There may be secondary infection by H. parasuis, P. multocida, A. pleuropneumoniae, M. hyopneumoniae, or S. suis-2.

Clinical Signs/Diagnosis   Animals appear very ill with anorexia, labored open-mouthed breathing, and a strong reluctance to move. The animals have fever, rhinitis, and nasal discharge, and during recovery, will cough. Despite the apparently severe clinical signs, the animals typically recover rapidly within 5–7 days of developing clinical signs. Morbidity is nearly 100% with less than 1% mortality. Clinical signs are similar between common swine serotypes (H1N1, H1N2, H3N2) (Van Reeth et al., 2012).

A definitive diagnosis can be made through isolation of the virus by swabbing nasal mucosa, or virus isolation from bronchoalveolar lavage, nasal, tonsil, or oropharyngeal swabs. Diagnosing weanling pigs via serology is difficult as maternal antibody persists up to 4 months, yet may still be infected and shed viral particles. The main differentials include bacterial pneumonias, porcine respiratory coronavirus, M. hyopneumoniae, and PRRSV.

Treatment   Although not field-tested, amantadine has been shown to reduce the febrile response and the shedding of virus in experimentally infected pigs. This drug is used for treatment and prevention of influenza in humans. Proper nursing care, avoidance of stress, and antibiotics to prevent secondary bacterial infections are recommended.

Prevention/Control   Currently, there are several vaccines licensed for use in the US and Europe. Other means of control include preventing influx of animals from unknown sources and preventing contact with birds and infected humans. PPE use by personnel in contact with pigs is quite important with this disease.

Necropsy   There is fibrinous to mucopurulent exudate in nasal passages, trachea, bronchi, and bronchioles (Thomson, 1988), and sharply demarcated dark-red to purple firm foci of consolidation in apical and cardiac lobes of the lung along with interlobular edema (Van Reeth et al., 2012). Microscopic lesions consist of a necrotizing bronchitis, bronchiolitis, and bronchointerstitial pneumonia, with airways filled with cell debris and neutrophils (Thomson, 1988).

Research Complications   SIV is primarily a pulmonary disease and may affect lung studies. It is a zoonotic disease as well as a reverse zoonosis in that personnel may infect research animals if they are carrying influenza virus.

i. Verminous Pneumonia (Verminous Bronchitis)

Etiology   Natural infections of swine with Metastrongylus spp. include one or more of M. salmi, M. pudendotectus, or M. elongates apri, with the latter being the most common. Adults are white, with males averaging 25mm in length and females, 50mm. Their eggs are oval, 40–50μm in diameter, and larvated.

Adult Ascaris suum (ascarids) are pinkish-yellow nematodes. Males are 15–25cm in length and females, 20–40cm. The eggs are oval, 40–60μm in width and 50–80μm in length, and have a rough or mammilated appearance (Greve, 2012). Both Metastrongylus spp. and A. suum may cause verminous bronchitis in pigs.

Epizootiology and Transmission   M. elongatus (lungworm) has an indirect life cycle and requires an earthworm as an intermediate host. Eggs are coughed up from the lungs, swallowed, and excreted in the feces. Swine eat an earthworm that contains infective larvae, which then migrate to the mesenteric lymph nodes and on to the right heart and lungs. They mature in the bronchi and bronchioles of the diaphragmatic lung lobes. The prepatent period is 28 days.

Ascarids have a direct life cycle and thus can be a problem even in indoor facilities. Ingested larvated eggs hatch in the small intestine and invade the wall of the cecum and colon. The larvae then migrate through the liver and lungs (Murrell *et al.*, 1997). In the lungs, the larvae enter the alveoli and migrate up the airways. They are coughed up and swallowed and then return to the small intestine where they molt into adults. The prepatent period ranges from 40 to 53 days. The presence and migration of these two parasites exacerbate the clinical signs and disease of other viral and bacterial pneumonias of swine.

Pathogenesis M. elongatus larvae migrate through the lung parenchyma, causing alveolar hemorrhage followed by inflammation and consolidation of the lungs. Maturing larvae migrate to the bronchioles and bronchi as they mature into adults, where they copulate and lay eggs which produce more irritation and inflammation (Jones and Hunt, 1983).

Migrating A. suum create liver lesions, which are seen grossly as white spots that peak at about 1 week post infection and heal in 3–8 weeks (Roepstorff, 1998). The pathogenesis of the lung lesions is similar to that of M. elongatus; however, the larvae are coughed up and then swallowed and mature into adults in the small intestine.

Clinical Signs/Diagnosis The clinical signs consist of dyspnea and decreased weight gain. Icterus can be seen if ascarids migrate into the common bile duct. An ELISA for anti-A. suum IgG is more sensitive and probably provides a more realistic assessment of the prevalence than fecal examination for oocysts (Roepstorff, 1998). Differentials should include all bacterial, mycoplasmal, and viral causes of pneumonia in swine.

Treatment M. elongatus is susceptible to doramectin, ivermectin, benzimidazoles, and levamisole (Logan *et al.*, 1996; Yazwinski *et al.*, 1997; Cowart, 1995). Antibiotic therapy may be indicated to treat primary or secondary bacterial pneumonia in swine showing respiratory signs.

A. suum is susceptible to numerous anthelmintics, including avermectins, ivermectin, benzimidazoles, pyrantel, piperazine, levamisole, dichlorvos, and hygromycin B (Logan *et al.*, 1996; Stewart *et al.*, 1996; Saeki *et al.*, 1997). Doramectin SQ has persistent activity of at least 7 days against a challenge with embryonated A. suum eggs (Lichtensteiger *et al.*, 1999).

Prevention/Control In indoor research facilities, the life cycles of both these parasites can be broken by frequent (minimize animal contact with infected feces) and thorough sanitation procedures (steam will kill the

eggs) (Stewart, 2007). Neopredisan (*p*-chloro-*m*-cresol) disinfectant has been shown to be a very efficacious ovicide and larvicide for A. suum (Mielke and Hiepe, 1998). This coupled with a strategic or continuous anthelmintic treatment program should eliminate clinical disease. If outdoor pens are utilized, housing on concrete or bringing the animals indoors to prevent access to earthworms and to facilitate sanitation and anthelmintic treatment is worthwhile. Feral *Sus scrofa* in the US and EU have A. suum and Metastrongylus spp. and are a potential reservoir in areas where contact is possible (Gipson *et al.*, 1999; Henne *et al.*, 1978).

Necropsy Adult M. elongatus can be found in the trachea, bronchi, or bronchioles, and larvae may be found in the lung parenchyma at necropsy (Jones and Hunt, 1983). Characteristically, mucoid plugs containing adults and eggs obstruct the bronchioles in the diaphragmatic lobes, producing atelectasis (Greve, 2012).

Adult A. suum are found in the small intestine, including the common bile duct, and white focal hepatic lesions (scarring) indicative of ascarid migration and sometimes called 'milk spots' are typically found at necropsy (Wagner and Polley, 1997). Larval migration through the lungs produces hemorrhage, inflammation, and emphysema, and may lead to secondary bacterial pneumonia (Greve, 2012).

Research Complications If untreated, these infections will damage the lungs, liver, and other tissues during migration. A. suum is a public health concern because it can cause visceral larval migrans. Appropriate PPE should be worn when staff work with potentially infected pigs (Stewart, 2007).

3. Gastrointestinal Diseases

Young swine commonly develop diarrhea associated with shipping stress, changes in diet, primary or mixed infection with a variety of enteric pathogens, or the perioperative use of antibiotics that may upset the balance of normal gut microbiota. The morbidity and mortality associated with enteritis make clinically affected pigs unsuitable for experimental use, and residual lesions in recovering animals may interfere with experimental assessment of the gastrointestinal tract. The following is a summary of the infectious diarrheas that may be encountered when young swine are managed within research facilities (Table 16.3).

a. Swine Dysentery

Swine dysentery is a severe mucohemorrhagic diarrhea of pigs of postweaning age.

Etiology B. hyodysenteriae, a gram-negative anaerobic spirochete, is the primary etiologic agent of swine dysentery and is one of six Brachyspira spp. known to infect swine (Boye *et al.*, 1998; Stanton, 2006). Because disease is less severe when gnotobiotic pigs are experimentally

TABLE 16.3 Common Infectious Causes of Enteritis in Swine (Newborn to Postweaning Age)[a]

Disease	Clinical signs	Age	Etiology	Gross lesions	Histological signs	Diagnosis
Colibacillosis	Acute death, clear watery to white–yellow or hemorrhagic, diarrhea	Newborn to postweaning	*Escherichia coli* ETEC, EPEC (AEEC), EHEC	Nonspecific dilation and congestion of small intestine, blood-tinged contents	Congestion, hemorrhage, acute inflammation, villous atrophy, adherent bacteria	Culture, serotyping
Swine dysentery	Watery, mucoid, and hemorrhagic diarrhea, rarely acute deaths	1 week and older	*Serpulina hyodysenteriae*	Large bowel edema, hyperemia, mucofibrinous exudate on mucosa	Mucosal edema, mucofibrinous enteritis with superficial erosions, hemorrhage	Culture, Warthin–Starry-positive spirochetes in colonic crypts, PCR
Proliferative enteropathy	Acute death, anorexia, loose watery to hemorrhagic diarrhea	Postweaning	*Lawsonia intracellularis*	Gross thickening of distal ileum, cecocolic junction; cecum, edema, exudate	Hyperplasia of glands and epithelium, intracellular bacteria on EM	In situhybridization, tissue culture isolation, electron microscopy
Clostridial enteritis	Acute death, pink mucoid to severe hemorrhagic diarrhea	Newborn to postweaning	*Clostridium perfringens*	Severe hemorrhagic involvement of small intestine, gas, bloody fluid in abdomen	Necrotic villi, adherent gram-positive bacilli, profuse hemorrhage	Culture, toxin assays on cecal contents, Gram stain of mucosal smears
Salmonella enterocolitis	Watery, yellow diarrhea with fever, anorexia, depression	Postweaning	*Salmonella typhimurium, S. choleraesuis*	Focal or diffuse necrotic typhlocolitis, enlarged mesenteric lymph nodes, other organ involvement	Necrosis of enterocytes, inflammatory infiltrates, thrombi, lymphoid atrophy or hyperplasia	Culture, clinical signs, necropsy lesions
Transmissible gastroenteritis	Vomiting, severe diarrhea, high mortality	Any age	TGE virus	Thin-walled small intestine distended with yellow fluid	Villous atrophy ulceration of Peyer's patch dome epithelium	Rising serum titers, viral isolation, PCR
Rotavirus	Profuse watery, white/yellow diarrhea, fever and vomiting	Most severe within days of birth	Porcine rotavirus	Nonspecific dilation of small and large intestine with yellow to gray watery fluid	Villous atrophy	Rising serum titers, viral isolation, PCR, *in situ* hybridization
Balantidiasis	Asymptomatic to severe ulcerative enterocolitis	Any age	*Balantidium coli*	Variable, secondary to other primary diseases	Ciliated trophozoites, flask-shaped ulcers	Histology, fecal direct smears
Giardiasis	Asymptomatic to anorexia with diarrhea	Any age	*Giardia intestinalis*	None to nonspecific enteritis	None to nonspecific enteritis, adherent comma-shaped	Histology, fecal direct smears
Coccidiosis	Asymptomatic to severe diarrhea	1–2 weeks of age	*Isospora suis*	None, severe cases may have fibrinonecrotic membrane in jejunum and ileum	Villous atrophy, villous fusion, hyperplasia of crypts, necrosis	Fecal flotation
Whipworms	Asymptomatic to severe mucoid or hemorrhagic diarrhea with mortality	Postweaning	*Trichuris suis*	Edema, nodules containing exudate, fibrinonecrotic membrane, hemorrhage, anemia, adult worms attached to mucosa	Migrating larva in submucosa, adult worms attached to mucosa	Fecal flotation, neropsy
Small intestinal threadworms	Asymptomatic to severe diarrhea with mortality	Nursing pigs	*Strongyloides ransomi*	Nonspecific, presence of adult worms in small intestine	Encysted larvae	Fecal flotation, necropsy

[a]*Fox* (2002).

infected, other microorganisms normally found in the lower bowel are believed to contribute to lesion development. Additionally, nutritional factors are important; diets rich in rapidly fermentable carbohydrates may exacerbate clinical signs whereas highly digestible diets, or those high in inulin are protective against disease (Pluske *et al.*, 1996; Hansen *et al.*, 2010; Thomsen *et al.*, 2007).

Epizootiology and Transmission   In natural outbreaks of swine dysentery, *B. hyodysenteriae* is transmitted by fecal–oral contact, either by direct contact between naive and infected pigs or by use of contaminated housing, equipment, or clothing. The organism can survive up to 60 days in moist ground or feces but is readily eliminated by disinfection in the absence of organic material. Recovered pigs may continue to shed *B. hyodysenteriae* in their feces.

Pathogenesis   *B. hyodysenteriae* is very efficient at penetrating mucus and attaching to the colonic epithelium. These organisms do not invade the gut wall below the lamina propria. The organism produces a hemolysin that is cytotoxic and an endotoxin. Diarrhea caused by *B. hyodysenteriae* is the result of colonic malabsorption from failure of colonic epithelial cells to transport sodium and chloride from the lumen to the blood (Argenzio *et al.*, 1980; Schmall *et al.*, 1983). The mechanism of diarrhea is therefore very different from that of *Salmonella, Shigella,* and *E. coli* (Schmall *et al.*, 1983). Dehydration and fluid loss are due to the failure to reabsorb endogenous secretions (Hampson, 2012).

Clinical Signs/Diagnosis   Rarely, swine dysentery may cause peracute death without premonitory signs. More commonly, severe diarrhea and fever with accompanying dehydration, weight loss, and weakness develop over several days. Diarrhea of acute onset is usually watery with large amounts of mucus accompanied by flecks of blood and white, mucofibrinous exudate. Pigs with chronic diarrhea may pass red to black soft stools that contain mucus. Nursing pigs are typically not affected but may develop catarrhal enteritis without hemorrhage. Mixed infections with *Yersinia pseudotuberculosis, S. enterica* ser. Typhimurium, or *B. pilosicoli* commonly result in more extensive lesions, affecting the cecum as well as the colon, and may prolong recovery time from swine dysentery (Thomson, 1988).

Diagnosis of *B. hyodysenteriae* infection can be confirmed by culture or PCR (Atyeo *et al.*, 1998). Hemorrhagic diarrhea in piglets that are newborn to several weeks of age could also be caused by *Clostridium perfringens*. In older pigs, other causes of hemorrhagic enteritis include *Salmonella, L. intracellularis,* and *Trichuris suis.*

Treatment   If indicated, therapy should consist of fluid and electrolyte replacement along with antibiotics. Carbadox, tiamulin, and lincomycin have all been reported to be effective in treatment and/or prevention of swine dysentery.

Prevention/Control   Swine dysentery is usually introduced to a facility by the purchase of an asymptomatic carrier pig. Wild rodents are also reservoirs. Pigs should be purchased from herds SPF for *B. hyodysenteriae* or alternatively, from herds in which drugs or vaccines that may only suppress infection are not used.

In the biomedical research setting, pigs affected with swine dysentery should be quarantined and treated or euthanized. Sanitation of the facility and associated equipment along with review of rodent control and vendor health status should be adequate to avoid reintroduction. Valuable pigs can be segregated by health status and treated with antibiotics. Nursing pigs are protected by colostrum from previously infected sows and can be a source of *Brachyspira*-free pigs if weaned early and housed in a clean facility.

Necropsy   Pigs that have died from swine dysentery are dehydrated and may have rough or fecal-stained coats. The gross lesions vary in distribution but are confined to the large bowel (Hughes *et al.*, 1977). Early lesions include reddening and edema of the gut wall, mucosa, and mesenteric lymph nodes, as well as a fibrinous, blood-flecked membrane covering the mucosa (Hampson, 2012). Older lesions are less edematous, but there is a thick mucosal pseudomembrane composed of fibrin, mucus, and blood (Hampson, 2012). Microscopic lesions consist of elongated colonic crypts, goblet cell hyperplasia, and necrosis of sheets of epithelial cells resulting in damage to exposed capillaries and exudation of fluid, fibrin, blood, and inflammatory cells from the lamina propria (Hughes *et al.*, 1977). Large numbers of spirochetes can be found in the crypts as well as in the lumen.

Research Complications   The morbidity and mortality associated with swine dysentery make clinically affected pigs unsuitable for experimental use.

b. *Brachyspira Pilosicoli*: Porcine Intestinal/Colonic Spirochetosis   New in this BB

Brachyspira pilosicoli is a relatively newly recognized species of pathogenic intestinal spirochete that causes porcine colonic spirochetosis, a nonfatal diarrheal disease that affects pigs during the growing and finishing stages (Duhamel *et al.*, 1998).

Etiology   *B. pilosicoli* was first identified in 1993 as *Anguillina coli* as a cause of porcine diarrhea and loss of condition (Lee *et al.*, 1993).

Epizootiology/Transmission   *B. pilosicoli* can be found in contaminated water and colonizes chickens, wild ducks, and immunocompromised humans. Transmission is fecal–oral.

Pathogenesis   Organisms attach only to mature apical enterocytes and not immature cells within crypts

(Trott *et al.*, 1996). Similar to *B. hyodysenteriae*, disease may be influenced by dietary factors. Non-pelleted diets result in reduced prevalence of disease, whereas pelleted diets increase the risk of colonization (Stege *et al.*, 2001; Lindecrona *et al.*, 2004).

Clinical Signs/Diagnosis Clinical signs develop soon after weaning or when swine are placed on a new diet (Duhamel *et al.*, 1998). Signs include loose stool in finishers, but younger animals often have watery green to brown mucoid diarrhea with flecks of blood (Duhamel *et al.*, 1998). Concurrent diseases that may lead to exacerbation include swine dysentery, salmonellosis, proliferative enteropathy, or PCV2 infection (Duhamel *et al.*, 1998).

Diagnosis is usually via specific PCR tests in conjunction with clinical signs consistent with the disease. Disease associated with *B. pilosicoli* may be concurrent with disease from *B. hyodysenteriae*, salmonellosis, *L. intracellularis*, *E. coli*, *Yersinia* spp., *T. suis*, PCV2, or nonspecific colitis which are all also differentials for *B. pilosicoli* (Duhamel *et al.*, 1998).

Treatment/Prevention/Control Treatment includes antimicrobials, decreasing stress within the animal's environment, and change of diet. Vaccines may ameliorate disease symptoms, but do not prevent infection.

Necropsy Gross lesions are limited to the cecum and colon, which are flaccid and fluid-filled, with enlarged associated lymph nodes. Serosal edema, congestion of the mucosa with erosions, and necrotic areas are common. Histological changes include dilated elongated crypts distended with mucus, cellular debris, degenerate inflammatory cells, and occasional Brachyspiral organisms (Jensen *et al.*, 2000). Organisms may also be found within goblet cells. The lamina propria is commonly distended with neutrophils and lymphocytes.

Research Complications This organism may colonize immunocompromised humans, so PPE is important when there is contact with pigs.

c. Proliferative Enteropathy

Based on the excessively proliferative lesions found at necropsy in the terminal ileum, proliferative enteropathy (PE) of the pig has historically been referred to as porcine intestinal adenomatosis, terminal or regional ileitis, intestinal adenoma, and porcine proliferative ileitis. Proliferative enteropathy affects multiple species (Cooper and Gebhart, 1998).

Etiology PE is associated with the presence of abundant intracellular organisms in enterocytes. The organisms are difficult to work with because they can be grown only in tissue culture. Koch's postulates have been fulfilled using a pure culture of the microaerophilic bacterium, *L. intracellularis* (Lawson *et al.*, 1993; McOrist *et al.*, 1995a). Variations in infectivity when attempting cross-species transmission suggest that two biovars exist

(Jasni *et al.*, 1994; Murakata *et al.*, 2008; McOrist and Gebhart, 2012).

Epizootiology and Transmission PE is present worldwide and affects many species, including the pig, hamster, dog, fox, ferret, horse, rat, and rabbit. Consequently, other animals, such as rodents, could be the sources of new infection. *Lawsonia* is shed in feces, and transmission is by fecal–oral contact. In endemic areas, 15–30% of the herds are estimated to be affected with a 5–20% infection rate within a herd. There is risk of environmental contamination, as *L. intracellulare* can remain viable in feces for at least 2 weeks (Collins *et al.*, 2000). *L. intracellulare* has also been reported in wild pigs which may also serve as a source of infection (Tomanova *et al.*, 2002).

Pathogenesis *L. intracellularis* is an obligate intracellular organism. Animals become infected as a result of consuming fecal-contaminated material (McOrist *et al.*, 1995a). *L. intracellularis* is endocytosed by cells via a vacuole which rapidly breaks down, liberating organisms which multiply freely within the cytoplasm (McOrist and Gebhart, 2012). The mechanism resulting in cells continuing to divide without maturing is currently unknown (McOrist and Gebhart, 2012). The organisms enter the immature, proliferating crypt epithelial cells and multiply within the apical cytoplasm with no discernible inflammatory reaction, and in fact, the number of CD8(+) T cells decreases within 14 days of infection (Macintyre *et al.*, 2003). The infected crypt cells fail to mature and are not shed, so the crypts become elongated and tortuous resulting in decreased nutrient absorption (McOrist and Gebhart, 2012). Pathogenesis for acute hemorrhagic proliferative enteropathy has not been fully elucidated.

Clinical Signs/Diagnosis Clinical disease attributed to PE is most often observed in postweaned pigs between 6 and 20 weeks of age. Clinical signs range from none to marked dullness, anorexia, and diarrhea. Diarrhea is typically moderate with loose to watery stools of normal color. Failure to grow at a normal rate may be the only clinical sign that is detectable *ante mortem*. Young adults may present with more severe hemorrhagic enteritis, acute death, or anemia secondary to acute hemorrhagic diarrhea, or a more chronic form associated with passage of black tarry feces. Pregnant animals may abort.

Diagnosis is achieved via fecal PCR or use of a specific antibody incorporated into a fecal immunoassay, serological diagnosis via ELISA, or demonstration of intracellular organisms in histological section using immunohistochemistry (McOrist and Gebhart, 2012). Differential diagnoses depend on the form of the disease presented, but include rotavirus, coronavirus, *S. enterica* ser. Typhimurium, *B. hyodysenteriae*, PCVAD, nutritional causes, and esophogastric ulceration.

Treatment Proliferative enteropathy can be self-limiting with spontaneous improvement after several weeks. Antibiotics are commonly used to control clinical signs. Treatment of this disease is problematic because of the lack of *in vivo* or *in vitro* data on antibiotic sensitivities of *Lawsonia*. In tissue culture, penicillin, erythromycin, difloxacin, virginiamycin, and chlortetracycline were the most effective antibiotics (McOrist *et al.*, 1995b). Tylosin phosphate can be effective for prevention and for treatment of PE (McOrist *et al.*, 1997).

Prevention/Control Swine should be purchased from a vendor with a herd-health history that is free of PE. Newly introduced pigs should be quarantined and housed separately to avoid contact with feces of other swine that may be shedding *Lawsonia*.

An oral, attenuated live vaccine is commercially available, provides protective immunity, and is effective at controlling disease and provides protective immunity (Kroll *et al.*, 2004). Clinically affected pigs should be quarantined and treated or euthanized, based on severity of disease and the intended use of the animal. Control efforts should include sanitation of equipment and the housing area, review of rodent control, and treatment with antibiotics of pigs at risk of clinical disease (McOrist *et al.*, 1996). Absence of clinical signs does not guarantee freedom from disease or infection with *L. intracellulare*.

Necropsy The gross lesions of PE are found in the ileum, cecum, and the most proximal one-third of the spiral colon and consist of a markedly thickened gut wall and mucosa containing multiple transverse or longitudinal folds (Fig. 16.19) (McOrist and Gebhart, 2012). In mild cases, the distal most 10 cm of the ileum is the most likely site of infection and should be examined carefully (McOrist and Gebhart, 2012). Microscopic lesions consist of markedly elongated branching crypts lined by immature epithelial cells and lack goblet cells (Fig. 16.20). Varying numbers of silver-staining organisms that also exhibit acid-fast staining with a modified Ziehl–Neelsen stain are found free in the apical cytoplasm of the lining cells (Fig. 16.21) (McOrist *et al.*, 1995a). Inflammatory response in the lamina propria may be minimal. In more severe cases, lesions may include coagulative necrotic enteritis with caseous mats adherent to the jejunal/ileal mucosa (McOrist and Gebhart, 2012).

The gross lesions of the hemorrhagic form of the disease are confined to the ileum and rarely involve the large bowel. These consist of a thickened, reddened mucosa that does not contain erosions but may be covered by a fibrinous membrane, and the lumen may contain

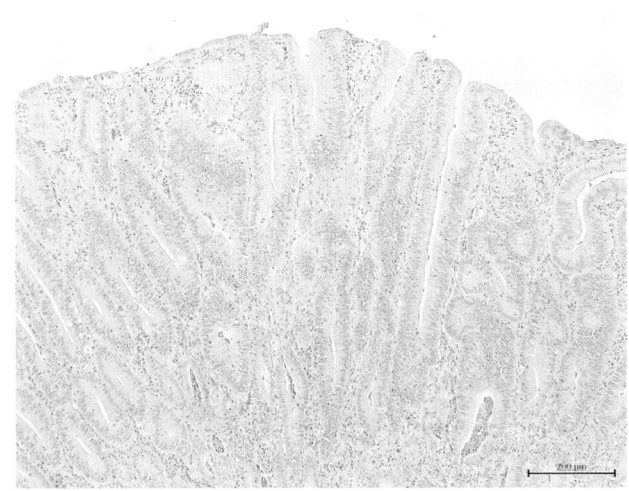

FIGURE 16.20 *Lawsonia intracellularis*, proliferative enteritis. Glands of the intestine are elongated. *Courtesy of J. Haruna.*

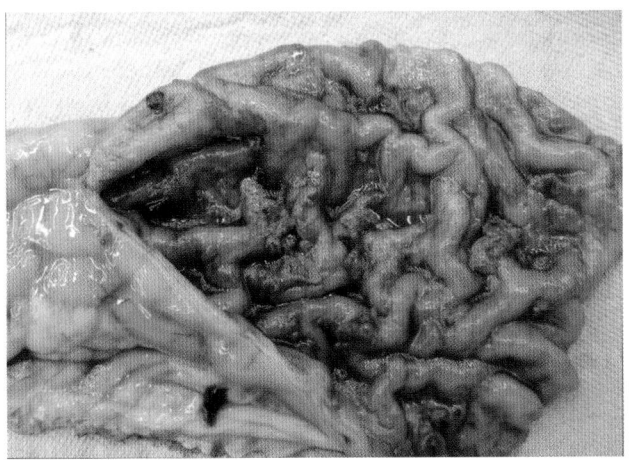

FIGURE 16.19 *Lawsonia intracellularis*, proliferative enteritis. The wall of the intestine is diffusely markedly thickened. *Courtesy of ISU Veterinary Diagnostic Laboratory.*

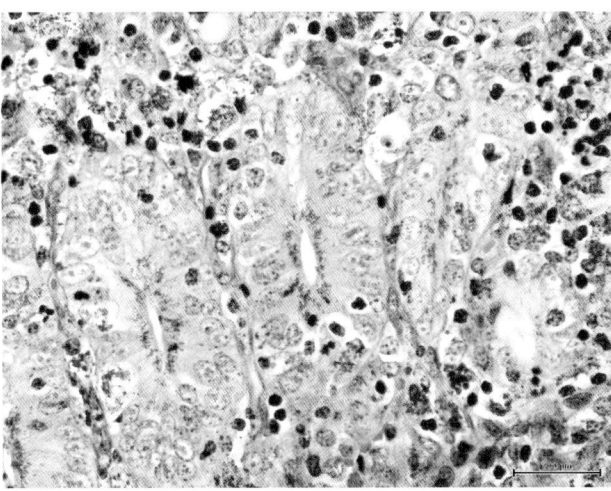

FIGURE 16.21 *Lawsonia intracellularis*, proliferative enteritis. Organisms are present within the apical cytoplasm of intestinal glandular enterocytes. *Courtesy of J. Haruna.*

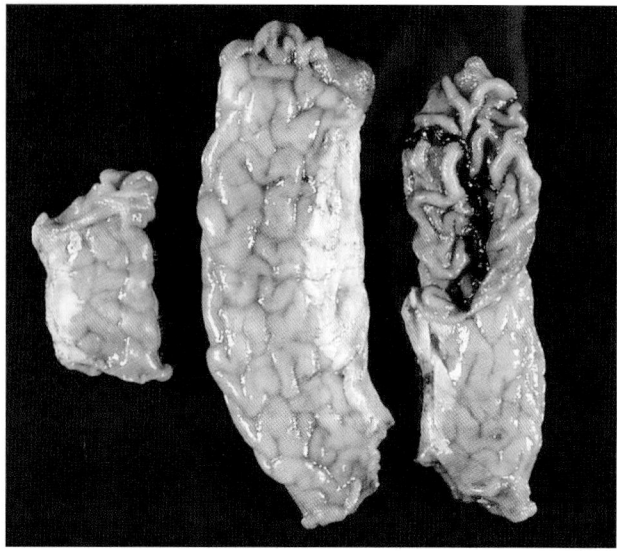

FIGURE 16.22   *Lawsonia intracellularis*, proliferative enteritis, hemorrhagic form. Intestinal wall is diffusely thickened with luminal hemorrhage present. *Courtesy of ISU Veterinary Diagnostic Laboratory.*

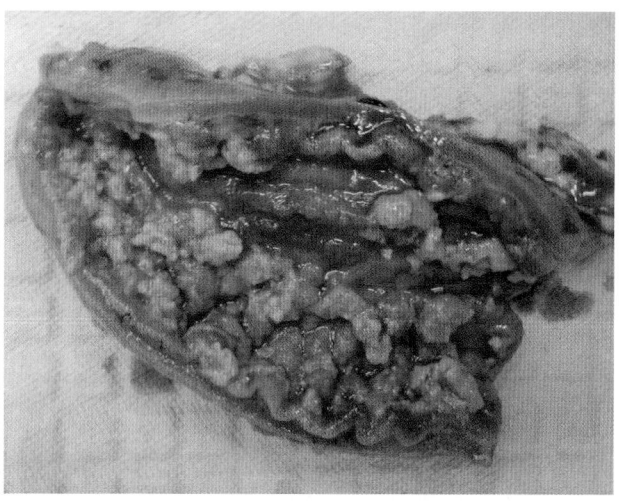

FIGURE 16.23   *Lawsonia intracellularis*, proliferative enteritis, fibrinonecrotic. The intestine is diffusely thickened and there is fibrinonecrotic debris adherent to the lumenal. *Courtesy of ISU Veterinary Diagnostic Laboratory.*

blood clots; colonic contents may be black and tarry (Figs 16.22, 16.23) (McOrist and Gebhart, 2012; Love and Love, 1979). Histologic findings include extensive degeneration and necrosis of the ileal epithelium, crypt abscesses, and extensive accumulation of proteinaceous fluids in the lamina propria of the villi, resulting in distortion of the villi (Love and Love, 1979).

Granulomatous inflammation has also been associated with *Lawsonia* infection (Segales, 2012).

Research Complications   The morbidity and mortality associated with PE make clinically affected pigs

unsuitable for experimental use. Although lesions typically resolve over time, the presence of clinical disease with lesions will impact research.

d. Colibacillosis

Enteric colibacillosis is the most important diarrheal disease of young swine (Fairbrother and Gyles, 2012). Diarrhea attributable to colibacillosis is commonly observed in neonates born to nonimmune sows or in piglets housed in heavily contaminated environments. Susceptible animals are those recently weaned and animals stressed by new housing, or dietary changes.

Etiology   Colibacillosis is caused by pathogenic *E. coli*, a gram-negative facultative anaerobic rod. *E. coli* are responsible for many diseases entities, the most important of which in pigs are postweaning diarrhea (PWD) and edema disease (ED). The species *E. coli* includes members that are normal gut flora as well as enteric pathogens that are further classified by antigenic serotype: somatic (O), capsular (K), flagellar (H), and fimbrial adhesins (F). Pathogenic *E. coli* also possess one or more virulence factors encoded on either the bacterial genome or plasmids. Various classifications associated with different modes of pathogenesis include enterotoxigenic strains of *E. coli* (ETEC), which produce heat-stable (ST) or heat-labile (LT) enterotoxins. Necrotoxic *E. coli* (NTEC) produce cytotoxic necrotic factors (CTF) which lead to diarrhea (De Rycke *et al.*, 1999; Toth *et al.*, 2000). Enteropathogenic *E. coli* (EPEC), also referred to as attaching and effacing strains (AEEC), attach to the enteric epithelium using fimbrial adhesins, and efface the microvilli and invade the epithelial cells. Strains of *E. coli* that cause hemorrhagic gastroenteritis are referred to as enterohemorrhagic *E. coli* (EHEC) (Tzipori *et al.*, 1989). ETEC is the most important of the *E. coli* in pigs. EPEC may also cause PWD. Shiga-toxin producing *E. coli* or ED associated *E. coli* (STEC/EDEC) are responsible for ED. This chapter will focus on causes of PWD and ED. Other conditions are beyond the scope of this publication but have been recently reviewed elsewhere (Kaper *et al.*, 2004; Croxen and Finlay, 2010).

Epizootiology and Transmission   Clinical disease results from interaction between the causative bacteria, adverse environmental conditions, and select host factors. Infections with *E. coli* are widespread and up to 25 different strains may be identified in the gastrointestinal tract of any one individual (Fairbrother and Gyles, 2012). Newborn pigs encountering large numbers of *E. coli* carrying the appropriate virulence factors will develop colibacillosis if colostrum is not available or if the sow is not immune to *E. coli*.

Pathogenesis   Some pigs are inherently resistant to colibacillosis because they lack receptors on their epithelial cell brush borders to which the fimbriae bind (Baker *et al.*, 1997).

The K1 polysaccharide enhances bacterial resistance to complement-mediated killing by inhibiting the alternative pathway to complement activation. The long O-chain polysaccharide chains in the cell wall bind the membrane attack complex resulting from complement activation distant from the cell membrane so that it cannot lyse the cell (Gyles, 1993). Specialized fimbriae, K88(F4), K99(F5), F6, and F41 permit the adherence and colonization of the enterocytes.

ETEC organisms produce toxins (STa, STb, LTI, LTII, and EAST-1) after attachment to the apical surface of enterocytes. These enterotoxins change the water–electrolyte flux in the small intestine which leads to diarrhea if the fluid is not resorbed in the large intestine. STa binds receptor leading to fluid/electrolyte secretion (Giannella and Mann, 2003). STb binds a receptor and increases cellular uptake of calcium inducing secretion of water and electrolytes (Harville and Dreyfus, 1995). LT is endocytosed and permanently activates adenylyl cyclase, which increases water and electrolyte secretion (Dorsey et al., 2006; Fairbrother and Gyles, 2012). EAST-1 acts similarly to STa (Fairbrother and Gyles, 2012).

ETEC have F4(K88) or F18 fimbrial adhesins. The fimbria produced determines where in the gastrointestinal tract the organism colonizes. When EPEC is involved in PWD, it causes attaching and effacing lesions via a complex secretion system. STEC/EDEC produce shiga toxins (also known as verotoxins). STEC/EDEC that secrete STx2e are most pathogenic of the STEC/EDEC and cause ED. STx2e damages blood vessel walls resulting in increased permeability and edema. STEC/EDEC often have F18 fimbrial adhesins.

Clinical Signs/Diagnosis Colibacillosis presents as diarrhea that varies in severity based on the virulence factors present and the age and immune status of the piglets. Severe dehydration, metabolic acidosis, and weight loss may accompany the diarrhea, or peracute death without diarrhea may be seen. Neonatal colibacillosis can develop within hours of birth and is characterized by either clear, watery diarrhea or loose stools that vary in color from white to brown. Litters born to gilts are more frequently affected versus litters born to sows. Severe outbreaks are associated with high morbidity and mortality in neonates; older pigs have less severe disease. Hemorrhagic gastroenteritis from colibacillosis can occur peracutely (sudden death) or acutely (rapid decline with severe diarrhea) in previously healthy, unweaned, or recently weaned pigs. The differential diagnoses for yellow to white, watery diarrhea in piglets that are newborn to several weeks of age should include salmonellosis, coronavirus, rotavirus, nematodiasis, and coccidiosis.

ED is characterized by swelling of the eyelids and forehead, and there is usually no diarrhea.

Treatment Administering broad-spectrum antibiotics should be started after confirming culture and sensitivity because sensitivity varies significantly amongst E. coli isolates (Fairbrother and Gyles, 2012). Most isolates are sensitive to aminoglycosides, potentiated sulfa drugs, and cephalosporins. Administration of phages against experimentally infected weaned piglets with O149:H10:F4 (ETEC) demonstrated that phages have a potential for prophylactic use against diarrhea and shedding of ETEC (Jamalludeen et al., 2009). Oral fluid therapy consisting of electrolyte replacement solutions containing glucose should be instituted to correct dehydration, energy depletion, and ongoing fluid and electrolyte losses.

Prevention/Control Farrowing management should be 'all in, all out' to provide for adequate sanitation between litters. In problem herds, gilts and sows should be immunized with a commercial vaccine or an autologous bacterin during gestation.

To minimize environmental stress, piglets should be kept warm, clean, and draft free. Nursing pigs will derive protection from colostrum feeding from immune sows.

Necropsy Lesions from animals with PWD are non-specific, but include dehydration, distended stomach with fundic hyperemia, and edema in the small intestine.

Gross lesions of ED may include marked edema of the mesenteric lymph nodes, mesocolon, mesentery, the wall of the stomach, large intestine, subcutaneous lymph nodes, eyelids, subcutaneous tissues, lungs, liver, and gallbladder. Degenerative angiopathy is present in above tissues as well as the brain (Fairbrother and Gyles, 2012).

Research Complications Morbidity and mortality from colibacillosis in neonatal pigs interfere with their experimental use. Once recovered, animals should be clinically normal.

Pigs can shed zoonotic EHEC and proper PPE should be worn when working with potentially or experimentally infected swine (Fairbrother and Gyles, 2012).

e. Clostridial Enteritis

Clostridial infection of the intestinal tract of young swine commonly results in necrotic enteritis with high mortality.

Etiology C. perfringens is an encapsulated, gram-positive bacillus that produces a variety of enterotoxins that are responsible for clinical signs and lesions (Buogo et al., 1995). C. perfringens type A is a normal inhabitant of the swine intestine but some strains cause enteric disease. In contrast, fatal necrotic enteritis is caused by C. perfringens type C. C. difficile is an emerging cause of porcine neonatal diarrhea.

Epizootiology and Transmission The bacillus is transferred from sow to pigs and between pigs by fecal–oral contact. C. perfringens exists in the environment as a vegetative form or as spores that persist for a least a year.

C. perfringens type C is usually introduced by a carrier sow in which the organism is a minor component, but when piglets ingest organism, they act as an amplifying vessel and are overwhelmed by toxins secreted from overgrowth of organisms.

Although disease is most common in pigs aged 12h to 7 days and peaks in incidence at 3 days of age, disease has also been observed in older pigs aged 2–4 weeks and in postweaning pigs. Disease is explosive, with 100% mortality in pigs born to nonimmune sows. Subsequent litters are protected by maternal immunity.

Pathogenesis Disease due to *C. perfringens* type A occurs when large numbers of organisms build up in the jejunum and ileum and produce a toxin (CPA) and may also produce CPB2 toxin. These organisms do not invade the enterocytes.

C. perfringens C attaches to the enteric epithelium at the apex of the villi leading to desquamation and proliferation of organisms along the basement membrane.

C. perfringens type C organisms produce a trypsin sensitive β-toxin that is responsible for much of the necrotizing lesions. The key factor is CPB toxin, although CPB2 toxin may also play a role. These organisms attach to enterocytes and result in initial loss of microvilli on the enterocytes at the tips of the villi and damage to terminal capillaries, with increased capillary permeability. This is followed by a rapid, progressive necrosis of the remaining villus enterocytes, the crypt cells, and mesenchymal structures in the lamina propria and muscularis mucosa (Niilo, 1993). Some organisms may penetrate to the muscle layers and produce emphysema of the gut wall and thrombosis of vessels (Frana, 2012).

C. difficile produces C. dif toxin A and C. dif toxin B, a cytotoxin and enterotoxin, respectively (Keel and Songer, 2006, 2011).

Clinical Signs/Diagnosis Clinical manifestations of infection with *C. perfringens* will depend on the immune status of the swine herd and the age of naive exposed piglets. Disease caused by *C. perfringens* Type A can develop within 48h of birth. Piglets have rough pelage, perineal staining, and creamy or pasty diarrhea which may become pink and mucoid and last up to 5 days (Songer, 2012). The majority of affected piglets recover but tend to develop slower. Clinical signs of *C. perfringens* type C include hemorrhagic diarrhea, weakness, and lethargy although the only sign may be peracute with death of piglets aged 12–36h. Acute disease is characterized by 2 days of reddish-brown diarrhea containing gray, necrotic debris, with death by 3 days of age. Subacute disease develops as persistent nonhemorrhagic diarrhea that is yellow initially and then changes to clear liquid with flecks of necrotic debris. Chronic enteritis may involve intermittent or persistent diarrhea for several weeks, with mucoid yellow–gray feces (Songer, 2012).

Diagnosis is difficult because *C. perfringens* A is normal flora. For *C. perfringens* C, ELISAs that detect the toxin in fecal matter, culture, examination of fecal smears, or histology may aid in diagnosis. Differentials for hemorrhagic diarrhea in newborn piglets to those several weeks of age should include *C. perfringens*, *B. hyodysenteriae*, *Salmonella*, *L. intracellularis*, and *T. suis*.

Treatment Once clinical signs develop, disease is extensive and often unresponsive to therapy. Oral antimicrobials such as ampicillin given soon after birth and repeated daily for the first 3 days of life may prevent clinical disease. Another prophylactic therapy is a combination of ceftiofur and bacitracin methylene disalicylate which may be given to sows before and after farrowing (Songer, 2012). Pigs with severe diarrhea should receive supplemental fluids containing glucose and electrolytes.

Prevention/Control Routine vaccination of sows will prevent disease (Kelneric *et al.*, 1996). Sows can be vaccinated with a toxoid at the time of breeding or midgestation and then again 2 weeks prior to farrowing. Piglets from immune sows will be protected by colostrum.

Clinically ill pigs should be isolated and treated and the premises sanitized. Individual piglets and pregnant swine that are at risk from recent exposure should be vaccinated with recombinant toxoids α and β (Salvarani *et al.*, 2013). Medicated feed has been shown to control clinical signs (Kyriakis *et al.*, 1996).

Necropsy *C. perfringens* A lesions consist of flaccid, thin-walled, intestine that is gas filled with watery contents, with necrosis of the superficial villus tip and fibrin.

White pasty fecal matter may be found in distended large intestines with no gross lesions. A large number of organisms may be found in the lumen and in lesions in the jejunum and ileum. *C. perfringens* C lesions are a segmental transmural necrosis with emphysema in the small intestine and sometimes in the cecum and proximal colon. The affected segments of gut vary from multifocal involvement to nearly diffuse involvement of the small intestine. The affected gut wall is dark red to black, and there may be gas bubbles. Enteric lymph nodes are red. The mucosa is dark red, and the intestinal contents in affected segments contain hemorrhagic and necrotic debris. The hallmark signs noted at necropsy are severe hemorrhage in the small intestines and blood-tinged peritoneal fluid (Songer, 2012). Microscopic lesions consist of severe necrosis of villi and crypts, and severe and extensive hemorrhages throughout the lamina propria and mucosa. There may be a necrotic membrane composed of bacteria, sloughed epithelium, fibrin, and inflammatory cells lying over the submucosa (Songer, 2012).

Research Complications Clostridial enteritis causes acute death and severe morbidity among survivors. Overgrowth of *C. perfringens* from perioperative use of antibiotics may cause acute losses and interrupt surgical studies.

f. Salmonella Enterocolitis

See *Polysystemic Diseases* (Section III, A, 1).

g. Transmissible Gastroenteritis

Transmissible gastroenteritis (TGE) is a highly contagious viral enteritis associated with vomiting, severe diarrhea, and high mortality in piglets less than 2 weeks old.

Etiology TGE is caused by a member of the species *Alphacoronavirus 1*, which are pleomorphic enveloped viruses containing a positive-sense, single-stranded RNA genome in the *Alphacoronavirus* genus, Coronavirinae subfamily of the Coronaviridae family (Viruses, 2013; Carstens, 2010). Alphacoronavirus-1 is historically known as transmissible gastroenteritis virus (TGEV). This is one of four members that naturally infect pigs: TGEV, hemagglutinating encephalomyelitis virus, porcine respiratory coronavirus (PRCV), and the emerging disease, porcine epidemic diarrhea virus (PEDV).

Epizootiology and Transmission Epizootic TGE can develop within days when the majority of animals are susceptible. A pattern of enzootic TGE will follow if viral challenge exceeds protection afforded by maternal immunity or as passive immunity wanes in the post-weaning period. In herds with enzootic TGE, older animals will be asymptomatic, but diarrhea will develop in 1- to 2-week-old pigs. Usually morbidity and mortality are lower, making diagnosis more difficult and requiring discrimination between other common causes of neonatal diarrhea, such as rotavirus and colibacillosis. PEDV has only recently been reported in the US, thus expanding its distribution (Service, 2013).

Pathogenesis TGEV uses the aminopeptidase-N receptor on porcine enterocytes to gain access to the cell. These receptors are only found on enterocytes with microvilli and only cells mid-villus to the tip and not in crypts (Perlman and Netland, 2009; Weingartl and Derbyshire, 1994). Enterocytes are replaced in the neonatal period when cell type changes from fetal to adult (Smith and Peacock, 1980). This accounts for neonates being primarily susceptible. The virus multiplies in mid-villus enterocytes, which are then sloughed leading to villar blunting and fusion of non-epithelialized basement membranes, thus decreasing digestive surface and enzymatic activity resulting in maldigestive/malabsorptive diarrhea.

Clinical Signs/Diagnosis Anorexia, vomiting, and/or diarrhea develop in 18–72h in susceptible animals of all ages, particularly in the winter (Saif *et al.*, 2012). Nursing pigs develop transient vomiting and profuse watery yellowish diarrhea, with dehydration and rapid weight loss. Malodorous diarrhea will contain milk curds. Piglets less than 2 weeks old experience high mortality secondary to dehydration from enteritis. Piglets over 3 weeks of age typically survive but their growth may be stunted (Saif *et al.*, 2012). Differential diagnoses for yellow to white watery diarrhea in piglets that are newborn to several weeks of age should include colibacillosis, rotavirus, coccidiosis, and nematodiasis.

Treatment There is no specific treatment for piglets infected with TGEV. Supportive care with fluids containing glucose and electrolytes is indicated. In piglets 2–5 weeks old, antibiotics are effective if there are concurrent primary or opportunistic bacterial pathogens.

Prevention/Control Swine intended for research should be purchased from a serologically negative herd. Naive swine should not be introduced into potentially contaminated environments or into established herds known to harbor enzootic TGEV. Vaccination of boars, gilts, and sows will moderately reduce clinical signs.

A moratorium on purchase of new animals and vaccination of reproductive stock will eventually contain an outbreak as the herd develops immunity. Stress exacerbates disease and should be minimized.

Necropsy Gross lesions are confined to the gastrointestinal tract and consist of a stomach distended with milk, gastric petechiation, and a distended, thin-walled small intestine, which is filled with watery material and curds of undigested milk. The piglets are usually severely dehydrated, and there is no chyle in the lymphatic channels in the mesentery (Hooper and Haelterman, 1966, 1969). The most striking microscopic lesion is severe villus atrophy in the jejunum and ileum (Fig. 16.24). The villus-to-crypt ratio of affected animals is 1:1, compared to a normal of about 7:1 (Hooper and Haelterman, 1966, 1969). The enterocytes are vacuolated and low-cuboidal or flattened, there is lymphoid depletion of Peyer's patches, and minimal inflammatory response in the lamina propria (Hooper and Haelterman, 1969). Virus particles can be found in the cytoplasm of villus enterocytes,

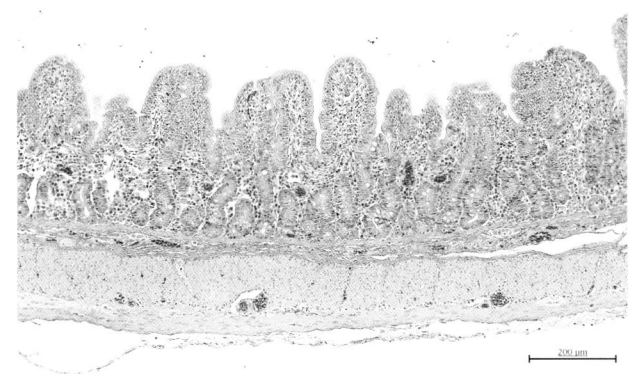

FIGURE 16.24 Porcine Coronavirus. Transmissible gastroenteritis. Villi of the small intestine are markedly shortened. *Courtesy of J. Haruna.*

M cells, lymphocytes, and macrophages within Peyer's patches (Saif et al., 2012).

Research Complications Clinical signs of TGEV are severe enough to make animals unsuitable for experimental use unless sufficient time is available for clinical recovery.

h. Porcine Epidemic Diarrhea Virus   *New this ed.*

Porcine epidemic diarrhea virus (PEDV) is an alphacoronavirus related to TGEV. Clinically, PEDV is very similar to TGEV, and laboratory tests are required to differentiate the viruses. This is not a new virus, but has recently (2013) been found in a small number of herds in the US and has quickly spread to 30 states as of April 5, 2014 (Practitioners, 2014). There are many variants of the virus, but this newly circulating virus in the US is particularly virulent with 90–95% mortality in suckling pigs and vomiting and diarrhea from all ages of pigs (Stevenson et al., 2013). Mice and cats can act as vectors of the virus (Truong et al., 2013). Vaccines are available in Asia, but not in the US or EU. Biosecurity is currently the best way to prevent the virus in facilities. In April 2014 it was declared a reportable disease by the USDA (Agriculture, 2014).

i. Porcine Rotavirus

Porcine rotavirus is a major cause of morbidity and mortality from acute diarrhea in very young pigs, particularly if piglets are colostrum-deprived or raised under gnotobiotic conditions in which the herd is free of natural infection (Bridger et al., 1998).

Etiology Rotaviruses are members of the family Reoviridae which are nonenveloped and contain a double-stranded RNA genome. Four (A, B, C, E) of seven serogroups (A–G) of rotavirus have been described in swine, with group A being the most commonly detected. Within these serogroups, rotaviruses fall into two major serotypes based on expression of two surface antigens, VP4 and VP7.

Epizootiology and Transmission Rotaviral infection is enzootic in most swine herds, and clinical disease is apparent only if viral challenge exceeds the capacity of passive maternal immunity. Piglets born to gilts are at greater risk than those farrowed by older sows, which are more likely to have naturally high virus neutralizing titers that protect the nursing piglets. Rotaviruses are stable in the environment and are relatively resistant to effects of temperature, pH, and disinfectants. Subclinical infection may persist in adult animals, with periodic shedding.

PATHOGENESIS Rotaviruses replicate in the cytoplasm of enterocytes and M cells overlying Peyer's patches (Buller and Moxley, 1988). Group A and C rotaviruses are responsible for diarrhea due to destruction of enterocytes on the tips of the villi and severe villous atrophy compared to groups B and E (Saif, 1999; Chang et al., 2012). An osmotic diarrhea ensues due to decreased resorption of sodium, water, and disaccharides in the jejunum and ileum, which causes intestinal contents to be hyperosmolar (Graham et al., 1984).

Clinical Signs/Diagnosis Disease is most severe in naive pigs first exposed at 1–5 days of age. Typical signs follow an 18- to 96-h incubation period and include anorexia, lethargy, vomiting, fever, and profuse watery diarrhea that is white to yellow in color and contains flocculent material. In pigs that will recover, consistency of feces slowly returns to normal after 3–5 days of diarrhea. Clinical signs and losses are less severe if exposure occurs after piglets are 7 days of age, and infection is commonly subclinical if it occurs after they are 21–28 days of age. Disease is usually mild and self-limiting if other enteric pathogens are absent. If rotaviral infection is detected in clinically ill pigs of postweaning age, mixed infection with other agents such as TGEV should be suspected. Severe diarrhea and 50–100% mortality is seen in 1- to 5-day-old gnotobiotic or colostrum-deprived pigs experimentally exposed to rotavirus. Differential diagnoses for yellow to white, watery diarrhea in piglets that are newborn to several weeks of age should include rotavirus, colibacillosis, TGE, coccidiosis, and nematodiasis.

Treatment No specific treatment is available. Supportive therapy should include replacement fluids containing glucose and electrolytes, antibiotics to treat or prevent secondary bacterial infections, and warm, clean housing.

Prevention/Control Because porcine rotavirus is enzootic in most herds, exclusion is difficult. Management should concentrate on minimizing the viral challenge for susceptible pigs through good sanitation and boosting passive immunity by exposing replacement gilts to feces from the herd prior to their first parturition. Modified live- and inactivated-virus vaccines are commercially available for immunization of sows and nursing pigs. However, immunity is serotype-specific, with unknown duration.

Necropsy Gross lesions are confined to the small bowel. The wall of the distal half of the small intestine is typically thin and dilated and contains watery material, while the mesenteric lymph nodes are tan and small (Chang et al., 2012). The cecum and colon are dilated, with watery contents similar to those in the small intestine. Gross lesions in pigs over 21 days of age are variable or absent. Microscopic lesions include degeneration and loss of enterocytes on the tips of the villi, which develop as early as 16h post inoculation, increased thickness of the lamina propria due to large numbers of neutrophils and mononuclear cells, reduction in villus height from the duodenum to the ileocecal juncture, and fusion of villi due to exposed lamina propria in villus cores (Pearson and McNulty, 1977).

Research Complications Morbidity and mortality of porcine rotaviral infection will impact studies using very young piglets and will probably be subclinical in postweaning animals.

j. Balantidiasis

Etiology Balantidiasis is caused by trophozoites of *Balantidium coli*, a ciliated protozoan that colonizes the cecum and anterior colon of swine, usually as a commensal. Trophozoites are large (25 × 150 μm), ciliated ovoid structures containing a macronucleus and micronucleus in addition to contractile and food vacuoles. Trophozoites of *B. coli* isolated from pigs affected by acute disease and from pigs with subclinical balantidiasis, as well as trophozoites cultured *in vitro*, have been shown to differ in nucleic acid content, suggesting that clinical disease may be associated with different strains of *B. coli* (Skotarczak and Zielinski, 1997).

Epizootiology and Transmission Infection with *B. coli* is contracted by ingestion of trophozoites or cysts that are shed in feces. Most infections are subclinical. If clinical enteritis is associated with *B. coli*, other infectious agents or management problems that may be cofactors in disease development should be investigated.

Pathogenesis Secondary invasion occurs when the integrity of the colonic mucosa is compromised.

Clinical Signs/Diagnosis Infection with *B. coli* may present as an acute typhlitis or colitis or more commonly, no apparent effect. Infection can cause severe ulcerative enterocolitis, which can be fatal. Clinical signs include weight loss, anorexia, weakness, lethargy, watery diarrhea, tenesmus, and rectal prolapse.

Treatment Balantidiasis can be successfully treated with antibiotics and oxytetracycline can eliminate *B. coli* (Stewart, 2007).

Prevention/Control Herd-health management that minimizes the risk of enteritis from any cause will help prevent clinical balantidiasis. Clinically ill pigs should be isolated and treated or necropsied to rule out other predisposing causes of enteritis.

Necropsy *B. coli* is not considered a primary pathogen in pigs, but has been shown to invade lesions caused by *Oesophagostomum* and *T. suis* (Bowman and Georgi, 2009; Beer and Lean, 1973).

Research Complications Although *B. coli* is usually nonpathogenic, severe ulcerative enterocolitis can develop. Because of zoonotic potential, it may be advisable to euthanize piglets shedding *B. coli* in high numbers.

k. Coccidiosis

While disease is commonly absent or subclinical, significant morbidity and mortality can result from severe diarrhea in neonatal piglets.

Etiology *Eimeria* spp., *Cryptosporidium parvum*, and *Isospora suis* are three genera of coccidia that infect swine and other mammals. There are eight species of *Eimeria* that infect up to 95% of the swine housed on dirt lots in the US. *Eimeria* spp. are considered to be nonpathogenic in swine. *C. parvum* typically causes subclinical infection in swine that are 6–12 weeks of age. Clinical neonatal coccidiosis is caused by the intracellular parasite, *I. suis*, and is the most important protozoal disease of nursing piglets that are 1–2 weeks of age (Lindsay *et al.*, 1997).

Epizootiology and Transmission The most common coccidia affecting swine are transmitted by fecal–oral contact. Warm temperatures and high humidity associated with indoor farrowing favor rapid sporulation of oocysts. Contaminated environments pose the greatest risk to naive piglets.

Pathogenesis Ingestion of sporulated oocysts by the pig permits development to sporozoites in the intestinal lumen. These invade enterocytes and form trophozoites, which then form merozoites, resulting in rupture of the cell membranes when they are released into the intestinal lumen.

Clinical Signs/Diagnosis *I. suis* causes clinical disease in nursing piglets that are 1–2 weeks old. Yellow to gray diarrhea that varies in consistency from watery to pasty develops and piglets will continue to nurse. Weight loss and dehydration secondary to coccidiosis can be exacerbated by concurrent infections with other parasites, bacteria, or viruses. The differential diagnoses should include colibacillosis, *C. perfringens*, TGE, rotavirus, and *Strongyloides ransomi*.

Treatment Piglets should be individually dosed orally with amprolium or furazolidone. Sulfonamides and trimethoprim-sulfa are also effective (Lindsay *et al.*, 1997). Drug therapy may only delay the onset of clinical signs. Electrolyte and water-balance disturbances should be treated with either oral or parenteral fluids.

Prevention/Control Piglets should be purchased from vendors with an established herd-health profile that is free of coccidiosis. Newly received piglets should be routinely quarantined and tested for coccidia by fecal flotation.

Coccidiosis can be controlled by 'all in, all out' husbandry and thorough cleaning of housing areas, including removal of organic debris, chemical disinfection, and steam cleaning.

Necropsy The gross lesions are confined to the jejunum and ileum and consist of necrotic enteritis involving the entire thickness of the mucosa. A yellow fibrinonecrotic pseudomembrane may be present over foci of mucosal ulceration. Microscopic lesions consist of moderate to severe segmental villous atrophy and necrotic enteritis. The variable reduction in villous heights ranges from slight to severe, and the villous enterocytes are flattened and irregularly shaped. There may be crypt epithelial hyperplasia, and the lamina propria is condensed and infiltrated with large numbers of mononuclear cells. The least involved sections of the mucosa contain varying stages of coccidia in vacuoles in the enterocytes of the distal two-thirds of the villi (Eustis and Nelson, 1981).

Research Complications Morbidity is high, but mortality is usually low to moderate in piglets affected by neonatal coccidiosis. Growth may be stunted.

l. Giardiasis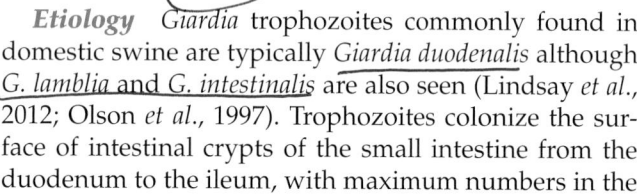

Etiology *Giardia* trophozoites commonly found in domestic swine are typically *Giardia duodenalis* although *G. lamblia* and *G. intestinalis* are also seen (Lindsay *et al.*, 2012; Olson *et al.*, 1997). Trophozoites colonize the surface of intestinal crypts of the small intestine from the duodenum to the ileum, with maximum numbers in the cranial part of the upper jejunum (Koudela *et al.*, 1991).

Epizootiology and Transmission *Giardia* exists as a commensal in the vast majority of domestic swine (Olson *et al.*, 1997). *Giardia* cysts are intermittently shed in feces and transmitted to other pigs by fecal–oral contact. Transmission is via the fecal–oral route.

Clinical Signs/Diagnosis Clinical signs include anorexia, depression, and formless feces. *Giardia* may be the primary cause of enteritis or may be found coincidental to other causes of enteritis (see Table 16.3). Fecal flotation using zinc sulfate is the most effective method of diagnosis.

Treatment Metronidazole is commonly used for 5 days to control giardiasis. Diagnostic steps to rule out other causes of enteritis are indicated.

Prevention/Control Sanitation protocols should include removing feces daily or housing pigs on slatted floors to minimize fecal contact. Clinical enteritis can be controlled by quarantine and treatment.

Necropsy No pathologic lesions were found in the small intestines of groups of pigs experimentally infected with *G. intestinalis* (Koudela *et al.*, 1991). Detection of organisms can be accomplished using Giemsa-stained fecal smears or histologic sections.

Research Complications Giardiasis can cause debilitation from diarrhea and dehydration but usually responds to both supportive and medical treatment. Giardiasis is a zoonotic disease.

m. Nematodiasis

Young swine can be infected with the nematodes *Hyostrongylus rubidus*, *Globocephalus urosubulatus*, *Macracanthorhynchus hirudinaceus*, *Oesophagostomum* spp., *Ascaris suum*, *T. suis*, and *Strongyloides ransomi* (Zimmerman *et al.*, 2012b). Only *T. suis* and *S. ransomi* will be discussed here because the other parasites are either discussed elsewhere (Ascaris), require intermediate hosts (*Macracanthorhynchus*), or infection by the parasite is associated with pasture maintenance (*Hyostrongylus,*

Globocephalus, Oesophagostomum spp.), which is unlikely to be an issue in laboratory animal research facilities.

i. TRICHURIS SUIS

Etiology The swine whipworm, *T. suis*, colonizes the small intestine and cecum, causing morbidity and possibly mortality in young, postweaning swine.

Epizootiology and Transmission Bipolar, thick-shelled eggs are intermittently shed in feces. After 3–4 weeks in the environment eggs are infective, and remain so, for as long as 6 years. Ingested eggs hatch in the small intestine and cecum, with newly released larvae penetrating cells lining the crypts. Larvae gradually migrate from the lamina propria into the submucosa over several weeks. After a series of molts, adult worms can be found with their anterior end buried in the mucosa and the posterior end free in the intestinal lumen. Prepatency is 6–7 weeks, and the life span of the adult worm is 4–5 months. Damage caused to the mucosa permits colonization by pathogenic bacteria and *B. coli*.

Clinical Signs/Diagnosis *T. suis* may cause anorexia, mucoid to hemorrhagic diarrhea, growth retardation, dehydration, and in severe infections, death (Batte *et al.*, 1977; Beer and Lean, 1973). Differential diagnoses for hemorrhagic diarrhea in piglets that are newborn to several weeks of age include colibacillosis, *C. perfringens*, and *B. hyodysenteriae*. In older pigs, *Salmonella* and *L. intracellularis* should be considered.

Treatment Effective anthelmintics for trichuriasis include fenbendazole, dichlorvos, and levamisole hydrochloride. Although ivermectin is considered to be efficacious for elimination of *Ascaris*, *Oesophagostomum*, and *Metastrongylus*, it is less effective for *Trichuris*.

Prevention/Control *T. suis* eggs passed in feces require 3–4 additional weeks to develop to an infectious stage; hence, indoor housing with good sanitation that includes regular removal of feces and organic debris should prevent environmental contamination and reinfection. Newly received swine should be tested for *Trichuris* by fecal flotation and treated with anthelmintics during the quarantine period. Housing areas and equipment should be steam-cleaned to destroy eggs and infective larvae.

Necropsy Gross lesions are found primarily in the cecum and colon. The wall of the large intestine is thickened, the mesentery may be thickened and appear as bands between coils of gut, and there may be foci of hemorrhages on the serosal surface (Beer and Lean, 1973). The mesenteric lymph nodes are enlarged and congested. The lumen of the gut is filled with bloody fluid, and there is a hemorrhagic catarrhal colitis and typhlitis, with portions of the mucosa being replaced by a yellow crumb-like, fibrinonecrotic membrane (Batte *et al.*, 1977; Beer and Lean, 1973). Microscopic examination reveals parasites embedded in the mucosa between villi and in crypts, which may be cystic, or they may penetrate to the muscularis mucosa and the lamina propria is infiltrated by large numbers of mononuclear cells (Batte and Moncol, 1972). Foci of hemorrhage may be found in the mucosa, as well as ulcers, which are covered by thick fibrinonecrotic material (Beer and Lean, 1973).

Research Complications Severe infection with *Trichuris* will cause bloody scours in young pigs, with associated morbidity and some mortality. *T. suis* is a potential human health hazard (Beer, 1976).

ii. STRONGYLOIDES RANSOMI

Etiology *S. ransomi* is the small intestinal threadworm of swine. It is most prevalent in warm climates and causes morbidity in suckling pigs (Greve, 2012).

Epizootiology and Transmission Larvae of *S. ransomi* can infect pigs *in utero* as well as by the oral, percutaneous, and transcolostral routes. Eggs shed in feces hatch within hours to release larvae that are directly infective within 24 h or develop into males and females that then reproduce, resulting in more larvae within 72 h.

Pathogenesis Larvae enter the bloodstream and are transported to the lungs where they are coughed up and swallowed.

Clinical Signs/Diagnosis Large numbers of *Strongyloides* can result in poor body condition, decreased weight gain, diarrhea, with secondary dehydration and death within the first 2 weeks of life. The differential diagnosis for nonhemorrhagic diarrhea in piglets aged upward of 14 days should include colibacillosis, salmonellosis, rotavirus, TGE, giardiasis, coccidiosis, and nematodiasis.

Treatment Young swine can be treated with paste formulations of thiabendazole. Other effective drugs are ivermectin and levamisole.

Prevention/Control Breeding animals should receive anthelmintics several weeks before farrowing to control the shedding of *S. ransomi* eggs and transmission through colostrum. Removing feces daily or housing on slatted floors should minimize exposure of neonates to infective larvae.

Necropsy Pigs may be dehydrated or may be stunted and unthrifty. Adult forms of the parasite are found in the small intestine, and ova are present in the feces.

Research complications *S. ransomi* is an important cause of parasitic debilitation in nursing pigs in the southeastern US. Routine diagnostic screening and timely use of anthelmintics should minimize any impact on research.

4. Circulatory Disease

a. Mycoplasma Suis

Etiology *M. suis* has been reclassified from *Eperythrozoon suis* based on 16S RNA and is the etiologic agent for this host-specific disease in swine (Neimark *et al.*, 2002). These are epicellular and membrane-bound intracellular, round to oval organisms that are found within or attached to the outer surface of erythrocytes and free within the plasma (Groebel *et al.*, 2009). They change size and shape as they mature, which gives the microscopic appearance of infection by two separate organisms. They stain well with Giemsa but not with Gram stain.

Epizootiology and Transmission The reservoir for *M. suis* is domestic swine, and serologic studies have not detected it in wild swine (Thacker and Minion, 2012). However, current serologic tests will not detect every latent carrier and some infected pigs never show disease. Transmission is mechanical by blood-sucking arthropods, primarily lice, or reuse of blood-contaminated needles, snares, and surgical or tattoo instruments. It can be directly transmitted orally when swine lick fresh wounds or any fluids containing blood. The organism can also be transmitted in utero (Henderson *et al.*, 1997).

Pathogenesis Acute disease is characterized by anemia which can be fatal, due to massive parasitism of host erythrocytes. Infected erythrocytes have altered membranes with increased fragility and are rapidly removed by the spleen. Endothelial cells are invaded and activated by the organism as well which further explains the range of clinical signs observed (Sokoli *et al.*, 2013).

Clinical Signs/Diagnosis Acute disease is usually seen in suckling or newly weaned piglets or other pigs that have been stressed, and consists of fever of 40–42°C, anemia, jaundice, pale mucous membranes, cyanosis of the ears, weakness, and poor weight gain. All ages of swine can be clinically affected, however, the very young are most likely to be. Acutely affected sows will become anorexic and febrile, and will have decreased milk production and poor maternal behavior. Vulvar and mammary gland edema may also be seen in sows.

The chronic form affects older pigs and is usually subclinical, but animals may show unthriftiness, pallor, and urticaria, or it may adversely affect reproductive parameters in sows (Messick, 2004; Groebel *et al.*, 2009). Reproductive problems include anestrus, low conception rates, abortions, weak piglets, and small litters. Mortality due to *M. suis* is extremely low.

PCR assays and ELISAs have been developed to detect and diagnose *M. suis* (Messick *et al.*, 1999). In acute cases, a fresh blood smear can be stained with Giemsa to visualize the organisms. Differentials include iron deficiency anemia and other causes of anemia in piglets and toxicity producing icterus or anemia.

Treatment Oxytetracycline either parenterally or in food or water will control the clinical signs but does not eliminate the organism. Iron dextran should be given to each clinically affected pig. In severely anemic animals, administration of whole blood may be beneficial. Additionally, any form of environmental, experimental, or physical stress should be eliminated.

Prevention/Control Control measures include eliminating ectoparasites, never reusing needles, and sterilizing surgical instruments thoroughly. The most satisfactory prevention is to allow only known *M. suis*-free swine into a facility.

Necropsy Gross findings include icterus, distended gallbladder filled with gelatinous bile, splenomegaly, pale mucous membranes, watery blood, swollen edematous lymph nodes, ascites, hydrothorax, and a swollen and yellow–brown liver (Splitter, 1950; Thacker and Minion, 2012).

One or more of the organisms can be found within RBCs in a smear of peripheral blood, where they appear as 0.8- to 1-μm diameter rings with a pale center (Thomson, 1988). Microscopic lesions in other organs include hemosiderosis in hepatocytes and Kupffer cells, fatty degeneration and centrilobular necrosis of hepatocytes, and hyperplastic bone marrow (Splitter, 1950; Thacker and Minion, 2012).

Research Complications *M. suis* causes an autoimmune hemolytic anemia, which will be precipitated or exacerbated by the stress of experimental protocols. This also predisposes affected animals to respiratory and gastrointestinal disease, which will further confound research protocols.

5. Skin Diseases

a. Exudative Epidermitis: Greasy Pig Disease

Etiology *Staphylococcus hyicus* is a gram-positive coccus considered to be normal flora on the skin of pigs.

Epizootiology and Transmission *S. hyicus* is present worldwide and in many herds does not cause disease. Outbreaks are seen upon introduction of naive animals. Newborn piglets are likely infected during parturition, and cross-contamination can occur when weanlings from different litters are group-housed. This bacterium is very persistent in the environment. Damage to the skin by abrasions from pen surfaces, fighting, mange mites, and concurrent vesicular disease facilitates entry of *S. hyicus*. Spread by other species is of little concern. Morbidity can reach 20%, with up to 80% mortality in affected piglets (Cowart, 1995). EE has also been associated with PCV2 (Kim and Chae, 2004).

Pathogenesis At least six antigenically distinct exfoliative toxins (ExhA, ExhB, ExhC ExhD, ShetA, ShetB) have been identified and are thought to correlate with clinical disease (Andresen, 1998; Sato *et al.*, 1999; Tanabe *et al.*, 1996). These toxins target the stratum granulosum in the epidermis and are similar to *S. aureus* toxins (Frana, 2012).

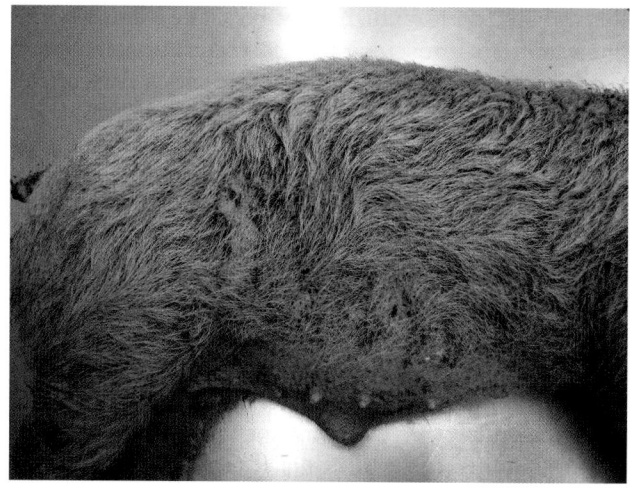

FIGURE 16.25 Staphylococcus hyicus, greasy pig disease. There is diffuse exudative dertmatitis covering the torso and legs primarily in haired areas. *Courtesy of ISU Veterinary Diagnostic Laboratory.*

Clinical Signs/Diagnosis The early clinical signs of EE are lethargy, depression, anorexia, and erythematous skin in a variable number of piglets in a litter. Pigs aged 5 days to 2 months are susceptible, and older pigs are more resistant. Lesions progress to an exudative dermatitis characterized by exfoliation and crusting, which begins in the groin, axillae, behind the ears, and on areas of damaged skin (Fig. 16.25). Within 24–48h lesions on the head expand, coalesce, and extend posteriorly. Haired areas are typically affected but lesions can also be seen on the tongue and oral mucosa. EE is generally self-limiting, lasting 2–3 months in most animals, but can last 12–18 months. Erosions at the coronary band of hooves and vesicles or ulcers in the mouth and on the tongue and snout are common findings. The dermatitis may progress to cover the majority of the body in 3–5 days and becomes exfoliative and crusty but non-pruritic. Severely affected members of the litter may die in 24h to 10 days, and others may or may not be affected or be chronically affected with small, localized patches of EE. Adult animals may be mildly affected with small areas of EE on their backs and sides (Frana, 2012; Cowart, 1995). *S. hyicus* has also been reported to be an etiologic agent for arthritis in piglets less than 12 weeks old (Hill *et al.*, 1996). Differential diagnoses should include swine pox, mange, ringworm, and pityriasis rosea.

Treatment Treatment with antibiotics is challenging due to resistance to beta lactams, erythromycin, streptomycin, tetracycline, and sulfonamide. The choice, therefore, should be based on sensitivity testing. Topical treatment of the affected skin with antibiotics and antiseptic shampoos or dips in conjunction with the antibiotics is beneficial. Treatment is most effective when started early in the course of the disease, and severely affected young piglets may be slow to recover (Cowart, 1995; Frana, 2012).

Prevention/Control Autogenous bacterins made from strains cultured from a particular herd and given to nonimmune sows are useful to protect the litters of newly introduced sows. The exfoliative toxin and the bacterial cells should be included as antigens when the vaccine is made. An indirect ELISA or phage typing can be utilized to select a toxigenic strain for vaccine production (Andresen, 1999). The sows can be washed with appropriate antibacterials (chlorhexidine or povidone–iodine shampoos) prior to parturition and checked for ectoparasites. Sharp or abrasive surfaces should be removed from the pens.

Necropsy The skin in the area of the erosive lesions may be reddened, edematous or thickened, and covered with an exudate composed of sebum, serum, and sweat (Jones, 1956). These lesions are most commonly found on the ears, around the eyes, on the ventral thorax, and on the abdomen. Microscopic findings are the presence of both a superficial and deep pyoderma that may extend to involve the subcutis, with multiple coalescing foci of necrosis of the stratum corneum, the presence of a brownish exudate, and the formation of rete pegs by the hyperplastic stratum germinativum (Jones, 1956; McGavin and Zachary, 2007; Frana, 2012).

Research Complications Exudative epidermitis will complicate most studies involving young piglets due to the potentially significant morbidity and mortality.

b. Swine Pox

Etiology Swine pox virus is the only member of the genus *Suipoxvirus*, family Poxviridae.

Epizootiology and Transmission The pig is the only known host of this virus, and although worldwide in distribution, it exists primarily in herds where poor sanitation is practiced. The reservoir is infected swine, as the virus is host-restricted. The virus may persist in an active form in dry skin scabs for up to 1 year. Although horizontal transmission may occur via nasal and oral secretions coming in contact with abraded skin, the primary method of transmission is mechanical via the pig louse. Flies and mosquitoes can also carry the viral particles. Once the virus is established within a herd, it usually persists. Outbreaks can result in high morbidity if young animals are present, although mortality is very low.

Pathogenesis The virus replicates in the cells of the stratum spinosum and is suspected to spread from initial site to secondary sites via an as yet undetected viremia (Delhon *et al.*, 2012). Viremia is also believed to be responsible for transplacental infection and disease in neonates.

Clinical Signs/Diagnosis The lesions associated with this virus mimic other pox diseases. Initially, macules form (reddening), followed by 1- to 6-mm-diameter papules (reddening with edema); transient vesicles (fluid within the lesion), then pustules (umbilicated, ischemic), and finally, crusts (brown to black in color). The progression of the lesions occurs over a 3- to 4-week period. Younger animals (less than 4 months old) are affected more severely than adults and may have lesions covering the entire body surface. Older animals tend to have lesions in more focal locations. If vector transmission has occurred, the location of the lesions follows the vector preferences, that is, the pig louse attacks the lower parts of the body, while flies feed predominantly over the top of the body. Adults have lesions primarily on their belly, udder, ears, snout, and vulva.

The diagnosis is primarily made by identifying the typical lesions in the typical locations. Differential diagnoses include any of the vesicular diseases, pityriasis rosea, allergic skin reactions, sunburn, or staphylococcal or streptococcal epidermitis. The presence of intracytoplasmic inclusion bodies along with central nuclear clearing in affected epithelial cells is a hallmark sign of this disease.

Treatment Supportive care should be given to prevent secondary bacterial skin infections.

Prevention/Control Affected animals should be isolated, and sanitation and pest control should be improved.

Necropsy Gross lesions are most commonly found on abdomen, chest, and legs, and only in severe cases involve the oral cavity and main airways. Early lesions consist of erythematous macules and papules, and later lesions progress to pustules and scabbing. Microscopic findings are related to viral replication in the stratum spinosum, causing hydropic degeneration, necrosis of epithelial cells, and formation of pustules that involves the full thickness of the epidermis with one to three eosinophilic intracytoplasmic poxvirus inclusion bodies in epithelial cells (Teppema and De Boer, 1975).

c. Mange (Scabies)

Etiology *Sarcoptes scabiei* var. *suis* from the family Sarcoptidae is the cause of sarcoptic mange in swine. This is probably the most significant ectoparasite of swine. This mite is 0.5 mm in length, has four pairs of legs, and completes its entire life cycle within the layers of the epidermis. The time necessary for an egg to hatch and develop into a mature egg-laying female is 10–25 days. This is one of the more common swine diseases, but it is frequently overlooked, probably because the clinical signs may be perceived as normal and losses are not readily apparent. Demodectic mange caused by *Demodex phylloides* can also occur in swine; however, it is a rarity.

Epizootiology and Transmission Mange infestations are fairly common in small conventional swine herds in the US. Nursing piglets obtain the mites from an infected sow through direct contact. Breeding sows with hyperkeratotic encrustations in their ears are the primary reservoirs of mites. Group housing of pigs, especially from various sources, will facilitate spread of mites although spread via environmental contamination is still possible, as mites can survive off the host for several days. Herd-to-herd transmission is by introduction of a carrier pig; other species are not known to harbor this mite.

Pathogenesis Young pigs or newly exposed older animals become pruritic due to a hypersensitivity response to the mites burrowing into the dermis and laying eggs (Davis and Moon, 1990). This generally occurs several weeks post infection. The first 3 weeks postinfection, the females burrow into the skin and a covering of keratinized encrustations develops which falls off after 7 weeks, after which the mites leave the burrows (Morsy *et al.*, 1989).

Clinical Signs/Diagnosis There are two clinical forms of sarcoptic mange in swine. The acute pruritic or allergic hypersensitive form affects younger, growing pigs. This is characterized by an intensely pruritic, erythematous papular dermatitis on the ventral abdomen, flank, and rump that develops 2–11 weeks after infection. Pigs with this form will rub the affected areas, often causing hair loss, abrasions, and thickened, keratinized skin. A reduced growth rate will be seen if the dermatitis is severe (Davies, 1995). It is difficult with this form to find the mites on skin scrapings.

The chronic or hyperkeratotic form is typically found in mature sows and boars. Thick, crusty scabs begin on the pinnae and spread to the neck and head, and contain numerous mites that are relatively easy to find on skin scrapings. Mortality is unlikely unless concurrent disease is severe.

An ELISA for serum antibody levels to *S. scabiei* can be used to diagnose along with periodic skin scrapings, and monitoring for prevalence of scratching and papular dermatitis lesions (Zimmermann and Kircher, 1998; Jacobson *et al.*, 1999; Wallgren and Bornstein, 1997; Bornstein and Wallgren, 1997; Hollanders *et al.*, 1997; Davies *et al.*, 1996). Differentials include causes of dermatitis in swine, such as exudative epidermitis, dermatomycosis, swine pox, parakeratosis, niacin and biotin deficiencies, sunburn, photosensitization, and insect bites (Greve and Davies, 2012).

Treatment Ivermectin is effective orally or subcutaneously and should be repeated in 14 days (Greve and Davies, 2012; Hollanders *et al.*, 1995). Doramectin intramuscularly has also been reported to be effective and has a greater persistent efficacy than ivermectin (Cargill *et al.*, 1996; Logan *et al.*, 1996; Saeki *et al.*, 1997; Yazwinski *et al.*, 1997; Arends *et al.*, 1999). Other acaricides, including amitraz, phosmet, and diazinon, are also effective. Two or more treatments at 1- to 2-week intervals are usually necessary to eliminate these mites.

Swine with unusually severe chronic hyperkeratosis should be culled from the group if possible. This should be followed by thorough cleaning of the environment.

Prevention/Control Allowing only mange-free SPF animals into the facility is the most effective and satisfactory method of prevention. Treatment of sows with a single dose of ivermectin 8 days prior to farrowing prevents transmission to piglets (Mercier *et al.*, 2002). It is feasible to maintain a herd free of *S. scabiei* if a good biosecurity and surveillance program is developed (Cargill *et al.*, 1997).

Necropsy Papular dermatitis is seen in growing swine with or without positive skin scrapings for the sarcoptid mites. The papules are manifestations of the hypersensitivity reaction, contain eosinophils, mast cells, and lymphocytes, and have an associated eosinophilic perivasculitis (Hollanders and Vercruysse, 1990; Greve and Davies, 2012). Histologic sections show mites in the deep stratum corneum and stratum malpighii, producing hyperkeratosis and acanthosis (Jones and Hunt, 1983).

Research Complications Sarcoptic mange should not result in direct loss of animals in a study since this disease is rarely associated with mortality unless there is concurrent disease. The intense rubbing is a potential threat to surgical incisions and implants in these models.

d. Lice (Pediculosis)

Etiology *Haematopinus suis* females are 4–6 mm in length and males, 3.5–4.75 mm. These are sucking lice and are the only species of louse that affects swine (Lapage, 1968).

Epizootiology and Transmission Transmission is by direct pig-to-pig contact, as this louse is host-specific and will not survive very long (less than 2–3 days) off the host. The life cycle is 23–32 days and is entirely in and on the skin of pigs. It is considered a vector for swine pox and *M. suis*.

Pathogenesis The three instars of the nymph stage and egg-laying females suck blood, causing irritation, pruritus, and anemia.

Clinical Signs/Diagnosis Young pigs may show pruritus, poor growth, and anemia. Lice can be found almost anywhere on the body but have a predilection for the skin on the flank area, neck, axilla, groin, and the inner ears. Their eggs, or nits, are 1–2 mm in length and attach to the hair shafts.

Treatment The same treatments that are effective for mites also work well for lice, including sprays, dips, dusts, and oral and injectable ectoparasiticides. Most are efficacious when given as two treatments 2 weeks apart. The avermectins (primarily doramectin) and ivermectin are available as oral or injectable treatments and are also effective for ascarids and lungworms (Logan *et al.*, 1996).

Prevention/Control The most reasonable and effective means of lice prevention is to allow only swine known to be lice-free into the research facility. Feral populations of *Sus scrofa* have been found to be reservoirs for *H. suis* (Gipson *et al.*, 1999), and certainly contact with domestic populations should be prevented.

Necropsy Adults can be visualized without special techniques. Allergic dermatitis and mechanically induced skin lesions with hemorrhage may be found on some affected pigs (Nickel and Danner, 1979).

Research Complications Severe infestations may cause anemia in young swine, and the rubbing may damage surgical incisions. Furthermore, the use of potentially toxic treatments to remove the lice may interfere with some research studies.

6. Reproductive Diseases

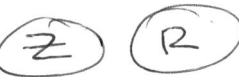

a. Brucellosis

Etiology *Brucella suis*, particularly biovars 1, 2, and 3, is the only species of *Brucella* that causes systemic infection and clinical disease, including infertility, in swine. Biovar 3 is currently the most common cause of this disease in swine. Morphologically, this genus is a nonmotile, non-spore-forming, small gram-negative, aerobic bacillus or coccobacillus.

Epizootiology and Transmission Domestic swine populations are the primary sources for *B. suis*. The European hare (*Lepus capinensis*) is a carrier for biovar 2 and has been linked to brucellosis in European swine facilities. Feral pigs are also reservoirs in areas where contact with domestic swine can occur (Heinritzi *et al.*, 1999). In the US, *B. suis* biovars 1 and 3 have been eradicated (Olsen *et al.*, 2012).

Transmission is most frequently via contaminated discharges or tissues from infected swine being ingested by a susceptible animal or via contaminated food or water. Contaminated tissues include aborted fetuses and fetal membranes. Additionally, nursing piglets frequently become infected while suckling infected sows. *B. suis* is present in semen of infected boars and can be spread by natural breeding or artificial insemination.

Pathogenesis After mucosal exposure to organisms, they enter through follicle-associated epithelial cells (M cells) or by phagocytosis, travel to the local lymph nodes, gain entrance to macrophages and neutrophils, and multiply. This is followed by a bacteremia with seeding of organisms in other lymph nodes, the genital tract, placenta, joint fluids, and bone marrow (Olsen *et al.*, 2012).

Clinical Signs/Diagnosis The clinical signs of *B. suis* infection vary with the herd and range from no obvious disease to the classical signs, which include abortion, infertility, metritis, orchitis, lameness, spondylitis, and posterior paralysis. Clinical disease in piglets of weaning age usually consists of spondylitis and posterior paralysis (Olsen *et al.*, 2012). Differentials include other causes of infertility and abortion in swine, such as PPV and leptospirosis.

Treatment Infected swine should be euthanized. Antimicrobials are unlikely to eliminate the bacteria from swine.

Prevention/Control The best prevention is to allow only brucellosis-free swine from validated herds into a facility. To date, available live bacteria vaccines are not effective in eradicating brucellosis but can create antibodies which could interfere with a serologic surveillance programs. Currently, the most effective control paradigm is to combine vaccination with test-and-removal procedures and sanitation measures. If a closed herd is maintained with a good biosecurity program, it is feasible to keep it brucellosis-free.

Necropsy Gross lesions are variable but generally consist of one or more abscesses, and there may be erosions of mucous membranes and seminal vesiculitis (Olsen *et al.*, 2012; Deyoe, 1967). Aborted fetuses may appear normal, or there may be edema or evidence of a suppurative placentitis. Microscopic lesions consist of granulomatous inflammation in the endometrium, uterine glands, and placenta. In the fetus, suppurative seminal vesiculitis; pyogranulomatous foci in the liver; caseous necrotic foci adjacent to growth plate cartilages in the vertebrae; and abscesses in the kidneys, spleen, ovaries, lungs, brain, and other tissues may be seen (Olsen *et al.*, 2012; Deyoe, 1967).

Research Complications Research protocols involving any aspect of swine reproduction are at highest risk for brucellosis. *B. suis* is one of the most common species implicated in cases of human brucellosis. Investigators and veterinarians performing necropsies on infected animals are at risk for becoming infected and BSL-3 containment is recommended for safely working with pathogenic strains of *B. suis* (Olsen *et al.*, 2012). Brucellosis is a zoonotic and reportable disease in the US (Olsen *et al.*, 2012). Since the US is considered Brucella free, health certificates from USDA-accredited veterinarians are needed for travel.

b. Leptospirosis

Etiology The etiologic agent for this disease in swine consists of several serovars of *Leptospira interrogans* and *L. borgpetersenii* (Ellis, 2012). All are gram-negative, motile aerobic spirochetes. The serovar *Pomona* is the most common cause of clinical leptospirosis in swine, and serovars *Bratislava* and *Muenchen* are commonly found in serologic surveys and are sometimes associated with clinical disease. There are several other serovars, which are typically maintained in other mammalian hosts but are occasionally found to infect swine. These include *Icterohaemorrhagiae, Sejroe, Hardjo, Canicola, Grippotyphosa*, and *Tarassovi* (Ellis, 2012; Cowart, 1995).

Epizootiology and Transmission Transmission from animal to animal is by direct or indirect contact with a carrier animal, which harbors the leptospires in the renal tubules or genital tract. Leptospires are shed from carrier animals in urine and genital fluids into the environment. Feral swine are potential sources of serovars *Pomona* and *Bratislava* for outdoor facilities where contact can occur (Saliki *et al.*, 1998; Mason *et al.*, 1998). Venereal transmission is thought to be the mode of spread for serovar *Bratislava* because sows and boars harbor it in the reproductive tract and urinary excretion is relatively low. Survival of the bacteria out of the host is favored by warm, moist conditions. The route of infection is believed to be via the mucous membranes of the mouth, nasal passages, eye, and vagina, although transmission via milk has not been shown experimentally (Ellis, 2012).

Swine are typically maintenance hosts for serovars of the serogroups *Pomona*, *Australis* (serovars *Bratislava* and *Muenchen*), and *Tarassovi*. Infection with other serovars is considered incidental. Typically, only a limited number of serovars will be endemic in a given area and host species (Ellis, 2012).

Pathogenesis A bacteremia develops that results in seeding of *Leptospira* organisms in most organs, including the liver, the pregnant uterus, and the proximal renal tubules, where they persist, multiply, and are voided for varying periods in the urine.

Clinical Signs/Diagnosis The acute form is characterized by a mild transient anorexia, listlessness, diarrhea, and pyrexia that resolves within a week and usually goes unrecognized. Rarely, piglets <12 weeks of age are infected with strains from the serogroup Icterohaemorrhagiae, and have hemoglobinuria, and jaundice. The chronic form is characterized by late-term abortions, stillbirths, and weak newborn piglets. This is particularly true of serovar *Pomona* infection. Infertility of the sow is seen following infections due to serovar *Bratislava*; however, reproductive performance following abortions due to *Pomona* is not affected (Ellis, 2012). The microscopic agglutination test is commonly utilized for serologic monitoring of herds. Diagnosis may also be via serological tests for antibodies to leptospires or via demonstration of leptospires within pig tissues. Differential diagnoses include parvovirus, brucellosis, and PRV.

Treatment Medicating feed for periods of 4 weeks or more with oxytetracycline or chlortetracycline will help control clinical signs until a vaccination program can be established. Individual dosing of pigs with dihydrostreptomycin-penicillin G, oxytetracycline, erythromycin, or tylosin may help eliminate serovar *Pomona* from the renal tubules (Ellis, 2012; Alt and Bolin, 1996).

Prevention/Control A biosecurity program that prevents potential vectors, such as rodents and feral swine, from making direct or indirect contact with the swine in the facility is essential to prevent introduction and minimize spread. Artificial insemination can be used to advantage to prevent spread or introduction of serovar *Bratislava*. Vaccination with bacterins will reduce the incidence of infection but not eliminate the disease from the herd. Immunity is short-lived, which necessitates revaccination at least every 6 months (Ellis, 2012; Cowart, 1995).

Necropsy In acute leptospirosis, few changes are present, but may include petechial or ecchymotic hemorrhages in the lungs and kidneys. In chronic disease, lesions are confined to the kidneys and consist of small gray lesions on the renal cortex. Glomeruli may be swollen or atrophic and cellular casts may be found in the lumen of renal tubules lined by atrophic epithelial cells (Ellis, 2012). The primary lesion is damage to endothelial cell membranes.

Research Complications Leptospirosis will interfere with studies involving swine reproduction or fetal surgery, due to the increased rate of late-term abortions associated with the chronic form of the infection.

c. Porcine Parvovirus

PPV is a disease of swine characterized by embryonic and fetal infection which is manifest as stillbirths, mummification, embryonic death, and infertility (SMEDI) when susceptible sows and gilts are exposed to the virus between 6 and 70 days of gestation. The infection typically causes no observable clinical signs in the infected female, and its major impact on animal health relates to the agent's ability to interfere with live births. Porcine parvovirus is one of the major infectious causes of embryonic and fetal death (Mengeling *et al.*, 1991).

Etiology The disease is caused by PPV-1, a single-stranded DNA virus classified in the genus *Parvovirus*, family Parvoviridae. Novel porcine parvoviruses recently identified include PPV2, hokovirus, PPV4, and PPV5, but the role of these viruses in pigs remains unclear (Xiao *et al.*, 2013).

Epizootiology and Transmission PV is ubiquitous among swine worldwide. In general, infection is enzootic in most herds, and with rare exception, sows are immune. Also, gilts usually contract PPV before conception and develop an active immunity that persists through life. Disease occurs when gilts do not have circulating antibody to the virus. Gilts are most commonly infected oronasally and prenatal pigs are infected transplacentally, although the exact mechanism remains unclear.

Nursing pigs absorb protective PPV antibody from colostrum. These titers diminish to levels that are not protective when the piglets are 3–6 months of age. The significance of the passively acquired antibody is that it interferes with the development of active immunity until the 3- to 6-month mark (Paul *et al.*, 1980).

The major reservoir for PPV is environmental. The virus is thermostable and resistant to many disinfectants. It has been shown that pigs transmit PPV in feces for about 2 weeks after exposure, but the pens they were housed in remained infectious for up to 4 months through which the virus may be transmitted to pigs via fomites (Truyen and Streck, 2012; Mengeling and Paul, 1986).

It is also possible that immunotolerant carriers of PPV, resulting from early *in utero* infection but not death, are carriers (Johnson, 1973). Boars may also play a role in dissemination of the disease. During acute infection with the agent, the virus can be shed in semen. Virus can also be isolated from scrotal lymph nodes up to 35 days post exposure.

Pathogenesis The virus replicates initially in tonsils after which it reaches the lymphatic system leading to cell-free viremia. Placental cells do not support porcine parvoviral infection nor can the virus cross the epitheliochorial placenta (Joo *et al.*, 1976). Current research points to the virus infecting fetal lymphocytes within the circulatory system of pregnant sows (Mengeling *et al.*, 2000; Rudek and Kwiatkowska, 1983). The virus requires the host DNA polymerase to replicate and thus can only produce viral particles in S-phase. The virus has a propensity to invade rapidly dividing cells.

Clinical Signs/Diagnosis Acute infection of both postnatal and pregnant dams is subclinical; however, the pigs will have a transient, mild leukopenia within 10 days after the initial exposure. Maternal reproductive failure is the major sign of infection and is the only clinical sequela to exposure. There is no evidence that PPV impacts either fertility or libido of boars (Thacker *et al.*, 1987).

Dams can cycle back into estrus, farrow fewer pigs per litter, or farrow a large proportion of mummified fetuses. Typically, an epizootic of PPV starts as a subclinical infection and culminates with the delivery of mummified fetuses, usually at or near term. Most of the infected fetuses have a crown–rump length of 17 cm or less because those infected after day 70 are able to respond to the viral assault and survive (Mengeling *et al.*, 1993). Infertility, abortion, stillbirth, neonatal death, prolonged gestations, and reduced neonatal viability have also been attributed to PPV. PPV is one of the primary diagnostic considerations when swine exhibit embryonic or fetal death. Gilts are the population primarily at risk. The lack of maternal illness, abortions, or fetal developmental anomalies differentiates this disease from other causes of reproductive failure. In addition, identifying mummified fetuses that have a crown–rump length of ≤17 cm is a strong indicator that PPV is the infectious agent at play.

The definitive diagnosis can be made by identifying viral antigen by immunofluorescent (IF) microscopy from sections of fetal tissues. Serologic testing for antibodies (i.e., ELISA) is recommended only when tissues from mummified fetuses are not available. Results from serum are of value if antibody is not detected or if samples are collected at intervals that document seroconversion for PPV. Since PPV is ubiquitous, the presence of antibody in a single sample is meaningless. Detection of antibody in sera of fetuses/stillborn before they nurse is evidence of *in utero* infection, as the maternal antibody does not cross the placenta (Chaniago *et al.*, 1978). Differential diagnoses should include PRRSV, brucellosis, leptospirosis, PRV, toxoplasmosis, and nonspecific uterine infection.

Prevention and Treatment There is no treatment for the reproductive failure associated with PPV. Prevention involves either naturally infecting gilts with PPV or vaccinating them with a modified live vaccine prior to pregnancy. Through herd-management practices, natural infections can be promoted. Seronegative gilts can be housed with seropositive sows. Vaccines are used extensively in the US. They are administered several weeks before conception but after the disappearance of passively acquired colostral antibody. In essence, the window for vaccination is small in herds keyed for production. Vaccination for boars is also recommended.

Necropsy Gross lesions are confined to the placenta, which may be edematous and have white, mineralized deposits and stunted fetuses with prominent blood vessels on their surfaces, petechial hemorrhages, edema, enlarged dark liver and kidneys, serosanguinous fluid in body cavities, and mummification (Joo *et al.*, 1977; Hogg *et al.*, 1977). Microscopic findings in the fetuses include vasculitis with hypertrophy of endothelial cells, and perivascular accumulations of mononuclear cells around vessels in the gray and white matter of the cerebrum, brainstem, and meninges, in the interstitial area around glomeruli, portal areas of the liver, and the placenta (Joo *et al.*, 1977; Hogg *et al.*, 1977).

d. Porcine Reproductive and Respiratory Syndrome

This disease was first identified in the US in the late 1980s. Hallmark signs include reproductive disorders, high piglet mortality, and respiratory disease seen in a wide age range of animals. The disease is known officially as PRRS (porcine reproductive and respiratory syndrome) but had been referred to in the literature as SIRS (swine infertility and respiratory syndrome). The disease is now endemic in many countries and has escalated into one of the major causes of reproductive losses and respiratory disease in swine.

Etiology The causative agent is a single-stranded RNA virus classified in the order *Nidovirales*, family Arteriviridae, and genus *Arterivirus*. This agent shares structural and functional organization with others in the genus, including lactate dehydrogenase-elevating virus, equine arteritis virus, and simian hemorrhagic fever virus. These viruses in general are known to have high rates of mutation. There are two distinct genotypes, Type

1 (Lelystad) found primarily in the EU and Type 2 (VR-2332), found primarily in the US, which have genomic and serologic differences. The US isolates differ genomically but cross-react serologically. Infections in vaccinated herds lend suspicion that immunization does not provide protection across all isolates and recent studies continue to show lack of vaccine protection from heterologous viruses (Geldhof et al., 2012). Likewise, if there is great enough antigen variation between strains, a new strain may cause disease in an enzootically infected herd (Tian et al., 2007; Li et al., 2007).

Epizootiology and Transmission This virus is spread predominantly through direct contact between infected and naive pigs, although the route of fetal PRRSV infection has not been identified. Once infected, pigs become persistently infected (Zimmerman et al., 2012a). The virus establishes a foothold by infecting macrophages located within mucosal surfaces. The virus is believed to be limited to domestic swine. The disease does persist in infected swine in a transmissible, viable state, often without stimulating antibody production, thereby making serologic screening for the disease inaccurate. Pigs subclinically infected with PRRSV are thought to be the key factor in disease transmission within herds, and shedding level varies depending on virus variant (Cho and Dee, 2006; Rossow, 1998). The virus has been found in serum, oropharyngeal fluids, semen, feces, and urine, and animals are susceptible via intranasal, intramuscular, oral, intrauterine and vaginal exposure (Rossow, 1998). Animals are extremely susceptible to infection via skin breaks, including tail docking and tattooing (Zimmerman et al., 2012a). Virus is inactivated by heat and drying, but remains infective in cool temperatures and high humidity. Transmission by aerosolization is possible, though routinely occurs only over short distances.

Pathogenesis The virus has been shown to enter via the nasal epithelium, bronchial epithelium, and tonsilar and pulmonary macrophages, followed by replication in alveolar macrophages, with a subsequent viremia and spread to lymphoid organs and lungs (Gomez-Laguna et al., 2010; Rossow et al., 1996a). PRRSV replicates in CD163(+)/sialoadhesin (+) macrophages, which include pulmonary alveolar macrophages, pulmonary intravascular macrophages, and lymphoid tissue macrophages (Zimmerman et al., 2012a). Migration of infected macrophages across the placenta may be one of the mechanisms for transplacental infection of fetuses. PRRSV induces increases in IL-10 which results in downregulation of cytokines involved in virus clearing (IFN-α, IFN-γ, TNF-α and IL-12p40) (Gomez-Laguna et al., 2010). Cytokines released in PRRS are thought to originate from septal macrophages, not the infected macrophages (Gomez-Laguna et al., 2010).

Clinical Signs/Diagnosis The clinical presentation of PRRSV infection depends on the age of the pig and the gestation status when infected. In addition, the clinical presentation can vary depending on complicating infections with viruses or bacteria. Late gestational abortions typically occur when animals are infected during the third trimester and can occur sporadically or sweep throughout the population of animals. Other reproductive manifestations that have been documented include delayed parturition and premature farrowing resulting in mummified or stillborn fetuses. Clinical signs in infected females vary from none to anorexia, fever, pneumonia, agalactia, red/blue discoloration of ears and vulva, subcutaneous edema, and a delayed return to estrus.

Clinical signs in PRRSV-infected newborn pigs also vary in frequency and severity. Dyspnea and tachypnea are the most characteristic clinical signs, with other signs including periocular and eyelid edema, conjunctivitis, blue discoloration of the ears, diarrhea, and CNS signs. Mortality can reach 100%. As the pigs reach postweaning age, the clinical signs shift to include fever, pneumonia, failure to thrive, and significant mortality caused by otherwise non-life-threatening concurrent bacterial infections. PRRSV should be suspected in litters delivered prematurely but after 100 days of gestation.

The susceptibility and resulting impact of secondary bacterial infections in pigs infected with PRRSV depends on the PRRSV isolate, the swine genetic composition, management practices, and environmental factors. Subclinical infections occur commonly as the pig continues to mature, with the only indication of infection being seroconversion to the virus. Occasionally, a transient fever and inappetence or loss of libido can be observed.

Hematologic parameters congruent with infection include a decrease in lymphocytes, neutrophils, and monocytes at 4 days post infection, with a concurrent increase in band neutrophils. Four-week-old pigs had decreased RBC counts, hemoglobin levels, and hematocrits (Rossow et al., 1994).

The viral infection is most accurately diagnosed through the demonstration of PRRSV by virus isolation, fluorescent antibody examination, immunohistochemistry, or PCR in concert with clinical signs and characteristic histologic lesions. Exposure to the virus can be documented through the use of serology testing for anti-PRRSV antibodies; however, if pigs are vaccinated with the modified live-PRRSV vaccine, the current serologic tests cannot differentiate between vaccine virus and field PRRSV isolates. It is also important to note that pigs vaccinated with the modified live vaccine can transmit vaccine virus to naive pigs, resulting in infection and seroconversion of the naive animal (Rossow, 1998).

The virus can most easily be located in lung tissue, lymphoid tissue, heart, brain, and nasal turbinates. Again, it is important to note that modified live-PRRSV vaccine virus can also be identified from these tissues, and pathogenic PRRSV isolates must be differentiated from the vaccine virus. Differential diagnoses include PPV, PRV, CSF, CMV, PCV2, SIV, and leptospirosis.

Treatment Once pigs show signs of disease, supportive therapy should be implemented. This can include antibiotics to control concurrent bacterial infections and vitamin and food supplements until animals regain their appetite.

Prevention/Control Vaccination of pigs with a modified live-PRRSV vaccine has protected pigs from clinical disease when the pigs were challenged with heterologous PRRSV isolates; yet, other reports have shown that the vaccine is not universally protective against all isolates of PRRSV. Efforts should be made to obtain pigs from sources that are free of PRRSV. Pigs coming from different sources should be isolated from each other.

Necropsy PRRSV-infected litters contain normal pigs, small weak piglets, fresh stillborn, autolyzed stillborn, and mummified fetuses. Gross lesions in young piglets include mottled lungs with tan foci of consolidation; lymphadenopathy of the mesenteric and middle iliac nodes, which are tan and may contain cysts, moderately enlarged and rounded hearts, and clear fluid in the pericardial space and abdominal cavity.

Microscopic lesions consist of a multifocal lymphohistiocytic myocarditis; an interstitial pneumonia with mononuclear cell infiltrates, resulting in septal thickening; peribronchial and peribronchiolar lymphohistiocytic cuffing; hypertrophy and hyperplasia of type II pneumocytes; and filling of alveolar spaces with necrotic and normal macrophages. There is also follicular hypertrophy, hyperplasia, and necrosis in lymphoid tissues, and a mild lymphohistiocytic choroiditis with cuffing of vessels in the meninges, choroid plexus, and brain (Halbur *et al.*, 1995). Lesions in fetuses consist of myocarditis with fibrosis, arteritis, and encephalitis (Rossow *et al.*, 1996b).

7. Vesicular Diseases

Vesicular diseases are important in swine and are presented here briefly.

a. Foot-and-Mouth Disease

Etiology Foot-and-mouth disease virus (FMDV) is in the family Picornaviridae, genus *Aphthovirus*.

Epizootiology/Transmission FMDV is enzootic in large parts of Africa, Asia, and the Middle East, and South America. FMDV affects members of the order Arteriodactyla. The virus is typically spread via contact of mucus membranes, abrasions or cuts in the skin, or ingestion of contaminated foodstuffs, but can also be transmitted over long distances via aerosol. All secretions and excretions from infected animals contain infectious virus. FMDV can remain infectious within the environment for extended periods.

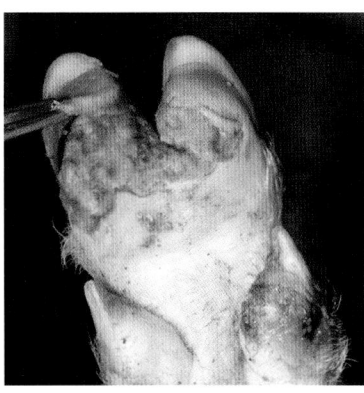

FIGURE 16.26 Foot-and-mouth disease virus. There is separation of the hoof keratin from underlying tissues. *Courtesy of ISU Veterinary Diagnostic Laboratory.*

Pathogenesis Typically, the pharynx is the primary site of infection, unless the virus enters the skin through a wound. The virus needs access to live cells on the surface and does not enter through cornified tissue (Alexanersen *et al.*, 2012). After initial replication, the virus enters the circulation and disseminates to the areas of amplification such as the skin, tongue, and mouth.

Clinical Signs/Diagnosis Pigs display fever and formation of vesicles in and around the mouth and feet (Fig. 16.26). Lesions on the feet are often interdigital, with the coronary band being especially predisposed due to the vascularity. Lesions on the feet result in the animal being lame and often 'dog-sitting'. Animals also show signs of depression and anorexia. If pregnant sows are infected with FMDV, they may abort.

Real-time RT-PCR is now used diagnostically to replace the combined ELISA/virus isolation system (Alexanersen *et al.*, 2012).

Treatment There is no treatment for foot-and-mouth disease in pigs. Euthanasia of all affected and susceptible animals at the infected site is recommended.

Prevalence/Control Increased biosecurity is paramount to preventing spread of this virus. Vaccines will not prevent infection, but may decrease clinical signs in those infected.

Necropsy Vesicles are often in and around the mouth and on the feet, but may also be present on the snout, teats, mammary gland, prepuce, vulva, and other sites. Oral lesions most commonly affect the tongue, and foot lesions are most often interdigital, at the heel bulb, and coronary bands. Lesions around coronary bands may lead to sloughing of claws. Histologically, there is ballooning degeneration in stratum spinosum of cornified stratified squamous epithelium. This is followed by intercellular edema, necrosis, and infiltration by mononuclear cells and granulocytes.

Research Complications The need to euthanize the animals results in loss of the colony. FMD is a reportable disease.

b. Swine Vesicular Disease

Etiology Swine vesicular disease virus is an *Enterovirus* in the family Picornaviridae.

Epizootiology/Transmission Transmission to new farms and animals is primarily through movement of animals, fomites, or feeding of contaminated waste food (Hedger and Mann, 1989). The virus can remain infectious for months. One major difference between SVDV and FMDV is that SVDV has not been shown to be transmitted via aerosol.

Pathogenesis The virus enters the pig via mucous membranes or abrasions of the skin.

Clinical Signs/Diagnosis Clinically, pigs have mild fever with rare lameness. Virus isolation and RT-PCR are used to diagnose the disease.

Treatment Treatment is not recommended as lesions are similar to FMD. Euthanasia is recommended.

Prevalence/Control SVD has only been isolated in Asia and Europe (Alexanersen *et al.*, 2012). It is on the OIE list because lesions caused by swine vesicular disease virus are indistinguishable from those caused by FMDV. Italy is one of only a few countries that actively screen for SVD antibodies, and recent outbreaks were detected via this screening (Alexanersen *et al.*, 2012). It is suspected that the virus is present in more countries than in which it has been reported.

Necropsy Vesicles are present at the coronary bands, snout, tongue, and lips. Lesions are indistinguishable from FMDV.

Research Complications Research is impacted by the loss of cohort or colony due to euthanasia. SVDV is a reportable disease.

c. Vesicular Exanthema of Swine

Vesicular exanthema of swine (VES) is caused by the vesicular exanthema of swine virus, genus *Vesivirus* in the Caliciviridae family (Knowles and Reuter, 2012). A disease indistinguishable from VES is present in wild sea lions in California, and occasionally in wildlife. After a fever, vesicles appear at snout, lips, tongue, oral mucosa, as well as sole, interdigital space and coronary band (McGavin and Zachary, 2007). This is a reportable disease.

d. Vesicular Stomatitis

Vesicular stomatitis (VS) infection in pigs is indistinguishable from FMD, and therefore is classified a notifiable disease (Health, 2013a). Vesicular stomatitis virus is in the genus *Vesiculovirus* and family Rhabdoviridae. Transmission is via aerosol or contact with experimental transmission via flies (Health, 2013a). Infection is localized to the site of inoculation. If the area is unhaired (oral

mucosa, snout, coronary bands), vesicles develop within 1–3 days, whereas if the area is haired, seroconversion with subclinical disease is seen (Swenson *et al.*, 2012). Clinical signs include excessive salivation, foot lesions with possible separation of the claw, and lameness. Virus detection is via tissue tags, vesicular fluid, or biopsy of affected area. Treatment is by supportive care and disinfection is crucial to prevent spread. VS is a zoonotic disease.

e. Classical Swine Fever

Etiology Classical swine fever (CSF) virus is in the family Flavivirus, genus *Pestivirus*. It is also known as hog cholera in the literature.

Epizootiology/Transmission Pigs are the only natural reservoirs of the virus, and it is included here for completeness, as it should be eradicated from all commercial breeding herds. The virus continues to circulate in China, Africa, Central America, and parts of South America (Kirkland *et al.*, 2012a). Transmission is oronasal, or by ingestion of infected material, although airborne transmission has been shown experimentally along with seminal transmission (Elbers *et al.*, 2001; Kirkland *et al.*, 2012a; De Smit *et al.*, 1999). The virus can survive in certain conditions for prolonged periods (Kirkland *et al.*, 2012a).

Pathogenesis Primary viral replication is in the tonsils followed by spread to lymph nodes, peripheral blood, and bone marrow. Not fully understood are the effects on immune system, endothelium, and epithelial cells, as well as thrombocytopenia and consumption coagulopathy followed by disseminated intravascular coagulation (Maxie and Jubb, 2007). Experimental infection of animals has shown platelet activation followed by macrophage activation and subsequent phagocytosis of platelets, which may explain the thrombocytopenia (Bautista *et al.*, 2002). Bone marrow megakaryocytic dysmegakaryocytopoiesis has also been described (Gomez-Villamandos *et al.*, 2003). Primary cytokines involved in this disease are TNF-α, IL-6, and IL-1α (Sanchez-Cordon *et al.*, 2005).

Clinical Signs/Diagnosis Animals with CSF have pyrexia, anorexia, lethargy, conjunctivitis, respiratory signs, and constipation followed by diarrhea (Kirkland *et al.*, 2012a). Signs are the same in acute and chronic forms; only the time course is different.

Virus isolation, RT-PCR, virus neutralization, and ELISA are all used to diagnose CSF. Differentials include African swine fever, BVDV, PRRSV, PCV2, salmonellosis, erysipelas, streptococcosis, leptospirosis, and coumarin poisoning.

Prevention and Control Some CSF-free areas try to maintain a 'no vaccination' policy and eradicate infected herds, while those in endemic areas vaccinate to prevent disease (Kirkland *et al.*, 2012a).

Confounding Factors Bovine viral diarrhea virus (BVDV) is usually only pathogenic for fetal pigs, but it can also infect pigs naturally, and pathological lesions can be indistinct from those of CSF (Maxie and Jubb, 2007; Kirkland *et al.*, 2012a). The primary problem with infection of pigs by BVDV is that it confounds accurate detection of CSF. Infection is typically cross-species, and BVDV lesions may be mistaken for CSF, thus complicating CSF detection and control.

Necropsy   The presence of lesions is variable, but most commonly hemorrhage of the peripheral lymph nodes and renal petechiae and ecchymoses are present, while splenic infarction is nearly pathognomonic for the disease (Maxie and Jubb, 2007). Lesions consistent with DIC may also be seen.

8. Newly Reported or Emerging Infectious Diseases/Agents

a. Nipah Virus

Etiology   Nipah virus is a single-stranded negative sense RNA virus in the family Paramyxovirus, genus *Henipavirus*. There are strain differences between isolates from different geographic regions.

Epizootiology/Transmission   Initially identified in Malaysia in 1999, the virus has since emerged in Bangladesh and India. Pigs are an amplifying host; however, bats are the reservoir host and secrete virus in urine where pigs may ingest items containing infectious viral particles and become infected (Williamson and Torres-Velez, 2010). Close contact is required for transmission (Fogarty *et al.*, 2008).

Pathogenesis   Vascular, nervous, and lymphoreticular systems are targets for the virus. The virus is able to circumvent the host interferon response (Williamson and Torres-Velez, 2010).

Clinical Signs   Pigs are asymptomatic or have acute febrile disease with respiratory/CNS signs (Kirkland *et al.*, 2012b).

Treatment   Euthanasia is the treatment of choice.

Prevention/Control   Recombinant vaccines have been used in pigs.

Necropsy   Enlarged lymph nodes, congestion and edema in meninges, pulmonary consolidation, and distended interlobular septa are associated with Nipah infection (Kirkland *et al.*, 2012b). Syncytial cells located in areas of interstitial pneumonia contain intracytoplasmic inclusion bodies (Torres-Velez, 2008).

Research Complications   Nipah is a BSL-4 agent and is zoonotic.

b. Porcine Lymphotropic Herpesviruses

Porcine lymphotropic herpesvirus (PLHV) has been associated with a porcine lymphotropic disease with high mortality, similar to that of human post-transplantation lymphoproliferative disease, in pigs immunosuppressed for transplantation studies

(Mettenleiter *et al.*, 2012; Huang *et al.*, 2001; Chmielewicz *et al.*, 2003; Ehlers *et al.*, 1999). There is also concern that pig–human xenotransplantation may result in human disease from this virus (Ehlers *et al.*, 1999; Goltz *et al.*, 2002).

Etiology   PLHV is in the Herpesviridae family, subfamily Gammaherpesvirinae, genus *Macavirus*, species *suid herpes-3,-4,-5. Suid herpesvirus-3,-4,-5* correspond to PLHV-1, -2, -3, respectively (Davison *et al.*, 2009).

Epizootiology/Transmission   PLHV appear to be present in pigs worldwide with no outward disease in healthy individuals (Goltz *et al.*, 2002).

Pathogenesis   PLHV predominantly infects B cells (Mettenleiter *et al.*, 2012).

Clinical Signs/Diagnosis   There is no known disease unless animals are immunosuppressed. In immunosuppressed minipigs, there was profound B-cell proliferation and the majority of animals died (Huang *et al.*, 2001). Clinical signs included lethargy, fever, anorexia, and enlarged lymph nodes (Huang *et al.*, 2001). Diagnosis is typically via PCR specific for each of the lymphotropic viruses (PLHV-1, -2,-3).

Prevention/Control   Caesarian derivation may reduce the prevalence of PLHVs (Tucker *et al.*, 2003).

Necropsy   Macroscopic findings included enlarged lymphoreticular organs, airway obstruction, and respiratory failure (Huang *et al.*, 2001). Disease is only manifest in immunocompromised individuals.

Research Complications   There is concern in xenotransplantation studies that lymphoproliferative disease due to PLHV will occur after immunosuppression of the host.

c. Ovine Herpesvirus-2

A naturally occurring disease similar to malignant catarrhal fever (MCF) has been reported in pigs, although rare and poorly documented (Alcaraz *et al.*, 2009; Loken *et al.*, 1998).

Etiology   The disease in pigs is caused by ovine herpesvirus 2 in the family Herpesviridae, subfamily Gammaherpesvirinae, genus *Macavirus* (Davison *et al.*, 2009). Porcine disease has not been associated with other viruses that cause MCF in cattle (Alcelaphine herpesvirus 1).

Epizootiology/Transmission   The mode of transmission is uncertain, but is suspected to be via nasal secretions. There have been reports of pigs becoming ill after having contact with sheep.

Clinical Signs/ Diagnosis   Pigs with MCF display high persistent fever, anorexia, depression, recumbency, foul-smelling nasal discharge, ocular discharge, bilateral corneal edema, keratoconjunctivitis, ataxia, tremors, and possible convulsions (Alcaraz *et al.*, 2009). Diagnosis is dependent on clinical signs, histology, and presence of virus-specific antibodies (Mettenleiter *et al.*, 2012). This disease can be mistaken for PRV, CSF, ASFV, porcine enterovirus, PCV2, and rabies.

Prevention/Control　There is currently no vaccine in pigs. Decreasing any interactions pigs may have with sheep will help prevent cross-species transmission.

Necropsy　There are multifocal cyanotic areas or petechiae on the skin, crusts on the skin, enlarged hyperemic lymph nodes, and mucopurulent exudate in airways. The spleen and liver are engorged (Alcaraz *et al.*, 2009). The most consistent and histological lesion is acute vasculitis in the CNS and other organs characterized by adventitial and transmural mononuclear cells with fibrinoid necrosis of vessel walls in many tissues. The myocardium, spleen, CNS, skin, and kidneys are commonly affected (panarteritis) (Mettenleiter *et al.*, 2012).

d. Hepatitis E

Hepatitis E is in the genus *Hepevirus* and there are four known genotypes of hepatitis E, of which genotypes 3 and 4 infect pigs (Temmam *et al.*, 2013). Infection in pigs is primarily without clinical signs. Genotype 3 infection of pigs leads to multifocal lympoplasmacytic hepatitis and focal necrosis, but no elevation of liver enzymes has been noted (Vasickova *et al.*, 2007; Krawczynski *et al.*, 2011). Transmission is typically fecal–oral (Vasickova *et al.*, 2007). Exposure of humans to infected swine can lead to transmission of the virus to humans (Temmam *et al.*, 2013). Swine veterinarians have been shown to have detectable antibody titers to the virus (Meng *et al.*, 2002).

e. Ebola Virus

Ebola viruses are in the family Filoviridae, genus *Ebolavirus*, species *Reston ebolavirus* (REBOV). Pigs showed signs consistent with severe form of PRRSV and were found to be infected with PRRSV, REBOV, and in some cases PCV2 (Barrette *et al.*, 2009). The primary differential is PRRSV (Rowland *et al.*, 2012). Pigs have also been experimentally infected with Zaire ebolavirus in which transmission to NHP has been demonstrated (Weingartl *et al.*, 2012).

REBOV is a subclinical disease in pigs, and only causes lesions if infection occurs via a systemic route (Marsh *et al.*, 2011). Current knowledge indicates that REBOV is involved in outward disease only if another agent is present.

f. Japanese Encephalitis

Japanese encephalitis virus (JEV) is a member of the family Flaviviridae, genus *Flavivirus*. While mosquitos transmit the agent, the pig is a natural reservoir of JEV (Grand, 2012). Clinical signs in pigs include testicular degeneration, infertility, mummified fetuses, and piglets with birth defects, reproductive failure, and still births (Grand, 2012). Reproductive failure is only seen when sows are infected before 60–70 days of gestation (Williams *et al.*, 2012). Experimental infection of 3-week-old piglets resulted in non-suppurative encephalitis of frontal and temporal lobes. The spinal cord was also affected (Yamada *et al.*, 2004). Differentials include PPV, PRV, PRRSV, toxoplasmosis, and leptospirosis. Virus isolation is required to diagnose the disease. Humans can also be infected by the virus, but only via a mosquito (Mackenzie *et al.*, 2004).

B. Metabolic/Nutritional Diseases

1. Porcine Stress Syndrome

Etiology　Porcine stress syndrome (PSS) refers to a cascade of physiologic events and clinical signs that occur in pigs that have a mutation in the calcium-release channel protein (ryanodine receptor [RYR]). This mutation results in a hypersensitive triggering mechanism of the calcium-release channel in skeletal muscle sarcoplasmic reticulum in response to various stressors, such as gas anesthetics or stressful environmental conditions. The lack of proper calcium control within the membranous portions of the sarcoplasmic reticulum and mitochondria is thought to initiate the cascade of events that results in the syndrome (O'Brien *et al.*, 1991; Fujii *et al.*, 1991). Stress-susceptible pigs are also known to overrespond to stressful stimuli, with excessive β-adrenergic receptor stimulation, lower rates of lactate, alanine, and aspartate conversion to carbon dioxide by the liver, abnormal phosphorus metabolism, and a much higher cortisol and thyroxine turnover rate.

Animals carrying the genetic defect in RYR had been found throughout the world. Genotypic analyses have indicated that the mutation arose from a single founder animal. The mutation is found in five major breeds of swine: Landrace, Yorkshire, Duroc, Pietrain, and Poland China and other breeds, including miniature potbellied pigs (Claxton-Gill *et al.*, 1993). The mode of inheritance is autosomal recessive with variable penetrance. With the advent of genetic testing, the disease due to the RYR mutation has largely been bred out of existence in research and production animals, but does remain in the show pig population (Woods and Tynes, 2012). However, a newly identified mutation (R1958W) in the dystrophin gene has recently been shown to be responsible for loss of animals due to transport stress (Nonneman *et al.*, 2012). This syndrome has also been reported in humans, dogs, cats, and horses.

Clinical Signs　In a laboratory setting, development of PSS has most commonly been associated with exposure to halothane and succinylcholine; however, methoxyflurane, enflurane, and isoflurane have all been shown to be capable of eliciting a reaction in susceptible swine. The course of the disease is variable, ranging from abatement of clinical signs when anesthesia is terminated to fatality.

Initial signs include tachycardia, tachypnea, muscle rigidity, and hyperthermia. Clinicopathologic changes include metabolic acidosis, myoglobinemia, hyperkalemia, and hyperglycemia. These metabolic derangements frequently lead to cardiovascular collapse and death. In addition to the typical manifestation, nonrigid and normothermic forms have been described. Signs of this disease are less pronounced in young pigs and those that are heterozygous for the trait. In non-anesthetized pigs, stressful situations will lead to the early signs of the disease, which include muscle and tail tremors. Progression of the syndrome leads to dyspnea, blanched and reddened areas on the skin, increased body temperature, and cyanosis. Muscle rigidity and cardiovascular collapse follow. This syndrome is also known as malignant hyperthermia.

Treatment Early recognition of the disease is the key to treatment. Anesthetic delivery should be discontinued immediately and 100% oxygen delivered. Additional treatment includes sodium bicarbonate to combat the metabolic acidosis and hyperkalemia. Active cooling of the animal may be done by ice packing and IV administration of cooled fluids, or by gastric and/or rectal lavage with iced saline. Dantrolene, an agent that prevents PSS by decreasing release of calcium from the sarcoplasmic reticulum while allowing calcium uptake to continue, is highly effective in stopping the progression of the syndrome when administered at the onset of signs. After the crisis is alleviated, the animal must be monitored closely for 48 h; redevelopment of the syndrome in response to minor stressors can occur. Dantrolene (3.5–5 mg/kg) can also be given as preventive therapy in animals known to be susceptible and to treat (Flewellen and Nelson, 1980; Ehler *et al.*, 1985).

Prevention/Control The disease is best controlled by identifying those animals that carry the genetic mutation and eliminating them from the breeding stock. A readily available, inexpensive DNA-based test can be used to screen for the mutation (O'Brien *et al.*, 1993). The RYR mutation has largely been bred out of swine herds.

Necropsy Pigs exhibiting this syndrome present with a very rapid development of rigor mortis. In addition, many of the animals will have muscles that appear very pale and are very soft, almost watery in texture, due to the high lactic acid content in muscles that occurs *post-mortem*. *Ante mortem* histologic changes have not been identified in these animals. Lesions in animals with the dystrophin mutations consist of cardiomyofiber degeneration (Nonneman *et al.*, 2012).

2. Salt Poisoning

Etiology Salt poisoning, also known as sodium ion toxicosis, is a condition that can easily occur in swine. It can be caused directly by the animal consuming excessive amounts of sodium. This happens infrequently, as animals are rarely presented with feed that has excessively high sodium content. However, feeding milk byproducts such as whey, which has high sodium content, has been shown to cause the disease. By far the most common initiator for the condition is water deprivation. Usually, signs are initiated after a minimum of 24 h of deprivation, but the condition can also occur after just a few hours of deprivation.

Pathogenesis Salt poisoning is caused by hyperosmolarity of the CNS. When the animal rehydrates, the osmotic pressure causes water to be drawn into the CNS, resulting in swelling and edema.

Clinical Signs/Diagnosis Initially, the animal presents as being very thirsty and constipated. CNS involvement, which may be delayed for several days after the insult, follows. The pigs will appear tense and apprehensive, with ears pricked and staring ahead with the head slightly elevated. The nose will then twitch, the eyes will close, and a rhythmic chomping of the jaws follows. Animals may also appear blind and deaf. Pigs near death may paddle continuously. If the condition occurs because of excessive salt consumption rather than water deprivation, vomiting and diarrhea may be part of the presentation.

The diagnosis can easily be made if the clinical signs are matched with known water deprivation. Supporting findings include gastritis, constipation, or enteritis. A laminar subcortical necrosis may occur if pigs are subacutely affected. The animal may present with hypernatremia; however, if the animal has had a chance to rehydrate, this finding will not be present. Differential diagnoses include PRV, hog cholera, and edema disease. Other causes of toxicosis, such as food poisoning, should also be considered.

Treatment Unfortunately, treatment is generally ineffective, and in fact, the condition is likely to be exacerbated by rehydration.

Pathology Histologic evaluation reveals eosinophilic cuffing of the meningeal and cerebral vessels.

3. Gastric Ulcers

Etiology Gastric ulceration in pigs refers to a condition in which ulceration of a specific region of the pig's stomach, the pars oesophagea, occurs. This condition has been diagnosed with increasing frequency since the 1950s, with the distribution being worldwide and varied in occurrence.

Pathogenesis To date, the pathogenesis of the disease remains speculative. However, a study has shown a relationship between the presence of *Helicobacter pylori*-like organisms, a high-carbohydrate diet, and gastric ulcers (Krakowka and Ellis, 2006).

Epizootiology Although this condition has been identified for decades, the definitive pathogenesis is still unknown. Fasted pigs exposed to stressful environmental conditions had a higher incidence of ulcers compared to controls. An increased incidence of ulceration was produced when pigs were fed finely ground diets. Many species of bacteria and fungi have been isolated from ulcer lesions, but none have been shown to be causative. One study investigated the prevalence of *Gastrospirillum suis* in pigs with gastric ulcer but found no correlation between its presence and the occurrence of ulceration (Barbosa *et al.*, 1995). Further investigations are needed to better define the etiology of this condition.

Clinical Signs/Diagnosis The clinical signs vary depending on duration of the ulceration. In the peracute form, apparently healthy animals are simply found dead. In the acute form, pigs will become pale and weak, with an increased respiratory rate. Vomiting of blood and passage of bloody, tarry feces are seen. In the subacute or chronic form, the animal will be anemic and anorexic, with passage of dark feces that may be intermittent or persistent. Occasionally, the only sign observed may be the passage of dark, hard feces. Pigs of either sex or any breed may be affected. Usually, single pigs are affected, and body temperature is normal or slightly subnormal. Anemia can be detected hematologically if the chronic/subacute form is present. Differential diagnoses include swine dysentery, *S. enterica* ser. Choleraesuis, TGE, and intestinal hemorrhagic syndrome. These diseases can be differentiated relatively easily, as they impact on groups of animals and, with the exception of the intestinal hemorrhagic syndrome, result in high body temperatures.

Treatment Early stages of ulceration are not typically identified, so treatment is often not initiated until the condition has progressed to a point where treatment is ineffective. Options include administering nonabsorbable antacids, and vitamin E and selenium, as well as H-2 blockers (cimetidine, Zantac, etc.).

Prevention Providing pigs with appropriate feed is a prudent measure to take toward disease prevention. The diet should be more coarsely ground (not less than 700 μm in size), not contain excessive unsaturated fatty acids, and have the right balance of vitamin E and selenium. Stressful conditions such as overcrowding, fasting, and unstable social groupings should be avoided.

Necropsy The pars oesophagea contains no glands and is covered by stratified squamous epithelium continuous with the esophagus. In a healthy animal, this surface appears white and smooth. Lesions can first be detected as a roughened, irregular surface. Ulceration follows, with a disruption in the epithelium that may be small, discrete, and single to multiple, large, and irregular. Blood or blood clots can be seen at the ulceration site, as well as in the stomach or in the gastrointestinal tract. If the subacute/chronic form of the condition is present, chronic ulceration usually ensues. This is characterized by the presence of fibrous tissue and the contraction of the area of ulceration.

In the early stages of the ulcer formation, parakeratosis of the epithelium occurs. Occasionally, infiltration of some polymorphonuclear cells occurs, but usually inflammatory cells are absent. The epithelium is weakened, and erosion of the tissue eventually occurs as a result of the parakeratosis. Once the underlying tissues are exposed to the gastric juices, diffuse necrosis and bleeding characteristic of any ulcer occur. Chronic ulcers develop as fibrous connective tissue forms in the underlying lamina propria. The muscularis mucosae may hypertrophy or may degenerate and be replaced by collagenized fibrous tissue. Occasionally, the ulcer may penetrate the serosa.

4. Melamine–Cyanuric Acid Toxicity

Melamine and cyanuric acids, when fed together, cause toxicity in animals. In 2007, there was a report in pigs in which they showed weight loss, pallor, rough coats, and increased mortality. Their kidneys were swollen with yellow discoloration. Histological examination revealed lesions in the proximal and distal tubules and collecting ducts with epithelial degeneration, necrosis, and crystals. The crystals were round, yellow to brown, and had radiating striations (Nilubol *et al.*, 2009).

C. Iatrogenic Diseases

1. Catheter Infections

Etiology A wide variety of either venous or arterial vascular-access lines are commonly used in swine and maintained for variable periods. Bacteria can be easily introduced into these lines if strict adherence to sterile technique is not observed during flushing. Improper maintenance of the catheter can also result in seeding of thrombi.

Pathogenesis Bacteremia with seeding of multiple organs can result in septic emboli in the lungs, kidney, spleen, and other sites. Thrombi dislodged from catheters during flushing can result in infarcts in multiple tissues, including the kidney.

Clinical Signs Swine with a catheter infection will be febrile, have decreased appetite, and have a discharge from around the vascular access port catheter exit site.

Differential Diagnosis The differential diagnosis should include foreign body reactions to the biomaterials.

Treatment Blood cultures or cultures taken from around the implant may identify the infectious agent responsible, and a sensitivity test should provide information needed to select appropriate antibiotics.

Prevention/Control Prevention and control consist of adequate flushing of lines, strict adherence to sterile technique in flushing, and use of flushes that have concentrations of anticoagulants adequate to prevent thrombus formation.

Necropsy A suppurative exudate may be present around the external access port or around subcutaneous implants. The entire catheter tract should be dissected to observe for any gross evidence of infection. Cultures should be taken of any suspicious sites. There may be a suppurative pneumonia with consolidation, suppurative emboli in multiple organs, renal infarcts, or infarcts in other organs. Microscopic lesions may include a cellulitis, myositis, suppurative pneumonia, suppurative emboli in one or more organs, or infarcts in the kidneys or other organs.

Research Complications Catheter infections are themselves research complications that may result in the animal being terminated from a study or euthanized due to persistent febrile state or compromised function of one or more organs.

D. Neoplastic Diseases

It has been touted that neoplasms occur with less frequency in pigs than in other domestic animals; however, this commonly held belief may be influenced by the fact that the majority of the pig population is slaughtered before reaching an age when cancer would normally appear with any significant incidence. The tumors that historically have been reported are those seen in young pigs, with the most common tumors being lymphosarcoma, embryonal nephroma, and melanoma. However, with the recent surge in popularity of potbellied pigs in the pet trade, more tumors are being found. A word of caution however, as these reports are from a single breed (Vietnamese potbellied) which may or may not be representative of the pig population at large.

A recent study of uteri from spayed miniature pigs (age 4 months to 14 years) found that 14/32 had smooth muscle tumors of the uterus or broad ligament (leiomyoma or leiomyosarcoma). One-third had adenoma or adenomyosarcoma (Ilha *et al.*, 2010). Another retrospective study found uterine leiomyomas in over 80% of samples and suggested similarities to human fibroids, proposing potbellied pigs as a model for this disease (Mozzachio *et al.*, 2004). Uterine adenocarcinoma has also been reported in mixed-breed research pigs (Cannon *et al.*, 2009).

Lymphosarcomas affect primarily younger animals but can affect mature animals of either sex. Most cases are classified as multicentric; thymic is the next most frequent classification. Infiltration of the liver, spleen, and kidney predominates. Histologically, pigs typically exhibit lymphocytic lymphosarcomas; however, lymphoblastic, histiocytic, and mixed types do occur. T-cell lymphosarcomas have also been found in aged potbellied pigs (Corapi *et al.*, 2011).

Embryonal nephromas affect pigs under 1 year of age, with predominance in females. The tumor arises in the kidney parenchyma, is typically unilateral, and may spread to the lungs and liver. Histologically, the classifications that occur most commonly are nephroblastic and epithelial.

Melanomas occur as congenital lesions with exceptionally high frequency in Sinclair miniature swine (85% incidence at 1 year of age) and in Duroc, Iberian, and Hormel breeds. The disease is occasionally seen in other breeds as well. The tumors can be single or multiple and may affect the skin only or may involve metastasis to multiple internal organs. Initially, the skin tumor appears as a flat black spot that becomes a raised nodule. The tumor initiates as a focus of melanocytic hyperplasia within the basal layer. Spontaneous regression, thought to be caused by the cytotoxic effects of infiltrated tumor-specific T lymphocytes, occurs in the vast majority of cases.

Investigators are also beginning to target specific genes in pigs to generate 'oncopigs' which are prone to specific tumors (Flisikowska *et al.*, 2013).

E. Miscellaneous

1. Thrombocytopenic purpura

Thrombocytopenic purpura has been reported in Gottingen pigs in both the US and EU. There is no sex predilection (Carrasco *et al.*, 2003; Dincer and Skydsgaard, 2012). Grossly, animals have extensive multifocal subcutaneous hemorrhage. They have thrombocytopenia and anemia, leading to subcapsular hemorrhage of lymph nodes and hemorrhages of the urinary bladder urothelium (Carrasco *et al.*, 2003). Other lesions include ulceration of the torus pyloricae and hemorrhages in numerous tissues (Carrasco *et al.*, 2003). Vascular lesions are consistently present in renal pelvis and coronary arteries, primarily within small to medium muscular arteries which display neointimal proliferation, thrombosis, and medial deposits of myxoid matrix (Maratea *et al.*, 2006). Renal glomeruli consistently have membranoproliferative lesions that label for immunoglobulins and C1q (Carrasco *et al.*, 2003). There are increased numbers of immature and apoptotic megakaryocytes within the bone marrow (Carrasco *et al.*, 2003). This is believed to be a Type III hypersensitivity reaction.

ACRONYMS USED IN CHAPTER

AHXR	Acute humoral xenograft rejection
APE	Acute pulmonary edema
APP	Actinobacillus pleuropneumoniae
AR	Atrophic rhinitis
ASFV	African swine fever virus
BM	Bone marrow

BVDV	Bovine viral diarrhea virus
CMV	Cytomegalovirus
CNS	Central nervous system
CSF	Classical swine fever
DNT	Dermonecrotic toxin – from *B. bronchiseptica*
ED	Edema disease
EE	Exudative epidermitis, greasy pig disease
ELISA	Enzyme-linked immunosorbent assay
EMCV	Encephalomyocarditis virus
EDEC	Edema disease associated *E. coli*
EHEC	Enterohemorrhagic *E. coli*
EPEC	Enteropathogenic *E. coli*
ETEC	Enterotoxigenic *E. coli*
EU	European Union
HAR	Hyperacute rejection
IBR	Inclusion body rhinitis (CMV)
IFA	Immunofluorescence assay
IFN	Interferon
Ig	Immunoglobulin
IHC	Immunohistochemistry
IL	Interleukin
MCF	Malignant catarrhal fever
MHC	Major histocompatibility complex
MPS	Mycoplasmal pneumonia of swine
NHP	Nonhuman primate
NPAR	Nonprogressive atrophic rhinitis (*B. bronchiseptica* alone)
PAN	PCV-2-associated neuropathy
PAR	Progressive atrophic rhinitis (*P. multocida* alone or in combination with *B. bronchiseptica*)
PCR	Polymerase chain reaction
PCV; PCV2	Porcine circovirus; porcine circovirus-2
PCVAD	PCV-associated disease
PDNS	Porcine dermatitis and nephropathy syndrome
PE	Proliferative enteropathy
PEDV	Porcine epidemic diarrhea virus
PHLV	Porcine lymphotropic herpesvirus
PMT	*P. multocida* toxin – from *P. multocida*
PMWS	Postweaning multisystemic wasting disease
PPV	Porcine parvovirus
PRDC	Porcine respiratory disease complex
PRRSV	Porcine reproductive and respiratory syndrome virus
PRV	Pseudorabies virus
PTV	Porcine teschovirus
PWD	Postweaning diarrhea
RT-PCR	Reverse transcriptase-polymerase chain reaction
RYR	Ryanodine receptor
SD	Swine dysentery
SE	Swine erysipelas
SIV	Swine influenza virus
SLA	Swine leukocyte antigen
SMEDI	Stillbirths, mummification, embryonic death, and infertility
SPF	Specific pathogen free
STEC	Shiga-toxin producing *E. coli*
TGE/TGEV	Transmissible gastroenteritis (coronavirus)/transmissible gastroenteritis virus
TNF	Tumor necrosis factor
TTV	Torque teno virus
US	United states

Acknowledgments

The authors acknowledge the input of the authors of the chapter in previous edition of this book: Drs. Kathy E. Laber, Mark T. Whary, Sarah A. Bingel, James A. Goodrich, and Alison C. Smith. Much of the current chapter is based on this influential work.

References

Aarestrup, F.M., Jorsal, S.E., Jensen, N.E., 1998a. Serological characterization and antimicrobial susceptibility of Streptococcus suis isolates from diagnostic samples in Denmark during 1995 and 1996. Vet. Microbiol. 60, 59–66.

Aarestrup, F.M., Rasmussen, S.R., Artursson, K., Jensen, N.E., 1998b. Trends in the resistance to antimicrobial agents of Streptococcus suis isolates from Denmark and Sweden. Vet. Microbiol. 63, 71–80.

Ackermann, M.R., Debey, M.C., Debey, B.M., 1991. Bronchiolar metaplasia and Ulex europaeus agglutinin I (UEA-I) affinity in Mycoplasma hyopneumoniae-infected lungs of six pigs. Vet. Pathol. 28, 533–535.

Ackermann, M.R., Register, K.B., Stabel, J.R., Gwaltney, S.M., Howe, T.S., Rimler, R.B., 1996. Effect of Pasteurella multocida toxin on physeal growth in young pigs. Am. J. Vet. Res. 57, 848–852.

Agriculture, U.S.D.O., 2008. Pseudorabies (Aujeszky's disease) and its eradication: a review of the U.S. experience. USDA.

Agriculture, U.S.D.O., 2014. Agriculture secretary Tom Vilsack announces additional USDA actions to combat spread of diseases among U.S. pork producers. Release No. 0066.14.

Alcaraz, A., Warren, A., Jackson, C., Gold, J., Mccoy, M., Cheong, S.H., et al., 2009. Naturally occurring sheep-associated malignant catarrhal fever in North American pigs. J. Vet. Diagn. Invest. 21, 250–253.

Alexanersen, S., Knowles, N.J., Dekker, A., Belsham, G.J., Zhang, Z., Koenen, F., 2012. Picornaviruses. In: Zimmerman, J.J., Karriker, L.A., Ramirez, A., Schwartz, K.J., Stevenson, G.W. (Eds.), Diseases of Swine, tenth ed. Wiley-Blackwell, Chichester, West Sussex.

Allan, G.M., Mc Neilly, F., Meehan, B.M., Kennedy, S., Mackie, D.P., Ellis, J.A., et al., 1999. Isolation and characterisation of circoviruses from pigs with wasting syndromes in Spain, Denmark and Northern Ireland. Vet. Microbiol. 66, 115–123.

Alt, D.P., Bolin, C.A., 1996. Preliminary evaluation of antimicrobial agents for treatment of Leptospira interrogans serovar pomona infection in hamsters and swine. Am. J. Vet. Res. 57, 59–62.

Amass, S.F., Scholz, D.A., 1998. Acute nonfatal erysipelas in sows in a commercial farrow-to-finish operation. J. Am. Vet. Med. Assoc. 212, 708–709.

Amass, S.F., Wu, C.C., Clark, L.K., 1996. Evaluation of antibiotics for the elimination of the tonsillar carrier state of Streptococcus suis in pigs. J. Vet. Diagn. Invest. 8, 64–67.

Andresen, L.O., 1998. Differentiation and distribution of three types of exfoliative toxin produced by Staphylococcus hyicus from pigs with exudative epidermitis. FEMS Immunol. Med. Microbiol. 20, 301–310.

Andresen, L.O., 1999. Development and evaluation of an indirect ELISA for detection of exfoliative toxin ExhA, ExhB or ExhC produced by Staphylococcus hyicus. Vet. Microbiol. 68, 285–292.

Anderson, M., 2006. Xenotransplantation: a bioethical evaluation. J. Med. Ethics 32, 205–208.

Aragon, V., Segales, J., Oliveira, S., 2012. Glasser's disease. In: Zimmerman, J.J., Karriker, L.A., Ramirez, A., Schwartz, K.J., Stevenson, G.W. (Eds.), Diseases of Swine, tenth ed. Wiley-Blackwell, Chichester, West Sussex.

Arends, J.J., Skogerboe, T.L., Ritzhaupt, L.K., 1999. Persistent efficacy of doramectin and ivermectin against experimental infestations of Sarcoptes scabiei var. suis in swine. Vet. Parasitol. 82, 71–79.

Argenzio, R.A., Whipp, S.C., Glock, R.D., 1980. Pathophysiology of swine dysentery: colonic transport and permeability studies. J. Infect. Dis. 142, 676–684.

Atyeo, R.F., Oxberry, S.L., Combs, B.G., Hampson, D.J., 1998. Development and evaluation of polymerase chain reaction tests as an aid to diagnosis of swine dysentery and intestinal spirochaetosis. Lett. Appl. Microbiol. 26, 126–130.

Bahls, M., Bidwell, C.A., Hu, J., Krueger, C.G., Reed, J.D., Tellez, A., et al., 2011. Gene expression differences in healthy brachial and femoral arteries of Rapacz familial hypercholesterolemic swine. Physiol. Genomics 43, 781–788.

Bahls, M., Bidwell, C.A., Hu, J., Tellez, A., Kaluza, G.L., Granada, J.F., et al., 2013. Gene expression differences during the heterogeneous progression of peripheral atherosclerosis in familial hypercholesterolemic swine. BMC Genomics 14, 443.

Baker, D.R., Billey, L.O., Francis, D.H., 1997. Distribution of K88 Escherichia coli-adhesive and nonadhesive phenotypes among pigs of four breeds. Vet. Microbiol. 54, 123–132.

Barbe, F., Atanasova, K., Van Reeth, K., 2011. Cytokines and acute phase proteins associated with acute swine influenza infection in pigs. Vet. J. 187, 48–53.

Barbosa, A.J., Silva, J.C., Nogueira, A.M., Paulino Junior, E., Miranda, C.R., 1995. Higher incidence of Gastrospirillum sp. in swine with gastric ulcer of the pars oesophagea. Vet. Pathol. 32, 134–139.

Barrette, R.W., Metwally, S.A., Rowland, J.M., Xu, L., Zaki, S.R., Nichol, S.T., et al., 2009. Discovery of swine as a host for the Reston ebolavirus. Science 325, 204–206.

Batte, E.G., Moncol, D.J., 1972. Whipworms and dysentery in feeder pigs. J. Am. Vet. Med. Assoc. 161, 1226–1228.

Batte, E.G., Mclamb, R.D., Muse, K.E., Tally, S.D., Vestal, T.J., 1977. Pathophysiology of swine trichuriasis. Am. J. Vet. Res. 38, 1075–1079.

Baumeister, A.K., Runge, M., Ganter, M., Feenstra, A.A., Delbeck, F., Kirchhoff, H., 1998. Detection of Mycoplasma hyopneumoniae in bronchoalveolar lavage fluids of pigs by PCR. J. Clin. Microbiol. 36, 1984–1988.

Baums, C.G., Verkuhlen, G.J., Rehm, T., Silva, L.M., Beyerbach, M., Pohlmeyer, K., et al., 2007. Prevalence of Streptococcus suis genotypes in wild boars of Northwestern Germany. Appl. Environ. Microbiol. 73, 711–717.

Bautista, M.J., Ruiz-Villamor, E., Salguero, F.J., Sanchez-Cordon, P.J., Carrasco, L., Gomez-Villamandos, J.C., 2002. Early platelet aggregation as a cause of thrombocytopenia in classical swine fever. Vet. Pathol. 39, 84–91.

Beach, N.M., Meng, X.J., 2012. Efficacy and future prospects of commercially available and experimental vaccines against porcine circovirus type 2 (PCV2). Virus Res. 164, 33–42.

Beer, R.J., 1976. The relationship between Trichuris trichiura (Linnaeus 1758) of man and Trichuris suis (Schrank 1788) of the pig. Res. Vet. Sci. 20, 47–54.

Beer, R.J., Lean, I.J., 1973. Clinical trichuriasis produced experimentally in growing pigs. I. Pathology of infection. Vet. Rec. 93, 189–195.

Beier, D., Gross, R., 2008. The BvgS/BvgA phosphorelay system of pathogenic Bordetellae: structure, function and evolution. Adv. Exp. Med. Biol. 631, 149–160.

Berthelot-Herault, F., Gottschalk, M., Labbe, A., Cariolet, R., Kobisch, M., 2001. Experimental airborne transmission of Streptococcus suis capsular type 2 in pigs. Vet. Microbiol. 82, 69–80.

Bertram, T.A., 1985. Quantitative morphology of peracute pulmonary lesions in swine induced by Haemophilus pleuropneumoniae. Vet. Pathol. 22, 598–609.

Bielaaski, A., Raeside, J.I., 1977. Plasma concentrations of steroid hormones in sows infected experimentally with Leptospira pomona or porcine enterovirus strain T1 in late gestation. Res. Vet. Sci. 22, 28–34.

Bobbie, D.L., Swindle, M.M., 1986. Pulse monitoring, intravascular and intramuscular injection sites in pigs. In: Tumbleson, M.E. (Ed.), Swine in Biomedical Research. Plenum Press, New York.

Bollen, P.J.A., Hansen, A.K., Alstrup, A.K.O., 2010. The Laboratory Swine. CRC Press/Taylor & Francis, Boca Raton, FL.

Bornstein, S., Wallgren, P., 1997. Serodiagnosis of sarcoptic mange in pigs. Vet. Rec. 141, 8–12.

Bosse, J.T., Janson, H., Sheehan, B.J., Beddek, A.J., Rycroft, A.N., Kroll, J.S., et al., 2002. Actinobacillus pleuropneumoniae: pathobiology and pathogenesis of infection. Microbes Infect. 4, 225–235.

Bouchet, B., Vanier, G., Jacques, M., Auger, E., Gottschalk, M., 2009. Studies on the interactions of Haemophilus parasuis with porcine epithelial tracheal cells: limited role of LOS in apoptosis and proinflammatory cytokine release. Microb. Pathog. 46, 108–113.

Bousquet, E., Morvan, H., Aitken, I., Morgan, J.H., 1997. Comparative in vitro activity of doxycycline and oxytetracycline against porcine respiratory pathogens. Vet. Rec. 141, 37–40.

Bousquet, E., Pommier, P., Wessel-Robert, S., Morvan, H., Benoit-Valiergue, H., Laval, A., 1998. Efficacy of doxycycline in feed for the control of pneumonia caused by Pasteurella multocida and Mycoplasma hyopneumoniae in fattening pigs. Vet. Rec. 143, 269–272.

Bowman, D.D., Georgi, J.R., 2009. Georgis' Parasitology for Veterinarians. Saunders/Elsevier, St. Louis, MO.

Boye, M., Jensen, T.K., Moller, K., Leser, T.D., Jorsal, S.E., 1998. Specific detection of Lawsonia intracellularis in porcine proliferative enteropathy inferred from fluorescent rRNA in situ hybridization. Vet. Pathol. 35, 153–156.

Brady, P.S., Ku, P.K., Ullrey, D.E., Miller, E.R., 1978. Evaluation of an amino acid–iron chelate hematinic for the baby pig. J. Anim. Sci. 47, 1135–1140.

Braun, W., 1993. Reproduction in miniature pet pigs. In: Reeves, D.E., Becker, H.N., American Association of Swine Practitioners, Care and Management of Miniature Pet Pigs: Guidelines for the Veterinary Practitioner, first ed. Veterinary Practice Pub. Co, Santa Barbara, CA.

Brenner, P., Reichenspurner, H., Schmoeckel, M., Wimmer, C., Rucker, A., Eder, V., et al., 2000. IG-therasorb immunoapheresis in orthotopic xenotransplantation of baboons with landrace pig hearts. Transplantation 69, 208–214.

Bridger, J.C., Tauscher, G.I., Desselberger, U., 1998. Viral determinants of rotavirus pathogenicity in pigs: evidence that the fourth gene of a porcine rotavirus confers diarrhea in the homologous host. J. Virol. 72, 6929–6931.

Brockmeier, S.L., Register, K.B., 2000. Effect of temperature modulation and bvg mutation of Bordetella bronchiseptica on adhesion, intracellular survival and cytotoxicity for swine alveolar macrophages. Vet. Microbiol. 73, 1–12.

Brockmeier, S.L., Register, K.B., Nicholson, T.L., Loving, C.L., 2012. Bordatellosis. In: Zimmerman, J.J., Karriker, L.A., Ramirez, A., Schwartz, K.J., Stevenson, G.W. (Eds.), Diseases of Swine, tenth ed. Wiley-Blackwell, Chichester, West Sussex.

Brooke, C.J., Riley, T.V., 1999. Erysipelothrix rhusiopathiae: bacteriology, epidemiology and clinical manifestations of an occupational pathogen. J. Med. Microbiol. 48, 789–799.

Brouard, S., Gagne, K., Blancho, G., Soulillou, J.P., 1999. T cell response in xenorecognition and xenografts: a review. Hum. Immunol. 60, 455–468.

Buettner, F.F., Konze, S.A., Maas, A., Gerlach, G.F., 2011. Proteomic and immunoproteomic characterization of a DIVA subunit vaccine against Actinobacillus pleuropneumoniae. Proteome. Sci. 9, 23.

Buller, C.R., Moxley, R.A., 1988. Natural infection of porcine ileal dome M cells with rotavirus and enteric adenovirus. Vet. Pathol. 25, 516–517.

Buogo, C., Capaul, S., Hani, H., Frey, J., Nicolet, J., 1995. Diagnosis of Clostridium perfringens type C enteritis in pigs using a DNA amplification technique (PCR). Zentralbl. Veterinarmed. B 42, 51–58.

Burton, P.J., Thornsberry, C., Cheung Yee, Y., Watts, J.L., Yancey Jr., R.J., 1996. Interpretive criteria for antimicrobial susceptibility testing of ceftiofur against bacteria associated with swine respiratory disease. J. Vet. Diagn. Invest. 8, 464–468.

Busque, P., Higgins, R., Caya, F., Quessy, S., 1997. Immunization of pigs against Streptococcus suis serotype 2 infection using a live avirulent strain. Can. J. Vet. Res. 61, 275–279.

Calsamiglia, M., Pijoan, C., Solano, G., Rapp-Gabrielson, V., 1999. Development of an oligonucleotide-specific capture plate hybridization assay for detection of Haemophilus parasuis. J. Vet. Diagn. Invest. 11, 140–145.

Cannon, C.Z., Godfrey, V.L., King-Herbert, A., Nielsen, J.N., 2009. Metastatic uterine adenocarcinoma in an 8-year-old gilt. J. Am. Assoc. Lab. Anim. Sci. 48, 795–800.

Cargill, C., Davies, P., Carmichael, I., Hooke, F., Moore, M., 1996. Treatment of sarcoptic mite infestation and mite hypersensitivity in pigs with injectable doramectin. Vet. Rec. 138, 468–471.

Cargill, C.F., Pointon, A.M., Davies, P.R., Garcia, R., 1997. Using slaughter inspections to evaluate sarcoptic mange infestation of finishing swine. Vet. Parasitol. 70, 191–200.

Carlson, S.A., Barnhill, A.E., Griffith, R.W., 2012. Salmonellosis. In: Zimmerman, J.J. (Ed.), Diseases of Swine, tenth ed. Wiley-Blackwell, Chichester, West Sussex.

Carrasco, L., Madsen, L.W., Salguero, F.J., Nunez, A., Sanchez-Cordon, P., Bollen, P., 2003. Immune complex-associated thrombocytopenic purpura syndrome in sexually mature Gottingen minipigs. J. Comp. Pathol. 128, 25–32.

Carstens, E.B., 2010. Ratification vote on taxonomic proposals to the International Committee on Taxonomy of Viruses (2009). Arch. Virol. 155, 133–146.

Chae, C., 2004. Postweaning multisystemic wasting syndrome: a review of aetiology, diagnosis and pathology. Vet. J. 168, 41–49.

Chae, C., 2005. A review of porcine circovirus 2-associated syndromes and diseases. Vet. J. 169, 326–336.

Chae, S.J., Kramer, A.D., Zhao, Y., Arn, S., Cooper, D.K., Sachs, D.H., 1999. Lack of variation in alphaGal expression on lymphocytes in miniature swine of different genotypes. Xenotransplantation 6, 43–51.

Chang, K.-O., Saif, L.J., Kim, Y., 2012. Reoviruses (rotaviruses and reoviruses). In: Zimmerman, J.J., Karriker, L.A., Ramirez, A., Schwartz, K.J., Stevenson, G.W. (Eds.), Diseases of Swine, tenth ed. Wiley-Blackwell, Chichester, West Sussex.

Chaniago, T.D., Watson, D.L., Owen, R.A., Johnson, R.H., 1978. Immunoglobulins in blood serum of foetal pigs. Aust. Vet. J. 54, 30–33.

Chiers, K., Haesebrouck, F., Van Overbeke, I., Charlier, G., Ducatelle, R., 1999. Early in vivo interactions of Actinobacillus pleuropneumoniae with tonsils of pigs. Vet. Microbiol. 68, 301–306.

Chirico, J., Eriksson, H., Fossum, O., Jansson, D., 2003. The poultry red mite, Dermanyssus gallinae, a potential vector of Erysipelothrix rhusiopathiae causing erysipelas in hens. Med. Vet. Entomol. 17, 232–234.

Chmielewicz, B., Goltz, M., Franz, T., Bauer, C., Brema, S., Ellerbrok, H., et al., 2003. A novel porcine gammaherpesvirus. Virology 308, 317–329.

Cho, J.G., Dee, S.A., 2006. Porcine reproductive and respiratory syndrome virus. Theriogenology 66, 655–662.

Cho, W.S., Jung, K., Kim, J., Ha, Y., Chae, C., 2005. Expression of mRNA encoding interleukin (IL)-10, IL-12p35 and IL-12p40 in lungs from pigs experimentally naturally infected with Actinobacillus pleuropneumoniae. Vet. Res. Commun. 29, 111–122.

Choi, C., Chae, C., 2001. Colocalization of porcine reproductive and respiratory syndrome virus and porcine circovirus 2 in porcine dermatitis and nephrology syndrome by double-labeling technique. Vet. Pathol. 38, 436–441.

Cino-Ozuna, A.G., Henry, S., Hesse, R., Nietfeld, J.C., Bai, J., Scott, H.M., et al., 2011. Characterization of a new disease syndrome associated with porcine circovirus type 2 in previously vaccinated herds. J. Clin. Microbiol. 49, 2012–2016.

Claxton-Gill, M.S., Cornick-Seahorn, J.L., Gamboa, J.C., Boatright, B.S., 1993. Suspected malignant hyperthermia syndrome in a miniature pot-bellied pig anesthetized with isoflurane. J. Am. Vet. Med. Assoc. 203, 1434–1436.

Collins, A., Love, R.J., Pozo, J., Smith, S.H., McOrist, S., 2000. Studies on the ex vivo survival of Lawsonia intracellularis. Swine Health Prod. 8, 211–215.

Cooper, D.M., Gebhart, C.J., 1998. Comparative aspects of proliferative enteritis. J. Am. Vet. Med. Assoc. 212, 1446–1451.

Corapi, W.V., Rodrigues, A., Lawhorn, D.B., 2011. Mucinous adenocarcinoma and T-cell lymphoma in the small intestine of 2 Vietnamese potbellied pigs (Sus scrofa). Vet. Pathol. 48, 1004–1007.

Cornell Veterinary Medicine, 2012. Dr. John M. King's necropsy show and tell [Online]. Available: <https://secure.vet.cornell.edu/nst/nst.asp> (accessed 13.09.13).

Cowart, R.P., 1995. An Outline of Swine Diseases: a Handbook. Iowa State University Press, Ames, IA.

Critser, J.K., Laughlin, M.H., Prather, R.S., Riley, L.K., 2009. Proceedings of the conference on swine in biomedical research. ILAR J. 50, 89–94.

Croxen, M.A., Finlay, B.B., 2010. Molecular mechanisms of Escherichia coli pathogenicity. Nat. Rev. Microbiol. 8, 26–38.

Czechowicz, J., Huaman, J.L., Forshey, B.M., Morrison, A.C., Castillo, R., Huaman, A., et al., 2011. Prevalence and risk factors for encephalomyocarditis virus infection in Peru. Vector Borne Zoonotic Dis. 11, 367–374.

Darwich, L., Mateu, E., 2012. Immunology of porcine circovirus type 2 (PCV2). Virus Res. 164, 61–67.

Darwich, L., Pie, S., Rovira, A., Segales, J., Domingo, M., Oswald, I.P., et al., 2003. Cytokine mRNA expression profiles in lymphoid tissues of pigs naturally affected by postweaning multisystemic wasting syndrome. J. Gen. Virol. 84, 2117–2125.

Davies, K.A., Chapman, P.T., Norsworthy, P.J., Jamar, F., Athanassiou, P., Keelan, E.T., et al., 1995. Clearance pathways of soluble immune complexes in the pig. Insights into the adaptive nature of antigen clearance in humans. J. Immunol. 155, 5760–5768.

Davies, P.R., 1995. Sarcoptic mange and production performance of swine: a review of the literature and studies of associations between mite infestation, growth rate and measures of mange severity in growing pigs. Vet. Parasitol. 60, 249–264.

Davies, P.R., Bahnson, P.B., Grass, J.J., Marsh, W.E., Garcia, R., Melancon, J., et al., 1996. Evaluation of the monitoring of papular dermatitis lesions in slaughtered swine to assess sarcoptic mite infestation. Vet. Parasitol. 62, 143–153.

Davis, D.P., Moon, R.D., 1990. Density of itch mite, Sarcoptes scabiei (Acari: Sarcoptidae) and temporal development of cutaneous hypersensitivity in swine mange. Vet. Parasitol. 36, 285–293.

Davis, W.C., Zuckermann, F.A., Hamilton, M.J., Barbosa, J.I., Saalmuller, A., Binns, R.M., et al., 1998. Analysis of monoclonal antibodies that recognize gamma delta T/null cells. Vet. Immunol. Immunopathol. 60, 305–316.

Davison, A.J., Eberle, R., Ehlers, B., Hayward, G.S., Mcgeoch, D.J., Minson, A.C., et al., 2009. The order herpesvirales. Arch. Virol. 154, 171–177.

Day, B.N., 1980. Parturition. In: Morrow, D.A. (Ed.), Current Therapy in Theriogenology: Diagnosis, Treatment, and Prevention of Reproductive Diseases in Animals. Saunders, Philadelphia, PA.

Delhon, G., Tulman, E.R., Afonso, C.L., Rock, D.L., 2012. Swinepox virus. In: Zimmerman, J.J., Karriker, L.A., Ramirez, A., Schwartz, K.J., Stevenson, G.W. (Eds.), Diseases of Swine, tenth ed. Wiley-Blackwell, Chichester, West Sussex.

Derbyshire, J.B., Arkell, S., 1971. The activity of some chemical disinfectants against Talfan virus and porcine adenovirus type 2. Br. Vet. J. 127, 137–142.

De Rycke, J., Milon, A., Oswald, E., 1999. Necrotoxic Escherichia coli (NTEC): two emerging categories of human and animal pathogens. Vet. Res. 30, 221–233.

De Smit, A.J., Bouma, A., Terpstra, C., Van Oirschot, J.T., 1999. Transmission of classical swine fever virus by artificial insemination. Vet. Microbiol. 67, 239–249.

De Vleeschauwer, A., Atanasova, K., Van Borm, S., Van Den Berg, T., Rasmussen, T.B., Uttenthal, A., et al., 2009. Comparative pathogenesis of an avian H5N2 and a swine H1N1 influenza virus in pigs. PLoS One 4, e6662.

Devriese, L.A., Haesebrouck, F., De Herdt, P., Dom, P., Ducatelle, R., Desmidt, M., et al., 1994. Streptococcus suis infections in birds. Avian Pathol. 23, 721–724.

Deyoe, B.L., 1967. Pathogenesis of three strains of Brucella suis in swine. Am. J. Vet. Res. 28, 951–957.

Didier, P.J., Perino, L., Urbance, J., 1984. Porcine Haemophilus pleuropneumonia: microbiologic and pathologic findings. J. Am. Vet. Med. Assoc. 184, 716–719.

Dincer, Z., Skydsgaard, M., 2012. Spontaneous/background pathology of Gottingen minipig. In: McAnulty, P., Dayan, A.D., Ganderup, N.-C., Hastings, K. (Eds.), The Minipig in Biomedical Research. CRC Press, Boca Raton, FL.

Dominick, M.A., Rimler, R.B., 1988. Turbinate osteoporosis in pigs following intranasal inoculation of purified Pasteurella toxin: histomorphometric and ultrastructural studies. Vet. Pathol. 25, 17–27.

Dorsey, F.C., Fischer, J.F., Fleckenstein, J.M., 2006. Directed delivery of heat-labile enterotoxin by enterotoxigenic Escherichia coli. Cell. Microbiol. 8, 1516–1527.

Dritz, S.S., Chengappa, M.M., Nelssen, J.L., Tokach, M.D., Goodband, R.D., Nietfeld, J.C., et al., 1996. Growth and microbial flora of nonmedicated, segregated, early weaned pigs from a commercial swine operation. J. Am. Vet. Med. Assoc. 208, 711–715.

Duhamel, G.E., Kinyon, J.M., Mathiesen, M.R., Murphy, D.P., Walter, D., 1998. In vitro activity of four antimicrobial agents against North American isolates of porcine Serpulina pilosicoli. J. Vet. Diagn. Invest. 10, 350–356.

Duncan, J.R., Ramsey, R.K., Switzer, W.P., 1966a. Pathology of experimental Bordetella bronchiseptica infection in swine: pneumonia. Am. J. Vet. Res. 27, 467–472.

Duncan, J.R., Ross, R.F., Switzer, W.P., Ramsey, F.K., 1966b. Pathology of experimental Bordetella bronchiseptica infection in swine: atrophic rhinitis. Am. J. Vet. Res. 27, 457–466.

Dwyer, K.M., Cowan, P.J., D'apice, A.J., 2002. Xenotransplantation: past achievements and future promise. Heart Lung Circ. 11, 32–41.

Edington, N., Smith, I.M., Plowright, W., Watt, R.G., 1976. Relationship of porcine cytomegalovirus and B bronchiseptica to atrophic rhinitis in gnotobiotic piglets. Vet. Rec. 98, 42–45.

Edington, N., Watt, R.G., Plowright, W., 1977. Experimental transplacental transmission of porcine cytomegalovirus. J. Hyg. (Lond) 78, 243–251.

Ehler, W.J., Mack Jr., J.W., Brown, D.L., Davis, R.F., 1985. Avoidance of malignant hyperthermia in a porcine model for experimental open heart surgery. Lab. Anim. Sci. 35, 172–175.

Ehlers, B., Ulrich, S., Goltz, M., 1999. Detection of two novel porcine herpesviruses with high similarity to gammaherpesviruses. J. Gen. Virol. 80 (Pt 4), 971–978.

Einarsson, S., 1980. Artificial inseminaiton. In: Morrow, D.A. (Ed.), Current Therapy in Theriogenology: Diagnosis, Treatment, and Prevention of Reproductive Diseases in Animals. Saunders, Philadelphia, PA.

Elbers, A.R., Stegeman, J.A., De Jong, M.C., 2001. Factors associated with the introduction of classical swine fever virus into pig herds in the central area of the 1997/98 epidemic in the Netherlands. Vet. Rec. 149, 377–382.

Ellis, E.A., 2012. Leptospirosis. In: Zimmerman, J.J., Karriker, L.A., Ramirez, A., Schwartz, K.J., Stevenson, G.W. (Eds.), Diseases of Swine, tenth ed. Wiley-Blackwell, Chichester, West Sussex.

Ellis, J., Hassard, L., Clark, E., Harding, J., Allan, G., Willson, P., et al., 1998. Isolation of circovirus from lesions of pigs with postweaning multisystemic wasting syndrome. Can. Vet. J. 39, 44–51.

Emery, D.W., Holley, K., Sachs, D.H., 1999. Enhancement of swine progenitor chimerism in mixed swine/human bone marrow cultures with swine cytokines. Exp. Hematol. 27, 1330–1337.

Enright, M.R., Alexander, T.J., Clifton-Hadley, F.A., 1987. Role of houseflies (Musca domestica) in the epidemiology of Streptococcus suis type 2. Vet. Rec. 121, 132–133.

Erickson, E.D., 1987. Streptococcosis. J. Am. Vet. Med. Assoc. 191, 1391–1393.

Eustis, S.L., Nelson, D.T., 1981. Lesions associated with coccidiosis in nursing piglets. Vet. Pathol. 18, 21–28.

Fairbrother, J.M., Gyles, C.L., 2012. Colibacillosis. In: Zimmerman, J.J., Karriker, L.A., Ramirez, A., Schwartz, K.J., Stevenson, G.W. (Eds.), Diseases of Swine, tenth ed Wiley-Blackwell, Chichester, West Sussex.

Fedorka-Cray, P.J., Kelley, L.C., Stabel, T.J., Gray, J.T., Laufer, J.A., 1995. Alternate routes of invasion may affect pathogenesis of Salmonella typhimurium in swine. Infect. Immun. 63, 2658–2664.

Fisher, T.F., 1993. Miniature swine in biomedical resarch: applications and husbandry considerations. Lab. Anim. 22, 47–50.

Flewellen, E.H., Nelson, T.E., 1980. Dantrolene dose response in malignant hyperthermia-susceptible (MHS) swine: method to obtain prophylaxis and therapeusis. Anesthesiology 52, 303–308.

Flisikowska, T., Kind, A., Schnieke, A., 2013. The new pig on the block: modelling cancer in pigs. Transgenic. Res. 22, 673–680.

Fogarty, R., Halpin, K., Hyatt, A.D., Daszak, P., Mungall, B.A., 2008. Henipavirus susceptibility to environmental variables. Virus Res. 132, 140–144.

Forum, M.R., 2013. Minipig Research Forum [Online]. Available: <http://minipigresearchforum.org/index.php?id=19> (accessed 13.09.13).

Fox, J.G., 2002. Laboratory Animal Medicine. Academic Press, Amsterdam, The Netherlands; New York.

Frana, T.S., 2012. Staphylococcosis. In: Zimmerman, J.J., Karriker, L.A., Ramirez, A., Schwartz, K.J., Stevenson, G.W. (Eds.), Diseases of Swine, tenth ed. Wiley-Blackwell, Chichester, West Sussex.

Friedman, T., Shimizu, A., Smith, R.N., Colvin, R.B., Seebach, J.D., Sachs, D.H., et al., 1999. Human CD4+ T cells mediate rejection of porcine xenografts. J. Immunol. 162, 5256–5262.

Fujii, J., Otsu, K., Zorzato, F., De Leon, S., Khanna, V.K., Weiler, J.E., et al., 1991. Identification of a mutation in porcine ryanodine receptor associated with malignant hyperthermia. Science 253, 448–451.

Galdiero, M., D'isanto, M., Vitiello, M., Finamore, E., Peluso, L., Galdiero, M., 2003. Monocytic activation of protein tyrosine kinase, protein kinase A and protein kinase C induced by porins isolated from Salmonella enterica serovar Typhimurium. J. Infect. 46, 111–119.

Gatlin, C.L., Jordan, W.H., Shryock, T.R., Smith, W.C., 1996. The quantitation of turbinate atrophy in pigs to measure the severity of induced atrophic rhinitis. Can. J. Vet. Res. 60, 121–126.

Geldhof, M.F., Vanhee, M., Van Breedam, W., Van Doorsselaere, J., Karniychuk, U.U., Nauwynck, H.J., 2012. Comparison of the efficacy of autogenous inactivated Porcine Reproductive and Respiratory Syndrome Virus (PRRSV) vaccines with that of commercial vaccines against homologous and heterologous challenges. BMC Vet. Res. 8, 182.

Giannella, R.A., Mann, E.A., 2003. E. coli heat-stable enterotoxin and guanylyl cyclase C: new functions and unsuspected actions. Trans. Am. Clin. Climatol. Assoc. 114, 67–85. discussion 85–6.

Gillespie, J., Opriessnig, T., Meng, X.J., Pelzer, K., Buechner-Maxwell, V., 2009. Porcine circovirus type 2 and porcine circovirus-associated disease. J. Vet. Intern. Med. 23, 1151–1163.

Gipson, P.S., Veatch, J.K., Matlack, R.S., Jones, D.P., 1999. Health status of a recently discovered population of feral swine in Kansas. J. Wildl. Dis. 35, 624–627.

Goltz, M., Ericsson, T., Patience, C., Huang, C.A., Noack, S., Sachs, D.H., et al., 2002. Sequence analysis of the genome of porcine lymphotropic herpesvirus 1 and gene expression during posttransplant lymphoproliferative disease of pigs. Virology 294, 383–393.

Gomez-Laguna, J., Salguero, F.J., Barranco, I., Pallares, F.J., Rodriguez-Gomez, I.M., Bernabe, A., et al., 2010. Cytokine expression by macrophages in the lung of pigs infected with the porcine reproductive and respiratory syndrome virus. J. Comp. Pathol. 142, 51–60.

Gomez-Villamandos, J.C., Salguero, F.J., Ruiz-Villamor, E., Sanchez-Cordon, P.J., Bautista, M.J., Sierra, M.A., 2003. Classical swine fever: pathology of bone marrow. Vet. Pathol. 40, 157–163.

Gottschalk, M., 2012a. Actinobacillosis. In: Zimmerman, J.J. (Ed.), Diseases of Swine, tenth ed. Wiley-Blackwell, Chichester, West Sussex.

Gottschalk, M., 2012b. Streptococcosis. In: Zimmerman, J.J., Karriker, L.A., Ramirez, A., Schwartz, K.J., Stevenson, G.W. (Eds.), Diseases of Swine, tenth ed. Wiley-Blackwell, Chichester, West Sussex.

Gottschalk, M., Segura, M., 2000. The pathogenesis of the meningitis caused by Streptococcus suis: the unresolved questions. Vet. Microbiol. 76, 259–272.

Gourlay, W.A., Chambers, W.H., Monaco, A.P., Maki, T., 1998. Importance of natural killer cells in the rejection of hamster skin xenografts. Transplantation 65, 727–734.

Graham, D.Y., Sackman, J.W., Estes, M.K., 1984. Pathogenesis of rotavirus-induced diarrhea. Preliminary studies in miniature swine piglet. Dig. Dis. Sci. 29, 1028–1035.

Gram, T., Ahrens, P., Nielsen, J.P., 1996. Evaluation of a PCR for detection of Actinobacillus pleuropneumoniae in mixed bacterial cultures from tonsils. Vet. Microbiol. 51, 95–104.

Grand, N., 2012. Diseases of minipigs. In: McAnulty, P.A., Dayan, A.D., Ganderup, N.-C., Hastings, K.L. (Eds.), The Minipig in Biomedical Research. CRC Press/Taylor & Francis, Boca Raton, FL.

Gray, J.T., Fedorka-Cray, P.J., Stabel, T.J., Kramer, T.T., 1996. Natural transmission of Salmonella choleraesuis in swine. Appl. Environ. Microbiol. 62, 141–146.

Greve, J.H., 2012. Internal parasites: Helminths. In: Zimmerman, J.J., Karriker, L.A., Ramirez, A., Schwartz, K.J., Stevenson, G.W. (Eds.), Diseases of Swine, tenth ed. Wiley-Blackwell, Chichester, West Sussex.

Greve, J.H., Davies, P., 2012. External parasites. In: Zimmerman, J.J., Karriker, L.A., Ramirez, A., Schwartz, K.J., Stevenson, G.W. (Eds.), Diseases of Swine, tenth ed. Wiley-Blackwell, Chichester, West Sussex.

Griesemer, A.D., Lamattina, J.C., Okumi, M., Etter, J.D., Shimizu, A., Sachs, D.H., et al., 2008. Linked suppression across an MHC-mismatched barrier in a miniature swine kidney transplantation model. J. Immunol. 181, 4027–4036.

Groebel, K., Hoelzle, K., Wittenbrink, M.M., Ziegler, U., Hoelzle, L.E., 2009. Mycoplasma suis invades porcine erythrocytes. Infect. Immun. 77, 576–584.

Gwaltney, S.M., Galvin, R.J., Register, K.B., Rimler, R.B., Ackermann, M.R., 1997. Effects of Pasteurella multocida toxin on porcine bone marrow cell differentiation into osteoclasts and osteoblasts. Vet. Pathol. 34, 421–430.

Gyles, C.L., 1993. Eschericia coli. In: Gyles, C.L., Thoen, C.O. (Eds.), Pathogenesis of Bacterial Infections in Animals, second ed. Iowa State University, Ames, IA.

Halbur, P.G., Paul, P.S., Frey, M.L., Landgraf, J., Eernisse, K., Meng, X.J., et al., 1995. Comparison of the pathogenicity of two US porcine reproductive and respiratory syndrome virus isolates with that of the Lelystad virus. Vet. Pathol. 32, 648–660.

Hamilton, T.D., Roe, J.M., Hayes, C.M., Webster, A.J., 1998. Effects of ammonia inhalation and acetic acid pretreatment on colonization kinetics of toxigenic Pasteurella multocida within upper respiratory tracts of swine. J. Clin. Microbiol. 36, 1260–1265.

Hamilton, T.D., Roe, J.M., Hayes, C.M., Jones, P., Pearson, G.R., Webster, A.J., 1999. Contributory and exacerbating roles of gaseous ammonia and organic dust in the etiology of atrophic rhinitis. Clin. Diagn. Lab. Immunol. 6, 199–203.

Hampson, D.J., 2012. Brachyspiral colitis. In: Zimmerman, J.J., Karriker, L.A., Ramirez, A., Schwartz, K.J., Stevenson, G.W. (Eds.), Diseases of Swine, tenth ed. Wiley-Blackwell, Chichester, West Sussex.

Hansen, M.S., Pors, S.E., Jensen, H.E., Bille-Hansen, V., Bisgaard, M., Flachs, E.M., et al., 2010. An investigation of the pathology and pathogens associated with porcine respiratory disease complex in Denmark. J. Comp. Pathol. 143, 120–131.

Hansen, M.S., Segales, J., Fernandes, L.T., Grau-Roma, L., Bille-Hansen, V., Larsen, L.E., et al., 2013. Detection of porcine circovirus type 2 and viral replication by in situ hybridization in primary lymphoid organs from naturally and experimentally infected pigs. Vet. Pathol.

Harris, I.T., Fedorka-Cray, P.J., Gray, J.T., Thomas, L.A., Ferris, K., 1997. Prevalence of Salmonella organisms in swine feed. J. Am. Vet. Med. Assoc. 210, 382–385.

Harville, B.A., Dreyfus, L.A., 1995. Involvement of 5-hydroxytryptamine and prostaglandin E2 in the intestinal secretory action of Escherichia coli heat-stable enterotoxin B. Infect. Immun. 63, 745–750.

Health, W.O.F.A., 2013a. Manual of Diagnostic Tests and Vaccines for Terrestrial Animals 2013 [Online]. OIE Organization Mondiale de la Sante Animale. Available: <http://www.oie.int/international-standard-setting/terrestrial-manual/access-online/> (accessed 12.02.14).

Health, W.O.F.A., 2013b. OIE-Listed Diseases, Infections and Infestations in Force in 2013 [Online]. OIE Organization Mondiale de la Sante Animale, Paris, France. Available: <http://www.oie.int/animal-health-in-the-world/oie-listed-diseases-2013/ (accessed 2.09.13).

Hedger, R.S., Mann, J.A., 1989. Swine vesicular disease virus. In: Pesaert, M.B. (Ed.), Virus Infection of Porcines, second ed. Elsevier Science Publishers BV, Amsterdam, The Netherlands.

Heinritzi, K., Aigner, K., Erber, M., Kersjes, C., Von Wangenheim, B., 1999. Brucellosis and Aujeszky's disease in a wild boar enclose. Case report. Tierarztl Prax Ausg. G Grosstiere Nutztiere 27, 41–46.

Helke, K.L., Swindle, M.M., 2013. Animal models of toxicology testing: the role of pigs. Exp. Opin. Drug Metab. Toxicol. 9, 127–139.

Henderson, J.P., O'hagan, J., Hawe, S.M., Pratt, M.C., 1997. Anaemia and low viability in piglets infected with Eperythrozoon suis. Vet. Rec. 140, 144–146.

Henne, E., Nickel, S., Hiepe, T., 1978. Parasites in the GDR.1. Studies on helminths occurrence in European wild pigs (Sus scrofa)]. Angew. Parasitol. 19, 52–57.

Hensel, A., Stockhofe-Zurwieden, N., Petzoldt, K., Lubitz, W., 1995. Oral immunization of pigs with viable or inactivated Actinobacillus pleuropneumoniae serotype 9 induces pulmonary and systemic antibodies and protects against homologous aerosol challenge. Infect. Immun. 63, 3048–3053.

Hill, B.D., Corney, B.G., Wagner, T.M., 1996. Importance of Staphylococcus hyicus ssp hyicus as a cause of arthritis in pigs up to 12 weeks of age. Aust. Vet. J. 73, 179–181.

Hodgins, D.C., Shewen, P.E., Dewey, C.E., 2004. Influence of age and maternal antibodies on antibody responses of neonatal piglets vaccinated against Mycoplasma hyopneumoniae. J. Swine Health Prod. 12, 10–16.

Hogg, G.G., Lenghaus, C., Forman, A.J., 1977. Experimental porcine parvovirus infection of foetal pigs resulting in abortion, histological lesions and antibody formation. J. Comp. Pathol. 87, 539–549.

Hollanders, W., Vercruysse, J., 1990. Sarcoptic mite hypersensitivity: a cause of dermatitis in fattening pigs at slaughter. Vet. Rec. 126, 308–310.

Hollanders, W., Harbers, A.H., Huige, J.C., Monster, P., Rambags, P.G., Hendrikx, W.M., 1995. Control of Sarcoptes scabiei var. suis with ivermectin: influence on scratching behaviour of fattening pigs and occurrence of dermatitis at slaughter. Vet. Parasitol. 58, 117–127.

Hollanders, W., Vercruysse, J., Raes, S., Bornstein, S., 1997. Evaluation of an enzyme-linked immunosorbent assay (ELISA) for the serological diagnosis of sarcoptic mange in swine. Vet. Parasitol. 69, 117–123.

Holman, J.E., Koestner, A., Kasza, L., 1966. Histopathogenesis of porcine polioencephalomyelitis in the germ free pig. Pathol. Vet. 3, 633–651.

Hooper, B.E., Haelterman, E.O., 1966. Growth of transmissible gastroenteritis virus in young pigs. Am. J. Vet. Res. 27, 286–291.

Hooper, B.E., Haelterman, E.O., 1969. Lesions of the gastrointestinal tract of pigs infected with transmissible gastroenteritis. Can. J. Comp. Med. 33, 29–36.

Horiguchi, Y., Okada, T., Sugimoto, N., Morikawa, Y., Katahira, J., Matsuda, M., 1995. Effects of Bordetella bronchiseptica dermonecrotizing toxin on bone formation in calvaria of neonatal rats. FEMS Immunol. Med. Microbiol. 12, 29–32.

Hormansdorfer, S., Bauer, J., 1998. Resistance of bovine and porcine Pasteurella to florfenicol and other antibiotics. Berl. Munch. Tierarztl. Wochenschr. 111, 422–426.

Horner, B.M., Randolph, M.A., Huang, C.A., Butler, P.E., 2008. Skin tolerance: in search of the Holy Grail. Transpl. Int. 21, 101–112.

Huang, C.A., Lorf, T., Arn, J.S., Koo, G.C., Blake, T., Sachs, D.H., 1999. Characterization of a monoclonal anti-porcine CD3 antibody. Xenotransplantation 6, 201–212.

Huang, C.A., Fuchimoto, Y., Gleit, Z.L., Ericsson, T., Griesemer, A., Scheier-Dolberg, R., et al., 2001. Posttransplantation lymphoproliferative disease in miniature swine after allogeneic hematopoietic cell transplantation: similarity to human PTLD and association with a porcine gammaherpesvirus. Blood 97, 1467–1473.

Huang, Y.Y., Walther, I., Martinson, S.A., Lopez, A., Yason, C., Godson, D.L., et al., 2008. Porcine circovirus 2 inclusion bodies in pulmonary and renal epithelial cells. Vet. Pathol. 45, 640–644.

Hughes, R., Olander, H.J., Kanitz, D.L., Qureshi, S., 1977. A study of swine dysentery by immunofluorescence and histology. Vet. Pathol. 14, 490–507.

Ierino, F.L., Gojo, S., Banerjee, P.T., Giovino, M., Xu, Y., Gere, J., et al., 1999. Transfer of swine major histocompatibility complex class II genes into autologous bone marrow cells of baboons for the induction of tolerance across xenogeneic barriers. Transplantation 67, 1119–1128.

Ilha, M.R., Newman, S.J., Van Amstel, S., Fecteau, K.A., Rohrbach, B.W., 2010. Uterine lesions in 32 female miniature pet pigs. Vet. Pathol. 47, 1071–1075.

Imada, Y., Goji, N., Ishikawa, H., Kishima, M., Sekizaki, T., 1999. Truncated surface protective antigen (SpaA) of Erysipelothrix rhusiopathiae serotype 1a elicits protection against challenge with serotypes 1a and 2b in pigs. Infect. Immun. 67, 4376–4382.

Institute of Laboratory Animal Resources (U.S.). Committee on Care and Use of Laboratory Animals, 2011. Guide for the Care and use of Laboratory Animals. NIH Publication, Bethesda, MD, The National Academies Press.

Iowa State University: The Center for Food Security and Public Health, 2014. Swine Diseases and Resources [Online]. Iowa State University: The Center for Food Security and Public Health. Available: <http://www.cfsph.iastate.edu/Species/swine.php> (accessed 10.04.14).

Jackson, P.G.G., Cockcroft, P.D., 2007. Haematology and blood biochemistry in the pig. In: Jackson, P.G.G., Cockcroft, P.D. (Eds.), Handbook of Pig Medicine. Saunders Elsevier, Amsterdam, The Netherlands.

Jacobs, A.A., Van Den Berg, A.J., Loeffen, P.L., 1996. Protection of experimentally infected pigs by suilysin, the thiol-activated haemolysin of Streptococcus suis. Vet. Rec. 139, 225–228.

Jacobson, M., Bornstein, S., Wallgren, P., 1999. The efficacy of simplified eradication strategies against sarcoptic mange mite infections in swine herds monitored by an ELISA. Vet. Parasitol. 81, 249–258.

Jamalludeen, N., Johnson, R.P., Shewen, P.E., Gyles, C.L., 2009. Evaluation of bacteriophages for prevention and treatment of diarrhea due to experimental enterotoxigenic Escherichia coli O149 infection of pigs. Vet. Microbiol. 136, 135–141.

Jasni, S., McOrist, S., Lawson, G.H., 1994. Reproduction of proliferative enteritis in hamsters with a pure culture of porcine ileal symbiont intracellularis. Vet. Microbiol. 41, 1–9.

Jensen, T.K., Boye, M., Hagedorn-Olsen, T., Riising, H.J., Angen, O., 1999. Actinobacillus pleuropneumoniae osteomyelitis in pigs demonstrated by fluorescent in situ hybridization. Vet. Pathol. 36, 258–261.

Jensen, T.K., Moller, K., Boye, M., Leser, T.D., Jorsal, S.E., 2000. Scanning electron microscopy and fluorescent in situ hybridization of experimental Brachyspira (Serpulina) pilosicoli infection in growing pigs. Vet. Pathol. 37, 22–32.

Jensen, T.K., Vigre, H., Svensmark, B., Bille-Hansen, V., 2006. Distinction between porcine circovirus type 2 enteritis and porcine proliferative enteropathy caused by Lawsonia intracellularis. J. Comp. Pathol. 135, 176–182.

Johnson, R.H., 1973. Isolation of swine papvovirus in Queensland. Aust. Vet. J. 49, 157–159.

Jones, L.D., 1956. Exudative epidermitis of pigs. Am. J. Vet. Res. 17, 179–193.

Jones, T.C., Hunt, R.D., 1983. Diseases caused by parasitic helminths and arthropods. In: Jones, T.C., Hunt, R.D., Smith, H.A. (Eds.), Veterinary Pathology, fifth ed. Lea & Febiger, Philadelphia, PA.

Joo, H.S., Donaldson-Wood, C.R., Johnson, R.H., 1976. Observations on the pathogenesis of porcine parvovirus infection. Arch. Virol. 51, 123–129.

Joo, H.S., Donaldson-Wood, C.R., Johnson, R.H., Campbell, R.S., 1977. Pathogenesis of porcine parvovirus infection: pathology and immunofluorescence in the foetus. J. Comp. Pathol. 87, 383–391.

Jung, T., Choi, C., Chae, C., 2002. Localization of swine influenza virus in naturally infected pigs. Vet. Pathol. 39, 10–16.

Kamp, E.M., Bokken, G.C., Vermeulen, T.M., De Jong, M.F., Buys, H.E., Reek, F.H., et al., 1996. A specific and sensitive PCR assay suitable for large-scale detection of toxigenic Pasteurella multocida in nasal and tonsillar swabs specimens of pigs. J. Vet. Diagn. Invest. 8, 304–309.

Kamp, E.M., Stockhofe-Zurwieden, N., Van Leengoed, L.A., Smits, M.A., 1997. Endobronchial inoculation with Apx toxins of Actinobacillus pleuropneumoniae leads to pleuropneumonia in pigs. Infect. Immun. 65, 4350–4354.

Kaper, J.B., Nataro, J.P., Mobley, H.L., 2004. Pathogenic Escherichia coli. Nat. Rev. Microbiol. 2, 123–140.

Kataoka, Y., Yamashita, T., Sunaga, S., Imada, Y., Ishikawa, H., Kishima, M., et al., 1996. An enzyme-linked immunosorbent assay (ELISA) for the detection of antibody against Streptococcus suis type 2 in infected pigs. J. Vet. Med. Sci. 58, 369–372.

Kawashima, K., Yamada, S., Kobayashi, H., Narita, M., 1996. Detection of porcine reproductive and respiratory syndrome virus and Mycoplasma hyorhinis antigens in pulmonary lesions of pigs suffering from respiratory distress. J. Comp. Pathol. 114, 315–323.

Keel, M.K., Songer, J.G., 2006. The comparative pathology of Clostridium difficile-associated disease. Vet. Pathol. 43, 225–240.

Keel, M.K., Songer, J.G., 2011. The attachment, internalization, and time-dependent, intracellular distribution of Clostridium difficile toxin A in porcine intestinal explants. Vet. Pathol. 48, 369–380.

Kelneric, Z., Naglic, T., Udovicic, I., 1996. Prevention of necrotic enteritis in piglets by vaccination of pregnant gilts with a Clostridium perfringens type C and D bacterin-toxoid. Vet. Med. (Praha) 41, 335–338.

Kelsey, D.K., Olsen, G.A., Overall Jr., J.C., Glasgow, L.A., 1977. Alteration of host defense mechanisms by murine cytomegalovirus infection. Infect. Immun. 18, 754–760.

Kim, B., Ahn, K.K., Ha, Y., Lee, Y.H., Kim, D., Lim, J.H., et al., 2009a. Association of tumor necrosis factor-alpha with fever and pulmonary lesion score in pigs experimentally infected with swine influenza virus subtype H1N2. J. Vet. Med. Sci. 71, 611–616.

Kim, H.B., Lyoo, K.S., Joo, H.S., 2009b. Efficacy of different disinfectants in vitro against porcine circovirus type 2. Vet. Rec. 164, 599–600.

Kim, J., Chae, C., 2004. A comparison of virus isolation, polymerase chain reaction, immunohistochemistry, and in situ hybridization for the detection of porcine circovirus 2 and porcine parvovirus in experimentally and naturally coinfected pigs. J. Vet. Diagn. Invest. 16, 45–50.

Kirkland, P.D., Le Potier, M.-F., Vannier, P., Finlaison, D., 2012a. Pestiviruses. In: Zimmerman, J.J. (Ed.), Diseases of Swine, tenth ed. Wiley-Blackwell, Chichester, West Sussex.

Kirkland, P.D., Stephano, A., Weingartl, H.M., 2012b. Paramyxoviruses. In: Zimmerman, J.J. (Ed.), Diseases of Swine, tenth ed. Wiley-Blackwell, Chichester, West Sussex.

Kirkwood, R.N., Althouse, G.C., Yaeger, M.J., Carr, J., Almond, G.W., 2012. Diseases of the reproductive system. In: Zimmerman, J.J., Karriker, L.A., Ramirez, A., Schwartz, K.J., Stevenson, G.W. (Eds.), Diseases of Swine, tenth ed. Wiley-Blackwell, Chichester, West Sussex.

Knowles, N.J., Reuter, G., 2012. Porcine caliciviruses. In: Zimmerman, J.J., Karriker, L.A., Ramirez, A., Schwartz, K.J., Stevenson, G.W. (Eds.), Diseases of Swine, tenth ed. Wiley-Blackwell, Chichester, West Sussex.

Kobayashi, E., Hishikawa, S., Teratani, T., Lefor, A.T., 2012. The pig as a model for translational research: overview of porcine animal models at Jichi Medical University. Transplant. Res. 1, 8.

Koenen, F., Vanderhallen, H., Castryck, F., Miry, C., 1999. Epidemiologic, pathogenic and molecular analysis of recent encephalomyocarditis outbreaks in Belgium. Zentralbl. Veterinarmed. B 46, 217–231.

Koestner, A., Kasza, L., Holman, J.E., 1966. Electron microscopic evaluation of the pathogenesis of porcine polioencephalomyelitis. Am. J. Pathol. 49, 325–337.

Kolber-Simonds, D., Lai, L., Watt, S.R., Denaro, M., Arn, S., Augenstein, M.L., et al., 2004. Production of alpha-1,3-galactosyltransferase null pigs by means of nuclear transfer with fibroblasts bearing loss of heterozygosity mutations. Proc. Natl. Acad. Sci. USA 101, 7335–7340.

Koudela, B., Nohynkova, E., Vitovec, J., Pakandl, M., Kulda, J., 1991. Giardia infection in pigs: detection and in vitro isolation of trophozoites of the Giardia intestinalis group. Parasitology 102 (Pt 2), 163–166.

Kozlowski, T., Ierino, F.L., Lambrigts, D., Foley, A., Andrews, D., Awwad, M., et al., 1998. Depletion of anti-Gal(alpha)1-3Gal antibody in baboons by specific alpha-Gal immunoaffinity columns. Xenotransplantation 5, 122–131.

Krakowka, S., Ellis, J., 2006. Reproduction of severe gastroesophageal ulcers (GEU) in gnotobiotic swine infected with porcine Helicobacter pylori-like bacteria. Vet. Pathol. 43, 956–962.

Krakowka, S., Ellis, J.A., Mcneilly, F., Ringler, S., Rings, D.M., Allan, G., 2001. Activation of the immune system is the pivotal event in the production of wasting disease in pigs infected with porcine circovirus-2 (PCV-2). Vet. Pathol. 38, 31–42.

Krakowka, S., Hartunian, C., Hamberg, A., Shoup, D., Rings, M., Zhang, Y., et al., 2008. Evaluation of induction of porcine dermatitis and nephropathy syndrome in gnotobiotic pigs with negative results for porcine circovirus type 2. Am. J. Vet. Res. 69, 1615–1622.

Krakowka, S., Allan, G., Ellis, J., Hamberg, A., Charreyre, C., Kaufmann, E., et al., 2012. A nine-base nucleotide sequence in the porcine circovirus type 2 (PCV2) nucleocapsid gene determines viral replication and virulence. Virus Res. 164, 90–99.

Krawczynski, K., Meng, X.J., Rybczynska, J., 2011. Pathogenetic elements of hepatitis E and animal models of HEV infection. Virus Res. 161, 78–83.

Kritas, S.K., Pensaert, M.B., Nauwynck, H.J., Kyriakis, S.C., 1999. Neural invasion of two virulent suid herpesvirus 1 strains in neonatal pigs with or without maternal immunity. Vet. Microbiol. 69, 143–156.

Kroll, J.J., Roof, M.B., McOrist, S., 2004. Evaluation of protective immunity in pigs following oral administration of an avirulent live vaccine of Lawsonia intracellularis. Am. J. Vet. Res. 65, 559–565.

Kulick, D.M., Salerno, C.T., Dalmasso, A.P., Park, S.J., Paz, M.G., Fodor, W.L., et al., 2000. Transgenic swine lungs expressing human CD59 are protected from injury in a pig-to-human model of xenotransplantation. J. Thorac. Cardiovasc. Surg. 119, 690–699.

Kyriakis, S.C., Sarris, K., Kritas, S.K., Tsinas, A.C., Giannakopoulos, C., 1996. Effect of salinomycin in the control of Clostridium perfringens type C infections in sucklings pigs. Vet. Rec. 138, 281–283.

Langohr, I.M., Stevenson, G.W., Nelson, E.A., Lenz, S.D., Wei, H., Pogranichniy, R.M., 2012. Experimental co-infection of pigs with Bovine viral diarrhea virus 1 and Porcine circovirus-2. J. Vet. Diagn. Invest. 24, 51–64.

Lapage, G., 1968. Order Phthiraptera. In: Lapage, G. (Ed.), Veterinary Parasitology, second rev. ed. Thomas, Springfield, IL.

Lawson, G.H., McOrist, S., Jasni, S., Mackie, R.A., 1993. Intracellular bacteria of porcine proliferative enteropathy: cultivation and maintenance in vitro. J. Clin. Microbiol. 31, 1136–1142.

Lee, C.A., Silva, M., Siber, A.M., Kelly, A.J., Galyov, E., Mccormick, B.A., 2000. A secreted Salmonella protein induces a proinflammatory response in epithelial cells, which promotes neutrophil migration. Proc. Natl. Acad. Sci. USA 97, 12283–12288.

Lee, J.I., Hampson, D.J., Lymbery, A.J., Harders, S.J., 1993. The porcine intestinal spirochaetes: identification of new genetic groups. Vet. Microbiol. 34, 273–285.

Leiner, G., Franz, B., Strutzberg, K., Gerlach, G.F., 1999. A novel enzyme-linked immunosorbent assay using the recombinant Actinobacillus pleuropneumoniae ApxII antigen for diagnosis of pleuropneumonia in pig herds. Clin. Diagn. Lab. Immunol. 6, 630–632.

Levonen, K., Frandsen, P.L., Seppanen, J., Veijalainen, P., 1996. Detection of toxigenic Pasteurella multocida infections in swine herds by assaying antibodies in sow colostrum. J. Vet. Diagn. Invest. 8, 455–459.

Levy, M.F., Crippin, J., Sutton, S., Netto, G., Mccormack, J., Curiel, T., et al., 2000. Liver allotransplantation after extracorporeal hepatic support with transgenic (hCD55/hCD59) porcine livers: clinical results and lack of pig-to-human transmission of the porcine endogenous retrovirus. Transplantation 69, 272–280.

Lewis, A.J., Southern, L.L., 2001. Swine Nutrition. CRC Press, Boca Raton, FL.

Li, H.W., Sykes, M., 2012. Emerging concepts in haematopoietic cell transplantation. Nat. Rev. Immunol. 12, 403–416.

Li, Y., Wang, X., Bo, K., Wang, X., Tang, B., Yang, B., et al., 2007. Emergence of a highly pathogenic porcine reproductive and respiratory syndrome virus in the Mid-Eastern region of China. Vet. J. 174, 577–584.

Lichtensteiger, C.A., Steenbergen, S.M., Lee, R.M., Polson, D.D., Vimr, E.R., 1996. Direct PCR analysis for toxigenic Pasteurella multocida. J. Clin. Microbiol. 34, 3035–3039.

Lichtensteiger, C.A., Dipietro, J.A., Paul, A.J., Neumann, E.J., Thompson, L., 1999. Persistent activity of doramectin and ivermectin against Ascaris suum in experimentally infected pigs. Vet. Parasitol. 82, 235–241.

Lindecrona, R.H., Jensen, T.K., Moller, K., 2004. Influence of diet on the experimental infection of pigs with Brachyspira pilosicoli. Vet. Rec. 154, 264–267.

Lindsay, D.S., Dubey, J.P., Blagburn, B.L., 1997. Biology of Isospora spp. from humans, nonhuman primates, and domestic animals. Clin. Microbiol. Rev. 10, 19–34.

Lindsay, D.S., Dubey, J.P., Santin-Duran, M., Fayer, R., 2012. Coccidia and other protozoa. In: Zimmerman, J.J., Karriker, L.A., Ramirez, A., Schwartz, K.J., Stevenson, G.W. (Eds.), Diseases of Swine, tenth ed. Wiley-Blackwell, Chichester, West Sussex.

Little, T.W., Harding, J.D., 1971. The comparative pathogenicity of two porcine haemophilus species. Vet. Rec. 88, 540–545.

Logan, N.B., Weatherley, A.J., Jones, R.M., 1996. Activity of doramectin against nematode and arthropod parasites of swine. Vet. Parasitol. 66, 87–94.

Loken, T., Aleksandersen, M., Reid, H., Pow, I., 1998. Malignant catarrhal fever caused by ovine herpesvirus-2 in pigs in Norway. Vet. Rec. 143, 464–467.

Love, D.N., Love, R.J., 1979. Pathology of proliferative haemorrhagic enteropathy in pigs. Vet. Pathol. 16, 41–48.

Macinnes, J.I., Desrosiers, R., 1999. Agents of the 'suis-ide diseases' of swine: Actinobacillus suis, Haemophilus parasuis, and Streptococcus suis. Can. J. Vet. Res. 63, 83–89.

Macintyre, N., Smith, D.G., Shaw, D.J., Thomson, J.R., Rhind, S.M., 2003. Immunopathogenesis of experimentally induced proliferative enteropathy in pigs. Vet. Pathol. 40, 421–432.

Mackenzie, J.S., Gubler, D.J., Petersen, L.R., 2004. Emerging flaviviruses: the spread and resurgence of Japanese encephalitis, West Nile and dengue viruses. Nat. Med. 10, S98–109.

Madsen, L.W., Svensmark, B., Elvestad, K., Jensen, H.E., 2001. Otitis interna is a frequent sequela to Streptococcus suis meningitis in pigs. Vet. Pathol. 38, 190–195.

Madsen, L.W., Svensmark, B., Elvestad, K., Aalbaek, B., Jensen, H.E., 2002. Streptococcus suis serotype 2 infection in pigs: new diagnostic and pathogenetic aspects. J. Comp. Pathol. 126, 57–65.

Makino, S., Yamamoto, K., Murakami, S., Shirahata, T., Uemura, K., Sawada, T., et al., 1998. Properties of repeat domain found in a novel protective antigen, SpaA, of Erysipelothrix rhusiopathiae. Microb. Pathog. 25, 101–109.

Mankertz, A., 2012. Molecular interactions of porcine circoviruses type 1 and type 2 with its host. Virus Res. 164, 54–60.

Maratea, K.A., Snyder, P.W., Stevenson, G.W., 2006. Vascular lesions in nine Gottingen minipigs with thrombocytopenic purpura syndrome. Vet. Pathol. 43, 447–454.

Marchant-Forde, R.M., Marchant-Forde, J.N., 2004. Pregnancy-related changes in behavior and cardiac activity in primiparous pigs. Physiol. Behav. 82, 815–825.

Marie, J., Morvan, H., Berthelot-Herault, F., Sanders, P., Kempf, I., Gautier-Bouchardon, A.V., et al., 2002. Antimicrobial susceptibility of Streptococcus suis isolated from swine in France and from humans in different countries between 1996 and 2000. J. Antimicrob. Chemother. 50, 201–209.

Marsh, G.A., Haining, J., Robinson, R., Foord, A., Yamada, M., Barr, J.A., et al., 2011. Ebola Reston virus infection of pigs: clinical significance and transmission potential. J. Infect. Dis. 204 (Suppl. 3), S804–S809.

Mason, R.J., Fleming, P.J., Smythe, L.D., Dohnt, M.F., Norris, M.A., Symonds, M.L., 1998. Leptospira interrogans antibodies in feral pigs from New South Wales. J. Wildl. Dis. 34, 738–743.

Mateusen, B., Maes, D.G., Van Soom, A., Lefebvre, D., Nauwynck, H.J., 2007. Effect of a porcine circovirus type 2 infection on embryos during early pregnancy. Theriogenology 68, 896–901.

Matsunari, H., Nagashima, H., 2009. Application of genetically modified and cloned pigs in translational research. J. Reprod. Dev. 55, 225–230.

Maurice, H., Nielen, M., Vyt, P., Frankena, K., Koenen, F., 2007. Factors related to the incidence of clinical encephalomyocarditis virus (EMCV) infection on Belgian pig farms. Prev. Vet. Med. 78, 24–34.

Maxie, M.G., Jubb, K.V.F., 2007. Cardiovascular system. In: Maxie, M.G., Robinson, W.F. (Eds.), Pathology of Domestic Animals, fifth ed. Elsevier Saunders, Edinburgh; New York.

McAnulty, P.A., 2012. The Minipig in Biomedical Research. CRC Press/Taylor & Francis, Boca Raton, FL.

McGavin, M.D., Zachary, J.F., 2007. Pathologic Basis of Veterinary Disease. Elsevier Mosby, St. Louis, MO.

McGregor, C.G., Davies, W.R., Oi, K., Teotia, S.S., Schirmer, J.M., Risdahl, J.M., et al., 2005. Cardiac xenotransplantation: recent preclinical progress with 3-month median survival. J. Thorac. Cardiovasc. Surg. 130, 844–851.

McOrist, S., Gebhart, C.J., 2012. Proliferative enteropathy. In: Zimmerman, J.J., Karriker, L.A., Ramirez, A., Schwartz, K.J., Stevenson, G.W. (Eds.), Diseases of Swine, tenth ed. Wiley-Blackwell, Chichester, West Sussex.

McOrist, S., Gebhart, C.J., Boid, R., Barns, S.M., 1995a. Characterization of Lawsonia intracellularis gen. nov., sp. nov., the obligately intracellular bacterium of porcine proliferative enteropathy. Int. J. Syst. Bacteriol. 45, 820–825.

McOrist, S., Mackie, R.A., Lawson, G.H., 1995b. Antimicrobial susceptibility of ileal symbiont intracellularis isolated from pigs with proliferative enteropathy. J. Clin. Microbiol. 33, 1314–1317.

McOrist, S., Morgan, J., Veenhuizen, M.F., Lawrence, K., Kroger, H.W., 1997. Oral administration of tylosin phosphate for treatment and prevention of proliferative enteropathy in pigs. Am. J. Vet. Res. 58, 136–139.

McOrist, S., Smith, S.H., Shearn, M.F., Carr, M.M., Miller, D.J., 1996. Treatment and prevention of porcine proliferative enteropathy with oral tiamulin. Vet. Rec. 139, 615–618.

Meerts, P., Van Gucht, S., Cox, E., Vandebosch, A., Nauwynck, H.J., 2005. Correlation between type of adaptive immune response against porcine circovirus type 2 and level of virus replication. Viral. Immunol. 18, 333–341.

Meng, X.J., Wiseman, B., Elvinger, F., Guenette, D.K., Toth, T.E., Engle, R.E., et al., 2002. Prevalence of antibodies to hepatitis E virus in veterinarians working with swine and in normal blood donors in the United States and other countries. J. Clin. Microbiol. 40, 117–122.

Mengeling, W.L., Paul, P.S., 1986. Interepizootic survival of porcine parvovirus. J. Am. Vet. Med. Assoc. 188, 1293–1295.

Mengeling, W.L., Lager, K.M., Zimmerman, J.K., Samarikermani, N., Beran, G.W., 1991. A current assessment of the role of porcine parvovirus as a cause of fetal porcine death. J. Vet. Diagn. Invest. 3, 33–35.

Mengeling, W.L., Paul, P.S., Lager, K.M., 1993. Virus-induced maternal reproductive failure of swine. J. Am. Vet. Med. Assoc. 203, 1268–1272.

Mengeling, W.L., Lager, K.M., Vorwald, A.C., 2000. The effect of porcine parvovirus and porcine reproductive and respiratory syndrome virus on porcine reproductive performance. Anim. Reprod. Sci. 60–61, 199–210.

Mercier, P., Cargill, C.F., White, C.R., 2002. Preventing transmission of sarcoptic mange from sows to their offspring by injection of ivermectin. Effects on swine production. Vet. Parasitol. 110, 25–33.

Messick, J.B., 2004. Hemotrophic mycoplasmas (hemoplasmas): a review and new insights into pathogenic potential. Vet. Clin. Pathol. 33, 2–13.

Messick, J.B., Cooper, S.K., Huntley, M., 1999. Development and evaluation of a polymerase chain reaction assay using the 16S rRNA gene for detection of Eperythrozoon suis infection. J. Vet. Diagn. Invest. 11, 229–236.

Mettenleiter, T.C., 2000. Aujeszky's disease (pseudorabies) virus: the virus and molecular pathogenesis – state of the art, June 1999. Vet. Res. 31, 99–115.

Mettenleiter, T.C., Ehlers, B., Muller, T., Yoon, K.-J., Teifke, J.P., 2012. Herpesviruses. In: Zimmerman, J.J., Karriker, L.A., Ramirez, A., Schwartz, K.J., Stevenson, G.W. (Eds.), Diseases of Swine, tenth ed. Wiley-Blackwell, Chichester, West Sussex.

Meyerholz, D.K., Stabel, T.J., 2003. Comparison of early ileal invasion by Salmonella enterica serovars Choleraesuis and Typhimurium. Vet. Pathol. 40, 371–375.

Meyerholz, D.K., Stabel, T.J., Ackermann, M.R., Carlson, S.A., Jones, B.D., Pohlenz, J., 2002. Early epithelial invasion by Salmonella enterica serovar Typhimurium DT104 in the swine ileum. Vet. Pathol. 39, 712–720.

Mezrich, J.D., Haller, G.W., Arn, J.S., Houser, S.L., Madsen, J.C., Sachs, D.H., 2003. Histocompatible miniature swine: an inbred large-animal model. Transplantation 75, 904–907.

Mielke, D., Hiepe, T., 1998. The effectiveness of different disinfectants based on p-chloro-m-cresol against Ascaris suum eggs under laboratory conditions. Berl. Munch. Tierarztl. Wochenschr. 111, 291–294.

Mikami, O., Nakajima, H., Kawashima, K., Yoshii, M., Nakajima, Y., 2005. Nonsuppurative myocarditis caused by porcine circovirus type 2 in a weak-born piglet. J. Vet. Med. Sci. 67, 735–738.

Minipigs, E.G., 2010. The Gottingen Minipig [Online]. Available: <http://minipigs.dk/thegottingenminipig/> (accessed 18.06.12).

Misinzo, G., Delputte, P.L., Meerts, P., Lefebvre, D.J., Nauwynck, H.J., 2006. Porcine circovirus 2 uses heparan sulfate and chondroitin sulfate B glycosaminoglycans as receptors for its attachment to host cells. J. Virol. 80, 3487–3494.

Moller, K., Jensen, T.K., Jorsal, S.E., Leser, T.D., Carstensen, B., 1998. Detection of Lawsonia intracellularis, Serpulina hyodysenteriae, weakly beta-haemolytic intestinal spirochaetes, Salmonella enterica, and haemolytic Escherichia coli from swine herds with and without diarrhoea among growing pigs. Vet. Microbiol. 62, 59–72.

Morandi, F., Ostanello, F., Fusaro, L., Bacci, B., Nigrelli, A., Alborali, L., et al., 2010. Immunohistochemical detection of aetiological agents of proliferative and necrotizing pneumonia in italian pigs. J. Comp. Pathol. 142, 74–78.

Morita, T., Sasaki, A., Kaji, N., Shimada, A., Kazama, S., Yagihashi, T., et al., 1998. Induction of temporary otitis media in specific-pathogen-free pigs by intratympanic inoculation of Mycoplasma hyorhinis. Am. J. Vet. Res. 59, 869–873.

Morita, T., Ohiwa, S., Shimada, A., Kazama, S., Yagihashi, T., Umemura, T., 1999. Intranasally inoculated Mycoplasma hyorhinis causes eustachitis in pigs. Vet. Pathol. 36, 174–178.

Morsy, G.H., Turek, J.J., Gaafar, S.M., 1989. Scanning electron microscopy of sarcoptic mange lesions in swine. Vet. Parasitol. 31, 281–288.

Mozzachio, K., Linder, K., Dixon, D., 2004. Uterine smooth muscle tumors in potbellied pigs (Sus scrofa) resemble human fibroids: a potential animal model. Toxicol. Pathol. 32, 402–407.

Mueller, N.J., Livingston, C., Knosalla, C., Barth, R.N., Yamamoto, S., Gollackner, B., et al., 2004. Activation of porcine cytomegalovirus, but not porcine lymphotropic herpesvirus, in pig-to-baboon xenotransplantation. J. Infect. Dis. 189, 1628–1633.

Mueller, Y.M., Davenport, C., Ildstad, S.T., 1999. Xenotransplantation: application of disease resistance. Clin. Exp. Pharmacol. Physiol. 26, 1009–1012.

Mulder, W.A., Pol, J.M., Gruys, E., Jacobs, L., De Jong, M.C., Peeters, B.P., et al., 1997. Pseudorabies virus infections in pigs. Role of viral proteins in virulence, pathogenesis and transmission. Vet. Res. 28, 1–17.

Muneta, Y., Minagawa, Y., Shimoji, Y., Nagata, R., Markham, P.F., Browning, G.F., et al., 2006. IL-18 expression in pigs following infection with Mycoplasma hyopneumoniae. J. Interferon Cytokine Res. 26, 637–644.

Murakata, K., Sato, A., Yoshiya, M., Kim, S., Watarai, M., Omata, Y., et al., 2008. Infection of different strains of mice with Lawsonia intracellularis derived from rabbit or porcine proliferative enteropathy. J. Comp. Pathol. 139, 8–15.

Murrell, K.D., Eriksen, L., Nansen, P., Slotved, H.C., Rasmussen, T., 1997. Ascaris suum: a revision of its early migratory path and implications for human ascariasis. J. Parasitol. 83, 255–260.

Murtaugh, M.P., 1994. Porcine cytokines. Vet. Immunol. Immunopathol. 43, 37–44.

National Research Council (U.S.). Committee on Nutrient Requirements of Swine, 2012. Nutrient Requirements of Swine. National Academies Press, Washington, DC.

Nauwynck, H.J., Sanchez, R., Meerts, P., Lefebvre, D.J., Saha, D., Huang, L., et al., 2012. Cell tropism and entry of porcine circovirus 2. Virus Res. 164, 43–45.

Neimark, H., Johansson, K.E., Rikihisa, Y., Tully, J.G., 2002. Revision of haemotrophic Mycoplasma species names. Int. J. Syst. Evol. Microbiol. 52, 683.

Nickel, E.A., Danner, G., 1979. Experimental studies on the course and the effects of pediculosis in domestic swine. Arch. Exp. Veterinarmed. 33, 645–649.

Nielsen, R., 1973. An outbreak of pleuropneumonia among a group of baconers. Pathological and bacteriological observations. Nord. Vet. Med. 25, 492–496.

Niilo, C.L., 1993. Enterotoxemic Clostridium perfringens. In: Gyles, C.L., Thoen, C.O. (Eds.), Pathogenesis of Bacterial Infections in Animals, second ed. Iowa State University, Ames, IA.

Nikolic, B., Gardner, J.P., Scadden, D.T., Arn, J.S., Sachs, D.H., Sykes, M., 1999. Normal development in porcine thymus grafts and specific tolerance of human T cells to porcine donor MHC. J. Immunol. 162, 3402–3407.

Nilubol, D., Pattanaseth, T., Boonsri, K., Pirarat, N., Leepipatpiboon, N., 2009. Melamine- and cyanuric acid-associated renal failure in pigs in Thailand. Vet. Pathol. 46, 1156–1159.

Nonneman, D.J., Brown-Brandl, T., Jones, S.A., Wiedmann, R.T., Rohrer, G.A., 2012. A defect in dystrophin causes a novel porcine stress syndrome. BMC Genomics 13, 233.

Ober, B.T., Summerfield, A., Mattlinger, C., Wiesmuller, K.H., Jung, G., Pfaff, E., et al., 1998. Vaccine-induced, pseudorabies virus-specific, extrathymic CD4 + CD8+ memory T-helper cells in swine. J. Virol. 72, 4866–4873.

O'Brien, P.J., Shen, H., Weiler, J., Ianuzzo, C.D., Wittnich, C., Moe, G.W., et al., 1991. Cardiac and muscle fatigue due to relative functional overload induced by excessive stimulation, hypersensitive excitation–contraction coupling, or diminished performance capacity correlates with sarcoplasmic reticulum failure. Can. J. Physiol. Pharmacol. 69 (262–8).

O'Brien, P.J., Shen, H., Cory, C.R., Zhang, X., 1993. Use of a DNA-based test for the mutation associated with porcine stress syndrome (malignant hyperthermia) in 10,000 breeding swine. J. Am. Vet. Med. Assoc. 203, 842–851.

O'Connor, B., Gauvreau, H., West, K., Bogdan, J., Ayroud, M., Clark, E.G., et al., 2001. Multiple porcine circovirus 2-associated abortions and reproductive failure in a multisite swine production unit. Can. Vet. J. 42, 551–553.

Oishi, E., Kitajima, T., Koyama, Y., Ohgitani, T., Katayama, S., Okabe, T., 1995. Protective effect of the combined vaccine prepared from cell-free-antigen of Actinobacillus pleuropneumoniae serotypes 1, 2 and 5 in pigs. J. Vet. Med. Sci. 57, 1125–1128.

Okada, M., Asai, T., Futo, S., Mori, Y., Mukai, T., Yazawa, S., et al., 2005. Serological diagnosis of enzootic pneumonia of swine by a double-sandwich enzyme-linked immunosorbent assay using a monoclonal antibody and recombinant antigen (P46) of Mycoplasma hyopneumoniae. Vet. Microbiol. 105, 251–259.

Olsen, S.C., Garin-Bastuji, G., Blasco, J.M., Nicola, A.M., Samartino, L., 2012. Brucellosis. In: Zimmerman, J.J., Karriker, L.A., Ramirez, A., Schwartz, K.J., Stevenson, G.W. (Eds.), Diseases of Swine, tenth ed. Wiley-Blackwell, Chichester, West Sussex.

Olson, L.B., Backstrom, L.R., 2000. The effect of tilmicosin in minimizing atrophic rhinitis, pneumonia, and pleuritis in swine. Swine Health Prod. 8, 263–268.

Olson, M.E., Thorlakson, C.L., Deselliers, L., Morck, D.W., Mcallister, T.A., 1997. Giardia and Cryptosporidium in Canadian farm animals. Vet. Parasitol. 68, 375–381.

Opriessnig, T., Halbur, P.G., 2012. Concurrent infections are important for expression of porcine circovirus associated disease. Virus Res. 164, 20–32.

Opriessnig, T., Langohr, I., 2013. Current state of knowledge on porcine circovirus type 2-associated lesions. Vet. Pathol. 50, 23–38.

Opriessnig, T., Wood, R.L., 2012. Erysipelas. In: Zimmerman, J.J., Karriker, L.A., Ramirez, A., Schwartz, K.J., Stevenson, G.W. (Eds.), Diseases of Swine, tenth ed. Wiley-Blackwell, Chichester, West Sussex.

Opriessnig, T., Thacker, E.L., Yu, S., Fenaux, M., Meng, X.J., Halbur, P.G., 2004. Experimental reproduction of postweaning multisystemic wasting syndrome in pigs by dual infection with Mycoplasma hyopneumoniae and porcine circovirus type 2. Vet. Pathol. 41, 624–640.

Opriessnig, T., Fenaux, M., Thomas, P., Hoogland, M.J., Rothschild, M.F., Meng, X.J., et al., 2006. Evidence of breed-dependent differences in susceptibility to porcine circovirus type-2-associated disease and lesions. Vet. Pathol. 43, 281–293.

Pallares, F.J., Halbur, P.G., Opriessnig, T., Sorden, S.D., Villar, D., Janke, B.H., et al., 2002. Porcine circovirus type 2 (PCV-2) coinfections in US field cases of postweaning multisystemic wasting syndrome (PMWS). J. Vet. Diagn. Invest. 14, 515–519.

Panepinto, L.M., 1986. Character and management of miniature swine. In: Stanton, H.C., Mersmann, H.J. (Eds.), Swine in Cardiovascular Research. CRC Press, Boca Raton, FL.

Panepinto, L.M., Phillips, R.W., Norden, S., Pryor, P.C., Cox, R., 1983. A comfortable, minimum stress method of restraint for Yucatan miniature swine. Lab. Anim. Sci. 33, 95–97.

Paul, P.S., Mengeling, W.L., Brown Jr., T.T., 1980. Effect of vaccinal and passive immunity on experimental infection of pigs with porcine parvovirus. Am. J. Vet. Res. 41, 1368–1371.

Paulin, S.M., Jagannathan, A., Campbell, J., Wallis, T.S., Stevens, M.P., 2007. Net replication of Salmonella enterica serovars Typhimurium and Choleraesuis in porcine intestinal mucosa and nodes is associated with their differential virulence. Infect. Immun. 75, 3950–3960.

Pearson, G.R., Mcnulty, M.S., 1977. Pathological changes in the small intestine of neonatal pigs infected with a pig reovirus-like agent (rotavirus). J. Comp. Pathol. 87, 363–375.

Pennington, L.R., Sakamoto, K., Popitz-Bergez, F.A., Pescovitz, M.D., Mcdonough, M.A., Macvittie, T.J., et al., 1988. Bone marrow transplantation in miniature swine. I. Development of the model. Transplantation 45, 21–26.

Perlman, S., Netland, J., 2009. Coronaviruses post-SARS: update on replication and pathogenesis. Nat. Rev. Microbiol. 7, 439–450.

Pescovitz, M.D., 1998. Immunology of the pig. In: Pastoret, P.-P. (Ed.), Handbook of Vertebrate Immunology. Academic Press, San Diego, CA.

Phaneuf, L.R., Ceccarelli, A., Laing, J.R., Moloo, B., Turner, P.V., 2007. Porcine dermatitis and nephropathy syndrome associated with porcine circovirus 2 infection in a Yorkshire pig. J. Am. Assoc. Lab. Anim. Sci. 46, 68–72.

Piffer, I.A., Ross, R.F., 1984. Effect of age on susceptibility of pigs to Mycoplasma hyopneumoniae pneumonia. Am. J. Vet. Res. 45, 478–481.

Pijoan, C., Fuentes, M., 1987. Severe pleuritis associated with certain strains of Pasteurella multocida in swine. J. Am. Vet. Med. Assoc. 191, 823–826.

Plumb, D.C., 2011. Plumb's Veterinary Drug Handbook. PharmaVet; Distributed by Wiley, Stockholm, Wis. Ames, Iowa.

Pluske, J.R., Siba, P.M., Pethick, D.W., Durmic, Z., Mullan, B.P., Hampson, D.J., 1996. The incidence of swine dysentery in pigs can be reduced by feeding diets that limit the amount of fermentable substrate entering the large intestine. J. Nutr. 126, 2920–2933.

Potgieter, L.N., Ross, R.F., 1972. Demonostration of Mycoplasma hyorhinis and Mycoplasma hyosynoviae in lesions of experimentally infected swine by immunofluorescence. Am. J. Vet. Res. 33, 99–105.

Potgieter, L.N., Frey, M.L., Ross, R.F., 1972. Chronological development of Mycoplasma hyorhinis and Mycoplasma hyosynoviae infections in cultures of a swine synovial cell strain. Can. J. Comp. Med. 36, 145–149.

Practitioners, A.A.O.S., 2014. Porcine Epidemic Diarrhea Virus (PEDV). American Association of Swine Veterinarians, Perry, IA.

Prideaux, C.T., Lenghaus, C., Krywult, J., Hodgson, A.L., 1999. Vaccination and protection of pigs against pleuropneumonia with a vaccine strain of Actinobacillus pleuropneumoniae produced by site-specific mutagenesis of the ApxII operon. Infect. Immun. 67, 1962–1966.

Ramjeet, M., Deslandes, V., Goure, J., Jacques, M., 2008. Actinobacillus pleuropneumoniae vaccines: from bacterins to new insights into vaccination strategies. Anim. Health Res. Rev. 9, 25–45.

Rasmussen, S.R., Aarestrup, F.M., Jensen, N.E., Jorsal, S.E., 1999. Associations of Streptococcus suis serotype 2 ribotype profiles with clinical disease and antimicrobial resistance. J. Clin. Microbiol. 37, 404–408.

Reeves, D.E., 1993. Neonatal care of miniature pet pigs. In: Reeves, D.E., Becker, H.N., American Association of Swine Practitioners (Eds.), Care and Management of Miniature Pet Pigs: Guidelines for the Veterinary Practitioner, first ed. Veterinary Practice Pub. Co, Santa Barbara, CA.

Register, K.B., Brockmeier, S.L., De Jong, M.C., Pijoan, C., 2012. Pasteurellosis. In: Zimmerman, J.J., Karriker, L.A., Ramirez, A., Schwartz, K.J., Stevenson, G.W. (Eds.), Diseases of Swine, tenth ed. Wiley-Blackwell, Chichester, West Sussex.

Rehm, T., Baums, C.G., Strommenger, B., Beyerbach, M., Valentin-Weigand, P., Goethe, R., 2007. Amplified fragment length polymorphism of Streptococcus suis strains correlates with their profile of virulence-associated genes and clinical background. J. Med. Microbiol. 56, 102–109.

Reimer, D., Frey, J., Jansen, R., Veit, H.P., Inzana, T.J., 1995. Molecular investigation of the role of ApxI and ApxII in the virulence of Actinobacillus pleuropneumoniae serotype 5. Microb. Pathog. 18, 197–209.

Roepstorff, A., 1998. Natural Ascaris suum infections in swine diagnosed by coprological and serological (ELISA) methods. Parasitol. Res. 84, 537–543.

Roop 2ND, R.M., Veit, H.P., Sinsky, R.J., Veit, S.P., Hewlett, E.L., Kornegay, E.T., 1987. Virulence factors of Bordetella bronchiseptica associated with the production of infectious atrophic rhinitis and pneumonia in experimentally infected neonatal swine. Infect. Immun. 55, 217–222.

Rose, N., Opriessnig, T., Grasland, B., Jestin, A., 2012. Epidemiology and transmission of porcine circovirus type 2 (PCV2). Virus Res. 164, 78–89.

Rosell, C., Segales, J., Domingo, M., 2000. Hepatitis and staging of hepatic damage in pigs naturally infected with porcine circovirus type 2. Vet. Pathol. 37, 687–692.

Ross, R.F., Switzer, W.P., Duncan, J.R., 1971. Experimental production of Mycoplasma hyosynoviae arthritis in swine. Am. J. Vet. Res. 32, 1743–1749.

Rossow, K.D., 1998. Porcine reproductive and respiratory syndrome. Vet. Pathol. 35, 1–20.

Rossow, K.D., Bautista, E.M., Goyal, S.M., Molitor, T.W., Murtaugh, M.P., Morrison, R.B., et al., 1994. Experimental porcine reproductive and respiratory syndrome virus infection in one-, four-, and 10-week-old pigs. J. Vet. Diagn. Invest. 6, 3–12.

Rossow, K.D., Benfield, D.A., Goyal, S.M., Nelson, E.A., Christopher-Hennings, J., Collins, J.E., 1996a. Chronological immunohistochemical detection and localization of porcine reproductive and respiratory syndrome virus in gnotobiotic pigs. Vet. Pathol. 33, 551–556.

Rossow, K.D., Laube, K.L., Goyal, S.M., Collins, J.E., 1996b. Fetal microscopic lesions in porcine reproductive and respiratory syndrome virus-induced abortion. Vet. Pathol. 33, 95–99.

Rowland, J.M., Geisbert, T.W., Rowland, R.R., 2012. Filovirus. In: Zimmerman, J.J., Karriker, L.A., Ramirez, A., Schwartz, K.J., Stevenson, G.W. (Eds.), Diseases of Swine, tenth ed. Wiley-Blackwell, Chichester, West Sussex.

Rudek, Z., Kwiatkowska, L., 1983. The possibility of detecting fetal lymphocytes in the maternal blood of the domestic pig, Sus scrofa. Cytogenet Cell. Genet. 36, 580–583.

Saadi, S., Platt, J.L., 1999. Role of complement in xenotransplantation. Clin. Exp. Pharmacol. Physiol. 26, 1016–1019.

Sablinski, T., Emery, D.W., Monroy, R., Hawley, R.J., Xu, Y., Gianello, P., et al., 1999. Long-term discordant xenogeneic (porcine-to-primate) bone marrow engraftment in a monkey treated with porcine-specific growth factors. Transplantation 67, 972–977.

Sachs, D.H., 2005. A knock-out punch? Nat. Med. 11, 1271.

Saeki, H., Fujii, T., Fukumoto, S., Kagota, K., Taneichi, A., Takeda, S., et al., 1997. Efficacy of doramectin against intestinal nematodes and sarcoptic manage mites in naturally infected swine. J. Vet. Med. Sci. 59, 129–132.

Safron, J., Gonder, J.C., 1997. The SPF Pig in Research. ILAR J. 38, 28–31.

Saif, L.J., 1999. Comparative pathogenesis of enteric viral infections of swine. Adv. Exp. Med. Biol. 473, 47–59.

Saif, L.J., Pensaert, M., Sestak, K., Yeo, S.-G., Jung, K., 2012. Coronaviruses. In: Zimmerman, J.J., Karriker, L.A., Ramirez, A., Schwartz, K.J., Stevenson, G.W. (Eds.), Diseases of Swine, tenth ed. Wiley-Blackwell, Chichester, West Sussex.

Sakamoto, K., Pennington, L.R., Popitz-Bergez, F.A., Pescovitz, M.D., Gress, R.E., Mcdonough, M.A., et al., 1987. Swine GVDH model and the effect of T cell deplestion of marrow by monocolonal antibodies. In: Gale, R.P., Champlin, R., Sandoz Inc. (Eds.), Progress in Bone Marrow Transplantation: Proceedings of the Fourth International UCLA Symposium on Bone Marrow Transplantation, held in Keystone, Colorado, April 13–18, 1986, Sponsored by Sandoz, Inc. UCLA Symposia on Molecular and Cellular Biology. Liss, New York.

Sakano, T., Okada, M., Taneda, A., Mukai, T., Sato, S., 1997. Effect of Bordetella bronchiseptica and serotype D Pasteurella multocida bacterin-toxoid on the occurrence of atrophic rhinitis after experimental infection with B. bronchiseptica and toxigenic type AP. multocida. J. Vet. Med. Sci. 59, 55–57.

Saliki, J.T., Rodgers, S.J., Eskew, G., 1998. Serosurvey of selected viral and bacterial diseases in wild swine from Oklahoma. J. Wildl. Dis. 34, 834–838.

Salvarani, F.M., Conceicao, F.R., Cunha, C.E., Moreira, G.M., Pires, P.S., Silva, R.O., et al., 2013. Vaccination with recombinant Clostridium perfringens toxoids alpha and beta promotes elevated antepartum and passive humoral immunity in swine. Vaccine 31, 4152–4155.

Sanchez-Cordon, P.J., Nunez, A., Salguero, F.J., Pedrera, M., Fernandez De Marco, M., Gomez-Villamandos, J.C., 2005. Lymphocyte apoptosis and thrombocytopenia in spleen during classical swine fever: role of macrophages and cytokines. Vet. Pathol. 42, 477–488.

Sandfoss, M.R., Deperno, C.S., Betsill, C.W., Palamar, M.B., Erickson, G., Kennedy-Stoskopf, S., 2012. A serosurvey for Brucella suis, classical swine fever virus, porcine circovirus type 2, and pseudorabies virus in feral swine (Sus scrofa) of eastern North Carolina. J. Wildl. Dis. 48, 462–466.

Sarli, G., Mandrioli, L., Panarese, S., Brunetti, B., Segales, J., Dominguez, J., et al., 2008. Characterization of interstitial nephritis in pigs with naturally occurring postweaning multisystemic wasting syndrome. Vet. Pathol. 45, 12–18.

Sarradell, J., Andrada, M., Ramirez, A.S., Fernandez, A., Gomez-Villamandos, J.C., Jover, A., et al., 2003. A morphologic and immunohistochemical study of the bronchus-associated lymphoid tissue of pigs naturally infected with Mycoplasma hyopneumoniae. Vet. Pathol. 40, 395–404.

Sato, H., Watanabe, T., Murata, Y., Ohtake, A., Nakamura, M., Aizawa, C., et al., 1999. New exfoliative toxin produced by a plasmid-carrying strain of Staphylococcus hyicus. Infect. Immun. 67, 4014–4018.

Sawatsky, J., 1993. Behavior of miniature pet pigs. In: Reeves, D.E., Becker, H.N., American Association of Swine Practitioners (Eds.), Care and Management of Miniature Pet Pigs: Guidelines for the Veterinary Practitioner, first ed. Veterinary Practice Pub. Co, Santa Barbara, CA.

Schmall, L.M., Argenzio, R.A., Whipp, S.C., 1983. Pathophysiologic features of swine dysentery: cyclic nucleotide-independent production of diarrhea. Am. J. Vet. Res. 44, 1309–1316.

Schoenbaum, M.A., Zimmerman, J.J., Beran, G.W., Murphy, D.P., 1990. Survival of pseudorabies virus in aerosol. Am. J. Vet. Res. 51, 331–333.

Schuurman, H.J., Graham, M.L., Spizzo, T., Patience, C., 2012. Xenotransplantation. In: McAnulty, P.A. (Ed.), The Minipig in Biomedical Research. CRC Press/Taylor & Francis, Boca Raton, FL.

Schwartz, K.J., 1991. Diagnosing and controlling Salmonella cholerasuis in swine. Vet. Med. (Praha) 86, 1041–1048.

Seeliger, F.A., Brugmann, M.L., Kruger, L., Greiser-Wilke, I., Verspohl, J., Segales, J., et al., 2007. Porcine circovirus type 2-associated cerebellar vasculitis in postweaning multisystemic wasting syndrome (PMWS)-affected pigs. Vet. Pathol. 44, 621–634.

Segales, J., 2012. Porcine circovirus type 2 (PCV2) infections: clinical signs, pathology and laboratory diagnosis. Virus Res. 164, 10–19.

Service, A.A.P.H.I., 2013. Technical Note: Porcine Epidemic Diarrhea (PED) [Online]. United States Department of Agriculture. Available: <http://www.aphis.usda.gov/animal_health/animal_dis_spec/swine/downloads/ped_tech_note.pdf> (accessed 23.09.13).

Sharing, U.N.F.O., 2013. United Network for Organ Sharing [Online]. Available: <http://www.unos.org/>.

Sheerar, M.G., Easterday, B.C., Hinshaw, V.S., 1989. Antigenic conservation of H1N1 swine influenza viruses. J. Gen. Virol. 70 (Pt 12), 3297–3303.

Shimizu, I., Smith, N.R., Zhao, G., Medof, E., Sykes, M., 2006. Decay-accelerating factor prevents acute humoral rejection induced by low levels of anti-alphaGal natural antibodies. Transplantation 81, 95–100.

Shimoji, Y., Mori, Y., Fischetti, V.A., 1999. Immunological characterization of a protective antigen of Erysipelothrix rhusiopathiae: identification of the region responsible for protective immunity. Infect. Immun. 67, 1646–1651.

Shryock, T.R., Losonsky, J.M., Smith, W.C., Gatlin, C.L., Francisco, C.J., Kuriashkin, I.V., et al., 1998. Computed axial tomography of the porcine nasal cavity and a morphometric comparison of the nasal turbinates with other visualization techniques. Can. J. Vet. Res. 62, 287–292.

Skjolaas, K.A., Burkey, T.E., Dritz, S.S., Minton, J.E., 2006. Effects of Salmonella enterica serovars Typhimurium (ST) and Choleraesuis (SC) on chemokine and cytokine expression in swine ileum and jejunal epithelial cells. Vet. Immunol. Immunopathol. 111, 199–209.

Skotarczak, B., Zielinski, R., 1997. A comparison of nucleic acid content in Balantidium coli trophozoites from different isolates. Folia Biol. (Krakow) 45, 121–124.

Smith, A.C., Swindle, M.M., 2006. Preparation of swine for the laboratory. ILAR J. 47, 358–363.

Smith, M.E., Gopee, N.V., Ferguson, S.A., 2009. Preferences of minipigs for environmental enrichment objects. J. Am. Assoc. Lab. Anim. Sci. 48, 391–394.

Smith, M.W., Peacock, M.A., 1980. Anomalous replacement of foetal enterocytes in the neonatal pig. Proc. R Soc. Lond. B Biol. Sci. 206, 411–420.

Sokoli, A., Groebel, K., Hoelzle, K., Amselgruber, W.M., Mateos, J.M., Schneider, M.K., et al., 2013. Mycoplasma suis infection results endothelial cell damage and activation: new insight into the cell tropism and pathogenicity of hemotrophic mycoplasma. Vet. Res. 44, 6.

Songer, J.G., 2012. Clostridiosis. In: Zimmerman, J.J., Karriker, L.A., Ramirez, A., Schwartz, K.J., Stevenson, G.W. (Eds.), Diseases of Swine, tenth ed. Wiley-Blackwell, Chichester, West Sussex.

Splitter, E.J., 1950. Eperythrozoon suis, the etiologic agent of icteroanemia or an anaplasmosis-like disease in swine. Am. J. Vet. Res. 11, 324–330.

Staats, J.J., Feder, I., Okwumabua, O., Chengappa, M.M., 1997. Streptococcus suis: past and present. Vet. Res. Commun. 21, 381–407.

Stanton, H.C., Mersmann, H.J., 1986. Swine in Cardiovascular Research. CRC Press, Boca Raton, FL.

Stanton, T.B., 2006. The genus Brachyspira. In: Dworkin, M., Falkow, S. (Eds.), The Prokaryotes: a Handbook on the Biology of Bacteria, third ed. Springer, New York; London.

Stege, H., Jensen, T.K., Moller, K., Baekbo, P., Jorsal, S.E., 2001. Risk factors for intestinal pathogens in Danish finishing pig herds. Prev. Vet. Med. 50, 153–164.

Stemke, G.W., 1997. Gene amplification (PCR) to detect and differentiate mycoplasmas in porcine mycoplasmal pneumonia. Lett. Appl. Microbiol. 25, 327–330.

Stevenson, G.W., Hoang, H., Schwartz, K.J., Burrough, E.R., Sun, D., Madson, D., et al., 2013. Emergence of Porcine epidemic diarrhea virus in the United States: clinical signs, lesions, and viral genomic sequences. J. Vet. Diagn. Invest. 25, 649–654.

Stewart, T.B., 2007. Parasites of swine. In: Baker, D.G. (Ed.), Flynn's Parasites of Laboratory Animals. Blackwell publishing, Ames, IA.

Stewart, T.B., Fox, M.C., Wiles, S.E., 1996. Doramectin efficacy against gastrointestinal nematodes in pigs. Vet. Parasitol. 66, 101–108.

Studdert, V.P., Gay, C.C., Blood, D.C., 2012. Saunders Comprehensive Veterinary Dictionary. New York, Saunders Elsevier, Edinburgh.

Swenson, S.L., Mead, D.G., Bunn, T.O., 2012. Rhabdoviruses. In: Zimmerman, J.J., Karriker, L.A., Ramirez, A., Schwartz, K.J., Stevenson, G.W. (Eds.), Diseases of Swine, tenth ed. Wiley-Blackwell, Chichester, West Sussex.

Swindle, M.M., 1986. Surgery and anesthesia. In: Tumbleson, M.E. (Ed.), Swine in Biomedical Research. Plenum Press, New York.

Swindle, M.M., 1998. Defining appropriate health status and management programs for specific-pathogen-free swine for xenotransplantation. Ann. NY Acad. Sci. 862, 111–120.

Swindle, M.M., 2007. Swine in the Laboratory:Surgery, Anesthesia, Imaging, and Experimental Techniques. CRC Press, Boca Raton, FL.

Swindle, M.M., Swindle, M.M., 2007. Swine in the Laboratory: Surgery, Anesthesia, Imaging, and Experimental Techniques. CRC Press, Boca Raton, FL.

Swindle, M.M., Thompson, R.P., Carabello, B.A., Smith, A.C., Hepburn, B.J., Bodison, D.R., et al., 1990. Heritable ventricular septal defect in Yucatan miniature swine. Lab. Anim. Sci. 40, 155–161.

Swindle, M.M., Moody, D.C., Phillips, L.D., 1992. Swine as Models in Biomedical Research. Iowa State University Press, Ames, IA.

Swindle, M.M., Smith, A.C., Laber-Laird, K., Dungan, L., 1994. Swine in biomedical research: management and models. ILAR J. 36, 1–5.

Swindle, M.M., Makin, A., Herron, A.J., Clubb Jr., F.J., Frazier, K.S., 2012. Swine as models in biomedical research and toxicology testing. Vet. Pathol. 49, 344–356.

Szeredi, L., Dan, A., Solymosi, N., Csagola, A., Tuboly, T., 2012. Association of porcine circovirus type 2 with vascular lesions in porcine pneumonia. Vet. Pathol. 49, 264–270.

Tanabe, T., Sato, H., Sato, H., Watanabe, K., Hirano, M., Hirose, K., et al., 1996. Correlation between occurrence of exudative epidermitis and exfoliative toxin-producing ability of Staphylococcus hyicus. Vet. Microbiol. 48, 9–17.

Temmam, S., Besnard, L., Andriamandimby, S.F., Foray, C., Rasamoelina-Andriamanivo, H., Heraud, J.M., et al., 2013. High prevalence of hepatitis E in humans and pigs and evidence of genotype-3 virus in swine, Madagascar. Am. J. Trop. Med. Hyg. 88, 329–338.

Teppema, J.S., DE Boer, G.F., 1975. Ultrastructural aspects of experimental swinepox with special reference to inclusion bodies. Arch. Virol. 49, 151–163.

Thacker, B.J., Joo, H.S., Winkelman, N.L., Leman, A.D., Barnes, D.M., 1987. Clinical, virologic, and histopathologic observations of induced porcine parvovirus infection in boars. Am. J. Vet. Res. 48, 763–767.

Thacker, E.L., Minion, F.C., 2012. Mycoplasmosis. In: Zimmerman, J.J., Karriker, L.A., Ramirez, A., Schwartz, K.J., Stevenson, G.W. (Eds.), Diseases of Swine, tenth ed. Wiley-Blackwell, Chichester, West Sussex.

Thacker, E.L., Halbur, P.G., Ross, R.F., Thanawongnuwech, R., Thacker, B.J., 1999. Mycoplasma hyopneumoniae potentiation of porcine reproductive and respiratory syndrome virus-induced pneumonia. J. Clin. Microbiol. 37, 620–627.

Thacker, E.L., Thacker, B.J., Young, T.F., Halbur, P.G., 2000. Effect of vaccination on the potentiation of porcine reproductive and respiratory syndrome virus (PRRSV)-induced pneumonia by Mycoplasma hyopneumoniae. Vaccine 18, 1244–1252.

Thacker, E.L., Thacker, B.J., Janke, B.H., 2001. Interaction between Mycoplasma hyopneumoniae and swine influenza virus. J. Clin. Microbiol. 39, 2525–2530.

Thanawongnuwech, R., Young, T.F., Thacker, B.J., Thacker, E.L., 2001. Differential production of proinflammatory cytokines: in vitro PRRSV and Mycoplasma hyopneumoniae co-infection model. Vet. Immunol. Immunopathol. 79, 115–127.

Thome, M., Hirt, W., Pfaff, E., Reddehase, M.J., Saalmuller, A., 1994. Porcine T-cell receptors: molecular and biochemical characterization. Vet. Immunol. Immunopathol. 43, 13–18.

Thomsen, L.E., Knudsen, K.E., Jensen, T.K., Christensen, A.S., Moller, K., Roepstorff, A., 2007. The effect of fermentable carbohydrates on experimental swine dysentery and whip worm infections in pigs. Vet. Microbiol. 119, 152–163.

Thomson, R.G., 1988. Special Veterinary Pathology. B.C. Decker; C.V. Mosby Co. distributor, Toronto; Philadelphia Saint Louis, Missouri.

Tian, K., Yu, X., Zhao, T., Feng, Y., Cao, Z., Wang, C., et al., 2007. Emergence of fatal PRRSV variants: unparalleled outbreaks of atypical PRRS in China and molecular dissection of the unique hallmark. PLoS One 2, e526.

Tischer, I., Mields, W., Wolff, D., Vagt, M., Griem, W., 1986. Studies on epidemiology and pathogenicity of porcine circovirus. Arch. Virol. 91, 271–276.

Tomanova, K., Bartak, P., Smola, J., 2002. Detection of Lawsonia intracellularis in wild pigs in the Czech Republic. Vet. Rec. 151, 765–767.

Torremorell, M., Calsamiglia, M., Pijoan, C., 1998. Colonization of suckling pigs by Streptococcus suis with particular reference to pathogenic serotype 2 strains. Can. J. Vet. Res. 62, 21–26.

Torres-Velez, F.J., 2008. Nipah virus. In: United States Animal Health Association. Committee on Foreign Animal Diseases, Foreign Animal Diseases, seventh ed. United States Animal Health Association, St. Joseph, MO.

Toth, I., Oswald, E., Mainil, J.G., Awad-Masalmeh, M., Nagy, B., 2000. Characterization of intestinal cnf1+ Escherichia coli from weaned pigs. Int. J. Med. Microbiol. 290, 539–542.

Trible, B.R., Rowland, R.R., 2012. Genetic variation of porcine circovirus type 2 (PCV2) and its relevance to vaccination, pathogenesis and diagnosis. Virus Res. 164, 68–77.

Trott, D.J., Huxtable, C.R., Hampson, D.J., 1996. Experimental infection of newly weaned pigs with human and porcine strains of Serpulina pilosicoli. Infect. Immun. 64, 4648–4654.

Truong, Q.L., Seo, T.W., Yoon, B.I., Kim, H.C., Han, J.H., Hahn, T.W., 2013. Prevalence of swine viral and bacterial pathogens in rodents and stray cats captured around pig farms in Korea. J. Vet. Med. Sci. 75, 1647–1650.

Truyen, U., Streck, A.F., 2012. Porcine parvovirus. In: Zimmerman, J.J., Karriker, L.A., Ramirez, A., Schwartz, K.J., Stevenson, G.W. (Eds.), Diseases of Swine, tenth ed. Wiley-Blackwell, Chichester, West Sussex.

Tucker, A.W., Mcneilly, F., Meehan, B., Galbraith, D., Mcardle, P.D., Allan, G., et al., 2003. Methods for the exclusion of circoviruses and gammaherpesviruses from pigs. Xenotransplantation 10, 343–348.

Tumbleson, M.E., 1986. Swine in Biomedical Research. Plenum Press, New York.

Turk, J.R., Fales, W.H., Maddox, C., Miller, M., Pace, L., Fischer, J., et al., 1992. Pneumonia associated with Salmonella choleraesuis infection in swine: 99 cases (1987–1990). J. Am. Vet. Med. Assoc. 201, 1615–1616.

Tzipori, S., Gibson, R., Montanaro, J., 1989. Nature and distribution of mucosal lesions associated with enteropathogenic and enterohemorrhagic Escherichia coli in piglets and the role of plasmid-mediated factors. Infect. Immun. 57, 1142–1150.

Uthe, J.J., Royaee, A., Lunney, J.K., Stabel, T.J., Zhao, S.H., Tuggle, C.K., et al., 2007. Porcine differential gene expression in response to Salmonella enterica serovars Choleraesuis and Typhimurium. Mol. Immunol. 44, 2900–2914.

Vahle, J.L., Haynes, J.S., Andrews, J.J., 1995. Experimental reproduction of Haemophilus parasuis infection in swine: clinical, bacteriological, and morphologic findings. J. Vet. Diagn. Invest. 7, 476–480.

Van Reeth, K., Nauwynck, H., Pensaert, M., 1998. Bronchoalveolar interferon-alpha, tumor necrosis factor-alpha, interleukin-1, and inflammation during acute influenza in pigs: a possible model for humans? J. Infect. Dis. 177, 1076–1079.

Van Reeth, K., Van Gucht, S., Pensaert, M., 2002. Correlations between lung proinflammatory cytokine levels, virus replication, and disease after swine influenza virus challenge of vaccination-immune pigs. Viral. Immunol. 15, 583–594.

Van Reeth, K., Brown, I.H., Olsen, C.W., 2012. Influenza virus. In: Zimmerman, J.J., Karriker, L.A., Ramirez, A., Schwartz, K.J., Stevenson, G.W. (Eds.), Diseases of Swine, tenth ed. Wiley-Blackwell, Chichester, West Sussex.

Vasickova, P., Psikal, I., Kralik, P., Widen, F., Hubalek, Z., Pavlik, I., 2007. Hepatitis E virus: a review. Veterinarni Medicina 52, 365–384.

Vazquez-Torres, A., Jones-Carson, J., Baumler, A.J., Falkow, S., Valdivia, R., Brown, W., et al., 1999. Extraintestinal dissemination of Salmonella by CD18-expressing phagocytes. Nature 401, 804–808.

Veterinarians, A.A.O.S., 2013. American Association of Swine Veterinarians: Increasing the Knowledge of Swine Veterinarians [Online]. Perry, IA. Available: <https://www.aasv.org/> (accessed 7.01.14).

Viruses, I.C.O.T.O., 2013. ICTV Taxonomy History for Alphacoroavirus-1 [Online]. Available: <http://www.ictvonline.org/taxonomyHistory.asp?taxnode_id=20123515&taxa_name= Alphacoronavirus%201> (accessed 30.09.13).

Vitiello, M., D'isanto, M., Finamore, E., Ciarcia, R., Kampanaraki, A., Galdiero, M., 2008. Role of mitogen-activated protein kinases in the iNOS production and cytokine secretion by Salmonella enterica serovar Typhimurium porins. Cytokine 41, 279–285.

Wagner, B., Polley, L., 1997. Ascaris suum prevalence and intensity: an abattoir survey of market hogs in Saskatchewan. Vet. Parasitol. 73, 309–313.

Wallgren, P., Bornstein, S., 1997. The spread of porcine sarcoptic mange during the fattening period revealed by development of antibodies to Sarcoptes scabiei. Vet. Parasitol. 73, 315–324.

Wang, F., Guo, X., Ge, X., Wang, Z., Chen, Y., Cha, Z., et al., 2009. Genetic variation analysis of Chinese strains of porcine circovirus type 2. Virus Res. 145, 151–156.

Wang, H., Verhalen, J., Madariaga, M.L., Xiang, S., Wang, S., Lan, P., et al., 2007. Attenuation of phagocytosis of xenogeneic cells by manipulating CD47. Blood 109, 836–842.

Wang, Q., Chang, B.J., Riley, T.V., 2010. Erysipelothrix rhusiopathiae. Vet. Microbiol. 140, 405–417.

Warrens, A.N., Simon, A.R., Theodore, P.R., Sachs, D.H., Sykes, M., 1998. Function of porcine adhesion molecules in a human marrow microenvironment. Transplantation 66, 252–259.

Weingartl, H.M., Derbyshire, J.B., 1994. Evidence for a putative second receptor for porcine transmissible gastroenteritis virus on the villous enterocytes of newborn pigs. J. Virol. 68, 7253–7259.

Weingartl, H.M., Embury-Hyatt, C., Nfon, C., Leung, A., Smith, G., Kobinger, G., 2012. Transmission of Ebola virus from pigs to non-human primates. Sci. Rep. 2, 811.

Wellenberg, G.J., Stockhofe-Zurwieden, N., De Jong, M.F., Boersma, W.J., Elbers, A.R., 2004. Excessive porcine circovirus type 2 antibody titres may trigger the development of porcine dermatitis and nephropathy syndrome: a case-control study. Vet. Microbiol. 99, 203–214.

Whary, M.T., Zarkower, A., Confer, F.L., Ferguson, F.G., 1995. Age-related differences in subset composition and activation responses of intestinal intraepithelial and mesenteric lymph node lymphocytes from neonatal swine. Cell Immunol. 163, 215–221.

Wiegand, M., Kielstein, P., Pohle, D., Rassbach, A., 1997. Examination of primary SPF swine after experimental infection with Haemophilus parasuis. Clinical symptoms, changes in hematological parameters and in the parameters of the cerebrospinal fluid. Tierarztl Prax. 25, 226–232.

Williams, D.T., Mackenzie, J.S., Daniels, P.W., 2012. Flaviviruses. In: Zimmerman, J.J., Karriker, L.A., Ramirez, A., Schwartz, K.J., Stevenson, G.W. (Eds.), Diseases of Swine, tenth ed. Wiley-Blackwell, Chichester, West Sussex.

Williamson, M.M., Torres-Velez, F.J., 2010. Henipavirus: a review of laboratory animal pathology. Vet. Pathol. 47, 871–880.

Wisselink, H.J., Reek, F.H., Vecht, U., Stockhofe-Zurwieden, N., Smits, M.A., Smith, H.E., 1999. Detection of virulent strains of Streptococcus suis type 2 and highly virulent strains of Streptococcus suis type 1 in tonsillar specimens of pigs by PCR. Vet. Microbiol. 67, 143–157.

Wood, R.L., 1984. Swine erysipelas – a review of prevalence and research. J. Am. Vet. Med. Assoc. 184, 944–949.

Woods, A.L., Tynes, V.V., 2012. Special considerations for show and pet pigs. In: Zimmerman, J.J., Karriker, L.A., Ramirez, A., Schwartz, K.J., Stevenson, G.W. (Eds.), Diseases of Swine, tenth ed. Wiley-Blackwell, Chichester, West Sussex.

Xiao, C.T., Halbur, P.G., Opriessnig, T., 2012. Complete genome sequence of a novel porcine circovirus type 2b variant present in cases of vaccine failures in the United States. J. Virol. 86, 12469.

Xiao, C.T., Gimenez-Lirola, L.G., Jiang, Y.H., Halbur, P.G., Opriessnig, T., 2013. Characterization of a novel porcine parvovirus tentatively designated PPV5. PLoS One 8, e65312.

Yaeger, M.J., 1995. Actinobacillus suis septicemia: an emerging disease in high health herds. Swine Health Prod. 3, 209–210.

Yamada, K., Yazawa, K., Shimizu, A., Iwanaga, T., Hisashi, Y., Nuhn, M., et al., 2005. Marked prolongation of porcine renal xenograft survival in baboons through the use of alpha1,3-galactosyltransferase gene-knockout donors and the cotransplantation of vascularized thymic tissue. Nat. Med. 11, 32–34.

Yamada, M., Nakamura, K., Yoshii, M., Kaku, Y., 2004. Nonsuppurative encephalitis in piglets after experimental inoculation of Japanese encephalitis flavivirus isolated from pigs. Vet. Pathol. 41, 62–67.

Yamamoto, K., Kijima, M., Yoshimura, H., Takahashi, T., 2001. Antimicrobial susceptibilities of Erysipelothrix rhusiopathiae isolated from pigs with swine erysipelas in Japan, 1988–1998. J. Vet. Med. B Infect. Dis. Vet. Public Health 48, 115–126.

Yamazaki, Y., Sato, H., Sakakura, H., Shigeto, K., Nakano, K., Saito, H., et al., 1999. Protective activity of the purified protein antigen of Erysipelothrix rhusiopathiae in pigs. Zentralbl. Veterinarmed. B 46, 47–55.

Yang, Y.G., Sykes, M., 2007. Xenotransplantation: current status and a perspective on the future. Nat. Rev. Immunol. 7, 519–531.

Yazwinski, T.A., Tucker, C., Featherston, H., Johnson, Z., Wood-Huels, N., 1997. Endectocidal efficacies of doramectin in naturally parasitized pigs. Vet. Parasitol. 70, 123–128.

Ye, Y., Niekrasz, M., Kosanke, S., Welsh, R., Jordan, H.E., Fox, J.C., et al., 1994. The pig as a potential organ donor for man. A study of potentially transferable disease from donor pig to recipient man. Transplantation 57, 694–703.

Yeatman, M., Daggett, C.W., Lau, C.L., Byrne, G.W., Logan, J.S., Platt, J.L., et al., 1999. Human complement regulatory proteins protect swine lungs from xenogeneic injury. Ann. Thorac. Surg. 67, 769–775.

Zheng, P., Zhao, Y.X., Zhang, A.D., Kang, C., Chen, H.C., Jin, M.L., 2009. Pathologic analysis of the brain from Streptococcus suis type 2 experimentally infected pigs. Vet. Pathol. 46, 531–535.

Zimmerman, J.J., Berry, W.J., Beran, G.W., Murphy, D.P., 1989. Influence of temperature and age on the recovery of pseudorabies virus from houseflies (Musca domestica). Am. J. Vet. Res. 50, 1471–1474.

Zimmerman, J.J., Benfield, D.A., Dee, S.A., Murtaugh, M.P., Stadejek, T., Stevenson, G.W., et al., 2012a. Porcine reproductive and respiratory syndrome virus (porcine Aterivirus). In: Zimmerman, J.J., Karriker, L.A., Ramirez, A., Schwartz, K.J., Stevenson, G.W. (Eds.), Diseases of Swine, tenth ed. Wiley-Blackwell, Chichester, West Sussex.

Zimmerman, J.J., Karriker, L.A., Ramirez, A., Schwartz, K.J., Stevenson, G.W., 2012b. Diseases of Swine. Wiley-Blackwell, Chichester, West Sussex.

Zimmermann, W., Kircher, P., 1998. Continuous serologic study and sanitation inspection of Sarcoptes scabiei var. suis infection: preliminary results. Schweiz Arch. Tierheilkd 140, 513–517.

CHAPTER

17

Nonhuman Primates

Elizabeth R. Magden, DVM, MS, DACLAM, cVMA[a], Keith G. Mansfield, DVM, DACVP[b], Joe H. Simmons, DVM, PhD, DACLAM[c] and Christian R. Abee DVM, MS, DACLAM[d]

[a]Department of Veterinary Sciences, Michale E. Keeling Center for Comparative Medicine and Research, The University of Texas MD Anderson Cancer Center, Bastrop, TX, USA [b]Discovery and Investigative Pathology, Novartis Institutes for Biomedical Research, Cambridge, MA, USA [c]Insight Diagnostics & Consulting, Pearland, TX, USA, [d]Department of Veterinary Sciences, Michale E. Keeling Center for Comparative Medicine and Research, The University of Texas MD Anderson Cancer Center, Bastrop, TX, USA

OUTLINE

Laboratory Animal Medicine, Third Edition
DOI: http://dx.doi.org/10.1016/B978-0-12-409527-4.00017-1

I. INTRODUCTION

Nonhuman primates are among the most expensive, complex, and demanding of species used in biomedical research. Their high cost, scarcity, and high level of sentience demand a specialized infrastructure and level of care that differs from other species used in research. Veterinary care must be balanced between colony management (colony health) and individualized care in such a way that individual animals are treated as patients within the animal care program. With the growing emphasis on translational science, nonhuman primates are often considered the ultimate translational research model due to their close phylogenetic relationship to human primates. Considering the high cost to carry out research using nonhuman primates, research must be vigorously justified based on the probability that the primate model will most closely recapitulate what would be observed in human beings. Their susceptibility to human infectious agents, similarities in physiological responses, developmental biology, and response to experimentally induced diseases are critically important to the advancement of biomedicine. Nonhuman primates are also among the most scarce, costly, and sentient of animal models used in research. During the past 40 years there has been a significant increase in our knowledge of the biology and care of these valuable animals. This chapter is intended to provide veterinarians, colony managers, and research scientists with an overview of the natural history, biology, clinical management, husbandry, and diseases of the eight most commonly used primate genera.

There are a number of nonhuman primate medical management, biology, and husbandry publications that should be examined when specific needs exceed the limits of this chapter (Keeling and Wolf, 1975; Richter *et al.*, 1984; Bennett *et al.*, 1998; Abee *et al.*, 2012). The chapter on primates in *Laboratory Animal Medicine* (Bernacky *et al.*, 2002) remains a valuable general reference to be consulted in conjunction with this chapter. More current American College of Laboratory Animal Medicine (ACLAM) series publications include the volumes titled *Nonhuman Primates in Biomedical Research: Biology and Management* (Abee *et al.*, 2012) and *Nonhuman Primates in Biomedical Research: Diseases* (Abee *et al.*, 2012). These publications together provide a comprehensive resource of information on the veterinary care, husbandry, and management of nonhuman primates used in research.

Although there are 200–300 species in the order Primates depending on the reference source and taxonomic scheme cited, this chapter emphasizes species within the eight genera most commonly used in research. Among the Old World primates, rhesus monkeys (*Macaca mulatta*), cynomolgus monkeys (*M. fascicularis*), baboons (*Papio* spp.), and African green

monkeys (*Chlorocebus* spp.); among the New World primates, squirrel monkeys (*Saimiri* spp.), owl monkeys (*Aotus* spp.), marmosets (*Callithrix* spp.), and tamarins (*Saguinus* spp.) are discussed in detail. One great ape, the common chimpanzee (*Pan troglodytes*), is also included. Although direct correlation cannot always be made, much of the information presented for these nonhuman primates may be applicable to other species that are closely related taxonomically.

During the last half-century, large numbers of nonhuman primates have been imported into the United States with 126,857 imported in 1968 (Johnsen, 1995) prior to the decision of the Indian government to cease exportation of rhesus monkeys. Over the years, much of the research that was carried out with rhesus monkeys was moved to cynomolgus monkeys with increases in importation of this species. Importation has gradually decreased over the years, but in the past 3 years an increase in importation of nonhuman primates has occurred with 16,071 imported in 2012, 19,678 in 2013, and 27,825 in 2014 (CDC, personal communication, Dr. Robert Mullan, 2014). Factors contributing to these fluctuations in import numbers include reductions in funding for biomedical research, placement of some primate species on the Endangered Species list, bans on exportation from countries of origin, and the efforts of animal activist groups to sway public opinion against the use of nonhuman primates in research. Other factors impacting importation include efforts to increase domestic production and efforts by the research community to more efficiently use nonhuman primate resources by incorporating the principles of the 3Rs as proposed by Russel and Burch (1959) (Tornqvist *et al.*, 2014). There has also been an international effort to minimize the number of nonhuman primates needed to accomplish research goals (NRC, 2011c). There has been a heightened sensitivity and more intense review of nonhuman primate studies by Institutional Animal Care and Use Committees. The University of Washington National Primate Research Center publication, *Primate Resource Referral Service* (formerly the Primate Supply Clearinghouse), has made significant contributions to conservation by listing primates that have become available from research facilities and suppliers within the United States. This has helped reduce the need to import animals from the wild or from breeding facilities in countries with indigenous primate species. Information obtained from USDA APHIS annual reports on the use of nonhuman primates in the United States indicate an increase in use from 2010 to 2013, with an increase from 71,317 to 107,014 (USDA, 2010, 2013). Today, most nonhuman primates originate from well-managed, limited production colonies within the countries of origin and domestic production colonies in the United States. The domestic breeding programs initiated in the 1970s have become either a major supply source or, in some cases, only source of Indian-origin rhesus monkeys, baboons, marmosets, African Green monkeys, owl monkeys, and squirrel monkeys. The United States has been dependent on existing colonies of chimpanzees since it became signatory to the Convention on International Trade in Endangered Species of Wild Fauna and Flora (CITES) treaty in 1975. Chimpanzee production from domestic breeding peaked in the late 1980s and early 1990s. The National Center for Research Resources (NCRR) chimpanzee breeding program recorded 381 births between 1986 and 1994 (NIH, 1994). In 1995, the NIH imposed a moratorium on breeding for all NIH-owned or NIH-supported chimpanzees (ILAR, 1997). This moratorium has remained in effect since, 1995. Additional restrictions and policies regarding the use of NIH-owned or NIH-supported chimpanzees were published in November 2013 (NIH NOT-OD-14-024) following recommendations published by the Institute of Medicine (IOM) regarding the need for chimpanzees in biomedical and behavioral research (NRC, 2011b).

The development of specific pathogen-free (SPF) production colonies of rhesus monkeys began in the late 1980s with support from the NIH, NCRR. SPF rhesus monkeys have become the preferred model for most studies that require this species. Despite increasing the cost of research using nonhuman primates, the engines driving these trends in domestic production of more well-defined nonhuman primates are personnel safety and the need for better-defined animals for sophisticated, molecular-based biomedical research. Such research demands high-quality nonhuman primate models free of pathogenic agents that can confound research and/or place laboratory personnel at greater risk of zoonotic infections.

In spite of efforts by groups opposed to the use of nonhuman primates in research, the contributions to date and future potential for improving human and animal health provide compelling justification for continued use of biologically defined and genetically characterized nonhuman primate models. Their close phylogenetic relationship to human beings, their similarity in susceptibility to diseases, and their subsequent similarity in immune responses place nonhuman primates in a unique position among currently available animal models. Public concerns as well as the concerns of veterinarians, primate caregivers, colony managers, and scientists over the use of nonhuman primates in biomedical research, combined with their high maintenance costs and relative scarcity, mandate high standards of care and judicious use of these species.

II. TAXONOMY

The taxonomic classification of nonhuman primates continues to change as new species are discovered. At least 41 new species of monkeys have been identified since 1980. As new species are identified and genetic and evolutionary relationships are redefined, new taxonomic classification schemes are proposed and debated.

Precise identification of primates in biomedical research is an essential part of their care and management. Because some laboratory species were obtained from the wild or are the offspring of animals obtained from importers many years ago, precise identification may not be documented or may not be correct. Thus, laboratory personnel should have a basic working knowledge of primate taxonomy. Identification is important for experimental reasons as well since some species and subspecies within the same genus respond differently to experimental procedures. Mixing species or subspecies within experimental groups could generate confounding variables leading to inaccurate data. Environmental and nutritional requirements also vary among primate species; therefore, identification may be important for optimizing husbandry, management, and veterinary care programs. Finally, some species are listed as endangered by the CITES treaty. Because the United States and most other countries are CITES signatories, all nonhuman primates must be precisely identified. There are strict regulations on export, import, movement, and use of some species as designated in the CITES appendices.

A. Characteristics Common to All Primates

The defining characteristics of taxa within the order Primates were first published by St. George Mivart in 1873. Mivart (1873) described a primate as "an unguiculate, claviculate, placental mammal with orbits encircled by bone; three kinds of teeth at least at one time of life; brain always with a posterior lobe and a calcarine fissure; the innermost digits of at least one pair of extremities opposable; hallux with a flat nail or none; a well-marked caecum; penis pendulous; testes scrotal; always two pectoral mammae." Nonhuman primates constitute the most diverse taxonomic group of those presented within the chapters of this text. They range in size from pygmy marmosets weighing about 100 g to gorillas weighing as much as 180 kg, and they are indigenous to all continents except Australia and Antarctica.

B. Geographic Distribution

With few exceptions, nonhuman primate species are found in the tropics, ranging from 25° north latitude to 30° south latitude. Habitats range from tropical rain forests to semiarid savannas to desert steppes. Primates are indigenous to regions within Africa, Asia, South America, Central America, and extreme southern Europe. Although most species are found primarily in tropical rain forest and savanna habitats, two species,

M. mulatta and *M. fuscata*, range as far north as Beijing, China, and the island of Honshu in Japan (approximately 41° north latitude) (Napier and Napier, 1967). A number of species and subspecies are now classified by the CITES as either threatened or endangered, primarily due to habitat encroachment from destructive agricultural practices, real estate development, and poaching. The most highly specialized species are most at risk because they have the most strict habitat requirements.

C.   Nomenclature

The classification of extant taxa of nonhuman primates continues to change as more information is accumulated, making classification increasingly complex as new species and subspecies are described. Members of some genera continue to be separated into new species or genera based on information obtained from tools such as those used by molecular geneticists. The classification of nonhuman primates from order to super families is summarized in Table 17.1. Prosimian, platyrrhine, and catarrhine primates are classified to the genus level in Table 17.2. The classification of genera most commonly used in biomedical research is found in Section III. The taxonomic classification of Wilson and Reeder (2005) and Groves (2001), are used by the CITES, the U.S. Fish and Wildlife Service, and international regulatory authorities. Therefore, we have primarily used these taxonomic references for classification in this chapter. However, there are some species names that have changed repeatedly and are subject to different opinions among primatologists. In some species classifications, we have used the more recent nomenclature and cited the associated reference(s).

D.   Comparative Primate Genomics

Much progress has been made in recent years in our understanding of the phylogeny of both human and nonhuman primates. Comparative primate genomics has provided a platform that uses molecular genetics to affirm, reform, and extend classical taxonomic classification that has primarily relied on morphological, adaptive, bio-geographical, reproductive, and behavioral traits for classification (Perelman *et al.*, 2011). Although much of this work has focused on human genetics and its association with diseases, comparative primate genomics has also provided important advances in resolving primate phylogeny and speciation and shows great promise in identifying new primate models of human disease (Fawcett *et al.*, 2011). Because precise identification of nonhuman primates can be critically important in biomedical research, these advances benefit biomedical scientists by helping to better define nonhuman primate models and reduce the number of animals needed to carry out studies. This is especially true of studies that model human diseases. In some cases, even subspecies differences in response to experimental manipulation could result in the failure of a study. With advances in genomics, it is now possible to more precisely identify species, subspecies, and specific genetic variants within a species that are relevant to human disease risk or susceptibility (Rogers and Gibbs, 2014). The identification of intraspecies specific single-nucleotide polymorphisms (SNPs) has been shown to be a useful tool in differentiating between macaques of Chinese *versus* Indian origin or confirming geographic origin in medical records of rhesus monkeys with uncertain origin (Ferguson *et al.*, 2007). Biomedical scientists are now able to request genetic testing that will provide confirmation of the species and geographic origin of macaques and other primate species.

E.   Terms Used in Identification of Primates

The following terms are frequently used by primatologists to describe primate groups.

Old World monkey and **New World monkey** are used to identify genera found in Africa and Asia or South and Central America, respectively. The term **neotropical primate** is considered to be interchangeable with New World monkey to describe primates indigenous to the Americas.
Prosimian is used to describe all taxa within the suborders Strepsirrhini and Haplorrhini, which include lemurs and tarsiers. The word *prosimian*, from the Latin root word meaning 'before monkeys,' refers to their phylogenetic position with respect to simian primates. Prosimian primates are not considered to be 'monkeys.'
Simian is used as an adjective or noun to describe monkeys and apes.
Tarsier is used to describe primates of the genus *Tarsius* that share characteristics of prosimians and simians. Like prosimians, tarsiers are nocturnal, have large eyes and mobile ears, have 'toilet claws' on the foot, and have a two-part mandible. Unlike prosimians, tarsiers lack a naked rhinarium and dental comb. Like anthropoids (simians), tarsiers have upright lower incisors and a dry, furry nose (Napier and Napier, 1985).
Monkey is the common name that describes all species of nonhuman primates except prosimians and apes. Monkeys are distinguished from apes by the presence of an external tail.
Macaque is the common name for primates belonging to the genus *Macaca*. This genus includes rhesus monkeys (*M. mulatta*) and cynomolgus monkeys (*M. fascicularis*), two of the most commonly used species in biomedical research.

TABLE 17.1 Classification of Nonhuman Primates[a]

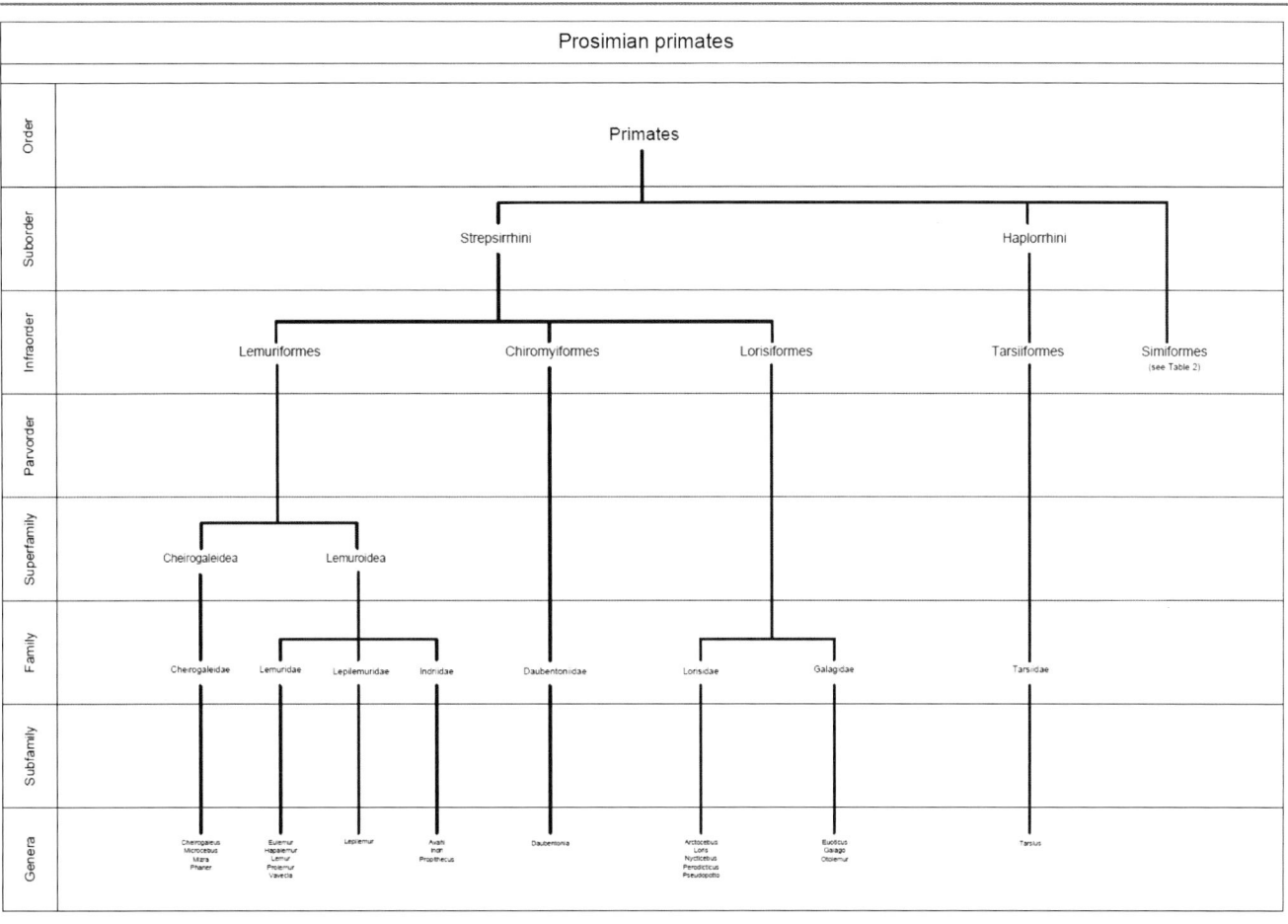

[a]*From Groves (2005).*

Baboon refers to primates belonging to the genus *Papio*.

Great ape is a term used to identify the apes within the family Hominidae. The great apes include chimpanzees, bonobos, gorillas, and orangutans. They are distinguished from monkeys by a number of anatomic features, including lack of tail. They are capable of bipedalism, although quadrupedal locomotion is common.

Lesser ape is a term used to identify members of the family Hylobatidae. Lesser apes include those species referred to as gibbons and siamangs. They are smaller than great apes and are almost entirely arboreal, whereas great apes such as chimpanzees and gorillas spend a large part of their time on the ground. They are true brachiators, using their arms to swing from branch to branch as their primary means of locomotion. They also lack an external tail.

Callitrichid is used as an adjective or noun to describe species in the subfamily Callitrichinae, which includes marmosets and tamarins.

Marmoset is the common name used to identify New World primates belonging to the genera *Callithrix* and *Callimico* within the subfamily Callitrichinae.

Tamarin is the common name used to identify New World primates belonging to the genera *Saguinus* and *Leontopithecus* within the family Callitrichidae.

Prehensile tail is found in some genera of new world monkeys. It has a tactile pad similar to that found on the tactile surface of fingers and palms of hands; it is used as an additional appendage for clinging and hanging from tree limbs. The primate can wrap and constrict its tail in a manner resembling that of an elephant's trunk. Prehensile tails are not found in any Old World monkey taxa.

A **pseudoprehensile** tail is found in some genera of new world monkeys. The term *pseudoprehensile tail* refers to the ability of the animal to grasp and cling with the tail; however, the tail does not possess a tactile pad.

TABLE 17.2   Classifications of Platyrrhine and Catarrhine Primates[a]

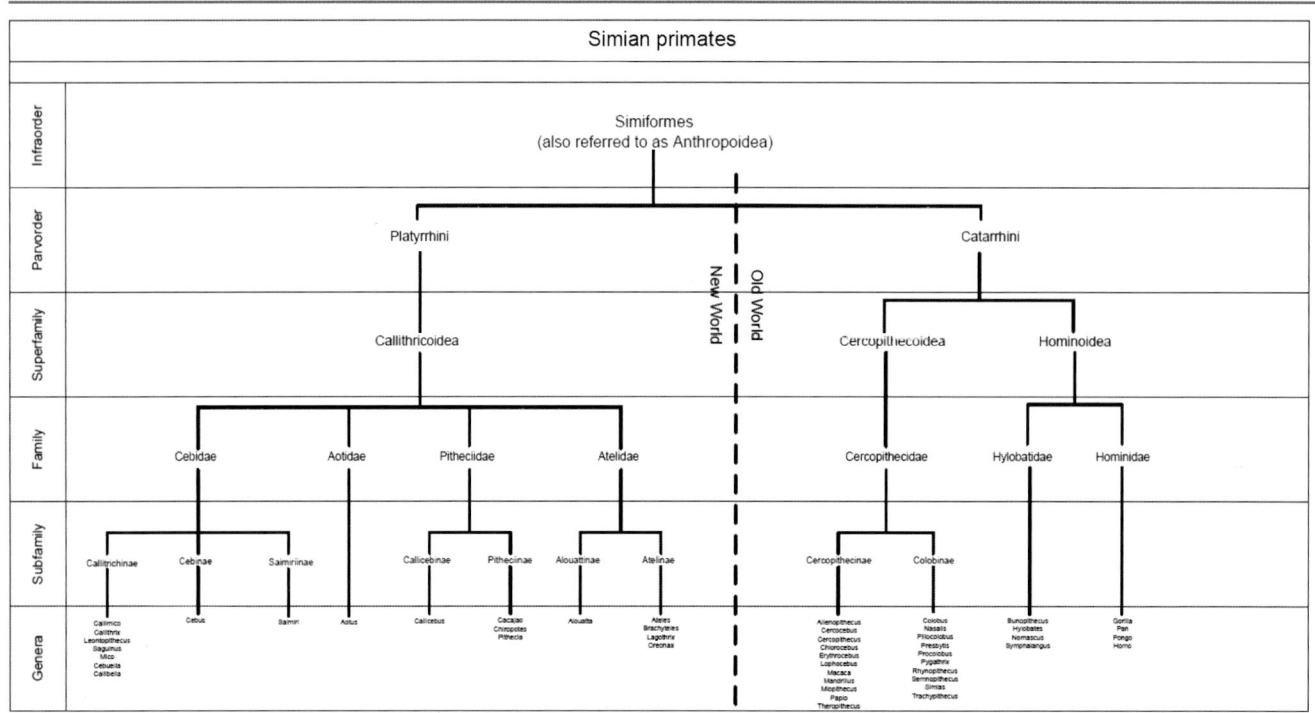

[a]From Groves (2005).

Cheek pouches are specialized pouches found in genera within the family Cercopithecidae. These specialized structures are extensions of the cheeks that extend below each ramus of the mandible. Cheek pouches allow the animal to quickly store food for eating at a later time.

Ischial callosities are specialized pads that cover the skin surface of the ischium and facilitate sitting. They are found in Old World monkeys and lesser apes. These structures are not found in New World monkeys.

Sex Skin is a term used to describe thickening and reddening of the skin in some species of Old World monkeys and apes. Areas affected most often are the perineal region and the upper legs, but it can be observed with almost any skin surface. Sex skin varies due to seasonality and cyclic hormonal fluctuations.

Perineal tumescence is a large cyclic swelling that occurs in some species of Old World monkeys and apes. It is most pronounced during the periovulatory phase of the menstrual cycle. This swelling can be confused with a pathologic process by those unfamiliar with this natural reproductive process.

F. Distinguishing Features of Old World and New World Primates

Nonhuman primates have been classified in part by phenotypic features such as pelage color, pattern and distribution, anatomic characteristics, and geographic distribution. The principal descriptors used to differentiate the parvorders Platyrrhini and Catarrhini are the spacing and orientation of the nares and geographic origin. The term *catarrhine*, meaning 'narrow, turned-down nose,' has been used extensively in the literature to describe Old World monkeys and apes. The term *platyrrhine*, meaning 'flat nose,' refers to the flattened muzzle with broadly spaced, laterally flared nares found in New World monkeys. Although these terms translated from the Latin root words literally refer to the nose, they actually describe the positioning of the nares or openings of the nostrils. Nonhuman primates do not possess a prominent bony, cartilaginous nose as do human beings. The following characteristics may be used to help differentiate prosimian, platyrrhine, and catarrhine primates.

1. Distinguishing features of prosimians
    1. Indigenous to Africa, India, and Southeast Asia.

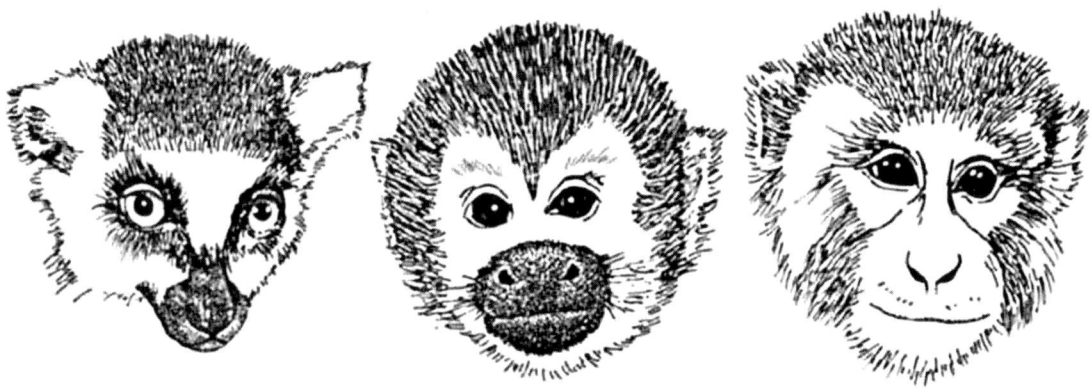

FIGURE 17.1 Distinguishing features of prosimians, New World monkeys, and Old World monkeys. Pictured from left to right are examples of a prosimian (*Lemur catta*), a New World monkey (*Saimiri* spp.), and an Old World monkey (*Macaca mulatta*). Note the rhinarium with a fissured, fixed upper lip in the lemur. The squirrel monkey has broadly spaced, laterally flared nares. The rhesus monkey has an elongate muzzle with narrowly spaced, turned-down nares.

2. Possess a naked, moist snout called a rhinarium with a fissured, fixed upper lip resembling the rhinarium of dogs and cats (Fig. 17.1).
3. All are nocturnal except the genera *Lemur, Varecia, Hapalemur, Indri*, and *Propithecus*.
4. Possess a 'toilet claw' on the second digit of the foot for grooming.
5. Possess a toothcomb for grooming, which is formed from the lower incisors.
6. Possess a sublingual structure for cleaning the toothcomb.
7. The mandible is in two parts joined at the midline by cartilage.
8. Dental formula: 4 incisors + 2 canines + 6 premolars + 6 molars × 2 = 36 (except Indridae with 30).
9. All have epitheliochorial placentas except Tarsiidae, which has hemochorial.

2. Distinguishing features of platyrrhine primates
    1. Indigenous to tropical South and Central America.
    2. Muzzle is flattened with broadly spaced, laterally flared nares (Fig. 17.1).
    3. Some species possess prehensile or pseudoprehensile tails.
    4. Do not possess cheek pouches or ischial callosities.
    5. Require vitamin D_3 in their diet; ingested vitamin D_2 is not bioavailable.
    6. All have estrous cycles, except *Cebus* spp., which menstruate.
    7. All are arboreal.
    8. All are diurnal except *Aotus* spp. (the only nocturnal simian primate).
    9. Dental formulas: Cebinae: 4 incisors + 2 canines + 6 premolars + 6 molars × 2 = 36 Callitrichinae: 4 incisors + 2 canines + 6

premolars + 4 molars × 2 = 32 (except genus *Callicebus* with 36 as in Cebinae).
    10. All have hemochorial placentas.
3. Distinguishing features of catarrhine primates
    1. Indigenous to Africa, Asia, and extreme southern Europe (introduced to Gibraltar).
    2. Muzzle is elongate (varying in degree among genera) with narrowly spaced, turned-down nares (Fig. 17.1).
    3. Some species possess ischial callosities for sitting.
    4. Cheek pouches for storing food are found in some genera of Cercopithecidae.
    5. All have menstrual cycles.
    6. Some species are adapted to terrestrial living while others are primarily arboreal.
    7. All can utilize vitamin D_2 in their diet.
    8. Dental formula: 4 incisors + 2 canines + 4 premolars + 6 molars × 2 = 32
    9. All are diurnal.
    10. All have hemochorial placentas.

III. BIOLOGY

A. Callitrichinae: Marmosets and Tamarins

1. Introduction

Marmosets and tamarins are New world monkeys that are distinguished from other nonhuman primates by their small size, which ranges from 100 to 850 g; their dental formula (2/2, 1/1, 3/3, 2/2); claws or falcula instead of nails on the digits; little to no sexual dimorphism; and a high frequency of twinning, approximately 80% (Gengozian *et al.*, 1978; Rensing and Oerke, 2005). They have a specialized nail on the first digit of each foot, the hallux, which is opposable, whereas the thumb is not. Callitrichids have two distinct scent-marking

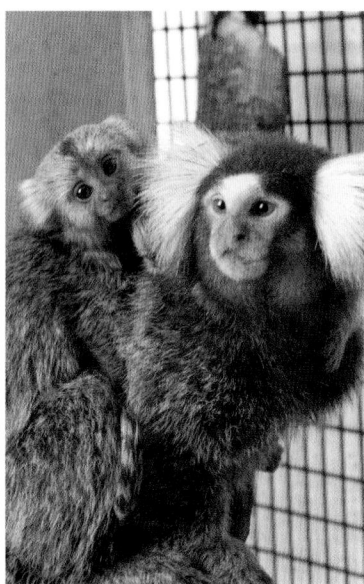

FIGURE 17.2   *Callithrix jacchus*, the common marmoset, with infant from Suzette Tardif, Texas Biomedical Research Institute, Southwest National Primate Research Center, San Antonio, Texas.

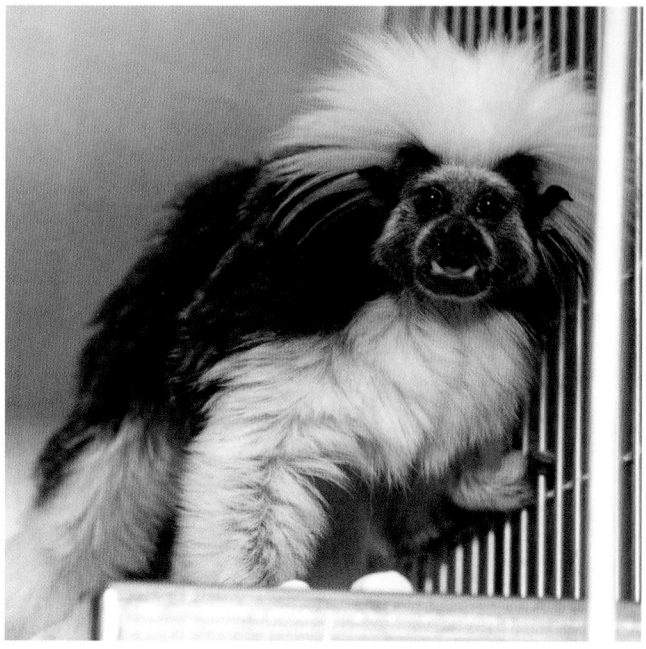

FIGURE 17.3   *Saguinus oedipus*, adult cotton-top tamarin, from David B. Elmore, D.V.M., New England National Primate Research Center, Southboro, Massachusetts.

glands. Circumgenital glands are well-developed sebaceous glands overlying enlarged apocrine glands that cover the labia majora and pudendum in the female and the scrotum in the male. Sternal glands are predominantly apocrine glands located on the anterior chest and may be focal or diffuse in structure (Epple *et al.*, 1993).

In general, marmosets are smaller than tamarins. Marmosets have procumbent incisor teeth that are the same length as the canine teeth. This dental arrangement enables them to gnaw holes in trees and eat gums and exudates, a staple of their diet. Tamarins have longer canine teeth, which can assist in differentiating the genera (NRC, 1998). This chapter will focus on the two most commonly used research species, marmosets of the genus *Callithrix* (Fig. 17.2) and tamarins of the genus *Saguinus* (Fig. 17.3).

Callithrix jacchus is one of six nonhuman primate species that was proposed for complete genome mapping (Abbott *et al.*, 2003). The marmoset genome has been sequenced by the Genome Institute at Washington University (St. Louis, MO) in collaboration with Baylor College of Medicine Human Genome Sequencing Center (BCM-HGSC) (Worley *et al.*, 2014).

2. Taxonomy

The Callitrichinae subfamily contains seven genera: *Callithrix*, *Mico*, *Cebuella*, *Callibella*, *Saguinus*, *Leontopithecus*, and *Callimico* (Cortés-Ortiz, 2009; Rylands and Mittermeier, 2009). A list of the *Callithrix*, *Mico*, and *Saguinus* species is found in Tables 17.3 and 17.4.

3. Natural History

Marmosets and tamarins prefer different habitats although their ranges may overlap. Marmosets are found throughout most of Brazil, primarily in savanna/forest habitats. The common marmoset (*C. jacchus*) prefers secondary or disturbed forests or edge habitats. Tamarins of the genus *Saguinus* are found throughout much of the lowland neotropical rain forest from Panama to Bolivia to northeastern Brazil and prefer primary or secondary forest. The size of territory varies considerably with species and within species: from 1 hectare for *C. jacchus* (Stevenson, 1977) to 30–50 hectares for *Saguinus nigricollis* (Izawa, 1978). Daily travel for a marmoset group is about 500–1000 m. Availability of food supply is probably the single most important determinant for group territory size. Callitrichids are territorial and may patrol and defend their territory vigorously from other groups (Dawson, 1977).

Group size ranges from 2 to 15, with the mean group size for most species falling in the range of four to seven individuals. Larger groups of 40+ are rarely seen and are assumed to be temporary associations of several family groups (Izawa, 1978). Group sizes vary due to emigration and immigration of transients, usually subadults (Dawson, 1977). Group composition is dependent on the species, and several compositions are possible. In *C. jacchus*, group composition may be multimale–multifemale, one male–multifemale, or one female–multimale (Scanlon *et al.*, 1988). Usually, common marmoset groups contain only one breeding pair, composed of

TABLE 17.3   Marmoset Taxonomy, CITES Status, and Distribution

Genus *Callithrix* or *Mico*	Common name(s)[a]	CITES[b] status	Distribution[c]
C. aurita	Buffy-tufted-ear marmoset	I	Brazil
C. flaviceps	Buffy-headed marmoset	I	Brazil
C. geoffroyi	Geoffroy's tufted-ear marmoset	II	Brazil
C. jacchus	Common marmoset	II	Brazil
C. kuhlii	Wied's black-tufted-ear marmoset	II	Brazil
C. penicillata	Black-tufted-ear marmoset	II	Brazil
M. acariensis	Rio Acarí marmoset	II	Brazil
M. argentatus	Silvery marmoset	II	Brazil
M. chrysoleucus	Golden-white tassel-ear marmoset	II	Brazil
M. cf. emiliae (rondoni)	Rondônia marmoset	?	Brazil
M. emiliae	Snethlage's marmoset	II	Brazil
M. humeralifer	Black and white tassel-ear marmoset	II	Brazil
M. intermedius	Aripuanã marmoset	II	Brazil
M. leucippe	Golden-white bare-ear marmoset	II	Brazil
M. manicorensis	Manicoré marmoset	II	Brazil
M. marcai	Marca's marmoset	II	Brazil
M. mauesi	Maués marmoset	II	Brazil
M. melanurus	Black-tailed marmoset	II	Bolivia, Brazil
M. nigriceps	Black-headed marmoset	II	Brazil
M. saterei	Sataré marmoset	II	Brazil

[a]Rylands and Mittermeier (2009).
[b]I, species listed in CITES Appendix I are threatened with extinction (endangered); II, species listed in CITES Appendix II are not currently threatened with extinction but may become so unless trade is strictly regulated. From CITES (20 June 2013).
[c]From IUCN Red List of Endangered Species (2013.1).

TABLE 17.4   Tamarin Taxonomy, CITES Status, and Distribution

Genus *Saguinus*	Common name(s)[a]	CITES[b] status	Distribution[c]
S. bicolor	Pied Bare-face tamarin	I	Brazil
S. fuscicollis	Saddle-back tamarin	II	Bolivia, Brazil, Colombia, Ecuador, Peru
S. geoffroyi	Geoffroy's tamarin	I	Colombia, Panama
S. imperator	Emperor tamarin	II	Bolivia, Brazil, Colombia, Peru
S. inustus	Mottled-faced tamarin	II	Brazil, Colombia
S. labiatus	Red-bellied tamarin	II	Bolivia, Brazil, Peru
S. leucopus	Silvery-brown tamarin	I	Colombia
S martinsi	Bare-face tamarin	I	Brazil
S. melanoleucus	Saddle-back tamarin	II	Brazil, Peru
S. midas	Golden-handed tamarin	II	Brazil, French Guiana, Guyana, Suriname
S. mystax	Mustached tamarin	II	Brazil, Peru
S. niger	Black-handed tamarin	II	Brazil
S. nigricollis	Black-mantle tamarin	II	Brazil, Colombia, Ecuador, Peru
S. oedipus	Cotton-top tamarin	I	Colombia
S. tripartitus	Golden-mantle saddle-back tamarin	II	Ecuador, Peru

[a]Rylands and Mittermeier (2009).
[b]I, species listed in CITES Appendix I are threatened with extinction (endangered); II, species listed in CITES Appendix II are not currently threatened with extinction but may become so unless trade is strictly regulated. From CITES (20 June 2013).
[c]From IUCN Red List of Endangered Species (2013.1).

the highest-ranking male and female within the group (Abbott *et al.*, 2003; Faulkes *et al.*, 2003). Although only the dominant male and female reproduce, all group members generally contribute to infant rearing (Abbott *et al.*, 2003; Faulkes *et al.*, 2003; Tardif, 1997). It has been shown that prolactin levels in fathers and older offspring of both sexes increase in association with the physical effort of raising the infants (da Silva Mota *et al.*, 2006). Tamarins have a multimale–multifemale social structure, and groups consist of unrelated and related adults and offspring (Garber, 1993; Savage *et al.*, 1996). The mating system is usually polyandry; multiple males copulate with the reproductive dominant female. Polygyny and monogamy also occur (Garber, 1993; Kinzey, 1997).

Group members sleep in huddles together in one of a number of familiar nesting trees within their territory (Caine, 1993). Callitrichids are diurnal; group activity usually begins 0–1.5 h after sunrise (Kantha and Suzuki, 2006). They will spend approximately 20% of the day traveling and 30–60% of the day foraging (Passamani, 1998; Rensing and Oerke, 2005).

Marmosets and tamarins are omnivorous, feeding on insects, fruits, nectars, buds and flowers, tree exudates (gum and sap), and whatever small animals they can capture. Many marmoset species spend considerable time consuming tree exudates and gums either by gnawing the bark or by consuming exudates released by other trauma to the tree (Coimbra-Filho and Mittermeier, 1977; ILAR, 1998). Tamarins eat more fruits but also consume tree exudates released by penetration of the bark (Garber, 1980). They lack the dentition to gnaw on trees to release sap, but use the sap exudate flows created by other animals (ILAR, 1998).

4. Reproduction

Callitrichids are unique in that usually only one adult female in an extended breeding group reproduces; subordinate females, usually offspring of the breeding female, may or may not have an estrous cycle, depending on the species. In general, nonbreeding females in the genuses *Callithrix* and *Saguinus* do not ovulate in the presence of the dominant female (Abbott *et al.*, 1981, 1993; Tardif, 1997), although exceptions have been noted (Savage *et al.*, 1997; Ziegler and Sousa, 2002). This suppression of cyclicity is thought to be caused by scent marking of the dominant female (Epple, 1970b; Epple *et al.*, 1993).

The ovarian cycle of the common marmoset has been reported to average 28.6 days (Saltzman *et al.*, 2011; Tardif *et al.*, 2012). The estrous cycle can be followed by changes in peripheral plasma hormone levels or hormone levels in urine or feces (Hodgen *et al.*, 1976; Hodges *et al.*, 1979). A marked rise in plasma progesterone within 1 day postovulation is a useful indicator of ovulation (Saltzman *et al.*, 2011). In the common marmoset there is no lactational anestrus, and Hearn and Lunn (1975) have reported that estrus occurs as early as 3

days postpartum. Ovulation occurs 9–11 days following parturition (Tardif *et al.*, 2012), and increased copulations are observed (Dixson and Lunn, 1987). The estrous cycle is slightly shorter in tamarins. In *S. fuscicollis*, the ovarian cycle lasts 25.7 days (Heistermann and Hodges, 1995) and in *S. oedipus*, 22.7 days (Saltzman *et al.*, 2011). Tamarins do not have a postpartum estrus, in contrast to marmosets (Savage *et al.*, 1997).

Gestation ranges and other reproductive parameters on selected species are provided in Table 17.5. Pregnancy can be diagnosed as early as 2 weeks by measurement of plasma or urine placental chorionic gonadotropin (Hodges *et al.*, 1979) or via measurement of the urinary progesterone metabolite, hydroxypregnanolone (Heger and Neubert, 1987). Diagnostic ultrasound is also used to diagnose pregnancy, follow prenatal growth, and estimate delivery date (Jaquish *et al.*, 1995; Oerke *et al.*, 1995). Female callitrichids are polyovulatory and dizygotic twinning is the rule, but singleton births, triplets, and even quadruplets occur (Tardif *et al.*, 2003, 2012). Blood chimerism occurs in callitrichids due to placental vascular anastomoses (Haig, 1999). Female callitrichid species avoid becoming freemartins *in utero* as often occurs with twinning in cattle via an effective aromatizing enzyme system, which converts androgens to estrone (Ryan *et al.*, 1961). Since many singletons are the result of a twin being resorbed, they are commonly chimeric; however, nonchimeric singletons can occur (Gengozian and Batson, 1975).

In most captive colonies of marmosets and tamarins there is no seasonality to births (Tardif *et al.*, 2012; Snowdon *et al.*, 1985), although these animals are seasonal breeders in the wild (McGrew and Webster, 1995). Most deliveries occur at night (Stevenson and Poole, 1976). Lactation lasts for 65–90 days in common marmosets, and infants begin to eat solid food at 30 days of age. Young are completely weaned by 100 days of age (Tardif *et al.*, 2012). Hand rearing of callitrichid infants may be attempted because of parental neglect (Pook, 1976) or for research purposes (Wolfe *et al.*, 1972). Hand rearing can be difficult with a high failure rate, behavioral abnormalities in surviving individuals, and low cost-effectiveness (Richter *et al.*, 1984).

Reproductive capacity of callitrichids exceeds that of any other simian primate because of postpartum estrus and twinning. Records of over 20 infants per reproductive female in several species have been reported (Richter *et al.*, 1984). Sex ratios of offspring are 1:1, and twins normally show the predicted 1:2:1 ratio (Gengozian *et al.*, 1977). First pregnancies may occur as early as 1 year of age; however, in view of normal growth and behavior requirements, planned mating at 1.5–2 years of age is preferable (Tardif *et al.*, 2012; Rensing and Oerke, 2005). There is a high rate of infant-rearing failure among primiparous captive-born females in some species. Most infant loss appears to be the result of failure of young

TABLE 17.5 Reproductive Parameters for Marmosets and Tamarins

Species	Gestation period (days)	Ovarian cycle length (days)	Age at sexual maturity (days)	Birth weights mean (g)	Interbirth interval (months)
Callithrix jacchus	148[a]	28.6[a]	F: 477[a]	29.68 ± 3.41[b]	6[a]
			M: 382[a]		
Saguinus oedipus	168[a]	22.7[a]	F: 548[a]	40[c]	7[a]
			M: 550[a]		
Saguinus fuscicollis	150–155[d]	25.7[e]	F: 398–631[f]	39.9[i]	6[i]
			M: 444–627[f]		
Saguinus labiatus	140–150[g]	–	–	42.3[i]	7–10[h]
Saguinus mystax	140–150[g]	–	F: 486[i]	46.9[i]	11[k]
			M: 540[i]		

[a]From Saltzman et al. *(2011)*.
[b]Tardif and Bales *(2004)*.
[c]Richter et al. *(1984)*.
[d]Rensing and Oerke *(2005)*.
[e]Heistermann and Hodges *(1995)*.
[f]Epple and Katz *(1980)*.
[g]From Goldizen *(1987)*.
[h]Coates and Poole *(1983)*.
[i]AnAge: The Animal Ageing and Longevity Database, *http://genomics.senescence.info/species/*.
[j]Tardif et al. *(1984)*.
[k]Löttker et al. *(2004)*.

females to accept and nurse their young (Rensing and Oerke, 2005).

5. Laboratory Management

Marmosets and tamarins are usually housed as pairs or in small family groups. Although multiple male and multiple female breeding groups occur in the wild, in captivity most are raised as extended families or monogamous pairs with a single breeding female (Layne and Power, 2003). If animals must be singly housed for research purposes, efforts should be made to allow visual, olfactory, and tactile (if possible) contact with compatible conspecifics (Rensing and Oerke, 2005).

Environmental temperatures for callitrichids in the laboratory may need to be relatively warm. Studies on thermoregulation in the cotton-top tamarin indicate that tamarins do not acclimate to a temperate environment and are metabolically stressed at an ambient temperature less than 32°C (89°F) (Stonerook et al., 1994). Cold stress associated with low ambient temperatures in captive environments has been proposed as a possible stressor leading to the development of chronic colitis in this species (Stonerook et al., 1994).

Large cages with branches, ropes, or other substrates for climbing are preferable and have been used successfully in breeding colonies (ILAR, 1998). Single, narrow high cages are preferable to wide, low cages placed over each other in a two-tiered system. Callitrichids spend little time on the floor of the cage, and it has been shown that animals housed in the lower cage of a two-tiered system are reported to have decreased activity levels and poorer reproductive performance than those housed in the upper tier (ILAR, 1998). Cages should be built with high vertical space for the monkeys to 'escape' above human eye level (Rensing and Oerke, 2005). Minimum cage space requirements can be found in both the *Animal Welfare Act* (USDA, 2013) and the *Guide for the Care and Use of Laboratory Animals* (NRC, 2011a); however, it is important to note that these are minimum requirements, and every effort should be made to exceed these minimum standards. Perches and nest boxes are often added to the cage for enrichment purposes. Callitrichids require a flat surface for sleeping and a nest box provides this flat surface where the animal can assume a curled posture to conserve body heat (Richter *et al.*, 1984). The nest box should have a viewing area at one end for observation and a closable opening into the cage. This configuration allows the nest box to serve as a capture box to isolate animals for procedures or cleaning purposes (Layne and Power, 2003). Nest boxes should be sanitized every other week, preferably on an alternate schedule from sanitization of the cages to allow for retention of social odor or scent marks (ILAR, 1998). Feeding areas or stations should be above the floor and multiple stations provided if more than one animal is in the cage. Lactating females may dominate feeding stations and consume most of the preferred food if additional feeding sites are not made available to accommodate other group members (Tardif and Richter, 1981).

Social, especially sexual, and territorial messages are conveyed by scent marking (Epple, 1973). Both sexes mark by rubbing the genitalia, pubis, or chest on the object being marked. Both sexes also mark with urine. Therefore, it is important to have materials within the cage, preferably wood or fiber, for scent marking. Wood or fiber structures, such as rope, can be replaced as they wear out in 2–3 months, or as necessary to maintain sanitation (ILAR, 1998). If the item for scent marking is to be sanitized, it should be on an alternate schedule from regular cage sanitation to allow some marked surfaces to remain within the living area at all times (ILAR, 1998).

In the wild, marmosets and tamarins are highly territorial. This natural behavior must be considered in captive housed callitrichids as they may display threatening behavior toward neighboring social groups. Incorporating visual barriers may decrease this aggressive behavior in group housed callitrichids (ILAR, 1998). Allogrooming and play are also part of normal callitrichid behavior. Allogrooming is observed more among sexually mature individuals, whereas play is seen among infants and subadults. Aggression can be seen among any family members, but is usually nondestructive (Wolters, 1977) and brief. Destructive agonistic behavior can result in injury and may require permanent separation of involved individuals. The introduction of mature adults into breeding groups in captivity is destabilizing and may result in fighting (Epple, 1970a).

6. Nutrition

Marmosets and tamarins have a high metabolic rate, shorter gastrointestinal transit times, and faster growth rates than other nonhuman primates. This correlates with a need for a high-energy diet. Many formulated New World primate diets contain 9–10% fat (increased during periods of lactation) and 20–25% protein (Layne and Power, 2003). Callitrichids also require a dietary source for vitamin D_3 and ascorbic acid. The National Research Council currently recommends at least 1000–3000 IU of vitamin D_3/kg of dry diet (2003); however, this nutritional issue has been addressed in commercial diet formulations (Ullrey et al., 1999). Dietary iron levels found in standard New World primate diets have traditionally been associated with the development of hepatic hemosiderosis in marmosets (Miller et al., 1997). While refinements to commercial diets have addressed this and decreased iron content, some may still be on the high end of the current recommendations (Kramer et al., 2014), and individual diet analysis should be considered.

Most callitrichid husbandry programs feed varied diets in an effort to improve general health status. These varied diets often consist of a commercially available canned or biscuit base (ZuPreem Marmoset Diet, Premium Nutritional Products, Inc., Mission, KS), with added supplements such as fresh or dried fruit, vegetables, vitamin C, and protein energy sources (Layne and Power, 2003). Variation in diet may be used as an enrichment tool but must be fed in a disciplined manner to ensure a nutritionally balanced diet. Individual monkeys need to be observed closely to determine that they eat a balanced diet and not only preferred items, such as fruit. Historically, some investigators have supplemented with high-protein foods such as cottage cheese, quail or chicken eggs, minced meat, and/or mealworms (ILAR, 1998; Layne and Power, 2003); however with balanced commercial diets such supplementation is not nutritionally required. Historically, feeding of neonatal mice was used as a protein source, but this is no longer in common use. This source of protein supplementation should be discouraged as it could be a potential source of pathogen transmission (Montali et al., 1993).

Callithrix jacchus are affected by a chronic inflammatory bowel disease (IBD) which affects primarily the small intestine resulting in villous atrophy and a maldigestion malabsorption syndrome. While often referred to as 'marmoset wasting disease', this term should be avoided as it has been linked to several distinct etiologies including protein deficiency (Brack and Rothe, 1981), food allergens (Gore et al., 2001) and chronic parasitism (Beglinger et al., 1988). This form of IBD is widespread throughout captive marmoset colonies and is characterized by weight loss, muscular atrophy, anemia, and hypoalbuminemia (Ludlage and Mansfield, 2003). Thus far, no effective treatment exists and prognosis is poor (Ludlage and Mansfield, 2003). Saguinus oedipus may also develop a form of IBD, but in this species lesions are present in the large intestine and characterized by chronic active inflammation with crypt abcessesation. Tamarin colitis has been used as a model of ulcerative colitis of man and may be modified by dietary, environmental, and genetic factors.

7. Normal Values

Normal daytime rectal temperature for callitrichids varies between 39.1°C and 40.6°C (Cilia et al., 1998; Rensing and Oerke, 2005). The wide range may reflect the excitability of the species, rigors involved in catching, and nocturnal torpor. Callitrichids develop a distinct torpor with hypothermia (34.0°C) during sleep (Hetherington, 1978). Normal hemogram and blood chemistry values for three species of callitrichids are given in Tables 17.6 and 17.7. Detailed hematologic and chemistry reference values are available for C. jacchus (McNees et al., 1982; Hawkey et al., 1982; Rensing and Oerke, 2005), S. oedipus (Shukan et al., 2012), and S. labiatus (Wadsworth et al., 1982). Small numbers of nucleated red blood cells are commonly seen in callitrichid blood smears (Rensing and Oerke, 2005).

8. Research Uses

Marmosets and tamarins are well suited for some types of research due to their relatively small body size,

TABLE 17.6 Marmoset and Tamarin Hemograms

Hemograms (mean values ±1 SD)

Value	Unit	*Callithrix jacchus*[a,b]	*Saguinus oedipus*[c]	*Saguinus labiatus*[d]
RBC	$\times10^6/\mu l$	F: 6.2 ± 0.7	F: 6.13 ± 0.35	F: 6.9 ± 0.5
		M: 6.7 ± 0.8	M: 6.42 ± 0.20	M: 7.0 ± 0.3
Hemoglobin	g/dl	F: 14.2 ± 1.8	F: 16.51 ± 1.06	F: 16.6 ± 1.4
		M: 15.5 ± 1.9	M: 17.50 ± 0.85	M: 17.4 ± 0.7
Hematocrit	%	F: 41 ± 6.5	F: 49.21 ± 3.03	F: 51 ± 4.0
		M: 44 ± 7.5	M: 52.19 ± 1.94	M: 52 ± 3.0
MCV	fl	F: 65 ± 6.0	F: 79.03 ± 4.93	F: 73 ± 3.5
		M: 66 ± 4.4	M: 81.33 ± 2.68	M: 74 ± 4.0
MCH	varies	25.8 ± 2.7 mg/dl	F: 26.91 ± 1.16 pg	F: 24 ± 1.4 pg
			M: 27.08 ± 1.33 pg	M: 25 ± 1.3 pg
MCHC	g/dl	34.2 ± 4.5	F: 33.56 ± 0.77	F: 33 ± 1.1
			M: 33.31 ± 1.16	M: 33 ± 1.0
WBC	$\times10^3/\mu l$	F: 12.0 ± 10.4	F: 7.41 ± 2.49	F: 13.0 ± 3.2
		M: 12.1 ± 10.8	M: 5.92 ± 1.85	M: 10.8 ± 3.5
Segmented neutrophils	$\times10^3/\mu l$	3.2 ± 1.5	F: 3.42 ± 1.16	F: 5.58 ± 3.02
			M: 2.88 ± 1.17	M: 4.48 ± 2.27
Lymphocytes	$\times10^3/\mu l$	3.0 ± 1.6	F: 2.96 ± 1.40	F: 6.85 ± 1.85
			M: 2.37 ± 1.09	M: 5.91 ± 2.75
Monocytes	$\times10^3/\mu l$	0.25 ± 0.18	F: 0.36 ± 0.21	F: 0.40 ± 0.18
			M: 0.38 ± 0.20	M: 0.27 ± 0.19
Eosinophils	$\times10^3/\mu l$	0.23 ± 0.14	F: 0.16 ± 0.14	F: 0.13 ± 0.18
			M: 0.18 ± 0.14	M: 0.08 ± 0.13
Basophils	$\times10^3/\mu l$	0.16 ± 0.15	F: 0.07 ± 0.06	F: 0.08 ± 0.12
			M: 0.06 ± 0.06	M: 0.08 ± 0.07
Platelets	$\times10^3/\mu l$	609 ± 200	F: 267.71 ± 63.98	F: 402 ± 82
			M: 253.94 ± 57.19	M: 428 ± 95
Prothrombin time	seconds	–	–	F: 7.1 ± 0.4
				M: 7.1 ± 0.5
Partial thromboplastin with kaolin	seconds	–	–	F: 32.7 ± 3.9
				M: 31.7 ± 3.4

RBC, red blood cell; MCV, mean corpuscular volume; MCH, mean corpuscular hemoglobin; MCHC, mean corpuscular hemoglobin concentration; WBC, white blood cell.
[a]*Rensing and Oerke (2005).*
[b]*McNees* et al. *(1982).*
[c]*Shukan* et al. *(2012).*
[d]*Wadsworth* et al. *(1982).*

more affordable housing and animal care costs, high reproductive capacity in captivity (especially true of marmosets), and earlier age of sexual maturity in comparison to macaque species. Marmosets and tamarins do not carry latent infections of macacine herpesvirus 1 (B virus) which makes handling safer than the more commonly used macaque species. One disadvantage of these species as animal models is that their small body size may limit sample size and collection frequencies (Mansfield, 2003).

C. jacchus, or common marmoset, is the callitrichid species most widely used in biomedical research and serves as an animal model in a variety of research

TABLE 17.7   Blood Chemistry Values for Marmosets and Tamarins

Parameter	Unit	Callithrix jacchus[a]	Saguinus oedipus[b]	Saguinus labiatus[c]
Glucose	Varies	177 ± 65 mg/dl	F: 262.95 ± 95.67 mg/dl	F: 8.0 ± 2.4 mmol/l
			M: 266 ± 96.34 mg/dl	M: 8.6 ± 2.5 mmol/l
Cholesterol	mg/dl	176 ± 73	F: 134.67 ± 31.04	–
			M: 153.94 ± 51.04	
Uric acid	mg/dl	0.5 ± 0.2	–	–
BUN	Varies	19 ± 5 mg/dl	F: 15.86 ± 3.35 mg/dl	F: 8.8 ± 1.9 mmol/l
			M: 14.35 ± 2.89 mg/dl	M: 8.5 ± 2.4 mmol/l
Creatinine	Varies	0.7 ± 0.2 mg/dl	F: 0.33 ± 0.09 mg/dl	F: 74 ± 9.4 μmol/l
			M: 0.41 ± 0.15 mg/dl	M: 83 ± 8.2 μmol/l
Fructosamine	μmol/l	–	F: 255.58 ± 47.62	–
			M: 255.79 ± 53.62	
Total bilirubin	Varies	0.2 ± 0.3 mg/dl	F: 0.14 ± 0.06 mg/dl	F: 9 ± 6.5 μmol/l
			M: 0.15 ± 0.07 mg/dl	M: 10 ± 5.7 μmol/l
Direct bilirubin	mg/dl	0.0 ± 0.0	–	–
Indirect bilirubin	mg/dl	0.1 ± 0.0	–	–
Total protein	g/dl	6.8 ± 1.0	F: 6.41 ± 0.35	F: 7.2 ± 0.76
			M: 6.24 ± 0.40	M: 7.1 ± 0.42
Albumin	g/dl	5.1 ± 0.6	F: 4.06 ± 0.31	F: 4.0 ± 0.42
			M: 3.97 ± 0.30	M: 3.9 ± 0.47
Globulin	g/dl	1.7 ± 0.5	F: 2.36 ± 0.27	–
			M: 2.27 ± 0.34	
ALP	U/l	125 ± 64	F: 116.19 ± 30.89	F: 519 ± 280
			M: 96.29 ± 14.76	M: 674 ± 832
ALT	U/l	13 ± 24	F: 44.43 ± 28.28	F: 33 ± 14.1
			M: 44.71 ± 29.67	M: 32 ± 14.6
AST	U/l	112 ± 112	F: 186.43 ± 68.16	F: 179 ± 41.4
			M: 198.13 ± 76.41	M: 184 ± 42.0
LDH	U/l	551 ± 429	–	–
CK	U/l	543 ± 0	F: 865.25 ± 421	F: 617 ± 1056
			M: 772.47 ± 354.08	M: 973 ± 1381
Calcium	varies	9.5 ± 1.1 mg/dl	F: 9.02 ± 0.50 mg/dl	F: 2.6 ± 0.17 mmol/l
			M: 8.69 ± 0.59 mg/dl	M: 2.5 ± 0.20 mmol/l
Phosphorus	mg/dl	5.3 ± 1.9 mg/dl	F: 2.81 ± 0.67	–
			M: 3.21 ± 0.64	
Sodium	mmol/l	147 ± 8	F: 150.50 ± 2.12	F: 156 ± 6.3
			M: 150.06 ± 2.54	M: 159 ± 5.0
Potassium	mmol/l	4.9 ± 2.6	F: 4.04 ± 0.44	F: 4.5 ± 0.78
			M: 4.25 ± 0.64	M: 4.0 ± 0.95
Chloride	mEq/l	103 ± 11	F: 106 ± 2.79	–
			M: 104.4 ± 2.35	
Magnesium	mg/dl	–	F: 1.97 ± 0.16	–
			M: 2.03 ± 0.16	
CO_2	mEq/l	–	F: 26.37 ± 2.67	–
			M: 24.75 ± 3.38	
Iron	mg/dl	129 ± 1	–	–

BUN, blood urea nitrogen; AST, Alanine aminotransferase; AST, Aspartate aminotransferase; ALP, Alkaline phosphatase; GGT, Gamma glutamyltransferase; LDH, lactate dehydrogenase;

[a]Rensing and Oerke (2005).
[b]Shukan et al. (2012).
[c]Wadsworth et al. (1982).

areas, including pharmacology, toxicology, neurophysiology, reproductive biology, and viral oncology, and as a model of infectious and noninfectious disease (Mansfield, 2003). Common marmosets have served as models of Parkinson's disease (Gibb *et al.*, 1987; Eslamboli, 2005), aging and age-related diseases (Tardif *et al.*, 2011a), and models of experimental allergic encephalomyelitis, which mimics several facets of multiple sclerosis in humans (Genain and Hauser, 1996, 1997; 't Hart *et al.*, 2007). They are also models for idiopathic hemochromatosis (Bulte *et al.*, 1997; Miller *et al.*, 1997). Research with tamarins has progressively decreased over the years due in part to classification of these species as endangered requiring a permit from the U.S. Fish and Wildlife Service before they can serve as research subjects. The cotton-top tamarin (*S. oedipus*), a critically endangered species (CITES Appendix I), is a research model of chronic colitis and colon cancer (Kirkwood *et al.*, 1986; Clap *et al.*, 1988; David *et al.*, 2009). *Saguinus labiatus*, the red-bellied tamarin, and *S. mystax*, the mustached tamarin, are used in viral hepatitis studies (Bukh *et al.*, 2001; Schlauder *et al.*, 1995), and more recently *S. mystax* has shown promise as a model for cardiomyopathy (Gozalo *et al.*, 2008, 2011).

B. *Aotus* spp.: Owl Monkeys

1. Introduction

Owl monkeys are small New world monkeys that weigh approximately 1 kg. Although there are a number of prosimian species that are nocturnal, the Owl monkey is the only nocturnal simian primate genus (Fernández-Duque *et al.*, 2010). Owl monkeys are an arboreal, monogamous genus living as pairs or in small family groups (Fig. 17.4).

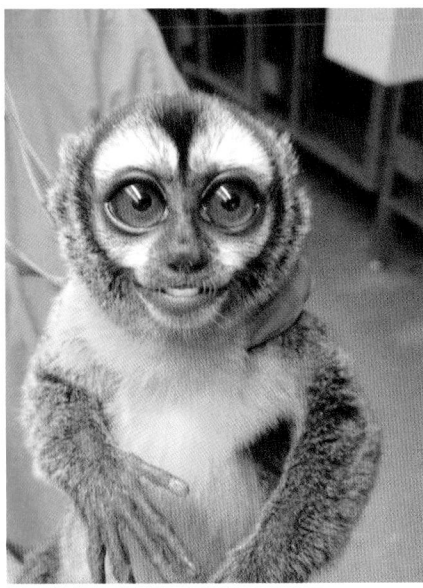

FIGURE 17.4   *Aotus nancymaae*, owl monkey adult.

They are not sexually dimorphic. The *Aotus* genus appears to have evolved from a diurnal ancestor because the eyes retain vestigial features characteristic of diurnal vision, such as a retinal fovea. *Aotus* spp. are superior to diurnal New World monkeys in seeing and following moving objects, and spatial resolution at low light levels. The eyes are large with a more spherical lens than found in diurnal monkeys, enabling refraction and focus of an image on the retina at low light levels. Unlike other nocturnal mammals, *Aotus* spp. lack a tapetum lucidum. The large retina contains both rods and cones, with a markedly decreased number of cones compared to other primates (Wright, 1989, 1994), but a comparatively increased number of rods (Finlay *et al.*, 2008).

Owl monkeys have a low basal metabolic rate, 18–24% below the predicted value for a 1-kg mammal (LeMaho *et al.*, 1981). The low basal metabolic rate is believed to be an adaptation of nocturnal mammals that allows survival with less energy consumption (Crompton *et al.*, 1978). In contrast, the squirrel monkey, a diurnal New World monkey of similar body size, has a metabolic rate 10% above the predicted value.

2. Taxonomy

Owl monkeys belong to a single genus, yet they have a wide variation in diploid chromosome number, from 46 to 56. Karyotypic variation may also occur within the species, as in *A. griseimembra*, *A. lemurinus*, and *A. vociferans* (Defler and Bueno, 2007). In the wild, some *Aotus* populations can experience a degree of chromosomal/karyotypic variation without speciation or cross-infertility. In particular, *A. lemurinus* and *A. vociferans* populations in Colombia and Panama, respectively, have chromosomal polymorphisms that do not pose a barrier to fertility or fitness (Ma, 1981; Ma *et al.*, 1985; Ma and Harris, 1989). *Aotus* species have a high degree of morphological similarities and karyotype is useful for more precise identification, an important consideration when conducting biomedical research or managing breeding colonies of *Aotus* spp. (Hershkovitz, 1983; Menezes *et al.*, 2010).

As with several species discussed in this chapter, there is debate about taxonomic designations for members of the genus *Aotus*. Due to the morphologic similarity of many *Aotus* spp., there have been many misidentifications based on phenotype. Investigations using nucleotide sequences have helped to define the phylogenic relationships of this genus (Menezes *et al.*, 2010). Hershkovitz (1983) described two phenotypic groups of *Aotus* composed of nine allopatric species distinguished by karyotype, pelage patterns, and neck color. However, a recent study by Menezes *et al.* (2010) challenges the division between red- and gray-necked species proposed by Hershkovitz (1983). Menezes *et al.* (2010) found that phylogenetic analysis using mtDNA indicated that the lineage leading to the gray-necked

TABLE 17.8 Owl Monkey Taxonomy, CITES Status, and Distribution

Genus *Aotus*	Common name	CITES[a] status	Distribution
RED-NECKED GROUP			
A. azarae[a]	Azara's night monkey	II	Argentina, Bolivia, Paraguay
A. miconax[b]	Andean night monkey	II	Peru
A. nancymaae[c]	Nancy Ma's night monkey	II	Brazil, Peru
A. nigriceps[d]	Black-headed night monkey	II	Brazil, Peru, Bolivia
GRAY-NECKED GROUP			
A. brumbacki[e]	Brumback's night monkey	II	Colombia
A. griseimembra[f]	Gray-handed night monkey	II	Colombia, Venezuela
A. jorgehernandezi[g]	Henández-Camacho's night monkey	II	Colombia
A. lemurinus[h]	Colombian night monkey	II	Colombia, Ecuador, Venezuela
A. trivirgatus[i]	Northern night monkey	II	Brazil, Venezuela
A. vociferan[j]	Spix night monkey	II	Brazil, Colombia, Ecuador, Peru
A. zonalis[k]	Panamanian night monkey	II	Colombia, Panama

[a]Fernández-Duque et al. (2008).
[b]Cornejo et al. (2008).
[c,d]Cornejo and Palacios (2008).
[e]Morales-Jiménez et al. (2008a).
[f,g]Morales-Jiménez and Link (2008).
[h]Morales-Jiménez and de la Torre (2008).
[i]Veiga and Rylands (2008).
[j]Morales-Jiménez et al. (2008b).
[k]Cuarón et al. (2008).

TABLE 17.9 Mean Adult Owl Monkey Body Weight[a]

Karyotype	Male	N	Female	N	Range
I	957 ± 124	130	885 ± 120	124	567–1232
II	880 ± 98	55	864 ± 111	48	531–1281
III	898 ± 109	52	907 ± 99	37	529–1237
V	838 ± 118	18	751 ± 91	17	572–1077

From Baer (1994).
[a]Data given in g (mean ± SD) listed by karyotype and sex. Data collected at Battelle Pacific Northwest Laboratories.

A. nancymaae and *A. vociferans* which are found both north and south of the river (Menezes *et al.*, 2010). Phenotypically, gray-necked owl monkeys have an agouti or gray neck identical in color to the dorsum and torso of the monkey, an intrascapular crest of hair, and elongate pectoral glands with feathering of the periglandular hair. Red-necked owl monkeys have monochromatic phelomelanin hairs (red neck) that are the same color as the ventrum of the body, an intrascapular whorl, and a rounded pectoral gland with surrounding hairs whorled (Hershkovitz, 1983).

In the wild, *Aotus* spp. live as monogamous pairs within an extended family that may include two to three offspring (Aquino and Encarnacíon, 1986; Aquino *et al.*, 1990; Fernández-Duque, 2011a), usually an infant, juvenile, and subadult (Wright, 1994). At approximately 3 years of age, the subadult leaves the family group to find a mate and establish its own territory. Aggression between the parents and subadult is not a primary cause of dispersement (Wright, 1994). In *A. nancymaae*, noncycling or breeding offspring of both sexes are tolerated within the family group, whereas in *A. vociferans*, only male offspring remain with the group (Aquino *et al.*, 1990). There is also some variation in body weight within the genus. *A. vociferans* is the smallest, weighing around 0.7 kg, and *A. azarai* is the largest at 1.25 kg (Huck *et al.*, 2011).

Owl monkeys lack sexual dimorphism and it can be difficult to differentiate the sexes as they grow at similar rates. In general, owl monkeys weigh between 0.8 and 1.3 kg (Fernández-Duque, 2011b), and average weights are listed in Table 17.9 (Baer, 1994). Nipple protrusion occurs in females greater than 5 years of age and can be used to sex animals at a distance (Huck *et al.*, 2011). The adult male and offspring actively participate in infant care, with males carrying the infant over 80% of the time (Fernández-Duque, 2009). In a monogamous species, males can be fairly certain of paternity, and it is likely that male participation in infant rearing will increase future reproductive opportunities (Smuts and Gubernick, 1992). Male participation in infant care may also increase survival of offspring and allow the females increased foraging opportunities (Tardif, 1994).

Owl monkeys are found in a wide variety of forest habitats from sea level up to 3000 m. Average territory

species, *A. trivirgatus*, is a sister lineage to that of one leading to a red-necked clade (*A. nigriceps, A. azarae*, and *A. infulatus*). The gray-necked species group of owl monkeys contains seven species and the red-necked owl monkeys are comprised of four separate species (Table 17.8) (Defler and Bueno, 2007; Menezes *et al.*, 2010).

3. Natural History

Owl monkeys are distributed widely from western Panama to northern Argentina. In general, the gray-necked group occurs north of the Amazon River and the red-necked group is found to the south, with the exception of size ranges from 5 to 9 hectares depending on whether the monkeys live in a tropical dry forest (5 hectares) or tropical rain forest (Wright, 1994). Owl monkeys travel at night. Available light affects night ranging patterns with monkeys traveling about twice as far on moonlit nights as on moonless nights (Wright, 1994). This observation is also supported by research from Fernández-Duque et al. (2010), who report decreased owl monkey activity during lunar eclipses. Owl monkeys are also more socially active on moonlit nights. The group exits the sleeping site at dusk and returns at dawn. They sleep as family groups within tree holes or vine tangles, and frequently use the same tree (Wright, 1994). While it is accepted that *Aotus* spp. are nocturnal, there is one species among the group that is not a strict nocturnal species. *A. azarai* has shown some diurnal activity patterns, likely in response to environmental factors (Fernández-Duque and Erkert, 2006). *Aotus* spp. defend their territory by vocalization, posturing, chases, and fights. Intergroup aggression occurs at bordering fruit trees and is preceded by loud whooping vocalization by both sexes (Moynihan, 1964). Whoops are accompanied by piloerection and stiff-legged jumping. Chases, wrestling, and fighting accompanied by whoops, followed by fights lasting no longer than 10 min, are typical for the species (Wright, 1978, 1994). Groups then retreat within their respective territories.

Owl monkeys utilize both urine and glandular secretions for scent marking and much of their communication is through olfactory cues. Owl monkeys will both drink their mates' urine and participate in urine-washing, although this communicatory mechanism is more likely territorial and does not appear to be associated with sexual activity (Wolovich and Evans, 2007). Owl monkeys posess apocrine glands on their face and brow region, sternal region, and most distinctly the subcaudal gland in the perianal region (Wolovich and Evans, 2007; MacDonald et al., 2008). Scent marking plays an important role in sexual recognition and inter-male aggression, but it has little effect on male sexual behavior (Dixson, 1983). Chemical analyses of subcaudal scent gland secretions have identified 300 distinct volatile chemicals, various levels and combinations of which likely communicate sex, age, and family group information through olfaction (MacDonald et al., 2008).

4. Reproduction

The owl monkey exhibits no change in external genitalia or predictable changes in vaginal cornification during the 15- 18-day estrous cycle (Cicmanec and Campbell, 1977; Bonney et al., 1980; Dixson, 1983; Wolovich et al., 2008). *A. azarai* have a slightly longer cycle at 22 days (Fernández-Duque, 2011b). Menstruation does not occur. Unlike the squirrel monkey in which copulations are limited to the day of ovulation when females are maximally receptive to males (Williams et al., 1988), female owl monkeys remain sexually receptive to males throughout the ovarian cycle (Dixson, 1983).

Estrone concentrations rise sharply from ovulation, peak 5 days later, and then decline to basal levels by day 13. Increases in plasma progesterone were observed 24 h after the estrone rise, peaking at day 8 and declining to basal levels by day 11. Urinary excretion of estrone and pregnanediol-3α-glucuronide (PdG), a major progesterone metabolite in the owl monkey, followed changes in the plasma levels of these hormones (Bonney et al., 1979). Peak plasma steroid levels during the cycle are extremely high (3.59 ± 0.066 ng/ml estrone; 250.48 ± 11.37 ng/ml progesterone), as is seen in other New World monkeys (Dixson, 1983). Levels of plasma testosterone in adult male owl monkeys have a circadian rhythm with peak levels occurring in the light of day (resting period), and lowest levels during the dark (active period) (Dixson and Gardner, 1981). These daily changes in testosterone are the opposite of those of macaques and lemurs in terms of light cycle, but the same in terms of activity cycles (Goodman et al., 1974; Dixson and Gardner, 1981).

There is some species variation in owl monkey gestation length. Based on one report of a timed pregnancy in *A. griseimembra*, the gestation period was 133 days (Hunter et al., 1979). Another study following four *A. nancymaae* females reported a mean gestation length of 117 ± 8 days, and one *A. azarai* was 121 days (Wolovich et al., 2008). Some estimates of the gestation length have been as high as 148–159 days (Elliot et al., 1976; Meritt, 1976). Urinary chorionic gonadotropin is detectable from 5 to 6 weeks following conception until 1 week before parturition (Hall and Hodgen, 1979). Corticotropin-releasing hormore (CRH) peaks during mid-gestation, at days 60–80 in owl monkeys (Power et al., 2010). Interbirth intervals reported by Dixson (1983) average 253 days and range from 166 to 419 days. Malaga et al. (1997) reported a diminishing interbirth interval in multiparous pairs with 11 months between the first and second births, 9.9 months until the third birth, and 8.8 months between subsequent parturitions. Interbirth interval also decreases with a higher frequency of food sharing from males to females (Wolovich et al., 2008). The mean time from pairing to first parturition was 14.6 ± 7.7 months (Malaga et al., 1997). There is no postpartum estrus. Unlike squirrel monkeys, captive owl monkeys have no seasonal breeding or birth seasons (Cicmanec and Campbell, 1977). However, in wild populations birth seasonality has been observed during May through September (Fernández-Duque et al., 2002). Pregnancy and fetus viability can be verified using transabdominal ultrasound. Gestational age can be determined by measuring biparietal diameter (BPD) via ultrasound (Schuler et al., 2010). Infants weigh 90–105 g at birth and have a well-developed pelage except for the abdomen and inner

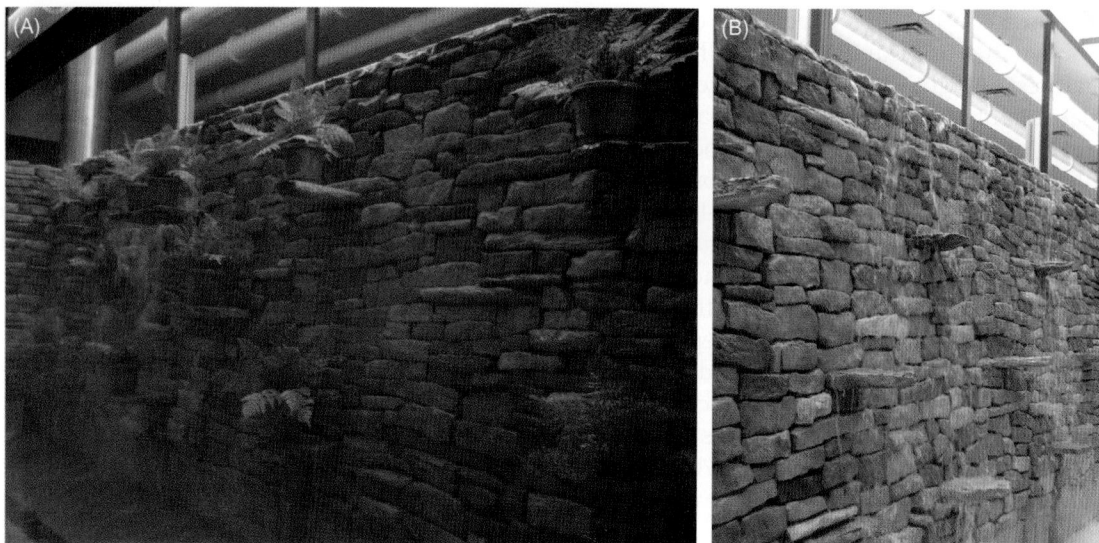

FIGURE 17.5   Waterfalls located in the owl monkey rooms at the Michale E. Keeling Center for Comparative Medicine and Research at the University of Texas MD Anderson Cancer Center, Bastrop, TX.

surface of the limbs. Most births are singletons; twinning occurs rarely. Most of the time, newborns cling to the parent in a ventrolateral position, climbing up to the nipple to suckle (Meritt, 1976; Cicmanec and Campbell, 1977; Dixson, 1983). Ventrolateral clinging is the major resting position of the infant until it reaches 3–4 weeks of age, at which time dorsal clinging becomes the preferred position (Dixson, 1983). Dorsal clinging and transfer from female to male parents may be observed as soon as the first day. Infants begin to get off the parents from 3 to 6 weeks of age, start to eat solid food at 35–60 days, and are weaned by 4–5 months (Dixson, 1983; Rotundo et al., 2005).

Puberty begins between 300 and 400 days of age in both males and females (Dixson et al., 1980; Dixson, 1983). A useful indicator of pubertal development is the growth of the sub-caudal scent-marking gland at the base of the tail. Growth of this gland corresponds to increasing testosterone levels in the male. Owl monkeys are sexually mature at 18–24 months of age. In family groups there is no increase in aggression as offspring progress through puberty. Male parents interact more frequently than female parents with older offspring, particularly in grooming behavior (Dixson, 1983).

5.   Laboratory Management

Housing and maintenance of the owl monkey should be designed to meet its unique needs as a nocturnal new world monkey. Room temperature should range from 75 to 80°F, with the higher temperature preferable. Provision of a tranquil setting with a minimum of extraneous noise appears to improve adaptation to captivity and survival. At the University of Texas MD Anderson Cancer Center,

Michale E. Keeling Center for Comparative Medicine and Research, owl monkeys are housed in a room with a waterfall running the center length of the room. The waterfalls serve a dual purpose. The white noise produced by the water helps to mask the more stressful husbandry sounds. Additionally, the waterfalls are a visual barrier, preventing the owl monkeys from visualizing other family groups. Because owl monkeys are highly territorial, contact with other family groups is not often encountered in the wild and any observation of other family groups is unnatural and likely increases stress. The waterfalls serve to minimize this stress (C. Abee, personal communication, 2013) (Fig. 17.5).

Red or gray filters are placed over light fixtures in many laboratories to provide diminished lighting. Owl monkeys are provided a 12:12h light–dark cycle that is offset from the normal day so that monkeys can be observed during the active 'night' cycle. Diminished illumination is better than absolute dark, as normal feeding, locomotion, and social behaviors occur more frequently when some illumination is present (Erkert, 1976; Wright, 1994). Provision of an automatic nightlight is an alternative to red-light illumination during the dark cycle.

Owl monkeys are sensitive to changes in routine and personnel. Unnecessary handling should be avoided by the use of transfer boxes or tunnels to facilitate cage changes. Owl monkeys are easily trained to jump into a transfer box or into a clean cage for cage transfers (Tardif et al., 2006). Handling and restraint are potentially upsetting not only to the animal being handled but also to others within the room. If necessary, owl monkeys may be captured within the nest box and the box and animal

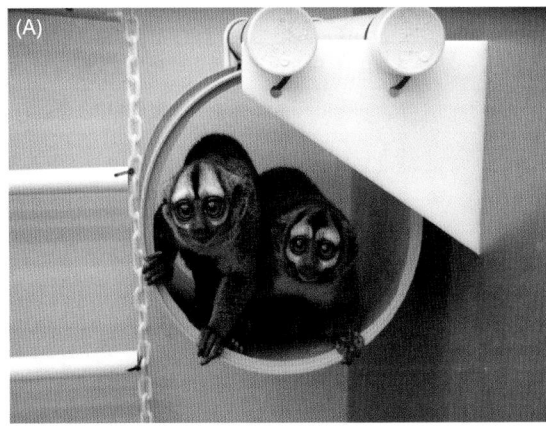
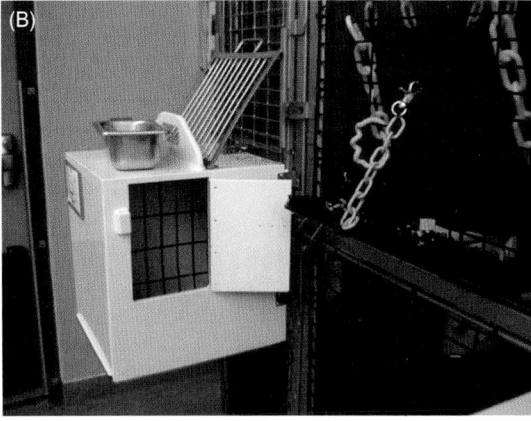

FIGURE 17.6 *Aotus* spp. thermoneutral resting structure using an 8-inch diameter polyvinyl chloride (PVC) pipe attached to a 2-inch PVC pipe perches (A). Nest box attached to caging unit for owl monkeys (B).

removed from the colony room. The animal can then be removed and handled in a separate room as warranted.

A nest box provides owl monkeys with a structure that simulates a tree-hole nest and can be placed in or attached to each cage. The presence of nest boxes also improves reproductive efficiency in owl monkeys (Obaldia *et al.*, 2011). Small animal airline transport cages in which the floor has been replaced with wire mesh, the door removed, and a perch provided are effective thermoneutral nest boxes that can be attached to the outside of the cage. Eighteen-inch sections of an 8-inch diameter polyvinyl chloride (PVC) pipe with access holes and an interior perch, or PVC T-sections, are inexpensive nest boxes that can be placed either on the floor or hung within the cage (Fig. 17.6). Nest box and cage sanitation should occur on alternate weeks. This provides stabilization of olfactory cues within the monkey's environment. In addition, because owl monkeys are scent markers, suitable pieces of hardwood may be used as perches within the cage. It is desirable that these perches also be sanitized on a different schedule than cages.

Owl monkeys are ideally housed as family groups, but may also be housed as pairs. Careful attention must be paid to juvenile animals to ensure that they are removed from family groups prior to any aggression. Usually, when pairs start to reject a juvenile animal, they will prevent it from entering the nest box. Attempts have been made with some success to house same-sex pairs together when breeding is undesirable (Weed and Watson, 1998).

6. Nutrition

Owl monkeys are principally frugivorous but consume a varied diet of fruits, young leaves, flowers, insects, and lesser amounts of bird eggs, small birds, and mammals. Composition of the diet can vary with the season and forest type. Increased amounts of fruit, flowers, and insects are eaten in the spring, and increased amounts of leaves

are eaten during the dry season (Wright, 1994; Fernández-Duque and Van der Heide, 2013). In captivity, owl monkeys require dietary supplementation with vitamins D_3 and C. In most owl monkey colonies, a balanced commercial New World monkey formulation is fed (Purina 5040 New World Primate Chow) (Malaga *et al.*, 1997). In some colonies, the commercial diet is moistened with fruit juice prior to feeding to soften the diet and increase its acceptance. Owl monkeys readily accept a variety of fruit and vegetables, including bananas, oranges, grapes, celery, squash, yams, carrots, green tomatoes, and green beans. These items should be fed to enrich, but not to replace the commercial monkey diet.

7. Normal Values

Normative hematologic and serum chemistry data for owl monkeys have been published by several authors (Porter, 1969; Sehgal *et al.*, 1980; Mrema *et al.*, 1987; Malaga *et al.*, 1990, 1995). Reported differences among laboratories are probably due to owl monkey karyotype, differences in husbandry and diet, and assay techniques. Tables 17.10 and 17.11 provide hematologic and clinical chemistry data on four karyotypes of owl monkeys maintained at the same facility under similar conditions (Baer, 1994). All monkeys tested were clinically healthy adults. Normal urine parameters can be referenced in Table 17.12 and are included due to the propensity for owl monkeys to develop renal disease when serving as subjects in malaria research.

8. Research Uses

Owl monkeys have been used extensively in the study of malaria, including maintenance of various malarial strains, antigen production, studies of host–vector relationships, parasite life-cycles, and potential therapeutics (Aikawa *et al.*, 1988; Herrera *et al.*, 2002; Ye *et al.*, 2013). Owl monkeys are susceptible to human and nonhuman

TABLE 17.10   Hematological Data for Owl Monkeys[a]

Analyte	K-I[b] (N = 254)		K-II (N = 62)		K-III (N = 55)		K-V (N = 35)	
	X	SD	X	SD	X	SD	X	SD
RBCs (10[6]/ml)	6.2	0.6	5.3	0.5	5.3	0.9	6.4	0.5
Hgb (g/dl)	16.3	1.6	14.3	1.5	14.0	2.3	17.1	1.3
VPRC (%)	49.7	4.4	43.6	4.2	43.6	7.0	52.2	–
Platelets (10[3]/ml)	431	119	342	–	333	117	295	90
MCV (μm[3])	79.8	3.5	82.6	3.0	82.3	4.0	81.3	4.1
MCH (pg)	26.2	1.6	27.0	1.4	26.5	1.6	26.6	1.6
MCHC (%)	32.8	1.1	32.8	0.9	32.2	0.8	32.8	0.6
WBC (10[3]/ml)	10.1	3.2	12.2	4.4	14.2	11.2	8.8	3.8
Segs (10[3]/ml)	3.0	2.0	3.4	1.8	4.3	2.2	2.6	1.2
Lymphs (10[3]/ml)	6.1	2.6	6.9	2.2	8.1	2.5	5.5	1.5
Monos (10[3]/ml)	0.4	0.3	0.3	0.3	0.3	0.2	0.3	0.3
Eosin (10[3]/ml)	0.4	0.5	1.4	1.1	1.4	1.5	1.6	1.1
Basos (10[3]/ml)	0.2	0.2	0.2	0.2	0.1	0.2	0.1	0.1

RBCs, red blood cells; Hgb, hemoglobin; MCV, mean corpuscular volume; MCH, mean corpuscular hemoglobin; MCHC, mean corpuscular hemoglobin concentration; WBC, white blood count; Segs, neutrophils; Lymphs, lymphocytes; Monos, monocytes; Eosin, eosinophils; Basos, basophils.
[a]From Baer (1994).
[b]Karyotype designation.

TABLE 17.11   Serum Chemistry Data for Owl Monkeys[a]

Analyte	K-I[b] (N = 254)		K-II (N = 57)		K-III (N = 53)		K-V (N = 35)	
	X	SD	X	SD	X	SD	X	SD
Total bilirubin (mg/dl)	0.8	0.4	0.5	0.2	0.5	0.2	0.7	0.2
Cholesterol (mg/dl)	150	46	91	34	111	44	99	34
Creatinine (mg/dl)	1.0	0.4	1.0	0.2	1.1	0.4	1.0	0.3
Glucose (mg/dl)	139	35	153	39	150	47	172	40
Calcium (mg/dl)	10.4	1.0	9.3	0.9	9.2	0.9	9.6	0.7
Alkaline phosphatase (IU/l)	494	469	183	151	143	87	364	381
Phosphorus (mg/dl)	4.0	1.5	4.4	1.5	4.6	1.5	4.8	1.5
ALT (IU/l)	47	37	44	34	49	35	59	34
SUN (mg/dl)	15	5.4	15	6.7	17	11	15	8.9
Total protein (g/dl)	8.3	0.9	8.0	0.7	8.1	1.1	8.2	0.5
Albumin (g/dl)	4.4	0.5	3.8	0.5	3.7	0.5	4.6	0.4
GGT (IU/l)	17	14	20	14	23	18	26	21
Sodium (mEq/l)	152	5	156	9	154	6	148	3
Potassium (mEq/l)	3.8	0.7	4.6	1.6	4.8	2.0	3.3	0.7

ALT, alanine aminotransferase; SUN, serum urea nitrogen; GGT, γ-glutamyltransferase.
[a]From Baer (1994).
[b]Karyotype designation.

TABLE 17.12   Normal Urine Parameters in Owl Monkeys[a]

Urine	Mean ± S.E.M.	Range
Specific gravity	1.010 ± 0.001	1.002–1.023
Volume (ml/kg/day)	81.9 ± 7.5	9–303

URINALYSIS SEMIQUANTITATIVE VALUES

Protein multistix	0–3+
Glucose	0–1+
Ketones	0–2+
Bilirubin	0
Urobilinogen	0
Occult blood	0–4+
pH	6–8.5
Appearance	Light-dark yellow; clear cloudy

Microscopic urinalysis	View
Red blood cells	Rare, few (3–5/hpf)
White blood cells	Rare, occasional
Epithelial cells	Rare, occasional squamous
Casts	Occasional granular
Crystals	Few, moderate triple phosphate; rare calcium oxalate
Miscellaneous	Occasional renal tubular epithelial cells

S.E.M., standard error of the mean.
[a]From Baer (1994).

primate malarias and can transmit these infections to mosquitoes. Differences in degree of susceptibility or immunity to experimental malarial infection and differences in serum proteins correspond to the red- or gray-necked group type. *Aotus griseimembra* is highly susceptible to *Plasmodium falciparum*; *A. nancymaae* is less susceptible to some strains and resistant to others (Schmidt, 1978). Both of these *Aotus* spp. are susceptible to *P. vivax* (Schmidt, 1978). While the owl monkey is an excellent animal model for human malaria and its treatment, it has also been identified as a model for studies of oncogenic viruses, particularly herpesviruses (Barhona *et al.*, 1976; Vernot *et al.*, 2005), and nononcogenic viruses such as hepatitis A (Asher *et al.*, 1995; Balayan, 1992), and it has shown potential as a model for Eastern equine encephalitis virus (Espinosa *et al.*, 2009) and dengue virus (Schiavetta *et al.*, 2003). Owl monkeys have also served as a model for cutaneous and visceral leishmaniasis (Chapman *et al.*, 1981; Broderson *et al.*, 1986), although a more recent study suggests that owl monkeys have developed resistance against *Leishmania infantum chagasi* via innate immune response mechanisms which may

limit its use with this pathogen (Carneiro *et al.*, 2012). In addition, the unique characteristics of the owl monkey eye have made it a valuable animal in vision research (Haefliger *et al.*, 1987; Silveira *et al.*, 2004).

C.   *Saimiri* spp.: Squirrel Monkeys

1.   Introduction

Squirrel monkeys (*Saimiri* spp.) have contributed much to the field of biomedical research. Although historically the squirrel monkey has been the most common New world monkey subject in biomedical research, in recent years the common marmoset has been cited more often in the scientific literature. The squirrel monkey continues to play an important role in biomedical research as the second most cited New world monkey genus.

Physical characteristics such as small size, ease of handling, and faster maturation contribute to their desirability as research subjects (Tardif *et al.*, 2011b). In general, the mean body weight of adult squirrel monkeys is less than 1 kg, although there is some variability among the species (Rowe, 1996). Some sexual dimorphism is observed in squirrel monkeys, although sex differences are less distinct than in many Old World primates. Male squirrel monkeys are 25–30% heavier than females, and canine teeth are larger and longer in males (Masterson and Hartwig, 1998).

Squirrel monkeys have a short, thick coat and all species have white coloration, or a mask, around their eyes and dark brown or black coloring around the muzzle. Although there is some species variation, in general squirrel monkeys have a gray–brown–colored crown, golden–orange coloration to their backs, legs, and arms, gray–brown shoulders and pelvis, and a black tipped tail (Fig. 17.7) (Rowe, 1996; Groves, 2001). One feature that may be useful in differentiating sex and age differences at a distance is the coloration of the peri-auricular hair coat. It has been shown that female monkeys greater than 5 years of age develop a black spot in the peri-auricular region, whereas males and young females have clear hair coats in this region (Goldschmidt *et al.*, 2009).

Large numbers of squirrel monkeys were imported to the United States in the 1960s (Cooper, 1968). However, the governments of South America began banning the export of primates indigenous to their countries in the 1970s. The exportation of the Bolivian squirrel monkey (*S. boliviensis boliviensis*), a species considered especially desirable for malaria vaccine studies, was banned by the Bolivian government in the 1980s. In the mid-1980s, only Peruvian squirrel monkeys (*S. boliviensis peruviensis*) were available from the wild (Abee, 1989). Currently, limited numbers of Guyanese squirrel monkeys

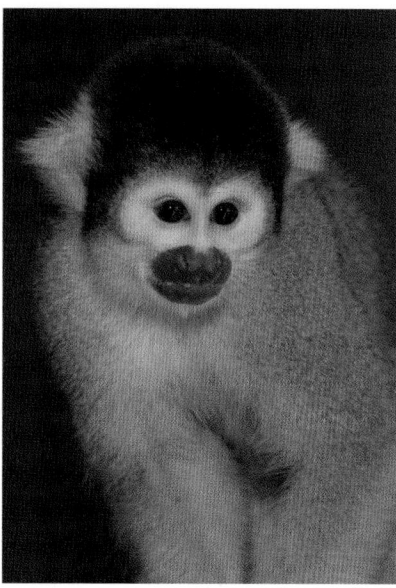

FIGURE 17.7 *Saimiri boliviensis boliviensis*, young adult female Bolivian squirrel monkey from Julio Ruiz, DVM, Michale E. Keeling Center for Comparative Medicine and Research at the University of Texas MD Anderson Cancer Center, Bastrop, TX.

TABLE 17.13 Squirrel Monkey Taxonomy, CITES Status, and Distribution

Genus *Saimiri*	Common name(s)[a]	CITES[b] status	Distribution
S. sciureus	Common squirrel monkey	II	Brazil, Colombia, Ecuador, French Guiana, Guyana, Peru, Suriname, Venezuela
S. s. sciureus	Guyanese squirrel monkey		
S. s. macrodon	Ecuadorian squirrel monkey		
S. s. cassiquiarensis	Humboldt's squirrel monkey		
S. s. albigena	Colombian squirrel monkey		
S. collinsi[c]	Collins' squirrel monkey	–	Brazil
S. boliviensis	Syn. *S. sciureus boliviensis*	II	Bolivia, Brazil, Peru
S. b. boliviensis	Bolivian squirrel monkey		
S. b. peruviensis	Peruvian squirrel monkey		
S. ustus	Golden-backed squirrel monkey	II	Brazil
S. oerstedii	Black-crowned Central American squirrel monkey	I	Costa Rica, Panama
S. o. oerstedii			
S. o. citrinellis	Red-backed squirrel monkey		
S. vanzolinii[d]	Black-headed squirrel monkey	II	Brazil

[a]IUCN 2014. IUCN Red List of Threatened Species. Version 2014.1. Available at: <www.iucnredlist.org>. Downloaded on 03 July 2014.
[b]I, species listed in CITES Appendix I are threatened with extinction (endangered); II, species listed in CITES Appendix II are not currently threatened with extinction but may become so unless trade is strictly regulated. From IUCN (2013) and Wilson and Reeder (1993); Groves (2001).
[c]From Mercês et al. (2014). Note: Recent research on morphological and mitochondrial phylogenetics has indicated S. collinsi should be considered a separate species; however, other publications still list this species as a subspecies of S. sciureus.
[d]From Groves (2001).

(*S. sciureus sciureus*) are also available for importation. Approximately 200–300 squirrel monkeys are imported from the wild each year. In addition to wild importations, there are two other sources of squirrel monkeys. One is through the captive breeding colony located at the University of Texas MD Anderson Cancer Center, Michale E. Keeling Center for Comparative Medicine and Research, in Bastrop, TX. The other is through an agreement with the Pan American Health Organization (PAHO) and NIH through the Peruvian Primatology Project, which provides small numbers of new world monkeys to the NIH (National Research Council (NRC), 2011a).

2. Taxonomy

Squirrel monkeys were once considered to be a single species (*S. sciureus*) with several geographically separated subspecies. However, karyotypic and phenotypic information gathered in the early 1980s led to the conclusion by Hershkovitz (1984) that squirrel monkeys should be classified as a single genus with four species and nine subspecies. More recent data has reclassified *S. vanzolinii* as its own species resulting in five distinct species and eight subspecies (Groves, 2001) (Table 17.13). There has been some debate on the subspecies under *S. sciureus* (*S. s. collinsi* and *S. s. macrodon*), and further gene sequencing studies are required (Lavergne *et al.*, 2010; Chiou *et al.*, 2011). The most commonly used phenotypic characteristic for species identification is the shape of the patch of nonpigmented hair above the eyes; squirrel

monkeys are divided into two groups based on this characteristic. Those belonging to the *S. sciureus*, *S. oerstedii*, and *S. ustus* groups are classified as 'gothic arch' squirrel monkeys as they possess a pointed arch of whitish hair above each eye (Fig. 17.8). Those belonging to the *S. boliviensis* and *S. vanzolinii* groups are referred to as 'roman arch' squirrel monkeys, characterized by more shallow, semicircular patterns above the eyes (Hershkovitz, 1984; Lavergne *et al.*, 2010; Zimbler-DeLorenzo and Stone, 2011). Additional phenotypic characteristics include differences in coloration of the hair on the head and body. These differences in coloration can range from subtle to

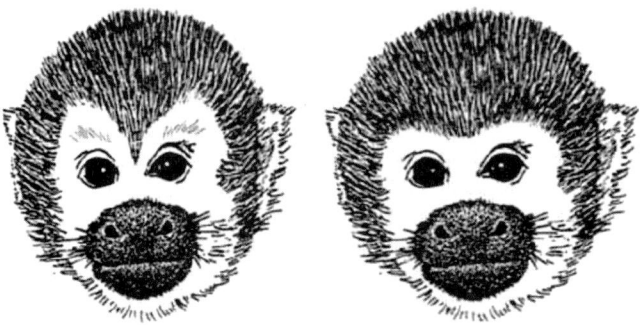

FIGURE 17.8 Phenotypic facial characteristics of *Saimiri* spp. A squirrel monkey with a 'gothic arch' phenotype typical of *S. sciureus* is pictured on the left. A 'roman arch' phenotype characteristic of *S. boliviensis* is featured on the right.

obvious. Squirrel monkeys of the 'roman arch' variety usually have black hair crowning their heads, though exceptions exist (Hershkovitz, 1984), whereas 'gothic arch' squirrel monkeys usually have a gray–green, agouti coloration. *Saimiri sciureus sciureus*, the Guyanese squirrel monkey, also possesses a pattern of pigmented hairs within the patch of whitish hair above each eye that resembles an eyebrow (Ariga *et al.*, 1978).

Precise identification of squirrel monkeys requires both phenotypic and karyotypic examination. All squirrel monkey species and subspecies have 44 (diploid) chromosomes; however, they vary in their number of acrocentric autosomes from five to seven. By counting the number of acrocentric autosomes and observing the periocular patches, more certain identification can be made (Ariga *et al.*, 1978). Such specific identification of the type of squirrel monkey to be used in a particular experiment is critical in that species and subspecies vary in their susceptibility to both naturally occurring and experimentally induced diseases (Portman *et al.*, 1980; Martin and McNease, 1982; Ausman *et al.*, 1985; Coe *et al.*, 1985). Furthermore, failure to identify and separate Peruvian, Bolivian, and Guyanese squirrel monkeys in breeding colonies may result in interbreeding. The karyotypic variations observed in squirrel monkeys are thought to be due to pericentric inversions in the ancestral karyotype (Jones *et al.*, 1973). Therefore, the progeny of squirrel monkeys that interbreed will be heterozygous for the inversion. This inversion heterozygosity can lead to the production of nonviable gametes due to crossovers at the inversion loop during meiosis. Theoretically, 50% of conceptions in hybrid squirrel monkeys could be nonviable, thus potentially reducing reproductive efficiency in breeding colonies. Also, mixing species and subspecies within experimental groups may create confounding variables caused by differences in responses to experimental manipulation, which could lead to difficulties in interpreting experimental results.

3. Natural History

Squirrel monkeys are found in the Amazon basin of South America and as isolated populations in Panama and Costa Rica. Geographic distributions are listed in Table 17.13. Squirrel monkeys are diurnal and arboreal. They inhabit most types of tropical forest, including wet and dry forest, continuous and secondary forest, mangrove swamps, riparian habitat, and forest fragments (Hernández-Camacho and Cooper, 1976; Terborgh, 1983; Baldwin, 1985; Boinski, 1987a). Their range includes altitudes from sea level to 2000 m. Squirrel monkeys are highly flexible in their adaptation to different environments; in some areas they have flourished in disturbed habitats (Konstant and Mittermeier, 1982; Boinski, 1987a).

Squirrel monkeys form large multimale–multifemale troops in the wild, numbering from 25 to 75 animals (Zimbler-DeLorenzo and Stone, 2011). Groups consist of adult females and offspring, subadult females, subadult males, and adult males. Female squirrel monkeys reach sexual maturity at 2.5–3.5 years of age. Males become subadults at 3.5–5 years of age (Boinski, 1987b; Zimbler-DeLorenzo and Stone, 2011). In Bolivian, Peruvian, and Guyanese squirrel monkeys, there is a low rate of female transfer and a high rate of male transfer from natal groups. However, in *S. oerstedii*, the male monkeys have strong bonds and it is the females who transfer from their natal groups at sexual maturity (Boinski *et al.*, 2005).

Social interactions between group members vary with the species groups. *S. oerstedii* integrate males into their egalitarian groups and intergroup aggression is very low. In social groups of *S. boliviensis*, females are dominant, males stay on the group periphery, and social aggression is common between both sexes. *S. sciureus* are intermediate: while males are integrated into the social groups, they are dominant and display a high level of male–male aggression (Boinski, 1999).

Squirrel monkeys are susceptible to predators such as raptors and wild felids (Mitchell *et al.*, 1991). They have a system of vocal calls consisting of 25–30 calls to alert of danger and communicate other social cues (Newman, 1985). Another predator avoidance technique is the close physical association between *Saimiri* and *Cebus* monkeys, as *Saimiri* spp. benefit from the extensive alarm call system of the *Cebus* monkeys (Sussman, 2000). Besides vocal calls, squirrel monkeys use postural displays and olfactory cues for communication. One of the most widely recognized is that of urine washing, when a male or female of any age urinates on their hands and feet and wipes the scent all over its body. This may help to mark trails or communicate sexual reproductive information (Boinski, 1992).

4. Reproduction

Squirrel monkeys are seasonal breeders. Both male and female squirrel monkeys undergo hormonally induced physiological changes during the breeding season, moving from periods of infertility or anestrus with low levels of circulating steroid hormones to fertility with high levels of hormones (Jarosz *et al.*, 1977). The breeding season is approximately 3 months in duration (December–March in the Northern Hemisphere) and consists of a cluster of ovulatory cycles varying between 6 and 12 days in length, with a mean cycle length of 9.5 days (Diamond *et al.*, 1984). Gestation is approximately 150 days, and the interbirth interval varies from 1 (*S. oerstedii*) to 2 (*S. boliviensis and S. sciureus*) years, depending on the species (Kerber *et al.*, 1977; Abee, 1989; Zimbler-DeLorenzo and Stone, 2011). The breeding season of female squirrel monkeys is characterized by elevations in circulating levels of estradiol and progesterone. Serum concentrations of estradiol in *S. boliviensis* increase dramatically in cycling females, from peak prebreeding season levels averaging less than 95 pg/ml to levels greater than 1000 pg/ml during the breeding season (Williams *et al.*, 1986). Estradiol levels are even higher in the hours immediately postmating, reaching levels in excess of 2000 pg/ml (Yeoman *et al.*, 1991). Although ovulatory cycles all occur at the same time of year, females do not cycle in synchrony with others in the same social group (Williams *et al.*, 1986). This makes the prediction of cyclic events within a breeding group difficult. Some adult females within breeding groups fail to cycle during portions of the breeding season, which further complicates management of a breeding colony. Ovulation can be verified by laparoscopy or serial ovarian hormone determinations (Aksel *et al.*, 1985; Alexander *et al.*, 1991).

Male squirrel monkeys experience seasonal enlargement of testes concomitant with spermatogenesis and undergo 'fatting' prior to breeding season. Males add approximately 15% to their body weight, primarily in the upper torso, in preparation for the breeding season (Fig. 17.9) (DuMond, 1968; Williams *et al.*, 1986; Zimbler-DeLorenzo and Stone, 2011). Behavior of male squirrel monkeys during the breeding season is characterized by a reduction in aggression and an increase in sexually related responses such as genital displays, anogenital inspection, and copulation. These responses correlate positively with elevations in circulating levels of androstenedione (Williams *et al.*, 1986). Copulations during the breeding season are associated specifically with ovulation; all copulations occur within 24 h of predicted ovulation, based on daily serum luteinizing hormone determinations (Williams *et al.*, 1986).

Hormone analysis of *S. b. boliviensis* show a peak elevation in follicle-stimulating hormone (FSH) during the late follicular stage that coincides with the luteinizing hormone (LH) surge, and a second FSH peak occurs during the luteal phase (Yeoman *et al.*, 2000). Serum concentrations of estradiol (E_2), progesterone (P), and squirrel monkey chorionic gonadotropin (SMG) can be

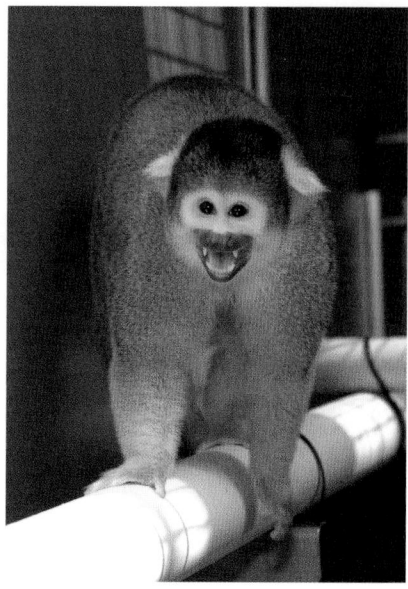

FIGURE 17.9   Fatted adult male Bolivian squirrel monkey, *Saimiri boliviensis boliviensis*. Note broad head and heavy shoulders. Photograph provided by Julio C. Ruiz, D.V.M., Michale E. Keeling Center for Comparative Medicine and Research at the University of Texas MD Anderson Cancer Center, Bastrop, TX.

used to diagnose early pregnancy in squirrel monkeys. In animals pregnant for less than 25 days, SMG levels are less than 300 pg/ml. After 30 days of pregnancy, concentrations increase and fluctuate between 700 and 2000 pg/ml. Pregnant squirrel monkeys have fluctuating concentrations of E_2 above 300 pg/ml and P above 150 ng/ml (Diamond *et al.*, 1987). During gestation, placental corticotropin-releasing hormone (CRH) stimulates the production of estrogens. CRH levels peak at days 45–70 of gestation, similar to findings in other New World monkeys, but in contrast to findings in humans and apes which show the highest CRH levels just prior to parturition (Power *et al.*, 2010).

Early abortions can be a serious problem in squirrel monkey breeding colonies because all females must conceive during the relatively narrow time span of a strict seasonal breeding pattern. Those that abort may not have another opportunity to conceive before the breeding season ends (Abee, 1989). Early, frequently occult abortions were documented in 25% of pregnancies in which pregnancy was diagnosed and followed by changes in circulating hormone levels (Diamond *et al.*, 1985). Another contributing factor to reduced reproductive efficiency in squirrel monkeys is the large fetal mass in comparison to maternal size. A term infant squirrel monkey weighs approximately 18% of the nonpregnant weight of the dam. Large fetal-to-dam size contributes to a high incidence of dystocia and resultant stillbirths in this species (Abee, 1989).

TABLE 17.14   Squirrel Monkey Birth Weights (*Saimiri* spp.)

Species	Weight ± SD (N)[a]		
	Female	Male	Average
Bolivian (*S. b. boliviensis*)	104 ± 14 (824)	109 ± 16 (830)	107 ± 15 (1654)
Peruvian (*S. b. peruviensis*)	108 ± 14 (74)	116 ± 15 (82)	112 ± 15 (156)
Guyanese (*S. sciureus*)	126 ± 14 (132)	133 ± 15 (134)	129 ± 15 (266)

[a]*Mean body weight in grams ± standard deviation (number of infants weighed). Unpublished data from Squirrel Monkey Breeding and Research Resource, Michale E. Keeling Center for Comparative Medicine and Research, University of Texas MD Anderson Cancer Center, 2014.*

Squirrel monkey infants are usually born in the summer months in the Northern Hemisphere. Normal squirrel monkey deliveries occur at night with labor lasting 1–2 h. The infant actively participates in delivery. Once the shoulders are free, the infant reaches up and grabs the ventrum of the dam and assists in pulling itself out (Hopf, 1967). Newborn infants weigh approximately 100 g (Table 17.14), and infants weighing less than 80 g rarely survive. During the first 2 weeks of life, the infant spends most of its time sleeping while clinging to the dorsum of the dam. At 1 month of age, the infant begins to move off the dam. Weaning age is variable between the species with *S. oerstedii* weaned at 4 months and *S. boliviensis* infants nursing for up to 18 months (Zimbler-DeLorenzo and Stone, 2011). The age of weaning of Bolivian squirrel monkeys maintained in the Squirrel Monkey Breeding and Research Resource has been determined to occur at approximately 90–120 days of age (Williams et al., 1994, 2002).

Male squirrel monkeys do not participate in infant care. Allomaternal care, or care provided to the infant by another female other than its dam, is provided by juvenile and adult females within the breeding group (Zimbler-DeLorenzo and Stone, 2011). Allomothering begins within the first 2 weeks of infant life and usually involves carrying the infant. Some females that have been unsuccessful during that reproductive year may also nurse the infant they allomother (Williams et al., 1994). *Saimiri* spp. have one of the highest infant care costs among small new world monkeys due to the carrying of a large infant relative to adult body size (Tardif, 1994).

5. Laboratory Management

As squirrel monkeys are New World monkeys with little body fat, a high metabolic rate, and a relatively large surface area, they need to be maintained in a warm laboratory environment, preferably at 80°F. Squirrel monkeys are prone to hypothermia and are stressed if placed in standard stainless steel cages at a room temperature

of 72°F. Thermoneutral perching, such as PVC pipe, is preferable to metal perches. It is important to provide perching that keeps the animals off the floor. Perches <¾ inch in diameter can cause pressure sores and eventually ulcers on the dorsum of the base of the tail. Squirrel monkeys routinely perch and sleep balancing on the base of the tail, with the tail wrapped around over the front and ventrum of the animal. They lack ischial callosities, so sitting puts considerable pressure on the base of the tail. Large-diameter perching will prevent the formation of tail-base ulcers (Abee, 1989).

Squirrel monkeys are social animals and every effort should be made to house them in social groups. It is possible to house squirrel monkeys as same-sex pairs; however, pairing of adult males must be carefully monitored. Squirrel monkeys do well in large pens or indoor–outdoor enclosures. It is important to provide multiple-level perches and multiple feeding areas in group cages. As arboreal animals, squirrel monkeys will use all levels of perching within the cage. Hide boxes can be used to provide escape areas for animals that are being chased or harassed. Small-to-large, mixed-sex groups work well in breeding situations with one to two males for 12–16 females. Single-male groups can also be effective in breeding when housed with no more than 12 females. Once established, mixed-sex groups are stable with minimal aggression or fighting, except at the beginning of the breeding season. New animals should not be added individually to established groups as aggression and serious injury will result (Williams et al., 2010).

Squirrel monkey infants may be reared successfully by foster dams or in a nursery, although nursery rearing should be considered a last resort if reintroduction to the dam and fostering are unsuccessful. At the Squirrel Monkey Breeding and Research Resource maintained at the Michale E. Keeling Center, orphaned infants are frequently reared by foster dams and this is the optimal rearing strategy if reintroduction to the biological dam is not possible. In the nursery environment, supplemental heat should be provided by a neonatal isolator or an enclosure placed over a water-recirculating heating pad. Ambient temperature should be maintained at 85°F for the first 2–3 weeks of life. Surrogates, such as a cylindrical fleece, that allow for the normal dorsal clinging posture of the infant on the back of the dam are desirable. Infant squirrel monkeys are inefficient in protein utilization and require approximately 13% of their calories as dietary protein (Ausman et al., 1979). Use of a dry formulation (Zoologic Milk Matrix, Pet-Ag., Inc., Hampshire, IL) that is mixed with powdered milk and water more closely approximates squirrel monkey milk, compared to human infant formulas, and is readily accepted by infants. Infants should be fed every hour initially for at least 14 h a day. The feeding interval can be extended as the infant gains weight. By 3–4 weeks of age the infant should be able to self-feed from a bottle, and at 1 month of age it can be started on moistened monkey chow. If an infant must be raised in a nursery setting, they should be socialized as soon as possible to prevent or minimize the development of behavioral abnormalities. Play times with other nursery infants or older, tolerant, nonreproductive females can be used to socialize the infant. Nursery infants can be introduced to a multiage social group by 6 months of age.

Squirrel monkeys are curious animals and will manipulate enrichment objects hung in their cage. Infant toys and PVC plumbing joints have been used both with and without food enrichment to increase activity levels (Williams et al., 2010). Some facilities have attempted to combine Saimiri–Cebus species to promote social enrichment and mimic the interactions that have been observed in the wild. Leonardi et al. (2010) suggested that the well-being of both species is enhanced by the interspecies association. However, as this is a relatively new undertaking, careful monitoring must be instituted while attempting this enrichment technique.

6. Nutrition

Squirrel monkeys are omnivorous, and their diet in the wild primarily consists of fruit and insects. Compared to other platyrrhines they consume a large amount of insects, spending 70–80% of their foraging time looking for insects (Zimbler-DeLorenzo and Stone, 2011). Squirrel monkeys also adapt well to commercial monkey diets specifically formulated for New World primates. Supplemental foods for dietary diversity and environmental enrichment include fresh vegetables, fresh fruit, and occasional meal worms (Williams et al., 2010). Because of a high basal metabolic rate and a gastrointestinal tract that is short compared to that of other monkeys, squirrel monkeys require a diet of high caloric density. Feed should always be present in the cage as they are susceptible to hypoglycemia.

Similar to other New World monkeys, squirrel monkeys have a dietary requirement for vitamin D_3 and vitamin C. As little as $1\,IU/g$ diet of vitamin D_3 is sufficient to prevent the development of rickets (Lehner et al., 1967). Ten milligrams per kilogram of body weight per day is sufficient ascorbic acid to correct signs of scurvy (Lehner et al., 1968). Squirrel monkeys have a high dietary requirement for folic acid, approximately $200\,pg$ per day. Megaloblastic anemia, low-birth weight infants, and stillbirths have been associated with folic acid deficiency in pregnant squirrel monkeys (Rasmussen et al., 1980).

7. Normal Values

Normal values for hematology and serum chemistry for Bolivian squirrel monkeys are presented in Tables 17.15 and 17.16. To reference normal hematological and serum biochemical values for pregnant and postpartum animals, refer to Suzuki et al. (1996). Normal adult body weights for Bolivian squirrel monkeys are presented in Table 17.17.

8. Research Uses

As one of the most common New World monkey research models, squirrel monkeys have helped to develop numerous research models. The squirrel monkey has served a valuable role in neuroscience research, including studies of the central nervous system (CNS), behavior/learning, and perception (Abee, 2000; Mowery et al., 2012; Gao et al., 2014). Squirrel monkeys are also valuable models in molecular studies of the cortisol receptor and the role of chaperone proteins due to their natural glucocorticoid resistance (Scammell, 2000; Tardif et al., 2011b). Their circulating levels of free or unbound cortisol are approximately 100 times greater than that found in humans or Old World primates (Klosterman et al., 1986). Squirrel monkeys have also contributed to studies of heart failure and cardiomyopathy due to their natural development

TABLE 17.15 Hematologic Data for Bolivian Squirrel Monkeys[a]

Parameter	Sample	Mean	SD	Minimum	Maximum	25th Percentile	50th Percentile	75th Percentile
WBCs ($\times10^3/mm^3$)	267	8.3	2.5	2.6	17.6	6.7	7.9	9.8
RBCs ($\times10^6/mm^3$)	267	6.4	0.8	2.9	7.96	6.2	6.7	6.9
Hgb (g/dl)	267	12.6	1.6	6.1	15.7	12.0	13.0	13.7
Hct (%)	267	38.5	5.5	15.4	49.8	36.2	39.7	42
MCV (fl)	267	60.0	3.2	50.3	70.8	58.0	60.0	62.2
MCH (pg)	267	19.8	2.4	13.7	49.1	18.7	19.6	20.7
MCHC (g/dl)	267	33.1	4.7	21.7	92.8	30.9	33.1	34.4

WBCs, white blood cells; RBCs, red blood cells; Hgb, hemoglobin; Hct, hematocrit; MCV, mean corpuscular volume; MCH, mean corpuscular hemoglobin; MCHC, mean corpuscular hemoglobin concentration.
[a]From Williams et al. (2010).

TABLE 17.16   Serum Chemistry Values for Bolivian Squirrel Monkeys[a]

Analyte	N	Mean	SD	Minimum	Maximum	25th Percentile	50th Percentile	75th Percentile
Alkaline phosphatase (μ/l)	153	389	159	98	1103	288	357	466
GGT (U/l)[b]	99	56.4	150.4	5	1329	21	29	42
Blood urea nitrogen (mg/dl)	256	34	10	18	147	30	34	38
Lactate dehydrogenase (U/l)[b]	99	123.2	111.9	9	721	60	91	149
AST (SGOT) (U/l)[b]	97	185.1	95.3	74	527	124	159	190
ALT (SGOT) c (μ/l)	52	181	78	82	502	128	171	211
Creatine phosphokinase (U/l)[b]	98	562	1379.8	54	9306	85	127.5	350
Amylase (μ/l)	203	54	96	10	943	31	37	46
Cholesterol (mg/dl)[b]	99	151.4	64.7	53	542	123	143	161
Triglycerides (mg/dl)[b]	86	74.9	32.7	28	208	51	66	95
Glucose (mg/dl)	256	109	28	51	201	89	104	129
Phosphorus (mg/dl)	128	4.6	1.5	1.6	9.0	3.3	4.3	5.5
Albumin (gm/dl)[b]	99	4.2	0.6	2.4	7.3	3.9	4.2	4.4
Globulin (gm/dl)	202	4.2	0.4	3.2	5.3	4.0	4.3	4.6
Total bilirubin (mg/dl)	243	0.4	0.2	0.1	1.3	0.3	0.4	0.5
Total protein (g/dl)	255	6.7	0.5	5.2	8.3	6.3	6.7	7.1
Calcium (mg/dl)	243	10.0	0.8	8.1	12.7	9.5	10.0	10.7
Creatinine (mg/dl)	256	0.6	0.2	0.2	1.5	0.4	0.6	0.7
Sodium (mmol/l)	256	149	6	130	170	145	149	153
Potassium (mmol/l)	252	5.3	1.0	3.0	9.8	4.7	5.4	6.0
CO_2[b]	96	11.1	3.9	1.2	20	8.8	11.3	14.5

GGT, γ-glutamyltransferase; AST, aspartate amino transferase; ALT, alanine aminotransferase.
[a]From Williams et al. (2010).
[b]Unpublished data from Squirrel Monkey Breeding and Research Resource, University of South Alabama, 2000.

TABLE 17.17   Adult Body Weights for Bolivian Squirrel Monkeys[a]

Adult	Time	Weight (g)		
		10th Percentile	Median	90th Percentile
Males (Nov–Feb)	Breeding season	870	1094	1362
Males (Mar–Oct)	Nonbreeding season	682	892	1062
Females	Nonpregnant	600	700	798

[a]From Brady (2000). Data from L.E. Williams, Squirrel Monkey Breeding and Research Resource, University of South Alabama, 2000. Weights obtained from Bolivian squirrel monkeys (Saimiri boliviensis boliviensis) that had been in captivity for at least 5 years.

of these conditions (Brady et al., 2003). They are also frequently used in infectious disease, genetics, pharmacology, behavioral pharmacology, drug addiction, and toxicology research (Tardif et al., 2011b; Myers et al., 2007; Brandler et al., 2012; Meyerson et al., 2014; Rowlett et al., 2005; Valdez et al., 2007; Achat-Mendes et al., 2012). However, some of their most valuable contributions have been in the fields of malaria research, transmissible spongiform encephalopathies, and pelvic organ prolapse. The squirrel monkey is an important model for malaria vaccine development because Plasmodium spp., which cause malaria, are host-specific. Animals used for studies of human malaria must be susceptible to the same strains of Plasmodium that cause disease in humans. The Bolivian squirrel monkey has been shown to be a superior model for studies of the pathogenesis of P. falciparum Indochina I (Whiteley et al., 1987), developing lesions and signs similar to those reported in the human disease. Bolivian, Peruvian, and Guyanese squirrel monkeys are susceptible to infection with different strains of P. vivax, but they respond differently depending on the strain of the parasite used (Galland, 2000). These differences in susceptibility to experimental malaria infections underscore the importance of species identification when using squirrel monkeys.

For many years, the squirrel monkey has been recognized as one of the most susceptible nonhuman primate species to experimental infection with Creutzfeldt–Jakob disease (CJD) and other transmissible spongiform encephalopathies (Zlotnik *et al.*, 1974; Brown *et al.*, 1994; Schätzl *et al.*, 1997; Piccardo *et al.*, 2012). The susceptibility of squirrel monkeys to experimental CJD infection is believed to be genetic; the squirrel monkey *PrP* gene sequence in squirrel monkeys is 93.8% homologous to the human *PrP* sequence, which is associated with increased susceptibility to infection in human beings (Schätzl *et al.*, 1997).

The squirrel monkey has been evaluated as a model for human labor and delivery and for pelvic organ prolapse (POP) (Bracken *et al.*, 2011). In women, the flexed position of the fetus and its rotating course through the birth canal are well documented. Fetal rotation resembling labor and delivery in women has been documented in the squirrel monkey (Stoller, 1995). The similarity of infant delivery in women and squirrel monkeys, and reports of lesions resembling POP in women and in squirrel monkeys (Coates *et al.*, 1995a) suggest that POP in the squirrel monkey may be of a similar etiology. POP afflicts older women, and it is associated with increased parity, with large infants, and with hormonal changes. Similarly, the incidence of POP in squirrel monkeys increases with age and parity, and the severity of the lesions is influenced by seasonal hormonal changes (Coates *et al.*, 1995b).

D. *Macaca* spp.: Rhesus and Cynomolgus Monkeys

1. *Introduction*

There are many species in the genus *Macaca*. However, the species that have contributed the most to biomedical research are *M. mulatta* and *M. fascicularis*, and it is these two species that will be discussed in the most depth here. Rhesus monkeys (*M. mulatta*) are among the least threatened and most biologically diverse monkeys in the world (Southwick and Lindburg, 1986). They are a sexually dimorphic, medium-sized Old World monkey, characterized as having brown to gray fur, lighter undersides, and a medium-length nonprehensile tail measuring between 20 and 23 cm (Fooden, 2000) (Fig. 17.10). Adult females range in weight from 4.4 to 10.9 kg and adult males from 5.5 to 12.0 kg. Their life span is approximately 29 years (Rowe, 1996).

Cynomolgus monkeys (*M. fascicularis*) are known as the long-tailed or crab-eating macaques. The species is sexually dimorphic and is described as having gray to red-brown fur, lighter underparts, a pointed crest to the crown of the head, females with a beard, and males with cheek whiskers (Rowe, 1996) (Fig. 17.11). The length of

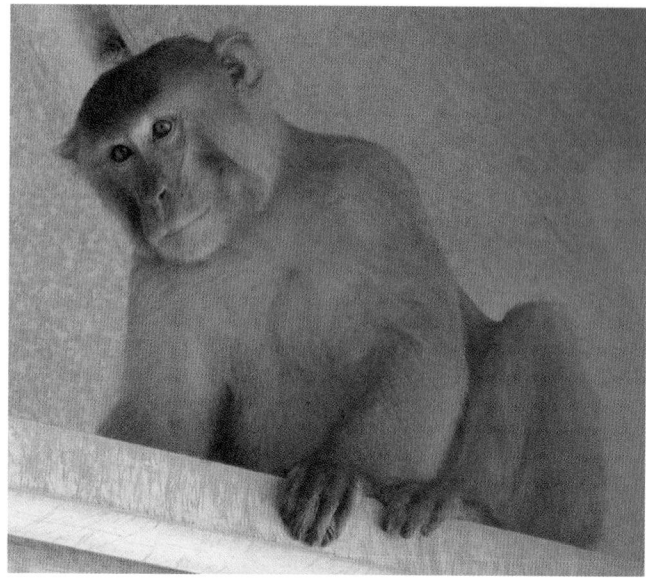

FIGURE 17.10   *Macaca mulatta*, adult rhesus macaque monkey.

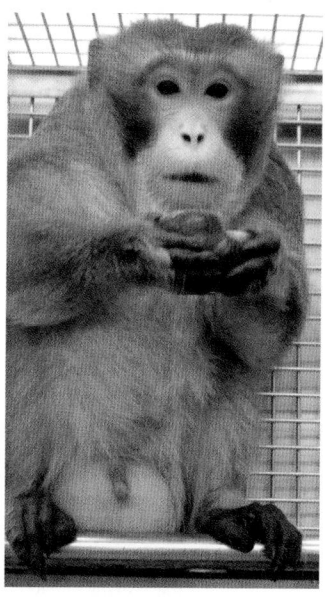

FIGURE 17.11   *Macaca fascicularis*, adult cynomolgus monkey.

the nonprehensile tail is longer than the rhesus, measuring approximately 47–54 cm (Fooden, 2006). The species is smaller than the rhesus monkey with adult females ranging in weight from 2.5 to 5.7 kg and males from 4.7 to 8.3 kg. The longest life span recorded is 37.1 years (Rowe, 1996).

Both rhesus and cynomolgus monkeys have a total of 32 teeth with a dental formula of 2-1-2-3. They have cheek pouches that allow storage of food for mastication at a later time. These pouches originate in the midbuccal area and extend toward the neck. Macaques are diurnal primates that can be both terrestrial and arboreal depending on their habitat (Seth and Seth, 1993), and they prefer to sleep in trees in the wild (Fooden, 2006). Both rhesus and cynomolgus macaques are known to be excellent swimmers, and the skill has been observed in rhesus macaques as young as 2 days of age (Rowe, 1996; Fooden, 2000, 2006).

2. Taxonomy

The genus *Macaca* is a diverse group composed of 20 species. Groves (2001) proposed dividing the species into six species groups, although there is some debate over whether *M. arctoides* should be included in the *M. fascicularis* species group (Fooden, 2006). *M. mulatta* are a species composed of six subspecies that are often divided based on their country of origin. The Chinese-derived rhesus macaques include *M. m. vestita*, *M. m. lasiota*, *M. m. sanctijohannis*, and *M. m. brevicauda*. The Indian-derived rhesus macaques include *M. m. mulatta* and *M. m. villosa* (Smith and McDonough, 2005). Cynomolgus monkey species contain ten subspecies: *M. f. fascicularis*, *M. f. aurea*, *M. f. umbrosa*, *M. f. atriceps*, *M. f. condorensis*, *M. f. fusca*, *M. f. lasiae*, *M. f. tua*, *M. f. karimondjawae*, and *M. f. philippinensis* (Groves, 2001). All have a genetic diploid number of 42. Taxonomy, CITES designation, and geographic distribution are presented in Table 17.18.

3. Natural History

Macaca spp. inhabit the widest geographical and environmental habitat of all nonhuman primates. Rhesus monkeys live in a wide altitude distribution from elevations surpassing 12,000 feet to lowland tropical rain forests and in geographical areas extending from Afghanistan to China, Hong Kong, and India. The rhesus monkey has prospered in part due to its commensal relationship with humans (Wang and Quan, 1986). It is not uncommon to find large groups of rhesus monkeys inhabiting towns, cities, and temples. Cynomolgus monkeys inhabit more subtropical climates (Fooden, 2006). They populate coastal, mangrove, swamp, and riverine forests, and can be found at elevations greater than 6000 feet (Rowe, 1996), although they are less cold tolerant than *M. mulatta* or *M. fuscata* (Lindburg, 1980). Cynomolgus macaques also thrive in human habitats such as temple sites and have been known to raid crops (Loudon *et al.*, 2006).

In the wild, both rhesus and cynomolgus monkeys exist primarily in male-dominated, multimale–multifemale groups ranging in size from 10 to 50 members, with a mean of 32 in rhesus macaques (Fooden, 2000) and a mean of 20 in cynomolgus macaques (Fooden, 2006). Rhesus females adhere to a strict hierarchical class system with the dominant male changing groups every few years (Rowe, 1996; Fooden, 2000). They are known as a belligerent species. Their most common threat behavior is a wide-open mouth with staring eyes. The submissive animal will scream and bare teeth, or will perform a silent bare-tooth display (Rowe, 1996). Cynomolgus macaques have a less stringent hierarchical dominance ranking and groups are often led by a number of high-ranking males (Rowe, 1996). Within the groups, infants of the same age tend to play together, as do infants born to higher-ranking adults. Tension among adults following an act of aggression typically is manifested by an increase in self-grooming, shaking, and scratching. Reconciliation between these adults is shown by the subservient member staring into the eyes and touching the genitals of the dominant member (Rowe, 1996). The main predators of rhesus and cynomolgus macaques include raptors, dogs, weasels, leopards, crocodiles, and tigers. The monkeys will alarm call at the site of these predators (Fooden, 2000; Fooden, 2006; Wheatley, 1999).

4. Reproduction

Rhesus monkeys are seasonal breeders. The breeding season in captivity is approximately 5 months (mid-September to mid-February in the Northern Hemisphere), and their gestation period is approximately 164 days (Rowe, 1996). Births are most common in the spring and summer (Fooden, 2000). Their menstrual cycle is 28 days with a mean estrous period of 9.2 days (Napier and Napier, 1967). The interbirth interval averages 360 days (Johnson-Delaney, 1994), and sexual maturity is achieved in females at 4.5 years of age and in males at approximately 6.5 years of age (Fooden, 2006). With vaginal delivery, infant birth weights average 476 g for females and 502.8 g for males (Fooden, 2000). Infants are generally weaned between 6 and 12 months of age (Fooden, 2000). In male infants, the testicles are generally in the scrotum at time of birth, then ascend into the inguinal region where they remain before returning to the scrotum between age 3–4 years (Fooden, 2000). In females the sexual skin begins to develop at age 2–3 years and it undergoes intermittent swelling and reddening that is maximal at the time of ovulation. The sexual skin extends beyond the vulva to tail, buttocks, thighs, nipples, and facial region to varying degrees in females (Fooden, 2000). Male rhesus macaques may also show a reddening on the skin of their face and hindquarters during breeding season (Fooden, 2006).

Cynomolgus monkeys are capable of mating and birthing throughout the year as they lack strong birth seasonality; however, there does appear to be a birth peak during late summer and early autumn (Fooden, 2006). Their gestation period is 163.5 days (Fooden, 2006). They also have a 28-day menstrual cycle with a mean estrus length of 11 days (Napier and Napier, 1967). The interbirth interval is approximately 390 days. Sexual maturity occurs at approximately 3.5 years of

TABLE 17.18   Macaque Taxonomy, CITES Status, and Distribution[a]

Genus *Macaca*	Common name(s)	CITES status	Distribution
1. M. SYLVANUS *GROUP*			
Monotypic	Barbary macaque	II	Morocco, Algeria
2. M. NEMESTRINA *GROUP*			
M. nemestrina	Pig-tailed macaque	II	Brunei, Indonesia, Malaysia, Thailand
M. leonina	Northern pig-tailed macaque	II	Bangladesh, Cambodia, China, Thailand, Vietnam, Myanmar
M. silenus	Lion-tailed macaque	I	India
M. pagensis	Pagai Island macaque	II	Mentawai Islands, Indonesia
3. SULAWESI *GROUP*			
M. maura	Moor macaque	II	Sulawesi
M. ochreata	Booted macaque	II	Sulawesi
M. tonkeana	Tonkean macaque	II	Sulawesi
M. hecki	Heck's macaque	II	Sulawesi
M. nigrescens	Gorontalo macaque	II	Sulawesi
M. nigra	Celebes crested macaque	II	Sulawesi
4. M. FASCICULARIS *GROUP*			
M. fascicularis	Crab-eating or Long-tailed macaque	II	Bangladesh, Brunei, India, Vietnam, Cambodia, Thailand, Indonesia, Laos, Myanmar, Phillipines, Singapore
M. arctoides	Stump-tailed macaque	II	Cambodia, China, India, Laos, Malaysia, Myanmar, Thailand, Vietnam
5. M. MULATTA *GROUP*			
M. mulatta	Rhesus monkey	II	India, Afghanistan, Kashmir, Vietnam, Nepal, Thailand, Bhutan, Bangladesh, China, Laos, Myanmar, Pakistan
M. cyclopis	Formosan rock macaque	II	Taiwan, China
M. fuscata	Japanese macaque	II	Japan
6. M. SINICA *GROUP*			
M. sinica	Toque macaque	II	Sri Lanka
M. radiata	Bonnet macaque	II	India
M. assamensis	Assam macaque	II	Bangladesh, Bhutan, China, India, Laos, Nepal, Thailand, Vietnam, Myanmar
M. thibetana	Tibetan macaque	II	China

From Groves (2001) and CITES (2013).
[a]I, species listed in CITES Appendix I are threatened with extinction (endangered); II, species listed in CITES Appendix II are not currently threatened with extinction but may become so unless trade is strictly regulated.

age for females and 5.5 years of age for males (Fooden, 2006). Infants are born black in color and transition to gray after the first few months (Rowe, 1996). Infant birth weights average 362 g for females and 402 g for males (Willes *et al.*, 1977). While the sexual skin is prominent in rhesus macaques, it is less obvious in cynomolgus macaques (Fooden, 2006).

5. Laboratory Management

Macaca spp. are very adaptable and do well in a laboratory setting. Cynomolgus macaques tend to be more passive and reserved in captivity compared to rhesus macaques (Winnicker *et al.*, 2013). There are also behavioral differences between Indian-origin and Chinese-origin rhesus monkeys. Starting as neonates, Chinese-origin rhesus monkeys were found to be more temperamental and irritable in comparison to Indian-origin rhesus macaques (Champoux *et al.*, 1994).

Whenever possible, it is preferable to house macaques in social groups or pair-housing to promote social enrichment and enhance their psychological wellbeing. Social housing encourages species-typical behavior (grooming, play, exercise, object manipulation) and decreases the risk of developing abnormal habits and behaviors (Segal, 1989; Schapiro *et al.*, 1996). When forming pairs or groups, consideration must be given to the behavioral influences of age, sex, social history, and individual temperament of the animals. Stress and aggression can occur when housing macaques socially, and thus social introductions must be closely monitored. These aggressive outcomes occur less frequently in cynomolgus compared to rhesus macaques (Winnicker *et al.*, 2013).

According to the *Guide for the Care and Use of Laboratory Animals*, social animals such as macaque species should be housed in pairs or groups of compatible animals unless they *must* be housed alone for experimental reasons, social incompatibility, or veterinary-related concerns (NRC, 2011a). When exceptions occur that necessitate individual housing, increased effort should be put into providing additional environmental enrichment options and providing positive social interactions with humans. Additional enrichment may include enhanced foraging opportunities, access to vertical space to enable macaques to naturally 'escape' perceived threats, and positive reinforcement training (PRT) (Reinhardt, 2008). These monkeys should also be provided opportunity for olfactory, auditory, and visual stimulation by being housed in rooms with other monkeys (Code of Federal Regulations (CFR), 1999).

Housing space minimums can be found in Appendix 1 of the *Guide for the Care and Use of Laboratory Animals* (NRC, 2011a) and in Subpart D, section 3.80 of the *Animal Welfare Act* (USDA, 2013). It should be stressed that these published values are minimum standards and every effort should be made to exceed these measurements

and provide an environment that allows the animals to display natural behavior. In the indoor environment, the recommended temperature range for nonhuman primates is 64–84°F, with a relative humidity between 30 and 70% (NRC, 2011a). The environmental lighting should be diffused throughout the animal area and generally provides a 12-h light–12-h dark cycle.

Orphaned infants can be fostered on a replacement dam, and while this is a preferred rearing technique, multiple factors can limit fostering success. Hand rearing of infants can be accomplished, but requires time-intensive care for the infant. The environment should be warm, especially during the first 2 weeks of life, and temperatures should be maintained between 80 and 90°F (the higher end used for newborns and premature infants). A surrogate, or soft structure to which an infant can cling, is an important addition to the nursery to promote socialization techniques (Anderson, 1986). For nutrition, the infant is fed 5–10% dextrose in water every 2 h for the first 24 h. This is followed by use of commercial formulas (Primilac, Enfamil, Similac), which can be diluted during the first couple days to help transition the infant to full-strength formula. During the first week, infants should be fed 20–30 ml per feeding every 2–3 h. Small pieces of solid moist food can be introduced between 5 and 14 days of age (Anderson, 1986).

6. Nutrition

In the wild, rhesus monkeys are mainly vegetarian. Their diet consists of fruit, seeds, flowers, leaves, shoots, roots, bark, fungi, and small invertebrates. The ingestion of soil has been noted to be both a source of nutrients and an aid in digestion (Lindburg, 1980; Fooden, 2000). The cynomolgus macaque diet is considered omnivorous due to the consumption of insects, frogs, and crabs, but they can also be highly frugivorous. In some instances, fruit has been noted to comprise 90% of their diet (Lindburg, 1980).

In captivity, both rhesus and cynomolgus macaques readily adapt to a commercial monkey chow diet. A standard diet used by multiple primate centers is Purina monkey chow #5038, which contains 3.45 kcal/g, 12% fat, 18% protein, 4.14% sugar carbohydrate, and 65.9% fiber (Reinhardt, 1993; Moore *et al.*, 2013). The stability of vitamin C in commercial diets has historically been a concern. It is still recommended that the commercial monkey diet be used within 90 days of being manufactured. Biscuits needing moisture should be soaked in fruit juice rather than water because of the propensity of water to deteriorate vitamin C (LabDiet Product Reference Manual, 1998). The typical daily ration of commercial biscuits for both male and female rhesus monkeys is approximately 2–4% of their body weight. They are usually fed twice daily to help prevent food waste.

Providing a variety of novel, supplemental food items is an important form of enrichment that promotes the well-being of rhesus monkeys (ILAR, 1998). Fruits, vegetables, legumes, and seeds are provided to mimic natural foraging substrates and promote species-typical behaviors. Seeds, grains, and legumes can be scattered among bedding substrates (hay, straw, grass) or used in food puzzles to encourage foraging behavior and possibly to reduce aggressive and stereotypic behaviors (Segal, 1989). In addition, macaques are susceptible to obesity with a sedentary lifestyle, and increasing foraging opportunities and food processing time will help to combat this nutritional issue (Winnicker et al., 2013).

7. Normal Values

Normative hematologic and serum chemistry data for the rhesus monkey have been published by Buchl and Howard (1997). Tables 17.19–17.22 provide data derived from 527 healthy, domestically bred and reared rhesus monkeys. Normal hematologic and chemistry data for the cynomolgus macaque is provided in Tables 17.23 and 17.24 and derived from a total of 917 healthy monkeys (Xie et al., 2013). For normal value comparisons on macaque monkeys with no anesthesia versus those receiving anesthesia, see Barnhart (2010).

8. Research Uses

Of all the species in the genus Macaca, rhesus monkeys have been cited most in research articles historically and have served as a model for the most biomedical research programs over the past 60 years. From the 1930s through the 1970s, research citing the use of rhesus monkeys referred to animals that were almost exclusively of Indian origin. As Indian-origin rhesus monkeys became more difficult to obtain following a ban on exports from India in 1978, other sources of rhesus monkeys were sought. Over the past 20 years, Chinese-origin rhesus monkeys have been imported and cited in numerous research articles. There are differences in morphology, allele frequencies, and population-specific differences in the allele distributions with both class I and II major histocompatibility complex (MHC) loci that indicate the two populations have distinct genetic characteristics that differ in these two subtypes of rhesus monkeys (Viray et al., 2001; Doxiadis et al., 2003). Genetic analysis using SNPs analysis has also revealed differences (Ferguson et al., 2007) and differences in disease progression following simian immunodeficiency virus (SIV) challenge have also been reported (Trichel et al., 2002). Although Indian-origin and Chinese-origin rhesus monkeys belong to the same genus and species, differences in phenotype and

TABLE 17.19 Normal Blood Values of Rhesus by Sex, Age, and Gravidity[a]

Age (years)	Sex	Gravidity	N	HCT (%)	HGB (g/dl)	WBC (×10³/±l)	RBC (×10⁶/±l)	MCV (fl)	MCH (pg)	MCHC (g/dl)
0.05–1	F		27	40.4 ± 2.5	12.8 ± 0.8	11.2 ± 4.3	6.04 ± 0.46	67.2 ± 3.9	21.3 ± 1.4	31.6 ± 0.7
0.05–1	M		27	41.4 ± 3.2	13.1 ± 0.8	9.5 ± 3.0	6.18 ± 0.56	67.1 ± 3.0	21.3 ± 1.1	31.7 ± 0.8
1–2	F		77	40.1 ± 2.4	12.9 ± 0.7	9.8 ± 3.4	5.75 ± 0.36	69.4 ± 4.2	22.4 ± 0.9	32.0 ± 1.2
1–2	M		30	40.0 ± 2.2	12.8 ± 0.7	9.8 ± 3.5	5.73 ± 0.39	69.8 ± 2.6	22.4 ± 1.0	32.0 ± 0.6
2–3	F		50	39.0 ± 2.5	12.6 ± 0.8	9.7 ± 3.3	5.49 ± 0.41	71.1 ± 2.6	23.0 ± 1.1	32.3 ± 0.6
2–3	M		27	39.7 ± 2.0	13.0 ± 0.6	8.9 ± 2.1	5.71 ± 0.31	68.4 ± 6.1	22.7 ± 0.9	32.7 ± 0.7
3–4	F		25	38.6 ± 2.3	12.5 ± 0.7	10.6 ± 3.3	5.56 ± 0.46	69.6 ± 2.9	22.6 ± 1.0	32.4 ± 0.7
3–4	F	Y	11	40.5 ± 2.3	13.0 ± 0.8	8.6 ± 1.8	5.73 ± 0.30	70.8 ± 3.1	22.8 ± 1.2	32.2 ± 0.5
3–4	M		30	40.2 ± 2.8	12.9 ± 0.7	10.5 ± 2.8	5.79 ± 0.42	69.5 ± 2.4	22.4 ± 1.1	31.9 ± 1.8
4–5	F		13	39.5 ± 2.5	12.8 ± 0.7	11.6 ± 3.1	5.85 ± 0.42	67.6 ± 2.5	22.0 ± 0.8	32.6 ± 0.5
4–5	F	Y	20	41.3 ± 3.2	13.3 ± 1.0	9.9 ± 3.0	5.91 ± 0.58	70.2 ± 3.1	22.6 ± 1.3	32.2 ± 0.6
4–5	M		44	41.1 ± 2.8	13.2 ± 0.8	10.4 ± 2.6	5.89 ± 0.35	69.7 ± 2.8	22.4 ± 0.9	32.2 ± 0.6
5–10	F		30	40.3 ± 2.6	12.9 ± 0.8	10.3 ± 3.3	5.75 ± 0.41	70.4 ± 3.6	22.4 ± 1.3	31.9 ± 0.6
5–10	F	Y	44	40.3 ± 2.2	12.9 ± 0.7	10.0 ± 2.8	5.79 ± 0.44	69.8 ± 3.5	22.4 ± 1.3	32.2 ± 1.0
5–10	M		21	42.4 ± 2.5	13.6 ± 0.7	11.8 ± 2.9	6.90 ± 0.34	70.7 ± 2.2	22.8 ± 0.9	32.2 ± 0.8
10+	F		29	42.1 ± 2.6	13.6 ± 0.9	9.6 ± 3.1	6.01 ± 0.72	70.0 ± 2.6	23.7 ± 1.1	32.4 ± 1.0
10+	F	Y	22	40.7 ± 3.1	13.5 ± 1.1	9.6 ± 2.2	6.81 ± 0.55	70.3 ± 2.5	23.3 ± 1.0	33.2 ± 0.8

WBC, white blood cells; RBC, red blood cells; HGB, hemoglobin; HCT, hematocrit; MCV, mean corpuscular volume; MCH, mean corpuscular hemoglobin; MCHC, mean corpuscular hemoglobin concentration.

[a]From MD Anderson Cancer Center, Department of Veterinary Sciences. Samples collected from clinically normal, colony-origin, SPF rhesus monkeys. SPF (specific-pathogen-free), no viral antibody titers to Macacine herpesvirus 1, simian immunodeficiency virus, simian retrovirus, or systemic T-lymphotrophic virus.

TABLE 17.20 Normal White Blood Cell Counts and Corresponding Absolute Values for Rhesus Monkeys[a]

Age (years)	Sex	Gravidity	N	WBC (×10³/µl)	SEG (µl)	Lymphocytes (µl)	Monocytes (µl)	Eosinophils (µl)	Band (µl)	Basophils (µl)
0.05–1	F		27	11.2 ± 4.3	5999 ± 3171	4749 ± 2665	261 ± 235	66 ± 101	109 ± 205	35 ± 76
0.05–1	M		27	9.5 ± 3.0	4794 ± 2490	4368 ± 1914	208 ± 165	29 ± 52	50 ± 92	19 ± 42
1–2	F		77	9.8 ± 3.4	5959 ± 3028	3439 ± 1729	277 ± 269	41 ± 81	82 ± 122	4 ± 17
1–2	M		30	9.8 ± 3.5	6369 ± 2861	2845 ± 1609	251 ± 249	29 ± 49	276 ± 476	5 ± 19
2–3	F		50	9.7 ± 3.5	5639 ± 2890	3400 ± 1711	324 ± 260	79 ± 121	163 ± 335	17 ± 38
2–3	M		27	8.9 ± 2.1	5118 ± 1705	3528 ± 1692	162 ± 151	29 ± 52	30 ± 43	6 ± 22
3–4	F		25	10.6 ± 3.3	6601 ± 2954	3630 ± 1540	185 ± 185	89 ± 150	35 ± 77	12 ± 58
3–4	F	Y	11	8.6 ± 1.8	5646 ± 1728	2491 ± 1226	343 ± 387	81 ± 109	37 ± 62	0 ± 0
3–4	M		30	10.5 ± 2.8	6034 ± 2316	3909 ± 1238	371 ± 391	119 ± 220	94 ± 132	5 ± 20
4–5	F		13	11.6 ± 3.1	7678 ± 2960	3588 ± 1102	191 ± 206	77 ± 105	97 ± 154	0 ± 0
4–5	F	Y	20	9.9 ± 3.0	7637 ± 2778	1832 ± 801	272 ± 159	43 ± 61	123 ± 191	2 ± 11
4–5	M		44	10.4 ± 2.6	6374 ± 2322	3587 ± 1589	288 ± 247	128 ± 203	55 ± 110	7 ± 28
5–10	F		30	10.3 ± 3.3	6922 ± 3160	3650 ± 4663	359 ± 258	117 ± 198	92 ± 172	14 ± 59
5–10	F	Y	44	10.0 ± 2.8	7301 ± 2823	2088 ± 712	324 ± 243	69 ± 84	137 ± 177	12 ± 34
5–10	M		21	11.8 ± 2.9	7911 ± 3580	3103 ± 1840	440 ± 296	144 ± 202	216 ± 333	3 ± 15
10+	F		29	9.6 ± 3.1	6536 ± 3262	2618 ± 1072	236 ± 237	162 ± 242	58 ± 96	16 ± 47
10+	F	Y	22	9.6 ± 2.2	6706 ± 2510	2210 ± 1201	326 ± 300	250 ± 225	30 ± 59	38 ± 70

WBC, white blood cells.

[a]From MD Anderson Cancer Center, Department of Veterinary Sciences. Samples collected from clinically normal, colony-origin, SPF rhesus monkeys. SPF (specific-pathogen–free), no viral antibody titers to Macacine herpesvirus 1, simian immunodeficiency virus, simian retrovirus, or systemic T-lymphotrophic virus.

TABLE 17.21 Normal Serum Biochemical Values for Rhesus Monkeys[a]

Age (years)	Sex	Gravidity	N	Bilirubin (mg/dl)	ALT (U/l)	AST (U/liter)	Alkaline phosphatase (U/l)	CR (mg/dl)	Glucose (mg/dl)	BUN (mg/dl)	Total protein (g/dl)	Albumin (g/dl)
0.05–1	F		27	0.2 ± 0.2	39 ± 9	48 ± 11	646 ± 136	0.6 ± 0.2	82 ± 16	18 ± 5	7.1 ± 0.3	4.3 ± 0.3
0.05–1	M		27	0.2 ± 0.2	42 ± 9	47 ± 10	727 ± 148	0.7 ± 0.2	88 ± 20	20 ± 5	7.3 ± 0.5	7.5 ± 18
1–2	F		77	0.1 ± 0.1	37 ± 10	49 ± 13	578 ± 149	0.7 ± 0.1	74 ± 15	21 ± 6	7.2 ± 0.8	4.5 ± 0.3
1–2	M		30	0.2 ± 0.1	38 ± 9	47 ± 13	527 ± 146	0.7 ± 0.1	74 ± 12	21 ± 5	7.0 ± 0.6	4.5 ± 0.3
2–3	F		50	0.2 ± 0.1	37 ± 10	44 ± 15	479 ± 136	0.7 ± 0.1	64 ± 14	21 ± 4	7.1 ± 0.3	4.5 ± 0.4
2–3	M		27	0.1 ± 0.1	35 ± 11	51 ± 13	529 ± 177	0.7 ± 0.1	60 ± 10	24 ± 5	7.0 ± 0.4	4.7 ± 0.4
3–4	F		25	0.2 ± 0.1	36 ± 14	43 ± 12	384 ± 121	0.8 ± 0.2	67 ± 14	19 ± 3	7.3 ± 0.4	4.5 ± 1.4
3–4	F	Y	11	0.2 ± 0.1	42 ± 42	32 ± 10	197 ± 58	0.7 ± 0.1	68 ± 7	12 ± 2	6.9 ± 0.4	3.8 ± 0.5
3–4	M		30	0.2 ± 0.1	37 ± 9	40 ± 13	541 ± 144	0.9 ± 0.1	73 ± 16	18 ± 3	7.3 ± 0.4	4.6 ± 0.3
4–5	F		13	0.2 ± 0.1	31 ± 8	38 ± 10	288 ± 71	0.9 ± 0.1	76 ± 18	21 ± 3	7.6 ± 0.4	4.6 ± 0.4
4–5	F	Y	20	0.1 ± 0.1	29 ± 8	31 ± 7	134 ± 56	0.9 ± 0.3	58 ± 11	15 ± 5	7.0 ± 0.5	3.6 ± 0.5
4–5	M		44	0.2 ± 0.1	41 ± 12	39 ± 13	456 ± 115	1.0 ± 0.2	77 ± 13	19 ± 5	7.5 ± 0.4	4.6 ± 0.4
5–10	F		30	0.2 ± 0.1	35 ± 7	32 ± 8	180 ± 63	0.9 ± 0.1	66 ± 13	19 ± 3	7.7 ± 0.5	4.5 ± 0.5
5–10	F	Y	44	0.2 ± 0.1	28 ± 13	29 ± 10	110 ± 64	0.8 ± 0.1	57 ± 12	12 ± 4	7.2 ± 0.5	3.3 ± 0.4
5–10	M		21	0.2 ± 0.2	33 ± 8	38 ± 10	203 ± 84	1.1 ± 0.1	67 ± 16	20 ± 3	7.8 ± 0.5	4.5 ± 0.4
10+	F		29	0.1 ± 0.1	40 ± 12	41 ± 11	118 ± 40	0.9 ± 0.2	74 ± 15	21 ± 4	7.8 ± 0.4	4.4 ± 0.6
10+	F	Y	22	0.2 ± 0.2	27 ± 10	42 ± 12	85 ± 58	0.8 ± 0.1	55 ± 18	15 ± 3	7.4 ± 0.5	3.3 ± 0.3

(Continued)

TABLE 17.21 (Continued)

Age (years)	Sex	Gravidity	N	Globulin (g/dl)	Cholesterol (mg/dl)	GGT (U/l)	Triglycerides (mg/dl)	Calcium (mg/dl)	PHOS (mg/dl)	CK (U/l)	LD (U/l)	UA (mg/dl)
0.05–1	F		27	2.8 ± 0.3	165 ± 30	75 ± 18	44 ± 14	10.5 ± 1.0	5.5 ± 1.2	386 ± 220	467 ± 186	0.2 ± 0.1
0.05–1	M		27	2.8 ± 0.5	179 ± 29	77 ± 14	52 ± 35	10.6 ± 0.8	6.4 ± 1.1	366 ± 147	427 ± 166	0.3 ± 0.3
1–2	F		77	2.8 ± 0.7	165 ± 30	71 ± 16	43 ± 11	10.5 ± 1.0	5.3 ± 1.0	436 ± 227	443 ± 180	0.2 ± 0.2
1–2	M		30	2.6 ± 0.5	161 ± 30	67 ± 19	41 ± 14	10.3 ± 0.5	5.1 ± 0.7	507 ± 297	422 ± 198	0.2 ± 0.1
2–3	F		50	2.6 ± 0.3	146 ± 27	59 ± 13	44 ± 16	10.1 ± 0.7	5.6 ± 1.0	446 ± 289	434 ± 211	0.1 ± 0.1
2–3	M		27	2.2 ± 0.5	151 ± 22	72 ± 13	46 ± 11	9.7 ± 0.7	6.2 ± 0.7	423 ± 276	542 ± 173	0.1 ± 0.1
3–4	F		25	2.8 ± 0.4	141 ± 20	47 ± 7	45 ± 16	10.4 ± 1.6	5.1 ± 0.9	544 ± 289	372 ± 129	0.1 ± 0.1
3–4	F	Y	11	3.2 ± 0.3	73 ± 35	46 ± 12	48 ± 16	9.8 ± 0.7	4.1 ± 0.7	305 ± 93	433 ± 197	0.1 ± 0.1
3–4	M		30	2.7 ± 0.4	138 ± 20	57 ± 20	50 ± 16	10.7 ± 0.6	5.2 ± 0.6	491 ± 250	427 ± 222	0.2 ± 0.1
4–5	F		13	2.9 ± 0.6	152 ± 30	49 ± 9	55 ± 23	10.4 ± 0.5	4.4 ± 1.1	447 ± 163	404 ± 139	0.2 ± 0.1
4–5	F	Y	20	3.4 ± 0.4	75 ± 18	42 ± 12	53 ± 21	9.8 ± 0.6	3.6 ± 0.9	444 ± 232	305 ± 61	0.1 ± 0.1
4–5	M		44	2.8 ± 0.4	143 ± 23	63 ± 17	45 ± 14	10.8 ± 0.8	4.7 ± 0.9	425 ± 184	381 ± 265	0.1 ± 0.1
5–10	F		30	3.3 ± 0.4	150 ± 34	77 ± 14	45 ± 19	10.7 ± 0.9	3.9 ± 0.9	446 ± 187	297 ± 83	0.1 ± 0.1
5–10	F	Y	44	3.8 ± 0.4	81 ± 33	45 ± 14	53 ± 22	9.2 ± 0.9	3.2 ± 0.6	420 ± 246	370 ± 143	0.1 ± 0.1
5–10	M		21	3.3 ± 0.5	155 ± 22	55 ± 16	43 ± 18	10.4 ± 0.9	3.6 ± 0.9	413 ± 163	363 ± 173	0.2 ± 0.2
10+	F		29	3.4 ± 0.6	180 ± 42	41 ± 6	58 ± 34	10.2 ± 1.1	3.5 ± 1.1	442 ± 231	393 ± 171	0.1 ± 0.1
10+	F	Y	22	4.1 ± 0.4	81 ± 24	41 ± 8	54 ± 21	8.8 ± 0.8	3.0 ± 1.4	286 ± 225	577 ± 229	0.1 ± 0.1

[a]From MD Anderson Cancer Center, Department of Veterinary Sciences. Samples collected from clinically normal, colony-origin, SPF rhesus monkeys.
SPF (specific-pathogen-free), no viral antibody titers to Macacine herpesvirus 1, simian immunodeficiency virus, simian retrovirus, or tystemic T-lymphotrophic virus.

TABLE 17.22 Normal Serum Electrolyte Values for Rhesus Monkeys[a]

Age (years)	Sex	Gravidity	N	Chloride (Cl⁻) (mEq/l)	Sodium (Na⁺) (mEq/l)	Potassium (K⁺) (mEq/l)
0.05–1	F		27	112 ± 3	148 ± 3	4.3 ± 0.6
0.05–1	M		27	113 ± 2	148 ± 3	4.3 ± 0.6
1–2	F		77	113 ± 4	148 ± 3	3.8 ± 0.6
1–2	M		30	114 ± 2	148 ± 2	4.0 ± 0.5
2–3	F		50	113 ± 2	148 ± 2	3.8 ± 0.4
2–3	M		27	112 ± 2	148 ± 2	3.7 ± 0.3
3–4	F		25	114 ± 2	147 ± 2	4.0 ± 0.3
3–4	F	Y	11	113 ± 2	144 ± 3	4.0 ± 0.4
3–4	M		30	113 ± 2	148 ± 3	4.0 ± 0.3
4–5	F		13	116 ± 3	147 ± 3	3.9 ± 0.2
4–5	F	Y	20	112 ± 3	142 ± 3	4.2 ± 0.6
4–5	M		44	113 ± 3	148 ± 3	4.0 ± 0.4
5–10	F		30	115 ± 3	148 ± 3	4.0 ± 0.5
5–10	F	Y	44	114 ± 3	143 ± 3	4.1 ± 0.4
5–10	M		21	113 ± 2	148 ± 3	3.9 ± 0.3
10+	F		29	116 ± 3	150 ± 2	4.0 ± 0.4
10+	F	Y	22	115 ± 2	145 ± 3	3.9 ± 0.3

[a]From MD Anderson Cancer Center, Department of Veterinary Sciences. Samples collected from clinically normal, colony-origin, SPF rhesus monkeys.
SPF (specific-pathogen-free), no viral antibody titers to Macacine herpesvirus 1, simian immunodeficiency virus, simian retrovirus, or systemic T-lymphotrophic virus.

TABLE 17.23 Normal Hematologic Values of *Macaca fascicularis* by Sex and Age[a]

Age (months)	Sex	N	HCT (%)	HGB (g/l)	WBCs (10^9/l)	RBCs (10^{12}/l)	MCV (fl)	MCH (pg)	MCHC (g/l)
13–24	F	162	44.6 ± 2.6	127.6 ± 7.9	13.3 ± 3.7	5.75 ± 0.40	77.6 ± 4.0	22.2 ± 1.2	287 ± 6.6
13–24	M	162	44.9 ± 2.8	129.5 ± 8.9	12.7 ± 2.2	5.78 ± 0.44	77.8 ± 4.1	22.4 ± 1.1	288 ± 7.6
25–36	F	178	45.8 ± 2.6	130 ± 7.8	13.7 ± 3.4	5.80 ± 0.37	79.0 ± 3.7	22.4 ± 1.2	284 ± 8.6
25–36	M	121	45.5 ± 3.0	131 ± 9.6	12.5 ± 2.7	5.86 ± 0.45	77.8 ± 3.6	22.3 ± 1.1	287 ± 7.5
37–48	F	72	45.8 ± 3.1	130 ± 9.0	14.4 ± 4.1	5.76 ± 0.44	79.8 ± 3.6	22.6 ± 1.0	284 ± 7.3
37–48	M	16	45.5 ± 2.5	130 ± 8.0	12.4 ± 1.5	5.87 ± 0.43	77.6 ± 2.8	22.3 ± 1.0	287 ± 7.6
49–60	F	84	44.4 ± 3.0	125 ± 9.0	13.7 ± 3.2	5.55 ± 0.48	80.1 ± 4.2	22.6 ± 1.3	282 ± 8.2
49–60	M	31	46.5 ± 4.2	132 ± 12.1	13.5 ± 2.2	5.89 ± 0.49	78.9 ± 3.4	22.4 ± 1.1	284 ± 7.5
61–72	F	47	42.9 ± 4.2	121 ± 12.2	12.4 ± 2.0	5.32 ± 0.48	80.8 ± 4.8	22.8 ± 1.4	282 ± 7.8
61–72	M	44	46.9 ± 2.6	133 ± 7.6	13.1 ± 2.3	5.90 ± 0.46	79.8 ± 4.1	22.7 ± 1.1	285 ± 7.5

Age (months)	Sex	N	Neutrophils (10^9/l)	Lymphocytes (10^9/l)	Monocytes (10^9/l)	Eosinophils (10^9/l)	Basophils (10^9/l)	Platelets (10^9/l)	Reticulocytes (10^9/l)
13–24	F	162	5.2 ± 3.3	7.1 ± 2.4	0.8 ± 0.3	0.2 ± 0.2	0.03 ± 0.2	370 ± 85	53 ± 23
13–24	M	162	4.2 ± 1.6	7.4 ± 2.0	0.9 ± 0.3	0.2 ± 0.2	0.03 ± 0.01	381 ± 95	54 ± 25
25–36	F	178	4.7 ± 2.3	7.7 ± 2.4	0.9 ± 0.4	0.4 ± 0.4	0.03 ± 0.02	358 ± 82	55 ± 28
25–36	M	121	3.9 ± 1.7	7.5 ± 2.4	0.9 ± 0.3	0.3 ± 0.3	0.02 ± 0.01	386 ± 116	47 ± 17
37–48	F	72	7.0 ± 3.8	6.1 ± 2.3	0.9 ± 0.3	0.4 ± 0.4	0.03 ± 0.02	377 ± 97	59 ± 23
37–48	M	16	4.5 ± 2.1	6.7 ± 1.6	0.9 ± 0.3	0.3 ± 0.3	0.02 ± 0.01	355 ± 127	43 ± 17
49–60	F	84	6.9 ± 3.2	5.7 ± 1.7	0.8 ± 0.3	0.4 ± 0.3	0.02 ± 0.01	366 ± 80	62 ± 32
49–60	M	31	5.6 ± 3.0	6.7 ± 1.9	0.9 ± 0.3	0.4 ± 0.3	0.02 ± 0.01	372 ± 130	47 ± 15
61–72	F	47	6.6 ± 3.1	5.0 ± 1.9	0.7 ± 0.2	0.3 ± 0.2	0.02 ± 0.01	386 ± 103	62 ± 31
61–72	M	44	4.9 ± 2.0	7.1 ± 2.0	0.9 ± 0.4	0.3 ± 0.2	0.02 ± 0.01	356 ± 84	53 ± 23

From Xie et al. (2013).
WBCs, white blood cells; RBCs, red blood cells; HGB, hemoglobin; HCT, hematocrit; MCV, mean corpuscular volume; MCH, mean corpuscular hemoglobin; MCHC, mean corpuscular hemoglobin concentration.
[a]*Value ranges given are ±2 standard deviations.*

genotype may impact the results of studies. Therefore, it is important to carefully consider the origin of rhesus monkeys prior to initiating studies.

In 1937, the rhesus monkey contributed to the identification of the red blood cell Rh factor (Lee, 1993). During the 1950s, they served as a model to investigate, develop, and produce the polio vaccine (Johnsen, 1995). They were also subjects in the comparative psychology research of maternal and social deprivation by Harry Harlow in the 1950s (Harlow *et al.*, 1965). During the 1970s and 1980s, they became the primate models of choice in drug safety and efficacy research and they continue to serve a valuable role in pharmacology studies (Rockwood *et al.*, 2008). Rhesus monkeys are one of the preferred models for studying the mechanisms of immunodeficiency diseases. Rhesus macaques' genetic homology to humans, based on nucleotide base sequences, is 93.45% (Gibbs *et al.*, 2007). This genetic similarity, coupled with a susceptibility to the SIV and their homology to the human MHC class I, II, and *TCR* genes (Knapp *et al.*, 1997), make them an excellent model for HIV vaccine research and development. Rhesus monkeys have also extensively contributed to research using the recombinant simian–human immunodeficiency virus (SHIV) (Carroll *et al.*, 2006). Other areas of research have included aging, atherosclerosis, alcoholism, diabetes, cancer, and myocarditis (Lee, 1993). A notable advancement for research involving rhesus macaques is the completion of genome sequencing in 2007 (Gibbs *et al.*, 2007). Having the entire rhesus macaque genome sequence available will substantially augment genetics research, comparative physiology, and basic biology studies (Gibbs *et al.*, 2007).

TABLE 17.24 Normal Chemistry Values of *Macaca fascicularis* by Sex and Age[a]

Age (months)	Sex	N	T bilirubin (mg/dl)	T protein (g/dl)	Albumin (g/dl)	Globulin (g/dl)	A/G	BUN (mg/dl)	Creatinine (mg/dl)
13–24	F	162	0.10 ± 0.03	7.2 ± 0.5	4.1 ± 0.4	3.1 ± 0.4	1.4 ± 0.2	21.7 ± 3.1	0.46 ± 0.09
13–24	M	162	0.10 ± 0.03	7.3 ± 0.5	4.1 ± 0.4	3.1 ± 0.3	1.3 ± 0.2	21.5 ± 3.1	0.49 ± 0.09
25–36	F	178	0.10 ± 0.04	7.5 ± 0.5	4.2 ± 0.4	3.3 ± 0.4	1.3 ± 0.2	19.8 ± 3.1	0.61 ± 0.13
25–36	M	121	0.10 ± 0.03	7.4 ± 0.6	4.1 ± 0.5	3.3 ± 0.3	1.3 ± 0.2	20.6 ± 3.2	0.58 ± 0.11
37–48	F	72	0.10 ± 0.04	7.5 ± 0.7	4.0 ± 0.6	3.5 ± 0.4	1.1 ± 0.2	19.1 ± 3.5	0.67 ± 0.14
37–48	M	16	0.10 ± 0.04	7.4 ± 0.4	4.1 ± 0.4	3.3 ± 0.4	1.3 ± 0.3	19.3 ± 2.6	0.71 ± 0.09
49–60	F	84	0.11 ± 0.04	7.7 ± 0.6	4.0 ± 0.4	3.7 ± 0.5	1.1 ± 0.2	17.5 ± 2.8	0.76 ± 0.14
49–60	M	31	0.10 ± 0.03	7.6 ± 0.9	4.0 ± 0.7	3.6 ± 0.4	1.1 ± 0.2	17.9 ± 2.9	0.85 ± 0.15
61–72	F	47	0.10 ± 0.03	7.7 ± 0.7	3.8 ± 0.7	3.9 ± 0.6	1.0 ± 0.2	17.8 ± 3.5	0.78 ± 0.11
61–72	M	44	0.09 ± 0.03	7.9 ± 0.6	4.2 ± 0.4	3.7 ± 0.4	1.2 ± 0.2	17.1 ± 2.6	1.01 ± 0.22

Age (months)	Sex	N	ALT (IU/l)	AST (IU/l)	ALP (IU/l)	GGT (IU/l)	LDH (IU/l)	Glucose (mg/dl)	Potassium (mmol/l)
13–24	F	162	56.5 ± 16.1	62.3 ± 13.2	752 ± 190	49.3 ± 15.2	655 ± 125	74.1 ± 22.0	5.6 ± 0.7
13–24	M	162	57.2 ± 17.1	60.2 ± 15.4	698 ± 198	48.1 ± 13.6	691 ± 134	76.9 ± 24.7	5.5 ± 0.7
25–36	F	178	46.0 ± 12.4	50.4 ± 11.0	650 ± 187	43.2 ± 15.7	537 ± 111	86.3 ± 24.9	5.7 ± 0.7
25–36	M	121	53.8 ± 18.0	54.6 ± 15.5	598 ± 182	46.7 ± 13.5	622 ± 142	87.2 ± 26.3	5.5 ± 0.6
37–48	F	72	45.0 ± 21.0	47.1 ± 11.4	424 ± 152	38.6 ± 12.0	519 ± 145	90.8 ± 25.9	5.5 ± 0.8
37–48	M	16	43.1 ± 10.1	49.3 ± 6.8	695 ± 265	48.2 ± 10.4	519 ± 125	78.2 ± 12.3	5.5 ± 0.8
49–60	F	84	44.8 ⊥ 19.3	45.0 ± 13.4	293 ± 139	35.5 ± 10.0	484 ± 132	92.3 ± 32.8	5.8 ± 0.7
49–60	M	31	44.5 ± 16.7	47.1 ± 12.0	547 ± 121	41.2 ± 11.8	533 ± 132	84.3 ± 22.9	5.7 ± 0.7
61–72	F	47	48.5 ± 29.1	42.2 ± 18.3	249 ± 117	37.4 ± 14.3	444 ± 101	90.6 ± 33.0	5.8 ± 0.5
61–72	M	44	42.6 ± 16.9	46.3 ± 12.6	423 ± 192	38.2 ± 8.9	454 ± 115	100.2 + 30.3	6.4 ± 0.8

Age (months)	Sex	N	Sodium (mmol/l)	Chloride (mmol/l)	Calcium (mg/dl)	Phosphorus (mg/dl)	Magnesium (mg/dl)	Cholesterol (mg/dl)	Triglyc. (mg/dl)
13–24	F	162	151.3 ± 2.7	108.0 ± 2.8	10.5 ± 0.4	7.0 ± 1.2	2.3 ± 0.2	127 ± 23	44.2 ± 17.7
13–24	M	162	150.0 ± 3.1	106.7 ± 2.5	10.2 ± 0.5	7.1 ± 1.1	2.2 ± 0.2	126 ± 24	50.4 ± 33.6
25–36	F	178	152.3 ± 3.3	108.0 ± 2.6	10.7 ± 0.6	6.5 ± 1.3	2.2 ± 0.2	126 ± 28	47.8 ± 18.6
25–36	M	121	150.8 ± 4.2	106.9 ± 2.8	10.3 ± 0.7	7.0 ± 1.3	2.2 ± 0.2	132 ± 29	43.4 ± 24.8
37–48	F	72	152.2 ± 3.8	108.3 ± 2.8	10.6 ± 0.6	6.3 ± 1.4	2.1 ± 0.2	133 ± 26	65.5 ± 67.3
37–48	M	16	153.4 ± 2.7	107.5 ± 2.5	10.5 ± 0.4	6.7 ± 1.2	2.0 ± 0.1	120 ± 22	62.8 ± 38.9
49–60	F	84	153.4 ± 3.6	108.3 ± 2.9	10.8 ± 0.6	6.2 ± 1.4	2.2 ± 0.2	126 ± 27	50.4 ± 25.7
49–60	M	31	152.9 ± 3.6	105.9 ± 2.4	10.5 ± 0.7	6.7 ± 1.1	2.0 ± 0.2	123 ± 24	54.0 ± 43.4
61–72	F	47	153.5 ± 3.3	107.6 ± 2.8	10.6 ± 0.6	6.2 ± 1.2	2.1 ± 0.2	124 ± 37	51.3 ± 26.5
61–72	M	44	155.8 ± 4.3	107.5 ± 2.8	10.9 ± 0.6	7.3 ± 1.6	2.2 ± 0.2	114 ± 22	46.9 ± 23.9

A/G, albumin/globulin; BUN, blood urea nitrogen; ALT, alanine aminotransferase; AST, aspartate aminotransferase; ALP, alkaline phosphatase; GGT, gamma glutamyltransferase; LDH, lactate dehydrogenase; Triglyc., triglycerides.

[a]From Xie et al. (2013). Note: publication values were converted from SI to conventional units. Value ranges given are ±2 standard deviations.

Just as with Indian- and Chinese-origin rhesus monkeys, cynomolgus monkeys that are cited in biomedical research have been imported from several geographically separate areas that include Mauritius, the Philippines, Indonesia, and Malaysia. Although all of these cynomologus monkeys are the same genus and species, there are differences that should be considered prior to initiating research projects. Mixing cynomolgus monkeys imported from different areas could create confounding variables that can be avoided by using monkeys from the same geographic origin. Cynomolgus monkeys have become the standard macaque model in pharmaceutical research in large part due to their availability through importers and the development of large breeding facilities in source countries (Ebeling *et al.*, 2011). In addition to their use in pharmaceutical safety testing, cynomolgus monkeys have contributed to reproductive biology research (Hendrickx and Dukelow, 1995). They have also served as a valuable model in behavioral research (Schapiro, 2008). Other research fields to which they have contributed include oncology, diabetes, cardiovascular disease, infectious disease, and retroviral studies (Lee, 1993; Wiseman *et al.*, 2007; Zou *et al.*, 2012). The whole genome for cynomolgus macaques has also been sequenced (Higashino *et al.*, 2012) and will likely lead to rapid advances in genomics and comparative studies.

There are other macaques in addition to rhesus and cynomolgus monkeys that have contributed to biomedicine. Pig-tailed macaques (*M. nemestrina*) continue to serve as a good model in HIV/SHIV research, gene therapy, and immunology studies (Peterson *et al.*, 2013; Xu *et al.*, 2013). Stumptail macaques (*M. arctoides*) have contributed to research on balding (Uno, 1986) and behavior studies (Santillán-Doherty *et al.*, 2010; Richter *et al.*, 2009). The bonnet macaque (*M. radiata*) has been used as a model for Kyasanur Forest disease (Kenyon *et al.*, 1992) and in reproduction biology (Nimbkar-Joshi *et al.*, 2012; Suresh *et al.*, 2011).

E.   *Papio* spp.: Baboons
1.   Introduction

Baboons are the largest Old World nonhuman primates (Fig. 17.12). Their large size is advantageous in that it allows biomedical devices made for humans, such as angioplasty catheters and vascular shunts, to be tested without modification of size. Baboons have marked sexual dimorphism; the male can be up to twice as large as the female. There is a wide range of color variations among the species of baboons. Olive baboons (*Papio anubis*) have a greenish-gray coat, yellow baboons (*Papio cynocephalus*) possess a yellow–brown coat color, and chacma baboons (*Papio ursinus*) are generally dark brown with yellow or black regions present on the upper body, hands, feet, and tail (Skinner and Smithers, 1990;

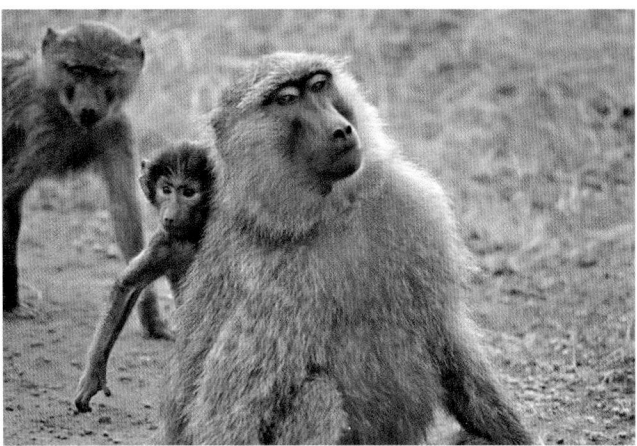

FIGURE 17.12   *Papio anubis*, adult female olive baboon with infant.

Rowe, 1996; Groves, 2001). Male hamadryas baboons (*Papio hamadryas*) have a unique silver–white coat coloration. Baboon species possess long tails and ischial callosities, the latter of which can be used to identify animal gender. Females have a separation between the two ischial callosities, while the two sides fuse below the anus in male baboons (Skinner and Smithers, 1990).

Baboons are diurnal and primarily terrestrial with some species also having an arboreal component. Their dental formula is the same as other old world primates: I2/2, C1/1, P2/2, and M3/3 (Skinner and Smithers, 1990). Baboons have long upper canine teeth, a feature especially prominent in males (Napier and Napier, 1985; Groves, 2001). They also have cheek pouches which they use to store foraged food (Rowe, 1996).

2.   Taxonomy

Due to the high rate of hybridization, and phenotypic and skeletal similarities between animals, there have been several proposals for speciation among the genus *Papio* (Groves, 2001). The method used in Table 17.25, and in this chapter, shows the genus divided into five species. Four of these species are considered savanna baboons: *P. anubis*, *P. cynocephalus*, *P. papio*, and *P. ursinus*. The remaining species, *P. hamadryas*, is sometimes referred to as a desert baboon.

3.   Natural History

Baboons are widely distributed throughout sub-Saharan Africa from Senegal and Sudan to the Cape of Good Hope, except for the main forested areas. Table 17.25 lists geographic information for each baboon species. Savanna baboons occupy a wide range of habitats, including semidesert, savanna, scrubland, woodlands, highland grass, and gallery forest (Aldrich-Blake *et al.*, 1971; Oates *et al.*, 2008a; Kingdon *et al.*, 2008a). Hamadryas baboons inhabit wooded or subdesert steppe, and mountains

TABLE 17.25 Baboon Taxonomy, CITES Status, and Distribution

Genus *Papio*	Common name(s)	CITES status[a]	Distribution
P. anubis[b]	Olive baboon	II	Benin, Brukina Faso, Burundi, Cameroon, Central African Republic, Chad, Democratic Republic of the Congo, Cote d'Ivoire, Eritrea, Ethiopia, Ghana, Guinea, Kenya, Mali, Mauritania, Niger, Nigeria, Rwanda, Sierra Leone, Somalia, Sudan, United Republic of Tanzania, Togo, Uganda
P. cynocephalus[b]	Yellow baboon	II	Angola, Democratic Republic of the Congo, Ethiopia, Kenya, Malawi, Mozambique, Somalia, United Republic of Tanzania, Zambia
P. hamadryas[c]	Hamadryas baboon	II	Djibouti, Eritrea, Ethiopia, Saudi Arabia, Somalia, Sudan, Yemen
P. papio[d]	Guinea baboon	II	Gambia, Guinea, Guinea-Bissau, Mali, Mauritania, Senegal
P. ursinus[e]	Chacma baboon	II	Angola, Botswana, Lesotho, Mozambique, Namibia, South Africa, Swaziland, Zambia, Zimbabwe

[a]*Species listed in CITES Appendix I are threatened with extinction (endangered); II, species listed in CITES Appendix II are not currently threatened with extinction but may become so unless trade is strictly regulated.*
[b]*Kingdon* et al. *(2008a).*
[c]*Gippoliti and Ehardt (2008).*
[d]*Oates* et al. *(2008a).*
[e]*Hoffmann and Hilton-Taylor (2008).*

bordering the Red Sea (Gippoliti and Ehardt, 2008). Availability of food, water, and elevated nesting sites may define the size of the home range or territory. For example, baboons in forest habitats where fruit is the major portion of the diet have smaller home ranges and higher population densities than baboons that feed on grass and roots in arid savanna habitats (Melnick and Pearl, 1987). Baboons prefer steep cliffs or closed-canopy trees as nesting sites since these sites provide protection from predators such as wild felids, hyenas, dogs, chimpanzees, crocodiles, hippos, and raptors (Hamilton, 1982; Cowlishaw, 1994; Barton *et al.*, 1996).

Baboons have strict social hierarchies. The savanna species have a multimale–multifemale social structure. Group sizes usually range from 20 to 130 animals and contain many more females than males. Females remain with their natal group and form the stable core of the social group with a linear type of dominance hierarchy (Altmann *et al.*, 1977; Skinner and Smithers, 1990). These groups contain more than one male, and there is competition for access to estrous females within the group. Males disperse from natal groups around puberty, and subsequently transfer groups several times during their lifespan to both prevent breeding with their offspring and to avoid dominance interactions with younger males (Packer, 1979; Sapolsky, 1996). Male–male interactions are usually more aggressive than affiliative, and mating access to estrous females is determined as much by the male's length of stay in the social group, alliances with females, and female choice as by male–male competition and dominance (Smuts and Watanabe, 1990; Williams and Bernstein, 1995).

In contrast, the hamadryas baboon forms a one-male social unit consisting of one male, several females, and their offspring. The male is the focus of attention in the one-male unit and receives most of the grooming. Males actively herd female members and prevent them from straying too far from the group. Several one-male units, usually two to three, may associate with each other to form a clan (Abegglen, 1984). Clans frequently travel and forage together. Several clans, one-male units, and single males can come together to form a stable social unit called a band. Social interactions are usually restricted to band members, and bands forage as an autonomous unit. (Kummer *et al.*, 1981; Sigg *et al.*, 1982; Abegglen, 1984; Colmenares *et al.*, 2006).

4. Reproduction

Baboons lack reproduction seasonality and female baboons are capable of breeding continuously throughout the year (Bercovitch and Harding, 1993). Sexual maturity generally occurs at 4–5 years of age for females and 4–7 years of age for males (Table 17.26). Gestation averages 6 months and interbirth intervals range from 1 to 3 years. The females have prominent perineal tumescence and sex skin, which allows assessment of both their ovarian function and their pregnancy status with relative ease. There is a menstrual cycle associated with swelling and color change of the sex skin. The initial turgescence or swelling takes an average of 4 days and is followed by increasing edematous distension until the sexual skin has no wrinkles and develops an intense red color (Hendrickx, 1971). Turgescence lasts 13–21 days depending on the species of baboon (Gauthier, 1999). Maximum turgescence is associated with the hormonal changes that occur with ovulation (Bercovitch, 1985). Initial deturgescence is characterized by loss of color, decreased swelling, and an increase in wrinkles in the perineum. A quiescent stage of about 12 days follows in which the sexual skin has many wrinkles, a dull surface, and little color (Hendrickx, 1971).

TABLE 17.26   Sexual Maturity, Gestation, and Interbirth Intervals of Baboons in the Wild and in Captivity

Species	Sexual maturity (years of age)		Gestation (days)	Interbirth interval (months)
	Male	Female		
Papio anubis[a]	5–7	4.5	180	12–34
P. cynocephalus[b]	4–7	5–6	175	21 (mean)
				11 (unsuccessful birth)
				22 (successful birth)
P. papio[c]		3.8 ± 0.8	182.2 ± 3.3 (SD)	11 (unsuccessful birth)
				13 (successful birth)
P. ursinus[d]		3.2	187	18–24
P. hamadryas[e]	4.7–6.8	4–5, 4.3 (mean)	172	12–36, 24 (mean)
P. hamadryas[f]		3.4	181 ± 1.0 (SD)	13

[a]*Wild population (Nicholson, 1982; Scott, 1984).*
[b]*Wild population (Altmann et al., 1977).*
[c]*Captive population (Gauthier, 1999).*
[d]*Wild population (Devore and Hall, 1965; Harvey et al., 1987).*
[e]*Wild population (Sigg et al., 1982; Harvey et al., 1987).*
[f]*Captive population (Birrell et al., 1996; Sunderland et al., 2008).*

The length of the menstrual cycle or intermenstrual interval varies among species, between individuals of each species, and with the age of the individual (Birrell *et al.*, 1996; Gauthier, 1999). Gauthier (1999) summarized several reports describing intermenstrual cycle length of wild and captive baboon species. Captive *P. papio* had the shortest intermenstrual interval, 29.8 ± 4.1 days, and feral *P. anubis* the longest, 40.1 ± 6.9 days. Birrell *et al.* (1996) reported that *P. hamadryas* females less than 5 years of age and females over 10 years of age had an increased average intermenstrual cycle length of 39 days, whereas animals of prime breeding age, from 5 to 10 years old, had an average cycle length of 34 days.

Ovarian cyclicity can be determined by monitoring menses, cyclic changes in sex skin, or hormone determinations of blood, urine, or feces. In singly caged animals, menses may be followed by visual examination of the external genitalia for fresh blood or by the use of vaginal swabs to obtain smears to examine for blood. Visual examination for blood is the least accurate method. Baboons can be trained to present for daily vaginal swabs, which will detect menstruation in approximately 95% of cycles (Hendrickx, 1971). Recording daily changes in the sex skin is a very accurate method of following the ovarian cycle and can be used in baboons that are singly or group-housed. Ovulation usually occurs on day 1–2 before deturgescence (Wildt *et al.*, 1977; Shaikh *et al.*, 1982); the third day prior to deturgescence is the optimal day for mating. Daily blood or urine collection for hormone determinations by enzyme immunoassay (EIA) or radio immunoassay (RIA) can provide a precise date for ovulation but are more time-consuming and

expensive methods of determining cyclicity. For investigators monitoring baboon troops in the wild, a combination of daily observation of sex skin, collection of individual fecal samples for future hormone evaluation, and behavioral observation of mounting and copulation can provide an accurate retrospective evaluation of cyclicity and even conception date (Wasser, 1996; Wasser *et al.*, 1998).

Pregnancy can be determined as early as gestation day (G.D.) 15–18 by detection of chorionic gonadotropin in plasma or urine (Hodgen and Neimann, 1975; Shaikh *et al.*, 1976; Fortman *et al.*, 1993). Detection of pregnancy is possible by ultrasound examination by G.D. 18–21 (Herring *et al.*, 1991) and by bimanual palpation by G.D. 20–21 (Hendrickx and Dukelow, 1995). During bimanual palpation, a gloved finger of one hand is inserted in the rectum while the other hand is placed on the abdomen, grasping the uterus. As with ultrasound, this procedure requires that the animal be anesthetized. Artificial insemination (Gould and Martin, 1986), *in vitro* fertilization (Clayton and Kuehl, 1984), and transfer of cryopreserved embryos (Pope *et al.*, 1986) have all resulted in normal pregnancy and live births in baboons.

Gestation length in the baboon is approximately 180 days (Sunderland *et al.*, 2008). Table 17.26 lists specific species statistics. Births are usually of singletons. The single discoid placenta is similar to that of humans. Reported birth weights range from 854 g (*P. cynocephalus*) to 1068 g (*P. anubis*) (Harvey *et al.*, 1987). Infants are carried in a ventral–ventral position by the dam when moving. There is no consistent alloparental behavior; on occasion, adult male hamadryas baboons have fostered infants if the dam has died. Infants are usually weaned at 6 months of age. Interbirth interval is decreased in individuals that have unsuccessful pregnancies.

One study by Cary *et al.* (2003) found an increase in reproductive success when baboons were moved from an all indoor enclosure to a larger indoor–outdoor enclosure. They found that moving to a larger enclosure with outdoor access resulted in a significant increase in breeding efficiency, as demonstrated by a decreased number of days measured for the following parameters: days from *postpartum* to first estrus, days from first estrus to conception, and days from conception to the next conception (Cary *et al.*, 2003).

5. Laboratory Management

Baboons adapt readily to a variety of housing situations, whether standard indoor laboratory cages, indoor/outdoor small-group housing, or large outdoor corrals. The preferred housing methods involve housing baboons in social groups with access to outdoor space. Animals moved from indoor single cages to outdoor social groups demonstrate decreased abnormal and self-directed behaviors, and increased locomotion, social, and enrichment-directed behavior (Kessel and Brent, 2001). If animals must be housed in single cages for specific research protocols, socialization opportunities can be maximized with the addition of grooming panels, which consist of cage dividers that allow limited physical access between two animals. Adaptation of single cages with grooming panels allows normal grooming behavior between individually housed baboons in adjacent but separate cages (Crockett and Heffernan, 1998). In these modified cages, the possibility of trauma between animals is reduced while contact is still permitted between animals with tethers, indwelling catheters, or other research requirements that preclude social housing.

Baboons are successful breeders in captivity. Large-scale breeding of savanna baboons in a 6-acre corral resulted in approximately 200 infants/year (Goodwin and Coelho, 1982) with an 81% live birth rate. Births occurred in all months of the year, with peak numbers occurring between June and December. Harem breeding has been used successfully in groups of baboons consisting of one to two adult males with 20–25 adult females in outdoor cages (Moore, 1975). Breeding groups required several days to establish a social structure. Although fighting occurred, wounds were minor. Pregnant animals were removed 3 weeks prior to delivery and placed in individual cages for delivery with a live birth rate exceeding 70%.

Hamadryas baboons are best housed as single-male–multifemale groups that mimic the one-male units of their social structure in the wild (Else *et al.*, 1986a; Birrell *et al.*, 1996). No maternal mortality occurred in these one-male units, unlike in hamadryas groups that had more than one male (Else *et al.*, 1986a). In this housing situation, the pregnancy rate was 90%. Abortions occurred in 20.5% of deliveries and stillbirths in 8%; the live birth rate was 71.5% (Birrell *et al.*, 1996).

Timed matings can be used to produce fetuses of known age and stage of development. Reported conception rates (number of conceptions/number of breedings) vary from 35% (Moore, 1975) to 48% when matings were performed on the third day following deturgescence (Hendrickx and Kraemer, 1969). The annual conception rate using timed matings usually exceeds 70%.

6. Nutrition

Savanna and hamadryas baboons are omnivorous feeders with diets consisting primarily of different parts and types of vegetation and fruit. They consume a variety of plant material, including fruit, roots, bulbs, tubers, rhizomes, flowers, leaves and grasses, twigs, bark, seeds, and tree gum. They also eat insects and small vertebrates such as reptiles, birds, hares, vervets, infant gazelles, and dik-diks (Stolz and Saayman, 1970; Strum, 1975). Olive baboons living near human agriculture have shown a preference for maize and sweet potato crops, although they were opportunistic and consumed other available agricultural crops as well (Naughton-Treves *et al.*, 1998). *P. ursinus* living near the sea have been known to consume crabs, mussels, and limpets (Rowe, 1996). In captivity, baboons readily adapt to commercialized diets consisting of a minimum of 15% protein, 4% fat, and 5% fiber (1999 Report of Progress, Southwest Foundation for Biomedical Research). As in other nonhuman primates, they require an exogenous source of vitamins C and D. Fresh fruits and vegetables can supplement the vitamin and mineral content of the ration and serve as enrichment.

7. Normal Values

The normal hematologic and clinical chemistry values for baboons can be found in Tables 17.27 and 17.28. For additional normal value information, including normal values for infant baboons, see Barnhart (2010). Adult body weights are listed in Table 17.29.

8. Research Uses

With a genetic similarity to humans of approximately 96% and a relatively large size capable of providing ample fluid and tissue samples, the baboon has served as an ideal experimental model for over three decades (Moore, 1975; Rogers and Hixson, 1997; Murthy *et al.*, 2006). Baboons serve as the model primate in approximately 6% of biomedical research projects involving nonhuman primates (Carlsson *et al.*, 2004). Known as the laboratory model for coronary heart and lung diseases, especially *Bordetella pertussis* or whooping cough

TABLE 17.27 Hematologic Reference Ranges in Baboons[a]

Value	Individual caged baboons				Gang-caged baboons				Corralled baboons			
	N	Mean	2 S.D.	2 S.D. range	N	Mean	2 S.D.	2 S.D. range	N	Mean	2 S.D.	2 S.D. range
White blood cell count (×10³)	c89	9.6	5.8	3.8–15.4	c62	9.3	6.5	2.8–15.8	c30	15.3	11.4	3.9–26.7
	M44	9.2	6.1	3.1–15.3	M24	8.1	4.8	3.3–12.9	M15	14.6	12.8	1.8–27.4
	F45	10.0	5.5	4.5–15.5	F38	10.1	6.9	3.2–17.0	F15	16.0	10.2	5.8–26.2
Red blood cell count (×10⁶)	c90	4.95	0.64	4.31–5.59	c62	4.88	0.78	4.10–5.66	c30	4.65	0.82	3.83–5.47
	M45	5.05	0.64	4.41–5.69	M24	4.99	0.80	4.19–5.79	M15	4.79	0.82	3.97–5.61
	F45	4.86	0.59	4.27–5.45	F38	4.82	0.75	4.07–5.57	F15	4.51	0.75	3.76–5.26
Hemoglobin (g/dl)	c89	12.6	1.7	10.9–14.3	c62	12.5	2.0	10.5–14.5	c30	11.9	2.2	9.7–14.1
	M44	12.9	1.5	11.4–14.4	M24	12.9	2.0	10.9–14.9	M15	12.4	2.1	10.3–14.5
	F45	12.3	1.7	10.6–14.0	F38	12.2	1.9	10.3–14.1	F15	11.3	1.8	9.5–13.1
Hematocrit (%)	c89	38.2	5.0	33.2–43.2	c62	38.3	5.5	32.8–43.8	c30	36.5	7.2	29.3–43.7
	M44	39.0	4.5	34.5–43.5	M24	39.3	5.6	33.7–44.9	M15	38.0	7.2	30.8–45.2
	F45	37.4	5.0	32.4–42.4	F38	37.7	5.2	32.5–42.9	F15	34.9	5.9	29.0–40.8
Mean cell volume (fl)	c90	77.0	5.8	71.2–82.8	c62	78.6	5.6	73.0–84.2	c30	78.4	6.7	71.7–85.1
	M45	76.9	5.2	71.7–82.1	M24	78.9	6.6	72.3–85.5	M14	80.0	3.3	76.7–83.3
	F45	77.1	6.3	70.8–83.4	F38	78.4	4.8	73.6–83.2	F15	77.5	6.9	70.6–84.4
Mean cell hemoglobin (pg)	c90	25.3	1.8	23.5–27.1	c62	25.5	2.1	23.4–27.6	c30	25.6	2.5	23.1–28.1
	M45	25.4	1.7	23.7–27.1	M24	25.9	2.4	23.5–28.3	M15	26.0	2.3	23.7–28.3
	F45	25.3	1.9	23.4–27.2	F38	25.3	1.8	23.5–27.1	F15	25.2	2.6	22.6–27.8
Mean cell hemoglobin concentration (g/dl)	c90	32.9	1.3	31.6–34.2	c62	32.5	1.4	31.1–33.9	c30	32.6	1.7	30.9–34.3
	M45	33.1	1.5	31.6–34.6	M24	32.8	1.1	31.7–33.9	M15	32.7	1.7	31.0–34.4
	F45	32.8	1.1	31.7–33.9	F38	32.3	1.4	30.9–33.7	F15	32.5	1.7	30.8–34.2
Red blood cell distribution width (%)	c90	12.8	1.6	11.2–14.4	c61	12.6	1.6	11.0–14.2	c30	13.4	3.0	10.4–16.4
	M45	12.7	1.5	11.2–14.2	M23	12.4	1.7	10.7–14.1	M14	12.7	1.7	11.0–14.4
	F45	13.0	1.7	11.3–14.7	F37	12.6	1.3	11.3–13.9	F15	13.8	2.7	11.1–16.5
Platelet count (×10⁶)	c89	316	165	151–481	c60	363	183	180–546	c30	320	205	115–525
	M44	279	115	164–394	M23	344	194	150–538	M15	274	170	104–444
	F44	348	173	175–521	F37	375	175	200–550	F15	367	199	168–566
Mean platelet volume (fl)	c89	8.3	1.9	6.4–10.2	c59	9.3	2.1	7.2–11.4	c30	10.2	2.2	8.0–12.4
	M45	8.2	1.9	6.3–10.1	M23	9.1	2.5	6.6–11.6	M15	10.0	2.0	8.0–12.0
	F44	8.4	1.9	6.5–10.3	F37	9.5	2.0	7.5–11.5	F15	10.5	2.4	8.1–12.9

(Continued)

TABLE 17.27 (Continued)

Value	Individual caged baboons				Gang-caged baboons				Corralled baboons			
	N	Mean	2 S.D.	2 S.D. range	N	Mean	2 S.D.	2 S.D. range	N	Mean	2 S.D.	2 S.D. range
Neutrophils (%)	c90	62	27	35–89	c62	49	37	12–86	c30	77	29	48–100
	M45	62	24	38–86	M24	49	35	14–84	M15	79	29	50–100
	F45	61	29	32–90	F38	48	39	9–87	F15	76	29	47–100
Bands (%)	c90	0	0	0	c62	0	0	0	c30	0	1	0–1
	M45	0	0	0	M62	0	0	0	M15	0	1	0–1
	F45	0	0	0	F62	0	0	0	F15	0	2	0–2
Lymphocytes (%)	c90	36	27	9–63	c62	49	37	12–86	c30	22	25	0–47
	M45	35	24	11–59	M24	48	34	14–82	M15	22	24	0–46
	F45	36	30	6–66	F38	49	39	10–88	F15	22	27	0–49
Monocytes (%)	c90	2	3	0–5	c62	2	3	0–5	c30	2	3	0–5
	M45	2	3	0–5	M24	2	3	0–5	M15	3	4	0–7
	F45	2	3	0–5	F38	2	3	0–5	F15	2	3	0–5
Eosinophils (%)	c89	1	2	0–3	c62	1	3	0–4	c29	0	1	0–1
	M44	1	2	0–3	M24	1	2	0–3	M15	0	1	0–1
	F45	1	2	0–3	F38	1	3	0–4	F15	0	2	0–2
Basophils (%)	c90	0	0	0	c62	0	1	0–1	c30	0	1	0–1
	M45	0	0	0	M62	0	1	0–1	M30	0	1	0–1
	F45	0	0	0	F62	0	1	0–1	F30	0	1	0–1

[a]From Hainsey et al. (1993); clinically normal, sedated adult female baboons, Papio spp.

TABLE 17.28 Clinical Chemical Reference Ranges in Baboons[a]

Value	N	Mean	2 S.D.	2 S.D. range	Value	N	Mean	2 S.D.	2 S.D. range
A/G ratio	c25	1.0	0.7	0.3–1.7	Creatine kinase (U/l)	c25	391	349	42–740
	M15	1.1	0.7	0.4–1.8		M15	400	330	70–730
	F10	0.9	0.5	0.4–1.4		F10	379	401	0–780
Albumin (g/dl)	c25	3.5	1.4	2.1–4.9	Creatinine (mg/dl)	c25	1.0	0.5	0.5–1.5
	M15	3.7	1.4	2.3–5.1		M15	1.1	0.4	0.7–1.5
	F10	3.2	1.4	1.8–4.6		F10	0.8	0.3	0.5–1.1
Alkaline phosphatase (U/l)	c25	248	303	0–551	Gamma GT (U/l)	c25	39	22	17–61
	M15	243	312	0–555		M15	43	20	23–63
	F10	254	306	0–560		FIO	32	21	11–53
ALT (SGPT) (U/l)	c24	45	22	23–67	Globulin (g/dl)	c25	3.6	1.1	2.5–4.7
	M15	49	20	29–69		M15	3.5	1.2	2.3–4.7
	F10	44	40	4–84		F10	3.7	0.9	2.8–4.6
Amyalse (U/l)	c25	243	155	88–398	Glucose (mg/dl)	c24	83	25	58–108
	M15	253	136	117–389		M15	83	18	65–101
	F10	228	183	45–411		F10	88	48	40–136
Anion gap (mmol/l)	c25	29	11	18–40	HDL cholesterol (mg/dl)	c25	56	45	11–101
	M15	29	11	18–40		M15	60	42	18–102
	F10	30	12	18–42		F10	50	48	2–98
AST (SGOT) (U/l)	c25	39	20	19–59	Iron (µg/dl)	c24	68	53	15–121
	M15	42	20	22–62		M15	64	60	4–124
	F10	34	16	18–50		F10	84	79	5–163
Bilirubin, direct (mg/dl)	c25	0.1	0.1	0.0–0.2	Lactate dehydrogenase (U/l)	c25	276	147	129–423
	M15	0.1	0.1	0.0–0.2		M15	271	167	104–438
	F10	0.1	0.1	0.0–0.2		F10	282	119	163–401
Bilirubin, total (mg/dl)	c25	0.2	0.2	0.0–0.4	Lipase (U/l)	c22	5	7	0–12
	M15	0.2	0.2	0.0–0.4		M14	7	12	0–19
	F10	0.2	0.1	0.1–0.3		F9	4	8	0–12
Blood urea, nitrogen (BUN) (mg/dl)	c25	14	5	9–19	Phosphorus (mg/dl)	c25	2.9	1.7	1.2–4.6
	M15	14	5	9–19		M15	3.1	1.5	1.6–4.6
	F10	14	6	7–20		F10	2.6	1.8	0.8–4.4
Calcium (mg/dl)	c25	9.0	1.2	7.8–10.2	Potassium (mmol/l)	c25	3.9	1.1	2.8–5.0
	M15	9.1	0.9	8.2–10.0		M15	4.0	1.1	2.9–5.1
	F10	8.9	1.5	7.4–10.4		F10	3.9	1.2	2.7–5.1
Carbon dioxide (mmol/l)	c25	24	5	19–29	Sodium (mmol/l)	c25	149	5	144–154
	M15	25	5	20–30		M15	151	3	148–154
	F10	22	5	17–27		F10	147	6	141–153
Chloride (mmol/l)	c24	99	8	91–107	Total protein (mg/dl)	c25	7.1	0.9	6.2–8.0
	M15	101	11	90–112		M15	7.1	0.8	6.3–7.9
	F10	99	10	89–109		F10	7.0	1.1	5.9–8.1
Cholesterol (mg/dl)	c25	99	57	42–156	Triglyceride (mg/dl)	c25	66	31	35–97
	M15	101	49	52–150		M15	65	29	36–94
	F10	97	70	27–167		F10	68	36	32–104

A/G, albumin/globulin; BUN, blood urea nitrogen; ALT, alanine aminotransferase; AST, aspartate aminotransferase.
[a]*From Hainsey et al., 1993; clinically normal, sedated* Papio *spp.*

TABLE 17.29   Adult Weights for *Papio* spp.

Species	Weight (kg)	
	Adult male	Adult female
P. anubis[a]	21	12
P. cynocephalus[a]	20	15
P. papio[a]	26	13
P. ursinus[a]	20.4	16.8
P. hamadryas[a]	21.5	9.4
P. hamadryas[b]	16.4–19.5	10.5–11.5

[a]From Harvey et al. (1987); feral animals.
[b]From Mahaney et al. (1993); captive animals ≥5 years of age; necropsy weights.

TABLE 17.30   *Chlorocebus* spp. Taxonomy, CITES Status, and Distribution

Genus *Chlorocebus*	Common names	CITES status	Distribution
C. sabaeus	Green monkey	II	Northwest Africa
C. aethiops	Grivet monkey	II	Ethiopia, Eritrea
C. djamdjamensis	Bale monkey	II	Bubbe Kersa, Gossa, Abera, Ethiopia
C. tantalus	Tantalus monkey	?	Nigeria, CAR, Ghana, Burkina Faso, Togo
C. pygerythrus	Vervet monkey	II	Uganda, Kenya, Ethiopia, Somalia, Zambia, Tanzania, South Africa
C. cynosuros	Malbrouck monkey	II	Angola, Zambia

Haus et al. (2013) (many instances of hybridization were noted in species in areas of close geographic contact); Butynski et al. (2008); Kingdon et al. (2008a,b); Kingdon and Butynski (2008); Kingdon and Gippoliti (2008).

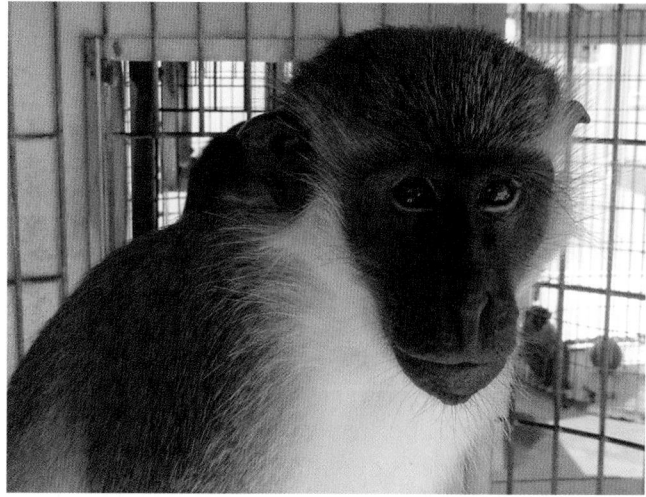

FIGURE 17.13   *Chlorocebus* spp.

(Eby *et al.*, 2013; Warfel *et al.*, 2014), the baboon has also served as a model in research involving atherosclerosis, hypertension, and osteopenia (Rogers and Hixson, 1997; 1999 Report of Progress, Southwest Foundation for Biomedical Research; Havill *et al.*, 2008; Northcott *et al.*, 2012; Shi *et al.*, 2013). Additionally, baboons have contributed to research on diabetes, genetics, stem cell therapies, and organ transplantation (Chen *et al.*, 2014; Cox *et al.*, 2013; Navara *et al.*, 2013; Tasaki *et al.*, 2014; Mohiuddin *et al.*, 2014). Currently, research utilizing baboons centers on reproductive physiology, vaccine development for HIV, hepatitis C, respiratory syncytial virus, and neonatal research (1999 Report of Progress, Southwest Foundation for Biomedical Research; Jeong *et al.*, 2004; Murthy *et al.*, 2006; Keenan *et al.*, 2013; Chege *et al.*, 2013; Papin *et al.*, 2013; Warfel *et al.*, 2014). Baboons have an immune system similar to humans in that they have the same immunoglobulin G (IgG) subclasses: 1, 2,

3, and 4 (Shearer *et al.*, 1999). This similarity makes them an excellent model for vaccine development.

The Baylor College of Medicine and the Human Genome Sequencing Center are currently working on sequencing the entire baboon (genus *Papio*) genome. A high-quality draft sequence is currently available at the following website: https://www.hgsc.bcm.edu/nonhuman-primates/baboon-genome-project. The definition of this genome sequence has and will continue to advance research on comparative genomics (Karere *et al.*, 2010).

F.   *Chlorocebus* spp.: African Green Monkeys

1.   Introduction

The genus *Chlorocebus*, also known as the African Green Monkey, includes several species as listed in Table 17.30. They are a medium-sized monkey with a greenish-golden coat and a white ventrum with a blue tinge to their abdominal region (Fig. 17.13). Black to dark-blue skin covers their face. The males have a distinct blue scrotum and red penis (Skinner and Smithers, 1990; Groves, 2001). Infants have a black coat with a pale-colored face, but transition to the adult colors within 12 weeks of birth (Lee, 1984) (Fig. 17.14).

The males and females of the genus *Chlorocebus* are sexually dimorphic, with wild adult males averaging 5.5 kg and wild females averaging 4.1 kg (Skinner and Smithers, 1990). The monkeys spend time both on the ground and in trees, making them semiterrestrial and semiarboreal (Fedigan and Fedigan, 1988). While their lifespan in the wild is around 11–13 years, their life span in captivity can exceed 25 years (Barrickman *et al.*, 2008).

African Green Monkeys are a popular model in biomedical research, and this popularity has been

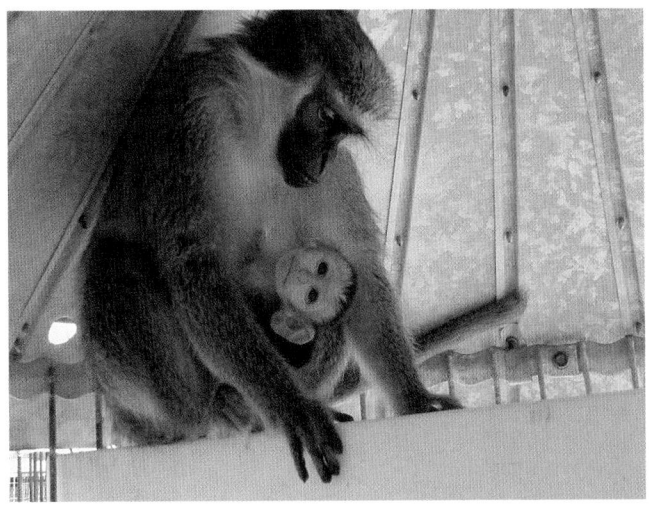

FIGURE 17.14   *Chlorocebus* spp., adult female with infant.

increasing. The increase is due in part to the abundance of animals located in the Caribbean. These animals were originally brought from Africa to the Caribbean islands by trading ships in the 1700s. Some escaped the ships and rapidly multiplied in the absence of natural predators, relatively abundant food sources, and favorable climate. Some of the qualities which make them good research subjects include their relatively small size, ease of handling, breeding success in captivity, and nonendangered status (Ervin and Palmour, 2003). They also may pose fewer health and safety risks than macaques (Baulu *et al.*, 2002). Although baboons and macaques have exactly the same karyotype with a diploid chromosome number of 42, *Chlorocebus* spp. differ with a diploid chromosome number of 60 (Freimer *et al.*, 2013).

2. Taxonomy

Chlorocebus spp. were previously listed in the genus *Cercopithecus*; however, genetic studies have separated them from *Cercopithecus* and reclassified them as genus *Chlorocebus* (Groves, 2001, 2005; Mekonnen *et al.*, 2010a, 2010b; Perelman *et al.*, 2011; Tosi *et al.*, 2002; Xing *et al.*, 2007). Although there is still some controversy on the species *versus* subspecies criteria (Elton *et al.*, 2010; Grubb *et al.*, 2003; Kingdon, 1997), the IUCN red list (2013) and Groves (2001) recognize six species: *Chlorocebus sabaeus, C. tantalus, C. aethiops, C. djamdjamensis, C. cynosuros,* and *C. pygerythrus.* Taxonomy, CITES status, and geographic distributions are listed in Table 17.30.

3. Natural History

In the wild, *Chlorocebus* spp. monkeys live in the savanna environment of Sub-Saharan Africa (Kingdon, 1997), ranging from Senegal and Ethiopia to the South African region. There are also several colonies located on the Caribbean islands of St. Kitts, Nevis, and Barbados,

consisting of approximately 40,000–50,000 animals (Ervin and Palmour, 2003).

Similar to other Old World monkeys, *Chlorocebus* spp. are diurnal and quadripedal, spending much of the time during the day foraging on the ground, and then sleeping in trees at night (Fedigan and Fedigan, 1988). They also possess cheek pouches for storing food (Rowe, 1996). Their adult dental formula is similar to other Old World nonhuman primate species: I 2/2, C 1/1, P 2/2, and M 3/3 (Skinner and Smithers, 1990).

The *Chlorocebus* social structure consists of multiple male/multiple female groups and they exhibit female philopatry, where the females remain with the social groups into which they were born, whereas the males migrate out at sexual maturity (Struhsaker, 1967). The average group size is 25 individuals (Struhsaker, 1967; Fedigan and Fedigan, 1988). They have a matrilinear dominance hierarchy, with the high-ranking females having access to the most preferred grooming partners and food sources (Isbell *et al.*, 1999). They are a territorial species and adult females will often attack young males emigrating from neighboring troops (Cheney and Seyfarth, 1983; Isbell *et al.*, 2002). When a male works his way up to alpha status, this position is generally held for a period of 3–5 years (Fairbanks and McGuire, 1986). Males of the species *C. aethiops* have been observed chest rubbing, which is believed to be a scent-marking behavior associated with higher ranking males (Freeman *et al.*, 2012). One threat gesture used by *Chlorocebus* spp. is the eyelid display, a brow contraction that reveals the paler skin of the eyelids. Depending on the social situation, the eyelid display can represent a defensive or aggressive threat behavior (Struhsaker, 1967; Skinner and Smithers, 1990).

Chlorocebus monkeys have a unique system of distinct and separate vocal predator calls. These calls serve as a communication tool to convey appropropriate predator responses in conspecific monkeys (Seyfarth *et al.*, 1980; Isbell and Enstam, 2002). Predators in the wild include leopards, eagles, and pythons. The attack methods from these predators differs (attacks from above *versus* below) and the distinct predator-specific vocal calls enable the monkeys to take cover from the specific harm (Seyfarth *et al.*, 1980).

4. Reproduction

In Chlorocebus monkeys, females are sexually mature at 3 years and males at 5–6 years of age (Ervin and Palmour, 2003). They are seasonal breeders and reports of the actual breeding season vary. Eley *et al.* (1986) reported that the breeding season generally lasts from July through September, while Ervin and Palmour (2003) observed a breeding season that lasted from October through March. Lee (1984) observed a copulatory season in the wild from May to June, with births primarily occuring between October and December. Either way, in captivity the monkeys do not follow the breeding season observed in the wild, and they instead tend to breed throughout their cycles (Rowell, 1971).

The cycle in females lasts 30–32 days and menstruation tends to be light and can be difficult to observe (Else *et al.*, 1986b, Eley *et al.*, 1989; Seier, 2005). Menstrual cycles in *Chlorocebus* spp. have a rise in estrogen midcycle, which causes a periovulatory LH surge approximately 12 days following the onset of menses. Ovarian histologic evaluation at late follicular phase reveals a large single Graafian follicle and examination at early luteal phase demonstrates a developing corpus luteum (Molskness *et al.*, 2007). Molskness *et al.* (2007) have found that Chlorocebus cyclicity is dependent on pituitary gonadotropin hormones and independent of a uterine luteolytic factor. These ovarian cycle characteristics are similar to that of human females and rhesus macaques (Molskness *et al.*, 2007).

Peak sexual activity occurs at day 13 of the cycle (Else *et al.*, 1986b, Eley *et al.*, 1989). Females do not have perineal swelling associated with peak fertility (Seier, 2005), and the lack of any visual cue of fertility is unique among cercopithecines living in multi-male groups (Melnick and Pearl, 1987). The lack of visual cues lends some confusion as to offspring paternity and may allow the lower-ranking males to sire a larger proportion of the offspring in comparison to species with obvious ovulatory cues (Heistermann *et al.*, 2001). This strategy may serve to decrease the risk of infanticide in the social group. If females do not become pregnant during the breeding season, anestrus reportedly occurs from March to October in the wild. During this anestrus period, the male testicle size also decreases (Ervin and Palmour, 2003).

Pregnancy can be detected via rectal palpation or ultrasound; however, it may be necessary to elevate the uterus toward the abdominal wall by digit insertion in the rectum in order to detect pregnancy via ultrasound (Seier *et al.*, 2000). Gestation spans 163–165 days (Eley *et al.*, 1986; Andelman, 1987). Births generally occur during the night or at dawn and typically last 15–20 min (Seier, 1986). The average birth weight of infants is 343 g for males and 318 g for females (Cho *et al.*, 2002). The incidence of twinning in *Chlorocebus* spp. is similar to humans at 1 in 88 births (Ervin and Palmour, 2003). The interbirth interval is 1–2 years, depending on the outcome of the previous year's birth/offspring. Females that have lost an infant are more likely to become pregnant the following year (Lee, 1984; Cheney *et al.*, 1988). Fertility in females decreases once they reach the age of 20 (Ervin and Palmour, 2003).

5. Laboratory Management

The territoriality observed in wild populations of African Green monkeys should be considered when housing them in captivity. Aggressiveness and fighting can commonly occur in harem groups consisting of single males and multiple females. Larger harem groups consisting of a single male and 5–10 females may exhibit more agonistic behavior than that observed in smaller groups of 2–6 females (Else, 1985; Kushner *et al.*, 1982). The highest infant survival rates are obtained when pregnant females are removed from the social groups and not returned until 2 weeks after they have given birth (Seier, 2005). Pair housing can also be used to house *Chlorocebus* spp. This method of housing leads to fewer conflicts and associated trauma, however it lacks juvenile interactions with other juveniles. This peer play has an important role in social development and the absence of peer play makes pair housing a less desirable option (Seier, 2005).

6. Nutrition

African Green monkeys are omnivorous with a varied diet that depends largely on the available seasonal food in the wild. Their diet includes leaves, seeds, nuts, fruits, flowers, gums, fungi, insects, eggs, and some small vertebrate species. The preferred foods, when available, are fruit and flowers (Harrison, 1984; Fedigan and Fedigan, 1988). When food availability is limited, visible signs of stress may appear, such as alopecia and skin hyperpigmentation (Isbell, 1995). In captivity, *Chlorocebus* spp. are generally fed a commercial Old World primate laboratory diet consisting of 18% protein, 13% fat, and 69% carbohydrates (LabDiet 5038, Purina Mills, St. Louis, MO) (Jorgensen *et al.*, 2013).

7. Normal Values

Normal hematology and clinical reference values for African Green monkeys are listed in Tables 17.31 and 17.32. These values are based on 331 male and female monkeys located at the St. Kitts Biomedical Research Foundation (SKBRF). The animals included both wild and captive-born monkeys that weighed between 1.5 and 7.5 kg. All animals were deemed healthy during physical exam prior to inclusion (Liddie *et al.*, 2010). For additional hematologic and serum biochemical values reported by age distribution using a smaller colony of African Green monkeys, refer to Sato *et al.* (2005).

8. Research Uses

There are several large colonies of Chlorocebus monkeys in the United States, derived primarily from small subsets of the Caribbean populations. African Green monkeys from St. Kitts and Nevis islands populated the large research colonies at New Iberia Research Center in Louisiana and the Vervet Research Colony (VRC) located at Wake Forest University Primate Center (relocated from its original location at UCLA) (Freimer *et al.*, 2013). There are also Chlorocebus research colonies on

TABLE 17.31   Hematology Reference Ranges in *Chlorocebus sabaeus*[a]

Value	N	Mean	SD	2 SD range	Value	N	Mean	SD	2 SD range
Hemoglobin (g/dl)	M 169	13.8	1.8	10.2–17.4	WBC (10^3/ml)	M 165	5.9	1.8	2.3–9.6
	F 77	12.2	1.2	9.8–14.7		F 72	6.8	1.7	3.4–10.2
Hematocrit (%)	M 169	43.9	5.4	33.2–54.7	Neutrophils (cells/ml)	M 164	2549.7	1152.8	244.0–4855.4
	F 77	39.7	4.4	30.9–48.5		F 72	2995.7	1261.2	473.4–5518.0
RBC (10^6/ml)	M 162	5.6	0.6	4.4–6.9	Lymphocytes (cells/ml)	M 163	2746.8	1132.6	481.7–5012.0
	F 77	5.2	0.5	4.1–6.3		F 74	3146.2	1127.1	891.9–5400.4
MCV (fl)	M 165	77.2	4.5	68.2–86.2	Monocytes (cells/ml)	M 165	226.7	153.3	0.0–533.2
	F 71	77.4	4.2	69.0–85.9		F 68	172.2	164.4	0.0–501.1
MCH (pg)	M 160	24.2	0.9	22.3–26.1	Eosinophils (cells/ml)	M 138	81.2	82.8	0.0–246.8
	F 72	23.7	0.9	21.9–25.6		F 55	54.2	74.8	0.0–203.7
MCHC (g/dl)	M 169	31.3	1.9	27.5–35.2	Basophils (cells/ml)	M 104	40.3	43.6	0.0–127.6
	F 77	30.9	1.7	27.4–34.3		F 52	33.9	41.5	0.0–116.9
Platelets (10^3/ml)	M 163	355.1	97.0	161.1–549.1	% Neutrophils	M 159	45.0	12.8	19.4–70.5
	F 74	368.4	99.7	169.0–567.9		F 72	45.0	12.8	19.4–70.7
PT (%)	M 39	12.6	0.8	11.0–14.3	% Lymphocytes	M 159	47.4	12.6	22.1–72.7
	F 35	12.9	0.8	11.3–14.6		F 73	47.5	13.3	20.8–74.1
PTT (%)	M 39	30.3	2.4	25.5–35.2	% Monocytes	M 163	3.7	2.5	0.0–8.6
	F 35	31.2	2.2	26.7–35.6		F 73	2.8	2.6	0.0–8.0
Fibrinogen (secs)	M 39	245.9	63.4	119.0–372.8	% Eosinophils	M 135	1.3	1.3	0.0–3.9
	F 35	217.3	61.5	94.2–340.3		F 55	0.8	1.0	0.0–2.8
					% Basophils	M 106	0.7	0.7	0.0–2.1
						F 54	0.5	0.6	0.0–1.7

RBC, red blood cells; MCV, mean corpuscular volume; MCH, mean corpuscular hemoglobin; MCHC, mean corpuscular hemoglobin concentration; PT, prothrombin time; PTT, partial thromboplastin time; WBC, white blood cells.
[a]*Liddie* et. al. *(2010), St. Kitts African green monkeys* (Chlorocebus sabaeus).

the islands of St. Kitts and Barbados that are utilized for research purposes (Redmond *et al.*, 2007; Lemere *et al.*, 2004; Gerald, 2002).

As with the baboon and rhesus macaque, genetic maps have been developed for *C. a. sabaeus* (Jasinska *et al.*, 2007). The development of these genetic linkage maps enhances the value of Chlorocebus monkeys as a research model by allowing comparative genome studies and identification of genetic factors in disease and behavior. Some of the many research areas include African trypanosomiasis infection (Ouwe-Missi-Oukem-Boyer *et al.*, 2006), vaccinology (Martín *et al.*, 2009), HIV/AIDS (Hatziioannou and Evans, 2012), hypertension (Ervin and Palmour, 2003), neurological disease (Lemere *et al.*, 2004; Harvey *et al.*, 2000), psychology and social behavior (Bailey *et al.*, 2007; Fairbanks *et al.*, 2004), atherosclerosis and metabolic syndrome (Rayner *et al.*, 2011; van Jaarsveld *et al.*, 2002), and leishmania (Olobo *et al.*,

2001). Vero cells, a cell line derived from the kidney epithelial cells of African Green monkeys, are also an important research contribution from this species. The use of this cell line continues to be widespread in biomedical research (Li *et al.*, 2013; Yurdakök and Baydan, 2013).

G.   *Pan* spp.: Chimpanzees

1.   *Introduction*

The chimpanzee is one of three members of the great apes, family Hominidae. Chimpanzees are large, primarily vegetarian nonhuman primates from the African continent. They are tailless, their arms are longer than their legs, they have protrusive lips and prominent ears, and there is a short opposable thumb (Fig. 17.15). The foot is short compared to trunk length, and the big toe is long and strong. Face and body skin coloration and

TABLE 17.32   Clinical Chemical Reference Ranges in *Chlorocebus sabaeus*[a]

Value	N	Mean	SD	2 SD range	Value	N	Mean	SD	2 SD range
A/G ratio	M 92	1.6	0.4	0.9–2.4	Creatine kinase (U/l)	M 173	1509.7	1666.7	0.0–4843.1
	F 95	1.4	0.4	0.5–2.3		F 90	2857.9	1872.4	140.0–6602.7
Albumin (g/dl)	M 170	4.1	0.4	3.3–4.9	Creatinine (mg/dl)	M 206	0.9	0.2	0.5–1.4
	F 94	4.0	0.5	3.1–4.9		F 116	0.7	0.2	0.3–1.1
Alkaline phosphatase (U/l)	M, 198	163.9	135.0	32.0–433.8	Gamma GT (U/l)	M 92	41.8	16.3	9.2–74.3
	F 117	273.3	163.5	56.0–600.2		F 96	40.3	16.7	6.9–73.7
ALT (SGPT) (U/l)	M 205	46.1	22.6	0.9–91.3	Globulin (g/dl)	M 171	2.9	0.6	1.6–4.1
	F 115	47.5	19.6	8.3–86.6		F 98	2.9	0.7	1.6–4.3
Amylase (U/l)	M 93	473.2	132.5	208.1–738.2	Glucose (mg/dl)	M, 198	81.7	18.0	45.6–117.8
	F 95	430.3	139.4	151.4–709.1		F 116	80.3	18.7	43.0–117.6
AST (SGOT) (U/l)	M 170	48.0	23.5	0.9–95.1	Lipase (U/l)	M 92	73.4	33.5	6.3–140.5
	F 96	62.2	26.5	9.2–115.2		F 97	74.2	30.1	14.0–134.5
Bilirubin, total (mg/dl)	M 204	0.8	0.6	0.1–1.9	Magnesium	M 94	1.6	0.2	1.1–2.1
	F 121	0.4	0.5	0.1–1.3		F 97	1.5	0.3	0.9–2.1
BUN (mg/dl)	M 206	19.8	4.4	10.9–28.7	Phosphorus (mg/dl)	M, 199	5.3	1.6	2.1–8.5
	F 114	20.1	5.1	9.9–30.3		F 112	5.2	1.6	2.0–8.4
BUN/creatinine	M 92	22.0	8.5	4.9–39.1	Potassium (mmol/l)	M 163	3.5	0.5	2.4–4.6
	F 92	32.6	12.3	7.9–57.3		F 95	3.8	0.7	2.5–5.1
Calcium (mg/dl)	M 205	9.1	0.6	7.8–10.3	Sodium (mmol/l)	M 168	151.7	5.0	141.8–161.7
	F 112	9.1	0.7	7.7–10.4		F 92	150.8	4.7	141.3–160.3
Chloride (mmol/l)	M 174	104.6	6.8	91.1–118.2	Total protein (mg/dl)	M, 198	6.9	0.5	5.9–8.0
	F 100	106.5	6.5	93.4–119.5		F 117	6.9	0.6	5.8–8.0
Cholesterol (mg/dl)	M 170	114.9	18.4	78.0–151.8	Triglyceride (mg/dl)	M 93	38.7	15.4	8.0–69.4
	F 90	131.7	18.9	94.0–169.5		F 95	46.5	18.1	10.3–82.7

ALT, alanine aminotransferase; AST, aspartate aminotransferase; BUN, blood urea nitrogen; GT, glutamyltransferase.
[a]*Liddie et al. (2010), St. Kitts African green monkeys (Chlorocebus sabaeus).*

pelage are unique for each species/subspecies; in captivity the facial coloration can vary between pink/tan, mottled, freckled, and black. The pelage is usually coarse, sparse, and predominantly black. Variation in age and sex will result in white hair tufts in the anal region and chin. The dental formula is 2–1–2–3 for 32 total teeth, with canines that are well developed. The stomach is simple, and the cecum has an appendix, similar to that of humans. Chimpanzees have extensive laryngeal (air) sacs in the neck and axillary spaces. A quadrupedal walk is used, interspersed with short distances of brachiating and standing upright, primarily to increase visual range. Chimpanzees choose to be arboreal 50–75% of the time; they sleep primarily in tree nests newly built each night and seldom less than 15 feet above the ground (Napier and Napier, 1967).

The chimpanzee has traditionally been the largest nonhuman primate research model in biomedical research. Due to the close phylogenetic relationship to human beings, the chimpanzee has been uniquely positioned to make important contributions to biomedical studies of human diseases and to contribute to expanding our understanding of the evolution of human behavior. Research with chimpanzees has been critical to the development of vaccines for hepatitis A and B and has resulted in important advances in our understanding of the pathogenesis of hepatitis C. The chimpanzee remains the only animal model that closely recapitulates hepatitis C virus infection and pathogenesis. Adenoviruses isolated from chimpanzees have recently shown considerable promise as vectors for vaccines for Ebola and malaria (Stanley *et al.*, 2014; Nébié *et al.*, 2014). The close phylogenetic relationship to human beings has also generated controversy regarding their participation in biomedical research. Despite refinements in research methods and strict oversight of all studies with chimpanzees, there are needed for critical studies of human diseases that can only be carried out with chimpanzees. The decision to select and limit the number of chimpanzees available for research to 50 animals is further complicated by the breeding moratorium that was begun in 1995. This will ultimately result in predominantly a geriatric chimpanzee population. It is predicted that by 2037, the federally funded captive chimpanzee population will cease to exist (NCRR, 2007; Cohen, 2007).

An additional challenge to fields of research in which chimpanzees serve as a model is a proposal by the U.S. Fish and Wildlife Service to reclassify captive chimpanzees as endangered rather than threatened. While wild chimpanzees have been classified as endangered since, 1990, captive chimpanzees have bred well in captivity and were not considered to be endangered, but instead, classified as 'threatened' (UFWS, 2013). The reclassification to endangered status along with the 2013 NIH Recommendations on the Use of Chimpanzees in NIH-Supported Research (NOT-OD-13-078, 2013) will likely result in a further decrease in chimpanzee research.

2. Taxonomy and Sources

There are two species (*Pan troglodytes* and *P. paniscus*) and four subspecies (*P. t. troglodytes*, *P. t. verus*, *P. t. schweinfurthii*, and *P. t. ellioti*) of chimpanzees (Table 17.33) (Prado-Martinez *et al.*, 2013). *P. troglodytes* has traditionally been known as the 'common chimpanzee' and has contributed the most to biomedical research. The bonobo (*P. paniscus*) has had more limited research use, primarily in the fields of behavior and cognition.

The normal diploid number for the chimpanzee is 48 compared to 46 for human beings. Hematology and serum chemistries are similar to those of the human. Blood types are also similar to the ABO typing system of the human; chimpanzees must be crossmatched before transfusions.

Although there are still wild populations of chimpanzees in the forested areas from Sierra Leone and Guinea eastward to the River Niger, the numbers continue to decline. It is believed that there are fewer than 200,000 chimpanzees remaining in the wild (Kormos *et al.*, 2003). As of May 2011, there were 937 chimpanzees housed in biomedical and/or behavioral research facilities with 612 of them supported by the NIH (NRC, 2011b). The NIH-supported chimpanzees are maintained at three facilities: the Alamogordo Primate Facility operated by Charles River Laboratories, the Michale E. Keeling Center for Comparative Medicine and Research at the University of Texas MD Anderson Cancer Center, and Texas Biomedical Research Institute in San Antonio, Texas. Yerkes National Primate Research Center at Emory University and the New Iberia Research Center at the University of Louisiana–Lafayette also maintain research colonies of chimpanzees (NRC, 2011b).

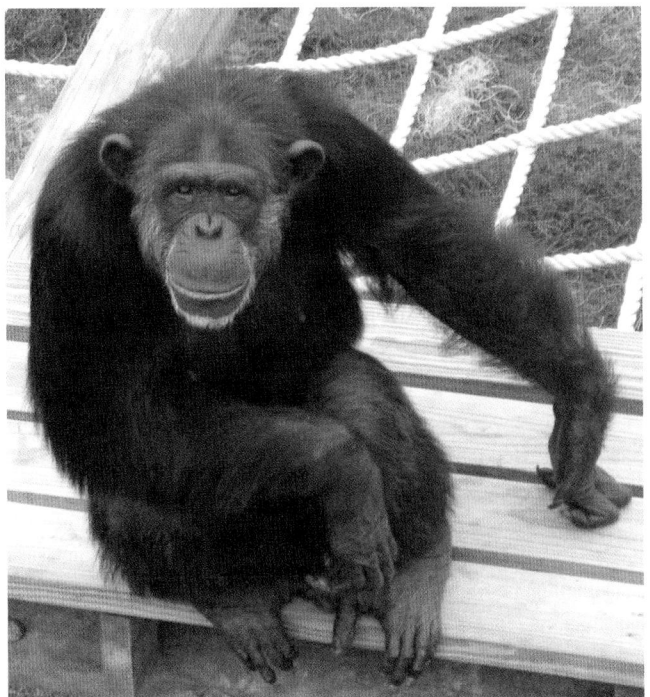

FIGURE 17.15   *Pan troglodytes*, adult female chimpanzee.

has been growing pressure from groups that oppose the use of animals in biomedical research to cease all research with chimpanzees. In 1995, the NIH instituted a moratorium on breeding NIH-owned or supported chimpanzees based on the fact that there were enough chimpanzees to meet research needs without breeding.

In December 2010, the NIH commissioned a study by the Institute of Medicine (IOM) to assess the need for chimpanzees in biomedical and behavioral research. This IOM report, published in December 2011 (NRC, 2011b), recommended stringent limits on the use of chimpanzees in biomedical and behavioral research. The report went on to recommend a set of principles and criteria that should be met in deciding whether to conduct research with chimpanzees. The NIH accepted this IOM report and charged a NIH Council of Councils Working Group to propose advice on implementing the recommendations of the IOM report and to provide recommendations on the size and placement of NIH-owned chimpanzee populations. On January 22, 2013, the Council of Councils accepted the recommendations of the Working Group. Following a period for public comment, the NIH accepted the majority of the recommendations made by the Working Group on June 26, 2013 (NIH NOT-OD-13-078, 2013).

The NIH decided to retire all but 50 NIH-owned chimpanzees from research. This decision was made based on the perceived reduced need for chimpanzees in research, but at the same time, recognized that some chimpanzees

TABLE 17.33   Chimpanzee Taxonomy, CITES Status, and Distribution[a]

Genus *Pan*	Common name(s)	CITES status	Distribution
P. paniscus[b]	Bonobo, dwarf chimpanzee, pygmy chimpanzee	I	Democratic Republic of the Congo
P. troglodytes	Chimpanzee	I	Angola, Burundi, Cameroon, Central African Republic, Congo, Cote d'Ivoire, Equatorial Guinea, Gabon, Ghana, Guinea, Guinea-Bissau, Liberia, Mali, Nigeria, Rwanda, Senegal, Sierra Leone, Sudan, Tanzania, Uganda
P. t. schweinfurthii	Eastern chimpanzee	I	Burundi, Central African Republic, Democratic Republic of the Congo, Rwanda, Sudan, Tanzania, United Republic of Uganda
P. t. troglodytes	Central chimpanzee	I	Angola, Cameroon, Central African Republic, Democratic Republic of the Congo, Equatorial Guinea, Gabon
P. t. verus	Western chimpanzee	I	Cote d'Ivoire, Ghana, Guinea, Guinea-Bissau, Liberia, Mali, Senegal, Sierra Leone
P. t. ellioti	Nigeria–Cameroon chimpanzee	I	Cameroon, Nigeria

I, species listed in CITES Appendix I are threatened with extinction (endangered).
[a]*Oates* et al. *(2008b).*
[b]*Fruth* et al. *(2008).*

3. Natural History

Chimpanzees are found in the wild across equatorial Africa and their geographical location by species can be found in Table 17.33. They live in a variety of different habitats ranging from savannah, rainforests, montane and swamp forests, and dry woodlands (Goodall, 1986; Poulsen and Clark, 2004). Their life span in the wild ranges from 15 to 19 years (Muller and Wrangham, 2014; Hill *et al.*, 2001). In captivity, their life span is significantly longer, and it is not uncommon for chimpanzees to live 40–50 years (Bloomsmith *et al.*, 1991). Chimpanzees are sexually dimorphic with males weighing an average of 40–60 kg and females weighing 32–47 kg (Rowe, 1996). Chimpanzees live in male-dominated fission–fusion social groups that favor male philopatry (Goldberg and Wrangham, 1997; Newton-Fisher, 2004; Emery Thompson, 2013). Most females will emigrate from their natal community 1–2 years following the onset of puberty (Emery Thompson, 2013).

The use of tools by chimpanzees has been well documented. They use sticks, bark, grass, stems to hunt for termites, and rocks to crack nuts, and they have been observed using a set of various sized sticks to extract honey (Mercader *et al.*, 2002; Boesch *et al.*, 2009; Stewart and Piel, 2014). Tool use by chimpanzees was first observed in 1960 by Jane Goodall and challenged the definition of 'man' at that time. Her many publications are recommended as essential reading for developing an appreciation of the natural history of the chimpanzee.

4. Reproduction

Puberty in the female chimpanzee is detected with the onset of cyclic swelling of the anogenital tissue. This swelling (perineal tumescence) may occur 1–1.5 years before menarche and is usually seen between 8 and 11 years of age. Sexual maturity in captivity can occur 2–3 years earlier due to enhanced nutrition (Emery Thompson, 2013). Although not strict seasonal breeders, geographically associated seasonal peaks in sexual receptivity have been observed (Emery Thompson, 2013). The chimpanzee menstrual cycle is approximately 37 days, slightly longer than that of women. Estrus or sexual receptivity coincides with a 5- to 6-day period of maximum swelling of the anogenital tissue. Ovulation occurs 1–6 days before detumescence of the anogenital tissue (Keeling and Roberts, 1972).

The chimpanzee normally has a 7.5- to 8-month gestation, approximately 227–235 days. Human pregnancy test kits are dependable in the chimpanzee, and as in women, amenorrhea is indicative of pregnancy. Another indication of pregnancy is a change in the sex-cycle swelling. Births are usually single; the twinning rate is comparable to that in humans. The onset of labor is rapid, and parturition usually takes only 30 min to a few hours (Brandt and Mitchell, 1971; Goodall and Athumani, 1980). Dystocia is rare because relative to the weight and pelvic dimensions of the female, the average infant birth weight is low (ILAR, 1973). The placenta should be produced within an hour of delivery, and placentophagia is not uncommon (Brandt and Mitchell, 1971; Goodall and Athumani, 1980). Chimpanzees achieve the highest reproductive rates between the ages of 15–30 years (Emery Thompson, 2013). Recent evidence suggests that chimpanzees reach follicular exhaustion, and a corresponding menopause, around 50 years of age (Emery Thompson, 2013; Herndon et al., 2012). This observation parallels human reproductive senescence.

Puberty in the male chimpanzee is approximately at 7 years of age (Marson et al., 1991). In captivity, viable sperm production and impregnation can occur earlier based on the male's exposure to and experience with sexually mature females. When socially housed, most sexually mature males will develop successful breeding skills, but their individual personalities, social histories, and experiences will heavily influence their long-term breeding proficiency and genetic pool contribution.

5. Laboratory Management

Chimpanzees are very intelligent animals that share biological, physiological, behavioral, and social characteristics with human beings (NRC, 2011b). These characteristics and ethical considerations, together dictate a more intense scrutiny of their care. Chimpanzees must be provided with an environment that ensures they are able to maintain a good quality of life. The past three decades have brought significant performance-based improvements in their maintenance, care, and welfare. Both the *Animal Welfare Act* and the *Guide for the Care and Use of Laboratory Animals* have published minimal standards for housing (USDA, 2013; NRC, 2011a). The goal of every institution housing chimpanzees is to exceed the minimum standards and provide an exceptional environment where chimpanzees can socialize and display species-typical behaviors.

Chimpanzees should be housed in compatible, multimale–multifemale social groups maintained in outdoor enclosures that have accessible shelters for protection from temperature extremes (Riddle et al., 1982). According to the *Recommendations on the Use of Chimpanzees in NIH-Supported Research*, any NIH-supported chimpanzees must be housed in social groups of no fewer than seven individuals with at least 20 feet of available vertical space (NIH NOT-OD-13-078, 2013). NIH-supported chimpanzees must also be housed at a maximum density of 250 ft^2 per animal (NIH NOT-OD-14-051, 2014). Chimpanzees not supported by the NIH must comply with the housing space requirements outlined in the *Animal Welfare Act* (USDA, 2013).

The formation of socially compatible groups of chimpanzees must be approached carefully and with knowledge of specific techniques of successful group formation (Fritz and Fritz, 1979). Group formation can take weeks, and in some instances, months, to be completely successful. Every effort should be made to socially house

chimpanzees. Most studies can be designed to allow chimpanzees to be socially housed. When this is impossible, modern housing and equipment almost always allow individually housed animals to see, smell, and hear other chimpanzees. In short-term studies in which individual caging is required, it should be large enough to provide for normal maintenance activity including brachiation. A vast array of environmental enrichment techniques have been developed for chimpanzees that must be individually housed. These include physical, food, and cognitive enrichment strategies (Bloomsmith et al., 1990, 1991).

PRT is an essential component of a captive chimpanzee care program. The cooperation between animals and husbandry staff that is accomplished with training reduces the daily stress that chimpanzees and husbandry personnel experience when performing routine procedures. The training also serves as an enrichment activity for the chimpanzee. PRT can also improve the veterinary care of chimpanzees. The animals can be trained to present and cooperate for many clinical procedures such as cardiac and respiratory auscultation, blood collections, close visual inspection of wounds, and acupuncture treatment (Lambeth et al., 2005; Magden et al., 2013). This reduces the need for animal sedations which benefits the animal, and also provides cost savings. Once established, PRT strengthens the efficiency and cost-effectiveness of routine chimpanzee husbandry and care.

6. Nutrition

In the wild, chimpanzees are primarily vegetarians, spending much of their day foraging. A large portion of their diet is fruit, but they also consume leaves, buds, seeds, bark, and supplement with insects, eggs, and vertebrate animals (Goodall, 1986). The most common mammalian prey is the red colobus monkey (*Procolobus badius*), which chimpanzees have hunted with such a preference that it has caused significant declines in the red colobus monkey population (Watts and Amsler, 2013).

Commercial diets in captivity provide all of their nutritional needs in a primate biscuit. The University of Texas MD Anderson Cancer Center, Keeling Center for Comparative Medicine and Research, feeds Harlan® Teklad Primate Diet #7775, a high-fiber diet with a minimum 20% protein. The staple biscuit diet is supplemented with a variety of fresh fruits, vegetables, and novel food items such as nuts, seeds, and cereals. These practices allow husbandry staff to provide foraging opportunities similar to the psychological rewards of food gathering in the wild.

The popularity of food enrichment strategies (types, delivery, puzzles) introduced in the 1980s continues today and is a well-recognized form of enrichment.

Feeding enrichment can encourage species-appropriate behavior by increasing foraging time and providing opportunities for tool use (Bloomsmith and Else, 2005). However, recent observations indicate that dietary moderation and good nutrition must be practiced with any enrichment strategy. In one study of a captive chimpanzee population, a 33–37% weight gain was observed per decade from 1985 to 2005 (Klimentidis *et al.*, 2011), which highlights the importance of moderation in preventing obesity and related adverse health conditions.

7. Normal Values

There is a substantial body of literature available for chimpanzee normal values. The most extensive volume of such information is the 1969 six-volume publication *The Chimpanzee*, edited by G.H. Bourne (Bourne, 1969). These volumes discuss anatomy, behavior, diseases, pathology, histology, physiology, hematology, serology, growth, reproduction, and captive maintenance. Normal hematology and serum chemistry values are provided in Tables 17.34 and 17.35 (Ihrig *et al.*, 2001). For additional information on normal flow cytometric values for cell surface immunophenotyping, refer to Stone *et al.* (2000).

8. Research Uses

The recent decision by the NIH to reduce the number of chimpanzees available for research is a reflection of the growing public unease with the use of chimpanzees in biomedical research. Although the current NIH plan will limit the availability of chimpanzees for future research, it is important to note that chimpanzees have contributed greatly to scientific discovery over the past several decades. Chimpanzees played a unique role in the aerospace research programs of the 1950s and 1960s, when 'Ham' the chimpanzee was the first hominidae launched into outer space on January 31, 1961 (Swenson *et al.*, 1966). In the 1960s, chimpanzees were used in the field of organ transplant immunology (Cooper, 2012). During the 1970s–1980s era, they were important animal models in cognition and language studies (Terrace *et al.*, 1979). From the 1970s to the mid-2010s, the chimpanzee has been a valuable model in investigating human infectious diseases (hepatitis A, B, C; respiratory syncytial virus; Ebola virus, malaria, and HIV) and associated vaccine development (Robertson *et al.*, 1994; Karron *et al.*, 1997; Prince and Brotman, 2001; Liang, 2013; De Groot and Bontrop, 2013; Nébié *et al.*, 2014; Stanley *et al.*, 2014). Other research areas that have benefited from chimpanzees in the 21st century include comparative genomics, neuroscience, immunology, and numerous behavioral studies (NRC, 2011b).

The chimpanzee genome sequence analysis was published in 2005 (Chimpanzee Sequencing and Analysis Consortium, 2005). The full sequence supports the genomic similarity of chimpanzees and humans. When examining just single-nucleotide divergence, the similarity is approximately 99%. When accounting for DNA insertion and deletion events, the genomic similarity decreases to approximately 96% (Varki and Altheide, 2005), with the major structure difference occurring on chromosome 2. The human chromosome 2 is a fused version of two ancestral ape chromosomes that remain separate in the chimpanzee. This results in 24 chromosome pairs for chimpanzees, compared to 23 pairs in humans (McConkey, 2004). This phylogenic similarity to humans has made chimpanzees an attractive and useful animal model in the past. However, the challenges involved with chimpanzee research must be considered. There are numerous ethical considerations involved to ensure that the research involving chimpanzees has strong scientific justification. An additional consideration is the long life expectancy of chimpanzees which requires forethought to their geriatric care.

IV. PRINCIPLES OF COLONY MANAGEMENT

A. Housing

The NIH, the USDA, and the biomedical research community have made a concerted effort to improve housing and standards of care for nonhuman primates. A relatively stable era using larger galvanized or stainless steel hanging cages was the result, and it brought improved sanitation, management, and health care. The 1985 Amendment to the Animal Welfare Act (Public Law 99–198) changed caging perspectives by challenging the research community to develop documents and follow an appropriate plan for environmental enhancement that would promote the psychological well-being of nonhuman primates. Social (group) housing was the most effective large-scale strategy for improving the psychological well-being of primates. This resulted in revolutionary new strategies for housing nonhuman primates. These creative, novel housing designs, strategies, and systems continue to improve how nonhuman primates are housed in research facilities.

The 2011 revision of the *Guide for the Care and Use of Laboratory Animals* ('*Guide*') (NRC, 2011a) effectively summarizes the contemporary vision for housing nonhuman primates. The primary enclosure for nonhuman primates varies depending on the species, age, size, use, social, and environmental needs. The 2011 *Guide* reinforces traditional primary enclosure considerations of allowing normal physical, physiological, and behavioral needs of the animal. The *Guide* also states that housing space should account for the social needs of the animal(s), and every effort should be made to socially house animals in pairs or larger groups unless

TABLE 17.34 Normal Chimpanzee Values: Hematology[a]

Value	N	Infant	N	Juvenile	N	Adolescent	N	Adult
WBC ($\times 10^3/\mu l$)	74	10.9 (6.64–16.0)	67	10.4 (6.93–16.3)	60	11.0 (6.4–16.2)	76	10.7 (7.2–14.8)
RBC ($\times 10^6/\mu l$)	57	5.1 (4.7–5.8)	56	5.0 (4.6–5.4)	43	5.1 (4.6–5.8)	76	5.2 (4.7–6.1)
Hgb (g/dl)	74	12.8 (11.5–14.7)	67	13.2 (11.9–15.2)	60	13.9 (12.8–16.4)	76	14.4 (12.2–16.8)
Hct (%)	74	39 (35–44)	67	40 (36–44)	60	42 (37–48)	76	43 (37–50)
MCV (fl)	58	75 (68–81)	57	79 (75–84)	44	81 (76–85)	76	81 (76–88)
MCH (pg)	58	25 (22–27)	57	26 (25–28)	44	27 (25–29)	76	27 (25–30)
MCHC (g/dl)	58	33 (32–34)	57	33.2 (32.0–34.3)	44	33.6 (32.5–34.6)	76	33.1 (32.1–34.1)
Platelet count ($\times 10^3/\mu l$)	57	319 (192–530)	56	320 (236–429)	43	279 (148–363)	76	240 (137–347)
Monocytes ($\times 10^3/\mu l$)	74	0.2 (0.0–0.6)	67	0.3 (49–539)	60	0.2 (0–443)	76	0.3 (69–504)
Lymphocytes ($\times 10^3/\mu l$)	74	5.6 (3.6–10.0)	67	4.0 (2179–6687)	60	3.9 (1995–7937)	76	4.3 (2001–6841)
Seg ($\times 10^3/\mu l$)	74	4.0 (1.9–9.7)	67	5.2 (2750–11101)	60	6.1 (2945–11016)	76	5.2 (3017–9026)
Bands ($\times 10^3/\mu l$)	74	0 (0.0–0.18)	67	0 (0–230)	60	0.2 (0–200)	76	0.4 (0–145)
Eosinophil ($\times 10^3/\mu l$)	74	0.1 (0.4–0.7)	67	0.1 (0–454)	60	0.2 (51–578)	76	0.2 (35–436)
Basophil ($\times 10^3/\mu l$)	74	0 (0–0.25)	67	0 (0–5)	60	0 (0–16)	76	0 (0–14)
Retic count (%)	74	0.7 (0.1–2.4)	67	0.10 (.1–2.0)	60	0	76	0.6 (0.1–1.5)
Sed rate (mm/h)	45	14 (2–36)	49	17 (5–36)	37	12 (4–47)	75	16 (3–60)

WBC, white blood cells; RBC, red blood cells; Hgb, hemoglobin; Hct, hematocrit; MCV, mean corpuscular volume; MCH, mean corpuscular hemoglobin; MCHC, mean corpuscular hemoglobin concentration; Seg, segmented neutrophils; Retic, reticulocyte; Sed, sedimentation. Absolute values are given for value ranges for juvenile, adolescent, and adult chimpanzees for monocytes through basophils.

[a]From Ihrig et al. (2001) and MD Anderson Cancer Center, Department of Veterinary Sciences; samples from clinically normal chimpanzees.

TABLE 17.35 Normal Chimpanzee Values: Serum Chemistries[a]

Value	N	Infant	N	Juvenile	N	Adolescent	N	Adult
Total bilirubin (mg/dl)	54	0.3 (0.10–0.60)	61	0.3 (0–7)	47	0.3 (.04–.76)	76	0.3 (0.21–0.58)
ALT (U/l)	73	33 (23–52)	67	40 (23–52)	60	30 (18–46)	76	29 (20–44)
AST (U/l)	73	24 (13–34)	67	22 (14–32)	60	19 (11–31)	76	21 (13–46)
Alkaline phosphatase (U/l)	73	600 (396–914)	67	508 (357–704)	60	375 (145–789)	76	85 (54–153)
Creatine (mg/dl)	55	0.6 (0.5–0.9)	62	0.6 (.5–.8)	50	0.8 (.6–1.7)	76	0.9 (0.8–1.3)
Glucose (mg/dl)	55	83 (68–125)	61	87 (65–120)	49	87 (61–115)	76	82 (66–108)
BUN (mg/dl)	73	11 (7–20)	67	14 (10–20)	60	14 (9–23)	76	12 (9–17)
Total protein (g/dl)	73	6.7 (6.0–7.6)	67	7.2 (6.4–7.8)	60	7.4 (6.8–8.0)	76	7.7 (6.7–8.3)
Albumin (g/dl)	73	3.7 (3.2–4.2)	67	3.9 (3.4–4.2)	60	3.9 (3.5–4.4)	76	3.7 (3.3–4.1)
Globulin (g/dl)	73	3.1 (2.4–3.7)	67	3.4 (2.7–4.1)	60	3.4 (2.7–4.1)	76	4.0 (3.2–4.7)
Cholesterol (mg/dl)	30	262 (178–357)	26	237 (190–285)	27	224 (162–298)	60	216 (170–288)
Gamma GT (U/l)	73	17 (9–114)	61	6 (1–20)	60	13 (13–24)	76	19 (10–35)
Triglycerides (mg/dl)	29	60 (32–135)	25	72 (49–124)	23	74 (40–108)	60	97 (56–164)
Calcium (mg/dl)	6	10.1 (9.6–11.9)	4	10.2 (8.7–11.7)	9	9.0 (8.8–9.4)	34	9.2 (8.1–10.2)
Phosphorus (mg/dl)	6	5.2 (4.7–7.7)	3	5.0 (1.6–6.1)	9	4.0 (1.9–5.3)	33	3.0 (1.8–4.3)
CPK (U/l)	6	113 (32–386)	3	156 (98–309)	9	139 (78–366)	34	313 (80–553)
LDH (U/l)	10	427 (216–553)	6	374 (230–435)	14	264 (125–408)	40	279 (203–503)
Chloride (mEq/l)	7	108 (100–115)	2	106 (104–120)	9	105 (93–119)	28	105 (93–115)
Sodium (mEq/l)	15	142 (130–146)	10	143 (129–146)	10	143 (95–147)	39	142 (136–148)
Potassium (mEq/l)	15	4.1 (2.9–6.0)	10	4.1 (3.6–4.7)	10	4.1 (3.6–4.5)	39	3.6 (3.2–4.4)
HDL (mg/dl)	25	80 (44–114)	23	66.5 (43–103)	21	64 (32.4–92.4)	59	51 (35–82)
LDL (mg/dl)	25	173 (98–242)	23	154 (119–195)	21	137 (109–174)	59	147 (106–209)

ALT, alanine aminotransferase; AST, aspartate aminotransferase; BUN, blood urea nitrogen; Gamma GT, gamma gutamyltransferase; CPK, creatinine phosphokinase; LDH, lactate dehydrogenase; HDL, high density lipoprotein, LDL, low density lipoprotein.

[a]From Ihrig et al. (2001) and MD Anderson Cancer Center, Department of Veterinary Sciences; samples from clinically normal chimpanzees.

experimental or incompatibility precludes such social arrangments (NRC, 2011a).

Individual space requirements vary between nonhuman primate species and can be found in the *Guide* (NRC, 2011a) and the *Animal Welfare Act* (USDA, 2013). The 2011 *Guide* recommendations differ from current Animal Welfare Regulations in that the *Guide* states that optimal cage measurements should not be based solely on floor space (engineering standards). Some nonhuman primates benefit more from vertical space (volume of primary enclosure), internal structures, and enrichment opportunities within the space (complexities) than from floor space. According to the *Guide*, space allowances should be derived from performance standards, professional judgment, and experience. An additional housing standard for NIH-owned or NIH-supported chimpanzees was published on April 7, 2014, stating that chimpanzees should have 250 ft^2 of space per animal in their housing enclosures (NIH NOT-OD-14-051, 2014). It should be emphasized that the housing space requirments in the documents listed above are minimum standards, and every effort should be made to exceed the minimum standards.

In Europe, housing standards in laboratory animal medicine are governed by the European Convention for the Protection of Vertebrate Animals used for Experimental and Other Scientific Purposes (ETS 123) and the European Union's Council Directive on the Approximation of Laws, Regulations and Administrative Provisions of the Member States Regarding the Protection of Animals Used for Experimental and Other Scientific Purposes EU 2010/63 (Directive). Species-specific minimum space requirements can be found in Appendix A of ETS 123 (http://conventions.coe.int/Treaty/EN/Treaties/PDF/123-Arev.pdf). This reference also contains detailed recommendations on ventilation, temperature, humidity, lighting, noise, environmental enrichment, breeding/weaning, and euthanasia (Bayne and Morris, 2012).

When selecting cage material and design, the dexterity, strength, and species-typical behavior of the species must be considered. The materials used should meet the needs of the animal and be easily sanitized and resistant to the accumulation of dirt, debris, and moisture. Surfaces should be smooth and resistant to rusting, chipping, cracking, and peeling. Materials that are often used include galvanized metal, stainless steel, aluminum, and plastics. Less durable material, such as wood, can provide a more comfortable tactile surfaces (perches, climbing structures, resting areas, nest boxes), but wooden items must be replaced periodically when sanitation becomes ineffective or damage to the wood structures occur.

Production colonies are housed in large outdoor enclosures (field cages, corncribs, corrals, runs,

Primadomes™) with great success. Successful outdoor housing necessitates providing an adequate acclimation period for the animals when first placed outdoors in advance of seasonal changes, grouping compatible animals in a species-appropriate social environment, training animals to enter cages or transfer tunnels to accommodate restraint and transport, and providing adequate security to protect the animals from intruders. Other considerations with outdoor housing are environmental enrichment, food and water, pest control, animal accessibility for health care, and frequent observation of animals. Ground surfaces in outdoor facilities may be native soil and grasses, vegetation or rock, gravel, and concrete. All surfaces must be cleaned periodically to maintain acceptable husbandry/sanitation standards. The benefits of elevated grid flooring are historically well established in individual cage design, and the same principle should benefit outdoor housing.

Poor cage design and construction can result in hazards to the primate occupants. Toxicity through the ingestion of caging material is possible. For example, leaded paints and galvanized steel have been implicated in inadvertent poisonings, along with certain indoor/outdoor plants, trees, and shrubs used to landscape holding areas (Obeck, 1978). The cage design and finish should eliminate sharp edges; protruding screws/bolts; and any ropes, chains, or cables that might pose a risk of strangulation.

B. Enrichment Programs

Since the 1985 amendments to the Animal Welfare Act, disciplines within the animal research community have struggled to promulgate minimum standards "for a physical environment adequate to promote the psychological well-being of primates" (CFR, 1999). Most successful and compliant enrichment program strategies do not depend upon tightly written engineering or prescriptive specifications. On the contrary, they have implemented performance-based strategies that rely heavily on professional judgment in interpreting and applying the regulatory recommendations. Personnel involved in developing, implementing, and evaluating an enrichment plan must have specialized knowledge, skills, and experience with nonhuman primates. Species-specific structures, devices, and foodstuffs can be used to create an environment conducive to normal health and expression of species-typical behaviors. Playscapes and structures for climbing stimulate normal physiologic development. Sight barriers such as crates and barrels allow lower-ranking animals to escape from aggressive encounters, thus reducing stress and trauma. Sticks, balls, chew toys, and other play items provide diversion and alleviate boredom. Nonhuman primates can forage as in nature if seeds, grains, fruits, vegetables, or other foods are distributed in a variety of substrates (hay, straw, artificial turf), or are presented in a puzzle feeder (NRC, 2003a). Social housing as a form of enrichment has been shown to be one of the most effective methods of preventing and reducing abnormal behavior (Lutz and Novak, 2005).

Numerous scientific publications have been designed to generate data for assessing enrichment strategies on individual species. One such reference is *A Guide to the Behavior and Enrichment of Laboratory Macaques* (Winnicker *et al.*, 2013), which contains expert summaries of recent laboratory-associated behavior and enrichment literature for macaque species. The 1998 National Research Council publication *The Psychological Well-Being of Nonhuman Primates* (ILAR, 1998) is an excellent overview of the principles and recommendations concerning a quality nonhuman primate enrichment program. In addition, the Animal Welfare Information Center (AWIC) maintains a database on *Environmental Enrichment for Nonhuman Primates Resource Guide* which covers literature published from 1999 to 2014, and is continually updated (AWIC, 2006).

PRT has been used as a nonhuman primate enrichment strategy. It is defined as a form of operant conditioning where an animal receives a reward for performing a desired behavior (Veeder *et al.*, 2009). PRT provides the animal with a choice, whether to participate in the training and receive a reward, or to not participate (Schapiro and Lambeth, 2007). Using this training technique, nonhuman primates have been trained to voluntarily comply with various husbandry procedures as well as various clinical procedures. Some clinical procedures can be performed cageside without sedation with appropriate animal training. Nonhuman primates have been trained to present for injections, blood/urine/semen collections, body temperatures, dental exams, cardiac and respiratory auscultations, wound treatments, cardiac and abdominal ultrasounds, acupuncture, and laser treatments (Laule *et al.*, 1996; Perlman *et al.*, 2003; Schapiro *et al.*, 2005; Coleman *et al.*, 2008; Magden *et al.*, 2013). The resulting benefits of this training are less stress which produces better scientific data (Lambeth *et al.*, 2006) and fewer animal sedations, and it allows the animal a level of control – they can choose to participate or not participate in the training (Laule *et al.*, 2003). Because this training involves positive reinforcement, it can be a very effective form of enrichment.

Developing environmental enrichment programs within a research facility with the constraints of various experimental protocols can be challenging. The Institutional Animal Care and Use Committee, the Institutional Biosafety Committee, the Personnel Health and Safety Program specialists, the principal investigator, the primate behaviorist, and the veterinarian should all be involved in risk assessments when the experiments involve infectious diseases, atypical rearing, physical restraint, minimally invasive procedures, surgery, multiple uses, conditions involving pain, and studies involving substance abuse or aggression. Even under these circumstances, creative and novel approaches can address some of the nonhuman primate needs for psychological well-being, and every effort should be made to socially house the animals.

In addition to providing an enriching environment, laboratory animal veterinarians have the added responsibility to ensure an appropriate quality of life for all laboratory animals. Traditionally, the veterinarian determines when an animal reaches a humane endpoint by assessing the clinical records and physical exam findings. However, it is beneficial to have multiple personell familiar with the animals to help interpret signs of pain or distress. To assist with humane endpoint considerations, the veterinarian can enlist the help of others with expertise in the care and behavior of the sick animal. One such approach involves the development of a Quality-of-Life (QOL) committee. The QOL committee is composed of a veterinarian, a veterinary pathologist, a veterinary technologist, a behaviorist, a colony manager, and an animal technician involved with the daily care of the animal. A QOL committee is formed when an animal is diagnosed with a life-threatening or debilitating chronic condition and requires more intense monitoring for pain or distress. An individual behavioral ethogram is developed for the animal that enables the QOL committee to quantitatively assess the loss of normal behaviors for the individual animal, and thus assist the veterinarian in making a more informed decision regarding the quality of life and whether euthanasia is appropriate (Lambeth *et al.*, 2013).

C. Environmental Controls

Nonhuman primates in indoor facilities should be protected from temperature extremes. The Animal Welfare Act requires that these temperatures not drop below 45°F or exceed 85°F for more than four consecutive hours. At temperatures above 85°F, provisions should be made for cooling or for increasing air movement. Temperature extremes, especially abrupt temperature excursions, can cause stress and can have a deleterious impact on animal wellbeing.

The recommended environmental temperature settings for most nonhuman primates is 64–84°F; however, consideration should be given to the animal's natural history and thermoneutral zone (NRC, 2011a). Due to their small size and how quickly they can lose body heat, particular care should be exercised with nonhuman primate species such as marmosets, tamarins, and smaller cebids to ensure that contact areas of cages are made from thermoneutral materials such as plastics

(Abee, 1989). Temperatures maintained within a facility will depend on a number of criteria: species, age, size, number, and health status of animals present. Sudden, prolonged temperature changes should be avoided if at all possible. Controlled environments should provide nonhuman primate holding rooms with nonrecirculated ventilation at a rate of 10–15 air changes per hour (NRC, 2011a).

Animals that are housed in outdoor facilities must be acclimated to outdoor air temperatures to avoid temperature-related stress and discomfort. Appropriately acclimated outdoor housed animals can often tolerate a wider range of temperatures than is recommended for nonacclimated animals. The deleterious effects of high temperature extremes can be lessened by providing housing areas with shade, misters, wading pools, or other devices and strategies to mitigate heat stress. Cold temperature extremes can be avoided by having secondary enclosures with supplemental heaters, windbreaks, and alternative bedding for the extreme cold.

For most species of nonhuman primates, the recommended range for relative humidity is 30–70% (NRC, 2011a). Some New World primates, such as tamarins and marmosets, require a minimum relative humidity of 50% (Southers and Ford, 1995). HVAC systems in indoor housing facilities should provide control of humidity levels; however, relative humidity should be considered when designing outdoor facilities. Conditions of low or high humidity may exacerbate problems associated with temperature extremes.

The regulations within the Animal Welfare Act require lighting (natural or artificial) of indoor facilities to be uniformly diffused throughout the enclosure. This allows for routine inspection of the primates, maintenance of acceptable husbandry standards, maintenance of physiologic and neuroendocrinologic stimulation, and improved personnel safety. The spectrum and intensity of light may have a physiologic impact on nonhuman primates; however, there are no conclusive studies available at this time to make an informed decision. For most primate species, a 12-h light–12-h dark diurnal cycle is sufficient to meet their needs (NRC, 2011a) and can be achieved by using a time-controlled lighting system. Facilities housing *Aotus* spp. or other nocturnal species may choose to provide a reverse light cycle. Red lighting during the animals' active part of the day provides illumination for husbandry practices and observation. White light can be provided during the evening and at night to encourage nesting behavior/sleep outside normal staff working hours.

Loud or sudden noises may be stressful to nonhuman primates (NRC, 2011a). Personnel working around animals should be educated to work quietly and minimize unnecessary noise to reduce overall stress levels. Service carts should be maintained with quiet casters and plastic or rubberized carts may also be used to reduce noise. Bedding, when used, should be from a high-quality source to minimize the potential for contamination, which may have a profound effect on the animals' health and well-being, and on research results.

D. Sanitation

To maintain a safe and healthy environment, a comprehensive sanitation program must be implemented. An understanding of possible sources of contamination and potential pathogens is essential when deciding on the materials and structures to be used in captive environments. Additionally, appropriate methods for sanitizing and the frequency of these procedures must be considered. As stated in the *Guide* (2011), effective sanitation is composed of two elements, cleaning and disinfecting. Cleaning is defined as the removal of dirt and waste products, while disinfection is the reduction or elimination of pathogenic microorganisms.

Providing a sanitary environment can be a challenge when nonhuman primates are group-housed. Solid floors in primary enclosures can increase the frequency of illnesses caused by fecal–oral transmission. Slatted or grid floors are preferable, since they allow waste products to fall away from the animal's environment. With decreased fecal contamination, the chance of fecal–oral transmission of pathogenic organisms can be reduced, even though food items are eaten from the cage floor.

Effective sanitation programs focus on a variety of target organisms. Parasites that can be harmful to nonhuman primates include arthropods, protozoa (such as amoebae and coccidia), and helminths (nematodes, cestodes, and trematodes). Bacteria that can cause gastrointestinal disease and deaths include *Salmonella*, *Campylobacter* spp., *Yersinia* spp., and *Shigella* spp. Transmissible viral agents that are of particular concern because they can cause gastrointestinal disease include rotaviruses, simian hemorrhagic fever virus, and measles virus (Brady and Carville, 2012).

Effective cleaning and disinfecting of both primary and secondary enclosures can be accomplished with water, detergents, bleach, phenolics, and quaternary ammonia compounds. The typical regime would begin with flushing of gross debris with water, followed by disinfecting with products that are bactericidal and virucidal. Tuberculocidal cleaning and disinfecting agents should be used during CDC mandated import quarantine or when otherwise warranted. Cleaning and disinfecting should be performed daily on primary enclosures, including perches, shelves, and enrichment devices. In a hospital setting, it is recommended that the primary enclosure be cleaned and disinfected twice daily (NRC, 2011a). In general, daily disinfection should be supplemented with biweekly sanitation of primary enclosures and their associated structures, such as cage racks and cage pans. Primary enclosures and food and water receptacles should be sanitized by live steam under pressure, 180°F water as found in a mechanical cage washer and soap or detergent, or washing all soiled surfaces with appropriate detergent solutions and disinfectants.

Primary enclosures with dirt floors or absorbent bedding should be spot-cleaned frequently enough to ensure that animals can move about without contacting their excrement. Cleaning and disinfection of animal rooms, treatment rooms, storage areas, cage-washing facilities, and corridors should be accomplished at a frequency that is consistent with their use and level of contamination (NRC, 2011a).

E.　Biosafety and Biosafety-Level Determination

Nonhuman primates pose unique zoonotic risks. Their care and use can present serious hazards to personnel that work directly with them, or with their tissues or body fluids. According to the Centers for Disease Control and Prevention (CDCP), research institutions that house nonhuman primates are obligated to provide their workers with established practices to ensure that appropriate levels of environmental quality and safety are maintained (CDCP/NIH, 2009). This obligation is driven by a series of federal regulations created for worker safety. Starting in the mid-1980s, the federal standard known as Hazard Communication ('Worker Right to Know') was developed by the Occupational Safety and Health Administration (OSHA) to create a work environment where hazards found in the specific work area are identified, their capabilities for related health problems are recognized, and the workers are given complete access to their respective laboratory results and medical records. This was followed in 1991 by the implementation by the OSHA of 29 CFR Part, 1910.1030, the Occupational Exposure to Bloodborne Pathogens: Final Rule, which states that blood, body fluids, and tissues infected with human disease agents must be handled in compliance with OSHA standards. Therefore, work practices associated with experimentally infected nonhuman primates must comply.

Nonhuman primate housing and research facilities must include a biosafety program with procedures and equipment for preventing exposure of personnel and animals to endemic or experimentally introduced pathogens. To determine these preventive measures, a risk assessment must be performed. This assessment addresses such specifics as the pathogenicity of the agent(s), its infectious dose, the route of transmission, the availability of an effective prophylactic regimen, and the experience of the at-risk personnel. Once the assessment is complete, the appropriate biosafety level can be assigned to limit the personnel and environmental exposure level. These potential exposures can then be reduced or eliminated through appropriate containment of the infectious materials. When working with nonhuman primates, the BSL should be set at a minimum of BSL-2. The decision to elevate beyond BSL-2 is based on an assessment of risks associated with the species, its documented pathogen status, and the research to be carried out. An effective biosafety program can prevent personnel exposures, infections, and other complications.

Simian foamy virus, likely transmitted through animal bites, has not been reported to cause disease in human beings, but it is the most frequently found zoonotic virus in occupationally exposed nonhuman primate caretakers (Switzer et al., 2004). Macacine herpesvirus 1 (McHV-1) also commonly referred to as herpes B virus, simian immunodeficiency virus (SIV, a retrovirus closely related to HIV-1 and HIV-2), tuberculosis, and bacterial gastroenteritis caused by Shigella, Salmonella, Yersinia, and Campylobacter spp. are some of the more serious pathogens that can be transmitted to personnel. The 1997 death of a national primate research center technician after an accidental, ocular-splash exposure to McHV-1 and an increase in research protocols that involve the use of pathogens such as HIV, SIV, SHIV, hepatitis B, and hepatitis C heightened the research community's awareness of the risks associated with nonhuman primates (NRC, 2003b; CDCP/NIH, 2009). Based on the information obtained from documented exposures to McHV-1, the recommended procedures following a bite or scratch were reassessed and subsequently published (Cohen et al., 2002). Table 17.36 lists recommendations from this report. Recommended PPE for working with nonhuman primates is provided in Table 17.37. Table 17.38 provides a list of zoonotic diseases, their mode of transmission, and the recommended biosafety precautions.

Chapter 27 of this textbook, *Working Safely with Experimental Animals Exposed to Biohazards*, contains additional information regarding recommended procedures for research with experimentally or naturally infected nonhuman primates.

F.　Medical Records

Effective recordkeeping systems are essential in order to adequately manage nonhuman primates in a research facility. A detailed record of the animal's prior experimental history and health is invaluable. It is common for nonhuman primates to have life spans in excess of 20 years and hence to be assigned to multiple research projects. The permanent animal record should contain relevant information pertaining to the animal's genetic, clinical, surgical, behavioral, reproductive, and research histories. Most research facilities have transitioned to

TABLE 17.36 Standard Operating Procedures for Macaque Monkey Bite, Scratch, and Mucosal Exposures[a]

1. Ocular, oral, and genital monkey secretions are all potentially infectious.
2. Routes of exposure to human beings include bites, scratches, needlestick injuries, and mucosal (including ocular) splash.
3. First aid
   a. Mucous membrane exposure: flush eye or mucous membranes with sterile saline or water for 15 min.
   b. Skin exposure: wash skin with a 0.25% hypochlorite (bleach) solution, followed by a wash with detergent soap (chlorhexidine or povidone-iodine) for 15 min.
4. Initial evaluation
   a. Human
      1. Health care provider to assess adequacy of cleansing, and repeat cleansing
      2. Determine date, time, location, and exposure description
      3. Evaluate general health and date of last tetanus booster
      4. Determine need for postexposure prophylaxis (antibiotics, rabies vaccine, etc.)
   b. Nonhuman primate
      1. Identify the monkey associated with the exposure, and the responsible veterinarian
      2. Assess general health (vaccination status, medications, past research involvement)
      3. Evaluate serologic history (including B virus status)
5. Examination and laboratory testing
   a. Human
      1. Physical examination (focus on site of exposure and neurological exam)
      2. Consider collecting serum samples for baseline serologic analysis
      3. Consider culture of wound site or exposed mucosal surface
   b. Nonhuman primate
      1. Examine animal for mucosal lesions (i.e. vesicles, ulcers), conjunctivitis, etc.
      2. Consider culture of lesions, conjunctiva, and buccal mucosa
      3. Consider serologic testing for B virus
6. Education and treatment
   a. Counsel patient on significance of injury
   b. Provide information on the signs and symptoms of B virus infection
   c. Ensure patient has a card to carry with information on B virus and emergency contact information
   d. Ensure the patient's supervisor and health care provider are notified.
   e. Review with patient and their supervisor safety precautions in place at time of exposure
   f. Schedule follow-up appointment
   g. Consider starting postexposure prophylaxis

[a]From Cohen et al. (2002).

TABLE 17.37 Personal Protective Equipment[a]

Laboratory clothing	Laboratory coats, smocks, gowns, total body suits, coveralls, two-piece scrub suits
Head coverings	Not required except in containment areas requiring a complete clothing change
	Simple cap, hoods, bouffant cap
Shoes and shoe covers	Sandals not allowed in biohazard areas
	For BSL-2 and BSL-3 areas, a change from street shoes is advised; shoe covers can be used when a complete change of clothes and dedicated shoes are not required
	Butyl rubber, neoprene, or PVC boots are advised in animal rooms when encountering large amounts of water
Gloves	Rubber, neoprene, latex, nitrile, PVC, polyvinyl alcohol, surgical
	Should extend to/beyond wrist
	Gauntlet-type leather gloves, Kevlar, or stainless steel liners for handling nonhuman primates
Respiratory protection	Single use, paper 'dust' mask can be worn in clean animal rooms; not for use where infectious aerosols present; allowed for necropsies of clean animals
	Areas where infectious aerosols present, use half-face or full-face respirators with HEPA filters recommended
	Particulate respirators allowed for BSL-3 areas
Eye or face protection	Areas of respirable aerosols or droplets, use full-face respirators or half-face respirators plus splash goggles
	Areas of McHV-1 (herpes B virus), use safety shields or face shields plus splash goggles
	Areas where McHV-1 not a concern, safety shields or face shields sufficient

McHV-1, Macacine herpesvirus 1; BSL, biosafety level; PVC, polyvinyl chloride.
[a]From Kuehne et al. (1995).

a computerized medical records system. A computerized system helps to organize not only animal health information, but also general colony information that can be quickly summarized for more efficient colony management. The facility veterinarian should have an oversight of the establishment, maintenance, and review of medical records (NRC, 2011a).

Animal records should document the nonhuman primate's individual permanent identification. This identification may include a tattoo with a uniquely assigned number or code applied to the chest or inner thigh, a simple technique that remains one of the most common methods of permanent animal identification (Dyke, 1995). Collars with attached identification tags are frequently used with baboons and squirrel monkeys. Subcutaneously placed microtransponders are also a common identification method. These transponders contain permanent identification information that can be read by a telemetry transceiver (Dyke, 1995).

TABLE 17.38 Zoonotic Diseases

Disease	Transmission[a]	Recommended precautions[a]
VIRAL		
Marburg	Aerosol, droplet, percutaneous	BSL-4
Ebola	Aerosol, droplet, percutaneous	BSL-4
Yellow fever	Arthropod vector, *Aedes* spp. mosquitoes, percutaneous	BSL-3
Dengue	Arthropod vector, *Aedes* spp. mosquitoes, percutaneous	BSL-2
West Nile virus	Arthropod vector, *Culex* spp. mosquitos, percutaneous	BSL-2
EEE, VEE, WEE (Eastern, Venezuelan, and Western equine encephalitis viruses)	Arthropod vector, multiple mosquito spp., percutaneous	BSL-3
McHV-1 (Herpesvirus simiae, herpes B)	Aerosol, droplet, percutaneous	BSL-2[b]
Hepatitis A	Ingestion	BSL-2; immunization
Hepatitis B	Droplet, percutaneous	BSL-2; immunization
Hepatitis C	Droplet, percutaneous	BSL-2
Hepatitis D	Droplet, percutaneous	BSL-2
Hepatitis E	Ingestion	BSL-2
Primate T-lymphotrophic virus 1	Droplet, percutaneous	BSL-2
HIV-1, HIV-2, SIV	Droplet, percutaneous	BSL-2
Monkeypox	Percutaneous	BSL-2 facilities with BSL-3 practices
Measles	Aerosol	BSL-2; Immunization
Influenza	Aerosol	BSL-2; Immunization
HPAI (Highly Pathogenic Avian Influenza)	Aerosol	BSL-3
Poliovirus	Percutaneous, ingestion	BSL-2; Immunization
Rabies	Droplet, percutaneous	BSL-2, Immunization
PRIONS		
Transmissible spongiform encephalopathy (TSE)	Percutaneous, aerosol	BSL-2
BACTERIAL		
Tuberculosis	Aerosol, percutaneous	BSL-3 if known
Mycobacterium tuberculosis		BSL-2 during quarantine
Campylobacteriosis	Ingestion	BSL-2
Campylobacter spp.		
Helicobacter	Ingestion	BSL-2
Helicobacter spp.		
Leptospirosis	Ingestion, droplet, Percutaneous	BSL-2
Leptospira spp.		

(Continued)

TABLE 17.38 (Continued)

Disease	Transmission[a]	Recommended precautions[a]
Shigellosis	Ingestion, percutaneous	BSL-2
Shigella spp.		
Salmonellosis	Ingestion, percutaneous	BSL-2
Salmonella spp.		
Yersinia enterocolitica	Ingestion	BSL-2
PARASITIC		
Nematodes		
Strongyloides spp.	Ingestion	BSL-2
Ancylostoma spp.	Percutaneous, ingestion	BSL-2
Trichuris spp.	Ingestion	BSL-2
Cestodes	Ingestion	BSL-2
Trematodes		
Schistosoma spp.	Contact	BSL-2
Malaria	Arthropod vector, percutaneous	BSL-2
Toxoplasmosis	Ingestion	BSL-2
Trypanosomiasis (Chagas disease)	Triatomine bug bite, percutaneous, aerosol, droplet	BSL-2
Trypanosoma cruzi		
Amebiasis		
Entamoeba histolytica	Ingestion	BSL-2
Balantidiasis	Ingestion	BSL-2
Balantidium coli	Ingestion	BSL-2
Giardia spp.	Ingestion	BSL-2
Cryptosporidiosis	Ingestion	BSL-2
FUNGAL		
Coccidoides immitis	Aerosol, percutaneous	BSL-2
Dermatophytes	Contact	BSL-2
Epidermophyton, *Trichophyton*, and *Microsporum* spp.		

BSL, biosafety level.
[a]*From CDCP/NIH (2009); for a more complete listing of zoonotic agents, refer to this reference.*
[b]*McHV-1 used in experimental infections of rhesus macaques are recommended BSL-4 containment.*

V. MEDICAL MANAGEMENT

A. Preventive Medicine

Laboratory animal veterinarians have the advantage of being able to employ all aspects of a preventive medicine program. The value of preventive medicine in maintaining healthy nonhuman primates far exceeds the benefits of the most sophisticated diagnostic laboratory capability or the most astute laboratory animal diagnostician. A comprehensive preventive medicine program not only involves preemptive immunizations, diagnostic capabilities, and prophylactic management strategies, but should permeate the entire health care and maintenance program. It includes good nutrition, parasite control, facility and primary enclosure design, quarantine and isolation policies, traffic patterns, experimental and social histories, sanitation, vermin control, and awareness of zoonoses.

1. Quarantine

All newly acquired primates must undergo a quarantine period appropriate to the species. The quarantine program provides for segregation of new animals for the time necessary to acclimate them to their new environment and carry out diagnostic procedures for the detection of adventitious infectious agents. Quarantined animals harboring undesirable agents may be treated without exposing other susceptible animals within the facility. Newly imported primates must be quarantined for a minimum of 31 days at a CDC-registered primate import facility (CDCP CFR 42 part 71.53, 2013).

Once animals have completed the required 31-day quarantine period, an additional quarantine period of 30 days or longer should be completed at the receiving research facility. Selecting the appropriate duration for quarantine depends on the source of the animal(s), facilities available, type of research, institutional policies, and the value and health status of the resident colony.

The quarantine facility location should allow complete separation from the resident colony. Supplies or equipment should be dedicated to the quarantine facility and should be thoroughly decontaminated before being transferred from the quarantine area to a 'clean area.' Personnel traffic patterns should always move from clean to dirty (quarantine). If staff must move from the quarantine to clean areas, they should shower and don clean clothing before entering the resident colony area.

On arrival, nonhuman primates should be allowed a 72-h acclimation period. After the acclimation period, a veterinarian should perform an entry medical examination. This should include creation of an individual animal record, blood collection for hematology and serology, body weight measurement, administration of anthelmintics, fecal parasitology exam, vaccinations as determined by the facility's preventive medicine program, thoracic radiographs (when appropriate), and a Mantoux tuberculin skin test (TST). The TST should be administered intradermally using Mammalian Old Tuberculin repeated every 2 weeks in alternating eyelids for the duration of the quarantine period. Each TST should be evaluated at 24, 48, and 72 h; however, since this test is an assessment of delayed type hypersensitivity, particular care should be paid to the 48- and 72-h time points. If there is any suspicious reactivity, the animal should be anesthetized and the palpebrum should be manually palpated as a more sensitive indicator of induration. In addition, the TST should be immediately repeated using the opposite eyelid or a shaved region of the abdomen near the umbilicus. Table 17.39 lists tuberculin test reaction grades, and an example of a positive TB test is shown in Fig. 17.16. Reactions in animals with tuberculosis can range from no reaction in anergic animals to slight enduration to extreme inflammation including ulceration of the skin. If one animal in

TABLE 17.39 Tuberculin Test Reaction Grades: Intradermal Intrapalpebral Test

Reaction grade	Description of changes
0	Negative: no reaction observed
1	Negative: bruise; extravasation of blood in eyelid from injection
2	Negative: varying degrees of erythema of palpebrum without swelling
3	Indeterminant: varying degrees of erythema of palpebrum with minimum swelling or slight swelling without erythema
4	Positive: obvious swelling of palpebrum with drooping of eyelid with varying degrees of erythema
5	Positive: swelling and/or necrosis with eyelid closed

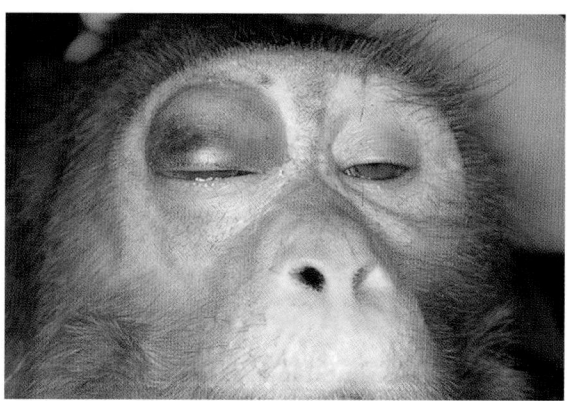

FIGURE 17.16 Positive tuberculin test reaction in a rhesus macaque (*Macaca mulatta*).

the group tests positive or reactive in the TST, all animals in the group must be considered exposed, and the testing and quarantine procedures should be extended (Martin, 1986). The animal(s) should be observed daily throughout the quarantine period. Key clinical parameters to evaluate include activity, appetite, and excreta. To ensure continuity, the same individual should perform these observations as frequently as possible. Once the quarantine period has been completed, the veterinarian should carry out an 'exit physical.' The veterinarian can release the animal(s) from quarantine or require an extension of the quarantine period.

2. Immunizations

Historically, various active and passive immunization agents and procedures have been used with nonhuman primates. The decision whether to administer conventional vaccines will depend on a risk–benefit assessment for each situation. While deleterious effects are uncommon, vaccination efficacy is rarely based on scientific data from nonhuman primates. Sometimes immunizations are contraindicated due to research design. Immunizations may serve as protection against introduction of a pathogen into a valuable research colony. Tetanus, rabies, and measles vaccines have been used in nonhuman primates; these may be indicated if animals are housed in large production colonies or outdoor facilities (Table 17.40).

Decisions about the frequency of boosting vaccines must be based on human protective titer literature and random titer sampling of the nonhuman primate colony. The new generations of pneumococcal vaccines do show promise for preventing pneumococcal meningitis in chimpanzees and should be considered when appropriate. Intensive efforts to develop vaccines effective against herpesviruses and retroviruses have been largely unsuccessful thus far. Should these types of vaccines become available, they could play an important role in protecting breeding colonies of nonhuman primates and preventing significant zoonoses. At this time, specific pathogen-free breeding colonies must depend on test-and-cull strategies. Although this technique has reduced the zoonotic risk of McHV-1, it cannot be relied upon for complete elimination of this virus. All management and handling techniques must be designed to protect against the remote possibility of latent McHV-1 transmission.

3. Diagnostic Testing

Management of nonhuman primates in biomedical research should include monitoring them for agents that are commonly found or that can potentially confound biomedical research results. This practice will reduce the risk of research interference or unintended introduction of new agents into the colony. Serodiagnostic testing forms the backbone of most laboratory animal health monitoring programs, and is often performed by easily automated, high throughput, techniques such as the indirect enzyme immunoassay (EIA) or multiplexed fluorometric immunoassay (MFIA). Diagnostic testing laboratories offer panels of diagnostic tests for common infectious agents. Some frequently utilized diagnostic panels for nonhuman primate species are shown in Table 17.41.

The ultimate goal of serodiagnostic testing is to mitigate the risks of adventitious infectious agents on research

TABLE 17.40 Vaccination Recommendations

Species	Vaccine	Age at initial immunization	Booster
Chimpanzee	Polio, MLV	1 year	None
	Rabies, killed[a]	2 year	q3 years
	MMR (measles, mumps, rubella), MLV[b]	1 year	annually
	Tetanus toxoid[a]	1 year	q5 years
Macaque	MMR, MLV[c]	3 months	At least 6 weeks after initial dose
	Rabies, killed[a]	1 year	q3 years
	Tetanus toxoid[a]	1 year	q5 years
Baboon	Rabies, killed[a]	1 year	q3 years
	Tetanus toxoid[a]	1 year	q5 years
Marmoset	MMR, MLV[b]	1 year	annually

MLV, modified live virus.
[a]Recommended for animals housed outdoors.
[b]Heatley and Musser (2014).
[c]Wachtman and Mansfield (2012).

TABLE 17.41 Diagnostic Testing Recommendations for Research Primates

		Macaque	African Green monkey	Baboon	Chimpanzee	New World monkey
Retrovirus		SIV	SIV	SIV	SIV	
		STLV	STLV	STLV	STLV	
		SRV 1–5				
Herpesvirus	Alpha	Macacine herpesvirus 1	Cercopithecine herpesvirus 2	Papiine herpesvirus 2	Human herpesvirus 1 and 2	Saimiriine herpesvirus 1
					Human herpesvirus 3	
	Beta		Cercopithecine herpesvirus 5	Cercopithecine herpesvirus 5	Panine herpesvirus 2	Squirrel monkey CMV
	Gamma				Panine herpesvirus 1	Saimiriine herpesvirus 2
Other		Measles	Measles	Measles	Measles	Measles

SIV, simian immunodeficiency virus; SRV, simian retrovirus; STLV, systemic T-lymphotrophic virus, CMV, cytomegalovirus.

and to use the information that is generated to make management decisions regarding the infection status of the animals. Diagnostic laboratories may take a multi-tiered approach to diagnostic testing. The first assay used is often an automated high-throughput assay such as an EIA or MFIA in which the assay performance parameters have been biased for high diagnostic sensitivity (DSn) to detect very early infections. The consequent result of biasing an assay for high diagnostic sensitivity is to decrease the assay's diagnostic specificity (DSp), which results in a higher number of false-positive (FP) results. A secondary assay with a very high diagnostic specificity (i.e., an assay that is very good at sorting out true positives from false positives), such as a western immunoblot (WIB) or indirect fluorescent antibody (IFA) test is then used to make a final positive or negative classification of the sample. However, because of the inherent limitations of assay performance, both false-negative (FN) and FP classifications occur even when using validated assays that have very good assay performance characteristics. One mistake that is commonly made when interpreting diagnostic testing results is to assume that an assay that has a DSn of 95% will result in 95 true-positive (TP) and five FN results for every 100 samples tested. And conversely, that an assay with a DSp of 95% will result in 95 true-negative (TN) and five FP results for every 100 samples tested. In fact, the number of TP, TN, FN and FP results cannot be calculated from the DSn and DSp unless the prevalence of the infection in the test population is known. If the prevalence of the infection in the test population is not known, it should be estimated based on the history and experience with the test population or based upon experience with similar populations of animals. Knowing the DSn, DSp, and prevalence in the target population allows for the calculation of the positive and negative predictive values (PPV and NPV) of the assay, i.e., the confidence that you can have in a positive or negative diagnostic test, respectively. For example, if an infectious agent has an expected prevalence of 25% in a population and the assay that is used to detect the agent has a DSn of 98% and a DSp of 95%, then the PPV is 86.7% and the NPV is 99.3%: i.e., you can have very good confidence in both the positive and the negative results. Now, what will happen if we take that same assay that gave excellent results when the prevalence of disease in the population was 25% and apply it to a SPF population? We can approximate an SPF population by assuming that the prevalence of disease in the population is 0.1%. If we now apply the same assay to this 'SPF' population, the PPV drops to 2% while the NPV increases to 100%. Thus, we can have very good confidence in the negative results from the SPF population, but only two out of every 100 animals that test positive are truly infected with the agent even though the assay is identical to the assay that gave outstanding results

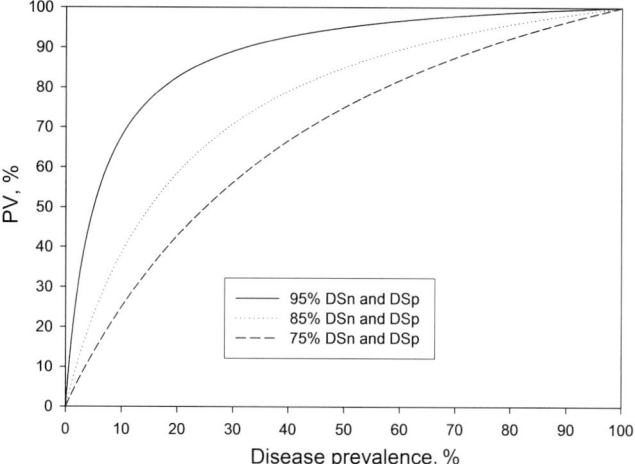

FIGURE 17.17   Calculated curves for the positive predictive value (PPV) of an assay *versus* the prevalence of disease in a population for assays with a diagnostic sensitivity (DSn) and diagnostic specificity (DSp) of 95%, 85% and 75%, respectively. These curves can be used to interpolate the PPV for an assay if the DSn, DSp, and disease prevalence in the population are either known or can be estimated with reasonable accuracy.

when the prevalence of disease in the target population was 25%.

These two examples demonstrate several critical issues that must be considered when interpreting sero-diagnostic test results. First, it is important to know the specific assay performance characteristics (DSn and DSp) for the assays that are being used in testing. Second, it is very important to either know the expected prevalence of the agent in the population being tested, or to be able to estimate the prevalence of the agent from previous experience, clinical impression, or analysis of potential risk of exposure. By knowing the DSn, DSp, and disease prevalence, one can calculate the positive and negative predictive values for the assay. As long as the DSn and DSp are above 50%, the predictive values for an assay follow the same trends: as the prevalence of an agent in a population falls to zero, so does the PPV (Fig. 17.17); however, at the same time, the NPV increases to 100% (Fig. 17.18). The converse is also true: as the prevalence of an agent in the population approaches 100% so does the PPV (Fig. 17.17); however, at the same time, the NPV falls to zero (Fig. 17.18). Because of these trends in the predictive value curves, if the DSn, DSp and disease prevalence can be estimated with reasonable accuracy, then the PPV and NPV for a given diagnostic test result can be interpolated using Figs 17.17 and 17.18, respectively.

This demonstrates the conundrum that confronts diagnostic laboratories and primate clinicians when interpreting unexpected positive test results in a population of animals with a low prevalence of disease or

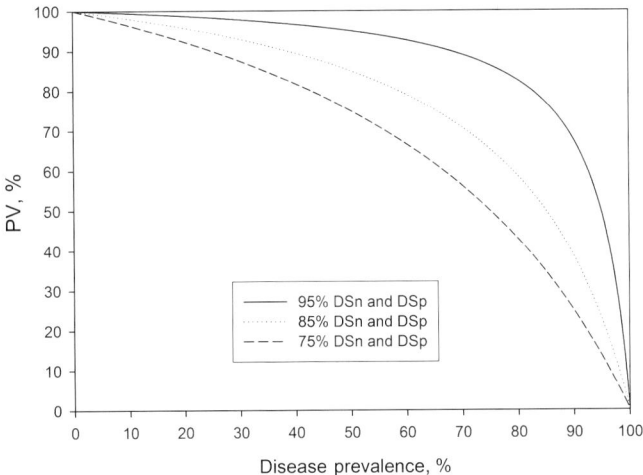

FIGURE 17.18 Calculated curves for the negative predictive value (NPV) of an assay *versus* the prevalence of disease in a population for assays with a diagnostic sensitivity (DSn) and diagnostic specificity (DSp) of 95%, 85%, and 75%, respectively. These curves can be used to interpolate the NPV for an assay if the DSn, DSp, and disease prevalence in the population either are known or can be estimated with reasonable accuracy.

one that is believed to be SPF. The PPV of the assay indicates that the result is most likely FP but there is a chance, albeit very small, that the result is correct. In this scenario, additional diagnostic testing using more specific diagnostic assays should be done so that the laboratory can attempt to sort out the true diagnostic test result. Additional serodiagnostic tests that often have greater DSp, and thus a lower rate of FP results, include IFA, WIB, hemagglutination inhibition, and polymerase chain reaction (PCR). Other information should be considered in the interpretation of the unexpected serodiagnostic test result as well. For example, was there a potential risk of exposure to the agent? How long has the colony been SPF and was the agent in question previously present in the population? Does a sporadic positive result fit with the expected biology of the virus or with the epidemiology of the agent in a naive population? All of this information should be considered in context with the diagnostic test results to make a final determination and classification of the unexpected result (Simmons, 2008).

4. Colony Surveillance

Frequent animal observations by caretakers, technicians, and veterinarians are a key element of an effective preventive medicine program. Serious illness can go undetected in some nonhuman primates because of their stoic nature. Animal care staff must be trained to recognize subtle physiologic and behavioral changes associated with early onset of disease.

Routine physical exams and supporting laboratory tests should be performed annually or more frequently based on the health status of the colony. The following elements are essential to a thorough physical examination:

1. History: should include reproductive parameters, cage location changes, participation in research, past disease diagnoses, and hospitalizations.
2. Body weight records: allow detection of subtle changes over time; the magnitude of weight loss may indicate a serious disorder.
3. Systems examined: to include cardiac, respiratory, ophthalmic, otolaryngeal, dermatologic, gynecologic, orthopedic, lymphatic, and digestive (dental, gastrointestinal).
4. Hematology: should include a complete blood count, serum chemistries and serology for McHV-1 for macaques, and retroviral surveillance for Old World monkeys.
5. Tuberculin test: 0.1 ml of full-strength, mammalian old tuberculin (MOT) in a 25- to 27-gauge ½-inch needle is injected intradermally into the upper eyelid. The test is read at 24, 48, and 72 h; Table 17.39 contains definitions of reaction grades.
6. Fecal examination: should include testing for nematodes, protozoa and apicomplexan parasites.
7. Vaccines: as indicated for the species, exposure history, and intended research assignment.
8. Radiology, ultrasonography: as needed.
9. Treatments: as needed. A formulary is given in Table 17.42.

5. Tuberculosis Testing

The significant mortality and zoonotic potential of tuberculosis in nonhuman primates, albeit rare, demands aggressive preventive measures (Garcia *et al.*, 2004a; Motzel *et al.*, 1999; Panarella and Bimes, 2010). Immunization techniques (e.g., BCG vaccination) are not practical and have many disadvantages in the United States, and vaccination makes it difficult to sort out protection against tuberculosis *versus* infection by routine diagnostic testing. A number of additional or adjunctive tests for tuberculosis have been developed with varying results including interferon-gamma releasing assays (IGRAs) (Garcia *et al.*, 2004b) and antibody assays (Lyashchenko *et al.*, 2007). However, the most effective means of identifying tuberculosis in nonhuman primates and preventing its spread to naive animals remains the tuberculin skin test, which is required during CDC mandated import quarantine. During quarantine, any positive or suspicious reactors should be identified and eliminated along with direct contact animals. The alarming rise in drug-resistant mycobacteria presents an additional serious consideration in diagnosing and

TABLE 17.42　Formulary

Compound	Macaque[a]	Chimpanzee[a]	Baboon[b]	New World monkey[c]	Dosage
ANTIBIOTICS					
Amoxicillin	20–40 mg/kg	250–500 mg/day	20 mg/kg		BID-QID
Ampicillin	25 mg/kg	500 mg	25 mg/kg		BID
Ceftriaxone	50 mg/kg	50–100 mg/kg			SID-BID; IM
Cephalexin	25–50 mg/kg/day	500–1000 mg	25 mg/kg		BID-TID
Cephapirin sodium				20 mg/kg	QID; IM, IV
Chloramphenicol	25 mg/kg	50 mg/kg/day	25 mg/kg	50 mg/kg	BID-QID; PO
Doxycycline	2.5 mg/kg	2–5 mg/kg	2.5 mg/kg		BID; PO
Enrofloxacin	2.5–10 mg/kg	2.5–10 mg/kg	5.0 mg/kg		SID-BID
Erythromycin	30–80 mg/kg/day	25–50 mg/kg/day	50 mg/kg		BID
Gentamicin	3–5 mg/kg	3–5 mg/kg	3 mg/kg	1–2 mg/kg	BID-TID; IM
Metronidazole	25–50 mg/kg	25 mg/kg	50 mg/kg		BID-TID
Penicillin G benzathine	30–60 kU/kg	900–1200 kU	30 kU/kg	15 kU	EOD; IM, SC
Penicillin G potassium				20 kU/kg	IV, IM, SC
Penicillin G procaine	20–40 kU/kg	600–1000 kU		15 kU	SID; SC
Tetracycline	25–50 mg/kg/day	25 mg/kg	25 mg/kg	15 mg/kg	BID; PO
Trimethoprim-sulfamethoxazole	4 mg/kg	800 mg	20 mg/kg	24 mg/kg	BID-TID; PO
ANALGESICS					
Acetaminophen	5–10 mg/kg	200–400 mg			TID; PO
Acetylsalicylic acid	10–20 mg/kg	325–650 mg	10.0 mg/kg		TID-QID; PO
Buprenorphine	0.01 mg/kg	0.01 mg/kg	0.01 mg/kg	0.01 mg/kg	BID; IM, SC
Butorphanol tartrate	0.05–0.10 mg/kg			0.02 mg/kg	QID; IM, SC
Carprofen	2 mg/kg	2 mg/kg			BID; PO
Flunixin meglumine	0.5–4 mg/kg		0.50 mg/kg		SID; IM
Meloxicam	0.1–0.2 mg/kg	0.1–0.2 mg/kg			SID; PO, IM
Naproxen	10 mg/kg	500 mg initial; then 250 mg			BID-TID
ANESTHETICS					
Acepromazine maleate	0.1–1.0 mg/kg				
Diazepam	1.0–5.0 mg	1.0–20.0 mg	5.0 mg		IM; PO
Ketamine hydrochloride	5–10.0 mg/kg	10.0 mg/kg	10.0 mg/kg	20–40 mg/kg,	IM
Midazolam hydrochloride				SC 0.225 mg	Prn; IV
				15–20 mg/kg	IV
Thiopental sodium	22–25 mg/kg				IM, IV
Tiletamine hydrochloride	3–6 mg/kg	3–5 mg/kg		1–2.5 mg/kg	IM, IV
Xylazine	0.25–0.5 mg/kg	0.5–1.0 mg/kg			IM, IV
Halothane w/50% O_2, 50% N_2	1–4% induction, 0.5–2.0% maintenance	1–4% induction, 0.5–2.0% maintenance	1–4% induction, 0.5–2.0% maintenance	4–8 mg/kg	SC
Isoflurane	1–2% induction, 0.5–1.5% maintenance	1–2% induction, 0.5–1.5% maintenance	1–2% induction, 0.5–1.5% maintenance	2–4% induction, 1–3% maintenance	

(Continued)

TABLE 17.42 (Continued)

Compound	Macaque[a]	Chimpanzee[a]	Baboon[b]	New World monkey[c]	Dosage
MISCELLANEOUS					
Atropine	0.05 mg/kg	0.02–0.2 mg/kg	0.05 mg/kg		IM
Dexamethasone	0.5–5 mg/day	5–15 mg/day	0.5 mg/kg		IM
Doxapram	2 mg/kg	2 mg/kg	2 mg/kg		IV
Epinephrine	0.1–0.5 mg	0.2–1.0 mg	0.1 mg		IM
Fenbendazole	50 mg/kg × 3 days	50 mg/kg × 3 days			PO
Furosemide	1–2 mg/kg	1–2 mg/kg	1 mg/kg		PO, IM
Ivermectin	200 µg/kg	200 µg/kg		200 µg/kg	PO, SC
Oxytocin	5–30 U	5–30 U		8 U	Prn, IM, SC
Stanozolol	10–50 mg/week				IM; ×2 weeks

Association of Primate Veterinarians (APV) Formulary (Lee, D.R. and Doane, C.J., Eds.) is also a reference for nonhuman primate dosages and can be found on the APV website: http://www.primatevets.org/education.
[a]From MD Anderson Cancer Center, Department of Veterinary Sciences.
[b]From Michelle Leland, Southwest Foundation.
[c]From Abee (1985) and Brady (2000).

treating nonhuman primates for tuberculosis. Currently, the greatest risk to this effective method of detection and control of tuberculosis in nonhuman primates is the availability of MOT. The very specialized, limited demand for this diagnostic product and its rigid manufacturing specifications make it impractical to manufacture in a cost-effective way. To date, its importance to the research community is appreciated, and its production is continuing.

6. Occupational Health Program

The potential exchange of diseases between humans and nonhuman primates requires that those managing the care of nonhuman primates develop, implement, and sustain a comprehensive personnel health program designed to meet the needs of their employees. Table 17.38 contains a preliminary list of the more common zoonotic agents to consider in a variety of commonly used species (NRC, 2003b; CDCP/NIH, 2009). In addition, the institution should have a standard operating procedure following suspected exposure to a zoonotic agent such as McHV-1 (B virus) (Cohen *et al.*, 2002). An example of a standard protocol is depicted in Table 17.36. Although policies vary between situations and facilities, there are certain basic elements that should be considered in any risk analysis. The 2003 NRC publication *Occupational Health and Safety in the Care and Use of Nonhuman Primates* is an excellent guide for developing an effective program (NRC, 2003b). A program must have oversight by occupational health specialists to protect personnel, along with a laboratory animal veterinary specialist who can provide input to the program regarding potential zoonotic agents. The veterinarian should also provide expertise regarding protection of nonhuman primates from human pathogens that could be transmitted to animals by the public, contract workers, students, caregivers, and investigators.

B. Clinical Techniques

With today's pediatric care devices, instrumentation, and biotechnology, there are few limitations to collecting biological samples, administering therapy, and carrying out clinical procedures on nonhuman primates. Based on body size, the New World monkeys are at times more challenging, but most investigative and animal care needs can be met if resources (financial, personnel, equipment) are available. Such constraints are more rare with Old World monkeys and chimpanzees. The techniques described in this section are applicable for delivering high-quality veterinary care as well as collecting data for biomedical research programs.

The list of zoonotic viral and bacterial pathogens continues to grow as more is learned about the SIV, simian retroviruses (SRVs), foamy viruses, Ebola virus, and recombinant/chimeric agents such as simian–human immunodeficiency virus (SHIV). Considering this level of risk, effective physical restraint, chemical restraint, and appropriate PPE are paramount to preventing human exposure. Bacterial infections have become increasingly resistant to many antibiotics requiring determination of the most appropriate antibiotics. Furthermore, bacterial resistance to antibiobics requires judicious use of these therapeutics. The recommended nonhuman primate dosages for anesthetics used in chemical restraint, analgesics, and antibiotics are given in Table 17.42.

Certain special techniques are beyond the scope of this chapter but are frequently used when working with nonhuman primates. For example, these special techniques may involve the use of Alzet osmotic pumps (ALZA Corporation, Palo Alto, California) or Ommaya reservoirs (Integra NeuroSciences, Plainsboro, New Jersey). The techniques addressed in this chapter are intended to aid the clinical veterinarian in the routine collection of body fluids or tissue and the most effective delivery of therapy. Techniques not addressed here have been documented elsewhere in the human and veterinary literature (Levin, 1995; Wolf and White, 2012).

1. Sample Collection

a. Blood

The most common site for venipuncture in the nonhuman primate is the femoral vein. In smaller species and infants, the venipuncture is 'blind,' aided by the anatomy of the femoral triangle. In larger species or adults, the femoral artery and adjacent vein can be palpated. In adult macaques, baboons, and chimpanzees, blood can also be collected from the saphenous or cephalic veins. The latter, however, are more commonly used for fluid administration. Venipuncture sites other than the femoral triangle in New World species include the saphenous veins and the bilateral tail veins (Abee, 1985). The jugular vein represents an alternative site for venipuncture in all species. The site of blood collection should be cleaned with 70% isopropyl alcohol. The maximum blood volume that can be safely taken during a sample collection is 10–15% of total blood volume, not taken more frequently than once every 2 weeks (Diehl et al., 2001). These estimates of blood volume that may be obtained should be carefully considered in the context of the animal's physical condition, previous blood collections, and current hematologic values. When all blood components are not required, blood samples can exceed the calculated limits if the plasma or red cells that were collected are returned to the animal after separation, along with appropriate fluid replacement. Blood collection guidelines have been adopted and published online by some institutional animal care and use committees. These online documents reference various publications in support of their guidelines. Prior to collection of large or repeated blood samples from nonhuman primates, it is advisable to determine whether institutional guidance documents are available.

In the research setting, nonhuman primates can be trained to allow voluntary hypodermic injection, urine collection, blood glucose testing, and venipuncture (Schapiro et al., 2005; Coleman et al., 2008; Reamer et al., 2014). Voluntary collection techniques are excellent for pharmacokinetic studies requiring repeated small blood samples without the complications of anesthetic drugs or the stress of physical restraint. Specialized equipment or cage modifications may be necessary to permit voluntary exteriorization of a limb, stabilization of the limb during venipuncture, and safety of animals and personnel (Schapiro, 2000). PRT is the most effective method for encouraging behaviors that allow primates to participate in these procedures (Coleman et al., 2008).

b. Urine

For routine urinalysis, urine can be collected from clean waste pans or via the free-catch method. The major disadvantage of these techniques is bacterial contamination. Catheterization of the urinary tract in both males and females can be done in many primate species. Cynomolgus and rhesus monkeys can be collected with 3.0–9.0 French catheters (Wickham et al., 2011; Veneziale et al., 2012; Wolf and White, 2012). A 3.0 French tomcat catheter may also be used for urethral catheterization of squirrel monkeys. Baboons can be catheterized with a 6–10 French Foley catheter (Sharma et al., 2011; Wolf and White, 2012). Aseptic catheterization of the urinary tract of both the male and female nonhuman primates is possible, but this usually requires physical or chemical restraint and experience overcoming anatomical differences. Cystocentesis is the preferred method for sterile urine collection. Cystocentesis by puncture of the surgically prepared suprapubic site using a 1.5- to 2.0-inch, 20- to 22-gauge needle is effective but may be difficult without experience (Keeling and Wolfe, 1975). Cystocentesis in the chimpanzee can be accomplished using a 2.0- to 3.0-inch, 20-gauge needle.

c. Cerebrospinal Fluid

Cerebrospinal fluid (CSF) can be collected from the cisterna magna or the lumbar area. When the subarachnoid space is to be entered, the animal must be anesthetized and the area surgically prepared. These procedures should be performed with either spinal needles or short bevel needles of appropriate size and length. Smith and Lackner (1993) detailed comparisons of fluid from the lumbar region to that of the cisterna magna, finding lumbar fluid to have higher concentrations of total protein, albumin, and IgG and lower concentrations of glucose and potassium. The report states that similar findings for total protein are seen in humans (Wolf and White, 2012).

Cisterna Magna CSF in the nonhuman primate should be collected at the junction of a line that bisects the cranial wings of the atlas and a line extending caudal from the external occipital protuberance (Bistner and Ford, 1995). In macaques, the procedure can be performed with a 1.5- to 2.0-inch, 22-gauge needle, whereas in chimpanzees, a 2.0- to 3.0-inch, 20-gauge spinal needle is used. Geretschlager *et al.* (1987) and Lipman *et al.* (1988) describe techniques for marmosets and cynomolgus monkeys, respectively.

Lumbar Collection of CSF by lumbar puncture is the most desirable approach as it involves less risk of complications. It is usually performed in lateral recumbency or in a sitting position with a slight flexion of the spine to facilitate the widening of the intervertebral space (Wolf and White, 2012). A horizontal line between both iliac crests will bisect the intervertebral space that should be entered. Based on the animal's size, the clinician should use an appropriately sized needle. If there is difficulty entering the vertebral space at the transverse plane of the iliac crests, either of the two spaces above can serve as alternate entry sites.

d. Skin Scraping

This diagnostic procedure involves abrading the skin with a scalpel blade, transferring the debris to a drop of mineral oil on a glass slide, and observing the debris microscopically to detect ectoparasites. Nonhuman primates are susceptible to skin parasites such as mites (*Sarcoptes* and *Demodex* spp.), fungal dermatophytes (*Microsporum* and *Trichophyton* spp.), and lice (Johnson-Delaney, 1994). An adequate skin scraping can confirm and differentiate ectoparasites. Scrapings should be collected from undisturbed and untreated areas (Bistner and Ford, 1995). For *Demodex* spp., a deep skin scraping is required which may cause some bleeding, and for *Sarcoptes* spp., large areas should be sampled. Dermatophyte scrapings can be used to inoculate culture media or a Wood's light can be used to detect microsporum fluorescence. The hair shafts collected from such scrapings can be examined for adult lice or eggs (Georgi, 1980).

e. Biopsy

The surgical removal of a small section of skin or other tissue may be needed when a differential diagnosis requires histopathology or impression smears. These samples can demonstrate the presence of bacterial, fungal, and parasitic organisms, and identify neoplastic or immune-mediated diseases (Crow and Walshaw, 1987).

Cutaneous Punch Biopsy The punch biopsy is a quick method of sampling a small core of skin for histopathological evaluation. The biopsy samples should include both diseased and normal tissues. It is not recommended to surgically prepare the skin in immune competent patients, as this can remove diagnostic indicators such as parasites and microorganisms, as well as the stratum corneum. Gentle hair clipping is sufficient in most circumstances, and an aseptic preparation is only indicated when entire masses are being removed. Lidocaine (1–2%) should be administered subcutaneously under each biopsy site. Punch biopsies offer a range of sizes, but the typical diameters are 2–8 mm (Seltzer, 2007). Skin sutures may be needed to close the biopsy site.

Cutaneous Wedge Biopsy When a large full-thickness skin biopsy is required, a cutaneous wedge biopsy may be a better option. A large wedge biopsy may result in an excisional biopsy of the entire lesion. If only a portion of the lesion is biopsied, an incisional biopsy is utilized (Bistner and Ford, 1995). With either technique, different stages of the lesion should be sampled with normal tissue (Crow and Walshaw, 1987). The biopsy should be performed under anesthesia and closed with sutures. When skin biopsies are collected, multiple samples will increase the likelihood of obtaining a diagnostic sample.

Organ Biopsy Liver biopsies may be necessary for diagnosis of hepatic diseases, such as hepatitis, amyloidosis, and neoplasia. A small biopsy sample can be obtained with a Tru-Cut® or Menghini needle. Ultrasound guidance can be used to sample focal liver lesions. For complete visualization of the liver prior to biopsy, a laparoscopic biopsy procedure can be performed. To obtain larger samples, a surgical procedure may be necessary with acquisition of a liver wedge biopsy. Complications can include gall bladder puncture and excessive hemorrhage. To minimize these complications, it is important to evaluate blood coagulation parameters prior to the biopsy and visually monitor the biopsy site following the procedure to ensure that hemostasis is achieved (Rothuizen and Twedt, 2009).

Kidney biopsies are most commonly performed for proteinuria or to diagnose renal disease. The same biopsy techniques that are employed for liver biopsies can also be used in the kidney. It has been shown that better diagnostic samples are obtained with a 14-gauge needle when compared to an 18-gauge needle (Rawlings *et al.*, 2003). While it is a fairly low-risk procedure, the most common complication is hemorrhage (Vaden *et al.*, 2005).

Lymph node biopsies are indicated when there is lymph node enlargement, generalized lymphadenopathy, or suspicion of tumor metastasis (Siedlecki, 2010). Lymph node samples can be collected by needle aspiration, punch biopsy, and excisional biopsy. The most accessible lymph nodes in nonhuman primates are the axillary and superficial inguinal nodes. During exploratory surgery, excisional biopsies are most frequently done on mesenteric and iliac lymph nodes (Boothe, 1990).

Bone Marrow   Needle aspiration is the most common technique used to collect samples from bone marrow in nonhuman primates. The preferred site is the iliac crest. While other sites can be used (trochanter of femur, tibial tuberosity, greater tubercle of the proximal humerus, sternum, rib, and ischial tuberosity), the iliac crest is usually an active site of marrow production (Perman *et al.*, 1974). In smaller species (marmosets, owl monkeys, and squirrel monkeys), the size of the marrow cavity may be small, and minimal aspiration will rupture vasculature in the space, resulting in a peripheral blood sample rather than a sample of bone marrow.

2.   *Administration of Fluids and Therapeutics*

a.   Intravenous Administration

Indwelling catheter placement is a frequently employed technique in nonhuman primates for extended intravenous (IV) fluid administration. IV delivery is the most efficient method for administering fluids and other therapeutics (Turner *et al.*, 2011). The cephalic or saphenous veins are frequently used for IV administration because needles or catheters can be more easily secured with tape at these sites and it leaves the femoral veins available for blood collection or other procedures requiring venous access. Numerous catheter systems can be used in combination with limb immobilization by splint and bandage or lightweight casting material. More sophisticated systems can be used by employing a jacket with tether or backpack equipment (McNamee *et al.*, 1984). For long-term vascular access associated with experimental protocols, vascular access ports (VAPs) can be placed to reduce the number of needle sticks and facilitate multiple sampling timepoints (Graham *et al.*, 2010).

b.   Subcutaneous Administration

Subcutaneous administration of fluids and therapeutics is a quick and easy route of administration. In an emergency, it is critical to provide fluid resuscitation quickly, and given the clinical condition of the patient, it may be difficult to place an IV catheter. Needle placement in the subcutaneous tissue space requires less time and skill to place when fluids must be delivered quickly. Only nonirritating isotonic substances may be administered via this route and absorption of fluids from the subcutaneous space is slower than IV routes (Turner *et al.*, 2011). One frequent area of administration in nonhuman primates is the dorsal surface; however, any area possessing loose skin can be utilized. The maximum amount that should be administered is 5 ml/kg per site (Turner *et al.*, 2011). Many drugs and/or vaccines can be delivered via the subcutaneous route. Care should be taken to ensure the needle is placed in the subcutaneous tissue space and not inadvertently placed intravenously. This is most easily accomplished by placing a gentle vacuum on the syringe barrel to observe whether blood is drawn.

c.   Intramuscular Administration

Intramuscular (IM) injections are a common drug administration route. There are abundant vascular structures in muscle tissue resulting in rapid absorption of substances (Turner *et al.*, 2011). Smaller volumes should be used in this location and it may be more difficult to administer substances via this route in smaller nonhuman primates. Possible side effects depend on the substance injected and can include muscle necrosis and nerve damage resulting in paresis or paralysis (Turner *et al.*, 2011).

d.   Intraosseous Administration

Intraosseous infusion of fluids may be used in severely debilitated, hypotensive animals when venous access is limited. The most accessible site in the owl monkey is the trochanteric fossa of the femur (Baer, 1994); however, the proximal anterior tibia is a common site in larger species (Fiorito *et al.*, 2005). The site is prepared aseptically, and the skin and periosteum are anesthetized with lidocaine. An 18-25 gauge needle is introduced aseptically into the medullary cavity. In small nonhuman primates, a hypodermic needle can be used, but larger species will require a spinal or bone marrow needle with a stylet. Fluid is administered through a standard infusion set; flow rate is limited because the bone marrow cavity cannot expand to accept increased volumes. The fluids directly enter the central venous circulation from the medullary venous sinuses. Potential complications include osteomyelitis, iatrogenic fracture, and growth plate injury (Turner *et al.*, 2011).

e.   Intraperitoneal Administration

While a commonly used administration route in rodents, intraperitoneal administration is rarely used in nonhuman primates. It can be used in smaller primate species to administer large volumes of fluid (maximum 10 mL/kg) safely when IV administration is not possible. Fluids or other therapeutics administered intraperitoneally are absorbed more slowly than IV administration because absorption occurs primarily via the mesenteric vessels, which closely resembles the pharmacokinetics of substances administered orally (Turner *et al.*, 2011).

f.   Nasogastric Intubation

Nasogastric intubation (5–8 French nasogastric tube) can be a rapid and effective means of delivering oral fluids and medication. The procedure is vital in relieving acute gastric dilation (bloat), and culture of gastric lavage has been used to confirm mycobacterial infection (Baron *et al.*, 1994). Because the orientation of the nares differs between Old World primates and New World primates, the techniques for placement of the nasogastric tube must be modified depending on the species being treated. New World primates have laterally flared nares that will require a lateral insertion, whereas Old World primates have a downward orientation of the nares that requires an upward insertion technique.

3. Restraint Techniques

Safe and effective restraint minimizes risk to both animals and staff, reduces animal stress, and improves the quality of research data by avoiding the altered physiological parameters that can be induced by stress-associated increases in cortisone, growth hormone, and glucagon (Brady, 2000). Proper restraint, whether by physical, chemical, or voluntary methods, requires well-trained personnel and well-equipped facilities. The appropriate use of personal protective equipment is essential (Table 17.34), as is the safe and effective use of restraint devices and equipment.

a. Physical Restraint

Numerous restraint devices are available for safe and effective physical restraint of nonhuman primates. Knowledge of species-typical behaviors can be utilized to make the restraint procedures less hazardous to personnel and less stressful to the animal. Restraint cages are an effective method of restraint that can be used on virtually all nonhuman primates, including the New World species (Klein and Murray, 1995). They allow brief procedures (e.g., reading tuberculin tests, treating wounds, and administrating medications) to be accomplished safely.

Restraint gloves (heavy leather or welder's-type gloves) can be used to effectively restrain small- to medium-sized nonhuman primates. Some gloves have Kevlar and/or stainless steel liners that increase personnel safety, and the gloves should extend above the elbows. Generally, hand capture with gloves can be performed on nonhuman primates that are not larger than a young adult female rhesus monkey. Adult male rhesus monkeys or animals of similar size should not be restrained with gloves only. Examples of procedures that can be performed on nonhuman primates restrained with gloves include injections, blood collection, wound treatment, subcutaneous fluid administration, and tuberculin testing (Sauceda and Schmidt, 2000).

Restraint nets are used when personnel need to maintain a safe distance from the animal being captured. Once the animal has been successfully netted, it can be hand-restrained with gloves or given an anesthetic or dissociative agent. Netting is very useful when capturing escaped animals or retrieving individual animals that are housed in social groups. Nets may be used to capture New World species and Old World monkeys up to 3.5 kg (Klein and Murray, 1995). The use of nets for capture and restraint requires experienced personnel to avoid injury to the animals being restrained or captured. Another method of restraint for larger nonhuman primates is the pole-and-collar method. The animal is fitted with a metal or plastic collar with a metal ring. The pole has a spring-activated clip that can be passed through the cage front and connected to the collar at the ring. To foster animal cooperation and minimize stress, the animals should be trained prior to using this restraint technique using PRT techniques (McMillan et al., 2014). Once a nonhuman primate has been trained to use this restraint system, they can be removed from the primary enclosure, restrained at a safe distance from the operator, and led to the procedure area. The advantages of the pole and collar include a reduction in opportunity for personnel and animal injury, and, once the animal is acclimated, a decreased level of stress for the nonhuman primate (Kennett, 1996).

Tether and vest restraint allows continuous physiologic monitoring, biological sampling, and infusion of drugs without the multiple restraint episodes typically associated with long-term studies. The tether device consists of a nylon-mesh vest or jacket and a flexible tether tube, with a swivel assembly connected to the back of the cage (Adams et al., 1988). The swivel assembly allows the animal freedom of movement within the cage, and sampling can take place without physical or chemical restraint (Coelho and Carey, 1990). The animals can be conditioned/trained to accept the tether and vest in as little as 1 week (Rennie and Buchanan-Smith, 2006). The advantages of the tether and vest include less animal stress, less animal handling, and less risk of injury to caregivers (McNamee et al., 1984; Rennie and Buchanan-Smith, 2006).

b. Chemical Restraint

Delivering chemical restraint for nonhuman primates can be accomplished through a variety of devices. Depending on the size of the animal and its primary enclosure, pole syringes, hand injection, CO_2 capture rifles or pistols, or blowpipes can be used. Pole syringes can be used effectively at distances up to 2 m. Hand injection can be successfully used with restraint cages, or when animals are trained to present for an injection (Schapiro et al., 2005). For distances greater than 20 m, CO_2-powered rifles are typically used, whereas CO_2-powered pistols suffice for distances less than 20 m (Kreeger, 1999). When CO_2-powered devices are used, the risk of animal injury increases as its size and distance from the device decreases. Bone fractures and internal organ injury can result from using too powerful a restraint device at too short a distance. Blowpipes work well at ranges up to 15 m with far less risk of injury than when the CO_2 or compressed air devices are used

(Klein and Murray, 1995). Safe-Capture® International, Inc. hosts workshops throughout the year that provide training on best practices for safely using chemical capture devices, immobilization drug pharmacology, and dosage recommendations.

The most commonly used drug for restraint of the nonhuman primate is the dissociative anesthetic, ketamine hydrochloride. The standard dose for Old World monkeys is 5–20 mg/kg body weight; higher dosages of 10–30 mg/kg are required for New World species, which provides 15–30 min of anesthesia (Popilskis *et al.*, 2008). Combinations of ketamine and xylazine or diazepam have been used successfully. A ketamine–xylazine combination can be used in a 3:1 volume ratio (3 parts ketamine:1 part xylazine) when the ketamine concentration is 100 mg/ml and the xylazine concentration is 20 mg/ml. Administered intramuscularly, this combination provides good anesthesia and analgesia at a dose of 0.1–0.2 ml/kg body weight (Klein and Murray, 1995). Acepromazine has been used with ketamine in the past to enhance sedation and muscle relaxation; however, it can also cause profound hypotension and has no analgesic properties, making other drugs preferred alternatives (Murphy *et al.*, 2012).

Telazol (tiletamine hydrochloride/zolazepam hydrochloride) has been used successfully for restraint, anesthesia, and procedures of short duration in a variety of nonhuman primates. The key ingredients (tiletamine, zolazepam) are chemically related to ketamine and diazepam, respectively (Plumb, 1995). An intramuscular injection of 2.5–6 mg/kg body weight provides immobilization and anesthesia for 45–60 min in chimpanzees, baboons, and macaques (Popilskis *et al.*, 2008).

For procedures that require greater than 45 min, inhalation anesthesia is indicated. Isoflurane is the most commonly used inhalation anesthetic in nonhuman primates. It is relatively inexpensive and has faster induction and recovery times compared to halothane (Murphy *et al.*, 2012). Isoflurane also has less catecholamine-sensitizing and cardiodepressive properties, making it a preferred inhalation anesthetic for hepatic and renal disease patients (Plumb, 1995). Sevoflurane has a lower solubility coefficient in comparison to isoflurane, which provides a quicker recovery from anesthesia. However, recovery in some cases can be too quick and it is recommended to taper sevoflurane dose following procedures to produce a smooth recovery (Murphy *et al.*, 2012). Desflurane produces the most rapid induction and recovery from anesthesia; however, its high cost and high vapor pressure make its use less common in veterinary medicine (Murphy *et al.*, 2012).

c. Voluntary Restraint

Animals can be trained to voluntarily present and hold positions using PRT techniques. This voluntary restraint can eliminate the need for physical or chemical restraint with some procedures, and has the benefit of reducing the stress associated with physical or chemical restraint (Lambeth *et al.*, 2006). The various procedures for which nonhuman primates have been successfully trained to cooperate with voluntary restraint are discussed previously in this chapter under *Principles of Colony Management, Enrichment Programs* (Section IV, B). Effective PRT can greatly reduce the amount of physical and chemical restraint necessary to carry out procedures (Schapiro, 2000).

4. Dental Procedures

Dental care is an essential component of the veterinary care program for nonhuman primates. This should include, at a minimum, routine cleaning and maintenance of teeth. The most common dental problems in nonhuman primates include tartar accumulation, gingivitis, tooth fractures, caries, periodontal disease, tooth abscesses, and osteomyelitis associated with tooth abscesses (Johnson-Delaney, 2008). Treatments involve scaling and polishing teeth, extractions, and/or root canal procedures (Wolf and White, 2012).

In the past, blunting or disarming the canine teeth of nonhuman primates was considered an acceptable management practice to reduce the risk of injury to social group members and personnel (Bass and Stark, 1980). However, the Animal Welfare Act, Animal Care Policy #3, states that non-medical canine tooth removal, or reduction that exposes the pulp cavity, is not considered appropriate veterinary care. The policy also states that in some behavioral or breeding situations it may be acceptable to reduce canine teeth as long as the pulp cavity is not exposed (USDA Policies, Veterinary Care, 2011). The American Veterinary Medical Association (AVMA) also issued a position statement, updated in 2007, stating that the removal of canine teeth must be medically or scientifically justified, or justified by animal or human safety concerns. The AVMA also recommends alternatives to the procedure such as behavior modification, environmental enrichment, or modifications to the social groups (AVMA, 2009).

C. Diagnostic Imaging

Various imaging modalities can be used in nonhuman primates for both research and diagnostic purposes. Radiography and ultrasound are commonly used for routine health care diagnostics in the clinic. However, these imaging techniques, along with more advanced imaging modalities such as endoscopy, magnetic resonance imaging (MRI), and computed tomography (CT) can also be utilized for investigative research. While these techniques are briefly covered in this chapter, a more detailed review is found in Winkelmann *et al.* (2012).

1. Radiology

Radiography is an important diagnostic tool in non-human primate medicine, disease model research, and morphometric primate anatomy studies (Xie *et al.*, 2014). Normal nonhuman primate radiographic anatomy has been published for rhesus macaques (Silverman and Morgan, 1980; Ji *et al.*, 2013), cynomolgus macaques (Schillaci *et al.*, 2010; Xie *et al.*, 2014), and marmosets (Wagner and Kirberger, 2005). Most institutions have transitioned to digital radiography. There are two types of detector systems that can be purchased with digital radiography systems: computed radiography (CR) and direct digital radiography (DR). CR systems use imaging plates to generate a digital image and they are generally less expensive than DR. While both CR and DR generate good quality images, DR has the benefit of greater speed of image generation (Wright, 2010).

Pulmonary diseases are common in nonhuman primates and radiography is an important diagnostic tool when tuberculosis or other pulmonary diseases are suspected. Thoracic radiography can also be used to assist in the diagnosis of cardiovascular disorders (Xie *et al.*, 2014). Although more advanced imaging modalities such as MRI and CT are available, plain film or digital radiography is the most cost-effective and time-efficient way to obtain images (Xie *et al.*, 2014). To be of greatest diagnostic value, nonhuman primate thoracic radiographs should be made with the animal in an upright posture, with images acquired during full inspiration (Puddy and Hill, 2007). Abdominal radiographs are most commonly performed to assist with the diagnosis of bowel obstruction, calculi, foreign bodies, intussusception, ascites, masses, pneumoperitoneum, or volvulus (Greene, 1986). Radiography with contrast (barium or other water soluable oral contrast) is useful in diagnosing full *versus* partial bowel obstructions and suspected perforations (Thompson, 2002). Various radiographic views (supine, anterior/posterior, posterior/anterior, and lateral) can capitalize on nonsupported, gravitational positioning of the organs.

2. Ultrasonography

Many clinical and diagnostic procedures are facilitated with ultrasound imaging. Fine-needle aspiration of organs and joints, as well as cavity and abscess drainage and centesis of abdominal, bladder, and thoracic regions, can be assisted with ultrasound guidance. Organs including the liver, kidney, and prostate are within reach for ultrasound-guided biopsies. Real-time ultrasonography can assess the form and function of the cardiovascular system. Ultrasonography of the reproductive system can detect prostate abnormalities, follicular and luteal changes, sex of a fetus, and gestational age (Blevins *et al.*, 1998). Morphological characteristics detected by fetal ultrasound (crown–rump length, biparietal diameter, head circumference, and femur length) have been determined for the rhesus monkey, baboon, squirrel monkey, owl monkey, and chimpanzee. Longitudinal growth curves established for these species can be used to predict estimated parturition dates (Nyland *et al.*, 1984; Herring *et al.*, 1991; Lee *et al.*, 1991; Lögdberg, 1993; Schuler *et al.*, 2010).

Preparation of the animal should include sedation or other appropriate restraint, and the region of interest may be clipped, shaved, and wiped with alcohol or soapy water. Acoustic gel is used as the interface between the animal's skin and the transducer. A 3.0- to 7.5-MHz transducer is adequate for most areas to be scanned, although most ocular ultrasonography requires a 10.0-MHz scan head (Blevins *et al.*, 1998).

3. Endoscopy

Endoscopy is a minimally invasive technique that allows direct visualization of internal organs and other structures. This technique is performed using either a rigid or a flexible endoscope attached to a fiberoptic light cable. Flexible endoscopes are used for visualization of stomach (gastroscopy), colon (colonoscopy), and bronchi (bronchoscopy). Rigid endoscopes can help visualize joints (arthroscopy), genitourinary structures (cystoscopy), the nasal cavity (rhinoscopy), and the abdominal cavity (laparoscopy). Benefits of endoscopy include the following: possible avoidance of surgery if a condition can be diagnosed and/or corrected endoscopically (e.g., removal of a gastrointestinal foreign body), a less invasive surgical procedure (e.g., laparoscopy), easier biopsy acquisition with more precise lesion targeting, and enhanced visualization of disease processes.

Endoscopic procedures require general anesthesia, and a gastrointestinal preparation may require fasting, laxatives, and an enema depending on the area to be visualized. For detailed procedural information on endoscopy, there are two excellent textbook references, *Small Animal Endoscopy*, 3rd ed. (Tams and Rawlings, 2011) and *Veterinary Endoscopy for the Small Animal Practitioner* (McCarthy, 2005).

4. Magnetic Resonance Imaging

MRI is an advanced imaging technique that uses a strong magnetic field to obtain detailed images via excitation of hydrogen protons. A greater signal is produced from tissues containing high amounts of hydrogen, such as fat and cerebrospinal fluid, and thus, MRI is preferred when obtaining images of soft tissue (Greenfield *et al.*, 1993; Elliot and Skerritt, 2010). MRI is less useful when the focus area consists of hydrogen-poor tissues such as the bone and lung (Elliot and Skerritt, 2010).

T1-weighted or T2-weighted tissue contrast can be used to enhance imaging depending on the lipid and water content of the target tissue (Elliot and Skerritt, 2010).

One advantage of MRI compared to CT is that MRI does not use ionizing radiation, and thus does not increase the risk for radiation-induced cancers. MRI is contraindicated with certain implants such as cardiac pacemakers and defibrillators (Mak and Truong, 2012). Intravenous contrast (gadolinium) appears bright white on T1-weighted images and can be used to help diagnose neoplasia and other disorders such as myocardial fibrosis, demyelination of nerve tissue, and vertebral disc herniation (Bell *et al.*, 2013; Goenka *et al.*, 2014; Löhr *et al.*, 2014). MRI has been used in research to study neurodegenerative disease in chimpanzees and macaques (Chen *et al.*, 2013), the effects of opioids in cynomolgus macaques (Kaufman *et al.*, 2013), and perfusion–diffusion mismatch stroke models in baboons (Wey *et al.*, 2011).

5. Computed Tomography

CT is another advanced imaging modality that uses X-rays to acquire images. The images obtained with CT are far superior to radiography due to a higher scan power, shorter rotation time, and smaller focal spots (Saunders and Ohlerth, 2011). CT is the preferred imaging technique for bone, thoracic structures, and certain masses/neoplasia (Even-Sapir, 2005; Subhawong *et al.*, 2010). In nonhuman primates, CT scans have been used to assess adipose tissue density (Murphy *et al.*, 2014) and orthopedic morphology and degeneration (Bagi *et al.*, 2011; Plate *et al.*, 2013), and in pharmacokinetic studies (Chin *et al.*, 2011).

D. Complementary Therapeutic Approaches

There are a number of promising new therapeutic approaches that are being introduced to veterinary care of nonhuman primates. Although these therapies are not new to medicine, they have not been routinely used in the care of nonhuman primates. However, these complementary, nonpharmaceutical treatments have found increasing utility in general veterinary medicine (Robinson, 2013). Complementary therapeutics are generally used in conjunction with conventional medical treatments. When using complementary therapies, the veterinarian must ensure that the treatments are supported by scientific literature. The laboratory animal veterinarian has an additional responsibility to ensure that the physiological changes elicited by these therapies do not confound experimental results. For example, some therapies have been shown to initiate anti-inflammatory actions, which could interfere with immune responses (Kavoussi and Ross, 2007). In studies that evaluate the effectiveness of these promising therapeutic approaches, nonhuman primates can serve as a valuable animal model as they lack a placebo effect that is often present in human studies.

1. Acupuncture

Acupuncture is used as a treatment for various conditions such as chronic pain, osteoarthritis, stress, nausea/vomiting, hypertension, and stroke (Chiu *et al.*, 1997; Middlekauff *et al.*, 2001; WHO, 2003; Mavrommatis *et al.*, 2012; Xie and Wedemeyer, 2012; Garcia *et al.*, 2013; Magden *et al.*, 2013; Robinson, 2013). Both the NIH and the World Health Organization have endorsed the therapeutic value of acupuncture for a variety of medical conditions (NIH Consensus Development Panel, 1998; WHO, 2003). Acupuncture is especially useful in research settings that maintain geriatric animals or in facilities that promote lifetime housing of animals, as is often the case in research facilities with colonies of nonhuman primates. For this reason, veterinarians providing care to nonhuman primates should consider the benefits of this therapy.

Acupuncture treatments use thin (0.12- to 0.30-mm diameter) sterile needles that are inserted into defined acupuncture points, which then stimulate physiologic processes through neural signaling (Robinson, 2007). There are 361 defined acupuncture points (anatomic sites), and these can be located using published acupuncture texts, charts, and anatomical landmarks (White *et al.*, 2008). The majority of defined acupuncture points correspond to neurovascular bundle locations (Dung, 1984; Ogay *et al.*, 2009; Robinson, 2009), and stimulation of these points generates a peripheral afferent signal that can initiate endogenous opioid release (Uchida *et al.*, 2003), release of vasodilation peptides (Dawidson *et al.*, 1999; Lundeberg, 1993), and/or stimulation of CNS that can influence hormonal regulation (Jedel *et al.*, 2011; Yang *et al.*, 2009). Nonhuman primates can be trained to accept acupuncture and laser therapy (see below) using PRT techniques. Chimpanzees have been trained to voluntarily present body parts for acupuncture therapy and hold a position for the time needed to complete the acupuncture treatment (Magden *et al.*, 2013) (Fig. 17.19). Rhesus monkeys, squirrel monkeys, and owl monkeys can be habituated to gentle restraint in order to administer acupuncture treatments (Zhao *et al.*, 2010; Magden, personal communication, 2014) (Fig. 17.20). Information on acupuncture techniques, neurological mechanisms, and determination of appropriate treatment schedules can be found in *An Introduction to Western Medical Acupuncture* by White *et al.* (2008). Training courses are available through the International Veterinary Acupuncture Society (IVAS), the Chi Institute, or Colorado State University's Medical Acupuncture for Veterinarians (MAV) certification program.

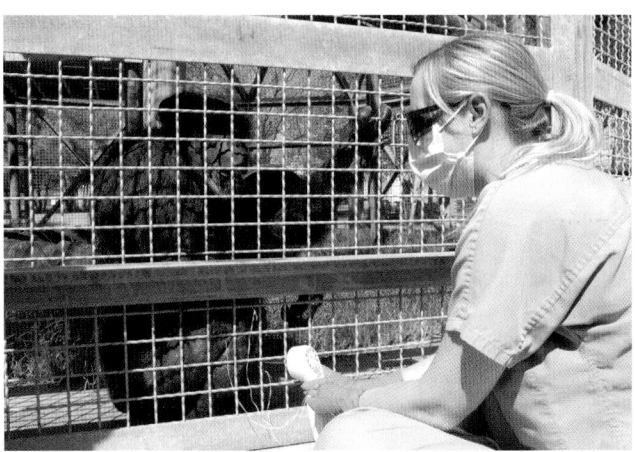

FIGURE 17.19   A chimpanzee (*Pan troglodytes*) voluntarily presenting and holding for acupuncture (points ST-34, ST-35, and ST-36) and laser therapy.

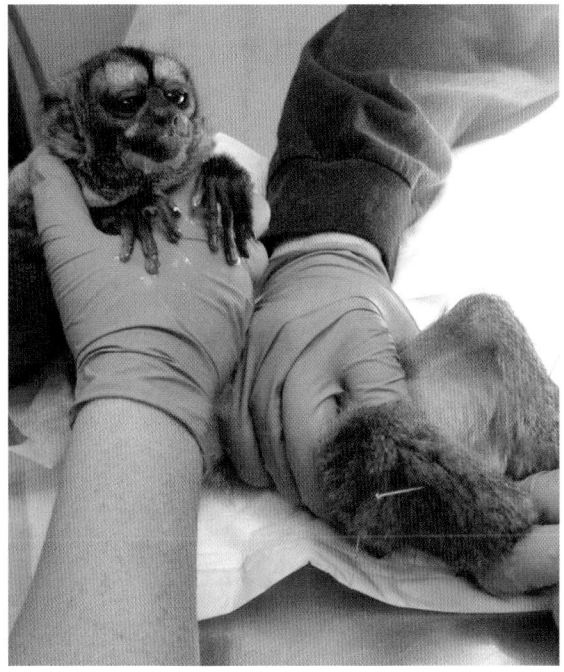

FIGURE 17.20   Owl monkey (*Aotus* spp.) receiving acupuncture (ST-34 and ST-36) therapy for stifle osteoarthritis using gentle manual restraint.

2. Laser

Low-level laser therapy (LLLT) involves the use of light energy (generally 600–1000 nm wavelength) to promote tissue healing, reduce inflammation, and relieve pain. The duration and frequency of therapy varies depending on the type of laser used and the condition being treated. Although fewer studies have been published supporting the efficacy of laser therapy in comparison to acupuncture, there are a number of randomized controlled clinical studies that support positive outcomes with the use of LLLT (Huang *et al.*, 2011). LLLT has been used to reduce pain associated with osteoarthritis (Hegedüs *et al.*, 2009; Ozdemir *et al.*, 2001; Stelian *et al.*, 1992), to improve wound healing (Gupta *et al.*, 1998; Woodruff *et al.*, 2004), and to reduce inflammation (Zhang *et al.*, 2014; Leal-Junior *et al.*, 2014). Huang *et al.* (2009) provide a good summary of the mechanisms of action for LLLT.

There are several possible variables when providing LLLT due to differences in laser types, dosimetry, irradiance, pulse structure, and concurrent medications (Huang *et al.*, 2009). Further studies are needed to more definitively elucidate the mechanism of action and the conditions that will benefit from this treatment modality. LLLT is currently being used to alleviate pain/inflammation and treat wounds in nonhuman primates at both the University of Texas MD Anderson Cancer Center, the Michale E. Keeling Center for Comparative Medicine and Research, and the Texas Biomedical Research Institute.

3. Physical and Massage Therapy

Physical and massage therapeutic techniques involve mechanical touch, cryotherapy, heat therapy, and range of motion exercises. These therapies are becoming a more accepted practice in veterinary medicine to help animals recover from trauma and surgical procedures (Rychel *et al.*, 2011). Physiotherapy has been shown to enhance mobility and prolong survival times in dogs with degenerative myelopathy (Kathmann *et al.*, 2006). Given the success of these therapies as nonpharmacological rehabilitation tools in other species, further investigation should be done to examine the possible benefits of these techniques in nonhuman primates.

VI.   DISEASES

A.   Bacterial Diseases

1.   Enteric

Enteric diseases of bacterial etiology are a primary cause of morbidity and mortality in both New and Old World monkeys, and apes. Determining the etiology of a bacterial diarrhea may be quite difficult. Commonly, two or more potentially pathogenic bacteria may be isolated from an individual with diarrhea. The clinician must ascertain the primary pathogen based upon clinical signs, bacterial culture results and colony history, and treat appropriately. A summary of bacterial enteric diseases by isolate and primate species is presented in Table 17.43.

a.   Shigellosis

Pathogenesis   *Shigella* spp. are among the most common enteric pathogens recovered from captive nonhuman primates, occurring most commonly in Old World

TABLE 17.43 Enteric Bacterial Infections

Agent	Primate	Clinical signs	Clinical pathology	Treatment
Shigella spp.	Macaque	Diarrhea ± blood ± mucus ± mucosal fragments Depression, hunched posture	Leukocytosis with left shift	Enrofloxacin 5 mg/kg[a,b] or multidrug therapy[c] Rehydrate
	Marmoset	Lethargy, dehydration, depression		Neomycin[d] in water for 10 days
	Tamarin	Pale mucous membranes Blood in feces		Quarantine
Campylobacter spp.	Macaque	Mucohemorrhagic diarrhea	Hyponatremia, hypochloremia acidosis	Usually self-limiting rehydrate
	Baboon	Chronic diarrhea		
	Marmoset	Watery or mucohemorrhagic diarrhea	Normal WBC to leukocytosis with left shift	Erythromycin 25 mg/day[e]
Escherichia coli	Chimpanzee	Mild-severe, watery diarrhea or dysentery		
	Squirrel monkey	Infant death		
	Owl monkey	Profuse, foul-smelling, blood-tinged diarrhea Dehydration, depression		Ampicillin, gentamicin, or trimethoprim-sulfamethoxazole[f] Intestinal protectant Rehydrate
	Tamarin	Watery diarrhea		
Salmonella spp.	Macaque	Diarrhea, pyrexia Infants: watery diarrhea ± blood ± mucus		Usually multidrug resistant; carrier state can develop
Yersinia spp.	Macaque	Diarrhea, vomition, bloodstained feces Depression, abdominal pain Dehydration Abortions/stillbirths	Leukocytosis Hyponatremia, hypochloremia, prerenal azotemia, hyperfibrinogenemia	Enrofloxacin, tetracycline, aminoglycosides
	Squirrel monkey	Weak, inactive, enlarged cervical lymph nodes		
	Owl monkey	Weakness, depression, diarrhea, abdominal distension, splenomegaly	Neutrophilia with left shift	Trimethoprim-sulfamethoxazole or gentamicin[f] Rehydrate[g] Oral intestinal protectant
Helicobacter spp.	Macaque	Gastric: anorexia, vomiting Intestinal: chronic diarrhea		Triple antibiotic therapy: amoxicillin, metranidazole, bismuth (other combinations also approved for humans)
	Cotton-top tamarin	Chronic diarrhea		
Lawsonia intracellularis	Macaque	Mild or transient diarrhea, abdominal distension Death, no clinical signs	Anemia	Tetracycline in horses

[a]*From Line et al. (1992).*
[b]*From Banish et al. (1993b).*
[c]*From Olson et al. (1986); therapy consisted of oral trimethoprim-sulfamethoxazole, erythromycin, and tetracycline.*
[d]*From Cooper and Needham (1976).*
[e]*From Pinheiro et al. (1993).*
[f]*Frorn Weller (1994); drug doses not provided in text.*
[g]*From Rosenberg et al. (1980).*

species such as macaques, baboons, and apes. *Shigella flexneri* is the most frequent isolate, including serotypes la, 2a, 3, 4, 5, 6, and 15 (Russell and DeTolla, 1993), with *S. sonnei* and *S. boydii* occurring less frequently. Endemic infections within colonies are maintained by asymptomatic carriers (Banish *et al.*, 1993b; Russell and DeTolla, 1993). Infection is spread by the fecal–oral route among primates within the same social group, by shared use of equipment, by movement of primates between groups, and through importation of new primates into an existing colony. Infection and disease with subsequent antibody production do not provide immunity, and animals may be reinfected (Banish *et al.*, 1993a). Overt disease, manifested by diarrhea or dysentery, may occur in endemically infected animals with a precipitating stressful event, such as social group disruption or formation or transport to a new facility.

Disease Bacillary dysentery is characterized by foul-smelling, liquid stool containing mucus, frank blood, and/or mucosal fragments. Anal atonia and rectal prolapse may also be observed. Affected monkeys are weak and moderately to severely dehydrated, and they require prompt medical treatment to correct life-threatening fluid and electrolyte imbalances. Bacillary dysentery may produce an epizootic of high morbidity and mortality when introduced into a naive population. A more common form of shigellosis is a subacute to chronic diarrhea with liquid to semisoft stool that may occur in colonies in which enzootic infections develop. Diarrhea is intermittent to episodic; occasionally animals will have firm, mucus-laden feces with streaks of fresh blood. These animals do not appear clinically ill, and clinical episodes may resolve spontaneously. Marked elevations in total neutrophil counts may be observed in otherwise normal animals. Such chronically infected animals may serve as a source of infection for other individuals within the colony. Gingivitis, abortion, and air sac infections are non-enteric forms of shigella infections that may occur in rhesus monkeys (McClure *et al.*, 1976).

A postinfective immune-mediated arthritis has been observed and generally occurs 3–4 weeks following resolution of intestinal signs (Urvater *et al.*, 2000). This particular aseptic arthritis often presents as a non-weight bearing lameness accompanied by high fever and responds to corticosteroids.

Pathology Lesions of enteric shigellosis occur primarily in the cecum and colon. The colonic mucosa is usually covered with a fibrinopurulent exudate that can progress to a pseudomembranous enterocolitis, and the intestinal wall is edematous and hemorrhagic with focal areas of ulceration. Neutrophilic infiltrates are commonly observed and in severe cases vasculitis may be present. Luminal contents vary from fluid mucus with fibrin and cellular debris to frank hemorrhage and mucus in the lumen (Lindsey *et al.*, 1971; Mulder, 1971).

Intussusception of the small intestine, rectal prolapse, splenomegaly, and mesenteric lymphadenopathy may occur. Gross lesions in marmosets and tamarins are confined to the cecum and colon (Cooper and Needham, 1976) and consist of multifocal ulceration and petechiation in the mucosa, with blood and fluid feces found throughout the large bowel.

Diagnosis and Treatment *Shigella* are fastidious bacteria and do not survive well if the period between collection and culture is prolonged; thus, direct plating or careful transport using transport medium and holding samples either refrigerated or frozen must be used to ensure success (Wells and Morris, 1981). *Shigella* are also segmentally produced in the lower gastrointestinal tract; thus, culture at a single time point can produce false-negative results. To reduce this possibility, sequential culture of samples taken from each of three successive days is recommended. *Shigella* can also be identified in clinical specimens by PCR of virulence genes such as *ipaH* that is carried by both pathogenic *Shigellas* and enteroinvasive *Escherichia coli* (EIEC), a pathogenic *E. coli* that causes diarrhea by a similar mechanism to *Shigella* (Vu *et al.*, 2004; Sethabutr *et al.*, 1994). Although *Shigella* spp. are considered primary pathogens, they can asymptomatically colonize up to 20–25% of clinically normal nonhuman primates.

Treatment for shigellosis should include antibiotic therapy based on culture and sensitivity testing in conjunction with aggressive correction of deficits in hydration, acid–base balance, and electrolytes. Empirical antibiotic therapy may be necessary in acute cases, based on colony history. Antibiotics that have been reported to be successful in treating shigella infections include enrofloxacin, 5 mg/kg body weight once a day (Line *et al.*, 1992; Banish *et al.*, 1993b), and combination therapy with oral trimethoprim-sulfamethoxazole, erythromycin, and tetracycline (Olson *et al.*, 1986). *Shigella* spp. were eliminated from a colony of callitrichids through quarantine procedures and administration of neomycin in the drinking water for 10 days (Cooper and Needham, 1976). An eradication and control program has been described in a rhesus macaque colony (Wolfensohn, 1998). Treatment of free-ranging colonies may be difficult but use of medicated feed containing trimethoprim-sulfamethoxazole has been successful. Shigellosis is a zoonotic disease and multiple antibiotic-resistent strains are commonly encountered. The organism has been transmitted from monkeys to children, pet owners, animal caretakers, and research technicians (Mulder, 1971; Fox, 1975; Tribe and Fleming, 1983; Kennedy *et al.*, 1993). Severe dysentery resulted from infection, and in one instance death occurred (Fox, 1975).

b. Campylobacteriosis

Pathogenesis *Campylobacter jejuni* and *C. coli* are the most frequent fecal bacterial isolates from subclinical

848 17. NONHUMAN PRIMATES *GULL WINGED SHAPE* ⌢

and clinically affected nonhuman primates (Tribe *et al.*, 1979; McClure *et al.*, 1986; Russell *et al.*, 1987). Infection usually occurs by the fecal–oral route. The presence of *Campylobacter* in the intestinal flora varies greatly, with some colonies reporting 100% prevalence (Russell *et al.*, 1988) and with positive cultures from clinically normal monkeys composing up to 81% of total isolations (Taylor *et al.*, 1989). Prevalence of infection in macaques increases with time in captivity, and varies by colony. In contrast, recently trapped tamarins had a higher prevalence of infection with *C. coli* initially than after they had been housed in the laboratory for 1 year (Gozalo *et al.*, 1991). Molecular markers of virulence are lacking and caution is advised before assigning disease causation to a specific isolate as campylobacters are frequently isolated from clinically normal Old World primate species.

Disease Campylobacter infection usually presents as watery diarrhea, although mucohemorrhagic diarrhea has also been reported (Paul-Murphy, 1993). Primates with diarrhea and campylobacter infection may have normal white blood cell counts or leukocytosis with a left shift (Paul-Murphy, 1993). Severe electrolyte abnormalities, including hyponatremia (Na <132 mEq/l), hypochloremia (Cl <93 mEq/l), acidosis, and a high anion gap occur in monkeys with campylobacter diarrhea (George and Lerche, 1990).

Pathology Gross lesions of *C. jejuni* or *C. coli* infection in cynomolgus monkeys were reported as thinning of the bowel wall, distension of the bowel with pasty-to-fluid yellow–gray feces, and wasting (Tribe *et al.*, 1979). Gross lesions observed in patas monkeys during surgical biopsy included thickening and rigidity of the terminal ileum, cecum, and proximal colon (Bryant *et al.*, 1983). The mucosal surfaces of biopsy specimens from the ileocecal junction and colon were covered with blood and mucus. Mesenteric and celiac lymph nodes were enlarged and there was a slight serosanguinous transudate in the abdominal cavity (Bryant *et al.*, 1983). Extraintestinal infections have been observed in rhesus macaques; however, these cases were associated with compromised immune function (Clemmons *et al.*, 2014).

Microscopic lesions in the small intestine of patas monkeys infected with *C. jejuni* included thickening and shortening of the villi, dilated lacteals, and infiltration of the lamina propria with macrophages, lymphocytes, and necrotic debris (Bryant *et al.*, 1983). The mucosal epithelium was low columnar to cuboidal. In the large intestine, lesions varied among animals and included mild to moderate hyperplasia of the epithelium, edema of the lamina propria or submucosa, and multifocal crypt abscesses (Bryant *et al.*, 1983). Spiral or comma-shaped bacteria were observed on the epithelial surface and in the lamina propria of the small and large intestine stained with Warthin–Starry silver stain.

Diagnosis Diagnosis of *C. jejuni* or *C. coli* is based on recovery of the organism from feces, rectal swabs, or intestinal biopsies or intestinal lesions at necropsy. Definitive identification can be made from a series of biochemical tests. *Campylobacter* spp. can be identified by their characteristic comma or spiral shapes when Gram stained. A novel species, *C. troglodytis*, has been recently cultured from wild, human-habituated chimpanizees (Kaur *et al.*, 2011).

Treatment Based on the reported electrolyte imbalances (see above), rehydration and replacement of electrolytes with normonatremic fluids such as lactated Ringer's solution or normal saline should be considered (George and Lerche, 1990). Because many infections are self-limiting and reinfection is frequent (Russell *et al.*, 1987), the efficacy of antibiotic treatment for campylobacter diarrhea is debatable and should be determined on a case-by-case basis. Erythromycin has been the antibiotic of choice; however, resistant campylobacter strains have been reported (Tribe and Fleming, 1983).

c. Colibacillosis

Pathogenesis Isolation of *E. coli* from a primate with diarrhea can be a diagnostic dilemma (Thomson and Scheffler, 1996), as it is a frequent normal fecal isolate. There are four recognized categories of diarrheagenic *E. coli*: Shiga toxin-producing *E. coli* (STEC), also known as enterohemorrhagic *E. coli* (EHEC), e.g., *E. coli* O157; enterotoxigenic *E. coli* (ETEC), which produces a heat labile or heat stable enterotoxin, or both; enteropathogenic *E. coli* (EPEC), which are associated with infantile diarrhea and are not known to produce enterotoxins or Shiga toxin; and EIEC, which invades cells of the colonic epithelium causing a watery and occasionally bloody diarrhea.

Disease Clinical signs of infection with a pathogenic *E. coli* vary with the primate species and the bacterial serotype. Young chimpanzees and an orangutan with pathogenic *E. coli* infection had mild to moderately severe watery diarrhea for 2–10 days. The stool was occasionally mucoid, and in one case contained small amounts of blood (McClure *et al.*, 1972). In squirrel monkey infants, death with no clinical signs occurred in infections with *E. coli* serotype O13 (Scimeca and Brady, 1990). Tamarins infected with a hemolytic *E. coli* developed a watery diarrhea (Potkay, 1992).

Common marmosets and Cotton-top tamarins are also susceptible to disease with EPEC. Marmosets often present with acute-onset diarrhea with severe hematochezia, hypotension, and hypothermia (Mansfield *et al.*, 2001; Ludlage and Mansfield, 2003). Animals respond rapidly to fluid replacement therapy and antibiotics with enrofloxacin a suitable empiric choice until sensitivity profiles are available.

EPEC has also been recognized as an important and common opportunistic pathogen of SIV-infected rhesus macaques (*M. mulatta*) with immune deficiencies. Retrospective analysis revealed that 27 of 96 (28.1%) animals with AIDS had features of EPEC infection, and EPEC was the most frequent pathogen of the gastrointestinal tract identified morphologically. Clinically, infection was associated with persistent diarrhea and wasting, and was more frequent in animals that died at less than 1 year of age (Mansfield *et al.*, 2001).

Pathology Gross lesions commonly include diffuse mucosal hemorrhage in the gastrointestinal tract, necrosis, acute inflammation in the colon, splenomegaly, congested and slightly enlarged mesenteric lymph nodes, and pulmonary hemorrhages and edema (McClure *et al.*, 1972; Scimeca and Brady, 1990). Tamarins with diarrhea had congestion, edema, and necrosis of the intestinal mucosa (Potkay, 1992).

Diagnosis and Treatment Isolation and identification of diarrheagenic *E. coli* requires bacterial culture, serotyping, and molecular characterization at a diagnostic laboratory, after other causes for disease have been ruled out. *E. coli* toxin genes can be readily detected by PCR (Tornieporth *et al.*, 1995); however, caution must be observed if this approach is used because these agents can be opportunistic pathogens carried asymptomatically in the gastrointestinal tracts of clinically normal animals. Animals respond rapidly to fluid replacement therapy and antibiotic treatment. Enrofloxacin is a suitable empiric choice until sensitivity profiles are available.

d. Salmonellosis

Recently, *Salmonella* nomenclature has undergone considerable revision and caution must be used when reviewing the abundant *Salmonella* literature as many of the species names have been changed. There are currently only two recognized species within the genus, *S. enterica* and *S. bongori*, with six main subspecies of *S. enterica*: *enterica* (I), *salamae* (II), *arizonae* (IIIa), *diarizonae* (IIIb), *houtenae* (IV), and *indica* (VI). Historically, serotype (V) was *bongori*, which is now considered its own species. Based on the Kauffman–White classification scheme, there are over 2500 serovars of *Salmonella* allowing members of the genus to be differentiated from one another.

Pathogenesis Using the historical naming scheme, the frequently reported serovars of *Salmonella* spp. from nonhuman primates have been *S. typhimurium*, *S. choleraesuis*, *S. anatum*, *S. stanley*, *S. derby*, and *S. oranienburg* (Good *et al.*, 1969; McClure, 1980; Potkay, 1992), all of which have been reclassified as subspecies of *S. enterica*. Salmonella infection usually occurs by fecal–oral transmission, and infection can result from ingestion of contaminated food, water, or fomites. Insects have served as mechanical vectors. Salmonellae can survive and multiply for relatively long periods in the environment.

The pathogenesis of experimental *Salmonella* infection has been described in the rhesus monkey. Eighty percent of rhesus monkeys inoculated orally with *S. typhimurium* developed diarrhea, which peaked in severity at 48–72 h postinoculation (Rout *et al.*, 1974). Mild morphologic changes occurred in the jejunum in animals with diarrhea, including shortening of villi, villous edema, mild elongation of crypts, reduction of mucus content in goblet cells, and an increase of mononuclear cells in the epithelium.

Reports of salmonella infection and disease within established primate colonies are rare; however, chronic carriers (Tanaka and Katsube, 1981) and severe outbreaks have been described in recently imported cynomolgus macaques (Takasaka *et al.*, 1988). *Salmonella* was isolated from 6% of enteric cultures from nonhuman primates with diarrhea at a primate research center (McClure, 1980); 21 of the isolates were *S. derby* recovered primarily from rhesus infants during a nursery outbreak (McClure, 1980). Clinical signs of enteric salmonellosis include watery diarrhea, sometimes with hemorrhage or mucus. Animals are often pyrexic (Paul-Murphy, 1993). Other signs include neonatal septicemia, abortion, osteomyelitis, and pyelonephritis (Thurman *et al.*, 1983; Klumpp *et al.*, 1986; Duncan *et al.*, 1994).

Pathology Clinical enteric salmonellosis is characterized by edema, hyperemia, and rare mucosal ulceration in the ileum and colon. Enlargement of the spleen and mesenteric lymph nodes may occur. Microabscesses are rarely found in colonic lymphoid tissue. In cases of septicemia, areas of focal necrosis can be found in the liver and spleen.

Diagnosis and Treatment Salmonellosis requires isolation of the organism from a rectal swab, stool culture, or culture from a lesion. Optimally, a recently passed uncontaminated stool sample of 1–2 g is rapidly placed in Gram-negative or selenite broth and incubated at 37°C. Cultures should be taken during the acute phase of illness. If transported prior to inoculation of culture media, the sample should be refrigerated. Serotyping has been useful in epidemiologic investigations due to the large number of *Salmonella* serovars.

Treatment for salmonella infections requires antibiotic therapy and supportive care to compensate for fluid loss and electrolyte and acid–base imbalances that result from diarrhea. Many isolates have multiple antibiotic resistance. Antibiotic therapy should be reserved for animals with severe diarrhea or septicemia.

e. Yersiniosis

Pathogenesis *Yersinia enterocolitica* and *Y. pseudotuberculosis* cause fulminating enteric and systemic disease in marmosets (*Callithrix* spp.), owl monkeys (*Aotus* spp.), squirrel monkeys (*Saimiri* spp.), and Old World monkeys. Infections are acquired by the fecal–oral route. Bacteria adhere to the cell membrane of intestinal epithelial cells and are subsequently ingested by bacterial endocytosis with vacuole formation; however, virulent strains resist phagocytosis by neutrophils and intracellular killing by macrophages. Virulent bacteria ultimately drain into the mesenteric lymph nodes resulting in systemic infections.

Disease Diarrhea, vomiting, severe abdominal pain, mild dehydration, and bloodstained feces were reported in macaques infected with *Y. pseudotuberculosis* (Bronson *et al.*, 1972; MacArthur and Wood, 1983). Leukocytosis due to neutrophilia, hyponatremia, hypochloremia, prerenal azotemia, and moderate hyperfibrinogenemia were reported in affected macaques by Rosenberg *et al.* (1980). Abortions and stillbirths occurred in some animals. *Yersinia*-infected squirrel monkeys had nonspecific clinical signs, such as inactivity, weakness, failure to cling to the dam, and cervical lymph node enlargement (Plesker and Carlos, 1992). Outbreaks of *Y. enterocolitica* may be seasonal with increased incidence observed in wet months in outdoor-housed animals (Skavlen *et al.*, 1985; Soto *et al.*, 2013).

Pathology *Yersinia* infections in nonhuman primates usually present with a triad of lesions at necropsy: multifocal hepatic and splenic necrosis or abscess formation, mesenteric lymphadenopathy, and ulcerative enterocolitis. Squirrel monkeys have an unusual presentation in that cervical lymph nodes are also markedly enlarged (Plesker and Carlos, 1992). Multifocal, purulent, and necrotizing hepatitis, splenitis, lymphadenitis, and ulcerative gastroenterocolitis are the characteristic microscopic lesions. Intestinal lesions range from focal mucosal necrosis with bacterial colonization to full-thickness mucosal necrosis with adherent intestinal contents, cellular debris and bacteria (McClure *et al.*, 1971; Baggs *et al.*, 1976), with ulcerative lesions overlying gut-associated lymphoid tissue (Bronson *et al.*, 1972). Often large bacterial colonies can be visualized in the center of necrotic regions and immunohistochemistry has recently been used to confirm their identity (Nakamura *et al.*, 2010).

Diagnosis and Treatment A presumptive diagnosis of *Yersinia* infection can be made from clinical presentation and lesions at necropsy. *Yersinia* can be recovered by rectal culture of monkeys presenting with diarrhea or from lesioned organs at necropsy. The organism grows well on a variety of media when it is the sole isolate; however, it is slow growing and cold enrichment of samples at 4–7°C may be necessary for recovery and isolation. Molecular diagnostic techniques can also be used to detect *Yersinia* virulence genes in both clinical and environmental samples, and these techniques have proven useful in epidemiologic review of suspected outbreaks (Thoerner *et al.*, 2003; Iwata *et al.*, 2008).

In many advanced cases of yersiniosis, treatment is ineffective. Supportive care including IV or oral fluid replacement, and antibiotic therapy has been successful. First-line antibiotics include aminoglycosides and trimethoprim-sulfamethoxazole. Other effective drugs include cephalosporins, tetracyclines, and fluoroquinolones.

f. *Helicobacter* spp.

A number of species within the genus *Helicobacter* have been identified as colonizing nonhuman primates; however, for many, disease association and causation have not been established. Isolation of *H. pylori* from stomachs of nonhuman primates, particularly macaques, has been reported by several authors, and the presence of *H. pylori* in the gastric mucosa of monkeys is often accompanied by persistent lymphocytic plasmacytic gastritis (Baskerville and Newell, 1988; Dubois *et al.*, 1994; Reindel *et al.*, 1999). This is a common incidental finding in cynomolgus macaques used in toxicological testing (Sato *et al.*, 2012) and has been described as a cause of epizootic gastritis in adolescent monkeys (Reindel *et al.*, 1999). Gastritis may or may not be present in monkeys infected with a related organism, *H. heilmannii* (Dubois *et al.*, 1991). Clinical signs of gastric helicobacter infection may include inappetence and occasional vomiting. This organism, now classified as *H. suis*, is commonly identified in many macaques. It is routinely diagnosed by silver stains or PCR-based assays (Haesebrouch *et al.*, 2009; Matsui *et al.*, 2014). Culture of the organism is difficult and seldom, if ever, successful. The rate of infection with gastric *Helicobacter* species may vary based upon geographic source (Drevon-Gaillot *et al.*, 2006). A serological assay has been developed for detection of *H. pylori* IgG responses in rhesus macaques, and in one study, 55 of 89 macaques were positive for antibodies for *H. pylori* (Kienesberger *et al.*, 2012).

A novel *Helicobacter* has been isolated and characterized from colons of cotton-top tamarins (*S. oedipus*), with inflammatory bowel disease (Saunders *et al.*, 1999). A specific serological response to this novel *Helicobacter* was also found in cotton-top tamarins with chronic colitis (Whary *et al.*, 1999). Similarly, novel *Helicobacter* spp. as well as *H. cinaedi* and recently identified *H. macacae* have been isolated from inflamed colons of rhesus monkeys (Fox *et al.*, 2001a,b; Fox *et al.*, 2007). Chronic, idiopathic, diffuse colitis is a well-recognized clinical and pathological entity in captive rhesus macaques that is characterized histologically by chronic, moderate to severe colitis and typhlitis, diffuse mononuclear inflammation of the lamina propria, reactive lymphoid hyperplasia, and multifocal microabscesses. Persistent infection of rhesus macaques with *H. macacae* associated with colonic adenocarcinoma has been described (Marini *et al.*, 2010; Lertpiriyapong *et al.*, 2014). The exact role of *Helicobacter* spp. in these disease entities has not been determined.

g. *Lawsonia intracellularis*

Klein *et al.* (1999) reported fatal proliferative enteritis in juvenile, colony-born, rhesus macaques resulting from infection with *L. intracellularis.* Affected monkeys were between 6 and 16 months of age. Clinical histories included depression, mild or transient diarrhea, and abdominal distension. Most animals were found dead or moribund with no clinical history. Moribund animals were hypothermic and anemic. The primary gross lesion was segmental thickening and pallor of the distal 5 cm of ileum. Distortion or loss of villous-crypt architecture, blunting and fusion of villi, and proliferation of pseudostratified tall columnar epithelial cells with varying degrees of inflammation were seen microscopically. Similar lesions have been identified in Japanese macaques (*M. fuscata*) (Wamsley *et al.*, 2005; Lafortune *et al.*, 2004).

2. *Respiratory and Nervous System Diseases*

Bacterial infections of the respiratory system frequently spread to the CNS in nonhuman primates and can progress to severe, life-threatening disease. Predisposing factors include recent shipping, overcrowding, and concomitant viral infections. Bacteria associated with respiratory and nervous system infections and the species affected are listed in Table 17.44.

a. *Streptococcus pneumoniae*

Pathogenesis By far, the most devastating respiratory pathogen in nonhuman primates is *Streptococcus pneumoniae.* Streptococcal infections are acquired by aerosol via the upper respiratory tract, middle ear, or mouth (Graczyk *et al.*, 1995). Stress-related factors including capture, transportation, and quarantine (Kaufmann and Quist, 1969a; Fox and Wikse, 1971), viral infection (Brendt *et al.*, 1974; Jones *et al.*, 1984), and decreased immunocompetence in neonates due to waning passive immunity (Graczyk *et al.*, 1995) predispose nonhuman primates to *S. pneumoniae* infection and disease.

Disease In macaques, disease is usually rapidly progressive; death may occur within hours of clinical onset (Gilbert *et al.*, 1987). In chimpanzees, clinical signs are initially those of an upper respiratory infection: coughing and a seromucoid to mucopurulent nasal discharge are followed by neurological signs (Keeling and McClure, 1974; Solleveld *et al.*, 1984). Duration of clinical illness can range from 2 to 14 days in chimpanzees.

Pathology The presence of degenerative neutrophils and phagocytized, encapsulated, Gram-positive diplococci in smears of cerebrospinal fluid provides a presumptive diagnosis of pneumococcal meningitis (Keeling and McClure, 1974; Solleveld *et al.*, 1984).

Gross lesions include engorgement of the meningeal vasculature, thickening and opacification of the leptomeninges, and purulent exudation over the cortex and/or the ventricles (Fox and Wikse, 1971; Solleveld *et al.*, 1984; Graczyk *et al.*, 1995). Lesions may extend to the spinal cord. In chronic disease, asymmetry of the cerebral hemispheres and severe malacia of the ventral frontal lobes of the brain may occur (Solleveld *et al.*, 1984). Congestion of the lungs, pulmonary edema, acute purulent bronchopneumonia, and consolidation of the ventral lung lobes have been reported in macaques, as well as diffuse, suppurative serositis with adhesions, suppurative arthritis, and panophthalmitis (Fox and Wikse, 1971; Herman and Fox, 1971). In chimpanzees, lesions have included purulent otitis interna, sinusitis, and tonsillitis (Solleveld *et al.*, 1984).

Microscopically, *S. pneumoniae* infection is characterized by fibrinopurulent leptomeningitis extending into the cerebral and cerebellar cortices (Fox and Wikse, 1971; Solleveld *et al.*, 1984). Necrotizing vasculitis and thrombosis due to fibrin deposition are common. Lung lesions range from acute serous inflammation with hyperemic congestion to exudative bronchopneumonia (Kaufmann and Quist, 1969a; Fox and Wikse, 1971).

Diagnosis Precise diagnosis may be made by recovery of *S. pneumoniae* from the blood, spinal fluid, upper respiratory tract, or affected organs at necropsy by bacterial culture. Commercial kits are available for the identification of streptococci and specific strains of *S. pneumoniae* can be differentiated by serotyping. Serotypes 2, 3, 6, 14, 18, and, 19 have been isolated from infections in nonhuman primates (Graczyk *et al.*, 1995; Jones *et al.*, 1984; Kaufmann and Quist, 1969a; Keeling and McClure, 1974). Definitive diagnosis can be made by amplifying regions of *S. pneumoniae*-specific genes including *lytA, ply*, spn9802, and spn9828 by PCR (Suzuki *et al.*, 2006).

Treatment *S. pneumoniae* remains sensitive to penicillin. Treatment of animals with advanced clinical signs indicating neurologic or systemic involvement is unlikely to be successful; however, prophylactic treatment of contact animals may be of benefit in preventing epizootics. In cases of pneumococcal meningitis, aggressive treatment with antibiotics, intravenous fluids and electrolytes, and diazepam (20–30 mg/day) to modulate seizure activity has been used in chimpanzees (Solleveld *et al.*, 1984).

A number of other members of the *Streptococcus* genus have been demonstrated to infect nonhuman primates including *S. pyogenes* resulting in a toxic shock like syndrome (Garcia *et al.*, 2006) and *S. equi zooepidemicus* resulting in severe bronchopneumonia (Mätz-Rensing *et al.*, 2009).

b. *Klebsiella pneumoniae*

Pathogenesis *Klebsiella pneumonia* is often found as part of the normal flora in the upper and lower

TABLE 17.44 Bacterial Respiratory and Nervous System Infections

Agent	Primate	Clinical signs and clinical pathology	Treatment/prevention
Streptococcus pneumoniae	Chimpanzee	**URI**	Penicillin 8×10^6 U/day and ampicillin 4 g/day and
		Slight cough, mucopurulent nasal discharge	diazepam 20–30 mg/day[a]
			or
			penicillin 2×10^5 U/day and
		Conjunctivitis	ampicillin 200–400 mg and chloramphenicol 25 mg/kg
		Pyrexia	TID[b]
			or
		Leukocytosis	ceftriaxone 50–100 mg/kg[c]
		Meningitis	
		Lethargy, vestibular signs	
		Head holding, lip droop	
		Seizures, dysphagia	
	Macaque	Panophthalmitis, conjunctivitis	
		Lethargy, incoordination, hypothermia	
		Depressed reflexes	
		Ataxia, muscle tremors, head pressing	
		Nuchal rigidity, nystagmus	
		Leukocytosis with left shift	
Klebsiella pneumoniae	Chimpanzee	Cough	
		Clear-mucopurulent nasal discharge	
		Rales	
		Pulmonary congestion	
	Macaque	Anorexia, adipsia	
		Listlessness, reluctance to move	
		Droopy eyelids	
		Leukocytosis due to neutrophilia	
	Squirrel monkey	Swollen throat, abscesses in throat, infant deaths	Autogenous bacterin[d]
			Two doses at 1-month interval
	Callitrichid	Death, no clinical signs	Autogenous bacterin[e]
			Tetracycline, 55 mg/kg body weight[f]
	Owl monkey	Death, no clinical signs	Autogenous bacterin[g]
			or
		Anorexia, pyrexia, sneezing, coughing, dyspnea	cephalothin, gentamicin
			Trimethoprim-sulfamethoxazole
			Amikacin or kanamycin[h]
		Cervical-mandibular swelling	
		Serous to mucopurulent nasal discharge	
		Facial edema; painful, distended abdomen	

(Continued)

TABLE 17.44 (Continued)

Agent	Primate	Clinical signs and clinical pathology	Treatment/prevention
Bordetella bronchiseptica	Marmoset	Mucopurulent nasal discharge	Oxytetracycline[i]
			Autogenous bacterin[f]
		Dyspnea during handling	
		Pyrexia, bright and alert	
		Deaths in animals <1 year old	
	Owl monkey	Serous to mucopurulent nasal and ocular discharges	Chloramphenicol, amoxicillin, or tetracycline[h]
		Dyspnea, depression, anorexia, weight loss	
		Usually self-limiting	
Pasteurella spp.	Squirrel monkey	Unsteady gait, circling	
		Nystagmus, head tilt	
		Edema of eyelids, serosanguinous discharge	
		from ears	
	Owl monkey	Lethargy, anorexia, depression, weight loss	Chloramphenicol
			Penicillin
		Dyspnea	Ampicillin[h]
		Seizures	
		Localized swelling and exudation associated	
		with abscesses	
	Baboon	Postsurgical air sacculitis, abscess from catheterization	Remove catheter
Nocardia spp.	Macaque	Dyspnea, epistaxis	
		Chronic weight loss, abdominal distension and discomfort	
		Chronic intermittent diarrhea	
		Lethargy, depression	
		Coma	
	Baboon	Cutaneous draining tract	Excision
	Squirrel monkey	Subcutaneous nodules	
Moraxella spp.	Cynomolgus	Epistaxis, mucohemorrhagic nasal discharge	Long-acting penicillin[j]

[a]*From Keeling and McClure (1974).*
[b]*From Solleveld et al. (1984).*
[c]*From Pernikoff and Orkin (1991).*
[d]*From Postal et al. (1988).*
[e]*From Gozalo and Montoya (1992).*
[f]*From Chalmers et al. (1983).*
[g]*From Obaldia (1991).*
[h]*From Weller (1994); drug doses not provided in text.*
[i]*From Baskerville et al. (1983).*
[j]*From VandeWoude and Luzarraga (1991).*

gastrointestinal tracts of many nonhuman primates. Pathogenic strains associated with the upper respiratory tract are usually heavily encapsulated. Many pathogenic strains possess fimbriae, which act as adhesins and a virulence factor that permits colonization of mucosal surfaces. The capsule also serves as a virulence factor by inhibiting phagocytosis. More virulent strains of *K. pneumoniae* with a hypermucoviscosity phenotype have been associated with severe disease in both human beings and nonhuman primates (Twenhafel *et al.*, 2008).

Disease *K. pneumoniae* infection can result in pneumonia, meningitis, air sacculitis, septicemia, peritonitis, and enteritis in New and Old World primate species, and in apes. New World monkeys in particular may die from septicemia or peritonitis with no clinical signs (Snyder *et al.*, 1970; Giles *et al.*, 1974; Gozalo and Montoya, 1991). Young animals are more frequently affected than adults (Campos *et al.*, 1981). A 64% incidence of infection has been reported for recently imported tamarins, and a 25–29% incidence of infection and disease has been reported for some owl monkey colonies (Snyder *et al.*, 1970). Pneumonia and septicemia due to *K. pneumoniae* caused mortality rates approaching 100% in young Guyanese squirrel monkeys. Maternal neglect, trauma, and failure of hand rearing predisposed infants to disease (Moisson and Gysin, 1994). Klebsiella infection in young chimpanzees has been a primary cause of respiratory disease deaths (Schmidt and Butler, 1971).

Recently, infections with invasive *K. pneumoniae* with a hypermucoviscous phenotype have been recognized (Twenhafel *et al.*, 2008). Asymptomatic and persistent infection of cynomolgus and rhesus macaques has been recognized in a research colony co-housing African green monkeys (Burke *et al.*, 2009).

Pathology Fibrinous lobar pneumonia, purulent peritonitis, and mesenteric lymphadenopathy are the primary lesions reported in callitrichids infected with *K. pneumoniae* (Gozalo and Montoya, 1991, 1992). Enteritis and hepatomegaly were reported in a colony of common marmosets by Campos *et al.* (1981). Purulent meningitis, consolidative pneumonia, intestinal hemorrhages, peritonitis, and air sacculitis occur in owl monkeys with *K. pneumoniae* infections (Gozalo and Montoya, 1991, 1992). Lesions in owl monkeys with acute air sacculitis range from diffuse hyperemia of the air sac mucosa to thickening with edema of the adventitia to suppurative bronchopneumonia and lymphadenitis (Giles *et al.*, 1974). Gross necropsy findings reported in rhesus macaques were exudative bronchopneumonia and hemopurulent meningitis (Good and May, 1971; Fox and Rohovsky, 1975). Chimpanzees had firm, inflated, red-purple lung lobes with yellow–white foci throughout the parenchyma (Schmidt and Butler, 1971). Baboons had thickened air sacs with suppurative to fibrinosuppurative exudate (Kumar *et al.*, 2012).

Microscopically, intense congestion with infiltrates of mononuclear and polymorphonuclear leukocytes occurred in affected organs of common marmosets (Campos *et al.*, 1981). Inflammation and suppuration of the Peyer's patches and cecal lymphoid tissue were observed in owl monkeys with *Klebsiella* septicemia (Gozalo and Montoya, 1991). Acute air sacculitis in owl monkeys was characterized by bacterial thromboembolism of the subepithelial vasculature of the air sac (Giles *et al.*, 1974). Diffuse fibrinopurulent bronchopneumonia, suppurative bronchitis, and pleuritis were reported in rhesus macaques by Fox and Rohovsky (1975), as well as fibrinopurulent meningitis, vasculitis, and thrombosis of meningeal vessels. Thickening of alveolar septae, congestion, alveolar

hemorrhage, and edema with mononuclear and neutrophilic inflammatory cell infiltrates characterized pneumonia in chimpanzees (Schmidt and Butler, 1971). Multifocal microabscesses and filling of bronchioles with necrotic debris and inflammatory cells were described.

Fatal multisystemic infection of African green monkeys resulted in abscess formation in the abdomen, liver, lungs, skin, and CNS. Often, abdominal masses were present entrapping and adhering to loops of bowel and were histologically characterized by chronic pyogranulomatous inflammation and fibrous adhesions (Twenhafel *et al.*, 2008).

Diagnosis and Treatment Diagnosis of *Klebsiella* infection depends on isolation of the organism from clinical specimens or at necropsy; however, *ante mortem* diagnosis is frequently not possible due to the acute course of the disease. Treatment of infections caused by *K. pneumoniae* has been difficult due to the fulminating course of disease (Fox and Rohovsky, 1975). Vaccination utilizing autogenous bacterins has been effective in preventing infection and disease in marmosets, and owl and squirrel monkeys (Postal *et al.*, 1988; Obaldia, 1991). *Klebsiella* infections can be treated with antibiotics, and Table 17.44 lists possible treatment options.

c. *Bordetella bronchiseptica*

Pathogenesis *Bordetella bronchiseptica* is carried as a commensal organism within the nasopharynx of many monkeys. Historically, disease has been associated with recent shipping, quarantine, poor condition, and overcrowding (Seibold *et al.*, 1970; Pinkerton, 1972), although outbreaks have occurred in established colonies of common marmosets in which the initiating factor was unknown (Baskerville *et al.*, 1983; Chalmers *et al.*, 1983).

Disease Clinical signs in affected common marmosets included bilateral mucopurulent nasal discharge, dyspnea during handling, and pyrexia. Marmosets usually remained bright and alert and in good body condition. Death occurred in marmosets less than 1 year of age, but adults survived (Baskerville *et al.*, 1983).

Pathology Bronchopneumonia affecting all lung lobes was the primary gross lesion (Baskerville *et al.*, 1983; Chalmers *et al.*, 1983). The typical microscopic pulmonary lesion was purulent bronchopneumonia with multifocal necrosis of the bronchiolar epithelium and filling of bronchioles with basophilic necrotic cellular debris, polymorphonuclear cells, and macrophages.

Diagnosis and Treatment Diagnosis of *B. bronchiseptica* infection is based upon isolation of the organism from clinical specimens, such as nasal or oropharyngeal swabs, or from lesioned tissues at necropsy. Molecular diagnostic techniques have been developed to identify *Bordetella* spp. in clinical specimens (Farrell *et al.*, 2000; Reizenstein *et al.*, 1993). While these assays are often developed to detect *B. pertusis* from human patients, they will often detect *B. bronchiseptica* due to shared virulence epitopes such as the pertusis toxin. Treatment of adult common marmosets with intramuscular oxytetracycline for 8 days resolved clinical disease, but it did not eliminate the organism from the nasal passages (Baskerville *et al.*, 1983). Use of an autogenous bacterin in marmoset colonies has been reported (Chalmers *et al.*, 1983).

d. *Pasteurella multocida*

Pasteurella multocida is a rarely described opportunistic pathogen of squirrel and owl monkeys affecting recently shipped animals and animals in poor condition (Greenstein *et al.*, 1965; Benjamin and Lang, 1971; Pinkerton, 1972). Squirrel monkeys presented with unsteady gait, nystagmus, head tilt, and circling. Meningitis, otitis media, lymphadenitis, and myocarditis were diagnosed at necropsy (Greenstein *et al.*, 1965). Pneumonia, pleuritis, and meningitis occurred in affected owl monkeys. Necrotizing, fibrinopurulent pneumonia with thrombosis of small blood vessels and severe, acute interstitial pneumonia with multifocal necrosis of alveolar septae were the primary microscopic lesions. Baboons have developed infections secondary to surgical procedures, chair restraint, and chronic catheterization (Bronsdon and DiGiacomo, 1993). Respiratory infection of wild chimpanzees has recently been recognized (Köndgen *et al.*, 2011).

e. *Nocardia* spp.

Nocardia spp. are aerobic actinomycetes found in richly fertilized soil as saprophytes on decaying vegetation. *Nocardia asteroides* is the most common isolate in nonhuman primates. Infection occurs following contact with skin wounds, inhalation, or ingestion. Clinical signs include dyspnea and epistaxis (McClure *et al.*, 1976), chronic weight loss, abdominal distension and discomfort (Liebenberg and Giddens, 1985), chronic intermittent diarrhea, lethargy or depression (Jones and Wyand, 1966), and coma (Al-Doory *et al.*, 1969). Radiographically, pulmonary lesions of nocardiosis cannot be distinguished from tuberculosis.

Gross pulmonary lesions include multinodular to diffuse red to gray areas of consolidation, pulmonary hemorrhage and edema, abscesses, and cavitary lesions. Disseminated nocardiosis with multifocal abscesses in the omentum, mesentery, liver, kidney, and stomach has been reported in macaques (Liebenberg and Giddens, 1985) in addition to hemorrhage and multifocal abscesses in the brain (Sakakibara *et al.*, 1984). Nocardiosis may also present as a draining multinodular cutaneous lesion (Boncyk *et al.*, 1975) or as subcutaneous nodules (Kessler and Brown, 1981). Multifocal to coalescing pyogranulomas containing sulfur granules with large colonies of filamentous bacteria are characteristic.

Multinucleated giant cells are found at the lesion periphery. There are no reports of successful treatment of nocardiosis in nonhuman primates; however, this is a rare disease.

f. *Moraxella catarrhalis*

Moraxella catarrhalis (formerly *Brahamella catarrhalis*) is a Gram-negative diplococcus associated with epistaxis and mucohemorrhagic nasal discharge in cynomolgus macaques (VandeWoude and Luzarraga, 1991). Clinical signs occur most commonly in dry winter months and may also include sneezing and occasionally, periorbital swelling. White blood cells, erythrocytes, and large diplococcal organisms are seen in nasal cytologic preparations. Treatment with long-acting penicillin may be effective (VandeWoude and Luzarraga, 1991), but recurrent infections are possible if low-humidity conditions persist. Recent work indicates that *M. catarrhalis* contains several genotypically distinct organisms. Sequencing of the 16S ribosomal RNA gene indicated that isolates from macaques were most closely related to *M. lincolnii* and rhesus macaques were resistant to infection with human strains of *M. catarrhalis* (Embers *et al.*, 2011).

3. *Tuberculosis and Mycobacteriosis*
a. Pathogenesis

Tuberculosis is an insidious disease capable of causing high morbidity and mortality within a nonhuman primate colony. Tuberculosis is caused by *Mycobacterium tuberculosis*, *M. bovis*, or *M. africanum* and is usually acquired though human or environmental contact. There is no apparent difference in tuberculous disease in nonhuman primates caused by *M. tuberculosis* or *M. bovis* (McLaughlin, 1978); distribution and character of the lesions are identical. Kaufmann *et al.* (1975) estimated that up to 10% of tuberculosis outbreaks in nonhuman primates were caused by *M. bovis*. While infections with *M. africanum* can be common in human beings, it is a rare *Mycobacterium* sp. isolate in nonhuman primates (Thorel, 1980; De Jong *et al.*, 2010).

Epizootic tuberculosis in nonhuman primates usually takes place by aerosol transmission, but transmission has occurred by ingestion, direct contact, and contact with fomites, including contaminated thermometers (Riordan, 1949) and a tattooing needle (Allen and Kinard, 1958). Although particular species may be more or less susceptible to disease, all nonhuman primates can develop tuberculosis. When cynomolgus macaques are infected with low doses of virulent *M. tuberculosis*, their disease course closely resembles that of human tuberculosis (Capuano *et al.*, 2003).

b. Disease

Infection may produce a variety of clinical signs including cough, dyspnea, diarrhea and lymphadenopathy, or infection may be asymptomatic. A common clinical sign of disease is progressive unexplained weight loss, leading to cachexia which is promoted by elevations of cytokines such as tumor necrosis factor (TNF)-α (Rook *et al.*, 1987; Beutler and Cerami, 1988). This can occur in the absence of overt respiratory signs. A summary of clinical signs associated with tuberculosis is presented in Table 17.45.

c. Pathology

Gross lesions of tuberculosis include caseous nodules in the hilar lymph nodes and lung, large cavitary and coalescing lesions within the lung, and tubercles extending into the thoracic pleura (Fig. 17.21). In advanced disease, there is secondary spread to the spleen, kidney, liver, and various lymph nodes with either multifocal miliary disease or larger nodular foci of caseation. Less

TABLE 17.45   Tuberculosis in Nonhuman Primates

Agent	Species	Clinical signs	Clinical pathology
Mycobacterium tuberculosis, M. bovis	Macaque	Persistent cough	Anemia, normocytic, normochromic
		Chronic fatigue	Leukocytosis
		Exertional dyspnea	Lymphopenia
		Anorexia, weight loss	Elevated serum globulins
		Peripheral lymph node enlargement ± draining tract	Elevated erythrocyte sedimentation rate
		Cutaneous abscesses	
		Enlarged liver or spleen on palpation	
	Baboon	Lethargy, emaciation	
	Squirrel monkey	Positive TB test ± clinical signs	
		Weakness, lethargy, paroxysmal cough	
	Owl monkey	Serous ocular and nasal discharge	
		Weight loss, dehydration, depression	
	Callitrichid	No clinical signs reported	

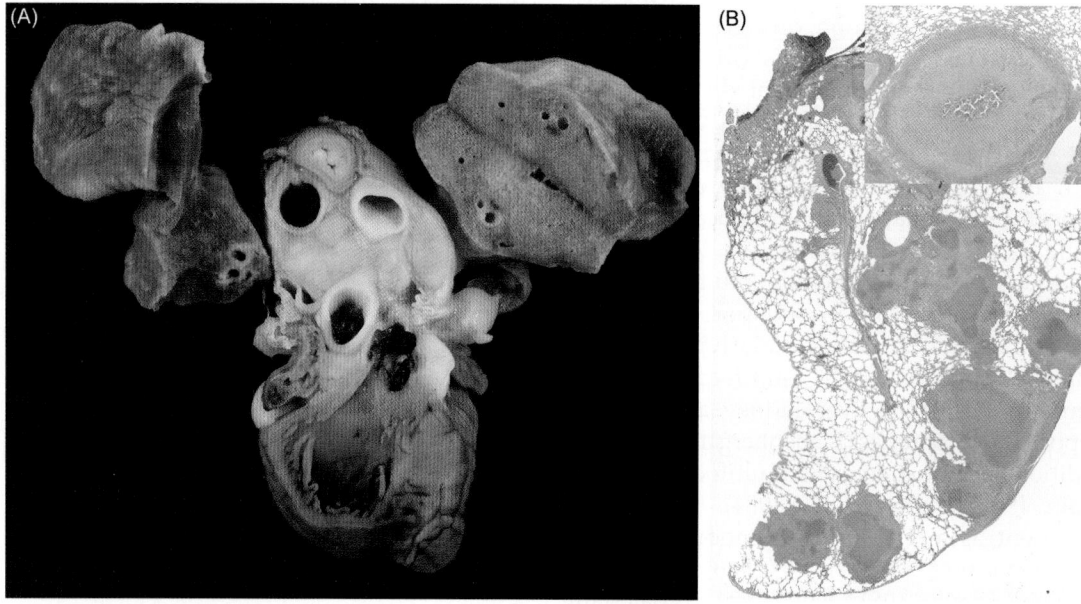

FIGURE 17.21   *Mycobacterium tuberculosis.* Lymphadenopathy of the tracheobronchiole lymph node in rhesus macaque (A). Granulomatous bronchopneumonia (B) with caseous necrosis (insert).

frequently, tuberculous nodules are found in the cerebrum (Machotka et al., 1975), spinal column, omentum, uterus and ovary (McLaughlin, 1978), peripheral lymph nodes, skin (Lindsey and Melby, 1966), mammary gland, or spinal vertebra (Fox et al., 1974). The typical microscopic lesions are un-encapsulated granulomas of varying size with a necrotic core. Surrounding the core is a layer of epithelioid macrophages and lesser numbers of neutrophils, with multinucleated Langhans' giant cells at the periphery. Mineralization is uncommon. Acid-fast bacilli (AFB) can be demonstrated within the lesions both intra- and extracellularly using an acid-fast stain; however, AFB are often rare or absent in clinical tuberculosis cases.

d. Diagnosis and Treatment

Ante mortem diagnosis of tuberculosis is based on the intradermal tuberculin test. Swelling, erythema, edema, and ptosis are indicative of a suspect or positive reaction (Table 17.39). McLaughlin and Marrs (1978) reported no advantage in using M. bovis purified protein derivative (PPD) over Mammalian Old Tuberculin (MOT) in the detection of monkeys infected with M. bovis; in fact, MOT was the superior diagnostic reagent and PPD should not be used. The tuberculin skin test is limited in its sensitivity in that animals with early or advanced disease may give false-negative reactions (Brusasca et al., 2003). Concomitant disease such as measles or measles vaccination may also result in a false-negative reaction due to immunosuppression. Therapy with isoniazid will invalidate the tuberculin skin test (Dillehay and Huerkemp, 1990). False positives may result from exposure to Freund's Complete Adjuvant (Pierce and Dukelow, 1988), trauma due to improper administration of the test, infection with atypical mycobacterium such as M. avium or M. kansasii, or nonspecific reactivity to the vehicle (Fox, 1975). Sensitivity and specificity of the intradermal skin test has recently been described as 84% and 87%, respectively (Garcia et al., 2004b). Despite issues with sensitivity and specificity, intradermal skin testing remains the standard diagnostic test for tuberculosis screening.

Thoracic radiography may provide confirmation of pulmonary disease but cannot distinguish between tuberculosis and other cavitary diseases of the lung, such as nocardiosis or cryptococcosis. Culture of M. bovis or M. tuberculosis may be difficult, especially early in the disease when there are low numbers of mycobacteria present, but culture remains the gold standard for diagnosing tuberculosis. Detection of infection by screening feces, sputum, or necropsy tissues using specific mycobacterial primers by PCR for mycobacterial DNA may provide a more rapid diagnosis of tuberculosis (Brammer et al., 1995). However, the sensitivity and specificity of PCR for the diagnosis of naturally acquired tuberculosis in nonhuman primates has not been determined and results should be interpreted with caution.

A number of alternative serology tests for the diagnosis of tuberculosis are currently under evaluation, such as the multiplex microbead immunoassay to detect specific mycobacterial antibodies (Khan et al., 2008), the ELISPOT assay, and interferon-gamma release assays (Lerche et al., 2008). Direct comparison of the whole-blood in vitro interferon-gamma assays (IGRAs) to intradermal skin testing suggests that the kinetics of positive results in infected animals may vary and that their combined use may improve diagnostic sensitivity (Garcia et al., 2004b).

4. Other Mycobacterial Infections

a. Mycobacterium avium-intracellulare

Pathogenesis Mycobacterium avium-intracellulare complex, also known as M. avium complex (MAC), consists of pathogenic, saprophytic, nontuberculous mycobacteria that are contracted through exposure to soil, water, or infected tissues. Entry into the body can be through the respiratory, oral, and cutaneous routes. A summary of nonhuman primate mycobacterioses is found in Table 17.46. Nonhuman primates are resistant to experimental infection with M. avium-intracellulare; however, macaques are highly susceptible to infection during progressive SIV infection and MAC represents the most common disseminated bacterial infection in simian AIDS (Mansfield et al., 1995).

Disease Disease primarily involves the gastrointestinal tract and reticuloendothelial system (Sesline, 1978; Holmberg et al., 1985) and can be acquired through potable water systems (Mansfield and Lackner, 1997). There are two reports of cutaneous manifestations (Latt, 1975; Bellinger and Bullock, 1988). Clinical signs of infection range from none (Sedgwick et al., 1970) to intermittent or continuous refractory diarrhea, accompanied by dramatic weight loss and generalized lymphadenopathy (Sesline, 1978).

Pathology In some macaques, no gross lesions were associated with M. avium infection (Sedgwick et al., 1970). Those with intestinal illness had mild to severe thickening of the intestinal wall from the distal small intestine through the cecum and colon (Sesline, 1978; Holmberg et al., 1985). Enlargement and edema of mesenteric lymph nodes and splenomegaly were frequently observed. Diffuse granulomatous inflammation of the terminal ileum and proximal colon due to infiltration of large, foamy macrophages into the mucosa and submucosa was characteristic. Numerous AFB were found in the cytoplasm of macrophages in Ziehl–Neelsen-stained intestinal sections (Fig. 17.22). An animal with a focal cutaneous lesion had numerous AFB-containing macrophages, epithelioid cells, and Langhans' giant cells, with granulation tissue (Bellinger and Bullock, 1988). This animal recovered spontaneously after removal of the lesion.

TABLE 17.46   Mycobacteriosis in Nonhuman Primates

Agent/species	Clinical signs	Clinical pathology
Mycobacterium	Intermittent-chronic diarrhea, refractory to treatment	Anemia, normocytic, normochromic
avium-intracellulare	Marked weight loss	Hypoalbuminemia
Macaques	General lymphadenopathy	Hypergammaglobulinemia
(Coinfection with SIV)	Draining fistula or ulcerated cutaneous lesions	
M. leprae	Self-mutilation hands and feet	None
Chimpanzee, sooty mangabey, cynomolgus macaque	Multiple, eroded nodular lesions face and ears	
	Nodules and papules along lateral extremities, scrotum, perineum	
M. kansasii	None, detected by TB test	None
Macaques, squirrel monkeys		
M. gordonae	None, detected by TB test	None
Squirrel monkeys, common marmoset		

Diagnosis Diagnosis of *M. avium-intracellulare* infection can be difficult. Responses to tuberculin skin testing, even when using avian tuberculin PPD, are variable (Sedgwick *et al.*, 1970; Holmberg *et al.*, 1985). Transitory erythema at 24-h postinoculation of MOT has been observed (Sedgwick *et al.*, 1970). Biopsy of colonic tissue or a suspected cutaneous site is a helpful diagnostic tool in that it can provide tissue for culture, histopathology, and PCR analysis for mycobacterial DNA. Culture of the organism from feces or lesions is time consuming. Treatment is not recommended because this organism has resistance to multiple drugs.

b. *Mycobacterium leprae*

Pathogenesis *Mycobacterium leprae* is the etiologic agent of leprosy or Hansen's disease. Leprosy is a chronic granulomatous disease affecting the skin and peripheral nerves with lesions preferentially occurring in cooler areas, i.e., the extremities, of the host. Naturally acquired infections with *M. leprae* have been reported in a sooty mangabey, *Cercocebus atys* (Meyers *et al.*, 1985), chimpanzees (Leininger *et al.*, 1978; Hubbard *et al.*, 1991; Alford *et al.*, 1996), and in a cynomolgus macaque (Valverde *et al.*, 1998).

Disease Multiple, eroded, nodular skin lesions of the face and ears occurred in chimpanzees with leprosy (Leininger *et al.*, 1978; Hubbard *et al.*, 1991; Alford *et al.*, 1996). One chimpanzee had a 10-year history of self-mutilation of the hands and feet (Alford *et al.*, 1996). In this individual and another chimpanzee at the same facility, nodular and papular lesions were also found on the lateral surfaces of the arms and legs, scrotum, perineum, and penis. The face and extremities appeared edematous and swollen, and many of the nodular lesions became ulcerated.

Pathology Microscopic lesions observed in biopsy or necropsy specimens revealed epidermal thinning and subepidermal clear zones (Leininger *et al.*, 1978; Meyers *et al.*, 1985; Hubbard *et al.*, 1991). Dermal inflammation was primarily histiocytic, with inflammatory cells localized around neurovascular channels. Large numbers of AFB were observed in histiocytes and lesser numbers within nerves.

Diagnosis and Treatment Diagnosis of leprosy is most commonly based upon clinical signs and symptoms. Skin smears with rod-shaped, AFB, which are diagnostic for the disease, may be seen in the smears taken from the affected skin and biopsy of affected tissues. A variety of different treatments have been used in primates with leprosy. The currently recommended multidrug chemotherapy for treating humans includes daily dapsone and clofazimine, with monthly rifampicin treatments (WHO, 1998).

c. *Mycobacterium kansasii* and *M. gordonae*

Pathogenesis Atypical mycobacteriosis due to *M. kansasii* infection has been reported in rhesus and squirrel monkeys (Valerio *et al.*, 1979; Brammer *et al.*, 1995). Similar lesions have been recognized in common marmosets associated with *M. gordonae* infection (Wachtman *et al.*, 2011). Unlike *M. tuberculosis* infection, there has been no evidence of animal-to-animal transmission.

Disease Gross lesions of *M. kansasii* infection in rhesus monkeys included one to two pulmonary nodules, some containing yellow–green caseous material, and tuberculous-type lesions in the mediastinal lymph nodes (Valerio *et al.*, 1979). Some monkeys had miliary lesions in the liver and/or spleen. Squirrel monkeys had enlarged bronchial, cervical, and/or mediastinal lymph nodes (Brammer *et al.*, 1995). Microscopic lesions were indistinguishable from those of tuberculosis.

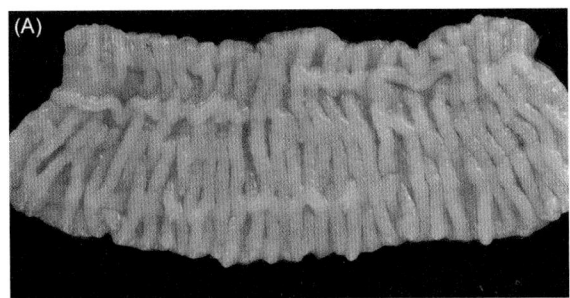

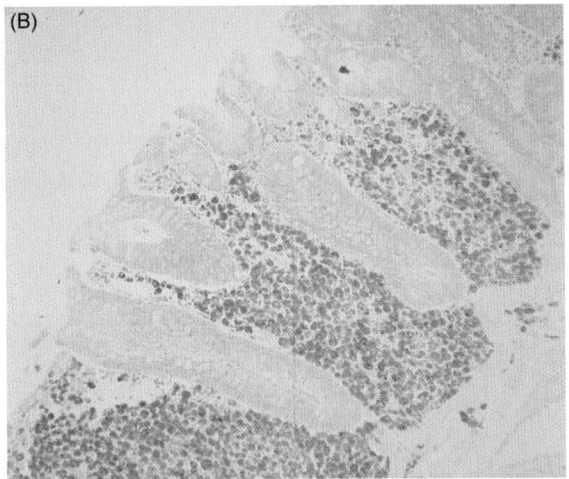

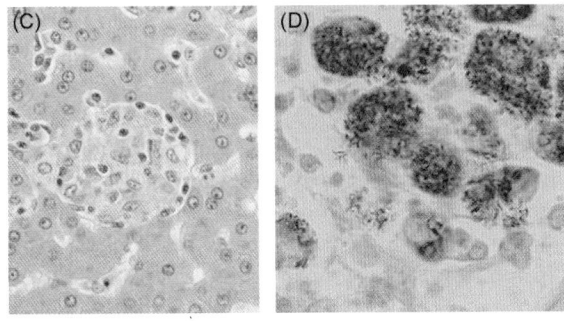

FIGURE 17.22 *Mycobacterium avium.* Granulomatous colitis (A) with myriads of AFB (B) in SIV-infected rhesus macaque. Hepatic microgranuloma (C) with histiocytes containing AFB (D).

Diagnosis In a breeding colony of rhesus monkeys, 71 monkeys developed positive tuberculin reactions, and 60 monkeys were culture positive for *M. kansasii* (Valerio *et al.*, 1979). Infection was initially detected by tuberculin skin test using MOT intradermally in both the eyelid and the abdomen. Minimal ptosis, with mild thickening of the eyelid and little or no hyperemia, was observed. A 1- to 2-cm area of blanched, thickened skin was found at the abdominal test site. Severity of tuberculin reactions became more pronounced in animals that were retested. Tuberculin testing with specific *M. kansasii* antigen or PPD was not diagnostically superior to testing with MOT (Valerio *et al.*, 1979). *M. kansasii* infection in squirrel monkeys was also detected by routine tuberculin testing (Brammer *et al.*, 1995). Diagnosis of *M. kansasii* infection was preliminarily confirmed by use of genus-specific probes for mycobacterial DNA in PCR testing of bronchial lymph nodes. The organism eventually was isolated from three of five animals with positive tuberculin skin tests.

Tuberculin testing of a colony of squirrel monkeys identified three positive animals (Soave *et al.*, 1981). Two monkeys were euthanized and necropsied. There were no gross or microscopic lesions, but *M. gordonae* was isolated from the mediastinal lymph nodes, spleen, and/or liver.

5. Other Bacterial Infections

Tetanus due to *Clostridium tetani* has been a cause of mortality in free-ranging or outdoor-housed monkeys. Tetanus occurred secondary to soil contamination of fight wounds or to parturition in rhesus macaques (DiGiacomo and Missakian, 1972; Rawlins and Kessler, 1982), bite wounds or other skin trauma in squirrel monkeys (Kessler and Brown, 1979), and frostbite lesions in baboons (Goodwin *et al.*, 1987). Clinical signs are summarized in Table 17.47. Tetanus is a clinical diagnosis because culture of the organism is difficult. Tetanus toxoid administered intramuscularly followed by a single booster was protective for rhesus macaques and baboons (Kessler *et al.*, 1988; Goodwin *et al.*, 1987) and immunization with tetanus toxoid is advised for populations at risk. Two doses of tetanus toxoid was highly effective at reducing mortality in a colony of free-ranging macaques on the island of Cayo Santiago. This immunization regimen elicited immune responses that persisted for at least 20 years in the majority of animals (Kessler *et al.*, 2006).

Naturally acquired leptospiral infections have been reported in tamarins, squirrel monkeys, baboons, and chimpanzees (Wilbert and Delorme, 1927; Fear *et al.*, 1968; Perolat *et al.*, 1992; Reid *et al.*, 1993). In squirrel monkeys and baboons, leptospirosis is associated with abortion. Squirrel monkeys may die without clinical signs or present with pyrexia, marked dehydration, and icterus (Perolat *et al.*, 1992). Gross necropsy lesions include jaundice of mucous membranes, subcutaneous tissues, and viscera; hemorrhagic pneumonia; renal necrosis and hemorrhage; and hepatomegaly (Perolat *et al.*, 1992; Reid *et al.*, 1993). Microscopic lesions include pulmonary hemorrhage and edema, multifocal hepatocellular degeneration and bile stasis, interstitial nephritis, tubular epithelial necrosis, and exudative glomerulopathy. Spirochetes can be seen with silver staining of renal tissues. Immunization with an inactivated vaccine was effective in eliminating leptospiral disease in a colony of squirrel monkeys (Perolat *et al.*, 1992).

Staphylococcus and *Pseudomonas* are bacteria genera associated with a variety of disease conditions, usually affecting individual animals. Staphylococci have been recovered from abscesses, ascitic fluid, ocular

TABLE 17.47   Tetanus (*Clostridium tetani*) in Primates

Species	History	Clinical signs	Treatment
Rhesus	Free-ranging	Torpor	None attempted; some obese animals recovered spontaneously
	Fight wounds	Unable to prehend food	
	Postpartum	Difficulty swallowing	
		Excessive thirst	
		Progressive stiffness, abduction pectoral limbs	
		Bipedal running and hopping	
		Piloerection	
		Trismus, opisthotonus, status epilepticus	
Baboon	Outdoor housing	Moribund	1500 units veterinary tetanus antitoxin
	Frostbite	Trismus and extensor rigidity	Acepromazine 3–5 mg QID × 4 weeks
			Valium 1.5 mg QID × 10 days[a]
Squirrel monkey	Outdoor housing	Slow, deliberate, stiff gait; reluctance to move	Treatment unsuccessful
	Bite wounds, trauma	Trismus, extensor rigidity, and opisthotonus	

[a]*From Goodwin* et al. *(1987).*

discharges, and fistulas of clinically ill owl monkeys (Weller, 1994) and from a tamarin with bronchopneumonia (Deinhardt *et al.*, 1967a). *Staphylococcus aureus* was isolated from macaques with clinical vaginitis or pyometra (Lang and Benjamin, 1969; Doyle *et al.*, 1991), and from a retrobulbar abscess in a rhesus infant (Rosenberg and Blouin, 1979). At Yerkes Regional Primate Research Center (Atlanta, GA), *S. aureus* was the most frequent isolate from external wounds and joint specimens from monkeys with arthritis, and a frequent isolate of blood cultures from clinical cases or necropsies (McClure *et al.*, 1986). Staphylococcal infection is a frequent problem with indwelling catheters; it can cause serious disease as well as reduce catheter life span by half (Taylor and Grady, 1998; Weese, 2010). In the report by Taylor and Grady, 64% of catheter infections in macaques were due to staphylococci, many of which were multiple-antibiotic resistant. Methicillin-resistant *S. aureus* (MRSA) infections have been observed in rhesus macaques that have undergone irradiation (Kolappaswamy *et al.*, 2008) and in association with an acute necrotizing stomatitis (Lee *et al.*, 2011).

Pseudomonas spp., including *P. aeruginosa*, have been recovered from monkeys with diarrhea, from skin wounds, blood cultures, and air sac infections (McClure, 1980). *Pseudomonas* spp. were associated with bronchopneumonia, empyema, vegetative endocarditis, pancarditis, and septicemia in marmosets and tamarins (Deinhardt *et al.*, 1967b; Cicmanec, 1977). *Pseudomonas aeruginosa* has been isolated from squirrel monkeys with meningitis, pododermatitis, cellulitis (Line *et al.*, 1984; Lausen *et al.*, 1986), and a maxillofacial abscess (Langner

et al., 1986), and also from a chimpanzee with suppurative nephritis (Migaki *et al.*, 1979). Treatment in all cases entailed aggressive antibiotic administration. Successful antibiotic regimens included intramuscular gentamicin (1.25 mg/kg every 12 h), procaine penicillin (50,000 U/kg every 12 h), and polymyxin B (12,500 IU/kg every 12 h) (Line *et al.*, 1984; Lausen *et al.*, 1986). More recent antibiotic recommendations in the human medical literature have included several combination therapies. However, a recent report comparing beta-lactam treatment alone to combination therapy with aminoglycoside antibiotics found monotherapy to be better because it reduced the risk of nephrotoxicity (Paul *et al.*, 2014).

B. Mycotic Diseases

1. *Pneumocystis* spp.

a. Pathogenesis

Historically known as *Penumocystis carninii*, phylogenetic analysis has revealed the genus to contain a large number of distinct but morphologically identical organisms which infect hosts in a highly species-specific fashion (Demanche *et al.*, 2001). The human pathogen is now known as *P. jirovecii*, whereas the rat pathogen is known as *P. carinii*; however, nomenclature for pneumocystis organisms identified in nonhuman primates is under review. Pneumocystis is ubiquitous in the environment and a recent study indicated that 70 of 74 (95%) healthy, asymptomatic, cynomolgus macaques had antibodies to the Pneumocystis HEX1 protein (Kling *et al.*, 2009). Pneumocystosis has been reported in nonhuman primates with debilitation due to recent importation, bacterial infection, neoplasia, or immuno-deficiency associated with retroviral infection (Poelma, 1975; Chandler *et al.*, 1976; Letvin *et al.*, 1983; Kestler *et al.*, 1990; Lowenstine *et al.*, 1992). *Pneumocystis* spp. infections have also occurred as an endemic infection within a colony of tamarins, *Saguinus fuscicollis* and *S. oedipus* (Richter *et al.*, 1978). Epizoological studies in SIV-infected macaques indicate that infection is usually acquired during progressive immunodeficiency from infected contacts rather than through reactivation of latent infections (Vogel *et al.*, 1993).

b. Disease

Clinical signs included progressive weight loss, anorexia, and failure to thrive. Chimpanzees with pneumocystosis and erythroleukemia developed anorexia, pyrexia, dyspnea, cyanosis, and pneumonia (Chandler *et al.*, 1976). Thoracic radiographs revealed extensive infiltrates in the lung lobes. A compensatory polycythemia may be recognized in immunodeficient rhesus macaques and often precedes the development of respiratory signs. Pneumocystosis should be considered in an immune-compromised animal with dyspnea or other indication of pulmonary disease. Overt dyspnea is a late manifestation of infection and is often preceded by elevations in hematocrit and progressive weight loss. Once dyspnea is recognized, disease is advanced.

c. Pathology

Gross lesions attributable to pneumocystosis include partial lung collapse; firm, rubbery lungs with multiple 1- to 2-mm gray nodules throughout the lungs; and multifocal or diffuse consolidation with subpleural hemorrhages (Chandler *et al.*, 1976; Richter *et al.*, 1978). Pneumocystosis is characterized by multiple foci in which alveoli are filled with granular, eosinophilic foamy material (Chandler *et al.*, 1976) accompanied by variable type II pneumocyte hyperplasia and is best confirmed by immunohistochemistry if needed (Mansfield *et al.*, 2014) (Fig. 17.23). Interstitial pneumonia with a mononuclear cell infiltrate occurred in chimpanzees and tamarins. Silver or periodic acid–Schiff stains revealed cystic *Pneumocystis* spp. within a honeycomb matrix. Organisms were dark brown to black, round, ovoid, or cup-shaped cysts, 4–6 μm in diameter.

d. Diagnosis and Treatment

Diagnosis and treatment of *Pneumocystis* infection is usually based upon characteristic histologic lesions as this pathogen represents the most common opportunistic infection in macaques infected with the simian immunodeficiency virus. *Ante mortem* diagnosis can be made by serology or PCR. Organisms can also be identified by silver or periodic acid–Schiff's stains of sputum or biopsy samples. Trimethoprim-sulfamethoxazole can be used in SIV-infected macaques to prevent overt disease but does not curtail colonization by the organism (Kling *et al.*, 2009).

2. *Dermatophytosis*

Dermatophytosis or ringworm occurs rarely in nonhuman primates and is caused by organisms of the genera *Microsporum* and *Trichophyton*. Lesions include baldness, typical circular or ring-shaped lesions, generalized scaly skin at lesion sites, and patchy hair loss to generalized alopecia (Al-Doory, 1972). *M. canis* has been isolated from New World monkeys (Kaplan *et al.*, 1957), a rhesus monkey (Baker *et al.*, 1971), and a chimpanzee (Klokke and deVries, 1963). *T. mentagrophytes* has been recovered from rhesus monkeys (Hauck and Klehr, 1977) and capuchins (Bagnall and Grunberg, 1972). An epizootic of ringworm caused by *T. violaceum* occurred in 60 baboons housed in the same cage in Sukhumi (Voronin *et al.*, 1948). The

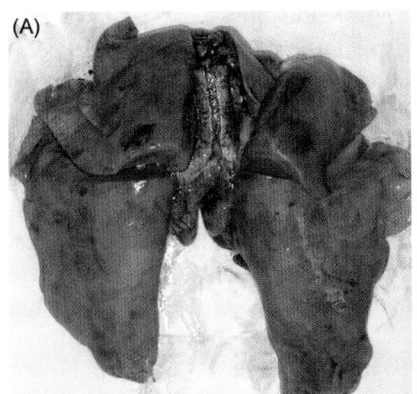
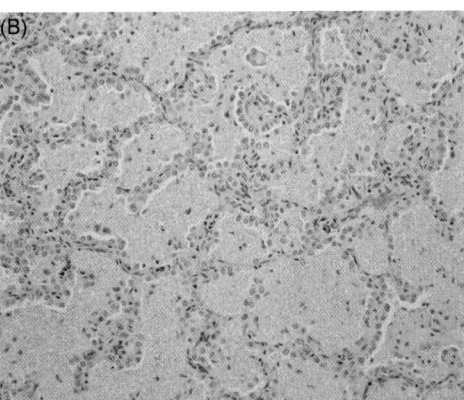
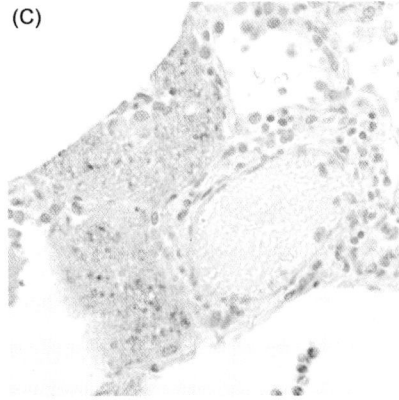

FIGURE 17.23 *Pneumocystis sp.* Diffuse interstitial pneumocystis pneumonia in SIV-infected rhesus macaque (A). Eosinophilic foamy material filling alveolar spaces with marked type 2 pneumocyte hyperplasia (B). Immunohistochemistry for pneumocystis demonstrating cysts within foamy material (C).

source of infection was believed to be dogs previously held in the cage.

3. Systemic

a. Coccidioidomycosis

Pathogenesis *Coccidiodes immitis* is commonly found in the soil in certain parts of the southwestern United States, northern Mexico, and parts of Central and South America. Infections with *C. immitis* have been reported in baboons, macaques, and apes (Migaki, 1986).

Disease Clinical signs associated with respiratory disease included nasal discharge, cough, and dyspnea. Vertebral *C. immitis* infection in a baboon resulted in lameness and reluctance to move (Rosenberg *et al.*, 1984); and in a rhesus monkey, characterized by altered gait leading to paralysis (Castleman *et al.*, 1980). In all reports, affected monkeys and apes had a history of outdoor housing in California, Texas, and Arizona (Hoffman *et al.*, 2007).

Pathology *C. immitis* infections usually result in disseminated disease, with lesions most frequently found in the lung and vertebrae (Migaki, 1986). Firm white nodules, partial or complete collapse of a lung lobe, pleural adhesions, and cavitations are common lesions (Breznock *et al.*, 1975; Castleman *et al.*, 1980; Bellini *et al.*, 1991). The hilar lymph nodes may be enlarged. Paravertebral masses or abscesses with invasion into the vertebrae and spinal cord were reported in monkeys with lameness or paralysis. Microscopic lesions are typically pyogranulomas bordered by multinucleated giant cells. Lesions contain thick-walled spherules 10–60 μm in diameter filled with 2- to 4-μm round endospores (Fig. 17.24).

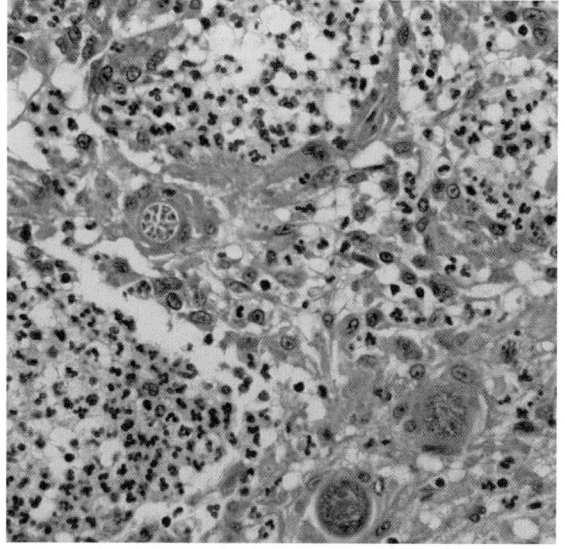

FIGURE 17.24 *Coccidioides immitis*: pyogranulomatous pneumonia with thick-walled fungal cysts in a rhesus macaque.

Diagnosis Radiography can reveal severe pulmonary disease with multiple cavitary lesions or lysis of vertebral bone. Serologic testing for specific antibody by complement fixation or tube precipitin test, or skin testing, may be helpful in reaching a diagnosis. A Gomori methenamine silver (GMS) stain can be used to confirm the presence of coccidioides organisms within the biopsy specimens.

b. Histoplasmosis

Spontaneous histoplasmosis due to *Histoplasma capsulatum* var. *capsulatum* has been reported in a squirrel monkey with granulomatous pneumonia, hepatitis, and splenitis (Bergeland *et al.*, 1970), an owl monkey (Weller *et al.*, 1990), and a rhesus monkey infected with SIV (Baskin, 1991). The owl monkey presented with weight loss and splenomegaly and had neutropenia, eosinophilia, hypercalcemia, hypercholesterolemia, and hypophosphatemia. The rhesus monkey had diarrhea, weight loss, anorexia, and dyspnea. Marked splenomegaly and enlargement of the mesenteric lymph nodes were found at necropsy (Baskin, 1991). In the rhesus monkey, there was diffuse histiocytosis of many organs, including intestines, mesenteric and peripheral lymph nodes, spleen, liver, adrenal gland, and bone marrow. Disseminated microgranulomas with multinucleated Langhans'-type giant cells were seen microscopically in affected abdominal viscera and lymph nodes of the owl and squirrel monkeys. Small yeasts, 2–4 μm in diameter, with a thin cell wall and a central basophilic structure, were found in the cytoplasm of macrophages or giant cells.

H. capsulatum var. *duboisii* is the etiological agent of African or large-form histoplasmosis. The agent is indigenous to Africa, but infection has been spread among feral-born and laboratory-born baboons in Texas (Butler and Hubbard, 1991). Direct contact with infected baboons through grooming or licking of skin lesions appeared to be the most likely mode of transmission in this epizootic. Lesions were usually confined to the skin, especially surfaces that contacted the ground, such as hands, buttocks, and tail, but also occurred on the face, ears, and scrotum. Papules, pustules 5–10 mm in diameter, or ulcerative granulomas 1–2 cm in diameter were common (Butler *et al.*, 1988; Butler and Hubbard, 1991). Radiography may reveal osteolytic lesions in the skull, digits, and vertebrae underlying affected areas of skin. Numerous discrete, elevated, and ulcerated skin lesions on the face, ears, hands, feet, tail and/or perineum, and rarely, the torso, were found at necropsy. Enlargement of superficial and retroperitoneal lymph nodes, particularly those draining areas with skin lesions, was also noted (Butler and Hubbard, 1991). Extension of cutaneous lesions to underlying bone resulted in osteolysis (Walker and

Spooner, 1960; Butler et al., 1988; Butler and Hubbard, 1991).

Pyogranulomatous inflammation of the dermis and subcutaneous tissues with marked histiocytic infiltrates, large numbers of both Langhans' and foreign body-type multinucleated giant cells, and neutrophils was reported by Butler and Hubbard (1991). Numerous intracellular and extracellular, 8- to 15-μm, uninucleate yeast cells were found throughout the lesions. Diagnosis of *H. capsulatum* var. *duboisii* can be made based on the characteristic appearance of the organism and resultant tissue inflammation (Butler and Hubbard, 1991). Antifungal therapy has been ineffective. Surgical excision of lesions was effective in eliminating infection from 13 baboons.

c. Candidiasis

Pathogenesis Candidiasis is caused by yeast of the genus *Candida*, usually *C. albicans*, a normal saprophytic inhabitant of the mucous membranes of the alimentary and genital tracts, and skin of nonhuman primates (Migaki et al., 1982). Predisposing factors for clinical candidiasis include antibiotic therapy, recent importation, retroviral infection, routine oral gavage, or parasitism (Migaki et al., 1982; Tucker, 1984; Lowenstine et al., 1992).

Disease Anorexia, dysphagia, open-mouth breathing due to ulcers of the hard palate, dehydration, and diarrhea are associated with candidiasis (Kaufmann and Quist, 1969b; Wikse et al., 1970; Weller, 1994). Onychomycosis, with shortening, erosion, and deformation of the nails, and balanitis have also been associated with candidiasis (Kerber et al., 1968; Wikse et al., 1970).

Pathology Pseudomembrane formation results from candidial overgrowth. White or creamy plaques are found on the tongue, buccal cavity, esophagus, and intestine. Large clusters of pseudohyphae and blastospores, 3–5 μm in diameter, are seen in the superficial portion of the epithelial mucosae (Migaki et al., 1982). Pseudomembranes are composed of degenerate and sloughed epithelial cells, neutrophilic infiltrates, and numerous yeasts. Necrosis and ulceration result from deep invasion of the epithelium and lamina propria.

Diagnosis and Treatment Because *Candida* are normal flora of the gastrointestinal and genital tract, culture alone is not sufficient for diagnosis. Wet mounts of scrapings from lesions in 10% NaOH, 20% KOH, or lactophenol cotton blue can be used to demonstrate yeasts and hyphae. Gram-stained smears from lesions reveal Gram-positive oval and budding yeast cells. Examination of tissue sections is most valuable for diagnosis in that tissue invasion can be demonstrated. Oral nystatin suspension is an effective treatment for lesions of the oral cavity or digestive system.

d. Cryptococcosis

Pathogenesis Cryptococcosis is a systemic infection of humans and animals caused by a yeast-like fungus, *Cryptococcus neoformans*. Transmission is usually by inhalation of spores but also occurs as a result of direct contact. Cryptococcosis has been described in New and Old World monkeys (Migaki et al., 1982).

Disease Clinical signs vary as infection is usually disseminated. CNS signs include depression (Miller and Boever, 1983), seizures, and blindness (Sly et al., 1977). A squirrel monkey developed a deforming mass of the lower jaw, weight loss, and leukopenia with lymphopenia and anemia (Roussilhon et al., 1987).

Pathology There are two general forms of gross lesions: a gelatinous mass loosely organized with no defined capsule, or a solid, granulomatous mass. Emaciation, splenomegaly, granulomatous pneumonia, and lymphadenopathy involving the hilar or peripheral lymph nodes are common features (Sly et al., 1977; Roussilhon et al., 1987). Histologically large, irregularly sized yeast cells with an abundant polysaccharide capsule occur singly, in small aggregates, or in large masses. The degree and type of inflammation ranges from none to acute or granulomatous.

Diagnosis Cytologic evaluation of cutaneous masses or spinal fluid can provide rapid diagnosis of cryptococcal infection. India-ink preparations allow visualization of the organism against a black background but are not diagnostic unless budding is observed.

C. Viral Diseases

1. DNA Viruses

The herpesviridae are double-stranded DNA viruses that include many important pathogens of primates. The family Herpesviridae is divided into three subfamilies: Alphaherpesvirinae, Betaherpesvirinae, and Gammaherpesvirinae.

a. Alphaherpesvirinae

Viruses in the subfamily Alphaherpesvirinae commonly cause subclinical infection in the natural host. Viral infections are persistent and latent resulting in lifelong infection. Clinical disease, when present, is usually self-limiting and consists of oral or genital vesicles that resolve over time (Table 17.48). Systemic, fatal disease occurs on rare occasion in the natural host. Disease is much more severe when an alphaherpesvirus infects an aberrant host; often infection is fulminating, systemic, and fatal. This is a common feature of infection of an aberrant host by a neurotropic simplex virus as nonhuman primates that are infected with a human herpes simplex virus often die from a fatal encephalitis (Hunt and Melendez, 1966; Huemer, et al., 2002; Mätz-Rensing

TABLE 17.48　Alphaherpesviruses: Disease in Host Species

	Host/reservoir	Synonyms	Lesions in host species
Macacine herpesvirus 1	Macaque	Herpes B, Herpes simiae, B virus	Common, usually subclinical, latent infection
			Virus shed in oral or genital secretions
			Transmitted by biting, sexual behavior, fomites
			Disease usually self-limiting with vesicles and ulcers of the oral and genital mucosa, resolved in 10–14 days
			Rare systemic infections are fatal
			Multifocal, necrotizing hepatitis[a]
			Hemorrhagic interstitial pneumonia[b]
			Intranuclear inclusion bodies in endothelial cells
Papiine herpesvirus 2	Baboon	Herpes papionus	Common subclinical, latent infection in baboons
		Herpesvirus papio 2	
Cercopithecine herpesvirus 2	African green monkey	SA 8	Virus shed in genital and oral secretions
			Venereal transmission[c]
			Small vesicles or pustules on genital or less commonly oral mucosa with primary infection or recrudescence
			Severe genital lesions may occur[c]
Cercopithecine herpesvirus 9	Unknown	Simian varicellovirus	Neutralizing antibodies found in stump-tailed macaques with no history of clinical disease[d]
	Macaque monkeys	Simian varicella	
Saimiriine herpesvirus 1	Squirrel monkey	Herpes tamarinus	Usually no clinical disease, latent infection, shed in saliva
		Herpes T	
		Herpes platyrrhinae	Ulcerative stomatitis[e]
Human herpesvirus 1, 2	Human	Herpes hominus	Common, symptomatic infection with latency
		Herpes simplex	HSV-1 oral lesions and/or encephalitis
			HSV-2 sexually transmitted, genital lesions in adults and disseminated disease in children

[a]From Simon et al. (1993).
[b]From Espana (1973).
[c]From Levin et al. (1988).
[d]From Mansfield and King (1998).
[e]From King et al. (1967).

et al., 2003) (Fig. 17.25). An exception to this is infection of apes with human herpesviruses 1, 2, or 3, which are usually self-limiting (McClure and Keeling, 1971; Mansfield and King, 1998). Clinical signs and lesions of alphaherpesvirus infection in aberrant primate hosts are found in Table 17.48.

I. SIMPLEX VIRUS

Pathogenesis Macacine herpesvirus 1 (McHV-1), also known as *Cercopithecine herpesvirus* 1, herpesvirus simiae, or B virus, causes a persistent, subclinical latent infection in macaques, the natural host species (Elmore and Eberle, 2008). B virus is horizontally transmitted among socially housed macaques by mucous membrane contact with contaminated oral, ocular, or genital secretions. The prevalence of B virus in an affected population increases in an age-dependent manner, with peak seroconversion occurring at 2–4 years of age (Weigler et al., 1990; Weigler, 1992).

Disease In the macaque host, primary infection may be associated with vesicular lesions at the site of exposure resulting frequently in stomatitis, conjunctivitis, vaginitis, or balanoposthitis. In most cases, this primary infection is rapidly controlled and the virus invades axons and is transported retrograde to the associated sensory ganglion where a lifelong infection is established. Reactivation of the latent infection may occur with axonal transport of the virus to a mucosal surface, and viral replication and shedding into the environment. This shedding may or may not be associated

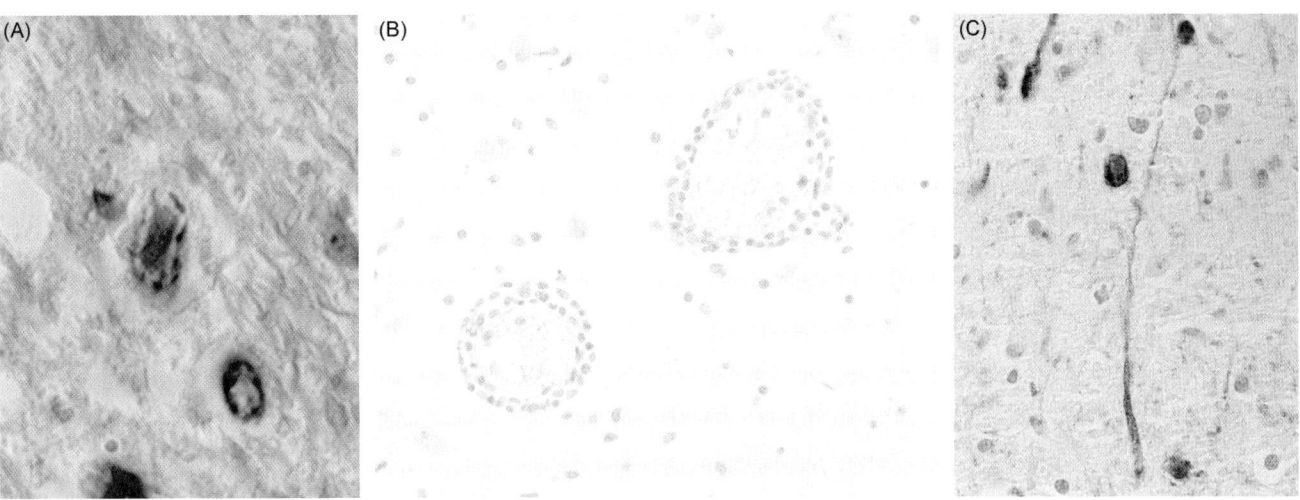

FIGURE 17.25   Human herpes virus 1 (herpes simplex virus 1). Intranuclear inclusion body within the CNS of a common marmoset (A) with nonsuppurative meningoencephalitis (B). Herpes simplex 1 antigen with neurons (C).

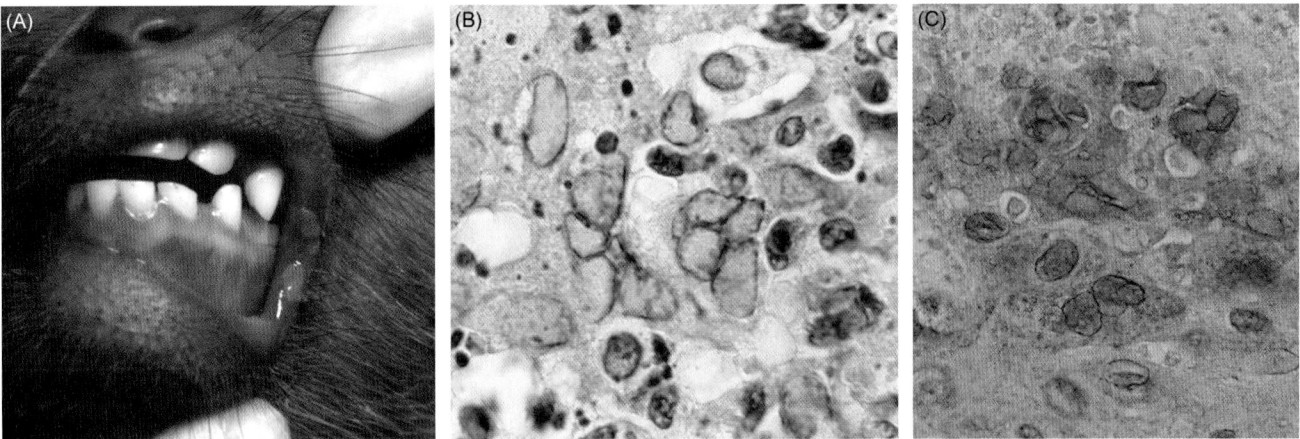

FIGURE 17.26   Macacine herpes virus 1 (monkey B virus). Thin-walled vesicles at the commissures of the lips of a pig tail macaque (A). Multinucleated syncytial cells with intranuclear inclusions (B) positive for alphaherpesvirus antigen (C).

with clinical signs. Rarely, severe infection may occur in neonates or immunocompromised animals (Anderson *et al.*, 1994; Chellman *et al.*, 1992). In such cases, dissemination to multiple organs including the lungs, liver, and CNS may occur. Dissemination without mucosal lesions has been described and presents a diagnostic challenge (Simon *et al.*, 1993). Histologically, necrosis with viral syncytia and intranuclear inclusions are observed (Fig. 17.26).

Diagnosis   Serological testing is commonly used in the diagnosis and management of B virus infection in macaques and may be performed with B virus whole virus antigens or recombinant proteins (Khan *et al.*, 2006; Katz *et al.*, 2012). Due to biosafety concerns, surrogate alphaherpesviruses can also be used as antigens for serology testing (Ohsawa *et al.*, 1999; Yamamoto *et al.*,

2005). Serological testing has high sensitivity for detection of B virus in groups of animals but must be interpreted with caution in individual animals. Serological results in an individual animal should be interpreted with knowledge of the serostatus of all contact animals. If seronegative animals have recently been housed with seropositive animals, all should be considered potentially infected. Culture of mucous membranes and PCR performed on secretions have value in the detection of shedding but have limited sensitivity in determining whether an individual animal is infected as false-negative test results are common.

Human Health Concern   B virus was first described in 1934 by Albert Sabin when the virus was cultured from tissues obtained from a young physician; Dr. W.B. died of encephalomyelitis approximately 2 weeks after being bitten by an apparently normal rhesus macaque (Sabin and Wright, 1934). Human infection by B virus is a major zoonotic concern when working with macaques as it causes a disseminated viral infection in humans, resulting in ascending paralysis, encephalitis, and death in about 70% of cases (Weigler, 1992; Cohen *et al.*, 2002; Huff *et al.*, 2003). Contact with monkey saliva, tissues, or tissue fluids is the most common route of transmission and transmission may occur through bites, scratches or fomites. Person-to-person transmission has been reported in one instance (CDCP, 1987). In 1997, death of a technician resulted from an ocular splash of material from a rhesus monkey (CDCP, 1998). Because of the number of human cases and the high fatality rate of this zoonotic disease, guidelines for protective clothing and procedures for handling macaques have been published (CDCP, 1987, 1998; Cohen *et al.*, 2002). In addition, specific postexposure procedures for wound cleansing, sample collection, risk assessment, and post- exposure prophylaxis have been listed in Table 17.36. All facilities that house macaque species or utilize their biological specimens should have a B virus prevention and control program in place. Of critical importance is risk assessment and postexposure management by a physician with knowledge and experience with B virus. Specific-pathogen-free (SPF) colonies of macaques have been developed that are free of B virus as well as several selected retroviruses (Buchl *et al.*, 1997; Hilliard and Ward, 1999). Separation of seronegative animals from the source colony at approximately 1 year of age and repeated quarterly testing has been used successfully (Morton *et al.*, 2008). However, all macaques regardless of their SPF status should be handled as if they are potentially infected with B virus and appropriate precautions must be taken.

II. VARICELLOVIRUS

Pathogenesis The species *Cercopithecine herpesvirus 9* composes a group of viruses in the genus *Varicellovirus* known as simian varicella that were first described in the late 1960s and early 1970s as a cause of severe epizootics in several species of African and Asian monkeys (Gray, 2010). The reservoir host has not been identified; however, serum-neutralizing antibodies have been detected in stump-tailed macaques (*Macaca arctoides*) with no history of clinical disease (Mansfield and King, 1998) and reactivation of latent infection has been demonstrated in immunocompromised macaques (Kolappaswamy *et al.*, 2007; Schoeb *et al.*, 2008).

Disease The disease in aberrant hosts, including African and Asian monkey species, is characterized by the development of a vesicular dermatitis progressing to death within 48 h. Involvement of the hands and feet is rare. Disseminated infection affects the lungs, liver, and gastrointestinal tract and is often associated with vesiculating hemorrhagic lesions (Table 17.49).

Pathology Histologically, vesicles in skin and mucosal surfaces are observed with viral syncytia and intranuclear inclusions evident (Fig. 17.27). In severe cases, vesicles may be blood filled and these changes are accompanied by multifocal to coalescing necrosis in the liver, lung, and lymphoid organs.

Diagnosis and Treatment Diagnosis of simian varicella can be accomplished by serologic assays for antibodies such as IFA, ELISA, or multiplexed fluorometric immunoassay (MFIA), or by demonstrating the presence of viral DNA by PCR. Immunohistochemistry can be used to visualize virus proteins in biopsy specimens. Acyclovir and interferon have been used to treat experimental disease and might be considered in epizootics (Soike *et al.*, 1984). Simian varicella has no known zoonotic potential but must be distinguished from alphaherpesviruses like B virus and members of the poxviridae family, which may have similar presentations.

b. Betaherpesvirinae

Within the subfamily Betaherpesvirinae, cytomegaloviruses (CMVs) commonly occur in humans and nonhuman primate species but rarely cause overt disease in the natural host. These viruses have a narrow host range, although interspecies transmission has been documented (Swack and Hsuing, 1982). Virus is transmitted horizontally in the blood, saliva, milk, urine, and semen (Asher *et al.*, 1974) and by 1 year of age, most animals will have asymptomatically acquired the infection and will be seropositive. Clinical disease is associated with intrauterine infection or immunosuppression (Haustein *et al.*, 2008). In macaques infected with SIV, rhesus CMV (Macacine herpesvirus 3) reactivation results in necrotizing encephalitis, enteritis, lymphadenitis, and/or interstitial pneumonia (Baskin, 1987). Reactivation of latent infection is common in animals on immunosuppressive therapy and results in fatal disseminated disease (Haustein *et al.*, 2008). Choice of immunosuppressive drugs may influence reactivation of the level of CMV viremia and valganciclovir may be used to prevent onset of severe disease (Han *et al.*, 2010). Histologically, neutrophilic infiltrates are observed with large cytomegalic cells containing intranuclear and intracytoplasmic viral inclusions (Hutto *et al.*, 2004) (Fig. 17.28). While these findings are diagnostic, immunohistochemistry may be used to confirm infection (Mansfield *et al.*, 2014).

c. Gammaherpesvirinae

The subfamily Gammaherpesvirinae includes two genera of interest, *Lymphocryptovirus* and *Rhadinovirus*, both of which contain species known to infect nonhuman primates.

I. LYMPHOCRYPTOVIRUSES

Pathogenesis The lymphocryptoviruses (LCVs) include a large number of viruses related to human

TABLE 17.49   Alphaherpesviruses: Disease in Aberrant Host Species

Virus	Species aberrantly infected	Disease and lesions
Macacine herpesvirus 1	Human[a]	Vesicular dermatitis ± pruritis at inoculation site 3–24 days post-exposure Lymphangitis and lymphadenopathy 'Flulike' symptoms: fever, conjunctivitis, paresthesia, muscle weakness Neurologic symptoms, coma, death and necrotizing encephalitis
Cercopithecine herpesvirus 2	None reported	
Cercopithecine herpesvirus 9	African green monkey[b] Patas monkey Macaque	Disseminated vesicular exanthema; death in 48h High morbidity and mortality; in some cases associated with recent importation Latent infection with reactivation demonstrated in African green monkeys[c] Disseminated infection with necrotizing lesions in the lung, liver, and gastrointestinal tract Cowdry type A intranuclear inclusion bodies
Saimiriine herpesvirus 1	Owl monkey[d] Marmoset Tamarin	Inadvertant exposure to host species Vesicular oral, labial, and/or dermal lesions 7–10 days post-infection Pruritis, anorexia, depression; with death in 24–48h; high morbidity and mortality Necrosis of epidermis, oral, and gastrointestinal mucosa; multifocal hepatic necrosis Cowdry type A intranuclear inclusion bodies; multinucleate giant cells in epidermis; modified live vaccine can cause outbreaks of disease[e]
Human herpesvirus 1, 2	Ape	Mild, usually self-limiting oral vesicular disease; fatal meningoencephalitis reported in gibbons[f]
	Owl monkey[g] Tamarin (experimental)[h]	Fatal, disseminated infection similar to that caused by Saimiirine herpesvirus 1, more common severe facial lesions, with blepharitis and stomatitis; encephalitis, more common Distinguish by virus isolation and identification Modified live vaccine developed and protective for owl monkeys[i]
Human herpesvirus 3 (may be simian in origin)	Ape[j]	Mild, self-limiting vesicular dermatitis

[a]*From McChesney* et al. *(1989) and Weigler (1992).*
[b]*From Clarkson* et al. *(1967), Felsenfeld and Schmidt (1975), Wenner* et al. *(1977).*
[c]*From Soike* et al. *(1984).*
[d]*From Hunt and Melendez (1966).*
[e]*From Asher* et al. *(1974).*
[f]*From Smith* et al. *(1969), Landolfi* et al. *(2005).*
[g]*From Melendez* et al. *(1970).*
[h]*From Felsburg* et al. *(1973).*
[i]*From Daniel* et al. *(1978).*
[j]*From McClure and Keeling (1971).*

Epstein–Barr virus (EBV) that infect both New and Old World primates. These viruses are species specific. As with the betaherpesviruses, subclinical infection with LCV is common by 1 year of age and seropositive animals remain infected for life.

Disease In immunocompromised animals, LCV may cause lymphoid and epithelial proliferative lesions (Table 17.50). Coinfections with rhesus LCV (Macacine herpesvirus 4) and SIV in macaques have been associated with malignant B cell lymphomas and oral lesions resembling hairy leukoplakia (Feichtinger *et al.*, 1992; Baskin *et al.*, 1995). A posttransplantation lymphoproliferative disorder has been described in cynomolgus macaques following renal transplantation and has a predilection for extranodal involvement (Schmidtko *et al.*, 2002; Page *et al.*, 2013).

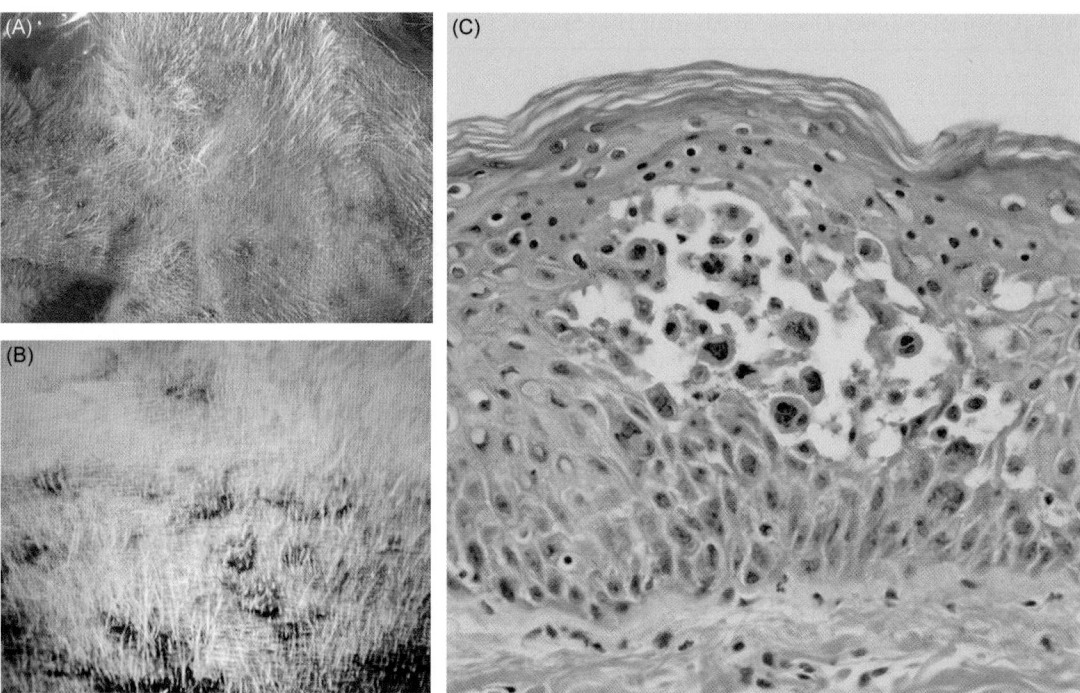

FIGURE 17.27   Cercopithicine herpesvirus 9 (simian varicella virus). Simian varicella virus cutaneous exanthema (A) with blood filled vesicles (B). Vesicle within haired skin demonstrating multinucleated syncytia and intranuclear inclusions (C).

Diagnosis   *Ante mortem* diagnosis can be made by serology or PCR assays of serum or whole blood, respectively. Immunohistochemistry for viral proteins EBNA2 and BZLF1 can be done on biopsy specimens to confirm infection and establish an etiologic diagnosis (Mansfield *et al.*, 2014).

II.   RHADINOVIRUSES *Rhadinovirus* is the second genus in the Gammaherpesvirinae subfamily that can infect nonhuman primates. Both rhesus rhadinovirus and retroperitoneal fibromatosis-associated herpesvirus (RFHV) are widespread in macaque colonies but are not often associated with disease (White *et al.*, 2009, 2011). RFHV has been detected in a mesenchymal proliferative disease termed retroperitoneal fibromatosis (RF) in association with SRV infections (Stromberg *et al.*, 1984; Bosch *et al.*, 1999) (Fig. 17.29). RF, once common in macaque colonies with high SRV infection rates, causes mesenchymal proliferations originating at the root of the mesentery and eventually engulfing the abdominal organs into a solid mass. This condition is now rare, likely due to the control of SRV in captive macaque colonies. RFHV has also been associated with gastrointestinal stromal cell-like tumors in SIV-infected macaques (Bruce *et al.*, 2006).

Rhadinoviruses have been found in New World monkeys. Herpesvirus saimiri (Saimiriine herpesvirus 2) and herpesvirus ateles (Ateline herpesvirus 2 and 3) cause limited disease in their natural hosts, the squirrel monkey and spider monkey (Fig. 17.30). Cross-species transmission to Callitrichids or owl monkeys results in the rapid onset of malignant lymphoma (Fig. 17.31).

d.   Poxviruses

The family Poxviridae contains a number of important viruses that infect nonhuman primates. The genus *Orthopoxvirus* contains the cowpox and monkeypox viruses, which are maintained in the environment in rodent reservoirs. Cross-species transmission to nonhuman primates resulting in epizootics, which may be of high morbidity and mortality, has been described (Damon, 2011). Recent outbreaks with cowpox have been recognized in New World monkeys housed in a zoological setting (Mätz-Rensing *et al.*, 2006). Clinical presentation includes the development of a papular rash progressing to umbilicated pox lesions often first observed on the extremities. In severe cases, dissemination to multiple organs including the lungs and gastrointestinal tract can be observed. The development of hemorrhage in association with these lesions is a poor prognostic sign and histologically infected cells contain large brightly eosinophilic intracytoplasmic inclusions termed Guarnieri bodies. Other genera within the poxviridae family produce distinct syndromes including the development of small to large skin masses with Yaba virus infection and small, raised proliferative lesions on the face as seen with molluscum contagiosum (Table 17.51). Primate poxviruses can be infectious to humans (Grace and Mirand, 1965; Hutin *et al.*, 2001; Reynolds,

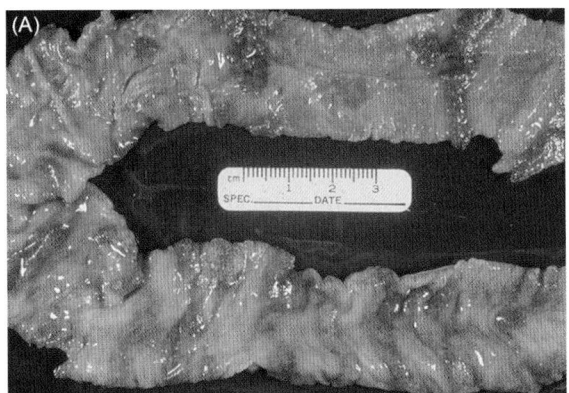

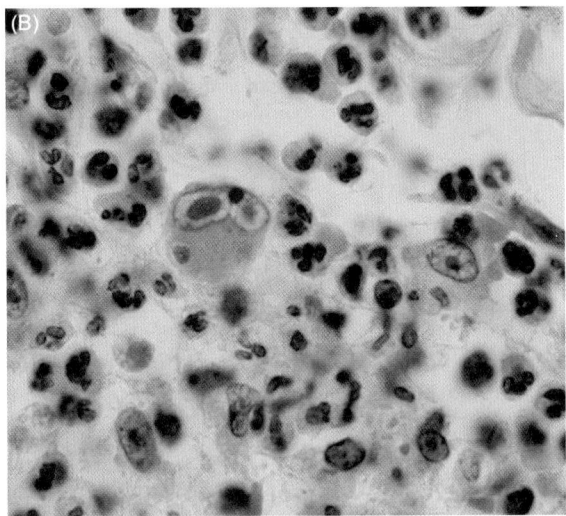

FIGURE 17.28 Rhesus cytomegalovirus (RhCMV) necrotizing colitis (A); cytomegalic cell with large intranuclear inclusions and neutrophilic infiltrates (B).

et al., 2007). Zoonotic disease is usually self-limiting; however, monkeypox infection has caused fatalities in children. Human-to-human transmission is rare.

e. Other DNA Viruses

Adenoviruses have been isolated from both apes and New and Old World monkeys, both from clinically affected and healthy animals (Wevers *et al.*, 2011). Subclinical infection is common in nonhuman primates. Clinical disease may be enteric or respiratory depending on viral tropism. Animals with enteric disease may develop diarrhea, which resolves in 10–14 days. Variably sized intranuclear inclusion bodies can be visualized in enterocytes (Fig. 17.32). Virus can be shed several weeks after clinical recovery. Severe disease may occur in immunocompromised animals and may disseminate to the liver and/or pancreas (Fig. 17.32). Adenovirus-induced necrotizing pancreatitis has been reported in immunocompromised macaques with natural or experimental retroviral infections (Chandler and McClure,

1982; Martin *et al.*, 1991). Diarrhea and death occurred in these monkeys. Sneezing, coughing, and rapid respiration can occur in clinical adenovirus respiratory tract infections with dyspnea and cyanosis developing in severe infections. Adults with respiratory disease usually recover in 7–10 days. Mortality is low except in neonates with secondary bacterial infections that contribute to mortality.

A member of the family Polyomaviridae, simian virus 40 (SV40), is a common latent viral infection of Asian macaques (Eddy *et al.*, 1961; Norkin, 1976; Strickler *et al.*, 1998). The virus was originally isolated from rhesus macaque kidney cell cultures used for production of polio vaccine (Strickler *et al.*, 1998). SV40 transforms cells *in vitro* and is oncogenic when inoculated into hamsters (Eddy *et al.*, 1961). Clinical disease in macaques is rare and results from reactivation of latent infection, usually due to immunosuppression associated with SIV infection or immunomodulatory therapy, where lesions of the CNS, kidney and/or lung may be observed (Horvath *et al.*, 1992). Lesions include demyelination in the cerebral white matter and subependymal areas, chronic tubulointerstitial nephritis with hypertrophy/hyperplasia of collecting tubule epithelium, and proliferative interstitial pneumonia (Mansfield and King, 1998). The CNS lesion resembles progressive multifocal leukoencephalopathy of human beings and is observed in SIV-infected rhesus macaques. Intranuclear inclusion bodies are found in affected areas.

Papillomavirus infections and associated dermal or oral lesions have been diagnosed in macaques and chimpanzees. In chimpanzees, focal epithelial hyperplasia, characterized by the development of multiple sessile well-circumscribed proliferative structures in the oral mucosa, is associated with papillomavirus infection. These masses are small (≤0.5 cm) and may persist for extended periods and then undergo spontaneous regression (Glad and Nesland, 1995). Papillomavirus infection of macaques is common and multiple serotypes may persist within colonies over time with at least 12 genotypes identified in macaques. These viruses tend to infect animals in an anatomically site-specific fashion and genital forms have been associated with cervical dysplasia and carcinomas in macaques and baboons (Wood *et al.*, 2004; Bergin *et al.*, 2012).

Three distinct members of the family Parvoviridae, and genus *Erythroparovirus* have been isolated from cynomolgus, rhesus, and pig-tailed macaques (*Macaca nemestrina*) with anemia (O'Sullivan *et al.*, 1994, 1996; Green *et al.*, 2000). Severe normocytic, normochromic anemia was reported for cynomolgus monkeys with parvovirus infection and concomitant SRV infection, and for cynomolgus monkeys with parvovirus infection in the high-dose test group of a drug safety study (O'Sullivan *et al.*, 1996). Similar lesions have been observed following

TABLE 17.50 Gammaherpesviruses

Virus	Synonym	Natural host	Aberrant host	Disease
Saimiriine herpesvirus 2	Herpesvirus saimiri 2	Squirrel monkey	Owl monkey Callitrichids Howler monkey Spider monkey	None Lymphoma or lymphocytic leukemia (experimental)[a] Naturally acquired disease rare in callitrichids T-cell origin Large, pleomorphic, histiocytic cells or well-differentiated lymphocytes
Ateline herpesvirus 2, 3	Herpesvirus ateles	Spider monkey	Owl monkey Callitrichids	None Lymphoma or leukemia (experimental)
Human herpesvirus 4	Epstein–Barr virus (EBV)	Human	New World monkeys	Asymptomatic or infectious mononucleosis Fever, pharyngitis, lymphadenopathy Circulating atypical lymphocytes Large cell lymphoma (experimental)[b] Callitrichids Malignant B-cell lymphoma (experimental)[e]
Panine herpesvirus 1	Chimpanzee herpes	Apes		None
Pongine herpesvirus 2	Orangutan herpes			
Gorilline herpesvirus 1	Gorilla herpes			
Macacine herpesvirus 4	Rhesus lymphocryptovirus		Rhesus	Subclinical infection common Coinfection with SIV: lymphoma in macaques or lesions resembling oral hairy leukoplakia[d]
Papiine herpesvirus 1	*Herpes papionis*		Baboon	Malignant lymphoma in baboons and macaques[c]
Cercopithecine herpesvirus 14	African green monkey EBV-like virus		Vervet	
Callitrichine herpesvirus 3	Marmoset lymphocryptovirus		Marmoset	Weight loss, inappetence and diarrhea. Firm mid-abdominal, B-cell lymphoma[f]

[a]From Melendez et al. (1970).
[b]From Cameron et al. (1987) and Neidobitek et al. (1994).
[c]From Deinhardt et al. (1978) and Rangan et al. (1995).
[d]From Baskin et al. (1995) and Feichtinger et al. (1992).
[e]From Miller et al. (1977).
[f]From Ramer et al.(2000) and Cho et al. (2001).

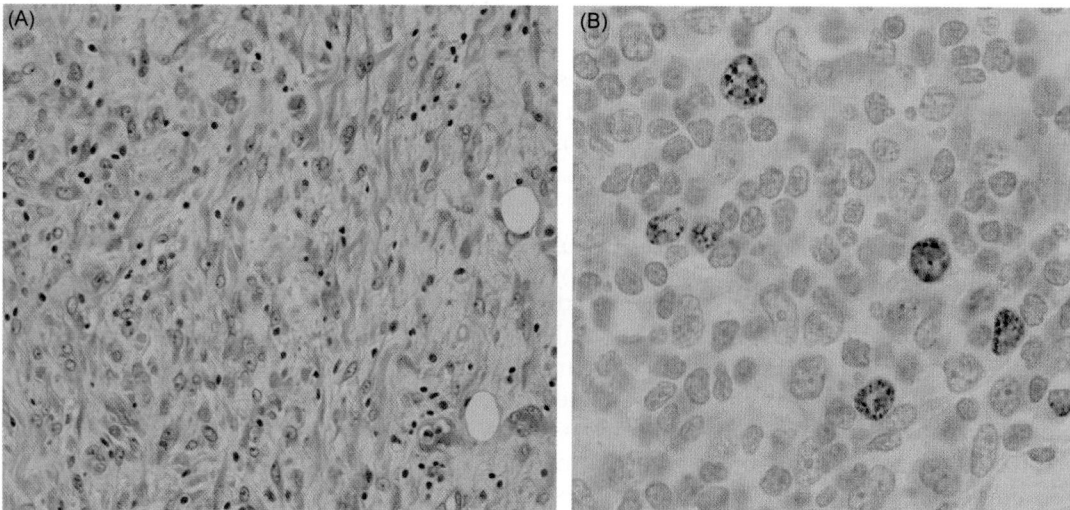

FIGURE 17.29 Rhesus retroperitoneal fibromatosis-associated herpes virus (RFHV). Pleomorphic spindle cells within retroperitoneal fibromatosis (A). RFHV-infected cells demonstrated by immunohistochemistry for latent nuclear antigen (LANA) (B).

the use of solid organ transplantation drug regimens (Schroder *et al.*, 2006). Experimental infection of cynomolgus monkeys with a parvovirus isolate resulted in mild anemia with destruction of erythroid cells in the bone marrow during peak viremia (O'Sullivan *et al.*, 1997). Rhesus parvovirus (RPV) can cause intranuclear inclusions within the erythroid precursors in bone marrow (Fig. 17.33).

2. RNA Viruses

a. Viruses Causing Hemorrhagic Fevers

Simian hemorrhagic fever virus (SHFV) is a highly contagious, fatal viral disease of macaques caused by an

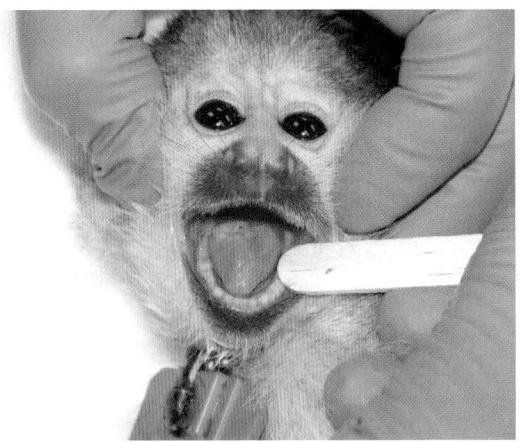

FIGURE 17.30 *Saimiri* spp. herpesvirus lesion by Julio C. Ruiz from the Michale E. Keeling Center for Comparative Medicine and Research at the University of Texas MD Anderson Cancer Center, Bastrop, TX.

arterivirus (Palmer *et al.*, 1968). Outbreaks have occurred in macaque colonies in the United States and Europe following exposure to infected blood or tissue from reservoir host species, usually patas monkeys (*Erythrocebus patas*). Infected macaques develop a bleeding diathesis that progresses to death. A lesion that distinguishes simian hemorrhagic fever from other hemorrhagic fevers in macaques is hemorrhagic necrosis of the proximal duodenum. Clinical and pathologic signs are summarized in Table 17.52.

Nonhuman primates serve as hosts for flaviviruses that can cause a hemorrhagic fever syndrome in human populations Carrion *et al.*, 2011). These diseases may be spread by arthropod vectors or be directly transmitted between mammalian hosts. Disease in the nonhuman primate host may be subclinical, or the host may develop fatal hemorrhagic disease (Table 17.53).

Two distinct groups of filoviruses are associated with hemorrhagic fever in humans and nonhuman primates (Table 17.54). In 1967, Marburg virus caused an outbreak of hemorrhagic fever in laboratory workers handling cell cultures from African green monkeys. Since then, small outbreaks of disease associated with this virus have been reported in Africa. Ebola virus is associated with hemorrhagic fever in humans, great apes and macaques. Four Ebola viruses, Zaire ebolavirus, Sudan ebolavirus, Bundibugyo ebolavirus, and Tai Forest ebolavirus have caused outbreaks in humans with mortality rates approaching 80%. The fruit bat (*Rousettus aegyptiacus*) is the likely reservoir species with primates and humans representing inadvertent hosts (Hayman *et al.*, 2010).

Reston ebolavirus was identified in newly imported cynomolgus macaques with high mortality due to

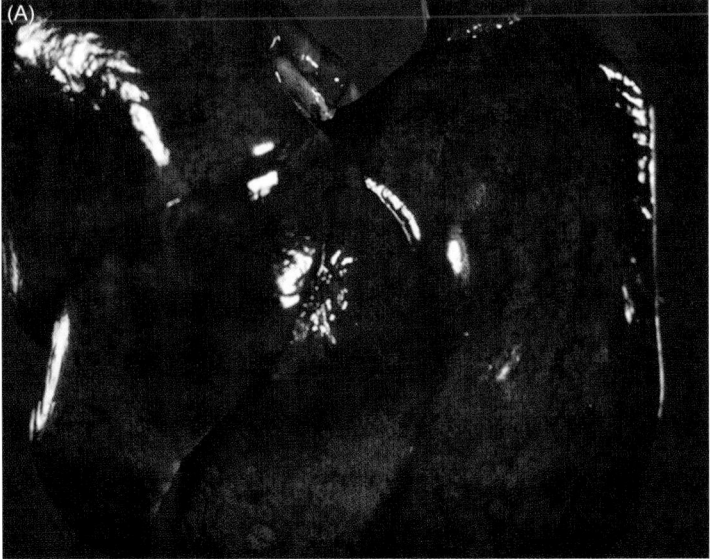
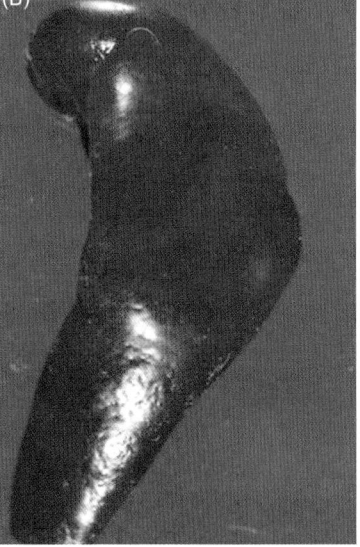

FIGURE 17.31 Saimiriine herpesvirus 2 (herpesvirus saimiri (HVS)): malignant lymphoma in the liver (A) and spleen (B) of HVS-infected owl monkey.

TABLE 17.51 Poxviruses

Virus	Host (naturally acquired disease)	Disease/lesions
Monkeypox	African green monkeys[a]	High prevalence of antibodies; no clinical disease
	Macaques[b]	Spread by aerosol, direct contact, and biting insects
	Apes	Viremia 3–4 days postinfection (pi); fever, anxiety, aggression
	Captive New World monkeys	Papules progress to vesicular rash 6–7 days pi with umbilication to classic pock lesion; buttocks, hands, and feet
		Dissemination to the lung, spleen, and mucous membranes
		Disease not always fatal, recovered monkeys immune
		Hemorrhagic necrosis of lungs
		Intracytoplasmic inclusion bodies
	Humans[c]	Sporadic outbreaks in Africa; human-to-human transmission rare
		Fatigue, fever, headache, back pain, lymphadenopathy
		Vesiculopapular rash over the face and body
		10–15% case fatality rate
		Vaccination against smallpox provides immunity
Yaba virus (Yaba monkey tumor virus)	Macaques, baboons[d]	Transmission unknown, suspect arthropod vector
		Subcutaneous masses of varying size on the feet, hands, and face
		Oral masses in baboons
		Large masses may ulcerate; masses regress in 6 weeks
		Nonencapsulated masses of large pleomorphic histiocytes ± large cytoplasmic inclusion bodies
	Humans	Pseudotumors ≤2 cm on the hands and feet
		Lymphadenopathy, fever
		Lesions regress in weeks
Tanapox	Humans[e]	Benign cutaneous skin infection in East Africa
		Fever for 2–3 days with headache, backache, and prostration
		One to two small papules on the face, extremities, or trunk; may umbilicate
	Macaques[f]	Small red papules develop 4–5 days pi on the face, thorax, and perineum
		Progress to 1 cm raised foci 14 days pi
		Papules become umbilicated, have red margins, and may ulcerate
		Resolve in 3–8 weeks
		Epidermal proliferation and ballooning degeneration
		Intracytoplasmic and intranuclear inclusion bodies
Marmoset poxvirus	*Callithrix jacchus*[g]	Papulovesicular disease lasting 4–6 weeks
		Not disseminated, not fatal
Molluscum contagiosum	Humans	Mildly contagious, chronic skin disease
		Multiple small skin tumors filled with waxy material
		Large central acanthocytes have cytoplasmic inclusion bodies
	Chimpanzees[h]	Small firm lesions with waxlike contents on the face and inguinal area
		Large intracytoplasmic inclusion bodies in lesions
Cowpox	*C. jacchus*[i]	Disseminated fatal infection
		Epidermal proliferation and ballooning degeneration
		Intracytoplasmic and intranuclear inclusion bodies

[a]*From Arita et al. (1972).*
[b]*From Mutombo et al. (1983).*
[c]*From McConnell et al. (1968), Arita et al. (1985), and Reynolds et al. (2007).*
[d]*From Downie (1974) and Bruestle et al. (1981).*
[e]*From Jezek et al. (1985), McNulty (1972).*
[f]*From Downie and Espana (1972).*
[g]*From Gough et al. (1982).*
[h]*From Douglas et al. (1967).*
[i]*From Mätz-Rensing (2006).*

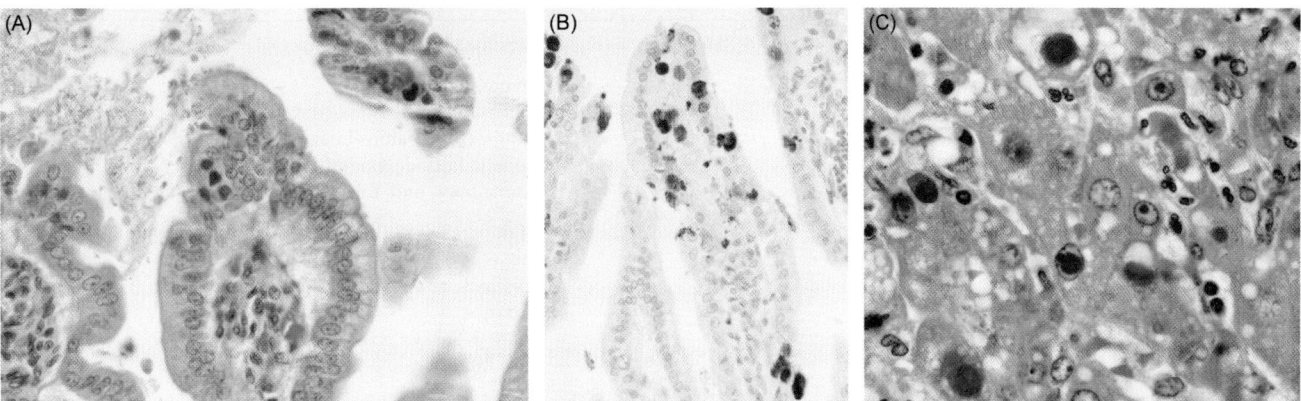

FIGURE 17.32   Adenoviral infection of the small intestine of a common marmoset demonstrating basophilic intranuclear inclusions within enterocytes of the villous tips (A) and corresponding adenoviral antigen (B). Hepatic necrosis with adenovirus intranuclear inclusions (C).

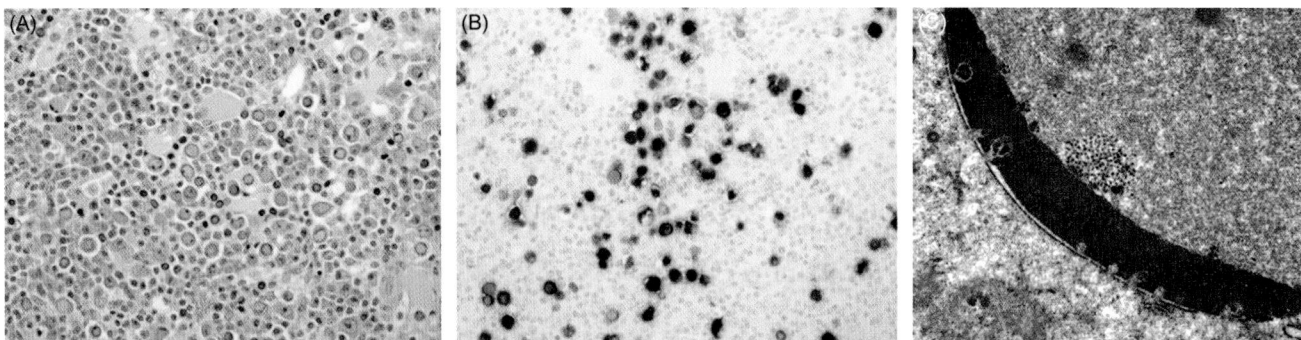

FIGURE 17.33   Rhesus parvovirus (RPV). Intranuclear inclusions within erythroid precursors of bone marrow in a rhesus macaque (A). *In situ* hybridization demonstrating RPV nucleic acid in the bone marrow (B). Electron microscopy demonstrating intranuclear viral particles (C).

TABLE 17.52   Simian Hemorrhagic Fever

Host	Disease
Reservoir: patas, African green monkey, baboon	Usually subclinical, may be persistently viremic[a]
Aberrant: Asian macaque	Fulminant, fatal hemorrhagic disease
	Initial spread by contact with blood/tissue of reservoir species
	Highly contagious among macaques once established
	Aerosol, direct contact, or fomite transmission[b]
	Fever, bleeding diathesis including ecchymoses and petechia
	Epistaxis, hematuria, melena
	Depression, photophobia, cyanosis, death[c]
	Hemorrhage and necrosis of proximal duodenum
	Random hemorrhage GI tract, liver, kidney, lung, subcutis
	Splenomegaly
	Lesions consistent with DIC, fibrin thrombi in glomeruli
	Necrosis of lymphoid tissue; cortical thymic necrosis[d]

DIC, disseminated intravascular coagulation; GI, gastrointestinal.
[a]*From Gravell* et al. *(1980).*
[b]*From Renquist (1990).*
[c]*From Palmer* et al. *(1968).*
[d]*From Zack (1993).*

TABLE 17.53   Flaviviruses

Virus	Host	Vector	Disease
Yellow fever	African monkeys	Mosquito	Subclinical, short-lived viremia
	New World monkeys		Severe, epizootic, fatal Icterus, multiple hemorrhages Multifocal hepatocellular necrosis Hepatic fatty degeneration Councilman and Torres bodies
	Humans[a]		High fever, chills, headache, backache, myalgia prostration, nausea, vomiting Epistaxis, oral bleeding, hematemesis Jaundice Death 3–7 days postinfection Case fatality rate 5–50%
Kyasanur Forest disease	Langurs	Ixodid tick	Pancytopenia, fever, bradycardia
	Bonnet macaques		Epistaxis and gastrointestinal hemorrhage Multifocal hepatocellular necrosis Hemorrhage adrenal, brain, kidney, lung Nonsuppurative encephalomyelitis
	Humans[a]		Fever, chills, lower back and leg pain, headache, insomnia, anorexia Stiff neck, tremors, confusion Fever lasts 1–1½ weeks Epistaxis, gastrointestinal hemorrhage (fatalities)
Dengue	Macaques	Mosquito	No clinical disease
	Langurs		High incidence of antibody titers
	Humans[b]		Fever, headache, myalgia, rash, nausea, vomiting Dengue hemorrhagic fever Increased vascular permeability Disseminated intravascular coagulation Thrombocytopenia Shock Fulminant hepatitis with encephalopathy

[a]Hugh-Jones et al. (1995).
[b]From Rigau-Perez et al. (1998), George and Lam (1997).

TABLE 17.54   Filoviruses

Virus	Strain	Reservoir host	Disease in human
Marburg		African green monkey	Fever, headache, muscle and joint aches, vomiting and diarrhea
			Maculopapular rash; gastrointestinal bleeding and epistaxis
			Hemorrhagic fever in technicians handling cell cultures
			Secondary and tertiary infections with human contacts
			28% fatalities in primary cases; no disease in monkeys
Ebola	Zaire Sudan	Unknown	Headache, fever, myalgia, and nausea
			Maculopapular rash, sore throat, vomiting, and diarrhea
			Epistaxis, melena, hematemesis, bloody diarrhea
			Hemorrhagic fever in humans with 86% mortality
			Spread to close contacts and medical personnel
			Lower mortality rate in contact cases suggests viral attenuation
	Cote d'Ivoire	Chimpanzee	Dengue-like disease following chimpanzee necropsy
	Ebola–Reston	*Rousettus amplexicaudatus*	No clinical signs of infection in animal handlers
			Handlers developed neutralizing antibodies indicating infection

hemorrhagic fever in 1989–1990. The monkeys were co-infected with SHFV (Dalgard *et al.*, 1992). Subsequent outbreaks of disease due to Ebola–Reston occurred in cynomolgus monkeys in 1992 and 1996 (Rollin *et al.*, 1999). Transmission occurred among macaques by direct contact, fomites, and aerosolization. Clinical signs included anorexia, lethargy, and death without premonitory clinical signs. In experimental disease, clinical signs included anorexia, lethargy, hypothermia, occasional nasal discharge, splenomegaly, facial petechia, and severe subcutaneous hemorrhages at venipuncture sites (Jahrling *et al.*, 1996). Disease progressed rapidly to cardiovascular collapse, severe depression, and coma. Elevated liver enzymes and lactate dehydrogenase were seen in the first outbreak. Gross lesions are similar to those reported for SHFV. Multifocal hepatocellular necrosis, multifocal necrosis within the zona glomerulosa of the adrenal gland, and mild interstitial pneumonia are microscopic lesions that distinguish Reston ebolavirus from SHFV (Dalgard *et al.*, 1992). Large eosinophilic or amphophilic intracytoplasmic inclusion bodies may be found in the liver and adrenal gland.

No Ebola-like disease has been reported in animal handlers or other personnel exposed to Reston ebolavirus-infected macaques or their tissues; however, detectable antibodies have been found in a small number of animal handlers, indicating that human infection with Reston ebolavirus does occur (Miranda *et al.*, 1999). Following the initial diagnosis of Reston ebolavirus in 1990, CDCP quarantine requirements for imported nonhuman primates became more stringent. Disease control measures emphasize protection of employees from exposure, prevention of spread among animals, and testing of all animals, in particular those that become ill or die during quarantine (DeMarcus *et al.*, 1999). The cases of imported cynomolgus macaque Reston ebolavirus were all linked to a single supplier and farm on the island of Mindanao in the Philippines, which has since stopped producing animals. More recently, three genotypes of Reston ebolavirus have been identified in pigs from this same geographic locality (Barrette *et al.*, 2009). Fruit bats are believed to represent the natural reservoir host.

b. Paramyxoviruses

Measles virus infection historically was a common and often severe infection of nonhuman primates. Serologic testing of primate populations indicates that infection may be subclinical in macaques (Kalter and Heberling, 1990), but severe disease may also occur (Willy *et al.*, 1999). Clinical signs and disease progression are detailed in Table 17.55. In addition to the typical skin lesions, clinical disease may be respiratory, GI, or neurologic (Fig. 17.34); abortions have also been reported (Renne *et al.*, 1973; Steele *et al.*, 1982, Roberts *et al.*, 1988). Measles infection induces immunosuppression in the

host (McChesney *et al.*, 1989) increasing susceptibility to secondary bacterial infections and concurrent infections may increase morbidity and mortality.

Measles infection in monkeys is usually acquired through contact with infected humans. Prevention of disease may be accomplished through screening of personnel to ensure adequate vaccination or measles infection history and/or vaccination of susceptible primate populations (Willy *et al.*, 1999). Vaccination using modified live measles vaccine has been shown to be safe and effective in some species of New and Old World nonhuman primates (Albrecht *et al.*, 1980; Willy *et al.*, 1999). Vaccination is most important in New World species, especially marmosets, as measles can cause a high mortality rate of 25–100% (Albrecht *et al.*, 1980; Levy and Mirkovic, 1971; Fahey and Westmoreland, 2012). Vaccination using canine distemper/measles virus vaccine has been reported to induce a measurable antibody response in rhesus monkeys (Staley *et al.*, 1995). However, measles vaccination with modified-live products can cause immunosuppression that interferes with intradermal skin testing for tuberculosis; the immune system of vaccinated monkeys may require up to 4–6 weeks to return to normal (Staley *et al.*, 1995). While measles is largely controlled in North America, periodic outbreaks in undervaccinated human populations may place animal colonies at risk. Recently, canine distemper virus has been described in China as a cause of a severe and massive epizootic in macaques associated with cutaneous and pulmonary lesions resembling measles (Qiu *et al.*, 2011).

Serologic surveys of wild and captive monkey and ape populations indicate that parainfluenza virus infections occur frequently (Kalter and Heberling, 1971, 1997). Transmission is by aerosol or direct contact with infected secretions. Clinical disease is usually self-limiting and ranges from mild upper respiratory disease to pneumonia. Morbidity within a primate population is usually high, with low mortality. Mortality is associated with secondary bacterial infections. The death of a juvenile chimpanzee has been attributed to respiratory syncytial virus infection (Clarke *et al.*, 1994).

c. Retroviruses

i. PRIMATE T-CELL LYMPHOTROPIC VIRUSES Simian T-cell lymphotrophic viruses (STLVs) and human T-cell lymphotrophic viruses (HTLVs) have a close molecular and phylogenetic relationship, and together these viruses compose the group referred to as primate T-cell lymphotropic viruses (PTLVs) (Van Dooren *et al.*, 2007). PTLVs are deltaretroviruses associated with lymphoproliferative disease in Old World monkeys, apes, and humans (Lee *et al.*, 1985; McCarthy *et al.*, 1990; Traina-Dorge *et al.*, 1992; Van Dooren *et al.*, 2007). In the natural host, infection is usually subclinical

TABLE 17.55   Paramyxoviruses

Genus	Virus	Species	Disease
Morbillivirus	Measles virus	Old World monkeys	6- to 10-day incubation[a]
		New World monkeys	Maculopapular rash, facial hyperemia, cough, conjunctivitis, coryza, epistaxis[b]
			May develop pneumonia
			Gastrointestinal signs may predominate[c]
			Secondary bacterial infections common
			Syncytia in skin, lung, and lymphoid tissues (Fig. 17.25) ± intracytoplasmic (IC) and intranuclear (IN) inclusion bodies
		Marmosets	Gastrointestinal disease, usually no rash[d]
			High mortality
			Necrotizing gastroenteritis
			Syncytia in gastrointestinal epithelium (Fig. 17.26) ± IC and/or IN inclusion bodies
	Canine distemper virus	Japanese macaque[e]	Respiratory signs
		Rhesus macaque[f]	Anorexia
		Cynomolgus macaque[g]	Pyrexia
			Thickening of the foot pad
			Maculopapular rash
			Encephalitis
	Paramyxovirus saguinus	Callitrichids	Anorexia, dehydration, diarrhea[h]
			10–100% mortality
			Necrotizing typhlocolitis
			Syncytia in crypt epithelium, pancreas, kidney, liver, and bile duct IC inclusion bodies
Paramyxovirus	Parainfluenza type 1 (Sendai virus)	Marmosets	Persistent sneezing, tachypnea, dyspnea
			Ocular and nasal discharge
			Depression, anorexia, piloerection
			High morbidity (50%), low mortality[i]
			Congestion and/or consolidation of lungs
			Interstitial pneumonia[j]
	Parainfluenza type 3 (simian agent 10)	Patas, gibbons	Upper respiratory tract infection
		Chimpanzees	Predisposed to streptococcal infection[k]
Pneumovirus	Respiratory syncytial virus	Chimpanzees	Upper respiratory tract infection
			Rhinorrhea, sneezing, coughing, fever
			Fatality in juvenile chimpanzee[l]

[a]*From Hall* et al. *(1971).*
[b]*From Willy* et al. *(1999).*
[c]*From Roberts* et al. *(1988).*
[d]*From Albrecht* et al. *(1980).*
[e]*From Yoshikawa* et al. *(1989).*
[f]*From Sun* et al. *(2010).*
[g]*From Sakai* et al. *(2013).*
[h]*From Fraser* et al. *(1978).*
[i]*From Flecknell* et al. *(1983).*
[j]*From Sutherland* et al. *(1986).*
[k]*From Churchill (1963), Martin and Kaye (1983), Jones* et al. *(1984).*
[l]*From Clarke* et al. *(1994).*

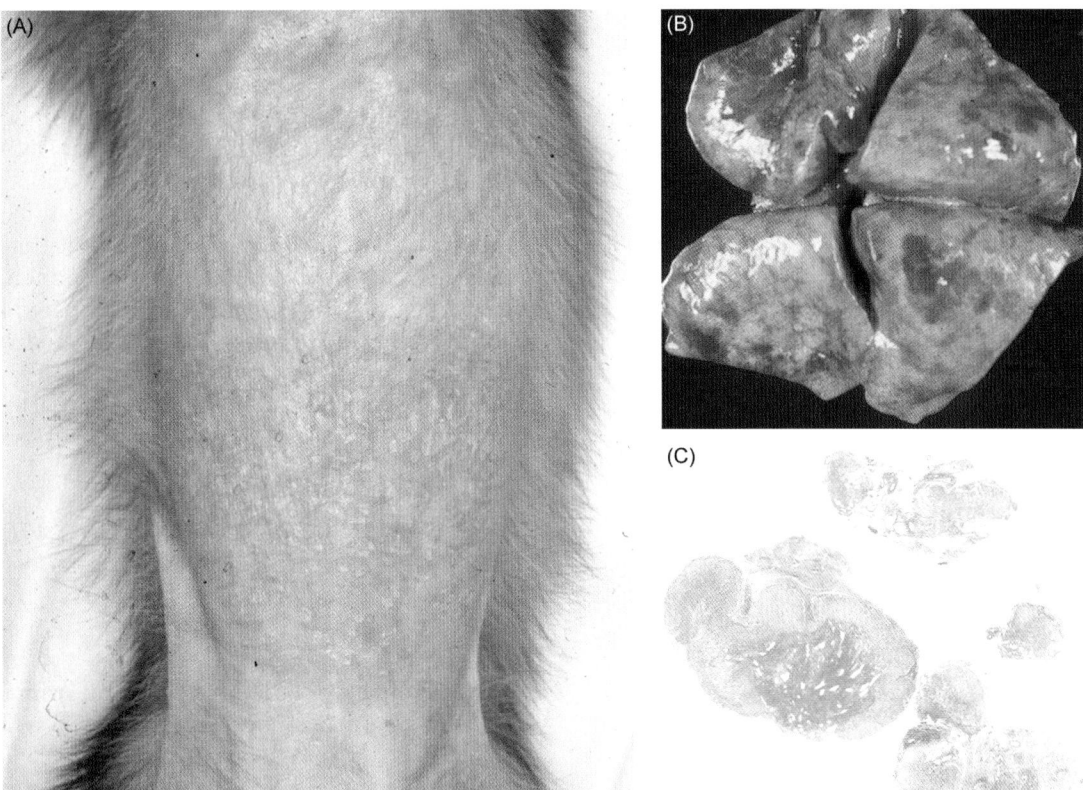

FIGURE 17.34 Measles virus viral exanthema in a juvenile rhesus macaque (A). Bronchointerstitial pneumonia in measles virus-infected macaque (B). Marked lymphoid depletion (C) can be a sequella of measles virus infection that may interfere with clinical testing that is dependent on immunological responses such as the intradermal tuberculosis test.

with a high rate of infection identified in feral and captive baboons, African green monkeys, and macaques. In baboons, leukemia/lymphoma associated with PTLV-1 resembles adult T-cell leukemia/lymphoma in humans. Clinical signs include anorexia, depression, lymph node enlargement, and hepatosplenomegaly. Overt leukemia occurs in greater than 50% of cases, and multilobulated, neoplastic lymphocytes are occasionally found in peripheral blood smears (McCarthy *et al.*, 1990). A high rate of pulmonary involvement was identified in an epizootic in baboons that was believed to have resulted from initial transmission from macaques (Voevodin *et al.*, 1996; d'Offay *et al.*, 2013). Cross-species transmission of PTLVs is believed common and wild primates are an important reservoir for human infections (Van Dooren *et al.*, 2001).

ii. SIMIAN BETARETROVIRUS

Pathogenesis   Endogenous simian betaretroviruses, historically known as the simian type-D retroviruses (SRVs), are a common natural cause of AIDS-like disease in macaques. SRV-1, 2, 4, and 5 are the primary cause of viral-induced immunodeficiency in captive macaque species (Montiel, 2010). SRV is endemic in several Asian macaque species, and prevalence can be high in captive

macaque colonies when efforts are not taken to eliminate it. The most likely mode of transmission is through inoculation with blood or saliva by biting (Lerche *et al.*, 1986); however, vertical transmission and horizontal transmission from the dam to infant during the perinatal or postnatal period has been documented (Tsai *et al.*, 1990).

Disease   Several clinical syndromes can occur with SRV infection: (1) persistent carrier state with no clinical disease with or without an antibody response; (2) severe immunodeficiency and viremia with or without an antibody response; (3) clearance of infection with an appropriate antibody response; (4) retroperitoneal or subcutaneous fibromatosis; or (5) persistent lymphadenopathy (Lowenstine, 1993). A case definition of simian AIDS induced by SRV is presented in Table 17.56. Immunosuppressed animals are particularly susceptible to pyogenic bacterial infections, disseminated CMV, candidiasis, intestinal cryptosporidiosis, and noma or cancrum oris (Lowenstine, 1993). Progressive diarrhea and weight loss with anemia is a frequent clinical presentation. Historically, SRV was the most common cause of naturally acquired immunosuppressive disease in captive macaques (Wachtman and Mansfield, 2008).

TABLE 17.56 Case Definition of Simian Betaretrovirus-Induced Simian AIDS[a]

Generalized lymphadenopathy and/or splenomegaly accompanied by at least four of the following clinical and laboratory findings:

Weight loss (>10%)

Fever (>103°F)

Persistent refractory diarrhea

Opportunistic infections

Noma (cancrum oris)

Retroperitoneal fibromatosis

Hematologic abnormalities

   Anemia (PCV <30%)

   Neutropenia (<1700)

   Lymphopenia (<1600)

   Thrombocytopenia (<50,000)

   Pancytopenia

Bone marrow hyperplasia

Characteristic lymph node lesions

[a]*From Lackner et al. (1988), Lerche and Osborn (2003).*

Pathology Proliferative lesions vary with virus serotype. Retroperitoneal fibromatosis is most frequently associated with SRV-2 infection and can present as a multinodular to coalescent mass originating from the ileocecal junction and involving the root of the mesentery, mesenteric lymph nodes, and gastrointestinal tract. Lesions range from small plaques or nodules spread across mesothelial surfaces to encasement of the gastrointestinal tract in a large fibrotic mass. Subcutaneous fibromatosis is more often associated with SRV-1 infection and is characterized by multiple nodules in the subcutis and oral cavity (Tsai *et al.*, 1985). These cases are believed to have resulted from concurrent infection with RFHV (Bryant *et al.*, 1986).

Microscopically, proliferative lesions are highly vascular with intersecting fascicles of spindle-shaped cells that infiltrate along serosal surfaces and encompass normal abdominal structures, usually accompanied by lymphoplasmacytic inflammation (Mansfield and King, 1998). In severely immunosuppressed animals, marked lymphoid depletion with effacement of normal architecture occurs in the spleen, thymus, and lymph nodes. Histiocytes replace depleted plasma cells and lymphocytes in the paracortex, and follicles contain hyalinized arterioles (Osborn *et al.*, 1984). Immunohistochemistry may be used to demonstrate RFHV latency-associated nuclear antigen (LANA) protein in these proliferative lesions (Mansfield *et al.*, 2014).

Diagnosis Establishment of SRV-free colonies by identification of SRV-negative animals is difficult because serologic testing is inadequate. Healthy seronegative monkeys with persistent infections can only be identified by virus isolation or PCR for proviral DNA. A colony screening protocol combining PCR and antibody screening must be used to identify all infected animals and has been successfully applied in the establishment of SPF colonies (Schroder *et al.*, 2000). Once common in domestic colonies, SRV has largely been eliminated from these sources. Infection may still be recognized in recently imported animals and a combination of PCR and serology should be used to identify these animals as infection represents a serious confounder of experimental work (Lerche and Osborn, 2003; Lerche, 2010).

iii. SIMIAN IMMUNODEFICIENCY VIRUS

Pathogenesis SIVs are lentiviruses closely related to human immunodeficiency viruses HIV-1 and HIV-2. Serologic studies have revealed that seropositive animals are frequently found among wild and captive African monkey populations. In Asian primate species, seropositive animals have been identified when housed near African primate species but not in wild populations of Asian primates (Gardner, 1996). SIV infection in African species is typically subclinical, but transmission to Asian species can result in an AIDS-like immunodeficiency disease (Hirsch *et al.*, 1995).

SIV isolates are identified by a subscript to indicate the species of origin, i.e., SIV_{mac} was isolated from a rhesus monkey and SIV_{cpz} from a chimpanzee. SIVs in African species are of relatively low pathogenicity in the natural host, sexual transmission is the most likely route of infection (Phillips-Conroy *et al.*, 1994), and transmission from dam to infant has also been proposed (Fultz *et al.*, 1990). SIV variants are divided into eight clades and have been shown to infect more than 40 species of African primates throughout Sub-Saharan Africa. In these species, the viruses replicate to high titers targeting lymphoid tissue and gut but fail to cause progressive loss of CD4 T lymphocytes. The viruses are readily transmissible leading to high seroprevalence in some populations and the founder effect has produced populations that are free of viral infection. Thus, African green monkeys from the island of St. Kitts have no evidence of infection while animals from sub-Saharan Africa demonstrate high seroprevalance rates.

SIV was first isolated from macaque colonies at several National Primate Research Centers in 1984 (Henrickson *et al.*, 1984; Osborn *et al.*, 1984). Subsequent sequence analysis of SIV_{mac} revealed a high degree of similarity to SIV_{sm} and HIV-2. SIVs are not identified as an indigenous infection of macaques and likely resulted through inadvertent transmission of SIV_{sm} from sooty mangabeys (Gardner, 1996). This cross-species transmission to an aberrant host results in progressive loss of CD4 T cells and the occurrence of an acquired immunodeficiency syndrome, which has been used extensively as an animal model to investigate aspects of HIV disease pathogenesis and prevention. Following experimental inoculation of macaques, different disease progression profiles may be observed depending on genetic and environmental cofactors. A normal disease progression profile is observed in about 75% of the cases in which peak viral loads of 10^7 genomic RNA copies/ml of plasma is observed at 2 weeks postinoculation. A humoral and cellular immune response is partially effective at controlling virus infection and lowering viral load, but a progressive loss of CD4 T cells usually continues with death at 18 months on average. In approximately 20% of cases, a rapid disease progression profile is observed. In these cases, humoral and cellular immune responses are blunted and not effective in controlling primary viremia. Animals progress to death in 3–4 months. Rarely, in approximately 5% of the cases, an elite controller profile is observed in which animals become infected but mount an effective immune response and clear the viremia (Wachtman and Mansfield, 2012).

Disease While opportunistic infections are common, viral-induced disease may also be observed including lymphoid hyperplasia/depletion, SIV enteropathy, giant cell pneumonia/lymphadenitis, SIV encephalitis, and SIV myocarditis. SIV encephalitis is a frequent disease entity in macaque species showing similarities to HIV encephalitis in human AIDS patients. The pathogenesis involves the recruitment and activation of infected macrophage/microglia to the CNS. These cells elaborate mediators of neuroinflammation that result in neuronal apoptosis and loss. Perivascular infiltrates of CD68 and viral positive macrophages and microglia with virally infected multinucleated syncytia are a hallmark of the disease.

Pathology Common lesions of uncomplicated SIV infection in macaques are listed in Table 17.57. Opportunistic infections occur with *Mycobacterium avium* complex, CMV, adenovirus, SV40, *Pneumocystis* spp., *Cryptosporidium* spp., *Cryptococcus neoformans*, toxoplasmosis, and candidiasis. Development of malignant B-cell lymphomas among SIV-infected macaque populations has been described and results from co-infection with rhesus LCV (Lowenstine *et al.*, 1992; Marr-Belvin *et al.*, 2008).

Diagnosis Unlike SRV infection, seronegative, viral-positive SIV infection in macaques is not common and generally leads to a rapidly progressive and fatal disease. Serologic testing of macaque colonies and removal of reactors is an effective way to eliminate infection from the population (Lowenstine *et al.*, 1986). Asian monkeys should not have direct contact with African species or their tissues. SIV is not a natural infection of macaques in

TABLE 17.57 Lesions Associated with SIV Infection in Macaques[a]

System	Comment
Lymphoid	Follicular hyperplasia
	Follicular involution ± expanded paracortical regions
	Depletion of follicular and paracortical regions
	Granulomatous (giant cell) lymphadenitis
	Generalized lymphoproliferative syndrome
Nervous	Nonsuppurative histiocytic meningoencephalitis
	Multifocal perivascular aggregates of giant cells and histiocytes
Gastrointestinal	Enteropathy; disseminated giant cell disease involving the lamina propria
Cardiopulmonary	Arteriopathy with medial and intimal proliferation of pulmonary arteries
	Thrombosis, hemorrhage, consolidation, and infarction of lung
Skin	Viral exanthema in experimental infections
	Perivascular lymphocytic dermatitis
Respiratory	Giant cell interstitial pneumonia

[a]Adapted from Mansfield and King (1998).

their home ranges and inadvertent infection of laboratory macaques has not been reported for many years.

d. Other RNA Viruses

Rabies has been reported in tamarins, marmosets, squirrel monkeys, macaques, and chimpanzees (Richardson and Humphrey, 1971; Fiennes, 1972; Favoretto *et al.*, 2001). Although current housing practices minimize the possibility of contact with carrier species, possible rabies exposure should be considered when primates are housed outdoors in rabies enzootic areas. Reported clinical cases in nonhuman primates are extremely rare. Clinical signs include irritability, self-mutilation, and paralysis of pharyngeal and pelvic muscles. Nonhuman primates may be vaccinated with killed vaccine; however, the efficacy of the vaccine is unknown. Use of attenuated rabies vaccine is contraindicated as vaccine-induced disease is believed to have occurred in New World species (McClure *et al.*, 1972).

Lymphocytic choriomeningitis virus (LCMV) infection, characterized by a rapidly progressive viral hepatitis, was reported in zoological collections of callitrichids by Montali *et al.* (1993). Infection has been shown to occur following feeding of neonatal mice infected with LCMV and is postulated to occur from consumption of naturally infected wild mice. Horizontal transmission between callitrichids does not occur; however, vertical transmission has been demonstrated. Clinical signs include anorexia, dyspnea, lethargy and weakness, ataxia or incoordination, and in some instances, seizures (Montali *et al.*, 1993). Affected animals may have icterus, elevated liver enzymes, bilirubin, and alkaline phosphatase levels. Mortality can be high, although serologic evidence of infection has been demonstrated in animals without history of clinical disease (Potkay, 1992). Gross lesions include hepatomegaly, splenomegaly, jaundice, subcutaneous and intramuscular hemorrhages, and pleural or pericardial effusions (Montali *et al.*, 1993). Liver lesions include multifocal hepatocellular necrosis with lymphocytic and neutrophilic infiltrates. Acidophilic apoptotic hepatocytes (Councilman bodies) are found within sinusoids and Kupffer's cells (Montali *et al.*, 1993). Necrosis of abdominal lymph nodes, adrenal glands, spleen, and gastrointestinal tract may be seen. Lymphocytic choriomeningitis is a zoonotic disease, and veterinarians in contact with infected marmosets developed antibody titers to LCMV (Montali *et al.*, 1995).

Hepatitis A virus infections have been diagnosed in chimpanzees, owl monkeys, African green monkeys, and cynomolgus monkeys. Serologic testing indicates that infection occurs in both wild and captive nonhuman primate populations, including many New and Old World species. Transmission is fecal–oral. Infection is usually self-limiting with no clinical disease. Elevated serum alanine aminotransferase and aspartate aminotransferase, 2–10 times above normal levels, with mild elevations of bilirubin are characteristic (Mansfield and King, 1998). Microscopic lesions include focal hepatocellular necrosis with nonsuppurative inflammatory infiltrates in the portal areas. Bile duct hyperplasia and necrosis of bile duct epithelium have been described in chimpanzees. Brack (1987) reported cases of human infection with hepatitis A virus contracted from nonhuman primates, particularly from chimpanzees.

Encephalomyocarditis viruses have been reported to produce fatal infections in owl and squirrel monkeys, baboons, rhesus macaques, and chimpanzees (Gainer, 1967; Blanchard *et al.*, 1987; Hubbard *et al.*, 1992; Baskin, 1993; Masek-Hammerman *et al.*, 2012). Wild rats are the primary reservoir hosts for this group of viruses, and fecal contamination of feed, water, or enclosures has been postulated as the source of infection in nonhuman primates. Death with no premonitory clinical signs is common in naturally infected monkeys. Pericardial effusion, white-tan mottling of the myocardium, and pulmonary congestion may be observed at necropsy. Nonsuppurative necrotizing myocarditis is the most important microscopic lesion. Placental infection and subsequent abortion can occur (Hubbard *et al.*, 1992). Elimination of feral rodents and cleaning of facilities are essential for prevention and control.

Poliovirus has been reported as a naturally occurring infection in great apes and rhesus monkeys. Infection may cause no clinical disease, or infected animals may develop paresis and paraplegia and then die. Lesions are located in the gray matter of the CNS and include perivascular inflammatory cell aggregates and meningeal infiltrates with neuronal necrosis and glial nodules. Vaccination of great apes with oral trivalent polio vaccine is recommended. Vaccination has been used effectively in wild chimpanzee populations to prevent disease (Morbeck *et al.*, 1991).

D. Parasitic Diseases

Nonhuman primates may be infested with a variety of external and internal parasites. Many of these infections are incidental or subclinical in nature and will not be presented in detail. Tables 17.58–17.65 list parasites that produce clinical disease in nonhuman primates; disease, pathology, diagnosis, and treatment are briefly described.

1. Chagas Disease

Chagas disease, also known as American trypanosomiasis, is caused by *Trypanosoma cruzi* and is a common hemoflagellate found distributed throughout South and Central America into the southwestern United States. Two forms of *T. cruzi* are observed in the host: the trypomastigote form is observed in the blood and the amastigote form is found in tissue pseudocysts. Some African primates are susceptible to additional trypanosomes (*Trypanosoma brucei gambiense* and *T. b. rhodesciense*) (Njiokou *et al.*, 2006; Thuita *et al.*, 2008). *T. brucei* has been reported in wild populations of African nonhuman primates at a frequency ranging from 8.3% to 19% (Jeneby *et al.*, 2002; Jeneby, 2011).

a. Pathogenesis

T. cruzi infections have been reported in a number of New World species including marmoset, squirrel, spider, cebus, and woolly monkeys, and Old World species including baboons, macaques, and great apes (Williams *et al.*, 2009; Andrade *et al.*, 2009; Mubiru *et al.*, 2014; Kunz *et al.*, 2002). Since New World monkeys may still be imported from South and Central America, or bred in the southern United States, chronic *T. cruzi* infection should remain in the differential diagnosis of animals with clinical signs consistent with trypanomomiasis (see section *Disease*). Transmission requires an intermediate triatomid host of the family Reduviidae, such as the kissing bug or assassin bug. Transmission occurs through bites or contamination of open wounds or mucous membranes with infected insect droppings, or by ingestion of contaminated fruits or infected triatomid insects. Elimination of the intermediate host will

TABLE 17.58 Enteric Protozoa

Parasite	Affected species[a]	Location	Clinical disease/ pathology	Diagnosis	Treatment
FLAGELLATES					
Giardia spp.	NWMs OWMs Apes	Small intestine	Frequently subclinical Diarrhea and vomiting ± steatorrhea	Saline wet mount, fresh feces Fecal concentration for cysts	Metronidazole[b,c] 30–50 mg/kg BID × 5–10 days; Tinidazole[b] 30–75 mg/kg PO once, repeat at 2 weeks (marmosets); Furozolidine[b] 1.5 mg/kg × 7 days (marmosets)
Trichomonas spp.	NWMs OWMs	Intestine Stomach, pelvic cavity (invasive disease in rhesus)	Diarrhea reported for callitrichids	Saline wet mount, fresh feces Rectal swab and culture	Metronidazole[d] 17.5–25 mg/kg BID × 10 days
AMOEBAS					
Entamoeba histolytica	NWMs OWMs Apes	Colon, cecum	Varies, more severe in young monkeys and NWMs Anorexia, vomiting Severe diarrhea ± hemorrhage Necroulcerative colitis Flask-shaped ulcers Amebic abscesses in the liver, lungs, or central nervous system	Saline wet mount Iodine, trichrome, or Giemsa stain Trophozoite 20–30 μm diameter Organism in lesioned organs Giemsa, trichrome, PAS stains	Metronidazole[c] 30 mg/kg TID × 5–10 days or in combination with Diiodohydroxyquin[c] 30–40 mg/kg TID Tetracycline[c] 25–50 mg/kg 5–10 days Chloroquin[c] 5 mg/kg × 14 days Chloramphenicol 50–100 mg/kg BID[e] Paromomycin[f] 12.5–15 mg/kg BID × 5–10 days
COCCIDIANS					
Isospora spp.	Callitrichids	Intestine	Diarrhea	Fecal flotation Saline wet mount	Sulfamethoxine[f] 50 mg/kg/day 1, then 25 mg/kg/day
Cryptosporidium spp.	Prosimians NWMs OWMs	Intestine Bile duct, pancreatic duct, conjunctiva, trachea, bronchioles in immunosuppressed animals	Intractable diarrhea Profuse, watery diarrhea Depression, weight loss Hypothermia, anorexia Dehydration Fluid and gas distension of intestine Mesenteric LN enlargement Blunting and fusion of villi/ Villous atrophy (Fig. 17.27) Increased mitotic index in crypts Hyperplasia of biliary and pancreatic duct epithelium; periductal fibrosis	Stain fecal smears or concentrates Flotation Direct or indirect FAS Stool antigen detection assay Formalin-fixed feces Histology 4–5-μm oocysts on brush border of enterocytes (Fig. 17.28)	Supportive care Replace fluid and electrolytes Antidiarrheals Antibiotics

(Continued)

TABLE 17.58   (Continued)

Parasite	Affected species[a]	Location	Clinical disease/ pathology	Diagnosis	Treatment
CILIATES					
Balantidium coli	NWMs OWMs Apes	Cecum, colon	Usually nonpathogenic Can cause severe, ulcerative colitis in apes Anorexia, weight loss, weakness, lethargy Watery diarrhea, tenesmus, rectal prolapse	Large ciliated ovoid organisms 30–150 × 25–120 μm	Metronidazole[c,g] 35–50 mg/kg/day divided doses TID Tetracycline[g] 40 mg/kg PO divided dose TID Diiodohydroxyquin[g] 40 mg/kg PO divided doses TID × 14–21 days

[a]NWMs, New World monkeys; OWMs, Old World monkeys.
[b]From Peisert et al. (1983), Kramer et al. (2009).
[c]From Lehner (1984).
[d]From Brady et al. (1988).
[e]From Renquist and Whitney (1987).
[f]From Wolff (1993).
[g]From Swenson et al. (1979).

TABLE 17.59   Hemoprotozoa

Parasite	Host[a]	Location	Clinical disease/pathology	Diagnosis	Treatment
Trypanosoma cruzi	NWMs OWMs Apes	Blood (trypomastigote) Skeletal and cardiac muscle, reticuloendothelial system (amastigote)	Subclinical Anemia, hepatosplenomegaly Lymphadenitis Generalized edema Anorexia, depression, weight loss Right bundle branch block-ECG Myocarditis Pseudocysts within myocardial fibers contain 1.5- to 4.0-μm round-to-oval organisms[b]	Smear, blood or body fluid, thick and thin Serology EIA or CF Histology	None
Plasmodium brazilianum, P. simium	NWMs	Erythrocytes	Usually persistent low parasitemia Can cause severe, fatal disease Anemia, cyclic pyrexia Hepatosplenomegaly Depression, death	Thick blood smear Serology (FA)	Chloroquine[c] 2.5–5 mg/kg IM × 4–7 days followed by Primaquine 0.75 mg/kg PO × 14 days
P. knowlesi, P. cynomolgi, P. fieldi, P. fragile, P. inui	Macaques Leaf monkeys	Erythrocytes	Usually subclinical unless splenectomized or immunosuppressed Anorexia, fever, weakness, splenomegaly		As above
P. pitheci, P. rodhairi, P. reichenowi, P. schwetzi	Great apes	Erythrocytes	Usually subclinical parasitemia Some strains cross-infective with humans		As above
P. hylobati, P. youngi, P. eylesi	Gibbons	Erythrocytes	Fever with parasitemia, pathogenic		As above

(Continued)

TABLE 17.59 (Continued)

Parasite	Host[a]	Location	Clinical disease/pathology	Diagnosis	Treatment
Hepatocystis spp.	OWMs Apes	Blood, liver	Subclinical infection Numerous, random, gray–white foci on surface of liver (merocyst) Eosinophilic granulomatous reaction to ruptured cysts Focal fibrosis when healed	Thick or thin blood smears Typical hepatic lesions Histology	None Vector control
Babesia pitheci	NWMs OWMs	Erythrocytes	Severe anemia, death with splenectomy Mild disease in intact monkeys	Blood smear Pyriform 2- to 6-μm organisms	None
Entopolypoides macacai	OWMs Apes	Erythrocytes	Usually subclinical Fever, anemia, monocytosis Hemolytic anemia and icterus following splenectomy or immunosuppression	Blood smear	None

[a]NWMs, New World monkeys; OWMs, Old World monkeys.
[b]EIA, enzyme-linked immunoassay; CF, complement fixation.
[c]From Lehner (1984).

TABLE 17.60 Disseminated Protozoal Infestations

Parasite	Host[a]	Location	Clinical disease/pathology	Diagnosis	Treatment
Toxoplasma gondii	Prosimians NWMs OWMs Apes	Lymph nodes, liver, lung, spleen, intestine, brain, heart	Death, no clinical signs Anorexia, listlessness, weakness Depression, somnolence Emesis, diarrhea Oculonasal discharges Dyspnea, tachypnea Neurologic signs Circling, head holding, head hitting, incoordination, paresis, convulsions Hepatosplenomegaly Ulcerative enteritis Lymphadenopathy Pulmonary edema	Serology (CF, IFA, HAI)[b] PCR[c] Impression smears of spleen, lung, lymph nodes Histology, Gram−, PAS− 4- to 8-μm banana-shaped tachyzooites in 60-μm cyst Animal inoculation	No treatment reported for nonhuman primates[d] Pediatric treatment regimen (humans) Sulfadiazine: 100 mg/kg/day; in divided doses BID × 1 month Pyrimethamine: load with 1 mg/kg/day × 2–4 days; then 1 mg/kg/day Folic acid: 1 mg/day to prevent bone marrow depression
Encephalitozoon cuniculi	Squirrel monkeys	Brain, kidney, lung, adrenal glands, liver, placenta	None or nonspecific, death Granulomatous inflammation	2.5 × 1.5 μm oval organisms in 60- to 120-μm pseudocysts in tissues Gram+, PAS+ Serology IFA, ELISA Organisms in urine	None

[a]NWMs, New World monkeys; OWMs, Old World monkeys.
[b]CF, complement fixation; IFA, indirect fluorescent antibody assay; HAI, hemagglutination inhibition test; PCR, polymerase chain reaction; ELISA, enzyme-linked immunosorbent assay.
[c]From Lin et al. (2000).
[d]From Lehner (1984).

TABLE 17.61 Acanthocephalans

Parasite	Host[a]	Location	Clinical disease/pathology	Diagnosis	Treatment
Prosthenorchis elegans, P. spirula	NWMs Prosimians	Ileum, cecum, colon	Anorexia, dehydration Abdominal distension Diarrhea Debilitation Weight loss Death	Fecal smears Formalin ether sedimentation (standard flotation not effective) Flexible fiberoptic proctoscopy Palpation of abdominal masses Necropsy	Insecticides and good sanitation to control intermediate hosts Dithiazine iodide has been effective; drugs that have been effective in pigs include loperamide hydrochloride 1.5 mg/kg BID q 3 days, fenbendazole 20 mg/kg daily q 5 days, or levamisole IM 0.3 mg/kg once[b]

[a]NWMs, New World monkeys.
[b]From Mehlhorn (2008).

TABLE 17.62 Scabies

Parasite	Host[a]	Clinical disease/pathology	Diagnosis	Treatment
Sarcoptes scablei	OWMs	Severe pruritis	Deep skin scrapings for parasites and eggs	Ivermectin 200 μg/kg; repeat in 3 weeks[b]
	Apes	Anorexia, weight loss, weakness		
		Tremors		
		Alopecia, scaling and thickening of skin		
		Self-mutilation		
		Bacterial dermatitis		
		Death		

[a]OWMs, Old World monkeys.
[b]From Toft and Eberhard (1998).

interrupt the cycle of infection. Congenital transmission has been reported in a squirrel monkey (Eberhard and D'Alessandro, 1982).

b. Disease

Clinical signs may be nonspecific and include lethargy, anorexia, and depression but are often secondary to cardiovascular involvement. Animals may present with peripheral edema, congestive heart failure (ascites, pulmonary edema), or cardiac dysrhythmias (first-degree heart block). A survey of serologically positive baboons suggests that functional deficits are common (Williams et al., 2009).

c. Pathology

Amastigotes are found in pseudocysts located in cardiac or skeletal muscle cells, or cells of the reticuloendothelial system. Pseudocysts containing characteristic

organisms may be found in vacuoles of infected cells. The organism must be differentiated from *Toxoplasma* which it may resemble; however, *T. gondii* does not contain a kinetoplast and the parasite pseudocyst of *T. gondii* is PAS positive. These are perhaps most easily recognized in the myocardium where degenerative cysts or cells are surrounded by areas of nonsuppurative inflammation and myocardial fibrosis. Histologically, myocardial edema and inflammatory cell infiltrates are recognized initially followed by diffuse or multifocal myocardial fibrosis (Kunz et al., 2002). Infection may also cause disruption of myocardial conduction resulting in death. Moreover, subclinical infection may complicate the interpretation of cardiac safety signals in preclinical toxicology studies (Pisharath et al., 2013).

d. Diagnosis

Ante mortem, Chagas disease can be diagnosed by serology or PCR; however, parasitemia can be transient, which can cause false negative test results. In chronic disease, it is difficult to demonstrate the presence of viable organisms in tissue sections by immunohistochemistry (IHC), *in situ* hybridization (ISH), or PCR in myocardial tissue and diagnosis may rely on serology and characteristic myocardial changes.

2. Toxoplasmosis

a. Pathogenesis

Toxoplasmosis is caused by the coccidian parasite *Toxoplasma gondii*, a member of the Sarcocystidae family. Various cat species (Felidae) serve as definitive hosts supporting the enteroepithelial phase and shed infectious oocytes into the environment, which are, in turn, ingested by the intermediate host. The organism then replicates in an extraintestinal phase in the intermediate host, which may transmit the organism if eaten as prey. *Toxoplasma* infection has been described in a variety of New and Old World primate species, but tamarins,

TABLE 17.63   Nematodes

Parasite	Host[a]	Location	Clinical disease/pathology	Diagnosis	Treatment
Strongyloides cebus	NWMs	Intestine	Usually none, eosinophilia Fatality in a woolly monkey	Fecal flotation, larvae, or larvated ova Necropsy, histology	**Ivermectin**[b] 200 µg/kg IM **Thiabendazole**[c] 50–100 mg/kg PO for 1, 2, or 5 days
S. fulleborni, S. stercoralis	OWMs Apes	Intestine Filariform larvae in lungs and other parenchymous organs	Diarrhea ± hemorrhage ± mucus Dermatitis, urticarial Vomiting, dehydration Debilitation, emaciation Cough, dyspnea Fatalities in apes, patas Enterocolitis—catarrhal, hemorrhagic, or necrotizing Peritonitis Pulmonary hemorrhage	Fecal flotation, larvae, or larvated ova Necropsy, histology	**Ivermectin**[b] 200 µg/kg IM, PO **Thiabendazole**[c] 50–100 mg/kg PO for 1, 2, or 5 days **Mebendazole**[d] 22 mg/kg/day PO or SQ × 2–3 days **Levamisole**[d] 10 mg/kg PO or SQ × 2–3 days **Pyrantel pamoate**[d] 11 mg/kg PO once
Trypanoxyuris sp.	NWMs	Cecum, colon	Usually subclinical Death in spider monkey due to overwhelming infestation	Observation of adults at the anus Perianal tape test or swab Fecal flotation for ellipsoid, asymmetric ova	**Thiabendazole**[e] 50–100 mg/kg PO
Enterobius vermicularis, E. anthropopitheci	OWMs Apes Chimpanzees	Cecum, colon	May be subclinical Anal pruritis and irritation Self-mutilation Aggressiveness Fatalities in chimpanzees Ulcerative colitis, peritonitis, lymphadenitis	Observation of adults at the anus Perianal tape test or swab Fecal flotation for ellipsoid, asymmetric ova	**Mebendazole**[d] 100 mg PO adult ape 10 mg/kg PO infant or smaller species **Pyrantel pamoate**[d] 11 mg/kg PO once
Oesophagostomum spp.	OWMs Apes	Cecum, colon	Weight loss, diarrhea Unthrifty Subserosal nodules 2–4 mm in colon and mesentery	Fecal flotation, hookworm like ova Identify larvae following stool culture	**Thiabendazole**[d] 25–100 mg/kg PO for 1–2 days **Levamisole**[d] 10 mg/kg PO or SQ once **Mebendazole**[d] 40 mg/kg PO, divided dose TID × 3–5 days Repeat all treatments at 10–14 days
Molineus elegans, M. torulosis	NWMs	Pylorus, duodenum Pancreatic ducts	M. elegans usually subclinical Ulcerative enteritis ± hemorrhage with M. torulosis Serosal nodules in duodenum Chronic pancreatitis	Fecal flotation Necropsy	None
Ascaris lumbricoides	OWMs Apes	Intestine	Usually subclinical Deaths associated with intestinal blockage due to heavy parasitism and migration to liver, bile ducts	Fecal flotation for roundworm ova	**Mebendazole**[f] 22 mg/kg PO × 3 days **Pyrantel pamoate**[f] 11 mg/kg PO once, repeat in 10–14 days
Trichospirura leptosoma	NWMs	Pancreatic ducts	Weight loss, wasting disease, acute/chronic pancreatitis, jaundice due to bile duct obstruction	Fecal flotation Thick-shelled, larvated ova	None

(Continued)

TABLE 17.63 (Continued)

Parasite	Host[a]	Location	Clinical disease/pathology	Diagnosis	Treatment
Pterygodermatites nycticebi, P. alphi	Prosimians NWMs Gibbons	Intestine	Watery diarrhea, anorexia, weakness (tamarins) Anemia, leukopenia, hypoproteinemia Pseudomembranous necrotizing enteritis	Fecal flotation, spirurid ova Adults, larvae in feces Necropsy, histology	**Ivermectin**[g] 0.5 µg/kg SQ × 3 days predilute in sterile water for smaller primates (marmosets) **Mebendazole**[g] 40 mg/kg × 3 days
Trichuris spp.	NWMs OWMs Apes	Cecum, colon	Anorexia, mucoid or watery diarrhea, and occasionally death may occur with heavy infestations	Fecal flotation Bipolar operculated ova	**Mebendazole**[d] 40 mg/kg PO BID × 5 days **Dichlorvos**[d] 10 mg/kg PO SID, 1–2 days **Levamisole**[h] 7.5 mg/kg SQ × 2 at 2-week interval **Flubendazole (5%)**[i] 27–50 mg/kg BID × 5 days (baboons)
Anatrichosoma cynomolgi	NWMs OWMs Apes	Nasal mucosa Secondary infestation of hands and feet (creeping eruption)	Subclinical nasal infestation or mild serous discharge Pruritis of hands and feet Vesicle/pustules in skin Regional lymph node enlargement	Nasal or epidermal swabs or scrapings – ova	**Fenbendazole**[j] 10–25 mg/kg PO SID × 3–10 days

[a]NWMs, New World monkeys; OWMs, Old World monkeys.
[b]From Brack and Rietschel (1986) and Battles et al. (1988).
[c]From Bingham and Rabstein (1964), Flynn (1973), Swenson et al. (1979), Lehner (1984), Abee (1985).
[d]From Swenson et al. (1979).
[e]From Lehner (1984).
[f]From Toft and Eberhard (1998).
[g]From Blampied et al. (1983).
[h]From Welshman (1985).
[i]From Kumar et al. (1978).
[j]From Harwell and Dalgard (1979).

TABLE 17.64 Cestodes

Parasite	Host[a]	Location	Clinical disease/pathology	Diagnosis	Treatment
Hymenolepis nana	All	Small intestine	Abdominal pain, tucked abdomen, crouching Anorexia, vomiting Catarrhal enteritis Abscessed mesenteric lymph node	Fecal flotation – ova Proglottids in feces Necropsy	**Niclosamide**[b] 100 mg/kg PO once **Bunamidine**[b] 25–100 mg/kg PO once **Praziquantel**[c] 0.1 mg/kg IM
LARVAL DISEASES					
Cysticercosis Taenidae	All	Abdominal or thoracic cavities Muscle Subcutaneous tissues Central nervous system (CNS)	Clinical signs dependent on number and location of cysticerci	Necropsy	None
Coenurosis *Multiceps* spp.	Prosimians OWMs	Subcutaneous tissue Peritoneal cavity Brain Liver	Dependent on number and location of coenuri Usually subclinical except in CNS	Radiography Palpation of mass in SQ tissues	None
Hydatidosis *Echinoccocus granulosus*	All	Abdominal or thoracic cavities Liver Lungs Retrobulbar Subcutaneous tissue	Usually subclinical, may mimic neoplasic disease Abdominal distension Exophthalmia Localized subcutaneous mass Anaphylactic shock, death following cyst rupture in lungs	Radiography Ultrasound Serology: intradermal skin test HA[d]	None

[a]All, all nonhuman primates; OWMs, Old World monkeys.
[b]From Swenson et al. (1979).
[c]From Welshman (1985).
[d]HA, hemagglutination assay.

TABLE 17.65   Trematodes

Parasite	Host[a]	Location	Clinical disease/pathology	Diagnosis	Treatment
Gastrodiscoides hominis	OWM	Cecum, colon	Mucoid diarrhea Mild chronic colitis	Ova in feces	None
Watsonius spp.	OWM	Intestine	Diarrhea, severe enteritis Death	Ova in feces	None
Paragonimus westermanii	OWM	Lung Ectopic sites include brain and liver	Cough, wheezing Blood in sputum Moist rales Progressive weight loss	Ova in feces Necropsy	None
Schistosoma mansoni, S. haematobium, S. matheei	NWM OWM	Mesenteric veins (S. mansoni and S. matheei)	Usually subclinical Fever, hemorrhagic diarrhea	Ova in feces or urine Necropsy, adults in veins	**Praziquantal** (56.8 mg/ml)[b] 0.2 cm^3/kg if <1 kg body weight; 0.1 cm^3/kg if >2 kg body weight
	Apes	Portal veins (S. haematobium)	Hematuria Ascites		

[a]NWMs, New World monkeys; OWMs, Old World monkeys.
[b]From Toft and Eberhard (1998).

marmosets, and owl monkeys appear to be particularly sensitive to severe disease (Dietz *et al.*, 1997; Epiphanio *et al.*, 2000).

b.   Disease

Initial clinical signs may be relatively nonspecific and include lethargy, anorexia, and weakness. Infection of Old World primates may be asymptomatic or reveal only mild clinical signs. In contrast, Neotropical primates may develop severe disease with progression of clinical signs to include seizures, diarrhea, fever, cough, and abortion.

c.   Pathology

Tachyzoites are found in various cells throughout the body and are recognized as crescent- or banana-shaped organisms that have a rounded and pointed end. They measure 4–8 × 2–4 μm in size and have an eccentrically placed nucleus. The organism initially is found in vacuoles within infected cells but may be released with cell death or necrosis (Fig. 17.35). Histologically, the organism may be observed in a variety of organs and is associated with necrosis and a mixed inflammatory cell infiltrate. Common organs involved in severe disease include the lungs, liver, and CNS, but also can include the gut, skeletal muscle, and lymphoid tissue. In the liver, multifocal hepatic necrosis is observed often with a neutrophilic infiltrate. The organisms may be visualized in these regions as small oval- to crescent-shaped bodies occasionally with an artifactual clear halo. Occasionally, organisms may be found in capillary endothelial cells.

d.   Diagnosis

Ante mortem diagnosis of *T. gondii* infection can be accomplished by serology. *Post mortem* diagnosis is often based upon histopathology, which can be confirmed by PCR.

While care should be given to excluding the definitive host from primate colonies, it can be particularly difficult to keep rodents and other small mammals out of outdoor primate enclosures. These feral animals may serve as vectors as they can be taken as prey and eaten by larger primates. Infectious oocysts can be carried by vectors such as cockroaches and may survive for short periods in water. Many epizootics in Neotropical primate colonies have been associated with the feeding of raw meat, thus uncooked meat should not be fed to NHPs (Cunningham *et al.*, 1992).

3.   Cryptosporidium parvum

a.   Pathogenesis

Cryptosporidium parvum is a common protozoal parasite of cold- and warm-blooded vertebrates. A number of genotypes have been described that may vary in their host species preference (Morgan *et al.*, 1999). Infection of a variety of New and Old World primates has been recognized. The organism is most common in macaque colonies where greater than 98% of animals will be seropositive by 2–3 years of age (Mansfield, personal communication, 2014). Transmission is by the fecal–oral route and is enzootic in Old World primate colonies. The organism is resilient to environmental conditions and may survive in water for prolonged periods (King and Monis, 2007).

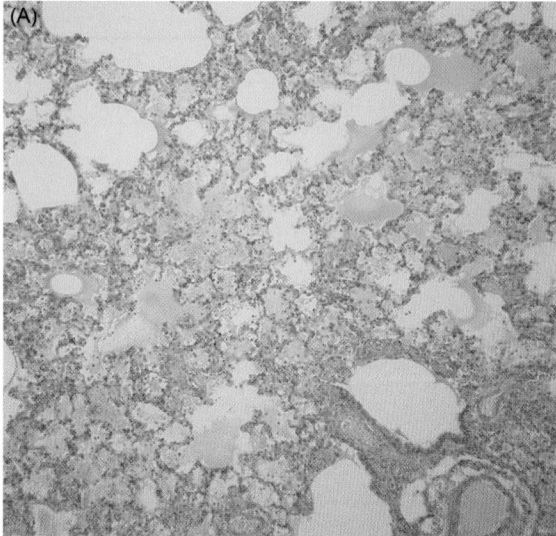

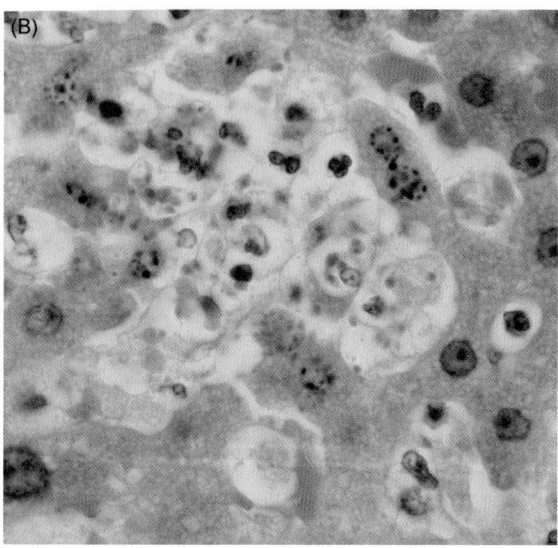

FIGURE 17.35   *Toxoplasma gondii*: severe interstitial pneumonia in a common marmoset due to toxoplasmosis (A); hepatic necrosis with small round to oval *Toxoplasma* tachyzoites (B).

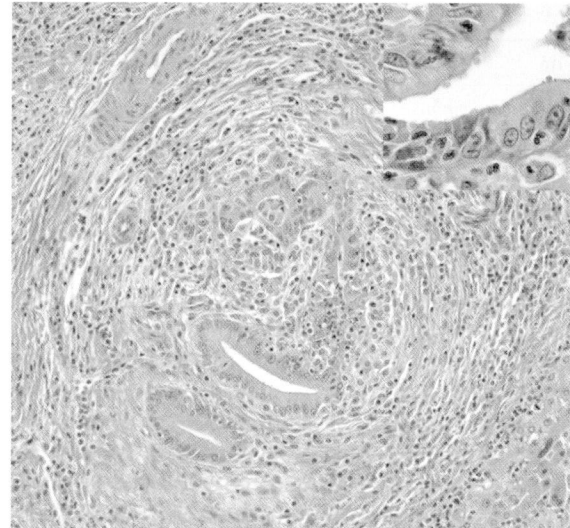

FIGURE 17.36   *Cryptosporidium parvum*: cyptosporidium induced necrotizing cholangitis with small basophilic organisms visible on the luminal surface of cholangiocytes (inset).

b. Disease

In most cases, clinical disease is mild and goes unrecognized in colony animals; however, in rare instances, more severe disease is seen and is characterized by protracted diarrhea, anorexia, and weight loss (Mansfield *et al.*, 2001). Disease is more severe in immunosuppressed or immunodeficient animals in which it may cause severe diarrhea and weight loss (Kaup *et al.*, 1998).

c. Pathology

The organism is most commonly found in the colon but may spread to the small intestine and is visualized as spherical 3- to 4-µm diameter basophilic bodies that

adhere to the apical surface of cells (Fig. 17.36). In severe cases, there is villous atrophy and epithelial cell hyperplasia within the gastrointestinal tract, where inflammatory changes are usually mild. In some cases, the organism may disseminate to multiple organs including liver and respiratory tract (Yanai *et al.*, 2000).

During immunosuppression, the organism commonly invades the biliary tree causing a cholangiohepatitis, cholecystitis, and choledochitis. There are often neutrophilic infiltrates surrounding and infiltrating bile ducts. Concentric fibrosis is evident and the involved biliary epithelium may take on a more squamous morphology from its normal cuboidal appearance, which is accompanied by epithelial cell necrosis. It can be difficult to visualize organisms in these areas and it is best to look in regions with less inflammation. Organisms may also disseminate to the trachea and lungs where they can be visualized on respiratory epithelium causing a necrotizing bronchiolitis. If doubt exists as to the identity of the basophilic organism, IHC can be used for confirmation (Mansfield *et al.*, 2014). Disease in Neotropical primate species is less frequent and sporadic. It may represent inadvertent introduction of the agent to colonies through contaminated food, water, or other fomites (Hahn and Capuano, 2010). Cryptosporidium is a zoonotic agent.

d. Diagnosis

Diagnosis may be made by examination of feces or biopsies. Fecal antigen capture tests are also a useful and sensitive method that combines detection of *C. parvum* with Giardia and Entamoeba.

4. *Plasmodium*

a. Pathogenesis

Malarial infections caused by the genus *Plasmodium* are a frequent cause of disease in primates that live in tropical environments. The plasmodium life cycle requires a female *Anopheles* mosquito.

Some of the common malarial parasites that infect NHPs include (1) *P. knowlesi*, a quotidian parasite that naturally infects *M. fascicularis* and *M. nemestrina* and may cause severe fatal infection of *M. mulatta*; (2) *P. cynomolgi*, a tertian parasite that naturally infects *M. fascicularis*, *M. nemestrina, M. cyclopis*, and several species of leaf monkeys and causes a disease in *M. mulatta* similar to *P. vivax* in man; (3) *P. simium*, a tertian parasite found in southern Brazil in spider and howler monkeys; and (4) *P. brazilianum*, a quartan parasite found naturally in spider, howler, capuchin, owl monkeys, and squirrel monkeys having a distribution from Mexico to Peru that is similar to *P. malariae* in man (Araüjo *et al.*, 2013). *Plasmodium* infection can be transmitted as a blood-borne pathogen from animals to human handlers and poses a serious zoonotic risk (Cox-Singh, 2012).

b. Disease

A large number of malarial species have been described that appear to infect primates in a species-specific fashion. For the most part, infection is not often associated with overt clinical signs in the immunocompetent host but may produce severe disease upon introduction to an aberrant host. For example, *P. knowlesi* is found in primates throughout Southeast Asia including *M. fascicularis* and *M. nemestrina* in which it causes relatively mild disease. In contrast, infection of *M. mulatta* causes severe and often fatal disease. Clinical signs may include anorexia, cyclic fever, and weight loss (Stokes *et al.*, 1983). Thrombocytopenia, leukopenia, and progressive anemia may also be observed. Fever develops at characteristic periods of parasite replication and may follow 24- (quotidian), 48- (tertian), or 72- (quartan) hour intervals. While disease can be relatively mild in the natural host, more severe disease may be precipitated during periods of stress, illness, or experimental manipulation (Donovan *et al.*, 1983). Splenectomy may exacerbate previous asymptomatic infection. The potential impact of concurrent malarial infection on experimental protocols should be considered and screening or prophylactic treatment employed if warranted.

c. Pathology

Plasmodium infection causes hepatosplenomegaly with hyperplasia of the lymphoid elements and macrophages in the liver, spleen, and bone marrow. Myeloid hyperplasia of the bone marrow may be seen in conjunction with erythropoiesis. Malarial hemazoin pigment deposition can be seen in Kupffer cells, bone marrow macrophages, and the red pulp of the spleen. Hemorrhages in the brain, splenic rupture, and necrosis of the lower nephron have also been reported. In contrast, the tissue phases of plasmodium infection are relatively harmless.

d. Diagnosis

The standard laboratory method for diagnosis of malaria infections in NHPs is microscopic examination of thick and thin blood smears stained with Giemsa or Wrights–Giemsa stains. A variety of additional techniques have been developed for malaria diagnosis including fluorescence microscopy, detection of hemozoin pigment with automated hematology analyzers, serodiagnostic assays, and PCR (Ameri, 2010). Most of these diagnostic techniques are for direct or indirect detection of circulating parasites, and false-negative diagnostic test results can occur.

E. Nutritional Diseases

Once common, nutritional diseases are now infrequently observed in laboratory-raised nonhuman primates. Issues may still occur in individual animals when prolonged illness leads to malnutrition through maldigestion/malabsorption or when food supplied as enrichment becomes a major source of nutrients resulting in an unbalanced diet. Errors can and have occurred during feed manufacture, and a specific batch of a commercial diet may be misformulated (Ratterree *et al.*, 1990; Eisele *et al.*, 1992) leading to deficiency and disease. Finally, detailed knowledge of the dietary requirements for many nonhuman primate species is not fully understood and requirements for individual nutrients have been based on extrapolation from human requirements. This may lead to a relative excess of specific nutrients, which may have unwanted health effects or potentially impact research (Penniston and Tanumihardjo, 2001). Common nutritional diseases of nonhuman primates are listed in Table 17.66.

1. Scurvy

Scurvy is a clinical condition produced by a deficiency of dietary ascorbic acid (vitamin C). While ascorbic acid is synthesized in the liver of most mammals, guinea pigs and most primates lack this capacity due to absence of the enzyme L-gulonolactone oxidase. Ascorbic acid is a cofactor required for the function of several hydroxylases. The absence of ascorbic acid reduces the function of prolyl hydroxylase, which is required to form hydroxyproline, an amino acid found in collagen but rarely found in other proteins. The presence of hydroxyproline in collagen stabilizes the collagen triple-helix structure by forming inter-strand hydrogen bonds. Collagen lacking hydroxyproline is more fragile and contributes to

TABLE 17.66   Nutritional Diseases

Condition	Common name	Species affected	Clinical signs	Lesions	Treatment
Hypovitaminosis A		Rhesus monkeys[a]	Abortion		Correct diet
Hypervitaminosis A		Callitrichids[b]	Musculoskeletal lameness, paresis cachexia, debilitation, alopecia[c]	Spinal hyperostosis and spinal ankylosis	Correct diet
Hypovitaminosis B_{12}	May contribute to 'cage paralysis'	Rhesus monkeys (experimental) Chimpanzees	Visual impairment Spastic paralysis of hindlimbs Decreased range of motion in knees Painful, swollen joints Contracted tendons Hand walking Megaloblastic anemia		Irreversible
Hypovitaminosis C	Scurvy	All primates (young animals most affected)	Reluctance to move Joint pain and tenderness Lameness, abnormal locomotion Gingival swelling, hyperemia, petechia Bruising Microcytic anemia	Subperiosteal hemorrhage Epiphyseal fracture Periodontal bone resorption Long bone fractures Periosteal elevation long bones	250 mg ascorbic acid IM × 2 days and oral 30–100 mg/kg/day[d] 25 mg/kg ascorbic acid IM BID × 5 days[e]
		Squirrel monkeys	Acute cephalohematoma	Periosteal elevation skull	50 mg ascorbic acid IM single dose[f] or 10 mg/kg body weight/day[g]
Hypovitaminosis D_2	Rickets	Old World monkeys	Failure to grow Wrists and knee enlargement Bowing of long bones	Cupping of epiphyses Decreased bone density	Provide D_2 in diet Ultraviolet light
Hypovitaminosis D_3	Rickets	New World monkeys (young animals)	Growth retardation Impaired ambulation Fractured long bones Masticatory weakness, difficulty chewing Inanition, death	Metaphyseal cupping and fraying of femur and tibia	1 IU/g diet D_3 preventive[h] Provide source of ultraviolet B radiation[i]
Folic acid deficiency		All primates	Megaloblastic anemia[j] Weight loss, petechia Anorexia, gingivitis, dehydration Diarrhea		Folic acid 109 μg/day Preventative
		Squirrel monkeys	Alopecia, scaly dermatitis Megaloblastic anemia of pregnancy[k]		
Hypovitaminosis E	Nutritional cardiomyopathy	Baboons[l]	Death, no clinical signs Heart failure, dyspnea	White areas of myocardium Acute myocytolysis, fibrosis	Vitamin E
	Vitamin E-responsive anemia	Owl monkeys[m] (gray-necked)	Weakness, pallor, heart murmur Icterus Hemolytic anemia, hematocrit ≤15	Splenomegaly	Vitamin E and selenium, O_2, supportive therapy, transfusion (rarely)

(Continued)

TABLE 17.66 (Continued)

Condition	Common name	Species affected	Clinical signs	Lesions	Treatment
	Contributes to marmoset wasting syndrome	Tamarins[n]	Weight loss, muscle atrophy Anemia	Myositis, steatitis	Not responsive to treatment but vitamin E was preventive
Calcium deficiency	Simian bone disease; osteomalacia	Prosimians and simians[o]	Decreased locomotion Impaired mobility	Kyphosis Bowing, fractured long bones Thickened jaw Dental displacement	Correct calcium: phosphorus in diet

[a]From O'Toole et al. (1974).
[b]From Demontoy et al. (1979).
[c]From Kark et al. (1974), Agamanolis et al. (1976).
[d]From Eisele et al. (1992).
[e]From Ratterree et al. (1990).
[f]From Kessler (1970).
[g]From Lehner et al. (1968).
[h]From Lehner et al. (1967).
[i]From Gacad et al. (1992).
[j]From Wixson and Griffith (1986).
[k]From Rasmussen et al. (1980).
[l]From Liu et al. (1984).
[m]From Sehgal et al. (1980), Weller (1994).
[n]From Baskin et al. (1983).
[o]From Krook and Barrett (1962), Snyder et al. (1980).

the clinical manifestations of scurvy, including vessel wall fragility. Osteoid matrix and dentin formation are defective and bone resorption is increased in vitamin C deficiency. Ascorbic acid functions as a reducing agent and as an antioxidant that is required for many physiologic functions, including folic acid metabolism and iron absorption.

The clinical manifestations of scurvy are primarily due to abnormal collagen synthesis. Clinical signs include weakness, depression, reluctance to move, gingival hemorrhage, and bruising. Physical examination may reveal swelling and instability involving the ends of long bones caused by physeal fractures. Affected bones often include the distal femur, proximal humerus, distal tibia/fibula, and distal radius/ulna. Anemia is a consistent finding likely related to the role of ascorbic acid in iron and folic acid absorption. Cephalohematomas are a pathognomonic finding in squirrel monkeys (Fig. 17.37). Morphologically, subperiosteal hemorrhage, epiphyseal fractures, periosteal bone resorption, long-bone fractures, and periosteal elevation of long bones are observed.

Therapy includes administration of ascorbic acid (250 mg IM BID or 30–100 mg/kg/day PO), cage rest, support bandages, and antibiotics if secondary bacterial infections are present. Post therapeutic radiographs may reveal large calcifying subperiosteal hematomas in epiphyseometaphyseal regions and are consistent with a diagnosis of scurvy. Clinical signs resolve within days of corrective vitamin C therapy. Cases have resulted from errors in the commercial manufacture of feed. Ascorbic

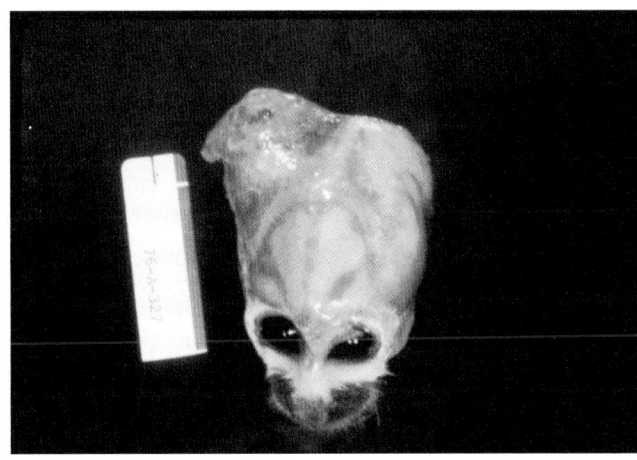

FIGURE 17.37 Hyperostosis of squirrel monkey skull subsequent to cephalohematoma from vitamin C deficiency.

acid is also labile and prolonged storage or exposure moisture can destroy dietary vitamin C (Ratterree et al., 1990; Eisele et al., 1992).

F. Noninfectious Diseases and Other Conditions

1. Cardiovascular Disease

Cardiac diseases are relatively uncommon in laboratory-housed nonhuman primates. While susceptible to dyslipidemias and atherosclerosis, this condition is relatively uncommon in animals fed standard laboratory diets. Myocardial fibrosis is a common incidental finding

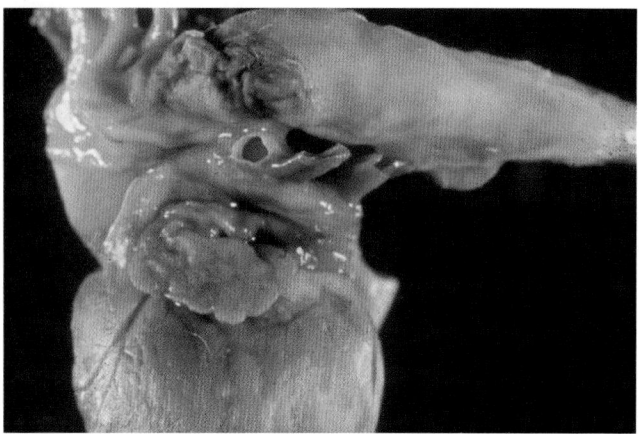

FIGURE 17.38   Aortic aneurysm in an owl monkey.

in macaques but is usually not associated with clinical signs. Several infectious agents such as encephalomyocarditis virus and *T. cruzi* can cause myocarditis and bacterial vegetative endocarditis can occur in immunocompromised animals or those with chronic indwelling catheters.

a. Aortic and Femoral Aneurysms

Femoral aneurysms and hematomas may occur infrequently as a sequella from trauma to the femoral artery during phlebotomy. Proper technique and appropriate hemostasis is critical in preventing this outcome. Animals may become anemic but the condition is usually not life threatening if recognized early. Proximal ligation of the femoral artery may be required and collateral circulation will provide adequate perfusion of the leg. Aortic aneurysms have also been recognized in several species of nonhuman primates. These aneurysms may occur secondary to atherosclerosis induced by high fat/high cholesterol diets (Borda *et al.*, 1994) and may also occur without known risk factors particularly in owl monkeys (Baer *et al.*, 1992) (Fig. 17.38). In this species, clinical signs may include anorexia, reluctance to move, systolic murmurs, palpable thrill, and lethargy. While the etiology is unknown, high blood pressure is recognized with some frequency and may mimic essential hypertension in man. Copper deficiency in other species may cause aortic aneurysms, but the role of copper deficiency or zinc excess in nonhuman primates has not been investigated. Treatment has not been attempted.

b. Congenital Heart Disease

Congenital defects have been rarely recognized in NHPs with ventricular septal defects, patent ductus arteriosis, and atrial septal defects being observed most frequently (Swindle *et al.*, 1986; Brandt *et al.*, 2002); however, other abnormalities have also been recognized (Koie *et al.*, 2007). Ultrasonography may be useful in diagnosis,

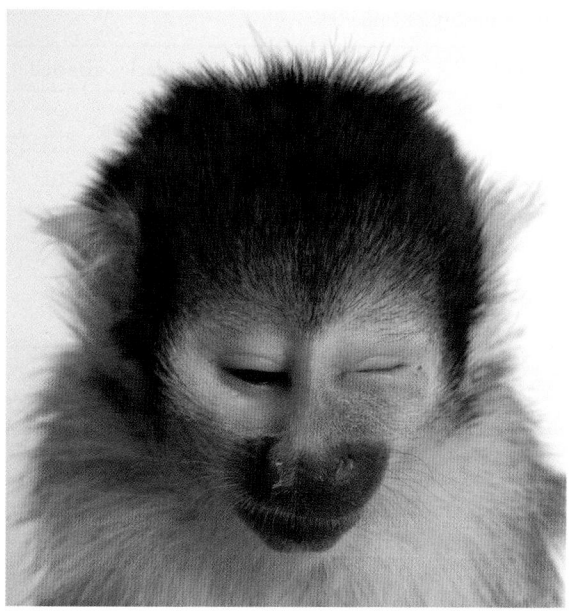

FIGURE 17.39   Swelling and cellulitis associated with a tooth abscess in a Bolivian squirrel monkey (*Saimiri boliviensis boliviensis*). By Julio C. Ruiz, D.V.M. from the Michale E. Keeling Center for Comparative Medicine and Research at the University of Texas MD Anderson Cancer Center, Bastrop, TX.

but in general, treatment is not attempted. Clinical signs may vary from a murmur with no other signs as observed with minor atrial septal defects, to failure-to-thrive and congestive heart failure. Patent ductus arteriosis is common and may be found in association with aortic hypoplasia, pulmonary valve defects, and aortic coarctation (narrowing of the aorta between the upper-body artery branches and the branches to the lower body). Cardiac malformations have been observed frequently in toxicologic experiments following administration of 13-cis retinoic acid, valproic acid, acetylsalicylic acid, thalidomide, and diphenylhydantoin (Hendrickx and Binkerd, 1990; Arpino *et al.*, 2000).

2. *Gastrointestinal*

a. Dental Disease

Severe wear and abscessation of teeth are common in adult squirrel monkeys and also occur in other species of nonhuman primates. Abscesses of the upper canine teeth often result from cracked or damaged teeth and present as swellings beneath the eye (Fig. 17.39). They will rupture and drain if left untreated. Abscessation of molar teeth in squirrel monkeys usually extends into the infraorbital region of the eye and can lead to exophthalmos and blindness (Abee, 1985). Enucleation of the eye may be required.

b. Acute Gastric Dilatation

Acute gastric dilatation or bloat in nonhuman primates has occurred following overeating and drinking, following alteration of gastric flora from antimicrobial therapy, or following anesthesia, transportation, or other change in routine (Soave, 1978; Stein et al., 1981). Bloat has been associated with gastric proliferation of *Clostridium perfringens* (Bennett et al., 1980; Stein et al., 1981), although a definitive causal relationship has not been proven. In one review, Bennett et al. (1980) reported that none of the monkeys involved had experienced a disruption in schedule nor had they been recently anesthetized or tranquilized. *C. perfringens* was isolated from gastric contents of 21 of the 24 monkeys and from monkey diet biscuits fed to the animals. Individual monkeys may have a predisposition for developing acute gastric dilatation and experience multiple episodes (Soave, 1978).

Early clinical signs include discomfort, as indicated by frequent grimacing and reduction in activity (Soave, 1978). As the disease progresses, monkeys may crouch or lie prone in the cage (Newton et al., 1971; Soave, 1978). Marked abdominal distension, shallow labored respiration, and coma occur terminally. Frequently, monkeys are found dead without prior clinical signs.

Acute gastric dilatation is a medical emergency and must be treated promptly. Soave (1978) reported the following procedures for treatment of bloat in macaques: sedation with ketamine hydrochloride (10–15 mg/kg body weight IM), gastric intubation to relieve intragastric pressure, administration of an agent to control gas formation, oral administration of ampicillin (30,000 IU/kg); intravenous administration of lactated Ringer's solution (20–30 ml/kg), and cortisone (1 mg/kg) administered IV or IM to counter shock.

c. Chronic Enteritides and Inflammatory Bowel Disease

Chronic diarrhea is one of the most frequent disease conditions and challenging diagnostic dilemmas encountered with captive nonhuman primates. Chronic diarrhea of more than 1 month in duration may have many causes including bacterial infections, dietary sensitivities/hypersensitivities, parasitism, dysbiosis, and neoplasia. It is often accompanied by progressive weight loss, and if not resolved, wasting of lean mass may lead to muscle contracture and permanent disability. Severe cases may require euthanasia for humane reasons. Protracted or recurrent episodes may predispose animals to systemic amyloidosis and intestinal carcinogenesis.

Facilities that house nonhuman primates should develop standard diagnostic and intervention approaches or algorithms to address chronic enteritides. These approaches should be based on the species of primate affected and known or suspected etiologic factors present within the colony. A diagnostic approach may include the use of serial fecal examinations, blood analysis, and endoscopic biopsies as well as interventions to exclude dietary sensitivities. Serial physical examinations and assignment of a body condition score to document body weight and body condition are helpful in monitoring the effectiveness of treatment. The laboratory tests used should be determined by the animal's signalment and facilities health surveillance program. Fecal examination may include direct smears, fecal flotation, antigen capture, and potentially, PCR to detect specific pathogens. Bacterial culture of fecal material can be a useful way to detect the presence of potential pathogens. In the future, next-generation sequencing technology may provide an opportunity to define the gastrointestinal metagenome and diagnose the full complement of commensal and pathogenic microbes within an individual animal (Handley et al., 2012). As this approach becomes more widely used, it may define additional etiologies as well as help direct therapy.

Intestinal biopsies may be of use in the diagnosis of chronic diarrhea and defining the severity of intestinal alterations. A number of pathogens have been identified as etiologic factors in chronic diarrheal disease including *Shigella* spp., *Campylobacter* spp., enteropathogenic *E. coli*, *Salmonella* spp., *Yersinia* spp., and *Helicobacter* spp. These are discussed in more detail in the enteric bacterial disease section of this chapter. Other chronic infectious and noninfectious processes may also lead to chronic diarrhea; examples include gastrointestinal neoplasias, malabsorption disorders, giardiasis and other protozoal parasites, and mycobacteriosis (Brady and Carville, 2012). Unfortunately, biopsies often reveal only nonspecific changes including inflammatory cell infiltrates, enterocyte or globlet hyperplasia, and altered mucosal architecture. These commonly observed changes are often lumped under the diagnosis of inflammatory bowel disease but provide little specificity as to the etiology or appropriate treatment. Rather than evidence of a single condition, these morphologic features should be viewed as an immune and regenerative response that may be initiated by a variety of often infectious causes and exacerbated by environmental, dietary and host genetic factors. Dietary factors, as well as environmental influences such as alterations in the metagenome, may be a source of antigenic stimulation that perpetuates intestinal inflammation following resolution of the initial insult to gastrointestinal mucosal integrity. The role of genetic influences has recently been investigated (Kanthaswamy et al., 2014).

Despite diagnostic efforts, the causes of chronic diarrhea often remain undetermined and treatment empiric. Initial treatment should be directed at stabilizing the animal. In severe cases, correction of fluid deficits and electrolyte imbalances may be necessary prior to further treatment. Separating these animals from conspecifics may also be indicated to prevent aggression toward the weakened animal and allow close monitoring and treatment. Once stabilized, treatment may include initiation of diets to avoid antigenic stimulation of intestinal immune responses, probiotics to alleviate dysbiosis, antibiotics against specifically identified pathogens, and immune modulators to dampen the host's enteric immune response. Dietary manipulations may be highly successful if initiated early in the disease course and can often be withdrawn once enteric inflammation and mucosal changes resolve. Several dietary alterations have been used including gluten-free, higher fiber, and semi-purified diets that may provide some benefit (Bethune *et al.*, 2008). Therapy directed at modulating intestinal immune responses include the use of antibiotics such as the macrolide tylosin (Blackwood *et al.*, 2008) and metronidazole as well as orally administered prednisolone.

d. Diverticulosis and Diverticulitis

Diverticular disease is a condition in which outpocketing or pouches occur in the colon wall. These blind pouches may increase with age and trap fecal matter predisposing animals to constipation and impaction (Bunton and Bacmeister, 1989). The most common clinical signs are bleeding, bloating, abdominal pain, and constipation. Occasionally, bleeding can be severe enough to cause life-threatening anemia (Azzam *et al.*, 2013; Sardana *et al.*, 2014). Diverticula may rupture causing pericolic abscess formation. Surgical resection of diverticula may be required in severe cases.

e. Rectal Prolapse Repair

Nonhuman primates of any age or sex can experience rectal prolapse, but it is most frequently diagnosed in young animals. Typically, rectal prolapse results from straining and severe diarrhea associated with enteritis or colitis. Other causes include social or management-related stress, rectal foreign bodies, lacerations, neoplasia of the rectum or distal colon, dystocia, urolithiasis, and prostatitis (Rubin, 2013; Brown and Swenson, 1995). The prolapse may be partial or complete. Partial prolapse involves only the rectal mucosa and appears as a red, swollen, doughnut-shaped mass. Complete prolapse appears as a cylindrically shaped, bright-red to purple edematous mass involving all layers of the rectal wall (Sherding, 1994).

Successful treatment involves reduction of the prolapse and identification of the underlying cause. Partial prolapses may reduce spontaneously or may require manual reduction using lubricants and hypertonic sugar compresses to reduce the associated edema. If manual reduction is not possible, an enema of lidocaine gel may be helpful. The gel aids in extending the tissue and relieves the urge to strain (Brown and Swenson, 1995). A perianal purse-string suture may be needed if straining is expected to occur while the primary cause is being treated. The suture should remain in place for 5–7 days.

If the viability of prolapsed tissue is questionable, then rectal resection and anastomosis should be performed. When the tissue is healthy but manual reduction fails after repeated attempts that include purse-string placement, a celiotomy and colopexy are advised (Rubin, 2013).

3. Inflammatory Diseases
a. Amyloidosis

Amyloidosis has been diagnosed in a variety of New and Old World primate species and may be localized or systemic. It is most frequently recognized in aged macaques and common marmosets (Ludlage *et al.*, 2005; Liu *et al.*, 2012; Rice *et al.*, 2013). AA or reactive 'secondary' amyloidosis is the most common systemic amyloid-associated disease found in mammals and nonmammalian species and results from the pathologic deposition of a ~76-residue N-terminal fragment of the serum amyloid A (SAA) protein. This precursor molecule is an acute-phase apolipoprotein reactant synthesized mainly by hepatocytes under control of certain cytokines, including interleukin (IL)-1 and IL-6, as well as TNF-α (Ludlage *et al.*, 2005). The etiology is unknown. In macaques systemic forms may be associated with inflammatory bowel disease, chronic catheterization, or chronic infections such as SRV. Systemic amyloidosis often involves the gastrointestinal tract (colon and small intestine), liver and spleen (Fig. 17.40). Renal disease may be seen in marmosets but is less frequent in macaques. Involvement of the gastrointestinal tract produces a maldigestion/malabsorption syndrome characterized by diarrhea and weight loss, steatorrhea, and hypoalbuminemia (Brady and Carville, 2012). Hyperglobulinemia may also be present. If total serum protein is low, systemic amylodosis may be accompanied by peripheral or pulmonary edema (Mansfield, personal communication, 2014).

Amyloid is recognized by characteristic tinctoral and ultrastructural features including a homogenous eosinophilic appearance on H&E-stained tissue sections, congophilia and green birefringence when examined under polarized light. By electron microscopy, amyloid is composed of ~10-nm-diameter fibrils. Immunohistochemical studies reveal cross-reactivity with a specific antihuman AA polyclonal antiserum (Ludlage *et al.*, 2005). Treatment with DMSO at 80 mg/kg for 6 months has been reported in macaques (Jayo *et al.*, 1990).

4. Metabolic
a. Diabetes, Metabolic Syndrome, and Obesity

Type 2 diabetes mellitus (T2DM) is a common clinical condition recognized in aging rhesus macaques found in association with obesity (Hansen, 1989; Kemnitz *et al.*, 1989). Affected macaques, primarily those with

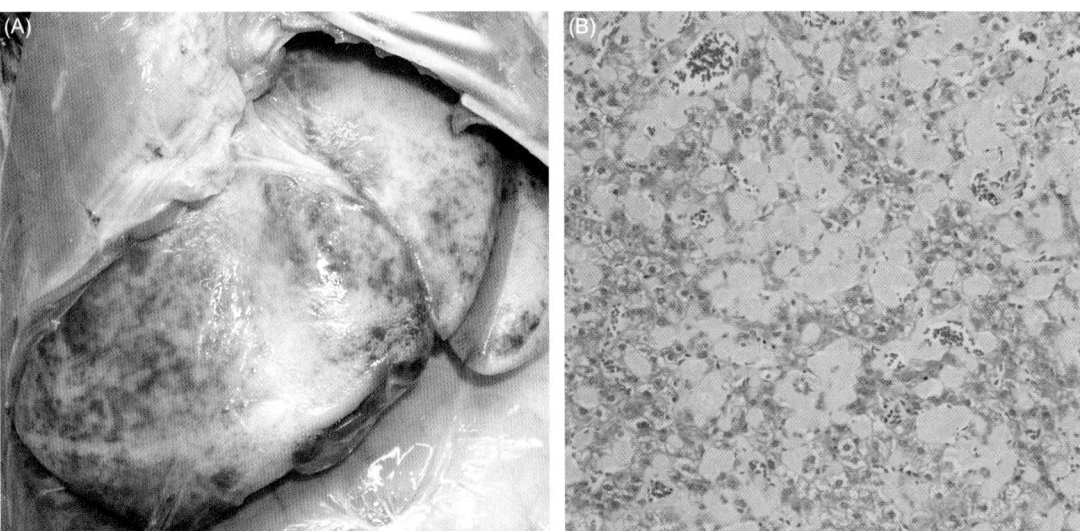

FIGURE 17.40   Hepatic amyloidosis demonstrating irregular coloration and waxy appearance (A). Hyalinized eosinophilic amyloid within space of Disse in a rhesus macaque (B).

increased adiposity and greater than age 10, demonstrate a syndrome characterized by altered fasting glucose, impaired glucose tolerance, insulin resistance (IR), and hyperinsulinemia. With progressive reductions in fasting insulin due to beta cell exhaustion and deposition of islet-associated amyloid, a subset of animals progress to overt diabetes. While prevalence is difficult to determine, of animals housed in captivity and fed standard *ad libitum* diets, approximately 35% will remain lean with normal carbohydrate and lipid profiles, 25% will develop overt T2DM, and a remaining 20–40% will manifest features of metabolic syndrome. This model has demonstrated utility in examining the pathogenesis of retinal disease and peripheral neuropathy, and in drug assessment of peroxisome proliferator-activated receptor (PPAR) agonists (Lebherz *et al.*, 2005; Cornblath *et al.*, 1989; Hansen *et al.*, 2011; Ding *et al.*, 2007). Early in disease, animals may show no overt clinical signs despite the occurrence of insulin resistance (IR). Animals may progress to overt T2DM with elevations in fasting blood glucose >110, polydyspsia, polyuria, and weight loss. Secondary sequelae may include atherosclerosis, renal disease, neuropathy, cardiomyopathy, and retinopathy. Animals may be more susceptible to bacterial infections.

An attribute of the rhesus macaque model of T2DM is the early development of IR that recapitulates the syndrome described in humans (Hansen and Bodkin, 1986). Progression from normal metabolism to IR and ultimately to overt T2DM represents a continuum of phenotypes with animals broadly categorized into four groups: those with normal insulin (NI) levels and normal glucose tolerance (NGT) that are aged and tending toward obesity (NI/NGT), those with compensatory hyperinsulinemia (HI) able to maintain normal glucose tolerance (HI/NGT), those with development of impaired glucose tolerance (IGT) characterized by reductions in glucose disappearance rates upon glucose challenge and modest increases in fasting glucose levels (HI/IGT), and those that have a progressive decrease in pancreatic beta cell capacity with normal or reduced levels of insulin production (NI/IGT). Animals in the later phases of IR, particularly following the development of IGT, begin to demonstrate dyslipidemias as evidenced by increased low-density lipoproteins (LDLs), decreased high-density lipoproteins (HDLs), and hypertriglyceridemia. Animals with HI and NGT may demonstrate only modest increases in triglycerides. In contrast, even in the earliest phases of IR (HI/NGT), animals are predisposed to a proinflammatory phenotype indicated by increased circulating leptin and decreased adiponectin. Morphologic changes may be few but initially will include hypertrophy of pancreatic islets during compensatory HI followed by amyloid deposition and islet exhaustion. It is during this later phase that fasting blood glucose levels rise and overt signs of diabetes develop. Prevention of obesity in macaques may help prevent T2DM as animals age (Hansen and Bodkin, 1993). In the early phases of IR, weight reduction and use of PPAR agonists may be useful. In the later stage, daily injections of insulin will help alleviate clinical signs.

b. Hypoglycemia

Squirrel monkeys, marmosets, and owl monkeys may develop hypoglycemia as a primary disorder. Hypoglycemia occurs more commonly in young animals, particularly infants, but can also be seen in older, debilitated animals. Predisposing factors include higher basal metabolic rates, lower percentage of body adipose tissue, limited glycogen reserves, limited gluconeogenic enzymes, and limited ability to utilize ketones or fatty acids (Abee, 1985; Baer, 1994). Separation from the social group, accidental feed deprivation, complications during weaning, prolonged research procedures, preanesthetic fasting, or anorexia due to an underlying disease condition can place monkeys at risk for hypoglycemia. Severity of clinical signs is related to the degree of hypoglycemia. Clinical signs include weakness, lethargy, disorientation, seizures, or unconsciousness (Baer, 1994). Glucose meters developed for human diabetics are useful in diagnosis as they require only one to two drops of blood to make a fast and accurate determination of blood glucose levels. Squirrel monkeys with blood glucose levels less than 40 mg/dl and owl monkeys with glucose levels less than 50 mg/dl are considered hypoglycemic. Conscious hypoglycemic animals can be given oral glucose, sucrose solutions, or fruit juice. Alternatively, warmed 5% dextrose solutions may be administered intravenously at 5–8 ml/100 g body weight (Abee, 1985; Baer, 1994). Use of concentrated dextrose solutions intravenously in New World monkeys is contraindicated (Brady, 2000). Treatment of unconscious squirrel monkeys with 20% dextrose orally by stomach tube at approximately 1 ml/100 g body weight is effective (Brady, 2000).

Hypoglycemia is not likely to be a primary disease condition in larger Old World monkeys. Treatment with an intravenous bolus of 10 ml of 50% dextrose is recommended for hypoglycemic animals weighing >5 kg (Rosenberg, 1995). If peripheral circulation and hydration are poor, then 10–20% dextrose solution can be administered intravenously. Solutions may be given by nasogastric tube or orally if the monkey has a good swallowing reflex.

c. Hypothermia/Hyperthermia

Primates housed outdoors are susceptible to hypothermia and hyperthermia associated with extremes in the weather. Particular care should be taken in the introduction of animals to outdoor housing; acclimatization should take place when temperatures are not extreme. Shelter and supplemental heat are required in areas where temperatures drop below freezing. Similarly, shade and shelter are necessary to provide relief during the summer. In areas with more severe summers, water misters may need to be provided to help keep animals cool. Temperature extremes may also occur in indoor housing due to a failure of environmental systems.

Hypothermia is frequently encountered in neonatal monkeys that have been separated from or rejected by the dam. These animals are also likely to be hypoglycemic.

Moribund infants may appear lifeless when discovered; vigorous toweling, gradual warming, and correction of hypoglycemia can revitalize them.

Treatment for hypothermia is best accomplished by placing the animal in a lukewarm water bath and monitoring body temperature every 4–5 min. Alternative methods of warming include use of recirculating water pads, warm air blankets, warmed fluid enemas, and warmed intravenous fluids, but they do not warm the animal as rapidly. Electric heating pads and heat lamps must be used with caution as extreme temperatures and subsequent burns or overheating of the animal can result. Treatment for hyperthermia is also best accomplished by a cool- to room-temperature water bath with frequent monitoring of body temperature.

d. Fatal Fasting Syndrome

Fatal fasting syndrome, also known as 'fat macaque syndrome' or 'fatal fatty liver syndrome', is an acute metabolic syndrome which may be precipitated by a variety of causes and which is seen most frequently in obese middle-aged female macaques (Bronson et al., 1982). Fatal fasting syndrome is associated with periods of anorexia or acute weight loss and can be observed in obese macaques of several species. While not always fatal, mortality rates may be greater than 50%. The pathogenesis is poorly understood but decreased food intake is thought to result in a shift to utilization of fatty acids as a primary energy source overwhelming the liver's ability to process these stores and resulting in severe hepatic lipidosis (Fig. 17.41). Affected monkeys generally have losses of 8–33% of body weight with a mean survival of 17 days. Azotemia is a common clinical pathologic finding. Clinical signs may include anorexia and lethargy and palpation may reveal hepatomegaly. Liver enzymes, total bilirubin, bile acids, creatine

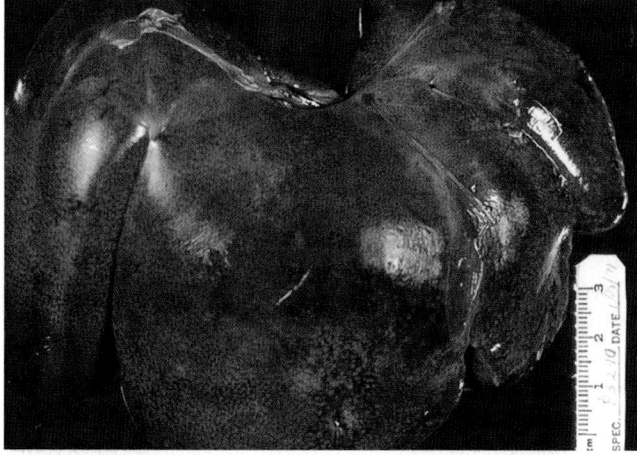

FIGURE 17.41   Hepatic lipidosis or steatosis may be a feature of the fatal fasting syndrome of macaques.

phosphokinase, creatinine, and blood urea nitrogen may be elevated. Glucose and albumin may be decreased. Less commonly, a nonregenerative anemia, neutrophilic leukocytosis, and bilirubinuria may be observed. Ultrasonography may indicate a diffuse increase in echogenicity and a liver biopsy can be diagnostic.

Gross findings at necropsy include enlarged, pale-yellow liver and pale-tan to yellow kidneys corresponding to severe hepatic lipidosis and severe fatty change of the proximal convoluted renal epithelium. Fatty change of the liver and kidney are the characteristic lesion found microscopically and may be accompanied by pancreatic ectasia, pancreatitis, or focal pancreatic necrosis often with fat necrosis. Females are more often affected than males. Animals may die with abundant remaining abdominal fat stores. Retrospective data suggests that obese animals are at risk if they become anorexic and body weight loss exceeds 0.1 kg/day. Predisposing factors include fecal impaction, traumatic lesions from fighting, and introduction to a new social group. Nutritional support through the use of parenteral nutrition may help reverse changes and improve survival (Christe and Valverde, 1999).

5. Neoplasia

Neoplasias are relatively uncommon in laboratory nonhuman primates unless they are maintained to advanced ages.

a. Adenocarcinoma of the Gastrointestinal Tract

Intestinal adenocarcinoma is the most frequent neoplasm in older rhesus macaques and has also been observed in cynomolgus macaques. A survey performed at the Wisconsin National Primate Research Center (WNPRC) indicated increasing frequency with age: 3.2% at 13–19 years, 9.2% at 20–25 years, 13.5% at 26–29 years, and 20.7% at 30–37 years (Uno et al., 1998). From 1999 to 2003 at WNPRC, 164 necropsies were performed on animals >15 years of age. In this cohort, neoplasia caused approximately 30% of the deaths, with 26% of the total (43 of 164) caused by enteric adenocarcinoma. The cause is unknown but may be associated with chronic inflammatory bowel disease.

Animals often present with anorexia and weight loss accompanied by constipation or hematochezia. An abdominal mass may be palpated but this can be difficult due to the small size of the mass and size of primate. Animals may have a microcytic hypochromic anemia, hypoproteinemia, and hypoalbuminemia. Intermittent fecal occult blood loss may be observed on testing in the absence of overt hematochezia and is the likely cause of anemia. The principal differential diagnosis in older female monkeys would be endometriosis.

Neoplasms are found most frequently in the cecum, ileocecal junction and transverse colon. Carcinomas may also be observed in ileum or distal jejunum. Tumorigenesis is not normally associated with polyps or polyposis, and histologically, tumors are characterized as mucinous adenocarcinomas. Early diagnosis and surgical resection of the tumor can extend the life of the affected macaque (Lertpiriyapong et al., 2014). Metastasis to the mesenteric lymph nodes may occur and there is often muscular invasion and a cirrhotic reaction causing a 'napkin ring' constriction of the colon. These tumors appear to metastasize slowly and resection may be attempted and can be curative. In general, clinical signs are recognized late in the course of disease.

b. Ampullary Carcinoma of Macaques

Ampullary carcinoma has been described in rhesus macaques (Usborne and Bolton, 2004). In humans, ampullary carcinoma is associated with the familial adenomatous polyposis (FAP) gene but the cause in macaques is unknown. Animals ranged from 20 to 35 years of age. The most common clinical sign is anemia followed by weight loss, lethargy, hepatomegaly, anorexia, and palpable mass. Icterus is infrequently observed. On serum chemistries, hypoalbuminemia and mild to moderate increases in alkaline phosphatase and γ-glutamyl transpeptidase were observed in some animals.

Gross lesions are characterized by thickening of the periampullary mucosal surface or formation of a discrete mass lesion associated with the ampullary orifice. The neoplasm consists of proliferation of epithelial cells with formation of papilliferous projections of fibrovascular stroma. These often form acini or glandular structures. These neoplasms tend to invade the underlying lamina propria and muscularis layer where they are associated with a cirrhotic reaction (desmoplasia). Cholangiohepatitis can be observed in a subset of animals. Treatment is difficult due to involvement of pancreatic duct and pancreas requiring pancreaticoduodenectomy.

c. Hepatocellular Carcinoma

Hepatocellular carcinomas (HCCs) have been recognized in a variety of nonhuman primate species including macaques, capuchin monkeys, African green monkeys, squirrel monkeys, and chimpanzees (Adamson, 1989). In a survey of 2000 cynomolgus macaques, two HCCs were recognized (Reindel et al., 2000). In another study HCCs were not identified in 373 aged control monkeys from a 32-year carcinogenicity study (Thorgeirsson et al., 1994). HCC and mixed hepatocellular carcinomas have been induced experimentally with orally administered carcinogens and found in association with schistosomiasis in the liver (Abe et al., 1993; Tabor, 1989).

Clinical signs may be nonspecific and include anorexia and weight loss. Jaundice may be seen on physical exam and alterations in liver function tests may be observed. Ultrasonography and biopsy may be used to confirm the diagnosis. Tumors may be solitary or multifocal. HCCs are characterized by solid sheets and trabeculae of neoplastic hepatocytes often partially surrounded by a fibrous capsule. Tumor cells are large but maintain many characteristics of hepatocytes including abundant eosinophilic cytoplasm and well-demarcated cell borders. Cellular pleomorphism may be pronounced. Cell nuclei are round to oval, of various sizes, enlarged, and vesicular, with prominent single or multiple nucleoli. Mitoses may be numerous and atypical. A key finding is interruption of the fibrous capsule and invasion into the surrounding hepatic parenchyma. Neoplastic cells stained positive for low-molecular-weight cytokeratin, cytokeratin (CK) 8, and CK18, and variably for carcinoembryonic antigen (CEA), glutathione *S*-transferase-*pi* (GST), and α-fetoprotein (AFP). They are reportedly negative for CK7. Treatment has not been attempted.

d. Squamous Cell Carcinoma

Squamous cell carcinoma (SCC) is the most common skin neoplasm in nonhuman primates (Kaspareit *et al.*, 2007). Etiologies include (1) exposure to sunlight, (2) papillomaviruses, (3) carcinogens such as *n*-methyl-*N*-nitrosourea that may experimentally induce SCCs in the digestive tract (esophagus), and (4) chronic inflammation at mucosal surfaces such as that induced by parasites or infection. Clinical signs relate to the site of involvement. SCCs may appear as solitary and ulcerated masses on haired skin. If involving the esophagus, they may induce dysphagia. Oral lesions may be associated with halitosis, swelling, and tooth loss. Tumors are locally invasive but metastasize slowly.

SCCs are characterized histologically by irregular cords and lobules of epithelial cells that invade surrounding tissue and disrupt the normal architecture. Neoplastic cells are round to oval with abundant eosinophilic cytoplasm and have a centrally located vesicular, round nucleus. The neoplastic cells often undergo keratinization forming keratin 'pearls' and form intercellular bridges (desmosomes). Solitary masses may be excised with wide excision.

6. Orthopedic Diseases

a. Osteoarthritis

A form of osteoarthritis or osteoarthrosis has been recognized in several species of macaques, gorillas, and chimpanzees. The etiology is unknown and study of large free-ranging primate colonies has shown that the occurrence of osteoarthritis is independent of common dietary and environmental factors (Kessler *et al.*, 1985; Rothschild and Woods, 1992). Radiographic features include narrowing of the joints, periarticular bone sclerosis and osteophyte formation. The process preferentially affects large joints and hands. Animals may develop gait abnormalities and hypertrophic deformation of the joints. At necropsy, softening of the cartilage, superficial fibrillation, and eventual erosion of the articular surface with eburnation of bone is observed. Treatment is symptomatic and may include the use of NSAIDs, opioids, and acupuncture (Dufour *et al.*, 2012; Schug, 2007; Magden *et al.*, 2013).

b. Reactive Arthritis

In humans, inflammatory or erosive arthritides may be divided into septic arthritis, rheumatoid arthritis, reactive arthritis, and inflammatory spondyloarthropathies. While the distinction between these latter entities may be clear in humans, clarity in nonhuman primates is lacking. These conditions may affect single joints including those of the spine. Animals often have a history of acute or chronic-active enterocolitis. The condition has been recognized in macaques, gorillas, baboons, and gibbons.

Reactive arthritis, secondary to previous *Shigella flexneri* infection, is the best characterized of these entities and is a well-recognized syndrome in macaques. Other infectious agents may also represent inciting events such as those seen in postreactive urethritis in man and should be considered. Increased risk for development of reactive arthritis is associated with specific MHC types in man (HLA-B27) but has not been identified in nonhuman primates. The Mamu-A*12 allele may be protective in rhesus macaques (Urvater *et al.*, 2000).

Reactive arthritis may present acutely in animals as a non-weight-bearing lameness affecting a single joint or limb and, if untreated, may become more generalized and chronic. In acute cases, a single joint may initially be involved which is swollen and warm on palpation. The animal or its cage mates may have a recent history of gastroenteritis, which resolved in the previous 3–4 weeks. Animals are often febrile and anorexic but respond quickly to corticosteroids. If left untreated, the animals have continued anorexia, lose considerable weight, show a reluctance to move, and have contracture of muscular tissue. Arthrocentesis may be used to evaluate joint fluid acutely and assist in diagnosis. In chronic cases, radiographic changes may be evident but definitive diagnosis may be difficult and distinguishing the different forms of inflammatory arthritides may not be possible.

Acutely, cytological evaluation of joint fluid reveals decreased viscosity and large numbers of nondegenerate neutrophils. Bacteria cannot be cultured from joint fluid and cytological evaluation of joint fluid is critical in making a timely diagnosis and in distinguishing reactive from septic arthritis. Chronically, changes may be nonspecific. At necropsy in advanced cases, erosion of articular surfaces may be observed with infiltration of synovium with a mixture of lymphocytes, plasma cells, and macrophages.

Rapid treatment with high doses of prednisolone (2 mg/kg) will induce remission of clinical signs and can be tapered over a 2- to 3-month period. With early recognition and treatment, animals respond quickly and can return to normal function. Treatment in chronic cases is more difficult and a response may be incomplete if treatment is delayed and significant damage has occurred to the articular surface.

c. Metabolic Bone Disease

Metabolic bone disease may have multiple etiologies dependent on the species and age of animals. Conditions considered to be metabolic bone disorders include rickets, osteomalacia, primary hyperparathyroidism, and secondary hyperparathyroidism such as renal osteodystrophy and iatrogenic hypercorticosteroidism. Nutritional causes include inadequate calcium or vitamin D, or excess phosphorus. New World primates have a requirement for vitamin D3 and easily develop rickets or osteomalacia if this need is not met. Clinical manifestations are dependent on the age, species, and etiology. In general, skeletal manifestations of metabolic bone disease in young growing animals are called rickets, and in older, mature animals they are called osteomalacia and fibrous osteodystrophy (Hunt et al., 1967). In growing animals, clinical signs relate to epiphyseal deformities and failure of bone to mineralize. In osteomalacia there is also a failure of osteoid to mineralize, which is often accompanied by increased fibrous tissue. In both cases, pathologic fractures may be evident.

All primates require adequate and balanced levels of calcium, phosphorus and vitamin D. Cholecaciferol or vitamin D3 is derived from animals and is hydroxylated in the liver to form 25(OH)D3 and is further hydroxylated in the kidney to form 1,25(OH)2D3 which is the active hormone. Differences exist in the requirement for vitamin D3 between New and Old World primates. New World primates have higher plasma levels of D3 and appear to have relative end-organ resistance to the effects of D3 compared to Old World primates and humans. While Old World primates are able to synthesize adequate D3 from D2, New World primates must have a dietary source of D3 to prevent metabolic bone disease. To further guard against the possibility of rickets and osteomalacia, some facilities provide vitamin D3 supplementation in addition to feeding diets formulated for these species.

Morphologically, rickets is characterized by deformation at epiphyseal plates, which appear enlarged and microscopically elongated. This elongation is associated with persistence of chondrocytes and accumulation of excess nonmineralized osteoid. Microfractures may occur at these sites with formation of transverse radiolucent ('Looser's') lines that may be recognized radiographically. Grossly, bones often show physeal cupping/widening and bowing. Enlargement of the costal cartilages (rachitic rosary) and dorsal kyphosis may also be observed.

In adults, osteomalacia is characterized by decreased mineralization and increased osteoid on trabecular bone. If accompanied by secondary hyperparathyroidism, increased fibrosis and numbers of osteoclasts may be observed. The clinical presentation of fibrous osteodystrophy similar to 'big head or bran disease' of horses may be observed in which the head appears swollen.

Diagnosis and treatment should be directed at understanding the underlying cause. If a nutritional etiology is responsible, corrective measures should be taken and appropriate vitamin supplementation given to reverse the deficiency. Enforced restricted activity should be considered to prevent further fractures and allow nondisplaced fractures to heal.

7. Reproductive

a. Endometriosis

Endometriosis is one of the most common gynecologic problems of Old World primates (Coe et al., 1998; Hadfield et al., 1997). It is a progressive disease characterized by the deposition and proliferation of endometrial tissue outside of the uterine cavity. This disorder is diagnosed in animals greater than 10 years old with an average age of detection being approximately 15–16 years. Endometriosis has been most thoroughly characterized in the rhesus and cynomolgus macaques as well as in baboons. It has also been reported in the African green and the pigtail macaque (Miller, 2012; DiGiacomo et al., 1977). Prevalence in aged baboons is ~8–27% and in rhesus is ~31% (Zondervan et al., 2004). In rhesus >20 years of age, prevalence may increase 10–45%. The incidence of endometriosis may be elevated in animals raised in captivity due to the number of reproductive cycles not resulting in pregnancy (for nonbreeding animals). A familial tendency has been reported in the rhesus macaque (Kennedy et al., 1997).

Retrograde menstruation is thought to play a contributing role in the development of endometriosis. Material containing endometrial cells is refluxed into the peritoneal cavity with viable endometrial cells implanting within the abdominal cavity. Contributing risk factors include radiation, treatment with estradiol implants, previous hysterotomy, and stress. Growth and maintenance of ectopic tissue may require presence of estrogen, growth factors, and active proto-oncogenes. Some suggest that a defective immune response to ectopic tissue contributes to maintenance of the condition. Along these lines, immunosuppression is thought to contribute to progression of disease. The disorder has also been induced experimentally in the common marmoset (Einspanier, et al., 2006). Surgical manipulation of the

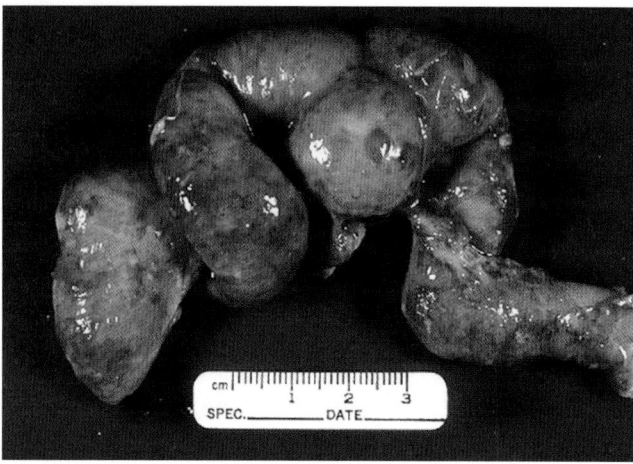

FIGURE 17.42   Large cysts on the serosal surface of the jejunum in a macaque with endometriosis.

myometrium is termed adenomyosis. The term adenomyoma is used to describe formation of a localized tumorlike mass composed of hyperplastic smooth muscle admixed with foci of endometrium. The presence of endometriosis may alter immunologic profiles and can result in research confounds. If animals are assigned to an experimental protocol, the effect that chronic inflammation caused by endometriosis may have on studies should be considered.

By the time endometriosis is diagnosed in macaques, treatment will often not restore fertility and is often palliative. Treatment options include ovariohysterectomy, resection of cysts, progesterone therapy, and leuprolide acetate (gonadotropin-releasing hormone analog). NSAIDs and analgesics should also be used (Mattison *et al.*, 2007) to reduce pain associated with this disease.

8. Trauma

a. Rhabdomyolysis Syndrome

Trauma is a common medical problem requiring treatment in pair- or group-housed primates. Aggression between animals can cause severe wounding or death. Trauma frequently involves injury to the skin or the underlying tissues. Associated tissue damage may require treatment for shock, sepsis, or multiple organ failure. Severely wounded animals require vigorous treatment, including intravenous fluid and electrolyte therapy.

Crush injuries to the skin are commonly associated with bite wounds. The extent of injury can easily be underestimated because there are no visible lacerations and external hemorrhage may be minimal or nonexistent. Laboratory values may be within normal limits. Several days later injured areas can develop ischemic necrosis characterized by dry, blackened, devitalized skin. Underlying tissues may be devitalized as well and require debridement. Secondary infection is common. In severe cases, damage to underlying tissues can result in myoglobinuria, myoglobin casts in the kidney, and resultant fatal acute renal disease. Accurate early diagnosis of crush injury and aggressive fluid therapy can ameliorate these sequelae.

Tail injuries due to tail chewing are a major problem in group-housed squirrel monkeys. Occasionally, one or two animals within a group will bite the tails of other members. Once injured, infection or irritation of the tail can lead to self-mutilation of the existing wound (Abee, 1985). Blood supply to the tail is poor, and gangrene and infection are frequent sequelae. Tail injuries may be self-inflicted; squirrel monkeys with abscessed teeth or other dental problems may gnaw the tail in order to alleviate the primary source of pain (Abee, 1985). Treatment of severely injured or infected tails is partial amputation of the tail to remove the damaged segment.

uterus may predispose animals to the development of endometriosis and this is a common history in affected animals.

While the disorder may be asymptomatic and discovered incidentally at necropsy, clinical signs include abdominal pain, cyclic anorexia, weight loss, irregular menstrual cycles, constipation, and anemia. Infertility results from the distortion of the pelvic organs and/or obstruction of the oviducts. Diagnosis is via palpation, imaging, or abdominal exploration. Ultrasonic guided aspiration of brownish fluid is highly suggestive of the presence of endometriosis.

Nonhuman primates have been proposed as a naturally occurring animal model for the human condition. Endometriosis in nonhuman primates is often very aggressive and in some respects may mimic carcinomatosis. Lesions may be found on visceral and peritoneal surfaces and is most commonly associated with the serosa of the uterus, bladder, omentum, colon, and uterine ligaments (Fig. 17.42). Abnormal tissue may less frequently be found dispersed widely throughout the abdominal cavity and associated with areas such as the diaphragm and liver. On gross examination, the abnormal tissue is adhered to a serosal surface and appears as a multichambered mass containing reddish-brown to brown raised cystic regions or 'chocolate cysts'. Adhesions may be present within the abdominal cavity. The histological appearance is characterized by ectopic endometrial glands and stroma adhered to serosal surfaces and occasionally penetrating surrounding tissue. Glands contain the blood and debris. Fibrosis, hemosiderosis, and variable degrees of inflammation are observed. This tissue undergoes cyclical changes in response to hormonal influences as occurs in the normal endometrium. Ectopic deposition of endometrial glands and stroma within the

b. Self-Injurious Behavior

Another cause of traumatic injury in macaques is self-mutilation or self-injurious behavior (SIB) and may be considered a severe form of maladaptive behavior on a continuum of whole-body or self-directed sterotypies. In its mildest form, SIB is expressed as hair pulling; head banging and self-biting are the more severe manifestations of SIB. From 5% to 12% of individually housed rhesuses, macaques have been reported to engage in SIB (Bayne et al., 1995; Novak et al., 1998). Wounds usually consist of bites or slashes to the skin and muscle. Episodes of self-biting behavior are more frequent than actual wounding.

On the continuum of stereotypic behaviors, a number of different therapeutic options are available including social housing, PRT, and nonsocial interventions such as providing additional space within the animal's primary enclosure and environmental enrichment. Depending on its severity, SIB may require immediate pharmacotherapy coupled with behavioral management and monitoring. A number of different therapeutics have been used including benzodiazepine (Tiefenbacher et al., 2005), L-tryptophan (Weld et al., 1998), fluoxetine (Fontenot et al., 2009), guanfacine (Macy et al., 2000), and cyproterone acetate (Eaton et al., 1999). While these treatments may provide some benefit during acute episodes, their long-term efficacy has not been rigorously evaluated. Moreover, recent evidence suggests that SIB subtypes may exist that respond differentially to pharmacotherapies (Major et al., 2009). Tieffenbacher et al. (2005) reported a bimodal response to diazepam in which the drug decreased self-wounding episodes in half of the rhesus macaques but had no effect or exacerbated wounding behavior in the remaining animals. Additional work will be required to identify behavioral or other biomarkers that may predict response to pharmacotherapies. Attempts to decrease the occurrence of SIB through environmental enrichment with puzzle feeders or other manipulanda have been mostly unsuccessful (Novak et al., 1998). There has been some success in reducing SIB behavior using various combinations of socialization techniques, environmental enrichment, and pharmacological interventions (Crockett and Gough, 2002; Honess and Marin, 2006; Bourgeois et al., 2007; Taylor et al., 2005). Cutting or blunting of the canine teeth decreases wounding but does not stop self-biting behavior (Bayne et al., 1995). Because of its severity and often refractory nature to treatment, prevention and reduction of the incidence of SIB is of primary importance. Research has indicated that early rearing husbandry practices may be very important in preventing behavioral pathologies and that providing infants with contact with conspecifics is critical to normal behavioral development (Lutz and Novak, 2005; Rommeck et al., 2009). In older primates, minimizing single housing of animals will also provide benefit (Lutz and Novak, 2005).

Acknowledgments

We acknowledge the hard work and contributions of many colleagues and staff who gave generously of their time and abilities to make this chapter possible. It is important to recognize the outstanding work of the authors of the original chapter that appeared in 2nd edition. The leadership, knowledge, experience, and scholarship of Drs. Susan V. Gibson, Michale E. Keeling, and Bruce Bernacky combined to create an outstanding chapter in the 2nd edition. Their work formed the foundation for this chapter. Although Drs. Gibson and Keeling are no longer with us, their intellectual and creative spirits remain alive in this chapter. Dr. Bruce Bernacky continues to make contributions to our field and his contributions as an author of the original chapter are acknowledged with appreciation. We also thank Dr. B. Taylor Bennett for his contributions and support in completing this chapter. Special thanks and appreciation are extended to Ms. Lindsey Saunders for her many hours of editing, formatting, wordprocessing, and scheduling the authors' many teleconferences. Ms. Saunders' hard work on this chapter significantly added to its clarity and quality. We also acknowledge the many hours of administrative support provided by Ms. Kathryn Meuth, whose hard work helped to initiate our collaborative efforts. It is also important to acknowledge our many colleagues who have helped us develop the knowledge and perspective to create a chapter that can serve the needs of not only laboratory animal veterinarians, but also colony managers, primate behaviorists, and scientists who carry out biomedical research with nonhuman primates.

References

1999 Report of Progress, Southwest Foundation for Biomedical Research. San Antonio, TX.

't Hart, B.A., Jagessar, S.A., Kap, Y.S., Brok, H.P.M., 2007. Preclinical models of multiple sclerosis in nonhuman primates. Exp. Rev. Clin. Immunol. 3 (5), 749+.

Abbott, D.H., McNeilly, A.S., Lunn, S.F., Hulme, M.J., Burden, F.J., 1981. Inhibition of ovarian function in subordinate female marmoset monkeys (Callithrix jacchus jacchus). J. Reprod. Fertil. 63, 335–345.

Abbott, D.H., Barrett, J., George, L.M., 1993. Comparative aspects of the social suppression of reproduction in female marmosets and tamarins. In: Rylands, A.B. (Ed.), Marmosets and Tamarins: Systematics, Behavior, and Ecology. Oxford University Press, New York, pp. 152–163.

Abbott, D.H., Barnett, D.K., Colman, R.J., Yamamoto, M.E., Schultz-Darken, N.J., 2003. Aspects of common marmoset basic biology and life history important for biomedical research. Comp. Med. 53, 339–350.

Abe, K., Kagei, N., Teramura, Y., Ejima, H., 1993. Hepatocellular carcinoma associated with chronic Schistosoma mansoni infection in a chimpanzee. J. Med. Primatol. 22, 237–239.

Abee, C.R., 1985. Medical care and management of the squirrel monkey. In: Rosenblum, L.A., Coe, C.L. (Eds.), Handbook of Squirrel Monkey Research. Plenum Press, New York, pp. 447–487.

Abee, C.R., 1989. The squirrel monkey in biomedical research. ILAR J. 31, 11–20.

Abee, C.R., 2000. Squirrel monkey (Saimiri spp.) research and resources. ILAR J. 41, 2–9.

Abee, C.R., Mansfield, K., Tardif, S.D., Morris, T., 2012. Nonhuman Primates in Biomedical Research: Biology and Management. Elsevier Saunders, San Diego, CA.

Abegglen, J.J., 1984. On Socialization in Hamadryas Baboons. Associated University Press, Cranbury, NJ.

Achat-Mendes, C., Platt, D.M., Spealman, R.D., 2012. Antagonism of metabotropic glutamate 1 receptors attenuates behavioral effects of cocaine and methamphetamine in squirrel monkeys. J. Pharmacol. Exp. Ther. 343, 214–224.

Adams, M.R., Kaplan, J.R., Manuck, S.B., Uberseder, B., Larkin, K.T., 1988. Persistent sympathetic nervous system arousal associated with tethering in cynomolgus macaques. Lab. Anim. Sci. 38, 279–281.

Adamson, R.H., 1989. Induction of hepatocellular carcinoma in non-human primates by chemical carcinogens. Cancer Detect. Prev. 14, 215–219.

Agamanolis, D.P., Chester, E.M., Victor, M., Kark, J., Hines, J.D., Harris, J.W., 1976. Neuropathy of experimental vitamin B_{12} deficiency in monkeys. Neurology 26, 906–914.

Aikawa, M., Broderson, J.R., Igarashi, I., Jacobs, G., Pappaioanou, M., Collins, W.E., et al., 1988. An Atlas of Renal Disease in Aotus Monkeys with Experimental Plasmodial Infection. American Institute of Biological Services, Arlington, VA.

Aksel, S., Diamond, E.J., Hazelton, J., Wiebe, R.H., Abee, C.R., 1985. Progesterone as a predictor of cyclicity in Bolivian squirrel monkeys (Saimiri sciureus) during the breeding season. Lab. Anim. Sci. 35, 54–57.

Albrecht, P., Lorenz, D., Klutch, M.J., Vickers, J.H., Ennis, F.A., 1980. Fatal measles infection in marmosets: pathogenesis and prophylaxis. Infect. Immun. 27, 969–978.

Al-Doory, Y., 1972. Fungal and bacterial diseases. In: Fiennes, R.N.T.-W. (Ed.), Pathology of Simian Primates. Karger, Basel and New York, pp. 206–241.

Al-Doory, Y., Pinkerton, M.E., Vice, T.E., 1969. Pulmonary nocardiosis in a vervet monkey. J. Am. Vet. Med. Assoc. 155, 1179–1180.

Aldrich-Blake, F.P.G., Bunn, T.K., Dunbar, R.I.M., Headley, P.M., 1971. Observations on baboons, Papio anubis, in an arid region in Ethiopia. Folia Primatol. 15, 1–35.

Alexander, S., Yeoman, R., Williams, L., Aksel, S., Abee, C.R., 1991. Confirmation of ovulation and characterization of LH and progesterone secretory patterns in cycling, iso-sexually housed Bolivian squirrel monkeys (Saimiri boliviensis boliviensis). Am. J. Primatol. 23, 55–60.

Alford, P.L., Lee, D.R., Binhazim, A.A., Hubbard, G.B., Matherne, C.M., 1996. Naturally acquired leprosy in two wild-born chimpanzees. Lab. Anim. Sci. 46, 341–346.

Allen, A.M., Kinard, R.F., 1958. Primary cutaneous inoculation of tuberculosis in Macaca mulatta monkeys. Am. J. Pathol. 34, 337–345.

Altmann, J., Altmann, S.A., Haufsfater, G., McCuskey, S., 1977. Life histories of yellow baboons: physical development, reproductive parameters, and infant mortality. Primates 18, 315–330.

Ameri, M., 2010. Laboratory diagnosis of malaria in nonhuman primates. Vet. Clin. Pathol. 39 (1), 5–19. http://dx.doi.org/10.1111/j.1939-165X.2010.00217.x.

American Veterinary Medical Association (AVMA), 2009. Removal or reduction of canine teeth in captive nonhuman primates or exotic and wild (indigenous) carnivores The Veterinarian's Role in Animal Welfare, Approved November 2003; revised April 2004, June 2007. p. 26.

AnAge: The Animal Ageing and Longevity Database, 2014. [online] Available at: <http://genomics.senescence.info/species/>.

Andelman, S.J., 1987. Evolution of concealed ovulation in vervet monkeys (Cercopithecus aethiops). Am. Nat. 129, 785–799.

Anderson, D.C., Swenson, R.B., Orkin, J.L., Kalter, S.S., McClure, H.M., 1994. Primary Herpesvirus simiae (B-virus) infection in infant macaques. Lab. Anim. Sci. 44, 526–530.

Anderson, J.H., 1986. Rearing and intensive care of neonatal and infant nonhuman primates. In: Benirschke, K. (Ed.), Primates: The Road to Self-Sustaining Populations. Springer, New York, pp. 747–762.

Andrade, M.C., Dick Jr., E.J., Guardado-Mendoza, R., Hohmann, M.L., Mejido, D.C., VandeBerg, J.L., et al., 2009. Nonspecific lymphocytic myocarditis in baboons is associated with Trypanosoma cruzi infection. Am. J. Trop. Med. Hyg. 81, 235–239.

Animal Welfare Information Center (AWIC), 2006. Environmental Enrichment for Nonhuman Primates Resource Guide. AWIC Resource Series No. 32. <http://www.nal.usda.gov/awic/pubs/Primates2009/primates.shtml>. Updated January 2014.

Aquino, R., Encarnacíon, F., 1986. Population structure of Aotus nancymae (Cebidae: Primates) in Peruvian Amazon lowland forest. Am. J. Primatol. 11, 1–7.

Aquino, R., Puertas, P., Encarnacíon, F., 1990. Supplemental notes on population parameters of northeastern Peruvian night monkeys, genus Aotus (Cebidae). Am. J. Primatol. 21, 215–221.

Araújo, M.S., Messias, M.R., Figueiró, M.R., Gil, L.H.S., Probst, C.M., Vidal, N.M., et al., 2013. Natural Plasmodium infection in monkeys in the state of Rondônia (Brazilian Western Amazon). Malar. J. 12, 180.

Arita, I., Gispan, R., Kalter, S.S., Wah, L.T., Marrenikova, S.S., Netter, R., et al., 1972. Outbreaks of monkeypox and serological surveys in non-human primates. Bull. W. H. O. 46, 625–631.

Arita, I., Jezek, Z., Khodakevich, L., Kalisa-Ruti, J., 1985. Human monkeypox: a newly emerged orthopox zoonosis in the tropical rainforests of Africa. Am. J. Trop. Med. Hyg. 34, 781–789.

Ariga, S., Dukelow, W.R., Emley, G.S., Hutchinson, R.R., 1978. Possible errors in identification of squirrel monkeys (Saimiri sciureus) from different South American points of export. J. Med. Primatol. 7, 129–135.

Arpino, C., Brescianini, S., Robert, E., Castilla, E.E., Cocchi, G., Cornel, M.C., et al., 2000. Teratogenic effects of antiepileptic drugs: use of an International Database on Malformations and Drug Exposure (MADRE). Epilepsia 41, 1436–1443.

Asher, D.M., Gibbs Jr., C.J., Lang, D.J., Gajdusek, D.C., 1974. Persistent shedding of cytomegalovirus in the urine of healthy rhesus monkeys. Proc. Soc. Exp. Biol. Med. 145, 794–801.

Asher, L.V., Binn, L.N., Mensing, T.L., Marchwicki, R.H., Vassell, R.A., Young, G.D., 1995. Pathogenesis of hepatitis A in orally inoculated owl monkeys (Aotus trivirgatus). J. Med. Virol. 47, 260–268.

Ausman, L.M., Gallina, D.L., Samonds, K.W., Hegsted, D.M., 1979. Assessment of the efficiency of protein utilization in young squirrel and macaque monkeys. Am. J. Clin. Nutr. 32, 1813–1823.

Ausman, L.M., Gallina, D.L., Nicolosi, R.J., 1985. Nutrition and metabolism of the squirrel monkey. In: Rosenblum, L.A., Coe, C.L. (Eds.), Handbook of Squirrel Monkey Research. Plenum Press, New York, pp. 349–378.

Azzam, N., Aljebreen, A.M., Alharbi, O., Almadi, M.A., 2013. Prevalence and clinical features of colonic diverticulosis in a Middle Eastern population. World J. Gastrointest. Endosc. 5, 391–397. http://dx.doi.org/10.4253/wjge.v5.i8.391.

Baer, J.F., 1994. Husbandry and medical management of the owl monkey. In: Baer, J.F., Weller, R.E., Kakoma, I. (Eds.), Aotus: The Owl Monkey. Academic Press, San Diego, CA, pp. 134–164.

Baer, J.F., Gibson, S.V., Weller, R.E., Buschbom, R.L., Leathers, C.W., 1992. Naturally occurring aortic aneurysms in owl monkeys (Aotus spp.). Lab. Anim. Sci. 42, 463–466.

Baggs, R.B., Hunt, R.D., Garcia, F.G., Hajema, E.M., Blake, B.I., Fraser, C.E.O., 1976. Pseudotuberculosis (Yersinia enterocolitica) in the owl monkey (Aotus trivirgatus). Lab. Anim. Sci. 26, 1079–1083.

Bagi, C.M., Berryman, E., Moalli, M.R., 2011. Comparative bone anatomy of commonly used laboratory animals: implications for drug discovery. Comp. Med. 61, 76–85.

Bagnall, B.G., Grunberg, W., 1972. Generalized Trichophyton mentagrophytes ringworm in capuchin monkeys (Cebus nigrivitatus). Br. J. Dermatol. 87, 655–670.

Bailey, J.N., Breidenthal, S.E., Jorgensen, M.J., McCracken, J.T., Fairbanks, L.A., 2007. The association of DRD4 and novelty seeking is found in a nonhuman primate model. Psychiatr. Genet. 17, 23–27.

Baker, H.J., Bradford, L.G., Montes, L.F., 1971. Dermatophytosis due to Microsporum canis in a rhesus monkey. J. Am. Vet. Med. Assoc. 159, 1607–1611.

Balayan, M.S., 1992. Natural hosts of hepatitis A virus. Vaccine 10 (Suppl. 1), S27–S31.

Baldwin, J.D., 1985. The behavior of squirrel monkeys (*Saimiri*) in natural environments. In: Rosenblum, L.A., Coe, C.L. (Eds.), Handbook of Squirrel Monkey Research. Plenum Press, New York, pp. 35–53.

Banish, L.D., Sims, R., Bush, M., Sack, D., Montali, R.J., 1993a. Clearance of *Shigella flexneri* carriers in a zoologic collection of primates. J. Am. Vet. Med. Assoc. 203, 133–136.

Banish, L.D., Sims, R., Sack, D., Montali, R.J., Phillips Jr., L., Bush, M., 1993b. Prevalence of shigellosis and other enteric pathogens in a zoologic collection of primates. J. Am. Vet. Med. Assoc. 203, 126–132.

Barhona, H., Melendez, L.V., Hunt, R.D., Daniel, M.D., 1976. The owl monkey (*Aotus trivirgatus*) as an animal model for viral diseases and oncologic studies. Lab. Anim. Sci. 26, 1104–1112.

Barnhart, K., 2010. Hematology of laboratory primates. In: Weiss, D.J., Wardrop, K.J. (Eds.), Schalm's Veterinary Hematology, sixth ed. Wiley Blackwell, Philadelphia, pp. 852–888.

Baron, E.J., Peterson, L.R., Finegold, S.M., 1994. Mycobacteria. In: Shanahan, J.P. (Ed.), Diagnostic Microbiology, Mosby, St. Louis, MO, pp. 596–597.

Barrette, R.W., Metwally, S.A., Rowland, J.M., Xu, L., Zaki, S.R., Nichol, S.T., et al., 2009. Discovery of swine as a host for the Reston ebolavirus. Science 325, 204–206.

Barrickman, N.L., Bastian, M.L., Isler, K., van Schaik, C.P., 2008. Life history costs and benefits of encephalization: a comparative test using data from long-term studies of primates in the wild. J. Hum. Evol. 54, 568–590.

Barton, R.A., Byrne, R.W., Whiten, A., 1996. Ecology, feeding competition and social structure. Behav. Ecol. Sociobiol. 38, 321–329.

Baskerville, A., Newell, D.G., 1988. Naturally occurring chronic gastritis and C. *pylori* infection in the rhesus monkey: a potential model for gastritis in man. Gut. 29, 465–472.

Baskerville, M., Wood, M., Baskerville, A., 1983. An outbreak of *Bordetella bronchiseptica* pneumonia in a colony of common marmosets (*Callithrix jacchus*). Lab. Anim. 17, 350–355.

Baskin, G.B., 1987. Disseminated cytomegalovirus infection in immunodeficient rhesus monkeys. Am. J. Pathol. 129, 345–352.

Baskin, G.B., 1991. Disseminated histoplasmosis in an SIV-infected rhesus monkey. J. Med. Primatol. 20, 251–253.

Baskin, G.B., 1993. Encephalomyocarditis virus infection, nonhuman primates. In: Jones, T.C. Mohr, U. Hunt, R.D. (Eds.), Monographs on Pathology of Laboratory Animals: Nonhuman Primates, vol. 2. Springer-Verlag, Berlin and New York, pp. 104–107.

Baskin, G.B., Roberts, E.D., Kuebler, D., Martin, L.N., Blauw, B., Heeney, J., et al., 1995. Squamous epithelial proliferative lesions associated with rhesus Epstein-Barr virus in simian immunodeficiency virus-infected rhesus macaques. J. Infect. Dis. 172, 535–538.

Baskin, G.B., Wolf, R.H., Worth, C.L., Soike, K., Gibson, S.V., Bieri, J.G., 1983. Anemia, steatitis, and muscle necrosis in marmosets (*Saguinus labiatus*). Lab. Anim. Sci. 33, 74–80.

Bass, F.G., Stark, D.M., 1980. A simplified technique for shortening canine teeth of rhesus monkeys. Lab. Anim. 9, 49–50.

Battles, A.H., Greiner, E.C., Collins, B.R., 1988. Efficacy of ivermectin against natural infection of *Strongyloides* in squirrel monkeys (*Saimiri sciureus*). Lab. Anim. Sci. 38, 474–476.

Baulu, J., Evans, G., Sutton, C., 2002. Pathogenic agents found in Barbados *Chlorocebus aethiops sabaeus* and in Old World Monkeys commonly used in biomedical research. Lab. Primate Newslett. 41, 4–6.

Bayne, K., Morris, T.H., 2012. Laws, regulations and policies relating to the care and use of nonhuman primates in biomedical research. In: Abee, C.R., Mansfield, K., Tardiff, S., Morris, T. (Eds.), Nonhuman Primates in Biomedical Research: Biology and Management, second ed. Academic Press, Elsevier, San Diego, CA, pp. 35–56.

Bayne, K., Haines, M., Dexter, S., Woodman, D., Evans, C., 1995. A retrospective analysis of the wounding incidence of nonhuman primates housed in different social conditions. Lab. Anim. Sci. 24, 40–44.

Beglinger, R., Illgen, B., Pfister, R., Heider, K., 1988. The parasite *Trichospira leptostoma* associated with wasting disease in a colony of common marmosets, *Callithrix jacchus*. Folia Primatol. 51, 45–51.

Bell, J.C., Qingwei, L., Gan, Y., Qiang, L., Liu, Y., Shi, F.-D., et al., 2013. Visualization of inflammation and demyelination in 2D2 transgenic mice with rodent MRI. J. Neuroimmunol. 264, 35–40.

Bellinger, D.A., Bullock, B.C., 1988. Cutaneous *Mycobacterium avium* infection in a cynomolgus monkey. Lab. Anim. Sci. 38, 85–86.

Bellini, S., Hubbard, G.B., Kaufman, L., 1991. Spontaneous fatal coccidioidomycosis in a native-born hybrid baboon (*Papio cynocephalus anubis/Papio cynocephalus cynocephalus*). Lab. Anim. Sci. 41, 509–511.

Benjamin, S.A., Lang, C.M., 1971. Acute pasteurellosis in owl monkeys (*Aotus trivirgatus*). Lab. Anim. Sci. 21, 258–262.

Bennett, B.T., Cuasay, L., Welsh, T.J., Belhun, F.Z., Schofield, L., 1980. Acute gastric dilatation in monkeys: a microbiologic study of gastric contents, blood, and feed. Lab. Anim. Sci. 30, 241–244.

Bennett, B.T., Abee, C.R., Henrickson, R.V., 1998. Nonhuman Primates in Biomedical Research: Diseases. Academic Press, San Diego, CA.

Bercovitch, F.B., 1985. Reproductive studies in adult female and adult male olive baboons. Ph.D. dissertation, University of California, Los Angeles, CA.

Bercovitch, F.B., Harding, R.S., 1993. Annual birth patterns of savanna baboons (*Papio cynocephalus anubis*) over a ten-year period at Gilgil, Kenya. Folia Primatol. (Basel) 61, 115–122.

Bergeland, M.E., Barnes, D.M., Kaplan, W., 1970. Spontaneous histoplasmosis in a squirrel monkey. Primate Surveillance Zoonosis Report 1, January–February, 1970, Center for Disease Control, Atlanta, pp. 10–11.

Bergin, I.L., Bell, J.D., Chen, Z., Zochowski, M.K., Chai, D., Schmidt, K., et al., 2012. Novel genital alphapapillomaviruses in baboons (*Papio hamadryas anubis*) with cervical dysplasia. Vet. Pathol. 50, 200–208.

Bernacky, B.J., Gibson, S.V., Keeling, M.E., Abee, C.R., 2002. Nonhuman Primates. In: Fox, J.G., Anderson, L.C., Loew, F.M., Quimby, F.W. (Eds.), Laboratory Animal Medicine, second ed. Elsevier, Academic Press, San Diego, CA.

Bethune, M.T., Borda, J.T., Ribka, E., Liu, M.X., Phillippi-Falkenstein, K., Jandacek, R.J., et al., 2008. A non-human primate model for gluten sensitivity. PLoS One 3, e1614. http://dx.doi.org/10.1371/journal.pone.0001614

Beutler, B., Cerami, A., 1988. Tumor necrosis, cachexia, shock, and inflammation: a common mediator. Annu. Rev. Biochem. 57, 505.

Bingham, G.A., Rabstein, M.M., 1964. A study of the effectiveness of thiabendazole in the rhesus monkey. Lab. Anim. Care 14, 357–365.

Birrell, A.M., Hennessy, A., Gillin, A., Horvath, J., Tiller, D., 1996. Reproductive and neonatal outcomes in captive bred baboons (*Papio hamadryas*). J. Med. Primatol. 25, 287–293.

Bistner, S.I., Ford, R.B., 1995. Kirk and Bistner's Handbook of Veterinary Procedures and Emergency Treatment. Saunders, Philadelphia.

Blackwood, R.S., Tarara, R.P., Christe, K.L., Spinner, A., Lerche, N.W., 2008. Effects of the macrolide drug tylosin on chronic diarrhea in rhesus macaques (*Macaca mulatta*). Comp. Med. 58, 81–87.

Blampied, N. LeQ., Allchurch, A.F., Tagg, J., 1983. Diagnosis, treatment, and control of *Pterygodermatites* (Mesopectines) *alphi* (Nematodes: Spirurida) in the collection of Callitrichidae and Callimiconidae at the Jersey Wildlife Preservation Trust. J. Jersey Wildl. Trust 20, 90–91.

Blanchard, J.L., Soile, K., Baskin, G.B., 1987. Encephalomyocarditis virus infection in African green and squirrel monkeys: comparison of pathologic effects. Lab. Anim. Sci. 37, 635–639.

Blevins, W.E., Widmer, W.R., Jakovljevic, S., Peter, A.T., 1998. A course for those new to diagnostic ultrasound. In: Veterinary Diagnostic

Ultrasound. School of Veterinary Medicine, Purdue University, West Lafayette, IN.

Bloomsmith, M.A., Keeling, M.E., Lambeth, S.P., 1990. Environmental enrichment for singly housed chimpanzees. Lab. Anim. 19, 42–46.

Bloomsmith, M.A., Else, J.G., 2005. Behavioral management of chimpanzees in biomedical research facilities: the state of the science. ILAR 46, 192–201.

Bloomsmith, M.A., Brent, L.Y., Schapiro, S.J., 1991. Guidelines for developing and managing an environmental enrichment program for nonhuman primates. Lab. Anim. Sci. 41, 372–377.

Boesch, C., Head, J., Robbins, M.M., 2009. Complex tool sets for honey extraction among chimpanzees in Loango National Park, Gabon. J. Hum. Evol. 56, 560–569.

Boinski, S., 1987a. Habitat use by squirrel monkeys (Saimiri oerstedii) in Costa Rica. Folia Primatol. 49, 151–167.

Boinski, S., 1987b. Mating patterns in squirrel monkeys (Saimiri oerstedi): implications for seasonal sexual dimorphism. Behav. Ecol. Sociobiol. 21, 13–21.

Boinski, S., 1992. Olfactory communication among Costa Rican squirrel monkeys: a field study. Folia Primatol. 59, 127–136.

Boinski, S., 1999. The social organizations of squirrel monkeys: implications for ecological models of social evolution. Evol. Anthropol. 3, 101–112.

Boinski, S., Kauffman, L., Ehmke, E., Schet, S., Vreedzaam, A., 2005. Dispersal patterns among three species of squirrel monkeys (Saimiri oerstedii, S. boliviensis, and S. sciureus): I. Divergent costs and benefits. Behaviour 142, 525–632.

Boncyk, L.H., McCullough, B., Grotts, D.D., Kalter, S.S., 1975. Localized nocardiosis due to Nocardia caviae in a baboon (Papio cynocephalus). Lab. Anim. Sci. 25, 88–91.

Bonney, R.C., Dixson, A.F., Fleming, D., 1979. Cyclic changes in the circulating and urinary levels of ovarian steroids in the adult female owl monkey (Aotus trivirgatus). J. Reprod. Fertil. 56, 271–280.

Bonney, R.C., Dixson, A.F., Fleming, D., 1980. Plasma concentrations of oestradiol-17B, oestrone, progesterone, and testosterone during the ovarian cycle of the owl monkey (Aotus trivirgatus). J. Reprod. Fertil. 60, 101–107.

Boothe, H.W., 1990. Exploratory laparotomy in small animals. Compend. Contin. Educ. Pract. Vet. 12, 1057–1066.

Borda, J.T., Ruiz, J.C., Sánchez-Negrette, M., 1994. Aortic aneurysm in a Cebus apella monkey with experimentally induced atherosclerosis. J. Med. Primatol. 23, 365–366.

Bosch, M.L., Harper, E., Schmidt, A., Strand, K.B., Thormahlen, S., Thouless, M.E., et al., 1999. Activation in vivo of retroperitoneal fibromatosis-associated herpesvirus, a simian homologue of human herpesvirus-8. J. Gen. Virol. 80, 467–475.

Bourgeois, S.R., Vazquez, M., Brasky, K., 2007. Combination therapy reduces self-injurious behavior in a chimpanzee (Pan troglodytes troglodytes): a case report. J. Appl. An. Welfare Sci. 10, 123–140.

Bourne, G.H., 1969. The Chimpanzee. S. Karger, New York.

Brack, M., 1987. Hepatitis viruses. In: Brack, M. (Ed.), Agents Transmissible from Simians to Man. Springer-Verlag, New York, pp. 83–89.

Brack, M., Rietschel, W., 1986. Ivermectin for the control of Strongyloides fulleborni in rhesus monkeys. Kleinter-Prax (Short communication) 31, 29. (in German), cited by Battles et al., 1988.

Brack, M., Rothe, H., 1981. Chronic tubulointerstitial nephritis and wasting disease in marmosets (Callithrix jacchus). Vet. Pathol. 18, 45–54.

Bracken, J.N., Reyes, M., Gendron, J.M., Pierce, L.M., Runge, V.M., Kuehl, T.J., 2011. Alterations in pelvic floor muscles and pelvic organ support by pregnancy and vaginal delivery in squirrel monkeys. Int. Urogynecol. J. 22, 1109–1116.

Brady, A.G., 2000. Research techniques for the squirrel monkey (Saimiri sp.). ILAR J. 41, 10–18.

Brady, A.G., Carville, A.A.L., 2012. Digestive system diseases of nohuman primates. In: Abee, C.R. Mansfield, K. Tardif, S. Morris, T. (Eds.), Nonhuman Primates in Biomedical Research: Diseases, vol. 2. Academic Press, San Diego, CA, pp. 599–606.

Brady, A.G., Pindak, F.F., Abee, C.R., Gardner, W.A., Jr., 1988. Enteric trichomonads of squirrel monkeys (Saimiri sp.): natural infestation and treatment. Am. J. Primatol. 14, 65–71.

Brady, A.G., Watford, J.W., Massey, C.V., Rodning, K.J., Gibson, S.V., Williams, L.E., et al., 2003. Studies of heart disease and failure in aged female squirrel monkeys (Saimiri sp.). Comp. Med. 53, 657–662.

Brammer, D.W., O'Rourke, C.M., Heath, L.A., Chrisp, C.E., Peter, G.K., Hofing, G.L., 1995. Mycobacterium kansasii infection in squirrel monkeys (Saimiri sciureus sciureus). J. Med. Primatol. 24, 231–235.

Brandler, S., Marianneau, P., Loth, P., Lacôte, S., Combredet, C., Frenkiel, M.-P., et al., 2012. Measles vaccine expressing the secreted form of west nile virus envelope glycoprotein induces protective immunity in squirrel monkeys, a new model of west nile virus infection. J. Infect. Dis. 206, 212–219.

Brandt, E.M., Mitchell, G., 1971. Parturition in primates: behavior related to birth. In: Rosenblum, L.A. (Ed.), Primate Behavior: Developments in Field and Laboratory Research, vol. 2. Academic Press, New York, pp. 178–223.

Brandt, R.R., Neumann, T., Neuzner, J., Rau, M., Faude, I., Hamm, C.W., 2002. Transcatheter closure of atrial septal defect and patent foramen ovale in adult patients using the Amplatzer occlusion device: no evidence for thrombus deposition with antiplatelet agents. J. Am. Soc. Echocardiogr. 15, 1094–1098.

Brendt, R.F., McDonough, W.E., Walker, J.S., 1974. Persistence of Diplococcus pneumoniae after influenza virus infection in Macaca mulatta. Infect. Immun. 10, 369–374.

Breznock, A.W., Henrickson, R.V., Silverman, S., Schwartz, L.W., 1975. Coccidioidomycosis in a rhesus monkey. J. Am. Vet. Med. Assoc. 167, 657–661.

Broderson, J.R., Chapman Jr., W.L., Hanson, W.L., 1986. Experimental visceral leishmaniasis in the owl monkey. Vet. Pathol. 23, 293–302.

Bronsdon, M.A., DiGiacomo, R.F., 1993. Pasteurella multocida infections in baboons (Papio cynocephalus). Primates 34, 205–209.

Bronson, R.T., May, B.D., Ruebner, B.H., 1972. An outbreak of infection by Yersinia pseudotuberculosis in nonhuman primates. Am. I. Path 69, 289–303.

Bronson, R.T., O'Connell, M., Klepper-Kilgore, N., Chalifoux, L.V., Sehgal, P., 1982. Fatal fasting syndrome of obese macaques. Lab. Anim. Sci. 32, 187–192.

Brown, B.G., Swenson, R.B., 1995. Surgical management. In: Bennett, B.T., Abee, C.R., Henrickson, R.V. (Eds.), Nonhuman Primates in Biomedical Research: Diseases. Academic Press, San Diego, CA, pp. 297–304.

Brown, P., Gibbs Jr., C.J., Rogers-Johnson, P., Asher, D.M., Sulima, M.P., Bacote, A., et al., 1994. Human spongiform encephalopathy: the National Institutes of Health series of 300 cases of experimentally transmitted disease. Ann. Neurol. 35, 513–529.

Bruce, A.G., Bakke, A.M., Bielefeldt-Ohmann, H., Ryan, J.T., Thouless, M.E., Tsai, C.C., et al., 2006. High levels of retroperitoneal fibromatosis (RF)-associated herpesvirus in RF lesions in macaques are associated with ORF73 LANA expression in spindleoid tumour cells. J. Gen. Virol. 87 (Pt 12), 3529–3538.

Bruestle, M.E., Golden, J.G., Hall, A., Bankneider, A.R., 1981. Naturally occurring Yaba tumor in a baboon (Papio papio). Lab. Anim. Sci. 31, 292–294.

Brusasca, P.N., Peters, R.L., Motzel, S.L., Klein, H.J., Gennaro, M.L., 2003. Antigen recognition by serum antibodies in non-human primates experimentally infected with Mycobacterium tuberculosis. Comp. Med. 53 (2), 165–172.

Bryant, J.L., Stills, H.F., Lentsch, R.H., Middleton, C.C., 1983. Campylobacter jejuni isolated from patas monkeys with diarrhea. Lab. Anim. Sci. 33, 303–305.

Bryant, M.L., Marx, P.A., Shiigi, S.M., Wilson, B.J., McNulty, W.P., Gardner, M.B., 1986. Distribution of type D retrovirus sequences in tissues of macaques with simian acquired immune deficiency and retroperitoneal fibromatosis. Virology 150 (1), 149–160.

Buchl, S.J., Howard, B., 1997. Hematologic and serum biochemical and electrolyte values in clinically normal domestically bred rhesus monkeys (Macaca mulatta) according to age, sex, and gravidity. Lab. Anim. Sci. 35, 528–533.

Buchl, S.J., Keeling, M.E., Voss, W.R., 1997. Establishing specific pathogen free (SPF) nonhuman primate colonies. ILAR 38, 22–27.

Bukh, J., Apgar, C.L., Govindarajan, S., Purcell, R.H., 2001. Host range studies of GB virus-B hepatitis agent, the closest relative of hepatitis C virus, in new world monkeys and chimpanzees. J. Med. Virol. 65, 694–697.

Bulte, J.W., Miller, G.F., Vymazal, J., Brooks, R.A., Frank, J.A., 1997. Hepatic hemosiderosis in non-human primates: quantifications of liver iron using different field strengths. Magn. Reson. Med. 37, 530–536.

Bunton, T.E., Bacmeister, C.X., 1989. Diverticulosis and colonic leiomyosarcoma in an aged rhesus macaque. Vet. Pathol. 26, 351–352.

Burke, R.L., Whitehouse, C.A., Taylor, J.K., Selby, E.B., 2009. Epidemiology of invasive Klebsiella pneumoniae with hypermucoviscosity phenotype in a research colony of nonhuman primates. Comp. Med. 59 (6), 589–597.

Butynski, T.M., Gippoliti, S., Kingdon, J., De Jong, Y., 2008. Chlorocebus djamdjamensis. In: IUCN 2013. IUCN Red List of Threatened Species. Version 2013.1. Available at: <www.iucnredlist.org>. Downloaded on September 25, 2013.

Butler, T.M., Hubbard, G.B., 1991. An epizootic of histoplasmosis duboisii (African histoplasmosis) in an American baboon colony. Lab. Anim. Sci. 41, 407–410.

Butler, T.M., Gleiser, C.A., Bernal, J.C., Ajello, L., 1988. Case of disseminated African histoplasmosis in a baboon. J. Med. Primatol. 17, 153–161.

Caine, N.G., 1993. Flexibility and co-operation as unifying themes in Saguinus social organization and behavior: the role of predation pressues. In: Rylands, A.B. (Ed.), Marmosets and Tamarins: Systematics, Behaviour, and Ecology. Oxford University Press, New York, pp. 210–211.

Cameron, K.R., Stamminger, T., Craxton, M., Bodemer, W., Honess, R.W., Fleckenstein, B., 1987. The 160, 000-Mr protein encoded at the right end of the herpesvirus saimiri genome is homologous to the 140, 000-Mr membrane encoded at the left end of the EBV genome. J. Virol. 61, 2063–2070.

Campos, M.E., Alvares, J.N., Arruda, M.F., do Vale, N.B., 1981. Surto epizootico por Klebsiella sp. num nucleo de reproducao de saguis (Callithrix jacchus), em cativiero. Rev. Bioterios 1, 95–99.

Capuano III, S.V., Croix, D.A., Pawar, S., et al., 2003. Experimental Mycobacterium tuberculosis infection of cynomolgus macaques closely resembles the various manifestations of human M. tuberculosis infection. Infect. Immun. 71 (10), 5831–5844.

Carlsson, H.E., Schapiro, S.J., Farah, I., Hau, J., 2004. Use of primates in research: a global overview. Am. J. Primatol. 63, 225–237.

Carneiro, L.A., Laurenti, M.D., Campos, M.B., de Castro Gomes, C.M., Corbett, C.E.P., Silveira, F.T., 2012. Susceptibility of peritoneal macrophage from different species of neotropical primates to ex vivo Leishmania (L.) infantum chagasi-infection. Rev. Inst. Med. Trop. Sao Paulo 54, 95–101.

Carrion, R., Ro, Y., Hoosien, K., Ticer, A., Brasky, K., de la Garza, M., et al., 2011. A small nonhuman primate model for filovirus-induced disease. Virology 420, 117–124.

Carroll, E.E., Hammamieh, R., Chakraborty, N., Phillips, A.T., Miller, S.-A.M., Jett, M., 2006. Altered gene expression in asymptomatic SHIV-infected rhesus macaques (Macaca mulatta). Virol. J. 3, 74–81.

Cary, M.E., Valentine, B., White, G.L., 2003. The effects of confinement environment on reproductive efficiency in the baboon. Contemp. Top. 42, 35–39.

Castleman, W.L., Anderson, J., Holmberg, C.A., 1980. Posterior paralysis and spinal osteomyelitis in a rhesus monkey with coccidioidomycosis. J. Am. Vet. Med. Assoc. 177, 933–934.

Centers for Disease Control and Prevention (CDCP), 1987. B virus infection in humans - Pensacola, Florida. Morb. Mortal. Wkly. Rep. 36, 289–290. 295–296, 680-682, 687-689.

Centers for Disease Control and Prevention (CDCP), 1998. Fatal cercopithecine herpesvirus 1 (B virus) infection following a mucocutaneous exposure and interim recommendations for worker protection. Morb. Mortal. Wkly. Rep. 47, 1073–1076. 1083.

Centers for Disease Control and Prevention/National Institutes of Health (CDCP/NIH), 2009. In: Chosewood, L.C., Wilson, D.E. (Eds.), Biosafety in Microbiological and Biomedical Laboratories, fifth ed. Government Printing Office, Washington, DC. HHS Publ. (CDC) 21-1112.

Centers for Disease Control and Prevention (CDCP), CFR 42 part 71.53. Final Rule on Regulations for the Importation of Nonhuman Primates. Effective April 16, 2013.

Chalmers, D.T., Murgatroyd, L.B., Wadsworth, P.F., 1983. A survey of the pathology of marmosets (Callithrix jacchus) derived from a marmoset breeding unit. Lab. Anim. 17, 270–279.

Champoux, M., Suomi, S.J., Schneider, M.L., 1994. Temperament differences between captive Indian and Chinese-Indian hybrid rhesus macaque neonates. Lab. Anim. Sci. 44, 351–357.

Chandler, F.W., McClure, H.M., 1982. Adenoviral pancreatitis in rhesus monkeys: current knowledge. Vet. Pathol. 19 (Suppl. 7), 171–180.

Chandler, F.W., McClure, H.M., Campbell Jr., W.G., Watts, J.C., 1976. Pulmonary pneumocystosis in nonhuman primates. Arch. Pathol. Lab. Med. 100, 163–167.

Chapman, W.L., Hanson Jr., W.L., Hendricks, L.D., 1981. Leishmania donovani in the owl monkey (Aotus trivirgatus). Trans. R. Soc. Trop. Med. Hyg. 75, 124–125.

Chege, G.K., Burgers, W.A., Stutz, H., Meyers, A.E., Chapman, R., Kiravu, A., et al., 2013. Robust immunity to an auxotrophic Mycobacterium bovis BCG-VLP prime-boost HIV vaccine candidate in a nonhuman primate model. J. Virol. 87, 5151–5160.

Chellman, G.J., Lukas, V.S., Eugui, E.M., Altera, K.P., Almquist, S.J., Hilliard, J.K., 1992. Activation of B virus (Herpesvirus simiae) in chronically immunosuppressed cynomolgus monkeys. Lab. Anim. Sci. 42, 146–151.

Chen, S., Bastarrachea, R.A., Roberts, B.J., Voruganti, V.S., Frost, P.A., Nava-Gonzalez, E.J., et al., 2014. Successful β cells islet regeneration in streptozotocin-induced diabetic baboons using ultrasound-targeted microbubble gene therapy with cyclinD2/CDK4/GLP1. Cell Cycle 13, 1145–1151. [Epub ahead of print].

Chen, X., Errangi, B., Li, L., Glasser, M.F., Westlye, L.T., Fjell, A.M., et al., 2013. Brain aging in humans, chimpanzees (Pan troglodytes), and rhesus macaques (Macaca mulatta): magnetic resonance imaging studies of macro- and microstructural changes. Neurobiol. Aging 34, 2248–2260.

Cheney, D.L., Seyfarth, R.M., 1983. Nonrandom dispersal in free-ranging vervet monkeys: social and genetic consequences. Am. Nat. 122, 392–412.

Cheney, D.L., Seyfarth, R.M., Andelman, S.J., Lee, P.C., 1988. Reproductive success in vervet monkeys. In: Clutton-Brock, T.H. (Ed.), Reproductive Success: Studies of Individual Variation in Contrasting Breeding Systems. University Chicago Press, Chicago (IL), pp. 384–402.

Chimpanzee Sequencing and Analysis Consortium, 2005. Initial sequence of the chimpanzee genome and comparison with the human genome. Nature 437, 69–87.

Chin, C.L., Carr, R.A., Llano, D.A., Barret, O., Xu, H., Batis, J., et al., 2011. Pharmacokinetic modeling and [123]5-IA-85380 single photon emission computed tomography imaging in baboons: optimization of dosing regimen for ABT-089. J. Pharmacol. Exp. Ther. 336, 716–723.

Chiou, K.L., Pozzi, L., Lynch Alfaro, J.W., Di Fiore, A., 2011. Pleistocene diversification of living squirrel monkeys (Saimiri spp.) inferred from complete mitochondrial genome sequences. Mol. Phylogenet. Evol. 59, 736–745.

Chiu, Y.J., Chi, A., Reid, I.A., 1997. Cardiovascular and endocrine effects of acupuncture in hypertensive patients. Clin. Exp. Hypertens. 19, 1047–1063.

Cho, F., Hiyaoka, A., Suzuki, M.T., Honjo, S., 2002. Breeding of African Green Monkeys (Cercopithecus aethiops) under indoor individually-caged conditions. Exp. Anim. 51, 343–351.

Cho, Y.-G., Ramer, J., Rivailler, P., Quink, C., Garber, R.L., Beier, D.R., et al., 2001. An Epstein–Barr-related herpesvirus from marmoset lymphomas. Proc. Natl. Acad. Sci. 98 (3), 1224–1229. http://dx.doi.org/10.1073/pnas.98.3.1224.

Christe, K.L., Valverde, C.R., 1999. The use of a percutaneous endoscopic gastrotomy (PEG) tube to reverse fatal fasting syndrome in a cynomolgus macaque (Macaca fascicularis). Contemp. Top. Lab. Anim. Sci. 38, 12–15.

Churchill, A.E., 1963. The isolation of parainfluenza 3 virus from fatal cases of pneumonia in Erythrocebus patas monkeys. Br. J. Exp. Pathol. 44, 529–537.

Cicmanec, J.C., 1977. Medical problems encountered in a callitrichid colony. In: Kleinman, D.G. (Ed.), The Biology and Conservation of the Callitrichidae. Smithsonian Institution Press, Washington, D.C, pp. 331–336.

Cicmanec, J.C., Campbell, A.K., 1977. Breeding the owl monkey (Aotus trivirgatus) in a laboratory environment. Lab. Anim. Sci. 27, 512–517.

Cilia, J., Piper, D.C., Upton, N., Hagan, J.J., 1998. A comparison of rectal and subcutaneous body temperature measurement in the common marmoset. J. Pharmacol. Toxicol. Methods 40, 21–26.

Clap, N.K., Henke, M.L., Lushbaugh, C.C., Humason, G.L., Gangaware, B.L., 1988. Effect of various biological factors on spontaneous marmoset and tamarin colitis: a retrospective histopathologic study. Dig. Dis. Sci. 33, 1013–1019.

Clarke, C.J., Watt, N.J., Meredith, A., McIntyre, N., Burns, S.M., 1994. Respiratory syncytial virus-associated bronchopneumonia in a young chimpanzee. J. Comp. Pathol. 110, 207–212.

Clarkson, M.J., Thorpe, E., McCarthy, K., 1967. A virus disease of captive vervet monkeys (Cercopithecus aethiops) caused by a new herpesvirus. Arch. Gersamte Virusforsch. 22, 219–234.

Clayton, O., Kuehl, T.J., 1984. The first successful in vitro fertilization and embryo transfer in a nonhuman primate. Theriogenology 21, 228.

Clemmons, E.A., Jean, S.M., Machiah, D.K., Breding, E., Sharma, P., 2014. Extraintestinal Campylobacteriosis in rhesus macaques (Macaca mulatta). Comp. Med. 64, 496–500.

Coates, K.W., Galan, H.L., Shull, B.L., Kuehl, T.J., 1995a. The squirrel monkey: an animal model of pelvic relaxation. Am. J. Obstet. Gynecol. 172, 588–593.

Coates, K.W., Gibson, S., Williams, L.E., Brady, A., Abee, C.R., Shull, B.L., et al., 1995b. The squirrel monkey as an animal model of pelvic relaxation: an evaluation of a large breeding colony. Am. J. Obstet. Gynecol. 173, 1664–1670.

Coates, A., Poole, T.B., 1983. The behavior of the Callitrichid monkey, Saguinus labiatus labiatus, in the laboratory. Internatl. J. Primatol. 4, 339–371.

Code of Federal Regulations (CFR), 1999. Title 9, Animals and Animal Products; Chapter 1, Animal and Plant Health Inspection Service, USDA; Subchapter A., Animal Welfare; Part 3, Standards, Subpart D. Office of the Federal Register, Washington, D.C.

Coe, C.L., Lemieux, A.M., Rier, S.E., Uno, H., Zimbric, M.L., 1998. Profile of endometriosis in the aging female rhesus monkey. J. Gerontol. A Biol. Sci. Med. Sci. 53, M3–M7.

Coe, C.L., Smith, E.R., Levine, S., 1985. The endocrine system of the squirrel monkey. In: Rosenblum, L.A., Coe, C.L. (Eds.), Handbook of Squirrel Monkey Research. Plenum Press, New York, pp. 191–218.

Coelho, A.M., Carey, K.D., 1990. A social tethering system for nonhuman primates used in laboratory research. Lab. Anim. Sci. 40, 388–394.

Cohen, J., 2007. The endangered lab chimp. Science 315, 450–452.

Cohen, J.I., Davenport, D.S., Stewart, J.A., Deitchman, S., Hilliard, J.K., Chapman, L.E., 2002. Recommendations for prevention of and therapy for exposure to B virus (Cercopithecine herpesvirus 1). Clin. Infect. Dis. 35 (10), 1191–1203.

Coimbra-Filho, A.F., Mittermeier, R.A., 1977. Tree-gouging, exudate-eating, and the short-tusked condition in Callithrix and Cebuella. In: Kleiman, D.G. (Ed.), The Biology and Conservation of the Callitrichidae. Smithsonian Institution Press, Washington, DC, pp. 105–115.

Coleman, K., Pranger, L., Maier, A., Lambeth, S.P., Perlman, J.E., Thiele, E., et al., 2008. Training rhesus macaques for venipuncture using positive reinforcement techniques: a comparison with chimpanzees. JAALAS 47, 37–41.

Colmenares, F., Esteban, M.M., Zaragoza, F., 2006. One-male units and clans in a colony of Hamadryas baboons (Papio hamadryas hamadryas): effect of male number and clan cohesion on feeding success. Am. J. Primatol. 68, 21–37.

Convention on International Trade in Endangered Species of Wild Fauna and Flora (CITES), 2000. Appendices I and II. CITES Secretariat, Geneva, Switzerland. Available at: <http://www.cites.org>.

Cooper, D.K.C., 2012. A brief history of cross-species organ transplantation. Proc. (Bayl. Univ. Med. Cent.) 25, 49–57.

Cooper, R.W., 1968. Squirrel monkey taxonomy and supply. In: Rosenblum, L.A., Cooper, R.W. (Eds.), The Squirrel Monkey. Academic Press, New York, pp. 1–29.

Cooper, J.E., Needham, J.R., 1976. An outbreak of shigellosis in laboratory marmosets and tamarins. J. Hyg. Camb. 76, 415–424.

Cornblath, D.R., Hillman, M.A., Striffler, J.S., Herman, C.N., Hansen, B.C., 1989. Peripheral neuropathy in diabetic monkeys. Diabetes 38, 1365–1370.

Cornejo, F., Palacios, E., 2008. Aotus nancymaae; Aotus nigriceps In: IUCN 2013. IUCN Red List of Threatened Species. Version 2013.1. Available at: <www.iucnredlist.org>. Downloaded on October 15, 2013.

Cornejo, F., Rylands, A.B., Mittermeier, R.A., Heymann, E., 2008. Aotus miconax. In: IUCN 2013. IUCN Red List of Threatened Species. Version 2013.1. Available at: <www.iucnredlist.org>. Downloaded on October 15, 2013.

Cortés-Ortiz, L., 2009. Molecular phylogenetics of the Callitrichidae with an emphasis on the marmosets and Callimico. In: Ford, S.M., Porter, L.M., Davis, L.C. (Eds.), The Smallest Anthropoids: The Marmoset/Callimico Radiation. Springer Publishing, New York, pp. 3–21.

Cowlishaw, G., 1994. Vulnerability to predation in baboon populations. Behaviour 131, 293–304.

Cox-Singh, J., 2012. Zoonotic malaria: Plasmodium knowlesi, an emerging pathogen. Curr. Opin. Infect Dis. 25, 530–536.

Cox, L.A., Comuzzie, A.G., Havill, L.M., Karere, G.M., Spradling, K.D., Mahaney, M.C., et al., 2013. Baboons as a model to study genetics and epigenetics of human disease. ILAR 54, 106–121.

Crockett, C.M., Gough, G.M., 2002. Onset of aggressive toy biting by a laboratory baboon coincides with cessation of self-injurious behavior. Am. J. Primatol. 57 (Suppl. 1), 39.

Crockett, C.M., Heffernan, K.S., 1998. Grooming-contact cages promote affiliative social interaction in individually housed adult baboons. Am. J. Primatol. 45, 176.

Crompton, A.W., Taylor, C.R., Jagger, J.A., 1978. Evolution of homeothermy in mammals. Nature 272, 333–336.

Crow, S.E., Walshaw, S.O., 1987. Manual of Clinical Procedures in the Dog and Cat. J. B. Lippincott, Philadelphia, PA.

Cuarón, A.D., Palacios, E., Morales, A., Shedden, A., Rodriguez-Luna, E., de Grammont, P.C., 2008. Aotus zonalis. In: IUCN 2013. IUCN Red List of Threatened Species. Version 2013.1. Available at: <www.iucnredlist.org>. Downloaded on October 15, 2013.

Cunningham, A.A., Buxton, D., Thompson, K.M., 1992. An epidemic of toxoplasmosis in a captive colony of squirrel monkeys (Saimiri sciureus). J. Comp. Pathol. 107, 207–219.

Dalgard, D.W., Hardy, R.J., Pearson, S.L., Pucak, G.J., Quander, R.V., Zack, P.M., et al., 1992. Combined simian hemorrhagic fever and Ebola virus infection in cynomolgus monkeys. Lab. Anim. Sci. 42, 152–157.

Damon, I.K., 2011. Status of human monkeypox: clinical disease, epidemiology and research. Vaccine 29 (Suppl 4), D54–D59.

Daniel, M.D., 1978. Prevention of fatal herpesvirus infections in owl and marmoset monkeys by vaccination In: Chivers, D.J., Ford, E.H.R. (Eds.), Recent Advances in Primatology, vol. 4 Academic Press, London, pp. 67–69.

da Silva Mota, M.T., Franci, C.R., Cordeiro de Susa, M.B., 2006. Hormonal changes related to paternal and alloparental care in common marmosets (Callithrix jacchus). Horm. Behav. 49, 293–302.

David, J.M., Dick, E.J., Hubbard, G.B., 2009. Spontaneous pathology of the common marmoset (Callithrix jacchus) and tamarins (Saguinus oedipus, Saguinus mystax). J. Med. Primatol. 38, 347–359.

Dawidson, I., Angmar-Månsson, B., Blom, M., Theodorsson, E., Lundeberg, T., 1999. Sensory stimulation (acupuncture) increases the release of calcitonin gene-related peptide in the saliva of xerostomia sufferers. Neuropeptides 33, 244–250.

Dawson, G.A., 1977. Composition and stability of social groups of the tamarin, Saguinus oedipus geoffroyi, in Panama: ecology and behavioral implications. In: Kleiman, D.G. (Ed.), The Biology and Conservation of the Callitrichidae. Smithsonian Institution Press, Washington, DC, pp. 23–37.

Defler, T.R., Bueno, M.L., 2007. Aotus diversity and the species problem. Primate Conserv. 22, 55–70.

Deinhardt, F., Falk, L.G., Wolf, A., Schudel, A., Nonyama, M., Lai, P., et al., 1978. Susceptibility of marmosets to Epstein-Barr virus-like baboon herpesviruses. Primate Med 10, 163–170.

Deinhardt, F., Holmes, A.W., Devine, J., Deinhardt, J., 1967a. Marmosets as laboratory animals. IV. The microbiology of laboratory-kept marmosets. Lab. Anim. Care 17, 48–70.

Deinhardt, J.B., Devine, J., Passavoy, M., Pohlman, R., Deinhardt, F., 1967b. Marmosets as laboratory animals. I. Care of marmosets in the laboratory, pathology, and outline of the statistical evaluation of data. Lab. Anim. Care 17, 11–29.

De Groot, N.G., Bontrop, R.E., 2013. The HIV-1 pandemic: does the selective sweep in chimpanzees mirror humankind's future? Retrovirology 10, 53. http://dx.doi.org/10.1186/1742-4690-10-53.

De Jong, B.C., Antonio, M., Gagneux, S., 2010. Mycobacterium africanum - Review of an important cause of human tuberculosis in West Africa. PLoS Negl Trop Dis., 4, e744. http://dx.doi.org/10.1371/journal.pntd.0000744.

Demanche, C., Berthelemy, M., Petit, T., Polack, B., Wakefield, A.E., Dei-Cas, E., et al., 2001. Phylogeny of Pneumocystis carinii from 18 primate species confirms host specificity and suggests coevolution. J. Clin. Microbiol. 39, 2126–2133. http://dx.doi.org/10.1128/JCM.39.6.2126-2133.2001.

DeMarcus, T.A., Tipple, M.A., Ostrowski, S.R., 1999. U.S. policy for disease control among imported nonhuman primates. J. Infect. Dis. 179 (Suppl), S281–S282.

Demontoy, M.C., Berthier, J.L., Letellier, F., 1979. Vitamin A et spondylose ankylosante chez des ouistitis. Erkrank, Zoot. Verhandlungsher Int. Symp. 21st (Berlin) 13, 33–35.

DeVore, I., Hall, K.R.L., 1965. Baboon ecology. In: Devore, I. (Ed.), Primate Behavior: Field Studies of Monkeys and Apes. Holt, Rinehart and Winston, New York.

Diamond, E.J., Aksel, S., Hazelton, J.M., Jennings, R.A., Abee, C.R., 1984. Seasonal changes in serum concentrations of estradiol and progesterone in Bolivian squirrel monkeys (Saimiri sciureus) during the breeding season. Am. J. Primatol. 6, 103–113.

Diamond, E.J., Aksel, S., Hazelton, J.M., Barnett, S.B., Williams, L.E., Abee, C.R., 1985. Serum hormone patterns during abortion in the Bolivian squirrel monkey. Lab. Anim. Sci. 35, 619–623.

Diamond, E.J., Aksel, S., Hazelton, J.M., Wiebe, R.H., Abee, C.R., 1987. Serum oestradiol, progesterone, chorionic gonadotrophin, and prolactin concentrations during pregnancy in the Bolivian squirrel monkey (Saimiri boliviensis). J. Reprod. Fertil. 80, 373–381.

Diehl, K.H., Hull, R., Morton, D., Pfister, R., Rabemampianina, Y., Smith, D., et al., 2001. A good practice guide to the administration of substances and removal of blood, including routes and volumes. J. Appl. Toxicol. 21, 15–23.

Dietz, H.H., Henriksen, P., Bille-Hansen, V., Henriksen, S.A., 1997. Toxoplasmosis in a colony of New World monkeys. Vet. Parasitol. 68, 299–304.

DiGiacomo, R.F., Missakian, E.A., 1972. Tetanus in a free-ranging colony of Macaca mulatta: a clinical and epizootiologic study. Lab. Anim. Sci. 22, 378–383.

DiGiacomo, R.F., Hooks, J.J., Sulima, M.P., Gibbs Jr., C.J., Gajdusek, D.C., 1977. Pelvic endometriosis and simian foamy virus infection in a pigtailed macaque. JAALAS 171, 859–861.

Dillehay, D.L., Huerkemp, M.J., 1990. Tuberculosis in a tuberculin-negative rhesus monkey (Macaca mulatta) on chemoprophylaxis. J. Zoo Wildl. Med. 21, 480–484.

Ding, S.Y., Tigno, X.T., Braileanum, G.T., Ito, K., Hansen, B.C., 2007. A novel peroxisome proliferator-activated receptor alpha/gamma dual agonist ameliorates dyslipidemia and insulin resistance in prediabetic rhesus monkeys. Metabolism 56, 1334–1339.

Dixson, A.F., 1983. The owl monkey. In: Hearn, J.P. (Ed.), Reproduction in New World Primates. MTP Press, Hingham, MA, pp. 69–113.

Dixson, A.F., Gardner, J.S., 1981. Diurnal variations in plasma testosterone in a male nocturnal primate, the owl monkey (Aotus trivirgatus). J. Reprod. Fertil. 62, 83–86.

Dixson, A.F., Lunn, S.F., 1987. Post-partum changes in hormones and sexual behavior in captive groups of marmosets (Callithrix jacchus). Physiol. Behav. 41, 577–583.

Dixson, A.F., Gardner, J.S., Bonney, R.C., 1980. Puberty in the male owl monkey (Aotus trivirgatus griseimembra): a study of physical and hormonal development. Int. J. Primatol. 1, 129–139.

d'Offay, J.M., Eberle, R., Wolf, R.F., Kosanke, S.D., Doocy, K.R., Ayalew, S., et al., 2013. Simian T-lymphotropic Virus-associated lymphoma in 2 naturally infected baboons: T-cell clonal expansion and immune response during tumor development. Comp. Med. 63, 288–294.

Donovan, J.C., Stokes, W.S., Montrey, R.D., Rozmiarek, H., 1983. Hematologic characterization of naturally occurring malaria (Plasmodium inui) in cynomolgus monkeys (Macaca fascicularis). Lab. Anim. Sci. 33, 86–89.

Douglas, J.D., Tanner, K.N., Prine, J.R., Van Riper, D.C., Derwelis, S.K., 1967. Molluscum contagiosum in chimpanzees. J. Am. Vet. Med. Assoc. 151, 901–904.

Downie, A.W., 1974. Serologic evidence of infection with Tana and Yaba pox viruses among several species of monkeys. J. Hyg. 72, 245–250.

Downie, A.W., Espana, C., 1972. Comparison of Tanapox and Yaba-like viruses causing epidemic disease in monkeys. J. Hyg. 70, 23–32.

Doxiadis, G.G., Otting, N., de Groot, N.G., de Groot, N., Rouweler, A.J., Noort, R., et al., 2003. Evolutionary stability of MHC class II haplotypes in diverse rhesus macaque populations. Immunogenetics 55, 540–551.

Doyle, L., Young, C.L., Jang, S.S., Hillier, S.L., 1991. Normal vaginal aerobic and anaerobic bacterial flora of the rhesus macaque (*Macaca mulatta*). J. Med. Primatol. 20, 409–413.

Drevon-Gaillot, E., Perron-Lepage, M.F., Clément, C., Burnett, R., 2006. A review of background findings in cynomolgus monkeys (*Macaca fascicularis*) from three different geographical origins. Exp. Toxicol. Pathol. 58, 77–88. Epub 2006 Sep 18.

Dubois, A., Tarnawski, A., Newell, D.G., Fiala, N., Dabros, W., Stachura, J., et al., 1991. Gastric injury and invasion of parietal cells by spiral bacteria in rhesus monkeys: are gastritis and hyperchlorhydria infectious diseases? Gastroenterology 100, 884–891.

Dubois, A., Fiala, N., Heman-Ackah, L.M., Drazek, E.S., Tarnawski, A., Fishbein, W.N., et al., 1994. Natural gastric infection with *Helicobacter pylori* in monkeys: a model for spiral bacteria infection in humans. Gastroenterology 106, 1405–1417.

Dufour, J.P., Phillippi-Falkenstein, K., Bohm, R.P., Veazey, R.S., Carnal, J., 2012. Excision of femoral head and neck for treatment of coxofemoral degenerative joint disease in a rhesus macaque (Macaca mulatta). Comp. Med. 62, 539–542.

DuMond, F.V., 1968. The squirrel monkey in a seminatural environment. In: Rosenblum, L.A., Cooper, R.W. (Eds.), The Squirrel Monkey. Academic Press, New York, pp. 87–145.

Duncan, M., Nichols, D.K., Montali, R.J., Thomas, L.A., 1994. An epizootic of *Salmonella enteritidis* at the National Zoological Park. Am. Assoc. Zoo Vet. Annu. Conf. Proc., Pittsburgh, USA, pp. 246–248.

Dung, H.C., 1984. Anatomical features contributing to the formation of acupuncture points. Am. J. Acupunct. 12, 139–143.

Dyke, B., 1995. Animal identification and record keeping: current practice and use. In: Bennett, B.T., Abee, C.R., Henrickson, R.V. (Eds.), Nonhuman Primates in Biomedical Research: Biology and Management. Academic Press, San Diego, CA, pp. 249–253.

Eaton, G.G., Worlein, J.M., Kelley, S.T., Vijayaraghavan, S., Hess, D.L., Axthelm, M.K., et al., 1999. Self-injurious behavior is decreased by cyproterone acetate in adult male rhesus (*Macaca mulatta*). Horm. Behav. 35, 195–203.

Ebeling, M., Kung, E., See, A., Broger, C., Steiner, G., Berrera, M., et al., 2011. Genome-based analysis of the nonhuman primate *Macaca fascicularis* as a model for drug safety assessment. Genome Res. 21, 1746–1756.

Eberhard, M., D'Alessandro, A., 1982. Congenital trypanosome cruzi infection in a laboratory-born squirrel monkey, Saimiri sciureus. Am. J. Trop. Med. Hyg. 31, 931–933.

Eby, J.C., Gray, M.C., Warfel, J.M., Paddock, C.D., Jones, T.F., Day, S.R., et al., 2013. Quantification of the adenylate cyclase toxin of *Bordetella pertussis* in vitro and during respiratory infection. Infect. Immun. 81, 1390–1398.

Eddy, B.E., Borman, G.S., Berkeley, W., Young, R.D., 1961. Tumors induced in hamsters by injection of rhesus monkey kidney cell extracts. Proc. Soc. Exp. Biol. 107, 191–197.

Einspanier, A., Lieder, K., Brüns, A., Husen, B., Thole, H., Simon, C., 2006. Induction of endometriosis in the marmoset monkey (*Callithrix jacchus*). Mol. Hum. Reprod. 12 (5), 291–299. http://dx.doi.org/10.1093/molehr/gal031.

Eisele, P.H., Morgan, J.P., Line, A.S., Anderson, J.H., 1992. Skeletal lesions and anemia associated with ascorbic acid deficiency in juvenile rhesus macaques. Lab. Anim. Sci. 42, 245–249.

Eley, R.M., Gulamhusein, N., Lequin, R.M., 1986. Reproduction in the vervet monkey (Cercopithecus aethiops): I. Testicular volume, testosterone, and seasonality. Am. J. Primatol. 10, 229–235.

Eley, R.M., Tarara, R.P., Worthman, C.M., Else, J.G., 1989. Reproduction in the vervet monkey (Cercopithecus aethiops): III. The menstrual cycle. Am. J. Primatol. 17, 1–10.

Elliot, I., Skerritt, G., 2010. Part one: physical principles of MRI Handbook of Small Animal MRI. Wiley-Blackwell, UK, pp. 1–29.

Elliot, M.W., Sehgal, P.K., Chalifoux, L.V., 1976. Management and breeding of *Aotus trivirgatus*. Lab. Anim. Sci. 26, 1037–1040.

Elmore, D., Eberle, R., 2008. Monkey B virus (Cercopithecine herpesvirus 1). Comp. Med. 58, 11–21.

Else, J.G., 1985. Captive propagation of vervet monkeys (Cercopithecus aethiops) in harems. Lab Anim. Sci. 35, 373–375.

Else, J.G., Tarara, R., Suleman, M.A., Eley, R.M., 1986a. Enclosure design and reproductive success in baboons used for reproductive research in Kenya. Lab. Anim. Sci. 36, 168–172.

Else, J.G., Eley, R.M., Wangula, C., Worthman, C., Lequin, R.M., 1986b. Reproduction in the vervet monkey (Cercopithecus aethiops): II. Annual menstrual patterns and seasonality. Am. J. Primatol. 11, 333–342.

Elton, S., Dunn, J., Cardini, A., 2010. Size variation facilitates population divergence but does not explain it at all: an example study from a widespread African monkey. Biol. J. Linn. Soc. 101, 823–843.

Embers, M.E., Doyle, L.A., Whitehouse, C.A., Selby, E.B., Chappell, M., Philipp, M.T., 2011. Characterization of a Moraxella species that causes epistaxis in macaques. Vet. Microbiol. 147, 367–375.

Emery Thompson, M., 2013. Reproductive ecology of female chimpanzees. Am. J. Primatol. 75, 222–237.

Epiphanio, S., Guimarães, M.A., Fedullo, D.L., Correa, S.H., Catão-Dias, J.L., 2000. Toxoplasmosis in golden-headed lion tamarins (*Leontopithecus chrysomelas*) and emperor marmosets (*Saguinus imperator*) in captivity. J. Zoo. Wildl. Med. 31, 231–235.

Epple, G., 1970a. Maintenance, breeding, and development of marmoset monkeys (Callitrichidae) in captivity. Folia Primatol. 12, 56–76.

Epple, G., 1970b. Quantitative studies on scent marking in the marmoset (*Callithrix jacchus*). Folia Primatol. 13, 48–62.

Epple, G., 1973. The role of pheromones in the social communication of marmoset monkeys (Callitrichidae). J. Reprod. Fertil. 19 (Suppl.), 447–454.

Epple, G., Katz, Y., 1980. Social influences on first reproductive success and related behaviors in the saddle-back tamarin (*Saguinus fuscicolli* Callitrichidae). Int. J. Primatol. 1, 171.

Epple, G., Belcher, A.M., Kuderling, I., Zeller, U., Scolnick, L., Greenfield, K.L., et al., 1993. Making sense out of scents: species differences in scent glands, scent-marking behavior, and scent-mark composition in Callitrichidae. In: Rylands, A.B. (Ed.), Marmosets and Tamarins: Systemics, Behaviour, and Ecology. Oxford University Press, New York, pp. 123–135.

Erkert, H.G., 1976. Beleuchtungsabhanglges aktivitalsoptimum bei nachtaffen (*Aotus trivirgatus*) (Light-induced activity optimum in night monkeys). Folia Primatol. 25, 186–192.

Ervin, F., Palmour, R., 2003. Primates for the 21st century biomedicine: the St. Kitts vervet (Chlorocebus aethiops, SK). In: [Anonymous]. International perspectives: the future nonhuman primate resources; 2002 Apr 17–19; Bogor, Indonesia. Washington, DC: Natl. Acad. Press, pp. 49–53.

Eslamboli, A., 2005. Marmoset monkey models of Parkinson's disease: which model, when and why? Brain Res. Bull. 68, 140–149.

Espana, C., 1973. Herpes simiae infection in *Macaca radiata*. Am. J. Phys. Anthropol. 38, 447–454.

Espinosa, B.J., Weaver, S.C., Paessler, S., Brining, D., Salazar, M., Kochel, T., 2009. Susceptibility of the Aotus nancymaae owl monkey to eastern equine encephalitis. Vaccine 27, 1729–1734.

Even-Sapir, E., 2005. Imaging of malignant bone involvement by morphologic, scintigraphic, and hybrid modalities. J. Nucl. Med. 46, 1356–1367.

Fahey, M.A., Westmoreland, S.V., 2012. Nervous system disorders of nonhuman primates and research models. In: Abee, C.R., Mansfield, K., Tardif, S., Morris, T. (Eds.), Nonhuman Primates in Biomedical Research: Diseases. Elsevier, Academic Press, San Diego, CA, pp. 734–782.

Fairbanks, L.A., McGuire, M.T., 1986. Age, reproductive value, and dominance-related behaviour in vervet monkey females: cross-generational influences on social relationships and reproduction. Anim. Behav. 34, 1710–1721.

Fairbanks, L.A., Newman, T.K., Bailey, J.N., Jorgensen, M.J., Breidenthal, S.E., Ophoff, R.A., et al., 2004. Genetic contributions to social impulsivity and aggressiveness in vervet monkeys. Biol. Psychiatry. 55, 642–647.

Farrell, D.J., McKeon, M., Daggard, G., Loeffelholz, M.J., Thompson, C.J., Mukkur, T.K., 2000. Rapid-cycle PCR method to detect *Bordetella pertussis* that fulfills all consensus recommendations for use of PCR in diagnosis of pertussis. J. Clin. Microbiol. 38, 4499–4502.

Faulkes, C.G., Arruda, M.F., Monteiro da Cruz, A.O., 2003. Matrilineal genetic structure within and among populations of the cooperatively breeding common marmoset. Callithrix Jacchus. Mol. Ecol. 12, 1101–1108.

Favoretto, S.R., de Mattos, C.C., Morais, N.B., Alves Araujo, F.A., de Mattos, C.A., 2001. Rabies in marmosets (*Callithrix jacchus*), Ceara, Brazil. Emerg. Infect. Dis. 7, 1062–1065.

Fawcett, G.L., Raveendran, M., Deiros, D.R., Chen, D., Yu, F., Harris, R.A., et al., 2011. Characterization of single-nucleotide variation in Indian-origin rhesus macaques (*Macaca mulatta*). BMC Genomics 12, 311.

Fear, F.A., Pinkerton, M.E., Cline, J.A., Kriewaldt, F., Kalter, S.S., 1968. A leptospirosis outbreak in a baboon (*Papio* sp.) colony. Lab. Anim. Care 18, 22–28.

Fedigan, L., Fedigan, L.M., 1988. Cercopithecus aethiops: a review of field studies. In: Gautier-Hion, A., Bourlière, F., Gautier, J.P., Kingdon, J. (Eds.), A Primate Radiation: Evolutionary Biology of the African Guenons. Cambridge University Press, Cambridge (UK), pp. 389–411.

Feichtinger, H., Li, S., Kaaya, E., Putkonen, P., Grunewald, K., Weyrer, K., et al., 1992. A monkey model of Epstein-Barr virus-associated lymphomagenesis in human acquired immunodeficiency syndrome. J. Exp. Med. 176, 281–286.

Felsburg, P.J., Heberling, R.L., Brack, M., Kalter, S.S., 1973. Experimental genital herpes infection of the marmoset. J. Med. Primatol. 2, 50–60.

Felsenfeld, A.D., Schmidt, N.J., 1975. Immunological relationship between delta herpesvirus of patas monkeys and varicella-zoster virus of humans. Infect. Immun. 12, 261–266.

Ferguson, B., Street, S.L., Wright, H., Pearson, C., Jia, Y., Thompson, S.L., et al., 2007. Single nucleotide polymorphisms (SNPs) distinguish Indian-origin and Chinese-origin rhesus macaques (*Macaca mulatta*). BMC Genomics 8, 43.

Fernández-Duque, E., 2009. Natal dispersal in monogamous owl monkeys (*Aotus azarai*) of the Argentinean Chaco. Behavior 146, 583–606.

Fernández-Duque, E., 2011a. The aotinae: social monogamy in the only nocturnal anthropoid. In: Campbell, C.J., Fuentes, A., MacKinnon, K.C., Panger, M., Bearder, S.K. (Eds.), Primates in Perspective Oxford University Press, Oxford, pp. 140–154.

Fernández-Duque, E., 2011b. Rensch's rule, Bergmann's effect and adult sexual dimorphism in wild monogamous owl monkeys (*Aotus azarai*) of Argentina. Am. J. Phys. Anthropol. 146, 38–48.

Fernández-Duque, E., Erkert, H.G., 2006. Cathemerality and lunar periodicity of activity rhythms in owl monkeys of the Argentinian Chaco. Folia Primatologica 77, 123–138.

Fernández-Duque, E., Van der Heide, G., 2013. Dry season resources and their relationship with owl monkey (*Aotus azarae*) feeding behavior, demography, and life history. Int. J. Primatol. 34, 752–769.

Fernández-Duque, E., Rotundo, M., Ramirez-Llorens, P., 2002. Environmental determinants of birth seasonality in night monkeys (*Aotus azarai*) of the Argentinian Chaco. Int. J. Primatol. 23, 639–656.

Fernández-Duque, E., Wallace, R.B., Rylands, A.B.,. 2008. Aotus azarae. In: IUCN 2013. IUCN Red List of Threatened Species. Version 2013.1. Available at: <www.iucnredlist.org>. Downloaded on October 15, 2013.

Fernández-Duque, E., de la Iglesia, H., Erkert, H.G., 2010. Moonstruck primates: owl monkeys (*Aotus*) need moonlight for nocturnal activity in their natural environment. PLoS One 5 (9), e12572. http://dx.doi.org/10.1371/journal.pone.0012572.

Fiennes, R.N., 1972. Rabies. In: Fiennes, R.N.T.-W. (Ed.), Pathology of Simian Primates. Karger, Basel and New York, pp. 646–662.

Finlay, B.L., Franco, E.C.S., Yamada, E.S., Crowley, J.C., Parsons, M., Muniz, J.A.P.C., et al., 2008. Number and topography of cones, rods, and optic nerve axons in New and Old world primates. Vis. Neurosci. 25, 289–299.

Fiorito, B.A., Mirza, F., Doran, T.M., Oberle, A.N., Cruz, E.C., Wendtland, C.L., et al., 2005. Intraosseous access in the setting of pediatric critical care transport. Pediatr. Crit. Care Med. 6, 50–53.

Flecknell, P.A., Parry, R., Needham, J.R., Ridley, R.M., Baker, H.F., Bowes, P., 1983. Respiratory disease associated with parainfluenza type I (Sendai) virus in a colony of marmosets (*Callithrix jacchus*). Lab. Anim. 17, 111–113.

Flynn, R.J., 1973. Parasites of Laboratory Animals. Iowa State University Press, Ames, IA.

Fontenot, M.B., Musso, M.W., McFatter, R.M., Anderson, G.M., 2009. Dose-finding study of fluoxetine and venlafaxine for the treatment of self-injurious and stereotypic behavior in rhesus macaques (*Macaca mulatta*). J. Am. Assoc. Lab. Anim. Sci. 48, 176–184.

Fooden, J., 2000. Systematic review of the rhesus macaque (Macaca mulatta). Zoology (Field Museum of Natural History) 96, 1–180.

Fooden, J., 2006. Comparative review of *Fascicularis*-group species of macaques (Primates: *Macaca*). Zoology (Field Museum of Natural History) 107, 1–43.

Fortman, J.D., Herring, J.M., Miller, J.B., Hess, D.L., Verhage, H.G., Fazleabas, A.T., 1993. Chorionic gonadotropin, estradiol, and progesterone levels in baboons (*Papio anubis*) during early pregnancy and spontaneous abortion. Biol. Reprod. 49, 737–742.

Fox, J.G., 1975. Transmissible drug resistance in *Shigella* and *Salmonella* isolated from pet monkeys and their owners. J. Med. Primatol. 4, 165–171.

Fox, J.G., Handt, L., Xu, S., Shen, Z., Dewhirst, F.E., Paster, B.J., et al., 2001b. Novel Helicobacter species isolated from rhesus monkeys with chronic idiopathic colitis. J Med Microbiol. 50, 421–429.

Fox, J.G., Rohovsky, M.W., 1975. Meningitis caused by *Klebsiella* spp. in two rhesus monkeys. J. Am. Vet. Med. Assoc. 167, 634–636.

Fox, J.G., Wikse, S.E., 1971. Bacterial meningoencephalitis in rhesus monkeys: clinical and pathological features. Lab. Anim. Sci. 21, 558–563.

Fox, J.G., Campbell, L.H., Snyder, S.B., Reed, C., Soave, O.A., 1974. Tuberculous spondylitis and Pott's paraplegia in a rhesus monkey. Lab. Anim. Sci. 24, 335–339.

Fox, J.G., Handt, L., Sheppard, B.J., Xu, S., Dewhirst, F.E., Klein, H., 2001a. *Helicobacter cinaedi* isolated from the colon, liver, and mesenteric lymph node of a rhesus monkey with chronic colitis and hepatitis. J. Clin. Microbiol. 50, 421–429.

Fox, J.G., Handt, L., Xu, S., Shen, Z., Dewhirst, F.E., Paster, B.J., et al., 2001b. Novel *Helicobacter* species isolated from rhesus monkeys with chronic idiopathic colitis. J. Med. Microbiol. 50, 421–429.

Fox, J.G., Boutin, S.R., Handt, L.K., Taylor, N.S., Xu, S., Rickman, B., et al., 2007. Isolation and Characterization of a Novel Helicobacter Species, 'Helicobacter macacae', from rhesus Monkeys with and without Chronic Idiopathic Colitis. J. Clin. Microbiol. 45, 4061–4063. http://dx.doi.org/10.1128/jcm.01100-07.

Fraser, C.E.O., Chalifoux, L., Sehgal, P., Hunt, R.D., King, N.W., 1978. A paramyxovirus causing fatal gastroenteritis in marmoset monkeys. In: Goldsmith, E.I., Moor-Janowski, J. (Eds.), Primates in Medicine. Karger, Basel, Switzerland, pp. 261–270.

Freeman, N.J., Pasternak, G.M., Rubi, T.L., Barrett, L., Henzi, S.P., 2012. Evidence for scent marking in vervet monkeys? Primates 53, 311–315. http://dx.doi.org/10.1007/s10329-012-0304-8.

Freimer, N., Dewar, K., Kaplan, J., Fairbanks, L. The importance of the Vervet (African Green Monkey) as a biomedical model. Accessed September 29, 2013: Available at: <http://www.genome.gov/

pages/research/sequencing/seqproposals/thevervetmonkeybio-medicalmodel.pdf.>

Fritz, P., Fritz, J., 1979. Resocialization of chimpanzees: ten years of experience at the Primate Foundation of Arizona. J. Med. Primatol. 8, 202–221.

Fruth, B., Benishay, J.M., Bila-Isia, I., Coxe, S., Dupain, J., Furuichi, T., et al., 2008. *Pan paniscus*. *In*: IUCN 2013. IUCN Red List of Threatened Species. Version 2013.2. Available at: <www.iucnredlist.org>. Downloaded on March 19, 2014.

Fultz, P.N., Gordon, R.P., Anderson, D.C., McClure, H.M., 1990. Prevalence of natural infection with SIVsmm and STLV-1 in a breeding colony of sooty mangabey monkeys. AIDS 4, 619–625.

Gacad, M.A., Deseran, M.W., Adams, J.S., 1992. Influence of ultraviolet radiation on vitamin D_3 metabolism in vitamin D_3-resistant New World primates. Am. J. Primatol. 28, 263–270.

Galland, G.G., 2000. Role of the squirrel monkey in parasitic disease research. ILAR J. 41, 37–43.

Gao, Y., Khare, S.P., Panda, S., Choe, A.S., Stepniewska, I., Li, X., et al., 2014. A brain MRI atlas of the common squirrel monkey. Proc. Soc. Photo Opt. Instrum. Eng. 9038, 90380C.

Gainer, J.H., 1967. Encephalomyocarditis virus infections in Florida, 1960–1966. J. Am. Vet. Med. Assoc. 151, 421–425.

Garber, P.A., 1980. Locomotor behavior and feeding ecology of the Panamanian tamarin (*Saguinus oedipus geoffroyi*) (Callitrichidae: Primates). Int. J. Primatol. 1, 185–201.

Garber, P.A., 1993. Feeding, ecology, and behaviour of the genus *Saguinus*. In: Rylands, A.B. (Ed.), Marmosets and Tamarins: Systematics, Behaviour, and Ecology. Oxford University Press, Oxford, pp. 273–295.

Garcia, A., Paul, K., Beall, B., McClure, H., 2006. Toxic shock due to *Streptococcus pyogenes* in a rhesus monkey (*Macaca mulatta*). J. Am. Assoc. Lab. Anim Sci. 45, 79–82.

Garcia, M.A., Bouley, D.M., Larson, M.J., Lifland, B., Moorhead, R., Simkins, M.D., et al., 2004a. Outbreak of *Mycobacterium bovis* in a conditioned colony of rhesus (*Macaca mulatta*) and cynomolgus (*Macaca fascicularis*) macaques. Comp. Med. 54, 578–584.

Garcia, M.A., Yee, J., Bouley, D.M., Moorhead, R., Lerche, N.W., 2004b. Diagnosis of tuberculosis in macaques, using whole-blood in vitro interferon-gamma (PRIMAGAM) testing. Comp. Med. 54 (1), 86–92.

Garcia, M.K., McQuade, J., Haddad, R., Patel, S., Lee, R., Yang, P., et al., 2013. Systemic review of acupuncture in cancer care: a synthesis of evidence. J. Clin. Oncol. 31, 952–960.

Gardner, M.B., 1996. The history of simian AIDS. J. Med. Primatol. 25, 148–157.

Gauthier, C.A., 1999. Reproductive parameters and paracallosal skin color changes in captive female guinea baboons. Papio Papio. Am. J. Primatol. 47, 67–74.

Genain, C.P., Hauser, S.L., 1996. Allergic encephalomyelitis in common marmosets: pathogenesis of a multiple sclerosis-like lesion. Methods 10, 420–434.

Genain, C.P., Hauser, S.L., 1997. Creation of a model for multiple sclerosis in Callithrix jacchus marmosets. J. Mol. Med. 75, 187–197.

Gengozian, N., Batson, J.S., 1975. Single-born marmosets without hemopoietic chimerism: naturally occurring and induced. J. Med. Primatol. 4, 252–261.

Gengozian, N., Batson, J.S., Smith, T.A., 1977. Breeding of tamarins (*Saguinus* spp.) in the laboratory. In: Kleiman, D.G. (Ed.), The Biology and Conservation of the Callitrichidae. Smithsonian Institution Press, Washington, DC, pp. 207–213.

Gengozian, N., Batson, J.S., Smith, T.A., 1978. Breeding of marmosets in a colony environment. Primates Med. 10, 71–78.

George, J.W., Lerche, N.W., 1990. Electrolyte abnormalities associated with diarrhea in rhesus monkeys: 100 cases (1986–1987). J. Am. Vet. Med. Assoc. 196, 1654–1658.

George, R., Lam, S.K., 1997. Dengue virus infection in the Malaysian experience. Ann. Acad. Med. Singapore 26, 815–819.

Georgi, J.R., 1980. Parasitology for Veterinarians. Saunders, Philadelphia, PA.

Gerald, M.S., 2002. The finding of an inverse relationship between social dominance and feeding priority among pairs of unfamiliar adult male vervet monkeys (*Cercopithecus aethiops sabaeus*). Primates 43, 127–132.

Geretschlager, E., Russ, H., Mihatsch, W., Przuntek, H., 1987. Suboccipital puncture for cerebrospinal fluid in the common marmoset (*Callithrix jacchus*). Lab. Anim. 24, 91–94.

Gibb, W.R., Lees, A.J., Wells, F.R., Barnard, R.O., Jenner, P., Marsden, C.D., 1987. Pathology of MPTP in the marmoset. Adv. Neurol. 45, 187–190.

Gibbs, R.A., et al., 2007. Evolutionary and biomedical insights from the Rhesus Macaque genome. Science 316, 222–234.

Gilbert, S.G., Reuhl, K.R., Wong, J.H., Rice, D.C., 1987. Fatal pneumococcal meningitis in a colony-born monkey (*Macaca fasicularis*). J. Med. Primatol. 16, 333–338.

Giles Jr., R.C., Hildebrandt, P.K., Tate, C., 1974. *Klebsiella* air sacculitis in the owl monkey (*Aotus trivirgatus*). Lab. Anim. Sci. 24, 610–616.

Gippoliti, S., Ehardt, T., 2008. *Papio hamadryas*. In: IUCN 2013. IUCN Red List of Threatened Species. Version 2013.2. Available at: <www.iucnredlist.org>. Downloaded on February 3, 2014.

Glad, W.R., Nesland, J.M., 1995. Focal epithelial hyperplasia of the oral mucosa in two chimpanzees (*Pan troglodytes*). Am. J. Primatol. 10, 83–89.

Goenka, A.H., Wang, H., Flamm, S.D., 2014. Cardiac magnetic resonance imaging for the investigation of cardiovascular disorders. Part 2: emerging applications. Tex. Heart Inst. J. 41, 135–143.

Goldberg, T.L., Wrangham, R.W., 1997. Genetic correlates of social behavior in wild chimpanzees: evidence from mitochondrial DNA. Anim. Behav. 54, 559–570.

Goldizen, A.W., 1987. Tamarins and marmosets: communal care of offspring. In: Smuts, B.B., Cheney, D.L., Seyfarth, R.M., Wrangham, R.W., Struhsaker, T.T. (Eds.), Primate Societies. University of Chicago Press, Chicago, pp. 34–43.

Goldschmidt, B., Mota-Marinho, A., Araújo-Lopes, C., Brück-Gonçalves, M.A., Matos-Fasano, D., Ribeiro-Andrade, M.C., et al., 2009. Sexual dimorphism in the squirrel monkey, Saimiri sciureus (Linnaeus, 1758) and Saimiri ustus (I. Geoffroy, 1844) (Primates, Cebidae). Braz. J. Biol. 69, 171–174.

Good, R.C., May, B.D., 1971. Respiratory pathogens in monkeys. Infect. Immun. 3, 87–99.

Good, R.C., May, B.D., Kawatomari, T., 1969. Enteric pathogens in monkeys. J. Bacteriol. 97, 1048–1055.

Goodall, J., 1986. The Chimpanzees of Gombe. Belknap Press of Harvard University Press, Cambridge, MA.

Goodall, J., Athumani, J., 1980. An observed birth in a free-living chimpanzee (*Pan troglodytes schweinfurthii*) in Gombe National Park, Tanzania. Primates 21, 545–549.

Goodman, R.L., Hotchkiss, J., Karsch, F.J., Knobil, E., 1974. Diurnal variations in serum testosterone concentrations in the adult male rhesus monkey. Biol. Repro. 11, 624–630.

Goodwin, W.J., Coelho Jr., A.M., 1982. Development of a large scale baboon breeding program. Lab. Anim. Sci. 32, 672–676.

Goodwin, W.J., Haines, R.J., Bernal, J.C., 1987. Tetanus in baboons of a corral breeding colony. Lab. Anim. Sci. 37, 231–232.

Gore, M.A., Brandes, F., Kaup, F.-J., Lenzner, R., Mothes, T., Osman, A.A., 2001. Callitrichid nutrition and food sensitivity. J. Med. Primatol. 30, 179–184.

Gough, A.W., Barsoum, N.J., Gracon, S.I., Mitchell, L., Sturgess, J.M., 1982. Poxvirus infection in a colony of common marmosets (*Callithrix jacchus*). Lab. Anim. Sci. 32, 87–90.

Gould, K.G., Martin, D.E., 1986. Artificial insemination of nonhuman primates. In: Benirschke, K. (Ed.), Primates: The Road to Self-Sustaining Populations. Springer-Verlag, New York, pp. 425–443.

Gozalo, A., Montoya, E., 1991. *Klebsiella pneumoniae* infection in a New World nonhuman primate center. Lab. Primate News 30, 13–15.

Gozalo, A., Montoya, E., 1992. Mortality causes in the moustached tamarin (*Saguinus mystax*) in captivity. J. Med. Primatol. 21, 35–38.

Gozalo, A., Block, K., Montoya, E., Moro, J., Escamilla, J., 1991. A survey for *Campylobacter* in feral and captive tamarins. Primatol. Today 13, 675–676.

Gozalo, A.S., Cheng, L.I., St Claire, M.E., Ward, J.M., Elkins, W.R., 2008. Pathology of captive moustached tamarins (*Saguinus mystax*). Comp. Med. 58, 188–195.

Gozalo, A.S., Ragland, D.R., St Claire, M.C., Elkins, W.R., Michaud, C.R., 2011. Intracardiac thrombosis and aortic dissecting aneurysms in mustached tamarins (Sanguinus mystax) with cardiomyopathy. Comp. Med. 61, 176–181.

Grace, J.T. Jr., Mirand, E.A., 1965. Yaba virus infection in humans. Exp. Med. Surg. 23, 213–216.

Graczyk, T.K., Cranfield, M.R., Kempske, S.E., Eckhaus, M.A., 1995. Fulminant *Streptococcus pneumoniae* meningitis in a lion-tailed macaque (*Macaca silenus*) without detected signs. J. Wildl. Dis. 31, 75–77.

Graham, M.L., Mutch, L.A., Rieke, E.F., Dunning, M., Zolondek, E.K., Faig, A.W., et al., 2010. Refinement of vascular access port placement in nonhuman primates: complication rates and outcomes. Comp. Med. 60, 479–485.

Gravell, M., Palmer, A.E., Rodriguez, M., London, W.T., Hamilton, R.S., 1980. Method to detect asymptomatic carriers of simian hemorrhagic fever virus. Lab. Anim. Sci. 30, 988–991.

Gray, W.L., 2010. Simian varicella virus: molecular virology. Curr. Top Microbiol. Immunol. 342, 291–308.

Green, S.W., Malkovska, I., O'Sullivan, M.G., Brown, K.E., 2000. Rhesus and pig-tailed macaque parvoviruses: identification of two new members of the erythrovirus genus in monkeys. Virology 269, 105–112.

Greene, C.S., 1986. Indications for plain abdominal radiography in the emergency department. Ann. Emerg. Med. 15, 257–260.

Greenfield, G.B., Arrington, J.A., Kudryk, B.T., 1993. MRI of soft tissue tumors. Skeletal Radiol. 22, 77–84.

Greenstein, E.T., Doty, R.W., Lowy, K., 1965. An outbreak of a fulminating infectious disease in the squirrel monkey (*Saimiri sciureus*). Lab. Anim. Care 15, 74–80.

Groves, C., 2001. Primate Taxonomy. Smithsonian Institution Press, Washington DC, 350 p.

Groves, C.P., 2005. Order primates, third ed. In: Wilson, D. Reeder, D. (Eds.), Mammal Species of the World: A Taxonomic and Geographic Reference, vol. 1. Johns Hopkins University Press, Baltimore, MD, pp. 111–184.

Grubb, P., Butynski, T.M., Oates, J.F., Bearder, S.K., Disotell, T.R., Groves, C.P., et al., 2003. Assessment of the diversity of African primates. Int. J. Primatol. 24, 1301–1357.

Gupta, A.K., Filonenko, N., Salansky, N., Sauder, D.N., 1998. The use of low energy photon therapy (LEPT) in venous leg ulcers: a double-blind, placebo-controlled study. Dermatol. Surg. 24, 1383–1386.

Hadfield, R.M., Yudkin, P.L., Coe, C.L., Scheffler, J., Uno, H., Barlow, D.H., et al., 1997. Risk factors for endometriosis in the rhesus monkey (*Macaca mulatta*): a case-control study. Hum. Reprod. Update. 3, 109–115.

Haefliger, E., Parel, J.M., Fantes, F., Norton, E.W., Anderson, D.R., Forster, R.K., et al., 1987. Accommodation of an endocapsular silicone lens (Phaco-Ersatz) in the nonhuman primate. Ophthalmology 94, 471–477.

Haesebrouck, F., Pasmans, F., Flahou, B., Chiers, K., Baele, M., Meyns, T., et al., 2009. Gastric Helicobacters in domestic animals and nonhuman primates and their significance for human health. Clin. Microbiol. Rev. 22, 202–223.

Hahn, N.E., Capuano 3rd, S.V., 2010. Successful treatment of cryptosporidiosis in 2 common marmosets (*Callithrix jacchus*) by using paromomycin. J. Am. Assoc. Lab. Anim. Sci. 49, 873–875.

Haig, D., 1999. What is a marmoset? Am. J. Primatol. 49, 285–296.

Hainsey, B.M., Hubbard, G.B., Leland, M.M., Brasky, K.M., 1993. Clinical parameters of the normal baboons (*Papio* species) and chimpanzees (*Pan troglodytes*). Lab. Anim. Sci. 43, 236–243.

Hall, R.D., Hodgen, G.D., 1979. Pregnancy diagnosis in owl monkeys (*Aotus trivirgatus*): evaluation of the haemagglutination inhibition test for urinary human chorionic gonadotropin. Lab. Anim. Sci. 29, 345–348.

Hall, W.C., Kovatch, R.M., Hermann, P.H., Fox, J.G., 1971. Pathology of measles in rhesus monkey. Vet. Pathol. 8, 307–319.

Hamilton III, W.J., 1982. Baboon sleeping site preferences and relationships to primate grouping patterns. Am. J. Primatol. 3, 41–53.

Han, D., Berman, D.M., Willman, M., Buchwald, P., Rothen, D., Kenyon, N.M., et al., 2010. Choice of immunosuppression influences cytomegalovirus DNAemia in cynomolgus monkey (*Macaca fascicularis*) islet allograft recipients. Cell Transplant. 19, 1547–1561.

Handley, S.A., Thackray, L.B., Zhao, G., Presti, R., Miller, A.D., Droit, L., et al., 2012. Pathogenic simian immunodeficiency virus infection is associated with expansion of the enteric virome. Cell. 151, 253–266.

Hansen, B.C., 1989. Pathophysiology of obesity-associated type II diabetes (NIDDM): implications from longitudinal studies of nonhuman primates. Nutrition 5, 48–50.

Hansen, B.C., Bodkin, N.L., 1986. Heterogeneity of insulin responses: phases leading to type 2 (non-insulin-dependent) diabetes mellitus in the rhesus monkey. Diabetologia 29, 713–719.

Hansen, B.C., Bodkin, N.L., 1993. Primary prevention of diabetes mellitus by prevention of obesity in monkeys. Diabetes 42, 1809–1814.

Hansen, B.C., Tigno, X.T., Bénardeau, A., Meyer, M., Sebokova, E., Mizrahi, J., 2011. Effects of aleglitazar, a balanced dual peroxisome proliferator-activated receptor α/γ agonist on glycemic and lipid parameters in a primate model of the metabolic syndrome. Cardiovasc. Diabetol. 10, 7. http://dx.doi.org/10.1186/1475-2840-10-7.

Harlow, H.F., Dodsworth, R.O., Harlow, M.K., 1965. Total social isolation in monkeys. Proc. Natl. Acad. Sci. USA. 54, 90–97.

Harrison, M.J.S., 1984. Optimal foraging strategies in the diet of the green monkey, Cercopithecus sabaeus, at Mt. Assirik, Senegal. Int. J. Primatol. 5, 435–471.

Harvey, P.H., Martin, R.D., Clutton-brock, T.H., 1987. Life histories in comparative perspective. In: Smuts, B.B., Cheney, D.L., Seyfarth, R.M., Wrangham, R.W., Struhsaker, T.T. (Eds.), Primate Societies. University of Chicago Press, Chicago, pp. 181–196.

Harvey, D.C., Laćan, G., Melegan, W.P., 2000. Regional heterogeneity of dopaminergic deficits in vervet monkey striatum and substantia nigra after methamphetamine exposure. Exp. Brain Res. 133, 349–358.

Harwell, G., Dalgard, D., 1979. Clinical *Anatrichosoma cutaneum* dermatitis in nonhuman primates. Annu. Proc. Am. Assoc. Zoo Vet., 83a–86a.

Hatziioannou, T., Evans, D.T., 2012. Animal models for HIV/AIDS research. Nat. Rev. Microbiol. 10, 852–867. http://dx.doi.org/10.1038/nrmicro2911.

Hauck, H., Klehr, N., 1977. Meerkatzenfavus als Ursache für die pilzinfektion eines menschen. Z. Allerg. Med. 53, 331–332.

Haus, T., Akom, E., Agwanda, B., Hofreiter, M., Roos, C., Zinner, D., 2013. Mitochondrial diversity and distribution of African Green monkeys. Am. J. Primatol. 75, 350–360.

Haustein, S.V., Kolterman, A.J., Sundblad, J.J., Fechner, J.H., Knechtle, S.J., 2008. Nonhuman primate infections after organ transplantation. ILAR J. 49, 209–219.

Havill, L.M., Levine, S.M., Newman, D.E., Mahaney, M.C., 2008. Osteopenia and osteoporosis in adult baboons (Papio hamadryas). J. Med. Primatol. 37, 146–153.

Hawkey, C.M., Hart, M.G., Jones, D.M., 1982. Clinical hematology of the common marmoset Callithrix jacchus. Am. J. Primatol. 3, 179–199.

Hayman, D.T., Emmerich, P., Yu, M., Wang, L.F., Suu-Ire, R., Fooks, A.R., et al., 2010. Long-term survival of an urban fruit bat seropositive for Ebola and Lagos bat viruses. PLoS One 5, e11978. http://dx.doi.org/10.1371/journal.pone.0011978

Hearn, J.P., Lunn, S.F., 1975. The reproductive biology of the marmoset monkey, *Callithrix jacchus*. In: Perkins, F.T., O'Donoghue, P.N. (Eds.), Breeding Simians for Developmental Biology. Laboratory Animals Ltd., London, pp. 191–202. Lab. Anim. Handbook No. 6.

Heatley, J.J., Musser, J., 2014. Overview of vaccination of exotic mammals. Available at: The Merck Veterinary Manual Online <http://www.merckmanuals.com/vet/exotic_and_laboratory_animals/vaccination_of_exotic_mammals/overview_of_vaccination_of_exotic_mammals.html>. Last full review/revision August 2014.

Hegedüs, B., Viharos, L., Gervain, M., Gálfi, M., 2009. The effect of low-level laser in knee osteoarthritis: a double-blind, randomized, placebo-controlled study. Photomed. Laser Surg. 27, 577–584.

Heger, W., Neubert, D., 1987. Determination of ovulation and pregnancy in the marmoset (*Callithrix jacchus*) by monitoring urinary hydroxypregnanolone excretion. J. Med. Primatol. 16, 151–164.

Heistermann, M., Hodges, J.K., 1995. Endocrine monitoring of the ovarian cycle and pregnancy in the saddle-backed tamarin (*Saguinus fuscicollis*) by measurement of steroid conjugates in urine. Am. J. Primatol. 35, 117–127.

Heistermann, M., Ziegler, T., van Schaik, C.P., Launhardt, K., Winkler, P., Hodges, J.K., 2001. Loss of oestrous, concealed timing of ovulation and paternity confusion in free-ranging Hanuman langurs. Proc. R. Soc. Lond. B Biol. Sci. 268, 2445–2451.

Hendrickx, A.G., Binkerd, P.E., 1990. Nonhuman primates and teratological research. J. Med. Primatol. 19 1981–1108.

Henrickson, R.V., Maul, D.H., Lerche, N.W., Osborn, K.G., Lowenstine, L.J., Prahalada, S., et al., 1984. Clinical features of simian acquired immunodeficiency syndrome (SAIDS) in rhesus monkeys. Lab. Anim. Sci. 34, 140–145.

Hendrickx, A.G., 1971. Embryology of the Baboon. University of Chicago Press, London.

Hendrickx, A.G., Dukelow, W.R., 1995. Reproductive biology. In: Bennett, B.T., Abee, C.R., Henrickson, R.V. (Eds.), Non-Human Primates in Biomedical Research: Biology and Management. Academic Press, San Diego, CA, pp. 147–191.

Hendrickx, A.G., Kraemer, D.C., 1969. Observation on the menstrual cycles, optimal mating time, and pre-implantation of embryos of the baboon, *Papio anubis* and *Papio cynocephalus*. J. Reprod. Fertil. 6, 119–128.

Herman, P.H., Fox, J.G., 1971. Panophthalmitis associated with diplococcic septicemia in a rhesus monkey. J. Am. Vet. Med. Assoc. 159, 560–562.

Hernández-Camacho, J., Cooper, R.W., 1976. The nonhuman primates of Colombia. In: Thorington Jr., R.W., Heltne, P.G. (Eds.), Neotropical Primates: Field Studies and Conservation. National Academy of Sciences, Washington DC, pp. 35–69.

Herndon, J.G., Paredes, J., Wilson, M.E., Bloomsmith, M.A., Chennareddi, L., Walker, M.L., 2012. Menopause occurs late in life in the captive chimpanzees (*Pan troglodytes*). Age (Dordr) 34, 1145–1156.

Herrera, S., Perlaza, B.L., Bonelo, A., Arevalo-Herrera, M., 2002. Aotus monkeys: their great value for anti-malaria vaccines and drug testing. Int. J. Parasitol. 32, 1625–1635.

Herring, J.M., Fortman, J.D., Anderson, R.J., Bennett, B.T., 1991. Ultrasonic determination of fetal parameters in baboons. Lab. Anim. Sci. 41, 602–605.

Hershkovitz, P., 1983. Two new species of night monkeys, genus *Aotus* (Cebidae, Plattyrrhini): a preliminary report on *Aotus* taxonomy. Am. J. Primatol. 4, 209–243.

Hershkovitz, P., 1984. Taxonomy of squirrel monkeys genus *Saimiri* (Cebidae, Platyrrhini): a preliminary report with description of a hitherto unnamed form. Am. J. Primatol. 7, 155–210.

Hetherington, C.M., 1978. Circadian oscillations of body temperature in the marmoset. Callithrix jacchus. Lab. Anim. 12, 107–108.

Higashino, A., Sakate, R., Kameoka, Y., Takahashi, I., Hirata, M., Tanuma, R., et al., 2012. Whole-genome sequencing and analysis of the Malaysian cynomolgus macaque (*Macaca fascicularis*) genome. Genome Biol. 13, R58. http://dx.doi.org/10.1186/gb-2012-13-7-r58.

Hill, K., Boesch, C., Goodall, J., Pusey, A., Williams, J., Wrangham, R., 2001. Mortality rates among wild chimpanzess. J. Hum. Evol. 40, 437–450.

Hilliard, J.K., Ward, J.A., 1999. B-virus specific-pathogen-free breeding colonies of macaques (*Macaca mulatta*): a retrospective study of seven years of testing. Lab. Anim. Sci. 49, 144–148.

Hirsch, V.M., Dapolito, G., Johnson, P.R., Elkins, W.R., London, W.T., Montali, R.J., et al., 1995. Induction of AIDS by simian immunodeficiency virus from an African green monkey: species-specific variation in pathogenicity correlates with the extent of in vivo replication. J. Virol. 69, 955–967.

Hodgen, G.D., Neimann, W.H., 1975. Application of the subhuman primate pregnancy test kit to pregnancy diagnosis in baboons. Lab. Anim. Sci. 25, 757–759.

Hodgen, G.D., Wolfe, L.G., Ogden, J.D., Adams, M.R., Descalzi, C.C., Hildebrand, D.F., 1976. Diagnosis of pregnancy in marmosets: hemagglutinin inhibition test and radioimmunoassay for urinary chorionic gonadotropin. Lab. Anim. Sci. 26, 224–229.

Hodges, J.K., Czekala, N.M., Lasley, B.L., 1979. Estrogen and luteinizing hormone secretion in diverse primate species from simplified urinary analysis. J. Med. Primatol. 8, 349–364.

Hoffman, K., Videan, E.N., Fritz, J., Murphy, J., 2007. Diagnosis and treatment of ocular coccidioidomycosis in a female captive chimpanzee (*Pan troglodytes*): a case study. Ann. NY Acad. Sci. 1111, 404–410.

Hoffmann, M., Hilton-Taylor, C., 2008. Papio ursinus. In: IUCN 2013. IUCN Red List of Threatened Species. Version 2013.2. Available at: <www.iucnredlist.org>. Downloaded on February 3, 2014.

Holmberg, C.A., Henrickson, R., Lenninger, R., Anderson, J., Hayashi, L., Ellingsworth, L., 1985. Immunologic abnormality in a group of *Macaca arctoides* with high mortality due to atypical mycobacterial and other disease processes. Am. J. Vet. Res. 46, 1192–1196.

Honess, P.E., Marin, C.M., 2006. Enrichment and aggression in primates. Neurosci. Behav. Rev. 30, 413–436.

Hopf, S., 1967. Notes on pregnancy, delivery, and infant survival in captive squirrel monkeys. Primates 8, 323–332.

Horvath, C.J., Simon, M.A., Bergsagel, D.J., Pauley, D.R., King, N.W., Garcea, R.L., et al., 1992. Simian virus 40-induced disease in rhesus monkeys with simian acquired immunodeficiency syndrome. Am. J. Pathol. 140, 1431–1440.

Huang, Y.-Y., Chen, A.C.-H., Carroll, J.D., Hamblin, M.R., 2009. Biphasic dose response in low level light therapy. Dose Response 7, 358–383.

Huang, Y.-Y., Sharma, S.K., Carroll, J.D., Hamblin, M.R., 2011. Biphasic dose response in low level light therapy – an update. Dose Response 9, 602–618.

Hubbard, G.B., Lee, D.R., Eichberg, J.W., Gormus, B.J., Xu, K., Meyers, W.M., 1991. Spontaneous leprosy in a chimpanzee (*Pan troglodytes*). Vet. Pathol. 28, 546–548.

Hubbard, G.B., Soike, K.F., Butler, T.M., Carey, K.D., Davis, H., Butcher, W.I., et al., 1992. An encephalomyocarditis virus epizootic in a baboon colony. Lab. Anim. Sci. 42, 233–239.

Huck, M., Rotundo, M., Fernández-Duque, E., 2011. Growth and development in wild owl monkeys (*Aotus azarai*) of Argentina. Int. J. Primatol. 32, 1133–1152.

Huemer, H.P., Larcher, C., Czedik-Eysenberg, T., Nowotny, N., Reifinger, M., 2002. Fatal infection of a pet monkey with Human herpesvirus. Emerg. Infect. Dis. 8 (6), 639–642.

Hugh-Jones, M.E., Hubbert, W.T., Hagstad, H.V., 1995. Zoonoses: Recognition, Control, and Prevention. Iowa State University Press, Ames, IA.

Hunt, R.D., Melendez, L.V., 1966. Spontaneous herpes-T infection in the owl monkey (*Aotus trivirgatus*). Vet. Pathol. 3, 1–26.

Hunt, R.D., Garcia, F.G., Hegsted, D.M., 1967. A comparison of vitamin D2 and D3 in New World Primates. I. Production and regression of osteodystraphia fibrosa. Lab. Anim. Care 17, 222–234.

Hunter, A.J., Martin, R.D., Dixon, A.F., Rudder, B.C., 1979. Gestation and inter-birth intervals in the owl monkey (*Aotus trivirgatus griseimembra*). Folia Primatol. 31, 165–175.

Hutin, Y.J., Williams, R.J., Malfait, P., et al., 2001. Outbreak of human monkeypox, Democratic Republic of Congo, 1996 to, 1997. Emerg. Infect. Dis. 7 (3), 434–438. http://dx.doi.org/10.3201/eid0703.010311.

Hutto, E.H., Anderson, D.C., Mansfield, K.G., 2004. Cytomegalovirus-associated discrete gastrointestinal masses in macaques infected with the simian immunodeficiency virus. Vet. Pathol. 41, 691–695.

IUCN, 2013. IUCN Red List of Threatened Species. Version 2013.1. Available at: <www.iucnredlist.org>. Downloaded on November 17, 2013.

IUCN, 2014. IUCN Red List of Threatened Species. Version 2014.1. Available at: <www.iucnredlist.org>. Downloaded on July 3, 2014.

Ihrig, M., Tassinary, L.G., Bernacky, B., Keeling, M.E., 2001. Hematologic and serum reference intervals for the chimpanzee (*Pan troglodytes*) characterized by age and sex. Comp. Med. 51, 30–37.

Institute of Laboratory Animal Resources (ILAR), 1973. Standards and Guidelines for the Breeding, Care, and Management of Laboratory Animals, second ed. National Academy of Sciences, Washington, DC.

Institute for Laboratory Animal Research (ILAR), 1997. Chimpanzees in Research, Strategies for Their Ethical Care, Management, and Use. National Academy Press, Washington, DC, A Report of the Institute for Laboratory Animal Research Committee on Long-Term Care of Chimpanzees.

Institute for Laboratory Animal Research (ILAR), 1998. The Psychological Weil-Being of Nonhuman Primates. National Academy Press, Washington, DC, A Report of the Institute for Laboratory Animal Research Committee on Well-Being of Nonhuman Primates, Publ. 98–40103.

Isbell, L.A., 1995. Seasonal and social correlates of changes in hair, skin, and scrotal condition in vervet monkeys (*Cercopithecus aethiops*) of Amboseli National Park, Kenya. Am. J. Primatol. 36, 61–70.

Isbell, L.A., Enstam, K.L., 2002. Predator (in)sensitive foraging in sympatric female vervets (*Cercopithecus aethiops*) and patas monkeys (*Erythrocebus patas*): a test of ecological models of group dispersion. In: Miller, L.E. (Ed.), Eat or Be Eaten: Predator Sensitive Foraging among Primates. Cambridge University Press, Cambridge (UK), pp. 154–168.

Isbell, L.A., Pruetz, J.D., Lewis, M., Young, T.P., 1999. Rank differences in ecological behavior: a comparative study of patas monkeys (*Erythrocebus patas*) and vervets (*Cercopithecus aethiops*). Int. J. Primatol. 20, 257–272.

Isbell, L.A., Cheney, D.L., Seyfarth, R.M., 2002. Why vervet monkeys (*Cercopithecus aethiops*) live in multimale groups. In: Glenn, M.E., Cords, M. (Eds.), The Guenons: Diversity and Adaptation in African Monkeys. Kluwer Academic Press/Plenum Press, New York, pp. 173–187.

Iwata, T., Une, Y., Okatani, A.T., Kato, Y., Nakadai, A., Lee, K., et al., 2008. Virulence characteristics of *Yersinia pseudotuberculosis* isolated from breeding monkeys in Japan. Vet. Microbiol. 129, 404–409.

Izawa, K., 1978. A field study of the ecology and behavior of the black-mantle tamarin (*Saguinus nigricollis*). Primates 19, 241–274.

Jahrling, P.B., Geisbert, T.W., Jaax, N.K., Hanes, M.A., Ksiazek, T.G., Peters, C.J., 1996. Experimental infection of cynomolgus macaques with Ebola-Reston filoviruses from the 1989–1900 U.S. epizootic. Arch. Virol. Suppl. 11, 115–134.

Jaquish, C.E., Toal, R.L., Tardif, S.D., Carson, R.L., 1995. Use of ultrasound to monitor prenatal growth and development in the common marmoset (*Callithrix jacchus*). J. Med. Primatol. 36, 259–275.

Jarosz, S.J., Kuehl, T.J., Dukelow, W.R., 1977. Vaginal cytology, induced ovulation and gestationin the squirrel monkey (*Saimiri sciureus*). Biol. Repro. 16, 97–103.

Jasinska, A.J., Service, S., Levinson, M., Slaten, M., Lee, O., Sobel, E., et al., 2007. A genetic linkage map of the vervet monkey (*Chlorocebus aethiops sabaeus*). Mamm. Genome. 18, 347–360.

Jayo, J.M., Sajuthi, D., Wagner, J.D., Bullock, B.C., McDole, G.K., 1990. Intestinal amyloidosis in a rhesus monkey responsive to treatment with dimthyl sulfoxide. Lab. Anim. Sci. 40, 548. JayJ.

Jedel, E., Labrie, F., Odén, A., Holm, G., Nilsson, L., Janson, P.O., et al., 2011. Impact of electroacupuncture and physical exercise on hyperandrogenism and oligo/amenorrhea in women with polycystic ovary syndrome: a randomized controlled trial. Am. J. Physiol. Endocrinol. Metab. 300, E37–E45.

Jeneby, M.M., Suleman, M.A., Gichuki, C., 2002. Sero-epizootiologic survey of Trypanosoma brucei in Kenyan nonhuman primates. J. Zoo Wildl. Med. 33, 337–341.

Jeneby, M.M., 2011. Haemoprotozoan parasites of nonhuman primates in Kenya. Studies on prevalence and characterization of haemoprotozoan parasites of wild-caught baboons, African green monkeys, and Syke's monkeys. Acta Universitatis Upsaliensis. Digit. Compr. Summ. Uppsala Dissertations Fac. Med. 663, 52. Uppsala.

Jeong, S.H., Qiao, M., Nascimbeni, M., Hu, Z., Rehermann, B., Murthy, K., et al., 2004. Immunization with hepatitis C virus-like particles induces humoral and cellular immune responses in nonhuman primates. J. Virol. 78, 6995–7003.

Jezek, Z., Arita, I., Szczeniowski, M., Paluku, K.M., Ruti, K., Nakanao, J.H., 1985. Human tanapox in Zaire: clinical and epidemiological observations on cases confirmed by laboratory studies. Bull. WHO 63, 1027–1035.

Ji, Y., Xie, L., Liu, S., Cheng, K., Xu, F., et al., 2013. Correlation of thoracic radiograph measurements with age in adolescent Chinese rhesus macaques (*Macaca mulatta*). J. Am. Assoc. Lab. Anim. 52, 1–5.

Johnsen, D.O., 1995. History. In: Bennett, B.T., Abee, C.R., Henrickson, R.V. (Eds.), Nonhuman Primates in Biomedical Research: Biology and Management. Academic Press, San Diego, CA, pp. 1–14.

Johnson-Delaney, C.A., 1994. Primates. Vet. Clin. North Am. Small Anim. Pract. 24, 121–156.

Johnson-Delaney, C.A., 2008. Nonhuman primate dental care. J. Exotic Pet Med. 17, 138–143.

Jones, A.M., Wyand, D.S., 1966. Pulmonary nocardiosis in the rhesus monkey: importance of differentiation from tuberculosis. Pathol. Vet. 3, 588–600.

Jones, E.E., Alford, P.L., Reingold, A.L., Russell, H., Keeling, M.E., Broome, C.V., 1984. Predisposition to invasive pneumococcal illness following parainfluenza type 3 virus infection in chimpanzees. J. Am. Vet. Med. Assoc. 185, 1351–1353.

Jones, T.C., Thorington, R.W., Hu, M.M., Adams, E., Cooper, R.W., 1973. Karyotypes of squirrel monkeys (*Saimiri sciureus*). Am. J. Phys. Anthropol. 38, 269–277.

Jorgensen, M.J., Aycock, S.T., Clarkson, T.B., Kaplan, J.R., 2013. Effects of a western-type diet on plasma lipids and other cardiometabolic risk factors in African Green Monkeys (*Chlorocebus aethiops sabaeus*). JAALAS 52, 448–453.

Kalter, S.S., Heberling, R.L., 1971. Comparative virology of primates. Bacteriol. Rev. 35, 310–364.

Kalter, S.S., Heberling, R.L., Cooke, A.W., Barry, J.D., Tian, P.Y., Northam, W.J., 1997. Viral infections of nonhuman primates. Lab. Anim. Sci. 47, 461–467.

Kalter, S.S., Heberling, R.L., 1990. Viral battery testing in nonhuman primate colony management. Lab. Anim. Sci. 40, 21–23.

Kantha, S.S., Suzuki, J., 2006. Sleep quantitation in common marmoset, cotton top tamarin and squirrel monkey by non-invasive actigraphy. Comp. Biochem. Physiol. 144, 203–210.

Kanthaswamy, S., Elfenbein, H.A., Ardeshir, A., Ng, J., Hyde, D., Smith, D.G., et al., 2014. Familial aggregation of chronic diarrhea disease (CDD) in rhesus macaques (Macaca mulatta). Am. J. Primatol. 76, 262–270. http://dx.doi.org/10.1002/ajp.22230.

Kaplan, W., George, L.K., Hendricks, S.L., Leeper, R.A., 1957. Isolation of Microsporum distortum from animals in the United States. J. Invest. Dermatol. 28, 449–453.

Karere, G.M., Glenn, J.P., VandeBerg, J.L., Cox, L.A., 2010. Identification of baboon microRNAs expressed in liver and lymphocytes. J. Biomed. Sci. 17, 54–61.

Kark, J.A., Victor, M., Hines, J.D., Harris, J.W., 1974. Nutritional vitamin B$_{12}$ deficiency in rhesus monkeys. Am. J. Clin. Nutr. 27, 470–478.

Karron, R.A., Wright, P.F., Crowe Jr., J.E., Clements-Mann, M.L., Thompson, J., Makhene, M., et al., 1997. Evaluation of two live, cold-passaged, temperature-sensitive respiratory syncytial virus vaccines in chimpanzees and in human adults, infants, and children. J. Infect. Dis. 176, 1428–1436.

Kaspareit, J., Friderichs-Gromoll, S., Buse, E., Habermann, G., 2007. Spontaneous neoplasms observed in cynomolgus monkeys (Macaca fascicularis) during a 15-year period. Exp. Toxicol. Pathol. 59, 163–169.

Kathmann, I., Cizinauskas, S., Dohrer, M.G., Steffen, F., Jaggy, A., 2006. Daily controlled physiotherapy increases survival time in dogs with suspected degenerative myelopathy. J. Vet. Intern. Med. 20, 927–932.

Katz, D., Shi, W., Patrusheva, I., Perelygina, L., Gowda, M.S., Krug, P.W., et al., 2012. An automated ELISA using recombinant antigens for serologic diagnosis of B virus infections in macaques. Comp. Med. 62, 527–534.

Kaufmann, A.F., Quist, K.D., 1969a. Pneumococcal meningitis and peritonitis in rhesus monkeys. J. Am. Vet. Med. Assoc. 155, 1158–1162.

Kaufmann, A.F., Quist, K.D., 1969b. Thrush in a rhesus monkey: report of a case. Lab. Anim. Care 19, 526–527.

Kaufmann, A.F., Moulthrop, J.I., Moore, R.M., 1975. A perspective of simian tuberculosis in the United States-1972. J. Med. Primatol. 4, 278–286.

Kaufman, M.J., Janes, A.C., Frederick, B.D., Brimson-Théberge, M., Tong, Y., McWilliams, S.B., et al., 2013. A method for conducting functional MRI studies in alert nonhuman primates: initial results with opioid agonists in male cynomolgus monkeys. Exp. Clin. Psychopharmacol. 21, 323–331.

Kaup, F., Mätz-Rensing, K., Kuhn, E., Hünerbein, P., Stahl-Hennig, C., Hunsmann, G., 1998. Gastrointestinal pathology in rhesus monkeys with experimental SIV infection. Pathobiology 66, 159–164.

Kaur, T., Singh, J., Huffman, M.A., Petrzelková, K.J., Taylor, N.S., Xu, S., et al., 2011. Campylobacter troglodytis sp. nov., isolated from feces of human-habituated wild chimpanzees (Pan troglodytes schweinfurthii) in Tanzania. Appl. Environ. Microbiol. 77, 2366–2373.

Kavoussi, B., Ross, B.E., 2007. The neuroimmune basis of anti-inflammatory acupuncture. Integr. Cancer Ther. 6, 251–257.

Keeling, M.E., McClure, H.M., 1974. Pneumococcal meningitis and fatal enterobiasis in a chimpanzee. Lab. Anim. Sci. 24, 92–95.

Keeling, M.E., Wolf, R.H., 1975. Medical management of the rhesus monkey. In: Bourne, G.H. (Ed.), The Rhesus Monkey, vol. 2 Academic Press, New York, pp. 11–96.

Keeling, M.E., Roberts, J.R., 1972. Breeding and reproduction of chimpanzees. In: Bourne, G.H. (Ed.), The Chimpanzee, vol. 5. Karger, Basel, Switzerland; University Park Press, Baltimore, MD, pp. 127–152.

Keeling, M.E., Wolfe, R.H., 1975. Medical management of the rhesus monkey. In: Bourne, G.H. (Ed.), The Rhesus Monkey, vol. 2. Academic Press, New York, pp. 11–96.

Kemnitz, J.W., Goy, R.W., Flitsch, T.J., Lohmiller, J.J., Robinson, J.A., 1989. Obesity in male and female rhesus monkeys: fat distribution, glucoregulation, and serum androgen levels. J. Clin. Endocrinol. Metab. 69, 287–293.

Keenan, K., Bartlett, T.Q., Nijland, M., Rodriguez, J.S., Nathanielsz, P.W., Zürcher, N.R., 2013. Poor nutrition during pregnancy and lactation negatively affects neurodevelopment of the offspring: evidence from a translational primate model. Am. J. Clin. Nutr. 98, 396–402.

Kennedy, F.M., Astbury, J., Needham, J.R., Cheasty, T., 1993. Shigellosis due to occupational contact with nonhuman primates. Epidemiol. Infect. 110, 247–251.

Kennedy, S., Hadfield, R., Barlow, D., Weeks, D.E., Laird, E., Golding, S., 1997. Use of MRI in genetic studies of endometriosis. Am. J. Med. Genet. 71, 371–372.

Kennett, M., 1996. Training shorts. ASLAP News 29, 20–21.

Kenyon, R.H., Rippy, M.K., McKee Jr., K.T., Zack, P.M., Peters, C.J., 1992. Infection of Macaca radiata with viruses of the tick-borne encephalitis group. Microb. Pathog. 13, 399–409.

Kerber, W.T., Reese, W.H., Van Natta, J., 1968. Balanitis, paronychia, and onychia in a rhesus monkey. Lab. Anim. Care 18, 506–507.

Kerber, W.T., Conaway, C.H., Smith, D.M., 1977. The duration of gestation in the squirrel monkey (Saimiri sciureus). Lab. Anim. Sci. 27, 700–702.

Kessel, A., Brent, L., 2001. The rehabilitation of captive baboons. J. Med. Primatol. 30, 71–80.

Kessler, M.J., Brown, R.J., 1979. Clinical description of tetanus in squirrel monkeys (Saimiri sciureus). Lab. Anim. Sci. 29, 240–242.

Kessler, M.J., Brown, R.J., 1981. Mycetomas in a squirrel monkey (Saimiri sciureus). J. Zoo Anim. Med. 12, 91–93.

Kessler, M.J., Berard, J.D., Rawlins, R.G., 1988. Effect of tetanus toxoid inoculation on mortality in the Cayo Santiago macaque population. Am. J. Primatol. 15, 93–101.

Kessler, M.J., London, W.T., Rawlins, R.G., Gonzalez, J., Martinez, H.S., Sanchez, J., 1985. Management of a harem breeding colony of rhesus monkeys to reduce trauma-related morbidity and mortality. J. Med. Primatol. 14, 91–98.

Kessler, M.J., Berard, J.D., Rawlins, R.G., Bercovitch, F.B., Gerald, M.S., Laudenslager, M.L., et al., 2006. Tetanus antibody titers and duration of immunity to clinical tetanus infections in free-ranging rhesus monkeys (Macaca mulatta). Am. J. Primatol. 68, 725–731.

Kestler, H., Kodama, T., Ringler, D., Marthas, M., Pederson, N., Lackner, A., et al., 1990. Induction of AIDS in rhesus monkeys by molecularly cloned simian immunodeficiency virus. Science 248, 1109–1112.

Khan, I.H., Mendoza, S., Yee, J., Deane, M., Venkateswaran, K., Zhou, S.S., et al., 2006. Simultaneous detection of antibodies to six nonhuman-primate viruses by multiplex microbead immunoassay. Clin. Vaccine Immunol. 13, 45–52.

Khan, I.H., Ravindran, R., Yee, J., Ziman, M., Lewinsohn, D.M., Gennaro, M.L., et al., 2008. Profiling antibodies to Mycobacterium tuberculosis by multiplex microbead suspension arrays for serodiagnosis of tuberculosis. Clin. Vaccine Immunol. 15, 433–438.

Kienesberger, S., Perez-Perez, G., Rivera-Correa, J., Tosado-Acevedo, R., Li, H., Dubois, A., et al., 2012. Serologic host response to Helicobacter pylori and Campylobacter jejuni in socially housed Rhesus macaques (Macaca mulatta). Gut Pathog. 4, 9.

King, B.J., Monis, P.T., 2007. Critical processes affecting Cryptosporidium oocyst survival in the environment. Parasitology 134, 309–323.

King, N.W., Hunt, R.D., Daniel, M.D., Melendez, L.V., 1967. Overt herpes-T infection in squirrel monkeys (Saimiri sciureus). Lab. Anim. Care 17, 413–423.

Kingdon, J., 1997. The Kingdon Field Guide to African Mammals. Academic Press, London, P. 496.

Kingdon, J., Butynski, T.M., 2008. Chlorocebus aethiops. In: IUCN 2013. IUCN Red List of Threatened Species. Version 2013.1. Available at: <www.iucnredlist.org>. Downloaded on September 25, 2013.

Kingdon, J., Butynski, T.M., De Jong, Y., 2008a. Papio anubis, Papio cynocephalus, In: IUCN 2013. IUCN Red List of Threatened Species. Version 2013.2. Available at: <www.iucnredlist.org>. Downloaded on February 3, 2014.

Kingdon, J., Gippoliti, S., Butynski, T.M., De Jong, Y., 2008b. *Chlorocebus pygerythrus*. In: IUCN 2013. IUCN Red List of Threatened Species. Version 2013.1. Available at: <www.iucnredlist.org>. Downloaded on September 25, 2013.

Kingdon, J., Gippoliti, S., 2008. Chlorocebus tantalus. In: IUCN 2013. IUCN Red List of Threatened Species. Version 2013.1. Available at: <www.iucnredlist.org>. Downloaded on September 25, 2013.

Kinzey, W.G., 1997. Saguinus. In: Kinzey, W.G. (Ed.), New World Primates: Ecology, Evolution, and Behavior. Aldine de Gruyter, New York, pp. 289–296.

Kirkwood, J.K., Pearson, G.R., Epstein, M.A., 1986. Adenocarcinoma of the large bowel and colitis in captive cotton-topped tamarins *Sanguinus o. Oedipus*. J. Comp. Pathol. 96, 507–515.

Klein, H.J., Murray, K.A., 1995. Medical management: restraint. In: Bennett, B.T., Abee, C.R., Henrickson, R.V. (Eds.), Nonhuman Primates in Biomedical Research: Biology and Management. Academic Press, San Diego, CA, pp. 286–295.

Klein, E.C., Gebhart, C.J., Duhamel, G.E., 1999. Fatal outbreaks of proliferative enteritis caused by *Lawsonia intracellularis* in young colony-raised rhesus macaques. J. Med. Primatol. 28, 11–18.

Klimentidis, Y.C., Beasley, T.M., Lin, H.-Y., Murati, G., Glass, G.E., Guyton, M., et al., 2011. Canaries in the coal mine: a cross-species analysis of the plurality of obesity epidemics. Proc. R. Soc. B. 278, 1626–1632.

Kling, H.M., Shipley, T.W., Patil, S., Morris, A., Norris, K.A., 2009. *Pneumocystis* Colonization in Immunocompetent and Simian Immunodeficiency Virus-Infected Cynomolgus Macaques. J. Infect. Dis. 199, 89–96. http://dx.doi.org/10.1086/595297.

Klokke, A.H., deVries, G.A., 1963. *Tinea capitis* in a chimpanzee caused by *Microsporum canis* Bodin, 1902 resembling *M. obesum* Conant, 1937. Sabaraudia 2, 268–270.

Klosterman, L.L., Murai, J.T., Siiteri, P.K., 1986. Cortisol levels, binding, and properties of corticosteroid-binding globulin in the serum of primates. Endocrinology 118, 424–434.

Klumpp, S.A., Weaver, D.S., Jerome, C.P., Jokinen, M.P., 1986. *Salmonella* osteomyelitis in a rhesus monkey. Vet. Pathol. 23, 190–197.

Knapp, L.A., Lehmann, E., Piekarczyk, M.S., Urvater, J.A., Watkins, D.I., 1997. A high frequency of Manu-A *01 in the rhesus macaque detected by polymerase chain reaction with sequence-specific primers and direct sequencing. Tissue Antigens 50, 657–661.

Koie, H., Abe, Y., Sato, T., Yamaoka, A., Taira, M., Nigi, H., 2007. Tetralogy of fallot in a Japanese macaque (*Macaca fuscata*). J. Am. Assoc. Lab. Anim. Sci. 46, 66–67.

Kolappaswamy, K., Mahalingam, R., Traina-Dorge, V., Shipley, S.T., Gilden, D.H., Kleinschmidt-Demasters, B.K., et al., 2007. Disseminated simian varicella virus infection in an irradiated rhesus macaque (*Macaca mulatta*). J. Virol. 81, 411–415.

Kolappaswamy, K., Shipley, S.T., Tatarov, I.I., DeTolla, L.J., 2008. Methicillin-resistant *Staphylococcus non-aureus* infection in an irradiated rhesus macaque (*Macaca mulatta*). J. Am. Assoc. Lab. Anim. Sci. 47, 64–67.

Köndgen, S., Leider, M., Lankester, F., Bethe, A., Lübke-Becker, A., Leendertz, F.H., et al., 2011. *Pasteurella multocida* involved in respiratory disease of wild chimpanzees. PLoS One 6, e24236.

Konstant, W.R., Mittermeier, R.A., 1982. Introduction, reintroduction, and translocation of neotropical primates: past experiences and future possibilities. Int. Zoo Yearbook 22, 69–77.

Kormos, R., Boesch, C., Bakarr, M.I., Butynski, T.M., 2003. West African Chimpanzees: Status survey and conservation action plan. IUCN, p. ix.

Kramer, J.A., Grindley, J., Crowell, A.M., Makaron, L., Kohli, R., Kirby, M., et al., 2014. The common marmoset as a model for the study of nonalcoholic fatty liver disease and nonalcoholic steatohepatitis. Vet. Pathol. 52, 404–413. Published online June 9, 2014, <http://www.dx.doi.org/10.1177/0300985814537839> .

Kramer, J.A., Hachey, A.M., Wachtman, L.M., Mansfield, K.G., 2009. Treatment of Giardiasis in Common Marmosets (Callithrix jacchus) with Tinidazole. Comp. Med. 59, 174–179.

Kreeger, T.J., 1999. Chemical restraint and immobilization of wild canids. In: Fowler, M.E., Miller, R.E. (Eds.), Zoo and Wild Animal Medicine: Current Therapy 4. Saunders, Philadelphia, PA, pp. 429–435.

Krook, L., Barrett, R.B., 1962. Simian bone disease – a secondary hyperparathyroidism. Cornell Vet. 52, 459–492.

Kuehne, R.W., Chatigny, M.A., Stainbrook, B.W., Runkle, R.S., Stuart, D.G., 1995. Primary barriers and personal protective equipment in biomedical laboratories. In: Fleming, D.O., Richardson, J.H., Tulis, J.J., Vesley, D. (Eds.), Laboratory Safety: Principles and Practices. ASM Press, Washington, DC, pp. 145–170.

Kumar, S., Fox, B., Owston, M., Hubbard, G.B., Dick Jr., E.J., 2012. Pathology of spontaneous air sacculitis in 37 baboons and 7 chimpanzees and a brief review of the literature. J. Med. Primatol. 41, 266–277.

Kumar, V., Ceulemans, F., De Meurichy, W., 1978. Chemotherapy of helminthiasis among wild animals. IV. Efficacy of flubendazole 5% (R 17889) against *Trichuris trichiura* infections of baboons, *Papio hamadryas* L. Acta Zool. Pathol. Antverp. 73, 3–9.

Kummer, H., Banaja, A.A., Abo-Khatwa, A.N., Ghandor, A.M., 1981. A survey of hamadryas baboons in Saudi Arabia. Fauna Saudi Arabia 3, 441–471.

Kunz, E., Mätz-Rensing, K., Stolte, N., Hamilton, P.B., Kaup, F.J., 2002. Reactivation of a *Trypanosoma cruzi* infection in a rhesus monkey (*Macaca mulatta*) experimentally infected with SIV. Vet. Pathol. 39, 721–725.

Kushner, H., Kraft-Schreyer, N., Angelakos, E.T., Wudarski, E.M., 1982. Analysis of reproductive data in a breeding colony of African green monkeys. J. Med. Primatol. 11, 77–84.

LabDiet Product Reference Manual, 1998. PMI Nutritional International, St. Louis, MO.

Lackner, A.A., Rodriguez, M.H., Bush, C.E., Munn, R.J., Kwang, H.S., Moore, P.F., et al., 1988. Distribution of a macaque immunosuppressive type D retrovirus in neural, lymphoid, and salivary tissues. J.Virol. 62, 2134–2142.

Lafortune, M., Wellehan, J.F., Jacobson, E.R., Troutman, J.M., Gebhart, C.J., Thompson, M.S., 2004. Proliferative enteritis associated with *Lawsonia intracellularis* in a Japanese macaque (*Macaca fuscata*). J. Zoo. Wildl. Med. 35, 549–552.

Lang, C.M., Benjamin, S.A., 1969. Acute pyometra in a rhesus monkey (*Macaca mulatta*). J. Am. Vet. Med. Assoc. 155, 1156–1157.

Lambeth, S.P., Perlman, J.E., Thiele, E., Schapiro, S.J., 2005. Changes in hematology and blood chemistry parameters in captive chimpanzees (*Pan troglodytes*) as a function of blood sampling technique: trained vs. anesthetized samples. Am. J. Primatol. 68, 245–256.

Lambeth, S.P., Hau, J., Perlman, J.E., Martino, M., Schapiro, S.J., 2006. Positive reinforcement training affects hematologic and serum chemistry values in captive chimpanzees (Pan troglodytes). Am. J. Primatol. 68, 245–256.

Lambeth, S.P., Schapiro, S.J., Bernacky, B.J., Wilkerson, G.K., 2013. Establishing 'quality of life' parameters using behavioral guidelines for humane euthanasia of captive non-human primates. Anim. Welfare 22, 429–435.

Landolfi, J.A., Wellehan, J.F., Johnson, A.J., Kinsel, M.J., 2005. Fatal human herpesvirus type 1 infection in a white-handed gibbon (*Hylobates lar*). J. Vet. Diagn. Invest. 17 (4), 369–371.

Langner, P.H., Brightman, A.H., Tranquilli, W.J., 1986. Maxillofacial abscesses in captive squirrel monkeys. J. Am. Vet. Med. Assoc. 189, 1218.

Latt, R.H., 1975. Runyon group III atypical mycobacteria as a cause of tuberculosis in a rhesus monkey. Lab. Anim. Sci. 25, 206–209.

Laule, G.E., Thurston, R.H., Alford, P.L., Bloomsmith, M.A., 1996. Training to reliably obtain blood and urine samples from a diabetic chimpanzee (*Pan troglodytes*). Zoo Biol. 15, 587–591.

Laule, G.E., Bloomsmith, M.A., Schapiro, S.J., 2003. The use of positive reinforcement training techniques to enhance the care, management, and welfare of primates in the laboratory. J. Appl. Anim. Welfare Sci. 6, 163–173. published online 4 June 2010.

Lausen, N.C., Richter, A.G., Lage, A.L., 1986. *Pseudomonas aeruginosa* infection in squirrel monkeys. J. Am. Vet. Med. Assoc. 189, 1216–1218.

Lavergne, A., Ruiz-García, M., Catzeflis, F., LaCote, S., Contamin, H., Mercereau-Puijalon, O., et al., 2010. Phylogeny and phylogeography of squirrel monkeys (genus *Saimiri*) based on cytochrome b genetic analysis. Am. J. Primatol. 72, 242–253.

Layne, D.G., Power, R.A., 2003. Husbandry, handling, and nutrition for marmosets. Comp. Med. 53, 351–359.

Leal-Junior, E.C., de Almeida, P., Tomazoni, S.S., de Carvalho Pde, T., Lopes-Martins, R.Á., Frigo, L., et al., 2014. Superpulsed low-level laser therapy protects skeletal muscle of mdx mice against damage, inflammation and morphological changes delaying dystrophy progression. PLoS One 9, e89453 http://dx.doi.org/10.1371/journal.pone.0089453.

Lebherz, C., Maguire, A.M., Auricchio, A., Tang, W., Aleman, T.S., Wei, Z., et al., 2005. Nonhuman primate models for diabetic ocular neovascularization using AAV2-mediated overexpression of vascular endothelial growth factor. Diabetes 54, 1141–1149.

Lee, D.R., 1993. Nonhuman Primate Models in Biomedical Research. Lecture at Baylor College of Medicine, Houston, Texas, November 10.

Lee, D.R., Kuehl, T.J., Eichberg, J.W., 1991. Real-time ultrasonography as a clinical and management tool to monitor pregnancy in a chimpanzee breeding colony. Am. J. Primatol. 24, 289–294.

Lee, J.I., Kim, K.S., Oh, B.C., Kim, N.A., Kim, I.H., Park, C.G., et al., 2011. Acute necrotizing stomatitis (noma) associated with methicillin-resistant Staphylococcus aureus infection in a newly acquired rhesus macaque (*Macaca mulatta*). J. Med. Primatol. 40, 188–193.

Lee, P.C., 1984. Early infant development and maternal care in free-ranging vervet monkeys. Primates 25, 36–47.

Lee, R.V., Prowten, W.M., Satchidanand, S., Srivastava, B.I.S., 1985. Non-Hodgkin's lymphoma and HTLV-1 antibodies in a gorilla. N. Eng. J. Med. 312, 118–119.

Lehner, N.D.M., 1984. Biology and diseases of the Cebidae. In: Fox, J.G., Cohen, B.G., Loew, F.M. (Eds.), Laboratory Animal Medicine. Academic Press, Orlando, FL, pp. 321–353.

Lehner, N.D.M., Bullock, B.C., Clarkson, T.B., Lofland, H.B., 1967. Biological activities of vitamin D_2 and vitamin D_3 for growing squirrel monkeys. Lab. Anim. Care 17, 483–493.

Lehner, N.D.M., Bullock, B.C., Clarkson, T.B., 1968. Ascorbic acid deficiency in the squirrel monkey. Proc. Soc. Exp. Biol. Med. 128, 512–514.

Leininger, J.R., Donham, K.J., Rubino, M.J., 1978. Leprosy in a chimpanzee: morphology of the skin lesions and characterization of the organism. Vet. Pathol. 15, 339–346.

LeMaho, Y., Goffart, M., Rochas, A., Feibabel, H., Chatonnet, J., 1981. Thermoregulation in the only nocturnal simian: the night monkey *Aotus trivirgatus*. Am. J. Physiol. 240, R156–R165.

Lemere, C.A., Beierschmitt, A., Iglesias, M., Spooner, E.T., Bloom, J.K., Leverone, J.F., et al., 2004. Alzheimer's disease Aß vaccine reduces' central nervous system Aß levels in a non-human primate, the caribbean vervet. Am. J. Pathol. 165, 283–297.

Leonardi, R., Buchanan-Smith, H.M., Dufour, V., MacDonald, C., Whiten, A., 2010. Living together: behavior and welfare in single and mixed species groups of capuchin (*Cebus apella*) and squirrel monkeys (*Saimiri sciureus*). Am. J. Primatol. 72, 33–47.

Lerche, N.W., 2010. Simian retroviruses: infection and disease - implications for immunotoxicology research in primates. J. Immunotoxicol. 7, 93–101. http://dx.doi.org/10.3109/15476911003657406.

Lerche, N.W., Osborn, K.G., 2003. Simian retrovirus infections: potential confounding variables in primate toxicology studies. Toxicol. Pathol. 31 (Suppl), 103–110.

Lerche, N.W., Osborn, K.G., Marx, P.A., Prahalda, S., Maul, D.H., Lowenstine, L.J., et al., 1986. Inapparent carriers of simian acquired immunodeficiency syndrome type D retrovirus and disease transmission with saliva. J. Nat. Cancer Inst. 77, 489–496.

Lerche, N.W., Yee, J.L., Capuano, S.V., Flynn, J.L., 2008. New approaches to tuberculosis surveillance in nonhuman primates. Ilar. J. 49 (2), 170–178.

Lertpiriyapong, K., Handt, L., Feng, Y., Mitchell, T.W., Lodge, K.E., Shen, Z., et al., 2014. Pathogenic properties of enterohepatic Helicobacter spp. isolated from rhesus macaques with intestinal adenocarcinoma. J. Med. Microbiol. 63, 1004–1016.

Letvin, N.L., Eaton, K.A., Aldrich, W.R., Sehgal, P.K., Blake, B.J., Schlossman, S.E., et al., 1983. Acquired immunodeficiency syndrome in a colony of macaque monkeys. Proc. Natl. Acad. Sci. USA. 80, 2718–2722.

Levin, J., 1995. Medical management: special techniques. In: Bennett, B.T., Abee, C.R., Henrickson, R.V. (Eds.), Nonhuman Primates in Biomedical Research: Biology and Management. Academic Press, San Diego, CA, pp. 304–316.

Levin, J.L., Hilliard, J.K., Lipper, S.L., Butler, T.M., Goodwin, W.J., 1988. A naturally occurring epizootic of simian agent 8 in the baboon. Lab. Anim. Sci. 38, 394–397.

Levy, B.M., Mirkovic, R.R., 1971. An epizootic of measles in a marmoset colony. Lab. Anim. Sci. 21, 33–39.

Li, R., Huang, L., Li, J., Mo, Z., He, B., Wang, Y., et al., 2013. A next-generation, serum-free, highly purified Vero cell rabies vaccine is safe and as immunogenic as the reference vaccine Verorab® when administered according to a post-exposure regimen in healthy children and adults in China. Vaccine 31, 5940–5947.

Liang, T.J., 2013. Current progress in development of hepatitis C virus vaccines. Nat. Med. 19, 869–878.

Liebenberg, S.P., Giddens, W.E., 1985. Disseminated nocardiosis in three macaque monkeys. Lab. Anim. Sci. 35, 162–166.

Liddie, S., Goody, R.J., Valles, R., Lawrence, M.S., 2010. Clinical chemistry and hematology values in a Caribbean population of African green monkeys. J. Med. Primatol. 39, 389–398. http://dx.doi.org/10.1111/j.1600-0684.2010.00422.x.

Lin, M.H., Chen, T.C., Kuo, T.T., Tseng, C.C., Tseng, C.P., 2000. Real-time PCR for quantitative detection of Toxoplasma gondii. J. Clin. Microbiol. 38 (11), 4121–4125.

Lindburg, D.G., 1980. The Macaques: Studies in Ecology, Behavior, and Evolution. Van Nostrand Reinhold, New York.

Lindsey, J.R., Melby Jr., E.C., 1966. Naturally occurring primary cutaneous tuberculosis in the rhesus monkey. Lab. Anim. Care 16, 369–385.

Lindsey, J.R., Hardy, P.H., Baker, H.J., Melby Jr., E.C., 1971. Observations on shigellosis and development of multiply resistant *Shigellas* in *Macaca mulatta*. Lab. Anim. Sci. 21, 832–844.

Line, S., Dorr, T., Roberts, J., Ihrke, P., 1984. Necrotizing cellulitis in a squirrel monkey. J. Am. Vet. Med. Assoc. 185, 1378–1379.

Line, A.S., Paul-Murphy, J., Aucoin, D.P., Hirsh, D.C., 1992. Enrofloxacin treatment of long-tailed macaques with acute bacillary dysentery due to multiresistant *Shigella flexneri* IV. Lab. Anim. Sci. 42, 240–244.

Lipman, B., Palmer, D., Noble, J., Haughton, V., Collier, D., 1988. Effect of lumbar puncture on flow of cerebrospinal fluid. Invest. Radiol. 23, 359–360.

Liu, S.K., Dolensek, E.P., Tappe, J.P., Stover, J., Adams, C.R., 1984. Cardiomyopathy associated with vitamin E deficiency in seven gelada baboons. J. Am. Vet. Med. Assoc. 185, 1347–1350.

Liu, D.X., Gilbert, M.H., Wang, X., Didier, P.J., Veazey, R.S., 2012. Reactive amyloidosis associated with ischial callositis: a report with histology of ischial callosities in rhesus macaques (*Macaca mulatta*). J. Vet. Diagn. Invest. 24, 1184–1188. http://dx.doi.org/10.1177/1040638712463919.

Lögdberg, B., 1993. Methods of timing for pregnancy and monitoring of fetal body and brain growth in squirrel monkeys. J. Med. Primatol. 22, 374–379.

Löhr, M., Lebenheim, L., Berg, F., Stenzel, W., Hescheler, J., Molcanyi, M., et al., 2014. Gadolinium enhancement in newly diagnosed patients with lumbar disc herniations are associated with inflammatory peridiscal tissue reactions – evidence of fragment degradation? Clin. Neurol. Neurosurg. 119, 28–34. <http://dx.doi.org/10.1016/j.clineuro.2014.01.008>. Epub Jan 18, 2014.

Löttker, P., Huck, M., Heymann, E.W., Heistermann, M., 2004. Endocrine correlates of reproductive status in breeding and nonbreeding wild female moustached tamarins. Int. J. Primatol. 25, 919–937.

Loudon, J.E., Howells, M.E., Fuentes, A., 2006. The importance of integrative anthropology: a preliminary investigation employing primatological and cultural anthropological data collectionmethods in assessing human-monkey coexistence in bali, indonesia. Ecol. Environ. Anthropol. (University of Georgia) 2, 1–13. (Paper 26).

Lowenstine, L.J., 1993. Type D retrovirus infection, macaques. In: Jones, T.C. Mohr, U. Hunt, R.D. (Eds.), Monographs on Pathology of Laboratory Animals: Nonhuman Primates, vol. 1. Springer-Verlag, Berlin and New York, pp. 20–32.

Lowenstine, L.J., Lerche, N.W., Yee, J.L., Uyeda, A., Jennings, M.B., Munn, R.J., et al., 1992. Evidence for a lentiviral etiology in an epizootic of immune deficiency and lymphoma in stump-tailed macaques (Macaca arctoides). J. Med. Primatol. 21, 1–14.

Lowenstine, L.J., Pedersen, N.C., Higgins, J., Pallis, K.C., Uyeda, A., Marx, P., et al., 1986. Seroepidemiologic survey of captive Old-World primates for antibodies to human and simian retroviruses, and isolation of a lentivirus from sooty mangabeys (Cercocebus atys). Int. J. Cancer 38, 563–574.

Ludlage, E., Mansfield, K., 2003. Clinical care and diseases of the common marmoset (Callithrix jacchus). Comp. Med. 53, 369–382.

Ludlage, E., Murphy, C.L., Davern, S.M., Solomon, A., Weiss, D.T., Glenn-Smith, D., et al., 2005. Systemic AA amyloidosis in the common marmoset. Vet. Pathol. 42, 117–124.

Lundeberg, T., 1993. Peripheral effects of sensory nerve stimulation (acupuncture) in inflammation and ischemia. Scand. J. Rehabil. Med. Suppl. 29, 61–86.

Lutz, C.K., Novak, M.A., 2005. Environmental enrichment for nonhuman primates: theory and application. ILAR 46, 178–191.

Lyashchenko, K.P., Greenwald, R., Esfandiari, J., Greenwald, D., Nacy, C.A., Gibson, S., et al., 2007. PrimaTB STAT-PAK Assay, a Novel, Rapid Lateral-Flow Test for Tuberculosis in Nonhuman Primates. Clin. Vaccine Immunol. 14, 1158–1164. http://dx.doi.org/10.1128/cvi.00230-07.

Ma, N.S.F., 1981. Chromosome evolution in the owl monkey. Aotus. Am. J. Primatol. 54, 293–303.

Ma, N.S., Harris, T.S., 1989. A putative homeolog of human chromosome 12 in the owl monkey. Cytogenet. Cell Genet. 50, 34–39.

Ma, N.S.F., Aquino, R., Collins, W.E., 1985. Two new karyotypes in the Peruvian owl monkey (Aotus trivirgatus). Am. J. Anthropol. 9, 333–341.

MacArthur, J.A., Wood, M., 1983. Yersiniosis in a breeding unit of Macaca fascicularis (cynomolgus monkeys). Lab. Anim. 17, 151–155.

Machotka, S.V., Chapple, F.E., Stookey, J.L., 1975. Cerebral tuberculosis in a rhesus monkey. J. Am. Vet. Med. Assoc. 167, 648–650.

MacDonald, E.A., Fernández-Duque, E., Evans, S., Hagey, L.R., 2008. Sex, age, and family differences in the chemical composition of owl monkey (Aotus nancymaae) subcaudal scent secretions. Am. J. Primatol. 70, 12–18.

Macy, J.D. Jr., Beattie, T.A., Morgenstern, S.E., Arnsten, A.F., 2000. Use of guanfacine to control self-injurious behavior in two rhesus macaques (Macaca mulatta) and one baboon (Papio anubis). Comp. Med. 50, 419–425.

Magden, E.R., Haller, R.L., Thiele, E.J., Buchl, S.J., Lambeth, S.P., Schapiro, S.J., 2013. Acupuncture as an adjunct therapy for osteoarthritis in chimpanzees (Pan troglodytes). JAALAS 52, 475–480.

Mahaney, M.C., Leland, M.M., Williams-Blangero, S., Marinez, Y.N., 1993. Cross-sectional growth standards for captive baboons: II. Organ weight by body weight. J. Med. Primatol. 7–8, 415–427.

Major, C.A., Kelly, B.J., Novak, M.A., Davenport, M.D., Stonemetz, K.M., Meyer, J.S., 2009. The anxiogenic drug FG7142 increases self-injurious behavior in male rhesus monkeys (Macaca mulatta). Life Sci. 85, 753–758.

Mak, G.S., Truong, Q.A., 2012. Cardiac CT: imaging of and through cardiac devices. Curr. Cardiovasc. Imaging Rep. 5, 328–336.

Malaga, C.A., Weller, R.E., Buschbom, R.L., Ragan, H.A., 1990. Hematology of the wild-caught karyotype I owl monkey (Aotus nancymaae). Lab. Anim. Sci. 40, 204–205.

Malaga, C.A., Weller, R.E., Buschbom, R.L., Ragan, H.A., 1995. Hematology of the wild-caught karyotype V owl monkey (Aotus vociferans). JAALAS 45, 574–577.

Malaga, C.A., Weller, R.E., Buschbom, R.L., Baer, J.F., Kimsey, B.B., 1997. Reproduction of the owl monkey (Aotus spp.) in captivity. J. Med. Primatol. 26, 147–152.

Mansfield, K.G., 2003. Marmoset models commonly used in biomedical research. Comp. Med. 53, 383–392.

Mansfield, K.G., King, N., 1998. Viral diseases. In: Bennett, B.T., Abee, C.R., Henrickson, R.V. (Eds.), Nonhuman Primates in Biomedical Research: Diseases. Academic Press, San Diego, CA, pp. 1–58.

Mansfield, K.G., Kuei-Chin, L., Newman, J., Schauer, D., MacKey, J., Lackner, A.A., et al., 2001. Identification of enteropathogenic Escherichia coli in simian immunodeficiency virus-infected infant and adult rhesus macaques. J. Clin. Microbiol. 39, 971–976.

Mansfield, K.G., Lackner, A.A., 1997. Simian immunodeficiency virus-inoculated macaques acquire Mycobacterium avium from potable water during AIDS. J. Infect. Dis. 175, 184–187.

Mansfield, K.G., Pauley, D., Young, H.L., Lackner, A.A., 1995. Mycobacterium avium complex in macaques with AIDS is associated with a specific strain of simian immunodeficiency virus and prolonged survival after primary infection. J. Infect. Dis. 172, 1149–1152.

Mansfield, K.G., Sasseville, V.G., Westmoreland, S.V., 2014. Molecular localization techniques in the diagnosis and characterization of nonhuman primate infectious diseases. Vet. Pathol. 5, 110–126.

Marini, R.P., Muthupalani, S., Shen, Z., Buckley, E.M., Alvarado, C., Taylor, N.S., et al., 2010. Persistent infection of rhesus monkeys with 'Helicobacter macacae' and its isolation from an animal with intestinal adenocarcinoma. J. Med. Microbiol. 59 (Pt 8), 961–969.

Marr-Belvin, A.K., Carville, A.K., Fahey, M.A., Boisvert, K., Klumpp, S.A., Ohashi, M., et al., 2008. Rhesus lymphocryptovirus type 1-associated B-cell nasal lymphoma in SIV-infected rhesus macaques. Vet. Pathol. 45, 914–921.

Marson, J., Meuris, S., Cooper, R.W., Jouannet, P., 1991. Puberty in the male chimpanzee: progressive maturation of semen characteristics. Biol. Repro. 44, 448–455.

Martin, D.P., 1986. Preventive medicine. In: Fowler, M.E. (Ed.), Zoo and Wild Animal Medicine. Saunders, Philadelphia, PA, pp. 667–669.

Martin, D.P., Kaye, H.S., 1983. Epizootic of parainfluenza-3 virus infection in gibbons. J. Am. Vet. Med. Assoc. 183, 1185–1187.

Martin, L.N., McNease, P.E., 1982. Genetically determined antigens of squirrel monkey (Saimiri sciureus) IgG. J. Med. Primatol. 11, 272–290.

Martin, B.J., Dysko, R.C., Chrisp, C.E., 1991. Pancreatitis associated with simian adenovirus 23 in a rhesus monkey. Lab. Anim. Sci. 41, 382–384.

Martín, J., Hermida, L., Castro, J., Lazo, L., Martínez, R., Gil, L., et al., 2009. Viremia and antibody response in green monkeys (Chlorocebus aethiops sabaeus) infected with dengue virus type 2: a potential model for vaccine testing. Microbiol. Immunol. 53, 216–223.

Masek-Hammerman, K., Miller, A.D., Lin, K.C., MacKey, J., Weissenböck, H., Gierbolini, L., et al., 2012. Epizootic myocarditis associated with encephalomyocarditis virus in a group of rhesus macaques (Macaca mulatta). Vet. Pathol. 49, 386–392.

Masterson, T.J., Hartwig, W.C., 1998. Degrees of sexual dimorphism in cebus and other new world monkeys. Am. J. Phys. Anthropol. 107, 243–256.

Matsui, H., Takahashi, T., Murayama, S.Y., Uchiyama, I., Yamaguchi, K., Shigenobu, S., et al., 2014. Development of new PCR primers by comparative genomics for the detection of *Helicobacter suis* in gastric biopsy specimens. Helicobacter 19, 260–271.

Mattison, J.A., Ottinger, M.A., Powell, D., Longo, D.L., Ingram, D.K., 2007. Endometriosis: clinical monitoring and treatment procedures in Rhesus Monkeys. J. Med. Primatol. 36, 391–398.

Mätz-Rensing, K., Jentsch, K.D., Rensing, S., Langenhuyzen, S., Verschoor, E., Niphuis, H., et al., 2003. Fatal Herpes simplex infection in a group of common marmosets (*Callithrix jacchus*). Vet. Pathol. 40 (4), 405–411.

Mätz-Rensing, K., Ellerbrok, H., Ehlers, B., Pauli, G., Floto, A., Alex, M., et al., 2006. Fatal poxvirus outbreak in a colony of New World monkeys. Vet. Pathol. 43, 212–218.

Mätz-Rensing, K., Winkelmann, J., Becker, T., Burckhardt, I., van der Linden, M., Köndgen, S., et al., 2009. Outbreak of *Streptococcus equi* subsp. *zooepidemicus* infection in a group of rhesus monkeys (*Macaca mulatta*). J. Med. Primatol. 38, 328–334.

Mavrommatis, C.I., Argyra, E., Vadalouka, A., Vasilakos, D.G., 2012. Acupuncture as an adjunctive therapy to pharmacological treatment in patients with chronic pain due to osteoarthritis of the knee: a 3-armed, randomized, placebo-controlled trial. Pain 153, 1720–1726.

McCarthy, T.C., 2005. Veterinary Endoscopy for the Small Animal Practitioner. Elsevier Saunders, St. Louis, MS, ISBN 0-7216-3653-5.

McCarthy, T.J., Kennedy, J.L., Blakeslee, J.R., Bennett, B.T., 1990. Spontaneous malignant lymphoma and leukemia in a simian T-lymphotrophic virus type 1 (STLV-1) antibody-positive olive baboon. Lab. Anim. Sci. 40, 79–81.

McChesney, M.B., Fujinami, R.S., Lerche, N.W., Marx, P.A., Oldstone, M.B., 1989. Virus-induced immunosuppression: infection of peripheral blood mononuclear cells and suppression of immunoglobulin synthesis during natural measles virus infection of rhesus monkeys. J. Infect. Dis. 159, 757–760.

McClure, H.M., 1980. Bacterial diseases of nonhuman primates. In: Montali, R.J., Migaki, G. (Eds.), The Comparative Pathology of Zoo Animals. Smithsonian Institution Press, Washington, DC, pp. 197–217.

McClure, H.M., Keeling, M.E., 1971. Viral diseases noted at the Yerkes Primate Center colony. Lab. Anim. Sci. 21, 1002–1010.

McClure, H.M., Weaver, R.E., Kaufmann, A.F., 1971. Pseudotuberculosis in nonhuman primates: infection with organisms of the *Yersinia enterocolitica* group. Lab. Anim. Sci. 21, 376–382.

McClure, H.M., Strozier, L.M., Keeling, M.F., 1972. Enteropathogenic *Escherichia coli* infection in anthropoid apes. J. Am. Vet. Med. Assoc. 161, 687–689.

McClure, H.M., Alford, P., Swenson, B., 1976. Nonenteric *Shigella* infections in nonhuman primates. J. Am. Vet. Med. Assoc. 169, 938–939.

McClure, H.M., Brodie, A.R., Anderson, D.C., Swenson, R.B., 1986. Bacterial infections of nonhuman primates. In: Benirschke, K. (Ed.), Primates: The Road to Self-Sustaining Populations. Springer-Verlag, New York, pp. 531–556.

McConkey, E.H., 2004. Orthologous numbering of great ape and human chromosomes is essential for comparative genomics. Cytogenet. Genome Res. 105, 157–158.

McConnell, S.J., Hickman, R.L., Wooding, W.L., Huxsoll, D.L., 1968. Monkeypox: experimental infection in chimpanzees and immunization with vaccinia virus. Am. J. Vet. Med. Res. 29, 1675–1680.

McGrew, W.C., Webster, J., 1995. Birth seasonality in cotton-top tamarins (Saguinus oedipus) despite constant food supply and body weight. Primates 36, 241–248.

McLaughlin, R.M., 1978. *Mycobacterium bovis* in nonhuman primates. In: Montali, R.J. (Ed.), Mycobacterial Infections in Zoo Animals. Smithsonian Institution Press, Washington, DC, pp. 151–155.

McLaughlin, R.M., Marrs, G.E., 1978. Tuberculin testing in nonhuman primates: OT vs. PPD. In: Montal, R.J. (Ed.), Mycobacterial

Infections in Zoo Animls. Smithsonian Institution Press, Washington, D.C, pp. 123–127.

McMillan, J.L., Perlman, J.E., Galvan, A., Wichmann, T., Bloomsmith, M.A., 2014. Refining the pole-and-collar method of restraint: emphasizing the use of positive training techniques with rhesus macaques (*Macaca mulatta*). JAALAS 53, 61–68.

McNamee, G.A., Wannemacher Jr., R.W., Dinterman, R.E., Rozmiarek, H., Montrey, R.D., 1984. A surgical procedure and tethering system for chronic blood sampling, infusion, and temperature monitoring in caged nonhuman primates. Lab. Anim. Sci. 34, 303–307.

McNees, D.W., Ponzio, B.J., Lewis, R.W., Stein, F.J., Sis, R.F., 1982. Hematology of common marmosets (*Callithrix jacchus*). Primates 23, 145–150.

McNulty, W.P., 1972. Pox diseases in primates. In: Fiennes, R.N.T.-W. (Ed.), Pathology of Simian Primates. Karger, Basel and New York, pp. 612–645.

Mehlhorn, H. (Ed.), 2008. Encyclopedia of Parasitology, (3rd ed. vol. 1). Springer-Verlag, Berlin.

Mekonnen, A., Bekele, A., Fashing, P.J., Hemson, G., Atickem, A., 2010a. Diet, activity patterns, and ranging ecology of the Bale monkey (*Chlorocebus djamdjamensis*) in Odobullu Forest, Ethiopia. Int. J. Primatol. 31, 339–362.

Mekonnen, A., Bekele, A., Hemson, G., Teshome, E., Atickem, A., 2010b. Population size and habitat reference of the vulnerable Bale monkey *Chlorocebus djamdjamensis* in Odobullu Forest and its distribution across the Bale Mountains, Ethiopia. Oryx 44, 558–563.

Melendez, L.V., Hunt, R.D., Daniel, M.D., Trum, B.F., 1970. New World monkeys, herpes viruses, and cancer. In: Balner, H., Beveridge, W.J.B. (Eds.), Infections and Immunosuppression in Subhuman Primates. Munksgaard, Copenhagen, Denmark, pp. 111–117.

Melnick, D.J., Pearl, M.C., 1987. Cercopithecines in multimale groups: genetic diversity and population structure. In: Smuts, B.B., Cheney, D.L., Seyfarth, R.M., Wrangham, R.W., Struhsaker, T.T. (Eds.), Primate Societies. University of Chicago Press, Chicago, pp. 121–134.

Menezes, A.N., Bonvicino, C.R., Seuánez, H.N., 2010. Identification, classification, and evoluation of owl monkeys (*Aotus*, Illiger 1811). BMC Evol. Biol. 10, 248.

Mercader, J., Panger, M., Boesch, C., 2002. Excavation of a chimpanzee stone tool site in the African rainforest. Science 296, 1452–1455.

Mercês, M.P., Lynch Alfaro, J.W., Ferreira, W.A., Harada, M.L., de Silva Júnior, J.S., 2014. Morphology and mitochondrial phylogenetics reveal that the Amazon River separates two eastern squirrel monkey species: *Saimiri sciureus* and *S. collinsi*. See comment in PubMed Commons below Mol. Phylogenet. Evol. pii: S1055-7903(14)00340-6. <http://dx.doi.org/10.1016/j.ympev.2014.09.020>.

Meritt, D.A., Jr., 1976. The owl monkey, *Aotus trivirgatus*: Husbandry, behavior, and breeding. In: Proceedings of the National Conference of AAZPA, pp. 107–123.

Meyers, W.M., Walsh, G.P., Brown, H.L., Binford, C.H., Imes Jr., G.D., Hadfield, T.L., et al., 1985. Leprosy in a mangabey monkey—naturally acquired infection. Int. J. Lepr. Other Mycobact. Dis. 53, 1–14.

Meyerson, N.R., Rowley, P.A., Swan, C.H., Le, D.T., Wilkerson, G.K., Sawyer, S.L., 2014. Positive selection of primate genes that promote HIV-1 replication. Virology 454–455, 291–298.

Middlekauff, H.R., Yu, J.L., Hui, K., 2001. Acupuncture effects on reflex responses to mental stress in humans. Am. J. Physiol. Regul. Integr. Comp. Physiol. 280, R1462–R1468.

Migaki, G., 1986. Mycotic infections in nonhuman primates. In: Benirschke, K. (Ed.), Primates: The Road to Self-Sustaining Populations. Springer-Verlag, New York, pp. 557–570.

Migaki, G., Asher, D.M., Casey, H.W., Locke, L.N., Gibbs Jr., C.J., Gajdusek, C., 1979. Fatal suppurative nephritis caused by *Pseudomonas* in a chimpanzee. J. Am. Vet. Med. Assoc. 175, 957–959.

Migaki, G., Schmidt, R.E., Toft, J.D. 2nd., Kaufmann, A.F., 1982. Mycotic infections of the alimentary tract of nonhuman primates: a review. Vet. Pathol. Suppl. 19, 93–103.

Miller, A.D., 2012. Neoplasia and proliferative disorders of nonhuman primates. In: Abee, C.R., Mansfield, K.M., Tardif, S., Morris, T. (Eds.), Nonhuman Primates in Biomedical Research. Elsevier, Academic Press, San Diego, CA, pp. 345–347.

Miller, R.E., Boever, W.J., 1983. Cryptococcosis in a lion-tailed macaque (*Macaca silenus*). J. Zoo Anim. Med. 14, 110–114.

Miller, G., Shope, T., Coope, D., Waters, L., Pagano, J., Bornkamm, G., et al., 1977. Lymphoma in cotton-topped marmosets after inoculation with Epstein-Barr virus: tumor incidence, histologic spectrum, antibody responses, demonstration of viral DNA, and characterization of viruses. J. Exp. Med. 145, 948–967.

Miller, G.F., Barnard, D.E., Woodward, R.A., Flynn, B.M., Bulte, J.W.M., 1997. Hepatic hemosiderosis in common marmosets, *Callithrix jacchus:* effect of diet on incidence and severity. Lab. Anim. Sci. 47, 138–142.

Miranda, M.E., Ksiazek, T.G., Retuya, T.J., Khan, A.S., Sanchez, A., Fulhorst, C.F., et al., 1999. Epidemiology of Ebola (subtype Reston) virus in the Philippines, 1996. J. Infect. Dis. 179 (S1), S115–S119.

Mitchell, C.L., Boinski, S., Van Schaik, C.P., 1991. Competitive regimes and female bonding in two species of squirrel monkeys (Saimiri oerstedi and S. sciureus). Behav. Ecol. Sociobiol. 28, 55–60.

Mivart, S.G., 1873. On *Lepilemur* and *Cheirogaleus* and on the zoological rank of the Lemuroidea. Proc. Zool. Soc. Lond., 484–510.

Mohiuddin, M.M., Singh, A.K., Corcoran, P.C., Hoyt, R.F., Thomas III, M.L., Lewis, B.G., et al., 2014. One-year heterotopic cardiac xenograft survival in a pig to baboon model. Am. J. Transplant. 14, 488–489. Epub 2013 Dec 11.

Moisson, P., Gysin, J., 1994. Reproductive performances and pathological findings in a breeding colony of squirrel monkeys (*Saimiri sciureus*) In: Anderson, J.R. Roeder, J.J. Thierry, B. Herrenschmidt, N. (Eds.), Current Primatology: Behavioral Neuroscience, Physiology, and Reproduction, vol. 3. University of Louis Pasteur, Strasbourg, France, pp. 263–272.

Molskness, T.A., Hess, D.L., Maginnis, G.M., Wright, J.W., Fanton, J.W., Stouffer, R.L., 2007. Characteristics and regulation of the ovarian cycle in vervet monkeys (Chlorocebus aethiops). Am. J. Primatol. 69, 890–900. http://dx.doi.org/10.1002/ajp.20395.

Montali, R.J., Scanga, C.A., Pernikoff, D., Wessner, D.R., Ward, R., Holmes, K.V., 1993. A common source outbreak of callitrichid hepatitis in captive tamarins and marmosets. J. Infect. Dis. 167, 946–950.

Montali, R.J., Connolly, B.M., Armstrong, D.L., Scanga, C.A., Holmes, K.V., 1995. Pathology and immunohistochemistry of callitrichid hepatitis, an emerging disease of captive New World primates caused by lymphocytic choriomeningitis virus. Am. J. Pathol. 147, 1441–1449.

Montiel, N.A., 2010. An updated review of simian betaretrovirus (SRV) in macaque hosts. J. Med. Primatol. 39, 303–314. http://dx.doi.org/10.1111/j.1600-0684.2010.00412.x.

Moore, C.J., Michopoulos, V., Johnson, Z.P., Toufexis, D., Wilson, M.E., 2013. Dietary variety is associated with larger meals in female rhesus monkeys. Physiol. Behav. 119, 190–194.

Moore, G.T., 1975. The breeding and utilization of baboons for biomedical research. Lab. Anim. Sci. 25, 798–801.

Morales-Jiménez, A.L., de la Torre, S., 2008. Aotus lemurinus. In: IUCN 2013. IUCN Red List of Threatened Species. Version 2013.1. Available at: <www.iucnredlist.org>. Downloaded on October 15, 2013.

Morales-Jiménez, A.L., Link, A., 2008. Aotus griseimembra; Aotus jorgehernandezi. In: IUCN 2013. IUCN Red List of Threatened Species. Version 2013.1. Available at: <www.iucnredlist.org>. Downloaded on October 15, 2013.

Morales-Jiménez, A.L., Link, A., Stevenson, P., 2008a. *Aotus brumbacki.* In: IUCN 2013. IUCN Red List of Threatened Species. Version 2013.1. Available at: <www.iucnredlist.org>. Downloaded on October 15, 2013.

Morales-Jiménez, A.L., Link, A., Cornejo, F., Stevenson, P., 2008b. *Aotus vociferans.* In: IUCN 2013. IUCN Red List of Threatened Species. Version 2013.1. Available at: <www.iucnredlist.org>. Downloaded on October 15, 2013.

Morbeck, M.E., Zihlman, A.L., Summner, D.R., Galloway, A., 1991. Poliomyelitis and skeletal asymmetry in Gombe chimpanzees. Primates 32, 77–91.

Morgan, U.M., Monis, P.T., Fayer, R., Deplazes, P., Thompson, R.C., 1999. Phylogenetic relationships among isolates of Cryptosporidium: evidence for several new species. J. Parasitol. 85, 1126–1133.

Morton, W.R., Agy, M.B., Capuano, S.V., Grant, R.F., 2008. Specific pathogen-free macaques: definition, history, and current production. ILAR J. 49, 137–144.

Motzel, S., Schachner, R., Kornegay, R., Fletcher, M., Kananaya, B., Gomez, J., et al., 1999. Assessment of methods for the diagnosis of tuberculosis in three species of nonhuman primates. Contemp. Top. Lab. Anim. Sci. 38, 28.

Mowery, T.M., Sarin, R.M., Elliot, K.S., Garraghty, P.E., 2012. Nerve injury-induced changes in $GABA_A$ and $GABA_B$ sub-unit expression in area 3b and cuneate nucleus of adult squirrel monkeys: further evidence of developmental recapitulation. Brain Res. 1415, 63–75.

Moynihan, M.A., 1964. Some behavior patterns of platyrrhine monkeys. 1. The night monkey (*Aotus trivirgatus*). Smithson. Misc. Collec. 146, 1–184.

Mrema, J.E., Caldwell, C.W., Stogsdill, P.L., Kelley, S.T., Green, T.J., 1987. Erythrocyte and erythrocyte morphologies of healthy and colony-born owl monkeys (*Aotus lemurinus griseimembra*). J. Med. Primatol. 16, 13–25.

Mubiru, J.N., Yang, A., Dick, E.J. Jr., Owston, M., Sharp, R.M., VandeBerg, J.F., et al., 2014. Correlation between presence of *Trypanosoma cruzi* DNA in heart tissue of baboons and cynomolgus monkeys, and lymphocytic myocarditis. Am. J. Trop. Med. Hyg. 90, 627–633.

Mulder, J.B., 1971. Shigellosis in nonhuman primates: a review. Lab. Anim. Sci. 21, 734–738.

Muller, M.N., Wrangham, R.W., 2014. Mortality rates among Kanyawara chimpanzees. J. Hum. Evol. 66, 107–114.

Murphy, K.L., Baxter, M.G., Flecknell, P.A., 2012. Anesthesia and analgesia in nonhuman primates. In: Abee, C.R., Mansfield, K., Tardif, S., Morris, T. (Eds.), Nonhuman Primates in Biomedical Research: Biology and Management, second ed. Academic Press, Elsevier, San Diego, CA, pp. 403–435.

Murphy, R.A., Register, T.C., Shively, C.A., Carr, J.J., Ge, Y., Heilbrun, M.E., et al., 2014. Adipose tissue density, a novel biomarker predicting mortality risk in older adults. J. Gerontol. A. Biol. Sci. Med. Sci. 69, 109–117.

Murthy, K.K., Salas, M.T., Carey, K.D., Patterson, J.L., 2006. Baboon as a nonhuman primate model for vaccine studies. Vaccine 24, 4622–4624.

Mutombo, W.M., Arita, I., Jezek, Z., 1983. Human monkeypox transmitted by a chimpanzee in a tropical rainforest of Zaire. Lancet 1, 735–737.

Myers, R.M., Greiner, S.M., Harvey, M.E., Griesmann, G., Kuffel, M.J., Buhrow, S.A., et al., 2007. Preclinical pharmacology and toxicology of intravenous MV-NIS, an oncolytic measles virus administered with or without cyclophosphamide. Clin. Pharmacol. Ther. 82, 700–710.

Nakamura, S., Hayashidani, H., Iwata, T., Namai, S., Une, Y., 2010. Pathological changes in captive monkeys with spontaneous yersiniosis due to infection by Yersinia enterocolitica serovar O8. J. Comp. Path. 143, 150–156. http://dx.doi.org/10.1016/j.jcpa.2010.01.017.

Napier, J.R., Napier, P.H., 1967. A Handbook of Living Primates. Academic Press, New York.

Napier, J.R., Napier, P.H., 1985. The Natural History of the Primates. MIT Press, Cambridge, MA.

National Center for Research Resources (NCRR), 2007. Report of the chimpanzee management plan working group. Available at: <http://ncrr.nih.gov/comparative_medicine/chimpanzee_management_program/ChimP05-22-2007.pdf>.

National Institutes of Health (NIH), 1994. In: NCRR Chimpanzee Breeding and Research Program Progress Report, July, 1994." National Institutes of Health, Washington, DC.

National Institutes of Health (NIH), 1998. NIH consensus development panel on acupuncture. JAMA 280, 1518–1524. http://dx.doi.org/10.1001/jama.280.17.1518.

National Institutes of Health (NIH), 2013. Announcement of Agency Decision: Recommendations on the Use of Chimpanzees in NIH-Supported Research, June 26, 2013. National Institutes of Health, Washington, DC (NOT-OD-13-078).

National Institutes of Health (NIH), 2014. Notice of Agency Decision: The Density of the Primary Living Space of Captive Chimpanzees Owned or Supported by the NIH or Used in NIH-Supported Research. National Institues of Health, Washington, DC, NOT-OD-14-051.

National Research Council (NRC), 1997. Occupational Health and Safety in the Care and Use of Research Animals. National Academy Press, Washington, D.C.

National Research Council (NRC), 1998. The Psychological Well-Being of Nonhuman Primate. National Academies Press, Washington, DC.

National Research Council (NRC), 2003a. Nutrient Requirements of Nonhuman Primates. National Academy of Sciences, Washington, DC.

National Research Council (NRC), 2003b. Occupational Health and Safety in the Care and Use of Nonhuman Primates. National Academy of Sciences, Washington, DC.

National Research Council (NRC), 2011a. Guide for the Care and Use of Laboratory Animals, eighth ed. National Academy Press, Washington, DC.

National Research Council (NRC), 2011b. Institute of Medicine (IOM) (US) and National Research Council (US) Committee on the use of chimpanzees in biomedical and behavioral research. In: Altevogt, B.M., Pankevich, D.E., Shelton-Davenport, M.K. (Eds.), Chimpanzees in Biomedical and Behavioral Research: Assessing the Necessity. National Academies Press, Washington DC. (2011). STUDY BACKGROUND AND CONTEXT. Available at: <http://www.ncbi.nlm.nih.gov/books/NBK91450/>.

National Research Council (US), 2011c. Institute for Laboratory Animal Research. Animal Research in a Global Environment: Meeting the Challenges. In: Proceedings of the November 2008 International Workshop. Washington DC: National Academies Press; International Coordination of Nonhuman Primates. Available at: <http://www.ncbi.nlm.nih.gov/books/NBK91512/>.

Naughton-Treves, L., Treves, A., Chapman, C., Wrangham, R., 1998.). Temporal patterns of crop-raiding by primates: linking food availability in croplands and adjacent forest. J. Appl. Ecol. 35, 596–606.

Navara, C.S., Hornecker, J., Grow, D., Chaudhari, S., Hornsby, P.J., Ichida, J.K., et al., 2013. Derivation of induced pluripotent stem cells from the baboon: a nonhuman primate model for preclinical testing of stem cell therapies. Cell Reprogram. 15, 495–502.

Nébié, I., Edwards, N.J., Tiono, A.B., Ewer, K.J., Sanou, G.S., Soulama, I., et al., 2014. Assessment of chimpanzee adenovirus serotype 63 neutralizing antibodies prior to evaluation of a candidate malaria vaccine regimen based on viral vectors. Clin. Vaccine Immunol. 21, 901–903.

Newman, J.D., 1985. Squirrel monkey communication. In: Rosenblum, L.A., Coe, C.L. (Eds.), Handbook of Squirrel Monkey Research. Plenum Press, New York, pp. 99–126.

Newton, W.M., Beamer, P.D., Rhoades, H.E., 1971. Acute bloat syndrome in stumptailed macaques (Macaca arctoides): a report of four cases. Lab. Anim. Sci. 21, 193–196.

Newton-Fisher, N.E., 2004. Hierarchy and social status in Budongo chimpanzees. Primates 45, 81–87.

Nicholson, N., 1982. Weaning and the Development of Independence in Olive Baboons. Ph.D. dissertation, Harvard University.

Niedobitek, G., Agathanggelou, A., Finerty, S., Tierney, R., Watkins, P., Jones, E.L., et al., 1994. Latent Epstein-Barr virus infection in cotton-top tamarins. Am. J. Pathol. 145, 969–978. 1999 Report of Progress, Southwest Foundation for Biomedical Research, San Antonio, TX.

Nimbkar-Joshi, S., Katkam, R.R., Chaudhari, U.K., Jacob, S., Manjramkar, D.D., Metkari, S.M., et al., 2012. Endometrial epithelial cell modifications in response to embryonic signals in bonnet monkeys (Macaca radiata). Histochem. Cell Biol. 138, 289–304.

Njiokou, F., Laveissiére, C., Simo, G., Nkinin, S., Grébaut, P., Cuny, G., et al., 2006. Wild fauna as a probable animal reservoir for Trypanosoma brucei gambiense in Cameroon. Infect. Genet. Evol. 6, 147–153.

Norkin, L.C., 1976. Rhesus monkeys kidney cells persistently infected with Simian Virus 40: production of defective interfering virus and acquisition of the transformed phenotype. Infect. Immun. 14, 783–792.

Northcott, C.A., Glenn, J.P., Shade, R.E., Kammerer, C.M., Hinojosa-Laborde, C., Fink, G.D., et al., 2012. A custom rat and baboon hypertension gene array to compare experimental models. Exp. Biol. Med. 237, 99–110.

Novak, M.A., Kinsey, J.H., Jorgensen, M.J., Hazen, T.J., 1998. Effects of puzzle feeders on pathological behavior in individually housed rhesus monkeys. Am. J. Primatol. 46, 213–227.

Nyland, T.G., Hill, D.E., Hendrickx, A.G., Henrickson, R., Anderson, J., Farver, T.B., et al., 1984. Ultrasonic assessment of fetal growth in the nonhuman primate (Macaca mulatta). J. Clin. Ultrasound 12, 387–395.

Oates, J.F., Gippoliti, S., Groves, C.P., 2008a. Papio papio. In: IUCN 2013. IUCN Red List of Threatened Species. Version 2013.2. <www.iucnredlist.org>. Downloaded on February 3, 2014.

Oates, J.F., Tutin, C.E.G., Humle, T., Wilson, M.L., Baillie, J.E.M., Balmforth, Z., et al., 2008b. Pan troglodytes. In: IUCN 2013. IUCN Red List of Threatened Species. Version 2013.2. Available at: <www.iucnredlist.org>. Downloaded on March 19, 2014.

Obaldia III, N., 1991. Detection of Klebsiella pneumoniae antibodies in Aotus I. lemurinus (Panamanian owl monkey) using an enzyme linked immunosorbent assay (ELISA) test. Lab. Anim. 25, 133–141.

Obaldia III, N., Otero, W., Marin, C., Aparicio, J., Cisneros, G., 2011. Long-term effect of a simple nest-box on the reproductive efficiency and other life traits of an Aotus lemurinus monkey colony: an animal model for malarial research. J. Med. Primatol. 40, 383–391.

Obeck, D.K., 1978. Galvanized caging as a potential factor in the development of the "fading infant" or "white monkey" syndrome. Lab. Anim. Sci. 28, 698–704.

Oerke, A.K., Einspanier, A., Hodges, J.K., 1995. Detection of pregnancy and monitoring patterns of uterine and fetal growth in the marmoset monkey (Callithrix jacchus) by real-time ultrasonography. Am. J. Primatol. 36, 1–13.

Ogay, V., Min, F., Kim, K.H., Kim, J.S., Bae, K.H., Han, S.C., et al., 2009. Observation of coiled blood plexus in rat skin with diffusive light illumination. J. Acupunct. Meridian Stud. 2, 56–65.

Ohsawa, K., Lehenbauer, T.W., Eberle, R., 1999. Herpesvirus papio 2: alternative antigen for use in monkey B virus diagnostic assays. Lab. Anim. Sci. 49 (6), 605–616.

Olobo, J.O., Gicheru, M.M., Anjili, C.O., 2001. The African Green Monkey model for cutaneous and visceral leishmaniasis. Trends Parasitol. 17, 588–592.

Olson, L.C., Bergquist, D.Y., Fitzgerald, D.L., 1986. Control of Shigella flexneri in Celebese black macaques (Macaca nigra). Lab. Anim. Sci. 36, 240–242.

Osborn, K.G., Prahalda, S., Lowenstine, L.J., Gardner, M.B., Maul, D.H., Henrickson, R.V., 1984. The pathology of acquired immunodeficiency syndrome in rhesus macaques. Am. J. Pathol. 114, 94–103.

O'Sullivan, M.G., Anderson, D.C., Fikes, J.D., Bain, F.T., Carlson, C.S., Green, S.W., et al., 1994. Identification of a novel simian parvovirus in cynomolgus monkeys with severe anemia. A paradigm of human B19 parvovirus infection. J. Clin. Invest. 93, 1571–1576.

O'Sullivan, M.G., Anderson, D.K., Lund, J.E., Brown, W.P., Green, S.W., Young, N.S., et al., 1996. Clinical and epidemiological features of simian parvovirus infection in cynomolgus macaques with severe anemia. Lab. Anim. Sci. 46, 291–297.

O'Sullivan, M.G., Anderson, D.K., Goodrich, J.A., Tulli, H., Green, S.W., Young, N.S., et al., 1997. Experimental infection of cynomolgus monkeys with simian parvovirus. J. Virol. 71, 4517–4521.

O'Toole, B.A., Fradkin, R., Warkany, J., Wilson, J.G., Mann, G.V., 1974. Vitamin A deficiency and reproduction in rhesus monkeys. J. Nutr. 104, 1513–1524.

Ouwe-Missi-Oukem-Boyer, O., Mezui-Me-Ndong, J., Boda, C., Lamine, I., Labrousse, F., Bisser, S., et al., 2006. The vervet monkey (Chlorocebus aethiops) as an experimental model for Trypanosoma brucei gambiense human African trypanosomiasis: a clinical, biological and pathological study. Trans. R. Soc. Trop. Med. Hyg. 100, 427–436.

Ozdemir, F., Birtane, M., Kokino, S., 2001. The clinical efficacy of low-power laser therapy on pain and function in cervical osteoarthritis. Clin. Rheumatol. 20, 181–184.

Packer, C., 1979. Inter-troop transfer and inbreeding avoidance in Papio anubis. Anim. Behav. 27, 1–36.

Page, E.K., Courtney, C.L., Sharma, P., Cheeseman, J., Jenkins, J.B., Strobert, E., et al., 2013. Post-transplant lymphoproliferative disorder associated with immunosuppressive therapy for renal transplantation in rhesus macaques (Macaca mulatta). Exp. Toxicol. Pathol. 65, 1019–1024.

Palmer, A.E., Allen, A.M., Tauraso, N.M., Shelokov, A., 1968. Simian hemorrhagic fever. I. Clinical and epizootiologic aspects of an outbreak among quarantined monkeys. Am. J. Trop. Med. Hyg. 17, 404–492.

Panarella, M.L., Bimes, R.S., 2010. A naturally occurring outbreak of tuberculosis in a group of imported cynomolgus monkeys (Macaca fascicularis). J. Am. Assoc. Lab. Anim. Sci. 49, 221–225.

Papin, J.F., Wolf, R.F., Kosanke, S.D., Jenkins, J.D., Moore, S.N., Anderson, M.P., et al., 2013. Infant baboons infected with respiratory syncytial virus develop clinical and pathological changes that parallel those of human infants. Am. J. Physiol. Lung Cell Mol. Physiol. 304, L530–L539.

Passamani, M., 1998. Activity budget of Geoffroy's Marmoset (Callithrix geoffroyi) in an Atlantic forest in Southeastern Brazil. Am. J. Primatol. 46, 333–340.

Paul, M., Lador, A., Grozinsky-Glasberg, S., Leibovici, L., 2014. Beta lactam antibiotic monotherapy versus beta lactam-aminoglycoside antibiotic combination therapy for sepsis. Cochrane Database of Systematic Reviews 2014, Issue 1. Art. No.: CD003344. http://dx.doi.org/10.1002/14651858.CD003344.pub3.

Paul-Murphy, J., 1993. Bacterial enterocolitis in nonhuman primates. In: Fowler, M. (Ed.), Zoo and Wild Animal Medicine: Current Therapy 3. Saunders, Philadelphia, PA, pp. 334–351.

Peisert, W., Taborski, A., Pawlowski, Z., Karlewiczowa, R., Zdun, M., 1983. Giardia infections in animals in Poznan Zoo. Vet. Parasitol. 13, 183–186.

Penniston, K.L., Tanumihardjo, S.A., 2001. Subtoxic hepatic vitamin A concentrations in captive rhesus monkeys (Macaca mulatta). J. Nutr. 131, 2904–2909.

Perelman, P., Johnson, W.E., Roos, C., Seúanez, H.N., Horvath, J.E., Moreira, M.A.M., et al., 2011. A molecular phylogeny of living primates. PLoS Genet. 7, e1001342.

Perlman, J.E., Bowsher, T.R., Braccini, S.N., Kuehl, T.J., Schapiro, S.J., 2003. Using positive reinforcement training techniques to facilitate the collection of semen in chimpanzees (Pan troglodytes). Am. J. Primatol. 60, 77–78.

Perman, V., Osborne, C.A., Stevens, J.B., 1974. Bone marrow biopsy. Vet. Clin. North Am. 4, 293–310.

Pernikoff, D.S., Orkin, J., 1991. Bacterial meningitis syndrome: an overall review of the disease complex and considerations of cross infectivity between great apes and man. Proc. Am. Assoc. Zoo. Vet, 235–241.

Perolat, P., Poingt, J., Vie, J., Jouaneau, C., Baranton, G., Gysin, J., 1992. Occurrence of severe leptospirosis in a breeding colony of squirrel monkeys. Am. J. Trop. Med. Hyg. 46, 538–545.

Peterson, C.W., Younan, P., Polacino, P.S., Maurice, N.J., Miller, H.W., Prlic, M., et al., 2013. Robust suppression of env-SHIV viremia in Macaca nemestrina by 3-drug ART is independent of timing of initiation during chronic infection. J. Med. Primatol. 42, 237–246.

Phillips-Conroy, J.E., Jolly, C.J., Petros, B., Allan, J.S., Desrosiers, R.C., 1994. Sexual transmission of SIVagm in wild grivet monkeys. J. Med. Primatol. 23, 1–7.

Piccardo, P., Cervenak, J., Yakovleva, O., Gregoril, L., Pomeroyl, K., Cook, A., et al., 2012. Squirrel monkeys infected with BSE develop Tau pathology. J. Comp. Pathol. 147, 84–93.

Pierce, D.L., Dukelow, W.R., 1988. Misleading positive tuberculin reactions in a squirrel monkey colony. Lab. Anim. Sci. 38, 729–730.

Pinheiro, E.S., Simon, F., Cassaro, K., Soares, M.E.G., 1993. Outbreak of diarrhea due to Campylobacter jejuni in lion-tamarins (Leontopithecus spp.) in captivity. Verh. Ber. Zootiere 35, 159–161.

Pinkerton, M., 1972. Miscellaneous organisms. In: T-W-Fiennes, R.N. (Ed.), Pathology of Simian Primates Part II: Infectious and Parasitic Diseases. Karger, Basel and New York, pp. 283–313.

Pisharath, H., Zao, C.L., Kreeger, J., Portugal, S., Kawabe, T., Burton, T., et al., 2013. Immunopathologic characterization of naturally acquired Trypanosoma cruzi infection and cardiac sequalae in cynomolgus macaques (Macaca fascicularis). J. Am. Assoc. Lab. Anim. Sci. 52, 545–552.

Plate, J.F., Bates, C.M., Mannava, S., Smith, T.L., Jorgensen, M.J., Register, T.C., et al., 2013. Age-related degenerative functional, radiographic, and histological changes of the shoulder in nonhuman primates. J. Shoulder Elbow Surg. 22, 1019–1029.

Plesker, R., Carlos, M., 1992. A spontaneous Yersinia pseudotuberculosis infection in a monkey colony. Zentrabi. Veterinarmed. B. 39, 201–208.

Plumb, D.C., 1995. Veterinary Drug Handbook. Iowa State University Press, Ames, IA, p. 604.

Poelma, F.G., 1975. Pneumocystis carinii infections in zoo animals. Z. Parasitenkd 46, 61–68.

Pook, A.G., 1976. Some Notes on the Development of Hand-Reared Infants of Four Species of Marmoset (Callitrichidae). 13th Annual Report, Jersey Wildlife Preservation Trust, pp. 38–46.

Pope, C.E., Pope, V.Z., Beck, L.R., 1986. Cryopreservation and transfer of baboon embryos. J. In Vitro Fertil. Embryo. Trans. 3, 33–39.

Popilskis, S.J., Lee, D.R., Elmore, D.B., 2008. Anesthesia and analgesia in nonhuman primates. In: Fish, R.E., Brown, M.J., Danneman, P.J., Karas, A.Z. (Eds.), Anesthesia and Analgesia in Laboratory Animals, second ed. Academic Press, Elsevier, San Diego, CA, pp. 335–363.

Porter Jr., J.A., 1969. Hematology of the night monkey. Aotus Trivirgatus. Lab. Anim. Sci. 19, 470–472.

Portman, O.W., Alexander, M., Tanaka, N., Osuga, T., 1980. Relationships between cholesterol, gallstones, biliary function, and plasma lipoproteins in squirrel monkeys. J. Lab. Clin. Med. 96, 90–101.

Postal, J.M., Gysin, J., Crenn, Y., 1988. Protection against fatal Klebsiella pneumoniae sepsis in the squirrel monkey Saimiri sciureus after immunization with a capsular polysaccharide vaccine. Ann. Inst. Pasteur. Immunol. 139, 401–407.

Potkay, S., 1992. Diseases of the callitrichidae: a review. J. Med. Primatol. 21, 189–236.

Poulsen, J.R., Clark, C.J., 2004. Densities, distributions, and seasonal movements of gorillas and chimpanzees in swamp forest in northern. Congo. Int. J. Primatol. 25, 285–306.

Power, M.L., Williams, L.E., Gibson, S.V., Schulkin, J., Helfers, J., Zorrilla, E.P., 2010. Pattern of maternal circulating CRH in laboratory-housed squirrel and owl monkeys. Am. J. Primatol. 72, 1004–1012.

Prado-Martinez, J., Sudmant, P.H., Kidd, J.M., Li, H., Kelley, J.L., Lorente-Galdos, B., et al., 2013. Great ape genetic diversity and population history. Nature 499, 471–475.

Prince, A.M., Brotman, B., 2001. Perspectives on hepatitis B studies with chimpanzees. ILAR 42, 85–88.

Puddy, E., Hill, C., 2007. Interpretation of the chest radiograph. Contin. Educ. Anaesth. Crit. Care Pain. 7, 71–75.

Qiu, W., Zheng, Y., Zhang, S., Fan, Q., Liu, H., Zhang, F., et al., 2011. Canine distemper outbreak in rhesus monkeys. China. Emerg. Infect. Dis. 17, 1541–1543.

Ramer, J.C., Garber, R.L., Steele, K.E., Boyson, J.F., O'Rourke, C., Thomson, J.A., 2000. Fatal lymphoproliferative disease associated with a novel gammaherpesvirus in a captive population of common marmosets. Comp. Med. 50, 59–68.

Rangan, S.R.S., Martin, L.N., Bozelka, B.E., Wang, N., Gomus, B.J., 1995. Epstein-Barr virus-related herpesvirus from a rhesus monkey (*Macaca mulatta*) with malignant lymphoma. Int. J. Cancer 38, 425–432.

Rasmussen, K.M., Thenen, S.W., Hayes, K.C., 1980. Effect of folic acid supplementation on pregnancy in the squirrel monkey (*Saimiri sciureus*). J. Med. Primatol. 9, 169–184.

Ratterree, M.S., Didier, P.J., Blanchard, J.L., Clarke, M.R., Schaeffer, D., 1990. Vitamin C deficiency in captive nonhuman primates fed commercial primate diet. Lab. Anim. Sci. 40, 165–168.

Rawlings, C.A., Diamond, H., Howerth, E.W., Neuwirth, L., Canalis, C., 2003. Diagnostic quality of percutaneous kidney biopsy specimens obtained with laparoscopy versus ultrasound guidance in dogs. JAALAS 223, 317–321.

Rawlins, R.G., Kessler, M.T., 1982. A five-year study of tetanus in the Cayo Santiago rhesus monkey colony: behavioral description and epizootiology. Am. J. Primatol. 3, 23–39.

Rayner, K.J., Esau, C.C., Hussain, F.N., McDaniel, A.L., Marshall, S.M., van Gils, J.M., et al., 2011. Inhibition of miR-33a/b in nonhuman primates raises plasma HDL and lowers VLDL triglycerides. Nature 478, 404–407. http://dx.doi.org/10.1038/nature10486.

Reamer, L.A., Haller, R.L., Thiele, E.J., Freeman, H.D., Lambeth, S.P., Schapiro, S.J., 2014. Factors affecting initial training success of blood glucose testing in captive chimpanzees (*Pan troglodytes*). Zoo. Biol. 33, 212–220.

Redmond Jr., D.E., Bjugstad, K.B., Teng, Y.D., Ourednik, V., Ourednik, J., Wakeman, D.R., et al., 2007. Behavioralimprovement in a primate Parkinson's model is associated with multiple homeostatic effects of human neural stem cells. Proc. Natl. Acad. Sci. USA 104, 12175–12180.

Reid, H.A., Herron, A.J., Hines Jr., M.E., Orchard, E.A., Altman, N.H., 1993. Leptospirosis in a white-lipped tamarin (*Saguinus labiatus*). Lab. Anim. Sci. 43 (3), 258–259.

Reindel, J.F., Fitzgerald, A.L., Breider, M.A., Gough, A.W., Yan, C., Mysore, J.V., et al., 1999. An epizootic of lymphoplasmacytic gastritis attributed to *Helicobacter pylori* infection in cynomolgus monkeys (*Macaca fascicularis*). Vet. Pathol. 36, 1–13.

Reindel, J.F., Walsh, K.M., Toy, K.A., Bobrowski, W.F., 2000. Spontaneously occurring hepatocellular neoplasia in adolescent cynomolgus monkeys (*Macaca fascicularis*). Vet. Pathol. 37, 656–662.

Reinhardt, V., 1993. Enticing nonhuman primates to forage for their standard biscuit ration. Zoo Biol. 12, 307–312.

Reinhardt, V., 2008. Taking Better Care of Monkeys and Apes. Animal Welfare Institute, Washington, DC.

Reizenstein, E., Johansson, B., Mardin, L., Abens, J., Mollby, R., Hallander, H.O., 1993. Diagnostic evaluation of polymerase chain reaction discriminative for *Bordetella pertussis*, *B. parapertussis*, and *B. bronchiseptica*. Diagn. Microbiol. Infect. Dis. 17, 185–191.

Renne, R.A., McLaughlin, R., Jenson, A.B., 1973. Measles virus-associated endometritus, cervicitis, and abortion in a rhesus monkey. J. Am. Vet. Med. Assoc. 163, 639–641.

Rennie, A.E., Buchanan-Smith, H.M., 2006. Refinement of the use of non-human primates in scientific research. Part III: refinement of procedures. Anim. Welfare 15, 239–261.

Renquist, D., 1990. Outbreak of hemorrhagic fever. J. Med. Primatol. 19, 77–80.

Renquist, D.M., Whitney, R.A., 1987. Zoonoses acquired from pet primates. Vet. Clin. North Am. Small Anim. Pract. 17, 219–240.

Rensing, S., Oerke, A.K., 2005. Husbandry and management of New World species: marmosets and tamarins. In: Wolfe-Coote, S. (Ed.), The Laboratory Primate. Elsevier, New York, pp. 145–162.

Reynolds, M.G., Davidson, W.B., Curns, A.T., Conover, C.S., Huhn, G., Davis, J.P., et al., 2007. Spectrum of infection and risk factors for human monkeypox, United States, 2003. Emerg. Infect. Dis. 13, 1332–1339.

Rhesus Macaque Genome Sequencing and Analysis Consortium, Gibbs, R.A., Rogers, J., Katze, M.G., Bumgarner, R., Weinstock, G.M., Mardis, E.R., et al., 2007. Evolutionary and biomedical insights from the Rhesus Macaque genome. Science 316, 222–234.

Rice, K.A., Chen, E.S., Metcalf Pate, K.A., Hutchinson, E.K., Adams, R.J., 2013. Diagnosis of amyloidosis and differentiation from chronic, idiopathic enterocolitis in rhesus (*Macaca mulatta*) and pig-tailed (*M. nemestrina*) macaques. Comp. Med. 63, 262–271.

Richardson, J.H., Humphrey, G.L., 1971. Rabies in imported nonhuman primates. Lab. Anim. Sci. 21, 1082–1803.

Richter, C.B., Humason, G.L., Godbold Jr., J.H., 1978. Endemic *Pneumocystis carinii* in a marmoset colony. J. Comp. Pathol. 88, 221–223.

Richter, C.B., Lehner, N.D.M., Henrickson, R.V., 1984. Primates. In: Fox, J.G., Cohen, B.J., Loew, F.M. (Eds.), Laboratory Animal Medicine. Academic Press, San Diego, CA, pp. 298–393.

Richter, C., Mevis, L., Malaivijitnond, S., Schülke, O., Ostner, J., 2009. Social relationships in free-ranging male *Macaca arctoides*. Int. J. Primatol. 30, 625–642.

Riddle, K.E., Keeling, M.E., Alford, P.L., Beck, T.F., 1982. Chimpanzee holding, rehabilitation, and breeding: facilities design and colony management. Lab. Anim. Sci. 32, 525–533.

Rigau-Perez, J.G., Clark, G.G., Gabler, D.J., Reiter, P., Sanders, E.J., Vorndam, A.V., 1998. Dengue and dengue hemorrhagic fever. Lancet 352, 971–977.

Riordan, J.T., 1949. Rectal tuberculosis in monkeys from the use of contaminated thermometers. J. Infect. Dis. 73, 93–94.

Roberts, J.A., Lerche, N.W., Markovits, J.E., Maul, D.H., 1988. Epizootic measles at the CRPRC. Lab. Anim. Sci. 38, 492.

Robertson, B.H., D'Hondt, E.H., Spelbring, J., Tian, H., Krawczynski, K., Margolis, H.S., 1994. Effect of postexposure vaccination in a chimpanzee model of hepatitis A virus infection. J. Med. Virol. 43, 249–251.

Robinson, N.G., 2007. Veterinary acupuncture: an ancient tradition for modern times. Altern. Complement. Ther. 13, 259–265.

Robinson, N.G., 2009. Making sense of the metaphor: how acupuncture works neurophysiologically. J. Equine Vet. Sci. 29, 642–644.

Robinson, N.G., 2013. Veterinary medical acupuncturists point to science. Vet. Pract. News Posted March 27, 2013. Available at: <http://www.veterinarypracticenews.com/vet-practice-news-columns/complementary-medicine/veterinary-medical-acupuncturists-point-to-science.aspx> .

Rockwood, G.A., Duniho, S.M., Briscoe, C.M., Gold, M.B., Armstrong, K.R., Moran, A.V., et al., 2008. Toxicity in rhesus monkeys following administration of the 8-Aminoquinoline 8-[(4-amino-1-methylbutyl)amino]-5-(1-hexyloxy)-6-methoxy-4-methylquinolone (WR242511). J. Med. Toxicol. 4, 157–166.

Rogers, J., Gibbs, R.A., 2014. Comparative primate genomics: emerging patterns of genome content and dynamics. Nat. Rev. Genet. 15, 347–359.

Rogers, J., Hixson, J.E., 1997. Baboons as an animal model for genetic studies of common human disease. Am. J. Hum. Genet. 61, 489–493.

Rollin, P.E., Williams, R.J., Bressler, D.S., Pearson, S., Cottingham, M., Pucak, G., et al., 1999. Ebola (subtype Reston) virus among quarantined nonhuman primates recently imported from the Philippines to the United States. J. Infect. Dis. 179 (S1), S108–S144.

Rommeck, I., Anderson, K., Heagerty, A., Cameron, A., McCowan, B., 2009. Risk factors and remediation of self-injurious and self-abusive behavior in rhesus macaques. J. Appl. An. Welfare Sci. 12, 61–72.

Rook, G.A., Taverne, J., Leveton, C., Steele, J., 1987. The role of γ-interferon, vitamin D3 metabolites and tumour necrosis factor in the pathogenesis of tuberculosis. Immunology 62, 229.

Rosenberg, D.P., 1995. Critical care. In: Bennett, B.T., Abee, C.R., Henrickson, R.V. (Eds.), Nonhuman Primates in Biomedical Research: Biology and Management. Academic Press, San Diego, CA, pp. 316–334.

Rosenberg, D.P., Blouin, P., 1979. Retrobulbar abscess in an infant rhesus monkey. J. Am. Vet. Med. Assoc. 175, 994–996.

Rosenberg, D.P., Lerche, N.W., Henrickson, R.V., 1980. *Yersinia pseudotuberculosis* infection in a group of *Macaca fascicularis*. J. Am. Vet. Med. Assoc. 177, 818–819.

Rosenberg, D.P., Gleiser, C.A., Carey, K.D., 1984. Spinal coccidioidomycosis in a baboon. J. Am. Vet. Med. Assoc. 185, 1379–1381.

Rothschild, B.M., Woods, R.J., 1992. Osteoarthritis, calcium pyrophosphate deposition disease, and osseous infection in old world primates. Am. J. Phys. Anthropol. 87, 341–347.

Rothuizen, J., Twedt, D.C., 2009. Liver biopsy techniques. Vet. Clin. Small Anim. 39, 469–480.

Rotundo, M., Fernandez-Duque, E., Dixson, A.F., 2005. Infant development and parental care in free-ranging *Aotus azarai azarai* in Argentina. Internation J. Primatol. 26, 1459–1473.

Roussilhon, C., Postal, J.M., Ravisse, P., 1987. Spontaneous cryptococcosis of a squirrel monkey (*Saimiri sciureus*) in French Guyana. J. Med. Primatol. 16, 39–47.

Rout, W.R., Formal, S.B., Dammin, G.J., Giannella, R.A., 1974. Pathophysiology of Salmonella diarrhea in the Rhesus monkey: intestinal transport, morphological and bacteriological studies. Gastroenterology 67 (1), 59–70.

Rowe, N., 1996. The Pictorial Guide to the Living Primates. Pogonias Press, New York.

Rowell, T.E., 1971. Organization of caged groups of cercopithecus monkeys. Anim. Behav. 19, 625–645.

Rowlett, J.K., Platt, D.M., Lelas, S., Atack, J.R., Dawson, G.R., 2005. Different GABAA receptor subtypes mediate the anxiolytic, abuse-related, and motor effects of benzodiazepine-like drugs in primates. Proc. Natl. Acad. Sci. USA 102, 915–920.

Rubin, S.I., 2013. Rectal Prolapse. In: The Merck Veterinary Manual, Available at: <http://www.merckmanuals.com/vet/digestive_system/diseases_of_the_rectum_and_anus/rectal_prolapse.html>.

Russell, R.G., DeTolla, L.J., 1993. Shigellosis. In: Jones, T.C. Mohr, U. Hunt, R.D. (Eds.), Nonhuman Primates, vol. 1. Springer-Verlag, Berlin, Germany, pp. 46–53.

Russell, R.G., Rosenkranz, S.L., Lee, L.A., Howard, H., DiGiacomo, R.F., Bronsdon, M.A., et al., 1987. Epidemiology and etiology of diarrhea in colony-born *Macaca nemestrina*. Lab. Anim. Sci. 37, 309–316.

Russell, R.G., Krugner, L., Tsai, C.-C., Ekstrom, R., 1988. Prevalence of *Campylobacter* in infant, juvenile, and adult laboratory primates. Lab. Anim. Sci. 38, 711–714.

Ryan, K.J., Benirschke, K., Smith, O.W., 1961. Conversion of androstenedione-4-^{14}C to estrone by the marmoset placenta. Endocrinology 69, 613–618.

Rychel, J.K., Johnston, M.S., Robinson, N.G., 2011. Zoologic companion animal rehabilitation and physical medicine. Vet. Clin. Exot. Anim. 14, 131–140.

Rylands, A.B., Mittermeier, R.A., 2009. The diversity of the new world primates (Platyrrhini): an annotated taxonomy. In: Garber, P.A., Estrada, A., Bicca-Marques, J.C., Heymann, E.W., Strier, K.B. (Eds.), South American Primates: Comparative Perspectives in the Study of Behavior, Ecology, and Conservation. Springer, New York, pp. 23–54.

Sabin, A.B., Wright, A.M., 1934. Acute ascending myelitis following a monkey bite, with the isolation of a virus capable of reproducing the disease. J. Exp. Med. 59 (2), 115–136. http://dx.doi.org/10.1084/jem.59.2.115.

Sakai, K., Nagata, N., Ami, Y., Seki, F., Suzaki, Y., Iwata-Yoshikawa, N., et al., 2013. Lethal canine distemper virus outbreak in cynomolgus monkeys in Japan in 2008. J. Virol. 87, 1105–1114. http://dx.doi.org/10.1128/JVI.02419-12.

Sakakibara, I., Sugimoto, Y., Takasaka, M., Honjo, S., 1984. Spontaneous nocardiosis with brain abscess caused by *Nocardia asteroides* in a cynomolgus monkey. J. Med. Primatol. 13, 89–95.

Saltzman, W., Tardif, S.D., Rutherford, J.N., 2011. Hormones and reproductive cyles in primates. In: Norris, D.O. Lopeze, K.H. (Eds.), Hormones and Reproduction of Vertebrates, vol. 5. Elsevier, London, pp. 291–328.

Santillán-Doherty, A.M., Cortés-Sotres, J., Arenas-Rosas, R.V., Márquez-Arias, A., Cruz, C., Medellín, A., et al., 2010. Novelty-seeking temperament in captive stumptail macaques (*Macaca arctoides*) and spider monkeys (*Ateles geoffroyi*). J. Comp. Psychol. 124, 211–218.

Sapolsky, R.M., 1996. Why should an aged male baboon ever transfer troops? Am. J. Primtol. 39, 149–155.

Sardana, N., Wallace, D., Agrawal, R., Aoun, E., 2014. Where's the ulcer? Spontaneous bleeding from Zenker's diverticulum. BMJ Case Rep. pii: bcr2014204677. doi:10.1136/bcr-2014-204677.

Sato, A., Fairbanks, L.A., Lawson, P.T., Lawson, G.W., 2005. Effects of age and sex on hematologic and serum biochemical values of vervet monkeys (*Chlorocebus aethiops sabaeus*). Contemp. Top. 44, 29–34.

Sato, J., Doi, T., Kanno, T., Wako, Y., Tsuchitani, M., Narama, I., 2012. Histopathology of incidental findings in cynomolgus monkeys (*Macaca fascicularis*) used in toxicity studies. J. Toxicol. Pathol. 25, 63–101. http://dx.doi.org/10.1293/tox.25.63.

Sauceda, R., Schmidt, M.G., 2000. Refining macaque handling and restraint techniques. Lab. Anim. 29, 47–49.

Saunders, J., Ohlerth, S., 2011. CT Physics and Instrumentation – Mechanical Design. In: Schwarz, T., Saunders, J. (Eds.), Veterinary Computed Tomography. Wiley-Blackwell, Chichester, pp. 1–8.

Saunders, K.E., Shen, Z., Dewhirst, F.E., Paster, B.J., Dangler, C.A., Fox, J.G., 1999. Novel intestinal *Helicobacter* species isolated from cotton-top tamarins (*Saguinus oedipus*) with chronic colitis. J. Clin. Microbiol. 37, 146–151.

Savage, A., Giraldo, L.H., Soto, L.H., Snowden, C.T., 1996. Demography, group composition, and dispersal in wild cotton-top tamarin (*Saguinus oedipus*) groups. Am. J. Primatol. 38, 85–100.

Savage, A., Shideler, S.E., Soto, L.H., Causado, J., Humberto Giraldo, L., Lasley, B.L., et al., 1997. Reproductive events of wild cotton-top tamarins (*Saguinus oedipus*) in Colombia. Am. J. Primatol. 43, 329–337.

Scammell, J.G., 2000. Steroid resistance in the squirrel monkey: an old subject revisited. ILAR J. 41, 19–25.

Scanlon, C.E., Chalmers, N.R., Monteiro da Cruz, M.A.O., 1988. Changes in the size, composition, and reproductive condition of wild marmoset groups (Callithrix jacchus jacchus) in North East Brazil. Primates 29, 295–305.

Schapiro, S.J., 2000. A few new developments in primate housing and husbandry. Scand. J. Lab. Anim. Sci. 27, 103–110.

Schapiro, S.J., 2008. Primates as models of behavior in biomedical research. In: Conn, P.M. (Ed.), Sourcebook of Models for Biomedical Research. Humana Press, New Jersey, pp. 259–262.

Schapiro, S.J., Bloomsmith, M.A., Suarez, S.A., Porter, L.M., 1996. Effects of social and inanimate enrichment of the behavior of yearling rhesus monkeys. Am. J. Primatol. 40, 247–260.

Schapiro, S.J., Perlman, J.E., Thiele, E., Lambeth, S., 2005. Training nonhuman primates to perform behaviors useful in biomedical research. Lab. Anim. 34, 37–42.

Schapiro, S.J., Lambeth, S.P., 2007. Control, choice, and assessments of the value of behavioral management to nonhuman primates in captivity. J. Appl. Anim. Welfare Sci. 10, 39–47.

Schätzl, H.M., Da Costa, M., Taylor, L., Cohen, F.E., Prusiner, S.B., 1997. Prion protein gene variation among primates. J. Mol. Biol. 265, 257.

Schiavetta, A.M., Harre, J.G., Wagner, E., Simmons, M., Raviprakash, K., 2003. Variable susceptibility of the owl monkey (Aotus nancymae) to four serotypes of dengue virus. Contemp. Top. Lab. Anim. Sci. 42, 12–20.

Schillaci, M.A., Lishchka, A.R., Karamitsos, A.A., Engel, G.A., Paul, N., et al., 2010. Radiographic measurement of the cardiothoracic ratio in a feral population of long-tailed macaques (Macaca fascicularis). Radiography 16, 163–166.

Schlauder, G.G., Dawson, G.J., Simons, J.N., Pilot-Matias, T.J., Gutierrez, R.A., Heynen, C.A., et al., 1995. Molecular and serologic analysis in the transmission of the GB hepatitis agents. J. Med. Virol. 46, 81–90.

Schmidt, L.H., 1978. Plasmodium falciparum and Plasmodium vivax infections in the owl monkey (Aotus trivirgatus). I. The courses of untreated infections. II. Responses to chloroquine, quinine and pyrimethamine. III. Methods employed in the search for new schizonticidal drugs. Am. J. Trop. Med. Hyg. 26, 671–737.

Schmidt, R.E., Butler, T.M., 1971. Klebsiella-Enterobacter infections in chimpanzees. Lab. Anim. Sci. 21, 946–949.

Schmidtko, J., Wang, R., Wu, C.L., Mauiyyedi, S., Harris, N.L., Della Pelle, P., et al., 2002. Posttransplant lymphoproliferative disorder associated with an Epstein-Barr-related virus in cynomolgus monkeys. Transplantation 73, 1431–1439.

Schoeb, T.R., Eberle, R., Black, D.H., Parker, R.F., Cartner, S.C., 2008. Diagnostic exercise: papulovesicular dermatitis in rhesus macaques (Macaca mulatta). Vet. Path. 45, 592–594.

Schroder, J.N., Daneshmand, M.A., Villamizar, N.R., Petersen, R.P., Blue, L.J., Welsby, I.J., et al., 2006. Heparin-induced thrombocytopenia in left ventricular assist device bridge-to-transplant patients. Ann. Thorac. Surg. 84, 841–845.

Schroder, M.A., Fisk, S.K., Lerche, N.W., 2000. Eradication of simian retrovirus type D from a colony of cynomolgus, rhesus, and stump-tailed macaques by using serial testing and removal. Contemp. Top. Lab. Anim. Sci. 39, 16–23.

Schug, S.A., 2007. The role of tramadol in current treatment strategies for musculoskeletal pain. Ther. Clin. Risk Manage. 3, 717–723.

Schuler, A.M., Brady, A.G., Tustin, G.W., Parks, V.L., Morris, C.G., Abee, C.R., 2010. Measurement of fetal biparietal diameter in owl monkeys (Aotus nancymaae). JAALAS 49, 560–563.

Scimeca, J.M., Brady, A.G., 1990. Neonatal mortality in the captive breeding squirrel monkey colony associated with an invasive Escherichia coli. Lab. Anim. Sci. 40, 546–547.

Scott, L.M., 1984. Reproductive behavior of adolescent female baboons (Papio anubis) in Kenya. In: Small, M.F. (Ed.), Female Primates: Studies by Female Primatologists. Alan R. Liss, New York.

Sedgwick, C., Parcher, J., Durham, R., 1970. Atypical mycobacterial infection in the pig-tailed macaque (Macaca nemestrina). J. Am. Vet. Med. Assoc. 157, 724–725.

Segal, E.F., 1989. Housing, Care, and Psychological Well-Being of Captive and Laboratory Primates. Noyes Publications, Park Ridge New Jersey.

Sehgal, P.K., Bronson, R.T., Brady, P.S., McIntyre, K.W., Elliot, M.W., 1980. Therapeutic efficacy of vitamin E and selenium in treating hemolytic anemia of owl monkeys (Aotus trivirgatus). Lab. Anim. Sci. 30, 92–98.

Seibold, H.R., Perrin Jr., E.A., Garner, A.C., 1970. Pneumonia associated with Bordetella bronchiseptica in Callicebus species primates. Lab. Anim. Care 20, 456–461.

Seier, J., 2005. Vervet monkey breeding. In: Wolfe-Coote, The Laboratory Primate. Academic Press Elsevier,, San Diego, CA, pp. 175–179.

Seier, J.V., 1986. Breeding vervet monkeys in a closed environment. J. Med. Primatol. 15, 339–349.

Seier, J.V., van der Horst, G., de Kock, M., Chwalisz, K., 2000. The detection and monitoring of early pregnancy in the vervet monkey (Cercopithecus aethiops) with the use of ultrasound and correlation with reproductive steroid hormones. J. Med. Primatol. 29, 70–75.

Seltzer, J.D., 2007. Skin biopsies in mammals. Lab. Anim. 36, 23–24.

Sesline, D.H., 1978. Mycobacterium avium enteritis in nonhuman primates. In: Montali, R.J. (Ed.), Mycobacterial Infections in Zoo Animals. Smithsonian Institution Press, Washington, DC, pp. 157–159.

Seth, P.K., Seth, S., 1993. Structure, function, and diversity of Indian rhesus monkeys, In: New Perspectives in Anthropology. MD Publications, Pvt. Ltd., New Delhi, India, pp. 47-82.

Sethabutr, O., Echeverria, P., Hoge, C.W., Bodhidatta, L., Pitarangsi, C., 1994. Detection of Shigella and enteroinvasive Escherichia coli by PCR in the stools of patients with dysentery in Thailand. J. Diarrhoeal Dis. Res. 12, 265–269.

Seyfarth, R.M., Cheney, D.L., Marler, P., 1980. Vervet monkey alarm calls: semantic communication in a free-ranging primate. Anim. Behav. 28, 1070–1094.

Shaikh, A.A., Allen-Rowlands, C., Dozier, T., Kraemer, D.C., 1976. Diagnosis of early pregnancy in the baboon. Contraception 14, 391–402.

Shaikh, A.A., Celaya, C.L., Gomez, I., Shaikh, S.A., 1982. Temporal relationship of hormonal peaks to ovulation and skin deturgescence in the baboon. Primates 23, 444–452.

Sharma, A.K., Bury, M.I., Marks, A.J., Fuller, N.J., Meisner, J.W., Tapaskar, N., et al., 2011. A nonhuman primate model for urinary bladder regeneration using autologous sources of bone marrow-derived mesenchymal stem cells. Stem Cells 29, 241–250.

Shearer, M.H., Dark, R.D., Chodosh, J., Kennedy, R.C., 1999. Comparison and characterization of Immunoglobulin G subclasses among primate species. Clin. Diag. Lab. Immunol. 6, 953–958.

Sherding, R., 1994. Anorectal diseases. In: Birchard, S.J., Sherding, R.C. (Eds.), Saunders Manual of Small Animal Practice. Saunders, Philadelphia, PA, pp. 777–786.

Shi, Q., Hornsby, P.J., Meng, Q., Vandeberg, J.F., Vandeberg, J.L., 2013. Longitudinal analysis of short-term high-fat diet on endothelial senescence in baboons. Am. J. Cardiovasc. Dis. 3, 107–119.

Shukan, E.T., Boe, C.Y., Hasenfus, A.V., Pieper, B.A., Snowdon, C.T., 2012. Normal hematologic and serum biochemical values of cotton-top tamarins (Saguinus oedipus). JAALAS 51, 150–154.

Siedlecki, C.T., 2010. Lymph node aspiration and biopsy, Ch. 102. In: Ettinger, S.J., Feldman, E.C. (Eds.), Textbook of Veterinary Internal Medicine, seventh ed. Elsevier, St. Louis, MO.

Sigg, H., Stolba, A., Abegglen, J.J., Dasser, V., 1982. Life history of hamadryas baboons: physical development, infant mortality, reproductive parameters, and family relationships. Primates 23, 473–487.

Silveira, L.C., Saito, C.A., Lee, B.B., Kremers, J., da Silva Filho, M., Kilavik, B.E., et al., 2004. Morphology and physiology of primate M- and P-cells. Prog. Brain Res. 144, 21–46.

Silverman, S., Morgan, J.P., 1980. Thoracic radiography of the normal rhesus macaque (Macaca mulatta). Am. J. Vet. Res. 41, 1704–1719.

Simmons, J.H., 2008. Development, application, and quality control of serology assays used for diagnostic monitoring of laboratory nonhuman primates. ILAR J. 49, 157–169.

Simon, M.A., Daniel, M.D., Lee-Parritz, D., King, N.W., Ringler, D.J., 1993. Disseminated B virus infection in a cynomolgus monkey. Lab. Anim. Sci. 43, 545–550.

Skavlen, P.A., Stills Jr., H.F., Steffan, E.K., Middleton, C.C., 1985. Naturally occurring Yersinia enterocolitica septicemia in patas monkeys (Erythrocebus patas). Lab. Anim. Sci. 35, 488–490.

Skinner, J.D., Smithers, R.H.N., 1990. The mammals of the southern African subregion, second ed. University of Pretoria, Pretoria, South Africa, 771 pp.

Sly, D.L., London, W.T., Palmer, A.E., Rice, J.M., 1977. Disseminated cryptococcosis in a patas monkey (Erythrocebus patas). Lab. Anim. Sci. 27, 694–699.

Smith, D.G., McDonough, J., 2005. Mitochondrial DNA variation in Chinese and Indian rhesus macaques (Macaca mulatta). Am. J. Primatol. 65, 1–25.

Smith, M.O., Lackner, A.A., 1993. Effects of sex, age, puncture site, and blood contamination on the clinical chemistry of cerebrospinal fluid in rhesus macaques (Macaca mulatta). Am. J. Vet. Res. 54, 1845–1850.

Smith, P.C., Yuill, T.M., Buchanan, R.D., Stanton, J.S., Chiacumpa, V., 1969. The gibbon (Hylobates lar); a new primate host for Herpesvirus hominia. I. A natural epizootic in a laboratory colony. J. Infec. Dis. 120, 292–297.

Smuts, B.B., Watanabe, J.M., 1990. Social relationships and ritualized greetings in adult male baboons (Papio cynocephalus anubis). Int. J. Primatol. 11, 147–172.

Smuts, B.B., Gubernick, D.J., 1992. Male-infant relationships in nonhuman primates: paternal investment or mating effort?. In: Hewlett, B.S. (Ed.), Father-Child Relations. Cultural and Biosocial Contexts. Aldine de Cruyter, New York, pp. 1–30.

Snowdon, C.T., Savage, A., McConnell, P.B., 1985. A breeding colony of cotton-top tamarins (Saguinus oedipus). Lab. Anim. Sci. 35, 477–480.

Snyder, S.B., Lund, J.E., Bone, J., Soave, O.A., Hirsch, D.C., 1970. A study of Klebsiella infection in owl monkeys (Aotus trivirgatus). J. Am. Vet. Med. Assoc. 157, 1935–1939.

Snyder, S.B., Omdahl, J.L., Law, D.H., Froelich, J.W., 1980. Osteomalacia and nutritional secondary hyperparathyroidism in a semi-free-ranging troop of Japanese monkeys. In: Montali, R.J., Migaki, G. (Eds.), The Comparative Pathology of Zoo Animals. Smithsonian Institution Press, Washington, DC, pp. 51–57.

Soave, O., 1978. Observations on acute gastric dilatation in nonhuman primates. Lab. Anim. Sci. 28, 331–334.

Soave, O., Jackson, S., Ghumman, J.S., 1981. Atypical mycobacteria as the probable cause of positive tuberculin reactions in squirrel monkeys (Saimiri sciureus). Lab. Anim. Sci. 31, 295–296.

Soike, K.F., Rangan, S.R.S., Gerone, P.J., 1984. Viral disease models in primates. Adv. Vet. Sci. Comp. Med. 28, 151–199.

Solleveld, H.A., van Zweiten, M.J., Heidt, P.J., van Eerd, P.M.C.A., 1984. Clinicopathologic study of six cases of meningitis and meningoencephalitis in chimpanzees (Pan troglodytes). Lab. Anim. Sci. 34, 86–90.

Soto, E., Griffin, M., Verma, A., Castillo-Alcala, F., Beierschmitt, A., Beeler-Marfisi, J., et al., 2013. An Outbreak of Yersinia enterocolitica

in a Captive Colony of African Green Monkeys (Chlorocebus aethiops sabaeus) in the Caribbean. Comp. Med. 63, 439–444.

Southers, J.L., Ford, E.W., 1995. Environmental controls. In: Bennett, B.T., Abee, C.R., Henrickson, R.V. (Eds.), Nonhuman Primates in Biomedical Research: Biology and Management. Academic Press, San Diego, CA, pp. 262–263.

Southwick, C.H., Lindburg, D.G., 1986. The primates of India: status, trends, and conservation. In: Benirschke, K. (Ed.), Primates: The Road to Self-Sustaining Populations. Springer-Verlag, New York, pp. 171–187.

Staley, E.C., Southers, J.L., Thoen, C.O., Easley, S.P., 1995. Evaluation of tuberculin testing and and measles prophylaxis procedures used in rhesus macaque quarantine/conditioning protocols. Lab. Anim. Sci. 45, 125–130.

Stanley, D.A., Honko, A.N., Aseidu, C., Trefry, J.C., Lau-Kilby, A.W., Johnson, J.C., et al., 2014. Chimpanzee adenovirus vaccine generates acute and durable protective immunity against ebolavirus challenge. Nat. Med. Available online 7 September 2014. http://dx.doi.org/10.1038/nm.3702.

Steele, M.D., Giddens Jr., W.E., Valerio, M., Sumi, S.M., Stetzer, E.R., 1982. Spontaneous paramyxoviral encephalitis in nonhuman primates (Macaca mulatta and M. nemestrina). Vet. Pathol. 19, 132–139.

Stein, F.J., Lewis, D.H., Stott, G.G., Sis, R.F., 1981. Acute gastric dilatation in common marmosets (Callithrix jacchus). Lab. Anim. Sci. 31, 522–523.

Stelian, J., Gil, I., Habot, B., Rosenthal, M., Abramovici, I., Kutok, N., et al., 1992. Improvement of pain and disability in elderly patients with degenerative osteoarthritis of the knee treated with narrowband light therapy. J. Am. Geriatr. Soc. 40, 23–26.

Stevenson, M.F., 1977. The behavior and ecology of the common marmoset (Callithrix jacchus jacchus) in its natural environment. Primate Eye 9, 5–6.

Stevenson, M.F., Poole, T.B., 1976. An ethogram of the common marmoset (Callithrix jacchus): general behavioural repertoire. Anim. Behav. 24, 428–451.

Stewart, F.A., Piel, A.K., 2014. Termite fishing by wild chimpanzees: new data from Ugalla, western Tanzania. Primates 55, 35–40.

Stokes, W.S., Donovan, J.C., Montrey, R.D., Thompson, W.L., Wannemacher, R.W. Jr., Rozmiarek, H., 1983. Acute clinical malaria (Plasmodium inui) in a cynomolgus monkey (Macaca fascicularis). Lab. Anim. Sci. 33, 81–85.

Stoller, M.K., 1995. The obstetric pelvis and mechanism of labor in nonhuman primates. Am. J. Phys. Anthropol. 101, 557–567.

Stolz, L.P., Saayman, G.S., 1970. Ecology and behavior of baboons in the northern Transvaal. Ann. Transvaal Mus. 26, 99–143.

Stone, G.A., Johnson, B.K., Druilhet, R., Garza, P.B., Gibbs Jr., C.J., 2000. Immunophenotyping of peripheral blood, ranges of serum chemistries and clinical hematology values of healthy chimpanzees (Pan troglodytes). J. Med. Primatol. 29, 324–329.

Stonerook, M.J., Weiss, H.S., Rodriguez, M.A., Rodriguez, J.V., Hernandez, J.I., Peck, O.C., et al., 1994. Temperature-metabolism relations in the cotton-top tamarin (Saguinus oedipus) model for ulcerative colitis. J. Med. Primatol. 23, 16–22.

Strickler, H.D., Rosenberg, P.S., Devesa, S.S., Hertel, J., Fraumeni Jr., J.F., Goedert, J.J., 1998. Contamination of poliovirus vaccines with simian virus 40 (1955-1963) and subsequent cancer rates. JAMA 279, 292–295.

Stromberg, K., Benveniste, R.E., Arthur, L.O., Rabin, H., Giddens Jr., W.E., Ochs, H.D., et al., 1984. Characterization of exogenous type D retrovirus from a fibroma of a macaque with simian AIDS and fibromatosis. Science 224, 289–292.

Struhsaker, T.T., 1967. Social structure among vervet monkeys (Cercopithecus aethiops). Behaviour 29, 83–121.

Strum, S.C., 1975. Life with the pumphouse gang: new insights into baboon behavior. Nat. Geog. 147, 672–691.

Subhawong, T.K., Fishman, E.K., Swart, J.E., Carrino, J.A., Attar, S., Fayad, L.M., 2010. Soft-tissue masses and masslike conditions: what does CT add to diagnosis and management? Am. J. Roentgenol. 194, 1559–1567.

Sun, Z., Li, A., Ye, H., Shi, Y., Hu, Z., Zeng, L., 2010. Natural infection with canine distemper virus in hand-feeding rhesus monkeys in China. Vet. Microbiol. 141 (3–4), 374–378. http://dx.doi.org/10.1016/j.vetmic.2009.09.024.

Sunderland, N., Heffernan, S., Thomson, S., Hennessey, A., 2008. Maternal parity affects neonatal survival rate in a colony of captive bred baboons (Papio hamadryas). J. Med. Primatol. 37, 223–228.

Suresh, P.S., Jayachandra, K.C., Medhamurthy, R., 2011. The effect of progesterone replacement on gene expression in the corpus luteum during induced regression and late luteal phase in the bonnet monkey (Macaca radiata). Reprod. Biol. Endocrinol. 3, 9–20.

Sussman, R.W., 2000. Primate Ecology and Social Structure. Volume 2, New World Monkeys. Pearson Custom, Needham Heights, MA, 207 pp.

Sutherland, S.D., Almeida, J.D., Gardner, P.S., Skarper, M., Stabton, J., 1986. Rapid diagnosis and management of parainfluenza 1 virus infection in common marmosets (Callithrix jacchus). Lab. Anim. 20, 121–126.

Suzuki, T., Suzuki, N., Shimoda, K., Nagasawa, H., 1996. Hematological and serum biochemical values in pregnant and postpartum femailes of the squirrel monkey (Saimiri sciureus). Exp. Anim. 45, 39–43.

Suzuki, N., Yuyama, M., Maeda, S., Ogawa, H., Mashiko, K., Kiyoura, Y., 2006. Genotypic identification of presumptive Streptococcus pneumoniae by PCR using four genes highly specific for S. pneumoniae. J. Med. Microbiol. 55 (Pt 6), 709–714.

Swack, N.S., Hsuing, G.D., 1982. Natural and experimental simian cytomegalovirus infections at a primate center. J. Med. Primatol. 11, 169–177.

Swenson, B., Strobert, E., Orkin, J., 1979. AALAS Workshop on Nonhuman Primate Parasitology. Emory University, Atlanta.

Swenson Jr., Loyd S., Grimwood, J.M., Alexander, C.C., 1966. This New Ocean: A History of Project Mercury. NASA History Series. National Aeronautics and Space Administration. OCLC 00569889. Retrieved 2014-04-07.

Swindle, M.M., Kan, J.S., Adams, R.J., Starr, F.L. 3rd, Samphilipo, M.A. Jr., Porter, W.P., 1986. Ventricular septal defect in a rhesus monkey. Lab. Anim. Sci. 36, 693–695.

Switzer, W.M., Bhullar, V., Shanmugam, V., Cong, M.E., Parekh, B., Lerche, N.W., et al., 2004. Frequent simian foamy virus infection in persons occupationally exposed to nonhuman primates. J. Virol. 78, 2780–2789.

Tabor, E., 1989. Nonhuman primate models for non-A, non-B hepatitis. Cancer Detect. Prev. 14, 221–225.

Takasaka, M., Kohno, A., Sakakibara, I., Narita, H., Honjo, S., 1988. An outbreak of salmonellosis in newly imported cynomolgus monkeys. Jpn. J. Med. Sci. Biol. 41, 1–13.

Tams, T.R., Rawlings, C.A., 2011. Small Animal Endoscopy, third ed. Elsevier, St. Louis, MO.

Tanaka, Y., Katsube, Y., 1981. Salmonella carriers in the imported cynomolgus monkeys (Macaca fascicularis). Nihon Juigaku Zasshi 43, 787–789.

Tardif, S.D., 1994. Relative energetic cost of infant care in small-bodied neotropical primates and its relation to infant-care patterns. Am. J. Primatol. 34, 133–143.

Tardif, S.D., 1997. The bioenergetics of parental behavior and the evolution of alloparental care in marmosets and tamarins. In: Solomon, N.G., French, J.A. (Eds.), Cooperative Breeding in Mammals. Cambridge University Press, New York, pp. 11–33.

Tardif, S.D., Bales, K., 2004. Relations among birth condition, maternal condition, and postnatal growth in captive common marmoset monkeys (Callithrix jacchus). Am. J. Primatol. 62, 83–94.

Tardif, S.D., Richter, C.B., 1981. Competition for a desired food in family groups of the common marmoset (Callithrix jacchus) and the cotton-top tamarin (Saguinus oedipus). Lab. Anim. Sci. 31, 52–55.

Tardif, S.D., Richter, C.B., Carson, R.L., 1984. Reproductive performance of three species of Callitrichidae. Lab. Anim. Sci. 34, 272–275.

Tardif, S.D., Smucny, D.A., Abbott, D.H., Mansfield, K., Shultz-Darken, N., Yamamoto, M.E., 2003. Reproduction in captive common marmosets (Callithrix jacchus). Comp. Med. 53, 364–368.

Tardif, S.D., Bales, K., Williams, L., Moeller, E.L., Abbott, D., Schultz-Darken, N., et al., 2006. Preparing new world monkeys for laboratory research. ILAR 47, 307–315.

Tardif, S.D., Mansfield, K.G., Ratnam, R., Ross, C.N., Ziegler, T.E., 2011a. The marmoset as a model of aging and age-related diseases. ILAR 52, 54–65.

Tardif, S.D., Abee, C.R., Mansfield, K.G., 2011b. Workshop summary: neotropical primates in biomedical research. ILAR 52, 386–392.

Tardif, S.D., Carville, A., Elmore, D., Williams, L.E., Rice, K., 2012. Reproduction and breeding of nonhuman primates. In: Abee, C.R. Mansfield, K. Tardif, S.D. Morris, T. (Eds.), Nonhuman Primates in Biomedical Research: Biology and Management, vol. 1. Academic Press, San Diego, CA, pp. 197–249.

Tasaki, M., Shimizu, A., Hanekamp, I., Torabi, R., Villani, V., Yamada, K., 2014. Rituximab treatment prevents the early development of proteinuria following pig-to-baboon xeno-kidney transplantation. J. Am. Soc. Nephrol. 25(4), 737–744. [Epub ahead of print].

Taylor, D.K., Bass, T., Flory, G.S., Hankenson, C.F., 2005. Use of low-dose chlorpromazine in conjuction with environmental enrichment to eliminate self-injurious behavior in a rhesus macaque (Macaca mulatta). Comp. Med. 55, 282–288.

Taylor, N.S., EUenberger, M.A., Wu, P.Y., Fox, J.G., 1989. Diversity of serotypes of Campylobacter jejuni and Campylobacter coli isolated in laboratory animals. Lab. Anim. Sci. 39, 219–221.

Taylor, W.M., Grady, A.W., 1998. Catheter-tract infections in rhesus macaques (Macaca mulatta) with indwelling intravenous catheters. Lab. Anim. Sci. 48, 448–454.

Terborgh, J., 1983. Five New World Primates. Princeton University Press, Princeton, NJ.

Terrace, H., Petitto, L.A., Sanders, R.J., Bever, T.G., 1979. Can an ape create a sentence. Science 206, 891–902.

Thoerner, P., Bin Kingombe, C.I., Bogli-Stuber, K., Bissig-Choisat, B., Wassenaar, T.M., Frey, J., et al., 2003. PCR detection of virulence genes in Yersinia enterocolitica and Yersinia pseudotuberculosis and investigation of virulence gene distribution. Appl. Environ. Microbiol. 69, 1810–1816.

Thompson, J.S., 2002. Contrast radiography and intestinal obstruction. Ann. Surg. 236, 7–8.

Thomson, J.A., Scheffler, J.J., 1996. Hemorrhagic typhlocolitis associated with attaching and effacing Escherichia coli in common marmosets. Lab. Anim. Sci. 46, 275–279.

Thorel, M.F., 1980. Isolation of Mycobacterium africanum from monkeys. Tubercle 61, 101–104.

Thorgeirsson, U.P., Dalgard, D.W., Reeves, J., Adamson, R.H., 1994. Tumor incidence in a chemical carcinogenesis study of nonhuman primates. Regul. Toxicol. Pharmacol. 18, 130–151.

Thuita, J.K., Kagira, J.M., Mwangangi, D., Matovu, E., Turner, C.M.R., Masiga, D., 2008. Trypanosoma brucei rhodesiense transmitted by a Single Tsetse Fly Bite in Vervet Monkeys as a Model of Human African Trypanosomiasis. PLoS Negl. Trop. Dis. 2, e238. http://dx.doi.org/10.1371/journal.pntd.0000238.

Thurman, J.D., Morton, R.J., Stair, E.L., 1983. Septic abortion caused by Salmonella heidelberg in a white-handed gibbon. J. Am. Vet. Med. Assoc. 183, 1325–1326.

Tiefenbacher, S., Fahey, M.A., Rowlett, J.K., Meyer, J.S., Pouliot, A.L., Jones, B.M., et al., 2005. The efficacy of diazepam treatment for the management of acute wounding episodes in captive rhesus macaques. Comp. Med. 55, 387–392.

Toft, J.D., Eberhard, M.L., 1998. Parasitic diseases. In: Bennett, B.T., Abee, C.R., Henrickson, R.V. (Eds.), Nonhuman Primates in Biomedical Research: Diseases. Academic Press, Orlando, FL, pp. 111–205.

Tornieporth, N.G., John, J., Salgado, K., de Jesus, P., Latham, E., Melo, M.C., et al., 1995. Differentiation of pathogenic Escherichia coli strains in Brazilian children by PCR. J. Clin. Microbiol. 33, 1371–1374.

Tornqvist, E., Annas, A., Granath, B., Jalkesten, E., Cotgreave, I., Oberg, M., 2014. Strategic Focus on 3R Principles Reveals Major Reductions in the Use of Animals in Pharmaceutical Toxicity Testing. PLoS One 9, e101638.

Tosi, A.J., Buzzard, P.J., Morales, J.C., Melnick, D.J., 2002. Y-chromosome data and tribal affiliations of *Allenopithecus* and *Miopithecus*. Int. J. Primatol. 23, 1287–1299.

Traina-Dorge, V., Balanchard, J., Martin, L., Murphey-Corb, M., 1992. Immunodeficiency and lymphoproliferative disease in an African green monkey dually infected with SIV and STLV-1. AIDS Res. Hum. Retroviruses 8, 97–100.

Tribe, G.W., Fleming, M.P., 1983. Biphasic enteritis in imported cyno-molgus (*Macaca fascicularis*) monkeys infected with *Shigella*, *Salmonella*, and *Campylobacter* species. Lab. Anim. 17, 65–69.

Tribe, G.W., MacKensie, P.S., Fleming, M.P., 1979. Incidence of thermo-philic *Campylobacter* species in newly imported simian primates with enteritis. Vet. Rec. 105, 333–337.

Trichel, A.M., Rajakumar, P.A., Murphey-Corb, M., 2002. Species-specific variation in SIV disease progression between Chinese and Indian subspecies of rhesus macaque. J. Med. Primatol. 31, 171–178.

Tsai, C.-C., Warner, T.F.C.S., Uno, H., Giddens Jr., W.E., Ochs, H.D., 1985. Subcutaneous fibromatosis associated with an acquired immune deficiency syndrome in pig-tailed macaques. Am. J. Pathol. 120, 30–37.

Tsai, C.-C., Follis, K.E., Snyder, K., Windsor, S., Thouless, M.E., Kuller, L., et al., 1990. Maternal transmission of type D simian retrovirus (SRV-2) in pig-tailed macaques. J. Med. Primatol. 19, 203–216.

Tucker, M.J., 1984. A survey of the pathology of marmosets (*Callithrix jacchus*). Lab. Anim. 18, 351–358.

Turner, P.V., Brabb, T., Pekow, C., Vasbinder, M.A., 2011. Administration of substances to laboratory animals: routes of administration and factors to consider. JAALAS 50, 600–613.

Twenhafel, N.A., Whitehouse, C.A., Stevens, E.L., Hottel, H.E., Foster, C.D., Gamble, S., et al., 2008. Multisystemic Abscesses in African Green Monkeys (*Chlorocebus aethiops*) with invasive *Klebsiella pneumoniae* – identification of the hypermucoviscosity phenotype. Vet. Path. 45, 226–231. http://dx.doi.org/10.1354/vp.45-2-226.

Uchida, Y., Nishigori, A., Takeda, D., Ohshiro, M., Ueda, Y., Ohshima, M., et al., 2003. Electroacupuncture induces the expression of Fos in rat dorsal horn via capsaicin-insensitive afferents. Brain Res. 978, 136–140.

Ullrey, D.E., Bernard, J.B., Peter, G.K., Lu, Z., Chen, T.C., Sikarskie, J.G., et al., 1999. Vitamin D intakes by Cotton-top tamarins (*Sanguinus oedipus*) and associated serum 25-hydroxyvitamin D concentrations. Zoo Biol. 18, 473–480.

Uno, H., 1986. The stumptailed macaque as a model for baldness: effects of minoxidil. Int. J. Cosmet. Sci. 8, 63–71.

Uno, H., Alsum, P., Zimbric, M.L., Houser, W.D., Thomson, J.A., Kemnitz, J.W., 1998. Colon cancer in aged captive rhesus monkeys (Macaca mulatta). Am. J. Primatol. 44, 19–27.

Urvater, J.A., McAdam, S.N., Loehrke, J.H., Allen, T.M., Moran, J.L., Rowell, T.J., et al., 2000. A high incidence of Shigella-induced arthritis in a primate species: major histocompatibility complex class I molecules associated with resistance and suscep-tibility, and their relationship to HLA-B27. Immunogenetics 51, 314–325.

Usborne, A.L., Bolton, I.D., 2004. Ampullary carcinoma in a group of aged rhesus macaques (*Macaca mulatta*). Comp. Med. 54, 438–442.

U.S. Department of Agriculture (USDA), 2010. Inspection Requirements Handbook, Riverdale, MD. Available at: <https://acissearch. aphis.usda.gov/LPASearch/faces/CustomerSearch.jspx>.

U.S. Department of Agriculture (USDA), 2011. Policies, Veterinary Care. Animal Care Resource Guide, Issue Date: March 25, 2011.

U.S. Department of Agriculture (USDA), 2013. Animal Welfare Act and Animal Welfare Regulations, U.S. Code Title 7, Chapter 54, Sections 2131-2159. Available at: <http://www.gpo.gov/fdsys/browse/collectionUScode.action?collectionCode=USCODE>.

U.S. Fish and Wildlife Services (UFWS), 2013. Federal Register, Vol. 78, No. 113, June 12, 2013. Available at: <http://www.fws.gov/policy/library/2013/2013-14007.pdf>.

Vaden, S.L., Levine, J.F., Lees, G.E., Groman, R.P., Grauer, G.F., Forrester, S.D., 2005. Renal biopsy: a retrospective study of meth-ods and complications in 283 dogs and 65 cats. J. Vet. Intern. Med. 19, 794–801.

Valdez, G.R., Platt, D.M., Rowlett, J.K., Rüedi-Bettschen, D., Spealman, R.D., 2007. Kappa agonist-induced reinstatement of cocaine seek-ing in squirrel monkeys: a role for opioid and stress-related mech-anisms. J. Pharmacol. Exp. Ther. 323, 525–533.

Valerio, D.A., Dalgard, D.W., Voelker, R.W., McCarrol, N.E., Good, R.C., 1979. *Mycobacterium kansasii* infection in rhesus monkeys. In: Montali, R.J. (Ed.), Mycobacterial Infections in Zoo Animals. Smithsonian Institution Press, Washington, DC, pp. 65–75.

Valverde, C.R., Canfield, D., Tarara, R., Esteves, M.I., Gormus, B.J., 1998. Spontaneous leprosy in a wild-caught cynomolgus macaque. Intl. J. Lepr. Other Mycobact. Dis. 66, 140–148.

VandeWoude, S.J., Luzarraga, M.B., 1991. The role of *Branhamella catarrhalis* in the "bloody-nose syndrome" of cynomolgus macaques. Lab. Anim. Sci. 41, 401–406.

Van Dooren, S., Salemi, M., Vandamme, A.M., 2001. Dating the origin of the African human T-cell lymphotropic virus type-i (HTLV-I) subtypes. Mol. Biol. Evol. 18, 661–671.

Van Dooren, S., Verschoor, E.J., Fagrouch, Z., Vandamme, A.-M., 2007. Phylogeny of primate T lymphotropic virus type 1 (PTLV-1) including various new Asian and African nonhuman primate strains. Infect. Genet. Evol. 7, 374–381.

van Jaarsveld, P.J., Smuts, C.M., Benadé, A., 2002. Effect of palm olein oil in a moderate-fat diet on plasma lipoprotein profile and aor-ticatherosclerosis in non-human primates. Asia Pac. J. Clin. Nutr. 11 (Suppl. 7), S424–S432.

Varki, A., Altheide, T.K., 2005. Comparing the human and chimpanzee genomes: searching for needles in haystacks. Genome Res. 15, 1746–1758.

Veeder, C.L., Bloomsmith, M.A., McMillan, J.L., Perlman, J.E., Martin, A.L., 2009. Positive reinforcement training to enhance the volun-tary movement of group-housed sooty mangabeys (Cercocebus atys atys). JAALAS 48, 192–195.

Veiga, L.M., Rylands, A.B., 2008. Aotus trivirgatus. In: IUCN 2013. IUCN Red List of Threatened Species. Version 2013.1. Available at: <www.iucnredlist.org>. Downloaded on October 15, 2013.

Veneziale, R.W., Kishnani, N.S., Nelson, J., Resendez, J.C., Frank, D.W., Cai, X.-Y., et al., 2012. Toxicity and exposure of an adenovirus con-taining human interferon alpha-2b following intracystic adminis-tration in cynomolgus monkeys. Gene Ther. 19, 742–751.

Vernot, J.-P., Perez-Quintero, L.A., Perdomo-Arciniegas, A.M., Quijano, S., Patarroyo, M.E., 2005. *Herpesvirus saimiri* immortalization of *Aotus* T lymphocytes specific for an immunogenically modified peptide of *Plasmodium falciparum* merozoite surface antigen 2. Immunol. Cell Biol. 83, 67–74.

Viray, J., Rolfs, B., Smith, D.G., 2001. Comparison of the frequencies of major histocompatibility (MHC) class-II DQA1 alleles in Indian and Chinese rhesus macaques (Macaca mulatta). Comp. Med. 51, 555–561.

Voevodin, A., Samilchuk, E., Schätzl, H., Boeri, E., Franchini, G., 1996. Interspecies transmission of macaque simian T-cell leukemia/

lymphoma virus type 1 in baboons resulted in an outbreak of malignant lymphoma. J. Virol. 70, 1633–1639.

Vogel, P., Miller, C.J., Lowenstine, L.L., Lackner, A.A., 1993. Evidence of horizontal transmission of Pneumocystis carinii pneumonia in simian immunodeficiency virus-infected rhesus macaques. J. Infect. Dis. 168, 836–843.

Voronin, L.G., Kanfor, I.S., Lakin, G.F., Tikh, N.N., 1948. Spontaneous diseases of lower monkeys, their prophylaxis, diagnosis, and treatment In: Experimentation on the Keeping and Raising of Monkeys at Sukhami. Academy Medical Science, Moscow, Russia.

Vu, D.T., Sethabutr, O., Von Seidlein, L., Tran, V.T., Do, G.C., Bui, T.C., et al., 2004. Detection of Shigella by a PCR assay targeting the ipaH gene suggests increased prevalence of shigellosis in Nha Trang, Vietnam. J. Clin. Microbiol. 42, 2031–2035.

Wachtman, L., Mansfield, K., 2012. Viral diseases of nonhuman primates Nonhuman Primates. In: Abee, C.R., Mansfield, K., Tardif, S., Morris, T. (Eds.), Biomedical Research Elsevier, San Diego, CA, pp. 46.

Wachtman, L.M., Mansfield, K.G., 2008. Opportunistic infections in immunologically compromised nonhuman primates. ILAR J. 49, 191–208.

Wachtman, L.M., Miller, A.D., Xia, D., Curran, E.H., Mansfield, K.G., 2011. Colonization with nontuberculous mycobacteria is associated with positive tuberculin skin test reactions in the common marmoset (Callithrix jacchus). Comp. Med. 61, 278–284.

Wadsworth, P.F., Hiddleston, W.A., Jones, D.V., Fowler, J.S.L., Ferguson, R.A., 1982. Haematological, coagulation, and blood chemistry data in red-bellied tamarins (Saguinus labiatus). Lab. Anim. 16, 327–330.

Wagner, W.M., Kirberger, R.M., 2005. Radiographic anatomy of the thorax and abdomen of the common marmoset (Callithrix jacchus). Vet. Radiol. Ultrasound 46, 217–224.

Walker, J., Spooner, E.T.C., 1960. Natural infection of the African baboon Papio papio with the large-cell form of Histoplasma. J. Pathol. Bacterial. 80, 436–438.

Wamsley, H.L., Wellehan, J.F., Harvey, J.W., Embury, J.E., Troutman, J.M., Lafortune, M., 2005. Cytologic diagnosis of Lawsonia intracellularis proliferative ileitis in a Japanese snow macaque (Macaca fuscata). Vet. Clin. Pathol 34, 57–60.

Wang, S., Quan, G., 1986. Primate status and conservation in China. In: Benirschke, K. (Ed.), Primates: The Road to Self-Sustaining Populations. Springer-Verlag, New York, pp. 213–220.

Warfel, J.M., Papin, J.F., Wolf, R.F., Zimmerman, L.I., Merkel, T.J., 2014. Maternal and neonatal vaccination protects newborn baboons from Pertussis infection. J. Infect. Dis. 210(4), 604–610. 14 Feb 12 [Epub ahead of print].

Wasser, S.K., 1996. Reproductive control in wild baboons measured by fecal steroids. Biol. Reprod. 2, 393–399.

Wasser, S.K., Norton, G.W., Rhine, R.J., Klein, N., Kleindorfer, S., 1998. Ageing and social rank effects on the reproductive system of free-ranging yellow baboons (Papio cynocephalus) at Mikumi National Park, Tanzania. Hum. Reprod. Update 4, 430–438.

Watts, D.P., Amsler, S.J., 2013. Chimpanzee-red colobus encounter rates show a red colobus population decline associated with predation by chimpanzees at Ngogo. Am. J. Primatol. 75, 927–937.

Weed, J., Watson, E.A., 1998. Pair housing of adult owl monkeys (Aotus sp.) for environmental enrichment. Am. J. Primatol. 45, 212.

Weld, K.P., Mench, J.A., Woodward, R.A., Bolesta, M.S., Suomi, S.J., Higley, J.D., 1998. Effect of tryptophan treatment on self-biting and central nervous system serotonin metabolism in rhesus monkeys (Macaca mulatta). Neuropsychopharmacology 19, 314–321.

Weese, J.S., 2010. Methicillin-resistant Staphylococcus aureus in animals. ILAR 51, 233–244.

Weigler, B.J., 1992. Biology of B virus in macaque and human hosts: a review. Clin. Infect. Dis. 14, 555–567.

Weigler, B.J., Roberts, J.A., Hird, D.W., Lerche, N.W., Hilliard, J.K., 1990. A cross sectional survey for B virus antibody in a colony of group housed rhesus macaques. Lab. Anim. Sci. 40, 257–261.

Weller, R.E., 1994. Infectious and noninfectious diseases of owl monkeys. In: Baer, J.F., Weller, R.E., Kakoma, I. (Eds.), Aotus: The Owl Monkey. Academic Press, San Diego, CA, pp. 178–215.

Weller, R.E., Dagle, G.E., Malaga, C.A., Baer, J.F., 1990. Hypercalcemia and disseminated histoplasmosis in an owl monkey. J. Med. Primatol. 19, 675–680.

Wells, J.G., Morris, G.K., 1981. Evaluation of transport methods for isolating Shigella spp. J. Clin. Microbiol. 13, 789–790.

Welshman, M.D., 1985. Management of newly imported primates. Ann. Technol. 36, 125–129.

Wenner, H.A., Abel, D., Barrick, S., Seshumurty, P., 1977. Clinical and pathogenetic studies of Medical Lake virus infections in cynomolgous monkeys (simian varicella). J. Infec. Dis. 135, 611–622.

Wevers, D., Metzger, S., Babweteera, F., Bieberbach, M., Boesch, C., Cameron, K., et al., 2011. Novel adenoviruses in wild primates: a high level of genetic diversity and evidence of zoonotic transmissions. J. Virol. 85, 10774–10784. http://dx.doi.org/10.1128/JVI.00810-11.

Wey, H.-Y., Kroma, G.M., Li, J., Leland, M.M., Jones, L., Duong, T.Q., 2011. MRI perfusion-diffusion mismatch in non-human primate (baboon) stroke: a preliminary report. Open Neuroimaging J. 5, 147–152.

Whary, M.T., Saunders, K.E., Esteves, M.I., Wood, J., Peck, O.C., Fox, J.G., 1999. A novel Helicobacter sp. isolated from inflamed colonic tissue in cotton-top tamarins is associated with a specific humoral immune response. Gastroenterology 116, A845.

Wheatley, B.P., 1999. The Sacred Monkeys of Bali. Waveland Press., Prospect Heights, IL, 189 p.

White, A., Cummings, M., Filshe, J., 2008. An Introduction to Western Medical Acupuncture. Churchill Livingstone, Elsevier, Philadelphia, PA.

White, J.A., Todd, P.A., Yee, J.L., Kalman-Bowlus, A., Rodgers, K.S., Yang, X., et al., 2009. Prevalence of viremia and oral shedding of rhesus rhadinovirus and retroperitoneal fibromatosis herpesvirus in large age-structured breeding groups of rhesus macaques (Macaca mulatta). Comp. Med. 59, 383–390.

White, J.A., Yang, X., Todd, P.A., Lerche, N.W., 2011. Longitudinal patterns of viremia and oral shedding of rhesus rhadinovirus and retroperitoneal fibromatosis herpesviruses in age-structured captive breeding populations of rhesus Macaques (Macaca mulatta). Comp. Med. 61, 60–70.

Whiteley, H.E., Everitt, J.I., Kakoma, I., James, M.A., Ristic, M., 1987. Pathologic changes associated with fatal Plasmodium falciparum infection in the Bolivian squirrel monkey (Saimiri sciureus boliviensis). Am. J. Trop. Med. Hyg. 37, 1–8.

Wickham, L.A., Kulick, A.A., Gichuru, L., Donnelly, M.J., Gai, C.L., Johnson, C.V., et al., 2011. Transurethral bladder catheterization of male rhesus macaques: a refinement of approach. J. Med. Primatol. 40, 342–350.

Wikse, S.E., Fox, J.G., Kovatch, R.M., 1970. Candidiasis in simian primates. Lab. Anim. Care 20, 957–963.

Wilbert, R., Delorme, M., 1927. Note sur la spirochetose icterohémorrhagique du chimpanzee. C.R. Soc. Bull. 98, 343–345.

Wildt, D.E., Doyle, L.L., Stone, S.C., Harrison, R.M., 1977. Correlation of perineal swelling with serum ovarian hormone levels, vaginal cytology, and ovarian follicular development during the baboon reproductive cycle. Primates 18, 261–270.

Willes, R.F., Kressler, P.L., Truelove, J.F., 1977. Nursery rearing of infant monkeys (Macaca fascicularis) for toxicity studies. Lab. Anim. Sci. 27, 90–98.

Williams, L.E., Bernstein, I.S., 1995. Study of primate social behavior. In: Bennett, B.T., Abee, C.R., Henrickson, R.V. (Eds.), Nonhuman Primates in Biomedical Research: Biology and Management Academic Press, San Diego, pp. 77–100.

Williams, J.T., Dick Jr., E.J., VandeBerg, J.L., Hubbard, G.B., 2009. Natural Chagas disease in four baboons. J. Med. Primatol. 38, 107–113.

Williams, L., Gibson, S., McDaniel, M., Bazzel, J., Barnes, S., Abee, C., 1994. Allomaternal interactions in the Bolivian squirrel monkey (*Saimiri boliviensis boliviensis*). Am. J. Primat. 34, 145–156. http://dx.doi.org/10.1002/ajp.1350340206.

Williams, L., Vitulli, W., McElhinney, T., Wiebe, R.H., Abee, C.R., 1986. Male behavior through the breeding season in *Saimiri boliviensis boliviensis*. Am. J. Primatol. 11, 27–35.

Williams, L.E., Abee, C.R., Barnes, S., 1988. Allomaternal behavior in *Saimiri boliviensis*. Am. J. Primatol. 14, 445.

Williams, L.E., Brady, A.G., Gibson, S.V., Abee, C.R., 2002. The squirrel monkey breeding and research resource: a review of *Saimiri* reproductive biology and behavior and breeding performance. Primatologie 5, 303–334.

Williams, L.E., Brady, A.G., Abee, C.R., 2010. Squirrel monkeys. In: Hubrecht, R., Kirkwood, J. (Eds.), The UFAW Handbook on the Care and Management of Laboratory and Other Research Animals, eighth ed. Wiley-Blackwell, West Sussex, pp. 564–578.

Willy, M.E., Woodward, R.A., Thornton, V.B., Wolff, A.V., Flynn, B.M., Heath, J.L., et al., 1999. Management of a measles outbreak among Old World nonhuman primates. Lab. Anim. Sci. 49, 42–48.

Wilson, D.E., Reeder, D.M., 1993. Mammal Species of the World: A Taxonomic and Geographic Reference, second ed. Smithsonian Institution Press, Washington, DC.

Wilson, D.E., Reeder, D.M., 2005. Mammal Species of the World. A Taxonomic and Geographic Reference, third ed. The Johns Hopkins University Press, Baltimore, MD.

Winkelmann, C.T., Krause, S.M., McCracken, P.J., Brammer, D.W., Gelovani, J.G., 2012. Imaging in research using nonhuman primates, second ed. In: Abee, C.R. Mansfield, K. Tardif, S. Morris, T. (Eds.), Nonhuman Primates in Biomedical Research: Diseases, vol. 2. Academic Press, Elsevier, San Diego, CA, pp. 795–815.

Winnicker, C., Honess, P., Schapiro, S.J., Bloomsmith, M.A., Lee, D.R., McCowan, B., et al., 2013. A Guide to the Behavior and Enrichment of Laboratory Macaques. Charles River Laboratories International, Inc. Newton, MA, ISBN 0-9835-4534-0, 978-0-9835-4534-7.

Wiseman, R.W., Wojcechowskyj, J.A., Greene, J.M., Blasky, A.J., Gopon, T., Soma, T., et al., 2007. Simian Immunodeficiency Virus SIVmac239 infection of major histocompatibility complex – identical Cynomolgus macaques from Mauritius. J. Virol. 81, 349–361.

Wixson, S.K., Griffith, J.W., 1986. Nutritional deficiency anemias of non-human primates. Lab. Anim. Sci. 36, 231–236.

Wolf, R.F., White, G.L., 2012. Clinical techniques used for nonhuman primates. In: Bayne, K., Turner, P.V. (Eds.), Nonhuman Primates in Biomedical Research: Biology and Management, second ed. Academic Press (Elsevier), San Diego, CA, pp. 323–336.

Wolfe, L.G., Ogden, J.D., Deinhardt, J.B., Fisher, L., Deinhardt, F., 1972. Breeding and hand-rearing marmosets for viral oncogenesis studies. In: Beveridge, W.I.B. (Ed.), Breeding Primates. Karger, Basel, Switzerland, pp. 145–157.

Wolfensohn, S., 1998. Shigella infection in macaque colonies: case report of an eradication and control program. Lab. Anim. Sci. 48 (4), 330–333.

Wolff, P.L., 1993. Parasites of New World primates. In: Fowler, M.E. (Ed.), Zoo and Wild Animal Medicine Current Therapy 3. Saunders, Philadelphia, PA, pp. 378–389.

Wolovich, C.K., Evans, S., 2007. Sociosexual behavior and chemical communication of *Aotus nancymaae*. Int. J. Primatol. 28, 1299–1313.

Wolovich, C.K., Evans, S., French, J.A., 2008. Dads do not pay for sex but do buy the milk: food sharing and reproduction in owl monkeys (*Aotus* spp.). Animal Behav. 75, 1155–1163.

Wolters, H.J., 1977. Some aspects of role taking behavior in captive family groups of the cotton-top tamarin *Saguinus oedipus oedipus*. In: Rothe, H. (Ed.), Biology and Behavior of Marmosets. Mecke-Druck, Duderstadt, Germany, pp. 259–278.

Wood, C.E., Borgerink, H., Register, T.C., Scott, L., Cline, J.M., 2004. Cervical and vaginal epithelial neoplasms in cynomolgus monkeys. Vet. Pathol. 41, 108–115.

Woodruff, L.D., Bounkeo, J.M., Brannon, W.M., Dawes, K.S., Barham, C.D., Waddell, D.L., et al., 2004. The efficacy of laser therapy in wound repair: a meta-analysis of the literature. Photomed. Laser Surg. 22, 241–247.

World Health Organization (WHO), 1998. WHO model Prescribing Information: Drugs Used in Leprosy. Geneva, WHO/DMP/DSI/98.1.

World Health Organization (WHO), 2003. Acupuncture: Review and Analysis of Reports on Controlled Clinical Trials. Zhang, X. (Ed.).

Worley, K.C., The Marmoset Genome Sequencing and Analysis Consortium, 2014. The common marmoset provides insight into primate biology and evolution. Nat. Genet. 46, 850–857.

Wright, P.C., 1978. Home range, activity pattern, and agonistic encounters of a group of night monkeys (*Aotus trivirgatus*) in Peru. Folia Primatol. 29, 43–55.

Wright, P.C., 1989. The nocturnal primate niche in the New World. J. Human Evol. 18, 635–658.

Wright, P.C., 1994. The behavior and ecology of the owl monkey. In: Baer, J.F., Weller, R.E., Kakoma, I. (Eds.), Aotus: The Owl Monkey. Academic Press, San Diego, CA, pp. 97–112.

Wright, M.W., 2010. Systematic approach to buying a digital radiography system. Vet. Pract. News, January 2010.

Xie, H., Wedemeyer, L., 2012. The validity of acupuncture in veterinary medicine. AJTCVM 7, 35–43.

Xie, L., Xu, F., Liu, S., Ji, Y., Zhou, Q., Wu, Q., et al., 2013. Age- and sex-based hematologic and biochemical parameters for Macaca fascicularis. PLoS One 8, 1–8.

Xie, L., Zhou, Q., Liu, S., Wu, Q., Ji, Y., et al., 2014. Normal Thoracic Radiographic Appearance of the Cynomolgus Monkey (*Macaca fascicularis*). PLoS One 9 (1), e84599. http://dx.doi.org/10.1371/journal.pone.0084599.

Xing, J., Wang, H., Zhang, Y., Ray, D.A., Tosi, A.J., Disotell, T.R., et al., 2007. A mobile element based evolutionary history of guenons (tribe Cercopithecini). BMC Biol. 5, 5.

Xu, Y., Fernandez, C., Alcantara, S., Bailey, M., De Rose, R., Kelleher, A.D., et al., 2013. Serial study of lymph node cell subsets using fine needle aspiration in pigtail macaques. J. Immunol. Methods 394, 73–83.

Yanai, T., Chalifoux, L.V., Mansfield, K.G., Lackner, A.A., Simon, M.A., 2000. Pulmonary cryptosporidiosis in simian immunodeficiency virus-infected rhesus macaques. Vet. Pathol. 37, 472–475.

Yang, J., Yang, Y., Wang, C.H., Wang, G., Xu, H., Liu, W.Y., et al., 2009. Effect of arginine vasopressin on acupuncture analgesia in the rat. Peptides 30, 241–247.

Ye, Z., Van Dyke, K., Rossan, R.N., 2013. Effective treatment with a tetrandrine/chloroquine combination for chloroquine-resistant falciparum malaria in Aotus monkeys. Malar. J. 12, 117.

Yamamoto, H., Ohsawa, K., Walz, S.E., Mitchen, J.L., Watanabe, Y., Eberle, R., et al., 2005. Validation of an enzyme-linked immunosorbent assay kit using herpesvirus papio 2 (HVP2) antigen for detection of herpesvirus simiae (B virus) infection in rhesus monkeys. Comp. Med 55, 244–248.

Yeoman, R.R., Williams, L.E., Aksel, S., Abee, C.R., 1991. Mating-related estradiol fluctuations during the estrous cycle of the Bolivian Squirrel Monkey (*Saimiri boliviensis boliviensis*). Biol. Repro. 44, 640–647.

Yeoman, R.R., Wegner, F.H., Gibson, S.V., Williams, L.E., Abbot, D.H., Abee, C.R., 2000. Midcycle and luteal elevations of follicle stimulating hormone in squirrel monkeys (*Saimiri boliviensis*) during the estrous cycle. Am. J. Primatol. 52, 207–211.

Yoshikawa, Y., Ochikubo, F., Matsubara, Y., Tsuruoka, H., Ishii, M., Shirota, K., et al., 1989. Natural infection with canine distemper virus in a Japanese monkey (*Macaca fuscata*). Vet. Microbiol. 20, 193–205.

Yurdakök, B., Baydan, E., 2013. Cytotoxic effects of Eryngium kotschyi and Eryngium maritimum on Hep2, HepG2, Vero and U138 MG cell lines. Pharm. Biol. 51, 1579–1585. [Epub ahead of print].

Zack, P.M., 1993. Simian hemorrhagic fever. In: Jones, T.C. Mohr, U. Hunt, R.D. (Eds.), Monographs on Pathology of Laboratory Animals: Nonhuman Primates, vol. 1. Springer-Verlag, Berlin and New York, pp. 118–131.

Zhang, Q., Zhou, C., Hamblin, M.R., Wu, M.X., 2014. Low-level laser therapy effectively prevents secondary brain injury induced by immediate early responsive gene X-1 deficiency. J. Cereb. Blood Flow Metab. 34, 1391–1401. (August May 21, 2014.) <http://www.dx.doi.org/10.1038/jcbfm.2014.95>. [Epub ahead of print].

Zhao, F., Fan, X., Grondin, R., Edwards, R., Forman, E., Moorehead, J., et al., 2010. Improved methods for electroacupuncture and electromyographic recordings in normal and parkinsonian rhesus monkeys. J. Neurosci. Methods 192, 199–206.

Ziegler, T.E., Sousa, M.B., 2002. Parent-daughter relationships and social controls on fertility in female common marmosets (Callithrix jacchus). Horm. Behav. 42, 356–367.

Zimbler-DeLorenzo, H.S., Stone, A.I., 2011. Integration of field and captive studies for understanding the behavioral ecology of the squirrel monkey (Saimiri sp.). Am. J. Primatol 73, 607–622.

Zlotnik, I., Grant, D.P., Dayan, A.D., Earl, C.J., 1974. Transmission of Creutzfeldt-Jakob disease from man to squirrel monkey. Lancet 2, 435–438.

Zondervan, K.T., Weeks, D.E., Colman, R., Cardon, L.R., Hadfield, R., Schleffler, J., et al., 2004. Familial aggregation of endometriosis in a large pedigree of rhesus macaques. Hum. Reprod. 19, 448–455.

Zou, C., Wang, J., Wang, S., Huang, F., Ren, Z., Chen, Z., et al., 2012. Characterizing the induction of diabetes in juvenile cynomolgus monkeys with different doses of streptozotocin. Sci. China Life Sci. 55, 210–218.

18

Biology and Diseases of Amphibians

Dorcas P. O'Rourke, DVM, MS, DACLAM[a] and
Matthew D. Rosenbaum, DVM, MS, DACLAM[b]

[a]Department of Comparative Medicine, East Carolina University, The Brody School of Medicine, Moye Blvd, Greenville, NC, USA [b]National Jewish Health, Biological Resource Center, Denver, CO, USA

I. INTRODUCTION

Amphibians are unique among vertebrate species in that many species transition from early aquatic life forms to terrestrial adults. In fact, the word *amphibian* is derived from the Greek 'amphibios,' which means 'double life.' This 'double life' describes the aquatic larval stage and postmetamorphic terrestrial lifestyle of many amphibians. This chapter presents an overview of amphibian biology and husbandry, followed by a specific section on *Xenopus* management, and concludes with a discussion of amphibian diseases.

A. Taxonomy

Class Amphibia is represented by over 7000 species (http://amphibiaweb.org) contained within three clades: Gymnophiona, Caudata, and Anura. Caecilians comprise the order Gymnophiona, and are legless, burrowing amphibians that inhabit wet, tropical areas of Asia, Africa, and the Americas. Most are less than 50 cm in length and resemble earthworms, with blunt, heavily ossified heads, degenerate eyes, and annular grooves along the body (Zug, 1993; Vitt and Caldwell, 2009). There are approximately 200 described species of caecilians; however, due to their secretive nature, little is known about caecilian biology (Wells, 2007). Caecilians are rarely used in a research setting.

Salamanders are in the order Caudata. There are over 650 species in Caudata, divided into three groups: sirens (eel-like amphibians), basal (primitive) salamanders (hellbenders and other related species), and derived salamanders (mudpuppies, amphiumas, axolotls, newts, and many terrestrial species) (Zug, 1993; Vitt and Caldwell, 2009). Sirens have external gills, no hindlimbs, and reduced forelimbs. They are totally aquatic and inhabit sluggish waterways of southern North America. There are two genera in the family Sirenidae, *Siren* and *Pseudobranchus*, each with two species (Vitt and Caldwell, 2009). There are two families of basal salamanders, Cryptobranchidae and Hynobiidae. Members of the family Cryptobranchidae include hellbenders (*Cryptobranchus* sp.) of the United States and the giant salamanders (*Andrias* sp.) of Asia. Cryptobranchids are primitive salamanders and exhibit paedomorphism (a condition where salamanders retain larval characteristics while becoming fully functional, reproducing adults; this was previously referred to as neotony). They are aquatic and live in cold mountain streams. Respiration is almost exclusively cutaneous, and the skin lies in extensive, fleshy folds on the sides of the body. The head and body are flattened. *Andrias* can reach a length of 1.5 m (5 feet); it is the largest salamander in the world. Hynobiidae, an exclusively Asian family comprising over 50 species, is the second family of basal salamanders. Most members of this group are smaller than the cryptobranchids, have stout bodies, and undergo complete metamorphosis (Conant and Collins, 1991; Zug, 1993; Vitt and Caldwell, 2009).

Six families make up the derived salamanders: Amphiumidae, Proteidae, Ambystomatidae, Rhyacotritonidae, Plethodontidae, and Salamandridae. Amphiumidae contains three species of *Amphiuma*, which superficially resemble sirens. *Amphiuma*, however, lack external gills and can reach an adult length of over 1 m. Proteidae contains two genera, *Proteus* and *Necturus*. *Proteus* is a cave-dwelling salamander found in Europe. *Necturus maculosus*, the mudpuppy, has a broad, flat head and well-developed external gills. Mudpuppies are aquatic and are found in east and central North America. There are two genera and over 37 species represented in Ambystomatidae. Several species demonstrate paedomorphism, including *Ambystoma mexicanum* (the axolotl) and *A. tigrinum* (the tiger salamander). Ambystomatids are predominantly terrestrial, with strong limbs and functional lungs. They are robust animals, and adults of many species can exceed 16 cm in length (Fig. 18.1). Rhyacotritonidae has a single genus (*Rhyacotriton*) with four species. These salamanders resemble the ambystomatids but are found in moist forests of the Pacific coast.

More than 400 species in North and South America, Mediterranean Europe, and Korea make up the family Plethodontidae. Plethodontids occur in a wide variety of sizes and shapes; however, all are lungless, quadrupedal, and possess a nasolabial groove. Among the multiple genera included in this family are *Plethodon*, *Desmognathus*, *Eurycea*, *Gyrinophilus*, *Pseudotriton*, *Aneides*, and *Batrachoseps*.

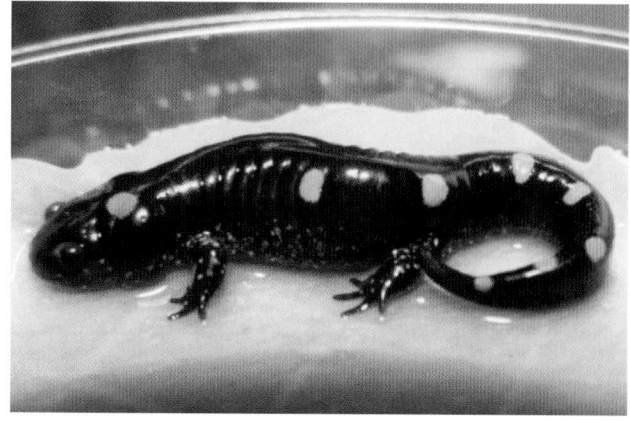

FIGURE 18.1 Ambystomatid salamanders are robust animals with strong limbs and functional lungs.

Members of the family Salamandridae share some characteristics with Plethodontidae; however, salamandrids possess lungs and have numerous poison glands in their skin. Additionally, they may be brightly colored, an advertisement of their toxicity. *Salamandra, Taricha,* and *Notophthalmus* are representative genera of this family. Newts (*Notophthalmus*) can have an aquatic larval stage, terrestrial juvenile period (during which the animals are termed 'efts'), and aquatic adult stage (Conant and Collins, 1991; Zug, 1993; Vitt and Caldwell, 2009).

There are over 6000 frog species in the order Anura, ranging from the Arctic Circle to extreme points in the southern hemisphere. Anurans are easily recognized by their common body plan, which is designed for jumping and allows movement an average of two to 10 times the body length. New species continue to be described in this widespread and diverse amphibian group. Application of molecular techniques has enabled taxonomists to add genetic information to existing classification methodologies, resulting in reclassification of many lineages of anurans. This process is ongoing, and scientific name changes will continue to occur (Conant and Collins, 1991; Zug, 1993; Vitt and Caldwell, 2009; amphibiaweb [http://amphibiaweb.org]). Familiar frog species include the fire-bellied toad, *Bombina orientalis*, and the midwife toad, *Alytes obstetricans*. Other commonly encountered species of anurans are found in the families Pipidae, Ranidae, Bufonidae, Dendrobatidae, Hylidae, Pyxicephalidae, and Ceratophryidae. The genera *Pipa, Xenopus* (including *X. laevis*), and *Silurana* (including *Silurana [Xenopus] tropicalis*) are in Pipidae. Bufonidae contains the true toads, including North American representatives of the genus *Anaxyrus* (e.g., *Anaxyrus [Bufo] americanus, Anaxyrus [Bufo] terrestris*). Toads have warty, thick skin with well-developed parotoid glands (a raised cluster of granular glands located on the head behind the eyes), and males have a Bidder's organ (ovarian tissue located on the cranial pole of the testis). The cane toad (*Rhinella marina [Bufo marinus]*) is a large, invasive bufonid. Poison dart frogs (e.g., *Dendrobates* and *Phyllobates*) are members of the family Dendrobatidae. They are small, active frogs with bright color patterns, which alert would-be predators to the presence of highly toxic alkaloid skin secretions (a characteristic termed aposomatism). These alkaloid secretions are derived from wild diets of arthropods, primarily ants, mites, and beetles (Saporito *et al.*, 2009), and toxins are greatly reduced in captive frogs eating typical diets of fruit flies and springtails. The family Hylidae contains over 840 species of the genus *Hyla* and their relatives. *Hyla* are tree frogs, recognizable by their slender bodies, their long limbs, and the expanded tips of their digits. *Ceratophrys*, the horned frogs of South America, are large animals with fleshy protuberances over the eyes and phenomenally wide mouths. These members of the family Ceratophryidae are voracious terrestrial predators (Zug, 1993). Ranidae ('true frogs') includes members of the genus *Rana (Lithobates)*. Species include *L. catesbeianus* (bullfrog), *L. grylio* (pig frog), *L. clamitans* (bronze frog), and *L. pipiens* (northern leopard frog). Ranids are medium to large frogs with smooth skin. In some species (bullfrog, pig frog, and bronze frog), the tympanum of the male is larger than the eye, while the tympanum of the female is the same diameter as the eye (Conant and Collins, 1991).

B. Use in Research

Amphibians have a long history of research use with *X. laevis*, the African clawed frog, being a a widely recognized example. *X. laevis* was originally used in pregnancy assays, when it was discovered that injection of a pregnant woman's urine into the dorsal lymph sac of a female *X. laevis* caused the frog to begin laying eggs. This method of pregnancy detection was soon replaced; however, the clawed frog remained popular with developmental biologists because of its ability to reproduce year-round when injected with commercially available hormones. *X. laevis* has also been used in cell and developmental biology research (Gurdon, 1996). Documentation of normal clawed frog development (Nieuwkoop and Faber, 1994) enabled *X. laevis* to be used in developmental toxicology investigations and standardized as the FETAX (frog embryo teratogenesis assay: *Xenopus*) system (Dumont *et al.*, 1983; Dawson and Bantle, 1987; Burkhart *et al.*, 1998). Currently, the most common use of *X. laevis* involves cell and molecular biology research (Sive *et al.*, 2000), such as identifying the molecular mechanisms underlying congenital heart disease (Kaltenbrun *et al.*, 2011).

The genome of *Silurana (Xenopus) tropicalis* has recently been sequenced. The combination of a small genome (10 chromosome pairs) and short generation time make this species a highly desirable animal model for genetic applications (Kashiwagi *et al.*, 2010).

The axolotl (*Ambystoma mexicanum*) is a commonly used amphibian research subject. Axolotls (*Ambystoma mexicanum*) and newts regenerate limbs, tail, jaws, skin, spinal cord, brain, and heart apex (Roy and Gatien, 2008; McCusker and Gardiner, 2011; Monaghan *et al.*, 2012) and therefore are excellent models for organ regeneration. Axolotls have also been used to study joint regeneration (Cosden *et al.*, 2011), blastema function (Kragl *et al.*, 2009), and scar-free healing (Seifert *et al.*, 2012). Axolotl oocytes have superior reprogramming ability and have been used in breast cancer research (Allegrucci *et al.*, 2011). A close relative of the axolotl, the tiger salamander (*Ambystoma tigrinum*), is used in vision and retinal research (Voss *et al.*, 2009). Mudpuppies (*Necturus* spp.) have traditionally been the subjects of comparative anatomy laboratories. Ranid frogs (typically bullfrogs [*Lithobates catesbeianus*] and leopard frogs [*Lithobates pipiens*]) have been extensively utilized in teaching physiology and in conducting physiology research (Karnes *et al.*, 1992; Williams, 1997). Because of their ability to regurgitate easily, these species have also been used to study the effects of antiemetics (Kawai *et al.*, 1994; Tai *et al.*, 1995). A leopard frog model was developed by Stevens (1992) and is widely used to test antinociceptive effects of analgesics. The pharmacologic and chemical properties of compounds secreted by amphibian skin are widely studied and characterized (Daly, 1995). Research into effects of environmental toxicants and endocrine disruptors often involves studying wild or captive populations of native amphibians. *Lithobates pipiens* and *Ambystoma tigrinum* have been used to study agrochemical and pesticide toxicity (Orton *et al.*, 2006; Henson-Ramsey *et al.*, 2008) (Fig. 18.2). Endocrine disrupter-induced gonadal abnormalities of the Bidder's organ in cane toad (*Rhinella marina*) populations from agricultural areas have been described (McCoy *et al.*, 2008), as has maternal-fetal

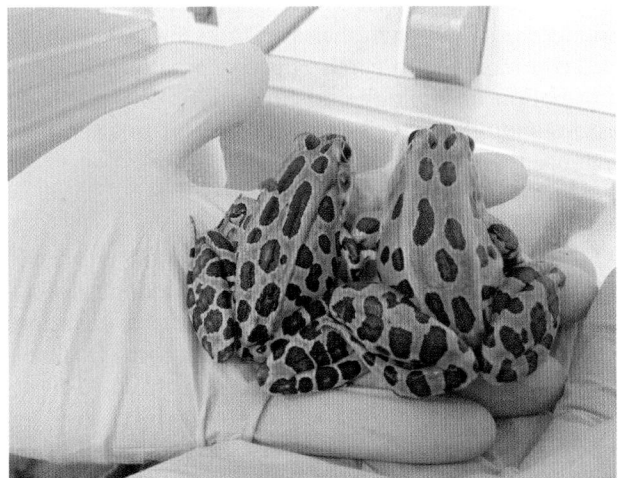

FIGURE 18.2 Leopard frogs (*Lithobates pipiens*) have been used extensively in physiology, pharmacology, and toxicology research.

transfer of heavy metals resulting from coal combustion (Metts *et al.*, 2013).

In addition to animal model and environmental toxicology research, amphibians are extensively studied in the laboratory and the field. Research focuses on ecology, behavior, conservation, and evolutionary biology (Brown *et al.*, 2010). This has become even more critically important as biologists strive to understand and address the worldwide decline of amphibian species. Laboratory animal veterinarians must have fundamental understanding of biology, husbandry, behavior, and medicine of amphibians in order to appropriately support these ongoing research efforts.

C. Availability and Sources

It is widely recognized that many amphibian populations throughout the world are drastically declining in numbers. Therefore, when choosing an amphibian as a model for teaching or research, special consideration should be given to acquiring animals that have been raised in captivity. Alternatively, animals could potentially be obtained from wild populations of invasive species. Colony-reared amphibians are available through commercial vendors such as NASCO, Xenopus Express, Xenopus I, Carolina Biological Supply, the National Xenopus Resource (http://www.mbl.edu/xenopus/), and the University of Kentucky *Ambystoma* Genetic Stock Center (http://www.ambystoma.org/genetic-stock-center). Using purpose-bred animals will protect wild populations and provide the researcher with a healthier, less stressed, and better-characterized animal model.

D. Laboratory Management and Husbandry

Amphibians occupy a variety of niches in the wild, and laboratory housing requirements are equally diverse. This section will describe general principles of amphibian husbandry, with emphasis on frogs and salamanders used commonly in research. Sources containing in-depth information on biology and husbandry of a particular species should always be consulted prior to attempting to house that species.

1. Primary Enclosures

Glass and acrylic aquaria work very well as primary enclosures for amphibians, especially aquatic species. Plastic shoe boxes and sweater boxes also provide appropriate housing and have the advantage of being stackable. Small terrestrial salamander species such as *Plethodon* have been successfully maintained in medium and large plastic petri dishes (Jaeger, 1992). Larger aquatic frogs and salamanders are frequently housed in stainless steel, fiberglass, and Plexiglas tanks. All cages should be constructed of impermeable, easily sanitized material, should

ideally be able to withstand multiple cage washings, and should not contain chemicals or toxic compounds that will leach into the animals' environment with constant exposure to water and humidity. Cages should be of adequate height to accommodate behavioral needs of climbing and jumping species, such as tree frogs and bullfrogs. Fitted, nonabrasive lids are necessary for most terrestrial and many aquatic species, to prevent escape. If tightly fitted lids are solid, small openings should be present to permit adequate airflow into the enclosure. Amphibians typically require a moist habitat with at least 70–80% relative humidity. Notable exceptions include species found in arid environments; however, most amphibians will rapidly desiccate if left in a dry environment. Terrestrial and semiaquatic species do well housed on natural substrates such as moistened sphagnum moss and coco fiber. To ensure moisture retention and create a natural biological filter, a bottom layer of gravel or lightweight expanded clay aggregate (LECA) can be covered by a substrate divider such as fine mesh fiberglass screen, then topped with sphagnum moss or coco fiber. Placing a drain in the tank bottom will facilitate flushing (Pramuk and Gagliardo, 2008). Alternatively, a rigid plastic structure such as an egg crate lighting diffuser can be supported by polyvinyl chloride (PVC) pipe, then covered with mesh screen and substrate to allow water drainage into the bottom of the tank (Fig. 18.3). Some authors suggest using a layer of heat-treated soil covered with leaves or sphagnum moss. Leaves can be frozen for several days

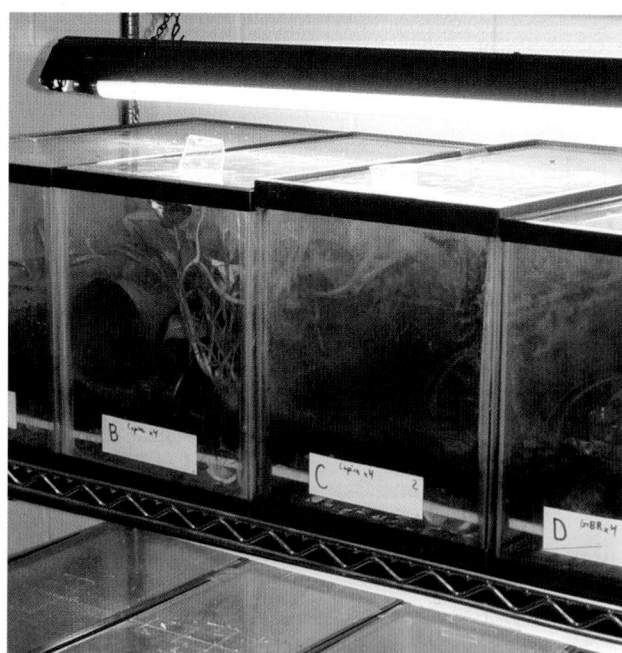

FIGURE 18.3   Terraria can be designed with substrate separated from water collection area at tank bottom by plastic egg crate diffusers supporting fiberglass mesh screen. Full-spectrum light should be provided to diurnal species.

to eliminate arthropod parasites (Wright, 1996). Natural substrates can harbor chytrid fungus and amphibian viruses; therefore it is essential to sterilize or disinfect all soils, mosses, and other fibers prior to use.

To reduce risk of introducing pathogens, artificial substrates may be used. For plethodontid salamanders, Jaeger (1992) recommended three layers of moistened filter paper for petri dish primary enclosures, and soft, moistened paper towels for larger containers. Paper towels and filter paper must not be abrasive or they will damage the animal's delicate skin. Others have used precut, fitted pieces of dechlorinated water-soaked foam or sponge on the tank bottom. These types of substrate can be discarded when soiled.

Substrate pH is important. In one study, the red-backed salamander (*Plethodon cinereus*) preferred the most basic pH range offered (pH 6–6.5). Juveniles avoided soils with a pH of less than 3.7. Very acidic pH ranges (pH 2.5–3) were acutely lethal, and a range of pH 3–4 caused death within 8 months (Wyman and Hawksley-Lescault, 1987).

Virtually all terrestrial salamander and frog species are very secretive and require visual barriers and retreats. Pieces of bark, coconut shell huts, PVC, or acetyl butyl styrene (ABS) pipe, plastic flower pots, artificial or natural plants, or other types of hiding places must be provided. St. Claire *et al.* (2005) recommend hardy live plants such as *Philodendron* and *Scindapsus aureus* (marble queen pothos) for terria housing dendrobatid frogs (Fig. 18.4). Living plants and the soil they are planted in should be free of chytrid fungus and other pathogens.

Many amphibians do not drink; water is absorbed through the skin (Pough, 1991). Water should be provided to terrestrial species in shallow dishes, through the moistened substrate, or by misting (Pough, 1991; Wright, 1996). Depending on species, aquatic amphibians may

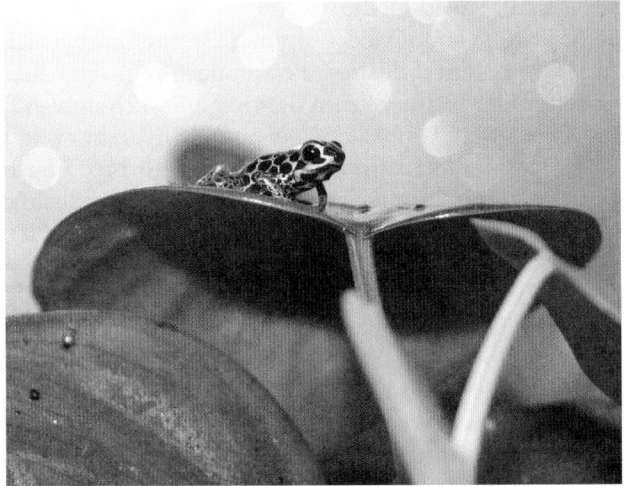

FIGURE 18.4 Dendrobatid frogs can be provided with hardy plants such as *Philodendron* or Pothos for perching and cover.

be housed with or without substrate. Gravel used for substrate in axolotl tanks should be greater than 3 cm diameter, to preclude accidental ingestion and potential gastrointestinal blockage (Gresens, 2004). Aquatic species should also be provided hiding places, such as PVC or ABS pipe or other submersible retreats. Semiaquatic frog and salamander species should be provided a sloping floor or other means of facilitating emergence from the water (Culley, 1992; Wright, 1996).

2. Water Quality

Fresh, dechlorinated/dechloraminated water is preferred for amphibians. Although some species may tolerate low levels of chlorine, many are quite sensitive and will die from exposure to chlorinated water. Allowing open containers of water to age for 24–48 h, aerating the water, adding sodium thiosulfate, and passing tap water through activated carbon filters are four methods of dechlorination. Chloramines may be used in place of chlorine in some municipal water systems. Chloramines can be more toxic than chlorine, do not readily evaporate from surface water, and are best removed with an unused, activated charcoal filter or sodium thiosulfate. When sodium thiosulfate is added to chloramines, ammonia will be released. Zeolites can be used to remove excess ammonia (Gratzek, 1992). An analysis of local water quality should always be obtained prior to establishing an amphibian housing facility.

Water is often treated by reverse osmosis prior to use. Reverse osmosis water or deionized water must be reconstituted with ions that are species-appropriate before use. Species that normally inhabit rainwater pools in leaf axils and ephemeral ponds should be housed in soft water, whereas species adapted to hard water (higher in calcium and magnesium salts) can develop edema and renal problems if chronically housed in soft water (Pramuk and Gagliardo, 2008). Axolotls originate from a brackish lake in Mexico; these animals should be housed in hard water or modified Holtfreter's solution. The University of Kentucky's Ambystoma Genetic Stock Center provides the following formula for a 40% Holtfreter's solution: 1 teaspoon KCl, 2.5 teaspoons $CaCl_2$, 2 tablespoons $MgSO_4.7H_2O$, 240 ml (add dry to beaker) NaCl in a 44-gallon barrel of water (Duhon, 2013). Other research programs modify chemical composition to varying degrees, but in general maintain animals at 40–50% Holtfreter's solution.

Copper is toxic to amphibians, and care should be taken to avoid use of pipes made with this metal. Maintaining correct pH of water in the tank or cage is very important. If the preferred pH of a given species is not known, Wright (1996) recommends starting with a pH of 6.8–7.1 (neutral to slightly acidic), then adjusting to a more basic pH if the animal appears irritated or is anorectic. Verhoeff-de Fremery *et al.* (1987) prefer housing amphibians at a pH of 7.5–8.5, and Horne and Dunson (1994) demonstrated that chronic exposure to low pH affected whole body water and sodium in a terrestrial salamander. Other major water quality factors that can affect amphibian health are dissolved oxygen, total gas levels, and ammonia. Test kits are commercially available to monitor water quality values such as pH and ammonia. Special equipment is needed for dissolved oxygen and total gas levels.

Amphibians can be housed in static, recirculating, or flow-through systems (Fleming, 1990; Sibold et al., 1993; Bartholomew et al., 1993; Stewart, 1994). Static systems work well for both small and large groups of animals, and many tanks can be plumbed to facilitate draining and refilling. A major disadvantage of this type of system is the need for frequent cleaning. Recirculating systems use filters to remove debris and nitrogenous waste from the water. Although less frequent cleaning is necessary with recirculating systems, filters can easily become overtaxed by high population densities and species that generate large amounts of waste. Flow-through systems run a constant stream of water into and out of the tank. Fresh water is always available with this method; however, a mechanism for dechlorination should be built in the line to assure removal of chlorine.

Appropriate water flow rates are critical for aquatic amphibians. Animals that are found in swift mountain streams do well with systems that provide high water flow rates. Conversely, species such as axolotls, which come from slow moving bodies of water, will suffer skin lesions when housed in systems which generate strong currents (Gresens, 2004). Microbial monitoring can be conducted on water sources, and ultraviolet sterilization systems (found in many modern recirculating systems) are important in keeping coliform counts low.

3. Temperature

Amphibians are ectothermic and rely on behavioral thermoregulation to maintain correct body temperatures. Therefore, provision of appropriate ambient temperatures is essential. Many species of salamanders spend their existence beneath leaf litter of forest floors or submerged in cool ponds and fast-moving streams. Consequently, most have preferred thermal zones lower than those of reptiles, and co-housing animals from these two classes is generally discouraged. Recommendations for temperature ranges for amphibians vary somewhat among experts. The Association of Zoos and Aquariums General Amphibian Husbandry guidelines (Pramuk and Gagliardo, 2008) recommend housing temperate species at 18–24°C (65–75°F), tropical lowland species at 24–30°C (75–85°F), tropical montane species at 18–24°C (65–75°F), and tropical hylids and dendrobatids at 25–27°C (77–80°F). Wright (1996) found that tropical species can be maintained at 21–29°C (70–85°F), while amphibians from

temperate regions do well at 18–22°C (65–72°F). Pough (1989) recommends lower ranges: 20–25°C (68–77°F) for tropical species, and 15–20°C (59–68°F) for temperate species. Animals from temperate zones may require seasonal decreases of 5–8°C (10–15°F) (Wright, 1996). Jaeger (1992) warns that temperatures in excess of 20°C (68°F) will prevent salamanders of the genus Plethodon from assimilating food rapidly enough to meet the needs of their increased metabolic rate. Mattison (1998) provides recommended temperatures for several species. Species-specific temperature recommendations include 22–26°C (72–79°F) for Dendrobates auratus (McRobert, 2003) and 15–18°C (59–64°F) for Ambystoma mexicanum (Duhon, 2013). Duhon also warns against exceeding 22°C (72°F) for axolotls. Tinsley (2010) recommends housing X. laevis at 18–22°C (64–72°F), while Green (2010) observes that most laboratories keep X. laevis at 21–22°C (70–72°F). Green et al. (2003) also describe thermal shock in X. laevis subjected to sudden increase in water temperature. Silurana tropicalis is typically housed at 24–25°C (75–77°F) (Green, 2010). Suboptimal temperatures also impact amphibian health and well-being. Tinsley (2010) stated that X. laevis housed at temperatures lower than 18°C (64°F) become immune suppressed, and animals housed at 10°C (50°F) have poor tolerance of routine husbandry activities such as water changes. Lithobates pipiens housed at 5°C (41°F) for several weeks demonstrated a decrease in T lymphocyte immune response (Maniero and Carey, 1997).

4. Lighting

Most amphibians live in cool, dark environments in the wild; therefore, direct exposure to bright light should generally be avoided. However, frog species that are diurnal and bask should have access to full-spectrum light (Pramuk and Gagliardo, 2008). For animal–room lighting, full-spectrum bulbs are suggested, especially if the particular needs of the species are not known (Wright, 1996). Shelter should be provided, so the animal may retreat from light if desired. Poison dart frogs have been housed under full-spectrum lighting on a 12 h light–12 h dark cycle (St. Claire et al., 2005), and this light cycle is satisfactory for many species. However, if breeding or mimicking the natural habitat of the animal is desired, light cycles will need to be manipulated accordingly.

5. Airflow

Amphibians require moist habitats, and relative humidities of about 80% work well for most species (Pough, 1991; Wright, 1996). Normal animal-room airflows tend to cause evaporation and dry out wet environments. To prevent this desiccation of habitat and animals, room airflows should be reduced. Alternatively, amphibians can be housed in primary enclosures which have minimal openings. These will retain moisture;

however, care should be taken to ensure that temperatures inside the primary enclosures do not rise to unacceptable levels.

6. Secondary Enclosures

Conventional animal rooms can be successfully adapted to house amphibians. Walls, floors, and ceilings should be impervious and easy to sanitize. Electrical outlets should be ground fault interrupted to prevent electrical shock, especially in rooms housing aquatic species. Individual light timers and thermostats are recommended for each room, since species have variable requirements. In cases where very cool and moist conditions are needed and cannot be achieved with normal room manipulations, environmental chambers can be utilized (Jaeger, 1992).

7. Sanitation

Routine sanitation of amphibian primary enclosures requires special consideration. Many terrestrial species, particularly salamanders, are territorial and mark their environments with pheromones. Excessive cleaning will disrupt normal behavior and can be stressful to the animal (Jaeger, 1992). However, allowing excess buildup of excreta will result in accumulation of toxic metabolites as well as overgrowth of bacteria and fungi. Animals then are placed in a more compromised and stressful environment and can easily succumb to disease. Singly housed, terrestrial animals with ample floor space can be changed every 2 weeks (Jaeger, 1992) and spot-cleaned as necessary. Group-housed animals require more frequent cleaning. Naturalistic environments with established biofilters should be assessed to determine bacterial stability and appropriate intervals for substrate change and system breakdown/cleaning. Enclosures for aquatic species may require cleaning on a daily, weekly, or less frequent basis, depending on stocking density, frequency of feeding, and type of system (filtration, flow-through, etc.). In general, tanks should be cleaned at appropriate intervals to prevent water from fouling.

Cleaning solutions should be carefully chosen, and extreme care must be taken to thoroughly rinse away chemical residues. Heat (60°C/140°F) and desiccation are effective against chytrid fungus, as are several chemicals, including 1% Virkon™ (oxidizing agent), 1% benzalkonium chloride, 2% bleach, and 70% ethanol (Johnson et al., 2003). Schmeller et al. (2011) recommends 1% Virkon™ for disinfecting because of its broad spectrum of efficacy and relatively low toxicity to amphibians. Chlorhexidine (0.75%), 3% bleach, and 1% Virkon™ were found to be effective against ranavirus with a 1-min contact time (Bryan et al., 2009). Amphibians are exquisitely sensitive to most compounds, and their permeable skin makes them particularly susceptible to toxins. Stoskopf et al. (1985) warn against use of iodine-based disinfectants with poison dart frogs. Phenolics are highly toxic and should never be used around amphibians.

8. Handling

Amphibians must be handled carefully, to avoid disrupting the protective mucus layer or causing excess secretion of toxins. Gloves should be worn when possible, and they must be free of powder and moistened with dechlorinated water. Cashins et al. (2008) reported morbidity and mortality in tadpoles following handling with both washed and unwashed latex and nitrile gloves; tadpoles did not show evidence of toxicity to well-rinsed vinyl gloves. Abrasive paper towels should never be used. Nets must be made of soft fine mesh, and should be an appropriate size to comfortably hold the animal. Aquatic species can be transferred or held in glass or plastic containers to prevent removal from water and to protect the sensitive gills. Small terrestrial amphibians can be manually restrained with one hand. Large salamanders should be firmly but gently grasped behind the head and around the pectoral girdle with one hand, and around the pelvic girdle with the other hand (Verhoeff-de Fremery et al., 1987; Crawshaw, 1993; Wright, 1996). Some species will release their tail as a predator-avoidance mechanism; therefore, the tail must not be used for restraint. Frogs, like salamanders, can be held around the pectoral girdle; however, the strong hindlegs must also be restrained to prevent kicking out and slipping through the handler's grasp. Most amphibians can bite, and some can inflict painful wounds. Additionally, many species secrete skin toxins, and in some species such as *Rhinella marina*, toxin can be ejected when the parotoid gland is pressed. Therefore, eye protection (Wright, 1996), gloves, and thorough hand washing is recommended when handling these animals.

9. Identification

Ferner (2010) presents a comprehensive review of amphibian marking techniques. Individual animals can be identified in a variety of ways. Adult animals with varying color patterns can be drawn or photographed and the patterns used as unique identifiers (Donnelly et al., 1994). Tattooing and freeze or chemical branding have been used, but can be nonpermanent. Glass or plastic beads have been used to identify individual frogs and salamanders (Verhoeff-de Fremery et al., 1987; Hoogstraten-Miller and Dunham, 1997). These beads are sewn to the animal using stainless steel or nonabsorbable suture. The suture must pass through a muscle mass in order to permanently anchor the beads; sewing to the skin can only result in sloughing within a few weeks.

Newer techniques for marking include passive integrated transponder (PIT) tags and visible injected or implanted elastomers. Transponders have been injected or implanted subcutaneously, in the dorsal lymph sac, and intracoelomically (Ferner, 2010; Hoogstraten-Miller and Dunham, 1997; McAllister *et al.*, 2004). Transponders can migrate after implanting and even exit the body, so consideration should be given to species and implant technique prior to using PIT tags. Visible fluorescent elastomers are safe for marking amphibians, including egg masses (Register and Woolsey, 2005). Heard *et al.* (2008) reported that visible implant alphanumeric tags did not affect frog survival or growth, and Schmidt and Schwarzkopf (2010) demonstrated that elastomer tagging had less impact on frogs and skinks than did toe clipping.

Toe clipping continues to be a primary means of amphibian field identification, and it continues to be fraught with controversy. Many amphibians regenerate digits, and this method may be less effective for those species. Studies supporting and decrying toe clipping have largely been based on recapture and survival estimates. Waddle *et al.* (2008) demonstrated variable effects between two closely related tree frog species, *Hyla cineria* and *Hyla squirella*. Toe clipping decreased survival in *Hyla cineria* but not in *Hyla squirella*. Grafe *et al.* (2011) confirmed these variable impacts among species, and further concluded that effects could be minimized by limiting the number of toes clipped to less than one toe per foot, and by avoiding specific toes on both front and hind feet that were critical to essential behavioral functions. Interestingly, fewer papers have addressed relevant animal health and welfare impacts. Concern regarding post-amputation inflammation, infection, and necrosis has been expressed by authors (Golay and Durrer, 1994; Wright, 1996). Phillott *et al.* (2011) recorded inflammation following toe clipping in stream dwelling hylid frogs, but cautioned that there was no data on how this procedure might affect other species in different habitats. Toe clipping should be performed with sterile instruments that are well-disinfected between animals, to guard against infection and spread of pathogens such as chytrid fungus. Anesthetics and analgesics should always be used whenever possible, to control stress documented with this procedure (Narayan *et al.*, 2011). Veterinarians and IACUCs must consider each request for toe clipping carefully, weighting factors such as proposed number and pattern of toes to be removed, species behavior and habitat, proper instrument handling and technique, appropriate pain and stress/distress management, potential for post-amputation sequelae, and availability of less invasive methods appropriate for the study under consideration.

10. Quarantine

All newly arrived amphibians, especially those that are wild-caught, should undergo a quarantine period. The animals must be housed separately from existing colonies, and their room should be serviced last. Implements should not be shared between quarantine and other rooms. Animals intended for long-term use should be screened and treated, if necessary, for parasites. Diseases should be diagnosed and treated accordingly. The length of quarantine will vary, depending on intended use of the amphibians. Animals for acute studies may be quarantined for shorter periods, but animals intended for long-term studies typically require at least a 4–6 week quarantine period. Green (2010) recommends quarantining *Xenopus* 2–3 months prior to introduction into existing colonies, if a sole source vendor is not used or if captive reared and wild-caught animals are co-housed. Longer periods may be necessary for wild-caught amphibians, due to their unknown health status.

11. Zoonoses/Allergies

Amphibians can potentially harbor zoonotic diseases. The most familiar amphibian zoonosis is atypical mycobacteriosis, caused primarily by *Mycobacterium marinum* (Martinho and Heatley, 2012). Other species that have been isolated include *M. fortuitum*, *M. xenopi*, *M. chelonae*, *M. gordonae*, *M. liflandi*, *M. avium intracellulare*, *M. ulcerans*, *and M. szulgai* (Green *et al.*, 2000; Sánchez-Morgado *et al.*, 2009; Mitchell, 2011; Martinho and Heatley, 2012). The disease in humans typically presents as self-limiting cutaneous lesions on the fingers and hands. Rarely, the disease may spread to involve lymph nodes and become severe. Immunocompromised individuals are more at risk and can develop severe systemic disease. The best precaution against atypical mycobacteriosis is to wear gloves, especially if there are pre-existing cuts or abrasions on the hands, and to wash hands after handling animals or animal habitats.

Salmonellosis has been reported in amphibians, but with much less frequency than in reptiles (Woodward *et al.*, 1997). In 2009, 85 cases of salmonellosis were linked to African dwarf frogs (*Hymenochirus* sp.) (Mitchell, 2011). Appropriate precautions include wearing gloves, washing hands thoroughly after handling amphibians or their surroundings, and screening animals periodically for *Salmonella*.

Chlamydiophila (Chlamydia) psittaci has been isolated from both *X. laevis* (Newcomer *et al.*, 1982; Wilcke *et al.*, 1983; Howerth, 1984) and *S. tropicalis* (Mitchell, 2011). *C. pneumoniae* was identified in a giant barred frog (Berger *et al.*, 1999). Although no reports have been identified that document amphibian-to-human transmission, both agents should be recognized as potential human pathogens and appropriate precautions taken.

There have been occasional reports of allergies to frog skin and secretions (Armentia and Vega, 1997; Holtz *et al.*, 1993). Individuals experiencing respiratory or cutaneous signs when working with frogs should seek medical advice concerning allergies.

II. BIOLOGY

A. Anatomy and Physiology

1. Integumentary System

Amphibian skin is typically smooth, moist, and glandular, and has multiple functions. Two primary types of skin glands are present in amphibians: mucous glands and granular glands. Mucous glands secrete a slimy protective layer, which prevents mechanical damage to the skin, facilitates retention of body fluids, and provides a barrier against pathogens. Granular glands synthesize and secrete a variety of compounds that protect against predators, as well as chemicals that have antibacterial and antifungal properties. Granular glands are usually found on the head and shoulders but can be scattered over the body (Zug, 1993; Clarke, 1997). The parotoid gland of toads (Bufonidae), located on the head behind the eyes, is a raised cluster of granular glands. Fire salamanders (*Salamandra salamandra*) and many other salamander species also have parotoid glands. Defensive compounds found in parotoid and other granular glands can have neurotoxic, cardiotoxic, myotoxic, hallucinogenic, hypotensive, and vasoconstrictive activity (Clarke, 1997). Highly toxic alkaloids found in poison dart frogs (Dendrobatidae), *Rhinella marina*, and other species of frogs and salamanders can cause vomiting, respiratory paralysis, and death. Granular gland secretions of extremely stressed *X. laevis* are reported to produce a milky secretion that caused gaping and yawning in snakes attempting to feed on the frogs (Barthalmus and Zielinski, 1998); this thick, milky secretion forms glutinous strands and has been reported to be toxic to the frogs themselves (Tinsley, 2010).

In addition to antipredator activity, granular glands of some species secrete peptides, which exhibit antimicrobial activity. The magainins, peptides secreted by *X. laevis*, inhibit growth of gram-positive and gram-negative bacteria, several fungi, and some protozoal species. Bombesin, caerulein, and bradykinin are among the peptides found in other amphibian species, including fire-bellied toads, midwife toads, and tree frogs. Skin secretions of bufonids have also demonstrated antibacterial and antifungal properties (Clarke, 1997).

Other chemical compounds secreted by granular glands of various species include pheromones used in courtship and mating; dermorphin, a potent opioid that may function as an endogenous analgesic; and bioadhesives, which allow temporary entrapment of predators (Clarke, 1997), or permit certain species of small male frogs to adhere to females during breeding (Zug, 1993).

Amphibians shed their skin in cycles, which may range from days to weeks. The skin commonly splits middorsally, and the animal uses its limbs to climb out of its skin. Shed skins are commonly eaten (Zug, 1993).

Males of several amphibian species develop keratinized epidermal thumb pads seasonally. These nuptial pads are typically shed and regrown in synchrony with each mating season (Vitt and Caldwell, 2009).

The permeability of amphibian skin causes these animals to be susceptible to water loss and dehydration; therefore, many hylid, bufonid, and ranid frogs have developed 'seat patches' (also called 'drink patches'). Seat patches are located on the ventral abdomen and hindlimbs. When pressed against a wet substrate, through the action of arginine vasotocin and aquaporins, seat patches increase permeability and facilitate absorption of water (Jorgensen, 1997; Viborg and Rosenkilde, 2004; Uchiyama and Norifumi, 2006; Ogushi et al., 2010; Shibata et al., 2011).

2. Musculoskeletal System

The amphibian skeleton has undergone several modifications. Salamander skeletons are largely cartilaginous. Ribs are absent or greatly reduced in most frogs. Anuran adaptations for jumping include fusion of postsacral vertebrae into an elongate bone, the urostyle, which articulates with the sacral vertebra and the ilium; and fusion of the tibia and fibula into a single, strong bone, the tibiofibula. The iliosacral joint of *X. laevis* articulates in a fashion that allows the joint to slide in a cranial-caudal direction along the vertebral column, thereby increasing hind limb propulsion both forward and backward (Videler and Jorna, 1985; Measey, 1998).

Many salamander species share a predator avoidance mechanism, tail autotomy. If the tail is grasped, it will break throught a fracture plane, and the animal can escape. Newts, axolotls, and other species also have the ability to regenerate limbs, jaws, and ocular tissues (Brockes, 1997).

3. Respiratory System

Larval amphibians breathe primarily through gills. Adult amphibians may retain and use gills, lose gills and develop lungs, breathe with both gills and lungs, or have neither and utlize cutaneous respiration mechansims. *X. laevis* tadpoles and axolotls have both gills and lungs and will gulp air at the water's surface. Axolotls flex their external gills to move fresh water over the filaments; this behavior increases when animals are housed in warm water with decreased oxygen content (Gresens, 2004). Adult plethodontids (lungless salamanders) lack both lungs and gills, and rely on cutaneous respiration. Skin, in fact, is the primary respiratory surface in most amphibians and must be kept moist. In species that use lungs for respiration, air is forced in and out of the lungs by movement of the buccopharyngeal floor (Zug, 1993). Lungs lack alveoli and are very fragile and easily ruptured (Wright, 1996) (Fig. 18.5). In many frog species, the trachea is short, and bifurcation occurs close to the

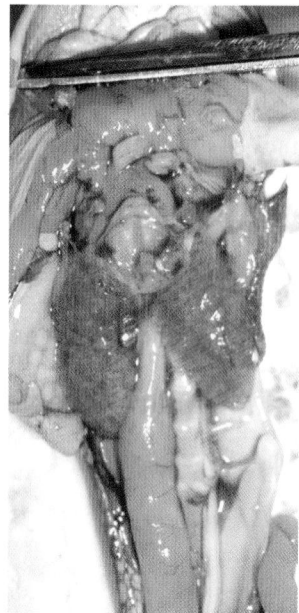

FIGURE 18.5   Amphibian lungs lack alveoli and are very fragile.

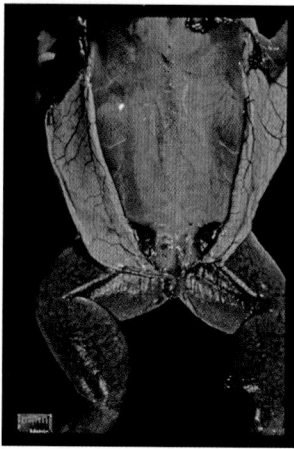

FIGURE 18.6   Dorsal surface of *X. laevis* with skin removed, showing lymph hearts that drain dorsal lymph sacs into venous system.

glottis; this anatomic feature must be taken into account when performing endotracheal intubation.

4. Cardiovascular System

Larval amphibians, like fish, have a two-chambered heart. Most adult amphibians have a three-chambered heart, consisting of paired atria and a single ventricle (plethodontid salamanders lack an atrial division, since they lack lungs). Hellbenders, mudpuppies, and sirens have a partial interventricular septum (Burggren and Warburton, 1994). Patterns of blood flow and mixing of oxygenated and deoxygenated blood vary among species, depending on degree of pulmonary respiration, physiological state, and anatomic structures (Zug, 1993; Vitt and Caldwell, 2009). Hepatic portal veins drain blood from the rear half of the amphibian's body; this may impact the pharmacokinetics of drugs with hepatic excretion (Wright, 1996). Plasma osmolarity of amphibians is 200mOsm/kg (Walker and Whitaker, 2000). This difference from mammalian osmolarity should be considered when preparing media for *in vitro* work with amphibian tissues, as well as when administering replacement fluids to dehydrated amphibians. Amphibian Ringer's solution contains 6.6g NaCl, 0.15g $CaCl_2$, and 0.2g $NaHCO_3$ per liter of water (Walker and Whitaker, 2000).

5. Lymphatic System

The lymphatic system of amphibians consists of sinuses and vessels and drains into the venous system. Large sinuses, collection sites for lymph, are found throughout the amphibian's body. At venous junctions, lymph hearts contract and force lymph from the sinuses

through lymphatic vessels into the veins. In frogs, a pair of these large sinuses lies subcutaneously over the sacral area, lateral to midline (Fig. 18.6). Substances injected into these dorsal lymph sacs will be transported directly to the venous circulation (Vitt and Caldwell, 2009).

6. Gastrointestinal System

Adult amphibians are carnivorous and therefore have a relatively short gastrointestinal tract. The tongue is attached rostrally and well developed in all species except pipids and is important for prehending food items. *Xenopus* and other pipids direct food items into the mouth with their front legs. Vomiting in amphibians is a common defensive mechanism, and it is not unusual for some frog species to evert part of the stomach during regurgitation (Bisazza *et al.*, 1998). Gastrointestinal contents empty into the cloaca, a common collecting chamber for the gastrointestinal, urinary, and reproductive tracts. Melanin is commonly found in the amphibian liver and other abdominal organs, and pronounced pigmentation is not unusual.

7. Excretory System

Salamanders and frogs have opisthonephric kidneys and lack the ability to concentrate urine in excess of plasma levels. Aquatic amphibians excrete ammonia, terrestrial amphibians excrete urea, and a few arboreal amphibians excrete uric acid. Most amphibians have a bladder, which functions in water conservation. Many frogs, when frightened, will release urine to deter predators (Wright, 1996).

8. Nervous System/Special Senses

Cerebral cortical structure in amphibians is dissimilar to that of higher vertebrates, and the function of the various areas is still controversial (Nieuwenhuys,

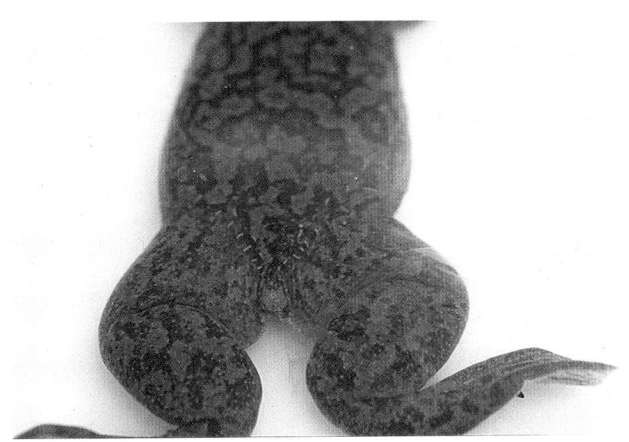

FIGURE 18.7 The lateral line system of *X. laevis* appears as a series of 'stitches' on the skin surface. Note the typical skin shedding on the right hindlimb.

1994; Bruce and Neary, 1995). Amphibians have 10 cranial nerves. The hypoglossal nerve (cranial nerve XII) is formed by branches of the first two spinal nerves (Anderson and Nishikawa, 1997). A lateral line system (similar to that of fish) is well developed in larval amphibians and is retained by adults of many aquatic species. The lateral line system is recognizable as a linear arrangement of neuromasts on the head and along the body of the animal; these appear as 'stitches' on the skin of *X. laevis* (Fig. 18.7). Neuromasts detect changes in water pressure and currents, and function in locating prey (Zug, 1993; Vitt and Caldwell, 2009). Amphibians can detect higher-frequency sound transmitted through the air to the tympanic membrane, but low-frequency vibration is transmitted through the forelimbs and the cranium to the ear. The amphibian eye has two types of rods, red and green, which detect the presence or absence of light. There are single and double cones for color reception (Vitt and Caldwell, 2009). A vomeronasal (Jacobson's) organ is responsible for odor detection. *X. laevis* has both terrestirial and aquatic olfactory receptors (Measey, 1998).

9. Normal Values

Longevity data are available for many amphibian species (Bowler, 1977; Kara, 1994; Smirina, 1994). Amphibians from northern climates tend to have longer life spans than those from southern latitudes, and larger aquatic salamanders live longer than their smaller, terrestrial counterparts. *X. laevis* have been documented to live 20 years (Tinsley, 2010); *A. mexicanum*, greater than 10 years (Gresens, 2004); *Bombina*, 11–13 years; *L. catesbeiannus*, 16 years; and newts, 9 years (Kara, 1994; Smirina, 1994). *Cryptobranchus* can exceed 25 years; *Desmognathus*, 10 years; and *Anaxyrus americanus*, 5 years (Zug, 1993). Age can be most accurately determined in amphibians by counting the layers in bone (Smirina, 1994).

Amphibian species have nucleated red blood cells and thrombocytes. Amphibian lymphocytes, monocytes, and thrombocytes function in a fashion similar to that of their higher vertebrate counterparts. Neutrophils appear to respond to infection in a manner similar to that of mammalian neutrophils and reptilian heterophils. Eosinophil and basophil function is largely unknown, and interpretation of elevated percentages of these cell types cannot be extrapolated from mammalian literature (Campbell, 1991).

Hematologic and serum chemistry values for amphibians can be affected by a number of variables, including season, sex, environmental factors, and method of sample processing. Cathers *et al.* (1997) found significant differences between male and female *L. catesbeiannus* for plasma proteins, sodium, and calcium. No differences were found in the remainder of the complete blood count (CBC) or serum chemistry values. Percentage of lymphocytes (63%) exceeded that of segmented neutrophils (22%). Pfeiffer *et al.* (1990) investigated hematologic changes in Japanese newts following tail amputation. They observed a decrease in hematocrit during the first 10 days postamputation; hematocrit was restored by day 30. A transient lymphocytosis was also noted in the first few days following amputation. Basophil percentages were consistently high (49–64%) throughout this study, in contrast to that of Jerrett and Mays (1973), who found no basophils in two populations of hellbenders. Forbes *et al.* (2006) observed that breeding male and female *Anaxyrus americanus* had an increased proportion of heretophils. Davis and Maerz (2008) investigated the effect of captive holding on paedomorphic *Ambystoma talpoideum*. Salamanders held in captivity for 10 days prior to bleeding demonstrated a higher neutrophil to lymphocyte ratio than animals wild-caught and immediately sampled. Wilson *et al.* (2011) conducted a robust study of hemotologic and serum chemistry values for *X. laevis* and found that values for this species were most consistent with those of *Cryptobranchus alleganiensis*. They reported variation between wild-caught and captive-raised *X. laevis*, and concluded that differences observed among groups sampled were likely due to temperature, water quality, and other physical parameters.

B. Nutrition

1. Adult

Adult amphibians are carnivorous, and many are opportunistic feeders. In the wild, salamanders feed on a variety of vertebrate and invertebrate species. *Ambystoma tigrinum* has been documented to ingest worms, insects, snails, young field mice, and lizards. *Plethodon cinereus* eats ants, spiders, flies, beetles, and other small invertebrates. *Notophthalmus viridescens* feeds on aquatic insects and mollusks. Adult amphibians will frequently cannibalize larvae of their own and other species. Large salamanders such as *Cryptobranchus* and *Amphiuma* eat crawfish, fish, frogs, and mammals. *Necturus* feeds on both small and large prey items (Petranka, 1998). Frogs also feed on a variety of invertebrates, and larger species such as *Lithobates catesbeianus* have been noted to eat salamanders, snakes, turtles, and small birds and mammals. *Rhinella marina* has been reported to eat dog food (Bartlett and Bartlett, 1996).

Most species will adapt to dietary modifications required for housing in a laboratory animal facility. Jaeger (1992) successfully kept several salamander species using a diet of *Drosophila* (wingless fruit flies) for smaller individuals, and crickets and earthworms for larger animals. Newts will eat chopped earthworms, fly larvae, and *Tubifex* worms. Many terrestrial and semi-aquatic frog species orient visually to prey and require moving food. *Lithobates*, *Anaxyrus*, *Bombina*, and most other frog species will take crickets, earthworms, and waxworms. Dendrobatid frogs can be fed *Drosophila*, *Collembola* (springtails), and juvenile crickets. Animals slow to adapt to captive feeding can be maintained on cricket/fruit fly puree delivered through a small feeding needle until they begin eating on their own (St. Claire *et al.*, 2005). Commercial insectivore and carnivore diets can also be used. Mudpuppies and axolotls have been maintained on diets of beef muscle and organ meat; however, vitamins and minerals should be supplemented if these are fed (Verhoeff-de Fremery *et al.*, 1987). Raw meat and organs should not be fed to young, growing amphibians, or calcium deficiency can result. *Salmonella* contamination is also a concern when feeding raw meat and organs, and *Chlamydiophila* outbreaks have been associated with feeding organ meat (Wright, 2001c). Axolotls will readily eat earthworms and adapt to commercially prepared diets, such as sinking pelleted salmon diet (Pramuk and Gagliardo, 2008) (Fig. 18.8). Gel diets can be prepared or formulated. Commericially prepared balanced diets are also available for *Xenopus*.

Most whole vertebrate prey items, if properly nourished, will constitute a balanced diet for larger amphibians. Bones provide calcium, phosphorus, and magnesium; liver and kidneys provide vitamins; pancreas provides zinc; and thyroids provide iodine. In contrast, the chitinous exoskeleton of many invertebrates is, for the most part, indigestible and contains little to no calcium or other nutrients (Donoghue, 1996). Because insects lack a calcium-rich skeletal structure, a calcium supplement should be dusted on the prey before feeding (Bartlett and Bartlett, 1996). Alternatively, insects can be fed a diet that is vitamin-mineral rich ('gut loaded') immediately before being fed to amphibians. Amphibian diets should also contain adequate levels of vitamin A (Dugas *et al.*, 2013).

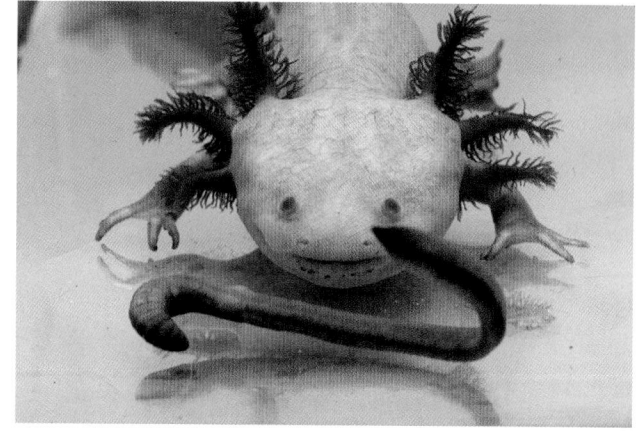

FIGURE 18.8   In addition to commercial pelleted diet, axolotls readily eat earthworms.

To avoid feeding prey items of poor nutritional quality, crickets, mealworms, and similar species can be raised in-house on nutritious diets. Crickets can be kept in a large, deep container on a substrate of sawdust, corncob bedding, or vermiculite. A shallow dish with moistened cotton balls or vermiculite serves as both a water source and a place to lay eggs. Crumpled newspaper, egg crates, or paper-towel tubes should be placed about the cage for hiding places. Crickets can be fed laying mash, rodent pellets, crushed dog food, or other suitable balanced diet. Vegetables such as broccoli, carrots, and alfalfa sprouts can be added, and food can be sprinkled with calcium. Mealworms can be raised in a ventilated container with a fitted lid. Laying mash or chick starter and bran can be used for substrate, and should be covered with a paper or cloth towel. Vegetables and fruit can be added to provide moisture. Food should be replenished periodically (Bartlett and Bartlett, 1996; Mattison, 1998). Nutritionally balanced cricket diets are also commercially available.

Adult amphibians should be fed any where from daily to twice weekly, depending on species, age of animal, and ambient temperature. Active species should eat at least three times a week (Pramuk and Gagliardo, 2008). *Xenopus* are typically fed to satiation two to three times per week (Green, 2010), although feeding intervals vary widely with this species. Conversely, axolotls thrive when fed small amounts on a daily basis (Gresens, 2004).

2. Larvae

Larval salamanders are carnivorous and eat a variety of prey items. *Ambystoma tigrinum* larvae in the wild consume aquatic mollusks, nematodes, insects, and eggs and larvae of their own and other amphibian species. Axolotl larvae eat freshly hatched brine shrimp, then can be transitioned on to sinking salmon pellets of increasing size as the larvae grow (Gresens, 2004). *Notophthalmus viridescens* larvae eat small invertebrates, including copepods, snails, and water mites. Hatchling *Cryptobranchus* have large yolk sacs and apparently rely on yolk for nutrition for the first few months of life (Petranka, 1998). In captivity, salamander larvae have been fed *Daphnia*, brine shrimp nauplii, blackworms, bloodworms, isopods, and chopped earthworms (Browne and Zippel, 2007).

Tadpoles tend to be more omnivorous than salamander larvae and species may have specific feeding mechanisms. Tropical fish food (Tetramin™) or fish pellets can be ground and placed into the water to feed many species. Sera Micron™ dried onto a microscope slide or Petri dish can be placed in the tank to feed grazing species (Pramuk and Gagliardo, 2008). Sera Micron™, blue-green algae (*Spirulina*), and nettle powder can be used for filter feeders such as *Xenopus* and some hylid tadpoles (Pramuk and Gagliardo, 2008; Tinsley, 2010).

Larval amphibians are voracious feeders and should be fed more frequently than adults. Some species require several small feedings throughout the day; others can be fed once or twice daily. Uneaten food must always be removed to prevent fouling of water.

C. Behavior

Many salamanders, particularly terrestrial species, are territorial and should not be housed together. Both males and females of *Plethodon cinereus* are territorial and will vigorously defend their habitats. Fecal pellets and granular gland secretions are routinely used to mark home ranges. If another animal is encountered, agonistic posturing such as raising the tail and trunk can result. Aggression can escalate to biting. *Plethodon cinereus* bites the nasolabial groove of its competitor, thereby decreasing that animal's ability to locate food, and ultimately affecting its survivability (Jaeger, 1981; Petranka, 1998). *X. laevis* establish hierarchies (Tinsley, 2010); small frogs feed after larger animals.

D. Reproduction

1. Reproductive Anatomy and Physiology

Sexual dimorphism exists in many amphibian species; this can be particularly evident during the breeding season. In general, female amphibians are larger than males. Male bullfrogs, pig frogs, and bronze frogs have a tympanum that is larger than the eye; the female counterpart is the same diameter as the eye (Fig. 18.9). Differences in coloration between males and females exist in some frog and salamander species (e.g., *Anaxyrus* and *Triturus*). The vocal sacs of male frogs become larger and more pigmented in breeding season. *Hyla* and related species often have yellowish vocal sacs, and the sacs of *Anaxyrus*

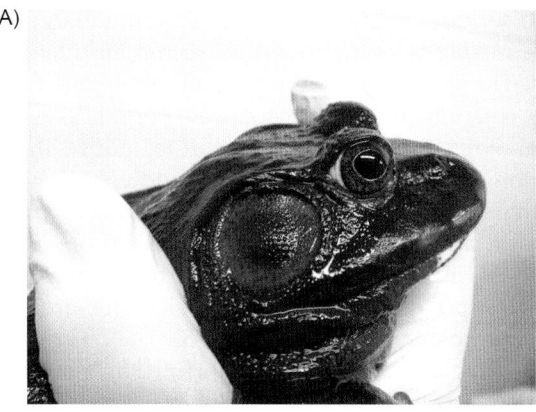
(A)

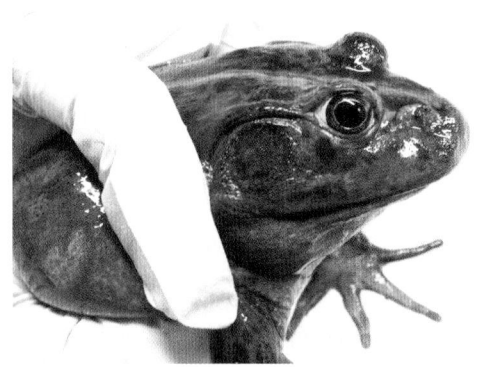
(B)

FIGURE 18.9 Male bullfrog tympanum is larger than eye diameter (A); female tympanum is approximately equal in diameter to eye (B).

tend to be blackish. Cloacal glands in male salamanders become swollen, resulting in enlarged cloacal lips. Male plethodontid salamanders develop enlarged hedonic glands on the chin; secretions of this gland are rubbed on the female during courtship. Most male frogs develop keratin pads on their thumbs to assist in gripping females during amplexus (a characteristic prolonged breeding embrace). Enlarged teeth can be found in certain frog and salamander males in breeding readiness. In some plethodontid species, these teeth are used to abrade the skin of females and allow introduction of chin gland secretions into the female's bloodstream (Conant and Collins, 1991; Zug, 1993; Petranka, 1998).

Courtship and reproduction in amphibians range from simple to very elaborate. Internal fertilization occurs in many salamander species. Salamanders may engage in ritual behavioral displays such as the 'hula' of *Notophthalmus viridescens*. In this dance, the male undulates his tail and body while swimming in front of a potential mate. If the female shows interest, the male deposits a spermatophore, and the female picks the packet up with her cloaca. *Plethodon cinereus* has a more complex courtship. Males use pheromone trails to locate receptive females. The male approaches the female, arches and undulates his tail, then rubs his hedonic gland secretions over her body (using his enlarged teeth to abrade her skin and introduce secretions into her system). The male next aligns himself along the female's body, keeping his tail arched and curled. The female places her chin on his dorsal surface above the vent, and the couple performs a 'tail-straddle walk.' Finally, the male deposits a spermatophore, the couple moves forward, and the female picks the packet up. The pair separates, the female deposits the fertilized eggs in clusters suspended by a pedicle, and she coils around the eggs until hatching (Petranka, 1998).

Frog courtship is no less colorful than that of salamanders. In general, frogs have external fertilization. In many species, males attract mates by vocalizing. When a receptive female is located, the male grasps her with his forelimbs in amplexus. The eggs are expelled, and the male releases sperm to fertilize them. Various adaptations of this basic plan include the courtship of the Surinam toad (*Pipa parva*), a relative of *Xenopus*. During amplexus, the pair swims in an upside-down circle, with the female releasing eggs at the top of the circle. The male releases sperm, and presses the fertilized eggs onto the back of the female The female's skin grows over the eggs, and the eggs are carried in this fashion until tadpoles hatch and emerge.

Nest guarding and egg brooding has been described in salamanders of the genera *Plethodon* and *Hemidactylum*. The midwife toad, *Alytes obstetricans*, exhibits another breeding strategy. After amplexus and fertilization, the male toad wraps the strands of eggs around his legs. He carries the eggs with him in this fashion, visiting ponds periodically to keep them moist until hatching (Mattison, 1998). Continued parental care is demonstrated by various amphibian species. *Pixicephalus adspersus* digs channels that permit tadpoles to travel from one body of water to another. Species of dendrobatid and hylid frogs that lay eggs in restricted pools with no available food, such as bromeliad axils, return to feed the tadpoles with trophic eggs. In some species, the tadpoles wriggle against the female in a begging behavior, which stimulates egg deposition (Vitt and Caldwell, 2009).

2. Husbandry

Many amphibian species have been successfully bred in the laboratory. Arginine vasotocin regulates reproductive behavior in amphibians (Boyd and Moore, 1992). In some species, temperature plays a more important role than photoperiod in certain aspects of reproduction (Paniagua *et al.*, 1990). Increasing day length in the axolotl light cycle will encourage breeding (Pramuk and Gagliardo, 2008).

3. Larval Amphibians and Metamorphosis

With few exceptions, larval amphibians are aquatic. Their skin is thin, fragile, and well vascularized to assist in respiration. Gills (internal or external) are typically present. All larvae lack eyelids. The skeleton is primarily to completely cartilaginous. Dorsal and ventral fins are present on the tail, and both the tail and body are heavily muscled for swimming. Lateral line systems are well developed in all amphibian larvae (Duellman and Trueb, 1986; Zug, 1993; Vitt and Caldwell, 2009).

Salamander larvae closely resemble adult animals, having four limbs and other common features. Premetamorphic tadpoles (frog larvae), in contrast, appear very different from adult frogs. Most tadpoles have a fleshy oral disc. This disc can be located dorsally, ventrally, or anteriorly, depending on method of feeding. Teeth are not present; tadpoles have horny beaks and denticles that rasp and cut. Gills are initially external but are soon covered, along with the forelimbs, by an operculum. Hindlimbs appear late in the larval period (Zug, 1993; Vitt and Caldwell, 2009).

Larvae should be housed in well-aerated aquaria in appropriate stocking densities. Care should be taken to separate large from small larvae, especially in cannibalistic species. Pfennig and Collins (1993) discovered that cannibalism develops more slowly if sibling larvae are housed together exclusively.

Metamorphosis requires the presence of thyroid hormone and iodine. Environmental factors such as crowding and reduced food availability can stimulate early thyroxine release and result in early metamorphosis (Vitt and Caldwell, 2009).

As larval development progresses (prometamorphosis) in tadpoles, external gills are resorbed and limbs develop. Immediately before emergence (metamorphic climax), the tail is resorbed, forelimbs break through the operculum, and the hindlimbs become functional (Duellman and Trueb, 1986; Zug, 1993).

Water levels should be decreased as larvae undergo metamorphic climax and prepare to emerge. In many cases, a ramp or other object should be placed on the water to facilitate emergence to a terrestrial existence. Newly transformed amphibians can drown if this assistance is not provided.

Metamorphosis is a time of immune stress in amphibians, and larvae that undergo metamorphosis at less-than-optimal size become immune-compromised (Rollins-Smith, 1998). Every effort should be made to prevent undue stressors and exposure to infectious agents during the metamorphic period.

E. Management and Reproduction of X. *laevis*

As previously noted, the African clawed frog, *X. laevis*, is used extensively in developmental, cellular, and molecular biology research. Current use of *X. laevis* has expanded largely due to its ease of maintenance, hardiness, adaptability to various housing arrangements, short generation time, and production of embryos with a high yield of genetic material. *X. laevis* is now a common resident in biomedical research facilities. (Gurdon, 1996).

1. Natural History

The African clawed frog belongs to the family Pipidae. There are 18 species of *Xenopus*, which occur throughout Africa. *Xenopus* used in research are exported from the Cape, South Africa (Tinsley, 2010). The clawed frog ranges from central to South Africa in a wide variety of habitats, including rivers, lakes, swamps, ditches, and wells. It appears to prefer still, opaque, vegetation-filled water, although populations are found in clear streams. In lakes devoid of fish, *Xenopus* has evolved to occupy the fish niche. This species occurs at altitudes up to 3000 meters (Tinsley *et al.*, 1996a).

Xenopus tolerates a fairly wide water-temperature range. Adults become stressed at prolonged temperatures less than 14°C (57°F) and greater than 26°C (81°F). At these extremes, a decrease in oocyte quality is observed (Wu and Gerhart, 1991). Individuals have been known to survive in ice-covered ponds and desert ponds. When temperatures become too hot (30°C, 86°F), *X. laevis* will excavate pits in the cool mud on the bottom of ponds. In drought conditions, it will estivate (Tinsley *et al.*, 1996a). In the wild, *Xenopus* will breed in both acidic and alkaline water (however, tadpole survival rates decrease in water with a pH of 5). *X. laevis* will also tolerate elevated salinity (40% seawater) for a short time (Tinsley *et al.*, 1996a).

2. Anatomy and Physiology

X. laevis has a yellowish to darker, spotted to marbled dorsal coloring. The frog's ventral surface is solid yellowish white to spotted. This species has a fifth toe that is much longer than the tibia. Female *X. laevis* are larger than males and average 110 mm in length (Kobel *et al.*, 1996). Females have large cloacal papillae, and males develop dark inner surfaces on their forearms (nuptial pads). The skin secretions of *Xenopus* include thyrotropin releasing hormone, caerulein, and xenopsin. Antimicrobial compounds (magainins) are also found in skin secretions (Kreil, 1996).

Xenopus lacks a tongue; when feeding, it lowers buccopharyngeal pressure and opens its mouth, suctioning prey in. *X. laevis* also shreds prey with its hind claws and uses its front feet to sweep food into its mouth (Tinsley *et al.*, 1996a; Carreño and Nishikawa, 2010). The eyes of the clawed frog are located more dorsally on the head, are lidless, have a convex cornea, and are adapted for vision in air rather than water. *Xenopus* floats at the water's surface, and vision is directed upward; therefore, objects passing above will elicit a hiding response from the frog. There are two separate olfactory cavities – one

for detecting scent in water, and one for airborne odors. The lateral line system is located dorsally and ventrally, and is retained in adult animals. The vocal apparatus of the clawed frog is designed for underwater sound production (Deuchar, 1975). Animals vocalize by clicking. *Xenopus* can be territorial and form dominant/subordinate hierarchies (Tinsley, 2010).

The lungs, heart, and liver of *Xenopus* are large, and the urinary bladder is spherical. *Xenopus* must come to the water's surface and gulp air, because cutaneous respiration is not as well developed as in other species. Even tadpoles develop and utilize lungs as well as gills for breathing (Deuchar, 1975).

During times of drought, *Xenopus* adapts physiologically by producing urea rather than ammonia. When ample water is available, the frog reverts to production of the more toxic ammonia, which is rapidly dissipated in the water (Tinsley *et al.*, 1996a).

Life span of *X. laevis* in the wild is reported to be greater than 10 years. In captivity, the clawed frog can live 20 years (Tinsley, 2010).

3. Housing and Husbandry

X. laevis are hardy frogs and can be kept successfully in a variety of housing situations. Tanks can be constructed of fiberglass, glass, plastic, or stainless steel. Unless the sides of the tank are tall, lids should be provided. Screen, metal grills, and perforated plastic lids are commonly used. *Xenopus* will jump out of tanks if water levels are low (such as during cleaning) and when they are startled. Commercial vendors, such as Aquatic Habitats, Inc.; Aquaneering, Inc.; and Techniplast, Inc. offer custom-designed *Xenopus* housing with recirculating systems. In the wild, *X. laevis* is commonly found in murky water. This dark water provides a visual barrier to predators (Tinsley *et al.*, 1996a). Although one study determined that *X. laevis* growth rates were unaffected by provision of cover (Gouchie *et al.*, 2008). Torreilles and Green (2007) demonstrated that addition of refuges resulted in decrease in bite wounds and cannibalism in group-housed *X. laevis*. Provision of refuges has included partially covered tanks, PVC or ABS pipe segments, stainless steel rabbit feeders, aquarium logs, round ceramic tiles, clay pots, and lily pads (Kaplan, 1993; Major and Wassersug, 1998; Brown and Nixon, 2004) (Fig. 18.10).

Both static and flow-through systems are also used. To prevent fouling of water, static systems should be changed after animals have fed. Inexpensive modified, nonrecirculating systems have been described (Dawson *et al.*, 1992; Rogers *et al.*, 1997). Recirculating systems may incorporate charcoal or sand filters to clean and reuse water. Flow-through systems frequently contain a standpipe to drain accumulated water and feces, and a hose or other constant-drip water source. Both flow-through and recirculating

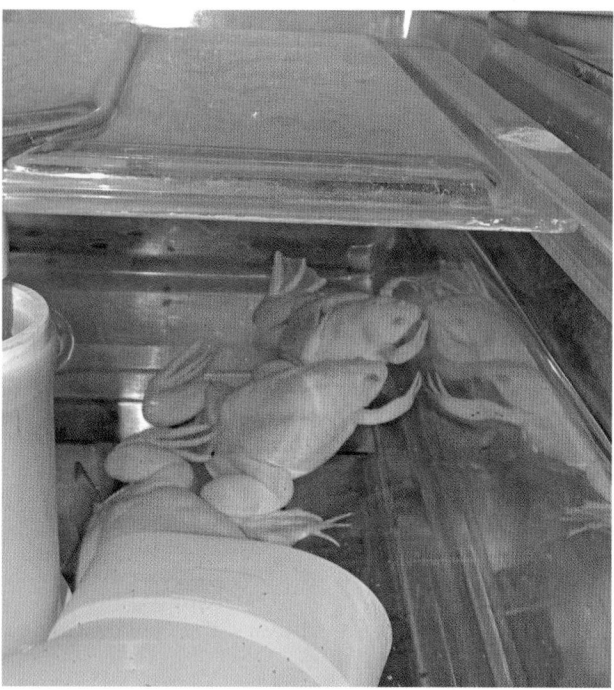

FIGURE 18.10	*X. laevis* group housed in commercial housing unit with PVC pipe for refuge.

systems are now commercially available through several companies. Regardless of the system, water should be dechlorinated before it is added to the tank.

Water depth can vary from 5 to 20 cm. One study concluded that although water that is too shallow will increase stress and escape response, no difference in growth was documented between water that was 5, 10, and 20 cm deep (Hilken *et al.*, 1995). This study, however, was limited by the small number of animals used, lack of detail about the study subjects, and a short study period. Tinsley (2010) prefers 30–50 cm water depth, but notes that captive reared animals can be housed adequately in 15 cm water depth.

Population density within the *Xenopus* tank is a critical factor in growth and productivity. Suggested stocking densities of adult breeding frogs range from one frog per 3 L to four frogs per 5–10 L (McBride, 1978; Dawson *et al.*, 1992; Hilken *et al.*, 1995; Major and Wassersug, 1998; Tinsley, 2010). Increase in stocking densities will cause decrease in growth. Most facilities house *X. laevis* at 21–22°C (Green, 2010). Some facilities keep *Xenopus* on a natural light cycle; however, most facilities use a constant 12 h light–12 h dark cycle, especially if breeding the frogs year-round (Major and Wassersug, 1998). Housing *Xenopus* directly under very bright light should be avoided (Hilken *et al.*, 1994).

Adult *Xenopus* should always be handled with soft nets or gloved hands to prevent skin abrasions and disruptions of the protective mucous layer.

4. Diet

In the wild, *Xenopus* eat a wide variety of prey items, including aquatic invertebrates, small crustaceans, and insects. Amphibians (including *Xenopus* tadpoles), small birds, and fish have also been documented as occasional prey items. Clawed frogs use olfaction rather then vision as the primary means of locating food; therefore, they will also scavenge carcasses (Tinsley *et al.*, 1996a). Groups of feeding *Xenopus* can become quite aggressive, resulting in bite wounds.

Laboratory-housed *Xenopus* are typically maintained on commercially prepared diets. Among those in use are salmon chow (Soft-Moist Salmon Diet, Rangen, Inc.), trout chow (Purina), and Frog Brittle (Nasco). Trout chow can be purchased in both floating and sinking forms, comes in various sizes, and does not break down in water. The amount of food per frog per feeding will vary depending on age, season, gender, and water temperature. Manufacturer-recommended volume of *Xenopus* frog brittle is 1 g/frog (Green, 2010).

Additional foods for clawed frogs have included earthworms, mealworms, chick embryos, *Tubifex* worms, goldfish, and crickets. Feeding chitin-containing animals (crickets, mealworms) excessively can result in intestinal obstruction.

Tanks should be cleaned after *Xenopus* are fed; however, care should be taken not to disturb the frogs for at least an hour, or they may regurgitate their food (Etheridge and Richter, 1978; McBride, 1978; Dawson *et al.*, 1992).

5. Reproduction

Under ideal conditions, *X. laevis* will undergo metamorphosis at 2 months and will reach sexual maturity within 8 months of hatching. Cooler temperatures will slow development. In the wild, the breeding cycle corresponds to the onset of the rainy season and subsequent prey abundance (Tinsley *et al.*, 1996a). Females reach optimum egg production at 2–3 years and continue producing for several years.

Females can be primed with HCG to induce egg laying. Green (2010) recommends resting ovulated females a minimum of 1–3 months. For natural matings, frogs should be bred in containers with false bottoms, to allow passage of the eggs and prevent ingestion by the parents. Each egg has an individual jelly capsule; therefore, eggs are less likely to clump as they do in other frog species. Larvae hatch 3 days after spawning.

6. Tadpole Biology

Xenopus tadpoles have functional lungs as well as gills, and will periodically surface to breathe. Tadpoles orient themselves parallel to one another and hover in a characteristic head-down fashion, using their undulating tails to direct food particles to their mouths (Fig. 18.11). They are very efficient filter feeders and eat materials

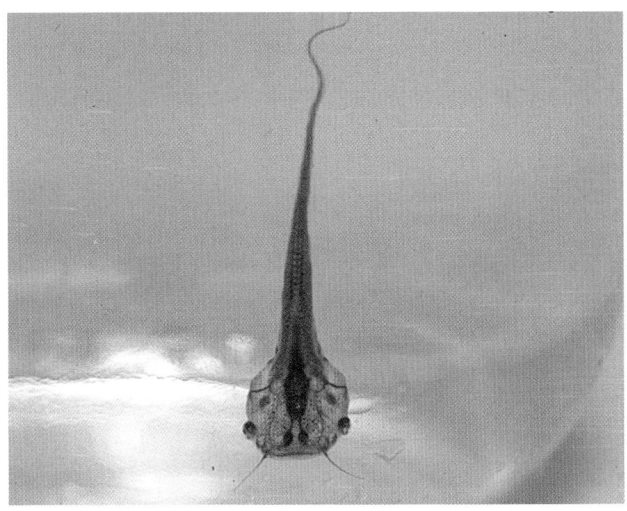

FIGURE 18.11 *X. laevis* tadpole hovering in characteristic head-down fashion.

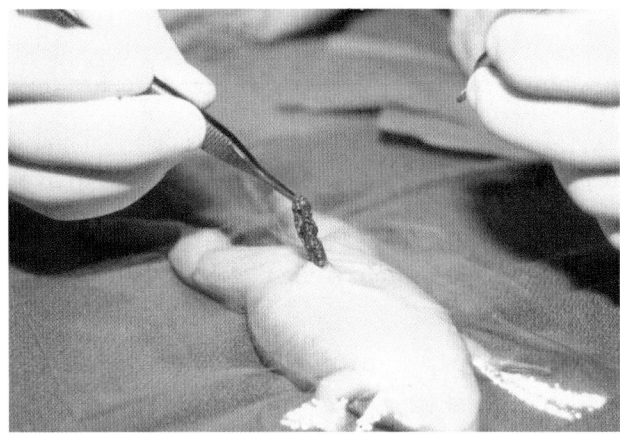

FIGURE 18.12 Surgical oocyte harvest in *X. laevis*.

suspended in the water. From hatching through day 4, tadpoles absorb yolk sac; they begin feeding on day 5. In the wild, plankton makes up the bulk of the diet of the *Xenopus* tadpole. In captivity, powdered tadpole food is commonly used. A pelleted tadpole diet can be fed to larger larvae. Tadpoles are generally fed twice weekly, and water should be changed after they feed. *Xenopus* tadpoles can be stocked at a density of 50/L initially, decreasing to 5/L at onset of metamorphosis (Green, 2010).

7. Oocyte Harvest

Buffered tricaine methane sulfonate (MS222) is used to anesthetize *Xenopus* for surgical oocyte harvest. Once anesthetized, the animal can be removed and anesthesia maintained if necessary by dripping the solution on the skin. Oocyte harvests can normally be completed in 30 min or less and should not require supplemental anesthesia. Once the procedure is concluded, the frog can be recovered from anesthesia by rinsing in clean, dechlorinated water or water from the primary enclosure and placing into a recovery tank with a very shallow water level. In order to reduce stress, the water used for both induction and recovery can be taken from the *Xenopus* tank. Frogs should be closely observed during induction and recovery, to ensure that drowning does not occur.

Aseptic technique must be used when harvesting oocytes surgically. A mask, sterile gloves, and sterile drapes should be used; impervious clear sterile drapes work well. Because *Xenopus* skin contains antimicrobial agents, a sterile saline prep can be used. Alternatively, dilute benzalkonium chloride or chlorhexidine solutions can be used sparingly for skin prep. Soaps and scrubs must not be used, for they will destroy the protective mucous layer.

The incision is made paramedian in the lower abdominal quadrant on either side (sides can be alternated in sequential surgeries to allow maximum healing time). Forceps are used to grasp the ovary and exteriorize the oocyte masses. The desired number of oocytes are excised, and the remainder carefully replaced in the coelomic cavity (Fig. 18.12). Muscle and skin layers are closed separately with 4–0 suture in a simple interrupted pattern. Absorbable suture can be used in the muscle layer. Tuttle *et al.* (2006) found monofilament nylon the least reactive for skin closure in amphibians, and warn that silk and chromic gut cause strong tissue reaction; gut also dehisces. Common analgesics that have been used in *Xenopus* or other frog species include buprenorphine, butorphanol, and meloxicam (Koeller, 2009; Minter *et al.*, 2011). Most doses are empirical for *Xenopus*, because pharmacokinetics have not been studied. After analgesic administration, care should be exercised to ensure that the frog's swimming and other motor functions are not impaired to the point of risking drowning. Once recovered, the frog can be returned to its home tank. Frogs are rested for at least a month between surgeries. Sutures should be removed in about 6 weeks if they have not sloughed out with shed skin.

F. Physical Examination and Techniques

1. Physical Examination

Physical examination of an amphibian should begin with observing the animal in its primary enclosure. Attitude, posture, equilibrium (especially if in water), locomotion, body color, respiration, and behavior should be noted. Axolotls that are stressed may float, rub, roll, or dart about the tank; these behaviors are abnormal in the typically sedentary bottom-dweller (Gresens, 2004). Sick *Xenopus* often float and are reluctant to dive (Green, 2010). The amphibian's enclosure should be checked for appropriate temperature, humidity, and cleanliness.

Presence and nature of feces and vomitus should be recorded. Once this initial assessment has been made, the animal can be removed from the cage for closer examination.

When restraining amphibians, care should always be taken to support the animal's entire body, and to avoid disrupting the protective mucous layer. When handling larger or more-aggressive amphibians, it is advisable to have one person restrain while the second performs the physical exam.

The surface of the skin should be thoroughly examined for ulcerations, abrasions, redness, or other lesions. Heart rate can be determined while examining the ventral body surface. Abdominal palpation can be attempted; however, many amphibians will inflate the abdomen as a defense mechanism, making palpation difficult. The corneas should be clear, and a blink reflex should be present (except in species such as *Xenopus*, which lack eyelids). Nares should be free of exudate. The mouth can be gently opened with a thin, flat plastic speculum, and the oral cavity examined for lesions, excessive salivation, or exudate. Care should be taken to avoid breaking the thin delicate maxillary bones. Withdrawal and righting reflexes can be tested (Raphael, 1993; Wright, 1996). The amphibian should be weighed and its body condition assessed before returning it to its enclosure. Body condition can be determined by observing the prominence of the skeletal system (particularly the pelvic bones in frogs), and by palpating muscles and abdominal contents (Crawshaw, 1993).

2. Blood Collection

Blood samples should be collected in lithium heparinized syringes. The midventral abdominal vein has been used to collect blood in both frogs and salamanders. A small-gauge needle appropriate for the amphibian's size (usually a 26- to 27-gauge) is inserted at a point midway between the sternum and pelvis in a cranial direction, and the sample is collected. The ventral caudal vein in salamanders can be used as a phlebotomy site. Frogs have a prominent lingual venous plexus situated beneath the tongue. The tongue can be gently drawn forward with a cotton-tipped applicator, the plexus punctured with a needle, and the blood sample collected in a heparinized capillary tube (Wright, 1996). Because *Xenopus* have neither tail nor tongue, and also lack a prominent midventral abdominal vein, cardiocentesis under anesthesia is the preferred method of terminal blood collection in this species (Green, 2010). Blood has been collected from the facial vein in some species (Forzán *et al.*, 2012).

3. Other Diagnostic Tests

Fecal examination is performed as for other species. Specimens collected for microbial culture and sensitivity should be incubated at both standard and room

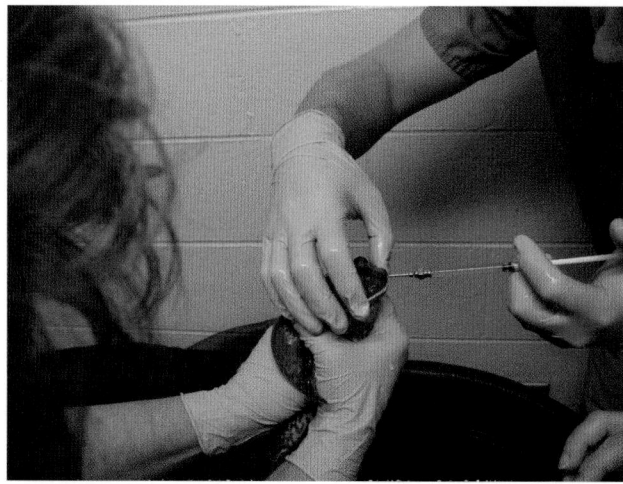

FIGURE 18.13   Drugs can be administered orally to frogs using gavage needles.

temperatures. Impression smears, skin scrapings, and abdominocentesis are performed as for other species. Biopsies can be taken under MS222 anesthesia, and the skin closed with nonabsorbable suture or tissue glue. Radiology is very useful in identifying foreign bodies, impactions, and pneumonia, and for assessing skeletal abnormalities. Digital dental radiography works well for small amphibians. Fluoroscopy, endoscopy, and transillumination (using an intense, cool light source) have also been used in amphibians (Crawshaw, 1993; Raphael, 1993; Wright, 1996).

4. Injections/Gavaging

Common routes of injection include intramuscular, intracoelomic, and dorsal lymph sac. The muscles of the forelimbs in frogs and the epaxial muscles in salamanders are locations for intramuscular injections (Wright, 1996). Intracoelomic injections should be given off midline in the lower abdomen, and dorsal lymph sac injections are given subcutaneously in the caudodorsal part of the frog's body (over the pelvic area). Gavaging can be accomplished using standard rodent stainless steel gavage tubes, or with IV Teflon catheters in small species (Wright, 1996) (Fig. 18.13).

5. Euthanasia and Necropsy

Euthanasia solutions such as sodium pentobarbital overdose can be injected IV or into the coelom or the dorsal lymph sacs of amphibians. Immersion or injection of buffered tricaine methane sulfonate (MS222), and immersion or topical application of benzocaine are also considered acceptable (AVMA, 2013). Torreilles *et al.* (2009) recommend following MS222 immersion with secondary physical methods. Detailed information on additional euthanasia methods can be found in the most current AVMA Guidelines for the Euthanasia of Animals (AVMA, 2013).

Normal anatomic features sometimes encountered during necropsy include Bidder's organ in male toads, which appear grossly in a grapelike cluster. Some animals have paravertebral lime sacs, which can appear as white structures along the vertebral column and within the skull; these are associated with calcium metabolism.

Normal reproductively active frog ovaries are typically black; black pigment is also found in liver of amphibians. However, antigenic stimulation and starvation will cause melanomacrophage stimulation and subsequent increase in black pigment.

Sample collection should always include multiple skin scrapings and wet mounts from various body surface areas, including seat patches and gills. Abdominal fluid should be collected for cytology. Heart blood, liver, spleen, and abdominal fluid can be collected for microbial culture. Other indicators of disease processes include rubbery, deformed bones associated with metabolic bone disease (MBD) and cloudy cornea and anterior chamber, associated with corneal lipidosis or secondary uveitis due to septicemia (Pessier and Pinkerton, 2003).

III. DISEASES

A. Infectious Diseases

1. *Bacterial*

a. Bacterial Septicemia (or Bacterial Infection)

Etiology Cutaneous manifestations of bacterial septicemia have been termed 'red leg' in the past and represent one of the more widely recognized syndromes in amphibians (Pessier, 2002). While red leg is historically considered a clinicial sign associated with bacterial dermatosepticemia (Densmore and Green, 2007), other underlying disease (e.g., ranavirus infection) can cause similar clinical signs. The first organism isolated from amphibians with red leg was *Aeromonas hydrophila*, a gram-negative bacterial rod. Other organisms that have also been reported as causative agents include *Proteus, Escherichia coli, Aerobacter, Pseudomonas, Citrobacter, Staphylococcus, Streptococcus, Enterobacter, Klebsiella,* and *Chryseobacterium*. Many of these are frequently found in the aquatic environment and are opportunistic pathogens (Hubbard, 1981; Hird et al., 1981; Green, 2010).

Epizootiology and Transmission Stress and subsequent immunosuppression predispose amphibians to colonization by opportunistic bacteria. Often, organisms are transmitted to susceptible animals through the tank water. Animals with this symptom have been associated with mass mortalities in both wild and captive

populations (Hubbard, 1981; Nyman, 1986; Rafidah et al., 1990). *Chryseobacterium* and *Aeromonas* have high epizootic potential (Klaphake, 2009).

Pathogenesis Bacterial sepsis often occurs following stress, injury, trauma, dehydration, parasites, systemic disease, or water quality problems. Waterborne bacteria can colonize the skin and visceral organs of frogs and salamanders. Course of the disease can be either acute or chronic and a single animal or many cohorts in a tank may show symptoms (Rafidah et al., 1990; Green, 2010).

Clinical Signs Signs of acute infection include petechiation, swelling, ecchymosis, and ulceration of the skin, particularly evident on the legs, digits, and abdomen (Fig. 18.14). Lethargy, anorexia, and ascites are also seen. Ocular and periocular inflammation is often noted with this disease. Chronically infected animals may exhibit ascites and neurologic signs (Hubbard, 1981; Nyman, 1986; Rafidah et al., 1990; Crawshaw, 1993; Williams and Whitaker, 1994; Wright, 1996; Green, 2010).

Necropsy Findings Hepatic necrosis, splenic congestion, and other lesions consistent with septic thrombi are commonly seen (Wright, 1996).

Differential Diagnoses Organisms that cause similar lesions include numerous other bacteria including *Chryseobacterium* (formerly *Flavobacterium*) (Crawshaw, 1993; Wright, 1996; Green, 2010). Cutaneous hyperemia can be associated with chlamydophilosis, systemic iridovirus infection, and *Batrachochytrium dendrobates* infection (chytridiomycosis) can mimic or be concurrent infections (Pessier, 2002; Hill et al., 2010).

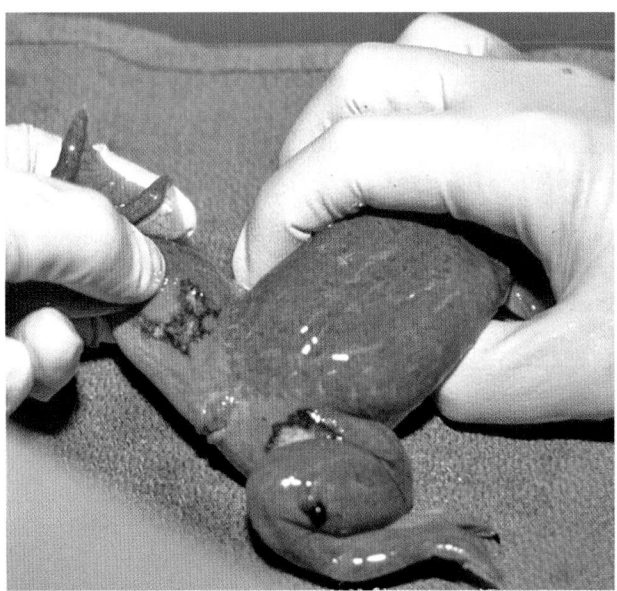

FIGURE 18.14 Ulcerated skin lesions can be one manifestation of bacterial septicemia and other systemic disease in amphibians.

Treatment Appropriate treatment is based on culture results, identification of the pathogen, and sensitivity. Identification and correction of husbandry issues may also play a critical role in treatment. Resolution may be complicated with concurrent disease processes. Treatment with systemic antibiotics may have limited success depending on simultaneous health status (Green, 2010). Many current antibiotic regimens are based on extrapolations from pharmacokinetic studies in terrestrial reptiles, semiaquatic frogs, and mammalian species (Howard *et al.*, 2010). Tetracycline (50 mg/kg PO BID) can be effective against *Aeromonas*. Valuable animals should be concomitantly treated with aminoglycosides (5 mg/kg IM q48 h). Chloramphenicol at 50 mg/kg IM, IP q24 h has also been effective against gram-negative bacteria (Raphael, 1993; Crawshaw, 1993; Wright, 1996). Stoskopf *et al.* (1987) found that gentamicin at 2.5 mg/kg IM q72 h provided therapeutic blood levels in *Necturus* housed at 3°C. Another study demonstrated that *Rana pipiens* required 3 mg/kg IM SID to achieve therapeutic levels when housed at 22°C (Teare *et al.*, 1991). Riviere *et al.* (1979) showed that immersion in a solution of gentamicin sulfate would provide therapeutic levels in *R. pipiens*; however, Teare *et al.* (1991) demonstrated that this concentration resulted in increasing serum levels and death after 120 h. Small lesions may be treated by housing animals singly in Ringer's Solution (changed SID) and topical application of Shield-X® on the affected area (Green, 2010). Caution should be used if adding antibiotics to water as it may kill microbiologic filters and may induce resistance to pathogens. Recently, pharmacokinetics of enrofloxacin were determined in *X. laevis* after a 10 mg/kg intramuscular or subcutaneous enrofloxacin injection. Plasma concentrations reached levels considered to be effective against common aquatic pathogens. Even in this instance, authors recommend changing the habitat water daily to prevent reabsorption of drug excretion (Howard *et al.*, 2010).

Control Affected animals should be isolated and husbandry practices reviewed to ensure that appropriate water quality, temperature, stocking density, and food are provided. The environment should be thoroughly cleaned and disinfected. Maintenance of the animal's slime coat layer of the skin is important.

Prevention Amphibians should be housed in clean, dechlorinated water with proper stocking density and temperature. When handling animals, gloves should be worn. Animals should be provided nutritious food on a feeding schedule appropriate for the species. Newly arrived animals must be quarantined separately and thoroughly examined before introduction into the existing colony. Animals should be colony-reared rather than wild-caught if at all possible.

Research Complications Bacterial infection can severely decimate research populations of adult and larval amphibians. The presence of this symptom may be indicative of other problems (Cunningham *et al.*, 1996a). Data can be affected by using chronically infected animals.

b. *Pseudomonas*

Etiology *Pseudomonas*, a gram-negative rod, is commonly found in the aquatic and terrestrial environment.

Epizootiology and Transmission The organism is a waterborne opportunist, which typically causes secondary infections in immunosuppressed animals. Experimental infections caused mortality in *Rana pipiens*, housed under suboptimal conditions (Taylor, 2001).

Pathogenesis In *Necturus*, the organism colonizes the gills (Anver and Pond, 1984). *Pseudomonas* has also been implicated in ulcerative disease in axolotls (Crawshaw, 1993).

Clinical Signs In axolotls and other amphibian species, *Pseudomonas* is associated with skin sloughing, discoloration, and ulceration. *Necturus* may become septicemic and die (Raphael, 1993; Anver and Pond, 1984).

Necropsy Findings Lesions in the mudpuppy include necrotic gray foci on the gills and cutaneous hyperemia (Anver and Pond, 1984).

Differential Diagnoses Other bacterial agents that may cause ulceration, skin sloughing, and hyperemia include *Aeromonas* and *Proteus*.

Treatment Gentamicin and chloramphenicol are the antibiotics of choice in treating *Pseudomonas*. Doses are the same as for *Aeromonas*.

Control Control is the same as for *Aeromonas* and other waterborne opportunistic bacteria.

Prevention Prevention is the same as for *Aeromonas*.

Research Complications As with *Aeromonas*, *Pseudomonas* can cause significant morbidity and mortality in research amphibians, thus preventing accurate data collection.

c. Mycobacteriosis

Etiology A number of *Mycobacterium* species have been detected and described in various amphibians (Martinho and Heatley, 2012; Hill *et al.*, 2010; Trott *et al.*, 2004; Godfrey *et al.*, 2007; Green *et al.*, 2000; Sánchez-Morgado *et al.*, 2009; Shrenzel, 2012). These include *M. marinum*, *M. chelonei*, *M. fortuitum*, *M. xenopi*, *M. avium intracellulare complex*, *M. liflandii*, *M. szulgai*, *M. gordonae*, *M. ulcerans*, and *Mycobacterium* sp. These acid-fast organisms are common saprophytes of soil and water (Wright, 1996; Klaphake, 2009). In captivity, both collections and laboratory models have been affected, including caecilians, anurans, and caudates. Generally, the organism is being reported in adult animals, after metamorphosis (Martinho and Heatley, 2012).

Epizootiology and Transmission Transmission of mycobacteriosis is most likely to amphibians through direct contact between infected individuals, contaminated water, and fomites.

Pathogenesis The organisms typically colonize amphibian skin from the water and may form nodules or ulcerations. They can also spread to the viscera and form granulomas in organs either with or without skin abnormalities (Crawshaw, 1993). *Rana pipiens* demonstrated chronic, nonlethal granulomatous disease in immunocompetent frogs; steroid-treated frogs developed an acute, lethal disease (Ramakrishnan *et al.*, 1997). It is typically a chronic, slow progressive disease in immunocompetent individuals, however in stressed or immunosuppressed, the course of infection is much more severe, leading to acute and systemic disease (Martinho and Heatley, 2012).

Clinical Signs Typically, amphibians suffering from mycobacteriosis will demonstrate wasting in spite of a good appetite. Pneumonia may develop. Nodules or ulcers may be seen on the skin surface. Extensive skin lesions can interfere with cutaneous respiration. As the disease progresses, animals become more debilitated and eventually die (Crawshaw, 1993; Raphael, 1993; Klaphake, 2009). Infected *X. laevis* have also presented with the loss of diving reflex and distended abdomens (Tarigo *et al.*, 2006).

Necropsy Findings Gross lesions include yellowish white dermal and visceral granulomas and ulcerations (Fig. 18.15) (Fremont-Rahl *et al.*, 2011). Visceral granulomas are most commonly found in the liver. Acid-fast organisms frequently are present in the granulomas (Anver and Pond, 1984). Chronic granulomatous inflammation is a hallmark of mycobacteriosis

(Fig. 18.16) (Densmore and Green, 2007). It is important to note that the clinical signs of mycobacteriosis vary based on the species of mycobacteria, the species of amphibian, and environmental conditions (Martinho and Heatley, 2012).

Differential Diagnoses Fungal infections can cause cutaneous ulcers and granulomas. Lesions can be cultured and examined histologically with acid-fast stains to distinguish between mycobacterial and mycotic infections. Other nodular skin diseases of amphibians include chromomycosis, neoplasia, abscesses, encysted metazoan parasites, and herpes-like infections (Pessier, 2002). Molecular methods such as PCR are now reliable and suitable for detecting Mycobacteria.

Treatment Occasional treatments have been reported in the literature (amputation of distal limbs and administration of azithromycin or clarithromycin) (Martinho and Heatley, 2012). Because of the zoonotic potential and possible spread of infection, most affected animals are culled.

Control Disease can be controlled by isolating and treating or culling affected animals, and by cleaning and disinfecting the environment. Identification of predisposing or contributory factors may also help.

Prevention Quarantine, good husbandry (clean environment, appropriate food and temperature, lack of abrasive objects in tank, and low stocking density) will help prevent mycobacteriosis.

Research Complications Debilitated animals are inappropriate as research subjects. Additionally, this disease is potentially zoonotic, therefore gloves should be worn when handling frogs, equipment, and water.

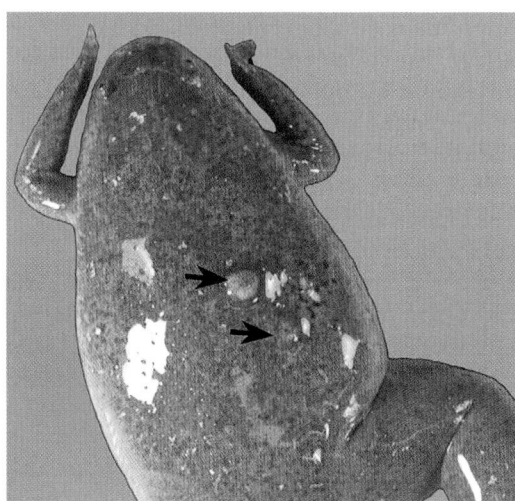

FIGURE 18.15 Skin; *Xenopus* (*Silurana*) *tropicalis* frog with *Mycobacterium liflandii* infection. Nodular, tan-red, discrete foci (arrows) on skin of the dorsum. *Modified from Fremont-Rahl et al.* (2011).

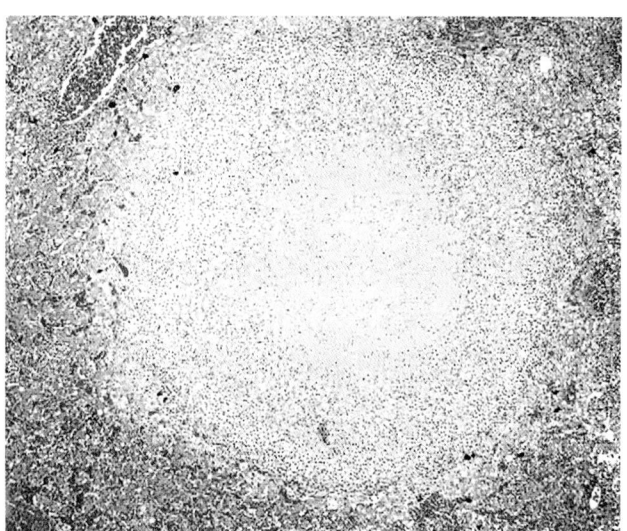

FIGURE 18.16 Liver; *Xenopus* (*Silurana*) *tropicalis* frog, hematoxylin and eosin. Focal, discrete, necrogranulomatous mycobacterium-induced lesion in liver with a central necrotic core bordered by a pale, cellular layer of inflammatory cells (macrophages). *Modified from Fremont-Rahl et al.* (2011).

d. Chryseobacterium (*Formerly* Flavobacterium)

Etiology *Chryseobacterium* are gram-negative, aerobic rods that are found in both soil and water. The organism is pigmented yellowish orange. Reports of this bacterial disease appear in the literature in association with both wild and captive amphibian populations, including anurans and caudates (Green *et al.*, 1999; Densmore and Green, 2007). These bacteria are highly resistant to antibiotics and chlorine/chloramines in certain conditions (Green, 2010).

Epizootiology and Transmission The organism is commonly present in aquatic environments and can enter through a wound or abrasion. Disease can occur in animals that are not stressed, however infection in immunosuppressed and stressed animals is the current thought (Olson *et al.*, 1992; Densmore and Green, 2007).

Pathogenesis *Chryseobacterium* can spread to multiple organs, ultimately causing septicemia. Some species are known to affect the nervous system (Olson *et al.*, 1992; Taylor *et al.*, 1993).

Clinical Signs Signs of *Chryseobacterium* infection resemble septicemia and may include weight loss, edema, ascites, petechia, dyspnea, uveitis, corneal edema, incoordination, or sudden death.

Necropsy Findings Histologic changes are vascular congestion and hemorrhage, panophthalmitis with conjunctival and corneal edema, cardiac and skeletal myositis, and hepatocellular degeneration and necrosis (Olson *et al.*, 1992). Other reported findings include panophthalmitis, meningitis, and otitis (Taylor *et al.*, 1993); macrophage and neutrophilic infiltration of liver, spleen, and kidney have also been described (Green *et al.*, 1999). Diagnosis can be made from microbial culture of blood, organs, coelomic fluid, environmental samples, and PCR (Green, 2010; Densmore and Green, 2007).

Differential Diagnoses Clinical signs and gross findings are nonspecific and include effusion in lymphatic sacs, hydrocoelom, corneal edema, petechiation and visceral congestion. These can closely resemble other bacterial infections (Densmore and Green, 2007).

Treatment Past literature references antibiotic therapy of trimethoprim sulfa, however treatment in *Xenopus* spp. is not recommended (Raphael, 1993; Green, 2010).

Control Sick animals should be isolated and the environment cleaned and disinfected, as for other bacterial diseases.

Prevention Husbandry practices used to prevent bacterial infections should help prevent outbreaks.

Research Complications This organism has epizootic potential and can seriously affect research colonies. It also has potential to be zoonotic, therefore diseased animals may pose a potential threat to researchers and animal-care staff.

e. Salmonella

Etiology The genus *Salmonella* contains two species, *S. bongori* which infects mainly poikilotherms and rarely, humans, and *S. enterica* which includes approximately 2500 serovars. *Salmonella* are properly designated using their serovar (which was often a species name formerly), so, for example, *S. enterica* subsp. *enterica* serovar Typhimurium (aka *S.* Typhimurium) and serovar Enteritidis (*S.* Enteritidis). (Miller and Pegues, 2000). *Salmonella* can infect many vertebrates, including numerous amphibians such as frogs, newts, and toads (Taylor *et al.*, 2001). Amphibians may carry pathogenic *Salmonella*, but are rarely clinically affected (Klaphake, 2009). Zoonotic concerns should be considered.

Epizootiology and Transmission The organism is most commonly shed by the fecal–oral route. Amphibians may be good reservoirs with high potential to contaminate aquatic environments (Klaphake, 2009).

Pathogenesis The organism colonizes the intestinal tract; it can also spread via the blood.

Clinical Signs Affected amphibians exhibit anemia, lethargy, anorexia, and diarrhea (Raphael, 1993; Crawshaw, 1993). Prevalence from clinically normal animals has been reported from 10–60% (Klaphake, 2009).

Necropsy Findings Gross and histopathologic lesions are consistent with enteritis and septicemia.

Differential Diagnoses Other bacteria that can cause septicemia. Blood or lymph cultures will identify the causative agent. Cloacal and/or fecal cultures will help determine the cause of diarrhea (Raphael, 1993).

Treatment Appropriate antibiotics should be selected based on culture and sensitivity results, however it is unlikely treatment will eliminate *Salmonella* from amphibians (Taylor *et al.*, 2001).

Control Isolation and disinfection of the environment should be done as for other bacterial agents. Certain *Salmonella* are zoonotic; care should be taken when handling infected animals.

Prevention Amphibians should be obtained from reliable, colony-bred sources; quarantined; and maintained in appropriate conditions.

Research Complications Anemia and diarrhea may affect results in physiologic and other types of studies. Clinically ill amphibians shedding *Salmonella* are most likely harboring a primary illness and underlying causes should be explored.

f. Chlamydia

Etiology *Chlamydophila* are gram-negative, obligate intracellular coccoid organisms. This agent has been commonly reported in birds and more recently in reptiles (Klaphake, 2009). *C. psittaci* and *C. pneumoniae* have been reported in *Xenopus* spp. and are the most frequently identified species associated with infection (Green, 2010).

Epizootiology and Transmission *C. psittaci* is most commonly transmitted through the fecal–oral route. The organism is commonly found in wild and captive populations of anurans.

Pathogenesis The organism colonizes the lung, liver, spleen, kidney, and heart of *Xenopus* and causes a pyogranulomatous inflammatory response.

Clinical Signs Signs include lethargy, bloating, dysequilibrium, subcutaneous edema, hydrocoelom, bloat, and erythema and patchy depigmentation of skin (Pessier, 2002). Infection has been reported to clinically appear similar to other systemic bacterial infections (Taylor *et al.*, 2001).

Necropsy Findings Gross lesions consist of hepatosplenomegaly, cutaneous petechiation and ulceration, gelatinous coelomic effusion, and edema. Dense, basophilic intracytoplasmic inclusions can be found in hepatocytes and splenocytes. Interstitial pneumonia, glomerulonephritis, and endocarditis have also been described (Newcomer *et al.*, 1982). African clawed frogs infected with *Chlamydophila* spp. often develop a necrotizing and granulomatous epicarditis and myocarditis (Heinz-Taheny, 2009).

Differential Diagnoses *Aeromonas, Chryseobacterium*, and iridovirus infections can produce cutaneous lesions similar to those of chlamydophilosis. Diagnosis can be made by ideally observing the following: typical chlamydial inclusions, microbial culture, PCR, immunohistochemistry, or evidence of histopathology with pathologic significance (Crawshaw, 1993; Wright, 1996; Klaphake, 2009; Green, 2010; Reed et al., 2000).

Treatment Tetracylines such as doxycycline at (10–50 mg/kg SID) are reported, however it is also recommended to cull affected animals (Green, 2010; Pessier, 2002; Densmore and Green, 2007).

Control Affected amphibians should generally be culled. Although treatment may be attempted with valuable animals. *Chlamydia* spp. are zoonotic; therefore, appropriate precautions should be taken. Proper sanitization of housing and equipment should be performed.

Prevention Amphibians should be purchased from reliable, disease-free sources. Appropriate husbandry should be provided, and sick animals should receive a thorough diagnostic workup to determine causative agents.

Research Complications This disease can cause significant animal loss, as well as interfere with physiologic and reproductive studies. Diseased animals pose a potential threat to researchers and animal-care staff.

2. Viral

a. Lucké Herpesvirus

Etiology The Lucké herpesvirus (ranid herpesvirus 1 or RaHV-1) has icosahedral morphology and is 95–110 nm in size. This oncogenic virus, a member of the family *Alloherpesviridae*, occurs spontaneously in the northern leopard frog, *Rana pipiens.* RaHV-1 has not been cultured in cell lines. RaHV-2 was isolated from urine of Lucké tumor bearing frogs and characterized negative for oncogenic activity (Davison *et al.*, 2006).

Epizootiology and Transmission The virus replicates during cool (hibernation) winter temperatures and is shed during spawning. When warmer temperatures of summer occur, viral replication ceases and tumor growth begins. If summer frogs are cooled down again, the inactive tumors will begin to demonstrate herpesvirus replication (Mizell, 1985; Williams *et al.*, 1996).

Pathogenesis The virus causes renal adenocarcinomas in *R. pipiens.* Tumor growth is rapid during the warm months of summer but stops during winter virus production. With warmer temperatures, tumor growth resumes, and most frogs die after spawning (Wright, 1996).

Clinical Signs Affected frogs may not show signs until disease is well advanced. Emaciation, lethargy, ascites, and death are most commonly seen.

Necropsy Findings At necropsy, one or more whitish tumors can be found on either or both kidneys. Tumors can be quite large and metastasize to other organs. Histologically, the tumor is a papillary adenocarcinoma. Ascitic fluid may contain neoplastic cells. In wintering frogs, eosinophilic intranuclear inclusions may be seen in renal cells (Anver and Pond, 1984; Wright, 1996).

Differential Diagnoses Lucké herpesvirus can be distinguished from other tumors by light and electron microscopy (Densmore and Green, 2007).

Treatment There is no treatment for this disease.

Control Affected frogs should be culled and not allowed to reproduce.

Prevention Purchase of laboratory-reared, disease-free *R. pipiens* will prevent this disease.

Research Complications Asymptomatic animals with early phase tumors can yield poor research data, particularly if renal physiology studies are being conducted.

b. Ranavirus

Etiology Ranavirus is in the family *Iridoviridae.* Iridoviruses are large double stranded DNA viruses identified by eosinophilic intranuclear inclusions in red blood cells or a basophilic intracytoplasmic inclusion in the stomach glands. Ranaviruses have been implicated in frog and salamander die offs (Fijan *et al.*, 1991; Drury *et al.*, 1995; Cunningham *et al.*, 1996a; Jancovich *et al.*, 1997; Klaphake, 2009).

Epizootiology and Transmission Infections tend to affect early life stages of amphibians (Green, 2010). Transmission has been documented via infected food, feces, water previously housing infected animals, and by handling. Cannibalism among larva or ingestion of affected animals has also been suspected (Pessier, 2002). Susceptibility may depend on species and age range.

Pathogenesis Initial lesions are found on the skin, with progression to viscera. Virulence is generally host specific, and highly virulent ranavirus species and strains are known to affect anurans and caudates (Densmore and Green, 2007).

Clinical Signs Disease presentation varies from sudden death with few or no clinical signs to high percentage of severely affected individuals. Affected wild frogs were found emaciated, with varying degrees of cutaneous erythema and ulcerations (Cunningham *et al.*, 1996a). Tiger salamanders initially developed small white polyps, which spread to cover most of the epidermis, then progressed to epidermal hemorrhaging, excess mucus production, sloughed skin, lethargy, and anorexia (Jancovich *et al.*, 1997).

Necropsy Findings Frog necropsies demonstrated petechial and ecchymotic hemorrhage of the skeletal muscle and viscera, dermal ulceration and necrosis, digit necrosis, organ discoloration, and erythema of the skin (Cunningham *et al.*, 1996a). In *Xenopus* spp., diffuse liver necrosis of the liver and hematopoietic tissues has been reported. Microscopic examination of salamander tissues showed hypertrophy of epidermal, gill, and liver cells, with evidence of viral infection (Jancovich *et al.*, 1997).

Differential Diagnoses Lesions may appear consistent with those of bacterial sepsis. Often times, bacteria are present in cases of iridoviral infection; however, Jancovich *et al.* (1997) were unable to reproduce disease using bacteria alone, and Cunningham *et al.* (1996a) postulate that the iridovirus causes the primary lesions, with secondary invasion by the opportunistic invaders. Diagnosis is confirmed by cell culture, PCR, and light and electron microscopy. Recently, non-lethal sampling techniques have been reported useful in ranavirus surveillance (Gray *et al.*, 2012).

Treatment Successful treatment of iridovirus infections in amphibians has not been documented. Secondary bacterial infections may be treated as described previously. Some have postulated that administering antivirals (acyclovir) might have clinical use (Densmore and Green, 2007).

Control Affected animals should be isolated if possible and given supportive care. Thorough disinfection of contaminated enclosures and quarantine-type animal handling practices are advisable in the face of an outbreak (Pessier, 2002). Special consideration should be given to wild-caught animals.

Prevention In laboratory populations, good quarantine and husbandry practices should help in prevention of outbreaks.

Research Complications Epizootics can decimate populations of amphibians and seriously impair accurate data collection.

3. Parasitic

Amphibians can normally host a variety of parasites, without exhibiting signs of disease (Poynton and Whitaker, 1994; Tinsley, 1995). Determination of a pathogenic state is made by identifying parasite burden, concomitant stressors, and the inherent pathogenicity of the parasite in question. Within *X. laevis*, virtually all the organ systems may provide habitat for parasites (Tinsley *et al.*, 1996b). Many species of parasites infest amphibians; the following are common examples from each of the major parasite groups. The decision to treat amphibians is multifactorial, depending not only on the type of parasite identified, but the number, presence of lesions, and/or the condition of the host. Special attention and care should be given if both captive and wild-caught animals are being co-housed. Avoiding use of wild-caught animals will reduce problems with many parasites (Pessier, 2002).

a. Protozoal

Etiology Protozoa frequently infect amphibians, however clinical disease is considered rare. Significant species include *Entamoeba ranarum*, *Trichodina*, *Oodinium*, *Piscinoodinium*, *Tetrahymena*, *Trypanosoma*, *Cryptosporidium*, and *Plistophora* (Microsporidea now possibly grouped with fungi). Relationships range from commensal to parasitic. Many protozoa appear to have co-evolved with amphibian hosts (Poynton and Whitaker, 2001; Green *et al.*, 2003; Pessier, 2002). External parasites may be seen on tadpoles.

Epizootiology and Transmission Fecal–oral transmission is common in enteric protozoal infestations. Species of pathogenic protozoa can be transmitted through water and from aquatic vegetation or feeder fish to amphibians.

Pathogenesis *Entamoeba* cysts are swallowed and directly colonize the colon. Trophozoites can spread to the kidney and liver. *Oodinium* and *Trichodina* are external parasites that affect the skin and gills of aquatic amphibians. Ingestion of infected fly larvae is the likely source of *Plistophora myotropica* in wild toads. *Trypanosoma* infects the blood of wild amphibians and has an indirect lifecycle and is unlikely pathogenic.

Clinical Signs Signs of amebiasis include dehydration, anorexia, and emaciation. Feces are loose and bloody; vomiting may also occur. Ascites may be noted with hepatic and renal involvement. *Oodinium* causes the skin and gills to become grayish in color. Debilitation occurs in chronic cases. Reddened gills and skin cloudiness and ulceration can be observed with *Trichodina* and other ciliates. Animals affected by trypanosomiasis may be asymptomatic or may die acutely. *Plistophora* causes anorexia, muscle wasting, and death. *Cryptosporidium* has been reported to cause emaciation in *X. laevis* (Green *et al.*, 2003).

Necropsy Findings *Entamoeba* causes lesions of the colonic mucosa, suppurative nephritis, and hepatic abscesses. Cysts may be found in the liver and kidney. Splenomegaly is seen in amphibians that die acutely from trypanosomiasis. Necropsy findings associated with *Plistophora* include muscle atrophy and pale streaks in myofibers.

Differential Diagnoses Enteric protozoa can be identified by fecal examination (though difficult and often unrewarding), PCR, or colonic wash. Skin scrapings and gill biopsies will demonstrate external protozoa. *Plistophora* sporocysts can be seen in histologic sections of degenerated myofibers. *Trypanosoma* and other hemoparasites can be identified on Wright–Giemsa-stained blood smears.

Treatment Amebiasis and other enteric protozoal infections can be treated with metronidazole (50 mg/kg PO SID for 3–5 days). Aquatic species may be treated with 50 mg/l bath for 24 h. Enteric ciliated protozoa may be treated with a combination of tetracycline (50 mg/kg PO BID) and paramomycin (50–75 mg/kg PO SID). Trypanosomiasis may respond to a quinine sulfate bath (30 mg/l for 1 h). *Oodinium*, *Trichodina*, and other external protozoa can be treated with salt baths (10–25 mg/l SID for 5–30 min) or acriflavin baths (constant 0.025% bath for 5 days). Copper sulfate has also been used, but this compound can be toxic in some amphibian species and is not recommended (Crawshaw, 1993; Raphael, 1993; Wright, 1996; Whitaker, 1999; Wright, 1999a). All treatments may not lead to total resolution, but instead a decrease in parasitic burden.

Control Affected animals should be separated from community groups; they should be handled last, and equipment should not be shared. Tanks should be cleaned and sanitized, and water should be changed more frequently. Attention to the environment and prevention of reinfection are important considerations. Vectors should be excluded from animal facilities (Densmore and Green, 2007).

Prevention Incoming animals should be quarantined and evaluated for presence of disease and/or pathogenic organisms. Food items and aquarium plants should be treated before introduction (short salt bath followed by thorough rinsing and 1- to 2-h acriflavin bath). Whenever possible, purchase colony-reared animals and food items from reliable sources.

Research Complications Subclinical infections of hemoparasites can confound hematologic and physiologic data. Overt protozoal disease can decrease research populations and render data questionable. Cryptosporidiosis infection of animal could cause health concerns for humans as well.

b. Nematodes

Etiology Disease with nematode infection is common in captivity, however rarely reported to cause endemics in the wild (Klaphake, 2009). The three most commonly described pathogenic nematodes of amphibians are *Pseudocapillaroides xenopi*, *Rhabdias*, and *Foleyella* (wild caught). *Pseudocapillaroides* is a major parasite of *X. laevis*; *Rhabdias* affects both frogs and salamanders; and *Foleyella* has been described in frogs (Crawshaw, 1993; Brayton, 1992). Strogyloides and cosmocerids have also been reported in tree frogs (Densmore and Green, 2007). Other nematodes may also be found in dendrobatids frogs and may or may not be pathogenic.

Epizootiology and Transmission *Pseudocapillaroides* is contracted when the eggs are ingested along with sloughed skin from a host frog. The life-cycle is direct, with the nematode living in the epidermis of *Xenopus* and shedding its eggs directly into the aquatic environment. *Rhabdias* larvae penetrate the host frog's skin and migrate to the lungs. Eggs are coughed up and swallowed; thus, eggs and larvae are found in the gastrointestinal tract. Larval *Foleyella* are found in the blood; adults live in the body cavity and lymph spaces.

Pathogenesis *Pseudocapillaroides xenopi* has a direct life-cycle and burrows into the epidermis, causing desquamation, debilitation, and secondary infection. Larval nematodes can be found in the kidney. *Rhabdias* causes damage to pulmonary tissue, and *Foleyella* can cause debilitation.

Clinical Signs *Xenopus* affected with *Pseudocapillaroides* have a rough, thickened, pitted appearance to the skin on their dorsal surface, and large patches slough. Burrows and parasites can sometimes be seen in the epidermis. Debilitation and invasion by opportunistic bacteria and fungi can follow. Pneumonia may be observed in frogs with heavy *Rhabdias* infection. *Foleyella* may be asymptomatic or cause weakness and general malaise (Stephens *et al.*, 1987; Crawshaw, 1993; Wright, 1996).

Necropsy Findings *Pseudocapillaroides xenopi* lesions are usually confined to the skin and consist of hyperkeratosis, vacuolation, and a mixed inflammatory cell infiltrate. Severe cases involve epithelial erosion and ulceration. Nematodes are present in the lesions. In severe cases, skin infection may lead to septicemia (Ruble *et al.*, 1995; Green, 2010). Larval nematodes are sometimes found in Bowman's spaces and wrapped around glomerular tufts in the kidneys (Brayton, 1992).

Differential Diagnoses *Pseudocapillaroides* can be diagnosed by wet-mount preparations of desquamated skin or skin scraping. Bipolar eggs and adults will be detectable with these methods. *Rhabdias* larvated eggs and larvae can be found by fecal examination, though presence does not always correlate to disease. Eggs can also be found in tracheal washes. *Foleyella* can be demonstrated in fresh blood smears or in Wright–Giemsa-stained samples.

Treatment *Pseudocapillaroides* was initially treated with thiabendazole, but efficacy problems coupled with reports of adverse reactions have resulted in reduction of its use (Ruble *et al.*, 1995; Iglauer *et al.*, 1997). Ivermectin (0.2 mg/kg into the dorsal lymph sac or IM; repeat in 14 days) has proven effective (Dawson *et al.*, 1992; Wright, 1999a). Levamisole has also been suggested as a treatment for *Pseudocapillaroides* (Cunningham *et al.*, 1996b; Iglauer *et al.*, 1997). Iglauer *et al.* (1997) recommend levamisole (12 mg/l water, with each frog having access to 4.17–6.25 l of treated water for a minimum of 4 days; treatment repeated in 10–14 days). Wright (1999a) recommends levamisole (8–10 mg/kg IM or intracoelomically q14–21 days or 100–300 mg/l bath for 24 h q7–14 days); however, he warns of toxicity problems (flaccid paralysis) at more prolonged exposures. *Rhabdias* and other nematodes can be treated with ivermectin (2.0 mg/kg topically q14 days, or 0.2–0.4 mg/kg IM or PO q14 days) (Letcher and Glade, 1992; Crawshaw, 1993; Wright, 1999a). Lower ivermectin doses given continually to treat life-cycles have had anecdotal success. Fenbendazole can also be used to treat nematodes (100 mg/kg PO q10–21 days or 50 mg/kg PO SID for 3–5 days; repeat in 14–21 days (Wright, 1999a). When housing in terrariums, many nematodes have direct life-cycles and may be difficult eradicate.

Control Isolation and treatment of affected animals, sanitation of environment, and elimination of vectors will help control nematodes in amphibians.

Prevention Prevention can be carried out as for protozoal diseases.

Research Complications Nematode-infested animals can be unthrifty to clinically ill, and therefore poor research subjects. Secondary bacterial infection and sepsis can be sequelae (Poll, 2009).

c. Trematodes and Cestodes

Etiology Amphibians can serve as hosts to both trematodes and cestodes. Most are usually larval forms in anurans that serve as intermediate hosts (Klaphake, 2009; Lemke *et al.*, 2008). *Polystoma* and *Gyrodactylus* are common trematodes of amphibians, and *Nematotaenia* is a frequently encountered cestode. Cercariae of the trematode *Ribeiroia* have been associated with limb abnormalities in Pacific tree frogs and a trematode from the genus *Clinostomum* was reported in a tiger salamander (Johnson *et al.*, 1999; Perpiñán *et al.*, 2010).

Epizootiology and Transmission *Polystoma* and *Gorgodera amplicava* are found in the bladder of frogs. *Gyrodactylus* is found on the skin and gills of aquatic species of amphibians. *Nematotaenia* is found in the

gastrointestinal tract of amphibians. Black nodules noted on the serosa of the stomach and intestinal serosa of bullfrogs consisted of granulomas surrounding multiple nematode larvae (*Contracaecum* sp.) (Fig. 18.17).

Pathogenesis Trematode and cestode infestations may be subclinical. High numbers of cestodes may cause mechanical obstruction of the gastrointestinal tract or wasting and debilitation of the amphibian. Most clinically relevant pathological change is associated with migration through tissues.

Clinical Signs and Necropsy Findings *Polystoma* is typically asymptomatic. *Gyrodactylus* can cause debilitation, dyspnea, anemia, and ulceration of the skin. *Nematotaenia* can cause unthriftiness and gastrointestinal obstruction. Scoliosis has been described in a tiger salamander found with encysted trematodes (Perpiñán *et al.*, 2010).

Differential Diagnoses *Polystoma* can be detected by urinalysis. *Gyrodactylus* requires skin scraping and gill biopsy, and *Nematotaenia* can be detected by fecal examination (Crawshaw, 1993; Whitaker, 1999; Wright, 1999a).

Treatment Praziquantel (8–24 mg/kg PO, SC, or intracoelomically q14–21 days or 10 mg/l bath for up to 3 h; repeat in 14–21 days) has been used to treat trematodes and cestodes in amphibians (Wright, 1996; Wright, 1999a; Pessier, 2002).

Control and Prevention Trematodes and cestodes can be controlled and prevented in the same manner as other parasites. Many pesticides and other chemicals amphibians may be exposed to can cause an increased problem with trematodes (Klaphake, 2009).

Research Complications Debilitated animals make inappropriate research subjects, and subclinical infestations may confound data.

d. Other

Etiology Acanthocephalans, copepods, leeches, trombiculid (chigger) mites, nasal mites, and toad flies are examples of other types of parasites that may infest amphibians (Tinsley *et al.*, 1996a; Pessier, 2002). Also, an unspecified cutaneous mite similar to the genus *Rhizoglyphus* has been reported to cause morbidity in laboratory *Xenopus* spp. (Ford *et al.*, 2004).

Epizootiology and Transmission Acanthocephalans have an indirect life-cycle and require an arthropod host. Copepods are seen in aquatic amphibians, and leeches may be found on wild-caught animals. Trombiculid mites are found in soil, moss, and leaf litter, and parasitize terrestrial species. Toad flies infest terrestrial anurans.

Pathogenesis Acanthocephalans inhabit the gastrointestinal tract; the other parasites are external. Toad flies lay eggs in the nasal cavity of frogs; larvae eat the nasal passages and the frog's face until the frog dies. Nasal

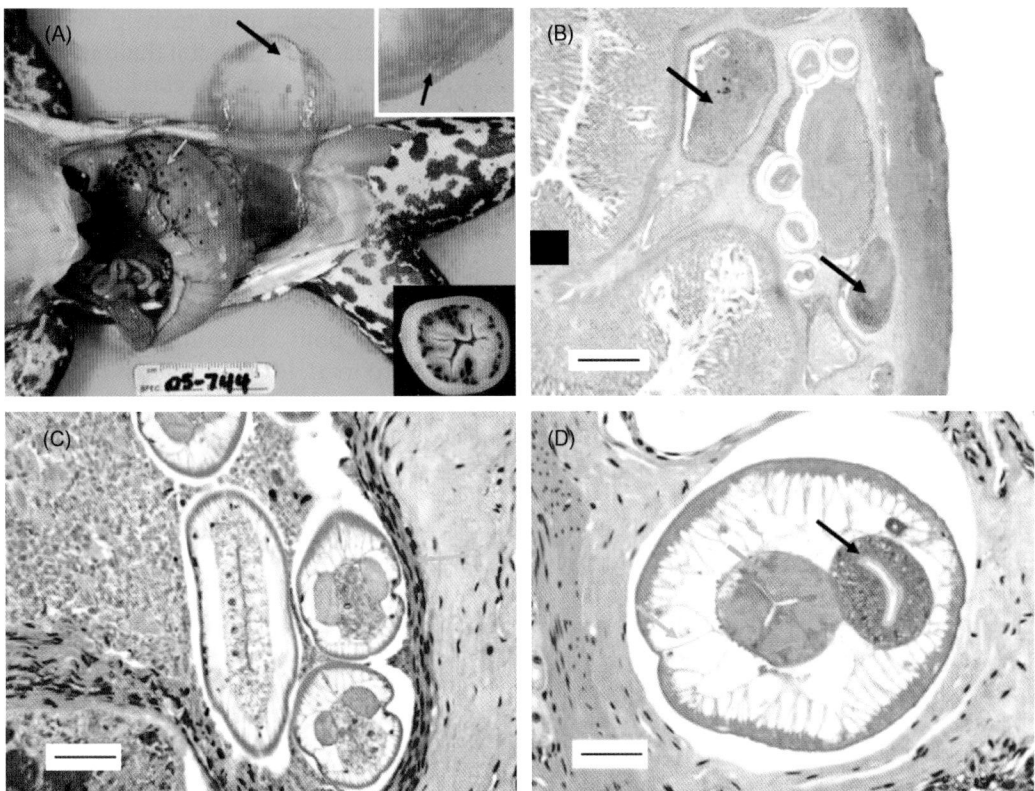

FIGURE 18.17 (A) Coelomic cavity of *Rana catesbiana*. Note the multifocal, 1- to 3-mm black nodules along the gastric wall (blue arrow). The bladder was distended with urine and contained yellow trematodes (*Gorgodera amplicava*, black arrow). Lower inset depicts a cross section of the stomach, highlighting the presence of the black nodules containing the nematodes (*Contracaecum* spp.) in the submucosa. (B) The black nodules in the gastric wall were consistent with granulomas surrounding multiple nematode parasites (black arrows). Hematoxylin and eosin stain; 500 μm. (C) Higher magnification of the verminous gastric granuloma. Note the peripheral layer of flattened epithelioid macrophages (blue arrow) that encircle central cellular debris, melanin pigment, admixed with nematode larvae (*Contracaecum* spp.). Hematoxylin and eosin stain; 50 μm. (D) Higher magnification of the *Contracaecum* larva in the stomach wall. Note the meromyarian musculature with prominent lateral cords (blue arrow). Within the pseudocoelom, triradiate esophagus (green arrow) abuts the intestine (black arrow). Gonads are lacking. Hematoxylin and eosin stain; 50 μm. *Modified from Lemke et al.* (2008).

mites, *Xenopacarus africanus*, found in *Xenopus* spp. can be considered commensal with no morbidity associated with its presence (Green, 2010).

Clinical Signs and Necropsy Findings Acanthocephalan infections may be subclinical; however, weight loss, coelomitis, perforation, and enteritis can be seen (Klaphake, 2009). If the intestinal wall is perforated, peritonitis will result. Leeches and copepods are visible externally. Trombiculid mites can cause erythematous vesicles on the skin of affected amphibians. Toad fly larvae can be seen in the nasal passages of affected frogs.

Differential Diagnoses Acanthocephalans are detected by fecal examination. Copepods can be detected on skin scrapings. Leeches, mites, and flies are readily visible.

Treatment Salt baths (10–25 g salt/l for 15–30 min) can be used to remove copepods and facilitate removal of leeches. Topical ivermectin may be effective in treating trombiculid mites. Treatment for toad flies and acanthocephalans is generally unrewarding (Crawshaw, 1993; Raphael, 1993; Wright, 1996; Whitaker, 1999).

Control and Prevention Excluding vectors and intermediate hosts is effective in controlling toad flies and acanthocephalans. Avoiding wild-caught animals will reduce problems with leeches and copepods (and many other parasites), and heat-treating or freezing leaf litter, soil, and other cage accouterments such as mosses, will eliminate trombiculid mites. Isolation of uninfected animals and thorough cleaning of the environment is necessary between treatments to eliminate the possibility of transmission or reinfection (Pessier, 2002).

Research Complications As in all parasitic infestations, compromised research animals are poor subjects and yield questionable data.

4. Fungal

a. Chytridiomycosis

Etiology An emerging infectious disease of amphibians is *Batrachochytrium dendrobates* (Bd), a keratinophilic fungus in the phylum Chytridiomycota discovered in the late 1990s. Named after the first species it was identified in the poison dart frog (*Dendrobates azureus* and *D. auratus*) and green tree frog (*Litoria caerulea*), this species' affected range has expanded to a wide variety of amphibians and is causing population declines (Klaphake, 2009). This is the only chytrid fungus known to infect vertebrates and the host list is increasing. Currently, it is considered an amphibian only disease, affecting both captive and wild animals (Densmore and Green, 2007, Padilla, 2011; Vredenburg *et al.*, 2013).

Epizootiology and Transmission Transmission occurs via flagellated, infective zoospores that require water or moist conditions for movement or direct contact of animals. Research suggests that the movement of *Xenopus* spp. throughout the world contributed to its spread. Though, the marine toad (*Bufo marinus*) and American bullfrog (*Rana catesbeiana*) have been implicated as subclinical carriers and spreaders (Klaphake, 2009; Green, 2010; Pessier, 2002). Typically the organism functions poorly at warmer temperatures. Recently, it was reported that Bd is present in wild *X. laevis* populations in California and supports the epidemic pathogen hypothesis in CA-Bd positive, non-native invasive species imported from Africa and released in CA are one of the possible means of spreading Bd to naïve amphibian hosts (Vredenburg *et al.*, 2013).

Pathogenesis Bd uses keratin as a substrate. Growth seems to be restricted to superficial layers of skin and other structures high in keratin. Cause of death has been attributed to disruption of the cutaneous homeostatic function (Pessier, 2002).

Clinical Signs Clinical signs include acute death, anorexia, general malaise, ventral edema, or petechial. Amphibian skin may shed, slough, become erythematous, display epidermal hyperplasia and discoloration, or become depigmented (Poll, 2009; Taylor, 2001; Pessier, 2002).

Necropsy Findings Mortality rates are high with Bd and it has caused hyperkeratosis associated with dysecdysis and evidence of secondary bacterial or fungal infections. Histologically, primary lesions are limited to keratinized epithelial cells. Acute infections are limited to the stratum corneum. In subacute to advanced cases, massive numbers of thalli will be found in retained layers of epidermis. Acanthosis also may be present. (Densmore and Green, 2007).

Differential Diagnoses PCR testing is now available and results should be interpreted cautiously. Since it is ubiquitous, a positive sample from the skin may not necessarily confer disease (Green, 2010). Routine sequencing of PCR positive samples should be done to confirm the positive finding. Other methodologies include immunohistochemistry, culture, or wet mount preparations with either Congo red, Dif-Quick, or periodic acid-Schiff stain to help identify the 7–20 µm spherical flask shaped fungal thalli within keratinocytes.

Treatment Treatment consists of itraconazole or miconazole baths, isolation, and culling. Heat treatment at 32.2°C for 72 hours in tolerant species is also reported (Poll, 2009). Recently, daily lower dose itraconazole baths (e.g., 100 mg/l for 3 days, followed by 5 mg/l for 6 days, and 50 mg/l for 1 day) for 10 days was reported to eliminate Bd infection (confirmed by Taqman PCR) in captive anurans, though may be toxic in some species (Jones *et al.*, 2012). Both chloramphenicol and amphotericin B were reported to significantly reduced Bd infection in naturally infected southern leopard frogs (*R. sphenocephala*), although neither drug was capable of complete fungal clearance (Holden *et al.*, 2014).

Control Disinfection of equipment and enclosures with disinfectants is an important control. Due to its transmission in moist environments, extreme care should be taken to isolate any potentially contaminated animals, enclosures, and equipment (Taylor, 2001).

Prevention Bd is presently thought to be a global threat to a broad host range of amphibians. Establishing adequate quarantine periods for any new animals (arriving or captured) is important. Also, using effective antifungal agents to prevent dissemination of the agent is vital (Poll, 2009). Currently, there is no known zoonotic potential (Padilla, 2011).

Research Complications Bd causes high morbidity and mortality to amphibians. Though successful treatments are reported in dendrobatid frogs, there are high risks of infecting other animals and effected animals acquiring secondary infections (Taylor, 2001).

b. Other Fungal/Mold Diseases

Etiology Most fungi and molds that affect amphibians are soil and water saprophytes; infection commonly occurs secondary to stress or disease. The mold/fungal infections most frequently identified in amphibians are saprolegniasis, chromomycosis, and phycomycosis.

Epizootiology and Transmission Saprolegniasis is caused by several fungi/molds, including *Saprolegnia* and other similar agents (*Achyla, Leptolegnia*, and *Aphanomyces*) (Densmore and Green, 2007; Pritchett and Sanders, 2007; Taylor, 2001). *Saprolegnia* is known to colonize already diseased skin and may affect external gills (Ford *et al.*, 2004). Various pigmented fungi cause chromomycosis, and *Basidiobolus* is the agent most commonly isolated from cases of phycomycosis.

Pathogenesis and Clinical Signs *Saprolegnia* colonizes pre-existing skin lesions in aquatic amphibians. A cottony mat of fungal hyphae cover the lesion. Paler tufts are indicative of acute infections, while darker mats indicate chronicity. Erythematous or ulcerated skin may be present. In salamanders (Crawshaw, 1993; Wright, 1996; Densmore and Green, 2007) lesions of chromomycosis are usually raised dark nodules; however, they may be ulcerated (Ackermann and Miller, 1992; Wright, 1996). Debilitation and weight loss may also be observed. Phycomycosis produces lesions similar to those of chromomycosis (Wright, 1996).

Necropsy Findings Lesions tend to remain cutaneous in saprolegniasis. Visceral granulomas can be seen in chromomycosis.

Differential Diagnoses Diagnosis can be made by wet mounts and fungal cultures. Mounts will show occasional branching, broad hyphae of varying widths without visible septa. Histologically, fungal filaments and zoospores are evident in lesions. (Poll, 2009).

Treatment Saprolegniasis can be treated with salt-water baths (10–25 g/l for 5–30 min SID), benzalkonium chloride (2 mg/l bath for 10–60 min), malachite green, new methylene blue, potassium permanganate, and copper sulfate (Wright, 1999a; Pessier, 2002; Densmore and Green, 2007). Groff *et al.* (1991) successfully treated *Basidiobolus ranarum* with benzalkonium chloride (2 mg/l bath for 30 min every other day for three treatments; repeat in 8 days). Several treatments for chromomycosis have been tried; results are unrewarding (Ackermann and Miller, 1992; Wright, 1996). Importantly, if the underlying disease condition is not addressed, prognosis is poor.

Control and Prevention Fungal infections can be minimized by keeping animals healthy and unstressed in a clean environment. Water molds are often secondary infections and are associated with poor water quality and the presence of abundant organic debris.

Research Complications Saprophytic fungi can colonize surgical wounds and other skin lesions, compromising the health of the research animals. *Xenopus* eggs and oocytes can become infected with Saprolegnia and diminish the quality (Green, 2010).

B. Metabolic/Nutritional Diseases/Other Conditions

Amphibians are susceptible to several metabolic and nutritional diseases, including MBD, lipid keratopathy, spindly leg, gas bubble disease, and dehydration. MBD is seen in both adult and larval amphibians that have been fed diets deficient in calcium or with an improper calcium–phosphorus ratio. Any amphibian with a diagnosis of a bone fracture should be evaluated for MBD, and appropriate supplementation of calcium and vitamin D begun immediately (Wright, 2001c). Tadpoles require significant amounts of calcium in their diet. Animals deficient in calcium will mobilize the mineral from bones in order to keep serum calcium levels normal. Adult frogs exhibit abdominal bloating and tetany following exertional movement. Diagnosis of MBD is based on clinical signs and radiographs (digital systems work well when radiographing small amphibians). Radiographic changes include decreased bone density and pathologic fractures. Treatment of MBD consists of appropriate calcium supplementation (daily 5% calcium gluconate baths, injectable vitamin D/calcium, oral supplementation with tropical fish food slurry), and change to an appropriate diet. The disease can be prevented by feeding larval and adult amphibians appropriate diets (Crawshaw, 1993; Wright, 1996).

Lipid keratopathy has been reported in some anurans (Shilton *et al.*, 2001; Heinz-Taheny, 2009). Affected animals have corneal thickening and opacity, with vascularization, superficial pigmentation, and cholesterol clefts. In some cases, xanthomatosis is associated with corneal changes. Possible etiologies include lipid and cholesterol mobilization associated with egg production, and high levels of dietary fat or cholesterol (Williams and Whitaker, 1994; Shilton *et al.*, 2001). Some have hypothesized that offering basking spots so that amphibians can raise their temperatures (above 39°C) may aid in fat metabolism.

Spindly leg (muscular underdevelopment) is seen in young frogs, particularly captive anurans (Wright, 2001b). Limbs develop abnormally, do not emerge properly at metamorphosis, are thin and poorly muscled, and have angular deformities. Etiology is unknown; theories include genetics, toxins, temperature, water quality, oversupplementation of vitamins, trauma, and malnutrition (vitamin deficiencies). The condition is untreatable, and euthanasia is recommended (Crawshaw, 1993; Wright, 1996, Wright, 2001b).

Gas bubble disease is produced by air supersaturation of water. Large amounts of gas accumulate in the vascular system, causing obstruction of blood flow and capillary hemorrhage. Commonly, nitrogen gases are the culprit rather than oxygen. Air bubbles are evident in webbing of feet and skin, and may permit entry of bacteria, resulting in septicemia. Other clinical signs include buoyancy problems, petechial hemorrhaging, and loss of mucous coats. Correcting the water imbalance can lead to recovery, however oftentimes morbidity and mortality are associated with secondary infections or poor egg production. To correct supersaturation, water must be degased by aeration and correcting any life support system problems. Progressively warming the housing water to ambient temperature of the room will also be of benefit. The disease can be prevented by ensuring that water is not supersaturated with air (Colt *et al.*, 1984; Crawshaw, 1993; Raphael, 1993; Wright, 1996; Densmore and Green, 2007; Green, 2010).

Amphibians require moist environments and are predisposed to dehydration. Signs of dehydration include dull, dark skin, sunken eyes, lethargy, and dry, sticky mucus. Desiccated animals may have wrinkly to leathery skin. Mild dehydration can be treated by immersion in clean, dechlorinated water (cool and well oxygenated). Animals in shock can be given dexamethasone (1–2 mg/kg intracoelomically) and hypotonic sterile fluids. Two parts saline to one part 5% dextrose is given intracoelomically at 2–5% of the animal's body weight. Subsequent fluid solutions should be nine parts saline to one part sterile water. Antibiotic baths are recommended if epidermis is damaged (Wright, 1999b). Amphibian Ringer's solution, artificial slime (Shield X®), and water conditioners have all been used for rehydrating amphibians (Green, 2010). However, if water loss exceeds a certain percentage of body weight, the excretory system may be damaged beyond the chance of recovery (Wright, 2006).

C. Traumatic Disorders

Traumatic lesions in amphibians are primarily bite wounds caused by cagemates, and abrasions from rough surfaces and cage tops (Fig. 18.18). Other instigators may include bites from live prey, rough or inappropriate substrate, or rough handling with dry or ungloved hands. Appropriate wound closure (if warranted) and antibiotic therapy are indicated (Wright, 1994; Wright, 2001a; Poll, 2009). Irrigating (sterile 0.9% saline solution) simple abrasions and lacerations with no signs of infection is effective. Intermedullary pins and amputation may be warranted if fractures are present, depending on the type (Gentz, 2007). Aggressive animals should be separated, and cages should be free of abrasive surfaces.

D. Toxins

Amphibians are exquisitely sensitive to a number of toxins, including chlorine and chloramine, nitrite,

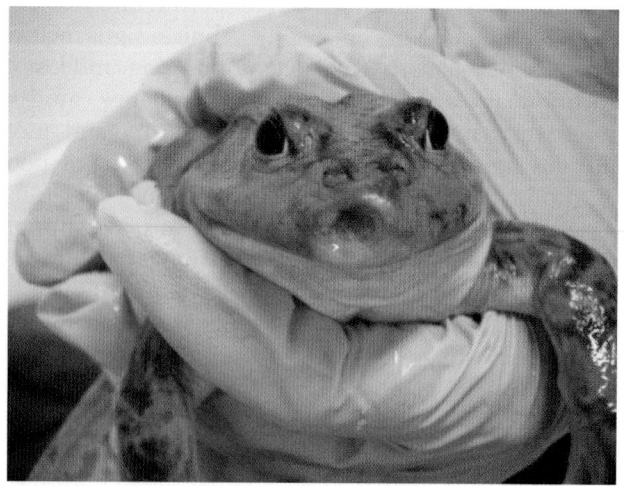

FIGURE 18.18 Nose abrasion in bullfrogs is commonly associated with jumping or rubbing against enclosure walls and tops.

ammonia, iodine, heavy metals (copper, lead, zinc), PVC adhesives, detergents or disinfectants, and pesticides (Whitaker, 1993; Stansley and Roscoe, 1996; Densmore and Green, 2007). Avoidance of metals use in enclosures and plumbing is highly recommended. Signs associated with toxicities include excess mucus production, irritability, dyspnea, convulsions, paralysis, petechiation, and regurgitation (Wright, 1996). In *Xenopus* spp., animals may present with eye irritation, skin sloughing, and acute death (Green, 2010). Animals displaying acute signs of toxicity should be removed immediately from their environment and placed in a clean, toxin-free enclosure. Following disinfection of enclosures, vigorous and thorough rinsing should be applied before use.

E. Neoplasms

Neoplastic disease, although reported and well documented among amphibians, is relatively uncommon. While the majority of documented cases come from captive amphibians, there are also reports from wild populations, including epidemics of neoplastic disease. Differential diagnoses include other causes of nodular skin lesions, especially granulomatous disease such as mycobacteriosis and chromomycosis (Pessier, 2002) Commonly reported neoplasms in amphibians are the Lucké renal carcinoma of northern leopard frogs and squamous cell papilloma in the Japanese fire bellied newt (Densmore and Green, 2007). Spontaneous tumors are reported more frequently in frogs, and frogs appear more sensitive than salamanders to carcinogen-induced tumors (Anver, 1992). Examples of spontaneous amphibian tumors include skin adenomas, papillomas, fibromas, pulmonary carcinomas, lymphangiosarcoma, lymphosarcoma, squamous cell carcinomas, melanophoromas, mastocytomas, and testicular tumors (Balls and Clothier, 1974; Gentz, 2007; Menger *et al.*, 2010). In *Xenopus*, melanophoroma and lymphosarcoma are the most commonly described tumors (Green, 2010). Diagnosis can be made by fine needle aspiration and cytology or excision and histopathology. Treatment depends on the type, size, and behavior of the tumor. Cryosurgery, radiosurgery, and diode laser surgery have been used for resection and ablation of cutaneous neoplasms in amphibians (Gentz, 2007).

References

Ackermann, J., Miller, E., 1992. Chromomycosis in an African bullfrog, *Pyxicephalus adspersus*. Bull. Assoc. Reptil. Amphib. Vet. 2, 8–9.
Allegrucci, C., Rushton, M.D., Dixon, J.E., Sottile, V., Shah, M., Kumari, R., et al., 2011. Epigenetic reprogramming of breast cancer cells with oocyte extracts. Mol. Cancer. 10, 7.
Anderson, C.W., Nishikawa, K.C., 1997. The functional anatomy and evolution of hypoglossal afferents in the leopard frog, *Rana pipiens*. Brain Res. 771, 285–291.

Anver, M.R., 1992. Amphibian tumors: a comparison of anurans and urodeles. In Vivo 6, 435–438.

Anver, M.R., Pond, C.L., 1984. Biology and diseases of amphibians. In: Fox, J.G., Cohen, B.J., Loew, F.M. (Eds.), Laboratory Animal Medicine Academic Press, Orlando, FL, pp. 427–447.

Armentia, A., Vega, J.M., 1997. Allergy to frogs. Allergy 52, 674.

AVMA Guidelines for the Euthanasia of Animals: 2013 Edition, Copyright © 2013 by the American Veterinary Medical Association, Schaumburg, IL 60173. Steven Leary, Wendy Underwood, Raymond Anthony, Samuel Cartner, Douglas Corey, Temple Grandin, Cheryl Greenacre, Sharon Gwaltney-Brant, Mary Ann. McCrackin, Robert Meyer, David Miller, Jan Shearer, Roy Yanong

Balls, M., Clothier, R.H., 1974. Spontaneous tumors in amphibia. Oncology 29, 501–519.

Barthalmus, G.T., Zielinski, W.J., 1998. Skin mucus induces oral dyskinesias that promote escape from snakes. Pharmacol. Biochem. Behav. 30, 957–959.

Bartholomew, J.L., Driessen, J.L., Walker-Harrison, P., Riggs, R.R., 1993. Continuous flow aquatic system for long-term housing of Xenopus laevis. Contemp. Top. Lab. Anim. Sci. 32, 37.

Bartlett, R.D., Bartlett, R.R., 1996. Frogs, Toads, and Treefrogs. Barron's Educational Series, Hauppauge, New York.

Berger, L., Volp, K., Matthews, S., Speare, R., Timms, P., 1999. Chlamydia pneumoniae in a free-ranging giant barred frog (Mixophyes iteratus) from Australia. J. Clin. Microbiol. 37, 2378–2380.

Bisazza, A., Rogers, L.J., Vallortigara, G., 1998. The origins of cerebral asymmetry: a review of evidence of behavioural and brain lateralization in fishes, reptiles, and amphibians. Neurosci. Biobehav. Rev. 22, 411–426.

Bowler, J.K., 1977. Longevity of Reptiles and Amphibians in North American Collections. Society for the Study of Amphibians and Reptiles, Oxford, Ohio.

Boyd, S.K., Moore, F.L., 1992. Sexually dimorphic concentrations of arginine vasotocin in sensory regions of the amphibian brain. Brain Res. 588, 304–306.

Brayton, C., 1992. Wasting disease associated with cutaneous and renal nematodes, in commercially obtained Xenopus laevis. Ann. N Y Acad. Sci. 653, 197–201.

Brockes, J.P., 1997. Amphibian limb regeneration: rebuilding a complex structure. Science 276, 81–87.

Brown, J.L., Morales, V., Summers, K., 2010. A key ecological trait drove the evolution of biparental care and monogamy in amphibian. Chicago J. 174, 436–446.

Brown, M.J., Nixon, R.M., 2004. Enrichment for a captive environment – the Xenopus laevis. Anim. Technol. Welfare 3, 87–95.

Browne, R.K., Zippel, K., 2007. Reproduction and larval rearing of amphibians. ILAR J. 48, 214–234.

Bruce, L.L., Neary, T.J., 1995. The limbic system of tetrapode: a comparative analysis of cortical and amygdalar populations. Brain Behav. Evol. 46, 224–234.

Bryan, L.K., Baldwin, C.A., Gray, M.J., Miller, D.L., 2009. Efficacy of select disinfectants at inactivating Ranavirus. Dis. Aquat. Org. 84, 89–94.

Burggren, W.W., Warburton, S.J., 1994. Patterns of form and function in developing hearts: contributions from non-mammalian vertebrates. Cardio. Sci. 5, 183–191.

Burkhart, J.G., Helgen, J.C., Fort, D.J., Gallagher, K., Bowers, D., Propst, T.L., et al., 1998. Induction of mortality and malformation in Xenopus laevis embryos by water sources associated with field frog deformities. Environ. Health Perspect. 106, 841–848.

Campbell, T.W., 1991. Hematology of exotic animals. Compendium 13, 950–957.

Carreño, C.A., Nishikawa, K.C., 2010. Aquatic feeding in pipid frogs: the use of suction for prey capture. J. Exp. Biol. 213, 2001–2008.

Cashins, S.D., Alford, R.A., Skerratt, L.F., 2008. Lethal effect of latex, nitrile, and vinyl gloves on tadpoles. Herpetol. Rev. 39, 298–301.

Cathers, T., Lewbart, G.A., Correa, M., Stevens, J.B., 1997. Serum chemistry and hematology values for anesthetized American bullfrogs (Rana catesbeiana). J. Zoo Wildl. Med. 28, 171–174.

Clarke, B.T., 1997. The natural history of amphibian skin secretions, their normal functioning, and potential medical applications. Biol. Rev. 72, 365–379.

Colt, J., Orwicz, K., Brooks, D., 1984. Gas bubble disease in the African clawed frog, Xenopus laevis. J. Herpetol. 18, 131–137.

Conant, R., Collins, J.T., 1991. A Field Guide to the Reptiles and Amphibians: Eastern and Central North America, third ed. Houghton Mifflin, Boston, MA.

Cosden, R.S., Lattermann, C., Romine, S., Gao, J., Voss, S.R., MacLeod, J.N., 2011. Intrinsic repair of full-thickness articular cartilage defects in the axolotl salamander. Osteoarthr. Cartilage 19, 200–205.

Crawshaw, G.J., 1993. Amphibian medicine. In: Fowler, M.E. (Ed.), Zoo and Wild Animal Medicine: Current Therapy 3 Saunders, Philadelphia, PA, pp. 131–139.

Culley, D.D., 1992. Managing a bullfrog research colony. In: Schaeffer, D.O., Kleinow, K.M., Krulisch, L. (Eds.), The Care and Use of Amphibians, Reptiles, and Fish in Research Scientists Center for Animal Welfare, Bethesda, MD, pp. 30–40.

Cunningham, A.A., Langton, T.E.S., Bennett, P.M., Lewin, J.F., Drury, S.E.N., Gough, R.E., et al., 1996a. Pathological and microbiological findings from incidents of unusual mortality of the common frog (Rana temporaria). Philos. Trans. R Soc. Lond. B Biol. Sci. 351, 1539–1557.

Cunningham, A.A., Sainsbury, A.W., Cooper, J.E., 1996b. Diagnosis and treatment of a parasitic dermatitis in a laboratory colony of African clawed frogs (Xenopus laevis). Vet. Rec. 138, 640–642.

Daly, J.W., 1995. The chemistry of poisons in amphibian skin. Proc. Natl. Acad. Sci. 92, 9–13.

Davis, A.K., Maerz, J.C., 2008. Comparison of hematological stress indicators in recently captured and captive paedomorphic mole salamanders, Ambystoma talpoideum. Capeoa 3, 613–617.

Davison, A.J., Cunningham, C., Sauerbier, W., McKinnell, R.G., 2006. Genome sequences of two frog herpesviruses. J. Gen. Virol. 87, 3509–3514.

Dawson, D.A., Bantle, J.A., 1987. Development of a reconstituted water medium and preliminary validation of the frog embryo teratogenesis assay – Xenopus (FETAX). J. Appl. Toxicol. 7, 237–244.

Dawson, D.A., Schultz, T.W., Schroeder, E.C., 1992. Laboratory care and breeding of the African clawed frog. Lab. Anim. 21, 31–36.

Densmore, C.L., Green, D.E., 2007. Diseases of amphibians. ILAR J. 48, 235–253.

Deuchar, E.M., 1975. Xenopus: The South African Clawed Frog. Wiley and Sons, London.

Donnelly, M.A., Guyer, C., Juterbock, J.E., Alford, R.A., 1994. Techniques for marking amphibians. In: Heyer, R.W., Donnelly, M.A., McDiarmid, R.W., Hayek, L.-A.C., Foster, M.S. (Eds.), Measuring and Monitoring Biological Diversity: Standard Methods for Amphibians Smithsonian Institution Press, Washington, D.C, pp. 277–284.

Donoghue, S., 1996. Veterinary nutritional management of amphibians and reptiles. J. Am. Vet. Med. Assoc. 208, 1816–1820.

Drury, S.E.N., Gough, R.E., Cunningham, A.A., 1995. Isolation of an iridovirus-like agent from common frogs (Rana temporaria). Vet. Rec. 137, 72–73.

Duellman, W.E., Trueb, L., 1986. Biology of Amphibians. McGraw-Hill, New York.

Dugas, M.B., Yeager, J., Richards-Zawacki, C.L., 2013. Carotenoid supplementation enhances reproductive success in captive strawberry poison frogs (Oophaga pumilio). Zoo Biol. 32, 655–658.

Duhon, S.T. Short guide to Axolotl husbandry. University of Kentucky SalSite, Lexington, KY. <http://www.ambystoma.org/education/guide-to-axolotl-husbandry> (accessed 12.05.13).

Dumont, J.N., Schultz, T.W., Buchanan, M., Kao, G., 1983. Frog embryo teratogenesis assay: Xenopus (FETAX) – a short-term assay applicable to complex environmental mixtures Symposium on the Application of Short-Term Bioassays in the Analysis of Complex Environmental Mixtures III. Plenum Press, New York.

Etheridge, A.L., Richter, M.A., 1978. Xenopus Laevis: Rearing and Breeding the African Clawed Frog. NASCO, Fort Atkinson, WI.

Ferner, J.W., 2010. Measuring and marking post-metamorphic amphibians. In: Dodd Jr., C.K. (Ed.), Amphibian Ecology and Conservation: A Handbook of Techniques Oxford University Press, New York, pp. 123–141.

Fijan, N., Matasin, Z., Petrinec, Z., Valpotic, I., Zwillenberg, L.O., 1991. Isolation of an iridovirus-like agent from the green frog (Rana esculenta L.). Veterinarski Arhiv. 61, 151–158.

Fleming, L.R., 1990. A standardized method for housing temperate region freshwater aquatic species. Lab. Anim. Sci. 40, 564.

Forbes, M.R., McRuer, D.L., Shutler, D., 2006. White blood cell profiles of breeding american toads (Bufo americanus) relative to sex and body size. Comp. Clin. Pathol. 15, 155–159.

Ford, T.R., Dillehay, D.L., Mook, D.M., 2004. Cutaneous Acariasis in the African clawed frog (Xenopus laevis). Comp. Med. 54, 713–717.

Forzán, M.J., Vanderstichel, R.V., Ogbuah, C.T., Barta, J.R., Smith, T.G., 2012. Blood collection from the facial (Maxillary)/Musculo-Cutaneous vein in true frogs (Family Ranidae). J. Wildlife Dis. 48, 176–180.

Fremont-Rahl, J.J., Ek, C., Williamson, H.R., Small, P.L.C., Fox, J.G., Muthupalani, S., 2011. Mycobacterium liflandii outbreak in a research colony of xenopus (Silurana) tropicalis frogs. Vet. Path. 48, 856–867.

Gentz, E.J., 2007. Medicine and surgery of amphibians. ILAR 48, 255–259.

Godfrey, D., Williamson, H., Silverman, J., Small, P.L.C., 2007. Newly identified mycobacterium species in a xenpopus laevis colony. Comp. Med. 57, 97–104.

Golay, N., Durrer, H., 1994. Inflammation due to toe-clipping in natterjack toads (Bufo calamita). Amphib. Reptil. 15, 81–83.

Gouchie, G.M., Roberts, L.F., Wassersug, R.J., 2008. Effect of available cover and feeding schedule on the behavior and growth of the juvenile African clawed frog (Xenopus laevis). Lab. Anim. 37, 165–169.

Grafe, U.T., Margaret, M.S., Lampert, K.P., Rodel, M.-O., 2011. Putting toe clipping into perspective: a viable method for marking anurans. J. Herp. 45, 28–35.

Gratzek, J.B., 1992. Getting started with aquaria. In: Gratzek, J.B., Matthews, J.R. (Eds.), Aquariology: The Science of Fish Healt Management Tetra Press, Morris Plains, NJ, pp. 3–19.

Gray, M.J., Miller, D.L., Hoverman, J.T., 2012. Reliability of non-lethal surveillance methods for detecting ranavirus infection. Dis. Aquat. Org. 99, 1–6.

Green, S.L., 2010. The Laboratory Xenopus sp. CRC Press, Boca Raton, FL.

Green, S.L., Bouley, D.M., Tolwani, R.J., Waggie, K.S., Lifland, B.D., Otto, G.M., et al., 1999. Identification and management of an outbreak of Flavobacterium meningosepticum infection in a colony of South African clawed frogs (Xenopus laevis). J. Am. Vet. Med. Assoc. 214, 1833–1838.

Green, S.L., Lifland, B.D., Bouley, D.M., Brown, B.A., Wallace Jr., R.J., Ferrell Jr., J.E., 2000. Disease attributed to Mycobacterium chelonae in South African clawed frogs (Xenpopus laevis). Comp. Med. 50, 675–679.

Green, S.L., Bouley, D.M., Josling, C.A., Fayer, R., 2003. Crypotosporidiosis associated with emaciation and proliferative gastritis in a laboratory-reared South African clawed frogs (Xenopus laevis). Comp. Med. 53, 81–84.

Gresens, J., 2004. An introduction to the Mexican axolotl (Ambystoma mexicanum). Lab. Anim. 33, 41–47.

Groff, J.M., Mughannam, A., McDowell, T.S., Wong, A., Dykstra, M.J., Frye, F.L., et al., 1991. An epizootic of cutaneous zygomycosis in cultured dwarf African clawed frogs (Hymenochirus curtipes) due to Basidiobolus ranarum. J. Med. Vet. Mycol. 29, 215–223.

Gurdon, J.B., 1996. Introductory comments: Xenopus as a laboratory animal. In: Tinsley, R.C., Kobel, H.R. (Eds.), The Biology of Xenopus. Clarendon Press, Oxford, pp. 3–8.

Heard, G.W., Scroggie, M.P., Malone, B., 2008. Visible implant alphanumeric tags as an alternative to toe-clipping for marking amphibians–a case study. Wildl. Res. 35, 747–759.

Heinz-Taheny, K.M., 2009. Cardiovascular physiology and diseases of amphibians. Vet. Clin. North Am. Exotic Anim. Pract. 12, 39–50.

Henson-Ramsey, H., Kennedy-Stoskopf, S., Levine, J.F., Taylor, S.K., Shea, D., Stoskopf, M.K., 2008. Acute toxicity and tissue distributions of malathion in Ambystoma tigrinum. Arch. Environ. Contam. Toxicol. 55, 481–487.

Hilken, G., Willmann, G.H.F., Dimigen, I., Iglauer, F., 1994. Preference of Xenopus laevis for different housing conditions. Scand. J. Lab. Anim. Sci. 21, 71–80.

Hilken, G., Dimigen, J., Iglauer, F., 1995. Growth of Xenopus laevis under different laboratory rearing conditions. Lab. Anim. 29, 152–162.

Hill, W.A., Newman, S.J., Craig, L., Carter, C., Czarra, J., Brown, J.P., 2010. Diagnosis of Aeromonas hydrophila, Mycobacterium species, and Batrachochytrium dendrobatidis in an African clawed frog (Xenpopus laevis). J. Am. Assoc. Lab. Anim. Sci. 49, 215–220.

Hird, D.W., Diesch, S.L., McKinnell, R.G., Gorham, E., Martin, F.B., Kurtz, S.W., et al., 1981. Aeromonas hydrophila in wild-caught frogs and tadpoles (Rana pipiens) in Minnesota. Lab. Anim. Med. 31, 166–169.

Holden, W.H., Ebert, A.R., Canning, P.F., Rollins-Smith, L.A., 2014. Evaluation of amphotericin B and chloramphenicol as alternative drugs for treatment of chytridiomycosis and their impacts on innate skin defenses. Appl. Environ. Microbiol. 80, 4034–4041.

Holtz, J., Frechelin, E., Noel, B., Savolainen, H., 1993. A case of frog allergy: antigenic skin protein. Int. Arch. Allergy Immunol. 101, 299–300.

Hoogstraten-Miller, S., Dunham, D., 1997. Practical identification methods for African clawed frogs (Xenopus laevis). Lab. Anim. 26, 36–38.

Horne, M.T., Dunson, W.A., 1994. Behavioral and physiological responses of the terrestrial life stages of the Jefferson salamander, Ambystoma jeffersonianum, to low soil pH. Arch. Environ. Contam. Toxicol. 27, 232–238.

Howard, A.M., Papich, M.G., Felt, S.A., Long, C.T., Mc Keon, G.P., Bond, E.S., et al., 2010. The pharmokinetics of enrofloxacin in adult African clawed frogs (Xenopus laevis). J. Am. Assoc. Lab. Anim. Sci. 49, 800–804.

Howerth, E.W., 1984. Pathology of naturally occurring chlamydiosis in african clawed frogs (Xenopus laevis). Vet. Pathol. 21, 28–32.

Hubbard, G.B., 1981. Aeromonas hydrophila infection in Xenopus laevis. Lab. Anim. Sci. 31, 297–300.

Iglauer, F., Willmann, F., Hilken, G., Huisinga, E., Dimigen, J., 1997. Anthelmintic treatment to eradicate cutaneous capillariasis in a colony of South African clawed frogs (Xenopus laevis). Lab. Anim. Sci. 47, 477–482.

Jaeger, R.G., 1981. Dear enemy recognition and the costs of aggression between salamanders. Am. Nat. 117, 962–974.

Jaeger, R.G., 1992. Housing, handling, and nutrition of salamanders. In: Schaeffer, D.O., Kleinow, K.M., Krulisch, L. (Eds.), The Care and Use of Amphibians, Reptiles, and Fish in Research Scientists Center for Animal Welfare, Bethesda, MD, pp. 25–29.

Jancovich, J.K., Davidson, E.W., Morado, J.F., Jacobs, B.L., Collins, J.P., 1997. Isolation of a lethal virus from the endangered tiger salamander Ambystoma tigrinum stebbinsi. Dis. Aquat. Org. 31, 161–167.

Jerrett, D.P., Mays, C.E., 1973. Comparative hematology of the hellbender, *Cryptobranchus alleganiensis* in Missouri. Copeia 2, 331–337.

Johnson, M.L., Berger, L., Philips, L., Speare, R., 2003. Fungicidal effects of chemical disinfectants, UV light, desicacation and heat on the amphibian chytrid Batrachochytrium dendrobatidis. Dis. Aquat. Org. 57, 255–260.

Johnson, P.T.J., Lunde, K.B., Ritchie, E.G., Launer, A.E., 1999. The effect of trematode infection on amphibian limb development and survivorship. Science 284, 802–804.

Jones, M.E.B., Paddock, D., Bender, L., Allen, J.L., Schrenzel, M.S., Pessier, A.P., 2012. Treatment of chytridiomycosis with reduced-dose itraconazole. Dis. Aquat. Org. 99, 243–249.

Jorgensen, C.B., 1997. 200 years of amphibian water economy: from Robert Townson to the present. Biol. Rev. 72, 153–237.

Kaltenbrun, E., Tandon, P., Amin, N.M., Waldron, L., Showell, C., Conlon, F.L., 2011. Xenopus: an emerging model for studying congenital heart disease. Birth Defect Res. 91, 495–510.

Kaplan, M.L., 1993. An enriched environment for the African clawed frog (*Xenopus laevis*). Lab. Anim. 22, 25–27.

Kara, T.C., 1994. Ageing in amphibians. Gerontology 40, 161–173.

Karnes, J.L., Mendel, F.C., Fish, D.R., 1992. Effects of low voltage pulsed current on edema formation in frog hindlimbs following impact injury. Phys. Ther. 72, 273–278.

Kashiwagi, K., Kashiwagi, A., Kurabayashi, A., Hanada, H., Nakajima, K., Okada, M., et al., 2010. Xenopus tropicalis: an ideal experimental animal in amphibia. Exp. Anim. 59, 395–405.

Kawai, T., Kinoshita, K., Koyama, K., Takahashi, K., 1994. Anti-emetic principles of *Magnolia obovata* bark and *Zingiber officinale* rhizome. Planta Med. 60, 17–20.

Klaphake, E., 2009. Bacterial and parasitic diseases of amphibians. Vet. Clin. North Am. Exotic Anim. Pract. 12, 597–608.

Kobel, H.R., Loumont, C., Tinsley, R.C., 1996. The extant species. In: Tinsley, R.C., Kobel, H.R. (Eds.), The Biology of *Xenopus*. Clarendon Press, Oxford, pp. 9–33.

Koeller, C.A., 2009. Comparison of buprenorphine and butorphanol analgesia in eastern red-spotted newt (Notophthalmus viridescens). J. Am. Assoc. Lab. Anim. Sci. 48, 171–175.

Kragl, M., Knapp, D., Nacu, E., Khattak, S., Maden, M., Epperlein, H.H., et al., 2009. Cells keep a memory of their tissue origin during axolotol limb regernation. Nature 460, 60–65.

Kreil, G., 1996. Skin secretions of *Xenopus laevis*. In: Tinsley, R.C., Kobel, H.R. (Eds.), The Biology of *Xenopus* Clarendon Press, Oxford, pp. 263–277.

Lemke, L.B., Dronen, N., Fox, J.G., Nambiar, P.R., 2008. Infestation of wild-caught American bullfrogs (*Rana catesbeiana*) by multiple species of metazoan parasites. J. Am. Assoc. Lab. Anim. Sci. 47, 42–46.

Letcher, J., Glade, M., 1992. Efficacy of ivermectin as an anthelmintic in leopard frogs. J. Am. Vet. Med. Assoc. 200, 537–538.

Major, N., Wassersug, R.J., 1998. Survey of current techniques in the care and maintenance of the African clawed frog (*Xenopus laevis*). Contemp. Top. Lab. Anim. Sci. 37, 57–60.

Maniero, G.D., Carey, C., 1997. Changes in selected aspects of immune function in the leopard frog, rana pipiens, associated with exposure to cold. J. Comp. Physiol. B 167, 256–263.

Martinho, F., Heatley, J.J., 2012. Amphibian mycobacteriosis. Vet. Clin. North Am. Exotic Anim. Pract. 15, 113–119.

Mattison, C., 1998. The Care of Reptiles and Amphibians in Captivity, rev. third ed. Blanford Press, London.

McAllister, K.R., Watson, J.W., Risenhoover, K., McBride, T., 2004. Marking and radiotelemetry of oregon spotted frogs (*Rana pretiosa*). Northwest. Nat. 85 (1), 20–25.

McBride, G., 1978. South African Clawed Frog *Xenopus laevis*. Ann Arbor Biological Center, Ann Arbor, MI.

McCoy, K.A., Bortnick, L.J., Campbell, C.M., Hamlin, H.J., Guillette, L.J., St Mary, C.M., 2008. Agriculture alters gonadal form and function in the toad Bufo marinus. Environ. Health Perspect. 116, 1526–1532.

McCusker, C., Gardiner, D.M., 2011. The axolotol model for regeration and aging research: a mini-review. Gerontology 57, 565–571.

McRobert, S.P., 2003. Methodologies for the care maintenance, and breeding of tropical poison frogs. J. Appl. Anim. Welf. Sci. 6, 95–102.

Measey, J., 1998. Terrestrial prey capture in Xenopus laevis. Copeia 3, 787–791.

Menger, B., Vogt, P.M., Jacobsen, I.D., Allmeling, C., Kuhbier, J.W., Mutschmann, F., et al., 2010. Resection of a large intra-abdominal tumor in the Mexican axolotl: a case report. Vet. Surg. 39, 232–233.

Metts, B.S., Buhlmann, K.A., Tuberville, T.D., Scott, D.E., Hopkins, W.A., 2013. Maternal transfer of contaminants and reduced reproductive success of southern toads (Bufo (Anaxyrus) terrestris) exposed to coal combustion waste. Environ. Sci. Technol. 19, 2846–2853.

Miller, S.I., Pegues, D.A., 2000. Salmonella species, including *Salmonella typhi*. In: Mandell, G.L., Bennett, J.E., Dolin, R. (Eds.), Principles and Practice of Infectious Diseases, fifth ed. Churchill Livingstone, Philadelphia, PA.

Minter, L.J., Clark, E.O., Gjeltema, J.L., Archibald, K.E., Posner, L.P., 2011. Effects of intramuscular meloxicam administration on prostaglandin E2 synthesis in the North American bullfrog (Rana catesbeiana). J. Zoo Wildl. Med. 42, 680–685.

Mitchell, M.A., 2011. Zoonotic diseases associated with reptiles and amphibians: an update. Vet. Clin. Exot. Anim. 14, 439–456.

Mizell, M., 1985. Lucké frog carcinoma herpesvirus: transmission and expression during early development. Adv. Viral. Oncol. 5, 129–146.

Monaghan, J.R., Athippozhy, A., Seifert, A.W., Putta, S., Stromberg, A.J., Maden, M., et al., 2012. Gene expression patterns specific to the regenerating limb of the Mexican oxolotl. Biol. Open. 10, 937–948.

Narayan, E.J., Molinia, F.C., Kindermann, C., Cockrem, J.F., Hero, J.-M., 2011. Urinary corticosone responses to capture and toe clipping in the cane toad (Rhinella marina) indicate that Toe- clipping is a stressor for amphibians. Gen. Comp. Endocrinol. 174, 238–245.

Newcomer, C.E., Anver, M.R., Simmons, J.L., Wilcke Jr., B.W., 1982. Spontaneous and experimental infections of *Xenopus laevis* with *Chlamydia psittaci*. Lab. Anim. Sci. 32, 680–686.

Nieuwenhuys, R., 1994. The neocortex. An overview of its evolutionary development, structural organization, and synaptology. Anat. Embryol. 190, 307–337.

Nieuwkoop, P.D., Faber, J., 1994. Normal Table of *Xenopus laevis* (Daudin): a Systematical and Chronological Survey of the Development from the Fertilized Egg Till the End of Metamorphosis. Garland Publ., New York.

Nyman, S., 1986. Mass mortality in larval *Rana sylvatica* attributable to the bacterium, *Aeromonas hydrophila*. J. Herpetol. 20, 196–201.

Ogushi, Y., Tsuzuki, A., Sato, M., Mochida, H., Okada, R., Suzuki, M., et al., 2010. The water-absorption region of ventral skin of several semiterrestrial and aquatic anuran amphibians identified by aquaporins. Am. J. Physiol. Regul. Integr. Comp. Physiol. 299, R1150–62.

Olson, M.E., Gard, S., Brown, M., Hampton, R., Morck, D.W., 1992. *Flavobacterium indologenes* infection in leopard frogs. J. Am. Vet. Med. Assoc. 201, 1766–1770.

Orton, F., Carr, J.A., Handy, R.D., 2006. Effects of nitrate and atrazine on larval development and sexual differentiation in the northern leopard frog Rana pipiens. Environ. Toxicol. Chem. 25, 65–71.

Padilla, L.R., 2011. Emerging fungal diseases of wild animal species Fungal Diseases An Emerging Threat to Human, Animal, and Plant Health 296–308. National Academy Press., Institute of Medicine, Workshop Summary.

Paniagua, R., Fraile, B., Sáez, F.J., 1990. Histol. Histopathol. 5, 365–378.

Perpiñán, D., Garner, M.M., Trupkiewicz, J.G., Malarchik, J., Armstrong, D.L., Lucio–Foster, A., et al., 2010. Scoliosis in a Tiger Salamander (Ambystoma tigrinum) associated with encysted digenetic trematodes of the genus clinostomum. J. Wildlife Dis. 46, 579–584.

Pessier, A.P., 2002. An overview of amphibian skin disease. Semin. Avian Exot. Pet. Med. 11, 162–174.

Pessier, A.P., Pinkerton, M., 2003. Practical gross necropsy and amphibians. Sem. Avian Exot. Pet. Med 12, 81–88.

Petranka, J.W., 1998. Salamanders of the United States and Canada. Smithsonian Institution Press, Washington, DC.

Pfeiffer, C.J., Pyle, H., Asashima, M., 1990. Blood cell morphology and counts in the Japanese newt (Cynops pyrrhogaster). J. Zoo Wildl. Med. 21, 56–64.

Pfennig, D.W., Collins, J.P., 1993. Kinship affects morphogenesis in cannibalistic salamanders. Nature 362, 836–838.

Phillott, A.D., McDonald, K.R., Skerratt, L.F., 2011. Inflammation in digits of unmarked and toe-tipped wild hylids. Wildlife Res. 38, 204–207.

Poll, C.P., 2009. Wound management in amphibians: etiology and treatment of cutaneous lesions. J. Exotic Pet. Med. 18, 20–35.

Pough, F.H., 1989. Amphibians: a rich source of biological diversity. In: Woodhead, A.D. (Ed.), Nonmammalian Animal Models for Biomedical Research CRC Press, Boca Raton, FL, pp. 245–278.

Pough, F.H., 1991. Recommendations for the care of amphibians and reptiles in academic institutions. ILAR News 33, S1–S21.

Poynton, S.L., Whitaker, B.R., 1994. Protozoa in poison dart frogs (Dendrobatidae): clinical assessment and identification. J. Zoo Wildl. Med. 25, 29–39.

Poynton, S.L., Whitaker, B.R., 2001. Protozoa and metazoa infecting amphibians. In: Wright, K.M., Whitaker, B.R. (Eds.), Amphibian Medicine and Captive Husbandry Krieger Publishing Company, Malabar, FL.

Pramuk J.B., Gagliardo R., 2008. General Amphibian Husbandry. Husbandry. Amphibian Husbandry Resource Guide. World Association of Zoos and Aquariums. pp. 4–42.

Pritchett, K.R., Sanders, G.E., 2007. Epistylididae ectoparasites in a colony of African clawed frogs (Xenpopus laevis). J. Am. Assoc. Lab. Anim. Sci. 46, 86–91.

Rafidah, J., Ong, B.L., Saroja, S., 1990. Outbreak of "red leg" – an Aeromonas hydrophila infection in frogs. J. Vet. Malaysia 2, 139–142.

Ramakrishnan, L., Valdivia, R.H., McKerrow, J.H., Falkow, S., 1997. Mycobacterium marinum causes both long-term subclinical infection and acute disease in the leopard frog (Rana pipiens). Infect. Immun. 65, 767–773.

Raphael, B.L., 1993. Amphibians. In: Quesenberry, K.E. Hillyer, E.V. (Eds.), The Veterinary Clinics of North America: Small Animal Practice, Vol. 23 Saunders, Philadelphia, PA, pp. 1271–1286.

Reed, K.D., Ruth, G.R., Meyer, J.A., Shukla, S.K., 2000. Chlamydia pneumonia infection in a breeding colony of African clawed frogs (Xenpopus tropicalis). Emerg. Infect. Dis. 6, 196–199.

Register, K.J., Woolsey, L.B., 2005. Marking salamender egg masses with visible fluorescent elastomer: retention time and effect on embryonic development. Am. Midl. Nat. 153, 52–60.

Riviere, J.E., Shapiro, D.P., Coppoc, G.L., 1979. Percutaneous absorption of gentamicin by the leopard frog, Rana pipiens. J. Vet. Pharmacol. Ther. 2, 235–239.

Rogers, W.P., Simpson, T.W., Jones, L.M., Renquist, D.M., 1997. An innovative aquatic non-recirculating system for use in housing African clawed frogs (Xenopus laevis). Contemp. Top. Lab. Anim. Sci. 36, 72–74.

Rollins-Smith, L.A., 1998. Metamorphosis and the amphibian immune system. Immunol. Rev. 166, 221–230.

Roy, S., Gatien, S., 2008. Regeneration in axolotls: a model to aim for. Exp. Geront. 43, 968–973.

Ruble, G., Berzins, I.K., Huso, D.L., 1995. Diagnostic exercise: anorexia, wasting, and death in South African clawed frogs. Lab. Anim. Sci. 45, 592–594.

Sánchez-Morgado, J.M., Gallagher, A., Johnson, L.K., 2009. Mycobacterium gordonae infection in a colony of African clawed frogs (Xenpopus tropicalis). Lab. Anim. 43, 300–303.

Saporito, R.A., Spande, T.F., Garraffo, M.H., Donnelly, M.A., 2009. Arthropod alkaloids in poison dart frogs: a review of the dietary hypothesis. Heterocycles 79, 277–297.

Schmeller, D.S., Loyau, A., Dejean, T., Milaud, C., 2011. Using amphibians in laboratory studies: precautions against the emerging infectious disease chytridiomycosis. Lab. Anim. 45, 25–30.

Schmidt, K., Schwarzkopf, L., 2010. Visible implant elastomer tagging and toe-clipping: effects of marking on locomoter performance of frogs and skinks. Herpetological J. 20, 99–105.

Seifert, A.W., Monaghan, J.R., Voss, S.R., Maden, M., 2012. Skin regeneration in adult axolotls: a blueprint for scar-free healing in vertebrates. PLoS One 7, e32875.

Shibata, Y., Takeuchi, H.A., Hasegawa, T., Suzuki, M., Tanaka, S., Hillyard, S.D., et al., 2011. Localization of water channels in the skin of two specis of desert toads, Anaxyrus (Bufo) punctatus and Incilius (Bufo) alvarius. Zoolog. Sci. 28, 664–670.

Shilton, C.M., Smith, D.A., Crawshaw, G.J., Valdes, E., Keller, C.B., Maguire, G.F., et al., 2001. Corneal lipid deposition in cuban tree frogs (Osteopilus septentrionalis) and its relationship to serum lipids: an experimental study. J. Zoo Wildlife Med. 32, 305–319.

Shrenzel, M.D., 2012. Molecular epidemiology of mycobacteriosis in wildlife and pet animals. Vet. Clin. Exotic Anim. 15, 1–23.

Sibold, A., Eickhoff, A., Bonner, R.A., 1993. Successful care and husbandry of the red-spotted newt, Notophthalmus viridescens. Contemp. Top. Lab. Anim. Sci. 32, 36.

Sive, H.L., Grainger, R.M., Harland, R.M., 2000. Early Development of Xenopus laevis: A Laboratory Manual. Coldspring Harbor Laboratory Press.

Smirina, E.M., 1994. Age determination and longevity in amphibians. Gerontology 40, 133–146.

Stansley, W., Roscoe, D.E., 1996. The uptake and effects of lead in small mammals and frogs at a trap and skeet range. Arch. Environ. Contam. Toxicol. 30, 220–226.

St. Claire, M., Kennett, M.J., Thomas, M.L., Daly, J.W., 2005. The husbandry and care of dendrobatid frogs. Contemp. Top. Lab. Anim. Sci. 44, 8–14.

Stephens, L.C., Cromeens, D.M., Robbins, V.W., Stromberg, P.C., Jardine, J.H., 1987. Epidermal capillariasis in South African clawed frogs (Xenopus laevis). Lab. Anim. Sci. 37, 341–344.

Stevens, C.W., 1992. Alternatives to the use of mammals for pain research. Life Sci. 50, 901–912.

Stewart, P.L., 1994. An efficient, economical multicompartment tank for housing Xenopus laevis. Lab. Anim. Sci. 33, A30.

Stoskopf, M.K., Winieski, A.P., Pieper, L., 1985. Iodine toxicity in poison-arrow frogs. In: Silberman, M.S., Silberman, S.D. (Ed.), Proceedings of the Annual Meeting of the American Association of Zoo Veterinarians, Philadelphia, American Association of Zoo Veterinarians, Philadelphia, PA, pp. 86–88.

Stoskopf, M.K., Arnold, J., Mason, M., 1987. Aminoglycoside antibiotic levels in the aquatic salamander Necturus necturus. J. Zoo Anim. Med. 18, 81–85.

Tai, T., Akita, Y., Kinoshita, K., Koyama, K., Takahashi, K., Watanabe, K., 1995. Anti-emetic principles of Poria cocos. Planta Med. 61, 527–530.

Tarigo, J., Linder, K., Neel, J., Harvey, S., Remick, A., Grindem, C., 2006. Reluctant to dive: coelomic effusion in a frog. Vet. Clin. Pathol. 35, 341.

Taylor, F.R., Simmonds, R.C., Loeffler, D.G., 1993. Isolation of *Flavobacterium meningosepticum* in a colony of leopard frogs (*Rana pipiens*). Lab. Anim. Sci. 43, 105.

Taylor, S.K., 2001. Mycoses. In: Wright, K.M., Whitaker, B.R. (Eds.), Amphibian Medicine and Captive Husbandry Krieger Publishing Company, Malabar, FL.

Taylor, S.K., Green, D.E., Wright, K.M., Whitaker, B.R., 2001. Bacterial diseases. In: Wright, K.M., Whitaker, B.R. (Eds.), Amphibian Medicine and Captive Husbandry Krieger Publishing Company, Malabar, FL.

Teare, J.A., Wallace, R.S., Bush, M.B., 1991. Pharmacology of gentamicin in the leopard frog (Rana pipiens). Proc. Am. Assoc. Zoo Vet. 128–129.

Tinsley, R., 2010. Amphibians, with special reference to xenopus. In: Hubrecht, R., Kirkwood, J. (Eds.), The UFAW Handbook on the Care and Mangament of Laboratory and Other Research Animals, eighth ed. Wiley-Blackwell, Oxford, UK.

Tinsley, R.C., 1995. Parasitic disease in amphibians: control by the regulation of worm burdens. Parasitology 111, S153–S178.

Tinsley, R.C., Loumont, C., Kobel, H.R., 1996a. Geographical distribution and ecology. In: Tinsley, R.C., Kobel, H.R. (Eds.), The Biology of *Xenopus* Clarendon Press, Oxford, UK.

Tinsley, R.C., Loumont, C., Kobel, H.R., 1996b. Parasites of Xenopus. In: Tinsley, R.C., Kobel, H.R. (Eds.), The Biology of Xenopus Oxford University Press, Oxford, UK.

Torreilles, S.L., Green, S.L., 2007. Refuge cover decreases the incidence of bite wounds in laboratory South African clawed frogs (Xenopus laevis). JAALAS 46, 33–36.

Torreilles, S.L., McClure, D.E., Green, S.L., 2009. Evaluation and refinement of euthanasia methods for Xenopus laevis. J. Am. Assoc. Lab. Anim. Sci. 48, 512–516.

Trott, K.A., Stacy, B.A., Lifland, B.D., Diggs, H.E., Harland, R.M., Khokha, M.K., et al., 2004. Characterization of a mycobacterium ulcerans-Like infection in a colony of African tropical clawed frogs (Xenpopus tropicalis). Comp. Med. 54, 309–317.

Tuttle, A.D., Law, J.M., Harms, C.A., Lewbart, G.A., Harvey, S.B., 2006. Evaluation of the gross and histological reactions to five commonly used suture materials in the skin of the African clawed frog (Xenopus laevis). J. Am. Assoc. Lab. Anim. Sci. 45, 22–26.

Uchiyama, M., Norifumi, K., 2006. Hormonal regulation of ion and water transport in anuran amphibians. Gen. Comp. Endocrin. 147, 54–61.

Verhoeff-de Fremery, R., Griffin, J., Macgregor, H.C., 1987. Urodeles (newts and salamanders). In: Poole, T.B. (Ed.), The UFAW Handbook on the Care and Management of Laboratory Animals, sixth ed. Churchill Livingstone, New York, pp. 759–772.

Viborg, A.L., Rosenkilde, P., 2004. Water potential receptors in the skin regulate blood perfusion in the ventral pelvic patch of toads. Physiol. Biochem. Zool. 77, 39–49.

Videler, J.J., Jorna, J.T., 1985. Functions of the sliding pelvis in *Xenopus laevis*. Copeia 1, 254–257.

Vitt, L.J., Caldwell, J.P., 2009. Herpetology: An Introductory Biology of Amphibians and Reptiles. Academic Press, San Diego, CA.

Voss, R.S., Epperlein, H.H., Tanaka, E.M., 2009. Ambrystoma mexicanum, the axolotl: a versatile amphibian model for regeneration, development, and evolution studies. Cold Spring Harbor Protocols 8 pdb.emo128.

Vredenburg, V.T., Felt, S.A., Morgan, E.C., McNally, S.V.G., Wilson, S., Green, S.L., 2013. Prevalence of Batrachochytrium dendrobatidis in Xenopus collected in Africa (1871–2000) and in California

(2001–2010). PLoS One 8 (5), e63791. Available from: http://dx.doi.org/10.1371/journal.pone.0063791

Waddle, J.H., Rice, K.G., Mazzotti, F.J., Percival, H.F., 2008. Modeling the effect of toe clipping on treefrog survival: beyond the return rate. J. Herp. 42, 467–473.

Walker, I.D.F., Whitaker, B.R., 2000. Amphibian therapeutics In: Fronefield, S.P.A. (Ed.), The Veterinary Clinics of North America: Exotic Animal Practic, vol. 3 Saunders, Philadelphia, PA, pp. 239–255.

Wells, K.D., 2007. The Ecology and Behavior of Amphibians. University of Chicago Press, Chicago.

Whitaker, B.R., 1993. The use of polyvinyl chloride glues and their potential toxicity to amphibians. Proc. Am. Assoc. Zoo Vet. 16–18.

Whitaker, B.R., 1999. Parasitic problems of amphibians. Proc. North Am. Vet. Conf. 801–803.

Wilcke Jr., B.W., Newcomer, C.E., Anver, M.R., Simmons, J.L., Nace, G.W., 1983. Isolation of *Chlamydia psittaci* from naturally infected African clawed frogs (*Xenopus laevis*). Infect. Immun. 41, 789–794.

Williams, D.L., Whitaker, B.R., 1994. The amphibian eye–a clinical review. J. Zoo Wild. Med. 25, 18–28.

Williams, J.H., 1997. Contractile apparatus and sarcoplasmic reticulum function: effects of fatigue, recovery, and elevated calcium. J. Appl. Physiol. 83, 444–450.

Williams III, J.W., Tweedell, K.S., Sterling, D., Marshall, N., Christ, C.G., Carlson, D.L., et al., 1996. Oncogenic herpesvirus DNA absence in kidney cell lines established from the northern leopard frog *Rana pipiens*. Dis. Aquat. Org. 27, 1–4.

Wilson, S., Felt, S., Torreilles, S., Howard, A., Behan, C., Moorhead, R., et al., 2011. Serum clinical biochemical and hematologic reference ranges of laboratory-reared and wild-caught Xenopus laevis. J. Am. Assoc. Lab. Anim. Sci. 50, 635–640.

Woodward, D.L., Khakhria, R., Johnson, W.M., 1997. Human salmonellosis associated with exotic pets. J. Clin. Microbiol. 35, 2786–2790.

Wright, K., 1994. Amputation of the tail of a two-toed amphiuma, *Amphiuma means*. Bull. Assoc. Reptil. Amphib. Vet. 4, 5.

Wright, K., 1999a. Common bacterial and fungal diseases of captive amphibians. Proc. North Am. Vet. Conf., 810–813.

Wright, K., 1999b. Fluid therapy for amphibians. Proc. North Am. Vet. Conf., 814–816.

Wright, K.M., 1996. Amphibian husbandry and medicine. In: Mader, D.R. (Ed.), Reptile Medicine and Surgery Saunders, Philadelphia, PA, pp. 436–459.

Wright, K.M., 2001a. Trauma. In: Wright, K.M., Whitaker, B.R. (Eds.), Amphibian Medicine and Captive Husbandry Krieger Publishing Company, Malabar, FL.

Wright, K.M., 2001b. Idiopathic syndromes. In: Wright, K.M., Whitaker, B.R. (Eds.), Amphibian Medicine and Captive Husbandry Krieger Publishing Company, Malabar, FL.

Wright, K.M., 2001c. Diets for captive amphibians. In: Wright, K.M., Whitaker, B.R. (Eds.), Amphibian Medicine and Captive Husbandry Krieger, Malabar, FL.

Wright, K.M., 2006. Overview of amphibian medicine. In: Mader, D.R. (Ed.), Reptile Medicine and Surgery, second ed. Saunders, Philadelphia, PA, pp. 941–971.

Wu, M., Gerhart, J., 1991. Raising *Xenopus* in the laboratory In: Kay, B.K. Peng, H.B. (Eds.), Methods in Cell Biology, vol. 36 Academic Press, San Diego, CA, pp. 3–18.

Wyman, R.L., Hawksley-Lescault, D.S., 1987. Soil acidity affects distribution, behavior, and physiology of the salamander *Plethodon cinereus*. Ecology 68, 1819–1827.

Zug, G.R., 1993. Herpetology: An Introductory Biology of Amphibians and Reptiles. Academic Press, San Diego, CA.

Biology and Diseases of Reptiles

Dorcas P. O'Rourke, DVM, MS, DACLAM[a] and
Kvin Lertpiriyapong, DVM, PhD[b]

[a]Department of Comparative Medicine, East Carolina University, The Brody School of Medicine,
Moye Blvd, Greenville, NC, USA [b]East Carolina University, The Brody School of Medicine,
Moye Blvd, Greenville, NC, USA

I. INTRODUCTION

Reptiles are the first group of vertebrates to evolve an amniotic, shelled egg, and thereby be freed of the requirement to reproduce in an aquatic environment. Like amphibians, reptiles are ectothermic, and several lizard species superficially resemble salamanders. These morphologic and physiologic similarities led scientists to traditionally consider reptiles and amphibians to be closely related. During the past two decades, however, emerging DNA technologies have allowed scientists to more accurately view genetic similarities, which resulted in major reclassification of these two groups, including realigning reptiles more closely evolutionarily and genetically with birds.

A. Taxonomy

There are currently over 9500 species of extant reptiles, the majority of which are lizards (59%) and snakes (35%). Turtles (3.4%), crocodilians (0.3%), amphisbaenians (2%), and tuataras (0.01%) comprise the remainder of this group (Pincheira-Donoso *et al.*, 2013). Based on skull characteristics, members of class Reptilia have been categorized into two lineages, Anapsida and Diapsida. Turtles, which lack skull fenestrae, were considered to be the only living anapsids. However, recent nuclear DNA analysis has determined that this condition is derived from the diapsid skull; therefore, turtles are now considered diapsids (Zardoya and Meyer, 2001; Vitt and Caldwell, 2009; Gilbert and Corfe, 2013). Extant reptiles are currently classified into the clades Archosauria or Lepidosauria. Although still controversial, most taxonomists place turtles in Archosauria with crocodilians and birds, rather than in Lepidosauria with tuatara and squamates (lizards, snakes, and amphisbeanians) (Vitt and Caldwell, 2009; Lu *et al.*, 2013). Furthermore, snakes and amphisbaenians evolved from lizards, making lizards paraphyletic.

Chelonians (turtles and tortoises) are divided into two broad taxonomic groups based on the method of head retraction. Pleurodira, or side-neck turtles withdraw the head and neck and fold it onto the shoulder. Three families of pleurodires are found in freshwater in the Southern Hemisphere: Pelomedusidae from Africa, Madagascar, and the Seychelles Islands; Podocnemidae from Madagascar and South America; and the Chelidae from South America, Australia, and New Guinea. The most familiar of the chelids is *Chelus fimbriatus*, the mata mata. This unusual turtle with fleshy head protuberances and pronounced keels on its shell inhabits the freshwater streams of South America (Ernst and Barbour, 1989; Zug, 1993).

Cryptodira comprises several families, all of which withdraw the neck into the shell in a vertical, S-shaped fashion. Members of this group can be found in terrestrial, freshwater, or marine habitats. Softshell turtles (Trionychidae) and pig-nosed turtles (Carettochelyidae) are sister taxa to the rest of the cryptodires. The remaining cryptodire groups include the mud and musk turtles (Kinosternidae), snapping turtles (Chelydridae), sea turtles (Cheloniidae and Dermochelyidae), and the clade Testudinoidea, which contains the 'pond' turtles (Emydidae) and the tortoises (Testudinidae). Representatives of Emydidae include the North American sliders (*Trachemys*), painted turtles (*Chrysemys*), box turtles (*Terrapene*), spotted turtles (*Clemmys*), wood turtles (*Calemys*), and diamondback terrapins (*Malaclemys*), Testudinidae includes the North American gopher tortoises (*Gopherus*), European Hermann's tortoise (*Testudo*), and South American yellow-footed and red-footed tortoises (*Chelonoidis [Geochelone]*) (Ernst and Barbour, 1989; Zug, 1993; Vitt and Caldwell, 2009).

Crocodilians are medium to large, quadrupedal reptiles adapted to an aquatic habitat. The phylogeny of Crocodylia is continuously undergoing revision. A recent report describes three clades within Crocodylia: Borealosuchus, Gavialidae, and Brevirostres (Holliday and Gardner, 2012). According to this scheme, all species of Borealosuchus are extinct; Gavialidae consists of only two living species, the narrow-snouted gharial, *Gavialis gangeticus*, and the false gharial, *Tomistoma schlegelii*; and Brevirostres includes Alligatoridae and Crocodylidae. The living species of Alligatoridae includes two species of alligators and six species of caimans. The common caiman (*Caiman crocodilus*) and American alligator (*Alligator mississippiensis*) have been most commonly used in

research. Crocodylidae is the largest family, consisting of at least 23 species (the exact number of species is still under rigorous debate), which occur throughout the world in tropical regions (Ross and Magnusson, 1989; Zug, 1993; McAliley *et al.*, 2006).

The remainder of reptiles are classified as lepidosaurs. Included in this group are the sphenodontidans and squamates. The tuatara, a unique, lizard-like reptile, is the sole representative of Sphenodontidae. This family contains one genus, *Sphenodon*, with two species, both confined to New Zealand. Lizard families comprising Squamata include, among others, Gekkonidae (geckos), Iguanidae (iguanas, anoles, fence lizards), Chamaeleonidae (chameleons), Helodermatidae (Gila monsters), Varanidae (monitors), Scincidae (skinks), and Teiidae (tegus and whiptail lizards) (Zug, 1993; Vitt and Caldwell, 2009).

Snake families commonly seen in research settings include Boidae (boa constrictors, anacondas), Pythonidae (reticulated pythons, Burmese pythons, ball pythons), Elapidae (coral snakes, mambas, sea snakes, cobras), Viperidae (rattlesnakes, copperheads, puff adders, Gaboon vipers), and Colubridae (king snakes, rat snakes, garter snakes, water snakes). Boas and pythons are primitive snakes with many large species, some of which can exceed lengths of 25 feet. Vipers are venomous snakes with large retractable fangs; elapids have smaller, fixed fangs. Colubridae is the largest family, with over 2000 species (Vitt and Caldwell, 2009). Most colubrids are nonvenomous; however, some venomous species, including the rear-fanged brown tree snake (*Boiga irregularis*), are members of this family (Zug, 1993; Greene, 1997; Vitt and Caldwell, 2009).

B. Use in Research

For many years, herpetologists have studied reptiles in the field as well as maintained captive populations in the research laboratory. In the field, these investigations have mainly focused on the natural history, behavior, and reproduction of animals in their native habitats. Specific questions that cannot be answered in the field are addressed by bringing specimens into the laboratory for more intensive study. Thus, a majority of research involving reptiles is dedicated to understanding and conserving the species themselves.

Reptiles have also been used as animal models and for teaching purposes. Striped-necked pond turtles (*Mauremys japonica*) have been used to investigate the effects of microgravity on orientation (Wassersug and Izumi-Kurotani, 1993). Red-eared sliders (*Trachemys scripta elegans*), known for anoxia tolerance, have been used to elucidate the mechanisms of neuroglobin (Nayak *et al.*, 2009). This species, along with the painted turtle (*Chrysemys picta*), is commonly used to teach physiology and anatomy (Fig. 19.1). Various species of lizards have been the subjects of investigations into stress, behavior,

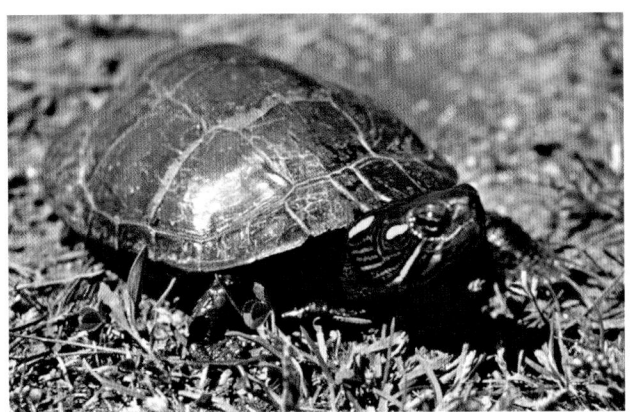

FIGURE 19.1 The painted turtle, *Chrysemys picta*, is commonly used in teaching and research.

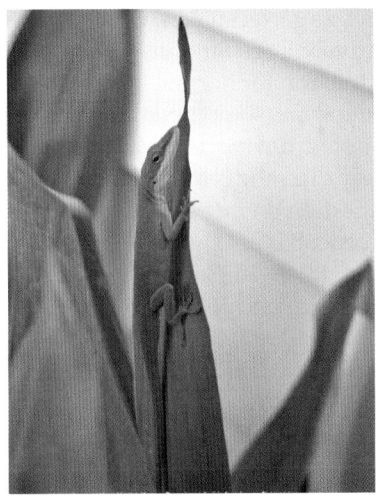

FIGURE 19.2 The green anole *Anolis carolinensis*, is a popular species for endocrinology and behavioral research.

and vertebrate evolutionary studies (Hews and Abell Baniki, 2013; Weiss *et al.*, 2013; Olsson *et al.*, 2013). The anole has been a model of reproductive morphology and behavior, locomotor performance, and hemoglobin biology (Lovern *et al.*, 2004; Storz *et al.*, 2011; Foster and Higham, 2012; Kerver and Wade, 2013) (Fig. 19.2). Due to the ability to regenerate its tail, the leopard gecko has been a model in regenerative research (McLean and Vickaryous, 2011). Fence lizards (*Sceloporus*) are used in toxicological investigations (Talent *et al.*, 2002; Brasfield *et al.*, 2004), and whiptails (*Aspidoscelis*) are models for investigating the mechanisms of parthenogenesis (Lutes *et al.*, 2010). Studies on tokay geckos have yielded insights into the adhesive property of the gecko toe that could lead to the invention of more effective and versatile synthetic fibrillar adhesives (Gillies *et al.*, 2013). Snakes are commonly used for chemoreception and behavior studies (Greenberg *et al.*, 1989). Snake venoms continue

to be extensively studied (Mackessy, 2010) and therapeutic startegies for envenomation investigated (Meggs *et al.*, 2010; Parker-Cote *et al.*, 2014). Venom research has resulted in development of models of conditions, such as myoglobinuria (Ponraj and Gopalakrishnakone, 1996), and contributed to discovery of novel therapeutic agents for diseases, such as diabetes (Furman, 2011). Crocodilians have been used in neuroanatomical and neurophysiological research, development of artificial blood and perfection of transmyocardial perfusion techniques (Dyer, 1995; Kohmoto *et al.*, 1997), stem cell research, mutagenic studies (Winston *et al.*, 1991; Wu *et al.*, 2013), and endocrine disrupter research (Crain and Guillette, 1998; Milnes and Guillette, 2008; Stoker *et al.*, 2008). With the advances in genomic research, genomes of a variety of reptile species have been sequenced, which has facilitated evolutionary biology studies and provided important insight into species-specific adaptive behavior (Castoe *et al.*, 2013; Tollis and Boissinot, 2014).

C. Availability and Sources

Acquisition of reptiles for research and teaching has traditionally involved capturing animals from the wild. Chronic overharvesting of species can result in severe declines of wild populations. When choosing a reptile species for research or teaching, reputable breeders should be used whenever possible. Animals purchased from these individuals are generally healthier and better adapted to captivity. Reptiles collected immediately after emergence from hibernation and held in suboptimal conditions are often susceptible to diseases resulting from stress and starvation. Many reptiles are captured in the wild by investigators and brought back to the laboratory for study. Alternatively, a species may be manipulated (sometimes rather extensively) in its natural habitat. Federal, state, and local permits may be required for collection and field studies, depending on location and the species involved. Investigators should be aware of and abide by all regulations governing the reptile they are studying (Greene, 1995; O'Rourke, 2014).

D. Laboratory Management and Husbandry

Reptiles represent a diverse group of animals with species-specific husbandry requirements. Several excellent references (cited throughout this chapter) address anatomy, physiology, behavior, reproduction, and captive maintenance of various species. These references should be routinely consulted prior to acquiring a given species of reptile.

1. *Primary Enclosures*

Reptiles can be maintained in a variety of primary enclosures. Glass aquaria are commonly used for housing. Aquaria are readily available, come in a variety of sizes, and are easily sanitized. The two major drawbacks to glass aquaria are that they are breakable and bulky. Plastic shoe and sweater boxes offer unbreakable alternatives to glass housing units. Durable brands can withstand repeated cage washing and do not warp if lids are placed back onto the cage immediately after removal from the cage washer. Perforations for ventilation can be made in the sides of the boxes, (often best done with a soldering iron under a fume hood to avoid cracking of the plastic) thereby allowing stacking of the plastic units while in use. Several types of reptile housing are commercially available; however, not all are sturdy enough to withstand cage washer temperatures. Cages can be purchased singly or in modular units. Some systems are constructed so that animals can be accessed from above, while others have front or back doors for access. When selecting a housing system, consideration should be given to which means of access is most suitable for the species being housed to avoid defensive or escape responses. Venomous reptiles should always be housed in unbreakable, lockable cages (Beaupre et al., 2004). Cages with central divider panels allow animal shifting for routine husbandry and minimize hazards associated with handling (Fig. 19.3). Despite the high thermal conductivity of metal, stainless steel cages can be adapted for larger species of reptiles, and turtles and crocodilians can be housed in galvanized stainless steel or fiberglass tanks. With few exceptions, reptiles are escape artists and must be housed in cages with secure lids. Lids can be made of screen or a solid impervious material that is partially screened or otherwise ventilated. Lids should fit snugly, and for many species, should be secondarily secured with latches.

Regardless of the type of primary enclosure, animals should be provided with adequate space to engage in natural behaviors and normal postural adjustments. Very active species with large home ranges will necessarily require larger cages than more sedentary species. Breeding animals may also require larger cage space. Substrate, visual barriers, climbing and perching surfaces, basking sites, and water sources add complexity to the cage and enhance physical and behavioral well-being. Substrates should be species-appropriate, absorbent, and nontoxic. Newspaper or brown paper works well and is easily removed and replaced, although not aesthetically pleasing and do not mimic a natural environment. Hardwood shavings and paper bedding are very absorbent, easy to spot-clean, and, most importantly, allow the animals to burrow. Indoor–outdoor carpet can be precut to fit cages, is easy to remove and sanitize, and works especially well for species such as garter snakes, which are very active and generate relatively large amounts of waste. Additionally, carpet offers traction for normal locomotion (Rossi, 1992). Hardwood chips are sometimes used but may inadvertently be ingested during feeding. Use of corncob bedding is strongly discouraged by many authors, because of accidental ingestion and development of gastrointestinal impaction. Corncob is also hygroscopic and will desiccate young animals. Likewise, kitty litter should not be used as a substrate (Page and Mautino, 1990; Anderson, 1991; Rossi, 1992; Boyer, 1991). Occasionally, a fastidious species may require a specific substrate, such as sand, small gravel, soil, sphagnum moss, bark, or mulch (Rossi, 1992), but care must be taken to ensure that sand and gravel are species-appropriate and will not be ingested and cause gastrointestinal impaction (Fig. 19.4). Sphagnum will

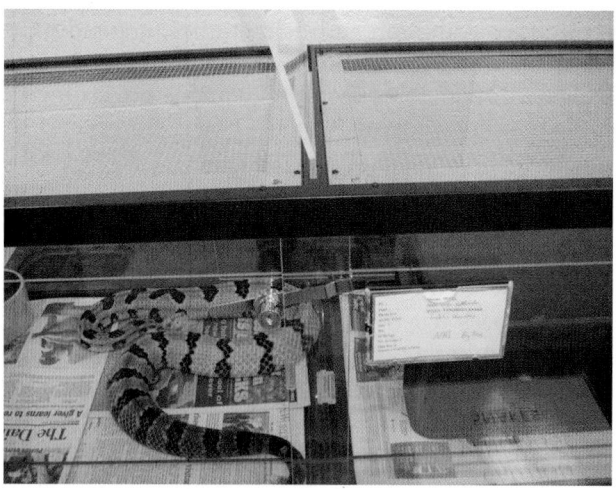

FIGURE 19.3 Venomous reptiles should be housed in unbreakable, lockable cages. Housing units with removable partitions allow animals to be shifted during husbandry.

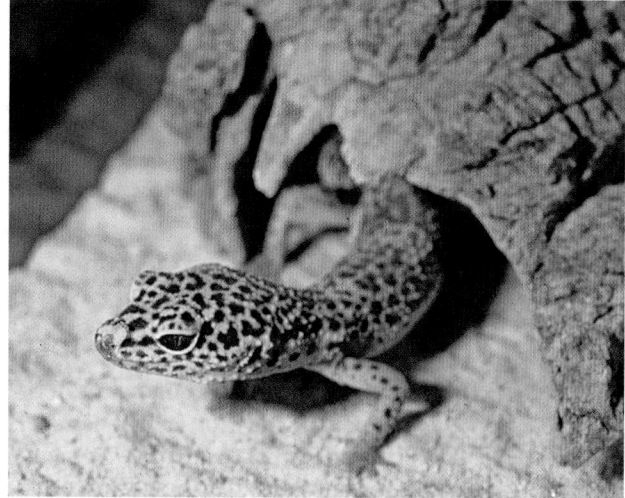

FIGURE 19.4 The leopard gecko is a desert species that can be housed on an appropriate sand substrate. Note the natural tree bark shelter that provides a visual barrier. Shelters should be provided for all species.

inhibit growth of pathogens; however, all natural substrates should be autoclaved, heat treated, or otherwise disinfected prior to use, to prevent potential introduction of pathogens. Most terrestrial reptiles should be provided with a water bowl. Species that lap drops of water from leaves in the wild should be misted in addition to being offered water in a container (Rossi, 1992). Water bowls should be shallow enough to allow easy access (especially for terrestrial turtles), heavy enough to prevent tipping, and wide enough to accommodate all occupants of the cage simultaneously. Most reptile species spend time soaking, particularly prior to shedding, and should have access to fresh water at all times.

In order to decrease stress and allow normal behavioral activity, reptile cages should contain certain accessories. Reptiles must be provided with a hide box or other shelter to serve as a retreat and visual barrier (Page and Mautino, 1990; Anderson, 1991; Boyer, 1991; Rossi, 1992). Stress and damage from trying to escape can also be minimized by making three sides of the cage opaque. A study conducted in aspic vipers indicated that shelter deprivation and low temperature are associated with increased corticosterone levels and decreased digestive performance (Bonnet et al., 2013). Environmental enrichment, such as a coconut shell on top of a branch to simulate a tree cavity, or a hide box containing moist sphagnum moss, has been shown to promote improvement in behavior of ratsnakes (Almli and Burghardt, 2006). Eastern box turtles raised in enriched enclosures containing cypress mulch substrate, shredded paper, and a hide box, had a lower heterophil to lymphocyte ratio (an indicator of chronic stress) and spent less time engaged in escape behavior compared to those housed in nonenriched enclosures (Case et al., 2004). Sanitizable, plastic hide boxes are available commercially in a variety of sizes. Polyvinyl chloride (PVC) pipe cut lengthwise in half works well, especially for larger species. Ceramic pots, heat-treated pieces of bark, and cardboard containers also make excellent refuges. Items that cannot be sanitized should be discarded when soiled. Arboreal (tree-dwelling) reptiles should be provided with branches or dowels on which to climb. Species that bask should be provided with basking platforms. This is particularly important for many aquatic reptiles. A haul-out area or platform, easily accessible from the water and large enough to comfortably hold all tank occupants, must be provided to aquatic species in order to allow normal drying and behavioral thermoregulation (Boyer and Boyer, 1992).

2. Water Quality

Aquatic reptiles are more tolerant than amphibians of chlorinated water; therefore, dechlorination of aquarium water is not necessary. In fact, chlorine may help retard growth of pathogens in the aquatic environment. When aquatic turtles are being housed, water should be at least as deep as the width of the shell; this will allow an overturned animal to right itself and not drown (Boyer and Boyer, 1992). Turtles and crocodilians generate significant amounts of waste; therefore, static systems with frequent complete water changes or flow-through systems are preferred over recirculating systems. If recirculating systems are used, water quality should be monitored on a routine basis.

3. Temperature

In general, reptiles prefer warmer temperatures than do amphibians. Warm temperatures are necessary for normal physiologic processes such as digestion, growth, reproduction, and immune function (Kanui et al., 1991; Dickinson and Fa, 1997). In general, each reptile species has an optimum temperature range in which it should be maintained (Mattison, 1998; Raske et al., 2012). Most reptiles possess the ability to raise and lower their body temperature in response to environmental fluctuations through behavioral and physiological mechanisms, such as basking, changes in posture, vascular shunting, metabolic heat production (limited to a few species), and changes in heart rate (hysteresis) (Seebacher and Franklin, 2005; Besson and Cree, 2010; Raske et al., 2012; Zhang et al., 2008). Some species, however, lack the capability to physiologically thermoregulate (Rice et al., 2006). Provision of a thermal gradient within a reptile's environment is dependent on individual species requirements (Beaupre et al., 2004). For terrestrial species, a thermal gradient can be provided by low-wattage incandescent bulbs focused over a basking area. For nocturnal or secretive species, heat pads or strips placed under part of the cage will result in a temperature gradient. Aquarium heaters will increase water temperature for aquatic species, and a haul-out with an overhead lamp will serve as a warm spot. 'Hot rocks' (electrically heated basking surfaces that directly contact the animal) can cause burns (Boyer, 1991; Barten, 1996a). Reptiles should never be allowed to come into direct contact with any heat source; life-threatening thermal burns can result.

4. Lighting

Many captive reptile species require exposure to ultraviolet light in the appropriate UVB spectrum (290–320 nm) in order to endogenously manufacture vitamin D_3 with the majority of conversion occurring around 290–300 nm (Gehrmann, 1996). Several species of active, diurnal lizards and turtles will develop metabolic bone disease (MBD) if deprived of ultraviolet light (Harcourt-Brown, 1996), particularly if an inappropriate diet (low in calcium or improper calcium–phosphorus ratio) is being fed. Conversely, too much light exposure can induce pathology (Gardiner et al., 2009). Information on specific species requirements are available (Barten and

Fleming, 2014; http://www.uvguide.co.uk/index.htm). These references additionally stress the importance of evaluating the levels of UVB produced by various light sources. Attention should also be given to composition of cage lids, as several materials will absorb UVB in the critical shorter wavelengths (Burger *et al.*, 2007). UV light diminishes rapidly with distance from the source and is easily filtered out by barriers; therefore, the ultraviolet light source should be placed close to the animal (generally less than 24 inches above the cage) with cage lids best being made of coarse mesh. Also, since bulb UV emittance diminishes with time, bulbs should be replaced approximately every 6 months (Divers, 1996). The biology, natural history, and nutritional requirements of a given species should always be carefully researched when deciding on whether or not to supplement with UV light.

Many reptiles do well with a 12h light–12h dark cycle. Animals on photoperiod-sensitive studies should have light cycles adjusted accordingly.

5. Airflow and Humidity

Reptiles are ectothermic and therefore have low metabolic rates and low oxygen demands. In fact, airflows appropriate for mammals can easily desiccate small reptiles due to their high surface to volume ratio.

Most reptiles (with the exception of some desert-dwelling species) do well in a relative humidity range of 30–70%, but humidity requirements can be very specific for some species. Low relative humidity can result in dysecdysis (difficulty with shedding), and humidity that is too high can result in 'blister disease' (Cooper, 2006).

6. Secondary Enclosures

Conventional animal rooms can be adapted for reptile housing. Temperature and light cycles should be controlled for each room, and airflow rates should not be excessive. Rooms housing aquatic species should be equipped with sinks and floor drains to facilitate tank flushing and cleaning.

7. Sanitation

Whenever possible, reptile cages should be sanitized in a cage washer. If this is not feasible, cages and tanks can be hand-sanitized with disinfectant. The choice should be based on safety to personnel and animals, accessibility of the compound, ease of application, and efficacy against pathogens. Bleach, chlorine dioxide, and hydrogen peroxides are effective against vegetative bacteria, *Mycoplasma*, enveloped and nonenveloped viruses, fungi, acid-fast bacteria, and some spores. However, these agents can be corrosive and concentrated solutions may be potentially harmful to respiratory systems. Quaternary ammonium compounds and chlorhexidine are effective against vegetative bacteria,

but not pseudomonads, acid-fast bacteria, and nonenveloped viruses. Iodines are effective against vegetative bacteria, pseudomonads, acid-fast bacteria, and bacterial spores, but are not effective against nonenveloped viruses. Alcohols are very effective against vegetative bacteria, Mycoplasmas, and pseudomonads, but ineffective against nonenveloped viruses and bacterial spores. Organic debris renders disinfectants less effective; therefore, debris should always be removed before application of disinfectant. For additional information on disinfection, consult the disinfection guidelines produced by the Center for Food Security and Public Health (http://www.cfsph.iastate.edu/Disinfection/). Phenolic compounds are extremely toxic to reptiles and must never be used around these animals, even to clean secondary enclosures (Page and Mautino, 1990; Anderson, 1991; Divers, 1996). In general, a 3% sodium hypochlorite solution (1 part commercial bleach and 29 parts water) works well for sanitizing cages, hide boxes, water bowls, indoor–outdoor carpet, and equipment. Regardless of disinfectant used, objects should be thoroughly rinsed and dried before being returned to cages. Sanitation frequency of terrestrial reptile primary enclosures depends on number of animals per enclosure, habitat type, feeding frequency, and other variables. Although reptiles produce less waste than mammals, infrequent cleanings can result in buildup of pathogens such as *Salmonella* and *Pseudomonas*. Some authors advocate prolonged intervals between cleanings, based on research demonstrating increased exploratory behavior (and presumably stress) following removal of feces and odor during cage cleaning (Conant, 1971; Pough, 1991). Other authors, however, have documented that the increased activity associated with being subjected to a clean environment or other novel stimuli can result in positive behaviors (Huff, 1980; Radcliffe and Murphy, 1983). Chiszar *et al.* (1980) demonstrated that the stimulus for increased exploratory behavior was the presence of a clean cage rather than the handling associated with the cleaning event. The most logical approach to maintaining a healthy environment is to sanitize at intervals frequent enough to prevent pathogen buildup, while spot-cleaning as necessary between complete cage changes. Assessing the effectiveness of cleaning and sanitizing at selected intervals will generate data driven performance standards for the species and housing conditions. As a rule of thumb, changing cages at 1- to 2-week intervals works well for most species of snakes. Cages for garter snakes and other reptiles that generate relatively large amounts of waste may need to be cleaned weekly. In contrast, desert species housed at low population densities in large enclosures may require more infrequent sanitation. Water bowls should be kept clean at all times, and changed upon contamination (some captive snakes preferentially defecate in water).

8. Handling

When handling a reptile, it is important to support the animal's body as much as possible. Reptiles should never be picked up or restrained by the tail. Autotomy, an escape mechanism involving tail loss through a fracture plane, is found in many lizard species. Lizards should have both the pectoral and pelvic girdles supported, with the tail gently held to prevent slapping. Very aggressive animals may have to be restrained behind the head to prevent defensive biting. Lizards typically bite and hold on, and even relatively small animals can inflict a painful wound. Many lizards also have long, sharp claws and can scratch the handler, as well as tail slap. Small crocodilians can be held much the same as lizards, with more attention focused on head and tail restraint (crocodilians can administer a very powerful slap with the tail). Crocodilians may also roll when being held, in an effort to escape, and rough scales with dermal bones on the dorsal surface of the crocodilian can abrade hands. Large crocodilians should never be handled by one person alone. Tape can be wrapped around the animal's snout (taking care to avoid the nares) to prevent biting. Crocodilians have powerful jaws for crushing prey, yet relatively weak muscles for opening the mouth; therefore, muzzles work well. Many turtles can be restrained by holding the sides of the shell. However, species such as snapping turtles, softshell turtles, and mud and musk turtles have exceptionally long necks and can reach around and bite. These animals should be held by the back of the shell, taking care to avoid being scratched by claws on the hind feet. When holding snakes, as much of the animal's body as possible should be supported. Many snakes are more comfortable if allowed to move about in the restrainer's hands. Snakes should never be held behind the head unless absolutely necessary. Grabbing a snake too tightly behind the head can damage tissues, restrict breathing, and elicit a much more panicked escape response. Many snakes are quite docile if approached quietly and restrained gently.

9. Identification

Reptiles can be identified in a variety of ways, including photographic documentation of unique color and scale patterns or physical anomalies; application of nontoxic paint or other temporary markers; shell notching, tail notching, scale clipping, and toe clipping; external tags and transmitters; and injected or surgically implanted passive integrated transponders (PIT tags) and radiotransmitters (Plummer and Ferner, 2012; Norton et al., 2014). Determination of the most appropriate method to use must take into consideration duration of study, potential damage/loss of external markers due to normal animal activities and environmental conditions, potential harm to animals from external markers entangling in objects, and potential migration and loss of internal markers (Norton et al., 2014). Knowledge of species behavior and habitat is essential when marking reptiles for release. Procedures involving notching or clipping that extend into dermal bone or tissues must be conducted with appropriate technique and involve adequate analgesia. Surgical procedures must be conducted aseptically, with appropriate anesthesia and analgesia. Toe clipping, a marking procedure widely used in lizards, remains controversial. One report indicated that toe clipping had no effect on locomotion speed of a scincid lizard (Borges-Landaez and Shine, 2003), while another described significant impact on clinging performance of Anolis carolinensis, and noted that increasing the number of toes removed dramatically reduced clinging performance (Bloch and Irschick, 2004). Toe clipping should be evaluated on a case-by case basis, with thorough consideration of species behavior, proper technique, appropriate pain mitigation, potential sequelae, and alternative marking methods.

10. Quarantine

All new reptiles entering a facility should be quarantined. Many animals purchased from vendors are in fact wild-caught, and, depending on the practices of the holding facility, could be more severely stressed and diseased than animals collected directly from the wild. Animals that are colony-bred are typically healthier; however, few reptiles arrive with complete health reports. Therefore, it is best to quarantine all animals prior to introduction into an existing colony. Jacobson (1993b) recommends a 90-day quarantine period for snakes. On arrival, animals should be weighed and receive physical examinations and appropriate diagnostic tests. External and internal parasites should be tested for and treated. Infectious disease should be diagnosed and treated. Feeding records should be kept, and any relevant observations recorded. A reptile with clinical signs of disease should never be introduced into an existing collection.

11. Zoonoses

Reptiles can harbor bacteria in their intestinal tracts, oral cavity, or skin that can be inadvertently transmitted to humans during handling. In many cases, these bacteria do not cause any clinical issues in humans; however, in immunocompromised individuals, the acquisition of these bacteria can manifest in serious clinical outcomes (Mitchell, 2011, 2012). Therefore, good hygiene and careful handling should always be practiced to prevent infection.

Among the bacteria harbored by reptiles, Salmonella is considered one of the most significant pathogens, causing serious disease in people (Mermin et al., 1997; Austin and Wilkins, 1998; Gong et al., 2013; Gorski et al., 2013). To date, numerous strains/serovars of Salmonella have been isolated from reptiles. Healthy turtles, snakes, and lizards can carry the organism in their gastrointestinal tracts and shed when stressed (Chiodini and Sundberg, 1981; Austin and Wilkins, 1998). Transmission to humans is through the fecal–oral route, and indirect transmission through handling contaminated objects is common. Signs of salmonellosis in humans include fever, vomiting, cramps, and diarrhea. Individuals who are immunosuppressed, elderly, very young (less than 1 year old), or taking medication to increase gastric pH are at greater risk of infection. The disease can progress and cause dehydration, meningitis, osteomyelitis, and sepsis (Anonymous, 1992, 1995; Austin and Wilkins, 1998). Treatment of reptiles to eliminate the carrier state has not been successful and can result in antibiotic-resistant strains of the organism (D'Aoust et al., 1990). Immunocompromised individuals, pregnant women, and children under 5 years of age should avoid contact with reptiles (Anonymous, 1992, 1995). A set of dedicated cleaning equipment and supplies should be used for reptiles, and hands must be washed thoroughly after contacting reptiles or equipment (Austin and Wilkins, 1998).

Aquatic species of reptiles have been implicated in cases of atypical mycobacteriosis (*Mycobacterium chelonae*) and *Edwardsiella tarda* infections. Although these infections are rare, the organisms may pose a health hazard, particularly for immunocompromised individuals or people with underlying diseases (Miller et al., 1990; Darrow et al., 1993). Humans often contract the disease during sanitation of the animal enclosure when contaminated water comes into contact with the skin. Appropriate precautions, such as avoiding direct contact with contaminated water (particularly if fingers and hands have preexisting injuries), wearing gloves, and washing hands thoroughly after handling aquatic reptiles or their caging and equipment, should help prevent disease transmission.

Recent evidence also suggests that reptiles may be a carrier of pathogenic bacteria such as *Chlamydia*, *Campylobacter fetus*, and vancomycin-resistant enterococcus species, all of which can cause diseases in humans (Mitchell, 2011). Crocodiles have been shown to carry West Nile virus. Pentastomes, *Crytosporidium pestis*, spargana, ticks, and mites (*Ophionyssus natricis*) of reptiles can also infect humans and cause mild to severe disease (Anantaphruti et al., 2011; Mitchell, 2011).

12. Venomous Species

Numerous snake species and two species of lizards are venomous. Venoms have been traditionally classified as hemotoxic and neurotoxic; however, extensive research into venom composition has identified complex mixtures of varying arrays of enzymes and toxins, including metalloproteinases, phospholipase 2 enzymes, serine proteases, three finger toxins, nucleases, disintegrins, fasiculins, hyaluronins, acetylcholinesterases, and

nerve growth factors (Mackessy, 2010). For this reason, it is essential to be thoroughly familiar with the biology, behavior, and toxicity of any venomous species housed in the laboratory animal facility. Essential considerations for management of venomous reptiles include limiting access to the housing room as much as possible; housing the animals in unbreakable, locked cages; use of equipment such as snake tongs, snake hooks, long forceps, large plastic garbage cans, and acrylic tubes for handling, feeding, and restraint; protocols for routine cage changing, animal handling, and accidental envenomation; and thorough training of all personnel involved with these species. Special caging can be designed for highly aggressive or specialized species (Mason et al., 1991; Greene, 1997), and venomous species can be housed in shift cages to minimize handling. General recommendations for housing and handling venomous species can be found in Beaupre et al. (2004).

II. BIOLOGY

A. Anatomy and Physiology

1. Integumentary System

Reptile skin consists of scales that include a β-keratin covering. The elastic form found in most vertebrates, α-keratin, covers the skin between the scales. Snakes and lizards have an epidermal structure with α-keratin on the inside and β-keratin on the outside covered by a thin layer consisting of mature very tough keratinized cells called Oberhauthcen (Zug, 1993; Mass, 2013). Both the scutes and sutures of many hard-shelled turtles contains only β keratin (Vitt and Caldwell, 2009), while the shell of softshell and leatherback sea turtles consists of an intricate mesh consisting of α-keratin and beta-proteins (β-keratin) (Alibardi et al., 2013). In crocodilians and turtles, epidermal growth is continuous, as is the shedding of pieces of skin. In contrast, lizards and snakes have a synchronized pattern of ecdysis (shedding). Germinal cells undergo a resting phase prior to synchronously beginning to divide. A second epithelial layer is formed beneath the original; this renewal phase takes 1–2 weeks. During this time, the skin is dull and the eyes appear cloudy (opaque) (Fig. 19.5). Lymph then diffuses between the layers and enzymatically cleaves them. The skin and eye opacities resolve, and shedding usually occurs 3–4 days following this clearing (Zug, 1993; Rossi, 1996; Fig. 19.5). In addition to its role in normal growth, ecdysis enables lizards and snakes to eliminate toxins and heavy metals (Jones et al., 2005). The frequency of shedding in snakes is increased by multiple factors, including increased temperature, feeding frequency, and injury.

Crocodilians, some lizards, and turtles have osteoderms (bony plates in the dermis); these are usually

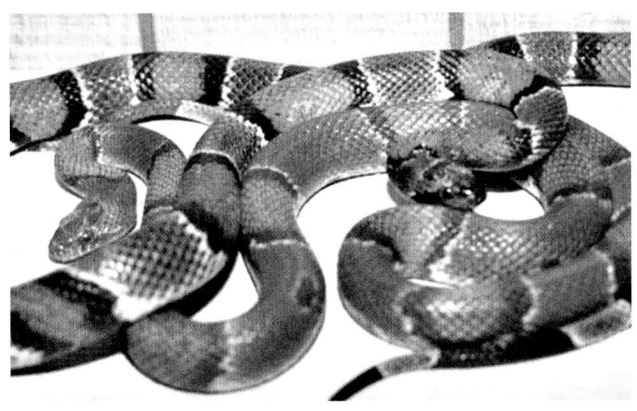

FIGURE 19.5 Two gray banded king snakes. The animal with the dull skin and eye coloration is in the process of generating a new epidermal layer, a stage often referred to as being 'opaque.' During the opaque phase, snakes may refuse to eat and become less visual and more defensive if handled.

found on the dorsal and lateral surfaces of the animals. Skin glands are present and have a variety of functions. Many turtles have Rathke's glands which open in the inguinal and axillary regions or on the bridge between the carapace (dorsal shell) and plastron (ventral shell) (Vitt and Caldwell, 2009; Mass, 2013). Male tortoises and both sexes of crocodilians have mental glands in the mandibular area; crocodilians also have cloacal glands. A linear array of secretory pores is evident on the inside of the thighs or cranial to the vent in male lizards of certain species; these are sexual scent glands. Snakes and some lizards have paired scent glands that empty through the cloaca and seem to function in defense and/ or sexual recognition. Salt glands are found in a variety of locations (tongue, orbit, nasal passage) in several species of marine and desert reptiles (sea snakes, crocodiles, some lizards, turtles). These glands excrete excess salt (Jacobson, 1984; Zug, 1993; Vitt and Caldwell, 2009).

2. Musculoskeletal System

Reptiles have undergone a variety of musculoskeletal adaptations during evolution. Crocodilians possess eight pairs of true ribs, each having an additional, floating rib, or gastralia, associated with it. The gastralia are actually dermal bones (Lane, 2006). Another notable feature of crocodilians is the bony and muscular arrangement that allows these animals to close their mouths with incredible crushing force. Refinement of cranial bones in snakes aid in feeding. Flexible ligaments, rather than a mandibular symphysis, connect the independently moving mandibles. Each mandible also has a joint in the middle, which permits outward bowing and expansion. Additionally, the mandibles are independently attached to outward-slanted, free-swinging quadrate bones (Greene, 1997). These adaptations allow snakes to swallow prey items much larger than their own heads.

Primitive snakes, such as boas and pythons, have remnants of pelvic girdles, which are visible radiographically. Boas and pythons also have residual hind limb bones which terminate in a claw on each side of the vent, These 'spurs' are used during courtship.

The vertebrae and ribs of turtles are fused with dermal bone to form a bony shell. The dorsal part is referred to as the carapace, and the ventral part of the shell is called the plastron. Box turtles have a hinge in the front part of the plastron, which closes to seal off access to the body when the legs and head are retracted.

Most iguanid lizard species have fracture planes in the more distal caudal vertebrae; these allow the tail to separate (autotomize) from the body if the animal's tail is seized by a predator. Cartilagenous rods, rather than bone, form the support structure for regrown tails (Barten, 2006).

3. Respiratory System

Compared to mammals, the glottis of reptiles is usually easy to visualize and access. This slitlike structure lies on the pharyngeal floor in all reptiles, and is typically closed (which allows reptiles to passively hold their breath). Its position in the cranial part of the mouth in snakes and many lizards enables them to hold large prey items in their mouth for prolonged periods while continuing to breathe. In turtles and crocodilians, the glottis can be found behind the base of the fleshy tongue. Crocodilians have a basihyal valve, a fold of tissue at the caudal aspect of the tongue, which meets the palate to form a watertight seal and permits these animals to hold prey in their mouths while submerged (Schaeffer, 1997).

The primary respiratory organ in reptiles is the lung. Most reptiles have paired lungs, although many snakes have an elongate right lung and either no or a small vestigal left lung. The lungs of snakes and many lizards are saclike structures with faveoli (small sacs) that radiate out from the lung wall and increase surface area for gas exchange. Lungs may end in rather extensive air sacs (Fig. 19.6). Advanced lizards, turtles, and crocodilians have multichambered lungs. In turtles, movement of the head and limbs causes air to be forced in and out of the lungs. Crocodilians have a muscular septum that functions like a mammalian diaphragm (Stoakes, 1992; Zug, 1993; Vitt and Caldwell, 2009). Both inspiration and expiration are active processes in squamates.

Many reptiles, particularly aquatic species, are tolerant of anoxia and can go for prolonged periods without breathing (Zug, 1993; Wasser et al., 1997; Hicks and Wang, 1998). This physiologic adaptation can significantly impact methods of anesthesia and euthanasia for these species.

Most reptiles do not routinely vocalize. Obvious exceptions are crocodilians, some species of turtles and lizards, and the pine snake, Pituophis melanoleucus. Pituophis is the first snake described to have a functional vocal cord (Young et al., 1995).

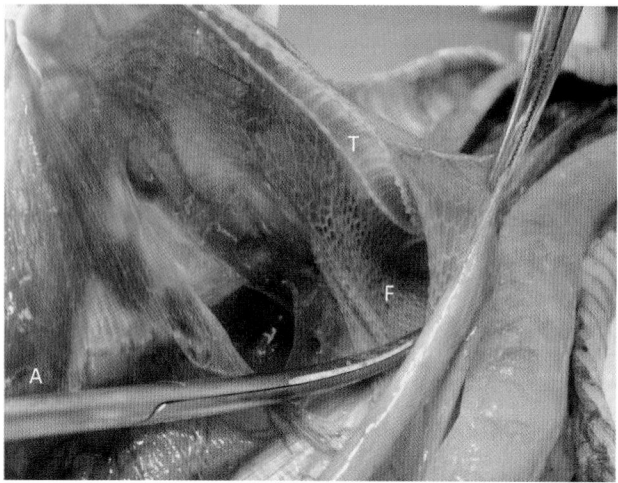

FIGURE 19.6   The lung of a snake. Note the incomplete tracheal rings (T), the faveoli (F) which increase surface area for gas exchange, and the posterior part of the lung terminating into the smooth walled air sac (A).

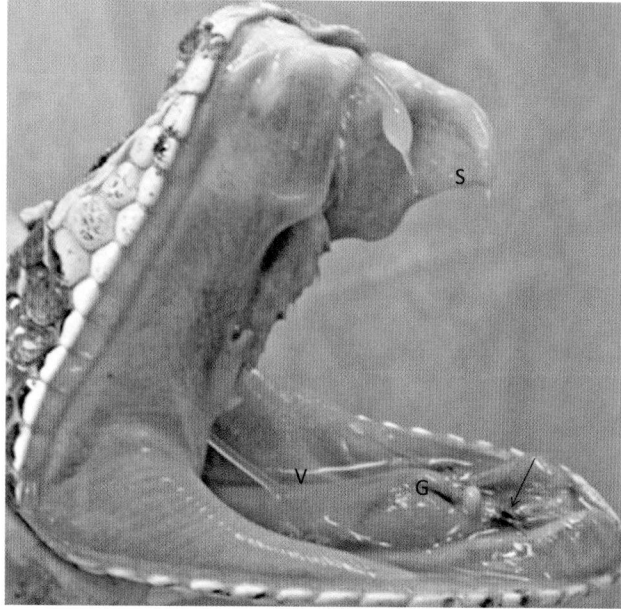

FIGURE 19.7   Vipers such as the rattlesnake have erectile fangs covered by a sheath (S). Note the glottis opening (G), forked tongue retracted into the tongue sheath (arrow), and pooled straw colored venom (V).

4. Cardiovascular System

No single anatomic model exists for the reptilian heart and circulation. Generally, with the exception of crocodilians, all reptiles have a three-chambered heart, consisting of paired atria and a single ventricle. Despite having only a single ventricle, presence of muscular ridges combined with timing of ventricular contraction sequences create functional separation of blood flow (Murray, 2006). Reptiles also have paired aortas.

Crocodilians have a four-chambered heart. However, the foramen of Panizza provides a connection between the two aortas that enables crocodilians to shunt blood to cephalic and coronary circulations during anoxic events such as diving (Axelsson *et al.*, 1991; Zug, 1993; Axelsson *et al.*, 1996; Vitt and Caldwell, 2009).

Lizards have a midventral abdominal vein that lies just inside the abdominal wall. This vein should be avoided when making surgical incisions (Barten, 1996b).

5. Gastrointestinal System

Snakes and a few lizard species demonstrate remarkable adaptation of the salivary glands. In these species, digestive enzymes have been modified into venoms. Vipers, elapids, and some other snakes have true venom glands, which secrete venom through ducts to a pair of fangs (generally fixed in elapids and retractable in viperids) (Fig. 19.7). Duvernoy's gland, composed of branched tubules, is present under the skin of the maxillary region, near the angle of the jaw. A duct connects Duvernoy's gland to a sometimes enlarged, grooved maxillary tooth. Duvernoy's gland is present in many species of colubrids (Greene, 1997). Venom production in Gila monsters and beaded lizards occurs in the enlarged salivary glands of the lower jaw, with venom entering the mouth through numerous ducts and then being transported up through groves in the teeth via capillary action; chewing enhances venom delivery in these species.

Crocodilians, snakes, and lizards have teeth; turtles have a keratinous jaw sheath (horny beak) that is used to bite off chunks of food.

The esophagus of snakes is thin-walled and distensible, to accommodate large prey. Crocodilian stomachs are round, muscular, and thick-walled, and often contain gastroliths to aid in digestion (Lane, 1996). Crocodiles have a number of connective tissue septa that separate the body cavity into several separate components (Van Der Merwe and Kotze, 1993; Mushonga and Horowitz, 1996). Unlike mammals, the pancreas in snakes is discrete and compact (Moscona, 1990). It is located caudal to the pylorus and closely associated with the gallbladder and spleen. The liver of snakes is elongate, in accordance with other anatomic features of this group. Alligators have fibrous trabeculae that course through the liver (Beresford, 1993). Some turtle species have pigmented cell aggregations in the spleen and liver; these are macrophages, which increase in number as animals age (Christiansen *et al.*, 1996).

Analogous to herbivorous mammals, the small intestine and colon tend to be larger in herbivorous species of reptiles (Jacobson, 1984; Barboza, 1995). In some snake species that eat infrequently, energy is conserved through atrophy of the small intestine and related organs between meals (Secor and Diamond, 1997). In all

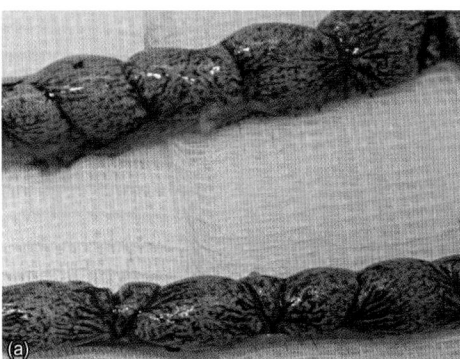
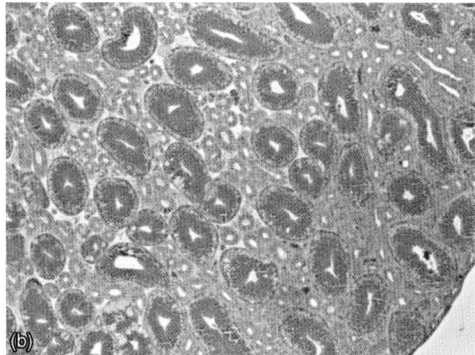

FIGURE 19.8   Reproductively active male snake kidneys can contain sexual segments that are grossly creamy pale colored (a) and histologically contain eosinophilic refractile granules (b). 4X magnification.

reptiles, products of the digestive, excretory, and reproductive tracts empty into the cloaca.

6. Excretory System

Reptiles have paired, metanephric kidneys. In many species of snakes, geckos, skinks, and iguanids, kidneys exhibit sexual dimorphic characteristics whereby reproductively active male kidneys develop accessory sex structures called sex segments. These segments appear creamy pale or yellowish (Fig. 19.8a) and contain eosinophilic refractile granules of lipids, enzymes, and proteins that are hypothesized to function as copulatory plugs (Holz and Raidal, 2006; Jacobson, 2007a; Sever et al., 2012) (Fig. 19.8b). This characteristic should not be mistaken for gout, as kidneys affected by gout and those that have sexual glands can appear quite similar. Functionally, the kidneys of aquatic species primarily excrete ammonia, semiaquatic species excrete urea, and terrestrial species excrete primarily uric acid (Coulson and Hernandez, 1983; Jacobson, 1984). *Pelodiscus sinensis*, the Chinese soft-shelled turtle, an inhabitant of brackish swamps and marshes, frequently lacks access to fresh water to enable urea secretion through the kidneys. Villiform processes inside the buccopharyngeal cavity have enabled this species to submerge its head under water and excrete urea through the mouth (Ip et al., 2013). A renal portal system that drains venous blood from the caudal half of a reptile's body directly through the kidneys has been described. Recent evidence, however, suggests that at least in some species, venous blood may be diverted past the kidneys directly to the liver in certain circumstances (Holz et al., 1997; Holz and Raidal, 2006). This should be taken into consideration when choosing routes of administration for drugs that undergo renal or hepatic metabolism and excretion (Mosley et al., 2011; Kummrow et al., 2008).

Many species of lizards and turtles have a urinary bladder. In lizards that lack a urinary bladder, urine is stored in the distal colon. Because urine is first drained into the urodeum of the cloaca before entering the bladder or colon, lizard urine is not sterile (Barten, 2006). In contrast, the ureters of turtles empty urine directly into the urinary bladder (Boyer and Boyer, 2006). Snakes and crocodilians do not have a urinary bladder, but can store urine in the distal colon.

7. Nervous System/Special Senses

The reptilian brain has cerebral hemispheres and 12 cranial nerves. The spinal cord extends to the tip of the tail and contains locomotor control centers, thereby allowing animals to respond at the spinal level (Davies, 1981; Lawton, 1992). Among the living reptile species, crocodilians appear to have the largest brain (Northcutt, 2013).

Most reptiles have lidded eyes and nictitating membranes. Snakes and some lizards (e.g., geckos) are an exception; in these species, the lids are transparent and have fused to permanently cover the eye as a spectacle. Snakes also lack nictitating membranes and scleral ossicles present in other reptiles (Millichamp and Jacobson, 1983; Vitt and Caldwell, 2009). Harderian glands are present in the orbits of many reptilian species and may function in vomerolfaction (Rehorek, 1997). Many reptiles have a vomeronasal organ, which is used to detect particulate odors (Zug, 1993; Vitt and Caldwell, 2009). In snakes and some lizards, particles of odor are picked up by a forked tongue and carried to the vomeronasal organ located in the palate.

Some species of snakes have pit organs that house infrared heat receptors. Certain boid species have pits scattered in the infralabial and supralabial scales. In pythons, a row of pits occurs in the labial (lip) scales; and, in pit vipers, a single organ is located on each side of the head in the loreal scale between the eye and nostril (Vitt and Caldwell, 2009). In pit vipers, coordination of the infrared sensing mechanism of pit organ and ocular function is essential for prey targeting (Chen et al., 2012).

Many lizard species have a parietal or 'third' eye, which contains photoreceptors that may permit enhanced detection at dawn and dusk (Solessio and Engbretson, 1993) and light dependent magnetoreceptive and orientation responses (Foà et al., 2009; Nishimura et al., 2010). Other lizards have dermal photoreceptors that may function in regulation of basking behavior (Tosini and Avery, 1996).

External ears are found only in crocodilians and some lizard species; other lizards and turtles possess tympana that are flush with the skin covering the head. Snakes lack external ears and tympanic membranes, and have significantly reduced to absent middle ear cavities (Vitt and Caldwell, 2006; Christensen et al., 2012). Detection of predators and prey is through vibration, transmitted through the body to the quadrate bone and then to the columella and inner ear (Greene, 1997; Christensen et al., 2012).

8. Normal Values

Hematology and plasma biochemistry analyses are routine diagnostic tests that can yield valuable information on the health status of reptiles. Normal values can vary considerably among and even within a species. Physiologic factors, such as age, sex, reproductive state, and body condition, will impact results, as will external factors such as captive versus wild state, and even sample purity and location of venipuncture site. Test results should always be interpreted in the context of these variables. Reptilian red blood cells are nucleated, as well as fewer in number and larger than red blood cells of mammals and birds. Lizards tend to have greater numbers of red blood cells than snakes, which have more than turtles. The normal packed cell volume (PCV) of reptiles is around 30% (Campbell, 2014). The white blood cells of reptiles include heterophils, eosinophils, basophils (granulocytes), thrombocytes, lymphocytes, monocytes, and in some species, azurophils (agranulocytes). In most species, heterophils have fusiform, eosinophilic cytoplasmic granules and function as phagocytic cells, similar to the neutrophils of mammals. Eosinophils resemble heterophils but have spherical brightly eosinophilic cytoplasmic granules. Basophils are small cells filled with basophilic granules, which frequently obscure the nucleus. Thrombocytes are the reptilian equivalent of platelets and are nucleated cells with elliptical to fusiform shape. Lymphocytes are round cells with a typically large nucleus to cytoplasm ratio. In some species, lymphocytes can closely resemble thrombocytes, but thrombocytes tend to have cytoplasmic vacuoles. Monocytes typically are the largest leukocytes, with vacuolated cytoplasm or azurophilic granules (azurophils). External variables can exert a significant impact on total leukocyte counts; therefore, numbers usually must exceed 30,000 cells/μl to be considered an inflammatory response to infection. Lymphocytes are typically

the predominant leukocyte in reptiles, and can comprise over 80% of a normal differential count in some species. Heterophils, likewise variable by species, can be up to 40% of a normal leukogram. Some turtle species can have up to 20% eosinophils, while lizards typically have lower numbers. Similarly, basophils are variable by species, and can reach up to 40%. Monocytes typically comprise up to 10% of the leukocyte count. Snake monocytes are often referred to as azurophils (Hawkey and Dennett, 1989; Campbell, 2014).

The most useful clinical chemistry tests for reptiles include aspartate aminotransferase (AST), calcium, glucose, phosphorus, total protein, and uric acid. Other useful tests include creatine and creatine kinase (CK). Tests used to detect renal disease include blood urea nitrogen (BUN), uric acid, and creatinine. Elevations in lactate dehydrogenase (LDH) and AST may be indicative of hepatocellular disease. Green-tinged plasma could be a sign of hepatobiliary disease, since biliverdin, not bilirubin, is the end product of reptilian hemoglobin catabolism in most species. Increased CK levels can be consistent with struggling or muscle damage. Normal plasma total protein values range between 3–7 g/dl; increases may indicate dehydration or chronic inflammatory disease. Conversely, hypoproteinemia can be associated with malnutrition and gastrointestinal parasitism, severe blood loss, and chronic hepatic or renal disease. Most reptiles have a normal blood glucose range between 60–100 mg/dl; sodium ranges between 120–170 mEq/l, and potassium typically ranges between 2–6 mEq/l, depending on species (Campbell, 2014).

B. Nutrition

Reptiles fill a wide variety of ecological niches and range in dietary habits from carnivorous to herbivorous. Regardless of diet, food should be fresh and nutritious. Prey items should be maintained on wholesome diets appropriate for that species. Crocodilians begin life preying on insects and other invertebrates, small frogs, and fish. As crocodilians grow, prey size increases and may include other reptiles, birds, and mammals. In captivity, small to medium crocodilians can be fed whole fish or rodents. Crocodilians can be adapted to dry chows; however, these should contain over 40% protein (Staton et al., 1990; Donoghue and Langenberg, 1996). Crocodilians do not digest or assimilate plant protein (Lane, 2006). Young crocodilians will eat daily; older animals can have longer intervals between meals.

Snakes are carnivorous and insectivorous, and several species have very specialized diets. Colubrids (king snakes, rat snakes) and boas feed readily on rodents; king snakes will also eat other snakes. Fish, frogs, and earthworms are common food items for garter snakes, and water snakes do well on fish. Specialized feeders among snakes include eastern hognose snakes, which subsist on toads and frogs; mud snakes, which eat amphiumas; and members of the genus *Regina*, which feed on crawfish. Whenever possible, snakes should be fed euthanized rodents to avoid prey-induced trauma and minimize distress in the prey animal. Frozen prey items should always be thawed to at least room temperature, to avoid putrefaction of food in the stomach (Fig. 19.9). Fish should be obtained from parasite-free sources or frozen for several days prior to feeding in order to prevent transmission of some parasites. Depending on species, most snakes will eat every 1–4 weeks; younger animals typically need to eat more frequently.

Many turtles are omnivorous or herbivorous. Box turtles are omnivores with carnivorous tendencies. In the wild, they will eat earthworms, slugs, insects, fish, frogs, and small birds and mammals, along with mushrooms,

tomatoes, berries, fruits, and vegetables (Fig. 19.10a). An example of a captive box turtle diet could include 50% animal protein (carnivore diet [trout chow] and whole prey), balanced with 50% plant material (75% dark leafy greens [mustard, collards, turnips, romaine, occasional cabbage, kale, spinach], vegetables [squash, sweet potatoes, carrots, mushrooms], 25% berries [raspberries, strawberries, blueberries], and fruit [tomatoes, bananas, apples, etc.]) (Boyer and Boyer, 2006). Herbivorous tortoises prefer thawed frozen mixed vegetables, fresh dark leafy greens, grasses, clover, dandelions, roses, hibiscus, carnations, legumes, soaked alfalfa pellets, squash, sprouts, and some fruit (Mattison, 1998; Boyer and Boyer, 2006) (Fig. 19.10b). Aquatic species such as the red-eared slider (*Trachemys scripta elegans*) and the painted turtle (*Chrysemys picta*) eat whole minnows, small chopped mice, trout chow, and earthworms (Mattison, 1998). For older animals, dark leafy greens and aquatic plants should also be offered (Parmenter and Avery, 1990; Boyer and Boyer, 2006). In general, small turtles should be fed daily, while larger animals can be fed two to three times per week.

Lizards range from total herbivores to strict carnivores. Green iguanas (*Iguana iguana*) are herbivorous and should be fed a plant-based diet that has adequate protein and calcium. Legumes, including alfalfa, clover, and bean sprouts; lima, snap, and green beans; and green, sugar, and snow peas are good sources of calcium and protein. Other plants with high protein content include mushrooms, dandelion, spinach, and romaine lettuce (Donoghue, 2006). One recommended diet for green iguanas includes calcium-rich leafy greens such as turnips, mustards, collards, parsley, and mint; equal amounts of other vegetables, such as beans, peas, squash, mushrooms, and yams; soaked alfalfa pellets; occasional fruits such as apples, peaches, figs, strawberries, and

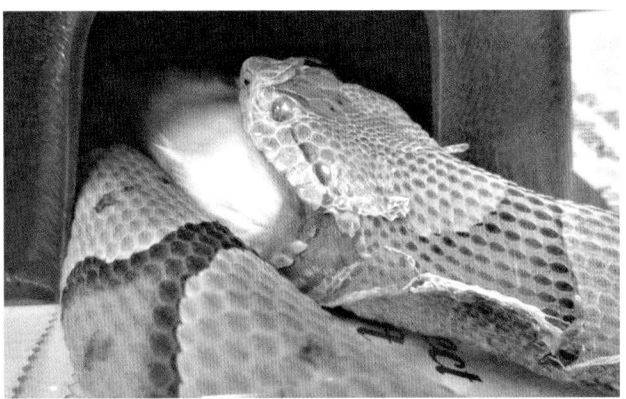

FIGURE 19.9 Copperhead swallowing pre-killed mouse. Snakes have flexible ligaments which permit mandibular expansion to swallow large prey items. Note the patchy, partially shed skin which is abnormal in snakes (dysecdysis) and indicative of environmental or health problems.

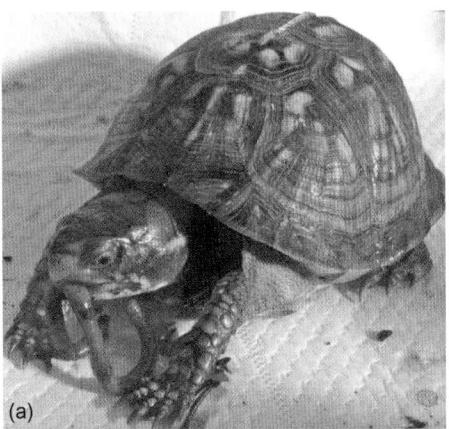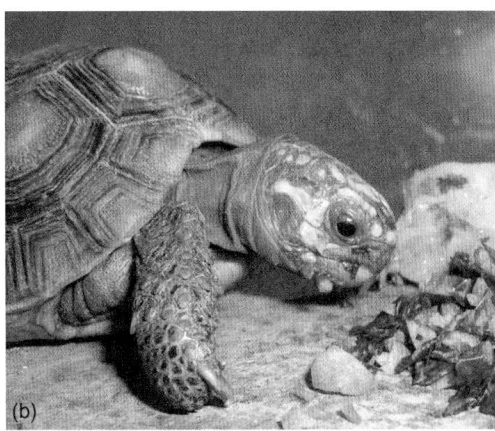

FIGURE 19.10 Box turtles are omnivores and relish earthworms (a). Tortoises are herbivorous and eat dark leafy greens such as collards, along with other vegetables and fruit (b).

bananas; and vitamin/mineral supplementation (Barten, 2006). Anoles are insectivorous and can be fed crickets, if the crickets are fed a nutritional diet prior to being offered to the lizard (Allen, 1997). Other insects that should be offered include mealworms, waxworms, and earthworms (Barten, 2006). Some species, such as the day geckos (genus *Phelsuma*), are primarily insectivorous but also eat ripe fruit (McKeown, 1984). Baby-food fruit can be substituted for fresh fruit (Henkel and Schmidt, 1995). Monitor lizards are carnivorous and opportunistic feeders, and do well on pre-killed whole prey items such as rodents. Vitamin/mineral supplements are recommended for herbivorous lizards. Young herbivorous lizards should be fed at least daily (Mattison, 1991); large carnivorous species can go longer between meals.

C. Reproduction

Sexual dimorphism can be very distinct in certain species of reptiles, making sex determination a relatively straightforward process; however, visual sex determination can be difficult or nearly impossible in certain species in which males and females have very similar morphological features. Sex determination in reptiles can be accomplished using several methods, with the preferred method varying among species. Male box turtles and tortoises of many species have a concaved plastron that serves to stabilize the male when he mounts the female during breeding. The tail of male turtles is longer and the vent more distally located on the tail than it is in females. Male red-eared sliders and other species have elongated claws on their forelegs; these claws are used to stroke the sides of the female's head during courtship. Males of several lizard species, such as iguanas, have a large row of femoral pores on the inside of the hindlegs. The femoral pores of females are smaller or absent. Male snakes have a longer, thicker, more gradually tapering tail than do females (Rossi and Rossi, 1995; Mattison, 1998). A single, fleshy penis is present in male turtles and crocodilians (Fig. 19.11a). Snakes and lizards have

paired, membranous hemipenes, which lie in the base of the tail and are everted during copulation (only one hemipenis is used during copulation) (Fig. 19.11b). In species such as the bearded dragon, the hemipenes may produce noticeable ventral bulges in the proximal tail that can often be used to distinguish male from female. Species with hemipenes can be sexed by gently inserting a smooth, blunt probe into the cloaca and directing the probe caudally. If the snake is a male, the probe will easily pass within the inverted hemipenis for a distance of 3–4 scale rows or more (Rossi and Rossi, 1995). Other sexing methods include manually everting the hemipenis of neonatal snakes, and injecting saline into the tail behind the hemipenes to hydrostatically evert them. Crocodilians can be sexed by digitally palpating the cloaca (Rossi and Rossi, 1995; DeNardo, 1996).

Reproductive strategies vary among reptile species. As breeding concludes, the male garter snake (*Thamnophis sirtalis*) leaves a solidified plug of ejaculate in the female's cloaca to prevent subsequent breeding by another male (Zug, 1993). The whiptail lizard, *Aspidoscelis uniparens*, is parthenogenetic. Postovulatory females act as surrogate males, courting preovulatory females and thereby stimulating ovulation and production of genetically identical offspring. All turtles and crocodilians lay eggs; some lizards and many snakes bear live young. Anoles lay one egg at a time throughout the breeding season, while iguanas lay 20–40 eggs in a single clutch. Rat snakes lay five to 44 eggs per breeding, and garter snakes deliver up to 80 live young at a time (Mattison, 1991; Rossi, 1992). Some species of day gecko (*Phelsuma* spp.) lay two eggs at a time. The female lies on her back and uses her hindlegs to roll the pliable eggs into spheres, which she presses together until they harden. She then hides the eggs in a selected hiding place to incubate (Henkel and Schmidt, 1995).

All female pythons provide protection as well as thermal and hydric benefits to their developing offspring by wrapping around their eggs. Certain python species shiver to produce metabolic heat and facilitate egg

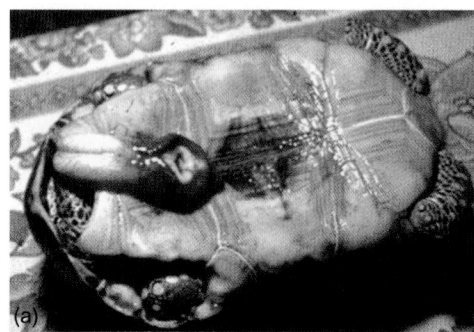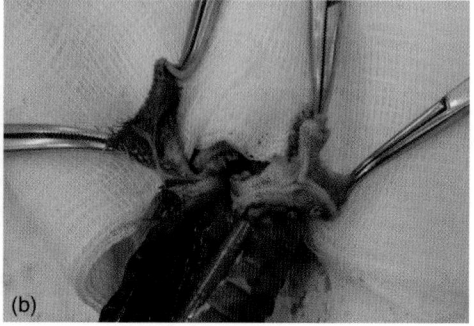

FIGURE 19.11   Male turtles have a single fleshy penis (a). Snakes have membranous paired hemipenes (b).

incubation (Stahlschmidt and DeNardo, 2010). Female crocodilians vigorously guard their nests throughout the incubation period. When the young are ready to emerge, they begin vocalizing. The female assists the young in digging out of the nest, and in some cases will pick them up and carry them to the water. Some females remain with their brood for up to 2 years and defend them from potential predators (McIlhenny, 1987; Lang, 1987; Burghardt and Layne, 1995).

Incubation temperature determines the sex of offspring in many reptile species. Alligator eggs incubated at lower temperatures produce females, and higher temperatures produce males. In the wild, temperature differentials across the nest result in a mixture of both sexes.

In the laboratory, most reptile eggs can be artificially incubated. The eggs should be removed and placed in an incubation chamber (usually a plastic shoe box with a loose-fitting lid), taking care to preserve their original orientation. A moist bed of sphagnum moss or vermiculite can serve as an incubation medium. Humidity should be about 90–100%, and temperatures should average about 30°C (Rossi, 1992). Alligators require slightly higher temperatures. Many snake eggs hatch 2–3 months after being laid (Fig. 19.12).

Neonatal reptiles are essentially miniature reproductions of adults, fully capable of surviving on their own. Some species may require diet modification; however, most eat essentially the same food type as the adults.

D. Behavior

Many species of turtles and snakes are not territorial and will tolerate being group-housed. Snakes that are group-housed must be fed separately. Snakes that are ophiophagic (snake-eating) should be housed individually. Young crocodilians are found in sibling groups in the wild and do well if kept together in the laboratory. Some lizard species are quite territorial, and males should never be housed together. In anoles, acute stress causes an epinephrine-induced dark eyespot to become visible (Greenberg and Wingfield, 1987). Chronic stress in alligators can cause chronic corticosteroid elevation and subsequent immunosuppression (Lance, 1990). Therefore, when maintaining reptiles in the laboratory, attention should be paid to providing the appropriate social as well as physical environment for these species.

E. Physical Examination and Diagnostic Techniques

When performing a physical exam on a reptile, the examiner should be familiar with the species (e.g., knowledge of the defense mechanism), and the size of the animal should be considered. Some snakes are relatively docile and can easily be examined and manipulated while moving through the examiner's hands. Aggressive snakes should be restrained gently behind the head while supporting the body. Snake hooks can be used to manipulate or transfer the snakes into a container. For larger animals, it is advisable to use two hooks to provide better support for the body. Transparent acrylic or plastic tubes are very useful for restraining snakes during visual examination, administration of injections, or collection of diagnostic specimens. Tubes can be customized with slits and holes through which injections can be given. These tubes are especially useful when dealing with venomous species.

Lizards, particularly large specimens, are capable of inflicting serious bite injuries. Some species will also use their tails as weapons. While most turtles and tortoises can be examined with minor physical restraint, the handler should be aware that they can inflict serious bites through their sharp beaks. Chelonians will retract into their protective shell, thereby making examination and treatment quite challenging. Chemical immobilization may be necessary to facilitate handling and to reduce stress to the turtle.

All crocodilians should be considered dangerous, and extreme care should be taken when handling members of this group. The mouth should be taped to prevent bites. Several people are necessary to safely restrain larger animals.

Reptiles may require chemical restraint or anesthesia to undergo a physical examination or diagnostic procedures. Knowledge of unique anatomic and physiologic features of the species is essential for successful anesthesia (Bennett, 1991, 1996; Schumacher, 1996a). Ketamine hydrochloride, in combination with drugs such as diazepam and butorphanol, and tiletamine/zolazepam can be

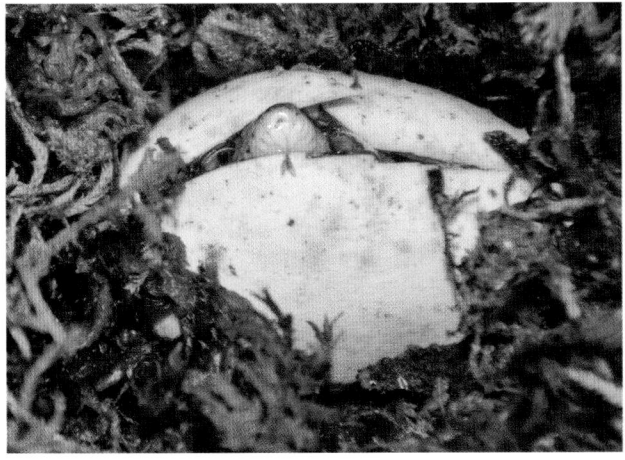

FIGURE 19.12   Many snake eggs hatch within 2–3 months after being laid. Eggs can be incubated in moist sphagnum moss. *Image courtesy of Fred Hawkins.*

used for chemical restraint and sedation in many species. Induction and recovery times may be prolonged with these injectable agents. Propofol, an ultra-short-acting nonbarbiturate agent, has rapid induction and recovery times; however, it must be given intravenously or intraosseously. Inhalation agents used in reptiles include isoflurane and sevoflurane, which can be administered for induction and maintenance of anesthesia. In most anesthetized reptiles of sufficient size, endotracheal intubation is easy to perform. Buprenorphine, butorphanol, carprofen, and meloxicam are analgesics that have been used in reptiles (Carpenter *et al.*, 2014), although doses are largely empirical.

1. Physical Examination

Prior to removing the animal from its enclosure and performing a physical examination, it is very helpful to observe it in the home cage. Behavior and attitude should be noted, as well as any signs of respiratory, musculoskeletal, or sensory abnormalities. The home cage should be checked for evidence of vomiting, diarrhea, or polyuria, and samples taken accordingly. When conducting a physical examination, a systematic approach is most helpful in identifying any abnormalities. The integument, including the shell of chelonians, should be inspected for the presence of lesions or abnormal growths, which may be indicative of infectious and/or metabolic disorders. This should be followed by inspection of the eyes (e.g., retained spectacles, periorbital abscesses), nares, and oral cavity. In many cases, the oral cavity should be examined last, as this procedure requires restraint and can stress the animal. Lizards, snakes, and crocodilians can be easily palpated, and knowledge of normal anatomy is essential in order to appreciate any abnormalities. Turtles can be palpated gently through the axillary and inguinal areas on either side of the bony bridge. The cloaca of all reptiles should be inspected for evidence of prolapsed tissue (e.g., reproductive or intestinal) or diarrhea.

2. Body Condition Assessment

Nutritional and hydration status should be noted since poor environmental conditions, such as excessively high or low humidity and temperatures outside the preferred temperature range, may contribute to poor feeding responses and inadequate hydration status. Incomplete shedding (dysecdysis), including retained spectacles, are commonly seen in sick reptiles and animals kept in suboptimal environmental conditions.

Muscle mass in snakes and lizards can best be assessed by examining the epaxial muscles in snakes and the pelvic region of lizards. The presence or absence of shell abnormalities in chelonians should also be recorded. In addition, the attitude of the reptile should be evaluated with consideration of the normal behavior of the

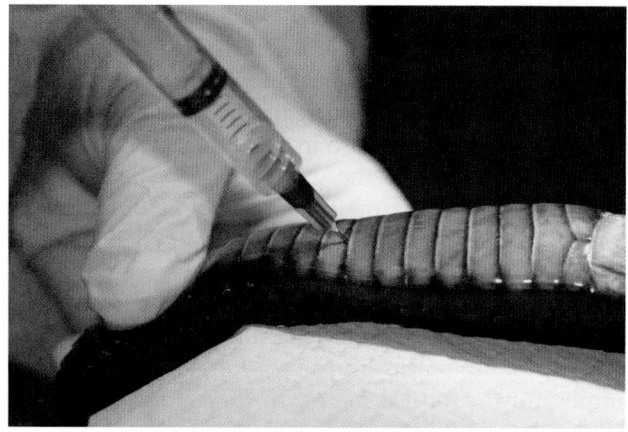

FIGURE 19.13   Blood can be collected from the ventral tail vein in snakes.

species or possibly even the individual as behavior can vary. An alert animal should be actively exploring its environment and not demonstrating signs of lethargy or weakness.

3. Blood Collection

Blood collection techniques, including sample handling and processing, have been reviewed by Jacobson (1993a). A venous blood sample can be collected from most reptile species using physical restraint alone. The volume of blood that can safely be withdrawn is determined by the size of the reptile. The total blood volume of reptiles ranges between 5–8% of total body weight, and 10% of the total blood volume can safely be collected from a reptile (Jacobson, 1993a). Snakes can be bled from the ventral tail vein (Fig. 19.13) or via cardiocentesis. In the latter technique, the sedated or anesthetized snake is positioned in dorsal recumbency, and the location of the heart is confirmed by either palpation or visualization of its beating and movement of the scales. The heart is stabilized between two fingers, and a small-gauge needle is inserted midline between the ventral scales. The needle is advanced at a 45° angle and aimed at the apex of the heart. When the needle is placed correctly, blood should fill the hub of the syringe with each heartbeat. Repeated attempts should be avoided to prevent excessive myocardial damage and hemorrhage. Depending on the species, turtles and tortoises can be bled from the dorsal or ventral tail vein, jugular vein, or subcarapacial site. Lizards can be bled from the ventral tail vein or from the ventral abdominal vein. Crocodilians are commonly bled from the ventral tail vein or from the occipital sinus (Hernandez-Divers, 2006). When bleeding, if lymph is aspirated into the needle, the sample should be discarded. Lithium heparin is used for blood collection for both hematologic and plasma chemistry analyses, because EDTA can lyse red blood cells in some turtle species; heparin also prevents loss of sample volume through entrapment by a clot, which can be significant if only small volumes are available for analysis (Campbell, 2014).

4. Injection Techniques

In certain species, such as red-eared sliders, femoral veins drain directly into the liver via the abdominal vein. Administration of a drug in the front limb of this species avoids reduction in drug bioavailability due to a hepatic first pass effect resulting from hind limb drug administration (Holz et al., 1997; Kummrow et al., 2008). In the green iguana, the majority of blood returning from the pelvic hindlimb enters the general circulation and bypasses the kidney; however, blood from the tail enters the renal portal system and goes directly to the kidney (Benson, 1999). This suggests that species-specific blood draining patterns exist. Therefore, drugs metabolized by the kidney and liver should be injected into the epaxial muscles of the cranial half of the body in snakes or the muscles of the front legs in chelonians, lizards, and crocodilians. If large volumes are to be administered, it may become necessary to divide it among multiple injection sites. Fluids and medications can also be administered intraosseously. In lizards and chelonians, an intraosseous catheter can be placed into the tibia. Intravenous injections can be challenging, particularly in small species. Depending on species, sites for IV injections can include the ventral tail vein, ventral abdominal vein, or the jugular vein.

5. Fecal Examination

Fecal samples for flotation, wet mounts, bacterial culture, and cytology can be collected from the cage. In order to obtain a fresh sample, a colonic lavage should be performed. A sterile, lubricated large diameter, flexible, round-tip catheter of appropriate size is carefully inserted into the cloaca and gently directed cranially toward the colon. Sterile saline (0.5–1.0 ml/100 g) is gently introduced into the colon and aspirated until fecal material is obtained (Hernandez-Divers, 2006).

6. Tracheal /Lung Lavage

Animals should be anesthetized and intubated with a sterile endotracheal tube to reduce contamination by oral flora. A sterile catheter is introduced, and 0.5 ml/100 g sterile saline infused and aspirated. Rotation or shifting the animal may facilitate collection of the aspirate (Hernandez-Divers, 2006). The collected material can then be submitted for microbiologic and cytologic evaluation.

7. Collection of Biopsy Specimens

Biopsy specimens should be obtained for histologic and microbiologic evaluation of skin, visceral organs, and masses. Biopsies can be collected by direct visualization (e.g., skin), by ultrasound guidance for visceral organs (e.g., kidneys), or by endoscopy (e.g., stomach). When biopsying skin, often removal of a single scale will permit evaluation of both epidermal and dermal components. Cortical bone biopsy instruments can be used to obtain turtle shell biopsies, but care must be taken to avoid deep biopsies penetrating into the coelomic cavity. The biopsy wound can be sealed with epoxy or acrylic (Hernandez-Divers, 2006).

8. Endoscopy

Endoscopy is a valuable tool for visualization of internal organs and collection of diagnostic specimens such as biopsies and cultures (Jenkins, 1996). The most commonly used endoscope for reptiles weighing 100 g to 20 kg is a 2.7-mm telescope system. For animals less than 500 g, a 1-mm semi-rigid endoscope can be used for tracheoscopy, and a 1.9-mm endoscope will work for tracheoscopy, gastroscopy, and coelioscopy of animals weighing 2–3 kg (Taylor, 2006; Divers, 2014).

9. Radiography/Ultrasound/CT/MRI

Imaging modalities are important diagnostic tools in the field of reptile medicine. In order to effectively use and interpret the images, it is essential to know the normal anatomy of the species being evaluated. Most reptiles do not require anesthesia for radiography. Snakes may be placed inside a plastic or acrylic tube to obtain dorsoventral and lateral views. Contrast studies are of diagnostic value in cases of gastrointestinal disease and for identification of foreign bodies and masses. Radiographs can be helpful in evaluating the respiratory and skeletal systems. Craniocaudal views are obtained in addition to the standard views in order to fully appreciate the respiratory tract. Ultrasound is used in reptiles to assess reproductive condition, diagnose abnormalities, and to guide organ biopsies. In snakes and lizards, linear transducers are recommended; sector or convex transducers are used in turtles. Ten to 18 MHz transducers are used for small lizards, 7.5–10 MHz for larger animals, and 2.5–5 MHz for very large species. Animals are typically restrained in dorsal recumbency or upright for the procedure; sedation may be necessary. Skin should be moistened with warm water and a generous amount of warm ultrasound gel used. When accessing the inguinal and axillary areas of turtles between the dorsal and ventral shells, excess air space can be filled by placing a warm water-filled exam glove in the void between the transducer and skin (Hochleithner and Holland, 2014).

Computer-assisted radial tomography (CT) is an excellent diagnostic tool for discerning details in bones, scutes, and airways. CT eliminates organ superimposition seen with radiographs. Images can be evaluated as two-dimensional sections, or reconstructed into three-dimensional images. Although the time required to perform a CT scan is typically short, many animals require anesthesia or sedation to prevent movement artifact. Contrast media can be used in reptiles; 2.5–3% of human pediatric concentrations are normally administered to reptiles (Wyneken, 2014).

Magnetic resonance imaging (MRI) is preferred over CT for imaging soft tissues, fluids, brain, and spinal cord. MRI images typically take much longer to obtain and therefore usually require anesthesia. Head, wrist, and knee coils enhance image quality in small animals. Like CT, MRI images can be viewed as two-dimensional slices or three-dimensional reconstructions. Functional MRI is used to detect increased blood flow in metabolically active areas (Wyneken, 2014).

10. Nutritional Support

Reptiles, especially those kept under suboptimal environmental conditions, often develop nutritional imbalances and/or diseases that may require nutritional support (Donoghue and Langenberg, 1996; Donoghue, 2006). Many reptiles diagnosed with noninfectious and infectious diseases are anorectic and require supportive care, including fluid therapy and nutritional support. Following identification and correction of environmental deficiencies and underlying disease processes, anorectic reptiles should receive assisted feeding. Care should be taken to ensure that the animal has a functional gastrointestinal tract. Reptiles with systemic disease or those kept in poor environmental conditions commonly have gastrointestinal stasis. Drugs that promote gastric emptying (e.g., cisapride, erythromycin, metoclopramide) have been used in reptiles. Most reptiles can be fed via a flexible orogastric feeding tube or stainless steel ball-tipped feeding needles, and medications can be added to the diet. If the animal requires long-term assisted feeding, placement of a pharyngostomy tube may be indicated (Donoghue, 2006).

11. Euthanasia

Sodium pentobarbital overdose (intravenously or intracoelomically; 60–100 mg/kg of body weight) is an effective means of euthanizing reptiles, although euthanasia by intracoelomic injection can take 30 min or longer. Many species are hypoxia-tolerant and therefore are resistant to physical methods of euthanasia such as CO_2 inhalation. Buffered tricane methane sulfonate (MS 222) can be injected into the coelomic cavity in a two-step process. First, 250–500 mg/kg of 0.7–1% buffered MS222 solution is injected, followed by 0.1–1.0 ml unbuffered 50% (v/v) MS222 solution (Conroy et al., 2009). General anesthesia with injectable combinations or inhalant anesthetics, followed by secondary, physical methods (exsanguination, decapitation, pithing) ensure death and remove concerns associated with hypoxia tolerance. Hypothermia is considered unacceptable for reptile euthanasia (2013 AVMA Guidelines).

III. DISEASES

A. Infectious Diseases

1. Bacterial

a. Gram-Negative and Gram-Positive Bacteria

Etiology Microbial organisms commonly affecting reptiles include Gram-negative bacteria (*Pseudomonas* spp., *Aeromonas* spp., *Chlamydia* spp., *Morganella* spp., *Klebsiella* spp., *Helicobacter* spp., *Salmonella*, *Vibrio* spp., *Proteus* spp., *Acinetobacter* spp., *Providencia* spp., *Shigella* spp., *Campylobacter* spp., *Escherichia coli*) and Gram-positive bacteria (*Micrococcus* spp., *Streptococcus* spp., *Staphylococcus* spp., and *Clostridium* spp.).

Epizootiology and Transmission Gram-negative and Gram-positive bacteria can be found ubiquitously throughout the environment and persistently colonize the skin and the gastrointestinal tract of apparently healthy captive reptiles (Goldstein et al., 1981; Tan et al., 1978; Blaylock, 2001; Ferrerira et al., 2010; Dipineto et al., 2014). In immunocompetent animals, these bacteria do not generally cause any clinical signs. However, during stressful conditions or when the immune system is compromised, overgrowth of these bacteria can occur and lead to severe clinical outcomes. Therefore, many bacteria found in reptiles likely act as secondary opportunisitic, rather than primary, pathogens (Joyner et al., 2006). Besides their ubiquitous presence, these bacteria can be found in invertebrates and other vertebrates, and reptiles can acquire these bacteria after consuming these infected animals.

Pathogenesis The precise pathogenic mechanisms of many bacteria in reptiles are unclear. However, in mammals, bacteria such as *E. coli*, *Clostridium* spp., *K. oxytoca*, *Vibrio* spp., and *Helicobacter* spp. can produce toxins and effector proteins that, once they enter the cell, induce cell death. They also contain a repertoire of genes that allows them to persistently colonize the host, thereby making them effective opportunistic organisms (Lertpiriyapong et al., 2012, 2014). It is likely that similar pathogenic mechanisms are employed by reptilian bacteria.

Clinical Signs Various clinical outcomes such as meningoencephalitis, stomatitis, pneumonia, conjunctivitis, upper respiratory tract disease, abscesses, osteoarthritis, septicemia, and gastrointestinal lesions have been associated with the above bacteria (Keymer, 1978; Hilf et al., 1990; Hetzel et al., 2003). In certain cases, affected animals may be found dead without prior clinical signs. *Pseudomonas* spp., *Aeromonas* spp., and *Klebsiella* spp. are associated with respiratory tract diseases in reptiles,

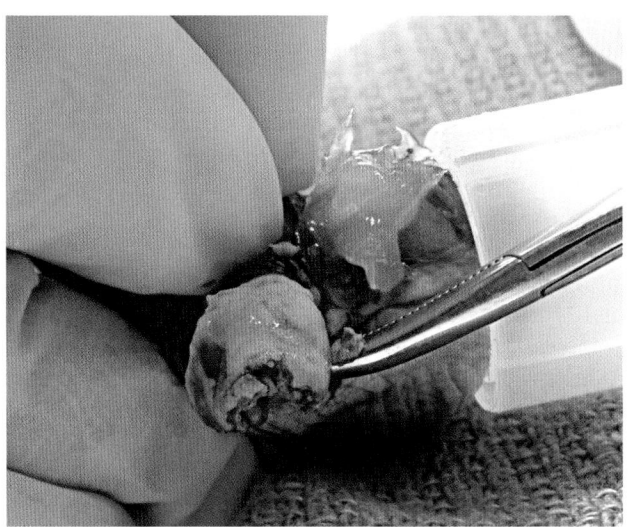

FIGURE 19.14 Aural abscesses are common in turtles, and are typically treated by surgical excision of the caseated material, followed by appropriate antibiotic therapy.

while *Serratia* spp. are most commonly isolated from subcutaneous abscesses. *Salmonella* was found to be the most common Gram-negative bacteria in snakes with pneumonia (Schmidt *et al.*, 2013). *Staphylococcus* spp., *Aeromonas hydrophila*, and *Vibrio alginolyticus* were isolated from salt gland abscesses and ulcerative dermatitis lesions of loggerhead sea turtles (Orós *et al.*, 2005, 2011). *Morganella morganii* has been associated with aural abscess in turtles (Joyner *et al.*, 2006) (Fig. 19.14). Among the anaerobic bacteria, *Bacteroides* spp. are the most commonly isolated species. *Clostridium* spp., including *C. glycolicum* and *C. perfriengen*, have been associated with gastrointestinal disease and endotoxemia in reptiles (Schumacher *et al.*, 1996c). The anaerobic bacteria, such as *Fusobacterium* spp. and *Peptostreptococcus* spp., can cause dermatitis following external injuries, such as bite lesions, scratches, and abrasions, or septicemia (Hellebuyck *et al.*, 2012). *Helicobacter* spp. have been identified in turtles with fatal septicemia and may be responsible for gastric lesions in this species (Stacy and Wellehan, 2010). *Providencia* spp. are associated with septicemia and meningoencephalitis in thermally stressed American alligators.

Necropsy Finding Since Gram-negative and Gram-positive bacteria can affect various organs, clinical signs can vary tremendously depending on the organ affected. Bacteremia can result in necrotizing enteritis, intestinal hemorrhage, fibrinous serositis, hepatitis, and pancreatitis. If the respiratory system is affected, pulmonary congestion and pleural effusion can be observed. In dermatitis cases, brown or red-spotted skin can often be detected on various regions of the body. Bacteria such as *Chlamydia* can cause granulomatous lesions in reptiles, while *Serratia* spp. can cause caseating abscesses.

Differential Diagnosis Bacterial infection can be a consequence of primary viral infection. Bacteria cultures from affected tissues should be performed if bacterial infection is suspected. Speciation can often be accomplished by a combination of biochemical characterization and PCR-based assays.

Treatment Culture and sensitivity testing should always precede antimicrobial treatment of bacterial diseases. In some cases, however, it may be necessary to administer broad-spectrum antimicrobials while culture and sensitivity results are pending (e.g., enrofloxacin 5mg/kg IM every 48h for 10 treatments; ceftazidime 20mg/kg IM every 72h for 10 treatments; amikacin 5mg/kg IM first dose, then 2.5mg/kg IM thereafter for 10 treatments). Selection of an appropriate antibiotic also depends on the size of the reptile, the route of administration, and the health status of the patient. Abscesses should be surgically debrided and allowed to heal by secondary intention (Murray, 2006).

Control Poor husbandry practices often lead to bacterial infection. If this is suspected, efforts should be made to identify the deficiencies, and changes in husbandry practices should be promptly instituted. Sick animals should be identified and isolated from healthy animals. Keeping animals at higher temperature that can be tolerated by the reptile, providing a balanced and appropriate diet, keeping water bowl clean, and administering an appropriate antimicrobial treatment should be part of this therapy.

Prevention Most commonly, stress and immunosuppression caused by improper environmental conditions have been associated with the development of bacterial diseases in reptiles. Thus, proper husbandry measures are important in preventing bacterial infection in reptiles.

Research Complication Treatment associated with bacterial infection affecting single or multiple organ systems in a reptile colony can be costly and labor intensive. Often times, treatment may fail to control the disease, resulting in a devastating loss of animals. This can be debilitating to any research endeavor. In venom studies, bacteria infection may interfere with venom production qualitatively or quantitatively (Ferreira *et al.*, 2010.)

b. Mycoplasmosis

Etiology Mycoplasmosis is caused by *Mycoplasma*, which are spherical to filamentous non-motile bacteria with no cell walls.

Epizootiology and Transmission Many species of *Mycoplasma* have been identified in reptiles, including lizards, crocodilians, tortoises, and turtles. *Mycoplasma iguana* and *M. insons* have been isolated from healthy green iguana and do not appear to cause any clinical issues in these species (May *et al.*, 2007; Brown *et al.*, 2007). *Mycoplasma agassizii* and *M. testiduneum* are associated with respiratory disease in snakes, tortoises, and turtles (Penner *et al.*, 1997; Jacobson *et al.*, 1991a; Sandmeier *et al.*, 2013; Guthrie *et al.*, 2013). Geographically, *M. testudineum* seems to have a similar distribution to, but a lower prevalence than, *M. agassizii* in desert and gopher tortoises across North America. Infection with *Mycoplasma* spp., including *M. alligatoris* and *M. crocodyli*, is associated with severe disease outcomes in alligators, caimans, and crocodiles (Brown *et al.*, 2001, 2004). *Mycoplasma* exhibits interspecies transmission, and cold weather has been shown to decrease the resistance of Mojave desert tortoises to infection (Sandmeier *et al.*, 2013). Frequent direct interaction with infected animals increases the chance of infection in naïve animals (Wendland *et al.*, 2010).

Pathogenesis Little is known about the pathogenesis of *Mycoplasma* in reptiles. However, *Mycoplasma* appears to contain a repertoire of genes, including hyaluronidase, sialidases, and mucinases that allows them to spread systemically (Brown *et al.*, 2004).

Clinical Signs In reptiles, *Mycoplasma* infection commonly leads to clinical signs associated with respiratory system dysfunction, although systemic signs have also been reported in some species. Affected turtles may have a clear to purulent nasal discharge, swollen eyelids, and, in advanced cases, occlusion of the upper airways. Upper respiratory problems caused by *Mycoplasma* appear to be chronic diseases. Infected snakes can have almost normal activity, but refuse to eat and display open-mouth breathing when handled. Clear mucous and bubbles can be observed on their labial scales. Some infected snakes can die acutely (Penner *et al.*, 1997). *Mycoplasma alligatoris* causes a lethal invasive disease in adult American alligators (*Alligator mississippiensis*) and closely related caimans (*Caiman latirostris*) (Brown *et al.*, 2001).

Necropsy Findings *Mycoplasma testidineum* infection is associated with the development of chronic rhinitis and conjunctivitis in desert tortoises and captive turtles (Brown *et al.*, 2004). In snakes, infection is associated with proliferative lymphocytic tracheitis and pneumonia (Penner *et al.*, 1997). Experimentally infected crocodiles have been shown to develop necrotizing pneumonia, severe pericarditis, necrotizing myocarditis, lymphocytic interstitial nephritis, lymphocytic periportal hepatitis, splenic hyperplasia, pyogranulomatous meningitis, necrotizing synovitis, and polyarthritis (Pye *et al.*, 2001; Brown *et al.*, 2001).

Differential Diagnosis Pneumonia and other signs of respiratory disease can be caused by other bacterial agents including the previously mentioned Gram-negative and Gram-positive bacteria. Toxin exposure, fungal infection, and primary viral infection, including paramyxoviral infection, should also be on the list of differentials. Diagnosis can be made by the presence of

clinical signs and serologic testing. An enzyme-linked immunosorbent assay (ELISA) has been developed for the detection of *M. agassizii*-specific antibodies. PCR-based assays and bacterial culture are also possible and can be used to determine the presence of *Mycoplama* spp. in the tissues (Schumacher *et al.*, 1993; Penner *et al.*, 1997; Guthrie *et al.*, 2013).

Treatment Treatment includes administration of antimicrobials (e.g., enrofloxacin 5 mg/kg IM every 48 h for 10 treatments) (Westfall *et al.*, 2006), supportive care, and isolation of affected animals. Antimicrobial sensitivity testing for each *Mycoplasma* isolate is highly recommended. Treatment with clarithromycin per rectum may be effective in desert tortoises (Wimsatt *et al.*, 2008).

Control When mycoplasmosis is suspected, efforts must be made to isolate sick animals to prevent further spread of the agents. Sick animals should be treated symptomatically. In severe cases, euthanasia is highly recommended.

Prevention Quarantine and testing of new animals should prevent introduction of the pathogen into the existing colony. Proper husbandry, including providing suitable temperature and diets, should be instituted to prevent stress that predisposes animals to infection.

Research Complication Mycoplasmosis can be associated with high morbidity and mortality in turtles and tortoises.

c. Mycobacteriosis

Etiology The causative agent of mycobacteriosis is *Mycobacteria*, which are slow-growing, slender, aerobic, acid-fast, Gram-positive rod bacteria. Species known to infect reptiles include *M. chelonae*, *M. szulgai*, *M. thamnopheos*, *M. marinum*, *M. fortuitum*, *M ulcerans*, *M. avium*, *M. lepraemuirum*, *M. terrae*, and *M. kansasii* (Mitchell, 2012).

Epizootiology and Transmission *Mycobacteria* can be found ubiquitously in the environment. Animals become infected via direct contact with contaminated water and food. Routes of entry include oral, skin, urogential, and inhalation. Although relatively uncommon in reptiles, cases of mycobacteriosis have been reported in snakes, lizards, turtles, and crocodilians. Among the reptile groups, chelonians appear to be the most susceptible. This is likely due to the aquatic nature of these species where water serves as an effective means of transmission. An annual incidence of 0.1–0.5% of mycobacteriosis has been reported in well-managed reptile colonies; however, without adequate environmental control, the incidence can be as high as 31.9% (Hernandez-Divers *et al.*, 2002; Maslow *et al.*, 2002). Thus, maintenance of appropriate environmental control is important in limiting the spread of disease.

Pathogenesis *Mycobacteria* can form biofilm that enables them to persist in the environment. The cell wall component of *Mycobacteria* is highly resistant to acids, alkalis, oxidative burst, and destruction by complement. Thus the organism can persist and incites strong inflammatory responses in the host. Certain species of *Mycobacteria*, such as *M. tuberculosis*, can secrete effector molecules that interfere with the host-pathogen degradration mechanisms, allowing them to establish persistence (Mehra *et al.*, 2013). Similar mechanisms may be employed by reptilian strains of *Mycobacteria*.

Clinical Signs   Clinical signs can vary depending on the organ affected. Systemic illness is often accompanied by non-specific signs such as anorexia, inappetence, lethargy, and wasting. When gastrointestinal and respiratory systems are involved, cloacal discharge and open-mouth breathing can be expected.

Necropsy Findings   *Mycobacteria* can affect any body system, and multiple organs can be affected at once. Stomatitis, subcutaneous granulomas, and granulomas in various organs including lung, viscera, bone, and joint have been reported in affected animals. In cases where the respiratory system is involved, serosanguinous fluid can be detected in the trachea accompanied by grayish-white nodules in the lungs. Affected intestines can have darkened mucosa with petechia and echymoses. Histologic lesions can vary from condensed clusters of macrophage containing intracytoplasmic acid-fast bacilli to caseating granuloma.

Differential Diagnosis   Differentials for mycobacteriosis includes bacteria infection (*Chlamydophila* spp., *Salmonella*, *Nocadia* spp.) and fungal infection (*Aspergillus* spp. and *Paecilomyces* spp.). Primary viral infection should also be ruled out. A diagnosis of mycobacteriosis can be made by demonstration of mycobacterial organisms by acid-fast and/or Ziehl–Neelsen staining of biopsy specimens, aspirates, or scrapings, although this method is asscociated with low sensitivity. PCR-based assays using infected tissue samples are also available.

Treatment   There is no effective treatment for reptile Mycobacteriosis, and, because of the zoonotic potential, euthanasia of infected animals should be considered.

Control   As with any other infectious agents, Mycobacteriosis suspects should be isolated. Practices that limit stress, including proper husbandry, should be implemented. Contaminated surfaces should be disinfected with sodium *o*-phenylphenol or sodium hypochlorite to limit the spread of the organism (Maslow *et al.*, 2002).

Prevention   Prevention of Mycobacteriosis includes a strict quarantine protocol, proper environmental conditions, and strict hygiene procedures. Routine microbiological culture and screening should be performed from dead or ill animals. Feeding of aquatic animals, which are a known reservoir of *Mycobacteria*, should be avoided to prevent introduction of bacteria into the existing colony.

2. Viral

A variety of DNA and RNA viruses have been described in reptiles. While most studies report a viral agent to be associated with a clinical or pathological condition in a single animal or a defined group of animals, few agents have actually been identified as disease-causing. Koch's postulates have been fulfilled in only a few cases. However, considering the relatively high number of reports of viral agents in reptiles and the limited number of studies being performed, viral infections likely play an important role in reptile disease processes. Reviews of viral agents detected in reptiles have been published elsewhere (Jacobson, 1986, 1993c; Schumacher, 1996b; Marschang, 2011). Only those agents strongly associated with clinical disease and with known important implications in captive collections of reptiles are reported here. It is also important to note that in some cases a single animal can be co-infected with multiple species of virus (Abbas *et al.*, 2011). Thus, caution should be exercised in interpreting diagnostic results.

a. Herpesvirus

Etiology   Herpesviruses (HVs) are large, enveloped viruses with cosahedral capsids and double-stranded DNA genomes. Current evidence suggests that reptilian HVs belong to the subfamily Alphaherpesvirinae (Wellehan *et al.*, 2005; Ackermann, 2012; Hughes-Hanks *et al.*, 2010). The pathogenetic properties of HVs have been demonstrated experimentally in turtles (Origgi *et al.*, 2004; Herbst *et al.*, 1999).

Epizootiology and Transmission   HVs have been detected in many species of lizards, snakes, chelonians, and crocodilians. It is likely that reptiles carry multiple genetically distinct HV strains (Marschang *et al.*, 2006). HV infection is usually subclinical; however, severe clinical signs are frequently observed in juvenile and immunocompromised animals. Marine turtles, particularly *Chelonia mydas*, appear to be highly susceptible to infection and to developing severe clinical signs. Recent genetic analyses suggest that HV strains causing skin lesions in green lizards (*Lacerta viridis*) are similar to those causing similar disease manifestations in sea turtles (Literak *et al.*, 2010), hinting at the possibility of interspecies transmission. The mode of HV transmission is unclear, but is most likely through the oral–fecal route or direct contact with oculonasal, respiratory secretions, and saliva. In sea turtles, marine leeches may serve as vectors for transmitting HVs (Greenblatt *et al.*, 2004; Ariel, 2011). Vertical and water-borne transmision are also possible (Curry *et al.*, 2000). HV transmission can be rapid among aquatic turtles. Typical of HVs, reptilian HVs can establish a lifelong latent infection and can be reactivated during stress or conditions that lead to immunosuprression. Latently infected animals can serve as an effective means to disseminate and propogate the virus in a colony through chronic shedding.

Pathogenesis Little is known about the pathogenic mechanisms of HVs in reptiles. Typical of DNA viruses, HVs exhibit nuclear replication.

Clinical Signs HV-infected turtles usually develop respiratory signs, including gasping, harsh respiratory sounds, inability to dive properly, buoyancy abnormalities, and the presence of caseous material on the eyes, glottis, and trachea. In juvenile sea turtles, fibropapillomatosis can develop on the carapace, plastron, eyes, epidermis, and, in severe cases, on the mucosal surface of internal organs. Such neoplastic lesions can regress with time (Machado *et al.*, 2013). In some species, such as some freshwater turtles, infected animals can die acutely, whereas other species develop chronic disease. HVs have been detected in the venom glands of snakes and are associated with decreased venom production (Simpson, 1979). In lizards, HV infection is associated with stomatitis and papillomas.

Necropsy Findings Hepatic necrosis has been observed in boas, whereas fibropapillomatosis as well as cutaneous, respiratory, oral, genital, and liver lesions are common among sea turtles and lizards (Stacy *et al.*, 2008; Literak *et al.*, 2010). Characteristic gross findings in turtles also include hepatomegaly and pulomonary edema. In tortoises, necrotizing lesions in the upper digestive tract are commonly observed (Jungwirth *et al.*, 2014). In lizards, development of papilloma-like growths on skin as well as, stomatitis, hepatitis, and enteritis have been reported (Literak *et al.*, 2010; Hughes-Hanks *et al.*, 2010). Intranuclear inclusion bodies were frequently observed in spleen, lung, kidney, pancreas, and hepatocytes of infected livers. HVs were also detected in cloacal lesions of American alligators. These lesions are characterized as submucosal lymphoid follicles with hyperemia and hemorrhage (Govett *et al.*, 2005). However, no inclusion bodies were observed within these lesions.

Differential Diagnosis Differentials for dermatitis and papillomatous lesions in reptiles include flavivirus, poxvirus, papillomavirus, bacterial, fungal, and ecto- or endoparasitic infection, as well as toxin exposures and burns. Methods for determining infection status in reptiles include serology testing via indirect ELISA, isolation and culture of HV, and amplification of HV genomic DNA via PCR (Jacobson *et al.*, 2012).

Treatment Treatment consists of debridement of lesions, prevention of secondary bacterial infections, and supportive care (fluids, nutritional support, heat, nebulization). Acyclovir and ganciclovir were reported to be effective when tested *in vitro* against one herpesvirus isolate (Marschang *et al.*, 1997) and can be used adjunctively. In California desert tortoises, 80 mg/kg of acyclovir given orally every 72 h was found to be effective (Ritchie, 2006).

Control Isolation of sick animals and strict biosecurity are important means to prevent the spread of HVs. As stress and poor husbandry can lead to virus activation in latently infected animals and an increase in susceptibility in naive animals, good husbandry and hygiene practices should be implemented. Bleach (1:10 dilution), phenolic, and quaternary ammonium compounds are recommended for disinfecting contaminated surfaces (Weber *et al.*, 1999).

Prevention Newly arrived animals should be quarantined for 3–6 months. Strict hygiene and proper husbandry practices should also be implemented to prevent spread of HVs and to promote health in latently infected animals.

Research Complication High morbidity and mortality associated with HV infection can be debilitating to any research endeavor.

b. Adenovirus

Etiology Adenoviruses are nonenveloped, linear, and double-stranded DNA viruses with icosahedral capsids. According to current taxonomy, reptilian adenoviruses belong to the genus *Atadenovirus*. Their pathogenicity has been demonstrated experimentally in one study involving boa constrictors (Jacobson *et al.*, 1985).

Epizootiology and Transmission Adenovirus infection is widespread among reptiles and can be found worldwide (Jacobson *et al.*, 1984; Jacobson and Gaskin, 1985; Jacobson and Gardiner, 1990; Schumacher *et al.*, 1994a; Schumacher *et al.*, 2012). Cases of infection have been reported in at least 28 species of reptile, including crocodilians, snakes, lizards, and turtles, but infection is most common in agamid (or dragon) lizards. It is recognized as a serious cause of mortality in captive bearded dragons, wild caught anoles, and tortoises (Hyndman and Shilton, 2011; Marschang, 2011; Schumacher *et al.*, 2012; Ascher *et al.*, 2013) Adenoviruses are highly stable in the environment and commonly spread through the fecal–oral route, but transmission via aerosol can also occur. These viruses are usually host-adapted; however, cross-species infection is very likely (Marschang, 2011; Ascher *et al.*, 2013). Young and immunocompromised animals are most vulnerable to infection and will often develop severe clinical signs, whereas adult immunocompetent animals frequently experience subclinical infection (Ascher *et al.*, 2013).

Pathogenesis Little is known about the pathogenic mechanisms of adenoviruses in reptiles. As with many DNA viruses, adenoviruses replicate inside the host nucleus, and the viruses are released when the infected cell lyses. Intranuclear inclusion bodies can often be detected in affected tissues and organs.

Clinical Signs Affected animals can die unexpectedly without any clinical signs. The most common clinical signs in bearded dragons are nonspecific and include weight loss, anorexia, and diarrhea. In snakes and turtles, anorexia, progressively declining body condition, diarrhea, mucosal erosion, and nasal or ocular discharge can be observed (Schumacher et al., 2012; Mahapatra et al., 2013). Signs associated with central nervous system (CNS) defects, such as head tilt, opisthotonus, and circling, as well as stomatitis and dermatitis have been described (Marschang, 2011). Secondary bacterial, fungal, parasitic, and other viral infections can occur and quickly worsen the condition. Infected anoles were reported to become lethargic and anorexic shortly after importation and died soon after.

Necropsy Findings At necropsy, signs of gastrointestinal disease can be noted and multiple organs can be affected. The most common histological change is hepatic necrosis, which is accompanied by liver enlargement, petechiation, and pale areas scattered throughout. Frequently, the intestine will be involved and changes include dilation of the duodenum and hyperemia of the mucosa. Basophilic or eosinophillic intranuclear inclusions are commonly observed, particularly in the hepatocytes of the necrotic liver, enterocytes, myocardial endothelial cells, spleen, renal epithelial cells, endocardium, epithelial cells of the lung, and glial and endothelial cells of the brain.

Differential Diagnosis Other viral pathogens and opportunistic bacteria infection commonly cause nonspecific and systemic clinical signs in reptiles, so they should be on the list of differentials. PCR-based assays and *in situ* hybridization to visualize the viral particles in tissues can be used to determine the infection status.

Treatment Treatment in all cases should consist of supportive care, including administration of antimicrobials (for secondary bacterial infection), which should be based upon culture and antimicrobial sensitivity testing, fluids, nutritional supplementation, and correction of environmental conditions.

Control Animals with clinical signs suspected of viral infection should be isolated and supportive care provided. Euthanasia should be considered in severe cases.

Prevention New additions should be quarantined. Proper husbandry and hygiene practices including regular disinfection of housing and used materials should be implemented to promote health. Since adenoviruses are stable in the environment, the current recommendation for disinfection includes removal of organic debris with soap and water followed by application of a 10% bleach solution on the contaminated surface, allowing at least a 10-min contact time. Direct unfiltered sunlight and other intense ultraviolet sources can aid disinfection (Latney et al., 2013).

Research Complication Considerable morbidity and mortality associated with adenovirus infection in some species can lead to specimen loss, and treatment can be time consuming and costly.

c. Poxvirus

Etiology Poxviruses are large, pleomorphic, enveloped, and double-stranded DNA viruses. In Nile crocodiles, the poxviruses belong to the subfamily *Chordopoxvirinae* (Afonso et al., 2006.)

Epizootiology and Transmission The first report of poxvirus-associated disease in reptiles was in captive caiman in the United States (Marschang, 2011). Since then, cases of poxvirus infection have been reported in a variety of reptile species, including a flap-necked chameleon, captive spectacled caiman, farmed Nile crocodiles, tegus, and tortoises (Jacobson et al., 1979; Jacobson and Telford, 1990; Pandey et al., 1990; Penrith et al., 1991; Orós et al., 1998; Huchzermeyer et al., 2009; Mass, 2013). Compared to other viral agents, reports of poxviral infection in reptiles are relatively rare and emphasis appears to be on crocodilians. Like any other viral agents, numerous strains of poxvirus appear to be present in crocodilians and are associated with distinct disease outcomes depending on the species involved. Juvenile and immunosuppressed animals are highly susceptible to the infection and usually develop the most severe clinical signs. Infection in adult animals are usually subclinical, but these individuals can serve as carriers shedding the virus during stressful condition. In general, poxviruses can be transmitted directly by contact with infected skin lesions or indirectly via contact with contaminated objects, insects, or water. The virus is highly stable outside of the host and can remain infectious for years in organic debris.

Pathogenesis Little is known about the pathogenic mechanisms of poxviruses in reptiles. However, they likely use mechanisms similar to those employed by poxvirus strains of mammals. Unlike many DNA viruses that replicate in the host's nucleus, poxvirus replicate within cytoplasmic viroplasms in infected epithelial cells. However, in chameleons, the poxvirus appears to target the monocyte.

Clinical Signs Poxvirus infection in crocodiles is associated with high morbidity, but low mortality. Affected animals develop skin lesions characterized by round grayish-white to brown lesions and either superficial or depressed foci that can coalesce to form large lesions. The lesions can be found throughout the entire body, are pruritic, and can cause the animals to rub their skin against the tank or other inanimate objects. Animals can lose a substantial amount of weight, and some can develop generalized edema due to protein deficiency. The skin lesions can persist for 5–6 months in affected crocodiles. As in crocodiles, infected tegus were reported to develop brown papules on various parts of the body (Marschang, 2011).

Necropsy Findings Lesions can be found predominantly around the head, including the mandible, maxilla, and palpebrae, and are characterized by hyperkeratosis and parakeratosis. In caiman, a typical grayish skin nodule was observed, whereas yellowish to brownish wart-like cutaneous nodules were observed in affected Nile crocodiles and tegus.

Differential Diagnosis Diagnosis can be made by histologic evaluation of skin samples and demonstration of typical eosinophillic intracytoplasmic inclusions and ballooning of epidermal cells (Huchzermeyer *et al.*, 2009). Currently, PCR-based assays targeting a conserved gene of poxviruses have been developed and can be used to detect the virus in tissues. However, a definitive diagnosis can be made solely by electron microscopy and demonstration of viral particles.

Treatment No effective strategies have been reported to eliminate poxvirus from infected crocodilians. Treatment should be tailored toward specific clinical signs. Skin lesions can be debrided, disinfected, and antimicrobial ointment can be applied. Systemic antibiotics are indicated for animals that exhibit systemic signs.

Control Strict hygiene practices, including decontamination of tools and equipment, and improvement of the nutritional quality of diet as well as provision of a low-stress environment appear to be effective in limiting transmission and reducing the incidence of infection. Animals that develop skin lesions should be quarantined and tested. Poxvirus appears to be resistant to many disinfectants. However, 1% KOH, steam and 2% NaOH, have been shown to be effective (Ritchie, 2006).

Prevention Quarantine and strict hygiene practices are paramount in preventing poxvirus introduction into the existing colony.

Research Complication In captive crocodilians, high morbidity among juvenile animals can complicate and limit the productivity of research.

d. Paramyxovirus

Etiology Paramyxoviruses (PMVs) are enveloped viruses with negative sense single-stranded RNA genomes. For many years, all reptilian PMVs have clustered within the genus, ferlavirus. However, a novel paramyxovirus genetically distinct from ferlavirus called Sunshine virus has been identified in an Australian python (Marschang, 2009; Hyndman *et al.*, 2013). At least three distinct genogroups (A, B, and C) of ferlaviruses have been identified. PMVs isolated from Aruba Island snakes induced pulmonary lesions in this species, demonstrating that PMVs is pathogenic in this species and likely in other reptile species (Marschang, 2011).

Epizootiology and Transmission Cases of PMV infection have been reported in several snake families (Jacobson *et al.*, 1992; Hyndman *et al.*, 2013) and are associated with major losses of specimen in captive collections. Most commonly, viperid snakes are affected. Compared to snakes, PMV infections have been described much less frequently in lizards and turtles. The first PMV outbreak in snakes, which occurred in a serpentarium in Switzerland, was described in 1976. The outbreak resulted in massive death in individual rooms. Ferlaviruses are transmitted through respiratory and oral secretion as well as through feces. Sunshine virus is transmitted via the fecal–oral route. Cross-species infection is possible (Marschang, 2009), but transmission by fomites appears to be insignificant in ferlaviruses. Vertical transmission appears unlikely. Age, species, and environmental factors play important roles in determining susceptibility. Whether PMVs can persistently infect reptiles or reptiles can be infected and clear the infection requires further investigation (Hyndman *et al.*, 2013).

Pathogenesis Ferlaviral infection may be immunosuppressive, most likely as a result of lymphoid depletion. Consequently, animals may be prone to secondary bacterial, protozoal, parasitic, fungal, or other viral infection, which can worsen the clinical signs.

Clinical Signs Infected snakes commonly show signs of respiratory tract disease, including open-mouth breathing, caseous material in the oral cavity, and respiratory sounds. The time from exposure to clinical disease is usually 6–10 weeks or more. Other clinical signs include brown or hemorrhagic nasal discharge, anorexia, and sudden death. CNS signs can often be observed, and these include opisthotonus and spasticity (Fig. 19.15). Sunshine virus infection is commonly associated with neurorespiratory disease in snakes. Non-specific clinical signs can be observed and include lethargy and inappetence (Hyndman *et al.*, 2012). In infected lizards, pneumonia, sudden death, and anorexia prior to death were reported. In turtles, skin lesions and respiratory signs have been reported (Oettle *et al.*, 1990; Zangger *et al.*, 1991.)

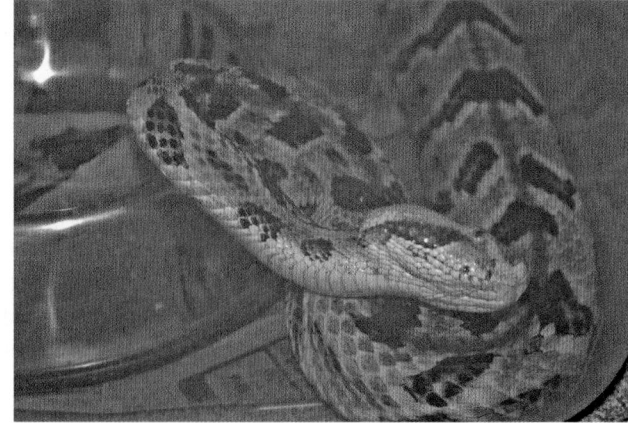

FIGURE 19.15 Neurological signs such as opisthotonus can be seen with paramyxovirus infections. Other diseases manifesting central nervous system signs include inclusion body disease, reovirus infection, and Mycoplasmosis.

Necropsy Findings There are no histological characteristics that are pathognomonic for ferlaviral infection. At necropsy, the main findings are frequently limited to the respiratory tract and include edematous lungs and fluid accumulation in all major airways. In many cases, obvious gross lesions may not be detected. Histologically, bronchointerstitial pneumonia with vacuolation and proliferation of epithelial cells lining the alveoli can be seen. Intracytoplasmic inclusions may be observed. Hindbrain white matter spongiosis and gliosis with neuronal necrosis have been reported in severe cases, particularly with Sunshine viruses (Hyndman *et al.*, 2012).

Differential Diagnosis Diagnosis can be made by serology, identification of virus in tissues using immunohistochemistry or *in situ* hybridization, PCR-based assays, and viral isolation from tissues and oral or cloacal swabs. Toxin, bacterial meningitis (e.g., mycoplasmosis), and other viral infectious agents (orthroreovirus, arenavirus) that can cause neurological and respiratory signs and chronic debilitation should be considered.

Treatment The prognosis in affected snakes is grave. There is no specific treatment, and isolation of suspected snakes with a strict quarantine protocol are highly recommended. Antimicrobial therapy instituted early in the course of infection may be helpful, but may not provide any improvement in already affected snakes. Seizure can be controlled with diazepam (0.5 mg/kg IM).

Control Affected animals should be separated or humanely euthanized. Reptiles suspected to be in direct or indirect contact with confirmed positive animals should be isolated and quarantined. Since virus transmission is considered airborne, no air exchange should occur between the quarantine or isolation room and the main collection. Bleach and Lysol® disinfectants have been proven effective against the virus and can be used to disinfect contaminated surfaces.

Prevention Quarantine of new animals (generally a minimum of 2–3 months; Bronson and Cranfield, 2006) with PCR screening on oral and cloacal swabs and transtracheal washes, serology testing, and/or hemagglutination assay should be instituted before and after addition to the established colony. Strict biosecurity and good sanitation and husbandry practices should be instituted. Ectoparasites can serve as a vector for transmission and must be eliminated from the colony.

Research Complication PMV infection can decimate a snake colony. Massive loss of experimental subjects can hinder research progress.

e. Arenavirus

Etiology For decades, inclusion body disease (IBD) has been attributed to infection with a retrovirus-like organism. However, recent evidence suggests that members of the family Arenaviridae are the most likely causative agent of this very important disease (Hetzel *et al.*, 2013). Arenaviruses are enveloped, single-stranded and negative-sense RNA viruses. Numerous genetically distinct strains have been isolated from snakes (Hetzel *et al.*, 2013).

Epizootiology and Transmission IBD affects many species of snakes including boas, vipers, and pythons; however, boid species, including boas and pythons, appear to be the most frequently reported species affected by the virus. Arenaviruses are highly infectious. Although the exact mode of transmission is currently unknown, the viruses appear to spread rapidly between animals, in particular among snakes showing concomitant infestation with mites, *Ophiomysus natricis* (Hetzel *et al.*, 2013). However, evidence supporting horizontal (direct) transmission is currently not available. Infected mice or rodents used to feed the snake may serve as a source of infection, although this possibility has not been investigated (Stenglein *et al.*, 2012). Inter-species transmission is possible. Subclinical cases have been reported, particularly in nonboid species. These animals can chronically shed and spread the virus throughout the colony.

Pathogenesis Currently, little is known about the pathogenic mechanisms of arenaviruses in reptiles.

Clinical Signs Animals with IBD can have varying clinical signs. Most commonly, affected animals will develop signs associated with CNS defects, including opisthotonus, loss of righting reflex, head tilt, disequilibrium, head tremors, and incoordination. Regurgitation is one of the first signs commonly observed in boas. Affected animals can also become bloated, be paralyzed, develop dysecdysis (incomplete shedding) and produce infertile eggs. Compared to boas, which can survive from months to many years after symptom onset, pythons succumb to the disease more rapidly (Stenglein *et al.*, 2012). Animals usually die from secondary bacterial, fungal (aspergillosis), and protozoal (amoebiasis) infections, and from neoplastic conditions such as lymphoma, which can occur concurrently with arenaviral infection (Schilliger *et al.*, 2011). Death can occur within weeks or months in highly susceptible reptile species.

Necropsy Findings Histologically, eosinophilic to amphophilic intracytoplasmic inclusions identified on hematoxylin-eosin-stained tissue sections can be observed in several organs, particularly in the brain, kidneys, pancreas, and liver.

Differential Diagnosis Infection with viruses, such as paramyxovirus and adenovirus, bacterial, fungal, and protozoal meningitis, as well as toxin exposure should be included in the list of differentials for CNS signs. One approach to detect the virus is RT-PCR using RNA purified from whole blood (Stenglein *et al.*, 2012). Other approaches include cell culture inoculation, electron microscopy to detect the virus, and immunoblotting

(Hetzel *et al.*, 2013). Use of specific anti-IBD protein to detect the virus in ante-mortem samples may also be possible (Chang *et al.*, 2013).

Treatment   Currently no treatments or vaccines are available. Supportive care may be provided, but this will not alter the course of the disease.

Control   Since no treatment or vaccines are available and the virus is highly infectious and can cause high morbidity and mortality in the affected colony, the current recommendation is euthanasia of infected animals to prevent further spread. During the outbreak, animals should be quarantined and strict hygiene practices should be implemented. The viruses are not very stable in the environment and can be easily inactivated by standard disinfectant practices. Since nonboid species can serve as carriers, they should be kept separate from boid species.

Prevention   New animals should be quarantined for at least 6 months and screened for the presence of the virus at the beginning and the end of the quarantine period. Strict hygiene and good husbandry practices should prevent spread of the disease and promote health and resistance to infection among the animals.

Research Complication   High morbidity and mortality associated with inclusion body disease can be debilitating to research due to extensive specimen loss.

f. Reovirus

Etiology   Reoviruses are nonenveloped, double-stranded, segmented RNA viruses. Currently, the strains known to infect reptiles have been placed in the genus *Orthoreovirus*. Experimental infection with clinical isolates of reovirus from beauty snakes and Moellendorff's ratsnakes induced severe clinical disease in juvenile black ratsnakes, confirming their pathogenic properties in these species and likely other species of reptiles (Lamirande *et al.*, 1999).

Epizootiology and Transmission   Reports of reovirus infection have been documented in various species of reptiles, including emerald tree boas, rough green snakes, Chinese vipers, rat snakes, iguanas, leopard geckos, green lizards, tortoises, and chameleons (Landolfi *et al.*, 2010; Marschang, 2011). Numerous strains of reovirus have been identified and appear to cause different clinical manifestations among different reptile species. While certain viral strains appear to be nonpathogenic, some strains are associated with high morbidity and mortality. Mode of transmission has not been clearly delineated in reptiles. However, in birds, transmission occurs via direct or indirect contact with contaminated feces. Interspecies infection may occur.

Pathogenesis   The precise pathogenic mechanisms of reoviruses in reptiles are unclear. As an RNA virus, reoviruses replicate in the cytoplasm of the infected cells. Reptilian reoviruses appear to mediate cell fusion to form syncitia from a small type III protein (Corcoran and Duncan, 2004).

Clinical Signs   Neurological signs, including incoordination, proprioceptive deficits, and convulsion, as well as pneumonia, stomatitis, and gastrointestinal signs, have been reported in animals infected with reoviruses (Vieler *et al.*, 1999; Lamirande *et al.*, 1999; Marschang and Divers, 2014). Infected green snakes were reported to develop papillomas (Marschang, 2011), while ratsnakes experimentally inoculated with reovirus were found dead 26 days post-inoculation (Lamirande *et al.*, 1999). In tortoises, infection can result in the development of tongue lesions, and animals can become cachectic.

Necropsy Findings   Proliferative tracheitis and interstitial pneumonia were the prominent lesions observed in experimentally inoculated ratsnakes. Microscopically, affected tissues can form syncytia. However, inclusions are not a distinct feature associated with reovirus infection. Some strains of reovirus are associated with hepatitis and pancreatitis. In snakes, reovirus infection is associated with the development of papillomas.

Differential Diagnosis   Differentials for CNS and respiratory signs include paramyxovirus infection and IBD, toxin exposure, as well as both bacteria (mycoplasmosis and mycobacteriosis) and fungal infection. PCR-based assays, virus isolation, and viral detection via electron microscopy can be used to determine the presence of the virus in tissues and feces.

Treatment   No effective treatment has been reported for reovirus infection. In severe cases, euthanasia is recommended.

Control   In birds, vertical transmission has been reported for reovirus, making eradication very difficult in an affected colony. A similar scenario may be expected for reovirus infection in reptiles. Consistent with their nonenveloped characteristic, reoviruses are stable in the environment and are resistant to many disinfectants, including pH3, 2% Lysol®, 3% formaldehyde, 1% hydrogen peroxide, quaternary ammonium, and heating to 56°C for 120 min. However, paracetic acid fogging has been shown to be effective in inactivating the virus in laboratories and facilities (Gregersen and Roth, 2012).

Prevention   As with other viral agents previously discussed, strict biosecurity, quarantine, and implementation of good hygiene practices should reduce the possibility of introducing the virus into the existing colony.

Research Complication   Reovirus infection is associated with high morbidity and mortality. Extensive loss of animals can hinder research progress.

g. Ranavirus

Etiology   As a member of family *Iridoviridae*, ranaviruses are nucleocytoplasmic large double-stranded DNA viruses. They can occur in enveloped or nonenveloped form, and both are considered infectious. Koch's postulates have been fulfilled when ranavirus isolates recovered from a Burmese star tortoise caused severe disease in box turtles and red-eared sliders (Johnson *et al.*, 2007).

Epizootiology and Transmission Ranaviruses have been identified in a number of reptile species, including brown and green anoles, leaf-tailed geckos, snakes, Asian glass lizards, Iberian mountain lizards, green iguanas, tortoises, turtles, green pythons, and bearded dragons (Stohr *et al.*, 2013; Johnson *et al.*, 2008); however, most cases have been described in chelonians. A mass mortality event associated with the infection was reported in a group of infected green-striped tree dragons (Behncke *et al.*, 2013). Multiple genetically distinct strains of reptilian ranavirus have been identified, and cross-species infection has been documented (Stöhr *et al.*, 2013). Reptilian ranaviruses are highly similar to *Frog virus 3* the type species of ranavirus, hinting at the possibility that the reptilian ranaviruses were transmitted from amphibians to reptiles and *vice versa*. Arthropods, such as crickets, can serve as reservoirs of the virus. Reptiles can become infected when contaminated arthropods are consumed. The virus is very stable outside the host and can remain infectious for months in water or organic debris.

Pathogenesis The pathogenic mechanisms of reptilian ranaviruses are largely unknown. Ranaviruses replicate in two stages. The first stage occurs in the nucleus, and the second stage occurs in the cytoplasm. It has been suggested that reptilian ranaviruses may be able to persist in the host. Subclinically infected animals develop clinical signs under stressful conditions or under conditions that lead to immunosuppression (Stohr *et al.*, 2013).

Clinical Signs Predominant signs observed in affected animals include ulcerative dermatitis with hyperkeratosis, nasal and ocular discharge, conjunctivitis, and diphtheroid-necrotic stomatitis. Other nonspecific signs associated with the infection include lethargy and anorexia. In some animals, subcutaneous cervical edema and 'red-neck disease' can develop. Secondary bacterial and fungal infection is often observed and can worsen the disease outcome.

Necropsy Finding Ulceration of nasal mucosa, necrotizing inflammation of the pharyngeal submucosa, esophagitis, vasculitis, splenitis, purulent to ulcerative-necrotizing dermatitis, tubulonephrosis, hepatitis, enteritis, and pneumonia are common histological findings among infected animals (Behncke *et al.*, 2013). Microscopically, fibrinoid vasculitis, and thrombin can be found in various organs. Skin lesions characterized by raised grayish skin alteration and intracytoplasmic inclusions can be observed.

Differential Diagnosis Differentials for skin lesions in reptiles should include other viral infections, such as papillomavirus, reovirus, poxvirus, and herpesvirus, bacterial infection, thermal and sun burn, toxin exposure, overcrowding, and poor nutrition. PCR-based assays targeting the DNA sequences encoding the viral capsid are available and can be used to determine the presence of the virus. DNA sequencing of the viral capsid gene can be performed to ascertain the identity of the virus. Virus isolation in established cell lines is also possible (Stohr *et al.*, 2013).

Treatment No vaccine is currently available. Treatment can be provided based on the clinical signs; however, due to high mortality associated with infection, euthanasia of positive animals is recommended.

Control Infected animals should be isolated from healthy animals. Quarantine and strict hygiene with the use of an appropriate disinfectant to decontaminate the vivarium should be implemented to prevent further spread of disease.

Prevention Quarantine of new animals and rigorous testing should be implemented at the beginning and end of quarantine. Since mass mortality has been observed in reptiles, particularly juvenile and immunocompromised ones, animals identified to be infected with ranavirus should be culled to prevent introduction of the virus into the colony. 0.75% Nolvasan, 3% bleach, and 1% Virkon S have been shown to be effective against ranavirus (Bryan *et al.*, 2009).

Research Complication Infection can cause substantial mortality in susceptible species.

h. Papillomavirus

Etiology Papillomaviruses are nonenveloped viruses from the family Papillomaviridae. They are approximately 55 nm in diameter and their genomes contain circular double-stranded DNA.

Epizootiology and Transmission Papillomavirus-associated skin lesions have been reported in reptiles, including Bolivian side-neck turtles, a Russian tortoise, green turtles, loggerhead turtles, snakes, and lizards (Jacobson *et al.*, 1982a; Manire *et al.*, 2008; Marschang, 2011; Gull *et al.*, 2012). The viruses are highly host-specific and tissue-restricted, although occasionally they can cross infect and cause lesions in related species (Marschang, 2011).

Pathogenesis Papillomaviruses target the epithelia of vertebrates. The viruses can transform normal epithelial cells into neoplastic cells and persist in the host without inducing any clinical signs.

Clinical Signs Affected turtles can be presented with generalized small, white, raised lesions in the mouth, by the neck, and on the shoulders, head, plastron, and flippers. In snakes, skin lesions are characterized by multiple black, papillated, exophytic proliferations. These lesions usually regress after several months.

Necropsy Findings Histologically, thickened stratum corneum, multifocal areas of hyperplasia, and abnormal nuclear morphology in the keratinocytes can be observed. Membrane-bound intracytoplasmic vacuoles and intranuclear inclusions have been reported in the epithelial cells of the skin (Manire *et al.*, 2008; Jacobson, 2007).

Differential Diagnosis Similar to papillomaviruses, herpesviruses and reoviruses can also cause papilloma-like lesions in reptiles. Papillomavirus infection can be diagnosed by electron microscopy and PCR-based assays (Marschang, 2011).

Treatment In snakes and turtles, regression of papillomavirus has been reported and usually occurs months after the initial presentation. Unless the lesions cause specific problems, papilloma lesions should be left untreated. In severe cases, radiosurgery can be performed or lasers can be used to remove the lesions. Treatment of lesions with salicyclic acid may also be useful (Ritchie, 2006).

Control Affected animals should be isolated and treated symptomatically.

Prevention Quarantine (at least 6 months) is recommended to help prevent the introduction of an infected animal to the existing colony (Ritchie, 2006).

Research Complication Severe papillomatous lesions can be debilitating and often lead to secondary infections that require extensive treatment.

3. Parasitic

Evaluation of reptiles for parasites is an important component of assessing the health status of the animal, especially wild-caught specimens. Proper quarantine procedures, including screening of fecal samples for parasites, should be followed, especially before introducing a new reptile into an existing colony. Parasite infestations often go undiagnosed due to nonspecific signs, including chronic weight loss, anorexia, regurgitation, and diarrhea. It is essential to collect proper samples (fresh fecal samples and biopsies, if necessary) to make an accurate diagnosis (Greiner and Schumacher, 1997; Jacobson, 1983).

a. Protozoan

ENTAMOEBA INVADENS

Etiology *Entamoeba invadens* is a small amoeboid protozoan with a single nucleus and a single lobose pseudopod.

Epizootiology and Transmission Although many species of protozoan can be found in reptiles, *E. invadens* is the most clinically important protozoan parasite. *Entamoeba invadens* is associated with high mortality in affected snakes and lizards (Donaldson *et al.*, 1975). Cases have also been reported in turtles and alligators (Bradford *et al.*, 2008). In chelonians, *E. invadens* is generally considered a commensal organism. The infective cysts are passed in the feces and are very stable in the environment. Transmission occurs by ingestion of infective cysts present in the feces. Due to the direct life cycle of this organism, a colony may rapidly be infected.

Pathogenesis The cyst is the main infective form. It releases the motile trophozoites after ingestion by the host. The trophozoites invade the intestine and liver and spread hematogenously through the portal vein. Proteolytic enzymes released by the parasite disrupt intestinal mucosa and the epithelial barrier facilitating tissue penetration (Chia *et al.*, 2009).

Clinical Signs Affected animals can become immobile, refuse to feed, regurgitate, and succumb to the disease. Gastrointestinal signs associated with the infection include dysentery with mucus and blood.

Necropsy Findings Intestinal and/or hepatic lesions are common. Intestinal lesions are characterized by hemorrhage, ulceration, and enteritis. The liver can become enlarged, and multiple irregular, discrete to coalescing friable white-yellow foci can be observed throughout the organ (Chia *et al.*, 2009). Severe granulomatous myositis and dermatitis have also been reported.

Differential Diagnosis Diagnosis can be made by demonstration of trophozoites in a direct smear of a fecal sample or infected tissues. *Entamoeba invadens*-specific PCR-based assays have also been developed and may be used (Bradford *et al.*, 2008).

Treatment Metronidazole (275mg/kg PO once) was proven to be rapidly effective and safe in snakes and lizards (Donaldson *et al.*, 1975).

Control Strict hygiene and disinfection of all contaminated cages and equipment, as well as isolation and treatment of infected and exposed animals, should be implemented to prevent further spread of the organism. Chlorine dioxide has been shown to be effective against many protozoa as well as their infective cysts, which are highly resistant in the environment (Dupuy *et al.*, 2014).

Prevention New animals should be quarantined, tested, and, if infected, treated before introduction into the existing colony.

Research Complication High mortality associated with *E. invadens* can result in a massive loss of research animals which can severely limit research productivity.

CRYPTOSPORIDIOSIS

Etiology Cryptosporidiosis is caused by numerous species of *Cryptosporidium*, a genus of protozoan belonging to the phylum Aplicomplexa. There are more than 25 species and greater than 60 genotypes of *Cryptosporidium* (Connelly *et al.*, 2013). It has an average size of 3.7μm (length) by 2.3μm (width). The oocyst is less than 8μm in diameter.

Epizootiology and Transmission Cryptosporidiosis is common among captive reptiles and can cause severe disease in susceptible animals. Over 80 species of reptiles have been reported to be infected by *Cryptosporidium*. *Cryptosporidium serpentine* and *C. varanii* (synonym *C. saurophylum*) are two of the most common species found in snakes and lizards, respectively. The zoonotic potential of these two species is questionable, although some reports suggest that they lack zoonotic potential (Rinaldi *et al.*, 2012). *Cryptosporidium serpentine* shows interspecies transmission, and all age groups appear to be susceptible to infection. In tortoises, a distinct species of *Cryptosporidium* similar to *C. ducismarci* has been described (Richter *et al.*, 2012). Latent infection can occur. Oocysts are considered transmission agents; reptile hosts become infected by ingesting contaminated feces containing the oocysts. *Cryptosporidium* oocysts are very stable in the environment due to the presence of a thick cell wall and can serve as a source of re-infection. Reptiles that are fed rodents infected with *Cryptosporidium*, which appears not to be infective in reptiles, can have the oocyst of rodent *Cryptosporidium* in their feces. This can often complicate the diagnosis.

Pathogenesis Compared to *C. serpentine*, which commonly infects snakes and colonizes their gastric glands, *C. varanii* has a predilection for lizards and appears to have a tropism for the small intestine in these species. Like *C. varanni*, *Cryptosporidium* spp. of tortoises also appears to induce intestinal pathology. After the sporozoites are released from the oocyst, they invade the enterocytes.

Clinical Signs Although clinical signs may be absent during the initial stage of disease in snake, chronic regurgitation, progressive weight loss, and a firm midbody swelling caused by gastric hypertrophy may be seen in advanced stages. Infected snakes can live for days to years. However, the disease is usually fatal in snakes. *Cryptosporidium varanii* can cause diarrhea in lizards. In turtles, cloacal prolapse and cystitis have been reported. Unlike mammals, disease in reptiles is not self-limiting.

Necropsy Finding Hypertrophic gastritis with a cobblestone appearance of the gastric mucosa can be observed in snakes, whereas enteritis can be seen in affected lizards and turtles. Intestinal lesions consist of heterophil, lymphocyte, and macrophage infiltration.

Differential Diagnosis Diagnosis can be challenging due to the intermittent shedding, but can be made by demonstration of oocysts in fecal smears of infected animals, by gastric lavage, or by collection of gastric and intestinal biopsies via gastroscopy for histopathology. PCR amplification of small subunit ribosomal RNA gene of *Cryptosporidium* can also be used to detect the organism. IFA can be used to detect oocytes and ELISA for determining exposure to the organism.

Treatment Hyperimmune bovine colostrum appears to be an effective treatment in many species of reptile (Graczyk *et al.*, 1998). Combined paromomycin (100 mg/kg body weight, orally once a day for 7 days and then twice a week for 3 months), spiramycin (160 mg/kg for 7 days and then twice a week for 3 months), and trimethoprim sulfa (20 mg/kg once a day for 14 days and one to three times weekly for 7 months) treatment appeared to improve clinical signs, but did not eliminate shedding (Richter *et al.*, 2012). Aminosidine, an aminoglycoside antibiotic, was also attempted in one report and appeared to reduce shedding but not eliminate the organism (Richter *et al.*, 2012).

Control Strict hygiene and good husbandry practices are important in controlling infection. Correction of husbandry practices and elimination of concurrent disease appear to be as effective as any anticryptosporidial medications.

Prevention Quarantine and testing along with good hygiene practices should prevent introduction of *Cryptosporidium* into the existing reptile colony. KENO™COX has been demonstrated to have a high efficacy against *C. parvum* oocysts (Naciri *et al.*, 2011). Other effective strategies include application of chlorine dioxide, ammonia (5%) and formal saline solution (10%) for 18 h at 4°C. Heating between 45°C and 60°C for 5–9 min appears to be effective for neutralizing the infectivity of oocysts.

Research Complication Cryptosporidiosis is usually fatal in snakes. Loss of animals due to infection can be detrimental to any research endeavor.

b. Nematodes

Etiology Numerous species of nematodes have been identified in reptiles, including hookworms, *Kalicephalus* spp.; lungworms, *Rhabdias* spp.; Microfilaria, *Macdonaldius oschei* and *Foleyella furcata*; and many round worm species, such as *Cyrtosomum penneri*, *Cosmocercoides* spp., *Anasakis* spp., *Sulcascaris sulcata*, *Augusticaecum* spp., *Trichinella* spp., *Serpinema* spp., *Spiroxys* spp., *Protractis* spp., *Chapiniella* spp., *Ozolaimus* spp., *Aleuris* spp., *Macdonaldius* spp., *Physaloptera* spp., *Paratrichosoma* spp., and *Capillaria* spp.

Epizootiology and Transmission Nematodes are commonly found in the gastrointestinal system of all orders of reptiles. A single animal can be infected with one or more species (Rataj *et al.*, 2011). Strongyles, especially the hookworm *Kalicephalus* spp., are important nematode parasites in snakes. Filarids and *Capillaria* spp. are commonly diagnosed in reptiles. Oxyurids are found frequently in lizards and less commonly in turtles, where the nematodes are thought to act as saprophytes in the colon (Johnson, 2004; Rataj *et al.*, 2011). Lungworm infection appears to be more common in snakes than lizards (Langford and Janovy, 2013); they can be transmitted via transport hosts and can survive in water for a long time (Langford and Janovy, 2009). Other nematodes can be transmitted by the fecal–oral route via consumption of contaminated feed including nematode-infected live feed.

Pathogenesis Different species of nematode have evolved strategies to effectively invade their hosts and exhibit distinct tissue and organ tropism. Some species of nematode can be transmitted to their respective reptile hosts via intermediate hosts, including amphibians and insects, which are consumed by the reptiles. *Kalicephalus* spp. have a direct life cycle and are most often found in the gastrointestinal tract. Unlike the amphibian lung-worms that penetrate the skin of their host, reptile lung-worms do not penetrate the skin, but the esophagus after ingestion (Langford and Janovy, 2009). After penetrating the esophagus, the parasites migrate to the fascia and the body cavity. Worms molt to adulthood and then penetrate the lung. The round worm *Cyrtosomum penneri* is transmitted venereally, but not orally (Langford *et al.*, 2013), and infection does not seem to be host specific. Physalopterid worms as well as *Dujardinascaris* spp., *Spiroxys* spp., *Chapiniella* spp., and *Sulcascaris sulcata* prefer to colonize the stomach (Jones, 1995). In contrast, the microfilarial worms have the propensity to invade the blood vessels (*Macdonaldius oschei*), subcutaneous tissues (*Foleyella furcata*), and connective tissues. Argasid ticks have been reported to serve as vectors for microfilarial worms.

Clinical Signs Heavy infection with ascarids may result in high morbidity and mortality. Extensive larval migration in the host may cause considerable damage to affected tissues and organs. While mild infections are subclinical, heavy infections have been associated with severe inflammatory responses in the mucosa of the esophagus and stomach. Secondary bacterial infections may also be present. Clinical signs associated with hook-worm infection include weight loss, wasting, and ano-rexia. Signs associated with lungworm infection include labored breathing, exudate within the oral cavity, and presence of secondary bacterial infections resulting in severe bacterial pneumonia. In contrast, signs of disease are usually absent with filarid and pinworm infection. If signs are present, they are nonspecific, consisting of anorexia, lethargy, and depression (Rideout *et al.*, 1987). In cases of heavy infection, death can occur 2–4 weeks after the onset of clinical signs (Johnson, 2004). The filarial worm *Macdonaldius oschei* can cause severe dermatitis in pythons; however, in the natural hosts, such as Mexican viperid and colubrid snakes, this parasite was found in the posterior vena cava and renal veins. In contrast, the parasite was identified in the mesenteric veins in pythons, where the parasite elicits a granulomatous response.

Necropsy Findings Hookworm infection has been associated with erosions and ulceration of intestinal lining. Lesions caused by lungworms have been reported to be restricted to the upper respiratory tree and are characterized by tracheal and bronchial epithelial hyperplasia and goblet cell hyperplasia (Manire *et al.*, 2012). Heavy filarial infestation can cause ischemic necrosis of skin and obstruction of vessels. Pinworm infection can lead to roughening and thickening of the mucosa of the cecum and colon and, in severe cases, tiny worms can be observed on the mucosal surface.

Differential Diagnosis Diagnosis of nematode infection can be done by observation of nematode eggs or larva in the fecal samples. Direct smear, sedimentation, or use of a Baermann apparatus appear to be more reliable methods for detecting nematodes than fecal floatation (Johnson, 2004). In ascarids, adult worms can sometimes be detected in regurgitated food. For micro-filarial species, diagnosis can be made by demonstration of microfilariae in a blood smear of an infected animal.

Treatment Generally, fenbendazole (50–100 mg/kg PO, repeat in 2 weeks or 100 mg/kg q 24h × 3 days) appears to be an effective treatment (Foronda *et al.*, 2007; Johnson, 2004). In certain cases, such as pinworm and filarial worm infection, treatment (e.g., ivermectin, 0.2 mg/kg, SC) is contraindicated as it appears to be ineffective and may be detrimental to the animal due to anaphylactic shock caused by the release of antigens from dead worms (Rideout *et al.*, 1987; Széll *et al.*, 2001). Ivermectin (0.05 mg/kg IM) appears to be effective in reducing the shedding of eggs and larvae in the feces, but fails to completely eliminate the parasites from the system. Dosages of ivermectin higher than 0.05 mg/kg may be more effective, but toxicosis and death have been observed in some species of turtles (Teare and Bush, 1983).

Control Infected animals should be isolated and treated accordingly. The contaminated area should be disinfected with appropriate disinfectant.

Prevention Strict quarantine and testing for nematodes should be performed on newly arrived animals.

Research Complication High morbidity and mortality associated with heavy infection can limit research productivity.

c. Cestodes

Etiology Cestodes, or tapeworms, are flatworms belonging to the phylum Platyhelmenthes. Numerous species, including *Proteocephalus* spp., *Acanthotaenia* spp., *Ophiotaenia* spp., *Crepidobothrium* spp., *Oochoristica* spp., *Australotaenia* spp., *Panceriella* spp., *Mesocestoides* spp., *Bothridium* spp., *Duthiersia* spp., and *Spirometra* spp. have been identified in reptiles.

Epizootiology and Transmission Cestodes have been reported in chelonians, lizards, and snakes, but rarely in crocodilians. Reptiles can serve as either definite or intermediate hosts. Within the order Proteocephalidea, the genus *Ophiotaenia* is most commonly seen in snakes following ingestion of frogs, which serve as the intermediate host. The genera *Bothridium* and *Botriocephalus* within the pseudophyllidean order are known to infect pythons. Tapeworms of the family Mesocestoidea can be found in all vertebrates.

Pathogenesis High numbers of cestodes can lead to gastrointestinal obstruction. The parasite also competes for the host's essential nutrients.

Clinical Signs Most infections in reptiles are subclinical; however, in severe cases, affected animals can become anorexic.

Necropsy Findings The genera *Bothridium* and *Botriocephalus* are associated with enteritis. *Mesocestoides* and *Tetrathyridia* infect snakes and lizards, causing subcutaneous nodules and the presence of many encysted larvae within the coelomic cavity.

Differential Diagnosis Diagnosis can be made by detection of eggs in the feces through fecal smear or fecal floatation. A fully formed oncosphere with six hooks should be observed in eggs of tapeworm recovered from reptiles (Greiner and Mader, 2006).

Treatment Treatment for cestode infections consists of praziquantel administration (8 mg/kg IM, PO, repeat in 2 and 4 weeks). A new combinatory drug therapy consisting of two anthelmintic compounds containing emodepside and praziquantel applied on the skin has been shown to be highly effective against cestodes as well as nematodes (Mehlhorn *et al.*, 2005).

Control Infected animals should be isolated and treated, and the contaminated area should be disinfected with an appropriate disinfectant.

Prevention Quarantine and testing of newly arrived animals should be performed. If positive animals are detected, treatment should be implemented with retesting at the completion of treatment to confirm eradication.

Research Complication In heavy infection, animals can become moribund. Loss of animals can limit research productivity.

d. Trematodes

Etiology Trematoda consists of a group of parasitic flatworms known as flukes. Numerous species of flukes including *Lophotaspis vallei*, *Haplometrema* spp., *Leardius* spp., *Carettacola* spp., *Ochestosoma* spp., *Dasymetra* spp., *Lechriorchis* spp., *Pneumatophilus* spp., *Zeugorchis* spp., *Stomatrema* spp., *Zeugorchis* spp., *Styphlodora* spp., and *Spirorchis* spp. can parasitize reptiles.

Epizootiology and Transmission The reptile hosts often acquire the parasite through ingestion of vertebrate intermediate hosts that contain encysted metacercariae. Trematodes are usually not considered to be major pathogens in reptiles. However, *Spirorchis* spp. and *Styphlodora* spp. have been reported to cause serious problems in marine turtles and snakes, respectively (Johnson *et al.*, 1998).

Pathogenesis Trematode species, such as *Spirorchis parvus*, are pathogenic, and adult flukes live in blood vessels and the heart where they lay eggs. Widespread deposition of eggs in blood vessels can cause blockage of small vessels leading to tissue ischemia and necrosis. *Spirorchis parvus* can also invade various tissues. *Styphlodora horrid* can invade the kidney causing severe nephritis in snakes (Kazacos and Fisher, 1977). Genera within the family Ochetosomatidae, including *Dasymetra*, *Lechriorchis*, *Seugorchis*, *Ochestosoma*, and *Plagiorchiidae* migrate from the oral cavity to the lungs and air sacs and can cause focal lesions in these organs (Jacobson, 2007a).

Clinical Signs Brain ischemia can cause neurologic signs in infected animals (Jacobson *et al.*, 2006). Captive boas infected with *Styphlodora* spp. can become anorexic and die. Members of digenetic trematodes, including the fluke Renifer, are associated with ulcerative lung lesions and predispose reptiles to secondary bacterial infections. Infected turtles may be lethargic, exhibit abnormal swimming behavior, and may develop skin ulcers and edematous limbs (Johnson, 2004).

Necropsy Finding Trematode eggs can be detected on the serosal surface of various organs, including heart, pancreas, kidney, and intestine, and granulomas can develop around the eggs causing widespread granulomatous lesions. In severe cases of *Styphlodora* spp. infection, interstitial nephritis with accumulation of cellular debris within tubules may be seen.

Differential Diagnosis Diagnosis is made by demonstration of eggs on fecal examination or within tissue sections. Renal flukes (*Styphylodora* spp.) can be found within renal tubules and ureters of snakes.

Treatment Intravascular or oral administration of praziquantel (8 mg/kg IM, PO, repeat in 2 and 4 weeks) appears to be an effective treatment for trematode infection.

Control Since many trematode species require an intermediate host to complete their life cycle, infection in captivity should be self-limiting when exposure to intermediate hosts is prevented.

Prevention The practice of feeding infected intermediate hosts to reptiles should be prevented to limit infection.

Research Complication Significant morbidity and mortality associated with trematode infection can compromise research.

e. Acanthocephalans

Etiology Acanthocephalans or thorny/spiny headed worms are parasitic worms belonging to the phylum Acanthocephala. Numerous species have been identified in reptiles including *Pseudoacanthocephalus smalesi*, *Pseudoacanthocephalus rhampholeontos*, *Acanthocephalus saurius*, *Corynosoma strumosum*, *Acracanthorynchus catulinus*, *Oncicola venezuelensis*, *Pachysentis canicola*, *Sphaerechinorhynchus ophiograndis*, *Centrorhynchus* spp.,

Porrorchis spp., *and Neoechinorhynchus* spp. (Tkach *et al.*, 2013; Bursey and Goldberg, 2003; Bolette, 1997a, b; Goldberg *et al.*, 1997).

Epizootiology and Transmission Acanthocephalans have a complex life cycle involving at least two hosts. The definitive host of spiny-headed worms is an amphibian. However, reptiles, including, snakes, chelonians, and mammalian species, can also serve as definitive hosts (Smales, 2007). They become infected upon consumption of intermediate hosts, such as fish and insects, including cockroaches (Nickol *et al.*, 2006).

Pathogenesis Some species, such as *Sphaerechinorhynchus serpenticola*, prefer to colonize the intestinal tract and the liver. Heavy infection can result in intestinal obstruction and induces a strong host inflammatory response that leads to colitis.

Clinical Signs Heavy infection can lead to emaciation and lethargy.

Necropsy Findings While most infections are subclinical, heavy infestations may result in granuloma formation and ulceration of intestinal lining. If larvae are present in unsuitable hosts, they may encyst in viscera, commonly the abdominal cavity and subcutaneous tissues. The worm can also be found within subcutaneous nodules.

Differential Diagnosis Diagnosis can also be made by demonstration of characteristic eggs in a direct fecal smear or fecal floatation.

Treatment While there appears to be no safe and effective treatment, administration of ivermectin (0.2 mg/kg IM, PO, repeat in 2 weeks) may be attempted. Ivermectin toxicity has been reported in turtles and skinks, thus the use of this drug is not advisable in these groups.

Control Positive animals with clinical signs should be isolated and treated. Contaminated surfaces should be disinfected with appropriate disinfectants.

Prevention Strict quarantine and testing should prevent introduction of this parasite into the existing colony.

Research Complication Treatment associated with infection can be costly and time consuming. Loss of animals associated with heavy infection can compromise research productivity.

f. Pentastomes

Etiology Pentastomids or tongue worms are worm-like endoparasites belonging to the phylum Pentastomida. Species known to infect reptiles includes *Armillifer* spp., *Raillietiella* spp., *Agema* spp., *Alofia* spp., *Leiperia* spp., *Porocephalus* spp., *Kiricephalus* spp., *Sebekia* spp., *Selfia* spp., and *Subtriquetra* spp.

Epizootiology and Transmission Tongue worms affect a variety of reptiles, including snakes, lizards, turtles, and crocodilians (Flach *et al.*, 2000; Junker *et al.*,

2006; Rataj, 2011; Kelehear *et al.*, 2011). An animal can be infected with multiple species of pentastomids. The prevalence can be high in susceptible populations, and hatchlings appear to be most susceptible. Inter-species infection can occur as anuran pentastomids appear to be able to cross infect reptiles and vice versa (Kelehear *et al.*, 2011).

Pathogenesis Mammals, such as rodents, as well as fish and insects can serve as intermediate hosts of pentastomids. The intermediate hosts become infected by ingesting eggs contained either in feces or in the sputum of the reptiles. Eggs hatch to larvae and then burrow to the abdominal cavity through the gut wall. The arthropod-like larvae mature to nymphs and get attached to the viscera in encysted forms. Reptiles become infected upon ingesting intermediate hosts containing the encysted nymphs. In the intestine, the nymphs excyst and migrate by various routes to the respiratory tract. Occasionally the parasites can bore through the body cavity and protrude from the skin. In the lung, adult worms deposit their eggs, which can be coughed up, ingested, passed through the intestinal tract, and excreted in feces.

Clinical Signs Minor infection may be asymptomatic, but heavy infection may cause pronounced inflammatory responses that lead to lung, air sac, and/or skin damage. The affected animals can present with oral and nasal discharge. Heterophilia and monocytosis may be noted in a differential count of blood cells (Brock *et al.*, 2012). Other nonspecific signs include vomiting after meals, lethargy, weight loss, and anorexia. Secondary fungal or bacterial infection can occur and, in severe cases, lead to death.

Necropsy Findings Pentastomid infection is associated with widespread pulmonary congestion, edema, and hemorrhage (Ayinmode *et al.*, 2010). Pale oral and conjunctival mucus membranes can also be observed. Live yellowish-white arthropod larvae can often be found on the surface of the lung and are associated with mucohemorrhagic lesions. Other lesions, such as hepatic necrosis and glomerulonephritis, can also be observed (Ayinmode *et al.*, 2010).

Differential Diagnosis Viral agents and pathogens, such as fungi, bacteria, and nematodes, that can infect the respiratory system and cause respiratory signs in reptiles should be included in the list of differentials. Diagnosis can be made by identification of pentastomid eggs or larva in a pulmonary wash.

Treatment Ivermectin (0.2 mg/kg S.C., repeated in 10 days) and supportive therapy have been shown to be effective as a treatment (Flach *et al.*, 2000). Pentastomes can also be removed from subcutaneous nodules by surgery or from the air sacs and lungs via endoscopy. Since pentastomids require intermediate hosts to complete their life cycles, preventive methods aimed at limiting exposure of reptiles to infected intermediate hosts should limit further infection, and treatment may not be needed.

Control Live fish, insects, and rodents can serve as carriers of the parasites, and their consumption has been associated with infection. Therefore, live feed, particularly of unknown health status, should be avoided if possible. Strict hygiene practices are also important in controlling the spread of the worms. Freezing of live infected fish at 10°C for 72 h appears to be effective in killing the parasites.

Prevention Quarantine and testing for the parasites should be performed in new animals before introduction into the existing colony. If the animals are found to be positive for the parasite, treatment should be implemented and animals retested at the completion of the treatment.

Research Complication High morbidity associated with heavy infection may require extensive treatment that can be costly and time consuming.

g. Mites and Ticks

Etiology More than 250 species of mites can parasitize reptiles. *Ophionyssus natricis* is common in snakes and *Ophionyssus acertinus* in lizards. Trombiculid or 'chiggers' can also affect reptiles. Reptiles can also be parasitized by several genera of ticks, including hard ticks (*Ixodes, Hyalomma, Haemaphysalis, Amblyomma,* and *Aponomma*) and soft ticks (*Argasidae* and *Ornithodoros*).

Epizootiology and Transmission Both mites and ticks are found in captive as well as wild reptiles. Mites may cause a major problem in captive collections of reptiles, especially snakes. Poor hygiene and/or introduction of infected reptiles into a collection are predisposing factors. Ticks and mites can rapidly establish dense populations due to their short life cycle (1–16 days), which depends on the temperature and humidity. The life cycle of the snake mite, *O. natricis,* consists of egg, larva, protonymph, deutonymph, and adult, with a molt occurring between the immature stages. Adult and protonymph stages are parasitic. The parasites feed on the blood of the reptiles. Ticks and mites can also serve as an effective means to spread reptilian bacterial and viral pathogens within the existing colony.

Pathogenesis Clinical signs associated with ticks and mites are skin injury due to their bites, which can be painful. Tremendous blood lost and anemia can also occur with heavy infestation. Many of the ticks are host specific. In snakes, some ticks can transmit parasitic worms and microbial pathogens from one snake to another.

Clinical Signs Infestations with ticks and mites can lead to a variety of clinical outcomes. The affected reptiles can become anorexic, inappetent, and dehydrated. In some cases, dermatitis, pruritis, dysecdysis, and retained eye caps can be observed. Behavioral change can also be observed, including frequent rubbing against the side of the enclosure or cage furniture or a long duration of soaking in water in an attempt to rid themselves of pests. The animals can also become anemic or septic.

Necropsy Findings Skin lesions indicative of dermatitis can often be seen along with persistent or recurrent dysecdysis.

Differential Diagnosis Mite infestation can be diagnosed by seeing them with the unaided eye on the skin or by skin scraping. Wiping a moist paper towel over the animal's skin can accumulate mites and mite feces (seen as reddish dots), easing the detection of a mite infestation. Ticks can also be identified on the skin of affected animals. The common location of mites and ticks include anterior axillae, on and around the elbow, between digits, in the gular fold, and around the cloaca and eyes.

Treatment Treatment of mite infestation is difficult; persistent and recurrent infestations are common. All infected and exposed reptiles, as well as the environment, should be included in the treatment regimen. Ivermectin (0.2 mg/kg IM, SQ, PO every 2 weeks; and topically, 0.5 ml of 10% solution/quart water for 10 days) has been recommended (Hellebuyck *et al.*, 2012). Carbaryl powder (5%) can be applied topically and should be rinsed off after 1 h. This should be repeated in 7 days. Other treatments include 0.03% pyrethrin spray, repeated in 14 days; 0.29% fipronils, repeated in 7 days. Organophosphate products (e.g., Vapona strip) for treatment of the environment should be used with caution due to potential toxic side effects. Treatment should not exceed 4 days. Ticks can be found on wild and captive reptiles and are best treated by manual removal.

Control Reptiles found to be positive for mites or ticks should be isolated and treated promptly. Animals should be maintained in quarantine for an additional 2–4 weeks past the time mites are last detected (Fitzgerald and Vera, 2006a). Room, cages that housed infested animals, and cage accessories should be thoroughly cleaned with hot water (>50°C or 122°F), 3% bleach, quaternary ammonia, or Roccal D. Cages should be allowed a minimum of 24 h to dry.

Prevention New animals should be quarantined for at least 3 months. During this time, the animals should be tested for the presence of the parasites and, if found to be positive, treated promptly. Since mites at certain developmental stage prefer to be in the environment (e.g., enclosure), the enclosure and the surrounding environment should be treated. Routine inspection of the animal, enclosures, and room for parasites should also be performed.

Research Complication Treatment of mite and tick infestation can be time consuming and costly. Loss of animals in heavily infected cases can limit research productivity.

4. Fungal

Etiology Both yeast and filamentous fungi have been incriminated in cutaneous and systemic diseases in many reptile species. While these fungal organisms have been isolated from clinical cases in reptiles, the majority of them, including *Aspergillus* spp., *Penicillium* spp., *Fusarium* spp., *Mucor* spp., *Trichosporon* spp., *Geotrichium* spp., *Nannizziopsis* spp., and *Candida* spp., can be found in the gastrointestinal tract, lung, and/or skin of healthy reptiles, indicating that many fungi likely act as opportunistic pathogens. Nevertheless, Koch's postulates were fulfilled with the Chrysosporium anamorph of *Nannizziopsis vriesii* (CANV), when dermatomycosis was induced in veiled chameleons (*Chamaeleo calyptratus*) experimentally inoculated with this organism. Therefore, certain fungal organisms, such as CANV, can act as primary pathogens. Of the numerous fungal species, those belonging to the genera *Aspergillus*, *Trichosporon*, *Geotichum*, and CANV have been repeatedly and reliably shown to induce diseases in reptiles. Numerous case reports on CANV infection have been described in different species of snakes, lizards, and turtles. *Chamaeleomyces granulomatis* has also been shown to induce disease in chameleon (Schmidt *et al.*, 2012). *Ophidiomyces ophiodiicola* is associated with fatal skin disease in captive and wild snakes, including timber rattlesnakes (Sigler *et al.*, 2013).

Epizootiology and Transmission Fungal organisms can be found ubiquitously in the environment, including water and soil, and as a normal flora on animal skin and organs. Fungal infections are often associated with suboptimal husbandry, including overcrowding, high humidity and temperature, poor hygiene, and other captivity-related stressors. Prolonged antimicrobial therapy may also predispose reptiles to fungal infection.

Pathogenesis Fungus invades through the epidermis and dermis and can spread locally or systemically.

Clinical Signs Mycotic dermatitis often manifests as skin lesions, characterized by hyperkeratosis, necrosis, or loss of pigmentation of the scales. In chelonians, lesions commonly occur on the shell and less often on the feet and skin. These lesions are characterized by coalescing, raised, grayish or yellowish to tan papules and plaques. Fatal cases have also been reported in turtle hatchlings and eggs. Systemic mycosis can be focal or disseminated and carries a graver prognosis than dermatomycosis. Clinical signs can range from subclinical infections to animals that are found dead unexpectedly. Pneumonia and disseminated granulomatous lesions are the most common manifestation of systemic mycosis in reptiles. The hallmark of CANV is keratinolytic activity, often seen as focal skin lesions characterized by crust formation, color change, and necrosis.

Necropsy Findings Snakes with cutaneous mycosis often develop single or multifocal, fluctuant to firm, caseous to granulomatous, subcutaneous nodules, a phenomenon that is less often observed in lizards. The cutaneous lesions may be indistinguishable from chronic bacterial abscesses or from tumors grossly. If left untreated, cutaneous lesions can progress to systemic disease.

Differential Diagnosis A positive fungal culture result provides support for fungi as a primary pathogen. Hypovitaminosis A and bacterial infection can also lead to similar clinical signs. Primary viral disease with subsequent immunosuppression should also be ruled out.

Treatment Supportive care, such as fluid therapy, as well as thermal and nutritional support, should be provided. Antibiotics should be given if concurrent bacterial infection is suspected. Vitamin A supplementation is recommended for turtles. Surgical excision of affected areas of skin can be performed as well as application of systemic and topical antifungal medications (Williams *et al.*, 2012). For aquatic species, such as turtles, medication may be mixed in a tub of water. Chlorhexidine-based solutions may be used for oral candidiasis. *In vitro* testing of filamentous fungi for drug susceptibility may be useful in selecting the right antifungal treatment. Voriconazole has extended activity against various molds, compared to other azoles. In one study, voriconazole (10 mg/kg q 24 h) was shown to be safe and effective in treating CANV infection in certain species of reptiles (Van Waeyenberghe *et al.*, 2010; Hellebuyck *et al.*, 2012). Fungal infections can also be treated with ketoconazole (15–30 mg/kg PO SID for 2–4 weeks), itraconazole (10 mg/kg PO SID for 4 weeks), nystatin for enteral fungal infections in tortoises (100,000 U/kg PO SID for 14 days), and malachite green (0.15 mg/l water, 1 h treatment for 14 days).

Control Since fungal disease in reptiles is often associated with underlying immunosuppression commonly caused by stress, critical assessment of captive conditions should be made and inadequacies corrected.

Prevention Good husbandry and hygiene practices should reduce fungal load in the environment and promote health and resistance to infection.

Research Complication Fungal infection can be associated with high morbidity and mortality. Massive loss of animals can be detrimental to any research.

B. Metabolic/Nutritional Diseases

1. Metabolic Bone Disease

MBD, often seen in herbivorous lizards and chelonians, is associated with a dietary deficiency of calicum and vitamin D, a negative calcium–phosphorus ratio in the diet, or a lack of exposure to ultraviolet UVB radiation (Barten, 1993; Boyer, 1996a). Metabolic bone disease is commonly seen in juvenile reptiles, but adult

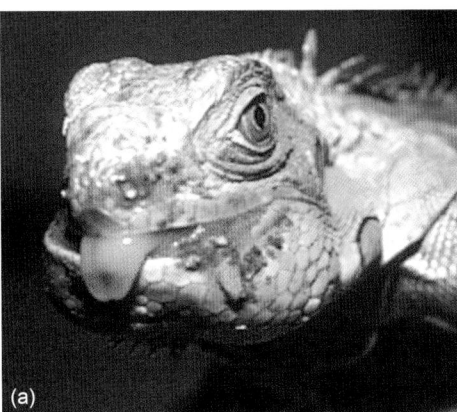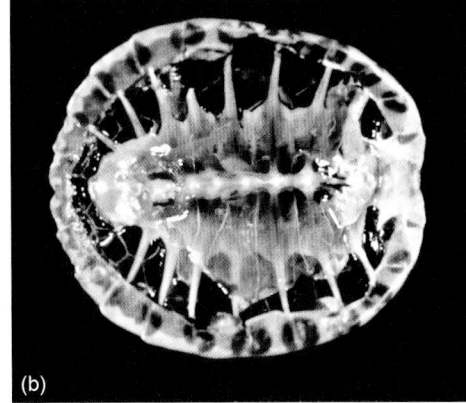

FIGURE 19.16   Cranial and facial deformities due to metabolic bone disease is common in young iguanas and other lizards due to calcium and vitamin D deficiency coupled with lack of exposure to ultraviolet B radiation (a). In turtles, these deficiencies manifest as bony abnormalities of the shell (b).

reptiles, particularly reproductively active females, can also develop the disease. In lizards, clinical signs include pliable mandibles, rounded skull, pathologic fractures (especially the humerus and femur), reluctance to move, and fibrous osteodystrophy of the long bones (Fig. 19.16a). In advanced cases, paresis, muscle tremors, and seizures may be present and carry a poor prognosis. Shell abnormalities are the most prominent clinical feature in chelonians (Fig. 19.16b). Radiographs are useful to determine the grade of MBD. Plasma concentration of 25-hydroxyvitamin D3 can be used to evaluate the level of vitamin D in the animal and thus assist in diagnosis. Treatment consists of dietary improvements, including administration of calcium-rich diets with a balanced calcium–phosphorus ratio, access to UVB radiation (natural sunlight is best), calcium and vitamin D supplementation, and supportive care. A successful treatment regimen has been reported (initial treatment: 400 IU/kg, IM, vitamin D₃, and 23 mg/kg calcium glubionate, PO, BID; a week later: 2nd dose of vitamin D₃ [400 IU/kg, IM] and calcium glubionate, calcitonin [50 IU/kg, IM]; 2 weeks later: a second dose of calcitonin [50 IU/kg IM]) (Mader, 2006a). Fractures of the long bones should be managed conservatively, including splinting and cage rest. The prognosis for MBD is good, especially in juvenile animals, if the disease is diagnosed and treated early. In general, the more advanced the disease, the poorer the prognosis for recovery. To prevent the occurrence of this disease, proper nutrition and exposure to sunlight or UVB light should be provided.

2. Hypovitaminosis A

Vitamin deficiency commonly arises in reptiles fed an unbalanced diet lacking adequate levels of vitamin A.

This condition is most commonly seen in chelonians, especially box turtles (Boyer, 1996b). Tortoises are generally not affected. Theoretically, any reptile is susceptible and this condition has also been observed in farm-raised crocodiles and captive green anoles (Miller *et al.*, 2001). Hyperkeratosis and squamous metaplasia of the respiratory, ocular, and gastrointestinal epithelia are most evident. The most prominent clinical signs are those involving the ocular system and upper respiratory tract, including cellular debris beneath the eyelids, and nasal and ocular discharges. Additional signs include anorexia, weight loss, and lethargy. Middle ear infections and egg retention are also common in box turtles. Kidney failure and fatty degeneration have also been noted in some species of reptiles. Diagnosis is made by evaluation of the diet, cytology of ocular discharge, or assay for serum or liver vitamin A concentrations. Normal liver vitamin A level has been reported to be >1000 IU/g in monitors and snakes. Retinol concentration can also be used for an assessment of vitamin A. Mean plasma retinol in tortoises ranges from 0.09–0.77 µg/ml (Raphael *et al.*, 1994). Treatment includes vitamin A injections (500–5000 IU/kg, SC, one or two treatments every 14 days), debridement of cellular debris from the eyes, treatment of secondary bacterial infections, and correction of dietary vitamin A deficiency. Nephrotoxic drugs should be avoided due to potential renal failure. Food rich in carotenes, especially the betacarotenes, consisting of dark leafy greens and yellow-colored or orange colored vegetables or fruits should be provided on a regular basis. Liver in whole mice or fish provides a good source of vitamin A for aquatic species. Commercial reptile diets are also available and are good sources of vitamin A.

3. Gout

Both articular gout and visceral gout are seen commonly and are associated with considerable morbidity and mortality in captive reptiles (Mader, 2006b; Mendyk et al., 2013). In most reptiles, uric acid is the end product of purine degradation. Uric acid and urate salts are insoluble in water and are cleared from the blood through renal tubules. In cases of hyperurecemia, uric acid forms insoluble crystals that are deposited in various organs. Gout may be primary, caused by an overproduction of uric acid, or secondary, due to conditions that affect normal balance between production and excretion of uric acid (e.g., chronic renal disease, hypertension, starvation, or use of diuretics and antibiotic, such as gentamycin, that interfere with normal kidney function). In reptiles, urate crystal deposits can be found in many organs, of which pericardial sac, kidney, liver, spleen, lungs, subcutaneous tissue, and other areas of soft tissues are the most common sites (Mader, 2006b). Diagnosis is based on history and clinical examination. In reptiles, blood urea nitrogen and creatinine often have little diagnostic value and laboratory samplings may or may not show hyperuricemia. Treatment of gout in reptiles follows the same principles as treatment of gout in humans. Drugs that lower serum uric acid levels (e.g., allopurinol) and promote urate excretion (e.g., probenecid) should be administered. The following treatments have been suggested to be effective in reptiles: allopurinol: 9.93 mg/kg q 24 h PO for 30 days followed by 3.31 mg/g PO for additional 90 days; allopurinol: 20 mg/kg q 24 h PO for 90 days, at 21 days into therapy, probenecid is added (250 mg q 12 h for 45 days) (Mader, 2006b). Anti-inflammatory drugs, such as corticosteroids, are indicated for management of arthritis. Treatment should also include dietary changes, improvement of environmental conditions, administration of antimicrobials, and adequate hydration. The prognosis for reptiles with severe gout is very poor, and treatment should include proper analgesic management of the reptile. Mild cases of gout can be managed long-term and reptile patients often do fine with the treatment.

4. Cloacal Prolapse

Prolapse of the cloaca is commonly seen in captive reptiles and is often associated with improper husbandry or infectious processes. There is always an underlying cause (e.g., bacterial enteritis, dystocia) for the prolapse, and successful treatment has to include correction of these conditions. If a reptile presents with a cloacal prolapse, it is most important to determine which organ has prolapsed: reproductive tract, colon, or urinary bladder. Once the tissue has been identified, it is necessary to evaluate the extent of tissue damage. Exposed tissue should be cleaned with antiseptic solution and lubricated to prevent drying. Necrotic tissue should be removed surgically. While some prolapses can be reduced manually, often a purse-string or transverse suture may be placed to prevent recurrence.

5. Dystocia

Dystocias are commonly diagnosed in captive reptiles. The dystocia etiology is multifactorial and may involve poor husbandry, improper nesting site and temperature, malnutrition, and dehydration (DeNardo, 2006). Infectious agents have also been found to cause dystocia. One has to differentiate between obstructive and nonobstructive dystocias. Obstructive dystocias result from oversized eggs or fetuses, or the inability of the female to pass the eggs because of anatomical abnormalities, infectious causes, or metabolic compromise. Nonobstructive dystocias are commonly seen in chelonians and lizards, especially green iguanas, and are characterized by the inability to pass normal-appearing eggs through a normal-appearing reproductive tract. In green iguanas and several other species of lizards, egg yolk coelomitis has also been reported.

A diagnosis of dystocia is sometimes difficult to make. Recent oviposition and presence of additional eggs within the reproductive tract are suggestive of dystocia in snakes. In lizards, behavioral changes help determine if the animal is truly egg bound. Gravid lizards (especially green iguanas) will normally not eat for up to 1 month. During this time, the animals remain alert and active. The presence of digging behavior followed by lethargy and weakness is an indicator of dystocia. Care should be taken to identify this crucial period since some lizards will start eating again, only to become ill within a short period of time. In chelonians, lack of a suitable nesting site and proper substrate may induce dystocia. Radiographs and ultrasonography are helpful to identify any egg abnormalities as well as to determine the stage of follicular development.

Once a diagnosis of dystocia is made, supportive care (including administration of fluids and calcium injections) is beneficial. Treatment to remove the retained eggs should be provided within 48 h after diagnosis. Hormonal stimulation may be successful in some species and a complete failure in others. Oxytocin (5–30 IU/kg, IM, or intracoelomically) or arginine vasotocin (0.01–1 μg/kg, IV, or intracoelomically) may be given. Since the action of oxytocin is potentiated by higher temperature, animals should be kept at or near their optimal temperature (DeNardo, 2006). Manual extraction may be attempted, but this procedure is oftentimes associated with deleterious outcome. If hormonal stimulation and manual extraction fail to produce oviposition, ovocentesis may be attempted. A sterile large-gauge needle is inserted into the egg, the content aspirated, and the egg subsequently passed. In cases where the egg is visible through the cloaca, the collapsed egg may be removed with forceps. This is easier to perform on soft-shelled eggs, while hard-shelled eggs must be handled carefully to avoid cuts and rupture of the oviduct by pieces of the shell. In some cases, general anesthesia and consequently better muscle relaxation of the reptile may help in manipulation and removal of the eggs.

If the above procedures fail, surgery is indicated. In snakes, multiple incisions may be necessary to facilitate removal of eggs. In lizards, a single paramedian incision is made to facilitate either salpingectomy or in cases where future breeding is not attempted, ovariosalpingectomy. In chelonians, an approach through the plastron or the inguinal region will facilitate removal of retained eggs.

The prognosis for recovery and future breeding depends on the condition of the reproductive tract at the time surgery is performed. Correction of improper environmental conditions will help future breeding attempts, but in general, reptiles diagnosed with dystocia have an increased likelihood of developing similar problems in the future.

6. Dehydration

Dehydration in reptiles is often the result of improper husbandry (low humidity, lack of water, and/or anorexia). Clinically, the skin may be wrinkled, the eyes may be sunken into the orbit, and mucous membranes may be dry. A definitive diagnosis of the degree of dehydration can be made only by collection of a venous blood sample and laboratory determinations, including plasma osmolality, PCV, total protein, and electrolyte concentrations. Fluid therapy should be initiated only with proof of volume depletion. In mild cases, soaking the animal in warm water may promote fluid intake. Oral administration of fluids is indicated in cases of mild dehydration. In cases of severe dehydration, the most effective way to administer fluids rapidly is through the intravenous and intraosseous routes. Intracoelomic fluid administration is an alternative route of fluid administration in cases of moderate dehydration. If low humidity is suspected, several different techniques, including using live plants, aerating water within the enclosure with an aquarium pump and air stones, or spraying the environment with water several times per day, can be used to increase the humidity. In general, the following range of humidity should be provided: desert species (25–50%); subtropical species (60–90%); tropical species (70–95%) (Mitchell, 2006).

7. Dysecdysis

Snakes shed their skins in one piece, while most lizards and chelonians shed in several pieces. Dysecdysis may be a result of improper husbandry, such as inadequate temperatures and humidity (low temperature and too dry or too moist environment), improper nutrition, and stress in the form of overcrowding, unsanitary cage, and improper photoperiods (Fitzgerald and Vera, 2006b)

(Fig. 19.9). Shedding problems may also be caused by heavy infestation with ectoparasites and bacterial and/or fungal dermatitis. The latter may also develop as a result of untreated shedding problems. Treatment consists of improving environmental conditions and removal of retained pieces of skin, especially retained eye caps. The animal should be soaked in warm water and loose skin carefully removed. Retained eye caps should also be removed carefully so as not to accidently remove the entire spectacle. The eye should be moistened with eyewash solutions and eye ointment. The eye cap should come off easily when gently pulled with blunt forceps. If in doubt, and the eye looks uninfected, one can also wait for the next shedding cycle, at which time the retained spectacle will often come off. In cases of bacterial or fungal dermatitis, systemic administration of antimicrobials or antifungal agents should be initiated. Cultures and sensitivity testing should be performed to assure appropriate drug selection. Scrapings of the skin or full-thickness skin biopsies can be submitted for microbiologic and histologic evaluation. Topical administration of antimicrobial ointments should accompany systemic antimicrobial treatment.

C. Traumatic Disorders

1. Bite Wounds

Bite wounds are most commonly inflicted by incompatible cagemates or prey animals. Care should be taken to become familiar with the social structure of the species of reptile kept in captivity. While immature reptiles can often be kept in a large community enclosure, adult, sexually mature animals will often display aggression to animals of the same sex. For example, juvenile iguanas can be kept together, whereas it is impossible to keep adult male iguanas together in one cage. Serious fights and injury may result. Females will often tolerate each other as long as there is enough space for each animal to establish its own territory. The same is true for most chelonians. Snakes may inflict serious bites to each other when not separated prior to feeding. Care should be taken not to house carnivorous reptiles of different sizes together, as cannibalism may occur. Prey animals should not be fed alive since they may inflict serious bite injuries to a snake or lizard. Rats in particular can cause significant trauma if left unattended with a snake that refuses to eat (Fig. 19.17). All bite wounds should be considered contaminated and appropriate treatment initiated. This will include sterile saline flushes and debridement of necrotic tissue. Bite wounds are best managed as an open wound and allowed to heal by granulation. Initially, wet to dry bandages are applied and changed daily until there is healthy granulation tissue present. Wound dressings and topical antibiotic ointments (e.g.,

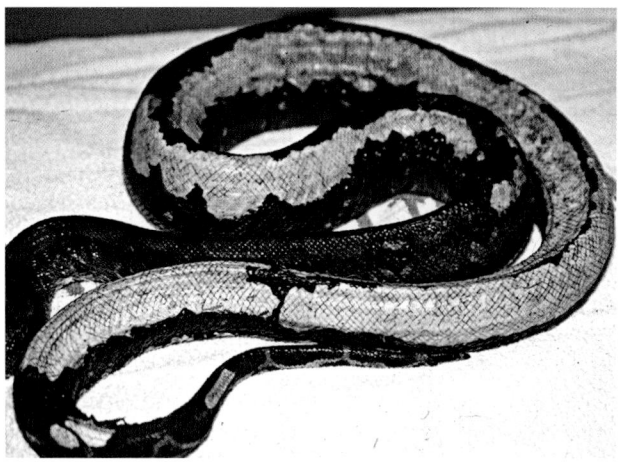

FIGURE 19.17   Live prey species such as rats can inflict fatal bite wounds to reptiles.

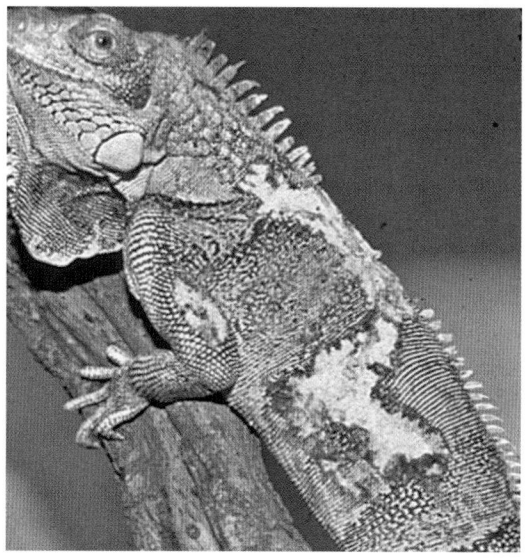

FIGURE 19.18   Iguana with scars from thermal burns caused by contact with a heat source.

Silvadene cream) should be applied to promote healing and prevent infection. In most cases, systemic administration of a broad-spectrum antibiotic (e.g., enrofloxacin) is recommended. During the healing process, which may take several months, particular attention should be paid to a clean environment for the animal.

2. Shell Fractures

Shell fractures in chelonians may result from improper handling. Radiographs should be taken in order to evaluate the extent of the fracture. Loose fragments of shell may be removed or may be incorporated into the shell repair if there is vascular supply. In general, the standard principles of wound management apply to shell fractures. Wounds should be cleaned with sterile saline and evaluated carefully to see if they penetrate into the coelomic cavity. While soft tissue injuries and the shell fracture should be managed as an open wound, it will greatly facilitate the healing process if the shell fragments can be stabilized with the use of wires. Holes can be drilled into the shell with a Dremel tool, and wires can be placed to reduce the fracture fragments. If at all possible, the wound should be treated as an open wound, including wet to dry bandages, followed by topical application of antimicrobial ointments. Epoxy and fiberglass materials should be used only if one is absolutely certain that there is no infection or contamination present and healthy granulation tissue is present. If not treated appropriately with broad-spectrum antimicrobials (e.g., enrofloxacin, amikacin, ceftazidime) prior to shell repair, abscess formation, septicemia, and death of the animal may result. A compromise is the use of epoxy and fiberglass materials in aquatic turtles, where it is necessary to place the animal back into its aquatic environment as soon as possible to prevent electrolyte imbalances.

3. Burns

Burns are often caused by improper functioning of heating devices such as hot rocks or inappropriately placed heating lamps (Fig. 19.18), as well as overexposure to sunlight particularly with nocturnal or albinistic individuals (Mass, 2013). In all cases, care should be taken to prevent the animal from direct contact with the heating device or over exposure to the sun. Heating tapes and lamps installed outside the enclosure or providing a thermal gradient in the enclosure (e.g., placing a heat lamp on one side of the cage and providing a shady area on the other side of the cage) are the safest solutions. In many cases, the burned area will become edematous, tissue will become necrotic, and secondary infections may develop. Proper wound care, including debridement of necrotic tissue, wet to dry bandages, and application of topical wound dressings, is essential for wound healing. Administration of systemic antimicrobials is also indicated in most cases to prevent secondary bacterial infections. In severe burn wounds that can lead to significant loss of fluids and electrolytes, supportive care, including fluid therapy should be initiated. Nutritional support should be implemented for animals that are inappetent.

4. Tail Injuries

Fractures of the tail are commonly seen with improper handling of some lizard species, such as green iguanas (Barten, 1993). A tail may break off if it hits a sharp object or if the animal is inappropriately restrained by holding its tail (Fig. 19.19). While some fractures may be splinted, loss of a segment of the tail should be treated conservatively. In species with tail autotomy, the wound should

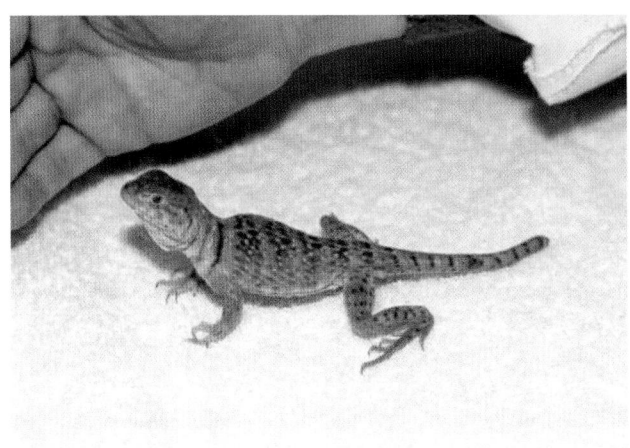

FIGURE 19.19 Tail fractures in lizards are commonly caused by inappropriate handling.

be treated as an open wound and never be sutured, so that the tail may regenerate. The treatment indicated in most cases is cleaning the wound with sterile saline, applying a topical antiseptic ointment, and providing a clean cage environment. In cases where the tail has to be amputated due to an infectious etiology (e.g., bacterial or fungal dermatitis, abscess formation) or neoplasia, systemic antimicrobial treatment is warranted.

D. Toxins

Toxins are often associated with improper use of pesticides (such as organophosphates) in the treatment of external parasites or with toxins on plant material fed to herbivorous reptiles. Some plants are toxic to reptiles, and one should consult with a knowledgeable source before feeding unknown plants. Improper use of drugs (e.g., metronidazole, ivermectin, gentamicin) has also been associated with toxicities. Clinical signs of affected reptiles may be nonspecific, such as lethargy and weakness, or may include tremors, convulsions, and seizures. Treatment consists of identification of the toxin or drugs; appropriate administration of an antidote, if available, and cessation of exposure; supportive care (administration of fluids, antiseizure drugs such as diazepam, and, if indicated, systemic antimicrobials to prevent secondary bacterial infections); and nutritional support.

E. Neoplastic Diseases

Neoplastic diseases are commonly seen in all orders of reptiles, especially chelonians, snakes, and lizards (Jacobson, 1981; Done, 1996). Most neoplastic diseases of domestic animals have also been reported in reptiles. Excellent reviews of neoplastic diseases in reptiles have been published (Hernandez-Divers and Garner, 2003; Garner et al., 2004; Sykes and Trupkiewicz, 2006)

and the reader is referred to these for more detailed descriptions of specific neoplasms. The etiology for most reptilian neoplasia is unknown, but viruses and environmental factors have been associated with development of tumors in reptiles. A diagnosis of neoplasia is always based on histopathologic or cytologic evaluation of suspected tissue. When performing a physical examination, care should be taken not to falsely misdiagnose a mass as a tumor. Granulomas, foreign bodies, or cysts may be falsely identified as tumors unless the examiner performs more diagnostic tests, such as radiography, ultrasonography, aspirates, and/or biopsies, which are submitted for cytologic and histopathologic evaluation.

In chelonians, tumors of the integumentary system include fibropapillomas and fibromas. Carcinomas of the gastrointestinal system and adenomas of the endocrine system have also been reported. In lizards, most commonly squamous cell carcinomas, fibrosarcomas, and lymphosarcomas have been reported. In snakes, lymphosarcomas and adenocarcinomas of the kidneys and gastrointestinal tract, as well as fibrosarcomas of the integumentary system, have been described.

Although some reports describing chemotherapy, radiation therapy, and photodynamic surgery in the treatment of reptile neoplasms have been published, none of these have proven to be successful. At present, standard surgical removal of the neoplasm, possibly combined with chemotherapy or radiation therapy, as well as supportive care, is the recommended treatment.

References

Abbas, M.D., Marschang, R.E., Schmidt, V., Kasper, A., Papp, T., 2011. A unique novel reptilian paramyxovirus, four atadenovirus types and a reovirus identified in a concurrent infection of a corn snake (*Pantherophis guttatus*) collection in Germany. Vet. Microbiol. 150, 70–79.

Ackermann, M., Koriabine, M., Hartmann-Fritsch, F., de Jong, P.J., Lewis, T.D., Schetle, N., et al., 2012. The genome of Chelonid herpesvirus 5 harbors atypical genes. PLoS One 7, e46623.

Afonso, C.L., Tulman, E.R., Delhon, G., Lu, Z., Viljoen, G.J., Wallace, D.B., et al., 2006. Genome of crocodilepox virus. J. Virol. 80, 4978–4991.

Alibardi, L., 2013. Immunolocalization of keratin-associated beta-proteins (beta-keratins) in pad lamellae of geckos suggest that glycine-cysteine-rich proteins contribute to their flexibility and adhesiveness. J. Exp. Zool. A Ecol. Genet. Physiol. 319, 166–178.

Allen, M.E., 1997. From blackbirds and thrushes to the gut-loaded cricket: a new approach to zoo animal nutrition. Br. J. Nutr. 78, S135–S143.

Almli, L.M., Burghardt, G.M., 2006. Environmental enrichment alters the behavioral profile of ratsnakes (Elaphe). J. Appl. Anim. Welf. Sci. 9, 85–109.

Anantaphruti, M.T., Nawa, Y., Vanvanitchai, Y., 2011. Human sparganosis in Thailand: an overview. Acta Trop. 118, 171–176.

Anderson, N.L., 1991. Husbandry and clinical evaluation of *Iguana iguana*. Compend. Contin. Educ. Pract. Vet. 13, 1265–1272.

Anonymous, 1992. Lizard-associated salmonellosis–Utah. Morb. Mortal. Wkly. Rep. 41, 610–611.

Anonymous, 1995. Reptile-associated salmonellosis-selected states, 1994–1995. Morb. Mortal. Wkly. Rep. 44, 347–350.

Ariel, E., 2011. Viruses in reptiles. Vet. Res. 42, 100.

Ascher, J.M., Geneva, A.J., Ng, J., Wyatt, J.D., Glor, R.E., 2013. Phylogenetic analyses of novel squamate adenovirus sequences in wild-caught *Anolis* lizards. PLoS One 8, e60977.

Austin, C.C., Wilkins, M.J., 1998. Reptile-associated salmonellosis. J. Am. Vet. Med. Assoc. 212, 866–867.

Axelsson, M., Franklin, C.E., Lofman, C.O., Nilsson, S., Grigg, G.C., 1996. Dynamic anatomical study of cardiac shunting in crocodiles using high-resolution angioscopy. J. Exp. Biol. 199, 359–365.

Axelsson, M., Fritsche, R., Holmgren, S., Grove, D.J., Nilsson, S., 1991. Gut blood flow in the estuarine crocodile, *Crocodylus porosus*. Acta Physiol. Scand. 142, 509–516.

Ayinmode, A., Adedokun, A., Aina, A., Taiwo, V., 2010. The zoonotic implications of pentastomiasis in the royal python (*python regius*). Ghana Med. J. 44, 115–118.

Barboza, P.S., 1995. Digesta passage and functional anatomy of the digestive tract in the desert tortoise (Xerobates agassizii). J. Comp. Physiol. B 165, 193–202.

Barten, S.L., 1993. The medical care of iguanas and other common pet lizards. In: Quesenberry, K.E., Hillyer, E.V. (Eds.), The Veterinary Clinics of North America, Small Animal Practice, Exotic Pet Medicine I. Saunders, Philadelphia, PA, pp. 1213–1249.

Barten, S.L., 1996a. Thermal burns. In: Mader, D.R. (Ed.), Reptile Medicine and Surgery. Saunders, Philadelphia, PA, pp. 419–421.

Barten, S.L., 1996b. Lizards. In: Mader, D.R. (Ed.), Reptile Medicine and Surgery. Saunders, Philadelphia, PA, pp. 47–61.

Barten, S.L., 2006. Lizards. In: Mader, D.R. (Ed.), Reptile Medicine and Surgery. Saunders, St. Louis, MO, pp. 59–77.

Barten, S.L., Fleming, G.J., 2014. Current herpetologic husbandry and products. In: Mader, D.R., Divers, S.J. (Eds.), Current Therapy in Reptile Medicine and Surgery. Saunders, St. Louis, MO, pp. 2–12.

Beaupre, S.J., Jacobson, E.R., Lillywhite, H.B., Zamudio, K., 2004. Guideline for use of Live and Reptiles in Field and Laboratory Research, second ed. American Society of Ichtyologists., revised by the Herpetological Animal Care and Use Committee.

Behncke, H., Stöhr, A.C., Heckers, K.O., Ball, I., Marschang, R.E., 2013. Mass-mortality in green striped tree dragons (*Japalura splendida*) associated with multiple viral infections. Vet. Rec. 173, 248.

Bennett, R.A., 1991. A review of anesthesia and chemical restraint in reptiles. J. Zoo Wildl. Med. 22, 282.

Bennett, R.A., 1996. Anesthesia. In: Mader, D.R. (Ed.), Reptile Medicine and Surgery. Saunders, Philadelphia, PA, pp. 241–247.

Benson, K.G., Forrest, L., 1999. Characterization of the renal portal system of the common green iguana (*Iguana iguana*) by digital subtraction imaging. J. Zoo Wildl. Med. 30, 235–241.

Beresford, W.A., 1993. Fibrous trabeculae in the liver of the alligator (*Alligator mississippiensis*). Ann. Anat. 175, 357–359.

Besson, A.A., Cree, A., 2010. A cold-adpated reptile becomes a more effective thermoregulator in a thermally challenging environment. Oecologia 163, 571–581.

Blaylock, R.S., 2001. Normal oral bacterial flora from some southern African snakes. Onderstepoort J. Vet. Res. 68, 175–182.

Bloch, N., Irschick, D.J., 2005. Toe-clipping dramatically reduces clinging performance in a pad-bearing lizard (*Anolis carolinensis*). J. Herp. 39, 288–293.

Bolette, D.P., 1997a. First record of *Pachysentis canicola* (Acanthocephal a:Oligacanthorhynchida) and the occurrence of Mesocestoides sp. tetrathyridia (Cestoidea:Cyclophyllidea) in the western diamond-back rattlesnake, *Crotalus atrox* (Serpentes:Viperidae). J. Parasitol. 83, 751–752.

Bolette, D.P., 1997b. *Sphaerechinorhynchus ophiograndis* n. sp. (Acanth ocephala:Plagiorhynchidae:Sphaerechinorhynchinae), described from the intestine of a king cobra, *Ophiophagus hannah*. J. Parasitol. 83, 272–275.

Bonnet, X., Fizesan, A., Michel, C.L., 2013. Shelter availability, stress level and digestive performance in the aspic viper. J. Exp. Biol. 216, 815–822.

Borges-Landaez, P.A., Shine, R., 2003. Influence of toe-clipping on running speed in *Eulamprus quoyii*, an Australian Scincid Lizard. J. Herp. 37, 592–595.

Boyer, T.H., 1991. Green iguana care. Am. Assoc. Reptil. Vet. 1, 12–14.

Boyer, T.H., 1996a. Metabolic bone disease. In: Mader, D.R. (Ed.), Reptile Medicine and Surgery. Saunders, Philadelphia, PA, pp. 385–392.

Boyer, T.H., 1996b. Hypovitaminosis A and hypervitaminosis A. In: Mader, D.R. (Ed.), Reptile Medicine and Surgery. Saunders, Philadelphia, PA, pp. 382–385.

Boyer, T.H., Boyer, D.M., 1992. Aquatic turtle care. Bull. Assoc. Reptil. Amphib. Vet. 2, 13–17.

Boyer, T.H., Boyer, D.M., 2006. Turtle, tortoises and terrapin. In: Mader, D.R. (Ed.), Reptile Medicine and Surgery. Saunders, St. Louis, pp. 78–99.

Bradford, C.M., Denver, M.C., Cranfield, M.R., 2008. Development of a polymerase chain reaction test for *Entamoeba invadens*. J. Zoo Wildl. Med. 39, 201–207.

Brasfield, S.M., Bradham, K., Wells, J.B., Talent, L.G., Lanno, R.P., Janz, D.M., 2004. Development of a terrestrial vertebrate model for assessing bioavailability of cadmium in the fence lizard (*Sceloporus undulatus*) and in ovo effects on hatchling size and thyroid function. Chemosphere 54, 1643–1651.

Brock, A.P., Gallagher, A.E., Walden, H.D., Owen, J.L., Dunbar, M.D., Wamsley, H.L., et al., 2012. *Kiricephalus coarctatus* in an Eastern Indigo Snake (*Drymarchon couperi*); endoscopic removal, identification, and phylogeny. Vet. Q. 32, 107–112.

Bronson, E., Cranfield, M.R., 2006. Paramyxovirus. In: Mader, D.R. (Ed.), Reptile Medicine and Surgery. Saunders, Philadelphia, PA, pp. 858–861.

Brown, D.R., Nogueira, M.F., Schoeb, T.R., Vliet, K.A., Bennett, R.A., Pye, G.W., et al., 2001. Pathology of experimental mycoplasmosis in *American alligators*. J. Wildl. Dis. 37, 671–679.

Brown, D.R., Wendland, L.D., Rotstein, D.S., 2007. Mycoplasmosis in green iguanas (*Iguana iguana*). J. Zoo Wildl. Med. 38, 348–351.

Brown, D.R., Zacher, L.A., Farmerie, W.G., 2004. Spreading factors of Mycoplasma alligatoris, a flesh-eating mycoplasma. J. Bacteriol. 186, 3922–3927.

Bryan, L.K., Baldwin, C.A., Gray, M.J., Miller, D.L., 2009. Efficacy of select disinfectants at inactivating Ranavirus. Dis. Aquat. Organ. 84, 89–94.

Burger, R.M., Gehrmann, W.H., Ferguson, G.W., 2007. Evaluation of UVB reduction by materials commonly used in reptile husbandry. Zoo Biol. 26, 417–423.

Burghardt, G.M., Layne, D.G., 1995. Effects of ontogenetic processes and rearing conditions. In: Warwick, C., Frye, F.L., Murphy, J.B. (Eds.), Health and Welfare of Captive Reptiles Chapman & Hall, London, pp. 165–185.

Bursey, C.R., Goldberg, S.R., 2003. *Acanthocephalus saurius* n. sp. (Acanthocephala: Echinorhynchidae) and other helminths from the lizard *Norops limifrons* (Sauria: Polychrotidae) from Costa Rica. J. Parasitol. 89, 573–576.

Campbell, T.W., 2014. Clinical pathology. In: Maders, D.R., Divers, S.J. (Eds.), Current Therapy in Reptile Medicine and Surgery. Saunders, St. Louis, MO, pp. 70–92.

Carpenter, J.W., Klaphake, E., Gibbons, P.M., 2014. Reptile formulary and laboratory normals. In: Mader, D.R., Divers, S.J. (Eds.), Current Therapy in Reptile Medicine and Surgery. Saunders, St. Louis, MO, pp. 382–410.

Case, B.C., Lewbart, G.A., Doerr, P., 2004. The physiological and behavioral impacts of and preference for an enriched environment in the eastern box turtle (*Terrapene Carolina carolina*). Appl. Anim. Behav. Sci. 92, 353–365.

Castoe, T.A., de Koning, A.P., Hall, K.T., et al., 2013. The Burmese python genome reveals the molecular basis for extreme adaptation in snakes. Proc. Natl. Acad. Sci. 110, 20645–20650.

Chang, L.W., Fu, A., Wozniak, E., Chow, M., Duke, D.G., Green, L., et al., 2013. Immunohistochemical detection of a unique protein within cells of snakes having inclusion body disease, a world-wide disease seen in members of the families Boidae and Pythonidae. PLoS One 10, e82916.

Chen, Q., Deng, H., Brauth, S.E., Ding, L., Tang, Y., 2012. Reduced performance of prey targeting in pit vipers with contralaterally occluded infrared and visual senses. PLoS One 7, e34989.

Chia, M.Y., Jeng, C.R., Hsiao, S.H., Lee, A.H., Chen, C.Y., Pang, V.F., 2009. *Entamoeba invadens* myositis in a common water monitor lizard (*Varanus salvator*). Vet. Pathol. 46, 673–676.

Chiodini, R.J., Sundberg, J.P., 1981. Salmonellosis in reptiles: a review. Am. J. Epidemiol. 113, 494–498.

Chiszar, D., Wellborn, S., Wand, M.A., Scudder, K.M., Smith, H., 1980. Investigatory behaviour in snakes II: cage cleaning and the induction of defaecation in snakes. Anim. Learn. Behav. 8, 505–510.

Christensen, C.B., Christensen-Dalsgaard, J., Brandt, C., Madsen, P.T., 2012. Hearing with an atympanic ear: good vibration and poor sound-pressure detection in the royal python, *Python regius*. J. Exp. Biol. 215, 331–342.

Christiansen, J.L., Grzybowski, J.M., Kodama, R.M., 1996. Melano-macrophage aggregations and their age relationships in the yellow mud turtle, *Kinosternon flavescens* (Kinosternidae). Pigment Cell. Res. 9, 185–190.

Conant, R., 1971. Reptile and amphibian management practices at Philadelphia Zoo. Int. Zoo Yearbook 11, 224–230.

Connelly, L., Craig, B.H., Jones, B., Alexander, C., 2013. Genetic diversity of *Cryptosporidium* spp. within a remote population of Soay Sheep on St. Kilda Islands, Scotland. Appl. Environ. Microbiol. 79, 2240–2246.

Conroy, C.J., Papenfuss, T., Parker, J., Hahn, N.E., 2009. Use of tricaine methanesulfonate (MS222) for euthanasia of reptiles. J. Am. Assoc. Lab. Anim. Sci. 48, 28–32.

Cooper, J.E., 2006. Dermatology. In: Mader, D.R. (Ed.), Reptile Medicine and Surgery. Saunders, Philadelphia, PA, pp. 196–216.

Corcoran, J.A., Duncan, R., 2004. Reptilian reovirus utilizes a small type III protein with an external myristylated amino terminus to mediate cell–cell fusion. J. Virol. 78, 4342–4351.

Coulson, R.A., Hernandez, T., 1983. Alligator Metabolism Studies on Chemical Reactions *In Vivo*. Pergamon Press, Oxford.

Crain, D.A., Guillette Jr., L.J., 1998. Reptiles as models of contaminant-induced endocrine disruption. Anim. Reprod. Sci. 53, 77–86.

Curry, S.S., Brown, D.R., Gaskin, J.M., Jacobson, E.R., Ehrhart, L.M., Blahak, S., et al., 2000. Persistent infectivity of a disease-associated Herpesvirus in green turtles after exposure to seawater. J. Wildl. Dis. 36, 792–797.

D'Aoust, J.-Y., Daley, E., Crozier, M., Sewell, A.M., 1990. Pet turtles: a continuing international threat to public health. Am. J. Epidemiol. 132, 233–238.

Darrow, M., Foulkes, G., Ayoub, M., 1993. Zoonotic transmission of turtle-borne *Edwardsiella tarda*. Compl. Surg. 12, 33–35.

Davies, P.M.C., 1981. Anatomy and physiology In: Cooper, J.E. Jackson, O.F. (Eds.), Diseases of the Reptilia, vol. 1 Academic Press, London.

DeNardo, D., 1996. Reproductive biology. In: Mader, D.R. (Ed.), Reptile Medicine and Surgery. Saunders, Philadelphia, PA, pp. 212–224.

DeNardo, D., 2006. Dystocias. In: Mader, D.R. (Ed.), Reptile Medicine and Surgery. Saunders, St. Louis, MO, pp. 787–792.

Dickinson, H.C., Fa, J.E., 1997. Ultraviolet light and heat source selection in captive spiny-tailed iguanas (*Oplurus cuvieri*). Zoo Biol. 16, 391–401.

Dipineto, L., Russo, T.P., Calabria, M., De Rosa, L., Capasso, M., Menna, L.F., et al., 2014. Oral flora of Python regius kept as pets. Lett. Appl. Microbiol. 58, 462–465.

Divers, S., 1996. Basic reptile husbandry, history taking, and clinical examination. In Prac. 18, 51–65.

Divers, S.J., 2014. Diagnostic Endoscopy. In: Maders, D.R., Divers, S.J. (Eds.), Current Therapy in Reptile Medicine and Surgery. Saunders, St. Louis, pp. 154–178.

Donaldson, M., Heyneman, D., Dempster, R., Garcia, L., 1975. Epizootic of fatal amebiasis among exhibited snakes: epidemiologic, pathologic, and chemotherapeutic considerations. Am. J. Vet. Res. 36, 807–817.

Done, L.B., 1996. Neoplasia. In: Mader, D.R. (Ed.), Reptile Medicine and Surgery. Saunders, Philadelphia, PA, pp. 125–141.

Donoghue, S., 2006. Nutrition. In: Mader, D.R. (Ed.), Reptile Medicine and Surgery. Saunders, St. Louis, MO, pp. 251–298.

Donoghue, S., Langenberg, J., 1996. Nutrition. In: Mader, D.R. (Ed.), Reptile Medicine and Surgery. Saunders, Philadelphia, PA, pp. 148–174.

Dupuy, M., Berne, F., Herbelin, P., Binet, M., Berthelot, N., Rodier, M.H., et al., 2014. Sensitivity of free-living amoeba trophozoites and cysts to water disinfectants. Int. J. Hyg. Environ. Health 217, 335–339.

Dyer, O., 1995. Crocodiles help to develop artificial blood. BMJ 310, 211.

Ernst, C.H., Barbour, R.W., 1989. Turtles of the World. Smithsonian Institution Press, Washington, DC.

Ferreira, R.S., Biscola, N.P., Campagner, M.V., Barraviera, B., 2010. How to raise snakes in capitivity. Vet. Microbiol. 141, 189.

Fitzgerald, K.T., Vera, R., 2006a. Acariasis. In: Mader, D.R. (Ed.), Reptile Medicine and Surgery. Saunders, Philadelphia, PA, pp. 720–738.

Fitzgerald, K.T., Vera, R., 2006b. Dysecdysis. In: Mader, D.R. (Ed.), Reptile Medicine and Surgery. Saunders, Philadelphia, PA, pp. 778–785.

Flach, E.J., Riley, J., Mutlow, A.G., McCandlish, I.A., 2000. In: Mader, D.R. (Ed.), Pentastomiasis in Bosc'Reptile Medicine and Surgery'. Saunders, Philadelphia, PA, pp. 463–465.

Foronda, P., Santana-Morales, M.A., Orós, J., Abreu-Acosta, N., Ortega-Rivas, A., Lorenzo-Morales, J., et al., 2007. Clinical efficacy of antiparasite treatments against intestinal helminths and haematic protozoa in Gallotiacaesaris (lizards). Exp. Parasitol. 116, 361–365.

Foà, A., Basaglia, F., Beltrami, G., Carnacina, M., Moretto, E., Bertolucci, C., 2009. Orientation of lizards in a Morris water-maze: roles of the sun compass and the parietal eye. J. Exp. Biol. 212, 2918–2924.

Foster, K.L., Higham, T.E., 2012. How forelimb and hindlimb function changes with incline and perch diameter in the green anole, Anoliscarolinensis. J. Exp. Biol. 215, 2288–2300.

Furman, B.L., 2011. The development of Byetta (exenatide) from the venom of the Gila monster as an anti-diabetic agent. Toxicon 59, 464–471.

Gardiner, D.W., Baines, F.M., Pandher, K., 2009. Photodermatitis and photokeratoconjunctivitis in a ball python (*Python regius*) and a blue-tongue skink (*Tiliqua* spp.). J. Zoo Wildl. Med. 40, 757–766.

Gehrmann, E.H., 1996. Evaluation of artificial lighting. In: Mader, D.R. (Ed.), Reptile Medicine and Surgery. Saunders, Philadelphia, pp. 463–465.

Garner, M.M., Hernandez-Divers, S.M., Raymond, J.T., 2004. Reptile neoplasia: a retrospective study of case submissions to a specialty diagnostic service. Vet. Clin.North Am. Exot. Anim. Pract. 7, 653–671.

Gilbert, S.F., Corfe, I., 2013. Turtle origins: picking up speed. Dev. Cell. 28, 326–328.

Gillies, A.G., Henry, A., Lin, H., Ren, A., Shiuan, K., Fearing, R.S., et al., 2014. Gecko toe and lamellar shear adhesion on macroscopic, engineered rough surfaces. J. Exp. Biol. 217, 283–289.

Goldberg, S.R., Bursey, C.R., Cheam, H., 1997. Helminths of *Anolis acutus* (Sauria: Polychrotidae) from St. Croix, U.S. Virgin Islands. J. Parasitol. 83, 530–531.

Goldstein, E.J., Agyare, E.O., Vagvolgyi, A.E., Halpern, M., 1981. Aerobic bacterial oral flora of garter snakes: development of normal flora and pathogenic potential for snakes and humans. J. Clin. Microbiol. 13, 946–954.

Gong, S., Wang, F., Shi, H., Zhou, P., Ge, Y., Hua, L., et al., 2014. Highly pathogenic *Salmonella Pomona* was first isolated from the exotic red-eared slider (*Trachemys scripta elegans*) in the wild in China: implications for public health. Sci. Total. Environ. 468–469, 28–30.

Gorski, L., Jay-Russell, M.T., Liang, A.S., Walker, S., Bengson, Y., Govoni, J., et al., 2013. Diversity of pulsed-field gel electrophoresis pulsotypes, serovars, and antibiotic resistance among Salmonella isolates from wild amphibians and reptiles in the California Central Coast. Foodborne Pathog. Dis. 10, 540–548.

Govett, P.D., Harms, C.A., Johnson, A.J., Latimer, K.S., Wellehan, J.F., Fatzinger, M.H., et al., 2005. Lymphoid follicular cloacal inflammation associated with a novel herpesvirus in juvenile alligators (*Alligator mississippiensis*). J. Vet. Diagn. Invest. 17, 474–479.

Graczyk, T.K., Cranfield, M.R., Helmer, P., Fayer, R., Bostwick, E.F., 1998. Therapeutic efficacy of hyperimmune bovine colostrum treatment against clinical and subclinical Cryptosporidium serpentis infections in captive snakes. Vet. Parasitol. 74, 123–132.

Greenberg, N., Burghardt, G.M., Crews, D., Font, E., Jones, R.E., Vaughn, G., 1989. Reptile models for biomedical research. In: Woodhead, A.D., Vivirito, K. (Eds.), Nonmammalian Animal Models for Biomedical Research. CRC Press, Boca Raton, FL, pp. 289–308.

Greenberg, N., Wingfield, J.C., 1987. Stress and reproduction: reciprocal relationships. In: Norris, D.O., Jones, R.E. (Eds.), Hormones and Reproduction in Fishes, Amphibians, and Reptiles. Plenum Press, New York, pp. 461–503.

Greenblatt, R.J., Work, T.M., Balazs, G.H., Sutton, C.A., Casey, R.N., Casey, J.W., 2004. The Ozobranchus leech is a candidate mechanical vector for the fibropapilloma-associated turtle herpesvirus found latently infecting skin tumors on Hawaiian green turtles (*Chelonia mydas*). Virology 30, 101–110.

Greene, H.W., 1995. Nonavian reptiles as laboratory animals. ILAR J. 37, 182–186.

Greene, H.W., 1997. Snakes: The Evolution of Mystery in Nature. Univ. of California Press, Berkeley, CA.

Gregersen, J.P., Roth, B., 2012. Inactivation of stable viruses in cell culture facilities by peracetic acid fogging. Biologicals 40, 282–287.

Greiner, E., Schumacher, J., 1997. Parasitology of reptiles. In: Ackerman, L. (Ed.), The Biology, Husbandry, and Health Care of Reptiles. TFH Publications, Neptune City, NJ, pp. 689–702.

Greiner, E.C., Mader, D.R., 2006. Parasitology. In: Mader, D.R. (Ed.), Reptile Medicine and Surgery. Saunders, Philadelphia, PA, pp. 343–364.

Gull, J.M., Lange, C.E., Favrot, C., Dorrestein, G.M., Hatt, J.M., 2012. Multiple papillomas in a diamond python, Morelia spilota spilota. J. Zoo Wildl. Med. 43, 946–949.

Guthrie, A.L., White, C.L., Brown, M.B., deMaar, T.W., 2013. Detection of Mycoplasma agassizii in the Texas tortoise (*Gopherus berlandieri*). J. Wildl. Dis. 49, 704–708.

Harcourt-Brown, F., 1996. Ultraviolet lights for reptiles. Vet. Rec. 138, 528.

Hawkey, C.M., Dennett, T.B., 1989. Color Atlas of Comparative Veterinary Hematology. Iowa State Univ. Press, Ames, IA.

Hellebuyck, T., Pasmans, F., Haesebrouck, F., Martel, A., 2012. Dermatological diseases in lizards. Vet. J. 193, 38–45.

Henkel, F.W., Schmidt, W., 1995. Geckoes. Krieger Pub. Co., Malabar, FL.

Herbst, L.H., Jacobson, E.R., Klein, P.A., Balazs, G.H., Moretti, R., Brown, T., et al., 1999. Experimental transmission of green turtle fibropapillomatosis using cell-free extracts. Dis. Aq. Org. 22, 1–12.

Hernandez-Divers, S.J., Shearer, D., 2002. Pulmonary mycobacteriosis caused by *Mycobacterium haemophilum* and *M. marinum* in a royal python. J. Am. Vet. Med. Assoc. 220, 1661–1663.

Hernandez-Divers, S.M., Garner, M.M., 2003. Neoplasia of reptiles with an emphasis on lizards. Vet. Clin. North Am. Exot. Anim. Pract. 6, 251–273.

Hernandez-Divers, S.J., 2006. Diagnostic techniques. In: Mader, D.R. (Ed.), Reptile Medicine and Surgery Saunders, St. Louis, pp. 490–532.

Hetzel, U., Sironen, T., Laurinmäki, P., Liljeroos, L., Patjas, A., Henttonen, H., et al., 2003. Isolation, identification, and characterization of novel arenaviruses, the etiological agents of boid inclusion body disease. Vet. Microbiol. 95, 283–293.

Hetzel, U., Sironen, T., Laurinmäki, P., Liljeroos, L., Patjas, A., Henttonen, H., et al., 2013. Isolation, identification, and characterization of novel arenaviruses, the etiological agents of boid inclusion body disease. J. Virol. 87, 918–935.

Hews, D.K., Abell Baniki, A.J., 2013. The breeding season duration hypothesis: acute handling stress and total plasma concentrations of corticosterone and androgens in male and female striped plateau lizards (*Sceloporus virgatus*). J. Comp. Physiol. B 183, 933–946.

Hicks, J.W., Wang, T., 1998. Cardiovascular regulation during anoxia in the turtle: an *in vivo* study. Physiol. Zoo. 71, 1–14.

Hilf, M., Wagner, R., Yu, V., 1990. A prospective study of upper airway flora in healthy boid snakes and snakes with pneumonia. J. Zoo Wildl. Med. 21 (3), 318.

Hochleithner, C., Holland, M., 2014. Ultrasonography. In: Maders, D.R., Divers, S.J. (Eds.), Current Therapy in Reptile Medicine and Surgery. Saunders, St. Louis, MO, pp. 107–127.

Holliday, C.M., Gardner, N.M., 2012. A new eusuchian crocodyliform with novel cranial integument and its significance for the origin and evolution of Crocodylia. PLoS One 7, e30471.

Holz, P., Barker, I.K., Crawshaw, G.J., Dobson, H., 1997. The anatomy and perfusion of the renal portal system in the red-eared slider (*Trachemys scripta elegans*). J. Zoo Wildl. Med. 28, 378–385.

Holz, P.H., Raidal, S.R., 2006. Comparative renal anatomy of exotic species. Vet. Clin. North Am. Exot. Anim. Pract. 9, 1–11.

Huchzermeyer, F.W., Wallace, D.B., Putterill, J.F., Gerdes, G.H., 2009. Identification and partial sequencing of a crocodile poxvirus associated with deeply penetrating skin lesions in farmed Nile crocodiles, *Crocodylus niloticus*. Onderstepoort J. Vet. Res. 76, 311–316.

Huff, T., 1980. Captive propagation of the subfamily Boinae with emphasis on the genus *Epicrates* In: Murphy, J.B. Collins, J.T. (Eds.), Reproductive Biology and Diseases of Captive Reptiles, vol. 1 Society for the Study of Amphibians and Reptiles, Oxford, pp. 125–134.

Hughes-Hanks, J.M., Schommer, S.K., Mitchell, W.J., Shaw, D.P., 2010. Hepatitis and enteritis caused by a novel herpesvirus in two monitor lizards (*Varanus spp.*). J. Vet. Diagn. Invest. 22, 295–299.

Hyndman, T., Shilton, C.M., 2011. Molecular detection of two adenoviruses associated with disease in Australian lizards. Aust. Vet. J. 89, 232–235.

Hyndman, T.H., Shilton, C.M., Doneley, R.J., Nicholls, P.K., 2012. Sunshine virus in Australian pythons. Vet. Microbiol. 161, 77–87.

Hyndman, T.H., Shilton, C.M., Marschang, R.E., 2013. Paramyxoviruses in reptiles: a review. Vet. Microbiol. 165, 200–213.

Ip, Y.K., Loong, A.M., Lee, S.M., Ong, J.L., Wong, W.P., Chew, S.F., 2013. The Chinese soft-shelled turtle, *Pelodiscus sinensis*, excretes urea mainly through the mouth instead of the kidney. Exp. Biol. 215, 3723–3733.

Jacobson, E.R., 1981. Neoplastic diseases In: Cooper, J.E. Jackson, O.F. (Eds.), Diseases of the Reptilia, vol. 2 Academic Press, San Diego, CA, pp. 429–468.

Jacobson, E.R., 1983. Parasitic diseases of reptiles. In: Kirk, R.W. (Ed.), Current Veterinary Therapy 8: Small Animal Practice Saunders, Philadelphia, PA, pp. 601.

Jacobson, E.R., 1984. Biology and diseases of reptiles. In: Fox, J.G., Cohen, B.J., Loew, F.M. (Eds.), Laboratory Animal Medicine. Academic Press, San Diego, CA, pp. 449–476.

Jacobson, E.R., 1993a. Blood collection techniques in reptiles: laboratory investigations. In: Fowler, M.E. (Ed.), Zoo and Wild Animal Medicine. Saunders, Philadelphia, PA, pp. 144–152.

Jacobson, E.R., 1993b. Snakes In: Quesenberry, K.E. Hillyer, E.V. (Eds.), The Veterinary Clinics of North America: Small Animal Practice, vol. 23. Saunders, Philadelphia, PA, pp. 1179–1212.

Jacobson, E.R., 1993c. Viral diseases of reptiles. In: Fowler, M.E. (Ed.), Zoo and Wild Animal Medicine. Saunders, Philadelphia, PA, pp. 153–159.

Jacobson, E.R., 2007a. Parasites and parasitic diseases of reptiles. In: Jacobson, E.R. (Ed.), Infectious Diseases and Pathology of Reptiles. CRC Press, Boca Raton, FL, pp. 571–607.

Jacobson, E.R., 2007b. Viruses and viral diseases of reptiles. In: Jacobson, E.R. (Ed.), Infectious Diseases and Pathology of Reptiles. CRC Press, Boca Raton, pp. 395–460.

Jacobson, E.R., Gardiner, C.H., 1990. Adeno-like virus in esophageal and tracheal mucosa of a Jackson's chameleon (Chameleo jacksonii). Vet. Pathol. 27, 210.

Jacobson, E.R., Gaskin, J.M., 1985. Adenovirus-like infection in a boa constrictor. J. Am. Vet. Med. Assoc. 187, 1226.

Jacobson, E.R., Telford, S.R., 1990. Chlamydial and poxvirus infections of circulating monocytes of a flap-necked chameleon (Chamaeleo dilepis). J. Wildl. Dis. 26, 527–572.

Jacobson, E.R., Popp, J., Shields, R.P., Gaskin, J.M., 1979. Pox-like virus associated with skin lesions in captive caimans. J. Am. Vet. Med. Assoc. 175, 937.

Jacobson, E.R., Gaskin, J.M., Clubb, S., Calderwood, M.B., 1982a. Papilloma-like virus infection in Bolivian side-neck turtles. J. Am. Vet. Med. Assoc. 181, 1325–1328.

Jacobson, E.R., Gardiner, C.H., Foggin, C.M., 1984. Adenovirus-like infection in two Nile crocodiles. J. Am. Vet. Med. Assoc. 185, 1421–1422.

Jacobson, E.R., Gaskin, J.M., Gardiner, C.H., 1985. Adenovirus-like infection in a boa constrictor. J. Am. Vet. Med. Assoc. 187, 1226–1227.

Jacobson, E.R., Gaskin, J.M., Roelke, M., 1986. Conjunctivitis, tracheitis, and pneumonia associated with herpesvirus infection in green sea turtles. J. Am. Vet. Med. Assoc. 189, 1020.

Jacobson, E.R., Gaskin, J.M., Brown, M.B., Harris, R.K., Gardines, C.H., La-Pointe, J.L., et al., 1991a. Chronic upper respiratory tract disease of free-ranging desert tortoises (Xerobates agassizii). J. Wildl. Dis. 27, 296–316.

Jacobson, E.R., Gaskin, J.M., Wells, S., Bowler, K., Schumacher, J., 1992. Epizootic of ophidian paramyxovirus in a zoological collection: pathological, microbiological, and serological findings. J. Zoo Wildl. Med. 23, 318.

Jacobson, E.R., Homer, B.L., Stacy, B.A., Greiner, E.C., Szabo, N.J., Chrisman, C.L., et al., 2006. Neurological disease in wild loggerhead sea turtle Caretta caretta. Dis. Aquat. Organ. 70, 139–154.

Jacobson, E.R., Berry, K.H., Wellehan Jr., J.F., Origgi, F., Childress, A.L., Braun, J., et al., 2012. Serologic and molecular evidence for Testudinid herpesvirus 2 infection in wild Agassiz's desert tortoises, Gopherus agassizii. J. Wildl. Dis. 48, 747–757.

Jenkins, J.R., 1996. Diagnostic and clinical techniques. In: Mader, D.R. (Ed.), Reptile Medicine and Surgery. Saunders, Philadelphia, PA, pp. 264–276.

Johnson, A.J., Pessier, A.P., Jacobson, E.R., 2007. Experimental transmission and induction of ranaviral disease in Western Ornate box turtles (Terrapene ornata ornata) and red-eared sliders (Trachemys scripta elegans). Vet. Pathol. 44, 285–297.

Johnson, A.J., Pessier, A.P., Wellehan, J.F., Childress, A., Norton, T.M., Stedman, N.L., et al., 2008. Ranavirus infection of free-ranging and captive box turtles and tortoises in the United States. J. Wildl. Dis. 44, 851–863.

Johnson, C.A., Griffith, J.W., Tenorio, P., Hytrek, S., Lang, C.M., 1998. Fatal trematodiasis in research turtles. Lab. Anim. Sci. 48, 340–343.

Johnson, J.H., 2004. Husbandry and medicine of aquatic reptiles. Semin. Avian Exot. Pet Med. 13, 223–228.

Jones, D.E., Gogal Jr., R.M., Nader, P.B., Holladay, S.D., 2005. Organochlorine detection in the shed skins of snakes. Ecotoxicol. Environ. Saf. 60, 282–287.

Jones, H.I., 1995. Pathology associated with physalopterid larvae (Nematoda: Spirurida) in the gastric tissues of Australian reptiles. J. Wildl. Dis. 31, 299–306.

Joyner, P.H., Brown, J.D., Holladay, S., Sleeman, J.M., 2006. Characterization of the bacterial microflora of the tympanic cavity of eastern box turtles with and without aural abscesses. J. Wildl. Dis. 42, 859–864.

Jungwirth, N., Bodewes, R., Osterhaus, A.D., Baumgärtner, W., Wohlsein, P., 2014. First report of a new alphaherpesvirus in a freshwater turtle (Pseudemys concinna concinna) kept in Germany. Vet. Microbiol. S0378–1135(14)00119–00119.

Junker, K., Boomker, J., 2006. Check-list of the pentastomid parasites crocodilians freshwater chelonians. Onderstepoort J. Vet. Res. 73, 27–36.

Kanui, T., Mwendia, C., Aulie, A., Wanyoike, M., 1991. Effects of temperature on growth, food uptake, and retention time of juvenile Nile crocodiles (Crocodylus niloticus). Comp. Biochem. Physiol. A Comp. Physiol. 99, 453–456.

Kazacos, K.R., Fisher, L.F., 1997. Renal styphlodoriasis in a boa constrictor. J. Am. Vet. Med. Assoc. 171, 876–878.

Kelehear, C., Spratt, D.M., Dubey, S., Brown, G.P., Shine, R., 2011. Using combined morphological, allometric and molecular approaches to identify species of the genus Raillietiella (Pentastomida). PLoS One 6, e24936.

Kerver, H.N., Wade, J., 2013. Seasonal and sexual dimorphisms in expression of androgen receptor and its coactivators in brain and peripheral copulatory tissues of the green anole. Gen. Comp. Endocrinol. 193, 56–67.

Keymer, I., 1978. Diseases of chelonians: necropsy survey of terrapins and turtles. Vet. Rec. 103, 577.

Kohmoto, T., Argenziano, M., Yamamoto, N., Vliet, K.A., Gu, A., DeRosa, C.M., et al., 1997. Assessment of transmyocardial perfusion in alligator hearts. Circulation 95, 1585–1591.

Kummrow, M.S., Tseng, F., Hesse, L., Court, M., 2008. Pharmacokinetics of buprenorphine after single-dose subcutaneous administration in red-eared sliders (Trachemys scripta elegans). J. Zoo Wildl. Med. 39, 590–595.

Lamirande, E.W., Nichols, D.K., Owens, J.W., Gaskin, J.M., Jacobson, E.R., 1999. Isolation and experimental transmission of a reovirus pathogenic in ratsnakes (Elaphe species). Virus Res. 63, 135–141.

Lance, V.A., 1990. Stress in reptiles. Prog. Clin. Biol. Res. 342, 461–466.

Landolfi, J.A., Terio, K.A., Kinsel, M.J., Langan, J., Zachariah, T.T., Childress, A.L., et al., 2010. Orthoreovirus infection and concurrent cryptosporidiosis in rough green snakes (Opheodrys aestivus): pathology and identification of a novel orthoreovirus strain via polymerase chain reaction and sequencing. J. Vet. Diagn. Invest. 22, 37–43.

Lane, T.J., 1996. Crocodilians. In: Mader, D.R. (Ed.), Reptile Medicine and Surgery. Saunders, Philadelphia, PA, pp. 78–94.

Lane, T.J., 2006. Crocodilians. In: Mader, D.R. (Ed.), Reptile Medicine and Surgery. Saunders, St. Louis, MO, pp. 100–117.

Lang, J.W., 1987. Crocodilian behaviour: implications for management. In: Webb, G.J.W., Manoles, S.C., Whitehead, P.J. (Eds.), Wildlife Management: Crocodiles and Alligators. Surrey Beatty and Sons, Australia, pp. 273–294.

Langford, G.J., Janovy Jr., J., 2009. Comparative life cycles and life histories of North American Rhabdias spp. (Nematoda: Rhabdiasidae): lungworms from snakes and anurans. J. Parasitol. 95, 1145–1155.

Langford, G.J., Janovy Jr., J., 2013. Host specificity of North American Rhabdias spp. (Nematoda: Rhabdiasidae): combining field data and experimental infections with a molecular phylogeny. J. Parasitol. 99, 277–286.

Langford, G.J., Willobee, B.A., Isidoro, L.F., 2013. Transmission, host specificity, and seasonal occurrence of Cyrtosomum penneri (Nematoda: Atractidae) in lizards from Florida. J. Parasitol. 99, 241–246.

Latney, L.V., Wellehan, J., 2013. Selected emerging infectious diseases of squamata. Vet. Clin. North Am. Exot. Anim. Pract. 16, 319–338.

Lawton, M.P.C., 1992. Neurological diseases. In: Beynon, P.H., Lawton, M.P.C., Cooper, J.E. (Eds.), Manual of Reptiles. British Small Animal Veterinary Assoc., Iowa State University Press, Ames, IA, pp. 128–137.

Lertpiriyapong, K., Gamazon, E.R., Feng, Y., Park, D.S., Pang, J., Botka, G., et al., 2012. Campylobacter jejuni type VI secretion system: roles in adaptation to deoxycholic acid, host cell adherence, invasion, and in vivo colonization. PLoS One 7, e42842.

Lertpiriyapong, K., Handt, L., Feng, Y., Mitchell, T.W., Lodge, K.E., Shen, Z., et al., 2014. Pathogenic properties of enterohepatic Helicobacter spp. isolated from rhesus macaques with intestinal adenocarcinoma. J. Med. Microbiol. [Epub ahead of print].

Literak, I., Robesova, B., Majlathova, V., Majlath, I., Kulich, P., Fabian, P., et al., 2010. Herpesvirus-associated papillomatosis in a green lizard. J. Wildl. Dis. 46, 257–261.

Lovern, M.B., Holmes, M.M., Wade, J., 2004. The green anole (Anolis carolinensis): a reptilian model for laboratory studies of reproductive morphology and behavior. ILAR J. 45, 54–64.

Lu, B., Yang, W., Dai, Q., Fu, J., 2013. Using genes as characters and a parsimony analysis to explore the phylogenetic position of turtles. PLoS One 8, e79348.

Lutes, A.A., Neaves, W.B., Baumann, D.P., Wiegraebe, W., Baumann, P., 2010. Sister chromosome pairing maintains heterozygosity in parthenogenetic lizards. Nature 464, 283–286.

Machado, G.S., Mas, G.H., Vidal, W.A., Monteiro-Neto, C., Lobo-Hajdu, G., 2013. Evidence of regression of fibropapillomas in juvenile green turtles Chelonia mydas caught in Niterói, southeast Brazil. Dis. Aquat. Organ. 102, 243–247.

Mackessy, S.P., 2010. The field of reptile toxinology: snakes, lizards, and their venoms. In: Mackessy, S.P. (Ed.), Venoms and Toxins of Reptiles. CRC Press, Boca Raton, FL, pp. 3–23.

Mader, D.R., 2006a. Metabolic bone disease. In: Mader, D.R. (Ed.), Reptile Medicine and Surgery. Saunders, St. Louis, MO, pp. 841–851.

Mader, D.R., 2006b. Gout. In: Mader, D.R. (Ed.), Reptile Medicine and Surgery. Saunders, St. Louis, MO, pp. 793–800.

Mahapatra, D., Reinhard, M., Naikare, H.K., 2013. Adenovirus and cryptosporidium co-infection in a corn snake (Elaphae guttata guttata). J. Zoo Wildl. Med. 44, 220–224.

Manire, C.A., Stacy, B.A., Kinsel, M.J., Daniel, H.T., Anderson, E.T., Wellehan Jr., J.F., 2008. Proliferative dermatitis in a loggerhead turtle, Caretta caretta, and a green turtle, Chelonia mydas, associated with novel papillomaviruses. Vet. Microbiol. 130, 227–237.

Manire, C.A., Kinsel, M.J., Anderson, E.T., Clauss, T.M., Byrd, L., 2012. Lungworm infection in three loggerhead sea turtles, Caretta caretta. J. Zoo Wild. Med. 39, 92–98.

Marschang, R.E., 2011. Viruses infecting reptiles. Viruses 3, 2087–2126.

Marschang, R.E., Divers, S.J., 2014. Reptile viruses. In: Maders, D.R., Divers, S.J. (Eds.), Current Therapy in Reptile Medicine and Surgery. Saunders, St. Louis, MO, pp. 369–381.

Marschang, R.E., Gravendyck, M., Kaleta, E.F., 1997. Herpesviruses in tortoises: investigations into virus isolation and the treatment of viral stomatitis in Testudo hermanni and T. graeca. Zentralbl. Veterinarmed. B 44, 385–394.

Marschang, R.E., Gleiser, C.B., Papp, T., Pfitzner, A.J., Böhm, R., Roth, B.N., 2006. Comparison of 11 herpesvirus isolates from tortoises using partial sequences from three conserved genes. Vet. Microbiol. 117, 258–266.

Marschang, R.E., Papp, T., Frost, J.W., 2009. Comparison of paramyxovirus isolates from snakes, lizards and a tortoise. Virus Res. 144, 272–279.

Maslow, J.N., Wallace, R., Michaels, M., Foskett, H., Maslow, E.A., Kiehlbauch, J.A., 2002. Outbreak of Mycobacterium marinum infection among captive snakes and bullfrogs. Zoo Biol. 21, 233–241.

Mason, R.T., Hoyt Jr., R.F., Pannell, L.K., Wellner, E.F., Demeter, B., 1991. Cage design and configuration for arboreal reptiles. Lab. Anim. Sci. 41, 84–86.

Mass, A.K., 2013. Vesicular, ulcerative, and necrotic dermatitis of reptiles. In: Fisher, P.G., Rupley, A.E. (Eds.), Veterinary Clinics of North America: Exotic Animal Practice. Elsevier, Philadelphia, PA, pp. 737–755.

Mattison, C., 1991. Keeping and Breeding Lizards. Blandford, London.

Mattison, C., 1998. The Care of Reptiles and Amphibians in Captivity. Blandford, London.

May, M., Ortiz, G.J., Wendland, L.D., Rotstein, D.S., Relich, R.F., Balish, M.F., et al., 2007. Mycoplasma insons sp. Nov., a twisted mycoplasma from green iguanas (Iguana iguana). FEMS Microbiol. Lett. 274, 298–303.

McAliley, L.R., Willis, R.E., Ray, D.A., White, P.S., Brochu, C.A., Densmore 3rd, L.D., 2006. Are crocodile really monophyletic?–Evidence for subdivisions from sequence and morphological data. Mol. Phylogenet. Evol. 39, 16–23.

McIlhenny, E.A., 1987. The Alligator's Life History. Ten Speed Press, Berkeley, CA.

McKeown, S., 1984. Management and propagation of the lizard genus. Phelsuma. Acta Zool. Pathol. Antverp. 78, 149–162.

McLean, K.E., Vickaryous, M.K., 2011. A novel amniote model of epimorphic regeneration: the leopard gecko, Eublepharis macularius. BMC Dev. Biol. 11, 50.

Meggs, W.J., Courtnery, C., O'Rourke, D., Brewer, K.L., 2010. Pilot studies of pressure-immobilization bandages for rattlesnake envenomations. Clin. Tox. 48, 61–63.

Mehlhorn, H., Schmahl, G., Frese, M., Mevissen, I., Harder, A., Krieger, K., 2005. Effects of a combinations of emodepside and praziquantel on parasites of reptiles and rodents. Parasitol. Res. 97 (Suppl. 1), S65–S69.

Mehra, A., Zahra, A., Thompson, V., Sirisaengtaksin, N., Wells, A., Porto, M., et al., 2013. Mycobacterium tuberculosis type VII secreted effector EsxH targets host ESCRT to impair trafficking. PLoS Pathog. 9, e1003734.

Mendyk, R.W., Newton, A.L., Baumer, M., 2013. A retrospective study of mortality in varanid lizards (Reptilia: Squamata: Varanidae) at the Bronx Zoo: implications for husbandry and reproductive management in zoos. Zoo Biol. 32, 152–162.

Mermin, J., Hoar, B., Angulo, F.J., 1997. Iguanas and Salmonella marina infection in children: a reflection of the increasing incidence of reptile-associated salmonellosis in the United States. Pediatrics 99, 399–402.

Miller, A.C., Commens, C.A., Jaworski, R., Packham, D., 1990. The turtle's revenge: a case of soft tissue Mycobacterium chelonae infection. Med. J. Aust. 153, 493–495.

Miller, E.A., Green, S.L., Otto, G.M., Bouley, D.M., 2001. Suspected hypovitaminosis A in a colony of captive green anoles (Anolis carolinensis). Contemp. Top. Lab. Anim. Sci. 40, 18–20.

Millichamp, N.J., Jacobson, E.R., 1983. Diseases of the eye and ocular adnexa in reptiles. J. Am. Vet. Med. Assoc. 18, 1205–1212.

Milnes, M.R., Guillette, L.J., 2008. Alligator tales: new lessons about environmental contaminants from a sentinel species. BioScience 58, 1027–1036.

Mitchell, M.A., 2006. Therapeutics. In: Mader, D.R. (Ed.), Reptile Medicine and Surgery. Saunders, St. Louis, MO, pp. 631–664.

Mitchell, M.A., 2011 Zoonotic diseases associated with reptiles and amphibians: an update. Vet. Clin. North Am. Exot. Anim. Pract. 14, 439–456.

Mitchell, M.A., 2012 Mycobacterial infections in reptiles. Vet. Clin. North Am. Exot. Anim. Pract. 1, 101–111.

Moscona, A.A., 1990. Anatomy of the pancreas and Langerhans islets in snakes and lizards. Anat. Rec. 227, 232–244.

Mosley, C., 2011. Pain and nociception in reptiles. Vet. Clin. North Am. Exot. Anim. Pract. 14, 45–60.

Murray, M.J., 2006. Aural abscesses. In: Mader, D.R. (Ed.), Reptile Medicine and Surgery. Saunders, St. Louis, MO, pp. 631–664.

Mushonga, B., Horowitz, A., 1996. Serous cavities of the Nile crocodile (*Crocodylus niloticus*). J. Zoo Wild. Med. 27, 170–179.

Naciri, M., Mancassola, R., Fort, G., Danneels, B., Verhaeghe, J., 2011. Efficacy of amine-based disinfectant KENO™COX on the infectivity of *Cryptosporidium parvum* oocysts. Vet. Parasitol. 30, 43–49.

Nayak, G., Prentice, H.M., Milton, S.L., 2009. Role of neuroglobin in regulating reactive oxygen species in the brain of the anoxia-tolerant turtle Trachemys scripta. J. Neurochem. 110, 603–612.

Nickol, B.B., Fuller, C.A., Rock, P., 2006. Cystacanths of *Oncicola venezuelensis* (Acanthocephala: Oligacanthorhynchidae) in Caribbean termites and various paratenic hosts in the U.S. Virgin Islands. J. Parasitol. 92, 539–542.

Nishimura, T., Okano, H., Tada, H., Nishimura, E., Sugimoto, K., Mohri, K., et al., 2010. Lizards respond to an extremely low-frequency electromagnetic field. J. Exp. Biol. 213, 1985–1990.

Northcutt, R.G., 2013. Variation in reptilian brains and cognition. Brain Behav. Evol. 82, 45–54.

Norton, T.M., Andrews, K.M., Smith, L.L., 2014. Techniques for working with wild reptiles. In: Maders, D.R., Divers, S.J. (Eds.), Current Therapy in Reptile Medicine and Surgery. Saunders, St. Louis, MO, pp. 310–340.

Olsson, M., Stuart-Fox, D., Ballen, C., 2013. Genetics and evolution of colour patterns in reptiles. Semin. Cell Dev. Biol. 24, 529–541.

Origgi, F.C., Romero, C.H., Bloom, D.C., Klein, P.A., Gaskin, J.M., Tucker, S.J., et al., 2004. Experimental transmission of a herpesvirus in Greek tortoise (*Testudo graeca*). Vet. Path. 41, 50–61.

Orós, J., Rodríguez, J.L., Déniz, S., Fernández, L., Fernández, A., 1998. Cutaneous poxvirus-like infection in a captive Hermann's tortoise (*Testudo hermanni*). Vet. Rec. 43, 508–509.

Orós, J., Torrent, A., Calabuig, P., Déniz, S., 2005. Diseases and causes of mortality among sea turtles stranded in the Canary Islands, Spain (1998–2001). Dis. Aquat. Organ. 25, 13–24.

Orós, J., Camacho, M., Calabuig, P., Arencibia, A., 2011. Salt gland adenitis as only cause of stranding of loggerhead sea turtles *Caretta caretta*. Dis. Aquat. Organ. 95, 163–166.

O'Rourke, D.P., 2014. Reptiles and amphibians in laboratory animal medicine. In: Mader, D.R., Divers, S.J. (Eds.), Current Therapy in Reptile Medicine and Surgery. Saunders, St. Louis, MO, pp. 290–295.

Page, C.D., Mautino, M., 1990. Clinical management of tortoises. Compend. Contin. Educ. Pract. Vet. 12, 221–228.

Pandey, G.S., Inoue, N., Ohshima, K., Okada, K., Chihaya, Y., Fujimoto, Y., 1990. Poxvirus infection in Nile crocodiles (*Crocodylus niloticus*). Res. Vet. Sci. 49, 171–176.

Parker-Cote, J.L., O'Rourke, D.P., Miller, S.N., Brewer, K.L., Rosenbaum, M.D., Meggs, W.J., 2014. Trypsin and rosmarinic acid reduce the toxicity of *Micrurus fulvis* venom in mice. Clin. Tox. 52, 118–120.

Parmenter, R.R., Avery, H.W., 1990. The feeding ecology of the slider turtle. In: Gibbons, J.W. (Ed.), Life History and Ecology of the Slider Turtle, pp. 257–266.

Penner, J.D., Jacobson, E.R., Brown, D.R., Adams, H.P., Besch-Williford, C.L., 1997. novel *Mycoplasma* sp. associated with proliferative tracheitis and pneumonia in a Burmese python (*Python molurus bivittatus*). J. Comp. Pathol. 117.

Penrith, M.L., Nesbit, J.W., Huchzermeyer, F.W., 1991. Pox virus infection in captive juvenile caimans (*Caiman crocodilus fuscus*) in South Africa. J. S. Afr. Vet. Assoc. 62, 137–139.

Pincheira-Donoso, D., Bauer, A.M., Meiri, S., Uetz, P., 2013. Global taxonomic diversity of living reptiles. PLoS One 8, e59741.

Plummer, M.V., Ferner, J.W., 2012. Marking reptiles. In: Reptile Biodiversity: Standard Methods for Inventory and Monitoring, pp. 143–150.

Ponraj, D., Gopalakrishnakone, P., 1996. Establishment of an animal model for myoglobinuria by use of a myotoxin from *Pseudechis australis* (king brown snake) venom in mice. Lab. Anim. Sci. 46, 393–398.

Pough, F.H., 1991. Recommendations for the care of amphibians and reptiles in academic institutions. ILAR News 33, S1–S23.

Pye, G.W., Brown, D.R., Nogueira, M.F., Vliet, K.A., Schoeb, T.R., Jacobson, E.R., et al., 2001. Experimental inoculation of broad-nosed caimans (*Caiman latirostris*) and Siamese crocodiles (*Crocodylus siamensis*) with *Mycoplasma alligatoris*. J. Zoo Wildl. Med. 32, 196–201.

Radcliffe, C.W., Murphy, J.B., 1983. Precopulatory and related behaviours in captive crotalids and other reptiles: suggestions for future investigations. Int. Zoo Yearbook 23, 163–166.

Raphael, B.L., Kelmens, M.W., Moehlman, P., Dierenfeld, E., Karesh, W.B., 1994. Blood values in free-ranging pancake tortoises (*Malacochersus tornieri*). J. Zoo Wildl. Med. 25, 63–67.

Raske, M., Lewbart, G.A., Dombrowski, D.S., Hale, P., Correa, M., Christian, L.S., 2012. Body temperatures of selected amphibian and reptile species. J. Zoo Wildl. Med. 43, 517–521.

Rataj, A.V., Lindtner-Knific, R., Vlahović, K., Mavri, U., Dovč, A., 2011. Parasite in pet reptile. Acta Vet. Scand. 53, 33.

Rehorek, S.J., 1997. Squamate Harderian gland: an overview. Anat. Rec. 248, 301–306.

Rice, A., Roberts IV, T.L., Dorcas, M.E., 2006. Heating and cooling rates of eastern diamondback rattlesnakes, *Crotalus adamanteus*. J. Thermal Biol. 31, 501–505.

Richter, B., Rasim, R., Vrhovec, M.G., Nedorost, N., Pantchev, N., 2012. Cryptosporidiosis outbreak in captive chelonians (*Testudo hermanni*) with identification of two Cryptosporidium genotypes. J. Vet. Diagn. Invest. 24, 591–595.

Rideout, B.A., Montali, R.J., Phillips, L.G., Gardiner, C.H., 1987. Mortality of captive tortoises due to viviparous nematodes of the genus Proatractis (Family Atractidae). J. Wildl. Dis. 23, 103–138.

Rinaldi, L., Capasso, M., Mihalca, A.D., Cirillo, R., Cringoli, G., Cacciò, S., 2012. Prevalence and molecular identification of Cryptosporidium isolates from pet lizards and snakes in Italy. Parasite 19, 437–440.

Ritchie, B., 2006. Virology. In: Mader, D.R. (Ed.), Reptile Medicine and Surgery. Saunders, Philadelphia, PA, pp. 391–417.

Ross, C.A., Magnusson, W.E., 1989. Living crocodilians. In: Ross, C.A. (Ed.), Crocodiles and Alligators Facts on File, New York, pp. 58–73.

Rossi, J.V., 1992. Snakes of the United States and Canada: Keeping Them Healthy in Captivity. Volume I: Eastern Area. Krieger Publ. Co., Malabar, FL.

Rossi, J.V., 1996. Dermatology. In: Mader, D.R. (Ed.), Reptile Medicine and Surgery. Saunders, Philadelphia, PA, pp. 104–117.

Rossi, J.V., Rossi, R., 1995. Snakes of the United States and Canada: Keeping Them Healthy in Captivity. Volume II: Western Area. Krieger Publ. Co., Malabar, FL.

Sandmeier, F.C., Tracy, C.R., Hagerty, B.E., DuPré, S., Mohammadpour, H., Hunter Jr., K., 2013. Mycoplasmal upper respiratory tract disease across the range of the threatened Mojave desert tortoise: associations with thermal regime and natural antibodies. Ecohealth 10, 63–71.

Schaeffer, D.O., 1997. Anesthesia and analgesia in nontraditional laboratory animal species. In: Kohn, D.F., Wixson, S.K., White, W.J., Benson, G.J. (Eds.), Anesthesia and Analgesia in Laboratory Animals. Academic Press, San Diego, CA, pp. 337–378.

Schilliger, L., Selleri, P., Frye, F.L., 2011. Lymphoblastic lymphoma and leukemic blood profile in a red-tail boa (*Boa constrictor constrictor*) with concurrent inclusion body disease. J. Vet. Diagn. Invest. 23, 159–162.

Schmidt, V., Plenz, B., Pfaff, M., Pees, M., 2012. Disseminated systemic mycosis in Veiled chameleons (*Chamaeleo calyptratus*) caused by *Chamaeleomyces granulomati*. Vet. Microbiol. 161, 145–152.

Schmidt, V., Marschang, R.E., Abbas, M.D., Ball, I., Szabo, I., Helmuth, R., et al., 2013. Detection of pathogens in Boidae and Pythonidae with and without respiratory disease. Vet. Rec. 172, 236.

Schumacher, I.M., Brown, M.B., Jacobson, E.R., Collins, B.R., Klein, P.A., 1993. Detection of antibodies to a pathogenic mycoplasma in desert tortoises (*Gopherus agassizii*) with upper respiratory tract disease. J. Clin. Microbiol. 31, 1454–1460.

Schumacher, J., 1996a. Reptile and amphibian anesthesia. In: Thurmon, J.C. (Ed.), Lumb and Jones' Veterinary Anesthesia. Williams and Wilkins, Baltimore, MD, pp. 670–685.

Schumacher, J., 1996b. Viral diseases. In: Mader, D.R. (Ed.), Reptile Medicine and Surgery. Saunders, Philadelphia, PA, pp. 224–234.

Schumacher, J., Papendick, R., Herbst, L., Jacobson, E.R., 1996c. Volvulus of the proximal colon in a hawksbill turtle (*Eretmochelys imbricata*). J. Zoo Wildl. Med. 27, 386–391.

Schumacher, J., Jacobson, E.R., Burns, R., Tramontin, R.R., 1994a. Adenovirus infection in two rosy boas (*Lichanura trivirgata*). J. Zoo Wildl. Med. 25, 461.

Schumacher, V.L., Innis, C.J., Garner, M.M., Risatti, G.R., Nordhausen, R.W., Gilbert-Marcheterre, K., et al., 2012. Sulawesi tortoise adenovirus-1 in two impressed tortoises (*Manouria impressa*) and a Burmese star tortoise (*Geochelone platynota*). J. Zoo Wildl. Med. 43, 501–510.

Secor, S.M., Diamond, J., 1997. Determinants of the postfeeding metabolic response of Burmese pythons. Python. Molurus. Physiol. Zool. 70, 202–212.

Seebacher, F., Franklin, C.E., 2005. Physiological mechanisms of thermoregulation in reptiles: a review. J. Comp. Physiol. B 175, 533–541.

Sever, D.M., Rheubert, J.L., Gautreaux, J., Hill, T.G., Freeborn, L.R., 2012. Observations on the sexual segment of the kidney of snakes with emphasis on ultrastructure in the yellow-bellied snake, *Pelamis platurus*. Anat. Rec. (Hoboken) 295, 872–885.

Sigler, L., Hambleton, S., Paré, J.A., 2013. Molecular characterization of reptile pathogens currently known as members of the Chrysosporium anamorph of Nannizziopsis vriesii complex and relationship with some human-associated isolates. J. Clin. Microbiol. 5, 3338–3357.

Simpson, C.F., Jacobson, E.R., Gaskin, J.M., 1979. Herpesvirus-like infection of the venom gland of Siamese cobras. J. Am. Vet. Med. Assoc. 175, 941–943.

Smales, L.R., 2007. *Acanthocephala* in amphibians (Anura) and reptiles (Squamata) from Brazil and Paraguay with description of a new species. J. Parasitol. 93, 392–398.

Solessio, E., Engbretson, G.A., 1993. Antagonistic chromatic mechanisms in photoreceptors of the parietal eye of lizards. Nature 364, 442–445.

Stacy, B.A., Wellehan Jr., J.F., 2010. Fatal septicemia caused by Helicobacter infection in a pancake tortoise (*Malacochersus tornieri*). J. Vet. Diagn. Invest. 22, 660–662.

Stacy, B.A., Wellehan, J.F., Foley, A.M., Coberley, S.S., Herbst, L.H., Manire, C.A., et al., 2008. Two herpesviruses associated with disease in wild Atlantic loggerhead sea turtles (*Caretta caretta*). Vet. Microbiol. 126, 63–73.

Stahlschmidt, Z.R., DeNardo, D.F., 2010. Parental care in snakes. In: Aldridge, R.D., Sever, D.M. (Eds.), Reproductive Biology and Phylogeny of Snakes. Science Publishers Inc., Enfield, NH, pp. 673–702.

Staton, M.A., Edwards Jr., H.M., Brisbin Jr., I.L., Joanen, T., McNease, L., 1990. Protein and energy relationships in the diet of the American alligator (*Alligator mississippiensis*). J. Nutr. 120, 775–785.

Stenglein, M.D., Sanders, C., Kistler, A.L., Ruby, J.G., Franco, J.Y., Reavill, D.R., et al., 2012. Identification, characterization, and in vitro culture of highly divergent arenaviruses from boa constrictors and annulated tree boas: candidate etiological agents for snake inclusion body disease. MBio. 3, e00180–12.

Stoakes, L.C., 1992. Respiratory system. In: Beynon, P.H., Lawton, M.P.C., Cooper, J.E. (Eds.), Manual of Reptiles. British Small Animal Veterinary Assoc., Iowa State University Press, Ames, IA, pp. 88–100.

Stöhr, A.C., Blahak, S., Heckers, K.O., Wiechert, J., Behncke, H., Mathes, K., et al., 2013. Ranavirus infections associated with skin lesions in lizards. Vet. Res. 44, 84.

Stoker, C., Beldomenico, P.M., Bosquiazzo, V.L., Zayas, M.A., Rey, F., Horacio, R., et al., 2008. Developmental exposure to endocrine disruptor chemicals alters follicular dynamics and steroid levels in *Caiman latirostris*. Gen. Comp. Endocrin. 156, 603–612.

Storz, J.F., Hoffmann, F.G., Opazo, J.C., Sanger, T.J., Moriyama, H., 2011. Developmental regulation of hemoglobin synthesis in the green anole lizard *Anolis carolinensis*. J. Exp. Biol. 214, 575–581.

Sykes, J.M., Trupkiewicz, J.G., 2006. Reptile neoplasia at the Philadelphia Zoological Garden 1901–2002. J. Zoo Wildl. Med. 37, 11–19.

Széll, Z., Sréter, T., Varga, I., 2001. Ivermectin toxicosis in a chameleon (*Chamaeleo senegalensis*) infected with Foleyella furcata. J. Zoo. Wildl. Med. 32, 115–117.

Talent, L.G., Dumont, J.N., Bantle, J.A., Janz, D.M., Talent, S.G., 2002. Evaluation of western fence lizards (*Sceloporus occidentalis*) and eastern fence lizards (*Sceloporus undulatus*) as laboratory reptile models for toxicological investigations. Environ. Toxicol. Chem. 21, 899–905.

Tan, R.J., Lim, E.W., Ishak, B., 1978. Intestinal bacterial flora of the household lizard, *Gecko gecko*. Res. Vet. Sci. 24, 262–263.

Taylor, W.M., 2006. Endoscopy. In: Mader, D.R. (Ed.), Reptile Medicine and Surgery. Saunders, St. Louis, pp. 549–573.

Teare, J.A., Bush, M., 1983. Toxicity and efficacy of ivermectin in chelonians. J. Am. Vet. Med. Assoc. 183, 1195–1197.

Tkach, V.V., Lisitsyna, O.I., Crossley, J.L., Binh, T.T., Bush, S.E., 2013. Morphological and molecular differentiation of two new species of *Pseudoacanthocephalus Petrochenko*, 1958 (Acanthocephala: Echinorhynchidae) from amphibians and reptiles in the Philippines, with identification key for the genus. Syst. Parasitol. 85, 11–26.

Tollis, M., Boissinot, S., 2014. Genetic variation in the green anole lizard (*Anolis carolinensis*) reveals island refugia and a fragmented Florida during the quaternary. Genetica 142, 59–72.

Tosini, G., Avery, R.A., 1996. Dermal photoreceptors regulate basking behavior in the lizard *Podarcis muralis*. Physiol. Behav. 59, 195–198.

Van Der Merwe, N.J., Kotze, S.H., 1993. The topography of the thoracic and abdominal organs of the Nile crocodile (*Crocodylus niloticus*). Onderstepoort J. Vet. Res. 60, 219–222.

Van Waeyenberghe, L., Baert, K., Pasmans, F., van Rooij, P., Hellebuyck, T., Beernaert, L., et al., 2010. Voriconazole, a safe alternative for treating infections caused by the *Chrysosporium anamorph* of Nannizziopsis vriesii in bearded dragons (*Pogona vitticeps*). Med. Mycol. 48, 880–885.

Vieler, E., Baumgärtner, W., Herbst, W., Köhler, G., 1999. Characterization of a reovirus isolate from a rattle snake, Crotalus viridis, with neurological dysfunction. Arch. Virol. 138, 341–344.

Vitt, L.J., Caldwell, J.P., 2009. Herpetology: An Introductory Biology of Amphibians and Reptiles. Elsevier, London.

Wallace, R., Michaels, M., Foskett, H., Maslow, E.A., Kiehlbauch, J.A., 2002. Outbreak of *Mycobacterium marinum* infection among captive snakes and bullfrogs. Zoo Biol. 21 (3), 233–241.

Wasser, J.S., Guthrie, S.S., Chari, M., 1997. *In vitro* tolerance to anoxia and ischemia in isolated hearts from hypoxia sensitive and hypoxia tolerant turtles. Comp. Biochem. Physiol. 118A, 1359–1370.

Wassersug, R., Izumi-Kurotani, A., 1993. The behavioral reactions of a snake and a turtle to abrupt decreases in gravity. Zoolog. Sci. 10, 505–509.

Weber, D.J., Barbee, S.L., Sobsey, M.D., Rutala, W.A., 1999. The effect of blood on the antiviral activity of sodium hypochlorite, a phenolic, and a quaternary ammonium compound. Infect. Control. Hosp. Epidemiol. 20, 821–827.

Weiss, S.L., Mulligan, E.E., Wilson, D.S., Kabelik, D., 2013. Effect of stress on female-specific ornamentation. J. Exp. Biol. 216, 2641–2647.

Wellehan, J.F., Johnson, A.J., Latimer, K.S., Whiteside, D.P., Crawshaw, G.J., Detrisac, C.J., et al., 2004. Varanid herpesvirus 1: a novel herpesvirus associated with proliferative stomatitis in green tree monitors (*Varanus prasinus*). Vet. Microbiol. 31, 83–92.

Wendland, L.D., Wooding, J., White, C.L., Demcovitz, D., Littell, R., Berish, J.D., et al., 2010. Social behavior drives the dynamics of respiratory disease in threatened tortoises. Ecology 91, 1257–1262.

Westfall, M.E., Demcovitz, D.L., Plourdé, D.R., Rotstein, D.S., Brown, D.R., 2006. *In vitro* antibiotic susceptibility of Mycoplasma iguanae proposed sp. nov. isolated from vertebral lesions of green iguanas (*Iguana iguana*). J. Zoo Wildl. Med. 37, 206–208.

Williams, S.R., Sims, M.A., Roth-Johnson, L., Wickes, B., 2012. Surgical removal of an abscess associated with Fusarium solani from a Kemp's ridley sea turtle (*Lepidochelys kempii*). J. Zoo Wildl. Med. 43, 402–406.

Wimsatt, J., Tothill, A., Offermann, C.F., Sheehy, J.G., Peloquin, C.A., 2008. Long-term and per rectum disposition of Clarithromycin in the desert tortoise (*Gopherus agassizii*). J. Am. Assoc. Lab. Anim. Sci. 47, 41–45.

Winston, G.W., Kirchin, M.A., Ronis, M.J.J., 1991. Microsomal activation of benzo[a]pyrene by *Alligator mississippiensis*: mechanisms, mutagenicity, and induction. Biochem. Soc. Trans. 19, 746–750.

Wu, P., Wu, X., Jiang, T.X., Elsey, R.M., Temple, B.L., Divers, S.J., et al., 2013. Specialized stem cell niche enables repetitive renewal of alligator teeth. Proc. Natl. Acad. Sci. 110, E2009–E2018.

Wyneken, J., 2014. Computed tomography and magnetic resonance imaging. In: Maders, D.R., Divers, S.J. (Eds.), Current Therapy in Reptile Medicine and Surgery. Saunders, St. Louis, MO, pp. 93–106.

Young, B.A., Sheft, S., Yost, W., 1995. Sound production in *Pituophis melanoleucus* (Serpentes: Colubridae) with the first description of a vocal cord in snakes. J. Exp. Zool. 273, 472–481.

Zardoya, R., Meyer, A., 2001. The evolutionary position of turtles revised. Naturwissenschaften 88, 193–200.

Zhang, Y., Westfall, M.C., Hermes, K.C., Dorcas, M.E., 2008. Physiological and behavioral control of heating and cooling rates in rubber boas, *Charina bottae*. J. Thermal. Biol. 33, 7–11.

Zug, G.R., 1993. Herpetology: An Introductory Biology of Amphibians and Reptiles. Academic Press, San Diego, CA.

CHAPTER

20

The Biology and Management of the Zebrafish

Michael Y. Esmail, VMD[a], Keith M. Astrofsky, DVM[b],
Christian Lawrence, MS[c] and Fabrizio C. Serluca, PhD[b]

[a]Division of Comparative Medicine, Massachusetts Institute of Technology, Cambridge, MA, USA
[b]Novartis Institutes for Biomedical Research, Cambridge, MA, USA [c]Aquatic Resources Program, Boston Children's Hospital, Boston, USA

OUTLINE

Laboratory Animal Medicine, Third Edition
DOI: http://dx.doi.org/10.1016/B978-0-12-409527-4.00020-1

1015

I. INTRODUCTION

A. Background

The zebrafish, *Danio rerio* (also referred to in the literature as *Brachydanio rerio* and the zebra danio), is currently emerging as an increasingly popular model of vertebrate embryonic development, gene function analysis, and mutagenesis (Fig. 20.1). Prior to the development of the zebrafish model in the 1970s, developmental geneticists relied on invertebrate models such as *Drosophila melanogaster* (fruit fly) and, more recently, *Caenorhabditis elegans* (nematode) for the investigation of early embryonic development. The prolific reproductive capacity of *Drosophila* and successful manipulation of its embryos combined to make embryo development and genetic analysis more practical in the laboratory. However, the application of this information to vertebrate embryonic development was limited. Since mouse embryos develop within an uterus and the African Clawed Frog (*Xenopus laevis)* has a slow reproductive capacity, neither of these more popular vertebrate models possess the characteristics that made *Drosophila* such a practical model (Kahn, 1994). Because of its high fecundity and external fertilization, the zebrafish possessed the attributes of these existing models without their inherent drawbacks.

Because the fundamental molecular mechanisms of embryonic development are similar for all vertebrates, the zebrafish has gradually become the lower vertebrate model of choice. Mutagenesis screens allow researchers to investigate uncharted areas of the genome without prior knowledge of the function of specific genes. Mice are utilized in more conventional laboratory techniques where knockout mutations of known genes of interest are created in order to study the effect of the gene in the resultant phenotype. Through the creation of mutant phenotypes via chemical mutagenesis, the functions of many genes associated with pigmentation, muscular, cardiovascular, and central nervous system development have been investigated extensively (Driever *et al.*, 1994; Postlethwait and Talbot, 1997).

In the early 1970s, George Streisinger (University of Oregon), a phage geneticist, identified the zebrafish as a vertebrate model to isolate mutations in genetic screens using systematic mutagenesis protocols. This line of work has been continued at the University of Oregon by several laboratories including that of Charles Kimmel who has also contributed much of the information involving the staging of early zebrafish embryo development. By the early 1990s, two laboratories (Christiane Nusslein-Volhard of the Max Planck Institute for Developmental Biology and Wolfgang Driever of Massachusetts General Hospital) began applying 'saturation mutagenesis' screens to identify mutant phenotypes in zebrafish (Kahn, 1994). Using this methodology, adult male zebrafish were treated with a chemical mutagen and the F3 generation was examined for developmental abnormalities. By observing mutant phenotypes in large numbers of developing zebrafish, the function of various disrupted genes could be identified. By 1996, these screens had produced over 2000 mutations in several hundred genes that are necessary for normal embryonic development (Driever *et al.*, 1996; Haffter *et al.*, 1996). In 1994, John Postlethwait (University of Oregon) published the first genetic map that identified approximately 400 markers in 29 linkage groups. By 1996, the genetic map had already grown to incorporate approximately 1200 markers (Postlethwait and Talbot, 1997).

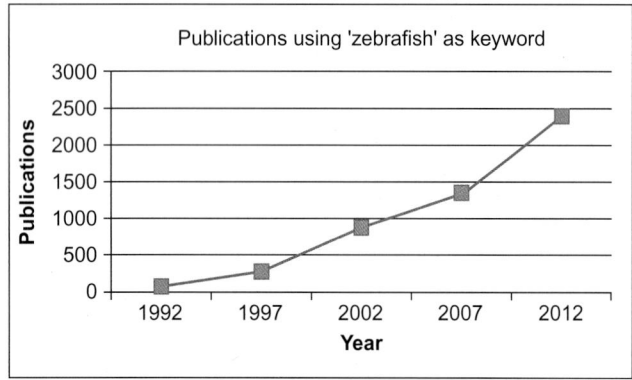

FIGURE 20.1 The zebrafish is a small vertebrate genetic model system which is rapidly gaining in popularity. Shown here are the number of publications in PubMed using 'zebrafish' as a keyword for the given year.

B. Natural History

The zebrafish is a freshwater species native to southern Asia and is widely distributed in freshwater habitats across much of India, Bangladesh, and lowland Nepal (Hamilton-Buchanan, 1822; Spence *et al.*, 2006; Engeszer *et al.*, 2007; Arunachalam *et al.*, 2013). The zebrafish is a member of the family Cyprinidae that includes the danios and barbs (Spence *et al.*, 2008). Adults are sexually dimorphic, with the females being slightly larger, more silvery, and slightly rounded. Adults usually do not exceed 3–4 cm in length. Males are more streamlined and usually more brightly colored than females. Healthy adults are usually a silver or gold (less common) tone with several bright blue/purple horizontal stripes extending from the operculum to the base of the caudal fin. Similarly colored stripes are frequently repeated on both the anal and dorsal fins. Dorsally, a dark yellowish-brown to olive tone is evident from the head to the caudal fin. The ventrum is usually a homogeneous, yellow–white tone. Two pairs of barbels are present on the lower jaw.

Selective breeding by the aquarium trade has produced a number of varieties including the veil-finned and the long-fin variants. Zebrafish are very active swimmers occupying the upper strata of the water column. They are omnivorous and have proven to be quite hardy and prolific breeders in captivity. Through good nutrition and by manipulation of the light–dark cycle, females can be readily induced to spawn in the laboratory. After a period of total darkness, the initial appearance of light and persistent rubbing of the female by the male induces the female to spawn into an egg collection chamber placed at the bottom of the containment unit. After inducing the female to spawn through tactile behavior, the males promptly fertilize the eggs. Egg collection devices or rows of glass beads and marbles placed at the bottom of the unit are necessary to prevent the adults from consuming their own fertilized eggs prior to collection. Improved understanding of zebrafish breeding behavior has led to the recent development of specialized spawning tanks that allow for the relatively facile collection of thousands of fertilized embryos within a period of minutes. For a more complete description of reproductive biology and behavior, see Spence *et al.* (2008).

II. ZEBRAFISH: THE EXPERIMENTAL MODEL IN BIOMEDICAL RESEARCH

A. Zebrafish as a Model System

1. Historical Perspective

The era of the zebrafish as a genetic model organism began with the pioneering work of George Streisinger and the production of homozygous diploid clones (Streisinger *et al.*, 1981). Methods for mutagenesis were subsequently developed using gamma ray irradiation as the mutagen. These mutagenesis protocols gave rise to the first series of experimentally induced mutations in the zebrafish (Walker and Streisinger, 1983). Mutations such as *no tail* (*ntl*) where embryos fail to develop a proper notochord and caudal structures, *spadetail* (*spt*) where mesodermal cells fail to gastrulate properly and *cyclops*, which prevents the formation of the floorplate in the neural tube, were all identified early on using these methods (Halpern *et al.*, 1993; Kimmel *et al.*, 1989; Hatta *et al.*, 1991). The early discovery that the *ntl* mutation (Fig. 20.2) disrupted a zebrafish ortholog of the mouse *brachyury* (*T*) gene provided evidence that homologous genes perform common functions and that discoveries made in the zebrafish could be translated to other vertebrate model systems including mammals (Schulte-Merker *et al.*, 1994).

More efficient mutagenesis protocols were later developed which used *N*-ethyl-*N*-nitrosourea (ENU) as a chemical mutagen (Mullins *et al.*, 1994). This method enabled the first large-scale genetic screens in zebrafish at the Max Planck Institute in Tuebingen, Germany, and Massachusetts General Hospital in Boston, Massachusetts (Driever *et al.*, 1996; Haffter *et al.*, 1996). The three-generation screen carried out provided researchers with over 2000 mutations, mostly recessive lethals, with clear embryonic development phenotypes. This endeavor proved to be a successful proof of concept

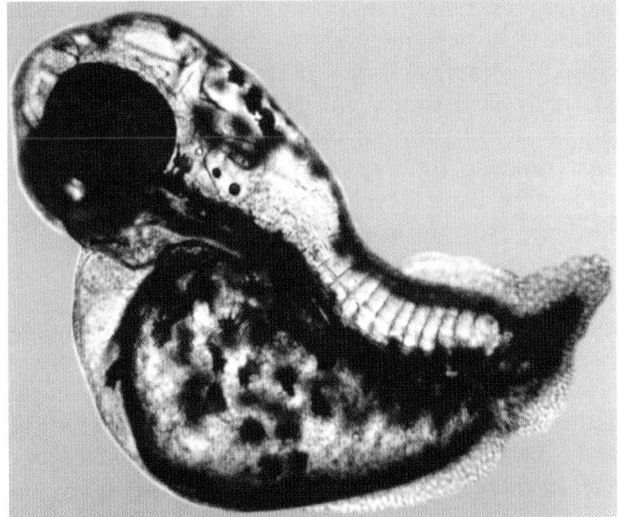

FIGURE 20.2 A mutant *no tail* (*ntl*) embryo at 2 days of development. Note the lack of tail structures caudal to the yolk and the compacted somatic muscle segments in the trunk. The *ntl* mutation was one of the first mutants isolated from large scale screens and was found to encode the zebrafish ortholog of the mouse *brachyury* (*T*) gene, providing evidence that discoveries made in zebrafish could be translated to other vertebrates. *Courtesy of Halpern Laboratory, Carnegie Institution for Science.*

as many other screens have been carried out in numerous laboratories since then. Mutations were identified that perturbed several aspects of embryonic development from the early steps of blastomere cleavage to the specific formation of an organ. The development of genetic mapping techniques enabled researchers to identify the precise molecular lesions in many of the mutations discovered in those original screens and beyond. With the establishment of newer more efficient methods, it is now possible to identify the mutations very quickly.

While much of the early work on the zebrafish as a model system focused on embryonic development, it is clear that this model system can be used to study other types of biology, including physiological phenomena such as diabetes and innate behaviors such as shoaling and schooling (Miller and Gerlai, 2012; Moss *et al.*, 2013).

2. Characteristics Making the Zebrafish an Attractive Model Organism

The zebrafish's small adult size permits large numbers of animals to be housed in less space than other vertebrate models. The maintenance requirements for a facility are relatively simple and automated systems exist for both life support and feeding of the zebrafish. Breeding adults can produce up to 200 or more fertilized eggs from single spawnings at weekly intervals. The large clutch size aids in the genetic mapping of mutations as more meiotic events yield greater resolution near the genetic lesion. Embryological approaches also benefit from the large clutch size as many phenotypic analyses resulting from an embryological manipulation require statistical methods to determine significance. Early developing embryos are transparent and develop externally in a simple salt solution facilitating observations of cell movements, organ development, and organ function. Embryos acquire a 'fishlike' appearance after only 24h of development as they have specified all three axes (rostro-caudal, dorso-ventral and left-right), possess a patterned rudimentary neural tube and eyes, and can be seen to twitch spontaneously. Pigment cells begin to develop shortly after this period and can obscure small local regions of the embryos. However, the zebrafish retain an overall transparent appearance as cardiac function and blood flow as well as gut motility can be directly observed using simple stereomicroscopes even in these later stages. Furthermore, there are now genetic strains of zebrafish that are completely transparent throughout their entire life span (White *et al.*, 2008). External development of the zebrafish embryo allows the researcher access to early stages not easily observable in vertebrates that develop *in utero*. Thus, manipulating development by introduction of genetic material such as DNA or RNA and gene knockdown reagents such as Morpholinos and chemical compounds is relatively easy

in this vertebrate. Indeed the small size of the zebrafish embryo as well as its external development make it ideally suited for medium- or high-throughput chemical screens as embryos can easily fit into the well of a 96- or 384-well plate and compound dosing by immersion can be partially automated.

3. Brief Overview of Zebrafish Development

After fertilization, the zebrafish embryo undergoes a series of rapid cleavages. At 28.5°C (the standard temperature for zebrafish maintenance) the first cleavage occurs 45 minutes after fertilization and the subsequent eight cleavages take place at regular 15-minute intervals. After the ninth cleavage, the cell cycle begins to lengthen and cell divisions become asynchronous. This marks the onset of the midblastula transition (MBT) at about 3 hours post-fertilization (hpf). One important aspect of the MBT is the activation of zygotic transcription; all processes taking place up to this point are regulated by maternal factors deposited in the egg. Gastrulation, the process whereby the three germlayers (endoderm, mesoderm, and ectoderm) take up their final positions in the embryo, begins after about 5.5hpf and is complete at 10hpf. Since the early cleavages do not bisect the yolk, the embryo proper sits as a ball of cells on top of the yolk until about 4.5hpf when the embryonic cells begin to spread down over the yolk. This process, termed epiboly, is also completed at 10hpf. During the period between 10 and 24hpf, the internal organs begin to form and morphological landmarks that preview adult structures become detectable. Over the next several days, the embryo continues to grow and internal organs complete their development. Embryos hatch from their chorions on day 3 or 4 and begin to feed shortly thereafter on day 4 or 5 (Kimmel *et al.*, 1995).

4. The Zebrafish as a Model for Human Disease

a. Cancer Models

The zebrafish has long been used as a model for evaluating the carcinogenicity of chemical agents (Pliss and Khudoley, 1975). Exposure to the commonly used mutagen ENU also induces tumors in zebrafish, mostly epidermal papillomas (Beckwith *et al.*, 2000). While the applications of carcinogens may well induce tumors, the tumor type and its state are variable. In an effort to directly model particular types of cancer, more recent studies have taken advantage of genetic causes to develop specific gain-of-function transgenic models. The underlying hypothesis of these models is that perturbation of the oncogenic pathway in the zebrafish will recapitulate certain molecular and cellular aspects of the tumors seen in humans. The oncogenic potential of the *c-myc* gene has been recognized for some time and its role in the development and progression of leukemias has been extensively reported upon. In order to create a zebrafish model, the *c-myc* oncogene was expressed in the zebrafish thymus using the *rag2* promoter. These transgenic animals develop T-cell acute lymphoblastic leukemia sharing several clinical features with the human disease (Langenau *et al.*, 2003).

Other groups have coupled genetic cancer models with one of the zebrafish's key attributes: its amenability to chemical screening. Yeh and colleagues developed an acute myelogenous leukemia (AML) model by creating a transgenic fish carrying the gene fusion product of the *AML1-ETO* translocation (Yeh *et al.*, 2008). This translocation is often seen in patients with AML and results in the *AML1* gene, important in hematopoiesis, being fused to the *ETO* gene involved in regulating gene regulation via its association with chromatin remodeling factors. The ectopic expression of this gene results in transgenic fish sharing several histopathological features with the human disease including a massive expansion of the myeloid lineage. As the zebrafish is particularly amenable to chemical screening, a screen for suppressors of the AML phenotype in zebrafish identified several compounds capable of suppressing or preventing the lymphoma-like state and these compounds pointed to prostaglandin E (PGE) and β-catenin signaling as key therapeutic nodes (Yeh *et al.*, 2009). These types of suppressor screens in zebrafish disease models may prove valuable in designing effective therapies for human patients.

Mutations in the *BRAF* gene, a signal transduction serine/thronine kinase, are strongly associated with melanomas (Davies *et al.*, 2002). A melanoma model in zebrafish was developed by expressing an oncogenic form of *BRAF*, often found in malignant melanomas (Fig. 20.3), in zebrafish melanocytes using the *mitfa* promoter (Patton *et al.*, 2005). This ectopic expression leads to a proliferation of melanocytes and the formation of nevi. When the animal model is coupled with a loss of function allele of the tumor suppressor gene *p53*, invasive melanomas which could be serially transplanted were observed in adult zebrafish.

Wild-type   *mitfa-BRAF;p53⁻/⁻*

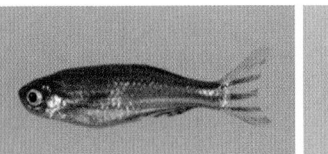 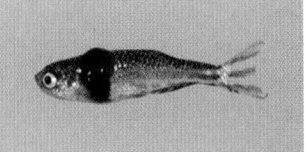

FIGURE 20.3   Melanoma models in zebrafish. Driving expression of an oncogenic form of *BRAF* (*BRAFV600E*) in melanocytes using the *mitfa* promoter in a *p53*-deficient genetic background is sufficient to drive melanomas in adult zebrafish. *Courtesy of Zon Laboratory, Children's Hospital, Boston, MA.*

b. Muscular Dystrophy Models

Many genes associated with disease in humans can give rise to similar abnormalities in zebrafish when mutated. These mutant zebrafish serve as a model for the disease and aid in deciphering disease mechanisms. Mutations in the zebrafish ortholog of the Duchenne muscular dystrophy (DMD) gene dystrophin lead to a progressive degeneration of muscle fibers (Bassett *et al.*, 2003). These animals display necrotic fibers, an inflammatory response with mono-nucleated cellular infiltrates and extensive fibrosis. A chemical screen for modulators of the DMD phenotype identified several candidates as potential suppressors of the phenotype (Kawahara *et al.*, 2011). One candidate in particular, aminophylline, implicated cyclic adenosine monophosphate (cAMP) signaling in disease progression and suggested phosphodiesterases as a therapeutic target. Screening drugs with known mechanisms of action provide the benefit of identifying key molecular pathways being affected by the drug and aids in the formulation of a therapeutic hypothesis.

c. Tissue Regeneration

Zebrafish have a great capacity for the regeneration of several tissues (recently reviewed in Gemberling *et al.*, 2013) and have served to identify new mechanisms for regeneration which may prove useful in mammals. The most well-studied regenerative process in zebrafish is that in fin regeneration. The distal part of the fin can be amputated and will regenerate over a 10–12-day period (Akimenko *et al.*, 1995). Within 1 or 2 days of the amputation, a regenerative blastema forms at the injury site and begins to proliferate. While these cells are morphologically similar, a fully patterned fin with fin rays, blood vessels, and connective tissue emerges at the end of the process, the patterning information being conserved throughout the process. More dramatic regeneration can be seen in the case of the zebrafish heart. Here, surgical resection of the distal (ventricular) apex of the adult heart leads to successive phases of cellular proliferation, cardiomyocyte and endothelial differentiation, and finally electrical coupling of the regenerated heart tissue (Poss *et al.*, 2002). It is interesting to note that not all methods of injury give rise to the same regenerative response. Genetic ablation of cardiac cells for example leads to a heart failure (HF)-like state but the heart eventually regenerates and the animals recover (Wang *et al.*, 2011).

Many other tissues are known to regenerate in the zebrafish, including retina, spinal cord, and kidney. One cell type that also possesses an intrinsic capacity for regeneration is the hair cell. Hair cells can be found in the ear and their depletion in older humans can cause gradual hearing loss. The apical surfaces of hair cells possess stereocilia, a high specialized structure capable of detecting sound vibrations. Hair cells can be found in zebrafish in the ear as well as the lateral line, a sensory organ along the rostro-caudal axis. Treatment of zebrafish larvae with high doses of neomycin, a known ototoxic agent, causes the loss of hair cells which can be regenerated within a period of two days (Harris et al., 2003). Research groups have taken advantage of this and carried out both chemical and genetic screens for agents that can prevent or suppress the damage caused by the antibiotic (Owens et al., 2008).

B. Commonly Used Experimental Methods

1. Genetic Methods

Genetic screens are an unbiased method for the identification of novel genes involved in a biological event. No assumptions need to be made with respect to a gene's mechanism of action, its localization of expression, nor its timing of expression. Early mutagenesis protocols utilized radiation to induce large-scale chromosomal rearrangements such as deletions, inversions, or translocations in the genome. More subtle changes, such as individual nucleotide point mutations or small (1- to 2-nucleotide) deletions can be induced by ENU. In this case, mutagenesis is accomplished by immersing adult male zebrafish in a solution of ENU for short periods of time for several days with 3- to 4-day recuperation periods in between each treatment (Solnica-Krezel et al., 1994). The mutations become fixed in the germline of the mutagenized males after several weeks and these are then used to generate the F1 generation which carry unique individual mutational events. The large-scale mutagenesis screens in the 1990s used a two-generation breeding approach with phenotypic scoring carried out in the third (embryonic F3) generation (Driever et al., 1996; Haffter et al., 1996).

Alternative screening approaches take advantage of parthenogenesis, which can be experimentally induced in zebrafish. In the haploid method, eggs from an F1 female are collected and fertilized in vitro with ultraviolet (UV)-irradiated sperm that cannot contribute any genetic material. The resulting F2 embryos develop from the maternal genetic component only and are thus haploid. The haploids' condition is eventually lethal with many embryos developing circulatory problems; however, screening for phenotypes affecting early embryonic decisions is possible. These haploid embryos can be made diploid through the use of either early pressure (EP) or heat shock (HS) to prevent chromosomal separation during the second meiotic division or first mitotic division, respectively.

The discovery of the precise genetic lesions that underlie each of the ENU phenotypes was aided by the resources made available shortly after the publication of the large-scale screens. Because the molecular changes

induced by ENU are subtle, finding the exact location of the mutation only became possible for the large number of mutants with the introduction of high-resolution genetic maps (Knapik et al., 1998). The zebrafish genome sequencing effort led by the Sanger Centre released its first draft (Zv1) in 2002. As of 2014, the current assembly is Zv9 and a reference genome containing over 26,000 protein-coding genes and over 6000 noncoding (RNA) genes has been published and made available to the zebrafish community (http://www.ensembl.org/Danio_rerio/Info/Index) (Howe et al., 2013).

Other viral-based mutageneis methods were also being developed contemporaneously (Lin et al., 1994). In this case, a viral genome would be randomly integrated into the zebrafish genome disrupting gene function. This is accomplished by directly microinjecting a pseudo-typed retrovirus into blastula-stage zebrafish embryos to create mosaic animals. As with the ENU protocol, breeding these animals to the F1 generation results in nonmosaic progeny that transmit the retroviral DNA in a mendelian fashion. Identification of the genetic lesion in this case is simplified as the viral DNA also functions as a 'tag' allowing the precise localization of the integration site and the identification of the affected gene.

2. Embryological Methods

As zebrafish develop externally, all embryonic stages are readily accessed by the researcher. As such it is an attractive model to study cell lineage and cell fate. Initially, techniques developed for use in amphibian embryology were adapted for use in zebrafish. Individual cells can be marked with a dye and observed throughout development to determine what cell type(s) arise from marked progenitors (Shih and Fraser, 1995). The marking of cells can also be accomplished through the use of caged fluorescent dyes and a laser. In this case, the caged dye is injected into early fertilized embryos alleviating the need for precise single blastomere microinjections. At the desired developmental stage, a laser can be used to uncage the dye rendering it fluorescent in a particular cell or group of cells (Serluca and Fishman, 2001). This tracer can be followed throughout the rest of development to create a fate map. Lasers can also be used to selectively ablate clusters of cells in a method adapted from C. elegans. This strategy proved useful in establishing the limits of particular organ fields such as the heart or kidney (Chan et al., 2001; Serbedzija et al., 1998).

Determining whether a particular mutation or a gene product functions within the affected cell (cell-autonomous) or if it can affect cells at a distance (cell-non-autonomous) can also be addressed using the cell transplantation techniques in zebrafish. Cells taken from blastula-stage embryos of a particular mutant genotype can be removed using aspiration with a glass capillary pipette and reintroduced into a second blastula-stage embryo of another genotype (Ho and Kane, 1990). Cell-transplantation can also be used in determining the role of one tissue on the development or patterning of another by using mutant strains that lack the original tissue source. The notochord, e.g., plays a key role in inducing neighboring cells to adopt the endothelial cell fate (Fouquet *et al.*, 1997). This technique is not limited to early embryonic stages as others have successfully transplanted primary motoneurons from one area of the spical cord to another (Eisen, 1991).

3. Transgenic and Molecular Methods

The study of gene function is typically accomplished by using gain-of-function and loss-of-function approaches. In the zebrafish, direct microinjection of either DNA or mRNA encoding a protein is easily accomplished at the one- to two-cell stage. Fertilized embryos are viewed under a stereomicroscope and the injection is accomplished using glass capillary needles and a standard micromanipulator. If desired, a tracer molecule such as a rhodamine dye or mRNA encoding green fluorescent protein (GFP) can be coinjected to monitor both injection efficiency and any dose-responsive component to the assay. The RNA injection approach is especially valuable if the gene in question acts very early in development prior to the onset embryonic transcription, but as the injected amounts are relatively small (in the nanoliter range), there can be variability in the dose injected from one individual to another.

Early transgenesis methods that relied on the random integration of microinjected DNA were plagued by low founder rates and gene silencing in later generations. The switch to a transposable element-based method provided a viable solution. The development of these transgenesis tools made use of the Tol2 transposon, originally from the medaka fish (*Oryzias latipes*). The modified transposon allows the introduction of a specific gene of interest and is coinjected with mRNA encoding the transposase enzyme that facilitates its integration into the genomic host DNA. The Tol2 method allows founder rates as high as 50% (Kawakami *et al.*, 2000; Kawakami, 2004). Use of a similar strategy has been used to generate enhancer trap lines where expression of a gene can be assayed through the use of a fluorescent reporter gene (Kawakami *et al.*, 2004).

Using stable transgenic lines instead of direct microinjection offers a number of advantages including less labor (as no microinjection step is required) and more uniform expression of the transgene as there is no variability in the copy number of the transgene.

While transgenesis methods provide a means to determine gene gain-of-function effects, the loss-of-function effect can be elucidated through the use of Morpholino antisense oligonucleotides (reviewed in Eisen and Smith, (2008)).

These antisense oligonucleotides are stable and can direct the knockdown of a particular gene by disrupting protein translation of transcriptional splicing. Antisense oligonucleotides allow the study of a particular gene for loss-of-function effects without the need of having a random ENU or retroviral allele. As these are directly microinjected into fertilized embryos, the Morpholino is diluted with every cell division resulting in potentially weaker knockdown efficiencies in later stage larvae.

4. Next-Generation Sequencing

The development of next-generation sequencing (NGS) technologies has allowed significant shortening of the time from phenotype to gene, easing a significant bottleneck in the process. Traditional methods of identifying ENU-induced mutated genes relied on genetic mapping and testing single-gene candidates for the presence of a mutation in the genomic DNA. NGS-based strategies combine the mapping and gene identification into one process (Obholzer *et al.*, 2012). In this method, the complete genome of mutants and wild-type siblings, both typically pooled, is sequenced. Linkage to a particular chromosomal location is indicated by regions of homozygosity in the mutant samples compared to the wild-type, where we would normally expect a random distribution at unlinked loci. The mapping of specific NGS reads onto the zebrafish reference genome allows the precise identification of candidate mutations once common polymorphisms have been filtered out and these can be tested and validated experimentally.

5. Genome Editing

Targeted mutation of particular genes has been a challenge. Embryonic stem cell technology as it is used in the creation of knockout mice has not been fruitful for the zebrafish system thus far. Recent advances in genomic editing techniques have allowed precise targeting of genes using a fusion protein consisting of a DNA recognition moiety and an endonuclease. In the case of zinc-finger nucleases (ZFNs), the DNA motif recognition is achieved using tandem zinc fingers selected to recognize a particular sequence (Doyon *et al.*, 2008). In a second method, the DNA editing is accomplished using transcription activator-like effector nucleases (TALENs) which are more flexible in the DNA motifs it can recognize (Cade *et al.*, 2012).

In both cases, however, each targeting event requires its own ZFN or TALEN protein to achieve modification of the genome. Recently, new methods using an RNA-guided endonuclease for genomic editing have proven to be successful (Hwang *et al.*, 2013a). The Clustered Regularly Interspaced Short Palindromic Repeats (CRISPR) method relies on the cas9 endonuclease from *Streptococcus pyogenes* (reviewed in Wiedenheft *et al.* (2012)) which uses an RNA molecule containing a 20-nucleotide guide sequence directing the endonuclease enzymatic activity to a stretch of DNA complementary to the sequence of the guide RNA (gRNA). The enzymatic activity of the endonuclease creates a DNA break which is repaired, often with errors leading to short insertion–deletion (indel) mutations. There is no need to design a specific nuclease fusion protein for each targeting event as with ZFNs and TALENs, specificity is achieved using RNA, while the nuclease component remains constant. The protocol is relatively straight forward: zebrafish embryos at the one- to four-cell stage are injected with the cas9/gRNA combination resulting in animals that are mosaic at the particular target locus. Breeding of these animals produces F1 animals heterozygous for the targeted modification and can transmit this change through to the next generation (Hwang *et al.*, 2013b). With the advent of this technology, it is estimated that nearly every protein coding gene can be targeted.

III. SIGNIFICANCES OF HEALTHY MANAGEMENT IN THE AQUATIC ANIMAL FACILITY

A. Health of the Aquatic Animal Model

Proper animal health will ensure vigorous animals, maximize reproductive yield, and minimize animal loss due to disease. Health is dependent not only on proper nutrition and animal selection, but also on proper water quality, water system/life support maintenance, and water system design. By operating closely monitored, well maintained water systems and implementing a preventive medicine program, fish hygiene can be maintained at a high level. This management approach will minimize losses in valuable animals, research time, and money due to water system failure or infectious disease (DeTolla *et al.*, 1995).

Unexpected loss of valuable aquatic research animals due to disease is one of the most common causes of research frustration when using aquatic animal models. Whether these losses occur due to slow, insidious mortality or by sudden, catastrophic loss due to an unexplained epizootic or life support system failure, diseases of aquatic animal models have adversely influenced the validity of statistics, confounded results, and disrupted research schedules. Preventative medicine programs tailored to the aquatic animal have as much validity in the modern zebrafish facility as these programs do in a rodent facility.

B. Host–Pathogen–Environment Interaction

Infection is always the result of a complex interaction of host, environment, and pathogen. All three factors may be out of balance in the highly artificial world of aquatic laboratory culture facilities. A primary goal of the aquatic animal manager is to maintain the aquatic system in a balanced state where host and potential pathogens coexist in the controlled laboratory environment (Fig. 20.4).

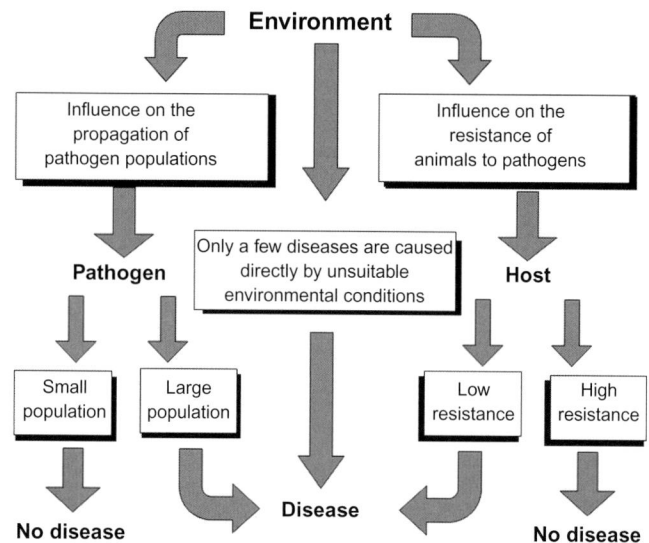

FIGURE 20.4 Host–pathogen–interaction diagram. The aquatic ecosystem maintains a delicate balance between fish, potential pathogens, and environmental parameters. While relatively few diseases are the direct result of environmental imbalances (e.g., temperature shock, gas bubble disease), the environment has a direct influence on potential pathogen populations and the host's resistance to disease (e.g., immunosuppression).

Because aquatic systems are very complex ecosystems, pathogen–host relationships are difficult to access in the artificial laboratory environment. Consequently, controlling disease outbreaks can be a difficult endeavor. Since primary pathogens can induce disease when other environmental factors are balanced, they must be distinguished from secondary or opportunistic pathogens that cause disease when other metabolic or environmental factors are suboptimal. Poor health is often a reflection of one or more marginal environmental variables such as improper temperature, pH, hardness/alkalinity, other water chemistry, nutrition, overstocking, biofouling, or bacterial overgrowth. Disease within the aquatic environment usually results when stresses within a marginal environment tip balance in favor of the pathogen.

Disease diagnosis can be viewed as the recognition of imbalance within the system. Prevention acts as a buffer to extend the limits of the balanced system. The aim of treatment is to restore balance to a disrupted system. Proper health management and disease control depend on effective implementation of all the above-mentioned laboratory practices: preventive medicine, diagnosis, and treatment.

C. Research Zebrafish Welfare

The vast majority of the efforts to care for research fish are dedicated to providing optimal environmental conditions, which mitigate stress, reduce research variability, and enhance welfare. Smith (2014) reviews aspects of and summarizes how laboratory fish welfare can be optimized in the zebrafish research environment: "1. Provide a balanced environment and social grouping that match as closely as possible those that the species favors in the wild…; 2. Maintaining high standards of management and care, including appropriate water quality parameters for the species; 3. Avoiding unnecessary, repetitive, or insensitive handling or restraint; 4. Using sedation or anesthesia for any potentially stressful situations, painful procedures, or activities that require prolonged restraint" (modified from Cooper (2004)). A well-run research zebrafish facility will address and assess these factors continuously, especially given that much is still unknown about the species-specific requirements for raising research zebrafish and the inherent difficultly in determining what may be painful, stressful, and distressful. Two factors are briefly covered here, but additional information regarding others can be found in this chapter and is reviewed in Smith (2014).

1. Social Housing

In the wild and captivity, the zebrafish is a shoaling species that typically prefers to associate in groups of varying size (Pritchard *et al.*, 2001; Wright *et al.*, 2003; Spence *et al.*, 2008; Engeszer *et al.*, 2007; Blaser and Gerlai, 2006). For captive zebrafish, the group size per unit area, otherwise known as housing density, has a profound impact on their social welfare. Density mediates many common behaviors (Harper and Lawrence, 2010). Zebrafish are territorial and readily establish dominance hierarchies that are mediated via various forms of aggression (chasing, biting, etc.) (Spence *et al.*, 2008). Fish engaging in these interactions tend to show increased cortisol levels, and growth and reproductive output may be decreased, especially in subordinate fish (Filby *et al.*, 2010; Pavlidis *et al.*, 2011, 2013). The frequency and intensity of these territorial behaviors is inversely correlated with density (Harper and Lawrence, 2010). Aggression is highest at low densities. As tank densities increase and it becomes progressively more difficult for dominance hierarchies to be maintained, the frequency and intensity of aggression and territoriality decreases. If the number of animals per space unit continues to increase to the point where conditions become crowded, stress levels increase, and performance may be impacted (Ramsay *et al.*, 2006; Harper and Lawrence, 2010).

2. Balanced Environment

The use of enrichment in the zebrafish tank is currently not as pervasive as it is in other laboratory species. Research in this area is still in its infancy and will likely expand in years to come. When making husbandry decisions on enrichment, zebrafish facility managers and caretakers should consider performance driven reports demonstrating the purported benefits (e.g., less

aggression, enhanced learning) and costs (e.g., growth reduction) of adding enrichment devices to the zebrafish tank under various conditions. For example, many research zebrafish users commonly use an artificial material, such as plastic plants, to encourage breeding. This action is supported by data published in the scientific literature; female fish have been shown to prefer to oviposit in vegetated areas (Spence *et al.*, 2007, 2008). Plastic plant materials are also commonly used to reduce the effects of aggression in low-density housing situations. While this latter approach has not yet been formally evaluated, one can readily observe that subordinate fish will utilize the structure as refuge from dominant tank mates. Emerging studies in this area will serve to inform and strengthen such practices in the future.

Zebrafish welfare can be assessed by behavioral, performance, or physiologic metrics. Behavioral indicators are the most readily available indicator of welfare. Abnormal or maladaptive behaviors include tight/cohesive shoaling, frequent or constant aggression, erratic activity bursts, freezing, and bottom-dwelling. Normal behavior includes loose shoaling, infrequent aggression, moderate activity levels, and occupying the entire water column (Smith, 2014). Performance metrics of the zebrafish include body size/condition, fecundity, egg and embryo uniformity, growth and survival rates, and age at maturity (Castranova *et al.*, 2011; Filby *et al.*, 2010). Physiologic metrics used in zebrafish include circulating levels plasma cortisol, sex steroids, cytokine profiles, and gene expression (Smith, 2014; Filby *et al.*, 2010). It should be noted that as with other animal species, increased performance metrics do not always correlate with welfare.

IV. ENVIRONMENTAL FACTORS IMPORTANT TO ZEBRAFISH HEALTH

A. Temperature

Temperature is critically important to the survival, development, growth, and successful reproduction of zebrafish. When the water temperature is abruptly raised or lowered, zebrafish, as do most poikilotherms, show an internal shock reaction. The magnitude of this effect depends on the strain, its recent thermal history, and the magnitude of the temperature change. As a general rule, a change in temperature should be limited to ±1.5°C/day although many aquatic organisms can tolerate larger shifts in temperature quite well after an initial shock and a brief period of acclimation. Indeed, zebrafish are among the most eurythermal fish species on record, displaying an acclimated thermal tolerance of 6.7–41.7°C (Schaefer and Ryan, 2006; Cortemeglia and Beitinger, 2005). The following generalizations may be useful in developing good laboratory practices that promote health. The optimal temperature for growing and breeding laboratory zebrafish appears to be between 75 and 82°F (24–28°C). Alterations in temperature affect tolerance to other factors. Increased temperature (within the tolerance range) speeds up metabolism and increases oxygen demand. As a general rule, metabolic rate doubles for each 10°C increase in temperature. Larvae are usually less temperature tolerant than their respective adult forms. Maintenance of the life support system at slightly lower temperatures in the laboratory will increase the available oxygen, reduce the need for food, and minimize losses due to accidental increases in temperature. However, lower temperatures will decrease rate of growth and development. The limits of temperature tolerance are highly variable among populations and between seasons. Temperature change (usually temperature increases) is often a factor in the initiation of reproductive activity or other hormonal induced activity.

The temperature of the water system should be monitored and recorded daily by the placement of a probe or thermometer into each independent system. Small shifts in the temperature either above or below the optimal range are usually not detrimental. However, sudden, large shifts in environmental temperature can shock and quickly become a major problem and should be avoided.

The ambient room temperature should also be maintained at least one or two degrees above that of the containment system water. Room air at a temperature of approximately 78–81°F (24–27°C) helps to prevent condensation of water on the external surfaces of aquaria, walls, and floors. Condensation on these surfaces can serve as a medium for the growth of mold or fungi and negatively impact air quality. Room temperatures of greater than 80°F (27°C) are generally not recommended due to the cost of maintaining such a high temperature, lower dissolved oxygen saturation associated with warmer water, higher metabolic rates of the fish, and laboratory worker discomfort.

B. Dissolved Oxygen

In water, a fish will asphyxiate when the dissolved oxygen content drops below a critical level. This level is species and strain specific, subject to adaptation, and temperature dependent. When a fish is taken out of water, the gill lamellae clump together because they lack sufficient skeletal support necessary for living in terrestrial environments. Since this dramatically reduces the surface area available for oxygen diffusion, the fish will ultimately die of asphyxiation unless returned to the water. Therefore, the length of time out of water due to periodic sampling for experiments or when transferring

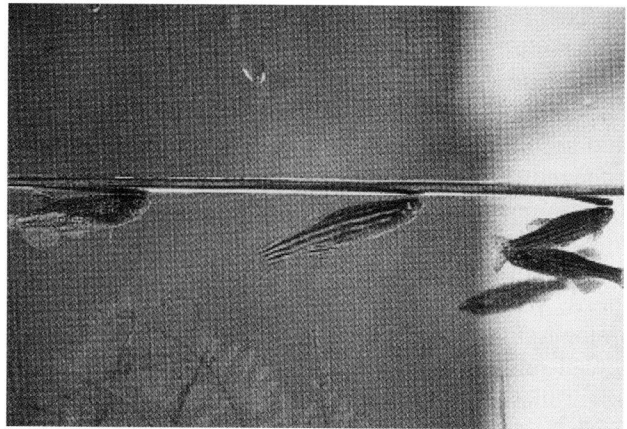

FIGURE 20.5 Zebrafish displaying abnormal surface breathing behavior due to low dissolved oxygen levels within the water. When low dissolved oxygen levels are present, fish will congregate in areas of highest saturation (e.g., air–water interface, water inflow ports). *Image courtesy of E. Scott Weber III.*

animals should be as brief as possible. Fish transfers should be done with water when possible.

Fish avoid areas where oxygen depletion develops. This can be an aid in the identification of oxygen deficient areas within water systems. Conversely, large numbers of fish gathered around aerators, air stones, or other points of air or water supply indicate serious oxygen depletion within the system. In the same manner, fish that appear to be 'gasping' or 'sipping' at the water surface also indicate oxygen deprivation (Fig. 20.5). This behavior is elicited because the oxygen saturation of the water is slightly higher at the air–water interface.

Although adequate oxygenation is essential, excess dissolved oxygen or other compressed gases such as nitrogen can be detrimental and even fatal if not corrected quickly. Massive aeration or the rapid heating of cold water can produce clouds of very fine bubbles. Also, improperly maintained equipment such as cavitating water pumps or air stones placed too close to the water pump inflow lines can compress room air to the point where the water becomes supersaturated with dissolved gas (Stoskopf, 2010; Noga, 2010). Supersaturation of dissolved gas can cause 'gas bubble disease' in zebrafish, which is discussed later in this chapter.

In general, sufficient aeration can be provided to the typical zebrafish holding tank by simply maintaining appropriate circulation of the water. Oxygen diffusion is adequate at depths of less than 4 inches of water. Appropriate flow rates for recirculating systems are variable, dependent on system vendor, research facilities, and fish life stage (Castranova *et al.* 2011). A lower flow rate can be utilized during the larval stages of development, and for adult fish that are being fed lightly, inactive, or maintained at water temperatures at the lower threshold of thermal tolerance for that strain. Dissolved oxygen should be monitored regularly, especially in systems where fish are being fed intensively and/or held at densities above 15 fish/l. A general rule for recirculating aquaculture systems is one complete turnover per hour (Helfrich, LA and Libey, G. 1990).

In many cases, compressed air is added to recirculating systems, usually at some point within the filtration zone. It is in some instances supplied directly to individual tanks, which can be beneficial when water flow is reduced or stopped due to mechanical failure. It should be noted that compressed air is often hot and dry, which tends to accelerate the evaporation of water within the system. Air bubbling into aquaria will produce a fine mist that can act as a fomite and aid in the transmission of pathogens (Kent et al., 2009). Mists can also result in the corrosion of metal components. The resulting 'scale' can build up and drop into tanks resulting in increased levels of metallic compounds that can be toxic. Therefore, all metallic components should be regularly evaluated for evidence of corrosion. Stainless steel can corrode or rust unless it is adequately maintained or sealed with an appropriate protectant or painted. These components should be either replaced or scraped routinely to prevent introduction of 'scale' or 'rust' into the water system.

C. pH

Zebrafish, like most freshwater species, perform well at a pH in the 7–8 range (Lawrence, 2007). As with temperature shifts outside the optimal range, sudden, drastic shifts in pH can be very detrimental to animal health. Higher pH (>8.0) also results in higher concentrations of toxic unionized ammonia (NH_3). Low pH (<5.0) inhibits the activity of nitrifying bacteria, required for biological filtration, which tends to increase total ammonia levels due to accumulation. In the wild, zebrafish can experience very wide swings in pH, and are therefore very tolerant of changes in this parameter (Spence et al., 2006, 2008). However, as with all environmental parameters, the management goal is stability within the preferred range.

In closed, recirculating water systems, the pH will gradually decrease due to the production of acids during the nitrification process as the bacteria within the biofilter convert ammonia to nitrate. The pH will also decrease in poorly aerated systems due to the production and accumulation of carbon dioxide (CO_2) created by respiring fish.

The pH of the water system has a direct influence on the susceptibility of fish to toxins. Common metallic contaminants such as zinc, copper, iron, and aluminum are more soluble in water under acidic conditions. Therefore, toxicity associated with exposure to these elements is more common in water systems maintained at a lower pH value.

D. Conductivity

Conductivity is an indicator of the total amount of dissolved ions in a solution which includes sodium and other ionized minerals. It is a direct measure of the amount of electric current that a particular aqueous solution can conduct. Since direct measurement of salinity is difficult, conductivity is a convenient method to imprecisely measure the salinity of the water system and allows monitoring of changes in salinity due to water changes or evaporative loss. Conductivity is usually measured in microseimens (μS). Most freshwater species have a salinity range for optimal growth and reproduction (Stoskopf, 2010; Noga, 2010). Zebrafish tolerate a wide range of salinities and can be maintained in the laboratory at conductivities between 125 and 2500 μS (Lawrence et al., 2012; Lawrence, 2007). Zebrafish larvae can be successfully reared at salinities of up to 5 g/l from day 5–10 postfertilization (Best et al., 2010). Again, as with other environmental parameters, stability within these ranges is more critical than maintaining at an absolute value.

E. Total Water Hardness

The amount of calcium and magnesium salts in the water is referred to as the water hardness. Other cations also contribute to the total hardness of the water, but these are usually only present in very small quantities within normal freshwater. Commercially available test kits tend to measure hardness in terms of how much calcium carbonate ($CaCO_3$) is present in the water. Water quality reports usually express hardness levels in terms of parts per million (ppm) or milligrams per liter (mg/l).

Zebrafish are generally considered to be a 'hard' water species with optimum calcium and magnesium levels between 80 and 200 ppm. Very soft water (0–10 ppm) can be detrimental to young developing fry since they rely on the water for essential mineral uptake during the early growing phases of life. Low water hardness or calcium levels have also been found to be associated with low embryo survival rates and increased susceptibility to other environmentally induced disease as a result of poor water quality (Piper et al., 1982).

When utilizing reverse osmosis (RO) or distilled water, some or all of the minerals that have been removed by the filtration process need to be replaced. Calcium can be added to the water in the form of $CaCO_3$ or by adding crushed coral or aragonite preparations (Lawrence, 2007).

F. Ammonia, Nitrite, and Nitrate

A thorough understanding of the major environmental inputs and ubiquitous microorganisms which metabolize proteins to form nitrogenous by-products by way of the nitrogen cycle is essential in evaluating or interpreting the levels of ammonia (NH_3), nitrite (NO_2), and nitrate (NO_3) within a water system.

1. Nitrogen or Nitrification Cycle

A fully functioning biological filter, or biofilter, should be capable of removing a large majority of toxic nitrogenous wastes produced within a closed system. The biofilter is populated by two distinct physiological groups of nitrifying bacteria: those that oxidize ammonia to nitrite and others that oxidize nitrite to nitrate (Fig. 20.6) (Bock and Wagner, 2006; Könneke et al., 2005). Within the fish system, the ammonia (NH_3) precursor primarily comes from fish excreta and uneaten, decaying food. Ammonia is first converted to nitrite (NO_2) by ammonia-oxidizing bacteria (AOB) in the biofilter. AOB identified in freshwater aquaria include *Nitrosomonas* spp., *Nitrospira* spp., and *Nitrosococcus* spp. (Burrell et al., 2001; Hovanec and Long, 1996; Noga, 2010). Interestingly, recently identified nonbacterial, archaea organisms have been shown to also oxidize ammonia in similar ways to that of AOB. These archaea organisms, which have been isolated in both marine and freshwater environments, are identified collectively as ammonia-oxidizing archaea (AOA) (French et al., 2012; Könneke et al., 2005; Stahl and de la Torre, 2012; Hatzenpichler, 2012). In some freshwater aquarium biofilters, AOA have been found to be the predominant ammonia-oxidizing microorganisms and outnumber AOB by orders of magnitude (Bagchi et al., 2014). AOB- and AOA-converted nitrite is then converted to nitrate (NO_3) by the action of nitrite-oxidizing bacteria (NOB), which includes primarily *Nitrospira* spp, but also *Nitrobacter* species (Hovanec et al., 1998; Hovanec, 1996; Abeliovich, 2006). Although these aforementioned chemotrophic bacteria are primarily responsible for the conversion of ammonia to nitrate, other bacterial species of the fish flora, including the potentially opportunistic heterotrophs, such as *Aeromonas* spp. and *Pseudomonas* spp., contribute to the conversion of nitrogenous wastes. These bacteria are also integral components of the normal flora of the fish and are constantly seeded into the biofilter through fish excretions (Castignettii and Hollocher, 1984).

It is important to realize that the biofilter is a dynamic population of many species of bacteria that have a significant impact on water quality and subsequently fish health. Any abrupt change in the aquatic environment can adversely affect the bacteria within the biofilter. The addition of too many new fish quickly or treatment of the water with unwarranted chemical agents, including antibiotics, can frequently result in disastrous shifts in the character of the bacterial flora within the biofilter. For example, prolonged administration of therapeutic levels of erythromycin in freshwater systems significantly disrupts the AOB and NOB populations (Collins et al., 1976). Hence, when populations of bacteria within the biofilter suddenly die off or 'crash,' significant and sudden changes in the pH of the water and levels of ammonia, nitrite, and nitrate frequently result. Mechanical disruption of a biofilter that dislodges the bacteria from the substrate can also compromise its performance.

While high levels of either ammonia or nitrite are very toxic to fish, nitrate is typically only toxic to fish at levels approaching or exceeding 200 mg/l (Camargo et al., 2005). However, maintaining lower levels of nitrate within the system is important to ensure proper health of the biofilter and to control the growth of algae. Therefore, periodic water changes are essential to prevent the accumulation of nitrate and other toxic metabolites within the environment. However, biofilter 'crashes' can also be precipitated by changing the system water too frequently or changing too large a volume of water during a scheduled water exchange.

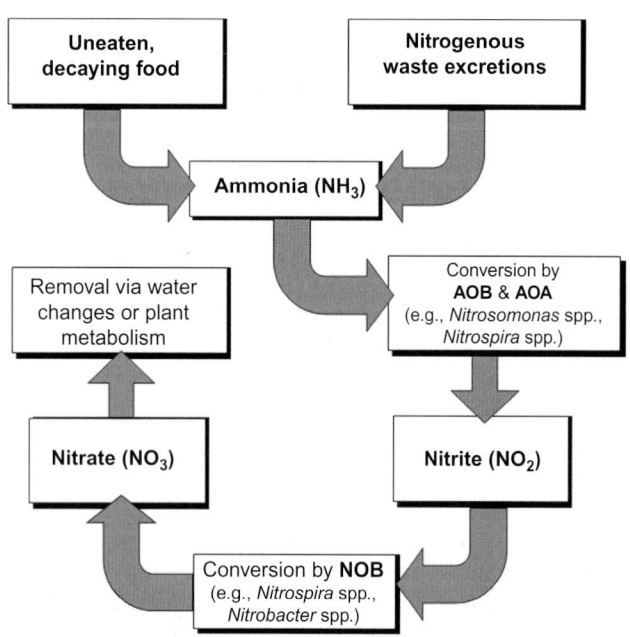

FIGURE 20.6　The nitrogen cycle. Decaying food and nitrogenous waste excretion are the primary sources of ammonia. Toxic ammonia is converted (oxidized) to nitrite by ammonia-oxidizing bacteria (AOB) and ammonia-oxidizing archaea (AOA). The toxic nitrite is then converted (oxidized) to relatively nontoxic nitrate by nitrite-oxidizing bacteria (NOB). Nitrate accumulates within the water unless removed by regular water changes (1–10% of system volume) or by resident plant metabolism.

V. GENERAL FEATURES OF LABORATORY ZEBRAFISH FACILITIES

A. Composition

Wall coverings, floor treatments, door thresholds, and ceilings should be of materials impervious to water or rendered water resistant as necessary. Epoxy-coated floors and epoxy-painted walls offer the advantages of easy sanitation and water resistance. Such surfaces should always also be slip-resistant. Doors should have thresholds that are bermed to prevent water leakage from the room and/or have floor trench drains located just inside the door.

B. Plumbing

Only 'food-grade' silicon sealer should be utilized to avoid the introduction of potentially toxic chemical leachates. Copper piping and lead-based solders should be avoided. Rooms should be provided with adequate drainage. This may require floor drains in several locations. Steeply angled flooring to a central drain should be avoided because this creates unstable footing for heavy aquarium racks.

Specialized drains are an important consideration. Discharges of water with infectious agents and or life stages of exotic (nonindigenous) species should not be released into surface waters. If outflow water is not plumbed to sanitary sewer lines with proper chlorine disinfection, UV disinfection, or ozone treatment, specialized systems to contain and treat contaminated waste water should be designed and constructed.

C. Lighting Systems

Photoperiod is of critical importance in maintaining normal physiological/environmental health in aquatic systems. Twelve to sixteen hours of light per day supplied by either natural or balanced fluorescent lights is most appropriate. Rooms should be equipped with overhead lighting with a timer control. Depending on the protocol, photoperiod control is then accomplished either by control of room lighting or by timers on individual aquaria. The installation of dimmer control ballasts that gradually phase lights on and off is recommended, infrastructure permitting (Harper and Lawrence, 2010).

In larger facilities with multiple modular rack systems extending from the floor to the ceiling, care must be given to the arrangement of lighting to ensure that adequate light penetrates to all tanks containing fish, especially those housed on the lower shelves near the floor. Conversely, fish housed on the top shelves too close to the light source may receive too intense light from overhead bulbs. Either too much or too little light can adversely influence the reproductive activity of the fish within the colony. In these facilities with rack-type shelving units, fluorescent lighting fixtures should be arranged parallel to the rows of shelving and directly over the aisles between two shelving units. This arrangement maximizes light penetration to fish housed on all levels of the shelving unit. The optimal light intensity

for laboratory zebrafish has not yet been determined, but a general recommendation is to provide between 5 and 30 ft candles or 54 and 354 lux at the water surface (Matthews *et al.*, 2002).

D. Heating, Ventilating, and Air Conditioning (HVAC)

The HVAC should provide adequate exchange rates of filtered air into and out of the animal housing and procedure areas (National Academies, 2011, p. 80). Humidity control should be considered for all rooms containing aquaria. Large numbers of aquaria containing water in range of 70–80°F can produce a significantly high degree of humidity, especially during summer months. Poorly circulated room air and high humidity could result in significant mold proliferation and corrosion of metallic components of equipment within the facility.

All rooms should be provided with a source of clean, compressed air of low or medium pressure plumbed appropriately to provide for air delivery to all tank areas (Harper and Lawrence, 2010). Overhead polyvinyl chloride piping with fittings for standard aquarium tubing provides for universal connection points for air stones that can be placed into aquaria when needed.

Care should be taken to ensure that the outdoor HVAC intake system is appropriately filtered, especially in agricultural areas in which the spraying of insecticides or herbicides can be common events. Similarly, air intakes for compressed air used in aeration of systems should be adequately filtered and protected from airborne contaminants as well. Pest control and abatement or physical plant activities (e.g., wall repair or painting) within or around a zebrafish facility should also be of concern. Facility managers should be aware of any physical plant maintenance scheduled inside, outside, or around the facility.

E. Electrical Service

All electrical services should ideally be supplied overhead and suspended from the ceiling by pendant or knuckle fixtures or permanent fixtures high along the walls (~4 ft) in waterproof conduits. All circuits or outlets should be ground fault interrupted (GFI) and of appropriate amperage and voltage. Outlets should have protective covers that are appropriate and functional for how they will or may be used. In general, most aquatic facilities never have enough properly installed outlet space. Plan ahead by designing for and installing greater than the standard numbers of outlets usually placed for a similar sized room scheme. Banks of electrical outlets should be provided for the location of life support equipment. An emergency power source should be provided for critical life support equipment supplying aeration, filtration, and lighting (CCAC, 2005). Loss of power can result in catastrophic losses within hours especially under the conditions of high water temperature and high stocking density that are encountered routinely in the laboratory setting.

F. Water Tanks and Support

Tank support should be carefully considered in terms of weight distribution and construction materials. Because one gallon of water (3.8l) weighs 8.34 lb (3.78 kg), a standard rack of 40 ten-gallon aquaria filled to capacity weighs nearly 2 tons (3,336 lb)! Support racks should be constructed of heavy duty plastic or powder-coated stainless steel. Unsealed wooden supports should be avoided since they tend to absorb moisture, harbor microorganisms, and cannot be routinely cleaned or disinfected effectively (National Academies, 2011, p. 82). Treated woods should also be avoided because of the potential for toxic leachates that could contaminate the water system. Even well-sealed or well-treated wood supports tend to degrade over time in the wet, high temperature, and high humidity environment of the aquatic facility. Nonleaching boric acid-treated wood or plastic may be a safe alternative if no other options exist. Various new products composed of plastics are emerging on the market and each should be evaluated thoroughly for chemical leachates associated with the product's composition or manufacturing process.

G. Water and Life Support System Design

The design of the aquatic environment within the laboratory should be a major concern when establishing or renovating a zebrafish facility (Lawrence and Mason, 2012). Animal health, system maintenance, cost of the system, and animal numbers/uses should be factors considered during the planning process. With the rapid increase in the number of aquatic species being housed routinely in the laboratory research community, a number of aquatic life support system manufacturers have emerged to offer an ever-increasing array of products to support the needs of the laboratory community.

The first element of facility design is water source. The operational goal is to provide a clean and stable template from which to operate life support systems (Harper and Lawrence, 2010). Ideally, deep wells are the best source of fresh water because they contain few infectious agents and toxic chemicals such as sewage or agricultural compounds; however, they can contain potentially toxic heavy metals. In most cases, municipal tap water must be treated for the removal of agents such as chlorine, copper, and chloramines that are toxic to fish. Deionized and/or Reverse Osmosis (RO) water systems may be used to remove these impurities. The advantage to the use of these filtration mechanisms is water purification via the removal of toxic chemicals and microorganism contaminants. However, the resultant water may have trace minerals removed completely (e.g., distilled) or significantly reduced (e.g., deionized or RO) by design. Since these compounds are extremely important to animal health and maintaining the buffering capacity of the water system, the water will then need to be properly conditioned by the addition of mineral compounds. The addition of commercially available conditioning preparations (i.e., Instant Ocean®, Sea Salts, etc.) to the purified water prior to use helps to prevent induced electrolyte deficiencies, osmoregulatory imbalances, and physiological problems of zebrafish or rapid, problematic shifts in pH within the water system. It is important to remember that with evaporative loss of system water, the salinity of the system will continue to increase. Therefore, the addition of salts/buffers to the water needs to be properly monitored to prevent exposure of the fish to a salinity or pH level beyond the range of normal tolerance.

Once water is made suitable to support aquatic life, it can be delivered to the chosen life support system. The modular life support system approach to facility design appears to offer the best advantages for most laboratories. These systems allow for the implementation of comprehensive health management protocols involving easy animal access and monitoring, disease surveillance, system maintenance, and cost-effective expansion of the facility as the need for more animals becomes necessary. Modular systems come in a variety of sizes and can be free standing or wall mounted. Custom modular systems can also be designed and constructed if fund limitations exist but proper research into design specifications is a necessity. Most systems are completely self-contained, closed recirculating water systems and incorporate mechanical, biological, and chemical filtration options (Fig. 20.7). Modular construction allows easy access to all pipes and mechanical components for routine maintenance and replacement service as well as in the case of system failure. With modular systems containing independent life support equipment, failure of one life support system will not result in catastrophic failure of the whole facility. As mentioned previously, these systems allow for expansion of a facility as necessary without the disruption of existing, established systems, provided that the potential for expansion is incorporated into original design. The modules also allow for maximum use of available space if limitations do exist (Fig. 20.7).

Within each modular rack system, the fish are housed in variable sized containment units. These containers can house anywhere between one and hundreds, if not thousands of zebrafish, depending on their size, and are usually composed of a high impact, transparent plastic or acrylic that allows for easy cleaning and visualization of the animals. Polycarbonate construction appears to be the best construction as acrylic frequently warps with

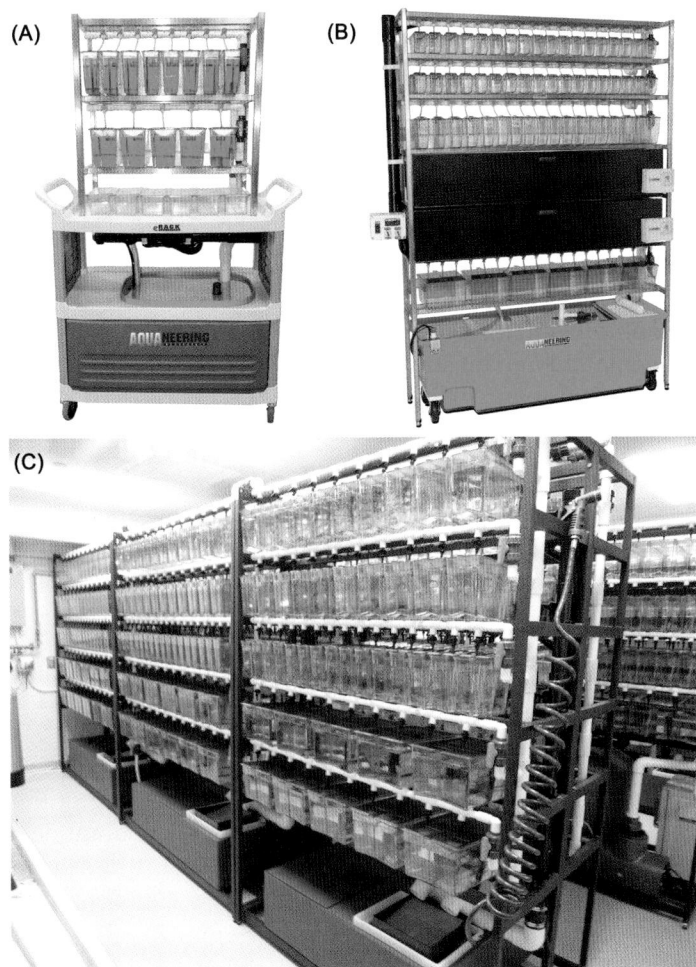

FIGURE 20.7   Examples of recirculating aquatic systems for zebrafish housing. A and B are modular recirculating systems containing filtration (particulate or mechanical filtration, biofiltration, carbon filtration) and disinfecting (UV) within the rack base. The rack pictured in A is portable, while the rack pictured in B provides light control for zebrafish behind dark panels. Pictured in C are multiple racks in a centrally filtered recirculating water system. *Top images courtesy of Wendy Porter-Francis, Aquaneering, Inc.; bottom image courtesy of Daniel A. Vinci, Aquatic Enterprises, Inc./Aquarius Fish Systems, LLC.*

age and repeated use. A limited number of manufacturers now produce containment units that are certified to be free of bisphenol A (BPA), a toxic component in many plastics that has been shown to cause reproductive problems in many animals, including zebrafish (Tse *et al.*, 2013; Saili *et al.*, 2012; Chung *et al.*, 2011).

Most commercially available units also employ some iteration of a 'self-cleaning' design that sweeps and/or siphons uneaten food and feces out of the unit through the outflow tract. In this system design, a directional current is created by the placement of the inflow/outflow tracts in the flow of water circulating by a baffle at the back of each individual container. It is important to remember that no tank is completely self-cleaning. The units need to be kept clean – by routine washing – to ensure proper function and reduce the risk of overflow from clogging.

Modular life support systems appear to be the most practical and economical choice in most circumstances.

However, individual, large volume (25l+) tanks still maintain utility in laboratory research colonies for a number of reasons. If a small colony is to be maintained, single aquaria offer an extremely inexpensive alternative and can be set up on the laboratory workbench if necessary. In infection studies requiring independent life support, multiple individual aquaria can be maintained for disease challenge in studies not involving large numbers of animals. For those studies involving multiple environmental parameters, it may be easier and more economical to maintain side-by-side aquaria than larger, multiple modular units. Even in a facility with multiple modular systems, individual aquaria are extremely useful as quarantine or 'hospital' units for treatment of fish in isolation from the rest of the facility.

In terms of disaster planning and prevention, the availability of backup or redundant power sources to integral system components (pumps, heaters, probes, filters, etc.)

can mean the difference between inconvenience and catastrophic loss (Lawrence and Mason, 2012). Especially in larger facilities or those housing valuable transgenic or mutant strains, backup equipment allows greater freedom to conduct routine maintenance on otherwise continuously operated equipment and allows for quicker reaction in the event of life support failure at an inopportune time. It is a virtual certainty that equipment will fail, and that operational errors will occur, multiple times in the life of a facility. Redundancy in equipment helps to reduce the chances of catastrophic loss in the event of such inevitable problems. Transgenic and mutant strains can also be 'backed up' as cryopreserved sperm in liquid nitrogen freezers at offsite locations (Yang *et al.*, 2007; Carmichael *et al.*, 2009).

On a regular basis, approximately 1–10% of the total volume of water in a recirculating water system should be removed and replaced with conditioned water. This regular input of a fresh volume of water helps to ensure the maintenance of adequate oxygen saturation, flushes excess nitrates, and replaces important trace mineral compounds. Prior to introducing fresh volumes of water from a reservoir tank to the system, the pH and temperature of the water should be equilibrated. Addition of large volumes of improperly buffered water or water of an inappropriate temperature can dramatically alter water chemistry and induce shock in the resident fish and biological filter. Reservoir water should be maintained at the same temperature as the current system water to avoid dramatic shifts during water changes.

H. Specialized Equipment

Rooms should be provided with an area where tanks can be cleaned, sanitized, and dried. In larger facilities especially, these cleaning areas should ideally be centralized. All equipment should be sanitized between each use, including housing tanks, breeding tanks, nets, or any other items that come into contact with fish or fish water. One goal of cleaning and disinfection practices is to prevent the spread of infectious agents within a room or among rooms of a larger facility. Clean, sanitized equipment should be available for use at all times. Following each use, each equipment component should be cleaned with a disinfectant solution (Clorox™, etc.) or sanitized by some other method that reduces the potential for transmission of potentially infectious agents at some predetermined level (Garcia and Sanders, 2011). Multiple disinfectants have been shown to reduce bacterial contamination, including freshly prepared 2% bleach (sodium hypochlorite) or 1% Virkon® Aquatic (potassium peroxymonosulfate + sodium chloride) (Collymore *et al.*, 2014b). Equipment should never be mixed among rooms, experiments, or especially with quarantine/isolation animals.

I. Specialized Areas

Some activities that routinely take place in aquatic facilities should be performed in designated, discrete areas, if at all possible. For example, space should be set aside to provide bench space for water quality analysis equipment. In large facilities, a water quality laboratory can be centralized. Depending on research goals, space can and should be allocated for other needs, including office work, storage, microscopy, imaging, surgical procedures, and behavioral analysis.

One function that absolutely requires specialized space is the importation of fish from outside entities. An isolation or 'quarantine' area should be provided and clearly designated for this purpose. This area can be a single designated use tank in small facilities or a designated quarantine area. Ideally, all facilities should designate a separate room for quarantine of incoming animals or treatment of sick in-house animals. All equipment and materials should be designated for quarantine use only and never be introduced back into the main facility. This room should be isolated from all other life support systems within the facility. Ideally, this room should be under negative pressure for containment purposes and be located in a noncentralized, low-traffic area. These precautions help to limit the number of people moving to and from the quarantine space and limit the possibility of inadvertent transfer of potentially contaminated equipment or animals.

J. The Use of Freshwater Snails

While some research laboratories routinely use freshwater snails (*Planorbella* spp.) to help control the unsightly growth of algae on tanks and maintain good water quality by consuming uneaten food and other organic debris, there are potential disadvantages to their use in the laboratory facility. Once introduced into an established water system, freshwater snails can reproduce quite readily and frequently out of control. As their numbers increase and the snails grow larger, they often migrate into the piping of the water system where the hard shells can disrupt and, in some instances, block the flow of water through the recirculating system. These conditions necessitate disruption of the established aquatic environment to remove snails from clogged piping. The control of algae and the accumulation of excess nitrogenous wastes can be better regulated by adjusting the amount of light and by decreasing the frequency and amount of feed introduced into the water system. One can also reduce the introduction of phosphorus by the use of acid-washed types of activated carbon.

Another potential and more problematic hazard of utilizing snails in the laboratory setting is that snails act as the intermediate host or vector for the larval stages of a number of parasitic organisms such as digenetic trematodes (Reno, 1998; Hoffman, 1999). Likewise, a limited number of reports indicate that invertebrates can carry bacterial pathogens such as *Mycobacterium* spp. (Michelson, 1961). Empirical evidence indicates that these freshwater snails could then act as a reservoir of infection once established within the water system. Although *Mycobacterium* spp. has been isolated from several species of freshwater snails (six species including *Helisoma* spp., *Australorbis* sp., *Rtomphalaria* spp.) under both experimental and natural infection studies, there has been as yet no report of invertebrate vectors transmitting *Mycobacterium* spp. to aquatic vertebrate organisms such as teleost fish. Lesions and acid-fast bacteria were associated with both natural and experimental infection of the snails (Michelson, 1961).

VI. NUTRITION AND FEEDING OF ZEBRAFISH

A. Diet Formulation

As with all other laboratory animal species, it is important to provide zebrafish with a complete and balanced diet. Because the precise nutritional requirements of the zebrafish are still largely undetermined (Watts *et al.*, 2012; Lawrence, 2007), this is not a straightforward endeavor. In most cases, laboratory zebrafish are fed a combination of live and formulated feeds. Live zooplanktons, such as brachionid rotifers and *Artemia*, are particularly effective in promoting high rates of growth and survival for larval and juvenile fish, especially during the first few days of feeding (Carvalho *et al.*, 2006; Harper and Lawrence, 2010; Best *et al.*, 2010). However, given that live diets are (1) often variable in their nutritional profiles (Cahu and Infante, 2001; Lavens and Sorgeloos, 1996), (2) a potential source of pathogens (Peterson *et al.*, 2013b), and (3) challenging to produce in large enough quantities to support demands beyond the juvenile stage, it is preferable to wean the fish onto processed diets as soon as possible. In general, fish show enhanced growth and reproductive output when maintained on formulated feeds from the sub-adult stage and beyond (Siccardi *et al.*, 2009; Lawrence *et al.*, 2012b). Furthermore, formulated feeds also afford the user greater levels of control over quantity, quality, and source of ingredients. All of these are advantages in a setting where eliminating experimental variation is of paramount importance (Watts *et al.*, 2012).

When formulated diets are utilized, it is especially important to ensure that the chosen feed contains adequate levels of essential fatty acids (Jaya-Ram *et al.*, 2008), and various vitamins (Ortuno *et al.*, 2003; Miller *et al.*, 2012; Kirkwood *et al.*, 2012). In particular, the ratio of n6:n3 fatty acids in the diet appears to have a significant effect on both growth and reproduction; with zebrafish displaying a dietary demand for higher levels of n6 fatty acids than do most species of cultured coldwater fish (Meinelt *et al.*, 1999, 2000). This last point is a critical one, since the great majority of commercially available fish feeds are formulated for coldwater species that generally require a much higher ratio of n3 fatty acids (Lawrence *et al.*, 2012b).

B. Feeding Interval

Feeding frequency is an important area of concern for the laboratory manager, especially in a zebrafish research facility setting where there can be thousands of individual tanks in a single room. In general, fish should not be fed more food than they can consume in 3–5 minutes. Food that is not readily eaten quickly sinks and is taken up by the recirculating water system where it fouls both mechanical and biological filters. Uneaten food quickly decays and is a major source of nitrogen waste in the water system. This decaying food can impact system function by clogging mechanical filters, and can adversely influence water quality by contributing large amounts of ammonia that can disrupt the biofilter and cause sudden pH shifts. Frequent or inappropriate feeding is a significant cause of poor water quality in terms of excess nitrogenous products, high bacteria counts, and pH fluctuation.

As with most species of cultured fish, the number of feedings per day for laboratory zebrafish should generally decrease as the fish age increases. Larval zebrafish need to eat nearly continuously to meet protein demands, so food needs to be presented in frequent, small doses. As the animals (and their digestive systems) mature and growth rates slow, they can be presented with less frequent but larger meals. Finally, once the fish have moved beyond the rapid phases of growth and become adults, they can be fed between 1 and 3 times daily to reach a consumption rate of 3–5% of body weight per day (Lawrence *et al.*, 2012b). In the event that fish undergo certain experimental procedures or other manipulations, feed amounts may be reduced further or even withheld completely for a short period. It is important to consider that there is no 'one-size-fits-all' prescription for feeding zebrafish. Feeding programs will often vary depending on the environment and experimental situation.

C. Feed Handling and Storage

The manner in which feeds are handled and stored is also critical to their success. Diets that are fed live, such as rotifers or *Artemia*, should be presented to the fish when they are alive to derive maximal benefit from their application. For larval fish especially, prey items should be moving slowly within the water column to maximize encounter rates with larvae (Best *et al.*, 2010). It is also important to remember that the nutritional value of live feeds will vary depending on how they are cultured and when they are collected/presented to fish. Rotifers should be fed out to fish when they are gut loaded with algae or whatever additive they are being 'enriched' with, and *Artemia* should be collected and presented as close to immediately after they have been hatched to ensure they are delivering maximal value to fish (Lawrence, 2007).

Dry, formulated feeds should be presented dry, and never mixed with water prior to delivery to the fish, as water-soluble vitamins and minerals will rapidly leach from these diets as soon as they are hydrated (Onal and Langdon, 2000). The rate of nutrient loss from diets will vary depending on their composition and formulation, but in general it is best to limit residence time in water.

The manner in which feed is stored is also very important to maintaining its integrity. In general, heat and moisture are the enemies of fish feeds, so they should always be stored in dry, cool environments. Each feed should be stored in strict accordance with manufacturer instructions. In general, long-term storage of formulated diets should be avoided.

VII. PATHOGEN CONTROL PROGRAM

Sources of pathogens in a new or established research zebrafish colony include imported and existing animals, personnel, water source, shared equipment, and food. Every research zebrafish colony should have a pathogen control program in place. A pathogen control program should address how risks associated with these sources are mitigated.

A. Acquisition and Quarantine

Efforts should be undertaken in established facilities to limit the introduction of fish from outside sources to those that are necessary. However, risks associated with fish importation can be mitigated by stringent quarantine and importing fish from quality zebrafish distributors or from facilities of research colleagues that implement, document, and follow a comprehensive fish health management protocol (Kent *et al.*, 2009).

The importance of obtaining zebrafish from a colony with a known disease history cannot be understated and will increase with our knowledge of the effects of latent, asymptomatic, and symptomatic infectious diseases (Lawrence *et al.*, 2012a). For example, subclinical disease presentations of microsporidosis or mycobacteriosis may contribute to nonprotocol variation of neurological or inflammation and neoplasia models in zebrafish, respectively (Kent *et al.*, 2009, Kent *et al.*, 2012a). Currently, the only commercial provider of specific pathogen-free (SPF) (free of *Pseudoloma neurophilia*) zebrafish is the Sinnhuber Aquatic Resource

Laboratory (SARL) at Oregon State University (Corvallis, OR) (Kent *et al.*, 2011). As of 2014, this particular colony has been free of *P. neurophilia* for over 6 years.

Much like mouse quarantine and rederivation programs, research zebrafish facilities should routinely quarantine incoming zebrafish with the goal of preventing the introduction of imported sub-adult or adult fish into the main zebrafish colony. Rather, progeny of imported animals should be introduced to the main colony. Quarantine strategies can be described as either 'refined' or 'traditional'. Both strategies involve the use of dedicated rooms and equipment, including, but not limited to, aquatic system, nets, and tanks, that are separate from main zebrafish colony. The 'refined' quarantine strategy imports only the progeny from previously imported surface disinfected embryos that were reared to adults and then spawned within the quarantine facility into the main zebrafish facility. The 'traditional' strategy imports surface-disinfected embryos from adult fish housed and spawned within the quarantine facility into the main zebrafish facility (Sanders, 2013).

In both strategies, imported animals are bred and their surface disinfected embryos are incorporated into the main zebrafish colony. Chorionated embryos are disinfected with dilute bleach (20–50 ppm buffered to pH 7.0) (Harper and Lawrence, 2010). Also, all quarantine animals should be continuously monitored for signs of clinical disease. Ill animals should be removed and tested for pathogens of interest based on clinical signs or diagnostic evaluations. It should be noted that pathogens that have true vertical transmission within the chorionated embryo, like *P. neurophilia*, can potentially circumvent current zebrafish quarantine procedures and will not be killed during surface bleach disinfection (Sanders *et al.*, 2013; Ferguson *et al.*, 2007).

1. Wild-Type Suppliers

It is important to consider that most of the retailers currently supplying wild-type zebrafish stocks to the laboratory research community are primarily suppliers of ornamental tropical fish to the aquarium pet trade. As a result, the significance placed on health management of fish within these farms varies greatly according to the individual companies. Therefore, never assume that all imported fish are completely healthy. While some suppliers will make an effort to identify and treat clinically observable disease in their fish stocks, fish with subclinical disease(s) obtained from suppliers with limited health monitoring could enter an established research facility undetected. Due to the limited ability of these retailers to implement a comprehensive health monitoring program for economic and practical reasons, it is extremely important to evaluate all incoming fish for latent or subclinical infection(s) before their introduction into a quarantine facility. Fish should never be directly imported into a colony's main system.

The acquisition of zebrafish from local pet stores for outcrossing is strongly discouraged. Due to the nature of the pet trade, local aquarium shops usually have a high degree of turnover in both incoming and outgoing animals. This usually results in little or no disease screening, overstocked aquaria, and fish stressed from shipping conditions. Pathogens that are either established in the system or that arrive with newly introduced fish can spread quickly among stressed or debilitated resident fish. Because of the high volume of fish within these shops, the fish frequently become infected with the more common aquatic pathogens, such as *Mycobacterium* spp., capillarid nematodes, and *Ichthyophthirius multifiliis*. Fish obtained from a local aquarium shop should be considered as high-risk candidates for harboring pathogens and should not be incorporated into an established research zebrafish colony.

2. Transfer Among Research Facilities

Due to the rapid expansion in the number and size of zebrafish facilities worldwide, the numbers of transgenic animals and their resultant phenotypes are dramatically increasing. Various research groups worldwide are constantly exchanging these transgenic fish among their

respective facilities. Therefore, it is important to ascertain the current health status of the facility from which you are obtaining fish. Establishing and continued use of a comprehensive health monitoring system among various institutions will allow for the safest and most expedient transfer of animals among facilities. Likewise, it is essential to share accurate colony health information with a facility to which you are sending fish. False, outdated, or inaccurate information concerning health status, especially with regard to infectious pathogens, can result in significant loss of valuable animals, research time, and funds for an unsuspecting facility receiving diseased animals.

B. Surveillance/Sentinel Program

A key component to a comprehensive health management program for the monitoring of animal health status is the monitoring of colony morbidity and mortality plus the maintenance of 'sentinel' animals within each aquatic system. The NIH Zebrafish International Resource Center (ZIRC) has developed a model sentinel fish program (ZIRC, 2009; Kent *et al.*, 2009). A surveillance program in recirculating systems utilizes fish exposed to pre- and postfiltration water (Fig. 20.8). Prefiltration, or 'dirty,'

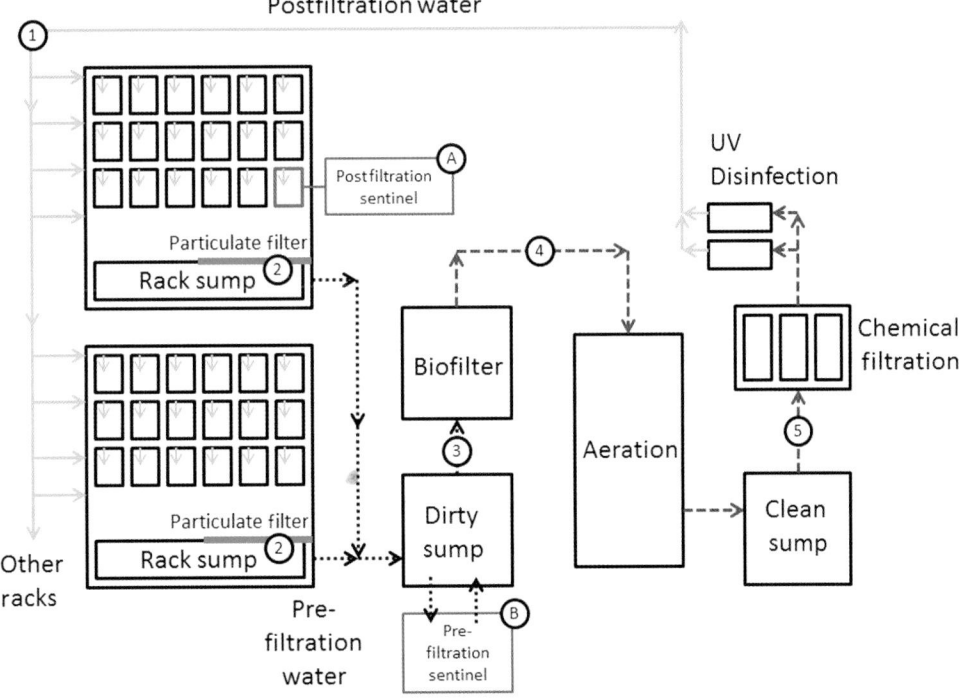

FIGURE 20.8 Schematic depicting the flow of water in centrally filtered recirculating system. System schematic varies depending on system manufacturer. The solid light-blue lines (1) indicate filtered water entering the modular racks of individual tanks. From individual tanks, waste water (2) passes through a particular filter, indicated by the solid green line, into the rack sump. Water leaves the rack sump to eventually enter (3) the biofilter. After biofiltration, water with less toxic oxidized nitrates travels to (4) aeration, (5) chemical filtration, and/or ultraviolet (UV) disinfecting units. The filtered and disinfected water then recirculates back into the tanks (1). Postfiltration sentinel fish are placed on the same rack as colony fish (A). Prefiltration sentinel fish require a flow of dirty sump water in and out of an isolated tank (B). Not indicated in this schematic are entry points for introduction of buffers and/or mineral salts.

water comes from a system sump containing fish waste and detritus, whereas post-filtration, or 'clean,' water comes from the system and is the same water that other fish in the system are exposed to. Placement of sentinel fish for at least 3 months is recommended to detect chronic infections like mycobacteriosis or *P. neurophilia* (Kent *et al.*, 2009). Choosing which diseases to survey is not trivial and requires consideration of disease pathogenicity and the impact of the disease on research models (Lawrence *et al.*, 2012a). In addition, you must have a reliable source of clean fish that are 'SPF' of the pathogen of interest. There are currently at least three commercial laboratories that test and screen for common fish pathogens in zebrafish. This fact further demonstrates the rationale for establishing a comprehensive health-management program including surveillance programs in research zebrafish facilities.

VIII. TECHNIQUES AND ANESTHESIA

A. Blood Collection and Parameters

A study on zebrafish blood was first published in 1963 describing the distribution of blood in embryos (Colle-Vandevelde, 1963). Since then, zebrafish have been used to model hematopoiesis, myelopoiesis, and hemostasis, with recent developments being driven by hematopoietic defects in mutant zebrafish (Carradice and Lieschke, 2008; Zang *et al.*, 2013). The primary hematopoietic organ of adult zebrafish is the head kidney (Al-Adhami and Kunz, 1977).

Blood collection in zebrafish is utilized more commonly for research than for clinical purposes. Blood diagnostics in fish are not routinely used, especially with smaller fish less than 8cm in length where blood withdrawal carries a high risk of death (Noga, 2010). The utility of blood diagnostics of research zebrafish for clinical purposes has not been extensively studied; however, hematological and chemistry parameters have been published for this species (Table 20.1) (Murtha *et al.*, 2003). Hematological and serum biochemical values across and within fish species are variable and should be compared to an established reference interval for a given machine and originating colony.

Blood smears demonstrate erythrocytes, thrombocytes, granulocytes, monocytes, and lymphocytes (Fig. 20.9) (Carradice and Lieschke, 2008; Murtha *et al.*, 2003). Zebrafish erythrocytes are $7 \times 10\,\mu m$ nucleated, elliptical cells with eosinophilic cytoplasm (Murtha *et al.*, 2003; Carradice and Lieschke, 2008). Adult zebrafish have at least two types of blood cells from granulocyte lineage (Lieschke, 2001; Jagadeeswaran *et al.*, 1999). The most abundant granulocyte in zebrafish blood are neutrophils, which are also referred to as heterophils. Mature neutrophils measure 9–10μm in diameter and have

TABLE 20.1 Blood Indices for Normal Adult Zebrafish

	Mean ± SD (%)	Range (%)
Lymphocytes	82.95 ± 5.47	71–92
Monocytes	9.68 ± 2.44	5–15
Neutrophils	7.10 ± 4.75	2–18
Eosinophils	0.15 ± 0.53	0–2
Basophils	0.13 ± 0.40	0–2

	Mean ± SD		Range	
Albumin	3.0 ± 0.2	g/dl	2.7–3.3	g/dl
ALP	2.0 ± 4.5[a]	U/l	0.0–10.0	U/l
ALT	367.0 ± 25.3	U/l	343.0–410.0	U/l
Amylase	2331.4 ± 520.6	U/l	1898.0–3195.0	U/l
Total bilirubin	0.38 ± 0.1	mg/dl	0.2–0.6	mg/dl
BUN	3.2 ± 0.4	mg/dl	3.0–4.0	mg/dl
Calcium	14.7 ± 2.3	mg/dl	12.3–18.6	mg/dl
Phosphorous	22.3 ± 1.5	mg/dl	20.3–24.3	mg/dl
Creatinine	0.7 ± 0.2	mg/dl	0.5–0.9	mg/dl
Glucose	82.2 ± 12.0	g/dl	62.0–91.0	g/dl
Potassium	6.8 ± 1.0	mEq/l	5.2–7.7	mEq/l
Total protein	5.2 ± 0.5	g/dl	4.4–5.8	g/dl
Globulin	2.1 ± 0.6	g/dl	1.3–2.8	g/dl

Table adapted from Murtha et al. (2003).
ALP, alkaline phosphatase; ALT, alanine transaminase; BUN, blood urea nitrogen.
[a]*ALP values were inconsistent and ranges from negative results to 10 U/l.*

two- to three-lobed segmented nucleus and carries cytoplasmic, multilamellated granules (Murtha *et al.*, 2003). Eosinophils are rare, have larger granules than neutrophils, and have shown to be increased during parasitic infection (Lieschke, 2001; Carradice and Lieschke, 2008; Balla *et al.*, 2010). Monocytes are 12–18μm in diameter with abundant, foamy, basophilic cytoplasm with irregularly shaped nuclei. Lymphocytes are 5–8μm in diameter and are round to ovoid with a large round nucleus and thin basophilic cytoplasmic rim (Murtha *et al.*, 2003; Carradice and Lieschke, 2008). Thrombocytes are 3–4μm in diameter nucleated cells with dense nuclear chromatin and frequently seen in aggregates in peripheral blood smear (Carradice and Lieschke, 2008; Murtha *et al.*, 2003).

There are a number of terminal blood collection techniques described in anesthetized zebrafish. Decapitation through the pelvic girdle severs the heart, allowing for 5–10μl of blood to be collected in a heparinized microcapillary tube (Eames *et al.*, 2010). Blood can also be terminally collected from the dorsal aorta by making a transverse incision between the anal and caudal fins

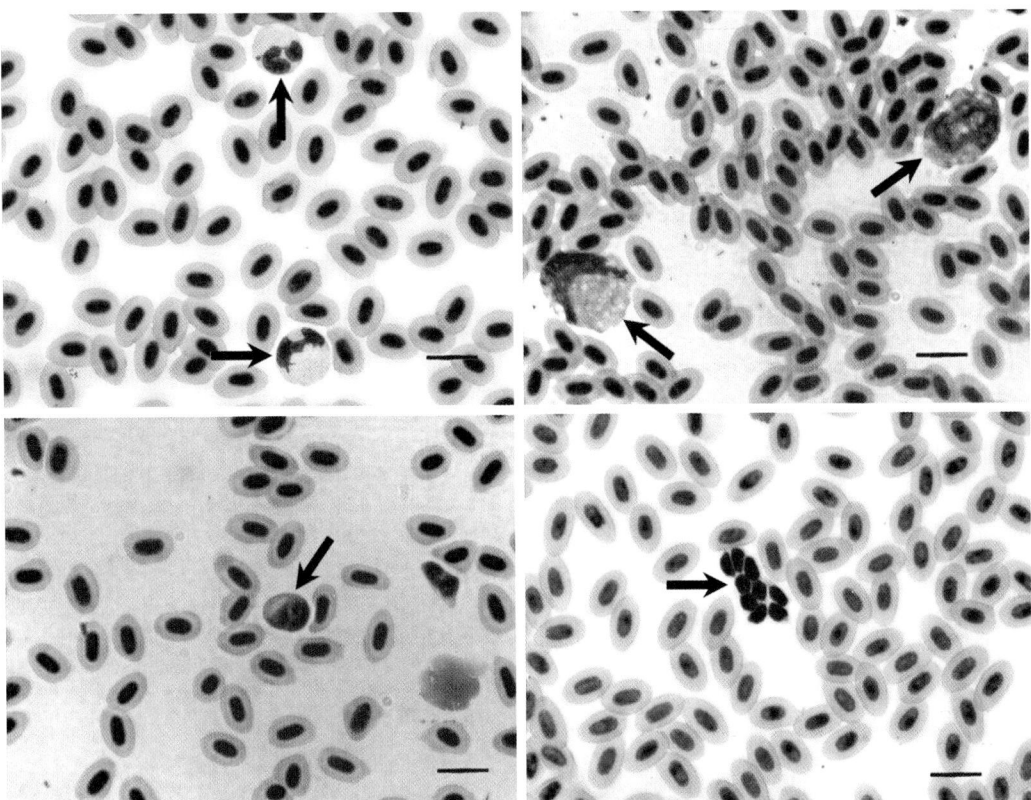

FIGURE 20.9 Blood smear photomicrographs demonstrating blood cell morphology (Murtha *et al.*, 2003). These three photomicrographs are Diff-Quik stains of blood smears from adult zebrafish. Arrows indicate blood cell types: neutrophil (top left), monocyte (top right), lymphocyte (bottom left), thrombocyte (bottom right). Bar = 10 µm (1000 × magnification). The other cells in this panels are nucleated red blood cells.

(Pedroso *et al.*, 2012; Velasco-Santamaría *et al.*, 2011; Jagadeeswaran *et al.*, 1999). Survival blood collection technique in zebrafish has a 2% mortality rate and can retrieve as much as 2% of body weight. Using a pulled glass micocapillary needle, blood can be withdrawn from the dorsal aorta and/or the posterior cardinal vein by aiming along the frontal plane body axis and posterior to the anus. To minimize blood loss anemia and hemorrhagic death, the maximum volume that is to be repeatedly collected is less than or equal to 1% of body weight every 2 weeks (Zang *et al.*, 2013). Regardless of technique, the blood volume retrieved from an individual zebrafish will be insufficient for most hematological or biochemistry assays, necessitating the use of pooled blood/serum samples. Microscopic evaluation of blood cell morphologies is best performed on cytospin blood samples (Spitsbergen, personal communication).

B. Oral Dosing

Oral dosing of adult zebrafish is useful for experimental administration of compounds or infectious organisms. While clinical treatment for large numbers of diseased fish is usually performed by mixing drugs with food or

directly into tank/system water, it may be advantageous to treat a fish directly. Placement of a flexible catheter on a 22-gauge needle tip into the mouth and intestinal tract of the zebrafish allows for accurate and relatively safe dosing of solutions of up to 5 µl (Collymore *et al.*, 2013). Use of gluten as a carrier molecule can also be used successfully to administer chemical compounds orally (Zang *et al.*, 2011).

C. Anesthesia

Although anesthetic protocols for zebrafish are extrapolated from other aquatic species, there is now substantial information gained regarding the effectiveness and safety of these anesthetic protocols. Indications for anesthesia in zebrafish are similar in other species, including potentially stressful or painful procedures. The most common route of administration of an anesthetic agent in zebrafish is immersion, although oral, intramuscular, intravenous, and intraperitoneal routes have been demonstrated in other fish species (Stoskopf and Posner, 2008).

Much like mammalian anesthesia, zebrafish anesthesia is described in four stages (Table 20.2) (Collymore *et al.*,

TABLE 20.2 Stages of Zebrafish Anesthesia

Stage	Plane	Level	General behavior	Voluntary locomotor activity	Equilibrium	Rate of opercular movement	Reflex response	Heart rate	Muscle tone	Examples of procedures
0		None	Normal	Normal	Normal	Normal	Normal	Normal	Normal	
I		Sedation	Disorientation	Decreased	Difficult to maintain	Normal	Reduced	Normal	Normal	ENU mutagenesis imaging
II		Excitation	Agitation	Increased	Lost	Increased	Increased	Increased	Normal	
III	1	Light anesthesia	Anesthetized	None	Lost	Decreased	Reduced	Regular	Decreased	Weighing, gill scrape, skin scrape
	2	Surgical anesthesia	Anesthetized	None	Lost	Shallow	None	Reduced	Decreased	Gill biopsy, tailfin clipping, recovery surgery
	3	Deep	Anesthetized	None	Lost	Rare movements	None	Reduced	Relaxed	Nonrecovery surgery
IV		Overdose	Apparently dead	None	Lost	None	None	Cardiac failure	None	

From Collymore et al., 2014a; Adapted from Ross and Ross, 2008; Stoskopf and Posner, 2008.

2014a; Ross and Ross, 2008; Stoskopf, 2010). Zebrafish in stage I of anesthesia (sedation) are disoriented and less responsive to stimuli but will have normal opercular movement. Following stage I, fish progress into stage II (excitatory) with a loss of equilibrium and a brief increase in opercular and voluntary movement. Stage III (surgical) anesthesia of zebrafish is broken down into three planes: light, surgical, and deep, where all voluntary movement is lost and muscle tone is decreased. Opercula movement decreases with plane depth, with deep plane anesthesia having rare opercula movement. Stage IV anesthesia (medullary collapse) where all opercula movement stops and muscle tone is lost. (Collymore et al., 2014a; Ross and Ross, 2008; Stoskopf, 2010). Level of anesthesia desired will be determined by the procedure being performed.

Refer to Chapter 23 for general anesthetic considerations and more information protocol regimens (MS-222 and metomidate) in other fish species. In addition, there is additional review of fish anesthesia in *ILAR* (Matthews and Varga, 2012) and in *Anesthesia and Analgesia of Laboratory Animals* (Stoskopf and Posner, 2008). Given the variation of fish species, it is critical to understand the physiological effects of commonly used protocols in zebrafish reviewed here.

1. Tricaine Methansulfonate (Also Known as MS-222, TMS, Tricaine-S®, Tricaine Mesylate)

MS-222 is a commonly described anesthetic agent for research zebrafish. Advantages for use include a moderate safety margin for short procedures, dose dependency, quick induction and recovery, and availability. Disadvantages include the need for buffering as MS-222 is acidic when dissolved in water and may be aversive even when buffered (Readman et al., 2013; Wong et al., 2014). The US Food and Drug Administration (FDA) currently approves Tricaine-S (Western Chemical, Inc., Ferndale, Washington, DC) as a fish anesthetic. MS-222 demonstrates variable efficacy based on age, with larvae showing an increased resistance relative to adults (Rombough, 2007). The immersion MS-222 dose to achieve a surgical plane of anesthesia for adult zebrafish ranges from 140 to 164 mg/l (Westerfied, 2000; Collymore et al., 2014a; Matthews and Varga, 2012; Huang et al., 2010). MS-222 anesthesia combined with isoflurane at 65 ppm each causes adult zebrafish to enter surgical plane of anesthesia within 90 s and remain there for significantly longer periods, and recovery more quickly than MS-222 alone (Huang et al., 2010). Isoflurane is not appropriate as a sole agent to achieve a surgical plane of anesthesia (Collymore et al., 2014a; Huang et al., 2010).

The related compound lidocaine hydrochloride is an effective anesthetic for adult zebrafish at immersion dose of 325 mg/l. Compared to MS-222, time to loss of equilibrium using lidocaine and recovery time is longer. Lidocaine hydrochloride may have a narrow safety margin, with 30% mortality seen at 350 mg/l (Collymore et al., 2014a).

2. Eugenol (Also Known as Clove Oil and Aqui-S® 20e)

Eugenol (4-allyl-2-methoxyphenol) is the active ingredient in clove oil and has emerged as an anesthetic used by hobby aquarists (Grush et al., 2004; Matthews and Varga, 2012). It is also sometimes used for laboratory zebrafish, including mutagenesis protocols (Rohner et al., 2011). Advantages include low cost, availability, wider safety margin than MS-222, quick induction, and rapid metabolism and excretion (Sánchez-Vázquez et al., 2011; Grush et al., 2004). Disadvantages include longer recovery times and the potential for it to elicit an aversive reaction in fish (Readman et al., 2013). Eugenol is not water soluble and is commonly mixed with ethanol in its preparation. The ethanol content in the 1:10 (eugenol:ethanol) stock does not have any detectable adverse effects on adult zebrafish. In adult zebrafish, immersion in eugenol at 2–5 ppm and 60–100 ppm causes sedation and surgical plane of anesthesia, respectively. (Grush et al., 2004).

3. Metomidate Hydrochloride

Metomidate hydrochloride is a common and safe anesthetic used in fish. The use of this compound in zebrafish for anesthesia is not extensively studied. In one report, metomidate provides sedation and light anesthesia at 6 mg/l immersion dose in adult zebrafish (Collymore et al., 2014a). In zebrafish and other fish, metomidate is considered to have a wide safety margin (Stoskopf and Posner, 2008).

4. Cooling

Gradual cooling, accomplished by gradually adding ice to achieve 10–12°C water, can be utilized for quick nonpainful procedures, and as such is not effective for invasive procedures considering the difficulty in maintaining fish at this temperature during the procedure (Collymore et al., 2014a; Stoskopf and Posner, 2008; Matthews and Varga, 2012). To minimize pain and injury, ice should not come into direct contact with fish. Rapid cooling to 0°C has been suggested as a safe method for anesthetizing embryo and larvae zebrafish, but produces high mortality in adults (Chen et al., 2014).

D. Euthanasia

Euthanasia of zebrafish is often accomplished by prolonged overdose of the aforementioned anesthetic compounds. Both the *ILAR* review (Matthews and Varga, 2012) and *Anesthesia and Analgesia of Laboratory Animals* textbook (Stoskopf and Posner, 2008) provide good literature reviews of fish euthanasia.

IX. SIGNIFICANT DISEASES OF LABORATORY ZEBRAFISH

In assessing colony health, it is important to evaluate the morbidity, mortality, appearance and behavior of zebrafish on a daily basis. Many clinical signs in diseased zebrafish are nonspecific, like coelomic distension (Fig. 20.10), but can often be useful in establishing an initial differential diagnosis (Table 20.3). Additional diagnostic tests must be performed to diagnose a particular etiologic agent.

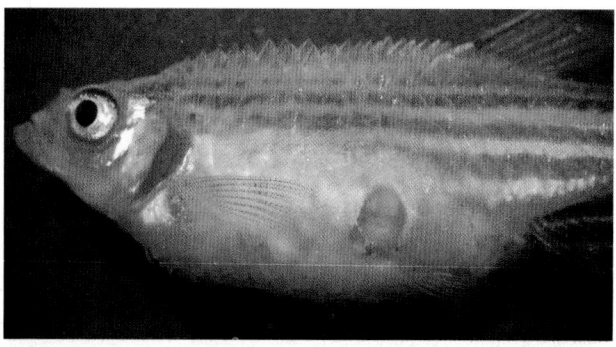

FIGURE 20.10   Zebrafish with nonspecific clinical sign of severe edema, or dropsy. Note focal epidermal ulceration, coelomic distension, and associated subcutaneous edema, causing the scales to be pushed up and away from body. *Image courtesy of Dr. Jennifer Matthews (Matthews, 2004).*

TABLE 20.3   Generalized Clinical Signs and Abnormal Behaviors Frequently Observed in Diseased Fish and Potential Differential Diagnoses That Should Be Considered

Generalized clinical signs	Differential diagnoses
Opercular flaring	Respiratory distress, parasites, disease
Sloughed mucus	Chemical irritation, parasites, mechanical trauma
Clamped fins	Parasites, disease, stress, pain
Petechiation or hemorrhage	Bacterial infection, parasites, mechanical trauma
Changes in body color	Bacterial infection, hormonal influence, disease, stress
Scale loss	Parasites, mechanical trauma, disease
Improper buoyancy	Baroregulatory (swim bladder) failure, disease
Lethargy	Disease, stress, starvation
Surface breathing	Oxygen depletion, respiratory distress
Sudden death	Chemical toxicity, abrupt change in water quality, disease
Flashing	Parasites

The following section contains information pertaining to significant and/or common pathogens that are of concern to the laboratory zebrafish facility. Within each disease section, information is given regarding the identification of clinical signs, diagnostic evaluation, and treatment options. The following list is a survey of pathogens that are largely naturally occurring in research zebrafish. In instances where pathogens or pathogenesis are not well documented in zebrafish, information extrapolated from other fish species is provided. At the time of this publication, there have been no documented naturally occurring zebrafish viral pathogen. Therefore, viruses are not covered here, but a review of teleost fish viruses and experimental viral infections of zebrafish are reviewed in Crim & Riley (2012). As the number of laboratory zebrafish facilities continues to increase, new, emerging diseases will continue to be characterized and, likewise, treatment and control options will increase.

A. Bacterial Infections

1. Mycobacteriosis (Fish Pseudo-Tuberculosis)

Etiology Naturally occurring zebrafish mycobacteriosis is caused by atypical, or environmental, *Mycobacterium* species, including *M. abscessus*, *M. chelonae*, *M. fortuitum*, *M. haemophilum*, *M. marinum, and M. peregrinum* (Astrofsky et al., 2000; Whipps et al., 2007; Kent et al., 2004; Watral and Kent, 2007). Mycobacteria are 1–10 μm long, pleomorphic, weakly gram-positive, acid-fast, aerobic, non-motile rod-shaped bacteria (Draper, 1971; Zheng and Roberts, 1999). Atypical mycobacteria are facultative pathogens and have been described in over 151 species of fishes, including freshwater and marine fishes from tropical to subartic altitudes (Gauthier and Rhodes, 2009; Talaat et al., 1997). Based on disease manifestation, mycobacteria can be broadly characterized as either pathogenic or opportunist in zebrafish (Whipps et al., 2012). Of the species reported in zebrafish, *M. haemophilum* and *M. marinum* are pathogenic and *M. abscessus*, *M. chelonae*, *M. fortuitum*, and *M. peregrinum* are opportunist (Table 20.3).

Epizootiology and Transmission Mycobacteriosis is a significant and commonly identified disease in zebrafish research facilities. The most common etiologic agents reported include *M. chelonae*, *M. haemophilum*, *M. abscessus*, *M. marinum*, and *M. fortuitum* (Kent et al., 2004; Astrofsky et al., 2000), with *M. chelonae* being the most commonly found mycobacteria in zebrafish submitted to diagnostic services (Dr. Mike Kent and Dr. Marcus Crim, personal communication). Most zebrafish mycobacteriosis is chronic with low-grade morbidity and mortality (Matthews, 2004).

Atypical mycobacteria can survive outside the host in surface biofilms, which contributes to its success to survive in and become a resident of microbial flora within

IX. SIGNIFICANT DISEASES OF LABORATORY ZEBRAFISH **1039**

a water system, including tanks and pipes (Kent *et al.*, 2011; Whipps *et al.*, 2008; Falkinham, 2009; Falkinham and Norton, 2001). *M. marinum* and *M. peregrinum* can be orally transmitted experimentally via immersion and oral inoculation of mycobacteria (Harriff *et al.*, 2007). Evidence of embryonal infection as early as 3 days post fertilization (dpf) with *M. marinum* has also been demonstrated upon experimental immersion inoculation (Davis *et al.*, 2002). Naturally acquired mycobacteriosis is therefore probably transmitted horizontally and orally by ingestion of shed bacteria from skin lesions and gastrointestinal tract, as well as infected fish tissue, food, and debris in water (Ross and Johnson, 1962; Nigrelli and Vogel, 1963). In addition, invertebrates, such as amoebae (Harriff *et al.*, 2007) and paramecia (Peterson *et al.*, 2013b) may be vectors of mycobacteria.

Pathogenesis and Predisposing Factors A major virulence characteristic of pathogenic mycobacteria is its ability to grow within the host macrophage. Once inside the host macrophage, most pathogenic mycobacteria will reside in vacuoles without fusing to lysosomes. The host macrophage is therefore unable to process and present mycobacteria antigen to the immune system (Cosma *et al.*, 2003; Russell, 2001). Macrophage phagocytosis is one of the first defense mechanisms of the 5 dpf zebrafish larvae experimentally exposed to *M. marinum* (Davis *et al.*, 2002). Three days after pathogenic mycobacteria infection, macrophage aggregates occur within the tissues and by day 4, differentiate into epithelioid and multinucleated cells ultimately forming granulomas. Therefore, the innate immune system is sufficient to drive *M. marinum* granuloma formation prior to development of adaptive immunity (Tobin and Ramakrishnan, 2008). Upon entering and colonizing the gastrointestinal tract, mycobacteria disseminates to other visceral organs, including swim bladder, liver, spleen, and kidney (Harriff *et al.*, 2007; Whipps *et al.*, 2008). As previously mentioned and discussed later, clinical disease is dependent on the species and even strain of mycobacteria.

Husbandry conditions (density, water quality, stress, etc.), immunological state, and genetic susceptibility are predisposing factors leading to opportunistic and pathogenic mycobacteriosis in laboratory-reared zebrafish (Astrofsky *et al.*, 2000; Ramsay *et al.*, 2009a; Murray *et al.*, 2011a). In particular, Tübingen (TU) and TAB5 line zebrafish show higher incidences of mycobacteriosis than AB and TAB14 (Murray *et al.*, 2011a).

Clinical Signs Clinical manifestation of mycobacteriosis in zebrafish varies in severity and onset time with *Mycobacterium* species and strain. Affected zebrafish can present with lethargy, decreased fecundity, emaciation, skin ulceration and hemorrhage/hyperemia, edema, or coelomic distension (Fig. 20.11). Of the *Mycobacterium* species isolated from zebrafish, *M. abscessus*, *M. chelonae*, *M. fortuitum*, and *M. peregrinum* cause low morbidity/

mortality and can cause clinical illness in stressed fish in suboptimal environmental and husbandry conditions. Pathogenic species *M. haemophilum* and *M. marinum* causes acute outbreaks of high morbidity and mortality. Of note, coelomic distension is associated with *M. marinum* infection, whereas severe emaciation is associated with *M. haemophilum*, although these are nonspecific clinical signs (Fig. 20.11) (Whipps *et al.*, 2012). Other uncommon clinical signs include skeletal and muscle deformities (Noga, 2010).

Diagnostic Findings In addition to external lesions previously described, other necropsy findings for mycobacteriosis include small, tan-colored nodules in visceral organs. Detecting acid-fast staining bacteria on wet mount smears of affected tissues, especially the spleen and kidney, can be quickly performed as part of diagnostic screening (Whipps *et al.*, 2012; Noga, 2010).

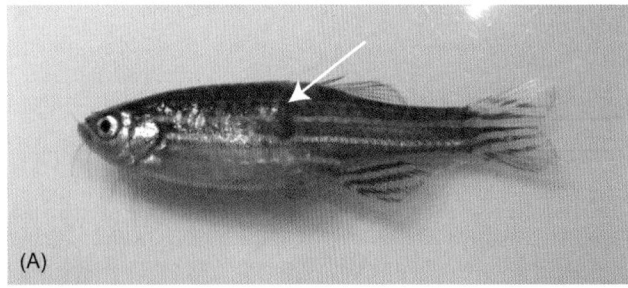

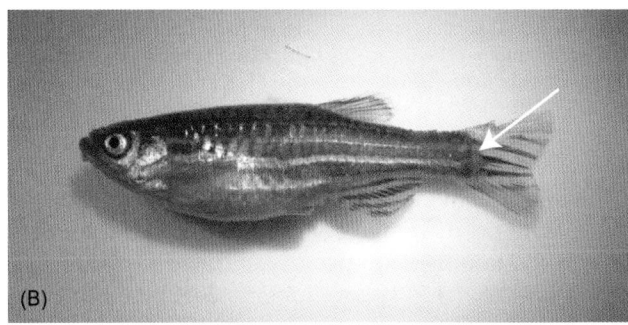

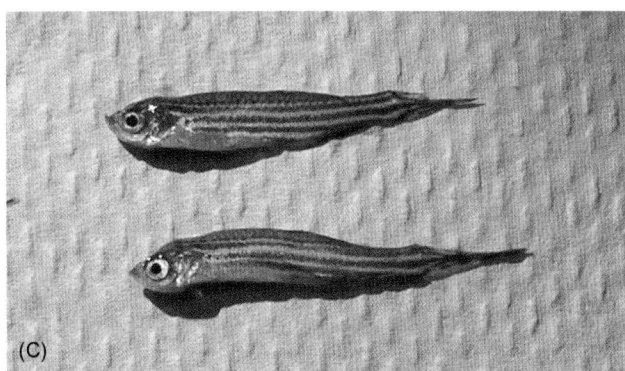

FIGURE 20.11 Different external appearances of zebrafish with mycobacteriosis with two different *Mycobacterium* spp. The top two panels indicate coelomic distension skin ulcerations (white arrow) in fish infected with *Mycobacterium marinum*. The bottom panel indicates severe emaciation in zebrafish infected with *Mycobacterium haemophilum* (Whipps *et al.*, 2012).

LABORATORY ANIMAL MEDICINE

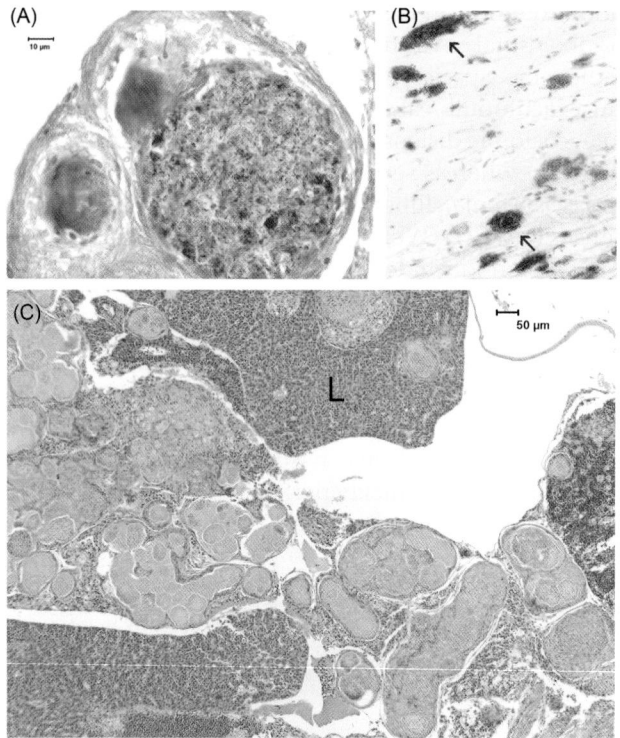

FIGURE 20.12 Histopathology of mycobacteriosis in zebrafish. (Kent *et al.*, 2004). (A) Ziehl-Neelsen acid-fast bacteria in typical granuloma formation. Bar = 10 μm. (B) Neurotropic mycobacteriosis from a fish infected with *M. haemophilum* in the spinal cord. Ziehl-Neelsen acid-fast. (C) Typical mycobacteriosis with granulomas throughout the visceral organs. The liver is marked. Hand E. Bar = 50 μm. Panel B *courtesy of Mike Kent*

Histological evidence of acid-fast bacteria highly correlates with positive mycobacteria culture. Mycobacteria are weakly staining gram-positive and acid-fast rods measuring 0.1–0.6 × 1.0–10 μm (Roberts, 2012). Granulomas containing acid-fast bacilli are identified in affected zebrafish, with varying severity and onset of accompanying inflammation (Fig. 20.12A). Confirmatory diagnosis to the species level is difficult by histology, but differences in presentation are seen depending on the *Mycobacterium* species. For example, *M. chelonae*-infected fish typically contain diffuse granulomatous inflammation in well-demarcated or poorly organized aggregates of macrophages with acid-fast bacilli (Whipps, 2008). *M. marinum*-infected fish will present with similar histologic findings, but lesions will generally be more aggressive (Watral and Kent, 2007). Infections with *M. haemophilum* present with massive numbers of bacteria in various organs, as this species is the only *Mycobacterium* spp. zebrafish infection that presents in a neurotropic form with colonies of acid-fast bacilli evident in the spinal cord and meninges (Fig. 20.12B). *M. fortuitum*-infected fish have multifocal necrosis in liver, spleen, and heart

(Whipps et al., 2007). Almost all organs of the zebrafish can be affected by *Mycobacterium* spp. infection (Fig. 20.12C, Table 20.4). Mycobacteriosis diagnosis via acid-fast technique may be hindered by some fixative and decalcification procedures. However, preservation in acidic fixatives such as Bouin's or Dietrich's and decalcification of embedded fixed whole zebrafish with 5% trichloroacetic acid does not affect acid-fast staining (Harriff *et al.*, 2007).

Atypical *Mycobacterium* species cultivation is difficult, but is best accomplished on Middlebrook 7H10 agar or Lowenstein–Jensen slants. Pathogenic *M. marinum* is considered a fast grower and can be cultured in less than 5 days. Other *Mycobacterium* spp. isolation may require more than 30 days to grow (Noga, 2010). Molecular techniques such as polymerase chain reaction (PCR) is a useful screening tool for genus-level detection using the 16s rRNA gene of *Mycobacterium* spp. (Talaat *et al.*, 1997). In recent years, heat shock protein 65 (*hsp65*) gene sequence has been shown to be more informative for species identification. PCR is performed either on DNA of cultured isolates or of tissues. The latter is particularly useful for fastidious bacteria such as *M. haemophilum* (Whipps *et al.*, 2007). Retrospective PCR identification can also be done from paraffin tissue blocks. Peterson *et al.* (2013a) were able to amplify sequence from zebrafish in paraffin blocks with mycobacteria about 50% of the time, regardless of the time in fixative.

Treatment There are no demonstrated effective treatments for zebrafish with mycobacteriosis. The primary goal after detection of clinically affected fish/ or and fish systems infected with *Mycobacterium* spp. should be remediation of any water quality issues, reduction of stress, improvement of husbandry procedures, and preventon of opportunistic infections. In one study, however, oral administration of erythromycin, rifampicin, or streptromycin increased the survival of experimentally infected yellowtail fish (*Seriola quinqueradiata*) (Kawakami and Kusuda, 1990).

Control and Prevention As with other zebrafish diseases, mycobacteria may colonize an aquatic system and infect its inhabitants under suboptimal conditions. In outbreak situations of pathogenic mycobacteriosis, complete eradication of fish and disinfection of system are required to remove mycobacteria (Astrofsky *et al.*, 2000). There are several preventative procedures that are effective at keeping mycobacteria from becoming a problem in a research zebrafish facility. Good importation practices via quarantine and appropriate surface disinfecting embryos will mitigate risk of spreading mycobacteria. Dilute bleach (neutral pH adjusted at 50 ppm for 10 minutes) has germicidal activity against *M. chelonae* (Whipps *et al.*, 2012). Prompt removal of sick and dead fish can reduce the amount of bacteria shed into water. Minimizing stress also decreases mycobacteria

TABLE 20.4   Summary of Characteristics of *Mycobacteria* spp. Infections Found in Research Zebrafish

Mycobacteria species	Culture growth	Disease category	Clinical signs	Enzootic characteristics	References
M. abscessus	Rapid (5 days)	Opportunistic	Subclinical	Chronic: low morbidity/mortality. Moderate disease in suboptimal environment	Astrofsky (2000), Watral and Kent (2007)
M. chelonae	Rapid (5 days)	Opportunistic	Subclinical	Chronic: low morbidity/mortality	Astrofsky (2000), Kent (2004), Whipps (2008)
M. fortuitum	Rapid (7 days)	Opportunistic	Incidental	No disease unless poor environment	Astrofsky (2000), Kent (personal communication)
M. haemophilum	Slow (6–8 weeks)	Pathogenic	Severe emaciation, lethargy	Persistent high morbidity/mortality outbreaks	Kent (2004), Whipps (2007)
M. marinum	Slow (10–14 days)	Pathogenic	Lethargy, coelomic distension, diffuse erythema, skin ulceration	High morbidity/mortality	Watral and Kent (2007)
M. peregrinum	Rapid	Opportunistic	Subclinical	Moderate mortality/morbidity in poor environment. Low mortality/morbidity in experimental exposure	Kent (2004), Watral and Kent (2007)

infections (Ramsay *et al.*, 2009a). Removal of biofilm and detritus in the system reduces the mycobacteria count in a system (Whipps *et al.*, 2012). Food sources can also be a route of entry for mycobacteria as it has been detected in *Artemia* fish feed in an ornamental fish breeding operation (Beran *et al.*, 2006). Recently, it has been shown that paramecia ingest mycobacteria and can transmit both *M. chelonae* and *M. marinum* to zebrafish larvae and subadults upon feeding with these 'infected' paramecia (Peterson *et al.*, 2013b).

Zoonosis   Most reports of human cutaneous mycobacteriosis from fish are associated with individuals who are in direct contact with aquaria or who work in aquaculture. *M. marinum* is the etiologic agent that causes human cutaneous mycobacteriosis, also known as 'fish tank granuloma' (Swift and Cohen, 1962). Major risk factors for contracting cutaneous *M. marinum* infection include immunosuppression and/or direct aquaria contact with compromised skin (Aubry *et al.*, 2002; Cheung *et al.*, 2010). In three studies, 34–84% of individuals with *M. marinum* infection had fish tanks at home or had fish-related occupations (Aubry *et al.*, 2002; Ang *et al.*, 2000; Chow *et al.*, 1987). The zoonotic potential of *M. marinum* from research zebrafish has not been reported in the literature. However, at two different academic institutions, a total of four cases of cutaneous mycobacteriosis have occurred in individuals working in zebrafish facilities. Three of the four became infected during the same time the zebrafish facility was experiencing a mycobacteriosis outbreak. *M. marinum* was the etiologic agent in the three human cases and the zebrafish outbreak (Christian Lawrence and Monte Matthews, personal communication).

2. Edwardsiellosis (Enteric Septicemia of Catfish)

Etiology   *Edwardsiella ictaluri*, a gram-negative rod, is the etiologic agent of Enteric Septicemia of Catfish (ESC) (Hawke *et al.*, 1981). Initially, this pathogen was considered to be host-specific for catfish species, but has recently been found in other non-catfish species, including research zebrafish (Noga, 2010; Hawke *et al.*, 2013). *E. ictaluri* is a member of the class Gammaproteobacteria, order Enterobacteriales, and family Enterobactericeae (Hawke *et al.*, 1981). Zebrafish have also been experimentally infected with *Edwardsiella tarda*, which is commonly isolated from Japanese flounder (*Paralichthys olivaceus*) (Pressley *et al.*, 2005).

Epizootiology and Transmission   Edwardsiellosis is an emerging naturally occurring disease in research zebrafish. *E. ictaluri* has been recognized to be associated with severe morbidity and mortality in several zebrafish research facilities (Hawke *et al.*, 2013). In these cases, natural outbreaks of disease associated with *E. ictaluri* had mortality rates ranging from 15–19%.

Transmission of *E. ictaluri* amongst channel catfish is horizontal via ingestion of shed bacteria by feces and/or cannibalism of infected fish (Klesius, 1994). In addition, zebrafish have been successfully infected with *E. ictaluri* after immersion in water containing viable bacteria (Hawke *et al.*, 2013; Petrie-Hanson *et al.*, 2007). *E. ictaluri* is considered to be an obligate pathogen requiring direct contact for transmission and does not persist in the environment (Hawke, 1979). There is, however, evidence suggesting that *E. ictaluri* may survive several days in 25°C water and longer in mud (Plumb and Quinlan, 1986).

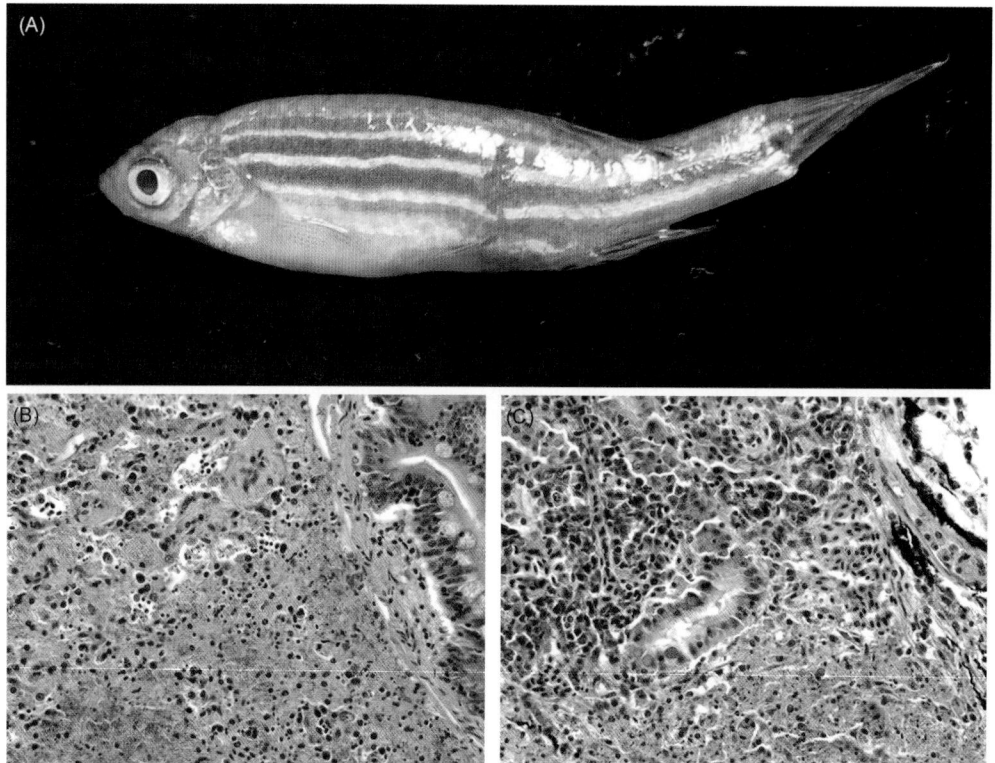

FIGURE 20.13   Gross and histological evaluation of zebrafish infected with *Edwardsiellia ictaluri*. (A) Note ulceration and erythema on ventral and lateral surface of coelomic cavity in the gross image (B) Photomicrograph demonstrating diffuse coagulative necrosis of the splenic parenchyma, with a myriad of bacterial rods and denerate inflammatory cells. A section of gastrointestinal tract is relatively unaffected (right). (C) Photomicrograph demonstrating severe caseous necrosis in the hematopoietic tissues of the kidney (bottom) with many rod bacteria present in debris, which extends into a nearby blood vessel (at right). The tubular epithelial cells contain hyaline eosinophilic droplets. *The gross photo is courtesy of John Hawke. The photomicrographs and interpretations are courtesy of Wes Baumgartner.*

Pathogenesis and Predisposing Factors
Edwardsiellosis is an acute disease in research zebrafish. Channel catfish infections with *E. ictaluri* usually present in an acute or chronic form, which is dependent on the routes of exposure. The acute form of *E. ictaluri* in catfish is usually acquired via the oral route and enters the bloodstream via the intestine and colonizes various visceral organs. The chronic infection of *E. ictaluri* is usually acquired via the nervous system by invading the olfactory organ via nasal opening, ultimately infecting the brain, meninges and skin, causing 'hole-in-the-head' lesions (Noga, 2010). Natural and experimental *E. ictaluri* infections in zebrafish have not clearly demonstrated these two forms of disease, but instead present acutely causing septicemia-related clinical signs.

In reported naturally acquired *E. ictaluri* zebrafish infections, predisposing/risk factors for outbreaks of clinical *E. ictaluri* infection include suboptimal water conditions and contact with infected imported fish (Hawke *et al.*, 2013). In channel catfish, ESC outbreaks occur in water temperatures of 24–28°C (Noga, 2010). Given that this temperature range is optimal for growth of both *E. ictaluri* and zebrafish, standard zebrafish husbandry conditions are favorable for propagation of this disease.

Clinical Signs   Clinical signs of *E. ictaluri* infection in zebrafish includes lethargy, raised scales, coelomic distension due to ascites, skin ulceration, hemorrhage in the skin near the eyes and opercula, base of fins, and ventral surface of abdomen (Fig. 20.13A) (Hawke *et al.*, 2013).

Diagnostic Findings   Zebrafish isolates of *E. ictaluri* are gram-negative rods that are non- to weakly motile via peritrichous flagella measuring $0.75 \times 1.25\,\mu m$ (Hawke *et al.*, 1981; Hawke *et al.*, 2013). Diagnosis of *E. ictaluri* infection is confirmed by culture isolation from lesions (Noga, 2010). Necropsy findings of *E. ictaluri*-infected zebrafish include pale gills and liver, and swollen spleen. Affected zebrafish present with severe, multifocally extensive to diffuse disease, most commonly in the kidney and spleen (Fig. 20.13B,C) (Hawke *et al.*, 2013). Kidneys contain areas of inflammation and necrosis as discrete expansive foci, with hematopoietic cords affected prior to glomerular necrosis. Splenic enlargement is accompanied by parenchymal necrosis with numerous apoptotic and necrotic (aponecrotic) macrophages with bacterial infiltration with and between cells. The nares contain extensive sheets of necrotizing chronic inflammation, which extend to and obliterate the olfactory rosettes. Other less common lesions include liver necrosis and inflammation, muscle necrosis with liquefaction, and dermatitis with epidermal ulceration (Hawke *et al.*, 2013). A hallmark histological character is the presence of numerous, large rods within phagocytes. Molecular analysis via PCR of affected tissues can aid in diagnosing *E. ictaluri* infection (Panangala *et al.*, 2005, 2007).

Treatment Florenfenicol medicated feed and enrofloxacin medicated feed curtailed mortality in two different zebrafish facilities with *E. ictaluri* outbreaks. All current zebrafish isolates of *E. ictaluri* show susceptibility to sulfadimethozine-ometoprim (Romet®), oxytetracycline, florfenical, and enrofloxacin (Hawke *et al.*, 2013).

Control and Prevention Appropriate use of a quarantine program is important for monitoring a number of fish diseases, including *E. ictaluri*. *E. ictaluri* has historically been considered an obligate pathogen and not persistent in the environment (Noga, 2010; Hawke *et al.*, 2013), but has been shown to remain viable in mud and water for up to 90 days outside the catfish host (Plumb and Quinlan, 1986). Given that zebrafish and *E. ictaluri* are grown best under similar water temperatures, care should be taken to sanitize equipment between uses and during an outbreak (Petrie-Hanson *et al.*, 2007). In addition, an *E. ictaluri* outbreak in a research zebrafish colony has been associated with imported pet store zebrafish, which underscores the importance of obtaining fish from reputable sources and the need for routine quarantine procedures (Hawke *et al.*, 2013).

3. Motile Aeromonad Septicemia (Ulcer Disease, Aeromoniasis, Red Sore, Motile Aeromonas Infection)

Etiology Motile Aeromonas Septicemia (MAS) in zebrafish is caused by *Aeromonas hydrophila* and *Aeromonas sobria* (Pullium *et al.*, 1999). In other freshwater species, other pathogenic aeromonads include *A. allosaccharophila* (Martinez-Murcia *et al.*, 1992), *A. sobria* (Toranzo *et al.*, 1989), *A. jandaei* (Esteve *et al.*, 1993), *A. bestiarum, A. caviae*, and *A. veronii* (Carnahan and Altwegg, 1996). These motile aeromonads are gram-negative opportunistic bacteria and are commonly isolated from mucosal surfaces and internal organs of clinical healthy fish (Harikrishnan and Balasundaram, 2005; Shotts *et al.*, 1976).

Epizootiology and Transmission Outbreak of MAS is characterized by high mortality in research zebrafish facilities (Pullium *et al.*, 1999; Rodríguez *et al.*, 2008). In freshwater fish, MAS outbreaks are limited to fish in suboptimal water conditions. In reports of MAS in largemouth bass, *A. hydrophila* infection is associated with infection of protozoan *Epistylis* (Hazen *et al.*, 1978; Esch and Hazen, 1980). While there is no evidence that zebrafish can be infected with *Epistylis*, *Tetrahymena* spp.

are ciliated protozoal organisms that are commonly found in zebrafish facilities. *Tetrahymena pyriformis* has been shown to facilitate the growth of *Aeromonas salmonicida* (King and Shotts, 1988; Astrofsky *et al.*, 2002a; Matthews, 2004).

Pathogenesis and Predisposing Factors Pathogenicity of motile aeromonads varies widely, with many being relatively weak pathogens. *A. hydrophila* virulence in zebrafish is associated with the presence of aerolysin, cytotoxic enterotoxin, and serine protease genes. *A. hydrophila* isolates expressing these genes are more pathogenic given the increased proteolytic, hemolytic, and cytotoxic activity in zebrafish (Li *et al.*, 2011).

Susceptibility to MAS in research zebrafish and other freshwater fish is associated with poor husbandry conditions, including stress, overcrowding, and suboptimal water parameters, including high temperatures, high nitrite levels, and hypoxia (Pullium *et al.*, 1999; Noga, 2010; Cipriano *et al.*, 1984). In addition, motile aeromonads can invade skin wounds (Noga, 2010).

Clinical Signs Clinical signs associated with MAS includes petechial hemorrhages of the skin, fins, oral cavity, and muscle (Pullium *et al.*, 1999). Other clinical signs associated with MAS in other freshwater fish species includes superficial to deep skin lesions, coelomic distension, and exophthalmos. Peracute signs are not typically associated with clinical signs (Noga, 2010).

Diagnostic Findings In freshwater species with MAS, hemorrhage may occur with necrosis on the skin near the base of the fins. Ulcers may extend deep into skeletal muscle. Necropsy findings include coelomic distension with serosanguineous fluid, visceral petechiation, and hemorrhage and swelling of the lower intestine and vent (Noga, 2010). Histologically, zebrafish with MAS have multiple areas of epidermal ulceration and mononuclear cell infiltrate. Multifocal necrogranulomatous myositis is also found in skeletal muscle. Aggregates of gram-positive bacteria are found observed beneath the surface of the skin and surrounding the outer aspect of the spinal cord (Pullium *et al.*, 1999).

Definitive diagnosis is made by culture isolation of organism and molecular characterization. Ascertaining that a motile aeromonad is the primary etiologic agent causing disease is difficult considering these bacteria will often migrate into tissues secondarily during illness or after death. Kidney tissues are commonly used for culture in freshwater fish diagnosis (Noga, 2010).

Treatment, Control, and Prevention Given that MAS is in an opportunistic infection, it is critical to eliminate the primary cause of environmental or husbandry stress when facing zebrafish illness. Removal of stressors will often suffice in resolving MAS outbreaks (Noga, 2010). The use of antibiotics should be based on culture/sensitivity results of isolates from affected fish. Antibiotics have been successfully used, in particular oxytetracycline and nifurpirinol, in freshwater fish outbreaks. Antibiotic resistance is a concern (Shotts *et al.*, 1976), with sulfadimethoxine-ormetoprim being used in oxytetracycline-resistant isolates (Noga, 2010).

Zoonosis Motile aeromonads can infect humans, but the risk of zoonotic infection is relatively low. Ingestion of infected fish or puncture wounds are routes of infection for motile aeromonads in immunocompetent humans, with some affected patients becoming septicemic. Immunocompromised individuals are most susceptible (Lehane and Rawlin, 2000).

4. Bacteria Gill Disease and Columnaris (Fin Rot, Cotton Wool Disease)

Etiology Bacterial gill disease and columnaris are caused by aerobic, opportunistic bacteria of the genus *Flavobacterium*. Bacterial gill disease is caused by *Flavobacterium branchiophilum*. Columnaris infection is caused by *Flavobacterium columnare* (formerly *Flexibacter columnare*) (Noga, 2010). These bacteria belong to the taxonomic Cytophaga-Flavobacterium-Bacteroides (CFB) group (Bernardet *et al.*, 1996). These two pathogens infect freshwater fish with similar, but not identical, clinical signs and pathologic findings. There is also variable pathogenicity amongst different strains of the same bacteria species (Moyer and Hunnicutt, 2007).

Epizootiology and Transmission *Flavobacterium* species are naturally occurring on healthy fish and in aquatic ecosystems as they are commonly isolated from these sources (Noga, 2010; Austin and Austin, 2007). Bacteria gill disease (BGD) has been reported in zebrafish as a result of shipping stress (Kent *et al.*, 2012b). It is one of the most important conditions affecting the salmonid industry as it causes explosive morbidity and mortality (Speare *et al.*, 1991). Pathogenic *F. branchiophilum* strains transmit horizontally in adult rainbow trout (*Oncorhynchus mykiss*) (Ferguson *et al.*, 1991).

Experimental introduction of *F. columnare* to zebrafish via superficial mechanical injury induces rapid, severe mortality that is similar to columnaris disease observed in other freshwater fish species (Moyer and Hunnicutt, 2007; Noga, 2010). In this same experiment, uninjured fish immersed in *F. columnare* produced no clinical disease, indicating compromise in the protective skin layer predisposes zebrafish to be infected with this bacteria (Moyer and Hunnicutt, 2007; Olivares-Fuster *et al.*, 2011).

Pathogenesis and Predisposing Factors In freshwater salmonids, *F. branchiophilum* targets only the gill epithelium and eventually disrupts respiratory and osmoregulatory functions in affected fish (Speare *et al.*, 1991). Secondary water mold infection and operculum damage may occur later in infection (Noga, 2010; Ostland *et al.*, 1990). Complete genome sequence analysis of *F. branchiophilum* indicates at least two genes that may play a role in its pathogenesis. *F. branchiophilum*

contains genes predicted to be involved with utilizing polysaccharide, which may explain this bacteria's predilection to mucopolysaccharide containing gill mucus. *F. branchiophilum* also encodes for a preprotein similar to heat-labile toxin (LTA), which is found in Enterotoxigenic *Escherichia coli* (ETEC) strains and provokes massive loss of water and electrolytes across the host intestinal cells of the host (Touchon *et al.*, 2011).

In zebrafish, *F. columnare* in the aquatic environment can infect and colonize damaged skin upon direct contact (Moyer and Hunnicutt, 2007). *F. columnare* will also infect the gill epithelium of uninjured zebrafish in bath immersion (Olivares-Fuster *et al.*, 2011). In freshwater fish, *F. columnare* is also primarily an epithelial disease, causing both gill and skin disease. *F. columnare* has been shown to adhere to gill mucus via lectin-mediated interactions (Decostere *et al.*, 1999). In addition, *F. columnare* has a greater chemotactic response to fish skin and gill mucus than intestinal mucus (Klesius *et al.*, 2008).

Both flavobacteria infections in zebrafish are primarily environmental and husbandry management diseases, as risk factors include stress, overcrowding, and shipping. Other risk factors for BGD in freshwater salmonids include high organic and ammonia loads in water, low oxygen, and high turbidity. Columnaris infection in zebrafish is more likely to occur if the mucus and skin layer is compromised (Moyer and Hunnicutt, 2007). Large amounts of uneaten feed can support growth of *F. columnare* (Noga, 2010).

Clinical Signs Zebrafish with BGD exhibit labored breathing and may swim closer to the surface of the water (Kent *et al.*, 2012b). Other freshwater salmonids with BGD also exhibit flared opercula and hypermic gills and swollen primary lamellae (Noga, 2010). Zebrafish with injured skin experimentally exposed to *F. columnare* via bath immersion exhibit a 'saddleback lesion' resulting in loss of pigment and scales around the dorsal fins (Moyer and Hunnicutt, 2007). Erosion of the fins occurs in fin and tail infections, known as fin and tail rot. Infected skin will appear white due to loss of overlying epidermis and exposure of dermis (Kent *et al.*, 2012b). In freshwater fish, skin disease may progress to skin ulcers which may penetrate into deeper tissues (Noga, 2010). *F. columnare* can cause erosive/necrotic skin and gill lesions, leading to sloughed epithelium (Noga, 2010).

Diagnostic Findings Wet mount microscopy of gills from infected fish can show fused secondary lamella due to epithelial hyperplasia. Filamentous bacteria in large quantities can be observed at surfaces of the gills. A rapid, presumptive diagnosis of BGD can be made via wet mount examination if excessive mucus production, gill epithelium hyperplasia, and/or large numbers of bacteria are present (Kent *et al.*, 2012b; Noga, 2010). Similarly, columnaris disease can be also identified on wet mount examination of lesions with large numbers of flexing or gliding bacteria. After several minutes,

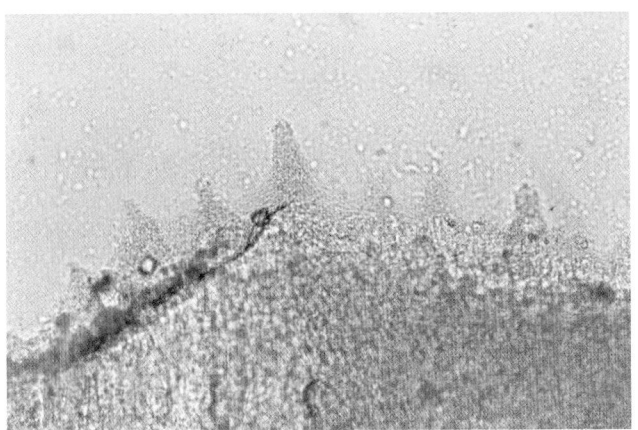

FIGURE 20.14 Wet mount image of 'haystack' formations of *Flavobacterium columnare*, the etiologic agent of columnaris disease, from koi fish. *Photograph courtesy of Jeff Wolf.*

bacteria in wet mounts may be arranged in a haystack formation (Fig. 20.14) (Noga 2010).

Histologic examination reveals severe epithelial hyperplasia of the gills accompanied by necrosis and colonies of bacteria on gill surface. Flavobacteria are long, thin rods (0.5–1.0 × 4–10 μm). In freshwater salmonids, severe disease may cause obliteration of the entire interlamellar space and may cause fusion of adjacent primary lamellae (Noga, 2010).

Culture of *Flavobacterium* species are possible, but are difficult and of limited clinical value, given bacteria are predictively susceptible to certain antiseptics or antibiotics. *F. columnare* is difficult to culture on standard bacteriological media.

Treatment There are no reports of treatment of zebrafish with *Flavobacterium* species infections. In other freshwater fish, columnaris disease has been successfully treated with antiseptic baths or prolonged immersion in potassium permanganate or copper sulfate. In advance cases of columnaris disease, treatment with antibiotics has been accomplished by oxytetracycline and/or nifurpirinol (Noga, 2010). In addition, higher salinity has been shown to reduce mortality associated in freshwater fish infected with *F. columnare* (Altinok and Grizzle, 2001).

Control and Prevention Removing the inciting stressor and/or environmental issue is the most important control measure for flavobacteria infections in zebrafish. Prevention may be accomplished by regular monitoring of water parameters of zebrafish tanks and minimizing injury due to handling.

B. Fungus-Like Infections

1. *Microsporidiosis*

Etiology Zebrafish microsporidiosis is caused by *Pseudoloma neurophilia* and *Pleistophora hyphessobryconis*;

however, *P. neurophilia* is more widely recognized (Sanders *et al.*, 2010; Kinkelin 1980; Matthews *et al.*, 2001). These organisms belong to the Microsporidia phylum, which has been reclassified into the Fungi kingdom upon molecular characterization (Hirt *et al.*, 1999; Hibbett *et al.*, 2007). *P. neurophilia* has been classified under class Microsporea, order Microsporida, and family Icthyosporidiidae (Cali *et al.*, 2011). Microsporidia are obligate intracellular parasites that generally undergo two developmental stages: merogeny and sporogeny. Spores are infective and enter the cell via sporoplasm injection or phagocytosis. Merogeny, or meront development, occurs in direct contact with host cell cytoplasm. During sporogeny, meronts differentiate into sporonts and undergo a number of morphological changes, including plasmalemma thickening (Monaghan *et al.*, 2009; Lom *et al.*, 2000). Sporonts mature into sporoblasts prior to becoming spores (Fig. 20.15A,B), which are liberated into the extracellular environment upon host cell death (Monaghan *et al.*, 2009).

Epizootiology and Transmission Microsporidiosis is the most common zebrafish disease with prevalence as high as 74% in research facilities tested by the ZIRC diagnostic service (Murray *et al.*, 2011b). In the zebrafish facility where *P. neurophilia* was first characterized and named, approximately 90% of emaciated fish and 30% of clinically normal fish were infected with *P. neurophilia* (Fig. 20.16) (Matthews *et al.*, 2001). Transmission of *P. neurophilia* has been shown to be both horizontal and vertical. Horizontal transmission is facilitated by ingestion of mature infective spores in the environment or in other infected live and dead fish (Kent and Bishop-Stewart, 2003; Murray *et al.*, 2011b; Sanders *et al.*, 2012). In addition, debris from tanks housing infected fish can infect fish in other tanks over the span of 7 weeks (Murray *et al.*, 2011b). Vertical transmission is supported by evidence of *P. neurophilia* spores in ovaries and within ova (Sanders *et al.*, 2012; Kent and Bishop-Stewart, 2003; Sanders *et al.*, 2013). Vertical transmission has been demonstrated by detection of *P. neurophilia* DNA and spores within embryos spawned from infected adults (Ramsay *et al.*, 2009b; Sanders *et al.*, 2013). It is currently unclear what role, if any, male sperm play in the role of embryo infection (Murray *et al.*, 2011b).

Pathogenesis and Predisposing Factors Evidence of *P. neurophilia* spores within the gut lumen and epithelium supports an oral route of transmission for microsporidiosis (Sanders *et al.*, 2012, 2014; Cali *et al.*, 2011). Exposure experiments of *P. hyphessobryconis* also supports ingestion as the route of transmission for this microsporidea (Sanders *et al.*, 2010). After oral ingestion, infective spores disseminate to other tissues, primarily infecting central nervous system but also muscle and ovarian tissues. After 4.5 days of experimental infection of zebrafish larvae, merogenic (proliferative) and

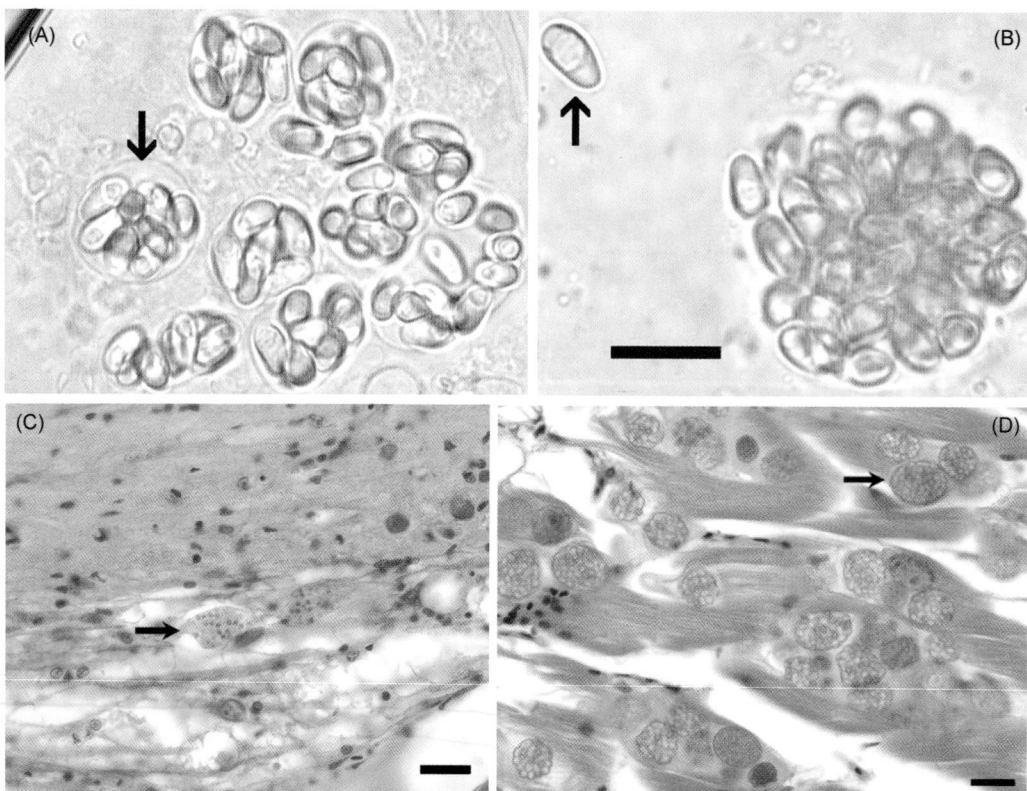

FIGURE 20.15   Wet mount and histological sections of *Pseudoloma neurophilia* and *P. hyphessobryconis*. (A) wet mount of 'bedroom slipper' spores of *P. neurophilia* within sporophorous vesicles (arrow). (B) wet mount of spores of *P. hyphessobryconis* from skeletal muscle. The arrow in this panel indicates organism with prominent round posterior vacuole. (C) H&E photomicrograph of *P. neurophilia* spores within the spinal tissue. (D) H&E photomicrograph of *P. neurophilia* spores within skeletal muscle. Panels A and B Bar = 10 μm (Sanders *et al.*, 2012). *Panels C and D courtesy of Justin Sanders, Oregon State University.*

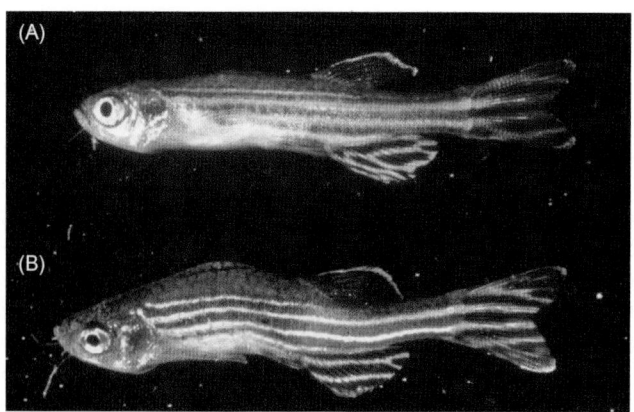

FIGURE 20.16   Gross images of fish infected with *Pseudoloma neurophilia*. Emaciation (A) and scoliotic changes (B) are associated with *P. neurophilia* infection in zebrafish. *Image courtesy of the Zebrafish International Resource Center (Kent et al., 2012b).*

sporogenic stages were detected in muscle tissue (Cali *et al.*, 2011). In clinical disease, *P. neurophilia* infection of spinal nerves can cause degenerative muscle atrophy, leading to scoliosis and emaciation (Fig. 20.16). Presence of mature spores in the musculature causes myositis and multifocal areas of atrophy in the epaxial musculature

(Sanders *et al.*, 2012). Unlike *P. neurophilia*, *P. hyphessobryconis* primarily develops within skeletal muscle (Fig. 20.15D) (Matthews *et al.*, 2001; Sanders *et al.*, 2010).

P. neurophilia infection severity is associated with husbandry stressors, including handling, high density, and transportation. Stressed infected zebrafish will develop the infection earlier than those infected fish housed in nonstressed conditions (Ramsay *et al.*, 2009b).

Clinical Signs Microsporidiosis is commonly known as 'skinny disease' because affected fish can become emaciated. *P. neurophilia* infection in zebrafish can range from subclinical to severe with emaciation, lordosis, scoliosis, and reduced growth (Fig. 20.16) (Matthews *et al.*, 2001), with severity of infection leading to increased clinical signs (Ramsay *et al.*, 2009b). The progression of this parasitic infection from subclinical to clinical disease is likely associated with stress, including environmental conditions, handling, and age of infection. Fish strain difference may be associated with severity of disease, with *P. neurophilia* infection reducing the size of TL strain versus AB strain fish (Ramsay *et al.*, 2009b). Severely infected *P. neurophilia* female fish have reduced fecundity lacking large numbers of eggs (Ramsay *et al.*, 2009b; Matthews *et al.*, 2001). Emaciation may not be due to anorexia as affected fish often contain food within their digestive tracts (Matthews *et al.*, 2001).

Diagnostics Gross necropsy findings are not commonly used to diagnose microsporidian infections. Instead, wet mount microscopy and histology are the most common and informative tests for *P. neurophilia* and *P. hyphessobryconis*. As previously mentioned, the primary site of infection of *P. neurophilia* is the central nervous system, specifically the hindbrain and spinal cord (Fig. 20.15C), but can also commonly infect nerve root ganglia, muscle, ovaries, and within eggs (Matthews *et al.*, 2001; Sanders *et al.*, 2013; Cali *et al.*, 2011).

Direct visualization of spores via tissue wet mount is diagnostic (Fig. 20.15A, B). Histological diagnosis of microsporidiosis includes direct visualization of spores within the tissue of fish, which can be accomplished by hematoxylin and eosin (H&E), Gram, Luna, periodic acid–Schiff (PAS), or Fungi-Fluor stains (Matthews *et al.*, 2001; Sanders *et al.*, 2012; Peterson *et al.*, 2011; Kent and Bishop-Stewart, 2003). Spores appear gram-positive and acid-fast, and are brick red under Luna stain. Spores are uninucleate ovoid- to pyriform-shaped. *P. neurophilia* are approximately 2.7 × 5.4 μm and *P. hyphessobryconis* are 4 × 6–7 μm in size.

P. neurophilia are found primarily in large aggregates of spores in the spinal cord, hindbrain, and muscle. These spore complexes have historically been called xenomas, but have recently been reassigned the term sporophorous vacuoles (SPOVs), since the outermost surface of the structure is parasite derived, not host derived. SPOVs are composed of uninucleate sporoblasts and spores (Fig. 20.15A) (Cali *et al.*, 2011; Matthews *et al.*, 2001). SPOVs found in neural and muscle tissue are usually not surrounded by host inflammation. Severe inflammation is usually seen in response to individual mature spores within other tissues, after expulsion from SPOVs (Ramsay *et al.*, 2009b). Spores have also been identified in the kidney, gut epithelium, and within follicles (Kent and Bishop-Stewart, 2003; Sanders *et al.*, 2013).

P. hyphessobryconis are found primarily in muscle tissue (Fig. 20.15D) and can illicit a severe inflammatory reaction. Spores of this parasite are also observed in the kidney, spleen, intestine, and ovaries (Sanders *et al.*, 2013).

Molecular diagnostics are sensitive and fast for detection (Fig. 20.15D) of *P. neurophilia*. Conventional PCR targets small subunit ribosomal DNA of *P. neurophilia* (Whipps and Kent, 2006). Real-time PCR has successfully targeted and amplified DNA of *P. neurophilia* from sonicated water, sperm, and eggs (Sanders and Kent, 2011).

Treatment There are no therapeutics described for zebrafish with microsporidiosis. Other antifungal agents, such as fumagillin, have been used in salmonids for treatment of other microsporidia, *Loma salmonae* (Speare *et al.*, 1999).

Control and Prevention Control and prevention of this disease is challenging given the high prevalence, transmission routes, and subclinical presentation of microsporidiosis. Limiting the source at the tank level can be accomplished by removing dead and moribund fish. Reducing environmental stressors, including high fish density, handling, and transportation, has been implied in reducing the severity of infection in fish with microsporidia (Ramsay *et al.*, 2009b). Monitoring microsporidia presence in zebrafish colonies can be accomplished by use of sentinel or surveillance zebrafish. Ideally, fish that are SPF for *P. neurophilia* would be used as sentinels exposed to waste tank water from individual tanks or sump water. It is recommended that zebrafish be held in sentinel tanks for at least 3 months to detect *P. neurophilia* (Kent *et al.*, 2009; Sanders and Kent, 2011). UV sterilization at 6 mJ/cm^2 (6,000 mWs/cm^2) is shown to be effective in inactivating other microsporidian parasites, such as *Encephalitozoon intestinalis* (Huffman *et al.*, 2002). Separating tanks that are known positive for *P. neurophilia* is an important control measure; however, transmission of *P. neurophilia* has been reported from infected tanks to adjacent noninfected tanks via aerosolization and/or splashing (Ramsay *et al.*, 2009b; Sanders *et al.*, 2012). Chlorine at 100 ppm that is buffered to pH 7.0 has been shown to be efficacious in inactivating >95% of *P. neurophilia* spores. While toxic for fish embryos (Kent *et al.*, 2014), this concentration may be efficacious in disinfecting equipment (Ferguson *et al.*, 2007). Current egg surface sterilization practices are insufficient in inactivating *P. neurophilia* spores on either outside or inside the zebrafish embryo.

Research Complications Given the subclinical presentation associated with microsporidiosis, nonprotocol variation of this disease should be considered in zebrafish research facilities (reviewed in Kent *et al.*, 2012a). Documented effects of microsporidiosis in fish includes reduced fecundity and decreased growth in some fish strains (Ramsay *et al.*, 2009b).

2. Water Molds (Saprolegniosis, Oomycete Infection, Winter Kill)

Etiology Water molds are composed of many genera of fungus-like organisms belonging to the class Oomycetes, also referred to as 'Pseudofungi,' that commonly infect freshwater fish. Class Oomycetes belongs to Chromista kingdom/supergroup, which has historically been included in Kingdom Protista (Hibbett *et al.*, 2007; Beakes *et al.*, 2012). There are three orders of class Oomycetes that can infect fish, including Saprolegniales, Leptomitales, and Peronosporales. Organisms within the family Saprolegniaceae are the most common fish pathogen (Noga, 2010). Reports of naturally occurring water mold infections in zebrafish include *Saprolegnia brachydanis* and *S. ferax*, identified via morphology

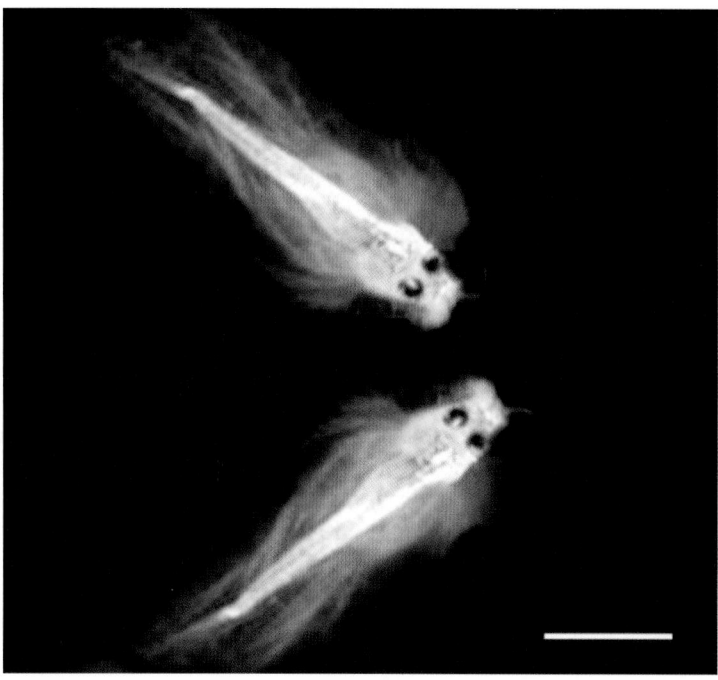

FIGURE 20.17   Gross image of zebrafish fry infected with *Saprolegnia spp.* Scale bar = 0.5 cm

and internal transcribed space (ITS) region (Fig. 20.17) (Ke *et al.*, 2009a, b). The two species most commonly isolated from other fish species are *S. parasicitica* and *S. diclina* (Noga, 2010; Pickering and Willouchby, 1977). Additionally, *Aphanomyces* spp. have been isolated from diseased zebrafish fry (Dykstra *et al.*, 2001).

Epizootiology and Transmission   Water molds are ubiquitous in aquatic water and soil. They feed saprophytically on dead or decaying organic matter and are transmitted as motile zoospores and spores. Most species of water molds do not routinely colonize healthy, living tissue. Pathogenicity varies between species of water mold (Noga, 2010; Roberts, 2012).

Pathogenesis and Predisposing Factors   Motile zoospores can germinate and grow on injured or immunocompromised fish. Lesions usually begin as small and focal, and can rapidly spread superficially across the body. Superficial damage of skin and gills can be fatal. *Saprolegnia* spp. infection in Brown Trout (*Salmo trutta* L.) causes significant reduction in serum electrolytes and protein, which is proportional to the amount of diseased skin and gills (Richards and Pickering, 1979). In addition to osmotic imbalance, secondary bacterial sepsis contributes to water mold infection mortality and morbidity. In salmonids infected with *Saprolegnia* spp., death can occur 36 hours after initial infection (Roberts, 2012).

Predisposing factors include skin wounds caused by mechanical trauma or other pathogens, handling, crowding, heavy feeding rates, immunosuppresion, and high organic loads (Tiffney, 1939; Swift and Cohen,

1962; Scott and O'Bier, 1962; Noga, 2010). These organisms frequently become established in mature biofilters (Astrofsky *et al.*, 2002b).

Clinical Signs   Clinical disease is identical amongst all Oomycetes organisms (Noga, 2010). Fish with water mold infections demonstrate thin, white filaments that build up to puffy, white, 'cottony' masses on the skin and gills. Upon removal of fish from water, the mass of fungal hyphae collapses and causes a glistening, matted appearance (Matthews, 2004; Noga, 2010).

Diagnostic Findings   Diagnosis of water mold infections can be made on wet mount with microscopic visualization of aseptate hyphae of variable width ~7–30 μm (Roberts, 2012; Matthews, 2004). Diagnostic samples should be taken from live or recently euthanized fish, as water molds will commonly invade dead tissue (Noga, 2010). *S. brachydanis* have dense mycelium near substratum with slender, sparingly branched hyphae measuring 18–55 μm in diameter at the base. Encysted zoospores are occasionally identified and are globose measuring 10–12 μm in diameter (Ke *et al.*, 2009a). Definitive diagnosis of the genus and species requires observation of asexual and sexual stages of the water mold, respectively, which requires special culture techniques (Noga, 2010).

Oomycete organism hyphae are usually present on H&E and are PAS positive on Gomori methenamine silver (GMS) stain. Hyphae do not usually penetrate deep to superficial muscle and illicit very little inflammatory response (Noga, 2010). Areas of degenerating tissue ranging from superficial dermal necrosis and edema to deep myofibrillar necrosis and extensive hemorrhage can be found under surface mats of mycelium in affected fish (Roberts, 2012).

Differential Diagnosis   Other pathogens, such as *Flavobacterium* spp. or *Epistylis* spp., may present with cottony, proliferative growths grossly, but can be distinguished easily microscopically. True fungal infections may also have a similar clinical presentation but can be differentiated by visualization of true fungal septate hyphae via wet mount microscopy (Noga, 2010).

Treatment and Prevention   Fish with large areas of the skin and gill infected with water mold carry a very poor prognosis. Treatment of water mold infection should focus on rectifying problems with and improving husbandry and environmental conditions, given that this disease is very difficult to successfully treat. Treatment of water mold infections in other fish species includes saltwater immersion at >3ppt (3 g salt in 1 l), which inhibits growth of the molds and can help counteract osmostic stress (Noga, 2010). Bronopol, a dehydrogenase enzyme inhibitor, at 20 mg/l is effective in successfully treating rainbow trout (*Oncorhynchus mykiss*) (Branson, 1997).

C. Protozoal

1. Piscinoodinium *spp. (Velvet Disease, Gold Dust Disease, Freshwater Velvet, Rust Disease, Pollularis Disease, Freshwater* Oodinium)

Etiology   Velvet disease is caused by a protozoal dinoflagellate of the genus *Piscinoodinium*. Members of the genus *Danio* are particularly susceptible to *P. pillulare* and *P. limneticum* (Westerfied, 2000). *Piscinoodinium* belongs to phylum Dinoflagellida, class Blastodiniphyceae, order Blastodiniales, and family Oodiniaceae (Noga and Levy, 2006).

Epizootiology and Transmission   *Piscinoodinium* spp. infection has become less common in zebrafish research facilities (Matthews, 2004). However, as researchers still obtain zebrafish from pet stores, this parasite is still a serious risk to research facilities. As a dinoflagellate, *P. pillulare* is highly adapted to the parasitic lifestyle and is transmitted horizontally. Trophonts feed directly on the skin or gill epithelium of fish. After feeding, the trophont detaches to form a reproductive cyst (tomont). The tomont undergoes several asexual divisions until it releases motile, infective dinospores. The life cycle is completed in 10–14 days under optimal conditions at 23–25°C. After infection of a dinospore, generation of a tomont occurs within 50–70h. Lower temperature slows the life cycle and results in larger dinospores (Noga and Levy, 2006).

Pathogenesis and Predisposing Factors   Damage to the host cell during trophont feeding is caused by epithelium invading trophont projections, or rhizocysts

which directly damages the epithelium (Noga and Levy, 2006). Damages to epithelial surfaces can also cause osmoregulatory impairment and secondary bacterial infections. The associated inflammatory and hyperplasia of the gill epithelium of trophont infection can cause hypoxia (Matthews, 2004).

Decreasing temperatures in tank-reared fish contributes to mass mortalities. *Piscinoodinium* infection is more pathogenic for young fish, which commonly die within 1–2 weeks after infection. Older fish may live for months with *Piscinoodinium* infection (Noga and Levy, 2006).

Clinical Signs   *Piscinoodinium* spp. colonizes and infests the skin and gills. Clinical signs include excess mucus production, skin darkening, anorexia, depression, decreased feeding, surface swimming, and labored breathing. Fish infected with *Piscinoodinium* spp. will also commonly flash, or flip over and rub against the side of the tank due to epithelial irritation/pruritus. Yellow or rusty sheen to the skin occurs in heavy infections (Fig. 20.18A) (Noga and Levy, 2006). In some cases, skin ulcerates and tattered, sloughing epithelium can be seen (Shaharom-Harrison *et al.*, 1990).

Diagnostic Findings   Microscopic visualization of the numerous, oval, opaque nonmotile trophonts can be seen in wet mount examination of the skin or gills. The trophonts measure approximately 9–12 × 40–90 μm (Kent *et al.*, 2012b). Gill histopathology includes separation of the respiratory epithelium, severe gill filament hyperplasia, degeneration, and/or necrosis (Fig. 20.18B). Skin histopathology includes deep, focal erosions of epithelium. Oval *Piscinoodinium* spp. can also be visualized on histopathology of affected tissues (Fig. 20.18C,D) (Noga and Levy, 2006; Kent *et al.*, 2012b).

Diagnosis of *Piscinoodinium* spp. infection is based on direct visualization of the organisms on wet mount or histopathology. Direct gross visualization of the organisms can be enhanced by directing a flashlight onto the dorsal aspect of the affected fish in a darkened room. A fine, dusty, granular effect will be evident (Matthews, 2004).

Treatment   While there are no reports of successful treatments of *Piscinoodinium* spp. in zebrafish, there are several treatment options for affected fish facilities. The safest and most effective treatment is prolonged immersion in saltwater solution of 1 gram per gallon of water. Immersion of heavily infected fish in saltwater bath concentration of 35 grams per liter of water for 3 minutes will dislodge trophonts (Noga, 2010). In the event of an outbreak in a system or systems, treatment of systems must be also taken into consideration. Removal of fish from affected systems will stop the *Piscoodinium* spp. life cycle within 2 weeks.

Control and Prevention   Given the source of *Piscinoodinium* spp. in a research zebrafish facility may

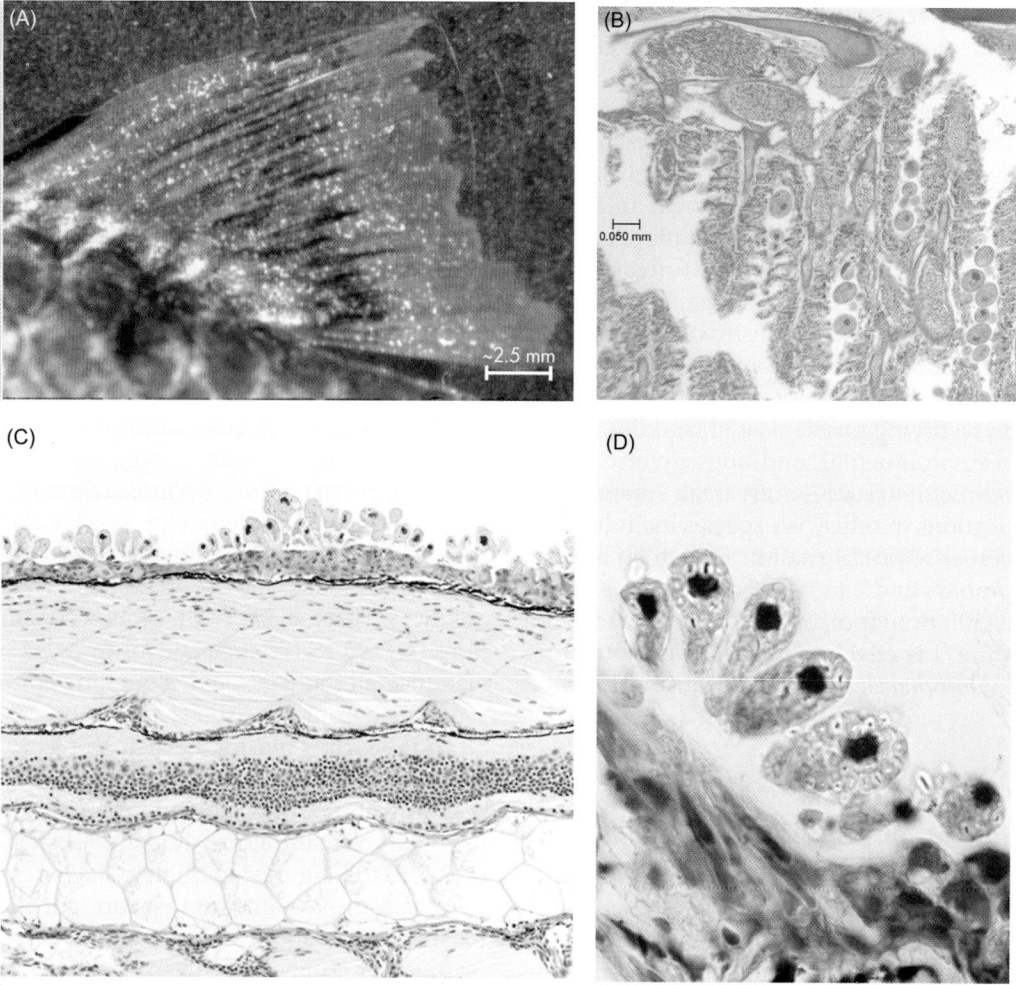

FIGURE 20.18 *Piscinoodinium* spp. infection in fish. (A) Gross image of the dust like covering of *P. pillulare* in tiger barb (Noga, 2010). (B) Photomicrograph of a H&E section of gills heavily infected with *Piscinoodinium* spp. (Matthews, 2004). (C,D) Photomicrographs of H&E sections of skin infected with trophonts on the skin of a zebrafish. Panel C and D photomicrographs taken at 200x and 1000x magnification. *Bottom panels are courtesy of Marcus Crim, IDEXX BioResearch.*

be incoming fish, preventing entry of this pathogen can be best accomplished by allowing only surface-sanitized (bleached) embryos into facility systems.

2. Ichthyophthirius multifilis (*White Spot Disease, Ich*)

Etiology White spot disease, or Ich, is caused by the ciliated protozoan parasite *Ichthyophthirius multifilis* (Ich). Zebrafish, along with most freshwater aquarium fishes, are susceptible to this parasite.

Ich has a similar life cycle to *Piscinoodinium* spp., in that it has both host and environmental life stages. The Ich trophont feeds within the epithelium fin, skin, and/or gills of the host fish. After feeding, Ich breaks through the epithelium, falls off the host, and forms a reproductive cyst (tomont). Unlike *Piscinoodinium* spp., the tomont secretes a sticky capsule that sticks to substrate. Binary fission occurs up to 10 times within the tomont

to produce tomites. Tomites next break through the nodule wall while differentiating into motile, infective $20 \times 50\,\mu m$ theronts. Over 1000 theronts can be produced from one trophont. The life cycle of Ich lasts 3–6 days at 25°C and increases in length as water temperature decreases (Noga, 2010; Dickerson, 2006).

Epizootiology and Transmission While mortality associated with this disease is high, this disease is rarely seen in research zebrafish facilities. However, it is an external parasite that is commonly found in fish from ornamental aquaculture and the pet fish trade. Outbreaks are usually associated in salmonids at high or low temperatures, or in overcrowded conditions (Noga, 2010).

Pathogenesis After differentiation from tomites, trophonts swim in the environment and attach to the epithelium surface of a host, where they penetrate to the basal layer of gill or skin epithelium within 5 minutes. As the parasite enters the skin, it becomes substantially

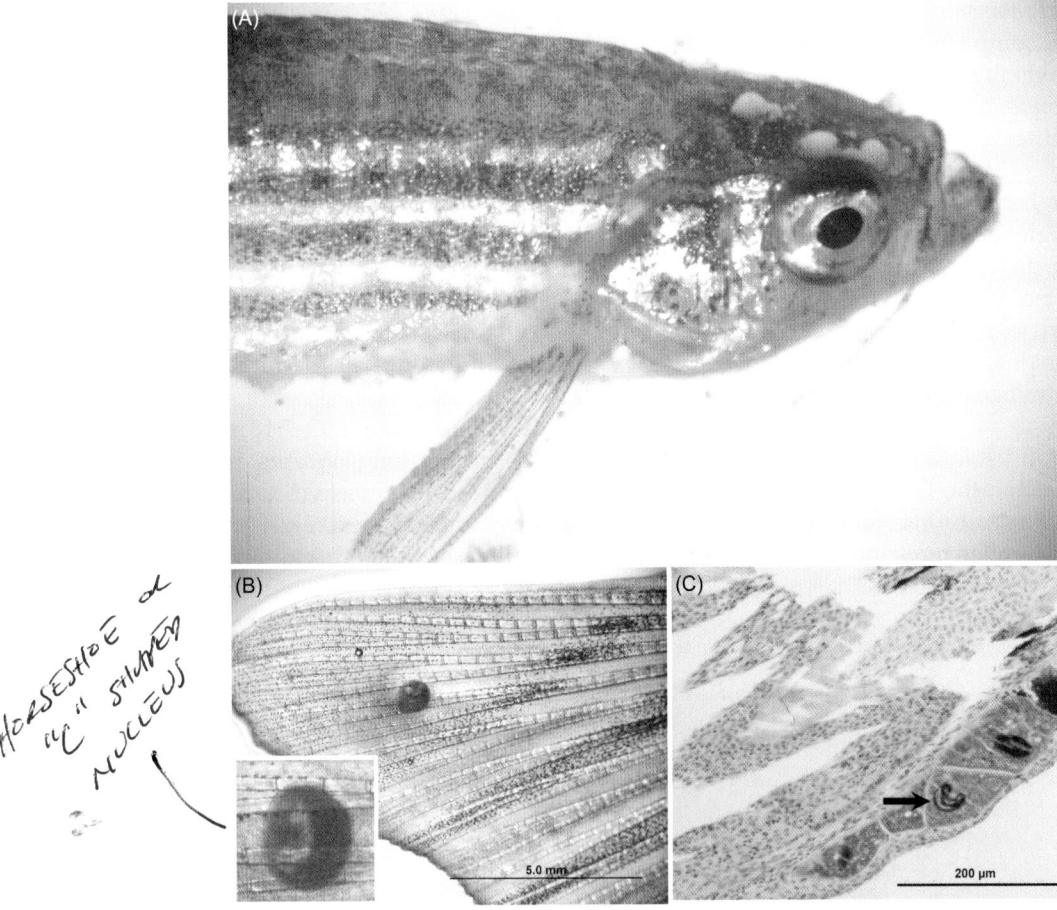

FIGURE 20.19   *Ichthyophthirius multifilis* infection. (A) Gross image of a zebrafish infected with numerous white, mucoid, spherical nodules along the external surface. (B) Photograph demonstrating a single trophont embedded within the caudal fin of a zebrafish. Note the C-shaped macronucleus. (C) Photomicrograph of an H&E section of skin. Infected with trophont of *I. multifilis. Images are courtesy of Marcus Crim, IDEXX BioResearch.*

larger and eventually creates a tissue space in the epithelium layers, which appears as a 1 mm white spot on the skin surface (Noga, 2010; Dickerson, 2006).

Clinical Signs   Affected fish develop multifocal, raised, white, 1 mm in diameter mucoid nodules on the skin and gills. The nodules contain trophont stage parasites (Fig. 20.19A). Other clinical signs include excessive mucus production, labored breathing, and lethargy (Kent *et al.*, 2012b; Noga, 2010).

Diagnostic Findings   Identifying a ciliate trophont encysted within the host's epithelium on a wet mount or microscopic examination is pathognomonic for Ich (Fig. 20.19B). Movement of cilia can be seen under microscope. The trophont also has a characteristic horseshoe-shaped macronucelus which is also visible on wet mount or histological section (Fig. 20.19B,C) (Noga, 2010). Histopathology findings of Ich include severe epithelial hyperplasia in the vicinity of the parasite (Kent *et al.*, 2012b).

Treatment   There are multiple treatment modalities for Ich in fish species. In addition to removing Ich from fish, efforts should be taken to remove Ich from the tank/system. Affected fish should be removed from the tank/

system and be placed into a clean tank. Some Ich isolates are susceptible to salt concentrations above 1 mg/l, but some may require higher concentrations of 5 mg/l of saltwater to treat successfully. Alternatively, prolonged formalin immersion is usually effective, with 25 ppm treatments on alternative days for 3 days. It is best to test the safety of treatment options on a few fish first before applying to all affected fish. The temperature of the water in the affected tank/system can be increased to hasten the life cycle of the parasite (Noga, 2010; Matthews, 2004).

Control and Prevention   Using UV light sterilizers can mitigate the risk of spread of infectious theronts. Theronts can be killed by UV light (100,000 µWs/cm^2) (Harper and Lawrence, 2010).

D. Metazoan

1. Intestinal Capillariasis (Nematode Infection, Roundworm Infection)

Etiology   *Pseudocapillaria tomentosa* is an intestinal nematode of zebrafish. Unlike some other capillarid nematodes of fishes, *P. tomentosa* does not require an intermediate host to complete a life cycle and can instead complete a direct life cycle with zebrafish (Kent *et al.*, 2002). *P. tomentosa*, however, could potentially use oligochaetes parenteric, or transport, hosts (Noga, 2010).

Epizootiology and Transmission   The incidence of intestinal capillariasis detected by the ZIRC diagnostic service is moderate with approximately 25% of facilities tested by ZIRC (Dr. Mike Kent, personal communication). Experimental exposure of zebrafish to other infected fish with intestinal capillariasis supports horizontal transmission, by ingestion of embryonated eggs (Kent *et al.*, 2002).

Pathogenesis   Adult *P. tomentosa* worms (Fig. 20.20A,C) are found within the lumen and gastrointestinal wall, which can cause chronic wasting. The adult worms can invade through the intestine, causing significant inflammation (Kent *et al.*, 2002).

Clinical Signs   In affected facilities, progressive wasting illness and reduced fecundity were associated with intestinal nematodes (Pack *et al.*, 1995). Clinical signs in affected zebrafish include emaciation, appearing darker in color, and reduced fecundity (Noga, 2010; Pack *et al.*, 1995; Kent *et al.*, 2002). A parasitic nematode similar to *P. tomentosa* causes emaciation, coelomic distension, and increased mortality ranging from 0.7% to 4.6% per month (Maley *et al.*, 2013).

Diagnostic Findings   In naturally occurring intestinal capillariasis, adult motile worms are observed within the epithelium and lamina propria of the intestines, which can be visualized in wet mount preparations. Male worms are 3.95–7.18 mm long and females are 7.30–12.04 mm long. Worms are thin and transparent and are locally invasive. Ova can be seen within the gravid female (Fig. 20.20A). Eggs have distinctive, bi-polar plugs, thin shell walls, and measure 27–35 × 57–68 µm (Fig. 20.20B) (Kent *et al.*, 2002).

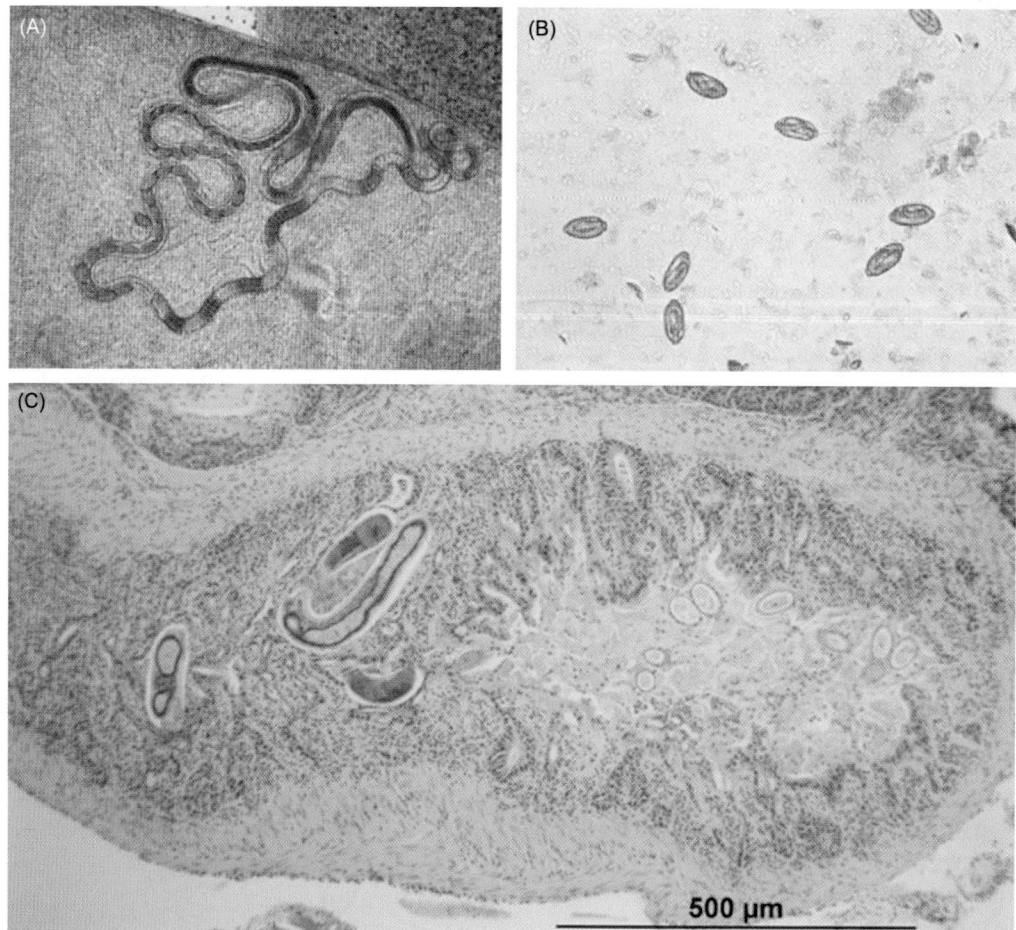

FIGURE 20.20   Images of *Pseudocapillaria tomentosa*. (A) Photo of a female worm. Note the striped anterior end with stichocysts. (B) Wet mount of embryonated eggs. (C) Photomicrograph of an H&E section of the gastrointestinal tract of a zebrafish infected with *P. tomentosa*. Note adult worms within the intestinal mucosa on the left and the associated eggs on the right. *The top panels are courtesy of Mike Kent and Virginia Watral. The bottom panel is courtesy of Marcus Crim, IDEXX BioResearch.*

Histologically, adult worms can be found within the lumen and the wall of the intestinal tract using H&E stain. The associated inflammation is variable, ranging from mild, locally extensive to diffuse, chronic granulomatous, transmural inflammation. Intestinal neoplasms near the intestinal–esophageal junction have also been identified in zebrafish with *P. tomentosa* infection, with worms often being associated directly with the locally extensive or multifocal tumor. Tumors are either intestinal cell carcinomas or mixed malignant tumors with epithelial and mesenchymal components (Kent *et al.*, 2002). Whereas *P. tomentosa* is likely a promoter of these tumors, the tumors occur in fish from many laboratories where the resident fish are not infected with the worm (Paquette *et al.*, 2013). Diagnosis of capillariasis is indicated upon findings adult worms inside the intestinal tract on H&E histological examination (Fig. 20.20C) or by identifying them grossly after dissecting the intestine (Matthews, 2004). Infection diagnosis can also be made by identification of bipolar eggs consistent with capillarid nematodes in fish excreta or aquarium detritus (Fig. 20.20B).

Treatment Successful treatment of zebrafish infected with intestinal nematodes can be accomplished safely by use of Emamectin (SLICE®, Merck) medicated pelleted diet or fenbendazole in *Artemia* feed suspension. Emamectin at 0.25–0.5 mg/kg daily for 7 days does not appear to affect behavioral observations, fecundity, or mortality, while significantly reducing infections and eliminating gravid female worms (Collymore *et al.*, 2014b). Fenbendazole solution (25 g/l) is added to a final concentration of 25 mg/l in *Artemia*, which zebrafish are allowed to feed to satiation while remaining off system circulation for 1 h. This regime is repeated twice a day for 3 days, which is repeated in 2 weeks. Fecundity of treated zebrafish 5 weeks after treatment is low, with nearly 50% of embryos in the first clutch being dead or malformed. Egg viability, however, returns to normal in subsequent clutches (Maley *et al.*, 2013).

Control and Prevention Effective control of established intestinal nematode infection can be accomplished by improving husbandry protocols, including using new nets per tank, regular disinfection of breeding containers, hand-washing for users, prompt removal of dead fish, and cleaning of system tanks every 3 weeks (Maley *et al.*, 2013).

Prevention can be accomplished by avoiding sources of infection, like oligochaete worms (*Tubifex tubifex*) feed sources (Kent *et al.*, 2002). Quarantine procedures and bleach-only egg procedures will mitigate the risk of importing intestinal nematodes into zebrafish systems (Harper and Lawrence, 2010).

Research Complications Zebrafish models of cancer, inflammation, or gastrointestinal disease may be impacted by the clinical presentation and *P. tomentosa*-associated intestinal neoplasia (Kent *et al.*, 2002, 2012a).

E. Fungal

1. Lecythophora mutabilis

Unlike water mold infections, fungal infections in fish are rare and are associated with localized epizootics. There is one report of a high mortality outbreak in a zebrafish facility of a true fungus *Lecythophora mutabilis*. *L. mutabilis* is an opportunistic, ubiquitous organism found in the environment. Zebrafish fry 5–24 dpf were affected with 'beards' of hyphae extending from oral cavity to opercula covering the gills. This outbreak is associated with a major renovation to the building water system. Other clinical signs include lethargy and decreased feeding behavior. Diagnosis was based on direct whole mounts of fish fry without staining. H&E or PAS-stained sections did not yield a consistent pattern of pathologic changes. Despite this, fungus was cultured and isolated, being characterized with cylindrical to slightly curved narrow conidia formed in wet clusters at the ends of short peg-like or needle-shaped phialides along the hyphae. In culture, the *L. mutabilis* isolate was found to be susceptible to antifungal drugs itraconazole, fluconazole, and amphotericin B (Dykstra *et al.*, 2001).

F. Water Quality Diseases

1. Gas Bubble Disease

Etiology Gas bubble disease (GBD) occurs as a result of gas supersaturation of tank/system water by nitrogen or oxygen, which is defined when the total pressure of gases in water is higher than ambient atmospheric pressure. The total pressure of gases in water is also dependent on temperature and salinity. In recirculating systems, supersaturation can be caused by a leaky pipe that leads to air injection, pumping water from deep wells without gas 'stripping,' and injection of air from filters upon water changes (Kent *et al.*, 2012b; Noga, 2010).

Epizootiology GBD will typically affect many zebrafish on a given system. Acute GBD can cause high mortality in minutes, but can also present less acutely. Morbidity and mortality rates are largely dependent on the degree of supersaturation and duration of exposure (Speare, 2010).

Pathogenesis Disease is caused by excess gas entering the bloodstream as emboli in various tissues. Cause of death is suggested to be vascular occlusion of the branchial vessels (Edsall and Smith, 1991; Smith, 1988).

Clinical Signs Severe, acute cases have gross appearances of gas bubbles, especially in the skin, fins, gills, or eyes (Fig. 20.21). Some fish may present with exophthalmia. Affected zebrafish can behave abnormally with hyperactivity and loss of equilibrium with rapid operculum movement, and will often accumulate at the bottom of the water column.

Diagnostic Findings The presence of gas emboli is pathognomonic for gas bubble disease. Diagnosis can be confirmed in the dead fish by squeezing bubbles from fin or gills while held under water (Noga, 2010). Gas bubbles can be visible in gill blood vessels, skin, or internal organs on wet mount. Histologic sections may reveal bubbles in the retrobulbar tissues and edema of the gill secondary lamella with degeneration of overlying epithelium. Air bubbles can be seen within blood vessels, causing thrombi and hemorrhage (Kent *et al.*, 2012b). It is important, however, to note that GBD can occur in the absence of macroscopic bubbles.

Treatment Elimination of excess gas in water is the primary treatment for GBD (Noga, 2010). Identifying and resolving the source of the problem in the system should be addressed immediately. If the source of air into the recirculation system is unknown, water circulation should be temporarily turned off to mitigate additional air entering the water. Most cases of gas supersaturation can be directly attributed to air becoming entrapped in the plumbing system through faulty or aging equipment such as piping, joint seals, or hose fittings usually on the suction side of the pump. Air trapped within a running pump will usually result in a 'gurgling or rattling' noise. Once the excess air is purged from the system and the cause of the gas supersaturation identified and remedied, the increased levels of dissolved gas within the water will equilibrate with the room air. However, this can be facilitated by the aeration of the water in the system or enclosures which will physically drive excessive dissolved gas out of solution at relevant atmospheric pressure.

Control and Prevention Supersaturated gases in water can be measured by saturometers and tensiometers. Less direct monitoring of oxygen in the water can be provided by dissolved oxygen or oxidation–reduction

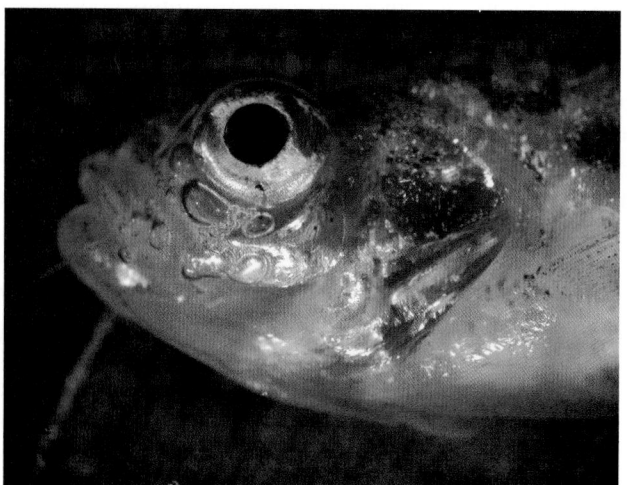

FIGURE 20.21 Gross image of zebrafish with pathognomonic signs of gas bubble disease. Note bubbles around the eye and under the skin of the head (Matthews, 2004).

potential meters. Zebrafish that survive GBD are susceptible to secondary infections and should be examined closely in the days after GBD resolution (Astrofsky *et al.*, 2000; Kent *et al.*, 2012b).

2. Ammonia Toxicity

Ammonia is the primary waste product of fish and is produced by uneaten food, unhatched *Artemia*, and fish decay. The unionized ammonia molecule, NH_3, is highly toxic to fish, whereas the ionized ammonium (NH_4^+) is much less toxic. The nitrogen cycle is covered earlier in this chapter in more detail. Ammonia is detoxified normally by biological filter microbes collectively called ammonia-oxidizing bacteria (AOB) and ammonia-oxidizing archaea (AOA). Disruptions in these microbe functions can be attributed to an excessive number of fish added to a new system, antibiotic-mediated obliteration of biofilter nitrifying bacteria, mechanical removal of nitrifying bacteria from biofilter's substrate, or inappropriate fish shipping and unloading (Harper and Lawrence, 2010). Clinical signs include behavioral abnormalities, including hyperexcitability, anorexia, and death (Daoust and Ferguson, 1984; Noga, 2010). Histologic presentation of chronic ammonia exposure includes gill hyperplasia and hypertrophy (Noga, 2010).

Diagnosing ammonia toxicity involves testing the water directly. The unionized ammonia in water is dependent on pH and temperature of the water. Table 20.5 lists the total ammonia nitrogen present in unionized form (in percent). For example, at a pH of 7.5 and temperature of 26°C, the total percent of unionized, or toxic, ammonia is 1.89%. The concentration of unionized ammonia can be calculated with a known quantity for total ammonia nitrogen, which can be measured easily using a commercially available kit. In this example, if, at 26°C, the total ammonia nitrogen measures 1 mg/l, then the unionized ammonia concentration (in mg/l) is equivalent to 1 mg/l × 0.0189. An unionized ammonia of 0.0189 mg/l is below the sublethal poisoning (0.02–0.05 mg/l (ppm)). The lethal limit of unionized ammonia can be as low as 0.5 mg/l (ppm); however, it should be maintained as close to 0 mg/l as possible (Matthews, 2004).

Correction of ammonia toxicity is the first step of treating affected fish. This is accomplished by reducing stocking density, increased water changes, addition of ammonia absorbing resins or binders, reduction pH, additional biologic filtration, and reduced feeding (Matthews, 2004; Noga, 2010). Any treatment option, however, should be part of a plan to establish a robust biological filter in the system (Noga, 2010).

3. Nitrite Toxicity

Nitrite toxicity occurs when fish are exposed to high levels of nitrite, which can be caused by similar circumstances noted in ammonia toxicity. Increased levels of nitrite are associated with inappropriate levels of nitrite-oxidizing bacteria (NOB), including *Nitrobacter* spp. and *Nitrospira* spp. that convert nitrite (NO_2) to nitrate (NO_3). In a new tank, nitrite spikes often occur after ammonia peaks, given chemotrophic, NOB require time to become active (Noga, 2010).

Active uptake of nitrite ions into the gills enters the bloodstream. Upon entry, nitrite oxidizes hemoglobin to methemoglobin, which carries oxygen inefficiently causing tissue hypoxia. Methemoglobin is brown, giving fish with nitrite poisoning a pale tan or brown gills. Clinical signs include lethargy, increased respiratory rate, and surface swimming. Diagnosis for nitrite toxicity can be made by combining clinical signs with nitrite concentration measures of the water (Noga, 2010).

Nitrite levels should be monitored regularly and be kept under 0.1 mg/l to avoid possible toxicity. Treatment modalities includes addition of chloride ions, which may competitively inhibit nitrite uptake across gills (Bowser *et al.*, 1983). Sodium chloride or calcium chloride can be added to tanks, but care should be taken in increasing salinity of water slowly. Using a 3-mg chloride to 1-mg nitrite ratio, channel catfish (*Ictalurus punctatus*) have been successfully treated for nitrite toxicity. Use of calcium chloride can be added at a concentration of less than 50 mg/l (Tomasso *et al.*, 1979). The goal of treatment should be the establishment of a stable, healthy biofilter.

4. Chlorine/Chloramine Toxicity

Both chlorine and chloramine are highly toxic to fish and are added to municipal water supplies to kill microorganisms. Municipal water systems require chlorine/chloramine concentrations of at least 0.2 mg/l, but may have up to 0.5–1.0 mg/l (Noga, 2010). Toxicity can lead to acute to subacute mortality following a new tank setup or use of tap water for a fresh water change. Chlorine reacts with gill tissue, causing acute necrosis and asphyxiation (Noga, 2010). Extensive mucous

secretion and gill epithelium hypertrophy can occur in chronic exposure (Leef *et al.*, 2007). Chlorine can be easily removed from water by allowing a 24-hour period of aeration or by adding a commercial dechlorinator. Acute chloramine exposures causes respiratory and acid-base disturbances. Chloramine cannot be removed by aeration, but must instead be filtered through activated carbon or treated with a chemical neutralizer, such as sodium thiosulfate. Near-boiling water can also remove chloramines (Noga, 2010). Treatment for acute chlorine poisoning includes eliminating chlorine/chloramine source water and supersaturated water with oxygen for several days (Noga, 2010).

Diagnosis of chlorine and chloramine toxicity is presumptive but can also be determined by using a commercially available test kit. Chlorine levels should be no higher than 0 mg/l (Noga, 2010).

5. Nephrocalcinosis

Nephrocalcinosis occurs in captive marine and freshwater fish and is seen commonly in research zebrafish (Roberts, 2012; Kent *et al.*, 2012b). This condition has been associated with high levels of carbon dioxide in the water (e.g., >12 mg/l) or unbalanced levels of diet calcium or magnesium (Smart *et al.*, 1979; Harrison, 1980). Use of calcium carbonate to maintain alkalinity in a recirculating aquaculture system is associated with moderate to severe nephrocalcinosis in nile tilapia (*Oerochromis niloticus*). Incidence of nephrocalcinosis decreased with replacement of calcium carbonate with sodium bicarbonate (Chen *et al.*, 2001). Increased CO_2 levels in water can be also caused by poor water exchange and increased housing density (Kent *et al.*, 2012b).

Zebrafish with nephrocalcinosis will normally present with incidental histological findings of basophilic, crystalline calcium urolith deposits in the kidney and collecting ducts. Unless the lesions are severe, there are usually no clinical signs of disease. In zebrafish, lesions are not typically grossly evident (Kent *et al.*, 2012b).

TABLE 20.5   Selected Percentage Values of Total Ammonia in Unionized Form (NH_3) Based on pH and Temperature of Water Tested

pH value	Temperature (°C)								
	22	23	24	25	26	27	28	29	30
6.0	0.046	0.049	0.053	0.057	0.061	0.065	0.070	0.075	0.080
6.5	0.145	0.156	0.167	0.180	0.193	0.207	0.221	0.237	0.254
7.0	0.457	0.491	0.527	0.566	0.607	0.651	0.697	0.747	0.799
7.5	1.430	1.540	1.650	1.770	1.890	2.030	2.170	2.320	2.480
8.0	4.390	4.700	5.030	5.380	5.750	6.150	6.560	7.000	7.460
8.5	12.700	13.500	14.400	15.300	16.200	17.200	18.200	19.200	20.300
9.0	31.500	33.000	34.600	36.300	37.900	39.600	41.200	42.900	44.600

Table taken from Matthews (2004) and adapted from Emerson et al. (1975).

G. Neoplasia

While zebrafish have been used extensively in oncology research, relatively little is known regarding basic cancer biology in spontaneous and induced tumors. Spontaneous neoplasia in zebrafish are common clinical findings, especially in older animals. Spitsbergen and colleagues (2012) provide a review of common neoplasia in zebrafish, with an emphasis on the role of nutrition and aquaculture system design. A brief overview of zebrafish neoplasia is given here.

1. Seminoma

Seminoma neoplasia is the most common spontaneous tumor seen in male zebrafish and one of the most common spontaneous tumors seen in zebrafish (Amsterdam et al., 2010; Spitsbergen et al., 2012). Males with seminomas present with distended coelomic cavities and are often older broodstock over 1.5 years of age. Grossly, the tumors are soft, white, and multilobulated and restricted to the testes. Microscopically, unlike human and dog seminoma, these are often characterized as being well-differentiated, maintaining normal testis structure, and containing multiple germ cell stages, not including sperm (Kent et al., 2012b).

2. Intestinal Neoplasia

Intestinal neoplasia is a commonly diagnosed disease in adult zebrafish over 1 year of age. This disease is commonly diagnosed as an incidental finding on histology. While intestinal neoplasia etiology is unclear, this disease is associated with P. tomentosa infection, with and without exposure to carcinogenic polycyclic aromatic hydrocarbon. In P. tomentosa infections, gut neoplasia develops in close proximity of the nematodes, which can occur at any site in the intestinal tract. Histologically, these tumors are epithelial- and mesenchymal-derived, primarily mucosal adenocarcinoma and small cell carcinomas located commonly in the anterior and mid-intestine (Kent et al., 2002; Paquette et al., 2013; Spitsbergen et al., 2012).

3. Ultimobranchial Neoplasia

The ultimobranchial gland is a paired midline organ located ventral to the esophagus in the transverse membrane separating the pericardial and coelomic cavities. This organ is analogous to the C cells of the mammalian thyroid gland by producing calcitonin (Menke et al., 2011; Busby et al., 2010; Alt et al., 2006). Ultimobranchial tumors are one of the most common neoplasia occurring spontaneously or after exposure to carcinogenic compounds, although the etiology is unknown (Spitsbergen et al., 2000; Spitsbergen et al., 2012). These tumors occur in older fish above 1.5 years of age and do not typically appear grossly, but are typically seen as incidental findings on histology examination (Kent et al., 2012b).

Ultimobranchial tumors can also be large enough to compromise venous return to the heart causing chronic passive congestion and gross enlargement of the spleen (Spitsbergen et al., 2012; Spitsbergen, personal communication). Histologically, ultimobranchial tumors are generally benign and consist of packets or monotonous sheets of ovoid to polygonal neuroendocrine cells. Malignant tumors consist of less differentiated epithelial cells invading through the gland fibrous capsule (Kent et al., 2012).

4. Spindle Cell Carcinoma

Spindle cell carcinoma is a term used to describe several tumors (fibrosarcoma, leiomyosarcoma, and malignant nerve sheath neoplasm) that are often difficult to differentiate grossly and histologically. These are relatively more common than hepatocellular carcinoma. Tumors can develop in the viscera, skeletal muscle, or behind the eye, with the latter causing exopthalmia. Diagnosis of this disease is usually done histologically (Kent et al., 2012b). These tumors become more common with exposure to mutagenic and carcinogenic compounds (Spitsbergen et al., 2012).

5. Hepatocellular Neoplasia

Hepatic neoplasia are one of the most common spontaneously occurring neoplasia in zebrafish. Grossly, tumors will appear as soft, white to tan within the liver. Histologically, most liver neoplasia are benign, but can also be malignant. Benign hepatocellular adenomas consist of well-differentiated hepatocytes and may compress surrounding hepatic parenchyma. Malignant hepatocellular carcinomas consist of anaplastic hepatocytes, which have lost organization and invade into surrounding normal hepatic tissue (Kent et al., 2012b).

H. Other Diseases

1. Egg-Associated Inflammation

Severe, chronic inflammation associated with degenerating eggs is a common finding of adult female zebrafish. This condition is anecdotally caused by egg retention and has not been found to be associated with a pathogenic agent. Clinical signs of egg-associated inflammation (EAI) are female zebrafish with distended or enlarged coelomic cavity and, on occasion, hyperplasia or papilloma of the vent. In some cases, the mass will adhere to the internal coelomic wall and extrude to the outside of the animal as an ulcer. Ovaries may appear as a solid, tumor like mass characterized with intact to degenerating eggs, fibrotic tissue, and, on occasion, prominent fibroplasia and fibrosarcoma. Given that egg retention is a potential cause, EAI prevention includes spawning females in a timely manner (Kent et al., 2012b).

Acknowledgment

The authors wish to offer their sincere gratitude to the following individuals for their input and evaluation of this chapter. Without the addition of their thoughts and personal experience, this chapter would be incomplete: Michael Kent, Oregon State University and George Sanders, University of Washington. In addition, we would like to thank the following individuals for the use of several photographs and figures: Leonard Zon, Boston Children's Hospital; Lucille B. Wilhelm, Massachusetts Institute of Technology; E. Scott Weber III; Wendy Porter-Fancis, Aquaneering, Inc.; Daniel A. Vinci, Aquatic Enterprises, Inc.; Jill Keller, University of Michigan; Chris M. Whipps, State University of New York-ESF; John Hawke, Louisiana State University; Wes Baumgartner, Mississippi State University; Justin Sanders, Oregon State University; Jeff Wolf, Experimental Pathology Laboratories, Inc.; Katy Murray, Zebrafish International Resource Center; Jianguo Wang, Chinese Academy of Sciences; Marcus Crim, IDEXX RADIL; Virginia Watral, Oregon State University; and Jennifer Matthews, Zebrafish International Resource Center.

References

Abeliovich, A., 2006. The nitrite oxidizing bacteria. In: Dworkin, M. (Ed.), The Prokaryotes, Volume 5: Proteobacteria: Alpha and Beta Subclasses. Springer, New York, pp. 861–872.

Akimenko, M.A., et al., 1995. Differential induction of four msx homeobox genes during fin development and regeneration in zebrafish. Development 121 (2), 347–357.

Al-Adhami, M.A., Kunz, Y.W., 1977. Ontogenesis of haematopoietic sites in brachydanio rerio (Hamilton-buchanan) (Teleostei). Dev. Growth Differ. 19 (2), 171–179.

Alt, B., et al., 2006. Analysis of origin and growth of the thyroid gland in zebrafish. Dev. Dyn. 235 (7), 1872–1883.

Altinok, I., Grizzle, J.M., 2001. Effects of low salinities on Flavobacterium columnare infection of euryhaline and freshwater stenohaline fish. J. Fish. Dis. 24, 361–367.

Amsterdam, A., et al., 2010. Zebrafish Hagoromo mutants upregulat fgf8 post-embryonically and develop neuroblastoma. Mol. Cancer Res. 7 (6), 841–850.

Ang, P., Rattana-Apiromyakij, N., Goh, C.L., 2000. Retrospective study of Mycobacterium marinum skin infections. Int. J. Dermatol. 39 (5), 343–347.

Arunachalam, M., et al., 2013. Natural history of zebrafish (Danio rerio) in India. Zebrafish 10 (1), 1–14.

Astrofsky, K.M., et al., 2000. Diagnosis and management of atypical Mycobacterium spp. infections in (Brachydanio rerio) facilities. Comp. Med. 50 (6), 666–672.

Astrofsky, K.M., Schech, J.M., et al., 2002a. High mortality due to Tetrahymena sp. infection in laboratory-maintained zebrafish (Brachydanio rerio). Comp. Med. 52 (4), 363–367.

Astrofsky, K.M., Bullis, R.A., Sagerstrom, C.G., 2002b. Chapter 19 Biology and Management of the Zebrafish. In: Fox, J.G. (Ed.), Laboratory Animal Medicine. Elsevier, pp. 861–883.

Aubry, A., et al., 2002. Sixty-three cases of mycobacterium marinum infection. Arch. Intern. Med. 162, 1746–1752.

Austin, B., Austin, D., 2007. Characteristics of the diseases. In: Austin, B., Austin, D.A. (Eds.), Bacterial Fish Pathogens: Diseases of Farmed and Wild Fish Springer Praxis Books, Dordrecht, pp. 15–46. Springer Netherlands.

Bagchi, S., et al., 2014. Temporal and spatial stability of ammonia-oxidizing archaea and bacteria in aquarium biofilters. PLoS One 9 (12), e113515.

Balla, K.M., et al., 2010. Eosinophils in the zebrafish: prospective isolation, characterization, and eosinophilia induction by helminth determinants. Blood 116 (19), 3944–3954.

Bassett, D.I., et al., 2003. Dystrophin is required for the formation of stable muscle attachments in the zebrafish embryo. Development 130 (23), 5851–5860.

Beakes, G.W., Glockling, S.L., Sekimoto, S., 2012. The evolutionary phylogeny of the oomycete "fungi." Protoplasma 249 (1), 3–19.

Beckwith, L.G., et al., 2000. Ethylnitrosourea induces neoplasia in zebrafish (Danio rerio). Lab. Invest. 80 (3), 379–385.

Beran, V., et al., 2006. Distribution of mycobacteria in clinically healthy ornamental fish and their aquarium environment. J. Fish. Dis. 29 (7), 383–393.

Bernardet, J., et al., 1996. Cutting a Gordian Knot: Emended Classification and Description of the Genus Flavobacterium, Emended Description of the Family Flavobacteriaceae, and Proposal of Flavobacterium hydatis. Int. J. of Syst. Bact 46 (1), 128–148.

Best, J., et al., 2010. A novel method for rearing first-feeding larval zebrafish: polyculture with Type L saltwater rotifers (Brachionus plicatilis). Zebrafish 7 (3), 289–295.

Blaser, R., Gerlai, R., 2006. Behavioral phenotyping in zebrafish: comparison of three behavioral quantification methods. Behav. Res. Methods 38, 456–469.

Bock, E., Wagner, M., 2006. Oxidation of inorganic nitrogen compounds as an energy source. In: Dworkin, M. (Ed.), The Prokaryotes, Volume 2: Ecophysiology and Biochemistry. Springer, New York, pp. 457–495.

Bowser, P.R., et al., 1983. Methemoglobinemia in channel catfish: methods of prevention. Prog. Fish Culturist 45 (3), 154–158.

Branson, E., 1997. Efficacy of bronopol against infection of the fungus Saprolegnia species. Vet. Rec. 151, 539–542.

Burrell, P.C., Phalen, C.M., Hovanec, T.A., 2001. Identification of bacteria responsible for ammonia oxidation in freshwater aquaria. Appl. Environ. Microbiol. 67 (12), 5791–5800.

Busby, E., Roch, G., Sherwood, N., 2010. Endocrinology of zebrafish: a small fish with a large gene pool. In: Perry, S. (Ed.), Fish Physiology, Vol. 29: Zebrafish, pp. 173–248.

Cade, L., et al., 2012. Highly efficient generation of heritable zebrafish gene mutations using homo- and heterodimeric TALENs. Nucleic. Acids Res. 40 (16), 8001–8010.

Cahu, C., Infante, J.Z., 2001. Substitution of live food by formulated diets in marine fish larvae. Aquaculture 200 (1–2), 161–180.

Cali, A., et al., 2011. Development, ultrastructural pathology, and taxonomic revision of the Microsporidial genus, Pseudoloma and its type species Pseudoloma neurophilia, in skeletal muscle and nervous tissue of experimentally infected zebrafish Danio rerio. J. Eukaryot. Microbiol. 59 (1), 40–48.

Camargo, J.A., Alonso, A., Salamanca, A., 2005. Nitrate toxicity to aquatic animals: a review with new data for freshwater invertebrates. Chemosphere 58, 1255–1267.

Carmichael, C., Westerfield, M., Varga, Z.M., 2009. Cryopreservation and in vitro fertilization at the zebrafish international resource center. Methods. Mol. Biol. 546, 45–65.

Carnahan, A., Altwegg, M., 1996. Taxonomy. In: Austin, B. (Ed.), The Genus Aeromonas John Wiley & Sons, Inc, West Sussex, England, pp. 1–38.

Carradice, D., Lieschke, G.J., 2008. Zebrafish in hematology: sushi or science? Blood 111 (7), 3331–3342.

Carvalho, A.P., Araujo, L., Santos, M.M., 2006. Rearing zebrafish (Danio rerio) larvae without live food: evaluation of a commercial, a practical and a purified starter diet on larval performance. Aquacul. Res. 37 (11), 1107–1111.

Castignettii, D., Hollocher, T.C., 1984. Heterotrophic nitrification among denitrifiers. Appl. Environ. Microbiol. 47 (4), 620–623.

Castranova, D., et al., 2011. The effect of stocking densities on reproductive performance in laboratory zebrafish (Danio rerio). Zebrafish 8 (3), 141–146.

Canadian Council on Animal Care, 2005. Guidelines on the care and use of fish in research, teaching and testing., Ottawa, Ontario.

Chan, J., et al., 2001. Morphogenesis of prechordal plate and notochord requires intact Eph/ephrin B signaling. Dev. Biol. 234 (2), 470–482.

Chen, C.-Y., et al., 2001. Nephrocalcinosis in nile tilapia from a recirculation aquaculture system: a case report. J. Aquat. Anim. Health. 13 (4), 368–372.

Chen, K., et al., 2014. The evaluation of rapid cooling as an anesthetic method for the zebrafish. Zebrafish 11 (1), 71–75.

Cheung, J.P., et al., 2010. Review article: mycobacterium marinum infection of the hand and wrist. J. Orthop. Surg. (Hong Kong) 18 (1), 98–103.

Chow, S.P., et al., 1987. Mycobacterium marinum infection of the hand and wrist: results of conservative treatment in twenty-four cases. J. Bone. Joint. Surg. 69 (October).

Chung, E., et al., 2011. Effects of bisphenol A and triclocarban on brain-specific expression of aromatase in early zebrafish embryos. Proc. Natl. Acad. Sci. 108, 17732–17737.

Cipriano, R.C., Bullock, G.L., Pyle, S.W., 1984. Aeromonas Hydrophila and Motile Aeromonad Septicemias of Fish.

Colle-Vandevelde, A., 1963. The blood anlage in teleostei. Nature 193, 1223.

Collins, M.T., et al., 1976. Effects of antibacterial agents on nitrification in an aquatic recirculating system. J. Fish. Res. Board Canada 33 (2), 215–218.

Collymore, C., Tolwani, A., et al., 2014a. Efficacy and safety of 5 anesthetics in adult zebrafish (Danio rerio). J. Am. Assoc. Lab. Anim. Sci. 53 (2), 198–203.

Collymore, C., Watral, V.G., et al., 2014b. Tolerance and efficiency of emamectin benzoate and ivermectin for the treatment of Pseudocapillaria tomentosa in laboratory zebrafish (Danio rerio). Zebrafish 11 (5).

Collymore, C., Rasmussen, S., Tolwani, R.J., 2013. Gavaging adult zebrafish. J. Vis. Exp. (78), e50691.

Cooper, J.E., 2004. Invertebrate care. Vet. Clin. North Am. Exot. Anim. Pract. 7 (2), 473–486. viii.

Cortemeglia, C., Beitinger, T.L., 2005. Temperature tolerances of wild-type and red transgenic zebra danios. Trans. Am. Fish. Soc. 134 (6), 1431–1437.

Cosma, C.L., Sherman, D.R., Ramakrishnan, L., 2003. The secret lives of the pathogenic mycobacteria. Annu. Rev. Microbiol. 57, 641–676.

Crim, M.J., Riley, L.K., 2012. Viral diseases in zebrafish: what is known and unknown. ILAR J. 53 (2), 135–143.

Daoust, P.-Y., Ferguson, H.W., 1984. The pathology of chronic ammonia toxicity in rainbow trout, Salmo gairdneri Richardson. J. Fish. Dis. 7 (3), 199–205.

Davies, H., et al., 2002. Mutations of the BRAF gene in human cancer. Nature 417 (6892), 949–954.

Davis, J.M., et al., 2002. Real-time visualization of mycobacterium–macrophage interactions leading to initiation of granuloma formation in zebrafish embryos. Immunity 17 (6), 693–702.

Decostere, A., et al., 1999. Characterization of the adhesion of Flavobacterium columnare (Flexibacter columnaris) to gill tissue. J. Fish. Dis. 22 (6), 465–474.

DeTolla, L.J., et al., 1995. Guidelines for the care and use of fish in research. ILAR. J. 37 (4), 159–173.

Dickerson, H.W., 2006. Ichthyophthirius multifiliis and Cryptocaryon irritans (Phylum Ciliophora). In: Woo, P.T.K. (Ed.), Fish Diseases and Disorders - Volume 1 Protozoan and Metazoan Infections CAB International, Oxfordshire, UK; Cambridge, MA, pp. 116–153.

Doyon, Y., et al., 2008. Heritable targeted gene disruption in zebrafish using designed zinc-finger nucleases. Nat. Biotechnol. 26 (6), 702–708.

Draper, P., 1971. The walls of Mycobacterium lepraemurium: chemistry and ultrastructure. J. Gen. Microbiol. 69 (3), 313–324.

Driever, W., et al., 1994. Zebrafish: genetic tools for studying vertebrate development. Trends Genet. 10 (5), 152–159.

Driever, W., et al., 1996. A genetic screen for mutations affecting embryogenesis in zebrafish. Development (Cambridge, England) 123, 37–46.

Dykstra, M.J., et al., 2001. High mortality in a large-scale zebrafish colony (Brachydanio rerio Hamilton and Buchanan, 1822) associated with Lecythophora mutabilis (van Beyma) W. Gams and McGinnis. Comp. Med. 51 (4), 361–368.

Eames, S.C., et al., 2010. Blood sugar measurement in zebrafish reveals dynamics of glucose homeostasis. Zebrafish 7 (2), 205–213.

Edsall, D.A., Smith, C., 1991. Oxygen-induced gas bubble disease in rainbow trout, Oncorhynchus mykiss (Walbaum). Aquacul. Fish. Manage. 22, 135–140.

Eisen, J.S., 1991. Determination of primary motoneuron identity in developing zebrafish embryos. Science 252 (5005), 569–572.

Eisen, J.S., Smith, J.C., 2008. Controlling morpholino experiments: don't stop making antisense. Development 135 (10), 1735–1743.

Emerson, K., et al., 1975. Aqueous ammonia equilibrium calculations: effects of pH and temperature. J. Fish. Res. Board Canada 32 (12), 2379–2383.

Engeszer, R.E., et al., 2007. Zebrafish in the wild: a review of natural history and new notes from the field. Zebrafish 4 (1), 21–40.

Esch, G.W., Hazen, T., 1980. The Ecology of Aeromonas hydrophila in Albemarle Sound, North Carolina. Water Resources Research Institute of the University of North Carolina, Raleigh, North Carolina.

Esteve, C., Biosca, E.G., Amaro, C., 1993. Virulence of Aeromonas hydrophila and some other bacteria isolated from European eels Anguilla anguilla reared in fresh water. Diseases of aquatic organisms 16, 15–20.

Falkinham, J.O., 2009. Surrounded by mycobacteria: nontuberculous mycobacteria in the human environment. J. Appl. Microbiol. 107 (2), 356–367.

Falkinham, J.O., Norton, C.D., 2001. Factors influencing numbers of Mycobacterium avium, Mycobacterium intracellulare, and other mycobacteria in drinking water distribution system, Journal of Applied and environmental Microbiology. 67(3), 1225–1231.

Ferguson, H.W., et al., 1991. Experimental production of bacterial gill disease in trout by horizontal transmission and by bath challenge. J. Aquat. Anim. Health. 3 (2), 118–123.

Ferguson, J.A., et al., 2007. Spores of two fish microsporidia (Pseudoloma neurophilia and Glugea anomala) are highly resistant to chlorine. Dis. Aquat. Organ. 76 (3), 205–214.

Filby, A.L., et al., 2010. Physiological and health consequences of social status in zebrafish (Danio rerio). Physiol. Behav. 101 (5), 576–587.

Fouquet, B., et al., 1997. Vessel patterning in the embryo of the zebra-fish: guidance by notochord. Dev. Biol. 183 (1), 37–48.

French, E., et al., 2012. Ecophysiological characterization of ammonia-oxidizing archaea and bacteria from freshwater. Appl. Environ. Microbiol. 78 (16), 5773–5780.

Garcia, R.L., Sanders, G.E., 2011. Efficacy of cleaning and disinfection procedures in a zebrafish (Danio rerio) facility. J. Am. Assoc. Lab. Anim. Sci. 50, 895–900.

Gauthier, D.T., Rhodes, M.W., 2009. Mycobacteriosis in fishes: a review. Vet. J. (London, England: 1997) 180 (1), 33–47.

Gemberling, M., et al., 2013. The zebrafish as a model for complex tissue regeneration. Trends. Genet. 29 (11), 611–620.

Grush, J., Noakes, D.L.G., Moccia, R.D., 2004. The efficacy of clove oil as an anesthetic for the zebrafish, Danio rerio (Hamilton). Zebrafish 1 (1), 46–53.

Haffter, P., et al., 1996. The identification of genes with unique and essential functions in the development of the zebrafish, Danio rerio. Development (Cambridge, England) 123, 1–36.

Halpern, M.E., et al., 1993. Induction of muscle pioneers and floor plate is distinguished by the zebrafish no tail mutation. Cell 75 (1), 99–111.

Hamilton-Buchanan, F., 1822. An Account of the Fishes Found in the River Ganges and Its Branches. George Ramsay and Co, Cheapside, London.

Harikrishnan, R., Balasundaram, C., 2005. Modern trends in aeromonas hydrophila disease management with fish. Rev. Fish. Sci. 13 (4), 281–320.

Harper, C., Lawrence, C., 2010. The Laboratory Zebrafish (Laboratory Animal Pocket Reference). CRC Press.

Harriff, M.J., Bermudez, L.E., Kent, M.L., 2007. Experimental exposure of zebrafish, Danio rerio (Hamilton), to Mycobacterium marinum and Mycobacterium peregrinum reveals the gastrointestinal tract as the primary route of infection: a potential model for environmental mycobacterial infection. J. Fish. Dis. 30 (10), 587–600.

Harris, J.A., et al., 2003. Neomycin-induced hair cell death and rapid regeneration in the lateral line of zebrafish (Danio rerio). J. Assoc. Res. Otolaryngol. 4 (2), 219–234.

Harrison, J.G., 1980. Nephrocalcinosis of Rainbow Trout (Salmo gairdneri Richardson) in Freshwater; a Survey of Affected Farms. In: Ahne, W. (Ed.), Fish Diseases: Third COPRAQ-Session Springer-Verlag, Berlin HeidelBerk New York, pp. 193–197.

Hatta, K., et al., 1991. The cyclops mutation blocks specification of the floor plate of the zebrafish central nervous system. Nature 350 (6316), 339–341.

Hatzenpichler, R., 2012. Diversity, physiology, and niche differentiation of ammonia-oxidizing archaea. Appl. Environ. Microbiol. 78 (21), 7501–7510.

Hawke, J.P., 1979. A Bacterium associated with disease of pond cultured channel catfish. J. Fish. Res. Board Canada 36 (12), 1508–1512.

Hawke, J.P., et al., 1981. Edwardsiella ictaluri sp. nov., the Causative Agent of Enteric Septicemia of Catfish. Int. J. Syst. Evol. Bacteriol. 31 (4), 396–400.

Hawke, J.P., et al., 2013. Edwardsiellosis caused by edwardsiella ictaluri in laboratory populations of zebrafish danio rerio. J. Aquat. Anim. Health. 25 (3), 171–183.

Hazen, T.C., et al., 1978. Ultrastructure of Red-Sore Lesions on Largemouth Bass. J. Protozool. 25 (3), 351–355.

Helfrich, L.A., Libey, G., 1990. Fish farming in recirculating aquaculture systems (RAS). Department of Fisheries and Wildlife, Virginia Tech, pp.19.

Hibbett, D.S., et al., 2007. A higher-level phylogenetic classification of the Fungi. Mycol. Res. 111 (5), 509–547.

Hirt, R.P., et al., 1999. Microsporidia are related to fungi: evidence from the largest subunit of RNA polymerase II and other proteins. Proc. Natl. Acad. Sci. USA. 96 (2), 580–585.

Ho, R.K., Kane, D.A., 1990. Cell-autonomous action of zebrafish spt-1 mutation in specific mesodermal precursors. Nature 348 (6303), 728–730.

Hoffman, G.L., 1999. Parasites of North American Freshwater Fishes. Cornell University Press.

Hovanec, T.A., DeLong, E.F., 1996. Comparative analysis of nitrifying bacteria associated with freshwater and marine aquaria. Appl. Environ. Microbiol. 62 (8), 2888–2896.

Hovanec, T.A., Long, E.F.D.E., 1996. Comparative analysis of nitrifying bacteria associated with freshwater and marine aquaria 62(8), 2888–2896.

Hovanec, T.A., Taylor, L.T., Blakis, A., 1998. Nitrospira-like bacteria associated with nitrite oxidation in freshwater aquaria. Journal of Applied and environmental Microbiology 64(1), 258–264.

Howe, K., et al., 2013. The zebrafish reference genome sequence and its relationship to the human genome. Nature 496 (7446), 498–503.

Huang, W.-C., et al., 2010. Combined use of MS-222 (tricaine) and isoflurane extends anesthesia time and minimizes cardiac rhythm side effects in adult zebrafish. Zebrafish 7 (3), 297–304.

Huffman, D.E., et al., 2002. Low- and medium-pressure UV inactivation of microsporidia Encephalitozoon intestinalis. Water Res. 36 (12), 3161–3164.

Hwang, W.Y., Fu, Y., Reyon, D., Maeder, M.L., Tsai, S.Q., et al., 2013a. Efficient genome editing in zebrafish using a CRISPR-Cas system. Nat. Biotechnol. 31 (3), 227–229.

Hwang, W.Y., Fu, Y., Reyon, D., Maeder, M.L., Kaini, P., et al., 2013b. Heritable and precise zebrafish genome editing using a CRISPR-Cas system. PLoS One 8 (7), e68708.

Jagadeeswaran, P., et al., 1999. Identification and characterization of zebrafish thrombocytes. Br. J. Haematol. 107 (4), 731–738.

Jaya-Ram, A., et al., 2008. Influence of dietary HUFA levels on reproductive performance, tissue fatty acid profile and desaturase and elongase mRNAs expression in female zebrafish Danio rerio. Aquaculture 277 (3–4), 275–281.

Kahn, P., 1994. Zebrafish hit the big time. Science (New York, N.Y.) 264 (5161), 904–905.

Kawahara, G., et al., 2011. Drug screening in a zebrafish model of Duchenne muscular dystrophy. Proc. Natl. Acad. Sci. USA. 108 (13), 5331–5336.

Kawakami, K., et al., 2004. A transposon-mediated gene trap approach identifies developmentally regulated genes in zebrafish. Dev. Cell. 7 (1), 133–144.

Kawakami, K., 2004. Transgenesis and gene trap methods in zebrafish by using the Tol2 transposable element. Methods Cell. Biol. 77 (201–22), 201–222.

Kawakami, K., Kusuda, R., 1990. Efficacy of rifampin, streptomycin and erythromycin against experimental Mycobacterium infection in cultured yellowtail. Bull. Jpn. Soc. Sci. Fish. 56 (1), 51–53.

Kawakami, K., Shima, A., Kawakami, N., 2000. Identification of a functional transposase of the Tol2 element, an Ac-like element from the Japanese medaka fish, and its transposition in the zebrafish germ lineage. Proc. Natl. Acad. Sci. USA. 97 (21), 11403–11408.

Ke, X.L., et al., 2009a. Saprolegnia brachydanis, a new oomycete isolated from zebra fish. Mycopathologia 167 (2), 107–113.

Ke, X.L., et al., 2009b. Morphological and molecular phylogenetic analysis of two Saprolegnia sp. (Oomycetes) isolated from silver crucian carp and zebra fish. Mycol. Res. 113 (5), 637–644.

Kent, M.L. et al., 2002. Pseudocapillaria tomentosa, a nematode pathogen, and associated neoplasms of zebrafish (Danio rerio) kept in research colonies. Comp. Med. 52(4), 354–358.

Kent, M.L., et al., 2004. Mycobacteriosis in zebrafish (Danio rerio) research facilities. Comp. Biochem. Physiol. C Toxicol. Pharmacol. 138 (3), 383–390.

Kent, M.L., et al., 2009. Recommendations for control of pathogens and infectious diseases in fish research facilities. Comp. Biochem. Physiol. Toxicol. Pharmacol. 149 (2), 240–248.

Kent, M.L., et al., 2011. Development and maintenance of a specific pathogen-free (SPF) zebrafish research facility for Pseudoloma neurophilia. Dis. Aquat. Organ. 95 (1), 73–79.

Kent, M.L., et al., 2014. Toxicity of chlorine to zebrafish embryos. Dis. Aquat. Organ. 107 (3), 235–240.

Kent, M.L., Bishop-Stewart, J.K., 2003. Transmission and tissue distribution of Pseudoloma neurophilia (Microsporidia) of zebrafish, Danio rerio. Journal of Fish Diseases, 26, 423–426.

Kent, M.L., Harper, C., Wolf, J.C., 2012a. Documented and potential research impacts of subclinical diseases in zebrafish. ILAR. J. 53 (2), 126–134.

Kent, M.L., et al., 2012b. Diseases of zebrafish in research facilities. ZIRC Health Services Zebrafish Disease Manual (April).

Kimmel, C.B., et al., 1989. A mutation that changes cell movement and cell fate in the zebrafish embryo. Nature 337 (6205), 358–362.

Kimmel, C.B., et al., 1995. Stages of embryonic development of the zebrafish. Dev. Dyn. 203 (3), 253–310.

King, C.H., Shotts, E.B., 1988. Enhancement of Edwardsiella tarda and A eromonas salmonicida through ingestion by the ciliated protozoan Tetrahymena pyrif ormis. FEMS. Microbiol. Lett. 51, 95–99.

Kinkelin, P., 1980. Occurrence of a microsporidian infection in zebra danio Brachydanio rerio (Hamilton-Buchanan). J. Fish. Dis. 3 (1), 71–73.

Kirkwood, J.S., et al., 2012. Vitamin C deficiency activates the purine nucleotide cycle in zebrafish. J. Biol. Chem. 287, 3833–3841.

Klesius, P., 1994. Transmission of edwardsiella ictaluri from infected, dead to noninfected channel catfish. J. Aquat. Anim. Health. 6 (2), 180–182.

Klesius, P.H., Shoemaker, C.A., Evans, J.J., 2008. Flavobacterium columnare chemotaxis to channel catfish mucus. FEMS. Microbiol. Lett. 288 (2), 216–220.

Knapik, E.W., et al., 1998. A microsatellite genetic linkage map for zebrafish (Danio rerio). Nat. Genet. 18 (4), 338–343.

Könneke, M., et al., 2005. Isolation of an autotrophic ammonia-oxidizing marine archaeon. Nature 437 (7058), 543–546.

Langenau, D.M., et al., 2003. Myc-induced T cell leukemia in transgenic zebrafish. Science 299 (5608), 887–890.

Lavens, P., Sorgeloos, P. 1996. Manual on the production and use of live food for aquaculture FAO Fisheries Technical Paper. No. 361. Rome, FAO. 295p.

Lawrence, C., 2007. The husbandry of zebrafish (Danio rerio): a review. Aquaculture 269 (1–4), 1–20.

Lawrence, C., Mason, T., 2012. Zebrafish housing systems: a review of basic operating principles and considerations for design and functionality. ILAR. J. 53 (2), 179–191.

Lawrence, C., et al., 2012. Generation time of zebrafish (Danio rerio) and medakas (Oryzias latipes) housed in the same aquaculture facility. Lab. Anim. (NY) 41 (6), 158–165.

Lawrence, C., Ennis, D.G., et al., 2012a. The challenges of implementing pathogen control strategies for fishes used in biomedical research. Comp. Biochem. Physiol. Toxicol. Pharmacol. 155 (1), 160–166.

Lawrence, C., Best, J., et al., 2012b. The effects of feeding frequency on growth and reproduction in zebrafish (Danio rerio). Aquaculture, 103–108. 368–369.

Leef, M.J., Harris, J.O., Powell, M.D., 2007. The respiratory effects of chloramine-T exposure in seawater acclimated and amoebic gill disease-affected Atlantic salmon Salmo salar L. Aquaculture 266 (1–4), 77–86.

Lehane, L., Rawlin, G.T., 2000. Topically acquired bacterial zoonoses from fish: a review. Med. J. Aust. 173 (5), 256–259.

Li, J., et al., 2011. Detection of three virulence genes alt, ahp and aerA in Aeromonas hydrophila and their relationship with actual virulence to zebrafish. J. Appl. Microbiol. 110 (3), 823–830.

Lieschke, G.J., 2001. Morphologic and functional characterization of granulocytes and macrophages in embryonic and adult zebrafish. Blood 98 (10), 3087–3096.

Lin, S., et al., 1994. Integration and germ-line transmission of a pseudotyped retroviral vector in zebrafish. Science 265 (5172), 666–669.

Lom, J., et al., 2000. Ultrastructural justification for the transfer of Pleistophora anguillarum Hoshina, 1959 to the genus Heterosporis Schubert, 1969. Dis. Aquat. Organ. 43 (3), 225–231.

Maley, D., et al., 2013. A simple and efficient protocol for the treatment of zebrafish colonies infected with parasitic nematodes. Zebrafish 10 (3), 447–450.

Martinez-Murcia, A., et al., 1992. Aeromonas allosaccharophila sp. nov., a new mesophili member of the genus Aeromonas. FEMS. Microbiol. Lett. 91, 199–206.

Matthews, J.L., 2004. Common diseases of laboratory zebrafish. Methods Cell. Biol. 77, 617–643.

Matthews, J.L., et al., 2001. Pseudoloma neurophilia n. g., n. sp., a new microsporidium from the central nervous system of the zebrafish (Danio rerio). J. Eukaryot. Microbiol. 48 (2), 227–233.

Matthews, M., Varga, Z.M., 2012. Anesthesia and euthanasia in zebrafish. ILAR. J. 53 (2), 192–204.

Matthews, M., Trevarrow, B., Matthews, J., 2002. A virtual tour of the Guide for zebrafish users. Lab. Anim. (NY) 3 (34–40).

Meinelt, T., et al., 1999. Dietary fatty acid composition influences the fertilization rate of zebrafish (Danio rerio Hamilton-Buchanan). J. Appl. Ichthyol. 15 (1), 19–23.

Meinelt, T., et al., 2000. Correlation of diets high in n-6 polyunsaturated fatty acids with high growth rate in zebrafish (Danio rerio). Comp. Med. 50 (1), 43–45.

Menke, A.L., et al., 2011. Normal anatomy and histology of the adult zebrafish. Toxicol. Pathol. 39 (5), 759–775.

Michelson, E.H., 1961. An acid-fast pathogen of fresh-water snails. Am. J. Trop. Med. Hyg. 10, 423–433.

Miller, G.W., et al., 2012. Zebrafish (Danio rerio) fed vitamin E-deficient diets produce embryos with increased morphologic abnormalities and mortality. J. Nutr. Biochem. 23, 478–486.

Miller, N., Gerlai, R., 2012. From schooling to shoaling: patterns of collective motion in zebrafish (Danio rerio). PLoS One 7 (11), e48865.

Monaghan, S.R., et al., 2009. Animal cell cultures in microsporidial research: their general roles and their specific use for fish microsporidia. In Vitro Cell. Dev. Biol. Anim. 45 (3–4), 135–147.

Moss, L.G., Caplan, T.V., Moss, J.B., 2013. Imaging Beta cell regeneration and interactions with islet vasculature in transparent adult zebrafish. Zebrafish 10 (2), 249–257.

Moyer, T.R., Hunnicutt, D.W., 2007. Susceptibility of zebra fish Danio rerio to infection by Flavobacterium columnare and F. johnsoniae. Dis. Aquat. Organ. 76 (1), 39–44.

Mullins, M.C., et al., 1994. Large-scale mutagenesis in the zebrafish: in search of genes controlling development in a vertebrate. Curr. Biol. 4 (3), 189–202.

Murray, K.N., Bauer, J., et al., 2011a. Characterization and management of asymptomatic Mycobacterium infections at the Zebrafish International Resource Center. J. Am. Assoc. Lab. Anim. Sci. 50 (5), 675–679.

Murray, K.N., Dreska, M., et al., 2011b. Transmission, diagnosis, and recommendations for control of Pseudoloma neurophilia infections in laboratory zebrafish (Danio rerio) facilities. Comp. Med. 61 (4), 322–329.

Murtha, J.M., Qi, W., Keller, E.T., 2003. Hematologic and serum biochemical values for zebrafish (Danio rerio). Comp. Med. 53 (1), 37–41.

National Academies, 2011. N.R.C. of The Guide for the Care and Use of Laboratory Animals, eighth ed. The National Academies Press, Washington, DC.

Nigrelli, R.F., Vogel, H., 1963. Spontaneous tuberculosis in fishes and in other cold-blooded vertebrates in special reference to mycobacterium fortuitum cruz from fish and human lesions. Zool. N. Y. Zool. Soc. 48 (9), 131–143.

Noga, E.J., 2010. Fish Disease: Diagnosis and Treatment, second ed.

Noga, E., Levy, M.G., 2006. Phylum Dinoflagellata. In: Woo, P.T.K. (Ed.), Fish Diseases and Disorders - Volume 1 Protozoan and Metazoan Infections CAB International, Oxfordshire, UK; Cambridge, MA, pp. 16–45.

Obholzer, N., et al., 2012. Rapid positional cloning of zebrafish mutations by linkage and homozygosity mapping using whole-genome sequencing. Development 139 (22), 4280–4290.

Olivares-Fuster, O., et al., 2011. Adhesion dynamics of Flavobacterium columnare to channel catfish Ictalurus punctatus and zebrafish Danio rerio after immersion challenge. Dis. Aquat. Organ. 96, 221–227.

Onal, U., Langdon, C., 2000. Characterization of two microparticle types for delivery of food to altricial fish larvae. Aquaculture Nutr. 6, 159–170.

Ortuno, J., Meseguer, J., Esteban, M.A., 2003. The effect of dietary intake of vitamins C and E on the stress response of gilthead seabream (Sparus aurata L.). Fish Shellfish Immunol. 2, 145–156.

Ostland, V.E., et al., 1990. Bacterial gill disease of salmonids; relationship between the severity of gill lesions and bacterial recovery. Dis. Aquat. Organ. 9, 5–14.

Owens, K.N., et al., 2008. Identification of genetic and chemical modulators of zebrafish mechanosensory hair cell death. PLoS Genet. 4 (2), e1000020.

Pack, M., et al., 1995. Intestinal capillariasis in zebrafish. Zebrafish Sci. Monit. 3 (4).

Panangala, V.S., et al., 2005. Analysis of 16S-23S intergenic spacer regions of the rRNA operons in Edwardsiella ictaluri and Edwardsiella tarda isolates from fish. J. Appl. Microbiol. 99 (3), 657–669.

Panangala, V.S., et al., 2007. Multiplex-PCR for simultaneous detection of 3 bacterial fish pathogens, Flavobacterium columnare, Edwardsiella ictaluri, and Aeromonas hydrophila. Dis. Aquat. Organ. 74 (3), 199–208.

Paquette, C.E., et al., 2013. A retrospective study of the prevalence and classification of intestinal neoplasia in zebrafish (danio rerio). Zebrafish 10 (2), 228–236.

Patton, E.E., et al., 2005. BRAF mutations are sufficient to promote nevi formation and cooperate with p53 in the genesis of melanoma. Curr. Biol. 15 (3), 249–254.

Pavlidis, M., et al., 2011. Adaptive changes in zebrafish brain in dominant–subordinate behavioral context. Behav. Brain. Res. 225, 529–537.

Pavlidis, M. et al., 2013. Husbandry of Zebrafish, Danio Rerio, and the Cortisol Stress Response. Zebrafish pp. 1–8.

Pedroso, G.L., et al., 2012. Blood collection for biochemical analysis in adult zebrafish. J. Vis. Exp. (63), e3865.

Peterson, T.S., et al., 2011. Luna stain, an improved selective stain for detection of microsporidian spores in histologic sections. Dis. Aquat. Organ. 95 (2), 175–180.

Peterson, T.S., Kent, M.L., et al., 2013a. Comparison of fixatives and fixation time for PCR detection of Mycobacterium in zebrafish Danio rerio. Dis. Aquat. Organ. 104 (2), 113–120.

Peterson, T.S., Ferguson, J.A., et al., 2013b. Paramecium caudatum enhances transmission and infectivity of Mycobacterium marinum and M. chelonae in zebrafish Danio rerio. Dis. Aquat. Organ. 106, 229–239.

Petrie-Hanson, L., et al., 2007. Evaluation of zebrafish Danio rerio as a model for enteric septicemia of catfish (ESC). J. Aquat. Anim. Health. 19 (3), 151–158.

Pickering, D., Willouchby, L.G., 1977. Epidermal lesions and fungal infection on the perch, Perca Jluviatilis L., in Windermere. 11, 349–354.

Piper, R.G. et al., 1982. Fish Hatchery Management, Washington, DC.

Pliss, G.B., Khudoley, V.V., 1975. Tumor induction by carcinogenic agents in aquarium fish. J. Natl. Cancer. Inst. 55 (1), 129–136.

Plumb, J.A., Quinlan, E.E., 1986. Survival of edwardsiella ictaluri in pond water and bottom mud. Prog. Fish Culturist 48 (3), 212–214.

Poss, K.D., Wilson, L.G., Keating, M.T., 2002. Heart regeneration in zebrafish. Science 298 (5601), 2188–2190.

Postlethwait, J.H., Talbot, W.S., 1997. Zebrafish genomics: from mutants to genes. Trends Genet. 13 (5), 183–190.

Pressley, M.E., et al., 2005. Pathogenesis and inflammatory response to Edwardsiella tarda infection in the zebrafish. Dev. Comp. Immunol. 29 (6), 501–513.

Pritchard, V.L., et al., 2001. Shoal choice in zebrafish, Danio rerio: the influence of shoal size and activity. Anim. Behav. 62, 1085–1088.

Pullium, J.K., Dillehay, D.L., Webb, S., 1999. High mortality in zebrafish (Danio rerio). Contemp. Top. Lab. Anim. Sci. 38 (3), 80–83.

Ramsay, J.M., et al., 2006. Whole-body cortisol is an indicator of crowding stress in adult zebrafish, Danio rerio. Aquaculture 258 (1–4), 565–574.

Ramsay, J.M., et al., 2009a. Husbandry stress exacerbates mycobacterial infections in adult zebrafish, Danio rerio (Hamilton). J. Fish. Dis. 32 (11), 931–941.

Ramsay, J.M., et al., 2009b. Pseudoloma neurophilia infections in zebrafish Danio rerio: effects of stress on survival, growth, and reproduction. Dis. Aquat. Organ. 88 (1), 69–84.

Readman, G.D. et al., 2013. Do fish perceive anaesthetics as aversive? Chapouthier, G. (Ed.), PLoS One, 8(9), e73773.

Reno, P.W., 1998. Factors involved in the dissemination of disease in fish populations. J. Aquat. Anim. Health. 10, 160–171.

Richards, R.H., Pickering, A.D., 1979. Changes in serum parameters of Saprolegnia-infected brown trout, Salmo trutta L. J. Fish. Dis. 2 (3), 197–206.

Roberts, R.J., 2012. In: Roberts, R.J. (Ed.), Fish Pathology, fourth ed. Wiley-Blackwell, Oxford.

Rodríguez, I., Novoa, B., Figueras, A., 2008. Immune response of zebrafish (Danio rerio) against a newly isolated bacterial pathogen Aeromonas hydrophila. Fish Shellfish Immunol. 25 (3), 239–249.

Rohner, N., Harris, M.P., Perathoner, S., 2011. Enhancing the Efficiency of N-Ethyl-N-Nitrosourea-Induced Mutagenesis in the Zebrafish. Journal of Zebrafish 8(3), 10–15.

Rombough, P.J., 2007. Ontogenetic changes in the toxicitiy and efficacy of the anaesthetic MS222 (tricaine methanesulfonate) in zebrafish (Danio rerio) larvae. Comp. Biochem. Physiol. A Mol. Integr. Physiol. 148 (2), 463–469.

Ross, A.J., Johnson, H.E., 1962. Studies of transmission of mycobacterial infections in chinook salmon. Prog. Fish Culturist. 147–149.

Ross, L., Ross, B., 2008. Anaesthetic and Sedative Techniques for Aquatic Animals, third ed., Oxford; Ames, Iowa: Blackwell.

Russell, D.G., 2001. Mycobacterium tuberculosis: here today, and here tomorrow. Nat. Rev. Mol. Cell. Biol. 2 (8), 569–577.

Saili, K.S., et al., 2012. Neurodevelopmental low-dose bisphenol A exposure leads to early life-stage hyperactivity and learning deficits in adult zebrafish. Toxicology 291, 83–92.

Sánchez-Vázquez, F.J., et al., 2011. Daily rhythms of toxicity and effectiveness of anesthetics (MS222 and eugenol) in zebrafish (Danio rerio). Chronobiol. Int. 28 (2), 109–117.

Sanders, G.E., 2013. Zebrafish housing, husbandry, and care. In Bioconference Live: International Laboratory Animal Science.

Sanders, J.L., et al., 2010. Pleistophora hyphessobryconis (Microsporidia) infecting zebrafish Danio rerio in research facilities. Dis. Aquat. Organ. 91 (1), 47–56.

Sanders, J.L., et al., 2013. Verification of intraovum transmission of a microsporidium of vertebrates: Pseudoloma neurophilia infecting the Zebrafish, Danio rerio. PLoS One 8 (9), e76064.

Sanders, J.L., Kent, M.L., 2011. Development of a sensitive assay for the detection of Pseudoloma neurophilia in laboratory populations of the zebrafish Danio rerio. Dis. Aquat. Organ. 96 (2), 145–156.

Sanders, J.L., Peterson, T.S., Kent, M.L., 2014. Early development and tissue distribution of pseudoloma neurophilia in the zebrafish, Danio rerio. J. Eukaryot. Microbiol. 61 (3), 238–246.

Sanders, J.L., Watral, V., Kent, M.L., 2012. Microsporidiosis in zebrafish research facilities. ILAR. J. 53 (2), 106–113.

Schaefer, J., Ryan, A., 2006. Developmental plasticity in the thermal tolerance of zebrafish Danio rerio (vol 69, pg 722, 2006). J. Fish. Biol. 69 (4), 1266.

Schulte-Merker, S., et al., 1994. No tail (ntl) is the zebrafish homologue of the mouse T (Brachyury) gene. Development 120 (4), 1009–1015.

Scott, W.W., O'Bier, A.H., 1962. Aquatic fungi associated with diseased fish and fish eggs. Prog. Fish Culturist 24 (1), 3–15.

Serbedzija, G.N., Chen, J.N., Fishman, M.C., 1998. Regulation in the heart field of zebrafish. Development 125 (6), 1095–1101.

Serluca, F.C., Fishman, M.C., 2001. Pre-pattern in the pronephric kidney field of zebrafish. Development 128 (12), 2233–2241.

Shaharom-Harrison, F.M., et al., 1990. Epizootics of Malaysian cultured freshwater pond fishes by Piscinoodinium pillulare (Schaperclaus 1954) Lom 1981. Aquaculture 86, 127–138.

Shih, J., Fraser, S.E., 1995. Distribution of tissue progenitors within the shield region of the zebrafish gastrula. Development 121 (9), 2755–2765.

Shotts, E.J., et al., 1976. Bacterial flora of aquarium fishes and their shipping waters imported from southeast asia. J. Fish. Res. Board Canada 33 (4), 732–735.

Siccardi, A.J. et al., 2009. Growth and Survival of Zebrafish (Danio rerio) Fed Different Commercial and Laboratory Diets. Zebrafish 6(3), 275–80.

Smart, G.R. et al., 1979. Nephrocalcinosis in rainbow trout Salmo gairdneri Richardson; the effect of exposure to elevated CO2 concentrations. Journal of Fish Diseases pp. 279–289.

Smith, C.E., 1988. Communications: histopathology of gas bubble disease in juvenile rainbow trout. Prog. Fish Culturist 50 (2), 98–103.

Smith, S.A., 2014. Welfare of laboratory fishes. In: Bayne, K., Turner, P.V. (Eds.), Laboratory Animal Welfare Elsevier, Waltham, MA, pp. 301–311.

Solnica-Krezel, L., Schier, A.F., Driever, W., 1994. Efficient recovery of ENU-induced mutations from the zebrafish germline. Genetics 136 (4), 1401–1420.

Speare, D.J., et al., 1991. Pathology of bacterial gill disease: sequential development of lesions during natural outbreaks of disease. J. Fish. Dis. 14 (1), 21–32.

Speare, D.J., et al., 1999. A preliminary investigation of alternatives to Fumagillin for the treatment of Loma somonae infection in rainbow trout. J. Comp. Pathol. 121 (3), 241–248.

Speare, D.J., 2010. Disorders associated with exposure to excess dissolved gases. In: Leatherland, J.F., Woo, T.K., Patrick, Fish Diseases and Disorders, Volume 2: Non-infectius Disorders, second ed. CAB International, Oxfordshire, UK; Cambridge, MA, pp. 342–356.

Spence, R., et al., 2006. The distribution and habitat preferences of the zebrafish in Bangladesh. J. Fish. Biol. 69 (5), 1435–1448.

Spence, R., et al., 2008. The behaviour and ecology of the zebrafish, Danio rerio. Biol. Rev. Camb. Philos. Soc. 83 (1), 13–34.

Spence, R., Ashton, R., Smith, C., 2007. Adaptive oviposition choice in the zebrafish, Danio rerio. Behavior 144, 953–966.

Spitsbergen, J.M., et al., 2000. Neoplasia in zebrafish (Danio rerio) Treated with N-methyl-N'-nitroN-nitrosoguanidine by three exposure routes at different developmental stages. Toxicol. Pathol. 28 (5), 715–725.

Spitsbergen, J.M., Buhler, D.R., Peterson, T.S., 2012. Neoplasia and neoplasm-associated lesions in laboratory colonies of zebrafish emphasizing key influences of diet and aquaculture system design. ILAR. J. 53 (2), 114–125.

Stahl, D.A., de la Torre, J.R., 2012. Physiology and diversity of ammonia-oxidizing archaea. Annu. Rev. Microbiol. 66, 83–101.

Stoskopf, M., 2010.. In: Stoskopf, M. (Ed.), Fish Medicine Volume I, second ed ART Sciences LLC, Apex, North Carolina.

Stoskopf, M., Posner, L.P., 2008. Anesthesia and restraint of laboratory fish. Anesth. Analg. Lab. Anim. 21, 519–534.

Streisinger, G., et al., 1981. Production of clones of homozygous diploid zebra fish (Brachydanio rerio). Nature 291 (5813), 293–296.

Swift, S., Cohen, H., 1962. Granulomas of the skin due to Mycobacterium baleni after abrasions from a fish tank. N. Engl. J. Med. 267 (24), 1244–1246.

Talaat, A.M., Reimschuessel, R., Trucksis, M., 1997. Identification of mycobacteria infecting fish to the species level using polymerase chain reaction and restriction enzyme analysis. Vet. Microbiol. 58 (2–4), 229–237.

Tiffney, W.N., 1939. The host range of saprolegnia parasitica. Mycologia 31 (3), 310–321.

Tobin, D.M., Ramakrishnan, L., 2008. Comparative pathogenesis of Mycobacterium marinum and Mycobacterium tuberculosis. Cell. Microbiol. 10 (5), 1027–1039.

Tomasso, J.R., Simco, B.A., Davis, K.B., 1979. Chloride inhibition of nitrite-induced methemoglobinemia in channel catfish (ictaluruspunctatus). J. Fish. Res. Board Canada 36 (9), 1141–1144.

Toranzo, A.E., et al., 1989. Association of aeromonas sobria with mortalities of adult gizzard shad, Dorosoma cepedianum Lesueur. J. Fish. Dis. 12 (5), 439–448.

Touchon, M., et al., 2011. Complete genome sequence of the fish pathogen Flavobacterium branchiophilum. Appl. Environ. Microbiol. 77 (21), 7656–7662.

Tse, W.K.F., et al., 2013. Early embryogenesis in zebrafish is affected by bisphenol A exposure. Biol. Open 2, 466–471.

Velasco-Santamaría, Y.M., et al., 2011. Bezafibrate, a lipid-lowering pharmaceutical, as a potential endocrine disruptor in male zebrafish (Danio rerio). Aquatic Toxicol. (Amsterdam, Netherlands) 105 (1–2), 107–118.

Walker, C., Streisinger, G., 1983. Induction of mutations by gamma-rays in pregonial germ cells of zebrafish embryos. Genetics 103 (1), 125–136.

Wang, J., et al., 2011. The regenerative capacity of zebrafish reverses cardiac failure caused by genetic cardiomyocyte depletion. Development 138 (16), 3421–3430.

Watral, V., Kent, M.L., 2007. Pathogenesis of mycobacterium spp. in zebrafish (Danio rerio) from research facilities. Comp. Biochem. Physiol. Toxicol. Pharmacol. 145 (1), 55–60.

Watts, S.A., Powell, M., D'Abramo, L.R., 2012. Fundamental approaches to the study of zebrafish nutrition. ILAR. J. 53 (2), 144–160.

Westerfied, M., 2000. The Zebrafish Book. A guide for the laboratory use of zebrafish (Danio rerio), fourth ed. University of Oregon Press, Eugene, OR.

Whipps, C.M., Kent, M.L., 2006. Polymerase chain reaction detection of pseudoloma neurophilia, a common microsporidian of zebrafish (Danio rerio) reared in research laboratories. J. Am. Assoc. Lab. Anim. Sci. 45 (1), 36–39.

Whipps, C.M., Dougan, S.T., Kent, M.L., 2007. Mycobacterium haemophilum infections of zebrafish (Danio rerio) in research facilities. FEMS. Microbiol. Lett. 270 (1), 21–26.

Whipps, C.M., Matthews, J.L., Kent, M.L., 2008. Distribution and genetic characterization of Mycobacterium chelonae in laboratory zebrafish Danio rerio. Dis. Aquat. Organ. 82 (1), 45–54.

Whipps, C.M., Lieggi, C., Wagner, R., 2012. Mycobacteriosis in zebrafish colonies. ILAR. J. 53 (2), 95–105.

White, R.M., et al., 2008. Transparent adult zebrafish as a tool for in vivo transplantation analysis. Cell. Stem. Cell. 2 (2), 183–189.

Wiedenheft, B., Sternberg, S.H., Doudna, J.A., 2012. RNA-guided genetic silencing systems in bacteria and archaea. Nature 482 (7385), 331–338.

Wong, D., et al., 2014. Conditioned place avoidance of zebrafish (Danio rerio) to three chemicals used for euthanasia and anaesthesia. PLoS One 9 (2), e88030.

Wright, D., et al., 2003. Inter and intra-population variation in shoaling and boldness in the zebrafish (Danio rerio). Naturwissenschaften 90, 374–377.

Yang, H., et al., 2007. Development of a simplified and standardized protocol with potential for high-throughput for sperm cryopreservation in zebrafish Danio rerio. Theriogenology 68 (2), 128–136.

Yeh, J.R., et al., 2008. AML1-ETO reprograms hematopoietic cell fate by downregulating scl expression. Development 135 (2), 401–410.

Yeh, J.R., et al., 2009. Discovering chemical modifiers of oncogene-regulated hematopoietic differentiation. Nat. Chem. Biol. 5 (4), 236–243.

Zang, L., et al., 2011. A novel protocol for the oral administration of test chemicals to adult zebrafish. Zebrafish 8 (4), 203–210.

Zang, L., et al., 2013. A novel, reliable method for repeated blood collection from aquarium fish. Zebrafish 10 (3), 425–432.

Zheng, X., Roberts, G., 1999. Diagnosis and Susceptibility Testing. In: Schlossberg, D. (Ed.), Tuberculosis and Nontuberculous Mycobacterial Infections W.B. Saunders Company, Philadelphia, PA, pp. 57–64.

ZIRC, 2009. Sentinel Fish Program. pp. 1–4. Available at: <http://zebrafish.org/zirc/documents/protocols/pdf/health_monitoring/sentinel_fish_program.pdf>.

21

Biology and Management of Laboratory Fishes

Michael K. Stoskopf, DVM, PhD, DACZM

Department of Clinical Sciences and Director of the Environmental Medicine Consortium, College of Veterinary Medicine, North Carolina State University, William Moore Dr. Raleigh, NC, USA

I. INTRODUCTION

A. Taxonomy

Fish is a broad term encompassing the most diverse and largest taxonomic grouping of the vertebrates. In common usage, the term includes all members of four taxonomic classes, the Myxini, Cephalaspidomorphi, Elasmobranchiomorphi, and Osteichthyes. More than 3800 species are known from the United States, Canada, and Mexico alone (Page *et al.*, 2013). The Osteichthyes alone, the class of the bony fishes, comprises more extant species than all of the mammals, birds, reptiles, and amphibians combined. This massive biodiversity is not a quirk of taxonomic whim. The anatomic and physiologic differences among species of fish are every bit as

Laboratory Animal Medicine, Third Edition
DOI: http://dx.doi.org/10.1016/B978-0-12-409527-4.00021-3

dramatic as the differences among mammalian species. This characteristic of fish offers tremendous opportunity for the researcher seeking a particular anatomic, physiologic, or disease model, but it also presents serious challenges for laboratory animal managers and veterinarians seeking to maintain the health and well-being of the animals selected. Fish welfare is as important a concern as for any other vertebrate animal (Smith, 2013). Although certain themes of medicine and health management transcend the species differences of the fishes, it is important to keep in mind the adage, 'A fish is not a fish.' This means all fish species are not equivalent in their basic biologic and husbandry needs. It is important to know what fish species you are dealing with when making a diagnosis or designing a health protocol.

Fish are susceptible to the entire range of infectious and noninfectious diseases known to affect terrestrial species, and the diversity of pathogens capable of causing disease in fish is at least as great as that of the terrestrial species familiar to most laboratory animal specialists. It is not possible to cover the vast array of diseases and their different manifestations among the broad diversity of all fishes within the confines of this chapter. There are major texts devoted to clinical medicine (Stoskopf, 2010; Noga, 2010), pathology (Roberts, 2012; Ferguson *et al.*, 2006), and more specialized disciplines such as virology (Wolf, 1988; Woo and Bruno, 2010) and bacteriology (Austin and Austin, 1999; Inglis *et al.*, 1993) of fishes. It is more appropriate for the reader to use these texts for more detailed and complete coverage of the wide range of disease manifestations affecting fishes and the therapeutic approaches employed. The zebrafish, a popular laboratory fish species bred for research use, and many of the common diseases of freshwater fishes are covered in Chapter 23 of this volume. The focus of this chapter will be on significant issues of health management of fishes in laboratory animal facilities, with particular attention to wild-caught or truly random-source fishes as laboratory animals. This unfortunately remains a common situation for many fish species used in research today.

B. Use in Research

The popularity of fish as laboratory animals continues to grow. They have become particularly useful in toxicology studies, in part because of their small size and the availability in large numbers of many species such as the Japanese medaka (*Oryzias latipes*) and the common guppy (*Poecilia reticulata*). The development of tumor-predisposed strains of zebrafish and swordtails (*Xiphophorus*) has resulted in useful fish models in the study of cancer. Ecological studies of aquatic environments need to evaluate fish, and some species, such as the mummichog (*Fundulus heteroclitus*), are serving as valuable monitors in pollution studies. In addition, there

has been a long tradition for the use of fish species in basic physiologic, biochemical, and molecular research.

The availability of laboratory fish is reasonably good, but by no means is the distribution network as extensive as that which exists for small rodents. Specialized fish strains can sometimes be obtained from individual laboratories that have developed the strains if collaborators or colleagues are aware of the work. However, the vast majority of research fish are obtained from animal wholesalers that specialize in aquatic life-forms. A few species, particularly freshwater tropical and ornamental species, are captive-reared in production facilities, but generally with no specialized containment or disease screening. The majority of species, particularly marine and estuary fish, are caught from the wild and undergo little or no acclimation to captive conditions prior to being shipped to laboratories. Prescreening for health problems or conditioning of these species remains rare.

The pressure for large numbers of inexpensive animals is what drives this predominance of non-conditioned animals in the teleost research world. More than unfortunate, it is an unacceptable situation that affects the quality of research that can be accomplished with fish models. It is interesting to consider where rodent research would be if the primary source of laboratory rodents was from extensive trapping in Midwestern granaries. Although the fish species commonly used in research are not directly threatened in the wild, it behooves the researcher and the laboratory animal veterinarian to seek out and demand captive-reared and acclimated fish from facilities with reasonable disease screening. Researchers and veterinarians should not be seduced to ignore massive inter-individual variability due to disease, variable conditioning, or even species and subspecies differences on the basis of low individual animal cost or the ability to use large numbers of animals at low cost. Fish models should be selected carefully, and all aspects of the three Rs (reduction, refinement, and replacement) should be applied to studies using these models.

II. FACILITY DESIGN

The best-conditioned fish will not thrive in a poorly designed or improperly operated facility (Stoskopf, 1988). The sophistication of laboratory animal facility design for fishes is beginning to reach that for mammals, and it should not surprise the laboratory animal veterinarian that the same principles are key to success in either type of facility design.

A. General Ergonomic and Safety Considerations

Human ergonomics is a major consideration in all laboratory animal facility design and certainly in the design of aquatic facilities. The controls and monitors for aquatic environmental systems must be easily accessible. Good visibility into the tanks from a comfortable position is critical. Tanks made entirely of glass usually provide excellent visibility, but larger tanks built with opaque materials often have large blind spots that thwart frequent censusing and daily observation of each animal. Technicians should be able to see all areas of the tank with ease from a safe position. Mirrors can be used to facilitate this in some complex installations.

Piscean ergonomics, or the consideration of the fish's needs, is also important in fish facility design. The life-support system should allow provision of appropriate light cycles, thermoregulation, space, and cover for the species being held. These factors are every bit as important for fishes as they are for mammalian laboratory species, and these conditions can be quite variable among fish species. Proper attention to the biological needs of the species being held will be possible in a multipurpose facility only if the controls and the tank configurations are sufficiently flexible to allow easy adjustment and modification.

A major design challenge is to provide adequate overhead clearance. It is tempting to pack as much water as possible into a vertical space. However, the minimum overhead clearance for any tank should exceed the depth of the tank. This allows the use of nets without impediment and facilitates handling of fish. This rule needs to apply to design of sophisticated rack-based multiple-tank systems as much as it does to larger individual tanks. Also, considerable time and irritation can be saved by making the top of a tank fully accessible. This usually means having completely removable tops, as well as lighting systems that do not interfere or are easily moved to allow complete access. Alternatively, in rack systems, pulling the tank out from any overhead obstructions for service is an important ergonomic feature. Good tank covers are an important safety feature. They prevent fish from jumping out of tanks unobserved and stop dropped objects from accidentally finding their way into the tanks.

The major safety hazard in aquatic facilities is electrocution. Ground-fault circuit breakers should be used throughout the facility, and all grounds should be properly wired. Electrical outlets should be positioned high on the wall (3–4 ft above the floor), to avoid their being shorted out in the event of flooding or inattentive use of hoses. Rubber gaskets to seal out moisture from outlets not in use help prolong the life of the outlets by reducing corrosion of the internal metal components. Employees should be trained in the safe use of electricity near water, and the floors and drains of the facility should not add to the hazard by retaining standing water. Nets with nonconducting handles should be used, and any form of exposed wiring should be avoided.

Ironically, a sudden failure of electrical power can threaten the survival of fish maintained in a system that depends on electrical pumps, heaters, and air generation. Emergency power generators should be provided that are of sufficient size to provide for emergency lighting for personnel, and air generation at the very minimum. It is better to be able to maintain water flow in all systems as well, preferably at normal operating levels, but at least at some rate of exchange to avoid anaerobiasis development. Though aeration is the most acute concern, impacting survival in some systems within hours, followed by water flow which becomes an issue within a day in some systems, temperature is another major concern. Temperature management is often very power intensive and may not be supportable on an emergency generator system through the normal means employed. However, emergency access to alternative approaches to water temperature management should be included in emergency response plans.

Another safety concern that may not be obvious to individuals inexperienced in the management of fish systems is the great weight of water (1l weighs approximately 1 kg). Even a relatively small 100-l tank (approximately 25 gallons) will weigh 100 kg (over 200 lb) when full. It is important to examine the materials and structural strength of any facility to ensure that it can safely support the cumulative weight of the water systems planned for it. It is also common for fish tanks and header tanks to be elevated above the floor. The support stands for these tanks must be able to safely support the weight of completely filled tanks with an adequate safety margin, and they should be secure from accidental tipping.

All systems should be designed so they can be drained completely without bailing buckets, mops, or sponges. Unfortunately, many bulkhead systems for installing bottom drains have a significant lip, which results in a tank that cannot be drained completely dry passively. The bottoms of these tanks may be built to minimize the amount of mopping and sponging required, or a tank design that does not require a bulkhead fitting may be used.

The general rule in plumbing fish facilities is to use gravity as much as possible to minimize the use of power pumps. This strategy reduces power consumption but means that careful attention must be paid to how water will move when a power failure occurs. It would be devastating for laboratory animals if accidental loss of power or equipment failure resulted in water draining from the holding system. The plumbing should be designed so that adequate water remains in the system for fish to survive when the system stops running for any reason. In routine operations, this means that the process of removing water from the tank should be limited by a standpipe or other device that protects the tank water level. If a pump fails, no siphons should allow the tank to continue to drain without return flow.

Pumps and compressors make a great deal of noise. This is particularly true of those used to manage large-water-volume systems. Fish holding facilities where the pumps and equipment are housed adjacent to the water systems often sound like an industrial factory. Technicians cannot be heard without raising their voices, and the continuous din makes it uncomfortable to remain in the facility for prolonged periods. This environment increases the likelihood of mistakes and minimizes the probability of good observation of the fish. Fish have complex sensory systems designed to gather information from waveforms in the water. They are quite sensitive to sound. Placing large pumps, compressors, and other life-support apparatuses in a separate room or enclosure to isolate the animal facility from their sound is an important design consideration. A good rule of thumb is that if you find that being in a room for prolonged periods is uncomfortable because of the noise levels, you can be certain that the fish are being affected by the noise.

Air handling and sources need to be carefully considered in the design of research fish facilities in addition to water sources and handling (see Section II, B). An improperly placed air intake can have serious consequences for a fish facility. In most fish systems, water is limited and aeration is used extensively to maintain reasonable oxygen concentrations and reduce carbon dioxide accumulation in the available water. In addition, airlifts are often used to effect the movement of water through components of the system. Large quantities of air are used in these processes, and even very low concentrations of impurities in the air can result in accumulations that can affect fish health or experimental results. Even more care should be exercised in the placement of air intakes for fish systems than is used in design of facilities for mammalian laboratory animals. In addition, care in handling the air, including the implementation of redundant systems, moisture traps, and constantly circulating loops, is very important to the long-term safety of the facility.

Regenerative blowers are used commonly to supply central air-delivery systems for fish facilities. Regenerative blowers have fewer moving parts than compressors and require much less service and maintenance. Although they deliver relatively low pressures, high pressures are not needed for most fish facility applications, and regenerative blowers deliver much higher volumes of air than similarly sized compressors. If the tanks in the facility are not going to be any deeper than 1 m water depth, the use of a regenerative blower rather than an air compressor should be strongly considered. Aeration can be critical to the viability of the fish in many systems, so duplication of the device driving the air supply is a wise investment.

The need for water exchanges in fish holding systems means that consideration of reserve water sources must have high priority in design. Reserve water systems should be thermally tempered and preferably designed to allow delivery of water of appropriate pH and hardness for an immediate 50% water exchange of every tank and system if necessary. This creates the ability to respond quickly to emergency situations and without delay for therapeutic interventions.

B. Water Sources and Handling

1. Recirculating Systems

The literature is replete with references to 'closed systems.' In truth, closed systems, in which no additional water or air are provided from external sources after the initial establishment of the system, are extremely rare and are not particularly useful for most research situations. What is more commonly meant by these references is a recirculating system where water is filtered through various means and reused. The selection and management of balanced filtration systems appropriate for the research being conducted are critical to the success of such systems and the health of the fish maintained in them.

2. Filter Selection

Three major types of filtration are used in aquatic design: mechanical, biological, and chemical, each with its own purpose and application. Mechanical filtration, sometimes referred to as primary filtration, removes suspended particles from water by passing it through a medium that obstructs the particles. The mesh of the medium is selected based on the size of the particulates that need to be removed and the amount of resistance that can be placed on the pump. As the mesh of the filter medium becomes finer, more pumping effort is required. Also, very fine-meshed filters occlude quickly and require frequent backwashing or replacement. A uniform medium with an effective size of 0.3 mm will remove about 95% of particles down to 6 μm in diameter. A coarser medium, 0.45 mm in diameter, will retain 15-μm particles. For complete retention of all bacteria, a mechanical filter must exclude particles down to 0.2 μm in diameter, a goal that is rarely practical in fish systems of any size (Hawkins, 1981; Wheaton, 1993).

Chemical filtration covers a wide range of methods for removing molecular contaminants (heavy metals, organic toxins, waste products) from water, including ion exchange, both specific (resins) and nonspecific (activated carbon), and oxidative systems (ozone). Foam fractionation by protein modification and ultraviolet filtration can also be considered methods of chemical filtration, because they rely on basic modifications of chemical structure to remove contaminants.

Activated carbon filters are the most commonly applied form of chemical filtration. This is sometimes described as absorption filtration but is actually a relatively nonspecific exchange filter. A finite number of binding sites are available on the carbon, which are capable of binding cations and anions with binding strengths that vary with the ion being bound. These ions undergo constant exchange with ions in the water at a rate inversely proportional to their binding strength to the carbon sites. Ions with strong binding affinity are effectively removed from the water. This works well until all of the binding sites are saturated and competitive binding between the more toxic compounds reaches a point where not all toxic ions can be bound simultaneously. At this point, some ions must be released by mass action. The filter also fails when a very strongly binding ion is introduced into the system and displaces more weakly bound toxic compounds from the binding sites. In either of these cases, the filter designed to remove toxic compounds can become a point source of toxic compounds. Deciding when to change an activated carbon filter can be challenging. Variations in the contaminant load of the water being filtered can make mass-action calculations based on infrequent sampling unreliable. One good strategy is to routinely monitor both the influent and the effluent water at the filter for a relatively common contaminant that is found in the influent water and has relatively low binding affinity for the carbon (usually total organic carbon [TOC]). When the effluent water begins to show a consistent spillover of the contaminant being monitored, while other factors such as flow rates, pH, and temperature remain stable, the carbon in the filter should be changed.

The term 'biological filtration' refers to the biological fixation of wastes into less toxic compounds or forms. Bacterial fixation of nitrogen is the most common form employed, but other forms of biological filtration are used, including the concentration of metals and certain toxic organics in algal scrubbers. A bacterial biological filter must maintain enough heterotrophic bacterial colonies to process the solid nitrogenous wastes of fish into soluble wastes such as ammonia. The ammonia from this process and that directly excreted by the fish are then converted by autotrophic bacteria to nitrite and then to nitrate. The surface area for bacterial growth is usually the limiting factor in biological filters, along with the ability to circulate the waste-laden water into contact with the bacteria responsible for nitrogen fixation. This is the principle behind the so-called undergravel filters. Containers filled with plastic-fluted spheres and cylinders that maximize surface area while minimizing flow impedance are often used to provide additional surface area for bacterial growth and easier water contact and are commonly referred to as biofilters. Biofilters need to provide adequate water turnover to avoid accumulation of toxic wastes in the system and to supply sufficient oxygenated water to maintain the aerobic processes of the filter. However, it is also important to provide enough contact time between the filter and waste-laden water to allow effective waste metabolism by the bacteria. An imbalance results in an ineffective biofilter.

3. Flow-Through Systems

Flow-through systems are also referred to as open systems. They are characterized by continuous addition of new water, with equal volumes being removed. Obviously the amount of flushing that occurs in the system is dependent on the rate of water addition and removal. There are several limitations, the first being the volume delivery limitations of the water source. A 2-h turnover time for a modest 4000-l system will require constant delivery from a source of 48,000l per day, or just over 32l per minute. Municipal water costs can easily be calculated for a 7-day week, and the expense can be quite surprising. Frequently, wells are used to reduce the maintenance costs through capital outlay to drill and plumb the well. It is important to have any wells tested for capacity by pumping down at least 24h before taking the flow measurements. The decision to draw water from a municipal system or from a well is a complex one. Other factors that need to be figured into the cost equations, beyond the simple cost per liter of water delivered, include the ongoing expense of removing municipal disinfectants, heating, and, for wells, the challenges of supersaturation and the risk of well failure.

If sufficient water is available, the next bottleneck for flow through systems is the tempering and conditioning of the water. Adjustments of water temperature take time and energy. The time can be reduced by increasing the energy, but this invariably increases costs. Finally, the fish themselves can provide limitations to the extent of flow-through operation that is acceptable. Rapid currents generated by high water turnover can force fish to swim more actively to maintain their position in the water column. It is possible to increase this effort to the point where the fish cannot eat enough food to maintain body condition and health over time. This is particularly a problem with sedentary species evolved to live in still waters. Unfortunately, many of the fish species prized for their ability to withstand fluctuations in oxygen tension, pH, and water quality in general have evolved these abilities to exploit still, calm waters.

4. Discharge

Disposal of effluent water from fish systems, especially when large quantities of water are involved, requires special consideration. This is true for recirculating systems as well as for flow-through systems. Certainly, if pathogens or toxins are being used in experiments, extra precautions must be taken to avoid discharging the pathogen or toxin with the water effluent. Even if no hazardous substances or pathogens are being used, very stringent nitrogen and other water-quality discharge limits may be enforced that require complex post-use modification of the water before discharge. If municipal waste facilities are intended to receive the discharged effluent, it will be important to establish the water quality, volume, and timing requirements for such discharges in order to avoid heavy fines and/or loss of permission to discharge through that mechanism. Similarly, settling and evaporating ponds and tanks are frequently heavily regulated by local as well as federal or state authorities and require specific attention to detailed design issues if they are employed.

5. Isolation

The same principles of isolation that have been successful in mammalian laboratory animal medicine apply to aquatic systems. All-in/all-out animal movements may be even more important with fish species because of the poor level of stock screening that currently exists. Any conjoined water system or air handling system should be considered a bridge across isolation barriers. Separation of species and other basic principles of laboratory animal medicine related to disease isolation all apply in aquatic systems.

The importance of the air systems deserves some further emphasis. Although it is intuitive to veterinarians that spread of infection through direct contact would occur in fish, and that fomite spread through use of implements shared between tanks or systems would be as much a problem as a shared water system, the importance of the air system in disease spread from fish tank to fish tank is often overlooked. Ideally, each system or tank would be housed in its own room. This is rarely practical but is the most effective way to eliminate aerosolization transfer of diseases. Fish don't sneeze, but the fine bubbles coming to the surface of tanks from airstones and airlifts cast millions of small aerosol droplets into the air. These droplets carry protozoa, bacteria, viruses, and fungal spores. All tanks should have tops, and preferably tops that minimize the chances for direct aerosolization into the room. If possible, tanks should be placed far enough apart to prevent the aerosolized droplets of one tank from settling on another. This distance is dependent on the type of top employed, the location of access openings in the top, and the degree of aeration and spray used in the tank system.

It is never a good idea to place a tank above another tank, but because of space considerations, it is often a necessity. When this occurs, every precaution should be taken to avoid splash or spill contamination of the lower tanks. If only tiered tank systems are used, fish with infectious disease should be kept in lower aquaria, not in top aquaria.

Disinfection of the complex surface areas involved in mechanical and chemical filter media is not recommended. The potential for transmitting disease from one group of fish to the next through incompletely disinfected media is high. In general, biological filters by their very nature cannot be disinfected easily.

For larger facilities, it may be practical to build a contact chamber for delivery of ozone or ultraviolet filtration to various aquarium systems in series to achieve a degree of disinfection. Before investing in this technology, it is best to arrange for a knowledgeable consultant. It will be critical that the contact chamber provide complete disinfection before returning the water to the fish holding tanks, or else disease transmission will be a major problem. Systems adequate to kill bacteria may not be adequate to kill protozoa or fungi.

Clearly, each system should have its own set of implements (nets, feeding sticks, tongs, etc.), which are used only in that system. Although disinfection of implements may seem a more economical approach initially, in the actual day-to-day rush of caring for the facility, disinfection often becomes impractical. In most applications, implements do not remain in contact with disinfectants long enough to be effective and hurried rinsing of 'disinfected' implements can expose fish to the disinfectant. Disinfection protocols can be effective if sufficient investment is made in redundant nets, buckets, and other implements to allow adequate exposure time to disinfectant and effective rinsing of the tools.

A major consideration in maintaining a fish facility is the disinfection and decontamination of the tanks and filter systems between experiments. Each time a tank and a filter are recycled for a new set of fish, they should be cleaned and sanitized to the degree appropriate, considering the known health status of the previous occupants. Most commonly, the water in a system is drained and replaced, perhaps after cleaning any visible dirt from the tank sides. Proponents of this approach argue that it saves time, presents less risk of accidental poisoning with disinfectants, and is cost-effective.

Spraying the walls of the tank (first cleaned of visible debris) with 70% ethanol or 2-propanol and allowing the alcohol to evaporate is another level of disinfection that has been used successfully for most bacterial diseases and enveloped viruses. This approach will not disinfect the plumbing or filtration systems. If disposable filters are being used, this may not be a major problem, but safer disinfection is accomplished by circulating disinfectant throughout the tank system. This process is time-consuming and usually reserved for systems that have held fish with highly infectious problems. The tank and system should be drained and cleaned of visible debris. Then the tank is refilled with a dilute chlorine or quaternary ammonium solution and circulated for 1 h or more. The tank is drained, and the system rinsed. A major concern is to be sure that all disinfectant is removed from the system before it goes back on line. Using removable or disposable filtration systems greatly aids in this process as disinfection, and removal of disinfectant from the complex surfaces of filters takes a great deal of time and is unreliable. If chlorine was used, the water can be tested for residual chlorine and thiosulfate added after the tank is refilled. Dilute vinegar solutions have also served as disinfectants of home aquarium systems. Considerable disinfection can be accomplished through merely altering the pH of the water running through the system and then discarding the water.

6. Facility Retrofits

As fish species become even more popular research models, retrofitting of mammalian facilities to house fish is much more common than the construction of new dedicated aquatic facilities. Retrofitting presents several challenges in addition to those faced in the design of new facilities. The same principles as for new facility design, outlined in Section II, B, 6, apply to the retrofitting of mammalian facilities for holding fishes. However, the constraints of the existing facilities usually dictate which fish species are appropriate, how many can be held, and, in some cases, the configurations of the water systems.

Preliminary assessment of facilities being considered for retrofitting to hold fish must include careful evaluation of all potential water sources and their reliability as well as quality. This includes an assessment of the existing water delivery infrastructure to identify potential sources of heavy metals and other toxic substances that may need to be dealt with by using specialized pre-use filtering. As a related issue, the drain and discharge system of the facility needs assessment. There must be somewhere for all of the water to go when it is disposed of, and the disposal ideally is accomplished in an ergonomic and cost-efficient way while preserving isolation principles.

Similarly, the electrical supply of the facility must be judged in light of the relatively high power consumption of aquatic laboratory animal space relative to that of routine mammal space. Electric resistance-based heaters, pumps, and lighting can, and usually do, double or triple the power requirements of the space being retrofitted. Besides increasing the power requirements, the addition of water to the space usually dictates an upgrade of the wiring to all ground-fault receptacles and to location of receptacles above splash points. Power-failure alarms and emergency power generators are a necessity for aquatic facilities and should support air supply pumps and generators as a first priority, along with emergency personnel safety lighting. Water recirculation is a second priority, followed by temperature maintenance if at all possible.

In most retrofits, air handling units are a fixed item beyond the scope of the budget, but it is important to recognize that aquatic facilities will load large amounts of moisture into the airhandling equation that may exceed the capabilities of the original equipment. This impact can be minimized by careful selection of the system design, including the configuration of tanks and the design of tank tops. The effects in the retrofitted space can also be reduced by careful selection of wall, floor, and ceiling surface coatings and the minimization of use of metal fixtures in the space. Sealed lights are a good investment, as are exterior, sealed light switches and receptacle boxes. Plastic laminate wall systems that provide a high degree of water seal will extend the life of the underlying structure of the building and are a cost-effective investment.

7. New Facility Design

The design of new facilities needs to balance flexibility with specialized concern for the immediate intended purpose of the facility. Important early considerations include whether the facility will hold freshwater species, marine species, or both. This will have a major impact on water system design and layout, which in turn greatly affects capitalization costs. It is also important to determine the temperature range of the fish intended for the facility. This range allows you to establish the limits of temperature variability as well as the preferred temperature setting of the facility and will also affect the feasibility of humidity control, an issue of significant concern in aquatic facilities. Finally, it is useful to know the size and, if possible, the species of fishes intended for the facility, as well as the number to be held. Clearly, this helps determine the number and size of primary enclosures as well as the scale of the water handling required.

Small tanks offer great flexibility for keeping large numbers of animals in a relatively small space. They are also economical if expensive drugs or chemicals are going to be used as water treatments. Unfortunately, small tanks are also inherently more volatile and must be watched much more carefully to avoid environmental problems that can be detrimental to research results. Large tanks offer a greater latitude with water quality and are less confining to the fish. Unfortunately, besides taking up space, large tanks take much more time to drain and refill for disinfection, and research treatments delivered in the water can become prohibitively expensive.

Round tanks allow continuous swimming patterns in pelagic species and can be manipulated to direct flow around the periphery of the tank, minimizing incidences of fish colliding with tank walls or rubbing in corners of the tank. Round tanks don't fit as neatly into rectangular rooms as do rectangular tanks, but if you choose rectangular tanks, remember, not all rectangles are created equal. The depth of the tank and the width-to-length ratio will be important. A fish must be able to turn around freely in its tank. It must also be able to make its normal vertical movements within the water column. From a husbandry standpoint, it is always best to have a working depth that allows the aquarist to reach the bottom of the tank with ease. Certainly, the issue of surface area for air exchange is also important.

8. Temperature Management

Many holding facilities for fish are designed to control temperature through regulation of the room air temperature. This design is energy efficient but requires careful attention to the dynamics of the heating and cooling system of the building. The human comfort range shifts seasonally. Although this change is not very large, it does occur on the edge of the temperature tolerance ranges of many tropical fish species. The difference between 20°C and 23°C can seriously affect research outcomes, and the lower temperatures can even be life-threatening to some fish. Many tropical fish need temperatures in the range of 24–26°C, and temperatures of 27°C are sometimes used when treating protozoal infections. By convention, zebrafish for embryologic studies are commonly maintained at 28°C during development, well above normal human indoor comfort zones. Facilities using air heating should be maintained at room temperatures in the 24–25°C range. Supplemental heaters should be available to boost temperatures in case of failure of the airhandling system. Glass-encased heaters are safer than metal enclosed heaters, particularly in marine systems. Selection of heater wattage is based on the volume of water that must be heated. A small heater in a large volume will be on a greater proportion of the time. A rule of thumb is 50–100W of heater for every 40l of water in the system. For larger systems, fused silica heaters may be required. Longer-barreled heaters have lower surface temperatures than shorter heaters of the same wattage and are, therefore, less liable to cause burns to fish caught up against them. Protective guard fences can be placed around heaters to keep fish away. Placing the heater horizontally near the bottom of the tank improves the convection dynamics of the heater but requires a sealed, submersible heater. Submersible heaters are easier to disinfect and may be preferable. If a facility has a large number of tanks, a worthwhile investment is a heater calibration bucket, a bucket or tank of water maintained at a desired temperature by a thermostatic heater. Other heaters can be placed in the tank and calibrated to roughly the temperature of the bucket, before being placed in a tank with fish.

The other side of temperature control is the cooling of water to maintain temperate or cold-water species. Refrigeration systems are expensive. They are a necessity if you are going to house cold-water fish. The most common refrigeration systems are heat exchangers driven by a compressible refrigerant. Heat exchangers constructed of a variety of materials are available. Titanium is the only metal proven suitable for heat exchangers used in marine systems. Coatings on coils of other metals are susceptible to scratching and other damage, resulting in toxicity problems from leached metals and serious corrosion problems in the chiller. These chillers can be used with some impunity in freshwater systems but are too dangerous for marine systems. Graphite exchange blocks are available but have yet to be adapted to aquarium systems and are not readily available commercially.

Occasionally, a clever designer will propose the use of temperature mixing valves in the design of the water supply system for a fish holding facility. This can be an important consideration and provides a means to temper replacement or makeup water to the temperatures the fishes are experiencing in their tanks. The selection and proper installation of temperature mixing valves are complex and not to be taken lightly. Many mixing valves require comparable water pressure from both hot and cold water systems in order to function properly. This state of balance rarely occurs without careful modification of the plumbing designs for the facility. Seasonal changes in water supply temperatures can also wreak havoc on automated tempering systems. Experienced plumbers and engineers are the best defense against a nonfunctional or even dangerous water tempering system.

9. Materials Selection

Fish holding systems can be constructed of almost anything that will retain water. However, only a few materials and designs are suitable for research fish facilities. For small systems, all-glass tanks are probably an ideal choice. They afford excellent visibility and are relatively chemically inert. Glass has certain advantages over plastic. It is harder and less easily scratched during maintenance than acrylic plastics, although plastic-coated safety plate is also readily scratched. Plastics require solvent sealing and cannot be properly sealed with silicone sealants, making construction and repair more difficult. Glass is also less expensive than high-quality clear acrylics. However, glass is more easily broken than most plastics and is difficult to drill for some plumbing applications.

Only aquaculture-grade or medical-grade silicone should be used in glass tank construction or repair. Low-grade, inexpensive silicone caulks contain heavy metals, cyanide, and organic toxins, which can kill fish. Systems larger than 200l require extremely thick glass. Complex plumbing is often more common in these systems, making plastic construction a major benefit.

Plastics cover a wide range of materials with diverse properties. Clear plastics used as glass substitutes are usually highly specialized acrylics. They are expensive, relatively soft, and susceptible to scratching. Acrylics have the advantage over glass in that acrylics can be molded in panes to fill very large spans. They are not subject to shattering with the same forces that affect glass, but they can be broken. Acrylic panes are subject to melting from the heat of photographic lights and can catch fire. Little is known about their interaction with chemicals and drugs used in the treatment of fish.

Opaque plastics are used as structural components of systems. New or unknown materials should be tested for toxicity with a bioassay before they are used in facility construction. Materials graded as acceptable for foodstuffs are usually acceptable for aquarium systems. Recycled plastics should be avoided or certainly tested rigorously, examining all lots being used.

Fiberglass has the highest tension loading capacity of the plastics. It is relatively inexpensive and probably the most commonly used structural plastic in aquarium construction. It is not suitable for construction of toxicological evaluation facilities, because of the variability of toxin leaching from the hardening resins. Newly constructed tanks incorporating fiberglass should be treated carefully to rid the system of polymerizing agents and trapped metals in the fiberglass resin. This can be accomplished by alternately running the filled system for a day with freshwater of pH 3.0 or lower, followed by freshwater of pH 11 or higher and, finally, by freshwater at pH 3.0, discarding the water after each pH shift. A final leaching with saltwater for an additional day should be performed if the tank is destined to be a marine aquarium. The entire treatment process is best facilitated by the use of warm water (37–40°C). A bioassay is still advisable before using such a system.

Vinyl is an inexpensive flexible plastic used in swimming pool liners. It can find its way into makeshift holding facilities. It is easily damaged and can have large residuals of toxic plasticizer and heavy metals trapped in the polymerization process. These leach out into the water. Dioctyl phthalate is a common contaminant, and although 10 days of soaking and etching is recommended for its removal, this is far from a certain procedure. Vinyl is a poor choice in any fish system.

High-density linear polyethylene and polypropylene tanks are relatively inert and can be stripped with the same protocol described for fiberglass, making them essentially free of heavy metal and plasticizer contaminants. They are expensive, opaque materials but are quite suited to use in research fish systems.

Polyvinyl chloride (PVC) generally is used not in tank construction but in the construction of the plumbing systems that operate tanks. PVC is basically inert to saltwater; however, it comes in several types or schedules which have different properties. High-impact or unplasticized PVC is most commonly used for plumbing applications but can contain trace amounts of metals, particularly lead, which can be leached in acid water systems. Acrylonitrile butadiene styrene (ABS) pipes are less likely to cause subtle toxicity problems and are recommended in construction of research systems.

Concrete is widely used for very large systems because of its durability, low cost, and formability. It is a consideration when constructing a facility for large fish and is used by aquaculture and display aquarium facilities. Concrete has a strong resistance to compression but lacks tensile strength and shear resistance, which must be provided by metal reinforcement buried in the concrete. Concrete is very alkaline because of free lime produced by hydration of the surface of the cement. It also contains small amounts of foreign materials, including chromates, which can leach out slowly over a long period after tank construction. Concrete structures should be thoroughly washed or leached with dilute muriatic acid, and then several coats of sodium silicate or other sealant should be applied before the structures are used for fish. A soaking period of several weeks, altering pH extremes and discarding water, is recommended.

In many instances, metals are required for the completion of a system where no other material will serve. The major problem with metals and water, particularly seawater, is corrosion. Corroded metals lose structural integrity and strength, and the metal being lost through corrosion is toxic to fish. Stainless steel is considered the most resistant metal to seawater corrosion, but its resistance is only relative. The most available stainless steel, AISI (American Iron and Steel Institute) type 316, is a high-molybdenum alloy, resistant to pitting and crevice corrosion. It is not a high-strength steel, and it will corrode. Where strength and maximal corrosion resistance are needed, titanium is preferred over stainless steel. Other common metals used in tank construction include galvanized fittings and brass or copper. Unfortunately, the galvanized coat placed on iron contains enough zinc to be lethal to fish within very short periods, even when calcium protection is in effect in seawater. Bronze can be a fatal source of zinc and copper. In fish research facility design, it is important to avoid the sublethal and lethal effects of heavy metals on fish behavior and physiology.

C. Monitoring

Fish systems can be designed to minimize most catastrophic events, but a program of careful environmental monitoring is necessary for any aquatic system. Three critical factors should be monitored essentially continuously: temperature, water level, and power failure. Electronic tank monitoring systems capable of measuring temperature, water level, and interruption in electrical supply are available commercially. Systems designed for monitoring incubators and laboratory equipment can be adapted for use in fish tanks. They can also be built from parts available in most electronics stores carrying burglar- or fire-alarm components. These systems can be programmed to call a prescribed telephone number and notify whoever answers that a problem exists. Many of such systems can even communicate what the problem is. These systems are extremely valuable security in lieu of staffing a fish facility 24 h a day.

III. MANAGEMENT AND HUSBANDRY

A. System Startup

It takes about 6 weeks to start a new or restart a disinfected biofilter and to have it working at full capacity. This is much too long for any practical research system to be down. One way to avoid the problem of downtime is not to use biofilters. Another is to have portable biofilters that are growing bacteria in a reserve system designed to keep the filters healthy. Strings of biorings or other plastic support media, suspended in the water, are a common approach (Spotte, 1979).

In a well-established reserve system, reseeding may require no more than placing the biofilter into the system. It may be beneficial to keep the disinfected biofilter downstream of and in close contact with well-seeded biofilters. It will take a minimum of 3 weeks to reseed the disinfected biofilter to a level that will be of any value in the research tank. This can be hastened somewhat by keeping the biofilter reserve system warmer; however, it is difficult to say whether this is a long-term benefit or not. The bacteria growing on the biofilters are susceptible to environmental changes, and a large drop in fixation efficiency can occur with just the careful transfer of a biofilter from the reserve system to a research tank. This loss is greater if the environmental conditions, including the water temperature, of the research tank and the reserve system are widely disparate.

It is important to feed biofilters while they are in the reserve system. This can be accomplished in a number of ways. Some aquarists maintain fish or invertebrates in the reserve system to provide metabolic waste material to feed the bacteria. This minimizes the work involved in operating the reserve system but has the obvious disadvantage of having potential reservoirs of infection in the reserve system itself. Another approach is to introduce ammonia into the system on a periodic or continuous basis. In marine systems, ammonium chloride solutions are often used for this purpose.

B. Water Management

The most critical issue in water management after certification and monitoring of the quality of the source is the water change procedure. Flow-through systems are constantly undergoing water change. Water is removed and new water enters the system continuously. The positioning of inflow and outflow pipes in these systems will have a major impact on the efficacy of this exchange. Ideally the flow dynamics and convection patterns of the tank would have only old water leave the system and all new water remain, but this is rarely achieved. Some degree of mixing of newly added water to old water nearly always occurs, reducing the effectiveness of the water change. It is important to avoid significant shunting of new water to the outflow, and it is advantageous to have a pattern of mixing in the tank that avoids 'dead spots,' or volumes of water that are never or only very slowly exchanged. In recirculating tanks the challenge of optimizing water mixing is not the primary concern. What is critical is to remove a volume of water prior to introducing the new water.

A frequent failure in recirculating systems is due to the misconception that 'topping off,' or the practice of adding water to compensate for evaporative losses, is equivalent to conducting water changes. Toxic compounds do not evaporate at the same rate as water, and most tend to accumulate in the system water if topping up is allowed to substitute for a true water change. The required rate of water change is dependent on the configuration of the tanks and the system, as well as the bioload of fish being maintained. A general rule of thumb of 0.75–1% per day is effective as a routine water exchange in a wide variety of systems. This approach of frequent small changes has the advantage of reducing the potential impact of temperature, pH, ionic, or other shocks that can occur if improperly tempered and conditioned water is used in larger volume exchanges. The issue of properly conditioning makeup water is particularly crucial when making 25–50% water changes, which are an excellent therapeutic and mitigative tool in fish health management.

C. Feeding

The problem of feeding is as complex for the laboratory animal veterinarian who manages fish as is the provision of suitable space and water. The breadth of laboratory fish species diversity contributes to the difficulty, but this difficulty is compounded by a lack of fundamental nutritional knowledge. Although diets that maintain and even support growth and reproduction are known for common laboratory fish species, these empirically derived diets are usually relatively undefined. Trace nutrient balance is rarely considered, and quality control, including component selection for these diets, is minimal. Protein sources can vary dramatically from lot to lot, as can processing and storage procedures. Relatively little is known about the natural diets of many commonly kept fish or about the effects of trace imbalances on fish physiology. These problems are all compounded by the relative plasticity of fish growth and development in adapting to nutrition availability.

A basic rule that would seem absurd in laboratory mammal management if it weren't so often ignored is that fish should be fed. Because fish can survive for relatively long periods without food, not feeding fish is sometimes seen as a way to circumvent the variability in food lots, difficulties in documenting individual intake in group-housed fish, or time constraints in acclimating fish to new diets. As a result, a large amount of knowledge of fish physiology and a considerable amount of disease model research are based on a catabolic animal. Fish entering a new system should be allowed time to acclimate to new diets before experiments are initiated. In experiments that depend on accurate assessment of individual food intake for interpretation of the results, fish should be housed and fed in a manner that makes this assessment feasible. Development of better diets, including certified standardized diets for laboratory fish, should be encouraged. Feeding patterns should try to mimic the natural feeding patterns of the fish (e.g., constant grazers *versus* opportunistic predators, crepuscular *versus* diurnal feeders, etc.).

D. Social Grouping Enrichment

Cover and substrates must allow a fish to be comfortable in the tank but not hinder capture or observation. Plastic piping can often be used to provide hiding places, and clear piping is often accepted by a fish, especially if tank lighting is kept subdued except during observation. Animals that need to burrow in sand can be easily observed through clear glass gravel placed in patches, in removable containers, or covering the entire bottom of the tank. Most laboratory fish are held in species isolation, which can simplify this issue. However, multiple-species housing in a primary enclosure is common in more generalized fish management, and inter- and intra-specific interactions among individuals must be managed appropriately when this is done. Not all fishes are cooperative, schooling species. Size differences, time-in-residence territoriality, gender interactions, and other social complexities can have important impacts on the physiology of the fishes being managed and the results of research (Pickering, 1981).

IV. MEDICAL PROTOCOLS

A. Health Screening

Considerable research is wasted every year through the use of diseased fish. The best solution to this problem is to deal with known and reliable suppliers of screened and/or SPF stock, but such commercial suppliers are rare. Random-source fish should be screened for disease prior to inclusion in research protocols. On-site screening at the source has a major advantage of reducing the probability of introducing a disease into the laboratory water systems, but few suppliers provide this service. Some research facilities send their own diagnostic specialists to screen stocks prior to purchase, but most facilities do not have the ability to accomplish this degree of security. Consultant companies are available to conduct screenings and are being used more frequently as investigators and laboratory animal managers realize the true costs of losing experiments to preventable diseases.

Alternatively, facilities with good quarantine capabilities are employing more in-house screening for diseases after fish arrive at the facilities. Sometimes in-house laboratories are capable of the screening, but more frequently, private fish health-screening consultants are contracted. Sampling for screening is always problematic, because essentially all currently used fish health screening techniques are lethal. Screening panels vary considerably, depending on the fish species in question and the research being conducted. Mycobacteriosis is an important problem and should be screened for in most widely used small tropical fish species. Microsporidian parasites of the brain and other tissues are a common problem in some of the marine species, including *Fundulus* spp., and can interfere with neurology and behavior studies. Common ciliate, flagellate, and monogenean ectoparasites can cause unexpected mortality when fish experience stressful conditions, confounding experimental results. Viral diseases have not been well studied in their ability to affect experimental results, and relatively few validated tests are available for viral screening, but this situation will change as the recognition of fish as laboratory animals continues to grow among researchers.

Sampling efficacy for fish health screening is ruled by the same statistical principles that dictate mammalian screening methods. For diseases with relatively high prevalences in infected populations, including *Ichthyophthirius multifilis*, *Ichthyobodo* spp., *Gyrodactylus* spp., and *Dactylogyrus* spp., relatively few fish need to be screened to establish, with reasonable confidence, whether a population is infected. Other problematic diseases such as mycobacteriosis can require sampling of 30 or more animals, depending on the size of the population being sampled, to detect low prevalences of the disease. Future development of nonlethal testing methods for the important laboratory fish diseases will greatly improve the acceptance of fish health screening in laboratory animal medicine.

B. Quarantine

The issue of quarantine for fish is closely coupled with the common use of random-source fish and the lack of validated specific screening tools. Quarantining and conditioning fish for 14–21 days avoids many problems, although longer isolation times may be appropriate in circumstances where all-in/all-out management is not practiced. Quarantines of 4–6 weeks are recommended for concerns about mycobacterial infections.

Fish in quarantine should be held in good water with filtration that maintains appropriate pH and nitrogen waste product levels. Fish should be given time to acclimate after arrival. Prophylactic treatments can be administered if the disease status of the supplying source is known, but generally a diagnostic workup of a subsample of the fish is a better approach. Lethal testing is the most common sampling approach used and allows bacterial cultures of internal organs and histologic examination of all organs. Nonlethal sampling procedures are used with extremely valuable fish and include skin impression smears and gill and fin biopsies taken under sedation or anesthesia and examined for the presence of protozoal and metazoal parasites. In larger fish, blood samples may be drawn for complete blood counts and selected serum chemistry determinations. Treatments are then instituted for the entire population, depending on the findings of the diagnostic screening. Quarantine duration is based on daily assessments of the condition and behavior of the fish population and the success of implemented therapies.

C. Pain

Equating pain in animals with that of humans is subjective. It is suggested that three stages of suffering should be recognized in animals: discomfort, stress, and pain. Discomfort may be characterized by such negative signs as poor condition, torpor, and diminished appetite. Stress is defined as a condition of tension or anxiety predictable or readily explicable from environmental causes or from or including physical causes. Finally, pain itself is recognized by more readily identifiable signs such as struggling, screaming or squealing, convulsions, or severe palpitations. Attempts to assess pain in animals are made more difficult by adaptive responses. It is well known that the fight-or-flight mechanism can override pain perception. Individual differences exist among various species in their ability to tolerate or react to pain. One theory for the perception of pain in higher animals involves the modulation of sensory cues that are normally controlled by specific cells in the spinal cord that operate a gating mechanism. The sensory input is relayed to central receptors by fast myelinated and slow unmyelinated fibers up the spinothalamic tract. An imbalance of input between these two sets of fibers is thought to be the cause of pain. There is a wealth of evidence that interruption of this tract, either by injury or disease, results in a loss of ability to feel pain.

A British Veterinary Association Fish Sub-Committee meeting in 1984 concluded that although the scientific evidence shows that fish do not have a spinothalamic pathway, there seems to be no way of showing whether or not another part of the brain has adapted to take over the function of the thalamus (Brown, 1985). In humans, parts of the nonspecific or association cortex have been shown to be concerned with nociceptive input. There are marked differences in cortical development among mammals, birds, reptiles, amphibia, and cartilaginous fishes, the simplest of which have no recognizable cerebral cortex, but despite many recent advances there remains a paucity of information available on centrally mediated reception of sensory cues in fish.

Fish physiologists argue that pain is probably not experienced as a strong sensation by fishes, though forceful or noxious physical or chemical stimuli evoke violent reactions. This contention still does not relieve laboratory animal professionals of the responsibility of giving animals the benefit of the doubt. Recent research largely counters the notion that fish do not experience pain as a strong sensation (Ashley et al., 2007; Dunlop and Laming, 2005; Jones et al., 2012). The main sensory cues to which fish respond in the aquatic environment are chemical, hydrodynamic, acoustic, thermal, electrical, light, and mechanical. The receptor sites for these stimuli vary from species to species. Physical changes in heat flow or touch are recognized by skin receptors, and visual cues are observed as changes in light intensity and/or quality. The inner ear and lateral line receive acoustic input, whereas chemical reception occurs in smell and taste organs located all over the body.

To summarize, we cannot definitively say whether fish perceive pain based on theoretical definitions, but we do know that sensory receptors are present for external environmental cues. Although the central reception of these sensory inputs is different in fish than in mammals, clinical signs of acute and chronic stress can be observed in fish, and we are able to determine physiological stress by several means, including assaying serum cortisol. Fish do act to remove themselves from an adverse stimulus. It is reasonable to postulate that fish need to be cognizant of their surroundings to react to stressors in their environment, which would suggest that fish should be considered susceptible to stress and pain.

D. Anesthesia

Anesthesia should be offered to fish for any painful or extremely stressful procedure and is required in fish for procedures that do not require it in other domestic animals. Immobilization, prolonged transport, and minor surgery for topical lesions all require some degree of tranquilization. General anesthesia is required for more complex surgery and sometimes even for injections. As fish are lifted out of the water, an attempt should be made to protect their eyes and reduce the physical abrasion of the net. Light and vibrational stimuli, including sound, should be reduced to a minimum during the examination. Fish anesthesia is covered extensively in a number of review publications and individual papers on specific methods (Neifer and Stamper, 2009).

Stressors should be removed as much as possible from the environment before a fish is anesthetized. Fish should not be harassed or chased around tanks prior to anesthesia. For smooth induction and recovery, anesthetic tanks for immersion anesthesia, and recovery tanks, should be prepared ahead of time. Anesthetic solutions should be properly buffered, and careful calculation of the anesthetic agent is important. Anesthetized fish should be handled carefully to avoid damage to the delicate epidermis. The hands of the operator should always be wet. For long procedures, a recirculating anesthesia machine can be used to deliver anesthetic for maintenance. When anesthetizing a group of fish of a new species, a small number should always be anesthetized first, and their recovery carefully monitored. This allows the dose to be assessed before all fish are involved. After anesthesia, the fish should be constantly monitored until the righting reflex returns and the fish is able to swim unaided in a coordinated manner. Intermittent monitoring should be continued for up to 24 h to make sure that no long-term side effects occur. When fish are under several of the anesthetic drugs, their blood oxygenation falls. Keeping the anesthetic water well aerated is critical but is not necessarily sufficient to ensure reasonable oxygenation of the fish's tissues. Considerable study is ongoing concerning the mechanism of the apparently hypoxic effects of drugs such as MS-222 and eugenol.

Most anesthetic agents for fish are administered by immersion. Other routes include parenteral, intramuscular, or intraperitoneal injection and oral ingestion. Although fish can survive for periods of several minutes in air and recover well in water, such an experience is physiologically stressful for them. If long operations are to be performed, constant recirculation systems must be used and the fish must be given access to oxygenated water at all times. Monitoring of anesthetic depth in fishes has been described following the stages and planes commonly used to describe depth of anesthesia in mammals (Stoskopf, 2010). As a fish becomes deeply sedated (stage I, plane 2), voluntary swimming stops and the respiratory rate (opercular movements) becomes slightly slower. The transition to stage II, plane 1, or light narcosis, may be preceded by a brief excitement period and an increase in respiratory rate. The fish loses equilibrium but works to right itself in the water. Deep narcosis (stage II, plane 2) is marked by a decrease in respiratory rate back to normal and total loss of equilibrium. This plane is suitable for external sampling, such as taking

fin or gill biopsies. Light anesthesia (stage III, plane 1) is characterized by a further decrease in the respiratory rate and near total loss of muscle tone. Minor surgeries are often performed at this stage and plane. Surgical anesthesia (stage III, plane 2) in fishes is usually characterized by a bradycardia, markedly low respiratory rate, and total loss of reactivity to manipulation. Stage IV, or medullary collapse, is characterized by total loss of gill movement followed in time by cardiac arrest.

1. Tricaine Methanesulfonate (MS-222)

Tricaine methanesulfonate, also called tricaine or MS-222, is the only FDA-approved anesthetic for use in fish in the United States and is one of the most widely used anesthetic agents for poikilotherms worldwide. A derivative of benzocaine, it has an additional sulfonate radical, rendering it more water-soluble and more acidic than its parent compound. Tricaine has no effect on ciliary action, but its effect on muscular activity is rapid. Recovery is also rapid. In weak solutions no long-term toxic effects have been reported in fish, so it is used for transporting fish long distances. Tricaine is a popular anesthetic agent because of its solubility in water. However, because tricaine is acid in aqueous solution, it should be buffered. Most commonly this is achieved with bicarbonate of soda. Tricaine has been noted by many authors to be a hypoxic agent. This characteristic is associated with several physiological changes, including bradycardia, an increase in resistance to blood flow through the gill lamellae, and erythrocyte swelling that impedes blood passage through the gills. Further physiological effects due to hypoxia during tricaine anesthesia can include increased concentrations of blood glucose, lactate, potassium, magnesium, hemoglobin, and hematocrit; increased urinary output; and electrolyte loss. These changes may persist for up to 4–7 days after anesthesia.

In general, a tricaine solution of 100 mg/l can be used for surgical anesthesia, whereas solutions of 20–30 mg/l are used for tranquilization and transport. Individual variation from fish to fish and between species can be very wide with this agent, so caution should be used when any dose is administered to species of fish the anesthetist has not had experience of anesthetizing.

2. Metomidate

Metomidate hydrochloride is an imidazole-based nonbarbiturate hypnotic agent with no analgesic properties in humans. Metomidate is effective in subduing fish, but long recovery times are common with this drug. Metomidate reduces plasma cortisol and glucose concentrations and increases fish pigmentation, presumably because of increased production of melanocyte-stimulating hormone on the same primary protein as adrenocorticotropic hormone (ACTH). Small adult rainbow trout can be tranquilized with metomidate at 5 mg/l. At these doses, total loss of reflexes does not occur. Channel catfish fingerlings have been tranquilized at 5 mg/l, although this dose may have been too high, because recovery times were reported to exceed 24 h. Muscle fasciculations are common with this drug, precluding its use in delicate procedures. Dosages generally used in freshwater and marine tropical species of fish vary from 2.5 to 5 mg/l. Doses reported for tropical marine fish for tranquilization or transportation are in the range of 0.06–0.20 mg/l.

3. Carbon Dioxide

Carbon dioxide is soluble in water at a dilution of 1:1.2 by volume at standard temperature and pressure. In humans, a CO_2 concentration above 7% causes headache, dizziness, mental confusion, palpitations, hypertension, and dyspnea. Concentrations above 10% cause unconsciousness. Excessive CO_2 in the blood can depress respiratory drive, so maintenance of sufficient aeration to sustain correct PO_2 levels in the fish is important. Bubbling CO_2 into the water is difficult to control, and PO_2 levels must be kept high to avoid severe acidosis and hypoxia.

4. Quinaldine

Quinaldine must be dissolved in acetone or ethanol in order to make it miscible with water. Quinaldine sulfate, however, is readily soluble in water but is acidic and should be buffered with sodium bicarbonate (0.45 g $NaHCO_3$ – 1 g quinaldine sulfate). Quinaldine is more potent in water with high pH. It irritates the gills and causes increased branchial mucous secretion. Although it produces a loss of equilibrium and depression of medullary centers in stage III anesthesia, the fish do not lose all reflex response, making it less than satisfactory for some delicate surgical procedures. The required solvents produce a noxious vapor that irritates the eyes of the surgeon. Analgesia with quinaldine is thought to be minimal, but quinaldine is popular for collecting fish from tidal pools and small lagoons. For warm-water species, generally 15–70 mg/l is used. The dose required to reach stage III anesthesia in many fish species is 16 mg/l. Doses of 50–1000 mg/l have been used in tilapia.

5. Euthanasia

Concerns about appropriate end points in experiments on fish are similar to those with mammals. Ideally euthanasia is achieved by appropriate application of anesthetic overdoses followed by cranial detachment or exsanguination. Many scientists are concerned about potential effects of anesthetic agents on their research data. These investigators should be encouraged to conduct pilot studies to document these effects. Ideally, quantifiable time-associated assessments of physiologic,

behavioral, or other appropriate responses should be used to judge the suitability of a proposed euthanasia methods for fishes. Though fish, as ectothermic vertebrates, are not covered by the U.S. Animal Welfare Act, they are covered under the U.S. Public Health Service regulations which are based on the *Guide for the Care and Use of Laboratory Animals*, produced, published, and maintained under contract by the ILAR Council of the National Academy of Sciences (National Research Council, 2011). The American Veterinary Medical Association (AVMA) also publishes specific guidelines for euthanasia that are widely accepted as authoritative by many institutional animal care and use committees (IACUCs). The AVMA euthanasia guidelines have recently undergone extensive review by an expert panel. Several methods of euthanasia of fishes that are popular with some investigators, such as dewatering (removal from the water and subsequent asphyxiation) or hypothermia, are not considered humane or appropriate methods of euthanasia for fishes by the AVMA. The physiologic impacts of dewatering with no adjunct procedure to hasten death should be obvious. Concerns about the use of ice or cold shock relate to the ability of neurons of cold-adapted poikilotherms to fire coherently at temperatures much lower than would cause loss of sensation in mammals. Decapitation without prior anesthesia is currently accepted by the AVMA as a humane method of euthanasia of fishes. Direct immersion of unanesthetized fish into fixatives is not considered appropriate, because of the reactions of the fish to the immersion and the prolonged times that fish can continue to gill in the fixatives.

V. ZOONOTIC CONSIDERATIONS

Although the number of reported outbreaks of fish-related diseases in the United States is increasing, the prevalences of fish-related diseases in humans remain relatively low. Increased awareness of disease symptoms and the increased prevalence of immunocompromising conditions appear to contribute to the increasing number of reported outbreaks. Nevertheless, zoonotic disease should be considered in the management of laboratory fish.

A. Bacterial Zoonoses

Bacterial diseases of fish with zoonotic potential are generally opportunistic. Development of disease in a human usually requires a compromised immune system. Exposures often result in mild gastroenteritis or localized infections of the skin and underlying tissues, but a few organisms are highly pathogenic and can produce high mortality in infected individuals.

Members of the genus *Streptococcus* have caused disease outbreaks in freshwater and saltwater fish in the southern United States and Japan. Many fish isolates are of the Lancefield's group B and D serotypes. *Staphylococcus* spp. occasionally produce disease in fish and have been isolated from aquarium water. The potential for human infection exists. *Streptococcus iniae* is an important zoonotic concern and this species is known to affect zebrafish and many other laboratory-maintained fishes.

Erysipelothrix rhusiopathiae (formerly *E. insidiosa*) appears not to cause disease in fish but is present in the external mucus of many fishes. Human infections with *E. rhusiopathiae* are prevalent among persons handling fish. Three forms of the disease are described: localized skin infections (erysipeloid, or 'fish rose'), usually involving the fingers or hands; diffuse cutaneous disease, when a localized infection spreads to adjacent tissues; and septicemia. Fish or shellfish are believed to be the source of infection in about a quarter of the reported cases in the United States in the past century.

Mycobacterium fortuitum, M. chelonei, and *M. marinum* are recognized pathogens of fish. Human infections with *M. chelonei* or *M. marinum* may not be detected, because incubation of human isolates is commonly done at 37°C, and the organisms generally do not grow well above 30°C.

Mycobacterium fortuitum has a wider temperature tolerance. In contrast to *M. avium* complex infections, few human infections with the three fish pathogens have been reported. Immunocompromised individuals may develop disseminated or respiratory disease, but immunocompetent patients more commonly develop circumscribed cutaneous lesions at sites of penetrating wounds.

Humans with *M. marinum* infections usually have a single granulomatous nodule, usually on the hands or fingers. However, a 'sporotrichoid' form of the disease, in which localized infection is followed by spread to nearby lymph nodes, can occur. The nodular form frequently resolves in weeks to months without treatment. The lack of spread to adjacent tissues is thought to be a result of the organism's intolerance of higher temperatures. When the organism occasionally spreads to adjacent tissues, a T-cell unresponsiveness is suspected. Individuals infected with human immunodeficiency virus (HIV) should be advised to avoid cleaning fish holding systems. It is important to keep in mind that human epidemics of granulomatous skin disease have occurred from swimming in infected waters and that this mode of human infection is much more common than infections from exposure to infected tropical fish tanks. Granulomas from *M. marinum* usually occur at sites of minor skin abrasions that become apparent 2–3 weeks after exposure.

Nocardia asteroides and *N. kampachi* have been isolated infrequently from tuberculoid lesions of fish and humans. These infections can be misdiagnosed as mycobacterial disease because of the similarity of clinical signs and the positive reaction to acid-fast staining.

Gram-negative bacteria have been incriminated in fish associated food-borne disease in humans, including *Vibrio cholerae* 0 group 1, *V. cholerae* non-01, *V. parahaemolyticus,* and *V. vulnificus.* None of these diseases should be considered a large risk in a facility that handles laboratory fish, but human infections with *V. vulnificus* have been the object of some study because of the high mortality associated with infection. Two clinical syndromes have been described. Most prominently described is a primary septicemia syndrome usually associated with eating raw oysters. Signs include fever, changes in mental status, ecchymotic hemorrhages, bulla formation, and pain in the lower extremities. The mortality rate is approximately 50%, even with prompt diagnosis and treatment. A prominent predisposing factor is pre-existing liver disease, especially cirrhosis, which is thought to adversely affect leukocyte migration.

The second clinical syndrome is more important in laboratory animal facilities and is a wound infection characterized by cellulitis, edema, hemorrhages, bulla formation, and extensive tissue necrosis. Despite prompt and aggressive treatment, the mortality rate ranges from 25 to 30% among affected individuals. In the majority of cases, infection is acquired by introduction of contaminated seawater into skin wounds, but cases with relatively freshwater exposure have been reported recently.

Aeromonas salmonicida, A. hydrophila, A. sobria, A. caviae, A. schubertii, and *A. veronii* are currently considered members of the motile *Aeromonas* complex and produce septicemia in infected fish. They are routinely found in the aquatic environment. The most commonly isolated species, *A. hydrophila,* is found worldwide in tropical and temperate freshwater and is considered to be part of the normal intestinal microflora of healthy fish. Despite the ubiquity of these organisms, motile aeromonads produce few human infections. Signs are variable in infected individuals, but gastroenteritis and localized wound infections are the most common manifestations. Wound infections can be superficial or can progress to cellulitis, deep muscle necrosis, or septicemia. The primary concern is with immunodeficient individuals who might acquire an aeromonad infection as a result of wound contamination.

Klebsiella spp. are found in aquatic environments, and *K. pneumoniae* septicemia has been reported as a consequence of handling contaminated fish. *Edwardsiella tarda* is a well-documented fish pathogen, and infections in humans through ingestion of contaminated water or fish or from contamination of a wound are known but are rare. Persons with serious pre-existing illnesses are predisposed to infection with *E. tarda,* and the mortality rate is high (44%) in those individuals. *Yersinia ruckeri* is highly pathogenic to fish, but human infection with this organism is rarely reported.

Three cases of *Leptospira icterohaemorrhagiae* infection in British fish farmers in 1981 caused concern that fish harbor leptospirosis and transmit the disease to humans. Studies of leptospirosis in aquatic species have concluded that fish can harbor the organism, but considerably more field and experimental data are needed to accurately determine the risk of human infection.

B. Parasitic Zoonoses

In the United States the prevalence of parasitic zoonoses attributable to fish is low, and most reported cases involve consumption of fish that serve as intermediate hosts for parasites of fish predators. Human infections with *Eustrongyloides* spp. generally cause an anisakiasis-like syndrome of acute abdominal pain. Infection has occurred after ingestion of live bait minnows and sushi, but of more interest to laboratory animal workers is an unusual case that involved the migration of a dracunculoid nematode (*Philometra* sp.) into an open hand wound (Deardorff *et al.*, 1986).

C. Fungal and Viral Zoonoses

No human infections with fish fungal pathogens have been well described. However, *Candida albicans* has been cultured from skin lesions of mullet, and human infection is considered possible. No human infections with fish viruses have been reported (Wolf, 1988). However, San Miguel sea lion virus, a calicivirus known to produce vesicular disease in both marine mammals and pigs, has been shown to elicit antibody production in humans and vesicular lesions in primates. The virus is believed to be transmitted by various marine fish, and it has been suggested that humans may become infected during handling of fish vectors.

D. Toxins

A large number of marine organisms produce toxic substances that can cause illness and death in humans. In most instances, however, poisonings caused by marine species occur as isolated events. The toxicology and clinical syndromes produced by these agents have been comprehensively reviewed (Halstead, 1988).

VI. DISEASES

A. Mycobacteriosis

Etiology   The mycobacterial species that infect fish are classed in Runyon group IV. They can be cultured successfully on standard tryptone soy agar and brain–heart infusion agar. More commonly, more specialized media, including Petragnani, Lowenstein–Jensen, Middlebrook 7H10, and Dorset egg media are used for isolation. *Mycobacterium fortuitum* and *M. marinum* are the most common mycobacterial isolates from affected laboratory fishes. *Mycobacterium chelonei* is also occasionally isolated from infected fish. Whether fish can be infected with other species of mycobacteria, including *M. tuberculosis*, is controversial. An interesting note is the apparently successful but unreplicated experimental infection of perch with *M. leprae* in 1951. '*Mycobacterium anabanti*' and '*M. platypoecilus*' are obsolete synonyms for *M. marinum*. '*Mycobacterium salmoniphilum*' is an archaic synonym for *M. fortuitum*. *Mycobacterium piscium* is in doubt taxonomically and is not currently accepted as a species.

Clinical Signs   Mycobacteriosis is a chronic progressive disease that can but does not necessarily take years to develop into a clinically apparent illness. Clinical manifestations include lethargy, anorexia, fin and scale loss, exophthalmia, emaciation, skin inflammation and ulceration, edema, peritonitis, and nodules in muscles that may deform the fish.

Epizootiology and Transmission   Mycobacteriosis is worldwide in distribution. All fish species should be considered susceptible. Mycobacteria are widespread in most waters. *Mycobacterium marinum* has been cultured from swimming pools, beaches, natural streams, estuaries, tropical fish tanks, and city tap water. Infection rates can be quite high in contaminated freshwater tropical fish production facilities.

Transmission may be from ingestion of contaminated food, as well as detritus and through cannibalism in poorly managed systems. Transovarian transmission has been established in Mexican platyfish and other viviparous fishes. Vertical transmission through eggs is not thought to occur in ovoviviparous fish, but more research is needed.

Necropsy Findings   *Postmortem* examination usually reveals gray or white nodules in the liver, kidney, heart, or spleen. Skeletal involvement can cause deformities. Diagnosis is usually based on clinical signs and the presence of acid-fast bacteria in tissue sections or smears.

Pathogenesis   Little information is available on the pathogenic mechanisms of mycobacterial infections in fish. Exotoxins are not thought to play a role. The possibility of a role for endotoxins is being investigated. The organisms' resistance host defense mechanisms is thought to be the primary factor in the pathogenesis of infection.

Differential Diagnosis   Mycobacteria are Gram-positive pleomorphic rods that are acid-fast and nonmotile. A major differential disease is nocardiosis, which shares some of the histologic characteristics of mycobacteriosis in fish.

Prevention No bacterins are available for prevention of the mycobacterial infection. Prevention is focused on careful lethal screening of incoming fish and effective isolation procedures.

Control Control is based on avoidance of excessive density or poor water conditions, removal of affected fish, and effective quarantines for periods of 4 or more weeks for incoming fish.

Treatment Usually mycobacteria that infect fish are resistant to commonly used antimycobacterial drugs such as isoniazid. Chloramine-B or chloramine-T, cyclosporin, doxycycline, ethambutol, ethionamide, isoniazid, kanamycin, minocycline, penicillin, rifampicin, streptomycin, sulfonamides, and tetracycline are all drugs that have been reported in therapeutic attempts. Multiple-drug therapy is generally more successful against these organisms than single-drug therapy. Doxycycline and rifampin are the drug combination frequently cited as effective against *M. marinum*. Many clinicians believe that the difficulty of treatment of this disease, and the risk of spread to other fishes or humans, are sufficient reasons to preclude attempts at therapy. Treatment probably should be reserved for particularly valuable animals in situations and facilities where isolation can be maintained.

Research Complications Usually a slowly developing disease, mycobacteriosis can be devastating to experiments that must maintain fish for prolonged periods. Granuloma formation can affect almost any organ, potentially affecting organ function. In addition, the granulomas can be mistaken for early neoplastic nodules in carcinogenesis studies.

B. *Ichthyophthirius multifiliis* Infestation

Etiology *Ichthyophthirius multifiliis* (Fig. 21.1) is a holotrichous ciliate that has a worldwide distribution and affects all freshwater fishes. A closely related organism, *Cryptocaryon irritans*, affects marine fishes.

Clinical Signs Predominant signs include small white spots widely distributed over the body and fins. In some cases, infestation is limited to the gills. A diagnosis can be confirmed by microscopic examination of biopsy material from skin or gills.

Epizootiology and Transmission These parasites have a complicated life cycle that includes stages on the host as well as in the environment. The white spot observed on the affected fish is called the trophont. It is the encysted feeding stage. Eventually, the trophont enlarges, breaks through the epithelium, and drops to the bottom of the aquarium, where it attaches to any object, such as gravel or tubing. At this point the organism is referred to as a tomont. The time taken for development on the fish is temperature-dependent and requires 3–4 days at 22°C, up to 11 days at 15°C, and nearly 30 days at 10°C.

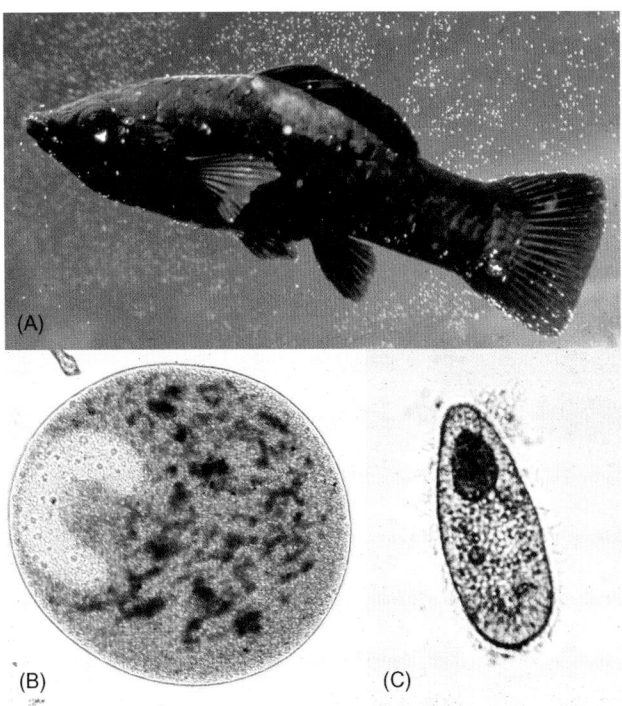

FIGURE 21.1 *Ichthyophthirius multifiliis*: Holotrichous ciliate parasites are a common health problem for teleosts maintained in closed systems. The clinical appearance is a varying number of classical round slightly raised spots on the fish. (A) Black molly with a few variably sized white spots caused by *Ichthyophthirius* cysts and the milky nature of the mucous coat that is seen in any condition where irritation causes excess mucus production. (B) *Ichthyophthirius* tomont with its characteristic horseshoe shaped nucleus as they frequently appear in a squash preparation or wet smear of affected tissues. These are highly variable in size, even in the same patient and they may vary from less than half a millimeter to nearly a millimeter in diameter. The rolling motion of the tomont aids in identification. (C) The much smaller free-swimming infective theront of *Ichthyophthirius*. These ciliated forms are elongated and are generally about 10 μm wide and 30–40 μm long.

The tomont attaches to bottom substrates or plants and begins to undergo mitosis (binary fission). Within 18–21 h at 23–25°C, this mitosis will result in hundreds of ciliated theronts that are released into the water. Theronts actively swim and, when they encounter a host fish, attach and actively penetrate skin or gill epithelium, where they enlarge until they are visible as a white spot. Free-swimming newly excysted ciliated theronts have only about 48 h in which to find a host before they die. The disease is usually observed several days after introducing new fish to an aquarium.

Necropsy Findings The characteristic white trophonts may not be visible on a dead fish. Routinely they excyst and drop from the fish very shortly after death of the fish. In wet mounts, trophonts appear round to oval and may be from 30 to 1000 μm in diameter. The organism moves slowly by means of cilia observable with a high-power objective. The motion is typically a rolling motion in which the parasite rotates across the field of view. The horseshoe-shaped nucleus is often visible and assists identification.

Pathogenesis The disease need not be fatal. Heavy infestations are thought to interfere with osmoregulation due to the disruption of the contiguous epithelium, but this is speculative and not based on solid research investigations.

Differential Diagnosis *Ichthyophthirius multifiliis* is one of the few fish parasites with cilia surrounding the entire organism. The free-swimming infective ciliated theronts are usually pear-shaped, actively motile, and about 30–45 μm in diameter.

Prevention Prophylactic treatments with saline baths or dilute copper are used on incoming fish during quarantine in some facilities. The immunocompromising impact of copper treatments is increasingly well documented. Maintenance of excellent water quality and minimization of stress are thought to reduce the likelihood of a clinical outbreak. Adequate water changes and cleaning of substrates are thought to help prevent accumulation of high numbers of infective tomonts.

Control Heavy filtration with diatomaceous earth or membrane filters will reduce the number of circulating theronts. Transferring fish to clean aquaria every day for 7 days will limit the infection by keeping one step ahead of theront reinfestation. Removal of theronts from the water can also be accomplished by making large daily water changes. This method, while efficacious, may stress fish excessively unless attention is paid to makeup water temperature and pH. Alternatively, fish can be removed from a system, and the parasites will eventually die for lack of a host. Elevating the temperature several degrees Celsius over normal temperatures accelerates this process. To ensure that all theronts are eliminated in a system, at least one complete water change should be made, along with removing debris from the gravel before returning fish to the system after leaving a tank or system fallow.

Treatment Currently available medications do not penetrate the encysted trophonts (Tomonts). All treatment is directed toward preventing reinfection of fish by killing free-swimming theronts. Formaldehyde at 25 ppm (1 ml/10 gallons) is effective if administered three times on alternate days. Water changes of up to 75% should be done 4–8 h after treatments. In addition to chemotherapy, management adjustments serve to control infestations. Elevating water temperatures several degrees Celsius over normal temperatures for 5–7 days will limit the infection by adversely affecting the heat-sensitive theronts as well as enhancing the immune response of the host.

Research Complications The most common complication associated with this disease is mortality. Certainly, affected fish become inappetent and lethargic, which can also affect experimental results.

C. *Ichthyobodo necator* Infestation

Etiology *Ichthyobodo necator*, formerly known as *Costia necatrix*, is a small flagellated protozoal parasite with wide distribution in freshwaters. It has been documented to survive and cause disease in marine fish as well, although similar marine-adapted organisms are also known.

Clinical Signs Fish affected with *Ichthyobodo* are often depressed, anorectic, and in respiratory distress. A whitish film from excess mucus production is commonly seen on the body surface. Some fish die without visible external signs. Diagnosis is confirmed by microscopic examination of wet mounts of skin or gills. The organisms are actively motile, small (7–15 μm long), and somewhat comma-shaped. They can be seen as free-swimming forms or as forms attached to cells by their flagellae. When detached, the parasites move in a characteristic circular fashion.

Epizootiology and Transmission These flagellates reproduce by simple binary fission. Transmission appears to be by direct contact or exposure to water that has held infected fish within several hours. The disease is found both in winter and summer months but is more serious in warmer water. Infestations are seen most frequently in fish that have recently been shipped from a primary producer. The organism survives only an hour or so off of the fish host.

Necropsy Findings Fish can die from ichthyobodiasis without showing characteristic lesions at necropsy. Epithelial sloughing, spongiosis, and hyperplasia and increased mucous cell production can be seen in other cases. The parasites leave a dead host quickly after death, making identification of the disease challenging unless affected fish are euthanized. Clinical diagnosis with skin or gill biopsies is generally more rewarding than necropsy in diagnosing this disease.

Pathogenesis The *Ichthyobodo* organism feeds directly on epithelial cells by a cytopharyngeal canal that protrudes into the host cell. The parasite can destroy gill and skin epithelium. Disease in older fish is usually associated with some sort of stress, often due to temperature fluctuations or transport.

Differential Diagnosis Identification of low numbers of these parasites does not necessarily mean they are the cause of morbidity observed in the fish. Ectocommensal bobonid flagellates that are nonpathogenic can also be found on the skin and gills of fish and can be confused with *Ichthyobodo*.

Prevention Prophylactic treatments with formalin baths or dilute copper are used on incoming fish during quarantine in some facilities. Maintenance of excellent water quality and minimization of stress are thought to reduce the likelihood of a clinical outbreak. Adequate water changes and cleaning of substrates are thought to help prevent accumulation of high numbers of infective free-swimming stages.

Control No vaccines are available, and prolonged prophylaxis is not generally recommended in laboratory fish. The disease is more severe in younger fish and is commonly associated with temperature fluctuations, so efforts to isolate young fish from older animals and careful attention to stable water temperatures appear to help control the disease.

Treatment This parasite is susceptible to most common antiprotozoal therapies. One treatment of 25 ppm of formaldehyde followed by a water change up to 75% in 4–8 h is usually effective in killing attached parasites, as well as those in the water column.

Research Complications This disease is of most concern to researchers studying early development of fish. It can be rapidly fatal, with high mortality rates, if introduced to naive animals or animals undergoing any stress.

D. Dactylogyridiasis

Etiology Dactylogyrid flukes are monogenean parasites common on freshwater fish and can infest species of all major fish groups. Pond-reared fish can be heavily infested.

Clinical Signs Fish in ponds or in the wild rarely exhibit clinical signs. Clinical disease is more common in small closed systems. Clinical signs include rapid respiratory movements, clamped fins, flashing, or rubbing. Fish may also become inactive and rest at the bottom of the aquarium. Death can result from heavy infestations. Diagnosis is confirmed by biopsies of the gills, where the parasites are readily visible. Dactylogyrid flukes have a four-pointed anterior end, a sucker near the anterior end, and four anterior eyespots. The caudal end has an attachment apparatus, or haptor, that consists of one or two large hooks surrounded by up to 16 smaller hooklets. The worms are approximately 400 μm long and have both testes and ovaries.

Epizootiology and Transmission Dactylogyrid flukes reproduce by mutual fertilization followed by release of eggs that develop off of the host. Eggs from some species hatch into ciliated forms as early as 60 h after being released. Other species require 4–5 days before hatching. The ciliated larvae attack suitable hosts, lose their cilia, and develop into adults. Transmission is greatly enhanced by overcrowding of fish. The parasite load per fish in a single aquarium, even within a single host species, can be quite variable. Immunocompetence may play a role in this variability.

Necropsy Findings These parasites disrupt the epithelial barrier of the fish and cause irritation and local disruption of tissues with variable inflammatory responses.

Pathogenesis Dactylogyrid flukes are usually found on the gills but can be found on the body. If present in sufficient numbers, they can cause hyperplasia, destruction of gill epithelium, and clubbing of gill filaments, which can lead to asphyxiation. It has been postulated that their feeding habits may aid in the introduction of pathogenic bacteria, in addition to their own impact on host physiology.

Differential Diagnosis Of the many genera of monogeneans that infest freshwater tropical fishes, the species of the genus Dactylogyrus are the most important. However, several related genera that are challenging for the average clinician to differentiate are also egg-laying monogeneans of freshwater fish capable of causing pathology.

Prevention No vaccines are available. Prevention involves careful prescreening and treatment of infected fish prior to introduction into the facility.

Control Control centers around careful management of water quality and avoiding overcrowding.

Treatment Specific treatments include long-duration exposure to formaldehyde or short-term baths. Saltwater baths have also been used. Organophosphates are used for freshwater fishes, but extended use of organophosphates can develop resistant strains of flukes. Praziquantel effectively removes monogeneans from gills and body surfaces when administered as a bath at 6 ppm. Low levels of formaldehyde (25 ppm) are effective.

Research Complications Affected fish can be energetically compromised through increased respiratory effort and may display erratic behavior related to attempts to scrape off the parasites. Heavy infestations seem to make fish more susceptible to other infections and toxic substances.

E. Gyrodactylidiasis

Etiology Many species of the genus *Gyrodactylus* are described. They infect a broad range of hosts, including most freshwater tropical fishes. Their distribution as a genus is most likely worldwide.

Clinical Signs Inapparent infections are common. The parasites feed on blood and epithelium by scraping and sucking the contents of host cells. Lesions can include localized hemorrhagic areas, excessive mucus, and localized ulcerations. Infected fish may have a ragged appearing tail from localized hyperplasia, necrosis, and loss of epithelial cells on the fins.

Epizootiology and Transmission Gyrodactylids are viviparous, and embryos with prominent hooks are commonly seen in adult parasites.

Necropsy Findings These parasites disrupt the epithelial barrier of the fish and cause local disruption of tissues and variable inflammatory responses.

Pathogenesis Secondary infections with bacteria (*Aeromonas* sp., *Flexibacter* sp.) are common. *Aeromonas hydrophila* has been isolated from gyrodactylids removed from goldfish, suggesting that the worms may actively transmit bacteria.

Differential Diagnosis Gyrodactylids are usually found on the skin but may occasionally be found on the gills. They can be up to 0.8 mm long, with two points at the anterior end. An anterior sucker is present, but no eyespots. An attachment organ, or haptor, with two large hooks surrounded by up to 16 hooklets is located at the caudal end.

Prevention No vaccines are available. Prevention involves careful prescreening and treatment of infected fish prior to introduction into the facility.

Control Control centers around careful management of water quality and avoiding overcrowding.

Treatment Praziquantel at 3 ppm in aquarium water will effectively remove gyrodactylids. Older treatments include addition of formaldehyde to aquaria at 25 ppm, saltwater baths (2.5–3%), or organophosphate baths. Extended use of organophosphates can result in development of resistant monogeneans. Because these monogeneans are live-bearing flukes, drug-resistant ova are not a problem. Single treatments can clear the infestation.

Research Complications Affected fish can be energetically compromised through increased flashing behavior related to attempts to scrape off the parasites. Secondary bacterial infections can result in mortality.

F. Nematode Infections

Etiology A number of genera of nematodes infect teleost fishes. Larval forms of *Eustrongyloides* spp. (Fig. 21.2) and adult forms of *Capillaria* sp. and *Camallanus* sp. affect a wide variety of freshwater fishes.

Clinical Signs Clinical signs vary with the species of worm and the species of fish infected. Syndromes range from emaciation and failure to thrive, with various intestinal parasites, to swellings and granulomas caused by larval worms, particularly those using the fish as an intermediate host. Infections by camallanids are usually initially noticed when a red worm protrudes from the anus of the fish.

Epizootiology and Transmission The life cycle of many nematode parasites involves an intermediate host such as an aquatic insect that harbors the larval stage of the nematode. Some forms use the fish as an intermediate host to reach a predatory final host. Nematodes that have direct life cycles such as *Capillaria* spp. Are more difficult to eradicate.

Necropsy Findings Adult or larval nematodes can be found within the lumen of the intestine, as free migratory forms in the coelomic cavity or as encysted forms

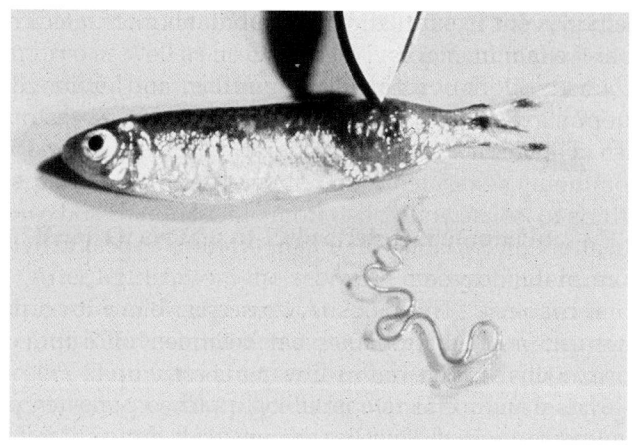

FIGURE 21.2 *Eustrongyloides* infection: teleost fish are infected by numerous forms of nematodes. Larval forms of *Eustrongyloides* are often observed as apparent swellings or 'tumors' on the surface of fish. Sharp dissection will reveal subcutaneous larval worms that use the fish as an intermediate host in their life cycle.

in internal organs or musculature. Larval *Eustrongyloides* spp. are usually found as encysted red worms in the muscles or peritoneum of the fish. Occasionally, cysts located close to the skin are confused with neoplasias.

Prevention Feeding insect larvae or free-swimming copepods to fish should be avoided, because these may carry immature stages of nematodes. Feeding of live foods may allow continuance of infestations, which would otherwise be self-limiting in an aquarium environment.

Treatment Adult nematodes can be treated with common nematicides in the food. Fenbendazole mixed with commercial food enhanced with cod liver oil and bound with gelatin controls *Camallanus* spp. Preparations such as Panacur can be used in food at the rate of 0.25% (250 ppm). Because fish may not accept medicated food immediately, but most will begin feeding after a few days, Panacur (equine formulation, containing 100 mg of active drug per milliliter) can be used at 2 ppm in aquarium water. This treatment should be repeated three times at weekly intervals. Carbon filters should be removed, and passing medication through undergravel beds should be avoided. A partial water change should be made 2–3 days after treatment, and then filtration should be resumed. Because fish are quick to refuse medicated food, withholding food for a few days prior to feeding medicated food may be beneficial. Piperazine in food is also effective against some intestinal nematodes. Ivermectin as a bath has been used to treat nematodes successfully; however, the margin of safety is low for many fish species.

Research Complications Fish farmers believe that *Capillaria* sp. infections can reduce reproductive potential and growth rates.

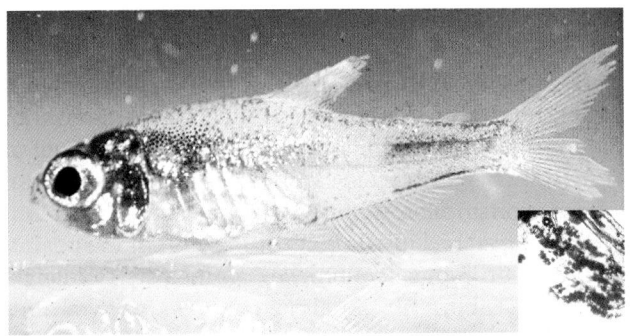

FIGURE 21.3 Pleistophoriasis: microsporidian infections are commonly found in teleost fish. One of the better-reported conditions is referred to as 'Neon Tetra Disease' because this species of fish is commonly affected. Clinically fish lose color and condition. On examination of squash preparations of muscles from infected fish, large numbers of space occupying spores are readily observed (inset).

G. Microsporidiosis

Etiology Members of the microsporidian genera *Glugea*, *Pleistophora*, and *Spraguea* (synonym *Nosema*) contain species that are highly pathogenic to teleost fishes (Fig. 21.3).

Clinical Signs Often no clinical signs are observed. Any signs are usually associated with the mechanical occupation of space in infected organs or disruption of the normal formation or function of organs and structures.

Epizootiology and Transmission Microsporidiosis can be fatal and highly contagious. Autogamy appears to initiate spore formation at the end of schizogonic activity. Oral ingestion is the mode of transmission. However, intermediate hosts, such as rotifers and planktonic crustaceans, may be required in the life cycle of the parasites.

Necropsy Findings The parasites are found in the intestines, pyloric ceca, bile ducts, liver, mesenteric lymph nodes, muscles, neural ganglia, subcutaneous tissues, testes, and ovaries. The microsporidian spore is ovoid and has a thick wall without any opening. In heavy infections, the gut wall can be largely supplanted by cysts. The intestine appears chalk white and pebbled and has a rigid, thickened, hard wall. The epithelium of the intestine is denuded and the lumen of the cecum may be almost occluded.

Pathogenesis The life cycle of a microsporidian species consists of two distinct phases: a multiplicative stage (schizogony) and a spore-forming stage (sporogony). The infection is invasive, with diffuse infiltration of tissues. The infective germ, the sporoplasm, is extruded to the exterior through a hollow, coiled polar tube that is everted after the spore has been ingested by a specific host. The sporoplasm is injected into the host cell and undergoes multiple binary fission, producing an

enormous number of cells. The parasites do not cause host cell degeneration but stimulate hypertrophy and abnormal development into a xenoparasitic complex, or xenoma. Mechanical distension of the intestinal tissue and starvation are thought to be the cause of death.

Differential Diagnosis Occasionally the presence of masses of the parasites has been mistaken for neoplasia.

Prevention Removal of ill or dying fish before cannibalism by other fish in the tank can occur greatly reduces the chance of transmission in closed systems not being fed live food.

Control and Treatment No effective chemotherapeutics have been identified for the treatment or control of these diseases.

Research Complications A common problem is the discovery that large portions of the organ system being studied have been displaced in infected fish. This is particularly a problem in studies of the central nervous system in which asymptomatic fish may be missing up to 50% of their brain tissue.

H. Myxosporidiosis

Etiology Classification of myxospores is based on the number of shell valves and the position of the polar capsules in the spore. Members of the order Bivalvulida have two spore wall valves, and Multivalvulida members have three or more valves in the spore wall. There are more than 1100 species of myxosporidia reported in literature, but only a few are described in laboratory fish species. All species of Multivalvulida and a few of Bivalvulida are important histozoic parasites that inflict serious injuries to the hosts.

Clinical Signs The function of the gallbladder, gill, muscle, and renal tissue can be impaired.

Epizootiology and Transmission Nearly all marine tropical fish collected from the wild harbor species of myxospores from the genera Ceratomyxa, Myxidium, or Leptotheca in their gallbladders. Transmission is assumed to be through ingestion of infective organisms that may be harbored in detritus or the carcasses of dead hosts.

Necropsy Findings In heavily infected fish, the bile appears cloudy and opaque, often with an amorphous cheese-like substance.

Pathogenesis These parasites generally infect the gallbladder and urinary tract (coelozoic) or are intercellular or intracellular parasites of muscle or connective tissue (histozoic). Trophozoites of coelozoic species attach to the transitional epithelium of the gallbladder and urinary bladder during their reproductive cycles, usually with no apparent damage to the host and without initiating a host reaction. Infected muscle fibers become enlarged and replaced by cysts filled with mature spores that may be encapsulated by the host's connective tissue. Muscular liquefaction is due to a proteolytic enzyme released by the parasites after the death of the host.

Prevention The life cycle of the myxosporidians has not been fully elucidated and requires future investigation. Existing evidence indicates that an intermediate host is needed.

Control and Treatment Satisfactory drugs to treat or control these infections are not available. Prescreening of entering fish and culling are the common approaches to control these infections, in addition to elimination of potential intermediate hosts.

Research Complications The most obvious impact on research is the loss of fish unexpectedly during experiments, but potentially far more hazardous is the probable impact on physiologic function of inapparently infected fishes.

I. Lymphocystis

Etiology Lymphocystis is caused by an iridovirus. The disease is recognized worldwide, occurring in at least 125 species of teleosts belonging to 34 families and nine orders. The disease occurs in warm-, cool-, and cold-water fish species from freshwater, estuarine, and marine environments.

Clinical Signs Lymphocystis is a chronic but seldom fatal disease. Fish with lymphocystis develop macroscopic nodules (0.3–2.0 mm or more in diameter) that occur primarily on the body surface but can also develop on the internal organs. The nodules appear cream-colored to pink or gray, depending on the condition of the overlying epithelium and the degree of vascularity of the lesion. They take a week to a year or more to develop, depending on the host species and the environmental conditions. The lesions eventually heal, leaving little scar tissue.

Epizootiology and Transmission The disease occurs with equal frequency in both sexes and can occur in fish of any age, although the prevalence appears higher in young fish. Lymphocystis can be experimentally transmitted with relative ease within a genus but with difficulty between families. This limited degree of host specificity may indicate that various types of lymphocystis virus exist.

In nature, lymphocystis virus appears to be transmitted by exposure of surface wounds to waterborne virus or by ingestion of virus or virus-infected cells. Lymphocystis can be transmitted experimentally by cohabitation, exposure to water containing virus, feeding lesion and lesion homogenate, and applying lesion homogenate to gills or scarified skin. The disease can also be experimentally transmitted by subcutaneous or intraperitoneal lesion implantation or by subdermal or intramuscular injection of lesion homogenate or medium from virus infected cell cultures.

Necropsy Findings Lymphocystis viral infection causes fibroblast hypertrophy. Infected cells do not divide, but the cytoplasm and nucleus become very large. Chromatin condensation and fragmentation are evident, and nucleoli are distorted or indistinct. Feulgen-positive inclusion bodies can be seen in the cytoplasm associated with icosahedral virus particles 150–250 nm in diameter. A thick hyaline capsule forms at the periphery of the cell, and proliferating fibroblasts isolate the infected cell. Plasma cells, lymphocytes, macrophages, and polymorphonuclear leukocytes accumulate at the periphery of the cell.

Pathogenesis The course of the disease is more rapid at warmer water temperatures. A month's timecourse is usual at 25°C, and 11 developmental stages have been described. Viral inclusion bodies generally appear about 8 days after infection of a susceptible cell, and virus is detectable as early as 15 days postinfection. The enlarged nucleus appears to be polyploid. Re-infection is possible, but lesions in second and third infections are usually smaller. Cell-mediated and humeral responses to the infection have been demonstrated late in the course of infection. Regression of lesions begins when precipitin reactions between host serum and lesion homogenates become demonstrable.

Differential Diagnosis Lymphocystis is usually differentiated from epitheliocystis on the basis of the cell type affected and the position of the nucleus of affected cells. The dermal fibroblasts affected by lymphocystis usually display a central nucleus, whereas the epithelial cells affected by epitheliocystis show distinctly peripheral nuclear placement.

Prevention No vaccines are available. Careful screening of fish stock sources is the only known prevention. Reduction of fish trauma through appropriate social and behavioral management and reduction of abrasions from harsh substrates or rough handling may help prevent the infection.

Control Lymphocystis virus is remarkably stable under a variety of storage conditions. Significant levels of infectivity were recovered after 15 years from infected tissue dried over P_2O_5 at 4°C. Lymphocystis virus is inactivated when exposed to ether or chloroform, heat (56–60°C), or pH 3.0. The virus is stable to multiple cycles of freezing and thawing.

Treatment Lesion-bearing fish should be removed. The antineoplastic drug 6-mercaptopurine inhibits virus-specific synthesis and the appearance of virus-induced cytopathic effects in cell culture, and has been used experimentally to control lymphocystis in fish. In cases where individually valuable fish are severely affected, surgical removal and cauterization of the wounds with dilute iodophor solution can be palliatively effective. Care should be taken to avoid burning the surrounding skin by prolonged exposure to the iodophor.

Research Complications Lymphocystis is a chronic, nonfatal disease. The lesions are unsightly and can affect fish energetics if severe enough to affect swimming dynamics and/or food prehension or ingestion.

J. Infectious Pancreatic Necrosis

Etiology Infectious pancreatic necrosis (IPN) is caused by IPN virus (IPNV), an aquatic birnavirus.

Clinical Signs Clinical signs vary with the species of fish affected. IPN and IPN-like viruses are often isolated from fish that show no clinical signs. Acute infection occurs in very young fish of some species and can result in cumulative mortality approaching 100%, particularly in salmonids. Older fish often develop subclinical or inapparent infection. Disease outbreaks in older fish are usually stress-activated in carrier animals. Affected fry and fingerlings swim by rotating on their long axis, or whirling. They are dark, often with exophthalmia, abdominal distension, and mucoid fecal pseudocasts. Anemia is a clinical feature of the disease.

Epizootiology and Transmission IPN and IPN-like viruses have been recovered from at least 65 species of fish and shellfish distributed essentially worldwide, including North America, South America, most of eastern and western Europe, and Asia. Horizontal transmission occurs with infected feces, urine, and sex products. Other animals can be mechanical vectors. IPN virus has been recovered from bird and mammals feces and from experimentally infected crayfish. Infectivity persisted in two protozoal species (*Miamiensis ovidus* and *Tetrahymena* sp.) that were fed virus-infected cells.

Vertical egg-associated transmission is suspected, and iodophor egg treatments are ineffective. The virus has been isolated from eyed eggs and transmitted to zebrafish eggs. The virus may be carried inside the egg with the sperm. The virus can be recovered from the shells of eyed eggs more than 3 weeks after infection and can be recovered from eggshells after hatching. Brood stock can possibly be infected with IPNV by injection of virus-contaminated pituitary extracts used to induce spawning. Experimentally, IPNV can be transmitted by injection, immersion, and feeding.

The virus probably gains access by contact with the gills, ingestion with food, or passage through the sensory pores of the lateral line system. Some survivors of infection become virus carriers and are reservoirs of infection. The carrier prevalence can exceed 90% of the survivors of an epizootic. The carrier state can continue for many years. The prevalence of the carrier state varies among species. Cross-species transmission occurs.

Stress factors and temperature affect IPNV infection. High, rapid mortality occurs between 10 and 14°C in salmonids, whereas high, protracted mortality occurs at lower temperatures. At higher temperatures, mortality is reduced. Similar patterns have not been identified in warm-water fishes. Recrudescence of infection in apparently healthy carrier fish stressed by transport, crowding, poor nutrition, increased temperature, or low oxygen concentration has been reported.

Necropsy Findings At *postmortem*, the liver and spleen are pale, and the stomach and intestines are empty of food and filled with mucoid fluid. Diffuse petechial hemorrhages throughout the pyloric and pancreatic tissues are characteristic. There is massive necrosis of pancreatic acinar cells and occasionally islet tissue with prominent intracytoplasmic inclusions. The pylorus, pyloric ceca, and anterior intestine also show extensive necrosis. Degenerative changes in renal and hepatic tissues are seen. Pancreatic and hepatic tissues are infiltrated by macrophages and polymorphonuclear leukocytes, and viral particles can usually be demonstrated by electron microscopy.

Differential Diagnosis Diagnosis is based on clinical signs and history. Confirmed diagnosis requires isolation and identification of the virus based on serological reactivity in neutralization, fluorescent antibody, immunoperoxidase, complement fixation, immunoelectrophoresis, coagulation, or enzyme-linked immunosorbent assay (ELISA) tests. Infectivity neutralization is the standard. Internal organs and sex products are the clinical samples of choice. Specimens should be assayed within 24 h of sampling. A variety of salmonid and non-salmonid cell lines support viral replication. The serological relations among the IPN and IPN-like viruses are complex, and multiple cross-reacting serotypes occur.

Prevention Water from surface water supplies should be disinfected, and wells should be protected from exposure to surface waters and from contamination by birds or mammals. Fish introduced into the facility should be assayed and determined to be specific pathogen-free for the virus. Eggs should originate from virus-free brood stock.

There is no evidence of maternally transferred immunity, but fry can be protected by passive transfer of antibody or interferon. Inactivated IPNV vaccines elicit a protective response when administered by injection and immersion but not by hyper-osmotic infiltration or feeding. Live-virus vaccines present diagnostic and regulatory problems. There are efforts to develop subunit vaccines by using cloned components from virulent strains of IPNV and from avirulent strains that cross-react with virulent strains, but care will need to be exercised in administering these vaccines across fish species.

Control Infectious pancreatic necrosis is most effectively controlled by preventing contact between the host and the virus. The incidence of acute IPN can also be reduced by controlling factors that promote physiological stress (e.g., high density, inappropriate feeding protocols, poor hygiene).

IPNV is not inactivated by exposure to ether, chloroform, or glycerol but is rapidly inactivated when exposed to chlorine, iodophor, ozone, or ultraviolet irradiation. With increasing water hardness, progressively higher concentrations and longer contact times are needed to inactivate the virus with chlorine or ozone. The virucidal activity of chlorine and iodophor is reduced by organic matter and at pH levels above 8.0. Exposure to ultraviolet irradiation (254 nm) causes rapid loss of infectivity at an intensity of $2000 \mu W/cm^2$. The virus is inactivated by prolonged exposure to beta-propiolactone, formalin, drying, heating at 60°C, or pH 2 or 9. Residual infectivity persists with exposure to low concentrations (1:4000) of formalin, but higher concentrations (1:200) at warm temperatures can completely inactivate the virus in 4 days. A contaminated facility can be disinfected by treatment with chlorine (200 mg/l for 1 h). Ozone and ultraviolet irradiation can be used to decontaminate large volumes of water.

Treatment No effective chemotherapeutic treatment is known for IPN. Virazole (1-n-ribofuranosyl-1,2,4-triazole-3-carboxsamide) inhibits IPNV replication in cell culture and may reduce mortality in infected fish. Interferon induction with tilorone is not protective. Polyvinylpyrrolidone-iodine, 8-aminocaproic acid, and tranexamic acid chemotherapy appears to reduce mortality but was not effective in experimental challenges.

Research Complications The obvious research problem of mortality in young fish is perhaps the most easily dealt with through careful screening of fish sources. The more subtle impacts of inapparent virus infection in carriers with the potential for recrudescence in stressful conditions can be devastating for a researcher.

References

Ashley, P.J., Sneddon, L.U., McCrohan, C.R., 2007. Nociception in fish: stimulus–response properties of receptors on the head of trout *Oncorhynchus mykiss*. Brain Res. 1166, 47–54.

Austin, B., Austin, D.A., 1999. Bacterial Fish Pathogens: Disease of Farmed and Wild Fish, third ed. Springer, London.

Brown, L.A., 1985. Pain in fish. In: Pain in Animals. British Veterinary Association, Animal Welfare Foundation Symposium. London.

Deardorff, T., Overstreet, R., Okihiro, M., Tam, R., 1986. Piscine adult nematode invading an open lesion in a human hand. Am. J. Trop. Med. Hyg. 35, 827–830.

Dunlop, R., Laming, P., 2005. Mechanoreceptive and nociceptive responses in the central nervous system of goldfish (*Carassius auratus*) and trout (*Oncorhynchus mykiss*). J. Pain 6, 561–568.

Ferguson, H.W., Bjerkas, E., Evensen, O., 2006. Systemic Pathology of Fish, A Text and Atlas of Normal Tissues in Teleosts and Their Response in Disease, second ed. Scottia Press, London.

Halstead, B., 1988. Poisonous and Venomous Marine Animals of the World. Darwin Press, Princeton, NJ.

Hawkins, A.D., 1981. Aquarium Systems. Academic Press, New York.

Inglis, V., Roberts, R.J., Bromage, N.R., 1993. Bacterial Diseases of Fish. Blackwell Science, Ames, IA.

Jones, S.G., Kamunde, C., Lemke, K., Stevens, E.D., 2012. The dose–response relation for the antinociceptive effect of morphine in a fish, rainbow trout. Vet. Pharmacol. Ther. 35, 563–570.

National Research Council, 2011. Guide for the Care and Use of Laboratory Animals, eighth ed. The National Academies Press, Washington, DC.

Neiffer, D.L., Stamper, M.A., 2009. Fish sedation, anesthesia, analgesia, and euthanasia: considerations, methods, and types of drugs. ILAR J. 50, 343–360.

Noga, E., 2010. Fish Disease; Diagnosis, and Treatment, second ed. Wiley, Blackwell and Sons, Ames, IA.

Page, L.M., Espinosa-Pérez, H., Findley, L.T., 2013. Common and Scientific Names of Fishes from the United States, Canada and Mexico, seventh ed. American Fisheries Society Special Publication 34, Bethesda, MD.

Pickering, A.D., 1981. Stress and Fish. Academic Press, New York.

Roberts, R.J., 2012. Fish Pathology, fourth ed. Wiley, Blackwell and Sons, Ames, IA.

Smith, S.A., 2013. Welfare of laboratory fishes. In: Bayne, K., Turner, P.T. (Eds.), Laboratory Animal Welfare. Academic Press, Waltham, MA, pp. 301–311.

Spotte, S., 1979. Seawater Aquariums: The Captive Environment. Wiley and Sons, New York.

Stoskopf, M.K. (Ed.), 1988. Tropical fish medicine Vet. Clin. North Am. Small Anim. Pract W.B Saunders, Philadelphia, PA.

Stoskopf, M.K., 2010. Fish Medicine, second ed. ART Sciences, printed by Lulu Press, Raleigh, NC.

Wheaton, F.W., 1993. Aquacultural Engineering. Krieger Publishing, Malabar, FL.

Wolf, K., 1988. Fish Viruses and Fish Viral Diseases. Cornell Univ. Press, Ithaca, NY.

Woo, P.T.K., Bruno, S.W., 2010. Fish Diseases and Disorders, Volume 3: Viral, Bacterial and Fungal Infections, second ed. CABI, Oxfordshire.

22

Japanese Quail as a Laboratory Animal Model

Janet Baer, DVM[a], Rusty Lansford, PhD[b] and
Kimberly Cheng, PhD[c]

[a]California Institute of Technology, Pasadena, CA, USA [b]Children's Hospital Los Angeles, Keck
School of Medicine at USC, Saban Research Institute, Department of Radiology, Los Angeles, CA,
USA [c]The University of British Columbia, Faculty of Land and Food Systems, Avian Research
Centre, Vancouver, BC, Canada

I. INTRODUCTION

Japanese quail (*Coturnix japonica*) are used as a laboratory animal model for multiple areas of scientific inquiry including, but not limited to developmental biology, endocrinology, aging, immunology, behavior studies, and a variety of human genetic disorders. The quail embryo is an amniote with early developmental patterns remarkably similar to those of humans; as such they present significant experimental advantages for the study of amniotes, e.g., rapid reproductive maturation, modest size of breeding adults, ease of breeding in laboratory animal facilities, resilience to research manipulations, availability of transgenic lines, a fully sequenced genome, and tools for molecular manipulations.

A. Ecology and Taxonomy

Japanese quail are terrestrial birds that generally live for 2–3 years in the wild (Ottinger, 2001). Their natural habitat consists of ever-dwindling grasslands, croplands, riversides, mountain slopes near water, and grass

Laboratory Animal Medicine, Third Edition
DOI: http://dx.doi.org/10.1016/B978-0-12-409527-4.00022-5

steppes in eastern Asia, including northern Mongolia, eastern Russia, northeastern China, Japan, South Korea, and North Korea (del Hoyo et al., 1994; Bump, 1971). They migrate seasonally; however, the migration pattern is complicated and not well understood. Some populations in Japan are year-round denizens, but most Japanese quail migrate south to winter in southern China, Vietnam, Laos, Myanmar, Cambodia, Bhutan, and northeastern India (del Hoyo et al., 1994; Pappas, 2002). Once thought to be common in China (del Hoyo et al., 1994), decreased quail populations seem to be occurring in Laos (Duckworth, 2009), Japan (Okuyama, 2004), and possibly throughout their habitat (del Hoyo et al., 1994; Duckworth, 2009). Endemic populations of Japanese quail are listed as 'Near Threatened' on the IUCN Red List (IUCN, 2013a) because they appear to have undergone an 80% population decline between 1973 and 2002, potentially owing to hunting (Okuyama, 2004), shifts in agriculture (Duckworth, 2009; IUCN, 2013b), contamination of the wild gene pool by escaped or released farm quail, and climate change. Research is urgently needed to establish population numbers and trends, as well as to determine the threats to naturally occurring wild populations of Japanese quail. Attempts to introduce them into the mainland of the United States as a gamebird, in a previous era when such transplants were considered a good idea, consistently failed due to a lack of understanding of their migratory tendencies (Standford, 1957). In contrast, introductions to the Hawaiian Islands were successful (Peterson, 1961).

Japanese quail belong to the order Galliformes, family Phasianidae, genus *Coturnix*, and species *japonica*. They are classified as Old World quail and are closely related to the European common quail, *Coturnix coturnix*. The two species are not thought to interbreed in native locations where they co-exist, so they are considered to be in an intermediate stage of speciation (Johnsgard, 1988; Pappas, 2002; Howard and Moore, 1984; Kano, 2006; Crawford, 1990; Union, 1983). However in captivity, *C. japonica* and *C. coturnix* will interbreed and produce fertile hybrids (Johnsgard, 1988).

B. Use in Research

1. Quail as a Model for Embryogenesis Studies

The understanding of myogenesis, vasculogenesis, angiogenesis, skeletogenesis, virology, immunology, endocrinology, and teratology has progressed significantly as a result of studies in avian embryos (Mizutani, 2002). In Japanese quail, embryogenesis progresses faster than in the chicken, yet closely mirrors that of the chicken. On average, incubation times for the quail and chicken are 16 days and 21 days, respectively. After Hamburger and Hamilton (Hamburger and Hamilton, 1951) established the prototype avian embryo staging system in the chicken, outlining the various developmental events that occur during each stage, Japanese quail embryos were similarly staged and registered (Padgett and Ivey, 1959, 1960; Zacchei, 1961; Ainsworth et al., 2010). More recently, developmental stages of the quail have been further delineated using modern imaging technologies (Ruffins et al., 2007). The accelerated ontogeny of quail embryos at mid- to late stages of gestation results in loss of precise registration with the chicken.

Developmental biologists have long used the differences between chicken and quail embryologic development to transplant tissue from one of these into the other (Le Douarin and Barq, 1969; Le Douarin and Kalcheim, 1999). Quail interphase nuclei have nucleoli with compact heterochromatin that stains intensely with Schiff's reagent, while chicken nucleoli are not stained (Le Douarin, 1973); thus permitting quail cells to be distinguished from chicken cells in chimeric embryos. The chick–quail chimera system has been effectively used for a myriad of cell lineage analyses (Le Douarin and Kalcheim, 1999). Similarly, quail cells and tissues have been reciprocally transplanted into other avian species, including ducks to generate quail–duck chimeras (i.e., qucks), and for heterochrony studies (Lwigale and Schneider, 2008).

The quail embryo can be imaged for minutes to days *in ovo* or *in vitro* using any number of imaging modalities, e.g., light microscopy, fluorescent microscopy, magnetic resonance imaging, and computer-assisted tomography. For light and fluorescent microscopy, the quail embryo is visible through a windowed egg for continuous imaging over several days (Kulesa et al., 2000; Bower et al., 2011). The quail embryo itself is also physically accessible, which permits cell and tissue transplantations and genetic manipulations. Differences between the preferred amniote model for molecular studies (mice), *versus* the best model for live imaging (avians), motivated the construction of transgenic, fluorescent protein-expressing Japanese quail as an experimental system using lentiviral vectors. Transgenic quail lines expressing fluorescently labeled cells in a ubiquitous or tissue-specific manner permit amniote embryogenesis to be dynamically recorded with subcellular resolution (Seidl et al., 2013; Sato et al., 2010; Sato and Lansford, 2013; Scott and Lois, 2005).

2. Quail as a Model for Health and Disease

Japanese quail are emerging as an animal model to study birth defects and diseases that affect human health (Cheng and Kimura, 1990; Mizutani, 2002; Tsudzuki, 2008), and a number of quail lines currently exist that recapitulate human hereditary diseases, malformations, and abnormalities. Quail have been used in studies addressing senescence in immunology, endocrinology, developmental (Dickman et al., 2004) and reproductive biology (Ottinger et al., 2004); hypercholesterolemia characterized by the development of vascular lesions and xanthomatosis (Hoekstra *et al.*, 1998; Murakami *et al.*, 2010; Yuan *et al.*, 1997); glycogen storage disease (Matsui *et al.*, 1983); and myotonic dystrophy and acid maltase deficiency, known as Pompe's disease (Kikuchi *et al.*, 1998; Mizutani, 2002). A neurofilament-deficient mutant of the Japanese quail, named 'Quiver,' exhibits widespread tremors (Hasegawa *et al.*, 1996); in this strain, neurofilament protein is lacking from neuronal axons and cell bodies. The noradrenaline and 5-hydroxytryptamine content in the neostriatum of the Quiver's brain differs from that in the normal quail, although disappearance of the three neurofilament proteins is observed in all areas of the Quiver's brain.

Japanese quail follow a predictable aging process with evidence of declining function in reproductive, metabolic, and sensory systems (Holmes and Ottinger, 2003), comparable to senescence in mammals. The use of Japanese quail to study aging provides two distinct advantages over mammalian models. First, hypothalamic systems in quail exhibit neuroplasticity; for example, aging males respond to testosterone replacement therapy with full recovery of sexual behavior (Ottinger *et al.*, 2004). Behavioral recovery is accompanied by the restoration of specific hypothalamic neuropeptide systems, which regulate both sexual behavior and gonadotropin-releasing hormone, thereby allowing identification of these neural systems. The male cloacal (proctodeal) gland, which is similar to the prostate gland in mammals, is androgen responsive. The second advantage to the quail model is that they exhibit a dynamic bone physiology. This is particularly true for females because their hollow bones serve as a reservoir for minerals used in egg production. Thus, aging female quail develop bone fragility and serve as a validated model for hormone effects on osteoporosis and the role of vitamin D (Takahashi *et al.*, 1983). Rescue of these systems via hormone replacement provides a tool for studying systems affected by aging and the restoration of their functions. Japanese quail have also been a model system for studying the genetics and neuroendocrine control of reproductive and social behavior (Ball and Balthazart, 2010; Nol *et al.*, 1996), including use as an animal model for testing the effects of endocrine-disrupting chemicals (Tattersfield *et al.*, 1997; Hutchinson *et al.*, 2000). Genetically unique strains of Japanese quail have been used to study the visual system; developmental pathology of the retina and optic nerve (Takatsuji *et al.*, 1984), spontaneous glaucoma (Takatsuji *et al.*, 1986, Weidner *et al.*, 1995), cataracts (Takatsuji *et al.*, 1985), and retinal degeneration (Zak *et al.*, 2010) are some of the topics that have been investigated.

Japanese quail are susceptible to pathogenic strains of bacteria such *Salmonella pullorum*, *Escherichia coli* (Woodard *et al.*, 1973), and *Mycobacterium avium* (Tell *et al.*, 2003), and have served as an animal model for understanding these pathogens in poultry. Recently Rundfeldt *et al.* (2013) employed quail to assess the efficacy of nanoparticulate itraconazole aerosolization against *Aspergillus fumigatus*.

II. BIOLOGY

A. Morphology and Physiology

Japanese quail measure ~17 cm in length, and males are slightly smaller than females. Whereas wild females weigh ~100 g and males weigh ~90 g, domesticated adult females weigh ~140 g and males weigh ~130 g. Some Japanese quail bred for meat production can weigh ~600 g. The birds have dark-brown feathers from the top of the head down to the nape of the neck with a tan streak over the eyes. Adults are sexually dimorphic, with females having light tan feathers and black speckling on their chest and throat and males characterized by a rusty brown throat and breast feathers (Fig. 22.1). Various plumage colors have been prized and selectively bred for over the past five centuries, e.g., rusty brown, Manchurian Gold, English Black, Barred, White, and A&M Giant White (Wetherbee, 1961; Roberts, 1999). Many plumage color mutants have also been developed and maintained for genetic studies (Cheng and Kimura, 1990) (Fig. 22.2).

The relatively small size and rapid growth rate of Japanese quail simplifies housing and production in laboratory animal facilities. Body weight at hatching ranges from 6 to 8 g with growth to 160–250 g by 5–6 weeks of age, depending on the sex and strain (Gerken and Mills, 1993) (Fig. 22.3). By 4–6 weeks post-hatch, males and females are sexually dimorphic and can be differentiated based on plumage coloration. Quail can be sexed within one day of hatching by cloacal examination; however, accuracy in performing this technique may take years to develop (Homma *et al.*, 1966). Life expectancy in commercial and laboratory settings ranges from 1.5 to 2.5 years, but individual birds have been reported to live up to 8 years (Cheng *et al.*, 2010).

The cloacal gland of adult male Japanese quail secretes a white foamy material (Adkins-Regan, 1999; Cheng *et al.*, 1989a,b); increased gland size correlates with an increased photoperiod (Sachs, 1969). Foam deposited during natural copulation can be retained by the female for more than 12 h and contributes to prolonged sperm motility (Biswas *et al.*, 2010). Cloacal gland size can be used as an external indicator of testicular function in male birds (Mohan *et al.*, 2002), while gland regression and decreased body weight has been associated with castration. Observation of foam following gentle manual pressure of the cloacal gland is also useful for differentiating males from females in strains that have a plumage color other than wildtype. In addition, foam production

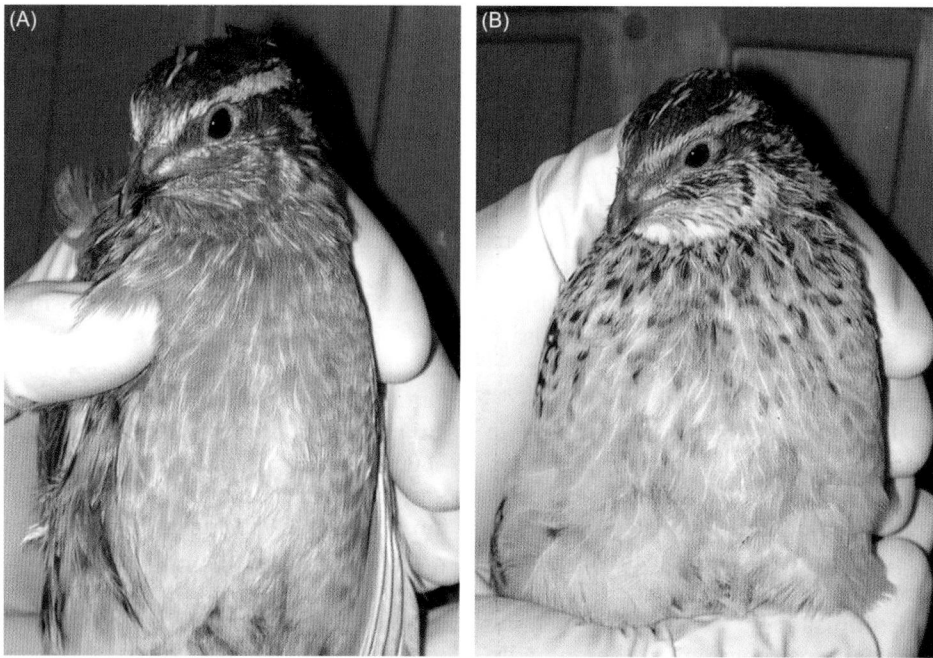

FIGURE 22.1   Wildtype plumage of a male (A) and female (B) adult Japanese quail (*Coturnix japonica*).

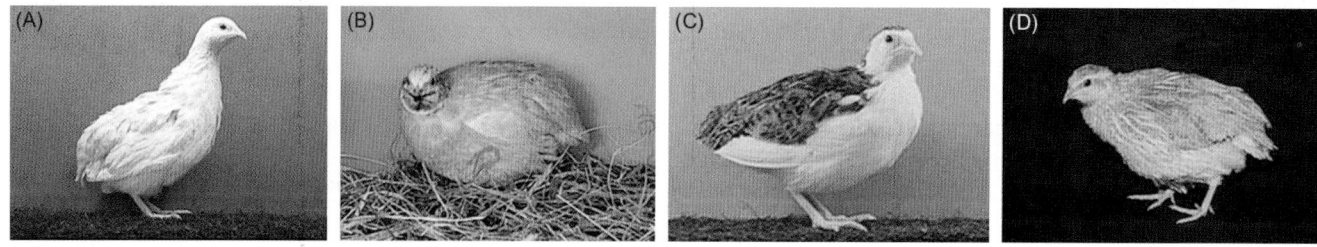

FIGURE 22.2   Japanese quail plumage color mutants developed for genetic studies: albino (A), yellow (B), white breasted (C), and silver (D).

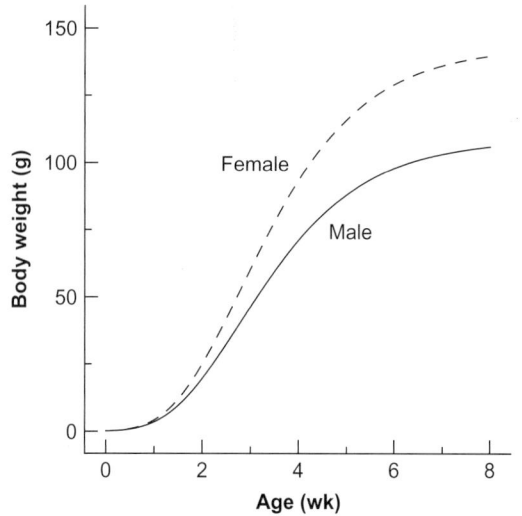

FIGURE 22.3   Growth curve for male and female domestic Japanese quail from hatching to 8 weeks of age. *Data from Aggrey (2003).*

has been related to the presence of bacteria in the cloacal gland. Treatment with fluoroquinolones has been demonstrated to result in decreased bacterial counts in the foam, decreased foam production, and decreased fertility (Mohan *et al.*, 2004).

Japanese quail have color vision, which appears to be more crucial than pattern or form for visual discrimination (Fidura, 1969). Similar to other ground-foraging birds, quail exhibit a lower field myopia that permits them to simultaneously focus on the ground while they forage and monitor the horizon and sky overhead for predators (Hodos and Erichsen, 1990). They exhibit greatest sensitivity in the auditory range between 1 and 4 kHz (Niemiec *et al.*, 1994). Young chicks (3–5 h post-hatch) show auditory discrimination learning, responding at greater frequency to a familiar sound than a novel sound (Evans and Cosens, 1977). Limited information is available regarding the senses of taste and smell in Japanese quail (Mills *et al.*, 1997).

TABLE 22.1 Standard Biological Data for Domestic Japanese Quail

BODY WEIGHT (G)

1 day	6–8
Adult male	100–130
Adult female	120–160

ORGAN WEIGHT (% BODY WEIGHT)

Liver	1.95
Heart	0.91
Kidney	0.73
Testes	2.88
Body temperature (°C)	40.7–43.2

PERFORMANCE AND LONGEVITY

Egg weight (g)	9–10
Egg number/100 bird days	80–90
Age at sexual maturity (d)	38–42
Life span (months)	24–26

BLOOD PRESSURE (MMHG)

Systolic

Adult male	151.8 ± 4.6[1]
Adult female	156.1 ± 4.7[1]

Diastolic

Adult male	158.1 ± 4.7[1]
Adult female	146.9 ± 4.2[1]

HEART RATE (BEATS/MIN)

Adult male	530.7 ± 17.7[1]
Adult female	489.5 ± 17.1[1]

ADULT FEED CONSUMPTION (G/DAY)   17.5–19.8

Modified from Cheng et al. (2010).
[1]Mean ± SE.

TABLE 22.2 Hematological[1] and Clinical Chemistry Values[2] for Adult Domestic Japanese Quail

	Adult male	Laying females
Erythrocytes (10^6/mm^3)	4.14 ± 0.07	3.81 ± 0.14
Packed cell volume (%)	53.1 ± 0.8	46.9 ± 1.3
Haemoglobin (g/100 ml)	15.8 ± 0.2	14.3 ± 0.5
Mean corpuscular volume (μm^3)	127.0 ± 2.0	124.0 ± 2.0
Mean corpuscular haemoglobin (ng)	38.5 ± 0.1	37.7 ± 0.7
Mean corpuscular haemoglobin concentration (%)	29.6 ± 0.3	30.4 ± 0.4
Reticulocytes (%)	7.0 ± 0.5	6.1 ± 0.4
Thrombocytes (10^3/mm^3)	117.0 ± 9.0	132.0 ± 17.0
Total leucocytes (10^3/mm^3)	19.7 ± 0.7	23.1 ± 1.0
Heterophils (%)	20.8 ± 1.9	21.8 ± 1.8
Eosinophils (%)	2.5 ± 0.04	4.3 ± 1.5
Basophils (%)	0.4 ± 0.1	0.2 ± 0.1
Lymphocytes (%)	73.6 ± 2.1	71.6 ± 1.
Monocytes (%)	2.7 ± 0.3	2.1 ± 0.3
Glucose (mmol/l)*	17.3 ± 0.6	14.4 ± 0.6
Uric acid (mmol/l)*	324 ± 21.5	320 ± 13.9
Total cholesterol (mmol/l)	6.7 ± 0.13	7.9 ± 0.26
Triglyceride (mmol/l)*	3.0 ± 0.2	23.5 ± 2.2
Bilirubin (μmol/l)	20.4 ± 1.00	8.9 ± 0.7
ASAT (U/l)	422 ± 9.5	402 ± 13
ALAT (U/l)	9.6 ± 0.6	6.5 ± 1.1
γ-GT (U/l)	1.7 ± 0.2	1.9 ± 0.1
Cholinesterase (kU/l)	4.8 ± 0.1	2.8 ± 0.1
Creatinine (μmol/l)*	4.0 ± 0.4	4.5 ± 0.3
Protein (g/l)	25.0 ± 1.0	33.6 ± 4.6
Albumin (g/l)	13.3 ± 0.2	15.3 ± 0.2
Phosphate (mmol/l)	1.2 ± 0.3	1.9 ± 0.4
Calcium (mmol/l)	2.3 ± 0.1	4.0 ± 1.3
Magnesium (mmol/l)	1.0 ± 0.04	1.2 ± 0.1
Iron (μmol/l)	12.5 ± 0.4	21.0 ± 2.8

Values given are mean ± SE.
*Significant daily patterns in concentration (Herichová et al., 2004).
[1]Data from Nirmalan and Robinson, 1971.
[2]Data from Faqi et al., 1997; Scholtz et al., 2009b.

Standard biological data for Japanese quail are presented in Table 22.1, while hematological and clinical chemistry values are given in Table 22.2. Sex related differences in serum chemistry reference values in adult Japanese quail have been reported (Scholtz et al., 2009a).

B. Behavior

Two studies (Nichols et al., 1991,1992) that compared the behavior of feral (considered wild because they were feral since the 1920s) and domesticated Japanese quail in a simulated natural environment found all but two of the courtship displays and behavioral components reported in the literature were exhibited by both groups. The differences in reproductive behavior between feral and domestic Japanese quail are shown in Table 22.3.

TABLE 22.3 Behavioral Differences between Feral and Domestic Japanese Quail in Outdoor Aviary with Simulated Natural Environment

Behavior	Feral[*]	Domestic
Male crowing	Less frequently; varied their crowing frequency during the female's laying cycle	More frequently with no temporal variation
Courtship displays	More	Less
Copulations	Less frequent	More frequent
Male aggression	More; toward both males and females	Less
Female aggression	Less	More; toward males
Pair bond duration	Paired for the whole breeding season	Shorter; frequently switched mates
Female laying	1 clutch of eggs for the season	Up to three clutches for the season

Data from Nichols (1991).
[*]Captured from the feral population on Hawaii. Japanese quail were released on Hawaii in the late 1920s.

The studies indicated that domestication was not 'degenerative,' but rather behavioral components are not expressed under conditions that lack the appropriate stimuli.

Because quail housed in a semi-natural environment spent approximately 8% of their activity budget on foraging behavior, including pecking and scratching, it is suggested that creating the opportunity for birds to perform this behavior will improve animal welfare (Schmid and Wechsler, 1997). A solid floor environment provided with a suitable substrate, e.g., wood chips, encourages foraging, and opportunities to forage can be created through scattering small seeds or grains in the bedding substrate or through providing other food items in the environment. In contrast, the same study found the birds spent little time on elevated structures; hence the provision of perches is likely of little value. Also of interest is that quail in semi-natural aviaries stayed under cover for a significant percentage of time (Schmid and Wechsler, 1997). Use of nest boxes with a small entrance but no other openings has been reported (Buchwalder and Wechsler, 1997). In outdoor aviaries, this type of nest box should be kept in the shade, especially in hot climates, as elevated nest box temperatures can be lethal to incubating females.

Captive Japanese quail engage in several dust bathing sessions daily when provided with a suitable material such as sand or cat litter (Schein and Statkiewicz, 1983). In the absence of such material, birds may exhibit 'vacuum dust bathing,' during which behavioral components of dust bathing are expressed, e.g., raking movements with the bill, scratching with the legs, tossing dust into the air with the wings while moving the body under the dust shower, accompanied by active feather ruffling and shaking (Mills et al., 1997). Dust bathing behavior occurs more frequently in the late afternoon compared to the early morning or early afternoon (Abdelfattah et al., 2012). In another report, the impact of four types of environmental enrichment (foraging opportunities, structural complexity, sensory stimulation/novelty, and social housing) were assessed (Miller and Mench, 2005). Use of foraging opportunities, structural complexity and dust bathing was observed in 29, 26, and 16% of activity budget scans, respectively, which supports a positive response to this type of enrichment. Social housing decreased the use of environmental enrichment and dust baths. Female Japanese quail co-housed with males in floor pens used environmental enrichment, foraged more, and were more active than the males.

Exposure to mild, unpredictable stressors during routine husbandry may impact the morphological and behavioral development of quail offspring. Chicks produced by laying hens exposed to mild daily stressors showed altered growth and behavioral responses. Potential stressors include sudden noise, sudden appearance of bright colored objects, or shaking the cages (Guibert et al., 2011).

The sexual behavior of captive Japanese quail ranges from polygamy to monogamy (Kovach, 1975; McKinney et al., 1983; Orcutt and Orcutt 1976). Females housed continuously with the same male had significantly higher egg hatching rates than females paired with a male every third day. When paired with a male every 3 days, females paired with the same male had fewer hatched eggs than females paired with a different male. Males were more receptive to females introduced into the male's cage than vice versa (Sullivan et al., 1992). A detailed review of social behavior, including courtship and vocalization types, rates, and patterns, has been published (Cheng et al., 2010).

Japanese quail show dominance through the development of a pecking order (Gerken and Mills, 1993); increased stocking density, and changes in group composition lead to more aggression and pecking-related injuries. In addition, adult females may outweigh males and will direct aggressive behavior toward smaller males. Maintenance of stable social groups over time improves animal welfare through reducing aggression associated with mixing social groups. Multi-male groups are associated with increased injuries due to aggressive pecking between males (Wechsler and Schmid, 1998). Provision of visual barriers, reducing the age at introduction, and changes in the male: female stocking density did not reduce male to male induced injuries. Importantly, reducing the light intensity decreased but did not eliminate pecking-related injuries.

C. Genetics

Both *C. japonica* and *Gallus domesticus*, the common chicken, have a diploid number of 78 chromosomes, most of which are orthological (Guttenbach *et al.*, 2003); numerous authors have concluded that quail and chicken lines diverged 35–46 million years ago (Jiang *et al.*, 2010; Kan *et al.*, 2010; Kayang *et al.*, 2006; Van Tuinen and Dyke, 2004; Van Tuinen and Hedges, 2001). The International Chicken Genome Sequencing Consortium has determined that chickens possess five pairs of macrochromosomes (>40 Mb), five pairs of intermediately sized chromosomes (20–40 Mb), and 28 pairs of microchromosomes (<20 Mb) (Hillier *et al.*, 2004; Wallis *et al.*, 2004); Japanese quail chromosomes are similar in this regard (Kawahara-Miki *et al.*, 2013). Chicken microchromosomes comprise about one-third of the total genome size (Wallis *et al.*, 2004), yet encode 50–75% of all genes (McQueen *et al.*, 1998; Burt, 2002), replicate earlier in the S phase than macrochromosomes (McQueen *et al.*, 1998), and have higher recombination rates than macrochromosomes (Wong *et al.*, 2004). It has been hypothesized that microchromosomes initiated as fragments of ancestral macrochromosomes, and conversely that macrochromosomes formed by aggregation of microchromosomes 100–250 million years ago (Fillon, 1998). In contrast to mammals, avian sex chromosomes are designated Z and W; males are ZZ and females are ZW and thus the ovum governs the sex of the offspring. There are no mutual genes between the avian ZW and mammal XY chromosomes, nor do the ZW and XY chromosomes seem to share a common origin (Stiglec *et al.*, 2007).

Recently, the female Japanese quail genome was sequenced using Illumina next-generation sequencing platforms and assembled against the chicken reference genome (Kawahara-Miki *et al.*, 2013). The Japanese quail genome is ~1.41 Gb in size (Kawahara-Miki *et al.*, 2013; Nakamura *et al.*, 2004; Tiersch and Wachtel, 1991). There are currently ~150 microsatellite markers identified for the Japanese quail based on the genome sequences (Kawahara-Miki *et al.*, 2013; Tadano *et al.*, 2014). The Japanese quail genome sequence and associated resources will offer essential genetic and genomic reference information, molecular tools for making improved primers and nucleic acid probes to use in polymerase chain reaction, multiplexed hybridization chain reaction-based RNA *in situ*, siRNA- and shRNA-based RNA inactivation, and CRIPR-Cas9 targeting approaches.

Considerable breeding in laboratory and commercial settings is carried out with quail lines that have been selected or screened for a particular phenotype or genotype, e.g., feather coloration, growth rate, mutant lines, transgenic lines. The most common method used to characterize the resulting phenotype is to observe the hatchlings for feather color, developmental abnormality, etc.

For genotypic analyses, the mesoderm-derived chorioallantoic membrane (CAM), a highly vascularized membrane in close contact with the pores of the eggshell to facilitate gas exchange, can be used to isolate and analyze the hatchling's genomic DNA. For example, transgenic founder lines that express markers such as fluorescent proteins or lacZ can be initially screened for transgene expression in the CAM cells or shell membrane cells of freshly hatched eggs, assuming the transgene is expressed by the cells being CAM cells. For instance, a ubiquitously expressed transgene or vascular-specific transgene (Sato *et al.*, 2010) is readily seen in the CAM cells when observed using a epifluorescence microscope; however, a transgene whose expression is restricted to the glial or adult kidney cells would not be expected to be visualized in CAM cells. Feather blood cells can also be visualized using a fluorescent microscope to assay transgene expression; in addition, genomic DNA can be analyzed by conventional recombinant DNA techniques to confirm a desired gene or transgene. Southern blot analysis will determine transgene copy number and genomic integration site (Sato *et al.*, 2010).

Japanese quail are very susceptible to inbreeding depression (Sittmann *et al.*, 1966), which reduces population fitness via decreased hatchability, viability, and fertility. Inbreeding increases genome homozygosity and preserves recessive mutations carried by a population (Frankham *et al.*, 2002; Keller and Waller, 2002). The inbred lines of quail that Sittmann *et al.* (Sittmann *et al.*, 1966) initiated by consecutive full-sibling matings only survived to the third generation. In another study, only five out of 17 full-sibling mating inbred lines survived to the fifth generation (Kulenkamp *et al.*, 1973). Using this standard approach, there is currently no record of any inbred Japanese quail line living past eight generations of consecutive full-sibling matings (Okimoto, R., University of Arkansas, personal communication to KC; Wada, M., Tokyo Medical and Dental University, personal communication to KC).

As in mice, the increase in genome homozygosity of inbred quail lines is useful for genome analysis and gene mapping (Hoti and Sillanpaa, 2006). At the Avian Research Centre at the University of British Columbia, a more relaxed inbreeding scheme was employed to generate an inbred Japanese quail line in order to estimate the inbreeding coefficient of a quail population and compare it to the inbreeding level that would be attained with full-sibling mating. The inbreeding scheme entailed mating full sibling sisters to full sibling brothers from a different (but related) family (Kim *et al.*, 2007). This quail line has now been inbred for 24 generations and still appears vigorous.

III. LABORATORY MANAGEMENT AND HUSBANDRY

A. Sources of Quail

Fertilized quail eggs can be ordered from a commercial supplier. However unlike for chickens, there is no vendor for particular quail strains with a known breeding history. Quail obtained from commercial farms may be heterogeneous genetically and may differ from batch to batch; this situation makes comparisons difficult between different experiments (Cheng and Nichols, 1992). Researchers desiring a specialized quail model usually obtain the birds from the laboratory that developed the model; however, two technical problems can be associated with such an acquisition. First of all, stringent and expensive quarantine procedures are required if the shipment has to cross national boundaries. Occasionally, there is also a tariff imposed. Importation regulations are country dependent and typically focus on avian-transmitted diseases such as avian influenza and salmonellosis, among others. It is hoped that adopting the practices used by commercial avian producers, such as the flock certification program provided by the US National Poultry Improvement Plan (NPIP), will facilitate the international transfer of eggs and birds.

Second, many specialized quail strains were not maintained beyond the researcher's tenure (Fulton and Delany, 2003), as maintaining bird colonies is expensive and budget allocation for conserving a population is not an administrative priority. Although until recently there was no practical procedure for the cryopreservation of avian germplasm, Liu and colleagues (Liu *et al.*, 2010, 2012a,b, 2013a–d) have pioneered such a procedure for Japanese quail gonadal tissue that shows great promise.

It is critical to use freshly laid eggs that come from a productive and healthy flock. Egg storage and shipping conditions can also contribute to egg fertility, e.g., low egg fertility levels may be observed if the eggs are exposed to high temperatures during transportation; transportation in cooled containers can mitigate this concern. Eggs should be stored immediately upon receipt in a refrigerator that is kept at ~13°C and humidified with an open tray of water; in contrast a 4°C refrigerator is too cold and will cause embryonic death.

B. Housing Systems

Housing systems for adult Japanese quail include commercially available poultry battery cages (Gerken and Mills, 1993) (Fig. 22.4), custom-built indoor floor pens (Gerken and Mills, 1993) (Fig. 22.5) and semi-natural outdoor aviaries (Schmid and Wechsler, 1997).

The type of housing system selected should take into consideration the anticipated use of the birds, as well as regulatory and animal welfare requirements. Housing design should accommodate ease of sanitation and maintenance.

Outdoor aviaries that provide a semi-natural environment encourage natural behaviors such as exercise, flight, social interaction, foraging and dust bathing (Schmid and Wechsler, 1997); access to ample vegetative

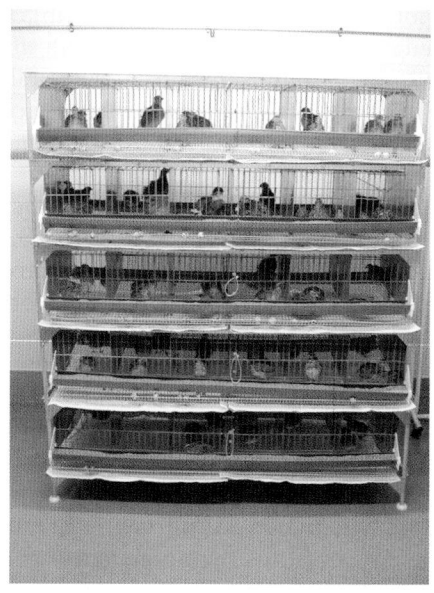

FIGURE 22.4   Commercial battery-cage housing Japanese quail.

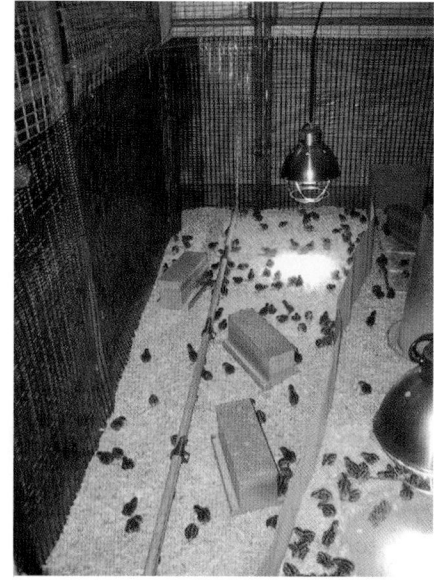

FIGURE 22.5   Custom-built indoor floor pen housing Japanese quail chicks.

cover is critical. In general, key features of a semi-natural environment are shelter from weather extremes, protection from predators, and ease of sanitation, egg collection, and capture. Similar to outdoor aviaries, indoor floor pens can promote the expression of natural behaviors and animal welfare through the provision of artificial cover and opportunities for exercise, foraging, dust bathing, and social behavior (RSPCA, 2001). Resource competition for food and water, as well as cover and dust baths, must be considered when housing quail in floor pens; provision of resources must be adjusted based on stocking density. Battery cages with sloped floors are widely used in commercial applications; these facilitate egg collection but result in an impoverished environment, i.e., decreased opportunities for exercise and other species-specific behaviors. The percentage of foot lesions, bone fractures, and beak deformities, as well as head and eye injuries resulting from aggressive pecking behavior, were increased in birds housed in battery cages compared to birds housed in deep litter floor pens (Abdelfattah et al., 2012). Because the same authors found that birds housed in deep litter floor pens demonstrated significantly increased cortisol levels and mortality attributed to increased disease, including parasitism, consideration should be given to increased health monitoring for infectious agents in quail housed in situations where routine sanitation may be difficult and substrates may remain damp for periods of time. The NRC Guide for the Care and Use of Laboratory Animals (2011) lists minimum space recommendations for quail as 0.25 feet^2 floor area/animal. Increased cage space resulted proportionally in significant improvement in body weight gain, age at 50% egg production, egg production, food conversion values, and decreased mortality (Nagarajan et al., 1991). Overall, aviary room temperatures of 22–25°C are considered ideal for quail.

It has been reported that the typical vertical escape response in quail may lead to serious head injuries if cage ceilings are too high; one study concluded that cage heights should be less than 25 cm to reduce head injuries associated with the escape response, but at least 20 cm to allow birds from heavy strains to stand up fully in a normal postural position (Gerken and Mills, 1993). In contrast, other experts (RSPCA, 2001) suggest that cages of 30 cm in height reduced or eliminated the problem of head injuries in quail; another proposed solution is cage roofs comprised of materials that do not cause head injuries, e.g., a flexible plastic grid. Because upward flight is part of the normal behavior repertoire for quail, further study into the topic of cage height would be useful. Environmental enrichment and habituation to human presence and environmental change can serve as amelioration strategies for panic reactions in quail (Mench and Blatchford, 2014).

Japanese quail may be housed on a number of different types of bedding substrates including wood shavings, chopped corn cobs, ground bark, and peanut hulls. Use of small, solid-bottom cages coupled with the type of food (i.e., wheat-based high gluten content) and bedding provided may result in accumulation of food on the digits (referred to as toe-balls) which may lead to trauma to the digits if left untreated. It should be appreciated that bedding substrates can be a source of contamination.

C. Food and Water

Food and water are typically provided *ad libitum* to quail; the delivery method for both is dependent on the type of housing and the age of the birds. Food receptacle design should encourage easy access while preventing the birds from soiling uneaten portions; for example, birds in cages with food dishes will often nest in the feeders, resulting in spillage and soiling. Placement of feed troughs outside of the cage reduces spillage, prevents soiling of the food, and facilitates ease of food provision. Trough feeders and waterers placed outside of the cage are commonly used in battery cages. Birds tend to actively investigate water sources, and cage floods can occur if the water source is placed inside a solid floor cage or pen. Quail readily adapt to use of an automatic drinking valve with an integral cup basin, whereas gravity-fed bell drinkers are commonly used for newly hatched chicks and juveniles. Grill screens, rubber rings, or pebbles should be used to reduce the available water drinking area for very young chicks, as otherwise they may drown (Randall and Bolla, 2008). Drinking devices should be inspected daily to ensure that they are working properly and not clogged with debris. Water consumption varies with age and strain, with 2-week-old chicks ingesting 23.3 ml daily, 4-week old birds drinking 30.0 ml per day (Farrell et al. 1982), and 7-week-old birds ingesting 40.9–62.1 ml/g per day (Visser et al., 2000; Cheng et al., 2010).

Wild quail are omnivorous, eating primarily seeds and plant matter but adding terrestrial invertebrates in the summer (del Hoyo et al., 1994). In captivity, the dietary requirements for Japanese quail vary depending on the age and genetic selection for meat or egg production (Table 22.4). In general, a commercial game bird or turkey starter diet with 24.0–26.0% crude protein should be provided for the first 6–8 weeks after hatching followed by a game bird or turkey finisher diet that contains less protein. The pelleted starter diet must be ground into a powder form for feeding chicks for the first two weeks post hatch. Facility staff should be aware that diets high in wheat content may mix with fecal material and stick to the digits of the birds. As expected, food consumption

TABLE 22.4   Diet Specifications for Japanese Quail (as Percentage or Unit per Pound of Diet)

Nutrient	Unit	Starter/grower 0–6 weeks	Finisher >6 weeks to market	Adult breeder
Crude protein	%	24.0–26.0	17.0–19.0	18.0–20.0
Metabolizable energy	kCal	1315	1315	1315
Calcium	%	1.80	0.70	2.50
Nonphytate phosphorus	%	0.30	0.25	0.35
Sodium	%	0.15	0.15	0.15
Methionine	%	0.50	0.42	0.45
Methionine + cystine	%	0.75	0.68	0.70
Lysine	%	1.30	0.90	1.00
Threonine	%	1.02	0.85	0.74
Tryptophan	%	0.22	0.20	0.19

Percentage amount per lb of diet				
Vitamins added per lb of diet		100%	80%	100%
Vitamin A	IU	3000		
Vitamin D	ICU[1]	1000		
Vitamin E	IU	18.0		
Vitamin K	mg	1.0		
Thiamin	mg	1.0		
Riboflavin	mg	2.8		
Niacin	mg	20.0		
Choline	mg	115		
Pyridoxine	mg	1.5		
Pantothenic acid	mg	7.0		
Folic acid	mg	1.0		
Vitamin B12	μg	5.0		
Biotin	μg	50.0		

Trace minerals added per lb of diet				
Manganese	mg	25.0		
Iron	mg	30.0		
Copper	mg	5.0		
Zinc	mg	30.0		
Iodine	mg	0.2		
Selenium	mg	0.136		

From http://www.aces.edu/pubs/docs/A/ANR-1343/index2.tmpl Alabama Cooperative Extension System ANR-1343.
[1]ICU = International Chick Unit.

and efficiency varies by age and gender (Table 22.5). Specially prepared diets may be purchased from feed companies, and a synthetic diet has been developed for Japanese quail used in research (Cheng et al., 2010). For experimental purposes, high-cholesterol diets have been used to induce atherosclerosis in Japanese quail (Cheng et al., 1997; Godin et al., 2001, 2003; Hoekstra et al., 2003, 2004). Game bird or turkey feeds incorporating coccidiostats (i.e., monensin sodium (Coban) and amprolium) and/or antibiotics are commercially available.

D. Common Procedures

Adults and chicks can be individually identified through the application of commercially available leg bands or wing tags. Plastic coil legs bands (Size 4) obtained in multiple colors (National Band and Tag Company, Newport, Kentucky, USA; www.national-band.com) can be used to identify chicks the day after hatching; however, the maximum diameter of these bands precludes their continued use once the birds reach 2–3 weeks of age. Colored aluminum leg bands in size 8 can be applied after the birds are 3 weeks of age. Wing tags are suitable for birds of all ages, but proper application in the propatagium of newly hatched chicks is difficult due to their small size. The wing tags must be positioned just behind the tendon along the leading edge of the wing, opposite the humeral–ulnar joint. Improper placement can result in traumatic damage to the musculature of the wing as the bird develops. Other recommendations are for the use of #5 fingerling tags (National Band and Tag Company) in hatchlings, and aluminum chick wing tags for adult birds. Rodent ear tags can also work as wing bands in chicks and adult birds.

Capture of caged Japanese quail can be achieved with relative ease; it should be performed calmly but quickly to avoid injuries during escape attempts. Chicks should be held carefully in the palm of the hand, using the thumb and forefinger for restraint. Adult birds should be restrained by pinning the wings against the body while allowing the legs to hang loose. Alternatively, the bird may be gently cupped around the wings using both hands. Attempts to restrain the bird by the legs can result in traumatic injury to the legs, and failure to restrain the wings may result in damage to the wings, including bone fractures. Capture of birds housed in large pens or aviaries usually requires netting of the birds.

When the suitability of five different sites (brachial, jugular, caudal tibial vein, external dorsal thoracic vein and the heart) was compared for blood sampling and intravenous injections in Japanese quail, the jugular vein was reported to be most successful (Arora, 1979). Small volumes of blood from the ulnar vein may be collected in microcapillary tubes.

TABLE 22.5 Body Weight, Cumulative Feed Consumption, and Feed Efficiency of Japanese Quail

Age (weeks)	Body weight (g)[1]		Feed consumption (g)		Feed efficiency (g:g)[2]	
	Male	Female	Male	Female	Male	Female
2	40	40	50	50	1.25	1.25
4	90	100	180	190	2.00	1.90
6	120	130	300	330	2.50	2.53
8	130	160	350	450	2.69	2.81
10	140	170	400	510	2.86	3.00

From http://www.aces.edu/pubs/docs/A/ANR-1343/index2.tmpl Alabama Cooperative Extension System ANR-1343.
[1]To convert gram values to pound units, divide by 454.
[2]Feed efficiency is the amount of feed required per unit of body weight.

Similar to other small avian species, Japanese quail can be anesthetized by exposure to an inhaled gas anesthetic (e.g., isoflurane) or through the administration of injectable anesthetics. Oral or intramuscular administration of ketoprofen at 2 mg/kg resulted in very low bioavailability and the drug exhibited a very short half-life in Japanese quail (Graham et al., 2005). Changes in complete blood count and serum chemistry were minimal but injection site muscle necrosis was observed in Japanese quail following intramuscular administration of 2 mg/kg meloxicam every 12 h for 14 days (Sinclair et al., 2010). Japanese quail can be euthanized by exposure to inhaled anesthetic gas (e.g., isoflurane) or CO_2; chicks and embryos that are beyond 50% incubation are acclimated to high CO_2 concentrations in the egg and thus require prolonged exposure to CO_2 for euthanasia. A high dose of an injectable anesthetic is also an effective method of euthanasia. Physical methods, including cervical dislocation (between the first and second vertebrae) or decapitation, are acceptable on the condition that personnel are properly trained and proficient in humane application of these techniques. Prolonged exposure to CO_2, cooling (<4°C for 4 h), or freezing is recommended for eggs at less than 50% incubation (AVMA, 2013).

IV. BREEDING AND REARING QUAIL

A. Reproduction

Reproduction in Japanese quail is strongly influenced by the photoperiod (Robinson and Follett, 1982; Yasuo et al., 2006), such that wild quail breed in spring and summer in response to increasing day length. When housed under artificial light with a day length of 12 h or more, Japanese quail will breed year round. Photoperiod influences sexual behavior, cloacal protrusion and cloacal foam production (Sachs, 1969). Changes

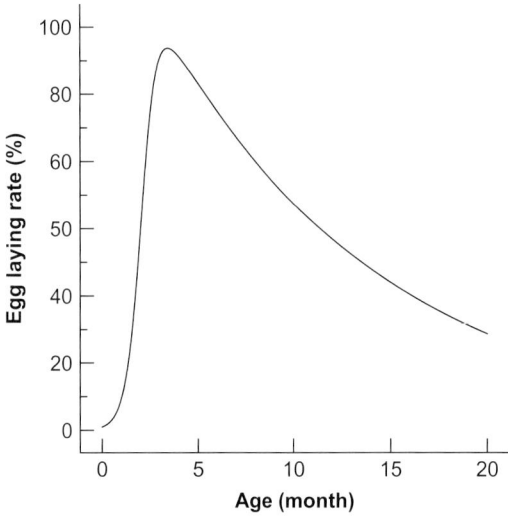

FIGURE 22.6 Egg production as a function of age in domestic Japanese quail. Data from Minvielle et al. (2000).

in photoperiod result in neuroendocrine changes in both male and female quail (Ball and Balthazart, 2010), and short day lengths result in gonadal regression and breeding cessation (Follet and Pearce-Kelly, 1990).

In general, Japanese quail reach sexual maturity at 6–8 weeks of age, but this is dependent on photoperiod and strain. Young quail raised under short-day lighting schemes, which mimic fall and winter days, either do not mature sexually or show delayed maturation (Delville et al., 1984). Lighting regimes for commercial producers vary but are typically designed with 16 h of light per day (Gerken and Mills, 1993). Hens typically begin to lay eggs consistently at ~8–10 weeks of age, with egg fertility rates quickly increasing over time; with time, egg production gradually declines (Fig. 22.6). Japanese quail exposed to continuous light gained weight faster and reached sexual maturity earlier than birds housed under 13h of daylight (De Jager, 2003). Female puberty, characterized by the average age of the first egg laid in a flock of Japanese quail maintained on a 16:8 day: night cycle, occurred at 48.8 days of age, while sexual maturity, characterized by the time at which egg production for the flock reached 50%, occurred at 54.2 days. Puberty in the male, defined by the first appearance of secondary sex characteristics like crowing and production of cloacal foam, occurred at 32.6 days of age; in contrast, sexual maturity in the cock, or the appearance of mating behavior and pronounced foam gland secretion, occurred by 42.4 days of age (Abdelfattah *et al.*, 2012). Maximum fertility in age-matched male and female group-housed birds maintained under a 16:8 day: night cycle was reached during the fourth month of age and then gradually declined (Abdelfattah *et al.*, 2012). Fertility in battery cage-housed Japanese quail is also influenced by the ratio of males to females. While a male: female ratio of 1:3 provided optimal fertility, a male: female ratio of 1:5 resulted in a significant decrease in fertility (Abdelfattah *et al.*, 2012). Fertility was also found to be significantly increased in birds housed in deep litter floor pens compared to birds in battery cages.

B. Egg Storage and Incubation

The average Japanese quail egg weighs 10–11 g, which corresponds to about 8% of the hen's body weight. Egg size, shape, and color patterns vary considerably based on the parent's strain; they are typically tan with brown speckles, but can also appear snowy white, mottled brown with a chalky blue covering, or other (Fig. 22.7). Each laying hen produces 10–12 eggs every 2 weeks year round in captivity under controlled light cycles. Wild populations typically lay eggs from late April to

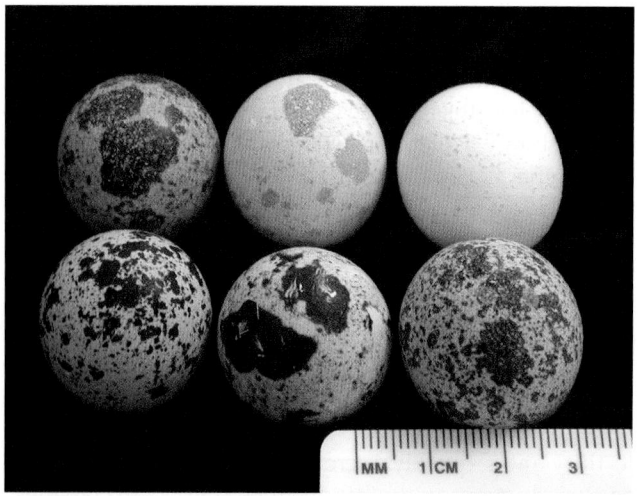

FIGURE 22.7 Japanese quail eggs exhibiting variation in size, shape, and color patterns.

early August in Russia, and from late May to August in Japan. Clutch sizes also vary, with 9–10 eggs per clutch in Russia and 5–8 in Japan. The female incubates the eggs in the wild (del Hoyo *et al.*, 1994); however, in captivity when males are co-housed with females, persistent male copulatory behavior prevents the hens from brooding (Cain and Cawley, 1972).

In the laboratory setting, quail eggs should be collected and stored daily. Egg collection is best performed early as most eggs are laid in the late afternoon or evening. Identification numbers can be recorded on the eggshell in permanent ink to facilitate tracking of egg numbers and fertility rates for different transgenic lines. As eggs are often soiled during egression, they should be washed with lukewarm water to remove debris and then air dried. Bacterial penetration across the eggshell is dependent on bacterial survival on the eggshell surface and egg storage conditions (Gole *et al.*, 2014). Once dry, eggs should be transferred to commercially available egg cartons designed to accommodate quail eggs. Fertilized quail eggs are best stored with their large end up or on their sides; these recommendations improve embryo development and orient the embryo in an experimentally desired position. Ideally, eggs should be stored in a refrigerator set to 13°C and equipped to provide 65% relative humidity. Turning eggs in their egg flats once daily improves hatchability. Eggs may be stored at ~11°C for up to 15 days, 21°C for up to 10 days, and 27°C for up to 5 days without a significant decrease in hatchability (Garip and Dere, 2011). Prior to incubation, refrigerated eggs should be maintained at room temperature until condensation on the shell has dried.

To optimize egg development, a quality egg incubator is essential. Many types and sizes of incubators can be purchased, and the best choice for a given situation will depend on the extent of planned experiments along with cost considerations. A forced-air incubator that utilizes an internal fan to circulate air inside the chamber is ideal. The egg incubator should include an automatic egg-turning option that is capable of tilting the egg trays through a 90° angle once an hour (Fig. 22.8). A separate hatching incubator equipped with hatching trays and matching wire mesh lids will be needed to hatch the eggs. Digital thermostats allow steady, consistent temperatures and humidity levels to be maintained in modern incubators. The incubator's internal temperature and relative humidity should be monitored at initial setup and daily during incubation with a high-quality, calibrated thermometer. Keeping a stock of numerous replacement parts is recommended to facilitate timely, in-house repairs. Incubators should be connected to electrical circuits with generator backup to ensure that power spikes or outages do not damage the eggs.

An incubation temperature of 38°C and 50–65% relative humidity results in optimal embryonic development.

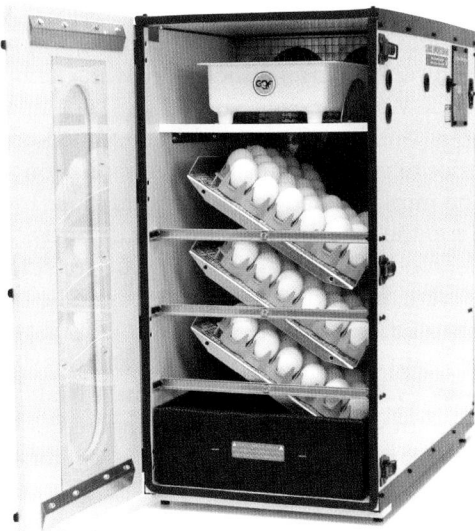

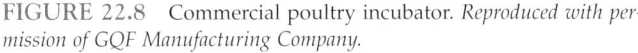

FIGURE 22.8   Commercial poultry incubator. *Reproduced with permission of GQF Manufacturing Company.*

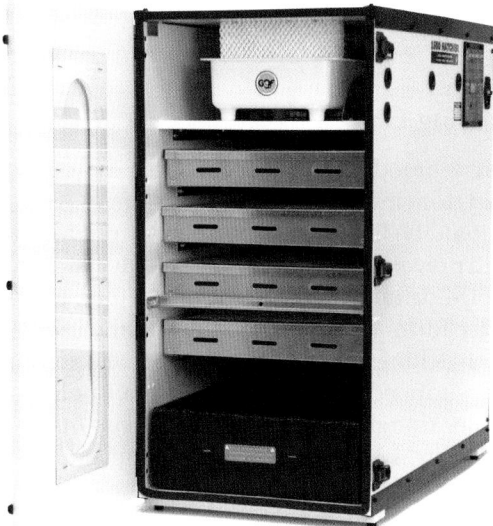

FIGURE 22.9   Commercial poultry hatching unit. *Reproduced with permission of GQF Manufacturing Company.*

The egg trays should be slowly rotated up to a total of 90° every hour until ~E13 to facilitate normal development. Eggs may be candled to inspect embryo viability using a standard commercial egg candler; however, caution is required to avoid overheating. Although staging early quail development by candling is difficult due to the blotchy colored eggshells (Fig. 22.6), viability can be reliably determined after about 7 days of incubation. Typical fertility ranges are from 90 to 95%, and peaks in embryonic mortality may occur during the first 3 and last 2 days of the 16–18 days of incubation.

Of interest is that quail embryos and chicks communicate with one another prior to hatching. This behavior is coincident with the onset of breathing, when quail embryos begin to acoustically communicate using clicking sounds which helps them synchronize their hatching times (Vince and Salter, 1967; Vince, 1964a,b). The same authors also reported that clicking sounds can accelerate or decelerate embryonic development and hatching times (Vince, 1966, 1968a,b, 1973; Vince *et al.*, 1984).

C. Hatching

On the 16th day of incubation, quail eggs should be transferred to an egg hatching incubator (Fig. 22.9), or hatchers, and placed on their sides in trays or compartments; the hatchers must be maintained at ~38°C and ~70% relative humidity. Trays of water should be placed in the incubator to maintain a high humidity, which will keep the chicks from adhering to their shell membranes during the hatching process. Relative humidity, the ratio of the current absolute humidity to the

highest possible absolute humidity (which depends on the current air temperature), can be measured using a wet bulb hygrometer. The trays should be covered with soft, absorbent paper to provide good traction for the hatchlings; if the lining material is too smooth or slick, hatchlings often develop splay leg. If the wire mesh is too large, the hatchlings can fall through or get their heads, wings, or legs stuck in the wire mesh. Once the hatchlings start to pip out the shell, the hatcher should be kept closed so the humidity levels remain high (~60–70%). Hatchling quail will typically emerge from their shells over the course of several hours.

In some cases, it may be important to keep hatchlings separated from one another if they are derived from distinct genetic or transgenic lines. If so, inexpensive separators can be made of plastic, cardboard, or other disposable material, and placed in the hatching trays to create separate cubicles. The design of hatching cubicles (each ~10 × 10 cm) can be such that each compartment has space for a single egg and its chick. This keeps the hatchling in the same container as its egg to ease phenotypic and genotypic analysis of both. Quail eggs lose approximately 13% of their 10- to 11-g starting weight via evaporation prior to hatching. The hatchlings typically weigh about 6–8 g and are brownish with yellow stripes. During the first 24 h in the hatcher, no food or water is necessary because the hatchlings obtain nutrition from their yolk sac that retracted into their coelom in the days prior to hatching. Understandably, hatched chicks are exhausted, but they typically gain strength and increase activity over 24 h. Within 24 h of hatching, the chicks should be transferred to a separate brooder that provides an auxiliary heat source during the first 4 weeks of life.

D. Rearing Chicks

Poultry brooders suitable for Japanese quail can be obtained from multiple commercial sources. The brooder floor should be lined with absorbent paper for the first 2 weeks to prevent leg injuries to the newly hatched chicks. Game bird or turkey starter diet should be ground into a powder form and sprinkled around the brooder floor for the hatchings to eat. Unrestricted access to water may be supplied through use of small bell jars fitted with water troughs; size appropriate glass marbles must be placed in the water troughs to prevent the hatchlings from falling into the water well and drowning. The temperature inside the brooder should be maintained at 37°C for the first week post-hatch. The heat source should be placed such that temperature gradients are established and chicks can select their desired temperature zone. Chick behavior should be observed daily or more frequently, and the temperature adjusted if they are huddled under the heat source (suggesting the heat source may be inadequate) or along the outer perimeter of the brooder (suggesting the heat source is providing too much warmth). The brooder temperature should be decreased 2–3°C every week for three weeks (Hodgetts, 1999). At 2 weeks post-hatch, the paper liner should be changed to a bedding substrate (paper chip, wood chip, or other suitable material). At 4 weeks post-hatch, the birds no longer need an external heat source. The diet should be changed to a game bird or poultry finisher/breeder diet when the birds are 5 weeks post-hatch.

V. DISEASES/WELFARE CONCERNS

A. Noninfectious

Japanese quail are susceptible to many common poultry diseases. Detailed reviews of diseases affecting quail, along with information on control, prevention, and treatment have been published (Barnes, 1987; Reed and Jack, 2013). As for other species, the implementation of biosecurity measures is critical to prevent introduction of infectious agents into a quail colony. Such measures include sanitation and quarantine practices; effective insect and rodent control programs; and the inspection of food, water, and bedding materials for potential contamination. A risk of disease transmission is reduced by the use of fumigated eggs rather than adult birds. The health status of the source flock should be carefully evaluated prior to transfer of eggs or birds. Ideally, egg incubation and hatching areas are physically separated from other areas, and human traffic always

flows from clean to dirty areas. Eggs from an external source should be carefully washed using a quaternary ammonium (250 ppm) solution and water temperature of 43–49°C. Washed eggs should be kept apart from soiled eggs, and egg flats should be cleaned and disinfected prior to use. A comprehensive sanitation program should be implemented for incubators and brooders as well as for the housing area for adult birds. Bedding substrate, food, and water must also be considered as a possible contamination source and should be evaluated and/or treated to reduce risk of pathogen transmission. Personnel with access to the housing facilities should not have contact with other birds for 72 h. A health surveillance program should also be implemented.

Trauma from conspecific pecking is one of the most frequently observed health concerns in laboratory colonies of Japanese quail. Head injuries from pecking are typically located toward the back of the head and neck areas (Fig. 22.10), while head injuries from bumping the cage ceiling are located more toward the top of the head. As these injuries commonly result from aggressive pecking in adult male quail, multi-male breeding groups are not generally recommended (Wechsler and Schmid, 1998). However multi-male breeding groups may be effective if (1) the male: female sex ratio is not too low (e.g., not less than 1 male:3 females), (2) the enclosure is adequately sized, (i.e., no high-density rearing), and (3) there are structures in the enclosure where birds can hide. A ratio of 1 male to 3 females is considered optimal in small, confined spaces. Even so, breeding groups with more space should be limited to a single male plus two to five females, as fertility will decrease if the sex ratio is higher than 1:5. Regardless, pecking injuries may still occur in single male breeding groups when females and males peck one another. In intensive breeding situations

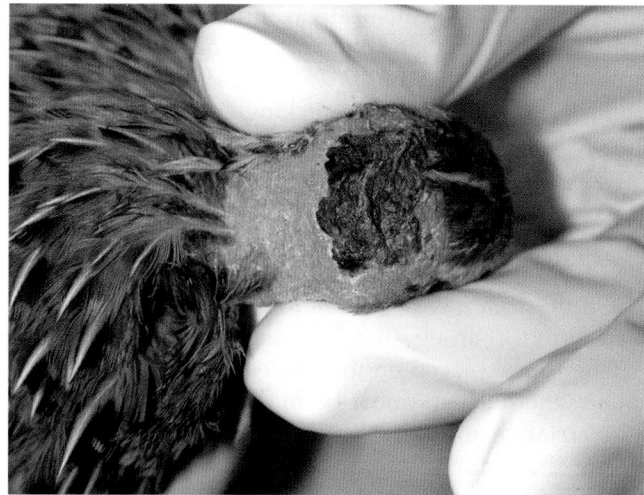

FIGURE 22.10 Head injury caused by aggressive pecking by cage mates.

with limited space and hiding areas, females may exhibit feather loss and occasional wounds to the back and head related to male mounting behavior. Misdirected copulation attempts by the male may result in head wounds and eye trauma of the female.

Depending on the anatomical location and severity of the trauma, the injured bird should be transferred to a separate enclosure and administered an anti-inflammatory drug such as ketoprofen (2–5 mg/kg IM). Birds with mild injuries can often be returned to the mating group once the injuries have healed. For birds raised in a laboratory setting, trimming the beak and nails with a conventional nail clipper every 4 weeks can reduce the number of pecking related-injuries. Kwik-Stop styptic powder (ARC Laboratories, Atlanta, GA) is effective in stopping bleeding that occurs coincident with beak and nail trimming. Alternatively, beak trimming can be performed through the use of a poultry hot-blade beak trimmer, which has an adjustable guard to keep from cutting too deep and also seals off blood vessels. However, hot-blade beak trimming is controversial due to the possibility for acute and chronic pain, as well as possible beak re-growth (Cheng, 2011). Infrared beak trimming performed on 1-day-old domestic chickens has been shown to be more effective at reducing beak re-growth and is associated with fewer side effects compared to hot-blade beak trimming (Dennis and Cheng, 2010). Animal welfare is enhanced when birds are housed in floor pens on natural substrate, as normal behaviors can negate the need for beak and nail trimming.

Foot injuries can be observed in battery-housed or deep-litter-housed quail. When housed in solid bottom cages or pens and fed a wheat-based (high gluten) diet, secretion from the male foam gland mixes with fecal matter and food and may adhere to the toes of birds

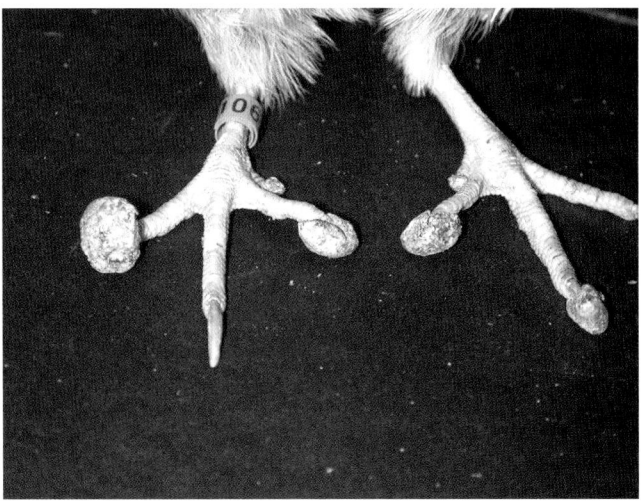

FIGURE 22.11 Accumulation of fecal material, food, and male cloacal gland foam on digits.

(Fig. 22.11). Once dried, the adhered material is often difficult to remove without injuring the bird's toes and nails. Pododermatitis in battery-caged quail (Abdelfattah *et al.* 2012) may also be associated with trauma due to abrasions caused by the wire bar floor. Provision of a solid resting surface can reduce foot lesions in battery-housed quail; nevertheless, scheduled monitoring of quail feet should be part of a routine health monitoring program established for Japanese quail.

Few neoplasms have been reported in Japanese quail. Sertoli cell tumors were reported in 9% of 3- to 5-year-old males kept in a laboratory colony for aging studies (Gorham and Ottinger, 1986). Leiomyomas were reported in the oviduct ligaments of rapidly growing Japanese quail (Foster *et al.*, 1989; Tuzcu *et al.*, 2010).

B. Infections

1. Viruses

Similar to other gallinaceous birds, Japanese quail are susceptible to a number of avian viral pathogens, most commonly quail bronchitis virus (QBV), Newcastle virus, and Eastern Equine Encephalomyelitis (Shivaprasad, 2002). Although a brief description of viral pathogens in Japanese quail is provided below, the reader can refer to more comprehensive information elsewhere, e.g., Swayne *et al.* (2013).

QBV, a type I avian adenovirus, has been documented to cause clinical disease in Japanese quail (Reed and Jack, 2013). The route of transmission is uncertain but likely via aerosolization. QBV is highly contagious in susceptible flocks, resulting in rapid morbidity and mortality; severe illness is most often observed in chicks of less than 6 weeks of age. Clinical signs include decreased appetite, ruffled feathers, open-mouth breathing, rales, sneezing, nasal and ocular discharge, and death. Older birds may remain asymptomatic. Gross necropsy findings include tracheal opacity, thickening of the trachea causing partial obstruction, and the presence of mucosal exudate. Histopathologic lesions are characterized by large basophilic intranuclear inclusions; necrotizing proliferative bronchitis; and hepatic, splenic, and cloacal bursa necrosis.

Newcastle disease, caused by avian paramyxovirus I, can infect Japanese quail (Usman *et al.*, 2008). Clinical signs range from subclinical infection to lethargy, ruffled feathers, dyspnea, torticollis, paralysis, and hemorrhagic diarrhea. Gross lesions include tracheal hemorrhage, inflamed and hemorrhagic Peyer's patches, pulmonary edema, hemorrhage of the proventriculus, and intestinal congestion. Transmission is horizontal via the fecal–oral route or by inhalation of contaminated dust.

Japanese quail are susceptible to Eastern Equine Encephalomyelitis, which is caused by an arbovirus

(Alphavirus, family Togaviridae); the virus may be transmitted by arthropod vectors, primarily the mosquito, *Culisetta melanura*, or through feather picking and cannibalism. Infected birds exhibit depression, tremor, paralysis, torticollis and death. A primary gross finding in a commercial quail flock was duodenal catarrhal enteritis (Eleazer *et al.*, 1978).

Duck Adenovirus A, also known as egg drop syndrome, has been reported in Japanese quail; it can be intermittently shed in feces as well as vertically transmitted, with viral particles on the external surface of the egg and internally. Clinical signs of decreased egg production, decreased eggshell pigment, and the production of thin or soft-shelled eggs have been described. To date, this virus has not been reported in the United States.

Hydropericardium syndrome in a commercial flock of Japanese quail has been attributed to infection with fowl adenovirus serotype 4 (FAV-4). Infection resulted in 4% mortality and was characterized by hydropericardium and mild-to-moderate hepatomegaly accompanied by splenic and kidney congestion (Roy *et al.*, 2004).

Natural outbreaks of Marek's disease, a lymphoproliferative disease caused by a cell-associated herpes virus, are relatively common in commercial flocks of Japanese quail (Nagarajan *et al.*, 2013). Transmission occurs through direct contact, and mortality in unvaccinated flocks may range from 10–20%. Gross lesions are observed in the proventriculus, spleen, and liver. Cooper *et al.* (2007) have presented a case report of Marek's disease in laboratory-housed Japanese quail. Clinical signs of disease included lethargy, anorexia, weight loss, soft feces, and lime-green urates.

Japanese quail have been shown to be more susceptible to infection with avian influenza virus than turkeys (Bonfante *et al.*, 2013); quail were readily infected with lower challenge doses and transmitted the virus to other birds without showing signs of clinical disease. Major influenza outbreaks in quail are uncommon (Perez *et al.*, 2003).

Natural infection with quail poxvirus has been reported in a commercial egg-laying flock of Japanese quail (Gulbahar *et al.*, 2005). Clinical signs of disease included weight loss, blepharitis, conjunctivitis, blindness, crusty papules at the commissures of the beak and around the external nares, decreased egg production, and impaired fertility. Infection was associated with 60% morbidity and 20% mortality. Quail pox is a distinct species of the genus Avipoxviridae, and vaccination with pigeon or fowl poxviruses does not provide protective immunity to quail.

Japanese quail are susceptible to avian encephalomyelitis virus, a member of the Picornaviridae family. Naturally occurring infection results from fecal–oral and vertical transmission. Clinical signs present in young birds, typically 1–2 weeks of age, include ataxia and tremors, especially of the head and neck. Morbidity among chicks is typically 40–60%. Depressed egg production, decreased hatchability and increased embryo mortality can be present in hens exposed as adults. Virus may be shed from 5 days in adult birds and up to 2 weeks in young birds. Gross necropsy lesions are often limited to whitish areas in the muscularis layer of the ventriculus, as a result of infiltrating lymphocytes. Histologic lesions include a disseminated, nonpurulent encephalomyelitis, ganglionitis of the dorsal root ganglia, and hyperplasia of lymphoid follicles in the proventriculus, ventriculus, and myocardium.

Reticulendotheliosis virus (REV) is a retrovirus found in a variety of domestic and wild birds; Japanese quail comprise a natural host for REV. Viral transmission occurs through direct contact. REV infection can result in immunosuppression, runting syndrome, high mortality, acute reticulum cell neoplasia, or T-cell and/or B-cell lymphomas. Histopathological lesions in REV infection are similar to those found in avian lymphoid leukosis and Marek's disease. Incidence of disease in commercial poultry flocks is sporadic.

2. Bacteria

Ulcerative enteritis or 'quail disease' is a fatal enteric disease caused by *Clostridium colinum*, primarily in captive quail but also in several other avian species; genetic susceptibility in Japanese quail may vary (Collins *et al.*, 1975). Young quail are most susceptible at 4–12 weeks of age, but disease may also occur in older birds. Transmission is via the fecal–oral route with contaminated food, water or litter being the most common source. Morbidity and mortality often depend on factors such as concurrent coccidiosis, overcrowding, food and water withdrawal, medication, and management. Clinical signs can be acute death with no premonitory signs, diarrhea, and emaciation. In young quail, 100% mortality can be seen. Gross necropsy findings include duodenal hemorrhagic enteritis with mucosal ulceration; the liver and the spleen may also exhibit pathological changes. Survivors may be carriers.

Japanese quail can be infected by two serovars of *Salmonella enterica*; these are often referred to as pullorum disease (*Salmonella pullorum*) and fowl typhoid (*Salmonella gallinarum*). Distribution is worldwide and, importantly, there is a potential for zoonotic transmission. Transmission is both horizontal via the fecal–oral route and vertical via transovarian infection. Chicks can present with weakness, decreased appetite, white chalky material on the vent, respiratory signs, joint swelling, anemia, and death. Adult birds may be subclinical or can exhibit generalized signs of disease, e.g., decreased appetite, diarrhea, depression, ruffled feathers, and decreased egg production. Gross lesions in quail include splenomegaly and hepatic lesions. Recovered birds are resistant to re-infection but may remain carriers. The bacterium is susceptible to common disinfectants.

Campylobacteriosis leads to acute gastroenteritis in birds, including Japanese quail, and humans (Maruyama and Katsube, 1988, 1990). It is caused by the gram-negative, microaerophilic bacteria *Campylobacter jejuni* and *C. coli*. Horizontal and vertical transmission are possible. Clinical signs may not be apparent or diarrhea can be present. Gross lesions are typically minimal, and confined to the gastrointestinal system. In one study, *C. jejuni* was reported to propagate in the spleen, liver, and lungs and to persist up to 17 days in orally inoculated Japanese quail (Maruyama and Katsube, 1988).

Worldwide, colibacillosis associated with avian pathogenic *Escherichia coli* infection is the most common infectious bacterial disease in poultry; the bacteria is responsible for significant economic losses in the poultry industry (Nolan *et al.*, 2013). Clinical signs include lameness, anorexia, dehydration, omphalitis, lethargy and mortality; histopathologic lesions can be localized, e.g., osteomyelitis, cellulitis, or systemic.

Pasteurella multocida, the causative agent of fowl cholera, is a contagious disease affecting a number of avian species, including quail. Clinical signs of acute disease may include fever, anorexia, oral discharge, diarrhea, dyspnea, and cyanosis. Birds with chronic disease may exhibit swollen joints including footpads, sternal bursae, wattles or sinuses, torticollis, and signs of respiratory impairment. Mortality due to acute septicemia has been reported in a quail colony bred for experimental use (Goto *et al.*, 2001).

Infection with *Bordetella avium* infection has been associated with a highly contagious upper respiratory tract disease in Japanese quail; the natural host for *B. avium* is the turkey. Clinical signs include sneezing, cough, nasal exudate, and dyspnea, and gross lesions are typically confined to the upper respiratory tract.

Naturally occurring infection with *Mycoplasma gallisepticum* and *M. synoviae* has been reported in Japanese quail. Transmission may be horizontal or vertical. Clinical signs of *M. gallisepticum* infection include nasal discharge, increased lacrimation and sinusitis. Sinusitis and arthritis has been attributed to *M. synoviae* infection in quail.

Chlamydiosis is caused by the bacterium *Chlamydia psittaci*; clinical signs and lesions in Japanese quail are similar to other avian species. Transmission results from inhalation or ingestion of contaminated material. Infected birds excrete the agent in feces and nasal discharge. *Chlamydia psittaci* is a zoonotic agent and is transmitted via infectious aerosols.

Japanese quail are likely susceptible to a number of other bacterial pathogens, such as *Mycobacterium avium*, *Staphylococcus* spp., *Streptococcus*, and *Listeria*. Reports of naturally occurring disease due to these organisms in quail are rare.

3. *Protozoa Agents*

Coccidiosis, caused by coccidian protozoa, *Eimeria* spp., has been diagnosed in Japanese quail (Teixeira *et al.*, 2004). In young quail chicks, infection is characterized by weight loss and diarrhea; it can be fatal or leave the bird with compromised digestion leading to malnutrition. Sulfonamides are an effective treatment.

Cryptosporidiosis, a diarrheal disease caused by infection with *Cryptosporidium* sp. has been reported in commercial quail colonies. Infected quail may have respiratory and intestinal involvement similar to chickens. The parasite is protected by an outer shell that allows survival outside the body for long periods and resistance to chlorine and many other disinfectants; however, it is killed by exposure to temperatures greater than 65°C.

4. *Fungi*

Infection with fungal agents is rare in quail. In some cases, transmission has been associated with contaminated litter and incubators. Aspergillosis caused by infection with *Aspergillis fumigatus* results predominantly in pulmonary disease, and may cause significant morbidity and mortality in young birds. Crop mycosis from *Candida albicans* is the most common fungal infection of the digestive tract. Zygomycosis and ochroconis are uncommon fungal infections in poultry. *Ochroconis gallopava* was reported as the causative agent in an outbreak of fungal encephalitis in Japanese quail chicks. Clinical signs were incoordination, loss of equilibrium, tremors, torticollis, paralysis, and death; histologically, fungal hyphae were apparent (Dykstra *et al.*, 2013). Histoplasmosis and cryptoccocosis result in rare infections in poultry species but are notable due to their zoonotic potential. Macrorhabdosis in quail and other avian species is caused by infection of the proventriculus and ventriculus with the yeast, *Macrorhabdus ornithogaster*. Clinical signs include emaciation, prostration, anorexia, cachexia, and death; whereas histopathologic lesions are marked lymphoplastic and heterophilic inflammation of the proventriculus and ventriculus.

5. *Parasites*

Like other gallinaceous birds, Japanese quail can host a number of internal and external parasites. Due to the limited scope of this chapter, readers are referred to a more complete review of these topics (Reed and Jack, 2013).

References

Abdelfattah, E., Karousa, M., El-Gendi, G., 2012. Effect of Some Managerial Factors on Behavior and Performance of Quail: Behavior, Management and Production of Japanese Quail (Coturnix Japonica). LAP LAMBERT Academic Publishing.

Adkins-Regan, E., 1999. Foam produced by male coturnix quail: what is its function? Auk 116, 184–193.

Aggrey, S.E., 2003. Dynamics of relative growth rate in Japanese quail lines divergently selected for growth and their control. Growth Dev. Aging 67, 47–54.

Ainsworth, S.J., Stanley, R.L., Evans, D.J.R., 2010. Developmental stages of the Japanese quail. J. Anat. 216, 3–15.

Arora, K.L., 1979. Blood sampling and intravenous injections in Japanese quail (Coturnix coturnix japonica). Lab. Anim. Sci. 29, 114–118.

AVMA, 2013. The AVMA Guidelines for the Euthanasia of Animals: 2013 Edition. American Veterinary Medical Association, Schaumburg, IL.

Ball, G.F., Balthazart, J., 2010. Japanese quail as a model system for studying the neuroendocrine control of reproductive and social behaviors. ILAR J. 51, 310–325.

Barnes, H.J., 1987. Diseases of quail. Vet. Clin. North. Am. Small. Anim. Pract. 17, 1109–1144.

Biswas, A., Ranganatha, O.S., Mohan, J., 2010. The effect of different foam concentrations on sperm motility in Japanese quail. Vet. Med. Int. 2010. Article ID 564921, http://dx.doi.org/10.4061/2010/564921.

Bonfante, F., Patrono, L.V., Aiello, R., Beato, M.S., Terregino, C., Capua, I., 2013. Susceptibility and intra–species transmission of the H9N2 G1 prototype lineage virus in Japanese quail and turkeys. Vet. Microbiol. 165, 177–183.

Bower, D.V., Sato, Y., Lansford, R., 2011. Dynamic lineage analysis of embryonic morphogenesis using transgenic quail and 4D multispectral imaging. Genesis 49, 619–643.

Buchwalder, T., Wechsler, B., 1997. The effect of cover on the behaviour of Japanese quail (Coturnix japonica). Appl. Anim. Behav. Sci. 54, 335–343.

Bump, G. 1971. The Coturnix or old world world. Game Bird Breeeders, Aviculturists, Zoologists and Conservationists' Gazette, 20, 13–16.

Burt, D.W., 2002. Origin and evolution of avian microchromosomes. Cytogenet. Genome. Res. 96, 97–112.

Cain, J.R., Cawley, W.O. 1972. Care Management Propagation: Japanese Quail (Coturnix). In: STATION, T. A. E. (ed.).

Cheng, H. 2011. Laying Hen Welfare Fact Sheet. In: Unit, A.R.S.M.A.L.B.R. (ed.). United States Department of Agriculture, Purdue University, IN.

Cheng, K.M., Aggrey, S.E., Nichols, C.R., Garnett, M.E., Godin, D.V., 1997. Antioxidant enzymes and atherosclerosis in Japanese quail: heritability and genetic correlation estimates. Can. J. Cardiol. 13, 669–676.

Cheng, K.M., Bennett, D.C., Mills, A.D., 2010. The Japanese quail. In: Hurbrecht, R., kirkwood, J. (Eds.), UFAW Handbook on the Care and Management of Laboratory Animals, eightth ed. Blackwell Scientific Publ, London.

Cheng, K.M., Hickman, A.R., Nichols, C.R., 1989a. Role of the proctodeal gland foam of male Japanese quail in natural copulations. Auk 106, 279–286.

Cheng, K.M., Kimura, M., 1990. Mutations and major variants in Japanese quail. In: Crawford, RD (Ed.), Developments in Animal and Veterinary Sciences, Vol 22. Poultry Breeding and Genetics Elsevier, Amsterdam, pp. 333–362.

Cheng, K.M., Mcintyre, R.F., Hickman, A.R., 1989b. Proctodeal gland foam enhances competitive fertilization in domestic Japanese quail. Auk 106, 287–291.

Cheng, K.M., Nichols, C.R., 1992. Japanese quail (Coturnix japonica): Conservation and management of genetic resources in Canada. Gibier Faune Sauvage 9, 667–676.

Collins, W.M., Hardiman, J.W., Urban, W.E., Corbett, A.C., 1975. Genetic differences in susceptibility to ulcerative enteritis in Japanese quail. Poult. Sci. 54, 2051–2054.

Cooper, C.S., Southard, T., Schultz, D., Scorpio, D., Dunn, J., Montali, R., 2007. A case of Marek's disease in Japanese quail (Coturnix japonica). J. Am. Assoc. Lab. Anim. Sci. 46, 106.

Crawford, R.D., 1990. Origins and History of Poultry Species. Elsevier, Amsterdam, the Netherlands.

De Jager, P.H., 2003. Effect of photoperiod on sexual development, growth and production of quail (Coturnix coturnix japonica). George Campus, Port Elizabeth Technikon, PhD.

Del Hoyo, J., Sargatal, J., Elliott, A., 1994. Handbook of the Birds of the World: New World Vultures to Guineafowl, Barcelona. Lynx Editions, Spain.

Delville, Y., Sulon, J., Hendrick, J.C., Balthazart, J., 1984. Effect of the presence of females on the pituitary-testicular activity in male Japanese quail (Coturnix coturnix japonica). Gen. Comp. Endocrinol. 55, 295–305.

Dennis, R.L., Cheng, H.W., 2010. A comparison of infrared and hot blade beak trimming in laying hens. Int. J. Poult. Sci. 9, 716–719.

Dickman, J.D., Huss, D., Lowe, M., 2004. Morphometry of otoconia in the utricle and saccule of developing Japanese quail. Hear. Res. 188, 89–103.

Duckworth, J.W. 2009. Recent observations of Galliformes in degraded parts of Laos. G@lliformed, 1, 18–20.

Dykstra, M.J., Charlton, B.R., Chin, R.P., Barnes, H.J., 2013. Fungal infections. In: Swayne, D.E., Glisson, J.R., Mcdougald, L.R., Nolan, L.K., Suarez, D.L., Nair, V. (Eds.), Diseases of Poultry, thirteenth ed. Wiley-Blackwell, Oxford.

Eleazer, T.H., Blalock, G., Warner, J.H., Pearson, J.E., 1978. Eastern equine encephalomyelitis outbreak in coturnix quail. Avian. Dis. 22, 522–525.

Evans, R.M., Cosens, S., 1977. Selective control of peep vocalizations by familiar sound in young Coturnix quail. Behaviour 62, 35–49.

Faqi, A.S., Solecki, R., Pfeil, R., Hilbig, V., 1997. Standard values for reproductive and clinical chemistry parameters of Japanese quail. Dtsch. Tierarztl. Wochenschr. 104, 167–169.

Farrell, D.J., Atmamihardja, S.I., Pym, R.A.E., 1982. Calorimetric measurements of the energy and nitrogen metabolism of Japanese quail. Br. Poult. Sci. 23, 375–382.

Fidura, F.G., 1969. Selective attention and complex discrimination learning in Japanese quail. Psychon. Sci. 15, 167–168.

Fillon, V., 1998. The chicken as a model to study microchromosomes in birds: a review. Genet. Sel. Evol. 30, 209–219.

Follet, B.K., Pearce-Kelly, K., 1990. Photoperiodic control of the termination of reproduction in Japanese quail (Coturnix coturnix japonica). Proc. Biol. Sci. 242, 225–230.

Foster, D.N., Nestor, K.E., Saif, Y.M., Bacon, W.L., Moorhead, P.D., 1989. Influence of selection for increased body weight on the incidence of leiomyomas and leiomyosarcomas in Japanese quail. Poult. Sci. 68, 1447–1453.

Frankham, R., Ballou, J.D., Briscoe, D.A., 2002. An Introduction to Conservation Genetics. Cambridge University Press, Cambridge, UK.

Fulton, J.E., Delany, M.E., 2003. Poultry genetic resources—operation rescue needed. Science 300, 1667–1668.

Garip, M., Dere, S., 2011. The effect of storage period and temperature on weight loss in quail eggs and the hatching weight of quail chicks. J. Anim. Vet. Adv. 10, 2363–2367.

Gerken, M., Mills, A.D., 1993. Welfare of domestic quail. In: Savory, C.J., Hughes, B.O. (Eds.), Proceedings of the Fourth European Symposium on Poultry Welfare. Universities Federation for Animal Welfare, Edinburgh.

Godin, D.V., Nichols, C.R., Hoekstra, K.A., Garnett, M.E., Cheng, K.M., 2001. Red cell and plasma antioxidant components and atherosclerosis in Japanese quail: a time-course study. Res. Commun. Mol. Pathol. Pharmacol. 110, 27–51.

Godin, D.V., Nichols, C.R., Hoekstra, K.A., Garnett, M.E., Cheng, K.M., 2003. Alterations in aortic antioxidant components in an experimental model of atherosclerosis: a time-course study. Mol. Cell. Biochem. 252, 193–203.

Gole, V.C., Chousalkar, K.K., Roberts, J.R., Sexton, M., May, D., Tan, J., et al., 2014. Effect of egg washing and correlation between eggshell characteristics and egg penetration by Various Salmonella Typhimurium Strains. PLoS One 9, e90987.

Gorham, S.L., Ottinger, M.A., 1986. Sertoli cell tumors in Japanese quail. Avian. Dis. 30, 337–339.

Goto, Y., Nakura, R., Nasu, T., Sawada, T., Shinjo, T., 2001. Isolation of Pasteurella multocida during an outbreak of infectious septicemia in Japanese quail (Cotunix coturnix japonica). Vet. Med. Sci. 63, 1055–1056.

Graham, J.E., Kollias-Baker, C., Craigmill, A.L., Thomasy, S.M., Tell, L.A., 2005. Pharmacokinetics of ketoprofen in Japanese quail (Coturnix japonica). J. Vet. Pharmacol. Ther. 28 (4), 399–402.

Guibert, F., Richard-Yris, M., Lumineau, S., Kotrschal, K., Bertin, A., Petton, C., et al., 2011. Unpredictable mild stressors on laying females influence the composition of Japanese quail eggs and offspring's phenotype. Appl. Anim. Behav. 132, 51–60.

Gulbahar, M.Y., Cabalar, M., Boynukara, B., 2005. Avipoxvirus infection in quails. Turk. J. Vet. Sci. 29, 449–454.

Guttenbach, M., Nanda, I., Feichtinger, W., et al., 2003. Comparative chromosome painting of chicken autosomal paints 1–9 in nine different bird species. Cytogenet. Genome. Res. 103, 173–184.

Hamburger, V., Hamilton, H.L., 1951. A series of normal stages in the development of the chick embryo. J. Morph. 88, 49–92.

Hasegawa, H., Murayama, T., Takahashi, A., Itakura, C., Nomura, Y., 1996. Changes of GTP binding proteins, not neurofilament-associated proteins, in the brain of the neurofilament-deficient quail, "Quiver." Neurochem. Int. 28, 221–229.

Herichová, I., Zeman, M., Juráni, M., Lamosová, D., 2004. Daily rhythms of melatonin and selected biochemical parameters in plasma of Japanese quail. Avian Poult. Biol. Rev. 15, 205–210.

Hillier, L.W., Miller, W., Birney, E., Warren, W., Hardison, R.C., Ponting, C.P., et al., 2004. Sequence and comparative analysis of the chicken genome provide unique perspectives on vertebrate evolution. Nature 432, 695–716.

Hodgetts, B., 1999. Quail production. In: Ewbank, R., Kim-Madslien, F., Hart, C.B. (Eds.), Management and Welfare of Farm Animals: The UFAW Farm Handbook, fourth ed. UFAW, Wheathampstead.

Hodos, W., Erichsen, J.T., 1990. Lower-field myopia in birds: an adaptation that keeps the ground in focus. Vision. Res. 30, 653–657.

Hoekstra, K.A., Nichols, C.R., Garnett, M.E., Godin, D.V., Cheng, K.M., 1998. Dietary cholesterol-induced xanthomatosis in atherosclerosis-susceptible Japanese quail (Cotunix japonica). J. Comp. Pathol. 119, 419–427.

Hoekstra, K.A., Godin, D.V., Kurtu, J., Cheng, K.M., 2003. Effects of oxidant-induced injury on heme oxygenase and glutathione in cultured aortic endothelial cells from atherosclerosis-susceptible and -resistant Japanese quail. Mol. Cell. Biochem. 254, 61–71.

Hoekstra, K.A., Godin, D.V., Cheng, K.M., 2004. Protective role of heme oxygenase in the blood vessel wall during atherogenesis. Biochem. Cell Biol. 82, 351–359.

Holmes, D.J., Ottinger, M.A., 2003. Birds as long-lived animal models for the study of aging. Exp. Gerontol. 38, 1365–1375.

Homma, K., Siopes, T.D., Wilson, W.O., Mcfarland, L.Z., 1966. Identification of sex of day old quail by cloacal examination. Poult. Sci. J. 45, 469–472.

Hoti, F., Sillanpaa, M.J., 2006. Bayesian mapping of genotype x expression interactions in quantitative and qualitative traits. Heredity (Edinb) 97, 4–18.

Howard, R., Moore, A., 1984. A Complete Checklist of the Birds of the World, revised ed. Macmillan, London.

Hutchinson, T.H., Brown, R., Brugger, K.E., Campbell, P.M., Holt, M., Länge, R., et al., 2000. Ecological risk assessment of endocrine disruptors. Environ. Health. Perspect. 108, 1007–1014.

IUCN. 2013a. IUCN Red List of Threatened Species.

IUCN. 2013b. Species factsheet: Coturnix japonica [Online]. BirdLife International. Available: <http://www.iucnredlist.org> (accessed 02.03.14 Downloaded from <http://www.birdlife.org> on 02/04/2014).

Jiang, F., Miao, Y., Liang, W., Ye, H., Liu, H., Liu, B., 2010. The complete mitochondrial genomes of the whistling duck (Dendrocygna javanica) and black swan (Cygnus atratus): dating evolutionary divergence in Galloanserae. Mol. Biol. Rep. 37, 3001–3015.

Johnsgard, P., 1988. The Quails, Partridges, and Francolins of the World. Oxford University Press, Oxford, UK.

Kan, X.Z., Li, X.F., Lei, Z.P., Chen, L., Gao, H., Yang, Z.Y., et al., 2010. Estimation of divergence times for major lineages of galliform birds: evidence from complete mitochondrial genome sequences. Afr. J. Biotechnol. 9, 3073–3078.

Kano, A. 2006. Study on the origin and phylogeny of domestic quail. Report of the Society for Researches on Native Livestock.

Kawahara-Miki, R., Sano, S., Nunome, M., Shimmura, T., Kuwayama, T., Takahashi, S., et al., 2013. Next-generation sequencing reveals genomic features in the Japanese quail. Genomics 101, 345–353.

Kayang, B.B., Fillon, V., Inoue-Murayama, M., Miwa, M., Leroux, S., Fève, K., et al., 2006. Integrated maps in quail (Coturnix japonica) confirm the high degree of synteny conservation with chicken (Gallus gallus) despite 35 million years of divergence. BMC Genomics 7, 101.

Keller, L.F., Waller, D.M., 2002. Inbreeding effects in wild populations. Trends. Ecol. Evol. 17, 230–241.

Kikuchi, T., Yang, H.W., Pennybacker, M., Ichihara, N., Mizutani, M., Van Hove, J.L., et al., 1998. Clinical and metabolic correction of pompe disease by enzyme therapy in acid maltase deficient quail. J. Clin. Investig. 101, 827–833.

Kim, S.H., Cheng, K.M., Ritland, C., Ritland, K., Silversides, F.G., 2007. Inbreeding in Japanese quail estimated by pedigree and microsatellite analyses. J. Hered. 98, 378–381.

Kovach, J.K., 1975. The behaviour of quail. In: Hafez, E.S.E. (Ed.), The Behaviour of Domestic Animals, third ed. Bailliere Tindall, London.

Kulenkamp, A.W., Kulenkamp, C.M., Coleman, T.H., 1973. The effects of intensive inbreeding (brother × sister) on various traits in Japanese quail. Poult. Sci. 52, 1240–1246.

Kulesa, P., Bronner-Fraser, M., Fraser, S., 2000. In ovo time-lapse analysis after dorsal neural tube ablation shows rerouting of chick hindbrain neural crest. Development 127, 2843–2852.

Le Douarin, N., 1973. A biological cell labeling technique and its use in experimental embryology. Dev. Biol. 30, 217–222.

Le Douarin, N., Barq, G., 1969. Use of Japanese quail cells as "biological markers" in experimental embryology. C. R. Acad. Sci. Hebd. Seances. Acad. Sci. D. 269, 1543–1546.

Le Douarin, N., Kalcheim, C., 1999. The Neural Crest. Cambridge University Press.

Liu, J., Song, Y., Cheng, K.M., Silversides, F.G., 2010. Production of donor-derived offspring from cryopreserved ovarian tissue in Japanese quail (Coturnix japonica). Biol. Reprod. 83, 15–19.

Liu, J., Cheng, K.M., Purdy, P.H., Silversides, F.G., 2012a. A simple vitrification method for cryobanking avian testicular tissue. Poult. Sci. 91, 3209–3213.

Liu, J., Cheng, K.M., Silversides, F.G., 2012b. Novel needle-in-straw vitrification can effectively preserve the follicle morphology, viability, and vascularization of ovarian tissue in Japanese quail (Coturnix japonica). Anim. Reprod. Sci. 134, 197–202.

Liu, J., Cheng, K.M., Silversides, F.G., 2013a. A model for cryobanking female germplasm in Japanese quail (Coturnix japonica). Poult. Sci. 92, 2772–2775.

Liu, J., Cheng, K.M., Silversides, F.G., 2013b. Production of live off-spring from testicular tissue cryopreserved by vitrification procedures in Japanese quail (Coturnix japonica). Biol. Reprod. 88, 124.

Liu, J., Cheng, K.M., Silversides, F.G., 2013c. Recovery of fertility from adult ovarian tissue transplanted into week-old Japanese quail chicks. Reprod. Fertil. Dev. 27, 281–284.

Liu, J., Robertson, M.C., Cheng, K.M., Silversides, F.G., 2013d. Chimeric plumage coloration produced by ovarian transplantation in chickens. Poult. Sci. 92, 1073–1076.

Lwigale, P.Y., Schneider, R.A., 2008. Other chimeras: quail–duck and mouse–chick. Methods Cell Biol. 87, 59–74.

Maruyama, S., Katsube, Y., 1988. Intestinal colonization of Campylobacter jejuni in young Japanese quails (Coturnix coturnix japonica). Jpn. J. Vet. Sci. 50, 569–572.

Maruyama, S., Katsube, Y., 1990. Isolation of Campylobacter jejuni from the eggs and organs in experimentally infected laying Japanese quails (Coturnix coturnix japonica). Jpn. J. Vet. Sci. 52, 671–674.

Matsui, T., Kuroda, S., Mizutani, M., Kiuchi, Y., Suzuki, K., Ono, T., 1983. Generalized glycogen storage disease in Japanese quail (Coturnix coturnix japonica). Vet. Pathol. 20, 312–321.

Mckinney, F., Derrickson, S.R., Mineau, P., 1983. Forced copulation in waterfowl. Behaviour 86, 250–294.

Mcqueen, H.A., Siriaco, G., Bird, A.P., 1998. Chicken microchromosomes are hyperacetylated, early replicating, and gene rich. Genome Res. 8, 621–630.

Mench, J.A., Blatchford, R.A., 2014. Birds as laboratory animals. In: Bayne, K., Turner, P.V. (Eds.), Laboratory Animal Welfare, first ed. Academic Press, San Diego, CA.

Miller, K.A., Mench, J.A., 2005. The differential use and effects of four types of environmental enrichment on the activity budgets, fearfulness, and social proximity preference of Japanese quail. Appl. Anim. Behav. Sci. 95, 169–187.

Mills, A., Crawford, L., Domjan, M., Faure, J.M., 1997. The behavior of the Japanese or domestic quail Corturnix japonica. Neurosci. Biobehav. Rev. 21, 261–281.

Minvielle, F., Coville, J.L., Krupa, A., Monvoisin, J.L., Maeda, Y., Okamoto, S., 2000. Genetic similarity and relationships of DNA fingerprints with performance and with heterosis in Japanese quail lines from two origins and under reciprocal recurrent or within-line selection for early egg production. Genet. Sel. Evol. 32, 289–302.

Mizutani, M., 2002. Establishment of inbred strains of chicken and Japanese quail and their potential as animal models. Exp. Anim. 51, 417–429.

Mohan, J., Moudgal, R.R., Sastry, K.V.H., Tyagi, J., Sing, R., 2002. Effects of hemicastration and castration on foam production and its relationship with fertility in male Japanese quail. Theriogenology 58, 29–39.

Mohan, J., Sastry, K.V.H., Tyagi, J.S., Singh, D.K., 2004. Isolation of E. coli from foam and effects of fluoroquinolones on E. coli and foam production in male Japanese quail. Theriogenology 62, 1383–1390.

Murakami, S., Sakurai, T., Tomoike, H., Sakono, M., Nasu, T., Fukuda, N., 2010. Prevention of hypercholesterolemia and atherosclerosis in the hyperlipidemia- and atherosclerosis-prone Japanese (LAP) quail by taurine supplementation. Amino. Acids. 38, 271–278.

Nagarajan, K., Thyagarajan, D., Balachandran, C., Pazhanivel, N., Arunkumar, S., 2013. Incidence of Marek's disease in Cotunix coturnix japonica in an organized farm. J. Food Agric. Vet. Sci. 3, 254–257.

Nagarajan, S., Narahari, D., Jayaprasad, I.A., Thyagarajan, D., 1991. Influence of stocking density and layer age on production traits and egg quality in Japanese-quail. Br. Poult. Sci. 32, 243–248.

Nakamura, H., Katahira, T., Sato, T., Watanabe, Y., Funahashi, J., 2004. Gain- and loss-of-function in chick embryos by electroporation. Mech. Dev. 121, 1137–1143.

National Research Council, 2011. Guide for the Care and Use of Laboratory Animals, eighth ed. National Academies Press.

Nichols, C.R. 1991. A comparison of the reproductive and behavioural differences in feral and domestic Japanese quail. MSc Thesis, University of British Columbia.

Nichols, C.R., Robinson, C.A.F., Cheng, K.M., 1992. Influence of domestication on fecundity and reproductive behaviour of Japanese quail (Coturnix japonica). Gibier Faune Sauvage 9, 743–755.

Niemiec, A.J., Raphael, Y., Moody, D.B., 1994. Return of auditory function following structural regeneration after acoustic trauma: Behavioral measures from quail. Hear. Res. 79, 1–16.

Nirmalan, G.P., Robinson, G.A., 1971. Haematology of the Japanese quail (Coturnix coturnix japonica). Br. Poult. Sci. 12, 475–481.

Nol, E., Cheng, K.M., Nichols, C.R., 1996. Heritability and phenotypic correlations of behaviour and dominance rank of Japanese quail. Anim. Behav. 52, 813–820.

Nolan, L.K., Barnes, H.J., Vaillancourt, J.P., Abdul-Aziz, T., Logue, C.M., 2013. Colibacillosis. In: Swayne, D., Glisson, J., McDougald, L., Nolan, L., Suarez, D., Nair, V. (Eds.), Diseases of Poultry Wiley-Blackwell, Oxford, pp. 751–806.

Okuyama, M., 2004. Current status of the Japanese Quail Coturnix japonica as a game bird. J. Yamashina Inst. Ornithology 35, 189–202.

Orcutt, F.S., Orcutt, A.B., 1976. Nesting and parental behavior in domestic common quail. Auk 93, 135–141.

Ottinger, M.A., 2001. Quail and other short-lived birds. Exp. Gerontol. 36, 859–868.

Ottinger, M.A., Abdelnabi, M., Li, Q., Chen, K., Thompson, N., Harada, N., et al., 2004. The Japanese quail: a model for studying reproductive aging of hypothalamic systems. Exp. Gerontol. 39, 1679–1693.

Padgett, C.A., Ivey, W.D., 1959. Coturnix quail as a laboratory research animal. Science 129, 267–268.

Padgett, C.S., Ivey, W.D., 1960. The normal embryology of the Coturnix quail. Anat. Rec. 137, 1–11.

Pappas, J., 2002. Coturnix japonica. Animal Diversity Web. <http://animaldiversity.ummz.umich.edu/accounts/Coturnix_japonica/>.

Perez, D.R., Lim, W., Seiler, J.P., Yi, G., Peiris, M., Shortridge, K.F., et al., 2003. Role of quail in the interspecies transmission of H9 influenza A viruses: molecular changes on HA that correspond to adaptation from ducks to chickens. J. Virol. 77, 3148–3156.

Peterson, R.T., 1961. A Field Guide to Western Birds. Houghton Mifflin Co, Boston, MA.

Randall, M., Bolla, G. 2008. Raising Japanese quail. State of New South Wales Department of Primary Industries. Prime Fact 602 2nd Edition.

Reed, W.M., Jack, S.W., 2013. Quail bronchitis. In: Swayne, D.E., Glisson, J.R., Mcdougald, L.R., Nolan, L.K., Suarez, D.L., Nair, V. (Eds.), Diseases of Poultry, thirteenth ed Wiley-Blackwell, Oxford.

Roberts, M., 1999. Quail, Past and Present. Bartlett and Son, Exeter.

Robinson, J.E., Follett, B.K., 1982. Photoperiodism in Japanese quail: the termination of seasonal breeding by photorefractoriness. Proc. R. Soc. Lond. B. Biol. Sci. 215, 95–116.

Roy, P., Vairamuthu, S., Sakthivelan, S.M., Purushothaman, V., 2004. Hydropericardium syndrome in Japanese quail (Coturnix coturnix japonica). Vet. Rec. 155, 273–274.

RSPCA, 2001. Quail: Good Practice for Housing and Care. Research Animals Department, West Sussex, UK, pp. 1–5.

Rundfeldt, C., Wyska, E., Steckel, H., Witkowski, A., Jeżewska-Witkowska, G., Wlaź, P., 2013. A model for treating avian aspergillosis: serum and lung tissue kinetics for Japanese quail (Coturnix japonica) following single and multiple aerosol exposures of a nanoparticulate itraconazole suspension. Med. Mycol. 51, 800–810.

Ruffins, S.W., Martin, M., Keough, L., Truong, S., Fraser, S.E., Jacobs, R.E., et al., 2007. Digital three-dimensional atlas of quail development using high-resolution MRI. Sci. World J. 7, 592–604.

Sachs, B., 1969. Photoperiod control of reproductive behavior and physiology of the male Japanese quail (Coturnix cotunix japonica). Horm. Behav. 1, 7–24.

Sato, Y., Lansford, R., 2013. Transgenesis and imaging in birds, and available transgenic reporter lines. Dev. Growth Differ. 55, 406–421.

Sato, Y., Poynter, G., Huss, D., Filla, M.B., Czirok, A., Rongish, B.J., et al., 2010. Dynamic analysis of vascular morphogenesis using transgenic quail embryos. PLoS One 5, e12674.

Schein, M.W., Statkiewicz, W.R., 1983. Satiation and cyclic performance of dust-bathing by Japanese quail (Coturnix coturnix japonica). Appl. Anim. Ethol. 10, 375–383.

Schmid, I., Wechsler, B., 1997. Behavior of Japanese quail (Coturnix japonica) kept in semi-natural aviaries. Appl. Anim. Behav. Sci. 55, 103–112.

Scholtz, N., Hale, J., Flachowsky, G., Sauerwein, H., 2009a. Serum chemistry reference values in adult Japanese quail (Coturnix coturnix japonica) including sex-related differences. Poult. Sci. 88, 1186–1190.

Scholtz, N., Halle, I., Flachowsky, G., Sauerwein, H., 2009b. Serum chemistry reference values in adult Japanese quail (Coturnix coturnix japonica) including sex-related differences. Poult. Sci. 88, 1186–1190.

Scott, B.B., Lois, C., 2005. Generation of tissue-specific transgenic birds with lentiviral vectors. Proc. Natl. Acad. Sci. U. S. A. 102, 16443–16447.

Seidl, A.H., Sanchez, J.T., Schecterson, L., Tabor, K.M., Wang, Y., Kashima, D.T., et al., 2013. Transgenic quail as a model for research in the avian nervous system: a comparative study of the auditory brainstem. J. Comp. Neurol. 521, 5–23.

Shivaprasad, H.L., 2002. Pathology of Birds – An Overview. C.L. Davis Foundation Conference on Gross Morbid Anatomy of Animals, Washington DC.

Sinclair, K.M., Church, M.E., Farver, T.B., Lowenstine, L.J., Owens, S.D., Paul-Murphy, J., 2012. Effects of meloxicam on hematologic and plasma biochemical analysis variables and results of histologic examination of tissue specimens of Japanese quail (Coturnix japonica). Am. J. Vet. Res. 73 (11), 1720–1727.

Sittmann, K., Abplanalp, H., Fraser, R.A., 1966. Inbreeding depression in Japanese quail. Genetics 54, 371–379.

Standford, J.A. 1957. A Progress Report of coturnix quail investigations in Missouri. Twenty-second North American Wildlife Conference.

Stiglec, R., Ezaz, T., Graves, J.A., 2007. A new look at the evolution of avian sex chromosomes. Cytogenet. Genome. Res. 117, 103–109.

Sullivan, J.P., Grasman, K.A., Scanlon, P.F., 1992. Effects of handling and pair management on reproduction in Japanese quail (Coturnix coturnix). Theriogenology 37, 877–883.

Tadano, R., Nunome, M., Mizutani, M., Kawahara-Miki, R., Fujiwara, A., Takahashi, S., et al., 2014. Cost-effective development of highly polymorphic microsatellite in Japanese quail facilitated by next-generation sequencing. Anim. Genet. 45, 881–884.

Takahashi, N., Shinki, T., Abe, E., Horiuchi, N., Yamaguchi, A., Yoshiki, S., et al., 1983. The role of vitamin D in the medullary bone formation in egg-laying Japanese quail and in immature male chicks treated with sex hormones. Calcif. Tissue. Int. 35, 465–471.

Takatsuji, K., Ito, H., Watanabe, M., Ikushima, M., Nakamura, A., 1984. Histopathological changes of the retina and optic nerve in the albino mutant quail (Coturnix coturnix japonica). J. Comp. Pathol. 94, 387–404.

Takatsuji, K., Iizuka, S., Nakatani, H., Nakamura, A., 1985. Morphology of the cataract in albino mutant quails (Coturnix coturnix japonica). Exp. Eye. Res. 40, 567–573.

Takatsuji, K., Sato, Y., Iizuka, S., Nakatani, H., Nakamura, A., 1986. Animal model of closed angle glaucoma in albino mutant quails. Invest. Ophthalmol. Vis. Sci. 27, 396–400.

Tattersfield, L., Matthiessen, P., Campbell, P.M., Grandy, N., Länge, R., 1997. SETAC Europe/OECD/EC Expert Workshop on Endocrine Modulators and Wildlife: Assessment and Testing (EMWAT). Brussels, SETAC Europe, Brussels, Belgium.

Teixeira, M., Teixeira Filho, W.L., Lopes, C.W.G., 2004. Coccidiosis in Japanese quails (Coturnix japonica): characterization of a naturally occurring infection in a commercial rearing farm. Rev. Bras. Cienc. Avic. 6, 129–134.

Tell, L.A., Woods, L., Foley, J., Needham, M.L., Walker, R.L., 2003. A model of avian mycobacteriosis: clinical and histopathologic findings in Japanese quail (Coturnix coturnix japonica) intravenously inoculated with Mycobacterium avium. Avian. Dis. 47, 433–443.

Tiersch, T.R., Wachtel, S.S., 1991. On the evolution of genome size of birds. J. Hered. 82, 363–368.

Tsudzuki, M., 2008. Mutations of Japanese quail (Coturnix japonica) and recent advances of molecular genetics for this species. J. Poult. Sci. 45, 159–179.

Tuzcu, M., Sahin, N., Ozercan, I., Seren, S., Sahin, K., Kucuk, O., 2010. The effects of selenium supplementation on the spontaneously occurring fibroid tumors of oviduct, 8-hydroxy-2′-deoxyguanosine levels, and heat shock protein 70 response in Japanese quail. Nutr. Cancer 62, 495–500.

Union, A.O. 1983. Check-List of North American Birds. sixth ed. Washington, DC.

Usman, B.A., Mani, A.U., El-Yuguda, A.D., Diarra, S.S., 2008. The effect of supplemental ascorbic acid on the development of Newcastle disease in Japaense quail (Coturnix coturnix Japonica) exposed to high ambient temperature. Int. J. Poult. Sci. 7, 328–332.

Van Tuinen, M., Dyke, G.J., 2004. Calibration of galliform molecular clocks using multiple fossils and genetic partitions. Mol. Phylogenet. Evol. 30, 74–86.

Van Tuinen, M., Hedges, S.B., 2001. Calibration of avian molecular clocks. Mol. Biol. Evol. 18, 206–213.

Vince, M.A., 1964a. Social facilitation of hatching in the bobwhite quail. Anim. Behav. 12, 531–534.

Vince, M.A., 1964b. Synchronisation of hatching in american bobwhite quail (Colinus virgineanus). Nature 203, 1192–1193.

Vince, M.A., 1966. Artificial acceleration of hatching in quail embryos. Anim. Behav. 14, 389–394.

Vince, M.A., 1968a. Effect of rate of stimulation on hatching time in Japanese quail. Br. Poult. Sci. 9, 87–91.

Vince, M.A., 1968b. Retardation as a factor in the synchronization of hatching. Anim. Behav. 16, 332–335.

Vince, M.A., 1973. Effects of external stimulation on the onset of lung ventilation and the time of hatching in the fowl, duck and goose. Br. Poult. Sci. 14, 389–401.

Vince, M.A., Salter, S.H., 1967. Respiration and clicking in quail embryos. Nature 216, 582–583.

Vince, M.A., Ockleford, E., Reader, M., 1984. The synchronisation of hatching in quail embryos: aspects of development affected by a retarding stimulus. J. Exp. Zool. 229, 273–282.

Visser, G.H., Boon, P.E., Meijer, H.A.J., 2000. Validation of the doubly labelled water method in Japanese quail Coturnix c. japonica chicks: is there an effect of growth rate? J. Comp. Physiol. 170, 365–372.

Wallis, J.W., Aerts, J., Groenen, M.A., Crooijmans, R.P., Layman, D., Graves, T.A., et al., 2004. A physical map of the chicken genome. Nature 432, 761–764.

Wechsler, B., Schmid, I., 1998. Aggressive pecking by males in breeding groups of Japanese quail (Coturnix japonica). Br. Poult. Sci. 39, 333–339.

Weidner, C., Repérant, J., Kirpitchnikova, E., Miceli, D., Desroches, A., Rio, J.P., 1995. Time course of degeneration of the visual system induced by spontaneous glaucoma in the albino quail (Coturnix coturnix japonica). Brain. Res. 419, 357–363.

Wetherbee, D.K., 1961. Investigations in the life history of the common Coturnix. Am. Midl. Nat. 65, 168–186.

Wong, G.K., Liu, B., Wang, J., Zhang, Y., Yang, X., Zhang, Z., et al., 2004. A genetic variation map for chicken with 2.8 million single-nucleotide polymorphisms. Nature 432, 717–722.

Woodard, A.E., Abplanalp, H., Wilson, W.O., Vohra, P., 1973. Japanese Quail Husbandry in the Laboratory. Department of Avian Sciences, University of California-Davis.

Yasuo, S., Watanabe, M., Iigo, M., Yamamura, T., Nakao, N., Takagi, T., et al., 2006. Molecular mechanism of photoperiodic time measurement in the brain of Japanese quail. Chronobiol. Int. 23, 307–315.

Yuan, Y.V., Kitts, D.D., Godin, D.V., 1997. Influence of dietary cholesterol and fat source on atherosclerosis in Japanese quail (Coturnix japonica). Br. J. Nutr. 78, 993–1014.

Zacchei, A.M., 1961. Archivio italiano di anatomia e di embriologia: Lo sviluppo embrionale della quaglia giapponese. Arch. Ital. Anat. Embriol. 66, 36–62.

Zak, P.P., Zykova, A.V., Trofimova, N.N., Abu Khamidakh, A.E., Fokin, A.I., Eskina, E.N., et al., 2010. The experimental model for studying of human age retinal degeneration (Japanese quail C. Japonica). Dokl. Biol. Sci. 434, 297–299.

CHAPTER

23

Zebra Finches in Biomedical Research

*Mary M. Patterson, MS, DVM, DACLAM[a] and
Michale S. Fee, PhD[b]*

[a]Division of Comparative Medicine, Massachusetts Institute of Technology, Cambridge, MA, USA
[b]Department of Brain and Cognitive Sciences, McGovern Institute, Massachusetts Institute of
Technology, Cambridge, MA, USA

I. INTRODUCTION

Zebra finches (*Taenopygia guttata*, formerly *Poephila guttata*) are small, colorful songbirds that have been favored by bird fanciers since the nineteenth century. In captivity, zebra finches are prolific breeders and robust 'easy keepers'; these characteristics, along with a diurnal activity pattern and the singing prowess of males, makes them an attractive model for biomedical researchers. Their increasing popularity resides especially in the fields of neurobiology, with a majority of investigations in the United States focusing on male vocal development, and behavior, such as the basis for mate preference and aggression. However, many other research applications,

as well as the production of transgenic birds, have also been pursued. The zebra finch genome is the second avian species to be sequenced (Warren *et al.*, 2010), after that of the chicken (*Gallus gallus domesticus*). Importantly, a high-resolution digital atlas of the zebra finch brain was recently published (Karten *et al.*, 2013), and detailed, current protocols for using zebra finches in research can be accessed online (Cold Spring Harbor Press, 2014). One review article determined there were considerably more articles about zebra finches in 2008 relative to other passerine species (Bateson and Feenders, 2010), while a tally of PubMed entries for the subject 'zebra finch' reveals a steady annual increase in publications that started to escalate during the 1980s.

Laboratory Animal Medicine, Third Edition
DOI: http://dx.doi.org/10.1016/B978-0-12-409527-4.00023-7

1109

II. HISTORY AND TAXONOMY

An overview of zebra finch history, taxonomy, and ecology can be found in a well-recognized treatise by Richard Zann (1996). Wild zebra finches live socially in flocks and cover large areas in search of their granivorous diet and other favorable conditions. Of two subspecies, *T. guttata guttata* occupying the Lesser Sundas archipelago of eastern Indonesia and *T. guttata castanotis* from continental Australia, members of the latter subspecies underwent early domestication in Europe. Offspring of these birds have given rise to the zebra finches commonly found in pet stores and used in research today. In general, captive populations have undergone so many generations without genetic input from wild stock that they likely constitute strains distinct from their native Australian forbears. Although the convention of most scientific articles is to refer to the caged zebra finch simply as *T. guttata*, an abbreviation for *T. guttata castanotis*, it should be appreciated that some bird specialists, e.g., in the *Handbook of Birds of the World*, Volume 15 (Payne, 2010), designate *T. castanotis* as the Australian zebra finch and its progeny, and not as a subspecies.

Phylogenetic classification schemes for zebra finches have evolved over the years. The Zann text (1996) placed them in the tribe Poephilini (grassfinches), subfamily Estrildinae (along with mannikins and waxbills), and family Passeridae. More recently (Payne, 2010), and based on mitochondrial genetics, zebra finches are assigned to the subfamily Lonchurinae (grassfinches, munias, and mannikins), family Estrildidae (waxbills), suborder Oscines (typical songbirds), and order Passeriformes (perching birds). Regardless, estrildid finches are from the Old World and do not share close taxonomic affinity with the 'true' finches (subfamily Fringillinae or family Fringillidae), e.g., house finches, goldfinches, and canaries. This distinction is noteworthy because some references cite information and data as pertaining broadly to 'finches,' with the actual species involved not specified; yet unrelated 'finches' may be dissimilar in important respects.

III. RESEARCH USES

Songbirds have provided a unique window for examining fundamental questions about the biology of complex social and motor behaviors; preeminent have been those related to acoustic communication (Beecher and Brenowitz, 2005). While many songbirds have been surveyed in the field (Marler, 1991), experimental studies have been confined to a relatively small number of species, such as the canary, *Serinus canarius* (Nottebohm *et al.*, 1976); the European starling, *Sturnus vulgaris* (Gentner *et al.*, 2006); and the zebra finch. Among these, zebra finches are most frequently used in the laboratory, where they breed well, attain sexual maturity as soon as 90 days after hatching, and exhibit a range of social, reproductive, and vocal behaviors considered typical of their wild relatives (Morris, 1954; Immelmann, 1969). Although neurobiological research is highlighted in this section, scientists in many other fields also employ the zebra finch model system; exemplary studies are cited throughout the chapter.

The striking similarity between songbird vocal learning and the learning of human speech (Brainard and Doupe, 2013, Doupe and Kuhl, 1999) has led researchers to characterize how male zebra finches learn songs by imitating the vocalizations of an adult conspecific tutor (Price, 1979), usually the father. Early singing in juveniles begins between 30–40 days post-hatch (dph) with babbling vocalizations called subsong (Veit *et al.*, 2011; Aronov *et al.*, 2011). During the subsequent plastic song stage, between roughly 45 and 75 dph, vocal patterns gradually become more structured. Variable but recognizable prototype syllables emerge, and over the course of several weeks, these differentiate into a number of distinct song syllables (Tchernichovski *et al.*, 2001; Lipkind and Tchernichovski, 2011). As male zebra finches approach adulthood (80–90 dph), the song crystallizes into a fairly stereotyped sequence of three to seven syllables, often sung in a repeated linear sequence referred to as a song motif (Fig. 23.1). During vocal learning, young males refine their songs until the majority of birds produce a good copy of the tutor song.

The zebra finch and other avian brains have been compared to the mammalian brain (Jarvis *et al.*, 2013). With similar striatal and pallidal cell types (Goldberg and Fee, 2010; Goldberg *et al.*, 2010), neurochemistry (Kubikova *et al.*, 2010), and circuit connections (Person *et al.*, 2008), the avian basal ganglia is considered homologous to the mammalian basal ganglia (Farries and Perkel, 2002). Zebra finch experiments have likewise revealed parallels between the avian pallium and the mammalian

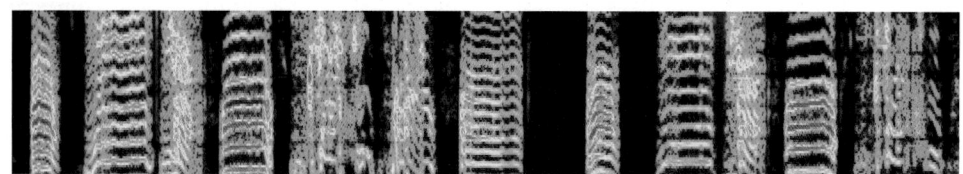

FIGURE 23.1   Example of a song from a male zebra finch at 90 dph; the frequency axis goes from 0 to 7 kHz and the recording is 2 s long.

neocortex (Dugas-Ford *et al.*, 2012), and have provided insights into the evolution of the vertebrate brain and neocortex (Jarvis *et al.*, 2013; Karten, 2013). Studies using zebra finches have helped identify specific premotor brain circuits for song production (Vu *et al.*, 1994); these include circuits that underlie the control of song timing (Hahnloser *et al.*, 2002; Long and Fee, 2008). Another set of brain areas, referred to as the anterior forebrain pathway, is necessary for vocal learning but not for adult song (Bottjer *et al.*, 1984; Scharff and Nottebohm, 1991). The similarity of the anterior forebrain pathway to cortical-basal ganglia-thalamocortical loops in mammals have made the zebra finch a valuable model for analyzing biophysical interactions in these areas (Goldberg and Fee, 2012; Kojima and Doupe, 2009; Leblois *et al.*, 2009).

Vocal learning and maintenance in zebra finches requires auditory feedback, similar to that observed in other songbirds (Lombardino and Nottebohm, 2000); this has been the motivation for numerous projects involving the zebra finch auditory system (Nagel *et al.*, 2011). Several studies have focused on functions related to song learning, e.g., the formation of auditory memories associated with storing the tutor song (Mello *et al.*, 1992; Jarvis *et al.*, 1998; London and Clayton, 2008), and in comparing the ongoing song with the tutor song (Keller and Hahnloser, 2009). The influence of periods of sleep on song development is being explored by other researchers (Dave and Margoliash, 2000; Deregnaucourt *et al.*, 2005; Shank and Margoliash, 2009).

Hormonal studies in the zebra finch have evaluated their role in regulating complex social relationships, along with the tight temporal control of song development. Brain areas important for song production and learning express receptors for androgens at a high density (Nottebohm and Arnold, 1976), and studies have shown that critical periods in vocal learning are under the control of these hormones, e.g., White *et al.* (1999). Vocal behaviors in zebra finches are sexually dimorphic, with the sexual differentiation of song-related brain regions under hormonal control (Remage-Healey *et al.*, 2010). In addition to song learning, researchers have assessed how hormones impact aggression in zebra finches (Arnold, 1975; Adkins-Regan, 1999; Goodson and Adkins-Regan, 1999).

Zebra finches are amenable to advanced neurobiological and genetic research techniques. Recordings from single neurons in freely behaving and singing zebra finches have been possible since the advent of extremely lightweight microdrives (Yu and Margoliash, 1996; Fee and Leonardo, 2001; Long *et al.*, 2010; Otchy and Ölveczky, 2012). Furthermore, recorded neurons can be identified by their projection targets using antidromic stimulation (Hahnloser *et al.*, 2006). Other newly developed methodologies, such as local drug infusion (Andalman and Fee, 2009; Charlesworth *et al.*, 2012),

viral infection (Roberts *et al.*, 2010; Scott *et al.*, 2012), and optogenetics (Knöpfel *et al.*, 2010; Roberts *et al.*, 2012), have allowed the manipulation of specific brain areas during singing and learning. Hypotheses about the role of specific genes in the development of vocal behaviors are also being tested with zebra finches. In humans, for example, mutations in the transcription factors FOXP2 and CNTNAP2 have been associated with speech and language disorders (Lai *et al.*, 2001; Alarcón *et al.*, 2008). These proteins in zebra finches are differentially expressed in song control brain regions, particularly in the song-related basal ganglia (Panaitof *et al.*, 2010). Direct knockdown of FOXP2 expression in the basal ganglia of zebra finches causes deficits in vocal learning (Haesler *et al.*, 2007) and disruptions in dopaminergic signaling (Murugan *et al.*, 2013). In the future, the completed sequencing of the zebra finch genome (Warren *et al.*, 2010), together with advances in creating transgenic zebra finches (Agate *et al.*, 2009), will create exciting new avenues for modifying brain circuits in experimental birds.

IV. BIOLOGY

Wild-type adult male zebra finches have orange cheek patches, fine black-and-white barring on the throat and upper breast with a subjacent solid black band, and chestnut-colored flanks speckled with white spots (Fig. 23.2); females are homogeneously gray in these areas.

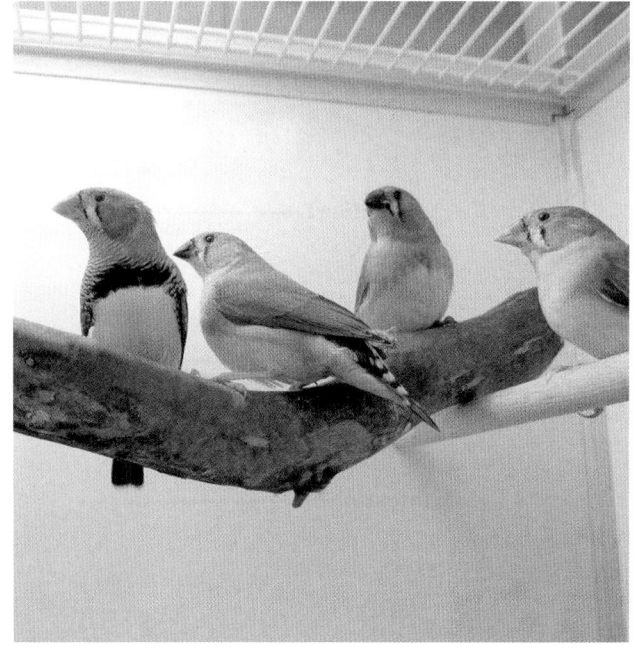

FIGURE 23.2   Wild-type adult male zebra finch on left, two juveniles in the center, and adult female on right.

Breeding by aviculturists has resulted in numerous color morphs, especially variations of fawn and white; nevertheless, even in these mutants, a faded cheek patch usually becomes visible in adult males. Their short, thick, and pointed bills are designed for dehusking seeds; beaks in mature males are more of a bright red color versus orange in females. Young zebra finches have black beaks, with a gradual change in coloring that starts around one month of age. Adults of both sexes are similar in size, about 10 cm in length, and usually weigh 14–16 g. Forstmeier *et al.* (2007) demonstrated that different stocks of zebra finches have variable body masses, e.g., European laboratory birds, as a result of selective breeding, were larger than North American birds, and both of these groups outweighed wild-caught and captive birds in Australia.

Heterogametes ZW are found in female zebra finches and ZZ in males, as for other birds; PCR analysis for these can be used to ascertain the gender of immature animals (Soderstrom *et al.*, 2007). Details about the embryological development of zebra finches have been published (Murray *et al.*, 2013), with the notable conclusion that many structural and temporal embryological features in zebra finches, which are completely altricial, differ from those in birds with precocious young, such as the domestic chicken. Approximate age classes (days post-hatch) for zebra finches are as follows: hatchling 1–20, fledgling 21–35, juvenile 36–65, young adult 66–90, adult 91–365, mature adult 366+. Under normal circumstances, male song learning takes place only during a particular phase of growth, such that a milestone for adulthood occurs around 90 days post-hatch when male songs have become stereotyped. Ninety days is also the age when domesticated females will start to lay eggs, which is later than their native counterparts in Australia (Nager and Law, 2010). Although most domesticated male zebra finches live 3 years and most females live 2, they have potential lifespans of 5–7 years under optimal circumstances. There are reports of individual birds reaching much more advanced ages.

Typical of the passerine group, the feet of zebra finches are anisodactylous, with three digits pointing forward and one backward. Their crop is smaller than in many other avian species, but ample seed in the crop of a healthy bird should be visible through its thin, almost transparent skin. The digestive tract contains a glandular proventriculus and a muscular ventriculus, or gizzard; a gall bladder is present. The spleen is an oblong and curved organ, approximately 5 mm in length. The nasal sinuses on either side do not communicate with one another (Sandmeier and Coutteel, 2006). In conjunction with highly elastic vibrating membranes and associated musculature, a complex syrinx is located at the distal end of the trachea where it divides into two bronchi; the right and left halves of the syrinx can be controlled independently. There are seven transparent air sacs, which function as bellows to ventilate the essentially nonexpansile lungs attached to the dorsal body wall. In female birds, only the left side of the reproductive tract develops. Some gross features of zebra finch anatomy are depicted in Fig. 23.3. As expected, zebra finches have very high basal metabolic rates; this is reflected in an average daytime body temperature of 41.8°C (close to 107°F) (Conover and Messmer, 1996).

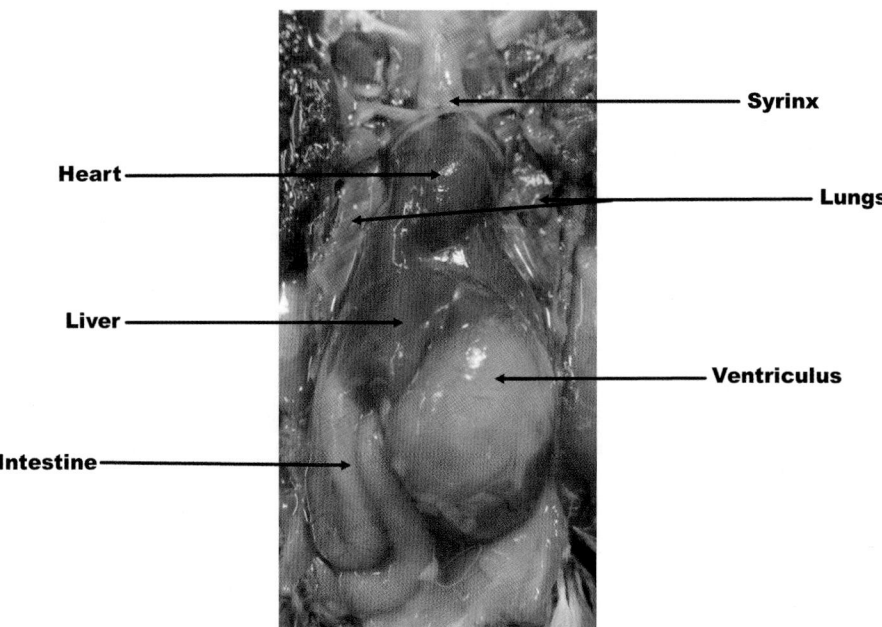

FIGURE 23.3   Photograph of zebra finch anatomy when keel and air sacs have been removed.

A. Normative Data

Limited hematological data, and perhaps no basic chemical parameters, are available specifically for laboratory zebra finches. A mean hematocrit of 51.2% (±3.6) in captive males was reported by Birkhead *et al.* (2006). Field researchers counted the number of each type of white blood cell per 1000 erythrocytes on blood smears obtained from wild-caught zebra finches (Tidemann *et al.*, 1992), while Ewenson *et al.* (2001) calculated differential leukocyte counts for zebra finches bred in an aviary for four generations. One chapter author (MP) sedated healthy-looking, adult zebra finches with isoflurane and collected cardiac blood prior to euthanasia. The heparinized blood samples were used for complete blood count and hematocrit determinations (Table 23.1), or for measuring select chemical analytes from plasma (Table 23.2). Because the number of birds sampled was limited ($n = 10$ per group), there is high variability for some values; nevertheless, general trends are evident. For example, Table 23.1 reveals that lymphocytes comprise the predominant leukocyte, with heterophils second; this relationship has been reported in some other passerines, and was also found by Ewenson *et al.* (2001) for zebra finches. As presented in Table 23.2, albumin and total protein levels are low in this species. Higher calcium values in females are presumably related to demands for egg production and would vary depending on reproductive status. Mean values of aspartate aminotransferase and creatine kinase are elevated, likely as a result of muscle activity when some of the birds struggled to avoid capture.

TABLE 23.1   Hematological Data for Adult Zebra Finches

	WBC* 10^3/μl	Hetero %	Lymph %	Mono %	Eos %	Baso %	HCT %
MALES (N = 10)							
Mean	6.7	16.0	74.7	0.8	0.1	2.4	53.0
Std Dev	2.4	10.2	10.3	0.6	0.3	2.6	5.5
Range	2.6–10.4	12–28	60–88	0–2	0–1	0–7	44–61
FEMALES (N = 10)							
Mean	6.9	32.5	59.5	0.5	0.2	7.3	51.5
Std Dev	4.0	15.5	14.2	0.7	0.4	4.2	6.1
Range	1.7–14.4	12–61	34–75	0–2	0–1	0–13	43–62
Lane**	3–8	20–65	20–65	0–1	0–1	0–5	45–62

*Each blood smear was assessed by a veterinary clinical pathologist specializing in avian medicine.
**Values reported for "finches" by Lane (1991), with no information as to finch species or collection technique.

TABLE 23.2   Chemistry Data for Adult Zebra Finches

	Alb g/dl	TP g/dl	BUN mg/dl	Glu mg/dl	Ca mg/dl	Uric acid mg/dl	Bile acids μmol/l	AST*** U/L	CK*** U/L
MALES (N = 10)									
Mean	0.9	2.3	2.8	395.9	7.1	13.8	27.8	480.3	995.4
Std Dev	0.1	0.3	1.2	33.6	0.4	4.1	8.5	181.0	497.4
Range	0.7–1.1	1.9–3	2–6	358–450	6.5–7.9	8–19.6	18.6–44.5	279–863	441–1704
FEMALES (N = 10)									
Mean	0.9	2.2	2.6	346.1	8.7	9.5	31.4	436.8	880.4
Std Dev	0.1	0.2	1.4	34.9	2.8	3.1	12.1	135.5	381.2
Range	0.7–1.1	1.9–2.5	0–5	293–403	6.5–14.7	4–13.2	12.8–51.1	226–601	477–1571
Lane**		3–5		200–450		4–12		150–350	

**Values reported for 'finches' by Lane (1991), with no information as to finch species or collection technique.
***AST and CK values are likely high as a result of muscle exertion during capture and restraint of birds.

B. Reproduction and Related Behavior

The male zebra finch sings a complex, learned song, and this is a major determinant for mate selection by females during courtship (reviewed by Riebel, 2009). Sexual preference likewise depends on appearance, in particular the redness of beaks in males (Burley and Coopersmith, 1987; Birkhead *et al.*, 1998; Simons and Verhulst, 2011; Simons *et al.*, 2012). Some studies have shown that females choose males with red leg bands versus green, along with black bands over blue (Burley *et al.*, 1982; Burley, 1986), but the effect of band color remains a topic of debate (Seguin and Forstmeier, 2012). Male social dominance is also considered to be an important criterion a female uses to select a mate (Ikebuchi and Okanoya, 2006).

Once formed, zebra finch pair bonds are very strong, and breeding occurs whenever a suitable environment is available. This results in potentially year-round breeding for captive birds; however, Williamson *et al.* (2008) found seasonal differences in clutch size and egg mass even when photoperiod, temperature, humidity, and diet were kept constant. Despite being physiologically ready to breed at 3 months of age, Nager and Law (2010) recommend waiting until a pair is at least 6–9 months old for optimal breeding results. Mutual preening and perching side-by-side can indicate a pair bond has been formed; an established pair will build and defend their nest together (Evans, 1970). Even so, given sexual attractiveness and opportunity, another male will mate with a paired female, so genetic monogamy is not a guarantee in the field or in an aviary setting with multiple birds of each sex (Burley *et al.*, 1996); extra-pair paternity in a captive setting was 10.2% in one recent study (Baran and Adkins-Regan, 2014). Conspecific brood parasitism, with an egg being cared for by other than its biological parents, is also common.

A typical zebra finch clutch will contain five white eggs (range 2–7); each egg measures 1 by 1.5 cm (Nager and Law, 2010) and weighs 1.1 g on average (Murray *et al.*, 2013). One egg is laid per day, early in the morning (Murray *et al.*, 2013), and the incubation period lasts 11–14 days from when the last egg is laid. There is biparental incubation of the eggs during the day, but only the female sits on the nest at night (Zann, 1996) and has a brood patch. In captivity, asynchronous hatching can occur because incubation may be initiated before the appearance of a final egg. After hatching, both parents will feed the nestlings and keep them warm. The crops of chicks that have been fed will be visibly distended with regurgitated seed; however, the frequency of nest visits does not reflect a parent's attentiveness to its offspring, as the young may be fed several times during one parental visit (Nager and Law, 2010). New hatchlings of domesticated birds weigh 0.6–0.9 g, compared to 10 g for fledglings, according to Zann (1996). At day 30–35, a fledgling is nutritionally independent and can be separated from its parents, but still needs to receive soft food. Personnel working with zebra finches should be aware that birds from small broods fare better in several areas of physiology and behavior compared to birds from larger broods (de Kogel and Prijs, 1996; Naguib *et al.*, 2004; Tschirren *et al.*, 2009).

V. LABORATORY MANAGEMENT AND HUSBANDRY

Most birds, including zebra finches, have received less attention from the laboratory animal community than many other animal species to date. However, a number of publications suggest a reversal of this trend; for example, a 2010 issue of the *ILAR Journal* was devoted to avian species used in research. The recent ACLAM *Laboratory Animal Welfare* text contains a chapter addressing birds as laboratory animals (Mench and Blatchford, 2014), and welfare considerations for housing all birds in captivity are discussed by Hawkins (2010). It is hoped a growing awareness has been fostered about the unique husbandry needs and clinical issues of birds.

A. Sources and Quarantine

Many researchers with zebra finches maintain a closed breeding colony in-house as much as possible, although this may come at a high economic cost (Schmidt, 2010). When birds need to be imported, they are procured from colleagues or from a limited number of pet bird dealers that, in turn, often buy zebra finches from 'backyard' breeders. The genetic makeup of birds from such vendors is unknown and not uniform (Schmidt, 2010); whereas if a research institution has maintained a closed colony for many generations, the degree of inbreeding could be important. Depending on the type of science involved, it has been recommended that research articles about zebra finches provide information on bird sources, as these could influence the outcome of particular experiments (Forstmeier *et al.*, 2007; Nager and Law, 2010).

Perhaps of greater consequence is that many commercial suppliers do little if any health monitoring of their birds prior to shipment to a research facility. In one study of 176 zebra finches, 23% of deaths occurred in the first week after arrival, while the birds were under quarantine (Prattis *et al.*, 1990). Because a given exporter might actually receive birds from various small breeding operations at different times, each individual shipment from the same vendor could be of a unique, or commingled, health status. Birds can arrive infected with diverse parasites, bacteria, and/or viruses, among other agents;

some of these have zoonotic potential. Depending on a myriad of factors, such as parasite burden, infections can stay subclinical, cause immediate morbidity or mortality, or be hidden until the eruption of an epizootic. Transport stress will also influence the health of incoming birds. Until vendors dedicated to providing 'specific pathogen-free' zebra finches become established, isolation and some diagnostic testing to characterize the birds' health profile is warranted before new zebra finches are allowed to join a resident colony. As particular research facilities may carry out limited diagnostic testing on their in-house birds, these shipments should not be exempt from a quarantine period at a new destination.

1. Health Monitoring During Quarantine

A limited, informal survey was undertaken (MP) by contacting the veterinary/research staff of 25 academic institutions using zebra finches in the United States; the objective was to learn about typical standard operating procedures for this species. Durations of quarantine are reported to last from 7 days to 6 months, but a 30-day quarantine period for zebra finches is common. In most instances, and regardless of the vendor, newly arrived zebra finches are tested for ectoparasites, e.g., feather mites, as well as for endoparasites, e.g., protozoa and helminths. Prophylactic treatment with ivermectin is frequently performed irrespective of test results; a high prevalence of feather mites in zebra finches justifies this practice. At some institutions, all incoming birds are dosed with other anthelminthics as well. Even though coccidia are frequently identified on fecal exams from zebra finches, there is little information about cases of clinical disease; hence whether antiprotozoal treatment is necessary in every instance remains unclear.

Additional quarantine testing is highly variable among the U.S. survey respondents, probably a reflection of previous experience and personal preference. Serology for viral agents, such as avian influenza and paramyxoviruses (PMVs), is submitted by an extremely limited number of groups working with zebra finches; even so, such test results have been reported as being negative overall. Only one institution reported routine testing for *Mycoplasma* spp. *Chlamydophila* and *Mycobacterium* spp. represent important zoonoses and are screened for more frequently, usually by PCR of cloacal samples; both *Mycobacterium genavense* and *M. avium* complex have been documented in laboratory populations of zebra finches according to the informal U.S. survey. Cloacal cultures are used to detect *Salmonella* sp. and other bacteria, while avian gastric yeast *(Macrorhabdus ornithogaster)* can be visualized with Gram's stains of fecal or crop samples. At the authors' institution, *Campylobacter jejuni* has been cultured using a microaerobic technique from newly arrived birds on many occasions, including

birds from different vendors and other research institutions, but associated signs of ill health have been absent. Nevertheless, positive findings for any potentially zoonotic agent necessitate occupational health training for research and husbandry staff. In addition, any bird that needs to be euthanized or dies in quarantine should undergo a complete evaluation. Depending on the size of a shipment, the necropsy of a healthy bird is warranted, as was suggested in a case report regarding suspect mycobacteriosis in a laboratory zebra finch (Asfaw and Sun, 2010).

B. Husbandry

Similar to other laboratory animals, the housing and care of captive zebra finches should mimic natural conditions for the species as much as is possible, and even simple enrichment has been shown to encourage more normal behavior (Jacobs et al., 1995). Because the ability to fly and roost is central to their behavioral repertoire, adequate space for flight and a variety of perches are critical to zebra finch welfare. It has been suggested that cage width can be sacrificed, if necessary, in exchange for more cage height and length that increase the distance available for free flight (Hawkins et al., 2001). Nager and Law (2010) commented that housing densities can be higher for the gregarious zebra finch than for some other bird species. Housing in isolation should be avoided, unless it is scientifically or medically justified. Specific aspects of husbandry will depend on the type of research being performed; for example, some institutions co-house zebra finches successfully with other avian species, such as society or Bengalese finches *(Lonchuria striata domestica)* and a variety of African finches, under aviary conditions.

1. Caging

ILAR's *Guide for the Care and Use of Laboratory Animals* (2011) does not address minimum cage space per bird for *T. guttata*. 'Common practice' space allowances for zebra finches, along with recommendations for 'good practice', as determined by the United Kingdom Joint Working Group (Hawkins et al., 2001), are presented in Table 23.3; guidelines from the Commission of the European Communities (2007), which have already been implemented in Germany (Poot et al., 2012), are comparable to the U.K.'s for 'good practice.' The U.K. dimensions pertain to standard and double canary cages for a breeding pair and up to six birds, respectively, and to aviary-type cages for larger groups. Those authors stress that aviary housing is preferred for zebra finches in most cases. A caveat to this suggestion would include situations where the birds need to be caught frequently, as capture is very stressful to all birds in the enclosure.

TABLE 23.3   Cage Parameters for Zebra Finches

	Minimum area (m²)		Minimum height (m)		Minimum cage volume (m³)/bird (assuming maximum number of birds in cage)	
	'Common practice'	'Good practice'	'Common practice'	'Good practice'	'Common practice'	'Good practice'
Breeding pair	0.3	0.5	0.3	0.3	0.045	0.075
Up to 6 birds	0.6	1	0.3	1	0.03	0.17
7–12 birds	1	1.5	1.5	2	0.125	0.25
12+ birds	1.5	2+	2	2	Not done	Not done

Adapted from Hawkins et al. (2001).

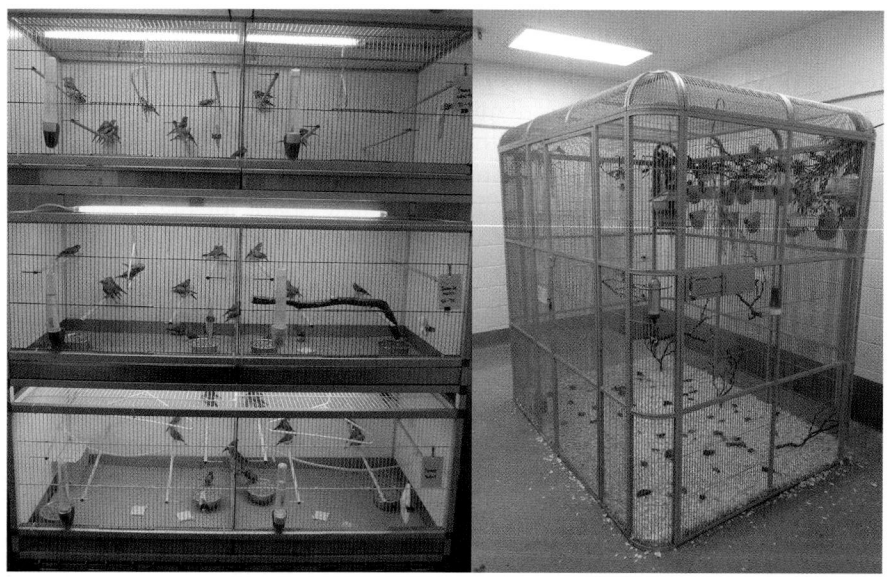

FIGURE 23.4   Examples of caging for zebra finches. *Picture on the right is courtesy of Dale Aycock.*

In U.S. research facilities as well, zebra finches are housed in various types of enclosures, ranging from small cages for a breeding pair, to flight cages and aviaries (Fig. 23.4). To give an indication of stocking densities for research zebra finches in the United States, cage volumes per bird were calculated for 40 cage types dispersed among 18 institutions (experimental cages not included) that were surveyed; of these cages, 45% (18/40) provided at least 0.03 m³ (1 ft³) cage volume per bird, which is the least amount of space given per bird in Table 23.3 and represents a reasonable minimum standard for U.S. facilities housing zebra finches, whenever feasible. Larger cages and lower population densities have been correlated with improved animal welfare (more flying, more vocalization, less stereotypic hopping, less aggression) in several studies (Jacobs *et al.*, 1995; Poot *et al.*, 2012). Indeed, conspecific aggression is the clinical issue most often reported by personnel working with zebra finches, and too little space is an important factor affecting the social dynamics within an enclosure. Also it must be noted that the data about cage dimensions given in Table 23.3 do not include how many offspring are allowed to remain in the home cage of a breeding pair, and for how long. Because juvenile males being tutored by their male parent is a common research paradigm, breeding cages can contain more than one generation of offspring at a time, leading to overcrowded conditions. Auxiliary housing for bird experiments, such as individual birds being kept in isolation chambers for song recording, should be described in an IACUC-approved protocol.

Zebra finches like to forage and eat off the ground, so their cages should have a solid floor that is covered with shavings, some type of paper liner, or other material. The floor covering will need to be changed twice a week or more in small breeding cages, but less often in spacious aviaries. The front of the enclosure, at least, should be open with a mesh or bars about 1 cm apart, and the

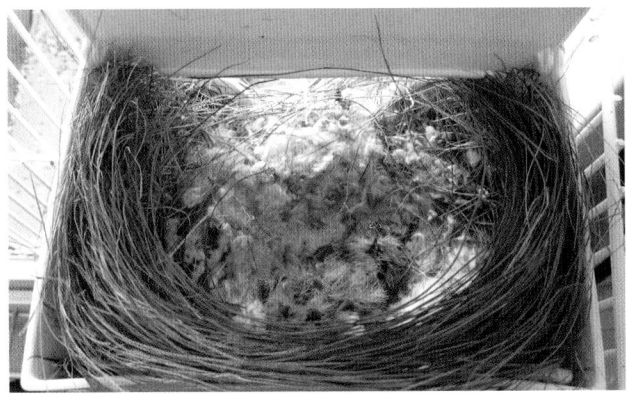

FIGURE 23.5 Zebra finch nest with hatchlings (nest box top has been opened).

cage should be constructed of a durable, nontoxic material that can withstand facility cagewash temperatures. Some institutions design their aviary cages in-house; in addition, there are a few companies specializing in customized caging for birds. Sanitation frequency for cages depends on size and stocking density, but monthly or bimonthly intervals are typical.

Nesting sites and suitable nesting materials are critical to promote successful breeding in zebra finches (Fig. 23.5). Plastic nest boxes attached outside the cage are advantageous because they can be checked without disturbing birds inside the cage itself. Popular nesting materials include sisal string, twine, coconut husk fiber, burlap squares, and cotton 'nestlets.' Loose threads that can entangle bird toes should be avoided; also Muth *et al.* (2013) determined that certain colors of nesting materials, e.g., blue, are preferred over others. One potential concern with nest boxes is that the breeding pair will line them with nesting material to the level of the entrance, which occasionally allows hatchlings and eggs to fall out. A second issue is that, in the interest of maximizing production and not interrupting parental care, investigator staff might be reluctant to have nests sanitized between clutches. Despite laboratory zebra finches being capable of breeding year round, rest periods should be imposed, e.g., two 30-day periods per year; these breaks are facilitated by the removal of all nest materials and boxes. When clutches are present, nest boxes should be opened infrequently.

2. Other Environmental Enrichment

Besides nesting sites, perches comprise an essential physical component of a zebra finch enclosure. Sufficient perches should be placed such that all birds can roost comfortably at one time, but they should not be so plentiful as to preclude the birds' flight. Installing perches at different heights, with some placed close to the top of the cage (about 15 cm from the top), is ideal (Hawkins *et al.*, 2001). Perches comprised of a mix of materials and

sizes gives each bird an opportunity to flex its toes and leg muscles. In addition to inflexible wooden dowels and more natural branches, e.g., commercially available manzanita products, plastic clothes hangers and swings made out of tubing or plastic-covered clothesline force the bird to keep balanced using its whole body. Such mobile perches are very popular; it is preferred they be long enough to allow two or more birds to co-habit them simultaneously. Perches with very rough surfaces can cause foot abrasions and should be used with caution. Commercial perches are available that are covered on both sides and the top, i.e., plastic 'stress' perches; these afford a respite from other birds. All perches should be easy to sanitize or disposable, and care staff should not position perches over feed or water containers.

Zebra finches enjoy bathing in shallow bowls of water, which encourages preening behavior. Many facilities place water baths in cages once a week or even daily; in some cases, they are removed after a few hours to prevent the accidental drowning of young birds. Sand baths for enrichment can be beneficial as well. Various toys for pet birds, such as 'bird pacifiers,' are often purchased to hang in finch cages. In aviary situations with group housing, hanging artificial vegetation or other kinds of visual barrier allows stressed or subordinate birds to shelter from conspecifics. However, whether providing an option for cover always improves the welfare of zebra finches is uncertain; in one study (Collins *et al.*, 2008), covering a third of a cage housing three males with an opaque cloth increased the birds' fearfulness of humans over time.

3. Food and Water

A good quality, mixed seed diet (especially red and white millet, and canary grass seed) is typically provided for zebra finches, with feeders scattered around the cage to prevent competition. The seed bowls need to be freshened or replaced frequently because of hull accumulation and inevitable spillage, albeit seed on the floor will encourage the birds to explore. Foraging behavior is also fostered by the placement of millet sprays. As a seed diet alone will not meet all of a bird's nutritional requirements (Harper and Skinner, 1998), e.g., for micronutrients, commercial seed mixes are often fortified with vitamins and minerals in the form of balls designed to taste and look like the seeds themselves. Concomitant protein deficiencies from seed-based diets, especially in breeding birds and juveniles on their own, can be addressed in various ways. For example, a mash of hard-boiled eggs mixed with water and a powder containing dehydrated greens, or some other high protein source, is one standard and palatable supplement to be given daily or on alternating days. Nutritionally adequate granular diets and powdered foods that can be mixed with water to form crumbles are also widely available. Other desirable foodstuff options include sprouted seeds and dark greens, e.g., kale; both of these should be rinsed well with water before use to minimize the risk of pathogen transmission. Slices of fruit or vegetables can be offered; these and leafy greens are excellent sources of carotenoids, which have been shown to affect bill color and overall health (McGraw et al., 2005). Live insects, such as mealworms, are alternative sources of protein and also serve as enrichment. All of these supplements should be fed in limited amounts if overeating and obesity are observed (Hawkins et al., 2001). Mean individual metabolizable energy intake for unfasted zebra finches on a seed diet has been determined (Harper et al., 1998), while Duerr (2008) offers dietary recommendations in the event that a zebra finch hatchling needs to be fed by hand.

Cuttlebones, essential as a source of calcium, should be available in every zebra finch cage. Whether grit is necessary for zebra finches is controversial, as they dehusk their seeds prior to ingestion. Dorrestein (2009b) cites a study in canaries where the presence or absence of grit, both soluble and insoluble, did not affect food intake or digestibility. If supplied, the amount of grit needs to be limited and monitored to prevent impaction resulting from engorgement.

Fresh water should always be present in the laboratory setting, albeit wild zebra finches without an external water source can survive for long periods and water deprivation for 2 days was less of an energetic challenge than food deprivation (Rashotte et al., 2001). Water can be provided via water dishes, bottles with sipper tubes, or water containers designed for birds; these options often need to be sanitized once a week because of algae growth. Automatic watering systems designed for birds are also suitable. It is important to prevent fecal contamination of food or water, and any change in diet or watering schedules should be implemented gradually to allow the birds to adjust (Prattis et al., 1990).

4. Environmental Monitoring

Wild counterparts of today's laboratory zebra finches inhabit the arid and semi-arid central zones of the Australian continent, i.e., all except borders in the tropical north and the wet, cool south; winter temperatures for these birds can drop to below freezing. This situation has been extrapolated to suggest laboratory zebra finches can tolerate very low temperatures, and Meijer et al. (1996) reported gradually decreasing temperatures in zebra finch enclosures from 20°C to 5°C. Although a cooler environment is safer than overheating, temperature extremes, especially sudden ones, are not advisable. Many zebra finch rooms in U.S. research institutions are kept at 70–80°F (21–27°C), and close to 75°F is optimal according to U.S. survey respondents. Likewise reported

humidity ranges are typically 30–70%. Cynx (2001) observed that egg laying and nest building decreased in indoor aviaries during the winter when the relative humidity was often below 10%, but does not mention the birds were otherwise impacted. When the humidity was experimentally increased to around 60–70%, males sang more and gathered more nest materials, whereas females were unaffected. It should be appreciated that the microenvironment of a small finch cage, with respiring birds and perhaps standing water bowls, will not be identical to the macroenvironment of the holding room. Conventional air change standards of 12–15 per hour are adequate for zebra finches.

With regard to photoperiod, zebra finches are typically maintained on a 12:12 or 14:10 hour light–dark cycle, and the lights should go on and off gradually to simulate natural conditions. Experiments by Meijer et al. (1996) showed that long photoperiods increased body mass and fat reserves in zebra finches, along with their readiness to breed; the effect of photoperiod was independent of the actual feeding period. Around 500 lux light levels are of adequate brightness for birds, as they are for humans; Nager and Law (2010) report that low light levels (under 20 lux) can be stressful. Zebra finches perceive light in the ultraviolet range, and this parameter affects how they react to the appearance of conspecifics, e.g., leg-band colors (Hunt et al., 1997). It is also hypothesized that birds have a higher temporal resolution compared to humans, so they may perceive the flicker emitted from typical low-frequency fluorescent lights (120 Hz in the United States). In experiments with European starlings, the females chose different mates under low-frequency versus high-frequency (over 30 kHz, when flicker is imperceptible) fluorescent lights (Evans et al., 2006). Thus the type of fluorescent tube used when housing zebra finches should be considered, and the high-frequency type with some UV component to mimic daylight is recommended (Nager and Law, 2010). In the event of a power failure, emergency lighting must be available as the birds will not consume food in the dark.

Care should be taken to avoid housing zebra finches where there are low frequency vibrations and white noise. Swaddle and Page (2007) showed that females' preference for their pair-bonded males, compared with extra-pair males, decreased significantly as the amplitude of environmental noise was increased. This result was presumably because the bonded males' pair-maintaining calls were masked or distorted. When zebra finches heard supplemental playback sounds from their own colony during the courtship period, the males sang more and the females had larger clutches (Waas et al., 2005). These studies indicate that acoustic 'social stimulation,' but not extraneous noise, is beneficial.

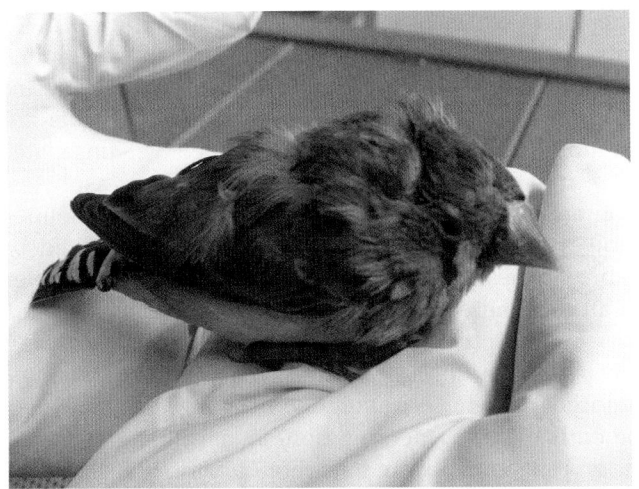

FIGURE 23.6   Adult female zebra finch with puffed feathers and immobile stance.

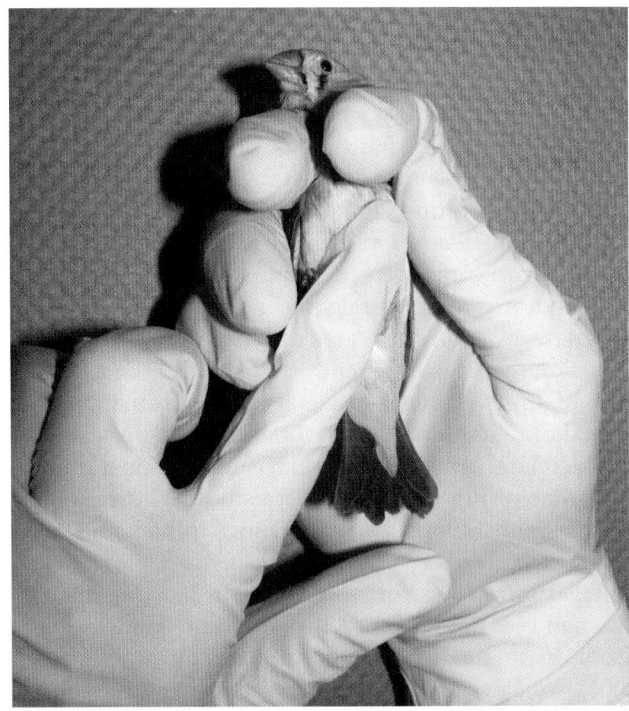

FIGURE 23.7   Recommended method for restraining a zebra finch.

C. Veterinary Care and Procedures

1. Evaluating an Unhealthy Bird

Personnel taking care of zebra finches should observe the birds unobtrusively in their enclosure for several minutes to assess whether an individual bird needs further attention. Signs for concern include obvious wounds, unexpected feather loss, partially closed eyes, open-mouth breathing, an irregular body contour, e.g., a swollen body part or ruffled feathers, an abnormal perch stance, and reluctance to move (Fig. 23.6). Abnormal droppings in the cage also need to be monitored: the fecal portion should be formed, with its color influenced by diet; urates should be white and somewhat moist; and discolored or unusual amounts of urine can reflect various disease states or be spurious, e.g., transient polyuria associated with excitement (Doneley, 2011). As both a bird being captured and its cagemates will be stressed by the procedure, this should be performed quickly and calmly. With some cage designs, a temporary divider can be inserted to reduce the area available for escape attempts. Using a flashlight to locate and grasp a particular bird after the room lights have been turned off is another strategy. Of interest is that zebra finches can become habituated to handling by humans if they are rewarded with a desirable food treat (Collins *et al.*, 2008).

During a physical examination, and whenever a zebra finch is restrained, its' respiratory movements must not be impeded. The method shown in Fig. 23.7 allows for inspection of the head and oropharynx, nares, crop contents, vent, wings and feet, feathers, skin and, importantly, the bird's body condition based on the pectoral musculature overlying the keel and ribs. Hydration status can be estimated by the moistness of mucous membranes, the presence of sunken eyes, and skin turgor. Coelomic contents are partially visible when warm saline or water is put on the midline and the feathers are parted. A sick finch can become totally decompensated with excessive handling, so the examination should be as rapid as possible and emergency supplies organized beforehand. Repeated short sessions, with periods of rest inbetween, are indicated when treating and obtaining diagnostic samples from a compromised patient.

2. Blood Sample Collection, Injections, and Treatments

A drop of blood for a blood smear or sex determination can be obtained from the right jugular or basilic vein using an insulin syringe; filling microhematocrit tubes from the hub of a needle inserted into the vein is an alternative method for collecting small amounts of blood (de Matos and Morrisey, 2005). Blood collection by clipping a toe is painful and unacceptable in perching birds such as zebra finches. If larger amounts of blood (500–800 μl) are required, cardiac puncture can be performed as a terminal event under anesthesia. Intramuscular injections should consist of small volumes administered into either pectoral muscle; a 27-gauge or smaller needle is suitable to minimize the risk of hemorrhage and muscle damage. Often subcutaneous injections are preferable; in zebra finches, medications given by this route are quickly absorbed. During an intracoelomic injection, the air sacs can be avoided by inserting the needle into the lower third of the body on the midline. Oral gavage needles designed for mice work well in zebra finches.

When warranted, fluid replacement therapy in zebra finches is most easily administered via the oral and/or subcutaneous routes. For intraosseous placement of a catheter in small birds, a 27-gauge needle in the distal ulna has been recommended (de Matos and Morrisey, 2005). A dehydrated bird should receive its calculated fluid deficit over 2–3 days, divided into two or more doses per day, along with maintenance fluids (50 ml/kg per day). Part of this volume can be given by crop gavage of crystalloid solutions or nutritious liquids designed for tube-feeding. The interscapular and inguinal regions are suitable sites for subcutaneous fluids; however, this route is not advised for a bird in hypovolemic shock where absorption will be poor (Doneley, 2011). More detailed guidelines for supportive and emergency care of small birds are provided by de Matos and Morrisey (2005), avian medical textbooks (Harrison and Lightfoot, 2006; Doneley, 2011), and other sources.

3. Anesthesia and Analgesia

Inhalational anesthetics, e.g., isoflurane, are most frequently used for zebra finches that undergo surgical procedures. When head fixation in a stereotaxic device is required, the isoflurane can be administered via a modified face mask or by taping a small (#5) French catheter just inside the oral cavity (Dr. Kvin Lertpiriyapong, personal communication); cannulation of an air sac for anesthetic gas delivery has also been described (Nilson et al., 2005). Parenteral drugs are less desirable because it is impossible to modulate anesthetic depth and recovery times are prolonged, but can be given if necessary, e.g., mixtures of ketamine and xylazine. When only deep sedation is required, 5–10 mg/kg diazepam IM provided a safe and dose-dependent duration of sedation that allowed minimally invasive procedures to be performed on zebra finches (Prather, 2012). Administration of the antagonist flumazenil at 0.3 mg/kg IM enabled the birds to recover from sedation and resume their normal activity rapidly. Schmidt (2010) summarizes how different anesthetics can influence neural response properties in songbirds. Buprenorphine (0.1 mg/kg IM) and carprofen (5–10 mg/ kg IM) are appropriate for analgesia and to reduce inflammation, respectively, although such drugs have not been critically evaluated in zebra finches or most other bird species (Machin, 2005; Hawkins and Paul-Murphy, 2011).

4. Euthanasia

According to the *AVMA Guidelines for Euthanasia* (2013), intracoelomic barbiturates and their congeners are acceptable for the euthanasia of avian species. At one point, the Guidelines state that the bird should be under anesthesia or unconscious when a barbiturate is given intracoelomically; nevertheless, the authors have found that 50 μl of a sodium pentobarbital solution injected medially into the caudal coelom causes no visible discomfort to an appropriately restrained yet unsedated bird. Inhaled anesthetics and carbon dioxide asphyxiation are acceptable with conditions per the Guidelines. However, aversive behavior is typically exhibited by zebra finches when carbon dioxide is introduced, even at an extremely low flow rate; isoflurane anesthesia followed by a physical method, in contrast, is much less stressful. The 2013 Guidelines require that unwanted embryos that have undergone over 50% of incubation be euthanized by decapitation, an anesthetic overdose, or prolonged exposure to carbon dioxide (over 20 min).

5. Bird Identification

Individual birds are often identified by the placement of metal or plastic leg bands. With leg band placement, staff should be cognizant of potential effects of different colored bands and band arrangements on sexual attractiveness (Burley et al., 1982; Burley, 1986; Swaddle and Cuthill, 1994; Hunt et al., 1997; Waas and Wordsworth, 1999). Leg bands have also been shown to affect male–male interactions, e.g., males with red bands were dominant over males with green bands (Cuthill et al., 1997). Toe clipping for identification purposes should not be permitted in zebra finches.

6. Routine Health Surveillance

The frequency at which routine health monitoring is performed on research zebra finches is unknown. If the colony is large (20 U.S. institutions supplying zebra finch colony information had daily censuses ranging from 50–1200 birds), a basic health monitoring program could be comprised of annual or semiannual fecal exams and fecal cultures on pooled samples, in addition to feather checks for ectoparasites. When other problems specific to the colony have been identified, the general scheme for testing should be modified appropriately.

VI. DISEASES/WELFARE CONCERNS

A. Noninfectious

1. Intraspecific Aggression

In contrast to many other avian species, zebra finches usually tolerate other individuals in close proximity; nonrelated conspecifics might keep themselves separated by small distances, but this is done by avoidance instead of by aggression (Caryl, 1975). Territorial behavior only involves defense of the nest itself, an area about 20 cm in diameter (Poot et al., 2012). The birds will fight over food (rare in captivity), nesting sites, desirable places to perch, and preferred mates (Caryl, 1975); levels of aggression are lower in non-breeding periods, when actual fighting is rare (Evans, 1970). Primary categories of agnostic interactions in zebra finches that are tracked by behaviorists include (Ardia *et al.*, 2010): bill fences – jabbing or pecking at the head of an opponent; displacement – driving an individual off of its perch; and chase – following an individual after it has been displaced; these behaviors are commonplace but usually not traumatic.

Comparatively more severe injuries, leading to wounds and/or feather loss from alloplucking, comprise the most common clinical issue involving zebra finch colonies according to U.S. survey respondents. An important factor influencing these incidents is overcrowding, as separating birds into smaller groups can solve the problem. Lack of nesting materials is also a potential trigger (Nager and Law, 2010). In German experiments comparing zebra finches in 'high density' versus 'low density' housing (given the cage volume per bird always surpassed European Commission standards per Table 23.3), the number of aggressive encounters (no injuries) was significantly higher in the 'high density' aviaries (Poot *et al.*, 2012). More enrichment in the cage might also reduce aggression, although controlled studies to investigate this subject are needed. Care staff should be aware that bald patches on birds can also result from self-plucking or molting; in addition, juveniles can experience irregular feather patterns as they transition to their full adult plumage.

Although females will also injure one another, cages with only male birds have been reported to have more aggressive encounters than cages with only female birds. A number of authors have correlated testosterone with aggression (Arnold, 1975; Adkins-Regan, 1999; Goodson and Adkins-Regan, 1999). In some zebra finch facilities, allowable housing densities for all-male cages are lower than for cages of females because of this gender effect. Another potentially aggressive situation is fledglings being attacked by the adult male, and occasionally by both parents, especially when several generations are housed in a small breeding cage. Zann (1996) considers parents driving off their young to be an artifact of confinement. Temporary or permanent separation of an injured bird may be necessary, as long as visual access to conspecifics is maintained.

2. Hatchling/Fledgling Loss

In the wild, a large proportion of hatched zebra finch eggs never reach adulthood. Hatchlings in captivity may fall out of a nest box if the bedding is too deep, while poor parenting behavior, especially by first-time breeders, can result in abandonment. Fledglings that leave the nest prematurely will often still be fed by the parents; regardless, extra food and water should be placed on the cage or aviary floor to support the immature birds. If neglected, chicks can be fed by hand; also society finches are sometimes used as surrogate parents for zebra finches.

3. Cage-Related, Individual Bird, and Iatrogenic Issues

Zebra finches are susceptible to 'bumblefoot' infections; these can originate from abrasions on the plantar surface in association with roughened perch surfaces. Wrapping of perches, e.g., with vet wrap, can prevent foot trauma or be part of a treatment regimen. Deformed beaks and claws that are overgrown need to be trimmed on a regular basis using sharp nail clippers or small scissors. While capturing young birds for cage transfers or other manipulations, attention should be paid to avoid their legs being caught in sliding doors, as fractures can result. Leg bands that are too tight need to be loosened or removed immediately to prevent tissue swelling and necrosis.

4. Miscellaneous Conditions – Reproductive, Neoplastic, Other

Female zebra finches can experience dystocia, or 'egg binding'; typically the bird will present with a swollen caudal coelom, tenesmus, and tail bobbing. Radiographs can be used to confirm the diagnosis, although an uncalcified egg would not be radiopaque. The bird should be put in a warm, moist, and quiet environment (incubator temperature of 85–95°F), and, if indicated, medical treatment initiated with Ca gluconate (10–100 mg/kg IM) diluted in saline every 3–6 hours (Doneley, 2011). Adequate hydration should be maintained with subcutaneous, oral, and/or intraosseous fluids. Because it is not the hormone responsible for uterine contractions in birds, the value of giving oxytocin (5 IU/kg SC or IM) is unclear; rather an intracloacal prostaglandin E2 gel, which produces sphincter dilation and straining within a few minutes, has been recommended (Doneley, 2011). Manual removal of the egg can be attempted if the bird is stable and medical intervention is unsuccessful (Sandmeier and Coutteel, 2006). In yolk coelomitis, a yellowish discoloration is often visible through the bird's skin (Fig. 23.8); euthanasia is likely indicated if large amounts of yolk are present. Such reproductive issues are more common in older birds.

Females with ovarian tumors can appear clinically similar to egg-bound females; one case at the authors' facility involved a bird over 7 years of age with a presumed ovarian carcinoma (Figs. 23.9–23.10). The cells comprising the mass were polyhedral with ill-defined borders and other neoplastic features, e.g., frequent mitotic figures. Although published reports about neoplasia in zebra finches are rare, avian researchers have established two zebra finch cell lines from spontaneous tumors (Itoh and Arnold, 2011). Malignant melanoma

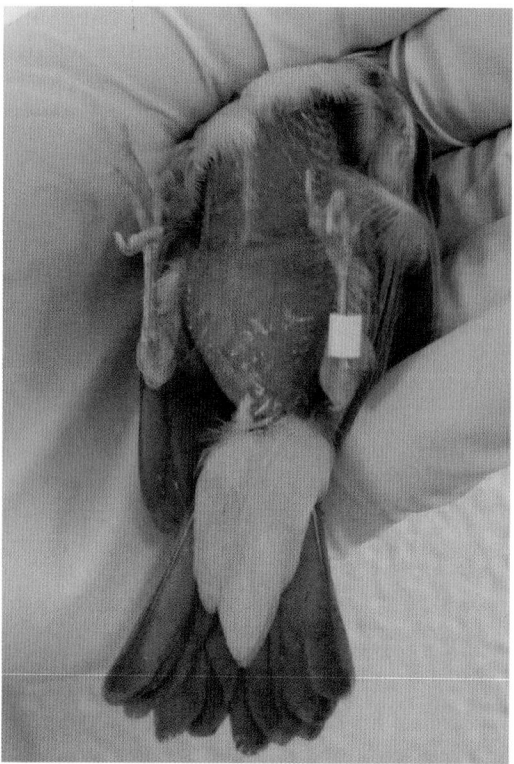

FIGURE 23.8   Female zebra finch with yolk coelomitis.

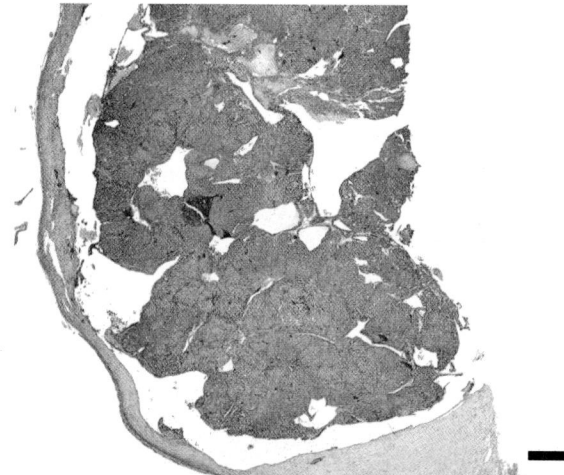

FIGURE 23.10   Ovarian tumor showing a highly cellular neoplastic mass that is lined by a thick fibrous stroma (H&E); bar is 400 μm.

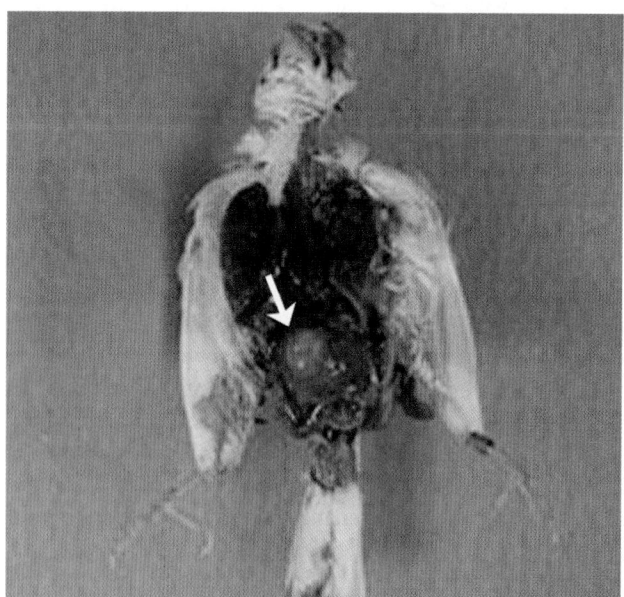

FIGURE 23.9   Ovarian mass (arrow) on gross necropsy of a female zebra finch.

has been diagnosed in the coelom of an adult male (Irizarry-Rovira *et al.*, 2007).

Personnel that work with zebra finches also encounter occasional cases of broken blood feathers, valgus

deformity (splay or spraddle leg), and general unthriftiness. Management of these and other conditions are discussed in general avian medicine and surgery texts, e.g., Harrison and Lightfoot, 2006; Doneley, 2011.

B. Infectious Diseases

Birds can be carriers of numerous zoonotic agents; these are summarized in a nonexhaustive but recent review (Boseret *et al.*, 2013). In the laboratory animal setting, the potential for transmission of infectious organisms from zebra finches to staff must be addressed as an ongoing concern. The infectious agents most frequently reported in zebra finch colonies by U.S. survey respondents were gastric yeast and subclinical mycobacteriosis, followed by various helminths and mites.

1. Viruses

Paramyxoviruses   Zebra finches are susceptible to a number of viruses. One group with potential impact is the paramyxoviruses (PMVs). In the United States, PMV-1 (Newcastle disease) is rare compared to PMV-3, which can cause clinical disease, e.g., neurologic signs, diarrhea, and occasionally respiratory signs, in psittacines and passerines (Shivaprasad, 1998). A case report of a PMV-3 outbreak in a California bird store described fatalities in parrots, canaries, and finches, but the particular finch species involved is not given (Loudis, 1999); no finches were presented for necropsy. Histopathology of several parrots with neurological signs revealed lymphoplasmacytic lesions in organs such as the spleen, pancreas, intestinal ganglia, and brain stem. PMV-3 infection can be diagnosed by serology and isolation in cell culture or inoculation of chick embryos. PMV-2 strains have also been reported in estrildid finches. At the authors' institution, serological samples from healthy birds in quarantine have been negative for PMV-1, -2, and -3, except for one positive PMV-2 sample over a decade ago; although the significance of the positive sample was unknown, the birds were healthy, used experimentally, and terminated shortly thereafter.

Avian Influenza Avian influenza, which is considered a zoonotic agent, can infect all bird species, causing sudden death, unthriftiness, respiratory and neurologic signs. Following the experimental infection of five bird species with a H5N1 strain of avian influenza, it was determined zebra finches were the most severely affected; anorexia, depression, and 100% mortality occurred within 5 days of inoculation (Perkins and Swayne, 2003). The zebra finches had no or mild gross lesions, but histologic changes and the corresponding viral antigen were found in multiple organs, especially the nasal cavity, brain, pancreas, spleen, adrenal glands, and ovary. Zebra finches, along with society finches, wild house sparrows (*Passer domesticus*), and parakeets (*Melopsittacus undulatus*), were inoculated with a human isolate of avian influenza H7N9 and all shed the virus from the oropharynx for several days (Jones *et al.*, 2014). The infected birds remained healthy in general, except for a sparrow and a zebra finch that were found dead; when these were necropsied, only the zebra finch had evidence of extrapulmonary virus. The authors propose that finches, sparrows, and parakeets can be intermediate hosts and sources of H7N9 for humans and other birds. To the authors' knowledge, no reports of naturally occurring cases of avian influenza in zebra finches have been published.

Polyomavirus Avian polyomavirus (APV) was diagnosed in a single bird at the authors' institution (Estrin *et al.*, manuscript in preparation). The adult female presented with unilateral periorbital swelling and discrete subcutaneous nodules, predominantly on the neck, thorax, and wings (Fig. 23.11). At necropsy, the surface of the crop, skeletal and cardiac muscles, intestine and mesentery were also involved. Histologically, the nodules were characterized by a highly cellular, unencapsulated, infiltrative neoplastic process comprising dense sheets of poorly differentiated, pleomorphic, neoplastic cells with mild fibrovascular stroma (Fig. 23.12). A polyomavirus etiology was suspected based on the histopathology, which included intranuclear inclusion bodies. Using PCR on frozen tissues, two avian polyomaviruses were sequenced that were unique but closest to the canary and crow strains. Some fecal samples from the colony were positive for both polyomaviruses based on qPCR of the sequenced fragment; however, signs of disease attributable to polyomavirus have not been observed except for the index case. This case was unusual because most APVs affect nestlings and do not cause tumors, e.g., an APV was associated with the deaths of nestling Gouldian finches (*Erythrura*

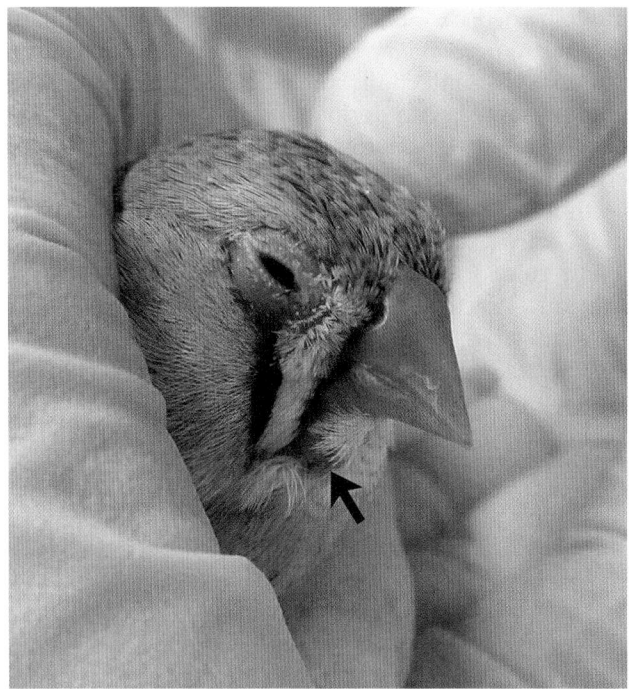

FIGURE 23.11 Female zebra finch with unilateral periorbital swelling and subcutaneous nodule under beak (arrow) associated with polyomavirus.

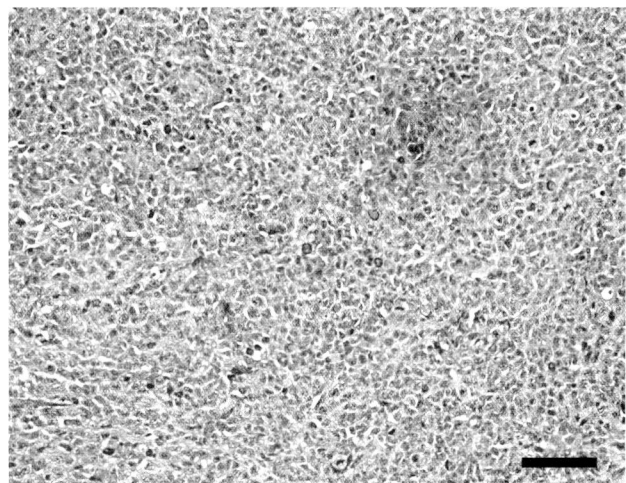

FIGURE 23.12 Histology of neoplastic nodule in a zebra finch, infected with polyomavirus, reveals dense sheets of poorly differentiated neoplastic cells (H&E); bar is 160 μm.

gouldiae) in New Zealand (Alley *et al.*, 2013). Earlier, anti-APV antibodies were identified in zebra finches as part of a report about a likely parrot polyomavirus affecting a green aracaris (Lafferty *et al.*, 1999).

Avipoxvirus Although spontaneously occurring cases have not been reported, the experimental inoculation of two wild avipoxvirus strains in zebra finches was successful (Ha *et al.*, 2013). A colony of wild-caught, gray-crowned rosy finches (*Leucosticte tephrocotis*) in an open-air rooftop aviary experienced 75% mortality from an avipoxvirus infection (Hukkanen *et al.*, 2003). Affected birds presented with dermal and mucosal lesions, anorexia, lethargy, emaciation, and sudden death; characteristic Bollinger body intracellular inclusion bodies and electron microscopy confirmed the diagnosis. The source of the virus remains unknown, but the likely route of introduction was through lice and mites acting as mechanical vectors. The authors comment that avipoxviruses can cross species and be transmitted horizontally.

2. Bacteria

Mycobacteriosis Mycobacteriosis affects birds throughout the world, and the species pathogenic to birds are considered ubiquitous environmental saprophytes (Tell *et al.*, 2001). Although *Mycobacterium avium* subsp. *avium* is the etiological agent reported in most birds with mycobacteriosis (Schrenzel *et al.*, 2008), *M. genavense* is known to predominate in psittacines and passerines (Dhama *et al.*, 2011; Shivaprasad and Palmieri, 2012). Older reports described acid-fast bacilli in birds with negative or inconclusive culture results; it is speculated these represent infections with *M. genavense*, a fastidious organism with special growth requirements (Tell *et al.*, 2001). A 20-year survey of companion birds attributed 23/24 cases of mycobacteriosis to *M. genavense*, including one of a zebra finch; the diagnoses were based on PCR and sequencing of an rRNA hypervariable region (Manarolla *et al.*, 2009). At least one earlier study also considered *M. genavense* to be the most prevalent species causing mycobacteriosis in pet birds (Hoop *et al.*, 1996).

In psittacines and passerines, mycobacterial infection most often affects the liver, spleen, and intestine (Shivaprasad and Palmieri, 2012); any of these organs can appear swollen. However, because gross lesions can be absent, detection of mycobacteriosis requires histopathology, acid-fast staining, culture, and/or PCR. Microscopic lesions in these bird groups, including canaries and finches, consist of a large number of epithelioid cells or foamy macrophages, plus or minus multinucleated giant cells, but without necrosis; thus the reaction is often 'lepromatous' instead of 'tuberculous' (Shivaprasad and Palmieri, 2012). Usually transmission is attributed to the fecal–oral, and perhaps the airborne, route. Clinical signs depend on the organ(s) involved; in one report, a pet zebra finch infected with *M. genavense* exhibited weakness, incoordination, and emaciation (Hoop *et al.*, 1993). When Sandmeier *et al.* (1997) necropsied zebra finches exhibiting central nervous system signs, acid-fast bacteria were demonstrated in the brain, liver, and intestines, and *M. genavense* was identified by PCR.

One article has been published concerning presumed mycobacteriosis in laboratory zebra finches

(Asfaw and Sun, 2010). Two months after its release from quarantine, an adult female displayed intermittent head-tossing behavior on several occasions, and was euthanized. Only microscopic lesions were observed, in particular many swollen, enlarged macrophages in the duodenum and lungs; the macrophages were packed with acid-fast-positive bacteria (Figs. 23.13–23.16). All zebra finches housed in the same room were depopulated and necropsied. Three additional animals were positive for *Mycobacterium*-like organisms, but further diagnostic tests were not performed. When U.S. veterinary/research personnel were queried about clinical issues in their zebra finch colonies, a number reported they either handled their birds as if they were positive for *Mycobacterium* spp. or they

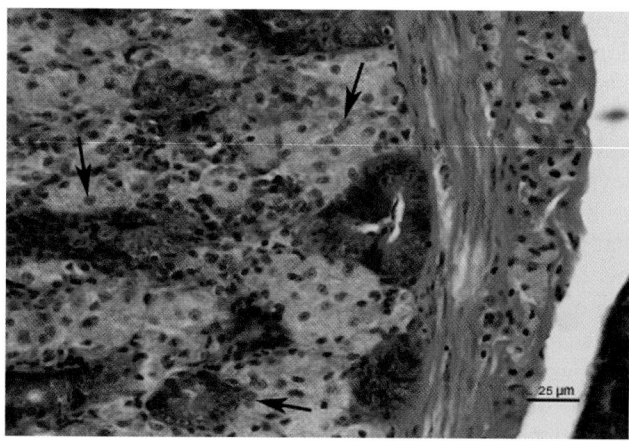

FIGURE 23.13 Zebra finch case of presumed mycobacteriosis. Many large, swollen macrophages (arrows) caused thickening of the lamina propria of the duodenal villi. Hematoxylin and eosin stain; bar, 25 μm. *Reprinted with permission from Asfaw and Sun (2010).*

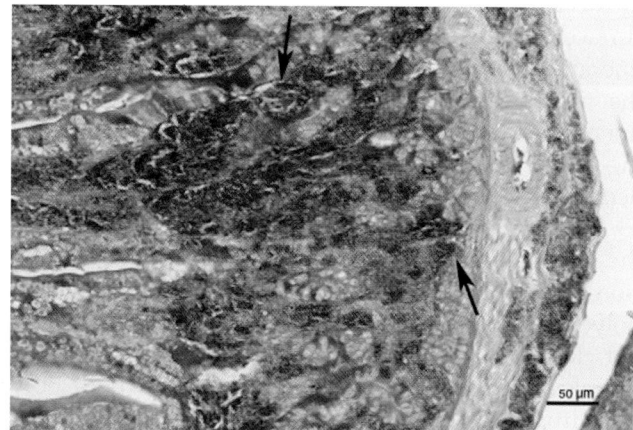

FIGURE 23.14 Acid-fast staining of duodenum revealed numerous intracellular, slender, rod-shaped, acid-fast–positive bacteria in macrophage cytoplasm (arrows) in case of presumed mycobacteriosis. Ziehl–Neelsen stain; bar, 50 μm. *Reprinted with permission from Asfaw and Sun (2010).*

considered mycobacteriosis to be endemic. Because *M. genavense* infection has been demonstrated in immunocompromised human patients, a concern for zoonotic transmission is valid and appropriate signage should be posted. Treatment of infected birds is not recommended. As the bacterium is stable in the environment for years, prevention relies on adequate cage sanitation and preventing contact with wild birds (Pollock, 2006).

Salmonellosis When a large-scale outbreak of fatal salmonellosis occurred in society finches in Japan, the causative organism was identified by culture, biochemistry, and serotyping as *Salmonella choleraesuis* subsp. *choleraesuis* serovar Typhimurium (Sato *et al.*, 1993). The livers of necropsied birds contained necrotic granulomatous lesions and cellular infiltrates. Zebra finches

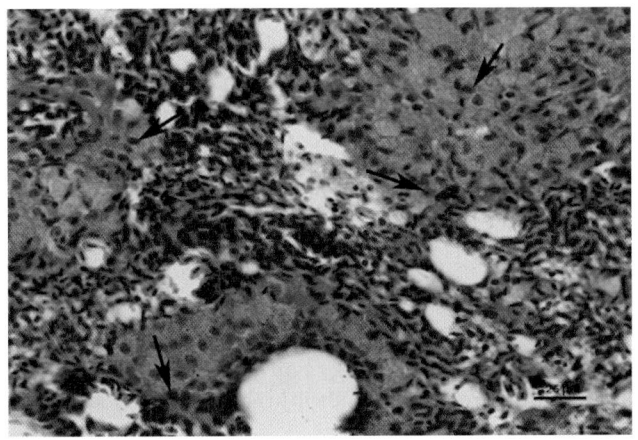

FIGURE 23.15 Zebra finch with presumed mycobacteriosis has lungs severely affected with a macrophage infiltrate (arrows) that is often oriented around the parabronchi. *Reprinted with permission from Asfaw and Sun (2010).*

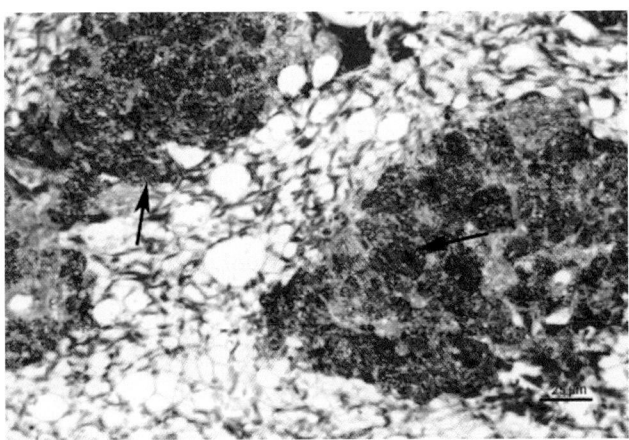

FIGURE 23.16 Acid-fast staining of lung revealed numerous intracellular, slender, rod-shaped, acid-fast–positive bacteria in the macrophage cytoplasm (arrows) in case of presumed mycobacteriosis. Ziehl–Neelsen stain; bar, 25 μm. *Reprinted with permission from Asfaw and Sun (2010).*

housed nearby were not affected at the time; however, some months later, 5/45 zebra finches died with signs that included ruffled feathers, severe diarrhea, and weakness (Sato and Wada, 1995). When a fecal sample from an apparently healthy zebra finch was cultured, *S.* Typhimurium was isolated that had the same antibiotic sensitivity and plasmids as were present in the original society finch sample. More than a year after control measures were instituted (ampicillin in the drinking water for 3 weeks, culling of sick birds, and disinfection of the premises), representative fecal samples were negative for *S.* Typhimurium; nevertheless, the authors emphasize being vigilant about chronic carriers. If warranted, a salmonellosis outbreak in a research colony of zebra finches could be treated with antibiotics chosen based on sensitivity results, often amoxicillin, trimethoprim-sulfa, or enrofloxacin, combined with proper sanitation and hygiene; 3–6 weeks after drug therapy, serial bacterial cultures should be carried out from pooled fecal samples in enriched media (Dorrestein, 2009a).

Campylobacteriosis *Campylobacter jejuni* is considered an important zoonotic pathogen that can affect juvenile estrildids, in particular (Dorrestein, 2009a; Boseret *et al.*, 2013). Society finches have been recognized as subclinical carriers. Potential clinical signs in birds are apathy, retarded molting, and formed or liquid feces that are yellow due to large amounts of undigested starch; in addition, whole seeds can be found in the droppings on occasion (Dorrestein, 2009a). Infected fledglings can experience high mortality.

Zebra finches in quarantine at the authors' institution, received from commercial vendors and from academic colleagues, have typically been culture-positive for *C. jejuni*, as have healthy birds in the resident colony during semiannual surveillance testing. Samples of the bacterium underwent 16S rRNA analysis to confirm the species. It should be stressed that *C. jejuni* requires a strict microaerobic environment for growth *in vitro*; Gram's stains of fecal samples to identify curved rods are not adequate to rule out its presence in laboratory birds. Genus-specific PCR screening for *Campylobacter* sp. can also be performed on fecal samples. *Campylobacter jejuni* is difficult to eradicate through antibiotic treatment, and subclinical carriers are common. If a colony is endemically infected, personnel should be informed of the zoonotic risk and need for proper hygiene practices.

Chlamydophilosis Psittacines are highly sensitive to *Chlamydophila psittaci*, but passerines can also be infected (Evans, 2011); infections in birds are often subclinical. Due to the zoonotic potential, cases of *C. psittaci* are reportable in most states. A few research institutions test zebra finches for *C. psittaci* in quarantine; however, there are no reports of confirmed cases in this species. Actual diagnosis of chlamydophilosis is challenging, especially in birds with no clinical signs. With sick birds, Evans (2011) recommends conjunctival and choanal swabs over feces for bacteriologic culture or PCR, as detectable levels of bacteria in feces can be absent; individual laboratories should be contacted for sample preferences and handling requirements. If warranted, doxycycline for 30–45 days is a historical treatment that is still being used to prevent an incomplete resolution of the infection; however, effective routes and durations of drug therapy for different avian species, as well as the use of other drugs like azithromycin, are being investigated (Evans, 2011).

Mycoplasmosis One U.S. research institution in the informal survey had newly acquired zebra finches test positive for *Mycoplasma* spp. by PCR on a single occasion; there were no associated clinical signs and no treatment was undertaken. In recent decades, conjunctivitis in North American house finches (*Haemorhous mexicanus*) has been related to infection with *M. gallisepticum*, a common pathogen in poultry (Hochachka et al., 2013); experimentally infected domestic canaries were similarly affected (Hawley et al., 2011). Because house finches and canaries are both in the family Fringillidae ('true' finches), it is unknown how zebra finches (family Estrildidae) might respond to a *Mycoplasma* infection. Ubiquitous wild house finches could serve as fomites for spreading infectious particles to any birds housed outdoors (Dorrestein, 2009a). *Mycoplasma* spp. are thought to respond to tetracyclines and enrofloxacin; house finches with mycoplasma-associated conjunctivitis were successfully treated with tylosin in the drinking water and ciprofloxacin ophthalmic ointment (Dorrestein, 2009a).

Other Bacteria A retrospective study was carried out on zebra finches in quarantine that exhibited clinical signs of disease and mortality (Prattis et al., 1990). *Staphylococcus aureus* and/or *S. epidermidis* were cultured from 25% of birds with respiratory or gastrointestinal signs. *Escherichia coli* and *Enterobacter* spp. were also isolated from 15% and 7% of clinically ill finches, respectively. The authors state that high numbers of gram-positive organisms and coliforms are abnormal in the respiratory and gastrointestinal tracts of healthy passerine birds, and that stress associated with shipping likely exacerbated the situation. Also of interest was that most of the sick birds had multiple nonspecific clinical signs (ruffled feathers, loose droppings, increased respiratory rate), and gross necropsy findings were not helpful in determining presumptive causes of death, i.e., serial cultures and histology are warranted in the face of colony-wide disease. The Enterobacteriaceae represent secondary pathogens in finches (species not defined) according to Dorrestein (2009a), and they are regularly cultured in passerine nestlings with diarrhea; sensitivity testing is required for treatment.

Dorrestein (2009a) associated abscesses, dermatitis, 'bumblefoot,' conjunctivitis, sinusitis, arthritis, pneumonia, and death in passerines with *Streptococcus* spp. and *Staphylococcus* spp. The same reference cited potential sources of *Pseudomonas* spp. and *Aeromonas* spp., including sprouted seeds that have not been washed adequately, in addition to contaminated drinking bowls and water baths.

3. Protozoa

Coccidiosis Coccidiosis occurs frequently in passerine birds. *Isospora* spp. (two sporocysts with four sporozoites) are more prevalent than *Eimeria* spp. (four sporocysts with two sporozoites) (Dorrestein, 2009a), but specific identification can be difficult. An older report describes the death of 7/24 zebra finches in a zoological park (Helman et al., 1984). At necropsy, most of the dead birds exhibited splenomegaly and two birds had hepatomegaly. Microscopic lesions, consisting of necrosis and granulomatous inflammation, were most severe in the liver and spleen. Macrophages contained oval to crescent-shaped organisms undergoing extraintestinal schizogony; however, oocysts were not visible in fecal examinations of the affected zebra finches. The authors attributed the mortalities to an *Isospora* or *Toxoplasma gondii* infection. Laboratory birds with coccidiosis can be administered coccidiostats such as amprolium (50–100 mg/l of drinking water for 5 days), if desired; cages should be changed near the end of the treatment period.

Cryptosporidiosis is rare in passerines. Fecal samples from 434 pet birds in China revealed 35 samples (8.1% prevalence) with *Cryptosporidium* oocysts (Qi et al., 2011). Out of 40 zebra finch samples, two were positive (5% prevalence); these were genotyped as *Cryptosporidium baileyi*. Among other passerines and psittacines, zebra finches could be infected with *Sarcocystis* sporocysts obtained from experimentally infected opossums (Box and Smith, 1982); in contrast, zebra finches resisted infection with *Neospora caninum* tachyzoites (McGuire et al., 1999).

Flagellates *Trichomonas* sp. is common in many avian species and not host specific. The flagellate can be identified in a bird, living or not, by staining a crop swab. An aviary owner in Canada lost 15/50 finches, of various types, within a few weeks of arrival; the birds developed respiratory distress and diarrhea (Chalmers, 1992). Four birds that were necropsied, including two society finches, exhibited mucosal ulceration accompanied by a yellow, caseous, adherent exudate in the pharynx and esophagus. *Trichomonas* sp. was identified by wet-mount smears of fresh material, as well as by histology. A 2006 report from the United Kingdom described an increase in trichomoniasis in wild finches associated with an increase in rainfall during the summer (Simpson and Molenaar, 2006).

Another flagellate, *Cochlosoma* sp., inhabits the intestinal tract of society finches and can cause deaths in zebra finches they have fostered (Dorrestein, 2009a). A survey of pet stores found *C. anatis*-like protozoa in several finch species (Filippich and O'Donoghue, 1997). Young zebra finches from 10 days to 6 weeks of age can exhibit debilitation, shivering from dehydration, and delayed moulting. Treatment using ronidazole (400 mg/kg in egg food or 400 mg/l drinking water) twice for 5 days, with a 2-day break inbetween, was efficacious and safe. Caution is warranted if treating with dimetridazole or metronidazole, as toxicity has been reported (Dorrestein, 2009a).

4. Fungi

Gastric Yeast The most consequential fungal disease in zebra finches is caused by *Macrorhabdus ornithogaster*, which was referred to as a 'megabacterium' but later classified definitively as a novel, anamorphic ascomycetous yeast (Tomaszewski *et al.*, 2003). Individual organisms are long, slender, and weakly gram positive; they take up periodic acid-Schiff and silver stains. In zebra finches, as in diverse other bird species, *M. ornithogaster* colonizes the luminal gastric surface, predominantly at the isthmus separating the proventriculus and ventriculus. Infections can be benign or a spectrum of diseases can develop (Phalen, 2005). A syndrome of emaciation and death was reported in canaries, budgerigars, and zebra finches (Martins *et al.*, 2006). Ulcerations and erosions of the ventriculus were evident during the necropsy of a zebra finch, and massive clumps of gastric yeast were visualized histologically.

A recent case report described an increase in morbidity and mortality over a one-month period in zebra finches maintained at an academic facility (Snyder *et al.*, 2013). In 4/6 necropsied birds, avian gastric yeast was present (Fig. 23.17), even though the birds had been treated prophylactically with amphotericin B (5 mg/ml in drinking water for 7 days, Megavac-S from Vetafarm in Australia) two months earlier. In addition, all six birds had evidence of enteritis and nephritis, and 5/6 had squamous hyperplasia of the oral and/or esophageal mucosa. An environmental assessment revealed that affected birds had been inadvertently exposed to continuous light; with correction of the light cycle and another round of amphotericin B, baseline mortality returned to normal. The severe disease outbreak was attributed to stress and immunosuppression associated with the disrupted photoperiod.

Several U.S. institutions that were surveyed commented that *M. ornithogaster* was a clinical concern and/or presence in their zebra finch colonies. Diagnosis

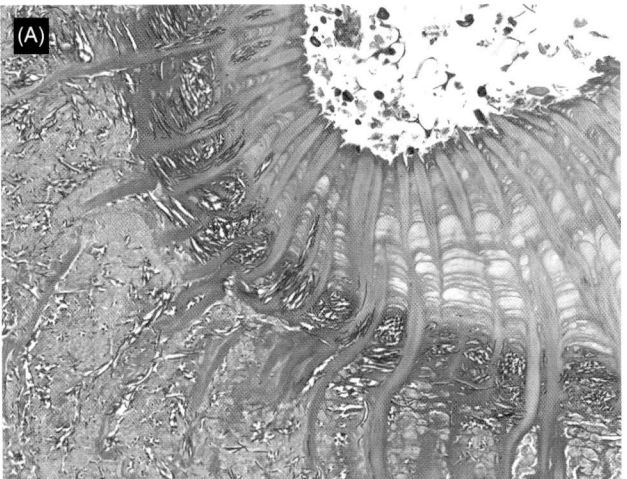

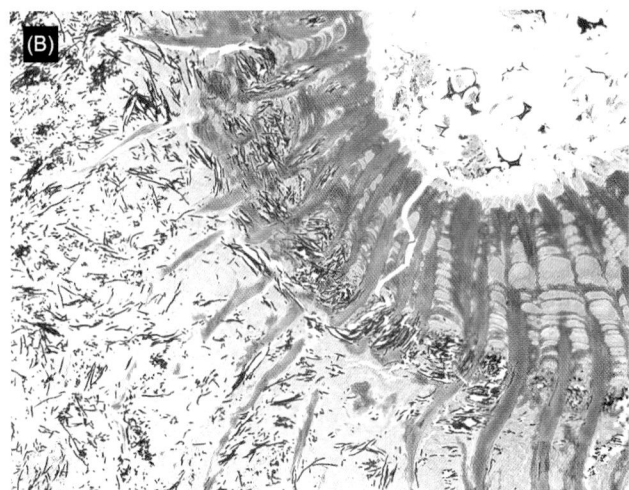

FIGURE 23.17 Ventriculus of a zebra finch infected with *Macrorhabdus ornithogaster*. (A) Periodic acid–Schiff stain. (B) Gomori methenamine silver stain. Note the abundant, long, rod-shaped organisms that stain magenta in panel A and black in panel B. Magnification, 20×. *Reprinted with permission from Snyder et al.* (2013).

can be achieved by using Gram's stain of a crop wash or fecal smear. Nevertheless, as the case report above implies, the organisms are often innocuous and in low numbers until there is an introduction of some stressor. Besides the administration of amphotericin B to treat gastric yeast, nystatin at 3,500,000 IU/l of drinking water for 2 days followed by 2,000,000 IU/l of water for 28 days was efficacious in a flock of budgerigars (Kheirandish and Salehi, 2011).

Candidiasis and Aspergillosis *Candida* spp. and *Aspergillus* spp. are associated with gastrointestinal and respiratory disease in pet birds, respectively; however, reports of infections in zebra finches are not available. Although these agents can infect humans as well as birds, evidence of transmission from birds to humans is lacking; instead humans acquire the fungi from environmental exposure (Evans, 2011).

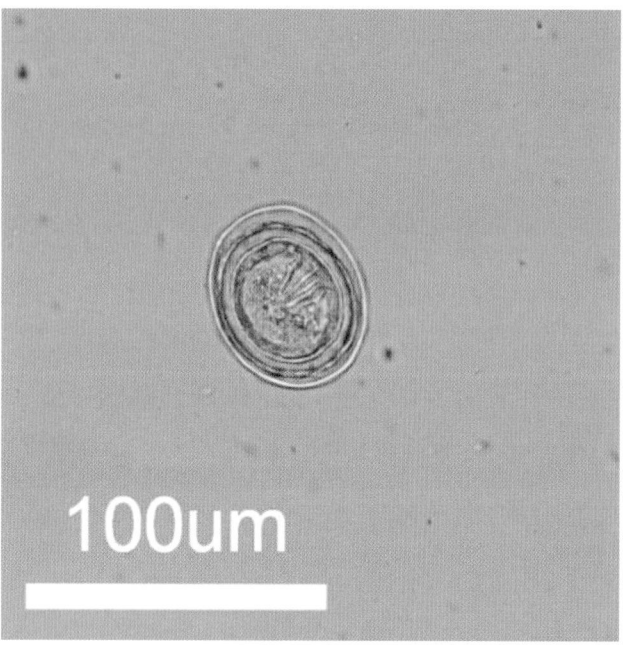

FIGURE 23.18   Tapeworm egg in a zebra finch fecal sample.

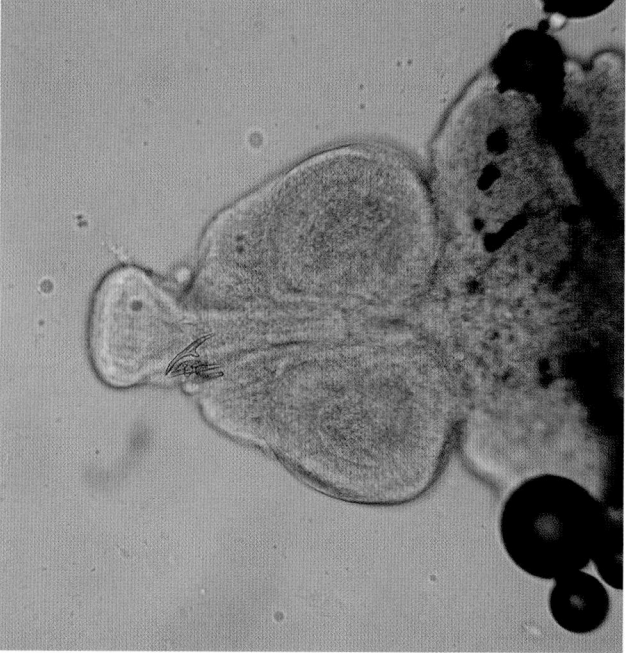

FIGURE 23.19   Scolex of *Choanotaenia* sp. found in a zebra finch. *Photograph is courtesy of Dr. Mike Kinsella.*

5. Helminths

Tapeworms   Despite a diet of predominately seeds, zebra finches can be infested with tapeworms, which generally require an insect or annelid host to complete their life cycle. At the authors' facility, several birds died or were euthanized because of ill health within 2 weeks of arrival from a vendor. At necropsy, one zebra finch was found to have its intestines impacted with worms; eggs containing hexacanth embryos were noted on fecal flotation exams (Fig. 23.18). The cestodes were identified as *Choanotaenia* sp. (courtesy of Dr. Mike Kinsella; Fig. 23.19); exact speciation was not possible because some taxonomic features, e.g., a complete ring of rostellar hooks, were lost during processing. Interestingly, there is a report of estrildid finches experiencing an infestation of *Choanotaenia* spp. in Australia about 30 years ago (McOrist *et al.*, 1984); the affected adult birds were depressed and had diarrhea prior to death. The two *Choanotaenia* spp. involved could not be determined, but one was similar to *C. infundibulum*, a tapeworm common in chickens and other birds (Morishita and Schaul, 2007), occasionally in insectivores and rodents, and at least once in a rhesus macaque (Jones *et al.*, 1980). Another U.S. research institution had zebra finches with tapeworms that were identified as *Raillietina* sp. (Dr. Larry Carbone, personal communication). Oral praziquantel (10 mg/kg in water by oral gavage weekly for 3 weeks) is effective in eliminating adult tapeworms. Most animal facilities would lack the intermediate hosts for their continued propagation.

Nematodes   Nematodes have been infrequently reported in captive finches; ivermectin (200 μg/kg) administered during quarantine would be expected to eliminate most of these. There are several reports of estrildid finch mortalities in Australia associated with the ventricular roundworm, *Acuaria skrjabini*, e.g., McOrist *et al.*, 1982; Hindmarsh and Ward, 1993, whereas *Dispharynx spiralis* was described from an adult finch, of undisclosed species, in California (Schock and Cooper, 1978). *Geopetitia aspiculata* resides in the proventriculus of several passerine species, including estrildids, and can lead to perforation of the proventricular wall (Dorrestein, 2009a). All of these are spiruroid worms with a two-host life cycle.

6. Arthropods

Dorrestein (2009a) enumerates a number of ectoparasites that can affect passerine birds, e.g., chewing and biting lice, blood-sucking mites (*Dermanyssus gallinae* and *Ornithonyssus sylviarum*; both can cause localized lesions and pruritus in humans), skin mites (*Backericheyla* spp. and *Neocheyletiella media*), and feather mites. Various quill mites have also been described in passerines. *Knemidocoptes pilae*, the scaly mite, causes hyperkeratotic lesions on the beak base and feet in finches; rarely, laboratory zebra finches have been infested with what was probably this species per U.S. survey respondents. In addition, air sac mites (*Sternostoma tracheacolum*) are reported to be

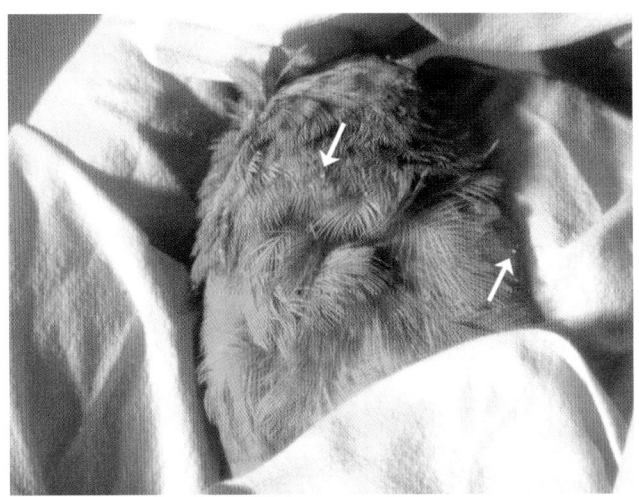

FIGURE 23.20 White specks observed on zebra finch infested with mites (arrows). *Reprinted with permission from Siddalls* et al. *(2015).*

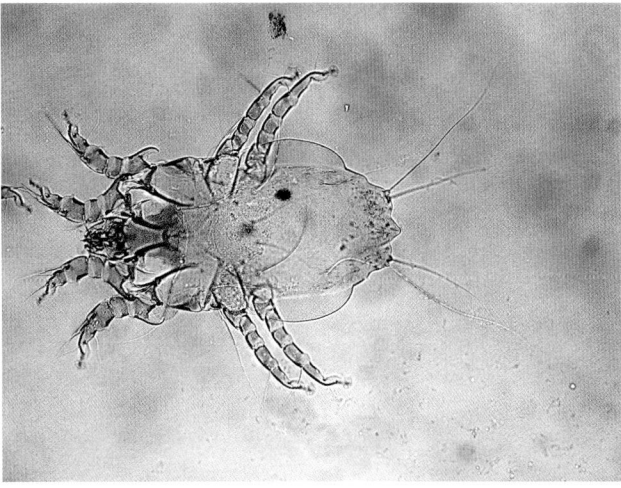

FIGURE 23.21 *Megninialges* sp. adult female. *Reprinted with permission from Siddalls* et al. *(2015).*

common in estrildid finches (Dorrestein, 2009a), with clinical signs that include respiratory distress, coughing and sneezing. The mites can be diagnosed on postmortem examination of the air sacs, lungs and/or the trachea; occasionally mites can be observed in live birds by transillumination of the trachea. Notably, an early report of *S. tracheacolum* in Gouldian finches and canaries (Riffkin and McCausland, 1972) commented that zebra finches were not affected with respiratory signs, thus leaving it equivocal regarding their susceptibility to respiratory acariasis.

Recently, two novel mite species were found on zebra finches at the authors' institution (Siddalls *et al.*, 2015). The index bird was heavily infested (Fig. 23.20) and housed in a research laboratory. A subsequent survey found mites on other birds, both in the laboratory and in the animal facility. One of the novel mite species was determined to be *Megninialges* sp. (Fig. 23.21), which represents a 'true' feather mite. The second novel mite species, in the family Cheyletidae and genus *Neocheyletiella*, was much more abundant (Figs. 23.22–23.23). Significantly, it constructs silken capsule-like nests on feathers (Fig. 23.24), in comparison to all its close relatives that are skin parasites and not known to construct nests; this mite has been given a scientific name, *Neocheyletiella parvisetosa* (Mertins and Bochkov, 2014). Multiple treatments with a pyrethrin spray were used to eradicate the mites, even though some estrildids are reported to be sensitive to this drug (Dorrestein, 2009a). Ivermectin treatment (200 µg/kg diluted in propylene glycol and applied topically) was later found to be more efficacious in treating such ectoparasites, and less labor intensive.

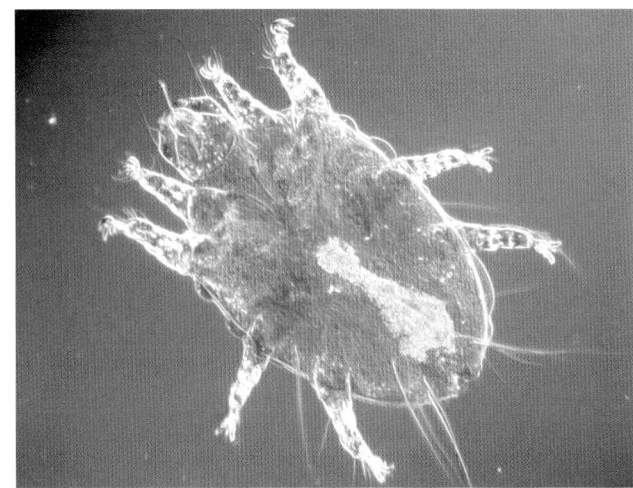

FIGURE 23.22 *Neocheyletiella parvisetosa*, adult female. *Reprinted with permission from Siddalls* et al. *(2015).*

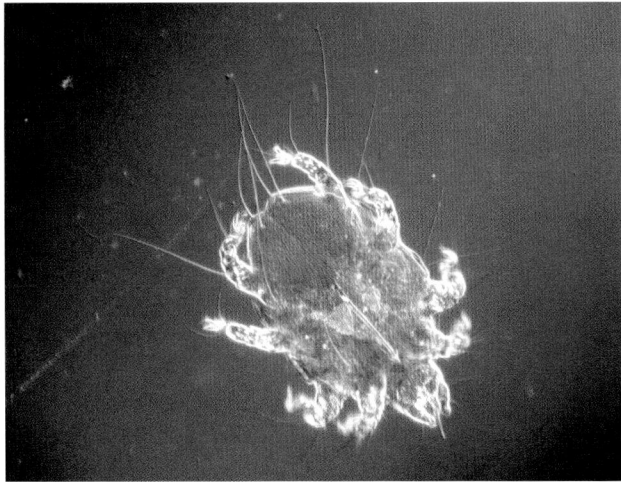

FIGURE 23.23 *Neocheyletiella parvisetosa*, adult male. *Reprinted with permission from Siddalls* et al. *(2015).*

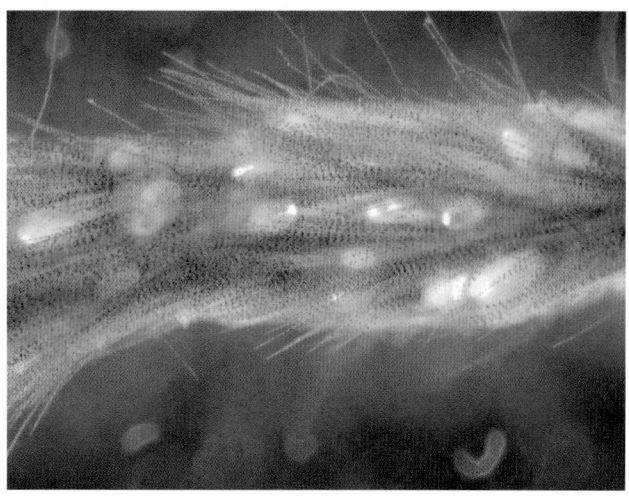

FIGURE 23.24 Silken nest capsules and various life stages of *Neocheyletiella parvisetosa*. *Reprinted with permission from Siddalls* et al. *(2015).*

References

Adkins-Regan, E., 1999. Testosterone increases singing and aggression but not male-typical sexual partner preference in early estrogen-treated female zebra finches. Horm. Behav. 35, 63–70.

Agate, R.J., Scott, B.B., Haripal, B., Lois, C., Nottebohm, F., 2009. Transgenic songbirds offer an opportunity to develop a genetic model for vocal learning. Proc. Natl. Acad. Sci. USA 106, 17963–17967.

Alarcón, M., Abrahams, B.S., Stone, J.L., Duvall, J.A., Perederiy, J.V., Bomar, J.M., et al., 2008. Linkage, association, and gene-expression analyses identify CNTNAP2 as an autism-susceptibility gene. Am. J. Hum. Genet. 82, 150–159.

Alley, M.R., Rasiah, I., Lee, E.A., How, L., Gartrell, B.D., 2013. Avian polyomavirus identified in a nestling Gouldian finch (Erythrura gouldiae) in New Zealand. N. Z. Vet. J. 61, 359–361.

Andalman, A.S., Fee, M.S., 2009. A basal ganglia-forebrain circuit in the songbird biases motor output to avoid vocal errors. Proc. Natl. Acad. Sci. USA 106, 12518–12523.

Ardia, D.R., Broughton, D.R., Gleicher, M.J., 2010. Short-term exposure to testosterone propionate leads to rapid bill color and dominance changes in zebra finches. Horm. Behav. 58, 526–532.

Arnold, A.P., 1975. The effects of castration and androgen replacement on song, courtship, and aggression in zebra finches (Poephila guttata). J. Exp. Zool. 191, 309–326.

Aronov, D., Veit, L., Goldberg, J.H., Fee, M.S., 2011. Two distinct modes of forebrain circuit dynamics underlie temporal patterning in the vocalizations of young songbirds. J. Neurosci. 31, 16353–16368.

Asfaw, Y.G., Sun, F.J., 2010. Presumed mycobacteriosis in laboratory zebra finch (Taeniopygia guttata). J. Am. Assoc. Lab. Anim. Sci. 49, 644–646.

AVMA, 2013. In: AVMA, AVMA Guidelines for the Euthanasia of Animals: 2013 Edition AVMA, Schaumburg, IL.

Baran, N.M., Adkins-Regan, E., 2014. Breeding experience, alternative reproductive strategies and reproductive success in a captive colony of zebra finches (Taeniopygia guttata). PLoS One 9 (2), e89808. doi:10.1371/journal.pone.0089808.

Bateson, M., Feenders, G., 2010. The use of passerine bird species in laboratory research: implications of basic biology for husbandry and welfare. ILAR J. 51, 394–408.

Beecher, M.D., Brenowitz, E.A., 2005. Functional aspects of song learning in songbirds. Trends Ecol. Evol. 20, 143–149.

Birkhead, T.R., Fletcher, F., Pellatt, E.J., 1998. Sexual selection in the zebra finch Taeniopygia guttata: condition, sex traits and immune capacity. Behav. Ecol. Sociobiol. 44, 179–191.

Birkhead, T.R., Pellatt, E.J., Matthews, I.M., Roddis, N.J., Hunter, F.M., McPhie, F., et al., 2006. Genic capture and the genetic basis of sexually selected traits in the zebra finch. Evolution 60, 2389–2398.

Boseret, G., Losson, B., Mainil, J.G., Thiry, E., Saegerman, C., 2013. Zoonoses in pet birds: review and perspectives. Vet. Res. 44, 36.

Bottjer, S.W., Miesner, E.A., Arnold, A.P., 1984. Forebrain lesions disrupt development but not maintenance of song in passerine birds. Science 224, 901–903.

Box, E.D., Smith, J.H., 1982. The intermediate host spectrum in a Sarcocystis species of birds. J. Parasitol. 68, 668–673.

Brainard, M.S., Doupe, A.J., 2013. Translating birdsong: songbirds as a model for basic and applied medical research. Annu. Rev. Neurosci. 36, 489–517.

Burley, N., 1986. Comparison of the band-colour preferences of two species of estrildid finches. Anim. Behav. 34, 1732–1741.

Burley, N., Coopersmith, C.B., 1987. Bill color preferences of zebra finches. Ethology 76, 133–151.

Burley, N., Krantzberg, G., Radman, P., 1982. Influence of colour-banding on the conspecific preferences of zebra finches. Anim. Behav. 30, 444–455.

Burley, N.T., Parker, P.G., Lundy, K., 1996. Sexual selection and extra-pair fertilization in a socially monogamous passerine, the zebra finch (Taeniopygia guttata). Behav. Ecol. 7, 218–226.

Caryl, P.G., 1975. Aggressive behaviour in the zebra finch Taeniopygia guttata. I. Fighting provoked by male and female social partners. Behaviour 52, 226–252.

Chalmers, G.A., 1992. Alberta. Trichomoniasis in finches. Can Vet. J. 33, 616–617.

Charlesworth, J.D., Warren, T.L., Brainard, M.S., 2012. Covert skill learning in a cortical-basal ganglia circuit. Nature 486, 251–255.

Cold Spring Harbor Protocols. 2014. Cold Spring Harbor Laboratory Press. <http://cshprotocols.cshlp.org/>.

Collins, S.A., Archer, J.A., Barnard, C.J., 2008. Welfare and mate choice in zebra finches: effect of handling regime and presence of cover. Anim. Welf. 17, 11–17.

Commission of the European Communities, 2007. Additional guidelines for housing and care of zebra finch, in stock and during procedures. Commission recommendation on guidelines for the accommodation and care of animals used for experimental and other scientific purposes. Official J. Eur. Union.

Conover, M.R., Messmer, T.A., 1996. Consequences for captive zebra finches of consuming tall fescue seeds infected with the endophytic fungus Acremonium coenophialum. Auk 113, 492–495.

Cuthill, I.C., Hunt, S., Clark, C., 1997. Colour bands, dominance, and body mass regulation in male zebra finches (Taeniopygia guttata). Proc. Biol. Sci. 264, 1093–1099.

Cynx, J., 2001. Effects of humidity on reproductive behavior in male and female zebra finches (Taeniopygia guttata). J. Comp. Psychol. 115, 196–200.

Dave, A.S., Margoliash, D., 2000. Song replay during sleep and computational rules for sensorimotor vocal learning. Science 290, 812–816.

de Kogel, C.H., Prijs, H.J., 1996. Effects of brood size manipulations on sexual attractiveness of offspring in the zebra finch. Anim. Behav. 51, 699–708.

de Matos, R., Morrisey, J.K., 2005. Emergency and critical care of small psittacines and passerines. Semin. Avian Exot. Pet Med. 14, 90–105.

Deregnaucourt, S., Mitra, P.P., Feher, O., Pytte, C., Tchernichovski, O., 2005. How sleep affects the developmental learning of bird song. Nature 433, 710–716.

Dhama, K., Mahendran, M., Tiwari, R., Dayal Singh, S., Kumar, D., Singh, S., et al., 2011. Tuberculosis in birds: Insights into the Mycobacterium avium infections. Vet. Med. Int. 2011, 712369.

Doneley, B., 2011. Avian medicine and surgery in practice. Companion and Aviary Birds. Manson Publishing Ltd, London.

Dorrestein, G.M., 2009a. Bacterial and parasitic diseases of passerines. Vet. Clin. North Am. Exot. Anim. Pract. 12, 433–451.

Dorrestein, G.M., 2009b. 8 – Passerines. In: Tully, T.N., Dorrestein, G.M., Jones, A.K., Cooper, J.E. (Eds.), Handbook of Avian Medicine, second ed. W.B. Saunders, Edinburgh.

Doupe, A.J., Kuhl, P.K., 1999. Birdsong and human speech: common themes and mechanisms. Annu. Rev. Neurosci. 22, 567–631.

Duerr, R., 2008. Passerines: hand-feeding diets. In: Gage, L.J., Duerr, R.S. (Eds.), Hand-Rearing Birds. Blackwell Publishing Ltd, Oxford, UK. doi:10.1002/9780470376393.ch34.

Dugas-Ford, J., Rowell, J.J., Ragsdale, C.W., 2012. Cell-type homologies and the origins of the neocortex. Proc. Natl. Acad. Sci. USA 109, 16974–16979.

Estrin, M.A., Coleman, J.K., Childress, A.L., Wellehan, J.F.X., Patterson, M.M., Muthupalani, S. Manuscript in preparation. Multisystemic, poorly differentiated neoplasia associated with two polyomaviruses in the zebra finch (Taeniopygia guttata).

Evans, E.E., 2011. Zoonotic diseases of common pet birds: psittacine, passerine, and columbiform species. Vet. Clin. North Am. Exot. Anim. Pract. 14, 457–476. vi.

Evans, J.E., Cuthill, I.C., Bennett, A.T.D., 2006. The effect of flicker from fluorescent lights on mate choice in captive birds. Anim. Behav. 72, 393–400.

Evans, S.M., 1970. Aggressive and territorial behaviour in captive zebra finches. Bird Study 17, 28–35.

Ewenson, E.L., Zann, R.A., Flannery, G.R., 2001. Body condition and immune response in wild zebra finches: effects of capture, confinement and captive-rearing. Naturwissenschaften 88, 391–394.

Farries, M.A., Perkel, D.J., 2002. A telencephalic nucleus essential for song learning contains neurons with physiological characteristics of both striatum and globus pallidus. J. Neurosci. 22, 3776–3787.

Fee, M.S., Leonardo, A., 2001. Miniature motorized microdrive and commutator system for chronic neural recording in small animals. J. Neurosci. Methods 112, 83–94.

Filippich, L.J., O'Donoghue, P.J., 1997. Cochlosoma infections in finches. Aust. Vet. J. 75, 561–563.

Forstmeier, W., Segelbacher, G., Mueller, J.C., Kempenaers, B., 2007. Genetic variation and differentiation in captive and wild zebra finches (Taeniopygia guttata). Mol. Ecol. 16, 4039–4050.

Gentner, T.Q., Fenn, K.M., Margoliash, D., Nusbaum, H.C., 2006. Recursive syntactic pattern learning by songbirds. Nature 440, 1204–1207.

Goldberg, J.H., Adler, A., Bergman, H., Fee, M.S., 2010. Singing-related neural activity distinguishes two putative pallidal cell types in the songbird basal ganglia: comparison to the primate internal and external pallidal segments. J. Neurosci. 30, 7088–7098.

Goldberg, J.H., Fee, M.S., 2010. Singing-related neural activity distinguishes four classes of putative striatal neurons in the songbird basal ganglia. J. Neurophysiol. 103, 2002–2014.

Goldberg, J.H., Fee, M.S., 2012. A cortical motor nucleus drives the basal ganglia-recipient thalamus in singing birds. Nat. Neurosci. 15, 620–627.

Goodson, J.L., Adkins-Regan, E., 1999. Effect of intraseptal vasotocin and vasoactive intestinal polypeptide infusions on courtship song and aggression in the male zebra finch (Taeniopygia guttata). J. Neuroendocrinol. 11, 19–25.

Guide for the Care and Use of Laboratory Animals: eighth ed., The National Academies Press, 2011.

Ha, H.J., Alley, M., Howe, L., Gartrell, B., 2013. Evaluation of the pathogenicity of avipoxvirus strains isolated from wild birds in New Zealand and the efficacy of a fowlpox vaccine in passerines. Vet. Microbiol. 165, 268–274.

Haesler, S., Rochefort, C., Georgi, B., Licznerski, P., Osten, P., Scharff, C., 2007. Incomplete and inaccurate vocal imitation after knockdown of FoxP2 in songbird basal ganglia nucleus Area X. PLoS Biol. 5, e321.

Hahnloser, R.H., Kozhevnikov, A.A., Fee, M.S., 2002. An ultra-sparse code underlies the generation of neural sequences in a songbird. Nature 419, 65–70.

Hahnloser, R.H., Kozhevnikov, A.A., Fee, M.S., 2006. Sleep-related neural activity in a premotor and a basal-ganglia pathway of the songbird. J. Neurophysiol. 96, 794–812.

Harper, E.J., Lambert, L., Moodie, N., 1998. The comparative nutrition of two passerine species: the canary (Serinus canarius) and the zebra finch (Poephila guttata). J. Nutr. 128, 2684S–2685S.

Harper, E.J., Skinner, N.D., 1998. Clinical nutrition of small psittacines and passerines. Semin. Avian Exot. Pet Med. 7, 116–127.

Harrison, G.J., Lightfoot, T.L. (Eds.), 2006. Clinical Avian Medicine. Volumes I and II. Spix Publishing, Palm Beach, FL.

Hawkins, P., 2010. The welfare implications of housing captive wild and domesticated birds. In: Duncan, I.J.H., Hawkins, P. (Eds.), The Welfare of Domestic Fowl and Other Captive Birds, Springer Science, pp. 53–102.

Hawkins, M.G., Paul-Murphy, J., 2011. Avian analgesia. Vet. Clin. North Am. Exot. Anim. Pract. 14, 61–80.

Hawkins, P., Morton, D.B., Cameron, D., Cuthill, I.C., Francis, R., Freire, R., et al., 2001. Finches, including the zebra finch, Taeniopygia guttata. Lab. Anim. 35, 126–131.

Hawley, D.M., Grodio, J., Frasca, S., Kirkpatrick, L., Ley, D.H., 2011. Experimental infection of domestic canaries (Serinus canaria domestica) with Mycoplasma gallisepticum: a new model system for a wildlife disease. Avian Pathol. 40, 321–327.

Helman, R.G., Jensen, J.M., Russell, R.G., 1984. Systemic protozoal disease in zebra finches. J. Am. Vet. Med. Assoc. 185, 1400–1401.

Hindmarsh, M., Ward, K., 1993. Mortality of finches (family Estrildidae) caused by Acuaria skrjabini. Aust. Vet. J. 70, 451–452.

Hochachka, W.M., Dhondt, A.A., Dobson, A., Hawley, D.M., Ley, D.H., Lovette, I.J., 2013. Multiple host transfers, but only one successful lineage in a continent-spanning emergent pathogen. Proc. Biol. Sci. 280 (1766), 20131068. doi:10.1098/rspb.2013.1068.

Hoop, R.K., Bottger, E.C., Ossent, P., Salfinger, M., 1993. Mycobacteriosis due to Mycobacterium genavense in six pet birds. J. Clin. Microbiol. 31, 990–993.

Hoop, R.K., Bottger, E.C., Pfyffer, G.E., 1996. Etiological agents of mycobacterioses in pet birds between 1986 and 1995. J. Clin. Microbiol. 34, 991–992.

Hukkanen, R.R., Richardson, M., Wingfield, J.C., Treuting, P., Brabb, T., 2003. Avipox sp. in a colony of gray-crowned rosy finches (Leucosticte tephrocotis). Comp. Med. 53, 548–552.

Hunt, S., Cuthill, I.C., Swaddle, J.P., Bennett, A.T.D., 1997. Ultraviolet vision and band-colour preferences in female zebra finches, Taeniopygia guttata. Anim. Behav. 54, 1383–1392.

Ikebuchi, M., Okanoya, K., 2006. Growth of pair bonding in zebra finches: physical and social factors. Ornithological Sci. 5, 65–75.

Immelmann, K. 1969. Song development in the zebra finch and other estrildid finches. In: Hinde, R.A. (Ed.), Bird Vocalizations. 61.

Irizarry-Rovira, A.R., Lennox, A.M., Ramos-Vara, J.A., 2007. Malignant melanoma in a zebra finch (Taeniopygia guttata): cytologic, histologic, and ultrastructural characteristics. Vet. Clin. Pathol. 36, 297–302.

Itoh, Y., Arnold, A.P., 2011. Zebra finch cell lines from naturally occurring tumors. In. Vitro. Cell. Dev. Biol. Anim. 47, 280–282.

Jacobs, H., Smith, N., Smith, P., Smyth, L., Yew, P., Saibaba, P., et al., 1995. Zebra finch behaviour and effect of modest enrichment of standard cages. Anim. Welf. 4, 3–9.

Jarvis, E.D., Scharff, C., Grossman, M.R., Ramos, J.A., Nottebohm, F., 1998. For whom the bird sings: context-dependent gene expression. Neuron 21, 775–788.

Jarvis, E.D., Yu, J., Rivas, M.V., Horita, H., Feenders, G., Whitney, O., et al., 2013. Global view of the functional molecular organization of the avian cerebrum: mirror images and functional columns. J. Comp. Neurol. 521, 3614–3665.

Jones, J.C., Sonnberg, S., Kocer, Z.A., Shanmuganatham, K., Seiler, Pl, Shu, Y., et al., 2014. Possible role of songbirds and parakeets in transmission of influenza A (H7N9) virus to humans. Emerg. Infect. Dis. 20, 380–385.

Jones, N.D., Brooks, D.R., Harris, R.L., 1980. Macaca mulatta – a new host for Choanotaenia cestodes. Lab. Anim. Sci. 30, 575–577.

Karten, H.J., 2013. Neocortical evolution: neuronal circuits arise independently of lamination. Curr. Biol. 23, R12–R15.

Karten, H.J., Brzozowska-Prechtl, A., Lovell, P.V., Tang, D.D., Mello, C.V., Wang, H., et al., 2013. Digital atlas of the zebra finch (Taeniopygia guttata) brain: a high-resolution photo atlas. J. Comp. Neurol. 521, 3702–3715.

Keller, G.B., Hahnloser, R.H., 2009. Neural processing of auditory feedback during vocal practice in a songbird. Nature 457, 187–190.

Kheirandish, R., Salehi, M., 2011. Megabacteriosis in budgerigars: diagnosis and treatment. Comp. Clin. Pathol. 20, 501–505.

Knöpfel, T., Lin, M.Z., Levskaya, A., Tian, L., Lin, J.Y., Boyden, E.S., 2010. Toward the second generation of optogenetic tools. J. Neurosci. 30, 14998–15004.

Kojima, S., Doupe, A.J., 2009. Activity propagation in an avian basal ganglia-thalamocortical circuit essential for vocal learning. J. Neurosci. 29, 4782–4793.

Kubikova, L., Wada, K., Jarvis, E.D., 2010. Dopamine receptors in a songbird brain. J. Comp. Neurol. 518, 741–769.

Lafferty, S.L., Fudge, A.M., Schmidt, R.E., Wilson, V.G., Phalen, D.N., 1999. Avian polyomavirus infection and disease in a green aracaris (Pteroglossus viridis). Avian Dis. 43, 577–585.

Lai, C.S., Fisher, S.E., Hurst, J.A., Vargha-Khadem, F., Monaco, A.P., 2001. A forkhead-domain gene is mutated in a severe speech and language disorder. Nature 413, 519–523.

Lane, R., 1991. Basic techniques in pet avian clinical pathology. Vet. Clin. North Am. Small. Anim. Pract. 21, 1157–1179.

Leblois, A., Bodor, A.L., Person, A.L., Perkel, D.J., 2009. Millisecond timescale disinhibition mediates fast information transmission through an avian basal ganglia loop. J. Neurosci. 29, 15420–15433.

Lipkind, D., Tchernichovski, O., 2011. Quantification of developmental birdsong learning from the subsyllabic scale to cultural evolution. Proc. Natl. Acad. Sci. USA 108 (Suppl. 3), 15572–15579.

Lombardino, A.J., Nottebohm, F., 2000. Age at deafening affects the stability of learned song in adult male zebra finches. J. Neurosci. 20, 5054–5064.

London, S.E., Clayton, D.F., 2008. Functional identification of sensory mechanisms required for developmental song learning. Nat. Neurosci. 11, 579–586.

Long, M.A., Fee, M.S., 2008. Using temperature to analyse temporal dynamics in the songbird motor pathway. Nature 456, 189–194.

Long, M.A., Jin, D.Z., Fee, M.S., 2010. Support for a synaptic chain model of neuronal sequence generation. Nature 468, 394–399.

Loudis, B.G. 1999. PMV-3 Outbreak–Presentation, diagnosis and management. Proceedings of the 1997 European Conference on Avian Medicine and Surgery, 223–227.

Machin, K.L., 2005. Avian pain: physiology and evaluation. Compend. Contin. Educ. Pract. Vet. 27, 98–109.

Manarolla, G., Liandris, E., Pisoni, G., Sassera, D., Grilli, G., Gallazzi, D., et al., 2009. Avian mycobacteriosis in companion birds: 20-year survey. Vet. Microbiol. 133, 323–327.

Marler, P., 1991. Song-learning behavior: the interface with neuroethology. Trends Neurosci. 14, 199–206.

Martins, N.R.S., Horta, A.C., Siqueira, A.M., Lopes, S.Q., Resende, J.S., Jorge, M.A., et al., 2006. Macrorhabdus ornithogaster in ostrich, rhea, canary, zebra finch, free range chicken, turkey, guinea-fowl, columbina pigeon, toucan, chuckar partridge and experimental infection in chicken, japanese quail and mice. Escola de Veterinária UFMG, 58.

McGraw, K.J., Adkins-Regan, E., Parker, R.S., 2005. Maternally derived carotenoid pigments affect offspring survival, sex ratio, and sexual attractiveness in a colorful songbird. Naturwissenschaften 92, 375–380.

McGuire, A.M., McAllister, M., Wills, R.A., Tranas, J.D., 1999. Experimental inoculation of domestic pigeons (Columbia livia) and zebra finches (Poephila guttata) with Neospora caninum tachyzoites. Int. J. Parasitol. 29, 1525–1529.

McOrist, S., Barton, N.J., Black, D.G., 1982. Acuaris skrjabini infection of the gizzard of finches. Avian Dis. 26, 957–960.

McOrist, S., Barton, N.J., Jones, A., 1984. Choanotaenia spp. infestation of Australian finches (Estrildidae). Avian Pathol. 13, 479–486.

Meijer, T., Rozman, J., Schulte, M., Stach-Dreesmann, C., 1996. New findings in body mass regulation in zebra finches (Taeniopygia guttata) in response to photoperiod and temperature. J. Zool. 240, 717–734.

Mello, C.V., Vicario, D.S., Clayton, D.F., 1992. Song presentation induces gene expression in the songbird forebrain. Proc. Natl. Acad. Sci. USA 89, 6818–6822.

Mench, J.A., Blatchford, R.A., 2014. Chapter 16 – Birds as Laboratory Animals. In: Bayne, K., Turner, P.V. (Eds.), Laboratory Animal Welfare Academic Press, Boston, MA.

Mertins, J.W., Bochkov, A.V., 2014. Key to the species of Neocheyletiella (Acariformes: Cheyletidae), with description of a new species. J. Med. Entomol. 51, 1116–1121.

Morishita, T.Y., Schaul, J.C., 2007. Parasites of Birds. In: Baker, D.G. (Ed.), Flynn's Parasites of Laboratory Animals, second ed. Wiley-Blackwell, Ames, IA.

Morris, D., 1954. The reproductive behavior of the zebra finch (Poephila guttata), with special reference to pseudofemale behavior and displacement activities. Behaviour 6, 271–322.

Murray, J.R., Varian-Ramos, C.W., Welch, Z.S., Saha, M.S., 2013. Embryological staging of the zebra finch, Taeniopygia guttata. J. Morphol. 274, 1090–1110.

Murugan, M., Harward, S., Scharff, C., Mooney, R., 2013. Diminished FoxP2 levels affect dopaminergic modulation of corticostriatal signaling important to song variability. Neuron 80, 1464–1476.

Muth, F., Steele, M., Healy, S.D., 2013. Colour preferences in nest-building zebra finches. Behav. Processes 99, 106–111.

Nagel, K., Kim, G., Mclendon, H., Doupe, A., 2011. A bird brain's view of auditory processing and perception. Hear. Res. 273, 123–133.

Nager, R.G., Law, G., 2010. The zebra finch. In: Hubrecht, R., Kirkwood, J. (Eds.), The UFAW Handbook on the Care and Management of Laboratory and Other Research Animals, eighth ed. Wiley-Blackwell.

Naguib, M., Riebel, K., Marzal, A., Gil, D., 2004. Nestling immunocompetence and testosterone covary with brood size in a songbird. Proc. Biol. Sci. 271, 833–838.

Nilson, P.C., Teramitsu, I., White, S.A., 2005. Caudal thoracic air sac cannulation in zebra finches for isoflurane anesthesia. J. Neurosci. Methods 143, 107–115.

Nottebohm, F., Arnold, A.P., 1976. Sexual dimorphism in vocal control areas of the songbird brain. Science 194, 211–213.

Nottebohm, F., Stokes, T.M., Leonard, C.M., 1976. Central control of song in the canary, Serinus canarius. J. Comp. Neurol. 165, 457–486.

Otchy, T.M., Ölveczky, B.P., 2012. Design and assembly of an ultra-light motorized microdrive for chronic neural recordings in small animals. J. Vis. Exp. 69, e4314. doi:10.3791/4314.

Panaitof, S.C., Abrahams, B.S., Dong, H., Geschwind, D.H., White, S.A., 2010. Language-related Cntnap2 gene is differentially expressed in sexually dimorphic song nuclei essential for vocal learning in songbirds. J. Comp. Neurol. 518, 1995–2018.

Payne, R.B., 2010. Family Estrildidae (Waxbills). In: Del Hoyo, J., Elliott, A., Christie, D.A. (Eds.), Handbook of the Birds of the

World, Volume 15. Weavers to New World Warblers Lynx Editions, Barcelona, Spain.

Perkins, L.E., Swayne, D.E., 2003. Varied pathogenicity of a Hong Kong-origin H5N1 avian influenza virus in four passerine species and budgerigars. Vet. Pathol. 40, 14–24.

Person, A.L., Gale, S.D., Farries, M.A., Perkel, D.J., 2008. Organization of the songbird basal ganglia, including area X. J. Comp. Neurol. 508, 840–866.

Phalen, D., 2005. Diagnosis and management of Macrorhabdus ornithogaster (formerly megabacteria). Vet. Clin. North Am. Exot. Anim. Pract. 8, 299–306.

Pollock, C.G., 2006. Chapter 28. Implications of mycobacteria in clinical disorders. In: Harrison, G.J., Lightfoot, T.L. (Eds.), Clinical Avian Medicine. Volume II. Spix Publishing, Palm Beach, FL.

Poot, H., ter Maat, A., Trost, L., Schwabl, I., Jansen, R.F., Gahr, M., 2012. Behavioural and physiological effects of population density on domesticated zebra finches (Taeniopygia guttata) held in aviaries. Physiol. Behav. 105, 821–828.

Prather, J.F., 2012. Rapid and reliable sedation induced by diazepam and antagonized by flumazenil in zebra finches (Taeniopygia guttata). J. Avian Med. Surg. 26, 76–84.

Prattis, S.M., Cioffee, C.J., Reinhard, G., Zaoutis, T.E., 1990. A retrospective study of disease and mortality in zebra finches. Lab. Anim. Sci. 40, 402–405.

Price, P.H., 1979. Developmental determinants of structure in zebra finch song. J. Comp. Physiol. Psychol. 93, 260.

Qi, M., Wang, R., Ning, C., Li, X., Zhang, L., Jian, F., et al., 2011. Cryptosporidium spp. in pet birds: genetic diversity and potential public health significance. Exp. Parasitol. 128, 336–340.

Rashotte, M.E., Sedunova, E.V., Johnson, F., Pastukhov, I.F., 2001. Influence of food and water availability on undirected singing and energetic status in adult male zebra finches (Taeniopygia guttata). Physiol. Behav. 74, 533–541.

Remage-Healey, L., London, S.E., Schlinger, B.A., 2010. Birdsong and the neural production of steroids. J. Chem. Neuroanat. 39 (2), 72. doi:10.1016/j.jchemneu.2009.06.009.

Riebel, K., 2009. Song and female mate choice in zebra finches: a review. In: Marc, N., Klaus, Z., Nicola, S.C., Vincent, M.J. (Eds.), Advances in the Study of Behavior. Academic Press.

Riffkin, G.G., McCausland, I.P., 1972. Respiratory acariasis caused by Sternostoma tracheacolum in aviary finches. N. Z. Vet. J. 20, 109–112.

Roberts, T.F., Gobes, S.M., Murugan, M., Olveczky, B.P., Mooney, R., 2012. Motor circuits are required to encode a sensory model for imitative learning. Nat. Neurosci. 15, 1454–1459.

Roberts, T.F., Tschida, K.A., Klein, M.E., Mooney, R., 2010. Rapid spine stabilization and synaptic enhancement at the onset of behavioural learning. Nature 463, 948–952.

Sandmeier, P., Coutteel, P., 2006. Chapter 39. Management of canaries, finches and mynahs. In: Harrison, G.J., Lightfoot, T.L. (Eds.), Clinical Avian Medicine. Volume II. Spix Publishing, Palm Beach, FL.

Sandmeier, P., Hook, R.K., Bosshart, G., 1997. Cerebral mycobacteriosis in zebra finches (Taeniopygia guttata) caused by Mycobacterium genavense. Proceedings of the 1997 European Conference on Avian Medicine and Surgery 119–122.

Sato, Y., Kumeta, A., Koyama, T., Takada, T., Aoyagi, T., Ichikawa, K., et al., 1993. An outbreak of Salmonella Typhimurium infection in bengalees, a variety of Lonchura striata. J. Vet. Med. Sci. 55, 1073–1076.

Sato, Y., Wada, K., 1995. Isolation of Salmonella Typhimurium from zebra finches (Poephila guttata). J. Vet. Med. Sci. 57, 137–138.

Scharff, C., Nottebohm, F., 1991. A comparative study of the behavioral deficits following lesions of various parts of the zebra finch song system: implications for vocal learning. J. Neurosci. 11, 2896–2913.

Schmidt, M.F., 2010. An IACUC perspective on songbirds and their use in neurobiological research. ILAR. J. 51, 424–430.

Schock, R.C., Cooper, R., 1978. Internal parasitisms in captive birds. Mod. Vet. Pract. 59, 439–443.

Schrenzel, M., Nicolas, M., Witte, C., Papendick, R., Tucker, T., Keener, L., et al., 2008. Molecular epidemiology of Mycobacterium avium subsp. avium and Mycobacterium intracellulare in captive birds. Vet. Microbiol. 126, 122–131.

Scott, B.B., Gardner, T., Ji, N., Fee, M.S., Lois, C., 2012. Wandering neuronal migration in the postnatal vertebrate forebrain. J. Neurosci. 32, 1436–1446.

Seguin, A., Forstmeier, W., 2012. No band color effects on male courtship rate or body mass in the zebra finch: four experiments and a meta-analysis. PLoS One 7, e37785.

Shank, S.S., Margoliash, D., 2009. Sleep and sensorimotor integration during early vocal learning in a songbird. Nature, 458. doi:10.1038/nature07615.

Shivaprasad, H.L., 1998. An Overview of Paramyxovirus 3 (PMV-3) Infection in Psittacines and Passerines. Proceedings of the 1998 Association of Avian Veterinarians 147–150.

Shivaprasad, H.L., Palmieri, C., 2012. Pathology of mycobacteriosis in birds. Vet. Clin. North Am. Exot. Anim. Pract. 15, 41–55. v–vi.

Siddalls, M., Currier, T.A., Pang, J., Lertpiriyapong, K., Patterson, M.M., 2015. Infestation of research zebra finch colony with two novel mite species. Comp. Med. 65, 51–53.

Simons, M.J., Briga, M., Koetsier, E., Folkertsma, R., Wubs, M.D., Dijkstra, C., et al., 2012. Bill redness is positively associated with reproduction and survival in male and female zebra finches. PLoS One 7, e40721.

Simons, M.J.P., Verhulst, S., 2011. Zebra finch females prefer males with redder bills independent of song rate – a meta-analysis. Behav. Ecol. 22, 755–762.

Simpson, V., Molenaar, F., 2006. Increase in trichomonosis in finches. Vet. Rec. 159, 606.

Snyder, J.M., Molk, D.M., Treuting, P.M., 2013. Increased mortality in a colony of zebra finches exposed to continuous light. J. Am. Assoc. Lab. Anim. Sci. 52, 301–307.

Soderstrom, K., Qin, W., Leggett, M.H., 2007. A minimally invasive procedure for sexing young zebra finches. J. Neurosci. Methods 164, 116–119.

Swaddle, J.P., Cuthill, I.C., 1994. Preference for symmetric males by female zebra finches. Nature 367, 165–166.

Swaddle, J.P., Page, L.C., 2007. High levels of environmental noise erode pair preferences in zebra finches: implications for noise pollution. Anim. Behav. 74, 363–368.

Tchernichovski, O., Mitra, P.P., Lints, T., Nottebohm, F., 2001. Dynamics of the vocal imitation process: how a zebra finch learns its song. Science 291, 2564–2569.

Tell, L.A., Woods, L., Cromie, R.L., 2001. Mycobacteriosis in birds. Rev. Sci. Tech. 20, 180–203.

Tidemann, S., Calley, M., Burgoyne, C., 1992. An investigation of blood smears from northern Australian finches. Emu 92, 114–117.

Tomaszewski, E.K., Logan, K.S., Snowden, K.F., Kurtzman, C.P., Phalen, D.N., 2003. Phylogenetic analysis identifies the 'megabacterium' of birds as a novel anamorphic ascomycetous yeast, Macrorhabdus ornithogaster gen. nov., sp. nov. Int. J. Syst. Evol. Microbiol. 53, 1201–1205.

Tschirren, B., Rutstein, A.N., Postma, E., Mariette, M., Griffith, S.C., 2009. Short- and long-term consequences of early developmental conditions: a case study on wild and domesticated zebra finches. J. Evol. Biol. 22, 387–395.

Veit, L., Aronov, D., Fee, M.S., 2011. Learning to breathe and sing: development of respiratory–vocal coordination in young songbirds. J. Neurophysiol. 106, 1747–1765.

Vu, E.T., Mazurek, M.E., Kuo, Y.C., 1994. Identification of a forebrain motor programming network for the learned song of zebra finches. J. Neurosci. 14, 6924–6934.

Waas, J.R., Colgan, P.W., Boag, P.T., 2005. Playback of colony sound alters the breeding schedule and clutch size in zebra finch (Taeniopygia guttata) colonies. Proc. Biol. Sci. 272, 383–388.

Waas, J.R., Wordsworth, A.F., 1999. Female zebra finches prefer symmetrically banded males, but only during interactive mate choice tests. Anim. Behav. 57, 1113–1119.

Warren, W.C., Clayton, D.F., Ellegren, H., Arnold, A.P., Hillier, L.W., Kunstner, A., et al., 2010. The genome of a songbird. Nature 464, 757–762.

White, S.A., Livingston, F.S., Mooney, R., 1999. Androgens modulate NMDA receptor-mediated EPSCs in the zebra finch song system. J. Neurophysiol. 82, 2221–2234.

Williamson, K., Gilbert, L., Rutstein, A.N., Pariser, E.C., Graves, J.A., 2008. Within-year differences in reproductive investment in laboratory zebra finches (Taeniopygia guttata), an opportunistically breeding bird. Naturwissenschaften 95, 1143–1148.

Yu, A.C., Margoliash, D., 1996. Temporal hierarchical control of singing in birds. Science 273, 1871–1875.

Zann, R.A., 1996. The Zebra Finch: A Synthesis of Field and Laboratory Studies. Oxford University Press, New York.

Multimodal analgesia options

DRUG	MECHANISM OF ACTION	ANALGESIC EFFECTS	REVERSIBLE	INDICATIONS	BENEFITS	PRECAUTIONS
Opioids Fentanyl (constant rate infusion [CRI], patch) Hydromorphone Oxymorphone Morphine Methadone Buprenorphine	Full μ receptor agonism Partial μ receptor agonism	Yes, potent	Yes, naloxone is a full opioid μ receptor antagonist	Peri- and postoperative, acute management of nonsurgical painful condition, premedication	Reliable, full mu agonists can be titrated to effect, good cardiovascular (CV) stability	Dose-dependent respiratory depression, vomiting
Benzodiazepines Diazepam Midazolam	Gamma-aminobutyric acid (GABA) receptor agonism	Not when used alone, synergistic effect with neuroleptanalgesia	Yes, flumazenil is a benzodiazepine antagonist	Sedation, tranquilization, anticonvulsant, muscle relaxation premedication when used with an opioid	Good CV and respiratory stability, anesthetic-sparing effects	Paradoxical excitation possible
Acepromazine	Phenothiazine, central dopamine receptor antagonism	Not when used alone, synergistic effect with neuroleptanalgesia	No	Tranquilization, premedication	Reliable neurolepsis	Vasodilatory, hypotension, long duration of action
NSAIDs Carprofen Robenacoxib Meloxicam	Cyclooxygenase (COX)-2 inhibition	Yes, anti-inflammatory effects	No	Analgesia due to inflammation in CV stable, hydrated patients, with good renal function	Only class of drugs with reliable anti-inflammatory effects	Patient selection required, vomiting, diarrhea, gastrointestinal (GI) ulceration, acute renal injury
α-2 adrenergic agonists Dexmedetomidine	α-2 receptor agonism	Yes, reliable	Yes, atipamezole is an α-2 receptor antagonist	Procedural sedation and analgesia, total intravenous anesthesia (TIVA) when combined with an opioid and ketamine	Good sedation and analgesia	CV depression, vomiting
Local anesthetics Lidocaine Bupivacaine	Na+ channel blockade of neuronal cell membrane	Yes, complete	No	Consider for use with every surgical procedure	Good safety, no systemic effects at therapeutic doses, analgesia and anesthetic-sparing effects, antimicrobial, and immunomodulating	Cats sensitive to toxic effects, dose-reduce or avoid use
Ketamine	Dissociative agent, N-methyl-D-aspartate (NMDA) receptor antagonism	Yes	No	Procedural sedation, trans- and postoperative pain management	Efficacy and safety at subanesthetic doses, TIVA when combined with an opioid and α-2 agonist	CV stimulatory, may increase intracranial pressure (ICP) and intraocular pressure (IOP), salivation, renal elimination in cats
Gabapentin	Weak anticonvulsant, analgesic properties may be through neuronal calcium channel down regulation	Yes	No	Neuropathic pain, "wind-up" pain, maladaptive pain	Wide safety profile, well-tolerated, acute and chronic pain management	Sedation, somnolence (usually resolves with patient acclimation)
Acetaminophen	Incompletely understood, possibly isoform nonspecific inhibition of COX	Yes, no significant anti-inflammatory effects	No	Adjunct analgesia in dogs only	Pain-modifying effect in dogs with orthopedic surgery	Contraindicated in cats at any dosage
Maropitant	Central antiemetic neurokinin-1 receptor antagonism, analgesic effects likely through substance-P binding blockade	Evidence in cats and dogs of anesthetic-sparing effects, may be non-inferior to morphine	No	Adjunct analgesia, anti-emetic effects may be desirable to treat vomiting due to premedication, brachycephalics	No CV or respiratory depression	May mask signs of GI obstruction

LABORATORY ANIMAL MEDICINE

CHAPTER

24

Preanesthesia, Anesthesia, Analgesia, and Euthanasia

Paul Flecknell, MA, VetMB, PhD, DECLAM, DLAS, DECVA, (Hon) DACLAM, (Hon) FRCVS[a], Jennifer L.S. Lofgren, DVM, MS, DACLAM[b], Melissa C. Dyson, DVM, DACLAM[b], Robert R. Marini, DVM[c], M. Michael Swindle, DVM[d] and Ronald P. Wilson, VMD, MS[e]

[a]Comparative Biology Medicine, Newcastle University, Newcastle Upon Tyne, UK [b]Unit for Laboratory Animal Medicine, University of Michigan Medical School, Ann Arbor, MI, USA [c]Division of Comparative Medicine, Massachusetts Institute of Technology, Cambridge, Massachusetts [d]Department of Comparative Medicine, Medical University of South Carolina, Charleston, SC, USA [e]Penn State College of Medicine, Department of Comparative Medicine, Hershey, PA, USA

I. INTRODUCTION

The purpose of this chapter is to provide practical advice for administering anesthetics, analgesics, and euthanasia agents to the most commonly used laboratory animal species. It is not meant to be an exhaustive review of all anesthetic and analgesic protocols used in these species. More detailed information is available in both specialist laboratory animal anesthesia texts, (e.g., Fish, 2008; Kohn *et al.*, 1997; Flecknell, 2009), and general veterinary anesthesia texts (e.g., Tranquilli *et al.*, 2007).

The most commonly used rodent species, rabbits, ferrets, pigs, small ruminants, and nonhuman primates were selected for inclusion in this chapter. These species encompass the overwhelming majority of laboratory animals that are currently utilized. References for in-depth discussion of anesthetic and analgesic protocols for each species are included within its particular section.

II. RODENTS

A. Introduction

Rodents, especially rats and mice, are the most numerous and arguably the most important group of animals used in research. Among the factors that differentiate anesthetic techniques used in rodents from those more commonly employed in larger species are the small size of the animals, the perceived and often real difficulties of vascular and airway access, and the frequent need to anesthetize large numbers of animals in a relatively short time. Trends that have combined to increase attention on the safe and appropriate anesthetic and analgesic delivery and monitoring for rodents include: humane concerns; scientific recognition of the effects of pain, anesthesia, and analgesia on experimental design; and the expense of generation or purchase of genetically altered rodents. This section will briefly discuss common anesthetic techniques for mice and rats, with comments on hamsters, gerbils, and guinea pigs. Drugs, techniques, and approaches to anesthesia and

analgesia for rodents are rapidly evolving. The reader is urged to consult laboratory animal anesthesia texts (Gaertner *et al.*, 2008; Flecknell, 2009) and journals for more complete and timely information.

B. Preoperative Assessment and Preparation

1. Preanesthetic Evaluation

No anesthetic regimen is universally safe or appropriate. Anesthetic protocols that are satisfactory for healthy animals can severely compromise or be fatal to unhealthy ones. A vigilant rodent health surveillance program is the first line of defense but cannot be expected to detect alterations in husbandry or experimental manipulations that may affect anesthesia outcomes. Preanesthetic considerations should include an assessment of appearance, behavior, and bodyweight for evidence of abnormality as well as for establishing doses for injectable agents. The history of the group of animals should be examined to identify experimental, housing, and strain-specific features that might affect choice of anesthesic agents and techniques. In addition, sex, age, and specific procedures may be expected to alter the effects of anesthesia, often to a surprising degree. A summary of anesthetic and analgesic variations among mice and rat stocks and strains is available in the chapter on Laboratory Rodents in the second edition of the text Anesthesia and Analgesia in Laboratory Animals (Gaertner *et al.*, 2008). Unless the anesthetic regimen is known to be safe and effective in the animals to be used, a pilot study should be conducted to assess and verify the effects of the proposed anesthetic and analgesic protocol (Flecknell, 2009). In all cases, it is important to allow adequate time for newly arrived animals to become acclimated to changes in housing, diet, and husbandry conditions and to recover from shipping stress. An acclimation period of at least 24–72h is recommended for rodents (Capdevila *et al.*, 2007; Obernier and Baldwin, 2006). Fasting is not usually necessary or recommended before anesthesia and surgery in rodents (Gaertner *et al.*, 2008).

2. Choice of Anesthetic Techniques

All anesthetics have undesirable properties, so a primary goal must be to select an anesthetic technique that has the least adverse effect on the animal and on the research. Thus, the goals of the research and the limitations this places on selection of the anesthetic agents must be taken into account in formulating an anesthetic protocol. For example, when prolonged stable anesthesia is required, the choice might favor an inhalation or continuous infusion method to avoid the variations that tend to occur with repeated bolus administration of drugs. A prolonged recovery period can further stress the animal and the resources of the facility, favoring selection of agents that have rapid recovery characteristics or agents that can easily be reversed, such as α_2-agonists, benzodiazepines, and some opioids. Finally, some techniques that meet all of the preceding criteria may be too technically demanding or simply too expensive for the proposed research. Inhalation anesthesia with modern agents requires the proper equipment and training. Precise intravenous infusion methods may require an infusion pump, as well as vascular access and experience with the technique. In many cases, only brief anesthesia may be needed, such as procedures that may not be extremely painful but require adequate restraint for the safety of the animal and the operator (e.g., bleeding, injections, or sampling of small amounts of tissue). Brief exposure to an inhalation agent is often selected to meet these needs.

In summary, selection of a suitable anesthetic technique must include professional and humane considerations, scientific requirements and restrictions, and recognition of technical and personnel limitations.

3. Preanesthetic Medications

Preanesthetic drugs are not commonly used in rodents. However, the advantages of sedation, analgesia, and reduced doses of the general anesthetic agent or agents apply equally well to rodents. The principal disadvantage of using a preanesthetic agent in rodents is the need to restrain and thus stress the animals twice rather than once for the induction of anesthesia. Drugs commonly used as preanesthetic agents in other species are frequently incorporated into anesthetic combinations for rodents. However, if postprocedural analgesia is needed following very short procedures, or if preemptive analgesia is desired, then some means of preanesthetic administration must be used. Preanesthetic administration of tranquilizers, including the phenothiazine derivatives, benzodiazepines, and pote-nt analgesics will all tend to substantially reduce the required dose of the principal anesthetic agent or agents.

C. Anesthetic Agents

A summary of commonly used drug doses is provided in Tables 24.1–24.5. These dosages should be used

TABLE 24.1 Selected Anesthetic and Analgesic Doses for Mice[a]

Drug	Dose	Route	Duration
ANESTHESTICS			
Barbiturates			
Pentobarbital	40–50 mg/kg	IP	20–40 min
EMTU (inactin)	80– mg/kg	IP	60–240 min
Dissociative agents and combinations			
Ketamine+	100 mg/kg	IP	20–30 min
acepromazine	5 mg/kg		
Ketamine+	50–75 mg/kg	IP	20–30 min
medetomidine	1–10 mg/kg		
Ketamine+	80–100 mg/kg	IP	20–30 min
xylazine	5–10 mg/kg		
Ketamine+	80–100 mg/kg	IP	30–40 min
Xylazine+	5–10 mg/kg		
acepromazine	3 mg/kg		
Neuroleptanesthetics			
Fentanyl-fluanisone (hypnorm)			
+midazolam	10.0 ml/kg[b]	IP	30–40 min
Fentanyl-fluanisone (hypnorm)	0.4 ml/kg		
+diazepam	5 mg/kg	IP	30–40 min
Inhalant agents			
Isoflurane	1–4%, to effect	Inhalant	
Other agents			
Propofol	12–26 mg/kg	IV	5–10 min
Tribromoethanol	125–300 mg/kg	IP	15–45 min
ANALGESICS			
Buprenorphine	0.05–0.1 mg/kg	SC, IP	6–12 h
Butorphanol	1–5 mg/kg	SC, IP	4 h
Morphine	2.5 mg/kg	SC, IP	2–4 h
Carprofen	5 mg/kg	SC, IP	24 h
Meloxicam	5 mg/kg	SC, IP	24 h[t]
Bupivacaine	Do not exceed 2 mg/kg	Local infiltration	1–2 h[t]
MISCELLANEOUS			
Atropine	0.04 mg/kg	SC, IP	[t]min
Yohimbine	0.2 mg/kg	IV	–
	0.5 mg/kg	IM	
Atipamezole	0.1–1 mg/kg	IM, IP, SC, IV	–

[a]Doses adapted with modifications from Gaertner et al. (2008) and Flecknell (2009).
[b]See Flecknell (2009) for mixing instructions.
[t]Uncertain duration.

TABLE 24.2   Rats: Drug Doses[a]

Drug	Dose	Route	Duration
ANESTHESTICS			
Barbiturates			
Pentobarbital	30–60 mg/kg	IP	20–60 min
EMTU (inactin)*	80–100 mg/kg	IP	60–240 min
Dissociative agents and combinations			
Ketamine+	75 mg/kg	IP	20–30 min
acepromazine	2.5 mg/kg		
Ketamine+	60–75 mg/kg	IP	20–30 min
medetomidine	0.5 mg/kg		
Ketamine+	40–80 mg/kg	IP	20–40 min
xylazine	5–10 mg/kg		
Ketamine+	40–50 mg/kg	IP	20–30 min
Xylazine+	2.5–8 mg/kg		
acepromazine	0.75–4 mg/kg		
Neuroleptanesthetics			
Fentanyl-fluanisone (hypnorm)			
+midazolam	2.7 ml/kg[b]	IP	30–40 min
Fentanyl-fluanisone (hypnorm)	0.4–0.6 ml/kg		
+diazepam	2.5 mg/kg	IP	20–40 min
Inhalant agents			
Isoflurane	1–4%, to effect	Inhalant	
Other agents			
Propofol	7.5–10 mg/kg	IV	5–10 min
ANALGESICS			
Buprenorphine	0.01–0.05 mg/kg	SC, IP	8–12 h
Butorphanol	2 mg/kg	SC, IP	4 h
Morphine	2.5 mg/kg	SC, IP	2–4 h
Carprofen	5 mg/kg	SC, IP	24 h
Ketoprofen	5 mg/kg*	SC, IP	24[t]
Meloxicam	1–2 mg/kg	SC, IP	24[t]
Bupivacaine	Do not exceed 2 mg/kg	Local infiltration	1–2 h[t]
MISCELLANEOUS			
Atropine	0.05 mg/kg	SC	
Atipamezole	0.1–1 mg/kg	IP, SC	
Yohimbine	0.2 mg/kg	IV	
	0.5 mg/kg	IM	

[a]Doses adapted with modifications from Gaertner et al. (2008) and Flecknell (2009).
[b]See Flecknell (2009) for mixing instructions.
*Use caution, reported to cause gastric ulceration at therapeutic doses (Lamon et al., 2008; Shientag et al., 2012).
[t]Uncertain duration.

TABLE 24.3   Drug Doses[a] for Hamsters

Drug	Dose	Route	Duration
ANESTHESTICS			
Dissociative agents and combinations			
Ketamine+	150 mg/kg	IP	45–120 min
acepromazine	5 mg/kg		
Ketamine+	75–100 mg/kg	IP	30–60 min
medetomidine	0.25–1 mg/kg		
Ketamine+	80–200 mg/kg	IP	30–60 min
xylazine	5–10 mg/kg		
Tiletamine-zolazepam+	20–30 mg/kg	IP	10–30 min
xylazine	10 mg/kg		
Neuroleptanesthetics			
Fentanyl-fluanisone (hypnorm)			
+midazolam	4.0 ml/kg[b]	IP	20–40 min
Fentanyl-fluanisone (hypnorm)	1 ml/kg		
+diazepam	5.0 mg/kg	IP	20–40 min
Inhalant agents			
Isoflurane	1–4%, to effect	Inhalant	
Other agents			
α-Chloralose (hypnosis only)*	80–100 mg/kg	IP	3–4 h
Urethane*	1000–2000 mg/kg	IP	6–8 h
ANALGESICS			
Buprenorphine	0.01–0.05 mg/kg	SC, IP	6–12 h
Butorphanol	1–5 mg/kg	SC, IP	4 h
Morphine	2.5 mg/kg	SC, IP	2–4 h
Meloxicam	1–2 mg/kg	SC, IP	24 h
Carprofen	5 mg/kg	SC, IP	24 h
Ketoprofen	5 mg/kg	SC, IP	24 h[t]
Bupivacaine	Do not exceed 2 mg/kg	Local infiltration	1–2 h[t]
MISCELLANEOUS			
Atropine	0.04 mg/kg	SC	
Yohimbine	0.2 mg/kg	IV	–
	0.5 mg/kg	IM	
Atipamezole	0.1–1 mg/kg	IM, IP, SC, IV	–

[a]Doses adapted with modifications from Gaertner et al. (2008) and Flecknell (2009).
[b]See Flecknell (2009) for mixing instructions.
*Terminal use only.
[t]Uncertain duration.

TABLE 24.4 Drug Doses[a] for Gerbils

Drug	Dose	Route	Duration
ANESTHESTICS			
Dissociative agents and combinations			
Ketamine+	75 mg/kg	IP	60–90 min
acepromazine	3 mg/kg		
Ketamine+	75 mg/kg	IP	20–30 min
medetomidine	0.5 mg/kg		
Ketamine+	50 mg/kg	IP	20–50 min
xylazine	2 mg/kg		
Neuroleptanesthetics			
Fentanyl-fluanisone (Hypnorm)			
+midazolam	8.0 ml/kg[b]	IP	20 min
Fentanyl-fluanisone (Hypnorm)	0.3 ml/kg		
+diazepam	5.0 mg/kg	IP	20 min
Inhalant agents			
Isoflurane	1–4%, to effect	Inhalant	
Other agents			
Fentanyl+	75 mg/kg	IP	20–30 min
medetomidine	0.5 mg/kg		
Tribromoethanol	250–300 mg/kg	IP	15–30 min
ANALGESIC			
Buprenorphine	0.01–0.05 mg/kg	SC, IP	6–12 h
Butorphanol	1–5 mg/kg	SC, IP	4 h
Meloxicam	1–2 mg/kg	SC, IP	24 h
Morphine	2.5 mg/kg	SC, IP	2–4 h
Carprofen	5 mg/kg	SC, IP	24 h
Ketoprofen	5 mg/kg	SC, IP	24 h[t]
Bupivacaine	Do not exceed 2 mg/kg	Local infiltration	1–2 h[t]
MISCELLANEOUS			
Atropine	0.04 mg/kg	SC	
Yohimbine	0.2 mg/kg	IV	–
	0.5 mg/kg	IM	
Atipamezole	0.1–1 mg/kg	IM, IP, SC, IV	–

[a]Doses adapted with modifications from Gaertner et al. (2008) and Flecknell (2009).
[b]See Flecknell (2009) for mixing instructions.
[t]Uncertain duration.

TABLE 24.5 Drug Doses[a] for Guinea Pigs

Drug	Dose	Route	Duration
ANESTHESTICS			
Barbiturates			
Pentobarbital	15–40 mg/kg	IP	60–90 min
Dissociative agents and combinations			
Ketamine+	100–125 mg/kg	IM/IP	45–120 min
acepromazine	5 mg/kg		
Ketamine+	40 mg/kg	IP	30–40 min
medetomidine	0.5 mg/kg		
Ketamine+	40 mg/kg	IP	30 min
xylazine	5 mg/kg		
Neuroleptanesthetics			
Fentanyl-fluanisone (hypnorm)			
+midazolam	8.0 ml/kg[b]	IP	45–60 min
Fentanyl-fluanisone (hypnorm)	1 ml/kg		
+diazepam	2.5 mg/kg	IP	45–60 min
Inhalant Agents			
Isoflurane	1–4%, to effect	Inhalant	
ANALGESICS			
Buprenorphine	0.01–0.05 mg/kg	SC, IP	6–12 h
Butorphanol	0.2–2 mg/kg	SC, IP	4 h
Codeine	25–40 mg/kg	SC, IP	4 h
Morphine	2–5 mg/kg	SC, IP	2–4 h
Meloxicam	0.1–0.3 mg/kg	SC, PO, IP	24 h
Carprofen	4 mg/kg	SC, IP	24 h
Ketoprofen	1 mg/kg	SC, IP	12–24 h
Bupivacaine	Do not exceed 2 mg/kg	Local infiltration	1–2 h[t]
MISCELLANEOUS			
Atropine	0.05 mg/kg	SC	
Yohimbine	0.2 mg/kg	IV	–
	0.5 mg/kg	IM	
Atipamezole	0.1–1 mg/kg	IM, IP, SC, IV	–

[a]Doses adapted with modifications from Gaertner et al. (2008) and Flecknell (2009).
[b]See Flecknell (2009) for mixing instructions.
[t]Uncertain duration.

as guidelines, not as firm recommendations. Although guidelines are useful starting points, final determination of optimum doses depends on careful observation of the animal's responses, consideration of experimental needs, and judicious fine tuning.

1. Injectable Anesthetics

Injectable agents, used singly or in combination, are common choices for rodent anesthesia. Their ease of use and apparent simplicity tend to conceal complex actions and side effects, but when correctly used, injectable agents are safe, effective, and convenient.

Many drugs used in rodent anesthesia are formulated for use in larger species, with the result that their concentration is often too high for accurate and convenient administration to rodents. Measurement errors that might be inconsequential in larger patients can have significant effects in small ones. Further, many drug mixtures are compounded extemporaneously by the user, sometimes without taking into account issues of measurement and dosing. These difficulties are addressed by diluting drugs to easily measurable concentrations. At the same time, final volumes can be adjusted to yield convenient dose rates, such as 0.2 ml per 100 gm body weight for a rat, or 0.10 ml per 10 gm body weight for a mouse. Thoughtful dilution and concentration adjustment increase not only the convenience but also the safety of drug administration in small rodents. Suitable diluents are sterile water for injection, U.S.P. (United States Pharmacopeia) or saline for injection, U.S.P. When producing these mixtures, it is important to establish that the combined components are compatible, stable, and safe.

Intraperitoneal (IP) injection is a commonly utilized route because of the relatively large potential space for injection and the ease and rapidity with which it can be carried out. It is important to consider the composition of injection to prevent irritation of abdominal contents due to pH or other factors. Additionally, this method requires training to ensure proper technique to prevent administration into abdominal organs or adipose tissues that could injure the animal or result in variable drug effects (Morton et al., 2001). Even with reduced volumes, intramuscular injection is unreliable and usually painful in conscious rodents, and intravenous injection is often difficult, with the possible exception of rat, and perhaps mouse, tail veins. Subcutaneous injection is also relatively straightforward and useful for some drugs and for perioperative fluid support.

a. Dissociative Agents

Ketamine and tiletamine are the two representatives of this class, for which phencyclidine is the parent compound. Drug combinations containing ketamine are the most commonly used injectable protocols in laboratory

rodents (Stokes et al., 2009). Ketamine produces a degree of analgesia and immobility without muscle relaxation. Used alone, it is generally considered to be adequate for restraint but not for anesthesia. For this reason, and because of its wide margin of safety, ketamine is often combined with various tranquilizers and sedatives to make a wide variety of anesthetic cocktails. The most commonly utilized combinations include ketamine with xylazine (± acepromazine) or dexmedetomidine (see further details in anesthetic adjuvant section). The analgesic effects of ketamine can be influenced by a number of factors but may be present 1–4 h after administration providing some short term postoperative pain relief (Wixson et al., 1987; Qian et al., 1996; Koizuka et al., 2005; Minville, 2010). Ketamine can be given orally, intramuscularly (IM), intravenously (IV), and subcutaneously (SC) but, for operator convenience and animal comfort, is usually given IP. Typical ketamine mixtures are given in the dose tables and mentioned under the specific species discussions following this section.

Tiletamine (Telazol) is available only in combination with zolazepam, a benzodiazepine. Telazol has been used alone or in combination with xylazine or butorphanol to produce anesthesia in rats and mice (Arras et al., 2001; Saha et al., 2007). Aside from a longer duration of effect, there seem to be few reasons to favor this more expensive combination in rodents over the various ketamine-based formulations (Saha et al., 2007).

b. Barbituates

Once the dominant drugs for rodent anesthesia, barbiturates have waned in popularity (Stokes et al., 2009). At sufficient doses these sedative hypnotics produce general anesthesia with muscle relaxation, loss of consciousness, and failure to respond to noxious stimuli. As a class, they have minimal analgesic effect independent of their ability to affect consciousness; therefore, if used for invasive recovery procedures, analgesia should also be provided. They also cause dose-related respiratory and cardiovascular depression, which worsens with time. As in other species, repeated doses of short-acting barbiturates are cumulative and will result in prolonged recovery. Barbiturates tend to have a narrow therapeutic window. In some species, such as hamsters and gerbils, the window is so narrow as to be a crevice, and considerable experience and finesse are required for safe use.

Sodium pentobarbital is the most frequently used barbiturate for rodent anesthesia, and it is usually given IP. If suitably diluted, it can be given IV in intermittent boluses or as a continuous infusion. Whereas dose requirements are somewhat predictable for rats, the effect of a given dose of pentobarbital in mice can be highly variable, depending on strain, sex, age, and housing conditions (Lovell, 1986a,b,c). Recovery can be lengthy, especially with longer surgical procedures, and is further prolonged by hypothermia. Anesthetic formulations of pentobarbital are currently not available in the USA and many other countries.

Sodium thiopental provides brief anesthesia following a single dose. It is probably best given IV, as in larger species, in which case other and safer agents would ordinarily be preferred. Like pentobarbital, thiopental is not currently available in the USA and other countries.

Inactin (EMTU, or ethylmalonyl urea) has a longer duration of effect than pentobarbital and is usually reserved for procedures requiring more than 3 h anesthesia in the rat (Buelke-Sam *et al.*, 1978). The primary advantage of inactin is a greater duration of stable anesthesia.

c. Alkylphenol Derivative: Propofol

Propofol is an alkylphenol derivative that should be administered IV. It produces respiratory and cardiovascular depression if administered too rapidly or if used as the sole means of achieving surgical anesthesia (Glen and Hunter, 1984; Brammer *et al.*, 1993). The vehicle supports microbial growth well, so careful aseptic technique is essential if an opened vial or bottle is to be kept for more than a brief period of time. In use, propofol resembles rapid-acting barbiturates, such as thiopental, with the important exception that recovery from propofol is relatively rapid, even following repeated boluses or infusion.

d. Tribromoethanol (Avertin)

Used properly, tribromoethanol is an adequate anesthetic for short surgical procedures in mice when given IP. For safety, it is essential that it be prepared, stored, and used properly. Tribromoethanol is not stable if stored at room temperature or if exposed to light and the resulting products of decomposition are irritant and toxic, resulting in significant morbidity and mortality (Papaioannou and Fox, 1993; Zeller *et al.*, 1998). The continued use of tribromoethanol has been questioned given the safety and effectiveness of alternative drugs or combinations (isoflurane or ketamine/xylazine combinations). Some recommend that it only be utilized for terminal procedures when given IP (Meyer and Fish, 2005), although there are anesthetic situations or procedures in which recovery procedures may be appropriate (see Special Anesthetic Considerations).

e. Neuroleptics

These drugs are combinations of potent opioids and butyrophenone tranquilizers. The two that have seen widespread use, Innovar-Vet (droperidol) and Hypnorm (fluanisone), are not available for use in the United States, but may be compounded by a pharmacy if necessary. Both products use fentanyl as the opioid

analgesic, albeit at different concentrations. In human practice these agents used alone would be termed neuroleptanalgesics. To produce neuroleptanesthesia, additional agents, such as nitrous oxide, would be added. In fact, the recommendations for Hypnorm in rats include the addition of a benzodiazepine, either diazepam or midazolam. The combination of hypnorm and a benzodiazepine is reported to reliably produce adequate to good anesthesia in mice, rats, and hamsters (Green, 1975; Flecknell and Mitchell, 1984; Richardson and Flecknell, 2005).

f. Miscellaneous Injectables

The drugs listed below are rarely used in modern rodent anesthesia as there are usually much safer and effective drugs available. However, there may be instances where these drugs or drug combinations are still being used for scientific or historical reasons.

α-Chloralose As a sedative hypnotic that provides minimal analgesia, α-chloralose is often used for studies involving autonomic reflexes. It is recommended that painful manipulations, such as surgical procedures, should be carried out under a more effective anesthetic, after which α-chloralose can be substituted to produce prolonged stable study conditions (Wixson and Smiler, 1997; Flecknell, 1996, 2009; Silverman and Muir, 1993). It is not considered suitable for survival procedures.

Chloral Hydrate As a sedative hypnotic, chloral hydrate at doses of 400 mg/kg IP can produce anesthesia for about 1–2 h in rats, causing respiratory, cardiovascular, and thermoregulatory depression. Chloral hydrate has been associated with peritonitis and adynamic ileus, apparently related more to concentration than to total dose. (Silverman and Muir, 1993; Field *et al.*, 1993; Vachon *et al.*, 1999).

Metomidate and Etomidate Metomidate and etomidate are imidazole 5-carbonic acid derivatives. Given IV, they produce rapid loss of consciousness, minimal analgesia, and good cardiovascular stability. Only etomidate (amidate) is available in the United States. When used in rodents, they are usually combined with a potent opioid (Wixson and Smiler, 1997; Flecknell, 2009; Green, 1975).

Urethane Ethyl carbamate, or urethane, provides greater analgesia than α-chloralose, as well as prolonged and relatively stable anesthesia in rats (Field *et al.*, 1993). It is sometimes used in conjunction with α-chloralose, to gain the advantage of increased analgesia. Urethane is carcinogenic and is unsuitable for recovery anesthesia.

2. Inhalation Anesthetics

Inhalation anesthesia circumvents many of the difficulties associated with injectable agents. Because the agents are used to effect, issues of dose calculation and variations in response do not arise. These agents are not controlled substances and also escape the burden of detailed record keeping required for barbiturates, opioids, benzodiazepines, and ketamine. Isoflurane and sevoflurane are the most widely used of the inhalant anesthetics for rodents. Ether is sympathomimetic and is not recommended because it is highly irritant and causes increased respiratory secretions. It also forms explosive mixtures with air and oxygen, resulting in storage and safety concerns. Pharmaceutical grade preparations of ether are not currently available. In general, the recommended inhalant agents are characterized by rapid induction and recovery. To varying degrees, all inhalation anesthetics cause dose-related cardiovascular and respiratory depression, but these effects are frequently less severe than equipotent doses of injectable agents. No currently produced inhalation agents are analgesic at subanesthetic doses. Currently, isoflurane probably possesses the best combination of properties in terms of expense and safety of personnel and patient. Sevoflurane is expensive but can provide a smoother and more rapid induction and recovery than isoflurane. There have been concerns about nephrotoxic effects in rats exposed to a product formed from sevoflurane in the presence of soda lime, called 'Compound A,' effects have been seen in low flow anesthesia when rats are exposed to high levels of sevoflurane (Kharasch et al., 2005; Morio et al., 1992).

The equipment needed for rodent anesthesia is relatively simple, comprising of a flowmeter, a vaporizer, an induction chamber, a delivery circuit, and some means of waste gas disposal. Face masks are commonly used in rodents, although endotracheal intubation, if mastered, permits assisted or controlled ventilation. The means of waste gas disposal varies with the facilities available. Because of increased interest in inhalation anesthesia for rodents, new equipment and innovative designs that more specifically address the needs of rodent anesthesia are becoming commercially available. Basic equipment and techniques for administration, including endotracheal intubation, are described in Flecknell (2009); Watanabe et al. (2009); Hamacher et al. (2008); Molthen (2006); and Turner et al. (1992).

Bell jar or anesthetic chambers may be used for induction of anesthesia with inhalant agents by allowing the anesthetic to vaporize within the ambient air into a closed jar or induction chamber. This 'open drop' or 'open circuit' method was developed when ether was the most widely used anesthetic agent. This type of administration is dangerously imprecise and requires careful monitoring due to the uncontrolled amount of gas to which the animal is exposed. Delivery of isoflurane in this way, for example, results in anesthetic concentrations of 20–25%, which can be rapidly lethal. It is not a suitable method for surgical anesthesia when using modern inhalant agent, however it is sometimes used for sedation prior to brief procedures. In this setting animals must be closely monitored and removed from the chamber rapidly upon loss of consciousness. Diluting isoflurane with propylene glycol can reduce the concentration of isoflurane vapor in an open circuit/nose cone setting and create a somewhat safer and more stable anesthetic without the use of a precision vaporizer. This method has been utilized in short-term surgical procedures with success (Itah et al., 2004). Fume hoods or scavenging systems must be used to prevent environmental contamination with these techniques (Flecknell, 2009).

Nitrous oxide is sometimes used to reduce the amount of potent inhalation anesthetic agent needed and to minimize respiratory and cardiovascular depression, but it is inadequate as a sole anesthetic. As with all inhalation agents, adequate scavenging is essential to avoid potential human health hazards. Scavenging systems that rely on activated charcoal are not effective for removing nitrous oxide.

3. Anesthestic Adjuvants

a. Local Anesthetics

Lidocaine, bupivacaine, and other local anesthetics are often used to supplement light levels of general anesthesia, as well as to provide some degree of postoperative analgesia. In rodents they are usually given by local infiltration or topical application prior to an invasive procedure. With care to assure adequate general anesthesia and to avoid toxicity, both short-acting (lidocaine) and longer-acting (bupivacaine) local anesthetics are useful. Discomfort from injection of local anesthetics in conscious animals can be reduced by buffering and warming the solution. Additional analgesia should be used if pain is expected to last more than a few hours due to the relatively short duration of action of these agents.

b. Opioids

As anesthetic adjuvants, opioid agonists provide potent analgesia and lower the required doses of anesthetic agents. Buprenorphine, a partial mu-agonist, is the preferred opioid for rodents as it is more potent than morphine and has a longer duration of action. In addition to buprenorphine, morphine, methadone, tramadol, butorphanol, fentanyl, and remifentanil have been found to reduce the isoflurane and sevoflurane minimum alveolar concentration (MAC) requirements in rats and mice (Criado and Gómez de Segura, 2000, 2003; Abreu et al., 2012; Smith et al., 2004). Opioids can be accompanied by bradycardia and respiratory depression, which may be balanced by lowering the dose of anesthetics. Additionally, atropine or glycopyrrolate can be used to counteract bradycardia but should be used with caution, if at all, when medetomidine is also a component of the anesthesia protocol, as correcting the bradycardia can

1143

result in a dangerous degree of hypertension. Opioid agonists can be effectively reversed by specific antagonists, such as naloxone, as well as by some partial agonists and mixed-function agonist–antagonists, such as butorphanol, nalbuphine, and buprenorphine, which are typically utilized for postoperative analgesia.

c. α₂-Adrenergic Agonists

Members of this group commonly used in rodent anesthesia include xylazine and medetomidine (or dexmedetomidine) (Stokes *et al.*, 2009). These drugs are anxiolytic, analgesic, and provide muscle relaxation. Another benefit of these agents is their ability to provide a brief period of analgesia (15–30 min, if co-administered with ketamine) beyond the period of surgical anesthesia (Gaertner *et al.*, 2008). They also cause hyperglycemia, bradycardia, peripheral vasoconstriction, hypothermia, and diuresis of variable severity in different species and with varying doses and drug mixtures (Hsu *et al.*, 1986; Gaertner *et al.*, 2008). Even so, the combination of ketamine and xylazine is generally reliable, safe, and convenient in laboratory rodents and enjoys wide popularity (Green *et al.*, 1981; Gaertner *et al.*, 2008; Stokes *et al.*, 2009). Ketamine can also be combined with medetomidine to provide similar effects (Nevlainen *et al.*, 1989). Some studies have noted increased anesthetic complications and death when using buprenorphine as a pre-medicant to ketamine/medetomidine combinations (Hedenqvist *et al.*, 2000b). If redosing is necessary for extended anesthetic effect, it is recommended that only ketamine be provided as additional dosing of xylazine or dexmedetomidine can cause bradycardia and cardiac arrest (Gaertner *et al.*, 2008). The sedation produced by α₂-adrenergics can be effectively antagonized by a number of drugs. Yohimbine is often used to reverse the sedation, diuresis, and cardiovascular effects produced by xylazine (Hsu *et al.*, 1986). Atipamezole was developed to antagonize α₂-adrenergics, especially medetomidine, more specifically and rapidly (Flecknell, 2009). The ability to reverse the effects of these drugs can be used to advantage to shorten recovery time, as well as to rescue the occasional patient that displays severe adverse reactions to the drugs. However, it should be noted that reversal of the effects of xylazine and dexmedetomidine also reduce the analgesic effect of the drugs, so additional analgesics may be necessary following reversal.

d. Benzodiazepines

Diazepam and midazolam are often used as adjuvants to anesthesia. They have similar effects, including anxiolysis, sedation, and muscle relaxation but are not analgesic. Midazolam is shorter-acting and is water-soluble, making it preferable for mixtures intended to provide short-term anesthesia. Midazolam paired with

fentanyl significantly reduced behaviors associated with distress during induction and reduced sevoflurane MAC by one-third (Cesarovic *et al.*, 2012). The effects of these agents can be quickly terminated by the reversal agent, flumazenil, however the effects of the antagonist are relatively brief, and repeated dosing may be needed.

e. Phenothiazine Tranquilizers

Acepromazine, and to a lesser extent promazine, are the most common phenothiazine tranquilizers utilized for rodent anesthesia. Phenothiazines produce sedation and potentiate the effects of anesthetics but do not provide analgesia. They also cause vasodilation, with some depression of blood pressure and body temperature, and should not be used in dehydrated or hemorrhaging patients.

In mice, acepromazine combined with ketamine and xylazine (KXA) has been shown to result in longer duration of anesthesia and immobility, as well as more stable physiologic parameters compared to ketamine/xylazine alone (Arras *et al.*, 2001; Buitrago *et al.*, 2008). The KXA combination has also been demonstrated to be effective for surgical anesthesia in rats (Welberg *et al.*, 2006).

f. Neuromuscular Blocking Agents

Paralytics may be required for specific experimental protocols, but their use must be justified as no anesthesia or analgesia is provided, and once the animal is paralyzed, it is difficult to assess depth of anesthesia. For this reason the anesthetic protocol should be demonstrated to be adequate for performance of the study procedures humanely without the use of neuromuscular blocking (NMB) agents. Controlled ventilation must be provided to paralyzed rodents and careful monitoring of blood pressure, heart rate, and end tidal CO_2, while imperfect indicators, may assist in assuring the patient is adequately anesthetized. Neostigmine and physostigmine may be used to reverse the effects of nondepolarizing NMB agents. The use of NMB agents in research has been reviewed by Gaertner *et al.* (2008).

D. Intraoperative Monitoring and Support

Monitoring anesthesia in rodents is often limited to observation of respiratory rate and character, color of the skin and mucus membranes (if the animal is an albino), and response to surgical stimulus. Depth of anesthesia may be estimated by pedal withdrawal response and eye reflexes but is probably most reliably indicated by response to surgical stimulus (Flecknell, 2009). While heart and respiratory rate, as well as oxygen saturation are more easily monitored in larger rodents, such as rats and guinea pigs, pulse oximeter options are now commercially available for use in mice and sensitive enough to be utilized for hypoxia research (Chodzyński et al., 2013). Electrocardiography is primarily used only as a research tool in rodents. Hypothermia will occur with all anesthetic protocols in rodents, and it is therefore important that body temperature is measured, and means of warming the animal are employed. Temperature can be monitored by using small rectal and surface probes. Thermal support utilizing circulating hot-water pads, homeothermic blankets, infrared warming pads, heating lamps, space blanket, or even bubble wraps are recommended. Fluid support in the form of warmed subcutaneous fluids is useful and simple, especially with prolonged procedures. As rodents do not close their eyes while anesthetized, lubrication to prevent corneal drying is an important step for all anesthetic events lasting more than a few minutes. Another undesirable side-effect of anesthesia, particularly with injectable agents, is modest to severe hypoxia and hypercapnia. Moderate hypercapnia can be tolerated by healthy animals for reasonable periods of time but if progressive may be difficult to correct without mechanical ventilation. Hypoxia, on the other hand, is often easily and inexpensively corrected by providing a low flow of oxygen by mask during anesthesia and surgery.

E. Special Anesthetic Considerations

1. Anesthesia for Transgenic Production and Pregnant Rodents

While appropriate preparation and storage are required, tribromoethanol has a long-standing history of successful use in transgenic mouse production. However, its use is waning as safer anesthetic options, ketamine/xylazine and isoflurane, have been shown to have equivalent minimal effects on fetal growth and pregnancy rates in mice as tribromoethanol (Thaete et al., 2013; Bagis et al., 2004). Similarly, the number of live mouse embryos, pups born and weaned from dams administered buprenorphine, flunixin meglumine, or a combination of buprenorphine and carprofen post-embryo transfer surgery were not significantly impacted by analgesic administration (Krueger and Fujiwara, 2008; Goulding et al., 2010; Parker et al., 2011). Providing supplemental heat overnight after embryo transfer surgery was shown to significantly increase rates of pregnancy and fetal implantation (Bagis et al., 2004). In rat dams undergoing embryo transfer, use of isoflurane and morphine resulted in significantly greater pregnancy rates and faster induction and recovery times compared to ketamine and xylazine; additionally, both anesthetic regimens resulted in comparable numbers of live pups (Smith et al., 2004). Regarding surgical manipulation of the fetus during gestation, the literature largely suggests that fetuses in utero are maintained in a sleeplike state of unconsciousness

and therefore are unable to experience conscious pain until after birth (Murrell et al., 2008).

Overall, suitability of an anesthetic protocol will depend to some extent on the stage of pregnancy and the species. Late pregnancy and the associated increased abdominal pressure may impede adequate respiration; therefore positioning the animal on its side, as well as provision of supplemental oxygen and possibly ventilation may be necessary (Flecknell, 2009). If surgical access to the fetus is required, inhaled anesthetics are preferred as they cause uterine relaxation and facilitate surgical manipulation of the uterus. Alpha-2 adrenergic agonists, on the other hand, reduce uterine blood flow and increase uterine contractility making them a less favorable choice for fetal surgery (Murrell et al., 2008). Local and regional analgesia, as well as preoperative administration of opioid analgesics can significantly reduce the anesthetic requirements (Murrell et al., 2008; Flecknell, 2009). General principles and approaches to anesthesia and analgesia in the pregnant dam are given in Murrell et al. (2008) and Flecknell (2009).

2. Neonatal Anesthesia

Inhalant anesthesia, primarily sevoflurane or isoflurane, is the preferred method of neonatal anesthesia due to the rapid induction and recovery; of note, neonates may require a higher concentration of gas anesthetic than adult rodents (Flecknell, 2009). Hypothermia can also be an effective anesthetic for altricial neonates when cooled to 5–10°C; though there is some debate as to possible discomfort during cooling and rewarming (Janus and Golde, 2014; Gaertner et al., 2008; Flecknell, 2009). Care must be taken not to expose neonates directly to ice to avoid tissue damage. Fentanyl plus fluanisone have also been used successfully for neonatal anesthesia (Clowry and Flecknell, 2000). Significant concerns with neonatal anesthesia include rapid development of hypoglycemia and hypothermia, which can contribute to subsequent maternal rejection or cannibalization. Where possible, analgesia for invasive procedures should be considered as unalleviated pain in the rodent neonate can affect response to pain and stress later in life (LaPrairie and Murphy, 2010; Sternberg et al., 2005; Victoria et al., 2013a,b, 2014). These alterations can be attenuated if preemptive analgesia is provided (LaPrairie et al., 2008; Walker et al., 2009), however there is little objective data on appropriate dose rates of analgesics for neonatal rodents.

3. Stereotactic and Neurosurgery

Anesthesia for stereotactic surgery has usually relied on the same anesthetics used for other purposes. Because placement of ear bars for fixation of the head is often more painful than the surgery itself, a relatively deep plane of anesthesia is needed. Lidocaine creams placed on the ear bars may reduce some of this discomfort. Removal of the

ear bars following surgery can result in an abrupt increase in the apparent depth of anesthesia (Gardiner and Toth, 1999). Face-mask adapters, used in place of the incisor bar, allow for more convenient use of inhalation techniques. Alternatively, intranasal cannulas with scavenging by snorkel or downdraft may facilitate delivery of gas anesthesia when use of a face-mask is not possible (Flecknell, 2009). Heat support can be challenging if the rodent is not in contact with a heated surface due to the stereotaxic positioning, thus possible options for preventing hypothermia include wrapping the animal in bubble wrap or pairing reflective foil with a thermogenic gel or circulating warm water blanket (Flecknell, 2009, Caro et al., 2013). Lastly, craniotomies and manipulation of the muscles of mastication may result in post-procedural discomfort when eating or drinking; early nutritional and fluid support has been demonstrated to significantly improve recovery after stereotactic craniotomy surgery (Hampshire et al., 2001). For minimally invasive nonsurvival studies involving measurement of autonomic reflexes, α-chloralose, with or without urethane, is sometimes used (Gaertner et al., 2008).

4. Anesthesia for Imaging Procedures

Imaging is an increasingly important tool for in vivo research, facilitating noninvasive longitudinal studies. Anesthesia plays a crucial role in reducing movement artifacts but can present challenges for monitoring, maintaining adequate anesthetic depth and preventing hypothermia. Bioluminescent imaging modalities frequently feature a heated stage and gas anesthetic delivery via face-masks. Other modalities, such as computed tomography (CT); micropositron emission tomography (MicroPET); single-photon emission CT (SPECT); and ultrasound permit use of a range of anesthetic agents, thermal support approaches, and associated monitoring. A shared complication is the often-long acquisition times requiring either inhalant or long acting injectable anesthesia. Anesthetic effect on tracer uptake and other physiological variables that may influence image quality should be considered (Alstrup and Smith, 2013). Where possible, monitoring should include basic respiratory parameters such as rate, depth and character, heart rate, temperature, mucous membrane color, muscle tone, and reflexes. If pre-imaging fasting is required, withholding food for up to 6h prior to imaging is sufficient for the stomach to clear ingesta (Tremoleda et al., 2012).

Magnetic resonance imaging (MRI) of rodents presents unique difficulties in terms of anesthetic administration, thermal support, and monitoring. For short procedures, any injectable method compatible with the study can be used. For longer procedures, inhalation anesthesia is the method of choice, but in its absence infusion techniques are also satisfactory. Although infusion pumps and conventional inhalation equipment must be kept at a safe distance, both can be effectively used. Long,

small-bore infusion lines can be used to deliver injectable agents. For inhalation techniques, rodents can be placed in plastic cylinders with fresh gas entering at one end of the cylinder and exiting at the opposite end to the scavenging system. If gating is necessary, the animal will likely need to be ventilated. Anesthetic monitoring may be limited to intermittent visual observations, but MRI-compatible pulse oximeters and capnographs may be used. Full commercial suites of MRI-compatible rodent monitoring, gating, and heating systems are available. Alternatively, a simple means of monitoring respiration rate is a thermistor placed near the nares, ET tube or face mask, which is sensitive for animals weighing more than 300g, or a pressure sensor (baby respiration sensor) to detect respiratory movements for animals weighing as little as 30g (Flecknell, 2009, Tremoleda et al., 2012). Heat support that will not interfere with the image, such as warm air or warmed fluid bags or gels, may be useful. A thorough review of anesthesia and physiological monitoring of in vivo imaging of rodents can be found in Tremoleda et al. (2012) and Gargiulo et al. (2012a,b).

F. Analgesic Therapy

The ethical and scientific value of relieving pain and distress in experimental animals is well accepted in principle but remains a challenging and often controversial topic in practice. Discussions regarding scientific justification for withholding of analgesics should be weighed with the behavioral, physiological, and immunological sequelae of untreated pain. In some models the untreated pain may be a greater variable than the analgesic (Piersma et al., 1999; Page, 2002; Page and Ben-Eliyahu, 2002; Franchi et al., 2007; Kolstad et al., 2012). Ideally the impact of analgesia versus unalleviated pain should be evaluated within each model to fully appreciate their individual contributions as variables on scientific outcomes.

1. Assessment of Pain/Discomfort

Species-specific signs of acute and chronic pain, approaches to pain recognition and to providing and monitoring analgesia are described in Karas and Cadillac (2008), Flecknell (2009), ACLAM Task Force Members (Kohn et al., 2006), ILAR Committee on Recognition and Alleviation of Pain in Laboratory Animals (National Research Council, 2009) as well as emerging behavioral assessments such as pain faces (grimace scores), burrowing and nest building behaviors, behavioral ethograms and even affective state (Matsumiya et al., 2012; Sotocinal et al., 2011; Jirkof et al., 2010, 2013a,b; Cesarovic et al., 2011; Roughan and Flecknell, 2003a; Wright-Williams et al., 2007, 2013; Roughan et al., 2009; Flecknell, 2010; Langford et al., 2010; Leach et al., 2012; Makowska et al., 2013; Rock et al., 2014). Carefully constructed scoring

systems, specifically adapted to the conditions of the protocol, are most useful in recognizing pain and monitoring analgesia in rodents. When planning for assessment and alleviation of postoperative and post-procedural pain, consider all sources of discomfort such as hypothermia, prolonged body positioning, ear bars, potential nausea, disorientation, etc.

2. Nonpharmacologic Methods

Almost invariably, the term *analgesia* is associated with drugs. But drugs cannot be substituted for meticulous surgical technique, nor for excellent nursing and husbandry. Comfortable bedding, ability to control light exposure and temperature with a shelter and/or appropriate nesting material, supplemental heat provided to a portion of the cage, easy access to palatable food and water, attention to wound care, as well as addressing issues of social deprivation will greatly improve the quality of postoperative and post-procedural recovery (Jirkof *et al.*, 2012; Van Loo *et al.*, 2007; Pham *et al.*, 2010; Gabriel *et al.*, 2009, 2010a,b). Of note, cryoanalgesia was recently found to provide effective local anesthesia for tail-tip biopsy in mice older than 21 days and may be a valuable alternative to isoflurane anesthesia; however cryoanalgesia was not recommended prior to toe clipping in mouse pups (Matthias *et al.*, 2013; Paluch *et al.*, 2014). Electroacupuncture has been demonstrated to be analgesic in several rodent pain models but veterinary use in rodents has yet to be explored (Kim *et al.*, 2010, 2011; Jiang *et al.*, 2013; Wang *et al.*, 2013).

3. Pharmacologic Methods

The major drugs used for analgesia include opioids, nonsteroidal anti-inflammatory drugs (NSAIDs), and local anesthesia. Optimal analgesia may be best achieved with a multimodal approach incorporating preemptive analgesia (Gaertner *et al.*, 2008; Zegre Cannon *et al.*, 2011; Flecknell, 2009; Penderis and Franklin, 2005; Schaap *et al.*, 2012). As with all drugs used in anesthesia and analgesia, these agents are generally safe and effective but are not completely free of adverse effects.

a. Opioids

For severe pain, pure opioid agonists, such as morphine, are preferred, despite a relatively brief period of effect (Gaertner *et al.*, 2008; Flecknell, 2009). Oxymorphone and hydromorphone also provide significant analgesia in mice and rats, but will likely only be useful for clinical applications if provided in sustained release formulations (Gillingham *et al.*, 2001; Krugner-Higby *et al.*, 2003; Smith *et al.*, 2006; Clark *et al.*, 2004; Leach *et al.*, 2010a; Schmidt *et al.*, 2011). For pain of moderate or lower intensity, partial opioid agonists and mixed-function agonist–antagonists, such as buprenorphine are often used (Curtin *et al.*, 2009; Guarnieri *et al.*,

2012). Due to their small size and high metabolic rate, rodents may require a buprenorphine dose frequency of 2–4 times daily (Gades *et al.*, 2008, 2000; Deng *et al.*, 2000; Roughan and Flecknell, 2002; Yu *et al.*, 2006). While lower doses are not associated with significant side effects, in the rat, pica and possibly long-term weight reductions have been reported at higher doses or with prolonged dosing schedules ((Schaap *et al.*, 2012; Bomzon, 2006). Strain and sex of rodents can also modulate response to opiates (Jablonski *et al.*, 2001; Avsaroglu *et al.*, 2007, 2008; Cotroneo *et al.*, 2012; Wright-Williams *et al.*, 2013). Although usually given as an injection, in some studies orally administered buprenorphine was efficacious in alleviating postoperative pain, however, its utility may be limited in duration of analgesia and by reliable consumption of the food stuffs or water into which it is compounded (Flecknell *et al.*, 1999a; Martin *et al.*, 2001; Jablonski and Howden, 2002; Thompson *et al.*, 2004, 2006; Jessen *et al.*, 2007; Goldkuhl *et al.*, 2010a,b; Leach *et al.*, 2010b; Kalliokoski *et al.*, 2011; Abelson *et al.*, 2012). Additionally, sustained release and transdermal formulations of buprenorphine are emerging as potentially viable and practical opiate delivery systems (Park *et al.*, 2008; Foley *et al.*, 2011; Carbone *et al.*, 2012a). Another opioid gaining attention is tramadol, particularly as it is not a controlled drug in some states. Data evaluating the therapeutic benefit of tramadol over buprenorphine or NSAID therapy is mixed (Cannon *et al.*, 2010; Zegre Cannon *et al.*, 2011; McKeon *et al.*, 2011; Rätsep *et al.*, 2013) and high dose tramadol may be associated with increased mortality in some mouse models of sepsis (Hugunin *et al.*, 2010).

b. Non-Steroidal Anti-Inflammatory Drugs

NSAIDs are sometimes preferable to opiates as they are less likely to induce behavioral changes, provide a longer duration of analgesia, and are not regulated controlled substances (Matsumiya *et al.*, 2012; Roughan and Flecknell, 2004; Roughan *et al.*, 2004; Bourque *et al.*, 2010; Brennan *et al.*, 2009). NSAIDs such as meloxicam, carprofen, ketoprofen, flunixin and indomethacin are potent and effective for moderate pain when injected subcutaneously or intraperitoneally (Stewart and Martin, 2003; Tubbs *et al.*, 2011; Roughan and Flecknell, 2001, 2004; Matsumiya *et al.*, 2012; Cooper *et al.*, 2005, 2008; Blaha and Leon, 2008). Carprofen but not meloxicam was found to reach therapeutic plasma levels if placed in drinking water 12–24h prior to a painful procedure (Ingrao *et al.*, 2013). However, neither carprofen nor ketoprofen administered orally in jelly resulted in significant decreases in postoperative pain (Flecknell *et al.*, 1999). A carprofen-infused diet gel is commercially available but has not been evaluated in the peer-reviewed literature at this time. Acetaminophen was shown by Cooper *et al.* (1997) to be effective in the rat when delivered intraperitoneally but was not efficacious when given SC (Matsumiya *et al.*, 2012). Acetaminophen had limited evidence of efficacy when administered in drinking water, predominantly due to neophobia and resulting decrease in fluid consumption (Cooper *et al.*, 1997; Speth *et al.*, 2001; Bauer *et al.*, 2003; Mickley *et al.*, 2006; Dickinson *et al.*, 2009). Sustained release NSAID formulations are on the horizon (Khurana *et al.*, 2013). When administering NSAIDs, attention must be paid to the patient's hydration status, blood pressure, and any other drugs being administered concurrently, as they may increase risk for renal tubular necrosis and/ or gastric ulceration (Lamon *et al.*, 2008; Shientag *et al.*, 2012; Jaquenod *et al.*, 1998; Kumar *et al.*, 2010). COX-2 specific NSAIDs such as Carprofen or Meloxicam offer analgesic efficacy with fewer renal and gastric side-effects (Flecknell, 2009; King *et al.*, 2009).

c. Local Anesthesia

Infiltration of incision sites can be used to decrease postoperative pain and topical application of a local anesthetic cream may minimize pain associated with needle sticks (Flecknell *et al.*, 1990; Leach *et al.*, 2012; Mert and Gunes, 2012; Kolesnikov *et al.*, 2004; Jones *et al.*, 2012). However, the duration of effect is relatively brief and may be more useful pre- or intraoperatively than in the postoperative period. The degree of analgesia provided by a local block alone is insufficient to control for visceral pain associated with laparotomy and therefore should be included as part of a multimodal analgesic approach (Hayes and Flecknell, 1999; Liles and Flecknell, 1993). Spinal and epidural administration of local anesthetics have not been reported for clinical use in rodents but efficacy data have been demonstrated in research evaluations (Tseng *et al.*, 2013; Sato *et al.*, 2008; Kroin *et al.*, 2012; Wada *et al.*, 2007; Bar-Yosef *et al.*, 2001; Morimoto *et al.*, 2001). Similarly, extended release formulations are being explored (Ickowicz, 2013).

d. Gabapentin

Originally developed as an antiepileptic, gabapentin is increasingly utilized to treat neuropathic pain and non-neuropathic pain from surgery, cancer, and arthritis in both human and veterinary patients. In rats, gabapentin decreased acetic acid-induced writhing and significantly attenuated paw incision-induced c-Fos activation, indicating reduced post-surgical stress (Feng *et al.*, 2003; Kazi and Gee, 2007). When combined with tramadol, gabapentin provided superior relief from footpad incisional pain than tramadol alone; however it did not outperform buprenorphine (McKeon *et al.*, 2011).

G. Species Considerations

Even within species, rodents manifest surprising variability in response to 'standard' doses of injectable agents and even inhalation agents. A pilot study is the best way to establish an acceptable anesthetic protocol with new techniques or agents. Published studies concerning anesthetic techniques in hamsters, gerbils, and guinea pigs are few compared with those for mice and rats, reflecting their relative numbers as research animals. To an even greater degree, information concerning analgesia efficacy is scarce. Commonly suggested agents and doses are given below and in dose tables, but the phrases 'to effect' and 'as needed' assume particular significance with these species (Tables 24.1–24.4).

1. Mice

Table 24.1 lists selected anesthetics and analgesia doses for mice. Both induction and maintenance with gas anesthesia, primarily isoflurane, produces the safest and most titratable anesthetic option. While endotracheal intubation requires training, a nose cone works well when paired with appropriate waste gas scavenging and air exchanges. Combinations of ketamine and xylazine, or dexmedetomidine, with or without acepromazine, may produce surgical anesthesia for up to 90 min, although depth of anesthesia may be variable (Burnside *et al.*, 2013). Reversal of xylazine or dexmedetomidine with atipamezole can significantly shorten the recovery period. Where available, fentanyl-fluanisone plus midazolam can be an excellent choice. Historically, tribromoethanol has served as the anesthetic of choice in transgenic production facilities, yielding effective surgical anesthesia for at least 15 min when properly used (Meyer and Fish, 2005; Papaioannou and Fox, 1993). Use of pentobarbital, where available, as an anesthetic in mice is decreasing with time but is still sometimes used for terminal procedures (Stokes *et al.*, 2009). Heat support and lubrication of the eyes remain important considerations for all anesthetic events lasting more than a few minutes. Commonly used analgesics include buprenorphine and/or NSAIDs via multiple routes including some oral, topical, and sustained release formulations, as well as local anesthesia.

2. Rats

Inhalation anesthesia has many advantages in the rat and is the preferred anesthetic for most research needs. While endotracheal intubation via transillumination or other visual techniques is common, blind oral endotracheal intubation techniques and novel devices such as a face mask and a supraglottic airway device have recently been described (Cheong *et al.*, 2010, 2013; Wang *et al.*, 2012). Ketamine with xylazine, or fentanyl-fluanisone with midazolam, if available, are the most commonly used injectable anesthetics in rats (see Table 24.2). Ketamine-xylazine intramuscular injection resulted in significant muscle necrosis; to a lesser degree lesions were identified in the abdominal musculature after IP injection (Smiler *et al.*, 1990; Wellington *et al.*, 2013). In comparison to ketamine-xylazine, ketamine-dexmedetomidine resulted in better local tissue tolerance when administered IP, while maintaining similar anesthetic properties (Wellington *et al.*, 2013). Pentobarbital, where available, is less reliable but can be useful for non-recovery applications. Buprenorphine is frequently employed for analgesia in rats. Its side-effects, such as pica, can be minimized by altering the dose schedule and utilizing a multimodal approach (Schaap *et al.*, 2012). NSAIDs, including meloxicam, carprofen, and ketoprofen, are also beneficial (Flecknell *et al.*, 1999b; Flecknell, 2009) but can be associated with gastric ulceration (Shientag *et al.*, 2012; Cooper *et al.*, 2008; Lamon *et al.*, 2008). Local anesthesia is a useful addition to multimodal analgesia (Wen *et al.*, 2012).

3. Hamsters

Inhalation anesthesia by nosecone or endotracheal intubation is safe and effective with the equipment and techniques used for other rodents (Gebhardt-Henrich *et al.*, 2007; Picazo *et al.*, 2009; Flecknell, 2009). As with rats, ketamine with xylazine or dexmedetomidine, or fentanyl-fluanisone with midazolam, are safe and reliable for procedures of moderate duration (see Table 24.3) (Payton *et al.*, 1993; Flecknell, 2009). A combination of Telazol and xylazine given IP was reported to produce surgical anesthesia (Forsythe *et al.*, 1992). Pentobarbital is reported to have a narrow margin of safety in hamsters and should be used with caution (Flecknell, 2009). Analgesics used in mice and rats can be similarly utilized in hamsters.

4. Gerbils

Inhalation anesthesia using isoflurane or sevoflurane is the safest and most reliable means of anesthetizing these small rodents, though gerbils may require a lower concentration of anesthetic gas than mice or rats (Henke *et al.*, 2004; de Segura *et al.*, 2009). Additionally, anesthesia in gerbils can be produced using a combination of fentanyl and metomidate, (see Table 24.4) (Flecknell, 2009; Pérez-García *et al.*, 2003). Alternatively, Telazol given IP resulted in surgical anesthesia but with a prolonged recovery time (Hrapkiewicz and Smiler, 1989). Pentobarbital should be used with caution. Gerbils are particularly sensitive to hypothermia during anesthesia and upon recovery may take several days to regain normal circadian rhythms (Weinandy *et al.*, 2005). Analgesics used in mice and rats can be similarly utilized in gerbils.

5. Guinea Pigs

Guinea pigs are considered to be among the more difficult laboratory animals to safely anesthetize. Guinea pigs can be quite neophobic, have few accessible peripheral vessels, unusually tough skin, and can be difficult to intubate.

Successful anesthesia and recovery require careful monitoring and perioperative support, as well as appropriate agents, dose and dosing routes (see Table 24.5). Over-the-endoscope or stylet, transillumination of the neck, use of an otoscope speculum, and even use of a purpose-made laryngoscope to facilitate intubation of guinea pigs have all been described (Johnson, 2010; Flecknell, 2009). In the absence of intubation, inhalation anesthesia is usually maintained by mask, using isoflurane or sevoflurane. Upon exposure to high concentrations of isoflurane in an induction box, guinea pigs frequently exhibit excessive lacrimation and salivation, which may be partially alleviated by preemptive application of sterile eye lubrication. Laboratory guinea pigs often have a considerable amount of pasty feed in their mouths, which can contribute to airway obstruction. This residue can be removed or reduced by gently rinsing the mouth with 10–20 ml of water before induction or swabbing gross debris out of the mouth with cotton swabs after induction.

Compared to alfaxolone/alfadolone (Saffan), pentobarbital either as a sole agent or in combination with droperidol and fentanyl (Innovar Vet), ketamine with xylazine had the least respiratory depressant effects in guinea pigs (Schwenke and Cragg, 2004). When given IP it will result in a surgical plane anesthesia for about 30 min but may require supplementation with an inhalant (Cetin *et al.*, 2005; Dang *et al.*, 2008). Fentanyl-fluanisone with midazolam is also effective for a similar period of time (Flecknell, 2009). A combination of tiletamine/zolazepam, xylazine, and butorphanol provided deep surgical, long-duration anesthesia in guinea pigs (Jacobson, 2001). In contrast, medetomidine and medetomidine in combination with ketamine was found to sedate but not anesthetize guinea pigs (Dang *et al.*, 2008; Nevlainen *et al.*, 1989). However, the combination of tiletamine-zolazepam and medetomidine was shown to induce a surgical plane of anesthesia (Buchanan *et al.*, 1998). Intramuscular administration of anesthetics in guinea pigs has been reported to cause self-mutilation and should be avoided (Leash *et al.*, 1973; Newton *et al.*, 1975). Judicious use of local anesthetics can reduce the risks of deep anesthesia and the dangers associated with repeated doses of injectable agents. Like other rodents, buprenorphine, meloxicam, and carprofen, as well as local anesthesia, are frequently utilized to reduce postprocedural pain (Flecknell, 2009; Aguiar *et al.*, 2013).

H. Euthanasia

Euthanasia methods must meet both experimental and humane criteria; a comprehensive review can be found in the Report of the ACLAM Task Force on Rodent Euthanasia and the AVMA Guidelines for the Euthanasia of Animals (2013) (Artwohl *et al.*, 2006; Leary *et al.*, 2013). Prior to euthanasia, activities that contribute to distress should be minimized; this may include euthanizing animals in their home cage to maintain established scent marks and not combining unfamiliar animals (Leary *et al.*, 2013). Injectable anesthetic overdose using a combination of xylazine, ketamine, or diazepam or a barbiturate, barbituric acid derivative, or barbiturate combination are acceptable methods of euthanasia of rodents (Leary *et al.*, 2013). Overdose with inhalant anesthetics or carbon dioxide are also acceptable, as long as death is confirmed by examination or via an adjunctive physical method. Carbon dioxide, the most common means of euthanasia for small rodents, should be administered from a compressed cylinder at a rate that will displace 10–30% of the cage volume per minute and not via prefilled chamber (Leary *et al.*, 2013). Additionally, altricial neonates require an extended period of CO_2 exposure, which may need to be followed by a physical adjunctive method of euthanasia (Klaunberg *et al.*, 2004; Pritchett-Corning, 2009). Automated carbon dioxide euthanasia systems have been validated and are commercially available (McIntyre *et al.*, 2007). There remains controversy regarding the recommended administration rate of CO_2 and the potential benefit for administration of isoflurane anesthesia or other gases or even injectable tranquilizers, sedatives, or anesthetics prior to, or in combination with, CO_2 (Hackbarth *et al.*, 2000; Niel and Weary, 2006, 2007; Makowska *et al.*, 2008, 2009; Chisholm *et al.*, 2013; Wong *et al.*, 2013; Leach *et al.*, 2002a,b, 2009; Valentine *et al.*, 2012; Makowska and Weary, 2009a,b; Makowska *et al.*, 2012; Niel *et al.*, 2008a,b; Thomas *et al.*, 2012a). Guinea pigs may struggle excessively when exposed to carbon dioxide. Pre-sedation, concurrent use of an inhalant anesthetic such as isoflurane or sevoflurane, and application of sterile eye lubricant may reduce distress associated with CO_2 euthanasia in guinea pigs. Cervical dislocation and decapitation of mice and rats less than 200 g can be rapid and humane if carried out by experienced operators, who were preferably trained on anesthetized animals, and as approved by the IACUC (Carbone *et al.*, 2012b; Cartner *et al.*, 2007; Golledge, 2012; Roustan *et al.*, 2012; Leary *et al.*, 2013).

III. RABBITS

A. Introduction

The rabbit remains an important research animal by virtue of its convenient size, ease of handling, definition in a number of experimental and teaching models, and availability at various ages and reproductive status. Rabbits have been considered difficult to anesthetize safely, a reputation earned when pentobarbital was in wide usage and rabbits were of questionable health status. With the development of newer anesthetic drugs and techniques, and with the availability of rabbits with

defined health status from quality vendors, this reputation has been dispelled. Although rabbits continue to be an anesthetic challenge because of individual variation in drug response and their timid nature, there now exist numerous methods for safe and effective induction and maintenance of anesthesia in the rabbit (Flecknell, 2009; Lipman *et al.*, 1997, 2008; Suckow *et al.*, 2012). The purpose of this section is to provide a basic guide to commonly used techniques.

B. Preoperative Assessment and Preparation

1. *Preoperative Evaluation*

Rabbits should be purchased specific pathogen-free for *Pasteurella multocida* and other infectious agents that might influence research. The two breeds most commonly used for research in the United States are the New Zealand White and the Dutch Belted. Rabbits that specifically model certain diseases, such as the Watanabe heritable hyperlipidemia rabbit, a model for familial hypercholesterolemia, may present additional challenges to the anesthetist. Rabbits within a particular study should be purchased from a single vendor as genetic differences will exist among stocks maintained by different vendors. Rabbits should be allowed acclimatization periods of a minimum of 72 h prior to use in a research project. Testing during the acclimatization period will be determined by the health status of the vendor colony, the duration of use, and the demands of the specific protocol.

There is no consensus on the requirement for overnight fasting for rabbits (Flecknell, 2009; Rees-Davies and Rees-Davies, 2003). Proponents argue that there is more consistent anesthesia and that the reduction in intragastric volume allows more effective diaphragmatic excursion with consequent improvements in ventilation. Opponents argue that coprophagia precludes complete gastric emptying and that the inability of the rabbit to vomit makes food withdrawal unnecessary. Rabbits under 3 kg should not have more than 12 h of food withdrawal; these rabbits may develop metabolic acidosis and a decline in blood glucose concentration (Bonath *et al.*, 1982).

2. *Choice of Anesthetic Technique*

Anesthetic regimens used in companion animal practice may differ from those used in the laboratory due to differences in objective and patient population. The choice of anesthetic technique is determined by the desired duration of anesthesia, the nature of the surgical stimulus, the physiologic effects of the technique, their potential impact on the variables studied, and the age and preoperative status of the animal. For example, the hyperglycemic effect of α_2-agonists such as xylazine, should be considered in studies where glucose concentration is important (Gleed, 1987).

3. Preoperative Medications

The use of preoperative medications may reduce the anesthetic requirement for maintenance agents, relieve patient apprehension, and facilitate handling. These agents may suffice for restraint when subjecting animals to non-invasive procedures like phlebotomy or mask induction with inhalants. Anticholinergics may be used to prevent vagal reflexes and to reduce salivary and tracheobronchial secretion that may compromise the airway during anesthesia. Atropine use may be ineffective in some rabbits because of high levels of atropinesterase, an enzyme that degrades atropine into inactive products (Ecobichon and Comeau, 1974). The enzyme may be present in up to 50% of New Zealand White rabbits, is highly variable by breed, and is heritable (Harrison *et al.*, 2006). Consequently, some authors have recommended very high doses of atropine, such as 1–2 mg/kg (Hall and Clarke, 1991), with frequent redosing, as often as every 15–20 min (Sedgwick, 1986). Glycopyrrolate is an effective parasympatholytic agent in the rabbit and produces 60 min of elevation of heart rate, prevention of ketamine/xylazine-associated bradycardia, and an antisialogogue effect when administered at a dose of 0.1 mg/kg IM (Olson *et al.*, 1994).

Tranquilizers used in rabbits include phenothiazines (principally acepromazine), benzodiazepines (diazepam and midazolam), opioids, and α_2-agonists (xylazine and dexmedetomidine). Dexmedetomidine has greater affinity and selectivity for α_2-receptors than does xylazine (Hellebrekers *et al.*, 1997). These agents may be used as sole agents in minor procedures such as echocardiography, radiology, physical examination, and phlebotomy. Benzodiazepine, opioids, and the α_2-agonists have specific antagonists that provide the anesthetist greater control over duration of sedation or anesthesia. Drug dosages are listed in Table 24.7.

C. Intraoperative Anesthesia

In this section, the most commonly used anesthetic agents will be described. Dosages are given in Tables 24.6 and 24.7.

1. Injectable Anesthetics

Injectables are useful for induction of anesthesia in preparation for the use of inhalants, as maintenance agents in short procedures, or as continuous infusions in balanced anesthetic techniques. Additional increments of the initial dosage may be used to prolong anesthesia. The popularity of injectables may be attributed to their ease of administration, predictability, and reasonable efficacy and safety. Many injectable combinations cause hypoxemia and supplemental oxygen should be used for those combinations that cause hypoxemia (Hellebrekers *et al.*, 1997; Peeters *et al.*, 1988).

TABLE 24.6   Drug Doses[a] in Rabbits

Drug	Dosage	Route
ANTICHOLINERGICS		
Atropine	0.04–2.0 mg/kg (0.5 mg/kg commonly recommended)	IM, SC
Glycopyrrolate	0.1 mg/kg	IM, SC
SEDATIVES/TRANQUILIZERS		
Diazepam	5–10 mg/kg	IM
	1–2 mg/kg	IM, IV
Midazolam	2 mg/kg	IP, IV
Acepromazine	0.75–10.0 mg/kg (0.75–1.0 mg/kg most frequently used)	IM
Xylazine	3–9 mg/kg	IM
Medetomidine	0.25 mg/kg	IM
Dexmedetomidine	20–80 µg/kg	IM, IV
BARBITURATES		
Thiopental	15–30 mg/kg	IV (1% solution) GTE[b]
	50 mg/kg	IV (2.5% solution) GTE
Thiamylal sodium	15 mg/kg	IV (1% solution) GTE
	29 mg/kg	IV (2% solution) GTE
EMTU	47.5 mg/kg	IV GTE
Methohexital	5–10 mg/kg	IV (1% solution) GTE
Pentobarbital	20–60 mg/kg	IV GTE
DISSOCIATIVES		
Ketamine	20–60 mg/kg	IM
Ketamine+	10 mg/kg	IV
xylazine	3 mg/kg	IV
Ketamine+	22–50 mg/kg	IM
xylazine (reverse with yohimbine)	2.5–10 mg/kg	
	0.2 mg/kg	IV
Acepromazine+	0.75–1.0 mg/kg	SC
ketamine+	35–40 mg/kg	IM
xylazine (preop. with atropine, 0.04 mg/kg IM)	3–5 mg/kg	
Ketamine+	75 mg/kg	IM
acepromazine	5 mg/kg	IM (given 30 min prior to ketamine)
Ketamine+	60–80 mg/kg	IM

(Continued)

TABLE 24.6 (Continued)

Drug	Dosage	Route
diazepam	5–10 mg/kg	IM (given 30 min prior to ketamine)
Ketamine+	25 mg/kg	IM
medetomidine	0.5 mg/kg	SC

NEUROLEPTANALGESICS

Fentanyl-fluanisone	0.2–0.6 ml/kg	IM, SC
Diazepam + fentanyl-fluanisone	1.5–5 mg/kg, 0.2–0.5 ml/kg (administer diazepam 5 min prior to fentanyl-fluanisone)	IM, IV, IP IM, SC IP, IV
Midazolam + fentanyl-fluanisone	2 mg/kg, 0.3 ml/kg (administer midazolam 5 min prior to fentanyl-fluanisone)	IM
Propofol	7.5–15 mg/kg	IV
Medetomidine + propofol	0.25 mg/kg followed in 5 min by 4 mg/kg	IM IV
medetomidine+	0.25 mg/kg	IM
midazolam+	0.5 mg/kg	IM
propofol	2 mg/kg	IV
α-Chloralose + urethane	32 mmol (10 gm)/ liter in saline	
	at dose of 258 µmol (80 mg)/kg	
	400–500 mg/kg (5.61 mmol/kg) in	IV (slowly)
	1 liter of saline (2.81 mol/liter)	
Urethane	1–1.6 gm/kg	IP
	1.5 gm/kg	IV

REVERSAL AGENTS

$α_2$-Antagonists

Yohimbine	0.2–1.0 mg/kg	IM, IV
Atipamezole	0.2–0.35 mg/kg	IV
Benzodiazepine antagonist: flumazenil	0.1 mg/kg	SC
Opioid antagonist: naloxone	0.001–0.1 mg/kg	IV

[a]Adapted from Lipman et al. (2008) and Wixson (1994).
[b]GTE, given to effect.

TABLE 24.7 Bolus or Infusion Regimens[a] in Rabbits

Drug	Dosage	Route
α-Chloralose + urethane	60 mg/kg	
	400 mg/kg followed by 1–3 ml	
	1% α-chloralose q30–50 min	IV
α-Chloralose + urethane	40–60 mg/kg	
	800 mg/kg, followed by 3–4 ml/h 1% α-chloralose	

SEDATION

Ketamine+	35 mg/kg	IM
xylazine	5 mg/kg	IM

MAINTENANCE

Ketamine+	1 mg/min	Continuous IV infusion
xylazine	0.1 mg/min	
Ketamine+	25 mg/kg	IV
xylazine	5 mg/kg	One-third bolus dose over 1 min, remainder over 4 min

SEDATION

Propofol	1.5 mg/kg	IV bolus

MAINTENANCE

Propofol	0.2–0.6 mg/kg/min	Continuous IV infusion

INDUCTION

Ketamine+	25 mg/kg	IM
xylazine	15 mg/kg	IM

MAINTENANCE

Propofol	0.6 mg/kg/min	Continuous IV infusion
Fentanyl	0.48 mg/kg/min	
Vecuronium	0.003 mg/kg/min	

Adapted from Lipman et al. (2008).
[a]*Intermittent bolus or continuous IV infusion regimens.*

2. Dissociatives

As a sole agent, ketamine can be used for restraint during noninvasive procedures. Endotracheal intubation can be achieved with ketamine combined with other agents (Lindquist, 1972; Green *et al.*, 1981).

Ketamine has been used with xylazine, medetomidine, dexmedetomidine, diazepam or midazolam, and myriad other agents. Ketamine/xylazine may be augmented with acepromazine or butorphanol to provide anesthesia of greater duration and depth (Lipman *et al.*, 1990; Marini *et al.*, 1992). These agents provide approximately 30–45 min of loss of the pedal withdrawal reflex. Physiologic effects of these combinations include depression of respiratory rate, hypoxemia, hypercarbemia, hypotension, and bradycardia. A constant-rate infusion (CRI) technique has also been described (Wyatt *et al.*, 1989). Procedures of moderate surgical stimulus intensity (such as carotid or iliac endarterectomy) may be performed with ketamine/xylazine. Accidental perineural injections of these combinations may lead to self-trauma.

Medetomidine/ketamine and dexmedetomidine/ketamine combinations are useful regimens for rabbit anesthesia (Lipman *et al.*, 2008). The physiologic effects of medetomidine/ketamine are similar to those observed with ketamine/xylazine; moderate hypoxemia, bradycardia, and respiratory rate reduction occur (Hellebrekers *et al.*, 1997). Arterial blood pressure is better preserved by the medetomidine combination in most studies. Reversal of medetomidine with atipamezole at doses once or twice that of medetomidine reduces arousal time and reverses physiologic changes dramatically (Kim *et al.*, 2004). Premedication of rabbits with buprenorphine (0.03 mg/kg SC) one hour before SC administration of ketamine (15 mg/kg)/medetomidine (0.25 mg/kg), significantly increased duration of anesthesia with only transient but physiologically benign depression of respiratory rate (Murphy *et al.*, 2010). Similarly, use of butorphanol (0.4 mg/kg SC) in ketamine/medetomidine-administered rabbits prolonged the duration of the loss of the ear pinch response and exacerbated respiratory rate depression but without influence on arterial blood gases (Hedenqvist *et al.*, 2002). Dexmedetomidine administered intravenously as a 10 min infusion at three different dosages (20, 80, or 320 μg/kg) caused dose-dependent depression of PaO_2 and heart and respiratory rates, and dose-dependent increase in sedation and $PaCO_2$ (Zornow, 1991). No significant change was observed in mean arterial blood pressure. Dexmedetomidine administered IM with subsequent IV ketamine produces approximately 20 min of surgical anesthesia.

The combination agent Telazol (Parke-Davis, Morris Plains, New Jersey), which contains the dissociative tiletamine and the benzodiazepine zolazepam, has been shown to be nephrotoxic in the rabbit and is best avoided (Doerning *et al.*, 1992). Tiletamine is the offending substance in this combination.

3. Neuroleptanesthesia–Neuroleptanalgesia

The most useful agent of the neuroleptanesthesia–neuroleptanalgesia class is a combination of fentanyl and fluanisone (Hypnorm; Vetapharma, United Kingdom) available in Europe (Flecknell *et al.*, 1983; Flecknell and Mitchell, 1984). It may be used for restraint or for sedation prior to administration of inhalation agents. The use of this agent after IV or IP diazepam or midazolam produces anesthesia of moderate duration; increments of hypnorm IM or diazepam IV will prolong anesthesia. Others administer fentanyl-fluanisone intramuscularly and follow with intravenous midazolam (Benato *et al.*, 2013). Premedication with parasympatholytics is important when using opioids. Other regimens that have been investigated include medetomidine-midazolam-fentanyl (Baumgartner *et al.*, 2010), and fentanyl-propofol (Baumgartner *et al.*, 2009). Significant cardiovascular and respiratory effects have been noted with both these combinations, making them less suitable for animals with impaired cardiovascular function.

Naloxone, doxapram, and various mixed agonist/antagonist opioids may be used to reverse fentanyl-induced respiratory depression. Use of mixed agonist/antagonist opioids for this purpose provides fentanyl reversal while preserving analgesia of various duration (DeCastro and Viars, 1968). When buprenorphine was used in this fashion to reverse hypnorm, it provided 420 min of analgesia while reversing depression of respiratory rate and effecting normalization of oxygenation and carbon dioxide elimination (Flecknell *et al.*, 1989).

a. Barbiturates

Pentobarbital was widely used in the past but has become prohibitively expensive and is no longer available as an anesthetic in some parts of the world. Physiologic effects may include respiratory depression or arrest, decreased arterial blood pressure, peripheral vasodilation, decreased cardiac output, depression of the vasopressor response to hemorrhage, and preservation of or increase in heart rate (Korner *et al.*, 1968; Warren and Ledingham, 1978; Morita *et al.*, 1987; Borkowski *et al.*, 1990). Pentobarbital may influence research variables. For example, it diminishes myocardial damage after coronary artery ligation when compared with halothane or α-chloralose (Chakrabarty *et al.*, 1991) and reduces plasma potassium ion concentration with consequent elevation of plasma renin and aldosterone concentrations (Robson *et al.*, 1981).

Thiamylal, thiopental, methohexital, and ethylmalonyl urea (EMTU) are other barbiturates that have been used in the rabbit. As with pentobarbital, these agents should be used as dilute solutions and injected slowly.

b. Propofol

The intravenously administered hypnotic agent propofol has been evaluated in several studies, the sum of which suggests that as a sole agent it is suitable only for induction and noninvasive procedures (Blake *et al.*, 1988; Ko *et al.*, 1992a,b; Aeschbacher and Webb, 1993a,b). Degree of sedation or anesthesia, as well as alteration of physiologic variables, depends upon infusion rate and time of day of administration. Ko used medetomidine/atropine and medetomidine/midazolam/atropine premedication prior to propofol induction and found the combination useful for anesthesia induction sufficient to achieve endotracheal intubation. Pedal withdrawal reflexes and preanesthetic levels of heart rate, respiratory rate, mean arterial pressure, and end tidal CO_2 were preserved (Ko et al., 1992). Propofol infusion in unsedated animals can be facilitated by catheterization of a marginal ear vein on which a lidocaine and prilocaine ointment (EMLA cream, Astra, Westborough, MA) has been applied. Allweiler et al. (2010) describe such administration to unsedated, pre-oxygenated rabbits. An initial infusion of 10 mg/kg IV over 60 s was followed by incremental doses (1–2 mg/kg) until relaxation adequate for endotracheal administration was achieved. The mean dosage required for intubation tolerance was 16 ± 5 mg/kg propofol; apnea did not occur. Rabbits were then maintained on sevoflurane for ovariohysterectomy. Excellent recovery and extubation within 2 min of termination of sevoflurane characterized this regimen. Pharmacokinetics and pharmacodynamics of propofol depend upon the time-of-day of administration. The degree of anesthesia achieved with 5 mg/kg propofol administered at different times-of-day, in order of greatest to least was 10:00 h, 22:00 h, and 16:00 h (Bienert et al., 2011). Medetomidine administered IM and followed by IV propofol provides approximately 11 min of surgical anesthesia with clinically acceptable preservation of physiologic variables (Hellebrekers et al., 1997). Electroencephalographic features of propofol infusions in rabbits have been described (Silva et al., 2011).

Propofol CRI has been evaluated in rabbits in two separate studies. Baumgartner et al. (2009) used propofol at 1.2–1.3 mg/kg/min IV after induction of anesthesia with 4–8 mg/kg IV. Intraosseus and intravenous infusion of propofol were evaluated by Mazaheri-Khameneh et al. (2012) who found both routes of administration to be similar with regard to physiologic variables and recovery times. Induction in this latter study was achieved with 12.5 mg/kg (1% propofol) and maintained with 1 mg/kg/min for 30 min.

c. Urethane

Urethane continues to be used alone and in combination with other agents (e.g., Tanaka et al., 2012). Among its characteristics are a long duration of action, excellent muscle relaxation, numerous endocrine effects, hemolysis, prolonged recovery, carcinogenic potential, and reduced response of vascular smooth muscle to norepinephrine (Bree and Cohen, 1965; Maggi et al., 1984). These features require its regulation by institutional safety personnel and restrict its use in animals to nonsurvival procedures. Chloralose combined with urethane

has historically been used by physiologists because of its reputation for preservation of baroreceptor reflexes (Sebel and Lowdon, 1989).

4. Inhalation Anesthesia

The inhalant agents are especially useful in rabbit anesthesia because of their reliability, efficacy, ease of manipulation of anesthetic depth, and reduction in recovery time when compared with many injectable agents. Invasive manipulations, especially those requiring prolonged surgical time, are best achieved through the use of inhalants. Isoflurane and sevoflurane are most commonly used. They may be administered via facemask or endotracheal tube. Rabbits should be sedated prior to face-mask inductions because the animals may struggle vigorously in this setting.

Endotracheal tubes of 3.0–4.0 mm internal diameter can be used in most rabbits. Both blind and visual orotracheal intubation techniques have been described and are summarized elsewhere (Lipman et al., 2008). A novel supraglottic device has been described as an alternative to endotracheal intubation (van Zeeland and Schoemaker, 2012). Another alternative is nasotracheal intubation using an endotracheal tube (inner diameter, 2.0–2.5 mm; length, 14.5 cm; Mallinckrodt Medical, St Louis, MO, and Rusch, Duluth, GA) inserted through the nares into the ventral nasal meatus. Factors facilitating placement and maintenance of such tubes are adequate anesthesia (complete relaxation), positioning the animal in dorsal recumbency but with dorsiflexion of the head during intubation, and securing the catheter to the dorsum of the nose by butterfly tape and sutures (Stephens DeValle, 2009). Anesthesia in rabbits may be maintained by using a chosen inhalant with oxygen as the carrier gas delivered via a Bain or other non-rebreathing circuit at 2–2.2 times the minute respiratory volume (Flecknell, 2009; Lipman et al., 1997, 2008). Inhalational anesthesia with isoflurane, enflurane, or halothane has been shown to protect the ischemic rabbit myocardium from infarction when compared with anesthesia with pentobarbital, propofol, or ketamine/xylazine (Cope et al., 1997).

a. Isoflurane

Isoflurane is currently the most commonly used inhalant for rabbit anesthesia. Cardiac safety, rapid induction and recovery, minimal hepatic transformation, and attendant reduction in viscerotoxicity are all features of this agent (Blake et al., 1991). Disadvantages of isoflurane include breath holding at first exposure, hypotension, and respiratory depression. Isoflurane has also been shown to decrease serum calcium and potassium concentration, and increase serum triglyceride, phosphorus and chloride concentrations (Gonzalez Gil et al., 2010). The MAC of isoflurane in rabbits is 2.05 ± 0.18%, 1.39 ± 0.32% for halothane, and 2.86 ± 0.18% for enflurane (Drummond, 1985). In another study evaluating the MAC-sparing effects of butorphanol, with or without meloxicam in rabbits, the MAC of isoflurane was determined to be 2.49 ± 0.07% (Turner *et al.*, 2006). Meloxicam did not have a direct sparing effect and did not influence the MAC-sparing effect of butorphanol. Both tramadol (4.4 mg/kg IV) and lidocaine (2 mg/kg IV followed by a CRI of 50 μg/kg/min) were shown in separate experiments to be MAC-sparing in the isoflurane-anesthetized rabbit (Egger *et al.*, 2009; Schnellbacher *et al.*, 2013). The physiologic effects of 1.3 MAC isoflurane in rabbits include increased heart rate, preservation of hepatic blood flow, and reduction in cardiac output, respiratory rate, mean arterial blood pressure and renal blood flow (Blake *et al.*, 1991). Isoflurane produces significantly less depression of myocardial contractility than does halothane of equivalent MAC concentration (1 MAC) (Marano *et al.*, 1997). Nitrous oxide may be used as a carrier gas at a ratio of 2:1 ($N_2O:O_2$), but concerns over waste gas pollution and recreational abuse have reduced the use of this agent. To avoid diffusion hypoxia when the technique includes N_2O, 10 min of pure O_2 should be administered at the completion of anesthesia.

b. Sevoflurane

Sevoflurane use in the rabbit has now been well-characterized (Scheller *et al.*, 1988; Allweiler *et al.*, 2010; Flecknell *et al.*, 1999). The MAC for this agent in rabbits as determined by tail clamp is 3.7% (Scheller *et al.*, 1988). In rabbits being ovariohysterectomized, propofol induction followed by sevoflurane maintenance (4.0 ± 0.5%) provided surgical anesthesia with cardiopulmonary stability and a return to sternal recumbency within 8 min of sevoflurane termination (Allweiler *et al.*, 2010). A number of studies have characterized the hemodynamic and ventilatory response of sevoflurane-anesthetized rabbits to infusion of various sedative-hypnotic (propofol, midazolam) and analgesic (remifentanyl, dexmedetomidine) agents (Nishizawa *et al.*, 2012; Chang *et al.*, 2009; Sazuka *et al.*, 2012; Koshika *et al.*, 2011).

D. Intraoperative Monitoring and Support

Intraoperative monitoring and support of rabbits are similar to those of other animals of similar size. Monitoring of reflexes, body temperature, and cardiopulmonary variables should be performed by trained personnel. The reflexes, ranked in descending order of usefulness and accuracy for determination of depth of anesthesia, are pinna, pedal withdrawal, corneal, and palpebral (Borkowski *et al.*, 1990; Hellebrekers *et al.*, 1997). Other indices of anesthetic depth, such as muscle tone, jaw tone, vocalization, and gross purposeful movement in response to surgical stimuli, may be used (Hellebrekers *et al.*, 1997).

Supplemental heat sources should be used judiciously both intraoperatively and postoperatively to reduce hypothermia and attendant changes in metabolism of injectable drugs and MAC reduction of inhalants. Drapes, circulating hot-water blankets, hot-water bottles, air blanket, fabric warmers, and use of warm IV and irrigation fluids should be considered, depending on the circumstances.

Conventional veterinary monitoring equipment may be used to monitor such cardiopulmonary variables as heart rate and rhythm, direct arterial blood pressure, oxygen saturation, and pulse rate. End tidal CO_2 may be evaluated but better reflects $PaCO_2$ when measured at the pulmonary tip of the endotracheal tube (Rich *et al.*, 1990). Arterial blood pressure measurement is facilitated by the presence of two large and percutaneously accessible peripheral arteries, the central auricular and saphenous arteries. Pulse oximetry is best performed using transmission clips on the tongue or reflectance probes intrarectally. Fluid infusion rate for most procedures of short to moderate duration is 10 ml/kg/h. The rate for neurosurgical procedures is 4 ml/kg/h (Hindman *et al.*, 1990).

Bispectral index (BIS) has been evaluated in rabbits anesthetized for laparotomy either by sevoflurane (1 MAC) or CRI (8 mg/kg IV over 60 s followed by 0.6 mg/kg/min IV) of propofol (Martín-Cancho *et al.*, 2006). Both agents reduced the BIS from a mean in conscious animals of approximately 98, to a value of 49.3 ± 2.2 for sevoflurane and 69.1 ± 6.0 for propofol CRI. All animals were adequately anesthetized as judged by traditional criteria. BIS of rabbits induced with thiopental has also been evaluated and found to correlate with loss of righting and other reflexes (Kazemi *et al.*, 2011).

E. Special Anesthetic Considerations

1. Spinal Anesthesia

Spinal anesthesia of the rabbit has been described in both clinical and research settings (Kero *et al.*, 1981; Hughes *et al.*, 1993). It has been used as a model for evaluating the pharmacology and toxicology of spinal anesthesia and analgesia. Both epidural and subarachnoid catheterization procedures have been described (Langerman *et al.*, 1990; Jensen *et al.*, 1992; Madsen *et al.*, 1993; Yamashita *et al.*, 2003). Although subarachnoid space cannulation requires exposure of the lumbar spinal column and incision of the ligamentum flavum, both surgical and percutaneous techniques have been described for epidural catheterization (Taguchi *et al.*, 1996; Malinosky *et al.*, 1997). The lumbosacral anatomy of the rabbit spinal cord makes inadvertent intrathecal administration of agents possible. In this regard, the spinal cord ends within the sacrum in the rabbit, and the epidural space is approximately 1 mm in width; even a short beveled spinal needle can pierce the dura. Moreover, a 'dry' tap does not guarantee placement in the epidural space after loss of resistance. In a study highlighting these issues, the use of minimum electrical threshold with an insulated spinal needle was not able to distinguish the epidural from the intrathecal space in the rabbit (Otero *et al.*, 2012). To the authors' knowledge, the use of analgesics administered through these routes has not been rigorously evaluated for the clinical setting in the rabbit.

2. Hypnosis

Hypnosis, or the immobility response or tonic immobility state, describes a constellation of physiologic and behavioral changes in rabbits effected by physical manipulation with or without incantation and reduced lighting (Danneman *et al.*, 1988; Klemm, 2001). Gentle head and neck traction appears to be commonly, but not uniformly, employed in this technique. Rabbits can be used as an animal model to study pain attenuation and other features of hypnosis of humans (Castiglioni *et al.*, 2009). The tonic immobility state in this latter report simply places animals in the supine position and immobilizes them for 15 min with gentle pressure. Hypnotized rabbits exhibit miosis, analgesia, increased depth of respiration, and reduced respiratory rate, heart rate, and blood pressure. The immobility response is not inhibited by naloxone. Although fascinating to the experimentalist, variation in response among rabbits limits the usefulness of this technique. It should not be considered a suitable surrogate for analgesia or anesthesia.

3. Long-Term Anesthetic Preparations

Long-term anesthesia in the setting of nonsurvival surgery in the rabbit requires rigorous attention to hydration, body temperature, adequacy of anesthetic depth, and monitoring of physiologic variables (Lipman *et al.*, 2008). For those techniques that include paralytics, guidelines described in the Guidelines for the Care and Use of Mammals in Neuroscience and Behavioral Research should be consulted (National Research council, 2003). A common technique is for surgery to be performed without paralytics, so that adequacy of analgesia may be determined; paralytics are then used in conjunction with anesthesia during the period of data collection. The use of paralytics with a high 'autonomic margin of safety' allow the experimentalist to use heart rate and blood pressure as indices of depth of anesthesia. Increases in these variables, suggestive of a symptho-adrenal response to anesthesia, should prompt administration of additional anesthetic. A typical regimen may include the following: induction and initial administration using an injectable technique, followed by maintenance with an inhalant or total IV infusion technique and pancuronium or vecuronium (Mills *et al.*, 1987; Hindman *et al.*, 1990; De Mulder *et al.*, 1997). These techniques have been reviewed by Lipman *et al.* (1997, 2008).

F. Acute and Chronic Analgesic Therapy

Preemptive administration of analgesia should be considered as part of the complete program of analgesia in rabbits subjected to surgery (see Table 24.8). In a report assessing analgesic administration to rabbits used in experimental surgery, Coulter *et al.* (2011) identified three areas in which perioperative care might be improved: pre- or peri-operative administration of agents in contrast to postoperative administration only; the use of multimodal technique in procedures likely to produce moderate or severe pain; and increasing the use of NSAIDs and adjunctive methods of analgesia (e.g., epidural analgesia). In their survey, the most commonly used agent was buprenorphine and opioid use exceeded NSAID use in two time periods evaluated (1995–1997 and 2005–2007).

Use of local infiltrative techniques in association with general anesthesia may also be used to enhance postoperative analgesia. Lidocaine and bupivacaine are commonly used. A liposomal formulation of bupivacaine has been evaluated for, and found safe to use in perineural application in the rabbit, but efficacy data were not reported (Richard *et al.*, 2012). Use of these formulations are associated with prolonged duration of nerve block in other species. Morphometric evaluation of the New Zealand White rabbit skull can assist in localization of nerves in regional anesthesia (Monfared, 2013). In ophthalmic procedures, topical and intracameral anesthetics should be considered as adjuncts to general anesthesia (Zemel *et al.*, 1995; Barquet *et al.*, 1999). During ocular manipulations in ophthalmic surgery, use of topical

TABLE 24.8 Analgesics[a] for Rabbits

Analgesic	Dosage
Aspirin	100 mg/kg per os
Ibuprofen	10–20 mg/kg, IV 4 h
Buprenorphine	0.01–0.05 mg/kg SC, IV q 6–12 hourly
Butorphanol	0.1–0.5 mg/kg IV, 4 hourly
Carprofen	5 mg/kg SC or PO q 24 hourly
Flunixin	1.1 mg/kg IM, q 24 hourly
Piroxicam	0.2 mg/kg per os, 8 hourly
Meloxicam	0.3–0.6 mg/kg SC or PO q 24 hourly
Meperidine	5–10 mg/kg SC, 2–3 hourly
Morphine	2.5 mg/kg SC, 2–4 hourly
Fentanyl	5–20 µg/kg, IV bolus
	15 µg/kg, continuous infusion over 2 h
Nalbuphine	1–2 mg/kg IV, 4–5 hourly
Pentazocine	5 mg/kg IV, 2–4 hourly

[a]*Adapted from Lipman et al. (2008) and Wixson (1994).*

anesthetics in rabbits anesthetized with propofol blocked the oculocardiac reflex (Singh *et al.*, 2010). In a study of peribulbar and retrobulbar anesthesia, Zhang *et al.* (2010) showed that full-strength bupivicaine can cause myonecrosis and degeneration of extraocular muscles in rabbits. Half- and quarter-strength formulations had fewer or no acute changes and were unassociated with untoward long-term effects. Finally, EMLA cream (Astra, Westborough, Massachusetts), a mixture of prilocaine and lidocaine that is administered topically, is useful for vasodilation and analgesia during venotomy and arteriotomy procedures (Flecknell *et al.*, 1990; Hellebrekers *et al.*, 1997; Keating *et al.*, 2012).

1. Assessment of Pain and Discomfort

The most frequently recognized signs of pain and discomfort in rabbits include inappetance, an unkempt appearance due to a failure to groom, and reduced activity. Postoperative evaluation for pain is greatly assisted by preoperative assessment of the demeanor of individual rabbits and their food and water consumption. Behavioral changes and facial expressions thought likely to be associated with pain in rabbits have been described (Keating *et al*, 2012).

2. Methods of Analgesic Drug Delivery

Parenteral analgesics may be administered IM, IV, SC, and epidurally or intrathecally (Table 24.8). Intravenous administration of µ-agonist opioids has been associated with muscle rigidity, opisthotonus, and oculogyric effects (Borkowski *et al.*, 1990; Marini *et al.*, 1993). Consequently, these drugs are best administered only after sedation with appropriate sedatives or as part of a neuroleptanesthetic or analgesic combination (Lipman *et al.*, 1997, 2008). Oral administration, although used in rabbits, has not been fully characterized for efficacy to the authors' knowledge. Patch administration of analgesics in rabbits has been described for the agents fentanyl (Foley *et al.*, 2001) and buprenorphine (Park *et al.*, 2008), but no efficacy data were presented.

3. Opioids

The opioid of choice in rabbits is buprenorphine, a partial agonist/antagonist with a long duration of action (8–12h) (Flecknell, 2009; Lipman *et al.*, 1997, 2008). This agent has only mild respiratory depressant properties, in contrast to the pure µ-agonists. A dose of 0.02–0.05 mg/kg IV, SQ, or IM produced 10h of analgesia when a thermal stimulus was used (Flecknell and Liles, 1990). Because onset of action is 30min, this agent should be administered intraoperatively or preoperatively.

Other opioid drugs that may be useful include morphine, which provides 2–4h of potent analgesia at doses of 2–5 mg/kg SC or IM (Wixson, 1994). It may cause sedation, respiratory depression, and moderate histamine release.

Butorphanol (0.1–0.5 mg/kg), a mixed agonist/antagonist agent, is useful in providing short-term analgesia in rabbits (4h). Butorphanol may be added to acepromazine or xylazine to effect both sedation and analgesia (Lipman *et al.*, 1997). It has a MAC sparing effect in the isoflurane-anesthetized rabbit (Turner *et al.*, 2006).

4. Non-Steroidal Anti-Inflammatory Drugs

Numerous NSAIDs have been advocated for rabbits, but rigorous data are lacking. Some of the agents that have been advocated are aspirin (10 mg/kg SQ), acetaminophen-codeine at 1 ml drug/100 ml water, meloxicam, and carprofen (Lipman *et al.*, 1997; 2008). In an experimental fracture model, both piroxicam and flunixin were shown to reduce limb swelling, but analgesic action was not independently evaluated (More *et al.*, 1989). The cyclooxygenase inhibitor ketorolac tromethamine (Toradol; Roche Laboratories, Nutley, New Jersey) has been evaluated in the rabbit at various doses because of its antithrombotic effect (Shufflebarger *et al.*, 1996; Delaporte-Cerceau *et al.*, 1998). Unfortunately, analgesic activity independent of investigation of these antithrombotic and anti-inflammatory effects appears lacking. In another study using a rabbit model of acute temporomandibular joint inflammation, intraperitoneal and intra-articular administration of 50 µg of ketorolac decreased the generation of the inflammatory mediators, prostaglandin E_2, and bradykinin (Swift *et al.*, 1998). The drug is well absorbed with no untoward effects related to ophthalmic, IM, or intranasal administration (Rooks *et al.*, 1985; Santus *et al.*, 1993). The COX-2 inhibitor meloxicam was evaluated for MAC-altering effects in isoflurane-anesthetized rabbits with or without concurrent butorphanol administration. No independent MAC-altering effects were observed, but meloxicam at 0.3 or 1.5 mg/kg augmented butorphanol-associated MAC reduction (Turner *et al.*, 2006).

IV. FERRETS

A. Introduction

The ferret is easily and reliably anesthetized using a variety of regimens (Ko and Marini, 2008, 2014). With practice, anesthetists can safely and reliably catheterize peripheral vessels, establish an airway by orotracheal intubation, and monitor anesthesia with instruments common in companion animal practice. Ferrets should be purchased from a quality vendor, be vaccinated against distemper and rabies, and be allowed an acclimation period of at least 3–7 days, depending on whether they will be used acutely or chronically. Facilities receiving ferrets during warm weather should recognize the limited heat tolerance of this species. Carriers and receivers should not allow animals to linger during transit, and animal technicians and veterinarians should be especially vigilant for signs of hyperthermia (e.g., prostration, panting etc.; Marini, 2014).

Quarantine testing should include, at a minimum, body weight, physical examination, fecal endoparasite flotation, and rectal culture for *Salmonella* spp., *Campylobacter* spp., *E. coli*, and other pathogens. Additional testing such as influenza virus status, complete blood count, and serum chemistry analysis is determined by experimental usage. Investigators studying vision and hearing should avoid the use of albino and white-headed ferrets in that these animals have deficits in both these senses (Hupfeld *et al.*, 2006; Morgan *et al.*, 1987; Moore and Kowalchuk, 1988).

B. Preoperative Assessment and Preparation

1. Preoperative Evaluation

Ferrets used in biomedical research are likely to have been purchased from breeding facilities with good animal health and conditioning standards. Young, experimentally naïve ferrets are good anesthetic subjects for which there are many acceptable regimens for anesthesia induction, maintenance, and monitoring. A thorough physical examination should be performed prior to anesthesia. Techniques for conscious restraint and physical examination have been reviewed elsewhere (Ko and Marini 2008; Marini, 2014). Normal physiologic variables evaluated during the physical examination include a heart rate of 180–300 bpm, a respiratory rate of 30–40 breaths per minute, and a body temperature of 100–104°F (37.7–40°C). Struggling may increase temperature. Particular attention should be paid to the pre-anesthetic size of the spleen, both because splenomegaly is common in ferrets but also because the ferret spleen enlarges during anesthesia with isoflurane, and presumably other inhalants as well. Clinicians must recognize that splenic sequestration of red blood cells and alteration of hematologic variables occurs during isoflurane and ketamine/xylazine anesthesia in ferrets (Jackson *et al.*, 1992; Marini *et al.*, 1997). Arrhythmias are common in ferrets, and can be appreciated during auscultation. The most common arrhythmias are second and third degree heart block (Malakoff *et al.*, 2012). These animals are best precluded from use.

Minimal preoperative blood work should include complete blood cell (CBC), blood glucose, and BUN. Adult ferrets have higher hematocrits (44–55%) than other laboratory animals. Blood transfusion should be considered in anemic ferrets with hematocrits less than 20–25%. The lack of discernable blood groups in ferrets obviates the need for cross matching prior to transfusion. Vulvar enlargement in jills is indicative of estrus, which,

if prolonged, may cause estrogen-induced pancytopenia and a tendency towards hemorrhage. Complete blood counts will help quantify risk in this context. BUN helps determine if higher hematocrits are associated with dehydration (pre-renal azotemia), and blood glucose determination helps identify the presence of an insulin-secreting pancreatic tumor (insulinoma), a very common disease in ferrets. Clinicians should consider screening ferrets over 18 months of age for both insulin-secreting islet cell-tumors and hyperadrenocorticism (adrenal-associated endocrinopathy). Bilaterally symmetric alopecia is a hallmark of the latter in ferrets. Vulvar enlargement in a spayed jill or prostatic enlargement in a hob may also be signs of this disease.

The sedated or anesthetized ferret is very prone to hypothermia due to its small size and correspondingly large surface area to body weight ratio. Great care is required to preserve body temperature, especially during preparation for surgery. Use of supplemental heating devices such as conductive fabric warmers, circulating hot-water blankets, forced air systems, and heated surgery or exam tables immediately upon onset of sedation or anesthetic induction helps to reduce heat loss. Ferrets also have short gastrointestinal transit times of approximately 3–4 h. Traditional fasting periods used in dogs and cats are far too long for ferrets and may result in hypoglycemia. Ferrets to be used in procedures scheduled for late morning should therefore have food withdrawn from early morning and not the previous evening.

2. Choice of Anesthetic Technique

As in other species, experimental objectives, age and condition of the subject, and investigator experience and expertise will help determine the choice of technique. Relatively short procedures of mild to moderate surgical intensity can be done with intermediate acting injectables, while longer, more complicated procedures should be done under inhalant anesthesia or a balanced technique. An example of the latter is a continuous infusion of propofol and ketamine in ferrets pre-medicated with medetomidine/atropine/buprenorphine/meloxicam. This regimen was designed and implemented as a consequence of severe, unresponsive bradycardia observed in ferrets undergoing bilateral cochlear implants maintained with other regimens (Hartley *et al.*, 2010), and might be suitable for a wide range of surgical procedures. Glycemic management in ferrets subjected to long procedures is critical; the authors typically use 5% dextrose in lactated Ringer's solution as a crystalloid maintenance fluid, infused at 10 ml/kg/h. Simple procedures in debilitated animals, and physical examination or sample collection in uncooperative animals can be achieved through face mask induction with isoflurane or sevoflurane. Ferrets will salivate copiously during mask induction, and should be premedicated with glycopyrrolate (0.01 mg/kg IM) or atropine (0.04 mg/kg IM). Pre-induction sedation is recommended for ferrets before mask induction. Chamber induction is associated with violent struggling and digging behaviors and is best avoided in the ferret.

3. Preoperative Medications

The use of preoperative medications may reduce the anesthetic requirement for maintenance agents, relieve patient apprehension, and facilitate handling. Injectable pre-anesthetic and anesthetic agents can be injected SC, IM, or IV. The typical site for subcutaneous injection is interscapular; those for intramuscular administration are the lateral thigh and epaxial musculatures. Most fully conscious ferrets will not tolerate the placement of an intravenous catheter, so premedicants and induction agents tend to be administered by other routes. In sedated ferrets, those anesthetized with injectable combinations, and those induced with inhalant agents via face-mask, 22–24 gauge, over the needle catheters can be placed in cephalic, lateral saphenous, or lateral tail veins. Piercing the skin with a 20-gauge needle facilitates intravenous catheterization of ferrets.

Premedication and anesthetic induction and maintenance have recently been reviewed (Ko and Marini, 2008; Ko and Marini, 2014). This section will present only a select number of those available. As in other species, ferrets may be premedicated with anticholinergics, analgesics, and neuroleptics of different classes. Among sedatives, acepromazine and the α_2-agonists are the most useful and commonly used. Acepromazine (0.01 mg/kg IM) produces rapid onset sedation, lateral recumbency, and immobilization adequate for minor procedures for approximately 40 min. Lower doses are unreliable while higher doses prolong recovery. Endotracheal intubation cannot be achieved with acepromazine alone and hypothermia and hypotension may occur due to α-adrenergic blockade. Acepromazine has no analgesic effect and should only be used in young, healthy, well-hydrated ferrets.

The α_2-agonists, xylazine, medetomidine, and dexmedetomidine are useful agents in ferrets. Xylazine (2 mg/kg IM) and dexmedetomidine (40 μg/kg IM) produce rapid immobilization, analgesia, and muscle relaxation sufficient for minor procedures but not for endotracheal intubation. Without reversal, xylazine and dexmedetomidine immobilization lasts 40–70 min and 150–200 min, respectively. Xylazine reversal can be achieved with yohimbine (0.5 mg/kg IM; Sylvina et al., 1990); dexmedetomidine by atipamezole (400 μg/kg IM; Ko et al., 1997). While heart rates of acepromazine-sedated ferrets remain within normal limits, those of α_2-agonist-sedated animals are significantly reduced. Xylazine causes hypotension, heart block, and ventricular arrhythmias in ferrets. These effects can be precluded or mitigated by preadministration with atropine or glycopyrrolate. Medetomidine and dexmedetomidine can produce hypertension in association with bradycardia.

Opioids can be used for pre-emptive analgesia, post-operative analgesia, or in combination with a neuroleptic in neuroleptanalgesia. Morphine, hydromorphone, buprenorphine, and butorphanol have been recommended as analgesics for use in ferrets (Ko and Marini, 2014). These agents may cause bradycardia and should be used with anticholinergics. Opioid use can also provide an anesthetic sparing effect (Murat and Housmans, 1988).

Morphine (0.5–0.75 mg/kg SC, IM) or hydromorphone (0.05–0.1 mg/kg SC, IM) provide analgesia and reduced resistance to manipulation in ferrets subjected to procedures such as bandage change and intravenous catheterization. Morphine doses lower than 0.5 mg/kg induce emesis in ferrets.

The opioid most commonly administered to ferrets is the partial μ agonist buprenorphine. It has a relatively slow onset (30 min) but a prolonged duration of action, the latter presumably as a result of the slow dissociation of this agent from μ receptors (Stoelting, 1987). Buprenorphine is only mildly sedative and is commonly used in postoperative pain management.

C. Intraoperative Anesthetics

In this section, the most commonly used anesthetic agents will be described. Dosages are given in Table 24.9.

1. Injectable Anesthetics

a. Dissociatives

Dissociative anesthetic combinations are effective anesthetic induction regimens and can be used both to induce and maintain anesthesia in procedures of mild to moderate surgical intensity and short duration. Ketamine and xylazine produce lateral recumbency and anesthesia adequate for endotracheal intubation, gastrointestinal endoscopy, and most minor procedures. Atropine pre-medication helps preclude cardiac arrhythmias. A combination of ketamine and medetomidine or dexmedetomidine produces immobilization, analgesia, and excellent muscle relaxation for 60 min (Ko et al., 1997). Atipamezole administration will reverse these effects. Another regimen providing 60–80 min of surgical anesthesia and intubation tolerance is ketamine, medetomidine (or dexmedetomidine), and butorphanol.

Telazol/xylazine, telazol/xylazine/butorphanol, and a telazol combination in which 2.5 ml of medetomidine (1 mg/ml) (or dexmedetomine; 0.5 mg/ml) and 2.5 ml of butorphanol (10 mg/ml) are used as diluents for the Telazol powder (Ko et al., 1998) are commonly used.

TABLE 24.9   Common Agents and Anesthetic Combinations and their Effects in Ferrets

Drug combinations (IM)	Time from injection to lateral recumbency (min)	Duration of dorsal recumbency (min)	Duration of endotracheal intubation (min)	Time from injection to complete mobilization (min)
Medetomidine (80 μg/kg)	3 ± 1	>120[a]	16 ± 14	>120
Medetomidine (80 mg/kg), butorphanol (0.1 mg/kg)	3 ± 1	>120[a]	91 ± 8[a]	>120
Medetomidine (80 mg/kg), butorphanol (0.1 mg/kg), ketamine (5 mg/kg)	2 ± 0.5	>180[a]	95 ± 0[a]	>180
Xylazine (2 mg/kg)	2 ± 0.9	68 ± 20	35 ± 17	71 ± 19
Xylazine (2 mg/kg), butorphanol (0.2 mg/kg)	2 ± 0.6	82 ± 4	69 ± 5	86 ± 9
Xylazine (2 mg/kg), butorphanol (0.2 mg/kg), ketamine (15 mg/kg)	1 ± 1	94 ± 13	81 ± 19	106 ± 13
Diazepam (3 mg/kg)	3 ± 1	43 ± 8	0	51 ± 12
Diazepam (3 mg/kg), butorphanol (0.2 mg/kg)	3 ± 1	79 ± 11	4 ± 9	85 ± 12
Diazepam (3 mg/kg), butorphanol (0.2 mg/kg), ketamine (15 mg/kg)	4 ± 5	75 ± 34	20 ± 25	95 ± 48
Acepromazine (0.1 mg/kg)	5 ± 3	49 ± 11	0	56 ± 12
Acepromazine (0.1 mg/kg), butorphanol (0.2 mg/kg)	5 ± 1	79 ± 11	16 ± 19	85 ± 12
Telazol (3 mg/kg), xylazine (3 mg/kg)	1.5 ± 0.9	103 ± 3	26 ± 29	117 ± 20
Xylazine (3 mg/kg)				

Adapted from Ko and Marini, 2014.
[a]*If not reversed with atipamezole. Medetomidine in this table can be replaced with 40 μg/kg of dexmedetomidine for the similar effects.*

A dose of 0.03–0.04 ml/kg of the latter cocktail enables intubation and provides a surgical plane of anesthesia for 30–50 min. Oxygen (>40%) should be provided when using these dissociative combinations, either by mask, intubation, or nasal catheter.

b. Propofol

Propofol can be used for induction, typically after sedation and establishment of vascular access, and must be given intravenously. The induction dose of 6–8 mg/kg should be reduced to 1–3 mg/kg in the sedated animals. Apnea, oxygen desaturation, and decreased myocardial contractility can all be observed, especially with rapid administration; rapid intubation and oxygen should be provided (Cook and Housmans, 1994). Hartley *et al.*, (2010) describe maintenance of anesthesia in bilateral cochlear implant surgery using a CRI of propofol and ketamine in 5% glucose/saline solution.

2. Inhalation Anesthesia

The inhalant anesthetics isoflurane and sevoflurane are the agents most often used for longer procedures of moderate to high levels of invasiveness in ferrets. Inhalants are best administered to the intubated ferret. Most adult ferrets can be intubated successfully with 2.5–3.0 mm endotracheal tubes and a straight Miller 0 or curved Macintosh 1 laryngoscope blade. Dorsiflexion of the head and moderate lingual traction facilitate intubation. Assistants may prefer to restrain the maxilla with roll gauze placed behind the incisor teeth. This makes operator injury less likely if the animal is too lightly anesthetized. Depressing the base of the tongue by downward displacement of the laryngoscope blade helps provide visualization of the glottis. Inhalants may also be administered in oxygen by face-mask, either for creating adequate depth to allow intubation or for anesthetic maintenance in the absence of endotracheal intubation. Glycopyrrolate or atropine premedication prevents hypersalivation associated with induction with either face-mask or dissociative agent.

Inhalants are administered via non-rebreathing systems such as the co-axial (Bain) circuit or Ayre's T-piece with Jackson-Rees modification. Flow rates of 2.2 × the minute respiratory volume will preclude re-breathing. Lower flows can be used in conjunction with capnography or capnometry to assure non-rebreathing. A surgical plane of anesthesia can be achieved in most ferrets with 2–2.25% isoflurane or with 2.5–4.5% sevoflurane. Both agents reduce peripheral vascular resistance and can therefore predispose the animal to hypothermia and hypotension (MacPhail *et al.*, 2004); sevoflurane better preserves blood pressure in closely-related species (Gaynor *et al.*, 1997). Moreover, sevoflurane has been associated with reduction of cardiac work and myocardial oxygen consumption, leading to increased cardiac efficiency at high doses.

D. Intraoperative Monitoring and Support

Intraoperative monitoring of body temperature, depth of anesthesia, and cardiovascular and respiratory function should be performed as in other species. Depth of anesthesia is reflected by palpebral and pedal withdrawal reflexes, eyelid aperture, ventral rotation of the eyeballs, reaction to surgical stimuli, muscle tone, and cardiorespiratory variables. Imai et al. (1999) showed that $PaCO_2$, eyelid aperture, and pupillary diameter all increased with increasing isoflurane dose.

In addition to traditional methods of observation and auscultation, cardiovascular and respiratory monitoring can be achieved in ferrets by indirect or direct blood pressure evaluation, ECG, pulse oximetry, blood gas analysis, and capnometry. Indirect blood pressure is most easily measured with an infant cuff (size 1) and an automated oscillometric device (e.g., BO-AccuGuard) placed on the distal fore or hind limb or base of the tail. A mean arterial pressure of >60mm Hg should be maintained. Electrocardiographic monitoring can be achieved with flattened ECG clips or with adhesive pediatric electrode pads. A traditional lead II or base apex lead with the RA and LL leads on the right side of the neck, and the LA lead on the left side of the thorax caudal to the heart can be used. The base apex lead is visualized using Lead I or Lead III of the monitor. Oxygenation can be monitored using pulse oximetry probes placed on the tongue, paw, ear, or tail tip; the authors find an intrarectal probe to provide the most stable measurements. Capnography can be used to evaluate ventilation (Olin et al., 1997; Ko and Marini, 2008, 2014).

E. Postoperative Recovery

Ferrets are robust surgical subjects, but their small size requires clinicians to be exceptionally mindful of management of heat, energy, and hydration. Intraoperative devices used to provide heat can be used postoperatively until recovery from anesthesia or normothermia has occurred. During postoperative recovery, ferrets can be provided with fabric tubes (snooze tubes) and will crawl into them upon recovery from anesthesia. Energy requirements can be managed by oral gavage of gruel in ferrets that are reluctant to eat and fluids can be provided either per os or by subcutaneous administration in ferrets without intravenous or intraosseus catheters. Ferrets object vigorously to subcutaneous administration of fluids. The authors prefer to administer warm crystalloids by placing the ferret into a deep sink and using a 12-inch butterfly infusion set with 21- to 25-gauge needles through which to inject the fluids. This protects the clinician and facilitates the process. Traditional methods of evaluating dehydration and replacement or maintenance volumes apply.

Oral medications can be administered in nutritive pastes such as Nutrical or Ferret-Cal. Ferrets can be trained as kits or adolescents to lick these pastes from a tongue depressor. If the animal objects to the taste of medication in the paste, it can be administered by placing it on the end of a Popsicle stick or longitudinally split tongue depressor, and scraping the medicated paste from the stick onto the lingual surface of the maxillary incisors. Ferrets restrained by the scruff typically yawn widely, and clinicians can use this phenomenon to time their drug administration or gavage.

F. Acute and Chronic Analgesic Therapy

1. Assessment of Pain and Discomfort

Activity level, food or water consumption, production of feces and urine, heart rate, respiratory rate and character, and incisional characteristics like integrity, touch-elicited pain and signs of inflammation, all inform the clinician of the adequacy of pain management. Ko has adapted the use of the Dynamic Interactive Visual Analog Scale (DiVas) used in dogs (Ko et al., 2011) to ferrets. Observation of ferrets in their enclosure and then as they interact with the observer, as well as food and water consumption, and fecal and urine production, are combined in this system with palpation of potentially painful sites. The use of a hand-held 'palpometer' for pressure-controlled palpation provides an objective measure of incisional or regional pain. Each observation and site palpation is assigned a score from zero (no pain) to 10 (severe pain), and the total score is used to direct clinical decisions.

2. Methods of Analgesic Drug Delivery

The current standard of care is the use of pre-emptive, multimodal pain management. Opioids, α_2-agonists, local anesthetics, and NSAIDs can all be used (Johnston, 2005; van Oostrom et al., 2011). The following are specific comments pertaining to the use of these agents in ferrets. Dosages are contained in Table 24.10.

3. Non-Steroidal Anti-Inflammatory Drugs

Non-steroidal anti-inflammatory drugs should be used with caution in ferrets because they are deficient in the glucuronidation pathway (Lichtenberger, 2006; Lichtenberger and Ko, 2007) and may manifest signs of toxicity (renal failure and gastrointestinal tract ulceration). One or more doses of the COX-2 inhibitors carprofen or meloxicam can be used safely, however, and improves the quality and duration of analgesia when combined with opioids or other analgesics. Always ensure adequate hydration in ferrets to which these agents are administered.

4. Epidural Analgesia

Both epidural anesthesia and analgesia have been described for use in ferrets (Sladsky et al., 2000; Eshar

TABLE 24.10 Analgesic Agents Used in Ferrets

	Dose/route	Effects	Duration	Indications
OPIOIDS				
Butorphanol	0.2–0.8 mg/kg, SC, IM or IV	Analgesia/sedation	1–2 h	For mild-to-moderate degree of pain
Morphine	0.25 – 1 mg/kg, SC, IM, or IV	Analgesia/sedation, may vomit, bradycardia may occur with doses higher than 0.5 mg/kg	3–4 h	For mild-to-severe degree of pain
Hydromorphone	0.025–0.1 mg/kg, SC, IM, or IV	Analgesia/sedation, occasionally vomit, bradycardia and respiratory depression may occur	1–2 h	For mild-to-severe degree of pain
Fentanyl	4–10 µg/kg, IM or IV	Analgesia; bradycardia and respiratory depression may occur	30 min	For immediate relief of severe pain
Buprenorphine	0.01–0.02 mg/kg, SC, IM, or IV	Analgesia, slow onset of effect	6–8 h	
ALPHA-2 AGONISTS				
Medetomidine	0.02–0.04 mg/kg, SC, IM, or IV	Analgesia–moderate sedation	30–60 min	Need sedation with analgesia
Dexmedetomidine	0.01–0.03 mg/kg SC, IM, or IV			
Xylazine	1–2 mg/kg	Analgesia–moderate sedation	30–50 min	Need sedation with analgesia
NSAID				
Ketoprefen	1–2 mg/kg, SC, IM, IV, or PO	Analgesia, anti-inflammation	24 h	In combination with opioids for severe pain with longer-lasting analgesia effect
Caprofen	2–4 mg/kg, SC, IM, IV, or PO	Analgesia, anti-inflammation	24 h	In combination with opioids for severe pain with longer lasting analgesia effect
Meloxicam	0.2 mg/kg, SC, IM, IV, or PO	Analgesia, anti-inflammation	24 h	In combination with opioids for severe pain with longer lasting analgesia effect

Adapted from Ko and Marini (2014).

and Wilson, 2010; Lichtenberger and Ko, 2007; Kleine and Quandt, 2012). The spinal cord of the ferret typically ends cranial to the site of administration, the lumbosacral space, and so intrathecal injection is unlikely. Nonetheless, if intrathecal injection is suspected, the dose rate of the agents used should be reduced.

G. Special Anesthetic Considerations

1. Long-Term Anesthetic Preparations

The use of ferrets in neuroscience and physiology research has necessitated the development of regimens for prolonged anesthesia. These regimens often involve balanced anesthetic techniques designed to maintain some critical physiologic function in an animal that has either just had surgery or is being imaged, and which therefore must remain anesthetized. The challenge is to maintain homeostasis, monitor and record anesthesia adequately and in accordance with approved animal use protocols, insure adequate anesthetic depth, and preserve the function of interest to the investigator. An example of such a regimen was published by Liu *et al.* (2008) who were able to preserve visually-evoked activity in ferrets used in functional MRI, by using a nitrous oxide/oxygen carrier gas mix with isoflurane (0.8–1.5% isoflurane with a N_2O to O_2 balance of 1:1.4). Other regimens include continuous infusions of short-acting intravenous anesthetics and these may also be combined with the use of NMB agents. Select regimens for prolonged anesthesia are found in Table 24.11.

2. Neonatal Anesthesia

Ferrets are used in neuroplasticity studies because much of neural development occurs postnatally (Sharma and Sur, 2014). In such studies, the normal course of development is altered for the purpose of evaluating hypothesized outcomes. A safe and efficacious method for providing anesthesia to neonates up until approximately day 5 is hypothermia. Kits are wrapped in moist gauze or placed in a latex sleeve (made from the finger

TABLE 24.11　Select Anesthetic Regimens for Prolonged Anesthesia

Induction	Maintenance	Comments
Pentobarbital 40 mg/kg IP	Pentobarbital 5 mg/kg/h IV	Auditory study, drug administered in 'dextrose-electrolyte' solution. Breathing unassisted
Ketamine 25 mg/kg IM Xylazine 1.5 mg/kg IM Atropine 0.04 mg/kg IM	Pentobarbital 1.5–2 mg/kg/h Gallamine triethiodide 10 mg/kg/h	Vision research CRI of a 1:1 mixture of 5% dextrose and lactated Ringer's solution
Ketamine 40 mg/kg IM Acepromazine 0.4 mg/kg IM Isoflurane 2%	Isoflurane in O_2 Vecuronium 0.2 mg/kg/h	Vision research
Ketamine 10 mg/kg IM Medetomidine 0.08 mg/kg IM Atropine 0.15 mg/kg IM	Isoflurane 1% in 1:1 $N_2O:O_2$ Pancuronium initial dose 0.15 mg/kg followed by 6 μg/kg/h	Vision research
Ketamine 10 mg/kg IM Medetomidine 0.08 mg/kg IM Atropine 0.1 mg/kg IM	Isoflurane 0.5% in 1:1 $N_2O:O_2$ Gallamine triethiodide 6 mg/kg/h IV	Vision research
Alphaxalone/alphadalone (Saffan) 6 mg/kg IV	Alphaxalone/alphadalone (Saffan) 6–8 mg/kg/h	Rate adjusted to pedal withdrawal reflex
Alphaxalone/alphadalone (Saffan) 2 ml/kg IM	5 ml/h of medetomidine (0.022 mg/kg/h) and ketamine (5 mg/kg/h) in saline and 5% glucose)	CRI of 0.5 mg/kg/h dexamethasone and 0.06 mg/kg/h atropine. Auditory study
Medetomidine 0.08 mg/kg IM Atropine 0.1 mg/kg IM Buprenorphine 0.05 mg/kg IM	Propofol 1 mg/kg/h Ketamine 5 mg/kg/h	Cochlear implantation Ventilated with air/O_2 mix
Isoflurane 1% in 1:1 $N_2O:O_2$	Isoflurane 1% in 1:1 $N_2O:O_2$ Pancuronium 0.6 mg/kg/h	Vision research

Adapted from Ko and Marini, 2014.

of a surgical glove), and then placed in a container of crushed ice until the cessation of spontaneous movement and respiration. Anesthesia is maintained in the anesthetized kit by placing it on a bed of crushed ice or a cold glass plate. The use of dry ice leads to frostbite and is unacceptable. Kits must be adequately warmed before return to the jill.

Two recent studies have departed from the use of hypothermia in kits (Mao and Pallas, 2012; Borrell, 2010). These studies used isoflurane from 1–5% delivered via customized face mask, to anesthetize kits from 12 h to 6 days of age. Warm SC saline and the respiratory stimulant doxapram (2 mg/kg SC) can promote survival. A more thorough discussion of issues pertaining to anesthesia and analgesia of neonates can be found in Ko and Marini (2014).

V. SWINE

A. Introduction

Research-oriented textbooks contain complete descriptions of anesthetic techniques and appropriate selection criteria for the various protocols specific to laboratory swine (Flecknell, 2009; Smith and Swindle, 2008; Swindle, 2007). Veterinary-oriented textbooks also contain useful information on anesthesia in swine, but care must be taken to consider the physiologic effects of the anesthetics on the research protocol (Riebold et al., 1995; Thurmon and Benson, 1986). Information on handling and selection of swine for surgical protocols is included in Chapter 16 in this text as well as in a textbook by Swindle (2007). The purpose of this section is to provide an abbreviated guide to the most commonly used techniques in a research setting.

B. Preoperative Assessment and Preparation

1. Preoperative Evaluation

Swine should be selected from sources with a known health status and standardized preventive health program. They should be stabilized and/or conditioned in the research institution for 5–7 days prior to performing anesthesia for survival surgery. Stabilization should include a physical exam as a minimum and, depending on the source and purpose of the research, laboratory tests, including a fecal exam, CBC count, and blood chemistry determination. Vaccination against common diseases may be appropriate for animals on long-term projects. A judgment should also be made in advance of the protocol on whether a particular breed or age of pig should be selected. The criteria for selection of swine for research projects and the differences between miniature and domestic farm breeds of swine are discussed in Chapter 16, as well as in Swindle (2007). Diseases of swine and their potential complications to research are also discussed in Chapter 16.

2. Choice of Anesthetic Technique

The choice of anesthetic technique should be based on the physiologic effects of the anesthetic protocol and the potential complications that a particular protocol may have on the research being conducted. Many swine are used in cardiovascular research; therefore, stable hemodynamics, which may be greatly influenced by the anesthetic protocol, are important for many projects. The basic criteria for selection of anesthetics for swine are similar to those for other species. Malignant hyperthermia, discussed in Chapter 15, is a unique genetic condition in certain breeds of domestic swine. Swine herds can be prescreened for this potential complication, which is triggered by many inhalant and injectable anesthetic agents, particularly halothane. Swine may also have congenital heart defects, such as ventricular septal defect (VSD) and patent foramen ovale (PFO) (Swindle *et al.*, 1992). Auscultation of swine prior to anesthesia is useful for detecting these conditions, as well as determining whether the animals have chronic respiratory diseases, which are common in some herds of domestic swine.

3. Preoperative Medications

Preoperative medications may be appropriate to relieve anxiety and decrease the amount of general anesthetic to be administered. Anticholinergics may also be useful in preventing the vagal reflex that may occur during endotracheal intubation and manipulation of the cardiovascular and pulmonary systems. Both atropine and glycopyrrolate have been utilized successfully as anticholinergics in swine. Atropine is also useful to counteract bradycardia associated with some protocols, such as those that use high-dose opioids.

Tranquilizers are mainly used to reduce anxiety, facilitate handling, and reduce the dosage of general anesthetics. The phenothiazine derivatives, especially acepromazine, have been widely used for this purpose. Benzodiazepine agents, such as diazepam and midazolam, are also used in swine for this purpose. Midazolam is used as a sole agent to provide approximately 20 min of relaxation to perform cardiovascular imaging techniques, such as echocardiography, with minimal effects on cardiovascular parameters (Swindle,

2007; Smith *et al.*, 1991). Drug dosages are provided in Table 24.12.

C. Intraoperative Anesthesia

In this section, the appropriate selection of anesthetics used in research protocols is discussed. The drug dosages are included in Table 24.12.

1. Injectable Anesthetics

Injectable anesthetics may be useful to induce anesthesia prior to administering an inhalant agent or for short-term procedures. Protocols that infuse these agents may be indicated in cases where inhalant anesthesia is not appropriate or is unavailable. Most injectable combinations only provide 20–30 min of surgical anesthesia. Consequently, it is preferable to administer continuous infusions of these injectable agents when longer anesthetic periods are required. Repeated bolus injections of these agents result in an unstable plane of anesthesia (Smith and Swindle, 2008; Swindle, 2007).

a. Dissociatives

The dissociative agents, when administered alone, are not sufficient to provide surgical anesthesia or relaxation for endotracheal intubation. Ketamine and tiletamine-zolazepam (telazol) are the two most widely used agents in swine. They are frequently combined with phenothiazine derivatives, benzodiazepines, and α_2-agonists.

Combinations include ketamine/acepromazine, ketamine/azaperone, ketamine/diazepam, ketamine/midazolam, ketamine/xylazine, ketamine/medetomidine, and telazol/xylazine (Thurmon *et al.*, 1988; Swindle, 2007; Smith and Swindle, 2008; Ko *et al.*, 1997; Flecknell, 1997, 2009; Portier and Slusser, 1985). These combinations typically require the addition of other agents, such as barbiturates, or the administration of inhalant agents via a face mask in order to provide enough relaxation for endotracheal intubation. All of the combinations provide 20–30 min of restraint when administered IM or SC. The combinations of ketamine/xylazine, ketamine/medetomidine, and telazol/xylazine are sufficient to provide anesthesia for minor surgical procedures. Ketamine/medetomidine may provide up to 45 min of chemical restraint as a single injection but rapidly induces hypothermia. None of the combinations are suitable for visceral analgesia unless provided as a continuous IV infusion. An infusion of ketamine/xylazine/guiafenesin is useful for providing stable hemodynamics for cardiovascular protocols (Thurmon, 1986). Ketamine/medetomidine is preferred when an α_2-agonist is indicated for a protocol, because it has less deleterious cardiovascular effects than xylazine. Telazol and telazol/xylazine may also be more cardiopressive than other dissociative combinations. Their usage in research protocols in swine should

TABLE 24.12   Drug Dosages[a] in Swine

Drug	Dosage	Route
DISSOCIATIVE AGENTS AND COMBINATIONS		
Ketamine[b]	11–33 mg/kg	IM, IV
	10–33 mg/kg/h	IV infusion
Ketamine+	22–33 mg/kg	IM
Acepromazine[b]	1.1 mg/kg	
Ketamine+	15 mg/kg	IM
Diazepam[b]	2 mg/kg	
Ketamine+	20 mg/kg	IM
xylazine	2 mg/kg	
Ketamine+	15 mg/kg	IM
azaperone	2 mg/kg	
Ketamine+	2 mg/kg	IV (2 × dose for IM)
xylazine+	2 mg/kg	
oxymorphone	0.075 mg/kg	
Ketamine+	20 mg/kg	IM
climazolam	5–1.0 mg/kg	
Tiletamine-zolazepam (Telazol)	4–6 mg/kg	IM
Tiletamine-zolazepam (Telazol)+	4–6 mg/kg	IM
xylazine	2.2 mg/kg	
BARBITURATES		
Pentobarbital	20–40 mg/kg	IV
	5–40 mg/kg/h	Continuous IV infusion
Thiopental	6.6–30 mg/kg	IV
	3–30 mg/kg/h	Continuous IV infusion
Thiamylal	6.6–30 mg/kg	IV
	3–30 mg/kg/h	Continuous IV infusion
MISCELLANEOUS INJECTABLE RESTRAINT AGENTS		
Azaperone	2–8 mg/kg	IM
α-Chloralose	55–100 mg/kg	IV
Etomidate[b]	4–8 mg/kg	IV
Etorphine/acepromazine (Imobilon)+	0.245 mg/10 kg	
Diprenorphine (Revivon)	0.3 mg/kg	
Ketamine xylazine glyceryl guaiacolate	1 ml/kg/h	See text for mixture
Midazolam[b]	100–500 μg/kg	IM
Metomidate	4 mg/kg	IV
Meperidine+	1 mg/lb	

(Continued)

TABLE 24.12   (Continued)

Drug	Dosage	Route
azaperone+	1 mg/lb followed in 20 min by	
ketamine+	10 mg/lb	
morphine	1 mg/lb	
Propofol	0.83–1.66 mg/kg	IV
	12–20 mg/kg/h	Continuous IV infusion
ANALGESICS		
Fentanyl	0.02–0.05 mg/kg	IM q2h
	30–100 mg/kg/h	IV drip
Sufentanil[b]	5–10 μg/kg	IM q2h
	10–30 mg/kg/h	IV drip
Buprenorphine[b]	0.05–0.1 mg/kg	IM q8–12h
Butorphanol	0.1–0.3 mg/kg	IM q4–6h
Meperidine	2–10 mg/kg	IM q4h
Oxymorphone	0.15 mg/kg	IM q4h
Pentazocine	1.5–3.0 mg/kg	IM q4h
Phenylbutazone	10–20 mg/kg	PO ql2h
Aspirin	10 mg/kg	PO q4h
Carprofen[b]	2.0–3.0 mg/kg	PO BID
MISCELLANEOUS		
Antiarrhythmics		
Bretylium tosylate	3.0–5.0 mg/kg	IV q30 min
Lidocaine	2–4 mg/kg	IV
	50 μg/kg/min	Continuous IV infusion
Calcium channel blocker: diltiazem	2–4 mg/kg	PO TID
Paralytic agents		
Pancuronium	0.02–0.15 mg/kg	IV
	5–6 μg/kg/min	Continuous IV infusion
Vercuronium	1.0 mg/kg	IV
Succinylcholine	1.1 mg/kg	IV
Coronary vasorelaxant: nitroglycerin	200 μg diluted in 2 ml saline	Infused slowly into coronary sinus
Anticholinergic: atropine	0.05 mg/kg	IM
	0.02 mg/kg	IV
Malignant hyperthermia treatment and prophylaxis: Dantrolene	5 mg/kg	IV

[a]See text for references. Only commonly used agents are listed here. The reference books cited in Section V, A provide complete information on drug dosages and administration techniques.
[b]Most commonly recommended anesthetics and analgesics.

be limited to single-dose administrations for chemical restraint or for protocols in which cardiovascular depression is unimportant. These agents have been shown to produce prolonged cardiovascular depression following a single injection (Lefkov and Mussig, 2007). Ketamine/ medetomidine and ketamine/midazolam have a protectant effect against cardiac arrhythmias and provide stable hemodynamics when administered as continuous IV infusions (Swindle, 2007; Smith and Swindle, 2008).

b. Propofol

Propofol is administered as a continuous IV infusion. Its use in research in swine is limited because of its minimal analgesic effects and significant cardiovascular depression in higher dosages. It must be administered in combination with analgesics or other agents in order to provide visceral analgesia. However, it may be useful as a continuous infusion for nonsurvival teaching protocols (Ramsey et al., 1993; Foster et al., 1992).

c. Barbiturates

The effects of the barbiturates in swine are similar to those in other species. Barbiturates are administered IV as bolus injections to facilitate endotracheal intubation or as continuous IV infusions for general anesthesia. Tranquilizers may be utilized as preanesthetics to reduce the IV dosage by one-third to one-half. The barbiturates are potent respiratory depressants in swine. Thiobarbiturates, such as thiopental, are less potent than pentobarbital and are shorter-acting; consequently, they are easier and safer to control. The thiobarbiturates are minimally metabolized by the liver, unlike pentobarbital, and are mainly excreted by the kidneys. The recovery time from thiobarbiturates may be as short as 20 min, whereas it may be hours for pentobarbital. For longer protocols the barbiturates should be administered as continuous IV infusions. They are most useful for nonsurvival teaching protocols, but thiobarbiturate infusions may be useful for providing a stable plane of cardiovascular hemodynamics when other agents are contraindicated (Smith et al., 1997; Swindle, 2007). Availability of these agents has greatly decreased and the cost has increased in recent years.

d. Opioids

Opioids may be used as analgesic adjuncts to other anesthetics to provide balanced anesthesia or may be administered in high-dose infusions for cardiovascular protocols. They have minimal effects on cardiac contractility and coronary blood flow when administered for those purposes. The opioids administered most commonly for cardiovascular protocols are fentanyl, sufentanil, and alfentanil. The latter two agents are more potent than fentanyl and consequently require lesser volumes for infusion; however, their potency may induce muscular rigidity, which can be controlled by starting the IV infusion first. The opioids induce bradycardia, especially when administered as IV boluses for induction of anesthesia. This bradycardia is transient but may be counteracted by atropine. For invasive surgical procedures, administration of low doses of inhalant agents is necessary during surgical manipulation. The analgesia provided by continuous infusions of these agents is adequate to provide a long-term stable plane of anesthesia and/or chemical restraint for cardiovascular measurements after the surgical manipulations are completed (Swindle, 2007).

e. Etomidate

Etomidate does not provide any advantage over other agents in research protocols in swine. It is relatively ineffective as a sole agent for any purpose other than short-term chemical restraint and it is a safe agent to use when cardiovascular compromise exists in the pig. It may be combined with azaperone or ketamine to provide anesthesia suitable for minor surgery (Worek et al., 1988; Smith and Swindle, 2008).

f. α_2-Agonists

Xylazine, dexmedetomidine, detomidine, and metomidine are the most commonly used α_2-agonists in swine. These agents are associated with blockage of the cardiac conduction system and with cardiovascular depression. Medetomidine has the fewest cardiovascular effects of this class of agents in swine. These agents are useful in combination with dissociative agents for short-term surgical analgesia or for inclusion in combination IV infusion protocols. They have minimal usage as sole agents for chemical restraint (Smith and Swindle, 2008; Swindle, 2007; Vainio et al., 1992; Riebold et al., 2007; Flecknell, 2009).

g. Miscellaneous Anesthetics

α-Chloralose was promoted in the past as an agent to provide anesthesia for cardiovascular hemodynamic measurements. However, it must be used at a high dosage or in combination with other agents in swine to provide analgesia, which minimizes its effectiveness for this purpose. α-Chloralose may be replaced by other IV infusion protocols, such as high-dose opioids or ketamine/ xylazine/guiafenesin, that provide adequate analgesia for these protocols (Silverman and Muir, 1993; Swindle, 2007; Thurmon, 1986).

2. Inhalational Anesthesia

Administration of general anesthesia using inhalational agents is the preferred method for swine for most protocols. However, proper administration of these agents requires an investment in equipment both for administration of the agents as well as monitoring of physiological parameters. Personnel must also be properly trained in the techniques involved in this form of anesthesia. Flow rates for gas delivery are variable between units, but as a general guideline 5–15 ml/kg/min is usually sufficient.

Nitrous oxide, halothane, and methoxyflurane have potential human health hazards when the vapors are inhaled on a chronic basis. No long-term health effects have been described for the minimally metabolized agents, such as isoflurane, desflurane, enflurane, and sevoflurane. However, arbitrary limits have been set for environmental exposure to these agents as well. An evacuation system to control waste gases and periodic monitoring of the operating room to check for leaks in the circuits are essential components of a program that uses inhalational anesthetics. Maintenance of equipment, including cleaning and calibration of the vaporizers and flowmeters as well as leak testing of anesthesia circuits, is also essential. The two primary inhalant agents used in swine are isoflurane and sevoflurane.

a. Nitrous Oxide

Nitrous oxide is ineffective as a sole agent for anesthesia in swine. However, it may be administered in combination with oxygen to reduce the amount of inhalational agent that must be administered. This reduces the dose-dependent cardiovascular depression associated with inhalational anesthetics in swine. Nitrous oxide is administered as an adjunct to oxygen in a 33–66% combination. Nitrous oxide–oxygen (2:1) provides blood gas measurements similar to those in unanesthetized swine and minimizes the amount of inhalant that must be administered (Swindle, 2007; Smith and Swindle, 2008). Diffusion hypoxia and the potential for abuse of the agent by personnel are considerations.

b. Halothane

Halothane has a MAC of 0.91–1.25% (Tranquilli et al., 1983; Smith et al., 1997). It is more cardiodepressant than the newer agents discussed below. Halothane is metabolized by the liver as well as being eliminated by the lungs. This agent is not widely available and its use should be discontinued in favor of the newer inhalant agents.

c. Isoflurane

Isoflurane is the least cardiodepressant of the inhalational agents commonly used in swine. Isoflurane has a MAC value of 1.58% (Smith and Swindle, 2008; Eisele et al., 1985). Less than 1% of this agent is metabolized by the liver. Isoflurane is generally used at concentrations of 2–4% for induction and 0.5–2.0% for maintenance of general anesthesia. When using nitrous oxide–oxygen 1:1 or 2:1 for delivery, the isoflurane concentration may be reduced to 0.5–1.0%. Isoflurane in nitrous oxide is commonly used for maintaining long-term anesthesia with physiological measurements.

d. Desflurane and Sevoflurane

Desflurane and sevoflurane have physiologic effects similar to those of isoflurane. They are not commonly used in swine, because of the increased expense (Weiskopf et al., 1992). Desflurane requires specialized equipment not commonly found in the research setting.

D. Intraoperative Monitoring and Support

Intraoperative monitoring and support of swine are similar to those of other large animal species. In order to monitor homeostasis, the following parameters should be monitored: muscular reflexes, ECG, heart rate, blood pressure, blood gas saturation values, and core temperature. Swine are susceptible to hypothermia because of their relatively hairless skin; consequently, the use of circulating hot-water blankets or heated air wraps and protection from stainless steel surfaces should be considered. Animals should be completely covered by drapes during surgery to prevent heat loss. Animals may be monitored by a variety of mechanical means. Pulse oximeters can monitor oxygen saturation and pulse rates. Surgical monitors may be obtained that monitor ECG, rectal temperature, and blood pressures. Blood pressure may be monitored either by invasive intravascular techniques or by use of blood-pressure cuffs on the tail, medial saphenous artery, or radial artery. Pulse oximetry finger cuffs can be attached to the tongue, ear, tail, or dewclaw. There will be some variability in the ability of the pulse oximetry cuff to function, depending on skin pigmentation and thickness of the body part. IV fluid maintenance rates are 5–10 ml/kg/h (Smith and Swindle, 2008; Swindle, 2007).

E. Special Anesthetic Considerations

1. Cardiac Anesthesia

Anesthesia for cardiac surgery requires that the protocol minimize effects on cardiovascular function. Parameters that need to be considered when selecting a protocol include cardiac contractility, cardiac output, blood pressure, myocardial oxygen consumption, and prevention of cardiac arrhythmias. Isoflurane or sevoflurane delivered in nitrous oxide–oxygen (2:1) minimizes cardiodepressant effects during surgery. If an inhalant agent is contraindicated, then high-dose opioid infusions may be used, especially if there is a requirement to maintain myocardial contractility and coronary blood flow. The physiologic effects of the various anesthetics should be reviewed prior to performing complex cardiac surgeries (Swindle, 2007).

Amiodarone and lidocaine infusions may be necessary as preventives for fatal cardiac arrhythmias. Paralytic agents, such as pancuronium and vercuronium, will be necessary to paralyze the diaphragm during cardiac manipulation and may be useful for providing increased exposure when using a lateral thoracotomy. Paralytic agents should not be administered until there is an assurance that adequate analgesia has been obtained. This can be ascertained by performing skin and muscular incisions prior to their administration. Heart rate and blood pressure should be monitored during surgical manipulation in a paralyzed animal to assure adequate anesthesia (Swindle, 2007).

Performing cardiopulmonary bypass (CPB) and extracorporeal membrane support (ECMO) procedures in swine is more difficult than in most species. In order to perform these techniques as survival procedures, a multidisciplinary team of personnel competent in these procedures is necessary. It is beyond the scope of this chapter to describe CPB and ECMO procedures; however, they are described elsewhere in a detailed stepwise fashion, which should be adequate for most research facilities to perform them successfully (Swindle, 2007; Smith, 1997).

2. Pediatric Anesthesia

Neonatal dosage rates are frequently different from dosage rates for adults. The dosage ranges given in this manuscript are safe for swine of all ages in our experience. Control of hypothermia during anesthesia is especially important in the neonate, particularly in the first week postnatally, when they are incapable of controlling their own body temperature adequately (Swindle et al., 1996).

3. Neuroanesthesia

Swine have not been used very often in neurosurgical research, and specific anesthetic protocols for neurosurgery have not been published. The general principles of neuroanesthesia for other species should be applied. For instance, all inhalant anesthetics increase blood flow to the brain in swine, and swelling of the tissue may result postsurgically after manipulation; therefore, techniques to reduce brain swelling, such as the use of diuretics and hypertonic glucose solutions, should be applied. Ventilation rates and volumes may also influence the oxygen supply to the central nervous system (Swindle, 2007).

4. Obstetrics and Gynecology

Most anesthetic agents will cross the epitheliochorial placentation of swine to affect the fetus. Transport across the placenta is enhanced if the agent is lipophilic, and some of these agents may reach a higher concentration in the fetus than in the sow. Tocolytic agents, such as terbutaline, may be useful if uterine contractions under anesthesia need to be controlled. Reviews of the special considerations and detailed protocols for performing fetal surgery in swine have been published (Swindle et al., 1996).

5. Anesthesia for Imaging Procedures (MRI and PET)

Specialized imaging procedures require that a long duration of anesthesia be provided without equipment that may be affected by the imaging equipment. Depending on the equipment and duration of the imaging procedure, the short-term (20–30 min) injectable protocols described above may be adequate for the procedure. Complete relaxation without paralysis is necessary to obtain clear images. The combinations of ketamine/midazolam and ketamine/medetomidine provide the best relaxation for these procedures. Infusion protocols with thiobarbiturates may be used if having an IV infusion is not contraindicated (Swindle, 2007).

F. Postoperative Recovery

Postoperative recovery procedures for swine are similar to those for other species. A complete description of these procedures and the emergency procedures for cardiopulmonary distress have been published. Extubation can be performed when the pig is moving into a sternal position and struggling against the endotracheal tube. It is best to let the air out of the cuff of the tube first and allow the pig to stabilize prior to removing the tube. Apnea frequently occurs when the tube is removed, and compressive manipulation of the chest or stimulation of the pharynx and epiglottis may have to be instituted to start spontaneous respiration. In some cases, the pig may have to be reintubated and respirated with a handheld respiratory bag. The apnea is more likely to occur with injectable anesthetics, such as the barbiturates, than with inhalants.

Monitoring of cardiopulmonary function during recovery can be provided by pulse oximetry and appropriate countermeasures taken when hypoventilation or cardiac emergencies occur. If pulse oximetry is not available, then the pulse and respiratory rates should be monitored either by auscultation or observation (Swindle, 2007; Smith, 1997).

G. Acute and Chronic Analgesic Therapy

If surgical procedures are performed, it is best to provide preemptive analgesia prior to making the skin incision or at least prior to removing the animal from general anesthesia if intraoperative administration of these agents is not possible (Smith, 1997; Swindle, 2007).

1. Assessment of Pain and Discomfort

Swine are generally sedentary animals that respond to the presence of humans only during manipulation or feeding activity. Pigs that are hyperactive and vocalizing tend to be in distress postsurgically. Incisional pain and abnormal posture are other reliable indicators of pain or distress. Pigs will readily eat, even after major surgical procedures, if they are comfortable. Consequently, swine that are not resting comfortably and responding to feeding are probably in pain or distress postsurgically (Swindle, 2007; Castel et al., 2014).

2. Methods for Analgesic Drug Delivery

Parenteral analgesics are usually administered IM or SC in the neck. IV administration is generally given by using indwelling catheters in the ear vein or one of the other cannulated vessels intraoperatively. Swine can readily be induced to take oral medication when the substance is placed in a food treat. Canned dog and cat food, apples, chocolate syrup, and sweets are usually successful when using this technique (Swindle, 2007).

3. Non-Steroidal Anti-Inflammatory Drugs

The newer-generation NSAIDs, such as ketorolac, ketoprofen, meloxicam, and carprofen, have been utilized successfully in postoperative analgesia protocols either by injection or *per os*. For some procedures they have been effective in BID dosages as sole agents, but usually they are combined with buprenorphine (see Section V, G, 5) in the lower dose range of each agent to maximize the effects of opioids and NSAIDs (Flecknell, 2009; Swindle, 2007).

4. Local, Regional, and Epidural Anesthesia

Local and regional anesthesia has not been commonly used in research settings and is typically used as an adjunct to analgesia rather than as the sole anesthetic (Smith and Swindle, 2008; Thurmon, 1986; St. Jean and Anderson, 1999). The most common areas are dorsal nerve root blocks in the intercostal spaces or lumbar regions as an adjunct to anesthesia and analgesia for dorsal–ventral surgical incisions, such as thoracotomies. Infiltration of the incision with local anesthetics is also performed prior to making the initial incision as a form of preemptive analgesia. Xylazine (2 mg/kg diluted in saline), xylazine (1 mg/kg) plus lidocaine (10 ml 10% solution), and medetomidine (0.5 mg/kg diluted in saline) have been utilized epidurally to provide analgesia during general surgery (St. Jean and Anderson, 1999; Ko et al., 1992a; Royal et al., 2013).

5. Opioids

Buprenorphine is generally considered to be the opioid analgesic of choice postoperatively. Preemptive analgesia with this agent preoperatively or intraoperatively reduces the course of postoperative analgesia and the dosage that may have to be given. There is a wide range of therapeutic effectiveness, depending on the procedure and time of administration. For major surgical procedures, such as thoracotomies or visceral transplantation, a dosage of 0.05–0.1 mg/kg may be needed in the initial stages. The dosage may be reduced by 50–75% of the initial dosage BID, depending upon the clinical condition of the animal. Buprenorphine may be combined with NSAIDs (see Section V, G, 3), such as ketoprofen, carprofen, meloxicam, or ketorolac, to reduce the dosage and get a synergistic effect.

Fentanyl and sufentanil have been used for both balanced anesthesia and as high-dose opioid infusions for cardiac surgery. These agents have a short half-life and are not good for postoperative analgesia when administered as bolus injections. Anecdotal accounts indicate that dermal patches of fentanyl may be used in swine, but a controlled study with blood levels of the agent has not been published to date. Effectiveness of fentanyl patches can be variable, depending upon housing conditions and such factors as moisture and heat. In our experience, it is possible to get analgesia using 50- to 100-pg patches, but animals may show signs of overdosage and have to be monitored. Until such time as a controlled study is available, the use of these patches should be considered experimental in swine.

H. Euthanasia

Most of the injectable forms of euthanasia utilized in other large animal species are suitable for swine. Pentobarbital overdose (>150 mg/kg) is the preferred form of parenteral euthanasia. It is acceptable to administer KCl injections or perform exsanguination while swine are under general anesthesia (Swindle, 2007).

VI. SMALL RUMINANTS

A. Introduction

According to the American Association of Small Ruminant Practitioners, the term small ruminants encompasses sheep, goats, camelids, elk, deer, and related species (AASRP, 2010). Sheep, goats, and calves are most often encountered in research, testing, or training, thus this review will be limited to those species. These animals are docile, adapt well to frequent handling, restraint, and chronic instrumentation that may be dictated by the research needs. They are readily available either as purpose-bred or farm-raised, conditioned animals. Historically, these species have been used in a number of areas of investigation including cardiovascular research, medical device implantation and testing, orthopedic research, fetal surgery, and pulmonary studies. Sheep and goats are often used for production of various reagents used in experimentation including red blood cells, sera and antibodies.

Relief of pain is a scientific imperative for any species used in biomedical research (NRC, 2011). Recognition and relief of pain is required by the Animal Welfare

Regulations when these species are used in biomedical research (USDA, 2008). Furthermore, use of anesthetics and analgesics for routine veterinary practices such as castration and dehorning, that in the past were often performed without the benefit of analgesics is now strongly encouraged (AVMA, 2012a,b). There is a growing body of literature on anesthesia, analgesia, and pain management specific to small ruminants (Gray and McDonell, 1986a, b; Carroll and Hartsfield, 1996; Lee and Swanson, 1996; Carroll et al., 1998b; Lin and Pugh, 2002; Swindle et al., 2002; Greene, 2003; Riebold, 2007; Abrahamsen, 2009a,c, 2013; Valverde and Doherty, 2009; Coetzee, 2013). In the research setting, anesthetic techniques and analgesic protocols often differ from those used in the field setting common to clinical practice and certain experimental surgical procedures may require complex anesthetic and analgesic regimens. For some procedures, empirical use of anesthetics and analgesics reportedly used in humans, companion animals, or other species may be adopted and modified for the small ruminant. Cardiovascular studies in particular may require use of cardiopulmonary bypass which is beyond the scope of clinical practice (Collan, 1970; Gerring and Scarth, 1974; Schauvliege et al., 2006; Carney et al., 2009). The attending veterinarian should be consulted for assistance in developing specific anesthetic protocols to meet study objectives.

The use of many anesthetic and analgesic drugs in small ruminants may constitute 'extra-label' use. Currently there are no analgesic drugs approved for the alleviation of pain in livestock in the United States (Coetzee, 2013; Smith, 2013). Only one anesthetic drug, 2% lidocaine, is approved for use in cattle in the US and one NSAID, flunixine meglumine, approved for use in livestock for the relief of pyrexia and inflammation, but not pain (Smith and Modric, 2013; Smith, 2013). Extra-label use of these drugs and its ramifications should be taken into consideration if there is the potential for return of ruminants used in research into the food supply through practices such as adoption, resale, or rendering.

Attention to the unique anatomical and physiologic characteristics of the ruminant and taking steps to minimize potential adverse effects these differences may have on anesthesia, surgery and recovery is paramount to a successful anesthetic and surgical outcome in these species. The unique challenges of anesthesia and surgery in ruminants not encountered in monogastric species is discussed below after which commonly used drugs and protocols for anesthesia and analgesia are presented (see also Table 24.13). Detailed information on all aspects of anesthesia and analgesia for ruminants in the research setting is beyond the scope of this section, however, readers are referred to the excellent review of this topic by Valverde and Doherty (2008).

B. Preoperative Evaluation and Preparation

1. Preoperative Evaluation

Prior to any surgical procedure, the ruminant animal should have a complete physical examination with special attention to the respiratory and gastrointestinal systems to determine if the animal is a suitable surgical candidate and to provide baseline data with which to compare the postoperative clinical condition. Laboratory diagnostics should include at a minimum, a hematocrit and measurement of blood urea nitrogen and creatinine levels. Additional tests, including CBC, chemistry panel and evaluation of fecal sample for ova and parasites are advisable, especially if the animals have been maintained on pasture.

2. Injection Sites and Venous Access

The preferred area for IM or SC injections in ruminants is a triangular area of the neck bordered by the nuchal ligament dorsally, the cervical vertebrae ventrally and the shoulder caudally (Diffay et al., 2002; Radositits et al., 2007). Other sites that may be used for IM injections include the epaxial muscles in the lumbar region, the quadriceps femoris, and the triceps (Diffay et al., 2002). The semimembranosus/semitendinosus muscle group can be used with caution to avoid injecting irritating drugs close to the sciatic nerve. The axillary region and chest wall may be used for SC injections in sheep and goats (Diffay et al., 2002).

The jugular vein is often used for administering drugs IV or blood collection. In sheep and goats the cephalic vein is readily available for IV administration and is easily accessed by having an assistant 'set up' the sheep on its rump and hold off the vein while venipuncture is made (Diffay et al., 2002). The saphenous vein may also be used for IV injection in the anesthetized or sedated animal.

Intravenous catheters can be placed in the jugular vein to provide continuous access for IV administration of fluids, drugs, or total intravenous anesthesia (TIVA). A 14-gauge, 5½ inch catheter can be used in most ruminants (Abrahamsen, 2009a). Smaller catheters can be used in the cephalic or saphenous veins or in lambs and kids. Jugular vein catheters should be placed in the cranial one-third of the jugular furrow to avoid interference with catheter function by the valves found in the distal jugular vein (Divers and Peek, 2008). The author often places double- or triple-lumen central venous catheters using the Seldinger technique after anesthesia induction. The additional lumens provide access for multiple infusions and for monitoring central venous pressure. The flexible design of most multi-lumen catheters leads to greater longevity and less complications if catheters are maintained long-term. Rigid catheters are more likely to fail, especially at the junction of the catheter with the

TABLE 24.13   Drug Dosages in Small Ruminants[a]

Drug	Dose	Route	Comments
ANTICHOLINERGICS			
Atropine	0.02 mg/kg	IV	Not recommended as a routine premedication. Indicated for treatment of bradyarrhythmias
Glycopyrrolate	0.005–0.01 mg/kg	IV	
SEDATIVE/TRANQUILIZERS			
Acepromazine	0.02 mg/kg	SC, IM, IV	
Xylazine	0.01–0.02 mg/kg; 0.02–0.04 mg/kg	IV	
		IM	
Medetomidine	0.01–0.03 mg/kg	IV, IM	
Dexmedetomidine	0.05 mg/kg	IV	Sheep
Diazepam	0.25–0.5 mg/kg	IV	
Midazolam	0.1–0.3 mg/kg	IV, IM	
α_2-ADRENERGIC ANTAGONISTS			
Yohimbine	0.1 mg/kg (cattle)	IV	
	1.0 mg/kg (sheep)		
Atipamezole	20–60 µg/kg	IV, IM	
Tolazoline	0.5–2.0 mg/kg	IV	
INDUCTION AGENTS			
Thiopental	10–16 mg/kg	IV	
Methohexital	3–5 mg/kg	IV	
Propofol	4–6 mg/kg	IV	Continuous rate infusion (0.3–0.5 mg/kg/min IV) for TIVA (see text).
Xylazine + ketamine	0.05–0.1 mg/kg X, followed by 3–5 mg/kg K	IV or IM IV	Xylazine and ketamine can be combined and administered concurrently.
Xylazine + ketamine	0.22 mg/kg X + 11 mg/kg K	IM	
Medetomidine + ketamine	0.005–0.01 mg/kg + 2 mg/kg K	IV or IM	
Dexmedetomidine + ketamine	0.005–0.015 mg/kg + 2m/kg K	IV or IM	
Ketamine + diazepam	5 mg/kg K + 0.3–0.5 mg/kg D	IV	Premedicate with xylazine, 0.03–0.05 mg/kg IM
Ketamine + midazolam	4 mg/kg K + 0.4 mg/kg M	IV	Midazolam can be administered IM followed by ketamine IV
ANALGESICS			
Morphine	0.1 mg/kg	IV	
Fentanyl	2.5–5 µg/kg	IV Transdermal	
	50 µg/h		
Butorphanol	0.05–0.1 mg/kg Q 4–6h	SC, IM, IV	
Buprenorphine	0.005–0.01 mg/kg Q 4–6h	SC, IM, IV	
Flunixin meglumine	1.1–2.2 mg/kg BID		Limit to total of 4 doses
Phenylbutazone	2–5 mg/kg	IV	Do not use chronically
	4–8 mg/kg	PO	
Carprofen	4 mg/kg Q 24h	SC, IM	
Meloxicam	0.5 mg/kg BID 1 mg/kg Q 24h	IM, IV, (sheep)	
		PO	

[a]See text for references and discussion.

luer-lock fitting from repeated flexion with movement of the animal.

3. Common Complications to Anesthesia and Prevention

The anatomy of the ruminant stomach coupled with the normal physiological functions of salivation, eructation, and regurgitation present unique challenges for anesthesia and surgery of the small ruminant. Common complications encountered in anesthetizing ruminants are directly associated with the effects of the digestive system on adequate ventilation and include regurgitation and aspiration, inadequate oxygenation, and bloating. Addressing these potential problems by proper preparation of the animal and preventive measures is the key to a successful surgical outcome irrespective of the anesthetic regimen used.

The stomach consisting of the rumen, reticulum, omasum, and abomasum is unique to ruminant species and is the site of production of volatile fatty acids, the primary energy source, through microbial fermentation (Leek, 2004). The ruminant stomach occupies approximately 75% of the abdominal cavity, filling most of the left half of the cavity and extending into the right half of the abdomen (Habel, 1975). The relative size of the four compartments of the stomach develop and change with age of the animal. In the newborn calf, the ruminoreticulum contains less than half the volume of the abomasum and remains functionless while the animal is on a milk diet (Nickel et al., 1973; Habel, 1975). The capacity of the ruminoreticulum is approximately equal to the abomasum by 8 weeks of age, double the capacity of the abomasum by 12 weeks, and in the adult the capacity is approximately 9:1 that of the abomasum (Habel, 1975). In lambs, the stomach represents 22% of total gastrointestinal wet tissue mass, but increases to 49% in adult sheep (Valverde and Doherty, 2008). In cattle, the volume of the stomach is approximately 115–150 l while in sheep and goats stomach volume is 15–18 l (Habel, 1975; Valverde and Doherty, 2008). The size and volume of the ruminant stomach can impede respiration and ventilation in the anesthetized animal by interfering with diaphragmatic excursion resulting in a reduction in functional residual capacity of the lung, thus interfering with effective pulmonary gas exchange (Lee and Swanson, 1996; Greene, 2003). Positioning of the anesthetized ruminant may further exacerbate hypoventilation as recumbency shifts the rumen mass leading to displacement of the diaphragm into the thoracic cavity. Cattle placed in lateral or dorsal recumbency developed significant hypoxemia and hypercapnea (Wagner et al., 1990; Jorgensen and Cannedy, 1996). Furthermore, the displaced rumen may interfere with venous return, predisposing to decreased cardiac output and low blood pressure (Jorgensen and Cannedy, 1996; Valverde and Doherty, 2008). For these reasons a key to successful anesthetic management and surgery of the small ruminant is preparation of the animal and taking preventive measures to minimize the potential for regurgitation and aspiration of stomach contents, prevent bloating and ensure adequate ventilation during anesthesia and surgery.

a. Fasting

Withholding food and water prior to surgery may decrease rumen volume, decreases the rate of fermentation and risk of regurgitation (Swindle et al., 2002). Recommendations on the duration of fasting prior to surgery vary widely ranging from a few hours to 48 h. Excessive fasting may lead to alterations in the rumen flora, reduced motility and rumen stasis resulting in a negative energy balance and complications during the postoperative period (Abrahamsen, 2009a, 2013). Furthermore, fasting may have adverse effects on acid base status sufficient to cause cardiac arryhythmias (Abrahamsen, 2009a, 2013). In cattle, a 48-h fast produced 20–30% reduction in heart rate which persisted for 48 h following recovery (Bednarski and McGuirk, 1986; McGuirk et al., 1990; Riebold, 2007). Fasting from food for 24–48 h and withholding water for 12–24 h in healthy sheep and goats resulted in better ventilation, less tympany and reduced incidence of regurgitation (Carroll and Hartsfield, 1996). Other authors recommend shorter periods of no more than 12–18 h fasting from food and either not withholding water or withholding for only 4–6 h (Swindle et al., 2002, Abrahamsen, 2009a, 2013). In the author's experience withholding food and water for 8–12 h before surgery and supporting fluid balance with intravenous maintenance fluids is sufficient while avoiding the complications of prolonged fasting. Young animals should not be fasted for longer than 12 h as at this age, they are transitioning from a functional monogastric to ruminant (Carroll and Hartsfield, 1996).

b. Intubation

Endotracheal intubation of the ruminant under general anesthesia is essential to protect the airway and assist in ventilating the animal. The long, narrow oral cavity of the ruminant requires use of laryngoscopes with longer blades than typically used in human or veterinary anesthesia. Cuffed, silicone endotracheal tubes in this size range are available for large animal applications (Cook, Surgivet, Pointe). Endotracheal tubes of 9.0–14.0 mm internal diameter (i.d.), 35–55 cm in length are used in adult sheep 50–80 kg body weight and tubes of 12.0–16.0 mm i.d., 50–75 cm in length are used in calves 50–100 kg body weight. The airway of goats is typically smaller than sheep and endotracheal tubes of 7.5–9.0 mm i.d. are recommended for goats of 50–70 kg body weight (Valverde and Doherty, 2008). For sheep and goats, a laryngoscope with a long, straight blade, such as a Miller #4 (20 cm in length) can be used to assist intubation; while the longer Rowson (35–45 cm in length) may be needed for larger sheep and calves (Carroll and Hartsfield, 1996). The entrance to the larynx is positioned obliquely and faces rostrodorsally relative to the oropharynx making intubation difficult (Fig. 24.1) (Valverde and Doherty, 2008). Positioning the animal in sternal recumbancy with the head and neck extended and flexed dorsally will bring the larynx in line with the oral cavity (Fig. 24.2). In addition,

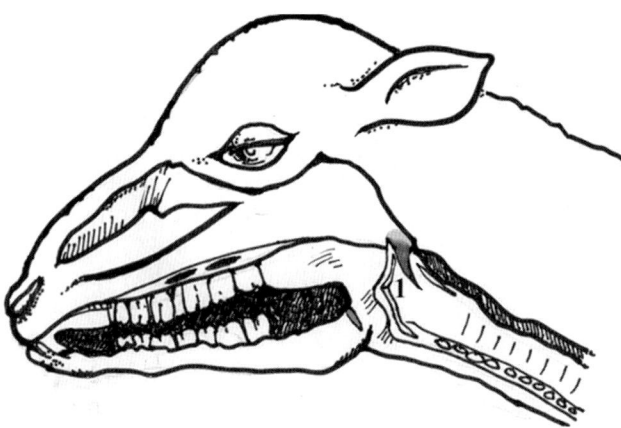

FIGURE 24.1   Lateral view of the head of a sheep showing the oral and nasal cavities. Note the rostrodorsal positioning of the epiglottis (1), which hinders the entrance to the laryngeal cavity making orotracheal intubation difficult. Valverde and Doherty (2008).

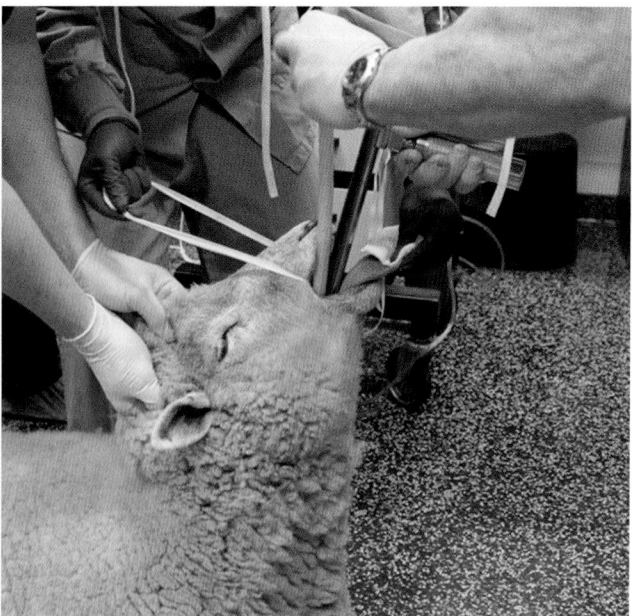

FIGURE 24.2   Endotracheal intubation of an adult sheep. Positioning of the sedated animal in sternal recumbancy with the head and neck extended aligns the oropharynynx, larynx, and trachea for easier intubation.

an assistant can apply gentle external pressure to the cricoid area of the neck to further align the laryngeal opening with the oropharynx. A plastic-coated malleable wire, or plastic, metal, or wooden rod can be used as a stylet to stiffen the endotracheal tube and assist intubation (Carroll and Hartsfield, 1996). Application of lidocaine gel or liquid to the arytenoids to obtund the laryngeal reflex will aid smooth intubation. Benzocaine-based sprays such as Cetacaine® should be avoided as they are reported to cause methemoglobinemia in sheep and goats (Lagutchik et al., 1992; Carroll and Hartsfield, 1996). Care should be taken in passing the endotracheal tube as the sharp points of the molar teeth can easily damage the tube. Once in place and intratracheal positioning confirmed, the endotracheal tube is secured with adhesive or cloth tape.

c. Preventing Regurgitation and Bloat

Regurgitation in the anesthetized ruminant may be either an active or passive process. Active regurgitation is most likely to occur due to inadequate or light anesthesia, whereas passive regurgitation results from increased transluminal pressure gradients and relaxed esophageal sphincters (Steffey, 1986; Jorgensen and Cannedy, 1996). In addition to fasting prior to anesthesia, induction techniques that quickly eliminate the gag reflex and positioning the animal in sternal recumbancy with the head elevated reduces the risk of regurgitation during intubation (Abrahamsen, 2009a, 2013). Intubation with an appropriately sized endotracheal tube with the cuff inflated will protect the airway if regurgitation occurs during surgery.

In the ruminant animal, gases in the form of carbon dioxide (60%) and methane (30–40%) are produced by the fermentation process in the rumen (Leek, 2004). The amount of gas production in adult cattle has been estimated to peak at a rate of 40 l/h, 2–4 h following a meal and accumulation of gas is normally eliminated by eructation which occurs every 1–2 min (Leek, 2004). Heavy sedation or general anesthesia inhibits ruminoreticular motility and impairs eructation (Valverde and Doherty, 2008). Placement of an orogastric tube into the rumen at the time of anesthesia induction will minimize accumulation of gas. A tube with an inflatable cuff such as a foal urethral tube will assist in positioning the end of the tube at the gas–liquid interface in the rumen so that primarily gas and not rumen fluid will be suctioned off (Swindle et al., 2002). Removal of large amounts of liquid from the rumen will not eliminate gas production and is likely to result in a dry mass of ingesta that can impair return to normal digestive function in the postoperative period. The orogastric tube may on occasion become clogged with ingesta or the wall of the rumen sucked on to the end of the tube causing it to no longer work. The authors have found that use of low pressures and intermittent vacuum is sufficient to minimize gas accumulation and avoid the problems of clogging or occlusion. If the tube ceases to function and gas accumulates during surgery, the gas cap can be cannulated percutaneously with a large bore (14–18 gauge) intravenous catheter connected to a sterile vacuum hose. The use of oral antibiotics such as neomycin prior to surgery to reduce fermentation will not significantly reduce the potential for regurgitation or bloating, can lead to problems with return to normal gastrointestinal function following surgery, and is not recommended.

4. Preoperative Medications

a. Anticholinergics

Pre-anesthetic medication with anticholinergics is controversial. Some authors recommend against their routine use as premedicants (Riebold, 2007; Abrahamsen, 2009a). Others recommend pretreatment with anticholinergics when administering xylazine to counteract its brachycardic effects (Plumb, 2011). Anticholinergics do not consistently reduce salivary secretions unless given at high doses which may cause tachycardia (Short, 1986; Carroll and Hartsfield, 1996; Ahern et al., 2010). Atropine has a shorter duration of action in ruminants compared to other species (Short, 1986). Sheep and goats require large and repeated doses of atropine to decrease salivation (Gray and McDonell, 1986a; Carroll and Hartsfield, 1996). Atropine reduces the aqueous fraction of secretions making any respiratory secretions more viscous and difficult to clear, potentially causing airway obstruction (Short, 1986; Carroll and Hartsfield, 1996; Abrahamsen, 2009a). Furthermore, atropine reduces gastrointestinal motility in ruminants (Abrahamsen, 2009a). The anticholinergics atropine (0.02 mg/kg IV) and glyocpyrrolate (0.005–0.01 mg/kg IV) are indicated when bradyarrhythmias occur (Carroll and Hartsfield, 1996; Riebold, 2007). Goats appear to require a higher dose of glycopyrrolate (0.01 mg/kg IV) than other species (Carroll and Hartsfield, 1996).

b. Sedatives and Tranquilizers

Sedatives may be used prior to anesthesia to minimize stress and anxiety and facilitate induction. Reducing stress and anxiety permits a greater portion of cardiac output to be directed to vital organs thus more of the induction agent is directed to the central nervous system rather than skeletal muscle (Abrahamsen, 2009a). This allows for smoother induction with less induction agent. Depending on the drug used, sedatives may also reduce the amount of anesthetic agent necessary for maintenance. Sedatives can be used for their calming and anxiolytic effects when regional anesthesia is used for minor procedures, and may be combined with analgesics for pain management (Swindle et al., 2002).

i. PHENOTHIAZINE TRANQUILIZERS Acepromazine maleate is the most commonly used phenothiazine tranquilizer in veterinary medicine. For sedation prior to anesthesia, a dose of 0.02 mg/kg SC, IM, or IV provides a slow onset of sedation with a slight decrease in respiratory rate but no change in heart rate (Valverde and Doherty, 2008). Acepromazine has a sparing effect on inhalant anesthetics, in one study reducing the MAC 36–45% in goats (Doherty et al., 2002a). It may also protect against the arryhthmogenic effects of anesthetics as observed in other species. Acepromazine (0.5 mg/kg, IV) inhibited epinephrine-induced arrhythmias in thiopental–halothane anesthetized sheep (Rezakhani et al., 1977).

ii. α₂-ADRENERGIC AGONISTS AND ANTAGONISTS Xyalzine, medetomidine, dexmedetomidine, detomidine, and romifidine have all been used in small ruminants as sole agents or in combination with other drugs for sedation, analgesia, or anesthesia. All α_2-adrenergics produce rapid, dose-dependent sedation in ruminants (Valverde and Doherty, 2008). A biphasic blood pressure response characterized by an initial hypertension due to increased vascular resistance is followed by hypotension secondary to decreased release of norepinephrine (Valverde and Doherty, 2008). Hypoxemia secondary to pulmonary edema has been reported in cattle, goats and sheep but is most severe in the latter species (Kumar and Thurmon, 1979; Celly et al., 1997, 1999). Xylazine, romifidine, detomidine and medetomidine can produce hypoxemia without a concomitant hypercapnia (Celly et al., 1997). Dexmedetomidine-induced hypoxemia with evidence of pulmonary edema and pulmonary vascular congestion has been reported in sheep (Kästner et al., 2007). For the purpose of this review, further discussion of the α_2 adrenergic agonists will be limited to the more commonly used xylazine, medetomidine and dexmedetomidine.

Xylazine is 10–20 times more potent in ruminants than other species with some breeds, e.g., the Brahman and Hereford breeds requiring only 1/10th the normal bovine dose for sedation (Greene and Thurmon, 1988; Kästner, 2006; Riebold, 2007). The difference in intraspecies sensitivity is likely due to G-protein binding affinity in ruminants compared to other species (Torneke et al., 2003). Within the small ruminants, the spectrum of sensitivity to the effects of xyalzine is goats > cattle> sheep (Riebold, 2007). Low doses of xylazine (0.01–0.02 mg/kg IV or 0.02–0.04 mg/kg IM) produce standing sedation in cattle suitable for short diagnostic or therapeutic procedures (Abrahamsen, 2013). Higher doses (0.1–0.2 mg/kg) of xylazine will induce heavy sedation, and possibly light planes of anesthesia (Riebold, 2007; Abrahamsen, 2008). Intramuscular administration of xylazine will typically double the duration of effect (Abrahamsen, 2013).

Xylazine may be used alone or combined with an opioid drug (i.e., butorphanol, morphine) as a premedicant prior to anesthesia, or administered with ketamine or tiletamine-zolazepam for anesthesia induction.

Medetomidine is a sedative-analgesic labeled for use in dogs that also produces dose-dependent analgesia of a degree similar to morphine in sheep (Muge et al., 1994). It is an equal mixture of two optical enantiomers, dexmedetomidine, the active drug, and levomedetomidine, the inactive drug, with a high affinity for α_2-adrenergic receptors (Lamont, 2009). Sedation produced by medetomidine is more rapid and longer lasting than xylazine (Carroll et al., 2005; Rioja et al., 2008). Its effects on the cardiovascular system are variable depending on species, the route of administration and concurrent administration with other drugs. Heart rate, mean arterial blood pressure, and pulmonary arterial blood pressure all increased following IV or IM administration of medetomidine in calves (0.03 mg/kg IV), sheep (0.01 mg/kg IV or 0.03 mg/kg IM), and goats (0.02 mg/kg IV) (Kästner et al., 2003; Carroll et al., 2005; Rioja et al., 2008). Medetomidine caused cardiovascular depression when administered epidurally or with midazolam (Raekallio et al, 1991; Mpanduji et al., 2000). In contrast to other species, medetomidine has significant effects on the stress response and tends to increase cortisol and glucose levels in ruminants (Carroll et al., 1998a, 2005; Ranheim et al., 2000b).

Dexmedetomidine, being the single enantiomer preparation of the dextrarotary form of medetomidine, is twice as potent as medetomidine (Plumb, 2011). As a sedative in sheep, 5 μg/kg IV of dexmedetomidine is equipotent to 10 μg/kg IV of medetomidine (Kästner et al., 2001b). As with other α_2-agonists, dexmedetomidine causes cardiopulmonary depression and may produce moderate to severe hypoxemia (Kästner et al., 2001b, Kästner et al., 2005, Kästner et al., 2007a, Kästner et al., 2007b). In sevoflurane-anesthetized goats, the adverse pulmonary effects may be mitigated by use of a CRI without loading dose (Kästner et al., 2007a). As with xylazine, medetomidine or dexmedetomidine may be used alone or combined with other drugs (e.g. ketamine) for sedation or anesthesia induction.

An advantage of the α_2-adrenergic agonists drugs is the ability to reverse sedation and some of their adverse effects with the α_2-adrenergic antagonists, yohimbine, tolazoline, atipamezole and idazoxan. Yohimbine (0.12 mg/kg IV) has variable efficacy in cattle for reversing α_2-adrenergic, while a higher dose (1.0 mg/kg IV) is necessary to reverse xylazine sedation in sheep (Thurmon et al., 1989; Riebold, 2007). Tolazoline (0.5–2.0 mg/kg IV) reverses xylazine-induced sedation in calves more rapidly than yohimbine (Thurmon et al., 1989; Young et al., 1989). At higher doses, tolazoline can cause hyperesthesia and transient bradycardia, sinus arrest, and hypotension (Riebold, 2007). Both tolazoline (2.2 μg/kg IV) and atipamezole (20–60 μg/kg IV or IM) were effective in reversing medetomidine–ketamine-induced sedation in calves (Raekallio et al., 1991; Lin et al., 1999). Re-sedation following atipamazole reversal of medetomidine, presumably due to redistribution or slower elimination from the central nervous system has been reported in dairy calves but not sheep (Ranheim et al., 1998, 2000a). Intramuscular administration of the antagonists is preferred because it reduces the risk of CNS excitement or cardiovascular complications (Abrahamsen, 2008). Dividing the dose of the reversal agent and administering a portion IM followed by IV can produce a more rapid recovery while avoiding return of sedation (Abrahamsen, 2008).

iii. BENZODIAZEPINES Diazepam and midazolam are the most commonly used benzodiazepine sedatives in small ruminants. For sedation, diazepam (0.25–0.5 mg/kg IV) or midazolam (0.1–0.3 mg/kg, IV or IM) can be administered to small ruminants (Swindle et al., 2002; Valverde and Doherty, 2008). Diazepam or midazolam are most often combined with other drugs, for example, ketamine or α_2-agonists, for the purposes of sedation, injectable anesthesia or anesthesia induction. Another benzodiazepine, zolazepam, combined with tiletamine is a component of the injectable sedative/anesthetic Telazol®. As a group, the benzodiazepines have minimal, transient effects on the cardiopulmonary systems and can be used alone for mild sedation and restraint of small ruminants (Valverde and Doherty, 2008). Diazepam is irritating to tissues and poorly absorbed following IM administration (Valverde and Doherty, 2008; Plumb, 2011). It should only be given by slow IV administration to avoid thrombogenesis (Plumb, 2011). Midazolam in contrast, is water soluble and can be administered by the IV or IM routes (Plumb, 2011). Midazolam is reported to have antinociceptive properties in a sheep model, presumably mediated by gamma-aminobutyric acid (GABA) receptors at the spinal level (Kyles et al., 1995; Valverde and Doherty, 2008).

iv. OPIOIDS In contrast to the α_2-adrenergic agonists and benzodiazepines, opioids are less commonly used in ruminant species for the purpose of sedation and premedication prior to general anesthesia. Butorphanol (0.05–0.1 mg/kg IV or IM) or morphine (0.05–0.1 mg/kg IV or IM) can be co-administered with an α_2-agonist to improve sedation and analgesia while reducing the total dose of the α_2-agonist, thereby minimizing unwanted side effects (Riebold, 2007; Abrahamsen, 2008, 2013). Intramuscular administration of butorphaonol is preferred as ataxia and dysphoria has been reported in sheep when the drug was given IV (Waterman et al., 1991a; Riebold, 2007).

5. Induction Techniques

a. Mask Induction

Anesthesia can be induced in tractable small ruminants weighing less than 100 kg with isoflurane or sevoflurane delivered through a large dog mask (Swindle et al., 2002; Riebold, 2007). In the opinion of the authors, mask induction is a less desirable method of inducing anesthesia in ruminants because it does not provide rapid control of the animal's airway and contamination of the immediate work environment with waste anesthetic gases will occur. Some authors recommend the use of nitrous oxide with the inhalant agent, taking advantage of the 'second gas effect' to hasten induction, however, nitrous oxide should be used with caution due to its propensity to diffuse into gas-filled spaces including the gastrointestinal tract causing distention and ruminal tympany (Trim, 1987; Borkowski and Allen, 1999; Riebold, 2007).

b. Barbiturates

Ultra-short acting barbiturates are often used for rapid induction of anesthesia, however availability of the drug can be problematic. Of the thiobarbiturates, thiamyl is no longer available and thiopental is currently not available in the United States at the time of writing. Thiopental (10–16 mg/kg IV) has been recommended for induction and intubation followed by maintenance with an inhalant agent (Carroll and Hartsfield, 1996; Lin and Pugh, 2002; Swindle et al., 2002). Methohexital sodium is a non-sulfur containing, ultra-short acting oxybarbiturate that has been used as an induction agent in calves and sheep (Stewart, 1965; Collan, 1970; Carney et al., 2009). A dose of 3–5 mg/kg IV is sufficient for induction of anesthesia and endotracheal intubation in calves, sheep, and goats (Thurmon and Benson, 1986). In the authors' experience, methohexital permits rapid induction and intubation with a minimum of upper airway secretions in comparison to ketamine combinations (Carney et al., 2009). Currently, methohexital is only available in the U.S. Barbiturates especially sulfur-containing drugs (i.e., thiopental) are not recommended in ruminants under 2–3 months of age (Trim, 1987; Carroll and Hartsfield, 1996). Due to the high alkalinity of the barbiturates, they should only be administered IV, preferably through a pre-placed catheter to avoid perivascular necrosis if extravasation occurs (Swindle et al., 2002).

c. Propofol

Propofol is a non-barbiturate, non-steroidal hypnotic agent labeled for use in cats and dogs (Plumb, 2011). It rapidly induces anesthesia in sheep, goats and calves (Waterman, 1988; Alves et al., 2003; Prassinos et al., 2005). A dose of 4–6 mg/kg IV is recommended for induction of anesthesia in ruminants (Reid et al., 1993; Carroll and Hartsfield, 1996; Riebold, 2007; Valverde and Doherty, 2008). Premedication of the animal with an α_2-agonist or fentanyl, reduces the dose of propofol necessary for induction (Kästner et al., 2006; Dzikiti et al., 2009). Unlike barbiturates, propofol is non-cumulative and does not depend on redistribution of the drug from body stores for elimination; therefore, it can be given by CRI for maintenance of anesthesia (Prassinos et al., 2005; Valverde and Doherty, 2008). In sheep, induction with propofol (6 mg/kg IV) followed by a CRI (0.5 mg/kg/min IV) resulted in stable, light anesthesia followed by recovery to standing within approximately 15 min (Lin et al., 1997). Because propofol has minimal analgesic properties, when it is used as the sole anesthetic agent, appropriate analgesic drugs should be administered when the potential for intraoperative or postoperative pain exists (Plumb, 2011). Carroll et al. reported that TIVA with propofol (induction, 3–4 mg/kg IV followed by 0.3 mg/kg/min IV infusion) in goats premedicated with detomidine and butorphanol provided adequate planes of surgical anesthesia for carotid artery translocation, castration or ovariectomy (Carroll et al., 1998b).

d. Ketamine

Ketamine is commonly used as an induction agent in small ruminants, and in combination with other sedatives or tranquilizers, may be suitable for short procedures (Riebold, 2007; Abrahamsen, 2009a). Ketamine induces a dissociative anesthetic state characterized by increased muscle tone and retention of peripheral reflexes, in particular, upper airway reflexes which may make intubation difficult (Valverde and Doherty, 2008). Because of these properties, ketamine should not be used as the sole agent for induction or short-term anesthesia and is most commonly used in conjunction with α_2-agonists and benzodiazepines. Ketamine and xylazine or the more selective α_2-agonists, medetomidine and dexmedetomidine have been used successfully for induction or short-term anesthesia in small ruminants (Raekallio et al., 1991; Caulkett et al., 1996; Lin et al., 1997; Kästner et al., 2001a; Swindle et al., 2002; Gogoi et al., 2003; Valverde and Doherty, 2008; Singh et al., 2010). The sympathomimetic effects of ketamine counteract the negative cardiovascular effects of xylazine and other α_2-agonists (Abrahamsen, 2009a). Xylazine (0.05–0.1 mg/kg, IV or IM) is administered initially, followed by ketamine (3–5 mg/kg IV or 5–10 mg/kg IM) when the animal becomes sedated or recumbent (Swindle et al., 2002; Valverde and Doherty, 2008; Abrahamsen, 2009a). Alternatively, xylazine (0.22 mg/kg) can be combined with ketamine (11 mg/kg) in the same syringe and administered IM (Swindle et al., 2002). Medetomidine (0.005–0.01 mg/kg, IV or IM) or dexmedetomidine (0.005–0.015 mg/kg, IV or IM) can be substituted for xylazine, however all three α_2-agonist can cause significant respiratory depression and hypoxemia especially when administered intravenously (Kästner *et al.*, 2001a; Valverde and Doherty, 2008).

The combination of ketamine with the benzodiazepines, diazepam, or midazolam, mitigates the increased muscle tone produced by ketamine alone with the advantage of minimal effects on the cardiorespiratory system (Valverde and Doherty, 2008). Due to poor absorption from tissues, diazepam is administered IV followed by ketamine, although midazolam may be administered IM (Stegmann, 1998; Swindle *et al.*, 2002). Equal volumes of ketamine (100 mg/ml) and diazepam (5 mg/ml) can be combined and the resultant mixture administered IV at the rate of 1 ml/18–22 kg body weight (Abrahamsen, 2009a). Midazolam (0.4 mg/kg IV or IM) can be substituted for diazepam and given with ketamine (4 mg/kg IV) (Stegmann, 1998). A classic induction protocol for small ruminants is to administer a low dose (0.03 mg/kg) of xylazine IM, followed 10–15 min later by induction with ketamine (5 mg/kg) mixed with diazepam (0.3–0.5 mg/kg) given IV to effect (Valverde and Doherty, 2008). Sedation with a low dose of xylazine prior to induction reduces anxiety in the ruminant patient directing a greater proportion of cardiac output to vital organs instead of skeletal muscle, thus intensifying and extending the effects of the induction bolus (Abrahamsen, 2009a).

6. Anesthesia Maintenance

a. Inhalant Anesthetics

Anesthesia in small ruminants is most often maintained with inhalant agents especially if the animals are intubated. Inhalant anesthetics provide the benefit of rapid adjustment of anesthetic depth and relatively rapid smooth recovery from anesthesia. Older inhalant anesthetics, methoxyflurane and halothane are off market and no longer available in most countries. New agents, including isoflurane, sevoflurane, and desflurane have been used successfully in small ruminants (Hikasa *et al.*, 1998; Greene *et al.*, 2002; Mohamadnia *et al.*, 2008; Sellers *et al.*, 2013).

For small ruminants <100 kg, anesthesia machines designed for humans or companion animals can be used. This equipment may not be able to support animals above 100 kg body weight. Anesthesia machines specifically designed for larger animals are available commercially and can provide the tidal volume and flow rates necessary to meet the ventilator requirements of these larger animals. High oxygen flow rates (5–10 L/min) are initially used to flush nitrogen from the circuit and animal and promote uptake of the inhalant agent (Abrahamsen, 2009a). Flow rates of 7–10 ml/kg (semi-closed system) or 2 ml/kg (closed system) are used for maintenance (Abrahamsen, 2009a). Very young animals may benefit from breathing 60–70% oxygen to

minimize adverse effects on the lungs (Carney *et al.*, 2009; Weiss *et al.*, 2012). For mechanical ventilation, respiratory rates of 6–10 breaths/min, tidal volumes of 10–22 ml/kg and peak pressures of 20–30 cm of water are typically used to minimize the effects of positive pressure ventilation on the cardiovascular system (Swindle *et al.*, 2002; Riebold, 2007).

The MAC, i.e., the concentration of the inhalant agent at the alveolus that inhibits purposeful movement in 50% of anesthetized animals in response to a noxiuous stimulus for the inhalant anesthetics in small ruminants is presented in Table 24.14. All inhalant anesthetics produce dose-dependent decreases in cardiac output, stroke volume, blood pressure, tidal volume and respiratory rate, and increases in $PaCO_2$ (Valverde and Doherty, 2008). The negative hemodynamic effects of inhalant agents may be exacerbated by intermittent positive pressure ventilation (IPPV) because mechanical ventilation suppresses venous return and cardiac function during the positive pressure phase (Valverde and Doherty, 2008; Abrahamsen, 2009a). Drugs used for premedication typically lower the MAC (see below) thus lessening the dose-dependent cardiorespiratory depression of the inhalant agents.

Both sevoflurane and desflurane are less soluble in blood than isoflurane. Therefore, induction, change in depth of anesthesia and recovery is more rapid than with isoflurane. There is little difference in cardiovascular and respiratory effects between the three agents (Hikasa

TABLE 24.14 Reported Minimum Alveolar Concentration of Inhalant Anesthetics in Small Ruminants

Inhalant agent	Cattle	Sheep	Goat
Halothane	0.76% (Valverde and Doherty, 2008)	0.69% (Valverde and Doherty, 2008)	0.96 ± 0.12% (Hikasa *et al.*, 1998)
			1.3 ± 0.1% (Antognini and Eisele, 1993)
Isoflurane	1.14 ± 0.01% (Cantalapiedra *et al.*, 2000)	1.19–1.53% (Valverde and Doherty, 2008)	1.31 ± 0.03% (Doherty *et al.*, 2002b)
			1.29 ± 0.11% (Hikasa *et al.*, 1998)
			1.5 ± 0.3% (Antognini and Eisele, 1993)
Desflurane	Not reported	9.5% (Lukasik *et al.*, 1998a)	Not reported
Sevoflurane	Not reported	3.3% (Lukasik *et al.*, 1998b)	2.33 ± 0.15% (Hikasa *et al.*, 1998)

MAC values for calves are assumed to be similar to adult cattle.

et al., 1998, 2002; Greene et al., 2002; Mohamadnia et al., 2008; Sellers et al., 2013). Because sevoflurane is approximately seven times the cost of isoflurane and a higher MAC is required for a surgical plane of anesthesia, any advantages of this agent may be outweighed by the cost per volume of inhalant needed (Sellers et al., 2013). More rapid recovery of the animal anesthetized with sevoflurane may be advantageous in specific situations such as anesthesia of pre-weanling lambs (Vettorato et al., 2012; Clutton et al., 2014).

Isoflurane, sevoflurane, and desflurane provide little to no post-recovery analgesia, therefore pain management must be provided by other drugs and techniques. Premedication or intra-operative use of analgesic drugs with inhalant anesthetics has the added benefit of reducing the amount of inhalant necessary to provide a surgical plane of anesthesia. Tiletamine-zolazepam administered as a premedicant or induction agent reduced the concentration of isoflurane needed to maintain anesthesia in goats (Doherty et al., 2002b). Similarly, acepromazine, but not butorphanol when administered as premedicants reduced isoflurane MAC 36–45% in anesthetized goats (Doherty et al., 2002a). CRIs of lidocaine alone or in combination with ketamine during anesthesia reduced the concentration of isoflurane necessary to maintain anesthesia in goats and calves (Doherty et al., 2007; Vesal et al., 2011).

b. Total and Partial Intravenous Anesthesia

TIVA refers to maintenance of an anesthetic plane by a combination of injectable anesthetic, sedative, and tranquilizer drugs most often administered by intermittent boluses or CRI. These injectable techniques are often used in the field where vaporizers and ventilators are not available or practical. Specific drug and dose recommendations for field anesthesia are provided in the published works of Abrahamsen (2008, 2009c). In the research setting, TIVA may be used for anesthetic maintenance where inhalant agents cannot be used, for example, heart–lung bypass procedures or MRI imaging studies. 'Triple drip,' i.e., adding xylazine (50mg) and ketamine (1–2g) to 1l of 5% guiafenesin and administering the drug combination at a rate of 1–2ml/kg/h has long been used for TIVA of ruminants (Lin et al., 1993; Greene, 2003). An advantage of this drug combination is the ability to partially reverse anesthesia with atipamezole (Yamashita et al., 1996).

Partial intravenous anesthesia (PIVA) is the administration of anesthetic, analgesic, and sedative drugs by CRI to supplement analgesia and reduce the inspired concentration of the inhalant, thereby lessening cardiorespiratory depression (Valverde and Doherty, 2008). CRI of low doses of ketamine (25–50µg/kg/min) with or without lidocaine (100µg/kg/min) reduced the MAC of isoflurane by approximately 30% in goats (Queiroz-Castro

et al., 2006; Doherty et al., 2007). In calves, infusion of lidocaine at 50µg/kg/min resulted in a 16.7% reduction in isoflurane MAC required for umbilical surgery (Vesal et al., 2011). Because small ruminants appear to clear lidocaine more rapidly than other species, Valverde and Doherty recommend higher infusion rates (150–200µg/kg/min) preceded by a loading dose of 2.5mg/kg administered over 5min (Valverde and Doherty, 2008).

7. Monitoring

As with any other species, monitoring of small ruminants is critical to ensure the appropriate level anesthesia and quickly detect and respond to any insult to the cardiovascular, respiratory, and other body systems. Due to the nature of anesthetic and surgical procedures typically encountered in biomedical research, the level of monitoring will often be more extensive than in the clinical setting. Most research facilities will have the equipment and capabilities to measure heart rate and rhythm, blood pressure, oxygenation, and end-tidal CO_2 levels. The American College of Veterinary Anesthesia and Analgesia (ACVAA) recommends routine assessment of circulation, oxygenation, ventilation, and body temperature on a routine basis every 5–10min during anesthesia (ACVAA, 2009). Guidelines for monitoring of small animal and equine patients can be adopted for monitoring of small ruminants.

Anesthetic depth is best assessed using several parameters, palpebral reflex, eye location, jaw tone, changes in ventilation, and response to surgical stimulation. Palpebral reflex decreases as anesthetic depth increases, being moderately brisk at lighter planes, obtunded at surgical planes and absent at deep planes of anesthesia (Riebold, 2007; Abrahamsen, 2009a). Position of the eye as an indicator of anesthetic depth can be misleading as the globe is centrally located on induction, moves ventrally as the plane of anesthesia deepens, moves from ventral toward a central location when a surgical plane is reached, and returns toward the ventral position at deep planes of anesthesia (Riebold, 2007; Abrahamsen, 2009a). Eye position is not a reliable indicator of anesthetic depth in sheep and goats (Riebold, 2007).

Cardiovascular function can be determined by monitoring electrocardiogram (ECG), pulse pressure and measurement of arterial pressure. Standard ECG limb leads (I, II, and III) are useful for measuring heart rate and detecting rhythm disturbances. Pulse pressure and quality can be determined by palpation of the common digital, auricular, radial and saphenous arteries, and the facial artery in young calves (Riebold, 2007). Direct measurement of blood pressure is most accurate. Non-invasive blood pressure monitoring is unreliable in small ruminants (Aarnes et al., 2013; Trim et al., 2013). For direct blood pressure monitoring, the auricular, saphenous, and common digital arteries can be catheterized

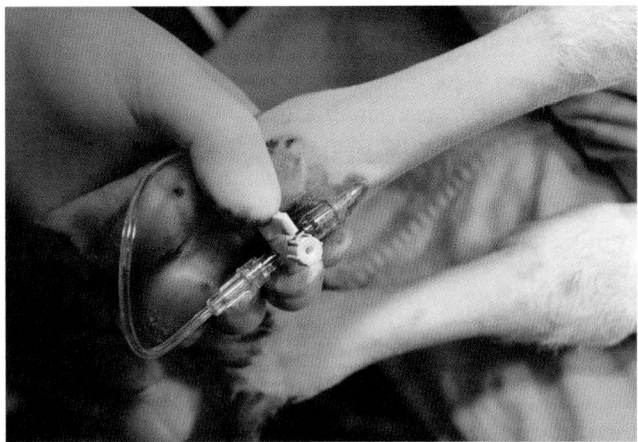

FIGURE 24.3 Catheterization of the common digital artery in the foreleg of an adult sheep for invasive blood pressure monitoring.

in most ruminant patients (Riebold, 2007). The median auricular branch of the rostral auricular artery located on the external surface of the ear can be easily cannulated with a 22- or 20-gauge over-the-needle Teflon catheter (Valverde and Doherty, 2008; Abrahamsen, 2009a). In animals for which the auricular artery cannot be catheterized, the common digital artery in the foreleg is an alternative site for direct blood pressure measurement (Fig. 24.3). The artery runs between the dewclaws, crossing over the palmer surface of the medial branch of the superficial flexor tendon, coursing rostrally to the medial side of the forelimb (Habel, 1978). An elongated pulsating bulge can be easily seen just proximal to the dewclaws and cannulated with a 20- or 18-gauge over-the-needle Teflon catheter. Central venous pressure is easily measured from a jugular catheter and the normal range is 5–10 cm H_2O (3–7 mmHg) (Riebold, 2007).

Inhalant anesthetics cause dose-dependent respiratory depression. In contrast to other species, respiratory rate is higher (20–40 breaths per min) and tidal volume lower in spontaneously breathing anesthetized ruminants (Riebold, 2007). Respiratory rate and/or tidal volume will decrease with deeper planes of anesthesia (Abrahamsen, 2009a). Hypoventilation is further exacerbated by pressure from the abdominal viscera reducing diaphragmatic excursions in the recumbent ruminant (Valverde and Doherty, 2008). It is preferable to support ventilation with intermittent positive pressure ventilation (IPPV) in anesthetized ruminants. For small ruminants, a tidal volume of 10–15 ml/kg at a rate of 8–12 breaths/min with a peak pressure not to exceed 30 cm H_2O is used (Valverde and Doherty, 2008).

Pulse oximetry provides a continuous estimation of oxygen saturation and should be >90%. Capnography in spontaneously breathing animals may not accurately reflect alveolar gas concentrations but is more accurate

during controlled ventilation (Riebold, 2007). End-tidal CO_2 in the mechanically ventilated animal should be in the range of 30–40 mmHg (4–5.3 kPa) (Valverde and Doherty, 2008). Furthermore, gas analyzers, especially those which measure the low infrared spectrum may erroneously report elevated inhalant agent concentrations due to detection of low levels of methane within the same spectrum (Moens and Gootjes, 1993; Dujardin et al., 2005; Turner et al., 2008). Arterial blood gas analysis provides the most accurate measure of the partial pressures of oxygen and carbon dioxide in the animal, and values in small ruminants are similar to other species (Riebold, 2007; Valverde and Doherty, 2008).

C. Postoperative Recovery and Pain Management

In addition to assessing respiration, heart or pulse rate, and temperature, ruminants must be monitored closely in the immediate postoperative period for regurgitation and bloating. If intubated, small ruminants should not be extubated until they exhibit full return of swallowing and upper airway reflexes. It is best to maintain the animal in sternal recumbency until it is able to stand. Bolsters or even hay bales can be placed alongside the animal to maintain the sternal position. If bloating occurs a stomach tube can be passed or in an emergency, a trocar placed percutaneously in the left dorsolateral fossa into the gas cap.

1. Assessment of Pain and Distress

Many small ruminants are docile and often stoic and may only exhibit subtle signs of pain. Pain is most often assessed in these species by observation and interpretation of changes from normal behavior. (Stasiak et al., 2003; Radositits et al., 2007; Anderson and Edmondson, 2013; Plummer and Schleining, 2013). Classic behavioral indicators of pain in large animals include rolling, pawing, crouching, moaning, grunting, or grinding of teeth (bruxism or odontoprisis) (Radositits et al., 2007). Bellowing by cattle or bleating in sheep and goats may also suggest pain and distress in these species (Radositits et al., 2007). However, more subtle signs such as subdued behavior, more time lying down, decreased appetite, and altered rumination may be the only signs of pain exhibited by small ruminants (Anderson and Edmondson, 2013; Plummer and Schleining, 2013). Physiologic responses to pain include increased heart rate, rapid shallow respirations and in extreme cases, dilated pupils (Swindle et al., 2002; Radositits et al., 2007). Assessment of small ruminants for pain following surgery should be frequent with comparison of behaviors observed in the postoperative period with normal behavior of the animal. Scoring systems have been developed for ruminants (Stasiak et al., 2003).

2. Opioids

Opioids can be administered preoperatively to provide pre-emptive analgesia, or administered intraoperatively or postoperatively to small ruminants. Opioids with μ receptor agonist activity, such as morphine can be used in ruminants, but with caution due to adverse effects on the GI system and behavioral side effects due to CNS stimulation. For these reasons, lower doses (0.1 mg/kg IV or IM) of morphine are recommended in ruminants (Abrahamsen, 2009b). Although GI side effects are minimized, rumen motility and contraction, and fecal output should be closely monitored and morphine discontinued if either parameter is decreased or absent.

Fentanyl, a potent μ-receptor agonist can be used in ruminants by either the IV or transdermal route of administration. The duration of activity when fentanyl is given IV is extremely short (about 20 min) and the half-life in sheep is 3 h and 1.2 h in goats (Carroll et al., 1999; Ahern et al., 2010). For these reasons, IV administered fentanyl is most appropriately used intra-operatively or in combination with other drugs as a CRI for management of postoperative pain. In the authors' experience, fentanyl has had little effect on gastrointestinal function and rumen motility.

For postoperative pain relief, fentanyl can be administered transdermally using a fentanyl patch, but their use has only been reported in sheep and goats (Dowd et al., 1998; Carroll et al., 1999; Ahern et al., 2009). Application of transdermal fentanyl patches (50 μg/h) to the skin of sheep prior to general anesthesia resulted in sustained plasma levels of fentanyl for 40 h (Ahern et al., 2010). In contrast, variable, potentially ineffective plasma concentrations of fentanyl were found in goats after application of transdermal fentanyl patches (Carroll et al., 1999). In sheep undergoing orthopedic surgery, postoperative pain management with transdermal fentanyl was judged to be superior to either oral phenylbutazone or IM buprenorphine (Dowd et al., 1998; Ahern et al., 2009).

Butorphanol, a synthetic κ- and σ-receptor agonist, μ receptor antagonist is three- to five-times more potent than morphine and has fewer GI and respiratory system side effects (Abrahamsen, 2009b, Plummer and Schleining, 2013). Butorphanol (0.05–0.1 mg/kg IV, IM, or SC) will relieve mild-moderate pain in small ruminants but duration is limited to 4–6 h (Abrahamsen, 2009b). Intravenous administration of butorphanol has been reported to cause negative behavioral side effects in goats and sheep (Waterman et al., 1991a; Doherty et al., 2002a). Intramuscular or SC administration results in lower peak serum concentrations than IV administration and less negative side effects (Plummer and Schleining, 2013). Administration of an NSAID with butorphanol provides greater analgesia than either drug alone and is efficacious in treating moderate levels of pain

in small ruminants (Abrahamsen, 2009b; Plummer and Schleining, 2013).

Buprenorphine (0.005–0.01 mg/kg) is effective in calves and sheep, although its duration of action appears to be shorter in ruminants compared to other species and may need to be dosed as frequently as every 4–6 h (Swindle et al., 2002; Ahern et al., 2009). Antinociception to thermal but not mechanical stimuli was observed for up to 3 h following a single IV dose (6 μg/kg) of buprenorphine in sheep (Nolan et al., 1987; Waterman et al., 1991b). In one study, in sheep undergoing orthopedic surgery, buprenorphine provided equally effective analgesia compared to piritramide, a μ receptor agonist, however in another report, transdermal fentanyl provided more effective analgesia than intermittent IM buprenorphine (Otto et al., 2000; Ahern et al., 2009). Buprenorphine may not be suitable for use as an analgesic in goats. Goats became agitated and ceased rumination after receiving IV or IM buprenorphine (Ingvast-Larsson et al., 2007).

3. Non-Steroidal Anti-Inflammatory Drugs

Flunixin meglumine (1.1–2.2 mg/kg) although labeled as an antipyrexic agent in cattle is often used effectively for control of postoperative pain. To minimize potential adverse effects such as renal toxicity and gastric hemorrhage, it should be given as needed every 12–24 h not to exceed 4 doses (Swindle et al., 2002). Other NSAIDs including phenylbutazone (2–6 mg/kg PO, IV), ketoprofen (2–3 mg/kg PO, IV), and aspirin (100 mg/kg PO) have been used for alleviation of pain following surgery in small ruminants, but none are approved for use in these species (Valverde and Doherty, 2008; Anderson and Edmondson, 2013; Plummer and Schleining, 2013). Both meloxicam and carprofen have been reported to provide effective analgesia in sheep and calves following husbandry procedures such as castration and dehorning (Heinrich et al., 2007; Paull et al., 2007; Stilwell et al., 2012; Glynn et al., 2013). In sheep, meloxicam is dosed at 0.5 mg/kg IV or 1.0 mg/kg PO, while in goats the recommended dose is 0.5 mg/kg IV, IM, or PO (Plummer and Schleining, 2013). Carprofen (4 mg/kg IM) was used effectively in combination with other analgesics for pain management in sheep following thoracotomy and aortic valve implantation (Schauvliege et al., 2006).

4. Local Anesthetics

The use of lidocaine and other local anesthetics for regional anesthesia and for blockade of specific nerves are well described and illustrated elsewhere (Skarda and Tranquilli, 2007). Used in conjunction with other analgesic drugs such as opioids and NSAIDs, local or regional anesthesia provides an effective regimen of multimodal analgesia (Schauvliege et al., 2006; Carney et al., 2009). Following thoracotomy in sheep and calves, the authors have used a diffusion catheter (Mila International) to deliver bupivacaine (0.25%, 5–12 ml q 8 h) at the thoracotomy incision (Carney *et al.*, 2009; Weiss *et al.*, 2012). Although CRI may be used with this method of drug delivery, intermittent boluses of local anesthetics delivered through a diffusion catheter appear to provide more effective local anesthesia (Hansen *et al.*, 2013).

D. Euthanasia

Most of the injectable euthanasia methods used in other species, with proper dosing are effective in small ruminants. An overdose (>150 mg/kg IV) of sodium pentobarbital or sodium pentobarbital-based euthanasia solutions is the preferred form of euthanasia in these species. To assist with IV administration of the euthanasia drug, reduce anxiety of the animal, and provide for the safety of personnel, sedation of the animal prior to euthanasia is highly recommended. It is acceptable to administer an overdose of potassium chloride or magnesium sulfate or perform exsanguination while small ruminants are under general anesthesia (AVMA, 2013).

VII. NONHUMAN PRIMATES

A. Introduction

Nonhuman primates are important models for a wide variety of biomedical and behavior research because of their phylogenetic proximity to humans. The range of species used include New World primates such as marmosets, tamarins, capuchins and squirrel monkeys; Old World primates such as macaques and baboons; and hominoids such as chimpanzees. The wide range of body sizes and weight of these different species needs to be considered when selecting anesthetic regimens, as does species variation in response to different agents. Extrapolation of anesthetic and analgesic doses from one primate species to another should be done with caution. The aim of this section is to provide a general guide to anesthesia and analgesia of nonhuman primates, indicate how this should be integrated into an overall plan of perioperative care, and highlight some of the specific issues arising when working with these species. Drug dosages are listed in Table 24.15.

B. Preoperative Assessment and Preparation

1. Preparations for Anesthesia

Larger primates pose a specific risk of physical injury when handling, and anesthetic regimens frequently incorporate initial immobilization with a sedative/tranquillizer. In addition, the ability to handle the animal safely during both anesthetic induction and the recovery period need be considered carefully. In addition to the

risk of physical injury, some primate species may be infected with potentially dangerous zoonotic infections. For example, macaques in many facilities may carry *Macacine herpesvirus* 1 (B virus), and personnel working with these animals need be provided with appropriate personal protective equipment (PPE), including gloves and face-shields. Anesthesia can pose an increased risk because of use of needles, production of aerosols of secretions (e.g., during endotracheal intubation), and the risk of bites and scratches during induction and recovery.

a. Preoperative Evaluation

Preoperative assessment is an important starting point that helps formulate the anesthetic plan. It usually includes history of previous use, physical examination, and pertinent laboratory data. Despite limitations associated with performing a thorough physical examination in nonhuman primates, signs of illness such as unusual posture, anorexia, and abnormal feces or urinary output can be readily identified. Laboratory animal handlers who have regular contact with individual animals can provide even more insight into an animal's unique characteristics that warrant more detailed evaluation. Routine laboratory tests should be performed while nonhuman primates are in quarantine and later as part of a preventive medicine program. It is usually not necessary nor is it practical to perform preoperative clinical laboratory testing in healthy animals. However, the nature of the surgical procedure should be taken into consideration. A baseline hematocrit may be desirable for animals undergoing surgical procedures that may produce vascular volume deficiencies.

Preoperative fasting is an accepted practice for nonhuman primates undergoing surgical procedures. Although it is conventional practice to fast primates for at least 12 h, members of the Callitrichidae (marmosets and tamarins) and other small species should be fasted only for 4–6 h, to avoid perioperative hypoglycemia. In situations requiring emergency surgery or in pregnant animals with delayed gastric emptying, inclusion of histamine 2 antagonists (cimetidine 10 mg/kg, ranitidine 1.5 mg/kg) may reduce the risk of aspiration pneumonia (Popilskis *et al.*, 1992). Metoclopromide (0.2 mg/kg SC or IM) can reduce the risk of vomiting and increase gastric emptying. It is always advisable to have suction available to clear the pharynx and airway during anesthetic induction and recovery, even in animals that have been fasted, since they may have ingested material from their cage environment.

2. Methods of Anesthetic Delivery

Intramuscular injection in nonhuman primates is commonly done into the caudal muscle of the thigh. For repeated IM injections, it is advisable to alternate the leg used to reduce the possibility of muscle or nerve

TABLE 24.15   Drug Doses[a] in Nonhuman Primates

OLD WORLD NONHUMAN PRIMATES (MACACA AND PAPIO SPECIES)

Drug	Dosage	Route
Dissociative agents and combinations		
Ketamine	5–20 mg/kg	IM
Ketamine+	7–10 mg/kg	IM
xylazine	0.15–0.5 mg/kg	IM
Ketamine+	5–10 mg/kg	IM
diazepam	0.3–1 mg/kg	IM
Ketamine+	5 mg/kg	IM
medetomidine	0.05 mg/kg	IM
Ketamine+	5–10 mg/kg	IM
Dexmedetomidine	0.01–0.03 mg/kg	IM
Tiletamine-zolazepam (Telazol)	2–6 mg/kg	IM
α_2-antagonist antipamezole	0.3–0.75 mg/kg	
Barbiturates		
Thiopentol	5–7 mg/kg	IV (induction)
	15–17 mg/kg/h	IV infusion (maintenance)
Pentobarbital	25–30 mg/kg	IV
Other injectable anesthetics		
Alphaxolone-alphadolone (Saffan)	18 mg/kg	IM (induction)
Alphaxalone	1–3 mg/kg	IV (after sedation with ketamine)
Propofol	2–6 mg/kg	IV (after sedation with ketamine)
	0.04–0.12 mg/kg/min	IV for maintenance
Etomidate	0.5 mg/kg	IV
	0.2 mg/kg boluses every 6–12 min	IV (repeated boluses)
Anticholinergics		
Atropine	0.02–0.05 mg/kg	IM
Glycopyrrolate	0.005–0.01 mg/kg	IM
MUSCLE RELAXANTS		
Pancuronium	0.04–0.1 mg/kg	IV
Vecuronium	0.04–0.06 mg/kg	IV
Inhalational anesthesia		
Halothane	1 MAC = 0.89–1.15%	

TABLE 24.15   (Continued)

Drug	Dosage	Route
Isoflurane	1 MAC = 1.28%	
Sevoflurane	1 MAC = 2%	
Analgesics		
Alfentanil	0.01–0.06 mg/kg/h	IV in combination with a volatile anesthetic or infusion of propofol
Fentanyl	5–10 µg/kg	IV in combination with a volatile anesthetic or infusion of propofol
Fentanyl	10–25 µg/kg/h	(as above)
Morphine	0.1–2 mg/kg	IM, SC
Morphine	0.1 mg/kg	Epidurally
Oxymorphone	0.15 mg/kg	IM
Buprenorphine	0.005–0.03 mg/kg	IM, SC
Opioid antagonist: naloxone	0.1–0.2 mg	IV as needed
Local anesthetic:		
Bupivacaine	1–2 mg/kg	Tissue infiltration or local nerve block
Lidocaine	4 mg/kg	As above
NSAIDs		
Carprofen	2–4 mg/kg	SC, IM
Meloxicam	0.1–0.2 mg/kg	SC, PO
Miscellaneous		
Antiarrhythmic: lidocaine	1–2 mg/kg IV 20–50 µg/kg/h	Continuous IV infusion
Vasoactive drugs and inotropes		
Dopamine	1–10 µg/kg/min	Continuous IV infusion
Norepinephrine	0.05–0.2 µg/kg/min	Continuous IV infusion
Dobutamine	2–10 µg/kg/min	Continuous IV infusion
Phenylephrine	1–2 µg/kg	IV bolus
	0.5–1.0 µg/kg/min	Continuous IV infusion

NEW WORLD NONHUMAN PRIMATES (SAIMIRI AND CALLITHRIX SPECIES)

Drug	Dosage	Route
Dissociative agents and combinations		
Ketamine	15–25 mg/kg	IM
Ketamine+	10–25 mg/kg	IM
xylazine	0.5–1 mg/kg	IM
Ketamine+	15–20 mg/kg	IM
diazepam	1 mg/kg	IM

(Continued)   *(Continued)*

TABLE 24.15   (Continued)

Drug	Dosage	Route
Tiletamine-zolazepam (Telazol)	2–5 mg/kg	IM
Other injectable anesthetics		
Alphaxolone-alphadolone (Saffan)	10 mg/kg	IM
Alphaxalone	2–5 mg/kg	IV
	0.16–0.18 mg/kg/min	IV infusion for maintenance
Propofol	2–8 mg/kg	IV
	0.3–0.6 mg/kg/min	IV infusion for maintenance
Medetomidine	100 μg/kg	IM, SC
Atipamezole	200 μg	IV
Fentanyl-fluanisone (Hypnorm)	0.3 ml/kg	IM, SC
Anticholinergics		
Atropine	0.04 mg/kg	IM
Analgesics		
Opioids		
Morphine	0.1–2 mg/kg	IM, SC
Oxymorphone	0.075 mg/kg	IM
Buprenorphine	0.005–0.03 mg/kg	IM, SC
Butorphanol	0.02 mg/kg	SQ
Opioid antagonist: naloxone	0.01–0.02 mg/kg	IV as needed

*a*See text for references.

irritation by drugs with low pH, such as ketamine. In nonhuman primates, SC injections into lateral thigh or dorsolateral sites in the back can be done with the help of 'squeeze-back' cages. The uptake of drugs from SC injection, and to lesser degree IM injection, can be variable and influenced by the rate of hydration and local perfusion. Chemical restraint is usually needed in primates for IV injections or blood withdrawal although animals can also be trained, using positive reinforcement methods, to accept these procedures. The cephalic and saphenous veins can be used both for venipuncture and administration of drugs, although in marmosets the tail vein may be more accessible. The femoral vein and artery are commonly used for the withdrawal of relatively large blood volumes. The femoral artery also offers a site for insertion of an indwelling catheter (20- to 22-gauge) to monitor direct blood pressure and in larger primates percutaneous catheter placement using a Seldinger technique is practicable. Whenever the femoral artery is used, manual pressure must be applied after blood sampling, for 1–2 min or longer, after removal of a percutaneous catheter, to prevent hematoma formation, especially if anticoagulants have been administered as part of the study protocol.

3. Preoperative Medication

Anticholinergic drugs are used to diminish salivary and bronchial secretions and prevent vagally induced bradycardia. These agents have a number of other effects, including predisposing animals to tachyarrythmias. For this reason they are now rarely used routinely in anesthesia, unless there is a particular risk of bradycardia, for example, when high doses of opioids are used as part of the anesthetic regimen. If required, atropine (0.02–0.05 mg/kg) or glycopyrrolate (0.01 mg/kg) can be administered.

C. Intraoperative Anesthesia

1. Injectable Anesthetics

a. Dissociatives

Ketamine has a wide margin of safety in many species of nonhuman primates, and it is widely used as an agent for chemical restraint and induction for subsequent administration of other injectable or gaseous anesthetics, particularly in Old World primates. At the dose of 5–20 mg/kg IM, onset of action is rapid and chemical restraint is provided for 15–30 min that is sufficient for minor procedures. Complete recovery occurs within 1 h, depending on the dosage used. The bite reflex is lost even at lower doses of ketamine, but laryngeal and pharyngeal reflexes are retained, even at high dose rates. This can be advantageous in providing protective reflexes should vomiting or regurgitation occur, but requires other agents to be administered to allow endotracheal intubation. Ketamine is usually administered by intramuscular injection, but lower doses can be administered intravenously to prolong the period of immobilization. The agent can also be administered orally if intramuscular injection is not possible. Oral ketamine is most rapidly absorbed if applied to the mucus membranes, and higher doses are needed to produce sedation. When injected into food items to sedate escaped animals, the effects are very unpredictable, and it is usually preferable to employ another technique, such as a blow-pipe or dart pistol to deliver the drug. Ketamine administration in marmosets can be associated with muscle damage because of the low pH (3–4), relatively small muscle mass, and the relatively high volume of drug needed in this species.

The influence of ketamine on hematologic, biochemical, and hormonal values should be considered in interpreting experimental data. Ketamine consistently reduces total leukocyte and absolute numbers of lymphocyte and monocytes (Bennett *et al.*, 1992; Fernie *et al.*, 1994). The red blood cell count, hemoglobin, and hematocrit are also significantly lower when ketamine is administered. When comparing the effects of ketamine on gender, higher values for lactate dehydrogenase (LDH) and creatine kinase (CK) are noted for males. In contrast, females tend to have higher values for amylase and cholesterol (Fernie *et al.*, 1994). Ketamine does not appear to alter the magnitude of endocrine responses even after multiple injections, thereby making it a suitable anesthetic for studies on hormonal change (Castro *et al.*, 1981; Malaivijitnond *et al.*, 1998).

Combining the α_2-agonists xylazine, medetomidine or dexmedetomidine, with ketamine provides muscular relaxation and analgesia sufficient for minor surgical procedures. These combinations may cause bradycardia and occasional heart-block, but as in other species, it is not advisable to attempt to correct this with atropine (Lewis, 1993; Vie *et al.*, 1998). Recovery times can be reduced by administration of atipamezole (300–750 μg/kg) which is a more specific α_2-antagonist than yohimbine, and has fewer side-effects.

A combination of ketamine (5–10 mg/kg) and diazepam (0.2–0.4 mg/kg) can be used to induce sedation and avoid perioperative excitement in Old World primates. In *Saimiri sciureus* and *Callithrix jacchus* the dose of diazepam required is higher (1 mg/kg IM). Although the duration of sedation is short, this combination is effective for minor procedures requiring muscle relaxation (Woolfson *et al*, 1980). Midazolam may cause less pain on injection than diazepam, and absorption may be more reliable. The shorter elimination half-life of midazolam makes it suitable for use as an infusion (0.05–0.15 mg/kg) in combination with ketamine (15 mg/kg IM) for various imaging techniques in *Macaca mulatta* and *Chlorocebus aethiops* (Jacobs *et al.*, 1993).

b. Tiletamine-Zolazepam (Telazol)

Telazol at 4–6 mg/kg IM has been reported to be useful as an anesthetic for minor procedures for about 45–60 min in various species of macaques (Cohen and Bree, 1978). New World primates require a higher dose of Telazol to produce immobilization; in *Saimiri sciureus* the dose is 10 mg/kg, and in *Alouatta seniculus* a dose of 22–30 mg/kg IM produces light to moderate anesthesia sufficient for restraint in wildlife conditions (Agoramoorthy and Rudran, 1994).

c. Miscellaneous Anesthetics

Although not available in the United States, alphaxolone-alphadolone (Saffan) has been reported to produce effective anesthesia in New World primates. A single IM injection of Saffan at 11.5–15.5 mg/kg provides up to 1 h of surgical anesthesia with good muscle relaxation in *Saimiri sciureus*. Rapid induction and uneventful recovery accompany Saffan anesthesia. However, respiratory depression and hypothermia are also noted (Logdberg, 1988). In macaques, effective surgical anesthesia can be produced with an IM injection of Saffan at 18 mg/kg, followed by 6–12 mg/kg IV as needed (Box and Ellis, 1973). This agent is no longer available commercially, however a new formulation consisting of alphaxalone (Alfaxan, Jurox) is marketed in Europe, Australia, and the USA. The single agent has similar effects to the combined steroid product.

d. Propofol

Propofol provides a smooth induction with adequate muscle relaxation sufficient for procedures of short duration. Because rapid clearance of propofol contributes to relatively fast awakening, repeated IV boluses of 2–5 mg/kg, or a continuous infusion IV can be administered to extend the duration of anesthesia without greatly delaying recovery. At 2.5 mg/kg IV, propofol provides good muscle relaxation sufficient for laparoscopy, with minimal effects on cardiovascular and respiratory functions in *Macaca fascicularis* (Sainsbury *et al.*, 1991) and has also been used successfully in marmosets and chimpanzees (Ludlage and Mansfield 2003; Sleeman, 2007). It can cause transient apnea if given rapidly, but this can be avoided by administering the initial dose slowly, over about 60 s. Supplemental oxygen via endotracheal tube or face mask is advisable, as with any injectable anesthetic regimen. The other potential problem associated with the infusion of propofol is a moderate hypotension. The hypotension is dose-dependent and can be partially corrected by adjusting the propofol infusion and by providing intravenous fluids and is rarely a significant problem in healthy animals.

e. Etomidate

Etomidate is an intravenous short-acting hypnotic agent that has been used in neuroanesthesia to monitor motor-evoked potentials after transcranial stimulation (Ghaly *et al.*, 1990). Because it is very short-acting, an initial dose of 0.5 mg/kg IV, followed by repeated boluses of etomidate 0.2 mg/kg every 6–12 min, is needed to maintain anesthesia in *Macaca fascicularis*.

f. Barbiturates

Thiopental provides short periods of anesthesia (5–10 min) and was widely used for anesthetic induction prior to intubation and maintenance of anesthesia with inhalational agents. One-half of the calculated dosage of 5–10 mg/kg IV is given as a bolus, followed by additional drug to effect. The dosage is reduced if the animal has received ketamine. Slow infusion of thiopental at 15–17 mg/kg/h provides satisfactory chemical restraint with stable physiological values for 90 min in

Papio ursinus. Animals were reported to recover uneventfully within 20 min after discontinuation of the infusion (Goosen *et al.*, 1984), however like most barbiturates, thiopental has greater cumulative effects than agents such as propofol and alphaxalone.

Despite its long history of use in research animal anesthesia, pentobarbital is now less frequently used as an anesthetic for survival procedures and commercially available anesthetic formulations of this agent are currently unavailable in the United States. Pronounced respiratory depression at the dosages required to produce adequate anesthesia, inability to modulate the depth of anesthesia, and a long period of recovery are additional shortcomings. Pentobarbital is better replaced by other agents, except for terminal (non-recovery) procedures such as perfusion–fixation, when the depressant effects of this drug are considered unimportant. The dose of pentobarbital in nonhuman primates is 25–30 mg/kg IV; however, in animals that have been chemically restrained with ketamine, the dose is reduced by about one-third to one-half.

g. Opioids

Opioids have been used in nonhuman primates to reduce the requirement for inhalational or injectable anesthetics and to enhance intraoperative analgesia during balanced anesthesia. Fentanyl, alfentanil, sufentanil, and remifentanil can all be used as anesthetic adjuncts, with infusion rates varying depending upon the dose rates of other agents that are administered (Table 24.1). Care must be taken to monitor and support respiratory function, as respiratory depression is common in nonhuman primates even after relatively small doses of opioids. Opioid administration can also cause a marked bradycardia, and if this results in a fall in blood pressure, then it should be corrected by administration of atropine.

2. Inhalational Anesthesia

a. Nitrous Oxide

Unlike the potent volatile anesthetics, nitrous oxide has high MAC (= 200%), preventing its use as a complete surgical anesthetic. Nitrous oxide has been used in combination with inhalational anesthetics such as isoflurane or sevoflurane because it allows for a lower concentration of these agents. This in turn results in a less pronounced circulatory depression, which may accompany the sole administration of isoflurane or sevoflurane. Administration of nitrous oxide should be terminated and 100% oxygen should be administered 10 min prior to extubation. This will preclude the development of diffusion hypoxia.

b. Isoflurane

Isoflurane has a MAC of 1.28% in *Macaca fascicularis* (Tinker *et al.*, 1977). It produces a dose-dependent decrease in blood pressure because it reduces systemic vascular resistance. Hypotension is especially pronounced during mask induction or when animals are maintained at or above 2%. Inclusion of fentanyl or another opioid allows the concentration of isoflurane to be reduced, which attenuates hypotension. Isoflurane produces direct dose-related cerebral vasodilatory effects. Although isoflurane-induced hypotension reduces cerebral blood flow, cerebral oxygenation is maintained (Enlund *et al.*, 1997). Isoflurane anesthesia does not influence the binding of dopamine receptor ligands, making it suitable for various positron emission tomography studies (Nader *et al.*, 1999). Isoflurane's effect on calcium metabolism in cynomolgus monkeys has been studied. Unexpectedly, isoflurane lowered ionized calcium, with secondary increases in parathyroid hormone and osteocalcin concentrations (Hotchkiss *et al.*, 1998). A cautious approach may be needed with respect to the use of isoflurane for studies of osteoporosis and the effects of various antiosteoporotic agents.

c. Sevoflurane

Sevoflurane has a lower blood/gas partition coefficient than isoflurane, making it useful for rapid induction and fast recovery from anesthesia. Because of its pleasant smell and lack of respiratory irritant properties, mask induction is a feasible alternative to other inhalant agents. However, it is degraded by carbon dioxide absorbents into an haloalkane known commonly as 'compound A.' Compound A at high doses has been shown to be nephrotoxic in nonhuman primates, causing proximal tubular necrosis (Kharasch, 1998). In common with other inhalational anesthetics, sevoflurane causes a dose-dependent cardiovascular depression. During sevoflurane anesthesia, cerebral blood flow is generally preserved; however, at 3% sevoflurane there was a clear inhibition of autoregulation of cerebral blood flow in rhesus monkeys (Yoshikawa *et al.*, 1997). Regardless, high concentrations of sevoflurane maintained oxygen consumption and delivery throughout the brain.

D. Intraoperative Monitoring and Support

Although primates can be maintained on a face mask, endotracheal intubation is advisable because of the high risk of vomiting or regurgitation, even for short procedures. Visualization of the larynx is relatively straightforward using an appropriately-sized curved or straight blade, and for small primates, rodent intubation equipment can be used (Thomas *et al.*, 2012b). It is advisable to spray the vocal cords with local anesthetic to prevent laryngospasm, and an introducer can be used to aid tube placement if this proves difficult.

As in other species, anesthetic monitoring is important even during brief periods of anesthesia. A range of electronic monitoring devices can be used successfully in larger primates. In marmosets, tamarins, and squirrel monkeys, the small body size of the animal may limit the use of some instruments, but specialist devices that function successfully in these smaller animals are now available. Maintenance of body temperature is particularly important and can be achieved using a range of different warming devices. In larger primates, forced air warming systems are particularly effective. Whichever method of maintaining temperature is employed, its efficacy should be monitored using electronic temperature probes.

Pulse oximetry is a quick and easy means of both detecting hypoxemia and monitoring heart rate, and should be routine in nonhuman primate anesthesia. Both main-stream and side-stream capnographs can be used in all species, although the accuracy of these instruments in detecting end-tidal carbon dioxide is reduced in small animals (<1 kg) which have low tidal volumes. Blood pressure can be measured non-invasively in nonhuman primates, with a suitable sized cuff placed on the upper or lower limb, or on the tail in marmosets. During prolonged procedures, it is advisable to remove the cuff, massage the limb, and replace or reposition on the contralateral limb, to avoid partial constriction of limb circulation. Invasive blood pressure measurement is possible in all species, with percutaneous placement of catheters practicable in larger animals (>3–4 kg). In smaller animals, surgical exposure of the vessel may be needed.

Anesthetic depth can be assessed using standard somatic reflex responses, coupled with loss of muscle tone (most easily assessed by evaluating jaw tone). The palpebral reflex is lost as anesthesia deepens, but in many species the eye remains relatively central rather than rotating downwards. Anesthetic depth can also be assessed by evaluating the EEG, or by use of bispectral index (BIS) monitors. Both techniques require careful interpretation. EEG changes are greatly influenced by the particular anesthetic agent used, and commercially available BIS monitors use an algorithm derived from human data. However there are reports of successful use of this technology in nonhuman primates (Izrailtyan et al., 2004).

E. Special Anesthesia Considerations

1. Imaging

Non-invasive imaging introduces a number of complications to anesthetic regimens in all species, and problems may become greater when the imaging process is prolonged. Nonhuman primates can be trained to remain immobile for imaging procedures, but frequently anesthesia is necessary to reduce the stress of prolonged immobility. The main anesthetic complications associated with imaging are due to the restricted access for clinical monitoring and intervention, and the lack of direct view of the animal. Use of electronic monitoring devices can help resolve these problems, but specially designed devices are required for MRI. Some instruments, such as side-stream capnographs, can be placed a safe distance from the magnet. However, this requires use of extensions to sampling tubing which can lead to instrument malfunction due to a loss of signal quality.

If delivering intravenous fluids, or maintaining anesthesia using continuous intravenous infusions, long extensions to the infusion tubing can increase resistance and cause pump failure due to activation of an occlusion alarm. Maintaining body temperature can be a particularly challenging problem during imaging, and warm air blowers and magnet-compatible heating devices, coupled with use of insulating materials, will be needed to maintain normothermia.

2. Neuroscience Procedures

Nonhuman primates are used in a range of neuroscience and neurosurgical studies, and surgical procedures may require placement in a stereotaxic frame. Although it is always advisable to intubate animals, care must be taken when positioning the animal, as flexing the neck may result in occlusion of the endotracheal tube. For non-recovery procedures, a tracheostomy can be carried out which avoids this problem. Use of an armored endotracheal tube (providing the animal will not be imaged in an MRI) prevents any risk of kinking of the tube. Pain caused by pressure from the ear bars of the stereotaxic frame can be reduced by filling the ear canals with local anesthetic cream (e.g., EMLA, Astra), and NSAIDs should be administered to reduce tissue inflammation (see below).

3. Obstetric Anesthesia

Physiologic changes during pregnancy (such as increased cardiac output and decreased requirements for inhaled anesthetics) can directly influence anesthesia management for obstetric surgery. Maintenance of anesthesia for obstetric procedures is usually achieved with isoflurane or sevoflurane. Low inspired concentrations of either agent, supplemented with at least 50–60% of inspired nitrous oxide, minimize cardiovascular depression. It has been shown that maintaining pregnant macaques at around 1.5% halothane reduces maternal blood pressure and cardiac output with consequential reduction in uterine blood flow (Eng et al., 1975; Sanders et al., 1991). This decreases fetal perfusion, resulting in fetal acidosis and hypoxia. Placing pregnant animals in a supine position may contribute to the hypotension because of compression of the caudal vena cava and abdominal aorta by the gravid uterus. Therefore the animal should be tilted to the left by placing a wedge under the right hip. Adequate fluid therapy is also indicated to prevent hypovolemia and hypotension. Placement of an urinary catheter allows one to monitor the effectiveness of fluid therapy. Because hypotension is the most common complication encountered during anesthesia, monitoring blood pressure should be routine during experimental procedures in pregnant nonhuman primates. If maternal hypotension persists despite hydration and positioning, consideration should be given to vasopressor therapy. Ephedrine (2.5–5.0 mg) can be used to correct maternal hypotension. Because of its predominant β-adrenergic activity, ephedrine will maintain arterial perfusion by increasing maternal cardiac output and restoring uterine blood flow without uterine arterial vasoconstriction.

Maternal normocapnia should be maintained during the intraoperative period because the effects of hypoventilation may be associated with premature ventricular contraction in macaques (Sanders *et al.*, 1991). Accordingly, controlled ventilation is the most efficient way of maintaining normal PCO_2.

4. Pediatric Anesthesia

There are important physiologic differences between adults and neonates. Neonatal cardiac output is heart rate-dependent. Therefore, one of the main goals of preanesthesia and induction is avoidance of heart rate reduction. Administration of ketamine and atropine provides protection against possible reduction in heart rate during the initial stages of anesthesia in pediatric primates.

Although mask induction is an accepted technique in pediatric animals, it must be recognized that isoflurane is pungent and produces airway irritation, which could possibly result in laryngospasm during induction, so use of sevoflurane is preferable. Smooth induction can be easily achieved with the IV propofol at 2–4 mg/kg. Because neonatal primates are usually allowed to nurse until anesthesia time, assisted ventilation during mask induction may lead to insufflation of the stomach with gases and put neonates at risk of aspiration. Cuffed or uncuffed tracheal tubes may be used in intubation of pediatric primates. Postintubation laryngeal edema is unlikely if the size of the tube in the trachea is such that slightly audible air leaks occur around it. Some operating theater pollution is inherent in this approach. Small tidal volume in pediatric primates requires the use of nonrebreathing systems such as modified Jackson-Rees and Bain. The fresh gas flow of twice minute volume (estimated as 7–10 ml/kg × respiratory rate) is adequate to prevent rebreathing during spontanous ventilation. Because isoflurane and sevoflurane depress spontaneous ventilation, controlled or assisted ventilation will prevent CO_2 accumulation. Because vasoconstrictive responses of neonates to hemorrhage are less than those

of adults, even moderate blood loss can result in a precipitous decline in blood pressure. Blood loss should be immediately replaced with three- to four-times the volume of crystalloid solution.

F. Postoperative Recovery

Although extubation is performed after the nonhuman primate regains the swallowing reflex, it may lead to gagging or vomiting. If vomiting occurs, the animal should be placed in a prone position with its head lowered to avoid aspiration of the vomitus, and the oropharynx should be suctioned. Gentle suctioning of the trachea prior to recovery from anesthesia is important in smaller primates because respiratory passages can be easily obstructed with bronchial secretions. Monitoring of cardiopulmonary functions in the immediate postoperative period will depend on the extent and type of procedure. Monitoring of arterial pressure is often needed until the nonhuman primate regains sufficient consciousness after cardiac or neurosurgical procedures. Maintaining a femoral arterial catheter helps to determine the status of arterial blood gases and avoid hypoxemia in the immediate postoperative period.

Postoperative hypothermia is frequently encountered during and after surgical procedures, particularly in young and small nonhuman primates. Hypothermia and associated shivering can be treated effectively with warming devices such as a Bair Hugger. Administering warm fluids will help avoid pronounced hypothermia.

1. Analgesic Therapy

Postoperatively, nonhuman primates often show little reaction to surgical procedures, and it should be recognized that the signs of pain may not be evident until the animal is in severe pain. Therefore, treating postoperative pain in a nonhuman primate in an effective and timely matter can be difficult to achieve. Many IACUCs may require the administration of analgesics before the surgical stimulus, i.e., in a pre-emptive fashion. Analgesics available for use in other species can be used safely and effectively in nonhuman primates (Table 24.15). However since there are no reliable means of pain assessment in these species, determining which analgesics are effective in the individual animal can be challenging. At present, attempts should be made to develop clinical scoring systems using well-defined signs that all personnel involved in the animal's care can recognize. Repeated assessment, particularly after analgesic administration and analgesic withdrawal, can help focus on those signs which are most related to an individual's pain.

Based on the invasiveness of the procedure, surgeons should administer opioid analgesics such as buprenorphine, either alone, or preferably in combination with an NSAID such as carprofen or meloxicam. The pharmacokinetics of a slow release formulation of buprenorphine have been reported (Nunamaker *et al.*, 2013) in macaques, and this agent may be useful for providing long-lasting analgesia in some circumstances.

Infiltration of the surgical site with local anesthetic prior to recovery from anesthesia can be a useful adjunct to the use of systemic analgesics. As in other species, use of a 50:50 mix of lidocaine and bupivacaine combines rapid onset, short duration effects with slower onset, longer duration effects. It is important to calculate the safe maximum dose to avoid inadvertent overdose.

Epidural analgesia using morphine is also practicable and effective in nonhuman primates (Popilskis *et al.*, 1994).

After less invasive procedures, use of NSAIDs alone may be sufficient. Following an initial dose intra-operatively, additional doses can be given by mouth 12–24h post-surgery. The veterinary oral formulation of meloxicam is readily taken by many animals in yogurt or mashed fruit.

G. Euthanasia

The preferred method of euthanasia in nonhuman primates is an overdose of pentobarbital (>100mg/kg) administered IV. Animals are commonly restrained with a dose of ketamine at 5–10mg/kg IM, after which IV pentobarbital or KCl is administered.

References

Aarnes, T.K., Hubbell, J.A., Lerche, P., Bednarski, R.M., 2013. Comparison of invasive and oscillometric blood pressure measurement techniques in anesthetized sheep, goats, and cattle. Vet. Anaesth. Analg.

AASRP, 2010. American association of small ruminant practitioners fact sheet. Available: <http://aasrp.org/associations/11223/files/AASRP%20Revised%20Fact%20Sheet.pdf>. (accessed 15.08.13).

Abelson, K.S.P., Jacobsen, K.R., Sundbom, R., Kalliokoski, O., Hau, J., 2012. Voluntary ingestion of nut paste for administration of buprenorphine in rats and mice. Lab. Anim. 46, 349–351.

Abrahamsen, E., 2008. Ruminant field anesthesia. Vet. Clin. North Am. Food Anim. Pract. 24, 429–441.

Abrahamsen, E., 2009a. Inhalation anesthesia in ruminants. In: Anderson, D., Rings, D. (Eds.), Current Veterinary Therapy Food Animal Practice, fifth ed. Elsevier, St. Louis, MO.

Abrahamsen, E., 2009b. Managing severe pain in ruminants. In: Anderson, D.E., Rings, D.M. (Eds.), Current Veterinary Therapy Food Animal Practice, fifth ed. Elsevier, St. Louis, MO.

Abrahamsen, E., 2013. Chemical restraint and injectable anesthesia of ruminants. Vet. Clin. North Am. Food Anim. Pract. 29, 209–227.

Abrahamsen, E.J., 2009c. Ruminant field anesthesia. In: Anderson, D.E., Rings, D.M. (Eds.), Current Veterinary Therapy: Food Animal Practice Saunders Elsevier, St. Louis, MO.

Abreu, M., Aguado, D., Benito, J., Gómez De Segura, I.A., 2012. Reduction of the sevoflurane minimum alveolar concentration induced by methadone, tramadol, butorphanol and morphine in rats. Lab. Anim. 46, 200–206.

ACVAA, 2009. Recommendations for monitoring anesthetized veterinary patients [Online]. (accessed 13.09.13.).

Adamson, T.W., Kendall, L.V., Goss, S., Grayson, K., Touma, C., Palme, R., et al., 2010. Assessment of carprofen and buprenorphine on recovery of mice after surgical removal of the mammary fat pad. J. Am. Assoc. Lab. Anim. Sci. 49, 610–616.

Aeschbacher, G., Webb, A.I., 1993a. Propofol in rabbits. 1. Determination of an induction dose. Lab. Anim. Sci. 43, 324–327.

Aeschbacher, G., Webb, A.I., 1993b. Propofol in rabbits. 2. Long-term anesthesia. Lab. Anim. Sci. 43, 328–335.

Agoramoorthy, G., Rudran, R., 1994. Field application of Telazol (tiletamine + zolazepam) immobilaze wild howler monkeys (Alouatta seniculus) in Venezuela. J. Wildl. Dis. 30 (3), 417–420.

Aguiar, J., Mogridge, G., Hall, J., 2013. Femoral fracture repair and sciatic and femoral nerve blocks in a guinea pig. J. Small. Anim. Pract.

Ahern, B., Soma, L., Boston, R., Schaer, T., 2009. Comparison of the analgesic properties of transdermally administered fentanyl and intramuscularly administered buprenorphine during and following experimental orthopedic surgery in sheep. Am. J. Vet. Res. 70, 418–422.

Ahern, B., Soma, L., Rudy, J., Uboh, C., Schaer, T., 2010. Pharmacokinetics of fentanyl administered transdermally and intravenously in sheep. Am. J. Vet. Res. 71, 1127–1132.

Allweiler, S., Leach, M.C., Flecknell, P.A., 2010. The use of propofol and sevoflurane for surgical anesthesia in New Zealand White rabbits. Lab. Anim. 44, 113–117.

Alstrup, A.K.O., Smith, D.F., 2013. Anaesthesia for positron emission tomography scanning of animal brains. Lab. Anim. 47, 12–18.

Alves, G.E.S., Hartsfield, S.M., Carroll, G.L., Santos, D.A.M.L., Zhang, S., Tsolis, R.M., et al., 2003. Use of propofol, isoflurane and morphine for prolonged general anesthesia in calves. Arquivo Brasileiro de Medicina Veterinária e Zootecnia 55, 411–420.

Anderson, D.E., Edmondson, M.A., 2013. Prevention and management of surgical pain in cattle. Vet. Clin. North Am. Food Anim. Pract. 29, 157–184.

Antognini, J.F., Eisele, P.H., 1993. Anesthetic potency and cardiopulmonary effects of enflurane, halothane and isoflurane in goats. Lab. Anim. Sci. 43, 607–610.

Arras, M., Autenried, P., Rettich, A., Spaeni, D., Rülicke, T., 2001. Optimization of intraperitoneal injection anesthesia in mice: drugs, dosages, adverse effects, and anesthesia depth. Comp. Med. 51, 443–456.

Artwohl, J., Brown, P., Corning, B., Stein, S., Force, A.T., 2006. Report of the ACLAM Task Force on Rodent Euthanasia. J. Am. Assoc. Lab. Anim. Sci. 45, 98–105.

AVMA Guidelines on the Euthanasia of Animals: 2013 Ed., 2013. <https://www.avma.org/KB/Policies/Documents/euthanasia.pdf>.

AVMA, 2012a. Castration and dehorning of cattle [Online]. Available: <https://www.avma.org/KB/Policies/Pages/Castration-and-Dehorning-of-Cattle.aspx>. (accessed 07.06.13).

AVMA, 2012b. Welfare implications of castration in cattle [Online]. Available: <https://www.avma.org/KB/Resources/Backgrounders/Documents/castration-cattle-bgnd.pdf 2013>.

Avsaroglu, H., Sommer, R., Hellebrekers, L.J., Van Zutphen, L.F.M., Van Lith, H.A., 2008. The effects of buprenorphine on behaviour in the ACI and BN rat inbred strains. Lab. Anim. 42, 171–184.

Avsaroglu, H., Van Der Sar, A.S., Van Lith, H.A., Van Zutphen, L.F.M., Hellebrekers, L.J., 2007. Differences in response to anaesthetics and analgesics between inbred rat strains. Lab. Anim. 41, 337–344.

Bagis, H., Odaman Mercan, H., Dinnyes, A., 2004. Exposure to warmer postoperative temperatures reduces hypothermia caused by anaesthesia and significantly increases the implantation rate of transferred embryos in the mouse. Lab. Anim. 38, 50–54.

Barquet, I.S., Soriano, E.S., Green, W.R., O'Brien, T.P., 1999. Provision of anesthesia with single application of lidocaine 2% gel. J. Cataract. Refract. Surg. 25, 626–631.

Bar-Yosef, S., Melamed, R., Page, G.G., Shakhar, G., Shakhar, K., Ben-Eliyahu, S., 2001. Attenuation of the tumor-promoting effect of surgery by spinal blockade in rats. Anesthesiology 94, 1066–1073.

Bauer, D.J., Christenson, T.J., Clark, K.R., Powell, S.K., Swain, R.A., 2003. Acetaminophen as a postsurgical analgesic in rats: a practical solution to neophobia. Contemp. Top. Lab. Anim. Sci. 42, 20–25.

Baumgartner, C., Bollerhey, M., Ebner, J., et al., 2010. Effects of medetomidine-midazolam-fentanyl IV bolus injections and its reversal by specific antagonists on cardiovascular function in rabbits. Can. J. Vet. Res. 74, 286–298.

Baumgartner, C.M., Koenighaus, H., Ebner, J.K., et al., 2009. Cardiovascular effects of fentanyl and propofol on hemodynamic function in rabbits. Am. J. Vet. Res. 70, 409–417.

Bednarski, R., McGuirk, S., 1986. Bradycardia associated with fasting in cattle. Vet. Surg. 15 458–458.

Benato, L., Chesnel, M., Eatwell, K., Meredith, A., 2013. Arterial blood gas parameters in pet rabbits anaesthetized using a combination of fentanyl-fluanisone-midazolam-isoflurane. J. Small. Anim. Pract. 54, 343–346.

Bennett, J.S., Gossett, K.A., McCarthy, M.P., Simpson, E.D., 1992. Effects of ketamine hydrochloride on serum biochemical and hematologic variables in rhesus monkeys (Macaca mulatta). Vet. Clin. Pathol. 21, 15–18.

Benson, G.J., Thurmon, J.C., 1986. Regional analgesia of food animals. In: Howard, J.L. (Ed.), Current Veterinary Therapy 2: Food Animal Practice. Saunders, Philadelphia, PA, pp. 71–83.

Bienert, A., Plotek, W., Zawidzka, I., et al., 2011. Influence of time of day on propofol pharmacokinetics and pharmacodynamics in rabbits. Chronobiol. Int. 28, 318–329.

Blaha, M.D., Leon, L.R., 2008. Effects of indomethacin and buprenorphine analgesia on the postoperative recovery of mice. J. Am. Assoc. Lab. Anim. Sci. 47, 8–19.

Blake, D.W., Jover, B., McGrath, B.P., 1988. Haemodynamic and heart rate reflex responses to propofol. Br. J. Anaesth. 61, 194–199.

Blake, D.W., Way, D., Trigg, L., Langton, D., McGrath, B.P., 1991. Cardiovascular effects of volatile anesthesia in rabbits: influence of chronic heart failure and enapril treatment. Anesth. Analg. 73, 441–448.

Bomzon, A., 2006. Are repeated doses of buprenorphine detrimental to postoperative recovery after laparotomy in rats? Comp. Med. 56, 114–118.

Bonath, K., Nolte, I., Schniewind, A., Sandmann, H., Failing, K., 1982. Food deprivation as precaution and aftercare measure for anaesthesia–the influence of fasting on the acid base status and glucose concentration in blood of rabbits. Berl. Munch. Tierarztl. Wochenschr. 95, 126–130.

Borkowski, G.L., Allen, M.J., 1999. The Laboratory Small Ruminant. CRC Press, Boca Raton, FL.

Borkowski, G.L., Danneman, P.J., Russell, G.B., Lang, C.M., 1990. Evaluation of three intravenous anesthetic regimens in New Zealand rabbits. Lab. Anim. Sci. 40, 270–276.

Borrell, V., 2010. In vivo gene delivery to the post-natal ferret cerebral cortex by DNA electroporation. J. Neurosci. Methods 186, 186–195.

Bourque, S.L., Adams, M.A., Nakatsu, K., Winterborn, A., 2010. Comparison of buprenorphine and meloxicam for postsurgical analgesia in rats: effects on body weight, locomotor activity, and hemodynamic parameters. J. Am. Assoc. Lab. Anim. Sci. 49, 617–622.

Box, P.G., Ellis, K.R., 1973. Use of CT 1341 anaesthetic (Saffan) in monkeys. Lab. Anim. 7, 161–170.

Brammer, A., West, C.D., Allen, S.L., 1993. A comparison of propofol with other injectable anesthetics in a rat model for measuring cardiovascular parameters. Lab. Anim. 27, 250–257.

Bree, M.M., Cohen, B.J., 1965. Effects of urethane anesthesia on blood and blood vessels in rabbits. Lab. Anim. Care. 15, 254–259.

Brennan, M.P., Sinusas, A.J., Horvath, T.L., Collins, J.G., Harding, M.J., 2009. Correlation between body weight changes and postoperative pain in rats treated with meloxicam or buprenorphine. Lab. Anim. (NY). 38, 87–93.

Buchanan, K.C., Burge, R.R., Ruble, G.R., 1998. Evaluation of Injectable Anesthetics for Major Surgical Procedures in Guinea Pigs. Contemp. Top. Lab. Anim. Sci. 37, 58–63.

Buelke-Sam, J., Hoson, J.F., Bazare, J.J., Young, J.F., 1978. Comparative stability of physiological parameters during sustained anesthesia in rats. Lab. Anim. Sci. 28 (2), 157–162.

Buitrago, S., Martin, T.E., Tetens-Woodring, J., Belicha-Villanueva, A., Wilding, G.E., 2008. Safety and efficacy of various combinations of injectable anesthetics in BALB/c mice. J. Am. Assoc. Lab. Anim. Sci. 47, 11–17.

Burnside, W.M., Flecknell, P.A., Cameron, A.I., Thomas, A.A., 2013. A comparison of medetomidine and its active enantiomer dexmedetomidine when administered with ketamine in mice. BMC. Vet. Res. 9, 48.

Cannon, C.Z., Kissling, G.E., Hoenerhoff, M.J., King-Herbert, A.P., Blankenship-Paris, T., 2010. Evaluation of dosages and routes of administration of tramadol analgesia in rats using hot-plate and tail-flick tests. Lab. Anim. (NY). 39, 342–351.

Cantalapiedra, A.G., Villanueva, B., Pereira, J.L., 2000. Anaesthetic potency of isoflurane in cattle: determination of the minimum alveolar concentration. Vet. Anaesth. Analg. 27, 22–26.

Capdevila, S., Giral, M., Ruiz De La Torre, J.L., Russell, R.J., Kramer, K., 2007. Acclimatization of rats after ground transportation to a new animal facility. Lab. Anim. 41, 255–261.

Carbone, E.T., Lindstrom, K.E., Diep, S., Carbone, L., 2012a. Duration of action of sustained-release buprenorphine in 2 strains of mice. J. Am. Assoc. Lab. Anim. Sci. 51, 815–819.

Carbone, L., Carbone, E.T., Yi, E.M., Bauer, D.B., Lindstrom, K.A., Parker, J.M., et al., 2012b. Assessing cervical dislocation as a humane euthanasia method in mice. J. Am. Assoc. Lab. Anim. Sci. 51, 352–356.

Carney, E.L., Clark, J.B., Myers, J.L., Peterson, R., Wilson, R.P., Weiss, W.J., 2009. Animal model development for the penn state pediatric ventricular assist device. Artif. Organs. 33, 953–957.

Caro, A.C., Hankenson, F.C., Marx, J.O., 2013. Comparison of thermoregulatory devices used during anesthesia of C57BL/6 mice and correlations between body temperature and physiologic parameters. J. Am. Assoc. Lab. Anim. Sci. 52, 577–583.

Carroll, G., Hartsfield, S., 1996. General anesthetic techniques in ruminants. Vet. Clin. North Am. Food Anim. Pract. 12, 627–661.

Carroll, G., Hartsfield, S., Champney, T., Slater, M., Newman, J., 1998a. Stress-related hormonal and metabolic responses to restraint, with and without butorphanol administration, in pre-conditioned goats. Lab. Anim. Sci. 48, 387–390.

Carroll, G., Hooper, R., Slater, M., Hartsfield, S., Matthews, N., 1998b. Detomidine-butorphanol-propofol for carotid artery translocation and castration or ovariectomy in goats. Vet. Surg. 27, 75–82.

Carroll, G., Hooper, R., Boothe, D., Hartsfield, S., Randoll, L., 1999. Pharmacokinetics of fentanyl after intravenous and transdermal administration in goats. Am. J. Vet. Res. 60, 986–991.

Carroll, G., Hartsfield, S., Champney, T., Geller, S., Martinez, E., Haley, E., 2005. Effect of medetomidine and its antagonism with atipamezole on stress-related hormones, metabolites, physiologic responses, sedation, and mechanical threshold in goats. Vet. Anaesth. Analg. 32, 147–157.

Cartner, S.C., Barlow, S.C., Ness, T.J., 2007. Loss of cortical function in mice after decapitation, cervical dislocation, potassium chloride injection, and CO2 inhalation. Comp. Med. 57, 570–573.

Castel, D., Willentz, E., Doron, O., Brenner, O., Meilin, S., 2014. Characterization of a porcine model of post-operative pain. Eur. J. Pain 18, 496–505.

Castiglioni, J.A., Russell, M.I., Setlowa, B., Younga, K.A., Welsha, J.C., Steele-Russell, I., 2009. An animal model of hypnotic pain attenuation. Behav. Brain Res. 197, 198–204.

Castro, M.I., Rose, J., Green, W., Lehner, N., Peterson, D., Taub, D., 1981. Ketamine-HCL as a suitable anesthetic for endocrine, metabolic, and cardiovascular studies in Macaca fascicularis monkeys. Proc. Soc. Exp. Biol. Med. 168, 389–394.

Caulkett, N.A., Duke, T., Cribb, P.H., 1996. Cardiopulmonary effects of medetomidine-ketamine in domestic sheep (ovis ovis) maintained in sternal recumbency. J. Zoo Wildl. Med. 27, 217–226.

Celly, C.S., McDonell, W.N., Young, S.S., Black, W.D., 1997. The comparative hypoxaemic effect of four alpha 2 adrenoceptor agonists (xylazine, romifidine, detomidine and medetomidine) in sheep. J. Vet. Pharmacol. Ther. 20, 464–471.

Celly, C.S., McDonell, W.N., Black, W.D., 1999. Cardiopulmonary effects of the alpha2-adrenoceptor agonists medetomidine and st-91 in anesthetized sheep. J. Pharmacol. Exp. Ther. 289, 712–720.

Cesarovic, N., Jirkof, P., Rettich, A., Arras, M., 2011. Implantation of radiotelemetry transmitters yielding data on ECG, heart rate, core body temperature and activity in free-moving laboratory mice. J. Vis. Exp.

Cesarovic, N., Jirkof, P., Rettich, A., Nicholls, F., Arras, M., 2012. Combining sevoflurane anesthesia with fentanyl-midazolam or s-ketamine in laboratory mice. J. Am. Assoc. Lab. Anim. Sci. 51, 209–218.

Cetin, N., Cetin, E., Toker, M., 2005. Echocardiographic variables in healthy guineapigs anaesthetized with ketamine-xylazine. Lab. Anim. 39, 100–106.

Chakrabarty, S., Thomas, P., Sheridan, D.J., 1991. Arrhythmias, haemodynamic changes, and extent of myocardial damage during coronary ligation in rabbits anaesthetized with halothane, alpha chloralose, or pentobarbitone. Int. J. Cardiol. 31, 9–14.

Chang, C., Uchiyama, A., Ma, L., 2009. A comparison of the effects on respiratory carbon dioxide response, arterial blood pressure, and heart rate of dexmedetomidine, propofol, and midazolam in sevoflurane-anesthetized rabbits. Anesth. Analg. 109, 84–89.

Cheong, S.H., Lee, K.M., Yang, Y.I., Seo, J.Y., Choi, M.Y., Yoon, Y.C., 2010. Blind oral endotracheal intubation of rats using a ventilator to verify correct placement. Lab. Anim. 44, 278–280.

Cheong, S.H., Lee, J.H., Kim, M.H., Cho, K.R., Lim, S.H., Lee, K.M., et al., 2013. Airway management using a supraglottic airway device without endotracheal intubation for positive ventilation of anaesthetized rats. Lab. Anim. 47, 89–93.

Chisholm, J., De Rantere, D., Fernandez, N.J., Krajacic, A., Pang, D.S.J., 2013. Carbon dioxide, but not isoflurane, elicits ultrasonic vocalizations in female rats. Lab. Anim. 47, 324–327.

Chodzyński, K.J., Conotte, S., Vanhamme, L., Van Antwerpen, P., Kerkhofs, M., Legros, J.L., et al., 2013. A new device to mimic intermittent hypoxia in mice. PLoS One, 8.

Clark, M.D., Krugner-Higby, L., Smith, L.J., Heath, T.D., Clark, K.L., Olson, D., 2004. Evaluation of liposome-encapsulated oxymorphone hydrochloride in mice after splenectomy. Comp. Med. 54, 558–563.

Clowry, G.J., Flecknell, P.A., 2000. The successful use of fentanyl/fluanisone ('Hypnorm') as an anaesthetic for intracranial surgery in neonatal rats. Lab. Anim. 34, 260–264.

Clutton, R.E., Vettoratto, E., Schoeffmann, G., Docherty, J., Burke, J.G., Gibson, A.J.N., 2014. The perioperative care of lambs and ewes when the former undergo major experimental (scoliotic) surgery. Lab. Anim. 48, 27–35.

Coetzee, J.F., 2013. A review of analgesic compounds used in food animals in the united states. Vet. Clin. North Am. Food Anim. Pract. 29, 11–28.

Cohen, B.J., Bree, M.M., 1978. Chemical and physical restraint of non-human primates. J. Med. Primatol. 7, 193–201.

Cook, D.J., Housmans, P.R., 1994. Mechanism of the negative inotropic effect of propofol in isolated ferret ventricular myocardium. Anesthesiology 80, 859–871.

Cooper, D.M., Delong, D., Gillett, C.S., 1997. Analgesic efficacy of acetaminophen and buprenorphine administered in the drinking water of rats. Contemp. Top. Lab. Anim. Sci. 36, 58–62.

Cooper, D.M., Hoffman, W., Wheat, N., Lee, H.-Y., 2005. Duration of effects on clinical parameters and referred hyperalgesia in rats after abdominal surgery and multiple doses of analgesic. Comp. Med. 55, 344–353.

Cooper, D.M., Hoffman, W., Tomlinson, K., Lee, H.Y., 2008. Refinement of the dosage and dosing schedule of ketoprofen for postoperative analgesia in Sprague-Dawley rats. Lab. Anim. (NY). 37, 271–275.

Cope, D.K., Impastato, W.K., Cohen, M.V., Downey, J.M., 1997. Volatile anesthetics protect the ischemic rabbit myocardium from infarction. Anesthesiology 86, 699–709.

Cotroneo, T.M., Hugunin, K.M.S., Shuster, K.A., Hwang, H.J., Kakaraparthi, B.N., Nemzek-Hamlin, J.A., 2012. Effects of buprenorphine on a cecal ligation and puncture model in C57BL/6 mice. J. Am. Assoc. Lab. Anim. Sci. 51, 357–365.

Coulter, C.A., Flecknell, P.A., Leach, M.C., Richardson, C.A., 2011. Reported analgesic administration to rabbits undergoing experimental surgical procedures. BMC. Vet. Res. 7, 12–18.

Coulthard, M.G., Flecknell, P., Orr, H., Manas, D., O'donnell, M., 2002. Renal scarring caused by vesicoureteric reflux and urinary infection: a study in pigs. Pediatr. Nephrol. 17, 481–484.

Criado, A.B., Gómez de Segura, I.A., 2003. Reduction of isoflurane MAC by fentanyl or remifentanil in rats. Vet. Anaesth. Analg. 30, 250–256.

Criado, A.B., Gómez de Segura, I.A., Tendillo, F.J., Marsico, F., 2000. Reduction of isoflurane MAC with buprenorphine and morphine in rats. Lab. Anim. 34, 252–259.

Curtin, L.I., Grakowsky, J.A., Suarez, M., Thompson, A.C., Dipirro, J.M., Martin, L.B.E., et al., 2009. Evaluation of buprenorphine in a postoperative pain model in rats. Comp. Med. 59, 60–71.

Dang, V., Bao, S., Ault, A., Murray, C., Mcfarlane-Mills, J., Chiedi, C., et al., 2008. Efficacy and safety of five injectable anesthetic regimens for chronic blood collection from the anterior vena cava of Guinea pigs. J. Am. Assoc. Lab. Anim. Sci. 47, 56–60.

Danneman, P.J., White, W.J., Marshall, W.K., Lang, C.M., 1988. Evaluation of analgesia associated with the immobility response in laboratory rabbits. Lab. Anim. Sci. 38, 51–56.

DeCastro, G., Viars, P., 1968. Anesthetie analgesique sequentielle, ou A.A.S. Arch. Med 23, 170–176.

Delaporte-Cerceau, S., Samama, C.M., Riou, B., Bonnin, P., Guillosson, J.J., Coriat, P., 1998. Ketorolac and enoxaparin affect arterial thrombosis and bleeding in the rabbit. Anesthesiology 88, 1310–1317.

De Mulder, P.A., Van Kerckhoven, R.J., Adriaensen, H.F., Gillebert, T.C., De Hert, S.G., 1997. Continuous total intravenous anesthesia using propofol and fentanyl in an open-thorax rabbit model: evaluation of cardiac contractile function and biochemical assessment. Lab. Anim. Sci. 47, 367–375.

Deng, J., St Clair, M., Everett, C., Reitman, M., Star, R.A., 2000. Buprenorphine given after surgery does not alter renal ischemia/reperfusion injury. Comp. Med. 50, 628–632.

De Segura, I.A.G., De La Víbora, J.B., Criado, A., 2009. Determination of the minimum alveolar concentration for halothane, isoflurane and sevoflurane in the gerbil. Lab. Anim. 43, 239–242.

Dickinson, A.L., Leach, M.C., Flecknell, P.A., 2009. The analgesic effects of oral paracetamol in two strains of mice undergoing vasectomy. Lab. Anim. 43, 357–361.

Diffay, B.C., McKenzie, D., Wolf, C., Pugh, D.G., 2002. Handling and examination of sheep and goats. In: Pugh, D.G. (Ed.), Sheep and Goat Medicine. Saunders, Philadelphia, PA.

Divers, T.J., Peek, S.F., 2008. Therapeutics and routine procedures. In: Divers, T.J., Peek, S.F. (Eds.), Rebhun's Diseases of Dairy Cattle, second ed. Saunders, St. Louis, MO.

Doerning, B.I., Brammer, D.W., Chrisp, C.E., Rush, H.G., 1992. Nephrotoxicity of tiletamine in New Zealand White rabbits. Lab. Anim. Sci. 42, 267–269.

Doherty, T., Redua, M.A., Queiroz-Castro, P., Egger, C., Cox, S.K., Rohrbach, B.W., 2007. Effect of intravenous lidocaine and ketamine on the minimum alveolar concentration of isoflurane in goats. Vet. Anaesth. Analg. 34, 125–131.

Doherty, T.J., Rohrbach, B.W., Geiser, D.R., 2002a. Effect of acepromazine and butorphanol on isoflurane minimum alveolar concentration in goats. J. Vet. Pharmacol. Ther. 25, 65–67.

Doherty, T.J., Rohrbach, B.W., Ross, L., Schultz, H., 2002b. The effect of tiletamine and zolazepam on isoflurane minimum alveolar concentration in goats. J. Vet. Pharmacol. Ther. 25, 233–235.

Dowd, G., Gaynor, J.S., Alvis, M., Salman, M., Turner, A.S., 1998. A comparison of transdermal fentanyl and oral phenylbutazone analgesia in sheep. Vet. Surg. 27, 168.

Drummond, J.C., 1985. MAC for halothane, enflurane, and isoflurane in the New Zealand White rabbit: and a test for the validity of MAC determinations. Anesthesiology 62, 336–338.

Dujardin, C.L.L., Gootjes, P., Moens, Y., 2005. Isoflurane measurement error using short wavelength infrared techniques in horses: influence of fresh gas flow and pre-anaesthetic food deprivation. Vet. Anaesth. Analg. 32, 101–106.

Dzikiti, T.B., Stegmann, G.F., Hellebrekers, L.J., Auer, R.E.J., Dzikiti, L.N., 2009. Sedative and cardiopulmonary effects of acepromazine, midazolam, butorphanol, acepromazine-butorphanol and midazolam-butorphanol on propofol anaesthesia in goats. J. S. Afr. Vet. Assoc. 80, 10–16.

Ecobichon, D.J., Comeau, A.M., 1974. Genetic polymorphism of plasma carboxylesterases in the rabbit: correlation with pharmacologic and toxicologic effects. Toxicol. Appl. Pharmacol. 27, 28–40.

Egger, C.M., Souza, M.J., Greenacre, C.B., et al., 2009. Effect of intravenous administration of tramadol hydrochloride on the minimum alveolar concentration of isoflurane in rabbits. Am. J. Vet. Res. 70, 945–949.

Eisele, P.H., Talken, L., Eisele, J.H., 1985. Potency of isoflurane and nitrous oxide in conventional swine. Lab. Anim. Sci. 35, 76–78.

Eng, M., Bonica, J.J., Alamatsu, T.J., Berges, P.U., Yuen, D., Ueland, K., 1975. Maternal and fetal responses to halothane in pregnant monkey. Acta. Anaesthesiol. Scand. 19, 154–158.

Enlund, M., Andersson, J., Hartvig, P., Valtysson, J., Wiklund, L., 1997. Cerebral normoxia in the rhesus monkey during isoflurane or propofol induced hypotension and hypocapnia, despite disparate blood-flow patterns. Acta. Anaesthesiol. Scand. 41 (8), 1002–1010.

Eshar, D., Wilson, J., 2010. Epidural anesthesia and analgesia in ferrets. Lab. Anim. (NY) 39, 339–340.

Feng, Y., Cui, M., Willis, W.D., 2003. Gabapentin markedly reduces acetic acid-induced visceral nociception. Anesthesiology 98, 729–733.

Fernie, S., Wrenshall, E., Malcolm, S., Bryce, F., Arnold, D.L., 1994. Normative hematological and serum biochemical values for adult and infant rhesus monkeys (Macaca mulatta) in a controlled laboratory environment. J. Toxicol. Environ. Health. 42, 53–72.

Field, K.J., White, W.J., Lang, C.M., 1993. Anaesthetic effects of chloral hydrate, pentobarbitone and urethane in adult male rats. Lab. Anim. 27, 258–269.

Fish, R.E., 2008. Anesthesia and Analgesia in Laboratory Animals. Elsevier/Academic Press, Amsterdam.

Flecknell, P.A., 1989. Rodent and rabbit anesthesia lecture. Paper presented at the 40th Annual American Association for Laboratory Animal Science Meeting, Little Rock, Arkansas.

Flecknell, P.A., 1996. Handbook of Rodent and Rabbit Medicine. Pergamon, Oxford; Tarrytown, NY.

Flecknell, P.A., 1997. Medetomidine and atipamezole: potential uses in laboratory animals. Lab. Anim. 26, 21–25.

Flecknell, P.A., 2001. Analgesia of small mammals. The veterinary clinics of North America. Exot. Anim. Pract. 4, 47–56. vi.

Flecknell, P.A., 2009. Laboratory Animal Anaesthesia, third ed. Academic Press, London.

Flecknell, P.A., 2010. Do mice have a pain face? Nat. Methods. 7, 437–438.

Flecknell, P.A., Mitchell, M., 1984. Midazolam and fentanyl-fluanisone: assessment of anaesthetic effects in laboratory rodents and rabbits. Lab. Anim. 18, 143–146.

Flecknell, P.A., Liles, J.H., 1990. Assessment of the analgesic action of opioid agonist–antagonists in the rabbit. J. Assoc. Vet. Anaesth. 17, 24–29.

Flecknell, P.A., John, M., Mitchell, M., Shurey, C., Simpkin, S., 1983. Neuroleptanalgesia in the rabbit. Lab. Anim. 17, 104–109.

Flecknell, P.A., Liles, J.H., Williamson, H.A., 1990. The use of lignocaine-prilocaine local anaesthetic cream for pain-free venepuncture in laboratory animals. Lab. Anim. 24, 142–146.

Flecknell, P.A., Roughan, J.V., Hedenqvist, P., 1999. Induction of anaesthesia with sevoflurane and isoflurane in the rabbit. Lab. Anim. 33, 41–46.

Flecknell, P.A., Roughan, J.V., Stewart, R., 1999a. Use of oral buprenorphine ("buprenorphine jello") for postoperative analgesia in rats– a clinical trial. Lab. Anim. 32 (2), 169–174.

Flecknell, P.A., Orr, H.E., Roughan, J.V., Stewart, R., 1999b. Comparison of the effects of oral or subcutaneous carprofen or ketoprofen in rats undergoing laparotomy. Vet. Rec. 144, 65–67.

Foley, P.L., Henderson, A.L., Bissonette, E.A., et al., 2001. Evaluation of fentanyl transdermal patches in rabbits: blood concentrations and physiologic response. Comp. Med. 51, 239–244.

Foley, P.L., Liang, H., Crichlow, A.R., 2011. Evaluation of a sustained-release formulation of buprenorphine for analgesia in rats. J. Am. Assoc. Lab. Anim. Sci. 50, 198–204.

Forsythe, D.B., Payton, A.J., Dixon, D., Meyers, P.H., Clark, J.A., Snipe, J.R., 1992. Evaluation of Telazol-xylazine as an anesthetic combination for use in Syrian hamsters. Lab. Anim. Sci. 42 (5), 497–502.

Foster, P.S., Hopkinson, K.C., Denborough, M.A., 1992. Propofol anaesthesia in malignant hyperpyrexia susceptible swine. Clin. Exp. Pharmacol. Physiol. 19, 183–186.

Franchi, S., Panerai, A.E., Sacerdote, P., 2007. Buprenorphine ameliorates the effect of surgery on hypothalamus-pituitary-adrenal axis, natural killer cell activity and metastatic colonization in rats in comparison with morphine or fentanyl treatment. Brain. Behav. Immun. 21, 767–774.

Gabriel, A.F., Marcus, M. a. E., Honig, W.M.M., Helgers, N., Joosten, E. a. J., 2009. Environmental housing affects the duration of mechanical allodynia and the spinal astroglial activation in a rat model of chronic inflammatory pain. Brain. Res. 1276, 83–90.

Gabriel, A.F., Marcus, M. a. E., Honig, W.M.M., Joosten, E. a. J., 2010a. Preoperative housing in an enriched environment significantly reduces the duration of post-operative pain in a rat model of knee inflammation. Neurosci. Lett. 469, 219–223.

Gabriel, A.F., Paoletti, G., Della Seta, D., Panelli, R., Marcus, M. a. E., Farabollini, F., et al., 2010b. Enriched environment and the recovery from inflammatory pain: social versus physical aspects and their interaction. Behav. Brain. Res. 208, 90–95.

Gades, N.M., Danneman, P.J., Wixson, S.K., Tolley, E.A., 2000. The magnitude and duration of the analgesic effect of morphine, butorphanol, and buprenorphine in rats and mice. Contemp. Top. Lab. Anim. Sci. 39 (2), 8–13.

Gades, N.M., Danneman, P.J., Wixson, S.K., Tolley, E.A., 2008. Effects of buprenorphine on body temperature, locomotor activity and cardiovascular function when assessed by telemetric monitoring in rats. Lab. Anim., 42.

Gaertner, D.J., Hallman, T.M., Hankenson, F.C., Batchelder, M.A., 2008. Chapter 10 – Anesthesia and analgesia for laboratory rodents. In: FIsh, E.F., Brown, J.B., Danneman, J.D., Karas, A.Z (Eds.), Anesthesia and Analgesia in Laboratory Animals, second ed. Academic Press, San Diego, CA.

Gardiner, T.W., Toth, L.A., 1999. Stereotactic surgery and long–term maintenance of cranial implants in research animals. Contemp. Top. Lab. Anim. Sci. 38 (1), 56–63.

Gargiulo, S., Greco, A., Gramanzini, M., Esposito, S., Affuso, A., Brunetti, A., et al., 2012a. Mice anesthesia, analgesia, and care, Part I: anesthetic considerations in preclinical research. ILAR. J. 53, E55–E69.

Gargiulo, S., Greco, A., Gramanzini, M., Esposito, S., Affuso, A., Brunetti, A., et al., 2012b. Mice anesthesia, analgesia, and care, Part II: anesthetic considerations in preclinical imaging studies. ILAR. J. 53, E70–E81.

Gaynor, J.S., Wimsatt, J., Mallinckrodt, C., Biggins, D., 1997. A comparison of sevoflurane and isoflurane for short-term anesthesia in polecats (Mustela eversmanni). J. Zoo Wildl. Med. 28, 274–279.

Gebhardt-Henrich, S.G., Fischer, K., Hauzenberger, A.R., Keller, P., Steiger, A., 2007. The duration of capture and restraint during anesthesia and euthanasia influences glucocorticoid levels in male golden hamsters. Lab. Anim. (NY). 36, 41–46.

Gerring, E.L., Scarth, S.C., 1974. Anesthesia for open-heart surgery in calf. Br. J. Anaesth. 46, 455–460.

Ghaly, R.F., Stone, J.M., Levy, W.J., Roccaforte, P., Brunner, E.B., 1990. The effects of etomidate on motor evoked potentials induced by transcranial magnetic stimulation in the monkey. Neurosurgery 27 (6), 936–942.

Gillingham, M.B., Clark, M.D., Dahly, E.M., Krugner-Higby, L.A., Ney, D.M., 2001. A comparison of two opioid analgesics for relief of visceral pain induced by intestinal resection in rats. Contemp. Top. Lab. Anim. Sci. 40, 21–26.

Gleed, R.D., 1987. Tranquilizers and sedatives. In: Short, C.E. (Ed.), Principles and Practice of Veterinary Anesthesia. Williams and Wilkins, Baltimore, MD, pp. 20–21. 384–386.

Glen, J.B., Hunter, S.C., 1984. Pharmacology of an emulsion formulation of ICI 35868. Br. J. Anaesth. 52, 617–626.

Glynn, H.D., Coetzee, J.F., Edwards-Callaway, L.N., Dockweiler, J.C., Allen, K.A., Lubbers, B., et al., 2013. The pharmacokinetics and effects of meloxicam, gabapentin, and flunixin in postweaning dairy calves following dehorning with local anesthesia. J. Vet. Pharmacol. Ther. 36, 550–561.

Gogoi, S.R., Sarma, B., Lahon, D.K., 2003. Clinical evaluation of medetomidine and medetomidine ketamine in goats. Indian J. Anim. Sci. 73, 271.

Goldkuhl, R., Hau, J., Abelson, K.S.P., 2010a. Effects of voluntarily-ingested buprenorphine on plasma corticosterone levels, body weight, water intake, and behaviour in permanently catheterised rats. In vivo (Athens, Greece) 24, 131–135.

Goldkuhl, R., Jacobsen, K.R., Kalliokoski, O., Hau, J., Abelson, K.S.P., 2010b. Plasma concentrations of corticosterone and buprenorphine in rats subjected to jugular vein catheterization. Lab. Anim. 44, 337–343.

Golledge, H.D.R., 2012. Response to Roustan et al. 'Evaluating methods of mouse euthanasia on the oocyte quality: cervical dislocation versus isoflurane inhalation': animal welfare concerns regarding the aversiveness of isoflurane and its inability to cause rapid death. Lab. Anim. 46, 358–359. author reply 360.

Gonzalez Gil, A., Silvan, G., Villa, A., et al., 2010. Serum biochemical response to inhalant anesthetics in New Zealand White rabbits. J. Amer. Assoc. Lab. Anim. Sci. 49, 52–56.

Goosen, D.J., Davies, J.H., Maree, M., Dormehl, I.C., 1984. The influence of physical and chemical restraint on the physiology of the chacma baboon (Papio ursinus). J. Med. Primatol. 13, 339–351.

Goulding, D.R., Myers, P.H., Goulding, E.H., Blankenship, T.L., Grant, M.F., Forsythe, D.B., 2010. The effects of perioperative analgesia

on litter size in Crl:CD1(ICR) mice undergoing embryo transfer. J. Am. Assoc. Lab. Anim. Sci. 49, 423–426.

Gray, P.R., McDonell, W.N., 1986a. Anesthesia and analgesia in goats and sheep 2. General anesthesia. Compendium on Continuing Education for the Practicing Veterinarian 8, S127–S135.

Gray, P.R., McDonell, W.N., 1986b. Anesthesia in goats and sheep 1. Local analgesia. Compend. Contin. Educ. Practicing Vet. 8, S33–S39.

Green, C.J., 1975. Neuroleptanalgesic drug combinations in the anaesthetic management of small laboratory animals. Lab. Anim. 9, 161–178.

Green, C.J., Knight, J., Precious, S., Simpkin, S., 1981. Ketamine alone and combined with diazepam or xylazine in laboratory animals: a 10 year experience. Lab. Anim. 15, 163–170.

Greene, S., 2003. Protocols for anesthesia of cattle. Vet. Clin. North Am. Food Anim. Pract. 19, 679–693.

Greene, S., Thurmon, J., 1988. Xylazine – a review of its pharmacology and use in veterinary-medicine. J. Vet. Pharmacol. Ther. 11, 295–313.

Greene, S.A., Keegan, R.D., Valdez, R.A., Knowles, D.K., 2002. Cardiovascular effects of sevoflurane in holstein calves. Vet. Anaesth. Analg. 29, 59–63.

Guarnieri, M., Brayton, C., Detolla, L., Forbes-Mcbean, N., Sarabia-Estrada, R., Zadnik, P., 2012. Safety and efficacy of buprenorphine for analgesia in laboratory mice and rats. Lab. Anim. (NY). 41, 337–343.

Habel, R.E., 1975. Ruminant digestive system. In: Getty, R. (Ed.), Sisson and Grossman's the Anatomy of the Domestic Animals, fifth ed. W.B. Saunders, Philadelphia, PA.

Habel, R.E., 1978. Applied Veterinary Anatomy. Edwards Brothers, Inc, Ann Arbor, MI.

Hackbarth, H., Küppers, N., Bohnet, W., 2000. Euthanasia of rats with carbon dioxide–animal welfare aspects. Lab. Anim. 34, 91–96.

Hall, L.W., Clarke, K.W., 1991. Veterinary Anaesthesia. Bailliere Tindall, London.

Hamacher, J., Arras, M., Bootz, F., Weiss, M., Schramm, R., Moehrlen, U., 2008. Microscopic wire guide–based orotracheal mouse intubation: description, evaluation and comparison with transillumination. Lab. Anim. 42, 222–230.

Hampshire, V.A., Davis, J.A., Mcnickle, C.A., Williams, L., Eskildson, H., 2001. Retrospective comparison of rat recovery weights using inhalation and injectable anaesthetics, nutritional and fluid supplementation for right unilateral neurosurgical lesioning. Lab. Anim. 35, 223–229.

Hansen, B., Lascelles, B., Thomson, A., DePuy, V., 2013. Variability of performance of wound infusion catheters. Vet. Anaesth. Analg. 40, 308–315.

Harrison, P.K., Tattersall, J.E.H., Gosden, E., 2006. The presence of atropinesterase activity in animal plasma. Naunyn Schmiedeberg's Arch. Pharmacol. 373, 230–236.

Hartley, D.E., Vongpaial, T., Xu, J., Shepherd, R.K., King, A.J., et al., 2010. Bilateral cochlear implantation in the ferret: a novel animal model for behavioral studies. J. Neurosci. Methods 190, 214–228.

Hayes, J.H., Flecknell, P.A., 1999. A comparison of pre- and post-surgical administration of bupivacaine or buprenorphine following laparotomy in the rat. Lab. Anim. 33, 16–23.

Hedenqvist, P., Orr, H.E., Roughan, J., et al., 2002. Anaesthesia with ketamine/medetomidine in the rabbit: influence of route of administration and the effect of combination with butorphanol. Vet. Anas. Anal. 29, 14–19.

Hedenqvist, P., Roughan, J.V., Flecknell, P.A., 2000a. Sufentanil and medetomidine anaesthesia in the rat and its reversal with atipamezole and butorphanol. Lab. Anim. 34, 244–251.

Hedenqvist, P., Roughan, J.V., Flecknell, P.A., 2000b. Effects of repeated anaesthesia with ketamine/medetomidine and of pre-anaesthetic administration of buprenorphine in rats. Lab. Anim. 34, 207–211.

Heinrich, A., Duffield, T., Lissemore, K., Squires, E.J., Millman, S.T., 2007. The efficacy of meloxicam at relieving the pain response to dehorning in dairy calves. J. Anim. Sci. 85 127–127.

Hellebrekers, L.J., de Boer, E.-J.W., van Zuylen, M.A., Vosmeer, H., 1997. A comparison between medetomidine-ketamine and medetomidine-propofol anaesthesia in rabbits. Lab. Anim. 31, 58–69.

Henke, J., Strack, T., Erhardt, W., 2004. Clinical comparison of isoflurane and sevoflurane anaesthesia in the gerbil (Meriones unguiculatus). Berl. Münch. tierärztl. Wochenschr. 117, 296–303.

Hikasa, Y., Okuyama, K., Kakuta, T., Takase, K., Ogasawara, S., 1998. Anesthetic potency and cardiopulmonary effects of sevoflurane in goats: comparison with isoflurane and halothane. Can. J. Vet. Res. 62, 299–306.

Hikasa, Y., Hokushin, S., Takase, K., Ogasawara, S., 2002. Cardiopulmonary, hematological, serum biochemical and behavioral effects of sevoflurane compared with isoflurane or halothane in spontaneously ventilating goats. Small Rumin. Res. 43, 167–178.

Hindman, B.J., Funatsu, N., Cheng, D.C.H., Bolles, R., Todd, M.M., Tinker, J.H., 1990. Differential effect of oncotic pressure on cerebral and extracerebral water content during cardiopulmonary bypass in rabbits. Anesthesiology 73, 951–957.

Hotchkiss, C.E., Bromage, R., Du, M., Jerome, C.P., 1998. The anesthetic isoflurane decreases ionized calcium and increases parathyroid hormone and osteocalcin in cynomolgus monkeys. Bone 23 (5), 479–484.

Hrapkiewicz, S., Smiler, K.L., 1989. A new anesthetic agent for use in the gerbil. Lab. Anim. Sci. 39 (4), 338–341.

Hsu, W.H., Bellin, S.I., Dellmon, H.D., 1986. Xylazine-ketamine induced anesthesia in rats and its antagonism by yohimbine. J. Am. Vet. Med. Assoc. 189 (9), 1040–1043.

Hughes, P.J., Doherty, M.M., Charman, W.N., 1993. A rabbit model for the evaluation of epidurally administered local anaesthetic agents. Anaesth. Intensive. Care. 21, 298–303.

Hugunin, K.M.S., Fry, C., Shuster, K., Nemzek, J.A., 2010. Effects of tramadol and buprenorphine on select immunologic factors in a cecal ligation and puncture model. Shock (Augusta, Ga.) 34, 250–260.

Hupfeld, D., Distler, C., Hoffmann, K.P., 2006. Motion perception deficits in albino ferrets (Mustela putorius furo). Vision Res. 46, 2941–2948.

Ickowicz, D.E., Golovanevski, L., Haze, A., Domb, A.J., Weiniger, C.F., 2013. Extended release local anesthetic agents in a postoperative arthritic pain model. J. Pharm. Sci. 103, 185–190.

Imai, A., Steffey, E.P., Farver, T.B., Ilkiw, J.E., 1999. Assessment of isoflurane-induced anesthesia in ferrets and rats. Am. J. Vet. Res. 60, 1577–1583.

Ingrao, J.C., Johnson, R., Tor, E., Gu, Y., Litman, M., Turner, P.V., 2013. Aqueous stability and oral pharmacokinetics of meloxicam and carprofen in male C57BL/6 mice. J. Am. Assoc. Lab. Anim. Sci. 52, 553–559.

Ingvast-Larsson, C., Svartberg, K., Hydbring-Sandberg, E., Bondesson, U., Olsson, K., 2007. Clinical pharmacology of buprenorphine in healthy, lactating goats. J. Vet. Pharmacol. Ther. 30, 249–256.

Itah, R., Gitelman, I., Davis, C., 2004. A replacement for methoxyflurane (Metofane) in open-circuit anaesthesia. Lab. Anim. 38, 280–285.

Izrailtyan, I., Glass, P., Fowler, J., Baumann, A., Benveniste, H.D., 2004. Bispectral Index (BIS) guidance of anesthesia decreases the interindividual variability of the maternal brain glucose uptake in non-human primates. Anesthesiology 101 (3).

Jablonski, P., Howden, B.O., 2002. Oral buprenorphine and aspirin analgesia in rats undergoing liver transplantation. Lab. Anim. 36, 134–143.

Jablonski, P., Howden, B.O., Baxter, K., 2001. Influence of buprenorphine analgesia on post-operative recovery in two strains of rats. Lab. Anim. 35, 213–222.

Jackson, L.R., Marini, R.P., Esteves, M.I., Andrutis, K.A., Goslant, C.M., Fox, J.G., 1992. The effect of anesthetics on hematology parameters in ferrets. Contemp. Top. Lab. Anim. Sci. 31 (4), 18.

Jacobs, B., Harris, G.C., Allada, V., Chugani, H.T., Pollack, D.B., Raleigh, M.J., 1993. Midazolam as an effective intravenous adjuvant to prolonged ketamine sedation in young rhesus (Macaca mulatta) and vervet (Cercopithecus aethiops sabaeus) monkeys: a preliminary report. Am. J. Primatol. 29, 291–298.

Jacobson, C., 2001. A novel anaesthetic regimen for surgical procedures in guineapigs. Lab. Anim. 35, 271–276.

Janus, C., Golde, T., 2014. The effect of brief neonatal cryoanesthesia on physical development and adult cognitive function in mice. Behav. Brain. Res. 259, 253–260.

Jaquenod, M., Ronnhedh, C., Cousins, M.J., Eckstein, R.P., Jordan, V., Mather, L.E., et al., 1998. Factors influencing ketorolac-associated perioperative renal dysfunction. Anesth. Analg. 86, 1090–1097.

Jensen, F.M., Dahl, J.B., Frigast, C., 1992. Direct spinal effect of intrathecal acetaminophen on visceral noxious stimulation in rabbits. Acta. Anaesthesiol. Scand. 36, 837–841.

Jessen, L., Christensen, S., Bjerrum, O.J., 2007. The antinociceptive efficacy of buprenorphine administered through the drinking water of rats. Lab. Anim. 41, 185–196.

Jiang, Y.-L., Yin, X.-H., Shen, Y.-F., He, X.-F., Fang, J.-Q., 2013. Low frequency electroacupuncture alleviated spinal nerve ligation induced mechanical allodynia by inhibiting TRPV1 upregulation in ipsilateral undamaged dorsal root ganglia in rats. Evid. Based Complement. Alternat. Med. 2013.

Jirkof, P., Cesarovic, N., Rettich, A., Nicholls, F., Seifert, B., Arras, M., 2010. Burrowing behavior as an indicator of post-laparotomy pain in mice. Front. Behav. Neurosci., 4.

Johnston, M.S., 2005. Clinical approaches to analgesia in ferrets and rabbits. Semin. Avian Exot. Pet. Med. 14, 228–235.

Johnson, D.H., 2010. Endoscopic intubation of exotic companion mammals. The veterinary clinics of North America. Exot. Anim. Pract. 13, 273–289.

Jones, C.P., Carver, S., Kendall, L.V., 2012. Evaluation of common anesthetic and analgesic techniques for tail biopsy in mice. J. Am. Assoc. Lab. Anim. Sci. 51, 808–814.

Jorgensen, J., Cannedy, A., 1996. Physiologic and pathophysiologic considerations for ruminant and swine anesthesia. Vet. Clin. North Am. Food Anim. Pract. 12, 481–500.

Kalliokoski, O., Jacobsen, K.R., Hau, J., Abelson, K.S.P., 2011. Serum concentrations of buprenorphine after oral and parenteral administration in male mice. Vet. J. (London, England: 1997) 187, 251–254.

Kästner, S.B., Boller, M., Kutter, A., Akens, M.K., Bettschart-Wolfensberger, R., 2001a. Clinical comparison of preanaesthetic intramuscular medetomidine and dexmedetomidine in domestic sheep. Dtsch. Tierarztl. Wochenschr. 108, 409–413.

Kästner, S.B., Wapf, P., Feige, K., Demuth, D., Bettschart-Wolfensberger, R., Akens, M.K., et al., 2003. Pharmacokinetics and sedative effects of intramuscular medetomidine in domestic sheep. J. Vet. Pharmacol. Ther. 26, 271–276.

Kästner, S.B.R., 2006. A(2)–agonists in sheep: a review. Vet. Anaesth. Analg. 33, 79–96.

Kästner, S.B.R., Boller, M., Kutter, A., Akens, M.K., Bettschart-Wolfensberger, R., 2001b. Clinical comparison of preanaesthetic intramuscular medetomidine and dexmedetomidine in domestic sheep. Deutsch. Tierärztl. Wochenschr. 108, 409–413.

Kästner, S.B.R., Kull, S., Kutter, A.P.N., Boller, J., Bettschart-Wolfensberger, R., Hu, M.K., 2005. Cardiopulmonary effects of dexmedetomidine in sevoflurane-anesthetized sheep with and without nitric oxide inhalation. Am. J. Vet. Res. 66, 1496–1502.

Kästner, S.B.R., Kutter, A.P.N., Rechenberg, B.V., Bettschart-Wolfensberger, R., 2006. Comparison of two pre-anaesthetic medetomidine doses in isoflurane anaesthetized sheep. Vet. Anaesth. Analg. 33, 8–16.

Kästner, S.B.R., Boller, J., Kutter, A.P.N., Pakarinen, S.M., Ramela, M.P., Huhtinen, M.K., 2007a. Comparison of cardiopulmonary effects of dexmedetomidine administered as a constant rate infusion without loading dose in sheep and goats anaesthetised with sevoflurane. Small Rumin. Res. 71, 75–82.

Kästner, S.B.R., Ohlerth, S., Pospischil, A., Boller, J., Huhtinen, M.K., 2007b. Dexmedetomidine-induced pulmonary alterations in sheep. Res. Vet. Sci. 83, 217–226.

Kazemi, A., Harvey, M., Cave, G., Lahner, D., 2011. The effect of lipid emulsion on depth of anaesthesia following thiopental administration to rabbits. Anaesthesia 66 (5), 373–378.

Kazi, J.A., Gee, C.F., 2007. Effect of gabapentin on c-Fos expression in the CNS after paw surgery in rats. J. Mol. Neurosci. 32, 228–234.

Keating, S.C.J., Thomas, A.A., Flecknell, P.A., Leach, M.C., 2012. Evaluation of EMLA cream for preventing pain during tattooing of rabbits: changes in physiological, behavioural and facial expression responses. PLoS One 7 (9), e44437.

Kero, P., Thomasson, B., Soppi, A.M., 1981. Spinal anaesthesia in the rabbit. Lab. Anim. 15, 347–348.

Kharasch, E.D., 1998. Compound A: toxicology and clinical relevance. Anaesthesist 47 (Suppl. 1), S7–S10.

Kharasch, E.D., Schroeder, J.L., Sheffels, P., Liggitt, H.D., 2005. Influence of sevoflurane on the metabolism and renal effects of compound A in rats. Anesthesiology 103, 1183–1188.

Khurana, S., Jain, N.K., Bedi, P.M.S., 2013. Development and characterization of a novel controlled release drug delivery system based on nanostructured lipid carriers gel for meloxicam. Life. Sci. 93, 763–772.

Kim, H.Y., Koo, S.T., Kim, J.H., An, K., Chung, K., Chung, J.M., 2010. Electroacupuncture analgesia in rat ankle sprain pain model: neural mechanisms. Neurol. Res. 32 (Suppl 1), 10–17.

Kim, J.H., Kim, H.Y., Chung, K., Chung, J.M., 2011. Electroacupuncture reduces the evoked responses of the spinal dorsal horn neurons in ankle-sprained rats. J. Neurophysiol. 105, 2050–2057.

Kim, M.S., Jeong, S.M., Park, J.H., et al., 2004. Reversal of medetomidine-ketamine combination anesthesia in rabbits by atipamezole. Exp. Anim. 53, 423–428.

King, J.N., Dawson, J., Esser, R.E., Fujimoto, R., Kimble, E.F., Maniara, W., et al., 2009. Preclinical pharmacology of robenacoxib: a novel selective inhibitor of cyclooxygenase-2. J. Vet. Pharmacol. Ther. 32, 1–17.

Klaunberg, B.A., O'malley, J., Clark, T., Davis, J.A., 2004. Euthanasia of mouse fetuses and neonates. Contemp. Top. Lab. Anim. Sci. 43, 29–34.

Kleine, S., Quandt, J.E., 2012. Anesthesia case of the month. J. Am. Vet. Med. Assoc. 241, 1577–1580.

Klemm, W.R., 2001. Behavioral arrest: in search of the neural control system. Prog. Neurobiol. 65, 453–471.

Ko, J.C., Freeman, L.J., Barletta, M., Weil, A.B., Payton, M.E., et al., 2011. Efficacy of oral transmucosal and intravenous administration of buprenorphine before surgery for postoperative analgesia in dogs undergoing ovariohysterectomy. J. Am. Vet. Med. Assoc. 238, 318–328.

Ko, J.C., Marini, R.P., 2008. Anesthesia and analgesia in ferrets. In: Fish, R.E., Danneman, P.J., Brown, M.J., Karas, A.Z. (Eds.), Anesthesia and Analgesia in Laboratory Animals, second ed. Academic Press, Boston, pp. 443–456. (Chapter 16).

Ko, J.C., Marini, R.P., 2014. Anesthesia. In: Fox, J.G., Marini, R.P. (Eds.), Biology and diseases of the ferret, third ed. Wiley and Sons, Ames, IA. (Chapter 12).

Ko, J.C., Nicklin, C.F., Montgomery, T., Kuo, W.C., 1998. Comparison of anesthetic and cardiorespiratory effects of tiletamine-zolazepam-xylazine and tiletamine-xylazine-butorphanol in ferrets. J. Am. Anim. Hosp. Assoc. 34, 164–174.

Ko, J.C.H., Thurmon, J.C., Benson, G.J., Gard, J., Tranquilli, W.J., Olson, W.A., 1992a. Evaluation of analgesia induced by epidural injection of detomidine or xylazine in swine. J. Vet. Anesth 19, 56–60.

Ko, J.C.H., Thurmon, J.C., Tranquili, W.J., Benson, G.J., Olson, W.A., 1992b. Comparison of medetomidine-propofol and medetomidine-midazolam-propofol anesthesia in rabbits. Lab. Anim. Sci. 42, 503–507.

Ko, J.C.H., Williams, B.L., McGrath, C.J., Short, C.E., Rogers, E.R., 1997. Comparison of anesthetic effects of Telazol-xylazine-xylazine, Telazol-xylazine-butorphanol, and Telazol-xylazine-azaperone combinations in swine. Lab. Anim. Sci. 35, 71–74.

Kohn, D.F., Wixson, S.K., White, W.J., Benson, G.J. (Eds.), 1997. Anesthesia and Analgesia in Laboratory Animals. Academic Press, New York.

Kohn, D.F., Martin, T.E., Foley, P.L., Morris, T.H., Swindle, M.M., Vogler, G.A., et al., 2006. ACLAM Task Force: Guidelines for the Assessment and Management of Pain in Rodents and Rabbits [Online]. Available: <http://www.aclam.org/Content/files/files/Public/Active/position_pain-rodent-rabbit.pdf>. (accessed 20.01.14).

Koizuka, S., Obata, H., Sasaki, M., Saito, S., Goto, F., 2005. Systemic ketamine inhibits hypersensitivity after surgery via descending inhibitory pathways in rats. Can. J. Anaesth. 52, 498–505.

Kolesnikov, Y., Cristea, M., Oksman, G., Torosjan, A., Wilson, R., 2004. Evaluation of the tail formalin test in mice as a new model to assess local analgesic effects. Brain Res. 1029, 217–223.

Kolstad, A.M., Rodriguiz, R.M., Kim, C.J., Hale, L.P., 2012. Effect of pain management on immunization efficacy in mice. J. Am. Assoc. Lab. Anim. Sci. 51, 448–457.

Korner, P.I., Uther, J.B., White, S.W., 1968. Circulatory effects of chloralose-urethane and sodium pentobarbitone anaesthesia in the rabbit. J. Physiol. 199, 253–265.

Koshika, K., Ichinhe, T., Kaneko, Y., 2011. Dose-dependent remifentanyl decreases oral tissue blood flow during sevoflurane and propofol anesthesia in rabbits. J. Oral. Maxillfac. Surg. 69, 2128–2134.

Kroin, J.S., Buvanendran, A., Tuman, K.J., Kerns, J.M., 2012. Safety of local anesthetics administered intrathecally in diabetic rats. Pain Med. (Malden, Mass.) 13, 802–807.

Krueger, K.L., Fujiwara, Y., 2008. The use of buprenorphine as an analgesic after rodent embryo transfer. Lab. Anim. (NY). 37, 87–90.

Krugner-Higby, L., Smith, L., Clark, M., Heath, T.D., Dahly, E., Schiffman, B., et al., 2003. Liposome-encapsulated oxymorphone hydrochloride provides prolonged relief of postsurgical visceral pain in rats. Comp. Med. 53, 270–279.

Kumar, A., Thurmon, J., 1979. Cardiopulmonary, hemocytologic and biochemical effects of xylazine in goats. Lab. Anim. Sci. 29, 486–491.

Kumar, G., Hota, D., Nahar Saikia, U., Pandhi, P., 2010. Evaluation of analgesic efficacy, gastrotoxicity and nephrotoxicity of fixed-dose combinations of nonselective, preferential and selective cyclooxygenase inhibitors with paracetamol in rats. Exp. Toxicol. Pathol. 62, 653–662.

Kyles, A.E., Waterman, A.E., Livingston, A., 1995. Antinociceptive activity of midazolam in sheep. J. Vet. Pharmacol. Ther. 18, 54–60.

Lagutchik, M.S., Mundie, T.G., Martin, D.G., 1992. Methemoglobinemia induced by a benzocaine-based topically administered anesthetic in eight sheep. J. Am. Vet. Med. Assoc. 201, 1407–1410.

Lamon, T.K., Browder, E.J., Sohrabji, F., Ihrig, M., 2008. Adverse effects of incorporating ketoprofen into established rodent studies. J. Am. Assoc. Lab. Anim. Sci. 47, 20–24.

Lamont, L., 2009. Alpha-2 agonists. In: Gaynor, J.S., Muir, W.W. (Eds.), Handbook of Veterinary Pain Management. Mosby Elsevier, St. Louis, MO.

Langerman, L., Chaimsky, G., Golomb, E., Tverskoy, M., Kook, A., 1990. Rabbit model for evaluation of spinal anesthesia: chronic cannulation of the subarachnoid space. Anesth. Analg. 71, 529–535.

Langford, D.J., Bailey, A.L., Chanda, M.L., Clarke, S.E., Drummond, T.E., Echols, S., et al., 2010. Coding of facial expressions of pain in the laboratory mouse. Nat. Methods 7, 447–449.

Laprairie, J.L., Murphy, A.Z., 2010. Long-term impact of neonatal injury in male and female rats: sex differences, mechanisms and clinical implications. Front. Neuroendocrinol. 31, 193–202.

Laprairie, J.L., Johns, M.E., Murphy, A.Z., 2008. Preemptive morphine analgesia attenuates the long-term consequences of neonatal inflammation in male and female rats. Pediatr. Res. 64, 625–630.

Leach, M.C., Bowell, V.A., Allan, T.F., Morton, D.B., 2002a. Aversion to gaseous euthanasia agents in rats and mice. Comp. Med. 52, 249–257.

Leach, M.C., Bowell, V.A., Allan, T.F., Morton, D.B., 2002b. Degrees of aversion shown by rats and mice to different concentrations of inhalational anaesthetics. Vet. Rec. 150, 808–815.

Leach, M.C., Allweiler, S., Richardson, C., Roughan, J.V., Narbe, R., Flecknell, P.A., 2009. Behavioural effects of ovariohysterectomy and oral administration of meloxicam in laboratory housed rabbits. Res. Vet. Sci. 87, 336–347.

Leach, M.C., Bailey, H.E., Dickinson, A.L., Roughan, J.V., Flecknell, P.A., 2010a. A preliminary investigation into the practicality of use and duration of action of slow-release preparations of morphine and hydromorphone in laboratory rats. Lab. Anim. 44, 59–65.

Leach, M.C., Forrester, A.R., Flecknell, P.A., 2010b. Influence of preferred foodstuffs on the antinociceptive effects of orally administered buprenorphine in laboratory rats. Lab. Anim. 44, 54–58.

Leach, M.C., Klaus, K., Miller, A.L., Scotto Di Perrotolo, M., Sotocinal, S.G., Flecknell, P.A., 2012. The assessment of post-vasectomy pain in mice using behaviour and the Mouse Grimace Scale. PLoS One 7, e35656.

Leary, S., Underwood, W., Anthony, R., Cartner, S., Corey, D., Grandin, T., et al., 2013. AVMA Guidelines for the Euthanasia of Animals: 2013 Edition [Online]. Available: <http://works.bepress.com/cheryl_greenacre/14> (accessed 20.01.14).

Leash, A.M., Beyer, R.D., Wilber, R.G., 1973. Self-mutilation following Innovar-Vet injection in the guinea pig. Lab. Anim. Sci. 23 (5), 720–721.

Lee, D., Swanson, C., 1996. General principles of anesthesia and sedation in food animals. Vet. Clin. North Am. Food Anim. Pract. 12, 473–480.

Leek, B.F., 2004. Digestion in the ruminant stomach. In: Reece, W.O. (Ed.), Duke's Physiology of Domestic Animals, twelfth ed. Cornell University Press, Ithaca, NY.

Lefkov, S.H., Mussig, D., 2007. Tiletamine-zolazepam and xylazine is a potent cardiodepressive combination: a case report. JAALAS 46, 42–43.

Lewis, J.C., 1993. Medetomidine-ketamine anaesthesia in the chimpanzee (Pan troglodytes). J. Vet. Anaesthesiol. 20, 18–20.

Lichtenberger, M., 2006. Shock, fluid therapy, anesthesia and analgesia in the ferret. Exot. DVM 7, 24–30.

Lichtenberger, M., Ko, J., 2007. Anesthesia and analgesia for small mammals and birds. Vet. Clin. North Am. Exot. Anim. Pract. 10, 293–315.

Liles, J.H., Flecknell, P.A., 1993. The influence of buprenorphine or bupivacaine on the post-operative effects of laparotomy and bile-duct ligation in rats. Lab. Anim. 27, 374–380.

Lin, H., Purohit, R.C., Powe, T.A., 1997. Anesthesia in sheep with propofol or with xylazine-ketamine followed by halothane. Vet. Surg. 26, 247–252.

Lin, H., Riddell, M.G., DeGraves, F.J., 1999. Comparison of three α2-antagonists, yohimbine, tolazoline, or atipamezole for reversing the anesthetic effects of medetomidine and ketamine in dairy calves. Bovine Pract. 33, 21–28.

Lin, H.C., Pugh, D.G., 2002. Anesthetic management. In: Pugh, D.G. (Ed.), Sheep and Goat Medicine. Saunders, Philadelphia, PA.

Lin, H.C., Tyler, J.W., Welles, E.G., Spano, J.S., Thurmon, J.C., Wolfe, D.F., 1993. Effects of anesthesia induced and maintained by continuous intravenous administration of guaifenesin, ketamine, and xylazine in spontaneously breathing sheep. Am. J. Vet. Res. 54, 1913–1916.

Lindquist, P.A., 1972. Induction of methoxyflurane anesthesia in the rabbit after ketamine hydrochloride and endotracheal intubation. Lab. Anim. Sci. 22, 898–899.

Lipman, N.S., Marini, R.P., Erdman, S.E., 1990. Comparison of ketamine/xylazine and ketamine/xylazine/acepromazine anesthesia in the rabbit. Lab. Anim. Sci. 40, 395–398.

Lipman, N.S., Marini, R.P., Flecknell, P.A., 1997. Anesthesia and analgesia in rabbits. In: Kohn, D.F., Wixson, S.K., White, W.J., Benson, G.J. (Eds.), Anesthesia and Analgesia in Laboratory Animals. Academic Press, New York, pp. 205–232.

Lipman, N.S., Marini, R.P., Flecknell, P.A., 2008. Anesthesia and analgesia in rabbits. In: Fish, R.E., Brown, M.J., Danneman, P.J., Karas, A.Z. (Eds.), Anesthesia and Analgesia in Laboratory Animals. Elsevier, London, pp. 299–333.

Liu, J.V., Sur, M., Moore, C.I., Sharma, J., 2008. Orientation maps in ferret visual cortex measured by multi-slice fMRI. Proc. Intl. Soc. Mag. Reson. Med. 16, 155.

Logdberg, B., 1988. Alphaxolone-alphadolone for anesthesia in squirrel monkeys of different ages. J. Med. Primatol. 17, 163–167.

Lovell, D.P., 1986a. Variation in pentobarbitone sleeping time in mice. 1. Strain and sex differences. Lab. Anim. 20, 85–90.

Lovell, D.P., 1986b. Variation in pentobarbitone sleeping time in mice. 2. Variables affecting test results. Lab. Anim. 20, 91–96.

Lovell, D.P., 1986c. Variation in pentobarbitone sleeping time in mice. 3. Strain X environment interactions. Lab. Anim. 20, 307–312.

Ludlage, E., Mansfield, K., 2003. Clinical care and diseases of the common marmoset (Callithrix jacchus). Comp. Med. 53 (4), 369–382.

Lukasik, V.M., Nogami, W.M., Morgan, S.E., 1998a. Minimum alveolar concentration and cardiovascular effects of desflurane in sheep. Vet. Surg. 27, 167.

Lukasik, V.M., Nogami, W.M., Morgan, S.E., 1998b. Minimum alveolar concentration and cardiovascular effects of sevoflurane in sheep. Vet. Surg. 27, 168.

MacPhail, C.M., Monnet, E., Gaynor, J.S., Perini, A., 2004. Effect of sevoflurane on hemodynamic and cardiac energetic parameters in ferrets. Am. J. Vet. Res. 65, 653–658.

Madsen, J., Jensen, F., Faber, T., Bill-Hansen, V., 1993. Chronic catheterization of the epidural space in rabbits: a model for behavioural and histopathologial studies–examination of meptazinol neurotoxicity. Acta. Anaesthesiol. Scand. 37, 307–313.

Maggi, C.A., Manzini, S., Parlani, M., Meli, A., 1984. Analysis of the effects of urethane on cardiovascular responsiveness to catecholamines in terms of its interference with Ca++ mobilization from both intra and extracellular pools. Experientia 40, 52–59.

Malakoff, R.L., Laste, N.J., Orcutt, C.J., 2012. Echocardiographic and electrocardiographic findings in client-owned ferrets: 95 cases (1994–2009). J. Am. Vet. Med. Assoc. 241, 1484–1489.

Makowska, I.J., Weary, D.M., 2009a. Rat aversion to induction with inhalant anaesthetics. Appl. Anim. Behav. Sci. 119, 229–235.

Makowska, I.J., Weary, D.M., 2009b. Rat aversion to carbon monoxide. Appl. Anim. Behav. Sci. 121, 148–151.

Makowska, I.J., Weary, D.M., 2013. Assessing the emotions of laboratory rats. Appl. Anim. Behav. Sci. 148, 1–12.

Makowska, I.J., Niel, L., Kirkden, R.D., Weary, D.M., 2008. Rats show aversion to argon-induced hypoxia. Appl. Anim. Behav. Sci. 114, 572–581.

Makowska, I.J., Vickers, L., Mancell, J., Weary, D.M., 2009. Evaluating methods of gas euthanasia for laboratory mice. Appl. Anim. Behav. Sci. 121, 230–235.

Makowska, J., Golledge, H., Marquardt, N., Weary, D.M., 2012. Sedation or inhalant anesthesia before euthanasia with CO2 does not reduce behavioral or physiologic signs of pain and stress in mice. J. Am. Assoc. Lab. Anim. Sci. 51, 396–397. author reply 397–399.

Malaivijitnond, S., Takenaka, O., Sankai, T., Yoshida, T., Cho, F., Yoshikawa, Y., 1998. Effects of single and multiple injections of ketamine hydrochloride on serum hormone concentrations in male cynomolgus monkeys. Lab. Anim. Sci. 48 (3), 270–274.

Malinosky, J.M., Bernard, J.M., Baudrimont, M., Dumand, J.B., Lepage, J.Y., 1997. A chronic model for experimental investigation of epidural anesthesia in the rabbit. Reg. Anaesth. 22, 80–85.

Mao, Y.T., Pallas, S.L., 2012. Compromise of auditory cortical tuning and topography after cross-modal invasion by visual inputs. J. Neurosci. 32, 10338–10351.

Marano, G., Formigari, R., Grigioni, M., Vergari, A., 1997. Effects of isoflurane versus halothane on myocardial contractility in rabbits: assessment with transthoracic two-dimensional echocardiography. Lab. Anim. 31, 144–150.

Marini, R.P., Avison, D.L., Corning, B.F., Lipman, N.S., 1992. Ketamine/xylazine/butorphanol: a new anesthetic combination for rabbits. Lab. Anim. Sci. 42, 57–62.

Marini, R.P., Hurley, R.J., Avison, D.L., Lipman, N.S., 1993. Evaluation of three neuroleptanalgesic combinations in the rabbit. Lab. Anim. Sci. 43, 338–345.

Marini, R.P., Callahan, R.J., Jackson, L.R., Jyawook, S., Esteves, M.I., et al., 1997. Distribution of technetium99-m-labeled red blood cells during isoflurane anesthesia in the ferret. Am. J. Vet. Res. 58, 781–785.

Marini, R.P., 2014. Physical examination, preventative medicine, and diagnosis in the ferret. In: Fox, J.G., Marini, R.P. (Eds.), Biology and diseases of the ferret. Wiley and Sons, Ames IA, pp. 235–258. (Chapter 11).

Martin, L.B., Thompson, A.C., Martin, T., Kristal, M.B., 2001. Analgesic efficacy of orally administered buprenorphine in rats. Comp. Med. 51, 43–48.

Martín-Cancho, M.F., Lima, J.R., Luis, L., Crisóstomo, V., Carrasco-Jiménez, M.S., Usón-Gargallo, J., 2006. Relationship of bispectral index values, haemodynamic changes and recovery times during sevoflurane or propofol anaesthesia in rabbits. Lab. Anim. 40, 28.

Matsumiya, L.C., Sorge, R.E., Sotocinal, S.G., Tabaka, J.M., Wieskopf, J.S., Zaloum, A., et al., 2012. Using the Mouse Grimace Scale to reevaluate the efficacy of postoperative analgesics in laboratory mice. J. Am. Assoc. Lab. Anim. Sci. 51, 42–49.

Matthias, N., Robinson, M.A., Crook, R., Lockworth, C.R., Goodwin Jr., B.S., 2013. Local cryoanalgesia is effective for tail-tip biopsy in mice. J. Am. Assoc. Lab. Anim. Sci. 52, 171–175.

Mazaheri-Khameneh, R., Sarrafzadeh-Rezaei, F., Asri-Rezaei, S., Dalir-Naghadeh, B., 2012. Comparison of time to loss of consciousness and maintenance of anesthesia following intraosseous and intravenous administration of propofol in rabbits. J. Am. Vet. Med. Assoc. 241, 73–80.

McGuirk, S., Bednarski, R., Clayton, M., 1990. Bradycardia in cattle deprived of food. J. Am. Vet. Med. Assoc. 196, 894–896.

Mcintyre, A.R., Drummond, R.A., Riedel, E.R., Lipman, N.S., 2007. Automated mouse euthanasia in an individually ventilated caging system: system development and assessment. J. Am. Assoc. Lab. Anim. Sci. 46, 65–73.

Mckeon, G.P., Pacharinsak, C., Long, C.T., Howard, A.M., Jampachaisri, K., Yeomans, D.C., et al., 2011. Analgesic effects of tramadol, tramadol-gabapentin, and buprenorphine in an incisional model of pain in rats (Rattus norvegicus). J. Am. Assoc. Lab. Anim. Sci. 50, 192–197.

Mert, T., Gunes, Y., 2012. Antinociceptive activities of lidocaine and the nav1.8 blocker a803467 in diabetic rats. J. Am. Assoc. Lab. Anim. Sci. 51, 579–585.

Meyer, R.E., Fish, R.E., 2005. A review of tribromoethanol anesthesia for production of genetically engineered mice and rats. Lab. Anim. (NY). 34, 47–52.

Mickley, G.A., Hoxha, Z., Biada, J.M., Kenmuir, C.L., Bacik, S.E., 2006. Acetaminophen self-administered in the drinking water increases the pain threshold of rats (Rattus norvegicus). J. Am. Assoc. Lab. Anim. Sci. 45, 48–54.

Mills, P., Sessler, D.I., Moseley, M., Chew, W., Pereira, B., James, T.L., et al., 1987. In vivo 19F nuclear magnetic resonance study of isoflurane elimination from the rabbit brain. Anesthesiology 67, 169–173.

Minville, V., Fourcade, O., Girolami, J.P., Tack, I., 2010. Opioid-induced hyperalgesia in a mice model of orthopaedic pain: preventive effect of ketamine. Br. J. Anaesth. 104, 231–238.

Moens, Y.P.S., Gootjes, P., 1993. The influence of methane on the infrared measurement of anesthetic vapor concentration. Anaesthesia 48, 270.

Mohamadnia, A.R., Hughes, G., Clarke, K.W., 2008. Maintenance of anaesthesia in sheep with isoflurane, desflurane or sevoflurane. Vet. Rec. 163, 210–215.

Molthen, R.C., 2006. A simple, inexpensive, and effective light- carrying laryngoscopic blade for orotracheal intubation of rats. J. Am. Assoc. Lab. Anim. Sci. 45, 88–93.

Monfared, A.L., 2013. Applied anatomy of the rabbit's skull and its clinical application during regional anesthesia. Global Vet. 10, 653–657.

Moore, D.R., Kowlachuk, N.E., 1988. An anomaly in the brainstem projections of hypopigmented ferrets. Hear Res. 35, 275–278.

Morgan, J.E., Henderson, Z., Thompson, I.D., 1987. Retinal decussation patterns in pigmented and albino ferrets. Neuroscience 20, 519–535.

More, R.C., Kody, M.H., Kabo, J.M., Dorey, F.J., Meals, R.A., 1989. The effects of two non-steroidal anti-inflammatory drugs on limb swelling, joint stiffness, and bone torsional strength following fracture in a rabbit model. Clin. Orthop. 247, 306–312.

Morimoto, K., Nishimura, R., Matsunaga, S., Mochizuki, M., Sasaki, N., 2001. Epidural analgesia with a combination of bupivacaine and buprenorphine in rats. J. Vet. Med. A. Physiol. Pathol. Clin. Med. 48, 303–312.

Morio, M., Fujii, K., Satoh, N., Imai, M., Kawakami, U., Mizuno, T., et al., 1992. Reaction of sevoflurane and its degradation products with soda lime. Toxicity of the byproducts. Anesthesiology 77, 1155–1164.

Morita, H., Nashida, Y., Uemura, N., Hosomi, H., 1987. Effect of pentobarbital anesthesia on renal sympathetic nerve activity in the rabbit. J. Auton. Pharmacol. 20, 57–64.

Morton, D.B., Jennings, M., Buckwell, A., Ewbank, R., Godfrey, C., Holgate, B., et al., 2001. Refining procedures for the administration of substances. Report of the BVAAWF/FRAME/RSPCA/UFAW Joint Working Group on Refinement. British Veterinary Association Animal Welfare Foundation/Fund for the Replacement of Animals in Medical Experiments/Royal Society for the Prevention of Cruelty to Animals/Universities Federation for Animal Welfare. Lab. Anim. 35, 1–41.

Mpanduji, D.G., Bittegeko, S.B., Mgasa, M.N., Batamuzi, E.K., 2000. Analgesic, behavioural and cardiopulmonary effects of epidurally injected medetomidine (domitor) in goats. J. Vet. Med. A 47, 65–72.

Murat, I., Housmans, P.R., 1988. Minimum alveolar concentration of halothane, enflurane, and isoflurane in ferrets. Anesthesiology 68, 783–786.

Murphy, K.L., Roughan, J.V., Baxter, M.G., et al., 2010. Anaesthesia with a combination of ketamine and medetomidine in the rabbit: effect of premedication with buprenorphine. Vet. Anaesth. Analg. 37, 222–229.

Murrell, J.C., Mellor, D.J., Johnson, C.B., 2008. Chapter 27 – Aneaesthesia and Analgesia in the Foetus and Neonate. In: Fish, E.F., Brown, J.B., Danneman, J.D., Karas, Z.K. (Eds.), Anesthesia and Analgesia in Laboratory Animals, second ed. Academic Press, San Diego, CA.

Nader, M.A., Grant, K.A., Gage, H.D., Ehrenkraufer, R.L., Kaplan, J.R., Mach, R.H., 1999. PET imaging of dopamine D2 receptors with [18] fluoroclebopride in monkeys: effects of isoflurane– and ketamine-induced anesthesia. Neuropsychopharmacology 21 (4), 589–596.

National Research council, 2003. Guidelines for the Care and Use of Mammals in Neuroscience and Behavioral Research. National Academies Press, Washington DC.

National Research Council, 2009. Recognition and Allevation of Pain in Laboratory Animals. The National Academies Press, Washington, DC.

Nevlainen, T., Pyhala, L., Voipio, H.M., Virtanen, R., 1989. Evaluation of anaesthetic potency of medetomidine-ketamine combination in rats, guinea-pigs, and rabbits. Acta. Vet. Scand. 85, 139–143.

Newton, W.M., Cusick, P.K., Raffe, M.R., 1975. Innovar–Vet-induced pathologic changes in the guinea pig. Lab. Anim. Sci. 25, 597–601.

Nickel, R., Schummer, A., Seiferle, E., Sack, W.O., 1973. The Viscera of the Domestic Mammals. Springer-Verlag, New York.

Niel, L., Weary, D.M., 2006. Behavioural responses of rats to gradual-fill carbon dioxide euthanasia and reduced oxygen concentrations. Appl. Anim. Behav. Sci. 100, 295–308.

Niel, L., Weary, D.M., 2007. Rats avoid exposure to carbon dioxide and argon. Appl. Anim. Behav. Sci. 107, 100–109.

Niel, L., Kirkden, R.D., Weary, D.M., 2008a. Effects of novelty on rats' responses to CO2 exposure. Appl. Anim. Behav. Sci. 111, 183–194.

Niel, L., Stewart, S.A., Weary, D.M., 2008b. Effect of flow rate on aversion to gradual-fill carbon dioxide exposure in rats. Appl. Anim. Behav. Sci. 109, 77–84.

Nishizawa, S., Ichinobe, T., Kaneko, Y., 2012. Tissue blood flow reductions induced by remifentanil and the effect of naloxone and phentolamine on these changes. J. Oral Maxillfac. Surg. 70, 797–802.

Nolan, A., Livingston, A., Waterman, A.E., 1987. Investigation of the antinociceptive activity of buprenorphine in sheep. Br. J. Pharmacol. 92, 527–533.

NRC, 2011. Guide for the Care and Use of Laboratory Animals. National Academies Press, Washington, DC.

Nunamaker, E.A., Halliday, L.C., Moody, D.E., Fang, W.B., Lindeblad, M., Fortman, J.D., 2013. Pharmacokinetics of 2 formulations of buprenorphine in macaques (Macaca mulatta and Macaca fascicularis). J. Am. Assoc. Lab. Anim. Sci. 52 (1), 48.

Obernier, J.A., Baldwin, R.L., 2006. Establishing an appropriate period of acclimatization following transportation of laboratory animals. ILAR. J. 47, 364–369.

Olin, J.M., Smith, T.J., Talcott, M.R., 1997. Evaluation of non-invasive monitoring techniques in domestic ferrets (Mustela putorius furo). Am. J. Vet. Res. 58, 1065–1069.

Olson, M.E., Vizzutti, D., Morck, D.W., Cox, A.K., 1994. The parasympatholytic effects of atropine sulfate and glycopyrrolate in rats and rabbits. Can. J. Vet. Res. 57, 254–258.

Otero, P.E., Portela, D.A., Brinkyer, J.A., Tarragona, L., Zaccagnini, A.S., Fuensalida, S.E., et al., 2012. Use of electrical stimulation to monitor lumbosacral epidural and intrathecal needle placement in rabbits. Am. J. Vet. Res. 73, 1137–1141.

Otto, K.A., Steiner, K.H.S., Zailskas, F., Wippermann, B., 2000. Comparison of the postoperative analgesic effects of buprenorphine and piritramide following experimental orthopaedic surgery in sheep. J. Exp. Anim. Sci. 41, 133–143.

Page, G.G., 2002. Analgesia administration attenuates surgery-induced tumor promotion. Reg. Anesth. Pain Med. 27, 197–199.

Page, G.G., Ben-Eliyahu, S., 2002. Indomethacin attenuates the immunosuppressive and tumor-promoting effects of surgery. J. Pain. 3, 301–308.

Paluch, L.R., Lieggi, C.C., Dumont, M., Monette, S., Riedel, E.R., Lipman, N.S., 2014. Developmental and behavioral effects of toe clipping on neonatal and preweanling mice with and without vapocoolant anesthesia. J. Am. Assoc. Lab. Anim. Sci. 53 (2), 132–140.

Papaioannou, V.E., Fox, J.G., 1993. Use and efficacy of tribromoethanol anesthesia in the mouse. Lab. Anim. Sci. 43 (2), 189–192.

Park, I., Kim, D., Song, J., In, C.H., Jeong, S.W., Lee, S.H., et al., 2008. Buprederm, a new transdermal delivery system of buprenorphine: pharmacokinetic, efficacy and skin irritancy studies. Pharm. Res. 25, 1052–1062.

Parker, J.M., Austin, J., Wilkerson, J., Carbone, L., 2011. Effects of multimodal analgesia on the success of mouse embryo transfer surgery. J. Am. Assoc. Lab. Anim. Sci. 50, 466–470.

Paull, D.R., Lee, C., Colditz, I.G., Atkinson, S.J., Fisher, A.D., 2007. The effect of a topical anaesthetic formulation, systemic flunixin and carprofen, singly or in combination, on cortisol and behavioural responses of merino lambs to mulesing. Aust. Vet. J. 85, 98–106.

Payton, A.J., Forsythe, D.B., Dixon, D., Myers, P.H., Clark, J.A., Snipe, J.R., 1993. Evaluation of ketamine-xylazine in Syrian hamsters. Cornell. Vet. 83, 153–161.

Peeters, M.E., Gil, D., Teske, E., Eyzenbach, V., van der Brom, W.E., Lumeij, J.T., et al., 1988. Four methods for general anesthesia in the rabbit: a comparative study. Lab. Anim. 22, 355–360.

Penderis, J., Franklin, R.J., 2005. Effects of pre- versus post-anaesthetic buprenorphine on propofol-anaesthetized rats. Vet. Anaesth. Analg. 32, 256–260.

Pérez-García, C.C., Peña-Penabad, M., Cano-Rábano, M.J., García-Rodríguez, M.B., Gallego-Morales, D., Ríos-Granja, M.A., et al., 2003. A simple procedure to perform intravenous injections in the Mongolian gerbil (Meriones unguiculatus). Lab. Anim. 37, 68–71.

Pham, T.M., Hagman, B., Codita, A., Van Loo, P.L.P., Strömmer, L., Baumans, V., 2010. Housing environment influences the need for pain relief during post-operative recovery in mice. Physiol. Behav. 99, 663–668.

Picazo, M.G., Benito, P.J., García-Olmo, D.C., 2009. Efficiency and safety of a technique for drawing blood from the hamster cranial vena cava. Lab. Anim. (NY). 38, 211–216.

Piersma, F.E., Daemen, M.A., Bogaard, A.E., Buurman, W.A., 1999. Interference of pain control employing opioids in in vivo immunological experiments. Lab. Anim. 33, 328–333.

Plumb, D.C., 2011. Plumb's Veterinary Drug Handbook. Wiley-Blackwell, Ames, IA.

Plummer, P.J., Schleining, J.A., 2013. Assessment and management of pain in small ruminants and camelids. Vet. Clin. North Am. Food Anim. Pract. 29, 185–208.

Popilskis, S., Daniel, S., Smiley, R., 1994. Effects of epidural versus intravenous morphine analgesia on postoperative catecholamine response in baboons. In: "Proceedings of the Fifth International Congress of Veterinary Anaesthesia," August 21–25, Guelph, Canada.

Popilskis, S.J., Danilo, P., Acosta, H., Kohn, D.K., 1992. Is preoperative fasting necessary? J. Med. Primatol. 21, 349–352.

Portier, D.B., Slusser, C.A., 1985. Azaperone: a review of a new neuroleptic agent for swine. Vet. Med. 80, 88–92.

Prassinos, N.N., Galatos, A.D., Raptopoulos, D., 2005. A comparison of propofol, thiopental or ketamine as induction agents in goats. Vet. Anaesth. Analg. 32, 289–296.

Pritchett-Corning, K.R., 2009. Euthanasia of neonatal rats with carbon dioxide. J. Am. Assoc. Lab. Anim. Sci. 48, 23–27.

Qian, J., Brown, S.D., Carlton, S.M., 1996. Systemic ketamine attenuates nociceptive behaviors in a rat model of peripheral neuropathy. Brain. Res. 715, 51–62.

Queiroz-Castro, P., Egger, C., Redua, M.A., Rohrbach, B.W., Cox, S., Doherty, T., 2006. Effects of ketamine and magnesium on the minimum alveolar concentration of isoflurane in goats. Am. J. Vet. Res. 67, 1962–1966.

Radositits, O.M., Gay, C.C., Hinchcliff, K.W., Constable, P.D., 2007. Veterinary Medicine. Saunders, Philadelphia, PA.

Raekallio, M., Kivalo, M., Jalanka, H., Vainio, O., 1991. Medetomidine/ketamine sedation in calves and its reversal with atipamezole. Vet. Anaesth. Analg. 18, 45–47.

Ramsey, D.E., Aldred, N., Power, J.M., 1993. A simplified approach to the anesthesia of porcine laparoscopic surgical subjects. Lab. Anim. Sci. 43, 336–337.

Ranheim, B., Arnemo, J.M., Stuen, S., Horsberg, T.E., 2000a. Medetomidine and atipamezole in sheep: disposition and clinical effects. J. Vet. Pharmacol. Ther. 23, 401–404.

Ranheim, B., Horsberg, T.E., Soli, N.E., Ryeng, K.A., Arnemo, J.M., 2000b. The effects of medetomidine and its reversal with atipamezole on plasma glucose, cortisol and noradrenaline in cattle and sheep. J. Vet. Pharmacol. Ther. 23, 379–387.

Ranheim, B., Soli, N.E., Ryeng, K.A., Arnemo, J.M., Horsberg, T.E., 1998. Pharmacokinetics of medetomidine and atipamezole in dairy calves: an agonist–antagonist interaction. J. Vet. Pharmacol. Ther. 21, 428–432.

Rätsep, M.T., Barrette, V.F., Winterborn, A., Adams, M.A., Croy, B.A., 2013. Hemodynamic and behavioral differences after administration of meloxicam, buprenorphine, or tramadol as analgesics for telemeter implantation in mice. J. Am. Assoc. Lab. Anim. Sci. 52, 560–566.

Rees Davies, R., Rees Davies, J.A.E., 2003. Rabbit gastrointestinal physiology. Vet. Clin. North. Am. Exot. Anim. Pract. 6 (1), 139–153.

Reid, J., Nolan, A.M., Welsh, E., 1993. Propofol as an induction agent in the goat: a pharmacokinetic study. J. Vet. Pharmacol. Ther. 16, 488–493.

Rezakhani, A., Edjtehadi, M., Szabuniewicz, M., 1977. Prevention of thiopental and thiopental-halothane cardiac sensitization to epinephrine in sheep. Can. J. Comp. Med. 41, 389–395.

Rich, G.F., Sullivan, M.P., Adams, J.M., 1990. Is distal sampling of end-tidal CO2 necessary in small subjects? Anesthesiology 73 (2), 265–268.

Richard, B.M., Newton, P., Ott, L.R., Haan, D., Brubaker, A.N., Richardson, C.A., et al., 2005. Anaesthesia and post-operative analgesia following experimental surgery in laboratory rodents: are we making progress? Altern. Lab. Anim. 33, 119–127.

Riebold, T.W., 2007. Ruminants. In: Tranquilli, W.J., Thurmon, J.C., Grimm, K.A. (Eds.), Lumb & Jones' Veterinary Anesthesia and Analgesia, fourth ed. Blackwell Publishing, Ames, IA.

Rioja, E., Kerr, C.L., Enouri, S.S., McDonell, W.N., 2008. Sedative and cardiopulmonary effects of medetomidine hydrochloride and xylazine hydrochloride and their reversal with atipamezole hydrochloride in calves. Am. J. Vet. Res. 69, 319–329.

Robson, W.L., Bayliss, C.E., Feldman, R., Goldstein, M.B., Chen, C.B., Richardson, R.M.A., et al., 1981. Evaluation of the effect of pentobarbital anaesthesia on the plasma potassium concentration in the rabbit and the dog. Can. Anaesth. Soc. J. 28, 210–216.

Rock, M.L., Karas, A.Z., Rodriguez, K.B., Gallo, M.S., Pritchett-Corning, K., Karas, R.H., et al., 2014. The Time-to-Integrate-to-Nest Test as an Indicator of Wellbeing in Laboratory Mice. J. Am. Assoc. Lab. Anim. Sci. 53, 24–28.

Rooks II, W.H., Maloney, P.J., Shott, L.D., Schuler, M.E., Sevelius, H., Strosberg, A.M., et al., 1985. The analgesic and anti-inflammatory profile of ketorolac and its tromethamine salt. Drugs. Exp. Clin. Res. 11, 479–492.

Roughan, J.V., Flecknell, P.A., 2001. Behavioural effects of laparotomy and analgesic effects of ketoprofen and carprofen in rats. Pain 90, 65–74.

Roughan, J.V., Flecknell, P.A., 2002. Buprenorphine: a reappraisal of its antinociceptive effects and therapeutic use in alleviating postoperative pain in animals. Lab. Anim. 36, 322–343.

Roughan, J.V., Flecknell, P.A., 2003a. Evaluation of a short duration behaviour-based post-operative pain scoring system in rats. Eur. J. Pain 7, 397–406.

Roughan, J.V., Flecknell, P.A., 2004. Behaviour-based assessment of the duration of laparotomy-induced abdominal pain and the analgesic effects of carprofen and buprenorphine in rats. Behav. Pharmacol. 15, 461–472.

Roughan, J.V., Flecknell, P.A., Davies, B.R., 2004. Behavioural assessment of the effects of tumour growth in rats and the influence of the analgesics carprofen and meloxicam. Lab. Anim. 38, 286–296.

Roughan, J.V., Wright-Williams, S.L., Flecknell, P.A., 2009. Automated analysis of postoperative behaviour: assessment of HomeCageScan as a novel method to rapidly identify pain and analgesic effects in mice. Lab. Anim. 43, 17–26.

Roustan, A., Perrin, J., Berthelot-Ricou, A., Lopez, E., Botta, A., Courbiere, B., 2012. Evaluating methods of mouse euthanasia on the oocyte quality: cervical dislocation versus isoflurane inhalation. Lab. Anim. 46, 167–169.

Royal, J.M., Settle, T.L., Bobo, M., Lombardini, E., Kent, M.L., Upp, J., et al., 2013. Assessment of postoperative analgesia after application of ultrasound-guided regional anesthesia for surgery in a swine femoral fracture model. J. Am. Assoc. Lab. Anim. Sci. 52, 265–276.

Saha, D.C., Saha, A.C., Malik, G., Astiz, M.E., Rackow, E.C., 2007. Comparison of cardiovascular effects of tiletamine-zolazepam, pentobarbital, and ketamine-xylazine in male rats. J. Am. Assoc. Lab. Anim. Sci. 46, 74–80.

Sainsbury, A.W., Eaton, B.D., Cooper, J.E., 1991. An investigation into the use of propofol (Rapinovet) in long-tailed macaques (Macaca fascicularis). J. Vet. Anaesthesiol. 18, 38–41.

Sanders, E.A., Gleed, R.D., Nathanielsz, R.W., 1991. Anesthetic management for instrumentation of the pregnant rhesus monkeys. J. Med. Primatol. 20, 223–228.

Santus, G., Rivolta, R., Bottoni, G., Testa, B., Canali, S., Peano, S., 1993. Nasal formulations of ketorolac tromethamine: technological evaluation–bioavailability and tolerability in rabbits. Farmaco 48, 1709–1723.

Sato, C., Sakai, A., Ikeda, Y., Suzuki, H., Sakamoto, A., 2008. The prolonged analgesic effect of epidural ropivacaine in a rat model of neuropathic pain. Anesth. Analg. 106, 313–320.

Sazuka, S., Matsuura, N., Ichinohe, T., 2012. Dexmedetomidine dose dependently decreases oral tissue blood flow during sevoflurane and propofol anesthesia in rabbits. J. Oral Maxillfac. Surg. 70, 1808–1814.

Schaap, M.W.H., Uilenreef, J.J., Mitsogiannis, M.D., Van 'T Klooster, J.G., Arndt, S.S., Hellebrekers, L.J., 2012. Optimizing the dosing interval of buprenorphine in a multimodal postoperative analgesic strategy in the rat: minimizing side-effects without affecting weight gain and food intake. Lab. Anim. 46, 287–292.

Schauvliege, S., Narine, K., Bouchez, S., Desmet, D., Van Parys, V., Van Nooten, G., et al., 2006. Refined anaesthesia for implantation of engineered experimental aortic valves in the pulmonary artery using a right heart bypass in sheep. Lab. Anim. 40, 341–352.

Scheller, M.S., Saidman, L.J., Partridge, B.L., 1988. MAC of sevoflurane in humans and New Zealand White rabbits. Can. J. Anaesth. 35, 153–156.

Schmidt, J.R., Krugner-Higby, L., Heath, T.D., Sullivan, R., Smith, L.J., 2011. Epidural administration of liposome-encapsulated hydromorphone provides extended analgesia in a rodent model of stifle arthritis. J. Am. Assoc. Lab. Anim. Sci. 50, 507–512.

Schnellbacher, R.W., Carpenter, J.W., Diane, E., Mason, D.E., KuKanich, B., Beaufrère, H., et al., 2013. Effects of lidocaine administration via continuous rate infusion on the minimum alveolar concentration of isoflurane in New Zealand White rabbits (Oryctolagus cuniculus). Amer. J. Vet. Res. 74.

Schwenke, D.O., Cragg, P.A., 2004. Comparison of the depressive effects of four anesthetic regimens on ventilatory and cardiovascular variables in the guinea pig. Comp. Med. 54, 77–85.

Sebel, P.S., Lowdon, J.D., 1989. Propofol: a new intravenous anesthetic. Anesthesiology 71, 250–277.

Sedgwick, C.J., 1986. Anesthesia for rabbits. Vet. Clin. North. Am. Food. Anim. Pract. 2, 731–736.

Sellers, G., Lin, H.C., Chamorro, M.F., Walz, P.H., 2013. Comparison of isoflurane and sevoflurane anesthesia in holstein calves for placement of portal and jugular vein cannulas. Am. J. Anim. Vet. Sci. 8, 1–7.

Sharma, J., Sur, M., 2014. The ferret as a model for visual system development and plasticity. In: Fox, J.G., Marini, R.P. (Eds.), Biology and diseases of the ferret. Wiley and Sons, Ames IA, pp. 711–734. (Chapter 30).

Shientag, L.J., Wheeler, S.M., Garlick, D.S., Maranda, L.S., 2012. A therapeutic dose of ketoprofen causes acute gastrointestinal bleeding, erosions, and ulcers in rats. J. Am. Assoc. Lab. Anim. Sci. 51, 832–841.

Short, C., 1986. Preanesthetic medications in ruminants and swine. Vet. Clin. North Am. Food Anim. Pract. 2, 553–566.

Shufflebarger, J.V., Doyle, J., Roth, T., Maguire, K., Rothkopf, D.M., 1996. The effect of ketorolac on microvascular thrombosis in an experimental rabbit model. Plast. Reconstr. Surg. 98, 140–145.

Silva, A., Campos, S., Monteiro, J., et al., 2011. Performance of anesthetic depth indexes in rabbits under propofol anesthesia. Anesthesiology 115, 303–314.

Silverman, J., Muir, W.W., 1993. A review of laboratory animal anesthesia with chloral hydrate and chloralose. Lab. Anim. Sci. 43 (3), 210–216.

Singh, J., Roy, S., Mukherjee, P., et al., 2010. Influence of topical anesthetics on oculocardiac reflex and corneal healing in rabbits. Int. J. Ophthalmol. 3, 14–18.

Skarda, R.T., Tranquilli, W.J., 2007. Local and regional anesthetic and analgesic techniques: ruminants and swine. In: Tranquilli, W.J., Thurmon, J.C., Grimm, K.A. (Eds.), Lumb and Jones' Veterinary Anesthesia and Analgesia, fourth ed. Blackwell Publishing, Ames, IA.

Sladsky, K.K., Horne, W.A., Goodrowe, K.L., Stoskopf, M.K., Loomis, M.R., et al., 2000. Evaluation of epidural morphine for postoperative analgesia in ferrets (Mustela putorius furo). Contemp. Top. Lab. Anim. Sci. 39, 33–38.

Sleeman, J., 2007. Great apes. In: Zoo Animal and Wildlife Immobilization and Anesthesia. pp. 387–394.

Smiler, K.L., Stein, S., Hrapkiewicz, K.L., Hiben, J.R., 1990. Tissue response to intramuscular and intraperitoneal injections of ketamine and xylazine in rats. Lab. Anim. Sci. 40, 60–64.

Smith, A.C., Swindle, M.M., 2008. Anesthesia and analgesia in swine. In: Fish, R., Danneman, P.J., Brown, M., Karas, A. (Eds.), Anesthesia and Analgesia in Laboratory Animals, second ed. Academic Press (Elsevier), New York, pp. 413–440.

Smith, A.C., Zellner, J.L., Spinale, F.G., Swindle, M.M., 1991. Sedative and cardiovascular effects of midazolam in swine. Lab. Anim. Sci. 41, 157–161.

Smith, A.C., Ehler, W., Swindle, M.M., 1997. Anesthesia and analgesia in swine. In: Kohn, D.F., Wixson, S.K., White, W.J., Benson, G.J. (Eds.), Anesthesia and Analgesia in Laboratory Animals Academic Press, New York, pp. 313–336.

Smith, E., Modric, S., 2013. Regulatory considerations for the approval of analgesic drugs for cattle in the united states. Vet. Clin. North Am. Food Anim. Pract. 29, 1–10.

Smith, G., 2013. Extralabel use of anesthetic and analgesic compounds in cattle. Vet. Clin. North Am. Food Anim. Pract. 29, 29–46.

Smith, J.C., Corbin, T.J., Mccabe, J.G., Bolon, B., 2004. Isoflurane with morphine is a suitable anaesthetic regimen for embryo transfer in the production of transgenic rats. Lab. Anim. 38, 38–43.

Smith, L.J., Valenzuela, J.R., Krugner-Higby, L.A., Brown, C., Heath, T.D., 2006. A single dose of liposome-encapsulated hydromorphone provides extended analgesia in a rat model of neuropathic pain. Comp. Med. 56, 487–492.

Sotocinal, S.G., Sorge, R.E., Zaloum, A., Tuttle, A.H., Martin, L.J., Wieskopf, J.S., et al., 2011. The Rat Grimace Scale: a partially automated method for quantifying pain in the laboratory rat via facial expressions. Mol. Pain., 7.

Speth, R.C., Smith, M.S., Brogan, R.S., 2001. Regarding the inadvisability of administering postoperative analgesics in the drinking water of rats (Rattus norvegicus). Contemp. Top. Lab. Anim. Sci. 40, 15–17.

St. Jean, G., Anderson, D.E., 1999. Anesthesia and analgesia in swine. In: Straw, B.E., D'Allaire, S., Mengeling, W.L., Taylor, D.J. (Eds.), Diseases of Swine Iowa State University Press, Ames, IA, pp. 1133–1154.

Stasiak, K.L., Maul, D., French, E., Hellyer, P.W., Vandewoude, S., 2003. Species-specific assessment of pain in laboratory animals. Contemp. Top. Lab. Anim. Sci. 42, 13–20.

Steffey, E., 1986. Some characteristics of ruminants and swine that complicate management of general–anesthesia. Vet. Clin. North Am. Food Anim. Pract. 2, 507–516.

Stegmann, G.F., 1998. Observations on the use of midazolam for sedation, and induction of anaesthesia with midazolam in combination with ketamine in the goat. J. S. Afr. Vet. Assoc. 69, 89–92.

Stephens DeValle, J.M., 2009. Successful management of rabbit anesthesia through the use of nasotracheal intubation. J. Amer. Assoc. Lab. Anim. Sci. 48, 166–170.

Sternberg, W.F., Scorr, L., Smith, L.D., Ridgway, C.G., Stout, M., 2005. Long-term effects of neonatal surgery on adulthood pain behavior. Pain 113, 347–353.

Stewart, L.S.A., Martin, W.J., 2003. Influence of postoperative analgesics on the development of neuropathic pain in rats. Comp. Med. 53, 29–36.

Stewart, W., 1965. Methohexital sodium brevane anesthesia for calves and sheep. J. Dairy. Sci. 48, 251.

Stilwell, G., Lima, M.S., Carvalho, R.C., Broom, D.M., 2012. Effects of hot-iron disbudding, using regional anaesthesia with and without carprofen, on cortisol and behaviour of calves. Res. Vet. Sci. 92, 338–341.

Stoelting, R.K., 1987. Opioids. In: Stoleting, R.K., Miller, R.D. (Eds.), Basics of Anesthesia, fifth ed. Churchill-Livingstone, London UK, pp. 112–122.

Stokes, E.L., Flecknell, P.A., Richardson, C.A., 2009. Reported analgesic and anaesthetic administration to rodents undergoing experimental surgical procedures. Lab. Anim. 43, 149–154.

Suckow, M.A., Stevens, K.A., Wilson, R.P., 2012. The Laboratory Rabbit, Guinea Pig, Hamster, and Other Rodents, first ed. Academic Press, New York.

Swift, J.Q., Roszkowski, M.T., Alton, T., Hargreaves, K.M., 1998. Effect of intra-articular versus systemic anti-inflammatory drugs in a rabbit model of temporomandibular joint inflammation. Int. J. Oral. Maxillofac. Surg. 56, 1288–1295.

Swindle, M.M., 2007. Swine in the Laboratory: Surgery, Anesthesia, Imaging, and Experimental Techniques. CRC Press, Boca Raton, FL.

Swindle, M.M., Thompson, R.P., Carabello, B.A., Smith, A.C., Green, C., Gillette, P.C., 1992. Congenital cardiovascular diseases. In: Swindle, M.M. (Ed.), Swine as Models in Biomedical Research. Iowa State University Press, Ames, IA, pp. 176–184.

Swindle, M.M., Wiest, D.B., Smith, A.C., Garner, S.S., Case, C.C., Thompson, R.P., et al., 1996. Fetal surgical protocols in Yucatan miniature swine. Lab. Anim. Sci. 46, 90–95.

Swindle, M.M., Vogler, G.A., Fulton, L.K., Marini, R.P., Popilskis, S., 2002. Chapter 22 – Preanesthesia, Anesthesia, Analgesia, and Euthanasia. In: James, G.F., Lynn, C.A., Franklin, M.L., Fred, W., Quimby – James, G., Fox, L.C.A., Fred, W.Q. (Eds.), Laboratory Animal Medicine, second ed. Academic Press, Burlington, VT.

Sylvina, T.J., Berman, N.G., Fox, J.G., 1990. Effects of yohimbine on bradycardia and duration of recumbency in ketamine/xylazine anesthetized ferrets. Lab. Anim. Sci. 40, 178–182.

Taguchi, H., Murao, K., Nakamura, K., Uchida, M., Shingu, K., 1996. Percutaneous chronic epidural catheterization in the rabbit. Acta. Anaesthesiol. Scand. 40, 232–236.

Tanaka, T., Matsumoto-Okano, S., Inatomi, N., et al., 2012. Establishment and validation of a rabbit model for In Vivo pharmacodynamic screening of tachykinin NK2 antagonists. J. Pharmacol. Sci. 118, 487–495.

Thaete, L.G., Levin, S.I., Dudley, A.T., 2013. Impact of anaesthetics and analgesics on fetal growth in the mouse. Lab. Anim. 47, 175–183.

Thomas, A.A., Flecknell, P.A., Golledge, H.D., 2012a. Combining nitrous oxide with carbon dioxide decreases the time to loss of consciousness during euthanasia in mice–refinement of animal welfare? PLoS One 7, e32290.

Thomas, A.A., Leach, M.C., Flecknell, P.A., 2012b. An alternative method of endotracheal intubation of common marmosets (Callithrix jacchus). Lab. Anim. 46, 71–76.

Thompson, A.C., Kristal, M.B., Sallaj, A., Acheson, A., Martin, L.B.E., Martin, T., 2004. Analgesic efficacy of orally administered buprenorphine in rats: methodologic considerations. Comp. Med. 54, 293–300.

Thompson, A.C., Dipirro, J.M., Sylvester, A.R., Martin, L.B.E., Kristal, M.B., 2006. Lack of analgesic efficacy in female rats of the commonly recommended oral dose of buprenorphine. J. Am. Assoc. Lab. Anim. Sci. 45, 13–16.

Thurmon, J.C., 1986. Injectable anesthetic agents and techniques in ruminants and swine. Vet. Clin. North Am. Food Anim. Pract. 2, 567–591.

Thurmon, J.C., Benson, G.J., Tranquilli, W.J., Olson, W.A., 1988. The anesthetic and analgesic effects of Telazol and xylazine in pigs: evaluating clinical trials. Vet. Med. 83, 841–845.

Thurmon, J.C., Tranquilli, W.J., Benson, G.J., 1986. Cardiopulmonary responses of swine to intravenous infusion of guaifenesin, ketamine, and xylazine. Am. J. Vet. Res. 47, 2138–2140.

Thurmon, J.C., Lin, H.C., Tranquilli, T.J., Benson, G.J., Olson, W.A., 1989. A comparison of yohimbine and tolazoline as antagonist of xylazine sedation in calves. Vet. Surg. 18, 170–171.

Tinker, J.H., Sharbrough, F.H., Michenfelder, J.D., 1977. Anterior shift of the dominant EEC rhythm during anesthesia in the Java monkey: correlation with anesthetic potency. Anesthesiology 46, 252–259.

Torneke, K., Bergstrom, U., Neil, A., 2003. Interactions of xylazine and detomidine with alpha2-adrenoceptors in brain tissue from cattle, swine and rats. J. Vet. Pharmacol. Ther. 26, 205–211.

Tranquilli, W.J., Thurmon, J.C., Benson, G.J., Steffey, E.P., 1983. Halothane potency in pigs–Sus scrofa. Am. J. Vet. Res. 44, 1106–1107.

Tranquilli, W.J., Thurmon, J.C., Grimm, K.A., 2007. Lumb and Jones' Veterinary Anesthesia and Analgesia, fourth ed. Wiley-Blackwell, Ames, Iowa.

Tremoleda, J.L., Kerton, A., Gsell, W., 2012. Anaesthesia and physiological monitoring during in vivo imaging of laboratory rodents: considerations on experimental outcomes and animal welfare. EJNMMI Res. 2.

Trim, C.M., 1987. Special anesthesia considerations in the ruminant. In: Short, C.E. (Ed.), Principles and Practice of Veterinary Anesthesia. Williams & Wilkins, Baltimore, MD.

Trim, C.M., Hofmeister, E.H., Peroni, J.F., Thoresen, M., 2013. Evaluation of an oscillometric blood pressure monitor for use in anesthetized sheep. Vet. Anaesth. Analg. 40, e31–e39.

Tseng, Y.-Y., Liao, J.-Y., Chen, W.-A., Kao, Y.-C., Liu, S.-J., 2013. Biodegradable poly([D,L]-lactide-co-glycolide) nanofibers for the sustainable delivery of lidocaine into the epidural space after laminectomy. Nanomedicine (London, England).

Tubbs, J.T., Kissling, G.E., Travlos, G.S., Goulding, D.R., Clark, J.A., King-Herbert, A.P., et al., 2011. Effects of buprenorphine, meloxicam, and flunixin meglumine as postoperative analgesia in mice. J. Am. Assoc. Lab. Anim. Sci. 50, 185–191.

Turner, M.A., Thomas, P., Sheridan, D.J., 1992. An improved method for direct laryngeal intubation in the guineapig. Lab. Anim. 26, 25–28.

Turner, P.G., Dugdale, A., Young, I.S., Taylor, S., 2008. Portable mass spectrometry for measurement of anaesthetic agents and methane in respiratory gases. Vet. J. 177, 36–44.

Turner, P.V., Kerr, C.L., Healy, A.J., Taylor, W.M., 2006. Effect of meloxicam and butorphanol on minimum alveolar concentration of isoflurane in rabbits. Am. J. Vet. Res. 67, 770–774.

USDA, 2008. Animal welfare act and animal welfare regulations, USDA Animal and Plant Health Inspection Service.

Vachon, P., Faubert, S., Blais, D., Comtois, A., Bienvenue, J.G., 1999. A pathophysiological study of abdominal organs following intraperitoneal injections of chloral hydrate in rats: comparison between two anaesthesia protocols. Lab. Anim. 34 (2), 84–90.

Vainio, O.M., Bloor, B.C., Kim, C., 1992. Cardiovascular effects of a ketamine-medetomidine combination that produces deep sedation in Yucatan mini swine. Lab. Anim. Sci. 42, 582–588.

Valentine, H., Williams, W.O., Maurer, K.J., 2012. Sedation or inhalant anesthesia before euthanasia with CO2 does not reduce behavioral or physiologic signs of pain and stress in mice. J. Am. Assoc. Lab. Anim. Sci. 51, 50–57.

Valverde, A., Doherty, T.J., 2008. Anesthesia and analgesia of ruminants. In: Fish, R.E., Brown, M.J., Danneman, P.J., Karas, A.Z. (Eds.), Anesthesia and Analgesia in Laboratory Animals, second ed. Academic Press, San Diego, CA.

Valverde, A., Doherty, T.J., 2009. Pain management in cattle and small ruminants. In: Anderson, D.E., Rings, D.M. (Eds.), Current Veterinary Therapy: Food Animal Practice, fifth ed. Saunders Elsevier, St. Louis, MO.

Van Loo, P.L.P., Kuin, N., Sommer, R., Avsaroglu, H., Pham, T., Baumans, V., 2007. Impact of 'living apart together' on postoperative recovery of mice compared with social and individual housing. Lab. Anim. 41, 441–455.

van Oostrom, H., Schoemaker, N.J., Uilenreef, J.J., 2011. Pain management in ferrets. Vet. Clin. North Am. Exot. Anim. Pract. 14, 105–116.

van Zeeland, Y.R.A., Schoemaker. N.J., 2012. A new supraglottic device as an alternative for rabbit endotracheal intubation. Association of Exotic Mammal Veterinarians. 11th Annual Conference. pp. 67–68.

Vesal, N., Spadavecchia, C., Steiner, A., Kirscher, F., Levionnois, O.L., 2011. Evaluation of the isoflurane-sparing effects of lidocaine infusion during umbilical surgery in calves. Vet. Anaesth. Analg. 38, 451–460.

Vettorato, E., Schöffmann, G., Burke, J.G., Gibson, A.J.N., Clutton, E.R., 2012. Clinical effects of isoflurane and sevoflurane in lambs. Vet. Anaesth. Analg. 39, 495–502.

Victoria, N.C., Inoue, K., Young, L.J., Murphy, A.Z., 2013a. Long-term dysregulation of brain corticotrophin and glucocorticoid receptors and stress reactivity by single early-life pain experience in male and female rats. Psychoneuroendocrinology 38, 3015–3028.

Victoria, N.C., Inoue, K., Young, L.J., Murphy, A.Z., 2013b. A single neonatal injury induces life-long deficits in response to stress. Dev. Neurosci. 35, 326–337.

Victoria, N.C., Karom, M.C., Eichenbaum, H., Murphy, A.Z., 2014. Neonatal injury rapidly alters markers of pain and stress in rat pups. Dev. Neurobiol. 74, 42–51.

Vie, J.C., DeThoisy, B., Fournier, P., Fournier-Chambrillon, C., Genty, C., Keravec, J., 1998. Anesthesia of wild red howler monkeys (Alouatta seniculus) with medetomidine/ketamine and reversal by atipamezole. Am. J. Primatol. 45 (4), 399–410.

Wada, H., Seki, S., Takahashi, T., Kawarabayashi, N., Higuchi, H., Habu, Y., et al., 2007. Combined spinal and general anesthesia attenuates liver metastasis by preserving TH1/TH2 cytokine balance. Anesthesiology 106, 499–506.

Wagner, A.E., Muir, W.W., Grospitch, B.J., 1990. Cardiopulmonary effects of position in conscious cattle. Am. J. Vet. Res. 51, 7–10.

Walker, S.M., Tochiki, K.K., Fitzgerald, M., 2009. Hindpaw incision in early life increases the hyperalgesic response to repeat surgical injury: critical period and dependence on initial afferent activity. Pain 147, 99–106.

Wang, Y., Hackel, D., Peng, F., Rittner, H.L., 2013. Long-term antinociception by electroacupuncture is mediated via peripheral opioid receptors in free-moving rats with inflammatory hyperalgesia. Eur. J. Pain (London, England) 17, 1447–1457.

Wang, Y.M., Fan, R., Li, J., Zhang, L.J., Shi, Q.X., Xu, X.Z., et al., 2012. Development of a rat respiratory mask and its application in experimental chronic myocardial ischaemia. Lab. Anim. 46, 293–298.

Warren, D.J., Ledingham, J.G.G., 1978. Renal vascular response to haemorrhage in the rabbit after pentobarbitone, chloralose-urethane, and ether anaesthesia. Clin. Sci. Mol. Med. 54, 489–494.

Watanabe, A., Hashimoto, Y., Ochiai, E., Sato, A., Kamei, K., 2009. A simple method for confirming correct endotracheal intubation in mice. Lab. Anim. 43, 399–401.

Waterman, A.E., 1988. Use of propofol in sheep. Vet. Rec. 122, 260.

Waterman, A.E., Livingston, A., Amin, A., 1991a. Analgesic activity and respiratory effects of butorphanol in sheep. Res. Vet. Sci. 51, 19–23.

Waterman, A.E., Livingston, A., Amin, A., 1991b. Further studies on the antinociceptive activity and respiratory effects of buprenorphine in sheep. J. Vet. Pharmacol. Ther. 14, 230–234.

Weinandy, R., Fritzsche, P., Weinert, D., Wenkel, R., Gattermann, R., 2005. Indicators for post-surgery recovery in Mongolian gerbils (Meriones unguiculatus). Lab. Anim. 39, 200–208.

Weiskopf, R.B., Holmes, M.A.A., Eger II, E.I., Yasuda, N., Rampil, I.J., Johnson, B.H., et al., 1992. Use of swine in the study of anesthetics. In: Swindle, M.M. (Ed.), Swine as Models in Biomedical Research. Iowa State University Press, Ames, IA, pp. 96–117.

Weiss, W.J., Carney, E.L., Clark, J.B., Peterson, R., Cooper, T.K., Nifong, T.P., et al., 2012. Chronic in vivo testing of the penn state infant ventricular assist device. Asaio J. 58, 65–72.

Welberg, L.A., Kinkead, B., Thrivikraman, K., Huerkamp, M.J., Nemeroff, C.B., Plotsky, P.M., 2006. Ketamine-xylazine-acepromazine anesthesia and postoperative recovery in rats. J. Am. Assoc. Lab. Anim. Sci. 45, 13–20.

Wellington, D., Mikaelian, I., Singer, L., 2013. Comparison of ketamine-xylazine and ketamine-dexmedetomidine anesthesia and intraperitoneal tolerance in rats. J. Am. Assoc. Lab. Anim. Sci. 52, 481–487.

Wen, Y.R., Lin, C.P., Tsai, M.D., Chen, J.Y., Ma, C.C., Sun, W.Z., et al., 2012. Combination of nerve blockade and intravenous alfentanil is better than single treatment in relieving postoperative pain. J. Formos. Med. Assoc. 111, 101–108.

Wixson, S.K., 1994. Anesthesia and analgesia for rabbits. In: Manning, P.J. (Ed.), The Biology of the Laboratory Rabbit. Academic Press, San Diego, CA, pp. 87–109.

Wixson, S.K., Smiler, K.L., 1997. Anesthesia and analgesia of rodents. In: Kohn, D.H., Wixon, S.K., White, W.J., Benson, G.J. (Eds.), Anesthesia and Analgesia in Laboratory Animals. Academic Press, New York, pp. 165–203.

Wixson, S.K., White, W.J., Hughes Jr., H.C., Marshall, W.K., Lang, C.M., 1987. The effects of pentobarbital, fentanyl-droperidol, ketamine-xylazine and ketamine-diazepam on noxious stimulus perception in adult male rats. Lab. Anim. Sci. 37, 731–735.

Wong, D., Makowska, I.J., Weary, D.M., 2013. Rat aversion to isoflurane versus carbon dioxide. Biol. Lett., 9.

Woolfson, M.W., Foran, J.A., Freedman, H.M., Moore, P.A., Shulman, L.B., Schnitman, P.A., 1980. Immobilization of baboons (Papio anubus) using ketamine and diazepam. Lab. Anim. Sci. 30, 902–904.

Worek, F.S., Blumel, G., Zeravik, J., Zimmerman, G.J., Pfeiffer, U.J., 1988. Comparison of ketamine and pentobarbital anesthesia with the conscious state in a porcine model of Pseudomonas aeruginosa septicemia. Acta Anaesthiol. Scand. 32, 509–515.

Wright-Williams, S., Flecknell, P.A., Roughan, J.V., 2013. Comparative effects of vasectomy surgery and buprenorphine treatment on faecal corticosterone concentrations and behaviour assessed by manual and automated analysis methods in C57 and C3H mice. PLoS One 8, e75948.

Wright-Williams, S.L., Courade, J.P., Richardson, C.A., Roughan, J.V., Flecknell, P.A., 2007. Effects of vasectomy surgery and meloxicam treatment on faecal corticosterone levels and behaviour in two strains of laboratory mouse. Pain 130, 108–118.

Wyatt, J.D., Scott, R.A.W., Richardson, M.E., 1989. Effects of prolonged ketamine-xylazine intravenous infusion on arterial blood pH, blood gases, mean arterial blood pressure, heart and respiratory rates, rectal temperature, and reflexes in the rabbit. Lab. Anim. Sci. 39, 411–416.

Yamashita, A., Matsumoto, M., Matsumoto, S., Itoh, M., Kawai, K., Sakabe, T., 2003. A comparison of the neurotoxic effects on the spinal cord of tetracaine, lidocaine, bupivacaine, and ropivacaine administered intrathecally in rabbits. Anesth. Analg. 97, 512–519.

Yamashita, K., Sasa, Y., Ikeda, H., Izumisawa, Y., Kotani, T., 1996. Total [general] intravenous anaesthesia in cows using a combination of guaifenesin, ketamine, and xylazine. J. Jpn. Vet. Med. Assoc. 49, 709–713.

Yoshikawa, T., Ochiaia, R., Kaneko, T., Takeda, J., Fukushima, K., Tsudaka, H., et al., 1997. The effect of sevoflurane on regional cerebral metabolism and cerebral blood flow in rhesus monkeys. Masui 46 (2), 237–243.

Young, D.B., Shawley, R.V., Barron, S.J., 1989. Tolazoline reversal of xylazine-ketamine anesthesia in calves. Vet. Surg. 189, 171.

Yu, S., Zhang, X., Sun, Y., Peng, Y., Johnson, J., Mandrell, T., et al., 2006. Pharmacokinetics of buprenorphine after intravenous administration in the mouse. J. Am. Assoc. Lab. Anim. Sci. 45, 12–16.

Zegre Cannon, C., Kissling, G.E., Goulding, D.R., King-Herbert, A.P., Blankenship-Paris, T., 2011. Analgesic effects of tramadol, carprofen or multimodal analgesia in rats undergoing ventral laparotomy. Lab. Anim. (NY). 40, 85–93.

Zeller, W., Meier, G., Bürki, K., Panoussis, B., 1998. Adverse effects of tribromoethanol as used in the production of transgenic mice. Lab. Anim. 32, 407–413.

Zemel, E., Loewenstein, A., Lazar, M., Perlman, I., 1995. The effects of lidocaine and bupivacaine on the rabbit retina. Doc. Ophthalmol. 90, 189–199.

Zhang, C., Phamonvaechavan, P., Rajan, A., et al., 2010. Concentration-dependent bupivacaine myotoxicity in rabbit extraocular muscle. J. AAPOS. 14, 323–327.

Zornow, M.H., 1991. Ventilatory, hemodynamic and sedative effects of the a-2 adrenergic agonist, dexmedetomidine. Neuropharmacology 30, 1065–1071.

CHAPTER

25

Techniques of Experimentation

Michael R. Talcott[a], Walter Akers, DVM, PhD[b] and
Robert P. Marini, DVM[c]

[a]Division of Comparative Medicine, Veterinary Surgical Services, Washington University School of
Medicine, St. Louis, Missouri, USA [b]Department of Radiology, Washington
University School of Medicine, St. Louis, Missouri, USA [c]Division of Comparative Medicine,
Massachusetts Institute of Technology, Cambridge, Massachusetts, USA

OUTLINE

Laboratory Animal Medicine, Third Edition
DOI: http://dx.doi.org/10.1016/B978-0-12-409527-4.00025-0

I. INTRODUCTION

Since the publication of the second edition of this text in 2004, the primacy of genetically engineered animals has been firmly established. The creation of transgenic and knockout mice with a wide variety of genotypes has revolutionized the study of many disease entities, some of which could previously be modeled only in larger animal species. The complete sequencing of a number of pertinent genomes, including the mouse, guinea pig, rabbit, and dog, along with the associated emerging fields of transcriptomics, proteomics, and metabolomics, has led to an increasingly insightful and focused inquiry into the nature of life and disease. A foundation for these inquiries is the enduring need to define and manipulate the animal model, and the comparative medicine scientist or clinician is the agent who develops and implements the techniques and procedures that are the essential tools for discovery.

The information presented in the literature covers a wide selection of animal species and a voluminous number of the experimental techniques. The reader should be aware of general reference texts that are available and that contain chapters on biomethods for individual species (Markowitz *et al.*, 1964; Gay, 1965–1986; UFAW Staff, 1976; Waynforth and Flecknell, 1992; Swindle and Adams, 1988; American College of Laboratory Animal Medicine Series; Queensberry and Carpenter, 2011, 2004; Laboratory Animal Pocket Reference Series; Swindle, 2007; Cramer *et al.*, 1993; Rigalli and Di Loreto, 2009; Bogdanske *et al.*, 2010; Hau and Schapiro, 2010; Field and Sibold, 1998; Flecknell, 2009; Martin, 1997; Mitchell and Tully, 2009; Sharp and LaRegina, 1998; Suckow, 1997; Suckow *et al.*, 2000; Terril-Robb, 1997). Readers are also encouraged to utilize the Internet-based mailing lists dealing with laboratory animals, especially COMPMED, available through the American Association for Laboratory Animal Science (AALAS), and the many other excellent Internet-based resources for comparative medicine.

The purpose of this chapter is to select and summarize the available information in an attempt to emphasize two major concepts: (1) the technique employed in animal experimentation is often the critical factor in determining the success or failure of a research protocol, and (2) a mastery of selected techniques is extremely useful to the veterinary clinician in performing diagnostic and therapeutic procedures.

This chapter discusses or outlines by organ system one or more of the following: (1) procedures for administration of drugs and collection of biological specimens; (2) collection of physiological data; (3) surgical procedures, postoperative care, and advantages and disadvantages of alternative ways of performing the same procedure; and (4) references for access to detailed descriptions for a described technique. An overview of imaging modalities completes the chapter. References are cited for complex techniques not described in this text.

Since anesthesia techniques are covered in depth in Chapter 24, anesthesia will not be discussed here as it relates to specific surgical procedures. Reference will be made to the type of anesthesia and instrumentation required when they are critical in the performance of the described technique. The authors have preserved historical information for techniques still in use and to provide a sense of the evolution of techniques of current interest and relevance.

II. IDENTIFICATION METHODS

Cage cards may be used to identify groups of rodents or individually housed animals. The information on the card should include the name and contact information of the responsible investigator; the approved protocol number under which the animals are being used; the source of the animal; the strain, stock and genotype information; and pertinent dates such as those of arrival or birth (*Guide for the Care and Use of Laboratory Animals*, 2011). Natural characteristics and coat coloration could be recorded and used to identify individual animals, but this process is cumbersome for large numbers of animals and impossible to use for animals identical in appearance. Table 25.1 lists some of the common markers for laboratory animal species. Cage cards may also incorporate barcodes or radiofrequency identification (RFID) chips that can be used to provide additional information regarding the animals, and they may also greatly facilitate routine colony management functions like census taking.

Animals may be easily marked by the application of dyes or ink to the fur or tail. Felt tip pens or markers work well, but the mark is not permanent.

Holes and notches may be placed in the ear with a commercially available ear punch or forceps (Roboz Surgical Instruments, Kent Scientific, and Braintree Scientific). A universal numbering system has been established and should be followed (Fig. 25.1) (Dickie, 1975). This method produces a permanent mark if the ear is not self-mutilated or altered by cagemates. Holes and notches may potentially close with time.

Amputation of toes with scissors according to an established code will produce a permanent identification (Kumar, 1979). The technique is more traumatic than ear notching (Fig. 25.1) and should be used only when no other method is feasible. It may be used for neonatal mice (less than 7 days) especially if this can be combined with genotyping (Castelhano-Carlos *et al.*, 2010; Schaefer *et al.*, 2010; *Guide*). Anesthesia should be used with toe amputation performed after 2 weeks of age (Hankenson *et al.*, 2008; *Guide*). This method of identification is

TABLE 25.1   Identification Markers

Animals	Marker[a]
Mouse, rat, hamster	Ear punch, toe clip, dye, tail tattoo, ear tags, SC chip
Guinea pig	Ear tags, dye, ear punch, ear tattoo, SC chip
Rabbit	Ear tattoo, ear tags, dye, SC chip
Dog	Collar with tags, tattoo, ear tag, SC chip
Cat	Collar with tags, tattoo, SC chip
Nonhuman primate	Tattoo, collar with tags, ear tag, SC chip

[a]SC, subcutaneous.

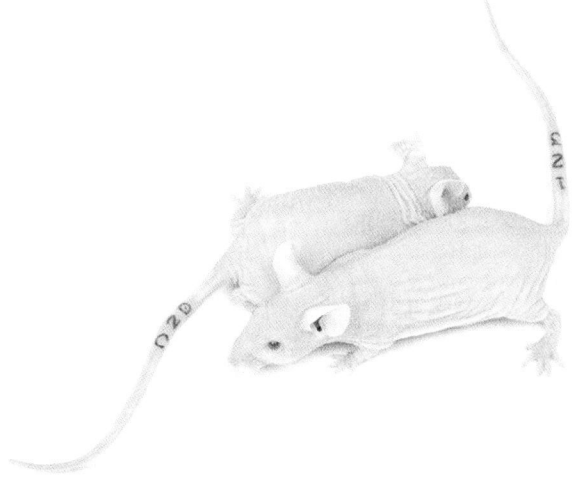

FIGURE 25.2   Mice tattooed with SoMark Industries LabStamp system. *SoMark Industries, St. Louis, MO.*

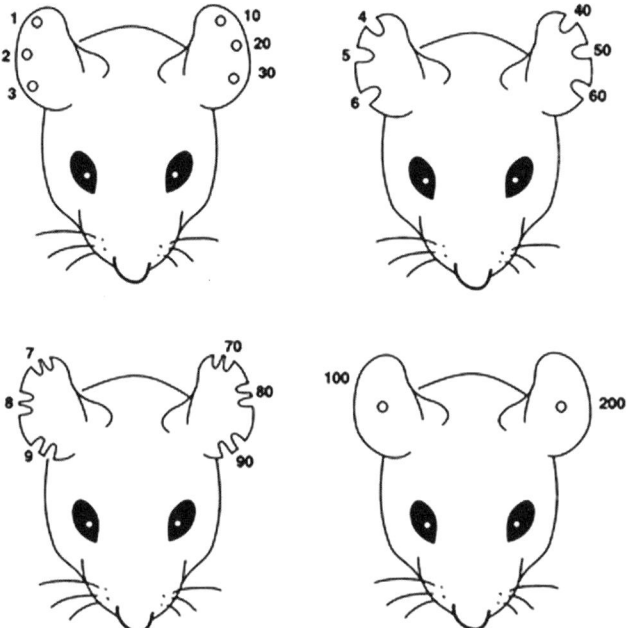

FIGURE 25.1   Ear notch code. *Adapted from Harkness and Wagner (1983).*

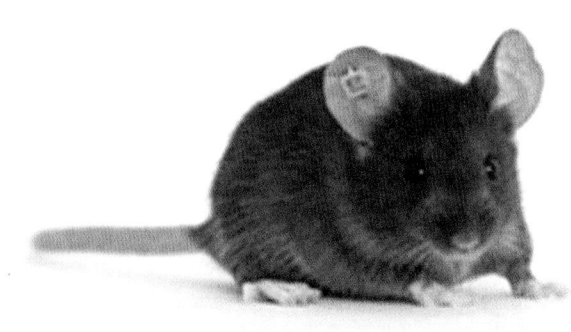

FIGURE 25.3   Ear tag with laser etched barcode.

prohibited by the U.S. Food and Drug Administration in Good Laboratory Practice studies (Federal Register, Vol. 54, No. 75, April 20, 1989 (Rule) 21 CFR Part 58).

Tattoos can be applied with pliers in large animals (Stone Manufacturing and Supply Co., Kansas City, MO), simple needles, electrovibrators, or automated applicators.

Tattoos may include various letter/number combinations, common with larger species such as rabbits and nonhuman primates, or colored dot patterns (Iwaki *et al.*, 1989). The tail and feet are the best sites for tattooing rats and mice (Fig. 25.2); specialized tattoo equipment and training are available for tattooing rodents (Avery and Spyker, 1977; Schoenborne *et al.*, 1977; Greenham, 1978). The inner surface of the ear can be tattooed in guinea pigs, rabbits, dogs, and cats. Nonhuman primates are usually tattooed on the abdomen, chest, inner arm or

thigh. The technique should be performed aseptically, and instruments must be disinfected after use on each animal.

A variety of ear tags are commercially available for all species of animals. Small aluminum ear studs are used in mice, rats, ferrets, and guinea pigs, and larger Ketchum tags are used in rabbits and dogs. RFID chips and laser-etched digital 2D barcodes have been incorporated into these tags for both rodent and non-rodent species (Fig. 25.3).

All tags should be placed in the ear according to the manufacturers' directions. It is essential that the tag is not too tight; otherwise, pressure necrosis and infection will occur. If the tag is too loose, it may easily be torn out.

Implantable transponders may be used in many species for rapid identification (Ball *et al.*, 1991; Mrozek *et al.*, 1995). These devices are miniature radio transponders capable of transmitting a unique identification number when queried using a low-power radiofrequency signal transmitter and reader. These small devices are individually packaged within a sterile large gauge needle and are implanted subcutaneously. Some transponders also are capable of providing additional physiologic information such as body temperature (BioMedic Data Systems, Inc., Maywood, NJ). Other techniques such as bead suturing and visual implant elastomere (VIE) tags have been used to identify amphibians and fish.

III. BLOOD COLLECTION AND INTRAVENOUS INJECTION

The techniques for obtaining blood from a variety of animal species are described in the following sections. Many studies now describe the use of indwelling catheters, swivels, and protective jackets and devices like subcutaneous access ports for repeated, long-term sampling of blood and the administration of drugs and other experimental substances (see Table 25.2 for a synopsis of sites and recommended volumes). Useful references regarding blood sampling from laboratory animals are McGuill and Rowan (1989), UFAW Joint Working Group on Refinement (1993), Diehl et al. (2001), and Hayward et al. (2006). Standard operating procedures are essential

for establishing best practices in blood collection and intravenous injection procedures. Preparation of all pertinent materials before performing techniques on awake either or anesthetized animals helps assure seamless operation. Systemic or local heating facilitates venipuncture in smaller rodents.

A. Rodents

Blood can be collected via cardiocentesis. From a humane perspective, cardiac puncture (Fig. 25.4A, B) should be performed only on anesthetized animals as a terminal procedure. It may be accomplished by inserting the needle through the ventral abdominal wall just lateral to the xiphoid process or through the lateral thoracic wall. The needle (23-gauge, 1 inch) is inserted at a 10–30° angle above the plane of the abdomen and directed cephalad toward the heart (Ambrus et al., 1951; Falabella, 1967; Krause, 1980; Simmons and Brick, 1970; Waynforth, 1980; Donovan and Brown, 2006). Frankenberg (1979) describes insertion of the needle through the thoracic inlet. Cardiocentesis in animals as large as a rabbit may be achieved through the ventral midline approach; needles should be 1.5″ long and 20 gauge. For animals larger than mice, the needle may be inserted through the

TABLE 25.2   Needle Sizes and Recommended Injection Volumes[a]

Species	Intravenous	Intraperitoneal	Intramuscular	Subcutaneous
Mouse	Lateral tail vein, 0.2 ml, 23–25 gauge	2–3 ml, 25–27 gauge	Quadriceps/posterior thigh, 0.05 ml, 25–27 gauge	Scruff, 2–3 ml, 23–25 gauge
Rat	Lateral tail vein, 0.5 ml, 22–25 gauge	5–10 ml, 25 gauge	Quadriceps/posterior thigh, 0.1 ml, 25 gauge	Scruff, back, 5–10 ml, 23–25 gauge
Hamster	Femoral or jugular vein (cut down), 0.3 ml, 25–27 gauge	3–4 ml, 23–25 gauge	Quadriceps/posterior thigh, 0.1 ml, 25 gauge	Scruff, 3–4 ml, 23–25 gauge
Guinea pig	Ear vein, 27 gauge saphenous vein, 0.5 ml, 25 gauge	10–15 ml, 23–25 gauge	Quadriceps/posterior thigh, 0.3 ml, <21 gauge	Scruff, back, 5–10 ml, 23–25 gauge
Rabbit	Marginal ear vein, 1–5 ml (slowly), 22–25 gauge	50–100 ml, 21–25 gauge	Quadriceps/posterior thigh, lumbar muscles, 0.5 ml, 23–25 gauge	Scruff, flank, 30–50 ml, 21–25 gauge
Cat	Cephalic vein, 2–5 ml (slowly), 21–25 gauge	50–100 ml, 21–23 gauge	Quadriceps/posterior thigh, 1 ml, 23 gauge	Scruff, back, 50–100 ml, 21–23 gauge
Dog	Cephalic vein, 10–15 ml (slowly), 21–23 gauge	200–500 ml, 21–23 gauge	Quadriceps/posterior thigh, 2–5 ml, 23 gauge	Scruff, back, 100–200 ml, 20–23 gauge
Pig (50 kg)	Ear vein, cephalic, cranial, abdominal, femoral, 10–50 ml, 20–21 gauge (1.5″ needle for cervical sites)	200–500 ml, 21–23 gauge	Lateral neck, lumbar epaxials, 5–10 ml, 20–23 gauge	Prefemoral fold, lateral neck 5–10 ml, 20–23 gauge
Primate (marmoset)	Lateral tail vein, 0.5–1 ml (slowly), 23–25 gauge	10–15 ml, 21–23 gauge	Quadriceps/posterior thigh, 0.3–0.5 ml, 23–25 gauge	Scruff, 5–10 ml, 21–25 gauge
Primate (baboon)	Cephalic vein, recurrent tarsal vein, jugular vein, 10–20 ml (slowly), 21–23 gauge	50–100 ml, 21–23 gauge	Quadriceps/posterior thigh, triceps, 1–3 ml, 21–23 gauge	Scruff, 100–200 ml, 21–25 gauge

[a]Modified from Flecknell (2009); AALAS (2013).

lateral thoracic wall in the region of maximum cardiac impulse (Burhoe, 1940; Moreland, 1965). As a terminal procedure in anesthetized mice, blood can be collected directly from the heart after removal of the sternum with scissors (Hayward *et al.*, 2006).

The technique of collecting blood from the orbital sinus or plexus is easily learned, requires minimal equipment, and reliably produces small blood samples (Fig. 25.5). The eye and health of the animal seem to be unaffected when the procedure is properly performed on an anesthetized subject (Cate, 1969; Grice, 1964; Pansky *et al.*, 1961; Simmons and Brick, 1970; Sorg and Buckner, 1964; Stone, 1954). In one study, hemorrhage was found in the puncture track, eye muscles, and periosteum immediately following blood sampling, but these lesions usually healed without scar formation following a single puncture. Four weeks following the procedure, no lesions were found (Van Herck *et al.*, 1992). The animal is

held on a flat surface, and the operator's thumb is used to apply pressure to the external jugular vein immediately caudal to the mandible, thus occluding venous return from the orbital sinus. The forefinger of the same hand is used to pull the dorsal eyelid back and produce slight exophthalmos (Fig. 25.5). Typically, a glass capillary tube or a 1- to 2-mm outer diameter borosilicate glass Pasteur pipette is used to penetrate the orbital conjunctiva and rupture the orbital sinus. Sorg and Buckner (1964) state that introduction of the tube into the lateral rather than the medial canthus reduces the incidence of epistaxis and eye trauma associated with the technique. Further anatomical studies by Timm (1989) have shown that this lateral approach should be used in the mouse, hamster, and gerbil. In an earlier publication, Timm (1979) describes the orbital venous anatomy of the rat and recommends directing the tube in a caudal and medial direction through the dorsal conjunctiva. This is necessary because the rat has an orbital plexus rather than a venous sinus, and the largest vein of this plexus is located deep within the orbit. Once the sinus or plexus has been ruptured, the blood will flow through and around the tube into a collection vessel. Slight withdrawal of the capillary tube will sometimes improve the flow of blood. Flow will cease when the tube is released and pressure is removed from the external jugular vein. Bleeding from this location may result in damage to the orbital structures. Retro-orbital hematoma, abscess, ocular injury, and phthisis bulbi may occur but are uncommon. Damage may be correlated with the experience and technique of the individual performing the procedure and the frequency of repetition. Operators should alternate eyes when performing serial bleeds.

Retrobulbar injection has been described in both adult and neonatal mice (Yardeni *et al.*, 2011). Anesthesia is

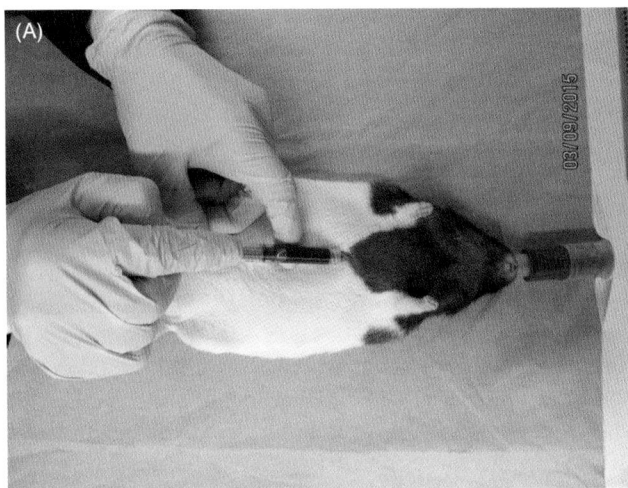

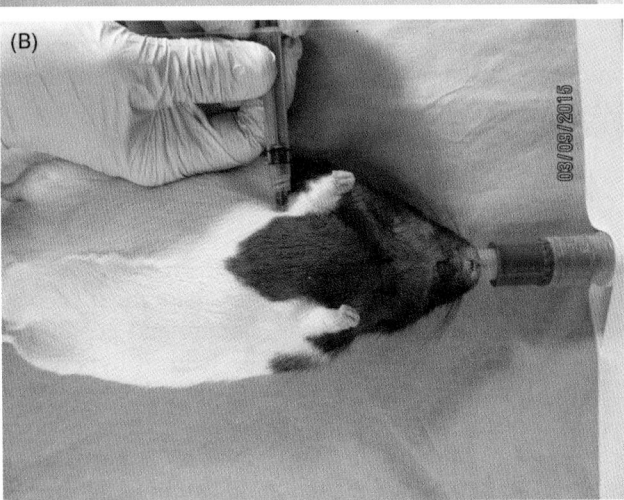

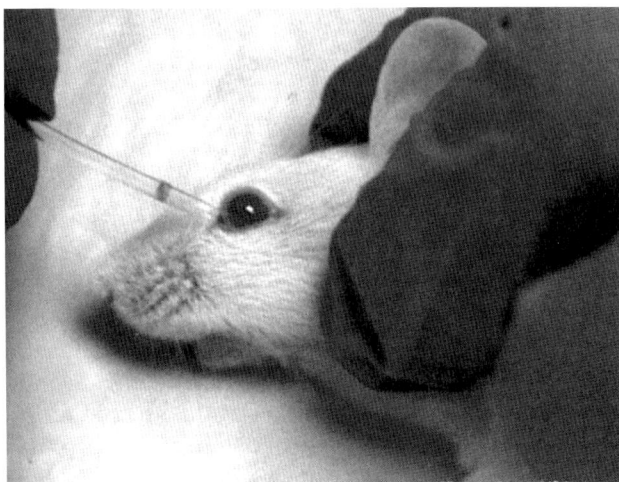

FIGURE 25.4   (A) Cardiac puncture in a rat. A 22- or 23-gauge needle is inserted through the right thoracic wall at the point of maximum heart palpitation. (B) A 22- or 23-gauge needle is inserted lateral to the xiphoid process.

FIGURE 25.5   Collection of blood from the orbital sinus of a mouse with a capillary tube. Note how traction applied by the forefinger produces exophthalmos.

required; the authors used isoflurane delivered by nose cone on a downdraft table. A hand warmer covered with gauze or paper towel is used to prevent hypothermia in the subject. Using a 27.5-gauge, 0.5-inch needle and insulin or tuberculin syringe, the right-handed operator inserts the needle bevel down, at a 30° angle to horizontal into the medial canthus of the right eye. Once the needle tip is at the base of the eye, the infusate is slowly delivered. After infusion, the operator waits momentarily before withdrawal. There should be little bleeding. For 1- to 2-day-old neonates, the technique is performed similarly, but pups are not anesthetized, and a 31-gauge, 0.3125-inch needle and 0.3-ml insulin syringe (BD Ultra-Fine II, Becton-Dickinson & Co., Franklin Lakes, NJ), a dissecting microscope, and light source are used. Without occluding venous return, the operator makes the injection into the area which will become the medial canthus (the 3 o'clock position). Tumor cells should not be administered with this technique in either adults or neonates.

Collection of blood from the tail is easily accomplished, and minimal equipment is required. Serial samples may be collected, bleeding can be controlled, and it is safe for the animal. Tail bleeding usually involves amputation of the tip of the tail or laceration of the blood vessel within the tail. If a vacuum apparatus is used, larger samples can be obtained (Levine et al., 1973; Nerenberg and Zedler, 1975; Stuhlman et al., 1972). The primary disadvantages of tail bleeding techniques which involve laceration or amputation of a portion of the tail are that blood may not flow freely from the wound, and a clot may form before a sample of adequate volume is obtained. Heparin or citrate solution may be applied directly to the wound to slow clot formation (Ambrus et al., 1951; Lewis et al., 1976). Serial samples can be collected by dislodging the clot on subsequent days. Abatan et al. (2008) describe clipping the distal 1–2 mm of the tail of mice and collection of two 20-µl samples using ethylenediaminetetraacetic acid (EDTA)-flushed capillary pipettes. Blood was collected serially on days 1, 3, 6, and 8 by simply disrupting the original wound. This technique compared favorably to saphenous venipuncture from the perspective of most behavioral reactions and corticosterone concentration. Saphenous venipuncture was associated with significantly more flinching and pulling than was tail clip. Mean total white blood cell (WBC) count was significantly lower with the saphenous blood collection technique. Rats and mice can be easily bled from the lateral caudal tail vein by using a 21-gauge butterfly set, after the animal is warmed in a 40°C chamber (Conybeare et al., 1988). Another technique is to partially lacerate the ventral artery of the tail with a sharp razor blade. This technique prevents constriction of the vessel and improves the yield of blood (Fields and Cunningham, 1976). Application of lidocaine-prilocaine

(EMLA) cream 30 min prior to incision may facilitate collection. Serial samples are collected by tail artery incision more proximally on the tail (Ott, 2009). Collection of five blood samples every 2–3 days by this method was not associated with variation in corticosterone concentrations over the sampling period (Dürschlag et al., 1996).

Proper restraint is essential for tail bleeding or injection, and effective restraint chambers are commercially available or may be constructed from a plastic syringe (Fumer and Mellett, 1975). Transillumination of the tail with a light source will improve visualization of the veins (Kaplan and Wolf, 1972; Keighley, 1966; Mylrea and Abbrecht, 1967), and occlusion of the veins at the base of the tail will also facilitate injection (Barrow, 1968). Omaye et al. (1987) described the use of a simple tourniquet on the tail to facilitate venous engorgement and blood sampling of rats. Another tourniquet fashioned from a 3-ml syringe has been described for use in mice (Joslin, 2009; Minasian, 1980). Compression of the lateral tail vein without compressing the middle coccygeal artery may be accomplished with a pair of forceps designed for wound clips (Bergstrom, 1971). A 27-gauge or smaller needle is used for venipuncture in the mouse, and a 19-gauge or smaller needle is used for the rat. Warming the tail (Ambrus et al., 1951; Fields and Cunningham, 1976; Levine et al., 1973) or warming the entire animal (Lewis et al., 1976; Stuhlman et al., 1972) increases the blood flow. Topical vasodilators like limonene and oil of wintergreen may facilitate the blood flow. It is essential that the tail be cleaned to remove all chemicals on completion. Disadvantages of the tail bleeding techniques include stimulation of the sympathetic nervous system, with resulting vasoconstriction (Carvalho et al., 1975). Significant differences were shown between samples obtained from the orbital sinus and tail of the same mouse; there was sample-to-sample variation of blood samples taken from the tail vessels in the same animal (Sakaki et al., 1961), and the mixing of venous and arterial blood plus extravascular tissue fluids in samples may occur.

Percutaneous puncture and bleeding from the jugular vein of rats and other rodents with a needle and syringe have been described (Kassel and Leviton, 1953; Phillips et al., 1973; Huneke, 2012; Hsu et al., 2012; Silverman, 2012). Because the technique is relatively safe, it can be used to collect serial samples. Success with the procedure is largely dependent on proper restraint and positioning of the animal. The neck should be held in hyperextension by fastening a strip of gauze behind the upper incisors and pulling the head back or to the side. Removal of hair from the ventral neck region by shaving or by use of a depilatory will make identification of landmarks easier. The site for venipuncture is just cephalad to the point where the external jugular vein passes between the pectoral muscle and the clavicle. If the needle is inserted through the pectoral muscle, it is stabilized better within the vein. Reliability of jugular vein techniques for blood collection can be improved by anesthetizing the animal and surgically exposing the vessel through a skin incision. Once the vessel is exposed, blood can be collected with a needle and syringe, by cannulation, or by severing the vessel and allowing blood to flow directly into a collection vial. Usually, one jugular vein is occluded while blood is collected from the opposite vein. Jugular blood collection from the unanesthetized rat and mouse has also been described (Covance, 2011; Adams et al., 2013). In the mouse, collection of 0.25 ml on three separate occasions within 40 h of the first collection was achieved without apparent adverse effects. Preshaving, alchohol prep, and traditional restraint technique, but with the mouse's head maintained slightly away from the jugular vein to be accessed, are required. A 25-gauge, ⅝-inch needle and 1 ml syringe is advanced cephalad, either cranial or caudal to the clavicle. Suction is applied once the skin has been pierced, and the needle is advanced until the blood appears in the hub (Adams et al., 2013).

Jugular venipuncture in the unanesthetized rat requires a restraint board, as well as a restrainer and phlebotomist (Covance, 2011). Essential to the success of this technique are optimal restraint and constant communication between the members of the venipuncture team. When properly restrained, the rat is in dorsal recumbency, with hindlimbs restrained at the hips and forelimbs secured by rope ties so that the limbs are perpendicular to the long axis of the body, and has its head restrained by a device made from a plastic cup, slit down the middle and perforated with breathing holes. The head is pulled opposite the venipuncture site. The phlebotomist inserts a 23-gauge, ¾-inch needle attached to a 1- to 3-ml syringe under the ventral aspect of the clavicle, keeping the syringe parallel to the restraint board, 1 cm lateral to the animal's midline, and advances the needle to a depth or 1 cm. After the needle has pierced the skin, the phlebotomist exerts gentle negative pressure; if bright-red blood appears, the needle is withdrawn and pressure is applied to the site.

The dorsal metatarsal vein in the rat (Nobonaga et al., 1966) is an excellent site for simple intravenous injection with a needle and syringe. When the animal's limb is grasped at the stifle joint, the vein is compressed and the leg is immobilized in extension. It is necessary to clip hair from the venipuncture site, and a 27-gauge or smaller needle is used. Other sites well suited for simple intravenous injection in rodents are the sublingual vein (Greene and Wade, 1967; Waynforth and Parkin, 1969) and the penile vein (Grice, 1964; Karlson, 1959). The animals must be anesthetized and venipuncture performed with a 26-gauge needle. In a more recent study, the sublingual vein of unanesthetized rats was used for blood collection (Kohlert, 2013). Advantages to this technique include the visibility of the vessel, the large volumes that can be collected, and its potential for serial use with quick

healing and minimal tissue damage. Two technicians are required, one to restrain the rat by its scruff and the other to pierce the vein. With one technician restraining the animal in a gavage hold, the other can force back the skin of the face so that the labial commissures are displaced caudally, causing the animal to 'smile.' The sublingual veins can then be visualized on either side of the tonque, and the blood can be collected by piercing the vein with a 25- or 23-gauge needle, depending on the volume required, tilting the rat so that its head is lower than its body, and allowing blood to drip into a collection tube. Thirty to forty-five seconds' hemostasis is required. Technical details that help ensure success with this technique can be found in Kohlert (2013). Snitily et al. (1991) have described a technique in which the interdigital space of the hindfoot of an anesthetized rat is punctured with a 20-gauge needle, yielding between 0.5 and 1.0 ml of blood. Oil of wintergreen is used to stimulate the blood flow to the foot beforehand. In the hamster, the cephalic vein may be used for intravenous injections (Ransom, 1984).

Decapitation may be used to collect the blood from smaller rodents, and the procedure may be accomplished with a commercially available guillotine or autopsy shears (Krause, 1980). Following decapitation, the blood flowing from the severed neck is collected in a funnel. The technique is aesthetically offensive and potentially dangerous for the operator, and electroencephalographic activity persists for a short period of time following decapitation (Mikeska and Klemm, 1975). Blood collected in this manner will also be contaminated with tracheal and salivary secretions. The American Veterinary Medical Association (AVMA) *Guidelines for the Euthanasia of Animals* (2013 edition) describes this technique as acceptable with conditions if required by the experimental design, approved by the Institutional Animal Care and Use Committee, and performed correctly by trained personnel.

Large quantities of blood may be obtained in terminal experiments using rodents by severing large vessels and exsanguinating the animal (Donovan and Brown, 2006). The inherent disadvantage of such a technique is that only one sample can be collected. Exsanguination techniques should be performed only on anesthetized animals. One to 1.5 ml of whole blood may be collected from mice by incising the brachial vessels (Young and Chambers, 1973). Large amounts of blood can be collected from the abdominal aorta by severing the vessel (Lushbough and Moline, 1961) or by aspirating with a needle and syringe (Grice, 1964). Terminal sampling from the caudal vena cava of mice can yield up to 2.5 ml of blood free from hemolysis and contamination (Adeghe and Cohen, 1986). In the rat, coagulation times in the blood obtained at euthanasia from the orbital venous plexus were abnormally prolonged, and serum magnesium and phosphorus levels were markedly lower than in the blood obtained from the posterior vena cava (Dameron et al., 1992).

Blood may be collected from fetal and newborn rodents by severing the jugular and carotid vessels (Smith and McMahon, 1977), by decapitation or amputation of an extremity (Grazer, 1958), or by cardiac puncture through the thoracic inlet (Gupta, 1973). Animals should be anesthetized, preferably by inhalant, prior to this procedure.

Blood collection and intravenous injection in the guinea pig are difficult because of the relatively small peripheral veins. Small amounts of blood can be collected by cutting a toenail close to the nail bed (Vallejo-Freire, 1951). Warming the animal in an incubator (40°C) tends to increase the blood flow. The veins of the ear may be punctured with a 25-gauge needle or lacerated with a scalpel blade, and small amounts of blood may be collected with a capillary tube (Bullock, 1983; Enta *et al.*, 1968; Grice, 1964). The auricular vein is also suitable for intravenous injection (Decad and Birnbaum, 1981). Blood can easily be aspirated from the medial saphenous vein of the anesthetized guinea pig (Carraway and Gray, 1989). A vacuum-assisted bleeding apparatus may be used to collect blood from the lateral or medial metatarsal veins. A small incision is made just distal to the malleolus, and a vacuum of 5 mmHg is applied (Dolence and Jones, 1975; Lopez and Navia, 1977; Rosenhaft *et al.*, 1971). The lateral metatarsal or lateral saphenous vein is also suitable for intravenous injection or blood sampling (Nau and Schunck, 1993). The dorsolateral vein of the penis may be used for both blood sampling and intravenous injection (Reuter, 1987). As noted previously, cardiac puncture by introduction of a needle (20- to 23-gauge, 1 inch) through the lateral thoracic wall in the region of maximum cardiac impulse may also be used to collect blood from anesthetized guinea pigs. Although not without some degree of postprocedural hemorrhage, the anterior vena cava may be accessed in a manner similar to that used to bleed domestic swine (Reuter, 1987). Guinea pigs should be anesthetized and placed in dorsal recumbency. Either shoulder flexion or extension can be used. A 23-gauge needle attached to a 3- to 6-ml syringe is inserted into the sternal notch under the first rib and directed toward the right hind leg. A 20–35° angle is used and the needle is inserted 1–1.5 cm into the thorax. If blood does not appear, the operator can redirect the needle toward the midline (Ott, 2009). Unanesthetized, restrained guinea pigs may be bled from the left jugular vein by inserting the needle in the hollow of the right shoulder above the clavicle and directing it toward the left hip (Shomer *et al.*, 1999).

Blood can be collected in the survival setting from hamsters by using the orbital sinus, cranial vena cava, and saphenous and cephalic veins (Ott, 2009). Orbital sinus bleeding is performed as in the mouse with the exception that the pipet or tube is placed in the lateral canthus in an orthogonally medial, and not rostromedial,

direction. The cranial vena cava technique is performed as in the rat. For nonsurvival blood collection, cardiocentesis using a 23-gauge, 1-inch needle inserted caudal and slightly to the left of the xiphoid process can be performed, and 3 ml of blood can be collected (Donovan and Brown, 2006).

Blood samples may be obtained from a number of sites in chinchillas, including the orbital sinus and a variety of peripheral veins, such as the auricular, femoral, cephalic, dorsal penile, saphenous, lateral abdominal, and tail veins (Tappa *et al.*, 1989; Hsu *et al.*, 2012). A technique utilizing the transverse sinus medial to the auditory bulla in anesthetized animals has been described. Samples of 0.5 ml were obtained at 3-day intervals (Boettcher *et al.*, 1990). By using a modification of the technique described by Boettcher, up to 10 ml of blood can be obtained from the transverse venous sinus (Paolini *et al.*, 1993).

Blood collection and intravenous injection techniques in a number of other rodents can be found in Colby *et al.* (2012).

B. Rabbits

Intravenous injection and blood collection techniques commonly utilize the auricular artery or marginal ear veins of the rabbit. Rabbits can be restrained using any of a number of commercially available restrainers. Blood collection from these sites may be facilitated by the topical application of a lidocaine–prilocaine local anesthetic cream 1 h prior to sampling (Flecknell *et al.*, 1990). Small amounts of blood may be collected from a puncture wound in the vessels produced by a 23-gauge needle. Collection of large amounts of blood and intravenous injection are facilitated if the blood vessels are dilated beforehand. This can be accomplished by the application of heat using a low-wattage bulb, the application of agents such as depilatories over the site of blood sampling, or topical application of 40% *d*-limonene to the posterior margin of the ear (Lacy *et al.*, 1987). These agents will dilate the vessels, and a 20-gauge needle may then be used. Vasodilatation may also be produced by the general administration of acepromazine or of a combination of acepromazine and butorphanol (Thulin, 1994), by multiple local injections of lidocaine along the marginal vein or medial artery (Paulsen and Valentine, 1984), or by topical use of EMLA cream. A vacuum apparatus (Hoppe *et al.*, 1969) or a miniperistaltic pump (Stickrod *et al.*, 1981) may be used to collect even larger quantities (30–50 ml) of blood. Cardiac puncture in the anesthetized rabbit is done as a terminal procedure with an 18-gauge, 1.5-inch needle (Kaplan and Timmons, 1979). The needle is inserted through the lateral chest wall at the site of maximal cardiac impulse or is inserted just caudal to the xiphoid cartilage, held at a 30° angle above the plane of the abdomen, and directed cranially (Bivin and Timmons, 1974). Once the needle is within the heart, blood may be collected by aspiration into a syringe by use of a miniperistaltic pump (Stickrod *et al.*, 1981) or by tubing directly into evacuated blood collection tubes or into a centrifuge tube (Kaplan and Timmons, 1979). Cranney and Zajac (1993) have described a technique for obtaining blood via jugular puncture in awake, restrained rabbits. Performance of the technique requires two people, and animals are restrained either in dorsal recumbency, or in ventral recumbency as in the cat. Dewlaps should be displaced if required (Ott, 2009). Sedation or anesthesia facilitates this procedure. Saphenous and cephalic veins can be used for venipuncture, but the ease of blood collection from the ear vessels makes these sites uncommonly used.

C. Ferrets and Mink

Small amounts of blood may be collected from the toenail of a ferret. The nail is clipped close to the nail bed, and blood is collected with a capillary tube. Larger amounts (3–5 ml) may be safely collected from the caudal artery of the tail (Bleakley, 1980). A 20- or 21-gauge needle is inserted into a groove in the ventral surface of the tail. The artery is superficially located, and care must be taken to prevent going through the artery. Blood may also be collected by cardiac puncture, using a syringe and a 20-gauge, 1.5-inch needle (Baker and Gorham, 1951). The needle is inserted on the midline just caudal to the xiphoid cartilage. Cardiac puncture should be done only in anesthetized animals as a terminal procedure. Other vessels from which blood may be collected or intravenous injection performed are the lateral saphenous and cephalic veins (Marini, 2014; Matchett *et al.*, 2012).

Jugular and cephalic venipuncture in mink and ferret has been described (Fletch and Wabeser, 1970; Otto *et al.*, 1993), as well as jugular vein cannulation (Bergman *et al.*, 1972; Mesina *et al.*, 1988). The jugular vein may be seen by occluding the vessel in the area between the sternum and the shoulder (Otto *et al.*, 1993). Ferrets may be conditioned to allow jugular venipuncture while awake. Towel and scruff restraint is used by an assistant while the animal is distracted with the nutritive paste Nutrical. A 20- to 25-gauge needle is required, depending on gender and size of the ferret. A cranial vena cava technique is commonly used for collection of a large volume of blood and may be performed in the conscious or anesthetized ferret. With the ferret in dorsal recumbency, a 25-gauge needle is inserted between the first and second ribs on the right side. The needle is inserted beneath the skin, suction is applied, and it is advanced at a 30° angle horizontal and toward the contralateral hip until blood appears (Quesenberry and Carpenter, 2011; Marini, 2014).

D. Dogs and Cats

Common sites for collection of blood from the dog and cat include the cephalic, recurrent metatarsal, jugular, and femoral veins. Collection of blood from the cephalic vein is usually accomplished while the animal is restrained in sternal recumbency on a table. The vein is stabilized and occluded by grasping the foreleg just behind the elbow. The vein may then be seen or palpated on the dorsal surface of the forelimb. As with the ear vein of the rabbit, the use of a topical anesthetic cream prior to sampling simplifies the process (Flecknell *et al.*, 1990). The recurrent metatarsal vein is located on the lateral surface of the hock joint. Collection of blood from the recurrent metatarsal vein is accomplished with the dog restrained in lateral recumbency. The vein is occluded by grasping the stifle joint and extending the limb. The vein is easily seen as it crosses the lateral surface of the hock joint, but venipuncture may be difficult because of a tendency for the vein to roll away from the needle.

The jugular vein is best for collection of blood from dogs with small peripheral veins and when large volumes are required. The animal is restrained with its neck extended and held slightly to one side. Pressure applied at the base of the neck will occlude the vein, which may then be visualized. Clipping the hair from the neck will aid in visualization of the vein. Two people are typically required for jugular venipuncture. Frisk and Richardson (1979), however, describe a technique that requires only one person. Femoral venipuncture is performed with the animal in lateral recumbency and the hindlimb extended. The vein is located just medial to the femoral pulse (Fig. 25.6).

E. Nonhuman Primates

Intravenous injection and blood collection techniques utilize the cephalic, saphenous, coccygeal, and femoral

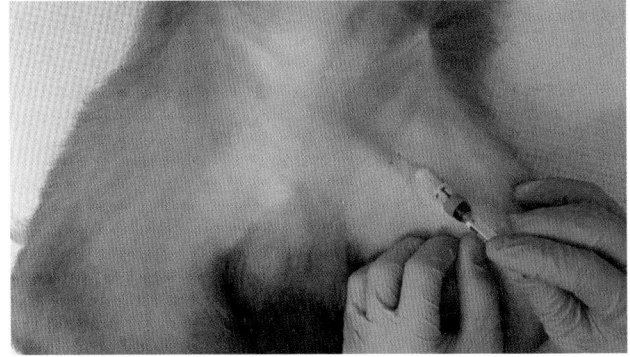

FIGURE 25.6 Femoral venipuncture in a rhesus monkey. The needle is inserted in the femoral triangle just medial to the femoral pulse. The legs of the animal can also be restrained by extending them straight back without hip abduction.

veins of nonhuman primates (Bowen *et al.*, 1976; Hall, 1966; Whitney *et al.*, 1973; Wolf and White, 2012). The femoral vein is most commonly used for blood collection; it lies within the femoral triangle just medial to the femoral artery and can be quite superficial in some species of primates (Fig. 25.6). If the femoral artery is inadvertently punctured, direct pressure must be applied to the site for a period of about 5 min in order to prevent excessive hemorrhage and hematoma formation. This is especially critical in New World monkeys (*Aotus trivirgatus*) (Loeb *et al.*, 1976). Blood can be collected from the jugular vein of a nonhuman primate if the animal is anesthetized. Small amounts of blood may be collected from neonatal primates by lancet puncture of a finger or toe or by superficial incision of the ear; however, the cellular indices may differ from those of a sample obtained from the femoral vein (Berchelman *et al.*, 1973).

F. Other Mammals

The laboratory opossum (gray short-tailed opossum, *Monodelphis domestica*) may be repeatedly bled via cardiac puncture under anesthesia (Robinson and VandeBerg, 1994). The common opossum (*Didelphis marsupialis virginiana*) may be bled from a number of sites, including the heart, lateral and ventral tail veins, femoral vessels, and pouch veins. Moore (1984) has described a method for obtaining blood from the brachiocephalic veins in a fashion similar to that used to bleed swine from the anterior vena cava. Daily samples ranging from 0.5 to 3.0 ml have been obtained from unanesthetized nine-banded armadillos (*Dasypus novemcinctus*) via puncture of the caudal tail vein between the second and third, or the third and fourth, bony tail segments. A modified piece of polyvinyl chloride (PVC) pipe is used for restraint (Herbst and Webb, 1988).

G. Birds

Common sites for blood collection and intravenous injection in avian species are the brachial veins of the wing, cutaneous ulnar, medial metatarsal (caudal tibial) vein, the jugular veins, and the heart (Evers, 2009; Kramer and Harris, 2010). The brachial vein can be easily seen on the medial surface of the wing if the feathers are plucked or separated at the region of the elbow joint. Venipuncture is easily accomplished in the brachial vein if the bird is not too small; however, hematoma formation is a common sequela (Fredrickson *et al.*, 1958). The right jugular vein, usually the largest in birds, is superficially located on the dorsolateral surface of the neck between the dorsal and ventral cervical feather tracts (Law, 1960; Stevens and Ridgeway, 1966). Occlusion of the vein may be accomplished by applying pressure to the base of the neck. Jugular venipuncture is safer than cardiac puncture, and hematoma formation rarely

occurs. Repeated collections may be done if venipuncture is done first at the base of the neck, and subsequent collections are made from sites nearer the head. Jugular venipuncture is the blood collection method of choice in Japanese quail (*Coturnix coturnix japonica*) (Arora, 1979). Cardiac puncture may also be used to collect blood from birds, and it has the advantage of yielding large amounts in a short period of time. The needle is inserted 1 inch lateral and 1 inch caudal to the point of the keel in chickens. The syringe and needle are held at a 45° angle above the body and directed toward the opposite shoulder. If the procedure is properly done, mortality rates are low (Hofstad, 1950). Garren (1959) constructed a vacuum apparatus that maintained constant negative pressure for bleeding from the wing vein or heart of chickens. Another vacuum-assisted technique of cardiac puncture has also been described (Foytik *et al.*, 1989). Cannulation of both the jugular and brachial veins may also be used for chronic blood sampling and intravenous infusion in the chicken (Cravener and Vasilatos-Younken, 1989; Zhou and Brown, 1988).

H. Unusual Species

Cooper (1993) has described a method for obtaining hemolymph from African land snails (*Achatina* spp.) that avoids perforation of the shell or incision of soft tissues by insertion of the needle at a variable distance below the pneumostome, depending on the size of the snail. Earthworms may constitute 60–80% of the animal biomass in some soils, and have been proposed as a surrogate species for vertebrates in toxicity studies related to environmental pollution. Such studies may require the collection of earthworm leukocytes (coelomocytes). Coelomic puncture using a sharpened Pasteur pipette is an invasive way to obtain such cells (Eyambe *et al.*, 1991). Such an invasive technique may injure the worm and frequently collects other cells in addition to the leukocytes. Two noninvasive methods have been described, which minimize contamination of the sample or injury to the worm (Eyambe *et al.*, 1991; Diogene *et al.*, 1997).

The limulus crab (*Limulus polyphemus*) is the source of amoebocyte collection for use in endotoxin assays (Armstrong and Conrad, 2008). Blood is collected from these animals by cardiocentesis; a large female crab can yield 200–400 ml of blood, whereas a small male will yield 50 ml. Crabs can be returned to the ocean immediately after use but if kept in an aquarium, can be re-bled every 1–2 months. Crabs are prechilled by keeping them in a 4°C room for 1–2 h prior to use and are restrained such that the operator holds the animal with its cranial dorsal carapace segment, the prostoma, at right angles to the middle section, the opisthosoma. The heart can be punctured using a 14-gauge needle placed in the hinge between these segments. The needle is advanced until blood flows. Successful harvest requires use of lipopoly-saccharide-free materials, sterile technique, immediate separation of cells from plasma, and the use of healthy uninjured animals (Armstrong and Conrad, 2008).

IV. VASCULAR CANNULATION

For short-term experiments, the animal may be anesthetized or physically restrained during infusion using one of the external vessels described above. For short-term administration, standard over-the-needle peripheral catheters, butterfly-type needle and catheters, or peripherally inserted central catheter (PICC) can be used. However, when the study requires repeated sampling or administration over an extended period of time, a more permanent access system may be preferable. Such a system may involve the implantation and exteriorization of chronic catheters, or the use of a variety of subcutaneous access port (Access Technologies, Skokie, IL; Instech-Solomon, Plymouth Meeting, PA; Ava Biomedical, Winnetka, IL; SAI Infusion Technologies, Lake Villa, IL) (Fitzgerald et al., 1996; Wojnicki et al., 1994; Swindle et al., 2005; Beck et al., 2009). If catheters are to be used for a long period of time, the technique of cannulation must provide for protection of the catheter and allow freedom of movement for the animal. To accomplish these objectives, many ingenious methods and apparati are described in the literature and will be briefly summarized here (Table 25.3). With the development of novel harnesses, form-fitting jackets, and tether and swivel systems, the need for chronic tail vein cannulations has decreased. Access to the vena cava and aorta from the lateral tail vein and the ventral tail artery in the rat (Fejes-Toth et al., 1984) and from the auricular arteries and veins in both rabbits and pigs (Fig. 25.7; Karnabatidis et al., 2006) have been reported, but chronic vascular access is commonly achieved by peripheral vessel (femoral artery/vein, carotid artery or jugular vein) access in most species.

The most common method of protecting the cannula is by creating a subcutaneous tunnel from the site of vessel cannulation to the dorsum of the neck. The

TABLE 25.3   Blood Vessel Cannulation

Species	Vessel	Reference(s)
Mouse	Tail vein	Conner et al. (1980); Plager (1972)
Rat	Tail vein	Born and Moller (1974); Rhodes and Patterson (1979); Saarni and Viikari (1976)
	Jugular vein	Terkel and Urbach (1974); Waynforth (1980)

(Continued)

TABLE 25.3   (Continued)

Species	Vessel	Reference(s)
	Dorsal aorta	Still and Whitcomb (1956)
	Carotid artery	Wixson et al. (1987)
	Cranial mesenteric vein	Zammit et al. (1979)
Ferret	Jugular vein	Mesina et al. (1988)
Guinea pig	Jugular vein	Christison and Curtin (1969)
	Carotid artery	Shrader and Everson (1968)
Rabbit	Jugular vein	Hall et al. (1974)
	Auricular vein	Knize and Weatherby-White (1974); Melich (1990)
	Carotid artery	Conn and Langer (1978)
	Renal, mesenteric, iliac, hepatic arteries; portal vein	Sils et al. (1994)
Dog	Jugular vein	Branham (1976); Dudrick et al. (1970); Foss and Barnard (1969); Goetz and Hermreck (1972); Platts et al. (1972); Engelhardt et al. (1993)
Nonhuman primate	Jugular vein	Craig et al. (1969)
	Coccygeal vein	Stickrod and Pruett (1979)
	Saphenous artery	Munson (1974)
	Saphenous vein	Conti et al. (1979)
	Aorta and vena cava	Scalese et al. (1990)
	Internal jugular vein (marmoset)	O'Byrne (1988)
Swine	Jugular vein	Ford and Maurer (1978); Wingfield et al. (1974); Zanella and Mendl (1992)
	Femoral artery and vein	Jackson et al. (1972)
	Portal vein	Knipfel et al. (1975)
	Anterior vena cava	Moritz et al. (1989)
	Inferior vena cava	Smith et al. (1992)
	Hepatic vein and artery	Drougas et al. (1996)
Sheep	Cervical arteriovenous fistula	Dennis et al. (1984)
Cattle	Jugular vein	Ladewig and Stribrny (1988)
Chicken	Brachial vein	Hamilton (1978); Zhou and Brown (1988)
	Jugular vein	Cravener and Vasilatos-Younken (1989)
Pigeon	Carotid artery	Wendt et al. (1982)
Atlantic salmon	Dorsal aorta	Pye-MacSwain et al. (1994)

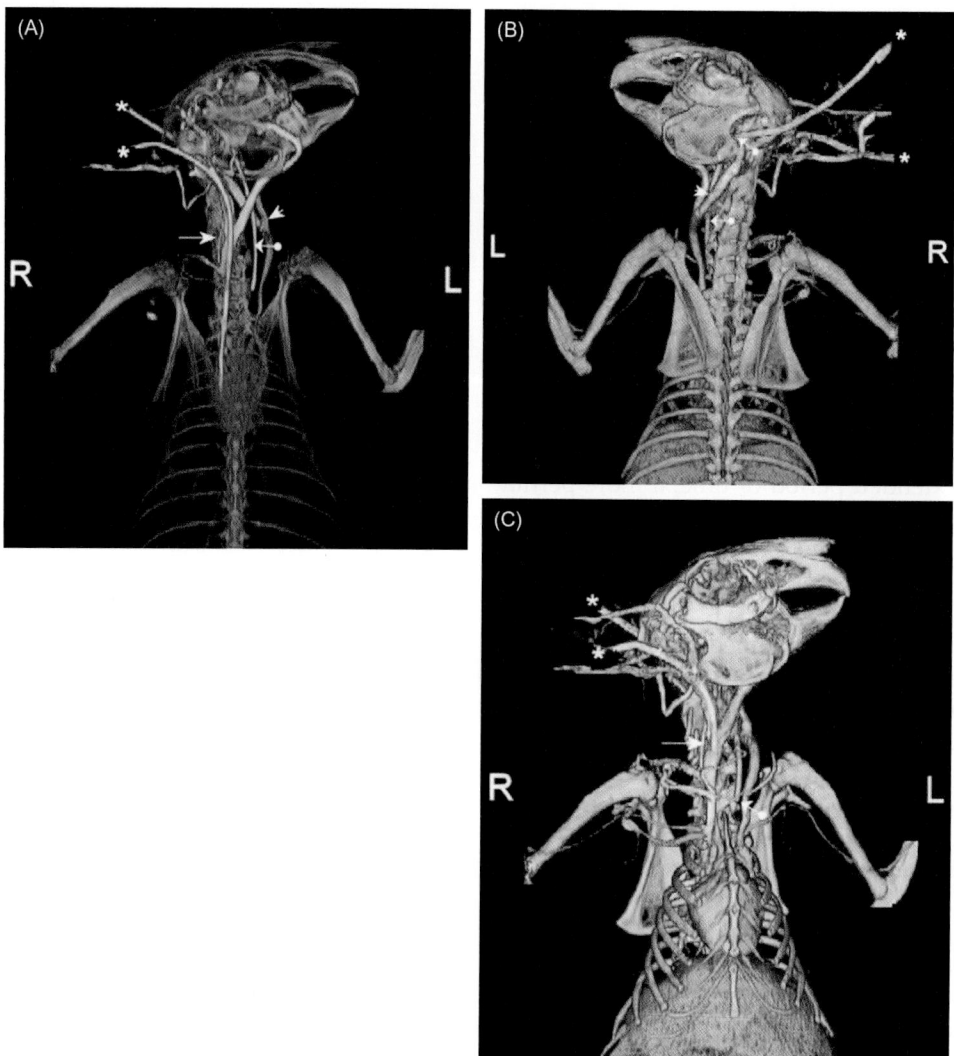

FIGURE 25.7   3D computed tomography (CT) angiography of a transauricular catheter in a rabbia. *Karnabatidis* et al. *(2006).*

tunnel may be formed by blunt dissection with scissors or with a modified intramedullary pin (Wingfield *et al.*, 1974) or trocars (both solid and hollow) designed to penetrate soft tissue and skin. Exiting the catheters from the dorsal surface of the neck minimizes the possibility of damage by the animal to the catheter or setup. Cloth sleeves made from stockinette or other suitable material can be placed over the neck to protect the infusion apparatus (Born and Moller, 1974; Wingfield *et al.*, 1974). Goetz and Hermreck (1972) and Zambraski and DiBona (1976) describe exteriorization devices for chronically implanted catheters that further protect the catheter and facilitate infusion. Skin buttons with Dacron patches for tissue ingrowth and silicon or metal sleeves can be placed at the exit site. These allow the catheter to exit and attach to a tether and swivel system or have luer adaptors for direct access. Implanted catheters can also be attached directly to a dental acrylic pedestal anchored on the skull in rodents allowing access to the catheter while eliminating the need for jackets or other restraint devices (Stripling, 1981).

Catheter materials can include silicone, polyurethane, polyethylene, and PVC. Materials vary in cost and physical attributes such as flexibility, strength, biocompatibility, and thrombogenicity (Table 25.4). Polyurethane has the additional advantage of accepting antithrombotic coatings that have been shown to decrease thrombosis of intravenous catheters (Foley *et al.*, 2002). Stiff catheters and sharp tip edges can cause irritation to the vascular intima which can promote tissue proliferation and microthrombi. Catheter materials that soften at body temperature and have tapered round openings cause less vessel trauma and remain patent longer (Wojnicki *et al.*, 1994).

Subcutaneous vascular access devices (VAPs) consist of a rigid reservoir (plastic or stainless steel) and a

TABLE 25.4   Characteristics of Catheter Materials

Characteristics	Silicone	Polyurethane	Polyethylene	Teflon/PTFE
ID Ratio	Thicker wall/ID smaller	Thinner wall/ID larger	Thicker wall	Thicker wall
Biocompatibility	Excellent	Excellent	Fair	Fair
Compatibility	Nonreactive	Nonreactive	Nonreactive	Non-reactive
Heat sensitivity	Excellent	Poor	Excellent	Excellent
Stiffness	Soft	Softens in body	Stiff	Stiff
Ease of insertion	More difficult	Moderately easy	Easy	Easy
Ease of modifying	Easy	Fair	Poor	Difficult
Memory	Excellent	Poor	Poor	Poor
Tensile strength	Fair	Excellent	Excellent	Excellent
Flexibility	Excellent	Moderate	Poor–rigid	Poor–rigid
Coefficient of friction	Fair	Excellent	Good	Excellent
Coating option	More difficult	Hydromer	n/a	n/a
Sterilization method	Autoclave or EtO	EtO	Autoclave or EtO	Autoclave or EtO

EtO, ethylene oxide; PTFE, polytetrafluorethylene.
From Access Technologies.

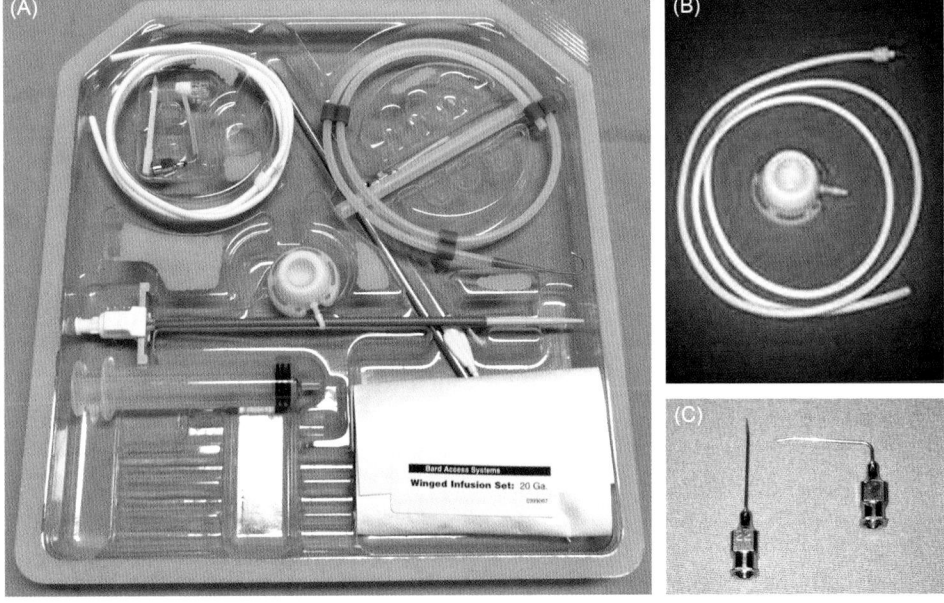

FIGURE 25.8   (A) Standard vascular access port kit. (B) Vascular access port. (C) Huber needles.

silicone septum buried beneath the skin so that it may be repeatedly punctured by a needle (Fig. 25.8A–C). Such devices give access to vascular or other structures to allow injections or withdrawal of blood without the risk of animal-induced damage or infections associated with catheters that perforate the skin. Such access ports are available in different sizes to accommodate most species, including rodents, rabbits (Perry-Clark and Meunier, 1991), cats (Webb *et al.*, 1995), swine (Bailie *et al.*, 1986; Swindle *et al.*, 2005), dogs (Polis *et al.*, 2002),

and nonhuman primates (Graham *et al.*, 2010). Accessing the port requires the use of a specialized noncoring needle or Huber needle that decreases damage to the septum. Swindle *et al.* (2005) provide a comprehensive overview of the use of vascular access ports in large animal species.

While catheters and access ports make blood sampling and vascular injections easier and less stressful for both animal and human, appropriate aseptic catheter maintenance techniques must be followed to prevent infection. Strict asepsis is necessary to prevent infection once these devices are in place and care must be taken to properly prepare the catheter or skin site prior to injection or sampling. Clipping the area free of hair and aseptic preparation of the site is recommended prior to accessing the port. Sterile supplies, including gloves to handle materials, needles, and solutions, should be used during the procedure. In conjunction with proper catheter handling, the installation of antibiotic and enzyme solutions into the catheter has been shown to be an effective way to prevent catheter-related sepsis (Palm *et al.*, 1991; O'Grady *et al.*, 2011; Chauhan *et al.*, 2012; Henderson *et al.*, 2003). Anticoagulants such as heparin, sodium citrate, sodium EDTA, and taurolidine citrate can be used as locking solutions; high-concentrate (50%) dextrose solution may be added to inhibit bacterial growth (Luo *et al.*, 2000; Stoll, 2009).

VAPs have been used for repeated blood sampling of woodchucks (Woolf *et al.*, 1989), desert tortoises (Wimsatt *et al.*, 1998), and a variety of nonhuman primates (Fitzgerald *et al.*, 1996; Wojnicki *et al.*, 1994). In dogs and ferrets, vascular access ports have been used to directly measure blood pressure (Mann *et al.*, 1987; Yao *et al.*, 1992). However, for studies in which blood pressure measurements may be required, there may be more variability when vascular access ports are used than when conventional catheters are used (Tartarini *et al.*, 1996). Protection of both exteriorized catheters and subcutaneously implanted devices including vascular access ports can be done using conventional bandaging and dressing, but close observation of the animal may be necessary to prevent damage to the site. Canvas and/or nylon vests and tight-fitted 'undershirts' that protect implanted catheters are commercially available for a variety of species (Fig. 25.9).

Such protective devices have been used in the ferret (Jackson *et al.*, 1988), dog (Foss and Barnard, 1969), rabbit (Knize and Weatherby-White, 1974), chicken (Hamilton, 1978), and different species of nonhuman primates, including macaques and African green monkeys (Bryant, 1980; McNamee *et al.*, 1984), baboons (Lukas *et al.*, 1982), and marmosets (O'Byrne, 1988). Tether systems are often incorporated into these protective jackets and attached to a swivel system and/or retractable springs or counterweighted pulleys to allow free movement of the animal around the cage to prevent catheter twisting or kinking. Tethers are generally constructed of hollow metal flexible tubing that protects catheters and other devices that are externalized from the animal and fixed to equipment outside of the cage. Use of tether systems of this type have been described by Conn and Langer (1978), Hamilton (1978), Desjardins (1986), and others. One commercially available tether system features a stationary tether with a rotating cage (http://www.basinc.com/products/culex/culex-L.html).

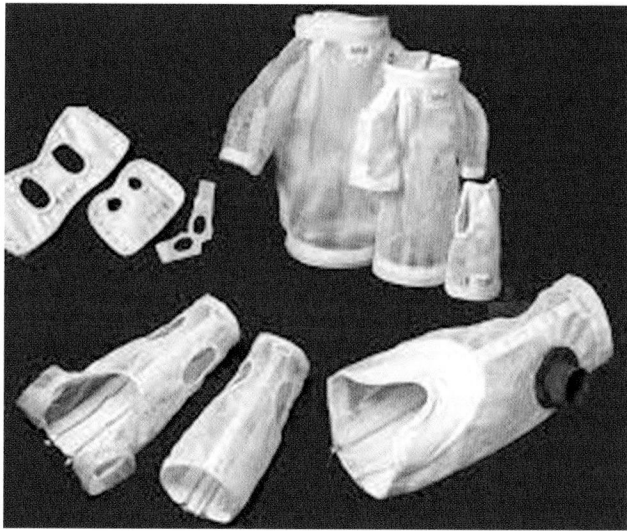

FIGURE 25.9   Nylon woven jackets can be custom designed for fitting for various animal species and sizes. *Courtesy of Lomir Biomedical.*

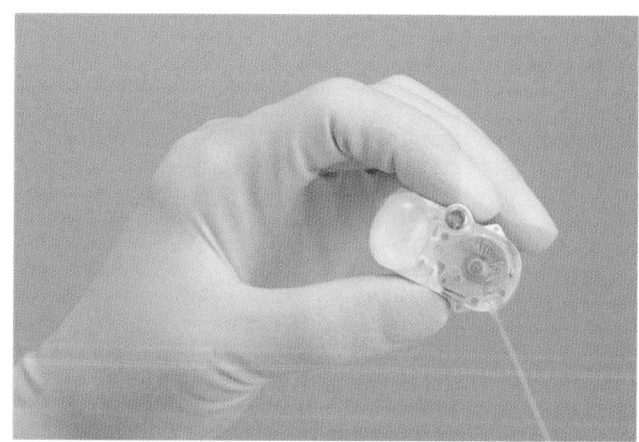

FIGURE 25.10   This micropump can be refilled and uniquely programmed for varying delivery rates. *With permission from www.lintoninst.co.uk or DSI.*

Electronically controlled infusion pumps have been used to deliver agents and can be fixed outside the cage and attached to jacket and tether systems Alternatively, battery-powered ambulatory pumps can be carried in pouches and jackets placed on the animal. An implantable micro-infusion pump has been developed (iPRECIO MicroInfusion Pump, Data Sciences International, St. Paul, MN) that can be surgically implanted in the subcutaneous space in rats and larger animals (Fig. 25.10; Tan *et al.*, 2011; Abe *et al.*, 2010). The pump is programmable and refillable, with a reservoir port similar to a VAP that allows emptying of the pump and refilling via subcutaneous injection. The pump can be connected to a catheter for administration of agents to body cavities, tissues, or vasculature.

Osmotic minipumps (Alzet osmotic pump, ALZA Corporation, Palo Alto, CA) are implantable devices that deliver a specified volume of fluid over a defined time period. These pumps have a flexible, impermeable reservoir chamber surrounded by a sealed layer containing an osmotic agent, all surrounded by a semipermeable membrane. When put into an aqueous environment (including subcutaneous or intraperitoneal implantation), the osmotic agent (high concentrated salt) imbibes water at a rate determined by the semipermeable membrane. The imbibed water generates hydrostatic pressure, which compresses the flexible reservoir chamber to produce a constant flow of the contained material. Numerous papers describe the use of these pumps to deliver drugs intravenously, intra-arterially, intrathecally, intraperitoneally, and subcutaneously. A limiting factor in the use of such pumps is the size of the pump relative to that of the animal to be used. Small animals can be implanted only with small pumps, which limits the volume, infusion rate, and duration of infusion. Infusion durations can last up to 6 weeks depending on the rate of infusion and the size of the pump. These cannot be refilled, but replacement pumps can be placed to extend the duration. One method to eliminate this difficulty has been described in marmosets. Whereas most applications require that the pump be implanted within the animal, a system has been described in marmosets in which the pump was contained in an aqueous chamber in an externally worn backpack. This device allowed continuous delivery of gonadotropin-releasing hormone over a period of 3 months by simply replacing the osmotic pump every 2 weeks (Ruiz de Elvira and Abbott, 1986).

V. INTRAPERITONEAL INJECTION

Intraperitoneal injection is a common method of administering drugs to rodents. The injection site should be in the lower left or right quadrant of the abdomen because vital organs are absent from this area. Many operators recommend restraining the animal in a 'head-down,' or Trendelenburg, position, ensuring that the viscera will be displaced cranially. Injection into the caudal abdominal quadrants of rodents restrained with the head lowered minimizes the risk of inadvertent injection into a viscus. As with injection in other sites, the operator should draw back the plunger of the syringe to determine that bowel contents, blood, or urine do not appear. Recommended volumes and needle sizes can be found in Table 25.2.

VI. SUBCUTANEOUS, INTRAMUSCULAR, AND INTRAOSSEOUS INJECTION

The preferred site for subcutaneous injection in most laboratory animals is the back or neck region. A fold of skin is held with one hand and 'tented' to create a potential space. The needle is inserted just under the skin at

the base of the fold. Lifting the needle slightly after its insertion in the skin helps ensure that it is properly placed. Subcutaneous injections in swine should be done in the flank fold or behind the ear where the skin can be tented in a similar fashion (Swindle, 2007). The thigh muscles are most commonly used for intramuscular injection. When large volumes of irritating substances are to be injected, the quadriceps group rather than the posterior thigh muscles should be used. The sciatic nerve lies posterior to the femur, and any substance injected into a fascial plane of the posterior thigh muscles may be carried directly to the nerve (Leash et al., 1973). Proper restraint is essential, and an assistant may be required for larger rodents. Needles should be advanced perpendicular to the skin and should not be driven so deep as to strike the bone. Alternative sites for injection in nonrodent species are the epaxial musculature of the rabbit, the triceps in most larger animal species, and the lateral neck of swine. Recommended volumes and needle sizes can be found in Table 25.2.

Intraosseous (IO) access can be used when conventional intravenous access cannot be achieved (Fettiplace et al., 2014). Standard sites for IO access include the medial tibia, humeral head, and sternum depending on the size of the animal. The most common site is the medial tibia due to the lack of vital vascular structures, nerves, and ease of placement. Access can be achieved through placement of manual devices (Fig. 25.11A, B; Cook I.O. needle, Cook Medical, Bloomington, IN; Baxter Jamshidi, Baxter Medical, Deerfield, IL) or mechanically assisted devices (Fig. 25.11C, E-Z IO, Vidacare, Shavano Park, TX; Bone Injection Gun (BIG), Implox Pty. Ltd., Keswick, Australia). For tibial placement, the needle should be set perpendicular to the shaft of the tibia and in the proximal third of the bone medial to the tibial plateau. The needle should be advanced until there is a reduction in resistance and the blood can be aspirated freely through the needle. This technique has been used in many species including dogs (Olsen et al., 2002), cats (Bukoski et al., 2010), rabbits (Korkmaz et al., 2013), swine (Hoskins et al., 2012), nonhuman primates, rats (Fettiplace et al., 2014), and others. IO techniques may cause pain, and analgesics should be considered.

VII. DIGESTIVE SYSTEM

The following techniques will be described in this section: oral examination, oral administration, tooth extraction, canine disarming, pulpectomy, cannulation of the common bile–pancreatic duct, biopsies of the liver and spleen, placement of intestinal cannulas, and formation of isolated intestinal loops.

Complex surgical procedures, including gastroscopy, gastric fistulas, pyloric cuff techniques, a denervated Heidenhain pouch, a Pavlov's pouch, repeated intestinal

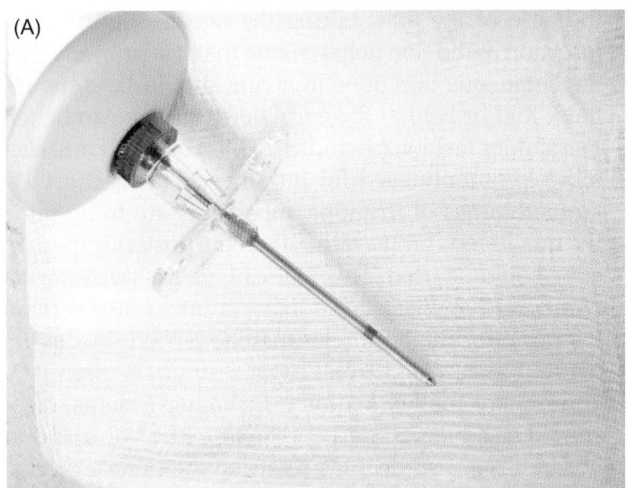

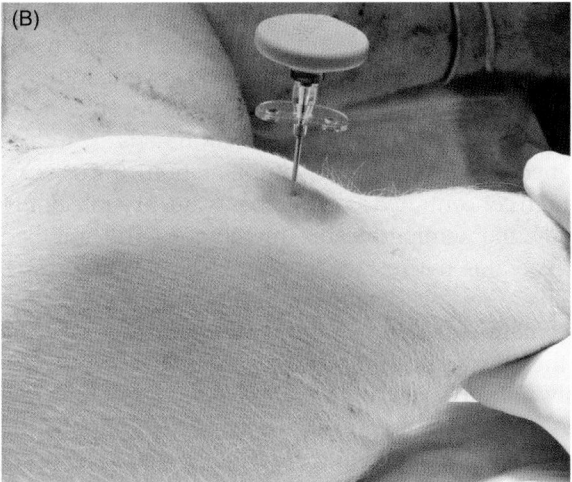

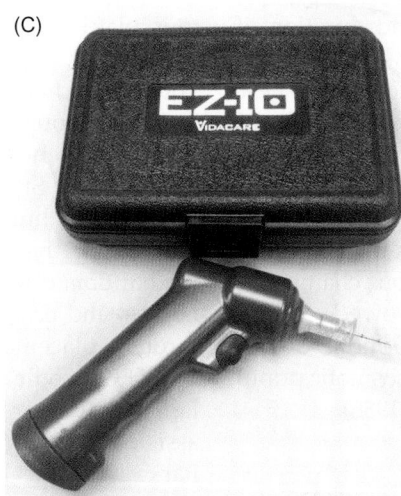

FIGURE 25.11   (A) Cook Biomedical Intraosseous needle (16 g). (B) Manual placement of an IO needle in the proximal medial tibia of a pig. (C) E-Z – IO drill with detachable 15-g needle.

biopsies, esophagogastroscopy, surgical removal of the pyloric antrum, and cecectomy, have been described in the literature (Markowitz *et al.*, 1964; Pare *et al.*, 1979; Pazin *et al.*, 1978; Cook and Williams, 1978; Bruckner-Kardoss and Worstmann, 1967; Harris and Decker, 1969; Houghton and Jones, 1977; Slatter, 2003) but will not be discussed in this text. Additional models are reviewed by Swindle and Adams (1988).

A. Oral Examination

Many types of specialized restraining devices for oral examination are described in the literature (Evans *et al.*, 1968; Davies and Grice, 1962; Redfern, 1971). A tubular device described by Macedo-Sobrinho *et al.* (1978) overcomes the difficulties created by the large diastema and small oral cavity of rodents. This device has proved to be reliable for intraoral examination of mice, rats, hamsters, and guinea pigs, even in the hands of inexperienced technical personnel. The bivalve nasal speculum from Welch Allyn is useful for oral exams (Welch Allyn®: 3.5v Bivalve Nasal Speculum Complete with 23557 Illuminator Model 26030 or 3.5v Bivalve Nasal Speculum Section Only Model 26035). A more sophisticated technique for examination of the oral cavity is dental endoscopy (Hernandez-Divers, 2008).

Certain species have unique anatomical adaptations that are utilized in research investigations. One example is the hamster cheek pouch. In order to expose this pouch, the hamster is held around the body with a thumb across its cheek. The fifth finger of the opposite hand is placed near the caudal end of the cheek pouch. By pushing cranially, while pulling gently at the corner of the hamster's mouth with the thumb of the free hand, the cheek pouch can be completely everted. This technique may be performed on an unanesthetized animal, the hamster does not bite its own everted cheek pouch, and traumatic instruments are not required (Haisley, 1980).

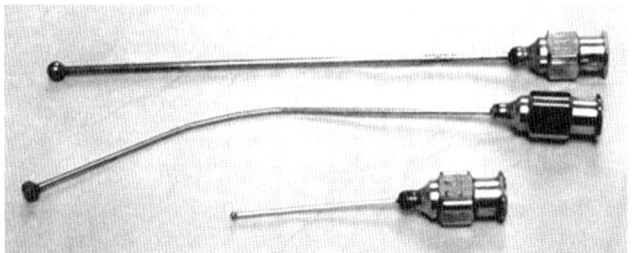

FIGURE 25.12   Stainless steel, ball-tipped needles used for gavage in rodents.

B. Oral Administration of Substances

Per os administration of solids and liquids to laboratory animals is an essential technique for a variety of experimental protocols, although voluntary consumption, if possible, is preferred. Gastric intubation ensures that all the material is administered. Flexible catheters may be used for gavage in small rodents, but durable, stainless steel, ball-tipped needles (Fig. 25.12), and semirigid disposable needles are used more frequently (animal feeding needles, Popper and Sons, New Hyde Park, NY). These needles minimize trauma to oropharyngeal tissues and make inadvertent endotracheal passage less likely. Common complications associated with gastric intubation are damage to the esophagus and administration of substances into the trachea. Careful and gentle passage of the gavage tube will greatly reduce these possibilities. In addition, introduction of the tube from the pharynx into the esophagus is best accomplished when the animal is in the act of swallowing. Usually, one can determine that the tube is not within the trachea by observing the tube's profile as it moves within the esophagus. Succesful gavage is facilitated by robust restraint, aligning the needle with the animal's body once the tip has reached the approximate location of the oropharynx, gentle oscillation of the tip to encourage swallowing, and counting to three before withdrawal to allow complete delivery of the dose (Heiser, 2013). Video training for nasal and oral administration of compounds is available (Machholz et al., 2012).

Even when compounds are administered appropriately by expert operators in rats, gavage-related reflux can occur. These events are sporadic and typically manifest as acute mortality or respiratory distress in single animals (Damsch et al., 2011). The recognition of gavage-related reflux is critical, in that it must be distinguished from untoward effects due to the test article. Risk factors for gavage-related reflux include materials administered at high volumes to fed animals, irritant or viscous compounds or those that delay gastric emptying, high concentrations of high-dose formulations, and the clinical condition of the animal (e.g., those with central nervous system (CNS) depression from the compound). To distinguish reflux-related pathological changes from those associated with the nature of compounds administered, complete histopathologic examination should be performed, with special attention given to the caudal nasal cavity, nasopharynx, and larynx (Damsch et al., 2011).

A method for administering gelatin capsules to awake guinea pigs using an intravenous catheter modified to contain a cup at one end has been described. The cup is sized to hold the gelatin capsule, such that, once passed into the stomach, the gelatin capsule can be pushed out of the cup by use of a wire through the catheter (DeBrant and Remon, 1991). Some species have anatomic variations that may cause difficulty in gastric intubation. Guinea pigs, chinchillas, and other hystricomorph rodents have a communication between the oropharynx and the pharynx on the dorsal midline of the soft palate termed the palatal ostium (Hargaden and Singer, 2012). Care must be taken to pass the needle or tube through this ostium to prevent damage to the adjacent velopharyngeal recess (Timm et al., 1987). Swine have a median cul-de-sac dorsal to the entrance to the esophagus termed the pharyngeal diverticulum that may also interfere with successful gastric or endotracheal intubation (Sisson and Grossman, 1966).

Oral specula such as those constructed from syringe cases or tongue depressors may be used to prevent the animal from chewing on gavage tubes when introduced into the oral cavity. Nasogastric intubation prevents tube damage, and it is easily accomplished in nonhuman primates or cats when the animals are anesthetized or severely depressed. For nonhuman primates, a mouth speculum has been described that minimizes the risk to the handlers. The device consists of a central stainless steel speculum tube with two stainless steel arms welded on either side (Halliday et al., 1998).

Surgically implanted gastric cannulas may also be used to deliver drugs to the stomach. As described in larger domestic animals like cats and dogs, pharyngostomy tubes may also be placed in rabbits (Rogers et al., 1988). In cats and other larger species, gastric cannulas may be placed endoscopically from the stomach through the body wall (Keshavarzian et al., 1989). Gastric cannulas may be placed during an abdominal laparotomy; the catheter may be tunneled subcutaneously to exit at the back, and the catheter may be maintained by using a protective sheath and jacket system, as previously described for vascular cannulas (Muller et al., 1992). Orogastric intubation is performed with suitably sized tubes as in companion animals. Nasogastric cannulae can be used for short periods in larger species.

C. Tooth Extraction

Because of their anatomical configuration, the teeth of some animals, such as the primate, are very difficult to remove. The technique of tooth extraction using the dental elevator involves (1) inserting the dental elevator between the alveolar bone and the tooth; (2) applying pressure on the elevator, using a rotating wrist action while directing it toward the apex of the root on all sides; and finally (3) attempting to pull the tooth only after all periodontal ligaments have been severed. Dental procedures may be adapted from those described from dogs and cats.

Canine tooth extraction and reduction in nonhuman primates appears less widely used than in the past, and policy statements by the AVMA and the U.S. Department of Agriculture (USDA) are in opposition to the practice if used for nonmedical reasons (http//www.avma.org/KB/Policies/Pages/Removal-or-Reduction-of-Teeth-in-Non-Human-Primates-and-Carnivores.aspx).

D. Bile Duct Manipulations

The common bile duct may be manipulated in a number of ways to accomplish various research goals. Complete biliary retention can be accomplished easily by ligation of the common bile duct, but this technique results in obstructive jaundice. Partial obstruction, to mimic disease conditions such as bile duct stricture, cholelithiasis, biliary tumors, or extrinsic compression of the bile duct, can be produced in the rat by ligation of the bile duct over a 0.5-mm rod, followed by removal of the rod (Sekas, 1990). Complete biliary retention without obstruction can be accomplished by implanting a catheter between the common bile duct and the venous return (Clements et al., 1985). This technique allows for studies of complete bile recirculation without the pathologic effects of complete obstruction.

Animal models in which bile can be sampled have many applications, especially in pharmacokinetic studies. Some techniques, such as that described by Spalton and Clifford (1979), involve the oral passage of a tube into the duodenum. After application of a vacuum for several minutes, the animal is given an intravenous injection of pancreozymic enzymes and cholecystokinin, which causes contraction of the gallbladder. Aspiration of the bile sample is carried out via the duodenal tube. In larger species such as dogs and pigs, endoscopic retrograde cholangiopancreatography (ERCP) can be done with placement of an 11-mm duodenoscope to collect bile and evaluate the biliary and pancreatic ductal system (Buscaglia et al., 2008; Spillmann et al., 2005; Swindle, 2007).

A simple, short-term method for collecting bile is direct surgical cannulation of the gallbladder and ligation of the common bile duct (Talbot and Hynd, 1985). In larger species, such as the dog, pig, and nonhuman primate, bile can be aspirated by cholecystocentesis under ultrasound guidance (Neel et al., 2006; Pekow et al., 1994). Cannulation of the common bile duct is described

by several authors in a variety of species including the rat (Tønsberg et al., 2011), mouse (Manautou and Chen, 2005), rabbit (West et al., 2002), guinea pig (Yu and Shen, 1991), pig (Faidley et al., 1991), and dog (Kissinger et al., 1998; Barringer et al., 1982; Soli and Birkeland, 1977; Knapp et al., 1971). Surgically modified, chronically catheterized mice, rats, and other species are commonly available from laboratory animal vendors. In mice and rats, a stereoscopic microscope may be used to identify the common bile–pancreatic duct. Once the junction between the hepatic ducts and the cystic duct is identified, the bile duct is closed immediately below their junction by a ligature. The common bile–pancreatic duct ends in an ampulla that connects it to the duodenal lumen. A small cut is made on the ampulla wall with Bellucci scissors, and a polyethylene cannula (internal diameter 150 pm) is inserted approximately 1 mm into the common bile–pancreatic duct lumen. This cannula is secured by a 7–0 nylon ligature. A calibrated capillary tube is placed in the free end of the cannula to collect the sample (Maillie et al., 1981). Chronic indwelling catheters for continuous collection of bile can be exteriorized through the skin at the base of the skull and protected by a metal coil covering (Balabaud et al., 1981).

Where maintenance of the enterohepatic recirculation of bile must be maintained during bile collection, a number of surgical techniques for catheter placement have been described in various species (Raggi et al., 1985; Rath and Hutchison, 1989; Rolf et al., 1991; Wang and Reuning, 1994; Clegg, 1997). Such techniques usually involve the insertion of two cannulas, one going proximally and the second distally in the bile duct or the duodenum, with both distal catheter ends being connected after exiting the body. The standard procedure involves creation of a choledo–choledocal biliary fistula. Through a midline laparotomy, the bile duct is exposed and dissected from the liver to the duodenal wall. Silicone catheters of appropriate size for the species are inserted into the bile duct. One is directed toward the liver, making sure that its end does not pass the cystic and secondary hepatic ducts. The other catheter is directed toward the duodeneum but is stopped short of the sphincter of Oddi. The catheters are then brought to the body surface through stab wounds in the lateral abdominal wall and may be connected by a 'U'-shaped cannula that can be detached to allow the bile samples to be taken and solutions infused. Bile may be collected by opening the connection between the catheters, aspirating the sample and then reinserting the connection.

A modification of this technique in swine used an external Y-connection between the two catheters, allowing aspiration without opening the system (Faidley et al., 1991). A method described in rats utilized an intraabdominally implanted reservoir with three catheters – two implanted proximally and distally in the bile duct,

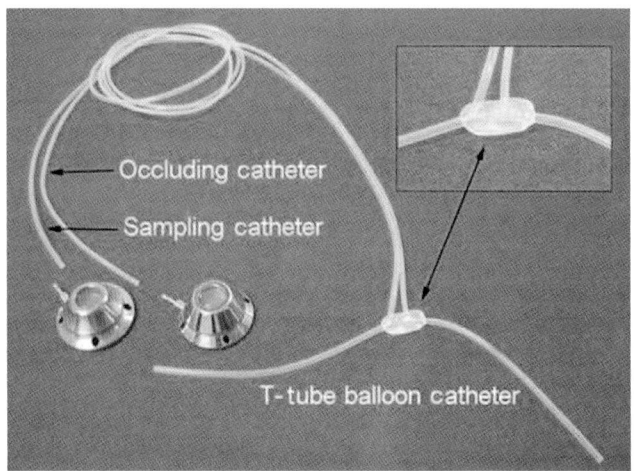

FIGURE 25.13   T-tube biliary catheter system (Access Technologies).

and a third exiting the body, through which samples could be collected (Heitmeyer and Powers, 1992). A procedure in dogs utilizes a T-piece with a central occluding diaphragm (Fig. 25.13). Each arm of the T-piece and the occluding chamber were connected to separate catheters. Both arms of the T-piece were implanted into the bile duct, with the three catheters exiting the body. With the central occluding diaphragm unexpanded, bile freely flowed through the T-piece, as it would through the normal bile duct. Expansion of the central diaphragm with saline occluded the cannula and allowed bile to flow through the collection catheter attached to the proximal arm of the T-piece for collection. Additionally, various solutions, uncontaminated with bile, could be injected through the infusion catheter attached to the distal arm of the T-piece (Kissinger et al., 1998).

E. Partial Hepatectomy and Liver Biopsy

In rodents, partial hepatectomy is performed to get sufficient tissue for certain types of studies or to remove a sufficient amount to induce regeneration with associated gene activation. Entire lobes may be removed relatively quickly with little hemorrhage by using hemoclips to ligate blood vessels (Schaeffer et al., 1994). More refined techniques specifically identifying the hepatic vasculature for individualized ligation (Madrahimov et al., 2006) or microsurgical isolation (Kubota, 1997) have been reported. Using this technique, Kubota identified that a minimum volume of 5–10% of the original liver is needed for survival. A comprehensive review of rodent hepatectomy models identifies the advantages and disadvantages of these various techniques (Martins et al., 2008).

The most straightforward method for performing liver biopsies involves a transcutaneous skin puncture.

Voss (1970) describes a simple, rapid, closed biopsy technique for primates utilizing a 16-gauge Klatskin needle and a subcostal approach. A similar method was used in swine by Washburn et al. (2005) for percutaneous liver biopsies using a Tru-cut (Allegiance Healthcare Corporation, McGraw Park, IL) and Courtney bovine liver biopsy instrument (Sontec Instruments Inc., Englewood, CO). Smaller gauge biopsy needles are used in a similar manner on rodent species and ducks (Varagona et al., 1991). Bacher et al. (1989) has described the use of a 6-mm Keyes skin punch for serial liver biopsies in Pekin ducks.

When larger tissue samples are needed, an open liver biopsy procedure may be required. Following anesthesia and surgical preparation of the abdominal area, a cranial midline abdominal incision is made to expose the liver. After identification of the area to be excised, a scalpel or scissors is used to remove the wedge of tissue. The incised area is then packed with a folded piece of absorbable gelatin sponge (Gelfoam, U.S.P., Upjohn Company, Kalamazoo, MI) (Voss, 1970). In Pekin ducks, an atraumatic cardiovascular clamp has been used to delineate the tissue to be removed (Carp et al., 1991). Large pieces of liver can also be removed by using the finger or ligature fracture technique. Using the fingers, the liver parenchyma is crushed along the line of tissue to be removed. The portal triads remain connected between the two segments and are easily double-ligated and separated. Similarly, an absorbable suture can be loosely tied around a segment of liver to be removed. When slowly tightened, the suture cuts through the liver parenchyma, isolating the portal triads, which are then ligated with the suture (Talcott and Dysko, 1991). Some authors have recommended the use of a TA-90 stapling gun (U.S. Surgical Corporation, Stamford, CT) or similar instrument. The advantage of this technique is that larger samples of biopsy material are provided and hemostasis of the severed liver lobe is excellent (Nolan and Conti, 1980). Laparoscopic biopsies of the liver and spleen have been described in the Schistosoma-infected baboon. Under halothane anesthesia, baboons had up to three biopsies obtained using an Olympus (Olympus, Tuttlingen, Germany: 0° 10 mm 29 cm telescope) laparoscope xenon light source in a three-trocar technique (Rawlings et al., 2000). Effective hemostasis is critical during laparoscopic liver biopsy procedures, and monopolar and bipolar electrosurgical devices have also been used in large animal species for liver biopsies. Ultrasonic scissors can seal and cut in a single process leading to faster tissue division, but maximum temperatures of 200°C or higher can lead to lateral thermal damage and potential injury to adjacent organs. The Harmonic ACE® scalpel (Ethicon Endo-Surgery, Cincinnati, OH) can safely seal vessels up to 5 mm and can be used on liver parenchyma to stop bleeding. Bipolar clamps like ENSEAL® (Ethicon

Endo-Surgery) and LigaSure V® (Valleylab Inc., Boulder, CO) can seal vessels of up to 7 mm and work with pulsed bipolar energy and a feedback control of the energy output during tissue coagulation. The heat production is lower leading to less thermal injury and inflammation of the surrounding tissue (Seehofer et al., 2012).

F. Pancreatic Exocrine and Endocrine Studies

Studies of pancreatic exocrine function may be performed in a variety of species by utilizing a number of techniques, which are well described by Sarr (1988) and Niebergall-Roth et al. (1997). Many of these older techniques involve the surgical creation of pancreatic fistulas, duodenal fistulas, or duodenal pouches. Other studies involve catheterization of the pancreatic duct (Niebergall-Roth et al., 1997; Naranjo et al., 1986). A study employing catheterization of a surgically created pancreatic fistula allowed studies to be done in conscious, freely mobile rats (Toriumi et al., 1994).

Models of pancreatic endocrine function largely involve study of diabetes mellitus (DM), especially type 1 DM. These models may be spontaneous, as in the non-obese-diabetic (NOD) mouse and BioBreeding (BB) rat, or can be induced. Induced models usually involve the chemical ablation of the pancreatic islets, using alloxan or streptozotocin (STZ), or surgical removal of the pancreas. Chemical induction techniques are based upon STZ's specific β-cell toxicity, a toxicity incumbent upon its use of the glucose transport protein GLUT2, which exists at higher concentrations in β cells. There are strain differences in the dose requirement of STZ in rodents and breed differences in pigs (Sakata et al., 2012). Multiple injections of low doses can yield a more stable and predictable diabetic state than single injections. Route of administration will also influence dose, as the intravenous dose in rodents is 90% that of the intraperitoneal dose. Chemical ablation is effective in mice, rats, rabbits, nonhuman primates, dogs, and pigs (Sakata et al., 2012; Hatchell et al., 1986; Litwak et al., 1998; Sarr, 1988; Miller, 1990). Cats are resistant to the diabetogenic effects of both alloxan and STZ, and surgical removal, or a combination of surgical and chemical techniques, is necessary (Hatchell et al., 1986; Reiser et al., 1987). In rats and swine, coadministration of nicotinamide and STZ can create a stable state of moderate post-prandial or fasting hyperglycemia (Musiello et al., 1998; Larsen et al., 2002). Alloxan has also been used, alone and in combination with STZ, in creating chemically induced models of diabetes (Sakata, 2012; Larsen and Rollins, 2004).

Pancreatectomy models can provide insights into DM caused by total pancreatectomy, islet autotransplantation, and allotransplantation, as well as immunosuppression protocols, bioengineered pancreas, and cell regeneration (Sakata et al., 2012; Rees and Alcolado, 2005).

Total pancreatectomy in dogs and swine is well described (Sarr, 1988; Stump et al., 1988). In laboratory rodents, surgical removal of the pancreas is very difficult because of its diffuse anatomy (Hatchell et al., 1986; Sarr, 1988; Miller, 1990). Still, the rat is used in pancreatic transplantation research, as reviewed by Mood et al. (2008). Numerous surgical models have been described and differ from one another in their method of vascular reconstruction and exocrine drainage. Heterotopic transplantation is more common than orthotopic. Microsurgical anastomosis of the extirpated pancreas to recipient sub-renal aorta and porto-portal venous drainage are most physiologic. Exocrine pancreatic drainage can be accomplished by diversion into the recipient intestine, urinary tract, or peritoneal cavity. All techniques have potential shortcomings, but enteric drainage is the more physiologic. Whatever trechnique is used, sophisticated microsurgical skills, close attention to reducing ischemia time in the graft, and prevention of hemorrhage and hypothermia in the recipient are required to improve graft survival and minimize postsurgical complications.

G. Intestinal Cannulation

There are many designs and materials used for insertion of rigid or flexible cannulas into alimentary tract fistulas of experimental animals. The choice of cannula depends on several factors, such as the size of the lumen of the organ to be fistulated, the particle size and viscosity of the material to be sampled or infused, the site of exteriorization of the cannula, and, in the case of reentrant fistulas, the volume and consistency of ingesta expected to flow through the cannulas to avoid producing excessive resistance to flow. Because of these variables, flexible plastic cannulas (polyvinyl chloride [PVC], Tygon, polyethylene, and silicone) may be preferable to rigid cannulas in some cases (Buttle et al., 1982; Banks et al., 1989; Rodhouse et al., 1988). Design modifications in the catheter tips have improved patency of intestinal catheters and includes formation of a slit or burp valve that allows infusion of materials while preventing ingesta from occluding the catheter. Many papers, however, still describe the use of rigid cannulas, often composed of stainless steel and plastic components (Carman and Waynforth, 1994; Maragos et al., 1990; Kloots et al., 1995; Hill et al., 1996; Swindle et al., 1998). These devices can be modified for longer patency by adding in barrel plugs to prevent ingesta from occluding the cannula (Wubben et al., 2001). The cannulas have also been used as access for repeated endoscopy and biopsy collections (Jacobson et al., 2001). Vascular access ports may be used for delivering drugs and solutions to various segments of the gastrointestinal tract without the problems associated with externalized catheters or cannulas (Meunier et al., 1993; Sutyak et al., 2000).

H. Intestinal Loop Isolation

Numerous research protocols for the study of gastro-intestinal physiology and pathology require segments of the digestive tract that have no continuity with the fecal stream. These segments are provided by preparation of isolated loops at different levels of the gut and are referred to as Thiry fistula (one end exteriorized) or Thiry–Vella loop fistula (both ends exteriorized) (Markowitz et al., 1964). The crucial stage in preparing such a segment is the method of anastomosis used on the intestinal wall. For most species, the preferred technique is the use of a simple, interrupted, approximating suture pattern that limits intestinal tissue trauma and minimizes luminal narrowing (Toofanian and Targowski, 1982). This is particularly true in smaller mammalian models such as the rat and guinea pig, because the small bowel of these species is highly friable. Anastomosis in these species requires using interrupted small gauge (6–0 and smaller) sutures meticulously placed 1 mm apart and 1 mm deep (Bett et al., 1980; Stenbäck, 2001). In addition, maintaining vascular viability is critical and tension should not be placed on the segment that could occlude the vasculature.

A technique called the RITARD (reversible intestinal tie–adult rabbit diarrhea) model allows temporary occlusion of a section of bowel for bacterial colonization studies in the rabbit. This technique utilizes sterile umbilical tape tied in such a way that the ligature can be loosened and removed by gentle traction on the ends that are exteriorized through the incision site (Spira et al., 1981; Kesel and Ellis, 1988). Recently, rabbit models have been utilized in vaccine development for prevention of Vibrio cholera (Eko et al., 2003; Bhowmick et al., 2009) using this technique. Although variations exist, all models are characterized by temporary small intestinal ligation and permanent cecal ligation at a site just distal to the sacculus rotundus. Occlusion of the cecum prevents absorption of fluids secreted from the small intestine.

VIII. URINARY SYSTEM TECHNIQUES

The techniques described in this section include methods of urine collection, exteriorization of the ureters, and implantation of the ureters into the intestine. Because meaningful descriptive techniques require extensive detail, the following procedures are referenced only: reconstructive surgery of the ureters, fistula of the urinary bladder, transposition of the kidney into the iliac fossa, and denervation and decapsulation of the kidney (Lopukhin, 1976). Renal allotransplantation and xenotransplantation procedures can be reviewed in Bernsteen et al. (2000) and Sprangers and Billiau (2008),

respectively. Studies for reduction of functional renal mass in hypertension studies are reviewed in Grossman (2010).

Urine is usually removed from the bladder by one of five methods: (1) collection during spontaneous micturition, (2) manual compression of the urinary bladder, (3) catheterization, (4) cystocentesis, and (5) use of metabolic cages (Khosho et al., 1985). With spontaneous collection and following manual expression, the first part of the urine stream should not be used for urinalysis or bacterial culture, because it may contain debris, bacteria, or exudate flushed from the urethra or genital tract. Manually restrained mice often urinate spontaneously; 50–500 µl can be collected in a 2-min period (Hayward et al., 2006). A collecting device to collect urine uncontaminated with feces during micturition in turkeys and chickens has been described by St. Cyr et al. (1987). In male rats, which are difficult to catheterize, urine may be collected by retraction of the prepuce and attachment of silicone tubing over the glans penis (White, 1971; Rahlmann et al., 1976). The urethra of male baboons is also difficult to catheterize. Gavellas et al. (1987) used an external condom catheter in restraint chair-trained male baboons to collect urine over a 24-h period.

Garvey and Alseth (1971) capitalized on the fact that abdominal muscle control is poorly developed in the newborn. Many females stimulate their newborn animals to urinate by stroking the lower abdomen. Although the technique is described for the rabbit, the investigator or clinician can collect urine samples from the newborn of several species by applying gentle strokes and pressure on the lower abdomen. Stroking and pressure are continued until the muscles relax and a drop of urine is observed; then pressure is applied over the bladder until the flow stops. Although there is individual variation, up to 5 ml of urine has been collected from newborn rabbits using this method (Garvey and Alseth, 1971). Success in obtaining urine by this method is often greater in females because of reduced urethral resistance. Other methods of urine collection have required the attachment of a modified pediatric urine bag to fully cover the vulva in swine and thus prevent fecal contamination (Galitzer et al., 1979) and the use of specialized metabolic cages, screens, and baffles to separate the urine and feces (Black and Claxter, 1979; Smith et al., 1981).

For some species, urethral and/or ureteral catheterization is the method of choice. Diagnostic catheterization is indicated for (1) collecting bladder urine for urinalysis or bacterial culture, (2) studying renal function, (3) instilling contrast media for radiography, (4) evaluating the urethral lumen for strictures and/or obstruction, and (5) surgically repairing the urethra and surrounding structures. These methods are routinely used for dogs and have also been described for calves (Allen, 1974), domestic fowl (Wideman and Braun, 1982), ferrets

(Marini *et al.*, 1994), and rats (Cohen and Oliver, 1964). In the female dog, visualization of the external urethral meatus aids in the placement of the catheter. A variety of devices have been used for this purpose.

Regardless of the specific procedure employed, a meticulous aseptic and gentle atraumatic technique should be used for catheterization of all species. Conscious patients should be restrained by an assistant in order to minimize contamination of the catheter as well as trauma to the urethra. The smallest diameter catheter that will permit catheterization should be used. If a stylet is used in the catheter, it should be lubricated before it is inserted into the lumen of the catheter. If it is not lubricated, difficulty may be encountered in removing the stylet after the catheter has been placed in the patient. Regardless of species or sex, the approximate distance from the external urethral orifice to the neck of the bladder should be determined and mentally transposed to the catheter. This step will minimize the likelihood of traumatizing the bladder wall due to insertion of an excessive length. Proper lubrication of the catheter with a liberal quantity of sterilized aqueous lubricant will minimize discomfort to the patient and catheter-induced trauma to the urethra. Although usually unnecessary, local anesthesia of the urethra may be provided with a topical anesthetic. Aseptic technique must be used in advancing the catheter into the urethra. If difficulty is encountered in inserting the catheter, the catheter should be withdrawn a short distance and inserted again while rotating. With unsuccessful catheterization, a smaller diameter catheter should be used. The tip of the catheter should be positioned so that it is located just beyond the junction of the neck of the bladder within the urethra. Verification of this position may be accomplished by injection of a known quantity of air through the catheter; inability to remove all of the air indicates improper positioning of the catheter. Proper positioning of the catheter facilitates removal of all of the urine from the bladder. Urine may be aspirated from the bladder with the aid of a syringe and two-way valve. Aspiration must be gentle to prevent trauma to the bladder mucosa as a result of sucking it into the eye of the catheter. Catheters that are to remain in the bladder for some time but that are not designed to permit self-retention may be sutured to the skin.

Potential complications associated with catheterization in all species include hematuria and infection. Although hematuria is usually self-limiting, it may interfere with interpretation of the urinalysis. Because of the risk of inducing infection of the bladder as a result of catheterization, this technique should be reserved for diagnostic or therapeutic purposes (Painter *et al.*, 1971; Goodpasture *et al.*, 1982). Procedures that may be used to reduce the incidence of infection following catheterization include (1) strict adherence to principles of asepsis, (2) administration of oral or parenteral antibiotics, (3) use of catheters impregnated with antibacterial agents, and (4) irrigation of the bladder with antibacterial solutions, such as neomycin or furacin (Osborne *et al.*, 1972).

Urine collection in rodents may be accomplished by one of the methods previously described. In mice, surgical catheterization of the bladder in association with subcutaneous port implants has been used for serial urine sampling with 5-week patency (Sessions *et al.*, 2002). The small size of the animals is one complicating factor; another is the unique reproductive system of some species. For example, catheterization of the male guinea pig can be accomplished rather easily; however, in almost all cases, the male will ejaculate as the catheter is passed, and the coagulum will quickly plug the catheter. Some success has been attained with urethral catheterization of the female rat using a No. 4 Coude urethral catheter that has a bend adjacent to the tip. This angulation allows the catheter to atraumatically slide by most obstructive areas in the urethra (Cohen and Oliver, 1964). Operators must recognize that female rats have distinct urethral and vaginal openings.

In order to avoid lower urinary tract infections and to facilitate renal function studies, techniques have been developed for catheterizing the ureter, urinary bladder (Black *et al.*, 1996), or urethra. Many studies describe the use of such catheters in the tethered, freely moving animal (Oz *et al.*, 1989; Mandavilli *et al.*, 1991). In some species, such as the rabbit, the ureters are very friable and subject to intraluminal bleeding. Reduced urine output during anesthesia, combined with bleeding tendencies, will often result in occlusion of the catheter with blood clots. In order to compensate for this problem, Harris and Best (1979) designed a double-lumen catheter. Irrigation of blood from the catheter is accomplished by perfusion of heparinized saline through a small inner catheter.

Other, still more invasive techniques have involved relocating or exteriorizing the ureters (Abernathy and Anderson, 1974). These procedures can be adapted from those described in textbooks on companion animal surgery (McLoughlin and Bjorling, 2003). The exteriorized ureter can then be cannulated, or it can be temporarily obstructed for research purposes. At times, resection of the ureters is required in order to facilitate a surgical procedure. If this is necessary, an elastic catheter with a diameter equal to or slightly smaller than the ureter is inserted into both ends of the transected ureter, and the ends are then approximated. Interrupted sutures are placed in the periureteral cellular tissue and muscular coat, with care taken not to enter the lumen. The catheter is removed through a lateral longitudinal incision in the ureter below the anastomosis. This incision is closed by using transverse interrupted sutures, taking care not to narrow the ureteral lumen (Lopukhin, 1976).

In swine, the proximal urinary tract can be easily accessed via a retroperitoneal approach (Parlett *et al.*, 1993; Bowen *et al.*, 1994). Uretero-ureteric anastomosis in swine using a robotic laparoscopy system has been described (Hubert *et al.*, 2003). Swine are also used to model dilated ureter associated with vesicoureteral reflux, ureteroneocystomy procedures, and many other urologic conditions (Dalmose *et al.*, 2000). Ureteral transplantation into the intestines or Heidenhain pouch has also been described (Lopukhin, 1976). Ureteral obstruction is used in mice to cause ipsilateral renal fibrosis (Tapmeier *et al.*, 2008).

IX. RESPIRATORY SYSTEM TECHNIQUES

This section will discuss the following techniques as useful tools in the diagnosis and treatment of respiratory diseases: collection of pharyngeal fluids, tracheobronchial washings, endotracheal inoculation and intubation, tracheal pouch formation, tracheostomy, bronchoscopy, and bronchopulmonary lavage. The references should be consulted for other techniques involving the lower respiratory system, including lobectomies (Nelson and Monnet, 2003; Bernstein and Agee, 1964; Markowitz *et al.*, 1964), bioinstrumentation of the thorax (Harvey and Jones, 1982), the development of chronic lung-lymph fistulas (Brown *et al.*, 1982); transplantation, isolated lung perfusion, and respiratory long-term facilitation (Jungraithmayr *et al.*, 2013; Bribriesco *et al.*, 2013; Tschernig *et al.*, 2013; Cypel and Keshavjee, 2012; Mateika and Sandhu, 2011). Because these techniques involve extensive protocols, a description could not be included in this chapter.

A. Collection of Pharyngeal Samples

A simple, effective, and inexpensive method for the collection of pharyngeal cultures from nonhuman primates without contamination by bacteria has been described (Snyder and Soave, 1970). A straight tube formed from a 1-ml tuberculin syringe is used as a speculum for the passage of sterile swabs into the pharynx. The transparent syringe barrel allows for easy visualization of the larynx. Commercial sources for sheathed applicator swabs are also available; however, the described technique can be performed in several species with materials readily available in the laboratory and at a much lower unit cost.

Oral and pharyngeal samples are routinely collected for polymerase chain reaction (PCR) and reverse transcription (RT)-PCR for detection of various diseases including BVD in cattle (Tajima *et al.*, 2008), West Nile virus in tree squirrels (Padgett *et al.*, 2007), rabies in bats and dogs (Shankar *et al.*, 2004; Wacharapluesadee *et al.*, 2012), and Pneumocystis in rats (Icenhour, 2001) as examples. Oral

swabs have also been used for genotyping transgenic mice using PCR (Zimmermann *et al.*, 2000).

B. Endotracheal Intubation

A patent airway is essential in reducing mortality during and after surgical procedures. A number of papers describe methods of intubating rodents with a variety of instruments. The simplest method described for anesthetized rats is a transillumination technique performed with the animals in dorsal recumbency on an inclined restraint board. With the superior incisors held by a rubber band, a 50-watt lighted bulb is placed 5 cm from the skin of the neck. A small curved spatula is then used like a laryngoscope to elevate the tongue, allowing easy visualization of the larynx because of the transillumination produced by the light bulb. A 16-gauge flexible intravenous catheter is then passed into the trachea (Cambron *et al.*, 1995).

Other techniques described for mice, hamsters, and guinea pigs use modified laryngoscope or otoscope specula to allow visualization of the larynx (Costa *et al.*, 1986; Tran and Lawson, 1986; Blouin and Cormier, 1987; Turner *et al.*, 1992). Another method of endotracheal intubation in rodents in dorsal recumbency is accomplished by retracting the upper jaw downward with a rubber band passed over the upper incisor teeth, retracting the tongue to one side, and observing the laryngeal region through a surgical microscope under 6× and 10× magnification. After the mucus is cleared with a cotton-tipped applicator to allow visualization of the epiglottis, glottis, and paired arytenoid cartilages, the endotracheal tube is inserted into the trachea. As the end of the tube is advanced past the larynx, water vapor is seen passing from the tube during expiration, indicating proper placement (Pena and Cabrera, 1980). Two commercially available products that use similar techniques for visualization of the larynx are the BioLITE Intubation Illumination System (Bioseb – In Vivo Research Instruments, Vitrolles, France) and Rodent Intubation Pack and Workstand (Hallowell EMC, Pittsfield, MA). Both products greatly facilitate endotracheal intubation in mice and rats.

Oral endotracheal intubation in the rabbit has been described by numerous authors, including Davis and Malinin (1974), Berthelot *et al.* (1970), Alexander and Clark (1980), Macrae and Guerreiro (1989), Bechtold and Abrutyn (1991), and Lipman *et al.* (2008). The present author believes that the 'blind' technique by Alexander and Clark (1980) is the simplest and most frequently used. The rabbit is anesthetized with gas administered via face mask and placed on a flat surface in an outstretched prone position. Anesthesia is continued until all laryngeal reflexes are abolished. The rabbit's head is tipped and extended into an upright position at right angles to the rest of the body. This position provides a straight passage from the lips to the larynx. A sterile, cuffed or uncuffed, nylon-reinforced, latex endotracheal tube (2.5–4.5 mm internal diameter) lubricated with a water-soluble sterile lubricant containing lidocaine is passed into the diastema over the tongue and positioned over, but not touching, the larynx. Correct positioning is ascertained by listening to the respiration through the tube, visualizing condensation within the tube and adjusting to obtain maximum ventilation. At inspiration, when the vocal cords are maximally opened, the endotracheal tube is inserted with a straight push to the desired depth (Alexander and Clark, 1980). Conlon *et al.* (1990) describe a technique in rabbits that utilizes an esophageal stethoscope attached to an uncuffed endotracheal tube. A small elliptical hole is cut in the end of the stethoscope to allow air to escape when the animal coughs. Under inhalant anesthesia, the rabbit is placed in a supine position and the neck is extended. The endotracheal tube is inserted into the mouth to the left of the incisor teeth, and by using the stethoscope to identify the inspiratory and expiratory phases of respiration, the tip of the tube can be placed precisely over the glottis. On the next inspiratory phase, the endotracheal tube is advanced into the trachea. Correct placement of the endotracheal tube in the trachea causes the rabbit to cough. Additional blind techniques include use of an endoesophageal tube (Kim and Han, 2000) and use of capnography during tube placement (Han *et al.*, 2000). Visual techniques require the use of laryngoscopes and laryngoscope blades of specific size (0–1 Wisconsin or Miller 1). Animals are restrained in sternal recumbency, dorsal cervical flexion, and lingual traction. The laryngoscope blade is inserted, and the tongue is depressed by the blade until the epiglottis is visualized. The tube is then advanced through the *aditus laryngis* and *rima glottidis* (Lipman *et al.*, 1997). Successful nasotracheal intubation in rabbits has recently been reported as an alternative to the standard blind methods of intubation (Stephens DeValle, 2009). An 'over-the-endoscope' intubation technique using a 30° rigid endoscope was described by Tran *et al.* (2001). Rabbits were sedated using standard procedures and the rabbit was placed in a supine position. A 2.5–4.5 cuffed or uncuffed endotracheal tube was placed over the endoscope (OD 0.4 cm × 18 cm length) which was passed through the diastema into the mouth. The epiglottis, arytenoids, and vocal cords were visualized and the endoscope was passed through the vocal cords into the trachea. Once positioned in the trachea, the endotracheal tube was advanced and the endoscope removed. Endoscopic assistance using both rigid and flexible endoscopes for direct observation of the larynx and airway and intubation of other species including cats, guinea pigs, hamsters, rats, and other small animals has been reported (Suckow *et al.*, 2012).

C. Tracheobronchial Washing and Inoculation

Tracheobronchial lavage or wash differs from a bronchoaveolar lavage based on the anatomical structure being evaluated. A tracheobronchial lavage assesses the upper airway exudate and cellular population, whereas a bronchoaveolar lavage concentrates on the lower airway structures. In some cases, such as *Rhodococcus* infections in horses and Bordetella infections in dogs, a tracheobronchial lavage may be more useful (Zietek-Barszcz and Gradzki, 2010). Tracheobronchial washing techniques have been described for the anesthetized primate. With the head tilted slightly off the edge of the table, the tongue is grasped with a gauze sponge and traction is applied. A pediatric laryngoscope permits easy visualization of the larynx and passage of the tubes. Tracheobronchial washings are obtained using a 3 French feeding tube, 40.6 cm long. A 5-ml syringe containing sterile saline is then attached to the feeding tube and used to infuse saline into the trachea. Saline is cleared from the tube using 2–3 ml of air. Aspirating the 5-ml syringe will generally yield 1–2 ml of foamy tracheobronchial fluid (Ilievski and Fleischman, 1981).

A second method is to use the transtracheal aspiration technique that involves passing a needle between the tracheal rings or cricothyroid membrane and into the tracheal lumen. A catheter is then directed through the needle and advanced to a bronchus. Sterile saline (10–15 ml for a macaque) is infused and aspirated through the catheter (Stills *et al.*, 1979). This technique, as with the previous technique, circumvents the potential problems of pharyngeal and laryngeal contamination. Transtracheal inoculation has been described in several species and used as an exposure technique for the evaluation of respiratory tract toxicity (Driscoll *et al.*, 2000).

Some experimental protocols require that chemical substances be administered intratracheally. If the animal already has an endotracheal tube in place, this procedure is quite simple. The material is injected directly through the tube. Other techniques for endotracheal inoculation in rodents have been described by Nicholson and Kinkead (1982), Yap (1982), and Pena and Cabrera (1980). The equipment required for intratracheal inoculation in small rodents includes two pairs of small curved forceps, a 100-μl microsyringe, a 38 × 1 mm diameter needle with a blunt tip bent at a 30° angle 10 mm from the end, and a laryngoscope made from a disposable polypropylene micropipette tip (Yap, 1982). The anesthetized rodent is placed on its back, and a pair of forceps is used to gently grasp the tongue and hold it to one side. The specially designed laryngoscope (Yap, 1982) is inserted, narrow end first, into the mouth. The inoculation needle, curved end uppermost, is then inserted through the laryngoscope. On entry, the syringe is held so that the portion of the inoculation needle up to the bend is parallel to the throat. With further insertion, the needle is gradually tilted upward, and when resistance is felt, the needle is withdrawn very slightly and tilted up further. On reinsertion, a give is felt when the epiglottis is passed (Yap, 1982). Another specialized speculum has been designed by Nicholson and Kinkead (1982) to facilitate intratracheal inoculations. This speculum is inserted into the rat's mouth, keeping the tongue flat beneath the blade and thus facilitating inoculation. Additional reports describe methods of acute intratracheal instillation in mice (Starcher and Williams, 1989), rats (Smith, 1991; Ruzinski et al., 1995; Wheeldon et al., 1992), and newborn rabbits (Venkatesh et al., 1988). Chronic, repeated intratracheal administration of materials may be performed through implanted catheters. Two such techniques have been described in laboratory rodents (Blouin et al., 1994) and ferrets (Chimes, 1993) and can likely be adapted to any species under study.

D. Tracheal Pouch Formation

The development of a model for studying tracheal secretions by using a surgically isolated segment of trachea with an intact nerve and blood supply, the tracheal pouch, was first described in the dog (Wardell et al., 1970). The technique involves resecting a segment of cervical trachea, with blood and nerve supply intact, and relocating this closed segment subcutaneously for ease in sampling. A more simplified technique for creating a tracheal pouch has been described in the ferret. Following anesthesia, an 8- to 10-cm ventral midline skin incision is made three cartilage rings caudal to the larynx to expose the trachea. The trachea is transected at two points between cartilage rings, being careful to preserve the dorsolateral recurrent laryngeal nerves and dorsal vascular supply. Pouches of eight cartilage rings in length can be made without causing discomfort. A stay suture is used to hold the tracheal segment away from the surgical field so that the ferret can easily breathe. Tracheal continuity is reestablished by anastomosis, using four 3–0 absorbable sutures. The cranial end of the tracheal segment is then sutured to the subcutis with four 3–0 nonabsorbable sutures. The caudal end is closed with three 3–0 absorbable sutures, thus forming a pouch (Olson, 1974; Barber and Small, 1977). A similar method has been described for rabbits (Goldstein et al., 1983). More recently, the tracheal pouch technique has been used to study nonadrenergic, non-cholinergic inhibitory (NANCI) neurotransmission in guinea pigs (Venugopalan et al., 1998; Krishnakumar et al., 2002), evaluation of mucolytic drops in miniature swine (Livingstone et al., 1990), and vasoactive intestinal peptide as a neurotransmitter of nonadrenergic inhibition of guinea pigs (Venugopalan et al., 1984).

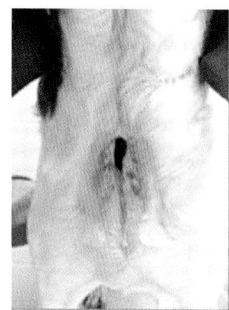

FIGURE 25.14 Permanent tracheostomy in a dog (the head is toward the top of the photo).

E. Tracheostomy

Permanent tracheostomies have been described in a number of species (Dalgard et al., 1979; Dueck et al., 1985; Eyibilen et al., 2011; Koc et al., 2012; Ritter, 1984). As with humans, some procedures create a permanent stoma into which a removable tracheostomy tube is inserted (Vogler et al., 1992). Although effective, this technique does necessitate daily management of the stoma and tube. A permanent tracheostomy has been developed for dogs that eliminates the need for the tracheostomy tube (Fig. 25.14). The procedure consists of dissecting portions of the cartilaginous rings free from the underlying tracheal mucosa, cutting through the mucosa, and suturing the mucosa to the skin. This procedure results in a permanent, maintenance-free, mucocutaneous stoma.

F. Bronchoscopy

Flexible fiberoptic bronchoscopy has been well established as a diagnostic and therapeutic tool in human medicine. With the development of smaller diameter bronchoscopes and improved optics, this technique can be applied to most species including rats (Nayci et al., 2003), rabbits (Nedeltchev et al., 2009), ferrets, and others. Endoscopes as small as 1.9 mm OD and working lengths of 115 mm are available and larger devices have multiple capabilities including high-definition optics (Olympus.com). Because the anatomy of the rhesus monkey is quite similar to that of the human, this technique has been utilized as a diagnostic and therapeutic tool in primate medicine. The monkey is anesthetized with ketamine or Telazol, and the vocal cords, larynx, and trachea are desensitized with supplemental topical anesthesia. Either a pediatric fiberoptic bronchoscope (outer diameter 4.5 mm; length 605 mm) or an adult bronchoscope (outer diameter 5.8 mm; length 605 mm) is used for inspection and photography (Strumpf et al., 1979). Rha and Mahony (1999) have provided a review of indications, instrumentation, and techniques of bronchoscopy in small animal medicine. Bronchoscopy of swine has been recommended for instruction of physicians in otolaryngology (Ram *et al.*, 1999). Sheep have been reported as an appropriate model for pulmonary physiology and respiratory diseases such as asthma and chronic obstructive pulmonary disease (Abraham, 2008) due to their similarity to human anatomy and respiratory physiology. Bronchoscopic procedures are routinely used for these studies.

G. Bronchoalveolar Lavage

Bronchoalveolar lavage is used as a therapeutic procedure in humans and as a means of recovering cells, surfactant, and inhaled particulates from the lungs of animals (Muggenberg and Mauderly, 1975; Brain and Frank, 1968; Myrvik *et al.*, 1961; Maxwell *et al.*, 1964; Medin *et al.*, 1976). For a more complete description of this procedure, the reader is referred to Singletary *et al.* (2008), in which bronchoalveolar lavage is performed by bronchoscopy. Highlights of the technique described by Singletary can be applied to rabbits, dogs, swine, and other larger species. The subject is deeply anesthetized and can be placed in a prone position. A mouth speculum can be placed behind the incisor teeth and an appropriately sized flexible endoscope or bronchoscope is advanced beyond the epiglottis and into the trachea. A saline-filled syringe can be attached to the working channel of the endoscope for instillation of lavage fluid. The volume of saline to be used for each wash is determined by individual pressure–volume measurements prior to lavage. In dogs and swine, the volume may range from 50 to 300 ml and larger animals (horses, sheep, etc.) may require larger volumes. In children, 3 ml/kg has been used and adult human volumes may be 10–300 ml (de Blic *et al.*, 2000; Singletary *et al.*, 2008). Lavage is accomplished by hyperventilating the subject, instilling the calculated volume of warmed normal saline, and immediately withdrawing the saline until a slight resistance is felt on the plunger. Various methods of fluid aspiration including manual suction, drainage by gravity, and mechanical suction at a judicious negative pressure (50–100 mmHg) have been described. Another syringe and the tracheal aspiration tube are used to clear residual fluid from the catheter, and the animal is then ventilated until effective spontaneous breathing is reestablished. For more specific localization, the bronchoscope can be wedged into a subsegmental bronchus to create a seal, which then allows fluid to be instilled and aspirated from the area of interest. The total volume of fluid should be reduced with this procedure to prevent peripheral lung damage. A total of three to four wash sequences will provide adequate sampling, taking care to drain as much fluid as possible from the lungs between washes. Additional methods for performing bronchoalveolar lavage in small laboratory rodents (mice, rats, guinea pigs) have been described (Moores *et al.*, 1989; Van Soolingen *et al.*, 1990; Tremblay *et al.*, 1990; Daubeuf and Frossard, 2012; Novak *et al.*, 2006).

X. REPRODUCTIVE SYSTEM

Many animal models have contributed to the voluminous literature on reproductive biology. In this section, the following techniques will be described or referenced: laparoscopy as an aid for ovarian biopsy, aspiration of follicle contents, ovarian injections, and artificial insemination; testicular biopsy; castration; vasectomy; semen collection; artificial insemination; pregnancy diagnosis; embryo transfer; and intrauterine fetal surgery. Many of these techniques have been developed either for maximizing reproductive potential in farm animals or for the purpose of creating genetically modified animals (Kent Lloyd, 2007; Gordon, 2004; Rodriguez-Martinez and Wallgren, 2011; Prentice and Anzar, 2010; Morrell and Rodriquex-Martinez, 2011; Bansal and Bilaspuri, 2010; Honaramooz and Yang, 2011). Comprehensive reviews of pertinent methodologies for rabbits (Fon and Watanabe, 2003), non-murine rodents (Suckow *et al.*, 2012), nonhuman primates (Tardif *et al.*, 2012), and ferrets (Sun *et al.*, 2014) are also available.

A. Laparoscopy

The earliest known report of endoscopy occurred in 1806 and described the projection of candlelight through a double-lumen urethral cannula. Traditionally, the basic research scientists have made discoveries and developed techniques that were then applied to clinical problems. Laparoscopy evolved in a reverse manner, with the extensive development of practical, clinically important techniques relating to ovarian biopsy, cyst removal, pregnancy diagnosis, implantation site quantification, recovery of uterine fluid, and sterilization by ligation of the oviducts in many laboratory animal species (Dukelow *et al.*, 1971; Dukelow and Ariga, 1976; Dukelow, 1978; Wildt *et al.*, 1975; Morcom and Dukelow, 1980). Laparoscopic ovariectomy in swine has been described by Boulton *et al.* (1995). The use of the laparoscope for examining the reproductive tracts of woodchucks and guinea pigs has also been described (Woolf and Curl, 1987; Porter *et al.*, 1997). Laparoscopy allows serial biopsy collections from the same animal and can reduce the overall number of animals needed for a particular study. Repeated laparoscopic examinations have been done safely in nonhuman primates for evaluation of experimentally induced endometriosis in several species including Japanese macaque, pigtailed macaque, rhesus monkeys, and baboons (Story and Kennedy, 2004; Harirchian *et al.*, 2012). There is decreased pain and tissue trauma resulting in shorter postsurgical recovery. Recent improvements in laparoscopic equipment and techniques have enabled the adaptation of laparoscopy for rodent procedures (Baran *et al.*, 2011; Divers, 2010).

The basic technique involves anesthetizing the animal and preparing the lower abdominal region for surgery. A Verres needle or cannula is attached to an insufflator, and the abdomen is inflated with either 5% carbon dioxide or 5% nitrogen. Sufficient abdominal insufflation is required to prevent collapse of the abdominal wall when the laparoscopic trocar is inserted. Several companies currently market this type of laparoscopy equipment (Ethicon Endo-Surgery, Cincinnati, OH; Stryker Medical, Kalamazoo, MI; Karl Storz Veterinary Endoscopy – America, Inc., Goleta, CA). The diameter of the endoscope sleeve will vary with the species under investigation and can range from 2.9 mm to 10 mm with various capabilities such as high definition and articulating optics. There is a marked difference in maneuverability and clarity of vision on the part of the investigator, depending on the instrument used.

Once the abdominal wall has been penetrated, a high-intensity light source and the prewarmed endoscope are inserted through the trocar. For ease in observation, the animal may be placed in a steep Trendelenburg (head down) position for access to abdominal and pelvic anatomy, while reverse Trendelenberg may be used for gastric, diaphragmatic, and hepatic procedures. Most procedures require the insertion of two or more trocars placed in a triangular manner to manipulate and displace organs or mesentery that are obstructing the view of the endoscope. Perfection of this technique has permitted visualization and color photography of the ovaries, ovarian biopsy, injections into the ovary, aspiration of follicle contents, and artificial insemination (Graham, 1976). Following laparoscopy, the skin incision is closed with a simple interrupted or mattress suture, and a systemic broad-spectrum antibiotic is administered (Dukelow *et al.*, 1971). Laparoscopy of experimental animals as a generalized technique has been used extensively for training of physicians (West *et al.*, 1999; Ravizzini *et al.*, 1999; Olinger *et al.*, 1999; Quintero *et al.*, 1994; Gutt *et al.*, 1998). The technique of manipulating these instruments and adapting to the eye–hand coordination necessary for observation of the abdominal organs requires repeated training in both animate and inanimate settings before a person becomes proficient. A laparoscopic trainer box setup for inanimate training is shown in Fig. 25.15.

In veterinary practice, laparoscopy may be used for examination of abdominal contents and peritoneal surfaces and for a range of procedures (Jones, 1990). Recently, fluorescent-guided laparoscopy or image-enhanced laparoscopy has been used to detect metastic

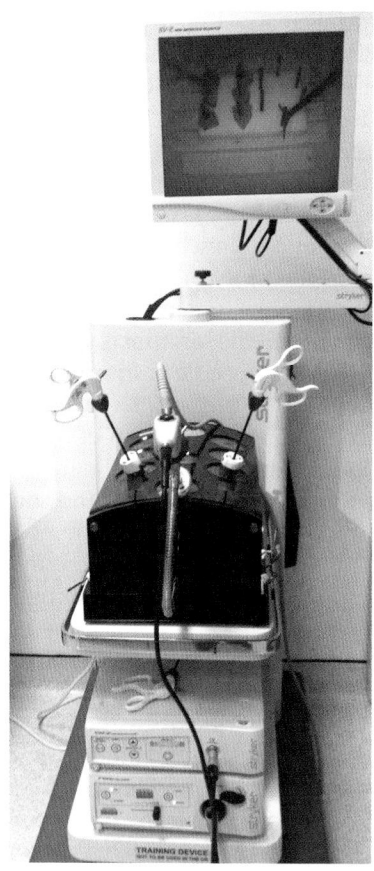

FIGURE 25.15 Laparoscopic trainer box setup for inanimate training.

ovarian cancer, endometrial tissue, thoracic and peritoneal metastatic tumors, and lymph node resection in mice, rats, and pigs (Metildi *et al.*, 2012; Matsui *et al.*, 2010; Collinet *et al.*, 2007). Using specifically designed fluorescent compounds and altering the light wavelength, various tissues can be identified including nerve, biliary channels, and ureters. Fluorescence laparoscopic detection of metastatic cancer in mice has been evaluated using a 3-mm 0° laparoscope. The mouse's abdomen is gently insufflated to 2 mmHg via a 22-gauge angiocatheter for visualization. All quadrants are evaluated in a systematic manner to identify primary tumor and detect metastasis using altered red, blue, and green components of the light-emitting diode light allowing simultaneous visualization of fluorescence-labeled tumor lesions of different wavelengths in the peritoneal cavity (Metildi *et al.*, 2012).

B. Testicular Biopsy

Existing methods of sampling testes include castration and biopsy. The most commonly used method of testis biopsy involves incision of the scrotum and tunica albuginea with subsequent removal of a small wedge of testis tissue (McFee and Kenelly, 1964; Simmons, 1952). Although this method is preferred over castration, it presents technical difficulties with small testes (Simmons, 1952) and has limited value in repeated sampling from the same individual. A procedure for obtaining multiple samples is described by Martin and Richmond (1972). The instrument for biopsy is constructed from a ¾-inch, 16-gauge needle and a 2-inch, 25-gauge needle. A small hook is made on the tip of the 25-gauge needle, which is then passed through the lumen of a 16-gauge needle. The animal is anesthetized, the scrotum is surgically scrubbed, and a sterile 16-gauge needle is introduced through the testis parenchyma. The sterile 25-gauge needle probe is then introduced through the lumen of the 16-gauge needle, and the hub is used to rotate the hook in the testis. As the 25-gauge needle is gently withdrawn, the tissue sample is extracted on the hook of the needle. Usually, one or two samples of seminiferous tubules provide an adequate sample for paraffin embedding (Martin and Richmond, 1972). The risk of damage by needle biopsy appears to be less than that from surgical excision. Semen quality and libido are not impaired by this technique. Liang et al. (1997) have described the use of a modified rotating cutting needle for obtaining testicular biopsy samples from cynomolgus monkeys (*Macacafascicularis*).

Tissue may be obtained from other portions of the reproductive tracts of male and female animals by *postmortem* harvest, laparotomy, and biopsy or with less invasive techniques. Olson and Sternfeld (1987) describe a percutaneous method of obtaining uterine biopsy samples from female rhesus monkeys (*Macaca mulatta*). Ultrasound-guided biopsy of the canine prostate is a relatively easy, minimally invasive procedure (Chang et al., 1996). Vaginal biopsy in the female canine and other species can be performed by using a vaginoscope and biopsy forceps (Schmitt, 1988). For smaller species, equipment modifications are necessary to make a vaginoscope of a size small enough to enter the vagina. An indwelling catheter system for obtaining repeated samples of uterine fluid in the cat has been described by Verhage et al. (1986) and could also be adapted to many other species. Laparascopic examination and biopsy may also be used.

C. Castration and Vasectomy

Castration has been well described for most domesticated species. Two techniques that may be of value to the surgeon for rabbits and guinea pigs are recorded by Hodesson and Miller (1964) and McGlinn et al. (1976). McGlinn's technique is unique in that it is designed to remove seminiferous tubules and Leydig's cells from the tunica albuginea, leaving the epididymis and its nerve and vascular supply intact. This technique is valuable in studies concerned with reproductive physiology of spermatozoa, the epididymis, and the vas deferens of many other mammals. For species with open inquinal canals, closure of scrotal approaches should include suturing the tunica albuginea and scrotal skin (Jenkins, 2000).

Vasectomy is performed most often to provide sterile but behaviorally normal animals to induce pseudopregnancy in recipient female mice for embryo transplant, and for the purpose of population control. In mice, the vas deferens can be accessed either through the scrotum or abdominally. In the abdominal approach, a transverse, 1.5-cm skin and body wall incision is made at the level of the proximal-most aspect of the legs, and a suture is placed through the abdominal musculature on one side. This facilitates finding the body wall for closure. Each testis is exteriorized by gentle traction on the testicular fat pad, the vas deferens is identified as a white tube with an associated blood vessel, and a 1-cm length of the vas is removed with scissors or red-hot forceps. Closure is routine. In the scrotal approach, a 1-cm skin incision is made along the midline raphe, a 5-mm incision is made into the tunica albuginea, the vas deferens is identified, and a 1-cm section is removed as described above. The skin is closed routinely (Behringer et al., 2014).

D. Semen Collection

Rectal probe ejaculation (RPE) and electrical stimulation of the penis have been utilized since the 1930s as means of obtaining semen from domestic agricultural animals, exotic animals, and some nonhuman primates (Seier et al., 1989). More recently, these techniques have been extended to common laboratory animals. It is also possible to use electroejaculation to obtain semen samples from woodchucks (Concannon et al., 1996). In some species, such as bulls, dogs, and rabbits, it is often more convenient to train individuals to serve an artificial vagina. Ejaculate volumes of 0.2–2 ml can be collected using an artificial vagina and a dummy doe made from a female rabbit hide (Pekow, 2012). This method eliminates the need to restrain or tranquilize the animal and also eliminates the risk of contamination of the ejaculate with urine (Fussell et al., 1973; Seager and Fletcher, 1972; Fayrer-Hosken et al., 1987; DeBoer and Krueger, 1991). In these species, RPE is more appropriately used for incidental collections from untrained animals. For a more complete description of the instrumentation and techniques required for RPE, the reader is referred to the works of Gould et al. (1978), Van Pelt and Keyser (1970), Lang (1967), and Fussell et al. (1967). Although the majority of the literature supports RPE as the preferred method of electroejaculation, some authors have indicated that direct stimulation of the penis is superior to RPE (Valerio et al., 1969). Collection of spermatozoa from male mice has usually been done as an *antemortem* or *post-mortem* procedure. With the increasing use of genetically manipulated mice, it may be useful to be able to obtain serial samples of spermatozoa from an individual male. Two techniques have been described, which involve the flushing of spermatozoa, post-coitus, from the uterine horns of a female mouse after euthanasia or the flushing of the uterus per vagina in the anesthetized female (King et al., 1994; Foxworth et al., 1996). RPE in mice results in secretion of both vesicular and coagulating glands. In the acute setting, spermatozoa can be collected via expression (milking) of the ductus deferens or mincing the epididymis in media (Hayward et al., 2006).

Collection of rete testis fluid is reported in monkeys (Waites and Einer-Jensen, 1974), rats (Cooper and Waites, 1974), and bulls and rams (Voglmayr et al., 1970). For a detailed description of catheter implantation of the rete testis in the ovine, the reader is referred to the works of Ellery and Kinnen (1981). Using this technique, up to 38 ml of rete testis fluid may be collected per testes for up to 3 weeks.

E. Artificial Insemination

Artificial insemination has long been recognized as a valuable technique in breeding domesticated mammals and poultry (Jones, 1971). Fresh semen, diluted fresh semen, or diluted stored semen can be used for artificial insemination. The osmotic tension, pH, buffer capacity, and electrolyte balance of the diluents must be compatible with the ejaculate. Many types of diluent have been tried, including tomato juice, coconut milk, glycerol, egg yolk, lactose, and skim milk solutions. Other diluent extenders have also included dimethyl sulfoxide (DMSO), commercial bovine extender, reconstituted dried skim milk, Locke's solution, and sodium chloride (Seager and Fletcher, 1972). Semen can be stored in frozen aliquots, and a number of studies have compared methods of freezing and thawing, safe storage duration, and reproductive efficiency in mice and other species (Nagy et al., 2003).

Prior to insemination, the female is determined to be in a receptive stage for implantation by examination of vaginal smears. The presence of well-defined cornified epithelial cells on the vaginal smear is indicative of ovulation in primates and most other species (Davis et al., 1975; Blakely et al., 1981; Hargaden and Singer, 2012). In contrast, cyclic changes in cytologic characteristics in rabbits can be highly variable (Quinn, 2012). Additional details in the rabbit can be found in Pekow (2012) and in the International Rabbit Production Group (2005) publication. Once the female has been determined to be in a receptive state, the insemination pipette is introduced into the cranial portion of the vagina or through the cervical canal. To ensure fertilization of most ova, the number of viable sperm inseminated should equal or exceed 10^6 (Stavy et al., 1978; Wolfe, 1967; Sojka et al., 1970).

In some species, such as swine, one can introduce the semen directly into the oviductal lumen by using laparoscopy. This procedure may have application for basic studies of sperm and egg physiology and may be adapted to other species (Morcom and Dukelow, 1980).

F. Pregnancy Diagnosis

Pregnancy diagnosis varies from observation of external appearance to digital palpation, radiographs, ultrasonography, and chemical tests. For the most part, rodent species are very receptive to mating, and if copulation does occur, a high percentage of the females will become pregnant. Therefore, it is a common practice either to observe copulation or to look for the vaginal plug that forms immediately following copulation. To ensure accuracy, vaginal smears may be obtained, and if sperm are found, the animal is designated as being in day 0 of pregnancy (Moler et al., 1979). A second method, developed primarily for use in primates, is digital palpation. Rectal bimanual palpation of the uterus in the rhesus macaque (Fig. 25.16) was described by Hartman (1932), with few improvements added to the technique in subsequent years. The palpator inserts a gloved lubricated index finger into the rectum (the 'pinky' finger is inserted into the smaller cynomolgus macaque (M. fascicularis). The cervix is encountered upon initial entry, but the finger must be inserted until the anterior free edge of the uterus is palpated (Van Pelt, 1974). The free hand is cupped on the caudoventral abdomen, and the uterus is immobilized between the thumb and first two fingers of the free hand ventrally or dorsally by the rectally positioned finger. The normal nonpregnant uterus may vary in width from 7 to 21 mm or more (Catchpole and van Wagenen, 1975). The first palpable sign of pregnancy is a dorsoventral rounding of the anterior aspect of the body of the uterus (Fig. 25.16)

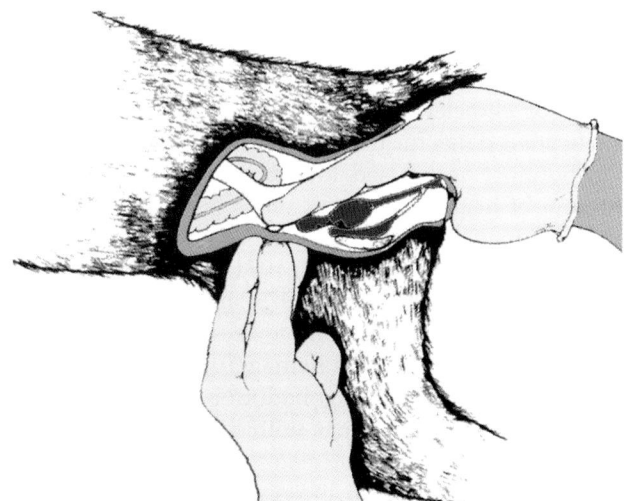

FIGURE 25.16 Rectal bimanual pregnancy palpation. This figure illustrates the positioning of the fingers for digital palpation of the female nonhuman primate reproductive tract. *Reprinted with permission from Van Pelt (1974).*

(Mahoney, 1975a, b). Individual animal records containing approximate uterine sizes on previous palpations, as well as menstrual cycle and breeding records, should be reviewed prior to palpating the animal (Moore, 1983).

Gloves should be changed and lubricated before palpating additional animals. Early embryonic abortions may occur if palpation is performed prior to implantation or if excess manipulation of the uterus occurs soon after implantation. Skilled, cautious palpators can determine pregnancy at 30 days from the onset of the last cycle, with a recheck performed 2 weeks after the initial positive palpation. Females should be palpated prior to assignment to breeding males to determine if they are in fact pregnant, thus freeing the male for use with another cycling female.

Rectal palpation in concert with daily cycle records aids in the evaluation of females as potential breeding stock. A long, 7-mm wide 'worm' uterus often indicates a poor breeding prognosis. Palpable adhesions of the uterus to abdominal structures may predict complications in future pregnancies. If spotting of blood is neither observed nor recorded in cycle records, either by technician error or 'personal hygiene' practice by the monkey, the female may be erroneously labeled as having irregular cycles. Review of cycle records should reveal the inconsistency with subsequent cycles occurring at the appropriate cycle interval for that female (Moore, 1983).

Sonographic measurements allow prediction or confirmation of gestational age using tables generated for cynomolgus and rhesus macaques (Tarantall and Hendrickx, 1988). Ultrasonic confirmation and characterization are the current standard for evaluating pregnancy in nonhuman primates. Radiographs have also been used to confirm pregnancy in its latter stages. This technique is most useful following calcification of the skeleton. Due to the variation in gestation periods among species, the effective date at which a diagnostic radiograph may be taken will vary. Therefore, the investigator or clinician needs to be knowledgeable of the calcification dates for the species under investigation.

Laboratory tests used for pregnancy determination are now of historical interest only. The nonhuman primate pregnancy test has been used for diagnosis in macaques (Hodgen and Ross, 1974), baboons (Hobson, 1976; Hodgen and Niemann, 1975), marmosets (Hodgen et al., 1976a, b, 1978), chimpanzees, and orangutans (Hodgen et al., 1977). This hemagglutination inhibition test for urinary chorionic gonadotropin uses an antiserum (H-26) that cross-reacts with the chorionic gonadotropin of a variety of primates and provides results within 2 h. Conventional bioassays and radioimmune assay systems are also useful procedures for detection of chorionic gonadotropin. The nonhuman primate pregnancy test, employed in conjunction with uterine palpation, is a useful method in most nonhuman primates (Hodgen et al., 1978; Lequin et al., 1981; Hall and Hodgen, 1979). In the domestic cat, abdominal palpation can determine pregnancy by 21–26 days of gestation, while serum progesterone levels are elevated as early as 6 days after breeding (Hammer and Howland, 1991). Ultrasound pregnancy diagnosis is a simple, commonly used technique for determining pregnancy in humans and a variety of animal species (Peter et al., 1990; Hammer and Howland, 1991).

G. Embryo Transfer and Cryopreservation

Embryo transfer, used extensively in research with laboratory animals, involves the removal of the developing embryo from the reproductive tract of one female and transferal to another. A technique commonly used for the production of transgenic and knockout mice, embryo transfer may also be used for the production of pathogen-free colonies (Rouleau et al., 1993). Experiments involving separation of maternal and fetal genetic effects are possible with this technique. The transfer of pre-implantation mouse embryos may be accomplished either surgically, by making an incision through the abdominal wall and exposing the uterus, or nonsurgically, by gaining access to the uterine lumen through the vagina. In the general technique, embryos can be transferred by oviductal (infundibular) or uterine transfer. A skin incision is made on the dorsal midline caudal to the costal arch. The incision is pushed to the left or right of the midline and the ovary or its fat pad is identified through the thin abdominal musculature. An incision through the body wall is made over the ovary and it is gently exteriorized and restrained using a serrefine. In the case of infundibular transfer, the ovarian bursa is incised, the infundibular opening identified, and the transfer pipette inserted. For uterine transfer, the uterine horn is exteriorized, a 26- to 30-g needle is used to pierce the horn, and the transfer pipette is inserted. After transfer is complete, the ovary or uterus is returned to the abdominal cavity, and the body wall and skin are sutured separately (Behringer et al., 2014). Embryo transfer has also been successful in rabbits (Prins and Fox, 1984), cats (Swanson and Godke, 1994), ferrets (Sun et al., 2014), and woodchucks (Concannon et al., 1997).

The creation and maintenance of archives of cryopreserved oocytes, ovaries, embryos, and spermatozoa are the necessary consequence of the study of mouse genomics (Glenister and Thornton, 2000). Mouse embryos may be collected and stored at −196°C. Successful cryoprotectants used for long-term storage of embryos include dimethyl sulfoxide, ethylene glycol, glycerol, and erythritol. Each cryoprotectant has an optimum freezing and thawing rate that must be followed in order to achieve the highest survivability of embryos (Leibo *et al.*, 1974; Kasai *et al.*, 1981; Guan *et al.*, 2012; Manno, 2010). Cryopreservation of a number of tissues has recently been reviewed (Sztein *et al.*, 1999; Pinkert, 1998; Nakagata, 2000; Rodriguez-Martinez and Wallgren, 2011).

H. Intrauterine Fetal Surgery

Surgical procedures performed on developing fetuses in a number of animal species have been excellent models for similar procedures in human fetuses and the study of maternal fetal physiology. At present, life-threatening congenital malformations, such as diaphragmatic hernia, obstructive uropathy, pulmonary hypoplasia, and some cardiovascular anomalies including aortic valve stenosis, have been corrected on human fetuses. Sheep have been the classic model for such studies because the developing lamb is close in size to the human fetus, and sheep usually have only one or two fetuses at a time (Emery *et al.*, 2007). Ultrasound may be used to confirm pregnancy and to determine the number of fetuses present in the uterus (Hoffman *et al.*, 1996; Keller-Wood *et al.*, 1998). Rabbits, swine, and nonhuman primates can also be used and may serve as excellent models for some disease conditions (Moise *et al.*, 1992; Kizilcan *et al.*, 1994; Swindle *et al.*, 1996; Stark *et al.*, 1989; Dewan *et al.*, 2000; Butler *et al.*, 1998).

XI. CARDIOVASCULAR TECHNIQUES

Animal models have been used to provide major insights into techniques of cardiovascular manipulation. Techniques have included developing surgical methods for organ transplants, vessel transplants and prostheses, arteriovenous shunts, blood pressure studies, electromagnetic flow probes, and microangiography (Bishop, 1980; Chung *et al.*, 1999; Zhong, 1999). Additional models are described in Simon and Rogers (2001).

A. Blood Pressure Techniques

Systolic and diastolic blood pressures can be difficult to monitor in animals because of the problems associated with physical restraint and the variability of cardiovascular parameters that can be caused due to the associated stress. Blood pressure can be monitored by direct or indirect measurement, each having advantages and disadvantages. Indirect blood pressure monitoring is usually done using a cuff system to identify changes in blood flow during cuff insufflation over a peripheral artery. Advantages include the noninvasiveness of the systems, the ability to do repeat measurements in

conscious animals, and relatively inexpensive equipment. Indirect measurements can detect larger differences in systolic pressures and are advantageous for screening larger groups of animals (Kurtz *et al.*, 2005). Disadvantages include the influences of restraint mechanisms during these measurements, inaccuracies due to measuring small sample sizes of cardiac cycles, and cuff size mismatches depending on the species. It is recommended that animals be exposed and acclimated to the measuring systems daily for 7–14 days prior to beginning experiments (Kurtz *et al.*, 2005). Sensing can be done using photoelectric, oscillometric, acoustic, or Doppler sensors. Tail cuff techniques generally are satisfactory in rats (Zatz, 1990; Ikeda *et al.*, 1991) and mice, and newer systems (CODA system, Kent Scientific; MRBP system, IITC Life Sciences) have been found to be comparable to invasive, telemetric blood pressure monitoring (Feng *et al.*, 2008). A tail cuff containing a photoelectric sensor has proven to be effective in miniature swine (Cimini and Zambraski, 1985). Using a commercial oscillometric pressure monitor in the baboon, Hartford *et al.* (1996) found no advantage in using the arm over the tail and concluded that such a device showed good correlation with, but not good agreement with, invasive measurements. In anesthetized dogs, Sawyer *et al.* (1991) showed that indirect blood pressure measurements were most accurate when the ratio of cuff width to limb circumference was between 0.4 and 0.6, and when systolic pressure was between 80 and 100 mmHg. Studies comparing indirect and direct blood pressure in ferrets have also been performed (Ko *et al.*, 1997; Olin *et al.*, 1997). Both studies found divergence in measured values.

Direct arterial blood pressure can be measured using radiotelemetry devices, fluid filled catheters, or high-fidelity pressure transducers (Millar Instruments, Houston, TX) placed directly into the vessel. Exteriorized catheters can be passed through the skin and placed in a protective jacket or passed through a swivel and tether system. Indwelling catheters (fluid-filled and high-fidelity) are the most accurate because of the ability to calibrate these over time. In addition, these allow for real-time, continuous, 24-h monitoring and data collection for weeks to months depending on the species. Indwelling catheters can be placed at varying locations including atrial and ventricular chambers and large vessels such as the pulmonary artery and aorta. A disadvantage of the fluid-filled catheter system is the potential for infection at the skin exit site or intravascular infections. These can also occlude due to clotting or fibrin deposition at the catheter tip and require strict aseptic techniques to maintain patency. Some infection complications can be avoided by attaching catheters to subcutaneous ports and accessing these via a Huber needle (see Section IV).

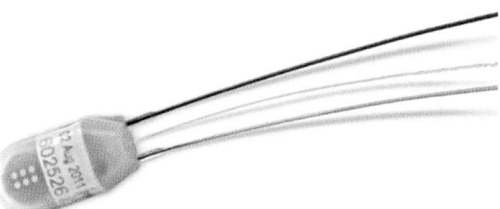

FIGURE 25.17   Multifunctional rodent telemetry device (HD-X11: Mouse Blood Pressure & ECG unit – Data Sciences International).

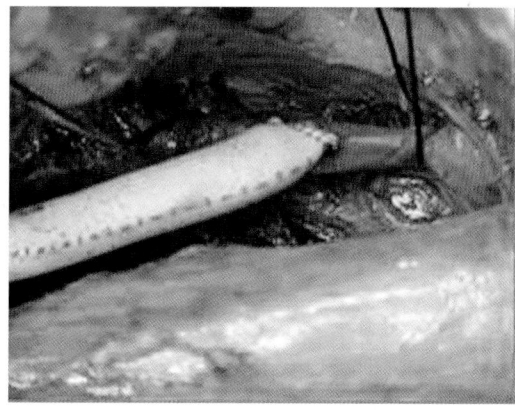

FIGURE 25.18   End-to-side anastomosis of PTFE graft to the jugular vein in a pig.

Radiotelemetry devices are also available that can be placed in virtually any species from mice to primates (Fig. 25.17). These are multifunctional units that have gel-filled catheters which are placed intravascularly to monitor blood pressure and have additional sensors for measuring body temperature, electrocardiogram (ECG), activity of the animal and other parameters (Integrated Telemetry Systems, Data Sciences International, St. Paul, MN). The primary advantage of these systems is that they allow continuous real-time measurements 24h a day without the use of jackets, restraint devices, or tethering systems. They have proven to be very accurate and reliable over long periods of time (Rey et al., 2012) and can be maintained for months depending on the species.

Other more invasive or direct methods have been used for direct arterial pressure measurements in sheep, cows, and horses including using the carotid artery loop procedure, which externalizes the carotid artery (Lagutchik et al., 1992; Orsini and Roby, 1997). In cardiopulmonary pathophysiology, the measurement of pulmonary arterial (PA) pressure is of considerable importance. This measurement is useful in studying the effects of drugs on pulmonary vasculature and in the diagnosis and treatment of lung and heart diseases. Using a bent-tip, 23-gauge light-wall Teflon catheter (PE-50) inserted into the right jugular vein, Carrillo and Aviado (1969) and Hayes and Will (1978) successfully catheterized the pulmonary artery of the rat. The Teflon catheter was inserted until the 'shepherd's crook' tip reached the right atrium and was then manipulated until its bent tip entered the pulmonary artery. Stinger et al. (1981) describe a similar method.

B. Carotid–Jugular Shunt

The carotid–jugular shunt technique has been used as an access site for obtaining repeated blood samples and for chronic vascular access (Belding et al., 1976). Larger species, including goats and dogs, have been used for carotid–jugular shunts. Following anesthesia, the carotid artery and jugular vein are surgically exposed. The jugular vein is tied off cranially with two strands of No. 2 surgical silk. Using a 20-cm-long and 6-mm-diameter

polytetrafluorethylene (PTFE) graft, end-to-side anastomoses were made between the jugular vein and the carotid artery following appropriately sized venotomy and arteriotomyincisions (Fig. 25.18).

The venous anastomosis is usually completed first followed by an end-to-side anastomosis to the carotid artery. The graft is then implanted subcutaneously in the cranial portion of the neck and the skin closed over the graft. Arteriovenous fistulas have been described in cats, rats (Korber and Flye, 1987), rabbits, and larger species (Desjardins, 1986). Arteriovenous shunts between the carotid artery and the jugular vein have been used in several species including rabbits (Miyamoto et al., 2004) and goats (Bolotin et al., 2002) to develop a volume overload hypertrophic cardiomyopathy and left ventricular hypertrophy models.

C. Microangiography

Microangiography is a technique in which blood vessels are visualized by the use of roentgen contrast medium and microradiographic techniques. It is a technique that can be used acutely or in the chronic (survival) setting and is applicable to a variety of experimental animals, including rodents, swine, dogs, rabbits, and rats, as well as many anatomical regions. For acute studies, the animal is placed under general anesthesia, an artery is cannulated by cutdown or percutaneous technique with an appropriate catheter, and 1mg of heparin per kilogram is administered. The level of cannulation and corresponding transection of vessels for the efflux of blood and the perfusion of finely ground barium sulfate for each species are well described by Erol et al. (1980). Following injection of the contrast medium, rapid film microradiographic techniques are employed.

In the survival setting, microangiography has been used in conjunction with more advanced technologies including magnetic resonance imaging (MRI), computed tomography (CT) and micro CT scan, and digital subtraction angiography (DSA) to provide information on vessel diameter and anatomy (Rhee *et al.*, 2006; Kumar *et al.*, 2009; Caldwell *et al.*, 2011), as well as functional information including changes in vessel diameter and blood flow with treatment or in different pathologic conditions (Schambach *et al.*, 2009, 2010a; Lin *et al.*, 2009; Figueiredo *et al.*, 2012). Image acquisition speed (temporal resolution), signal or contrast-to-noise ratio (CNR), volumes of contrast agents required (contingent on their inherent contrast, clearance time, and the circulation time of the patient), and spatial resolution vary by imaging modality, technique and instrumentation within a modality, and study objective (Schambach *et al.*, 2010a,b). Micro CT provides very good contrast for bone but relatively poor soft tissue contrast, necessitating the use of contrast agents for angiography. In rodents, iodinated compounds are cleared very rapidly, and the circulation time is so short that the first pass of a contrast medium bolus cannot be visualized. Blood-pool contrast agents have therefore been developed that bind to plasma proteins and have a much longer duration within the blood. These agents have a lower level of contrast and so are useful only for vessels of large caliber but allow serial evaluation of the vasculature within an individual animal. Longer scan times also produce higher CNR. Newer, liposome-based blood-pool contrast agents provide better visualization of smaller anatomical structures (Schambach *et al.*, 2010b). In a comparison of micro CT, DSA, and magnetic resonance angiography in evaluation of mouse cerebrovascular circulation, Figueiredo showed that micro CT and DSA provided better spatial (16 × 16 × 16 µm and 14 × 14 µm, respectively) and temporal resolution than time-of-flight (ToF) magnetic resonance (MR), but the latter had better CNR. The temporal resolution of DSA was such (30 frames per second) that cerebrovascular blood flow could be analyzed. Micro CT angiography required 20–40 s, whereas ToF MR angiography required 57 min for completion. The use of MR contrast agents shortens this time, increases the CNR, and can also evaluate perfusion. Commercially available instruments and software were used in their study. In a separate evaluation, DSA images were used to statistically derive blood flow metrics that were then correlated to physiologic techniques (Fick effect and thermodilution) for calculating cardiac output in rats (Lin *et al.*, 2009).

XII. ENDOCRINE SYSTEM TECHNIQUES

Studies involving mechanisms of the endocrine system often require the sacrifice of large numbers of experimental animals in the experimental protocol. Therefore, the rodent species have assumed a major role of importance in these studies. Endocrine techniques discussed in this section include hypophysectomy, pinealectomy, adrenalectomy, thyroidectomy, and parathyroidectomy.

A. Hypophysectomy

Rodents possess an almost flat sella turcica that positions the hypophysis for rapid and easy removal (Sato and Yoneda, 1966). The position of the hypophysis under the midbrain is directly on the midline at a point perpendicular to a line joining openings of the auditory canals. As the rat grows older, the hypophysis becomes displaced rostrally. The transauricular technique of Falconi and Rossi (1964) and its modification by Sato and Yoneda (1966) have been supplanted by the parapharyngeal approach described by Nakanishi and Nagasawa (1976). A recent modification of the classical approach includes the use of ketamine/xylazine/isoflurane anesthesia, eliminating the use of tracheotomy, and stabilization of the mouse in a 'V'-shaped trough (Hoff *et al.*, 2006). In this technique, a 1-cm ventral midline incision is made in the neck, followed by intermittent, lateral retraction of the salivary glands, omohyoid muscle and trachea, and removal of the periosteum from a 4- to 6-mm area centered at the occipitosphenoidal synchondrosis. A burr hole is made at the synchondrosis with a dental drill and the hypophysis is gently aspirated. Survival rates improved when 5% glucose or tetracycline is used for 3 days postoperatively. Drinking water should be supplemented with 5–10% glucose for the duration of the study (Charles River Laboratories, 2006; Hoff *et al.*, 2006). A parapharyngeal method has also been described in the rat (Waynforth and Flecknell, 1992). Hypophysectomies have been performed in the dog by an extracranial route through the oral cavity (transsphenoidal), by an intracranial route through the anterior or middle cranial fossa, and by the pharynrecess. These techniques are described by Lopukhin (1976) and Markowitz *et al.* (1964). Other techniques described include a paraoccular approach for the rabbit (Lopukhin, 1976) and a combination of the transtemporal and parapharyngeal approaches for hypophysectomizing calves (Whipp *et al.*, 1970).

B. Pinealectomy

The rodent pineal body is a median epithalamic structure originating from the dorsal diencephalon and extending dorsally to the superior sagittal sinus (Peterborg *et al.*, 1980). The first technique for pinealectomy was presented in 1910 (Baker *et al.*, 1980). Subsequent techniques were described by Hoffman and Reiter (1965), Bliss and Bates (1973), and, most recently, Kuszak and Rodin (1977) and Jurek (1977). The most recent technique is described by Foley (2005) and involves the following: the anesthetized animal is placed in a stereotaxic device; a 1.5-cm longitudinal skin incision is made over the cranium; periosteum is scraped from the area to be drilled; and a dental drill is used to create a burr hole over the right cerebral hemisphere at the junction of the saggital and lamboid sutures. The dura is incised; the superior saggital vein is doubly ligated (if necessary), and then resected to expose the gland. The pineal gland is then freed and removed using a blunt-tipped, curved, iris scissor. This technique has the advantage of being more direct, produces a minimal amount of hemorrhage, and allows for a perfect sham operation because no sympathectomy is required. Pohlmeyer *et al.* (1994) have described pinealectomy in rats.

C. Adrenalectomy

Adrenalectomy is the surgical removal of one or both adrenal glands. Removal of both glands causes severe physiologic changes that are difficult to correct with replacement therapy. Therefore, in clinical practice, it is a rarely used technique, with the exception of use in the ferret, in which adrenal gland tumors are prevalent and in which staged unilateral adrenalectomies and subtotal bilateral adrenalectomies are established techniques. However, from a research standpoint, this technique has proved to be very valuable (Lang, 1976).

The technique of adrenalectomy for the dog is well described by Lang (1976) and Lopukhin (1976). Hoar (1966) cites several references indicating the difficulties of performing this procedure in guinea pigs. He also describes a technique for the guinea pig that is shorter, simpler, and less traumatic than other similar procedures. A brief description of his procedure is as follows: surgical preparation of the thoracoabdominal region, incision of the skin over the penultimate intercostal space, incision of the intercostal muscles (avoiding cutting the peritoneum), incision of the peritoneum using a blunt-nosed scissors, and use of saline-soaked gauze to pack off the intestines and liver for exposure of the kidney and adrenal. Mobilization of the adrenal is a four-step procedure: (1) the cranial pole of the kidney is freed, (2) the loosened fascia attached to the adrenal is freed from the diaphragm, (3) the adrenal is now freed by blunt dissection, and (4) the fascial connections between the liver and posterior vena cava are dissected free. When the gland is adequately freed, the adrenal vein is clamped off and the gland removed. A Gelfoam sponge is used to control hemorrhage over the severed stump of the adrenal vein (Hoar, 1966). If required, removal of the opposite adrenal is usually accomplished at a later date.

In mice, adrenalectomy is achieved using a dorsal midline incision at the level of the first through third lumbar vertebrae (Charles River Laboratories, 2006). In a fashion similar to that used for ovarian access, the incision is moved laterally to expose the paracostal

musculature. An incision is made caudal to the caudalmost rib, and the adrenal on either side is visualized by lateral retraction of the spleen (left side) or cranial retraction of the liver (right side). The adrenal and its associated fat pad are identified, and the vessels supplying the gland are crushed with two pairs of hemostats. The gland is removed by section between the clamps. No other hemostasis is required. Bilaterally adrenalectomized mice require normal saline as a water source (Hayward *et al.*, 2006; Charles River Laboratories, 2006).

An adrenalectomy procedure using a paralumbar approach has been described in the rat (Waynforth and Flecknell, 1992). Adrenalectomy techniques in the ferret utilize both ventral abdominal and paralumbar approaches (Marini and Fox, 1988; Mehler, 2014).

D. Thyroidectomy and Parathyroidectomy

The role of the thyroid in reproduction, metabolism, myocardial enzyme activity, and tissue catalase activity has been investigated in several species (Kromka and Hoar, 1975; Lopukhin, 1976; Lang, 1976). The thyroid gland in most species consists of two lobes connected centrally by an isthmus. It can be removed surgically or destroyed by radio-iodine administration (Hayward *et al.*, 2006). The murine thymus is in the cranioventral cervical region, deep into the cervical musculature and directly superficial to the cricoid cartilage and first four tracheal rings. The surgical approach requires a 1.5- to 2.0-cm ventral midline incision extending from the clavicle cranially. Surgical resection requires crushing associated vasculature and preserving the recurrent laryngeal nerves; the latter cross the dorsal surface of the gland. As some parathyroids are invariable removed, mice should receive 2% calcium lactate solution for at least 7 days postoperatively. Alternatively, parathyroids can be dissected free from the thyroid gland and reimplanted in the potential space created by the absent thyroid (Charles River Laboratories, 2006; Taconic, 2014; Hayward *et al.*, 2006).The parathyroid glands are critical for the body to maintain the proper calcium and phosphorus metabolism. Although references to thyroparathyroidectomy procedures are scattered throughout the literature, they are difficult to find and generally are lacking in details necessary for surgical proficiency. The anatomy of the thyroid differs from species to species and should be reviewed prior to surgery. The following technique is described for guinea pigs by Kromka and Hoar (1975). The animal is anesthetized, and the ventral neck area is surgically prepared. A 2.5-cm skin incision is made just caudal to the larynx. With the aid of a dissecting microscope, the infrahyoid musculature is separated on a midline exposing the trachea. Retractors are used to visualize the thyroids and parathyroids on either side of the trachea. The thyroids and/or parathyroids are dissected free, being careful not to damage the recurrent laryngeal nerve as it passes deep and medial to the thyroids. Cautery is helpful in freeing the gland to expose the vascular bed, which lies on the medial aspect of the cranial pole. This vasculature is then ligated and/or cauterized to free the thyroid and parathyroid glands. Surgical thyroidectomy is enough to produce a temporary hypothyroid state, but long-term experimentation requires the additional use of ^{131}I to destroy developing thryoid rests (Kromka and Hoar, 1975). The parathyroids are not always attached to the thyroids in guinea pigs, so care should be taken to identify these organs before excising (Peterson et al., 1952). The number and the location of the parathyroids vary in each species. In mice, a variable number of glands exist and are located anywhere from the dorsolateral border of the thyroids to the thymic septa (Hummel et al., 1975). Moreover, the glands are not easily distinguished from surrounding tissue unless they are from strains in which melanoblasts are contained in the parathyroids. Complete surgical removal is difficult, therefore, and thyroidectomy may only affect partial parathyroidectomy. Parathyroid glands which can be identified appear as minute white areas on the anterior surface of the thyroid and can be removed by electrocautery (Taconic, 2014). Reduction in serum Ca^{2+} concentration is considered a biomarker for successful parathyroidectomy (Hayward et al., 2006; Taconic 2014; Charles River Laboratories, 2006). Parathyroidectomy has also been described for the dog by Lang (1976) and Lopukhin (1976) and for the rat by Waynforth and Flecknell (1992).

XIII. ORTHOPEDIC PROCEDURES FOR LABORATORY ANIMALS

The need for surgical correction of clinical fractures, tendon, or cartilage injuries in laboratory animals is usually determined through a thorough physical examination and/or diagnostic imaging (Fig. 25.19; MRI, CT, or digital radiography).

The advisability of injury repair should be determined by suitability of the animal for further study, the severity of the injury, and other considerations. Fracture repair and stabilization techniques should be adapted from procedures described for companion animals (Richards et al., 1972; Anson, 1993; DeYoung et al., 1993; Egger, 1993; DeCamp, 1993; Piermattei et al., 2006). Current orthopedic research using animals tends to be directed toward issues such as fracture healing, tendon repair, and cartilage replacement and regenerative medicine using various stem cell therapies. A lumbar spinal fusion in a goat model is shown in Fig 25.20.

Recent studies have focused on the use of growth-enhancing materials (bone morphogenic protein;

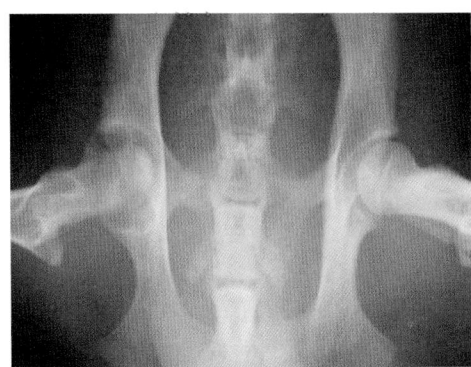
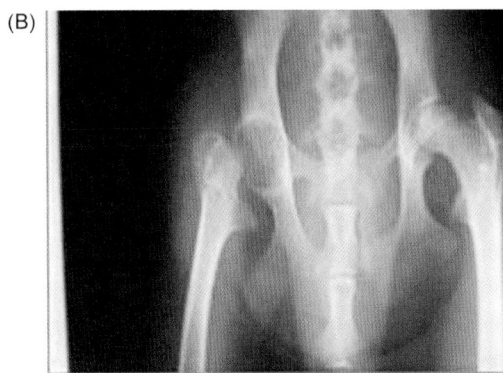

FIGURE 25.19 Legg–Perthes in a cynomolgus macaque. (A) Avascular necrosis of the right femoral head. Note the osteolysis of the femoral head. (B) Femoral head and neck osteotomy. *Images courtesy of Drs. Chad Faulkner and Michael Talcott (2013).*

low-level electromagnetic stimulation) to speed the healing of bone fractures, the continuing search for safe and effective prosthetic materials, and methods to speed healing in the presence of antineoplastic drugs. Many of the techniques used in these studies are well described by Adams (1988) and by An and Freidman in *Animal Models of Orthopedic Research* (1998).

XIV. NEUROSURGICAL TECHNIQUES

A. Surgical Procedures

1. Lumbar Sympathectomy

Lumbar sympathectomy has been used for conditions of humans such as Raynaud's disease, arteriosclerosis, and thromboangiitis obliterans. In experimental animals the technique involves anesthesia; surgical preparation of the abdomen; a midline incision; use of a self-retaining retractor; packing off the small intestine with warmed, saline-soaked sterile towels; and exposure of the lumbar sympathetic chain with subsequent sympathectomy or excision of the hypogastric nerve. Cold allodynia and hyperalgesia are frequent clinical findings in patients with neuropathic pain. Rats undergoing lumbar sympathectomy were found to have attenuated

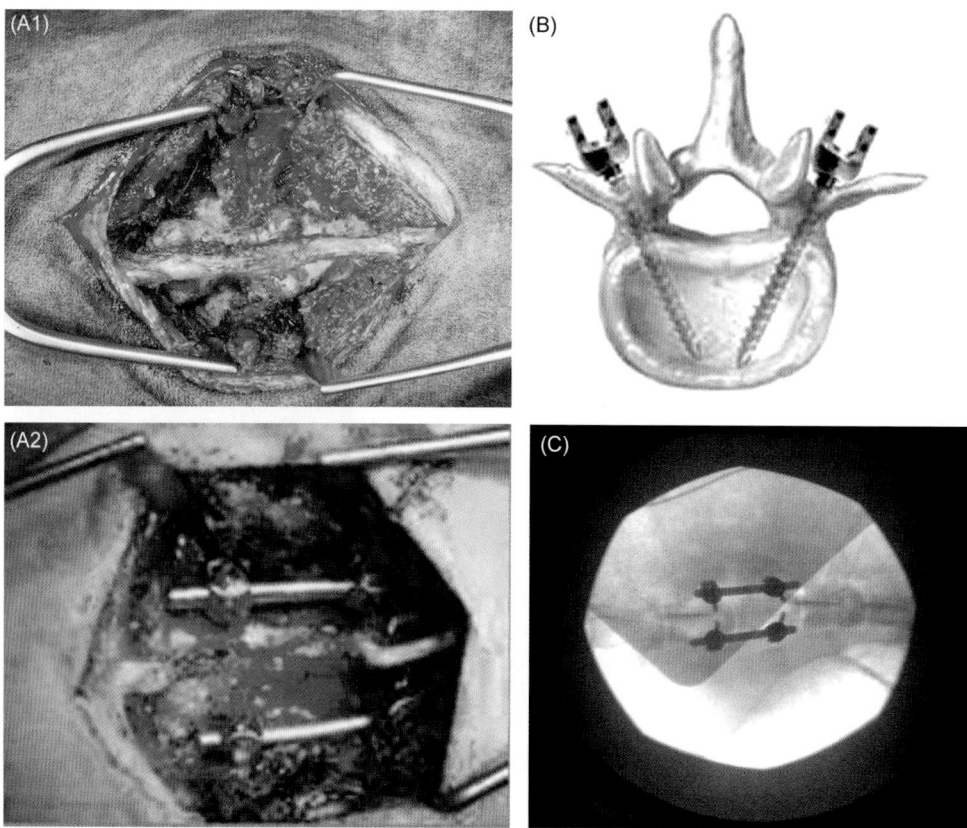

FIGURE 25.20   Lumbar spinal fusion in a goat model. (A) Surgical exposure of the dorsal spinous processes and lumbar vertebra; (B) placement of bilateral pedicle screws and rods; (C) radiographic confirmation of adequate placement of stabilization devices. *Images courtesy of Dr. Michael Talcott, 2011; www.jedpwebermd.com.*

response to cold allodynia and have been used in the assessment of sympathetic pain states (Zhao *et al.*, 2007; Murata *et al.*, 2006). Renal sympathectomy is theoretically a sound operation for chronic glomerulonephritis, especially before there is too much destruction of the renal parenchyma. It should be noted that there is regeneration of the excised sympathetic chain in most species. Total extirpation of the sympathetic chains in cats, dogs, and monkeys does not seem to affect the life of the animal (Markowitz *et al.*, 1964). Catheter-based interventional strategies that interrupt the renal sympathetic nervous system have shown promising results in providing better blood pressure control in patients with resistant hypertension. Dogs (Lu *et al.*, 2012), pigs (Linz *et al.*, 2013), and rats (Intapad *et al.*, 2013) have been used to investigate the effect of renal sympathetic denervation on the development of hypertension and associated cardiac disease including the development of atrial fibrillation and other arrhythmias.

Sympathectomy has been used in swine to investigate the effect of vasospasm on restenosis following angioplasty (Lamawansa *et al.*, 1999) and in dogs to investigate blood flow to the cauda equina following compression injury (Onda *et al.*, 2004). Bilateral lumbar sympathectomy was performed in swine subjected to femoral balloon endarterectomy. Although sympathectomy did not inhibit intimal thickening, it did result in an increase in luminal area. Lumbar sympathectomy has been used in a rat model of chronic limb ischemia (Van Dielen *et al.*, 1998) and in the rat model of neuropathic pain induced by ligation of the L5 spinal nerve (Ringkamp *et al.*, 1999).

2. Exposure of the Cerebrum, Cerebellomedullar Region, and the Skull Base

Techniques have been established in smaller laboratory animals to approach areas of the brain and skull base without damage to associated structures. Exposure of the cerebral cortex has been performed in many species using a standard craniotomy (replacement of the bone flap) or craniectomy (bone flap is not replaced) for craniofacial procedures (Eufinger *et al.*, 2007) and numerous neurosurgical procedures, including deep brain stimulation (Katada *et al.*, 2008; Johnson *et al.*, 2008). Pigs and rabbits have also served as models for evaluating biomaterials for dural replacements (Fig. 25.21) (Chaplin *et al.*, 1999).

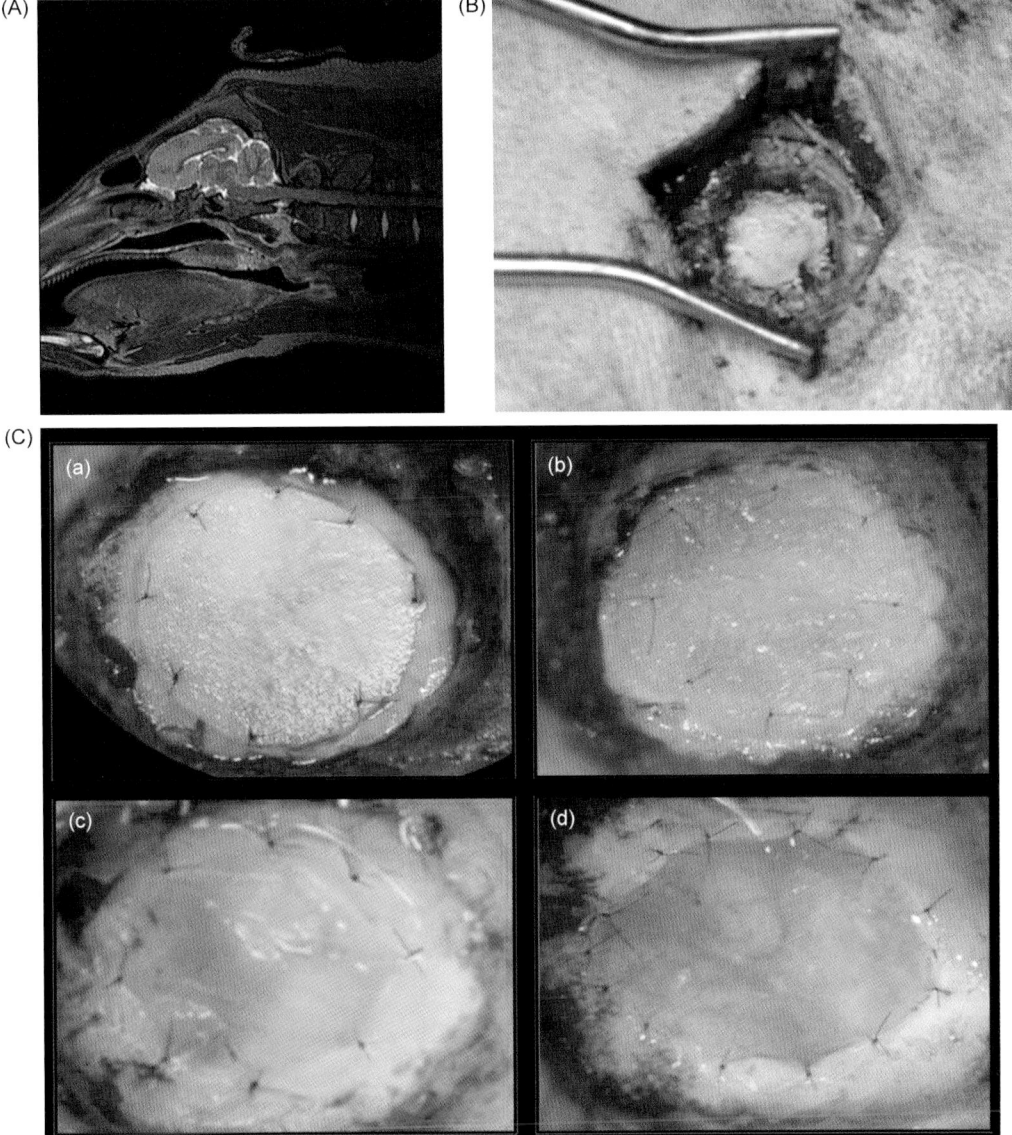

FIGURE 25.21 (A) MR image of swine head identifying cranial vault; (B) 1-cm craniotomy of parietal bone exposing cerebrum; (C) duroplasty using various biomaterials in the pig.

Renella and Hussein (1986) have described a microsurgical approach to the cerebellomedullary region of the rat, which provides access to the medulla and basal cerebellum. The spheno-occipital synchondrosis located in the posterior basicranium is important for normal craniofacial growth. Experimental studies in laboratory animals have helped define the importance of this area. Surgical exposure in the neonatal rat (Reidenberg and Laitman, 1990b) and the rabbit (Haworth *et al.*, 1992) has been described. Rabbits have been used to investigate craniosynostosis which can be associated with calvarial and midfacial abnormalities and leads to optic nerve compression, blindness, and mental retardation (Putz *et al.*, 2002; Fellows-Mayle *et al.*, 2006).

3. Spinal Laminectomy

Spinal laminectomy is a relatively common procedure to expose the spinal cord in larger laboratory animals. With the increase in the availability of genetically manipulated mice, surgical access to the spinal cord for various neuromuscular studies has been developed and refined. Ellegalla *et al.* (1996) have described the approach to the thoracolumbar spinal cord in mice by using fine-toothed forceps rather than rongeurs for removing the dorsal spinal lamina. The spinal motoneuron provides a good model system in mice for studying neural function and recent studies have reported performing intracellular recordings of motoneurons *in vivo* and the force developed by their muscle targets allowing identification of different types of motoneurons based on their force profile (Manuel and Heckman, 2012).

4. Intracerebral Implantation and Injection

A number of experiments have been designed to demonstrate the effects of the direct action of neonatal hormones on a mammal's developing brain (Hayashi and Gorski, 1974). The instruments required for this technique in the rat include a converted 5-ml syringe that can be attached to a stereotaxic instrument. The syringe has a central threaded metal rod that is fitted with a clip to hold the steel wire of the implanting stylet. The stylet (27-gauge hypodermic needle) tubing and wire are attached to the syringe, and the wire is firmly held by the clip. A hormone implant is fused to the end of the wire, and as the wire is pulled through the tubing, the implant is left unattached to the apparatus. This technique of implantation in the gerbil involves anesthetizing the animal; making a scalp incision; placing the head in a stereotaxic apparatus; and, using coordinates, drilling a hole into the skull. The stylet is now lowered to the proper depth and the implant is detached. The stylet is then removed and the wound is closed with collodion (Holman, 1980). Other methods for neurological examination in the gerbil include the implantation of platinum wire-recording electrodes and the implantation of a chronic ventricular infusion cannula (Herndon and Ringle, 1969).

Mice are commonly used for neurologic studies investigating infectious diseases, pharmacological agents, and cancer therapies. Intracerebral injections are used to administer compounds directly into the brain at various locations based on the study needs. Orthotopic tumor implantation is generally performed through a dorsal approach using bregma as a landmark for locating the desired region of the brain to be targeted. Mice are placed in a standard stereotaxic apparatus (Stoelting, Inc.) following anesthesia. A small incision is made through the skin and a small drill hole is made in the desired location for the injection using standard stereotaxic coordinates (Paxinos and Franklin, 2012). Figure 25.22 shows the location of bregma and lambda as defined by Dr. George Paxinos (Paxinos and Watson, 1998).

An alternative method for delivering compounds through the postglenoid foramen in the mouse has been developed and found to be precise, less invasive, and a safe alternative to standard stereotaxic procedures (Iwami et al., 2012).

5. Stereotaxic Electrode Implantation and Headplate Attachment

Stereotaxic brain electrode implantation involves the use of an instrument for immobilizing the animal's head and calibrated to identify coordinates in the brain for placement of electrodes in premapped structures. The coordinates are read from horizontal, coronal, and sagittal planes. Stereotaxic atlases are available for most common laboratory animals and may be developed for others (Cain and Dekergommeaux, 1979; Harris and Walker, 1980; Paxinos and Franklin, 2012). The zero point for the coordinate system may be alternately the intersection of the coronal and sagittal skull sutures – bregma – or the middle of an interaural line. Atlases have been developed based on these two zero systems. Bregma zero points have the advantage of being grossly visible and introducing less error with different-sized heads. Stereotaxic devices come with varying frame sizes for different-sized animals but have interchangeable coordinate bars so that one frame might be used on mouse-through dog-size heads and another on goats. Parts include a cranial–caudal adjustment for coronal planes,

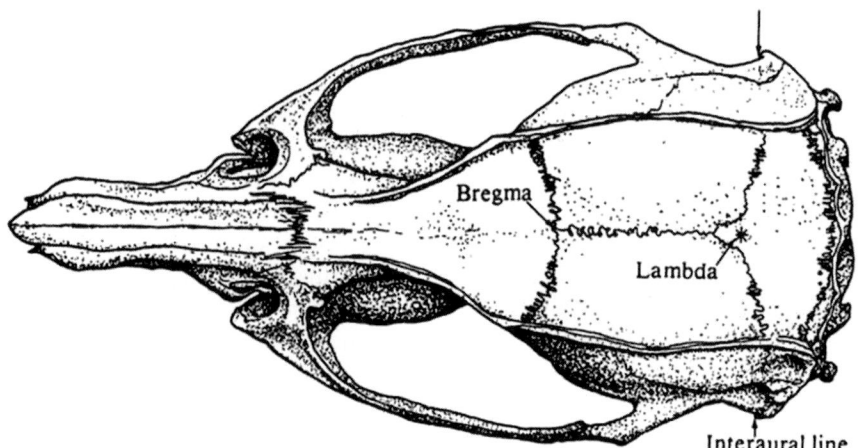

FIGURE 25.22   Location of bregma and lambda as defined by Dr. George Paxinos. *George Paxinos and Charles Watson: The Rat Brain in Stereotaxic Coordinates, Academic Press, New York, 1998, p. 11. Courtesy of Academic Press.*

lateral adjustment for sagittal planes, depth adjustment for horizontal planes, and electrode holder, ear bars, incisor bars, nose clamp, and infraorbital bars for dogs, cats, and monkeys. For stereotaxic electrode implantation in the rat brain, the rat is anesthetized and atropine is given at 1 mg/kg to reduce airway secretions. The shaved head is steadied in a stereotaxic device by the ear bars placed in each auditory meatus, and the incisor bar is fitted behind the front incisors with a nose clamp over the snout. Placement must be precise for symmetric alignment of the brain between these points. Sterile ophthalmic ointment (petrolatum ointment) is placed in both eyes to keep them moist and protect them from noxious materials such as antiseptics or dental acrylic. The scalp is appropriately prepped, and a midline scalp incision is made from between the eyes to between the ears and to the end of the external occipital crest. The incision is extended to the skull, and the periosteum is reflected back with a bone curette or periosteal elevator. The periosteum is held back with hemostats on each side of both ends of the incision. Bleeding is controlled with cotton swabs and pressure. An electrode drill is attached to the electrode carrier. The skull is leveled visually or by making horizontal readings at bregma (intersection of sagittal and coronal sutures) and lambda (intersection of sagittal and lambdoidal sutures). Different atlases may specify various horizontal readings above or below zero. If bregma is not used as the zero, this point will have to have been established prior to positioning the ear bars on the rat to get the right interaural depth reading for zero. The coordinates for electrode placement are read from an atlas for the structure being examined as millimeters from zero in each plane. If bregma is zero in the atlas, the coordinates of bregma are read from the stereotaxic device on the rat to an accuracy of 0.1 mm, using a Vernier scale. The structure site for implantation is identified in the serial sections of an atlas at its largest size, and the coordinates of the atlas are added or subtracted from the coordinates attributed to the zero reading in the rat being implanted. Only the bony skull is drilled, with the dura left intact. Additional smaller holes are drilled in four corners of the skull within the incision line for placing jeweler's screws to help anchor the dental acrylic cap. The holes should not be placed in the relatively weak suture lines or too close to the electrode hole. The dura is slit with a sterile needle, and the jeweler's screws are placed 1 mm into the calvarium, avoiding the dura and brain surface. The electrode is placed, using either the surface of the brain or the surface of the skull as a reference point for depth. Atlas readings for depth or structures are generally from the brain surface. One millimeter is added for skull thickness if this is used for reference (Cooley and Vanderwolf, 1978). A small piece of Gelfoam dipped in saline and pressed nearly dry is placed around the electrode to keep toxic

dental acrylic off the brain (Skinner, 1971). The electrode is fixed in dental cement. Powder and solvent are mixed to syrupy consistency and allowed to harden around the electrode and jeweler's screws. The electrode end(s) are fitted with contacts that attach to a connector base, and they are incorporated in additional dental acrylic layers applied over the skull to create a secure cap. Acrylics and bone cements generate heat during curing; these materials should be applied in thin laminae to avoid thermal injury to subjacent tissue. The connector base eases connection of the electrodes to electrical recording instruments. The acrylic cap should be free of sharp edges that could hinder incision healing. The bottom of the connector base should be as close as possible to the skull, to preclude dislodgement of the implant cap. Skin closure is made with simple interrupted sutures, bringing the skin tight against the cement cap. The rat is removed from the stereotaxic device and allowed to recover (Skinner, 1971).

Headplates are commonly attached to the skull of laboratory animals to protect implanted electrodes, to provide a point of restraint to prevent head movement, and to hold and protect cephalic cylinders used to provide repeated access to various structures of the brain. Gardiner and Toth (1999) provide extensive description of methods to place and maintain cranial implants in rats. These techniques are readily adaptable to other laboratory species and are commonly used in nonhuman primate neuroanatomy studies. A comprehensive review of common neurosurgical procedures in primates including application of head restraint posts, implantation of multi-electrode arrays and eye coils, and creation of cranial recording chambers can be found in *Nonhuman Primates in Biomedical Research: Biology and Management, Surgery in Nonhuman Primates* (Niekrasz and Wardrip, 2012). Headplates often consist of a combination of a stainless steel or titanium implant with dental acrylic, such that the device is affixed to the skull with screws and then partially covered with dental acrylic. Rabbits have a well-developed sagittal crest that prevents the attachment of some types of headplates. Rickards and Mitchell (1992) have described a headplate that has been modified to eliminate this problem. Headplates and access cylinders require meticulous care to minimize infection (Lee *et al.*, 1998).

B. Spinal Catheters

Catheterization of the spinal canal is done for both therapeutic and experimental purposes. Epidural administration of analgesics is a commonly performed practice in humans for relief of pain associated with a variety of surgical procedures and medical conditions and is becoming more common for pain control in surgically manipulated large laboratory animal species such as dogs. In laboratory animals, such catheters are more likely used for the delivery of drugs for experimental reasons, as in a recent study evaluating the epidural anesthetic effect of an 8% emulsified isoflurane infusion in rabbits (Chai et al., 2008). Such studies may be directed at investigating the effects of a drug on the spinal cord or at studying the effects of such drugs on the fetus. Epidural catheters may be inserted surgically or percutaneously. In the guinea pig, epidural catheters can be inserted surgically by performing a dorsal laminectomy in the L3–L4 space to expose the dura. The catheter is then carefully inserted in the epidural space and implanted subcutaneously for future access (Eisele et al., 1994). In another study, intrathecal administration of indomethacin was achieved using a P-10 caliber microcatheter placed at the L2–L3 interspace. The catheter was attached to an Alzet osmotic minipump which was then placed subcutaneously (Guavera-Lopez et al., 2006). In the rabbit, Arkan et al. (1996) describe the placement of an epidural catheter by amputating the tail and inserting the catheter through the exposed epidural space. Chai et al. (2008) removed the dorsal spinous process of L6 to facilitate ligamentum flavum incision and epidural placement of a polyethylene catheter (diameter 0.8 mm). Rosenquist et al. (1996) report the placement of an epidural catheter in the rabbit via percutaneous puncture of the L5–L6 space. Epidural cooling catheter placement has been described in spinal cord protection studies using both rabbits and swine (Yoshitake et al., 2007; Inoue et al., 2013). An intrathecal catheter was inserted 7 cm cephalad after incision of the dura at the L6 level (Malinovsky et al., 2002). No catheter-induced spinal cord lesions were observed in 10 control animals.

Subarachnoid catheter placement in both lumbar and thoracic spinal cord of mice requires a surgical approach, although the lumbar technique involves only the skin (Poon et al., 2011; Wu et al., 2004). The size of the catheter is important, as less postoperative motor dysfunction was observed with PU-10 (OD 0.25 mm) compared to PE-5 (OD 0.51 mm). The PU catheter is also more pliant and less likely than PE to impale or damage structures (Poon et al., 2011). Surgical access in placement of the thoracic catheter required removal of the paravertebral musculature from T11 through L1, and removal of dorsal interspinous and interspinous ligaments between T12 and T13. The intervertebral space was accessed next, the epidural fat removed, and the dura mater slit with a 30-gauge needle. The catheter was inserted and secured with tissue glue. In the PU-10 group, all mice surviving anesthesia and the immediate postoperative period had no motor deficits (Poon et al., 2011). Similar approaches and procedures are described in the rat. A variation on the approach involves drilling a 2 × 2 mm hole in the left T13 lamina proper, and subsequent insertion of a custom modified PE-10 catheter. Tissue glue and a silicon

bead affixed to the catheter help stabilize it to the vertebra (Poon et al., 2005). A 4-0 suture serves as a stylet for the catheter; a 1-cm, L-shaped hook placed at the insertion end assists in placement of the catheter into the laminotomy space. Ehlert et al. (2010) review procedures that access the intracranial subarachnoid space of the rat and describe the placement of a catheter into the subarachnoid space at the cerebro-cerebellar fissure. Access is achieved by trepanation just rostral to the occipital-interparietal suture. The subarachnoid space within the skull is accessed to model subarachnoid hemorrhage or to infuse agents onto cerebral arteries (Ehlert et al., 2010).

Remedios and Duke (1993) described the surgical placement of an epidural catheter attached to a vascular access port in the L4–L7 region of the cat. The dorsal lamina of the selected spinal segment was exposed by dissection of the overlying musculature. By use of a handheld drill chuck, an intramedullary pin was used to create a hole through the dorsal lamina into the epidural space though which the catheter was inserted. Percutaneous insertion of an epidural catheter attached to a vascular access port through the L7–S1 site has been described in the rhesus macaque (DeWeert et al., 1995). Proper placement of the catheter is determined by a loss of resistance during insertion and is confirmed by contrast radiography.

C. Cerebrospinal Fluid Sampling

The collection of ventricular and cisternal cerebrospinal fluid (CSF) has been described for cattle (Cox and Littledike, 1978), swine (Boogeerd and Peters, 1986), goats (Peregrine and Mamman, 1993), rhesus monkeys (Snead and LaCroix, 1977; Wolf and White, 2012), marmosets (Geretschlager et al., 1987), horses (Spinelli et al., 1968), rats (Brakkee et al., 1979; Waynforth and Flecknell, 1992; Kusaka et al., 2004), guinea pigs (Suckling and Reiber, 1984), dogs (Elias and Brown, 2008), and rabbits (Kusumi and Plouffe, 1979). These techniques should be performed aseptically in anesthetized animals. In dogs, the animal is placed in lateral recumbency and the neck is flexed so that the head is approximately at a right angle to the body. A line is drawn on the dorsal midline joining the external occipital protuberance and the dorsal spine of the axis; another line is drawn at the cranial extremity of the wings of the atlas. The spinal needle must be perfectly parallel to the mandible, and, at least to start, orthogonal to the dorsal cervical surface. A 20- to 22-gauge, 1.5-inch spinal needle is inserted at the intersection of this line and advanced 2–3 mm at a time until a sudden loss of resistance, the characteristic 'pop,' is felt. As the needle is advanced, the operator periodically removes the stylet and checks for the presence of fluid by wiping it against the sterile gloved hand. Once fluid appears in the needle hub or is discerned by wiping the stylet, cerebrospinal fluid (CSF) can be collected by allowing it to drop from the needle or can be gently aspirated by syringe. One milliliter of CSF can be withdrawn for every 5 kg body weight of the patient (Elias and Brown, 2008). A 23- or 25-gauge butterfly catheter can be used for cats.

For obtaining rabbit CSF, the rabbit is anesthetized, and the dorsal cervical area and occipital area of the skull are shaved. The rabbit is positioned in lateral recumbency, and with the ears firmly secured, the neck is flexed to expose the base of the skull. This area is aseptically prepared, and a 22-gauge, 3.81-cm (1.5-inch) needle (Stoelting, Chicago) is inserted with the free hand approximately 2 mm caudal to the external occipital protuberance. The needle is kept parallel to the table and is advanced slowly toward the animal's mouth. At times, a slight rotation of the head is needed to raise the anterior skull segments to allow this alignment. The needle is advanced through the caudal spinous muscle until a slight decrease in resistance is felt upon entering the fourth ventricle (cisterna magna). The stylet is then removed, and 1.5–2 ml of CSF can be collected (Fig. 25.23). This procedure may be accomplished in less than 5 min following anesthesia (Kusumi and Plouffe, 1979).

Catheters may be percutaneously inserted into the subdural space in the L4–L7 location and pushed cranially into the cisterna magna for CSF sampling in the rabbit (Haslberger and Gaab, 1986). The chronic catheterization of the cisterna magna, or third ventricle of the brain, has been used to obtain CSF in rabbits (Glue et al., 1988; Vistelle et al., 1994); rats (Shapiro et al., 2012; Sarna et al., 1983); swine, sheep, and goats (Prelusky and Hartin, 1991; Forte et al., 1989; Eisenhauer et al., 1994);

and rhesus monkeys (McCully et al., 1990; Bacher et al., 1994).

CSF collection in macaques and rhesus monkeys is performed in the Telazol-anesthetized animal in ventral recumbency. The neck is flexed and prepared aseptically, the foramen magnum is palpated, and a 23-gauge, 1.5-inch needle is inserted, perpendicular to the skin, into the cisterna magna (Wolf and White, 2012). A distinctive release of resistance ('pop') is felt as the needle passes into the cisterna. A 1-ml syringe is used to gently aspirate the fluid (Fahey and Westmoreland, 2012). A similar technique describing cisternal aspiration of CSF and subsequent infusion of test article suggests the use of extension tubing attached to the spinal or hypodermic needle. This reduces the chance of altering the position of the needle during syringe transfer (Clingerman et al., 2010). In smaller nonhuman primates, the animal is anesthetized, restrained seated or upright, prepared aseptically, and a 25-gauge, ⅝-inch needle is used to access the cisterna. Lumbar collection of CNS in larger nonhuman primates can be achieved using the L4–L5 or L5–L6 interspaces.

CSF may be obtained from mice and rats following surgical exposure of the atlanto-occipital region of the spine (Vogelweid and Kier, 1988; Hudson et al., 1994). Serial collection of CSF at 2- to 3-month intervals from mice can also be achieved though a surgical approach in the same animal if approved by an Institutional Animal Care and Use Committee (IACUC) (Liu and Duff, 2008). With the mouse positioned in a stereotaxic device, a skin incision is made caudal to the occipital protuberance. The dorsal neck muscles are bluntly dissected and retracted. The mouse's body and head are positioned

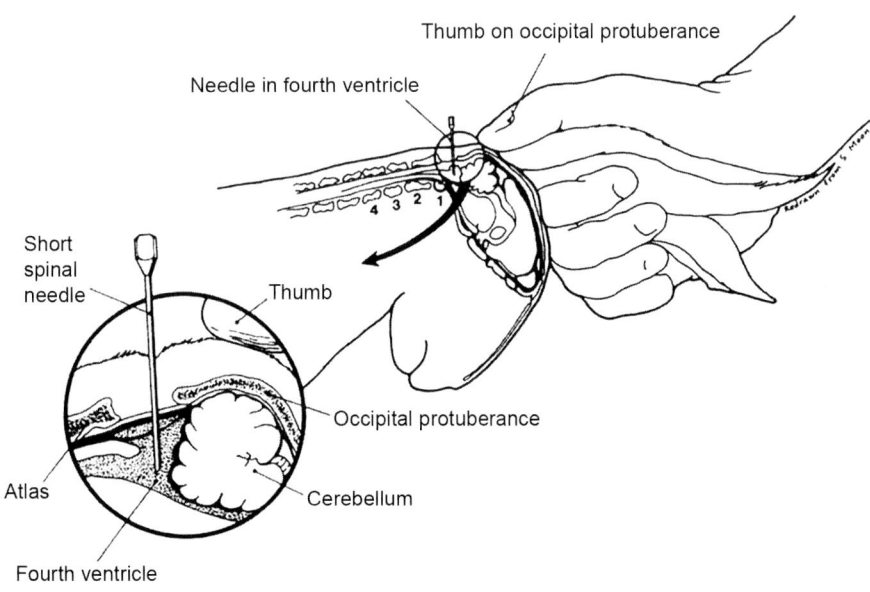

FIGURE 25.23 Landmarks for CSF sampling in the rabbit. *Reprinted with permission from Kusumi and Plouffe (1979).*

so that a 135° angle is created (equivalent to a 45° ventral deflection of the snout). A dissecting microscope is used to insert a glass capillary tube, pulled to an ID of 0.5 mm, through the atlanto-occipital membrane and into the cisterna magna. The insertion site should be lateral to the midline dorsal spinous artery. Seven to 8 μl of CSF can be collected. Similar surgical techniques have been described in the rat (Pegg et al., 2010; Liu et al., 2012). Both these studies require an anesthetized animal and stereotaxic restraint. Liu et al. (2012) position rats with a 45° angle deflection as described in mice. After dissection to expose the atlanto-occipital membrane, a 21-gauge needle, customized to have a 90° angle bend of its distal tip away from the bevel, is used to produce a longitudinal slit in the membrane, exposing the dura. A 30-gauge needle attached to a 1-ml syringe is then advanced with bevel up at a 30° angle into the dura from a caudal direction. When the end of the bevel is at the level of the dura, the bevel is rotated downward, so that it faces the spinal cord, it is inserted another millimeter, and gentle aspiration collects the CSF. Typical volumes of 50–150 μl are collected. Only one of nine animals had blood contamination of the sample with this technique; no animals experienced behavioral or motor deficits. Liu et al. (2012) describe a similar dissection, except that the atlantooccipital membrane is not dissected independently, and the animal is positioned such that its body is perpendicular to the horizontal axis of the stereotaxic device, and the needle, attached to polyurethane tubing, is attached to an electrode holder with a 90° bend at its distal end. The needle thus restrained is then advanced using the holder arm. It pierces the atlantooccipital membrane and enters the cisterna magna; CSF flows into the tubing and is collected by gentle aspiration. Collection volumes varied from 150 to 200 μl in a 5-min period. Serial samples of 100 μl on each of three occasions at weekly intervals were taken in a subset of rats; the third sample was collected acutely. Muscles were sutured after each sampling. No behavioral or ambulatory abnormalities were noted (Liu et al., 2012).

Techniques not requiring surgical exposure have also been described for CSF collection in rats. Mahat et al. (2012) achieved serial sampling for 4 weeks and collected an average volume of 150 μl. Anesthesia and stereotaxic restraint were used as in the surgical approaches, but animals were positioned with the dorsum of their heads at a 110° angle to the horizontal plane of the stereotaxic base (conversely, with the ventral aspect of their heads at a 70° angle to the horizontal plane), and their bodies raised by a platform to a height of 3 cm above the base. This positioning and the use of the platform allowed access to the cisterna magna while diminishing the potential for respiratory obstruction. A 21-gauge needle with a silicon bead 4–6 mm from its beveled end was attached to an electrode holder and used to access

the cisterna. In this technique, the needle is advanced using the electrode holder and the coordinates A–P: 1.5 ±1 mm; M–L 0 mm; the needle is advanced until the bead rests on the skin. The authors report the use of this technique in 150 rats with a 97% rate of success (samples uncontaminated with blood) (Mahat et al., 2012). The use of ultrasound to collect CSF percutaneously from rats has also been described (Lu et al., 2013).

Lumbar collection of CSF from rats requires surgery to assist placement of the needle. Contamination of taps with blood occurred in 25% of samples of 30–50 μl taken from animals accessed through the L5–L6 interspace (De la Calle and Paino, 2002), and in 11% of samples taken through L6–S1 (Wang et al., 2005). The latter study succeeded in collecting CSF 96% of the time, compared to 90% in the former study. The Wang study was considerably more invasive, however, and required removal of the dorsal spinous process of S1 and the interspinous ligament to accurately access the subarachnoid space. A 27-gauge needle, bent at a 60° angle, was used.

XV. TUMOR TRANSPLANTATION

A number of excellent reviews of mouse models of cancer are available and explore not only transplantable tumors but those involving genetically engineered animals and administration of carcinogens (Molecular Oncology, 2013; Borowsky et al., 2003; Galvez et al., 2004; Cheon and Orsulic, 2011). Additionally, the Mouse Models of Human Cancers Consortium of the National Cancer Institute website (http://www.nih.gov/science/models/mouse/resources/hcc.html) provides considerable information on mouse models of cancer with links to animal sources and other databases. Select definitions concerning transplantation are found in Table 25.5.

Since 1965, stable lines of transplantable tumors have been developed that are well characterized in terms

TABLE 25.5 Transplantation, Select Definitions

Term	Definition
Autograft	A graft of tissue from one site to another on the same individual. Rejection is rare.
Allograft	A graft between genetically dissimilar animals of the same species. This graft may undergo rejection.
Xenograft	A graft between animals of different species. Rejection may be quite violent.
Heterotopic	A graft of tissue or organ from its normal anatomic site in the donor to another anatomic site in the recipient.
Orthotopic	A transplant of tissue or organ from its normal anatomic site in the donor to its normal anatomic site in the recipient.

of speed of growth, size, morphology, histology, local invasiveness, tendency to metastasize or regress, and response to chemotherapeutic agents (Roberts, 1969). The athymic (nude) mouse was the traditional recipient of these tumor tissues, either allograft or xenograft, and was typically placed heterotopically (ectopically). The *In Vivo* Hollow Fiber Assay, in which varying numbers of semipermeable hollow fibers, each fiber filled with a different tumor cell line, is implanted in a nude mouse, derived from this common practice (http://www.dtp.nci.nih.gov/branches/btb/hfa.html) (Zhang *et al.*, 2007). The most common site of tumor transplantation has traditionally been the subcutis, although intraperitoneal and subrenal capsule implantation are also used.

It is now recognized, however, that with some notable exceptions these heterotopically placed tumor cell lines neither accurately model the pathophysiologic features of the parent tumor nor predict clinical responsiveness to therapeutics (Ruggeri *et al.*, 2014). Tumors derived from cell lines tend to be undifferentiated and homogenous, with a diminished capacity for metastasis (Kelland, 2004). In contrast, tumors derived from primary sources like patient biopsies better maintain their original morphology. It has been suggested that the selection pressures exerted on tumor cells in culture are responsible for the phenotypic differences between tumors resulting from original and cell line-derived cells (Ruggeri *et al.*, 2014; Kelland, 2004). The virtues of orthotopic xenotransplants have made tumor site-specific implantation far more common than in the past. The advantage of the orthotopic transplant is that it can exploit the microenvironmental and stromal factors on which phenotypic development, growth, and metastatic potential of the parent tumor depend (Singh *et al.*, 2004; Sano and Myers, 2009).

One of the most important aspects of ensuring a long-lasting transplant take is proper selection and/or preparation of the host to prevent a host-*versus*-graft reaction (Festing, 1980). The mouse has been the model of choice for xenotransplantation due to availability of mutant or genetically engineered animals with varying degrees of pertinent immunodeficiency. The use of immunodeficient rodents in tumor transplantation is reviewed in *Immunodeficient Rodents* (NRC, 1989) and elsewhere (Barbacid and Berns, 2013). *In vivo* xenotransplantation has been traditionally performed in nude (athymic), severe combined immunodeficient (SCID), or recombinase-activating gene-mutant (Rag) mice. The generation of mice lacking the common cytokine receptor gamma chain (γc), for example, NOD, scid, γ (NSG) mice, or Rag $2^{-/-}$ $γc^{-/-}$ mice, has improved engraftment of human xenografts (Konantz *et al.*, 2012). In the case of NSG mice, they have defective macrophage and dendritic cells (innate immune system), the *scid* mutation, thereby lacking T and B cells, and a null mutation of the γc chain, rendering natural killer (NK) cells nonfunctional (JAX website). Humanization of immunodeficent mice can theoretically improve the relevance of studies of human xenografts.

Another animal model of xenotransplantation which is growing in acceptance is the zebrafish. In comparison with the mouse, the zebrafish has shorter time to engraftment of human cells, less engraftment heterogeneity among animals, and the ability to image small numbers of engrafting cells (Konantz *et al.*, 2012). Fish can be immunosuppressed by irradiation or dexamethasone administration if receiving transplants as adults, but do not require immunosuppression if receiving xenotransplants prior to the development of adaptive immunity (blastocyst to 48 h postfertilization). Embryonic development *ex utero*, and the transparency of embryos and the existence of transparent lines of fish, allows easy visualization of small numbers of prelabeled tumor cells. Zebrafish have been used in studies of invasiveness, metastasis, and tumor-induced angiogenesis, and as a tool for drug discovery (Konantz *et al.*, 2012).

The physical techniques involved with tumor transplantation are fairly simple. Careful selection of tumor and host combination are necessary. Healthy host animals must be chosen, and the transplant should be an actively dividing, nonulcerated tumor if possible. High standards of sterile technique are mandatory. For animal donors, the donor is anesthetized or euthanized, and the tumor is removed to a sterile Petri dish. Chilled sterile saline or refrigerated culture medium is used to moisten the tissue, and nonhemorrhagic, nonnecrotic areas are aseptically minced into 2- to 3-mm fragments. If tumor cells are being grown by tissue culture, the cells are dispersed by using 0.02% EDTA in phosphate-buffered saline. Cell viability is determined using trypan blue staining. The amount of media necessary to adjust the viable cells to $10^6/0.2$ ml is added (Kyriazis *et al.*, 1982). For optimal results, transplantation should occur quickly following removal from the donor. Donor tissue from noninstitutional sources should be tested prior to transplant for murine adventitious agents and agents hazardous to personnel.

Subcutaneous inoculation is the oldest and most commonly used site for transplantation. If tumor fragments are being utilized, a 3- to 5-mm fragment is inoculated subcutaneously, using a trocar. Alternatively 10^6–10^7 tumor cells may be injected. Growth is measured using calipers. The tumor should not be palpated, because of the danger of fatal hemorrhage from highly vascular tissues. Newer cell-labeling techniques now allow the evaluation of tumor cell 'takes' before tumors are of adequate size for palpation. Green fluorescent protein and firefly luciferase are two of the reporter vectors used for tracking labeled xenograft cells (Zhang *et al.*, 2007). Such noninvasive imaging also allows for the evaluation of tumor progression, drug response, metastasis, cure, or relapse (Baiocchi *et al.*, 2010). Strict criteria and endpoints should be established by the IACUC for guidance concerning clinical intervention and euthanasia endpoints in tumor studies.

For orthotopic evaluation of intracranial cancer, xenotransplants or allotransplants are delivered via stereotaxic injection through cranial burr holes. The most commonly evaluated tumor is gliobastoma multiforme, the most malignant of the glioma class of tumor. Approximately 10^5–10^6 cells are required for successful engraftment in the nude mouse (Houchens *et al.*, 1983). Cells characterized and isolated as cancer stem cells (CSCs), however, require as few as 100 cells to produce a tumor capable of generating adequate mass to be used subsequently as an allograft (Singh *et al.*, 2004). The use of CSCs resulted in the development of intracranial tumors in 16 of 19 NOD-SCID mice injected with $CD133^+$ cells from patients with gliobastoma or medulloblastoma. CSC research is now actively engaged in determining strategies for treatment and prevention of recurrence (Pointer *et al.*, 2014).

Due to the rich vascular supply of renal tissue, implantation of tumors under the renal capsule may be desirable for enhanced tumor growth. Fragments of $1\,mm^3$ are implanted (Bogdon *et al.*, 1979). The subrenal capsule site provides a better microenvironment for tumor growth than the subcutis. Normal, primary human cells grown in culture can develop into fully vascularized, functional tissue in this site, and can also undergo malignant transformation, as demonstrated in cultured primary human fibroblast cells (2×10^6 cells) transduced by oncogenes and implanted below the renal capsule in Rag $2^{-/-}\,\gamma c^{-/-}$ mice (Sun *et al.*, 2005). Bladder cancer models can be established by intravesicular or intramural methods. The technique described by Edwards *et al.* (1978) is typical of the intravesicular approach, in that instillates are placed transurethrally. The bladder is infused with the antiseptic Cetavlon, which is left in for 30 min. The bladder is then emptied, irrigated with 0.9% saline, and filled with tumor suspension. This method is very effective for induction of bladder tumors in rabbits and rats. Disadvantages of intravesicular approaches include seeding of the tumor cells in extravesicular sites like the ureter or urethra. Rats will also show renal tumor growth, because of a species-characteristic vesicoureteral reflux. The intramural methods have the advantage of visualization of the placement of the tumor inoculum, either directly, when a laparotomy is performed, or ultrasonically or laparoscopically. A technique for ultrasonographic intramural inoculation of tumor cells into the bladders of nude mice has been recently described (Jäger *et al.*, 2014). Progression can be evaluated by ultrasound or by chemiluminescence if reporter genes are used.

XVI. IMAGING TECHNIQUES

Diagnostic and imaging techniques routinely used in human medicine include plain and contrast radiography; fluoroscopy, X-ray CT; ultrasonography, nuclear scintigraphy, MRI, positron emission tomography (PET), single-photon emission CT (SPECT), and endoscopy. As the technologies have been refined and new technologies developed, higher sensitivity and resolution have also provided significant benefits, such as reduction in the number of subjects needed for many research studies involving laboratory animals (Koba *et al.*, 2011), for research involving laboratory animals Anesthesia is generally required for restraint during procedures, both to minimize animal stress and to reduce motion artifacts during image acquisition.

Radiography is a standard diagnostic tool that uses X-rays' attenuation by body tissues to produce an image. The development of thin screen phosphor films enables high-resolution digital imaging of small animals using low-energy X-ray sources (Pizzonia *et al.*, 2012). Fluoroscopy is a modification of X-ray examination that is used to visualize the continuous movement of internal structures. In many instances, a contrast medium, such as barium or an iodinated compound, is administered to provide more definition of the soft tissue in the area of interest (e.g., gastrointestinal system, urinary tract, CNS, or cardiovascular system). X-ray CT involves acquisition of many X-ray views which can be later reconstructed into 3D images. CT is particularly useful for musculoskeletal investigations, with resolution of 50 μm in living animals (Koba *et al.*, 2013).

Ultrasonography detects surface reflection of physical vibrations (echoes) produced by high-frequency sound waves to create visual images of internal structures. It requires direct contact of transducer probes with tissue surfaces and generally requires fluid interface for optimal signal contrast. It is commonly used for diagnostic purposes in both humans and animals to discriminate cystic *versus* solid masses; to interrogate body cavities filled with fluids that prohibit radiographic techniques; to discriminate the texture of suspected solid masses; to locate nonradiopaque calculi within organs; to evaluate cardiovascular physiology (echocardiography), muscle, and tendon tissues; to diagnose pregnancy; and to provide biopsy guidance for biopsy of internal masses and fluids (e.g., cystocentesis, amniocentesis). High-frequency ultrasound (HFUS) systems enable imaging laboratory animals with very high spatial (30 μm) and temporal (1000 fps) resolution (Gregg and Butcher, 2012). It is used primarily to visualize tissue blood flow and cardiovascular physiology in rodents (Moran *et al.*, 2013).

MRI is a common diagnostic tool in human medicine and is becoming more commonly used in domestic and laboratory animal diagnosis and experimental techniques. It provides excellent intrinsic tissue contrast for 3D, whole-body imaging, without radiation, by detecting small differences in bulk physical properties of hydrogen nuclei aligned in high-strength magnetic fields. Dynamic contrast enhancement with magnetic (iron) and paramagnetic agents (gadolinium) are used to assess blood flow kinetics and vascular permeability in various diseases. MRI contrast and resolution are dependent on magnetic field strength. Clinical MRI scanners are most commonly used for imaging larger animals, such as rabbits, cats, dogs, and nonhuman primates. While clinical MRI systems use magnetic field strengths of 1.5 or 3 Tesla (T), laboratory animal studies benefit from smaller bore, higher field systems, now up to 21 T. High-field MRI systems are very expensive, but newer technology in permanent magnets enables bench top low-field magnets (1 T) which are used for good mouse MRI (Rotman et al., 2011).

PET and SPECT are two methods for whole-body imaging using radioactive tracers (Koba et al., 2013). Validation of new radiotracers for selective targeting of disease-specific molecular mechanisms is performed in mouse and rat models prior to use in humans. Instruments for PET and SPECT also include CT to provide anatomical information for signal localization. The small size of mice enables new imaging geometries such as parallel plate PET for high-throughput imaging with a small footprint (Herrmann et al., 2013).

Optical imaging is a pillar in biomedical research from super-resolution microscopy to whole-body imaging in animal models (Zhang et al., 2012; Ntziachristos and Razansky, 2013). Optical imaging techniques for imaging beyond 1 mm deep in tissue face significant barriers as resolution of light-based imaging decreases rapidly with depth due to scattering and absorption. Despite these challenges, laboratory animal optical imaging systems are now prevalent for in vivo detection of genetic reporters (luciferase, fluorescent proteins, galactosidase). These technologies enable translation of cell-based assays into living animals. With bioluminescent reporters, as few as 1000 cells can be detected noninvasively after implantation. Fluorescent proteins have expanded from the original GFP through protein engineering to span the visible wavelength range (Brogan et al., 2012; Drummen, 2012). This is particularly important for animal imaging studies as longer wavelength light (<650 nm) penetrates deeper in tissues for improved sensitivity (Zhang et al., 2012).

Hybrid imaging methods include optoacoustic (a.k.a. photoacoustic) imaging which combines optical and ultrasound imaging to provide the sensitivity of optical contrast with the depth of ultrasound detection (Ntziachristos and Razansky, 2013). Conversion of light energy to localized heat upon absorption of light causes an elastic expansion that can be detected by ultrasound transducers. Tissue

chromophores such as hemoglobin and melanin provide natural contrast, while synthetic dyes and nanomaterials can be administered for enhancing tissue specific contrast. As with optical imaging, photoacoustic imaging resolution scales with depth, providing micrometer resolution at depths less than 1 mm and millimeter resolution at 1 cm. Optoacoustic imaging is frequently paired with ultrasound imaging for anatomic information.

XVII. RADIOTELEMETRY

Radiotelemetry combines a physiologic sensor with a radio transmitter and receiver to allow the acquisition of data from a freely moving animal without the need for any type of restraint (such as tether and jacket) (DataSciences International, St. Paul, MN; Mini-Mitter Company, Inc., Sunriver, OR; Biomedic Data Systems, Seaford, DE; Konigsberg Instruments, Pasadena, CA; Star Medical Arakawa-ku, Tokyo, Japan). Current devices now have batteries that can be turned on and off magnetically to extend their life and battery life has been improved considerably. Such devices can simultaneously transmit data on body temperature, ECG, blood pressure, blood flow, activity, electromyogram (EMG), electroencephalogram (EEG), and pH, although the parameters that can be transmitted vary by device. A surgical procedure is needed to implant the device and to connect the catheters or wires to the structures to be monitored. Transmitters are typically inserted subcutaneously or intraperitoneally. Advances in miniarization and the use of genetically engineered animals allow considerable sophistication in experimental design. Telemetry to obtain physiologic data has been described in most laboratory animal species, including rodents (Kramer and Kinter, 2003), rabbits (Varosi et al., 1990; Brackee et al., 1995; Ronisz et al., 2013), ferrets (Percie du Sert et al., 2009), swine (Myrie et al., 2012), marmosets (Schnell and Wood, 1995), rhesus monkeys (Sadoff et al., 1992), and baboons (Pearce et al., 1989; Crean et al., 2007).

Radiotelemetry eliminates restraint-associated artifacts and collects a large amount of data with high precision. Moreover, sensor catheters and leads do not require maintenance and implanted animals can be reused with approval of the IACUC. In the industrial setting, general toxicity and safety data can be achieved in the same animals, and animal number can be further reduced if changes in physiologic variables identify dose-limiting toxicity (Kramer and Kinter, 2003).

XVIII. THYMECTOMY

Investigators may require thymectomized neonatal or adult mice for studies involving T-cell maturation or

ALFALFA IN FEED CAN CAUSE AUTO FLORESCENCE — USE ALFALFA FREE CHOW IN RODENTS requiring transplant tolerance. The murine thymus is an asymmetrically bilobed, mediastinal organ lying from the thoracic inlet to the heart base. Commercial vendors providing thymectomized mice use a thoracotomy procedure to remove the thymus. The pneumothorax created in this approach requires reestablishment of negative pressure after thymic removal. This is achieved simply by compression of the chest during surgical closure with wound clips or suture (Taconic, 2014; Charles River Laboratories, 2006; Hayward *et al.*, 2006). Procedures which do not require thoracotomy typically involve incision and dissection of the thoracic inlet, elevation of the manubrium, and suction removal of each thymic lobe with a 2.2-mm glass aspiration cannula. Procedures for thymectomy have been recently reviewed (Hayward *et al.*, 2006).

Acknowledgments

The authors recognize the contribution of Robert J. Adams, W. Sheldon Bivin, and Gerald D. Smith to previous versions of this chapter.

References

AALAS (American Association for Laboratory Animal Science), 1990.

Abatan, O.I., Welch, K.B., Nemzek, J.A., 2008. Evaluation of saphenous venipuncture and modified tail-clip blood collection in mice. J. Am. Assoc. Lab. Anim. Sci. 47, 8–15.

Abe, C., Tanaka, K., Iwata, C., Morita, H., 2010. Vestibular-mediated increase in central serotonin plays an important role in hypergravity-induced hypophagia in rats. J. Appl. Physiol. 109, 1635–1643.

Abernathy, R.E., Anderson, C.B., 1974. Exteriorized ureters in the dog. Lab. Anim. Sci. 24, 946–947.

Abraham, W.M., 2008. Modeling of asthma, COPD and cystic fibrosis in sheep. Pulm. Pharmacol. Ther. 21, 743–754.

Adams, C.L., Riehl, T.B., Johnson, T.L., 2013. Hand-held jugular vein phlebotomy technique for non-anesthetized mice. AALAS Poster.

Adams, R.J., 1988. Musculoskeletal system. In: Swindle, M.M., Adams, R.J. (Eds.), Experimental Surgery and Physiology: Induced Animal Models of Human Disease. Williams and Wilkins, Baltimore, MD, pp. 10–41.

Adeghe, A.J.-H., Cohen, J., 1986. A better method for terminal bleeding of mice. Lab. Anim. 20, 70–72.

Alexander, D.J., Clark, G.C., 1980. A simple method of oral endotracheal intubation in rabbits (*Oryctolagus cuniculus*). Lab. Anim. Sci. 30, 871–873.

Allen, S.A., 1974. A method for bladder catheterization of the male calf. Lab. Anim. Sci. 24, 96–98.

Allen, M.J., Borkowski, G.L., 1999. The Laboratory Small Ruminant. Laboratory Animal Pocket Reference Series. CRC Press, Boca Raton, Florida.

Ambrus, J.L., Ambrus, C.M., Harrison, P.W.E., Leonard, C.A., Moser, C.E., Cravitz, H., 1951. Comparison of methods for obtaining blood from mice. Am. J. Pharm. 123, 100–104.

American College of Laboratory Animal Medicine Series. Academic Press, Orlando, FL.

An, Y.H., Freidman, R.J., 1998. Animal Models in Orthopaedic Research. CRC Press.

Anson, L.W., 1993. Emergency management of fractures, second ed. In: Slatter, D. (Ed.), Textbook of Small Animal Surgery, vol. 2 Saunders, Philadelphia, PA, pp. 1603–1610.

Arkan, A., Kucukguclu, S., Kupelioglu, A., Maltepe, F., Gokel, E., 1996. New technique for catheterization of the sacral canal in rabbits. Contemp. Top. 35, 96–98.

Armstrong, P., Conrad, M., 2008. Blood collection from the American horseshoe crab, Limulus polyphemus. J. Vis. Exp. 20, e958.

Arora, K.L., 1979. Blood sampling and intravenous injections in the Japanese quail. Lab. Anim. Sci. 29, 114–118.

Avery, D.L., Spyker, J.M., 1977. Foot tattoo of neonatal mice. Lab. Anim. Sci. 27, 110–112.

Bacher, J., Kassianides, C., Moskal, T.J., Mathews, D.M., Hoofnagle, J.H., 1989. A technique for liver biopsy in Pekin ducks. Lab. Anim. Sci. 39, 67–68.

Bacher, J.D., Balis, F.M., McCully, C.L., Godwin, K.S., 1994. Cerebral subarachnoid sampling of cerebrospinal fluid in the rhesus monkey. Lab. Anim. Sci. 44, 148–152.

Bailie, M.B., Wixson, S.K., Landi, M.S., 1986. Vascular-access-port implantation for serial blood sampling in conscious swine. Lab. Anim. Sci. 36, 431–433.

Baiocchi, M., Biffoni, M., Ricci-Vitiani, L., Pilozzi, E., De Maria, R., 2010. New models for cancer research: human cancer stem cell xenografts. Curr. Opin. Pharmacol. 10, 380–384.

Baker, G.A., Gorham, J.R., 1951. A technique for bleeding ferrets and mink. Cornell Vet. 41, 235–236.

Baker, H.J., Lindsey, J.R., Weisbroth, S.H. (Eds.), 1979–1980. "The Laboratory Rat," vol. 1, "Biology and Diseases" (1979); vol. 2, "Research Applications" (1980). Academic Press, NY.

In: Baker, H.J. Lindsey, J.R. Weisbroth, S.H. (Eds.), The Laboratory Rat, vol. 2. Academic Press, New York.

Balabaud, C., Saric, J., Gonzales, P., Deiphy, C., 1981. Bile collection in free moving rats. Lab. Anim. Sci. 31, 273–275.

Ball, D.J., Argentieri, G., Krause, R., Lipinski, M., Robison, R.L., Stoll, R.E., et al., 1991. Evaluation of a microchip implant system used for animal identification in rats. Lab. Anim. Sci. 41, 185–186.

Banks, R.E., Roy, M., Hellems-Lewis, G., Hadick, C., 1989. Antigen delivery to gut associated lymphoid tissue of rabbits. Lab. Anim. Sci. 39, 582–586.

Bansal, A.K., Bilaspuri, G.S., 2010. Impacts of oxidative stress and antioxidants on semen functions. Vet. Med. Int.

Baran, S.W., Perret-Gentil, M.I., Johnson, E.J., Miedel, E.L., Kehler, J., 2011. Rodent laparoscopy: refinement for rodent drug studies and model development, and monitoring of neoplastic, inflammatory and metabolic diseases. Lab. Anim. 45 (4), 231–239.

Barbacid, M., Berns, A., 2013. Mouse models of cancer: essential tools for better therapies. Mol. Oncol. 7, 143–296.

Barber, H.W., Small Jr., P.A., 1977. Construction of an improved tracheal pouch in the ferret. Am. Rev. Respir. Dis. 115, 165–169.

Barringer, M., Sterchi, J.M., Jackson, D., Meredith, J., 1982. Chronic biliary sampling via a subcutaneous system in dogs. Lab. Anim. Sci. 32, 283–285.

Barrow, M.V., 1968. Modified intravenous injection technique in rats. Lab. Anim. Care 18, 570–571.

Bechtold, S.V., Abrutyn, D., 1991. An improved method of endotracheal intubation in rabbits. Lab. Anim. Sci. 41, 630–631.

Beck, J.M., Preston, A.M., Wilcoxen, S.E., Morris, S.B., Sturrock, A., Paine, R. I.I.I., 2009. Critical roles of inflammation and apoptosis in improved survival in a model of hyperoxia-induced acute lung injury in Pneumocystis murina-infected mice. Infect. Immun. 77, 1053–1060.

Behringer, R., Gertsenstein, M., Nagy, K.V., Nagy, A., 2014. Surgical Procedures Manipulating the Mouse Embryo, fourth ed. Cold Spring Harbor Press, Cold Spring Harbor NY, pp. 251–285.

Belding, R.C., Quarles, J.M., Beaman, T.C., Gerhardt, P., 1976. Exteriorized carotid-jugular-shunt for hemodialysis of the goat. Lab. Anim. Sci. 26, 951–954.

Berchelman, M.L., Kolter, S.S., Britton, H.A., 1973. Comparison of hematologic values from peripheral blood of the ear and venous blood of infant baboons (*Papio cynocephalus*). Lab. Anim. Sci. 23, 48–52.

Bergman, R.K., Lodmel, D.L., Hadlow, W.J., 1972. A technique for multiple bleedings or intravenous inoculations of mink at prescribed intervals. Lab. Anim. Sci. 22, 93–95.

Bergstrom, A., 1971. A simple device for intravenous injection in the mouse. Lab. Anim. Sci. 21, 600–601.

Bernsteen, L., Gregory, C.R., Kyles, A.E., Wooldridge, J.D., Valverde, C.R., 2000. Renal transplantation in cats. Clin. Tech. Small Anim. Pract. 15, 40–45.

Bernstein, L.I., Agee, J., 1964. Successful lobectomy in the guinea pig. Lab. Anim. Care 14, 519–523.

Berthelot, P., Erlinger, S., Dhumeaux, D., Pavaux, A.M., 1970. Mechanism of phenobarbital induced hypercholeresis in the rat. Am. J. Physiol. 219, 809–813.

Bett, N.J., Hynd, J.W., Green, C.J., 1980. Successful anesthesia and small-bowel anastomosis in the guinea pig. Lab. Anim. Care 14, 225–228.

Bhowmick, T.S., Koley, H., Das, M., Saha, D.R., Sarkar, B.L., 2009. Pathogenic potential of vibriophages against an experimental infection with Vibrio cholerae O1 in the RITARD model. Int. J. Antimicrob. Agents 33, 569–573.

Bishop, S.P., 1980. Cardiovascular research In: Baker, H.J. Lindsey, J.R. Weisbroth, S.H. (Eds.), The Laboratory Rat, vol. 2. Academic Press, New York, pp. 168–173.

Bivin, W.S., Timmons, F.H., 1974. Basic biomethodology. In: Weisbroth, S.H., Flatt, R.F., Kraus, A.L. (Eds.), The Biology of the Laboratory Rabbit. Academic Press, New York, pp. 73–90.

Black, D., Claxter, M., 1979. A simple reliable and inexpensive method for the collection of rat urine. Lab. Anim. Sci. 29, 253–254.

Black, K.W., Roberts, P.R., Zaloga, G.P., 1996. New urine collection technique for monitoring acute changes in renal function of the rat. Contemp. Top. 35, 69–70.

Blakely, G.B., Beamer, T.W., Dukelow, W.R., 1981. Characteristics of the menstrual cycle in nonhuman primates. IV. Timed mating in *Macaca nemestrina*. Lab. Anim. 15, 351–353.

Bleakley, S.P., 1980. Simple technique for bleeding ferrets (*Mustela putorius furo*). Lab. Anim. 14, 59–60.

Bliss, D.K., Bates, P.L., 1973. A rapid and reliable technique for pinealectomizing rats. Physiol. Behav. 11, 111–112.

Blouin, A., Cormier, Y., 1987. Endotracheal intubation in guinea pigs by direct laryngoscopy. Lab. Anim. Sci. 37, 244–245.

Blouin, A., Kingma, I., Boutet, M., 1994. An innovative technical approach for repetitive intratracheal instillation without anesthesia in small animals. Lab. Anim. Sci. 44, 274–279.

Boettcher, F.A., Bancroft, B.R., Salvi, R.J., 1990. Blood collection from the transverse sinus in the chinchilla. Lab. Anim. Sci. 40, 223–224.

Bogdanske, J.J., Hubbard-Van Stelle, S., Riley, M.R., Schiffman, B.M., 2010. Laboratory Mouse Procedural Techniques: Manual and DVD. CRC Press, Boca Raton, FL.

Bogdon, A.E., Haskell, P.M., Le Page, D.L., Kelton, D.E., Cobb, W.R., Esber, H.J., 1979. Growth of human tumor xenografts implanted under the renal capsule of normal immunocompetent mice. Exp. Cell. Biol. 47, 281–293.

Boiti, C., 2005. International rabbit reproduction group. Recommendations and guidelines for applied reproduction trials with rabbit does. World Rabbit Sci. 13, 147–164.

Bolotin, G., Lorusso, R., Schreuder, J.J., Nesher, N., Kaulbach, H., Uretzky, G., et al., 2002. Perioperative hemodynamic and geometric changes of the left ventricle during cardiomyoplasty in goats with dilated left ventricle. Chest 121, 1628–1633.

Boogeerd, W., Peters, A.C.B., 1986. A simple method for obtaining cerebrospinal fluid from a pig model of herpes encephalitis. Lab. Anim. Sci. 36, 386–388.

Born, C.T., Moller, M.L., 1974. A simple procedure for long-term intravenous infusion in the rat. Lab. Anim. Sci. 29, 78.

Borowsky, A.D., Munn, R.J., Galvez, J.J., Cardiff, R.D., 2003. Comparative pathology of mouse models of human cancers. Comp. Med. 53, 248–258.

Boulton, E.P., Gould, A.V., Shwaery, G.T., 1995. Laparoscopic ovariectomy of miniature swine. Contemp. Top. 34, 78–82.

Bowen, J., Cranley, J., Glough, D., 1994. The flank approach to the porcine upper urinary tract: safe and reliable. Lab. Anim. 29, 204–206.

Bowen, W.H., Coid, C.R., T-W-Fiennes, R.N., Mahoney, C.J., 1976. Primates. In: UFAW Staff, The UFAW Handbook on the Care and Management of Laboratory Animals, fifth ed. Churchill Livingstone, Edinburgh, pp. 377–427.

Brackee, G., Young, E., Coffey, T., Perry, R., Bankneider, R., 1995. Technique for telemetric determination of blood pressure and heart rate in the conscious, pregnant rabbit. Contemp. Top. 34, 90–92.

Brain, J.D., Frank, N.R., 1968. Recovery of free cells from rat lungs by repeated washings. J. Appl. Physiol. 25, 63–69.

Brakkee, J.H., Wiegant, V.M., Gispen, W.H., 1979. A simple technique for rapid implantation of a permanent cannula into the rat brain ventricular system. Lab. Anim. Sci. 29, 78–81.

Branham, G.W., 1976. A device for continuous intravenous fluid injections in dogs. Lab. Anim. Sci. 26, 75–77.

Bribriesco, A.C., Li, W., Nava, R.G., Spahn, J.H., Kreisel, D., 2013. Experimental models of lung transplantation. Front Biosci. (Elite Ed) 5, 266–272.

Brogan, J., Li, F., Li, W., He, Z., Huang, Q., Li, C.Y., 2012. Imaging molecular pathways: reporter genes. Radiat Res. 177 (4), 508–513.

Brown, M.J., Erichsen, D.F., Helgerson, R., Will, J.A., 1982. A modification for preparing the chronic lung-lymph fistula in sheep. J. Appl. Physiol. Respir. Environ. Exerc. Physiol. 52 (6), 1664–1666.

Bruckner-Kardoss, F., Worstmann, B.S., 1967. Cecectomy in germfree rats. Lab. Anim. Care 17, 542–546.

Bryant, J.M., 1980. Vest and tethering system to accommodate catheters and temperature monitors for nonhuman primates. Lab. Anim. Sci. 30, 706–708.

Bukoski, A., Winter, M., Bandt, C., Wilson, M., Shih, A., 2010. Original study: comparison of three intraosseous access techniques in cats. J. Vet. Emerg. Crit. Care 20, 393–397.

Bullock, L.P., 1983. Repetitive blood sampling from guinea pigs. Lab. Anim. Sci. 33, 70–71.

Burhoe, S.O., 1940. Methods of securing blood from rats. J. Hered. 31, 445–448.

Butler, P.E., Sims, C.D., Randolph, M.A., Van de Water, A.P., Lee, W.P., 1998. Prolonged survival in fetal rabbit surgery. J. Invest. Surg. 11 (1), 57–61.

Buscaglia, J.M., Shin, E.J., Clarke, J.O., Giday, S.A., Ko, C.W., Thuluvath, P.J., et al., 2008. Endoscopic retrograde cholangiopancreatography, but not esophagogastroduodenoscopy or colonoscopy, significantly increases portal venous pressure: direct portal pressure measurements through endoscopic ultrasound-guided cannulation. Endoscopy 40, 670–674.

Buttle, H.L., Clapham, C., Oldham, J.D., 1982. A design for flexible intestinal cannulas. Lab. Anim. 16, 307–309.

Cain, D.P., Dekergommeaux, S.E., 1979. Electrode implantation in small rodents for kindling and long-term brain recording. Physiol. Behav. 22, 799–801.

Caldwell, B., Flores, R., Lowery, J., Brown, A.T., Culp, W.C., 2011. Variations in the circle of Willis in the New Zealand white rabbit. J. Vasc. Interv. Radiol. 22, 1188–1192.

Cambron, H., Latulippe, J.-F., Nguyen, T., Cartier, R., 1995. Orotracheal intubation of rats by transillumination. Lab. Anim. Sci. 45, 303–304.

Carman, R.J., Waynforth, H.B., 1994. Chronic fistulation and cannulation of the rabbit cecum. Lab. Anim. 18, 258–260.

Carp, N.Z., Saputelli, J., Halbherr, T.C., Mason, W.S., Jilbert, A.R., 1991. A technique for liver biopsy performed in Pekin ducks using anesthesia with Telazol. Lab. Anim. Sci. 41, 474–475.

Carraway, J.H., Gray, L.D., 1989. Blood collection and intravenous injection in the guinea pig via the medial saphenous vein. Lab. Anim. Sci. 39, 623–624.

Carrillo, L., Aviado, D.M., 1969. Monocrotaline induced pulmonary hypertension and p-chlorophenylalanine (PCPA). Lab. Invest. 20, 243–248.

Carvalho, J.S., Shapiro, R., Hopper, P., Page, L.B., 1975. Methods for serial study of renin–angiotensin system in the unanesthetized rat. Am. J. Physiol. 228, 369–375.

Castelhano-Carlos, M.J., Sousa, N., Ohl, F., Baumans, V., 2010. Identification methods in newborn C57BL/6 mice: a developmental and behavioural evaluation. Lab. Anim. 44, 88–103.

Catchpole, H.R., van Wagenen, G., 1975. Reproduction in the rhesus monkey, Macaca mulatta In: Bourne, G.H. (Ed.), The Rhesus Monkey, vol. 2. Academic Press, New York, pp. 118–140.

Cate, C.C., 1969. A successful method for exsanguinating unanesthetized mice. Lab. Anim. Care 19, 256–258.

Chai, Y.F., Yang, J., Liu, J., Song, H.B., Yang, J.W., Liu, S.L., et al., 2008. Epidural anaesthetic effect of the 8% emulsified isoflurane: a study in rabbits. Br. J. Anaesth. 100, 109–115.

Chang, S.S.C., Anthony, S., Koder, P.C., Brown, S.G., 1996. Transrectal ultrasound guided manipulation of the canine prostate with minimum intervention. Lab. Anim. 31, 219–224.

Chaplin, J.M., Costantino, P.D., Wolpoe, M.E., Bederson, J.B., Griffey, E.S., Zhang, W.X., 1999. Use of an acellular dermal allograft for dural replacement: an experimental study. Neurosurgery 45 (2), 320–327.

Charles River Laboratories (CRL), 2006. Surgical Services: soft tissue procedures. (www.criver.com).

Chauhan, A., Lebeaux, D., Decante, B., Kriegel, I., Escande, M.C., Ghigo, J.M., et al., 2012. A rat model of central venous catheter to study establishment of long-term bacterial biofilm and related acute and chronic infections. PLoS One 7, e37281.

Cheon, D.J., Orsulic, S., 2011. Mouse models of cancer. Annu. Rev. Pathol. 6, 95–119.

Chimes, M.J., 1993. A technique for catheterization of ferrets for chronic intratracheal material administration. Lab. Anim. Sci. 43, 346–349.

Christison, G.E., Curtin, R.M., 1969. A simple venous catheter for sequential blood sampling from unrestrained pigs. Lab. Anim. Care 19, 259–262.

Chung, W.S., Cho, C., Kim, S., Wang, Y., Lee, S., Tarin, T., et al., 1999. Review of significant microvascular surgical breakthroughs involving the heart and lungs in rats. Microsurgery 19, 71–77.

Cimini, C.M., Zambraski, E.J., 1985. Non-invasive blood pressure measurement in Yucatan miniature swine using tail cuff sphygmomanometry. Lab. Anim. Sci. 35, 412–416.

Clegg, J.M., 1997. A practical in-house method for bile duct cannulation of rats. Contemp. Top. 36, 49–50.

Clements, D., Iqbal, S., Mills, C., Elias, E., 1985. A new method of complete biliary retention. Lab. Anim. 19, 277–278.

Clingerman, K.J., Spray, S., Flynn, C., Fox, H.S., 2010. A technique for intracisternal collection and administration in a rhesus macaque. Lab. Anim. (NY) 39, 307–311.

Cohen, E., Oliver, M., 1964. Urethral catheterization of the rat. Lab. Anim. Sci. 29, 781–784.

Colby, L.A., Rush, H.G., Mahoney, M.M., Lee, T.M., 2012. Other rodents. In: Suckow, M.A., Stevens, K.A., Wilson, R.P. (Eds.), The Laboratory Rabbit, Guinea Pig, Hamster, and Other Rodents. Academic Press, San Diego, CA.

Collinet, P., Sabban, F., Cosson, M., Farine, M.O., Villet, R., Vinatier, D., et al., 2007. Laparoscopic photodynamic diagnosis of ovarian cancer peritoneal micro metastasis: an experimental study. Photochem. Photobiol. 83, 647–651.

Concannon, P., Roberts, P., Parks, J., Bellezza, C., Tennant, B., 1996. Collection of seasonally spermatozoa-rich semen by electroejaculation of laboratory woodchucks (Marmota monax), with and without removal of bulbourethral glands. Lab. Anim. Sci. 46, 667–675.

Concannon, P., Roberts, P., Ball, B., Schlafer, D., Yang, J., Baldwin, B., et al., 1997. Estrus, fertility, early embryo development, and autologous embryo transfer in laboratory woodchucks (Marmota monax). Lab. Anim. Sci. 47, 63–74.

Conlon, K.C., Corbally, M.T., Bading, J.R., Brennan, M.F., 1990. Atraumatic endotracheal intubation in small rabbits. Lab. Anim. Sci. 40, 221–222.

Conn, H., Langer, R., 1978. Continuous long-term intraarterial infusion in the unrestrained rabbit. Lab. Anim. Sci. 28, 598–602.

Conner, M.K., Dombroske, R., Cheng, M., 1980. A simple device for continuous intravenous infusion of mice. Lab. Anim. Sci. 30, 212–214.

Conti, P.A., Nolan, T.E., Gehret, J., 1979. Immobilization of a chronic intravenous catheter in the saphenous vein of African green and rhesus monkeys. Lab. Anim. Sci. 29, 234–236.

Conybeare, G., Leslie, G.B., Angles, K., Barrett, R.J., Luke, J.S.H., Gask, D.R., 1988. An improved simple technique for the collection of blood samples from rats and mice. Lab. Anim. 22, 177–182.

Cook, R.W., Williams, J.F., 1978. Surgical removal of the pyloric antrum in weanling rats. Lab. Anim. Sci. 28, 437–439.

Cooley, R.K., Vanderwolf, C.H., 1978. Stereotaxic Surgery in the Rat: A Photographic Series, second ed. A. J. Kirby Co., Ontario, Canada.

Cooper, J.E., 1993. Bleeding of pulmonate snails. Lab. Anim. 28, 277–278.

Cooper, T.G., Waites, G.M.H., 1974. Testosterone in rete testis fluid and blood of rams and rats. J. Endocrinol. 62, 619–629.

Costa, D.L., Lehmann, J.R., Harold, W.M., Drew, R.T., 1986. Transoral tracheal intubation of rodents using a fiberoptic laryngoscope. Lab. Anim. Sci. 36, 256–261.

<http://www.covance.com/industry-solutions/drug-development/services/research/research-models/surgical-technical-services.html>.

Cox, P., Littledike, E.T., 1978. Techniques for sampling ventricular and cisternal cerebrospinal fluid from unanesthetized cattle. Lab. Anim. Sci. 28, 465–469.

Craig, D.J., Trost, J.G., Talley, W., 1969. A surgical procedure for implantation of a chronic, indwelling jugular catheter in a monkey. Lab. Anim. Care 19, 237–239.

Cramer, D.V., Podesta, L.G., Makowka, L., 1993. Handbook of animal models in transplantation research. CRC Press, Boca Raton.

Cranney, J., Zajac, A., 1993. A method for jugular blood collection in rabbits. Contemp. Top. 32, 6.

Cravener, T.L., Vasilatos-Younken, R., 1989. A method for catheterization, harnessing, and chronic infusion of undisturbed chickens. Lab. Anim. 23, 270–275.

Crean, R.D., Davis, S.A., Taffe, M.A., 2007. Oral administration of (+/−)3,4-methylenedioxymethamphetamine and (+)methamphetamine alters temperature and activity in rhesus macaques. Pharmacol. Biochem. Behav. 87, 11–19.

Cypel, M., Keshavjee, S., 2012. Isolated lung perfusion. Front. Biosci. (Elite Ed) 4, 2226–2232.

Dalgard, D.W., Marshall, P., Fitzgerald, G.H., Rendon, F., 1979. Surgical technique for a permanent tracheostomy in beagle dogs. Lab. Anim. Sci. 29, 367–370.

Dalmose, A.L., Hvistendahl, J.J., Olsen, L.H., Eskild-Jensen, A., Djurhuus, J.C., Swindle, M.M., 2000. Surgically induced urologic models in swine. J. Invest. Surg. 13, 133–145.

Dameron, G.W., Weingand, K.W., Duderstadt, J.M., Odioso, L.W., Dierckman, T.A., Schwecke, W., et al., 1992. Effect of bleeding site on clinical laboratory testing of rats: orbital venous plexus versus posterior vena cava. Lab. Anim. Sci. 42, 299–301.

Damsch, S., Eichenbaum, G., Tonelli, A., Lammens, L., Van den Bulck, K., Feyen, B., et al., 2011. Gavage-related reflux in rats: identification, pathogenesis, and toxicological implications (review). Toxicol. Pathol. 39, 348–360.

Daubeuf, F., Frossard, N., 2012. Performing bronchoalveolar lavage in the mouse. Curr. Protoc. Mouse Biol. 2, 167–175.

Davies, L., Grice, H.C., 1962. A device for restricting the movements of rats suitable for a variety of procedures. Can. J. Comp. Med. Vet. Sci. 26, 62.

Davis, L., Malinin, T.I., 1974. Rabbit intubation and halothane anesthesia. Lab. Anim. Sci. 24, 617–621.

Davis, R.H., Kramer, D.L., Sackman, J.W., Kyriazis, G., 1975. A simple staining method for vaginal smears using red ink. Lab. Anim. Sci. 25, 319–320.

de Blic, J., Midulla, F., Barbato, A., Clement, A., Dab, I., Eber, E., et al., 2000. Bronchoalveolar lavage in children. ERS Task Force on bronchoalveolar lavage in children. European Respiratory Society. Eur. Respir. J. 15, 217–231.

DeBoer, K.F., Krueger, D., 1991. A simplified artificial vagina for use in rabbits and other species. Lab. Anim. Sci. 41, 187–188.

DeBrant, V., Remon, J.P., 1991. A simple method for the intragastric administration of drugs to fully conscious guinea pigs. Lab. Anim. 25, 308–309.

Decad, G.M., Birnbaum, L.S., 1981. Noninvasive techniques for intravenous injection of guinea pigs. Lab. Anim. Sci. 31, 85–86.

DeCamp, C.E., 1993. External coaptation, second ed. In: Slatter, D. (Ed.), Textbook of Small Animal Surgery, vol. 2 Saunders, Philadelphia, PA, pp. 1661–1676.

De la Calle, J.L., Paino, C.L., 2002. A procedure for direct lumbar puncture in rats. Brain Res. Bull. 59, 245–250.

Dennis, M.B., Cole, J.J., Jensen, W.M., Scribner, B.H., 1984. Long-term blood access by catheters implanted into arteriovenous fistulas of sheep. Lab. Anim. Sci. 34, 388–392.

Desjardins, C., 1986. Indwelling vascular cannulas for remote blood sampling, infusion, and long term instrumentation of small laboratory animals. In: Gay, W.I. Heavner, J.E. (Eds.), Methods of Animal Experimentation, vol. 7. Academic Press, Orlando, FL, pp. 143–194.

Dewan, P.A., Ehall, H., Edwards, G.A., MacGregor, D., 2000. The development of a pig model to study fetal vesico-ureteric reflux. BJU Int. 86, 1054–1057.

DeWeert, T.M., Golub, M.S., Kaaekuahiwi, M.A., 1995. Long-term epidural catheterization of rhesus macaques: loss of resistance technique. Lab. Anim. Sci. 45, 94–97.

DeYoung, D.J., Probst, C.W., Pardo, A.D., 1993. Methods of internal fracture fixation. Chap. 122, 1610–1640, second ed. In: Slatter, D. (Ed.), Textbook of Small Animal Surgery, vol. 2. Saunders, Philadelphia, PA, pp. 1610–1640.

Dickie, M.M., 1975. Keeping records. In: Green, E.L. (Ed.), Biology of the Laboratory Mouse, third ed. Dover, New York, pp. 23–27.

Diehl, K.H., Hull, R., Morton, D., Pfister, R., Rabemampianina, Y., Smith, D., et al., 2001. A good practice guide to the administration of substances and removal of blood, including routes and volumes. J. Appl. Toxicol. 21, 15–23.

Diogene, J., Dufour, M., Poirier, G.G., Nadeau, D., 1997. Extrusion of earthworm coelomocytes: comparison of the cell populations recovered from the species Lumbricus terrestris, Eisenia fetida, and Octolasion tyrtaeum. Lab. Anim. 31, 326–336.

Divers, S.J., 2010. Exotic mammal diagnostic endoscopy and endosurgery. Vet. Clin. North Am. Exot. Anim. Pract. 13, 255–272.

Dolence, D., Jones, H.F., 1975. Pericutaneous phlebotomy and intravenous injection in the guinea pig. Lab. Anim. Sci. 25, 106–107.

Donovan, J., Brown, P., 2006. Blood collection. Curr. Protoc. Immunol. 73, 1.7.1–1.7.9.

Driscoll, K.E., Costa, D.L., Hatch, G., Henderson, R., Oberdorster, G., Salem, H., et al., 2000. Intratracheal instillation as an exposure technique for the evaluation of respiratory tract toxicity: uses and limitations. Toxicol. Sci. 55, 24–35.

Drougas, J.G., Barnard, S.E., Wright, J.K., Sika, M., Lopez, R.R., Stokes, K.A., et al., 1996. A model for the extended studies of hepatic hemodynamics and metabolism in swine. Lab. Anim. Sci. 46, 648–655.

Drummen, G.P., 2012. Fluorescent probes and fluorescence (microscopy) techniques – illuminating biological and biomedical research. Molecules 17 (12), 14067–14090.

Dudrick, S.J., Steiger, E., Wilmore, D.W., Vars, H.M., 1970. Continuous long-term intravenous infusion in unrestrained animals. Lab. Anim. Care 20, 521–529.

Dueck, R., Davidson, T.M., Rathbun, M., 1985. Intermittent tracheostomy in sheep. Lab. Anim. Sci. 35, 509–512.

Dukelow, W.R., 1978. Laparoscopic research techniques in mammalian embryology. In: Daniel Jr., J.C. (Ed.), Methods in Mammalian Reproduction. Academic Press, New York, pp. 437–460.

Dukelow, W.R., Ariga, S., 1976. Laparoscopic techniques for biomedical research. J. Med. Primatol. 5, 82–99.

Dukelow, W.R., Jarosz, S.J., Jewett, D.A., Harrison, R.M., 1971. Laparoscopic examination of the ovaries in goats and primates. Lab. Anim. Sci. 21, 594–597.

Dürschlag, M., Würbel, H., Stauffacher, M., Von Holst, D., 1996. Repeated blood collection in the laboratory mouse by tail incision--modification of an old technique. Physiol. Behav. 60 (6), 1565–1568.

Edwards, L., Rosin, D., Leaper, M., Swedan, M., Trott, P., Vertido, R., 1978. The induction of cystitis and the implantation of tumours in rats and rabbit bladders. Br. J. Urol. SO, 502–504.

Egger, E.L., 1993. External skeletal fixation, second ed. In: Slatter, D. (Ed.), Textbook of Small Animal Surgery, vol. 2. Saunders, Philadelphia, PA, pp. 1641–1661.

Ehlert, A., Tiemann, B., Elsner, J., Puschel, K., Manthei, G., 2010. Long-term subarachnoid catheter placement in the middle cranial fossa of the rat. Lab. Anim. (NY) 39, 352–359.

Eisele, P.H., Kaaekuahiwi, M.A., Canfield, D.R., Golub, M.S., Eisele, J.H., 1994. Epidural catheter placement for testing of obstetrical analgesics in female guinea pigs. Lab. Anim. Sci. 44, 486–490.

Eisenhauer, C.L., McCullen, A.H., Ichimura, W.M., Claybaugh, J.R., 1994. Technique for placement of chronic third cerebroventricular cannula in female goats (Capra hircus). Lab. Anim. Sci. 44, 55–59.

Eko, F.O., Schukovskaya, T., Lotzmanova, E.Y., Firstova, V.V., Emalyanova, N.V., Klueva, S.N., et al., 2003. Evaluation of the protective efficacy of Vibrio cholerae ghost (VCG) candidate vaccines in rabbits. Vaccine 21, 3663–3674.

Elias, A., Brown, C., 2008. Cerebellomedullary cerebrospinal fluid collection in the dog. Lab. Anim. (NY) 37, 457–458.

Ellegalla, D.B., Tassone, J.C., Avellino, A.M., Pekow, C.A., Cunningham, M.L., Kliot, M., 1996. Dorsal laminectomy in the adult mouse: a model for nervous system research. Lab. Anim. Sci. 46, 86–89.

Ellery, A., Kinnen, L., 1981. Operative procedures for the collection of rete testis fluid from conscious sheep. Lab. Anim. 15, 187–188.

Emery, S.P., Kreutzer, J., Sherman, F.R., Fujimoto, K.L., Jaramaz, B., Nikou, C., et al., 2007. Computer-assisted navigation applied to fetal cardiac intervention. Int. J. Med. Robot 3, 187–198.

Engelhardt, J.A., Zeilinga, M.J., Phelps, J.O., Turner, D.A., 1993. Chronic jugular vein cannulation in beagles. Contemp. Top. 32, 7–9.

Enta, T., Lockey Jr., S.D., Reed, C.F., 1968. A rapid safe technique for repeated blood collection from small laboratory animals. The farmer's wife methods. Proc. Soc. Exp. Biol. Med. 127, 136–137.

Erol, O.O., Spira, M., Levy, B., 1980. Microangiography: a detailed technique of perfusion. J. Surg. Res. 29, 406–413.

Eufinger, H., Rasche, C., Lehmbrock, J., Wehmollder, M., Weihe, S., Schmitz, I., et al., 2007. Performance of functionally graded implants of polylactides and calcium phosphate/calcium carbonate in an ovine model for computer assisted craniectomy and cranioplasty. Biomaterials 28, 475–485.

Evans, C.S., Smart, J.L., Stoddart, R.C., 1968. Handling methods for wild house mice and wild rats. Lab. Anim. 2, 29.

Evers, D.C., 2009. Protocol for sampling bird and mammal tissue for blood contaminant analysis.United States Fish and Wildlife Service. Appendix IV. Sampling Protocol. Report BRI 2009-01, BioDiversity Research Institute.

Eyambe, G.S., Goven, A.J., Fitzpatrick, L.C., Venables, B.J., Cooper, E.L., 1991. A non-invasive technique for sequential collection of earthworm (*Lumbricus terrestris*) leukocytes during subchronic immunotoxicity studies. Lab. Anim. 25, 61–67.

Eyibilen, A., Güven, M., Aladağ, I., Kesici, H., Koç, S., Gürbüzler, L., et al., 2011. Does mitomycin-C increase collagen turnover as a modulator of wound healing in tracheostomyzed rats? Kulak Burun Bogaz Ihtis Derg 21, 154–158.

Fahey, M.A., Westmoreland, S., 2012. Nervous system disorders of non-human primates and research models. In: Abee, C.R., Mansfiled, K., Tardif, S., Morris, T. (Eds.), Nonhuman Primates in Biomedical Research. Elsevier, Waltham, MA, pp. 733–782.

Faidley, T.D., Galloway, S.T., Luhman, C.M., Foley, M.K., Beitz, D.C., 1991. A surgical model for studying biliary bile acid and cholesterol metabolism in swine. Lab. Anim. Sci. 41 477–450.

Falabella, F., 1967. Bleeding mice: a successful technique of cardiac puncture. J. Lab. Clin. Med. 70, 981–982.

Falconi, G., Rossi, G.L., 1964. Transauricular hypophysectomy in rats and mice. Endocrinology 74, 301–303.

Fan, J., Watanabe, T., 2003. Transgenic rabbits as therapeutic protein bioreactors and human disease models. Pharmacol. Ther. 99, 261–282.

Fayrer-Hosken, R.A., Brackett, B.G., Brown, J., 1987. Reversible inhibition of rabbit sperm-fertilizing ability by cholesterol sulfate. Biol. Reprod. 36, 878–883.

FDA, 2005. Good Laboratory Practices for Conducting Nonclinical Laboratory Studies 21CFR58. Available from: <http://www.accessdata.fda.gov/scripts/cdrh/cfdocs/cfcfr/CFRSearch.cfm?CFRPart=58&showFR=1>.

Fejes-Toth, G., Naray-Fejes-Toth, A., Ratge, D., Frolich, J.C., 1984. Chronic arterial and venous catheterization of conscious, unrestrained rats. Hypertension 6, 926–930.

Fellows-Mayle, W., Hitchens, T.K., Simplaceanu, E., Horner, J., Barbano, T., Losee, J.E., et al., 2006. Testing causal mechanisms of nonsyndromic craniosynostosis using path analysis of cranial contents in rabbits with uncorrected craniosynostosis. Cleft. Palate Craniofac. J. 43, 524–531.

Feng, M., Whitesall, S., Zhang, Y., Beibel, M., D'Alecy, L., DiPetrillo, K., 2008. Validation of volume–pressure recording tail-cuff blood pressure measurements. Am. J. Hypertens. 21, 1288–1291.

Festing, M.W.F., 1980. Inherited immunological defects in laboratory animals. In: Castro, J.E. (Ed.), Immunodeficient Animals for Cancer Research. Oxford University Press, London.

Fettiplace, M.R., Ripper, R., Lis, K., Feinstein, D.L., Rubinstein, I., Weinberg, G., 2014. Intraosseous lipid emulsion: an effective alternative to IV delivery in emergency situations. Crit. Care Med. 42, e157–e160.

Field, K., Sibold, A.L., 1998. The Laboratory Hamster and Gerbil.

Fields Jr., B.T., Cunningham, D.R., 1976. A tail artery technique for collecting one-half milliliter of blood from a mouse. Lab. Anim. Sci. 26, 505–506.

Figueiredo, G., Brockmann, C., Boll, H., Heilmann, M., Schambach, S.J., Fiebig, T., et al., 2012. Comparison of digital subtraction angiography, micro-computed tomography angiography and magnetic resonance angiography in the assessment of the cerebrovascular system in live mice. Clin. Neuroradiol. 22 (1), 21–28.

Fitzgerald, A.L., Dillon, L.M., Altrogge, D.M., Bleavins, M.R., Breider, M.A., 1996. Use of subcutaneous vascular access ports in common marmosets (*Callithrix jacchus*). Contemp. Top. 35, 57–59.

Flecknell, P.A., 2009. Laboratory Animal Anesthesia, third ed. Elsevier, San Diego, CA.

Flecknell, P.A., Liles, J.H., Williamson, H.A., 1990. The use of lignocaine–prilocaine anaesthetic cream for pain-free venipuncture in laboratory animals. Lab. Anim. 24, 142–146.

Fletch, S.M., Wabeser, G., 1970. A technique for safe multiple bleedings, or intravenous injections in mink. Can. Vet. J. 11, 33.

Foley, P.L., 2005. Common surgical procedures in rodents. In: Reuter, J.D., Suckow, M.A. (Eds.), Laboratory Animal Medicine and Management. International Veterinary Information Service, Ithaca, NY.

Foley, P.L., Barthel, C.H., Brausa, H.R., 2002. Effect of covalently bound heparin coating on patency and biocompatibility of long-term indwelling catheters in the rat jugular vein. Comp. Med. 52, 243–248.

Ford, J.J., Maurer, R.R., 1978. Simple technique for chronic venous catheterization of swine. Lab. Anim. Sci. 28, 615–618.

Forte Jr., V.A., Devine, J.A., Cymerman, A., 1989. A reusable adapter for collection of cerebrospinal fluid in chronically cannulated goats. Lab. Anim. Sci. 39, 433–436.

Foss, M.L., Barnard, R.J., 1969. A vest to protect chronic implants in dogs. Lab. Anim. Care 19, 113–114.

Foxworth, W.B., Carpenter, E., Kraemer, D.C., Kier, A.B., 1996. Nonsurgical and nonlethal retrieval of mouse spermatozoa. Lab. Anim. Sci. 46, 352–354.

Foytik, J.E., Satterfield, W.C., Bailey, J.W., Keeling, M.E., 1989. Vacuum-assisted cardiac puncture in chickens. Lab. Anim. Sci. 39, 626–628.

Frankenberg, L., 1979. Cardiac puncture in the mouse through the anterior thoracic aperture. Lab. Anim. 13, 311–312.

Fredrickson, T.N., Chute, H.L., O'Meara, D.C., 1958. Simple improved method for obtaining blood from chickens. J. Am. Vet. Med. Assoc. 132, 390–391.

Frisk, C.S., Richardson, M.R., 1979. Rapid methods for jugular bleeding of dogs requiring one technician. Lab. Anim. Sci. 29, 371–373.

Fumer, R.L., Mellett, L.B., 1975. Mouse restraining chamber for tail-vein injection. Lab. Anim. Sci. 25, 648–649.

Fussell, E.N., Roussel, J.D., Austin, C.R., 1967. Use of the rectal probe method for electrical ejaculation of apes, monkeys, and a prosimian. Lab. Anim. Care 17, 528–530.

Fussell, E.N., Franklin, L.E., Frantz, R.C., 1973. Collection of chimpanzee semen with an artificial vagina. Lab. Anim. Sci. 23, 252–255.

Galitzer, J., Hayes, R.H., Oehme, F.W., 1979. A simplified urine collection method for female swine. Lab. Anim. Sci. 29, 404–405.

Galvez, J.J., Cardiff, R.D., Munn, R.J., Borowsky, A.D., 2004. Mouse models of human cancers (Part 2). Comp. Med. 54, 13–15.

Gardiner, T.W., Toth, L.A., 1999. Stereotaxic surgery and long-term maintenance of cranial implants in research animals. Contemp. Top. 38, 56–63.

Garren, H.W., 1959. An improved method for obtaining blood from chickens. Poult. Sci. 38, 916–918.

Garvey, J.S., Alseth, B.L., 1971. Urine collection from newborn rabbits. Lab. Anim. Sci. 21, 739.

Gavellas, G., Disbrow, M.R., Hwang, K.H., Hinkle, D.K., Bourgoignie, J.J., 1987. Glomerular filtration rate and blood pressure monitoring in awake baboons. Lab. Anim. Sci. 37, 657–662.

Gay, W.I. (Ed.), Methods of Animal Experimentation, vols. 1–7. Academic Press, New York.

Geretschlager, E., Russ, H., Mihatsch, W., Przuntek, H., 1987. Suboccipital puncture for cerebrospinal fluid in the common marmoset (*Callithrix jacchus*). Lab. Anim. 21, 91–94.

Glenister, P.H., Thornton, C.E., 2000. Cryoconservation – archiving for the future. Mamm. Genome 11, 565–571.

Glue, P., Bacher, J.D., Nutt, D.J., 1988. A technique for chronic catheterization of the cisterna magna in rabbits. Lab. Anim. Sci. 38, 740–742.

Goetz, K.L., Hermreck, A.S., 1972. A simple, inexpensive,diaphragm-type skin connectorfor implanted catheters. Lab. Anim. Sci. 22, 538–540.

Goldstein, H., Klein, N.I., Rubinstein, A., 1983. Construction of a tracheal pouch in rabbits. Lung 161, 207–211.

Goodpasture, J.C., Cianci, J., Zanefeld, L.J.D., 1982. Long-term evaluation of the effect of catheter materials on urethral tissue in dogs. Lab. Anim. Sci. 32, 180–182.

Gordon, I.R., 2004. Reproductive Technologies in Farm Animals. CABI Publishing, Cambridge, MA.

Gould, K.G., Warner, H., Martin, D.F., 1978. Rectal probe ejaculation in primates. J. Med. Primatol. 7, 213–222.

Graham, C.E., 1976. Technique of laparoscopy in the chimpanzee. J. Med. Primatol. 5, 111–123.

Graham, M.L., Mutch, L.A., Rieke, E.F., Dunning, M., Zolondek, E.K., Faig, A.W., et al., 2010. Refinement of vascular access port placement in nonhuman primates: complication rates and outcomes. Comp. Med. 60, 479–485.

Grazer, F.M., 1958. Technique for intravascular injection and bleeding of newborn rats and mice. Proc. Soc. Exp. Biol. Med. 99, 407–409.

Greene, F.E., Wade, A.F., 1967. A technique to facilitate sublingual vein injection in the rat. Lab. Anim. Care 17, 604–606.

Greenham, L.W., 1978. Tattooing newborn albino mice in life-span experiments. Lab. Anim. Sci. 28, 346.

Gregg, C.L., Butcher, J.T., 2012. Quantitative in vivo imaging of embryonic development: opportunities and challenges. Differentiation 84 (1), 149–162.

Grice, H.C., 1964. Methods for obtaining blood and for intravenous injections in laboratory animals. Lab. Anim. Care 14, 483–493.

Grossman, R.C., 2010. Experimental models of renal disease and the cardiovascular system. Open Cardiovasc. Med. J. 4, 257–264.

Guan, M., Marschall, S., Raspa, M., Pickard, A.R., Fray, M.D., 2012. Overview of new developments in and the future of cryopreservation in the laboratory mouse. Mamm. Genome 23, 572–579.

Guavera-Lopez, U., Covarrubias-Gomez, A., Gutierrez-Acar, H., Aldrete, J.A., Lopez-Munoz, F.J., Martinez-Benitez, B., 2006. Chronic subarachnoid administration of 1-(4chlorobenzoyl)-5methoxy-2methyl-1H-indole-3 acetic acid (indomethacin): an evaluation of its neurotoxic effects in an animal model. Anesth. Analg. 103, 99–102.

Guide for the Care and Use of Laboratory Animals, 2011., eighth ed. National Academies Press, Washington DC.

Gupta, B.N., 1973. Technique for collecting blood from neonatal rats. Lab. Anim. Sci. 23, 559.

Gutt, C.N., Riemer, V., Brier, C., Berguer, R., Paolucci, V., 1998. Standardized technique of laparoscopic surgery in the rat. Dig. Surg. 15, 135–139.

Haisley, A.D., 1980. A technique for cheek pouch examination of Syrian hamsters. Lab. Anim. Sci. 30, 107–109.

Hall, A.S., 1966. Methods and techniques of manipulating laboratory primates. Lab. Anim. Dig. 2, 3–5.

Hall, L.L., DeLopez, O.H., Roberts, A., Smith, F.A., 1974. A procedure for chronic, intravenous catheterization in the rabbit. Lab. Anim. Sci. 24, 79–83.

Hall, R.D., Hodgen, R.D., 1979. Pregnancy diagnosis of owl monkeys (Aotus trivirgatus): evaluation of the hemagglutination inhibition test for urinary chorionic gonadotropin. Lab. Anim. Sci. 29, 345–348.

Halliday, L.C., Fortman, J.D., Bennett, B.T., 1998. A mouth speculum for orogastric administration of compounds to nonhuman primates. Contemp. Top. 37, 76–77.

Hamilton, R.M.G., 1978. Intravenous cannulation of hens for long-term infusion. Lab. Anim. Sci. 28, 746–750.

Hammer, J.G., Howland, D.R., 1991. Use of serum progesterone levels as an early, indirect evaluation of pregnancy in the timed pregnant domestic cat. Lab. Anim. Sci. 41, 42–45.

Han, J.S., Kim, J.S., Lee, J.J., 2000. Intubation in rabbits using capnography. Contemp. Top. Lab. Anim. Med. 39, 80.

Hankenson, F.C., Garzel, L.M., Fischer, D.D., Nolan, B., Hankenson, K.D., 2008. Evaluation of tail biopsy collection in laboratory mice (Mus musculus): vertebral ossification, DNA quantity, and acute behavioral responses. JAALAS 47, 10–18.

Hargaden, M., Singer, L., 2012. Guinea pigs: anatomy, physiology, and behavior. In: Suckow, M.A., Stevens, K.A., Wilson, R.P. (Eds.), The Laboratory Rabbit, Guinea Pig, Hamster, and Other Rodents. Academic Press, Waltham, MA, pp. 576–602.

Harirchian, P., Gashaw, I., Lipskind, S.T., Braundmeier, A.G., Hastings, J.M., Olson, M.R., et al., 2012. Lesion kinetics in a non-human primate model of endometriosis. Hum. Reprod. 27, 2341–2351.

Harkness, J.E., Wagner, J.F., 1983. The Biology and Medicine of Rabbits and Rodents. Lea & Febiger, Philadelphia, PA, p. 3.

Harris, D.L., Decker, W.J., 1969. A method for obtaining repeated serial intestinal biopsies from the dog. Lab. Anim. Care 19, 849–852.

Harris, D.V., Walker, J.M., 1980. A semi-chronic electrode implant for very small animals. Brain Res. Bull. 5, 479–480.

Harris Jr., R.H., Best, C.F., 1979. Ureteral catheter system for renal function studies in conscious rabbits. Lab. Anim. Sci. 29, 781–784.

Hartford, C.G., Marcos, E.F., Rogers, G.G., 1996. Noninvasive versus invasive blood pressure measurement in normotensive and hypotensive baboons. Lab. Anim. Sci. 46, 231–233.

Hartman, C.G., 1932. Studies in the reproduction of the monkey Macacus (pithecus) rhesus with special reference to menstruation and pregnancy. Contrib. Embryol. Carnegie Inst. 23, 1–161.

Harvey, R.G., Jones, E.F., 1982. A technique for bioinstrumentation of the thorax of miniature swine. Lab. Anim. Sci. 32, 94–96.

Haslberger, A.G., Gaab, M.R., 1986. A technique for repeated sampling of pure cerebrospinal fluid from the conscious rabbit. Lab. Anim. Sci. 36, 181–182.

Hatchell, D.L., Reiser, H.J., Bresnahan, J.E., Whitworth Jr., U.G., 1986. Resistance of cats to the diabetogenic effect of alloxan. Lab. Anim. Sci. 36, 37–40.

Hau, J., Schapiro, S.J., 2010. Essential principles and practices, third ed. Handbook of Laboratory Animal Science, vol. I. CRC Press, Boca Raton, FL.

Haworth, R.D., Rosenberg, P.H., Hoffman, L.A., Latrenta, G., 1992. Anterior cervical microsurgical approach to the cranial base in the rabbit: technical note. Lab. Anim. 26, 196–199.

Hayashi, S., Gorski, R.A., 1974. Critical exposure time for androgenization by intracranial crystals of testosterone proprionate in neonatal female rats. Endocrinology 94, 1161–1167.

Hayes, B.E., Will, J.A., 1978. Pulmonary artery cathetenzation in the rat. Am. J. Physiol. 235, H452–H455.

Hayward, A.M., Lemke, L.B., Bridgeford, E.C., Theve, E.J., Jackson, C.J., Cunliffe-Beamer, T.L., et al., 2006. Biomethodology and surgical techniques The Mouse in Biomedical Research. Academic Press, Elsevier, Boston, MA.

Heiser, A., 2013. Training ideas and procedures (TIPS) for successful mouse gavage. Lab. Anim. Sci. Prof., 49–50.

Heitmeyer, S.A., Powers, J.F., 1992. Improved method for bile collection in unrestrained conscious rats. Lab. Anim. Sci. 42, 312–315.

Henderson, K.K., Mokelke, E.A., Turk, J.R., Rector, R.S., Laughlin, M.H., Sturek, M., 2003. Maintaining patency and asepsis of vascular access ports in Yucatan miniature swine. Contemp. Top Lab. Anim. Sci. 42 (6), 28–32.

Herbst, L.H., Webb, A.I., 1988. A simple technique for sampling blood from fully conscious nine-banded armadillos. Lab. Anim. Sci. 38, 335–336.

Hernandez-Divers, S.J., 2008. Clinical technique: dental endoscopy of rabbits and rodents. J. Exot. Pet Med. 17, 87–92.

Herndon, B.L., Ringle, D.A., 1969. Methods for neurological experimentation in the Mongolian gerbil, Merionesunguiculatus. Lab. Anim. Care 19 (2), 240–243.

Herrmann, K., Dahlbom, M., Nathanson, D., Wei, L., Radu, C., Chatziioannou, A., et al., 2013. Evaluation of the Genisys4, a bench-top preclinical PET scanner. J. Nucl. Med. 54 (7), 1162–1167.

Hill, R.C., Ellison, G.W., Burrows, C.F., Bauer, J.E., Carbia, B., 1996. Ileal cannulation and associated complications in dogs. Lab. Anim. Sci. 46, 77–80.

Hoar, R.M., 1966. A technique for bilateral adrenalectomy in guinea pigs. Lab. Anim. Care 16, 410–416.

Hobson, B.M., 1976. Evaluation of the subhuman primate tube test for pregnancy of primates. Lab. Anim. 10, 87–89.

Hodesson, S., Miller, J.N., 1964. Testis and popliteal lymph node removal from the living rabbit using aseptic techniques and other anesthesia. Lab. Anim. Care 14, 494–498.

Hodgen, G.D., Niemann, W.H., 1975. Application of the subhuman primate pregnancy test kit to pregnancy diagnosis in baboons. Lab. Anim. Sci. 25, 757–759.

Hodgen, G.D., Ross, G.T., 1974. Pregnancy diagnosis by a hemagglutination inhibition test for urinary macaque chorionic gonadotropin (mCG). J. Clin. Endocrinol. Metab. 3, 927–930.

Hodgen, G.D., Wolfe, L.G., Ogden, J.D., Adams, M.R., Descalzi, C.C., Hildebrand, D.F., 1976a. Diagnosis of pregnancy in marmosets: hemagglutination inhibition test and radio immunoassay for urinary chorionic gonadotropin. Lab. Anim. Sci. 26, 224–229.

Hodgen, G.D., Niemann, W.H., Turner, C.K., Chen, H.C., 1976b. Diagnosis pregnancy in chimpanzees using the nonhuman primate pregnancy test kit. J. Med. Primatol. 5, 247–252.

Hodgen, G.D., Turner, C.K., Smith, E.E., Bush, R.M., 1977. Pregnancy diagnosis in the orangutan (Pongo pygmaeus) using the subhuman primate pregnancy test. Lab. Anim. Sci. 27, 99–101.

Hodgen, G.D., Stolzenberg, S.J., Jones, D.C.L., Hildebrand, D.F., Turner, C.K., 1978. Pregnancy diagnosis in squirrel monkeys: hemagglutination test, radio immunoassay, and bioassay of chorionic gonadotropin. J. Med. Primatol. 7, 59–64.

Hoff, J.B., Dysko, R., Kurachi, S., Kurachi, K., 2006. Technique for performance and evaluation of parapharyngeal hypophysectomy in mice. J. Am. Assoc. Lab. Anim. Sci. 45, 57–62.

Hoffman, K.M., Timmel, G.B., Meuli-Simmen, C., Meuli, M., Yingling, C.D., Adzick, N.S., 1996. Experimental fetal neurosurgery: the normal neurology of neonatal lambs and abnormal findings after in utero manipulation. Contemp. Top. 35, 53–56.

Hoffman, R.A., Reiter, R.J., 1965. Rapid pinealectomy in hamsters and other small rodents. Anat. Rec. 153, 19–21.

Hofstad, M.S., 1950. A method of bleeding chickens from the heart. J. Am. Vet. Med. Assoc. 66, 353–354.

Holman, D., 1980. A method for intracerebrally implanting crystalline hormones into neonatal rodents. Lab. Anim. 14, 263–266.

Honaramooz, A., Yang, Y., 2010. Recent advances in application of male germ cell transplantation in farm animals. Vet. Med. Int. 2011.

Hoppe, P.C., Laird, C.W., Fox, R.R., 1969. A simple technique for bleeding the rabbit ear vein. Lab. Anim. Care 19, 524–525.

Hoskins, S.L., do Nascimento Jr., P., Lima, R.M., Espana-Tenorio, J.M., Kramer, G.C., 2012. Pharmacokinetics of intraosseous and central venous drug delivery during cardiopulmonary resuscitation. Resuscitation 83, 107–112.

Houchens, D.P., Ovejera, A.A., Riblet, S.M., Slagel, D.E., 1983. Human brain tumor xenografts in nude mice as a chemotherapy model. Eur. J. Cancer Clin. Oncol. 19, 799–805.

Houghton, P.W., Jones, C.L., 1977. A chronic gastrostomy and test system for evaluation of gastric secretion in rhesus monkeys. Gastroenterology 73, 252–254.

Hsu, C.C., Briscoe, J.A., Keffer, A.B., 2012. Chinchillas. Basic Experimental Methods.. In: Suckow, M.A., Stevens, K.A., Wilson, R.P. (Eds.), The Laboratory Rabbit, Guinea Pig, Hamster, and Other Rodents Academic Press, Boston, pp. 977–990. (Chapter 41).

Hubert, J., Feuillu, B., Mangin, P., Lobontiu, A., Artis, M., Villemot, J.P., 2003. Laparoscopic computer-assisted pyeloplasty: the results of experimental surgery in pigs. BJU Int. 92, 437–440.

Hudson, L.C., Hughes, C.S., Bold-Fletcher, N.O., Vaden, S.L., 1994. Cerebrospinal fluid collection in rats: modification of a previous technique. Lab. Anim. Sci. 44, 358–361.

Hummel, K.P., Richardson, F.L., Fekete, E., 1975. Anatomy. In: Green, El (Ed.), Biology of the Laboratory Mouse Dover, New York, pp. 257–307.

Huneke, R.B., 2012. Basic experimental methods. In: Suckow, M.A., Stevens, K.A., Wilson, R.P. (Eds.), The Laboratory Rabbit, Guinea Pig, Hamster, and Other Rodents Academic Press, Boston, pp. 621–635. (Chapter 22).

Icenhour, C.R., Rebholz, S.L., Collins, M.S., Cushion, M.T., 2001. Widespread occurrence of Pneumocystiscariniiin commercial rat colonies detected using targeted PCR and oral swabs. J. Clin. Microbiol. 39 (10), 3437–3441.

Ikeda, K., Nara, Y., Yamori, Y., 1991. Indirect systolic and mean blood pressure determination by a new tail cuff method in spontaneously hypertensive rats. Lab. Anim. 25, 26–29.

Ilievski, V., Fleischman, R.W., 1981. A technique for obtaining tracheobronchial washings from rhesus monkeys (Macaca mulatta). Lab. Anim. Sci. 31, 524–525.

Immunodeficient Rodents. A guide to their immunobiology, husbandry and use, 1989. National research Council. National Academy press, Washington DC.

Inoue, S., Mori, A., Shimizu, H., Yoshitake, A., Tashiro, R., Kabei, N., et al., 2013. Combined use of an epidural cooling catheter and systemic moderate hypothermia enhances spinal cord protection against ischemic injury in rabbits. J. Thorac. Cardiovasc. Surg. 146, 696–701.

Intapad, S., Tull, F.L., Brown, A.D., Dasinger, J.H., Ojeda, N.B., Fahling, J.M., et al., 2013. Renal denervation abolishes the age-dependent increase in blood pressure in female intrauterine growth-restricted rats at 12 months of age. Hypertension 61, 828–834.

Iwaki, S., Matsuo, A., Kast, A., 1989. Identification of newborn rats by tattooing. Lab. Anim. 23, 361–364.

Iwami, K., Momota, H., Natsume, A., Kinjo, S., Nagatani, T., Wakabayashi, T., 2012. A novel method of intracranial injection via the postglenoid foramen for brain tumor mouse models. J. Neurosurg. 116, 630–635.

Jackson, I., Cook, D.B., Gill, G., 1972. Simultaneous intravenous infusion and arterial sampling in piglets. Lab. Anim. Sci. 22, 552–555.

Jackson, R.K., Kieffer, V.A., Sauber, J.J., King, G.L., 1988. A tethered-restraint system for blood collection from ferrets. Lab. Anim. Sci. 38, 625–628.

Jacobson, M., Lindberg, J.E., Lindberg, R., Segerstad, C.H., Wallgren, P., Fellstrom, C., et al., 2001. Intestinal cannulation: model for study of the midgut of the pig. Comp. Med. 51, 163–170.

Jäger, W., Moskalev, I., Janssen, C., Hayashi, T., Gust, K.M., Awrey, S., et al., 2014. Minimally invasive establishment of murine orthotopic bladder xenografts. J. Vis. Exp. 84, e51123.

Jenkins, J.R., 2000. Surgical sterilization in small mammals. Spay and castration. Vet. Clin. North Am. Exot. Anim. Pract. 3, 617–627, v.

Johnson, M.D., Franklin, R.K., Gibson, M.D., Brown, R.B., Kipke, D.R., 2008. Implantable microelectrode arrays for simultaneous electrophysiological and neurochemical recordings. J. Neurosci. Methods 174, 62–70.

Jones, B.D., 1990. Laparoscopy. Vet. Clin. North Am. Small Anim. Pract. 20, 1243–1263.

Jones, R.C., 1971. Uses of artificial insemination. Nature (Lond.) 229, 534–537.

Joslin, J.O., 2009. Blood collection techniques in exotic small mammals. J. Exotic Pet. Med. 18, 117–139.

Jungraithmayr, W., Jang, J.H., Schrepfer, S., Inci, I., Weder, W., 2013. Small animal models of experimental obliterative bronchiolitis. Am. J. Respir. Cell Mol. Biol. 48, 675–684.

Jurek, F.W., 1977. Antigonadal effect of melatonin in pinealectomized and intact male hamsters. Proc. Soc. Exp. Biol. Med. 155, 31–34.

Kaplan, A., Wolf, I., 1972. A device for restraining and intravenous injection of mice. Lab. Anim. Sci. 22, 223–224.

Kaplan, H.M., Timmons, F.H., 1979. The Rabbit: A Model for the Principles of Mammalian Physiology and Surgery. Academic Press, New York.

Karlson, A.G., 1959. Intravenous injections in guinea pigs via veins of the penis. Lab. Invest. 8, 987–989.

Karnabatidis, D., Katsanos, K., Diamantopoulos, A., Kagadis, G.C., Siablis, D., 2006. Transauricular arterial or venous access for cardiovascular experimental protocols in animals. J. Vasc. Interv. Radiol. 17, 1803–1811.

Kasai, M., Neva, K., Tritani, A., 1981. Effects of various cryoprotective agents on the survival of unfrozen and frozen mouse embryos. J. Reprod. Fertil. 63, 175–180.

Kassel, R., Leviton, S., 1953. A jugular technique for the repeated bleeding of small animals. Science 118, 563–564.

Katada, A., Van Himbergen, D., Kunibe, I., Nonaka, S., Harabuchi, Y., Huang, S., et al., 2008. Evaluation of a deep brain stimulation electrode for laryngeal pacing. Ann. Otol. Rhinol. Laryngol. 117, 621–629.

Keighley, G., 1966. A device for intravenous injection of mice and rats. Lab. Anim. Care 16, 185–187.

Kelland, L.R., 2004. Of mice and men: values and liabilities of the athymic nude mouse model in anticancer drug development. Eur. J. Cancer 40, 827–836.

Keller-Wood, M., Cudd, T.A., Norman, W., Caldwell, S.M., Wood, C.E., 1998. Sheep model for study of maternal adrenal gland function during pregnancy. Lab. Anim. Sci. 48, 507–512.

Kesel, M.L., Ellis, R.P., 1988. A reversible-tie technique of the rabbit gut for bacterial colonization and toxin production. Lab. Anim. Sci. 38, 621–623.

Keshavarzian, A., Schoenau, G., Isaac, R., 1989. Percutaneous endoscopic gastrostomy tube placement in cats. Lab. Anim. Sci. 39, 459–461.

Khosho, F.K., Kaufmann, R.C., Amankwah, K.S., 1985. A simple and efficient method for obtaining urine samples from rats. Lab. Anim. Sci. 35, 513–514.

Kim, J.S., Han, J.S., 2000. Endoesophageal intubation for controlled ventilation in rabbits: a rapid and easy technique to establish a patent airway. Contemp. Top. Lab. Anim. Med. 39, 80.

King, W.W., St. Amant, L.G., Lee, W.R., 1994. A technique for serial spermatozoa collection in mice. Lab. Anim. Sci. 44, 295–296.

Kissinger, J.T., Garver, E.M., Schnell, M.A., Schantz, J.D., Coatney, R.W., Meunier, L.D., 1998. A new method to collect bile and access the duodenum in conscious dogs. Contemp. Top. 37, 89–93.

Kizilcan, F., Tanyel, F.C., Buyukpamukcu, N., Hicsonmez, A., 1994. Fetal survival after in-utero experimentation in the rabbit. Lab. Anim. Sci. 44, 144–147.

Kloots, W.J., van Amelsvoort, J.M.M., Brink, E.J., Ritskes, J., Remie, R., 1995. Technique for creating a permanent cecal fistula in the rat. Lab. Anim. Sci. 45, 588–591.

Knapp, W.C., Leeson, G.A., Wright, B.J., 1971. An improved technique for the collection of bile in the unanesthetized rat. Lab. Anim. Sci. 21, 403–405.

Knipfel, J.E., Peace, R.W., Evans, J.A., 1975. Multiple vascular and gastric cannulations of swine for studies of gastrointestinal, liver, and peripheral tissue metabolism. Lab. Anim. Sci. 25, 74–78.

Knize, D.M., Weatherby-White, R.C.A., 1974. Restraint of rabbits during prolonged administration of intravenous fluids. Lab. Anim. Sci. 19, 394–397.

Ko, J.C.H., Harrison, J.M., Maldelach, C.H., 1997. Comparison of invasive and non-invasive cardiopulmonary monitoring techniques in ferrets. Vet. Anesth. 26, 160. (Abstract).

Koba, W., Jelicks, L.A., Fine, E.J., 2013. MicroPET/SPECT/CT imaging of small animal models of disease. Am. J. Pathol. 182 (2), 319–324.

Koba, W., Kim, K., Lipton, M.L., Jelicks, L., Das, B., Herbst, L., et al., 2011. Imaging devices for use in small animals. Semin. Nucl. Med. 41 (3), 151–165.

Koc, S., Kiyici, H., Sogut, E., Eyibilen, A., Ekici, A., Salman, N., 2012. Effect of pentoxifylline and 5-fluorouracil/triamcinolone on laryngotracheal stenosis developing as a complication of tracheostomy: study in rats. Eur. Arch. Otorhinolaryngol. 269, 1813–1820.

Kohlert, D.J., 2013. Unanesthetized sublingual blood collection in rats. Lab. Anim. Sci., 32–35.

Konantz, M., Balci, T.B., Hartwig, U.F., Dellaire, G., Andre, M.C., Berman, J.N., et al., 2012. Zebrafish xenografts as a tool for in vivo studies on human cancer. Ann. N.Y. Acad. Sci. 1266, 124–137.

Korber, K.E., Flye, M.W., 1987. Arteriovenous shunt construction for vascular access in the rat. Microsurgery 8, 245–246.

Korkmaz, T., Atalgin, S.H., Kilicgun, H.A., Bugra, O., Kahramansoy, N., 2013. The efficacy of intraosseous blood and ringer lactate in a rabbit model of hemorrhagic hypovolemia. Clin. Med. Res. 2, 18–23.

Kramer, K., Kinter, L.B., 2003. Evaluation and applications of radiotelemetry in small laboratory animals. Physiol. Genomics 13, 197–205.

Kramer, M.H., Harris, D.J., 2010. Avian blood collection. J. Exotic Pet Med. 19 (1), 82–86.

Krause, A.L., 1980. Research methodology In: Baker, H.J. Lindsey, J.R. Weisbroth, S.H. (Eds.), The Laboratory Rat, vol. 2. Academic Press, New York, pp. 1–42.

Krishnakumar, S., Holmes, E.P., Moore, R.M., Kappel, L., Venugopal, C.S., 2002. Non-adrenergic non-cholinergic excitatory innervation in the airways: role of neurokinin-2 receptors. Auton. Autacoid. Pharmacol. 22, 215–224.

Kromka, M.C., Hoar, R.M., 1975. An improved technique for thyroidectomy in guinea pigs. Lab. Anim. Sci. 25, 82–84.

Kubota, K., 1997. Measurement of liver volume and hepatic functional reserve as a guide to decision-making in resectional surgery for hepatic tumors. Hepatology 26 (5), 1176–1181.

Kumar, N., Lee, J.J., Perlmutter, J.S., Derdeyn, C.P., 2009. Cervical carotid and circle of willis arterial anatomy of macaque monkeys: a comparative anatomy study. Anat. Rec. (Hoboken) 292, 976–984.

Kumar, R.K., 1979. Toe clipping procedure for individual identification of rodents. Lab. Anim. Sci. 29, 679–680.

Kurtz, T.W., Griffin, K.A., Bidani, A.K., Davisson, R.L., Hall, J.E., 2005. Recommendations for blood pressure measurement in animals: summary of an AHA scientific statement from the council on high blood pressure research, professional and public education subcommittee. Arterioscl. Thromb. Vasc. Biol. 25, 478–479.

Kusaka, G., Calvert, J.W., Smelley, C., Nanda, A., Zhang, J.H., 2004. New lumbar method for monitoring cerebrospinal fluid pressure in rats. J. Neurosci. Methods 135, 121–127.

Kusumi, R.K., Plouffe, J.F., 1979. A safe and simple technique for obtaining cerebrospinal fluid from rabbits. Lab. Anim. Sci. 29, 681–682.

Kuszak, J., Rodin, M., 1977. A new technique for the pinealectomy of adult rats. Experientia 33, 283–284.

Kyriazis, A.P., Kyriazis, A.A., Scarpelli, D.G., Fogh, J., Rao, S., Lepers, L., 1982. Human pancreatic adenocarcinoma line Capan-1 in tissue culture and the nude mouse. Am. J. Pathol. 106, 250–260.

Laboratory Animal Pocket Reference Series. CRC Press, Boca Raton, Florida. <https://www.crcpress.com>.

Lacy, M.J., Kent, C.R., Voss, E.W., 1987. d-Limonene: an effective vasodilator for use in collecting rabbit blood. Lab. Anim. Sci. 37, 485–486.

Ladewig, J., Stribrny, K., 1988. A simplified method for stress free continuous blood collection in large animals. Lab. Anim. Sci. 38, 333–335.

Lagutchik, M.S., Sturgis, J.W., Martin, D.G., Bley, J.A., 1992. J. Invest. Surg. 5, 79–89.

Lamawansa, M.D., Wysocki, S.J., House, A.K., Norman, P.E., 1999. The changes seen in balloon-injured porcine femoral arteries following sympathectomy. Cardiovasc. Surg. 7, 526–531.

Lang, C.M., 1967. A technique for the collection of semen from squirrel monkeys (Saimiri sciureus) by electroejaculation. Lab. Anim. Care 17, 218–221.

Lang, C.M., 1976. Animal Physiologic Surgery. Springer-Verlag, Berlin, Germany, pp. 107–120.

Larsen, M.O., Rolin, B., 2004. Use of the Göttingenminipig as a model of diabetes, with special focus on type 1 diabetes research. ILAR J. 45 (3), 303–313.

Larsen, M.O., Wilken, M., Gotfredsen, C.F., Carr, R.D., Svendsen, O., Rolin, B., 2002. Mild streptozotocindiabetes in the Göttingenminipig. A novel model of moderate insulin deficiency and diabetes. Am. J. Physiol. Endocrinol. Metab. 282 (6), E1342–E1351.

Law, G.R.J., 1960. Blood samples from jugular vein of turkeys. Poult. Sci. 39, 1450–1452.

Leash, A.M., Beyer, R.D., Wilber, R.G., 1973. Self-mutilation following Innovar-Vet injections in the guinea pig. Lab. Anim. Sci. 23, 720–721.

Lee, G.E., Danneman, P.J., Rufo, R.D., Kalesnykas, R.P., Eng, V.M., 1998. Use of chlorine dioxide for antimicrobial prophylactic maintenance of cephalic recording devices in rhesus macaques (Macaca mulatta). Contemp. Top. 37, 59–63.

Leibo, S.P., Mazur, P., Jackowski, S.C., 1974. Factors affecting survival of mouse embryos during freezing and thawing. Exp. Cell Res. 89, 79–88.

Lequin, R.M., Elvers, L.H., Bertens, A.P.M.G., 1981. Early detection of pregnancy in rhesus and stumptailed macaques (Macaca mulatta and Macaca arctoides). J. Med. Primatol. 10, 189–198.

Levine, G., Lewis, L., Cember, H., 1973. A vacuum-assisted technic for repetitive blood sampling in the rat. Lab. Anim. Sci. 26, 211–213.

Lewis, V.J., Thacker, W.L., Mitchell, S.H., Baer, G.M., 1976. A new technique for obtaining blood from mice. Lab. Anim. Sci. 26, 211–213.

Liang, J.-H., Sankai, T., Yoshida, T., Yoshikawa, Y., 1997. Use of a modified rotating cutting needle for testicular biopsy in cynomolgus monkeys (Macaca fascicularis). Contemp. Top. 36, 77–79.

Lin, M., Marshall, C.T., Qi, Y., Johnston, S.M., Badea, C.T., Piantadosi, C.A., et al., 2009. Quantitative blood flow measurements in the small animal cardiopulmonary system using digital subtraction angiography. Med. Phys. 36, 5347–5358.

Linz, D., Wirth, K., Ukena, C., Mahfoud, F., Poss, J., Linz, B., et al., 2013. Renal denervation suppresses ventricular arrhythmias during acute ventricular ischemia in pigs. Heart Rhythm. 10, 1525–1530.

Lipman, N.S., Marini, R.P., Flecknell, P.A., 1997. Anesthesia and Analgesia in Laboratory Animals, first ed. Academic Press, San Diego, Chapter 10, pp. 205–232, 299–333.

Lipman, N.S., Marini, R.P., Flecknell, P.A., 2008. Chapter 11 - Anesthesia and Analgesia in Rabbits Anesthesia and Analgesia in Laboratory Animals, second ed. Academic Press, San Diego, pp. 299–333.

Litwak, K.N., Cefalu, W.T., Wagner, J.D., 1998. Streptozotocin-induced diabetes mellitus in cynomologus monkeys: changes in carbohydrate metabolism, skin glycation, and pancreatic islets. Lab. Anim. Sci. 48, 172–178.

Liu, L., Duff, K., 2008. A technique for serial collection of cerebrospinal fluid from the cisterna magna in mouse. J. Vis. Exp. 21, 960.

Liu, M., Shen, L., Begg, D.P., D'Alessio, D.A., Woods, S.C., 2012. Insulin increases central apolipoprotein E levels as revealed by an improved technique for collection of cerebrospinal fluid from rats. J. Neurosci. Methods 209, 106–112.

Livingstone, C.R., Andrews, M.A., Jenkins, S.M., Marriott, C., 1990. Model systems for the evaluation of mucolytic drugs: acetylcysteine and Scarboxymethylcysteine. J. Pharm. Pharmacol. 42, 73–78.

Loeb, W.F., Ciemanec, J.L., Wickum, M., 1976. A coagulopathy of the owl monkey (Aotus trivirgatus) associated with high antithrombin III activity. Lab. Anim. Sci. 26, 1084–1086.

Lopez, H., Navia, J.M., 1977. A technique for repeated collection of blood from the guinea pig. Lab. Anim. Sci. 27, 522–523.

Lopukhin, Y.M., 1976. Experimental Surgery. M.I.R. Publishers, Moscow, Russia, pp. 191–236, 271–308, 350–366.

Lu, C.Z., Liu, J., Xia, D.V., Zhao, X.D., Chen, X., Yu, X., et al., 2012. Efficacy of catheter-based renal denervation in mongrel neurogenic hypertensive dogs. Zhonghua Xin Xue Guan Bing Za Zhi 40, 14–17.

Lu, Y.G., Wei, W., Wang, L., Tao, K.M., Sun, Y.M., You, Z.D., et al., 2013. Ultrasound-guided cerebrospinal fluid collection from rats. J. Neurosci. Methods 215, 218–223.

Lukas, S.E., Griffiths, R.R., Bradford, D., Brady, J.V., Daley, L., 1982. A tethering system for intravenous and intragastric drug administration in the baboon. Pharm. Biochem. Behav. 17, 823–829.

Luo, Y.S., Luo, Y.S., Ashford, E.B., Morin, R.R., White, W.J., Fisher, T.F., 2000. Comparison of catheter lock solutions in rats. Charles River Laboratories, Wilmington, MA.

Lushbough, C.H., Moline, S.W., 1961. Improved terminal bleeding method. Proc. Anim. Care Panel 11, 305–308.

Macedo-Sobrinho, B., Roth, G., Grellner, T., 1978. Tubular device for intraoral examination of rodents. Lab. Anim. 12, 137–139.

Machholz, E., Mulder, G., Ruiz, C., Corning, B.F., Pritchett-Corning, K.R., 2012. Manual restraint and common compound administration routes in mice and rats. J. Vis. Exp. 67, e2771.

Macrae, D.J., Guerreiro, D., 1989. A simple laryngoscopic technique for the endotracheal intubation of rabbits. Lab. Anim. 23, 59–61.

Madrahimov, N., Dirsch, O., Broelsch, C., Dahmen, U., 2006. Marginal hepatectomy in the rat: from anatomy to surgery. Ann. Surg. 244, 89–98.

Mahat, M.Y., Fakrudeen Ali Ahamed, N., Chandrasekaran, S., Rajagopal, S., Narayanan, S., Surendran, N., 2012. An improved method of transcutaneous cisterna magna puncture for cerebrospinal fluid sampling in rats. J. Neurosci. Methods 211, 272–279.

Mahoney, C.J., 1975a. The accuracy of bimanual rectal palpation for determining the time of ovulation and conception in the rhesus monkey (Macaca mulatta). In: Perkins, F.T., O'Donoghue, P.N. (Eds.), Breeding Simians for Developmental Biology. Laboratory Animals Handbook 6. Laboratory Animals Ltd., London, pp. 127–138.

Mahoney, C.J., 1975b. Practical aspects of determining early pregnancy, stage of fetal development, and imminent parturition in the monkey (Macaca fascicularis). In: Perkins, F.T., O'Donoghue, P.N. (Eds.), Breeding Simians for Developmental Biology. Laboratory Animal Handbook 6. Laboratory Animals Ltd., London, pp. 261–274.

Maillie, A.J., Calvo, F.L., Vaccaro, M.I., Caboteau, L.I., Pivetta, O.H., 1981. An experimental model to study bile and exocrine pancreatic secretion from mice. Lab. Anim. Sci. 31, 707–709.

Malinovsky, J.M., Charles, F., Baudrimont, M., Pereon, Y., Le Corre, P., Pinaud, M., et al., 2002. Intrathecal ropivacaine in rabbits: pharmacodynamic and neurotoxicologic study. Anesthesiology 97, 429–435.

Manautou, J.E., Chen, C., 2005. Collection of bile and urine samples for determining the urinary and hepatobiliary disposition of xenobiotics in mice. Curr. Protoc. Toxicol. 5, 5.7.

Mandavilli, U., Schmidt, J., Rattner, D.W., Watson, W.T., Warshaw, A.L., 1991. Continuous complete collection of uncontaminated urine in conscious rodents. Lab. Anim. Sci. 41, 258–261.

Mann, W.A., Landi, M.S., Horner, E., Woodward, P., Campbell, S., Kinter, L.B., 1987. A simple procedure for direct blood pressure measurements in conscious dogs. Lab. Anim. Sci. 37, 105–108.

Manno III, F.A., 2010. Cryopreservation of mouse embryos by vitrification: a meta-analysis. Theriogenology 74, 165–172.

Manuel, M., Heckman, C.J., 2012. Simultaneous intracellular recording of a lumbar motoneuron and the force produced by its motor unit in the adult mouse in vivo. J. Vis. Exp. e4312.

Maragos, C.M., Fubini, S.L., Hotchkiss, J.H., 1990. A two stage cannula for gastic fistulation of swine. Lab. Anim. Sci. 40, 217–219.

Marini, R.P., 2014. Physical examination and diagnosis. In: Fox, J.G., Marini, R.P. (Eds.), Biology and Diseases of the Ferret. Wiley-Blackwell, Ames, IO, pp. 235–259.

Marini, R.P., Fox, J.G., 1988. Anesthesia, surgery, and biomethodology. In: Fox, J.G. (Ed.), Biology and Diseases of the Ferret. Williams and Wilkins, Baltimore, MD, pp. 449–484.

Marini, R.P., Esteves, M.I., Fox, J.G., 1994. A technique for catheterization of the urinary bladder in the ferret. Lab. Anim. 28, 155–157.

Markowitz, J., Archibald, J., Downie, H.G., 1964. Experimental Surgery, fifth ed. Williams and Wilkins, Baltimore, MD, pp. 326–352, 332–381, 581–598, 630–643.

Martin, B.J., 1997. The Laboratory Cat.

Martin, K.H., Richmond, M.E., 1972. A method for repeated sampling of testis tissue from small mammals. Lab. Anim. Sci. 22, 541–545.

Martins, P.N., Theruvath, T.P., Neuhaus, P., 2008. Rodent models of partial hepatectomies. Liver Int. 28, 3–11.

Masiello, P., Broca, C., Gross, R., Roye, M., Manteghetti, M., Hillaire-Buys, D., et al., 1998. Experimental NIDDM. Development of a new model in adult rats administered streptozotocin and nicotinamide. Diabetes 47, 224–229.

Matchett, C.A., Marr, R., Berard, F.M., Cawthon, A.G., Swing, S.P., 2012. Experimental methodology. The Laboratory Ferret. CRC Press, Boca Raton, FL, pp. 63–86.

Mateika, J.H., Sandhu, K.S., 2011. Experimental protocols and preparations to study respiratory long term facilitation. Respir. Physiol. Neurobiol. 176, 1–11.

Matsui, A., Tanaka, E., Choi, H.S., Winer, J.H., Kianzad, V., Gioux, S., et al., 2010. Real-time intra-operative near-infrared fluorescence identification of the extrahepatic bile ducts using clinically available contrast agents. Surgery 148, 87–95.

Maxwell, K.W., Dietz, T., Marcus, S., 1964. An *in situ* method for harvesting guinea pig alveolar macrophages. Am. J. Vet. Med. Res. 37, 237–238.

McCully, C.L., Balis, F.M., Bacher, J., Phillips, J., Poplack, D.G., 1990. A rhesus monkey model for continuous infusion of drugs into cerebrospinal fluid. Lab. Anim. Sci. 40, 520–525.

McFee, A.F., Kenelly, J.J., 1964. Evaluation of a testicular biopsy technique in the rabbit. J. Reprod. Fertil. 8, 141–144.

McGlinn, S.M., Shepherd, B.A., Martan, J., 1976. A new castration technique in the guinea pig. Lab. Anim. Sci. 26, 203–205.

McGuill, M.W., Rowan, A.N., 1989. Biological effects of blood loss: implications for sampling volumes and techniques. ILAR News 31, 5–20.

McLoughlin, M.A., Bjorling, D.E., 2003. Ureters. In Textbook of Small Animal Surgery, third ed. Elsevier Science (USA), Philadelphia, pp. 1,690–1,628.

McNamee, G.A., Wannemacher, R.W., Dinterman, R.E., Rozmiarek, H., Montrey, R., 1984. A surgical procedure and tethering system for chronic blood sampling, infusion, and temperature monitoring in caged nonhuman primates. Lab. Anim. Sci. 34, 303–307.

Medin, N.I., Osebold, J.W., Zee, Y.C., 1976. A procedure for pulmonary lavage in mice. Am. J. Vet. Res. 37 273–238.

Mehler, S.J., 2014. Surgical diseases of the ferret Biology and Diseases of the Ferret, third ed. Elsevier, Boston, MA.

Melich, D., 1990. A method for chronic intravenous infusion of the rabbit via the marginal ear vein. Lab. Anim. Sci. 40, 327–328.

Mesina, J.E., Sylvina, T.S., Hotaling, L.C., Pecquet Goad, M.E., Fox, J.G., 1988. A simple technique for chronic jugular catheterization in ferrets. Lab. Anim. Sci. 38, 89–90.

Metildi, C.A., Kaushal, S., Lee, C., Hardamon, C.R., Snyder, C.S., Luiken, G.A., et al., 2012. An LED light source and novel fluorophore combinations improve fluorescence laparoscopic detection of metastatic pancreatic cancer in orthotopic mouse models. J. Am. Coll. Surg. 214, 997–1007, e2.

Meunier, L.D., Kissinger, J.T., Marcello, J., Nichols, A.J., Smith, P.L., 1993. A chronic access port model for direct delivery of drugs into the intestine of conscious dogs. Lab. Anim. Sci. 43, 466–470.

Mikeska, J.A., Klemm, W.R., 1975. EEG evaluation of humaneness of asphyxia and decapitation euthanasia in the laboratory rat. Lab. Anim. Sci. 25, 175–179.

Miller, D.L., 1990. Experimental diabetes: effect of streptozotocin on the golden Syrian hamster. Lab. Anim. Sci. 40, 539–540.

Minasian, A., 1980. A simple tourniquet to aid mouse tail venipuncture. Lab. Anim. 14, 205.

Mitchell, M.A., Tully, T.N., 2009. Rabbits Manual of Exotic Pet Practice. Saunders Elsevier, St. Louis, MO.

Miyamoto, T., Takeishi, Y., Tazawa, S., Inoue, M., Aoyama, T., Takahashi, H., et al., 2004. Fatty acid metabolism assessed by 125I-iodophenyl 9-methylpentadecanoic acid (9MPA) and expression of fatty acid utilization enzymes in volume-overloaded hearts. Eur. J. Clin. Invest. 34, 176–181.

Moise Jr., K.J., Hesketh, D.E., Belfort, M.M., Saade, G., Van den Veyver, I.B., Hudson, K.M., et al., 1992. Ultrasound-guided blood sampling of rabbit fetuses. Lab. Anim. Sci. 42, 398–401.

Moler, T.L., Donahue, S.E., Anderson, G.B., 1979. A simple technique for nonsurgical embryo transfer in mice. Lab. Anim. Sci. 29, 353–356.

Mood, Z.A., Mehrabi, A., Schmied, B.M., Müller, S.A., Engelmann, G., Schemmer, P., et al., 2008. Review of various techniques of pancreas transplantation in rat model. J. Surg. Res. 145 (2), 205–213.

Moore, D.M., 1983. Dept. of Comparative Medicine, UTHSC Medical School at Houston, Texas. Unpublished paper.

Moore, D.M., 1984. A simple technique for blood collection in the opossum (*Didelphis virginiana*). Lab. Anim. 18, 52–54.

Moores, H.K., Janigan, D.T., Hajela, R.P., Luner, S.J., 1989. Use of a fluid dispensing apparatus for bronchoalveolar lavage in mice. Lab. Anim. Sci. 39, 149–152.

Moran, C.M., Thomson, A.J., Rog-Zielinska, E., Gray, G.A., 2013. High-resolution echocardiography in the assessment of cardiac physiology and disease in preclinical models. Exp. Physiol. 98 (3), 629–644.

Morcom, C.B., Dukelow, W.R., 1980. A research technique for the oviductal insemination of pigs using laparoscopy. Lab. Anim. Sci. 30, 1030–1031.

Moritz, M.M., Dawe, E.J., Holliday, J.F., Elliott, S., Mattei, J.A., Thomas, A.L., 1989. Chronic central vein catheterization for intraoperative and long-term venous access in swine. Lab. Anim. Sci. 39, 153–155.

Morrell, J.M., Rodriguez-Martinez, H., 2011. Vet. Med. Int. 2011 Article ID 894767, 9 pages http://dx.doi.org/10.4061/2011/894767.

Mrozek, M., Fischer, R., Trendelenburg, M., Zillmann, U., 1995. Microchip system used for animal identification in laboratory rabbits, guinea pigs, woodchucks, and in amphibians. Lab. Anim. 29, 339–433.

Muggenberg, B.A., Mauderly, J.L., 1975. Lung lavage using a single lumen endotracheal tube. J. Appl. Physiol. 38, 922–926.

Muller, G., Schaarschmidt, K., Stratmann, U., 1992. A new device for long-term continuous enteral nutrition of rats by elementary diet via gastrostomy, following extensive oesophageal or lower gastrointestinal surgery. Lab. Anim. 26, 9–14.

Munson, E.S., 1974. Arterial cannulation in awake restrained monkeys. Lab. Anim. Sci. 24, 793–795.

Murata, Y., Olmarker, K., Takahashi, I., Takahashi, K., Rydevik, B., 2006. Effects of lumbar sympathectomy on pain behavioral changes caused by nucleus pulposus-induced spinal nerve damage in rats. Eur. Spine J. 15, 634–640.

Mylrea, K.C., Abbrecht, P.H., 1967. An apparatus for tail vein injection in mice. Lab. Anim. Care 17, 602–603.

Myrie, S.B., McKnight, L.L., King, J.C., McGuire, J.J., Van Vliet, B.N., Bertolo, R.F., 2012. Effects of a diet high in salt, fat, and sugar on telemetric blood pressure measurements in conscious, unrestrained adult Yucatan miniature swine (Sus scrofa). Comp. Med. 62, 282–290.

Myrvik, Q.N., Leake, E.S., Fariss, B., 1961. Studies on pulmonary alveolar macrophages from the normal rabbit: a technique to produce them in a high state of purity. J. Immunol. 86, 128–132.

Nagy, A., Gertsensstein, M., Vintersten, K., Behringer, R., 2003. Manipulating the Mouse Embryo. Cold Spring Harbor Laboratory Press, Cold Spring harbor.

Nakagata, N., 2000. Cryopreservation. Mamm. Genome 11, 572–576.

Nakanishi, Y., Nagasawa, H., 1976. Improved method for hypophysectomy of the mouse (author's translation]. Jikken Dobutsu. 25, 13–17.

Naranjo, J.A., Valverde, A., Martinez de Victoria, E., Manas, M., Moreno, M., 1986. Surgical preparation for the study of pancreatic exocrine secretion in the conscious preruminant goat. Lab. Anim. 20, 231–233.

Nau, R., Schunck, O., 1993. Cannulation of the lateral saphenous vein – a rapid method to gain access to the venous circulation in anaesthetized guinea pigs. Lab. Anim. 27, 23–25.

Nayci, A., Atis, S., Talas, D.U., Ersoz, G., 2003. Rigid bronchoscopy induces bacterial translocation: an experimental study in rats. Eur. Respir. J. 21, 749–752.

Nedeltchev, G.G., Raghunand, T.R., Jassal, M.S., Lun, S., Cheng, Q.J., Bishai, W.R., 2009. Extrapulmonary dissemination of mycobacterium bovis but not mycobacterium tuberculosis in a bronchoscopic rabbit model of cavitary tuberculosis. Infect. Immun. 77, 598–603.

Neel, J.A., Tarigo, J., Grindem, C.B., 2006. Gallbladder aspirate from a dog. Vet. Clin. Pathol. 35, 467–470.

Nelson, A.W., Monnet, E., 2003. Lungs. In: Slatter, D.H. (Ed.), Textbook of Small Animal Surgery., third ed. Saunders, Philadelphia, pp. 880–889.

Nerenberg, S.T., Zedler, P., 1975. Sequential blood samples from the tail vein of rats and mice obtained with modified Liebig condenser jackets and vacuum. J. Lab. Clin. Med. 85, 523–526.

Nicholson, J.W., Kinkead, E.R., 1982. A simple device for intratracheal injections in rats. Lab. Anim. Sci. 32, 509–510.

Niebergall-Roth, E., Teyssen, S., Singer, M.V., 1997. Pancreatic exocrine studies in intact animals: historic and current methods. Lab. Anim. Sci. 47, 606–614.

Niekrasz, M.A., Wardrip, C.L., 2012. Chapter 14 – Surgery in Nonhuman Primates. In: Morris, C.R.A.M.T. (Ed.), Nonhuman Primates in Biomedical Research, second ed. Academic Press, Boston, MA, pp. 339–358.

Nobonaga, T., Nabamura, K., Imamichi, T., 1966. A method for intravenous injection and collection of blood from rats and mice without restraint and anesthesia. Lab. Anim. Care 16, 40–49.

Nolan, T.E., Conti, P.A., 1980. Liver wedge biopsy in chimpanzees (Pan troglodytes) using an automatic stapling device. Lab. Anim. Sci. 30, 578–580.

Novak, Z., Petak, F., Banfi, A., Toth-Szuki, V., Barati, L., Kosa, L., et al., 2006. An improved technique for repeated bronchoalveolar lavage and lung mechanics measurements in individual rats. Respir. Physiol. Neurobiol. 154, 467–477.

Ntziachristos, V., Razansky, D., 2013. Optical and opto-acoustic imaging. Recent Results Cancer Res. 187, 133–150.

O'Byrne, K.T., 1988. Long-term blood sampling technique in the marmoset. Lab. Anim. 22, 151–153.

O'Grady, N.P., Alexander, M., Burns, L.A., Dellinger, E.P., Garland, J., Heard, S.O., et al., 2011. Summary of recommendations: guidelines for the prevention of intravascular catheter-related infections. Clin. Infect. Dis. 52, 1087–1099.

Olin, J.M., Smith, T.J., Talcott, M.R., 1997. Evaluation of noninvasive monitoring techniques in domestic ferrets. Am. J. Vet. Res. 58, 1065.

Olinger, A., Pistorius, G., Lindemann, W., Vollmar, B., Hlidebrandt, U., Menger, M.D., 1999. Effectiveness of a hands-on training course for laparoscopic spine surgery in a porcine model. Surg. Endosc. 13, 118–122.

Olson, G.A., 1974. A method for surgical construction of a tracheal pouch in the ferret. Lab. Anim. Dig. 9, 47–49.

Olsen, D., Packer, B.E., Perrett, J., Balentine, H., Andrews, G.A., 2002. Evaluation of the bone injection gun as a method for intraosseous cannula placement for fluid therapy in adult dogs. Vet. Surg. 31 (6), 533–540.

Olson, L.C., Sternfeld, M.D., 1987. A percutaneous method for obtaining uterine biopsies. Lab. Anim. Sci. 37, 663–664.

Omaye, S.T., Skala, J.H., Gretz, M.D., Schaus, E.E., Wade, C.E., 1987. Simple method for bleeding the unanesthetized rat by tail venipuncture. Lab. Anim. 21, 261–264.

Onda, A., Yabuki, S., Iwabuchi, M., Anzai, H., Olmarker, K., Kikuchi, S., 2004. Lumbar sympathectomy increases blood flow in a dog model of chronic cauda equina compression. J. Spinal Disord. Tech. 17, 522–525.

Orsini, J.A., Roby, K.A., 1997. Modified carotid artery transposition for repetitive arterial blood gas sampling in large animals. J. Invest. Surg. 10, 125–128.

Osborne, C.A., Low, D.G., Finco, D.R., 1972. Canine and Feline Urology. Saunders, Philadelphia, PA, pp. 28–30.

Ott Johnson, J., 2009. Blood collection techniques in exotic small mammals. J. Exotic Pet Med. 18 (2), 117–139.

Otto, G., Rosenblad, W.D., Fox, J.G., 1993. Practical venipuncture techniques for the ferret. Lab. Anim. 27, 26–29.

Oz, M.C., Popilskis, S.J., Morales, A., Nowygrod, R., 1989. Long term catheterization of the rat ureter. Lab. Anim. Sci. 39, 349–350.

Padgett, K.A., Reisen, W.K., Kahl-Purcell, N., Fang, Y., Cahoon-Young, B., Carney, R., et al., 2007. West Nile virus infection in tree squirrels (Rodentia: Sciuridae) in California, 2004–2005. Am. J. Trop. Med. Hyg. 76 (5), 810–813.

Painter, N.W., Borski, A.A., Trevino, G.S., 1971. Urethral reaction to foreign objects. J. Urol. 106, 227–230.

Palm, U., Boemke, W., Bayerl, D., Schnoy, N., Juhr, N.-C., Reninhardt, H.W., 1991. Prevention of catheter-related infections by a new, catheter-restricted antibiotic filling technique. Lab. Anim. 25, 142–152.

Pansky, B., Jacobs, M., House, E.L., 1961. The orbital region as a source of blood samples in the golden hamster. Anat. Rec. 39, 409.

Paolini, R.V., Rossman, J.E., Patel, V., Stanievich, J.F., 1993. A reliable method for large volume blood collection in the chinchilla. Lab. Anim. Sci. 43, 524–525.

Pare, W.P., Vincent, G.P., Isom, K.E., 1979. Comparison of pyloric ligation and pyloric cuff techniques for collecting gastric secretion in the rat. Lab. Anim. Sci. 29, 218–220.

Parlett, W.R., George III, T.F., Bley, J.A., 1993. A paramedian retroperitoneal approach to the kidney and ureter in pigs. Lab. Anim. Sci. 43, 520–523.

Paulsen, R., Valentine, J.L., 1984. A procedure for intravenous administration of drugs and repeated arterial blood sampling in the rabbit. Lab. Anim. 13, 34–36.

Paxinos, G., Franklin, K.B.J., 2012. Paxinos and Franklin's the Mouse Brain in Stereotaxic Coordinates, fourth ed. Academic Press, New York.

Paxinos, G., Watson, C., 1998. The Rat Brain in Stereotaxic Coordinates. Academic Press, New York.

Pazin, G.J., Wu, B.A., Van Theil, D.H., 1978. Fiberoptic esophagogastroscopy, brushings, and biopsy in rabbits. Lab. Anim. Sci. 28, 733–736.

Pearce, P.C., Halsey, M.J., Ross, J.A.S., Luff, N.P., Bevilacqua, R.A., Maclean, C.J., 1989. A method of remote physiological monitoring of a fully mobile primate in a single animal cage. Lab. Anim. 23, 180–187.

Pegg, C.C., He, C., Stroink, A.R., Kattner, K.A., Wang, C.X., 2010. Technique for collection of cerebrospinal fluid from the cisterna magna in rat. J. Neurosci. Methods 187, 8–12.

Pekow, C.A., 2012. Basic experimental methods in the rabbit. In: Suckow, M.A., Stevens, K.A., Wilson, R.P. (Eds.), The Laboratory Rabbit, Guinea Pig, Hamster, and Other Rodents. Academic Press, Waltham, MA, pp. 243–258.

Pekow, C.A., Weller, R.E., Kimsey, B.B., Allen, M.K., 1994. Ultrasound-guided cholecystocentesis in the owl monkey. Lab. Anim. Sci. 44, 365–369.

Pena, H., Cabrera, C., 1980. Improved endotracheal intubation technique in the rat. Lab. Anim. Sci. 30, 712–713.

Percie du Sert, N., Chu, K.M., Wai, M.K., Rudd, J.A., Andrews, P.L., 2009. Reduced normogastric electrical activity associated with emesis: a telemetric study in ferrets. World J. Gastroenterol. 15, 6034–6043.

Peregrine, A.S., Mamman, M., 1993. Pharmacology of diminazene: a review. Acta. Trop. 54, 185–203.

Perry-Clark, L.M., Meunier, L.D., 1991. Vascular access ports for chronic serial infusion and blood sampling in New Zealand White rabbits. Lab. Anim. Sci. 41, 495–497.

Peter, A.J., Bell, J.A., Manning, D.D., Bosu, W.T.K., 1990. Real-time ultrasonographic determination of pregnancy and gestational age in ferrets. Lab. Anim. Sci. 40, 91–92.

Peterborg, L.J., Philo, R.C., Reiter, R.J., 1980. The pineal body and pinealectomy in the cotton rat (*Sigmodon hispidus*). Acta Anat. 107, 108–113.

Peterson, R.R., Webster, R.C., Rayner, B., 1952. The thyroid and reproductive performance in the adult male guinea pig. Endocrinology 5, 504–518.

Phillips, W.A., Stafford, W.W., Stunt, J., 1973. Jugular vein technique for serial blood sampling and intravenous injection in the rat. Proc. Soc. Exp. Biol. Med. 143, 733–735.

Piermattei, D.L., Flo, G.L., DeCamp, C.E., 2006. Brinker, Piermattei and Flo's Handbook of Small Animal Orthopedic and Fracture Repair, fourth ed. Elsevier.

Pinkert, C.A., 1998. Mouse sperm cryopreservation: a legacy in the making. Lab. Anim. Sci. 48, 224.

Pizzonia, J., Holmberg, J., Orton, S., Alvero, A., Viteri, O., McLaughlin, W., et al., 2012. Multimodality animal rotation imaging system (Mars) for in vivo detection of intraperitoneal tumors. Am. J. Reprod. Immunol. 67 (1), 84–90.

Plager, J.E., 1972. Intravenous, long-term infusion in the unrestrained mouse-method. J. Lab. Clin. Med. 79, 669–672.

Platts, R.G.S., Wilson, P., Shaw, K.M., 1972. Design for a chronic right ventricular catheter for dogs. Lab. Anim. Sci. 22, 900–903.

Pohlmeyer, G., Reuss, S., Baum, A., 1994. An improved technique for visually controlled pinealectomy in the rat. J. Exp. Anim. Sci. 36, 84–88.

Pointer, K.B., Clark, P.A., Zorniak, M., Alrfaei, B.M., Kuo, J.S., 2014. Glioblastoma cancer stem cells: biomarker and therapeutic advances. Neurochem. Int. 71C, 1–7.

Polis, I., Moens, Y., Gasthuys, F., Tshamala, M., Risselada, M., 2002. Arterial catheterization and vascular access port implantation for blood sampling and continuous blood pressure measurement in dogs. Vlaams Diergeneesk. Tijdschr. 71, 404–410.

Poon, Y.Y., Chang, A.Y., Ko, S.F., Chan, S.H., 2005. An improved procedure for catheterization of the thoracic spinal subarachnoid space in the rat. Anesth. Analg. 101, 155–160.

Poon, Y.Y., Chang, A.Y., Ko, S.F., Chan, S.H., 2011. Catheterization of the thoracic spinal subarachnoid space in mice. J. Neurosci. Methods 200, 36–40.

Porter, K.B., Tsibris, J.C.M., Porter, G.W., O'Brien, W.F., Spellacy, W.N., 1997. Use of endoscopic and ultrasound techniques in the guinea pig leiomyoma model. Lab. Anim. Sci. 47, 537–539.

Prelusky, D.B., Hartin, K.E., 1991. A technique for serial sampling of cerebrospinal fluid from conscious swine and sheep. Lab. Anim. Sci. 41, 481–485.

Prentice, J.R., Anzar, M., 2010. Cryopreservation of mammalian oocyte for conservation of animal genetics. Vet. Med. Int. http://dx.doi.org/10.4061/2011/146405.

Prins, J.-B., Fox, R.R., 1984. A successful technique for the preservation of rabbit embryos. Lab. Anim. Sci. 34, 484–487.

Putz, D.A., Weinberg, S.M., Smith, T.D., Burrows, A.M., Cooper, G.M., Losken, H.W., et al., 2002. Coronal suturectomy does not cause acute postoperative displacement in the cranial bases of craniosynostotic rabbits. J. Craniofac. Surg. 13, 196–201.

Pye-MacSwain, J.K., Cawthorn, E.G., Rainnie, D.J., Johnson, G.R., 1994. Modification of the cannulation for the dorsal aorta of Atlantic salmon (*Salmo salar*). Lab. Anim. Sci. 44, 540–541.

Quesenberry, K.E., Carpenter, J.W., 2004. Ferrets, Rabbits, and Rodents: Clinical Medicine and Surgery, third ed. Saunders, St. Louis.

Quesenberry, K.E., Carpenter, J.W., 2011. Ferrets, Rabbits, and Rodents: Clinical Medicine and Surgery, third ed. Saunders, St. Louis.

Quinn, R.H., 2012. Rabbits: rabbit colony management and related health concerns. In: Suckow, M.A., Stevens, K.A., Wilson, R.P. (Eds.), The Laboratory Rabbit, Guinea Pig, Hamster, and Other Rodents. Academic Press, Waltham, MA, pp. 218–242.

Quintero, R.A., Puder, K.S., Bardicef, M., Rossman, K., Acosta, L., Esclapes, M., et al., 1994. Hydrolaparoscopy in the rabbit: a fine model for the development of operative fetoscopy. Am. J. Obstet. Gynecol. 171, 1139–1142.

Raggi, L.A., Manas, M., Martinez de Victoria, E., Lupiani, M.J., Mataix, F.J., 1985. Biliary secretion in the conscious preruminant goat: use of a reentrant cannula. Lab. Anim. 19, 35–38.

Rahlmann, D.F., Mains, R.C., Kodama, A.M., 1976. A urine collection device for use with the male pigtail macaque (*Macaca nemestrina*). Lab. Anim. Sci. 26, 829–831.

Ram, B., Oluwole, M., Blair, R.L., Mountain, R., Dunkley, P., White, P.S., 1999. Surgical simulation: an animal tissue model for training in therapeutic and diagnostic bronchoscopy. J. Laryngol. Otol. 113, 149–151.

Ransom, J.H., 1984. Intravenous injection of unanesthetized hamsters (*Mesocricetus auratus*). Lab. Anim. Sci. 34, 200–201.

Rath, L., Hutchison, M., 1989. A new method of bile duct cannulation allowing bile collection and re-infusion in the conscious rat. Lab. Anim. 23, 163–168.

Ravizzini, P.I., Shulsinger, D., Guarnizo, E., Pavlovich, C.P., Marion, D., Sosa, R.E., 1999. Hand-assisted laparoscopic donor nephrectomy versus standard laparoscopic donor nephrectomy: a comparison study in the canine model. Tech. Urol. 5, 174–178.

Rawlings, C.A., Van Lue, S., King, C., Freeman, L., Damian, R.T., Greenacre, C., et al., 2000. Serial laparoscopic biopsies of liver and spleen from *schistosoma*-infected baboons (*Papio spp.*). Comp. Med. 50 (5), 551–555.

Redfern, R., 1971. Techniques for oral intubation of wild rats. Lab. Anim. 5, 169–172.

Rees, D.A., Alcolado, J.C., 2005. Animal models of diabetes mellitus. Diabet Med. 22 (4), 359–370.

Reidenberg, J.S., Laitman, J.T., 1990a. A new method for radiographically locating upper respiratory and upper digestive tract structures in rats. Lab. Anim. Sci. 40, 72–76.

Reidenberg, J.S., Laitman, J.T., 1990b. A new surgical approach to the skull base in rats. Lab. Anim. Sci. 40, 312–315.

Reiser, H.J., Whitworth Jr., U.G., Hatchell, D.L., Sutherland, F.S., Nanda, S., McAdoo, T., et al., 1987. Experimental diabetes in cats induced by partial pancreatectomy alone or combined with local injection of alloxan. Lab. Anim. Sci. 37, 449–452.

Remedios, A.M., Duke, T., 1993. Chronic epidural implantation of vascular access catheters in the cat lumbosacrum. Lab. Anim. Sci. 43, 262–264.

Renella, R.R., Hussein, S., 1986. Microsurgical approach to the cerebellomedullar region in rat. Lab. Anim. 20, 210–212.

Report of the AVMA Panel on Euthanasia, 2001. J. Am. Vet. Med. Assoc. 218, 669–696.

Reuter, R.E., 1987. Venipuncture in the guinea pig. Lab. Anim. Sci. 37, 245–246.

Rey, M., Weber, E.W., Hess, P.D., 2012. Simultaneous pulmonary and systemic blood pressure and ECG Interval measurement in conscious, freely moving rats. J. Am. Assoc. Lab. Anim. Sci. 51, 231–238.

Rha, J.Y., Mahony, O., 1999. Bronchoscopy in small animal medicine: indications, instrumentation, and techniques. Clin. Tech. Small Anim. Pract. 14, 207–212.

Rhee, T.K., Park, J.K., Cashen, T.A., Shin, W., Schirf, B.E., Gehl, J.A., et al., 2006. Comparison of intraarterial MR angiography at 3.0 T with X-ray digital subtraction angiography for detection of renal artery stenosis in swine. J. Vasc. Interv. Radiol. 17, 1131–1137.

Rhodes, M.L., Patterson, C.E., 1979. Chronic intravenous infusion in the rat: a nonsurgical approach. Lab. Anim. Sci. 29, 82–84.

Richards, D.A., Hinko, P.J., Morse, E.M., 1972. Orthopaedic procedures for laboratory animals and exotic pets. J. Am. Vet. Med. Assoc. 161, 729–732.

Rickards, E.S., Mitchell, G., 1992. Improved stereotaxic headplates for rabbits. Lab. Anim. Sci. 42, 81–82.

Rigalli, A., Di Loreto, V., 2009. Experimental Surgical Models in the Laboratory Rat, first ed. CRC Press, Boca Raton, FL.

Ringkamp, M., Eschenfelder, S., Grethel, E.J., Habler, H.J., Meyer, R.A., Janig, W., et al., 1999. Lumbar sympathectomy failed to reverse mechanical allodynia- and hyperalgesia-like behavior in rats with L5 spinal nerve injury. Pain 79, 143–153.

Ritter, J.W., 1984. Permanent tracheostomy for expired air collection in conscious dogs. Lab. Anim. Sci. 34, 79–81.

Roberts, D.C., 1969. Transplanted Tumors of Rats and Mice: An Index of Tumors and Host Strains. Laboratory Animals, London.

Robinson, E.S., VandeBerg, J.L., 1994. Blood collection and surgical procedures for the laboratory opossum (*Monodelphis domestica*). Lab. Anim. Sci. 44, 63–68.

Rodhouse, S.L., Herkelman, K.L., Veum, T.L., Zinn, G.M., 1988. A flexible T-cannula for ileal cannulation of 10 to 20 kg pigs. Lab. Anim. Sci. 38, 92–94.

Rodriguez-Martinez, H., Wallgren, M., 2011. Advances in boar semen cryopreservation. Vet. Med. Int. 2011, Article ID 396181.

Rogers, G., Taylor, C., Austin, J.C., Rosen, C., 1988. A pharyngostomy technique for chronic oral dosing of rabbits. Lab. Anim. Sci. 38, 619–620.

Rolf Jr., L.L., Bartels, K.E., Nelson, E.C., Berlin, K.D., 1991. Chronic bile duct cannulation in laboratory rats. Lab. Anim. Sci. 41, 486–492.

Ronisz, A., Delcroix, M., Quarck, R., 2013. Measurement of right ventricular pressure by telemetry in conscious moving rabbits. Lab. Anim. 47, 175–183.

Rosenhaft, M.E., Bing, D.H., Knudson, K.C., 1971. A vacuum-assisted method for repetitive blood sampling in guinea pigs. Lab. Anim. Sci. 21, 598–599.

Rosenquist, R.W., Bunte, R.M., Artwohl, J.E., 1996. Percutaneous spinal catheterization in the rabbit. Contemp. Top. 35, 76–78.

Rotman, M., Snoeks, T.J., van der Weerd, L., 2011. Pre-clinical optical imaging and MRI for drug development in Alzheimer's disease. Drug Discov. Today Technol. 8 (2-4), e117–e125.

Rouleau, A.M.J., Kovacs, P.R., Kunz, H.W., Armstrong, D.T., 1993. Decontamination of rat embryos and transfer to specific pathogen-free recipients for the production of a breeding colony. Lab. Anim. Sci. 43, 611–615.

Ruggeri, B.A., Camp, F., Miknyoczki, S., 2014. Animal models of disease: pre-clinical animal models of cancer and their applications and utility in drug discovery. Biochem. Pharmacol. 87, 150–161.

Ruiz de Elvira, M.-C., Abbott, D.H., 1986. A backpack system for long-term osmotic minipump infusions into unrestrained marmoset monkeys. Lab. Anim. 20, 329–334.

Ruzinski, J.T., Skerrett, S.J., Chi, E.Y., Martin, T.R., 1995. Deposition of particles in the lungs of infant and adult rats after direct intratracheal administration. Lab. Anim. Sci. 45, 205–210.

Saarni, H., Viikari, J., 1976. A simple technique for continuous intravenous infusion under neuroleptic tranquillization. Lab. Anim. 10, 69–72.

Sadoff, D.A., Fischel, R.J., Carroll, M.E., Brockway, B., 1992. Chronic blood pressure radiotelemetry in rhesus macaques. Lab. Anim. Sci. 42, 78–80.

Sakaki, K., Tanaka, K., Hirasawa, K., 1961. Hematological comparison of the mouse blood taken from the eye and the tail. Exp. Anim. 10, 14–19.

Sakata, N., Yoshimatsu, G., Tsuchiya, H., Egawa, S., Unno, M., 2012. Animal Models of Diabetes Mellitus for Islet Transplantation. Exp. Diabetes Res. 2012 Article ID 256707, 11 pages, 2012. http://dx.doi.org/10.1155/2012/256707.

Sano, D., Myers, J.N., 2009. Xenograft models of head and neck cancers. Head Neck Oncol. 1, 32.

Sarna, G.S., Hutson, P.H., Tricklebank, M.D., Curzon, G., 1983. Determination of brain 5-hydroxytryptamine turnover in freely moving rats using repeated sampling of cerebrovascular fluid. J. Neurochem. 40, 383–388.

Sarr, M.G., 1988. Pancreas. In: Swindle, M.M., Adams, R.J. (Eds.), Experimental Surgery and Physiology: Induced Animal Models of Human Disease. Williams and Wilkins, Baltimore, MD, pp. 204–216.

Sato, M., Yoneda, S., 1966. An efficient method for transauricular hypophysectomy in rats. Acta Endocrinol. (Copenhagen) 51, 43–48.

Sawyer, D.C., Brown, M., Striler, E.L., Durham, R.A., Langham, M.A., Rech, R.H., 1991. Comparison of direct and indirect blood pressure measurement in anesthetized dogs. Lab. Anim. Sci. 41, 134–138.

Scalese, R.J., DeForrest, J.M., Hammerstone, S., Parente, E., Burkett, D.E., 1990. Long term vascular catheterization of the cynomolgus monkey. Lab. Anim. Sci. 40, 530–532.

Schaefer, D.C., Asner, I.N., Seifert, B., Burki, K., Cinelli, P., 2010. Analysis of physiological and behavioural parameters in mice after toe clipping as newborns. Lab. Anim. 44, 7–13.

Schaeffer, D.O., Hosgood, G., Oakes, M.G., St. Amant, L.G., Koon, C.E., 1994. An alternative technique for partial hepatectomy in mice. Lab. Anim. Sci. 44, 189–190.

Schambach, S.J., Bag, S., Groden, C., Schilling, L., Brockmann, M.A., 2010a. Vascular imaging in small rodents using micro-CT. Methods 50, 26–35.

Schambach, S.J., Bag, S., Schilling, L., Groden, C., Brockmann, M.A., 2010b. Application of micro-CT in small animal imaging. Methods 50, 2–13.

Schambach, S.J., Bag, S., Steil, V., Isaza, C., Schilling, L., Groden, C., et al., 2009. Ultrafast high-resolution in vivo volume-CTA of mice cerebral vessels. Stroke 40 (4), 1444–1450.

Schmitt, P.-J., 1988. Vaginal biopsy in long-term toxicity studies of beagle dogs. Lab. Anim. Sci. 38, 86–88.

Schnell, C.R., Wood, J.M., 1995. Measurement of blood pressure and heart rate by telemetry in conscious unrestrained marmosets. Lab. Anim. 29, 258–261.

Schoenborne, B.M., Schrader, R.E., Canolty, N.L., 1977. Tattooing newborn mice and rats for identification. Lab. Anim. Sci. 27, 110.

Seager, S.W.J., Fletcher, W.S., 1972. Collection, storage, and insemination of canine semen. Lab. Anim. Sci. 22, 177–182.

Seehofer, D., Mogl, M., Boas-Knoop, S., Unger, J., Schirmeier, A., Chopra, S., et al., 2012. Safety and efficacy of new integrated bipolar and ultrasonic scissors compared to conventional laparoscopic 5-mm sealing and cutting instruments. Surg. Endosc. 26, 2541–2549.

Seier, J.V., Fincham, J.E., Menkveld, R., Venter, F.S., 1989. Semen characteristics of vervet monkeys. Lab. Anim. 23, 43–47.

Sekas, G., 1990. A technique for creating partial obstruction of the common bile duct in the rat. Lab. Anim. 24, 284–287.

Sessions, A., Eichel, L., Kassahun, M., Messing, E.M., Schwarz, E., Wood, R.W., 2002. Continuous bladder infusion methods for studying voiding function in the ambulatory mouse. Urology 60, 707–713.

Shankar, V., Bowen, R.A., Davis, A.D., Rupprecht, C.E., O'shea, T.J., 2004. Rabies in a captive colony of big brown bats (*Eptesicusfuscus*). J. Wildl. Dis. 40 (3), 403–413.

Shapiro, J.S., Stiteler, M., Wu, G., Price, E.A., Simon, A.J., Sankaranarayanan, S., 2012. Cisterna magna cannulated repeated CSF sampling rat model – effects of a gamma-secretase inhibitor on Abeta levels. J. Neurosci. Methods 205, 36–44.

Sharp, P., LaRegina, M., 1998. The Laboratory Rat.

Shomer, N.H., Astrofsky, K.M., Dangler, C.A., Fox, J.G., 1999. Biomethod for obtaining gastric juice and serum from unanesthetized guinea pigs (*Cavia porcellus*). Contemp. Top. 38, 32–35.

Shrader, R.E., Everson, G.J., 1968. Intravenous injection and blood sampling using cannulated guinea pigs. Lab. Anim. Care 18, 214–219.

Sils, I.V., Szlyk-Modrow, P.C., Tartarini, K.A., Hubbard, L.J., Glass, E., Caretti, D.M., et al., 1994. Chronic implantation of nonocclusive catheters and flow probes in the splanchnic and hindlimb vasculature of the rabbit. Lab. Anim. Sci. 44, 319–323.

Silverman, J., 2012. Biomedical research techniques. In: Suckow, M.A., Stevens, K.A., Wilson, R.P. (Eds.), The Laboratory Rabbit, Guinea Pig, Hamster, and Other Rodents. Academic Press, Waltham, MA, pp. 779–793.

Simmons, F.A., 1952. Correlation of testicular biopsy material with semen analysis in male infertility. Ann. N. Y. Acad. Sci. 5, 643–656.

Simmons, M.L., Brick, J.O., 1970. The Laboratory Mouse – Selection and Management. Prentice-Hall, Englewood Cliffs, NJ.

Simon, D.I., Rogers, C., 2001. Vascular Disease and Injury: Preclinical Research. Humana Press, Totowa, NJ.

Singh, S.K., Hawkins, C., Clarke, I.D., Squire, J.A., Bayani, J., Hide, T., et al., 2004. Identification of human brain tumour initiating cells. Nature 432, 396–401.

Singletary, M.L., Phillippi-Falkenstein, K.M., Scanlon, E., Bohm Jr., R.P., Veazey, R.S., Gill, A.F., 2008. Modification of a common BAL technique to enhance sample diagnostic value. J. Am. Assoc. Lab. Anim. Sci. 47, 47–51.

Sisson, S., Grossman, J.D., 1966. The Anatomy of the Domestic Animals. Saunders, Philadelphia, PA, p. 489.

Skinner, J.E., 1971. Neuroscience: A Laboratory Animal. Saunders, Philadelphia, PA.

Slatter, D., 2003. Textbook of Small Animal Surgery. Saunders, Philadelphia.

Smith, C.J., McMahon, J.B., 1977. Method for collecting blood from fetal and neonatal rats. Lab. Anim. Sci. 27, 112–113.

Smith, C.R., Felton, J.S., Taylor, R.T., 1981. Description of a disposable individual mouse collection apparatus. Lab. Anim. Sci. 31, 80–82.

Smith, G., 1991. A simple non-surgical method of intrabronchial instillation for the establishment of respiratory infections in the rat. Lab. Anim. 25, 46–49.

Smith, D.M., Lieberman, R.P., Stribley, J.A., Sharp, J.G., 1992. Chronic catheterization of the inferior venacva in Yucatan miniature swine. Lab. Anim. Sci. 42, 602–606.

Snead III, O.C., LaCroix, J.T., 1977. Lumbar puncture obtaining cerebrospinal fluid in the rhesus monkey (*Macaca mulatta*). Lab. Anim. Sci. 27, 1039–1040.

Snitily, M.U., Gentry, M.J., Mellencamp, M.A., Preheim, L.C., 1991. A simple method for collection of blood from the rat foot. Lab. Anim. Sci. 41, 285–287.

Snyder, S.B., Soave, O.A., 1970. A method for the collection of throat specimens for laboratory primates for the rapid identification of respiratory infection. Lab. Anim. Care 20, 518–520.

Sojka, N.J., Jennings, L.L., Hamner, C.E., 1970. Artificial insemination in the cat (*Felis catus*). Lab. Anim. Care 20, 198–204.

Soli, N.E., Birkeland, R., 1977. A method for collection of bile in conscious sheep. Acta Vet. Scand. 18, 221–226.

Sorg, D.A., Buckner, B., 1964. A simple method for obtaining venous blood from small laboratory animals. Proc. Soc. Exp. Biol. Med. 115, 1131–1132.

Spalton, P.N., Clifford, J.M., 1979. Nasogastric intubation technique for bile sampling in the baboon, *Papio ursinus*. Lab. Anim. Sci. 29, 237–239.

Spillmann, T., Happonen, I., Kahkonen, T., Fyhr, T., Westermarck, E., 2005. Endoscopic retrograde cholangio-pancreatography in healthy Beagles. Vet. Radiol. Ultrasound 46, 97–104.

Spinelli, J., Holliday, T., Homer, J., 1968. Technical notes: collection of large samples of cerebrospinal fluid from horses. Lab. Anim. Care 18, 565–567.

Spira, W.M., Sack, R.B., Froehlich, J.L., 1981. Simple adult rabbit model for *Vibrio cholerae* and enterotoxigenic *Escherichia coli* diarrhea. Infect. Immun. 32, 739–747.

Sprangers, B., Billiau, A.D., 2008. Xenotransplantation: where are we in 2008? Kidney Int. 74, 14–21.

Starcher, B., Williams, I., 1989. A method for intratracheal instillation of endotoxin into the lungs of mice. Lab. Anim. 23, 234–240.

Stark, R.I., Daniel, S.S., James, L.S., MacCarter, G., Morishima, H.O., Niemann, W.H., et al., 1989. Chronic instrumentation and long term investigation in the fetal and maternal baboon: tether system, conditioning procedures, and surgical techniques. Lab. Anim. Sci. 39, 25–32.

Stavy, M., Terkel, J., Marder, U., 1978. Artificial insemination in the European hare (*Lepus europaeus syriacus*). Lab. Anim. Care 28 (2), 163–166.

St. Cyr, J., Bianco, R., Judd, D., Pierpont, M.E., Staley, N., Noren, G., et al., 1987. A new method of urine collection in turkeys and chickens. Lab. Anim. Sci. 37, 366–367.

Stenbäck, A., Meurling, S., Lundholm, M., Wallander, J., Johnsson, C., 2001. A model for bacterial translocation from small bowel in the rat. Transplant Proc. 33 (4), 2473.

Stephens Devalle, J.M., 2009. Successful management of rabbit anesthesia through the use of nasotracheal intubation. J. Am. Assoc. Lab. Anim. Sci. 48 (2), 166–170.

Stevens, R.W.C., Ridgeway, G.J., 1966. A technique for bleeding chickens from the jugular vein. Poult. Sci. 45, 204–205.

Stickrod, G., Pruett, D.K., 1979. Multiple cannulation of the primate superficial lateral coccygeal vein. Lab. Anim. Sci. 29, 398–399.

Stickrod, G., Ebaugh, T., Garnett, C., 1981. Use of a miniperistaltic pump for collection of blood from rabbits. Lab. Anim. Sci. 31, 87–88.

Still, J.W., Whitcomb, E.A., 1956. Techniques for long-term intubation of rat aorta. J. Lab. Clin. Med. 48, 152.

Stills Jr., H.F., Balady, M.A., Liebenberg, S.P., 1979. A comparison of bacterial flora isolated by transtracheal aspiration and pharyngeal swabs in *Macaca fasicularis*. Lab. Anim. Sci. 29, 229–233.

Stinger, R.B., Iacopino, V.J., Alter, I., Fitzpatrick, T.M., Rose, J.C., Kot, P.A., 1981. Catheterization of the pulmonary artery in the closed-chest rat. J. Appl. Physiol. 51, 1047–1050.

Stoll, L.J., Sept. 2009. Taurolidine-Citrate as a Venous Access Port Lock Solution: A Review. ASR Newsletter.

Stone, S.H., 1954. Method for obtaining venous blood from the orbital sinus of the rat or mouse. Science 109, 100.

Story, L., Kennedy, S., 2004. Animal studies in endometriosis: a review. ILAR J. 45, 132–138.

Strumpf, I.R., Bacher, J.D., Gadek, J.E., Morin, M.L., Crystal, R.G., 1979. Flexible fiberoptic bronchoscopy of the rhesus monkey (*Macaca mulatta*). Lab. Anim. Sci. 29, 785–788.

Stripling, J.S., 1981. A simple intravenous catheter for use with a cranial pedestal in the rat. Pharmacol. Biochem. Behav. 15, 823–825.

Stuhlman, R.A., Packers, J.T., Rose, S.D., 1972. Repeated blood sampling of *Mystromys albicaudatus*. Lab. Anim. Sci. 22, 268–270.

Stump, K.C., Swindle, M.M., Saudek, C.D., Strandberg, J.D., 1988. Pancreatectomized swine as a model of diabetes mellitus. Lab. Anim. Sci. 38, 439–443.

Suckling, A.J., Reiber, H., 1984. Cerebrospinal fluid sampling from guinea pigs: sample volume-related changes in protein concentration in control animals and animals in the relapsing phase of chronic relapsing experimental allergic encephalomyelitis. Lab. Anim. 18, 36–39.

Suckow, M.A., 1997. The Laboratory Rabbit.

Suckow, M.A., Danneman, P., and Brayton, C., 2000. The Laboratory Mouse.

Suckow, M.A., Stevens, K.A., Wilson, R.P., 2012.. In: Suckow, M.A., Stevens, K.A., Wilson, R.P. (Eds.), The Laboratory Rabbit, Guinea Pig, Hamster, and Other Rodents. Academic Press, Boston, MA.

Sun, B., Chen, M., Hawks, C.L., Pereira-Smith, O.M., Hornsby, P.J., 2005. The minimal set of genetic alterations required for conversion of primary human fibroblasts to cancer cells in the subrenal capsule assay. Neoplasia 7, 585–593.

Sun, X., Yan, Z., Liu, X., Olivier, A.K., Engelhardt, J.F. 2014. Genetic engineering in the ferret. In: Fox, Marini (Eds) Biology and Diseases of the Ferret, 3ed., John Wiley and Sons, Inc.

Sutyak, J.P., Lee, Y.H., Perry, B.A., Stern, W., Makhey, V., Sinko, P.J., 2000. Improved longevity and functionality of a canine model providing portal vein and multi-site intestinal access. Comp. Med. 50, 167–174.

Swanson, W.F., Godke, R.A., 1994. Transcervical embryo transfer in the domestic cat. Lab. Anim. Sci. 44, 288–291.

Swindle, M.M., 2007. Swine in the Laboratory: Surgery, Anesthesia, Imaging, and Experimental Techniques, second ed. CRC Press, Boca Raton, FL.

Swindle, M.M., Adams, R.J. (Eds.), 1988. Experimental Surgery and Physiology: Induced Animal Models of Human Disease. Williams and Wilkins, Baltimore, MD.

Swindle, M.M., Wiest, D.B., Smith, A.C., Garner, S.S., Case, C.C., Thompson, R.P., et al., 1996. Fetal surgical protocols in Yucatan miniature swine. Lab. Anim. Sci. 46, 90–95.

Swindle, M.M., Harvey, R.B., Kasari, E., Buckley, S.A., 1998. Chronic cecal cannulation in Yucatan miniature swine. Contemp. Top. 37, 68–69.

Swindle, M.M., Nolan, T., Jacobson, A., Wolf, P., Dalton, M.J., Smith, A.C., 2005. Vascular access port (VAP) usage in large animal species. Contemp. Top. Lab. Anim. Sci. 44, 7–17.

Sztein, J.M., McGregor, T.E., Bedigian, H.J., Mobraaten, L.E., 1999. Transgenic mouse strain rescue by frozen ovaries. Lab. Anim. Sci. 49, 99–100.

Taconic Biosciences. http://www.taconic.com/prepare-your-model/preconditioning-solutions/surgical-services/surgical-models.

Tajima, M., Ohsaki, T., Okazawa, M., Yasutomi, I., 2008. Availability of oral swab sample for the detection of bovine viral diarrhea virus (BVDV) gene from the cattle persistently infected with BVDV. Jpn. J. Vet. Res. 56 (1), 3–8.

Talbot, R.W., Hynd, J.W., 1985. Intermittent sampling of portal venous blood and bile from guinea pigs. Lab. Anim. 19, 173–176.

Talcott, M.R., Dysko, R.C., 1991. Partial lobectomy via a ligature fracture technique: a method for multiple hepatic biopsies in nonhuman primates. Lab. Anim. Sci. 41, 476–480.

Tan, T., Watts, S.W., Davis, R.P., 2009. Drug delivery: enabling technology for drug discovery and development. iPRECIO® micro infusion pump: programmable, refillable and implantable. Front. Pharmacol. 2, 1–13.

Tapmeier, T.T., Brown, K.L., Tang, Z., Sacks, S.H., Sheerin, N.S., Wong, W., 2008. Reimplantation of the ureter after unilateral ureteral obstruction provides a model that allows functional evaluation. Kidney Int. 73 (7), 885–889.

Tappa, B., Amao, K.W., Takahashi, K.W., 1989. A simple method for intravenous injection and blood collection in the chinchilla (*Chinchilla laniger*). Lab. Anim. 23, 73–75.

Tarantal, A.F., Hendrickx, A.G., 1988. Use of ultrasound for early pregnancy detection in the rhesus and cynomolgusmacaque (Macacamulatta and Macacafascicularis). J. Med. Primatol. 17 (2), 105–112.

Tardiff, S., Carville, A., Elmore, D., Williams, L.E., Rice, K., 2012. Reproduction and breeding of nonhuman primates. In: Abee, C., Mansfield, K., Tardiff, S., Morris, T. (Eds.), Nonhuman Primates in Biomedical Research, two-volume set, second ed. Academic Press, San Diego.

Tartarini, K.A., Sils, I.V., Szlyk-Modrow, P.C., 1996. Comparison of blood pressure measurements using vascular access ports and conventional catheters. Contemp. Top. 35, 57–61.

Terkel, L., Urbach, L., 1974. A chronic intravenous cannulation technique adapted for behavioral studies. Horm. Behav. 5, 141–148.

Terril-Robb, L., 1997. The Laboratory Guinea Pig.

Thulin, J., 1994. Re: Vasodilator for rabbit blood collection. COMPMED, AALAS.

Timm, K.I., 1979. Orbital venous anatomy of the rat. Lab. Anim. Sci. 29, 636–638.

Timm, K.I., 1989. Orbital venous anatomy of the Mongolian gerbil with comparison to the mouse, hamster, and rat. Lab. Anim. Sci. 39, 262–264.

Timm, K.I., Jahn, S.E., Sedgwick, C.J., 1987. The palatial ostium of the guinea pig. Lab. Anim. Sci. 37, 801–802.

Tønsberg, H., Holm, R., Mu, H., Boll, J.B., Jacobsen, J., Mullertz, A., 2011. Effect of bile on the oral absorption of halofantrine in polyethylene glycol 400 and polysorbate 80 formulations dosed to bile duct cannulated rats. J. Pharm. Pharmacol. 63, 817–824.

Toofanian, F., Targowski, S., 1982. Small intestinal anastomosis and preparation of intestinal loops in the rabbit. Lab. Anim. Sci. 32, 80–82.

Toriumi, Y., Samuel, I., Wilcockson, D.P., Joehl, R.J., 1994. A new model for study of pancreatic exocrine secretion: the tethered pancreatic fistula rat. Lab. Anim. Sci. 44, 270–273.

Tran, D.Q., Lawson, D., 1986. Endotracheal intubation and manual ventilation of the rat. Lab. Anim. Sci. 36, 540–541.

Tran, H.S., Puc, M.M., Tran, J.L., Del Rossi, A.J., Hewitt, C.W., 2001. A method of endoscopic endotracheal intubation in rabbits. Lab. Anim. 35 (3), 249–252.

Tremblay, G., Gagnon, L., Cormier, Y., 1990. Sequential bronchoalveolar lavages by endotracheal intubation in guinea pigs. Lab. Anim. 24, 63–67.

Tschernig, T., Thrane, L., Jorgensen, T.M., Thommes, J., Pabst, R., Yelbuz, T.M., 2013. An elegant technique for ex vivo imaging in experimental research – Optical coherence tomography (OCT). Ann. Anat. 195, 25–27.

Turner, M.A., Thomas, P., Sheridan, D.J., 1992. An improved method for direct laryngeal intubation in the guinea pig. Lab. Anim. 26, 25–28.

UFAW (Universities Fund for Animal Welfare) Joint Working Group on Refinement, 1993. Removal of blood from laboratory mammals and birds. Lab. Anim. 27, 1–22.

UFAW Staff, The UFAW Handbook on the Care and Management of Laboratory Animals, fifth ed. Churchill-Livingstone, Edinburgh.

Valerio, D.A., Ellis, E.B., Clark, M.L., Thompson, G.E., 1969. Collection of semen from macaques by electroejaculation. Lab. Anim. Care 19, 250–252.

Vallejo-Freire, A., 1951. A simple technic for repeated collection of blood samples from guinea pigs. Science 114, 524–525.

Van Dielen, F.M., Kurvers, H.A., Dammers, R., Oude Egbrink, M.G., Slaaf, D.W., Tordoir, J.H., et al., 1998. Effects of surgical sympathectomy on skin blood flow in a rat model of chronic limb ischemia. World J. Surg. 22, 807–811.

Van Herck, H., Baumans, V., Van der Craats, N.R., Hesp, A.P.M., Meijer, G.W., Van Tintelen, G., et al., 1992. Histological changes in the orbital region of rats after orbital puncture. Lab. Anim. 26, 53–58.

Van Pelt, L.F., 1974. Clinical assessment of reproductive function in female rhesus monkeys. Lab. Anim. 8, 199–212.

Van Pelt, L.F., Keyser, P.E., 1970. Observations on semen collection and quality in macaques. Lab. Anim. Care 20, 726–733.

Van Soolingen, D., Moolenbeek, C., Van Loveren, H., 1990. An improved method of bronchoalveolar lavage of lungs of small laboratory animals: short report. Lab. Anim. 24, 197–199.

Varagona, G., Ellis, L.A., Moore, D., Penney, D., Dusheiko, G.M., 1991. A percutaneous liver biopsy technique in ducks (Anas platyrhynchos) experimentally infected with duck hepatitis B virus. Lab. Anim. 25, 254–257.

Varosi, S.M., Brigmon, R.L., Besch, E.L., 1990. A simplified telemetry system for monitoring body temperature in small animals. Lab. Anim. Sci. 40, 299–302.

Venkatesh, V.C., Whyte, H.E.A., Read, S.E., 1988. A simple technique for repeated intratracheal instillation of foreign material in newborn rabbits. Lab. Anim. Sci. 38, 618–619.

Venugopalan, C.S., Said, S.I., Drazen, J.M., 1984. Effect of vasoactive intestinal peptide on vagally mediated tracheal pouch relaxation. Respir. Physiol. 56, 205–216.

Venugopalan, C.S., Krautmann, M.J., Holmes, E.P., Maher, T.J., 1998. Involvement of nitric oxide in the mediation of NANC inhibitory neurotransmission of guinea-pig trachea. J. Auton. Pharmacol. 5, 281–286.

Verhage, H.G., Murray, M.K., Brown, M.J., Bennett, B.T., 1986. An indwelling catheter for the collection of cat uterine fluids. Lab. Anim. Sci. 36, 71–73.

Vistelle, R., Jaussaud, R., Trenque, T., Wiczewski, M., 1994. Rapid and simple cannulation technique for repeated sampling of cerebrospinal fluid in the conscious rabbit. Lab. Anim. Sci. 44, 362–364.

Vogelweid, C.M., Kier, A.B., 1988. A technique for the collection of cerebrospinal fluid from mice. Lab. Anim. Sci. 38, 91–92.

Vogler, G.A., Yagi, K., Frank, P.A., Baudendistel, L.J., 1992. Permanent tracheostomy in goats. Contemp. Top. 31, 15–17.

Voglmayr, J.K., Larsen, L.H., White, I.G., 1970. Metabolism of spermatozoa and composition of fluid collected from the rete testis of living bulls. J. Reprod. Fertil. 21, 449–460.

Voss, W.R., 1970. Primate liver and spleen biopsy procedures. Lab. Anim. Care 20, 995–997.

Wacharapluesadee, S., Tepsumethanon, V., Supavonwong, P., Kaewpom, T., Intarut, N., Hemachudha, T., 2012. Detection of rabies viral RNA by TaqMan real-time RT-PCR using non-neural specimens from dogs infected with rabies virus. J. Virol. Methods 184 (1–2), 109–112.

Waites, G.M.H., Einer-Jensen, N., 1974. Collection and analysis of rete testis fluid from macaque monkeys. J. Reprod. Fertil. 41, 505–508.

Wang, X., Kimura, S., Yazawa, T., Endo, N., 2005. Cerebrospinal fluid sampling by lumbar puncture in rats – repeated measurements of nitric oxide metabolites. J. Neurosci. Methods 145, 89–95.

Wang, Y.-M.C., Reuning, R.H., 1994. A comparison of two surgical techniques for preparation of rats with chronic bile duct cannulae for the investigation of enterohepatic circulation. Lab. Anim. Sci. 44, 479–485.

Wardell Jr., J.R., Chakrin, L.W., Payne, B.J., 1970. The canine tracheal pouch: a model for use in respiratory mucus research. Am. Rev. Respir. Dis. 101, 741–754.

Washburn, K.E., Powell, J.G., Maxwell, C.V., Kegley, E.B., Johnson, Z., Fakler, T.M., 2005. A successful method of obtaining percutaneous liver biopsy samples of sufficient quantity for trace mineral analysis in adult swine without the aid of ultrasound. J. Swine Health Prod. 13, 126–130.

Waynforth, H.B., 1980. Experimental and Surgical Technique in the Rat. Academic Press, New York.

Waynforth, H.B., Flecknell, P.A., 1992. Experimental and Surgical Technique in the Rat, second ed. Academic Press, New York.

Waynforth, H.B., Parkin, R., 1969. Sublingual vein injection in rodents. Lab. Anim. 3, 35–37.

Webb, A.I., Bliss, J.M., Herbst, L.H., 1995. Use of vascular access ports in the cat. Lab. Anim. Sci. 45, 110–113.

Wendt, D.J., Normile, H.J., Dawe, E.J., Trumpeter, T., Barraco, R.A., 1982. Chronic intracarotid cannulation of pigeons for administration of behaviorally active peptides. Lab. Anim. 16, 335–338.

West, D.A., Rallo, M.C., Moore, R.G., Vogler, G.A., Niehoff, M., Parra, R.O., et al., 1999. Laparoscopic v. laparoscopy-assisted donor nephrectomy in the porcine model. J. Endourol. 13, 513–515.

West, W.L., Cheatham, L.R., Gaillard, E.T., Wright, M., 2002. A chronic bile duct and intravenous cannulation model in conscious rabbits for pharmacokinetic studies. J. Invest. Surg. 15, 81–89.

Wheeldon, E.B., Walker, M.E., Murphy, D.J., Turner, C.R., 1992. Intratracheal aerosolization of endotoxin in the rat: a model of the adult respiratory distress syndroms (ARDS). Lab. Anim. 26, 29–37.

Whipp, S.C., Littledike, E.T., Wangsness, S., 1970. A technique of hypophysectomy of calves. Lab. Anim. Care 20, 533–538.

White, W.A., 1971. A technique for urine collection from anesthetized male rats. Lab. Anim. Sci. 21, 401–402.

Whitney Jr., R.A., Johnson, D.J., Cole, W.C., 1973. Laboratory Primate Handbook. Academic Press, New York.

Wideman, R.F., Braun, E.J., 1982. Urethral urine collection from anesthetized domestic fowl. Lab. Anim. Sci. 32, 298–301.

Wildt, D.E., Morcom, C.B., Dukelow, W.R., 1975. Laparoscopic pregnancy diagnosis and uterine fluid recovery in swine. J. Reprod. Fertil. 44, 301–304.

Wimsatt, J., Johnson, J.D., Mangone, B.A., 1998. Use of a cardiac access port for repeated collection of blood samples form desert tortoises (Gopherus agassizii). Contemp. Top. 37, 81–83.

Wingfield, W.E., Tumbleson, M.E., Hicklin, K.W., Mather, E.C., 1974. An exteriorized cranial vena caval catheter for serial blood sample collection from miniature swine. Lab. Anim. Sci. 24, 359–361.

Wixson, S.K., Murray, K.A., Hughes, H.C., 1987. A technique for chronic arterial catheterization in the rat. Lab. Anim. Sci. 37, 108–111.

Wojnicki, F.H.E., Bacher, J.D., Glowa, J.R., 1994. Use of subcutaneous vascular access ports in rhesus monkeys. Lab. Anim. Sci. 44, 491–494.

Wolf, R.F., White, G.L., 2012 2012. Clinical techniques used for nonhuman primates. In: Abee, C., Mansfield, K., Tardiff, S., Morris, T. (Eds.), Nonhuman Primates in Biomedical Research, two-volume Set, second ed. Academic Press, San Diego. (Chapter 13).

Wolfe, H.G., 1967. Artificial insemination of the laboratory mouse (Mus musculus). Lab. Anim. Care 17, 426–432.

Woolf, A., Curl, J.L., 1987. A technique for laparoscopic examination of woodchuck ovaries. Lab. Anim. Sci. 37, 664–665.

Woolf, A., Curl, J., Gremillion-Smith, C., 1989. The use of subcutaneous ports in the woodchuck (Marmota monax). Lab. Anim. Sci. 39, 620–622.

Wu, W.P., Xu, X.J., Hao, J.X., 2004. Chronic lumbar catheterization of the spinal subarachnoid space in mice. J. Neurosci. Methods 133, 65–69.

Wubben, J.E., Smiricky, M.R., Albin, D.M., Gabert, V.M., 2001. Improved procedure and cannula design for simple-T cannulation at the distal ileum in growing pigs. Contemp. Top. Lab. Anim. Sci. 40, 27–31.

Yao, Z., Adler, A., Kovar, P., Kleinert, H., 1992. A restraint device for blood sampling and direct blood pressure measurement in conscious ferrets. Contemp. Top. 31, 19–21.

Yap, K.L., 1982. A method for intratracheal innoculation of mice. Lab. Anim. 16, 143–145.

Yardeni, T., Eckhaus, M., Morris, H.D., Huizing, M., Hoogstraten-Miller, S., 2011. Retro-orbital injections in mice. Lab. Anim. (NY) 40, 155–160.

Yoshitake, A., Mori, A., Shimizu, H., Ueda, T., Kabei, N., Hachiya, T., et al., 2007. Use of an epidural cooling catheter with a closed countercurrent lumen to protect against ischemic spinal cord injury in pigs. J. Thorac. Cardiovasc. Surg. 134, 1220–1226.

Young, L., Chambers, T., 1973. A mouse bleeding technique yielding consistent volume with minimal hemolysis. Lab. Anim. Sci. 23, 428–430.

Yu, H.Y., Shen, Y.Z., 1991. Pharmacokinetics of valproic acid in guinea-pigs with biliary abnormality. J. Pharm. Pharmacol. 43 (7), 470–474.

Zambraski, E.J., DiBona, G.F., 1976. A device for the cutaneous exteriorization of chronic intravascular catheters. Lab. Anim. Sci. 26, 939–941.

Zammit, M., Toledo-Pereya, L.H., Malcom, S., Konde, W.N., 1979. Long-term cranial mesenteric vein cannulation in the rat. Lab. Anim. Sci. 29, 364–366.

Zanella, A.J., Mendl, M.T., 1992. A fast and simple technique for jugular catheterization in adult sows. Lab. Anim. 26, 211–213.

Zatz, R., 1990. A low cost tail-cuff method for the estimation of mean arterial pressure in conscious rats. Lab. Anim. Sci. 40, 198–201.

Zhang, G.J., Chen, T.B., Bednar, B., Connolly, B.M., Hargreaves, R., Sur, C., et al., 2007. Optical imaging of tumor cells in hollow fibers: evaluation of the antitumor activities of anticancer drugs and target validation. Neoplasia 9, 652–661.

Zhang, Y., Hong, H., Engle, J.W., Yang, Y., Theuer, C.P., Barnhart, T.E., et al., 2012. Positron emission tomography and optical imaging of tumor CD105 expression with a dual-labeled monoclonal antibody. Mol. Pharm. 9 (3), 645–653. http://dx.doi.org/10.1021/mp200592m Epub 2012 Jan 31.

Zhao, C., Chen, L., Tao, Y.X., Tall, J.M., Borzan, J., Ringkamp, M., et al., 2007. Lumbar sympathectomy attenuates cold allodynia but not mechanical allodynia and hyperalgesia in rats with spared nerve injury. J. Pain 8, 931–937.

Zhong, R., 1999. Organ transplantation in mice: current status and future prospects. Microsurgery 19, 52–55.

Zhou, C., Brown, L.A., 1988. Intravenous cannulation of chickens for blood sampling. Lab. Anim. Sci. 38, 631–632.

Zietek-Barszcz, A., Gradzki, Z., 2010. The suitability of selected methods of nucleic acid extraction for detecting Rhodococcusequi DNA in tracheobronchial wash fluid using PCR. Pol. J. Vet. Sci. 13 (3), 409–413.

Zimmermann, K., Schwarz, H.P., Turecek, P.L., 2000. Deoxyribonucleic acid preparation in polymerase chain reaction genotyping of transgenic mice. Comp. Med. 50 (3), 314–316.

26

Gnotobiotics

Trenton R. Schoeb, DVM, PhD, DACVP[a]
and Richard J. Rahija, DVM, PhD, DACLAM[b]

[a]Department of Genetics, Comparative Pathology Laboratory, Animal Resources Program, UAB
Gnotobiotic Facility, University of Alabama at Birmingham, Birmingham, AL, USA
[b]Animal Resources Center, St. Jude Children's Research Hospital, Memphis, TN, USA

I. INTRODUCTION

The microbial cells that populate the human body (the microbiota), the largest mass of which occupies the lower bowel, outnumber the cells of the body itself by an order of magnitude (Savage, 1977), and the number of genes in the collective genome of the microbiota (the microbiome) exceeds that of human genes by nearly 2 orders of magnitude (Qin *et al.*, 2010). Only in about the past two decades have the tremendous complexity of the microbiota and the depth of interdependence between the microbiota and the host become apparent, but the

developing understanding of the role of the microbiota in health and disease that has emerged in that time is revolutionary. That period might be considered to have begun with the report that interleukin (IL)-10-deficient mice spontaneously developed enterocolitis, which became less severe when the mice were made specific pathogen-free (SPF) (Kuhn *et al.*, 1993). Subsequently, mice with various induced mutations in genes related to immune, inflammatory, and epithelial function were found to spontaneously develop colitis. The crucial discovery was that such mice did not develop colitis when germfree, but did so when reconstituted with various autochthonous bacteria, showing that colitis was dependent on the intestinal microbiota (Lorenz *et al.*, 2005; Peloquin and Nguyen, 2013; Podolsky, 1997; Sartor, 2005). Research using such mice provided fundamental, and previously unobtainable, insights into the pathogenesis of inflammatory bowel diseases (Crohn's disease and ulcerative colitis), leading to the well-accepted concept that, fundamentally, these diseases result from dysregulated immune and inflammatory responses to specific antigens of certain autochthonous intestinal bacteria (Elson and Cong, 2012; Peloquin and Nguyen, 2013).

Development of high-throughput techniques for taxonomic analysis of complex microbial populations allowed comprehensive characterization of intestinal bacterial microbiota, showing not only that intestinal bacteria were much more diverse than previously understood, but also that their composition varied with diet and other factors, including disease states. It is now clear the intestinal microbiota affect energy metabolism and have substantial potential roles in obesity and development of type 2 diabetes, hypertension, and atherosclerosis (Backhed, 2011, 2012; Backhed *et al.*, 2004, 2007; Caesar *et al.*, 2010; Cani *et al.*, 2007, 2008, 2012; Cani and Delzenne, 2009; Everard *et al.*, 2013; Fei and Zhao, 2013; Hooper *et al.*, 2002; Kallus and Brandt, 2012; Karlsson *et al.*, 2012; Ley, 2010; Ley *et al.*, 2005; Ley *et al.*, 2006; Liou *et al.*, 2013; Manco *et al.*, 2010; Mendelsohn and Larrick, 2013; Musso *et al.*, 2011; Ridaura *et al.*, 2013; Tang *et al.*, 2013; Tremaroli and Backhed, 2012; Turnbaugh *et al.*, 2006). Evidence is also accumulating that the microbiota have roles in cancer, asthma, and other immune-mediated diseases such as type 1 diabetes, necrotizing enterocolitis, *Clostridium difficile* disease, chronic hepatitis, periodontal disease, bone metabolism, neurological development and behavior, and preterm birth (Bultman, 2014; Carlisle and Morowitz, 2013; Grishin *et al.*, 2013; Hara *et al.*, 2013; Hyman *et al.*, 2013; Kim, 2014; Liu *et al.*, 2013; Mabrok *et al.*, 2012; Ou *et al.*, 2013; Plottel and Blaser, 2011; Seki and Schnabl, 2012; Sjogren *et al.*, 2012; Sommer and Backhed, 2013; Wang *et al.*, 2013; Wu and Wu, 2012; Yoshimoto *et al.*, 2013; Zhu *et al.*, 2011).

Investigating the role of the microbiota in health and disease requires the ability to manipulate and define the microbiota, that is, the capability to not only house germfree and defined-microbiota animals, but also derive new genotypes germfree and colonize them with specific microbiota. Thus, there has been a tremendous increase in interest among research institutions in establishing gnotobiotic facilities or expanding existing facilities. In this chapter, we focus on principles and practical guidance related to establishing and operating a gnotobiotic mouse facility. Most of the information is also applicable to rats. General principles apply to larger animals such as pigs, but different equipment is required.

II. TERMINOLOGY

Definitions are provided to familiarize the reader with the terminology found in the literature and used by scientists in the field.

Associated animal: Animal that harbors one or more microorganisms of known identity. Any intentional introduction of a known organism to a germfree animal. Synonymous with defined microbiota or defined flora.

Axenic or germfree: From the Greek *a*, meaning 'without', and *xenos*, meaning 'strangers'. An animal that is free of all foreign life forms apart from itself, including bacteria, viruses, fungi, protozoa, and other saprophytic or parasitic life forms. The germfree state is thought to be a hypothetical because of the presence of indigenous viruses or other heretofore uncharacterized life forms that have integrated into the host genome. Some specialists in the field believe that since these organisms have incorporated into the host genome and cannot be removed, they are part of the animal itself and are no longer a 'stranger.'

Conventional animal: An animal reared in an animal room environment with an unknown microbiota and therefore with an unknown disease status.

Defined microbiota (flora) animal: A gnotobiote maintained in an isolator or equivalent environment and intentionally associated with one or more known life forms, usually microorganisms. Also referred to as an associated animal.

Ex-germfree animal: An animal born or delivered under germfree conditions that has subsequently been removed from the germfree state and therefore acquires an unknown microbiota from its environment.

Gnotobiotics: The field of investigation concerned with the rearing of animals that are free of all microorganisms or associated only with known species. The term includes the basic husbandry of the animals and the characterization of any biological phenomena arising in the animal as a result of the elimination of microorganisms or the association with specific microorganisms.

Gnotobiote or gnotobiotic animal: From the Greek *gnotos*, meaning 'known or well known', and *bios*, meaning 'life'. An animal stock or strain that has been derived by aseptic hysterotomy or hysterectomy, embryo transfer, or sterile hatching of eggs, and continuously maintained using sterile technique in an isolator where the microbial status of the animal is fully defined. An animal in which all life forms have been completely defined. Gnotobiotic animals include both germfree and defined flora animals.

Isolation technology: The equipment and procedures used to create and maintain a sealed sterile environment for the isolation of gnotobiotic animals.

Microbiome: The collective genome of a host's microbiota.

Microbiota: A community of microorganisms harbored by a host. The largest consortium of microbiota are found in the gastrointestinal tract.

Monoxenic or dixenic animals: Gnotobiotes that have been associated with one (monoxenic) or two (dixenic) species of organism, usually microbial.

Pathobiont: An organism associated with the host that has the potential to cause dysregulated inflammation and disease under certain environmental conditions.

Restricted flora or microbiota: A gnotobiotic animal that has been associated with a defined microbiota, such as altered Schaedler flora (ASF), and that has been removed from the isolator into a maximum barrier room where it becomes colonized by additional organisms, but continues to be free of both primary pathogens and opportunistic pathogens. A restricted flora animal is therefore the highest level of SPF animal since it is free of all adventitious pathogenic agents.

Specific pathogen free (SPF): Animals free from a specified list of pathogens and potential pathogens or opportunists, but otherwise having an undefined microbiota.

Symbiosis: From the Greek *syn*, meaning 'together with', and *bios*, meaning 'life'. Close biological relationship between organisms. Types of symbiosis most relevant here include commensalism, in which one organism benefits and the other is unaffected; mutualism, in which both organisms benefit; and parasitism, in which one organism benefits and the other is harmed.

III. HISTORY

The history of gnotobiotics has been thoroughly reviewed elsewhere (Carter and Foster, 2005; Coates and Gustafsson, 1984; Foster, 1980; Lindsey and Baker, 2005; Luckey, 1963; Pleasants, 1974; Rahija, 2007; Trexler, 1983; Trexler and Orcutt, 1999; Wostmann, 1996). The advances of greatest significance in the context of this chapter are noted here, those that enabled widespread practical use of gnotobiotic rodents. A major obstacle was the necessity of deriving every germfree animal via hysterectomy or hysterotomy and hand-rearing, until the essential nutrients normally supplied by the microbiota were understood and nutritionally adequate autoclavable diets were developed that allowed self-sustaining reproduction and indefinite maintenance

of germfree rats (Gustafsson, 1947, 1948; Reyniers *et al.*, 1946) and mice (Pleasants, 1959). Another barrier was that the isolators originally developed at the Laboratories of Bacteriology, University of Notre Dame (LOBUND) Institute, the University of Lund in Sweden, and Nagoya University in Japan were very expensive, complex items of equipment custom manufactured of stainless steel, often incorporating an integral autoclave, that were beyond the means of most research institutions. This was alleviated by development of the flexible film isolator by Trexler (Trexler and Reynolds, 1957) and use of peracetic acid for sterilization of the isolator and ports (Barrett, 1959; Trexler, 1963).

By the early 1960s, germfree rat and mouse colonies were well established at the LOBUND Institute, and animals were made available for distribution to the scientific community. Trexler held a workshop at the LOBUND Institute to educate commercial animal suppliers and the laboratory animal science community about the application of gnotobiotic technology for producing SPF mice (Trexler, 1961). At the time, most commercially available mice and rats used in biomedical research were infected with pathogenic or potentially pathogenic bacteria, mycoplasmas, parasites, and murine viruses (Weisbroth *et al.*, 1998). Animal suppliers recognized that gnotobiotics could be used to develop and maintain nucleus colonies of mice and rats that could be expanded to SPF production colonies. Thus, one of the most important contributions of gnotobiotics was the technology-enabling production and maintenance of disease-free laboratory animals for biomedical research (Foster, 1959; Weisbroth *et al.*, 1998; White *et al.*, 1998).

IV. CHARACTERISTICS OF GNOTOBIOTES

Characteristics of gnotobiotic animals have also been reviewed previously (Carter and Foster, 2005; Coates and Gustafsson, 1984; Foster, 1980; Gordon, 1960; Lindsey and Baker, 2005; Luckey, 1963; Pleasants, 1974; Rahija, 2007; Trexler, 1983; Wostmann, 1996). Pertinent publications that have appeared since are too numerous for review here; interested readers can access them via PubMed search statements such as "(germfree [TIAB] OR germ-free [TIAB] OR gnotobiotic [TIAB])" and narrowing the search results by filtering for reviews or ANDing this statement with specific topics.

Investigators working with germfree mice should be aware of the potential for spontaneous mutations and subline divergence in colonies of mice maintained for multiple generations under germfree conditions. Subline divergence should be considered when designing experiments and interpreting the results from studies involving gnotobiotic mice and their conventional counterparts.

V. ESTABLISHING A GNOTOBIOTIC FACILITY

A. General Considerations

It is imperative that prospective operators, investigators, and administrators, particularly those who may be providing financial support, understand the major requirements and constraints inherent in a gnotobiotic facility before undertaking an effort to establish one.

1. Budget

The first consideration is, of course, funding, which must be adequate to purchase isolators and associated items such as sterilizing cylinders, as well as meeting continuing operational costs, including personnel salaries; isolator replacement parts such as gloves, filters or filter medium, port caps, and transfer sleeves; consumables such as sterilant and microbiological media; autoclave maintenance; and *per diem* charges. Costs can vary widely, depending on factors such as the type, model, and manufacturer of isolator, institutional salary scales and *per diem* rates, and methods and frequency of microbiological monitoring, but, based on our experience, a facility with 20 breeding and experimental isolators probably would require total annual direct cost expenditures of at least $100,000.

2. Space

Space is a major limitation in a gnotobiotic facility. Typical isolator housing is very inefficient. In roughly the same floor space as a ventilated rack holding over 100 cages, two plastic film isolators such as those shown in Fig. 26.1 might hold 24 cages, and the practical limits for stacked semirigid isolators such as those shown in Figs 26.2 and 26.3 are about 48 in each case. Although isolators can be constructed to hold larger numbers of cages (Fig. 26.4), most facilities in research institutions will use larger numbers of smaller isolators, for several reasons. First, users will need breeding populations of mice of different genotype and microbial status, and each stock, or combination of genotype and microbial status, requires separate isolator housing. Second, it is impossible to totally prevent contamination, so at least two breeding isolators for each stock must be maintained to minimize the risk that the stock will be lost due to contamination, and more mice will be lost if larger isolators are used. Third, gnotobiotic mice, especially germfree mice, frequently do not reproduce as well as mice with normal microbiota, and therefore require a larger number of breeding cages. Finally, isolators also must be available for conducting experiments, at least one for each microbial status, and preferably one for each combination of genotype and microbial status. A single experiment can occupy two to four isolators, possibly for weeks, for example, in the case of colitis studies to model

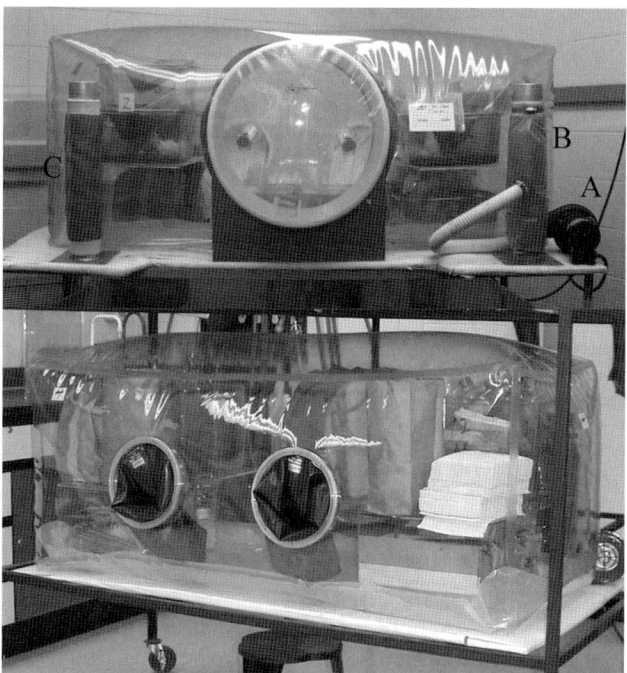

FIGURE 26.1 Plastic film isolators assembled from parts purchased from Controlled Environment Products division of Standard Safety Equipment Co. PVC port and supporting rack were fabricated by the UAB Research Machine Shop. Padded plywood support was fabricated in the facility. Top, port side. A, blower; B, inlet filter; C, outlet filter. Filters are of the wrapped, reusable type. Bottom, glove side. One-piece full-length gloves attached via two-piece aluminum compression rings.

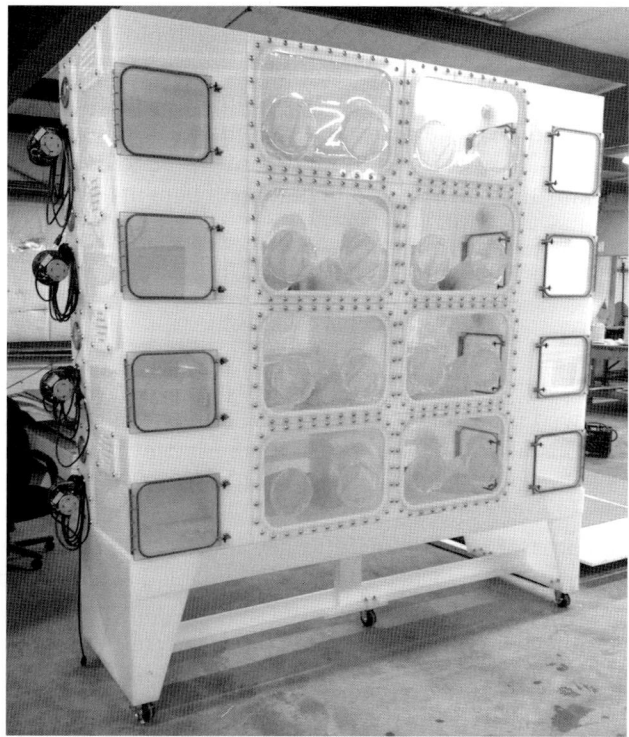

FIGURE 26.2 Eight Mini-Q™ semirigid isolators stacked on a mobile table. *Courtesy of Park Bioservices LLC.*

of microbiota from significant numbers of patients and controls, as, for example, in studies related to obesity, fecal microbiota transplantation, or colon cancer.

The dimensions of rooms in which isolators will be placed and the overall dimensions of the isolators will be used should be considered together. Small or narrow rooms limit the ways in which isolators can be arranged and allow access, and thus may not be suitable for larger or stacked isolators.

3. Autoclave

The autoclave is the single most important item of equipment in any gnotobiotic facility that does not rely completely on irradiation for sterilization. Even if commercial irradiated food and bedding are used, it may still be necessary for other supplies and items used in isolators to be sterilized by autoclaving. Different conditions are required for steam sterilization of food, water, materials such as bedding and paper towels, and other items such as cages and water bottles, so the autoclave must be capable of suitable cycles for each, including high vacuum or pulse pressure vacuum preconditioning and post-sterilization vacuum-drying steps. The autoclave must be large enough to hold at least one supply cylinder, if these are used, and must be maintained to ensure correct operation. Steam quality problems can cause sterilization failure in even the most carefully maintained autoclave (Sedlacek and Rose, 1985); thus, institutional support in the form of proper installation, maintenance, and repair of building steam supplies is an important factor in successful facility operation. We also recommend that, if at all possible, the facility have an autoclave dedicated to its own use and that only trained facility personnel operate it, so as to avoid conflicts and delays in daily use as well as maintenance and repairs. It also is advisable to identify a backup autoclave that has the necessary capabilities and monitor it regularly, even if it is rarely used.

4. Personnel

Selection of personnel for gnotobiotic technician positions is critical. A high level of education is not required, but it is essential that personnel be diligent, reliable workers, able and willing to follow procedures exactly, every time, and equally well whether the supervisor is present or not. One might say, without much exaggeration, that a combination of obsessive–compulsive disorder and paranoia is desirable. Certainly, hiring the wrong person can be disastrous. Some people simply cannot do the job and will have endless trouble with contamination.

5. Standard Operating Procedures

We recommend that the facility develop a manual or set of standard operating procedures (SOPs) describing all procedures in detail, as well as keeping logs of all autoclaving, sterilization monitoring, and isolator

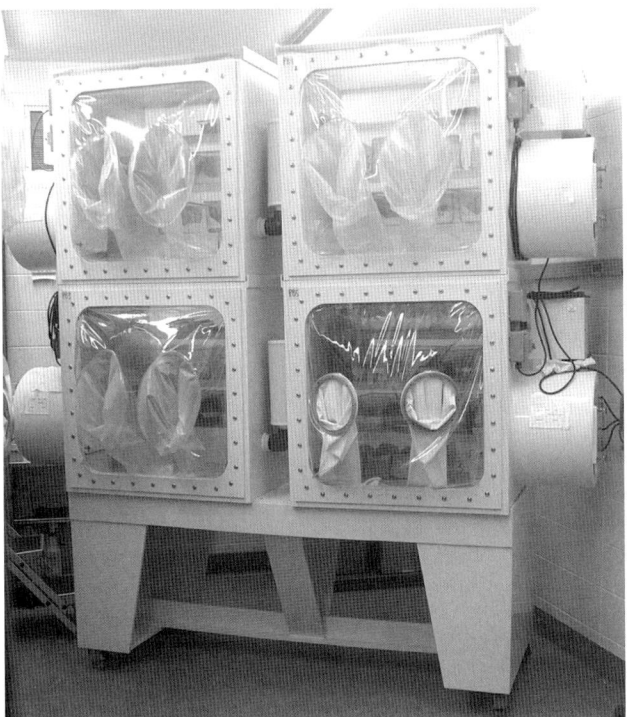

FIGURE 26.3 Four stacked semirigid isolators manufactured by Park Bioservices LLC with cylindrical ports for use with transfer sleeves. The bottom right isolator has one-piece full-length gloves installed with compression rings by the user. The others have original manufacturer supplied flexible front panels with integral glove sleeves.

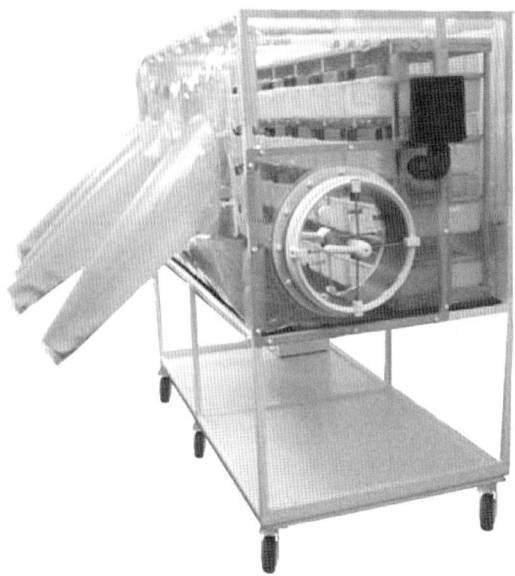

FIGURE 26.4 Harlan Isotec™ flexible film isolator with Quadro-Lock™ port, cartridge-type outlet filter, and rigid external frame. This model holds 50 mouse cages. *Courtesy of Harlan Laboratories.*

inflammatory bowel disease. Thus, space needs tend to increase rapidly with the number of investigators supported. This is particularly so if research is anticipated in which germfree mice are to be 'humanized' with samples procedures. These greatly facilitate training employees, troubleshooting problems, and ensuring continuity in the event of personnel changes.

6. Work Area

It is advisable to have a separate work area or workshop with a workbench, basic hand tools, and storage for tools, parts, and supplies. Tasks such as wrapping filter medium onto filters and sterilizing cylinders, preparing cylinders for sterilization, and making up supply packs are far easier and more efficient in an appropriately equipped work area.

7. Microbiology Laboratory Support

Monitoring for contamination is an essential activity in a gnotobiotic facility and consumes significant amounts of time and resources. Thus, access to a microbiology laboratory is very valuable, especially a laboratory equipped with an anaerobic bacteriology chamber. An experienced micriobiologist can help optimize monitoring protocols and is more likely to be able to identify contamination with slow-growing or fastidious organisms, or extremely oxygen-sensitive anaerobic bacteria. It also is very helpful for microbiological monitoring using polymerase chain reaction (PCR) techniques to be available, both to screen for contamination and to verify presence of members of limited microbiota. If such services are not available, basic procedures such as Gram staining and inoculating solid and liquid media and inspecting them for growth can be done by personnel with moderate laboratory skills, and commercial laboratories can be used for identification of cultured contaminants.

B. Isolator Construction

Isolators can be of differing size and construction, but the basic components of each are the chamber, air supply, transfer port, and gloves (Figs 26.1–26.7). Before purchasing isolator equipment, it is advisable to discuss with manufacturers and users how isolators of differing construction might best meet anticipated research needs.

1. Chamber

Isolators having rigid, semirigid, or flexible film chambers made of plastic or stainless steel are commercially available in a variety of sizes to accommodate the needs of the research to be conducted, the biological needs of the animals that will be used, and ergonomic and safety needs of personnel. Plastic semirigid and flexible film isolators are most widely used.

Flexible film isolators are made of optically clear polyvinyl chloride (PVC) film that is cut into sheets and joined by thermo-welded seams. The chief advantage of flexible film isolators is that they are less expensive to construct than rigid or semirigid isolators. Also, the

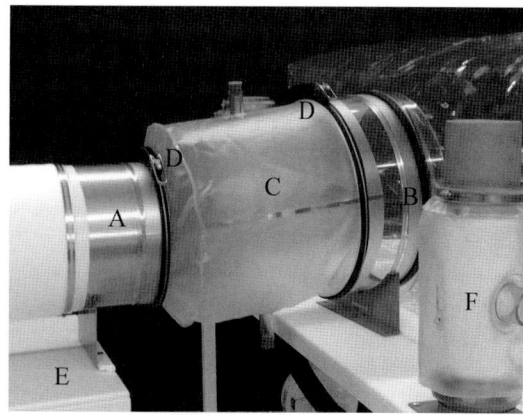

FIGURE 26.5   Class Biologically Clean flexible film isolator. Supply cylinder (A) is connected to transfer port (B) via reducing diameter transfer sleeve (C) and patented clamps (D). Cylinder is supported by stand (E). F, outlet filter of the wrapped, reusable type. *Courtesy of Class Biologically Clean.*

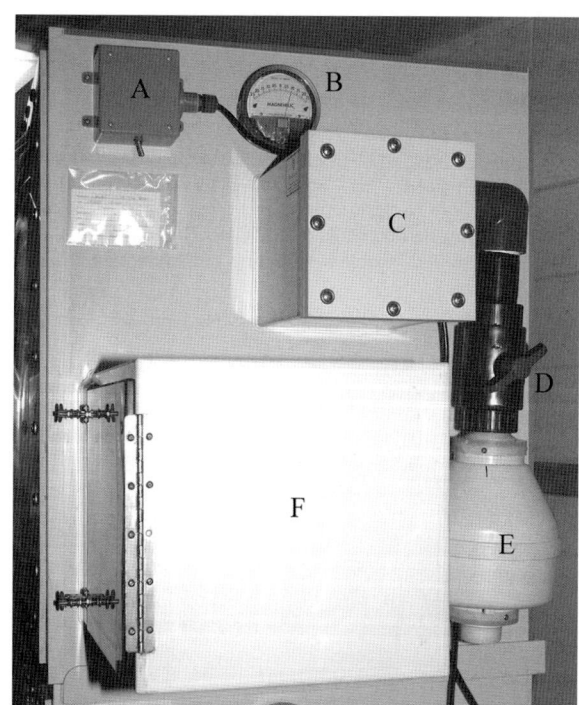

FIGURE 26.6   Parts of a Park Bioservices LLC semirigid isolator. A, light switch; B, differential pressure gauge; C, chamber containing cartridge-type inlet air filter; D, inlet air damper valve; E, blower; F, rectangular transfer port.

flexibility of PVC chambers allows persons of small stature to more easily reach all areas of the chamber interior than is possible with rigid isolators of similar size and shape. PVC is tough, and although it can be damaged by sharp objects and by some organic solvents, small punctures are easily and permanently repaired with PVC patches and appropriate cement, such as that sold for repair of vinyl swimming pools.

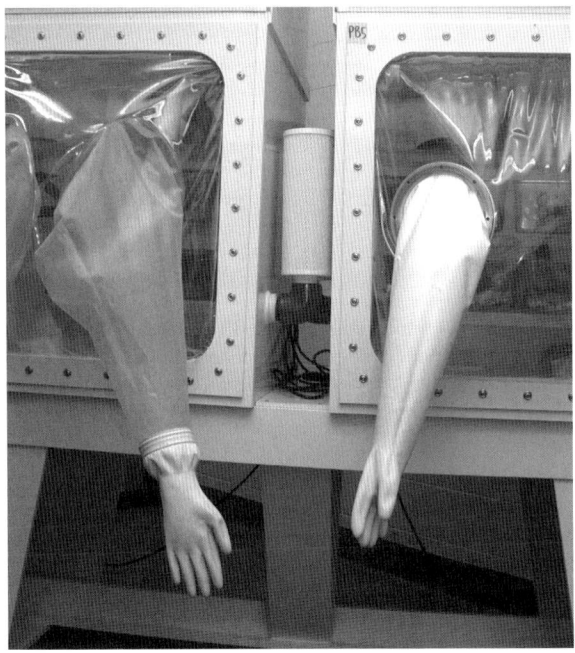

FIGURE 26.7   Hypalon™ gloves fitted to Park Bioservices LLC semirigid isolators. Left, original equipment sleeve; right, user installed one-piece glove and compression ring. A cartridge-type pleated air outlet filter is visible between the two isolators.

Flexible film isolators require a working surface to support the floor of the chamber and a rack or table to support the isolator, its port, and its air blower and filters (Fig. 26.1). A rigid frame is sometimes used to help maintain the shape of the chamber (Fig. 26.4). Such isolators are available as complete assemblies or as individual parts that are assembled by the user. The lower cost of the latter approach can be attractive; however, it requires that the user have the knowledge and skills to properly assemble the parts, and it may be necessary to fabricate parts such as padded plywood supports. These are readily made by anyone who can safely use a circular saw and jigsaw, but items such as isolator supporting racks and supply cylinder stands will require the services of a metal working shop if they are not to be purchased ready-made.

Semirigid isolators are made from panels of natural polypropylene, a translucent white rigid plastic, welded together, with a clear flexible film front panel to which the gloves are attached. One advantage of this type is that if biohazardous work is anticipated, they can be operated at negative pressure. For most gnotobiotic work; however, their chief advantage in our view is that smaller units can be stacked so as to take advantage of vertical space to the extent that facility ceiling height allows (Figs 26.2, 26.3). Some users consider semirigid isolators to have a greater risk of contamination than flexible film isolators, due to the gasket seals of the transfer port doors and between the front panel

and the chamber, which are subject to distortion, deterioration, and leakage, and to the fact that the cartridge-type air filters used on some such isolators are not autoclavable. However, we have not found this to be the case.

Rigid stainless steel isolators have the advantage of amenability to negative pressure operation for containment and operator protection from biohazardous agents. They are rarely used today for non-biohazardous gnotobiotic work, largely because of their costly construction.

2. Air Supply

The air supply of an isolator is provided by an electric blower that forces air through the chamber via high-efficiency particulate air (HEPA) filters at the chamber inlet and outlet. Air can be supplied by a dedicated fan for each chamber, as in typical university research facilities, or through a central air supply system, as in a commercial setting in which large numbers of isolators are in use. Blowers of rigid and semirigid isolators typically can be operated so as to maintain internal pressure either positive or negative to ambient. Positive pressure helps prevent introduction of airborne contaminants through leaks such as damage to gloves and flexible film, and, in the case of flexible film isolators, is necessary to keep the chamber from collapsing, unless a supporting framework is used. Maintenance and experimental use of gnotobiotic animals are done under positive pressure unless they are inoculated with biohazardous agents. If it is necessary that an isolator be temporarily disconnected from the building electrical supply, for example, to move it from one location to another in a vehicle, the fan can be operated from an automotive battery by use of an inverter. Alternatively, fans that run on 12-volt direct current may be available.

It is highly advisable that the facility be provided with emergency electrical power, as animals in isolators will suffocate within hours if power is lost. We also suggest that standard three-prong electrical plugs and receptacles serving isolator blowers be replaced with twist lock plugs and receptacles to guard against accidental disconnection. One or two spare blowers should be kept on hand. Blowers can last for many years of continuous operation, but they do occasionally fail. Most are not repairable or are not cost-effective to repair.

Inlet and outlet filters are of two general types. One is constructed of a perforated steel or stainless steel cylinder with a supporting base and a fitting that connects to the isolator (Figs 26.1, 26.5). Filter medium is wrapped around the cylinder and taped or otherwise fastened in place; the opening of the fitting is closed with Mylar™ film or tape, which is punctured and torn away after the isolator is assembled and sterilized; and the assembly is sterilized by autoclaving. The cylindrical frame can be rewrapped and reused indefinitely. Originally, spun glass fiber (glass wool) was used as the filter medium. Although it withstands repeated autoclaving well, it is easily damaged, is susceptible to being rolled too tightly to allow adequate air flow, and may entail safety concerns. Spun polyurethane lacks these disadvantages and is thus superior, although it does gradually deteriorate with autoclaving, so the wrapping of sterilizing cylinders must be replaced periodically. The other filter type is the pleated cartridge (Figs 26.4, 26.7). These are not repairable and are replaced when damaged or clogged by dust.

Semirigid isolators typically are fitted with a damper to adjust air flow and chamber pressure and with a differential air pressure gauge to monitor air pressure within the chamber and the resistance of the exhaust filter. Some flexible film isolators are similarly equipped; others rely simply on the resistance of the inlet and outlet filters to maintain sufficient positive pressure while permitting adequate air exchange. The air exchange rate in an isolator is determined by the size of the isolator chamber; the output of the blower; the setting of the inlet air damper, if one is used; and particulate accumulation on the filters, particularly the outlet filter, which eventually can accumulate considerable food and bedding dust. However, most isolators are designed to provide at least 30 air changes per hour, so unless the damper is set too restrictively, or the filters are severely clogged, an air exchange rate higher than that in animal rooms is expected.

Although excessive heat and humidity are possible in large isolators housing many cages of mice, or in isolators housing larger animals, they seldom occur in isolators housing mice in typical research settings. Blowers of modern isolators draw little current and generate little heat, and thus rarely affect maintenance of proper room temperature.

3. Transfer Port

The transfer port is an airlock that provides a means of transferring materials and animals into and out of the isolator while protecting the materials and the isolator from contamination. Ports are either cylindrical or cuboid rectangular. The most important difference is that cylindrical ports allow the use of transfer sleeves to enter supplies from sterilizing cylinders and to pass animals from one isolator to another (Fig. 26.5), whereas rectangular ports require either use of an adapter (Fig. 26.8) providing a cylindrical opening to which a transfer sleeve can be attached, or that supplies be sterilized and transferred using wrapped packages and animals be transferred in a sterilizable container (Fig. 26.9) that is proof against contamination.

Cylindrical ports as used on flexible film isolators are of stainless steel or plastic, usually either 12 or 18 inches in diameter, and typically about 12 inches long, but they can be made larger if necessary to accommodate special equipment. Plastic construction is preferable to stainless steel, as liquid sterilants are corrosive to stainless steel, resulting in increased maintenance and the need

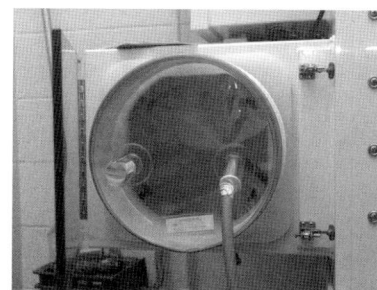

FIGURE 26.8   Circular adapter attached to rectangular port. A PVC outer port cap is taped to the adapter and an air hose is passed through one nipple for spraying the isolator interior with sterilant.

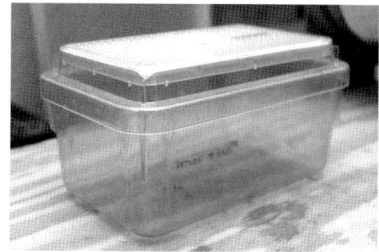

FIGURE 26.9   Transfer cage.

to monitor for pinhole leaks. The inner and outer caps of the port are made of flexible film, with the outer cap having one or two 1-inch plastic nipples for introduction of sterilant (Fig. 26.1). Originally, the outer cap was secured with vinyl tape, and the inner cap retained with a large rubber band. This method is still used, but is labor intensive and requires a significant expenditure for tape. Other methods, such as circular clamps (Fig. 26.5) to retain the caps, or ports having rigid plastic doors (Fig. 26.4), are available today and, although they are more expensive to purchase, require less personnel time to operate and obviate the need for tape.

Semirigid isolators can be made with cylindrical (Fig. 26.3) or rectangular (Figs 26.2 and 26.6) ports, or both. Rectangular ports have clear plastic doors that seal via silicon foam rubber gaskets and have latches that apply clamping pressure when closed. The ports are often made with a small opening, closed with a threaded plug that can be used to introduce sterilant. If cylindrical ports are to be used with transfer sleeves, the exterior end should be closed with a plastic film cap, or the hinges of the exterior door should be such that the door can be lifted off the hinge pins; otherwise, the door can interfere with use of the sleeve. Consideration should also be given to the ergonomics of passing materials and animals into and out of semirigid isolators using transfer sleeves. Depending on the location and geometry of the ports in relation to the position of the gloves, the dimensions of the glove sleeves, and the curvature of the flexible front panel, it can be very difficult to get materials out of a sterilizing cylinder, through the sleeve, and into the port where they can be reached from inside the chamber. Such difficulties can be alleviated by use of transfer sleeves with glove sleeves installed by the manufacturer or user.

4. Gloves

Manipulation of animals and supplies in isolators is awkward compared to such activities in ordinary animal room housing. Well-chosen gloves can help minimize this, whereas poorly chosen ones can make these activities much more difficult than necessary. (Glove selection is discussed in Section VI, A.) Whatever gloves are chosen, operators must bear in mind that the gloves are the most vulnerable part of the isolator, and that damaged gloves are common causes of contamination. Thus, while in use, gloves must be frequently inspected for damage, which is most easily detected when the gloves are light colored and kept clean. The gloves also must be changed at short enough intervals to minimize the risk of damage due to wear or deterioration. This will vary according to the type and thickness of material and the frequency and type of usage, but we recommend that even the most robust gloves be replaced at least annually.

5. Individually Ventilated Cages

Studies involving transfer of large numbers of human microbiota samples could require larger numbers of separate housing units than is practical or possible to manage in most gnotobiotic facilities. In such situations, positive pressure individually ventilated caging systems could provide an acceptable alternative to isolator housing (Clough et al., 1995; Stehr et al., 2009). All manipulations would have to be conducted in a biosafety cabinet, with very careful technique. Experience with such systems, though modest as yet, indicates that success is possible (C. Vowles, personal communication, May 2014).

C. Ancillary Equipment

Unless one relies entirely on wrapped packs for sterilization and entry of food, bedding, and other materials and supplies, sterilizing cylinders (Fig. 26.10) are used for such materials. Use of supply cylinders requires a cart or stand to position the cylinder at the correct height to be connected to the isolator port with a transfer sleeve (Fig. 26.5). These can be purchased ready-made or fabricated locally.

A V- or U-shaped dip tank or dunk trap will be needed for hysterectomy derivation of new germfree mice (Fig. 26.11). Such a device is easily fabricated of plastic materials by a university research machine shop, a local fabrication shop, or even a knowledgeable

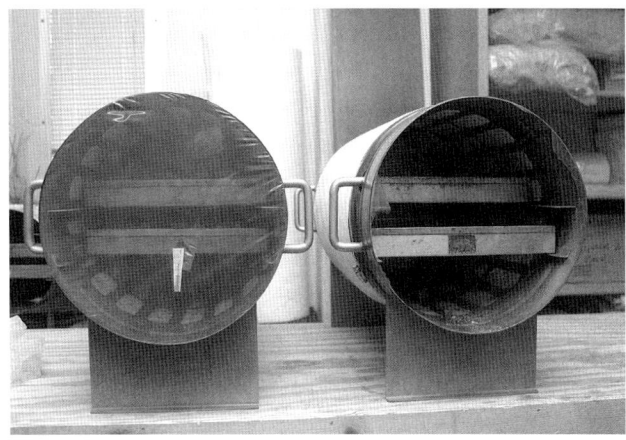

FIGURE 26.10 Supply cylinders from Class Biologically Clean made to hold removable food trays. Left cylinder is closed with Mylar™, with a SteriGage™ chemical integrator taped to the inside, ready for autoclaving.

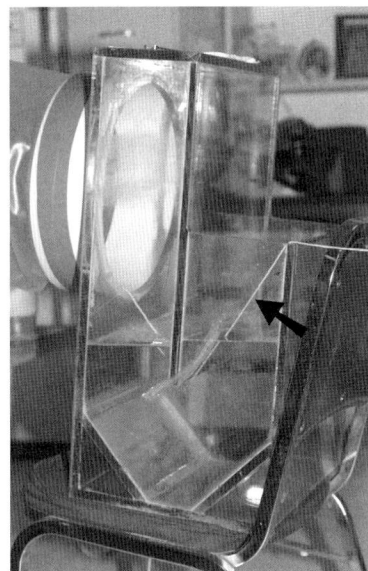

FIGURE 26.11 Sterilant trap connected to isolator in preparation for hysterectomy derivation. String (arrow) leads to forceps that will be used to bring the gravid uterus into the isolator through the sterilant.

handyman. Such traps can also be used to pass waste and other materials out of isolators in which biohazardous agents are used.

We recommend use of a compressed air atomizer (Fig. 26.12) for applying liquid sterilant to facilitate thorough coverage and generate a dense mist of sterilant. In old buildings, compressed air lines can contain enough rust to clog sprayers frequently. If this occurs, filters can be installed to remove particulate debris from the air supply. Alternatively, or if building compressed air is not available, a small portable electric compressor can be used. Some of these are quite noisy, but acceptably

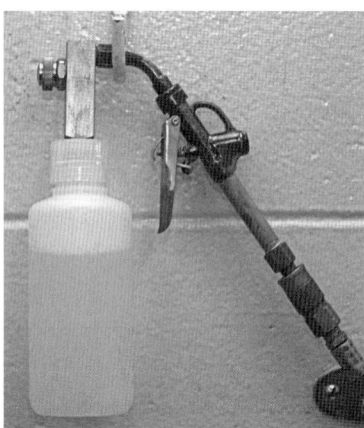

FIGURE 26.12 Model 5870 chlorine sprayer from Spraying Systems Co. fitted with a 500-ml bottle and an automotive air hose connector.

quiet ones are available. Another alternative is to use compressed nitrogen cylinders. If these are used, oil-free gas should be specified. The disadvantage of gas cylinders is the well-documented risk of injury if the valve is broken, as the escape of high-pressure gas can cause the cylinder to spin with great force or even become a projectile. Thus, it is imperative that cylinders be properly secured. In our view, cylinder gas should be used only if there is no alternative.

D. Sterilization

It is crucially important that those selecting and developing sterilization methods and procedures understand the principles, strengths, and limitations of each method. All sterilization procedures must be validated by testing with biological indicators before introduction of gnotobiotic animals is attempted and must be constantly monitored thereafter.

1. Liquid Chemical

Peroxyacetic, or peracetic, acid was the first germicide used to sterilize isolators and is still used because of its effectiveness, low cost, and compatibility with most plastics. It is effective at low concentrations and temperatures, and, in liquid form, in the presence of organic matter, although it does not penetrate parasite cysts and arthropod eggs (van der Gulden and van Erp, 1972). It is available from laboratory chemical suppliers as a liquid containing 40% peracetic acid. A major advantage of peracetic acid is that it is effective in vapor and liquid phases (Block, 2001; Trexler, 1984). The vapor generated when a 1–2% solution is sprayed at room temperature will inactivate the most resistant bacteria and mold spores within 15 min, and direct application of the liquid achieves the same action within 1 min (Trexler, 1984). Peracetic acid is sometimes used at a concentration

of 4%, but there is no evidence from actual gnotobiotic applications that this is more effective than 1% (R. Orcutt, personal communication, March 2014). Optimal sporicidal activity in the vapor phase is achieved at 80% relative humidity. Peracetic acid solution should always be prepared immediately before use, because it loses about half of its strength within 24 h. Thirty minutes of contact time is sufficient. Peracetic acid is corrosive, and it is irritating to the eyes, skin, and respiratory tract. Personnel using peracetic acid should wear gloves, disposable clothing, and a full-face respirator with chemical filter cartridges. Peracetic acid is not considered a carcinogen by the Environmental Protection Agency, Occupational Safety and Health Administration, or the National Toxicology Program, and it is not genotoxic or mutagenic (Malchesky, 2001), although it can be a tumor promoter.

Combining peracetic acid with hydrogen peroxide results in synergistic antimicrobial activity (Block, 2001). Spor-Klenz™ (Steris Life Sciences), a ready-to-use sterilant solution containing 1% hydrogen peroxide and 0.08% peracetic acid, has broad sporicidal efficacy and completely inactivates Mycobacterium spp. after 20 min of contact time at 20°C (Rutala et al., 1991). It has become an accepted sterilant for gnotobiotics. A contact time of 1 h is recommended. Other products combining peracetic acid and hydrogen peroxide are available, as noted below.

Chlorine dioxide in liquid form is now the most commonly used sterilant in gnotobiotics. It is highly effective against all microorganisms, and, like peracetic acid, is effective in both gaseous and liquid phases (Jeng and Woodworth, 1990; Knapp and Battisti, 2001; Orcutt et al., 1981; Pell-Walpole and Waller, 1984). It is 1075 times more sporicidal in the gaseous state than ethylene oxide (Jeng and Woodworth, 1990). Liquid chlorine dioxide sterilants include Exspor™ (Ecolab Inc.) and Clidox-S™ (Pharmacal Research Laboratories). These are composed of two parts, a base solution of sodium chlorite and an acidic activator, which are combined and mixed with water immediately before application to form a solution of chlorous acid and chlorine dioxide. A contact time of at least 30 min is recommended. Such products can corrode stainless steel.

Steriplex™ SD (sBioMed) is a two-part product utilizing silver, peracetic acid, and ethanol (0.015%, 0.15%, and 10%, respectively, in the activated product). It is sold as a disinfectant, not a sterilant, for hospital and other applications. However, it is stated by the manufacturer to be sporicidal, bactericidal, fungicidal, and viricidal; to rapidly inactivate Clostridium difficile and Bacillus subtilis spores; to be nonirritating; and to have a shelf life of 60 days after activation (Robison, 2012; sBioMed, 2013a, b, c). Steriplex™ SD has begun to be adopted for gnotobiotic use (C. Bell, personal communication, January 2014).

In our tests, Steriplex™ SD killed *Geobacillus stearothermophilus* 10^6 spore strips in 10 min and *Bacillus atropheus* 10^6 strips in 30 min.

Other liquid sterilant and 'high-level' disinfectant products include Actril™ (0.08% peracetic acid and 1.0% hydrogen peroxide; Mar Cor Purification), Cidexplus™ 28-Day Solution (3.4% glutaraldehyde; Johnson & Johnson), Minncare™ (4.5% peracetic acid and 22.0% hydrogen peroxide; Minntech BV), PeridoxRTU™ (4.0–4.8% hydrogen peroxide and 0.17–0.29% peracetic acid; Contec Inc.), Vimoba™ (chlorine dioxide; Quip Laboratories), Sanosil S010™ (5% hydrogen peroxide and 0.01% silver nitrate; Sanosil International), Sporgon™ (7.35% hydrogen peroxide and 0.23% PAA; Decon Laboratories), and Wavicide-01™ (2.65% glutaraldehyde; Medical Chemical Corporation). We are not aware of reports of evaluation of any of these products for use in gnotobiotics.

There is a large volume of literature on testing liquid sterilant and disinfectant procedures in health care and food processing; unfortunately, however, there is little information regarding comparative effectiveness or standardized testing as applied directly to gnotobiotics. Users should be aware that results of standardized testing methods can vary considerably. Organisms on surfaces are almost always more difficult to kill than those in suspension (Berube *et al.*, 2001; Gibson *et al.*, 1995; Sagripanti and Bonifacino, 1999, 2000; Springthorpe and Sattar, 2005; van Klingeren *et al.*, 1998), and, in surface tests, different materials can yield different results (Thorn *et al.*, 2013). Moreover, results of standardized tests do not necessarily indicate effectiveness in the environment in which sterilants and procedures will actually be used (Gibson *et al.*, 1995; R. Orcutt, personal communication, March 2014). In our view, using standard laboratory tests to compare products well established to be effective sterilants when properly used is of far less value than determining that a sterilant's *applications* – that is, the procedures in which it is used – are effective and reliable. Methods we use are described in relevant places in this chapter. A final recommendation is that although one chooses to verify liquid sterilization, it is important to determine that sterilization is real and not merely apparent due to growth inhibition. This can be done by use of dilution techniques, neutralizing media, or combinations of these. Dey–Engley neutralizing broth works well with chlorine dioxide and peracetic acid sterilants (Espigares *et al.*, 2003; Sutton *et al.*, 2002; Terleckyj and Axler, 1987). However, in our hands it did not neutralize Steriplex SD™.

Gnotobiotic facility personnel are advised to work with their institutional environmental health and safety personnel regarding the use of aerosolized sterilants. A work hazard assessment should be conducted to implement the use of the appropriate personal protective equipment (chemical respirator, gloves, goggles, face shield, etc.) and engineering controls such as exhaust air to scavenge chemical vapors away from personnel.

2. Gas and Vapor Chemical

Various methods of gas and vapor chemical sterilization have been developed. Ethylene oxide is widely used in health care facilities to sterilize items that cannot be autoclaved (Joslyn, 2001, Rutala *et al.*, 2008). It has been used to sterilize isolator chambers (Dennis *et al.*, 1985), food (Charles *et al.*, 1965; Luckey, 1963) and bedding (Reyniers *et al.*, 1964), but it is not ordinarily used in gnotobiotics except to sterilize non-autoclavable items. Ethylene oxide is carcinogenic and otherwise hazardous (Joslyn, 2001; Rutala *et al.*, 2008). Occurrence of tumors in germfree mice exposed to ethylene oxide-treated bedding has been reported (Reyniers *et al.*, 1964).

Chlorine dioxide gas, vaporized hydrogen peroxide, and formaldehyde gas generators are used for facility decontamination and processing of drugs and medical devices (Block, 2001; Coles, 1998; Joslyn, 2001; Rutala *et al.*, 2008). Although these could be used to sterilize isolator chambers, the equipment is expensive and formaldehyde is considered a carcinogen.

3. Steam

Steam sterilization is the chief method of sterilization of supplies and other materials in most gnotobiotic facilities. The combination of moisture and heat, in the form of saturated steam under pressure, is highly effective (McDonnell, 2007; Perkins, 1969; Rutala *et al.*, 2008). However, to ensure complete sterilization, the necessary conditions must be attained, for sufficient time, in the most challenging location in the load. Those conditions are determined by steam quality, temperature, and pressure. To most efficiently transfer heat and moisture to the materials to be sterilized, the steam must be dry saturated steam with no more than 3% entrained water. Steam that is too dry (superheated) or too wet does not transfer heat and moisture as well. The most commonly used steam temperatures are 121°C (250°F) and 132°C (270°F). The pressure of the steam is necessary to maintain its temperature; otherwise, it does not contribute to sterilization. Killing of microorganisms occurs rapidly under direct contact with steam of the proper temperature and moisture content, but air entrapped by any sort of container, or within porous materials such as food, bedding, and paper towels, inhibits sterilization by retarding steam penetration and reducing steam temperature. Sterilization time is thus dependent on the method of replacing the air in the load with steam, the nature of the materials to be sterilized, and how the materials are packed and loaded. Air removal by gravity displacement does not effectively remove air from porous materials such as food, bedding, and paper products (McDonnell, 2007); thus, gravity displacement autoclave cycles are unsuitable for use in gnotobiotics. Before more modern autoclaves became available, gravity displacement autoclaves were sometimes modified for use with sterilizing cylinders that connected to the chamber discharge so that steam exiting the chamber flowed through the cylinder. The process is difficult to control, requires constant operator attention, and leaves the cylinder filters and contents wet. Newer autoclaves utilize preconditioning steps to remove most of the air from the load and preheat it, greatly shortening the sterilization time required.

Wrapping, packing, and loading affect air removal and steam penetration, and consequently sterilization, to a considerable extent. In general, supplies should be packed and loaded so as to facilitate steam penetration as much as possible. For example, water bottles and packs should not be closely packed against one another. Although directed toward hospital use rather than gnotobiotics, Chapter 9 of Perkins (1969) provides good guidance. The Bowie–Dick test can be used to evaluate air removal from test or challenge packs, and kits are commercially available. However, we prefer to directly monitor steam sterilization with biological indicators containing 10^6 G. stearothermophilus spores. They should be used to test and validate sterilization procedures, and should be included in every supply cylinder or pack, with every load of water, and in all other materials to be sterilized for isolator use. Indicators should be placed in the most challenging locations, generally in the center or densest part of the load, and in the part closest to the coolest area of the chamber, usually nearest the steam discharge. Some users employ electronic temperature data loggers to monitor autoclave performance, or include test or challenge packs with every load, and determine the biological indicators to be sterile by culture for at least 48h before the supplies are passed into isolators.

Autoclaves should be serviced regularly by a qualified technician to ensure proper operation. It is advisable to 'map' the autoclave chamber for 'cold' spots with the various loads that may be used. This can be done by the technician with thermocouples and by users with data loggers or biological indicators in test packs. Steam quality must be adequate, or sterilization failures are likely no matter how well the autoclave is maintained and operated (Sedlacek and Rose, 1985). Malfunctioning condensate separators are common causes of steam that is too wet for effective sterilization.

4. Dry Heat

Materials that are difficult or impossible for steam to penetrate, such as oils, greases, and powders, cannot be sterilized effectively by autoclaving (Perkins, 1969). In gnotobiotics, the need to sterilize such materials is uncommon, but does arise occasionally, in which case dry heat or irradiation must be used. Microorganisms are much more resistant to dry heat than to moist heat. G. stearothermophilus spores, for example, can survive 121°C (250°F) dry heat for 2h (Perkins, 1969). In the presence of oil or grease, sterilization can require 160°C (320°F) for up to 4h. Recommendations for dry heat sterilization of some common materials, such as mineral oil, can be found via literature or web searches. Otherwise, the required conditions will have to be determined using suitable biological indicators. Glass ampoule indicators cannot be used because the spores are suspended in aqueous medium.

5. Ionizing Radiation

Gamma irradiation offers advantages in economy and convenience over autoclaving and has been used to sterilize food and bedding for gnotobiotic animals for many years (Barc et al., 2004; Cahenzli et al., 2013; Caulfield et al., 2008; Cherbuy et al., 2010; Corpet et al., 1989; Gianni F, personal communication, October 2013; Hartmann et al., 2000; Hirayama et al., 2007; Hudcovic et al., 2009; Ley et al., 1969; Luckey, 1963; Mabrok et al., 2012; Matsumoto et al., 1988; Mwangi et al., 2010; Paterson and Cook, 1971; Rabot et al., 2010; Respondek et al., 2013; Trexler, 1983; Wrzosek et al., 2013; Yamanaka et al., 1977). Many users also consider irradiation to be more reliable than autoclaving, especially with difficult materials such as pelleted chow, and a few have replaced autoclaving entirely with irradiation (F. Gianni, personal communication, January 2014).

Irradiated food and bedding are available commercially in prepackaged form. The key requirement with such products is that the dose of radiation used be adequate to ensure consistent complete sterilization. Although doses appropriate for decontaminating feeds of certain pathogens have been established, no broadly accepted standard or minimum dose for sterilizing chow for gnotobiotic rodents exists. Doses reported in the above publications range from 30 kGy to 59 kGy, but in the United States feed manufacturers are limited by federal regulation to 50 kGy (21 CFR § 579.22). Only chow closest to the radiation source will receive that dose; packages farther away will receive less. Thus, the minimum dose, rather than the maximum, must be determined to be adequate to ensure sterilization.

As with all sterilization methods, sterilization by irradiation must be monitored. Bacterial resistance to sterilization by irradiation has been linked to microbiological burden, moisture level, oxygen content, and temperature of the product (Halls, 1992; Hanson and Shaffer, 2001). Contamination of germfree mice fed irradiated diet has been attributed to incomplete sterilization because the target dose of 50 kGy was not attained in some parts of the load (Taylor, 1985). Vitamin deficiencies also have been reported with irradiated diets (Caulfield *et al.*, 2008, Hirayama *et al.*, 2007). Thus, sterilization of each product, and the manufacturer's specifications and guarantee, should be carefully evaluated.

6. Filtration

Hydropac™ systems have begun to be used to supply water for gnotobiotic mice without autoclaving (B. Bakos, personal communication, December 2013; F. Gianni, personal communication, October 2013 and December 2013; D.K. Johnson, personal communication, December 2013). These systems automatically form 8-oz. or 13-oz. pouches from continuous rolls of plastic film, fill them with filtered water, and seal them. Sterile disposable valves are inserted into the pouches to provide water for mice and rats. Water is sterilized by use of optional 1.2-µm, 0.2-µm, and 0.1-µm filters and by including 5–10 ppm free chlorine in the water (F. Gianni, personal communication, December 2013). The pouches are transferred into isolators by dunking and spraying with sterilant (B. Bakos, personal communication, December 2013). For facilities having access to the equipment, this offers the potential for a substantial savings in labor.

7. Sterilization Monitoring

Monitoring sterilization of isolators, ports, and supplies is discussed at various points in this chapter under each respective topic. In general, each procedure must be validated when protocols are being developed or modified, and monitored during regular use thereafter. Validation and monitoring should challenge the procedure by a significant margin so that minor deviations from requirements are unlikely to result in sterilization failure. For additional information, one should consult sources such as Berube *et al.* (2001), Humphreys (2011), McDonnell (2007), Perkins (1969), ANSI/AAMI ST34 Guideline for the Use of Industrial Ethylene Oxide and Steam Biological Indicators (AAMI, 2009), ANSI/AAMI ST79 Comprehensive guide to steam sterilization and sterility assurance in health care facilities (AAMI, 2013), and Standard Test Method for Quantitative Sporicidal Three-Step Method (TSM) to Determine Sporicidal Efficacy of Liquids, Liquid Sprays, and Vapor or Gases on Contaminated Carrier Surfaces (ASTM International, 2005).

VI. OPERATION

A. Isolator Setup

1. Cleaning and Inspection

Isolators should be thoroughly inspected for damage, especially to filters, flexible film parts, and glove sleeves, including new isolators for damage that might have occurred during shipping. Isolators must be scrupulously cleaned before being sterilized, including new ones as well as isolators that have been in use and require refurbishing. In the case of semirigid isolators, this is greatly simplified by removing the front panel. Inasmuch as the front panel is attached by a number of large screws, removing it is much easier and faster with an electric driver. A compact 12-volt driver is handy and has more than enough torque. The driver should allow the torque to be adjusted, and the operator should take care to adjust the torque setting to avoid stripping the threads when replacing the screws. Dust and loose debris should be removed with a vacuum and the interior thoroughly cleaned with hot water and detergent, including all corners and around door latches and hinges, then rinsed and wiped dry.

Semirigid isolators should be inspected for proper adjustment and closure of both inner and outer transfer port doors. Maintenance and adjustment of the inner door is difficult, but possible, with the front panel installed. Door gaskets should be inspected for complete contact with the door. Closing and latching the door on a paper strip and pulling on the strip is a simple way to check gasket contact. If the gasket does not make full contact, the door latches may need adjustment. New gaskets that do not make full contact usually can be adjusted by removing them and carefully replacing them in the groove so as to avoid lengthwise stretching or compression, which can cause uneven protrusion of the gasket. Old gaskets eventually lose elasticity and must be replaced.

Before installing the flexible front panel of a semirigid isolator that is being refurbished, the panel and the glove sleeves should be thoroughly inspected for discoloration, stiffness, or other evidence of deterioration. Although the materials are tough and durable, they are susceptible to aging and eventually need to be replaced, even if they appear undamaged. The manufacturer should be consulted for guidelines regarding frequency of replacement.

Air filters also should be inspected for damage, and, in the case of outlet filters of isolators that have been in use, clogging by food and bedding dust. We are not aware of gnotobiotic facilities that routinely HEPA certify air filters, in the manner of biological safety cabinets. (According to U.S. government standards, a HEPA filter must remove 99.97% of particles 0.3 µm in diameter and larger from the air passing through it.) The major reason for this is probably that the equipment required is expensive, as is paying someone having the equipment to do it on a per-filter basis. Such costs would be difficult to justify for most gnotobiotic work, unless required by institutional occupational health and safety officials for studies with human microbiota. One manufacturer recommends checking filters for leakage using a particle counter of the type used to determine airborne particulate counts in work environments (F. Razzaboni, personal communications, August 2013). These are available from industrial and safety equipment suppliers for under $2000. In any case, it is advisable to visually inspect filters after shipment and periodically thereafter. This is facilitated by illuminating the filter interior in a darkened room. If there is any doubt as to the condition of a cartridge type filter, it should be replaced. Wrapped cylindrical filters are routinely rewrapped and resterilized whenever the isolator is refurbished.

2. Gloves

An important part of isolator setup is installing properly selected gloves, unless the original manufacturer-installed gloves have been determined to be satisfactory. Gloves suitable for isolator use are available from several sources in different sizes, materials, thicknesses, methods of attachment to the isolator, and as two-piece or full-length designs.

Glove size is a very important consideration if any, but the simplest cage maintenance tasks are to be done. The gloves must be sized to accommodate the operator having the largest glove size. However, if another operator has much smaller hands, working in the isolator will be much more difficult for that person, especially if the gloves are of thick or stiff material. It can be helpful to consider whether operators should be assigned to particular isolators having the appropriate size gloves installed, but someone must always be available who can get into the gloves to care for the animals if the primary operator is absent.

Materials used for isolator gloves include neoprene, nitrile rubber, chlorosulfonated polyethylene rubber (CSP, Hypalon™), polyurethane, and bonded layers of CSP and polyurethane. These differ in flexibility, durability, and cost. Bonded CSP–polyurethane offers a very good combination of durability and flexibility, but is quite costly; a single pair of gloves can cost several-hundred dollars. Neoprene has been used for isolator gloves for a long time and is relatively inexpensive, but in our experience is somewhat less durable than more modern materials, being more prone to cracking with age. CSP and polyurethane gloves are tough and flexible, less costly than those of bonded materials, and the choice of many users.

Gloves are available in different thicknesses. Thickness affects flexibility and durability. Choice of thickness should be balanced according to both the need for dexterity and the risk of damage. Gloves thinner than 15 mil (0.015 inches) probably should not be used unless really necessary, as they could be too easily damaged. Thirty mil gloves are very tough, but they can also be rather stiff and seem somewhat more prone to cracking than thinner gloves of the same material.

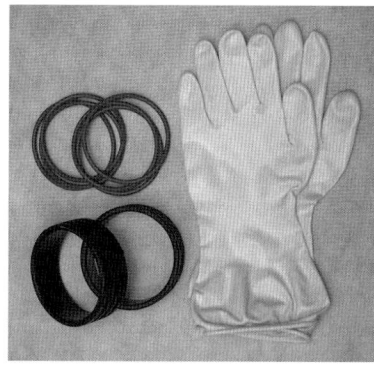

FIGURE 26.13 Hypalon™ gloves with plastic cuffs and silicone rubber O-rings used to attach the gloves to glove sleeves.

Gloves can be of full-length, one-piece design, or have separate sleeves and gloves (Fig. 26.7). In the latter case, the sleeve and glove are joined via a grooved plastic cuff with rubber O-rings used to hold the gloves and sleeves together and provide sealing pressure (Fig. 26.13). Vinyl tape can be applied over the O-rings for additional security. Two-piece gloves offer the advantage that gloves can be replaced while the isolator is in operation. This is accomplished by everting the glove and sleeve and then closing off the sleeve either by twisting and taping or with a padded clamp. After the old glove is removed, a liberal amount of sterilant is poured into the sleeve and the new glove attached. The glove and sleeve are manipulated to thoroughly distribute the sterilant inside the glove and sleeve. After the requisite contact time, the clamp is removed, or the sleeve untwisted, the glove and sleeve are inverted back into the chamber, and the sterilant residue is mopped up with paper towels. It also is possible to replace such gloves inside the isolator (Trexler, 1983), but it is not easy to do. A disadvantage of two-piece gloves is that, because the assembled glove and sleeve must be long enough to allow the operator to reach the most distant areas of the chamber, shorter individuals may find the cuffs frequently sliding down over their hands and getting in the way. For that reason, some users prefer one-piece full length gloves, but of course these cannot be replaced while the isolator is in operation.

Gloves can be attached to the chamber by either of two general methods (Fig. 26.7). In the case of two-piece gloves, the sleeve can be made of PVC, polyurethane, or blended PVC–polyurethane permanently bonded to the isolator chamber of flexible film isolators, or to the flexible front panel of semirigid isolators. Alternatively, the sleeve can be attached via a rigid ring assembly (Figs 26.1, 26.3, 26.7), which is the method used to attach one-piece gloves. The advantage of permanently attached sleeves is that they can be made with a larger diameter at the upper arms than is usually available with rigid rings, allowing somewhat improved ergonomics for the operator. Shorter operators may find that this does not outweigh the inconvenience of the cuffs of two-piece gloves and prefer full-length gloves attached with rigid rings. Rigid ring assemblies of the two-piece compression type provide a very secure attachment, but they require considerable care to assemble properly so that a complete seal is formed between the glove and chamber.

The O-rings used to attach gloves to sleeves are made of either silicone or nitrile rubber. These are available from industrial suppliers in a wide range of sizes and are inexpensive if purchased in quantity. In our experience, silicone ones seem to be somewhat more durable, as well as more elastic and thus easier to apply. Some operators find the O-rings supplied by isolator manufacturers excessively tight and difficult to apply. This is easily alleviated by using O-rings of slightly larger diameter.

In sum the optimal choice of gloves involves several factors. We suggest a relatively robust glove, such as 20- or 30-mil CSP, when dexterity is not an overriding concern, such as breeding isolators, in which the main task is routine cage maintenance. In that situation, we recommend glove replacement annually. For experimental isolators in which a higher degree of dexterity is needed, such as performing injections or gavages or collecting blood samples, 15-mil or 18-mil neoprene gloves work well. They are less robust and thus need to be replaced more frequently, but gloves suitable for use with separate sleeves can be obtained inexpensively. CSP gloves of 15 mil thickness are appropriate general-purpose gloves.

3. Leak Testing

The isolator must be tested for leakage before it is sterilized and stocked for use. The most common method is to use a gas detector. Detectors are available for a variety of gases, such as helium and carbon dioxide, but we recommend using a handheld multipurpose gas detector of the type capable of detecting refrigerants and solvent vapors (Fig. 26.14), which are available from industrial, safety equipment, and test instrument suppliers for $150–400. These can detect the propellant gas from inexpensive and safe aerosol can dust removal products sold by office, photographic, and scientific suppliers. The general procedure is similar for isolators of all construction types. The transfer port is closed and the air outlet is plugged. Duster gas is introduced into the isolator either by triggering the can inside the isolator or through an aperture that is then plugged. The gloves are everted and the blower run until the gloves stand out to indicate positive internal pressure. The air inlet is then closed or plugged. The gas detector is turned on and adjusted for sensitivity according to the manufacturer's instructions. (Some care is needed, as

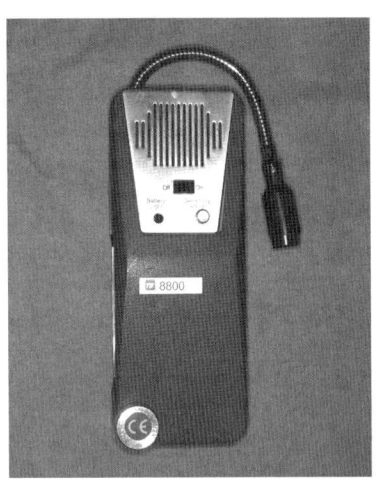

FIGURE 26.14 Gas detector for leak testing.

it is possible to adjust the detector to be too sensitive and give false-positive results.) The detector wand is slowly passed over all joints, seams, and welds. Sealing of the gaskets of the transfer port inner door and the front panel of semirigid isolators should receive especially careful attention, and gloves, including new ones, also should be checked thoroughly. Any leaks must be repaired as required. Semirigid isolator front panels having dart seams at the corners to provide the curvature of the panel are sometimes difficult to seal, and one cannot simply tighten the screws to try to get them to seal, as this risks cracking the rigid plastic. An effective remedy is to remove the front panel, apply silicone sealant to the gasket where it contacts the seam, replace the panel, and repeat the leak test after the sealant has set. Good-quality silicone caulking applied with a caulking gun, available from home improvement suppliers, works well. If this is done, it is advisable first to apply a thin film of silicone spray lubricant, light silicone grease, or paste wax to the gasket and surrounding area to act as a release agent, so the panel can be easily removed in the future, and, when removing the panel, to use a thin-bladed putty knife with rounded corners to free the panel without damaging the gasket.

4. Sterilization

Sterilant can be applied with a hand sprayer, but we prefer a compressed air atomizer such as the model 5870 chlorine sprayer manufactured by Spraying Systems Co. (Fig. 26.12). When equipped with a 500-ml bottle, this sprayer holds enough sterilant to thoroughly wet the interior of a 60-inch flexible film isolator or 30-inch semirigid isolator and fill the interior with a dense sterilant mist. We suggest replacing the length of tubing that forms the handle of the sprayer with a 2-inch or 3 × 1/4-inch brass or stainless steel pipe nipple and installing a male brass automotive air hose connector on the nipple and a female brass fitting on the air hose to permit the sprayer to be disconnected from the air hose easily.

The UAB Gnotobiotic Facility uses the following procedure for sterilizing flexible film isolators. The operator places the sprayer inside the chamber, dons the gloves, and sprays the inside of the chamber, including the gloves, inside the filter nipples, and around the glove rings and the junction of the chamber and port, repeatedly until all surfaces are thoroughly wet and sterilant has begun to pool in the bottom of the isolator. The sprayer is then removed from the chamber. Using a new heavy-duty paper towel or new clean sponge, the operator thoroughly wets all surfaces of the floor mat, cage shelves, and inner port cap with Exspor™ and places them in the isolator. Rubber bands, forceps, and stoppers are dunked in sterilant and placed in the isolator. (Some authorities recommend autoclaving rubber items because of the possibility that such materials could be porous and thus entrap microorganisms. This is probably the best practice, but autoclaving can accelerate deterioration of such items, and we consider the risk to be small.) Wearing gloves, the operator unwraps the autoclaved cage bottoms and places them in the isolator. (This avoids having to transfer cages a few at a time through the port after the isolator is sterilized.) The operator again dons the gloves and arranges the items inside the chamber so as to maximize exposure to the sterilant, with the cage shelves on edge, cages separated and set with their bottoms on the floor of the chamber, and the floor mat draped over the cages and shelves. The gloves are left stretched out inside the isolator. The operator tapes the outer cap on the port and sprays sterilant through one nipple into the chamber until it is filled with sterilant fog and fog issues from the other nipple. One nipple is stoppered and taped, and sterilant is sprayed into the chamber until the chamber is fully inflated and the gloves turn inside out. The operator dons the gloves, venting the chamber slightly if necessary, and secures the inner port cap. The port is sprayed and fogged and the remaining outer cap nipple is stoppered and taped. When the job is completed, there should be a substantial amount of liquid sterilant in the bottom of the isolator. The isolator is allowed to stand overnight, then sterile paper towel packs are passed in, as much as possible of the sterilant is wiped up, the Mylar™ film over the filter fittings is torn away, and the blower turned on to dry the chamber interior.

The procedure for sterilizing semirigid isolators is similar, but incorporates measures to sterilize the inlet and outlet filters, which are not autoclavable. The operator places the cage bottoms and sprayer filled with 500 ml of sterilant inside the chamber. An adapter is installed on the outer port opening that provides a cylindrical opening to which a plastic film outer port cap with nipples is secured with tape. The air hose is inserted through one nipple and taped in place, and the other nipple is stoppered and taped (Fig. 26.8). The operator reverses the blower and turns it on, opens the air inlet damper, dons the gloves, and sprays sterilant into the inlet opening for 60 s. The blower is returned to the positive pressure position and sterilant is sprayed into the outlet filter opening for 60 s. The operator turns the blower off and sprays the entire isolator interior, including the bottom surfaces of the shelves, all corners, the hinges and latches of the inner door, the junction of the inner door with its gasket, the light fixture enclosure, and all surfaces of the cages. This is done repeatedly until about 50 ml of sterilant remains. At that point, the air inlet damper is closed and the outlet air filter covered with a plastic bag secured with tape or elastic cord. The chamber is sprayed until there is modest positive pressure in the chamber, and the sprayer is passed out, the inner door is closed, the port outer door adapter is removed, and the port is sprayed and fogged. The next day, the plastic bag is removed from the outlet filter, the air inlet damper is opened, the blower is turned on, towel packs are passed in, and the sterilant is wiped from the chamber interior. The air damper is opened completely to dry the chamber interior, after which it is adjusted to the specified internal pressure.

A commonly used approach to verifying the chamber sterilization procedure is to take multiple swabs of the isolator interior and culture them using nonselective agar and broth media able to support growth of fastidious organisms. We recommend use of spore strips containing 10^6 *G. stearothermophilus* or *B. atropheus* spores for establishing isolator sterilization procedures. These can be attached with masking tape at various points in the isolator interior prior to application of sterilant. After sterilization, the strips are transferred using aseptic technique to tubes of neutralizing broth.

B. Sterilization and Entry of Supplies

After the isolator is sterilized, cage tops, water bottles, and sipper tubes must be entered, and the isolator must be stocked with food, water, bedding, and various other items. Consumable items must be replaced while the isolator is in operation, and used bedding and other waste and empty water bottles must be removed. It is crucial that the sterilization procedure for each item be determined to be adequate and that sterilization of each item be monitored.

1. Sterilizing Cylinders and Packs

Supplies can be sterilized and transferred into isolators by use of sterilizing cylinders, wrapped packs, or, in the case of water bottles and solid items that cannot be autoclaved, spraying or dipping in sterilant. Although use of sterilizing cylinders and transfer sleeves poses the least risk of contamination, in our experience these methods work about equally well, if procedures are adequate and carefully followed.

Sterilizing cylinders are typically 12 or 18 inches in diameter, made of perforated stainless steel sheet metal, with one end open and the other closed, and are wrapped with filter medium to exclude microorganisms and allow for steam penetration during autoclaving (Fig. 26.10). These are available commercially and can be made with removable perforated trays for sterilizing food. (The 18-inch cylinders can be quite heavy when loaded.) After the cylinder is loaded, the open end of the cylinder is covered with polyethylene terephthalate polyester (Mylar™) plastic film. The sterilized cylinder is attached to the transfer port with a transfer sleeve (Fig. 26.5), and the sleeve and port are then sterilized with a chemical sterilant. Using dressing forceps, the operator then breaks the Mylar™ cover from inside the isolator and brings the contents of the cylinder through the transfer sleeve and transfer port into the isolator chamber. Transfer sleeves are available either straight 12 or 18 inches diameter or 12 inches at one end and 18 at the other to accommodate various combinations of port and sterilizing cylinder diameter.

Food and other autoclavable solid items and materials can be sterilized in packs using disposable autoclaving wraps. Packs should be of such size and weight that they will fit readily into the port and can be handled securely. The pack is prepared with an inner and outer wrap, the outer wrap being closed in the manner of a surgical pack, which allows the operator to grasp the corners and fold it back without touching the inner wrap. To enter a pack into an isolator, the operator sprays the port with sterilant, then, with the pack either held in one hand or placed on a clean level surface, reflects the outer wrap so that the pack can be held by the bottom, which remains protected by the outer wrap, and placed in the port. The outer wrap is withdrawn. If the procedure is done properly, the inner pack is never touched by anything that is not sterile, other than the bottom of the port, which already has been sprayed with sterilant. The port is then fogged and allowed to stand for the requisite time before bringing the pack into the isolator.

The filter material of supply cylinders is a greater impediment to steam penetration than the wrapping of supply packs. Therefore, sterilization protocols for the same materials in cylinders and packs require separate validation. Spore strips or self-contained biological indicators, such as Attest™ (3M) and Verify™ (Steris Life Sciences), should be used to monitor sterilization of 'dry goods.' We suggest placing a chemical integrator, such as the Comply™ SteriGage™ (3M), on each pack, or taped to the inside of the Mylar™ of sterilizing cylinders (Fig. 26.10), to provide a readily visible indication that the pack or cylinder has been autoclaved.

2. Food

Food poses the greatest difficulty in steam sterilization. Chow contains large numbers of bacteria, and pelleted food is dense and difficult for steam to penetrate, even with optimal preconditioning. In the UAB Gnotobiotic Facility, we found that spore strips placed inside food pellets may not be sterilized under conditions in which biological indicator vials adjacent to the test pellets were consistently sterilized. Autoclavable diets are highly fortified to ensure that adequate amounts of labile nutrients remain after autoclaving, but the length of time to which the food can be subjected to steam sterilization conditions is still limited. Steam that is too wet can fail to sterilize pelleted chow even after prolonged sterilization times (Sedlacek and Rose, 1985).

Extruded diets may be preferable to pelleted ones (F. Gianni, personal communication, October 2013). They are processed at higher temperatures than pelleted diets, and thus may be expected to contain fewer viable bacteria. They also are more porous than pelleted diets, which should facilitate steam penetration. Whichever diet is chosen, it is advisable to determine the sterilization time the diet will withstand and retain adequate amounts of the most labile nutrients, such as thiamine, vitamin A, and vitamin K. Thirty minutes is a typically recommended sterilization time, but analysis of samples autoclaved using different sterilization times or temperatures may show that it is possible to use longer times or higher temperatures, and thus help ensure consistent sterilization while retaining adequate amounts of labile nutrients.

Another factor affecting food sterilization is the method of packaging. Food packaged in paper bags several inches in each dimension is more difficult to sterilize than food in the shallow perforated trays used in food-sterilizing cylinders. Food sterilization cycles should include a preconditioning step to purge air from the load before sterilization and a drying step after sterilization. Each food cylinder or load of food packs should be accompanied by a test or challenge pack containing test pellets and/or biological indicators that are determined to be sterile by culture for at least 48 h before the food is passed into an isolator. Inasmuch as the test pack does not directly monitor the interior of the cylinder or food pack, we also recommend that biological indicators or food test pellets be included in each cylinder or pack of food. These should be placed in locations most difficult for steam to penetrate, such as the center of food packages in the center of a cylinder and near its closed end. These are passed out after the food is entered into the isolator and incubated to verify sterilization.

3. Water

Water is sterilized using a liquid autoclaving cycle, with typical sterilization times of 90–120 min. Commonly used water containers include 2-liter borosilicate glass bottles with vented rubber caps and ordinary quart mason jars. The borosilicate glass bottles are rather expensive and can be somewhat awkward to handle for persons with small hands. Mason jars are inexpensive and easier to handle, but they are more easily broken. To 'spray in' water bottles, the port and bottles are thoroughly sprayed with sterilant, the bottles are placed in the port, and the port is fogged. If mason jars are used, the ring is unscrewed and the threads on the jar and the inside of the ring are sprayed. Water sterilization is monitored using glass *G. stearothermophilus* biological indicator ampoules. These are hung in the center of water bottles, using cotton thread, dental floss, or similar material, in various places in each load. After the bottles have cooled, the ones containing the biological indicators are opened and the indicators are cultured for at least 48 h before the bottles are transferred into isolators.

4. Other Materials and Supplies

Cage tops, water bottles, sipper tubes with stoppers, bedding, nesting material, 10- or 12-inch dressing forceps, paper towels, paper bags, gauze sponges, culture swabs and tubes, and other items according to personal preference or experimental objective will be needed. Any sterilizable contact bedding can be used; however, it is advisable to choose a product that contains or produces little dust, as food and bedding dust accumulates in air outlet filters and can eventually clog them. Porous materials such as bedding, paper products, gauze pads, swabs, and nesting material should be autoclaved using preconditioning and drying steps. Sterilization of bedding should be rigorously validated, as bedding can contain large numbers of bacteria. Because sterilization can be affected by the arrangement of items in cylinders and packs, we recommend that a few standard supply loads be developed and the sterilization cycle necessary to reliably sterilize each be determined by use of biological indicators placed in the most challenging locations, such as the center of bedding and towel packages and the interior of water bottles. Inasmuch as materials such as those listed above do not undergo deterioration during autoclaving, sterilization times can be increased to provide an additional margin of safety. Nonetheless, biological indicators placed in challenging locations should be included in each cylinder or pack.

Cages and water bottles should be new or in like new condition. Clouding and mineral deposits interfere with monitoring the animals and water levels in the bottles, and rough handling during cage washing can cause chips and burrs on cages and cage tops that can damage gloves.

Occasionally, a research protocol requires weighing animals inside isolators. Some users sterilize mechanical scales by autoclaving or by dunking in liquid sterilant. Others have sterilized electronic scales with ethylene oxide (Teah, 1984; S. McBride, personal communication, September 2013). We have used a small digital scale inside a heavy-duty zip-lock plastic bag. An Archimedes scale accurate enough to weigh mice also can be fashioned from graduated cylinders (attributed to J. Pleasants by E. Vieira and L. Vieira, personal communication, January 2014).

Some users keep writing materials in their isolators. Ordinary lead pencils are most commonly used, although some use felt-tip laboratory markers (S. Cormier, personal communication, January 2014; S. McBride, personal communication, January 2014). Whether the interior of such markers can be effectively sterilized by steam can be questioned, but it seems unlikely that microorganisms could survive the solvent. Medi-Dose™ surgical skin markers also can be used (B. Thompson, personal communication, January 2014). They are available in sterile packages. We do not use such items in our isolators, as we mark materials such as sample tubes before passing them in, and we identify mice via ear punches or tags, or by microchip devices.

We advise against unquestioned trust in sterile labeling and packaging of medical products. These should be treated by filtration, autoclaving, or other appropriate method to independently ensure sterility.

5. Port Sterilization

The transfer port and interior of the transfer sleeve, if used, must be sterilized to allow supplies to be passed into the isolator. This is done by spraying all surfaces with sterilant and waiting the required contact time. We prefer to use a compressed air atomizer and to fog the port with sterilant mist after spraying. The port must be kept scrupulously clean and free of particles of food, bedding, or other debris that could inhibit sterilization. The port sterilization procedure must be verified to reliably sterilize the port by culture or use of spore strips as described above for verification of isolator chamber sterilization. We have found spore strips to provide a stringent test. Strips that are not thoroughly wetted with Exspor™ can still contain viable spores after an hour, whereas thoroughly wetted strips are reliably killed in 30 min. Thus, the procedure in the UAB facility is to spray all interior surfaces, including the doors and door gaskets, repeatedly for a minimum of 1 min. Coverage must be such that sterilant is visibly dripping or running down vertical surfaces. The port is then fogged for a minimum of 30 s with the sprayer directed so as to swirl the mist inside the port. Liquid sterilant must be visible in the bottom of the port. Contact time is as long as practicable but a minimum of 1 h. The procedure for preparing to transfer materials using a transfer sleeve is similar.

C. Introduction and Transfer of Animals

Sterile conditions should be verified after all required materials have been transferred into the isolator but before animals are transferred in. This is typically done by culturing swabs of the isolator interior, in some cases at intervals for up to 3 weeks (Roesch, 2012). Another method is to transfer one or two mice of known germfree status into the isolator and, after a week or so, testing the isolator according to the standard monitoring procedure before introducing breeding or experimental mice.

Shipment of gnotobiotic mice from a vendor or other source requires a special shipping container to maintain their microbiological status. In many cases, this will be by commercial shipment in a shipper available from Taconic (Taconic, 2006). The shipper is a sleeve constructed of flexible film with filtered openings for ventilation that can accommodate up to three cages of mice. After the mice are transferred into the shipper, it is closed via a Mylar™ diaphragm, which is pressed into place and secured by an external wrapping of vinyl tape. The open end of the sleeve, which is left wet with sterilant, is rolled up and taped in place. After arrival, the mice are transferred into an isolator by connecting the sleeve to the isolator port. The sleeve of the shipper is 12 inches in diameter and designed to be connected directly to a standard 12-inch port. A 12-inch ring of PVC plastic or stainless steel can be used to connect the shipper to an 18-inch port using an 18- to 12-inch reducing-diameter transfer sleeve. After sterilizing the sleeve and port, the operator removes the tape holding the diaphragm in place and 'massages' the diaphragm by external manipulation to turn it 90°, which allows it to be pulled out of the sleeve. The cages are then transferred, also by external manipulation of the shipper, into the sleeve or port where they can be reached from inside the isolator.

It is frequently necessary to move animals from one isolator to another for experiments, to establish new breeding isolators, or to empty an isolator that requires maintenance or repair. One method is similar to transferring supplies from a sterilizing cylinder using a transfer sleeve. A sleeve of appropriate diameter is used to connect the two isolators. This is most easily done if the isolators are at the same height, but longer sleeves formed with angles and integral gloves are available to allow transfer between isolators at different heights. Flexible film isolators can be moved to different positions on supporting racks to facilitate connection, but this can be quite awkward, requires at least two persons, and invites accidents. In any case, after the connected ports and sleeves are sterilized, the mice to be moved are placed in a paper bag, transfer cage, or other container and placed in the port. The inner openings of both isolators are never opened at the same time. The mice are moved through the sleeve into the port of the second isolator and brought inside, after which the sleeve is disconnected and the ports are closed and sterilized.

It is possible to purchase or fabricate a small isolator or transfer chamber on a cart or stand, which can have height adjustments, for transferring animals. This is useful if it is necessary to move animals between rooms, floors, or even buildings.

Animals also can be transferred without connecting the two isolators by use of a transfer cage. These are commercially available, although any container of suitable size that provides secure closure and is sterilizable could be used. In the UAB facility, we use filter-top cages of the type with a raised plastic top with a replaceable filter and that has a substantial lip that extends over the cage bottom in the manner of a Petri dish lid (Fig. 26.9). The original glass fiber filter is replaced with DW4 filter material sealed at the edges with silicone sealer. Cages with tops are kept wrapped and autoclaved ready for use. The cage is passed into the first isolator by the same procedure used to transfer supplies in wrapped packs. After spraying the port, the cage, including the filter top, is thoroughly wetted with sterilant before being placed in the port by an operator wearing sterile gloves. After the required contact time, the cage is passed into the isolator and the mice to be moved are placed inside. The cage is passed out of the isolator and into the second isolator by the same procedure, except that the contact time is reduced to 15 min. Although this may seem riskier than using transfer sleeves, it works well if procedures are followed, as one begins with a sterile transfer cage that is never touched by anything not sterile or thoroughly wet with sterilant, and the cage itself is kept wet with sterilant and is exposed to the room environment only briefly.

D. Working in Isolators

Working in isolators is quite different from working in an open animal room. Routine tasks such as changing cages, filling water bottles, and moving materials in and out of the chamber are subject to limitations on movement and dexterity imposed by the gloves, limited space within the isolator, and, to a lesser extent, reduced visibility. Thus, ergonomic considerations are very important in designing a gnotobiotic facility and selecting the isolators that will be used. This will not only help prevent injuries but also reduce the risk of contamination, as operators who are uncomfortable could tend to cut corners to reduce the amount of time spent working in the isolator.

There are inherent practical limits on lifting and arm movement within the isolator chamber. The maximum length of the gloves, whether of one- or two-piece design, is about 30 inches from the fingertips to the juncture of the glove or its sleeve with the isolator. While the position of the glove opening can be varied somewhat, the ability of the operator to reach all areas of the isolator interior is barely adequate in most flexible film and semirigid isolators, and is even more limited for short persons. The effect of this can be reduced by measures to optimally position the operator relative to the isolator to allow the maximum arm reach and comfort, such as isolator stands that have adjustable legs, and step stools and platforms that allow the operator to select a comfortable height and position. If the facility uses isolators stacked so that the upper units are several feet above the floor, electrically operated hydraulic personnel lifts are available that provide greater safety in addition to more flexible height adjustment.

Thoughtful and efficient organization will help reduce the number of awkward and repetitive movements and associated injuries, as well as the time required to complete necessary tasks. Efficient operation of an isolator requires balancing the needs for space for cages and supplies, and performing tasks such as changing cages. In general, one should position objects that are heavy or used frequently where they can be easily reached and objects that are light or handled infrequently in other locations. Packaging food and bedding in rectangular packages that can be efficiently stacked helps conserve space. Positioning materials in the same place in each isolator reduces wasted motion, and good organization helps minimize the number of times materials must be passed into the isolator, which helps reduce the risk of contamination. Also, personnel should handle loaded sterilizing cylinders carefully, especially those containing food, as they can be heavy and awkward.

Conducting animal procedures, such as giving injections, performing gastric gavages, collecting blood and tissue samples, and identifying animals via ear punches or tags, can be challenging. However, such procedures are manageable with careful glove selection, proper instruction, and experience. Sharps, of course, must be handled very carefully.

E. Monitoring for Contamination

It is essential that a gnotobiotic facility has an adequate monitoring program to verify that the mice remain free of microbial contaminants. Major considerations are summarized below.

1. Sources of Contamination

The most common causes of contamination are damaged gloves and incomplete sterilization of supplies, especially chow. The most commonly identified contaminants are aerobic bacteria that grow readily on standard media. The identity of contaminants can suggest possible sources. Spore-forming bacilli often come from inadequately autoclaved food or bedding. Non-spore-forming organisms of types common in the environment of animal facilities are likely to gain entry via damaged gloves or as a result of inadequate coverage with liquid sterilant in the port, or inadequate contact time. Organisms such as *Staphylococcus* spp. that are carried on human skin or in the respiratory tract suggest glove damage. Fungi can come from inadequately sterilized food or from growth on filter material (Pleasants, 1974). In recently derived mice, vertical transmission, or introduction during the derivation procedure, should also be considered. It should be expected that a source cannot be definitively identified in many cases of sporadic contamination, but episodes of multiple isolator contamination indicate a serious problem, such as autoclave malfunction or poor steam supply quality. In one instance, it was found via steam calorimetry that the steam supply sometimes contained 5% or more entrained water, and when this occurred, autoclaving pelleted chow for 60 min at 126°C did not sterilize it consistently (Sedlacek and Rose, 1985). Malfunctioning steam line condensate separators are likely culprits, so any such devices in the steam supply to the autoclave should be inspected by a qualified technician. Such episodes also can accompany personnel changes, indicating poor adherence to procedures.

2. Inspection and Observation

Operators should develop the habit of inspecting each isolator frequently. All flexible parts, especially gloves and glove sleeves, should be visually inspected for damage. Gloves should be either donned or everted and closely inspected for cracks, pinholes, and tears. Cracks most often occur between the fingers. Two-piece gloves often develop perforations at the junction of the glove with the cuff, and one-piece gloves commonly do so at the attachment rings. Applying tension can make small defects easier to see. Any damaged glove should be immediately twisted or clamped off and samples should be collected for monitoring. If the isolator has not become contaminated, the damaged glove can be replaced while the isolator is in operation if it is separate from the sleeve, but if the gloves are one piece, it will be necessary to move the animals to another isolator. To help reduce the occurrence of glove damage, all items placed in isolators, especially cages and cage tops, should be inspected for burrs and chipping before use. It is best to obtain such items new rather than from the cage wash area, where they are frequently damaged.

The odor of the isolator exhaust air should be checked frequently. The exhaust air from an isolator containing germfree mice or mice colonized with ASF should have very little odor. Any change signals possible contamination and the need for immediate microbiological testing. For example, urease-producing bacteria convert urea in urine to ammonia, which is readily detected in the exhaust air, and some contaminants produce substances with a putrefactive odor.

Food and water should be inspected for mold growth. Contaminating mold readily grows on food unless it is very dry. In fact, some users monitor for mold contamination by placing a few food pellets in a shallow dish or the bottom of an empty cage and keeping them damp with water. 'Water mold' (oomycete) contamination is evident in water bottles as a fine, cotton-like growth.

The majority of germfree mice found dead probably will be found to have torsion of the cecum, but occasionally a contaminating microorganism can cause germfree mice to become ill and even die. Thus, any sick or dead mice should be subjected to necropsy examination and cultured for contaminants. Organs should be prepared for histopathologic examination unless they are cannibalized or severely autolyzed.

3. Microbiological Monitoring

Although protocols vary, a combination of direct fecal examination and culture methods typically is employed (Carter and Foster, 2005; Foster, 1980; Fuller, 1984; ILAR, 1970; Luckey, 1963; Pleasants, 1974; Rahija, 2007; Roesch, 2012; Trexler, 1983). Molecular methods may be used in addition. Major considerations are summarized below.

a. Sampling

Typical samples include fresh fecal pellets, water from in-use water bottles, and swabs from inside sipper tubes and various locations in the isolator interior. We recommend using simple wood shaft cotton swabs and glass screw-top microbiology tubes autoclaved with other supplies. Some users prefer commercial sampling devices having an integral capsule of transport medium, but we advise against using prepackaged sterile medical products that cannot be independently sterilized by the user. Swabs, fecal pellets, and water samples can be kept separate or placed together in sample tubes. If anaerobic cultures are to be done, fecal pellets should be as fresh as possible. Pellets can be collected by stimulating the perianal area of a mouse with a swab or by placing the mouse in an empty cage, in which it will almost invariably deposit one or more pellets within a minute or less. Pellets should be placed in an airtight tube with transport medium immediately after collection and transported to the laboratory without delay. It is not necessary to sample every cage, as mice kept in unfiltered cages readily exchange microorganisms. Samples are typically collected monthly, although some facilities monitor every 2 weeks or even weekly.

Some facilities also monitor retired breeder or surplus weanling mice. The mice are removed from the isolator in a transfer cage or sealed container and aseptically sacrificed and dissected in the laboratory in a class II biological safety cabinet. Typically, the contents of the gastrointestinal tract are examined and cultured as described below, but it may be advisable to include other organs if contamination with organisms that colonize the skin, respiratory tract, or other organs, or induce bacteremia, is suspected.

b. Fecal Wet Mounts and Gram Staining

Direct examination of feces suspended in broth or saline is a rapid method of screening for contamination. Samples should be examined both as wet mounts, using phase microscopy, and dried on slides and stained with Gram stain or a simple direct stain such as crystal (gentian) violet. Proficiency with any of these techniques requires some practice, and findings must be interpreted in light of the results of cultural procedures and molecular tests. The residue of the diet contains many small debris particles that resemble Gram-negative bacteria, and commercial diets can contain large numbers of bacteria, some of which, particularly large Gram-positive rods, are usually evident.

Interpretation of preparations from ASF-colonized mice requires that one distinguishes contaminants from the ASF organisms. Common isolator contaminants include cocci and blunt-ended rods, whereas ASF includes Gram-positive short rod lactobacilli, a Gram-negative Bacteroides-like bacillus, the tiny spirilliform Mucispirillum schaedleri, and four fusiform Gram-positive rods (Table 26.1).

One might assume that a contaminant would proliferate to large numbers in the intestine of germfree mice and thus be readily visible. In our experience, that is often the case, but it is by no means a consistent finding. We have experienced instances in which contaminating bacteria readily demonstrated by culture could not be identified by direct examination of feces.

c. Culture

Recommendations of several sources (Carter and Foster, 2005; Foster, 1980; Fuller, 1984; ILAR, 1970; Luckey, 1963; Pleasants, 1974; Rahija, 2007; Roesch, 2012; Trexler, 1983) can be summarized as follows: Fresh feces or swabs collected in the isolator should be put in liquid thioglycollate medium without resazurin dye. Inoculation can be done in the isolator, or the samples can be transferred to the medium in the laboratory. Aerobic organisms grow near the surface, whereas anaerobes that are not extremely oxygen sensitive grow at the bottom of the tube where oxygen tension is low. (Extremely oxygen-sensitive anaerobes must be cultivated in an anaerobic chamber.) Samples also should be plated on general-purpose agar media suitable for anaerobic and aerobic conditions, such as brain–heart infusion agar with 5% sheep blood. Incubation at 25°C and 37°C is recommended. Sabouraud's agar incubated at 25°C is

TABLE 26.1   Altered Schaedler Flora

Organism		Morphology[a]	Growth[b,c]
ASF 356	*Clostridium* cluster XIV, *Bacillus–Clostridium* group (Firmicutes phylum); most closely related to *Clostridium propionicum*[d]	Gram-positive large tapered rod	EOS[e] anaerobic
ASF 360	Probably *Lactobacillus intestinalis*[f] (previously identified as *L. acidophilus*)	Gram-positive rod (Schaedler's 'rhizoid' lactobacillus)	Facultative
ASF 361	Probably *Lactobacillus murinus*[c,d,g] (previously identified as *L. salivarius*)	Gram-positive rod	Facultative
ASF 457	*Mucispirillum schaedleri* (Deferribacteres phylum)[h]	Gram-negative slender curved or spiral	Anaerobic
ASF 492	*Eubacterium plexicaudatum* (*Clostridium* cluster XIV, *Bacillus–Clostridium* group)[d]	Gram-positive large tapered rod, less tapered than ASF 356, subpolar tuft of flagella	EOS[e] anaerobic
ASF 500	Probably *Pseudoflavonifractor* sp. (Clostridiales)[i,j]	Gram-positive long thin tapered rod	EOS[e] anaerobic
ASF 502	*Clostridium* cluster XIV, *Bacillus–Clostridium* group; most closely related to *Ruminococcus gnavus*[d]	Gram-positive medium tapered rod, about 1/2 the length of ASF 356, some cells have round swellings	EOS[e] anaerobic
ASF 519	Probably *Parabacteroides goldsteinii*[k] (previously identified as *Bacteroides distasonis*)	Gram-negative rod, bipolar staining	Anaerobic

[a]See Schaedler and Orcutt (1983). Figure 5a on p. 333 is ASF 356, and Figures 5c, d, and e are ASF 492, ASF 502, and ASF 500, respectively.[b]
[b]Orcutt (2006b).
[c]Sarma-Rupavtarm et al. (2004).
[d]Dewhirst et al. (1999).
[e]Extremely oxygen sensitive.
[f]Park and Itoh (2005).
[g]ASF 361, Lactobacillus murinus, and Lactobacillus animalis are probably the same species.[d] Lactobacillus murinus Hemme et al. 1982, sp. nov. would take precedence over Lactobacillus animalis Dent and Williams 1983, sp. nov.
[h]Robertson et al. (2005).
[i]Duca et al. (2014), supplementary data [online]. Available at <http://diabetes.diabetesjournals.org/content/suppl/2014/01/14/db13-1526.DC1/DB131526SupplementaryData.pdf> (Accessed 06.09.14).
[j]Sequence AF157051 in EzTaxon (Kim et al., 2012) [online]. Available at <http://www.ezbiocloud.net/eztaxon/hierarchy?m=browse&k=AF157051&d=1>(Accessed 06.09.14).
[k]Momose et al. (2011).

recommended for fungal culture. Use of selective media may be indicated to isolate particular microorganisms or to inhibit growth of members of defined microbiota. For example, the lactobacilli in ASF will grow aerobically on blood agar plates. Usually, they are easily distinguished from contaminants by colony morphology and Gram staining, but if, for example, contamination with a Gram-negative organism is suspected, a medium selective for such organisms, such as MacConkey's, can be used. Samples incubated at 37°C should be held for 5–7 days before being discarded. Those incubated at room temperature should be held for 10 days to 2 weeks.

d. Molecular Methods

PCR methods targeting bacterial 16S ribosomal RNA sequences are used to detect bacteria and analyze bacterial microbiota in a wide range of settings (Bibiloni et al., 2005; Sontakke et al., 2009; Weisburg et al., 1991; Wilson et al., 2006; Zucol et al., 2006). Such methods can be valuable techniques for monitoring gnotobiotic mice and offer the important advantage of being able to detect contaminants that are difficult or impossible to culture. Sequencing technology is now economical enough that amplicon sequencing can be used routinely to identify contaminants and verify the presence of members of defined microbiota. Packey et al. (2013) describe the use of quantitative PCR using universal 16S rRNA primers, amplicon sequencing, and random amplification of polymorphic DNA for monitoring gnotobiotic rodents and found that these methods more accurately detected and identified isolator contamination than culturing and Gram-staining feces. PCR methods targeting specific organisms are useful for verifying members of defined microbiota such as ASF (Alexander et al., 2006; Dewhirst et al., 1999; Ge et al., 2006; Sarma-Rupavtarm et al., 2004). Commercial laboratories offer rapid and sensitive methods to screen newly derived mice for agents such as *Mycoplasma* spp., *Helicobacter* spp., and *Pneumocystis murina*. Commercial PCR testing also is available for rodent viruses.

As is the case for any diagnostic method, the limitations of the technology must be recognized. Negative results are not conclusive evidence of the absence of contaminants, as there are various technical reasons why a reaction may not produce detectable amplification product even though target sequences are present. (One of the authors experienced an instance in which 'broad-range' 16S rRNA PCR did not detect a readily cultured contaminant.) In the case of 'broad-range' primers, not all taxa are necessarily amplified with equal efficiency, and relatively rare sequences may not be detected in the presence of highly abundant ones. Conversely, false-positive results can be obtained due to dead bacteria present in food and bedding. This is less likely with methods targeting the entire 16S rRNA gene, or large portions of it, because of fragmentation due to autoclaving, but it is a significant possibility with methods targeting shorter sequences.

High-throughput methods for analyzing microbial diversity have been developed (Andersson et al., 2008; Caporaso et al., 2011; DeSantis et al., 2007; Zoetendal et al., 2008). Although these are very powerful tools for that purpose, their utility for monitoring gnotobiotic animals is as yet unclear. Using the Illumina Genome Analyzer IIx™ platform, the UAB Microbiome Core has analyzed samples from UAB Gnotobiotic Facility mice. In some cases, known contaminants were detected, but detection of members of the ASF was inconsistent. However, the most striking finding was the number of reads that were present in all samples of feces from taxa that were prevalent in samples of autoclaved food.

e. Serologic Testing

Serologic testing, available from several commercial laboratories, is used to detect infections with viruses and a few other organisms such as *Mycoplasma pulmonis*. In general, the risk of viral contamination of isolator-housed mice is very low, with the exception of mice newly derived from a stock of unknown health status or one known to harbor a virus that can be transmitted vertically. Testing requires either collection of blood samples inside the isolator, or removing one or more mice from the isolator to obtain the samples. Obviously, collecting blood samples, or any other activity involving use of sharps inside an isolator, must be done with great care, but it is quite feasible if appropriate precautions are taken. Though somewhat cumbersome, injectable anesthetics, hypodermic syringes and needles, pipettes, and sample tubes routinely used for blood collection can also be used in isolators. These should be sterilized by the user, rather than relying on sterile packaging and labeling. We have found that submandibular vein puncture using a lancet (Golde et al., 2005) is very satisfactory for collecting blood samples for most purposes and does not require anesthesia.

4. Frequency of Monitoring

There are no strict guidelines for frequency of monitoring. Using historical contamination data from one commercial vendor, Selwyn and Shek (1994) developed a probability model for estimating the frequency of testing isolators and barriers. The rate of contamination among 94 isolators was used to predict contamination over time, with the result that the probability that an isolator that tested negative 1 week would be contaminated 4 weeks later was 8%, or about 2% per week. Based on the results of the study and the assumptions used to apply the model, the authors recommend that the frequency of testing be adjusted in accordance with changes in the historical contamination rate and the estimated risk of contamination. However, facilities typically monitor breeding populations monthly. Scheduling of monitoring of experimental isolators should take into account the manipulations that will be required and the frequency with which supplies, experimental samples, and other materials will be passed into and out of the isolator, as these will affect the risk of contamination. In general, monitoring should be done before the start of an experiment, periodically during the experiment, and at the end of the experiment.

5. Summary

Facility operators and users must recognize that no method or combination of methods is 100% sensitive and 100% specific. Any of those described above can fail and should be expected to do so on occasion. Second, there is a practical limit on the degree of certainty that can be attained. As efforts to attain greater confidence increase, costs in time and resources increase in a diminishing-returns manner. The goal therefore should be to develop a program that provides the optimal level of assurance that can be had with the available resources. We suggest that in doing so, facility managers and investigators consult operators of other facilities, as well as a qualified practical microbiologist experienced in isolating and identifying anaerobic and aerobic bacteria and fungi. The standard routine monitoring protocol used in the UAB Gnotobiotic Facility was devised in this manner and begins with fresh fecal pellets, swabs of sipper tubes and isolator interior, and water from an in-use water bottle placed together in a screw-cap culture tube inside the isolator. Tubes are transported to the laboratory as soon as possible, where they are vortexed to form a suspension. A slide is prepared for Gram staining, and *Brucella* blood agar plates, brain–heart infusion broth, and Sabouraud slants are inoculated. The plates and broth tubes are incubated at 37°C and the slants at room temperature. The plates are incubated for 5 days before discarding, broth tubes 7 days, and Sabouraud slants at least 2 weeks. An aliquot of suspension is extracted for 'broad-range' bacterial 16S rRNA PCR. Cultured contaminants are identified by a commercial laboratory. Samples are archived frozen for future analysis if indicated. This is done monthly. When a retired breeder or surplus weanling mouse is available, the mouse is brought to the laboratory in a transfer cage, sacrificed, and immediately passed into an anaerobic bacteriology chamber. Samples of ingesta are aseptically collected from the cecum and colon and cultured using pre-reduced nonselective anaerobic media.

Finally, it is important to have a response plan in the event of frequent contamination or episodes of multiple isolator contamination. Possible sources of contamination should immediately and thoroughly be investigated, and autoclave function and sterilization procedures should be revalidated as necessary. If autoclave malfunction is suspected, all autoclaved supplies that have not been entered into isolators should be discarded and replaced with supplies sterilized after proper autoclave function has been established, or using a backup autoclave if one is available. More frequent monitoring should be instituted until the extent of contamination has been determined and contaminated isolators have been closed down.

VII. DERIVATION OF GERMFREE MICE

Today, the primary, if not exclusive, methods of deriving germfree mice are by hysterectomy and embryo transfer. Each has advantages and disadvantages. Hysterectomy derivation can be done by anyone with the capability to operate a gnotobiotic facility, but maintaining a stock of germfree foster mice consumes resources, and hysterectomy derivation entails some risk of failing to eliminate microorganisms that can be transmitted via the placenta. Embryo transfer avoids that risk, but not all institutions performing embryo transfer have, or are willing to develop, the capacity to do it under sterile conditions, and such services available commercially are expensive.

Some facilities have found hysterectomy derivation to be inefficient and to result in too few pups weaned relative to embryo transfer (Faith *et al.*, 2010). Our success rate with hysterectomy derivation was low initially, but improved greatly with experience and with use of progesterone to delay parturition as described below. Thereafter, we have been successful with one or two attempts per genotype, and have weaned up to 27 pups per attempt. In any case, neither method is free of occasional frustration.

Newly derived mice should be monitored intensively for contamination. We suggest that monitoring be done weekly beginning the first week after derivation and continuing until the mice are established in breeding isolators. We also recommend that serologic and PCR testing for rodent pathogens be included.

A. Hysterotomy and Hysterectomy

The first germfree mice were derived by hysterotomy (Pleasants, 1959). This method utilizes an isolator having a panel or window of thin plastic membrane. The abdomen of the donor female, shaved and scrubbed as for surgery, is placed in direct contact with the membrane. The operator cuts through the membrane, abdominal wall, and uterus to bring the pups into the isolator. In hysterectomy derivation, the gravid uterus is removed and passed into the isolator via immersion in a germicidal dip (Fig. 26.11). This is easily done using a hemostat forceps and attached cotton string, which are autoclaved and passed into the derivation isolator. The forceps is passed out through the dip tank, leaving the end of the string inside. After the uterus is removed, it is clamped in the forceps and drawn by the string through the dip tank and into the isolator. The pups are then removed from the uterus and gently cleaned and massaged to stimulate breathing. In either case, the newly derived neonates are fostered on germfree mothers. Complete descriptions of these procedures are provided by Foster (1959, 1980).

Elements critical to success by these methods include timing of the matings of the donor and foster mice, timing of the derivation procedure, selection of foster mice, and measures to minimize the risk of contamination by agents that can be transmitted via the placenta. Although the average gestation period in mice is 19.5 days, it can vary from 19 to 21 days. Pups will not survive if they are removed from the uterus too early. Therefore, if the gestation period of the donor mice is not known, it must be determined by pair mating, checking for vaginal plugs, and recording the interval until birth for several litters. Matings of donor and foster mice are then timed so that the foster mothers will have delivered their litters 1–2 days before the donor mice are due to deliver theirs. In the UAB Gnotobiotic Facility, we have found that the likelihood of success is greatly increased by use of progesterone to delay parturition in the donor mice. Donor mice are mated for one night; the next day is thus day 0.5 of gestation. In the case of mice whose average gestation is 19–19.5 days, the derivation is scheduled for the morning of day 19.5, and the donor mothers are given 1 mg progesterone subcutaneously the morning of day 18.5. Thus, the derivation is scheduled to allow the full gestation period to be reached, and progesterone treatment ensures that the pups will not be delivered before the time of the derivation.

Success also is facilitated by use of foster mice that lactate well and readily accept fostered pups. In our experience, germfree Swiss Webster mice available from Taconic are excellent in these respects, as they routinely wean large litters of vigorous pups and rarely reject fostered pups. The proportion of donor mice that become pregnant via timed matings can be increased by estrus synchronization with injections of progesterone and cloprostenol (Pallares and Gonzalez-Bulnes, 2009). We have not found the increase to be as great as described, but it is worthwhile nonetheless.

Some infectious agents of mice, including lymphocytic choriomeningitis virus, lactate dehydrogenase elevating virus, *Pasteurella pneumotropica*, and *Mycoplasma* spp., can be transmitted transplacentally (Baker, 1998) and thus might not be eliminated by hysterotomy or hysterectomy derivation. Fortunately, these agents are likely to be detected by the comprehensive health surveillance protocols employed by most research institutions, and they rarely are encountered in contemporary SPF mice. Mice of unknown pathogen status should be subjected to thorough health assessment before being used as donors. If agents such as the above are found to be present, derivation by embryo transfer should be considered instead. In the case of bacterial or *Pneumocystis* infections, donor females could be treated with broad-spectrum antibiotics during gestation.

B. Embryo Transfer

Embryo transfer is increasingly being used to derive germfree mice. The embryo transfer procedure itself is described by Hogan *et al.* (1994) and by Jackson and Abbott (2000). Its use under sterile conditions to derive mice is reported by Okamoto and Matsumoto (1999), Inzunza *et al.* (2005), and Faith *et al.* (2010). This requires a biological safety cabinet or surgical isolator equipped with a microscope for vasectomizing germfree males and implanting embryos into germfree pseudopregnant recipient females. The success rate varies among donor mice. On average, about half of the transferred embryos can be expected to survive to weaning.

Although there appear to be no published reports of use of *in vitro* fertilization or artificial insemination to produce germfree mice, both are technically feasible, and could be useful to derive germfree mice that they reproduce poorly.

C. Defined Microbiota

Development of germfree mice was quickly accompanied by recognition that they had a number of abnormalities that complicated their use in research. The cecum of germfree mice is greatly enlarged, and, as a result, prone to volvulus or torsion about the base, resulting in strangulation of the organ and death of the mouse (Orcutt, 2006a). Germfree mice often reproduce poorly compared with mice of the same genotype having normal microbiota. This has been attributed to restriction by the enlarged cecum of abdominal space available for the gravid uterus, but this is unlikely to be the sole, or even the major, factor. Some germfree mice, for example, the Swiss Webster mice available from Taconic and commonly used as foster mice, have large litters and reproduce about as well as their non-germfree counterparts despite their large ceca. Germfree mice that do

reproduce poorly have prolonged diestrus, reduced frequency of estrus and thus copulation, and decreased implantation rates (Shimizu *et al.*, 1998). This is likely related to differences in enterohepatic estrogen recirculation. Whether glucuronidated estradiol is recycled after secretion into the intestine via the bile is dependent on intestinal bacterial glucuronidases. Thus, deconjugation does not occur in germfree mice, which alters the estrogen peak reaching the pituitary and hypothalamus, leading to altered secretion of luteinizing hormone and follicle-stimulating hormone (S. Barnes, personal communication, November 2013; Shapira *et al.*, 2013). Germfree mice are also susceptible to morbidity and mortality resulting from colonization with opportunistic environmental bacteria when removed from the isolator (Orcutt, 2006a), which is a result of loss of the colonization resistance imparted by the normal microbiota (Vollaard and Clasener, 1994). This was a significant problem when commercial vendors began using germfree technology to produce SPF mice. Consequently, efforts were begun to develop defined limited microbiota to improve reproductive performance and resistance to opportunistic pathogens.

1. Altered Schaedler Flora

Most cultivable bacteria in the gastrointestinal tract of conventional mice were found to be facultative anaerobes and obligate anaerobes, including *Lactobacillus* spp., *Enterococcus* spp., *Enterobacter* spp., *Bacteroides* spp., and *Clostridium* spp. (Dubos *et al.*, 1965; Schaedler *et al.*, 1965b). However, at least 90% of the microscopically visible bacteria in the lower bowel were fusiform or tapered rods that could not be cultured until improved anaerobic methods were developed (Gordon and Dubos, 1970; Lee *et al.*, 1968, 1971; Schaedler and Orcutt, 1983). Schaedler isolated aerobic and anaerobic bacteria from pathogen-free mice and colonized germfree mice with them in various combinations (Orcutt, 2006a; Schaedler *et al.*, 1965a; Schaedler and Orcutt, 1983). These 'cocktails' were provided to commercial animal vendors as defined microbiota with which to associate germfree mice to establish pathogen-free breeding populations. One 'cocktail,' for example, included *E. coli* var. *mutabilis*, *Streptococcus fecalis*, *Lactobacillus acidophilus*, *Lactobacillus salivarius*, group N *Streptococcus*, *Bacteroides distasonis*, an unidentified *Clostridium* spp., and another unidentified organism, 'fusiform bacterium #356' (Schaedler and Orcutt, 1983). It reduced cecal volume, not to that of conventional mice but enough to eliminate cecal torsion, and restored reproductive performance.

It soon became apparent that there were disadvantages to the presence of certain bacteria in Schaedler's 'cocktails' (Orcutt, 2006a). For example, *S. fecalis* was morphologically similar to staphylococci, which can contaminate isolators as a result of glove damage, and it overgrew aerobic plates, complicating or preventing isolation and identification of slower growing organisms. Moreover, various different 'cocktails' were in use, and there were no criteria for standardizing them, making it difficult for the National Cancer Institute (NCI) to monitor the microbiota used by the different vendors with which it had production contracts. Thus, in 1978 the NCI sought development of a standard defined microbiota. Criteria were that anaerobic organisms be included, as they are the dominant members of the intestinal microbiota (Trexler and Orcutt, 1999). Cocci and blunt-ended spore-forming rods could not be included to facilitate detection of contaminants. The selected combination had to reduce cecal volume and promote normal reproduction. Finally, it could include no more than eight bacteria. Extensive investigations by Orcutt et al. (1987) led to the ASF (Table 26.1), which is now used worldwide by most commercial rodent vendors, as well as by researchers as a standard limited intestinal microbiota. Current understanding of the taxonomy of the ASF organisms is based on 16S rRNA sequence analysis (Dewhirst et al., 1999; Duca et al., 2014; Momose et al., 2011; Park and Itoh, 2005; Robertson et al., 2005). Draft genome sequences of all eight species recently have become available (Wannemuehler et al., 2014) and will significantly improve understanding of their biology.

Germfree mice can be colonized with ASF by inoculation with either cultured individual ASF organisms or feces and intestinal content of ASF-colonized mice (Orcutt, 2006c). Methods for cultivating each organism under anaerobic conditions and with appropriate media are described by Orcutt (2006b). The lactobacilli and Bacteriodes-like ASF 519 are given first, via gavage, to establish the low oxygen tension environment in the intestine necessary to allow the oxygen-sensitive spirilliform and fusiform organisms, which are given by gavage 2 days later, to survive and grow. More commonly, however, germfree mice are given ASF by withholding water overnight and, the next morning, mixing fresh feces from an ASF-colonized mouse with drinking water and placing the bottle on the cage. This is repeated daily for 2 more days, except that on the last day, the ASF-colonized mouse is sacrificed. The cecum and large intestine are quickly removed, coarsely minced, and mixed with the drinking water. In our experience, this consistently results in colonization with all eight ASF organisms.

ASF-colonized mice are monitored for contamination by culture and examination of fecal Gram stains and wet mounts as described for germfree mice, taking into account the organisms that should be present. Each ASF organism has characteristic morphology, best appreciated by use of phase-contrast microscopy (Orcutt et al., 1987). Culture of ASF organisms is described by Orcutt (2006b) and by Dewhirst et al. (1999). The lactobacilli grow modestly on blood agar plates and in brain–heart infusion broth under aerobic conditions; contaminants are identified by colony morphology, Gram staining, and subculturing using selective media as needed. Positive anaerobic cultures are examined for organisms of morphology other than that of Bacteroides, fusiform bacilli, or spirochetes and subcultured if indicated. Monitoring for presence of individual ASF organisms is considerably facilitated by development of quantitative PCR methods (Alexander et al., 2006; Sarma-Rupavtarm et al., 2004). Although ASF is stable indefinitely under most circumstances, the ASF 360 lactobacillus has been observed to be lost from mice fed a semi-synthetic diet (Dubos and Schaedler, 1962).

2. Other Limited Microbiota

Numerous studies have been conducted using gnotobiotic mice colonized with single or limited numbers of microbial species to study the role of the microbiota in physiology, immunity, colonization resistance, and disease pathogenesis. Selected highlights are discussed below.

Studies of mice with limited microbiota were instrumental in advancing the understanding of the pathogenesis of inflammatory bowel diseases. Beginning in the early 1990s, mice with induced mutations in cytokine genes and other genes related to immune, inflammatory, and epithelial function were found to develop colitis spontaneously, which was shown to be dependent on presence of the intestinal microbiota (Lorenz et al., 2005; Peloquin and Nguyen, 2013; Podolsky, 1997; Sartor, 2005). It soon became apparent that different organisms and combinations of organisms had different effects, and that those effects often varied among mice of different genotypes and even according to the laboratory conducting the study. In the case of IL-10-deficient mice, Sellon et al. (1998) reported that the mice had minimal colitis when monocolonized with Bacteroides vulgatus or with a combination of B. vulgatus, group D Streptococcus faecium, E. coli, Peptostreptococcus productus, Eubacterium contortum, and Streptococcus avium, whereas Balish and Warner (2002) and Kim et al. (2005) found that colonization with Enterococcus faecalis alone induced colitis, and Kim et al. (2007) reported that colitis induced by E. fecalis was exacerbated by co-colonization with E. coli. Sydora et al. (2005) reported that IL-10-deficient mice colonized with viridans group Streptococcus, Clostridium sordellii, or both B. vulgatus and C. sordellii did not develop colitis. Bifidobacterium animalis was shown to cause duodenitis and colitis in monoassociated IL-10-deficient mice (Moran et al., 2009). Whary et al. found that monocolonization with Lactobacillus reuteri or Helicobacter hepaticus did not induce intestinal inflammation in IL-10-deficient mice, whereas colonization with both organisms caused signficant cecocolitis, an unexpected result because *L. reuteri* was previously reported to have anti-inflammatory properties (Whary *et al.*, 2011).

Similar studies have been conducted using IL-2-deficient mice (*E. coli* strains, *B. vulgatus*) (Bohn *et al.*, 2006; Waidmann *et al.*, 2003), TCRα-deficient mice (*Lactobacillus plantarum*, *Streptococcus faecalis*, *S. faecium*, *E. coli*) (Dianda *et al.*, 1997), and HLA-B27/β2 microglobulin transgenic rats (*S. faecium*, *E. coli*, *S. avium*, *E. contortum*, *P. productus*, *B. vulgatus*) (Rath *et al.*, 1996, 1999). In severe combined immunodeficient (SCID) mice, transfer of CD45RB(high) T cells induced colitis in mice colonized with *H. hepaticus* and ASF, but not ASF without *H. hepaticus* (Cahill *et al.*, 1997); with *H. muridarum*, but not segmented filamentous bacteria (SFB), *Ochrobactrum anthropi*, nonpathogenic *Listeria monocytogenes*, or *Morganella morganii* (Jiang *et al.*, 2002); and with SFB with a combination of 12 bacteria from SPF mice, but not the 12 species without SFB; monocolonization with SFB, *E. faecalis*, *Fusobacterium mortiferum*, *Bacteroides distasonis;* or combinations of SFB and *F. mortiferum* or SFB and *B. distasonis* (Stepankova *et al.*, 2007). In immunocompetent mice colonized with ASF, *Helicobacter bilis* induced colitis associated with immune responses to antigens of the ASF (Jergens *et al.*, 2006, 2007), and *H. hepaticus* altered the distribution of ASF organisms (Ge *et al.*, 2006).

The intestinal microbiota has a major role in development of immunity, as described in recent reviews (Bengmark, 2013; Chu and Mazmanian, 2013; Hansen *et al.*, 2012; Hooper *et al.*, 2012; Kamada and Nunez, 2013; Kamada *et al.*, 2013; Purchiaroni *et al.*, 2013). Evidence is accumulating from studies of gnotobiotic mice that particular bacterial species have specific effects. For example, *Bacteroides fragilis* induces development of Foxp3+ regulatory T (Treg) cells that produce IL-10 in the intestine, effects that are mediated by polysaccharide A (Round and Mazmanian, 2010). Treg cells also are induced by certain clostridia of human microbiota (Atarashi *et al.*, 2013). SFBs, which based on 16S rRNA sequence analysis, are related to group I clostridia (Snel *et al.*, 1995), induce Th17 cells, CD4+ T-helper cells that produce IL-17 and IL-22 in the lamina propria, and enhance resistance to *Citrobacter rodentium* (Ivanov *et al.*, 2009). SFBs also were found to promote appearance of TCRαβ intraepithelial lymphocytes, induce epithelial MHC class II expression, increase IgA production, and activate Peyer's patch lymphocytes (Klaasen *et al.*, 1993; Talham *et al.*, 1999; Umesaki *et al.*, 1995, 1999).

Studies of mice with limited microbiota have begun to elucidate the roles of individual bacterial species on other physiologic and pathologic processes. For example, *Bacteroides thetaiotaomicron*, a major member of the intestinal microbiota of both mice and humans, affects expression of genes related to intestinal maturation, vascular development, metabolism of xenobiotics, barrier function, and absorption of nutrients (Hooper *et al.*,

2001). A strain of *Enterobacter cloacae* isolated from an obese volunteer induced obesity, insulin resistance, and systemic inflammation in mice fed a high fat diet (Fei and Zhao, 2013), and some *E. coli* strains promoted macrophage accumulation and inflammation and impaired insulin and glucose tolerance in white adipose tissue of monocolonized mice (Caesar *et al.*, 2012). Strains of *Klebsiella pneumoniae* and *Proteus mirabilis* participate in induction of colon cancer in *Tbx21* (T-bet) and *Rag2* null ulcerative colitis (TRUC) mice (Garrett *et al.*, 2010).

It appears from the literature, and it has been our experience, that establishing limited microbiota in germfree mice is usually straightforward and can be done by oral inoculation, gastric gavage, enema, or a combination of these. Monocolonization with extremely oxygen-sensitive anaerobes, however, can be difficult to accomplish, due to the lack of prior colonization with facultative anaerobes (Lee *et al.*, 1971; Orcutt, 2006c). In such cases, the odds of success can be increased by addition of 2% cysteine and 3% ascorbic acid to the dosing medium (K. Garden, personal communication, 2008).

3. *Human Microbiota*

'Humanized' mice – gnotobiotic mice colonized with microbiota of patient and control volunteers – have provided important tools with which to investigate the relationships among the microbiota, diet, and metabolism (Liou *et al.*, 2013; Marcobal *et al.*, 2013; Respondek *et al.*, 2013; Turnbaugh *et al.*, 2009). The rapidly developing interest in understanding the role of the microbiota in normal homeostasis and in obesity-related disease, cancer, immune-mediated and infectious diseases, and other disease states is certain to drive increasing investigations using such mice. Transfer of human fecal microbiota to mice is readily accomplished and is stable after transfer, although the presence and distribution of phylotypes in recipient mice differs to various degrees from that of the human donor (Hirayama, 1999; Hirayama *et al.*, 1995; Turnbaugh *et al.*, 2009; Wos-Oxley *et al.*, 2012).

VIII. RESOURCES

A. Recommended Reading

1. *Gnotobiotics*

Carter, P.B., Foster, H.L., 2005. Gnotobiotics. In: Suckow, M.A., Weisbroth, S.H., Franklin, C.L. (Eds.), The Laboratory Rat, second ed. Elsevier Academic Press, San Diego, CA, pp. 693–710.

Coates, M.E., Gustafsson, B.E. (Eds.), 1984. Laboratory Animal Handbooks 9. The Germfree Animal in Biomedical Research. Laboratory Animals Ltd., London.

Lindsey, J.R., Baker, H.J., 2005. Historical foundations. In: Suckow, M.A., Weisbroth, S.H., Franklin, C.L. (Eds.), The Laboratory Rat. Elsevier Academic Press, San Diego, CA, pp. 1–52.

Luckey, T.D., 1963. Germfree Life and Gnotobiology. Academic Press, New York.

Rahija, R.J., 2007. Gnotobiotics. In: Fox, J.G., Barthold, S., Davisson, M.T., Newcomer, C.E., Quimby, F.W., Smith, A. (Eds.), The Mouse in Biomedical Research, Vol. 3: Normative Biology, Husbandry, and Models, second ed. Academic Press, New York, pp. 217–233.

Trexler, P.C., 1983. Gnotobiotics. In: Foster, H.L., Small, J.D., Fox, J.G. (Eds.), The Mouse in Biomedical Research. Vol. III. Normative Biology, Immunology, and Husbandry. Academic Press, New York, pp. 1–16.

Trexler, P.C., Orcutt, R.P., 1999. Development of gnotobiotics and contamination control in laboratory animal science. In: Mcpherson, C.W. (Ed.), 50 Years of Laboratory Animal Science. American Association for Laboratory Animal Science, Memphis, TN, pp. 121–128.

Wostmann, B.S., 1996. Germfree and Gnotobiotic Animal Models: Background and Applications. CRC Press, Boca Raton, FL.

2. Sterilization

Block, S.S. (Ed.), 2001. Disinfection, Sterilization and Preservation. Lippincott Williams & Wilkins, Philadelphia, PA.

McDonnell, G.E., 2007. Antisepsis, Disinfection, and Sterilization: Types, Action, and Resistance. ASM Press, Washington, DC.

Perkins, J.J., 1969. Principles and Methods of Sterilization in Health Sciences, second ed. Charles C. Thomas, Springfield, IL.

Rutala, W.A., Weber, D.J., Weinstein, R.A., et al., 2008. Guideline for Disinfection and Sterilization in Healthcare Facilities. Centers for Disease Control and Prevention, Atlanta, GA.

B. Online

LinkedIn Gnotobiotic Technology Group (http://www.linkedin.com/groups?gid=4128592&trk=myg_ugrp_ovr)

Gnotobiotics E-mail List (https://listserv.uab.edu/scgi-bin/wa?A0=GNOTOBIOTICS)

C. Manufacturers

Ansell Limited (gloves)
Red Bank, NJ
800 800 0444
http://www.ansellpro.com/index.asp

Class Biologically Clean Ltd. (isolators and associated equipment)
Madison, WI
608 273 9661
http://www.cbclean.com/

Controlled Environment Products (isolators)
Division of Standard Safety Equipment Co.
McHenry, IL
815 363 8565
http://www.controlledenvironmentproducts.com/

Harlan Laboratories, Inc. (isolators)
Indianapolis, IN
800 793 7287
http://www.harlan.com/products_and_services/research_models_and_services/flexible_film_isolators

Hydropac (watering system)
Seaford, DE
800 526 0469
http://www.hydropac.net/

Innovative Technology, Inc. (gloves)
Amesbury, MA
978 462 4415
http://www.isolatorgloves.com/

North by Honeywell (gloves)
Honeywell Safety Products
Smithfield, RI
800 430 5490
http://www.honeywellsafety.com/USA/Brands/North.aspx

Park Bioservices, LLC (isolators)
Groveland, MA
800 947 5226
http://www.parkbio.com/index.htm

Piercan USA, Inc. (gloves)
San Marcos, CA
760 599 4543
http://www.piercanusa.com/gloves/glovesisolatorssleeves.html

Renco Corp. (gloves)
Manchester, MA
800 257 8284
http://www.rencogloves.com/index.html

Spraying Systems Co. (sterilant sprayer)
Wheaton, IL
630 665 5000
http://www.spray.com/contact/world_hq.aspx

Tecniplast USA (Isocage™ positive pressure individually ventilated cage system)
Exton, PA
877 669 2243
http://www.tecniplast.it/us/product/isocage-isolator-at-cage-level.html

D. Laboratories

Accugen Laboratories
Willowbrook, IL
800-282-7102
http://www.accugenlabs.com/

Antech GLP
Morrisville, NC
800 872 1001
http://www.antechglp.com/index.htm

Charles River Laboratories Health Monitoring & Diagnostic Services
Wilmington, MA
877 274 8371
http://www.criver.com/products-services/basic-research/health-monitoring-diagnostic-services

IDEXX RADIL Lab Animal and Biological Materials Diagnostic Testing
Columbia, MO
800 669 0825, 573 499 5700
http://www.idexxbioresearch.com/radil

References

AAMI/ISO 14161, 2009. Sterilization of Health Care Products – Biological Indicators – Guidance for the Selection, Use, and Interpretation of Results. Association for the Advancement of Medical Instrumentation, Arlington, VA.

Alexander, D.A., Orcutt, R.P., Henry, J.C., Baker Jr., J., Bissahoyo, A.C., Threadgill, D.W., 2006. Quantitative PCR assays for mouse enteric flora reveal strain-dependent differences in composition that are influenced by the microenvironment. Mamm. Genome 17, 1093–1104.

Andersson, A.F., Lindberg, M., Jakobsson, H., Backhed, F., Nyren, P., Engstrand, L., 2008. Comparative analysis of human gut microbiota by barcoded pyrosequencing. PLoS One 3, e2836.

ANSI/AAMI ST79, 2013. Comprehensive Guide to Steam Sterilization and Sterility Assurance in Health Care Facilities. Association for the Advancement of Medical Instrumentation, Arlington, VA.

ASTM International Standard E2414, 2005. Standard Test Method for Quantitative Sporicidal Three-Step Method (TSM) to Determine Sporicidal Efficacy of Liquids, Liquid Sprays, and Vapor or Gases on Contaminated Carrier Surfaces. ASTM International, West Conshohocken, PA.

Atarashi, K., Tanoue, T., Oshima, K., Suda, W., Nagano, Y., Nishikawa, H., et al., 2013. Treg induction by a rationally selected mixture of clostridia strains from the human microbiota. Nature 500, 232–236.

Backhed, F., 2011. Programming of host metabolism by the gut microbiota. Ann. Nutr. Metab. 58 (Suppl. 2), 44–52.

Backhed, F., 2012. Host responses to the human microbiome. Nutr. Rev. 70 (Suppl. 1), S14–S17.

Backhed, F., Ding, H., Wang, T., Hooper, L.V., Koh, G.Y., Nagy, A., et al., 2004. The gut microbiota as an environmental factor that regulates fat storage. Proc. Natl. Acad. Sci. USA 101, 15718–15723.

Backhed, F., Manchester, J.K., Semenkovich, C.F., Gordon, J.I., 2007. Mechanisms underlying the resistance to diet-induced obesity in germ-free mice. Proc. Natl. Acad. Sci. USA 104, 979–984.

Baker, D.G., 1998. Natural pathogens of laboratory mice, rats, and rabbits and their effects on research. Clin. Microbiol. Rev. 11, 231–266.

Balish, E., Warner, T., 2002. *Enterococcus faecalis* induces inflammatory bowel disease in interleukin-10 knockout mice. Am. J. Pathol. 160, 2253–2257.

Barc, M.C., Bourlioux, F., Rigottier-Gois, L., Charrin-Sarnel, C., Janoir, C., Boureau, H., et al., 2004. Effect of amoxicillin-clavulanic acid on human fecal flora in a gnotobiotic mouse model assessed with fluorescence hybridization using group-specific 16S rRNA probes in combination with flow cytometry. Antimicrob. Agents. Chemother 48, 1365–1368.

Barrett Jr., J.P., 1959. Sterilizing agents for Lobund flexible film apparatus. Proc. Anim. Care Panel 9, 127–133.

Bengmark, S., 2013. Gut microbiota, immune development and function. Pharmacol. Res. 69, 87–113.

Berube, R., Oxborrow, G.S., Gaustad, J.W., 2001. Sterility testing: validation of sterilization processes and sporicide testing. In: Block, S.S. (Ed.), Disinfection, Sterilization, and Preservation, fifth ed. Lippincott Williams & Wilkins, Philadelphia, PA, pp. 1361–1372.

Bibiloni, R., Simon, M.A., Albright, C., Sartor, B., Tannock, G.W., 2005. Analysis of the large bowel microbiota of colitic mice using PCR/DGGE. Lett. Appl. Microbiol. 41, 45–51.

Block, S.S., 2001. Peroxygen compounds. In: Block, S.S. (Ed.), Disinfection, Sterilization and Preservation, fifth ed. Lippincott Williams & Wilkins, Philadelphia, PA, pp. 185–204.

Bohn, E., Bechtold, O., Zahir, N., Frick, J.S., Reimann, J., Jilge, B., et al., 2006. Host gene expression in the colon of gnotobiotic interleukin-2-deficient mice colonized with commensal colitogenic or noncolitogenic bacterial strains: common patterns and bacteria strain specific signatures. Inflamm. Bowel. Dis. 12, 853–862.

Bultman, S.J., 2014. Emerging roles of the microbiome in cancer. Carcinogenesis 35, 249–255.

Caesar, R., Fak, F., Backhed, F., 2010. Effects of gut microbiota on obesity and atherosclerosis via modulation of inflammation and lipid metabolism. J. Intern. Med. 268, 320–328.

Caesar, R., Reigstad, C.S., Backhed, H.K., Reinhardt, C., Ketonen, M., Lunden, G.O., et al., 2012. Gut-derived lipopolysaccharide augments adipose macrophage accumulation but is not essential for impaired glucose or insulin tolerance in mice. Gut 61, 1701–1707.

Cahenzli, J., Koller, Y., Wyss, M., Geuking, M.B., McCoy, K.D., 2013. Intestinal microbial diversity during early-life colonization shapes long-term IgE levels. Cell Host Microbe. 14, 559–570.

Cahill, R.J., Foltz, C.J., Fox, J.G., Dangler, C.A., Powrie, F., Schauer, D.B., 1997. Inflammatory bowel disease: an immunity-mediated

condition triggered by bacterial infection with *Helicobacter hepaticus*. Infect. Immun. 65, 3126–3131.

Cani, P.D., Delzenne, N.M., 2009. Interplay between obesity and associated metabolic disorders: new insights into the gut microbiota. Curr. Opin. Pharmacol. 9, 737–743.

Cani, P.D., Amar, J., Iglesias, M.A., Poggi, M., Knauf, C., Bastelica, D., et al., 2007. Metabolic endotoxemia initiates obesity and insulin resistance. Diabetes 56, 1761–1772.

Cani, P.D., Bibiloni, R., Knauf, C., Waget, A., Neyrinck, A.M., Delzenne, N.M., et al., 2008. Changes in gut microbiota control metabolic endotoxemia-induced inflammation in high-fat diet-induced obesity and diabetes in mice. Diabetes 57, 1470–1481.

Cani, P.D., Osto, M., Geurts, L., Everard, A., 2012. Involvement of gut microbiota in the development of low-grade inflammation and type 2 diabetes associated with obesity. Gut Microbes 3, 279–288.

Caporaso, J.G., Lauber, C.L., Walters, W.A., Berg-Lyons, D., Lozupone, C.A., Turnbaugh, P.J., et al., 2011. Global patterns of 16S rRNA diversity at a depth of millions of sequences per sample. Proc. Natl. Acad. Sci. USA 108 (Suppl. 1), 4516–4522.

Carlisle, E.M., Morowitz, M.J., 2013. The intestinal microbiome and necrotizing enterocolitis. Curr. Opin. Pediatr. 25, 382–387.

Carter, P.B., Foster, H.L., 2005. Gnotobiotics. In: Suckow, M.A., Weisbroth, S.H., Franklin, C.L. (Eds.), The Laboratory Rat, second ed. Elsevier Academic Press, San Diego, CA, pp. 693–710.

Caulfield, C.D., Cassidy, J.P., Kelly, J.P., 2008. Effects of gamma irradiation and pasteurization on the nutritive composition of commercially available animal diets. J. Am. Assoc. Lab. Anim. Sci. 47, 61–66.

Charles, R.T., Stevenson, D.E., Walker, A.I., 1965. The sterilisation of laboratory animal diet by ethylene oxide. Lab. Anim. Care 15, 321–324.

Cherbuy, C., Honvo-Houeto, E., Bruneau, A., Bridonneau, C., Mayeur, C., Duee, P.H., et al., 2010. Microbiota matures colonic epithelium through a coordinated induction of cell cycle-related proteins in gnotobiotic rat. Am. J. Physiol. Gastrointest. Liver Physiol. 299, G348–G357.

Chu, H., Mazmanian, S.K., 2013. Innate immune recognition of the microbiota promotes host–microbial symbiosis. Nat. Immunol. 14, 668–675.

Clough, G., Wallace, J., Gamble, M.R., Merryweather, E.R., Bailey, E., 1995. A positive, individually ventilated caging system: a local barrier system to protect both animals and personnel. Lab. Anim. 29, 139–151.

Coates, M.E., Gustafsson, B.E. (Eds.), 1984. Laboratory Animal Handbooks 9. The Germ-Free Animal in Biomedical Research. Laboratory Animals Ltd., London.

Coles, T., 1998. Isolation Technology: A Practical Guide. Interpharm Press, Inc., Buffalo Grove, IL.

Corpet, D.E., Lumeau, S., Corpet, F., 1989. Minimum antibiotic levels for selecting a resistance plasmid in a gnotobiotic animal model. Antimicrob. Agents. Chemother. 33, 535–540.

Dennis, E.D., Matthews, P.J., Jensen, M.T., 1985. Ambient pressure ethylene-oxide sterilization of flexible film germ free isolators. Prog. Clin. Biol. Res. 181, 69–72.

DeSantis, T.Z., Brodie, E.L., Moberg, J.P., Zubieta, I.X., Piceno, Y.M., Andersen, G.L., 2007. High-density universal 16S rRNA microarray analysis reveals broader diversity than typical clone library when sampling the environment. Microb. Ecol. 53, 371–383.

Dewhirst, F.E., Chien, C.C., Paster, B.J., Ericson, R.L., Orcutt, R.P., Schauer, D.B., et al., 1999. Phylogeny of the defined murine microbiota: altered Schaedler flora. Appl. Environ. Microbiol. 65, 3287–3292.

Dianda, L., Hanby, A.M., Wright, N.A., Sebesteny, A., Hayday, A.C., Owen, M.J., 1997. T cell receptor-alpha beta-deficient mice fail to develop colitis in the absence of a microbial environment. Am. J. Pathol. 150, 91–97.

Dubos, R., Schaedler, R.W., Costello, R., Hoet, P., 1965. Indigenous, normal, and autochthonous flora of the gastrointestinal tract. J. Exp. Med. 122, 67–76.

Dubos, R.J., Schaedler, R.W., 1962. The effect of diet on the fecal bacterial flora of mice and on their resistance to infection. J. Exp. Med. 115, 1161–1172.

Duca, F.A., Sakar, Y., Lepage, P., Devime, F., Langelier, B., Dore, J., et al., 2014. Replication of obesity and associated signaling pathways through transfer of microbiota from obese-prone rats. Diabetes 63, 1624–1636.

Elson, C.O., Cong, Y., 2012. Host–microbiota interactions in inflammatory bowel disease. Gut Microbes 3, 332–344.

Espigares, E., Bueno, A., Fernandez-Crehuet, M., Espigares, M., 2003. Efficacy of some neutralizers in suspension tests determining the activity of disinfectants. J. Hosp. Infect. 55, 137–140.

Everard, A., Belzer, C., Geurts, L., Ouwerkerk, J.P., Druart, C., Bindels, L.B., et al., 2013. Cross-talk between *Akkermansia muciniphila* and intestinal epithelium controls diet-induced obesity. Proc. Natl. Acad. Sci. USA 110, 9066–9071.

Faith, J.J., Rey, F.E., O'Donnell, D., Karlsson, M., McNulty, N.P., Kallstrom, G., et al., 2010. Creating and characterizing communities of human gut microbes in gnotobiotic mice. ISME J. 4, 1094–1098.

Fei, N., Zhao, L., 2013. An opportunistic pathogen isolated from the gut of an obese human causes obesity in germfree mice. ISME J. 7, 880–884.

Foster, H.L., 1959. A procedure for obtaining nucleus stock for a pathogen-free animal colony. Proc. Anim. Care Panel 9, 135–142.

Foster, H.L., 1980. Gnotobiology. In: Baker, H.J., Lindsey, J.R., Weisbroth, S.H. (Eds.), The Laboratory Rat. Vol. II. Research Applications. Academic Press, New York, pp. 43–57.

Fuller, R., 1984. Microbiological monitoring of gnotobiotic isolators. In: Coates, M.E., Gustafsson, B.E. (Eds.), The Germ-Free Animal in Biomedical Research. Laboratory Animals Ltd., London, pp. 111–116.

Garrett, W.S., Gallini, C.A., Yatsunenko, T., Michaud, M., DuBois, A., Delaney, M.L., et al., 2010. Enterobacteriaceae act in concert with the gut microbiota to induce spontaneous and maternally transmitted colitis. Cell. Host. Microbe. 8, 292–300.

Ge, Z., Feng, Y., Taylor, N.S., Ohtani, M., Polz, M.F., Schauer, D.B., et al., 2006. Colonization dynamics of altered Schaedler flora is influenced by gender, aging, and *Helicobacter hepaticus* infection in the intestines of Swiss Webster mice. Appl. Environ. Microbiol. 72, 5100–5103.

Gibson, H., Elton, R., Peters, W., Holah, J.T., 1995. Surface and suspension testing: conflict or complementary. Int. Biodeterior. Biodegrad. 36, 375–384.

Golde, W.T., Gollobin, P., Rodriguez, L.L., 2005. A rapid, simple, and humane method for submandibular bleeding of mice using a lancet. Lab. Anim. (NY) 34, 39–43.

Gordon, H.A., 1960. The germ-free animal. Its use in the study of "physiologic" effects of the normal microbial flora on the animal host. Am. J. Dig. Dis. 5, 841–867.

Gordon, J.H., Dubos, R., 1970. The anaerobic bacterial flora of the mouse cecum. J. Exp. Med. 132, 251–260.

Grishin, A., Papillon, S., Bell, B., Wang, J., Ford, H.R., 2013. The role of the intestinal microbiota in the pathogenesis of necrotizing enterocolitis. Semin. Pediatr. Surg. 22, 69–75.

Gustafsson, B.E., 1947. Germ-free rearing of rats. Preliminary report. Acta Anat. (Basel) 2, 376–391.

Gustafsson, B.E., 1948. Germfree rearing of rats. Acta Pathol. Microbiol. Scand. 73 (Suppl), 1–130.

Halls, N., 1992. The microbiology of irradiation sterilization. Med. Device. Technol. 3, 37–45.

Hansen, C.H., Nielsen, D.S., Kverka, M., Zakostelska, Z., Klimesova, K., Hudcovic, T., et al., 2012. Patterns of early gut colonization shape future immune responses of the host. PLoS One 7, e34043.

Hanson, J.M., Shaffer, H.L., 2001. Sterilization and preservation by radiation sterilization. In: Block, S.S. (Ed.), Disinfection, Sterilization and Preservation, fifth ed. Lippincott Williams & Wilkins, Philadelphia, PA, pp. 729–746.

Hara, N., Alkanani, A.K., Ir, D., Robertson, C.E., Wagner, B.D., Frank, D.N., et al., 2013. The role of the intestinal microbiota in type 1 diabetes. Clin. Immunol. 146, 112–119.

Hartmann, L., Taras, D., Kamlage, B., Blaut, M., 2000. A new technique to determine hydrogen excreted by gnotobiotic rats. Lab. Anim. 34, 162–170.

Hirayama, K., 1999. Ex-germfree mice harboring intestinal microbiota derived from other animal species as an experimental model for ecology and metabolism of intestinal bacteria. Exp. Anim. 48, 219–227.

Hirayama, K., Miyaji, K., Kawamura, S., Itoh, K., Takahashi, E., Mitsuoka, T., 1995. Development of intestinal flora of human-flora-associated (HFA) mice in the intestine of their offspring. Exp. Anim. 44, 219–222.

Hirayama, K., Uetsuka, K., Kuwabara, Y., Tamura, M., Itoh, K., 2007. Vitamin K deficiency of germfree mice caused by feeding standard purified diet sterilized by gamma-irradiation. Exp. Anim. 56, 273–278.

Hogan, B., Beddington, R., Constantini, F., Lacy, E., 1994. Manipulating the Mouse Embryo: A Laboratory Manual, second ed. Cold Spring Harbor Press, New York.

Hooper, L.V., Wong, M.H., Thelin, A., Hansson, L., Falk, P.G., Gordon, J.I., 2001. Molecular analysis of commensal host–microbial relationships in the intestine. Science 291, 881–884.

Hooper, L.V., Midtvedt, T., Gordon, J.I., 2002. How host–microbial interactions shape the nutrient environment of the mammalian intestine. Annu. Rev. Nutr. 22, 283–307.

Hooper, L.V., Littman, D.R., Macpherson, A.J., 2012. Interactions between the microbiota and the immune system. Science 336, 1268–1273.

Hudcovic, T., Kozakova, H., Kolinska, J., Stepankova, R., Hrncir, T., Tlaskalova-Hogenova, H., 2009. Monocolonization with *Bacteroides ovatus* protects immunodeficient SCID mice from mortality in chronic intestinal inflammation caused by long-lasting dextran sodium sulfate treatment. Physiol. Res. 58, 101–110.

Humphreys, P.N., 2011. Testing standards for sporicides. J. Hosp. Infect. 77, 193–198.

Hyman, R.W., Fukushima, M., Jiang, H., Fung, E., Rand, L., Johnson, B., et al., 2013. Diversity of the vaginal microbiome correlates with preterm birth. Reprod. Sci. 21, 32–40.

Institute of Laboratory Animal Resources, National Research Council, 1970. Gnotobiotes. Standards and Guidelines for the Breeding, Care, and Management of Laboratory Animals: A Report. National Academies Press, Washington, DC.

Inzunza, J., Midtvedt, T., Fartoo, M., Norin, E., Osterlund, E., Persson, A.K., et al., 2005. Germfree status of mice obtained by embryo transfer in an isolator environment. Lab. Anim. 39, 421–427.

Ivanov, I.I., Atarashi, K., Manel, N., Brodie, E.L., Shima, T., Karaoz, U., et al., 2009. Induction of intestinal Th17 cells by segmented filamentous bacteria. Cell 139, 485–498.

Jackson, I.J., Abbott, C.M., 2000. Mouse Genetics and Transgenics. A Practical Approach. Oxford University Press, Oxford.

Jeng, D.K., Woodworth, A.G., 1990. Chlorine dioxide gas sterilization under square-wave conditions. Appl. Environ. Microbiol. 56, 514–519.

Jergens, A.E., Dorn, A., Wilson, J., Dingbaum, K., Henderson, A., Liu, Z., et al., 2006. Induction of differential immune reactivity to members of the flora of gnotobiotic mice following colonization with *Helicobacter bilis* or *Brachyspira hyodysenteriae*. Microb. Infect. 8, 1602–1610.

Jergens, A.E., Wilson-Welder, J.H., Dorn, A., Henderson, A., Liu, Z., Evans, R.B., et al., 2007. *Helicobacter bilis* triggers persistent immune reactivity to antigens derived from the commensal bacteria in gnotobiotic C3H/HeN mice. Gut 56, 934–940.

Jiang, H.Q., Kushnir, N., Thurnheer, M.C., Bos, N.A., Cebra, J.J., 2002. Monoassociation of SCID mice with *Helicobacter muridarum*, but not four other enterics, provokes IBD upon receipt of T cells. Gastroenterology 122, 1346–1354.

Joslyn, L.J., 2001. Gaseous chemical sterilization. In: Block, S.S. (Ed.), Disinfection, Sterilization and Preservation, fifth ed. Lippincott Williams & Wilkins, Philadelphia, PA, pp. 337–359.

Kallus, S.J., Brandt, L.J., 2012. The intestinal microbiota and obesity. J. Clin. Gastroenterol. 46, 16–24.

Kamada, N., Nunez, G., 2013. Role of the gut microbiota in the development and function of lymphoid cells. J. Immunol. 190, 1389–1395.

Kamada, N., Seo, S.U., Chen, G.Y., Nunez, G., 2013. Role of the gut microbiota in immunity and inflammatory disease. Nat. Rev. Immunol. 13, 321–335.

Karlsson, F.H., Fak, F., Nookaew, I., Tremaroli, V., Fagerberg, B., Petranovic, D., et al., 2012. Symptomatic atherosclerosis is associated with an altered gut metagenome. Nat. Commun. 3, 1245.

Kim, J.H., 2014. Necrotizing enterocolitis: the road to zero. Semin. Fetal Neonatal. Med. 19, 39–44.

Kim, O.S., Cho, Y.J., Lee, K., Yoon, S.H., Kim, M., Na, H., et al., 2012. Introducing EzTaxon-e: a prokaryotic 16S rRNA gene sequence database with phylotypes that represent uncultured species. Int. J. Syst. Evol. Microbiol. 62, 716–721.

Kim, S.C., Tonkonogy, S.L., Albright, C.A., Tsang, J., Balish, E.J., Braun, J., et al., 2005. Variable phenotypes of enterocolitis in interleukin 10-deficient mice monoassociated with two different commensal bacteria. Gastroenterology 128, 891–906.

Kim, S.C., Tonkonogy, S.L., Karrasch, T., Jobin, C., Sartor, R.B., 2007. Dual-association of gnotobiotic Il-10−/−mice with 2 nonpathogenic commensal bacteria induces aggressive pancolitis. Inflamm. Bowel Dis., 1457–1466.

Klaasen, H.L., Van der Heijden, P.J., Stok, W., Poelma, F.G., Koopman, J.P., Van den Brink, M.E., et al., 1993. Apathogenic, intestinal, segmented, filamentous bacteria stimulate the mucosal immune system of mice. Infect. Immun. 61, 303–306.

Knapp, J.E., Battisti, D.L., 2001. Chlorine dioxide. In: Block, S.S. (Ed.), Disinfection, Sterilization and Preservation, fifth ed. Lippincott Williams & Wilkins, Philadelphia, PA, pp. 215–227.

Kuhn, R., Lohler, J., Rennick, D., Rajewsky, K., Muller, W., 1993. Interleukin-10-deficient mice develop chronic enterocolitis. Cell 75, 263–274.

Lee, A., Gordon, J., Dubos, R., 1968. Enumeration of the oxygen sensitive bacteria usually present in the intestine of healthy mice. Nature 220, 1137–1139.

Lee, A., Gordon, J., Lee, C.J., Dubos, R., 1971. The mouse intestinal microflora with emphasis on the strict anaerobes. J. Exp. Med. 133, 339–352.

Ley, F.J., Bleby, J., Coates, M.E., Paterson, J.S., 1969. Sterilization of laboratory animal diets using gamma radiation. Lab. Anim. 3, 221–254.

Ley, R.E., 2010. Obesity and the human microbiome. Curr. Opin. Gastroenterol. 26, 5–11.

Ley, R.E., Backhed, F., Turnbaugh, P., Lozupone, C.A., Knight, R.D., Gordon, J.I., 2005. Obesity alters gut microbial ecology. Proc. Natl. Acad. Sci. USA 102, 11070–11075.

Ley, R.E., Turnbaugh, P.J., Klein, S., Gordon, J.I., 2006. Microbial ecology: human gut microbes associated with obesity. Nature 444, 1022–1023.

Lindsey, J.R., Baker, H.J., 2005. Historical foundations. In: Suckow, M.A., Weisbroth, S.H., Franklin, C.L. (Eds.), The Laboratory Rat. Elsevier Academic Press, San Diego, CA, pp. 1–52.

Liou, A.P., Paziuk, M., Luevano Jr., J.M., Machineni, S., Turnbaugh, P.J., Kaplan, L.M., 2013. Conserved shifts in the gut microbiota due to gastric bypass reduce host weight and adiposity. Sci. Transl. Med. 5 178ra41.

Liu, Z., Cao, A.T., Cong, Y., 2013. Microbiota regulation of inflammatory bowel disease and colorectal cancer. Semin. Cancer Biol. 23, 543–552.

Lorenz, R.G., McCracken, V.J., Elson, C.O., 2005. Animal models of intestinal inflammation: ineffective communication between coalition members. Springer Semin. Immunopathol. 27, 233–247.

Luckey, T.D., 1963. Germfree Life and Gnotobiology. Academic Press, New York.

Mabrok, H.B., Klopfleisch, R., Ghanem, K.Z., Clavel, T., Blaut, M., Loh, G., 2012. Lignan transformation by gut bacteria lowers tumor burden in a gnotobiotic rat model of breast cancer. Carcinogenesis 33, 203–208.

Malchesky, P.S., 2001. Medical applications of peracetic acid. In: Block, S.S. (Ed.), Disinfection, Sterilization and Preservation, fifth ed. Lippincott Williams & Wilkins, Philadelphia, PA, pp. 979–996.

Manco, M., Putignani, L., Bottazzo, G.F., 2010. Gut microbiota, lipopolysaccharides, and innate immunity in the pathogenesis of obesity and cardiovascular risk. Endocr. Rev. 31, 817–844.

Marcobal, A., Kashyap, P.C., Nelson, T.A., Aronov, P.A., Donia, M.S., Spormann, A., et al., 2013. A metabolomic view of how the human gut microbiota impacts the host metabolome using humanized and gnotobiotic mice. ISME J. 7, 1933–1943.

Matsumoto, T., Ando, K., Koike, S., 1988. Significance of bacterial flora in abdominal irradiation-induced inhibition of lung metastases. Cancer. Res. 48, 3031–3034.

McDonnell, G.E., 2007. Antisepsis, Disinfection, and Sterilization: Types, Action, and Resistance. ASM Press, Washington, DC.

Mendelsohn, A.R., Larrick, J., 2013. Dietary modification of the microbiome affects risk for cardiovascular disease. Rejuvenation Res. 16, 241–244.

Momose, Y., Park, S.H., Miyamoto, Y., Itoh, K., 2011. Design of species-specific oligonucleotide probes for the detection of Bacteroides and Parabacteroides by fluorescence in situ hybridization and their application to the analysis of mouse caecal Bacteroides–Parabacteroides microbiota. J. Appl. Microbiol. 111, 176–184.

Moran, J.P., Walter, J., Tannock, G.W., Tonkonogy, S.L., Sartor, R.B., 2009. *Bifidobacterium animalis* causes extensive duodenitis and mild colonic inflammation in monoassociated interleukin-10-deficient mice. Inflamm. Bowel. Dis. 15, 1022–1031.

Musso, G., Gambino, R., Cassader, M., 2011. Interactions between gut microbiota and host metabolism predisposing to obesity and diabetes. Annu. Rev. Med. 62, 361–380.

Mwangi, W.N., Beal, R.K., Powers, C., Wu, X., Humphrey, T., Watson, M., et al., 2010. Regional and global changes in TCRalphabeta T cell repertoires in the gut are dependent upon the complexity of the enteric microflora. Dev. Comp. Immunol. 34, 406–417.

Okamoto, M., Matsumoto, T., 1999. Production of germfree mice by embryo transfer. Exp. Anim. 48, 59–62.

Orcutt, R.F., 2006a. A brief history of the use of microfloras in gnotobiotic rodents. Taconic Tech. Libr. [online]. Available at: <http://www.taconic.com/wmspage.cfm?parm1=290> (accessed 30.09.13).

Orcutt, R.F., 2006b. Culturing members of the altered Schaedler flora from stock vials. Taconic Tech. Libr. [online]. Available at: <http://www.taconic.com/wmspage.cfm%3Fparm1=288> (accessed 03.01.14).

Orcutt, R.F., 2006c. Protocols for colonizing axenic rodents with the altered Schaedler flora (ASF). Taconic Tech. Libr. [online]. Available at: <http://www.taconic.com/wmspage.cfm?parm1=289> (accessed 02.07.13).

Orcutt, R.F., Otis, A.P., Alliger, H., 1981. Alcide: an alternative sterilant to peracetic acid. In: Sasaki, S., Ozawa, A., Hashimoto, K. (Eds.), Recent Advances in Germfree Research. Proceedings of the VIIth International Symposium on Gnotobiology. Tokyo University Press, Tokyo, Japan, pp. 79–81.

Orcutt, R.P., Gianni, F.J., Judge, R.J., 1987. Development of an "Altered Schaedler Flora" for NCI gnotobiotic rodents. Microecol. Ther. 17, 59.

Ou, J., Carbonero, F., Zoetendal, E.G., Delany, J.P., Wang, M., Newton, K., et al., 2013. Diet, microbiota, and microbial metabolites in colon cancer risk in rural Africans and African Americans. Am. J. Clin. Nutr. 98, 111–120.

Packey, C.D., Shanahan, M.T., Manick, S., Bower, M.A., Ellermann, M., Tonkonogy, S.L., et al., 2013. Molecular detection of bacterial contamination in gnotobiotic rodent units. Gut Microbes 4, 361–370.

Pallares, P., Gonzalez-Bulnes, A., 2009. A new method for induction and synchronization of oestrus and fertile ovulations in mice by using exogenous hormones. Lab. Anim. 43, 295–299.

Park, S.H., Itoh, K., 2005. Species-specific oligonucleotide probes for the detection and identification of Lactobacillus isolated from mouse faeces. J. Appl. Microbiol. 99, 51–57.

Paterson, J.S., Cook, R., 1971. Utilization of diets sterilized by gamma irradiation for germfree and specific-pathogen-free laboratory animals, in Defining The Laboratory Animal. IV Symposium, International Committee on Laboratory Animals. Organized by the International Committee on Laboratory Animals and the Institute of Laboratory Animal Resources, National Research Council. National Academy of Sciences, Washington, DC, pp. 586–596.

Pell-Walpole, C., Waller, M., 1984. Effective sterilization of a plastic film rack isolator with 'Alcide.' Lab. Anim. 18, 349–350.

Peloquin, J.M., Nguyen, D.D., 2013. The microbiota and inflammatory bowel disease: insights from animal models. Anaerobe 24, 102–106.

Perkins, J.J., 1969. Principles and Methods of Sterilization in Health Sciences, second ed. Charles C Thomas, Springfield, IL.

Pleasants, J.R., 1959. Rearing germfree cesarean-born rats, mice, and rabbits through weaning. Ann. N Y Acad. Sci. 78, 116–126.

Pleasants, J.R., 1974. Gnotobiotics In: Melby Jr., E.C. Altman, N.H. (Eds.), Handbook of Laboratory Animal Science, vol. I. CRC Press, Cleveland, OH, pp. 119–174.

Plottel, C.S., Blaser, M.J., 2011. Microbiome and malignancy. Cell Host Microbe. 10, 324–335.

Podolsky, D.K., 1997. Lessons from genetic models of inflammatory bowel disease. Acta Gastroenterol. Belg. 60, 163–165.

Purchiaroni, F., Tortora, A., Gabrielli, M., Bertucci, F., Gigante, G., Ianiro, G., et al., 2013. The role of intestinal microbiota and the immune system. Eur. Rev. Med. Pharmacol. Sci. 17, 323–333.

Qin, J., Li, R., Raes, J., Arumugam, M., Burgdorf, K.S., Manichanh, C., et al., 2010. A human gut microbial gene catalogue established by metagenomic sequencing. Nature 464, 59–65.

Rabot, S., Membrez, M., Bruneau, A., Gerard, P., Harach, T., Moser, M., et al., 2010. Germ-free C57BL/6J mice are resistant to high-fat-diet-induced insulin resistance and have altered cholesterol metabolism. FASEB J. 24, 4948–4959.

Rahija, R.J., 2007. Gnotobiotics. In: Fox, J.G., Barthold, S., Davisson, M.T., Newcomer, C.E., Quimby, F.W., Smith, A. (Eds.), The Mouse in Biomedical Research, Vol. 3: Normative Biology, Husbandry, and Models, second ed. Academic Press, New York, pp. 217–233.

Rath, H.C., Herfarth, H.H., Ikeda, J.S., Grenther, W.B., Hamm, T.E.J., Balish, E., et al., 1996. Normal luminal bacteria, especially Bacteroides species, mediate chronic colitis, gastritis, and arthritis in HLA-B27/human beta2 microglobulin transgenic rats. J. Clin. Invest. 98, 945–953.

Rath, H.C., Wilson, K.H., Sartor, R.B., 1999. Differential induction of colitis and gastritis in HLA-B27 transgenic rats selectively colonized with Bacteroides vulgatus or Escherichia coli. Infect. Immun. 67, 2969–2974.

Respondek, F., Gerard, P., Bossis, M., Boschat, L., Bruneau, A., Rabot, S., et al., 2013. Short-chain fructo-oligosaccharides modulate intestinal microbiota and metabolic parameters of humanized gnotobiotic diet induced obesity mice. PLoS One 8, e71026.

Reyniers, J.A., Trexler, P.C., Ervin, R.F., 1946. Rearing Germfree Albino Rats: Lobund Report 1. University of Notre Dame Press, Notre Dame, IN.

Reyniers, J.A., Sacksteder, M.R., Ashburn, L.L., 1964. Multiple tumors in female germfree inbred albino mice exposed to bedding treated with ethylene oxide. J. Natl. Cancer Inst. 32, 1045–1057.

Ridaura, V.K., Faith, J.J., Rey, F.E., Cheng, J., Duncan, A.E., Kau, A.L., et al., 2013. Gut microbiota from twins discordant for obesity modulate metabolism in mice. Science 341, 1241214.

Robertson, B.R., O'Rourke, J.L., Neilan, B.A., Vandamme, P., On, S.L., Fox, J.G., et al., 2005. Mucispirillum schaedleri gen. nov., sp. nov., a spiral-shaped bacterium colonizing the mucus layer of the gastrointestinal tract of laboratory rodents. Int. J. Syst. Evol. Microbiol 55, 1199–1204.

Robison, R.A., 2012. Efficacy v. B. subtilis endospores [online]. Available at: <http://www.stericleanway.com/app/download/756045273/Efficacy+v.+B.+subtilis+endospores.pdf> (accessed 30.12.13).

Roesch, P.L., 2012. Microbial monitoring of GF isolators 2013 [online]. Available at: <http://www.taconic.com/user-assets/Documents/Media/Validating_Equipment_and_Supplies_4262013.pdf> (accessed 02.01.14).

Round, J.L., Mazmanian, S.K., 2010. Inducible Foxp3+ regulatory T-cell development by a commensal bacterium of the intestinal microbiota. Proc. Natl. Acad. Sci. USA 107, 12204–12209.

Rutala, W.A., Cole, E.C., Wannamaker, N.S., Weber, D.J., 1991. Inactivation of Mycobacterium tuberculosis and Mycobacterium bovis by 14 hospital disinfectants. Am. J. Med. 91, 267S–271S.

Rutala, W.A., Weber, D.J., Weinstein, R.A., Siegel, J.D., Pearson, M.L., Chinn, R.Y.W., et al., 2008. Guideline for disinfection and sterilization in healthcare facilities. Centers for Disease Control and Prevention, Atlanta, GA.

Sagripanti, J.L., Bonifacino, A., 1999. Bacterial spores survive treatment with commercial sterilants and disinfectants. Appl. Environ. Microbiol. 65, 4255–4260.

Sagripanti, J.L., Bonifacino, A., 2000. Resistance of Pseudomonas aeruginosa to liquid disinfectants on contaminated surfaces before formation of biofilms. J. AOAC Int. 83, 1415–1422.

Sarma-Rupavtarm, R.B., Ge, Z., Schauer, D.B., Fox, J.G., Polz, M.F., 2004. Spatial distribution and stability of the eight microbial species of the altered Schaedler flora in the mouse gastrointestinal tract. Appl. Environ. Microbiol. 70, 2791–2800.

Sartor, R.B., 2005. Role of commensal enteric bacteria in the pathogenesis of immune-mediated intestinal inflammation: lessons from animal models and implications for translational research. J. Pediatr. Gastroenterol. Nutr. 40 (Suppl. 1), S30–S31.

Savage, D.C., 1977. Microbial ecology of the gastrointestinal tract. Annu. Rev. Microbiol. 31, 107–133.

sBioMed, 2013a. Steriplex® SD Activated Solution EPA Claims Sheet [online]. Available at: <http://www.stericleanway.com/app/download/756045246/Activated+Solution+EPA+Claims+Sheet.pdf> (accessed 30.12.13).

sBioMed, 2013b. Steriplex® SD DNA Decon [online]. Available at: <http://www.steriplex.com/pdf/STERIPLEX%20SD%20DNA%20DECON.pdf> (accessed 30.12.13).

sBioMed, 2013c. Steriplex® SD Efficacy: Disinfecting [online]. Available at: <http://www.steriplex.com/products/steriplex_sd_sporicide_efficacy_disinfecting.php#.UsGY7bQgrHs> (accessed 30.12.13).

Schaedler, R.W., Dubos, R., Costello, R., 1965a. Association of germfree mice with bacteria isolated from normal mice. J. Exp. Med. 122, 77–82.

Schaedler, R.W., Dubos, R., Costello, R., 1965b. The development of the bacterial flora in the gastrointestinal tract of mice. J. Exp. Med. 122, 59–66.

Schaedler, R.W., Orcutt, R.P., 1983. Gastrointestinal microflora. In: Foster, H.L., Small, J.D., Fox, J.G. (Eds.), The Mouse in Biomedical Research. Vol. III. Normative Biology, Immunology, and Husbandry. Academic Press, Inc., New York, pp. 327–345.

Sedlacek, R.S., Rose, E.F., 1985. Steam quality and effective sterilization. Prog. Clin. Biol. Res. 181, 65–68.

Seki, E., Schnabl, B., 2012. Role of innate immunity and the microbiota in liver fibrosis: crosstalk between the liver and gut. J. Physiol. 590, 447–458.

Sellon, R.K., Tonkonogy, S., Schultz, M., Dieleman, L.A., Grenther, W., Balish, E., et al., 1998. Resident enteric bacteria are necessary for development of spontaneous colitis and immune system activation in interleukin-10-deficient mice. Infect. Immun. 66, 5224–5231.

Selwyn, M.R., Shek, W.R., 1994. Sample sizes and frequency of testing for health monitoring in barrier rooms and isolators. Contemp. Top. Lab. Anim. Sci. 33, 56–60.

Shapira, I., Sultan, K., Lee, A., Taioli, E., 2013. Evolving concepts: how diet and the intestinal microbiome act as modulators of breast malignancy. ISRN Oncol., 693920.

Shimizu, K., Muranaka, Y., Fujimura, R., Ishida, H., Tazume, S., Shimamura, T., 1998. Normalization of reproductive function in germfree mice following bacterial contamination. Exp. Anim. 47, 151–158.

Sjogren, K., Engdahl, C., Henning, P., Lerner, U.H., Tremaroli, V., Lagerquist, M.K., et al., 2012. The gut microbiota regulates bone mass in mice. J. Bone Miner. Res. 27, 1357–1367.

Snel, J., Heinen, P.P., Blok, H.J., Carman, R.J., Duncan, A.J., Allen, P.C., et al., 1995. Comparison of 16S rRNA sequences of segmented filamentous bacteria isolated from mice, rats, and chickens and proposal of "Candidatus Arthromitus." Int. J. Syst. Bacteriol. 45, 780–782.

Sommer, F., Backhed, F., 2013. The gut microbiota – masters of host development and physiology. Nat. Rev. Microbiol. 11, 227–238.

Sontakke, S., Cadenas, M.B., Maggi, R.G., Diniz, P.P., Breitschwerdt, E.B., 2009. Use of broad range16S rDNA PCR in clinical microbiology. J. Microbiol. Methods 76, 217–225.

Springthorpe, V.S., Sattar, S.A., 2005. Carrier tests to assess microbicidal activities of chemical disinfectants for use on medical devices and environmental surfaces. J. AOAC Int. 88, 182–201.

Stehr, M., Greweling, M.C., Tischer, S., Singh, M., Blocker, H., Monner, D.A., et al., 2009. Charles River altered Schaedler flora (CRASF) remained stable for four years in a mouse colony housed in individually ventilated cages. Lab. Anim. 43, 362–370.

Stepankova, R., Powrie, F., Kofronova, O., Kozakova, H., Hudcovic, T., Hrncir, T., et al., 2007. Segmented filamentous bacteria in a defined bacterial cocktail induce intestinal inflammation in SCID mice reconstituted with CD45RBhigh CD4+ T cells. Inflamm. Bowel. Dis. 13, 1202–1211.

Sutton, S.V., Proud, D.W., Rachui, S., Brannan, D.K., 2002. Validation of microbial recovery from disinfectants. PDA J. Pharm. Sci. Technol. 56, 255–266.

Sydora, B.C., Tavernini, M.M., Doyle, J.S., Fedorak, R.N., 2005. Association with selected bacteria does not cause enterocolitis in IL-10 gene-deficient mice despite a systemic immune response. Dig. Dis. Sci. 50, 905–913.

Taconic, 2006. Taconic Germfree Shipper [online]. Available at: <http://www.taconic.com/wmspage.cfm?parm1=301> (accessed 02.01.14).

Talham, G.L., Jiang, H.Q., Bos, N.A., Cebra, J.J., 1999. Segmented filamentous bacteria are potent stimuli of a physiologically normal state of the murine gut mucosal immune system. Infect. Immun. 67, 1992–2000.

Tang, W.H., Wang, Z., Levison, B.S., Koeth, R.A., Britt, E.B., Fu, X., et al., 2013. Intestinal microbial metabolism of phosphatidylcholine and cardiovascular risk. N. Engl. J. Med. 368, 1575–1584.

Taylor, D.M., 1985. Monocontamination of germ-free mice by a fastidious unidentified anaerobe. Lab. Anim. 19, 251–254.

Teah, B.A., 1984. Weighing problems in germfree environment. In: Wostmann, B.S., Pleasants, J.R., Pollard, M., Teah, B.A., Wagner, M. (Eds.), Germfree Research. Microflora Control and Its Application to the Biomedical Sciences. Alan R. Liss, Inc., New York, pp. 59–60.

Terleckyj, B., Axler, D.A., 1987. Quantitative neutralization assay of fungicidal activity of disinfectants. Antimicrob. Agents Chemother. 31, 794–798.

Thorn, R.M., Robinson, G.M., Reynolds, D.M., 2013. Comparative antimicrobial activities of aerosolized sodium hypochlorite, chlorine dioxide, and electrochemically activated solutions evaluated using a novel standardized assay. Antimicrob. Agents Chemother. 57, 2216–2225.

Tremaroli, V., Backhed, F., 2012. Functional interactions between the gut microbiota and host metabolism. Nature 489, 242–249.

Trexler, P.C., 1961. Report of the gnotobiotic workshop for laboratory animal breeders. Proc. Anim. Care Panel 11, 249–253.

Trexler, P.C., 1963. The Design, Development, and Study of Germfree Isolators for use with Patients and in Research. U.S. Department of Defense, Washington, DC.

Trexler, P.C., 1983. Gnotobiotics. In: Foster, H.L., Small, J.D., Fox, J.G. (Eds.), The Mouse in Biomedical Research. Vol. III. Normative Biology, Immunology, and Husbandry. Academic Press, Inc., New York, pp. 1–16.

Trexler, P.C., 1984. Equipment. In: Coates, M.E., Gustafsson, B.E. (Eds.), Laboratory Animal Handbooks 9. The Germ-Free Animal in Biomedical Research. Laboratory Animals Ltd., London, pp. 11–32.

Trexler, P.C., Orcutt, R.P., 1999. Development of gnotobiotics and contamination control in laboratory animal science. In: McPherson, C.W. (Ed.), 50 Years of Laboratory Animal Science. American Association for Laboratory Animal Science, Memphis, TN, pp. 121–128.

Trexler, P.C., Reynolds, L.I., 1957. Flexible film apparatus for the rearing and use of germfree animals. Appl. Microbiol. 5, 406–412.

Turnbaugh, P.J., Ley, R.E., Mahowald, M.A., Magrini, V., Mardis, E.R., Gordon, J.I., 2006. An obesity-associated gut microbiome with increased capacity for energy harvest. Nature 444, 1027–1031.

Turnbaugh, P.J., Ridaura, V.K., Faith, J.J., Rey, F.E., Knight, R., Gordon, J.I., 2009. The effect of diet on the human gut microbiome: a metagenomic analysis in humanized gnotobiotic mice. Sci. Transl. Med. 1, 6ra14.

Umesaki, Y., Okada, Y., Matsumoto, S., Imaoka, A., Setoyama, H., 1995. Segmented filamentous bacteria are indigenous intestinal bacteria that activate intraepithelial lymphocytes and induce MHC class II molecules and fucosyl asialo GM1 glycolipids on the small intestinal epithelial cells in the ex-germ-free mouse. Microbiol. Immunol. 39, 555–562.

Umesaki, Y., Setoyama, H., Matsumoto, S., Imaoka, A., Itoh, K., 1999. Differential roles of segmented filamentous bacteria and clostridia in development of the intestinal immune system. Infect. Immun. 67, 3504–3511.

van der Gulden, W.J., van Erp, A.J., 1972. The effect of paracetic acid as a disinfectant on worm eggs. Lab. Anim. Sci. 22, 225–226.

van Klingeren, B., Koller, W., Bloomfield, S.F., Böhm, R., Cremieux, A., Holah, J., et al., 1998. Assessment of the efficacy of disinfectants on surfaces. Int. Biodeterior. Biodegrad. 41, 289–296.

Vollaard, E.J., Clasener, H.A., 1994. Colonization resistance. Antimicrob. Agents Chemother. 38, 409–414.

Waidmann, M., Bechtold, O., Frick, J.S., Lehr, H.A., Schubert, S., Dobrindt, U., et al., 2003. *Bacteroides vulgatus* protects against *Escherichia coli*-induced colitis in gnotobiotic interleukin-2-deficient mice. Gastroenterology 125, 162–177.

Wang, J., Qi, J., Zhao, H., He, S., Zhang, Y., Wei, S., et al., 2013. Metagenomic sequencing reveals microbiota and its functional potential associated with periodontal disease. Sci. Rep. 3, 1843.

Wannemuehler, M.J., Overstreet, A.M., Ward, D.V., Phillips, G.J., 2014. Draft genome sequences of the altered schaedler flora, a defined bacterial community from gnotobiotic mice. Genome Announc. 2, 1–2.

Weisbroth, S.H., Peters, R., Riley, L.K., Shek, W., 1998. Microbiological assessment of laboratory rats and mice. ILAR J. 39, 272–290.

Weisburg, W.G., Barns, S.M., Pelletier, D.A., Lane, D.J., 1991. 16S ribosomal DNA amplification for phylogenetic study. J. Bacteriol. 173, 697–703.

Whary, M.T., Taylor, N.S., Feng, Y., Ge, Z., Muthupalani, S., Versalovic, J., et al., 2011. *Lactobacillus reuteri* promotes *Helicobacter hepaticus*-associated typhlocolitis in gnotobiotic B6.129P2-IL-10(tm1Cgn) (IL-10(−/−)) mice. Immunology 133, 165–178.

White, W.J., Anderson, L.C., Geistfeld, J., Martin, D.G., 1998. Current strategies for controlling/eliminating opportunistic microorganisms. ILAR J. 39, 291–305.

Wilson, K.H., Brown, R.S., Andersen, G.L., Tsang, J., Sartor, B., 2006. Comparison of fecal biota from specific pathogen free and feral mice. Anaerobe 12, 249–253.

Wos-Oxley, M., Bleich, A., Oxley, A.P., Kahl, S., Janus, L.M., Smoczek, A., et al., 2012. Comparative evaluation of establishing a human gut microbial community within rodent models. Gut Microb. 3, 234–249.

Wostmann, B.S., 1996. Germfree and Gnotobiotic Animal Models: Background and Applications. CRC Press, Boca Raton, FL.

Wrzosek, L., Miquel, S., Noordine, M.L., Bouet, S., Joncquel Chevalier-Curt, M., Robert, V., et al., 2013. *Bacteroides thetaiotaomicron* and *Faecalibacterium prausnitzii* influence the production of mucus glycans and the development of goblet cells in the colonic epithelium of a gnotobiotic model rodent. BMC Biol. 11, 61.

Wu, H.J., Wu, E., 2012. The role of gut microbiota in immune homeostasis and autoimmunity. Gut Microb. 3, 4–14.

Yamanaka, M., Nomura, T., Kametaka, M., 1977. Influence of intestinal microbes on heat production in germ-free, gnotobiotic and conventional mice. J. Nutr. Sci. Vitaminol. (Tokyo) 23, 221–226.

Yoshimoto, S., Loo, T.M., Atarashi, K., Kanda, H., Sato, S., Oyadomari, S., et al., 2013. Obesity-induced gut microbial metabolite promotes liver cancer through senescence secretome. Nature 499, 97–101.

Zhu, Y., Michelle Luo, T., Jobin, C., Young, H.A., 2011. Gut microbiota and probiotics in colon tumorigenesis. Cancer Lett. 309, 119–127.

Zoetendal, E.G., Rajilic-Stojanovic, M., de Vos, W.M., 2008. High-throughput diversity and functionality analysis of the gastrointestinal tract microbiota. Gut 57, 1605–1615.

Zucol, F., Ammann, R.A., Berger, C., Aebi, C., Altwegg, M., Niggli, F.K., et al., 2006. Real-time quantitative broad-range PCR assay for detection of the 16S rRNA gene followed by sequencing for species identification. J. Clin. Microbiol. 44, 2750–2759.

27

Working Safely with Experimental Animals Exposed to Biohazards

James R. Swearengen, DVM, DACLAM, DACVPM^a and
Calvin B. Carpenter, DVM, DACLAM^b

^{a}National Biodefense Analysis and Countermeasures Center, Research Plaza, Fort Detrick, MD, USA
^{b}Animal Resources, Alcon Research Ltd., South Freeway, Fort Worth, TX, USA

I. INTRODUCTION

When the term is used generically, a biological hazard (biohazard) may constitute a variety of hazards that are encountered in an animal facility. It could incorporate such risks as zoonotic diseases inherent to the species of animals being housed, allergens, or experimentally related infectious agents or biological toxins. This chapter will focus on experimentally related infectious agents and toxins of biological origin that are hazardous to both animals and humans and require biological containment

(biocontainment) to prevent their inadvertent release into the environment. Since it is not possible to adequately cover in this chapter all of the topics related to this subject, the authors have concentrated on areas that they consider key issues for safely and ethically managing an animal care and use program and vivaria that involve these types of biohazards. There has been a significant increase in research scope and number of facilities conducting research in this area due to heightened concerns by state and federal governments about both bioterrorism and emerging infectious diseases. While the rapid

Laboratory Animal Medicine, Third Edition
DOI: http://dx.doi.org/10.1016/B978-0-12-409527-4.00027-4

expansion of research in these areas has created some challenges, it has also provided some excellent advances as a new generation of professionals has looked at many old issues with a new set of eyes. The authors hope some of these newer ideas and approaches are captured in this chapter and will be useful for those just entering this field of research and those whose tireless efforts have contributed to the current knowledge and development of practices, equipment, and techniques that have allowed the safe and humane use of animals exposed to biohazards.

II. RISK ASSESSMENT

The tremendous importance of risk assessment is evidenced by its pervasiveness in nearly every current guidance publication that applies to working with biohazards or animals. For example, *Section II – Biological Risk Assessment* of the National Institutes of Health (NIH) publication *Biosafety in Microbiological and Biomedical Laboratories* (BMBL) contains a detailed discussion on the process and importance of conducting an effective biological risk assessment (CDC-NIH, 2009). The *Guide for the Care and Use of Laboratory Animals* (*Guide*) stresses the importance of risk assessment in mitigating hazards associated with the experimental use of animals, and specifically discusses the need for assessing hazards associated with animal experimentation involving hazardous agents (NRC, 2011a). Since the basic components of the risk assessment process are universal, it can be applied to most any situation involving potential exposure to a hazard. When working with biohazards, a common approach is to use an agent- and activity-based risk assessment that involves the following components: identification of the hazard, identification of the activities that can result in exposure to a hazard, the likelihood of the hazard to cause harm upon exposure; and determination of the possible consequences (CDC-NIH, 2009). The information provided by the risk assessment is then used to establish the appropriate biosafety levels and safeguards to protect at-risk personnel from exposure to biohazardous agents. The risk assessment for work with biohazards must take into account not only the agents but also the worker's health status and the environment (Fleming, 2006). When working with animals, it is critical that the additional risks the animals and related experimental activities bring are factored into the risk assessment equation. It is important to realize that risks change, especially when working with animals, and ongoing risk assessments should be conducted. One example of this situation could be changes in an animal's disposition brought on by illness. Evaluating changes in disposition to include signs of aggressiveness should be noted daily and shared with other personnel that

may come into contact with the animal for any reason. Most safety and biosafety professionals are adept at performing very thorough risk assessments, but oftentimes the risks associated with the animal related activities go unidentified and hence, the opportunity is missed for the in-depth analysis the risk assessment process affords. This overlooks the opportunity to identify additional safeguards that can be put into place to protect research, veterinary, and animal care personnel that come into contact with exposed/infected animals. Examples of these types of mitigation strategies will be discussed later in the chapter.

The risk assessment process can be effectively utilized to address other issues related to the use of animals and biohazards that are not directly related to determining appropriate biosafety levels and practices, safety equipment, and facility safeguards. For example, the process can be applied to determining the need for immunization(s). In determining the need for immunizations for at-risk personnel, there should be a well-defined risk assessment process that considers both the pros and cons of receiving prophylactic immunizations. While vaccination may provide an additional element of personal protection, the benefits and risks should be considered with equal rigor and the decision to immunize an employee should be made because of a clearly defined, recognized risk (NRC, 1997). Since several of the vaccines associated with biodefense research in particular are only approved as investigational new drugs (INDs) and have not received full licensure by the United States Food and Drug Administration (FDA), the risks associated with these vaccines due to their investigational status need to be fully considered. The IND vaccines should be offered to laboratory workers on a voluntary basis, subject to risk assessment and informed consent (NRC, 2011b). In the determination of any immunization recommendation, whether fully licensed or an IND, the inclusion of appropriate subject matter experts and safety and health professionals is critical. Veterinarians are frequently active participants in decision making regarding immunization programs for animal care and research workers (Weigler *et al.*, 2012). In general, the areas that should be evaluated prior to recommending any prophylactic immunization should include the following: the identification of hazards to which personnel are exposed; the health risks associated with those hazards; the history of laboratory acquired infections with the agent; an evaluation of facility design, traffic flow, and engineering safeguards in place; an evaluation of the proficiency of the staff with regard to safe practices and the type and integrity of any safety equipment being used; the health risks associated with the vaccines under consideration; and a review of published guidance on vaccine recommendations. The Advisory Committee on Immunization Practices (ACIP) provides expert advice

TABLE 27.1   A Matrix Commonly Used in the Risk Assessment Process When Determining the Level of Risk

Severity of the outcome	Probability of the event occurring				
	Frequent	Likely	Occasional	Seldom	Unlikely
Catastrophic	Extremely high	Extremely high	High	High	Moderate
Critical	Extremely high	High	High	Moderate	Low
Marginal	High	Moderate	Moderate	Low	Low
Negligible	Moderate	Low	Low	Low	Low

to U.S. government agencies and is the only entity in the federal government that makes such recommendations. The ACIP is a group of medical and public health experts that develop recommendations on how to use vaccines to control disease in the United States. These recommendations include specific advice for vaccination of laboratory and health care workers against several of the biohazards used in research (ACIP, 2013). All of these factors and resources can be used to determine vaccine recommendations for both direct work with an agent and, in some cases, entry into a particular area or room where an agent is used. Once a risk assessment has been performed and a decision made, the process should be handled through the appropriate legal and occupational health programs to ensure the vaccine recipients' legal rights and personal health status are considered prior to receiving an immunization.

A risk assessment matrix is a common tool used to visualize and quantify the overall risk and can be utilized for most any situation. The United States Army Medical Research Institute of Infectious Diseases (USAMRIID) has utilized such a tool for many years when conducting biosafety risk assessments (Table 27.1). Having a formalized and thoughtful risk assessment process that involves the appropriate professionals that are familiar with the risks and consequences of working with a biohazard is critical for ensuring appropriate safeguards are identified that protect both people and the environment.

III. MANAGING AN ANIMAL BIOCONTAINMENT PROGRAM

A. Basic Principles of Biohazard Containment

A fundamental objective of any biosafety program is the containment of potentially hazardous biological agents and toxins, and the term 'biocontainment' is used to describe safe methods, facilities, and equipment for managing infectious materials and biological toxins in the laboratory environment where they are being handled or maintained (CDC-NIH, 2009). Within

an animal biocontainment facility, hazardous material also includes animals exposed to pathogenic organisms or biological toxins, their tissues, and associated waste. A quality animal biocontainment program (BCP) will make every effort to reduce or eliminate exposure of laboratory workers, animal care staff, and the outside environment to hazardous materials. A biocontainment animal facility should have a single person who has both responsibility and authority for all animal-related activities conducted within the biocontainment envelope. While this typically is a laboratory animal veterinarian, other qualified staff can serve as the biocontainment animal facility manager. The manager will need to work closely with the principal investigator, biological safety professionals, and facility personnel to develop the animal biocontainment program, coordinate safety training, and provide oversight of the activities involving hazardous agents within the animal facilities.

As part of the BCP, the manager should initially develop or adopt a biosafety manual that identifies the hazards that will or may be encountered, and specifies equipment, practices, and procedures designed to minimize or eliminate exposures to these hazards. When standard laboratory practices are not sufficient to control the hazards associated with a particular agent or laboratory procedure, additional measures may be needed. In those cases, safety practices and techniques must be supplemented by appropriate facility design and engineering features, safety equipment, personal protective equipment, and management practices.

The manager is responsible for ensuring that animal care personnel receive appropriate training in the practices and operations specific to the animal facility, such as animal husbandry procedures, potential hazards present, manipulations of animals exposed to infectious agents, and necessary precautions to prevent potential exposures. Individuals must demonstrate a high level of proficiency in standard and special microbiological practices, and experimental techniques before entering the biocontainment facility or working with animals exposed to infectious agents. There should be standard operating procedures (SOPs) for working with biohazards and infected animals, and each person having contact with the agent or infected animal should understand the SOPs, know the clinical signs and symptoms associated with the agent in use, be adequately trained in handling exposed animals, be determined competent to perform all procedures, and be properly supervised. Each person providing care for the animals or carrying out experimental procedures must be alert to the hazards and understand how to perform the procedures properly and safely. Before a project is started that involves the use of an agent, it is important to seek consultation on safety requirements and SOPs from people experienced in working with the microorganism. A scientist, or a principal investigator, who is trained and knowledgeable in appropriate laboratory techniques, safety procedures, and hazards associated with handling infectious agents must be responsible for work with any infectious agents or materials. This is especially true if a project is proposed that involves the use of an agent that has not been previously used in the facility or has not been studied in animals. Conducting a formal risk assessment that takes all of these issues into consideration is an important part of the ability to effectively identify and mitigate potential risks. As the study progresses, regular safety meetings with all involved staff will help to identify and resolve new risks and issues as they arise. Even changes in an animal's disposition can be an important factor in a biocontainment environment and is information that should be shared with others working with, or caring for, the animals.

B. Animal Facility Considerations

Facilities in which biohazards are used should meet or exceed the standards set forth in the most recent edition of the BMBL. Table 27.2 summarizes the containment equipment and procedures recommended by the BMBL for research involving infected vertebrates. Four animal biosafety levels (ABSL-1, 2, 3, and 4) are identified, with ABSL-1 being the lowest level and ABSL-4 being the highest. In addition to the four ABSLs, the United States Department of Agriculture (USDA) has developed additional requirements for handling agents of agricultural significance. Appendix D of the BMBL includes a discussion on BSL-3 Agriculture (BSL-3-Ag). The determination of the appropriate ABSL requires experience and professional judgment and should be made in consultation with a biosafety professional, and based on a thorough risk assessment of the agent and how it is going to be used. All work with hazardous agents should be reviewed and approved by the appropriate committees. Even different projects involving the same microorganism or toxin might have a different level of risk because of the animal species involved and the activities or procedures being performed. For example, hantavirus studies in rodents which do not excrete the

virus can be conducted in ABSL-2 facilities with ABSL-2 practices. Studies involving tissue from animals infected with hantavirus can be conducted safely at ABSL-2 or at ABSL-2 with ABSL-3 practices. However, if the study is being conducted in a rodent species permissive for chronic infection, it requires ABSL-4.

An important facility consideration is the heating, ventilation, and air conditioning (HVAC) system. For biocontainment facilities, the HVAC system is considered secondary containment and must be able to maintain the facility under negative pressure, thereby containing the hazardous agents and preventing any accidental release into the environment. This is usually accomplished using HVAC systems that have automated controls on the intake and exhaust valves creating directional airflow from areas that do not have pathogens to areas that do. Their use is particularly important at ABSL-3 and ABSL-4 because the agents assigned to those levels may transmit disease by the inhalation route and can cause life-threatening disease. Directional airflow is dependent on the operational integrity of the laboratory's HVAC system. HVAC systems require careful monitoring and periodic maintenance to sustain operational integrity. Loss of directional airflow compromises safe laboratory operation and HVAC systems should be redundant and designed to prevent positive pressurization from occurring during an HVAC failure. ABSL-4 containment facilities require more complex safeguards that necessitate significant expertise to design and operate.

C. Safety Equipment

One of the basic principles of biosafety is the concept of primary and secondary barriers. Safety equipment is considered a primary barrier and may include enclosed containers and other engineering controls designed to minimize exposure to hazardous biological materials. Primary barriers may also include items worn for personal protection, such as gloves, gowns, shoe covers, respirators, and eye protection. Secondary barriers are incorporated into the design and construction of the facility and may include features such as autoclaves, specialized ventilation that provides directional airflow, air filtration, controlled access zones, or airlocks located at laboratory entrances (CDC-NIH, 2009).

The biological safety cabinet (BSC) is the principal device used to contain biohazards and is considered to be a primary barrier. To be effective, a BSC must be well maintained and regularly tested and certified using the appropriate National Sanitation Foundation standard (NSF, 2004). Personnel must be trained to use them properly. According to the BMBL, those procedures that involve the manipulation of infectious materials must be conducted within BSC or other physical containment devices that provide the same level of

TABLE 27.2 RABSLs for Activities in Which Experimentally or Naturally Infected Vertebrate Animals Are Used[a]

Animal biosafety level	Agents	Practices	Primary barriers and safety equipment	Facilities (Secondary barriers)
1	Not known to consistently cause disease in healthy adults	Standard animal care and management practices, including appropriate medical surveillance programs	As required for normal care of each species • PPE: laboratory coats and gloves; eye and face protection, as needed	Standard animal facility: • No recirculation of exhaust air • Directional air flow recommended • Hand-washing sink is available
2	• Agents associated with human disease • Hazard: percutaneous injury, ingestion, mucous membrane exposure	ABSL-1 practices plus: • Limited access • Biohazard warning signs • Sharps precautions • Biosafety manual • Decontamination of all infectious wastes and animal cages prior to washing	ABSL-1 equipment plus primary barriers: • Containment equipment appropriate for animal species • PPE: Laboratory coats, gloves, face, eye, and respiratory protection, as needed	ABSL-1 plus: • Autoclave available • Hand-washing sink available • Mechanical cage washer recommended • Negative airflow into animal and procedure rooms recommended
3	Indigenous or exotic agents that may cause serious or potentially lethal disease through the inhalational route of exposure	ABSL-2 practices plus: • Controlled access • Decontamination of clothing before laundering • Cages decontaminated before bedding is removed • Disinfectant footbath, as needed	ABSL-2 equipment plus: • Containment equipment for housing animals and cage dumping activities • Class I, II, or III BSCs available for manipulative procedures (inoculation, necropsy) that might create infectious aerosols • PPE: appropriate respiratory protection	ABSL-2 facility plus: • Physical separation from access corridors • Self-closing, double-door access • Sealed penetrations • Sealed windows • Autoclave available in facility • Entry through anteroom or airlock • Negative airflow into animal and procedure rooms • Hand-washing sink near exit of animal or procedure room
4	• Dangerous/exotic agents which pose high risk of aerosol transmitted laboratory infections that are frequently fatal, for which there are no vaccines or treatments • Agents with a close or identical antigenic relationship to an agent requiring BSL-4 until data are available to redesignate the level • Related agents with unknown risk of transmission	ABSL-3 practices plus: • Entrance through change room where personal clothing is removed and laboratory clothing is put on; shower on exiting • All wastes are decontaminated before removal from the facility	ABSL-3 equipment plus: • Maximum containment equipment (i.e., Class III BSC or partial containment equipment in combination with full-body, air-supplied positive pressure personnel suit) used for all procedures and activities	ABSL-3 facility plus: • Separate building or isolated zone • Dedicated supply and exhaust, vacuum, and decontamination systems • Other requirements outlined in the text (CDC-NIH, 2009)

PPE, personal protective equipment.
[a]From CDC-NIH (2009).

protection. There are three classes of BSCs: I, II, and III. A full description of these cabinets can be found in the BMBL in Appendix A: Primary Containment of Biohazards: Selection, Installation, and Use of Biological Safety Cabinets (CDC-NIH, 2009). Biosafety cabinets are designed to protect the individual using the cabinet and the environment through the use of directional air flow and high-efficiency particulate air (HEPA) filtration. Always consult with a biosafety professional to ensure that you have the correct type of BSC for the agent,

animal species, and activities that you are performing. For example, Class I BSCs are not designed to protect the product (e.g., culture, animal, or agent) in the cabinet from contaminated air that may be pulled into the BSC from the surrounding environment.

D. Animal Housing and Movement

As stated above, working with hazardous agents is usually done within a BSC, which is the primary device

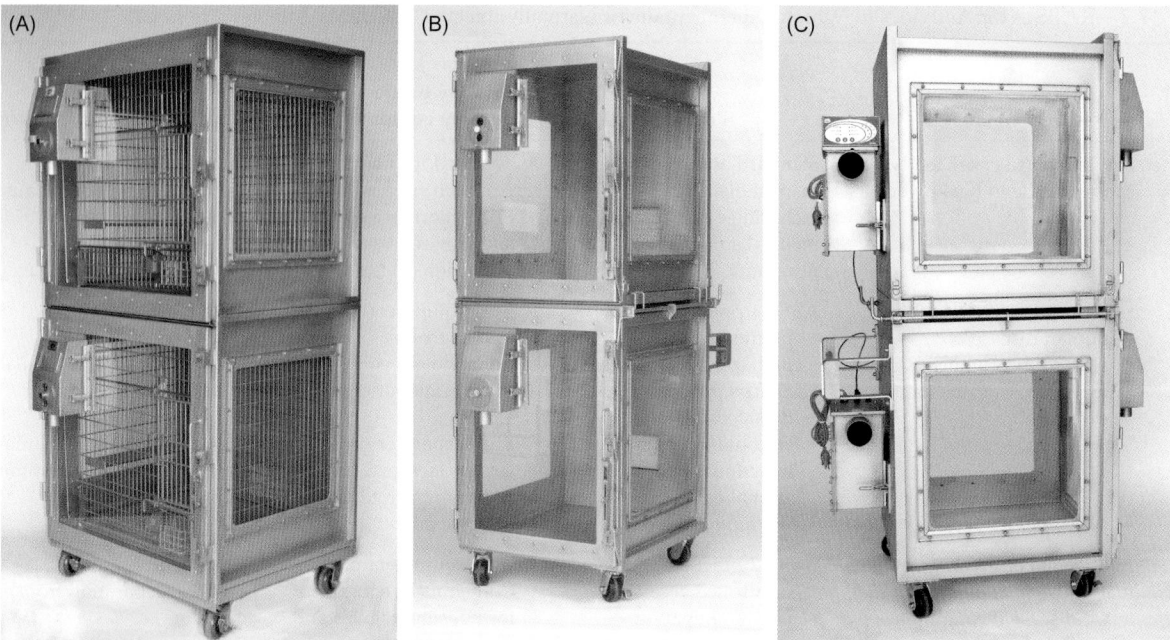

FIGURE 27.1   The primary containment cage shown is designed to house nonhuman primates. The clear Lexan® panels allow plentiful light penetration and a HEPA filtered air inlet box in the front of the cage (A) has a connection for a controlled warming system for animals recovering from anesthesia, or that otherwise become hypothermic. Cages are easily removed for cleaning the interior of the primary containment envelope (B). The blower motors and HEPA-filtered exhaust boxes are located on the back of each cage (C). *Photos provided courtesy of Carter Systems, Inc.*

used to contain the hazard. When infected animals are considered the 'hazardous agent,' a primary concern is how to then contain the hazard. Procedures, such as cage changes or inoculations which may generate aerosols, should be performed in a BSC. However, the animals themselves are rarely housed in BSCs. Instead, they may be housed in static microisolator, negative pressure individually ventilated, or other caging systems that provide a primary barrier. Caging systems that provide a primary barrier between the infected animals and the room in which they are housed are commonly referred to as primary containment caging (Fig. 27.1). A clear understanding of the agent, its infectivity, and the route(s) of transmission in the species of animal being utilized is critical in determining the best way to manage the hazard.

According to the BMBL, facilities that house animals at ABSL-3 can reduce the risk of infectious aerosols from infected animals or their bedding if animals are housed in primary containment caging systems. At ABSL-4, the BMBL states that infected animals must be housed in ventilated enclosures with inward directional airflow and HEPA-filtered exhaust and infected animals that require manipulation outside the primary containment cage should be handled within a primary barrier, such as a Class II BSC or other containment system.

The recommendations in the BMBL differ somewhat regarding the need for primary containment caging for high-consequence livestock pathogens. The

management of risk is based primarily on the potential economic impact of animal morbidity and mortality in the nation's agricultural population and the resultant impact on international trade. The containment category of BSL-3-Ag is unique to agriculture because of the necessity to protect the environment from high-consequence livestock pathogens and accomodate studies that are conducted with large agricultural animals for which primary containment caging is neither practical nor available. A key difference between BSL-3 and BSL-3-Ag is that for BSL-3Ag the facility barriers (i.e., secondary barriers) act as the primary barriers when housing large animals that cannot be readily housed in primary containment cages (e.g., cattle, horses, sheep). BSL-3-Ag facilities that cannot readily house animals in primary containment caging systems require the features for an ABSL-3 facility with enhancements typical of BSL-4 facilities (CDC-NIH, 2009).

Individually ventilated caging is commonly used in conventional animal facilities to house animals with the cages maintained under positive pressure relative to the animal room in order to protect the animals from exposure to disease causing agents, but many of these systems can also be used under negative relative pressure to maintain animals that have been exposed to a hazardous agent. Usually, the air being supplied and the air being discharged from the cage are filtered and the air being exhausted into the room is HEPA filtered or connected to the building ventilation system, protecting the room

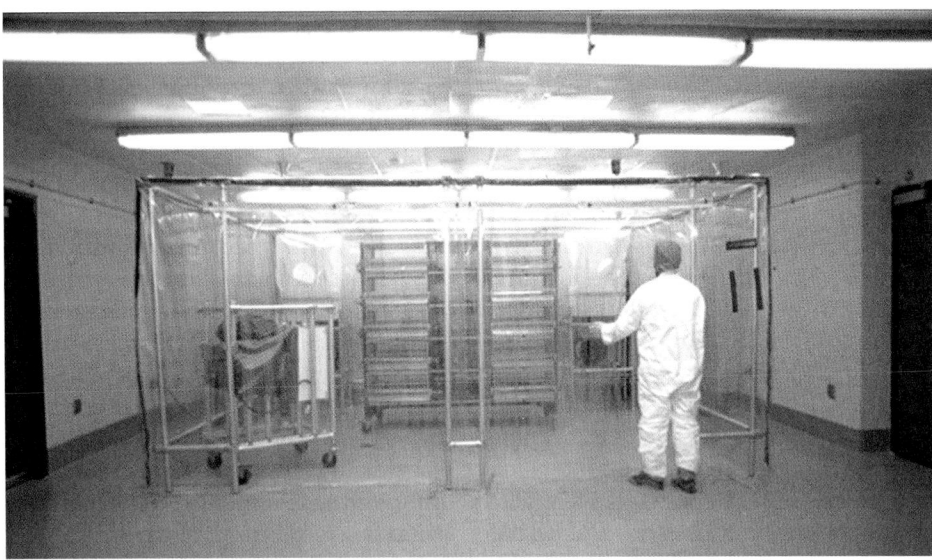

FIGURE 27.2   Negative pressure freestanding bioBUBBLE® enclosure. This unit is designed to be used for avian research requiring a primary containment system. Cages are located in the center of the enclosure and a bioBUBBLE® bedding disposal system is located in the front left corner of the enclosure. The disposal system is used for control of dust and allergens during cage waste disposal procedures. Two HEPA-filtered blower motors are present, one located in each of the back corners of the enclosure. *Photo provided courtesy of bioBUBBLE®.*

environment, other animals, and the workers. In either case, the rack should be designed to 'fail safe' by going neutral or static to prevent exposure in the event that the power supply is disrupted. Actively ventilated caging systems must be designed to prevent the escape of infectious agents from the cage and the exhaust plenums should be sealed to prevent escape of microorganisms if the ventilation system becomes static. The system should also be alarmed to indicate operational malfunctions. Cages should only be open or changed in a biosafety cabinet to prevent exposure to the agent or waste. HEPA filters on ventilated cage systems should be tested on a regular basis to certify their effectiveness.

Biocontainment caging has been developed by a number of caging manufacturers to house animals exposed to highly infectious agents and is available for both rodent and large animal species. Biocontainment caging provides a high level of protection for personnel and the environment when used properly. Some systems use cages that are completely sealed, and in the event of a power outage or motor failure may have a limited air supply. Having backup emergency power to the outlets supplying these units, or a battery backup system internal to the caging system itself, is an important consideration. Other considerations for using some types of primary containment caging for larger animals involve worker safety, animal handling, cage sanitation, and singly housing animals. Single housing of social species limits social interaction and should be thoroughly justified based on experimental requirements or veterinary-related concerns about animal well-being (NRC, 2011a). The challenge of balancing the scientific needs of the

study, worker safety, and the social preferences of the animals requires thoughtful consideration and deliberation. Additional considerations for other forms of environmental and behavioral enrichment may be needed to help address the animals' needs when pair or group housing is not possible.

An alternative to individually ventilated, primary containment caging or housing systems is the use of flexible film isolators or panels that surround the cage and/or rack (Fig. 27.2). These units are maintained under negative pressure using exhaust motors with HEPA filters to exhaust back into the room or by attaching to the facility HVAC and exhausting to the outside. These units have historically been used in combination with conventional caging systems and/or when housing multiple species or agents within the same area.

Movement of infected animals within a biocontainment facility should be performed with careful coordination and risk assessment. The main concern is the containment of the hazard and animal located within the primary barrier in order to prevent inadvertent release, including escape, and to prevent exposure of the surrounding environment to the hazard. Transport devices may be used to provide containment of the animal and the associated hazard during movement. A number of devices have been utilized, from using filtered rodent microisolator caging to transport small animals to specialized mobile HEPA-filtered enclosures for multiple cages of rodents and larger animals. The primary containment transport device should be a durable, leak-proof container that can be secured for transport, allows sufficient air exchange to support the physiological needs of the animal(s), and can be surface decontaminated. The interior and exterior of the containment devices should be easily disinfected.

The U.S. Department of Health and Human Services (DHHS) and the USDA have established lists of infectious agents and toxins that could threaten public health and safety. The possession or use of these agents and toxins is governed by federal law (see Section VI.A.3), and are designated as biological select agents and toxins. It is very important to fully understand both the regulatory requirements that apply to an animal exposed to a select agent or toxin and the regulatory requirements that apply to the agent/toxin to which the animal is exposed. For example, animals exposed to select toxins in the laboratory do not have to be housed in Centers for Disease Control and Prevention (CDC)-registered space, but if the toxin is brought into the animal housing space for administration to the animals, the space must be registered with the CDC for use of the toxin. Animals exposed to infectious select agents must be housed in CDC-registered space and tracked as part of the select agent inventory. Also, biological samples obtained from animals exposed to infectious select agents are subject to the same regulatory requirements, unless the agent can be shown to be inactivated (Kastenmayer, 2012). Removal of biological materials that are to remain in a viable or intact state from the biocontainment facility must be placed in a nonbreakable, sealed primary container and then enclosed in a nonbreakable, sealed secondary container (CDC-NIH, 2009).

IV. STANDARD PRACTICES

A. Personal Protective Equipment

While engineering controls provide a barrier between the individual and a hazard, the use of personal protective equipment (PPE) is the final physical barrier used to prevent exposures to hazardous materials and should not be used in lieu of appropriate engineering controls. Many types of PPE are available and their use should be risk-based and determined through a risk assessment process that takes into consideration specific knowledge of the potential hazards, activities being performed, engineering controls in place, experience, and sound professional judgment. Requirements for PPE in any given situation should not be written generically (e.g., PPE will be worn) as the type of PPE should be specified and must be consistent with the hazard and the required level of containment (Fontes, 2008).

PPE comes in many forms and some common items include scrubs, solid-front laboratory gowns, jumpsuits, sleeve covers, hair bonnets, safety glasses, shoe covers, examination gloves, respiratory protection, and a multitude of specialty safety items. While PPE comes in many forms and each item serves an important purpose, working with animals, sharps, and infectious agents and toxins together makes gloves and respiratory protection critical considerations (Copps, 2005). Glove material must provide an adequate barrier against the expected hazard. For example, the choice of latex or nitrile gloves may depend on the ability of a solvent or chemical being used to penetrate the glove material, and the use of additional bite or cut-resistant outer gloves may be necessary when handling animals that pose a bite or scratch risk, respectively (NRC, 1997). The use of Kevlar® sleeve protectors can be useful in preventing scratches to the wrist and forearms when handling larger animals, like rabbits that pose a significant scratch risk from the combination of powerful hind legs and toenails that can easily penetrate most standard PPE, such as scrubs, lab coats, or Tyvek® coveralls. People subject to a risk of an aerosol exposure to infectious agents or toxins must be provided appropriate respiratory protection. When the use of a respirator is required, the institution must implement a respiratory protection program and have a dedicated program administrator (CFR, 2007). Personnel required to wear a respirator must be enrolled in a respiratory protection program that includes medical clearance to wear a respirator, fit testing, and training on its proper use and disposal, or disinfection, maintenance, and storage if reusable.

B. Sharps

Working with animals frequently requires the use of syringe needles and other sharps. Good sharps handling practices and the use of integral needle safety technologies, such as self-retracting needles and no-touch sheath covering devices, can help prevent inadvertent needle sticks. When working with highly hazardous agents or toxin, using a pair of forceps to remove needle caps provides an additional level of safety for personnel. It is imperative to always have an appropriately sized sharps container positioned within arm's reach and in a manner that prevents crossing over of arms or hands to dispose of sharps. If more than one person is working with sharps nearby or within the same biosafety cabinet, each person should have their own sharps container. Needles should not be recapped, especially in a high-hazard environment. If procedures necessitate the repeated use of a single syringe and needle, a plastic tube (e.g., 50-ml Falcon tube) or a small plastic beaker can be used to safely cover the sharp end of a needle if needed between uses (Fontes, 2008). These items are also useful to keep close to the work zone should an unexpected occurrence arise with the animal that necessitates securing a loaded syringe and needle after the needle cap has been removed and before it can be injected.

Sharps containers should be discarded when they are {2/3} to {3/4} full. Performing necropsies on infected animals requires special consideration for hand protection, such as cut-resistant outer gloves, due to the high risk that comes from frequent use of scalpels and other sharp instruments. Retractable scalpels can reduce the risk of injury if used as designed to cover the scalpel blade when not in use.

C. Waste Disposal

Waste streams must be clearly identified to ensure the proper decontamination and disposal of all types of waste generated in animal rooms and support areas within a containment envelope. The types of waste streams can vary from institution to institution based on the activities being performed; therefore, each institution should identify and define their waste streams and implement appropriate decontamination and disposal procedures for each stream. The regulations governing the disposal of biohazards are complex and can have multiple layers of state and local regulations in addition to federal requirements. Some of the federal agencies with regulations that apply to biohazardous waste include the United States Occupational Health and Safety Administration (OSHA), Department of Transportation (DOT), Environmental Protection Agency (EPA), and the FDA. Knowledge of the multiple federal, state and local regulations that apply to the identification of waste streams, decontamination, handling, transportation, and disposal of biohazard waste is critical to ensure compliance. The use of commercial hazardous waste disposal companies to help with navigating the myriad of regulatory requirements for waste disposal has become a common practice. These companies can be an excellent resource for obtaining training on identifying waste streams and for help with developing internal waste handling procedures that meet regulatory requirements.

D. Sanitation Procedures

In animal husbandry, sanitation is the maintenance of environmental conditions conducive to the health and well-being of the animal, and involves bedding changes, cleaning, and disinfection (NRC, 2011a). Environmental conditions include both the primary and secondary environments in which animals are maintained. Maintenance of those conditions involves such activities as changing cages and bedding (contact and noncontact), and routine sanitation of animal caging, racks, and the secondary environment. Cleaning and disinfection are important aspects of any sanitation program and the difference between the two methods should be understood in a biocontainment environment. Cleaning is the removal of excessive amounts of gross contamination caused by animal waste, dirt, and debris, while disinfection is the reduction or elimination of unacceptable concentrations of microorganisms (NRC, 2011a). Neither method is designed to sterilize the environment. These activities in biocontainment may be slightly altered to achieve the same goals of a conventional area while adhering to biosafety requirements. For example, in most biocontainment facilities, the cage wash is located outside of the biocontainment area, so caging and waste must be sterilized prior to removal from the containment area.

Changing contact bedding involves decontamination of the cage and bedding prior to removal from the biocontainment area, preferably leaving the bedding in the caging system to reduce the potential of aerosolizing the agent (CDC-NIH, 2009). Noncontact bedding is placed in leak-proof containers and decontaminated prior to removal from the biocontainment area. After decontamination and removal from the biocontainment area, bedding may be disposed of and the cage sanitized using conventional methods. Disposable caging for rodents is available, which may reduce the complexity of cage sanitation in a biocontainment environment. The convenience of disposable caging can be weighed against the associated costs in determining its practicality for use in each situation.

Cleaning in biocontainment may be complicated by the need to clean in place due to facility and/or protocol constraints, the use of complex biocontainment caging, and the requirement to minimize aerosol formation. Some caging, such as biocontainment caging for larger, non-rodent species, may have to be partially disassembled to allow for adequate cleaning. Cleaning in biocontainment is usually performed by hand without the use of a mechanical washer. Caging should be adequately rinsed after cleaning to prevent exposure of the animals to residual chemicals. When using handwashing to clean cages in lieu of a mechanical washer, evaluating the effectiveness of the sanitation procedures is recommended (NRC, 2011a).

Disinfection of primary and secondary enclosures in containment usually involves the use of chemical disinfectants during the conduct of the study and chemical, gas, or vapor disinfectants between studies. The type of chemical disinfectant to use must be carefully considered since it must be effective against both those microorganisms that are naturally occurring and those that are used experimentally. There are some disinfectants that have been approved for use against the more common organisms or classes of organisms. In those cases, the manufacturer's directions should be followed. However, there is limited information on the effectiveness of most disinfectants against all infectious disease agents, especially in the cases of new or uncommon agents. Appendix B of the BMBL provides guidance on classes of disinfectants and selection of the type of disinfectant to use (CDC-NIH, 2009). Ultimately, a biosafety professional should be involved in the selection of an appropriate disinfectant for use in your facility based on a risk assessment. Validation studies may be required to verify the effectiveness of the disinfectant and the appropriate contact time.

E. Animal Handling and Restraint

Animals exposed to infectious diseases present a concern to individuals handling the animal due to the risk of transmission of the agent from the animal to the handler. Transmission could occur by a variety of methods, including bites, scratches, needle sticks, mucous membrane exposure, or aerosol transmission. The use of physical restraint devices, chemical restraint, additional PPE as previously described, and practices that reduce the risk of exposure during animal manipulations should be used whenever possible. According to the BMBL, all procedures involving the manipulation of infectious materials (either the infectious agent or tissues from infected animals), handling of infected animals or the generation of aerosols must be conducted within BSCs or other physical containment devices when practical. BSCs are commonly used with small rodents, but present a challenge when handling larger animals, such as rabbits or nonhuman primates, and are impractical for agricultural animals. When a procedure cannot be performed within a biosafety cabinet, a combination of personal protective equipment and other devices or methods must be used. Other devices or methods may include the use of squeeze cages, or other types of mechanical restraint, and chemical restraint. Depending on the species of animal and/or procedure being performed, more than one person may be required to work safely.

V. VETERINARY CARE

The American College of Laboratory Animal Medicine's (ACLAM) position statement on adequate veterinary care (http://www.aclam.org/education-and-training/position-statements-and-reports) states that the essential components of an adequate veterinary care program for laboratory animals includes one or more qualified veterinarians and veterinary technical staff; authority to implement the veterinary care program and provide oversight of related aspects of the institutional animal care and use program; disease prevention, diagnosis, and control programs; guidance for research staff in animal methods and techniques; and the promotion of animal well-being. Several challenges exist in applying these concepts to an animal care and use program in which biohazards are introduced as part of the research requirement.

It can be difficult to find veterinary care staff that have experience working with animals exposed to biohazards and can also meet the strict security requirements that oftentimes accompany having access to select agents and toxins, or animals that are exposed to them. While these challenges apply to all professional and technical positions, the relative shortage of husbandry and veterinary care staff with experience in biocontainment and with select agents usually means that these specialized skill sets are attained through formal mentoring programs and on-the-job training. To avoid problems postemployment, clear and frequent communication with potential hires during the interview process about the strict security standards required for these positions is very important and should be clearly defined in written preemployment job requirements.

Provision of veterinary care to animals housed in a containment environment can present new challenges in diagnosis, detection, and treatment of ill or injured animals. Novel approaches can be used to overcome a sometimes significant decrease in sensory perception resulting from the type of personal protective equipment required. For example, in instances where encapsulating positive pressure suits or powered air-purifying respirators (PAPRs) prevent the use of conventional stethoscopes, digital recording stethoscopes can be used to record heart, lung, or abdominal sounds. These recordings can then be downloaded to a computer inside the containment envelope and transferred to another computer in a noncontainment environment for diagnostic interpretation. Providing a complete diagnostic evaluation of animals that may unexpectedly become ill for reasons unrelated to experimental manipulations has historically been difficult due to the obvious restrictions of moving diagnostic samples outside of the containment envelope for analysis and the high cost of purchasing and maintaining large, complicated blood analyzers inside containment. The development of hand-held, point-of-care diagnostic blood analyzers that can provide rapid and reliable evaluation of hematological and serum chemistry parameters can be a valuable resource for performing diagnostics in a containment environment. Remote physiological monitoring, often referred to as biotelemetry, is an advancing technology that allows real-time monitoring of single or multiple physiological parameters simultaneously. While most biotelemetry is used for gathering experimental data, the information it provides can many times be used in cases where veterinary intervention may be needed. Currently, biotelemetry systems have the ability to record and collect detailed data on the function and status of a variety of physiological systems such as cardiovascular, respiratory, neurological, and thermoregulation. This data is transmitted through a wireless system and can be viewed from a remote site outside of the containment envelope. This results in less stress to the animal to collect the data and increased safety of personnel, since the animal does not have to be anesthetized or handled and the containment envelope does not have to be entered. If biotelemetry is used as part of a research project, it can be a very useful adjunct should diagnostic veterinary care be required.

The provision of veterinary care to animals housed in a containment environment should meet the criteria outlined in the ACLAM position statement on veterinary care. Careful planning and resourcefulness can ensure the appropriate level of veterinary care is provided to all animals regardless of the containment level in which they are housed.

VI. OTHER CONSIDERATIONS

A. Oversight of Animal Research Involving Biohazards

Research involving hazardous agents, including pathogenic organisms, toxins, biological materials from infected animals, and recombinant or synthetic nucleic acid molecules, requires careful consideration during the review process. To ensure compliance with all applicable laws and regulations, research involving hazardous agents may be reviewed by a number of different groups prior to the conduct of the study. The review includes the Institutional Animal Care and Use Committee (IACUC) if animals are involved and the Institutional Biosafety Committee (IBC) if biohazardous agents are involved. Outside agencies may also be involved such as the NIH Office of Biotechnology Activities (OBA) for certain activities with recombinant or synthetic nucleic acid molecules or the Select Agent Program if select agents are used.

While this chapter focuses primarily on infectious agents and toxins of biological origin, animal research has begun to incorporate new risks involving nontraditional microscopic hazards that increase the need for a thorough process of risk assessment and oversight. Examples of two microscopic hazards of significance that have moved into the animal research realm include prions and nanoparticles. Prions are small proteinaceous particles with no detectable nucleic acid. The use of prions has brought with them several new considerations for research involving animals. Due to their involvement in a number of neurological diseases and extreme resistance to conventional inactivation procedures, including irradiation, boiling, dry heat, and chemicals, special consideration must be given for handling infected animals and tissues, decontamination procedures, and waste disposal (Richmond et al., 2003). A nano-object is a material with one, two, or three external dimensions in the 1- to 100-nm size range (ISO, 2008). Nano-objects are frequently incorporated into a larger matrix known as a nonmaterial. Nanoparticles are a specific type of nano-object, with all three external dimensions at the nanoscale. Experimental studies in animals have shown that there is a potential risk of internalizing nanoparticles through inhalation, ingestion, dermal exposure, and even the possibility of movement from the nose to the brain through the blood–brain barrier (Behrens et al., 2002; Duffin et al., 2007; Elder et al., 2006; Ryman-Rasmussen et al., 2006). Guidance on safe practices for working with engineered nanomaterials in a research environment is available from the National Institute for Occupational Safety and Health (NIOSH, 2012).

1. Institutional Animal Care and Use Committee

The ultimate responsibility for review and approval of animal use protocols lies with the IACUC (CFR, 2000; PHS, 2002; NRC, 2011a). It is important that there are members of the IACUC that has the background and experience to adequately review protocols involving possible biohazards. The committee should have access to a biosafety professional who is knowledgeable about the biohazards that will be used. Many institutions have someone from the institutional biosafety program serve as a member of the IACUC. Alternatively, an appropriate biosafety professional could serve as an *ad hoc* reviewer for the committee. During the review process, it is important to have adequate information about the biohazard and protective measures. Many institutions have adopted the use of a biohazard appendix to the protocol form to assist in the review process. The biohazard appendix is tailored to the needs of the institution.

Beyond the initial review and approval of the animal use protocol by the IACUC, institutions are required by federal regulations and other guidance to conduct a continuing assessment of ongoing animal activities (CFR, 2000; PHS, 2002; NRC, 2011a). This oversight can be provided in a variety of ways, including the use of formal postapproval monitoring programs that involve dedicated staff that evaluate the accuracy of compliance with IACUC-approved activities; conducting annual protocol reviews by the IACUC; performing laboratory inspections (conducted either during regularly scheduled semiannual IACUC facility inspections or separately); observation of selected procedures by IACUC members or veterinary staff; observation of animals by animal care, veterinary, and IACUC staff and members; and external regulatory inspections and assessments (NRC, 2011a). Providing oversight of ongoing activities in a biocontainment facility can provide additional challenges to the IACUC and external regulatory and oversight groups. Personnel entering the facility will need to comply with all of the entry requirements, which may include vaccinations, respirator, and medical clearance and training. Other requirements may apply if entering areas that are registered with the CDC for use of select agents or toxins. In certain cases, alternatives to entering biocontainment facilities by oversight entities may include the use of security cameras for real-time visual access or date/time-stamped photos or videos to view the room conditions and observe animals and procedures.

2. Institutional Biosafety Committee

Institutions have safety offices and committees that review the use of hazardous agents, including chemicals, biological agents, and radioactive materials. Institutions that receive federal funding from the NIH to work with recombinant or synthetic nucleic acid molecules are required to comply with the NIH Guidelines for Research Involving Recombinant or Synthetic Nucleic Acid Molecules (*NIH Guidelines*) (NIH, 2013). The *NIH Guidelines* are administered by the NIH Office of Biotechnology Activities. A requirement of the *NIH Guidelines* is the establishment of an IBC that includes individuals with experience and expertise in recombinant or synthetic nucleic acid technology, biosafety, and physical containment. The committee must also have a biological safety officer if work is being conducted at ABSL-3 or ABSL-4 and a member with expertise in animal containment if experiments with animals are being performed. The *NIH Guidelines* provide guidance on physical and biological containment practices for recombinant or synthetic nucleic acid molecule research involving etiological agents and animals. Experiments with recombinant or synthetic nucleic acid molecules and animals could include the creation of transgenic or 'knockout' animals as well as the use of manipulated biological agents in animals. Either situation makes the risk assessment and review more difficult because the disease process and pathogenesis in the animal may be changed. In such cases, serious consideration should be given to increasing the containment conditions from what is recommended for the unmanipulated agent.

3. Select Agent Program

Concerns regarding the ease with which disease-causing agents could be obtained led Congress to pass the Antiterrorism and Effective Death Penalty Act of 1996 (PL 104–132, 1996). This Act directed the DHHS to establish a list of biological agents and toxins that could threaten public health and safety, procedures for governing the transfer of those agents, and training requirements for entities working with these agents, designated biological select agents and toxins. The Division of Select Agents and Toxins (DSAT) in the CDC Office of Public Health Preparedness and Response was created to implement this program. The *Public Health Security and Bioterrorism Preparedness and Response Act of 2002* (PL 107–188, 2002)

strengthened the regulatory authorities of DHHS and granted comparable regulatory authorities to the USDA over select agents that pose a severe threat to animal and plant health or products. The Agriculture Select Agent Program (ASAP) was created in the USDA's Animal and Plant Health Inspection Service (APHIS) to implement the program. The combination of the DSAT and ASAP constitutes the Federal Select Agent Program. The Federal Select Agent Program select agent regulations for the possession, use, and transfer of select agents and toxins are published in the Federal Register (CFR, 2012a; CFR, 2012b; CFR, 2012c). Individuals or entities possessing, using, or transferring select agents and toxins are required to be registered with the Federal Select Agent Program and comply with the select agent regulations.

B. Occupational Health

Institutions have a responsibility for ensuring worker safety. An essential part of an institution's safety program is an occupational health and safety program (OHSP) that is consistent with federal, state, and local regulations and focuses on maintaining a safe and healthy workplace. An effective OHSP takes into consideration all facets of the research program including facilities, personnel, research activities, biohazards, and animal species, and includes careful coordination with members of the research, animal care and use, occupational health, safety, and administration groups. There are a number of references to utilize when establishing an OHSP for personnel working with hazardous agents. For general guidance, there are the *Guide for the Care and Use of Laboratory Animals* (NRC, 2011a) and the National Research Council's Publication *Occupational Health and Safety in the Care and Use of Research Animals* (NRC, 1997). For those facilities working with infectious agents and biological toxins, guidance is provided in the BMBL (CDC-NIH, 2009) and the *Guidelines for Research Involving Recombinant and Synthetic Nucleic Acid Molecules* (NIH, 2013). For species specific guidance, the Occupational Health and Safety in the Care and Use of Nonhuman Primates (NRC, 2003), is available. Components of an occupational health program include preplacement medical evaluations, vaccines, periodic medical evaluations, and medical support for occupational illnesses and injuries (CDC-NIH, 2009).

1. Preplacement Medical Evaluations

Workers who may be exposed to biohazardous agents and toxins should be enrolled in an OHSP and receive a preplacement/preassignment medical evaluation (CDC-NIH, 2009; Fontes, 2008; NRC, 1997). Individuals with access to Tier 1 Select Agents are required to be enrolled in an occupational health program (CFR, 2012a). Health care providers should be cognizant of potential hazards encountered by the worker and have an understanding of the potential health hazards present in the work environment. Optimally, there should be ready access to an infectious disease physician with understanding of the hazards presented by the agents used within the facility. As part of the medical evaluation, the health care provider should review any previous and ongoing medical problems, current medications, allergies, and prior immunizations in order to determine an individual's medical fitness to perform the duties of a specific position and what medical services are needed to permit the individual to safely assume the duties of the position. Criteria for fitness for duty should be established based upon the occupational health hazards identified from a site-specific comprehensive risk assessment (CDC, 2013a).

2. Vaccines

Commercial vaccines should be made available to workers to provide protection against infectious agents to which they may be occupationally exposed. Animal care personnel are routinely vaccinated against tetanus (NRC, 1997) and preexposure immunization is offered to people at risk of infection or exposure to specific agents such as rabies virus (e.g., if working with susceptible species) or hepatitis B virus (e.g., if working with human blood or human tissues, cell lines, or stocks) (NRC, 2011a). As part of the risk assessment, it should be determined if there are vaccines available for the agents present in the workplace. And if warranted, vaccination should be provided for those biohazardous agents for which effective vaccines are available. In the event, an FDA-licensed vaccine does not exist for a biohazardous agent, but a vaccine in an IND status is available, the IND vaccine should be offered to those at risk of infection by or exposure to the agent, if deemed appropriate during the risk assessment. The BMBL and the CDC ACIP provide general vaccination and vaccine-specific recommendations (CDC, 2011b).

3. Periodic Medical Evaluations

Routine, periodic medical evaluations may be a part of an OHSP for personnel working with hazardous agents, and medical clearances may be required for specific circumstances (e.g., respirator usage). Based on the needs of the program, the frequency and methods of medical evaluation may vary. Routine medical evaluations may be done through the use of questionnaires or through physical evaluations, depending on the level of risk present in the workplace and the health of the individual. In the interim between evaluations, it is important that individuals working in facilities with hazardous agents self-report changes in their health status that may impact their ability to work safely with the agents. It is also important to note that in special circumstances, it may be appropriate to offer periodic laboratory testing to workers with substantial risk of exposure to infectious agents to detect preclinical or subclinical evidence for an occupationally acquired infection (NIH-CDC, 2009).

4. Medical Support for Occupational Illnesses and Injuries

As part of the OHSP, plans for addressing potential exposures to hazardous agents should be in place. Proper and timely postexposure response is supported by having agent and exposure-specific protocols readily available that define the appropriate first aid, potential postexposure prophylaxis options, recommended diagnostic tests, and sources of expert medical evaluation (CDC, 2013a). Potential exposures are not always obvious, such splashes with infectious material, but can present days later with signs that are similar to common respiratory diseases. Workers should be encouraged to seek medical evaluation for symptoms that can be associated with infectious agents in their work area. It is always better to be cautious because infections are more difficult to treat and have greater morbidity and mortality if treatment is delayed. Fatal occupational infections have resulted from apparently unknown exposures (CDC, 2011a).

C. Training and Competency

Working with animals in a hazardous environment increases the level of risk to personnel over standard *in vitro* laboratory activities through the introduction of the potential for bites, scratches, and kicks; the frequent movement of heavy equipment; and the frequent need for use of sharps for injection, phlebotomy, and necropsy procedures. The increase in risk factors requires that personnel are highly skilled in performing all the needed tasks and can operate safely in the hazardous environment. Training on task-specific activities and general biosafety are both of critical importance in order for staff to maintain a high level of safety. While training is often thought of as an answer to this need, other factors of equal or greater importance must be considered in this type of high-risk environment. In addition to training, one must also include knowledge, competence, and performance in order to evaluate the effectiveness of training when working with animals in a hazardous environment. Definitions of each of these components include the following: training provides the necessary information and instruction; knowledge is how well students understand what is being taught; competence is demonstrating how to accomplish each task successfully under controlled circumstances; and performance is what is done under actual work conditions in the laboratory or animal facility (Foshay and Tinkey, 2007). There are many approaches to implementing an effective training program and most institutions use a combination of activities. Training will often use didactic sessions, online modules, or personal mentoring to relay the necessary information, and quizzes are oftentimes used to assure a minimum level of knowledge was attained from the training materials. The initial determination of competency and the ongoing monitoring of performance in the laboratory setting are performed by an experienced mentor. The training program should also have a process for providing routine refresher training and ensuring that training is documented in accordance with the many regulatory agencies and guidelines that apply to the type of work being performed (Pritt and Duffee, 2007). It is important that all personnel that have access to areas in which hazardous materials are used are included in the appropriate aspects of the training program. In one survey of biocontainment laboratories in the United States, only 59% of the respondents from institutions with BSL-3/ABSL-3 laboratories indicated that custodial or maintenance workers were required to receive biosafety training (Chamberlain et al., 2009).

With the designation of many microorganisms and biological toxins as select agents/toxins by the CDC, training in aspects of biosecurity is also now required when personnel have access to animals exposed to select agents/toxins. Information on training and operational requirements for working with select agents/toxins can be found on the APHIS/CDC National Select Agent Registry website (http://www.selectagents.gov/index.html). The list of training for working with animals exposed to any hazardous agent can be considerable and can include OSHA requirements; agent-specific hazards; BMBL requirements; use of biosafety cabinets; use of recombinant or synthetic nucleic acid molecules; occupational health; standard precautions; reporting of spills and potential exposures; risk identification and assessment; engineering controls; select agent regulations; task-specific activities; and many others depending on the type of work being performed (Pritt et al., 2007). Ensuring that all the regulatory requirements are met for training of staff involved in a research animal care and use program involving hazardous materials requires personnel with experience and extensive knowledge in the appropriate areas.

D. Emergency/Disaster Planning

The need to prepare for emergencies and disasters for animal facilities is universally prescribed by professional organizations, such as the American Veterinary Medical Association (AVMA), regulatory agencies (e.g., USDA), and those oversight bodies that use the Guide as their primary standard for evaluating animal care and use programs, such as the Association for the Assessment and Accreditation of Laboratory Animal Care International

and the NIH Office of Laboratory Animal Welfare (AVMA, 2008; CFR, 2012; NRC, 2011a). The Guide requires that institutions develop disaster plans that take into account the well-being of animals and personnel during unexpected events and that location-based risk should be accounted for in the disaster plan. The BMBL states that biocontainment facilities should give advance consideration to emergency and disaster recovery plans, as a contingency for man-made or natural disasters, and describes additional requirements that are mandated for institutions using select agents and toxins. By federal regulation, the CDC requires all entities using select agents and toxins to have an incident response plan (IRP) that is designed to address physical security concerns that may occur during a disaster by conducting analyses of the likelihood of various disasters and the resulting damage (CDC, 2002). While federal regulations do not explicitly address animals exposed to select agents and toxins, such animals are subject to the same requirements as a select agent/toxin for the purposes of reporting a theft, loss, or release (APHIS-CDC, 2010). Additionally, the IRP checklist provided by the CDC states that incident response procedures must account for hazards associated with the select agent and toxin and appropriate actions to contain such select agent or toxin, including any animals (including arthropods) or plants intentionally or accidentally exposed to or infected with a select agent (CDC, 2013b). Animals exposed to select agents/toxins must be incorporated into the IRP in order to better protect their security and health, the health of the public, and the environment in the event of a disaster (Swearengen et al., 2010). In all cases, it is prudent to conduct a thorough site-specific risk assessment based on location-specific natural disasters and common emergency situations to minimize any potential harm to animals, the environment, or the public when hazardous materials are involved.

VII. SUMMARY

The ability to work safely with research animals exposed to biohazards depends on multiple factors, several of which are presented in this chapter for consideration. It is critical that anyone working in this field be knowledgeable, well trained, and highly engaged in the risk assessment process and how it applies to a wide variety of situations. Working in, or managing an animal biocontainment program, requires a thorough understanding of the basic principles of containment, including both the engineering and procedural controls necessary to protect both personnel and the animals with which they work. One must also be fully aware of the highly regulated environment that accompanies this type of work and the serious consequences of non-compliance.

Providing a high level of care to research animals in a biocontainment environment requires perseverance and ingenuity to overcome some of the challenges that may be encountered along the way, but the rewards for the animals' well-being and one's own professional fulfillment can be great. While this chapter is not a comprehensive review of all the aspects of working with animals exposed to biohazards, it should provide a basis for understanding the complexity of the environment and provide additional reference materials for anyone working in this area or considering it as a career path.

References

ACIP (Advisory Committee on Immunization Practices), 2013. Vaccination Recommendations. Available from: <http://www.cdc.gov/vaccines/acip/index.html> (12 September 2013).

APHIS-CDC (Animal and Plant Health Inspection Service – Center for Disease Control and Prevention), 2010. Select Agents and Toxins Theft, Loss and Release Information Document. Available from: <www.selectagents.gov/TLRForm.html> (12 September 2013).

AVMA (American Veterinary Medical Association), 2008. The AVMA Emergency Preparedness and Response Guide, Schaumburg, IL.

Behrens, I., et al., 2002. Comparative uptake studies of bioadhesive and non-bioadhesive nanoparticles in human intestinal cell lines and rats: the effect of mucus on particle adsorption and transport. Pharm. Res. 19 (8), 1185–1193.

CDC, 2002. Laboratory security and emergency response guidance for laboratories working with select agents. Morb. Mortal. Wkly. Rep. 51 (RR–19), 1–6.

CDC, 2011a. Fatal laboratory–acquired infection with an attenuated Yersinia pestis Strain, Chicago, Illinois, 2009. Morb. Mortal. Wkly. Rep. 60 (7), 201–205.

CDC, 2011b. National center for immunization and respiratory diseases. general recommendations on immunization: recommendations of the Advisory Committee on Immunization Practices (ACIP). Morb. Mortal. Wkly. Rep. 60 (2), 1–64.

CDC, 2013a. Occupational Health Program Guidance Document for Working with Tier 1 Select Agents and Toxins. Available from: <www.selectagents.gov/Occupational_Health_Program_Guidance_Document.html> (12 September 2013).

CDC, 2013b. Inspection Checklist for Incident Response. Available from: <http://www.selectagents.gov/resources/2013_Incident_Response_Checklist.pdf> (12 September 2013).

CDC-NIH (Centers for Disease Control and Prevention-National Institutes of Health), 2009. Biosafety in Microbiological and Biomedical Laboratories. In: Chosewood, L.C., Wilson, D.E. (Eds.), fifth ed. Government Printing Office, Washington, DC.

CFR (Code of Federal Regulations), 2000. Title 9, Animals and Animal Products; Chap. 1: Animal and Plant Health Inspection Service, Department of Agriculture; Subchap. A: Animal Welfare; Parts 1, 2, 3, and 4. Office of the Federal Register, Washington, DC, Available from: <http://www.gpo.gov/fdsys/pkg/CFR-2000-title9-vol1/pdf/CFR-2000-title9-vol1-toc-id2.pdf> (17 September 2013).

CFR, 2007. Title 29, Labor; Part 1910, Occupational Safety and Health Standards; Subpart I, Personal Protective Equipment; Section 1910.134, Respiratory Protection. Office of the Federal Register, Washington, DC. Available from: <http://www.ecfr.gov/cgi-bin/text-idx?c=ecfr&tpl=/ecfrbrowse/Title29/29cfr1910_main_02.tpl> (12 September 2013).

CFR, 2012. Title 9, Handling of Animals; Contingency Plans, Final Rule: Animal and Plant Health Inspection Service, Department of Agriculture; Federal Register, volume 77, number 250. Parts 2 and 3. Available from: <http://www.gpo.gov/fdsys/pkg/FR-2012-12-31/pdf/2012-31422.pdf> (12 September 2013).

CFR, 2012a. Title 42-Public Health, Part 73. Select Agents and Toxins. Office of the Federal Register, Washington, DC. Available from: <http://www.ecfr.gov/cgi-bin/retrieveECFR?gp=1&SID=86d42d0c66832c85e43bfb1bf20e11fe&ty=HTML&h=L&n=42y1.0.1.6.61&r=PART> (12 September 2013).

CFR, 2012b. Title 7-Agriculture, Part 331. Possession, Use, and Transfer of Select Agents and Toxins. Office of the Federal Register, Washington, DC. Available from: <http://www.ecfr.gov/cgi-bin/retrieveECFR?gp=1&SID=86d42d0c66832c85e43bfb1bf20e11fe&ty=HTML&h=L&n=7y5.1.1.1.9&r=PART> (15 September 2013).

CFR, 2012c. Title 9-Animals and Animal Products, Part 121.: Possession, Use, and Transfer of Select Agents and Toxins. Office of the Federal Register, Washington, DC. Available from: <http://www.ecfr.gov/cgi-bin/retrieveECFR?gp=1&SID=86d42d0c66832c85e43bfb1bf20e11fe&ty=HTML&h=L&n=9y1.0.1.5.58&r=PART> (15 September 2013).

Chamberlain, A.T., et al., 2009. Biosafety training and incident-reporting practices in the United States: a 2008 survey of biosafety professionals. Appl. Biosaf. 14 (3), 135–143.

Copps, J., 2005. Issues related to the use of animals in biocontainment research facilities. ILAR J. 46 (1), 34–43.

Duffin, R., Tran, L., Brown, D., Stone, S., Donaldson, K., 2007. Proinflammogenic effects of low-toxicity and metal nanoparticles in vivo and in vitro: highlighting the role of particle surface area and surface reactivity. Inhalation Toxicol. 19 (10), 849–856.

Elder, A., et al., 2006. Translocation of inhaled ultrafine manganese oxide particles to the central nervous system. Environ. Health Perspect. 114 (8), 1172–1178.

Fleming, D.O., 2006. Risk assessment of biological hazards. In: Fleming, D.O., Hunt, D.L. (Eds.), Biological Safety: Principles and Practices. ASM Press, Washington, DC, pp. 81–91.

Fontes, B., 2008. Institutional responsibilities in contamination control for research animals and in occupational health and safety for animal handlers. ILAR J. 49 (3), 326–337.

Foshay, W.R., Tinkey, P.T., 2007. Evaluating the effectiveness of training strategies: performance goals and testing. ILAR J. 48 (2), 156–162.

Kastenmayer, R.J., 2012. Select agent and toxin regulations: beyond the eighth edition of the guide for the care and use of laboratory animals. J. Am. Assoc. Lab. Anim. Sci. 51 (3), 333–338.

ISO (International Organization for Standardization)/TS 27687, 2008. Nanotechnologies–terminology and definitions for nano-objects–nanoparticle, nanofibre and nanoplate. Available from: <https://www.iso.org/obp/ui/#iso:std:44278:en> (22 April 2015).

NIH, 2013. Office of Biotechnology Activities. Guidelines for Research Involving Recombinant or Synthetic Nucleic Acid Molecules. United States Department of Health and Human Services, Washington, DC. Available from: <http//www.oba.od.nih.gov/rdna/nih_guidelines_oba.html> (12 September 2013).

NIOSH (National Institute for Occupational Health and Safety), 2012, General safe practices for working with engineered nanomaterials in research laboratories. Publication No. 2012-147. Available from: <http://www.cdc.gov/niosh/docs/2012-147/pdfs/2012-147.pdf> (22 April 2015).

NRC, 1997. Occupational Health and Safety in the Care and Use of Research Animals. National Academies Press, Washington DC, p. 132.

NRC, 2003. Occupational Health and Safety in the Care and Use of Nonhuman Primates. National Academies Press, Washington, DC.

NRC, 2011a. Guide for the Care and Use of Laboratory Animals, eighth ed. National Academies Press, Washington, DC.

NRC, 2011b. Protecting the Frontline in Biodefense Research: The Special Immunizations Program. Committee on Special Immunizations Program for Laboratory Personnel Engaged in Research on

Countermeasures for Select Agents. National Academies Press, Washington DC, p. 131.

NSF (National Science Foundation), 2004. NSF International; American National Standards Institute (ANSI). NSF/ANSI Standard 49-2004. Class II (laminar flow) biosafety cabinetry, Ann Arbor, MI.

PHS (Public Health Service), 2002. Office of Laboratory Animal Welfare, National Institutes of Health. Public Health Service Policy on Humane Care and Use of Laboratory Animals. Available from: <http://grants.nih.gov/grants/olaw/olaw.htm> (12 September 2013).

PL (Public Law) 104–132, 1996. Antiterrorism and Effective Death Penalty Act of 1996.

PL 107–188, 2002. Public Health Security and Bioterrorism Preparedness and Response Act of 2002. Enhanced Control of Certain Biological Agent and Toxins Section 201(a) (42 U.S.C. 262a), and the Agricultural Bioterrorism Protection Act of 2002 Section 212, (7 USC 8401).

Pritt, S., Duffee, N., 2007. Training strategies for animal care technicians and veterinary technical staff. ILAR J. 48 (2), 109–119.

Pritt, S., Hankenson, F.C., Wagner, T., Tate, M., 2007. The basics of animal biosafety and biocontainment training. Lab. Anim. 36 (6), 31–38.

Richmond, J.Y., Hill, R.H., Weyent, R.S., Nesby-O'Dell, S.L., Vinson, P.E., 2003. What's hot in animal biosafety? ILAR J. 44 (1), 20–27.

Ryman-Rasmussen, J.P., et al., 2006. Penetration of intact skin by quantum dots with diverse physicochemical properties. Toxicol. Sci. 91 (1), 159–165.

Swearengen, J.R., et al., 2010. Disaster preparedness in biocontainment animal research facilities: developing and implementing an incident response plan (IRP). ILAR J. 51 (2), 120–126.

Weigler, B.J., et al., 2012. Risk-based immunization policies and tuberculosis screening practices for animal care and research workers in the United States: survey results and recommendations. J. Am. Assoc. Lab. Anim. Sci. 51 (5), 561–573.

28

Selected Zoonoses

James G. Fox, DVM, MS, DACLAM[a], Glen Otto, DVM[b] and Lesley A. Colby, DVM, DACLAM[c]

[a]Division of Comparative Medicine, Massachusetts Institute of Technology, Cambridge, MA, USA, [b]Animal Resources Ctr University Texas Austin, Austin, TX, USA, [c]Department of comparative Medicine University of Washington, Seattle, WA, USA

I. INTRODUCTION

Human risks of acquiring a zoonotic disease from animals used in biomedical research have declined over the past decade because higher quality research animals have defined microbiologic profiles. Even with diminished risks, the potential for exposure to infectious agents still exists, especially from larger species such as nonhuman primates, which may be obtained from the wild, and from livestock, dogs, ferrets, and

Laboratory Animal Medicine, Third Edition
DOI: http://dx.doi.org/10.1016/B978-0-12-409527-4.00028-6

cats, which are generally not raised in barrier facilities and are not subject to the intensive health monitoring performed routinely on laboratory rodents and rabbits. Additionally, when laboratory animals are used as models for infectious disease studies, exposure to microbial pathogens presents a threat to human health. Also, with the recognition of emerging diseases, some of which are zoonotic, constant vigilance and surveillance of laboratory animals for zoonotic diseases are still required.

Transmission of zoonotic agents between animals and personnel is either by direct contact with the infected animal or by indirect contact by exposure to contaminated equipment or supplies. Many activities performed in laboratories and animal facilities result in the formation of small particles or droplets that are suspended and transferred in air currents, and this aerosolization of infectious material is a principal means of disease transmission. However, direct inoculation through bites and scratches, skin or mucous membrane exposure to contaminated surfaces, and accidental ingestion can also result in agent transmission.

As in a microbiologic laboratory or an infectious disease ward of a hospital, safety procedures can minimize potential zoonotic disease transmission to associated personnel in the biomedical laboratory. Some examples of sound procedures to follow in the control of exposure to zoonotic pathogens are (1) purchase of pathogen-free animals; (2) quarantine of incoming animals to detect any zoonotic pathogens; (3) appropriate treatment of infected animals or their removal from the facility; (4) vaccination of animal carriers and high-risk contacts if/when vaccines are available; (5) use of specialized containment caging or facilities and protective clothing; and (6) regular surveillance.

It is not within the scope of this chapter to discuss these issues in detail. A number of sources are available that offer additional information. In particular, the Centers for Disease Control and Prevention (CDCP) in conjunction with the National Institutes of Health (NIH) has published a monograph, *Biosafety in Microbiological and Biomedical Laboratories* (CDCP-NIH, 2009). The National Academy of Sciences (NAS) has published *Occupational Health and Safety in the Care and Use of Research Animals* (National Research Council, 1997). *Occupational Medicine: State of the Art Reviews*, dealing with animal handlers (Langley, 1999), is also available. All of these are important resources available for use in designing protective programs for personnel involved in biomedical research using animals.

The discussion that follows is a brief overview of select viral, rickettsial, chlamydial, bacterial, fungal, protozoal, and parasitic diseases shared by humans and the animals that are commonly used in biomedical laboratories.

II. VIRAL DISEASES

A. Poxviruses

Numerous poxviruses are capable of zoonotic transmission from laboratory animals to humans. While many poxviruses are predominantly of historical interest, some may be encountered in the research setting and are of increasing concern in the United States (Reid and Dagleish, 2011). The poxviruses associated with zoonosis are classified within three genera, *Orthopoxvirus*, *Parapoxvirus*, and *Yatapoxvirus*, with the nonhuman primate serving as host for the majority of the potentially zoonotic poxviruses species. In humans, these infections are usually characterized by the development of proliferative cutaneous or subcutaneous self-limiting lesions and, in a laboratory animal setting, most frequently result from a nonhuman primate or small ruminant exposure. Fomite transmission is also of concern as most poxviruses can persist for prolonged periods in the environment and sloughed scab material.

1. Nonhuman Primate Poxvirus Infections

The zoonotic poxviruses most likely to infect nonhuman primates bred or captured for use in research include monkeypox virus, Yaba-like disease virus, and Yaba virus, although the incidence of infection is low.

a. Monkeypox

Reservoir and Incidence Monkeypox is an *Orthopoxvirus* causing sporadic cases of human disease in Africa. Natural outbreaks of monkeypox have been recorded in nonhuman primates in the wild and in laboratory settings (CDCP-NIH, 2009; Essbauer et al., 2010). Two clades of the virus are recognized: the Congo Basin clade and the West African clade. Disease severity in both humans and nonhuman primates differs with the West African clade causing a milder disease with lower mortality and rare person-to-person transmission (Wachtman and Mansfield, 2012).

The virus is naturally occurring in animals only on the continent of Africa where infection has been documented in at least 10 nonhuman primate species and four squirrel species. Squirrels are believed to be the major disease reservoir in Africa (Reid and Dagleish, 2011). The virus has a broad host range of Asian, African, and South American nonhuman primates including select apes, and New and Old World monkeys (Wachtman and Mansfield, 2012). Most of the infections of captive nonhuman primates have involved Asian macaques (Fenner, 1990).

Mode of Transmission Within susceptible nonhuman primate populations, the disease spreads rapidly with high morbidity and variable mortality. Suspected modes of transmission between nonhuman primates include aerosol, direct contact, and biting insects (Wachtman and

Mansfield, 2012). Transmission of monkeypox from captive nonhuman primate populations to humans has not been recorded. The first reported case of human monkeypox outside of Africa occurred in the Midwestern United States in June 2003 following the importation of 800 West African small rodents for the pet trade, six of which (two rope squirrels (*Funisciurus* spp.), one Gambian giant rat (*Cricetomys* spp.), and three dormice (*Graphiurus*)) were later shown to be infected with the West African clade of monkeypox virus (CDC, 2003; Guarner *et al.*, 2004). The infected rodents were co-housed with black-tailed prairie dogs (*Cynomys ludovicianus*) who contracted the disease and then served as the source of a human monkeypox disease outbreak with 87 reported (37 laboratory-confirmed) human cases (CDC, 2003; Parker *et al.*, 2007). Infection was also identified in hamsters (*Cricetus* spp.), gerbils (*Gerbillus* spp.), and chinchillas (*Chinchilla* spp.) cohoused with the infected animals (Parker *et al.*, 2007). As a result of this outbreak, U.S. importation of African rodents and interstate transportation of prairie dogs and select African rodents was banned. Human-to-human and zoonotic transmission of this agent is low and has occurred presumably through close contact with active lesions, recently contaminated fomites, or respiratory secretions (CDC, 1997; Damon, 2011; Ligon, 2004).

Clinical Signs Clinical signs in the nonhuman primate host include fever followed in 4–7 days by cutaneous eruptions, usually on the limbs and face and less frequently on the trunk. The disease may be fatal in nonhuman primates although subclinical infections are common in endemically infected populations. Fatal infections do occur in humans, predominantly in children, the malnourished, or immunocompromised individuals.

Monkeypox in humans is primarily of interest and importance because it produces a disease similar to smallpox (variola virus). Following a 7- to 19-day incubation period, monkeypox infection of humans is characterized by fever, malaise, headache, severe backache, prostration, and occasional abdominal pain (Damon, 2011; Sejvar *et al.*, 2004). Subsequent signs include lymphadenopathy of the neck, inguinal, and axillary region (a condition not normally observed with smallpox (Parker *et al.*, 2007)), as well as a maculopustular skin rash characterized by papules, vesicles, peduncles, scabs, and desquamation (Fig. 28.1). Encephalitis rarely develops. A severe fulminating disease with an approximate 10% fatality rate is observed in individuals infected with the Congo Basin clade and not vaccinated against smallpox (Reid and Dagleish, 2011).

Control and Prevention As is characteristic of *Orthopoxviruses*, monkeypox infection does not normally produce a carrier state or latent infection. Unlike most other poxviruses, monkeypox has a wide host range. It is endemic in some wild populations whose geographic ranges increasingly overlap with encroaching human

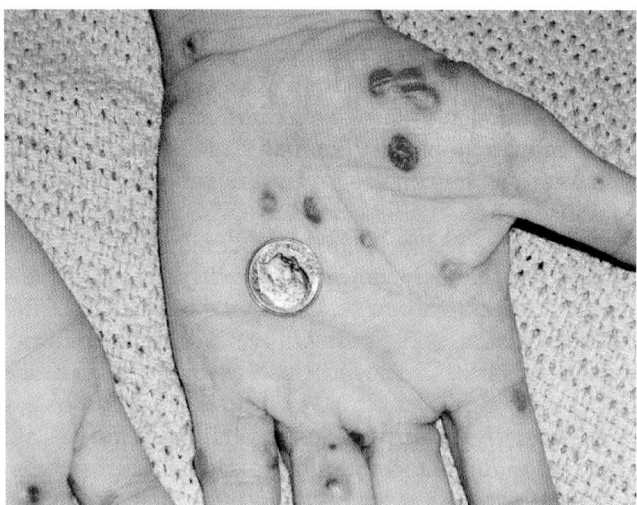

FIGURE 28.1 Photograph of skin lesions on patient A. Hemorrhagic-appearing palmar lesions are depicted. *JID, 2004: Human Monkeypox Infection: A Family Cluster in the Midwestern United States.*

populations, many of which have increasingly high numbers of immunocompromised individuals. These factors increase the potential for human transmission (Parker *et al.*, 2007). Within human populations, infections occur in small clusters, not larger outbreaks as is typical with smallpox (Reid and Dagleish, 2011). Smallpox vaccination provides partial and limited-term protection against the development and severity of monkeypox disease in both humans and nonhuman primates (Reynolds *et al.*, 2012).

Aside from the direct health impact of human infection, the monkeypox virus holds significant public health importance given its clinical similarity to smallpox in both human and animal populations. While smallpox, a zoonotic *Orthopoxvirus*, was once a significant cause of human morbidity and mortality throughout the world, the virus was declared eradicated in 1980 by the World Health Organization. Nonhuman primates are susceptible to experimental smallpox virus infection and have been shown to contract the virus from infected humans. It is considered unlikely that nonhuman primates in the wild could serve as a natural reservoir of the disease. Current concern regarding smallpox relates to its potential use as a bioterrorism agent given the public panic and high human mortality rate likely to occur in an outbreak.

Monkeypox virus (excluding the West African clade) is classified as a 'Select Agent' in the United States. Although human and animal clinical smallpox disease does not occur, an awareness of the clinical disease and diagnostic methods to rule out its presence is still relevant.

b. Yaba-Like Disease Virus

Yaba like disease virus (YLDV), previously known as benign epidermal monkeypox (BEMP) and OrTeCa poxvirus, is a *Yatapoxvirus* that has been zoonotic in the laboratory environment on numerous occasions. YLDV was once believed to be identical to tanapox. Subsequent genetic analysis has shown YLDV and tanapox to be two strains of the same virus with YLDV causing disease predominantly in nonhuman primates and tanapox causing disease (a benign cutaneous infection) in humans in East Africa (Wachtman and Mansfield, 2012).

Reservoir and Incidence   Natural infections with YLDV have been documented in African but not New World primates. In 1967, an outbreak of YLDV occurred in macaque colonies of three U.S. primate facilities during which human handlers were also affected. The source of this outbreak was never identified.

Mode of Transmission   The rapid spread of YLDV among nonhuman primates housed in gang cages suggests direct viral transmission. Infections in animal handlers were attributed to viral contamination of skin abrasions.

Clinical Signs   YLDV infection of nonhuman primates is characterized by the development of circumscribed, oval-to-circular, elevated red lesions usually on the eyelids, face, body, or genitalia that regress spontaneously in 3–4 weeks. The localization of YLDV lesions in the epidermis and adnexal structures differentiates them histologically from Yaba lesions, but similar to Yaba, eosinophilic intracytoplasmic inclusion bodies are present (Kupper *et al.*, 1970). Clinical disease in humans is characterized by a short febrile illness and lymphadenopathy followed by the development of pock lesions (Wachtman and Mansfield, 2012).

Control and Prevention   Appropriate personal protective equipment employed (PPE) while working with nonhuman primates is believed sufficient to prevent the zoonotic transmission of this agent.

c. Yaba

Yaba monkey tumor virus is an oncogenic member of the genus *Yatapoxvirus* that was reported initially in a colony of rhesus macaques (*Macaca mulatta*) housed outdoors in Yaba, Nigeria (Bearcroft and Jamieson, 1958). There have been subsequent outbreaks and experimental studies of the agent, as well as sporadic incidental cases of the disease in laboratory-housed nonhuman primates.

Reservoir and Transmission   Natural cases of the disease have been reported in the rhesus macaque and the baboon (*Papio* spp.) while experimental studies have expanded the host range to include pigtail macaques (*Macaca nemestrina*), stumptail macaques (*Macaca arctoides*), cynomolgus (*Macaca fascicularis*), African green (*Chlorocebus aethiops*), sooty mangabey (*Cercocebus atys*), and patas monkeys (*Erythrocebus patas*) (Ambrus and Strandstrom, 1966; Ambrus *et al.*, 1969). Many African monkeys apparently originate from areas with endemic infection and are immune to the agent, and New World nonhuman primate species are resistant to infection

(Ambrus and Strandstrom, 1966). The route(s) of transmission are not yet known; arthropod vectors, tattoo needles, and trauma are suspected (Wachtman and Mansfield, 2012). Experimental studies in macaques have demonstrated aerosol transmission of the agent. Thus, aerosolized Yaba virus must be considered a potential hazard to humans.

Clinical Signs   Infected animals consistently develop subcutaneous masses 5–7 days after viral exposure that reach a maximum size of approximately 2–5 cm in 3 weeks with spontaneous regression by 6–8 weeks postexposure. Mass development may not be synchronous and may occur over several months, so masses at varying stages of development may be observed (Blanchard and Russell-Lodrigue, 2012). Larger masses may ulcerate (Wachtman and Mansfield, 2012). Natural mass regression confers immunity to reinfection (Niven *et al.*, 1961), and the surgical removal of a Yaba mass in a baboon prior to natural regression was associated with subsequent susceptibility and reinfection with Yaba virus.

Six human volunteers have been inoculated experimentally with Yaba virus and developed similar, but smaller masses than those seen in monkeys; mass regression was also earlier. Yaba mass induction has been recorded as a result of accidental self-inoculation (needlestick) in a laboratory worker using the virally infected cells. Complete mass resection was curative.

2. Orf Virus (Contagious Ecthyma)

Orf virus is a *Parapoxvirus* disease of sheep, goats, and wild ungulates characterized by epithelial proliferation and necrosis of the skin and mucous membranes of the urogenital and gastrointestinal tracts.

Reservoir and Incidence   Orf virus disease is an endemic infection in many sheep flocks and goat herds throughout the United States and worldwide. The disease affects all age groups although young or immunocompromised animals are most frequently and most severely affected. Mortality may be high in lambs (10%) and kids (93%) often partially due to anorexia resulting from severe oral lesions or secondary infections (Hosamani *et al.*, 2009). In sheep, orf virus infection does not reliably confer protection against reinfection with different strains of virus, aiding in viral persistence within a population (Haig *et al.*, 1997). Recently, orf virus infections have been reported in multiple other ungulate species (Hosamani *et al.*, 2009).

Mode of Transmission   Orf virus is transmitted to humans by direct contact with scabs and exudates from viral-laden lesions. Scabs may remain infectious in the environment for years. External lesions are not always readily apparent. Transmission of this agent by fomites or other animals contaminated with the virus is also possible due to the extended environmental persistence of the virus. Although the virus requires a break in the skin for entry, rare cases of person-to-person transmission have been recorded (Chin, 2000).

Clinical Signs Orf virus produces proliferative, pustular encrustations on the lips, nostrils, and mucous membranes of the oral cavity and urogenital orifices of infected animals. Internal organs may also be affected.

The disease in humans is usually characterized by a 3- to 7-day incubation period followed by the development of a solitary lesion on the hands, arms, or face (Fig. 28.2). Initially, the lesion is maculopapular or pustular but then progresses to a weeping proliferative nodule with central umbilication. Occasionally, several nodules are present, each measuring up to 3 cm in diameter and persisting for 3–6 weeks, followed by spontaneous regression with minimal residual scarring. Regional adenitis is uncommon, and progression to generalized disease is considered a rare event although severe disease may develop in immunocompromised individuals. Previous infection does not confer protection as reinfection can occur in both humans and animals (Chin, 2000; Reid and Dagleish, 2011).

Control and Prevention Personnel should wear gloves and hand wash, as well as launder clothing and disinfect boots, after contact with sheep and goats. Current herd management practices in endemic areas can involve the use of live attenuated orf virus vaccines that provide only short-term (approximately 6 months), partial protection and contribute to the perpetuation of environmental contamination. The vaccines also pose some risk to the individuals handling the vaccine product, and there is currently no effective human vaccine. Next generation approaches, such as the development of recombinant subunit vaccines or the use of DNA vaccines, may be able to improve this situation in the future (Hosamani *et al.*, 2009; Mercer *et al.*, 1997; Zhao, *et al.*, 2011).

B. Hemorrhagic Fevers

The hemorrhagic fever viruses constitute a group of RNA viruses that produce a clinical syndrome in humans characterized by high fever, epistaxis, ecchymosis, diffuse hemorrhage in the gastrointestinal tract and other organs, hypotension, and shock. These diseases often are spread to humans by mosquitoes, ticks, or other arthropod vectors; by direct contact with the excreta of infected rodents; or by the contaminated blood and bodily fluids of other infected animals. These viral agents have taken on increased importance in recent years and are receiving considerable attention within the context of emerging infections potentially impacting the United States and other regions of the globe. Contemporary society has catalyzed the process of emerging infections by introducing ecological disturbances affecting host and vector availability and distribution, by developing rapid means of international transportation, and through the increased proportion of immunocompromised individuals within

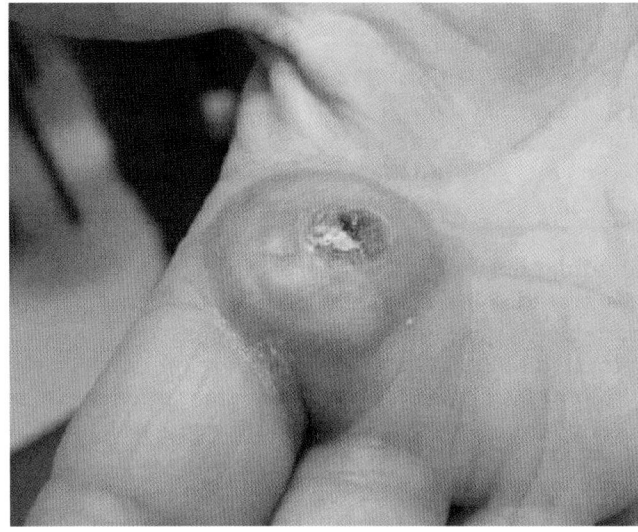

FIGURE 28.2   Bulla caused by orf virus infection after puncture by a bone of a recently slaughtered goat – Pennsylvania, 2009. *MMWR – Human Orf Virus Infection from Household Exposures – United States, 2009–2011.*

many populations (e.g., secondary to endemic human immunodeficiency virus (HIV) infections), thereby enhancing the potential dissemination and dispersion of these agents (Bengis *et al.*, 2004; Jones *et al.*, 2013).

Nonhuman primates serve as reservoirs of and are susceptible to numerous zoonotic viral hemorrhagic diseases (e.g., yellow fever, dengue, Marburg virus disease, and Ebola) as well as to viral hemorrhagic diseases that are not considered zoonotic (e.g., simian hemorrhagic fever). The zoonotic viral hemorrhagic diseases are not likely to be encountered in programs that follow an appropriate quarantine/importation process and are involved in the conventional care of nonhuman primates in indoor facilities. The salient features of natural and experimental infections by these agents in nonhuman primates have been reviewed in detail (Blanchard and Russell-Lodrigue, 2012; Wachtman and Mansfield, 2012) but will be discussed only briefly in this section. Rodent hantavirus infections have resulted in serious and fatal human infection in association with laboratory animal studies and field studies involving wild animals and are covered in more detail.

1. Flaviviruses – Yellow Fever and Dengue

Reservoir, Incidence, and Transmission Yellow fever, caused by an RNA flavivirus, is endemic in the tropical regions of the Americas and Africa where the mosquito serves as the reservoir host. The virus is not naturally transmitted directly between humans or between nonhuman primates. Although multiple genuses of mosquitos can be infected and transmit the disease, the *Aedes* spp. (*Stegomyia* spp.) mosquito is of primary importance due to its feeding habits and the ability of the virus to persist in the insect over the dry season by transovarian transmission (Wachtman and Mansfield, 2012).

Two forms of the disease are recognized based on the cyclic transmission between vertebrate hosts and mosquito vectors. In the jungle (sylvatic) form, disease transmission occurs most commonly between tree-hole breeding mosquitoes (e.g., *A. africanus* in Africa, *Haemagogus* spp. in Central and South America) and nonhuman primates residing in the forest canopy. Virus transmission to humans occurs where the human and mosquito ranges overlap such as during forestry activities that disrupt mosquito feeding preferences. Once introduced into a human population, the urban (rural) form of disease transmission may develop in which the virus is transmitted between individuals by peridomestic mosquitoes (predominantly *Aedes aegypti)* which breed well in urban settings and feed on humans (Blanchard and Russell-Lodrigue, 2012; Monath and Staples, 2011).

There are four serotypes of dengue virus, any of which can cause dengue hemorrhagic fever in humans. Dengue is endemic in tropical and subtropical Asia, Africa, Oceania, Australia, and the Americas, and is widespread in the Caribbean basin. Dengue is regarded as one of the most significant emerging diseases in the United States. The virus persists in nonhuman primate–mosquito and human–mosquito cycles involving *A. aegypti* and *A. albopictus.* While *A. aegypti* have been present in the southern United States for many years, the more aggressive *A. albopictus* was only introduced into the United States in 1985 but has quickly expanded its range to at least 18 states (Blanchard and Russell-Lodrigue, 2012). Dengue virus is passed transovarially in the mosquito vector (Chin, 2000).

Clinical Signs   Most nonhuman primates are susceptible to yellow fever although disease severity varies significantly across species, with some species exhibiting no clinical signs despite an active infection. African monkeys apparently acquire yellow fever infection as young animals and develop a mild and brief form of the disease with subsequent immunity and induced antibody titers. The disease in both New World nonhuman primates and humans is most frequently fulminating and severe, characterized by fever, vomiting, anorexia, yellow to green urine, icterus, and albuminuria. In humans, a hepatic-induced coagulopathy may develop with gingival hemorrhage, epistaxis, petechiae, hematemesis, melena, or blood oozing from the skin. At necropsy, the internal organs are hemorrhagic, necrotic, and bile-stained. The classic lesion is massive, midzonal necrotizing hepatitis with necrotic hepatocytes containing characteristic eosinophilic, intracytoplasmic inclusion bodies, or 'Councilman bodies' (Gardner and Ryman, 2010; Monath and Staples, 2011).

Immune response to the dengue virus has been demonstrated in a wide range of free roaming nonhuman primate species, indicating that they can be naturally infected with the virus. However, the significance of infection in nonhuman primates is unknown (Wachtman and Mansfield, 2012). Experimental infection of nonhuman primates can induce mild to severe clinical signs. Human dengue infection is characterized by the abrupt onset of fever, intense headache, myalgia, arthralgia, retro-orbital pain, anorexia, gastrointestinal disturbances, and rash. In some, the disease progresses to include a generalized hemorrhagic syndrome with increased vascular permeability, thrombocytopenia, unusual bleeding manifestations, and death.

Diagnosis and Control   Yellow fever is diagnosed by identification of the virus in the blood, a specific antibody response, or histopathology. The variable expression of yellow fever in African *versus* New World nonhuman primates decreases the reliability of clinical signs as indicators of active infection. Consequently, imported monkeys should have a certificate that they have originated from a yellow fever-free area; have been maintained in double-screened, mosquito-proof enclosures; or have been vaccinated for yellow fever. The same general principles apply to the prevention of introduction of dengue virus in newly imported nonhuman primates.

The Centers for Disease Control and Prevention (CDC), which regulates nonhuman primate importation facilities, stipulates specific record-keeping procedures, and requires the prompt (within 24h) reporting of any disease in a nonhuman primate suspected of being infected with yellow fever, Marburg, monkeypox, or Ebola disease (filovirus). This reporting requirement also applies to any illness among staff members that may have been acquired from nonhuman primates. Nonhuman primates that die during primary import quarantine must be necropsied and evaluated for characteristic lesions of yellow fever or other zoonotic diseases (42 CFR 71.53).

Control of human yellow fever is centered on eradication of the *A. aegypti* mosquito as well as human vaccination with the live-attenuated 17D vaccine strain (Gardner and Ryman, 2010). Dengue disease prevention also emphasizes control of the mosquito vector. Human vaccines are being developed.

2. Marburg Virus Disease

Marburg virus is a single-stranded RNA virus (genus *Marburgvirus,* family Filoviridae) that is the etiologic agent of Marburg hemorrhagic fever in humans and nonhuman primates (Mehedi *et al.,* 2011). The first outbreak occurred simultaneously in 1967 in Marburg, Frankfurt, and Belgrade with 31 human cases, 7 of which were fatal. The outbreak was traced to one shipment of African green monkeys originating from Uganda, held in an airport exotic animal quarantine facility in London and then shipped to Marburg, Frankfurt, and Belgrade for use in vaccine production. Primary infections were traced to humans exposed to tissues, blood, or primary cell cultures derived from infected African green monkeys or infected humans. Secondary infection occurred in additional persons in contact with one or more primary cases. No animal handlers were infected. Although African green monkeys are not now believed to serve as a reservoir of the virus, Marburg virus disease is often referred to as African green monkey disease or vervet monkey disease due to the initial association between this nonhuman primate species and virus.

Reservoir and Incidence Between the initial 1967 outbreak and 2013, there have been 10 recognized outbreaks of human Marburg virus infection. In these, the number of identified cases ranged from 1 to 252 cases with the case fatality rate in the four larger outbreaks ranging from 22% to 90%. While most cases are confined to Africa, human cases have been diagnosed in Europe, the Netherlands, and the U.S. Each has been linked to travel in or animal importation from Africa (Centers for Disease Control and Prevention, n.d.-a, n.d.-b).

The natural reservoir for the Marburg disease agent has not been definitively identified, although African fruit bats (*Rousettus aegyptiacus*) are considered highly likely (Towner *et al.*, 2007). Experimental studies in nonhuman primates and other laboratory animals have shown that the virus produces a 100% fatal infection in African green monkeys, rhesus monkeys, squirrel monkeys, guinea pigs, and hamsters. Although African green monkeys were clearly incriminated in the original outbreak, the high fatality rate observed following the experimental infection of African green monkeys and other nonhuman primate species suggests that nonhuman primates are not a likely natural reservoir of the disease (Mehedi *et al.*, 2011).

Mode of Transmission In humans, disease transmission is most commonly traced to mucous membrane or skin exposure to tissues or bodily fluids during the clinical care of infected patients or in handling of their bodies for burial. Parental transmission has occurred and sexual transmission has been suspected in at least one case. Studies in nonhuman primates have demonstrated lethal infections following experimental aerosol exposure. Although human epidemiologic data does not suggest a high risk of aerosol transmission during the clinical care of infected individuals, respiratory transmission has been suspected from inhalation of infected bat excreta. Significant concern exists regarding the potential use of Marburg virus as a bioterrorism agent (Lloyd, 2011; Mehedi *et al.*, 2011). As such, Marburg virus as been classified as a Tier 1 Select Agent (CDC, n.d.-c).

Clinical Signs The incubation period for Marburg disease is 2–21 days in humans and 4–20 days in nonhuman primates (Lloyd, 2011). The disease in humans includes systemic viral replication, immunosuppression, and abnormal inflammatory response, and is manifested by the abrupt onset of fever, chills, myalgia,

headache, anorexia, and conjunctival suffusion. In fatal cases, progressive involvement of the gastrointestinal tract with severe pain and gastrointestinal bleeding, maculopapular rash, severe coagulation abnormalities with uncontrolled hemorrhage, renal dysfunction, multiorgan failure, and shock often occurs (Mehedi *et al.*, 2011). The clinical course is very similar in nonhuman primates (Schou and Hansen, 2000) although severity varies across species. Treatment of Marburg virus disease consists of intensive supportive therapy and pain management.

Diagnosis and Prevention Disease diagnosis is possible through virological, serological, and molecular methods, with polymerase chain reaction (PCR) and antigen detection enzyme-linked immunosorbent assay (ELISAs) most commonly employed (Mehedi *et al.*, 2011). Biosafety level 4 (BSL4) containment is required for any procedures involving potentially contaminated substances (e.g., blood, saliva, urine, breast milk). Irradiation and heat can be used to inactivate the virus in some samples to allow their safe handling at lower containment levels. In a recent study, a live, attenuated recombinant vaccine was shown to protect rhesus macaques from development of Marburg virus infection when administered soon after experimental challenge. It is hoped that a similar treatment could be developed for use in humans (Geisbert *et al.*, 2010). No Marburg virus disease vaccines are currently approved for human use.

3. Ebola Hemorrhagic Fever

Reservoir and Incidence Ebola and Marburg viruses share many similarities. Morphologically identical but antigenically distinct, they are members of the family Filoviridae. Human cases of Ebola are rare and have been confined to the continent of Africa. Ebola was first detected in Sudan and the Democratic Republic of Congo in 1976. Since that time, multiple virus subtypes have been identified. All induce clinical, often fatal disease in humans with the exception of Ebola-Reston. Hospital case fatality rates range from 42% to 88% (Gire *et al.*, 2012). The subtypes are, in approximate decreasing degree of human disease severity (based on case fatality rates), Zaire, Sudan, Bundibugyo, Ivory Coast, and Reston.

Ebola-Reston is unique as it is the only subtype of Asian (not African) origin and is not known to induce human disease, although human infection can occur. Ebola-Reston was first identified in 1989 in cynomolgus macaques soon after their importation into the United States from an export facility in the Philippines. The infected monkeys died of an acute hemorrhagic disease. It is unknown what influence their coinfection with the immunosuppressive simian hemorrhagic fever virus played in the animals' deaths. Clinical disease was not recognized in animal technicians who handled the infected animals and who developed filovirus-specific serum antibodies (CDC, 1990;- Dalgard *et al.*, 1992). Nevertheless, the disease outbreak in this nonhuman primate colony within the United States garnered significant public health concerns, ultimately resulting in the development and ongoing enforcement of nonhuman primate importation and handling guidelines (42 CFR Part 71.53). Since the 1989 nonhuman primate outbreak, Ebola-Reston has been identified in additional cynomolgus monkeys associated with the same Philippine export facility as well as on a pig farm in the Philippines where viral transmission, but not disease, occurred in humans (CDC, n.d.-c).

The natural reservoir(s) for the Ebola virus is still debated. Nonhuman primates are not likely natural disease reservoirs (Dalgard *et al.*, 1992). African fruit bats are the leading reservoir candidate of Ebola subtypes of African origin (Leroy *et al.*, 2005). The reservoir for Ebola-Reston is suspected to be a mammal native to Asia.

Mode of Transmission   As with Marburg virus, transmission appears in most cases to be from direct contact with infected tissues or close contact with humans or animals shedding the organism. Oral and conjunctival transmission of Ebola-Zaire in macaques has also been confirmed experimentally (Jaax *et al.*, 1996). However, in the natural outbreak of Ebola-Reston infection in a laboratory colony of nonhuman primates, transmission occurred among animals without apparent direct intimate contact, suggesting the possibility of airborne or aerosol transmission. Three of six animal technicians working with these animals developed antibody response to Ebola-Reston virus, but the details of transmission were not determined in all cases. One of these individuals was infected during *postmortem* examination of an infected monkey (Ksiazek *et al.*, 1999). Epidemiologic findings in animal caretakers working in the Philippine-source colony for Ebola-Reston-infected nonhuman primates suggest that the transmission of Ebola-Reston to humans is rare (Miranda *et al.*, 1999).

Clinical Signs   In experimental nonhuman primate infections with Ebola-Zaire or Sudan, animals rapidly develop a febrile, debilitating illness characterized by high-titer viremia; virus dissemination and replication in multiple organs producing tissue necrosis, effusions, coagulopathy, and hemorrhage; and death. Although less virulent than the Sudan or Zaire strains of Ebola virus in nonhuman primates, Ebola-Reston produces a hemorrhagic disease in macaques involving multiple organ systems, resulting in death in 8–14 days. Clinical signs in humans vary somewhat by infecting Ebola subtype. With the exception of Ebola-Reston, humans develop a pattern of infection similar to that of nonhuman primates manifested by acute illness, fever, chills, headache, myalgia, and anorexia with progressive deterioration to vomiting, abdominal pain, and sore throat with or without obvious bleeding abnormalities (Feldmann and Geisbert, 2011).

Diagnosis and Prevention   The gross and histopathologic findings of Ebola infection have been reported in numerous nonhuman primate species including chimpanzees (Wyers *et al.*, 1999), baboons, African green monkeys (Ryabchikova *et al.*, 1999), and macaques (Dalgard *et al.*, 1992). In macaques, intracytoplasmic inclusion bodies associated with hepatocellular necrosis, adrenal necrosis, and patchy pulmonary interstitial infiltrates were noted in cases of Ebola-Reston infection and considered useful for the differentiation of this disease from simian hemorrhagic fever (Dalgard *et al.*, 1992).

Diagnostic tests commonly used for human infection include reverse transcriptase PCR (RT-PCR), antigen capture ELISA testing, ELISAs for IgM and IgG antibody levels, and virus isolation. A human vaccine is not yet available. Most current vaccine candidates are based on recombinant technologies.

Due to effective importation procedures mandated by the CDC (CDC, 1990), only those personnel employed in nonhuman primate facilities involved in animal importation should have the potential for Ebola virus exposure. These personnel should become familiar with the equipment and procedures used to minimize the potential for Ebola virus transmission in the event of an outbreak. Neither vaccination nor antiviral pharmaceuticals are available for the treatment of Ebola virus infection. Experimental drugs are being tested in an attempt to curb the African Ebola outbreak in 2014. Recently, 16/16 macaques experimentally infected with Marburg virus, a close filovirus relative of Ebola virus, have been protected by administering a small interfering RNA molecule, encapsulated in a lip nanoparticle (Tekmira drug — TKM-Marburg) on day 3 postinfection, when clinical signs begin to manifest. Infected monkeys not receiving the drug died between days 7 and 9 (Thi *et al.*, 2014). It is recommended that BSL 4 containment be employed with Ebola virus (CDCP-NIH, 2009).

4. Hantaviruses (Hemorrhagic Fever with Renal Syndrome; Hantavirus Pulmonary Syndrome)

Reservoir and Incidence   Within the family Bunyaviridae, the genus *Hantavirus* is composed of at least 20 viruses known to naturally infect a wide range of mammalian species including numerous wild rodents that serve as disease reservoirs. Unlike other members of the Bunyaviridae family, hantaviruses are maintained in vertebrate–vertebrate cycles without arthropod vectors (Maclachlan *et al.*, 2011a). Antibodies against hantaviruses have been detected in multiple species including domestic and wild cats, dogs, pigs, cattle, deer, and nonhuman primates. Evidence exists that cats and pigs may serve as a reservoir of infection for humans for at least one hantavirus (Zeier et al., 2005). Other animal species may also serve as disease reservoirs for human infection. In the United States, serological surveys have detected evidence of hantavirus infection in urban and rural areas involving *Rattus norvegicus, Peromyscus maniculatus, P. leucopus, Microtus pennsylvanicus, Tamias* spp., *Sigmodon hispidus, Reithrodontomys megalotis, Oryzomys palustris,* and *Neotoma* spp. (CDCP-NIH, 2009; Schmaljohn and Hjelle, 1997; Tsai et al., 1985).

In humans, hantaviruses are responsible for two recognized disease syndromes, hemorrhagic fever with renal syndrome (HFRS) and hantavirus pulmonary syndrome (HPS). The severity of the disease produced depends on the specific virus involved (LeDuc, 1987; Maclachlan et al., 2011a; Schmaljohn and Hjelle, 1997). Old World (Asia and Europe) hantaviruses are responsible for HFRS, whereas New World (the Americas) hantaviruses are responsible for HPS. Rodent reservoir species typically remain asymptomatic despite persistent infection and viral shedding in the saliva, urine, and feces (Maclachlan et al., 2011a).

Over 200,000 human cases of HFRS are reported yearly throughout the world with most cases in China, Russia, and Korea (Maclachlan et al., 2011a). At least four hantaviruses are involved (Hantaan, Seoul, Puumala, and Dobrava), each with a specific reservoir rodent host.

Multiple hantaviruses can induce HPS. In 1993, the first cases of HPS were diagnosed in the Four Corners area of the United States with an over 50% case fatality rate (CDC, n.d.-f; Schmaljohn and Hjelle, 1997). The genetically distinct hantavirus responsible for this outbreak was subsequently named Sin Nombre virus (Zeier et al., 2005). Since the initial outbreak, cases of HPS have been reported in 34 U.S. states (36% case fatality rate) and Central and South America including a 2012 outbreak in Yosemite National Park. About three-quarters of identified cases have been from rural areas and half have been from areas outside of the Four Corners area (CDC, n.d.-f). Hantavirus pulmonary syndrome has been reported in the United States in persons associated with outdoor activities and occupations that place them in close proximity to infected wild rodents and their excrement (Hjelle et al., 1996; Jay et al., 1996; Schmaljohn and Hjelle, 1997). Cases of clinical disease and/or seroconversion has been recognized in individuals involved in field research studies (Torres-Perez et al., 2010), but whether this is directly attributable to wild animal handling or could be associated with contamination of the living quarters associated with fieldwork is not always clear (Kelt et al., 2007).

Numerous cases of hantavirus infection have occurred among laboratory animal facility personnel following exposure to infected rats (*Rattus*), including outbreaks in Korea, Japan, Belgium, France, and England (LeDuc, 1987). Infected individuals exhibited clinical signs consistent with HFRS.

Mode of Transmission The transmission of hantavirus infection is through the inhalation of infectious aerosols; brief exposure times (5 min) have resulted in human infection. Rodents shed the virus in their respiratory secretions, saliva, urine, and feces for many months (Tsai, 1987). Transmission of the infection can also occur through an animal bite or from disturbing dried materials contaminated with rodent excreta, allowing wound contamination, conjunctival exposure, or ingestion to occur (CDCP-NIH, 2009). Infection of animal caretakers and research personnel has resulted from the introduction of infected wild rodents into the laboratory animal facility environment as well as biologics derived or contaminated by them. Person-to-person transmission is rare, but has been documented with select hantaviruses (Schmaljohn and Hjelle, 1997).

Clinical Signs Clinical signs are related to the hantavirus species involved and are largely a result of the target cell of infection, endothelial cells (Zeier et al., 2005). The classical pattern of HFRS is characterized by fever, headache, myalgia, and hemorrhagic manifestations including petechiae, anemia, gastrointestinal bleeding, oliguria, hematuria, severe electrolyte abnormalities, and shock (Lee and Johnson, 1982). Common clinical signs and laboratory abnormalities of HPS include a febrile prodrome, headache, thrombocytopenia (usually without overt hemorrhage), and leukocytosis. In addition, patients may develop a non-productive cough and shortness of breath that can rapidly proceed to respiratory failure due to capillary leakage into the lungs, followed by shock and cardiac complications (CDCP-NIH, 2009; Schmaljohn and Hjelle, 1997).

Diagnosis and Prevention Both antigenic and genetic methods have been used for the characterization of the hantaviruses. RT-PCR, antigen capture ELISA, and immunohistochemistry are most commonly used (Maclachlan et al., 2011a). Additional information about hantavirus serological testing is available through the Special Pathogens Branch, Division of Viral and Rickettsial Diseases, Centers for Disease Control and Prevention. Treatment is based on provision of supportive care. Administration of the antiviral drug ribavirin can be beneficial in the treatment of HFRS, but not HPS (Bi et al., 2008). No vaccine is currently available.

Hantavirus infections should be prevented through the detection of infection in rodents and rodent tissues prior to their introduction into resident laboratory animal populations and facilities (Maclachlan et al., 2011a). Rodent tumors and cell lines can be tested for hantavirus contamination with PCR and immunofluorescence assays. Also, wild rodent intrusions into animal facilities must be prevented. Animal BSL 4 (ABSL4) guidelines are recommended for animal studies involving hantavirus infections in permissive hosts such as *P. maniculatus*. Wild-caught rodents brought into the laboratory that are susceptible to hantaviruses producing HPS or HFRS should also be handled according to these guidelines (CDCP-NIH, 2009).

C. Lymphocytic Choriomeningitis Virus

Lymphocytic choriomeningitis virus (LCMV) infections in rodents (e.g., mice, hamsters) are of particular interest and concern as the virus can be transmitted from asymptomatic, infected animals to humans with relative ease. While some estimate that up to 5% of the U.S. population has been infected with LCMV, seriously debilitating and fatal human infections are uncommon (case fatality rate <1%), but do occur (Childs *et al.*, 1997; Fischer *et al.*, 2006; Morita *et al.*, 1996; Smith *et al.*, 1993; Stephensen *et al.*, 1992). In parallel with the persistent and emerging importance of arenaviruses for humans with wild rodent contact, LCMV has remained an important natural infection of laboratory animals (Bowen *et al.*, 1975; Dykewicz *et al.*, 1992; Jahrling and Peters, 1992; Rousseau *et al.*, 1997).

Reservoir and Incidence   LCMV is a member of the family Arenaviridae, which are single-stranded RNA viruses with a predilection for rodent reservoirs. Other members of the family are important zoonoses that produce a hemorrhagic fever syndrome, including Lassa fever (in Africa) and Argentine and Bolivian hemorrhagic fevers (in South America).

The house mouse, *Mus musculus*, is the recognized natural reservoir host of LCMV with infected wild mouse populations present throughout most of the world. LCMV infections have also been noted in multiple common laboratory animal species including rats, hamsters, guinea pigs, rabbits, swine, dogs, and nonhuman primates. LCMV is especially well adapted to the mouse, living in a symbiotic relationship characterized by asymptomatic infection with lifelong virus shedding. The mouse, and in certain well-defined outbreaks, the hamster, has remained the species of primary concern as zoonotic reservoirs in the laboratory as evidenced by a recent outbreak of LCMV in humans (Dykewicz *et al.*, 1992). Athymic and other immunodeficient mouse strains may pose a special risk by harboring silent, chronic infections (CDCP-NIH, 2009; Dykewicz *et al.*, 1992).

An LCMV variant has been identified as the etiologic agent of the disease marmoset (callitrichid) hepatitis (Stephensen *et al.*, 1995). First reported in the 1980s at 11 North American zoos, epizootics of the disease have occurred in zoological parks in both the United States and England, often with high case fatality rates in marmosets and tamarins (Montali *et al.*, 1989, 1995). Rodent infestations are common in zoos and mice, as known carriers of LCMV are the probable source of infection in

these outbreaks. Some outbreaks have been traced to the feeding of neonatal mice ('pinkies') from enzootically infected mouse populations to callitrichids (Montali *et al.*, 1993). Interestingly, two veterinarians involved in the care of infected callitrichids seroconverted to the agent but did not develop clinical signs of disease (Blanchard and Russell-Lodrigue, 2012). The pathologic lesions observed in LCMV-infected callitrichids share many similarities with those of humans infected with another *Arenavirus* in sub-Saharan Africa, Lassa hemorrhagic fever virus. As a result, callitrichids have been proposed as an animal model of human Lassa disease.

Mode of Transmission   The course of LCMV infection of the laboratory mouse is influenced by host factors and the organotrophism of the LCMV strain (Baker, 1998). Under some circumstances, LCMV produces a pantropic infection and may be copiously present in the blood, cerebrospinal fluid, urine, nasopharyngeal secretions, feces, and tissues of natural hosts and possibly humans. In endemically infected mouse and hamster colonies, the infection is transmitted *in utero* or early in the neonatal period, producing a tolerant infection characterized by chronic viremia and viruria without significant clinical disease. Thus, bedding material and other fomites contaminated by LCMV-infected animals can be important sources of infection for humans, as demonstrated in numerous outbreaks among laboratory animal technicians (Dykewicz *et al.*, 1992; Newcomer and Fox, 2007; CDC, 2012b). Exposure of adult, immunocompetent mice most frequently results in a transient infection with seroconversion although persistent infection with wasting may develop following immune exhaustion (Maclachlan *et al.*, 2011b). This differs from the hamster that may remain persistently infected regardless of the age at exposure.

The experimental passage of tumors and cell lines appears to pose one of the biggest threats for the introduction of LCMV into animal facilities at the present time. Spread of LCMV among animals by contaminated tumors and cell lines has been widely recognized (Bhatt *et al.*, 1986; Dykewicz *et al.*, 1992; Nicklas *et al.*, 1993). Transmission by infected, bloodsucking ectoparasites has been demonstrated experimentally, and LCMV has been recovered from cockroaches. However, these sources for LCMV infection have not been shown to play a significant role in any of the LCMV infections (human or animal) in laboratory animal facilities to date.

Infection in humans may be by parental inoculation, inhalation, or contamination of mucous membranes or broken skin with infectious tissues or fluids from infected animals as may occur with bites. Airborne transmission is well documented. In human LCMV infections associated with infected pet hamsters, the infection rate correlated with cage type and cage location in the household. Open wire cages were correlated with the highest rate of infection, whereas deep boxes and aquariums were associated with a lower human infection rate. Similarly, cage placement in an area of high human activity was associated with infection, but cages located away from areas of frequent human activity (e.g., the basement) did not result in infection of occupants (Biggar et al., 1975). Also, infections are known to occur in individuals who have not had direct physical contact with infected hamsters but who had simply entered the room housing the animals (Hinman et al., 1975). These findings suggest that airborne transmission plays an important role in human infection. Human-to-human transmission has been documented through maternal–fetal transmission and solid organ transplantation (CDC, 2008; Fischer et al., 2006; Macneil et al., 2012).

Clinical Signs LCMV was so named due to the lymphocytic choriomeningitis induced in multiple species following experimental intracerebral inoculation. Clinical signs are not usually evident in immunocompetent mice naturally infected as fetuses or neonates, although signs (e.g., body condition wasting, weakness, tremors) may develop if immunotolerance wanes ('late-onset disease') or if mice are infected a few days after birth. Hamsters infected as adults typically remain asymptomatic, while hamsters infected early in life may fail to thrive and display growth retardation, weakness, conjunctivitis, dehydration, and/or tremors (Maclachlan et al., 2011b).

Humans usually develop a transient flu-like illness characterized by fever, myalgia, headache, and malaise following an incubation period of 1–3 weeks (Table 28.1). However, more serious disease manifestations may develop in patients including photophobia, vomiting, nuchal rigidity, central nervous system disease (e.g., septic meningitis, meningoencephalitis), and rarely pneumonitis, myocarditis, orchitis, dermatitis, and pharyngitis (Bonthius, 2012; Maclachlan et al., 2011b). Fatal human cases have been characterized by severe pharyngitis, fever, bleeding abnormalities, pneumonia, and hepatic triaditis. In the last decade, at least five clusters of deaths in human transplant recipients have resulted from the implantation of solid organs from donors later known or presumed to be infected with LCVM (Macneil et al., 2012; Schafer et al., 2014). A hemorrhagic fever-like disease was noted in some of these individuals (CDC, 2008). It is postulated that the severity of disease in transplant recipients is largely influenced by their induced immunosuppression (Fischer et al., 2006). Intrauterine infection has resulted in fetal and neonatal death, hydrocephalus, and chorioretinitis (Maclachlan et al., 2011b).

Diagnosis and Prevention ELISAs and immunofluorescence assays are most commonly employed to screen mice that may have been exposed to the virus after the neonatal period. These assays are not useful to diagnose persistently infected, immune tolerant mice, as

circulating antibodies may not be present at detectable levels. RT-PCR should be used in these circumstances and to screen biologic materials (e.g., cell lines, tumors, serum). The virus does grow easily in many cell types but produces minimal cytopathic effects. Therefore, cell cultures must be assayed for antigen detection (Charrel and de Lamballerie, 2010; Maclachlan et al., 2011b). Depopulation of infected colonies is highly recommended. Prevention of this disease in animal facilities is achieved through the periodic serological surveillance of both new animals with inadequate disease profiles and resident animal colonies at risk. Screening all biologics intended for animal passage for the presence of LCMV is another crucial element in the program to prevent the introduction of LCMV into established animal colonies. The exclusion of wild rodent vermin and the elimination of ectoparasites and insect vectors from animal facilities are part of the overall scheme for LCMV disease prevention and are expected of modern laboratory animal facilities.

Human infection is most frequently diagnosed through a combination of serologic testing, virus isolation from the blood or cerebrospinal fluid, PCR testing, and immunohistochemistry. Treatment consists of supportive care as no specific antiviral medications are recommended.

TABLE 28.1 Symptoms of Persons with Positive Titers for Lymphocytic Choriomeningitis

Symptom	Number of cases	
	49[a]	11[b]
None recognized	3	1
Fever	44	9
Headache	42	7
Myalgia	39	8
Pain on moving eyes	29	7
Nausea	26	9
Vomiting	17	9
Biphasic illness	12	NR[c]
Sore throat	12	NR
Photophobia	12	7
Cough	9	1
Swollen glands	8	NR
Diarrhea	8	1
Rash	6	1
Upper respiratory tract symptoms	6	NR
Orchitis	1	NR

[a]From Biggar et al. (1975).
[b]From Maetz et al. (1976).
[c]NR, None recognized.

D. B Virus Infection (*Macacine herpesvirus 1*)

Many animal species commonly maintained in a research setting are susceptible to natural infections with herpesviruses (e.g., saimiriine herpesvirus 1 and 2, suid herpesvirus 1, porcine lymphotrophic herpesvirus 1). While few animal herpesviruses are proven zoonotic agents, there is great concern that at least some may crossover to the human population, especially into immunocompromised individuals or in association with xenotransplantation. However, macacine herpesvirus 1 (formerly *Cercopithecine herpesvirus 1* and *herpesvirus simiae* and often referred to as herpes B, monkey B virus, and herpesvirus B) stands alone as a documented hazard with devastating potential for humans working with select nonhuman primate species.

Reservoir and Incidence   First described by Gay and Holden following a cluster of human cases in 1932, B virus produces a life-threatening disease of humans that has resulted in approximately 40 reported human cases with a greater than 70% case fatality rate (CDC, 1987, 1989a,c, 1998; Huff and Barry, 2003). Only macaque monkeys (e.g., rhesus, cynomolgus, and pig-tailed macaques) are known to naturally harbor B virus (Cohen et al., 2002). The virus has been detected in the saliva, urine, feces, and nervous tissue of infected macaques as well as cell cultures derived from their tissues. The virus persists latently in the trigeminal and lumbosacral ganglia of the macaque with occasional reactivation of viral shedding from peripheral sites in asymptomatic animals in response to physical or psychological stressors or during periods of immunosuppression (Estep et al., 2010; Simmons, 2010). The infection is transmitted between macaques by virus-laden secretions through close contact involving primarily the oral, conjunctival, and genital mucous membranes (Weigler et al., 1995). Infection of other nonhuman primate species can be fatal although select Old World monkey species have been shown to be seropositive to B virus, indicating that they may also be potential disease reservoirs (Kalter et al., 1997).

In an endemically infected domestic macaque production colony, the incidence of B virus infection was shown to increase with animal age, approaching 100% by the end of their first breeding season (Weigler et al., 1993). Wild-caught rhesus macaques have also exhibited a high (near 100%) seroconversion rate following their capture. Consequently, B virus should be considered endemic among Asian monkeys of the genus *Macaca*.

Three genotypes of B virus have been identified through molecular and phylogenetic analysis with each genotype represented by isolates from the presumed macaque species of origin: rhesus and Japanese macaques, cynomolgus macaques, and pigtail macaques (Smith et al., 1998). Nearly all humans diagnosed with B virus infection have had known contact with rhesus macaques in a research setting and all recovered human isolates have been of the rhesus viral genotype (Smith et al., 1998; Weigler, 1992). As a result, the strain common in rhesus macaques is suspected to be more pathogenic for humans (Huff and Barry, 2003).

Mode of Transmission   The transmission of B virus to humans primarily occurs through exposure to contaminated saliva through bites and scratches. Exposure by the airborne route may have played a role in several human cases (Palmer, 1987), and exposure of ocular mucous membranes to biological material, possibly fecal, has been confirmed in one human fatality (CDC, 1998). Other confirmed routes of B virus transmission to humans include needle stick injury (Benson et al., 1989) and exposure to infected nonhuman primate tissues (Wells et al., 1989). The possibility of fomite transmission through an injury obtained in handling contaminated caging warrants consideration in an institution's hazard assessment and risk analysis. One case of human-to-human transmission has been documented (CDC, 1987). In this case, the spouse of an infected animal handler contracted B virus infection after applying ointment to herpetic skin lesions on her husband and then to an area of dermatitis on her own hand (Cohen et al., 2002).

Clinical Signs   In macaques, the natural disease reservoir, infection is asymptomatic or results in only a mild clinical disease similar to human herpes simplex virus infection. During primary infection, macaques develop vesicles or ulcers on the mucous membranes or skin that generally heal within a 1- to 2-week period; keratoconjunctivitis or corneal ulcer may also be noted. Recovery is usually uneventful.

In humans, the period between initial exposure and onset of clinical signs ranges from 2 days to, more frequently, 2–5 weeks. However, in one case, an individual developed severe clinical disease from B virus 10 years after his last known exposure to the agent. Researchers in the field have also suggested that asymptomatic human B virus infection may occur (Benson et al., 1989), but it is not known whether viral reactivation resulting in severe clinical disease can occur later.

Disease progression is influenced by the number of inoculated infectious viral particles as well as the anatomic site of exposure. In most cases, following exposure by bite, scratch, or other local trauma, humans may develop a herpetiform vesicle at the site of inoculation. In the B virus fatality resulting from ocular exposure, the patient did not develop a dendritic corneal lesion typical of ocular herpes infections; rather, she developed a swollen, painful orbit with conjunctivitis (CDC, 1998). As the clinical signs in this patient progressed, she developed retro-orbital pain, photophobia, anorexia, nausea, and abdominal pain. Other early clinical signs of B virus include myalgia, fever, headache, and fatigue followed by progressive neurological disease characterized by numbness, hyperesthesia, paresthesia, diplopia, ataxia, confusion, urinary retention, convulsions, dysphagia, and an ascending flaccid paralysis resulting in respiratory failure. Central nervous system involvement signals a grave prognosis even with aggressive treatment (Huff and Barry, 2003).

Diagnosis and Prevention Direct virus isolation is the 'gold standard' in B virus disease diagnosis, although it cannot detect latent infections *pre-mortem*. Serologic assays are often used to detect an immunological response to infection. However, immunologic response is delayed for some period of time after infection. Both virus isolation and the conduct of select serologic assays require BSL4 containment as they involve manipulation of live, infectious virus. More recently, PCR methods and serologic assays with recombinant technology have been developed that do not require BSL4 containment, thus simplifying disease diagnosis (Huff and Barry, 2003; Katz *et al.*, 2012).

A key provision to prevent B virus exposures within an institution's animal care and use program concerns the utilization of macaques as research subjects. Macaques should be used only when there are no suitable alternative animal models. Efforts to acquire and maintain macaques free of B virus infection should be pursued whenever feasible. Efforts have been made to produce macaque colonies free of B virus (Weir *et al.*, 1993). While the incidence of disease in these colonies is significantly lower than in conventional colonies, all macaques must be considered potentially infected with B virus and handled accordingly.

Following a 1987 outbreak of B virus infection in monkey handlers, guidelines were developed to prevent B virus infection in humans (CDC, 1987). Additional provisions for protection against B virus exposure via ocular splash were adopted following the death of a young woman exposed by this route (CDC, 1998). Readers should refer to these sources or other detailed reviews before engaging in studies involving macaques or developing institutional programs for the prevention and control of B virus among monkey handlers (Blanchard and Russell-Lodrigue, 2012; Cohen *et al.*, 2002). Briefly, these recommendations emphasize the need for nonhuman primate handlers to conform fully with a written comprehensive PPE program based on a thorough hazard assessment of all work procedures, potential routes of exposure, and potential adverse health outcomes (CDC, 1998).

Approaches to hazard assessment and the development of occupational health and safety programs for research animal facilities have been reviewed extensively in other sources (ILAR, 1997). Use of protective clothing, including protective gloves or long-sleeved garments and barriers to mucous membrane exposure (e.g., goggles, mask), is essential to prevent exposure to infectious secretions. The use of a face shield is insufficient as the sole method for protection against ocular exposure because droplet splashes to the head may drain into the eyes and infectious materials may enter via the gap along the margins of the shield. The use of examination gloves alone for hand protection should be reserved for the handling of monkeys under full chemical restraint. Chemical restraint or specialized restraining devices should be used whenever possible to reduce personnel injuries.

The outcome of a human exposure is heavily influenced by the time until treatment initiation. Patients should have direct and immediate access to local medical consultants knowledgeable about B virus and versed in current B virus treatment recommendations as prescribed by the Centers for Disease Control and Prevention and the B Virus Working Group (Cohen *et al.*, 2002). Prompt and thorough cleaning of the exposure site is vital after which serum samples and cultures should be obtained for serology and viral isolation from both the patient and the macaque. Antiviral therapy (e.g., valacylovir or acyclovir) may also be warranted based on the nature of the exposure (e.g., deep puncture bite, mucosal exposure), the interval between exposure and cleaning of the exposure site, and a positive culture of B virus from the patient or nonhuman primate (Cohen *et al.*, 2002). However, antiviral therapy is not without risk to the patient and may complicate diagnostic testing. The administration of antiviral therapy in patients diagnosed with B virus infection is controversial because increasing antibody titer has been demonstrated in a patient following its discontinuation (Cohen *et al.*, 2002). The determination of the most efficacious antiviral(s) for use is ongoing (Krug *et al.*, 2010). Physicians should consult the National Center for Immunization and Respiratory Disease, Division of Viral Diseases, Centers for Disease Control and Prevention, for assistance in case management. Additional information about B virus diagnostic resources is available through the National B Virus Resource Center, Georgia State University, Atlanta, Georgia.

E. Rabies

Rabies is an acute, almost invariably fatal disease caused by a virus in the genus *Lyssavirus* of the family *Rhabdoviridae* (Banyard and Fooks, 2011).

Reservoir and Incidence Rabies occurs worldwide with the exception of a few countries, generally island nations and other regions that have excluded the disease through animal importation and control programs with the aid of geographic barriers. Bats and terrestrial carnivores are the natural hosts of the rabies virus; however, most mammals are susceptible to infection (CDCP-NIH, 2009). Historically, most human rabies cases resulted from contact with infected domestic animals including pets and agricultural species. This has slowly changed such that now most human cases result from contact with infected wildlife.

The grand majority of confirmed animal rabies cases in the United States are reported in wildlife species with raccoons, bats, skunks, and foxes predominating (Dyer *et al.*, 2013). Only two laboratory-acquired human rabies cases have been documented in the United States, neither involving direct animal exposure (CDC, 1977; Winkler *et al.*, 1973). Among the rodent and lagomorph species maintained in the laboratory, the wild-caught groundhog and rabbit appear to represent a risk of transmitting rabies (Childs *et al.*, 1997; Karp *et al.*, 1999). In addition, other rabies-susceptible wildlife species studied in the field or introduced into the laboratory have the potential to harbor rabies virus (Fitzpatrick *et al.*, 2014). Because the incidence of rabies in wildlife in the United States is high and continues to increase, the possibility of rabies transmission to dogs, cats, or other species with uncertain vaccination histories and originating from an uncontrolled environment must be considered.

Mode of Transmission   Rabies virus is transmitted by the bite of a rabid animal or by the introduction of virus-laden saliva into a fresh skin wound or intact mucous membrane. Transmission through urine and feces exposure is technically possible, but considered to be of low risk (Banyard and Fooks, 2011). Of particular concern is the risk of aerosol transmission of the rabies virus, although the true risk of this means of transmission has been questioned (Gibbons, 2002). Most human cases are associated with bat variant rabies virus infection contracted either during an unrecognized exposure incident or following an exposure incident for which the individual did not seek prompt medical care (Dyer *et al.*, 2013). The virus has also been transmitted through corneal and organ transplants from individuals with undiagnosed central nervous system disease.

Clinical Signs   While there are no pathognomonic signs of animal rabies cases, most infected animals will develop either the 'furious' or 'dumb' form of the disease. The furious form is characterized by progressive neurologic signs often including hyperexcitability, parasthesia occasionally with self-mutilation, and death secondary to respiratory arrest and organ failure. In contrast, the dumb form is characterized by lethargy, incoordination, and ascending paralysis (Banyard and Fooks, 2011).

In humans, the timing until disease onset as well as the speed of disease progression is influenced by many variables including the anatomic site of exposure, the quantity of virus inoculated, virus strain, and host age and immune status (Banyard and Fooks, 2011). The disease course proceeds through several phases: incubation, prodrome state, acute neurologic period, coma, and death (CDC, 2010a). The incubation period in humans is ordinarily 1–3 months but may vary from 9 days to over 8 months. During the 2- to 4-day prodromal stage, patients experience a period of apprehension and develop headache, malaise, and fever. An abnormal, indefinite sensation at the exposure site is the first specific symptom. Patients may also develop intermittent periods of excitation, nervousness, or anxiety interspersed with quiet periods when the mental state appears normal. Further progression of the disease is marked by paresis or paralysis, inability to swallow, hydrophobia, delirium, convulsions, and coma. Few individuals recover from rabies infection; once clinical signs develop, the disease is almost invariably fatal from an acute viral encephalomyelitis followed by respiratory paralysis (Banyard and Fooks, 2011; Hemachudha *et al.*, 2013).

Diagnosis and Prevention   Rabies should be considered as a differential diagnosis in any wild-caught or random-source laboratory animal of unknown vaccination history exhibiting encephalitic signs. Any wild animal that has bitten a human should be submitted for rabies examination in a manner that permits definitive identification of the species for epidemiologic purposes if the species is not already known.

No reliable *pre-mortem* diagnostic test is available for use in animals. In human patients, multiple methods are most frequently used in combination to diagnose the disease. These include virus isolation, molecular techniques (e.g., RT-PCR), and antibody or antigen detection techniques.

The definitive diagnosis of rabies requires identification of the virus in any part of the brain via the direct fluorescent antibody (DFA) test and therefore is conducted *postmortem*. Most commonly, at least two brain regions are examined with the brain stem and cerebellum preferred. In the absence of the DFA test, histologic examination of brain tissue or molecular evaluation of other tissues or fluids can be useful but must be interpreted with caution and have not been widely adopted for use by diagnostic laboratories.

Preventing or minimizing disease development following a potential rabies virus exposure is heavily influenced by a person's pre-exposure rabies vaccination status as well as the speed at which the exposure site is thoroughly cleaned and additional postexposure prophylaxis (PEP) is provided. Rabies vaccines, administered in a series of injections as a component of pre-exposure prophylaxis, are highly efficacious and should be available to personnel at high risk for encountering the virus including veterinarians, personnel involved in the care of high-risk or inadequately characterized animals, field biologists working in rabies-endemic areas, and scientists working directly with the virus. The need for periodic booster vaccinations is determined by an individual's subsequently measured rabies serum antibody titer (Banyard and Fooks, 2011).

General guidelines for PEP administration are published and periodically updated by the CDC's Advisory

Committee on Immunization Practices. In addition to prompt cleaning and wound care, the guidelines call for application of human rabies immune globulin at and around the exposure site of individuals without prior vaccination as well as multiple parental administrations of rabies vaccine. The number of recommended vaccine doses, administered at a defined interval, varies based on the individual's pre-exposure vaccination status and presumed general immunocompetence (CDC, 2010a).

Whenever possible, animals brought into the laboratory should have histories that preclude their exposure to rabies or assure that they have been previously vaccinated for this disease. Serologic assays have been developed to help identify vaccinated animals. Vaccine titers should not be used to determine the timing of booster vaccinations (Banyard and Fooks, 2011; Brown et al., 2011).

F. Viral Hepatitis Infections

Many of the nonhuman primate zoonoses causing systemic infections in humans include hepatitis as one component of the disease. However, of the viral infections that target the liver as the primary site of involvement, only hepatitis A virus (HAV) has proven to be a significant zoonotic pathogen in the laboratory animal facility environment. Nonhuman primates are important experimental hosts in viral hepatitis research and have been used to study hepatitis A, B, C, D, and E infections (Vitral et al., 1998). Other viruses known to induce hepatitis in naturally acquired infections of laboratory animal species include the coronavirus, mouse hepatitis virus; the adenovirus, infectious canine hepatitis virus; and the hepadnavirus, woodchuck hepatitis virus. None of these are recognized zoonotic agents.

1. Hepatitis A

Reservoir and Incidence　HAV is a human enterovirus belonging to the family Picornaviridae. The primary reservoirs for HAV infection are humans, with nonhuman primate infections resulting from contact with infected humans or other infected nonhuman primates. However, more than 100 cases of HAV infection in humans have been associated with newly imported chimpanzees (Dienstag et al., 1976; Hinthorn et al., 1974). There are also many other nonhuman primate species naturally susceptible to HAV, including tamarins, owl monkeys (*Aotus trivirgatus*), African green monkeys, cynomolgus (*M. fascicularis*) and rhesus macaques, and that could serve as sources for human HAV infection (Burgos-Rodriguez, 2011; Lemon et al., 1990; Shevtsova et al., 1988; Wachtman and Mansfield, 2012).

Mode of Transmission　HAV can be isolated from the blood and is shed in the feces during the prodromal

phase of the disease. It is transmitted by the fecal–oral route, most commonly via contaminated food or water. Aerosol transmission is not suspected (CDCP-NIH, 2009).

Clinical Signs　The disease in nonhuman primates is much less severe than in humans and is frequently subclinical. Clinical disease develops in the chimpanzee, owl monkey, and several marmoset species, and is characterized by malaise, vomiting, jaundice, and elevated serum levels of hepatic enzymes.

The disease in humans varies from a mild illness lasting less than 2 months to a severely debilitating illness lasting up to 6 months. Following an incubation period of approximately 1 month, patients experience an abrupt onset of fever, malaise, anorexia, nausea, joint pain, and abdominal discomfort followed within a few days by jaundice (Fig. 28.3). Children often have mild disease without jaundice, whereas HAV infections in older patients may be fulminant and protracted with prolonged convalescence. However, protracted HAV infection is considered an acute infection that is ultimately resolved by the patient; a chronic hepatitis A carrier state has never been shown to exist. Infection confers lifelong immunity (ACIP, 2006).

Diagnosis and Prevention　Infection is diagnosed by demonstration of elevated IgM-specific anti-HAV or total combined IgM and IgG anti-HAV antibodies in the serum or plasma. Alternatively, detection of HAV RNA in the blood or feces is considered diagnostic of active infections. The presence of IgG anti-HAV antibodies is useful in detecting previous infection (ACIP, 2006).

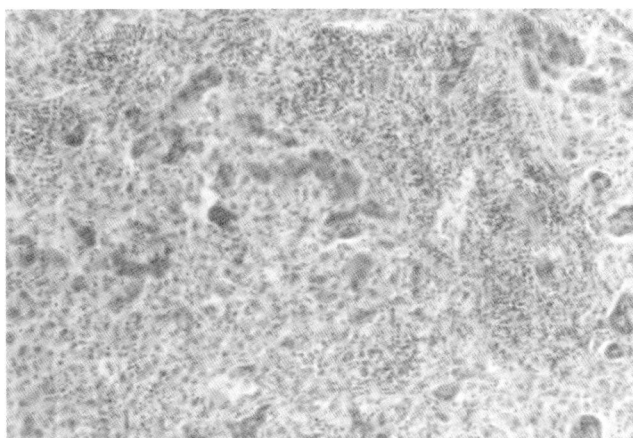

FIGURE 28.3　Under a magnification of 100×, this hematoxylin and eosin photomicrograph depicts the cytoarchitectural changes found in a liver tissue specimen extracted from a hepatitis A patient. In this particular view, note that there are several layers of hepatic parenchyma, which are still recognizable in the midst of massive necrosis. There is no fatty change, but there is an extensive inflammatory infiltrate. *Source: PHIL Library ID# 13020.*

A safe, effective multidose hepatitis A vaccine is available in the United States and is recommended for individuals at high risk for exposure to HAV infection, such as persons involved with the care of nonhuman primates used in experimental HAV infection studies. Passive protection of such persons can also be undertaken through the intramuscular administration of specific immune serum globulin (ISG). Passive protection should be given before experimental animal HAV infection studies begin because infected animals start shedding HAV at 7–11 days postinoculation and continue shedding for several weeks. Two different dosages of ISG are recommended, each providing differing durations of passive protection (1–2 months *versus* 3–5 months) (ACIP, 2006). PEP can be administered following suspected virus exposure. PEP recommendations varies with the age and prior vaccination history of the exposed individual and may include administration of a single-antigen hepatitis A vaccine and/or ISG within 2 weeks of exposure (ACIP, 2007). The use of protective clothing, personal hygiene, and appropriate sanitation practices for equipment and facilities will also minimize the potential for zoonotic transmission.

2. Hepatitis E Virus

Hepatitis E virus (HEV) is unique among the major hepatitis viruses (A, B, C, and D) in that animals serve as natural reservoirs of the virus (Pavio *et al.*, 2010). HEV is classified in the genus *Hepevirus* and is currently subdivided into at least four major genotypes, although additional genotypes are proposed (Maclachlan *et al.*, 2011c). Genotypes 1 and 2 infect only humans; genotypes 3 and 4 can infect both humans and a range of other species involved in zoonotic transmission of the virus. HEV infects people worldwide, causing a sometimes fatal viral hepatitis (Lhomme *et al.*, 2013). Its detection in animal populations has steadily risen in the recent past, thereby prompting increased concern of its zoonotic potential.

Reservoir and Incidence In humans, a large proportion of the enterically transmitted acute viral hepatitis cases in developing countries in Asia, Africa, and Mexico are due to HEV infections. In industrialized countries, serologic evidence of HEV exposure is high and widespread, although clinical HEV infection is only sporadically diagnosed. Hepatitis E may be disproportionally fatal in pregnant women, with over a 25% case fatality rate as compared to 1% in the general population (Meng, 2005). However, it is unclear what role other underlying health factors may have played in this increased fatality rate (Meng, 2010a). In industrialized countries, identified cases usually occur sporadically, presumably due to zoonotic transmission from one or more animal reservoirs or following consumption of contaminated meat or shellfish (Lhomme *et al.*, 2013; Meng, 2010a). In contrast, outbreaks most commonly

occur in developing countries secondary to fecal contamination of food or water (Maclachlan *et al.*, 2011c; Meng, 2005). Direct human-to-human transmission is rare (Pavio *et al.*, 2010).

Domestic pigs can be naturally infected with HEV and shed large quantities of virus in their feces. Under experimental conditions, swine HEV strains are infectious for nonhuman primates and the human strains of HEV are infectious to pigs. In addition, pig handlers (e.g., swine veterinarians, swine farmers) have a significantly higher rate of seroconversion to HEV than does the general population (Huang *et al.*, 2002). Swine infection is widespread and worldwide. In the United States, the seroprevalence rate of swine HEV infection ranges between 50 and 100% in some herds (Lhomme *et al.*, 2013). Infection occurs in farmed pigs between 2 and 4 months of age, presumably by fecal–oral transmission, with a transient viremia followed by fecal shedding (Huang *et al.*, 2002; Meng, 2011). Given this, domestic pigs are recognized as likely reservoirs of HEV for the human population.

An avian strain of HEV exists with a high incidence of seroconversion in farmed chickens. The virus is now believed to be the etiologic agent of big liver and spleen disease (hepatitis-splenomegaly syndrome) of chickens. However, disease has not resulted following experimental transmission of the avian virus to other species including nonhuman primates, suggesting that the avian strain does not present a significant zoonotic threat. Other animals including farmed rabbits, wild rats, wild boar, bats, mongeese, and deer are susceptible to HEV infection and are being evaluated as potential sources of human disease (Cossaboom *et al.*, 2011; Lhomme *et al.*, 2013; Meng, 2011). Of these, rabbit HEV is of greatest concern as antibody titers, suggestive of infection, have been detected in rabbit farms in the United States and China, and experimental infection of pigs has been demonstrated (Cossaboom *et al.*, 2012). Some species (e.g., tamarins, owls monkeys, and cynomolgus monkeys) are susceptible to experimental infection and antibody response to HEV has been detected in wild-caught macaques. Nonhuman primates are not considered likely disease reservoirs although disease transmission from nonhuman primates to humans should not be discounted (Wachtman and Mansfield, 2012).

Mode of Transmission In human populations, hepatitis E was originally believed to result most commonly from human fecal contamination of drinking water in areas endemic for the disease. Recent research has focused on the role that many animal species may play in zoonotic disease transmission from the feces of infected animals and the consumption of undercooked, contaminated animal tissues (meat and liver) (Lhomme *et al.*, 2013). Aerosol transmission is not suspected. Given the suspected routes of virus transmission to humans, the risk within an animal facility should be minimal. Nevertheless, personnel are advised to observe proper PPE practices to prevent possible HEV exposure.

Clinical Signs Disease is frequently self-limiting and asymptomatic, although an acute hepatitis can develop with classical signs of liver involvement including jaundice, anorexia, and hepatomegaly. A fulminant, fatal hepatitis of pregnant women has been attributed to HEV infection, although this disease course has not been observed in naturally or experimentally infected pigs or experimentally infected rhesus macaques (Lhomme et al., 2013; Meng, 2010b). Chronic disease may develop in the immunocompromised including transplant recipients (Zhou et al., 2013). Infected pigs most frequently appear clinically normal despite microscopic lesions of hepatitis (Meng et al., 1997).

Diagnosis and Prevention Propagation of HEV in cell culture has been problematic, hindering its evaluation and development of diagnostic tests. Disease diagnosis in both humans and pigs is based on the detection of anti-HEV antibodies or the presence of HEV RNA in serum or feces (Pavio et al., 2010). Treatment is limited to provision of supportive care.

A hepatitis E vaccine is not currently available.

3. Other Viral Hepatitis Agents

Humans are considered natural hosts for viral hepatitis types B, C, and D, all of which are transmitted parenterally by exposure to blood or other bodily fluids. Hepatitis B virus (HBV), caused by a human hepadnavirus, has been widely studied experimentally in the chimpanzee although the gibbon, orangutan, and wooly monkey are known to be susceptible (MacDonald et al., 2000). Natural HBV infection was first noted by demonstration of HBV surface antigen in cynomologus in 1985 (Kornegay et al., 1985). Recently, wild-living cynomolgus macaques from Mauritius Island were diagnosed with natural, chronic infection of a genotype of HBV distinct from the human genotype. The disease appears relatively benign in the infected animals. The zoonotic risk of the cynomolgus genotype is yet unknown (Dupinay et al., 2013). It is postulated that infected cynomolgus monkeys may serve as a useful animal model of the disease. Other natural hepadnavirus infections of animals (woodchuck, ground squirrel, and duck) are used as animal models of HBV infection, but none are transmissible to humans (Blanchard and Russell-Lodrigue, 2012). The chimpanzee has been used as an experimental model for the study of hepatitis C and D viruses. Thus, the concern for hepatitis B, C, and D as zoonoses is minimal in the laboratory animal facility environment except where these agents are used in experimental animal studies. In these cases, personnel should adhere to appropriate precautions when handling nonhuman primates.

G. Retroviruses

In the wake of the human acquired immunodeficiency syndrome (AIDS) epidemic, there has been an intense, multifaceted interest in the study of human and comparative retrovirology. The zoonotic potential for animal retroviruses has been clearly identified. Retroviruses are RNA viruses with a high mutation rate, facilitating the virus' adaptation to novel hosts. It is currently postulated that all human retroviral pathogens have evolved from simian retroviral precursors (Huang et al., 2012). HIV-1 and HIV-2 evolved from simian immunodeficiency virus (SIV) strains originating in the chimpanzee (*Pan troglodytes troglodytes*) and sooty mangabey (*Cercocebus atys*), respectively (Chen et al., 1996; Gao et al., 1999). In addition, human T-cell lymphotropic virus type 1 (HTLV-1) appears to have evolved in humans following interspecies transmission of an earlier form of the virus (simian Tcell leukemia virus) from nonhuman primates (Gessain et al., 2013). These findings have heightened the concerns of zoonotic retroviral transmission, particularly in connection with the use of nonhuman primates as potential xenograft donors to humans requiring organ transplantation. Similar concerns have been raised about the pig as a donor for xenotransplants to humans because the porcine endogenous retrovirus has been demonstrated to grow in human cells *in vitro* (Wilson et al., 1998). However, although there are numerous retrovirus infections of wild, laboratory, and domestic animal species, the transmission of these agents from their natural host to humans under laboratory conditions has been infrequent but consistently involves nonhuman primates as source species. Four simian retroviruses have crossed species to infect humans: SIV, simian retrovirus, simian T-cell leukemia virus, and simian foamy virus (SFV). Each is detailed below although it must be noted that there is concern that additional simian retroviruses may adapt and become zoonotic agents.

When working with any nonhuman primates or associated tissues or fluids, personnel should be instructed to observe applicable PPE requirements, operational procedures, and safe syringe/needle-handling practices. Potential virus exposure sites should be immediately cleansed and/or disinfected and medical attention sought. Follow-up medical evaluations with periodic monitoring for infection may be warranted. Supervisory personnel should be informed of the incident. Written institutional policies should be in place to address confidentiality, counseling, and other issues related to potential retrovirus exposure. Those with evidence of retroviral infection should not donate blood or tissues.

1. Simian Immunodeficiency Virus

Reservoir and Incidence SIV is a lentivirus known to infect over 45 species of nonhuman primates in Africa in which it is endemic in many nonhuman primate populations. Seroprevalence rates increase with animal age and may be as high as 76% (Murphy *et al.*, 2006) in naturally infected, wild populations. A unique species-specific SIV strain has been identified in 33 infected nonhuman primate species (Kalish *et al.*, 2005), although cross-species transmission does occur. To date, infection has not been detected in Asian or South American nonhuman primates in the wild (Hayami *et al.*, 1994; Locatelli and Peeters, 2012).

Most SIV strains can grow in human cells *in vitro*. Seroconversion to the virus has been detected in multiple individuals with occupational exposure to nonhuman primates or their tissues. Occupational exposures have included an individual with active dermatitis of the hands who handled SIV-infected primate samples and cultures while not wearing gloves. SIV was successfully isolated from this individual. Seroconversion has also been documented in two other individuals, each of which suffered accidental needlesticks while working with samples from SIV-infected macaques. One individual remained seropositive for only a short time, whereas the second individual remained seropositive for 11 years. SIV was not isolated from either individual (Khabbaz *et al.*, 1994; Murphy *et al.*, 2006).

Mode of Transmission The blood, cerebrospinal fluid, secretions (e.g., semen, saliva, urine, milk), and tissues of SIV-infected monkeys should be presumed to be infectious. Both horizontal (via sexual contact and fight wounds) and vertical virus transmission occurs between nonhuman primates (Locatelli and Peeters, 2012). Aerosol transmission is not suspected.

Clinical Signs Initially, it was presumed that SIV infections were nonpathogenic in natural hosts despite their persistent, lifelong infection. However, an acquired immunodeficiency disease with chronic wasting has rarely developed in some naturally infected animals after prolonged infection. Disease does develop in nonhuman primate species that are not natural hosts of the virus following natural or experimental infection. In these animals, an acute infection or a chronic, latent infection may occur. Asian nonhuman primates, including rhesus macaques, may develop an especially severe form of the disease that closely resembles human AIDS including immunosuppression and increased susceptibility to opportunistic infections. Clinical signs have not been recorded in any cases of human SIV infection.

Diagnosis and Prevention A combination of serologic (e.g., ELISA, Western blot) and molecular assays (PCR) as well as virus isolation are employed to detect infection in both humans and nonhuman primates. Testing samples can include blood, urine, feces, and tissues. However, the selection and interpretation of specific diagnostic assays must be made with consideration of the numerous, genetically diverse strains

of SIV identified and the knowledge that cross-species transmission may occur (Murphy *et al.*, 2006). African species may not develop antibody titers despite infection. To prevent inadvertent disease transmission, Asian macaques should not be allowed direct contact with African species.

2. Simian Retrovirus

Reservoir and Incidence Simian retrovirus (SRV) was first identified in the 1980s soon after which it was detected in nonhuman primate colonies in several U.S. regional primate research centers. SRV, an oncogenic betaretrovirus and formally designated the Mason-Pfizer monkey virus, is now known to exist in at least seven serotypes. Some serotypes have been confirmed to be endogenous retroviruses, resulting in germline transmission with no easily detectable, induced serologic immune response. Up to 90% of some wild and captive nonhuman primate populations are infected. Serologic evidence of human infection exists in West African populations as well as those with occupational exposure to nonhuman primates. In addition, the virus has been isolated from one patient with AIDS and lymphoma but with no known nonhuman primate contact (Murphy *et al.*, 2006; Wachtman and Mansfield, 2012). Overall, the degree of the risk for zoonotic transmission of SRV remains unclear.

Mode of Transmission Blood, urine, and bodily fluids can be infectious, and both horizontal (via bite wounds and sexual contact) and vertical transmission occurs in nonhuman primates (Burgos-Rodriguez, 2011). Human infection may result from contact with infectious substances such as through wound contamination, mucous membrane exposure, and needlestick injuries. Aerosol transmission is not suspected at this time.

Clinical Signs New World primates appear resistant to SRV infection, whereas other species (e.g., macaques) may develop immunodeficiency with chronic wasting, increased susceptibility to opportunistic infections, necrotizing gingivitis, retroperitoneal fibromatosis, persistent diarrhea, hematologic abnormalities, and sudden death (Burgos-Rodriguez, 2011; Murphy *et al.*, 2006; Wachtman and Mansfield, 2012). No clinical signs have been noted in humans with serologic evidence of infection.

Diagnosis and Prevention In nonhuman primates, severe disease may exist in the absence of a serologic antibody response, whereas an antibody response may be detectable in the absence of clinical signs. Therefore, attempts at virus isolation, molecular assays (e.g., PCR), and direct visualization of the virus in fixed tissue are necessary to help rule out infection. Chronic wasting and/or clinical signs related to a specific opportunistic infection may be the first indication of SRV infection (Wachtman and Mansfield, 2012). Prevention of disease transmission in an occupational setting is based on strict observance of practices and procedures designed to limit human exposure to infected nonhuman primates and their tissues.

3. Simian T-Cell Leukemia Virus

Reservoir and Incidence Human T-cell leukemia virus subtypes 1–3 (HTLV-1, HTLV-2, and HTLV-3) are believed to have developed following multiple instances of transmission of the oncogenic *Deltaretrovirus* primate T-lymphotropic virus subtypes 1–3 (PTLV-1, PTLV-2, and PTLV-3) from African nonhuman primates to humans. A simian analog of HTLV-4 has not yet been identified, nor has a human analog been identified for the recently discovered PTLV-5 of macaques. HTLV is a significant disease of humans, infecting approximately 10–20 million people worldwide. PTLV infections have been documented in over 33 species of Old World monkeys and apes in Africa and Asia, with seroprevalence increasing with age. Some subtypes have species specificity in natural infections of wild populations with PTLV-2 currently found only in bonobos (*Pan paniscus*) and PTLV-3 found only in African nonhuman primates. Infection with multiple PTLV subtypes does occur (Locatelli and Peeters, 2012). Some New World primates are susceptible to experimental infection, but natural infection has not been identified in their wild populations (Murphy *et al.*, 2006).

Mode of Transmission Within nonhuman primate species, PTLV disease transmission occurs through sexual contact and fight wounds, and possibly through the nursing of young. Human infection with PTLV has occurred in Africa in individuals exposed to blood, bodily fluids, or tissues of infected nonhuman primates. Infection of persons with occupational exposure to nonhuman primates or their fluids has not been documented.

Clinical Signs Nonhuman primates infected with PTLV-1 infrequently develop a lymphoproliferative disease with persistent lymphocytosis and T-cell abnormalities; lymphoma and leukemia with accompanying skin lesions; hepatosplenomegaly; or, in gorillas only, chronic wasting (Murphy *et al.*, 2006). Clinical signs are not observed in nonhuman primates infected with PTLV-2 or PTLV-3 (Burgos-Rodriguez, 2011).

Diagnosis and Prevention Infection is diagnosed through serologic assays employing ELISA, IFA, Western blot, and PCR assays. Subtype differentiation requires sequence analysis (Murphy *et al.*, 2006; Wachtman and Mansfield, 2012).

4. SFV Infection

Natural infections of foamy viruses have been identified in many species including nonhuman primates, cats, cows, and horses. *In vitro*, foamy viruses cause cytopathic effects in many cell types, yet in their natural host, foamy viruses do not induce pathologies and remain lifelong persistent infections (Murray and Linial, 2006).

Reservoir, Incidence, Transmission, and Clinical Signs The SFVs are complex retroviruses (genus *Spumavirus*) that have been isolated from a number of New and Old World nonhuman primates (Wachtman and Mansfield, 2012). Infection rates in many wild and captive nonhuman primate colonies approach 100% with transmission suspected to occur through exposure to saliva (e.g., contamination of deep fight wounds) and possibly blood. A wide range of animal species have been experimentally infected with SFV. No evidence of pathogenicity has been detected in these species or the natural nonhuman primate hosts although lifelong, stable virus persistence is suspected (Khan, 2009). Human infection with SFV has been documented with no apparent ill effects. The virus has recently been detected in the saliva of infected humans (Huang *et al.*, 2012). Human-to-human transmission has not been detected, suggesting that humans may serve as dead-end hosts. In Africa and Asia, human infection is believed to result from contact with infected wild nonhuman primates, especially during their hunting, butchering, or consumption (Khan, 2009). It is debatable if a human foamy virus variant exists. However, foamy virus infections have been confirmed on multiple occasions. The first was reported in 1971 from the cell culture of an East African patient with nasopharyngeal carcinoma. The isolated foamy virus was, based on immunologic and sequence data, judged to be closely related to a chimpanzee foamy virus (Heneine *et al.*, 1998; Schweizer *et al.*, 1997). The second case involved an animal handler employed at a research institute for over 20 years and who had suffered multiple bite wounds from African green monkeys. The worker became seropositive for foamy virus within 6 years of employment. African green monkey foamy virus DNA was later detected in his peripheral blood mononuclear cells, indicating persistent yet asymptomatic infection (Schweizer *et al.*, 1997). A subsequent survey of U.S. and Canadian workers with occupational exposure to nonhuman primates revealed evidence of SFV infection via serology, proviral DNA detection, and/or virus isolation in 4 of the 231 individuals tested. Each of the four was employed at different institutions. Three individuals were infected with SFV of baboon origin, one with SFV of African green monkey origin. Infection was asymptomatic in all four individuals and evidence of infection was not found among their close contacts, including the three spouses tested (Heneine *et al.*, 1998). From these and other confirmed cases of human infection (Gessain *et al.*, 2013; Switzer *et al.*, 2004), it is now assumed that human infections with SFV result in a latent, asymptomatic infection with minimal risk for human-to-human transmission.

Prevention Those with occupational exposure to nonhuman primates are at a significantly increased risk of SFV infection. The risk that SFV may have yet unseen, long-term effects or could mutate into a human-adapted, pathologic form should not be dismissed. Infected humans are advised to not donate blood or other tissues (Boneva *et al.*, 2002; Heneine *et al.*, 1998; Khan and Kumar, 2006). The use of PPE as described in connection with the prevention of SIV transmission to humans should be applied when handling SFV-infected nonhuman primates.

H. Measles Virus (Rubeola)

Reservoir and Incidence Measles virus, a paramyxovirus (genus *Morbillivirus*), infects millions of people worldwide and can have devastating effects on nonhuman primate colonies. In the United States, approximately 60 human measles cases are reported each year although that number has been significantly higher in the most recent past (CDC, 2013). A small number of human measles infections are postulated to have resulted from contact with infected macaques during one large-scale measles outbreak at a U.S. primate center (Roberts *et al.*, 1988). The virus can infect both Old World and New World monkeys and apes although it is not naturally found in wild populations removed from human contact. Humans are the natural disease reservoir and serve as the reservoir for nonhuman primates (Wachtman and Mansfield, 2012).

Measles outbreaks within U.S. and European domestically born nonhuman primate colonies are infrequent, but do occur (Willy *et al.*, 1999). In these domestic colonies, the source of the virus is infected humans or the importation of infected animals. Outbreaks frequently occur in geographic regions where naïve nonhuman primate populations may come into close association with endemically infected human populations. Within these nonhuman primate populations, the seroprevalence of infection may, depending on animal species, approach 100%. With the current emphasis on and success of domestic nonhuman primate production, it has become more likely that institutions will develop large populations of susceptible nonhuman primates that could contract measles and then transmit the disease to susceptible humans.

Mode of Transmission Measles is a highly communicable disease that is transmitted by infectious aerosols, contact with nasal or throat secretions, or contact with fomites freshly contaminated with infectious secretions. Viral shedding can occur prior to clinical signs and continues until after rash onset. (CDC, 2012a).

Clinical Signs The clinical course of the disease differs significantly between nonhuman primate species. Macaques and other species of Old World primates commonly develop a mild upper respiratory infection although asymptomatic infections occur. Clinical signs most frequently seen in Old World monkeys include nasal and ocular discharge, conjunctivitis, facial edema, blepharitis, and a maculopapular skin rash. The rash first develops on the ventral body surface then becomes generalized before ultimately progressing to a dry and scaly desquamative dermatitis. Immunosuppression is common. Occasionally, measles infection progresses to depression, anorexia, coughing, and dyspnea in conjunction with giant cell pneumonia. Abortions and neurologic signs have also been reported. Koplik's spots inconsistently appear on the buccal mucosa (Wachtman and Mansfield, 2012). Morbidity is high and mortality, caused by secondary bacterial infections, is low in Old World monkeys. The disease is much more severe in marmosets, owl monkeys, and colobines in which hemorrhagic gastroenteritis and immunosuppression predominate and respiratory tract lesions and the skin rash are absent or less significant. To mitigate the possibility of introducing the virus into a susceptible monkey population, personnel working with these primates should have a measles virus antibody titer to assess their immunity to the virus.

The clinical signs observed in humans (CDC, 2012a) closely resembles those seen in macaques.

Diagnosis and Prevention Characteristic clinical signs can be highly suggestive of the disease. Diagnostics include serology to detect virus-specific antibodies, virus isolation, and molecular assays. Treatment of animals at high risk for virus exposure with human gamma globulin may be useful in controlling disease during epizootics (Roberts *et al.*, 1988). A monovalent human measles vaccine is effective in protecting both Old World and New World monkeys from the disease. A less expensive monovalent vaccine designed for use in dogs has been shown to be equally effective. However, production of this vaccine has been suspended and an alternate monovalent vaccine has not yet been validated for use in nonhuman primates. Polyvalent vaccines may be shown to be efficacious in measles prevention; however, they may produce an immune response that interferes with select research.

A current measles vaccination or evidence of immunity should be assured for all handlers of nonhuman primates.

I. Newcastle Disease Virus

Reservoir and Incidence Newcastle disease is caused by a paramyxovirus that can infect possibly all bird species and results in a wide range of disease outcomes ranging from unapparent infection to 100% mortality (CDCP-NIH, 2009). Virus strains are classified into five pathotypes based upon the clinical signs they induce in chickens. The five pathotypes are as follows: viscerotropic velogenic, neurotropic velogenic, mesogenic, lentogenic, and asymptomatic (OIE, n.d.). The zoonotic potential of this agent in the laboratory environment has been realized on numerous occasions (Barkley and Richardson, 1984).

Mode of Transmission The virus is shed in the respiratory secretions and feces of infected birds. Disease transmission between birds occurs via aerosol exposure or ingestion of contaminated food or water. Transmission to humans occurs via aerosols (usually in a laboratory setting) or by direct or indirect inoculation of the eyes as may occur during handling of infected animals, their tissues, or contaminated fomites during necropsy or at poultry processing plants. Human-to-human transmission is not suspected although human-to-bird transmission is possible (Maclachlan *et al.*, 2011d; Swayne and King, 2003).

Clinical Signs The severity of the disease in birds depends on the pathogenicity of the infecting strain. Highly pathogenic strains have largely been excluded from flocks within the United States. Moderately pathogenic strains produce anorexia and respiratory disease in adult birds and neurologic signs in young birds. In humans, the disease is characterized by a mild-to-moderate self-limiting conjunctivitis with orbital pain without corneal involvement that resolves without complications and without therapy. Mild fever and respiratory involvement may rarely develop in humans, most frequently following aerosol exposure (Swayne and King, 2003) although some question the true frequency of this occurrence (Goebel *et al.*, 2007). One fatal case has been documented in a severely immunosuppressed individual (Goebel *et al.*, 2007).

Diagnosis and Prevention Virus isolation and characterization from avian tracheal, oropharyngeal, or cloacal samples is the preferred diagnostic method although molecular assays and serologic tests (e.g., hemagglutination, hemagglutination inhibition, and ELISA) are also frequently utilized (OIE, n.d.). This disease can be prevented in the laboratory environment by immunizing birds susceptible for this disease or obtaining birds from flocks known to be free of this agent. Live, inactivated, and recombinant vaccine strains are used. Personal hygiene practices should also be in place to prevent zoonotic transmission. Select virulent strains of Newcastle disease virus are designated as Select Agents (CDC, n.d.-c) due to their potential use as an agribioterrorism agent.

J. Influenza Virus

Influenza viruses are RNA orthomyxoviruses that are categorized into three types (A, B, and C) based upon antigenic variation, host specificity, and pathogenicity. Type A influenza naturally infects humans as well as a wide range of avian and mammalian species including swine, horses, ferrets, dogs, large felids, domestic cats, mink, and seals, and is further subclassified into subtypes based upon two viral surface glycoproteins: hemagglutinin and neuraminidase. Type B and C influenza viruses infect only humans (Harder and Vahlenkamp, 2010; Mak *et al.*, 2012).

Reservoir and Incidence Humans are considered the reservoir for human influenza virus infections. Animals, however, are thought to play a significant role in the emergence of new human strains of influenza virus and may serve as disease reservoirs. Animals can be infected with influenza strains that then undergo mutational and reassortment events resulting in the emergence of a novel, pathogenic virus transmissible to humans. Pigs are well-known examples and are believed to serve as 'mixing vessels' during the adaptation of avian influenza viruses to human hosts, although their full role in this capacity is still unknown (De Vleeschauwer *et al.*, 2009; Mak *et al.*, 2012; Webster, 1997). In the laboratory, ferrets are highly susceptible to human influenza and often are used as experimental models of influenza infection (Belser *et al.*, 2011). Recently, concern of avian-to-mammalian transmission has intensified, as such transmissions are presumed to have occurred resulting in human fatalities such as in the 1997 H5N1 influenza outbreak in Hong Kong. In addition, the human influenza viruses from the 1918, 1957, and 1968 pandemics are believed to have originated in avian species (CDCP-NIH, 2009).

Mode of Transmission Transmission occurs by airborne spread of the virus and by direct contact through droplet spread or contact with infectious tissues, feces (in select avian species), or secretions. The transmission of animal influenza strains from animals to humans is an uncommon occurrence, but one of increasing concerns due to perceived significant public health implications. Pigs experimentally infected with influenza virus in the laboratory have been shown to directly and readily spread the virus to persons working with these animals (Wentworth *et al.*, 1997). Ferrets housed in the laboratory will develop epizootic infection concomitant with human outbreaks of the disease. Ferret-to-human transmission of the virus has been documented (Marini *et al.*, 1989).

Clinical Signs In humans, influenza is an acute disease of the respiratory tract characterized by fever, headache, myalgia, prostration, coryza, sore throat, and cough. Viral pneumonia and gastrointestinal involvement manifested by nausea, vomiting, and diarrhea may also develop, especially in children.

Diagnosis and Prevention Poultry may remain asymptomatic or only mildly affected with reduced weight gain or egg production although some will develop neurologic symptoms (e.g., ataxia, torticollis, and seizures). In contrast, waterfowl infected with highly pathogenic avian influenza may exhibit sudden death or develop lethargy; diarrhea; and edema and cyanosis of the comb, wattles, and legs with near 100% mortality (Kalthoff *et al.*, 2010).

Diagnostic tests include virus isolation, rapid antigen tests, and molecular assays (Mak *et al.*, 2012). Personnel should wear proper protective clothing including respiratory protection and practice appropriate personal hygiene measures when contacting experimentally infected animals or with animals suspected of having natural influenza infection (e.g., ferrets, pigs, birds). Vaccination of personnel may be indicated.

Select influenza strains (e.g., reconstructed replication competent forms of the 1918 pandemic influenza virus and highly virulent avian influenza virus) are classified as Select Agents due to their potential use as a bioterrorism or agribioterrorism agent.

III. RICKETTSIAL DISEASES

A. Murine Typhus (Endemic Typhus)

Murine typhus is caused by *Rickettsia typhi*. Although this flea-borne disease has been recognized for centuries, it was not until the 1920s that it was distinguished from louse-borne or epidemic typhus. The absence of louse infestation in humans, seasonal occurrence, and sporadic nature help differentiate murine typhus from epidemic typhus, which is caused by *R. prowazekii* and is seen only in the eastern United States in association with flying squirrels (Reynolds *et al.*, 2003).

Reservoir and Incidence Murine typhus is worldwide, and in the United States, it is usually diagnosed in southeastern or Gulf Coast states and in areas along the northern portion of the Mississippi River and southern California. It is also associated with human populations subjected to areas of high-density wild rat colonies, such as ports, granaries, farms, or rat-infested buildings in inner cities. Laboratory personnel have been infected with this agent when inoculating rodents and handling infected animals.

Since the 1970s, there has been a shift in the distribution of human cases of murine typhus to more rural locales in southern California and central and south Texas (Adams *et al.*, 1970). Southern California was considered an unusual locale because the area was considered a wealthy region where rat infestation and the associated flea (*Xenopsylla cheopis*) were uncommon. Epidemiologic studies indicated that opossums had a high seropositivity to murine typhus, and some of the cat fleas (*Ctenocephalides felis*) infesting the opossums were infected with a newly recognized rickettsia eventually named *R. felis* (Adams *et al.*, 1990; Williams *et al.*, 1992).

Follow-up studies have confirmed the presence of both *R. typhi* and *R. felis* in California, Texas, and other southern locales, helping explain the spread of flea-borne murine rickettsia into rural areas in the United States (Boostrom *et al.*, 2002; Eremeeva *et al.*, 2012). Human cases of disease caused by *R. felis* have been identified throught the world, establishing the zoonotic potential of this organism that is grouped with the spotted fever group of Rickettsia based on genetic analysis (Perez-Osorio *et al.*, 2008).

Mode of Transmission Murine typhus is primarily a disease of rats, with its principal vectors being the oriental rat flea, *X. cheopis*, and the flea *Nasopsyllus fasciatus*. These fleas will also naturally colonize the mouse *M. musculus*. The cat flea, *Ctenocephalides felis*, (as well as seven other species of fleas) has also been implicated in the spread of the disease. Rickettsiae are ingested by a blood meal of the flea, where they multiply in the gut, and are subsequently passed out in the dejecta of the flea. Infection in the rat and the human is the result of contamination of the puncture wound by flea feces (Farhang-Azad *et al.*, 1985). Experimental evidence indicates that a flea bite can also directly transmit the infection (Farhang-Azad *et al.*, 1985). *R. typhi* are resistant to drying and remain infectious for up to 100 days in rat feces.

Clinical Signs After infection with rickettsia, the incubation period is 7–14 days. Because murine typhus is difficult to differentiate either clinically or anatomically from other rickettsial diseases, specific serological tests or PCR-based assays are extremely important in making the correct diagnosis (Farhang-Azad *et al.*, 1985). The acute febrile disease is usually characterized by general malaise, headache, rash, and chills, with signs ranging from mild to severe. An encephalitic syndrome can also occur (Mushatt and Hyslop, 1991). In one report, 25% of 180 patients with the disease had delirium, stupor, or coma. Fortunately, these findings resolve with lowering of the febrile response. Fatality rate for all ages is about 2% but increases with age. Proper antibiotic therapy is the most effective measure to prevent morbidity or mortality due to rickettsial infections and has been shown to be effective in hastening recovery and preventing neurologic sequelae, such as deafness due to eighth cranial nerve involvement (Mushatt and Hyslop, 1991). Doxycycline, tetracycline, and chloramphenicol are considered agents of choice.

Diagnosis and Control Recovery of rickettsial organisms or antigens from biological specimens is inconsistent and is not routinely done except in labs equipped to process and identify these samples. It must be stressed that manipulation of rickettsia in the laboratory is hazardous and has accounted for numerous infections of laboratory personnel. Serological diagnosis via the IFA technique has been considered to be the standard reference test, but the classical assay is not species-specific and does not distinguish epidemic from endemic typhus. Differentiation between IgM and IgG antibodies or evidence of a rising titer on serial samples can be used to confirm recent, active infections. Species-specific ELISA and PCR tests are becoming available and can be used to differentiate between the rickettsia.

Fleas can be controlled by applying insecticides as residual powders or sprays in areas where rats nest or traverse. It is imperative that insecticides be applied prior to using rodenticides; this will prevent fleas from leaving the dead rodents and feeding on human hosts (Beaver and Jung, 1985). This disease should not be encountered in rat colonies in well-maintained research vivaria. However, with the cat flea being a newly recognized vector of rickettsial disease, its presence on random-source dogs, cats, and opossums raises the risk of transmission to personnel working with these flea-infested animals.

B. Rickettsial Pox

A variety of rodents are infected with other rickettsial diseases. *M. musculus* is the natural host for the causative agent of rickettsial pox, *Rickettsia akari*, a member of the spotted fever group of rickettsia (Chin, 2000). This organism is also isolated from *Rattus rattus* and *R. norvegicus*, and the rat under certain circumstances may transmit the disease to humans. The disease is transmitted by the mite *Liponyssoides* (*Allodermanyssus*) *sanguineus* and has been diagnosed in New York City and other eastern cities, as well as in Russia, Egypt, and South Africa (Chin, 2000). The incubation period is approximately 10–24 days, and the clinical disease is similar to that noted in murine typhus. The rash of rickettsial pox commences as a discrete maculopapular rash, which then becomes vesicular. The palms and soles are usually not involved. About 90% of affected persons develop an eschar, with a shallow ulcer covered by a brown scab (Farhang-Azad *et al.*, 1985; Chin, 2000) (Fig. 28.4). Although headaches are common and may be accompanied by stiff necks, lumbar cerebrospinal fluid samples are normal. Pulmonary and gastrointestinal involvement also are almost never encountered. Diagnosis, treatment, and control are similar to those described for murine typhus and *Yersinia pestis*.

As discussed above with the emerging pathogen *R. felis*, the recognized geographical and host ranges of rickettsia are likely to continue to grow. Serological evidence of exposure to *R. akari* or an antigenically related rickettsia has been found in humans in southern California, and associated animal screening identified serological evidence of prior exposure in rodents of the genera *Mus*, *Rattus*, *Peromyscus*, and *Neotoma* (Bennett *et al.*, 2007).

C. *Coxiella burnetii* Infection (Q Fever)

Reservoir and Incidence   *Coxiella burnetii*, the causative agent of Q fever, has a worldwide distribution perpetuated in two intersecting cycles of infection composed of domestic or wild animals and their associated ticks (Babudieri, 1959; Marrie, 1990). The domestic animal cycle involves mainly sheep, goats, and cattle. The prevalence of the infection among sheep is high throughout the United States, and sheep have been the primary species associated with disease outbreaks associated with research animal facilities (Anderson *et al.*, 2013). However, human cases of the disease have also been associated with nonruminants, such as pregnant cats (Langley *et al.*, 1988; Kopecny *et al.*, 2013) and wild rabbits (Marrie *et al.*, 1986). Thus, a broad range of domestic and wild animal species, including birds, should be given consideration as potential sources for Q fever infection in animal care and use activities (To *et al.*, 1998). A survey of other domestic animals performed as part of the investigation into a major goat-related outbreak in the Netherlands found evidence of the agent in dog and horse placentas (Roest *et al.*, 2013).

Mode of Transmission   *C. burnetii* are shed in the urine, feces, milk, and especially placental tissues of domestic ungulates that generally are asymptomatic. The organism is highly infectious with possibly as few as 10 organisms inducing infection, which is significant considering that the placenta of infected ewes can contain up to 10^9 organisms per gram of tissue, and milk may contain 10^5 organisms per gram (Chosewood and Wilson, 2009). The primary method of transmission is through infectious aerosols. The organism produces a spore-like form that is resistant to desiccation and persists in the environment for long periods of time, contributing to the widespread dissemination of infectious aerosols and resulting in infections miles from the original organism source (Franz *et al.*, 1997; Tissot-Dupont *et al.*, 1999). The importance of these factors was

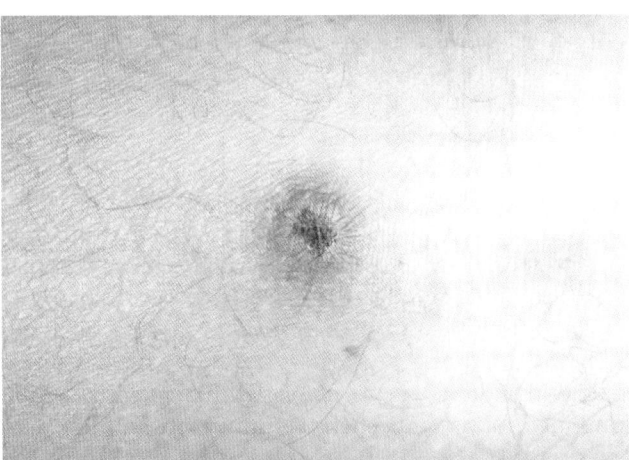

FIGURE 28.4   Eschar on posterior right calf of patient with rickettsial pox. *Source: Emerg Infect Dis – "Rickettsial pox in North Carolina: A Case Report."*

illustrated in outbreaks of the disease associated with the use of pregnant sheep in research facilities in the United States (Bernard *et al.*, 1982). In these outbreaks, personnel who did not have direct contact with infected sheep but who worked along the transport routes for these animals became serologically positive for Q fever (Bernard *et al.*, 1982; Reimer, 1993). Also, five of nine laundry workers without direct sheep contact but who processed linens soiled during sheep surgery developed serological evidence of infection.

Clinical Signs, Susceptibility, and Resistance in Humans Q fever in humans varies in duration and severity, and asymptomatic infection may occur. The disease often presents as an acute flu-like illness with fever, frontal headache with retro-orbital pain, and chest pain with a nonproductive cough and pneumonia, resolving within 2 weeks of infection. However, serious extrapulmonary complications, such as acute or chronic hepatitis, nephritis, epicarditis, and endocarditis, may also occur. Individuals with valvular heart disease should not work with *C. burnetii* due to the prospect of serious, chronic, relapsing infection (Asher, 1989; Chosewood and Wilson, 2009). A linkage between Q fever and a chronic fatigue syndrome is also suspected (Ayres *et al.*, 1998).

Diagnosis, Prevention, and Control Whenever possible, male or nonpregnant sheep should be used in research programs; however, many research applications specifically call for the use of pregnant animals. Multiple commercial vendors now supply sheep from closed, SPF flocks that have been serologically negative for an extended period. Although serological status is not a reliable indicator of organism shedding in an individual sheep, many institutions have elected to use these animals, reasoning that cumulative and consistent negative Q fever serology on a herd basis provides a reasonably strong assurance of Q fever-free status. Advances in PCR methods have improved the sensitivity of *C. burnetii* detection over that of the antigen capture ELISA, as well as improved the speed, safety, and convenience of the assay. The PCR method allows for the assessment of organism shedding, which may provide an option to minimize the potential risk of Q fever outbreaks in animal facilities (Lorenz *et al.*, 1998; Yanase *et al.*, 1998). However, shedding can be sporadic, and diagnostic samples such as amniotic fluid and placenta are not readily available *antemortem*. A combination of colony health components such as acquisition from a 'clean' flock, serological testing of incoming animals with follow-up *postmortem* PCR screening can be combined for a comprehensive program to minimize Q fever risks.

Sheep and other animals known to harbor Q fever infections (e.g., experimentally infected animals) should be maintained under ABSL3 conditions to prevent the transmission of the organism in the research animal facility environment (Chosewood and Wilson, 2009). Additional detailed recommendations have been published concerning sheep handling in biomedical research programs (Bernard *et al.*, 1982; Anderson *et al.*, 2013). In many institutions, ABSL3 compliant physical containment for sheep may prove to be unachievable as a preventative measure for sheep held under agricultural conditions for food and fiber production or utilized for instructional exercises. The use of enhanced personal protective equipment such as N95-type respirators and protective face shields should be considered in those settings, especially if pregnant ruminants are involved. The extracellular form of the organism is very resistant to inactivation and nearly sporicidal treatments are required for decontamination.

An effective Q fever vaccine is licensed in Australia (Q-Vax), but the only vaccines that have been utilized in the United States are experimental and have seen very limited distribution.

IV. CHLAMYDIAL INFECTIONS

A. Chlamydiosis (Psittacosis, Ornithosis, or Parrot Fever)

Reservoir and Incidence The taxonomy for the order Chlamydiales has been extensively revised and re-revised in the past two decades based upon evolving genotopic and phenotypic information. A proposal to split a number of species into the new genus *Chlamydophila* has been published (Everett *et al.*, 1999), but it has not been uniformly adopted by the scientific community and the latest edition of Bergey's Manual retains the designation of these species as *Chlamydia* spp. (Kuo *et al.*, 2010). Chlamydial species are widely distributed among birds and mammals worldwide and occur naturally among many laboratory animal species, including birds, mice, guinea pigs, hamsters, rabbits, ruminants, swine, cats, ferrets, muskrats, and frogs (Storz, 1971; Newcomer *et al.*, 1982). Of these host species, birds with *Chlamydia psittaci* infection, particularly psittacines, have proven to be the most frequent sources of virulent human infection (CDCP, 1997); however, infections with *C. abortus* in ruminants (Hyde and Benirschke, 1997; Jorgesen, 1997) and *C. felis* in cats (Cotton and Partridge, 1998) also have the potential to cause human disease. The most common human chlamydial infection, *C. trachomatis*, is not naturally transmissible to animals but is used to produce experimental infections in nonhuman primates. *C. muridarium* occurring in the mouse and *C. suis* occurring in the pig are closely related to *C. trachomatis* but are not infectious for humans. *C. caviae* has been isolated from the guinea pig. *C. pecorum* produces intestinal infection in ruminants and other animals but not in humans. *C. pneumoniae* produces respiratory infections in humans and related biovars have been isolated from the koala, horse, frog, and reptiles (Bodetti, *et al.*, 2002). Zoonotic infections from animal-related biovars of *Chlamydia pneumoniae* have not been recorded, but genomic studies suggest that one or more animal-to-human transmission events led to the establishment of the human *C. pneumonia* biovar (Roulis *et al.*, 2013).

Mode of Transmission The organism is spread to humans from infectious material present in exudates, secretions, or desiccated fecal material by direct contact or the aerosol route. Latent infection is an important feature of epizootology of the *C. psittaci* infection in birds; stress can reactivate enteric shedding of the organism and clinical signs (Storz, 1971).

Clinical Signs, Susceptibility, and Resistance in Humans Chlamydiae produce a diverse spectrum of animal disease, including conjunctivitis, pneumonitis, air sacculitis, pericarditis, hepatitis, enteritis, arthritis, meningoencephalitis, urethritis, endometritis, and abortion. Zoonotic infections in humans are characterized mainly by upper and lower respiratory tract complaints; however, conjunctivitis, thrombophlebitis, myocarditis, hepatitis, and encephalitis have also been reported (Smith, 1989; Leitman *et al.*, 1998). Although *C. psittaci* is considered to be more pathogenic for humans than are the mammalian species, as mentioned above the occurrence of ovine strain-related (*C. abortus*) human gestational infections and feline pneumonitis strain-related (*C. felis*) conjunctivitis, pneumonia, and extrapulmonary infection (Cotton and Partridge, 1998) emphasizes the zoonotic potential of a variety of reservoir hosts.

Diagnosis and Control The diagnosis of *C. psittaci* in birds can be made by the identification of inclusions in tissue specimens or impression smears, by actual isolation of the organism, or by using ELISA-based fecal antigen tests. PCR can also detect the organism in blood, cloacal or throat swabs, and environmental samples. A variety of serological tests are available, but differentiation between active infection and previous exposure can be difficult. Whenever possible, birds used in research animal facilities should be acquired from flocks free from *C. psittaci* infection. Prophylactic antibiotic treatment should be considered for wild-caught birds or birds of unknown disease status, and therapeutic antibiotics may be useful when treating mammals or amphibians diagnosed with chlamydial infection. Personnel protection adhering to ABSL-2 procedures along with respiratory protection is generally adequate when dealing with known infections, but ABSL-3 procedures are warranted for research activities with the high potential for droplet or infectious aerosol production, such as necropsy of known-infected birds (Chosewood and Wilson, 2009).

V. BACTERIAL DISEASES

A. Trauma-Associated Bacterial Diseases

1. Bites and Scratches

Several million Americans, with up to 2% of the population, annually suffer animal bites, which continues to be a major health problem in the United States and accounts for approximately 1% of emergency room visits. Dogs and cats are responsible for 90% of the recorded bites (Weber and Hansen, 1991; Talan *et al.*, 1999). The majority of these bites are due to dog bites, with up to 4.7 million sustaining injury and approximately 800,000 requiring some form of medical care annually (CDC, n.d-g). Each year dog attacks account for 10–20 deaths in the United States (Sacks *et al.*, 2000). It is estimated that 400,000 persons in the United States are bitten or scratched by cats annually. According to one report, approximately 40,000 rat bites are recorded annually (Committee on Urban Pest Management, 1980). As with bites from dogs and cats, the majority of rat bites occur in children. It is estimated that 2% of rat bites become infected (Ordog, 1985). The hand is the most likely anatomic site to develop infection and long-term disability (Thomas and Brook, 2011). One report notes that up to 40% of hand bites become infected (Oehler *et al.*, 2009).

Veterinarians, animal control officers, and presumably animal care personnel in research facilities as well as in municipal pounds are at higher risk of bites than the general population. Although rabies is the most serious public health threat from bites and scratches, the risk of bacterial infection from dog bites is lower (approximately 3–18%) than that from cat bites, which is reported to be approximately 28–80% (Weber and Hansen, 1991).

Animals in general have a complex oral microflora consisting of numerous bacterial species; both aerobic and anaerobic bacteria are therefore routinely isolated from traumatic bite wounds inflicted by domestic and wild animals. Common organisms isolated from dog bites include *Staphylococcus* species, *Streptococcus* species, including *S. canis* and a variety of anaerobes, and *Pasteurella multocida* (Takeda *et al.*, 2001; Bert and Lambert-Zechovsky, 1997). Also, a case of zoonotic transmission of *S. equi* subsp. *zooepidemicus* from a dog to its handler, via wound infection or aerosols, has been recently reported (Abbott *et al.*, 2010). In a comprehensive multicenter study, 60% of dog bite wounds were punctures, 10% were lacerations, and 30% were a combination of both. This compared to 85% of cat bite wounds being punctures, 3% lacerations, and 12% a combination of both. In this study, 39% of 57 patients with cat bites presented as purulent wounds, whereas abscesses were present in 19% of the cases reviewed (Talan *et al.*, 1999). Of the 50 patients with dog bites, 58% had purulent wounds, 30% were nonpurulent, and 12% were noted to have abscesses. Dog and cat bites had a mean of five bacterial species per wound; 63% of the cat bites analyzed compared to 48% of dog bites had a mixed anaerobic and aerobic population (Talan *et al.*, 1999). Only aerobes grew in 36% of the cases (42% of dog bites and 32% cat bites), whereas anaerobes were the only species grown in 1% of the cases. *Capnocytophaga canimorsus*, an invasive organism, was recovered from 4.7% of the wounds. It should be noted that if fever occurs in immunocompromised patients (including asplenic individuals) after a bite wound, this organism should be considered in the differential diagnosis. *Erysipelothrix rhusiopathiae* was isolated from two cat bite wounds, whereas *Pasteurella* spp. were present in the wounds 75% of the time in cats and 50% in dogs. Geographic locale is also important in defining bacterial flora of bites and scratches. In a study conducted in the southwestern and central United States, 17 of 1041 (1.6%) of the cases of tularemia in humans diagnosed from 1981 to 1987 were associated with cat scratches or bites (Taylor *et al.*, 1991).

Several bacterial pathogens have been isolated from rat bites, including *Leptospira interrogans*, *P. multocida*, and *Staphylococcus* species; however, the most commonly isolated pathogens are *Streptobacillus moniliformis* and *Spirillum minus* (Fox, 2009). Bite wounds from primates and ferrets (and other laboratory animals) can also result in bacterial infection. For example, a chronic *Mycobacterium bovis* infection on the hand of a human resulted from a ferret bite that had occurred 22 years previously (Jones *et al.*, 1993). The greatest concern from macaque bites still remains the threat of B virus infection.

Thorough cleaning and debridement (if necessary) is required for all bite wounds. Determination of tetanus vaccination and radiologic assessment are critically important in bite wound management. Amoxicillin/Clavulanate is considered the standard oral antibiotic therapy to empirically treat mammalian bite wound infections (Thomas and Brook, 2011).

2. Atypical Mycobacteriosis

Reservoir and Incidence The rapidly growing mycobacteria (RGM) *Mycobacterium fortuitum*, *M. chelonae*, and *M. abscessus* are ubiquitous, being found in soil throughout the world. *M. chelonae* was first isolated from sea turtles; *M. fortuitum* from frogs (originally called *ranae*); and *M. abscessus*, as the name implies, from soft tissue abscesses of a patient. Of the nontuberculosis mycobacterium belonging to Runyon group I, *M. marinum* is by far the most common. The organism was first isolated from cutaneous lesions in 1826 and was responsible for the death of saltwater fish in a Philadelphia aquarium 100 years later; the authors named the mycobacterium *M. marinum*.

Mode of Transmission The RGM most commonly are associated with a traumatic injury with potential soil contamination and result in skin, soft tissue, or bone disease. *M. marinum* is pathogenic only on abraded skin; a disruption of the epidermis must be present for development of disease. Because this organism is recognized as a pathogen in zebrafish, it can be a source of infection in personnel working with this species in a research environment.

Clinical Signs *M. marinum* is a free-living mycobacterium that causes disease in fresh-water and saltwater fish and occasionally in humans. Initially called swimming pool granuloma, it is now commonly named fish tank granuloma because of the association with this environmental exposures and human infections. Importantly, *M. marinum*, because of its optimum growth at 30–32°C, is primarily localized to skin infections. However, it can extend to deeper tissues, including joints and tendons. For individuals exposed to diseased fish and/or their environment, the lesions are in general located on the backs of hands or fingers or forearms (Baiano and Barnes, 2009). Infections have also resulted from the bite of a dolphin (Flowers, 1970).

Diagnosis and Control Identification for the common RGM and *M. marinum* has been given low priority and is only performed routinely in reference laboratories. Fortunately, however, PCR-based assays have become available for rapid diagnosis of atypical mycobacteria.

3. Rat-Bite Fever

Rat-bite fever (RBF) can be caused by either of two microorganisms: *Streptobacillus moniliformis* or *Spirillum minus*. *S. moniliformis* causes the diseases designated as streptobacillary fever, streptobacillary RBF, or streptobacillosis (McEvoy *et al.*, 1987; Rupp, 1992; Heymann, 2008; Fox, 2009). Haverhill fever and epidemic arthritic erythema are diseases associated with ingestion of water, food, or raw milk contaminated with *S. moniliformis*. Sodoku is derived from the Japanese words for rat (*so*) and poison (*doku*), and is used to designate infection with *S. minus*. Spirillosis and spirillary RBF are other names given to the infections caused by *S. minus*.

Reservoir and Incidence These organisms are present in the oral cavity and upper respiratory passages of asymptomatic rodents, usually rats (Wilkins *et al.*, 1988). *S. moniliformis* has been isolated as the predominant microorganism from the upper trachea of laboratory rats in one study (Paegle *et al.*, 1976). Other surveys indicate isolation of the organism in 0/15, 7/10, 2/20, and 7/14 laboratory rats and 4/6 wild rats (Geller, 1979). The incidence of *S. moniliformis* is probably lower in high-quality, commercially reared specific pathogen-free rats. Surveys in wild rats indicate 0–25% infection with *S. minus* (Hull, 1955) or 50–100% for *S. moniliformis*.

TABLE 28.2   Clinical Signs of RBF[a]

Clinical features	Streptobacillary fever (*Streptobacillus moniliformis*)	Spirillosis (*Spirillum minus*)
Incubation period	2–10 days	1–6 weeks
Fever	+++	+++
Chills	+++	+++
Myalgia	+++	+++
Rash	++	++
	Morbilliform, petechial	Maculopapular
Lymphadenitis	+	++
Arthralgia, arthritis	++	±
Indurated bite wound	–	+++
Recurrent fever/constitutional signs (untreated)	Irregular periodicity	Regular periodicity

[a]*Modified from Lipman (1996).*

Mode of Transmission   The bite of an infected rat is the usual source of infection. In some cases, bites from other animals, including mice, gerbils, squirrels, weasels, ferrets, dogs, and cats, or rare traumatic injuries unassociated with animal contact cause the infection.

Clinical Signs   RBF is not a reportable disease, which makes its prevalence, geographic location, racial data, and source of infection in humans difficult to assess. The disease, though uncommon in humans, has nonetheless appeared among researchers or students working with laboratory rodents, particularly rats (Anderson *et al.*, 1983). Historically, bites from wild rats and subsequent illness (usually in small children) relate to poor sanitation and overcrowding (Hull, 1955). One survey of rat bites in Baltimore tabulated RBF in 11 of 87 cases (Brooks, 1973). The disease can also occur in individuals who have no history of rat bites but reside or work in rat-infested areas. Exposure to dogs and cats who prey on wild rodents may also be the source of the organism. Ingestion of milk, food, or water contaminated with rat feces can result in RBF (CDC, 1995).

The incubation period for *S. moniliformis* infection varies from a few hours to 2–10 days, whereas the incubation period for *S. minus* infection, most commonly seen in Asia, ranges from 1 to 6 weeks (Table 28.2). Fever is present in either form. Inflammation associated with the bite and lymphadenopathy are frequently accompanied by headache, general malaise, myalgia, and chills. The discrete macular rash that often appears on the extremities may generalize into pustular or petechial sequelae. Arthritis occurs in 50% of all cases of *S. moniliformis*

but is less common in *S. minus*. *S. moniliformis* may be cultured from serous to purulent effusion that is recovered from affected larger joints. The organism should be considered in the list of differential diagnosis in cases of septic arthritis, particularly with synovial fluid with high inflammatory cell counts (Dendle *et al.*, 2006).

Most cases of RBF resolve spontaneously within 14 days; however, 13% of untreated cases are fatal (Sens *et al.*, 1989). Prophylactic efficacy of antibiotic treatment following rat bites has not been thoroughly investigated. If antibiotic treatment (intravenous penicillin for 5–7 days, followed by oral penicillin for 7 days) is not instituted early, complications such as pneumonia, hepatitis, pyelonephritis, enteritis, and endocarditis may develop (Anderson *et al.*, 1983). If endocarditis is present, the penicillin should be given parenterally at doses of 15–20 million units daily for 4–6 weeks. Streptomycin and tetracyclines are also effective antibiotics for those individuals with penicillin-associated allergies. Death has occurred in cases of *S. moniliformis* involving pre-existent valvular disease. The recent reports of fatalities due to *S. moniliformis* in adults working in a pet store and having rats as pets highlight the need to be vigilant in recognizing the clinical manifestations of RBF in patients with a history of rat bites or intimate exposure to rats (CDC, 2005).

Diagnosis and Prevention   *S. minus* does not grow *in vitro* and requires inoculation of culture specimens into laboratory animals, with subsequent identification of the bacteria by dark-field microscopy. Streptobacillary RBF can be diagnosed only by blood culture. *S. moniliformis* grows slowly on artificial media, but only in the presence of 15% blood and sera, usually 10–20% rabbit or horse serum incubated at reduced partial pressures of oxygen (Fox, 2009). Because of its properties as a bacterial growth promoter, sodium polyanethol sulfonate, which is sometimes found in blood-based media, should not be used due to its inhibitory effects on *S. moniliformis*. Growth on agar consists of 1–2 mm gray, glistening colonies. The API ZYM diagnostic system can be used for rapid biochemical analysis and diagnosis. Unfortunately, no serological test is available. Acute febrile diseases, especially if associated with animal bites, are routinely treated with penicillin or other antibiotics.

4. Cat Scratch Disease

Both viruses and chlamydia had been suspected as a cause of cat scratch fever (CSF) until histopathologic examination of lymph nodes from 39 patients with clinical criteria for cat scratch disease (CSD) revealed pleomorphic, gram-negative bacilli in 34 of the 39 nodes. Organisms in lymph node sections exposed to convalescent serum from three patients and to immunoperoxidase stained equally well with all three samples. The authors concluded that the bacilli appear to be the causative agents of CSD (Wear *et al.*, 1983). The following year, using the same staining protocol, researchers demonstrated identical organisms in skin biopsies taken from CSF inoculation papules (Margileth *et al.*, 1984). *Bartonella henselae*, a fastidious gram-negative bacteria, is now recognized as the primary cause of CSD. *B. henselae* has been isolated from lymph nodes of CSD patients, and elevated serological titers to *B. henselae* are also noted in these individuals (Dolan *et al.*, 1993; Zangwill *et al.*, 1993). A second organism, *Afipia felis*, has also been isolated from CSD lesions but is not considered the common etiologic agent of CSD.

Reservoir and Incidence   An estimation of 22,000 cases of CSD in the United States, of which approximately 2000 require hospitalization, is based on an analysis of three databases (Jackson *et al.*, 1993). Almost all *B. henselae* infections are associated with exposure or ownership of cats; however, not all cases of CSD are associated with a scratch or bite.

Mode of Transmission   Patients with CSD commonly have a history of exposure to a cat, and of these patients, the majority have either been bitten or scratched. Most of the patients are under 20 years of age. It is now known that cat fleas are infected with *B. henselae*. It is suspected that the organism is shed in the feces of the flea and can result in the transmission of the organism from cat to cat and from cat to human via mucous membrane or skin contact. Subsequently there is self-inoculation by scratching the flea bite, or alternatively by having the contaminated claws or teeth of cats inoculate the organism into traumatized skin. Importantly, several surveys have shown that cats can be chronically infected with *B. henselae*, with the organism capable of being isolated from blood of asymptomatic cats over an extended period of time (Koehler *et al.*, 1994; Goldstein and Greene, 2009). Impounded or stray cats are more likely to be chronically infected than cats maintained in a household long term.

Clinical Signs   The natural course of CSD, which consists of a mild or absent fever, few systemic sequelae, and localized lymphadenitis with little or no discomfort, probably results in a large number of unrecognized cases. A primary lesion will develop in 50% of the cases about 10 days after a cat bite or scratch; the erythematous pustule will usually persist for 1–2 weeks. A regional lymphadenopathy develops 14 days after the initial lesion in most cases. Lymphadenitis regresses in about 6 weeks, with 30–50% of the nodes becoming suppurative. Of the approximately 65% of people who develop systemic illness, fever and malaise are the symptoms most often noted. Occasionally observed are generalized lymphadenopathy. Other clinical syndromes include ocular granuloma, thrombocytopenia, encephalitis, osteolytic lesions, pneumonia, liver and spleen abscesses, and erythema nodosum. The disease is benign, and most patients recover spontaneously without sequelae within 2 months, although lymphadenopathy can persist for up to a year. In immunocompromised individuals, CSD is manifested by an unusual vascular growth seen on the skin and given the name bacillary epithelioid angiomatosis (LeBoit *et al.*, 1988; Kemper *et al.*, 1990). Systemic disease involving the spleen and liver also occurs in these patients.

Diagnosis and Control   If lymphadenitis is present, three of the four following criteria should be fulfilled to diagnose CSD: (1) positive serology for *B. hensalae*; a positive titer of 1:64 or greater by IFA assay is considered positive; a recently developed modified IFA has been described with a sensitivity of 85% and specificity of 98% for both IgG and IgM (Metzkor-Cotter *et al.*, 2003); (2) history of contact with a cat; (3) characteristic histopathologic changes present in involved lymph node biopsy; (4) absence of other disease; and (5) growth of the organism on rabbit, horse, or sheep blood agar in 5% CO_2. However, growth on human blood agar appears superior (Goldstein and Greene, 2009).

Prevention is based on flea control as well as thorough cleansing of cat bites and scratches.

5. Pasteurella *spp.*

Reservoir and Incidence   *Pasteurella* species, particularly *P. multocida*, are considered one of the most prevalent bacterial species known to colonize the upper respiratory tract and oral mucosa of domestic and wild animals (Dewhirst *et al.*, 2012).

Mode of Transmission   Zoonotic transmission of *P. multocida* most often occurs through animal bites and scratches, or contact with respiratory secretions (Wilson and Ho, 2013). *Pasteurella* species are cultured from infections resulting from 50% of dog bites and 75% of cat bites (Freshwater, 2008; Talan *et al.*, 1999; Rempe *et al.*, 2009). Other contact, such as kissing infected animals or the animals licking skin abrasions or mucosal surfaces (eyes, mouth, and nose), or exposure to respiratory secretions of infected animals can also account for zoonotic transmission of *Pasteurella* spp. (Myers *et al.*, 2012). Immunocompromised, elderly, pregnant individuals, those administrating palliative care, and children are particularly vulnerable to acquiring *P. multocida* from animals' respiratory secretions or contact of patients' skin lesions (through licking).

Clinical Signs   Bite wound infections linked to *Pasteurella* spp. infections can be clinically apparent as early as 8–12 hours, and are aggressive in presentation with skin and soft tissue swelling, erythema, local lymphadenopathy, fever, pain, and swelling (Fig. 28.5). Osteomyelitis can also occur in bone underlying the wound, and septicemia can result on occasion (Hombal and Dincsoy, 1992). Cat scratches have also resulted in *P. multocida*-associated corneal ulceration and keratitis

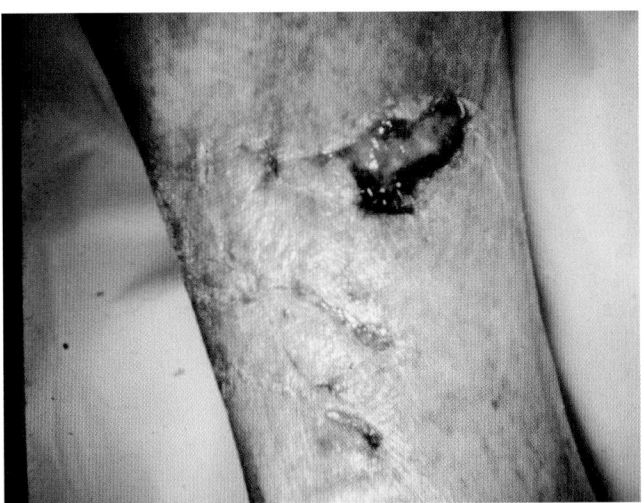

FIGURE 28.5 *Pasteurella multocida*-associated dog bite wound. *Source: John Moses, M.D.*

(Ho and Rapuan, 1993). Routine, prompt prophylactic treatment with broad spectrum antibiotics of animal bite wounds probably accounts for pasteurellosis being a relatively uncommon cause of mortality in humans. Mortality rates, though uncommon, of 25–30% have been reported in human cases of pasteurellosis due to bite wounds, with bacteremia being commonly reported, and to a lesser extent meningitis (Kimura *et al.*, 2004; Myers *et al.*, 2012).

Diagnosis and Control Bacterial culture of the wound is undertaken prior to local cleansing and antisepsis of the traumatic site of injury. The bacteria are gram-negative rods that grow readily on blood agar.

6. Streptococcus iniae

Reservoir and Incidence *Streptococcus iniae* is now recognized as a cause of high mortality in rainbow trout and tilapia (members of the cichlid group of fish) being raised in fish farming environments. *S. iniae* was recognized as a pathogen in 1976 when the bacteria was first cultured from cutaneous abscesses in aquaria-maintained Amazon freshwater dolphins (Pier and Madin, 1976).

Mode of Transmission Many infected patients sustain an injury to the hand when preparing infected fish for consumption. The organism can be readily cultured from these infected fish (Goh *et al.*, 1998).

Clinical Signs *S. iniae* was identified as a zoonotic agent in 1995–1996 when a cluster of cases presented with fever and lymphangitis in individuals handling whole or live fish purchased in Toronto, Canada (CDCP, 1995; Weinstein *et al.*, 1997). *S. iniae* was cultured from the blood of each of these patients.

Diagnosis and Control The organisms are gram-positive cocci, B-hemolytic on 5% sheep blood agar and are nonreactive in the Lancefield sero-grouping system.

Unfortunately, *S. iniae* currently is not included in commercial and clinical databases and diagnostic kits, making it likely that human infections are underreported (Fulde and Valentin-Weigand, 2013). A nested PCR assay specific for the 16S–23S ribosomal intergenic spacer and a chaperonin 60 (cpu 60) gene identification method are two molecular techniques that provide accurate, rapid, and specific diagnosis of this organism (Berridge *et al.*, 1998; Goh *et al.*, 1998). Infected individuals respond to parenteral antibiotics within 2–4 days after initiation of treatment.

Other *Streptococcus* spp. associated with zoonosis include *S. canis*, *S. zooepidemicus*, and *S. suis* (Fulde and Valentin-Weigand, 2013) (Fig. 28.6). *S. zooepidemicus* has been recently transmitted from guinea pigs to their owners, resulting in clinical septicemia (Gruszynski *et al.*, 2015).

B. Systemic Diseases

1. Brucellosis

Reservoir and Incidence Of the *Brucella* spp., *Brucella canis* is the most likely zoonotic agent in the laboratory animal facility due to the frequent use of random-source and laboratory-bred dogs in comparison with other large domestic animals known to be infected with other *Brucella* spp.

Mode of Transmission In one study, investigators considered the zoonotic transmission of *B. canis* unlikely, as evidenced by negative serological tests among 12 individuals exposed to five infected dogs. Since 1967, when the first human *B. canis* infection was identified, more than 35 natural and laboratory-acquired infections have been reported; most resulted from contact with aborting bitches (Lucero *et al.*, 2010). Fortunately, humans are relatively resistant to infection; however, *B. canis* is not a reportable disease, and prevalence data are not available. Although *B. canis* is particularly well adapted to dogs and is not readily transmitted to other species, susceptibility has been reported in several wild species of Canidae (Greene and Carmichael, 2011).

Clinical Signs Bacteremia occurred in several infections; other systemic involvement included painful generalized lymphadenophathy and splenomegaly. Additional signs include fever, headache, chills, sweating, weakness, malaise, myalgia, nausea, and weight loss. Rare complications include endocarditis, meningitis, hepatitis, and arthritis. Although *B. canis*-produced clinical disease in humans is similar to that caused by other *Brucella* spp., it is generally not as severe. Seroconversion to *B. canis* has been reported in 0.5% of asymptomatic military personnel who had contact with infected dogs, indicating that inapparent infection may occur (Polt *et al.*, 1982).

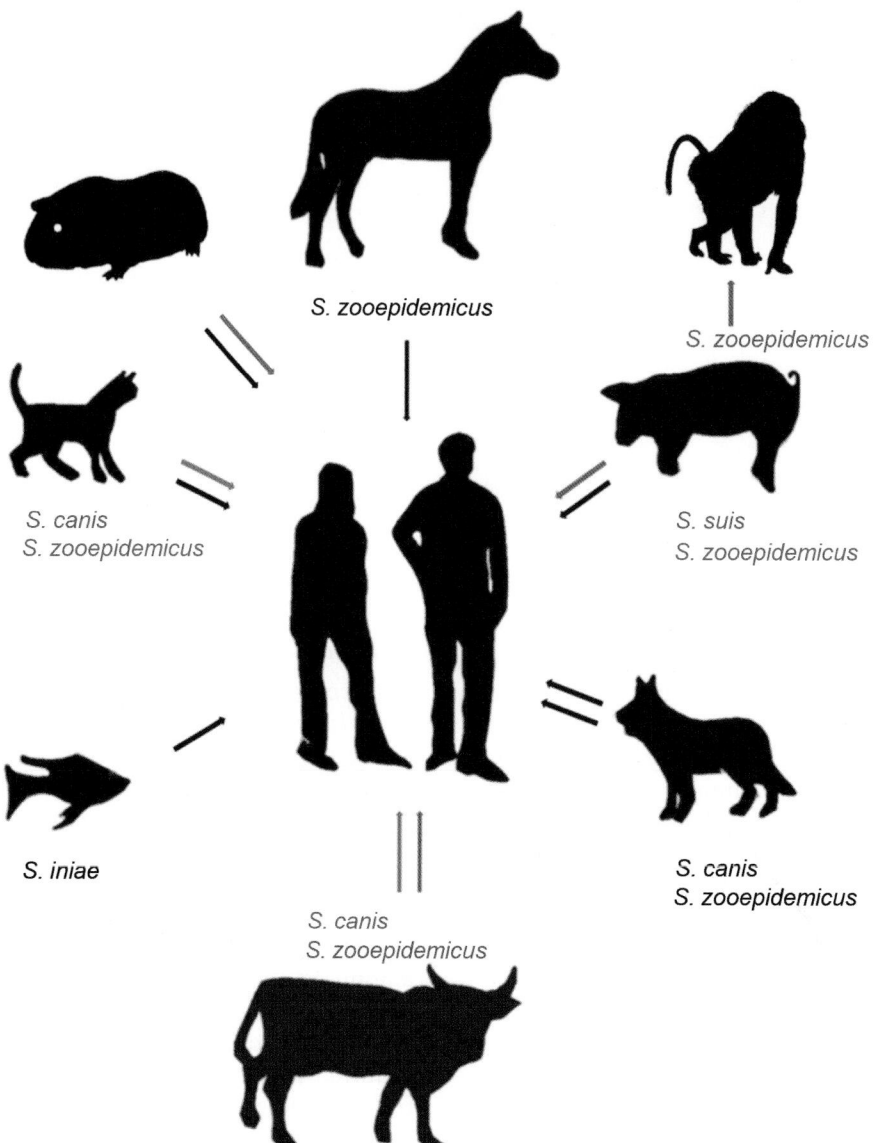

FIGURE 28.6 Schematic figure representing host–pathogen relations of zoonotic streptococci. Black arrows indicate the transmission to one individual, whereas red arrows illustrate the origin of outbreaks. An identification of zoonotic species in animals without a proven transmission to humans is colored blue. *Adapted from Fulde and Valentin-Weigand (2013).*

Diagnosis and Control When a canine's history includes abortions, infertility, testicular abnormalities, and poor semen quality, infection should be considered. A rapid slide agglutination test that produces presumptive diagnostic information is commercially available. To confirm the results of the slide test, one should perform blood cultures and additional serological tests, such as the tube agglutination test (Polt *et al.*, 1982; Serikawa *et al.*, 1989). There have not been any large-scale efforts to eradicate *B. canis* in the general canine population as there have been with *Brucella* spp. of large domestic animals (Forbes and Pantekoek, 1988). Because of the intracellular location of *B. canis*, efficacy of antibiotic therapy is variable, and failures or relapses after therapy are reported in dogs. Ultimate control of *B. canis* in humans relies on elimination of dogs with the disease.

2. Plague

Human infections due to *Yersinia pestis*, a gram-negative coccobacillus, in the United States are sporadic and limited, usually resulting from infected flea or rodent contact. Since 1924–1925, when a plague epidemic ravaged Los Angeles, neither urban plague nor rat-borne plague has been diagnosed in the United States (Craven and Barnes, 1991). All reported cases since then have occurred in states located west of the 101st meridian.

Reservoir and Incidence Although plague has occurred repeatedly in recorded history, by the fourteenth century the disease had appeared in the Far East, spread to Asia Minor, and followed the trade routes to Europe. Plague, however, did not make its arrival in the United States until the disease appeared in California in the early 1900s, where it still exists endemically in the ground squirrel and chipmunk.

Wild rat populations still act as the primary reservoir in many parts of the world and remain a continued threat in the United States. Sciurid rodents (rock squirrels, California ground squirrels, chipmunks, and prairie dogs) account for the primary plague reservoir in the western parts of the United States (Kaufman *et al.*, 1980; Rosner, 1987). Cricetid rodents, such as the wood rat, are occasionally cited as reservoir hosts. The oriental rat flea, *X. cheopis*, the common vector of plague, is well established throughout the United States, particularly in the southern states and southern California. It is important to remember that more than 1500 species of fleas and 230 species of rodents are infected with *Y. pestis*. Only 30–40 rodent species, however, are permanent reservoirs of the infection (Macy, 1999). Plague is infrequently reported in the United States, with a low of one case in 1972 and a high of 40 cases in 1983 (Craven and Barnes, 1991). Ninety percent of the cases have been diagnosed in New Mexico, Colorado, and California. Urban development (particularly in New Mexico) encroached into plague-enzootic rodent habitats, placing human populations at increased risk of contracting the disease. In addition to rodent epizootics, dogs, and increasingly cats, either have served as passive transporters of the disease or have been actively infected (Rosner, 1987). The disease has seasonal peaks, with the highest proportion occurring May through September.

Mode of Transmission An individual is usually infected by the bite of an infected flea, but infection can also occur via cuts or abrasions in the skin or via infected aerosols coming into contact with the oropharyngeal mucous membrane.

Primary pneumonic plague historically occurred by inhalation of infectious droplets from a pneumonic plague patient. However, in the past several decades, this form of the disease has occurred from exposure to infected animals (usually cats) that have developed secondary pneumonia due to septicemic spread of the organism (Rosner, 1987; Craven and Barnes, 1991). Personnel attending these sick animals are then infected by inhaling infected aerosols.

Clinical Signs Bubonic plague in humans is usually characterized by fever (2–7 days postexposure) and the formation of large, tender, swollen lymph nodes, or buboes. If untreated, the disease may progress to severe pneumonic or systemic plague. Inhaled infective particles, particularly from animals with plague pneumonia, may also result in the pneumonic form of the disease.

Diagnosis and Control A presumptive diagnosis can be made by visualizing bipolar-staining, ovoid, gram-negative rods on the microscopic examination of fluid from buboes, blood, sputum, or spinal fluid; confirmation can be made by culture. Complement fixation, passive hemagglutination, and immunofluorescence staining of specimens can be used for serological confirmation.

Mortality without antibiotic therapy, particularly in cases of pneumonic plague, exceeds 50% in untreated cases. Although *Y. pestis* is susceptible to a wide variety of antibiotics, multiple antibiotic-resistant strains are being isolated with increasing frequency (Dennis and Hughes, 1997). Aminogylcosides, such as streptomycin and gentamicin, are the most effective antibiotics *in vivo* against *Y. pestis.* Chloramphenicol is the drug of choice for treating plague meningitis and endophthalmitis (Craven and Barnes, 1991; Mushatt and Hyslop, 1991). In people exposed to *Y. pestis*, prophylactic therapy with tetracycline for a 7-day period is often prescribed.

An inactivated plague vaccine is available for laboratory personnel working with the organism and in high-risk individuals working in areas where the disease is endemic (e.g., wildlife management employees, Peace Corps volunteers) and where they are exposed to plague reservoirs.

Rodent and flea control, particularly in endemic areas, is an indispensable part of containing exposure to plague, as is restricting certain locales for recreational use. Animal facilities should be constructed and maintained to prevent wild rodent egress. Furthermore, feral or random-source animals acquired from plague-endemic areas should be quarantined and treated with appropriate insecticides to kill fleas.

3. Leptospirosis

Leptospirosis is solely a zoonotic disease of livestock, pet and stray dogs, and wildlife, including wild rodents. Human-to-human transmission is extremely rare. *Leptospira interrogans* (comprising >200 serovars) has been isolated worldwide. Although particular serotypes usually have distinct host species, most serotypes can be carried by several hosts. *Leptospira* spp. are well adapted to a variety of mammals, particularly wild animals and rodents. Recent molecular analysis of *Leptospira* spp. has classified these bacteria into over 15 species. In clinical practice, however, *Leptospira* spp. continue to be identified by serotype and importantly used for epidemiological studies (Bharti *et al.*, 2003; Levett, 2001).

Reservoir and Incidence Leptospira icterohaemorrhagiae was first recovered in 1918 in the United States from wild rats sampled in New York City. In the 1950s, in a study conducted in Baltimore, 45.5% of 1643 rats were infected with *Leptospira*; higher prevalence rates occurred in older rats (approximately 60%). In the late

1970s, more than 90% of adult Brown Norway rats sampled in Detroit were infected with *L. icterohaemorrhagiae* (Thiermann, 1977). Other studies confirm the high prevalence of this organism in wild rats inhabiting U.S. cities (Alexander, 1984; Sanger and Thiermann, 1988). Rodent reservoir hosts of leptospirosis, in addition to rats, include mice, field moles, hedgehogs, gerbils, squirrels, rabbits, and hamsters (Torten, 1979; Fox and Lipman, 1991). Livestock serve as a significant source of primary long-term shedding of at least three serovars. Cattle are the natural carriers of the serotype *L. hardjo*, whereas swine carry *L. pomona* and *L. bratislava*; each animal can shed the organism for extended periods in their urine. Dogs also commonly harbor two other serotypes; feral dogs harbor *L. icterohaemorrhagiae* as well as serve as natural carrier hosts of *L. canicola*. Sheep, goats, and horses can also be infected with a variety of serotypes. Raccoons are reservoirs of *L. autumnalis* and *L. grippotyhosa*, whereas rats, mice, and other wild rodents are common animal hosts for another serotype, *L. ballum*. In wild mice, the infection can persist unnoticed for the animal's lifetime and can also be harbored by laboratory mice, although their carrier rates in the United States are unknown (Torten, 1979). There was, however, a report of leptospirosis in a research colony of mice in the United States in the early 1980s (Alexander, 1984). In several European laboratories, personnel have contracted leptospires from laboratory rats (Geller, 1979).

Mode of Transmission Infection with *Leptospira* most frequently results from handling infected animals (contaminating the hands with urine) or from aerosol exposure during cage cleaning or through exposure to contaminated water or soil. Skin abrasions or mucous membrane exposure may serve as the portal of entry in humans. All secretions and excretions from infected animals should be considered infective. In one instance, a father apparently was infected after his daughter used his toothbrush to clean a contaminated pet mouse cage. Handling infected wild rats increases the risk of contracting leptospires (Luzzi *et al.*, 1987). Also, a young man died of acute leptospirosis by falling into a heavily polluted river contaminated with *L. icterohaemorrhagiae* (Sanger and Thiermann, 1988). In addition, rodent bites can transmit the disease. Children living in rat-infested tenements may be at increased risk of infection. For example, children from inner-city Detroit had significantly higher *L. icterohaemorrhagiae* antibody titers when compared to those of children living in the Detroit suburbs (Demers *et al.*, 1983). It is important to note that leptospirosis can infect hosts on a chronic basis, by colonizing their kidney tubules. Outbreaks of leptospirosis in humans with varying mortality in underdeveloped countries have been documented in 1995–1998.

Clinical Signs The disease may vary from inapparent to severe infection and death. Individuals infected

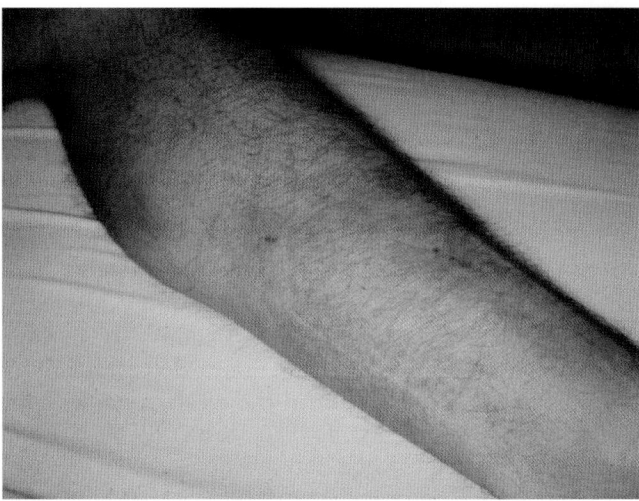

FIGURE 28.7   Leptospirosis causing diffuse redness on a leg of a veterinarian after visiting sick lamb. *Source: John Moses, M.D.*

with *Leptospira* spp. experience a biphasic disease (Sanger and Thiermann, 1988; Faine, 1991). They become suddenly ill with weakness, headache, myalgia, malaise, chills, and fever, and usually exhibit leukocytosis. During the second phase of the disease, which is immunologically mediated, conjunctival suffusion and a rash may occur (Fig. 28.7). On examination, renal, hepatic, pulmonary, and gastrointestinal findings may be abnormal. The most severe form of the diseases, known as Weil's disease, is characterized by hepatic and renal dysfunction, hemorrhage, and circulatory collapse (Bharti *et al.*, 2003; Levett, 2001). Treatment of the disease is controversial given the disease is self-limiting. Penicillin is the drug of choice in treating early onset of leptospirosis infection (Vinetz, 2003). Comparison of penicillins to ceftriaxone, cefotaxime, and doxycycline in cases of severe leptospirosis indicated that all of these antibiotics were equally efficacious in reducing fever and clinical complications (Vinetz, 2003). Ampicillin and doxycycline have also been effective in treating people with leptospirosis.

Diagnosis and Control Leptospirosis in humans is often difficult to diagnose; therefore, the low incidence of reported infection in humans may be misleading. Outbreaks have been documented in the United States from personnel working with laboratory mice (Stoenner and Maclean, 1958; Barkin *et al.*, 1974). In one study, 8 of 58 employees handling infected laboratory mice (80% of breeding females were excreting L. *ballum* in their urine) contracted leptospirosis (Stoenner and Maclean, 1958). Personnel performing field research may be predisposed to developing leptospirosis and other zoonotic diseases, since occupational exposure to wild animal habitats is a work-related risk factor (Adjemian *et al.*, 2012). Because of the variability in clinical symptoms and lack of pathognomonic findings in humans and animals, serological diagnosis or actual isolation of leptospires is imperative (Bharti *et al.*, 2003; Levett, 2001). As an aid to diagnosis, leptospires can sometimes be observed by examination or direct staining of body fluids or fresh tissue suspensions. The definitive diagnosis in humans or animals is made by culturing the organisms from tissue or fluid samples. Culture media with long-chain fatty acids with 1% bovine serum albumin are routinely used as a detoxicant (Faine, 1991). Serological assessment is accomplished by indirect hemagglutination, agglutination analysis, complement fixation, microscopic agglutination, and fluorescent antibody techniques (Faine, 1991). Growth of the organism is slow, and cultures should be incubated in the dark for 6 weeks at 30°C (Goldstein, 1991; Collins and Lorber, 2009). The serological test most frequently used is the microscopic agglutination test, which employs dark-field microscopy. Titers of 1:100 or greater are considered significant. When comparing serological assays, ELISA and dot ELISA have the highest sensitivities and specificities (Goldstein, 1991; Collins and Lorber, 2009). PCR-based assays are also available for diagnosis (Smythe *et al.*, 2002). Personnel hygiene and protective garments that minimize exposure to infected urine and other infected animal tissue are important for control of zoonotic infection with leptospires.

C. Enteric Diseases

1. Campylobacteriosis

Campylobacter spp. have been known as a pathogenic and commensal bacterium in domestic animals for decades. During the past several years, *C. jejuni* and *C. coli* have gained recognition as a leading cause of diarrhea in humans.

Reservoir and Incidence *C. jejuni, C. coli, C. upsaliensis*, and *C. helveticus* have been isolated from a variety of laboratory animals, including dogs, cats, guinea pigs, hamsters, ferrets, nonhuman primates, poultry, and rabbits (Fox, 1982a; Engvall *et al.*, 2003) and also from healthy swine, sheep, and cattle. *Campylobacter* spp. commonly cause abortion in livestock. They can be shed in the stool for variable periods of time in asymptomatic carriers, and multiple species of *Campylobacter* spp. as well as *Helicobacter* spp. can be isolated from the feces of a single individual or animal (Allos *et al.*, 1995; Shen *et al.*, 1999; Fox, 2011).

Mode of Transmission In most reports citing pet-to-human transmission of *C. jejuni*, diarrheic puppies or kittens recently obtained from animal pounds were the source of the infection (Blaser *et al.*, 1980; Deming *et al.*, 1987; Tenkate and Stafford, 2001). People who live with dogs are at increased risk of acquiring campylobacter infections. In a laboratory animal setting, personnel

performing husbandry chores have become infected when handling *Campylobacter*-infected animals (Fox *et al.*, 1989b). Prevalence studies of dogs, cats, newly imported primates, or animals housed in groups suggest that younger animals more easily acquire the infection and, hence, commonly shed the organism. More recently, *C. upsaliensis* and *C. helveticus* have been isolated from dogs and cats. *C. upsaliensis* has also been associated with diarrheal disease in humans (Fox, 2011).

Clinical Signs The clinical features of campylobacter enteritis in humans are usually consistent with an acute gastrointestinal illness. Diarrhea – sometimes watery – with or without blood and leukocytes, abdominal pain, and constitutional symptoms, especially fever, occur routinely. The severity of the illness can be variable, but in most cases it is brief and self-limiting. Complications of *C. jejuni* infections include reactive arthritis, Guillian–Barre syndrome, and rarely myocarditis. In protracted or severe cases, antimicrobial therapy (e.g., erythromycin) is instituted. Erythromycin eliminates *C. jejuni* from the intestine of most infected patients within 72 hours.

Diagnosis and Control There are multiple *C. jejuni/coli* serotypes; the use of serotyping schemes and restriction enzyme analysis of isolates aids in confirming zoonotic spread of the organism (Russell *et al.*, 1990). Additional molecular techniques also can be used to discriminate strain identity. Because animals can be asymptomatic carriers of Campylobacters, protective measures preventing fecal contamination and inadvertent oral ingestion are important for prevention of infection.

2. Enteric Helicobacteriosis

Reservoir and Incidence *Helicobacter cinaedi* is primarily recovered from immunocompromised individuals; the organism is also recovered from chronic alcoholics as well as immunocompetent men and women. The hamster is suspected to be the reservoir host for *H. cinaedi* (Gebhart *et al.*, 1989). Even though *H. canis, H. cinaedi, H. fennelliae*, and *H. rappini* (now classified as *H. bilis*) have been isolated from both dogs and humans, *H. canis* and *H. cinaedi* from cats, and *H. cinaedi* from rhesus monkeys (Fox, 2002; Fox *et al.*, 2001), additional investigations will be required to ascertain whether these enteric helicobacters in dogs, cats, hamsters, non-human primates, and other unrecognized mammalian hosts constitute a potential reservoir for zoonotic transmission to people. Although there are a multitude of *Helicobacter* spp. in rodents, no zoonotic link, other than hamsters, has been associated with these enteric helicobacters (Whary and Fox, 2006). Recently, however, *H. pullorum*, isolated from poultry and humans, has also been cultured from commercially raised mice (Turk *et al.*, 2012).

Mode of Transmission Fecal–oral transmission is the likely route of infection. *H. cinaedi*, a fastidious microaerophile, has been recovered from blood and fecal specimens of children and of a neonate with septicemia and meningitis. The mother of the neonate had cared for pet hamsters during the first two trimesters of her pregnancy (Orlicek *et al.*, 1993). Because *H. cinaedi* has been isolated from normal intestinal flora of hamsters, it was suggested that the pet hamsters served as a reservoir for transmission to the mother. The mother had a diarrheal illness during the third trimester of pregnancy; the newborn was likely to have been infected during the birthing process, although this was not proven (Orlicek *et al.*, 1993). Furthermore, the hamster has been suggested as possibly infecting other humans with *H. cinaedi* (Gebhart *et al.*, 1989). Studies are needed to confirm zoonotic risk of handling *H. cinaedi*-infected hamsters (Gebhart *et al.*, 1989). Also of interest is the isolation, based on cellular fatty acid and biochemical identification, and molecular analysis, of *H. cinaedi* from the feces of dogs, cats, and nonhuman primates. *H. canis* has also been isolated from blood of a bacteremic 7 month-old child living with a cat (Prag *et al.*, 2007).

Clinical Signs   *H. cinaedi* (previously *Campylobacter cinaedi*) was first isolated from the lower bowel of homosexuals with proctitis and colitis. It has also been isolated from the blood of homosexual patients with HIV as well as children and adult women (Orlicek *et al.*, 1993). In a retrospective study of 23 patients with *H. cinaedi*-associated illness, 22 of the cases had the organism isolated from blood by using an automated blood culture system in which a slightly elevated growth index was noted (Kiehlbauch *et al.*, 1994). This study also described a new *H. cinaedi*-associated syndrome consisting of bacteremia and fever, and accompanied by leukocytosis and thrombocytopenia. Recurrent cellulitis and/or arthritis are also noted in a high percentage of infected immunocompromised patients (Kiehlbauch *et al.*, 1994; Burman *et al.*, 1995). Other enteric helicobacters, *H. canis*, *H. pullorum*, *H. bilis*, *H. fenneliae*, *H. canadensis*, and *H. westmeadii*, have been isolated from diarrheic patients as well as bacteremic immunocompromised individuals (Fox, 2002).

Diagnosis and Control   It should be stressed that many hospital and veterinary laboratories have difficulty isolating this organism. Because of the slow growth of *H. cinaedi* and other enteric helicobacters, laboratory diagnosis is unlikely if blood culture procedures that rely on visual detection of the culture media are used (Kiehlbauch *et al.*, 1994; Burman *et al.*, 1995; Kiehlbauch *et al.*, 1995). Use of dark-field microscopy or acridine orange staining of blood culture media, rather than gram staining, increases likelihood of seeing the organism. Likewise, fecal isolation is difficult; selective antibiotic media are required, and recovery is facilitated by passing fecal homogenates through a 0.45-pm filter (Gebhart *et al.*, 1989). In one study, several strains of both *H. cinaedi* and *H. fennelliae* were inhibited by concentrations of cephalothin and cetazolin used frequently in selective media for isolation of enteric microaerophilic bacterium. These organisms also require an environment rich in hydrogen for optimum *in vitro* growth. Until diagnostic laboratories embark on routine isolation attempts of *Helicobacter* spp. from feces, the extent of their presence in companion and pocket pets and their zoonotic potential will be unknown.

3. Gastric Helicobacter Infections

Reservoir and Incidence   Because gastric helicobacter-like organisms (GHLOs) (i.e., '*H. heilmannii*' (now classified as *H. suis*) or *H. felis*, and *H. bizzozeronii* in dogs) cause a small percentage of gastritis in humans and no environmental source for these bacteria has been recognized, various animals, particularly dogs and cats, have been implicated in zoonotic transmission. In colony-reared dogs, cats, and nonhuman primates, GHLO infection may approach 100%. *H. pylori*, the primary gastric pathogen in humans, has been isolated from only one colony of commercial cats and macaque species. If *H. pylori*, as demonstrated in commercially reared cats (Handt *et al.*, 1994; Fox *et al.*, 1996), is isolated from pet cats, the zoonotic potential of helicobacteriosis from cats would obviously increase substantially. *H. pylori* infection is an important cause of human gastritis; however, most epidemiologic studies do not incriminate animal contact as a cause of human infection. An epidemiologic survey conducted in Germany did not show an increased risk of *H. pylori* because of cat ownership. In a serological survey measuring antibodies to *H. pylori*, lower socioeconomic status, and not pet ownership or day care, was associated with seropositivity (Staat *et al.*, 1996).

Mode of Transmission   Oral–oral transmission is likely, but fecal–oral transmission may also occur. In one case study, a researcher performing physiologic studies with cat stomachs developed an acute gastritis, presumably resulting from *H. felis* on the basis of electron microscopy (EM) (Lavelle *et al.*, 1994). Gastric spiral bacteria were demonstrated in gastric mucosa of cats being used by this scientist. In Germany, a survey of 125 individuals infected with GHLOs provided information in a questionnaire regarding animal contact. Of these patients, 70.3% had contact with one or more animals compared with 37% in the clinically healthy control population (Stolte *et al.*, 1994).

Clinical Signs   Infection with GHLOs in animals (although associated with gastritis in the majority of humans) does not cause characteristic clinical illness with any consistency or reproducibility. In people with GHLO infections, bismuth subsalicylate, amoxicillin, tetracycline, and metronidazole in various combinations successfully eradicated GHLOs from the gastric mucosa with resolution of gastritis (Heilmann and Borchard, 1991). No systematic antibiotic trials have been conducted in dogs and cats to test for efficacy in eradicating either '*H. heilmannii*' or *H. felis* from gastric mucosa.

Diagnosis and Control A diagnosis of chronic gastritis in animals, as in humans, cannot be made by gross visual examination of the gastric mucosa by endoscopy. Histologic evaluation of gastric biopsy samples is required, utilizing a special silver stain or modified Giemsa stain to reveal the presence of GHLOs. Unfortunately, *H. bizzozeronii* is the most common spiral organism in dogs and cats, and it has been extremely difficult to culture on artificial media (Hanninen *et al.*, 1996). '*H. heilmannii*,' (now *H. suis*) also common in primates, has been cultured successfully from pigs and humans (Baele *et al.*, 2008). *H. felis* is also difficult to isolate. In practice, histological findings of inflammatory changes accompanied by gastric spiral organisms on the gastric mucosa or in the gastric mucous layer have been used for diagnosis. *H. felis* cannot be distinguished from '*H. heilmannii*' by histologic examination; EM evaluation is necessary.

Because oral bacteria and bacteria refluxed from the duodenum may overgrow the fastidious *Helicobacter* species, selective antibiotic media are available for isolation. Helicobacters, like campylobacters, require special environmental and cultural conditions for their growth. The organisms are thermophilic and grow at 37°C, and some species at 42°C. Growth on chocolate or blood agar takes 3–5 days (Hanninen *et al.*, 1996). For *H. bizzozeronii* isolation, incubation requires 5–10 days. A provisional diagnosis of gastric helicobacters takes advantage of a biochemical feature of these organisms: the ability to produce large quantities of urease. Gastric biopsy samples can be placed in a urea broth containing a pH indicator (phenol red) and a preservative (sodium azide). A similar test is available commercially. Serological assays are being employed to diagnose *H. pylori* in humans (Staat *et al.*, 1996; Fox and Megraud, 2007), as are *H. pylori* antigen-based fecal assays. However, serological tests currently do not provide a reliable, noninvasive diagnostic test for gastric helicobacter infection in dogs and cats or primates.

4. Salmonellosis

The genus *Salmonella* are gram-negative bacteria of which there are two species, *S. bongori* which infects mainly poikilotherms and rarely humans, and *S. enterica* which includes approximately 2500 serovars. *Salmonella* are properly designated using their serovar (which was often formerly a species name), for example, *S. enterica* subsp. *enterica* serovar Typhimurium (aka *S. Typhimurium*) and serovar Enteritidis (*S. Enteritidis*). Nontyphoidal salmonellosis is caused by any of these serotypes. *Salmonella* are flagellated, nonsporulating, aerobic gram-negative bacilli that can be readily isolated from feces on selective media designed to suppress bacterial growth of other enteric bacteria.

Reservoir and Incidence Salmonellosis occurs worldwide and is important in humans and animals. *Salmonella* isolates, because of molecular taxonomics, are now divided between *S. enterica* and *S. bongori*. Salmonellae are pathogenic to a variety of animals.

Although the reported prevalence of *Salmonella* in laboratory animals has decreased in the past several decades because of management practices (e.g., pasteurizing animal feeds), environmental contamination with *Salmonella* continues to be a potential source of infection for these animals and for the personnel handling them. Until all animal feeds in the United States and Europe are *Salmonella*-free and animals are procured from *Salmonella*-free sources, laboratory animal-associated cases of salmonellosis in humans will continue. The increasing number of recalls due to *Salmonella*-contaminated, commercially available dog and cat food, presumably manufactured in facilities with improper quality control procedures, is particularly of concern (CDC, 2012c). Endemic salmonellosis in commercially raised guinea pigs as well as dogs, cats, and nonhuman primates has also been a source of infection in personnel working with these animals. Prevalence data from eight studies conducted worldwide indicated that a wide range (0.6–27%) of cats were culture positive for *Salmonella*, and a conservative estimate for the U.S. canine population would be 10%. Rats are extremely susceptible to infection with *Salmonella*. In studies performed in the 1920s through 1940s, the prevalence of *Salmonella* in wild rats surveyed in the United States varied from 1% to 18%, compared to 19% in Europe (Geller, 1979; Weisbroth, 1979; Alexander, 1984). In experimental studies, when rats were dosed orally with *Salmonella*, 10% shed the organism in the 2 months after inoculation, and a few remained carriers when examined 5 months after experimental challenge. These rats, when placed with other naive rats, were capable of initiating new epizootics. Fortunately, the disease in laboratory rats, although common prior to 1939, has been isolated rarely in U.S. commercially reared rats since that time. Birds and reptiles are particularly dangerous sources of *Salmonella*; as much as 94% of all reptiles harbor *Salmonella*. (Chiodini and Sundberg, 1981). Turtles have received a great deal of zoonotic attention and in 1970 alone may have caused 280,000 human cases of salmonellosis. In the late 1960s, with annual sales of 15 million turtles, zoonotic salmonellosis became a growing problem. In 1972, the U.S. Food and Drug Administration (FDA) banned importation of turtles and turtle eggs and the interstate shipment of turtles that were not certified as free of *Salmonella* or *Arizona hinshawii* in their state of origin. However, the unreliable effectiveness of this method forced the FDA in 1975 to rule against the sale of viable turtle eggs or live turtles with a carapace length less than 10.2 cm, with exceptions made for educational or scientific institutions and marine turtles. Subsequently, there was a substantial decrease in turtle-associated salmonellosis, indicating the efficacy of this regulation. These restrictions are difficult to enforce, and other reptiles, e.g., iguanas, are increasingly cited in zoonotic outbreaks of salmonellosis, particularly in children. Also of note, because of repeated reports of chick- and duckling-associated salmonellosis, some states have also restricted their sale as pets.

An outbreak of multidrug resistant *S. enterica* serovar Typhimurium associated with commercially distributed pet rodents, including rats, mice, and hamsters, was recently reported (Swanson *et al.*, 2007). Twenty-eight matching isolates identified by PFGE of *S. enterica* serotype Typhimurium from humans were identified from humans; 13 (59%) had previously had contact with rodents purchased from retail pet stores and 2 patients (9%) had secondarily acquired the infection from a patient who had been exposed to an infected rodent. These 15 patients whose median age was 16 years (neonate-43) resided in 10 different states. No single source of rodents was common in all cases and each case household had purchased the rodents from a different retail pet store. It was ascertained that several of the rodent breeders and distributors routinely used antimicrobials (e.g., spectinomycin, leptomycin, tetracycline, and nitrofurazone) in the drinking water as a preventative measure for nonspecific rodent enteritis. Interestingly, all human animal and environmental samples of *S. enterica* serovar Typhimurium isolates tested in this outbreak were uniformly resistant to ampicillin, chloramphenicol, streptomycin, sulfisoxazole, and tetracycline (R-type ACSSuT). Patients infected with multiple antibiotic resistant strains of *S. enterica* serotype Typhimurium have higher hospitalization rates than patients infected with susceptible strains (Martin, 2004; Varma, 2005). There are also reports of increased risk of septicemia, treatment failure, and mortality associated with multidrug resistant *S. enterica* serotype Typhimurium (Helms *et al.*, 2002). The spread of these multiple antibiotic resistant strains in rodents may have been facilitated by the widespread use of antibiotics as a prophylactic measure in the pocket pet retail industry. Indeed treatment with oral antibiotics may eliminate normal enterobacteriacae enteric flora and facilitate colonization with antibiotic resistant *Salmonella*, as observed in mice treated with antimicrobials (Que, 1985; van der Waaij, 1968; van der Waaij *et al.*, 1971. The authors of this outbreak urged heightened disease surveillance in pet retail facilities, as well as increased hygiene and husbandry practices to minimize the need for prophylactic antimicrobial therapy. Individuals purchasing rodents as pets or for food consumption by reptiles should be alerted to the possibility that these animals' feces are potentially infectious. For example, additional outbreaks of Salmonellosis have been traced to households that have pet snakes. The source of *Salmonella* infection in humans, particularly children, was caring for the pet snakes that, as part of their diet, were fed *Salmonella*-infected frozen rats and mice sold commercially in the United States, as well as the United Kingdom (Fuller, 2008; Harker *et al.*, 2011). Aquatic frogs, particularly African dwarf frogs, can also be a source of *Salmonella* infection (CDC, 2010b; CDC, 2011). This highlights the importance of ascertaining pet status of prospective animal technicians who have applied for positions in vivaria. Another multistate outbreak of *S. enterica* serovar Typhimurium has been recently reported due to exposure to infected pet hedgehogs (Marsden-Haug *et al.*, 2013). The increased incidence of *Salmonella* infections can be reduced by hand washing with soap and water after handling of rodents, their cages, and bedding.

Mode of Transmission   *Salmonella* spp. are ubiquitous in nature and are routinely found in water or food contaminated with animal or human excreta. Fecal–oral transmission is the primary mode for spread of infection from animal to animal or to humans. Rat feces can remain infective for 148 days when maintained at room temperature. *Salmonella* is routinely associated with food-borne disease outbreaks, is a contaminant of sewage, and is found in many environmental water sources. Transmission is enhanced by crowding and poor sanitation.

Both humans and animals can be asymptomatic carriers and periodic shedders; they may have mild, unrecognized disease, or they may be completely asymptomatic. In the biomedical laboratory, asymptomatic animals can easily infect other animals, technicians, and investigators. Personnel at veterinary hospitals are at increased risk because of outbreaks of salmonellosis in hospitalized animals (Ikeda *et al.*, 1986). The prevalence of human salmonellosis acquired from laboratory animals or *vice versa* is unknown; however, the literature is replete with examples of cases of this infection obtained from pets; this is particularly true for exotic pets such as iguanas, turtles, sugar gliders, and hedgehogs (Woodward *et al.*, 1997).

Clinical Signs   Clinical signs of salmonellosis in humans include acute sudden gastroenteritis, abdominal pain, diarrhea, nausea, and fever. Diarrhea and anorexia may persist for several days. Organisms invading the intestine may create septicemia without severe intestinal involvement; most clinical signs are attributed to hematogenous spread of the organisms. As with other microbial infections, the severity of the disease relates to the serotype of the organism, the number of bacteria ingested, and the susceptibility of the host. In experimental studies with volunteers, several serovars induced a spectrum of clinical disease, from brief enteritis to serious debilitation. Incubation varied from 7 to 72h. Cases of asymptomatic carriers, persisting for several weeks, were common (Hull, 1955).

Salmonella gastroenteritis is usually mild and self-limiting. With careful management of fluid and electrolyte balance, antimicrobial therapy is not necessary. In humans, antimicrobial therapy may prolong rather than shorten the period that *Salmonella* is shed in the feces (Nelson *et al.*, 1980; Pavia and Tauxe, 1991). In one double-blind placebo study of infants, oral antibiotics did not significantly affect the duration of *Salmonella* carriage. Bacteriological relapse after antibiotic treatment occurred in 53% of the patients, and 33% of these suffered a recurrence of diarrhea, whereas none of the placebo group relapsed (Nelson *et al.*, 1980). Also of interest is the fact that in outbreaks of DT104 *S. enterica* serotype Typhimurium infection, a high percentage of patients had been recently on antibiotics before becoming infected with the *S. enterica* serovar Typhimurium strain DT104 (Molba *et al.*, 1999).

Diagnosis and Control As with other fecal–oral transmitted diseases, control depends on eliminating contact with feces, food, or water contaminated with *Salmonella* or animal reservoirs excreting the organism. *Salmonella* survive for months in feces and are readily cultured from sediments in ponds and streams previously contaminated with sewage or animal feces. Fat and moisture in food promote survival of *Salmonella*. Pasteurization of milk and proper cooking of food (56°C for 10–20 min) effectively destroy *Salmonella*. In the laboratory, control and prevention of salmonellosis depends on the rapid detection, removal, or treatment of both acute and chronic animal infections, particularly during the quarantine period. Multiple antibiotic resistance is commonly encountered in *Salmonella* strains. For example, multiple-resistant *S. enterica* serotype Typhimurium strain DT104 has been increasingly cited (in Europe and recently in the United States) as a cause of human infections (Tauxe, 1999). Importantly, this organism has been isolated from farm animals, cats, wild birds, rodents, foxes, and badgers. It definitely has been transmitted from cattle and sheep to humans and has caused epizootic gastroenteritis and fatal bacteremia in dairy cattle (Besser *et al.*, 1997).

5. Shigellosis

Reservoir and Incidence Shigellosis is a significant zoonotic disease in nonhuman primates (Fox, 1975; Richter *et al.*, 1984). *Shigella flexneri*, *S. sonnei*, and *S. dysenteriae* are the most common species found in nonhuman primates. Humans are the main reservoir of the disease, which occurs worldwide. Nonhuman primates acquire the disease following capture and subsequent contact with other infected primates or contaminated premises, food, or water. Shigellosis is one of the most commonly identified causes of diarrhea in nonhuman primates.

Mode of Transmission *Shigella* organisms may be shed from clinically ill as well as asymptomatic humans and nonhuman primates. In humans, transmission occurs by ingestion of fecally contaminated food or water, or by direct contact (even if only minimal) with infected animals. Pet monkeys shedding *Shigella* are a particular threat to owners, and pet store proprietors, unless cautious, can contract the disease (Fox, 1975).

Clinical Signs Humans are generally susceptible to shigellosis, although it is much more severe in children than in adults. The disease varies from completely asymptomatic to a bacillary dysentery syndrome characterized by blood and mucus in the feces, abdominal cramping, tenesmus, weight loss, and anorexia. Usually, the disease presents only as a clinically mild diarrhea. However, fatal shigellosis has been reported in children and adults who have had contact with infected pet or zoo monkeys (Fox, 1975); survivors can remain asymptomatic carriers. The clinical disease in nonhuman primates is similar to that in humans but may be associated with higher mortality rates.

Diagnosis and Control When humans or nonhuman primates experience acute diarrhea (especially if traced with blood or mucus), *Shigella* spp. may be the cause (Richter *et al.*, 1984; Dupont, 2000). A definitive diagnosis requires the isolation of the organism from inoculation of fresh feces or gingival swabs onto selective media. An identification can be confirmed by agglutination with polyvalent *Shigella* antisera. Because many *Shigella* spp. from nonhuman primates have plasmid-mediated antibiotic resistance markers, determination of antibiotic sensitivities of these isolates is mandatory before instituting treatment.

To prevent shigellosis in the laboratory, quarantine and screening of all newly arrived primates to detect carriers of *Shigella* spp. are required. As in the treatment of the disease in humans, trimethoprim and sulfamethodoxazole can be effective in eliminating the *Shigella* spp. carrier state in rhesus monkeys. Enrofloxacin is also used to eliminate subclinical *Shigella* spp. in macaques.

D. Respiratory Infections

1. Bordetella bronchiseptica

Bordetella bronchiseptica, a gram-negative bacteria, is commonly recovered from the respiratory tract of dogs, cats, rabbits, and a variety of laboratory rodents. Despite its widespread occurrence in animals, it is seldom cultured from diseased tissues of humans, with few cases reported in the literature. Its isolation is often from immunocompromised patients (Woolfrey and Moody, 1991) who have pneumonia and/or bacteremia, or cystic fibrosis (Spilker *et al.*, 2008). It has also been isolated from AIDS patients (Ng *et al.*, 1992). In children with respiratory infection due to *B. bronchiseptica*, a 'whooping cough'-like syndrome is described. This is not surprising given that *B. bronchiseptica* produces a dermatonecrotoxin, tracheal cytotoxin, and adenylate cyclase similar to that isolated from *B. pertussis*. In one interesting report, three children with *B. bronchiseptica* infection developed whooping cough-like symptoms; both their pet rabbits and cats subsequently died of *B. bronchiseptica* pneumonia (Kristensen and Lautrop, 1962). Fluoroquinolones have been used successfully to treat the disease in humans (Carbone *et al.*, 1999; Spilker *et al.*, 2008).

2. Tuberculosis

Reservoir and Incidence   Tuberculosis is an important zoonosis associated with laboratory animals and a potential concern in wildlife research programs or when wild-caught animals are brought into the laboratory. It is caused by acid-fast bacilli of the genus *Mycobacterium*. Natural reservoir hosts for the etiologic agent of this disease correspond to the three most common species of *Mycobacterium*: *M. bovis*, *M. avium* complex, and M. *tuberculosis*. Although cattle, birds, and humans are the major reservoir hosts, many animals, including swine, sheep, goats, monkeys, cats, dogs, and ferrets, are susceptible and contribute to the spread of disease (Marini *et al.*, 1989; Fox and Marini, 2014; Swennes and Fox, 2014). This susceptibility varies according to the immune response of the host and to the particular *Mycobacterium* spp. infecting the host. In nonhuman primates, outbreaks of tuberculosis still occur, particularly in the Old World species of monkeys. They initially contract the disease in the wild through human contact, and then the organism is transmitted from monkey to monkey (Richter *et al.*, 1984).

Mode of Transmission   *Mycobacterium* bacilli are transmitted from infected animals or tissue samples via the aerosol route. The disease is spread beyond the natural host range through animal-to-animal and human-to-human contact, usually by airborne infectious particles. Laboratory workers have the highest risk of contracting the disease when caring for or performing autopsies on infected animals. In the laboratory, certain situations can enhance disease transmission, such as exposure to (1) dusty bedding of infected animals, (2) aerosolized organisms from a high-pressure water sanitizer, and (3) the coughing of clinically affected animals. The disease may also be contracted by direct ingestion of bacilli. Reports have documented an increase of tuberculin skin conversion in personnel working with primates infected with *Mycobacterium* spp. (Kalter *et al.*, 1978).

Clinical Signs   Clinical signs of tuberculosis in humans are dependent on the organ system or systems involved. Most familiar are the signs related to the pulmonary form. Although this form of the disease often remains asymptomatic for months or years, it may eventually produce a cough with sputum and hemoptysis. In addition, general symptoms include anorexia, weight loss, lassitude, fatigue, fever, chills, and cachexia (Division of Tuberculosis Elimination, 2000).

Diagnosis and Control   A positive diagnosis is often quite difficult to obtain. Three widely used tools for a presumptive diagnosis are the intradermal tuberculin test, radiographic analysis, and positive acid-fast-stained sputum smears. Serological assays for diagnosis of tuberculosis have been recently introduced as an adjunct or replacement for intradermal testing (Mazurek *et al.*, 2010). A more definitive diagnosis of the organisms from body fluids or biopsy specimens is obtained by culture, PCR analysis, and confirmation using standard biochemical techniques.

Control of tuberculosis infection, particularly within the biomedical research arena, requires a multifaceted approach. This includes personnel education, a regular health surveillance program for personnel and nonhuman primates, isolation and quarantine of suspect animals, and rapid euthanasia and careful disposal of confirmed positive animals. Vaccination or chemoprophylaxis may be considered, but certain precautions are necessary (Division of Tuberculosis Elimination, 2000). Vaccination with Bacillus Calmette–Guerin (BCG), a strain of *M. bovis*, is an effective means of preventing active tuberculosis. Vaccination is suggested in high-risk groups. However, this vaccine often elicits a positive tuberculin test, thereby negating the best diagnostic indicator of early disease. Vaccination in the United States is therefore reserved for demonstrated high-risk individuals and children in locations where 20% or more of school-age children are tuberculin-positive (Division of Tuberculosis Elimination, 2000).

Chemoprophylaxis with effective antituberculosis agents used to treat humans, such as isoniazid, rifampin, and ethambutol, has been used to treat valuable nonhuman primates (Wolf *et al.*, 1988). A well-conceived tuberculosis control program will include some or all of the above methods tailored to the needs and special circumstances of individual animal resource programs.

VI. FUNGAL DISEASES

The superficial mycoses are commonly referred to as ringworm due to the characteristic circular erythematous lesion found on the skin of the host. The most common of the fungi responsible for disease in animals and humans are the three genera of the dermatophytes:

Microsporum, Epidermophyton, and *Trichophyton.* Species of dermatophytes are subcategorized as anthropophilic (primarily infect humans), geophilic (soil inhabitants), and zoophilic (parasitic on animals). The zoophilic dermatophytes are known to infect humans.

Reservoir and Incidence Dermatophytes are distributed worldwide, with particular species found more frequently in specific geographic regions. Ringworm in laboratory animals is common, particularly among random-source animals, such as dogs, cats, and livestock. *Microsporum canis* is the common isolate from dogs and cats, whereas *Trichophyton verrucosum* and *T. equinum* are the species usually isolated from ruminants and horses. *T. mentagrophytes* is the most common isolate from laboratory rodents, and human transmission has occurred (Hironaga *et al.,* 1981; Kraemer *et al.,* 2013).

Mode of Transmission Transmission to humans occurs from direct or indirect contact with symptomatic or asymptomatic carrier animals; contaminated bedding, caging, or other equipment; or fungal contamination of the environment. The resultant disease in humans, tinea, is frequently self-limiting and often goes unnoticed. When lesions occur, they are generally on the extremities, particularly on the arm or hand. Lesions are focal, annular, scaling, and erythematous with central clearing resembling a ring. Occasionally, vesicles or fissures are reported. In contrast with anthropophilic species, zoophilic dermatophytes generally produce more eczematous and inflammatory lesions, which regress rapidly.

Clinical Signs Generally, dermatophytes grow only in dead, keratinized tissue. Advancing infection is halted when contact with live cells and inflammation occurs. Dermatophytes are species-adapted and rarely cause severe inflammatory lesions in the specific-host species. When zoophilic species infect humans, the inflammatory response usually restricts the progress of the infection. Contact with the dermatophyte does not necessarily result in infection in the animal or human host. A number of factors, including but not limited to age; immune, hormonal, and nutritional status; and prior exposure, all are important in disease expression.

When observed, disease in animals is often mild and goes undetected. Disease in cats, usually seen in kittens, is quite variable. Lesions, generally seen on and around the head, are crusting and mildly erythemic. The areas may be alopecic with numerous broken hairs. In dogs, lesions consist of circular, alopecic, crusting patches. In laboratory rodents, lesions are generally absent. Presence of the organism may not be detected until personnel become infected and manifest lesions (Fig. 28.8).

Diagnosis and Control Diagnosis in humans and animals is similar, and is best approached by a combination of direct microscopy on hairs and skin scrapings, Wood's lamp examination (approximately 50% of *Microsporum canis* isolates fluoresce when examined

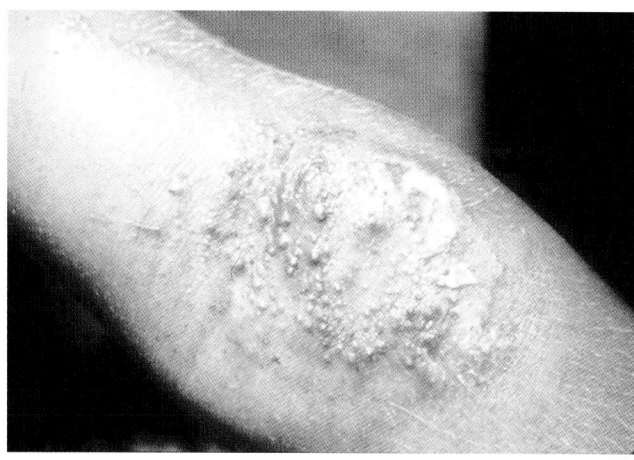

FIGURE 28.8 Ringworm on the forearm. Note the circumscribed lesion with multiple vesicles.

with a cobalt-filtered ultraviolet lamp) and fungal culture (Bond, 2010). Specialized dermatophyte test media (DTM) or Sabouraud's agar may be used.

The risk of zoonotically acquired dermatophytosis can be reduced among laboratory and animal care personnel by wearing protective garments, specifically long-sleeved clothing or laboratory coats; practicing effective personal hygiene; handling random-source animals with disposable gloves; screening newly acquired animals for suggestive lesions; and isolating and treating animals with lesions.

Treatment consists of either systemic therapy with griseofulvin or topical therapy with any one of a number of antifungal agents, such as miconazole. Infectious spores will persist on the animal despite successful treatment of active lesions. Eradication of spores is generally unfeasible, as it may require extensive depilation and the use of sporicidal dips.

VII. PROTOZOAL DISEASES

A. Enteric Diseases

1. Amebiasis

Amebiasis is a parasitic infection of the large intestine caused by the protozoan parasite *Entamoeba histolytica* (Ravdin, 1995).

Reservoir and Incidence The disease occurs worldwide in humans, with a greater prevalence in tropical areas. The parasite is found routinely in clinically normal monkeys and anthropoid apes but may occasionally cause severe clinical disease in these species. The reported incidence of *E. histolytica* has ranged from 0–21% in rhesus monkeys, 2–67% in chimpanzees, and up to 30% in other nonhuman primates. Molecular techniques can be used to characterize potentially virulent strains found in captive primates (Rivera *et al.*, 2010; Tachibana *et al.*, 2009).

Mode of Transmission   *E. histolytica* exists as either resistant cysts or the more fragile trophozoites (Visvesvar and Stehr-Green, 1990). Cysts are the infectious form of the parasite and are usually found in the normal stool of asymptomatic carriers or humans with mild disease (Ravdin, 2000). Cysts may remain viable in moist, cool conditions for over 12 days and in water for up to 30 days. Epidemics of amebiasis in humans usually result from ingestion of fecally contaminated water containing amebic cysts. Laboratory animal workers handling nonhuman primates are potentially exposed to infection from infected fecal matter transferred through the workers' skin or clothing. The infective cyst forms may be subsequently ingested.

Clinical Signs   Most human infections with *E. histolytica* have few or no detectable symptoms (Ravdin, 2000). Clinical signs result when trophozoites invade the large bowel wall causing an amebic colitis. Signs begin with a mild, watery diarrhea with bad-smelling stool, which is frequently preceded by constipation in early stages. There may be gas, abdominal cramps, and tenderness progressing to an acute fulminating bloody or mucoid dysentery with fever, chills, and muscle ache. The disease may have periods of remission and exacerbation over months to years (Ravdin, 2000). Rarely, extraintestinal amebic abscesses may form in the liver, lung, pericardium, or central nervous system. Involvement of the liver may lead to tenderness in the right abdomen and can progress to jaundice.

Diagnosis and Control   The diagnosis of amebiasis is commonly made via the microscopic identification of trophozoites or cysts in fresh stool specimens. The organism must be carefully measured to differentiate it from other nonpathogenic amebas. As is the case with many infectious agents potentially present in stool samples, PCR screening methods have also been developed (Rivera *et al.*, 2010). Control measures to prevent amebiasis should include strict adherence to sanitation and personal hygiene practices. Water supplies should be protected from fecal contamination since usual water purification chlorine levels do not destroy the cysts (Chin, 2000). A chlorine concentration of 10 ppm is necessary to kill amebic cysts (Ravdin, 2000). Cysts may also be killed by heating to 50°C. Nonhuman primates should be screened during quarantine to identify carriers of *E. histolytica* and should be appropriately treated. Nonhuman primates with acute diarrhea or dysentery should also have stool examined for the presence of *E. histolytica* and should be treated as necessary. Recommended drugs for treatment of *E. histolytica* infection include metronidazole, paromomycin, emetine, and iodoquinol (diiodohydroxyquin). The benzoate salt of metronidazole does not posess the bitterness inherent in standard preparations and is useful for oral regimens. Both asymptomatic carriers and symptomatic patients should be treated (Ravdin, 2000).

2. Balantidiasis

Balantidiasis is a zoonotic disease caused by the large ciliated protozoan *Balantidium coli.*

Reservoir and Incidence   *Balantidium coli* is distributed worldwide and is common in domestic swine. It may also be found in humans, great apes, and several monkey species. The incidence in nonhuman primate colonies has ranged from 0 to 63%. These infections are usually asymptomatic in most animals, although clinical disease characterized by diarrhea or dysentery may occur.

Mode of Transmission   Infection usually results from the ingestion of trophozoites or cysts from the feces of infected animals or humans. Transmission may also occur from ingestion of contaminated food or water.

Clinical Signs   Balantidiasis may cause ulcerative colitis characterized by diarrhea or dysentery, tenesmus, nausea, vomiting, and abdominal pain. In severe cases, blood and mucus may be present in the stool. Humans apparently have a high natural incidence, and infections are often asymptomatic (Chin, 2000).

Diagnosis and Control   Balantidiasis is diagnosed by the detection of trophozoites or cysts in fresh fecal samples. Control measures to prevent balantidiasis should be directed at maintaining good sanitation and personal hygiene practices in nonhuman primate and swine colonies. Water supplies should be protected from fecal contamination, especially since usual water chlorination does not destroy cysts (Chin, 2000). Nonhuman primates exhibiting acute diarrhea should be examined for the presence of *B. coli* organisms in the feces. Positive animals should be isolated and the infection appropriately treated. Tetracyclines, metronidazole, and paromomycin have been used successfully to eliminate *B. coli* infections (Teare and Loomis, 1982) and iodoquinol is also used in humans.

3. Cryptosporidiosis

Cryptosporidiosis was first described in the mouse. The genus *Cryptosporidium* now contains over 10 named species (Levine, 1980), many of which have been incriminated as opportunistic, pathogenic parasites (Angus, 1983). Cryptosporidiosis, once considered an infrequent, inconsequential protozoan infection in mammals and reptiles, is now considered a significant enteric pathogen. *Cryptosporidium parvum* and *C. hominis* are considered the human pathogens, but a variety of species and genotypes have been identified and mixed infections can occur (Ng-Hublin *et al.*, 2013).

Reservoir and Incidence *Cryptosporidium* spp. are coccidian parasites known to infect a variety of mammals, including humans, monkeys, livestock, ferrets, pigs, guinea pigs, mice, fish, reptiles, and birds. Neonates of mammalian domestic species are uniquely susceptible to this infection, in comparison with the adults, who are resistant. In humans, however, both children and adults are susceptible. The host-specificity of cryptosporidia isolated from mammals is controversial (Monis and Thompson, 2003), but it is clear that the bovine strains are zoonotic (Levine *et al.*, 1988). Bovine cryptosporidia from calves can also cause infection in newborn pigs, lambs, chicks, mice, rats, and guinea pigs.

Mode of Transmission The life cycle of cryptosporidia is direct, with infection generally limited to the small intestine; however, infections of the respiratory tract, stomach, and conjunctiva have been reported. The life cycle of cryptosporidia is similar to that of other coccidia except that cryptosporidial oocysts do not require time outside the host to sporulate but are infectious at the time of excretion. Large epidemics have occurred in humans ingesting the organism in contaminated municipal drinking water. Sporulated oocysts can exist in the intestine before being excreted. Disease transmission is through ingestion of infectious oocysts. The organisms are small (4–5 pm in diameter) and are located on the apical surface of the parasitized epithelial cell, where they protrude from the brush border. The organisms are intracellular, as the plasma membrane of the host cell envelops the parasite.

Clinical Signs Recorded cases of this disease generally occur in children, particularly in developing countries with poor sanitation, and in immunosuppressed (compromised) individuals. Zoonotic disease has been reported among animal handlers and veterinary students working with neonatal ruminants, principally calves, infected before 6 weeks of age (Levine *et al.*, 1988). Another transmission was recorded in an individual who became infected performing a survey of *Cryptosporidium* spp. in calves (Reese *et al.*, 1982). In this patient, clinical remission occurred by day 13, and oocytes of cryptosporidium were no longer apparent on fecal flotation (Fig. 28.9). Disease in neonatal ruminants may be subclinical or may present with protracted watery diarrhea, very similar to what occurs in humans. Symptoms in humans occur 1–2 weeks after contact with infected calves, and diarrhea may be accompanied by vomiting, severe abdominal cramps, lassitude, fever, and headache. Disease is generally self-limiting except in immunocompromised individuals (Fayer and Ungar, 1986). Most of the recorded cases of protracted human cryptosporidiosis have occurred in immunodeficient individuals, particularly AIDS patients, and are regarded as opportunistic infections (Chin, 2000). Disease in these individuals produced low-grade fever, malaise, anorexia, nausea, abdominal cramps, and a protracted, watery diarrhea. Repeated intestinal biopsies in a patient have documented indigenous cryptosporidial stages for as long as 1 year; clinical signs also persisted in this patient.

Diagnosis and Control Diagnosis is made by examination of feces for the characteristic oocysts. Direct wet mounts may be satisfactory in heavy infections; the organism can be concentrated by the Sheather sugar

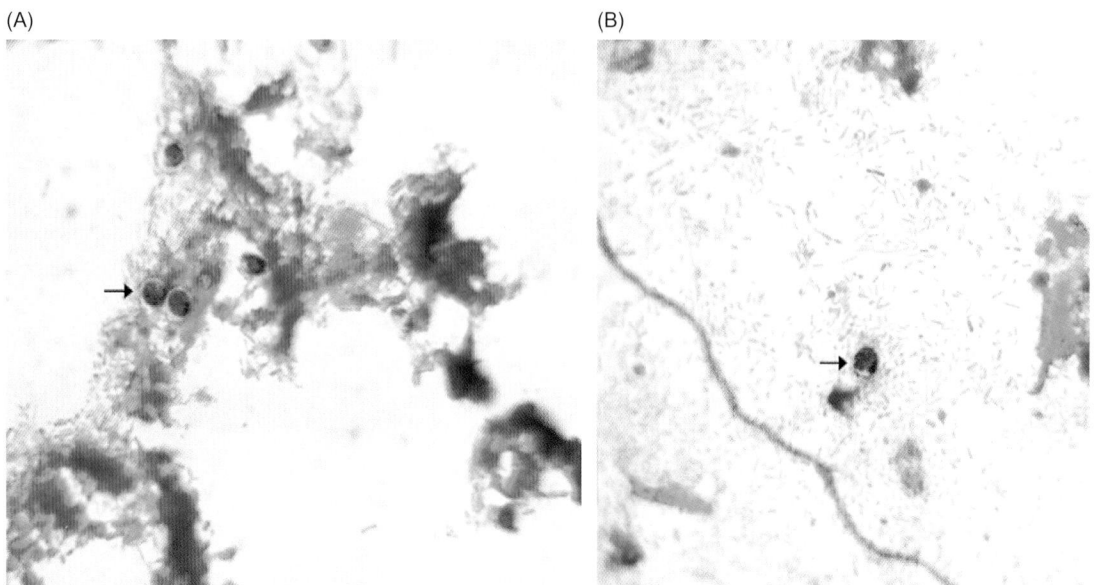

FIGURE 28.9 *Cryptosporidium* oocysts in calf (A) and human (B) feces stained with cold modified Ziehl–Neelsen staining method. *Source: Jafari et al., JRHS 2013; 13(1): 86–89.*

flotation or the formalin-ethyl acetate method. A modified acid-fast stain can be used to detect oocytes in fecal specimens or biopsies. Histologic evaluation of intestinal and rectal biopsies can also be used for diagnosis. Fecal antigen IFA and PCR tests have also been developed. Currently, no pharmaceutic agent is considered completely effective in treating cryptosporidiosis, but agents such as paramomycin and nitazoxanide may have some utility and are used in human treatment. The infection is considered to persist until the host's immune response clears the parasite, which may never occur in severely immunocompromised patients.

4. Giardiasis

Giardiasis is usually a mild intestinal illness, caused by the protozoan parasite *Giardia duodenalis* (syn. *G. lamblia*). The parasite can be found in the feces of infected animals (dogs, cats, beavers, and rodents).

Reservoir and Incidence   *Giardia* spp. are found worldwide among all classes of vertebrates and occur among numerous laboratory animals. Historical classification schemes have speciated *Giardia* based on host origin, since the recovered cysts are for the most part morphologically indistinguishable. However, based on experimental infections, it is known that cross-species transmission can occur. Considering the cosmopolitan distribution of the parasite in wild and domestic animals, the potential for zoonotic transmission appears significant. When infected beavers were identified in the watersheds associated with human waterborne outbreaks, this circumstantial evidence led to supposition that beavers were the cause (Dykes *et al.*, 1980; Keifer *et al.*, 1980) and resulted in the disease being referred to as 'beaver fever.' Experimental transmission studies showed that cysts from a beaver source can infect dogs as well as human volunteers (Davies *et al.*, 1979). However, further studies comparing the infectious dose of homologous and heterologous isolates determined that host-adapted strains are more readily transmitted, and the significantly higher innolum required for cross-species transmission in some cases is enough to lend some doubt to the likelihood of natural transmission (Erlandsen *et al.*, 1988). Wildlife giardiasis may be a reverse zoonosis whereby human contamination of the environment leads to animal infection (Thompson *et al.*, 2011). To paraphrase a veterinary school lecture comment by parasitologist Dr. W.J. Bemrick (attended by author GO), "Show me a stream where humans contracted giardiasis and I'll show you a stream contaminated by humans."

Nonhuman primates have also been implicated in human disease, and theoretically primate-to-man cross-transmission could be more likely due to the close genetic similarity. A clinically ill gibbon was presumed to be the source of infection for three zoo attendants and six apes that subsequently developed clinical giardiasis (Armstrong and Hertzog, 1979). Dogs (and puppies in particular) are often considerd sources of human infection, and a cross-sectional survey of laboratory animal workers resulted in self-reporting of giardiasis associated with canine exposure (Weigler *et al.*, 2005). Ruminants are another potential source of human contamination.

Advanced classification methods for *G. duodenalis* isolates based on genetic techniques have now established a classification consisting of various assemblages (genotypes) which has provided evidence that certain assemblages are more commonly associated with particular species (Feng *et al.*, 2011). The addition of genetic studies to future epidemiologic investigations may shed more light on the comparative risks of zoonotic transmission, but at this time the genetic studies suggest that zoonotic risks may be lower than previously thought (Yoder *et al.*, 2012).

Mode of Transmission   The life cycle of *Giardia* is direct, with trophozoites, the feeding stage of the organism, residing in the upper gastrointestinal tract. They multiply and develop into infective cysts that are shed in the feces and ingested by subsequent hosts (Fig. 28.10).

Clinical Signs   The disease in humans and animals is often similar. Giardiasis in humans is characterized by chronic or intermittent diarrhea, bloating, abdominal cramping, anorexia, fatigue, and weight loss. The stool

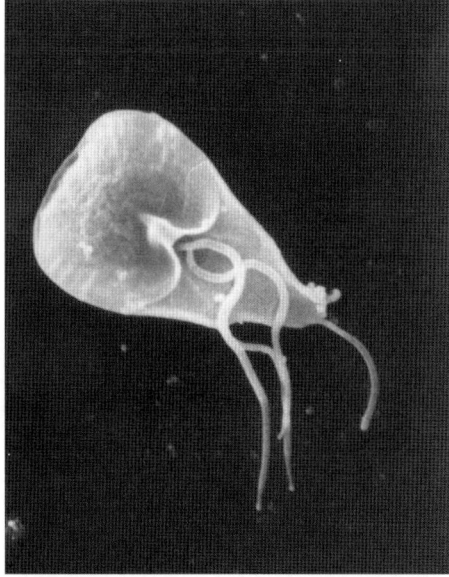

FIGURE 28.10 Scanning electron micrograph (SEM) revealing some of the external ultrastructural details displayed by a flagellated *Giardia lamblia* protozoan parasite. *G. lamblia* is the organism responsible for causing the diarrheal disease 'giardiasis.' Once an animal or person has been infected with this protozoan, the parasite lives in the intestine and is passed in the stool. Because the parasite is protected by an outer shell, it can survive outside the body and in the environment for long periods of time. *Source: PHIL 8698.*

frequently is mucus-laden, light-colored, and soft, but not watery. Symptoms may persist for several weeks and then resolve spontaneously. Fever is usually not present, and many persons infected with *Giardia* may have no symptoms at all. Individuals with the disease are contagious for the entire period of infection and may recover without treatment.

Prevention and Control Although many species of domesticated laboratory animals can be infected experimentally with *Giardia* pathogenic for humans, the majority have not been demonstrated to harbor human-related assemblages naturally. *Giardia* infections of non-human primates and wild-caught species may present a greater public health risk. Isolation and treatment of symptomatic shedders is certainly indicated, and personnel handling these animals should take appropriate safety measures. Metronidazole is commonly used for treatment, but quinacrine, furazolidone, and paromomycin are also used. The risk and benefit of attempted eradication when dealing with asympomatic carriers should be considered before initiating prophylactic treatment.

B. Systemic Infections

First discovered in 1908, toxoplasmosis is caused by infection with a microscopic parasite called *Toxoplasma gondii*. Toxoplasmosis has been found in humans and most warm-blooded animals. An estimated 500 million humans have been infected with the organism, and nearly one-third of all adult humans in the United States and in Europe have antibodies to toxoplasma, which provides evidence that they have been exposed to this parasite.

Reservoir and Incidence The life cycle of *T. gondii* consists of definitive and intermediate hosts. *Toxoplasma* infection has spread throughout the animal kingdom to include hundreds of species of mammals and birds as its intermediate hosts. Mice, rats, hamsters, guinea pigs and other rodents, rabbits, dogs, sheep, cattle, and nonhuman primates include some of the laboratory animals that could serve as intermediate hosts (Teutsch *et al.*, 1979; Wright, 1985). These laboratory animal hosts have not been shown to be important in zoonotic infection by *T. gondii* in the laboratory environment because the organism replicates only asexually in extraintestinal sites (Parker and Holliman, 1992; Herwaldt and Juranek, 1993). Serological surveys conducted in the United States have demonstrated *T. gondii* infection in 30–80% of cats with the highest prevalence in stray or outdoor cats (Ladiges *et al.*, 1982; Dubey *et al.*, 2002). Presumably, all serologically positive cats have shed *Toxoplasma* oocysts and could again shed organisms by reinfection or by reactivation.

Mode of Transmission Domestic and wild felids develop extraintestinal invasion with *T. gondii* analogous to that of the nonfelid hosts. In addition, as the definitive hosts in the *T. gondii* life cycle, felines develop intestinal infection, with the shedding of oocysts. Thus, the domestic cat is the primary reservoir for the zoonotic transmission of *T. gondii* in the laboratory environment. The three common modes of transmission are congenital infection, ingestion of *T. gondii*-infected tissue, and ingestion of toxoplasma oocytes or from direct exposure and consumption of contaminated food or water (Dubey, 1998). Most postnatally acquired infections in cats are asymptomatic and have a variable prepatent period and pattern of oocyst shedding. The prepatent period can be as brief as 3 days if the cat has ingested mice or meat containing *T. gondii* cysts, or it can be as long as several weeks if oocysts have been ingested. Shedding of oocysts in the feces occurs for 1–2 weeks, during which time cats are considered a public health risk (Dubey, 1998). Oocysts become infectious after sporulation, which occurs in 1–5 days. Oocysts survive best in warm, moist soil. Oocyst shedding is less likely to occur if the cat was infected by oocysts or tachyzoites than if infection resulted from the ingestion of *Toxoplasma* cysts. Oocyst shedding can be reactivated by induction of hypercorticism or by superinfection with other feline microorganisms, such as *Isospora felis* (Chessman, 1972). Oocysts of *T. gondii* have been observed infrequently in the feces of naturally infected cats (Ladiges *et al.*, 1982), and shedding usually precedes the development of antibody titers to *T. gondii*. The oocyst is very hardy and can survive freezing and as much as several months of extreme heat and dehydration. Importantly, high IgG titers do not prove recent or active infection (Dubey *et al.*, 1995).

Clinical Signs *Toxoplasma* infection in humans and animals is very common, but clinical disease occurs only sporadically and has a low incidence. In addition to sporadic clinical cases, occasional epidemics can occur when humans are exposed to oocyst-contaminated environments (Teutsch *et al.*, 1979). Populations at high risk of infection are pregnant women and immunodeficient individuals. Congenital infection in humans results in systemic disease, frequently with severe neuropathological changes. Postnatal infection results in disease that is less severe and commonly presents as nondescript, consisting of fever, myalgia, and generalized lymphadenopathy that may resolve without treatment in a few weeks. Asymptomatic infection may recrudesce with encephalitis if patients become immunocompromised. Although rare, serious systemic toxoplasmosis can be acquired by older individuals. This is manifested by fever, maculopapular eruption, malaise, myalgia, arthralgia, posterior cervical lymphadenopathy, pneumonia, myocarditis, and meningoencephalitis. Ocular toxoplasmosis, usually chorioretinitis, is commonly seen in postnatal infections but can also occur in infections of older individuals. Clinically severe and progressive illness is most likely to develop in immunocompromised individuals. As high as 10% of AIDS patients have toxoplasmosis (Gill and Stone, 1992). These patients develop neurologic disease and can experience convulsions, paralysis, or coma or even die from toxoplasmosis, even after treatment is administered. Infection in these cases is considered in most cases to be reactivation of tissue cysts from a chronic infection.

Diagnosis and Control Diagnosis can be made by histopathologic demonstration of the organisms, demonstration of serum antibody, testing for antigenemia, or skin test. Chemotherapeutic treatment is indicated in patients with diagnosed clinical disease, active ocular lesions, or congenital infection, and in immunocompromised individuals with disease suggestive of toxoplasmosis. The preferred therapy in humans is pyrimethamine administered in combination with a sulfa drug. Laboratory-acquired infections are likely restricted to the use and handling of laboratory cats (DiGiacomo *et al.*, 1990). Rigorous sanitation should effectively prevent human toxoplasmosis from occurring in the laboratory environment. Since oocysts must sporulate before they are infectious, daily cleaning of litter plans will prevent accumulation of infectious oocysts. Personnel should wear gloves when handling litter pans and wash their hands thoroughly before eating. Pregnant women should completely avoid contact with cat feces. Most cats acquire infection shortly after weaning and shed the oocysts for a short period of time (<3 weeks). Nevertheless, unsporulated oocysts are more susceptible to proper disinfection, and control of exposure should be centered around disinfection of litter pans at this stage.

VIII. HELMINTH INFECTIONS

Many of the helminth parasites common to animals and humans have an indirect life cycle that is interrupted in the laboratory environment, thus precluding cross-infection of animals and humans. Although numerous helminths of laboratory animals should be regarded as zoonotic (Soulsby, 1969; Flynn, 1973), the risk of human infection from laboratory-housed animals appears to be minimal. One exception may be the dwarf tapeworm of humans, *Hymenolepis* (*Rodentolepis*) *nana*, a common parasite of house mice and occasionally diagnosed in mice used for research. It is conservatively estimated that over 20 million people (mostly children) are infected with this parasite (Markell *et al.*, 1999). *H. (Rodentolepis) nana* is unique among cestodes in that the adult worm develops following ingestion of the egg by humans and does not require an intermediate host for its life cycle (Table 28.3).

Nematodes in aberrant hosts are a potential cause of visceral and ocular larval migrans. Ingested eggs of several nematode larvae may be shed in the feces and ingested by humans. These ingested eggs hatch in the abnormal host and migrate into deep tissues, but development proceeds no further. Larvae may persist in the visceral organs or the eyes and cause granulomatous lesions, resulting in hepatosplenomegaly, fever, and eosinophilia (visceral larval migrans) (Edelglass *et al.*, 1982; Davies *et al.*, 1993) or leucocoria, eye pain, strabismus, or loss of vision (ocular larval migrans) (Bathrick, 1981). The most frequent cause of these diseases is *Toxocara canis* (dog) (Wolfrom *et al.*, 1995) and *T. cati* (cat) (Glickman and Magnava, 1993), but *Baylisascaris procyonis* in the raccoon is much more aggressive and therefore more pathogenic (Fox *et al.*, 1988). Fatal or severe central nervous system disorders have been documented for mice, woodchucks, pigeons, domestic quail, turkeys, captive prairie dogs, and armadillos, and two human fatalities have been reported. Several other animal parasites have been associated with larval migrans-like syndromes. These include *Ascaris suum* (swine), *Capillaria hepatica* (rat), *Angiostrongylus cantonensis* (rat), *Gnathostoma spinigerum* (dogs and cats) (Bathrick, 1981), and *Angiostrongylus costaricensis* (cotton rats) (Levine, 1980). Human involvement has been reported with each of the above.

The practices encountered in a properly managed animal facility are not conducive to the transmission of these parasites. Proper quarantine, surveillance, and treatment procedures drastically reduce the endoparasitic burden of laboratory animals. Routine sanitation eliminates most parasitic ova before they have undergone the embryonation necessary for infectivity. Education of personnel on standard hygiene practices further reduces the likelihood of zoonotic infection.

Laboratory-housed nonhuman primates are presumed to be the most likely, although infrequent, source of parasitic infection for animal handlers (Orihel, 1970; Nasher, 1988). However, literature reports of captive primate-to-human transmission are restricted to exposures to pet animals, not laboratory primates.

IX. ARTHROPOD INFESTATIONS

Health hazards to humans due to ectoparasite infestations from arthropods associated with laboratory animals are most often mild and limited to manifestations of allergic dermatitis. However, arthropods can serve as vectors to systemic illnesses such as rickettsial pox, tularemia, and Lyme disease. Those working with laboratory animals, particularly those species arriving directly from their natural habitat, should be familiar with the arthropods capable of transmitting these diseases.

TABLE 28.3 Zoonotic Helminth Parasites in the Laboratory Environment

Disease	Etiology	Natural host(s)	Aberrant hosts	Comments
Cestodiasis	*Hymenolepis (Rodentolepsis) nana*	Rats, mice, hamsters, nonhuman primates	Humans	Intermediate host is not essential to the life cycle of this cestode. Direct infection and internal autoinfection can also occur. Heavy infections result in abdominal distress, enteritis, anal pruritis, anorexia, and headache.
Strongyloidiasis	*Strongyloides stercoralis, S. fulleborni*	Nonhuman primates, dogs, cats, humans, Old World nonhuman primates	Humans	Oral and transcutaneous infections can occur in animals and humans. Heavy infections can produce dermatitis, verminous pneumonitis, enteritis. Internal autoinfection can occur.
Ternidens infection	*Ternidens deminutus*	Old World primates	Humans	Rare and asymptomatic
Ancylostomiasis	*Ancylostoma duodenale*	Humans	Nonhuman primates, pigs	Oral and transcutaneous routes of infection occur. Heavy infections produce transient respiratory signs during larval migration followed by anemia due to gastrointestinal blood loss.
	Necator americanus	Humans	Nonhuman primates, pigs	
Trichostrongylosis	*Trichostrongylus colubriformis, T. axei*	Ruminants, pigs, dogs, rabbits, Old World nonhuman primates	Humans	Heavy infections produce diarrhea.
Oesophagostomiasis	*Oesophagostomum* spp.	Old World primates	Humans	Heavy infections result in anemia. Encapsulated parasitic granulomas are usually an inocuous sequella to infection.
Ascariasis	*Ascaris lumbricoides*	Old World primates	Humans	Infection occurs by ingestion of embryonated eggs only. Embryonation, requiring 2 or more weeks, ordinarily would not occur in laboratory. Heavy infections can produce severe respiratory and gastrointestinal tract disease.
Enterobiasis	*Enterobias vermicularis*	Humans	Old world primates	Oral and inhalational infection can occur. Disease in humans characterized by perianal pruritis, irritability, and disturbed sleep.
Trichuriasis	*Trichuris trichiura*	Humans	Old world primates	Three-week embryonation makes laboratory infection highly unlikely. Heavy infection in humans results in intermittent abdominal pain, bloody stools, diarrhea, and occasionally rectal prolapse.
Larval migrans (viscera)	*Toxocara canis*	Dogs and other canids	Humans	Chronic eosinophilic granulomatous lesions distributed throughout various organs. Should not be encountered in laboratory.
	T. cati	Cats and other felids	Humans	
	T. leonina	Dogs, cats, wild canids, felids	Humans	
	Baylisascaris procyonis	Raccoons	Humans and other animals	Infections in aberrant host produce granulomas in visceral organs with a predilection for the central nervous system.
Larval migrans (cutaneous)	*Ancylostoma caninum*	Dogs	Humans	Transcutaneous infection causes a parasitic dermatitis called 'creeping eruption'.
	A. braziliense	Dogs, cats	Humans	
	A. duodenale	Dogs, cats	Humans	
	Uncinarla stenocephala	Dogs, cats	Humans	
	N. americanus	Dogs, cats	Humans	

(A)

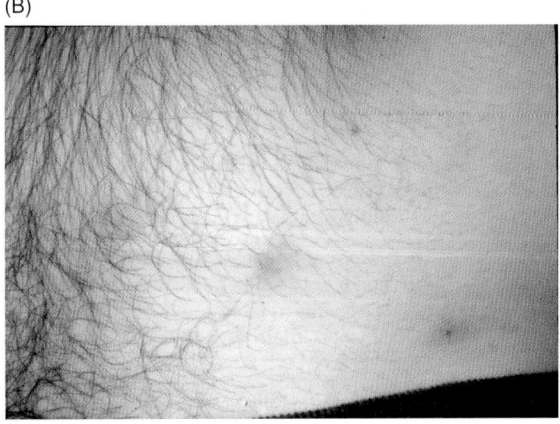

(B)

FIGURE 28.11 (A) Tropical rat mite (*Ornithonyssus bacoti*). (B) Tropical rat mite dermatitis. Note the three bites, referred to as 'breakfast, lunch, and dinner.' *Beck, 2009 Travel Medicine and Infectious Disease "Occurrence of a house-infesting Tropical rat mite (Ornithonyssus bacoti) on murides and human beings"; and Fox et al., 2009 Arch Derm.)*

Mites probably pose the greatest health hazard, not only because they are the most common inhabitants in number and variety of species, but because they also readily transmit agents from almost every major group of pathogens: bacteria, chlamydia, rickettsia, viruses, protozoa, spirochetes, and helminths (Yunker, 1964). In addition, most of these mites are capable of producing severe allergic papular dermatitis in humans (Fox and Reed, 1978; Fox, 1982b) (Fig. 28.11). Control of mite infestation is primarily dependent on their habitats. Some,

such as *Sarcoptes* spp. and *Notoedres* spp., are obligate parasites that require treatment of the host. Other mites, such as *Ornithonyssus bacoti*, which live most of the time off the animal, require treatment of the environment with appropriate insecticides (Markell *et al.*, 1999; Fox, 2009, Fox, 1982b).

Ticks, with the exception of those in newly arrived dogs or wild animals brought into the laboratory, are rarely found in the well-managed animal facility. The brown dog tick, *Rhipicephalus sanguineus*, is an exception. It readily infests kennels and vivaria. Ticks, like mites, can transmit a variety of diseases, including Rocky Mountain spotted fever, tick-borne typhus, Lyme disease, and others (Table 28.4). Lyme borreliosis is a commonly reported tick-borne infection in Europe and North America. The illness is caused by a spirochete, *Borrelia burgdorferi*, which is transmitted during the blood feeding of ticks of the genus *Ixodes*. The larvae and nymphs feed readily on a wide range of hosts, including birds, and an abundance of reservoir hosts exists, usually small and medium-sized animals. Larger animals, such as deer, sheep, cows, or horses, must be present for the maintenance of the tick population since adult ticks only engorge successfully on larger animals. Transmission occurs through salivation during the feeding process on a host. Control of ticks indoors is aimed primarily at the resting places of the unattached ticks and proper treatment of newly arrived animals, which are noted for harboring ticks.

Fleas are notorious for their ability to transmit disease to humans, particularly plague and murine typhus. Three rodent fleas, *X. cheopis*, *Nasopsyllus fasciatus*, and *Leptopsylla segnis*, have been found in a high percentage of urban dwellings in certain areas of the United States and are potential transmitters of disease in the laboratory. Apparently, *X. cheopis* in the past was readily established in animal facilities. At a Midwestern U.S. university, it inhabited rooms housing laboratory mice, where on two separate occasions fleas bit students (Yunker, 1964). *L. segnis*, the mouse and rat flea, bites humans and is a vector for plague and typhus, serious diseases in humans. *L. segnis* can also serve as an intermediate host for the rodent tapeworms *H. (Rodentolepsis) nana* and *H. diminuta*, both of which can infect humans (Markell *et al.*, 1999). The flea bite can be irritating and can cause allergic dermatitis. The cat flea, *Ctenocephalides felis*, is the most common flea in and around human dwellings in the United States. This flea is capable of experimentally transmitting plague and murine typhus, and therefore, the potential exists for transmitting the disease to humans. Control of fleas consists of treatment of infested areas as well as the primary host; in the case of rodent fleas, the animal facility must be free of feral rodents and their entry to prevent introduction of these arthropods.

TABLE 28.4   Ectoparasites[a,b]

Species	Disease in humans	Animal host	Agent
Mites			
Obligate skin mites			
Sarcoptes scabiei subspecies	Scabies	Mammals	
Notoedres cati	Mange	Cats, dogs, rabbits	
Nest-inhabiting parasites			
Ornithonyssus bacoti	Dermatitis, murine typhus	Rodents and other vertebrates, including birds	WEE,[c] ShE[d] virus Rickettsia mooseri
O. bursa	Dermatitis	Birds	WEE, EEE,[e] SLE viruses
O. sylviarum	Dermatitis, encephalitis	Birds	
Dermanyssus gallinae	Dermatitis, encephalitis	Birds	
Allodermanyssus sanguineus	Dermatitis, rikettsialpox	Rodents, particularly *Mus musculus*	*Rickettsia mooseri*
Ophionyssus natricis	Dermatitis	Reptiles	
Haemogamasus pontiger	Dermatitis	Rodents, insectivores, straw bedding	
H. casalis	Dermatitis	Birds, mammals, straw, hay	
Eulaelaps stabularis	Dermatitis, tularemia	Small mammals, straw bedding	*Francisella tularensis*
Glycyphagus cadaverum	Dermatitis, psittacosis	Birds	*C. psittaci*
Acaropsis docta	Dermatitis, psittacosis	Birds	*C. psittaci*
Trixacarus caviae	Dermatitis	Guinea pigs	
Facultative mites			
Cheyletiella spp.	Dermatitis	Cats, dogs, rabbits, bedding	
Dermatophagoides scheremtewskyi	Dermatitis, urinary infections, pulmonary acariasis	Feathers, animal feed, bird nests	
Eutrombicula spp.	Human pest (chiggers), local pruritis	Chickens, occasional mammals obtained from natural habitat	
Laelaps echidninus			Potential Argentine hemorrhagic fever
Ixodids (ticks)			
Rhipicephalus sanguineus	Irritation, RMSF,[f] tularemia, other diseases	Dogs	*Rickettsia rickettsii, Francisella tularensis*
Dermacentor variabilis	Irritation, RMSF,[f] tularemia tick paralysis, other diseases	Wild rodents, cottontail rabbits, dogs from endemic areas	See above
D. andersoni	Irritation, Colorado tick fever, Q fever, RMSF,[f] other diseases	Small mammals, uncommon on dogs	See above Ungrouped rhabdoviruses
D. occidentalis	Irritation, Colorado tick fever, RMSF,[f] tularemia	Small mammals, uncommon on dogs	See above
Ambylomma americanum	Irritation, RMSF,[f] tularemia	Wild rodents, dogs	
Ixodes scapularis	Irritation, possible tularemia	Dogs, wild rodents	
Ixodes spp.	Lyme disease	Dogs, cats, wild rodents	*Borrelia burgdonferi*
Omithodorus spp.	Irritation, relapsing fever	Captive reptiles, wild animals, pigs	*B. recurrentis*
Argas persicus	Irritation, seldom bites humans, but can transmit anthrax, Q fever	Domestic fowl	*B. recurrentis*

(Continued)

TABLE 28.4 (Continued)

Species	Disease in humans	Animal host	Agent
Fleas			
Ctenocephalides felis	Dermatitis, vector of *Hymenolepis diminuta*, *Dipylidium caninum*	Dogs, cats	
C. canis (cat and dog fleas)			
Xenopsylla cheopis	Dermatitis, plague vector, *Hymenolepis nana*, *H. diminuta*	Mouse, rat, wild rodents	*Yersinia pestis*
Nasopsyllus fasciatus	Dermatitis, plague vector,		
	Hymenolepis nana, *H. diminuta*, murine typhus	Mouse, rat, wild rodents	*Y. pestis*
Leptopsylla segnis	*Hymenolepis diminuta*, *H. nana*, murine typhus vector	Rat	Harbors salmonella
Echidnophaga gallinacea (sticktight flea)	Potential plague vector	Poultry	
Pulex irritans	Irritation	Domestic animals (especially pigs) and humans	

[a]Found in laboratory animals that cause allergic dermatitis or from which zoonotic agents have been recovered in nature.
[b]Modified from Fox et al. (1984).
[c]WEE, Western equine encephalitis.
[d]SLE, St. Louis encephalitis.
[e]EEE, Eastern equine encephalitis.
[f]RMSF, Rocky Mountain spotted fever.

Acknowledgments

The authors wish to acknowledge the work of the second edition authors, Christian E. Newcomer and Harry Rozmiarek, for the previous contributions to this chapter.

References

Abbott, Y., Acke, E., Khan, S., Muldoon, E.G., Markey, B.K., Pinilla, M., et al., 2010. Zoonotic transmission of Streptococcus equi subsp. zooepidemicus from a dog to a handler. J. Med. Microbiol. 59, 120–123.

Adams, W.H., Emmons, R.W., Brooks, J.E., 1970. The changing ecology of murine (endemic) typhus in southern California. Am. J. Trop. Med. Hyg. 19, 311–318.

Adams, J.R., Schmidtmann, E.T., Azad, A.F., 1990. Infection of colonized cat fleas, Ctenocephalides felis (Bouche), with a rickettsia-like microorganism. Am. J. Trop. Med. Hyg. 43, 400–409.

Adjemian, J., Weber, I.B., Mcquiston, J., Griffith, K.S., Mead, P.S., Nicholson, W., et al., 2012. Zoonotic infections among employees from Great Smoky Mountains and Rocky Mountain National Parks, 2008–2009. Vector Borne Zoonotic Dis. 12, 92–431.

Advisory Committee on Immunization Practices (ACIP), 2006. Prevention of hepatitis a through active or passive immunization: recommendations of the Advisory Committee on Immunization Practices (ACIP). MMWR 55, 1–23.

Advisory Committee on Immunization Practices (ACIP), 2007. Update: prevention of hepatitis a after exposure to hepatitis a virus and in international travelers. Updated recommendations of the Advisory Committee on Immunization Practices (ACIP). MMWR 56, 1080–1084.

Alexander, A.D., 1984. Leptospirosis in laboratory mice. Science 224, 1158.

Allos, B.M., Lastovica, A.J., Blaser, M.J., 1995. Atypical campylobacters and related microorganisms. In: Blaser, M.J., Smith, P.D., Ravdin, J.I., Greenberg, H.B., Guerrant, R.L. (Eds.), Infections of the Gastrointestinal Tract. Raven Press, New York, pp. 849–865.

Ambrus, J.L., Strandstrom, H.V., 1966. Susceptibility of Old World monkeys to Yaba virus. Nature 211, 876.

Ambrus, J.L., Strandstrom, H.V., Kawinski, W., 1969. "Spontaneous" occurrence of a Yaba tumor in a monkey colony. Experimentia 25, 64–65.

Anderson, A., Bijlmer, H., Fournier, P.E., Graves, S., Hartzell, J., Kersh, G.J., et al., 2013. Diagnosis and management of Q fever-United States, 2013: recommendations from CDC and the Q fever working group. MMWR Recomm. Rep. 62 (RR-03), 1–30.

Anderson, L.C., Leary, S.L., Manning, P.J., 1983. Rat-bite fever in animal research laboratory personnel. Lab. Anim. Sci. 33, 292.

Angus, K.N., 1983. Cryptosporidiosis in man, domestic animals, and birds: a review. J. R. Soc. Med. 76, 62–70.

Armstrong, J., Hertzog, R.E., 1979. Giardiasis in apes and zoo attendants, Kansas city, Missouri. Vet. Public Health Notes 1, 7–8.

Asher, M.S., 1989. Rickettsial diseases. In: Schmidt, N.J., Emmons, R.W. (Eds.), Diagnostic Procedures for Viral, Rickettsial, and Chlamydial Infections. American Public Health Association, Washington, DC, pp. 1141–1164.

Ayres, J.G., Flint, N., Smith, E.G., Tunnicliffe, W.S., Fletcher, T.J., Hammond, K., et al., 1998. Post-infection fatigue syndrome following Q fever. QJM 91, 105–123.

Babudieri, B., 1959. Q fever: a zoonosis. Adv. Vet. Sci. 5, 82–182.

Baele, M., Decostere, A., Vandamme, P., Ceelen, L., Hellemans, A., Mast, J., et al., 2008. Isolation and characterization of Helicobacter suis sp. nov. from pigs stomachs. Int. J. Syst. Evol. Microbiol. 58, 1350–1358.

Baiano, J.C., Barnes, A.C., 2009. Towards control of Streptococcus iniae. Emerg. Infect. Dis. 15, 1891–1896.

Baker, D.G., 1998. Natural pathogens of laboratory mice, rats, and rabbits and their effects on research. Clin. Microbiol. Rev. 11, 231–266.

Balayan, M.S., 1997. Epidemiology of hepatitis E virus infection. J. Viral Hepat. 4, 155–165.

Banyard, A., Fooks, A., 2011. Rabies and rabies-related lyssaviruses. In: Palmer, S.R., Soulsby, L., Torgerson, P., Brown, D. (Eds.), Oxford Textbook of Zoonoses: Biology, Clinical Practice, and Public Health Control Oxford University Press, New York, pp. 398–422.

Barkin, R.M., Guckian, J.C., Glosser, J.W., 1974. Infections by *Leptospira ballum:* a laboratory-associated case. South Med. J. 67, 155–176.

Barkley, W.E., Richardson, J.H., 1984. The control of biohazards associated with the use of experimental animals. In: Fox, J.G., Cohen, B.J., Loew, F.M. (Eds.), Laboratory Animal Medicine. Academic Press, Orlando, FL, pp. 595–602.

Bathrick, M.E., 1981. Intraocular gnathostomiasis. Ophthalmology 99, 1293–1295.

Bearcroft, W.G.C., Jamieson, M.F., 1958. An outbreak of subcutaneous tumors in rhesus monkeys. Nature 182, 195–196.

Beaver, P.C., Jung, R.C., 1985. Animal Agents and Vectors of Human Disease, fifth ed. Lea & Febiger, Philadelphia, PA.

Belser, J.A., Katz, J.M., Tumpey, T.M., 2011. The ferret as a model organism to study influenza a virus infection. Dis. Model. Mech. 4, 575–579.

Bengis, R.G., Leighton, F.A., Fischer, J.R., Artois, M., Mörner, T., Tate, C.M., 2004. The role of wildlife in emerging and re-emerging zoonoses. Rev. Sci. Tech. Int. Off. Epizoot. 23, 497–511.

Bennett, S.G., Comer, J.A., Smith, H.M., Webb, J.P., 2007. Serologic evidence of a Rickettsia akari-like infection among wild-caught rodents in Orange County and humans in Los Angeles County, California. J. Vec. Ecol. 32, 198–201.

Benson, P.M., Malane, S.L., Banks, R., Hicks, C.B., Hilliard, J., 1989. B virus (*Herpesvirus simiae*) and human infection. Arch. Dermatol. 125, 1247–1248.

Bernard, K.W., Parham, G.L., Winkler, W.G., Helmick, C.G., 1982. Q fever control measures: recommendations for research facilities using sheep. Infect. Control 3, 461–465.

Berridge, B.R., Fuller, J.D., de Azavedo, J.C., Low, D.E., Bercovier, H., Frelier, P.F., 1998. Development of specific nested oligonucleotide PCR primers for the *Streptococcus iniae* 16S-23S ribosomal DNA intergenic spacer. J. Clin. Microbiol. 36, 2778–2781.

Bert, F., Lambert-Zechovsky, N., 1997. Septicemia caused by *Streptococcus canis* in a human. J. Clin. Microbiol. 35, 777–779.

Besser, T.E., Gay, C.C., Gay, J.M., Hancock, D.D., Rice, D., Pritchett, L.C., et al., 1997. Salmonellosis associated with *S. typhimurium* DT104 in the USA [letter; comment]. Vet. Rec. 140, 73.

Bharti, A.R., Nally, J.E., Ricaldi, J.N., Mathhias, M.A., Diaz, M.M., Lovett, M.A., et al., 2003. Leptospirosis: a zoonotic disease of global importance. Lancet Infect. Dis. 3, 757–771.

Bhatt, P.N., Jacoby, R.O., Barthold, S.W., 1986. Contamination of transplantable murine tumors with lymphocytic choriomeningitis virus. Lab. Anim. Sci. 36, 136–139.

Bi, Z., Formenty, P.B.H., Roth, C.E., 2008. Hantavirus infection: a review and global update. J. Infect. Dev. Ctries. 2, 3–23.

Biggar, R.J., Woodall, J.P., Walter, P.D., Haughie, G.E., 1975. Lymphocytic choriomeningitis outbreak associated with pet hamsters. J. Am. Vet. Med. Assoc. 232, 494–500.

Blanchard, J.L., Russell-Lodrigue, K.E., 2012. Biosafety in laboratories using nonhuman primates. In: Abee, C.R., Mansfield, K., Tardif, S.D., Morris, T. (Eds.), Nonhuman Primates in Biomedical Research: Biology and Management. Elsevier, pp. 437–492.

Blaser, M.J., LaForce, F.M., Wilson, N.A., Wang, W.L.L., 1980. Reservoirs for human campylobacteriosis. J. Infect. Dis. 141, 665–669.

Bodetti, T.J., Jacobson, E., Wan, C., Hafner, L., Pospischil, A., Rose, K., et al., 2002. Molecular evidence to support the expansion of the hostrange of Chlamydophila pneumoniae to include reptiles

as well as humans, horses, koalas and amphibians. Syst. Appl. Microbiol. 25, 146–152.

Bond, R., 2010. Superficial veterinary mycoses. Clin. Dermatol. 28, 226–236.

Boneva, R.S., Grindon, A.J., Orton, S.L., Switzer, W.M., Shanmugam, V., Hussain, A.I., et al., 2002. Simian foamy virus infection in a blood donor. Transfusion 42, 886–891.

Bonthius, D.J., 2012. Lymphocytic choriomeningitis virus: an underrecognized cause of neurologic disease in the fetus, child, and adult. Semin. Pediatr. Neurol. 19, 89–95.

Boostrom, A., Beier, M.S., Macaluso, J.A., Macaluso, K.R., Sprenger, D., Hayes, J., et al., 2002. Geographic association of Rickettsia felis-infected opossums with human murine typhus, Texas. Emerg. Infect. Dis. 8, 549–554.

Bowen, G.S., Calisher, C.H., Winkler, W.G., Kraus, A.L., Fowler, E.H., Garmon, D.W., et al., 1975. Laboratory studies of lymphocytic choriomeningitis virus outbreak in man and laboratory animals. Am. J. Epidemiol. 102, 233–240.

Brooks, J.E., 1973. A review of commensal rodents and their control. Rev. Eviron. Control 3, 405–453.

Brown, C.M., Conti, L., Ettestad, P., Leslie, M.J., Sorhage, F.E., Sun, B., 2011. Compendium of animal rabies prevention and control. J. Am. Vet. Med. Assoc. 239, 609–617.

Burgos-Rodriguez, A.G., 2011. Zoonotic diseases of primates. Vet. Clin. North Am. Exot. Anim. Pract. 14, 557–575.

Burman, W.J., Cohn, D.L., Reves, R.R., Wilson, M.L., 1995. Multifocal cellulitis and monoarticular arthritis as manifestations of *H. cinaedi* bacteremia. Clin. Infect. Dis. 20, 564–570.

Carbone, M., Fera, M.T., Pennisi, M.G., Masucci, M., De Sarro, A., Macri, C., 1999. Activity of nine fluoroquinolones against strains of *Bordetella bronchiseptica*. Int. J. Antimicrob. Agents 12, 355–358.

Centers for Disease Control and Prevention (CDC), n.d.-a. Known Cases and Outbreaks of Ebola Hemorrhagic Fever, in Chronological Order [online]. Available at: <http://www.cdc.gov/ncidod/dvrd/spb/mnpages/dispages/ebola/ebolatable.htm>(accessed 08.09.13).

Centers for Disease Control and Prevention (CDC), n.d.-b. Known Cases and Outbreaks of Marburg Hemorrhagic Fever, in Chronological Order [online]. Available at: <http://www.cdc.gov/ncidod/dvrd/spb/mnpages/dispages/marburg/marburg-table.htm>(accessed 08.09.13.).

Centers for Disease Control and Prevention (CDC), n.d.-c. National Select Agent Registry, Select Agents and Toxins List [online] Available at: <http://www.selectagents.gov/Select%20Agents%20and%20Toxins%20List.html>(accessed 08.09.13).

Centers for Disease Control and Prevention (CDC), n.d.-f. Reported Cases of HPS – Hantavirus [online]. Available at: <http://www.cdc.gov/hantavirus/surveillance/index.html>(accessed 09.09.13).

Centers for Disease Control and Prevention (CDC), n.d.-g. Dog Bite: Fact Sheet [online]. Available at: <http://www.cdc.gov/homeandrecreationalsafety/dog-bites/dogbite-factsheet.html>(accessed 11.11.13).

Centers for Disease Control and Prevention (CDC), 1977. Rabies in a laboratory worker. MMWR 26, 183–184.

Centers for Disease Control and Prevention (CDC), 1987. Guidelines for the prevention of *Herpesvirus simiae* (B virus) infection in monkey handlers. MMWR 36, 680–689.

Centers for Disease Control and Prevention (CDC), 1989a. Epidemiologic notes and reports B virus infections in humans – Michigan. MMWR 38, 453–454.

Centers for Disease Control and Prevention (CDC), 1989b. Ebola virus infection in imported primates – Virginia. MMWR 38, 831–832.

Centers for Disease Control and Prevention (CDC), 1989c. Epidemiologic notes and reports B virus infections in humans – Michigan. MMWR 38, 453–454.

Centers for Disease Control and Prevention (CDC), 1990. Update: Ebola-related filovirus infection in nonhuman primates and interim guidelines for handling nonhuman primates during transit and quarantine. MMWR 39, 22–30.

Centers for Disease Control and Prevention (CDC), 1992a. Anonymous survey for simian immunodeficiency virus (SIV) seropositivity in SIV-laboratory researchers–United States. MMWR 41, 814–815.

Centers for Disease Control and Prevention (CDC), 1995. Outbreak of acute febrile illness and pulmonary hemorrhage – Nicaragua. MMWR 44, 841–843.

Centers for Disease Control and Prevention (CDCP), 1996. Invasive infection due to *Streptococcus iniae* – Ontario, 1995–1996. MMWR 45, 650–653.

Centers for Disease Control and Prevention (CDCP), 1997. Human monkeypox – Kasai Oriental, Democratic Republic of Congo, February 1996–October 1997. MMWR 46, 1168–1171.

Centers for Disease Control and Prevention (CDCP), 1998. Fatal *cercopithecine herpesvirus* 1 (B virus) infection following a mucocutaneous exposure and interim recommendations for worker protection. MMWR 47, 1073–1076.

Centers for Disease Control and Prevention (CDC), 2003. Update: multistate outbreak of monkeypox – Illinois, Indiana, Kansas, Missouri, Ohio, and Wisconsin, 2003. MMWR 52, 561–564.

Centers for Disease Control and Prevention (CDC), 2005. Fatal Rat-Bite Fever – Florida and Washington, 2003. MMWR 53, 1198–1202.

Centers for Disease Control and Prevention (CDC), 2008. Brief report: lymphocytic choriomeningitis virus transmitted through solid organ transplantation – Massachusetts, 2008. MMWR 57, 799–801.

Centers for Disease Control and Prevention (CDC), 2010a. Use of a reduced (4-dose) vaccine schedule for postexposure prophylaxis to prevent human rabies-recommendations of the advisory committee on immunization practice. Ann. Emerg. Med. 56, 64–67.

Centers for Disease Control and Prevention (CDC), 2010b. Multistate outbreak of human salmonella typhimurium infections associated with aquatic frogs – United States, 2009. MMWR 58, 1433–1436.

Centers for Disease Control and Prevention (CDC), 2011. Notes from the field: update on human salmonella typhimurium infections associated with aquatic frogs – United States, 2009–2011. MMWR 60, 628.

CDC. Human Orf virus infection from household exposures – United States, 2009–2011. MMWR Morb Mortal Wkly Rep. 2012 Apr 13;61(14):245–8.

Centers for Disease Control and Prevention (CDC), 2012a. Measles. In: Atkinson, W., Wolfe, C., Hamborsky, J. (Eds.), Epidemiology and Prevention of Vaccine – Preventable Diseases, twelfth ed. Public Health Foundation, Washington DC, pp. 173–192. second printing.

Centers for Disease Control and Prevention (CDC), 2012b. Notes from the field: lymphocytic choriomeningitis virus infections in employees of a rodent breeding facility – Indiana, May–June 2012. MMWR 61, 622–623.

Centers for Disease Control and Prevention (CDC), 2012c, Multistate Outbreak of Human *Salmonella Infantis* Infections Linked to Dry Dog Food (Final Update) [online]. Available at: <http://www.cdc.gov/salmonella/dog-food-05-12/>.

Centers for Disease Control and Prevention (CDC), 2013. Measles – United States, January 1–August 24, 2013. MMWR 62, 741–743.

Centers for Disease Control and Prevention–National Institutes of Health (CDCP–NIH), 2009. Biosafety in Microbiological and Biomedical Laboratories, fifth ed. U.S. Government Printing Office, Washington, DC, HHS Publ. (CDC) 21–1112.

Charrel, R.N., de Lamballerie, X., 2010. Zoonotic aspects of arenavirus infections. Vet. Microbiol. 140, 213–220.

Chen, Z., Telfier, P., Gettie, A., Reed, P., Zhang, L., Ho, D.D., et al., 1996. Genetic characterization of new West African simian immunodeficiency virus SIVsm: geographic clustering of household-derived SIV strains with human immunodeficiency virus type 2 subtypes and genetically diverse viruses from a single feral sooty mangabey troop. J. Virol. 70, 3617–3627.

Chessman, B.S., 1972. Reactivation of toxoplasm oocyst production in the cat by infection with *Isospora felis*. Br. Vet. J. 128, 33–36.

Childs, J.E., Colby, L., Krebs, J.W., Strine, T., Feller, M., Noah, D., et al., 1997. Surveillance and spatiotemporal associations of rabies in rodents and lagomorphs in the United States, 1985–1994. J. Wildl. Dis. 33, 20–27.

Chin, J. (Ed.), 2000. Control of communicable diseases manual: an official report of the American Public Health Association. American Public Health Association, Washington, DC.

Chiodini, R.J., Sundberg, J.P., 1981. Salmonellosis in reptiles: a review. Am. J. Epidemiol. 113, 494.

Chosewood, L.C., Wilson, D.E., 2009. Biosafety in Microbiological and Biomedical Laboratories. U.S. Department of Health and Human Services, Public Health Service, Centers for Disease Control and Prevention, National Institutes of Health, Washington, DC.

Cohen, J.I., Davenport, D.S., Stewart, J.A., Deitchman, S., Hilliard, J.K., Chapman, L.E., 2002. Recommendations for prevention of and therapy for exposure to B virus (*Cercopithecine Herpesvirus* 1). Clin. Infect. Dis. 35, 1191–1203.

Collins, J.M., Lorber, B., 2009. With man's best friend. In: Schlossberg, D. (Ed.), Infections of Leisure, fourth ed. ASM Press, Washington, DC, pp. 127–153.

Committee on Urban Pest Management, 1980. Urban Pest Management. National Academies Press, Washington, DC.

Cossaboom, C.M., Córdoba, L., Dryman, B.A., Meng, X.J., 2011. Hepatitis E virus in rabbits, Virginia, USA. Emerg. Infect. Dis. 17, 2047–2049.

Cossaboom, C.M., Córdoba, L., Sanford, B.J., Piñeyro, P., Kenney, S.P., Dryman, B.A., et al., 2012. Cross-species infection of pigs with a novel rabbit, but not rat, strain of hepatitis E virus isolated in the United States. J. Gen. Virol. 93, 1687–1695.

Cotton, M.M., Partridge, M.R., 1998. Infection with feline *Chlamydia psittaci*. Thorax 53, 75–76.

Craven, R.B., Barnes, A.M., 1991. Plague and tularemia in animal associated human infections. Infect. Dis. Clin. North Am. 1, 165–175.

Dalgard, D.W., Hardy, S.L., Pearson, G.J., Pucak, G.J., Quander, Z., Zack, P.M., et al., 1992. Combined simian hemorrhagic fever and Ebola virus infection in cynomolgus monkeys. Lab. Anim. Sci. 42, 152–159.

Damon, I.K., 2011. Status of human monkeypox: clinical disease, epidemiology and research. Vaccine 29 (Suppl. 4), D54–D59.

Davies, H.D., Sakuls, P., Keystone, J.S., 1993. Creeping eruption. A review of clinical presentation and management of 60 cases presenting to a tropical disease unit. Arch. Dermatol. 129, 588–591.

Davies, R.B., Hibler, C.P., 1979. Animal reservoirs and cross-species transmission of Giardia. In: Jakubowski, W., Hoff, J.C. (Eds.), Waterborne Transmission of Giardiasis. Environmental Protection Agency, Cincinnati, OH, pp. 104–126.

Demers, R.Y., Thiermann, A., Demers, P., Frank, R., 1983. Exposure to *Leptospira icterohaemorrhagiae* in inner-city and suburban children: a serologic comparison. J. Fam. Prac. 17, 1007–1011.

Deming, M.S., Tauxe, R.V., Blake, B.A., Dixon, S.E., Fowler, B.S., Jones, T.S., et al., 1987. *Campylobacter* enteritis at a university: transmission from eating chicken and from cats. Am. J. Epidemiol. 126, 526–534.

Dendle, C., Woolley, I.J., Korman, T.M., 2006. Rat-bite fever septic arthritis: illustrative case and literature review. Eur. J. Clin. Microbiol. Infect. Dis. 25, 791–797.

Dennis, D.T., Hughes, J.M., 1997. Multidrug resistance in plague. N. Engl. J. Med. 337, 702–704.

De Vleeschauwer, A., Atanasova, K., Van Borm, S., van den Berg, T., Rasmussen, T.B., Uttenthal, A., et al., 2009. Comparative pathogenesis of an avian H5N2 and a swine H1N1 influenza virus in pigs. PLoS One 4, e6662.

Dewhirst, F.E., Klein, E.A., Thompson, E.C., Blanton, J.M., Chen, T., Miella, L., et al., 2012. The canine oral microbiome. PLoS One 7, e36067.

Dienstag, J.L., Davenport, F.M., McCollum, R.W., Hennessy, A.V., Klatskin, G., Purcell, R.H., 1976. Nonhuman primate-associated viral hepatitis type A. Serologic evidence of hepatitis a virus infection. JAMA 236, 462–464.

DiGiacomo, R.F., Harris, N.V., Huber, N.L., Cooney, M.K., 1990. Animal exposures and antibodies to *Toxoplasma gondii* in a university population. Am. J. Epidemiol. 131, 729–733.

Division of Tuberculosis Elimination, 2000. Core Curriculum on Tuberculosis: What the Clinician Should Know, fourth ed. Centers for Disease Control and Prevention, Atlanta, GA.

Dolan, M.J., Wong, M.T., Regnery, R.L., Jorgensen, J.H., Garcia, M., Peters, J., et al., 1993. Syndrome of *Rochalimaea henselae* adenitis suggesting cat scratch disease. Ann. Intern. Med. 118, 331–336.

Dubey, J.P., 1998. Advances in the life cycle of *Toxoplasma gondii*. Int. J. Parasitol. 28, 1019–1024.

Dubey, J.P., Lappin, M.R., Thulliez, P., 1995. Long-term antibody responses of cats fed *Toxoplasma gondii* tissue cysts. J. Parasitol. 81, 887–893.

Dubey, J.P., Saville, W.J., Stanek, J.F., Reed, S.M., 2002. Prevalence of Toxoplasma gondii antibodies in domestic cats from rural Ohio. J. Parasitol. 88, 802–803.

Dupinay, T., Gheit, T., Roques, P., Cova, L., Chevallier-Queyron, P., Tasahsu, S.I., et al., 2013. Discovery of naturally occurring transmissible chronic hepatitis B virus infection among *Macaca fascicularis* from Mauritius Island. Hepatolology 58, 1610–1620.

Dupont, H.L., 2000. *Shigella* species (bacillary dysentery). In: Mandell, G.L., Bennett, J.E., Dolin, R. (Eds.), Practices and Principles in Infectious Diseases. Churchill Livingston, Philadelphia, PA, pp. 2363.

Dyer, J.L., Wallace, R., Orciari, L., Hightower, D., Yager, P., Blanton, J.D., 2013. Rabies surveillance in the United States during 2012. J. Am. Vet. Med. Assoc. 243, 805–815.

Dykes, A.C., Juranek, D.D., Lorenz, R.A., Sinclair, S., Jakubowski, W., Davies, R., 1980. Municipal waterborne giardiasis: an epidemiologic investigation. Beavers implicated as a possible reservoir. Ann. Intern. Med. 92, 165–170.

Dykewicz, C.A., Dato, V.M., Fisher-Hoch, S., Horwath, M.V., Perez-Oronoz, G., Ostroff, S.M., et al., 1992. Lymphocytic choriomeningitis outbreak associated with nude mice in a research institute. J. Am. Med. Assoc. 267, 1349–1353.

Edelglass, J.W., Douglass, M.C., Stiefler, R., Tessler, M., 1982. Cutaneous larva migrans in northern climates. A dream vacation. J. Am. Acad. Dermatol. 7, 353–358.

Engvall, E.O., Brandstrom, B., Andersson, L., Baverud, V., Trowald-Wigh, G., Englund, L., 2003. Isolation and identification of thermophilic *Campylobacter* species in faecal samples from Swedish dogs. Scand. J. Infect. Dis. 35, 713–718.

Eremeeva, M.E., Karpathy, S.E., Krueger, L., Hayes, E.K., Williams, A.M., Zaldivar, Y., et al., 2012. Two pathogens and one disease: detection and identification of flea-borne Rickettsiae in areas endemic for murine typhus in California. J. Med. Entomol. 49, 1485–1494.

Erlandsen, S.L., Sherlock, L.A., Januschka, M., Schupp, D.G., Schaefer III, F.W., Jakubowski, W., et al., 1988. Cross-species transmission of Giardia spp.: inoculation of beavers and muskrats with cysts of human, beaver, mouse, and muskrat origin. Appl. Environ. Microbiol. 54, 2777–2785.

Essbauer, S., Pfeffer, M., Meyer, H., 2010. Zoonotic poxviruses. Vet. Microbiol. 140, 229–236.

Estep, R.D., Messaoudi, I., Wong, S.W., 2010. Simian herpesviruses and their risk to humans. Vaccine 28 (Suppl. 2), B78–B84.

Everett, K.D., Bush, R.M., Andersen, A., 1999. Emended description of the order Chlamydiales, proposal of Parachlamydiaceae fam.

nov. and Simkaniaceae fam. nov. each containing one monotypic genus, revised taxonomy of the family Chlamydiaceae, including a new genus and five new species, and standards for the identification of the organisms. Int. J. Syst. Bacteriol. 49, 415–440.

Faine, S., 1991. Leptospirosis. In: Evans, A.S., Brachman, P.S. (Eds.), Bacterial Infections of Humans. Plenum Medical Book Co., New York, pp. 367–393.

Farhang-Azad, A., Traub, R., Baqar, S., 1985. Transovarial transmission of murine typhus, rickettsiae in *Xenopsylla cheopis* fleas. Science 227, 543–545.

Fayer, R., Ungar, B.L.P., 1986. *Cryptosporidium* spp. and cryptosporidiosis. Microbiol. Rev. 50, 458.

Feldmann, H., Geisbert, T.W., 2011. Ebola haemorrhagic fever. Lancet 377, 849–862.

Feng, Y., Xiao, L., 2011. Zoonotic potential and molecular epidemiology of Giardia species and giardiasis. Clin. Microbiol. Rev. 24, 110–140.

Fenner, F., 1990. Poxviruses of laboratory animals. Lab. Anim. Sci. 40, 469–480.

Fischer, S.A., Graham, M.B., Kuehnert, M.J., Kotton, C.N., Srinivasan, A., Marty, F.M., et al., 2006. Transmission of lymphocytic choriomeningitis virus by organ transplantation. N. Engl. J. Med. 354, 2235–2249.

Fitzpatrick, J.L., Dyer, J.L., Blanton, J.D., Kuzmin, I.V., Rupprecht, C.E., 2014. Rabies in rodents and lagomorphs in the United States, 1995–2010. JAVMA 245, 333–337.

Flowers, D.J., 1970. Human infection due to *Mycobacterium marinum* after a dolphin bite. J. Clin. Pediatr. 23, 475–477.

Flynn, R.J., 1973. Parasites of Laboratory Animals. Iowa State University Press, Ames, IA.

Forbes, L.B., Pantekoek, J.F., 1988. *Brucella canis* isolates from Canadian dogs. Can. Vet. J. 29, 149.

Fox, A.S., Kazacos, K.R., Gould, N.S., Heydemann, P.T., Thomas, C., Boyer, K.M., 1988. Fatal eosinophilic meningoencephalitis and visceral larva migrans caused by the raccoon ascarid *Baylisascaris procyonis*. N. Engl. J. Med. 312, 1619.

Fox, J.G., 1975. Transmissible drag resistance in *Shigella* and *Salmonella* isolated from pet monkeys and their owners. J. Med. Primatol. 4, 164.

Fox, J.G., 1982a. Campylobacteriosis – a "new" disease in laboratory animals. Lab. Anim. Sci. 32, 625.

Fox, J.G., 1982b. Outbreak of tropical rat mite dermatitis in laboratory personnel. Arch. Dermatol. 118, 676–678.

Fox, J.G., 2002. The non-*H. pylori* helicobacters: their expanding role in gastrointestinal and systemic diseases. Gut 50, 273–283.

Fox, J.G., 2009. With man's worst friend: the rat. In: Schlossberg, D. (Ed.), Infections of Leisure, fourth ed. ASM Press, Washington, DC, pp. 221–251.

Fox, J.G., 2011. *Campylobacter* infections. In: Greene, C.E. (Ed.), Infectious Diseases of the Dog and Cat, second ed. Elsevier-Saunders, St. Louis, MO, pp. 370–373.

Fox, J.G., Lipman, N.S., 1991. Infections transmitted from large and small laboratory animals. In: Weinberg, A., Weber, D. (Eds.), Infectious Diseases of North America. Saunders, Philadelphia, PA, pp. 131–163.

Fox, J.G., Marini, R.P., 2014. Biology and Diseases of the Ferret, third ed. Wiley-Blackwell, Ames, IA.

Fox, J.G., Megraud, F., 2007. Helicobacter. In: Murray, P.R., Baron, E.J., Jorgensen, J.H., Landry, M.L., Pfaller, M.A. (Eds.), Manual for Clinical Microbiology, ninth ed. ASM Press, Washington, DC, pp. 947–962.

Fox, J.G., Reed, C., 1978. Cheyletiella infestation of cats and their owners. Arch. Dermatol. 117, 1233–1234.

Fox, J.G., Taylor, N.S., Penner, J.L., Shames, B., Gurgis, R.V., Thomson, F.N., 1989b. Investigation of a zoonotically acquired *Campylobacter jejuni* enteritis with serotyping and restriction endonuclease DNA analysis. J. Clin. Microbiol. 27 (11), 2423–2425.

Fox, J.G., Perkins, S., Yan, L., Shen, Z., Attardo, L., Pappo, J., 1996. Local immune response in *Helicobacter pylori* infected cats and identification of *H. pylori* in saliva, gastric fluid, and feces. Immunology 88, 400–406.

Fox, J.G., Handt, L., Sheppard, B.J., Xu, S., Dewhirst, F.E., Motzel, S., et al., 2001. Isolation of Helicobacter cinaedi from the colon, liver and mesenteric lymph node of a rhesus monkey with chronic colitis and hepatitis. J. Clin. Microbiol. 39, 1580–1585.

Franz, D.R., Jahrling, P.B., Friedlander, A.M., McClain, D.J., Hoover, D.L., Bryne, W.R., et al., 1997. Clinical recognition and management of patients exposed to biological warfare agents. J. Am. Med. Assoc. 278, 399–411.

Freshwater, A., 2008. Why your housecat's trite little bite could cause you quite a fright: a study of domestic felines on the occurrence and antibiotic susceptibility of *Pasteurella multocida*. Zoonoses Public Health 55, 507–513.

Fulde, M., Valentin-Weigand, P., 2013. Epidemiology and pathogenicity of zoonotic streptococci. Curr. Top. Microbiol. Immunol. 368, 49–81.

Fuller, C., 2008. A multi-state *Salmonella* Typhimurium outbreak associated with frozen vacuum-packed rodents used to feed snakes. Zoonoses Public Health 55, 481–487.

Gao, F., Bailes, E., Robertson, D.L., Chen, Y., Rodenburg, C.M., Michael, S.F., et al., 1999. Origin of HIV-1 in the chimpanzee (*Pan troglodytes troglodytes*). Nature 397, 436–441.

Gardner, C.L., Ryman, K.D., 2010. Yellow fever: a reemerging threat. Clin. Lab. Med. 30, 237–260.

Gebhart, C.J., Fennell, C.L., Murtaugh, M.P., Stamm, W.E., 1989. *Campylobacter cinaedi* is normal intestinal flora in hamsters. J. Clin. Microbiol. 27, 1692–1694.

Geisbert, T.W., Hensley, L.E., Geisbert, J.B., Leung, A., Johnson, J.C., Grolla, A., et al., 2010. Postexposure treatment of Marburg virus infection. Emerg. Infect. Dis. 16, 1119–1122.

Geller, E.H., 1979. Health hazards for man. In: Baker, H.J., Lindsey, J.R., Weisbroth, S.H. (Eds.), The Laboratory Rat. Academic Press, New York, p. 402.

Gessain, A., Rua, R., Betsem, E., Turpin, J., Mahieux, R., 2013. HTLV-3/4 and simian foamy retroviruses in humans: discovery, epidemiology, cross-species transmission and molecular virology. Virology 435, 187–199.

Gibbons, R.V., 2002. Cryptogenic rabies, bats, and the question of aerosol transmission. Ann. Emerg. Med. 39, 528–536.

Gill, D.M., Stone, D.M., 1992. The veterinarian's role in the AIDS crisis. J. Am. Vet. Med. Assoc. 201, 1683–1684.

Glickman, L.T., Magnava, J.F., 1993. Zoonotic roundworm infections. Infect. Dis. Clin. North Am. 7, 717–732.

Goebel, S.J., Taylor, J., Barr, B.C., Kiehn, T.E., Castro-Malaspina, H.R., Hedvat, C.V., et al., 2007. Isolation of avian paramyxovirus 1 from a patient with a lethal case of pneumonia. J. Virol. 81, 12709–12714.

Goh, S.H., Driedger, D., Gillett, S., Low, D.E., Hemmingsen, S.M., Amos, M., et al., 1998. *Streptococcus iniae*, a human and animal pathogen: Specific identification by the chaperonin 60 gene identification method. J. Clin. Microbiol. 36, 2164–2166.

Goldstein, E.J.C., 1991. Household pets and human infections. Infect. Dis. Clin. North Am. 5, 117–130.

Goldstein, E.J.C., Greene, C.E., 2009. Around cats. In: Schlossberg, D. (Ed.), Infections of Leisure, fourth ed. ASM Press, Washington, DC, pp. 153–173.

Greene, C.E., Carmichael, L.E., 2011. Canine brucellosis. In: Greene, C.E. (Ed.), Infectious Diseases of the Dog and Cat. Elsevier-Saunders, St. Louis, MO, pp. 398–411.

Gruszynski, K., Young, A., Levine, S.J., Garvin, J.P., Brown, S., Turner, L., et al., 2015. Streptococcus equi subsp. zooepidemicus infections associated with guinea pigs. Emerg. Infect. Dis. 21 (January).

Guarner, J., Johnson, B.J., Paddock, C.D., Shieh, W.J., Goldsmith, C.S., Reynolds, M.G., et al., 2004. Monkeypox transmission and pathogenesis in prairie dogs. Emerg. Infect. Dis. 10, 426–431.

Haig, D.M., McInnes, C., Deane, D., Reid, H., Mercer, A., 1997. The immune and inflammatory response to orf virus. Comp. Immunol. Microbiol. Infect. Dis. 20, 197–204.

Handt, L.K., Fox, J.G., Dewhirst, F.E., Fraser, G.J., Paster, B.J., Yan, L., et al., 1994. *Helicobacter pylori* isolated from the domestic cat: public health implications. Infect. Immun. 62, 2367–2374.

Hanninen, M.L., Happonen, I., Saari, S., Jalava, K., 1996. Culture and characteristics of *Helicobacter bizzozeronii*, a new canine gastric *Helicobacter* sp. Int. J. Syst. Bacteriol. 46, 160–166.

Harder, T.C., Vahlenkamp, T.W., 2010. Influenza virus infections in dogs and cats. Vet. Immunol. Immunopathol. 134, 54–60.

Harker, K.S., Lane, C., De Pinna, E., Adak, G.K., 2011. An outbreak of Salmonella Typhimurium DT191a associated with reptile feeder mice. Epidemiol. Infect. 139, 1254–1261.

Hayami, M., Ido, E., Miura, T., 1994. Survey of simian immunodeficiency virus among nonhuman primate populations. Curr. Top. Microbiol. Immunol. 188, 1–20.

Heilmann, K.L., Borchard, F., 1991. Gastritis due to spiral shaped bacteria other than *Helicobacter pylori*: clinical, histological, and ultrastructural findings. Gut 32, 137–140.

Helms, M., Vastrup, P., Gerner-Smidt, P., Molbak, K., 2002. Excess mortality associated with antimicrobial drug-resistant *Salmonella* Typhimurium. Emerg. Infect. Dis. 8, 490–495.

Hemachudha, T., Ugolini, G., Wacharapluesadee, S., Sungkarat, W., Shuangshoti, S., Laothamatas, J., 2013. Human rabies: neuropathogenesis, diagnosis, and management. Lancet Neurol. 12, 498–513.

Heneine, W., Switzer, W.M., Sandstrom, P., Brown, J., Vedapuri, S., Schable, C.A., et al., 1998. Identification of a human population infected with simian foamy viruses. Nat. Med. 4, 391–392, 644–645.

Herwaldt, B.L., Juranek, D.D., 1993. Laboratory acquired malaria, leishmaniasis, trypanosomiasis, and toxoplasmosis. Am. J. Trop. Med. Hyg. 48, 313–323.

Heymann, D.L. (Ed.), 2008. Control of Communicable Diseases. Manual American Public Health Association, Washington, DC.

Hinman, A.R., Fraser, D.W., Douglas, R.D., Bowen, G.S., Krause, A.L., Winkler, W.G., et al., 1975. Outbreaks of lymphocytic choriomeningitis infection in medical center personnel. Am. J. Epidemiol. 101, 103–110.

Hinthorn, D.R., Foster Jr., M.T., Bruce, H.L., Aach, R.D., 1974. An outbreak of chimpanzee associated hepatitis. J. Occup. Med. 16, 388–391.

Hironaga, M., Fujigaki, T., Watanabe, S., 1981. Trichophyton mentagrophytes skin infections in laboratory animals as a cause of zoonosis. Mycopathologia 73, 101–104.

Hjelle, B., Torrez-Martinez, N., Koster, F.T., Jay, M., Ascher, M.S., Brown, T., et al., 1996. Epidemiologic linkage of rodent and human hantavirus genomic sequences in case investigation of hantavirus pulmonary syndrome. J. Infect. Dis. 173, 781–786.

Ho, A.C., Rapuan, C.J., 1993. *Pasteurella multocida* keratitis and corneal laceration from a cat scratch. Ophthalmic. Surg. 24, 346–348.

Hombal, S.M., Dincsoy, H.P., 1992. *Pasteurella multocida* endocarditis. Am. J. Clin. Pathol. 98, 565–568.

Hosamani, M., Scagliarini, A., Bhanuprakash, V., McInnes, C.J., Singh, R.K., 2009. Orf: an update on current research and future perspectives. Expert Rev. Anti. Infect. Ther. 7, 879–893.

Huang, F., Wang, H., Jing, S., Zeng, W., 2012. Simian foamy virus prevalence in *Macaca mulatta* and Zookeepers. AIDS Res. Hum. Retroviruses 28, 591–593.

Huang, F.F., Haqshenas, G., Guenette, D.K., Halbur, P.G., Schommer, S.K., Pierson, F.W., et al., 2002. Detection by reverse transcription-PCR and genetic characterization of field isolates of swine hepatitis E virus from pigs in different geographic regions of the United States. J. Clin. Microbiol. 40, 1326–1332.

Huff, J.L., Barry, P.A., 2003. B-virus (*Cercopithecine herpesvirus* 1) infection in humans and macaques: potential for zoonotic disease. Emerg. Infect. Dis. 9, 246–250.

Hull, T.G., 1955. Diseases Transmitted from Animals to Man, fourth ed. Thomas, Springfield, IL.

Hyde, S.R., Benirschke, K., 1997. Gestational psittacosis: case report and literature review. Mod. Pathol. 10, 602–607.

Ikeda, J.S., Hirsch, D.C., Jang, S.S., Biberstein, E.L., 1986. Characteristics of *Salmonella* isolated from animals at a veterinary medical teaching hospital. Am. J. Vet. Res. 47, 232–235.

Institute of Laboratory Animal Resources (ILAR), Committee on Occupational Safety and Health in Research Animal Facilities, 1997. Occupational Health and Safety in the Care and use of Research Animals. National Academies Press, Washington, DC.

Jaax, N.K., Davis, K.J., Geisbert, T.J., Vogel, P., Jaax, G.P., Topper, M., et al., 1996. Lethal experimental infection of rhesus monkeys with Ebola-Zaire (Mayinga) virus by the oral and conjunctival route of exposure. Arch. Pathol. Lab. Med. 120, 140–155.

Jackson, L.A., Perkins, B.A., Wenger, J.D., 1993. Cat scratch disease in the United States: an analysis of three national databases. Am. J. Public Health 83, 1707–1711.

Jahrling, P.B., Peters, D.J., 1992. Lymphocytic choriomeningitis virus, a neglected pathogen of man. Arch. Pathol. Lab. Med. 116, 486–488.

Jay, M., Hjelle, B., Davis, R., Ascher, M., Baylies, H.N., Reilly, K., et al., 1996. Occupational exposure leading to hantavirus pulmonary syndrome. Clin. Infect. Dis. 22, 841–844.

Jones, B.A., Grace, D., Kock, R., Alonso, S., Rushton, J., Said, M.Y., et al., 2013. Zoonosis emergence linked to agricultural intensification and environmental change. Proc. Natl. Acad. Sci. USA 110, 8399–8404.

Jones, J.W., Pether, J.V.S., Rainey, H.A., Swinburn, C.R., 1993. Recurrent *Mycobacterium bovis* infection following a ferret bite [letter]. J. Infect. 26, 225–226.

Jorgesen, D.M., 1997. Gestational psittacosis in a Montana sheep rancher. Emerg. Infect. Dis. 3, 191–194.

Kalish, M.L., Wolfe, N.D., Ndongmo, C.B., McNicholl, J., Robbins, K.E., Aidoo, M., et al., 2005. Central African hunters exposed to simian immunodeficiency virus. Emerg. Infect. Dis. 11, 1928–1930.

Kalter, S.S., Milstein, C.H., Bocyk, L.H., Cummins, L.B., 1978. Tuberculosis in nonhuman primates as a threat to humans. Dev. Biol. Stand. 41, 85–91.

Kalter, S.S., Heberling, R.L., Cooke, A.W., Barry, J.D., Tian, P.Y., Northam, W.J., 1997. Viral infections of nonhuman primates. Lab. Anim. Sci. 47, 461–467.

Kalthoff, D., Globig, A., Beer, M., 2010. (Highly pathogenic) avian influenza as a zoonotic agent. Vet. Microbiol. 140, 237–245.

Karp, B.E., Ball, N.E., Scott, C.R., Walcoff, J.B., 1999. Rabies in two privately owned domestic rabbits. J. Am. Vet. Med. Assoc. 215, 1824–1827.

Katz, D., Shi, W., Patrusheva, I., Perelygina, L., Gowda, M.S., Krug, P.W., et al., 2012. An automated ELISA using recombinant antigens for serologic diagnosis of B Virus infections in macaques. Comp. Med. 62, 527–534.

Kaufman, A.F., Boyce, J.M., Martone, W.J., 1980. Trends in human plague in the United States. J. Infect. Dis. 141, 522.

Kawamata, J., Yamanouchi, T., Dohmae, K., Miyamoto, H., Takahaski, M., Yamanishi, K., et al., 1987. Control of laboratory acquired hemorrhagic fever with renal syndrome (HFRS) in Japan. Lab. Anim. Sci. 37, 431–436.

Keifer, A., Lynch, G., Conwill, D., 1980. Water-borne giardiasis–California, Colorado, Pennsylvania, Oregon. MMWR 29, 121–123.

Kelt, D.A., Van Vuren, D.H., Hafner, M.S., Danielson, B.J., Kelly, M.J., 2007. Threat of hantavirus pulmonary syndrome to field biologists working with small mammals. Emerg. Infect. Dis. 13, 1285–1287.

Kemper, C.A., Lombard, C.M., Deresinki, S.C., Tompkins, L.S., 1990. Visceral bacillary epithelioid angiomatosis: possible manifestations of disseminated cat scratch disease in the immunocompromised host: a report of two cases. Am. J. Med. 89, 216–222.

Khabbaz, R.R., Heneine, W.M., George, J.R., Parekh, B.S., Rowe, T., Woods, T., et al., 1994. Brief report: infection of a laboratory worker with simian immunodeficiency virus. N. Engl. J. Med. 330, 172–177.

Khan, A.S., 2009. Simian foamy virus infection in humans: prevalence and management. Expert Rev. Anti. Infect. Ther. 7, 569–580.

Khan, A.S., Kumar, D., 2006. Simian foamy virus infection by whole-blood transfer in rhesus macaques: potential for transfusion transmission in humans. Transfusion 46, 1352–1359.

Kiehlbauch, J.A., Tauxe, R.V., Baker, C.N., Wachsmuth, I.K., 1994. *Helicobacter cinaedi-associated* bacteremia and cellulitis in immunocompromised patients. Ann. Intern. Med. 121, 90–93.

Kiehlbauch, J.A., Brenner, D.J., Cameron, D.N., Steigerwalt, A.G., Makowski, J.M., Baker, C.N., et al., 1995. Genotypic and phenotypic characterization of *H. cinaedi* and *H. fennelliae* strains isolated from humans and animals. J. Clin. Microbiol. 22, 2940–2947.

Kimura, R., Hayashi, Y., Takeuchi, T., 2004. *Pasteurella multocida* septicemia caused by close contact with a domestic cat: case report and literature review. J. Infect. Chemother. 10, 250–252.

Koehler, J.E., Glaser, C.A., Tappero, J.W., 1994. *Rochalimaea henselae* infection: new zoonosis with the domestic cat as reservoir. J. Am. Med. Assoc. 271, 531–535.

Kopecny, L., Bosward, K.L., Shapiro, A., Norris, J.M., 2013. Investigating *Coxiella burnetii* infection in a breeding cattery at the centre of a Q fever outbreak. J. Feline Med. Surg. 15, 1037–1045.

Kornegay, R.W., Giddens Jr., W.E., Van Hoosier Jr., J.L., Morton, W.R., 1985. Subacute nonsuppurative hepatitis associated with hepatitis B virus infection in two cynomolgus monkeys. Lab. Anim. Sci. 35, 400–404.

Kraemer, A., Hein, J., Heusinger, A., Mueller, R.S., 2013. Clinical signs, therapy and zoonotic risk of pet guinea pigs with dermatophytosis. Mycoses 56, 168–172.

Kristensen, K.H., Lautrop, H., 1962. A family epidemic caused by the whooping cough bacillus *Bordetella bronchiseptica* (Danish). Ugeskr. Laeger 124, 303–308.

Krug, P.W., Schinazi, R.F., Hilliard, J.K., 2010. Inhibition of B Virus (*Macacine herpesvirus* 1) by conventional and experimental antiviral compounds. Antimicrob. Agents Chemother. 54, 452–459.

Krusell A, Comer JA and Sexton DJ. Rickettsialpox in North Carolina: A Case Report. Emerg Infect Dis. [serial on the Internet]. 2002 Jul. Available from: <http://wwwnc.cdc.gov/eid/article/8/7/01-0501>.

Ksiazek, T.G., West, C.P., Rollin, P.E., Jahrling, P.B., Peters, C.J., 1999. ELISA for the detection of antibodies to Ebola viruses. J. Infect. Dis. 179, S192–S198.

Kuo, C.-C., Stephens, R., 2010. Phylum XXIV. Chlamydiae Garrity and Holt 2001. In: Krieg, N., Staley, J., Brown, D. (Eds.), Bergey's Manual® of Systematic Bacteriology. Springer, New York, pp. 843–877.

Kupper, J.L., Casey, H.W., Johnson, D.K., 1970. Experimental Yaba and benign epidermal monkeypox in rhesus monkeys. Lab. Anim. Care 20, 979–988.

Ladiges, W.C., DiGiacomo, R.F., Yamaguchi, R.A., 1982. Prevalence of *Toxoplasma gondii* antibodies and oocytes in pound source cats. J. Am. Vet. Med. Assoc. 180, 1334–1335.

Langley, J.M., Marrie, T.H., Covert, A., 1988. Poker player's pneumonia: an urban outbreak of Q fever following exposure to a parturient cat. N. Engl. J. Med. 319, 354–356.

Animal handlersLangley, R.L. (Ed.), 1999. Occupational Medicine: State of the Art Reviews. Hanley and Belfus, Philadelphia, PA.

Lavelle, J.P., Landas, S., Mitros, F.A., Conklin, J.L., 1994. Acute gastritis associated with spiral organisms from cats. Dig. Dis. Sci. 39, 744–750.

LeBoit, P.E., Berger, T.G., Egbert, B.M., Yen, T.S.B., Stoler, M.H., Bonfiglio, T.A., et al., 1988. Epithelioid haemangioma-like vascular proliferations in AIDS: manifestation of cat scratch disease bacillus infection? Lancet 1, 960–963.

LeDuc, J.W., 1987. Epidemiology of Hantaan and related viruses. Lab. Anim. Sci. 37, 413.

Lee, H.W., Johnson, K.M., 1982. Laboratory acquired infections with Hantaan virus, the etiologic agent of Korean hemorrhagic fever. J. Infect. Dis. 146, 645–651.

Leitman, T., Brooks, D., Moncada, J., Schachter, J., Dawson, D., Dean, D., 1998. Chronic follicular conjunctivitis associated with *Chlamydia psittaci* or *Chlamydia pneumoniae*. Clin. Infect. Dis. 26, 1335–1340.

Lemon, S.M., Binn, K.N., Marchwicki, R., Murphy, P.C., Ping, L.H., Jansen, R.W., et al., 1990. *In vivo* replication and reversal to wild type of a neutralization resistant antigenic variant of hepatitis a virus. J. Infect. Dis. 161, 7–13.

Leroy, E.M., Kumulungui, B., Pourrut, X., Rouquet, P., Hassanin, A., Yaba, P., et al., 2005. Fruit bats as reservoirs of Ebola virus. Nature 438, 575–576.

Levett, P.N., 2001. Leptospirosis. Clin. Microbiol. Rev. 14, 296–326.

Levine, J.E., Levy, M.G., Walker, R.L., Crittenden, S., 1988. Cryptosporidiosis in veterinary students. J. Am. Vet. Med. Assoc. 193, 1413–1414.

Levine, N.D., 1980. Nematode Parasites of Domestic Animals and of Man. Burgess Publishing Co., Minneapolis, MN.

Lhomme, S., Dubois, M., Abravanel, F., Top, S., Bertagnoli, S., Guerin, J.L., et al., 2013. Risk of zoonotic transmission of HEV from rabbits. J. Clin. Virol. 58, 357–362.

Ligon, B.L., 2004. Monkeypox: a review of the history and emergence in the Western hemisphere. Semin. Pediatr. Infect. Dis. 15, 280–287.

Lipman, N.S., 1996. Rat bite fevers. In: Schlossberg, D. (Ed.), Current Therapy of Infectious Disease. Mosby-Yearbook, Philadelphia, PA, pp. 451–455.

Lloyd, G., 2011. Marburg and Ebola viruses. In: Palmer, S.R., Soulsby, L., Torgerson, P.R., Brown, W.G.B. (Eds.), Oxford Textbook of Zoonoses: Biology, Clinical Practice, and Public Health Control. Oxford University Press, New York, pp. 353–368.

Locatelli, S., Peeters, M., 2012. Cross-species transmission of simian retroviruses: how and why they could lead to the emergence of new diseases in the human population. AIDS 26, 659–673.

Lorenz, H.J., Cornelie, J., Willems, H., Baljer, G., 1998. PCR detection of *Coxiella burnetii* from different clinical specimens, especially bovine milk, on the basis of DNA preparation with silica matrix. Appl. Environ. Microbiol. 64, 4234–4237.

Lucero, N.E., Corazza, R., Almuzara, M.N., Reynes, E., Escobar, G.I., Boeri, E., et al., 2010. Human *Brucella canis* outbreak linked to infection in dogs. Epidemiol. Infect. 138, 280–285.

Luzzi, G.A., Milne, L.W., Waitkins, S.A., 1987. Rat-bite acquired leptospirosis. J. Infect. 15, 57–60.

MacDonald, D.M., Holmes, E.C., Lewis, J.C., Simmonds, P., 2000. Detection of hepatitis B virus infection in wild-born chimpanzees (*Pan troglodytes verus*): phylogenetic relationships with human and other primate genotypes. J. Virol. 74, 4253–4257.

Maclachlan, N.J., Dubovi, E.J., Fenner, F., 2011a. Bunyaviridae Fenner's Veterinary Virology. Elsevier Academic Press, Boston, MA, pp. 371–384.

Maclachlan, N.J., Dubovi, E.J., Fenner, F., 2011b. Arenaviridae Fenner's Veterinary Virology. Elsevier Academic Press, Boston, MA, pp. 385–392.

Maclachlan, N.J., Dubovi, E.J., Fenner, F., 2011c. Other Viruses: Hepeviruses, Hepadnaviridae, Deltaviruses, Anelloviruses, and Unclassified Viruses Fenner's Veterinary Virology. Elsevier Academic Press, Boston, MA, pp. 483–488.

Maclachlan, N.J., Dubovi, E.J., Fenner, F., 2011d. Paramyxoviridae Fenner's Veterinary Virology. Elsevier Academic Press, Boston, MA, pp. 299–324.

Macneil, A., Ströher, U., Farnon, E., Campbell, S., Cannon, D., Paddock, C.D., et al., 2012. Solid organ transplant-associated lymphocytic choriomeningitis, United States, 2011. Emerg. Infect. Dis. 18, 1256–1262.

Macy, D.W., 1999. Plague. In: Greene, C.E. (Ed.), Infectious Diseases of the Dog and Cat, second ed. Saunders, Philadelphia, PA.

Maetz, H.M., Sellers, C.A., Bailey, W.C., Hardy Jr., G.E., 1976. Lymphocytic choriomeningitis from pet hamster exposure: a local public health experience. Am. J. Public Health 66, 1082–1085.

Mak, P.W.Y., Jayawardena, S., Poon, L.L.M., 2012. The evolving threat of influenza viruses of animal origin and the challenges in developing appropriate diagnostics. Clin. Chem. 58, 1527–1533.

Margileth, A.W., Wear, D.J., Hadfield, T.L., Schlagel, C.J., Spigel, G.T., Muhlbauer, J.E., 1984. Cat-scratch disease. Bacteria in skin at the primary inoculation site. JAMA 252, 928–931.

Marini, R.P., Adkins, J.A., Fox, J.G., 1989. Proven or potential zoonotic diseases of ferrets. J. Am. Vet. Med. Assoc. 195, 990.

Markell, E.K., John, D.T., Krotoski, W.A., 1999. Medical Parasitology, eighth ed. Saunders, Philadelphia, PA.

Marrie, T.J., 1990. Epidemiology of Q fever. In: Marrie, T.J. (Ed.), Q Fever: The Disease. CRC Press, Boca Raton, FL, pp. 49–70.

Marrie, T.J., Williams, J.C., Schlech, W.F., Yates, L., 1986. Q fever pneumonia associated with exposure to wild rabbits. Lancet 1, 427–429.

Marsden-Haug, N., Bidol, S.A., Culpepper, W., Behravesh, C.B., Morris, J., Anderson, T.A., 2013. Multistate outbreak of human *Salmonella* typhimurium infections linked to contact with pet hedgehogs – United States, 2011–2013. MMWR 61, 73.

Martin, L.J., Fyfe, M., Doré, K., 2004. Increased burden of illness associated with antimicrobial-resistant *Salmonella enterica* serotype Typhimurium infections. J. Infect. Dis. 189, 377–384.

Mazurek, G.H., Jereb, J., Vernon, A., LoBue, P., Goldberg, S., Castro, K., 2010. Updated guidelines for using interferon gamma release assays to detect mycobacterium tuberculosis infection – United States, 2010. MMWR Recomm. Rep. 59, 1–25.

McEvoy, M.B., Noah, N.D., Pilsworth, R., 1987. Outbreak of fever caused by *Streptobacillus moniliformis*. Lancet 2, 1361–1363.

Mehedi, M., Groseth, A., Feldmann, H., Ebihara, H., 2011. Clinical aspects of Marburg hemorrhagic fever. Future Virol. 6, 1091–1106.

Meng, X.J., 2005. Hepatitis E virus: cross-species infection and zoonotic risk. Clin. Microbiol. Newsl. 27, 43–48.

Meng, X.J., 2010a. Recent advances in hepatitis E virus. J. Viral Hepat. 17, 153–161.

Meng, X.J., 2010b. Hepatitis E virus: animal reservoirs and zoonotic risk. Vet. Microbiol. 140, 256–265.

Meng, X.J., 2011. From barnyard to food table: the omnipresence of hepatitis E virus and risk for zoonotic infection and food safety. Virus Res. 161, 23–30.

Meng, X.J., Purcell, R.H., Halbur, P.G., Lehman, J.R., Webb, D.M., Tsareva, T.S., et al., 1997. A novel virus in swine is closely related to the human hepatitis E virus. Proc. Natl. Acad. Sci. USA 94, 9860–9865.

Mercer, A., Fleming, S., Robinson, A., Nettleton, P., Reid, H., 1997. Molecular genetic analyses of parapoxviruses pathogenic for humans. Arch. Virol. Suppl. 13, 25–34.

Metzkor-Cotter, E., Kletter, Y., Avidor, B., Varon, M., Golan, Y., Ephros, M., et al., 2003. Long-term serological analysis and clinical follow-up of patients with cat scratch disease. Clin. Infect. Dis. 37, 1149–1154.

Miranda, M.E., Ksiazek, T.G., Retuya, T.J., Khan, A.S., Sanchez, A., Fulhorst, C.F., et al., 1999. Epidemiology of Ebola (subtype Reston) in the Philippines, 1996. J. Infect. Dis. 179, S115–S119.

Molba, K., Baggesen, D.L., Aarestrup, F.M., Ebbesen, J.M., Engberg, J., Frydendahl, K., et al., 1999. An outbreak of multidrug-resistant, quinolone-resistant *Salmonella enterica* serotype *typhimurium* DT104. N. Engl. J. Med. 341, 1420–1425.

Monath, T.P., Staples, J.E., 2011. Yellow fever. In: Palmer, S.R., Soulsby, L., Torgerson, P., Brown, D. (Eds.), Oxford Textbook of Zoonoses: Biology, Clinical Practice, and Public Health Control. Oxford University Press, New York, pp. 443–453.

Monis, P.T., Thompson, R.C., 2003. Cryptosporidium and Giardia-zoonoses: fact or fiction? Infect. Genet. Evol. 3, 233–244.

Montali, R.J., Ramsay, E.C., Stephensen, C.B., Worley, M., Davis, J.A., Holmes, K.V., 1989. A new transmissible viral hepatitis of marmosets and tamarins. J. Infect. Dis. 160, 759–765.

Montali, R.J., Scanga, C.A., Pernikoff, D., Wessner, D.R., Ward, R., Holmes, K.V., 1993. A common-source outbreak of callitrichid hepatitis in captive tamarins and marmosets. J. Infect. Dis. 167, 946–950.

Montali, R.J., Connolly, B.M., Armstrong, D.L., Scanga, C.A., Holmes, K.V., 1995. Pathology and immunohistochemistry of callitrichid hepatitis, an emerging disease of captive New World primates caused by lymphocytic choriomeningitis virus. Am. J. Pathol. 147, 1441–1449.

Morita, C., Tsuchiya, K., Ueno, H., Muramatsu, Y., Kojimahara, A., Suzuki, H., et al., 1996. Seroepidemiological survey of lymphocytic choriomeningitis virus in wild house mice in China with particular reference to their subspecies. Microbiol. Immunol. 40, 313–315.

Murphy, H.W., Miller, M., Ramer, J., Travis, D., Barbiers, R., Wolfe, N.D., et al., 2006. Implications of simian retroviruses for captive primate population management and the occupational safety of primate handlers. J. Zoo Wildl. Med. 37, 219–233.

Murray, S.M., Linial, M.L., 2006. Foamy virus infection in primates. J. Med. Primatol. 35, 225–235.

Mushatt, D.M., Hyslop, N.E., 1991. Neurologic aspects of North American zoonoses. Infect. Dis. North Am. 5, 703–731.

Myers, E.M., Ward, S.L., Myers, J.P., 2012. Life-threatening respiratory pasteurellosis associated with palliative pet care. Clin. Infect. Dis. 54, e55–e57.

Nasher, A.K., 1988. Zoonotic parasitic infections of the Arabian sacred baboon *Papio hamadryas arabicus*, Thomas in Asir Province, Saudi Arabia. Ann. Parasitol. Hum. Comp. 63, 448–454.

National Research Council, 1997. Occupational Health and Safety in the Care and Use of Research Animals. National Academies Press, Washington, DC, p. 154.

Nelson, J.D., Kusmiesz, H., Jackson, L.H., Woodman, E., 1980. Treatment of *Salmonella* gastroenteritis with ampicillin, amoxicillin, and placebo. Pediatrics 65, 1125–1130.

Newcomer, C.E., Anver, M.R., Simmons, J.L., Wilcke, B.W., Nace, G.W., 1982. Spontaneous and experimental infections of *Xenopus laevis* with *Chlamydia psittaci*. Lab. Anim. Sci. 32, 680–686.

Newcomer, C.E., Fox, J.G., 2007. Zoonoses and other human health hazards. In: Fox, J.G., Barthold, S., Davisson, M., Newcomer, C.E., Quimby, F.W., Smith, A. (Eds.), The Mouse in Biomedical Research: Diseases. Elsevier, Boston, MA, pp. 719–745.

Ng, V.L., Boggs, J.M., York, M.K., Golden, J.A., Hollander, H., Hadley, W.K., 1992. Recovery of *Bordetella bronchiseptica* from patients with AIDS. Clin. Infect. Dis. 15, 376–377.

Ng-Hublin, J.S., Combs, B., Mackenzie, B., Ryan, U., 2013. Human cryptosporidiosis diagnosed in Western Australia: a mixed infection with *Cryptosporidium meleagridis*, the *Cryptosporidium* mink genotype, and an unknown *Cryptosporidium* species. J. Clin. Microbiol. 51, 2463–2465.

Nicklas, W., Kraft, V., Meyer, B., 1993. Contamination of transplantable tumors, cell lines, and monoclonal antibodies with rodent viruses. Lab. Anim. Sci. 43, 296–300.

Niven, S.J.F., 1961. Subcutaneous "growths" in monkeys with Yaba pox virus. J. Pathol. Bacteriol. 81, 1–14.

Oehler, R.L., Velez, A.P., Mizrachi, M., Lamarche, J., Gompf, S., 2009. Bite-related and septic syndromes caused by cats and dogs. Lancet Infect. Dis. 9, 439–447.

Ordog, G.J., 1985. Rat bites: fifty cases. Ann. Emerg. Med. 14, 126.

Orihel, T.C., 1970. The helminth parasites of nonhuman primates and man. Lab. Anim. Care 20, 395–401.

Orlicek, S.L., Welch, D.F., Kuhls, T.L., 1993. Septicemia and meningitis caused by *Helicobacter cinaedi* in a neonate. J. Clin. Microbiol. 31, 569–571.

Paegle, R.D., Tweari, R.P., Bernhard, W.N., Peters, E., 1976. Microbial flora of the larynx, trachea, and large intestine of the rat after long-term inhalation of 100 percent oxygen. Anesthesiology 44, 287–290.

Palmer, A.E., 1987. *Herpesvirus simiae:* historical perspective. J. Med. Primatol. 16, 99–130.

Parker, S., Holliman, R.E., 1992. Toxoplasmosis and laboratory workers: a case control assessment of risk. Med. Lab. Sci. 49, 103–106.

Parker, S., Nuara, A., Buller, R.M.L., Schultz, D.A., 2007. Human monkeypox: an emerging zoonotic disease. Future Microbiol. 2, 17–34.

Pavia, A.T., Tauxe, R.V., 1991. Salmonellosis: nontyphoidal. In: Evans, A.S., Brachman, P.S. (Eds.), Bacterial Infections of Humans. Epidemiology and Control, second ed. Plenum Press, New York, pp. 573–592.

Pavio, N., Meng, X.J., Renou, C., 2010. Zoonotic hepatitis E: animal reservoirs and emerging risks. Vet. Res. 41, 46.

Perez-Osorio, C.E., Zavala-Velazquez, J.E., Arias Leon, J.J., Zavala-Castro, J.E., 2008. *Rickettsia felis* as emergent global threat for humans. Emerg. Infect. Dis. 14, 1019–1023.

Pier, G.B., Madin, S.H., 1976. *Streptococcus iniae* sp. nov., a beta-hemolytic streptoccus isolated from an Amazon freshwater dolphin, *Inia geoffrensis*. Int. J. Syst. Bacteriol. 26, 545–553.

Polt, S.S., Dismukes, W.E., Flint, A., Schaefer, J., 1982. Human brucellosis caused by *Brucella canis*: clinical features and immune response. Ann. Intern. Med. 97, 717–719.

Prag, J., Blom, J., Krogfelt, K.A., 2007. *Helicobacter canis* bacteraemia in a 7-month old child. FEMS Immun. Med. Microbiol. 50, 264–267.

Ravdin, J.L., 1995. Amebiasis. Clin. Infect. Dis. 20, 1453–1466.

Ravdin, J.I., 2000. Entamoeba histolytica. In: Mandell, G.L., Bennett, J.E., Dolin, R. (Eds.), Principles and Practice of Infectious Diseases. Churchill Livingstone, Philadelphia, PA, pp. 2798–2810.

Reese, N.C., Current, W.L., Ernst, J.V., Barley, W.S., 1982. Cryptosporidiosis of man and calf: a case report and results of experimental infections in mice and rats. Am. J. Trop. Med. Hyg. 31, 226–229.

Reid, H.W., Dagleish, M.P., 2011. Poxviruses. In: Palmer, S.R., Soulsby, L., Torgerson, P., Brown, D. (Eds.), Oxford Textbook of Zoonoses: Biology, Clinical Practice, and Public Health Control. Oxford University Press, New York, pp. 380–385.

Reimer, L.G., 1993. Q fever. Clin. Microbiol. Rev. 6, 193–198.

Rempe, B., Aloi, M., Iskyan, K., 2009. Evidence-based management of mammalian bite wouds. Pediatr. Emerg. Med. Pract. 6, 1–22.

Reynolds, M.G., Krebs, J.S., Comer, J.A., Sumner, J.W., Rushton, T.C., Lopez, C.E., et al., 2003. Flying squirrel-associated typhus, United States. Emerg. Infect. Dis. 9, 1341–1343.

Reynolds, M.G., Carroll, D.S., Karem, K.L., 2012. Factors affecting the likelihood of monkeypox's emergence and spread in the post-smallpox era. Curr. Opin. Virol. 2, 335–343.

Richter, C.P., Lehner, N.D.M., Henrickson, R.V., 1984. Primates. In: Fox, J.G., Cohen, B.J., Loew, F.M. (Eds.), Laboratory Animal Medicine. Academic Press, Orlando, FL, p. 298.

Rivera, W.L., Yason, J.A., Adao, D.E., 2010. Entamoeba histolytica and *E. dispar* infections in captive macaques (*Macaca fascicularis*) in the Philippines. Primates 51, 69–74.

Roberts, J.A., Lerche, N.W., Markowits, J.E., Maul, D.H., 1988. Epizootic measles at the CRPRC. Lab. Anim. Sci. 38, 492.

Roest, H.I., van Solt, C.B., Tilburg, J.J., Klaassen, C.H., Hovius, E.K., Roest, F.T., et al., 2013. Search for possible additional reservoirs for human Q fever, The Netherlands. Emerg. Infect. Dis. 19, 834–835.

Rosner, W.W., 1987. Bubonic plague. J. Am. Med. Assoc. 191, 406–409.

Roulis, E., Polkinghorne, A., Timms, P., 2013. *Chlamydia pneumoniae*: modern insights into an ancient pathogen. Trends Microbiol. 21, 120–128.

Rousseau, M.C., Saron, M.F., Brouqui, P., Boureade, A., 1997. Lymphocytic choriomeningitis in France: four case reports and a review of the literature. Eur. J. Epidemiol. 13, 817–823.

Rupp, M.E., 1992. *Streptobacillus moniliformis* endocarditis: case report and review. Clin. Infect. Dis. 14, 769–772.

Russell, R.G., Sarmiento, J.I., Fox, J.G., Panigrahi, P., 1990. Evidence of reinfection with multiple strains of *C. jejuni* and *C. coli* in *Macaca nemestrina* housed under hyperendemic conditions. Infect. Immun. 58, 2149.

Ryabchikova, E.I., Kolesnikova, L.V., Luchko, S.V., 1999. An analysis of features of pathogenesis in two animal models of Ebola virus infection. J. Infect. Dis. 179, S199–S202.

Sacks, J.J., Sinclair, L., Gilchrist, J., Lockwood, R., 2000. Breeds of dogs involved in fatal human attacks in the United States between 1979 and 1998. J. Am. Vet. Med. Assoc. 217, 836–840.

Sanger, J.G., Thiermann, A.B., 1988. Leptospirosis. J. Am. Vet. Med. Assoc. 193, 1250–1254.

Schafer, I.L., Miller, R., Strother, U., Knust, B., Nichol, S.T., Rollin, P.E., 2014. Notes from the field: a cluster of lymphocytic choriomeningitis virus infections transmitted through organ transplantation. MMWR 63, 249.

Schmaljohn, C., Hjelle, B., 1997. Hantaviruses: a global disease problem. Emerg. Infect. Dis. 3, 95–104.

Schou, S., Hansen, A.K., 2000. Marburg and Ebola virus infections in laboratory non-human primates: a literature review. Comp. Med. 50, 108–123.

Schweizer, M., Falcone, V., Gange, J., Turek, R., Neumann-Haefelin, D., 1997. Simian foamy virus isolated from an accidentally infected human individual. J. Virol. 71, 4821–4824.

Sejvar, J.J., Chowdary, Y., Schomogyi, M., Stevens, J., Patel, J., Karem, K., et al., 2004. Human monkeypox infection: a family cluster in the midwestern United States. J. Infect. Dis. 190, 1833–1840.

Sens, M.A., Brown, E.W., Wilson, L.R., Crocker, T.P., 1989. Fatal *Streptobacillus moniliformis* infection in a two month old infant. Am. J. Clin. Pathol. 91, 612–616.

Serikawa, T., Iwaki, S., Mori, M., Muraguchi, T., Yamada, J., 1989. Purification of *Brucella canis* cell wall antigen using immunosorbent columns and use of the antigen in enzyme-linked immunosorbent assay for specific diagnosis of canine brucellosis. J. Clin. Microbiol. 27, 837–842.

Shen, Z., Feng, Y., Fox, J.G., 1999. Co-infection with enteric *Helicobacter* spp. and *Campylobacter* spp. in cats. J. Clin. Micro. 39, 2166–2172.

Shevtsova, Z.V., Lapin, B.A., Doroshenko, N.V., Krilova, R.L., Korzaja, L.I., Lomovskaya, I.B., et al., 1988. Spontaneous and experimental hepatitis A in Old World monkeys. J. Med. Primatol. 17, 177–194.

Simmons, J.H., 2010. Herpesvirus infections of laboratory macaques. J. Immunotoxicol. 7, 102–113.

Smith, A.L., Singleton, G.R., Hansen, G.M., Shellam, G., 1993. A serologic survey for viruses and *Mycoplasma pulmonis* among wild house mice (*Mus domesticus*) in southeastern Australia. J. Wildl. Dis. 29, 219–229.

Smith, A.L., Black, D.H., Eberle, R., 1998. Molecular evidence for distinct genotypes of monkey B virus (*Herpesvirus simiae*) which are related to the macaque host species. J. Virol. 72, 9224–9232.

Smith, T.F., 1989. Chlamydia. In: Schmidt, N.J., Emmons, R.W. (Eds.), Diagnostic Procedures for Viral, Rickettsial and Chlamydial Infections. American Public Health Association, Washington, DC, pp. 1335–1340.

Smythe, L.D., Smith, I.L., Smith, G.A., Dohnt, M.F., Symonds, M.L., Barnett, L.J., et al., 2002. A quantitative PCR (TaqMan) assay for pathogenic *Leptospira* spp. BMC Infect. Dis. 2, 13–19.

Soulsby, E.J.L., 1969. Helminths, Arthropods, and Protozoa of Domesticated Animals, sixth ed. Williams & Wilkins, Baltimore, MD.

Spilker, T., Liwienski, A.A., LiPuma, J.J., 2008. Identification of *Bordetella* spp. in respiratory specimens from individuals with cystic fibrosis. Clin. Microbiol. Infect. 14, 504–506.

Staat, M.A., Kruszon-Moran, D., McQuillan, G.M., Kaslow, R.A., 1996. A population-based serologic survey of *Helicobacter pylori* infection in children and adolescents in the United States. J. Infect. Dis. 174, 1120–1123.

Stephensen, C.B., Blount, S.R., Lanford, R.E., Holmes, K.V., Montali, R.J., Fleenor, M.E., et al., 1992. Prevalence of serum antibodies against lymphocytic choriomeningitis virus in selected populations from two U.S. cities. J. Med. Virol. 38, 27–31.

Stephensen, C.B., Park, J.Y., Blount, S.R., 1995. cDNA sequence analysis confirms that the etiologic agent of callitrichid hepatitis is lymphocytic choriomeningitis virus. J. Virol. 69, 1349–1352.

Stoenner, H.G., Maclean, D., 1958. Leptospirosis (ballum) contracted from Swiss albino mice. Arch. Intern. Med. 101, 706–710.

Stolte, M., Wellens, E., Bethke, B., Ritter, M., Eidt, H., 1994. *Helicobacter heilmannii* (formerly *Gastrospirillum hominis*) gastritis: an infection transmitted by animals? Scand. J. Gastroenterol. 29, 1061–1064.

Storz, J., 1971. Chlamydia and Chlamydia-Induced Diseases. Thomas, Springfield, IL.

Swanson, S., Snider, C., Braden, R., 2007. Multidrug-resistant *Salmonella enterica* serotype Typhimurium associated with pet rodents. NEJM 356, 21–28.

Swayne, D.E., King, D.J., 2003. Avian influenza and Newcastle disease. J. Am. Vet. Med. Assoc. 222, 1534–1540.

Swennes, A.G., Fox, J.G., 2014. Bacterial and Mycoplasmal Diseases. In: Fox, J.G., Marini, R.P. (Eds.), Biology and Diseases of the Ferret. Wiley-Blackwell, Ames, IA.

Switzer, W.M., Bhullar, V., Shanmugam, V., Cong, M.E., Parekh, B., Lerche, N.W., et al., 2004. Frequent simian foamy virus infection in persons occupationally exposed to nonhuman primates. J. Virol. 78, 2780–2789.

Tachibana, H., Yanagi, T., Akatsuka, A., Kobayashi, S., Kanbara, H., Tsutsumi, V., 2009. Isolation and characterization of a potentially virulent species *Entamoeba nuttalli* from captive Japanese macaques. Parasitology 136, 1169–1177.

Takeda, N., Kikuchi, K., Asano, R., Harada, T., Totsuka, K., Sumiyoshi, T., et al., 2001. Recurrent septicemia caused by *Streptococcus canis* after a dog bite. Scand. J. Infect. Dis. 33, 927–928.

Talan, D.A., Citron, D.M., Abrahamian, F.M., Moran, G.R., Goldstein, E.J.C., 1999. Bacteriologic analysis of infected dog and cat bites. N. Engl. J. Med. 340, 85–92.

Tauxe, R.V., 1999. *Salmonella enteritidis* and *Salmonella typhimurium* DT104: successful subtypes in the modern world. In: Scheld, W.M., Craig, W.A., Hughes, J.M. (Eds.), Emerging Infections 3. ASM Press, Washington, DC, pp. 37–52.

Taylor, J.P., Istre, G.R., McChesney, T.C., Satalowich, F.T., Parker, R.L., McFarland, L.M., 1991. Epidemiologic characteristics of human tularemia in the southwest-central states, 1981–1987. Am. J. Epidemiol. 133, 1032–1038.

Teare, J.A., Loomis, M.R., 1982. Epizootic of balantidiasis in lowland gorillas. J. Am. Vet. Med. Assoc. 181, 1345–1347.

Tenkate, T.D., Stafford, R.J., 2001. Risk factors for *Campylobacter* infections in infants and young children: a matched case-control study. Epidem. Infect. 127, 399–404.

Teutsch, S.M., Juranek, D.D., Sulzer, A., Dubey, J.P., Sikes, R.K., 1979. Epidemic toxoplasmosis associated with infected cats. N. Engl. J. Med. 300, 695–699.

Thi, E.P., Mire, C.E., Ursic-Bedoya, R., Geisbert, J.B., Lee, A.C.H., Agans, K.N., et al., 2014. Marburg virus infection in nonhuman primates: therapeutic treatment by lipid-encapsulated siRNA. Sci. Transl. Med. 6, 250ra116.

Thiermann, A.B., 1977. Incidence of leptospirosis in the Detroit rat population. Am. J. Trop. Med. Hyg. 26, 970–974.

Thomas, N., Brook, I., 2011. Animal bite-associated infections: microbiology and treatment. Expert Rev. Anti. Infect. Ther. 9, 215–226.

Thompson, R.C., Smith, A., 2011. Zoonotic enteric protozoa. Vet. Parasitol. 182, 70–78.

Tissot-Dupont, H., Torres, S., Nezri, M., Raoult, D., 1999. Hyperendemic focus of Q fever related to sheep and wind. Am. J. Epidemiol. 150, 67–74.

To, H., Sakai, R., Shirota, K., Kano, C., Abe, S., Sugimoto, T., et al., 1998. Coxiellosis in domestic and wild birds from Japan. J. Wildl. Dis. 34, 310–316.

Torres-Perez, F., Wilson, L., Collinge, S.K., Harmon, H., Ray, C., Medina, R.A., et al., 2010. Sin Nombre virus infection in field workers, Colorado, USA. Emerg. Infect. Dis. 16, 308–310.

Torten, M., 1979. Leptospirosis. In: Steele, J.H. (Ed.), CRC Handbook Series in Zoonoses, 1. CRC Press, Cleveland, OH, pp. 363–421.

Towner, J.S., Pourrut, X., Albariño, C.G., Nkogue, C.N., Bird, B.H., Grard, G., et al., 2007. Marburg virus infection detected in a common African bat. PLoS One 2, e764.

Tsai, T.F., 1987. Hemorrhagic fever with renal syndrome: mode of transmission to humans. Lab. Anim. Sci. 37, 428.

Tsai, T.F., Bauer, S.P., Sasso, D.R., Whitfield, S.G., McCormick, J.B., Caraway, T.C., et al., 1985. Serological and virological evidence of a hantaan virus-related enzootic in the United States. J. Infect. Dis. 152, 126–136.

Turk, M.L., Cacioppo, L.D., Ge, Z., Shen, Z., Whary, M.T., Parry, N., et al., 2012. Persistent *Helicobacter pullorum* colonization in C57BL/6NTac mice: a new mouse model for an emerging zoonosis. J. Med. Microbiol. 61, 720–728.

van der Waaij, D., 1968. The persistent absence of Enterobacteriaceae from the intestinal flora of mice following antibiotic treatment. J. Infect. Dis. 118, 32–38.

van der Waaij, D., Berghuis-de Vries, J., Lekkerkerk-van der Wees, J., 1971. Colonization resistance of the digestive tract in conventional and antibiotic-treated mice. J. Hyg. (Lond.) 69, 405–411.

Varma, J.K., Molbak, K., Barrett, T.J., Beebe, J.L., Jones, T.F., Rabatsky-Ehr, T., et al., 2005. Antimicrobial-resistant nontyphoidal *Salmonella* is associated with excess bloodstream infections and hospitalizations. J. Infect. Dis. 191, 554–561.

Vinetz, J.M., 2003. A mountain out of a molehill: do we treat acute leptospirosis, and if so, with what? Clin. Infect. Dis. 36, 1514–1515.

Visvesvar, G.S., Stehr-Green, J.K., 1990. Epidemiology of free-living amoebae infections. J. Protozool. 37, 25S–33S.

Vitral, C.L., Yoshida, C.F., Gaspar, A.M., 1998. The use of non-human primates as animal models for the study of hepatitis viruses. Braz. J. Med. Biol. Res. 31, 1035–1048.

Wachtman, L., Mansfield, K., 2012. Viral diseases of nonhuman primates. In: Abee, C.R., Mansfield, K., Tardif, S.D., Morris, T. (Eds.), Nonhuman Primates in Biomedical Research: Biology and Management. Elsevier, pp. 1–104.

Wear, D.J., Margileth, A.M., Hadfield, T.L., Fischer, G.W., Schlagel, C.J., King, F.M., 1983. Cat stratch disease: a bacterial infection. Science 221, 1403–1405.

Weber, D.J., Hansen, A.R., 1991. Infections resulting from animal bites In: Weinber, A., Weber, D. (Eds.), Infectious Disease Clinics of North America, vol. 5. Saunders, Philadelphia, PA, pp. 663–677.

Webster, R.G., 1997. Influenza virus: transmission between species and relevance to the emergence of the next human pandemic. Arch. Virol. 13, 105–113.

Weigler, B.J., 1992. Biology of B virus in macaque and human hosts: a review. Clin. Infect. Dis. 14, 555–567.

Weigler, B.I., Hird, D.W., Hilliard, J.K., Lerche, N.W., Roberts, J.A., Scott, L.M., 1993. Epidemiology of *cercopithecine herpesvirus* 1 (B virus) infection and shedding in a large breeding cohort of rhesus macaques. J. Infect. Dis. 167, 257–267.

Weigler, B.J., Scinicareillo, F., Hilliard, J., 1995. Risk of venereal B virus (cercopithecine herpes virus 1) transmission on rhesus monkeys using molecular epidemiology. J. Infect. Dis. 171, 1139–1143.

Weigler, B.J., Di Giacomo, R.F., Alexander, S., 2005. A national survey of laboratory animal workers concerning occupational risks for zoonotic diseases. Comp. Med. 55, 183–191.

Weinstein, M.R., Litt, M., Kertesz, D.A., Wyper, P., Rose, D., Coulter, M., et al., 1997. Invasive infections due to a fish pathogen, *Streptococcus iniae*. N. Engl. J. Med. 337, 589–594.

Weir, E.C., Bhatt, P.N., Jacoby, R.O., Hilliard, J.K., Morgenstern, S., 1993. Infrequent shedding and transmission of *Herpesvirus simiae* from seropositive macaques. Lab. Anim. Sci. 43, 541–544.

Weisbroth, S.H., 1979. Bacterial and mycotic diseases In: Baker, H.J. Lindsey, J.R. Weisbroth, S.H. (Eds.), The Laboratory Rat, vol. 1. Academic Press, New York, pp. 194–230.

Wells, D.L., Lipper, S.L., Hilliard, J., 1989. *Herpesvirus simiae* contamination of primary rhesus monkey kidney cell cultures: CDC recommendations to minimize risks to laboratory personnel. Diagn. Microbiol. Infect. Dis. 12, 333–335.

Wentworth, D.E., McGregor, M.W., Macklin, M.D., Neumann, V., Hinshaw, V.S., 1997. Transmission of swine influenza virus to humans after exposure to experimentally infected pigs. J. Infect. Dis. 175, 7–15.

Whary, M.T., Fox, J.G., 2006. Detection, eradication and research implications of *Helicobacter* infections in laboratory rodents. Lab. Anim. 35, 25–36.

Wilkins, E.G.L., Millar, J.G.B., Cockcroft, P.M., Okubadejo, O.A., 1988. Rat-bite fever in a gerbil breeder. J. Infect. 16, 177.

Williams, S.G., Sacci Jr., J.B., Schreifer, M.E., Andersen, E.M., Fujioka, K.K., Sorvillo, F.J., et al., 1992. Typhus and typhus-like rickettsiae associated with opossums and their fleas in Los Angeles County, California. J. Clin. Microbiol. 30, 1758–1762.

Willy, E.M., Woodward, R.A., Thorton, V.B., Wolff, A.V., Flynn, B.M., Heath, J.L., et al., 1999. Management of a measles outbreak among Old World nonhuman primates. Lab. Anim. Sci. 49, 42–48.

Wilson, B.A., Ho, M., 2013. *Pasteurella multocida:* from Zoonosis to cellular microbiology. Clin. Microbiol. Rev. 26, 631–655.

Wilson, C.A., Wong, S., Muller, J., Davidson, C.E., Rose, T.M., Burd, P., 1998. Type C retrovirus released from porcine primary peripheral blood mononuclear cells infects human cells. J. Virol. 72, 3082–3087.

Winkler, W.G., Fashinell, T.R., Leffingwell, L., Howard, P., Conomy, P., 1973. Airborne rabies transmission in a laboratory worker. J. Am. Med. Assoc. 226, 1219–1221.

Wolf, R.H., Gibson, S.V., Watson, E.A., Baskin, G.B., 1988. Multidrug chemotherapy of tuberculosis in rhesus monkeys. Lab. Anim. Sci. 38, 25–33.

Wolfrom, E., Chene, G., Boisseau, H., Beylot, C., Geniaux, M., Taieb, A., 1995. Chronic urticaria and *Toxocara canis* [letter]. Lancet 345, 196.

Woodward, D.L., Khakhria, R., Johnson, W.M., 1997. Human salmonellosis associated with exotic pets. J. Clin. Microbiol. 35, 2786–2790.

Woolfrey, B.F., Moody, J.A., 1991. Human infections associated with *Bordetella bronchiseptica*. Clin. Microbiol. Rev. 4, 243–255.

Wright, W.H., 1985. Laboratory-acquired toxoplasmosis. Am. J. Clin. Pathol. 28, 1.

Wyers, M., Formenty, P., Cherel, Y., Guigand, L., Fernandez, B., Boesch, C., et al., 1999. Histopathological and immunohistochemical studies of lesions associated with Ebola virus in a naturally infected chimpanzee. J. Infect. Dis. 179, S54–S59.

Yanase, T., Muramatsu, Y., Inouye, I., Okabayashi, T., Ueno, H., Morita, C., 1998. Detection of *Coxiella burnetii* from dust in a barn housing dairy cattle. Microbiol. Immunol. 42, 51–53.

Yoder, J.S., Gargano, J.W., Wallace, R.M., Beach, M.J., 2012. Giardiasis surveillance – United States, 2009–2010. MMWR Surveill. Summ. 61, 13–23.

Yunker, C.E., 1964. Infections of laboratory animals potentially dangerous to man: ectoparasites and other arthropods, with emphasis on mites. Lab. Anim. Care 14, 455–465.

Zangwill, K.M., Hamilton, D.H., Perkins, B.A., Regnery, R.L., Plikaytis, B.D., Hadler, J., et al., 1993. Cat scratch disease in connecticut: epidemiology, risk factors, and evaluation of a new diagnostic test. N. Engl. J. Med. 329, 8–13.

Zeier, M., Handermann, M., Bahr, U., Rensch, B., Müller, S., Kehm, R., et al., 2005. New ecological aspects of hantavirus infection: a change of a paradigm and a challenge of prevention – a review. Virus Genes 30, 157–180.

Zhao, K., He, W., Gao, W., Lu, H., Han, T., Li, J., et al., 2011. Orf virus DNA vaccines expressing ORFV 011 and ORFV 059 chimeric protein enhances immunogenicity. Virol. J. 8, 562.

Zhou, X., de Man, R.A., de Knegt, R.J., Metselaar, H.J., Peppelenbosch, M.P., Pan, Q., 2013. Epidemiology and management of chronic hepatitis E infection in solid organ transplantation: a comprehensive literature review. Rev. Med. Virol. 23, 295–304.

29

Xenozoonoses: The Risk of Infection after Xenotransplantation

Marian G. Michaels, MD, MPH

Professor of Pediatrics and Surgery Children's Hospital of Pittsburgh of UPMC,
Division of Infectious Diseases, Pittsburgh, PA, USA

I. INTRODUCTION

Immunological and technical advances have led to tremendous increases in the number of people potentially able to benefit from allotransplantation. Ironically, it is the success of the field that has led to a renewed interest in xenotransplantation during the past several decades. To a large part, this has occurred because of the great scarcity of human organ and tissue donors. However, it has expanded to include the use of cells from animals into humans such as porcine islet cells for diabetes or extracorporeal perfusion of human blood through animal organs or cells. Similar to allotransplantation, issues regarding transmission of infections from the graft to the human recipient were brought up for consideration with these procedures in the 1990s (Michaels and Simmons, 1994; Chapman et al., 1995; Hammel et al., 1998; Fishman et al., 1998). A risk for infection exists with the use of any biologic agent regardless of whether it is from a human or an animal source. Accordingly, transmission of infections from human organs, tissues, or cells is a well-recognized cause of disease after allotransplantation (Ison and Grossi, 2013; Green and Michaels, 2012). As the human graft shortage continues, newer cellular therapies are explored. Thus, attention continues to be given to the potential use of xenogeneic organs, tissues, or cells for human maladies through xenotransplantation. The potential for novel zoonotic infections to emerge because of xenotransplantation (xenozoonoses or xenosis) led to a debate on whether the field should be permitted to progress. This chapter reviews the issues of xenotransplantation related to infections from animals to humans. Lessons learned from infections with prior nonhuman primate xenotransplantation and human allotransplantation are used to help inform about risks with newer xenogeneic procedures. In addition, information on known zoonoses is reviewed to better develop constructs to decrease the hazard of infection with these novel procedures.

II. LESSONS FROM ALLOTRANSPLANTATION/HISTORICAL PERSPECTIVE

While the field of allotransplantation has advanced significantly over the years, infections remain a substantial cause of morbidity and mortality. The major risk factor for severe infections is the use of nonspecific immunosuppression to prevent rejection of the new graft. In xenotransplantation, where systemic immunosuppression is even more intense than in allotransplantation, risks of infection by commensal or opportunistic pathogens are significant. Sources of microbes can be from the recipient's endogenous flora, the environment, or organisms harbored within the donated organ, tissues, or cells (Ison and Grossi, 2013; Green and Michaels, 2012). The first two sources, the environment and the recipient's endogenous flora, are the same regardless of if a person undergoes an allo- or xenotransplant. These contributed to the deaths of five of six recipients that received a baboon or chimpanzee kidney xenotransplant in two separate series from the early 1960s (Reemtsma et al., 1964; Starzl et al., 1964). Similarly, the first baboon-to-human liver xenotransplant recipient died from aspergillus, an environmental pathogen after receiving aggressive immunosuppression (Starzl et al., 1993). A second recipient of a baboon liver xenotransplant also succumbed to infection, dying with multiorgan failure 26 days after transplantation largely due to sepsis from his endogenous intraabdominal bacteria secondary to an anastomotic leak (Starzl et al., 1994). These human clinical trials using animal organs identified infections that were caused by immunosuppression and surgical complications.

However, it is possible that the graft may lead to novel infections. Some donor-associated infections are often predictable. These agents are often maintained in a quiescent intracellular state and are asymptomatic in the donor. They can potentially be transmitted via the graft organ or the accompanying hematopoietic cells (Ison and Grossi, 2013; Green and Michaels, 2012; Michaels and Simmons, 1994). Examples include blood-borne pathogens such as hepatitis B virus (HBV), hepatitis C virus (HCV), and retroviruses, along with some herpesviruses and parasites. Similar classes of organisms are of concern with animal organ transplantation and are worth examining more fully. Human herpesviruses, in particular, human cytomegalovirus (HCMV) and Epstein–Barr virus (EBV) are important donor-associated infections after allotransplantation. Their transmission from donors was first suspected by epidemiologic evidence and later confirmed using molecular techniques (Chou, 1986; Cen et al., 1991). Both HCMV and EBV cause more severe disease in naive hosts who undergo primary infection after transplantation (Rubin, 1990; Ho et al., 1985). In particular, seronegative recipients of organs from seropositive donors are at highest risk. However, even patients with previous immunity to HCMV or EBV can be reinfected with donor strains of these viruses (Chou, 1986; Cen et al., 1991; Rubin, 1990; Ho et al., 1985). Thus, it is unlikely that complete protection from analogous animal viruses after xenotransplantation will occur.

Some latent donor herpesviruses are not generally transmitted by transplantation. For example, herpes simplex virus (HSV) and varicella zoster virus (VZV) are latent in sensory ganglia and, as such, are not usually present in the blood or the transplanted graft. Consequently, they represent a very low risk of donor transmission and highlight the concept of relative risk for donor-associated infection based upon microbial tropism and individual properties of the organism. Other donor viruses outside the herpesvirus family can be transmitted. Blood-borne pathogens such as human immunodeficiency virus (HIV), HBV, and HCV have all been unintentionally transmitted after allotransplantation (Ison and Grossi, 2013; Green and Michaels, 2012; Pereira et al., 1991; Dummer et al., 1989). Usually, this happened when viruses were missed or screening tests were unavailable (Pereira et al., 1991; Dummer et al., 1989). However, even in the era of universal screening, transmission still occurs. Transmission of HIV from a single donor to four organ recipients and three of four bone marrow recipients was reported. The patient had had a negative HIV screening (Simonds et al., 1992; Ison et al., 2011). Retrospective analysis concluded that the donors were infected before a detectable antibody response could be mounted, emphasizing the inherent limitations of all screening tests. Even as improved screening tools become available, including nucleic acid testing (NAT), false-positive and false-negative results still occur (Humar et al., 2010).

Nonviral infections can also be transmitted during allotransplantation. Parasites such as Toxoplasma gondii are transmissible if the donor has organisms within the transplanted graft. T. gondii is an example of a donor-graft-specific infection. Naive heart transplant recipients are at highest risk because of the protozoa's tropism for cardiac muscle (Wreghitt et al., 1989; Campbell et al., 2006). On rare occasions, acute bacteremia or viremia is unrecognized in a donor and is transmitted to the new recipient. Prevention of disease relies largely on screening of donors. Except in the case of living related donation, donor screening is limited by substantial time constraints and the inability to retest serial samples. Prophylaxis and surveillance of recipients are important. The process should be dynamic in applying new protocols for screening and surveillance being developed.

Similarly, protocols for xenozoonoses will be invaluable to help in preventing infections from animals.

III. POTENTIAL MECHANISMS FOR CROSS-SPECIES INFECTIONS

Transmission of an animal pathogen could occur by several mechanisms (Michaels and Simmons, 1994; Chapman et al., 1995). First, an organism could be infectious to both the animal donor and the human recipient (T. gondii is an example). Second, animal viruses that are similar to human viruses, even if not currently known to be zoonotic, could infect humans with this novel access to human cells. This has been postulated for animal herpesviruses such as cytomegalovirus (CMV) and EBV (Michaels and Simmons, 1994; Michaels et al., 1994). Third, a nonpathogenic animal microbe could cause disease after xenotransplantation due to immunosuppression. Fourth, a viral recombination between animal and human viruses leading to a virulent recombinant strain is of concern. It is also possible that latent animal viruses present in the graft can reactivate, and without infecting the human, cause graft failure. Likewise, it is possible that human viruses may infect the animal graft and induce its failure. These latter concerns are particularly germane for xenotransplantation because the human recipient's immune system will not recognize porcine MHC receptors.

The concept of 'species specificity' deserves a more thorough discussion. If true, it is possible that xenotransplantation carries less risk of donor-transmitted infections than allotransplantation. However, examples of transmission of viruses that were considered to be species-specific can be found where the consequences are severe, such as with the herpesvirus family. The alpha herpesvirus of macaques, macacine herpesvirus 1 (B virus) is well established as a virus that is capable of being more pathogenic after crossing species lines (Artenstein et al., 1991; Cohen et al., 2002; Hilliard et al., 1989). Transmission to humans is rare, but usually lethal. Furthermore, and of public health concern, is documentation of a husband secondarily infecting his wife after he was infected by direct contact with infectious monkey secretions (Cohen et al., 2002). This example of a virus harmless in one species but causing more severe disease in another species with potential for secondary transmission is of major concern in xenotransplantation (Michaels and Simmons, 1994; Chapman et al., 1995; Hammel et al., 1998; Fishman et al., 1998; Institute of Medicine, 1996; Public Health Service, 2001; Kennedy, 1996; Sgroi et al., 2010; Archidiacono et al., 2010). Alpha herpesvirus such as macacine herpesvirus 1 is latent in nerve endings rather than in organ tissue or hematopoietic cells. Accordingly, similar to HSV, this alpha herpesvirus is anticipated to be of low risk for transmission

via xenotransplantation; however, its disease severity makes any risk unacceptable.

During the past 20 years, only baboons and pigs have been used as source animals for attempted whole-organ xenotransplants, whereas a variety of animal sources including baboons, swine, rabbits, cows, sheep, and hamster have been used for tissue and cellular xenografts into humans (Sgroi et al., 2010). While nonhuman primates are no longer used as a source, they are still used as recipients in nonhuman experimental xenotransplant models; thus, lessons learned from when they were used are still valuable. Most information on potential pathogens is available for baboons and swine. Neither baboons nor swine harbor macacine herpesvirus 1, but they do have analogous alphaherpesviruses, Simian agent 8 (cercopithecine herpesvirus 2) (SA8) and pseudorabies, respectively (Michaels et al., 1994). Thus far, active surveillance has not found transmission of SA8 to humans. Pseudorabies can cause fatal disease in sheep, dogs, and cattle but has not been proven to be infectious to nonhuman primates (Sawitzky, 1997). However, an anecdotal report noted three immunocompetent humans with transient fever, weakness, and neurologic abnormalities to test positive for pseudorabies antibodies suggesting transmission between swine and humans (Archidiacono et al., 2010).

As noted, members of the alpha herpesvirus family show that infections across species' lines can be dangerous, but these viruses are unlikely to be easily transmitted. However, both baboons and swine harbor beta and gammaherpesviruses that are likely to be in tissues, cells, or organs (Michaels et al., 1994; Edington et al., 1988; Falk, 1976).

Transmission of CMV or EBV between disparate species has been suggested. The Towne strain of human CMV replicates in cultures of chimpanzee skin fibroblasts and baboon CMV replicates in human fibroblasts (Perot et al., 1992; Michaels et al., 1997). In addition, neurologic disease in two humans has been attributed to primate CMV (Huang et al., 1978; Charamella et al., 1973; Martin et al., 1994, 1995). In the first case, the Colburn CMV strain was reportedly isolated from a brain biopsy of an encephalopathic child and was homologous to African green monkey CMV (strain GR2757) (Huang et al., 1978; Charamella et al., 1973). In the second case, an African green monkey-like CMV was repeatedly isolated from a woman diagnosed with chronic fatigue syndrome (Martin et al., 1994, 1995). Both cases suggest potential transmission of a simian CMV to humans, but neither provides evidence for how the transmission may have transpired. More direct implications for xenotransplantation were found with the isolation of baboon CMV from a blood specimen of a recipient of a baboon liver 1 month after transplantation but not subsequently (Michaels et al., 2001). Swine CMV has been less extensively investigated; thus far, it has not grown in human cell lines *in vitro*. Few studies on cross-species transmission of gammaherpesviruses such as EBV are available, although it has long been known that human EBV is able to infect marmoset lymphocytes in the laboratory (Miller, 1990). Our studies have also found variable cross-reactivity of antibody tests directed against human EBV antigens with antibodies found in baboons. Commercial tests for EBV viral capsid antigen found a high seropositivity rate in a baboon colony, whereas the majority of paired specimens were negative when tested for antibody against EBV nuclear antigen (EBNA). This finding may be related to differences in the conservation of some sites of gammaherpesviruses (Falk *et al.*, 1976).

Human organs, blood, and tissues have been vehicles for transmitting retroviruses, such as HIV. Retroviruses are often species restricted, but similar to herpesviruses, can cross species barriers. For example, simian immunodeficiency virus (SIV) appears to be benign in its natural host, the African green monkey, but progresses to an acquired immunodeficiency syndrome (AIDS)-like disease when inoculated into macaques (Benveniste *et al.*, 1988). Transmission is variable in other nonhuman primates. SIV and HIV type 2 are genetically similar (Benveniste *et al.*, 1988). Probable transmission to two humans who were exposed to SIV has been documented (Khabbaz *et al.*, 1992, 1994). One individual remained asymptomatic and gradually lost antibody against SIV over a 2-year period. The other person had SIV isolated from peripheral blood cells documenting an ongoing active infection albeit without clinical symptoms (Khabbaz *et al.*, 1994). SIV strains of chimpanzees have been identified as the origin of HIV type 1 and responsible for the human AIDS epidemic (Gao *et al.*, 1999). Little is however known about lentiviruses in pigs.

Retroviruses other than lentiviruses may be transmissible during xenotransplantation. It is particularly problematic when using nonhuman primates. Examples include simian T-lymphotropic virus (STLV) which is an oncogenic retrovirus found in many nonhuman primate populations. Genetically, STLV has homologous sequences with human T-lymphotropic virus, type 1 (HTLV). HTLV has been associated with leukemia in humans (Homma *et al.*, 1984). Foamy viruses are another class of retroviruses found in nonhuman primates named for a foamy cytopathic effect that was found in primary monkey cell lines that are used in virology laboratories. Surveillance of workers with occupational exposure to nonhuman primates have found several to be infected with foamy virus although no disease has been noted (Schweizer *et al.*, 1997; Anonymous, 1997). The exact timing of infection could not be elicited but was felt to have been at least 16–20 years prior to testing in one case. Family members remained seronegative (Schweizer *et al.*, 1997). Polymerase chain reaction (PCR) studies found DNA from foamy virus in two human recipients of

baboon liver transplants (Allan *et al.*, 1998). The virus was not able to be isolated despite multiple cultures; likewise, serologic studies on the human recipients remained negative after transplantation. Accordingly, the interpretation of the finding of DNA from foamy virus in these human xenografts recipients is unclear; it may represent microchimerism rather than true infection of human cells. Despite the problems with interpretation in these two cases, the risk of infection appeared to be high albeit the proof of clinical relevance remained unknown. Exogenous retroviruses of swine are less well characterized than those of non-human primates. Some pig retroviruses reactivate after exposure to radiation and therefore may be at risk for reactivation under the influence of immunosuppressive drugs (Frazier, 1985). While it may prove to be laborious, it would seem prudent to screen potential swine donors that are considered for xenotransplantation that harbor exogenous retroviruses.

Endogenous retroviruses, normal genetic elements encoded in the chromosome, have been raised as concerns for xenotransplantation in particular because they cannot be removed from source animal populations by current rearing methods. These viruses have long been recognized but only with the renewal of interest in clinical xenotransplantation have more in-depth studies of endogenous retroviruses begun to be conducted. All strains of pigs studied carry porcine endogenous retroviruses (PERVs) within their genome (Patience *et al.*, 1997; Le Tissier *et al.*, 1997; Martin *et al.*, 1998; Wilson *et al.*, 1998; Takeuchi *et al.*, 1998). Likewise, baboon endogenous virus (BaEV) is found in baboon genomes. *In vitro* studies show both PERV and BaEV capable of infecting human cell lines (Patience *et al.*, 1997; Le Tissier *et al.*, 1997; Martin *et al.*, 1998; Wilson *et al.*, 1998; Takeuchi *et al.*, 1998; Huang *et al.*, 1989). A human who received baboon bone marrow for experimental treatment of HIV-1 had transient presence of BaEV detected at day 5 after transplantation but not subsequently (Michaels *et al.*, 2004). The finding was in conjunction with finding baboon mitochondria, again limiting interpretation as to whether this represented chimerism versus true infection. The largest review to date evaluated 160 people who had various pig tissue transplants up to 12 years earlier (Paradis *et al.*, 1999). No patient was found to have detectable viremia. In addition, no persistent PERV infection could be found; 23 patients had evidence of microchimerism up to 8 years after exposure to pig tissues. Likewise, more recent studies looking at other groups of patients exposed to porcine cells over time have not shown infection with PERV (DiNicuolo *et al.*, 2010). Long-term follow-up of eight patients surviving treatment with porcine cell-based Academic Medical Center bioartificial liver found no evidence of PERV DNA in peripheral blood mononuclear cells (PBMCs) nor RNA in plasma or PBMC samples (DiNicuolo *et al.*,

2010). Extensive reviews on the subject likewise failed to find viremia, but caution remains about the potential risk particularly with recombination of PERV-A and PERV –C strains (Denner and Tonjes, 2012; Fishman *et al.*, 2012).

Other virus classes have been transmitted after allotransplantation and may likewise cause disease after xenotransplantation. For example, unrecognized acute viremia with adenovirus has caused graft failure after human liver transplantation (Varki *et al.*, 1990). Since adenovirus can infect many animal species similar concerns may exist. Alternatively, it is possible that xenotransplantation may cause less of a risk for this type of transmission of acute infectious agents because animals can be reared under much more stringent conditions where surveillance for infections or unwellness could be detected.

HBV and HCV have been transmitted after allotransplantation and bring up another area where xenotransplantation has been suggested as a superior alternative to human grafts. Baboons appeared to be resistant to infection with HBV (Starzl *et al.*, 1993, 1994; Michaels *et al.*, 1996). Accordingly, livers from baboons were used in an attempt to transplant two patients with end-stage HBV liver disease (Starzl *et al.*, 1993, 1994). Subsequent research showed that under experimental conditions HBV could actually infect baboon livers and alternative strategies to xenotransplantation using antiviral agents in combination with hepatitis B immunoglobulin have permitted successful allotransplantation for people with HBV infection. Some hepatitis viruses are not species-specific and could pose a risk for xenotransplantation; related strains of hepatitis E virus have been found to cross species barriers (Meng *et al.*, 1998).

Numerous other viruses, some long recognized and others newly recognized, in animal populations can be added to the growing lists of potential xenozoonotic infections. Examples include reoviruses, circoviruses, and paramyxoviruses (Public Health Service, 2001; Philbey *et al.*, 1998; Halpin *et al.*, 1999). Menangle virus is a paramyxoviral zoonosis infecting pigs and humans in Australia and believed to be harbored by flying foxes (Halpin *et al.*, 1999). Coronaviruses in particular can cross species lines with fatal results as found with severe acute respiratory syndrome (SARS) and more recently the Middle East respiratory syndrome (MERS) (Peiris *et al.*, 2003; Reusken *et al.*, 2013). It is imperative that animal sources are maintained under strict rearing methods and issues of rodent, insect, or other animal infestation considered. For more information, please refer to The Public Health Service guideline on infectious disease in xenotransplantation (Public Health Service, 2001) and other relevant reviews (Denner and Tonjes, 2012; Fishman *et al.*, 2012).

In addition to infection of a xenotransplant recipient with an animal virus, consideration must also be given to the possibility of recombination (Chou, 1989; Halliburton *et al.*, 1977; Isfort *et al.*, 1992). Mixed-strain isolates of human CMV can recombine *in vitro* with passage (Chou, 1989). Mouse studies have demonstrated that infection with two avirulent HSV can lead to recombinations that are lethal (Halliburton *et al.*, 1977). *In vitro* integration of reticuloendotheliosis virus (an avian retrovirus) into an avian herpesvirus (Marek disease virus) can lead to lethal recombinant strains (Isfort *et al.*, 1992). Consideration should also be given to whether it is possible for avian influenza to gain access to swine tissue within a xenotransplant recipient leading to mixing of influenza within a human host. In addition, as mentioned earlier, consideration for infection of porcine or other xenogeneic tissue with human viruses could lead to graft dysfunction (Millard and Mueller, 2010).

IV. NONVIRAL AGENTS

Nonviral agents may also cause xenogeneic infections if present in tissues being transplanted such as toxoplasma cysts in the cardiac muscle of a transplanted heart, regardless of the donor species. Throughout the world, commercial herds of swine are commonly seropositive for *T. gondii* (Hill and Dubey, 2013). Parasites normally confined to the gastrointestinal tract could be a problem if extra-intestinal infection occurs as is possible for *Entamoeba histolytica* and some schistosoma species. Local epidemiologic considerations will influence the types of parasites considered. Source animal populations should be raised in protected environments, where parasitic infestation is avoided.

Bacterial and fungal diseases, while less likely to be latent, still require consideration. For example, mycobacterium species can infect animals including baboons and swine which may not manifest clinical symptoms until disseminated end-stage disease. Often the source of tuberculosis in animal populations is from human caretakers; accordingly, serial tuberculin skin testing of human caregivers and source animals should be routine. Prions likewise need to be considered when using animal neurogenic cells for diseases such as Parkinson's disease, although prion disease has not been found thus far in swine.

V. DEVELOPMENT OF SPF HERDS

Many concerns for xenozoonoses could be diminished if source animals could be raised under germ-free conditions. Small laboratory animals have been raised in gnotobiotic environments. Pigs have also been raised under these conditions to a lesser extent, but have problems after several months of age because of their size and waste (stool and urine) production. These environments also preclude the typical colonization of the gastrointestinal tract with normal microbial agents that help with the digestion of food. For this reason, pigs raised in germ-free conditions are less robust and may not be ideal organ sources (Michaels and Simmons, 1994; Chapman, 1995; Public Health Service, 2001; Fishman, 1994). Consideration therefore turned to raising source animals under controlled environments in which specific pathogens have been eliminated and the introduction of outside pathogens is guarded against (Michaels and Simmons, 1994; Chapman, 1995; Public Health Service, 2013; Fishman et al., 2012; Fishman, 1994). Vigilance against the accidental introduction of microbes to an established colony must be strictly maintained from human caretakers or outside animals. In addition, concern remains for the possibility of xenogeneic infection from microbes that are currently not identified and therefore not screened out of the population.

Decisions regarding which microbial agents to be screened out of a source animal population need to be reviewed and periodically updated as new infections information is available. For example, the protocol designed for screening a baboon to be used for a bone marrow xenotransplant to attempt to reconstitute the immune system in a person with AIDS-classified microbes into one of four groups: (1) absolute contraindications, (2) relative contraindications, (3) treatable microbes, or (4) unavoidable microbes (Michaels et al., 2004). Absolute contraindications included microbial agents that were known to be zoonotic and dangerous to humans, even if they were not anticipated to be found in baboons that were born and raised in the United States. For example, SIV, STLV, filoviruses, T. gondii, M. tuberculosis, and herpes B virus were put in this category, even though SIV and herpes B were not anticipated in baboon populations at all. Relative contraindications consisted of microbes that were hypothesized to be xenozoonotic but were unproven or with uncertain consequence. Examples included baboon herpesviruses and foamy virus. Treatable infections were microbes that could be identified and eradicated prior to bone marrow harvest such as Babesia species or gastrointestinal pathogens. The fourth category, 'unavoidable organisms' included BaEV and microbes that exist but were as yet unrecognized and thus clearly of indeterminate risk (Michaels et al., 2004). The categories were developed with the most up-to-date information available but also with the recognition that future protocols might move some of the infectious agents into different classes. The same is true for screening lists for swine and other species considered for source animals. In addition to developing protocols for which organisms should be evaluated, it is important to determine which testing method will be

used and to be prepared to change these methods as more sophisticated techniques are developed (Fishman et al., 2012). As noted previously, not all testing methods are equivalent. For example, a serologic survey of baboons raised in the United States demonstrated great variability in identifying baboons with evidence of H. papio, the EBV analog (Michaels et al., 1994). This highlights the need to develop more sensitive techniques specific to the agent being evaluated. One approach to increase the sensitivity of screening was used when screening baboons for liver transplantation; paired sera samples from potential source animals were sent to two laboratories using different techniques to look for a wide variety of viruses; any positive finding was classified as a true positive (Michaels et al., 1994). Also recognizing that serologic surveys have the potential to miss an immunologic response to a recently encountered agent, selected animals that tested negative initially were quarantined and retested over time for these same potential pathogens.

Swine can be reared efficiently in controlled environments, which makes screening somewhat easier. However, prospective considerations for the types of screening are still necessary (Public Health Service, 2011; Fishman et al., 2012; Fishman, 1994; Ye et al., 1994). One study evaluated 10 newborn piglets that were reared in a brucellosis, pseudorabies virus, atrophic rhinitis, and Mycoplasma hyponeumonia (Ye et al., 1994). The investigators cultured the skin, urine, feces and nasal swabs for bacteria and examined the tissues for fungi and parasites. Further testing included bacterial blood culture commercial serologic tests for antibody against human CMV, HBV, HCV, HIV, T. pallidum, and T. gondii. Tests were performed serially and at necropsy. No pathogens were identified which the investigators considered as a risk for xenotransplantation. However, 2 of the 10 pigs had positive enzyme-linked immunosorbent assay (ELISA) tests for HIV at one point in time. Further investigation revealed them to be negative, but this again emphasizes limitations that can exist with screening techniques.

VI. POTENTIAL BENEFITS OF XENOTRANSPLANTATION AND OTHER INFECTIOUS DISEASE ISSUES

It is possible that xenotransplantation may decrease the risk of some infections after transplantation. For example, in the 1980s allotransplantation was not an ideal treatment for humans with HBV or HIV because the virus would infect the new organ or hematopoietic cells. The resistance of baboon livers to HBV was the rationale for xenotransplantation in two patients with end-stage liver disease from HBV (Starzl et al., 1993, 1994). Likewise, the rationale of attempting to reconstitute the immune system of a patient with HIV through xenotransplantation was again because of the natural resistance of the baboon to HIV-1 (Michaels *et al.*, 2004). Newer strategies for treating both viruses emerged, and accordingly the risk benefit weighed against the use of xenotransplantation for these particular diseases but conceptually an animal organ may still have this type of benefit. As noted previously, xenotransplantation may avoid many donor-transmitted infections by permitting source animals to be reared in controlled, SPF environments and surveyed against acute infections. Performing transplants as elective surgery rather than as emergency procedures which is often required with allotransplantation would also decrease postoperative infectious complications.

VII. ISSUES AFTER XENOTRANSPLANTATION

SPF-controlled and well-regulated environments are critical to decrease the risk of xenozoonoses, but will not eliminate it completely. For this reason, it is important for any recipient of xenogeneic tissue to undergo counseling about the potential risks and surveillance for new infections after xenotransplantation. In this fashion, the true epidemiology and risks of xenotransplant infections will be recognized. Serial samples from the recipient and transplanted tissues should be collected for cultures and/or assays to look for agents that were known or suspected to be in the source animal, such as endogenous viruses. These recommendations were added into the guidelines recommended by the United States Public Health Services (PHS) and World Health Organization (WHO) (Public Health Service, 2001; Fishman *et al.*, 2012). However, as noted, current techniques for screening may ultimately prove inadequate. Accordingly, archiving samples for future studies are important and should be maintained for a minimum of 50 years (Public Health Service, 2001; FDA, 2003). Shared or centralized registries and repositories for archived specimens may help with evaluating potential infectious agents; however, at this time they are not available. Initially, the Department of Health and Human Services formed a Secretary's Advisory Committee on Xenotransplantation as well as the FDA Biological Response Modifiers Advisory Committee (BRMAC) to consider the complexities of xenotransplantation and to help with ongoing review of these procedures. However, xenogeneic activity is now directly under the auspices of the FDA Cell, Tissue and Gene Therapies Advisory Committee (CTGTAC), which coordinate and participate with global groups such as the WHO (FDA, 2003).

All biologic agents have an inherent risk for transmitting infections and our ability to recognize and prevent these infections is continuously growing. Xenotransplantation has the potential to offer life-saving tissues and grafts to a number of people who currently die because of the absence of available human donors; as the field grows, it is imperative that new techniques be developed to help identify and prevent novel infections.

References

Allan, J.S., Broussard, S.R., Michaels, M.G., et al., 1998. Amplification of simian retroviral sequences from human recipients of baboon liver transplants AIDS. Res. Hum. Retrov. 14, 821–824.

Anonymous, 1997. Nonhuman primate spumavirus infections among persons with occupational exposure – United States, 1996. JAMA 277, 783–785.

Archidiacono, J.A., Evdokimov, E., Lee, M.H., et al., 2010. Regulation of xenogeneic porcine pancreatic islets. Xenotransplantation 17, 329–337.

Artenstein, A.W., Hicks, C.B., Goodwin Jr, B.S., Hilliard, J.K., 1991. Human infection with B virus following a needle stick injury. Rev. Infect. Dis. 13, 288–291.

Benveniste, R.E., Morton, W.R., Clark, E.A., et al., 1988. Inoculation of baboons and macaques with SIV/mne, a primate lentivirus closely related to HIV 2. Virology 2 (6), 2091–2101.

Campbell, A.L., Goldberg, C.L., Magid, M.S., Gondolesi, G., Rumbo, C., Herold, B.C., 2006. First case of toxoplasmosis following small bowel transplantation and systematic review of tissue-invasive toxoplasmosis following noncardiac solid organ transplantation. Transplantation 81, 408–417.

Cen, H., Breinig, M.C., Atchinson, R.W., Ho, M., McKnight, J.L.C., 1991. Epstein–Barr virus transmission via the donor organs in solid organ transplantation: polymerase chain reaction and restriction fragment length polymorphism analysis of IR2, IR3 and IR4. J. Virol. 65, 976.

Chapman, L.E., Folks, T.M., Salomon, D.R., Patterson, A.P., Eggerman, T.E., Noguchi, P.D., 1995. Xenotransplantation and xenogeneic infections. N. Engl. J. Med. 333, 1498.

Charamella, L.J., Reynolds, R.B., Ch'ien, L.T., Alford Jr., C.A., 1973. Biologic characterization of an unusual human cytomegalovirus isolated from the brain. ABST V 373, Ann Meetings of Amer. Soc. Med. 256.

Chou, S., 1986. Acquisition of donor strains of cytomegalovirus by renal-transplant recipients. Engl. J. Med. 314, 1418.

Chou, S., 1989. Reactivation and recombination of multiple cytomegalovirus strains from individual organ donors. J. Infect. Dis. 160, 11–15.

Cohen, J.I., Davenport, D.S., Stewart, J.A., Deitchman, S., Hilliard, J.K., Chapman, L.E., 2002. Recommendations for prevention of and therapy for exposure to B virus (Cercopithecine herpesvirus 1) B virus working group. Clin. Infect. Dis. 35, 1191–2003.

Denner, J., Tonjes, R.R., 2012. Infection barriers to successful xenotransplantation focusing on porcine endogenous retroviruses. Clinl. Microbiol. Rev. 25 (2), 318–343.

DiNicuolo, G., D'Alessandro, A., Andria, B., et al., 2010. Long-term absence of porcine endotenous retrovirus infection in chronically immunosuppressed patients after treatment with the porcine cell-based Academic Medical Center bioartifical liver. Xenotransplantation 17, 431–439.

Dummer, J.S., Erb, S., Breinig, M., et al., 1989. Infection with human immunodeficiency virus in the Pittsburgh transplant population. Transplantation 47, 134.

Edington, N., Wrathall, A.E., Done, J.T., 1988. Porcine cytomegalovirus (PCMV) in early gestation. Vet. Micro. 17, 117–128.

Falk, L., Deinhardt, F., Nonoyama, M., Wolfe, L.G., Bergholz, C., 1976. Properties of a baboon lymphotropic herpesvirus related to Epstein–Barr virus. Int. J. Cancer 18, 798–807.

FDA, 2003. Guidance for Industry: Source animals, product, preclinical and clinical issues concerning the use of xenotransplantation products in human. Available at: <http://www.fda.gov/Biologics BloodVaccines/GuidanceComplianceRegulatoryInformation/ Guidances/xenotransplantation/ucm074354.htm> (Accessed 8.12.13).

Fishman, J., Sachs, D., Shaikh, R. (Eds.), 1998. Xenotransplantation: Scientific Frontiers and Public Policy, Annals of the New York Academy of Sciences, vol. 862, pp. 1–25.

Fishman, J.A., 1994. Miniature swine as organ donors for man: strategies for prevention of xenotransplant infections. Xenotransplantation 1, 47–57.

Fishman, J.A., Scobie, L., Takeuchi, Y., 2012. Xenotransplantation-associated infectious risk: a WHO consultation. Xenotransplantation 19, 72–81.

Frazier, M.E., 1985. Evidence for retrovirus in miniature swine with radiation-induced leukemia or metaplasia. Arch. Virol. 83, 83–97.

Gao, F., Bailes, E., Robertson, D.L., et al., 1999. Origin of HIV-1 in the chimpanzee Pan troglodytes troglodytes. Nature 397, 436–441.

Green, M., Michaels, M.G., 2012. Infections in solid organ transplant recipients. In: Long, S.S., Prober, C.G., Pickering, L.K. (Eds.), Principles & Practice of Pediatric Infectious Diseases, fourth ed. Churchill Livingstone, New York.

Halliburton, I.W., Randall, R.E., Killington, R.A., Watson, D.H., 1977. Some properties of recombinants between type 1 and type 2 herpes simplex viruses. J. Gen. Virol. 36, 471–484.

Halpin, K., Young, P.L., Field, H., Mackenzie, J.S., 1999. Newly discovered viruses of flying foxes. Vet. Med. 68, 83–87.

Hammel, J.M., Prentice, E., Fox, I.J., 1998. Current status of xenotransplantation. Probl. Gen. Surg. 15, 189–201.

Hill, D.E., Dubey, J.P., 2013. Toxoplasma gondii prevalence in farm animals in the United States. Int. J. Parasitol. 43 (2), 107–113.

Hilliard, J.K., Black, D., Eberle, R., 1989. Simian alphaherpesviruses and their relation to the human herpes simplex viruses. Arch. Virol. 109, 83–102.

Ho, M., Miller, G., Atchinson, R.W., et al., 1985. Epstein–Barr virus infections and DNA hybridization studies in post-transplantation lymphoma and lymphoproliferative lesions: the role of primary infection. J. Infect. Dis. 152, 876.

Homma, T., Kanki, P.J., King, N.W., et al., 1984. Lymphoma in macaques: association with virus of HTLV family. Science 225, 716–718.

Huang, E., Kilpatrick, B., Lakeman, A., Alford, C.A., 1978. Genetic analysis of a cytomegalovirus-like agent isolated from human brain. J. Virol. 26, 718–723.

Huang, L., Silberman, J., Rothschild, H., Cohen, J.C., 1989. Replication of baboon endogenous virus in human cells. J. Biol. Chem. 264, 8811–8814.

Humar, A., Morris, M., Blumberg, E., et al., 2010. Nucleic Acid Testing (NAT) of organ donors: is the "best" test the right test? a consensus conference report. Am. J. Transpl. 10 (4), 889–899.

Institute of Medicine. Xenotransplantation: Science, ethics and public policy, 1996. National Academy Press, Washington, DC.

Isfort, R., Jones, D., Kost, R., Witter, R., Kung, H., 1992. Retrovirus insertion into herpesvirus in vitro and in vivo. Proc. Natl. Acad. Sci. USA 89, 991–995.

Ison, M.G., Grossi, P., 2013. Donor-derived infections in solid organ transplantation. Am. J. Transpl. 13, 22–30.

Ison, M.G., Llata, E., Conover, C.S., et al., 2011. Transmission of human immunodeficiency virus and hepatits C virus from an organ donor to four transplant recipients. Am. J. Transpl. 11, 1218–1225.

Kennedy, I. 1996. Advisory Group on Ethics of Xenotransplantation. Animal tissue into humans, Department of Health, United Kingdom, ISBN 011 321866 4, London, Publications Center.

Khabbaz, R.F., Rowe, T., Murphey-Corb, M., et al., 1992. Simian immunodeficiency virus needle stick accident in a laboratory worker. Lancet 340, 271–273.

Khabbaz, R.F., Heneine, W., George, J.R., 1994. Brief report. Infection of a laboratory worker with Simian immunodeficiency virus. N. Engl. J. Med. 330, 172–177.

Le Tissier, P., Stoye, J.P., Takeuchi, Y., Patience, C., Weiss, R.A., 1997. Two sets of human-tropic pig retrovirus. Nature 389, 681–682.

Martin, U., Kiessig, V., Blusch, J.H., et al., 1998. Expression of pig endogenous retrovirus by primary porcine endothelial cellls and infection of human cells. Lancet 352, 692–694.

Martin, W.J., Zeng, L.C., Ahmed, K., Roy, M., 1994. Cytomegalovirus-related sequence in an a typical cytopathic virus repeatedly isolated from a patient with chronic fatigue syndrome. Am. J. Pathol. 145, 440–451.

Martin, W.J., Ahmed, K., Zeng, L.C., Olsen, J., Seward, J.G., Seehrai, J.S., 1995. African green monkey origin of the atypical cytopathic "stealth virus" isolated from a patient with chronic fatigue syndrome. Clin. Diag. Virol. 4, 93–103.

Meng, X.J., Halbur, P.G., Shapiro, M.S., et al., 1998. Genetic and experimental evidence for cross-species infection by swine hepatitis E virus. J. Virol. 72, 9714–9721.

Michaels, M.G., Simmons, R.L., 1994. Xenotransplant-associated zoonoses. Transplantation 57, 1.

Michaels, M.G., McMichael, J., Brasky, K., Kalter, S., Peters, R.L., Starzl, T.E., et al., 1994. Screening donors for xenotransplantation: the potential for xenozoonoses. Transplantation 57, 1462–1465.

Michaels, M.G., Lanford, R., Demetris, A.J., Chavez, D., Brasky, K., Fung, J., et al., 1996. Lack of susceptibility of baboons to infection with hepatitis B virus. Transplantation 61, 350–351.

Michaels, M.G., Alcendor, D., St George, K., Rinaldo Jr., C.R., Ehrlich, G., Becich, M.J., et al., 1997. Distinguishing baboon CMV from human CMV: importance for xenotransplantation. J. Infect. Dis. 176, 1476–1483.

Michaels, M.G., Jenkins, F., St George, K., et al., 2001. Detection of infectious baboon cytomegalovirus after baboon to human liver transplantation. J. Virol. 75, 2825–2828.

Michaels, M.G., Kaufman, C., Volberding, P.A., Gupta, P., Switzer, W.M., Heneine, W., et al., 2004. Baboon bone marrow xenotransplant in a patient with advanced HIV disease: case report and eight-year follow-up. Transplantation 78, 1582–1589.

Millard, A.L., Mueller, N.J., 2010. Critical issues related to porcine xenografts exposure to human viruses: lessons from allotransplantation. Curr. Opin. Org. Transpl. 15, 230–235.

Miller, G., 1990. Epstein–Barr virus: biology, pathogenesis, and medical aspects. In: Fields, B.N., Knipe, D.M. (Eds.), Virology, second ed. Raven Press, New York, pp. 1921.

Paradis, K., Langford, G., Long, Z., et al., 1999. Search for cross-species transmission of porcine endogenous retrovirus in patients treated with living pig tissue. Science 285, 1236–1241.

Patience, C., Takeuchi, Y., Weiss, R.A., 1997. Infection of human cells by an endogenous retrovirus of pigs. Nat. Med. 3, 282–286.

Peiris, J.S.M., Yuen, K.Y., Osterhause, A.D., Stohr, K., 2003. The severe acute respiratory syndrome. N. Engl. J. Med. 349, 2431–2441.

Pereira, B.J.G., Milford, E.L., Kirkman, R.L., Levey, A.S., 1991. Transmission of hepatitis C virus by organ transplantation. N. Engl. J. Med. 325, 454.

Perot, K., Walker, C.M., Spaete, R.R., 1992. Primary chimpanzee skin fibroblast cells are fully permissive for human cytomegalovirus replication. J. Gen. Virol. 73, 3281–3284.

Philbey, A.W., Kirkland, P.D., Ross, A.D., et al., 1998. An apparently new virus (family Paramyxoviridae) infectious for pigs, humans and fruit bats. Emerging Infect. Dis. 4, 269–271.

Public Health Service guideline on infectious disease issues in xenotransplantation (2001). Available at: <http://www.fda.gov/ BiologicsBloodVaccines/GuidanceComplianceRegulatory Information/Guidances/xenotransplantation/ucm07427.htm>. (Accessed 30.11.13).

Reemtsma, K., McCracken, B.H., Schlegel, J.U., et al., 1964. Renal Heterotransplantation in man. Ann. Surg. 160, 384–410.

Reusken, C.B., Haagmans, B.L., Muller, M.A., et al., 2013. Middle East respiratory syndrome coronavirus neutralising serum antibodies in dromedary camels: a comparative serological study. Lancet Infect. Dis. 13 (10), 859–866.

Rubin, R.H., 1990. Impact of cytomegalovirus infection on organ transplant recipients. Rev. Infect. Dis. 12 (Suppl. 7), S754–S766.

Sawitzky, D., 1997. Transmission, species specificity, and pathogenicity of Aujeszky's disease virus. Arch. Virol. Suppl. 13, 201–206.

Schweizer, M., Falcone, V., Gange, J., Turek, R., Neumann-Haefelin, D., 1997. Simian foamy virus isolated from an accidentally infected human individual. J. Virol. 71, 4821–4824.

Sgroi, A., Buhler, L.H., Morel, P., Sykes, M., Noel, L., 2010. International human xenotransplantation inventory. Transplantation 90, 597–603.

Simonds, R.J., Holmberg, S.D., Hurwitz, R.L., et al., 1992. Transmission of human immunodeficiency virus type I from a seronegative organ and tissue donor. N. Engl. J. Med. 326, 726.

Starzl, T.E., Marchioro, T.L., Peters, G.N., et al., 1964. Renal heterotransplantation from baboon to man: experience with 6 cases. Transplantation 2 (6), 752–776.

Starzl, T.E., Fung, J., Tzakis, A., et al., 1993. Baboon-to-human liver transplantation. Lancet 341, 65–71.

Starzl, T.E., Tzakis, A., Fung, J.J., et al., 1994. Prospects of clinical xeno-transplantation. Transpl. Proc. 26 (3), 1082–1088.

Takeuchi, Y., Patience, C., Magre, S., et al., 1998. Host-range and interference studies of three classes of pig endogenous retroviruses. J. Virol. 72, 9986–9991.

Varki, N.M., Bhuta, S., Drake, T., Porter, D.D., 1990. Adenovirus hepatitis in two successive liver transplants in a child. Arch. Pathol. Lab. Med. 114, 106.

Wilson, C.A., Wong, S., Muller, J., Davidson, C.E., Rose, T.M., Burd, P., 1998. Type C retrovirus released from primary peripheral blood mononuclear cells infects human cells. J. Virol. 72, 3082–3087.

Wreghitt, T.G., Hakim, M., Gray, J.J., et al., 1989. Toxoplasmosis in heart and heart and lung transplant recipients. J. Clin. Pathol. 42, 194.

Ye, Y., Niekrasz, M., Kosanke, S., et al., 1994. The pig as a potential organ donor for man. Transplantation 57, 694–703.

CHAPTER

30

Occupational Health of Laboratory Animal Workers

Peter M. Rabinowitz, MD MPH[a], Rafael Y. Lefkowitz, MD MPH[b], Lisa A. Conti, DVM MPH, Dipl ACVPM, CPM, CEHP[c], Carrie A. Redlich, MD MPH[b] and Benjamin J. Weigler, DVM MPH PhD[d]

[a]University of Washington Center for One Health Research, Department of Environmental and Occupational Health Sciences, University of Washington School of Public Health, Seattle, WA, USA
[b]Yale Occupational and Environmental Medicine Program, Yale University School of Medicine, New Haven, CT, USA [c]Global Health Solutions, Tallahassee, FL, USA [d]Washington National Primate Research Center, University of Washington, Seattle, Washington, USA

OUTLINE

Laboratory Animal Medicine, Third Edition
DOI: http://dx.doi.org/10.1016/B978-0-12-409527-4.00030-4

I. INTRODUCTION

Workers engaged in the care and handling of laboratory animals perform tasks in a variety of indoor and outdoor settings on behalf of the civil and uniformed services, academic institutions, hospitals and non-profit entities, contract research organizations, pharmaceutical and biotechnology companies, diagnostic facilities, and animal breeding facilities, among others. The vivarium environment is one where both animals and human workers spend extended time in close proximity, and can involve both terrestrial and aquatic animals of highly diverse species for in-life as well as *post-mortem* stages of research, teaching, and testing. In these environments, workers may encounter exposures to a wide range and intensity of biological, physical, chemical, and psychosocial health hazards. Managers of laboratory animal facilities therefore need to simultaneously consider the health and well-being of the animals as well as that of the animal handlers and other staff in the facility. In many laboratory animal settings, however, preventive programs for animal care workers have been less developed and comprehensive than those for workers in other industries (McMurry and Key, 1999).

One challenge in the provision of occupational health services has been the broad range of job types that involve ongoing or periodic contact with animals in these settings, requiring each institution to self-identify the groups of personnel (research staff, visiting scientists, animal care staff, students, support staff, etc.) who should appropriately be encompassed within their preventive medicine programs (National Research Council, 2011). Health and safety programs for laboratory animal workers often span several recognized occupational categories that may involve a variety of species-specific as well as research project-related hazards, themselves varying by location within institutions and over time, depending upon the type and purpose of active study. The U.S. Department of Labor's Bureau of Labor Statistics defines laboratory animal caretakers within broad categories that are not specific to the vivarium and exclude veterinarians and other research staff participants, compliance and quality-assurance specialists, site managers, facilities maintenance support staff, students, and nonaffiliated members of the Institutional Animal Care and Use Committee (IACUC), among others, who devote significant amounts of work effort in areas where laboratory animals are held and used (Weigler *et al.*, 2005). As a result, it can be difficult to assemble an accurate estimation of the extent of occupational illnesses and injuries within this diverse workforce with exposure to the laboratory animal setting.

This chapter will review the identification and control of occupational exposure risks in laboratory animal facilities and outline the basic structure of occupational health services for animal care workers that can help detect, prevent, and manage such risks. The scope of material presented here is intended to broadly apply to persons who engage in a number of job- or educational-related functions involving animal contact, involving all indoor and outdoor areas where laboratory animals of any species are held and used. In this chapter we will use the generic term 'laboratory animal workers,' to refer to all such workers regardless of their employment category or duration of association with the institution.

II. OCCUPATIONAL ILLNESS AND INJURY IN LABORATORY ANIMAL WORKERS

This section reviews current knowledge about the health of laboratory animal workers. Although the scientific literature remains limited concerning the general health of animal workers, published surveys of health have revealed significant rates of allergy and respiratory disease, particularly among persons exposed to laboratory rodents and rabbits. Additional evidence suggests that animal care workers may also be at increased risk for psychosocial distress and illness and injury resulting from physical and chemical hazards.

A. Laboratory Animal Allergy

An allergy is an immune system reaction to exposure to a substance (often a protein) that does not have the same effect on most other people. Laboratory animal allergy (LAA) involves the development of a number of allergic symptoms in workers exposed to allergenic high-molecular-weight proteins related to laboratory animals and the laboratory animal environment, including animal urine, dander, and saliva as well as to bedding, feed, mold, and insects. Symptoms of LAA can include sneezing, rhinitis, nasal discharge, conjunctivitis and tearing, eyelid swelling, itching, and dermatitis. Laboratory animal-induced asthma can develop as a complication of allergy (see below), often following the development of rhinitis (Acton and McCauley, 2007; Corradi *et al.*, 2013). Cases of life-threatening anaphylaxis have been reported related to exposure to animal allergens (Leng *et al.*, 2008), and severe skin reactions may also occur (Bhabha and Nixon, 2012).

A number of studies have reported on the risk of LAA among animal workers, and estimates of the prevalence of animal allergy among animal handlers as high as 33% have been reported (Massachusetts Department of Health, 1999), particularly for persons occupationally exposed to laboratory rodents and rabbits (Venables *et al.*, 1988a). Fewer data exist to demonstrate a substantially increased risk for LAA among workers whose main job-related exposures involve other species used in research, including nonhuman primates, agricultural species, and aquatic animals. The majority of studies of LAA have been cross-sectional surveys of workers who have already been working for a number of years. Such surveys can underestimate the incidence and prevalence of occupational allergy due to the 'healthy worker effect' whereby sensitized workers who develop symptoms leave the workplace for other employment, resulting in a lower rate of disease in the remaining workers and diluting the association between exposure and effect; this healthy worker phenomenon has been reported in the laboratory animal setting (Hollander *et al.*, 1997). Estimates of the annual incidence of LAA vary between studies: a longitudinal study of workers in the pharmaceutical industry estimated an annual incidence of LAA symptoms of approximately 2 per 100 person-years, with some groups such as younger workers and those not previously exposed demonstrating higher rates (Elliott *et al.*, 2005). The risk level may vary by geographic region depending on differences in work practices and exposures; a survey of laboratory animal handlers in Brazil found evidence of occupational allergy in 16% of workers, while only 25% of respondents reported receiving orientation training in the prevention of animal allergy (Ferraz *et al.*, 2013). Other reasons for the variability in prevalence and incidence seen between studies include different criteria for diagnosis, with some studies being based on skin allergy testing, others using blood testing for IgE antibodies to specific animal allergens, and still others based largely on symptom reports.

Animal allergy typically develops within the first several years after employment. A retrospective cohort study of 99 workers in the Netherlands followed workers who were asymptomatic at the time of hire for approximately 10 years on average and reported that almost 20% of them developed animal allergy symptoms as determined by questionnaire, with atopic individuals developing symptoms more quickly (mean 45 months) compared to non-atopic individuals (mean time to symptoms 109 months) (Kruize *et al.*, 1997). In addition, after developing an allergy to one type of allergen (primary LAA), workers may develop a secondary allergy to a different type of animal allergen (secondary LAA) – a 10-year follow up study found annual incidence rates of primary and secondary LAA to be 1.34 and 11 per 100 person-years, respectively (Goodno and Stave, 2002). Reported risk factors for the development of LAA include a history of atopy, allergy to other furred pets, smoking (Venables *et al.*, 1988b), and physician-diagnosed hay fever or asthma (Pacheco, 2007).

B. Asthma and Other Respiratory Disease

A serious manifestation of LAA is the development of asthma, characterized by airway hyper-responsiveness and inflammation. Symptoms include shortness of breath,

wheezing, dry cough, and chest tightness. Symptoms may awaken the individual at night (Corradi *et al.*, 2013). The National Institute for Occupational Safety and Health has published an alert regarding the risk of asthma in animal handlers and estimated that up to 10% of animal handlers will develop occupational asthma (Massachusetts Department of Health, 1999; NIOSH, 1998). Over the first 4 years of employment, increased rates of decline in airway function including forced expiratory volume in 1 second (FEV1) and forced vital capacity (FVC) have been reported in animal workers, with the greatest decline occurring in sensitized individuals who continued to have contact with animals (Portengen *et al.*, 2003). While exposure to allergens may account for a good deal of such respiratory disease, other studies have found that exposure to airborne endotoxin, present in animal bedding and other dusts in an animal facility (see below), may play an important role in the development of airway disease and decline of respiratory function, with genetic susceptibility also playing an important role (Pacheco *et al.*, 2010). Other reported risk factors for work-related respiratory disease in animal workers include age, smoking, atopy, and skin test reactivity to non-animal allergens (Fuortes *et al.*, 1996).

C. Infectious Diseases

Zoonotic disease (infections transmitted between animals and humans) remains an occupational concern for laboratory animal workers (Hankenson *et al.*, 2003), who are considered to be at elevated risk for such infections compared to other groups of workers (Haagsma *et al.*, 2012). Veterinarians surveyed regarding infectious disease risks have reported that, at most laboratory animal facilities, programs are in place to assess and reduce the risk of vaccine-preventable infections in lab animal workers (Weigler *et al.*, 2012). A national survey of 1367 lab animal workers estimated the risk of occupational zoonoses at 45 cases per 10,000 worker-years at risk, which was similar to the rate for nonfatal occupational illnesses in the agricultural production–livestock industry and for those employed in the health services. In this survey, almost one-fourth of respondents indicated that they had been medically evaluated by a doctor or nurse for exposure to a zoonotic disease related to their laboratory animal work during the past 5 years. Only 23 persons in the sample, however, believed they were actually infected with a zoonotic agent during the same time period, with six of these cases being medically confirmed. The most frequent type of case involved dermatophytes causing ringworm, with exposure to dogs, cats, rabbits, and cattle being implicated (nine cases, four of which were medically confirmed). B virus (Macacine herpesvirus 1) was implicated in two disease incidents, although neither was medically confirmed. Some of the other reported suspected zoonotic agents in this survey included Q fever from sheep, *Giardia* spp.

from a dog, *Pasteurella* spp. related to a bite wound and a needlestick exposure, cat scratch disease, ectoparasite contact from a mouse and a rabbit, influenza from ferrets and pigs, rhinovirus from a chimpanzee, *Mycobacterium* spp. from a guinea pig, and simian foamy virus from a baboon, among others (Weigler *et al.*, 2005). Survey respondents also reported that over a third of suspected zoonotic disease cases were not reported to the employee's supervisor. Anecdotal explanations for underreporting these events included a minimization of acceptance of the perceived risks of zoonotic diseases, fear of retaliation in the workplace, the time required for medical follow-up, and lack of faith in the quality of some institutional occupational health programs (Weigler *et al.*, 2005). These findings suggest the need for significant programmatic efforts to overcome these real or perceived barriers to care.

D. Noise-Induced Hearing Loss

Elevated noise levels have been reported in animal facilities from sources such as cage cleaning and power equipment. Preventive programs for hearing conservation in workers have been recommended in such facilities, but there are few reports documenting the extent of hearing loss in this population (Randolph *et al.*, 2007). At the same time, hearing loss has been reported in other occupational groups caring for animals and using high pressure washing equipment (Kristensen and Gimsing, 1988) that may resemble noise exposures to laboratory animal workers from cage cleaning equipment.

E. Injuries

While limited information is available about the extent of physical injuries in laboratory animal workers, studies of workers caring for nonhuman primates have reported an overall injury incidence of 43.5–65.5 per 100,000 person-work-days, with higher rates for particular injuries such as bites and scratches, and higher rates of injury in particular subgroups such as veterinary residents and persons with less than 2 years of experience. At the same time, many such injuries may not be reported (bin Zakaria *et al.*, 1996). In addition to acute injuries, workers may experience cumulative trauma disorders including tendonitis from performing repetitive tasks such as cage cleaning.

F. Psychosocial Distress

In considering the overall occupational health of laboratory animal workers, their emotional and behavioral needs must be considered (Wolfle, 1985). The impact on mental health of working in laboratory animal facilities has been examined less frequently than other health outcomes such as LAA, but some have raised concerns about the emotional toll of this work on animal workers.

Particular concerns revolve around the process of becoming desensitized to euthanasia and the performing of experimental procedures, uneasiness about the value of the research being performed, difficulty discussing their work with others who may be critical of animal experimentation, and developing emotional bonds with animals that make performing some work tasks such as invasive procedures more difficult (Arluke, 1999; Halpern-Lewis, 1996). Working in nonhuman primate research facilities may be particularly stressful, particularly when animals are ill or die (Coleman, 2011). Little is known, however, about the extent and significance of such effects. Strong emotional bonds can develop between caretakers and animals in research environments (Bayne, 2002), and emotional distress has been reported among persons who regularly euthanize animals (Rohlf and Bennett, 2005).

III. OCCUPATIONAL HEALTH APPROACH

A. Occupational Health Concept

Occupational health care is a preventive medicine approach that seeks to maximize both the health and the function of workers by providing services that address individual worker concerns and health issues as well as the health-promoting aspects of the workplace. The National Research Council document *Occupational Safety and Health in the Care and Use of Research Animals* (Institute of Laboratory Animal Resources, 1997) outlines the basic components of an occupational health and safety program for animal research facilities. A similar text has been created that addresses specific occupational health issues for workers caring for nonhuman primates in research (National Research Council, 2003). Box 30.1 shows the components of an occupational health approach that begins with an effort to identify potential hazards and, whenever possible, to control or eliminate such hazards at the source. For hazards that cannot be completely controlled, screening of workers at baseline and periodically thereafter can help detect the presence of unacceptable exposures that require preventive intervention.

Beyond 'diagnosis and treatment' of the work environment, occupational health services involve assessing and managing individual worker host factors that place them at increased risk of work-related injury or illness or otherwise affect their occupational functioning. Such services include 'pre-placement' medical screening of workers for the presence of conditions that could affect the ability to work safely in the animal care environment and those that may require special accommodation. An example would be the presence of immunocompromising conditions that could predispose to zoonotic disease transmission. Another would be active infection that could pose a risk to the animals in the facility or coworkers. The administration of vaccines helps promote immune resistance to particular infectious agents, while training and education improve the ability of workers to function with the highest degree of safety as well as the optimal psychosocial approach to workplace stressors. Occupational medical surveillance involves baseline and periodic screening for the development of work-related conditions or evidence of exposure to workplace hazards. When workers suffer acute injury or illness, there is a need for prompt and effective medical management as well as consideration and recognition that the injury or illness is related to workplace exposures and constitutes a 'sentinel health event,' indicating the presence of a workplace hazard and/or a breakdown in the system of workplace exposure controls. Management of the injured or ill worker also requires consideration of particular work restrictions on work, including job modification, or, in some circumstances, removal from the workplace. All of these services need to be provided in a manner that protects worker confidentiality, including the management and safekeeping of occupational health records.

B. Occupational Health Team: Roles and Responsibilities

A unique challenge of occupational health in the animal care setting is that it involves the health of the workers, the animals, and the shared work environment. These interrelationships require a systems-based, comprehensive approach that seeks to simultaneously maximize human, animal, and environmental health. This concept is increasingly recognized as a 'One Health' approach requiring interdisciplinary cooperation between multiple types of professionals. Professionals that could contribute to such a One Health 'team' for occupational health in animal care settings include human health care providers, veterinarians, industrial hygienists, and engineers.

Improving animal workers' occupational health and safety is a challenge that requires collaboration among the occupational health team. One Health occupational health services include enhancing surveillance to detect exposure events; assessing infection risk in specific tasks; reducing risk through animal disease control; and interrupting transmission pathways by appropriate use of engineering controls, work practices, and personal protective equipment. To ensure that steps are taken in such a way as to maximize both human and animal health, input from all team members – human, animal, and environmental health/industrial hygiene – is crucial in these efforts.

1. Occupational Health Care Providers

Health care services for laboratory animal workers are often delivered by a team of providers that may include physicians, advanced practice nurses, physician associates, licensed nurses, and medical assistants. The composition of the health care team may vary widely depending on the size of the facility and the type of services required. Some animal care facilities have an on-site clinic, while others rely on off-site providers or facilities. Physicians providing occupational health services to laboratory animal workers may be board certified in Occupational and Environmental Medicine by the American Board of Preventive Medicine (ABPM), but many other physicians providing such services may be general internists, family physicians, infectious disease specialists, or others. Likewise, nurses may have received training and certification in occupational health nursing (OHN) including advanced practice training, but many nurses in occupational health facilities have not gone through such training. Therefore, the background and training in the principles of occupational medicine, including the special problems faced by laboratory animal workers, may vary widely between physicians and other human health care provider members of the occupational health team. In the case of work with nonhuman primates of the genus *Macaca*, it is essential for programs to have medical consultants available who are knowledgeable about B virus (Macacine herpesvirus 1) and other hazards associated with these species for appropriate prompt and follow-up care of persons with potential exposure (Cohen *et al.*, 2002).

2. Veterinary Staff

Veterinarians working in the laboratory animal setting may complete internships, residencies, such as comparative medicine and pathology residencies, and further specialize in their field of practice to focus on the laboratory animal environment. Specialty board certification of veterinarians in the American College of Laboratory Animal Medicine (ACLAM) demonstrates their expertise in this field and thus ACLAM diplomats are frequently considered core members of the occupational health team. Veterinary and research support technicians may or may not be licensed, depending upon the hiring institution and the state's requirements. Because they deal with animal diseases and the necessary procedures involved in animal care and handling, veterinary and research support staff members play an important role in the development of occupational safety and health strategies for animal workers.

3. Industrial Hygienist

Industrial Hygiene (also known as Occupational Hygiene or Environmental Exposure Assessment and Control) is the practice of preventing and controlling environmental factors in the workplace which may cause impaired health or significant discomfort among workers. Industrial hygienists may have a baccalaureate, masters, and/or graduate degree. Certified Industrial hygienists (CIH) have completed academic training, accumulated 4 years of work experience, passed a certification exam, and are re-certified every 5 years. Industrial hygienists monitor and analyze workplace hazards – chemical, physical, biological, or psychosocial – and devise engineering, work practice controls, and other methods to control these hazards.

4. Infection Control/Biosafety Officer

Many institutions have designated officials who oversee infection control policies and procedures. A Biosafety officer (BSO) is an individual appointed by an institution to oversee management of biosafety risks. Institutions are required to have a BSO if they are funded by the U.S. National Institutes of Health and engage in basic or clinical research with recombinant or synthetic nucleic acid molecules designated for use in Biosafety level 3 or Biosafety Level 4 containment procedures, or engage in research or production activities with large amounts (greater than 10 liters) of this type of material. Biosafety officers are involved in biosafety in laboratories involving animals as well as those handling specific pathogens. These officials can help ensure that workable policies and procedures are in place for the reduction of infectious risk to workers. They can evaluate the biosafety risks involved with particular pathogens, animal species and experimental procedures, recommend particular hazard controls to reduce exposure risks (see below), and oversee and conduct training of workers in specific procedures to reduce chances of microbial contamination.

5. Laboratory Animal Care Workers

The animal care workers themselves form a critical part of the occupational health team for animal care

facilities. Technical certification of animal care workers by the American Association for Laboratory Animal Science demonstrates alignment with professional standards for the field and is used to help ensure levels of competence, including topics involving occupational health and safety. Feedback from workers is helpful in identifying new hazards as well as innovative methods for control of such hazards.

6. Animal Care and Use Committee

Most institutions that engage in animal research, teaching, or testing have ongoing, internal oversight by their appointed IACUC which is charged with overseeing all aspects of the institution's animal care and use program. An undetermined number of smaller institutions in the United States may have LAA without the benefit of IACUC oversight depending upon the species held, the type of institution, the location where animals are used, and the source of their funding, but this is considered unusual under contemporary standards of care. IACUC activities include reviewing proposed animal care and use protocols and considering the impacts on both animal health and well-being. IACUC review, at least in the case of institutions receiving federal funding and/or those which are accredited by the Association for Assessment and Accreditation of Laboratory Animal Care International), may also include consideration of potential occupational risks to the laboratory animal workers engaged in the protocol. If such occupational health risks are identified, the matter may be referred to other health and safety committees or offices.

IV. HAZARD IDENTIFICATION

Workplace hazards can be categorized into four major categories: physical, chemical, biological, and psychosocial. The physical, chemical, and biological hazards are often more apparent, yet psychosocial hazards are increasingly recognized. All types of hazards must be identified and managed by coordinated efforts of the laboratory occupational health and safety team.

A. Biological Hazards

Biological hazards in animal laboratories include zoonoses (covered in more detail in Chapter 25), allergens, genetically altered or wild-type pathogens in experimental protocols, and contaminant pathogens in cultured cell media, bacterial toxins, and recombinant genetic material. Genetically altered pathogens may have more or less pathogenicity to animals or humans than the wild-type, and exposures to such pathogens may present the possibility of unique health risks.

Biohazard exposures can occur through inhalation, ingestion, parenteral, ocular and other mucus membrane, and cutaneous routes. Examples of inhalational exposure risks include *Mycobacterium tuberculosis*, influenza viruses, hantaviruses, Q fever, and others depending on the animals species. Risk of unintentional ingestion of bacterial zoonotic agents (e.g., *Shigella*, *Salmonella*, and *Campylobacter*) depends on the species handled (see Chapter 25), and may result in gastrointestinal illness and infection in lab workers. Injury with contaminated sharps, including needles or scalpels, or wounds sustained from animal bites and scratches may result in parenteral inoculation of pathogens such as *Pasteurella*, B virus, and *Bartonella henselae*. Infection may result from direct skin, eye, or mucous membrane exposure, and cutaneous exposures may also result in transmission of dermatophytes and zoonotic species of ectoparasites, as well as contact allergy. Animal studies involving human blood, patient-derived tumor xenografts, AIDS-related models of human disease, and other potentially infectious material which are subject to OSHA's Bloodborne Pathogens standards, present additional recognized biohazard risks from human pathogens including HIV and hepatitis B (Zel, 2003). The magnitude of occupational risk from biohazards can be classified based on pathogenicity and treatment availability in case of human disease (Choosewood and Wilson, 2009).

1. Allergens

As described above, LAA is one of the most prevalent occupational conditions affecting laboratory animal workers. In addition to exposures in the workplace, studies of the homes of laboratory animal workers have revealed significant levels of animal allergen in mattress dust, suggesting that workers can bring animal allergens home in uncovered hair and clothes and potentially expose family members and others in the community (Krop *et al.*, 2007).

Mouse and rat urinary allergens are a major source of inhalable allergenic protein for laboratory animal worker exposure. Air sampling during work tasks has revealed that washing and cleaning cages and number of mice handled daily can be determinants of personal exposures to mouse urinary allergen (Glueck *et al.*, 2012). At the same time, a study of workers at a mouse facility found that the day-to-day variability of exposure levels to mouse allergen was a significant predictor of skin-test positivity to this allergen, suggesting that peak exposures may play an important role in addition to average daily exposure (Peng *et al.*, 2011). While the levels of exposure to animal allergens appear to correlate with the development of allergies, there is evidence that atopic individuals working in animal facilities in jobs that do not involve direct contact with animals (such as office workers) may also be at significant risk for development

of LAA through indirect exposure to lower levels of allergen (Jang *et al.*, 2009).

In addition to concern about low-level exposure to allergens, the dose–response relationship between allergen exposure levels and development of allergy may be complex. Some investigators have postulated that exposure to high allergen levels can induce production of immunoglobulin G4 antibodies which may play a protective role in attenuating the risk of allergic sensitization (Matsui *et al.*, 2005). As a result, some studies show the highest rates of sensitization in workers exposed at moderate levels of allergen (Pacheco, 2007). Genetic susceptibility of the individual also plays an important role in allergic sensitization (Jones, 2008).

There is evidence that allergenicity of animal allergens varies between species. A large study of animal workers found that allergy symptoms were higher for those exposed to rabbits compared to mouse, rats, and guinea pigs, and that hamsters were unlikely to be associated with allergic symptoms (Elliott *et al.*, 2005). In addition, male rodents have been reported to cause greater degrees of allergen sensitization than female rodents, since males excrete higher levels of urinary protein antigens compared to females (Renströ *et al.*, 2001). Insects may be a significant source of allergen in workers as well (Lopata *et al.*, 2005). Allergy to nonhuman primates appears to be rare (Jeal *et al.*, 2010).

In addition to specific animal allergens, there is evidence from chamber studies of individuals with LAA that other allergens such as dust mites may play a role in the development of occupational rhinitis and other allergies in the laboratory animal environment (Ruoppi *et al.*, 2004, 2005).

2. Endotoxin

Another biological exposure that may cause symptoms that resemble LAA is endotoxin that may be aerosolized during work with rodents and other species. Daily endotoxin exposure has been found to correlate with respiratory and skin symptoms in non-mouse sensitized lab animal workers (Pacheco *et al.*, 2003).

B. Physical Hazards

Physical hazards facing the laboratory animal worker depend on the particular lab and experimental protocols, but may include heat, noise, vibration, ultraviolet light, and ionizing radiation. Unique exposures of concern in an animal lab would include bites, scratches, and other musculoskeletal strain from lifting and handling larger animals for daily care and research procedures, such as some species of nonhuman primates, livestock, and laboratory dogs. In addition, lifting and pushing heavy bags of feed and bedding, racks of water bottles, and animal cages may provoke back injury or other musculoskeletal strains or sprains. Slips, trips, and falls may occur when working on wet or slippery surfaces (Langley, 1999). Repetitive tasks in animal care, such as water bottle handling, cage cleaning, and cage washing, may cause tendonitis or other soft-tissue musculoskeletal injuries.

Cage wash and surgical facilities typically have steam autoclaves which can present substantial risks of burn injuries for dry or liquid loads. Glass bead sterilizers used for small surgical instruments and hot water and steam lines common in animal facilities present additional burn injury hazards. Facilities with cage/rack washers and bulk sterilizers, which personnel enter for loading and unloading, can become entrapment hazards with dire consequences, thus it is essential that they are equipped with functioning safety devices that are readily available for staff to activate (National Research Council, 2011).

Instrumentation presents its own set of hazards, including scalpel and needle-stick injuries. Use of sharp objects such as the guillotine for small animal decapitation has inherent danger (AVMA Panel on Euthanasia, 2013). Performing euthanasia using captive bolt stunners or gunshot may also pose injury risks to the operator or assistant (Morrow, 1999).

Noise levels in animal facilities have been found to represent a potential hazard to worker hearing. High noise levels for laboratory animal workers include exposure to the vocalization for some species such as dogs and swine (Kristensen and Gimsing, 1988). Other noise sources include cage cleaning and decontamination equipment (Pate et al., 2013). Because of differences in hearing ranges, humans may be more susceptible to the harmful effects of certain noise sources compared to the laboratory animals (Reynolds et al., 2010).

C. Chemical Hazards

Depending on the particular use and task performed, exposure to chemicals can occur through inhalation, ingestion, mucocutaneous contact, or percutaneous inoculation. The broad spectrum of chemical hazards reflects the multiple uses of chemicals in labs. Sterilants and disinfectants are needed for many laboratory hygiene tasks, and commonly include ethanol, isopropyl alcohol, formaldehyde, glutaraldehyde, orthophthalaldehyde, phenol and phenolic compounds, hydrogen peroxide, potassium permanganate, ethylene oxide, sodium hypochlorite, and chlorine dioxide. These chemicals may be used for decontaminating lab surfaces, sterilizing equipment, or cleaning animal cages. Many of these compounds are acutely irritating to the eyes, upper respiratory tract, and skin. Ethanol and isopropyl alcohol present a flammable hazard.

Formaldehyde and glutaraldehyde are sensitizers, and can cause allergic symptoms and occupational asthma. Phenol, formaldehyde (or formalin, a solution of formaldehyde with methanol stabilizer), and potassium permanganate are examples of common animal laboratory disinfectants that can cause severe effects in cases of significant overexposure. Phenol exposure can cause neurologic, respiratory, and cardiac toxicity, and death. Concentrated potassium permanganate is corrosive and can cause severe burns to exposed skin, and in case of ingestion, severe gastritis and perforation. Anesthesia and euthanasia agents are other commonly encountered chemical hazards (Meyer, 1999). Exposures to nitrous oxide or halogenated gases may occur during administration of these gaseous agents. While many historical studies of the health effects of occupational anesthesia exposures have been methodologically challenging, occupational exposure to nitrous oxide has been associated with fertility problems, including spontaneous abortions and decreased fertility (Rowland et al., 1992, 1995). If anesthetic gases are used, waste gas scavenging techniques are essential to reducing the hazard (Flecknell, 1996). OSHA has not yet specified permissible exposure limits for isoflurane and sevoflurane and both are commonly used volatile anesthetics in this field. These agents generally cannot be detected by odor until room air concentrations are high, so leak testing of equipment and emission monitors should be used in assessing these hazards through various applications with laboratory animals. Highly effective methods to help mitigate anesthetic pollution generated from their use in various contexts with laboratory rodents have been described (Smith and Bolon, 2006; Taylor and Mook, 2009; Todd et al., 2013). Injectable anesthetics and tranquilizers including ketamine, etomidate, barbiturates, opioids, and paralytics, may induce dose-related effects on animals and administering humans alike. Some animal tranquilizers are extremely potent and acute loss of consciousness has been reported with minimal percutaneous exposure (Meyer, 1999). Gases used in euthanasia are generally the same as those used for anesthesia, but are administered at higher doses and duration, typically in conjunction with a secondary method to ensure animal death. Therefore, the same hazards exist. Euthanasia by gaseous agents should be performed with particular caution due to the possibility of higher concentrations of exposure in the administering worker. In addition, euthanasia procedures may utilize different gases, such as carbon dioxide, carbon monoxide, nitrogen, or argon. Carbon monoxide is an odorless, tasteless gas, and causes dose-related acute central nervous system toxicity (including unconsciousness and death at high doses). Chronic exposure can cause neuropsychiatric and cardiovascular disease (Raub *et al.*, 2000) and defects in the developing fetus, which is more sensitive to the effects than the pregnant mother (Ernst and Zibrak, 1998). Pesticides may be used in laboratory animal facilities to control ticks, fleas, and other insects, and these carry unique risks depending on the specific agent (Meggs, 1999). As for other health-related professions, institutions should remain vigilant to the potential for substance abuse by laboratory animal workers where controlled drugs and other pharmaceutical agents are used in their veterinary care and research-related programs. Laboratory euthanasia agents also pose a risk of use by laboratory animal workers to commit suicide, as has been reported among veterinary workers (Bartram and Baldwin, 2010).

D. Psychosocial Hazards

Minimizing psychosocial hazards is vital to maintaining a healthy and productive workplace environment. Occupational psychosocial hazards include a broad range of work-related stressors, including job demand, job control, and relationships between employees. In the case of animal workers, the relationship between employees and animals would be an additional domain of occupational psychosocial hazards. The human–animal relationship in a research laboratory is complex, and may revolve around the psychological dissonance of lab animals as pets to be loved *versus* objects to be used (Arluke, 1988; Herzog, 1989). Emotional bonds between laboratory workers and animal subjects result from a variety of normal work circumstances and activities, including close and frequent contact and animal care staff as sole providers for animal needs. A sense of unique attachment may develop with animals felt to have more personality (more friendly, intelligent, courageous, etc.) (Bayne, 2002). Stress and feelings of isolation have been reported and further investigation into the emotional effects of working with laboratory animals is underway (Davies and Lewis, 2010).

Maintaining animal enclosures, capturing wild animals, or euthanizing animals for experimental purposes can cause significant psychological distress for some individuals. Laboratory workers should be aware of early signs of mental illness in themselves or their colleagues, which may include depression, lethargy, appetite change, insomnia, irritability, decreased concentration, labile mood, and impaired relationships. Persistent symptoms may be due to true disease states of depression or anxiety. Such symptoms can lead to loss of work, high staff turnover, low morale, and decreased productivity (American Association for Laboratory Animal Science, 2013), as well as significant health consequences including risk of severe depression and suicide.

V. HAZARD CONTROLS

In controlling workplace hazards, a hierarchy of methods has been employed to successfully control hazards in a wide variety of workplaces. This hierarchy is shown in Figure 30.1. The basic concept is that controlling hazards at the source (represented as the top of the hierarchy) is potentially more effective and protective than control measures at the bottom, and leads to an inherently safer workplace.

As Figure 30.1 shows, elimination of a hazard is the most effective form of control, whereas the least effective form of hazard control involves use of personal protective equipment. Table 30.1 outlines different levels of controls for particular classes of hazards in laboratory animal care.

A. Control of Biological Hazards

Control of biological hazards can be performed using the hierarchy of controls described above. Elimination of allergy risk may involve finding an alternative to the use of a particular animal model. Substitution can involve use of less allergenic species. Engineering controls include the use of individually ventilated HEPA-filtered caging systems in conjunction with HEPA-filtered cage change and bedding dump enclosures (particularly for laboratory rodents), high-efficiency particulate air-filtered room ventilation, increased room air exchanges, dust-free bedding, and use of filter-top cages. Work practice controls include limiting animal density, implementing wet-shaving practices, performing high-risk tasks in a biological safety hood (Sharpe, 2009), altering work processes using robotics and other techniques to reduce required animal handling, and establishment of regular housecleaning routines. Other recommended control steps include the use of masks and gloves as well as overalls and head coverings (Table 30.1). A program at a

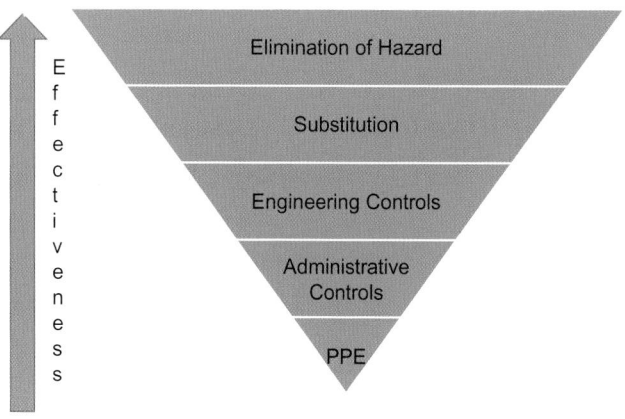

FIGURE 30.1 Hierarchy of controls (http://www.cdc.gov/niosh/topics/engcontrols/).

TABLE 30.1   Control of Occupational Hazards in Laboratory Animal Facilities

Hazard	Elimination	Substitution	Engineering controls	Administrative/work practice controls, training	Personal protective equipment
BIOLOGICAL					
Laboratory animal allergens/ endotoxin	Eliminate need for a particular source of allergen or endotoxin	Use less allergenic species, change type of bedding	Individually ventilated cages, negative pressure, HEPA filtration, filter-top cages	Perform high-risk task in a safety hood, or using robotics, restrict sensitized workers from further exposure, consider special measures for atopic workers, control animal density	Head covering, N95 masks, gloves, dedicated shoes or shoe covers, respirators where indicated, protective gowns/clothing which are not worn beyond the boundary of the work area
Zoonoses	Reduce pathogens in animals through rederivation of colonies to pathogen-free status, quarantine, vaccination	Choose species and sources with less zoonotic pathogen potential	Ventilation, work surfaces easy to disinfect, isolate sick animals, animal housing and use within HEPA filtered enclosures, sharps injury protection, and needleless systems	Regular use of disinfectants, hand hygiene, avoid eating and drinking in animal areas, sanitize items coming out of animal areas, consider restriction for pregnant, immunocompromised workers	Head covering, gloves, N95 masks, dedicated shoes or shoe covers, facial protection for spray or splash exposures, respirators or PAPRs where indicated, arm protectors where indicated
CHEMICAL					
Disinfectants, cleaners		Less toxic cleaners	Adequate ventilation during cleaning		Gloves, chemical respirators, eye protection when indicated
Anesthetic gases		Less toxic agents	Adequate ventilation/ scavenging systems	Waste gas monitors	Gloves, respirators
PHYSICAL					
Slips, trips, falls		Less slippery floor material selection, cleaner selection		Control access to areas with slip and fall hazards, training, signage	Non-slip boots or covers in wet floor areas
Repetitive motion injury	Elimination or automation of task	Modification of task	Improved design of tools and equipment to minimize ergonomic risks	Limitation of task duration, institution of rest periods and staff rotation	Wrist protectors, other local measures
Radiation			Adequate radiological shielding	Training in radiation safety measures, work restriction for pregnant workers	Lead radiation shielding (gloves, aprons)
Noise	Eliminate noisy machines and processes	Substitute less noisy machines or tools	Noise shielding	Training about avoidance of excessive noise	Hearing protection
Heat			Emergency shut off and de-energizing mechanisms for cage/rack washers and bulk sterilizers	Training in burn prevention and in cage/rack washer and bulk autoclave safety devices	Heat resistant gloves and gauntlets for autoclaves and rack washers
PSYCHOLOGICAL					
Stress	Eliminate certain stressful procedures	Change protocols for euthanasia or other stressful procedures		Counseling for workers, training, restrict workers who are experiencing acute distress	

pharmaceutical company used a combination of worker training and education, modification of work practices, engineering controls, and use of personal protective equipment, including mandatory respiratory protection and medical surveillance, to significantly reduce the annual incidence of LAA (Fisher *et al.*, 1998). Despite such reports of success in individual programs, a national survey of institutional officials at NIH-identified laboratory animal facilities found wide differences between institutional programs to reduce animal allergy and that, while 80% required use of uniforms and gloves, only 25% required the use of N95 respirators (which offer greater protection than dust masks) (Stave and Darcey, 2012).

In recent decades, the virtual elimination of most zoonotic diseases and other communicable agents from commercial breeders and vendors of commonly used species, designated within the domain of specific pathogen-free colonies, has greatly benefited the control of zoonotic pathogen biohazards for laboratory animal workers. Ongoing surveillance for zoonotic disease through microbiological monitoring programs of animal colonies, avoidance and exclusion of high-risk species such as wild and feral animals (unless they are the subject for field biology studies), biosafety measures including use of fume hoods and HEPA-filtered cabinets to reduce inhalation exposures, prevention of contact with body fluids of a potentially infected animal, bite, scratch, and splash prevention programs, prompt post-exposure response action including wound cleansing and medical follow-up, vector control, sharps and needlestick prevention, use of personal protective equipment which should not leave the animal facility, strict measures of waste control, and high standards of sanitation for animal facility surfaces and housing and use equipment.

B. Control of Physical Hazards

Physical hazards in the laboratory should be minimized in order to prevent worker injury. Exposure modification should also be accompanied by appropriate training in use of equipment, with particular attention to equipment that is potentially unsafe. Such equipment may include cages, collars, traps, and harnesses. Laboratory workers should be educated in the behavior of the animals they will handle, in order to foster healthy laboratory human–animal interactions that reflect the handler's patience and proficiency and promote animal tractability. In addition, all personnel should be instructed in the proper techniques of approaching and handling animals to avoid kicks, bites, and scratches to the extent possible. Personal protective equipment may include non-penetrable and heat-resistant gloves or gauntlets, arm sleeves, slip-resistant footwear, coats or coveralls, and eye and face protection as appropriate to the species and tasks involved. Use of proper ergonomic technique is advised to minimize stress and strain on joints and soft tissues that may occur in performing both less stressful routine repetitive tasks with risk of cumulative trauma, as well as more intermittent tasks with higher stress and strain. Administrative controls, such as rest periods and task rotation between technicians, may also help reduce repetitive motion injuries by decreasing frequency of exposure to such physical hazards.

C. Control of Chemical Hazards

Training in proper storage, use, and disposal of laboratory chemicals is essential for workplace safety. Proper containment and sequestration of gases, including use of specialized anesthesia chambers and effective waste scavenging methods, is recommended to reduce chronic occupational exposures to these anesthetic gases, thereby reducing health risk to workers. Use of properly stored, unexpired equipment is recommended to avoid mechanical failure while administering such potent pharmacological compounds (Flecknell, 1996). Material safety data sheets (MSDS, or the new standard Safety Data Sheets, SDS) on all chemicals used in the laboratory must be accessible to all workers (OSHA, 2011) and persons responsible for using chemicals must be trained in how to properly interpret those documents for safe practices, including spill clean-up. All workers must be informed regarding the location and proper operation of safety information and location of eye washes, showers, and other safety procedures in the event of acute exposures. Essential safety equipment such as eye-wash stations should be tested periodically to ensure it is functioning properly. The proper selection and use of personal protective equipment, including the correct model and material of gloves, eye, and face protection relative to the type of task, should be guided by experienced professionals. Chemical waste-disposal methods must be consistent with regulatory standards, and room ventilation parameters should be conducive to worker safety during use of volatile chemicals in addition to meeting research animal environmental requirements. Storage and methods for dispensing of controlled substances and other drugs subject to abuse should be closely scrutinized and aligned with regulatory standards of diversion control, including disposal of waste and expired volumes.

D. Control of Psychosocial Hazards

Administrative controls should include implementing practices that help in coping with job responsibilities, which may include assisting coworkers in more difficult tasks (e.g., euthanasia), avoiding particularly distressful situations (euthanizing favorite animals), maintaining a laboratory pet, or implementing workplace rituals or memorials for animal subjects (Arluke, 1999; Iliff, 2002). Education, including initial training on the mechanisms of humane euthanasia, has been suggested to help lower the risk of emotional dissonance (American Association for Laboratory Animal Science, 2013). Training laboratory animals for routine procedures can reduce stress in both the laboratory personnel performing the procedure as well as the animals (Bayne, 2002).

VI. OCCUPATIONAL MEDICINE SERVICES

A. Pre-Placement Evaluations

An occupational pre-placement evaluation is a medical examination conducted following an offer of employment to a new worker. The purpose of the evaluation is to determine whether there are any disabilities or other medical conditions that will require accommodation in the workplace in order for an employee to work safely without danger to themselves or others. This examination is also an opportunity for preventive services, including an assessment of occupational risks in the job, health and safety training, necessary vaccinations, and consideration of baseline testing. In general, there are no standard regulations for the content of such pre-placement evaluations; however, recommended components include a face-to-face physical examination and medical history, completion of a risk questionnaire, and consideration of additional diagnostic testing (such as baseline spirometry) as indicated (Nicholson *et al.*, 2010).

The pre-placement evaluation should begin with a review of the worker's basic medical and occupational history. The examiner should enquire as to prior work experience with animals, including specific species and any health problems related to this work. Past medical conditions related to laboratory work exposures should be carefully documented. A history of allergies or asthma in the worker would prompt additional allergy work-up and may necessitate closer monitoring (see below). Reported risk factors for development of LAA include a history of allergies or atopy. While the association between smoking and development of lab animal allergy is uncertain, smoking predisposes to lung disease and should be assessed, as should a previous history of asthma or other lung disease (Corradi *et al.*, 2013). Specific tasks of the job, including grooming, feeding, and procedures involving animals, should be reviewed in detail. The examination should assess for any deficiencies in ability to perform essential duties of the job. In addition, vaccination history should be reviewed, with particular attention to any vaccines required or recommended for pathogens that may be present in the animals or laboratory.

The history should also include current medical problems, including medical conditions that could increase the susceptibility of the worker to infections. Such conditions could include pregnancy, cancer, use of steroids or other immunosuppressive medications, or HIV infection. Female workers of child-bearing age should be counseled during the preplacement visit to consult with a medical provider if they are contemplating pregnancy or if they become pregnant, and all workers should be counseled to notify the occupational medicine service if they develop a new medical condition that could affect their immune status. The history should also screen for risk factors for occupational allergy, including a history of asthma or hay fever. If latex is present in the facility, the clinician should take a careful history for any history of latex allergy. The physical examination should focus on signs of atopy or allergy, including a careful examination of the head and neck, skin, and lungs. If a respirator will be worn, assessing physical barriers to the use of a respirator such as a beard or facial deformity is part of a medical clearance for such use under the OSHA respirator standard (OSHA, 2011). Use of a screening questionnaire helps ensure that the history is comprehensive and standardized for all workers; an example of such a baseline screening questionnaire is included as Appendix 30.1. If an N-95 or other type of respirator will be used, OSHA requires completion of a medical screening questionnaire as well (OSHA, 2011, Appendix C).

1. Risk Assessment

Based on the results of history and physical exam, and with knowledge of the hazards faced by workers in a particular job, the clinician should perform a risk assessment and determine whether the worker can safely perform the proposed job with or without particular accommodations. One suggested approach to risk assessment for biohazards and microbial contamination in laboratory animal medicine is based on consideration of the five 'Ps.' This is a mnemonic for Pathogens, the proposed experimental Procedure (including the species involved), the Personnel involved, the Protective equipment and work practices used, and factors related to the Place or facility (Fontes, 2008). An example would be a worker who has a documented allergy to a particular animal, such as a cat, and who may be at increased risk of developing allergy to other species as well. Another example would be a worker with cardiac disease who may be at increased risk from endocarditis due to Q-fever and therefore may need to be restricted from work with high-risk animals such as pregnant sheep. In performing the risk assessment, the clinician may wish to consult with other members of the team such as veterinarians and industrial hygienists in order to better understand the hazard and discuss whether special measures will be necessary to reduce risk for an individual.

It is important that this risk assessment process and determination of necessary accommodations, if any, be conducted with safeguards for the confidentiality of the medical information regarding the employee, in order to prevent workplace discrimination. For example, if work restrictions are necessary, this can be communicated to a supervisor without disclosing details about the medical condition.

The Pregnant Worker

In assessing occupational risk for a pregnant worker, clinicians must consider risks to both the mother and fetus. Pregnancy has been considered a period of relative immunocompromise and fetuses are at increased susceptibility to a number of occupational exposures. The complexity of the maternal immune response relative to the fetal/placental unit is being re-examined, which could impact appropriate prophylaxis or therapeutic measures (Mor and Cardenas, 2010). Anesthetic gases represent one occupational hazard with particular risks in pregnancy, as do exposures to particular therapeutic agents. Pregnant women are at increased risk of infection with *Coxiella burnetti*, the etiologic agent for Q fever. Referral to a genetic counselor or the patient's treating obstetric provider may be necessary to review specific pregnancy risks.

The Immunocompromised Worker

An individual may have compromised immune system function due to a medical condition or medications. Immune-compromising conditions include malignancy, chemotherapy-induced immunosuppression, biopharmaceutical-induced immunosuppressants, HIV infection, and congenital immunodeficiencies. Such individuals may need special counseling about risks of infection from their job, such as the risk of Lymphocytic Choriomeningitis Virus (LCMV) infection; salmonella, shigella, and other enteric agents from various species; and research-related hazards including radioisotopes, chemicals, and etiological agents used in animal models of human disease.

2. Baseline Testing

As stated above, there are no regulatory requirements for baseline testing of laboratory animal workers, and therefore testing should be customized to the types of species and other exposures that will be encountered.

If there are concerns about pathogen exposures, testing for antibodies to specific pathogens is indicated, such as hepatitis B surface antibody for workers who will be working with this agent. Rigorous programs for *Mycobacterium tuberculosis* (TB) surveillance are indicated for workers who enter or use facilities housing nonhuman primates. These typically involve intradermal skin testing of workers using purified protein derivative, or

interferon-γ release assays, symptom questionnaires, radiographic tests, or a combination of the above. Motivation for such programs has been principally directed at reducing the risk for non-human primate colonies due to their susceptibility to *Mycobacterium tuberculosis* complex (MTBC) agents, including *M. tuberculosis*, *M. bovis*, and others. Outbreaks of MTBC agents among nonhuman primate research colonies continue to occur, most commonly among recently imported groups (Panarella and Bimes, 2010). Tuberculosis research workers involving other species of animals should also be included in these programs, and some workplace settings (e.g., research hospitals) may require TB testing of all staff for reasons independent of animal contact. Documentation of recent immunization or sufficient immunity to measles virus (rubeola) among persons who work with nonhuman primates is likewise important as part of the medical clearance process for laboratory animal workers due to the high susceptibility of many nonhuman primate species to infection with significant sequelae (Willy *et al.*, 1999) and the possibility of bidirectional transmission between non-immune humans and animals.

For baseline assessment of the risk of LAA and asthma, some authorities have recommended baseline testing for particular animal allergens by serum IgE antibody testing or pinprick allergy testing (OSHA, 2011). Others have recommended baseline spirometry testing of lung function (Nicholson *et al.*, 2010), although rigorous evidence to support such screening on a routine basis is lacking.

In some facilities, baseline serology is collected and banked to assess possible seroconversion due to exposure to infectious agents in the future. At present, however, there is no consensus about the value of such serum banking, such banking poses logistical challenges including storage and cost, and it is not currently routinely performed in most laboratory animal facilities.

B. Vaccines

Similar to testing decisions, recommendations for vaccination of laboratory animal workers are often based on the species or biological agents they will be working with. In general, immunization programs for laboratory animal workers should follow the recommendations of the Advisory Committee on Immunization Practices for the U.S. civilian population, including tetanus toxoid boosters every 10 years (CDC, 2013). Persons with occupational exposures subject to OSHA's Bloodborne Pathogens standards should be offered hepatitis B vaccination, and the extent to which that applies to laboratory animal workers is appropriately guided by the occupational health providers and the institutional biosafety officer. Rabies laboratory research workers or animal workers encountering wildlife species or non-purpose bred dogs and cats with uncertain rabies immunization histories should be considered for pre-exposure rabies vaccination (Lang, 2005). The use of non-highly attenuated strains of vaccinia virus as recombinant vector systems for animal-based research in infectious diseases, cancer, and other areas of study may dictate the performance and documentation of satisfactory vaccination of laboratory animal workers with potential exposure. Additional vaccines may be necessary depending on the particular biological agents used in the lab and should be directed by occupational risk assessment methods applicable to each institution's program of care.

C. Training and Education

Resources for the technical training and certification of laboratory animal workers by the American Association for Laboratory Animal Science are noted above, and several other specialty organizations and scientific resources exist to help bridge communication about occupational health issues applicable to this field. National surveys have reported that in many organizations, awareness of the prevalence and incidence of LAA varies widely, suggesting the need for better evidence-based training and education (Stave and Darcey, 2012). Laboratory workers should take all required safety and biosafety training from their institution in order to safely perform work tasks. Such training should be completed at baseline and there should be periodic refreshers. Completion of such training should be documented for each worker. Training should cover a review of specific hazards in the workplace and the availability of resources, including material safety data sheets and access to professional advice regarding specific issues. Educational materials should be appropriate to the literacy level and language of the learners. Particular points to cover in training include the early recognition of symptoms that could indicate development of an allergic condition, work-related infectious disease or other work-related condition, and how to seek help in such a situation.

D. Monitoring and Surveillance

Pre-placement and periodic health assessments should be focused on ascertaining and minimizing risk of occupational illness and injury in the animal laboratory worker. These examinations should be viewed as opportunities to recognize occupational health interventions that may improve the health and productivity of the workers.

Surveillance examinations should screen for occupational illnesses that may have developed over the course of time. In addition, the examiner should enquire if there were any injuries related to work. The surveillance examination is also an appropriate opportunity to screen for development of anxiety, depression, or general concerns related to animal handling in the laboratory. Any change in laboratory animal species or specific pathogens that enter the lab should trigger an updated health assessment for the laboratory workers. Any other changes in work tasks should be documented and assessed for potential health risks; the examination should again focus on fitness to perform the essential functions of the job. If the laboratory requires the use of respirators (even if just for specific tasks), then respirator program review, including OSHA questionnaires to workers, should be administered on an annual basis.

1. Screening for Animal Allergies

Surveillance for animal allergies should be prioritized in the first 2–3 years of employment, when many cases develop (Moscato et al., 2011). One basic way to screen for the development of LAA is to administer a periodic questionnaire that asks about the development of new symptoms or worsening of existing symptoms: an example of such a questionnaire is provided as Appendix 30.2. If workers complain about potentially allergic symptoms such as rhinitis, conjunctivitis, or dermatitis, an in-person evaluation by a clinician is indicated, and further testing may include repeat serum or skin prick testing for IgE allergy. In evaluating workers with symptoms such as rhinitis, clinicians should keep in mind that such symptoms may be due to exposure to airborne irritants including chemicals and endotoxin as well as allergens (Ruoppi et al., 2004; Zhao and Shusterman, 2012).

2. Screening for Occupational Asthma

The use of a symptom questionnaire as described above to identify potential cases of occupational asthma has been found to have equivalent value to screening workers with serial lung testing (spirometry) (Allan et al., 2010). If a worker complains of symptoms consistent with asthma including wheezing, shortness of breath, cough, or chest tightness on a questionnaire such as is shown in Appendix 30.2, or if the worker is seen by a medical provider with such complaints, further medical evaluation is indicated (Tarlo et al., 2008). This evaluation could include spirometry testing of lung function, with bronchodilator response testing if the baseline spirometry shows a decrease in FEV1, or methacholine challenge if the spirometry appears normal. The employee can be provided with a peak flow meter and keep a serial peak flow diary to detect variability in airway function and determine whether work exposures are associated with a decrease in peak flows. Management of individuals suspected of having occupational asthma is described below.

3. Screening for Zoonotic Diseases

In addition to screening for allergy, the periodic questionnaire should also enquire about symptoms consistent with infectious disease, including episodes of fever, pneumonia, and diarrhea. Tuberculosis status can be monitored with annual or semiannual yearly skin testing by one or more methods, as already detailed. If particular infectious diseases are suspected on such screening, serological testing, or direct exam (e.g., stool cultures or other assays in the case of enteric infections) can be performed, and referral to an infectious disease specialist may be indicated. The medical management of acute exposures to herpes B virus (Macacine herpesvirus 1) is addressed below.

4. Screening for Hearing Loss

Under the 1983 OSHA noise standard, workers exposed to occupational noise of 85 dBA or greater averaged over an 8-hour work shift (8 h TWA) should be enrolled in a hearing conservation program that includes noise control, training, use of hearing protection, and annual audiometric testing (Randolph et al., 2007; Rogers et al., 2009). If a worker demonstrates loss of hearing on a surveillance audiogram, they need to be notified, counseled, and referred as necessary. In addition, such events should prompt a review of noise monitoring and whether noise from particular animal housing areas, cage decontamination equipment or other noise sources are being adequately controlled.

E. Management of Occupational Injuries and Illnesses

When a laboratory worker experiences an acute injury or illness due to exposures in the workplace, there may be specific measures that the treating medical provider needs to take to ensure effective management of the condition. At the same time, the occurrence of such an injury or illness often represents a 'sentinel event' indicating that workplace safety and health controls may not be functioning adequately. It is therefore important that the acute medical care and follow-up of work-related conditions in workers in animal facilities take place in coordination with the involvement of the occupational health provider for the facility, as well as other members of the occupational health team described above, as necessary.

1. Acute Infections: Animal Bites and Other Exposures

B virus, found in macaques, is described in Chapter 25. Workers caring for macaques can be exposed to the virus through bites, scratches, or body fluid exposures, and should be considered for emergency prophylaxis with antiviral medication. Specific risk-based post-exposure antiviral prophylaxis guidelines exist to assist in the evaluation and care of persons potentially exposed to B virus (Cohen et al., 2002). Breeding colonies of macaques free from evidence of B virus and other agents are increasingly available for use in research, which should result in reduced likelihoods of transmission events to laboratory animal workers (Morton et al., 2008). Nonetheless, vigilance for this potentially fatal infection must remain high due to the limited timelines for the recommended wound cleansing or mucous membrane flushing and initiation of antiviral therapy.

Laboratory animal workers bitten by small laboratory rodents should be instructed to thoroughly cleanse their wound, apply a light bandage, and monitor the site for the possibility of developing infections such as rat bite fever and, rarely, LCMV. Such workers with bite exposures should report fevers, local signs of infection, or other new symptoms to the medical care provider.

Bites from other animals such as cats should be evaluated for risk of local infections with agents such as P. multocida. The health care provider treating a laboratory animal worker for an acute bite should be provided with information about the species of animal involved as well as any suspected zoonotic pathogens associated with that species. One way to do this is to have an exposure card listing such exposure risks that can be carried by the worker and given to a treating health care professional. The occurrence of animal bites and scratches to laboratory animal workers could indicate that training or retraining in methods of animal handling and restraint are indicated to help mitigate future recurrences.

2. Other Occupational Injuries

Other injuries such as slips and falls, cuts, and back injuries should receive prompt and appropriate treatment. In follow-up there should be an assessment of the workplace circumstances of the injury in order to identify ergonomic solutions and other means of preventing future injuries.

3. Acute Allergic Conditions

Acute allergic symptoms may range from mild rhinitis to life-threatening episodes of anaphylaxis and asthmatic reactions. A low threshold for referral to an adequate medical facility should be maintained in any circumstances where allergic symptoms appear to be developing rapidly.

4. Management of Specific Medical Conditions
Management of the Worker Who Has Developed Animal Allergies

The development of new or worsening allergic conditions may be detected either through periodic screening or after an acute disease episode. It is then important to identify the causative agents responsible for the allergic symptoms, and to decide on a management strategy. Such management may be carried out in conjunction with or under the direction of a specialist in allergic diseases. Medical management may include the use of antihistamines and corticosteroids. Importantly, reduction of further exposure to the allergen is critical. It is possible that an individual sensitized to one animal species may tolerate exposure to a different species; however, the individual who has developed animal allergies will require close monitoring and possible work restrictions. A particular concern is the development of secondary allergy to another allergen, which studies have found can be a significant occurrence (Goodno and Stave, 2002). A component of such monitoring is determining whether more serious conditions such as occupational asthma are developing.

Recognition and Management of Work-Related Asthma in Laboratory Animal Workers

Work-related asthma (WRA) can be divided into two categories. The first is new-onset asthma that develops in an individual who previously did not have a history of asthma (occupational asthma or OA). The second category of WRA involves a worsening of an asthmatic condition in an individual who has previously been found to have asthma (work-exacerbated asthma or WEA). The cause of occupational asthma can be either allergic, as in the case of reaction to mouse or cat antigens, or irritant, as in the case of high dose or repeated exposure to chemical irritants such as cleaning chemicals. Likewise, work-exacerbated asthma may be due to re-exposure of an allergic individual to known allergens or to exposure to airborne irritants including dusts and chemicals. The clinician caring for a laboratory animal worker who has developed asthmatic symptoms needs to be aware of these distinctions since they will affect the type of management necessary in the workplace. Irritant-induced asthma may be managed with relatively straightforward methods to reduce irritant exposures, while asthma due to allergic sensitization may require removal from any further exposure to the offending allergen.

The decision to allow a worker to keep operating in an area where they have developed new or worsening asthmatic symptoms is a complex one that may involve other members of the occupational health team as well as a specialist in allergy or pulmonary medicine. Close monitoring of such workers with serial spirometry and/or peak flow testing may be necessary, and early removal or transfer from a workplace considered if symptoms continue to worsen.

Psychosocial Distress

Workers who report development of symptoms consistent with depression or anxiety or other mood disorders should be referred for counseling and a careful review of the psychosocial stressors associated with their job activities performed. Such workers may need additional support and be able to seek such help in a confidential setting.

Other Work Restrictions and Return to Work Decisions

In addition to the work-related conditions described above, workers may develop new medical conditions that require time away from work or a change in work abilities. Such events should trigger a reevaluation of their job exposures and risks similar to that performed during the pre-placement evaluation. The occupational medical provider for the animal care facility should ideally be involved in the medical decisions regarding return to work for such individuals as well as possible work restrictions.

F. Records Management

A key aspect of occupational health services for animal care workers is the need for confidential management of medical information. Such information, even if an electronic medical record, needs to be maintained in a secure location with access restricted to only the medical providers. When communicating with supervisors and other management personnel regarding particular work restrictions or fitness for duty issues, confidential medical information should not be disclosed. Ensuring such confidentiality encourages openness during medical encounters between employees and the occupational medical provider and helps ensure adequate screening, prevention and management of occupational health issues.

APPENDIX 30.1

Occupational Risk Assessment and Medical Questionnaire
Laboratory Animal Worker

Name:_____ Today's Date: _____/___/_____

Gender: ☐ Male ☐ Female Date of Birth: _____/___/_____

Job Title: _____ Brief description of work:

_____

Location/building/lab:

_____

_____

Work assignment (check all that apply): ☐ BSL-3 lab ☐ BSL-2 lab ☐ Insectary ☐ Field work ☐ other: _____

Species you work with (list all):

☐ Amphibians ☐ Birds ☐ Rabbits ☐ Mice☐ Rats ☐ Other rodents ☐ insects ☐ non-human primates ☐ serum / tissue only (species):

☐ Dog☐ Ferret ☐ Cat ☐ Mice ☐ Pigs ☐ Sheep ☐ Goat ☐ Horse ☐ Fish ☐ wildlife (species): _____

Average frequency of interaction with animals:

☐ daily ☐ weekly ☐ monthly ☐ other: _____

Major animal-related tasks:

☐ feeding ☐ grooming ☐ handling animals ☐ cleaning cages ☐ change bedding ☐ sedation ☐ euthanasia

☐ capture/restrain wild animals (species): _____ ☐ other: _____ ☐ no animal - related tasks

Other hazardous exposures:

☐ human blood / tissue ☐ anesthetic gases (e.g. isoflurane) ☐ temperature extremes ☐ other chemicals (please list):

_____

☐ Experimental Infectious Agents (specify): _____ ☐ Radioisotopes ☐ dust ☐ noise ☐ radiation ☐ heavy lifting ☐ other (please specify): _____

Non-occupational animal exposures (e.g. pets, other): Please state if outside of work you have exposure to any of the following

☐ Dog☐ Bird ☐ Cat ☐ Ferret☐ Fish ☐ Horse ☐ other (species): _____

Medical History: Please indicate if you have ever had any of the following medical conditions:

Symptoms: Please check if you have had any of the following symptoms:

	Yes	If yes, please describe or explain
Asthma		
Seasonal allergies		
Sinusitis		
Chronic respiratory infection		
Conjunctivitis		
Eczema		
Poison ivy		
Other skin disease		
Heart murmur		
Hepatitis		
Back problems		
Hernia		
Joint pains or arthritis		
Other musculoskeletal problems		
Depression or anxiety		
Diabetes		
Cancer		
Lyme disease		
Recurrent infections		
Medical conditions that could compromise the immune system		
Other		

	Current	Please describe or explain
Cough		
Shortness of breath		
Wheezing		
Chest tightness		
Runny/itchy eyes		
Runny/itchy/congested nose/sneezing		
Skin rash or hives		
Muscle pain		
Persistent diarrhea		
Weight loss		
Unexplained fevers		
Depression		
Anxiety		
Problems with co-workers		
Work-related concerns		

Please list known allergies to medications, animals, or other environmental allergens, and reactions:_____

_____

APPENDIX 30.1 (Continued)

Have you ever worked in a laboratory before? ☐ Yes   ☐ No _____
_____

Have you ever worked with animals, ticks, or insects before? ☐ Yes   ☐ No _____
_____

Have you ever received immunosuppressive therapy (e.g. steroids, chemotherapy, radiation)? ☐ Yes   ☐ No _____
_____

Please list current medications (prescription, over the counter, and supplements):_____
_____

Do you use tobacco products? ☐ Yes   ☐ No If yes, how much and how often?_____
_____

Are you currently being cared for by another health provider? ☐ Yes   ☐ No (name): _____
_____

Prior laboratory and/or animal work injuries or illness (if applicable):

	Yes	No	Comments
Muscle sprain or strain			
Animal bite			
Animal scratch			
Needle stick or scalpel injury			
Laceration or cut on animal cage or equipment			
Infection acquired from animal			
Lyme disease or other tick-borne illness			
Reaction to chemicals			
Other			

Do you have any concerns about your health related to your current job? (if so, please elaborate):_____
_____
_____

Do you have any other concerns about your work exposures? (if so, please elaborate):_____
_____
_____

Immunizations:
Please state your most recent immunizations and date:

Immunization	Yes	No	Unknown	If yes, date of vaccination
Tetanus				
Rabies				
Influenza				
Hepatitis B				
Hepatitis A				
Measles				
Yellow Fever				
Vaccinia				
Other Vaccines (list)				

When is the last time you were tested for tuberculosis? (Month, year): _____
How were you tested for tuberculosis? (Circle one): Skin Test   IGRA blood test   X-Ray   Other

Is there anything we should know about your health that has not already been mentioned? (if so, please elaborate):_____
_____
_____

Physician/Clinician comments:

Reviewed by (sign and print name):_____   Date:_____

APPENDIX 30.2

Annual Surveillance Questionnaire
Laboratory Animal Worker

Name:_____   Today's Date: _____/___/_____

Gender: ☐ Male ☐ Female   Date of Birth: _____/___/_____

Job Title: _____   Brief description of work:

Location/building/lab:
_____
_____

Work assignment (check all that apply):   ☐ BSL-3 lab   ☐ BSL-2 lab   ☐ Insectary   ☐ Field work   ☐ other:
_____

List of Species you work with:
☐ Amphibians ☐ Birds ☐ Rabbits ☐ Mice☐ Rats ☐ Other rodents ☐ insects ☐ non-human primates   ☐ serum / tissue only (species):
☐ Dog☐ Ferret ☐ Cat ☐ Mice ☐ Pigs ☐ Sheep ☐ Goat ☐ Horse   ☐ Fish ☐ wildlife (species): _____

Average frequency of interaction with animals:
☐ daily ☐ weekly ☐ monthly ☐ other: _____

Major animal-related tasks:
☐ feeding   ☐ grooming   ☐ handling animals   ☐ cleaning cages   ☐ change bedding   ☐ sedation   ☐ euthanasia
☐ capture/restrain wild animals (species): _____   ☐ other: _____   ☐ no animal - related tasks

Other hazardous exposures:
☐ human blood / tissue   ☐ anesthetic gases (e.g. isoflurane)   ☐ temperature extremes   ☐ other chemicals (please list):
_____

☐ dust ☐ noise ☐ radiation ☐ heavy lifting ☐ other (please specify):
_____

Non-occupational animal exposures (e.g. pets,
*other):*_____

Personal protective equipment you regularly use (check all that apply):
☐ gloves ☐ mask ☐ eye protection ☐ lab coat ☐ respirator ☐
other:_____

Medical History: Please indicate if you have ever had any of the following medical conditions:

Symptoms: Please check if you have had any of the following symptoms:

	Yes	If yes, please describe or explain
Asthma		
Seasonal allergies		
Sinusitis		
Chronic respiratory infection		
Conjunctivitis		
Eczema		
Poison ivy		
Other skin disease		
Heart murmur		
Hepatitis		
Back problems		
Hernia		
Joint pains or arthritis		
Other musculoskeletal problems		
Depression or anxiety		
Diabetes		
Cancer		
Lyme disease		
Recurrent infections		
Medical conditions that could compromise the immune system		
Other		

	Current	Please describe or explain
Cough		
Shortness of breath		
Wheezing		
Chest tightness		
Runny/itchy eyes		
Runny/itchy/congested nose/sneezing		
Skin rash or hives		
Muscle pain		
Persistent diarrhea		
Weight loss		
Unexplained fevers		
Depression		
Anxiety		
Problems with co-workers		
Work-related concerns		

In the past year,

APPENDIX 30.2 (Continued)

A) Have you been treated for any major medical illnesses? _____ _____

B) Have you had any changes in existing medical conditions? _____ _____

C) Have you been hospitalized? _____ _____

D) Have you been advised to avoid contact with animals for medical reasons? _____ _____

E) Have you left work for an extended period of time (i.e. more than two weeks)? _____ _____

F) Have you had any accidental injuries or exposures while at work? _____ _____

G) If female, are you currently pregnant or contemplating pregnancy in the near future? _____ _____

Please list known allergies to medications, animals, or other environmental allergens, and reactions:_____ _____

Have you ever worked in a laboratory before? ☐ Yes ☐ No _____ _____

Have you ever worked with animals, ticks, or insects before? ☐ Yes ☐ No _____ _____

Have you ever received immunosuppressive therapy (e.g. steroids, chemotherapy, radiation)? ☐ Yes ☐ No _____ _____

Please list current medications (prescription, over the counter, and supplements):_____ _____

Do you use tobacco products? ☐ Yes ☐ No If yes, how much and how often?_____ _____

Are you currently being cared for by another health provider? ☐ Yes ☐ No (name): _____ _____

Do you have any concerns about your health related to your current job? (if so, please elaborate):_____ _____

Do you have any other concerns about your work exposures? (if so, please elaborate):_____ _____

Immunizations:
Please state your most recent immunizations and date:

Immunization	Yes	No	Unknown	If yes, date of vaccination
Tetanus				
Rabies				
Influenza				
Hepatitis B				
Hepatitis A				
Measles				
Yellow Fever				
Vaccinia				
Other Vaccines (list)				

When is the last time you were tested for tuberculosis? (Month, year): _____
How were you tested for tuberculosis? (Circle one): Skin Test   IGRA blood test   X-Ray   Other
Is there anything we should know about your health   that has not already been mentioned? (if so, please elaborate):_____
_____ _____

Physician/Clinician comments:

Reviewed by (sign and print name):_____   Date:_____ _____

References

Acton, D., McCauley, L., 2007. Laboratory animal allergy: an occupational hazard. AAOHN J. 55 (6), 241–244.

Allan, K.M., Murphy, E., Ayres, J.G., 2010. Assessment of respiratory health surveillance for laboratory animal workers. Occup. Med. (Lond.) 60 (6), 458–463. http://dx.doi.org/10.1093/occmed/kqq055

American Association for Laboratory Animal Science, (2013). Cost of caring: human emotions in the care of laboratory animals.

Arluke, A.B., 1988. Sacrificial symbolism in animal experimentation: object or pet? Anthroz Multidiscip. J. Interact. People Anim. 2 (2), 98–117.

Arluke, A.B., 1999. Uneasiness among laboratory technicians. Occup. Med. (Philadelphia, PA) 14 (2), 305–316.

AVMA Panel on Euthanasia, 2013. AVMA Guidelines for the Euthanasia of Animals. 2013 Edition. American Veterinary Medical Association, Schaumburg, IL.

Bartram, D., Baldwin, D., 2010. Veterinary surgeons and suicide: a structured review of possible influences on increased risk. Vet. Rec. 166 (13), 388–397.

Bayne, K., 2002. Development of the human-research animal bond and its impact on animal well-being. ILAR J. 43 (1), 4–9.

Bhabha, F.K., Nixon, R., 2012. Occupational exposure to laboratory animals causing a severe exacerbation of atopic eczema. Australas. J. Dermatol. 53 (2), 155–156. http://dx.doi.org/10.1111/j.1440-0960.2011.00754.x

bin Zakaria, M., Lerche, N.W., Chomel, B.B., Kass, P.H., 1996. Accidental injuries associated with nonhuman primate exposure at two regional primate research centers (USA): 1988–1993. Lab. Anim. Sci. 46 (3), 298–304.

CDC, 2013. Advisory Committee on Immunization Practices (ACIP) recommended immunization schedule for adults aged 19 years and older—United States, 2013. Morb. Mortal. Wkly. Rep. 62 (1), 1–19.

Choosewood, L.C., Wilson, D.E. (2009). Biosafety in Microbiological and Biomedical Laboratories. HHS Publication No. (CDC) 21-1112, (fifth ed.).

Cohen, J.I., Davenport, D.S., Stewart, J.A., Deitchman, S., Hilliard, J.K., Chapman, L.E., et al., 2002. Recommendations for prevention of and therapy for exposure to B virus (Cercopithecine Herpesvirus 1). Clin. Infect. Dis. 35 (10), 1191–1203.

Coleman, K., 2011. Caring for nonhuman primates in biomedical research facilities: scientific, moral and emotional considerations. Am. J. Primatol. 73 (3), 220–225. http://dx.doi.org/10.1002/ajp.20855

Corradi, M., Ferdenzi, E., Mutti, A., 2013. The characteristics, treatment and prevention of laboratory animal allergy. Lab. Anim. (NY) 42 (1), 26–33.

Davies, K., Lewis, D., 2010. Can caring for laboratory animals be classified as emotional labour? Anim. Technol. Welfare 9 (1), 1–6.

Elliott, L., Heederik, D., Marshall, S., Peden, D., Loomis, D., 2005. Incidence of allergy and allergy symptoms among workers exposed to laboratory animals. Occup. Environ. Med. 62 (11), 766–771. http://dx.doi.org/10.1136/oem.2004.018739

Ernst, A., Zibrak, J.D., 1998. Carbon monoxide poisoning. N. Engl. J. Med. 339 (22), 1603–1608.

Ferraz, E., Arruda, L.K., Bagatin, E., Martinez, E.Z., Cetlin, A.A., Simoneti, C.S., et al., 2013. Laboratory animals and respiratory allergies: the prevalence of allergies among laboratory animal workers and the need for prophylaxis. Clinics 68 (6), 750–759. http://dx.doi.org/10.6061/clinics/2013(06)05

Fisher, R., Saunders, W.B., Murray, S.J., Stave, G.M., 1998. Prevention of laboratory animal allergy. J. Occup. Environ. Med. 40 (7), 609–613.

Flecknell, P.A., 1996. Laboratory Animal Anaesthesia: A Practical Introduction for Research Workers and Technicians. Academic Press, London; San Diego, CA.

Fontes, B., 2008. Institutional responsibilities in contamination control for research animals an in occupational health and safety for animal handlers. ILAR J. 49 (3), 326–337.

Fuortes, L.J., Weih, L., Jones, M.L., Burmeister, L., Thorne, P.S., Pollen, S., et al., 1996. Epidemiologic assessment of laboratory animal allergy among university employees. Am. J. Ind. Med. 29, 67–74.

Glueck, J.T., Huneke, R.B., Perez, H., Burstyn, I., 2012. Exposure of laboratory animal care workers to airborne mouse and rat allergens. J. Am. Assoc. Lab. Anim. Sci. 51 (5), 554–560.

Goodno, L.E., Stave, G.M., 2002. Primary and secondary allergies to laboratory animals. J. Occup. Environ. Med. 44 (12), 1143–1152. http://dx.doi.org/10.1097/01.jom.0000044117.59147.2d

Haagsma, J.A., Tariq, L., Heederik, D.J., Havelaar, A.H., 2012. Infectious disease risks associated with occupational exposure: a systematic review of the literature. Occup. Environ. Med. 69 (2), 140–146. http://dx.doi.org/10.1136/oemed-2011-100068

Halpern-Lewis, J.G., 1996. Understanding the emotional experiences of animal research personnel. Aalas Contemp. Top. Lab. Anim. Sci. 35 (6), 58–60.

Hankenson, F.C., Johnston, N.A., Weigler, B.J., Di Giacomo, R.F., 2003. Zoonoses of occupational health importance in contemporary laboratory animal research. Comp. Med. 53 (6), 579–601.

Herzog, H., 1989. Tangled lives: human researchers and animal subjects. Anthrozoos 3 (2), 80–82.

Hollander, A., Heederik, D., Doekes, G., 1997. Respiratory allergy to rats: exposure–response relationships in laboratory animal workers. Am. J. Respir. Crit. Care. Med. 155, 562–567.

Iliff, S.A., 2002. An additional "R": remembering the animals. ILAR J. 43 (1), 38–47.

Institute of Laboratory Animal Resources, C.o.O.S.H.i.R.A.F., 1997. Occupational Health and Safety in the Care and Use of Research Animals. National Academy Press, Washington, DC.

Jang, J.H., Kim, D.W., Kim, S.W., Kim, D.-Y., Seong, W.K., Son, T.J., et al., 2009. Allergic rhinitis in laboratory animal workers and its risk factors. Ann. Allergy Asthma Immunol. 102, 373–377.

Jeal, H.L., Jones, M.G., Cullinan, P., 2010. Epidemiology of laboratory animal allergy. In: Occupational Asthma, pp. 33–55.

Jones, M.G., 2008. Exposure–response in occupational allergy. Curr. Opin. Allergy. Clin. Immunol. 8, 110–114.

Kristensen, S., Gimsing, S., 1988. Occupational hearing impairment in pig breeders. Scand. Audiol. 17 (3), 191–192.

Krop, E.J., Doekes, G., Stone, M.J., Aalberse, R.C., van der Zee, J.S., 2007. Spreading of occupational allergens: laboratory animal allergens on hair-covering caps and in mattress dust of laboratory animal workers. Occup. Environ. Med. 64 (4), 267–272. http://dx.doi.org/10.1136/oem.2006.028845

Kruize, H., Post, W., Heederik, D., Martens, B., Hollander, A., van der Beek, E., 1997. Respiratory allergy in laboratory animal workers: a retrospective cohort study using pre-employment screening data. Occup. Environ. Med. 54, 830–835.

Lang, Y.C., 2005. Animal exposure surveillance: a model program. AAOHN J. 53 (9), 407–412.

Langley, R., 1999. Physical hazards of animal handlers. Occup. Med. (Philadelphia, PA) 14 (2), 181–194.

Leng, K., Wiedemeyer, K., Hartmann, M., 2008. Anaphylaxis after mouse bite. J. Dtsch. Dermatol. Ges. 6 (9), 741–743. http://dx.doi.org/10.1111/j.1610-0387.2008.06616.x

Lopata, A.L., Fenemore, B., Jeebhay, M.F., Gade, G., Potter, P.C., 2005. Occupational allergy in laboratory workers caused by the African migratory grasshopper Locusta migratoria. Allergy 60 (2), 200–205. http://dx.doi.org/10.1111/j.1398-9995.2005.00661.x

Massachusetts Department of Health. (1999). Asthma in Animal Handlers. SENSOR Occupational Lung Disease Bulletin.

Matsui, E.C., Diette, G.B., Krop, E.J., Aalberse, R.C., Smith, A.L., Curtin-Brosnan, J., et al., 2005. Mouse allergen-specific immunoglobulin G and immunoglobulin G4 and allergic symptoms in immunoglobulin E-sensitized laboratory animal workers. Clin. Exp. Allergy 35 (10), 1347–1353. http://dx.doi.org/10.1111/j.1365-2222.2005.02331.x

McMurry, F.G., Key, T.J., 1999. Medical surveillance of animal handlers. Occup. Med. 14 (2), 317–336.

Meggs, W.J., 1999. Chemical hazards faced by animal handlers. Occup. Med. (Philadelphia, PA) 14 (2), 213–224.

Meyer, R.E., 1999. Anesthesia hazards to animal workers. Occup. Med. (Philadelphia, PA) 14 (2), 225–234.

Mor, G., Cardenas, I., 2010. The immune system in pregnancy: a unique complexity. Am. J. Reprod. Immunol. 63 (6), 425–433.

Morrow, W.E., 1999. Euthanasia hazards. Occup. Med. (Philadelphia, PA) 14 (2), 235.

Morton, W.R., Agy, M.B., Capuano, S.V., Grant, R.F., 2008. Specific pathogen-free macaques: definition, history, and current production. ILAR J. 49 (2), 137–144.

Moscato, G., Pala, G., Boillat, M.A., Folletti, I., Gerth van Wijk, R., Olgiati-Des Gouttes, D., et al., 2011. EAACI position paper: prevention of work-related respiratory allergies among pre-apprentices or apprentices and young workers. Allergy 66 (9), 1164–1173. http://dx.doi.org/10.1111/j.1398-9995.2011.02615.x

National Research Council, 2003. Occupational Health and Safety in the Care and Use of Nonhuman Primates. The National Academies Press, Washington, DC.

National Research Council, 2011. Guide for the Care and Use of Laboratory Animals. The National Academies Press, Washington, DC, (eighth ed.).

Nicholson, P.J., Mayho, G.V., Roomes, D., Swann, A.B., Blackburn, B.S., 2010. Health surveillance of workers exposed to laboratory animal allergens. Occup. Med. (Lond.) 60 (8), 591–597. http://dx.doi.org/10.1093/occmed/kqq150

NIOSH, 1998. Preventing Asthma in Animal Handlers.

OSHA, 2011. 1910.134 Respiratory Protection Standard.

Pacheco, K.A., 2007. New insights into laboratory animal exposures and allergic responses. Curr. Opin. Allergy. Clin. Immunol. 7, 156–161.

Pacheco, K.A., McCammon, C., Liu, A.H., Thorne, P.S., O'Neill, M.E., Martyny, J., et al., 2003. Airborne endotoxin predicts symptoms in non-mouse-sensitized technicians and research scientists exposed to laboratory mice. Am. J. Respir. Crit. Care. Med. 167 (7), 983–990. http://dx.doi.org/10.1164/rccm.2112062

Pacheco, K.A., Rose, C.S., Silveira, L.J., Van Dyke, M.V., Goelz, K., MacPhail, K., et al., 2010. Gene–environment interactions influence airways function in laboratory animal workers. J. Allergy Clin. Immunol. 126 (2), 232–240. http://dx.doi.org/10.1016/j.jaci.2010.04.019

Panarella, M.L., Bimes, R.S., 2010. A naturally occurring outbreak of tuberculosis in a group of imported cynomolgus monkeys (Macaca fascicularis). J. Am. Assoc. Lab. Anim. Sci. 49 (2), 221–225.

Pate, W., Charlton, M., Wellington, C., 2013. Measurement and analysis of 8-hour time-weighted average sound pressure levels in a vivarium decontamination facility. Arch. Environ. Occup. Health. 68 (3), 173–179. http://dx.doi.org/10.1080/19338244.2012.676104

Peng, R.D., Paigen, B., Eggleston, P.A., Hagberg, K.A., Krevans, M., Curtin-Brosnan, J., et al., 2011. Both the variability and level of mouse allergen exposure influence the phenotype of the immune response in workers at a mouse facility. J. Allergy Clin. Immunol. 128 (2), 390–396. e397. http://dx.doi.org/10.1016/j.jaci.2011.04.050

Portengen, L., Hollander, A., Doekes, G., de Meer, G., Heederik, D., 2003. Lung function decline in laboratory animal workers: the role of sensitisation and exposure. Occup. Environ. Med. 60, 870–875.

Randolph, M.M., Hill, W.A., Randolph, B.W., 2007. Noise monitoring and establishment of a comprehensive hearing conservation program. J. Am. Assoc. Lab. Anim. Sci. 46 (1), 42–44.

Raub, J.A., Mathieu-Nolf, M., Hampson, N.B., Thom, S.R., 2000. Carbon monoxide poisoning—a public health perspective. Toxicology 145, 1–14.

Renströ, A., Karlsson, A.-S., Malmberg, P., Larsson, P.H., van Hage-Hamsten, M., 2001. Working with male rodents may increase the risk of allergy to laboratory animals. Allergy 56, 964–970.

Reynolds, R.P., Kinard, W.L., Degraff, J.J., Leverage, N., Norton, J.N., 2010. Noise in a laboratory animal facility from the human and mouse perspectives. J. Am. Assoc. Lab. Anim. Sci. 49 (5), 592–597.

Rogers, B., Berryman, P., Lukes, E., Meyer, D., Summey, C., Scheessele, D., et al., 2009. What makes a successful hearing conservation program? AAOHN J. 57 (8), 321–335. http://dx.doi.org/10.3928/08910162-20090716-02.

Rohlf, V., Bennett, P., 2005. Perpetration-induced traumatic stress in persons who euthanize nonhuman animals in surgeries, animal shelters, and laboratories. Soc. Anim. 13 (3), 201–219.

Rowland, A.S., Baird, D.D., Weinberg, C.R., Shore, D.L., Shy, C.M., Wilcox, A.J., 1992. Reduced fertility among women employed as dental assistants exposed to high levels of nitrous oxide. N. Engl. J. Med. 327 (14), 993–997.

Rowland, A.S., Baird, D.D., Shore, D.L., Weinberg, C.R., Savitz, D.A., Wilcox, A.J., 1995. Nitrous oxide and spontaneous abortion in female dental assistants. Am. J. Epidemiol. 141 (6), 531–538.

Ruoppi, P., Koistinen, T., Susitaival, P., Honkanen, J., Soininen, H., 2004. Frequency of allergic rhinitis to laboratory animals in university employees as confirmed by chamber challenges. Allergy 59, 295–301.

Ruoppi, P., Koistinen, T., Pennanen, S., 2005. Sensitisation to mites in laboratory animal workers with rhinitis. Occup. Environ. Med. 62 (9), 612–615. http://dx.doi.org/10.1136/oem.2004.015685

Sharpe, D., 2009. Implementing a medical surveillance program for animal care staff. Am. Biotechnol. Lab. 27 (6), 20.

Smith, J.C., Bolon, B., 2006. Isoflurane leakage from non-rebreathing rodent anaesthesia circuits: comparison of emissions from conventional and modified ports. Lab. Anim. (NY) 40 (2), 200–209. http://dx.doi.org/10.1258/002367706776318999

Stave, G.M., Darcey, D.J., 2012. Prevention of laboratory animal allergy in the United States: a national survey. J. Occup. Environ. Med. 54 (5), 558–563. http://dx.doi.org/10.1097/JOM.0b013e318247a44a

Tarlo, S.M., Balmes, J., Balkissoon, R., Beach, J., Beckett, W., Bernstein, D., et al., 2008. Diagnosis and management of work-related asthma. Chest 134 (3), 1–41.

Taylor, D.K., Mook, D.M., 2009. Isoflurane waste anesthetic gas concentrations associated with the open-drop method. J. Am. Assoc. Lab. Anim. Sci. 48 (1), 61–64.

Todd, E.T., Morse, J.M., Casagni, T.J., Engelman, R.W., 2013. Monitoring and mitigating isoflurane emissions during inhalational anesthesia of mice. Lab. Anim. (NY) 42 (10), 371–379.

Venables, K.M., Tee, R.D., Hawkins, E.R., Gordon, D.J., Wale, C.J., Farrer, N.M., et al., 1988a. Laboratory animal allergy in a pharmaceutical company. Br. J. Ind. Med. 45, 660–666.

Venables, K.M., Upton, J.L., Hawkins, E.R., Tee, R.D., Longbottom, J.L., Newman Taylor, A.J., 1988b. Smoking, atopy, and laboratory animal allergy. Br. J. Ind. Med. 45 (10), 667–671.

Weigler, B.J., Di Giacomo, R.F., Alexander, S., 2005. A national survey of laboratory animal workers concerning occupational risks for zoonotic diseases. Comp. Med. 55 (2), 183–191.

Weigler, B.J., Cooper, D.R., Hankenson, F.C., 2012. Risk-based immunization policies and tuberculosis screening practices for animal care and research workers in the United States: survey results and recommendations. J. Am. Assoc. Lab. Anim. Sci. 51 (5), 561–573.

Willy, M.E., Woodward, R.A., Thornton, V.B., Wolff, A.V., Flynn, B.M., Heath, J.L., et al., 1999. Management of a measles outbreak among old world nonhuman primates. Lab. Anim. Sci. 49 (1), 42–48.

Wolfle, T., 1985. Laboratory animal technicians. Their role in stress reduction and human–companion animal bonding. Vet. Clin. North Am. Small Anim. Pract. 15 (2), 449–454.

Zel, P., 2003. Human xenograft transplantation in animal research: risk assessment and hazard control for animal care workers. Contemp. Top. Lab. Anim. Sci. 42 (6), 64–65.

Zhao, Y.A., Shusterman, D., 2012. Occupational rhinitis and other work-related upper respiratory tract conditions. Clin. Chest. Med. 33 (4), 637–647. http://dx.doi.org/10.1016/j.ccm.2012.09.004

CHAPTER

31

Genetic Monitoring of Laboratory Mice and Rats

Marjorie C. Strobel, PhD[a], Laura G. Reinholdt, PhD[b],
Rachel D. Malcolm, MS, BA[c] and Kathleen Pritchett-Corning,
DVM, DACLAM, MRCVS[d]

[a]JAX Mice & Clinical Research Services, The Jackson Laboratory, Bar Harbor, ME, USA
[b]The Jackson Laboratory, Bar Harbor, ME, USA [c]The Jackson Laboratory, Diagnostic & GQC
Laboratories, Bar Harbor, ME, USA [d]Office of Animal Resources, Harvard University Faculty of Arts
and Sciences, and Department of Comparative Medicine, University of Washington

OUTLINE

I. INTRODUCTION

In the early days of research involving mice and rats, the importance of both genetic and health quality and monitoring of that quality was not recognized. The health quality of animals was quickly reflected in sick animals that could not be used for research, so immediate strides were made to ensure animal health in the research environment. Recognition of and efforts to maintain genetic quality lagged behind as laboratory animal genetics was initially only important to geneticists. As detailed investigations into genetics and immunology

Laboratory Animal Medicine, Third Edition
DOI: http://dx.doi.org/10.1016/B978-0-12-409527-4.00031-6

began, the inbred mouse and more recently, the rat, arose as genetic models of disease (Malakoff, 2000) and with those came the challenge of maintaining genetic homogeneity. Human error and genetic drift are ever-present sources of unwanted genetic heterogeneity, which ultimately lead to experimental irreproducibility. Genetic monitoring and colony maintenance quality control are necessary measures to detect and remove unwanted genetic heterogeneity. This chapter will discuss the rationale for genetic homogeneity and monitoring, the history of genetic monitoring from its inception to today, and current and historical means by which this may be accomplished. Also addressed in the chapter are current monitoring paradigms, or genetic quality control (GQC), for mice and rats, including inbred, congenic, outbred, and genetically engineered strains, as well as the role of breeders, vivaria, and end users in GQC. Finally, the future of genetic monitoring and GQC will be discussed.

II. HISTORY OF GENETIC MONITORING

In 1909, Clarence Cook Little created the first inbred mouse strain, DBA, at the Bussey Institute at Harvard University while at the same time, Helen Dean King created the first inbred rat strain, PA, at The Wistar Institute (Jacob and Kwitek, 2002). Since then, the number of genetically modified animals used in research has risen exponentially and their use has spread far beyond genetics and oncology research into almost every aspect of science and medicine. Today, scientists routinely use inbred, outbred, congenic, conplastic, recombinant inbred (RI), spontaneous mutant, and genetically engineered animals, as well as various combinations of the different types (Tables 31.1 and 31.2).

Loss of genetic homogeneity is a fairly routine occurrence throughout the history of the inbred mouse and rat. Human mistakes and mismanagement, murine size and abilities, and the genetics of coat colors, have all led to the inadvertent mixing of murine genetic material that researchers were attempting to separate and define. In 1974, the importance of genetic monitoring in commercial strains was demonstrated by Festing using mandibular measurements to determine genetic background (Festing, 1974). Roderick et al., in 1971 proposed using isoenzyme alleles to genetically monitor animals. Although contaminations certainly occurred before then (see the history of the C57BL/Ks [Naggert et al., 1995] and Groen's 1977 studies [Groen, 1977] for examples), the issue of genetic contamination of inbred mouse strains became a reality to many scientists in 1982 with a publication reporting contaminated BALB/c mice (Kahan et al., 1982). Festing reported several additional previously unpublished strain contaminations (Festing, 1982), including contaminated AKR mice, 'inbred' rats

TABLE 31.1   Common Rodent Strains/Lines/Stocks

Strain	Description
Inbred	Strain established by a minimum of 20 consecutive generations of sister × brother matings (sib matings)
	Maintained by sib mating (http://research.jax.org/grs/type/inbred/index.html)
Outbred	Stock/line established and maintained by strict avoidance of sib mating
	Commonly, maintained using a defined breeding scheme and multiple breeding lines
F1 hybrid	Created by mating mice of two inbred strains in a defined direction – i.e., the B6D2F1 hybrid mouse line is produced by mating a C57Bl/6 female to a DBA/2 male at each generation (http://research.jax.org/grs/type/hybrid/index.html)
F2 hybrid	Created by mating two F1 hybrid mice – i.e., B6D2F2 is produced by mating 2 B6D2F1 animals
Recombinant inbred	Lines established by inbreeding of the progeny of individual F2 hybrid sibling pairs for at least 20 generations (http://www.jax.org/smsr/ristrain.html)
Congenic	Introduction of a mutation onto a defined inbred strain background by 5–10 or more generations of matings back to the inbred strain with selection for the mutation (backcrossing)
	Established congenic strains generally are maintained by purely sibling mating
Consomic	An inbred strain that carries one chromosome from another inbred strain
	Ten generations of backcrossing and selection for the donor chromosome is required for a fully consomic strain
	Mouse consomic panels generally consist of 21 strains, each carrying a different donor chromosome (1–19, plus X or Y) on a single host inbred strain background (http://research.jax.org/grs/type/consomic.html)
Conplastic	An inbred strain that carries the nuclear genome of one inbred strain and the cytoplasm and cytoplasmic (mitochondrial) genome of another
	Since the egg contributes the embryonic cytoplasm, 10 generations of backcrossing inbred females to an inbred male recipient is required for a fully conplastic strain (http://research.jax.org/grs/type/conplastic.html)

that were not histocompatible, and NZB mice contaminated within a research facility. More recently, Dahl salt-sensitive and Buffalo rats were found to be contaminated by other rat strains (Jones et al., 1994; Lewis et al., 1994; St Lezin et al., 1994) and the 129 family of mouse strains was discovered to be extensively genetically contaminated (Threadgill et al., 1997). Additional contaminations in mice have been reported in 101, SJL, and C57BL/6N (Benavides, 1999; Nitzki et al., 2007; West et al., 1985). Genetic contamination is not limited to inbred strains,

TABLE 31.2 Common Mutations Maintained in Rodent Colonies

Mutation type	Description
Spontaneous	Genomic alterations that arise generally from errors in the normal cellular processes, such as DNA replication, mitosis, or meiosis, chromosome structure changes, etc.
Induced	Genomic alterations that arise from intentional exposure to agents that can affect the normal cellular processes or genome structure, such as mutagenic chemicals or various forms of radiation
Genetically engineered – transgenic	Random insertion of DNA sequences into the rodent genome
	Transgenic rodents generally are created by microinjecting purified DNA into the nucleus of a fertilized egg; the introduced DNA contains all or part of a gene's coding sequence, usually with gene expression control elements
	Commonly generated to examine the expression of a foreign gene or overexpression an endogenous mouse or rat gene
Genetically engineered – gene targeted	Precise integration of DNA sequences into the rodent genome by homologous recombination
	Gene targeted rodents are commonly created by introducing DNA with targeted changes into embryonic stem (ES) cell genome in vitro, then microinjecting altered ES cells into host blastocysts to create a chimeric mouse
	Gene targeting can be used to ablate a gene ('knock-out'), to replace a gene ('knock-in'), or to regulate the temporal or spatial expression of a gene ('conditional mutation') by placing it under control of inducible elements
DNA sequence-specific genomic editing	Sequence targeted genomic alterations (point mutations, insertions, deletions, etc.) created directly in cells, embryonic stem cell or fertilized eggs by using zinc finger nucleases (ZFNs), sequence specific RNA-guided endonucleases (CRISPR-Cas9) or transcription activator-like effector nucleases (TALENs)
	These technologies decrease the requirement for extensive breeding to establish a mutant mouse strain on a consistent genetic background (http://jaxmice.jax.org/news/2014/CRISPR_Onestep.html)

however, as contaminations have been reported in MHC-congenic mice and RI mice as well (Marshall *et al.*, 1992, Nandakumar and Holmdahl, 2005). These incidences of genetic contamination, and the many others that go unnoticed or unpublished, underscore the need for standardized genetic monitoring.

One of the oldest methods of genetic monitoring, and one in use to this day, is simply verification of normal characteristics for the strain in question. Examples of observable, expected phenotypes include coat color, body size and shape, reproductive performance, and behavior. To use coat color as an easily accessible example, it is easy to confirm that inbred albino animals, which are by definition homozygous for recessive *Tyr* alleles, have not been contaminated by a pigmented strain (e.g., this colony of BALB/c mice is comprised entirely of albino animals, therefore there has not been a contamination with a pigmented strain). Scientists and veterinarians should know the basic phenotypes of the strains with which they work, or know where to quickly obtain this information if abnormal phenotypes are seen and genetic contamination is suspected.

Beyond simple monitoring of observable, expected phenotypes, more sophisticated means of GQC were developed as the use of laboratory rodents expanded into various fields of study. Soon after the discovery of the major histocompatibility complex, tail skin grafting was developed as a way to ensure that animals were genetically identical (Whitmore *et al.*, 1996; Bailey and Usama, 1960). Animals were anesthetized and skin grafts between animals of the same sex (or female to male animals; the reverse being ineffective due to the presence of antigens produced by genes on the Y chromosome) were placed on the ventral surface of the tail. If animals rejected the skin grafts, then there were major or minor histocompatibility differences and, therefore, they were not the same strain or substrain. For those who wanted to monitor genetic quality of their animals but did not want to perform surgery, morphometry, most specifically mandibular measurements taken after the animals were euthanized, was also used to ensure that animals were genetically identical (Lovell *et al.*, 1984; Festing, 1972, 1993).

From 1960, when the inbred strains were known only by coat colors and MHC, to 1971, when the use of biochemical markers began to be widespread, inbred strain characteristics became more clearly defined. Biochemical loci rarely showed more than two or three allelic forms in inbred mice and by monitoring the forms of isoenzymes, a biochemical 'fingerprint' for each strain could be easily determined using blood, tissue extracts, and urine. Although more than 25 different standard biochemical markers were devised, The Jackson Laboratory found that a panel of approximately 10, combined with coat color, could distinguish one strain from the approximately 100 others maintained in their Foundation Stocks colony (see Fig. 31.1; Fox *et al.*, 2007). The weakness of this approach is its lack of granularity; although the isoenzymes examined allowed for strain discrimination for these biochemical variants, more subtle differences or contaminations might not be detected. In addition, animals must be euthanized to examine biochemical markers and tissue. However, no reasonable option was available until direct examination of DNA became feasible on a large scale.

In some cases, especially for some immunologic congenic strains, where the only difference between animals

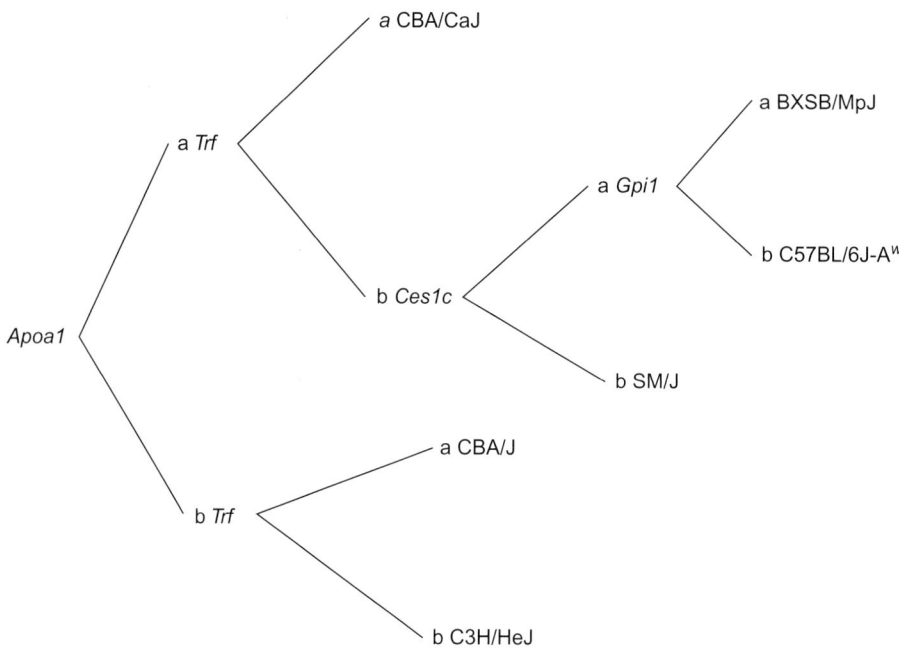

FIGURE 31.1   An illustration of how isoenzymes can be used to differentiate a group of mice with the same coat color. Isoenzyme genes and alleles are in italics; mouse strain names are in normal text. Based on the alleles present, animals can be differentiated–for example, a CBA/J will have *Apoa1^b* and *Trf^a*, while a C3H/HeJ will have *Apoa1^b* but *Trf^b*. This is a minimal amount of information or a critical subset of isoenzymes necessary to differentiate between the strains in the colony. Redrawn from Fox *et al.* (2007).

might be at the histocompatibility locus, immunologic markers are still in use. In immunologic tests, hemagglutination, in which the coagulation of red blood cells demonstrates the presence of incompatible alloantibodies, may be used to demonstrate that mice are expressing different red blood cell antigens than expected. A titer is determined by testing constant numbers of cells against serial dilutions of antisera and reporting the lowest dilution at which agglutination can be recognized. The primary means of demonstrating alloantibodies, however, is usually by examining white blood cells. If they are lysed or otherwise damaged by the presence of alloantibodies, they lose their ability to exclude a dye (Gorer and O'Gorman, 1956) or they refract glycerine differently (Shiroishi *et al.*, 1981). In some cases, there is only one assay that can distinguish one mouse from another. For example, only the hemolytic complement (Hc) assay can distinguish between the two congenic strains B10. D2-*Hc^1H2^dT18^c*/nSnJ and B10.D2-*Hc^0H2^dT18^c*/nSnJ, as the former expresses Hc while the latter does not.

Advances in the ability to manipulate DNA led to further sophistication in the way in which animals were monitored for genetic uniformity. The first method described was the use of DNA fingerprinting, or DNA profiling, to distinguish inbred strains (Russell *et al.*, 1993). DNA fingerprinting originally relied on the use of restriction fragment length polymorphism (RFLP), in which DNA was isolated, digested using bacterial restriction enzymes, and then Southern blotting was used to detect the RFLPs. This

technique was effective, but cumbersome. With the discovery and widespread adoption of PCR as a tool for DNA investigation, RFLP analysis was quickly supplanted by PCR amplification of microsatellite repeats, short repeating sequences of 2–6 base pairs of DNA (also known as simple sequence length polymorphisms [SSLPs] or short tandem repeats [STRs]). Microsatellite panels were developed for mice and rats, and the use of SSLPs to analyze murine DNA for genetic contamination was widespread until recently and is still in use today (Montagutelli *et al.*, 1991; Hirayama *et al.*, 1994; Kloting *et al.*, 1995).

Current genetic monitoring using DNA relies on single nucleotide polymorphisms (SNPs) (Wiltshire *et al.*, 2003; Petkov *et al.*, 2004a,b; Fox *et al.*, 2007; Bothe *et al.*, 2011; Zurita *et al.*, 2011). This method of monitoring for genetic contamination was moved from theoretical to practical in 2004, with a publication by researchers at The Jackson Laboratory, aided by KBiosciences (Petkov *et al.*, 2004a). Petkov *et al.* developed a panel of 1638 SNPs, and then determined that a minimal panel of 29 SNPs was sufficient to monitor the genotypes of over 300 strains of mice maintained at The Jackson Laboratory (Petkov *et al.*, 2004b). The identification of SNPs has proceeded at a rapid pace since then, and commercial suppliers of SNP testing routinely offer panels of thousands of SNPs for genetic monitoring and linkage mapping. SNPs are also being routinely used to distinguish substrains as seen in Zurita *et al.* (Zurita *et al.*, 2011) and to monitor rats for genetic contamination (Nijman *et al.*, 2008; Saar *et al.*, 2008;

Bothe *et al.*, 2011) SNP testing offers several advantages when compared to classical isoenzyme and tissue evaluations, including the sheer number of described variants, the ability to collect samples from living animals, and SNP analysis' ability to detect subtle genomic changes. In addition, SNPs can provide good genomic coverage and can be tailored quite closely to chromosomes or chromosomal portions of interest with high resolution.

While classical genetic monitoring paradigms are useful to detecting inadvertent, contaminating alterations in an animal's or strain's genome, an animal's or colony's genome can change over time for other reasons, such as the accumulation and fixation of spontaneous mutations and the resulting genetic drift (Casellas, 2011). Genetic monitoring may not be useful in these situations, unless the drifted or mutated region randomly coincides with a monitored locus or results in a detectable phenotype change. In the case of outbred animals, genetic monitoring is useful to ensure that the colony is maintaining heterozygosity over time. Genetic monitoring of outbred animals, however, would not necessarily detect every possible inbred strain contamination, since inbred strains and outbred stocks often originate from the same predecessors (Beck *et al.*, 2000; Chia *et al.*, 2005). Where genetic monitoring excels is in the detection of contamination of one inbred strain by another or an inbred strain by mutant strain.

For commercial breeders, the challenge is to ensure each colony conforms to genetic and phenotype expectations, while realistically being able to monitor only a subset of animals from a large production colony. Typically, breeders organize their colonies in a pyramidal fashion (Figure 31.2), for which only very small

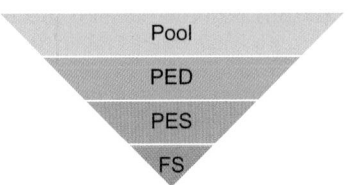

FIGURE 31.2 Organization of a large commercial production rodent colony. FS – foundation stocks: small number of pedigreed sibling pair matings, derived from cryopreserved stocks or progeny derived from a prior generation of FS matings; for individual strains, FS colonies are organized into multiple sibling-mated lineages; all FS breeders are genotyped for strain background and expected mutations, if applicable. PES – pedigree expansion stocks: expansion of pedigreed lineages by sibling pair matings of FS progeny, as well as progeny derived from a prior generation of PES matings. PED – production pedigree stocks: further expansion of pedigree lineages by two female × one male trio matings of FS, PED, and PED lineages. Pool or distribution colony: single generation of matings of progeny from FS, PES or PED colonies, all progeny placed into inventory. The illustrated colony plan can be adjusted to meet demands. Every strain/line/stock colony should have at least a pedigreed FS (or a supply of lineage-identified frozen animals) and a distribution colony. PES or PES/PED colonies are required only to generate the number of Pool colony breeders to ensure the desired supply of experimental or inventory animals.

number of pedigreed founder animals can be sequentially expanded to generate breeding units that may not be pedigreed, to breeding animals selected arbitrarily from a large group. Genetic contamination at the bottom of this pyramid potentially will affect many more animals and, in turn, researchers than genetic contamination at the top of the pyramid. Therefore, all foundation stock breeders should be rigorously tested for their strain background and expected mutations, while smaller numbers of breeders and progeny animals are examined in the downstream colonies. Through the use of modern DNA testing methodology, as few as eight animals would detect a contamination present in 30% of a large breeding colony with a 95% confidence interval (ILAR, 1976; Dubin and Zeitz, 1991), if certain assumptions are made.

III. RODENT STRAINS: GENETIC HOMOGENEITY OR GENETIC DIVERSITY

During cell division, spontaneous mutations naturally occur primarily during DNA synthesis due to incomplete replication-dependent repair. When spontaneous mutations occur in the germ line, the change is heritable and is the underlying cause of genetic drift. For the mouse, Drake *et al.* (1998) calculated a spontaneous mutation rate of 1.8×10^{-10} per base pair per replication, equivalent to 0.9 mutations per gamete per sexual generation. This natural genetic drift results in the acquisition of new alleles and phenotypes, previously not recognized in the strain.

To address the inevitability of spontaneous mutations and genetic drift, each commercial animal producer and rodent researcher should employ breeding schemes to ensure each strain, stock, or line remains consistent with genetic expectations. Does the colony's breeding plan conserve genetic homogeneity by limiting genetic drift or permit, even enhance, genetic heterogeneity by fostering genetic drift? In the simplest view, a spontaneous mutation creates a recessive, loss-of-function allele with no or little detectable phenotype expression when heterozygous. What is the impact of this heterozygosity on different mating schemes? Inbreeding decreases genetic diversity through the routine mating of siblings, expected to be among the most genetically homogenous individuals. However, sib matings also can enhance the probability of a heterozygous mutation becoming homozygous through the generations, eventually resulting in its detection as an overt or deleterious phenotype. A detectable phenotype permits the elimination of the new mutation from the colony by removing any affected and related individuals. By contrast, outbreeding or any approach that purposefully avoids the mating of related individuals will permit heterozygous spontaneous mutation to be carried in the colony with little chance of phenotypic detection, promoting the genetic heterogeneity of an outbred population.

However, the greatest source of potential genetic divergence in any rodent colony is genetic contamination, incorrect matings or other undetected deviations. A GQC monitoring program should be designed to discover these natural and introduced errors before they are perpetuated by assessing not only the strain/stock/line genetic background, but also the presence and zygosity of specific alleles expected in specific colonies or individual mutant strains.

IV. SNP ANALYSIS: TESTING STRAIN BACKGROUND

For monitoring the strain background, the selection of SNP testing panels must take into account the extent of 'genetic insurance' that is acceptable and required. What depth and breadth of genomic coverage meets the reasonableness test by balancing the risk of genetic contamination with the colony's management procedures and practices, the effective deployment of resources, and the available analytical tools? In general, low-density SNP panels are most applicable for routine screening of a substantial number of large colonies. For example, all new breeders in The Jackson Laboratory's foundation colonies are screened with a panel of ~35 SNPs: these SNPs cover all the laboratory mouse autosomes and the X chromosome, with at least one diagnostic SNP per chromosome. This approach provides only a genetic snapshot of each colony, but a sufficient picture to differentiate all common inbred strains and most substrains. By contrast, high-density SNP panels are required for genome scanning, as well as for gene and quantitative trait locus (QTL) identification. The Mouse Universal Genotyping Array (MUGA, ~7851 SNPs) (Collaborative Cross Consortium, 2012), MegaMUGA (~80,000 SNPs; http://csbio.unc.edu/CCstatus/index.py?run=GeneseekMM), and the Mouse Diversity Array (~623,000 SNPs) (Yang et al., 2009) are among the panels available for detailed genomic analysis. A variety of diagnostic SNP panels are available from commercial vendors or have been reported in the research literature. Further, community resources, such as the International Mouse Genome Informatics (MGI) website (http://www.informatics.jax.org/strains_SNPs.shtml) or the Rat Genome Database (http://rgd.mcw.edu/) catalog the SNP differences between inbred mouse and rat strains. Using these data, SNP panels can be developed to efficiently discriminate strains, lines or stocks or to conduct genome analyses.

When selecting a SNP panel, researchers must define their experimental goals, then balance the analytical costs against their desired outcome. The mapping of a mutation or phenotype to a specific gene or discrete chromosomal region likely will require high-density SNP panels or even genomic sequencing, whereas lower-density SNP panels generally will suffice to determine whether a strain is genetically contaminated.

When examining a strain, stock, or line's genetic background, it is critical to assess whether discrimination among inbred strain background is sufficient or whether the evaluation must be refined to differentiate among common inbred substrains. Substrains arise when animals from a common ancestor pair (i.e., an inbred strain) are independently sister × brother bred for at least 20 generations. For example, the development of the C57BL inbred strain began in 1921; by 1970, numerous C57BL substrains were recognized (Bailey, 1978). During the generations of independent breeding, a substrain accumulates a unique repertoire of spontaneous mutations and alleles, leading to substrain-distinct phenotypes. The widely used C57BL/6J and C57BL/6N substrains were separated in 1951 at generation F32, when The Jackson Laboratory transferred mice to the National Institutes of Health. The independent inbreeding of these mice at NIH resulted in the 'N' substrain. In 1984, NIH cryopreserved this substrain at generation F124: the present C57BL/6NJ substrain is derived from the 1984 cryostock. By contrast, the present cryostock of C57BL/6J is at generation F226. Given that these two substrains have been independently maintained for ~300 generations, not all C57BL/6 mice are genetically or phenotypically equivalent and these differences can affect experimental results. Specifically, Simon et al. (2013) identified 36 coding sequence differences, as well as significant phenotypical differences, between the C57BL/6J and C57BL/6N substrains, two substrains separated for approximately 60 years.

V. ALLELE-SPECIFIC GENOTYPING: TESTING MUTANT STRAINS

For strains carrying known spontaneous, induced, or genetically engineered mutations, routine analysis of the presence and copy number of the mutant alleles is essential. Individual mutant strains, historically, were identified by an easily recognized phenotype, such as coat color. With the development of genetically engineered rodent strains, molecular confirmation of the presence and zygosity of engineered mutations became a critical GQC step, using a routine genotyping protocol is determined by the colony breeding requirements. Breeder genotype confirmation generally is sufficient for monitoring strains/lines bred homozygote × homozygote. By contrast, strains/stocks or lines with segregating mutations require genotyping of each progeny animal to identify the appropriate animals for subsequent breeding or experiments.

TABLE 31.3 Suggested Mating Schemes and Genetic Monitoring Strategies for Various Types of Animals Where Ensuring That Homozygosity and Genetic Uniformity Is Retained

Genetically homogenous

Strain type	Mating scheme	Options for genetic quality control testing		
		Which animals to test	Strain background assays	Allele-specific assays
Inbred	Sister × Brother (sib mating)	Breeders	Homozygous for strain/substrain-specific SNPs	Can test for strain/substrain-specific alleles
Congenic or isogenic	Hom × Hom	Breeders	Homozygous for strain/substrain-specific SNPs	Homozygous for mutant allele
	Hom × Het (or reciprocal)	Progeny, including presumptive breeders		Homozygous or heterozygous for mutant allele
	Het × Het	Progeny, including presumptive breeders		Homozygous, heterozygous or wild-type for mutant allele
	Wild-type from colony (or inbred) × Heterozygous or hemizygous carrier (or reciprocal)	Progeny, including presumptive breeders		Heterozygous/hemizygous or wild-type for mutant allele
F1 hybrid	Inbred 1 × Inbred 2	Breeders	As for inbreds	As for inbreds
Established recombinant inbred (RI) lines	Sister × Brother (sib mating)	Breeders	Homozygous for line-specific SNPs	

VI. MAINTAINING STRAINS

Tables 31.3 and 31.4 provide options for maintaining common laboratory rodent strains/stocks/lines to ensure the desired genetic homogeneity or heterogeneity in the population, as well as for conducting GQC analysis to confirm colony status (see Berry and Linder (2007) for a comprehensive review).

A. Inbred Strains

Strains maintained by inbreeding provide the greatest assurance of genetic identity through sib mating at each generation. A strain is considered inbred after a minimum of 20 generations (F20) of sib matings; however, with continual inbreeding, the genetic homogeneity of the inbred strain background is further increased by 40 generations of inbreeding, a strain is mathematically 99.98% homozygous (Green, 1981; Silver, 1995). The common inbred laboratory mouse strains (C57BL/6, DBA/1, DBA/2, BALB/c, CBA, C3H) were developed early in the last century (1909–1921) and are presently at F200 or greater generations of inbreeding. The primary GQC consideration is genetic consistency of the inbred strain background. Inbred strain SNP analysis should exhibit homozygosity for all markers; however, strain/substrain specific alleles can be tested for a higher level of confidence and discrimination.

TABLE 31.4 Suggested Mating Schemes and Genetic Monitoring Strategies for Various Types of Animals Where Ensuring Heterozygosity Is Retained Is Paramount

Genetically heterogenous

Strain type	Mating scheme	Options for genetic quality control testing	
		Which animals to test	Assays to monitor background
F2 Hybrid	F1 × F1	Progeny	Random distribution of grandparental inbred strain/substrain-specific SNPs
Established advanced intercross recombinant inbred (RI) lines	Sister × Brother	Breeders	Homozygous for line-specific SNPs
Outbred	Various (avoid sib matings)	Any	Random distribution of stock-specific SNPs
Random bred	Randomly generated among lines (avoid sib matings)	Any	Random distribution of population-specific SNPs

An additional approach to ensure the long-term genetic consistency of inbred strains is to combine sib mating with the cyclic reintroduction of cryopreserved animals and rebuilding of foundation colonies with pedigreed, cryopreserved embryos, thus ensuring downstream colonies and inventory mice are as genetically consistent as possible with the foundation stocks and substrains have not inadvertently arisen within the colony. The Jackson Laboratory's Genetic Stability Program (GSP, US patents 7,592,501 [2010] and 8,110,721 [2012]) provides a colony management approach for maintaining breeding colonies within a defined generation interval for many years or decades, thus limiting genetic drift and avoiding substrain divergence.

B. Isogenic Strains

Isogenic (coisogenic) strains differ from their parental inbred strain at a single locus, generally due to fixation of a spontaneous mutation initially recognized by an observable phenotype. When these mutant mice are inbred separately from their parental strain, the isogenic mice will retain their mutant phenotype, but will acquire background mutations not found in the parental strain. It is recommended that the mutant strain background is refreshed by backcrossing to the parental inbred strain approximately every 10 generations to ensure the mutant strain remains truly isogenic with the original parent strain. An alternative approach is to develop a stock of cryopreserved embryos derived from backcrossed animals and periodically refresh colonies with cryorecovered embryos (Taft *et al.*, 2006). When properly maintained, an isogenic colony will exhibit an identical strain background to its parental inbred strain, deviating only at the specific mutant allele. The mutant allele can be confirmed by the distinctive phenotype or by directly testing for the specific genomic change that created the mutant allele.

C. Congenic Strains

Congenic (and consomic) strains contain a discrete DNA region derived from another strain (for consomic strains, this region is an entire chromosome; Table 31.1). Historically, congenic mice were developed by the repeated backcrossing of strain-specific alleles onto another strain background with the selection of the desired allele/region at each backcross generation. With genetically engineered mutations, initially generated either by embryonic stem cell-mediated gene targeting or by the introduction of transgenic DNA constructs, the generation of congenic mice has accelerated, facilitating the characterization of individual mutations on a well-defined strain background and eliminating potential ambiguities due to variable strain background effects.

Generally, 10 generations of backcrossing is considered the standard for congenic strain development. Theoretically, with each backcross, the mutant stock acquires 50% of the inbred backcross partner's DNA sequences. By the 10th backcross generation (N10), 99.99% of the congenic strain background will be from the recipient inbred; only the congenic interval, the genomic region flanking the introduced allele, is essentially unchanged from the donor strain (Berry and Linder, 2007). However, theory and practice may not be in accordance and a genome scan is recommended to quantify the congenic strain background – the contributions of the donor and recipient strains – after repeated backcrosses. Marker-assisted backcrossing can accelerate the development of fully congenic strains by SNP analysis of progeny at each backcross generation and the selection of next-generation breeders for their content of recipient strain sequences (Berry and Linder, 2007; Wakeland *et al.*, 1997).

The optimal mating scheme for individual congenic lines will vary, generally determined by the phenotype of the introduced allele. The congenic strain background will remain isogenic with the recipient inbred strain, if the congenic colony is refreshed by periodic backcrossing or by the introduction of cryopreserved, backcrossed stocks. To ensure congenic strain identity, however, the presence and zygosity of the mutant allele should be routinely confirmed.

D. Genetically Modified Strains

Genetically modified strains (Table 31.2) are created through microinjection of DNA constructs (transgenic strains), targeted embryonic stem (ES) cells (gene targeted strains) or genomic editing through the injection of programmable endonucleases (e.g., zinc finger nucleases [ZFN], TALEN, CRISPR/Cas9) into embryos (Hsu *et al.*, 2014; Joung and Sander, 2013). Recent advances in embryonic stem cell derivation technology and site-specific nuclease technologies now make it possible to genetically engineer any murine strain. Genetic monitoring of the engineered alleles by PCR is essential to successfully maintaining these strains. However, additional GQC is recommended depending on the type of engineered strain.

Transgenic alleles generated by microinjection of DNA into embryos can be unstable because the injected DNA randomly integrates into the genome, frequently in multiple copies organized into an array. The stability of these arrays varies across generations; therefore, it is important to monitor transgene copy number and expression periodically. It is also important to perform GQC on engineered strains when they are first developed or acquired. This quality control depends on the nature of the engineered allele. A common quality control issue faced by mouse repositories involves conditional alleles. Conditional alleles containing loxP sites require cre-mediated recombination, which is usually provided through a cross of the strain carrying the conditional allele with a strain carrying a tissue specific cre (usually a transgenic strain). Subsequent breeding, assisted by a cre-specific PCR assay, is required to remove the cre, but this step is often neglected and unwanted cre alleles remain segregating in the colony.

The development of mutant mice has been revolutionized by the use of programmable endonucleases to generate sequence-specific mutations *in vivo*. By microinjecting targeting vectors/nucleases directly into inbred strain zygotes (fertilized eggs or single cell embryos), specific mutations can be created on a defined strain background, obviating the requirement for repeated backcrossing to introduce the mutant allele onto a defined genetic background. However, researchers should be cautious in evaluating these progeny: initially, they may be mosaic for the introduced mutation or carry unwanted second-site mutations due to target sequence similarities. Therefore, sib mating, coupled with genotyping for the precise targeted mutation and survey of the strain background, are recommended to ensure these mice conform to desired expectations.

E. F1 Hybrids

F1 hybrid animals are generated by the mating of two different inbred strains at each generation, using the same the maternal and paternal inbred parents. The F1 animals are genetically homogeneous and heterozygous at every locus, with 50% of their genomes derived from each parent. While these animals cannot be maintained as continuously breeding strains, F1 hybrid progeny provide the advantage of heterosis or hybrid vigor with larger litters and larger pups with generally more robust constitution than either inbred parent. F1 hybrids, therefore, can provide a consistent genetic background for studying potentially deleterious mutations or detrimental agents. Since F1 hybrid progeny require the repeated mating of two inbred strains, the genetic identity of parental inbred strains must be unequivocal.

F. F2 Hybrids

F2 hybrid progeny arise from the mating of two F1 hybrid animals. As a result of meiotic recombination, F2 hybrid progeny are not genetically homogeneous; rather each F2 animal is genetically heterogeneous with an assortment of alleles, SNPs or other molecular markers derived from their inbred grandparents. F2 hybrid mice are often used as approximate controls for mutant stocks that are not fully congenic.

G. Recombinant Inbreds

RI lines are developed by the mating of randomly selected F2 hybrid progeny followed by sib mating to establish individual inbred lines. After 20 generations of inbreeding, individual RI lines will be genetically homogenous, but a family of related RI lines will exhibit considerable genetic diversity, reflecting the genetic backgrounds of F2 hybrid line founders (Crow, 2007). A family of related RI lines can provide a unique resource for mapping genes and QTLs (Pollard, 2012). The analytical power of related RI lines lies in their diversity, but care must be taken in ensuring individual RI lines remain genetically homogeneous by careful colony maintenance and GQC/SNP testing to ensure each line retains its distinctive strain genetic background. Periodic analysis for the expected strain parameters of individual RI lines should be conducted to elucidate whether each line maintains its anticipated characteristics or has acquired new phenotypes or acquired detectable genotype changes.

H. Advanced Intercross Lines

Historically, RI lines were developed by inbreeding F2 progeny derived from grandparent of two distinct inbred strains. More recently, the RI strategy has been augmented by the use of breeding schemes to maximize meiotic recombination in the RI population (Rockman and Kruglyak, 2008) or by using multiple inbred strains to create the hybrid founder animals (Aylor *et al.*, 2011; Philip *et al.*, 2011).

In 2002, the International Collaborative Traits Consortium began the development of RI lines that combined the genomes of eight inbred laboratory mice strains by using a funnel-breeding scheme (The Complex Traits Consortium, 2004; Collaborative Cross Consortium, 2012). Following three generations of funneled, 'hybrid' matings, individual RI lines were established by classic inbreeding for 20 generations, creating the Collaborative Cross (CC) RI lines. When fully inbred, each CC RI line is genetically homogenous, but individual lines contain a unique genome, incorporating contributions from the eight original inbred founders.

The chromosomes of each advanced intercross line contain a combination of alleles or chromosomal regions randomly derived from the founder lines through meiotic recombination. The use of high-density SNP panels and advanced analytical tools generally are required to develop a genomic map for each chromosome of individual inbred advanced intercross line, identifying which chromosomal regions and alleles are derived from each original founder lines. Periodic reconfirmation by high-density SNP analysis of continuously bred lines can determine whether the initial genomic map remains essentially unchanged. Since any continuously bred line/stock will acquire spontaneous genomic changes, cryopreservation and recovery of the initially characterized lines can ensure genetic stability of individual lines. By comparisons among individual lines, specific traits can be mapped to specific chromosomal regions and, ultimately, correlated with founder line-specific alleles, strikingly illustrating the power of advanced intercross genomes for mapping genes, complex traits, and QTLs.

I. Non-Inbred Stocks (Outbred and Random-Bred Rodent Populations)

Rodents from outbred or non-inbred stocks are widely used for a variety of research applications that require animals with the greatest possible genetic variation (Aldinger et al., 2009; Chia et al., 2005; White and Lee, 1998; Hartl, 2001). When maintaining an outbred colony, the greatest challenge is ensuring the population, which may be split into several locations, truly retains its heterozygosity. The tendency of a closed colony built from a finite number of founder animals is to lose heterozygosity by the fixation of alleles over generations of continual mating: with increasing allele homozygosity, an outbred stock will become inbred. Therefore, outbred colonies must be maintained by a systematic breeding program optimized for breeding unrelated individuals (Nomura and Yonezawa, 1996; White, 1999) and by using methodology such as genomic scans employing high-density SNP panels to evaluate the extent of genetic heterozygosity. In general, outbreeding strategies require a large number of independent breeding lines with multiple breeding units for each line, unbiased breeder selection, and the routine infusion into the closed colony of animals from an independently maintained colony or cryopreserved stocks.

Another way in which heterozygosity and genetic diversity can be retained in colonies of outbred mice separated by space is by a scheme in which animals migrate to and from a founder colony (Charles River, 2011). In this means of preserving diversity, any drift or new mutations are retained and distributed to other colonies by means of the foundation colony. Animals from outlying colonies are rederived into the foundation colony at a rate of 5% of the foundation colony each year, and incorporated into the existing breeding scheme. The foundation colony is maintained through rotational mating. Each outlying colony also periodically receives 25% of its male breeders from the foundation colony as an efficient way of rotating alleles through a large population.

Random breeding provides another option for maintaining a population's genetic diversity (Aldinger et al., 2009; Churchill et al., 2012; Rockman and Kruglyak,

2008). The mating pairs at each generation are selected by use of a random number program, coupled with the exclusion of any randomly generated sib matings. The J:DO (Jax Diversity Outbred) mouse stock (Churchill et al., 2012; Svenson et al., 2012) is maintained by such a random mating scheme: the DO population was founded by the random mating of 144 partially inbred Collaborative Cross RI lines to establish 175 DO lines, which are randomly propagated at each generation. High-density SNP genome scans of DO progeny have confirmed the significant diversity of alleles among individual genomes and the utility of this stock for high resolution genetic mapping (Logan et al., 2013; Svenson et al., 2012).

VII. PHENOTYPE QUALITY CONTROL

GQC alone does not ensure a rodent model will meet experimental expectations and requirements. It is critical to know the expected phenotypes of any research strain and the impact of environmental or other factors on these phenotypes. Caging, diet, water, bedding, husbandry practices, and microbiome all may have a dramatic impact on phenotype. Both commercial providers and researchers should assess the physiological and biochemical parameters of the animals raised in their facilities and the potential impact of environmental changes on these variables. It is recommended that anyone receiving animals into a new location allow them to acclimate to their new environment prior to their use in experiments.

Commercial rodent provider public websites may provide basic phenotype information as well as other resources on the responses and experimental applications of individual research strains. The animal research community, moreover, has developed a wealth of databases that archive strain or mutation-specific genotypes and phenotypes. Among these are the Mouse Phenome database (http://phenome.jax.org/), the International Mouse Phenotyping Consortium (http://www.mouse-phenotype.org/), Mouse Genome Informatics database (http://www.informatics.jax.org/), the Rat Genome Database (http://rgd.mcw.edu/), and The National Bio Resource Project (http://www.anim.med.kyoto-u.ac.jp/nbr/phenome.aspx).

VIII. THE FUTURE OF GQC

The advent of high-throughput sequencing has revolutionized the field of genetics in innumerable ways. The sequencing and assembly of the mouse genome representing a single inbred strain, C57BL6, was completed in 2002 (Mouse Genome Sequencing Consortium, 2002) after a three-year effort based on dideoxy or chain termination sequencing (a.k.a. Sanger sequencing). In 2011, The Sanger Mouse Genomes project published the whole genome sequence of 17 inbred strains using high-throughput/massively parallel sequencing demonstrating the power of this sequencing technology to generate DNA sequencing data on a scale that is orders of magnitude over earlier methods. Today, a single mouse genome can be re-sequenced to a depth of 30× coverage for less than $5000 using this technology (Yalcin et al., 2012). Select regions of the genome can be subjected to high-throughput sequencing by applying any number of techniques that allow for enrichment of specific regions of interest. Selective sequencing is most commonly accomplished using a pool of DNA probes that share homology with the regions of interest. Enrichment for those regions is accomplished by probe hybridization to total genomic DNA in solution, followed by capture of the DNA hybrids and high-throughput sequencing. The most common application is selective sequencing of the coding portion of the genome or exome sequencing. Exome sequencing can be accomplished for as little as $900 and provides sufficient coverage to confidently genotype the coding portion of the mouse genome, which is ~50 Mb (Fairfield et al., 2011). This method captures all of the variation within the annotated coding portion of the genome and can provide significant baseline data for any mouse strain. In fact, this approach is now used routinely as follow up GQC for spontaneous mutations that confer clinically interesting phenotypes in mouse colonies at The Jackson Laboratory (Fairfield et al., 2011). Identification of spontaneous mutations also allows for the design of genotyping assays that can then be used to selectively remove these unwanted alleles from breeding colonies. While this approach is not yet cost effective for routine GQC, the race for the $1000 genome (Hayden, 2014) is driving costs down making high-throughput sequencing an eventuality that could have a significant impact on GQC options in the future.

IX. GQC: PRACTICAL ASPECTS

Genetic monitoring of rodent colonies focuses on molecular markers, biochemical or immunological assays to assess the allelic diversity within a colony, as well as individual genotypes. While these techniques provide qualitative and quantitative evidence of a colony's genetic constitution, the foundation of any GQC program lies with basic colony management and animal husbandry. These approaches are simple in concept and execution, but produce huge dividends in insurance of a colony's genetic status.

- Employ consistent, tested husbandry practices designed to avoid cross contamination between individual cages or strains.
- Segregate strains/lines/stocks by coat color or another observable phenotype.
- Use appropriate colony nomenclature and separate colonies with similar names. For example, separate C57BL/6J from C57BL/6N, BALB/c from BALB/cBy, etc.
- Consistently use distinct cage cards for each strain and separate strains with similar cage cards. Use the colony-specific cage cards for all cages, both breeders and weaned progeny. Employ colony management software coupled with bar-coded cage cards or other card or animal identification method. Among the available animal ID methods are standard ear notching or ear tags, bar-coded ear tags, microchip implants, or permanent tattoos.
- Consider maintaining pedigreed colonies: for inbred, isogenic, congenic or established RI lines, sibling breeder units are established at weaning, and each mating is recorded by family lineage in colony management software, on cage cards and in pedigree books or charts. While potentially far more complex, similar records should be kept for non-inbred colonies.
- Not only do pedigreed colonies reduce potential mating errors, but also lineage tracking provides an unambiguous record for tracking the ancestry of any phenotypic deviations, spontaneous mutations, or potential genetic contamination.
- Maintain physically separated colonies for each strain/stock/line. Commercial animal providers maintain their breeding colonies with several subcolonies (Figure 31.2): foundation stocks (FS) provide the breeders to expansion stocks that, in turn, send breeders to the distribution colonies. With independent colonies, spontaneous mutations or genetic contaminations can be limited to and eliminated from a single colony.
- Maintain cryopreserved stocks of each strain or population, using these stocks either to routinely replenish your foundation colonies, thus limiting genetic drift and substrain development, or to provide a source of new breeder stock in the event of genetic contamination or widespread fixation of new mutations (Wiles and Taft, 2010). Know the expected deviations of your strains, then detect, track and eliminate all phenotypic deviants whether expected or unexpected. Be on the alert for the recurrence of an unexpected phenotype within a strain or line.
- Animals exhibiting abnormal, unexpected phenotypes can result from the expression of a spontaneous mutation, a genetic contamination or

a developmental, often not heritable, mutation. The analysis of phenotypic deviants and their parents can elucidate the heritability and origin of the phenotype, facilitating the removal of undesirable contaminants before they become fixed in the colony.

- Supplement your colony management program with a consistent, statistically significant GQC program. For any colony, monitor the genetic background to ensure the desired composition is retained; for strains carrying mutations, monitor both the genetic background and the expected mutant allele(s).

When monitoring for spontaneous, induced, or engineered mutations,

- Employ allele-specific assays. While generic assays for drug resistance markers, Cre or green fluorescent protein provide a convenient option for routine genotype analysis, they do not provide the highest level of discrimination when a colony contains numerous similar strains or single strains carrying multiple alleles.
- Ensure allele-specific assays can unambiguously differentiate homozygotes from heteterozygotes from wild-type.
- For transgenic strains, for which the extent of a phenotype may be a function of the expression of multiple transgene copies, detection of the transgene alone may not be sufficient to ensure the strain's conformity to phenotype expectations. The use of assays to assess the transgene copy number may be essential to ensuring the stability and reproducibility of a transgenic model.
- Only accept unequivocal assay results, ascribable to individual animals. If any result is questionable, resample and repeat the allele-specific assay or remove the animal from your colony.
- Assess your process: where are the greatest vulnerabilities for breeding or using an incorrect animal? The greatest chance for confusion of individual animals or strains lies when animals move or are shipped from one location to another. Therefore, it is recommended that the identity of animals is confirmed when they arrive at their final destination or employ unambiguous animal or strain identification methods prior to movement.

X. CONCLUSIONS

Careful genetic monitoring of laboratory mouse and rat strains maintains genetic homogeneity, which is critical (with the exception of strains that are intentionally heterogeneous) for reproducibility in animal studies. Therefore, it is essential that the vivarium design and

implement rigorous GQC protocols. GQC methods vary in their sensitivity and specificity as well as their cost; choice and implementation of GQC methods should be guided by the nature of the strains to be monitored. Finally, the responsibility of proper GQC is not only the responsibility of the vivarium, it should be carefully considered during strain development and by the end user to ensure responsible laboratory animal stewardship and high-quality scientific results.

References

Aldinger, K.A., Sokoloff, G., Rosenberg, D.M., Palmer, A.A., Millen, K.J., 2009. Genetic variation and population substructure in outbred CD-1 mice: implications for genome-wide association studies. PLoS One 4, e4729.

Aylor, D.L., Valdar, W., Foulds-Mathes, W., Buus, R.J., Verdugo, R.A., Baric, R.S., et al., 2011. Genetic analysis of complex traits in the emerging Collaborative Cross. Genome Res. 21, 1213–1222.

Bailey, D.W., 1978. Sources of subline divergence and their relative importance for sublines of six major inbred strains. In: Morse III, J.D. (Ed.), Origins of Inbred Mice. Academic Press, New York.

Bailey, D.W., Usama, B., 1960. A rapid method of grafting skin on tails of mice. Transplant. Bull. 25, 424–425.

Beck, J.A., Lloyd, S., Hafezparast, M., Lennon-Pierce, M., Eppig, J.T., Festing, M.F., et al., 2000. Genealogies of mouse inbred strains. Nat. Genet. 24, 23–25.

Benavides, F.J., 1999. Genetic contamination of an SJL/J mouse colony: rapid detection by PCR-based microsatellite analysis. Contemp. Top. Lab. Anim. Sci. 38, 54–55.

Berry, M.L., Linder, C.C., 2007. Breeding systems: considerations, genetic fundamentals, genetic background, and strain types. In: Fox, J.G., Barthold, S.W., Davisson, M.T., Newcomer, C., Quimby, F.W., Smith, A.L. (Eds.), The Mouse in Biomedical Research. Academic Press, New York.

Bothe, G.W., Gray, J.L., Rusconi, J.C., Festin, S.M., Perez, A.V., 2011. A Panel of 96 single nucleotide polymorphisms for genetic monitoring of rats. J. Am. Assoc. Lab. Anim. Sci. 50 797–797.

Casellas, J., 2011. Inbred mouse strains and genetic stability: a review. Animal 5, 1–7.

Charles River. 2011. International Genetic Standardization (IGS) Program. <http://www.criver.com/files/pdfs/rms/rm_rm_r_igs.aspx>.

Chia, R., Achilli, F., Festing, M.F., Fisher, E.M., 2005. The origins and uses of mouse outbred stocks. Nat. Genet. 37, 1181–1186.

Churchill, G.A., Gatti, D.M., Munger, S.C., Svenson, K.L., 2012. The diversity outbred mouse population. Mamm. Genome 23, 713–718.

Collaborative Cross Consortium, 2012. The Genome Architecture of the Collaborative Cross Mouse Genetic Reference Population. Genetics 190 389–U159.

Crow, J.F., 2007. Haldane, Bailey, Taylor and recombinant-inbred lines. Genetics 176, 729–732.

Drake, J.W., Charlesworth, B., Charlesworth, D., Crow, J.F., 1998. Rates of spontaneous mutation. Genetics 148, 1667–1686.

Dubin, S., Zeitz, S., 1991. Sample size for animal health surveillance. Lab. Anim. (NY) 20, 29–33.

Fairfield, H., Gilbert, G.J., Barter, M., Corrigan, R.R., Curtain, M., Ding, Y., et al., 2011. Mutation discovery in mice by whole exome sequencing. Genome Biol. 12, R86.

Festing, M., 1972. Mouse strain identification. Nature 238, 351–352.

Festing, M.F., 1974. Genetic reliability of commercially-bred laboratory mice. Lab. Anim. 8, 265–270.

Festing, M.F.W., 1982. Genetic contamination of laboratory animal colonies: an increasingly serious problem. ILAR News 25, 6–10.

Festing, M.F.W., 1993. Genetic quality control in laboratory rodents. Aging Clin. Exp. Res. 5, 309–315.

Fox, R.R., Wiles, M.V., Petkov, P.M., 2007. Genetic monitoring. In: Fox, J.G., Barthold, S.W., Davisson, M.T., Newcomer, C., Quimby, F.W., Smith, A.L. (Eds.), The Mouse in Biomedical Research. Academic Press, New York.

Gorer, P.A., O'Gorman, P., 1956. The cytotoxic activities of isoantibodies in mice. Transplant. Bull. 3, 142–143.

Green, E.L., 1981. Genetics and Probability in Animal Breeding Experiments. Macmillan, London.

Groen, A., 1977. Identification and genetic monitoring of mouse inbred strains using biochemical polymorphisms. Lab. Anim. 11, 209–214.

Hartl, D.L., 2001. Genetic management of Gold Standard outbred laboratory populations.

Hayden, E.C., 2014. Technology: The $1,000 genome. Nature 507, 294–295.

Hirayama, N., Kuramoto, T., Kondo, Y., Yamada, J., Serikawa, T., 1994. Genetic profiles of 12 inbred rat strains for 46 microsatellite loci selected as genetic monitoring markers. Exp. Anim. 43, 129–132.

Hsu, P.D., Lander, E.S., Zhang, F., 2014. Development and Applications of CRISPR-Cas9 for Genome Engineering. Cell 157, 1262–1278.

ILAR, 1976. Long-term holding of laboratory rodents. ILAR News 19, L1–L25.

Jacob, H.J., Kwitek, A.E., 2002. Rat genetics: attaching physiology and pharmacology to the genome. Nat. Rev. Genet. 3, 33–42.

Jones, R.E., Weinberg, A., Bourdette, D., 1994. Evidence for genetic contamination of inbred Buffalo rats (Rt-1(B)) obtained from a commercial vendor. J. Neuroimmunol. 52, 215–218.

Joung, J.K., Sander, J.D., 2013. TALENs: a widely applicable technology for targeted genome editing. Nat. Rev. Mol. Cell Biol. 14, 49–55.

Kahan, B., Auerbach, R., Alter, B.J., Bach, F.H., 1982. Histocompatibility and isoenzyme differences in commercially supplied "BALB/c" mice. Science 217, 379–381.

Kloting, I., Voigt, B., Vogt, L., 1995. 47 polymorphic microsatellite loci in different inbred rat strains. J. Exp. Anim. Sci. 37, 42–47.

Lewis, J.L., Russell, R.J., Warnock, D.G., 1994. Analysis of the genetic contamination of salt-sensitive Dahl/Rapp rats. Hypertension 24, 255–259.

Logan, R.W., Robledo, R.F., Recla, J.M., Philip, V.M., Bubier, J.A., Jay, J.J., et al., 2013. High-precision genetic mapping of behavioral traits in the diversity outbred mouse population. Genes Brain Behav. 12, 424–437.

Lovell, D.P., Totman, P., Johnson, F.M., 1984. Variation in the shape of the mouse mandible. 1. Effect of age and set on the results obtained from the discriminant functions used for genetic monitoring. Genet. Res. 43, 65–73.

Malakoff, D., 2000. The rise of the mouse, biomedicine's model mammal. Science 288, 248–253.

Marshall, J.D., Mu, J.L., Cheah, Y.C., Nesbitt, M.N., Frankel, W.N., Paigen, B., 1992. The AXB and BXA set of recombinant inbred mouse strains. Mamm. Genome 3, 669–680.

Montagutelli, X., Serikawa, T., Guenet, J.L., 1991. PCR-analyzed microsatellites – data concerning laboratory and wild-derived mouse inbred strains. Mamm. Genome 1, 255–259.

Mouse Genome Sequencing Consortium, 2002. Initial sequencing and comparative analysis of the mouse genome. Nature 420, 520–562.

Naggert, J.K., Mu, J.L., Frankel, W., Bailey, D.W., Paigen, B., 1995. Genomic analysis of the C57BL/Ks mouse strain. Mamm. Genome 6, 131–133.

Nandakumar, K.S., Holmdahl, R., 2005. A genetic contamination in MHC-congenic mouse strains reveals a locus on chromosome 10 that determines autoimmunity and arthritis susceptibility. Eur. J. Immunol. 35, 1275–1282.

Nijman, I.J., Kuipers, S., Verheul, M., Guryev, V., Cuppen, E., 2008. A genome-wide SNP panel for mapping and association studies in the rat. BMC Genomics 9.

Nitzki, F., Kruger, A., Reifenberg, K., Wojnowski, L., Hahn, H., 2007. Identification of a genetic contamination in a commercial mouse strain using two panels of polymorphic markers. Lab. Anim. 41, 218–228.

Nomura, T., Yonezawa, K., 1996. A comparison of four systems of group mating for avoiding inbreeding. Genet. Sel. Evol. 28, 141–159.

Petkov, P.M., Cassell, M.A., Sargent, E.E., Donnelly, C.J., Robinson, P., Crew, V., et al., 2004a. Development of a SNP genotyping panel for genetic monitoring of the laboratory mouse. Genomics 83, 902–911.

Petkov, P.M., Ding, Y.M., Cassell, M.A., Zhang, W.D., Wagner, G., Sargent, E.E., et al., 2004b. An efficient SNP system for mouse genome scanning and elucidating strain relationships. Genome Res. 14, 1806–1811.

Philip, V.M., Sokoloff, G., Ackert-Bicknell, C.L., Striz, M., Branstetter, L., Beckmann, M.A., et al., 2011. Genetic analysis in the Collaborative Cross breeding population. Genome Res. 21, 1223–1238.

Pollard, D.A., 2012. Design and construction of recombinant inbred lines. In: Rifkin, S.A. (Ed.), Quantitative Trait Loci (QTL): Methods in Molecular Biology. Humana Press.

Rockman, M.V., Kruglyak, L., 2008. Breeding designs for recombinant inbred advanced intercross lines. Genetics 179, 1069–1078.

Russell, R.J., Festing, M.F., Deeny, A.A., Peters, A.G., 1993. DNA fingerprinting for genetic monitoring of inbred laboratory rats and mice. Lab. Anim. Sci. 43, 460–465.

Saar, K., Beck, A., Bihoreau, M.T., Birney, E., Brocklebank, D., Chen, Y., et al., 2008. SNP and haplotype mapping for genetic analysis in the rat. Nat. Genet. 40, 560–566.

Shiroishi, T., Sagai, T., Moriwaki, K., 1981. A Simplified Micro-Method for Cytotoxicity Testing Using a Flat-Type Titration Plate for the Detection of H-2 Antigens. Microbiol. Immunol. 25, 1327–1334.

Silver, L.M., 1995. Mouse Genetics. Oxford University Press, New York.

Simon, M.M., Greenaway, S., White, J.K., Fuchs, H., Gailus-Durner, V., Wells, S., et al., 2013. A comparative phenotypic and genomic analysis of C57BL/6J and C57BL/6N mouse strains. Genome Biol. 14.

St Lezin, E.M., Pravenec, M., Wong, A., Wang, J.M., Merriouns, T., Newton, S., et al., 1994. Genetic contamination of Dahl SS/Jr rats. Impact on studies of salt-sensitive hypertension. Hypertension 23, 786–790.

Svenson, K.L., Gatti, D.M., Valdar, W., Welsh, C.E., Cheng, R., Chesler, E.J., et al., 2012. High-resolution genetic mapping using the mouse diversity outbred population. Genetics 190, 437–447.

Taft, R.A., Davisson, M., Wiles, M.V., 2006. Know thy mouse. Trends Genet. 22, 649–653.

The Complex Traits Consortium, 2004. The Collaborative Cross, a community resource for the genetic analysis of complex traits. Nat. Genet. 36, 1133–1137.

Threadgill, D.W., Yee, D., Matin, A., Nadeau, J.H., Magnuson, T., 1997. Genealogy of the 129 inbred strains: 129/SvJ is a contaminated inbred strain. Mamm. Genome 8, 390–393.

Wakeland, E., Morel, L., Achey, K., Yui, M., Longmate, J., 1997. Speed congenics: a classic technique in the fast lane (relatively speaking). Immunol. Today 18, 472–477.

West, J.D., Lyon, M.F., Peters, J., 1985. Genetic differences between substrains of the inbred mouse strain 101 and designation of a new strain 102. Genet. Res. 46, 349–352.

White, W.J., 1999. Genetic evaluation of outbred rats from a breeder's perspective. In: National Research Council (US) International Committee of the Institute for Laboratory Animal Research editor, Microbial Status and Genetic Evaluation of Mice and Rats: Proceedings of the 1999 US/Japan Conference. National Academies Press, Washington, DC, pp. 51–64.

White, W.J., Lee, C.S., 1998. The development and maintenance of the Crl:CD(SD) IGS rat breeding system. In: Matsuzawa, T., Inoue, H. (Eds.), Biological Reference Data on CD(SD) IGS Rats Charles River, Yokohama, Japan.

Whitmore, S.P., Gilliam, A.F., Hendren, R.W., Lewis, S.E., Rao, G.N., Whisnant, C.C., 1996. Genetic monitoring of inbred rodents from controlled production colonies through biochemical markers and skin grafting procedures. Lab. Anim. Sci. 46, 585–588.

Wiles, M.V., Taft, R.A., 2010. The sophisticated mouse: protecting a precious reagent. Methods Mol. Biol. 602, 23–36.

Wiltshire, T., Pletcher, M.T., Batalov, S., Barnes, S.W., Tarantino, L.M., Cooke, M.P., et al., 2003. Genome-wide single-nucleotide polymorphism analysis defines haplotype patterns in mouse. Proc. Natl. Acad. Sci. USA 100, 3380–3385.

Yalcin, B., Adams, D.J., Flint, J., Keane, T.M., 2012. Next-generation sequencing of experimental mouse strains. Mamm. Genome 23, 490–498.

Yang, H., Ding, Y.M., Hutchins, L.N., Szatkiewicz, J., Bell, T.A., Paigen, B.J., et al., 2009. A customized and versatile high-density genotyping array for the mouse. Nat. Methods 6 663–U55.

Zurita, E., Chagoyen, M., Cantero, M., Alonso, R., Gonzalez-Neira, A., Lopez-Jimenez, A., et al., 2011. Genetic polymorphisms among C57BL/6 mouse inbred strains. Transgenic Res. 20, 481–489.

CHAPTER

32

Genetically Modified Animals

Kathleen R. Pritchett-Corning, DVM, DACLAM, MRCVS[a] and Carlisle P. Landel, PhD[b]

[a]Harvard University Faculty of Arts and Sciences, Office of Animal Resources and Department of Comparative Medicine, University of Washington, Seattle, Washington, USA
[b]Department of Microbiology, Immunology and Molecular Genetics, Transposagen Biopharmaceuticals Inc., University of Kentucky, Lexington, KY, USA

I. INTRODUCTION

For most of the 20th century, increasing numbers of genetically defined laboratory mice have been described and incorporated into biological research; this trend has accelerated in the 21st century. Initially, research using inbred strains was limited mostly to basic genetic studies in which biochemical or visual phenotypic expression patterns were observed. With the advent of molecular genetics in the 1960s, laboratory mice developed into critical research tools in which the genomic basis of disease and mutation could be examined at the level of individual genes. By the 1970s, the prospect of intentionally modifying the murine genome by the addition of new

functional DNA was at hand (Jaenisch, 1976; Jaenisch and Mintz, 1974). By the early 1980s, the persistence of microinjected laboratory-derived DNA within the cells of live-born mice (Gordon and Ruddle, 1981) and the functional expression of transgenes in mice (Brinster *et al.*, 1981; Costantini and Lacy, 1981) were reported. Within a few years, major universities, medical schools, and pharmaceutical and biotechnology companies had created in-house transgenic mouse laboratories and genetic modification technologies had been expanded to other species. Genetically modified (GM) *C. elegans*, *Drosophila*, zebrafish, mice, and rats have been used in biomedical research for studies of basic genetics and gene function, as well as for modeling human disease.

Laboratory Animal Medicine, Third Edition
DOI: http://dx.doi.org/10.1016/B978-0-12-409527-4.00032-8

1417

GM cattle, goats, and sheep have been used to produce proteins in milk (Schnieke et al., 1997), while GM pigs have been used as large animal models of certain diseases and as potential xenotransplantation donors (Lai et al., 2002). The mouse remains the primary choice for transgenic experimentation due to the relative ease of embryo and adult manipulation and the unparalleled depth of murine genetic knowledge, although rats may have more utility for some purposes (Zheng et al., 2012). Today, GM mice are produced as models of human disease, to study basic gene function and regulation, and as in vivo systems in which mammalian (and nonmammalian) genetic expression may be investigated.

The creation and production of GM animals entails an intensive sequence of procedures involving genetics, molecular biology, embryology, and animal science. For details on how to perform many of the procedures discussed in this chapter, *Manipulating the Mouse Embryo: A Laboratory Manual, Fourth Edition* by Behringer et al. is a valuable resource for veterinarians and gene manipulation facilities alike (Behringer et al., 2014). This chapter will not discuss in depth the development or maintenance of GM animal colonies, as there are texts that discuss this in detail (Pritchett-Corning et al., 2011; Flurkey et al., 2009). This chapter will not discuss the individual special husbandry needs of GM animals, as those are potentially as diverse as the disruption of each gene in a species might allow. Instead, this chapter will attempt to give the reader an overview of genetic modification technologies currently and historically in use, how each is accomplished, their advantages, and their disadvantages, were known. In addition, while many of these technologies have been used in varying species (Table 32.1), this review will focus mainly on rats and mice, since those animals are the vast majority of those used in biomedical research.

II. MANIPULATING ANIMALS FOR GENETIC MODIFICATION

Genetic modification of rodents is accomplished by either mutagenizing the germline of intact animals with radiation or chemical mutagens, altering the genome of the 1-cell embryo, or by manipulating the genome of cells (ESCs) that can give rise to an animal in some manner. In the latter case, these cells include embryonic stem cells, induced pluripotent stem (iPS) cells, somatic cells and spermatogonial stem cells (SSCs).

A. Mutagenizing the Genome of Intact Animals

One of the first means of generating GM animals was through the deliberate induction of mutations in male germplasm. Spermatogonia, with their short lifespan, continuous division, and abundant production, are ideal

targets for mutagenic effects. Ionizing radiation was one of the first mutagens used in mice to produce heritable phenotypes and allow scientists to investigate the mutations and their patterns of heritability. The fact that ionizing radiation had an effect on DNA had been shown by George Snell and his colleagues, and then further refined by William and Lee Russell, working at the Oak Ridge National Laboratories, using the T stock mouse. This mouse, which carried seven recessive mutations, all viable, all affecting different traits, was hugely important in the discovery of mutation rates induced by radiation and the effects of dose and type of radiation on mutations in mice (Russell et al., 1958). Radiation is rarely used as a primary means of mutation induction today.

Until recently, chemical mutagenesis was employed for large-scale mouse mutagenesis projects (Nolan et al., 2000). The idea was to mutagenize males, mate them to wild-type animals, and screen F1 and N2 offspring for desired phenotypes. The mutagen of choice was ENU (N-ethyl-N-nitrosurea; Fig. 32.1). This compound was discovered to be a potent mutagen by William and Lee Russell, working at Oak Ridge National Laboratories (Russell et al., 1979). ENU targets the SSC in males and can induce one mutation in every 175–4500 loci (Davis and Justice, 1998). Effective doses vary between mouse stocks and strains (Justice et al., 1999), but a typical dose is 100 mg/kg given three times, each a week apart. Doses too high will kill animals or render them permanently sterile. Doses of ENU recorded as successfully inducing mutations in SD rats were 60 mg/kg given in two doses (Zan et al., 2003). Fertility recovery can take place in as little as 10 weeks, but is more typically recovered 12–20 weeks after the last injection.

After the males have recovered their fertility, they are mated with females, either from the same strain as the injected males, or for mapping purposes, a different strain. A tester strain can also be used as mates for the mutagenized males. Dominant mutations compatible with life are revealed in the first generation (G1), as offspring require only one copy of the mutated allele to exhibit a phenotype. For efficiency's sake, male offspring showing no phenotype are typically saved from G1, and then outcrossed to the inbred strain used earlier to generate G2 mice. G2 females are saved, then mated back to the male G1 parent. G3 offspring or embryos are then evaluated for recessive mutations (Fig. 32.2). Depending on the mutation, if one is interested in the mutation's ability to modify the expression of other genes, other breeding and monitoring schemes may be undertaken (Hrabe de Angelis et al., 2007).

ENU mutagenesis is a useful tool in the genetic modification arsenal as it generates point mutations in a manner that is completely unbiased by a preconceived notion of the nature of a gene and instead searches for a resulting phenotype. Thus, a mutant allele can occur

TABLE 32.1 A List of Commonly Used Research Animals That Have Been Genetically Modified

Animal	GM technologies reported	Example references
C. elegans	Irradiation, ENU, transgenesis, homologous recombination, programmable nucleases	Cheng et al. (2013); Radman et al. (2013); Chen et al. (2013); Barstead et al. (2012); Stewart et al. (1991); De Stasio and Dorman (2001); Frokjaer-Jensen et al. (2010); Katic and Grosshans (2013)
D. melanogaster	Irradiation, ENU, transgenesis, homologous recombination, programmable nucleases	Liu et al. (2012); Beumer et al. (2006); Gratz et al. (2013); Hagmann et al. (1998); Tosal et al. (1998); Bibikova et al. (2002); Gloor et al. (1991); Hanson and Winkleman (1929)
D. rerio	Irradiation, ENU, transgenesis, homologous recombination, programmable nucleases	Hwang et al. (2013); Doyon et al. (2008); Cade et al. (2012); Hagmann et al. (1998); Grunwald and Streisinger (1992); Ma et al. (2001)
A. mexicanum	Transgenesis, programmable nucleases	Sobkow et al. (2006); Khattak et al. (2013); Flowers et al. (2014)
X. laevis and X. tropicalis	Transgenesis, homologous recombination, programmable nucleases	Blitz et al. (2013); Tran and Vleminckx (2014); Young et al. (2011); Lei et al. (2012); Nakajima et al. (2012); Ju et al. (1997); Nakajima et al. (2013); Kroll and Amaya (1996)
Laboratory mice	Irradiation, ENU, transgenesis, homologous recombination, programmable nucleases	See text
R. norvegicus	Irradiation, ENU, transgenesis, homologous recombination, programmable nucleases	See text
O. cuniculagus	Transgenesis, programmable nucleases	Hirabayashi et al. (2001); Hammer et al. (1985); Flisikowska et al. (2011)
G. gallus	Transgenesis, homologous recombination	Schusser et al. (2013); Lillico et al. (2005)
C. familiaris	Transgenesis	Kim et al. (2011)
C. cattus	Transgenesis	Yin et al. (2008)
Callithrix jaccus	Transgenesis	Sasaki et al. (2009)
Macaca spp.	Transgenesis, programmable nucleases	Chan et al. (2001); Yang et al. (2008); Niu et al. (2014)
Ovis aries	Transgenesis	Schnieke et al. (1997); Hammer et al. (1985)
Capra aegagrus hircus	Transgenesis	Baldassarre et al. (2003); Tan et al. (2013)
Sus scrofa	Transgenesis, homologous recombination, programmable nucleases	Hirabayashi et al. (2001); Lutz et al. (2013); Bao et al. (2014); Xin et al. (2013); Hai et al. (2014); Lai et al. (2002); Hammer et al. (1985); Bultmann et al. (2012); Tan et al. (2013); Carlson et al. (2012)
Bos primigenius	Transgenesis, programmable nucleases	Xu et al. (2013); Tan et al. (2013); Carlson et al. (2012); Clark and Whitelaw (2003)

The list of means of genetic modifications for each animal may not be complete, although an effort was made to only include reports where the genetic modification was transmissible to offspring. Transgenesis is the insertion of foreign DNA through pronuclear injection or viral vectors. Homologous recombination refers to the induction of targeted mutations using gene targeting vectors in either embryonic stem cells or other cells. Programmable nucleases include zinc-finger nucleases (ZFN), transcription activator-like effector nucleases (TALENs), and clustered regularly interspaced short palindromic repeat-associated systems (CRISPR).

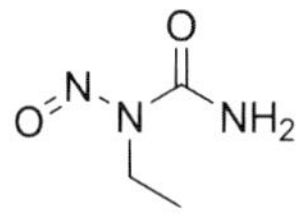

FIGURE 32.1 The chemical structure of ENU, N-ethyl-N-nitrosurea. Its chemical formula is $C_3H_7N_3O_2$. It is an alkylating agent that has a preference for inducing A- > T base transversions and AT- > GC transitions in DNA.

in a previously unsuspected region of importance that affects gene expression rather than in the recognized coding or control regions of a gene (Justice et al., 1999). On the other hand, this method fell out of favor because of the difficulty of actually identifying the physical mutation that is causative for the observed phenotype and was replaced by large-scale, high-throughput methods targeting all known coding genes. However, ENU has been used more recently in a target-directed high-throughput mutagenesis scheme, where offspring were screened for useful mutations in a selected set of genes (Smits et al., 2006).

B. Mutagenizing the Embryo

In the case of manipulating the embryo directly, it is fairly straightforward: nucleic acids (DNA and/or RNA) or perhaps enzymes are microinjected into the embryo or delivered to the embryo with a virus. The embryo is

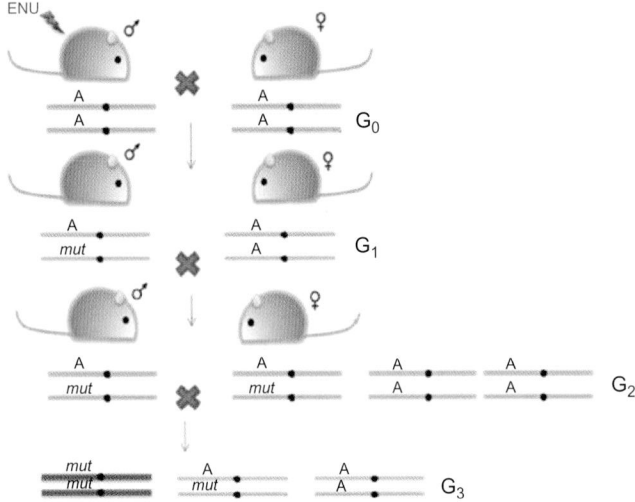

FIGURE 32.2 Steps in evaluation of animals generated through ENU mutagenesis (a conventional or genome-wide screen). Other means of identifying mutated genes or regions are possible. These are termed region-specific screens and focus on generating a series of alleles in the region of interest. *"Conventional screenfig1," via Wikipedia: http://en.wikipedia.org/wiki/File:Conventional_screenfig1.JPG#mediaviewer/ File:Conventional_screenfig1.JPG.*

then surgically implanted into a foster mother that carries the embryo to term, and the resultant pups are simply screened for the presence of the induced mutation. (Obtaining the requisite embryos and foster mothers are described later in the chapter.)

Embryos for microinjection are obtained as follows. Male mice are mated with young, superovulated female mice (see later in this chapter for details). The females are euthanized the next morning (0.5 days post-conception, or DPC) and embryos are harvested from the oviduct and placed in medium. They are then injected through the use of a microinjection apparatus (Fig. 32.3) and the injected embryos are transferred into the oviducts of a 0.5 DPC pseudopregnant recipient. The entire process is diagrammed in Figure 32.4. The females then give birth to offspring that may have integrated the foreign DNA into their genomes. The offspring are screened, and if any are positive, breeding is attempted to further the new transgenic lines just created.

C. Mutagenizing Cells

1. Embryonic Stem Cells

ESC are derived from the very early (blastocyst-stage) pre-implantation embryo, when the embryo is a hollow ball of trophectoderm cells enclosing a group of cells

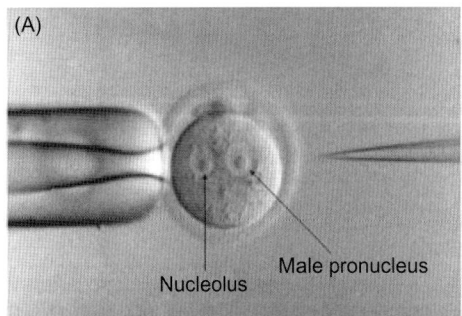
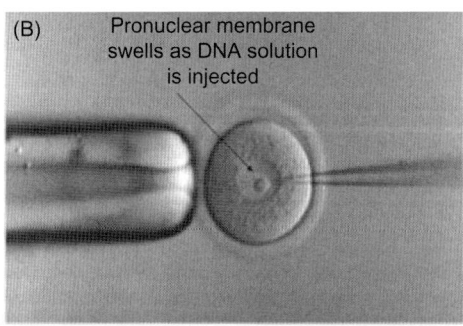
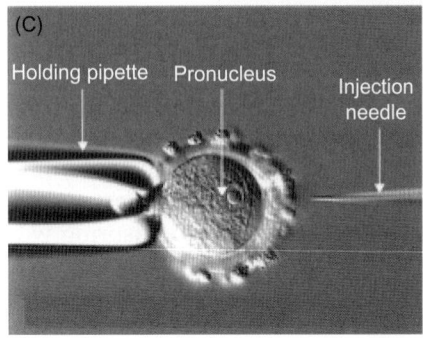
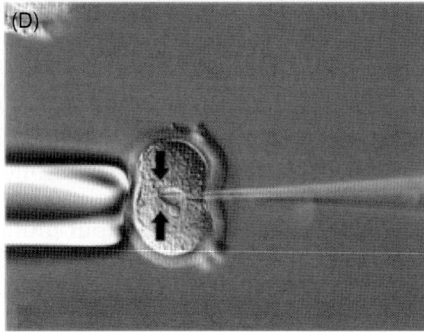
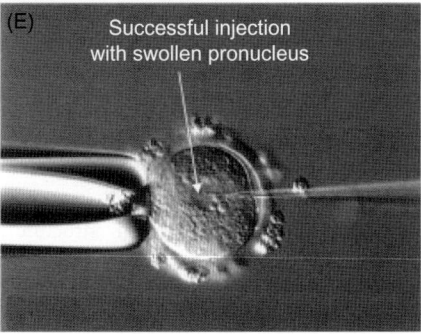

FIGURE 32.3 Pronuclear injection of mouse (A, B) and rat (C, D, E) single-celled embryos (day 0.5 post-conception). The fertilized embryo is held in place by the holding pipette seen on the left while the DNA injection needle can be seen on the right. (A) Mouse embryo before microinjection showing the larger male pronucleus and nucleolus. (B) Microinjection has been successful, as indicated by the swollen pronucleus. (C) Rat embryo before microinjection. The pronuclei are difficult to distinguish when compared to the mouse embryo. In this photo, a cumulus cell is still attached to the rat embryo. (D) Insertion of injection needle without successful penetration of the cell membrane. Arrows show the tip of the injection needle not yet within the embryo. (E) Successful penetration of the cell membrane and pronuclear membrane showing swelling of the pronucleus as the DNA is injected. Magnification ×200. *Source: White et al. (2014).*

known imaginatively as the inner cell mass and a fluid-filled cavity known as the blastocoel (Fig. 32.5). The trophectoderm is fated to become only extra-embryonic membrane, while the inner cell mass is totipotent, that is, will develop not only into extra-embryonic membrane

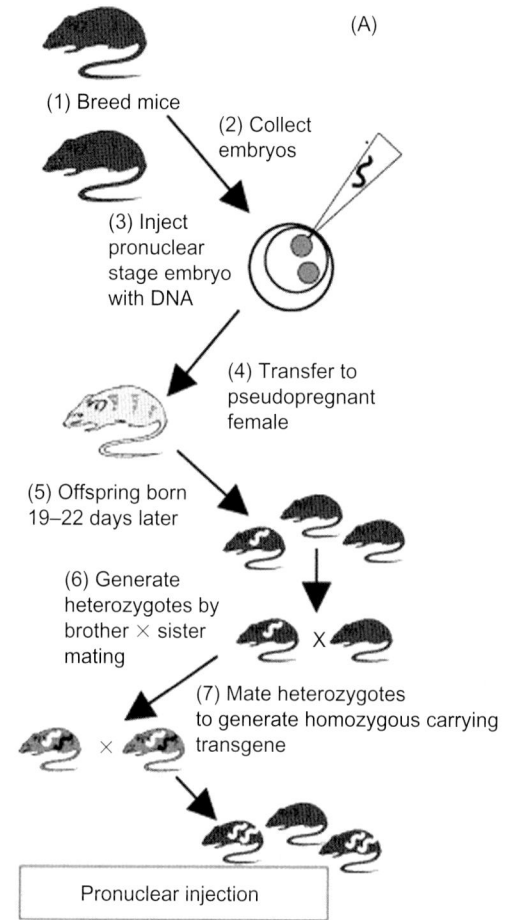

(A)

(1) Breed mice

(2) Collect embryos

(3) Inject pronuclear stage embryo with DNA

(4) Transfer to pseudopregnant female

(5) Offspring born 19–22 days later

(6) Generate heterozygotes by brother × sister mating

(7) Mate heterozygotes to generate homozygous carrying transgene

Pronuclear injection

FIGURE 32.4   Process of creating mice or rats through pronuclear injection. *Source: Hickman-Davis and Davis (2006).*

but also all the cell types of the animal *including the germ cells.* Like all cell lines, one can manipulate the genome *in vitro,* as we will discuss later. Furthermore, they will divide and replicate indefinitely *in vitro.* However, when these cells are combined with a morula or injected into the blastocoel of a host embryo, they will combine with that embryo that will then, after it is again implanted to a foster mother and brought to term, result in a chimeric animal, that is one that is a combination of cells derived from both the host embryo and the ESC. If the ESC contribute to the germline, this animal will then produce offspring that carry the induced mutation. It is important to note that this contribution cannot be reliably controlled, and thus it is important to generate many chimeras with high ESC contribution in order to ensure that animals are capable of transmitting the ESC mutation, although this last drawback may have been solved in mice (Taft *et al.,* 2013).

The morula forms at 2.5 DPC, and the blastocyst forms at 3.5 DPC. The embryos are again obtained from superovulated embryo donors that are euthanized at the appropriate time after mating, and cells are microinjected under the zona pellucida of the morula or into the blastocoel using a microinjection apparatus.

There are some interesting details to the methodology. The first concerns the strains used. Until recently, the only mouse strain for which ESC could be reliably generated were those in the 129 family as well as B6129F1s. A few lines existed also for C57BL/6, but in general, other strains were refractory to the production of ESC, primarily because the cells would rapidly lose totipotency during culture. (Interestingly, many 129 strains are predisposed to produce spontaneous teratomas at high frequency, which probably contributes to their ability to also form ESCs.) However, recent developments in ESC culture media enabled the reliable isolation of ESCs from many strains of mice and also from rats (Lee *et al.,* 2012; Hirabayashi *et al.,* 2010). The second strain consideration involves the strain used as host embryos,

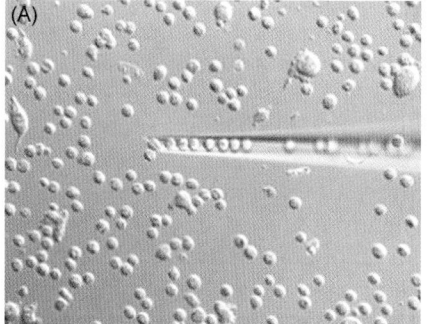
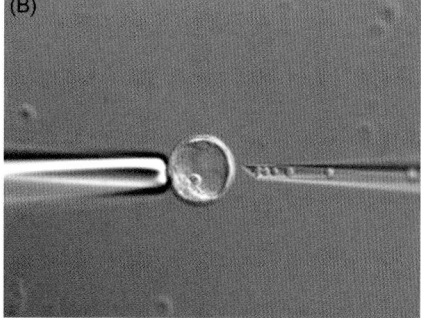
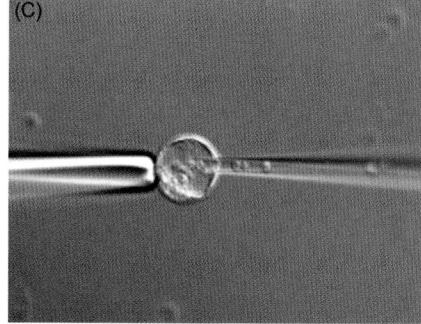

FIGURE 32.5   Injection of mouse blastocysts with genetically modified mouse embryonic stem cells. (A) Loading of embryonic stem cells (ESCs) into microinjection needle. (B) Blastocyst prior to microinjection, with holding pipette to the left and microinjection needle with ESC to the right. The bore of a microinjection needle used for ESC injection is much larger than that used to inject DNA. (C) Successful microinjection of ESCs, with needle in blastocoel and deposition of ESCs. Magnification ×200. *Source: White et al. (2014).*

and not unexpectedly, the strain used matters here too. Given that during embryogenesis there is essentially a competition to populate the germline with the ESC-derived primordial germ cells, some hosts are more or less robust. Thus utilizing inbred strains as hosts results in a larger contribution of the ESCs to the adult animal than using F1 strains, which in turn are less effective than outbred lines, such that it is unlikely that an outbred host will result in a germline chimera, i.e., one that has ESC contribution to the germline. Naturally, there is variation even among inbred lines in this measure, and in practice it is C57BL/6 that is most often used as a host. The exception is when aggregating the ESCs with morulae rather than injecting them into blastocysts, in which case host strain is seemingly unimportant. In this case, the accepted explanation is that since the ESCs are from a more advanced embryologic stage (recall that they are derived from blastocysts), they already have a 'head start' in populating the inner cell mass and eventually the majority of the animal.

A second detail concerns sex. Almost all ESC lines are XY for a very simple reason: these will produce sperm, and one can generate many more offspring from a male founder than from a female. When the ESCs are combined with a female embryo, the result will depend on the relative contributions of the ESCs and the host the offspring: if the female host predominates, the animals will be female and the male germ cells cannot produce oocytes (unless nondisjunction results in an XO karyotype), while if the ESCs predominate, a male will result and the host germ cells cannot produce sperm; equal contribution will result in a sterile intersex animal.

Finally, ESCs, like all cell lines, can undergo chromosomal changes *in vitro* that will destroy their totipotency. Thus any ESC clone has a significant potential to fail to produce germline chimeras, so it is common to use multiple independently targeted clones to generate the desired mutant animal.

2. iPS Cells

Recent technical advances have made it possible to alter primary cells so that they have the phenotype of ESCs (Schnabel *et al.*, 2012). These induced pluripotent stem cells can then be used exactly like ESCs to generate GM animals.

3. Somatic Cells

In animals, it is possible to genetically modify certain somatic cells, isolate the nuclei, and then transfer these to enucleated oocytes, which are then activated to trigger development. Again, the embryos are transplanted to foster mothers to obtain the animals. This somatic cell nuclear transfer (SCNT) is technically demanding and relatively inefficient and as such is performed rarely in rodents except for specialized research into the technique

itself; it is instead utilized for other species (Kim *et al.*, 2011; Schnieke *et al.*, 1997; Xu *et al.*, 2013; Yin *et al.*, 2008).

4. Spermatogonial Stem Cells

SSCs are isolated from immature male rats or mice, and under the appropriate culture conditions are capable of self-renewal *in vitro*. However, once transplanted into the seminiferous tubules of weanling, sterile males that have been treated with busulfan, they will populate the niche and produce sperm derived from the SSCs (Nagano *et al.*, 2001).

III. GENETIC MODIFICATION AND TECHNOLOGIES

Genetic modification strategies can be thought of in two ways: random, in which the genetic target is not specified, or targeted, in which specific genes of interest are mutated. Examples of the former are the aforementioned whole-animal mutagenesis using radiation or chemicals and the insertion of fragments of DNA into the genome; the latter include altering a particular locus to produce either a random change at that locus or a defined mutation. These defined mutations can include the alteration of single nucleotides, the deletion of varying amounts of sequence and/or the insertion of specific DNA sequences.

A. Random Mutagenesis

1. Generation of Transgenic Animals by Pronuclear Injection

The ability to insert exogenous DNA sequences into the genome was the first step in the revolution in genetic modification of animals that underlies much of modern genetics. This was done by the microinjection of an artificial DNA construct (a transgene) into the pronucleus of the single-cell embryo; this DNA then randomly inserts into the genome, resulting in a transgenic animal.

Pronuclear injection technology was first discovered by Lin, who showed that mouse zygotes could withstand the insertion of a fine glass needle (Lin, 1966), and further developments by Jaenisch *et al.* ushered in the era of the transgenic mouse (Jaenisch and Mintz, 1974; Jaenisch, 1976). Further developments in the technology by several other groups were able to accomplish the microinjection of laboratory-derived DNA into the zygotic pronucleus and obtain live-born mice and functionally expressing the transgene in mice (Costantini and Lacy, 1981; Gordon and Ruddle, 1981; Brinster *et al.*, 1981). In pronuclear injection, genetic material, usually DNA, is injected into the male pronucleus of a single-celled embryo. A transgenic mouse is one that contains within its genome DNA sequences coding for all or part of a foreign gene. These genes can be from prokaryotes or eukaryotes, may result in gain or loss of function, may be conditional on treatment or withdrawal of treatment of a compound, or expressed with tissue- or developmental stage-specific promoters, or any combination of the above.

Using the example of a simple DNA construct, the basic concepts of transgenesis through pronuclear injection can be explained. The DNA of interest is cloned within a bacterial plasmid and propagated in *E. coli*. The construct in its simplest form is a promoter sequence, a start sequence, the cloned gene (including an intron, necessary for proper expression), a stop sequence, and the vector backbone (Jackson and Abbott, 2000). The transgene itself is isolated away from vector sequences, which otherwise would inhibit transgene expression, and injected into the pronucleus of 0.5 DPC embryos.

Pronuclear injection is a relatively simple way to integrate foreign DNA into the genome of a mouse or rat. Successful integration is relatively low, however, with 1–5% of injected zygotes successfully integrating the foreign DNA (Rülicke and Hübscher, 2000; Hirabayashi et al., 2001). The DNA integrates randomly, which means that the phenotype seen may not be related to the transgene, but rather the disruption of another gene through the random integration of the transgene (Jaenisch et al., 1983; Cases et al., 1995). In addition, the transgene integrates as a head-to-tail array (a 'concatamer') containing multiple copies of the transgene; the number of copies in a concatamer cannot be controlled and phenotype may also be related to the number of foreign DNA copies integrated, as well as the site of integration (Ganss et al., 1994). Finally, the site where the transgene integrates may not be transcriptionally active, so that it is not expressed; this occurs in roughly 15% of founders. For these reasons, it is important to generate several (at least three) founder animals to ensure that a phenotype is not the result of insertional mutagenesis; ideally, several different lines will share a common phenotype.

Making these lines from the founders carrying the independent insertion events is a matter of simple breeding, for the most part (Wilkie et al., 1986). However, there are some wrinkles. Between 10 and 30% of transgenic founders may be mosaic due to integration of the transgene concatamers at the two-cell stage or later. These animals thus may exhibit a relatively reduced frequency of gene transmission to the F1 generation, reflecting mosaicism of the germline (Overbeek, 2014). Therefore, a founder (i.e., transgene-positive tail DNA Overbeek, 2014) may produce one or more completely nontransgenic litters. Another complication reflects the reality that the transgene insertion is a mutation event, and this insertion may be in an essential gene, affecting the ability to produce homozygous animals when breeding.

Finally, incorporation is completely random, so if 15% of all pups from microinjected embryos are founders, 15% of the transgenic founders will carry a second, independent insertion event. In this case, when breeding the founders, these transgenic arrays will independently assort among this founder's offspring, and 75% of them will be carriers. More details on breeding founders are provided later in this chapter.

2. Alternative Methods of Transgenesis Using the Embryo

A method using intracytoplasmic injection of sperm delivering exogenous DNA to the oocyte while also fertilizing it has also been described. This method may be more effective in ensuring integration of large constructs, but will not be discussed further (Lloyd, 2007).

Successful viral delivery of foreign genetic material in mice was first described in 1976 by Jaenisch (Jaenisch, 1976) using the Moloney leukemia virus. Jaenisch infected preimplantation mouse embryos with the virus and then bred them, showing that the virus integrated into the genome and converted to an endogenous retrovirus; however, expression of this DNA was silenced during embryogenesis. In 2002, Lois et al. used lentiviral vectors to successfully infect single-celled mouse and rat embryos with green fluorescent protein driven by both ubiquitous and tissue-specific promoters (Lois et al., 2002), while also in 2002, Hamra et al. generated transgenic rats via lentiviral transduction of spermatagonic cells (Hamra et al., 2002). This method has also been used to modify mouse spermatozoa to allow for generation of transgenic mice (Chandrashekran et al., 2014). Viral delivery of foreign DNA using lentiviruses is reviewed by Cockrell and Kafri (2007).

Lentiviruses are extremely efficient transgene delivery systems, inserting single copies of the transgene into the genome. In fact, depending on the viral concentration used, each and every embryo can undergo multiple infection and integration events. Therefore, 100% of the offspring are founders, but by the same token, downstream breeding to stabilize the number of copies in a line become problematic. In addition, lentivirus can infect almost all cell types including humans, so use of this technology comes with considerable biosafety concerns.

3. Gene Traps

A high-throughput method for randomly targeting genes was developed known as 'gene trapping.' Taking advantage of the fact that randomly inserted DNA fragments themselves cause mutations, the strategy was as follows. Transgenes were developed expressing a selectable marker such as drug resistance or a fluorescent protein in such a way that the marker would be expressed only when the transgene inserted within a gene and also inactivated ('knocked out') the interrupted gene. After selecting for survival after drug treatment or by fluorescence-activated cell sorting, clones would be grown from these cells and the DNA sequence surrounding the insertion site(s) in each clone would be determined, thereby identifying the disrupted genetic locus. (Hansen et al., 2003, 2008). First described in 1991 (Friedrich and Soriano, 1991), the technique became the backbone of high-throughput, large-scale international efforts to collect mutations in every gene in the mouse genome once the sequence of the mouse genome was elucidated, allowing the easy identification of the insertion sites (Hansen et al., 2003, 2008). A wide variety of gene trap vectors were developed that, in theory, could target any gene, and a number of large-scale gene trapping efforts eventually were centralized into the International Knockout Mouse Consortium. In this effort, large numbers of clones were isolated, processed to identify the target locus, and banked for future use in producing mice. Interestingly, not all genes were amenable to this kind of targeting, so that some loci were targeted multiple times while others were not targeted in this random effort. The project, now centralized under the International Mouse Phenotyping Consortium (www.mousephenotype.org), is now attempting to use targeted mutagenesis to target these remaining genes with a priority based on expressed interest by the scientific community. ESC clones carrying gene-trapped alleles are available from the consortium can be ordered by local microinjection facilities to produce mice carrying the mutation; the consortium will also produce the mice upon request. The IMPC's eventual goal "is to discover functional insight for every gene by generating and systematically phenotyping 20,000 knockout mouse strains."

B. Targeted Mutagenesis

The ability to mutate a specific genetic locus was the second landmark event in the genome modification revolution; indeed, this development garnered the Nobel Prize in Physiology and Medicine in 2007 for Mario Capecchi, Martin Evans, and Oliver Smithies. The approach pioneered by these laboratories was rapidly adopted worldwide, allowing the precise engineering of genes in ESCs via homologous recombination. Much more recently, targeted mutagenesis has been vastly simplified by the development of targeted double-stranded DNA nucleases to harness the cell's DNA repair machinery to again introduce specific mutations in the genome.

1. Homologous Recombination in ES (and Other) Cells

When DNA is introduced into a cell, it usually integrates into a random location in the genome, but if that DNA has is homologous to the cellular DNA it will on occasion integrate by recombination into the

cellular locus. This was the breakthrough pioneered by the Capecchi, Evans, and Smithies laboratories (Bradley et al., 1984; Doetschman et al., 1987; Evans and Kaufman, 1981; Koller and Smithies, 1989; Mansour et al., 1988; Robertson et al., 1986; Thomas and Capecchi, 1987). They demonstrated that a DNA construct with arms homologous to a targeted locus would insert DNA flanked by these arms into the genome. Because this recombination event is so rare, this payload DNA includes a selectable marker to select for cells that incorporate the targeting vector, and one of the arms is itself flanked by a negative selection marker (usually the Herpes Simplex Virus thymidine kinase gene) that allows selection against cells that have randomly incorporated the vector, leaving those that have targeted the locus by homologous recombination (Fig. 32.6). The payload can be designed to 'knock-out,' or inactivate a gene, or it can be designed to 'knock-in,' or insert, some desired sequence into the genome. The creations of knock-in mutations allow insertions as fine as a single nucleotide to recapitulate or correct a mutation or as long as an entire protein coding sequence, for example, to place the expression of a protein under the control of an endogenous promoter so that protein is expressed in a particular cell type or tissue or at a particular time in development. Even more complex types of knock-ins are routinely engineered, such as creating conditional alleles of a gene to ablate expression in particular developmental lineages and/ or at particular times, inserting elements that allow the creation of large-scale duplications or deletions of chromosomal regions. Once the desired mutation is created in ESCs, it is a straightforward matter to then generate mice with the desired mutation (Fig. 32.7). In addition, this methodology can be applied to any of the other cell types described above.

2. Targeted Mutagenesis Using Programmable DNA Nucleases

When a double-stranded break (DSB) occurs in cellular DNA, the cell repairs this event via one of two mechanisms. The first, known as non-homologous end joining (NHEJ), simply re-attaches the broken ends using an error-prone process that tends to introduce small deletions and/or insertions of DNA at the break site known as indels. The second, known as homologous repair (HR) or homology-directed repair (HDR), utilizes the homologous chromosome or sister chromatid as a template for error-free repair using the recombination machinery (Fig. 32.8). Thus if one could target a DSB to a particular locus in the genome, NHEJ will result in mutations that will, in most cases, be frame-shift mutations that introduce stop codons, usually resulting in a null mutation. In-frame mutations can be silent or may be hypomorphic mutation, i.e, mutations that reduce gene activity. Conversely, one can introduce an exogenous

Homologous recombination

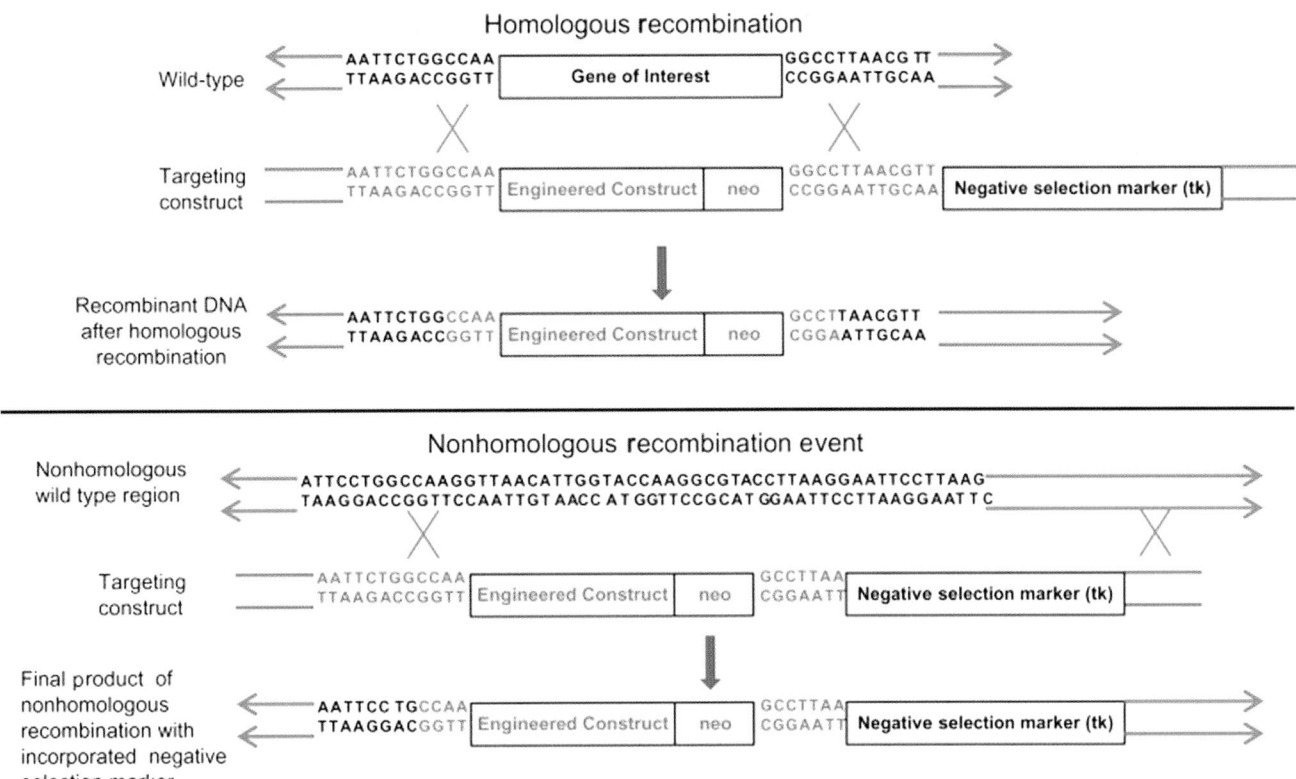

FIGURE 32.6 Homologous recombination. A targeting construct containing the engineered construct and *neo* resistance gene cassette are incorporated into wild-type embryonic stem cells (ESCs) via electroporation. In electroporation, an electrical field is applied to the ESCs, changing the permeability of the cell membrane and allowing for entry of the construct. Homologous recombination can occur between the engineered construct and the targeted gene. This event is relatively rare. In this figure, the sequences surrounding the gene of interest and the engineered construct are the homologous regions. Crosses indicate the areas of recombination. Successful homologous recombination is shown as the construct incorporated into the ESC genome. *Source: White et al. (2014).*

targeting vector, and harness HDR to produce knockins. The development of the programmable nucleases made this targeting a reality that has revolutionized genome engineering.

The first of these engineered nucleases to be developed for practical use were the zinc-finger nucleases (ZFNs). ZFNs are artificial enzymes composed of a sequence-specific DNA-binding zinc-finger domain joined to the nuclease domain from the restriction endonuclease Fok1 (Kim *et al.*, 1996). Sequence specificity of ZFNs is mediated by the zinc-finger domain. Each zinc-finger recognizes a specific 3-base-pair DNA sequence and zinc-fingers are bound together to form a domain that binds to 9–18 base pairs (Wolfe *et al.*, 2000). A ZFN pair is designed to a pair of binding sites that flank a spacer sequence; when the ZFN is bound to DNA, the Fok1 nuclease domains dimerize and cleave the DNA in the spacer (Fig. 32.9). Although each zinc-finger binds a trinucleotide, binding is context dependent, that is, binding also depends on surrounding sequence. As a result, not all sequences can be targeted, but in practice targets can be identified at densities of one target every 100–1000 nucleotides, depending on the system

used. Further, ZFNs are prone to cutting elsewhere in the genome (Kim and Kim, 2014).

TALENs were the second artificial enzyme developed, again with a sequence-specific DNA-binding domain coupled to a Fok1 nuclease domain, but they differ from ZFNs in their DNA-binding domains. TALEN DNA-binding domains are derived from DNA binding proteins of *Xanthomonas* spp., a plant pathogen, known as TALEs (transcription activator-like effectors) (Mussolino and Cathomen, 2012). These consist of a set of 33–35 amino acid repeat sequences known as effector-binding elements (EBEs), each of which recognizes a single base pair (Boch *et al.*, 2009) in the folded protein groove (Deng *et al.*, 2012). Again, a set of EBEs are assembled to bind to a pair of specific sequences of 15–18 bases flanking a spacer sequence, so that the Fok1 nuclease cleaves the DNA in the spacer (Fig. 32.10). Because the binding of each EBE is not dependent on context, TALENs can be designed to target any sequence. Typically constructed TALENs cannot bind and cut methylated DNA (Bultmann *et al.*, 2012), although a way to engineer TALENs that can manage this feat has been described (Valton *et al.*, 2012). Because TALENs cut with a higher

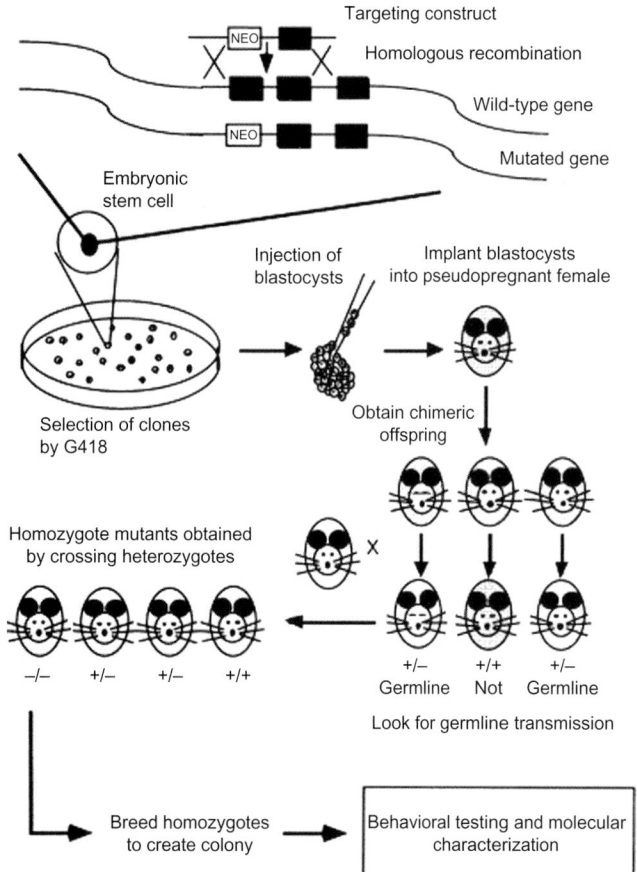

FIGURE 32.7   Process of mouse or rat production through targeted mutation of embryonic stem cells. *Source: Sibille and Hen (2001).*

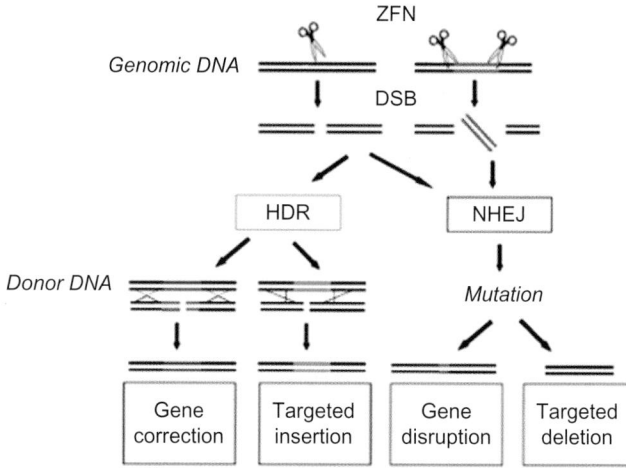

FIGURE 32.8   Illustration of programmable endonuclease methods of action, using ZFN-mediated genome editing. After binding to the target site a ZFN creates a DNA double-strand break (DSB), which will be repaired by one of the two major DNA repair pathways: homology-directed repair (HDR) or non-homologous end-joining (NHEJ). In the presence of high concentrations of donor DNA, which contains homologous sequences to the genomic target locus, HDR is preferentially initiated to repair the induced DSB. Depending on the structure of the donor DNA either gene correction or targeted insertion can be achieved. In the absence of a template DNA, the two DNA ends are re-ligated by the error-prone NHEJ pathway, which inserts small insertions and deletions (indels) at the target site. If the DSB is created in the coding region of a gene, these mutations will lead to disruption of the open reading frame. A targeted deletion can be obtained if two pairs of ZFNs create simultaneous DSBs at adjacent sites on a chromosome. *Source: Bobis-Wozowicz et al. (2011).*

target density and are simpler to generate, and because ZFN intellectual property rights were so restrictive, TALENs quickly replaced ZFNs for pronuclear targeting.

The most recent of these programmable nucleases are the RNA guided nucleases, known as RGNs or by the names CRISPR/Cas or Crisprs (Fig. 32.11). These were derived from a bacterial system that uses RNA homologous to invading phage or plasmids to target digestion of foreign DNA. Thus, unlike the ZFNs and TALENs, they are a ribonucleoprotein complex consisting of a protein, Cas9, and a guide RNA (gRNA) that both binds Cas9 and guides it to the DNA to bind at a stretch of complementary target sequence in the DNA. This complementary sequence is 17–10 bases long and terminates in a protospacer adjacent motif (PAM), usually NGG. The protein cuts the target at the NGG. The target density is lower than that of the TALENs, but much higher than that of the nucleases, and engineering an RGN is extremely easy: it only requires plugging a short piece of DNA corresponding to the target site into an existing backbone that encodes the gRNA. Although they may have significantly more off-target cutting (though this is controversial) than ZFNs and TALENs, they are also more active (at least in mice) and thus the current programmable nuclease of choice.

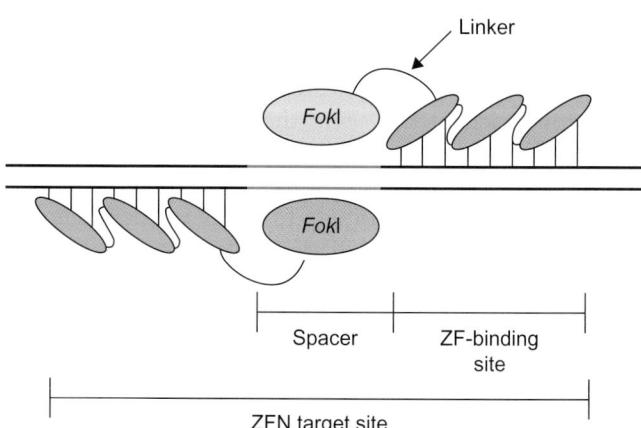

FIGURE 32.9   Structure of a zinc-finger nuclease (ZFN). A ZFN is composed of two subunits that bind to the target site in a tail-to-tail orientation. The two target half sites are separated by a five- to six-nucleotide 'spacer' sequence. Each subunit usually contains three to four fingers in a tandem array and each individual finger recognizes ~3 nucleotides of the target DNA. The zinc-finger array, which constitutes the specific DNA-binding domain, is fused to the catalytic domain of the FokI endonuclease by a short 'linker' sequence. *Source: Bobis-Wozowicz et al. (2011).*

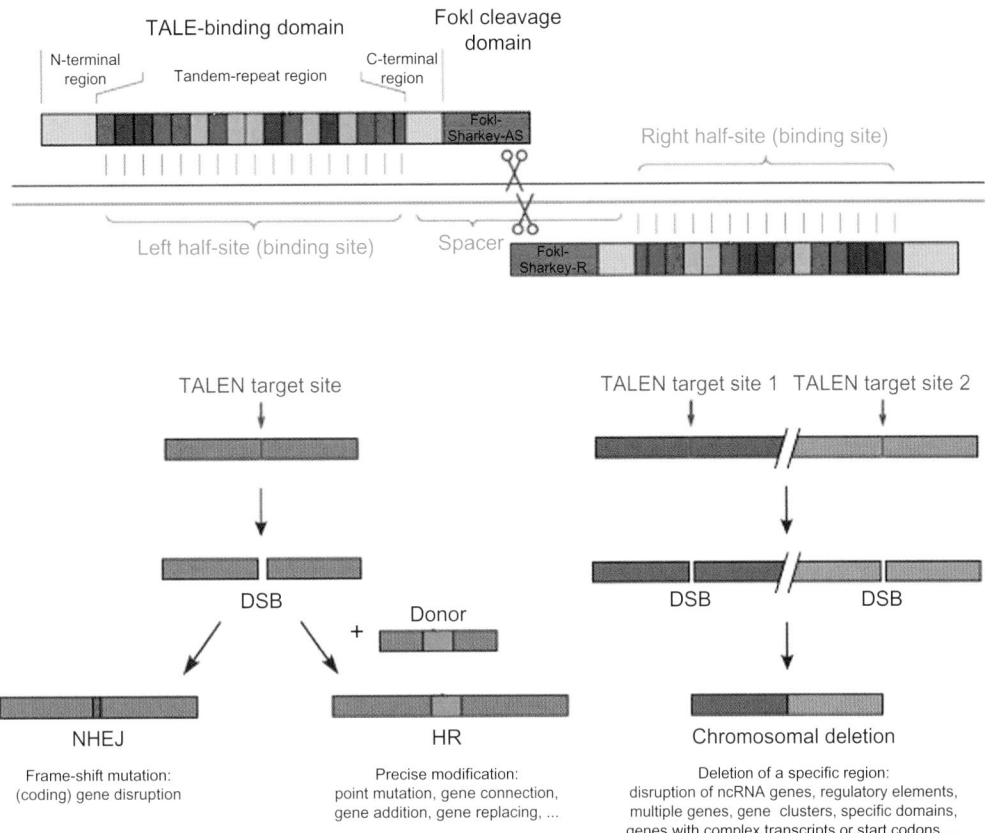

FIGURE 32.10   Binding sites of transcription activator-like effector nucleases and the resultant cleavage of DNA. Schematic diagram of the application of TALENs. (A) Schematic diagram of the TALEN dimer and the target site. Each TALEN monomer comprises a TALEN DNA-binding domain and a FokI DNA-cleavage domain. The binding domains recognize the left and right half-sites in different strands of the target site, and the dimer of FokI cleavage domains cleavages DNA at the spacer and generates a DSB. (B) Schematic diagram of three strategies of genomic manipulation mediated by TALENs. Small NHEJ indels can be mediated by a DSB induced by a pair of TALENs; precise genome modification by HR can be mediated by a DSB with a donor construct provided; chromosomal deletion can be mediated by two DSBs induced by two pairs of TALENs. *Source: Huang et al. (2014).*

Programmable nucleases have been used in a variety of systems to modify endogenous genes, including viruses, bacteria, nematodes, insects, plants, frogs, fish, mammals such as rats, mice, rabbits, non-human primates, pigs, and human stem cells (Gaj et al., 2013; Segal and Meckler, 2013; Kim and Kim, 2014; Hai et al., 2014; Flisikowska et al., 2011; Niu et al., 2014). Each programmable nuclease has its advantages and disadvantages, such as varying success rates (24–99%; much higher than any other genetic engineering method used previously), target densities, mutation rates (10–20%), and off-target effects (Kim and Kim, 2014).

The main advantage to the programmable nucleases, though, is their simplicity, specificity, and versatility when compared to other genome engineering methods (Wang et al., 2013). Because the programmable nucleases cut so efficiently, this methodology has largely supplanted ESCs as the route to targeted mutagenesis in mice and rats. One can simply microinject the nucleases as either plasmids or as mRNA into the pronucleus and obtain knockout animals in the offspring at rates as high as 80–90%, depending on the locus. One can even include targeting vectors in this microinjection and obtain knock-ins, and CRISPRs are efficient enough that multiple alleles can be targeted simultaneously (Fujii et al., 2014). This is clearly faster than modifying ESCs *in vitro*, then making chimeric animals that must then be bred another generation to produce founder animals. In addition, one is not limited to modifying only those strains for which ESCs exist, as embryos of any inbred strain or line can be targeted in this manner.

IV. COLONY MANAGEMENT FOR GM MICE AND RATS

The most important factor in realizing the potential of a study involving GM animals involves the choice of genetic background used for the initial embryology and for the follow-on breeding strategies. Individual

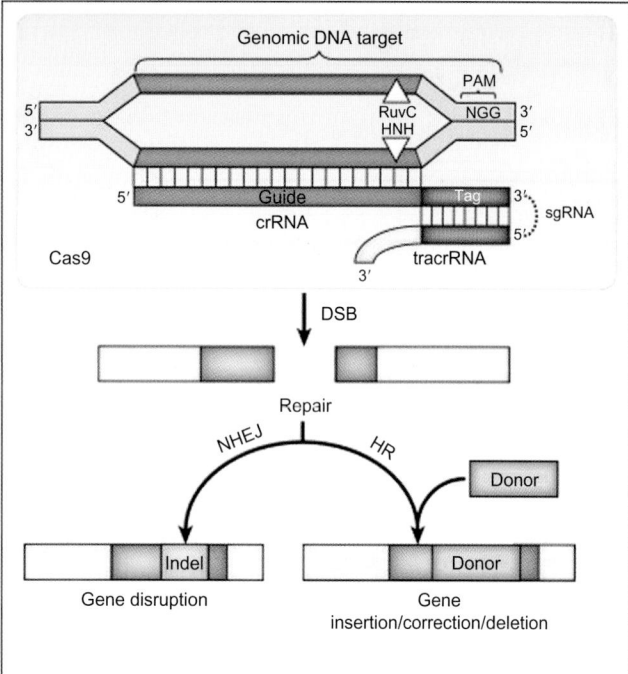

FIGURE 32.11 Binding sites of clustered regularly interspaced short palindromic repeat-associated system nucleases and the resultant cleavage of DNA. RNA-programmable genome editing by Type II Cas9 CRISPR-Cas systems. The Cas9 endonuclease (yellow) has two nuclease active sites (RuvC and HNH) that cleave opposing strands of a DNA molecule to generate a blunt-ended, double-strand DNA break (DSB). The cleavage is directed by the associated CRISPR (cr)RNA that contains a guide region that recognizes one strand of the target sequence by base-pairing. The enzyme requires a short protospacer adjacent motif (PAM) immediately adjacent to the region of homology as an auxiliary target identification signal. Cas9 activity also requires a second RNA (trans-activating crRNA (tracrRNA)) that base-pairs with the repeat-derived tag of the crRNA. The crRNA and tracrRNA can be combined through covalent linkage into a single-guide RNA (sgRNA). In human and many other cell types, the Cas9-induced, DSBs undergo repair by either nonhomologous end joining (NHEJ) or homologous recombination (HR). NHEJ repair results in indels (short insertions or deletions) and provides a means to selectively disrupt or inactivate target genes. When provided with a homologous donor DNA, HR repair can affect sequence replacement to insert, modify, or delete sequence at the site. *Source: Terns and Terns (2014).*

laboratories frequently rely on the use of favorite strains based on many factors, including what strains other investigators in the field are working with, known mutations or modifying genes, cost, availability, health history, and reproductive characteristics. Investigators should review the frequencies of specific pathologies reported for well-known inbred and outbred strains (Sellers *et al.*, 2012; Treuting *et al.*, 2012). Exceptional strain-dependent tumor frequencies or metabolic deficiencies should be avoided for specific predicted genetic modification phenotypes (Pettan-Brewer and Treuting, 2011). The reproductive and nurturing nature of the recipient pseudopregnant females and their coat-color

genetics also should be considered carefully. Because different strains exhibit different average litter sizes, this factor should also be considered in the choice of embryo transfer recipient strains.

The following questions should be reviewed before proceeding with a mouse or rat genetic modification program. In the case of rats, some of this information may not be known, since rats are relative newcomers to genetic manipulation.

- *Is the genetic background critical to the experiment?* If a defined genetic background is desired, an inbred strain with the appropriate genetics should be selected. Predictability of the effects of background genetics on the genetic modification minimizes the variability in expression or phenotype between animals. If genetics is not apparently critical to the project, then hybrid (a cross between two inbred strains) animals with above-average vigor and breeding characteristics may be selected. Compared to inbred strains, many hybrids yield larger numbers of oocytes than either parental strain in response to superovulation, and these embryos may also exhibit increased survival to implantation following manipulation. Hybrid animals also usually exhibit more reliable fertility characteristics and fairly large litter sizes.
- *What are the behavioral characteristics of the parental strains?* Are they exceptionally aggressive? Do they frequently cannibalize or neglect their newborn litters? Are they attentive mothers?
- *What are the reproductive characteristics of the potential parental strains?* What are the average litter sizes? Do the females respond well to superovulatory stimulation? Are gestation times usually predictable?
- *What types of pathologies normally occur in the strains being considered?* Could these pathologies mask the expected expression of the transgene? Could endogenous pathologies enhance, accentuate, or confound the predicted transgenic phenotype?
- *Is coat color important or useful in the project?*
- *What is the minimal acceptable health status for the project and within the facility?*

The inbred mouse strains most frequently used in GM animal creation are C57BL/6, FVB/N, and 129/SvEv, while in rats, DA, F344, and Wistar rats are commonly used. For embryo transfer procedures, outbred Swiss albino (CD1, ICR) or Sprague Dawley (CD, SD) origin stocks are very widely employed as recipients of GM embryos. Some characteristics of these strains are listed in Table 32.2. The C57BL/6 is the most widely used inbred strain for GM animals. The genetics and phenotypic variation of this mouse strain have been well characterized over several decades. The reproductive

TABLE 32.2 Strains Commonly Used in Mouse and Rat Transgenic and Knockout Production

Strain	Litter size	Superovulation response	General comments
FVB/N	8–9	Good	Albino, excellent mothers, large pronuclei for injection
C57BL/6	6–7	Good	Black, poor mothers, most commonly used inbred background in biomedical research, ESC lines from B6N, also albino B6 available for chimera creation on one genetic background
B6D2F1	n/a[a]	Good	Black, hybrid animals, also used for pronuclear injection
129S6/SvEv	6	Poor	White-bellied agouti, many ESC lines of 129 lineage
DA	6	?	Agouti, docile, first rat ESC line from these animals
SD	10–12	Good	Albino, excellent mothers, large litters, large body size, docile
WI	9–11	Good	Albino, rat ESC have been described from these outbred animals
F344	8	Good	Albino, smaller inbred animal, moderate ease of handling

Any strain may be used for ENU mutagenesis, as well as for ZFN, TALEN, and CRISPR technology.
[a]F1 hybrids are not self-perpetuating.

and maternal characteristics of this mouse are only fair to average, but the response of females to injected exogenous hormones is above average; relatively high yields of pronuclear embryos may be collected following superovulation and mating. For knockout mouse studies, C57BL/6 blastocysts have been used almost exclusively as recipients of genetically engineered ESCs. These blastocysts reliably give rise to ESC chimeras, and coat-color genetics usually facilitates analysis of the live-born mice.

The FVB/N is another popular strain for pronuclear microinjection because many researchers assert that the pronuclei of the zygotes are somewhat larger and more distinctive than those collected from comparable strains (Taketo et al., 1991). These albino mice yield relatively large numbers of embryos and are excellent mothers. FVB males, however, are extremely aggressive toward conspecifics and are usually housed singly by 8 weeks of age to avoid the severe injuries caused by fighting.

The 129S6/SvEv mouse has favorable reproductive traits and many of the available ESC lines are derived from 129S6/Sv substrains, so chimeric animals may be crossed onto 129S6/SvEv mice. The ESC lines derived from 129S6/Sv mice are reputed to have a high incidence of germline transmission and are easily maintained in culture. Chimeric, knockout-positive mice produced from these cells may be mated to 129S6/SvEv inbred mice to increase and preserve the inbred background of the knockout line. Considerable genetic variation has been reported in the 129 substrains (Simpson et al., 1997).

The DA or Dark Agouti strain is an inbred rat homozygous at the agouti locus (A/A). This strain is the first rat from which pluripotent ESC were isolated (Li et al., 2008; Buehr et al., 2008). F344 are a widely used inbred albino rat. These have been used to generate blastocysts for rat chimera formation. F344s are relatively good

breeders for inbred rats. Outbred Wistar females have also been used to generate rat ESC lines (Hirabayashi et al., 2010).

To produce GM mice and rats, it is necessary to maintain four different types of animals within the production colony. The four different types of mice or rats required may be generated in-house or more commonly, purchased commercially as needed to conserve valuable facility space: (i) embryo donor females (superovulated), (ii) fertile stud males (proven breeders), (iii) embryo transfer recipient females (pseudopregnant), and (iv) sterile stud males (vasectomized). To create embryos for genetic manipulation, the embryo donor females are superovulated, mated with proven breeder males, then euthanized, often by cervical dislocation, for embryo collection in order to preserve embryo quality, although this may not be necessary (Howell et al., 2003). Superovulation protocols for various strains and stocks may be found in the literature, most notably in Popova et al. (2005) and Byers et al. (2006). The embryos produced by superovulation are then manipulated in the laboratory, and transferred surgically to females made pseudopregnant by mating with vasectomized males. Generally, the production of 30–40 embryos for implantation (15–20 per side) will allow for implantation in one recipient female. Numbers fewer than that are less likely to result in a successful pregnancy by the recipient female.

The effort involved in the creation and characterization of GM animals is significant. Protein overexpression or gene knockout frequently results in phenotypic and genotypic characteristics that challenge colony-management skills. Animals may need precisely timed doses of compounds in order to exhibit phenotype without lethality. Depending on the specific nature and location of the modification, GM animals may exhibit infertility, immune incompetence, infection-promoting skin disorders, or a specific disease process or syndrome, among other phenotypical aberrations. Any of these phenotypes may affect health, longevity, or reproductive performance. Therefore, the management of colonies of GM animals is more delicate than the management of genetically unmodified animals. Four major support systems should be established when investigators or facilities begin to work with GM animals (and it is never too late to establish the systems if work has already begun):

- an established facility health program, including explicit methods for the importation of animals from other facilities;
- explicit and well-documented breeding strategy standard operating procedures (SOPs) and guidelines;
- a fastidious record-keeping system for reproductive and phenotypic data;
- access to an internal or external embryo or sperm cryopreservation program.

These systems and procedures must be supported and managed by well-trained personnel.

A. Health Profile

An animal genetic modification program should always use specific pathogen-free animals for production, for breeding, and for fostering, where available. For best results, pathogens and adventitious agents should be excluded by using high-quality animals, by carefully managing importation of new animals into the facility, and most important, by adhering to stringent animal care and husbandry SOPs. In addition, diligent health-monitoring protocols and smooth, rapid strategies for dealing with potential discoveries of unwanted agents within the facility must be in place and understood by all animal care personnel and researchers. The barrier should be monitored on a regular schedule for all undesirable agents, using wild-type sentinel animals or immune-incompetent animals produced within the colony (see Shek et al. Chapter 11, in this volume for more information on health monitoring).

The animal health risks associated with a genetic modification facility are more challenging than those in a facility using only wild-type animals from vendors, especially if that facility also performs rederivations. Animals from a variety of sources are imported frequently, usually on a weekly basis. The health profiles of all imported animals must be reviewed carefully because 'clean' animals from different vendors or laboratories will have different lists of excluded agents and testing frequencies. Mice and rats received from academic laboratories should absolutely be quarantined and assayed for excluded agents before inclusion into a

breeding program. Some institutions require rederivation of all animals, regardless of source, as a means of minimizing risk. Transfer of animals – and personnel – between colonies or barriers must be regulated stringently. Research animals that leave the colony should not be returned to the colony. The genetic modification production and breeding units should preferably be maintained within a barrier separated from research animal housing, which may be managed as a conventional facility to make investigator access and use simpler, if the health of the animals will not be affected. Perhaps the most challenging aspect of GM animal management involves the long-term breeding strategies of important lineages. Maintaining animal health quality during continuous, possibly multiyear, breeding programs of critical animals presents a formidable task. When an unwanted agent enters this type of operation, it is extremely difficult to eradicate it without a hiatus in production, rederivation of the valuable founder animals, depopulation of replaceable animals, and thoroughly cleaning and disinfecting the facility. Fostering of neonates, hysterectomy rederivations, and embryo transfer procedures can be critical to save important lines after disease has been discovered.

B. Colony Breeding Strategies

With all lines of GM animals, only a single animal, the founder, is initially available for production. There may be multiple founders from one construct's pronuclear injection or one ESC transfection, but each founder is unique and has unique characteristics (an example may be seen in Feng et al. (2000)) and occasionally many lines are bred before the most useful one is selected. Therefore, it is imperative to perpetuate the line by breeding this founder as rapidly as possible. Obviously, colonies may be generated from male founders through polygamous and repeated mating within a relatively short time. Well-planned and reliably executed mouse-breeding strategies are critical to fully understanding and appreciating the effects of genetic modification on the phenome of an animal. Table 32.3 reviews the time frames of various components of a GM mouse program. Staff in the genetic modification facility should be clear with researchers about the timelines involved. Expected phenotypic patterns and possible effects on health, behavior, or fertility should be reviewed by the researcher and the genetic modification staff with the veterinary and animal care staff. Other topics that should be discussed include the importance of record keeping, potential sex-influenced expression and imprinting, and key early indicators of modification-mediated pathology. The specific goals of the breeding program should be documented and reviewed by all relevant personnel. Priorities must be explicitly clear because the number of GM breeding

TABLE 32.3   Time Frames for Components of Transgenic and Knockout Mouse Production and Breeding Programs

Procedures	Time frame (may be additive)	Goal
Construct creation/ESC transfection and selection	?	Successful integration of construct into vector or homologous recombination into ESC

CREATION AND IDENTIFICATION OF GENETICALLY MODIFIED MICE

(a) Manipulation of embryos and implantation into pseudopregnant females	Time 0	Obtain live-born litters
(b) Birth of genetically modified pups	3 weeks	Survival to weaning for DNA analysis
(c) Tissue biopsy	2–3 weeks	Weaning, DNA analysis
(d) Identification of founders	1–2 weeks depending on lab and assay development	Identification of founders

BREEDING FOR COLONY EXPANSION OF TRANSGENICS

(a) Mating pairs from founders set up	3 weeks	Most animals should be at least 6 weeks old for successful mating
(b) Birth of F1 generation	3 weeks	Obtain live-born pups
(c) Tissue biopsies and genetically modified F1 animals identified	3 weeks	Biopsies taken at 2–3 weeks of age; survival to weaning
(d) Sibling matings set up	3 weeks	Identified F1 animals should be mated to obtain homozygous animals; mating at ~6 weeks
(e) F2 animals delivered	3 weeks	Obtain live-born pups, check for litter size to determine possible embryonic lethality in homozygotes
(f) Identification of F2 genetically modified animals	3–4 weeks	Biopsies taken at 2–3 weeks of age; survival to weaning

BREEDING TO DETERMINE IF CHIMERIC ANIMALS HAVE GONE GERMLINE

(a) Chimeric potential founders identified	3 weeks	Evaluate animals at weaning when coat fully in
(b) Test matings set up with strain of interest	3 weeks	Most animals should be at least 6 weeks old for successful mating
(c) Offspring evaluated for germline transmission	6 weeks	Pregnancy is 3 weeks, full coat color in at 2 weeks after birth, tissue biopsies usually taken 2–3 weeks after birth

Adapted from Monastersky and Geistfeld (2002).
Rats would be materially quite similar in terms of time, but other animals might take more or less time to reach these goals.

animals almost always will be the key rate-limiting factor for the progress of the research program. Goals of the breeding program may include the following:

- stabilization of the genetic modification on a specific genetic background by backcrossing to an inbred strain;
- breeding to homozygosity (especially for knockouts);
- utilization of sibling crosses to stabilize genetic and phenotypic expression;
- expansion of the colony to provide animals for research;
- production of embryos or sperm for cryopreservation;
- surgical rederivation of the line.

When a founder animal is identified, it is important to expand the line as rapidly as possible by mating with wild-type mates. This procedure is more easily accomplished when the founder is a male because he can breed several females each week. The wild-type mates are usually from the parental strain of the founder (or one of the parental strains in the case of hybrid embryo injection). In most programs and for most lineages, it is advisable to mate to produce homozygous offspring as soon as possible (Table 32.4). For knockout heterozygotes, production of the homozygous (i.e., null) genotype is absolutely required. The evaluation of dominant genotypes and Y chromosome-linked gene insertions may not require homozygous study. A transgenic founder always is *hemizygous* (He) for the transgene, since there

TABLE 32.4 Mating Schemes for Generation of Genetically Modified Animals of Differing Zygosities and the Advantages and Disadvantages of These Mating Schemes

Zygosity of parent[a]	Zygosity of parent[b]	Zygosity of offspring[a,b]	Advantages	Disadvantages
TRANSGENIC ANIMALS				
Hemizygous (+/tg)	Wild-type (+/+)	50% hemizygous (+/tg)	Useful when homozygosity is lethal and hemizygotes are suitable experimental subjects.	No homozygotes produced.
		50% wild-type (+/+)	Generates littermate controls.	
Hemizygous (+/tg)	Hemizygous (+/tg)	25% homozygous (tg/tg)	Useful when phenotype varies with zygosity.	Can generate large numbers of unusable animals.
		50% hemizygous (+/tg)	Generates littermate controls.	
		25% wild-type (+/+)	Useful when homozygotes are infertile/ do not survive to breeding age.	
Homozygous (tg/tg)	Wild-type (+/+)	100% hemizygous (+/tg)	Useful when hemizygous animals are experimental subjects, but only one homozygous sex is fertile.	No wild-type littermate controls.
Homozygous (tg/tg)	Hemizygous (+/tg)	50% homozygous (tg/tg)	Useful when phenotype varies with zygosity.	No wild-type littermate controls.
		50% hemizygous (+/tg)	All animals produced may be useful experimental subjects.	
Homozygous (tg/tg)	Homozygous (tg/tg)	100% homozygous (tg/tg)	Simplicity of breeding and genotyping.	No wild-type littermate controls.
			All animals produced are useful experimental subjects.	
SEX-LINKED GENETIC MODIFICATIONS				
Hemizygous (tg/X)	Wild-type (X/Y)	25% X/Y	Same sex littermate controls generated.	Can generate large numbers of unusable animals.
		25% tg/Y		
		25% X/X		
		25% tg/X		
Homozygous (tg/tg)	Wild-type (X/Y)	50% tg/X	All males generated are experimental subjects.	Only possible if female tg/tg and male tg/Y animals are fertile.
		50% tg/Y		

A '+' in classical genetics terminology indicates the wild-type allele and a '−' indicates a mutant allele. 'tg' is used here in the case of hemizygous transgenic animals to avoid confusion. For knockout/knockin animals, substitute '−' for 'tg' and 'heterozygous' for 'hemizygous.' All other percentages and considerations apply.
[a]*All percentages are approximate over large numbers of offspring. Individual litters may contain different distributions.*
[b]*Assuming no embryonic/perinatal lethality associated with genes involved.*

is no corresponding DNA on the complementary chromosome. Although breeding to homozygosity is usually attempted for most transgenic lines within the first 6 months after a founder is born, homozygosity may not always be realized due to potential homozygous lethality, infertility resulting from certain transgenes, or problems with sperm resulting in wild-type sperm outcompeting other types. In all transgenic experiments, multiple lines expressing the same construct at different integration loci must be assessed to discount the impact of potential insertional mutations on expression patterns or embryonic survival. If homozygotes are not obtained after several litters of *He × He* matings within a single lineage have been examined, it may be assumed that the homozygous genotype somehow impairs embryonic or fetal development. In these cases, insertional mutation cannot be ignored as a possible factor, and studies for these lines must be restricted to analysis of *He* animals. Transgenic expressions related to endocrine or glandular (e.g., uterine) functions may also affect maternal transgenic female capabilities to support gestation. If homozygous breeders are available and fertile, significant time and expense can be saved since there will be no need for test mating or genotyping. Breeding homozygous animals, however, does not result in the production of littermate controls, which are often desired. It is usually wise to maintain a few backcross matings in case the homozygotes exhibit challenged reproduction

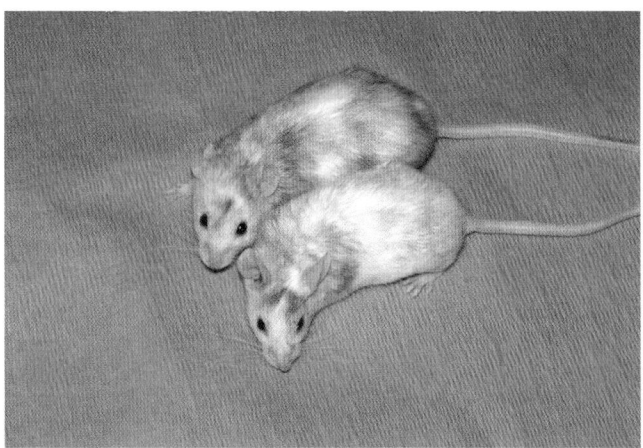

FIGURE 32.12 Chimeric animals, exhibiting coat colors from both the albino recipient blastocyst and the agouti donor embryonic stem cells (ESC). Animal coat color can be used as a rough guide to the amount of the animal that is composed of the ESC. Generally, the more of the ESC coat color visible, the more likely the animal is to have germ cells composed of the ESC, allowing for transmission of the genetic modification.

due to phenotype and/or morbidity or – in the extreme case – excessive mortality.

With chimeric mice produced using ESC, it is important to confirm germline transmission of the transgenic insertion as soon as possible after sexual maturity of the founder animal. Phenotypic evidence, most commonly a chimeric coat-color pattern, is not necessarily predictive of germline transmission, but may offer a clue (Fig. 32.12). Polymerase chain reaction (PCR) amplification assay for knockout gene-specific sequence may be performed with ejaculated sperm from a male knockout founder (i.e., collected from postcoital vaginal lavage), if desired. Chimeric mice may occasionally be sterile hermaphrodites (Shomer et al., 1997). Because most ES cell lines have an XY karyotype, the sex ratio of chimeric mice is skewed toward males (Robertson et al., 1986). As a rule, any chimeric mouse with more than 50% chimeric coat coloring should be test-bred to confirm transgene transmission. Since the knockout phenotype can vary on different genetic backgrounds, it may be useful to evaluate a mutation on at least one inbred and one outbred background. Because the ESCs modified by homologous recombination are heterozygous for the inserted DNA sequence, generally only 50% of the offspring of a successful germline chimera × wild-type mating will carry the mutation (biallelic disruptions are possible, but less common than monoallelic disruptions). Therefore, the genotypes of all offspring should be tested. Choice of ESC line will determine the coat color of animals in which the ESC have formed the reproductive tissue and gone germline. With chimeric animals, a minimum of three litters should be produced before a chimera is

determined to have no germline contribution from the injected ESC. As discussed previously, homozygous null knockout mice should be produced to assess the true effects of the loss-of-gene function.

C. Genotype Analysis of GM Animals

Regardless of which particular breeding strategies are selected for the study of a lineage, molecular genotype analysis must be performed for breeders. Performance of this genetic quality-control program will provide great peace of mind because record-keeping errors and unplanned matings may occur in the best programs. Occasionally, especially with homozygous knockout mice, zygosity may be determined by phenotypic characteristics by observing either visual or biochemical markers of gene expression.

However, molecular analyses of DNA from a putatively GM animal remain the most reliable methods of genotypic analysis. At the time of construct assembly, and before the construct is used for genetic modification, all assays potentially used by the researcher to confirm the mutation/transgene should be optimized. Losing animals due to age while the assay to determine which are founders is worked out is all too common. All GM breeders, especially founders, should be analyzed by either a Southern blot hybridization assay or by PCR amplification. Either of these assays will confirm the presence of modification-specific sequences and, with appropriate expertise and equipment, may be employed to detect zygosity for certain transgenes. The subsequent confirmation of zygosity by test mating is highly recommended. Test mating of a transgenic mouse must be performed carefully. A minimum of 10 offspring from each transgenic animal should be evaluated in order to confirm homozygosity. It is not uncommon to perform a minimum of three test matings to determine the gene transmittance frequency for chimeric animals.

D. Special Circumstances

The specific characteristics of an acquired line of GM mice must be understood upon receipt. It is important to discuss the line with the creator or vendor before using the animals in experiments or breeding programs. When the animals are newly created in-house, understanding the potential effects of gene disruption are just as important. It is imperative that the idiosyncrasies of rare or expensive GM animals are familiar so that their care and breeding are performed expediently and efficiently. For example, the probable need for foster mothers, dietary supplementation, or an exceptionally sterile environment must be incorporated into the husbandry protocols. The altered immune competence and associated environmental requirements of certain lines may be critical, and the survival and/or experimental performance of these animals may require stringent barrier procedures and specially prepared husbandry supplies. Other characteristics that could affect the care and use of the animals would include highly aggressive behavior or a tendency for cannibalism. All animal care staff must be trained to detect the onset of specific phenotypic events such as tumor growth, hair loss, arthritis, or optic pathologies. Life-threatening syndromes potentially associated with genetic modification, such as diabetes, respiratory disorders, or intestinal blockage, must be expected and managed professionally. The welfare and comfort of the animals and the ultimate success of the research program depend on the training, attention, and performance of the daily animal care technicians. Extra care needs to be taken during the first year of existence of a colony to ensure survival until expansion breeding and embryo cryopreservation can be completed. If a particular line has difficulty eating pelleted feed, softened feed may have to be provided. Sufficient nesting material should be used to protect the pups from hypothermia, especially when a ventilated caging system is utilized.

E. Colony Record Keeping

Transgenic animal production, genotype assessment, colony management, and phenotype observation generate an enormous amount of data that must be recorded properly and accurately so that they may be used to support the scientific conclusions of the research using the animals. The origin, breeding history, and individual characteristics of each line of GM animals in a colony must be documented clearly and must be accessible. If these data are not kept, or not kept in an organized fashion, important research aims may not be met and valuable animals may be lost.

The maintenance of a written or computer-based pedigree for each individual lineage is mandatory. The pedigree should note any changes in breeding strains and the dates and types of disposition of animals in a clearly understandable notation. This tool permits the easy correlation of inheritance and expression patterns, based on generation and sex, with phenotypic patterns and genotype analyses. Pedigree charts can be maintained in laboratory notebooks, using genealogy software for humans or mice, or using mouse-specific databases, such as the free, MS Access-based JAX Colony Management System (http://colonymanagement.jax.org/). Each individual member of a GM lineage should be physically marked, using subcutaneous transponders, ear tags, or tattoos. All animal care and investigative staff must be aware that critical retrospective analysis of the expression pattern of a line may depend on accurate records of common events, including reproductive performance, litter sex ratios, life span, causes and dates of death, and the timing of phenotypic characteristics. Coat-color patterns and imprinting phenomena must also be reported.

For each lineage, the molecular biology information, including construct data and genotype analysis records, must be accessible whenever required. For each individual animal, recorded information should include the date of birth, sex, generation and identification number, line code, genotype, coat color, phenotypic expression data, genotype and phenotype sample information, backcrossing information, and the date of final disposition (i.e., death, experiment, shipment to collaborator). Production information may include plugging data, number and size of litters, gestation times and parturition dates, lost and cannibalized litters, and the number of weaned pups produced. The use and retention of well-maintained cage cards is mandatory. Cards should contain all normal mouse data in addition to proper nomenclature of the GM animal and any treatment dates and the dates of any exceptional phenotypic events. Backcrossing and breeding notes must specify the sexes and genotypes of all animals and the ratio of males to females bred. The use of different-colored cage cards for each lineage is helpful.

F. Nomenclature for GM Animals

Nomenclature for GM animals is a moving target, changing as new technologies become available to manipulate genomes. Some basic principles apply, however, and these are related to the naming of inbred and outbred animals and to the naming of mouse and rat genes. The most recent rules associated with mouse and rat gene and animal nomenclature are available on the web at: http://www.informatics.jax.org/mgihome/nomen/index.shtml (for mice) and http://rgd.mcw.edu/nomen/nomen.shtml (for rats; many links refer to pages available on the mouse page as the nomenclature rules are often identical). This overview of mouse and rat nomenclature will be brief and cover only the basics.

As with any other animal, when first discussing the animal, the binomial nomenclature or Latin name is often used. For rats, this is simple, as domesticated laboratory rats are *Rattus norvegicus*. For laboratory mice, however, it is more complicated as they are a mix of several different species and subspecies (Didion and de Villena, 2013) and they are properly called 'laboratory mice', not *Mus musculus musculus* or *Mus musculus domesticus*.

Inbred strains of mice and rats are predominantly used in research today and they are often interrelated (Beck *et al.*, 2000; Lindsey and Baker, 2005). Mice and rats are considered inbred when certain criteria are met, namely that they are sibling mated, have been sibling mated for 20 or more consecutive generations, and members of the strain descend from a single ancestral pair at the 20th or subsequent generation (International Committee on Standardized Genetic Nomenclature for Mice and Rat Genome and Nomenclature Commitee, 2013). Most inbred mice and rats used in research today have been inbred for more than 100 generations. Inbred mice and rats should be named with a short, unique series of capital letters and numbers, beginning with a letter. Note that some older strains do not follow this naming convention: the 'c' in BALB/c should be lowercase, and all 129 strains begin with numbers. A standard list of abbreviations of inbred strains exists and should be used when called for in other nomenclature situations, such as congenic (genes and flanking DNA transferred through mating from one strain to another) or hybrid (a cross of two inbred strains) animals.

Once an inbred strain is established, given time it may genetically diverge either through residual heterozygosity in incompletely inbred animals, normal DNA replication errors (genetic drift), or through deliberate or inadvertent mixing with other strains. Inbred substrains are formed when animals are separated after 20 but before 40 generations of inbreeding, if they are separated for more than 20 generations from a common ancestor, or if genetic differences are shown between members of a strain by genetic analysis (Threadgill et al., 1997). Substrain designations are indicated by a forward slash followed by the substrain designation. Substrain designations may be numeric or alphabetic. Alphabetic substrain designations are usually lab codes, which are one- to five-letter codes, registered by a laboratory, facility, or investigator with ILAR (http://dels.nas. edu/global/ilar/Lab-Codes). Examples of some inbred strains and their substrains are given as Table 32.5.

Outbred mice and rats, called stocks, not strains, are also in use, especially in toxicology and drug development. Outbred animals are animals bred to maintain as much genetic diversity as possible within a closed colony and many of them have similar origins as the inbred mice and rats in use (Chia et al., 2005; Lindsey and Baker, 2005). Many originate from inbred lines which were subsequently bred to maximize any remaining heterozygosity and others are more inbred than would be apparent from their nomenclature, due to events such as rederivation for disease. Outbred animals are usually managed in closed colonies and with a system of mating to avoid breeding close relatives such as siblings or cousins. Outbred stocks are also named with short, unique series of capital letters and numbers, also beginning with a letter. In the case of outbred animals, however, the laboratory code is listed first, followed by a colon, and then the stock name. If known, the origin of the stock follows the stock name in parentheses. The origin may be a lab code or a strain/stock name, so capitalization may vary. Examples of outbred stock nomenclature are given as Table 32.6.

TABLE 32.5 Examples of Inbred Strains and Their Substrains

Inbred strain	Examples of substrains
C57BL	C57BL/6J
	C57BL/10
	C57BL/6N
	C57BL/6By
	C57BL/NTac
BN	BN/Rj
	BN/SsN
	BN/Crl
C3H	C3H/HeJ
	C3H/HeNCrl
	C3H/HeOuJ
F344	F344/Arc
	F344/NHsd
	F344/NSlc

TABLE 32.6 Examples of Outbred Stock Nomenclature

Common name	Examples of correct nomenclature
CD-1	Crl:CD1(Icr)
Swiss Webster	Tac:SW
Sprague Dawley	Hsd:SD
Wistar	RjHan:WI

Gene names in rats and mice are coordinated between species and with human genetic nomenclature, meaning that in many cases, homologous genes in all three organisms will have the same name and symbol. Mouse and rat full gene names are not italicized, and neither are the names of the proteins produced by the genes. Mouse and rat gene symbols are usually three to five characters (but no more than 10) and are italicized in print. Gene symbols typically begin with capital letters, unless the gene symbol is that of a mutation known only by a phenotypic name, in which case the gene symbol begins with a lowercase letter. When the new gene denoted with solely a phenotypic designation is cloned, it is assigned a function-based symbol. The most common allele of a gene in the population is typically called the 'wild-type' and is the gene name without any allelic designation. Alleles of genes are denoted by the addition of superscripts to the genes and are often named for the phenotypes they induce in animals. Alleles beginning with capital letters are dominant; alleles beginning with lowercase letters are recessive. New allelic forms of genes can be created by genetic engineering or occur

Mouse or rat gene:	*Lepr*
Spontaneous mutant allele in mouse or rat:	*Lepr^{ob}*
Transgenic mouse or rat with human leptin receptor gene inserted:	Tg(LEPR)1Lab
Knockout mouse or rat:	*Lepr^{tm1Lab}*
Knock-in mouse or rat with leptin gene inserted:	*Lepr^{tm1(Lep)Lab}*
Mouse or rat mutation induced by programmable nucleases:	*Lepr^{em1Lab}*

FIGURE 32.13 Examples of nomenclature for mouse or rat genes. For the purposes of illustration, one gene, the leptin receptor (*Lepr* in mouse genetic nomenclature) has been chosen. Animals with these genetic modifications may not actually exist.

through natural processes. Congenic animals are created when alleles, whether natural or human-modified, are transferred between inbred genetic backgrounds.

Finally, in mice and rats, genes are modified by humans. In transgenic mice, the mouse is named, then the newly inserted gene is named, preceded by 'Tg.' This gene name is not italicized, as this is not the mouse or rat's own genetic material. In the case of endogenous genetic material modified by technology, the gene modified is in italics and the information on the modification is contained in an allelic superscript (through genetic modification, an allele has been created). Modifications made through homologous recombination in ESC are denoted as 'tm' while those made through the use of programmable endonucleases are denoted 'en.' If a gene has been knocked-in, its name is present in the allele in parentheses. Some examples of simple gene modification nomenclature are given in Figure 32.13.

G. Preservation of GM Animals

The cryopreservation of preimplantation embryos collected from GM animals allows the long-term storage of valuable lines for an infinite period of time and the subsequent ability to regenerate a colony of live animals in the future (Guan *et al.*, 2012). Cryopreserved embryos are protected from genetic mutation and drift and genetic contamination as well as most facility catastrophes and husbandry expenses are avoided. Cryopreserved embryos may also be used for future support of patent claims, avoidance of international animal quarantine restrictions, and relatively cost-effective embryo transfer rederivation (Reetz *et al.*, 1988). Liquid nitrogen is not sterile, however, and animals reconstituted from cryopreserved germplasm should always be

TABLE 32.7 Some Resources Available Online to Locate Genetically Modified Mice and Rats, Mouse ESC, and Information on Mouse and Rat Genes, Mouse Phenomes, and Sources of Genetically Modified Mice and Rats

Name	URL	Data
Rat Genome Database	http://rgd.mcw.edu/	Genome tools, rat strain and stock information, phenotype data, rat gene, allele, and mutation information.
The National BioResource Project for the Rat in Japan	http://www.anim.med.kyoto-u.ac.jp/nbr/	Rat strain/stock depot for Japan, information on phenotypes of deposited strains/stocks, SSLP information on deposited strains/stocks. Includes photos of most animals.
Mouse Genome Informatics	http://www.informatics.jax.org/	Mouse gene, allele, and mutation information. Vast resource. Also information on nomenclature of mice, rats, and their genes and alleles.
Mouse Phenome Database	http://phenome.jax.org/	Curated phenome datasets from classical inbred mouse strains, other strains with fixed genotypes, and populations where data may be openly acquired.
International Mouse Phenotyping Consortium	https://www.mousephenotype.org/	Generation and phenotyping of 20K+ knockout mouse strains.
International Mouse Strain Resource	http://www.findmice.org/	Massive international searchable online database of mouse ESC, strains, and stocks. Includes mutant and genetically engineered strains.

This is not an exhaustive list.

quarantined and tested for excluded agents before being released into a colony. Valuable lines that are not in current or imminent demand should be cryopreserved as soon as feasible, preferably as homozygotes to facilitate the future analysis and breeding of reconstituted lines. When cryopreserving embryos, embryos from the batch should always be reconstituted, implanted, and live mice produced to prove that this is possible, before the cryopreservation is considered successful. Major rodent vendors offer this service, as do many genetic modification cores at various institutions. The ability to freeze and recover viable, motile, fertilization-capable mouse sperm is another simple way to preserve valuable animals against change or disaster (Nakagata, 2000). Kits are available from many major mouse vendors. Costs for cryopreservation of embryos or sperm are low compared to the costs of recreating a GM mouse or rat and all the research associated with it. Researchers should be strongly encouraged to cryopreserve animals that are essential to their research.

V. FINDING MOUSE AND RAT RESOURCES

Investigators are often interested in acquiring animals or ESC or that may not be available from commercial vendors or information on genes, alleles, or phenotypes of animals. Resources are available online for many of these items, and some of the more prominent are listed and their functions explained briefly in Table 32.7. These have also been reviewed in Ringwald and Eppig (2011) and Donahue et al. (2012).

References

Baldassarre, H., Wang, B., Kafidi, N., et al., 2003. Production of transgenic goats by pronuclear microinjection of in vitro produced zygotes derived from oocytes recovered by laparoscopy. Theriogenology 59, 831–839.

Bao, L., Chen, H.D., Jong, U.M., et al., 2014. Generation of ggta1 biallelic knockout pigs via zinc-finger nucleases and somatic cell nuclear transfer. Sci. China–Life Sci. 57, 263–268.

Barstead, R., Moulder, G., Cobb, B., et al., 2012. Large-scale screening for targeted knockouts in the caenorhabditis elegans genome. G3–Genes Genomes Genet. 2, 1415–1425.

Beck, J.A., Lloyd, S., Hafezparast, M., Lennon-Pierce, M., Eppig, J.T., Festing, M.F., et al., 2000. Genealogies of mouse inbred strains. Nat. Genet. 24, 23–25.

Behringer, R., Gertsenstein, M., Vintersten Nagy, K., Nagy, A., 2014. Manipulating the Mouse Embryo: A Laboratory Manual, fourth ed. Cold Spring Harbor Press, Cold Spring Harbor, NY.

Beumer, K., Bhattacharyya, G., Bibikova, M., Trautman, J.K., Carroll, D., 2006. Efficient gene targeting in drosophila with zinc-finger nucleases. Genetics 172, 2391–2403.

Bibikova, M., Golic, M., Golic, K.G., Carroll, D., 2002. Targeted chromosomal cleavage and mutagenesis in drosophila using zinc-finger nucleases. Genetics 161, 1169–1175.

Blitz, I.L., Biesinger, J., Xie, X.H., Cho, K.W.Y., 2013. Biallelic genome modification in f-0 xenopus tropicalis embryos using the crispr/cas system. Genesis 51, 827–834.

Bobis-Wozowicz, S., Osiak, A., Rahman, S.H., Cathomen, T., 2011. Targeted genome editing in pluripotent stem cells using zinc-finger nucleases. Methods 53, 339–346.

Boch, J., Scholze, H., Schornack, S., Landgraf, A., Hahn, S., Kay, S., et al., 2009. Breaking the code of DNA binding specificity of tal-type iii effectors. Science 326, 1509–1512.

Bradley, A., Evans, M., Kaufman, M.H., Robertson, E., 1984. Formation of germ–line chimeras from embryo–derived teratocarcinoma cell-lines. Nature 309, 255–256.

Brinster, R.L., Chen, H.Y., Trumbauer, M.E., 1981. Mouse oocytes transcribe injected xenopus 5s-RNA gene. Science 211, 396–398.

Buehr, M., Meek, S., Blair, K., Yang, J., Ure, J., Silva, J., et al., 2008. Capture of authentic embryonic stem cells from rat blastocysts. Cell 135, 1287–1298.

Bultmann, S., Morbitzer, R., Schmidt, C.S., Thanisch, K., Spada, F., Elsaesser, J., et al., 2012. Targeted transcriptional activation of silent oct4 pluripotency gene by combining designer tales and inhibition of epigenetic modifiers. Nucl. Acids Res. 40, 5368–5377.

Byers, S.L., Payson, S.J., Taft, R.A., 2006. Performance of ten inbred mouse strains following assisted reproductive technologies (arts). Theriogenology 65, 1716–1726.

Cade, L., Reyon, D., Hwang, W.Y., et al., 2012. Highly efficient generation of heritable zebrafish gene mutations using homo- and heterodimeric talens. Nucl. Acids Res. 40, 8001–8010.

Carlson, D.F., Tan, W.F., Lillico, 2012. Efficient talen-mediated gene knockout in livestock. Proc. Natl. Acad. Sci. U S A 109, 17382–17387.

Cases, O., Seif, I., Grimsby, J., Gaspar, P., Chen, K., Pournin, S., et al., 1995. Aggressive-behavior and altered amounts of brain-serotonin and norepinephrine in mice lacking maoa. Science 268, 1763–1766.

Chan, A., Chong, K.-Y., Martinovich, C., Simerly, C., Schatten, G., 2001. Transgenic monkeys produced by retroviral gene transfer into mature oocytes. Science 291, 309–312.

Chandrashekran, A., Sarkar, R., Thrasher, A., Fraser, S.E., Dibb, N., Casimir, C., et al., 2014. Efficient generation of transgenic mice by lentivirus-mediated modification of spermatozoa. FASEB J. 28, 569–576.

Chen, C.C., Fenk, L.A., De Bono, M., 2013. Efficient genome editing in caenorhabditis elegans by crispr-targeted homologous recombination. Nucl. Acids Res. 41.

Cheng, Z., Yi, P.S., Wang, X.M., et al., 2013. Conditional targeted genome editing using somatically expressed talelens in C. elegans. Nat. Biotechnol. 31, 934 – +.

Chia, R., Achilli, F., Festing, M.F., Fisher, E.M., 2005. The origins and uses of mouse outbred stocks. Nat. Genet. 37, 1181–1186.

Clark, J., Whitelaw, B., 2003. A future for transgenic livestock. Nat. Rev. Genet. 4, 825–833.

Cockrell, A.S., Kafri, T., 2007. Gene delivery by lentivirus vectors. Mol. Biotechnol. 36, 184–204.

Costantini, F., Lacy, E., 1981. Introduction of a rabbit beta-globin gene into the mouse germ line. Nature 294, 92–94.

Davis, A.P., Justice, M.J., 1998. An oak ridge legacy: the specific locus test and its role in mouse mutagenesis. Genetics 148, 7–12.

Deng, D., Yan, C.Y., Pan, X.J., Mahfouz, M., Wang, J.W., Zhu, J.K., et al., 2012. Structural basis for sequence-specific recognition of DNA by tal effectors. Science 335, 720–723.

De Stasio, E.A., Dorman, S., 2001. Optimization of enu mutagenesis of caenorhabditis elegans. Mutat. Res.–Gen. Toxicol. Environ. Mutagen. 495, 81–88.

Didion, J.P., De Villena, F.P.M., 2013. Deconstructing mus gemischus: advances in understanding ancestry, structure, and variation in the genome of the laboratory mouse. Mamm. Genome 24, 1–20.

Doctschman, T., Gregg, R.G., Maeda, N., Hooper, M.L., Melton, D.W., Thompson, S., et al., 1987. Targeted correction of a mutant hprt gene in mouse embryonic stem-cells. Nature 330, 576–578.

Donahue, L., Hrabe De Angelis, M., Hagn, M., Franklin, C., Lloyd, K.C.K., Magnuson, T., et al., 2012. Centralized mouse repositories. Mamm. Genome 23, 559–571.

Doyon, Y., Mccammon, J.M., Miller, J.C., et al., 2008. Heritable targeted gene disruption in zebrafish using designed zinc-finger nucleases. Nat. Biotechnol. 26, 702–708.

Evans, M.J., Kaufman, M.H., 1981. Establishment in culture of pluripotential cells from mouse embryos. Nature 292, 154–156.

Feng, G., Mellor, R.H., Bernstein, M., Keller-Peck, C., Nguyen, Q.T., Wallace, M., et al., 2000. Imaging neuronal subsets in transgenic mice expressing multiple spectral variants of gfp. Neuron 28, 41–51.

Flisikowska, T., Thorey, I.S., Offner, S., Ros, F., Lifke, V., Zeitler, B., et al., 2011. Efficient immunoglobulin gene disruption and targeted replacement in rabbit using zinc finger nucleases. PLoS One 6, e21045.

Flowers, G.P., Timberlake, A.T., Mclean, K.C., Monaghan, J.R., Crews, C.M., 2014. Highly efficient targeted mutagenesis in axolotl using cas9 RNA-guided nuclease. Development 141, 2165–2171.

Flurkey, K., Currer, J.M., Leiter, E.H., Witham, B. (Eds.), 2009. The Jackson Laboratory Handbook on Genetically Standardized Mice. The Jackson Laboratory, Bar Harbor, ME.

1438 32. GENETICALLY MODIFIED ANIMALS

Friedrich, G., Soriano, P., 1991. Promoter traps in embryonic stem-cells-a genetic screen to identify and mutate developmental genes in mice. Genes. Dev. 5 (9), 1513–1523. http://dx.doi.org/10.1101/gad.5.9.1513.

Frokjaer-Jensen, C., Davis, M.W., Hollopeter, G., et al., 2010. Targeted gene deletions in c. Elegans using transposon excision. Nat. Methods 7, 451. U57.

Fujii, W., Onuma, A., Sugiura, K., Naito, K., 2014. One-step generation of phenotype-expressing triple-knockout mice with heritable mutated alleles by the crispr/cas9 system. J. Reprod. Develop. 60, 324–327.

Gaj, T., Gersbach, C.A., Barbas, C.F., 2013. Zfn, talen, and crispr/cas-based methods for genome engineering. Trends Biotechnol. 31, 397–405.

Ganss, R., Montoliu, L., Monaghan, A., Schütz, G., 1994. A cell-specific enhancer far upstream of the mouse tyrosinase gene confers high level and copy number-related expression in transgenic mice. EMBO J. 13, 3083.

Gloor, G.B., Nassif, N.A., Johnsonschlitz, D.M., Preston, C.R., Engels, W.R., 1991. Targeted gene replacement in drosophila via p-element-induced gap repair. Science 253, 1110–1117.

Gordon, J.W., Ruddle, F.H., 1981. Integration and stable germ line transmission of genes injected into mouse pronuclei. Science 214, 1244–1246.

Gratz, S.J., Cummings, A.M., Nguyen, J.N., et al., 2013. Genome engineering of drosophila with the crispr RNA-guided cas9 nuclease. Genetics 194, 1029 – +.

Grunwald, D.J., Streisinger, G., 1992. Induction of recessive lethal and specific locus mutations in the zebrafish with ethyl nitrosourea. Genet. Res. 59, 103–116.

Guan, M., Marschall, S., Raspa, M., Pickard, A., Fray, M., 2012. Overview of new developments in and the future of cryopreservation in the laboratory mouse. Mamm. Genome 23, 572–579.

Hagmann, M., Bruggmann, R., Xuc, L., et al., 1998. Homologous recombination and DNA-end joining reactions in zygotes and early embryos of zebrafish (danio rerio) and drosophila melanogaster. Biol. Chem. 379, 673–681.

Hai, T., Teng, F., Guo, R.F., Li, W., Zhou, Q., 2014. One-step generation of knockout pigs by zygote injection of crispr/cas system. Cell Res. 24, 372–375.

Hammer, R.E., Pursel, V.G., Rexroad, C.E., et al., 1985. Production of transgenic rabbits, sheep and pigs by microinjection. Nature 315, 680–683.

Hamra, F.K., Gatlin, J., Chapman, K.M., Grellhesl, D.M., Garcia, J.V., Hammer, R.E., et al., 2002. Production of transgenic rats by lentiviral transduction of male germ-line stem cells. Proc. Natl. Acad. Sci. 99, 14931–14936.

Hansen, G.M., Markesich, D.C., Burnett, M.B., Zhu, Q.H., Dionne, K.M., Richter, L.J., et al., 2008. Large-scale gene trapping in c57bl/6n mouse embryonic stem cells. Genome Res. 18, 1670–1679.

Hansen, J., Floss, T., Van Sloun, P., Fuchtbauer, E.M., Vauti, F., Arnold, H.H., et al., 2003. A large-scale, gene-driven mutagenesis approach for the functional analysis of the mouse genome. Proc. Natl. Acad. Sci. U S A 100, 9918–9922.

Hanson, F.B., Winkleman, E., 1929. Visible mutations following radium irradiation in drosophila melanogaster. J. Hered. 20, 277–286.

Hickman-Davis, J.M., Davis, I.C., 2006. Transgenic mice. Paedia. Respir. Rev. 7, 49–53.

Hirabayashi, M., Takahashi, R.-I., Ito, K., Kashiwazaki, N., Hirao, M., Hirasawa, K., et al., 2001. A comparative study on the integration of exogenous DNA into mouse, rat, rabbit, and pig genomes. Exp. Anim. 50, 125–131.

Hirabayashi, M., Kato, M., Kobayashi, T., Sanbo, M., Yagi, T., Hochi, S., et al., 2010. Establishment of rat embryonic stem cell lines that can participate in germline chimerae at high efficiency. Mol. Reprod. Develop. 77, 94. 94.

Howell, R.L., Donegan, C.L., Pinkert, C.A., 2003. Mouse embryo yield and viability after euthanasia by co2 inhalation or cervical dislocation. Comp. Med. 53, 510–513.

Hrabe De Angelis, M., Michel, D., Wagner, S., Becker, S., Beckers, J., 2007. Chemical mutagenesis in mice. In: Fox, J., Barthold, S., Davisson, M., Newcomer, C., Quimby, F., Smith, A. (Eds.), The Mouse in Biomedical Research: Normative Biology, Husbandry, and Models, second ed. Academic Press, New York.

Huang, P., Xiao, A., Tong, X., Zu, Y., Wang, Z., Zhang, B., 2014. Talen construction via 'unit assembly' method and targeted genome modifications in zebrafish. Methods. http://dx.doi.org/10.1016/j.ymeth.2014.02.010.

Hwang, W.Y., Fu, Y., Reyon, D., et al., 2013. Efficient genome editing in zebrafish using a crispr-cas system. Nat. Biotechnol. 31, 227–229.

International Committee on Standardized Genetic Nomenclature for Mice, Rat Genome and Nomenclature Commitee, 2013. Guidelines for nomenclature for mouse and rat strains [Online]. Mouse Genome Informatics website: The Jackson Laboratory, Bar Harbor, ME. Available from: <http://www.informatics.jax.org/mgihome/nomen/strains.shtml> (accessed July 2014).

Jackson, I.J., Abbott, C.M. (Eds.), 2000. Mouse Genetics and Transgenics: A Practical Approach. Oxford University Press, Oxford.

Jaenisch, R., 1976. Germ line integration and mendelian transmission of the exogenous moloney leukemia virus. Proc. Natl. Acad. Sci. 73, 1260–1264.

Jaenisch, R., Mintz, B., 1974. Simian virus 40 DNA sequences in DNA of healthy adult mice derived from preimplantation blastocysts injected with viral DNA. Proc. Natl. Acad. Sci. 71, 1250–1254.

Jaenisch, R., Harbers, K., Schnieke, A., Lohler, J., Chumakov, I., Jahner, D., et al., 1983. Germline integration of moloney murine leukemia-virus at the mov13 locus leads to recessive lethal mutation and early embryonic death. Cell 32, 209–216.

Ju, W., Xu, W.M., Hwang, Y.W., Brown, W.T., Zhong, N., 1997. Molecular pathogenetic studies of the fragile x syndrome: double knockouts of fmr1 and fxr1 affect early development of xenopus oocytes. Am. J. Hum. Genet. 61, A33. A33.

Justice, M.J., Noveroske, J.K., Weber, J.S., Zheng, B., Bradley, A., 1999. Mouse enu mutagenesis. Hum. Mol. Genet. 8, 1955–1963.

Katic, I., Grosshans, H., 2013. Targeted heritable mutation and gene conversion by cas9-crispr in caenorhabditis elegans. Genetics 195, 1173–1176.

Khattak, S., Schuez, M., Richter, T., et al., 2013. Germline transgenic methods for tracking cells and testing gene function during regeneration in the axolotl. Stem Cell Rep. 1, 90–103.

Kim, H., Kim, J.S., 2014. A guide to genome engineering with programmable nucleases. Nat. Rev. Genet. 15, 321–334.

Kim, M.J., Oh, H.J., Park, J.E., Kim, G.A., Hong, S.G., Jang, G., et al., 2011. Generation of transgenic dogs that conditionally express green fluorescent protein. Genesis 49, 472–478.

Kim, Y.G., Cha, J., Chandrasegaran, S., 1996. Hybrid restriction enzymes: zinc finger fusions to fok i cleavage domain. Proc. Natl. Acad. Sci. U S A 93, 1156–1160.

Koller, B.H., Smithies, O., 1989. Inactivating the beta-2-microglobulin locus in mouse embryonic stem-cells by homologous recombination. Proc. Natl. Acad. Sci. U S A 86, 8932–8935.

Kroll, K.L., Amaya, E., 1996. Transgenic xenopus embryos from sperm nuclear transplantations reveal fgf signaling requirements during gastrulation. Development 122, 3173–3183.

Lai, L.X., Kolber-Simonds, D., Park, K.W., Cheong, H.T., Greenstein, J.L., Im, G.S., et al., 2002. Production of alpha-1,3-galactosyltransferase knockout pigs by nuclear transfer coning. Science 295, 1089–1092.

Lee, K.H., Chuang, C.K., Guo, S.F., Tu, C.F., 2012. Simple and efficient derivation of mouse embryonic stem cell lines using differentiation inhibitors or proliferation stimulators. Stem. Cells Dev. 21, 373–383.

Lei, Y., Guo, X.G., Liu, Y., et al., 2012. Efficient targeted gene disruption in xenopus embryos using engineered transcription activator-like effector nucleases (talens). Proc. Natl. Acad. Sci. U S A 109, 17484–17489.

Li, P., Tong, C., Mehrian-Shai, R., Jia, L., Wu, N., Yan, Y., et al., 2008. Germline competent embryonic stem cells derived from rat blastocysts. Cell 135, 1299–1310.

Lillico, S.G., Mcgrew, M.J., Sherman, A., Sang, H.M., 2005. Transgenic chickens as bioreactors for protein-based drugs. Drug Discov. Today 10, 191–196.

Lin, T.P., 1966. Microinjection of mouse eggs. Science 151, 333 –&.

Lindsey, J.R., Baker, H.J., 2005. Historical foundations. In: Suckow, M.A., Weisbroth, S.H., Franklin, C.L. (Eds.), The Laboratory Rat, second ed. Academic Press, New York.

Liu, J.Y., Li, C.Q., Yu, Z.S., et al., 2012. Efficient and specific modifications of the *drosophila* genome by means of an easy talen strategy. J. Genet. Genomics 39, 209–215.

Lloyd, K.C.K., 2007. Gamete and embryo manipulation. In: Fox, J., Barthold, S., Davisson, M., Newcomer, C., Quimby, F., Smith, A. (Eds.), The Mouse in Biomedical Research: Normative Biology, Husbandry, and Models, second ed. Academic Press, New York.

Lois, C., Hong, E.J., Pease, S., Brown, E.J., Baltimore, D., 2002. Germline transmission and tissue-specific expression of transgenes delivered by lentiviral vectors. Science 295, 868–872.

Lutz, A.J., Li, P., Estrada, J.L., et al., 2013. Double knockout pigs deficient in n-glycolylneuraminic acid and galactose alpha-1,3-galactose reduce the humoral barrier to xenotransplantation. Xenotransplantation 20, 27–35.

Ma, C.G., Fan, L.C., Ganassin, R., Bols, N., Collodi, P., 2001. Production of zebrafish germ-line chimeras from embryo cell cultures. Proc. Nat. Acad. Sci. U S A 98, 2461–2466.

Mansour, S.L., Thomas, K.R., Capecchi, M.R., 1988. Disruption of the proto-oncogene int-2 in mouse embryo-derived stem-cells – a general strategy for targeting mutations to non-selectable genes. Nature 336, 348–352.

Monastersky, G.M., Geistfeld, J.G., 2002. Transgenic and knockout mice. In: Fox, J.G., Anderson, L.C., Lowe, F.M., Quimby, F.W. (Eds.), Laboratory Animal Medicine, second ed. Academic Press, New York, pp. 1127–1141. http://dx.doi.org/10.1186/Scrt121 Vol 3:30.

Mussolino, C., Cathomen, T., 2012. Tale nucleases: tailored genome engineering made easy. Curr. Opin. Biotechnol. 23, 644–650.

Nagano, M., Brinster, C.J., Orwig, K.E., Ryu, B.Y., Avarbock, M.R., Brinster, R.L., 2001. Transgenic mice produced by retroviral transduction of male germ-line stem cells. Proc. Natl. Acad. Sci. U S A 98, 13090–13095.

Nakagata, N., 2000. Cryopreservation of mouse spermatozoa. Mamm. Genome 11, 572–576.

Nakajima, K., Nakajima, T., Takase, M., Yaoita, Y., 2012. Generation of albino xenopus tropicalis using zinc-finger nucleases. Dev. Growth Differ. 54, 777–784.

Nakajima, K., Nakai, Y., Okada, M., Yaoita, Y., 2013. Targeted gene disruption in the xenopus tropicalis genome using designed tale nucleases. Zool. Sci. 30, 455–460.

Niu, Y.Y., Shen, B., Cui, Y.Q., Chen, Y.C., Wang, J.Y., Wang, L., et al., 2014. Generation of gene-modified cynomolgus monkey via cas9/RNA-mediated gene targeting in one-cell embryos. Cell 156, 836–843.

Nolan, P.M., Peters, J., Vizor, L., Strivens, M., Washbourne, R., Hough, T., et al., 2000. Implementation of a large-scale enu mutagenesis program: towards increasing the mouse mutant resource. Mamm. Genome 11, 500–506.

Overbeek, P.A., 2014. Factors affecting transgenic animal production. In: Pinkert, C.A. (Ed.), Transgenic Animal Technology, *third ed.* Elsevier, London, pp. 71–107.

Pettan-Brewer, C., Treuting, P.M., 2011. Practical pathology of aging mice. Pathobiol. Aging Age Relat. Dis. 1. http://dx.doi.org/10.3402/pba.v1i0.7202.

Popova, E., Bader, M., Krivokharchenko, A., 2005. Strain differences in superovulatory response, embryo development and efficiency of transgenic rat production. Transgenic. Res. 14, 729–738.

Pritchett-Corning, K.R., Chou, S., Conour, L.A., Elder, B.J., 2011. Guidebook on Mouse and Rat Colony Management. Charles River, Wilmington, MA.

Radman, I., Greiss, S., Chin, J.W., 2013. Efficient and rapid *c. Elegans* transgenesis by bombardment and hygromycin b selection. PLoS One 8.

Reetz, I.C., Wullenweberschmidt, M., Kraft, V., Hedrich, H.J., 1988. Rederivation of inbred strains of mice by means of embryo transfer. Lab. Anim. Sci. 38, 696–701.

Ringwald, M., Eppig, J.T., 2011. Mouse mutants and phenotypes: accessing information for the study of mammalian gene function. Methods 53, 405–410.

Robertson, E., Bradley, A., Kuehn, M., Evans, M., 1986. Germ-line transmission of genes introduced into cultured pluripotential cells by retroviral vector. Nature 323, 445–448.

Rülicke, T., Hübscher, U., 2000. Germ line transformation of mammals by pronuclear microinjection. Exp. Physiol. 85, 589–601.

Russell, W.L., Kelly, E.M., Hunsicker, P.R., Bangham, J.W., Maddux, S.C., Phipps, E.L., 1979. Specific-locus test shows ethylnitrosourea to be the most potent mutagen in the mouse. Proc. Natl. Acad. Sci. U S A 76, 5818–5819.

Russell, W.L., Russell, L.B., Kelly, E.M., 1958. Radiation dose rate and mutation frequency. Science 128, 1546–1550.

Sasaki, E., Suemizu, H., Shimada, A., et al., 2009. Generation of transgenic non-human primates with germline transmission. Nature 459, 523–527.

Schnabel, L.V., Abratte, C.M., Schimenti, J.C., Southard, T.L., Fortier, L.A., 2012. Genetic background affects induced pluripotent stem cell generation. Stem Cell Res. Ther. 3 (4), 30. http://dx.doi.org/10.1186/Scrt121.

Schnieke, A.E., Kind, A.J., Ritchie, W.A., Mycock, K., Scott, A.R., Ritchie, M., et al., 1997. Human factor ix transgenic sheep produced by transfer of nuclei from transfected fetal fibroblasts. Science 278, 2130–2133.

Schusser, B., Collarini, E.J., Yi, H., et al., 2013. Immunoglobulin knockout chickens via efficient homologous recombination in primordial germ cells. Proc. Natl. Acad. Sci. U S A 110, 20170–20175.

Segal, D.J., Meckler, J.F., 2013. Genome engineering at the dawn of the golden age. Ann. Rev. Genomics Hum. Genet. 14 (14), 135–158.

Sellers, R.S., Clifford, C.B., Treuting, P.M., Brayton, C., 2012. Immunological variation between inbred laboratory mouse strains: points to consider in phenotyping genetically immuno-modified mice. Vet. Pathol. 49, 32–43.

Shomer, N.H., Foltz, C.J., Li, X., Fox, J.G., 1997. Diagnostic exercise: infertility in two chimeric mice. Lab. Anim. Sci. 47, 321.

Sibille, E., Hen, R., 2001. Combining genetic and genomic approaches to study mood disorders. Eur. Neuropsychopharmacol. 11, 413–421.

Simpson, E.M., Linder, C.C., Sargent, E.E., Davisson, M.T., Mobraaten, L.E., Sharp, J.J., 1997. Genetic variation among 129 substrains and its importance for targeted mutagenesis in mice. Nat. Genet. 16, 19–27.

Smits, B.M.G., Mudde, J.B., Van De Belt, J., Verheul, M., Olivier, J., Homberg, J., et al., 2006. Generation of gene knockouts and mutant models in the laboratory rat by enu-driven target-seletted mutagenesis. Pharmacogenet Genomics 16, 159–169.

Sobkow, L., Epperlein, H.H., Herklotz, S., Straube, W.L., Tanaka, E.M., 2006. A germline gfp transgenic axolotl and its use to track cell fate: dual origin of the fin mesenchyme during development and the fate of blood cells during regeneration. Dev. Biol. 290, 386–397.

Stewart, H.I., Rosenbluth, R.E., Baillie, D.L., 1991. Most ultraviolet-irradiation induced mutations in the nematode *caenorhabditis elegans* are chromosomal rearrangements. Mutat. Res. 249, 37–54.

Taft, R.A., Low, B.E., Byers, S.L., Murray, S.A., Kutny, P., Wiles, M.V., 2013. The perfect host: a mouse host embryo facilitating more efficient germ line transmission of genetically modified embryonic stem cells. PLoS One 8, e67826.

Taketo, M., Schroeder, A.C., Mobraaten, L.E., Gunning, K.B., Hanten, G., Fox, R.R., et al., 1991. Fvb/n – an inbred mouse strain preferable for transgenic analyses. Proc. Natl. Acad. Sci. U S A 88, 2065–2069.

Tan, W.F., Carlson, D.F., Lancto, C.A., et al., 2013. Efficient nonmeiotic allele introgression in livestock using custom endonucleases. Proc. Natl. Acad. Sci. U S A 110, 16526–16531.

Terns, R.M., Terns, M.P., 2014. Crispr-based technologies: prokaryotic defense weapons repurposed. Trends Genet. 30, 111–118.

Thomas, K.R., Capecchi, M.R., 1987. Site-directed mutagenesis by gene targeting in mouse embryo-derived stem-cells. Cell 51, 503–512.

Threadgill, D.W., Yee, D., Matin, A., Nadeau, J.H., Magnuson, T., 1997. Genealogy of the 129 inbred strains: 129/svj is a contaminated inbred strain. Mamm. Genome 8, 390–393.

Tosal, L., Comendador, M.A., Sierra, L.M., 1998. N-ethyl-n-nitrosourea predominantly induces mutations at at base pairs in pre-meiotic germ cells of *drosophila* males. Mutagenesis 13, 375–380.

Tran, H.T., Vleminckx, K., 2014. Design and use of transgenic reporter strains for detecting activity of signaling pathways in xenopus. Methods 66, 422–432.

Treuting, P.M., Clifford, C.B., Sellers, R.S., Brayton, C.F., 2012. Of mice and microflora: considerations for genetically engineered mice. Vet. Pathol. 49, 44–63.

Valton, J., Dupuy, A., Daboussi, F., Thomas, S., Marechal, A., Macmaster, R., et al., 2012. Overcoming transcription activator-like effector (tale) DNA binding domain sensitivity to cytosine methylation. J. Biol. Chem. 287, 38427–38432.

Wang, H., Yang, H., Shivalila, C.S., Dawlaty, M.M., Cheng, A.W., Zhang, F., et al., 2013. One-step generation of mice carrying mutations in multiple genes by crispr/cas-mediated genome engineering. Cell 153, 910–918.

White, K.E., Koller, D.L., Corbin, T., 2014. Chapter 8 – skeletal genetics: from gene identification to murine models of disease. In: Burr, D.B., Allen, M.R. (Eds.), Basic and Applied Bone Biology. Academic Press, San Diego, CA.

Wilkie, T.M., Brinster, R.L., Palmiter, R.D., 1986. Germline and somatic mosaicism in transgenic mice. Dev. Biol. 118 (1), 9–18. http://dx.doi:10.1016/0012-1606(86)90068-0

Wolfe, S.A., Nekludova, L., Pabo, C.O., 2000. DNA recognition by cys(2)his(2) zinc finger proteins. Ann. Rev. Biophys. Biomol. Struct. 29, 183–212.

Xin, J.G., Yang, H.Q., Fan, N.N., et al., 2013. Highly efficient generation of ggta1 biallelic knockout inbred mini-pigs with talens. PLoS One 8.

Xu, Y.N., Uhm, S.J., Koo, B.C., Kwon, M.S., Roh, J.Y., Yang, J.S., et al., 2013. Production of transgenic korean native cattle expressing enhanced green fluorescent protein using a fiv-based lentiviral vector injected into mii oocytes. J. Genet. Genomics 40, 37–43.

Yang, S.-H., Cheng, P.-H., Banta, H., et al., 2008. Towards a transgenic model of huntington/'s disease in a non-human primate. Nature 453, 921–924.

Yin, X.J., Lee, H.S., Yu, X.F., Choi, E., Koo, B.C., Kwon, M.S., et al., 2008. Generation of cloned transgenic cats expressing red fluorescence protein. Biol. Reprod. 78, 425–431.

Young, J.J., Cherone, J.M., Doyon, Y., et al., 2011. Efficient targeted gene disruption in the soma and germ line of the frog xenopus tropicalis using engineered zinc-finger nucleases. Proc. Natl. Acad. Sci. U S A 108, 7052–7057.

Zan, Y., Haag, J.D., Chen, K.-S., Shepel, L.A., Wigington, D., Wang, Y.-R., et al., 2003. Production of knockout rats using enu mutagenesis and a yeast-based screening assay. Nat. Biotech. 21, 645–651.

Zheng, S., Geghman, K., Shenoy, S., Li, C., 2012. Retake the center stage – new development of rat genetics. J. Genet. Genomics 39, 261–268.

CHAPTER

33

Factors That Can Influence Animal Research

*David G. Baker, DVM, PhD, MS, MPA, DACLAM[a] and
Neil S. Lipman, VMD, DACLAM[b]*

[a]Division of Laboratory Animal Medicine, Louisiana State University, School of Veterinary Medicine,
Baton Rouge, LA, USA, [b]Center of Comparative Medicine and Pathology, Memorial Sloan Kettering
Cancer Center and the Weill Medical College of Cornell University, New York, NY, USA

I. INTRODUCTION

Animal research involves the collection of data from carefully designed experiments. The validity of the research and the conclusions drawn from the data are influenced by many factors. Some of these factors can confound experimental results and therefore must be carefully considered and, where possible, controlled. Otherwise, distortions can result that lead to false observations or erroneous conclusions. Recent evidence indicates that some of these factors can even have epigenetic effects, influencing future research in a transgenerational manner.

This chapter describes many known or potential confounders of research as described in the scientific literature. There are certainly additional factors which have not yet been recognized, as well as interactions among factors that may also influence experimental outcomes. The chapter has been divided into two principal sections: *intrinsic considerations* are those inherent to the animal itself, such as its genotype, and *extrinsic considerations* are those external to the animal that can influence its response. Finally, the chapter is intenationally weighted toward the effects on laboratory rodents *versus* non-rodent laboratory animal species. In order to obtain reliable, meaningful results, an attempt should be made

Laboratory Animal Medicine, Third Edition
DOI: http://dx.doi.org/10.1016/B978-0-12-409527-4.00033-X

to control or standardize all known biological, environmental, and social factors when conducting experiments involving animals.

II. INTRINSIC CONSIDERATIONS

Experimental animals vary among one another based on their genetic constitution, age, sex, health, and nutritional and immune status, as well as on other biological factors such as the immune-modulating effects of commensal flora and fauna. Although animals with genetic uniformity are available and often used, other intrinsic factors must also be considered to ensure reproducible research results.

A. Genetics

The genotype of an animal is an important consideration in designing an experimental protocol, as genetic differences clearly exist between species, breeds, and strains. Both inbred and outbred animals are widely used in biomedical research, each having advantages and limitations. For outbred animals, the breeding colony from which they are obtained must be large enough to maintain heterogeneity, and management techniques must be employed to ensure genetic variability. Heterogeneity can be monitored by using computer models; analyzing biochemical, genetic, phenotypic, and immunologic markers; and examining physiologic variables (Katoh et al., 1990; Shang et al., 2008; Vaickus et al., 2010; Williams-Blangero, 1993). Even within an outbred stock, populations of animals housed at different locations can experience genetic and phenotypic drift over time and so must be periodically monitored so that heterogeneity is maintained, or that subtle changes are detected and accounted for or eliminated (Rex et al., 2007).

The development and availability of inbred strains permit researchers to address specific questions while generating reproducible and comparable data. However, it is important to understand that the genetic integrity of an animal is not necessarily guaranteed by its nomenclature. As noted above for outbred stocks, genetic drift is common and can result in variation among the same strain or even substrain, thus potentially altering experimental data (Fanning et al., 2009; Wahlsten et al., 2006; Zurita et al., 2011). Genetic differences between individuals of the same inbred strain from the same colony can be the result of incomplete inbreeding, mismatings, inadvertent outcrossings with other strains, spontaneous mutations, chromosomal aberrations, or residual heterozygosity (Casellas and Medrano, 2008; Stevens et al., 2007). Thus, inbred animals must be monitored and homogeneity maintained or differences recognized. Commercial rodent vendors diligently control and monitor genetic integrity and carefully manage breeding practices for inbred and F_1 hybrid colonies using genetic, immunologic, and biochemical markers (Nitzki et al., 2007).

When using animals generated by gene targeting, additional details must be considered. Choosing the best genetic strain or stock of mice when developing targeted mutant mice requires an extensive knowledge of their endogenous traits (Orr et al., 2013). In transgenic animals, the number of copies and site of gene integration may not be known. Additionally, in 'knockout' or 'knockin' animals, the integrated or deleted gene(s) can interact with other genes and extrinsic factors, producing unexpected results that may compromise the interpretation of the mutant phenotype (Kurima et al., 2011). Importantly, understanding the normal phenotype of the strain in which a mutation will be analyzed can avoid overinterpretation of the mutant phenotype. As with inbred animals, comprehensive genetic monitoring, including monitoring the inserted gene and copy number, determining the site of integration, and the influence of cis-acting elements should be performed to maintain these unique resources and to verify the presence and zygosity of the genotype.

Species and strains of animals can metabolize xenobiotics differently as a result of inherent quantitative and qualitative variations in constitutive and inducible enzymes (Dalvie et al., 2013). Quantitative variations include differences in cytochrome P450 isoenzymes, cytochrome P450 concentrations, and competing isoenzyme reactions within the host (Malenke et al., 2012). Qualitative variations generally involve differences in metabolic pathways or in their regulation, or both (Greenberg et al., 2011). Variations in xenobiotic metabolism can result from defective or absent enzymes, the ability of a species to conduct unique enzymatic reactions, or environmentally induced perturbations in metabolic regulation. Therefore, species and strain selection of an animal can have profound effects on experimental results.

B. Age

The age of an animal can affect research outcomes and has been shown to be a source of variability in studies involving a variety of body systems. Virtually all body systems continue to develop after birth. The immune system undergoes considerable maturation (Rothkötter et al., 2002); gonadal steroid and other hormonal systems become more active (Nugent et al., 2012); changes occur in brain stem–spinal cord connections, which influence pain processing (Hathway et al., 2009); and the gastrointestinal system matures, influencing digestion and absorption of nutrients (Klein, 1986). Development also occurs in the musculoskeletal and cardiopulmonary systems, and others. These developmental changes can profoundly impact research results. Other reported age differences include metabolic changes in demand for oxygen, respiratory rate, renal tubular concentrating and diluting capabilities, and the ability to thermoregulate (Nichelmann and Tzschentke, 2002). Finally, the ability to biotransform xenobiotics is severely limited in fetuses and neonates due to the immaturity of their hepatic microsomal enzymes (Unüvar and Büyükgebiz, 2012). Similarly, aging processes can result in declining metabolic and physiologic function throughout the body. For example, aging is associated with diminished immune function (Chinn et al., 2012; Molano et al., 2012); joint mobility declines due to loss of viscoelasticity in the chondrocytes (Duan et al., 2012); the ability to detect and eliminate cancerous cells diminishes (de Magalhães, 2013); and reproductive function declines (Kong et al., 2012). The aging animal experiences reduced cardiac output (Singh et al., 2012); redistribution of body fat (Caso et al., 2013); changes in vascular resistance (Davis et al., 2013); and other biochemical and physiologic changes that can influence experimental results.

C. Sex

Animal sex, expressed through epigenetic mechanisms, such as X-inactivation, can influence experimental outcomes (Gabory et al., 2012; Isensee and Ruiz Noppinger, 2007). For example, marked differences in pharmacologic and toxicologic responses to a variety of xenobiotics have been demonstrated in male and female rats. Compared to males, female Sprague–Dawley rats have reduced hepatic detoxification capacity due to reduced expression of the inducible antioxidant enzyme, NAD(P)H:quinone oxidoreductase 1, which plays a major role in protection against free radical damage and oxidative stress. Similar hepatic sexual dimorphism was not observed in August Copenhagen × Irish (ACI) rats (Augustine et al., 2008). Additional examples of sex-related differences have been observed to include the effects of early life stress as a dysregulator of the hypothalamic–pituitary–adrenal axis (Bourke et al., 2013); the incidence of certain types of tumors in male *versus* female rats (Rogers et al., 2007); the greater expression of the CYP2C11 isoform of cytochrome P450 in male *versus* female rats (Thangavel et al., 2007); the suppression of immune responses in male but not female mice after trauma-induced blood loss (Samy et al., 2001); and the increased responsiveness of the male rat brain to steroid-mediated phosphorylation pathways involved in differentiation (Auger, 2003).

D. Immune Status

The immune status of an experimental animal can have profound effects on the experimental outcome,

depending on the nature of the research. The immune system has many functions, including homeostasis of leukocyte differentiation and maturation, immunoglobulin production, and immune surveillance, providing the host with a defense system against microbes, neoplastic cells, and environmental agents. Because the response capabilities of the immune system are to a large extent genetically determined and heritable, it comes as no surprise that laboratory animals, even of the same species, can differ considerably in susceptibility, response, and resistance to infectious agents, as well as in associated outcomes such as pathologic changes and/or healing (Baker, 2005; Fowell and Locksley, 1999). Many examples can be cited of differential susceptibility to infectious diseases among inbred strains and outbred stocks of mice, rats, and other laboratory animals (Baker, 2003). The functional basis for these differences lies in the various cellular, humoral, and pattern recognition components of the innate and adaptive immune systems, which are capable of responding to specific antigens, epitopes, and ligands (McCullough and Summerfield, 2005). In addition to normal immune responses, immunologic dysfunction, including hypersensitivity and allergy, autoimmunity, and immunodeficiency, can profoundly influence experimental outcome. Lastly, there are a wide variety of agents and activities that alter immune function, including chemicals, drugs, food additives, metals, microbes, adverse stressors and experimental manipulations, endogenous compounds, sleep, and exercise (Hertz-Picciotto et al., 2008; Procaccini et al., 2012).

E. Nutritional Status

An animal's nutritional status is dependent on the type(s) of food provided, method and amount of feeding, appetite, general body condition, intestinal microbial status, and age (Donini et al., 2003; Stubbs, 1999; van't Land et al., 2011). Changes in nutritional status can alter specific research outcomes. For example, various dietary conditions, such as mineral, vitamin, and protein deficiencies; lipid composition; and the composition of the diet, alter the biotransformation of xenobiotics (Guengerich, 1995). Nutritional status is also known to influence the development of neoplasia and thus impact research involving cancer development or prevention. Mechanisms associated with tumor development and that are subject to alteration include those regulating chromatin structure and dynamics, epigenetic processes such as DNA methylation and histone posttranslational modification, transcription factors, and noncoding RNA (Ross, 2010). The sex ratio of offspring in a number of species, including rodents, can be skewed by nutritional factors (Rosenfeld and Roberts, 2004). Outbred Swiss mice fed a diet high in saturated fats but low in carbohydrates gave birth to significantly more male than female offspring when fed to 20-week-old *versus* 10-week-old females (Rosenfeld *et al.*, 2003; Rosenfeld and Roberts, 2004).

Excessive caloric intake can have a significant impact on health and experimental results as dietary restriction has been documented to be beneficial to the host for resisting effects of aging, degeneration and infectious diseases, neoplasia, and the toxicity of chemical agents (Fernandes, 2008; Keenan *et al.*, 1996; Martin, 2011; Masoro, 1992; National Toxicology Program, 1997; Spindler, 2005).

F. Circadian Rhythms

Circadian rhythms are endogenous rhythms that influence nearly all physiologic functions (Zee *et al.*, 2013). They have a periodicity of approximately 24 h and are synchronized to the physical environment by the 'central clock' in the suprachiasmatic nucleus and by peripheral clocks in various metabolic tissues such as the liver, pancreas, and intestine, with influence from photic and nonphotic factors (Stenvers *et al.*, 2012). Many behavioral, biochemical, metabolic, and physiologic parameters display rhythmic cyclicity, with minima and maxima occurring at specific times of the day and night. These cycles can be altered, thereby confounding research results, by disturbances in the circadian rhythm. For example, disruption of the normal circadian rhythm can result in alterations in sleep and arousal; food intake; activities of the gastrointestinal, cardiovascular, endocrine, gustatory, hematopoietic, and immune systems; changes in glucose, protein, and lipid metabolism; metabolism of xenobiotics, susceptibility to neoplasia, as well as in other biologic functions (Bass, 2012; Bollinger *et al.*, 2010; Krupp and Levine, 2010; Modric and Martinez, 2011; Morris *et al.*, 2012; Payne, 2011; Stenvers *et al.*, 2012; Yasenkov and Deboer, 2012).

G. Endocrine Factors

The endocrine system, in conjunction with the circadian central clock, is perhaps the principal control system of the body, producing hormones that regulate a wide range of both cellular and metabolic functions (Kalsbeek *et al.*, 2011). The endocrine system interacts with virtually all other body systems. Therefore, disruptions in the endocrine system caused by internal or external stressors, such as those discussed in this chapter, have the potential to interfere with other bodily functions and introduce experimental variability. Hormones are produced by eight endocrine glands within the body. These include the pituitary, pineal, thyroid, parathyroid, and adrenal glands; thymus; pancreas; and gonads (ovaries and testes). In addition, other organs within the body contain endocrine cells, including the hypothalamus, duodenum, stomach, liver, kidneys, heart, skin, adipose, and placenta.

Several intentional or unintentional experimental manipulations or alterations in the animal or in its research environment can disturb the endocrine system. Among the most common are environmental and psychologic stressors such as those discussed in this chapter, and gonadectomy. For a discussion of the former, the reader is referred elsewhere in this chapter. Concerning the latter, loss of sex hormones through neutering can profoundly alter an animal's physiology and therefore research outcomes. A few examples should suffice to illustrate the importance of sex hormones on maintenance of behavioral, metabolic, and physiologic processes. Gonadectomy increases the incidence of estrogen-secreting adrenal tumors in ferrets (Bielinska *et al.*, 2006); reduces stress-associated acetylcholine release in the dorsal hippocampus (Mitsushima *et al.*, 2009); alters body composition (Dušková and Pospíšilová, 2011); reduces growth hormone secretion (Jansson *et al.*, 1985); reduces the incidence of hypertension and chronic renal disease (Kittikulsuth *et al.*, 2013); and reduces cognitive performance and memory (Hill and Boon, 2009). The effects of gonadectomy are often sex-specific. For example, orchiectomy decreases food intake in male rodents, whereas ovariectomy increases food intake in females (Asarian and Geary, 2006).

III. EXTRINSIC CONSIDERATIONS

A. Physical Factors

The provision of a stable environment for the conduct of animal research is essential to ensure the integrity of both the animals and the results obtained. The environment to which the animals are exposed must be considered from two perspectives, the *macroenvironment* of the room in which the animals are housed and the cage *microenvironment* with which the animals have direct and prolonged contact. Dependent on the species housed and the caging system utilized, macro- and microenvironmental conditions may be vastly dissimilar. The principal factors influencing the microenvironment include the macroenvironment, caging system, bedding, if used, and the animals.

Extensive effort is devoted to maintaining the temperature, relative humidity, and air quality within the macroenvironment. Guidelines have been established for these parameters to ensure the animal's well-being is met, as well as providing a stable environment (National Research Council, 2011). Alterations and fluctuations of environmental conditions are well recognized to influence results in a variety of disciplines. For example, the effect of environment on mouse behavior was examined in a variety of inbred strains and a targeted mutant mouse line. Despite using animals of the exact genotype, the same experimental setup and procedures, the same caging, and controlling for the effects of shipment, differences in results were observed and attributed to environmental influences including differences in air handling and humidity (Crabbe *et al.*, 1999). Facility-associated differences in behavioral test responses were shown to be task dependent in that locomotor activity, responses in an elevated plus maze, and cocaine activation were observed to differ by facility, whereas ethanol preference and water escape learning did not (Wahlsten *et al.*, 2003). Differences in airway responsiveness in a murine asthma model were attributed to unknown environmental factors and these phenotypic differences were shown to be of greater significance than substrain-associated genetic variation (Chang *et al.*, 2012).

1. Temperature

The animal's thermoneutral zone (TNZ) is the temperature at which homeotherms are subject to minimal thermal stress. When animals are exposed to temperatures above or below the TNZ, both behavioral and physiologic adjustments are made to ensure homeostasis, including postural adjustments, huddling, piloerection, peripheral vascular dilatation or constriction, alterations in the respiratory rate and pattern, and food consumption. If alterations in ambient temperature persist or the adaptive adjustments are inadequate, changes in the animal's basal metabolic rate result (Clough, 1982; Newton, 1978). However, the TNZ is not necessarily identical with the temperature range providing optimal development, comfort, reactivity, and adaptability, or for particular species such as the rat, even the animal's thermal preference (Gordon *et al.*, 1991; Overton, 2010; Weihe, 1965). The TNZ is dependent on the animal's physical environment and can vary broadly based on housing condition; the TNZ is also influenced by relative humidity, temperatures to which the animals are acclimated, whether the animal has fur or is glabrous, air velocity, barometric pressure, as well as contact with the housing structure and its conductive properties (Gwosdow and Besch, 1985; Romanovsky *et al.*, 2002; Székely and Mercer, 1999). Alterations in ambient temperature have greater impact on small mammals, such as rodents, because of their large surface area-to-body weight ratios. Importantly, metabolic adaptation can occur within minutes of temperature change (Hart, 1963).

The confounding influence of environmental temperature on research has been recognized for years. However, most reports reflect the effects of temperature extremes; few describe more subtle changes expected to occur in modern animal holding facilities. In mice and rabbits, both the onset and severity of hypoglycemia and associated seizures were observed to differ with ambient temperature when the biological effects of insulin were assayed (Chen *et al.*, 1943; Johlin, 1944). The influence of temperature on studies of drug-induced toxicity is well recognized. The toxicity of sympathomimetic amines, such as amphetamine, increases with a rise in ambient temperature, whereas others, e.g., ephedrine, decrease (Chance, 1957). Malberg and Seiden (1998) demonstrated that an environmental temperature change of only 2°C, from 20 to 22°C, resulted in a drop in core body temperature in 3,4-methylenedioxymethamphetamine (MDMA)-treated rats. Not only is the temperature at which a study is conducted important, but the animals' thermal history plays an important role. Mice exposed to cold (4°C) for 7 days prior to evaluation of the β-agonist, isoproterenol, at 24°C demonstrated enhanced toxicity (up to 10,000 times) when compared to mice maintained at 24°C for the entire test period (Balazs *et al.*, 1962). Weihe (1973) has suggested that differences in drug toxicity attributed to high cage population density may actually have resulted from difficulty in thermoregulation. Reductions in temperature, as well as its elevation, are also of importance. Hypothermia resulting from housing rats in isolation has been attributed to a decrease in systemic clearance of antipyrine, a marker compound for hepatic oxidative metabolism and for the estimation of total body water (Brunner *et al.*, 1994).

Three drug toxicity curves have been described with respect to environmental temperature: (1) a V- or U-shaped curve with minimal toxicity observed at or near the TNZ with increasing toxicity observed above or below thermal neutrality, which characterizes many centrally acting drugs affecting the thermoregulatory system; (2) a linear relationship between toxicity and increasing temperature, as exemplified by sympathomimetic amines which stimulate heat production; and (3) a skewed relationship in which no change in toxicity is obtained until the TNZ is exceeded, after which a linear relationship is observed (Fuhrman and Fuhrman, 1961).

Effects of temperature are not limited to drug toxicity. Macroenvironmental temperature elevation to 31.6°C in a rat production colony for 2 days resulted in death of 33% of the animals. Twenty-five percent of the surviving males, 4–66 days of age at time of exposure, were sterile as a result of bilateral testicular atrophy (Pucak *et al.*, 1977). The time rats spend in REM sleep is reduced significantly when their ambient housing temperature is increased by 5°C (Szymusiak and Satinoff, 1981). Periods of mild hyperthermia in which core body temperature increased to 39°C or 40°C, as compared to 37°C, significantly increased the contusion area and volume as well as cell death and axonal injury in Sprague–Dawley models of mild and moderate to severe traumatic brain injury (Suzuki *et al.*, 2004; Sakurai *et al.*, 2012). Rabbits whose dams were exposed to elevated temperatures (33°C) 14 days pre-partum responded differently to cold exposure, endotoxin administration, and noradrenalin infusion, than those whose dams were maintained in a stable environment (Cooper *et al.*, 1980). Reported effects on lactation include reduced latency to first milk ejection and reduction in the quantity of milk produced by directly impacting the activity of the mammary alveolae in rats (Jans and Woodside, 1987; Yagil *et al.*, 1976). Exposure to elevated environmental temperatures for extended periods during rearing can influence morphological features by increasing tail, ear, paw, and salivary gland size in rodents (Caputa and Demicka, 1995; Clough, 1982). Reductions in growth rate, litter size, responsiveness to nursing young, maternal aggression, and neonate viability as well as an increase in anogenital distance in female offspring, which may extend into subsequent generations, have been reported in rodents exposed to low temperatures (Barnett, 1965, 1973; Benderlioglu *et al.*, 2005). Kokolus *et al.* (2013) have recently shown that housing several widely used murine cancer models at their TNZ (30–31°C) *versus* a standard temperature (22–23°C) had a significant effect on antitumor adaptive immunity. Housing mice at their TNZ reduced tumor volumes and delayed postimplantation growth, as well as resulted in fewer metastases and an increased percentage of tumor-free animals, dependent on the model.

The provision of appropriate macroenvironmental conditions is equally critical for poikilothermic vertebrates. Of the various environmental conditions affecting fish, temperature exerts the most significant influence (Sfakianakis *et al.*, 2012). In zebrafish, a gonochoristic species which goes through a stage of juvenile hermaphroditism, the water temperature in which larvae are reared significantly influences the sex ratio of offspring with male-biased populations produced at lower temperatures (22°C) and female-biased ones at higher temperatures (31°C) (Sfakianakis *et al.*, 2012). Water temperature, as well as light cycle length, has also been shown to have a significant impact on the influence of endocrine disruptors in zebrafish. Rising temperatures and increasing photoperiod length increased the transcription of estrogen-responsive genes, making it necessary to assess toxicological responses in fish under different environmental conditions (Jin *et al.*, 2010).

2. Relative Humidity

Both high and low relative humidity (RH) have the potential to affect research. Elevation in RH directly impacts the animals' ability to thermoregulate, as evaporative heat loss is essential for core body temperature control in homeotherms. Rats consume approximately 5% more food when maintained at the same temperature but at 35% as compared to 75% RH (Weihe *et al.*, 1961). These findings may be of relevance to studies in which test agents or chemicals are administered in the food or in which the amount of food consumed is critical. Baer *et al.* (1997) observed body weight increases in Swiss–Webster mice housed in cages with elevated microenvironmental

RH. The authors presumed that these changes were the result of decreased activity as food intake remained unaffected. Abnormally low and high RH increases preweaning mortality (Clough, 1982). Low humidity has also been shown to delay sexual maturity (Drickamer, 1990a).

Environmental moisture impacts the viability and transmission of infectious microorganisms. Most organisms have greater transmission efficiencies from porous and nonporous surfaces to fingers at high (40–65%) RH (Lopez *et al.*, 2013). Transmission of Sendai virus (SV) is enhanced by high RH, whereas transmission of influenza virus is reduced (Noti *et al.*, 2013; van der Veen *et al.*, 1972). In general, the viability of microorganisms appears to be lowest when RH is 50% (Anderson and Cox, 1967).

RH has a dramatic impact on the generation of intracage ammonia, especially in static rodent isolator cages (Corning and Lipman, 1991; Gamble and Clough, 1976). In these cages, microenvironmental RH may be elevated by as much as 38% as compared to macroenvironmental RH.

RH has implications for skin absorption studies, particularly when animals devoid of fur are used (Chang and Riviere, 1991; Chang *et al.*, 1994). Increased environmental temperature and RH generally increase absorption of topically applied substances by altering evaporative rates, the animals' peripheral circulation, and the material's viscosity (Clough, 1982). Variation would also be expected when test substances are administered as aerosols.

Ringtail in rats, which in part is genetically determined and influenced by both caging and nutrition, is characterized by annular constrictions and swellings along the length of the tail, which may lead to tail sloughing. The incidence of ringtail increases when the RH falls below 25% and the environmental temperature is below the animal's TNZ (Flynn, 1959; Njaa *et al.*, 1957; Crippa *et al.*, 2000). The syndrome is observed most frequently in young animals. Histopathologic findings from affected suckling rats have led to speculation that epidermal acanthosis and hyperkeratosis are the main and primary developmental events (Crippa *et al.*, 2000). Ringtail has also been observed in mice and *Mystromys albicaudatus* (Nelson, 1960; Stuhlman and Wagner, 1971).

Microenvironmental RH could induce or exacerbate cutaneous disorders and affect research protocols influenced by epidermal structure and function. Transepidermal water loss is markedly decreased and epidermal DNA synthesis, stratum granulosum cell lamellar body number and exocytosis, stratum corneum dry weight, and total lipid content all are increased when hairless mice are housed at an RH less than 10% or when suddenly moved from a more humid (>40% RH) to a dry environment (<10% RH) (Denda *et al.*, 1998; Sato *et al.*, 1998, 2002).

3. Air Exchange and Composition

Small laboratory animals breathe considerable quantities of air. It is estimated that a mouse breathes approximately 35 l of air per day under normal conditions (Clough, 1982). The composition of the air is important, not only to the animal, but also the researcher because of the potential implications for research. The quality of air to which an animal is exposed is dependent on a multitude of factors including, but not limited to, geographic location, particularly with respect to proximity to heavy industry and urban populations; the scope of its treatment by the HVAC system; and the location of air intake(s), especially in consideration to building exhaust locations and automobile traffic. Air may contain particulates and/or volatile substances, which may be injurious to the respiratory system, skin, and mucous membranes, or may be absorbed and cause systemic effects. Microenvironmental pollutants, principally the metabolic waste gases such as ammonia and carbon dioxide, may be of major importance. In addition, cage components, feed, and bedding may potentially off-gas undesirable substances (Perkins and Lipman, 1995; Vessel et al., 1976; Wade et al., 1968).

The quality of microenvironmental air is influenced by the caging system employed; the sex, strain, stock, and weight of the animal(s) housed; housing density; cage change frequency; bedding type, volume, and processing method; and macroenvironmental conditions (Choi et al., 1994; Corning and Lipman, 1991; Domer et al., 2012; Hasenau et al., 1993; Memarzadeh et al., 2004; Perkins and Lipman, 1995; Reeb et al., 1998; Reeb-Whitaker et al., 2001; Rosenbaum et al., 2009; Silverman et al; 2009; Smith et al., 2004; Vogelweid et al., 2011). Although of concern for all laboratory-housed species, poor microenvironmental air quality is of particular concern for rodents maintained in isolator caging. Static isolator caging systems used to house rodents significantly impede air exchange leading to accumulation of gaseous pollutants, notably ammonia (NH_3) and carbon dioxide (CO_2) (Corning and Lipman, 1991; Gamble and Clough, 1976; Keller et al., 1989; Memarzadeh et al., 2004; Silverman et al., 2009).

Considerable intercage variability in microenvironmental conditions is frequently observed when housing animals of the same strain and biomass in identical caging (Corning and Lipman, 1991). Ammonia is formed by urease-producing bacteria or bedding containing heat-labile urealytic and urease-activating enzymes, which convert urea in urine and feces into ammonia. Microenvironmental NH_3 may reach 350 ppm within 7 days, when housing the maximum number of mice prescribed in the Guide (Perkins and Lipman, 1996). This concentration exceeds, by as much as 14-fold, limits of 25 ppm established as an 8-h time-weighted average (TWA) by the American Conference of Governmental Industrial Hygienists (ACGIH) for human exposure in the workplace (ACGIH, 2013). Physiologic alterations and interference with research may occur at NH_3 concentrations which can be observed in static isolator cages. NH_3 is a potent respiratory irritant which can induce morphologic changes including reduction in the number of cilia of the respiratory epithelium, hyperplasia of epithelial cells, and formation of glandular crypts in respiratory and olfactory epithelium (Broderson et al., 1976; Gamble and Clough, 1976). In addition, exposure of Mycoplasma pulmonis-infected rats to NH_3 concentrations observed in isolator cages (2–250 ppm) enhances M. pulmonis isolation and severity of infection (Broderson et al., 1976; Schoeb et al., 1982). Pneumocystosis and a variety of immunosuppressive effects have also been attributed to elevations in NH_3 (Gordon et al., 1980; Targowski et al., 1984; Walzer et al., 1989). It has also been suggested that NH_3 inhibits select components of the hepatic microsomal enzyme (HME) system and is a contributing factor in the development of corneal opacities in a variety of inbred and F_1 hybrid mouse strains (Van Winkle and Balk, 1986; Vessel et al., 1976).

CO_2 concentrations may also be significantly elevated in static isolator cages (Corning and Lipman, 1991; Huerkamp and Lehner, 1994; Silverman et al., 2009). Concentrations up to 4000 ppm higher than those observed in the macroenvironment, when housing the maximum biomass permissible in the Guide, have been reported (Perkins and Lipman, 1995). However, maximum reported concentrations do not exceed ACGIH exposure limits of 5000 ppm established as an 8-h TWA (ACGIH, 2013). As a result, minimal concern has been raised with its elevation. However, decreased heart rate and blood pressure have been observed in rats exposed to as little as 3% and 5% CO_2, respectively (Krohn et al., 2003).

Microenvironmental oxygen was shown to be reduced 0.5% in individually ventilated cages (IVC) containing four mice as compared to housing in open cages with wire bar lids (York et al., 2012). IVC-housed mice had higher platelet and red blood cell counts, increased hematocrit and hemoglobin concentrations, as well as saccharin preference and fluid consumption, but lower white blood cell counts. Differences in water consumption, body weight, and cage location preference have also been observed when comparing different IVC types (Kostomitsopoulos et al., 2012). Mice were also observed to prefer IVCs with reduced cage ventilation rates and air supplied through the cage lid, although the former could be counteracted by providing nesting material (Baumans et al., 2002).

The potential for other microenvironmental contaminants must also be considered. Bolon et al. (1991) questioned the presence of an uncharacterized pollutant in isolator cages while evaluating the inhalational effects of methyl bromide on F344 rats. Although elevated ammonia concentrations were contributory to the nasal lesions induced by methyl bromide, the olfactory sensory cell loss observed could not be attributed to either agent. In another study, acetic acid (0.86 ppm) was determined to have been off-gassed from corn cob bedding in isolator cages, although no adverse effects are known to occur at the concentrations observed (Perkins and Lipman, 1995).

Volatile chemicals used for research purposes, such as gas anesthetics and agents used for sanitization and environmental control (e.g., disinfectants and pesticides), have the potential to influence the air the animals breathe. The effects of aromatic hydrocarbons released from cedar and pine bedding on induction of hepatic microsomal enzymes have been well documented (Vessel et al., 1976; Wade et al., 1968). Similarly pesticides, used intentionally or introduced inadvertently, and a variety of room deodorizer constituents may similarly alter hepatic microsomal enzyme function (Cinti et al., 1976; Conney and Burns, 1972; Hodgson et al., 1980; Jori et al., 1969; Robacker et al., 1981). Modern pesticides frequently contain organophosphates or carbamates which may alter mammalian cholinergic transmission, even at low levels of exposure. Pesticides, applied as a spray in an oil base or an aqueous carrier, are likely to result in concentrations in ambient air which increase the risk of direct animal contact (Pakes et al., 1984). They are known to induce immune cell dysfunction, act as tumor promoters, be toxicants, act as antiandrogens, alter hippocampus-dependent novel object recognition, modulate expression of the N-methyl-D-aspartate receptor (NMDA) receptor and neurotrophins, and induce renal copper accumulation when dietary copper or zinc is high or low (Kelce and Wilson, 1997; Panemangalore and Bebe, 2005; Rought et al., 1999; Win-Shwe et al., 2013). Odorants, such as citrus fragrance used in cleaning products as well as lemon and rose scent found in cosmetics, have been observed to restore stress-induced immunosuppression, decrease locomotor activity during open field testing, alter pentobarbital-induced sleeping time and sleep latency, and reduce total immobility time in a forced swimming test (Komori et al., 1995a,b, 2006). Because of their high volatility, sufficient amounts of vapor from odorants or other volatile chemicals may drift into animal holding rooms from corridors or storage sites (Lindsey et al., 1978).

4. Noise

The impact of intense noise of frequencies detectable by humans, on both the physiology and behavior of laboratory animals, has been recognized for many decades (Peterson, 1980). However, the effects of noise of lower intensity and ultrasound have received considerably less attention. Noise can induce auditory effects, principally destruction of auditory structures and degradation of

hearing (Basner et al., 2014). Of considerable importance are the nonauditory effects attributed to exposure to sounds of particular intensities and frequency. The hearing range of species used in the laboratory overlaps only partially with that of humans. Among laboratory animal species, rodents, cats, dogs, and small primates can detect ultrasounds (>20 kHz) which are outside of man's hearing range. While the human ear is most sensitive to sounds at 2 kHz, many rodents have peak auditory sensitivities in the range of 30–60 kHz (Bell, 1974; Heffner and Heffner, 1980). Ultrasounds are used for communication in rodents, small primates, anurans, and possibly cats (Bell et al., 1972; Brown, 1976; Milligan et al., 1993; Portfors, 2007; Sales and Pye, 1974; Shen et al., 2011). Ultrasound communication is important to a number of intraspecies interactions in rodents including those between dam and pup, establishing dominance hierarchies, alerting conspecifics of danger, and mating (Hofer and Shair, 1978; Kim et al., 2010; Portfors, 2007; Sales and Pye, 1974; Sales and Smith, 1980; White and Barfield, 1987).

Low-frequency sounds (≤20 kHz) have been demonstrated to alter water consumption; blood pressure; blood corticosteroid, glucose, insulin, cholesterol and epinephrine concentrations; reproductive performance; body weight; eosinophil counts; small intestinal eosinophil infiltrates; immune responsiveness; tumor resistance; histology of the pituitary gland; sleep–wake cycles; microvascular integrity; intestinal mast cell degranulation; embryo production; behavioral responses; grooming activity; learning ability; gastric secretion; balance; hippocampal structure; as well as induce adrenal and cardiac hypertrophy and hypertension in rodents (Anthony and Harclerode, 1959; Armario et al., 1985; Baldwin et al., 2006; Baldwin and Bell, 2007; Buckley and Smookler, 1970; Clough, 1982; Diercks et al., 2010; Fay, 1988; Fink and Iturrian, 1970; Friedman et al., 1967; Geber, 1970; Guha et al., 1976; Jensen and Rasmussen, 1970; Lockett, 1970; Morseth et al., 1985; Rabat et al., 2004; Rabat, 2007; Schmid et al., 1989; Tamura et al., 2012; Uran et al., 2012; Wolstenholme and O'Connor, 1967; Zondek and Tamari, 1967). Noise can induce effects which remain long after it is removed. Barlow (1972) observed that pups born to mice stressed by sound during pregnancy had reduced learning ability.

Ultrasound has been observed to reduce fertility and productivity, cause diuresis and increased urinary sodium secretion, induce audiogenic seizures, reduce locomotor activity, and destroy auditory structures in rodents (Fink and Iturrian, 1970; Lockett, 1970; Peterson, 1980; Pye, 1973; Sales, 1991; Zondek and Tamari, 1967). Structural damage to the auditory system can occur even though subjective (conditioned) responses to sound stimuli remain normal (Catlin, 1986). The direct application of ultrasound to the body wall of the rat, at power similar to that used for human echography, resulted in a significant decrease in fetuses detectable at day E-15, may produce harmful effects in the fetal liver and brain, and induced apoptosis and ultrastructural changes in the fetal heart which disappeared after birth (Bologne *et al.*, 1983; Jia *et al.*, 2005; Karagöz *et al.*, 2007). Ultrasound has also been shown to alter behavior in cattle, horses, poultry, sheep, and swine (Algers, 1984). Sound has also been demonstrated to entrain circadian rhythms in several species (Menaker and Eskin, 1966; Mrosovsky, 1988; Richter, 1968).

The ability of sound to induce audiogenic seizures, a model for human epilepsy, has been well studied. Audiogenic seizure activity has been studied principally in mice, rats, and gerbils, although a variety of other species are susceptible (Pierson and Liebman, 1992; Clough, 1982). Genetically susceptible strains of mice include the AKR, BALB/c, SJL, CBA, SM, RF, LP, 129, and DBA/2 (Fuller *et al.*, 1967), although weanlings of any murine strain can be made susceptible if they are audio-conditioned between 15 and 21 days of age when they are most sensitive (Clough, 1982). Some mouse strains remain susceptible to seizure activity for several months after conditioning (Clough, 1982; Seyfried *et al.*, 1999). Both Sprague–Dawley and Wistar rats can be made epileptogenic by noise exposure as neonates, although the severity of seizures and the age dependence of maximum severity differ among stocks and epilepsy prone substrains (Pierson and Liebman, 1992).

Anthony (1962) recommended that noise levels in animal facilities not exceed 85 dB, a level equivalent to the current 8-h TWA established for human occupational exposure to noise (ACGIH, 2013). The noise generated by the daily activity of animal facility personnel and the use of equipment routinely employed to meet animal husbandry and research needs, as well as by particular species such as rabbits, dogs, and swine, may be of sufficient intensity to result in behavioral and physiological alterations. Milligan *et al.* (1993) examined sound pressure levels in animal holding rooms housing a variety of species at five institutions at both low (0.01–12.5 kHz) and high (12.5–70 kHz) frequencies for periods up to 24 h. The authors concluded that high sound levels were most frequently generated by human activity at frequencies within the audible range of animals, but often outside the human audible range. Another study undertaken to determine the presence and source of ultrasound in laboratories and animal holding facilities demonstrated that 24 of 39 sources monitored, including cage washers, oscilloscopes, and video display terminals, emitted ultrasonic sound, as did running water taps and rotating glass stoppers (Sales *et al.*, 1988). Of particular concern was the finding that some equipment produced only ultrasound and were silent to man. Concerns regarding the activation of fire alarm annunciators and the effect of the noise generated by them on animals led to the development of an annunciator which produces noise below the auditory frequency threshold of mice and rats (Clough and Fasham, 1975).

Construction noise ranging between 70 and 100 dB at 50–2000 Hz has been demonstrated to alter changes *ex vivo* in γ-aminobutyric acid (GABA) release and uptake in rat amygdoloid and hippocampal slices (Fernandes and File, 1993). Rasmussen *et al.* (2009) measured the intensity and frequency of construction-associated noise and the effects of noise on murine reproductive efficiency. Ambient noise levels in mouse rooms were between 61 and 63 dBA L_{eq} with spikes of 80–87 dBA L_{max} associated with personnel activity. Use of a jackhammer generated noise well within the mouse hearing range at intensities over 80 dB, although the building structure attenuated the noise at sites away from its generation. They also observed that Swiss mice implanted with B6CBAF1 embryos and exposed to 70- and 90-dBA concrete saw-cutting noise during select gestational time points had increased stillbirths and smaller litter sizes.

5. Light

The impact of light, including its periodicity, intensity, and wavelength, on the reproduction, behavior, and physiology of mammalian species is well documented. Light is an important synchronizer of circadian rhythm. In the absence of light, the cycle length of diurnal rhythms deviates more than an hour from the usual 24-h period (Weihe, 1976). The time during which the nadir or peak of a specific parameter occurs shifts with an alteration of the light:dark (L:D) cycle. The synchronizing effect of light on the 24-h clock and the amplitude of the cycle are closely associated with its intensity. The direction of amplitude shift frequently depends upon whether the species is nocturnal or diurnal.

Intensity of lighting affects reproductive physiology. The incidence of anestrus increases significantly when hamsters are exposed to light at an intensity less than 15 lux and fecundity rates are highest when rats are housed at 250 lux as compared to six other ambient light intensities (Weihe *et al.*, 1969). Additionally, light intensity has been reported to affect the mean vaginal opening time; ovarian and uterine weights; estrus cycle length; preweaning mortality; heart rate, both in undisturbed rats and those subject to stressful procedures; and defecation rates in rodents (Azar *et al.*, 2008; Donnelly and Saibaba, 1993; Hautzinger and Piacsek, 1973; Porter *et al.*, 1963; Weihe *et al.*, 1969; Williams, 1971). Aschoff (1960) demonstrated that hamster nocturnal wheel running activity decreased as light intensity increased.

Phototoxic retinopathy occurs in man and a variety of animal species. It is most commonly reported in rodents, especially albino rat stocks and strains. Light intensity well below that which causes thermal epidermal burns leads to retinal damage (Case and Plummer, 1993). In addition to light intensity and albinism, other variables including photoperiod duration, body temperature, nocturnality, the light level under which the animals were raised, age, genotype, hormone status, and time of day during light exposure all affect the extent of photic damage (Duncan and O'Steen, 1985; Lanum, 1978; Organisciak et al., 2003; Sanyal and Hawkins, 1986; Semple-Rowland and Dawson, 1987a,b; Vaughan et al., 2002; Weihe, 1976). Continuous illumination as low as 110 lux for 7–10 days can damage photoreceptor cells in rats (Noell and Albrecht, 1971). Numerous studies indicate that retinal degeneration may occur at illumination levels observed in standard animal holding rooms (Bellhorn, 1980; La Vail, 1976; O'Steen and Anderson, 1972; O'Steen et al., 1973; Shear et al., 1973). Current recommendations for illumination at the cage level of between 130 and 325 lux are recommended to prevent photoreceptor degeneration in sensitive species. Animals raised at extremely low (6 lux) light levels may require lower light levels to prevent damage (National Research Council, 2011; Semple-Rowland and Dawson, 1987a,b).

The location of cages on a rack is important as light intensity decreases with the square of the distance from its source. The intracage light intensity may differ by as much as 80-fold in transparent plastic cages from the top to the bottom of a rack, while differences up to 20-fold have been observed within a single cage (Weihe et al., 1969). Variation is lowest in cages furthest away from the light source (Clough, 1982). Greenman et al. (1982) concluded that differences in retinal morphology observed in BALB/c mice used in a chronic toxicity study were due to cage position. The caging system utilized, as well as the shelf, rack, and room positions in which the cages are located, should be rotated to reduce complications induced by light (Clough, 1982; Weihe et al., 1969).

Photoperiodicity is an important stimulant and regulator of reproduction. Complex neuroendocrine pathways initiated at the retinal photoreceptors result in the release of hypothalamic hormones including the gonadotrophins (Brainard et al., 1997). Many, but not all, commonly used laboratory species remain highly sensitive to changes in photoperiod. A decline in hamster reproductive performance with shortening of the light phase, accompanied by a regression of the size and activity of their gonads, is well established (Nelson and Zucker, 1987). The marked increases in body weight associated with increased testicular size, elevations in plasma testosterone, and spermatogenesis in male squirrel monkeys are also photoperiod dependent (Baldwin, 1968; DuMond and Hutchinson, 1967; Mendoza et al., 1978). When species are maintained in the laboratory under constant photoperiod, many of these seasonal reproductive changes disappear; however, seasonal fluctuations in fecundity, sex ratios of litters, body

weight at weaning, and age at sexual maturation are observed in rodents (Drickamer, 1977, 1984, 1990b; Lee and McClintock; 1986).

The optimal photoperiod is unknown for most species. A 12-h light:12-h dark cycle is used for most species; however, longer photoperiods (14L:10D) are used by many laboratories for rodent and zebrafish breeding (Harper and Lawrence, 2011; Mulder, 1971). Estrus cycle length has been shown to increase in Sprague–Dawley rats from a 4- to ≥ 5-day cycle when photoperiod is increased from 12L to 16L (Hoffman, 1973). Heart rate and blood pressure decrease in rats when the light phase of the photoperiod is decreased from 12H to 8H (Azar et al., 2008; Zhang et al., 2000). Significant differences in melanopsin gene expression were observed in zebrafish when the light phase of the photoperiod was extended from 14L to 18L (Matos-Cruz et al., 2011). Shifting of the light:dark cycle reduced pregnancy success in mice with advancement of the cycle having the greatest negative impact (Summa et al., 2012). Phase shifts also adversely altered cognition in mice as assessed by contextual fear conditioning (Loh et al., 2010). Interruption of the photoperiod (3L:3D) for 8 weeks led to obesity, glucose intolerance and hyperglycemia, and increased diabetic markers, expression of hepatic gluconeogenic regulatory genes, and serum and hepatic cholesterol in mice (Oishi, 2009; Oishi and Itoh, 2013). As strain differences in circadian re-entrainment have been reported, the impact of light cycle change disruption may be strain dependent (Legates et al., 2009). Locomotion of zebrafish larva is sensitive to both the time of day in which the assessment is performed and lighting conditions (MacPhail et al., 2009). Similarly, the regenerative response of the caudal fin as well as the toxicity and effectiveness of both MS-222 and clove oil in zebrafish are also dependent on timing with respect to the circadian clock (Idda et al., 2012; Sánchez-Vázquez et al., 2011). Photoperiod length as well as water temperature increased gene transcription and influenced the effects of endocrine disruptors in zebrafish (Jin et al., 2010). Lopez-Olmeda et al. (2010) reported that scheduled feeding is a potent synchronizer and may be a more important zeitgeber than light in zebrafish.

Contamination with as little as 0.2 lux light exposure during the dark phase of the light cycle can reset the circadian rhythm and increase the growth of the transplantable Morris hepatoma, N-nitrosomethylurea (NMU)-induced mammary tumors, and human xenografted MCF-7 human breast cancer cells in rats by inhibiting melatonin secretion and its suppression of tumor linoleic acid uptake and metabolism to 13-hydroxyoctadecadienoic acid; the latter amplifies the activity of the epidermal growth factor receptor/ mitogen-activated protein kinase pathway leading to cell proliferation (Blask et al., 2002; Brainard et al., 1983;

Dauchy *et al.*, 1997, 1999). Exposure to 5 lux during the night may increase depressive-like responses and brain-derived neurotrophic factor (BDNF) expression and impairs cognition in rodents (Fonken *et al.*, 2012; Fonken and Nelson, 2013).

The function of time-controlled lighting systems should be carefully monitored. Although continuous dark cycles are highly unlikely to go undetected, the provision of continuous illumination for varying periods may not be noticed, unless monitored. Continuous lighting has an overstimulating effect on reproduction, leading to cessation of cycling, permanent vaginal cornification, and the development of excess ovarian follicles in rodents (Sawada and Kosaka, 1981; Weihe, 1976). Constant light also enhances the growth and metabolism of some transplantable and spontaneous tumors and leads to splenic hypertrophy as well as increased expression of serotonin transporter in the corpus striatum and hippocampus in mouse pups whose dams were exposed to constant light during late gestation through suckling and an immediate reduction of rhythmic suprachiasmatic nuclei pacemaker activity, increased food intake, decreased energy expenditure, and body weight gain (Anisimov *et al.*, 2004; Blask *et al.*, 2002; Coomans *et al.*, 2013; Dauchy *et al.*, 1997; Popovich *et al.*, 2013; Yajima *et al.*, 2013). Zebrafish reared under CL from fertilization to 6 DPF had significantly lower visual acuity as compared to those raised under 14L:10D (Bilotta, 2000).

The wavelength and hence the color of light have been shown to alter both behavioral and physiological parameters in many species. Light wavelength, including the color generated by fluorescent lights, has been shown to alter voluntary wheel-running activity, the time of vaginal opening, reproductive organ weights, body weight, submandibular gland development, sexual maturity, and the development of dental caries in various rodent species (Hautzinger and Piacsek, 1973; Saltarelli and Coppola, 1979; Sharon *et al.*, 1971; Spalding *et al.*, 1969a,b; Wurtman, 1975).

6. Radiation

Electromagnetic and ionizing are the two principal forms of radiation. Electromagnetic radiation consists of oscillating electric and magnetic fields composed of different wavelengths or frequencies. Ultraviolet, visible, and infrared light, and micro- and radiowaves are forms of electromagnetic radiation. The ever-increasing exposure of humans to electromagnetic radiation from cell phones, Wi-Fi networks, power lines, magnetic imaging instruments, and so on has led to numerous studies on their health effects, often with conflicting results. Electromagnetic radiation has been shown to alter cellular stress responses by activating heat shock proteins and stress-activated protein kinases, the blood–brain barrier, the circadian secretion of melatonin, plasma levels of total cholesterol and phospholipids, macrophage activity, numbers of ovarian follicles, expression of several genes including the upregulation of the transforming growth factor β (TGF-β) superfamily and downregulation of diacylglycerol acyltransferase (DGAT) 2, sperm motility and mortality, *in vivo* neurogenesis, the seizure induction threshold, and performance in a variety of behavioral tests (Cuccurazzu *et al.*, 2010; Fadakar *et al.*, 2013; Frahm *et al.*, 2006; Gaestel, 2010; Gul *et al.*, 2009; Hori *et al.*, 2012; Izmerov, 1985; Kumlin *et al.*, 2005; Lai *et al.*, 1998; Lai, 2004; Nittby *et al.*, 2008; Wilkening and Sutton, 1990; Yan *et al.*, 2007). An increased level of ultraviolet B (UV-B) radiation in the environment due to ozone depletion has increased the risks of ocular damage, immunosuppression, immune modulation as well as neoplasia (Goettsch *et al.*, 1994; Longstreth *et al.*, 1998; Selgrade *et al.*, 1997). The induction of a cataract in mice by UV-B exposure of one eye predisposes the other eye to inflammatory damage (Meyer *et al.*, 2013). UV-A and UV-B exposure each independently alters leukocyte and platelet counts as well as epidermal, erythrocytic, and hepatic enzymes (Svobodová *et al.*, 2011). In animal studies, UV-related immunosuppression has had an effect on the outcome of some infectious diseases and cancers (Brown *et al.*, 2001; Denkins and Kripke, 1993; Garssen *et al.*, 2000, 2001; Goettsch *et al.*, 1994; Longstreth *et al.*, 1998). Wireless local area networks are becoming commonplace in vivaria and research laboratories. Whole-body exposure of a triple transgenic mouse (3 × Tg-AD) to 2.4-GHz Wi-Fi signals improved their cognitive ability in a variety of behavioral tests (Banaceur *et al.*, 2013).

Exposure of laboratory animals to electromagnetic fields has been associated with various neoplasms, including lymphomas, pulmonary sarcomas, hepatotomas, and mammary and skin tumors; however, other animal studies have found no carcinogenic effects (Harris *et al.*, 1998; Repacholi, 1997; Repacholi *et al.*, 1997). Exposure to sinusoidal bipolar oscillating magnetic fields has been reported to cause malformations in chicken embryos (Bryan and Gildersleeve, 1988). Phillips *et al.* (2013) demonstrated, using a four-arm water maze, that B6 mice have a well-developed magnetic compass similar to that which has been described in amphibians and migratory birds. These findings raise the question of potential impact of housing or conducting experiments in proximity to a powerful magnetic source, e.g., magnetic resonance imaging (MRI).

Ionizing radiation is the result of rays and particles producing enough energy to release free electrons from atoms leaving the atom electrically charged or ionized. Gamma rays, X-rays, and atomic particles (alpha and beta) are types of ionizing radiation. They can cause harmful biological effects, including damage of DNA resulting in genetic, teratogenic, and somatic effects, e.g., death and increases in neoplasms (Burkart *et al.*,

1999; USNRC Regulatory Guide 8.13, 1999; USNRC Regulatory Guide 8.29, 1996).

7. Caging and Housing-Related Issues

Modern caging is generally manufactured from stainless steel or synthetic polymers. These materials differ dramatically in their thermal conductivity. Metabolic rate, evaporative water loss, response to a psychoactive drug, MDMA, and colon temperatures were altered when rats are housed in cages with floors made from metal or plastic for periods as short as 60 min (Gordon and Fogelson, 1994). Cage design is also recognized to influence animal health. As an example, pododermatitis can occur in rats housed for extended periods on wire caging (Anver and Cohen, 1979). Wire caging has also been associated with an increased incidence and severity of urologic syndrome in AKR mice (Everitt et al., 1988). Bisphenol A, an endocrine disruptor and the principal component of many thermoplastics used in rodent cages, animal drinking bottles, and aquatic tanks, can leach from new, aged, and improperly processed thermoplastic cage components (Howdeshell et al., 2003). It has been shown to cause meiotic chromosomal abnormalities including oocyte aneuploidy and proliferation of human breast cancer cells (Hunt et al., 2003). In addition, exposure to bisphenol A has been shown to cause alteration in neuroendocrine levels and behaviors in a transgenerational manner (up to F_4) mediated by epigenetic effects (Wolstenholme et al., 2011). Similar epigenetic effects are seen with other endocrine-disrupting compounds such as the herbicide atrazine (Skinner et al., 2011).

Bedding may, in addition to its impact on the cage microenvironment and cytochrome P450 enzymes previously described, induce physical trauma (hardwood chip) that is exacerbated by the use of running wheels; increase ultrasonic (50 kHz) vocalizations indicative of a positive affective state (hardwood chip); alter baseline and cyclic adenosine monophosphate (cAMP)-stimulated rates of acidification of rat liver endosomes (hardwood chip); alter core body temperature dependent on bedding type and amount as well as light cycle phase (hardwood chip and pine shavings); contain an isomeric mixture of linoleic acid derivatives containing a tetrahydrofuran ring and two hydroxyl groups (THF-diols) that act as endocrine disruptors that impede mating and cause acyclicity in both male and female rats and stimulate estrogen receptor-positive and receptor-negative breast and prostate cancer cell lines and prostate cancer cell xenografts (corncob); contain high levels of fungal spores (hardwood and corncob) resulting in fungal-induced rhinitis (corncob); reduce the amount of time spent in slow-wave sleep (corncob); influence the intestinal immune response increasing the number of Peyer's patches as well as total and virus-specific IgA production (hardwood chip as compared to cotton);

impede the generation of intracage ammonia (corncob, hardwood chip, and hardwood chip/alpha cellulose); and alter ascorbic acid levels in rat cardiac tissue (vermiculite) (Beaulieu and Reebs, 2009; Buddaraju and Van Dyke, 2003; Gordon, 2004; Leys et al., 2012; Mani et al., 2005; Markaverich et al., 2002a,b; Mayeux et al., 1995; Natusch and Schwarting, 2010; Perkins and Lipman, 1995; Potgieter et al., 1996; Royals et al., 1999; Sanford et al., 2002; Smith et al., 2004). Additionally, high levels of endotoxin can be found in corncob, hardwood, or a corncob–paper mixture as compared to paper bedding products (Whiteside et al., 2010).

The provision of a complex cage environment to rodents, in lieu of housing in barren shoebox cages, may enhance cell proliferation and improve response in behavioral tests following implantation of intracerebral grafts and lesions of the hippocampus and cortex (Galani et al., 1997; Kelche et al., 1988; Kempermann et al., 1998); can result in increased weight gain without altering food intake; modify ethanol consumption in an ethanol-preferring inbred rat strain (Adams and Oldham, 1996); alter responses in a variety of behavioral tests as well as activity and stereotypic and exploratory behaviors (Anderson et al., 2012; Augustsson et al., 2003; Marques and Olsson, 2007; Olsson and Sherwin, 2006; Tsai et al., 2003); increase variation in hematologic parameters and responses in open field and food drive tests (Tsai et al., 2002); lower the percentage of CD4 and CD8 cells in male ABG mice (Marashi et al., 2004); reduce arterial pathology in a genetically engineered knockout (fibulin-4 +/−) mouse model (Cudilo et al., 2007); and reduce resistance to challenge with Babesia microti in CFLP mice (Barnard et al., 1996). Cage enrichment, especially when providing nest boxes or modifications that provide spatial and visual separation, also may result in the loss of stable dominance hierarchies, leading to increased aggression and neuroendocrine alterations that are dependent upon the individual animal's social position (Haemisch and Gärtner, 1997). Provision of a complex cage environment has been shown to have beneficial effects on animals, especially rodents, as demonstrated in various animal models including learned helplessness (Richter et al., 2013), Alzheimer's disease (Pardon et al., 2009), and age-related changes in cognitive function (Frick et al., 2003).

Numerous studies have reported on the influence of cage size and/or housing density. The febrile response to lipopolysaccharide (LPS) is reduced when hamsters are housed in cages providing 200 cm^2 of floor space as compared to cages providing 1815 cm^2. The author theorized the diminished response was a result of the stress from housing in a small cage, as glucocorticoids and other stress hormones alter the response to LPS (Kuhnen, 1997, 1998). In examining play activity in young rats, Siegel and Jensen (1986) determined that animals housed in smaller cages exhibited greater social play as defined by

1453

pinning behavior. When housed in groups of three in shoebox caging providing 32.2, 64.5, 96.8, or 129 cm² per mouse, C57BL/6 mice provided the least floor area consumed or wasted more water and responded more vigorously to a T-cell mitogen than mice provided greater space (Fullwood et al., 1998). However, an increase in aggressive behavior as well as adrenal gland weight and plasma glucocorticoid concentration were observed as progressively more space was provided. Van Loo et al. (2001) observed a similar effect in male BALB/cJ mice. Provision of greater floor space to male mice alters the animal's dominance rank (Poole and Morgan, 1976). Examining the effects of housing density and cage floor space on male and female mice of three inbred strains, BALB/cJ, NOD/LtJ, and FVB/NJ, Smith et al. (2005) observed that cage size affected the age of aggression onset in FVB/NJ male mice as increased aggression was noted in the smaller and larger of the three cage sizes evaluated. They also measured urinary testosterone output and observed that it decreased with increasing density only in BALB/cJ males. Female BALB/cJ mice were heavier and had increased lymphocyte blastogenesis to phytohemagglutinin when housed at 32 cm² versus 129 cm² per mouse (McGlone et al., 2001). Cage size was not observed to significantly influence the behavior or physiology of dogs and rhesus monkeys (Hite et al., 1977; Line et al., 1989); however, the provision of larger, more complex cages to the common marmoset resulted in increased activity and variation in specific behaviors while decreasing stereotypies (Kitchen and Martin, 1996).

The use of ventilated caging for rodent housing may potentially alter research findings. Although intracage ventilation improves microenvironmental conditions, excessive intracage ventilation, especially when air is supplied at the level of the cage, may lead to chilling and dehydration, with neonates and hairless mutants being particularly sensitive. Intracage air velocities as high as 100 linear feet per minute (lfpm) have been measured in a commonly used caging system (Tu et al., 1997). As 20°C air moving at 60 lfpm has a cooling effect of 7°C, exposure of animals to a ventilated cage may alter behavioral and physiologic responses (Weihe, 1971). Ventilated caging systems may cause pheromone dilution and alter breeding, and dependent on the location within the cage from which air is supplied and exhausted, can alter nest building and cage location preferences impacting other microenvironmental variables such as light intensity exposure (Baumans et al., 2002; Ferguson and Bailey, 2013). A comparison of behavioral responses of mice housed in IVCs as compared to static isolator cages revealed a number of behavioral differences in C57Bl/6JArc mice. IVC-raised female mice demonstrated increased anxiety in the elevated plus maze and both sexes had greater social interaction and demonstrated increased sensitivity to drug-induced locomotor activity (Logge et al., 2013).

Housing mice in ventilated cages can also affect behavioral responses in a strain-specific manner (Mineur and Crusio, 2009; Kallnik et al., 2007). Kallnik et al. (2007) observed differences in the acoustic startle response and fear potentiated startle tests as well as grooming latency in C57BL/6J and C3HeB/FeJ mice. A negative synergistic effect has been reported between ventilated cages and the use of automatic watering systems resulting in increased mouse pup mortality (Huerkamp et al., 1994). The generation of noise and vibration by these systems are additional considerations that may influence experimental findings (Lipman, 1999).

Our understanding of the impact of husbandry as a confounding research variable continues to expand. The manner in which food is provided to Maudsley reactive and nonreactive inbred rats was shown to influence ethanol consumption in this genetically vulnerable rat strain. Ethanol consumption was higher when food was provided in a hopper than when placed loosely on the cage floor (Adams et al., 2000). The relocation of mice to a clean cage has been shown to increase systolic arterial pressure, heart rate, and locomotor activity for as long as 105 minutes and the changes were greater in females and were of a magnitude similar to those associated with collection of blood via a tail nick or rectal temperature determination (Gerdin et al., 2012). The frequency of cage change, weekly versus biweekly, did not further influence the magnitude of change. The authors recommended that a 2-h acclimatization period be implemented after cage changing before evaluating cardiovascular parameters. Similarly, rats exhibit a stress response consisting of elevated serum corticosterone and prolactin levels, as well as increases in heart rate and systolic, diastolic, and mean arterial blood pressures, when their cages were changed (Sharp et al., 2003). Behavioral changes associated with cage changing included increases in locomotion, grooming, rearing, digging, and climbing (Armario et al., 1986; Duke et al., 2001; Saibaba et al., 1996; Sharp et al., 2002). Changes in heart rate and arterial blood pressure persisted up to 180 min and, in contrast to mice, decreased cage change frequency (every 2 weeks as compared to weekly) resulted in earlier and more robust cardiovascular changes (Duke et al., 2001). Wilson and Baldwin (1999) observed that housing rats in a holding room with high levels of personnel activity induced stress that resulted in mast cell degranulation, activation of goblet cells as well as changes in the capillary endothelial ultrastructure and epithelial cell morphology of the intestinal mucosa.

8. Vibration

Vibration is motion characterized by an oscillatory cycle around an equilibrium position. It consists of two components, amplitude, measured in acceleration, and frequency, both of which influence the distance vibration travels and the resulting damage. The effect of vibration on animals has been subject to limited evaluation, but it is known to be important in interspecies communication, predator–prey interactions, and maternal–young relationships. The impact of vibration on an object (animal) is dependent upon its resonance frequency (RF). The object's RF is the frequency that causes the object to vibrate more readily and often increases its amplitude of displacement. Vibration frequencies near the RF are perceived more strongly and cause greater adverse effects (Wasserman, 1987). In humans and animals, RF differs by anatomical location. The RF of the rat's head is 75–80 Hz, thorax is 225–230 Hz, and abdomen is 27–29 Hz, all considerably higher than reported in humans (MacMillian, 2009; Ushakov et al., 1983). There are no published RFs for mice, but Norton et al. (2011) have provided estimates.

There is limited literature on the effects of vibration on animals. Cardiovascular function, bone formation and osteoclast activity, lipid metabolism, electrolyte and trace element concentration, acid–base balance and reproductive function, hypothalamic–pituitary–adrenal axis, body weight, and gastric emptying have all been shown to be altered in mammals exposed to whole-body vibration (WBV) (Edwards et al., 1972; Shenaeva, 1990; Tzvetkov, 1993; Wenger et al., 2010; Xie et al., 2006). For example, swine (20–25 kg) exposed to WBV of 2–18 Hz at 1–3 m/s^2 for 2 h, to simulate vibration during transport, displayed an immediate increase in both plasma adrenocorticotropic hormone (ACTH) and cortisol, the latter remaining elevated until 1 h after vibration ceased (Perremans et al., 2001). In mice, exposure to brief periods of low-magnitude WBV at 2 m/s^2 and 90 Hz for 15 weeks inhibited adipogenesis and decreased hepatic triglycerides and nonesterified free fatty acids, whereas exposure at 3 m/s^2 and 90 Hz for 5 weeks increased bone formation in 7-month-old mice (Lynch et al., 2010; Rubin et al., 2007). Congenital malformations and reduced pup weight have been associated with exposure of pregnant mice to WBV during gestation (Bantle, 1971).

With the increasing use of ventilated caging systems, many of which contain blower systems mounted directly on the rack, the possibility of continuous long-term exposure to low levels of vibration should be considered. Norton et al. (2011) measured vibration in cages housed in an IVC system with rack-mounted blowers. Vibration, although low, was significantly higher at 0.035 m/s^2 as compared to ambient at 0.024 m/s^2. Vibration was highest at lower frequencies, the frequency at which rodents are more sensitive, and decreased as frequency increased to 12.5 Hz. They concluded that the RF range, a measure of the potential that the vibration will be perceived and have a physical affect, for rats and mice is increased by ventilated rack blowers. They also measured the intracage vibration and noise associated with various types of noise- and vibration-generating construction equipment, e.g., jackhammers and shot blasters, which may be used to make repairs within an operational vivarium at various distances from an IVC rack. The most potentially damaging vibration measured affected the rat's thorax and mouse's head and, even when generated at modest distances away from the rack, vibrations were detectable by the animals. They concluded that the vibration generated by the equipment would be of greater concern than the associated noise. Other laboratories have described construction-associated research effects caused by vibration, noise, or both, including alteration of energy balance, i.e., decreased food consumption and body weight; increased stillbirths and pup mortality; and a marked stress response resulting in elevation of plasma ACTH, corticosterone, and aldosterone (Dallman et al., 1999; Raff et al., 2011; Rasmussen et al., 2009).

Even less is understood about the effects of vibration on aquatic vertebrate species. Low-frequency vibrations have been demonstrated to impact embryos of both Xenopus and Danio species in a frequency-, waveform-, and direction-specific manner causing heterotaxia, resulting from altered cytoplasmic cytoskeletal dynamics and tight junctions in the early embryo, neural tube defects (Xenopus sp.), and tail morphogenesis (Danio sp.) (Vandenberg et al., 2011, 2012). Construction (jackhammer)-generated noise and vibration appeared to disrupt the mechanoreceptive function of the lateral line hair cells in adult Xenopus laevis resulting in overstimulation of the noxious feeding response, regurgitation, and eversion of the stomach and distal esophagus causing bloating and suffocation as a result of airway obstruction (Felt et al., 2012).

9. Miscellaneous

Sanz et al. (1988) attributed anomalies detected while evaluating the molecular mechanism of toxic substances to meteorologic (storms), geologic (earthquakes), and astronomic (lunar phase) events. Montenegro et al. (1995) replicated the characteristics of a large earthquake and aftershocks that occurred in Santiago, Chile, in 1985, and reported a marked increase in cleft palates in A/Sn but not in CB7BL/10 mice as well as resorbed embryos in both strains. Interestingly, behavioral tests that were ongoing concurrent with a 2008 earthquake in Wenchang, China, revealed that changes in geomagnetic intensity resulted in dramatic decreases in locomotor activity in six of eight mice being tested beginning 3 days prior to the earthquake (Li et al., 2009).

B. Chemical Factors

1. Xenobiotics (Other Than Pharmaceuticals)

Xenobiotics are chemicals or compounds that are foreign to a biologic system. Exposure to xenobiotics may occur via the air, water, diet, bedding, caging, and/or equipment, or may be pharmacologic agents intentionally introduced as part of the routine conditioning or experimental procedure. The effect or toxicity of a xenobiotic is based on the dose and disposition. Absorption, distribution, biotransformation, and excretion all affect xenobiotic disposition (Parkinson et al., 2013). In addition, host barriers, i.e., the skin, lungs, and alimentary tract, and the physical and chemical composition of the xenobiotic also affect its toxicity. The xenobiotic or its metabolites may cause physiologic alterations in the animal and thus affect the outcome of the experiment by altering immune function, and by acting as a mutagen and/or a teratogen (Kaplan et al., 2013; Parkinson et al., 2013). Examples include aflatoxins; phytoestrogens; endocrine disruptors; heavy metals such as lead, mercury, and cadmium; organochlorine insecticides; and commonly administered anesthetic agents (Cheng et al., 2006; Gerber et al., 1980; Thaete et al., 2013; Thigpen et al., 2013; Whiteside et al., 2010; Wogan et al., 2012).

Inter-animal or inter-colony response variability to xenobiotics may be attributable to differences in the intestinal microbiome of individual animals or colonies as microbiotia may affect chemical metabolism by altering biotransforming enzymatic activity, enterohepatic circulation, absorption, direct chemical activation, the bioavailability of antioxidants and environmental chemicals from feed, as well as gut motility (Clayton et al., 2009; Meinl et al., 2009; Sczesny et al., 2009; Snedeker and Hay, 2012), epigenetic mechanisms (Ingelman-Sundberg et al., 2014), as well as genetic polymorphisms, gender and age (Zanger and Schwab, 2013).

a. Biotransformation

Xenobiotic biotransformation is determined by the physiochemical properties of the compound, as well as the dose, route of administration, protein binding ability, and a variety of host factors, including species, strain, age, sex, time of exposure, microbiome, state of its biotransforming enzymes, nutritional and disease status, and environmental factors (Meinl et al., 2009; Parkinson et al., 2013).

b. Diet

In many cases, the diet is the principal source of xenobiotic exposure (Torronen et al., 1994). Ideally, laboratory animal diets should not contain compounds that can alter experimental response. However, many animal diets contain natural and synthetic chemical compounds, which may have significant effects upon physiologic processes and thus alter the experimental outcome, especially in pharmacology and toxicology studies (Schecter et al., 1996; Thigpen et al., 2013; Torronen et al., 1994). Diets may contain various inducers, suppressors, activators, inhibitors, and substrates, all of which may influence hepatic microsomal enzyme levels (Stott et al.,

2004; Torronen et al., 1994; Yang et al., 1992). Potential feed contaminants include chlorinated hydrocarbons, organophosphates, polychlorinated biphenyls, heavy metals, mycotoxins, nitrates, nitrosamines, and estrogenic compounds (Edwards et al., 1979; Kozul et al., 2008; Newberne and McConnell, 1980; Schecter et al., 1996; Silverman and Adams, 1983; Thigpen et al., 1987, 1998, 1999, and 2007; Waldemarson et al., 2005; Weiss et al., 2005). Certified diets are commonly used in toxicology studies to avoid these potential contaminants. Many contaminants are found naturally in plant materials or are agricultural residues. Diets may also be contaminated during storage or formulation. Examples include aflatoxin or other mycotoxin contamination of corn, wheat, and other cereals during storage; the presence of phytoestrogens in dietary constituents; and contamination of diets with estrogenic compounds during formulation (Hadlow et al., 1955; Wogan, 1968; Wright and Seibold, 1958; Thigpen et al., 1999).

The presence of significant levels of phytoestrogens (isoflavonoids and coumestans), particularly the flavonoids genistein and daidzein, in natural plant-based diets is well recognized. Phytoestrogens have been shown to have the potential to significantly influence studies in a broad array of disciplines including cancer development and biology, reproductive biology, central nervous system structure and function and its association with learning and behavior, models of neurologic disease and obesity, skeletal biology, especially bone mineral density, and toxicology (Jensen and Ritskes-Hoitinga, 2007; Ju et al., 2002; Kurzer and Xu, 1997; Lakshman et al., 2008; Lephart et al., 2002; Odum et al., 2001; Thigpen et al., 2013; Westmark et al., 2013). As examples, Stott et al. (2004) examined the effects of diet (standard versus phytoestrogen-free) on the constitutive and benzo(a)pyrene-induced activity of a various drug-metabolizing enzymes and observed significant diet-associated differences that could potentially alter the toxicity of numerous chemicals. The inability to define the no observed adverse effect level in humans for bisphenyl A, an endocrine disruptor found in numerous plastic products, can be attributed, in part, to inconsistent results obtained from rodent studies in which exogenous phytoestrogens confounded results (Thigpen et al., 2013). Soybean meal and alfalfa are the principal offending dietary ingredients and diets free of these constituents have trace or undetectable phytoestrogen levels and may be necessary for specific studies (Brown and Setchell, 2001; Heindel and vom Saal, 2008; Stroud et al., 2006; Thigpen et al., 1987, 1999, 2007). The epigenetic impact of dietary phytoestrogens may be transgenerational as dietary supplementation of mice during gestation with genistein altered DNA methylation and gene expression in offspring that persisted into adulthood (Dolinoy et al., 2006). While most attention has been given to the presence of phytoestrogens in cereal-based rodent diets, they may also be present in high concentrations in diets fed to nonhuman primates and fish (Inudo *et al.*, 2004; Stroud *et al.*, 2006). Inudo *et al.* (2004) detected daidzein and genistein in all 15 fish diets examined from the United Kingdom and Japan, although there were over 20-fold differences detected between diets. Hepatic vitellogenin values were significantly higher in male medaka fish fed a diet with high phytoestrogen levels (Inudo *et al.*, 2004).

Variations in the constituents and formulation of the diet result in a wide variety, type, and concentration of chemical contaminants as well as nutrient quality (Newberne and McConnell, 1980; Wise, 1982). In mice, purified diets have been shown to reduce the number of lactobacilli and organic acids in the stomach, which allowed for sustained colonization with *Candida albicans* after experimental inoculation (Yamaguchi *et al.*, 2005). Variations in dietary constituents may alter the toxicity of chemical contaminants and potentially affect animal responses to specific drugs or chemicals (Parkinson *et al.*, 2013). Post-milling feed processing may also impact dietary constituents and increase the concentrations of unwanted chemicals. Steam sterilization is well recognized to reduce the concentrations of heat-labile dietary constituents, such as certain vitamins, and these nutrients must be supplemented in autoclavable diets. Twaddle *et al.* (2004) demonstrated that autoclaving a standard rodent diet increased the concentration of acrylamide, a neurotoxin and carcinogen, by 14-fold. Further, the acrylamide in the autoclaved diet was bioavailable and metabolically activated to its genotoxic metabolite, glycidamide, when fed to rats. Gamma irradiation of a dry cat diet reduced vitamin A and elevated peroxide concentrations, inducing feline leukoencephalomyelopathy, which had been previously reported in animals fed irradiated diets (Cassidy *et al.*, 2007; Caulfield *et al.*, 2009). Caulfield *et al.* (2008) also evaluated the impact of gamma irradiation on pelleted dog, cat, and rodent diets at two irradiation doses (typical: 28.9–34.3 kGy; and high: 38.4–48.7 kGy). The changes were limited to alterations in vitamin A and peroxide concentrations, as noted above, and were dose dependent. The high dose of irradiation reduced the vitamin A concentration in the rodent diets, whereas both doses reduced vitamin A levels in the cat diet and neither dose affected the canine diet. Irradiation increased the peroxide concentration of all three diets in a dose-dependent manner resulting in increases up to 25-fold.

The protein and fat content of a diet may have profound effects on physiologic processes and on the toxicity of certain xenobiotics. Olovson (1986) demonstrated dramatically increased breeding efficiency, decreased mortality, and increased body weight gain in both male and female cats when dietary fat content was increased from 15% to 27% in a conventional cat-breeding colony.

In inbred rats, both diet and strain strongly influence the number, size, and hemoglobin content of red blood cells (Hackbarth *et al.*, 1983). In rats, aflatoxin B1-induced hepatic neoplasms were more significant when corn oil was the source of dietary fat compared to beef fat (Newberne *et al.*, 1979). In comparing a cereal-based and a purified diet, rats, mice, and hamsters fed the cereal-based diet had decreased blood levels of cholesterol and phospholipid. The differences were attributed to the level and composition of the fiber fraction of the cereal-based diet (Rutten and de Groot, 1992). Additionally, transgenic mice expressing a human breast cancer oncogene, c-neu, fed a diet containing fiber from nonpurified cereal ingredients had delayed development of mammary tumors (Rao *et al.*, 1997).

Variations in the quantity or availability of essential vitamins and trace minerals may alter drug-metabolizing systems, affect membrane integrity, or predispose to the affects of carcinogens (Newberne and McConnell, 1980). Deficiencies in calcium, copper, iron, magnesium, and zinc have been shown to decrease cytochrome P450 enzyme levels and redox reactions (Parkinson *et al.*, 2013). Hypervitaminosis A has been associated with teratogenic effects in rabbits including fetal resorptions, abortions, and stillbirths (DiGiacoma *et al.*, 1992). Miller *et al.* (1997) demonstrated that the amount of dietary iron intake in common marmosets can affect liver iron content and health. Diets high in iron (350–500 ppm) can lead to hepatic hemosiderosis with subsequent effects including death.

Laboratory diets may be contaminated by carcinogenic nitrosamines (Edwards *et al.*, 1979; Walker *et al.*, 1979) and nitrates (Newberne and McConnell, 1980), which can be converted to nitrosamines in the gastrointestinal tract. Recent studies have shown a widely used closed-formula commercial rodent diet to be contaminated with arsenic and methylmercury (Kozul *et al.*, 2008; Weiss *et al.*, 2005). In rodents, exposure to heavy metals, such as lead and cadmium, has been shown to suppress disease resistance, alter the effects of endotoxin; cause immunosuppression, influence reproductive performance, and may be carcinogenic (Cheng *et al.*, 2006; Gerber *et al.*, 1980; Goyer, 1991; Hanson *et al.*, 2012; Hemphill *et al.*, 1971; Koedrith *et al.*, 2013; Lukacinova *et al.*, 2012; Sengupta and Bishayi, 2002). The type and quantity of feed provided to rats may cause differences in central nervous system responsiveness and function (Kacew *et al.*, 1998). In cats, increased dietary cysteine promotes higher methionine, homocysteine, glutathione, and oxidized glutathione concentrations in the blood (Fettman *et al.*, 1999). Aged female beagle dogs fed a diet with *n*-6-to-*n*-3 fatty acid ratio of 1:4 had increased total lymphocyte and CD4+ T-cell counts and a decreased CD4+-to-CD8+ ratio after vaccination with a keyhole limpet hemocyanin suspension (Hall *et al.*, 1999). Finally, food deprivation can have a dramatic effect on the outcome of toxicology studies as deprivation can induce hepatic microsomal enzymes and reduce the concentration of cofactors and conjugating agents (Parkinson *et al.*, 2013).

c. Water

Animal drinking water is generally supplied from a local potable water source which meets standards applied to human consumption. Depending on geographic location; area geology; the use of surface or well water; proximity to industrial, agricultural, or urban centers; and the type of water treatment used, the water consumed is subject to considerable variation. Drinking water may be contaminated by microbial agents, pesticides, heavy metals, radionuclides, various chemicals including polychlorinated biphenyls (PCBs), perchlorates, endocrine disruptors, and other compounds which may produce biological effects (Blount *et al.*, 2010; Cantor, 2010; Reynolds *et al.*, 2008; Surbeck, 1995). A variety of pharmaceuticals, including antibiotics, analgesics, antiseptics, beta-blockers, and psychoactive and cholesterol-lowering drugs have been detected in the drinking water supply in various North American municipalities (Watts, 2011; Ritter *et al.*, 2002; Thomas and Klaper, 2012).

There is epidemiologic evidence of an association between drinking water contaminants, including pesticides, arsenic, volatile organics, asbestiform fibers, and radionuclides, and the formation of one or more types of neoplasms in humans (Cantor, 2010). Nitrogen fertilizers and pesticides have been used worldwide since the 1960s and pesticide contamination of drinking water supplies has been increasing (Morales *et al.*, 1993; Ritter *et al.*, 2002; Shapiro, 1980; Taets *et al.*, 1998). Perchlorates found in drinking water in certain regions of the United States inhibit thyroid uptake of iodide (Trumbo, 2010). Kligerman *et al.* (1993) demonstrated cytogenic damage in splenocytes of male F344 rats and female B6C3F1 mice following exposure to simulated California groundwater contaminated with a mixture of pesticides and the fertilizer, ammonia nitrate. Herbicides have also been shown to cause chromosomal damage to Chinese hamster ovary (CHO) cells *in vitro* (Taets *et al.*, 1998).

Heavy metals such as arsenic, lead, copper, cadmium, nickel, and silver may contaminate drinking water. In humans, chronic arsenic exposure can lead to serious health effects including cancer, melanosis, hypopigmentation, hyperkeratosis, restrictive lung disease, peripheral vascular disease, respiratory disease, diabetes mellitus, hypertension, and ischemic heart disease (Otleş and Cağindi, 2010), whereas *in utero* exposure to low-dose arsenic in mice alters lung mechanics (Ramsey *et al.*, 2013). Kozul-Horvath *et al.* (2012) exposed C57BL/6J pups to 10ppb arsenic, the current U.S. drinking water standard, administered in the dam's drinking water and observed impaired growth in the F_1 offspring and

decreased nutrient content of the dam's milk. Ronis *et al.* (1998a,b) evaluated chronic lead exposure in pregnant Sprague–Dawley rats. Pregnant rats exposed at E-5 to lead acetate, 0.05–0.45% w/v, in drinking water had a dose–response-related decrease in neonatal birth weights and crown-to-rump lengths with a subsequent delay in sexual maturity. The disruptions in reproductive physiology were accompanied by a significant decrease in neonatal sex steroids and suppression of sex hormones during puberty. Zheng *et al.* (1996) exposed weanling, male Sprague–Dawley rats to lead acetate in drinking water, at 0, 50, or 250µg/ml, and demonstrated a dose-related decrease in production of choroid plexus transthyretin, a major cerebrospinal fluid protein manufactured by the choroid plexus responsible for the transport of thyroid hormones to the developing brain. Although low-level *in utero* and early postnatal exposure (E-18 to PND-21) of Long Evans rats to lead reduced hippocampal neurogenesis in these rats as adults, no significant impact on spatial learning was detected (Gilbert *et al.*, 2005).

Water treatment can be used to minimize microbial contamination; however, many forms of treatment result in physiologic alterations that can affect experimental data or the formation of disinfection by-products which have adverse effects (Fidler, 1977; Hall *et al.*, 1980; Hermann *et al.*, 1982; Homberger *et al.*, 1993; Richardson *et al.*, 2007). Chlorine can cause alterations in the immune response or react with organic matter, man-made contaminants, bromide and iodide, resulting in the formation of carcinogenic, genotoxic, and mutagenic by-products (Exon *et al.*, 1987; Hermann *et al.*, 1982; Koivusalo and Vartiainen, 1997; Morris *et al.*, 1992; Richardson *et al.*, 2007). Trihalomethanes are formed as a result of interactions between chlorine or bromine with methane groups from natural organic materials. Chloroform, a trihalomethane, is found in relatively high concentrations in water and has demonstrated biological impact including cytotoxicity, increased DNA synthesis, and carcinogenesis (Lee *et al.*, 1998; Lipsky *et al.*, 1993; Vessel *et al.*, 1976).

The processing and delivery system of water in a laboratory animal facility can affect water constituents. Hall *et al.* (1980) evaluated the effects of acidified drinking water on select biologic phenomena of normal and immunosuppressed male mice. Depending on the pH of the water and the acid (hydrochloric *versus* sulfuric) used for acidification, there can be a decrease in weight gain, water consumption, and number of bacteria species isolated from the terminal ileum, with more pronounced changes noted in immunosuppressed mice. The authors concluded that the acidification of drinking water was not innocuous and it should be evaluated as an environmental variable. Exposure of rats to acidified water (pH 2.0) leads to extensive enamel and dental erosion of molar teeth (Karle *et al.*, 1980; Tolo and Erichson, 1969). Lohmiller and Lipman (1998) documented increases in water silicon concentration and the formation of silicon crystals from in glass water bottles that underwent autoclaving. The increase in silicon and variations from bottle to bottle in silicon concentration could cause alterations in experimental variables. Renal lesions have been induced in guinea pigs following the experimental administration of silica-containing compounds (Dobbie and Smith, 1982). Kennedy and Beal (1991) evaluated rubber water bottle stoppers for mineral content and mineral leaching ability in both deionized and acidified-deionized drinking water. Minerals were present in all three types of stoppers evaluated. Acidified-deionized drinking water typically leaches more minerals from the stoppers. The authors concluded that certain types of stoppers can be more suitable for particular nutritional and toxicologic studies. Nunamaker *et al.* (2013) evaluated the heavy metal content and the effects of water acidification (pH 2.23) and autoclaving on stainless steel sipper tubes, polysulfone water bottles, as well as rubber and neoprene stoppers after a week of contact. They determined that the sipper tubes and stoppers all had varying levels of multiple heavy metals and leaching was promoted by both acidification and autoclaving.

Ensuring appropriate water quality is essential for laboratory-maintained aquatic species. Many of the environmental drinking water contaminants described previously have the potential to affect the health and biology of aquatic species. Particular attention has been paid to endocrine disruptors because of their increasing environmental presence. They have been shown to influence gonadal differentiation in fish and amphibia. Exposure to estrogenic compounds leads to female-biased development, whereas the opposite is true following exposure to androgens (Baumann *et al.*, 2013; Larsen *et al.*, 2009; Larsen and Baartrup, 2010; Olmstead *et al.*, 2010; Santos *et al.*, 2006).

2. Pharmaceuticals

Pharmaceutical agents are administered to laboratory animals for a variety of reasons. For example, pharmaceuticals are administered to induce and maintain anesthesia, for pain relief, to prevent or treat microbial disease, or to activate an inducible promoter, which turns on or off specific genes. In general, their administration is necessary but can be ancillary to the primary experimental goal. Pharmaceuticals can result in physiological changes, distinct from those expected from their principal mechanism of action, or they can alter the metabolism of other chemicals and therefore alter experimental results. Importantly, effects induced by pharmaceutical agents can frequently be dose and species dependent.

a. Anesthetics, Tranquilizers, and Analgesics

The induction and maintenance of general anesthesia leads to significant physiological alterations principally of the cardiovascular, pulmonary, neuroendocrine, immune, and nervous systems. Tranquilizers, anesthetics, and analgesic combinations are usually selected which minimize physiologic disturbance of the system under study, and appropriate controls are utilized to reduce their impact as a confounding factor. This choice is most critical when experimentation is conducted while the animal is under anesthesia, as most significant cardiopulmonary alterations return to normal following recovery. However, some anesthetics can induce physiologic and behavioral changes distinct from their cardiopulmonary effects, which can persist long after the animal has recovered from anesthesia. As an example, brain protein-level expression was aletered in rats exposed to 1 minimum alveolar concentration (MAC) sevoflurane for as long as 28 days postanesthetic exposure (Kalenka *et al.*, 2007).

Anesthetics can be directly toxic and the state of anesthesia may also result in adverse consequences in research animals. Anesthetics such as tribromoethanol, xylazine, the combination of ketamine and xylazine, and various inhalational anesthetics have been shown to induce tissue injury when administered at clinically relevant doses. Pulmonary parenchymal, lymphocyte and Kupffer cell damage, muscle necrosis, peritonitis, ileus, corneal calcium deposition and ulceration, and keratoconjunctivitis sicca have been reported in animals undergoing anesthesia (Celly *et al.*, 1999; Gaertner *et al.*, 1987; Guillet *et al.*, 1988; Kufoy *et al.*, 1989; Lieggi *et al.*, 2005; Reid *et al.*, 1999; Smiler *et al.*, 1990; Thompson *et al.*, 2002; Turner and Albassam, 2005, Zeller *et al.*, 1998). Methoxyflurane is nephrotoxic in F344 rats causing a dose-related diabetes insipidus syndrome (Mazze *et al.*, 1973). During metabolism of desflurane, enflurane, halothane, and isoflurane, tissue acetylation occurs creating neo-antigens against which an antibody-mediated immune response may occur, leading to hepatic toxicity (Reichle and Conzen, 2003). Halothane is associated with the highest risk. Plasma inorganic fluoride concentrations are increased after sevoflurane anesthesia (Reichle and Conzen, 2003). Compound A, a haloalkene degradant of sevoflurane following its interaction with CO_2 absorbent, is nephrotoxic to both rats and nonhuman primates (Kharasch, 1998). Inhaled concentrations of compound A are highest at low flow rates and high sevoflurane concentrations, and are higher with barium hydroxide *versus* soda lime absorbent.

Various anesthetics, including isoflurane, nitrous oxide, propofol, sevoflurane, and the sedative midazolam, have been shown to be neurotoxic in neonatal mice and rats (Istaphanous *et al.*, 2013; Jevtovic-Todorovic *et al.*, 2003; Krzisch *et al.*, 2013; Zheng *et al.*, 2013). The stage of brain development at the time of exposure, as well as frequency and the cumulative dose of anesthetic, was shown to impact neuroapoptosis as well as synaptic development. While there are species differences in age susceptibility, even within the same species, different brain regions are susceptible to anesthetic-related damage at different developmental timepoints (Jevtovic-Todorovic et al., 2013). Conversely, anesthetics including dexmedetomidine, halothane, isoflurane, ketamine, pentobarbital, and propofol can be neuroprotective by modulating ion channels either directly or indirectly, in some cases, downstream signaling molecules, which are components of cell toxicity and survival pathways (Karmarkar et al., 2010).

Tribromoethanol, ketamine/xylazine cocktails, isoflurane, meloxicam, and buprenorphine, drugs commonly administered to mice during gestation, were shown to significantly reduce fetal growth (Thaete et al., 2013). In addition, buprenorphine increased the incidence of microphthalmia nearly eightfold. Anesthetics can enhance or inhibit the toxicity of other agents. Barbiturates and xylazine induce hepatic cytochrome P450 metabolizing enzymes, which can influence the metabolism of other chemicals (Nossaman et al., 1990). Enflurane, halothane, and methoxyflurane have been shown to inhibit cytochrome P450-dependent type I substrates (Rice and Fish, 1987). The authors speculated that methoxyflurane, because of its high lipid solubility, could have long-lasting effects.

The effects of anesthetics on the immune system are well recognized. Inhalational anesthetics, including methoxyflurane, halothane, isoflurane, sevoflurane, and desflurane, and injectable agents, including including tribromoethanol, ketamine-xylazine mixtures, chloral hydrate, pentobarbital, and urethane, have been shown to reduce the responsiveness of lymphocytes to mitogens and decrease their chemotactic, phagocytic, and transforming capabilities, as well as their ability to synthesize RNA and protein; inhibit cell-mediated cytotoxicity, neutrophil and monocyte chemotaxis, and neutrophil phagocytosis; and influence T-cell adhesion properties as well as their inflammatory response (Bette et al., 2004; Bruce, 1972, 1975; Cullen, 1974, Cullen et al., 1972, 1976; Moudgil, 1986; Puig et al., 2002). A variety of anesthetic agents and opioid analgesics, including tribromoethanol, fentanyl, halothane, isoflurane, ketamine/xylazine, morphine, sufentanil, and sevoflurane, may reduce the cytotoxic activity of natural killer (NK) cells in the postoperative period (Beilin et al., 1989; Markovic and Murasko, 1990, 1991, 1993; Markovic et al., 1993). NK-cell hyporesponsiveness lasts for at least 11 days after anesthesia (Markovic et al., 1993). Following anesthesia, NK cells fail to respond normally to interferon (INF) or poly I:C, an inducer of endogenous INF synthesis (Markovic and Murasko, 1990, 1991; Markovic et al., 1993). Anesthetic-induced NK-cell activity depression strongly accelerated progression of spontaneous lung metastasis produced by the 3LL Lewis lung carcinoma

and B16 melanoma (Katzav et al., 1986; Shapiro et al., 1981). Ketamine and thiopental have anti-inflammatory effects in the face of endotoxemia. They have been shown to inhibit the production of endogenous proinflammatory cytokines, including tumor necrosis factor-α (TNF-α), interleukin (IL)-1, IL-6, and IL-8, and increase the production of the anti-inflammatory cytokine, IL-10 (Taniguchi and Yamamoto, 2005).

The administration of local anesthetics inhibits lymphocyte capping; depresses adhesion, phagocytosis, and the production of superoxide anions and hydrogen peroxide in neutrophils; reduces both the number and function of CD4+ and CD 19+ cells; alters lymphocyte secretion of INF, TNF, IL-1, and soluble IL-2 receptor following stimulation by a variety of mitogens; and increases plasma endothelin-like immunoreactivity (Azuma et al., 2000; Brand et al., 1998; Corsi et al., 1995; Kutza et al., 1997; Sato et al., 1996; Shirakami et al., 1995). Local anesthetics including procaine, lidocaine, butacaine, tetracaine, and dibucaine have been shown to enhance the toxicity of the bleomycin derivative, peplomycin (Mizuno and Ishida, 1982).

The effects of anesthetics on cardiovascular function are well known. At concentrations used clinically, most volatile anesthetics and many injectable anesthetics depress myocardial contractivity. The mechanisms underlying the negative inotropic effects of these agents partially involve the effect of calcium on the myofibrillar apparatus (Gare et al., 2001). Volatile anesthetics, including halothane, isoflurane, and sevoflurane, have an inhibitory effect upon both vascular and tracheal smooth muscle, leading to both vascular and airway dilatation (Kai et al., 1998; Mercier and Denjean, 1996; Zhang and List, 1996). These agents attenuate and prevent airway smooth muscle constriction when exposed to allergen and leukotriene-D4 (Tudoric et al., 1995). These effects are mediated by influencing calcium sensitivity (Kai et al., 1998; Zhang and List, 1996).

Select anesthetic agents may have effects which, while although clinically inapparent, can be of critical importance to experimental outcome. The application of the topical anesthetic benzocaine is associated with methemoglobinemia in a variety of species (Davis et al., 1993). A 2-s burst of anesthetic spray or direct application of 56 mg of benzocaine increased methemoglobin concentrations sufficiently to substantially alter cardiovascular and pulmonary function (Davis et al., 1993; Lagutchik et al., 1992). The widely used α2-adrenergic agonist, xylazine, lowers basal plasma insulin concentrations and abolishes the rise in insulin following glucose administration resulting in elevations in fasting glucose and glucose intolerance in multiple species (Brockman, 1981; Goldfine and Arieff, 1979; Hsu, 1988; Koppel et al., 1982). Ketamine–xylazine combinations administered prior to isolation of guinea pig heart were shown to impact cardiac ischemia–reperfusion injury, with a higher dose improving hemodynamic performance (Sloan *et al.*, 2011). Hematologic parameters can be markedly altered following anesthesia. As examples, a 30-min exposure to isoflurane leads to a 15.4% reduction in circulating white blood cells, a 26.9% reduction in neutrophils, and a 11.2% reduction in platelets when measured 48h after anesthesia in C3H mice, whereas in New Zealand white rabbits, plasma biochemistry parameters can increase or decrease in association with the specific agent used to anesthetize the animal for sample collection (Gil *et al.*, 2004; Jacobsen *et al.*, 2004). Ketamine and pentobarbital both affect the circadian secretion of melatonin as well as influence locomotor activity in rats, depending on the specific phase of the light cycle during which each anesthetic is administered (Mihara *et al.*, 2012).

Anesthetics have been shown to exert effects on the neuroendocrine system. Reported anesthetic-induced alterations include both increased and decreased cortisol and catecholamine secretion; increased concentrations of serum ACTH, growth hormone, thyroxine, antidiuretic hormone, and renin; and decreased secretion of luteinizing hormone, aldosterone, and testosterone (Dispersyn *et al.*, 2009; Gould, 2008; Oyama, 1973; Pettinger *et al.*, 1975; Xu *et al.*, 2012; Zaretsky *et al.*, 2010).

Anesthetics and analgesic agents can also influence behavior. High doses of the analgesic drug, buprenorphine, are associated with pica in rats (Clark *et al.*, 1997). Volatile anesthetics have been demonstrated to affect cognitive performance, either impairing and enhancing behavior in assays of cognitive function. The performance of rats, previously trained to complete a spatial memory task, was impaired for up to 2 weeks after isoflurane–nitrous oxide anesthesia, whereas acquisition of a new task was impaired for only 2 days (Culley *et al.*, 2003, 2004a,b; Crosby *et al.*, 2005). Mice repeatedly exposed to isoflurane had a decrease in cognitive performance (Bianchi *et al.*, 2008). However, other studies showed performance was enhanced in mice 24h, but not 7 days, after exposure to either isoflurane and sevoflurane (1 MAC for 2h) in a test of visuospatial behavior, which was thought to result from upregulation of specific NMDA receptor subunits (Rammes *et al.*, 2009; Haseneder *et al.*, 2013).

b. Euthanasia Agents

There are limited studies examining the effects of euthanasia technique on experimental results. Butler *et al.* (1990) observed differences in prostacyclin production in aortic tissue and response of aortic and colonic smooth muscle to acetylcholine when rabbits and rats were sacrificed using methoxyflurane, carbon dioxide, and pentobarbital. Cervical dislocation, with or without methoxyflurane or pentobarbital anesthesia and CO_2, and halothane overdose were observed

to alter both mitogen induced lymphoproliferation and the induction of alloantigen-specific cytolytic T lymphocytes in mice (Howard *et al.*, 1990). Administration of various concentrations of CO_2 (70% and 100%) resulted in slight increases in several hematologic parameters (MCV and MCH), the percentage of circulating cytotoxic T lymphocytes, and affected spontaneous leukocyte blastogenesis in the blood and spleen (Pecaut *et al.*, 2000). Decapitation has been associated with dramatic increases in plasma catecholamine concentrations in rats, presumably caused by environmentally induced changes in sympathoadrenalmedullary activity (Popper *et al.*, 1977).

Isoflurane used as an euthanasia agent reduced both the number and the motility of spermatazoa in Sprague–Dawley rats as compared to CO_2, purportedly a result of the agent's inhibitory effect on vas deferens smooth muscle (Campion *et al.*, 2012). In contrast, no difference in motility was observed between CO_2, two commercially available euthanasia solutions, and four volatile anesthetics, including isoflurane in rats (Stutler *et al.*, 2007). CO_2 inhalation, dependent on concentration, has varying effects on brain excitability, causes acidosis, decreases the cerebral concentrations of both sodium and potassium, increases brain glutamate levels, decreases enzymes responsible for branched-chained amino acid degradation, increases c-Fos gene expression, increases plasma norepinephrine, and markedly decreases hepatic glycogen levels *postmortem* (Borovsky *et al.*, 1998; Brodie and Woodbury, 1958; Brooks *et al.*, 1999; Gos *et al.*, 2002; Kc *et al.*, 2002; Woodbury *et al.*, 1958). It also is reported to cause tissue petechiation, particularly in the lungs, and in mice, *antemortem* respiratory acidosis leading to artifactual hyperkalemia, a decrease in blood pH, and lactic acidemia (Traslavina *et al.*, 2010). The euthanasia method, including exsanguination, impacted inflammatory cytokine profiles in a rat scald-burn injury model (Al-Mousawi *et al.*, 2010). Administration of isoflurane immediately before decapitation had the least impact on cytokine profile dampening.

The euthanasia agent, T-61, causes intravascular hemolysis which interferes with serum hexosaminidase measurements and artifactual damage of the pulmonary parenchyma characterized by congestion, edema, and endothelial necrosis, as well as endothelial swelling of the renal glomerular tufts (Doughty and Stuart, 1995; Port *et al.*, 1978; Prien *et al.*, 1988). The pulmonary architecture is extremely sensitive to effects of a variety of euthanasia techniques (Feldman and Gupta, 1976). Most euthanasia techniques are unsuitable to maintain the integrity of enzymatically labile neurochemicals; therefore, microwave irradiation is utilized by neuroscientists to fix brain neurochemicals and metabolites *in vivo* while maintaining the brain's anatomic integrity (Stavinoha, 1993).

c. Antimicrobials

The potential for antimicrobial compounds to influence physiologic responses is well established. As they are commonly administered to animals used in biomedical research, it is imperative to recognize the nature and scope of their potential side effects. Antibiotic administration can be toxic to a variety of laboratory animals. For example, vancomycin is known to cause nephrotoxicity. While the exact mechanism is undefined, studies in laboratory animals incriminate oxidative effects on the proximal tubule renal tubule (Elyasi et al., 2012). Aminoglycoside antibiotics, including gentamicin, amikacin, and dihydrostreptomycin/streptomycin, are also nephrotoxic, ototoxic, can induce neuromuscular blockade, and can produce negative inotropic effects in both cardiac and arterial muscle (Adams, 1976; Hanberger et al., 2013; Tabuchi et al., 2011; Wightman et al., 1980). Procaine, used in some penicillin formulations, is toxic to guinea pigs, mice, and rabbits (Galloway, 1968). Some penicillins, sulfamethoxazole/trimethoprim, erythromycin, and several other macrolides are hepatotoxic (Hautekeete, 1995). Some fluoroquinolones are known to damage cartilage (Maślanka et al., 2004) and can cause hepatotoxicity (Shaw et al., 2010). Lincomycin at high doses disrupts myocardial conductance and is arrhythmogenic in dogs (Daubeck et al., 1974). Some antibiotics can affect the endocrine system. Sulfamethoxazole (SMZ), commonly administered to immunocompromised rodents to prevent pneumocystosis, induces thyroid hyperplasia and hypertrophy in mice, rats, and dogs, and causes a decrease in free thyroxine (T4) in dogs and mice (Altholtz et al., 2006; Swarm et al., 1973). Altholtz et al. (2006) demonstrated a marked elevation in thyroid-stimulating hormone and a decrease in circulating T4 after feeding mice a commercially available rodent diet impregnated with trimethoprim-SMZ for as little as 2 weeks.

Lastly, several classes of antibiotics can influence immune function. These include tetracyclines (Ingham et al., 1991), aminoglycosides (Metcalf and Wilson, 1987), fluoroquinolones (Jimenez-Valera et al., 1995), trimethoprim-SMZ, and chloramphenicol (Hauser and Remington, 1982).

Other antibiotics indirectly induce toxicity by altering the normal (commensal) flora of the gastrointestinal tract (Levy, 2000). Commensal bacteria are important in modulating the host innate immune system (Hooper et al., 2003), suppressing inflammatory responses, promoting immune tolerance (O'Hara and Shanahan, 2006), and altering the course of autoimmune and allergic diseases, as well as inflammatory bowel disease (Clemente et al., 2012). Commensal bacteria may also influence the development of various physiologic conditions, such as obesity and diabetes, and can affect neural function and behavioral response (Cryan and Dinan, 2012). Antibiotic use can eliminate commensal bacteria, opening niches that allow for colonization and overgrowth of harmful bacteria. For example, guinea pigs, hamsters, gerbils, and rabbits may develop fatal enterotoxemias, when treated orally with antibiotics, such as penicillins, permitting colonization and proliferation of either toxin-producing Clostridium difficile or C. spiroforme, dependent on the animal species, the route of administration, and the dose (Bergin et al., 2005; Borriello, 1995).

Whether by direct or indirect action, antibiotics can also influence the pharmacokinetics and metabolism of other agents. For example, the fluoroquinolones compete with GABA receptors and therefore can interfere with studies involving the central nervous system (De Sarro and De Sarro, 2001). Bacitracin, gentamicin, and nystatin alter cecocolonic motility and increase fecal excretion of dry matter and water in rats, and amoxicillin-clavulanate alters intestinal motility in humans (Cherbut et al., 1991). Macrolide antibiotics can inhibit hepatic metabolism of some compounds by forming complexes with them, they can directly inactivate cytochrome P450, or they can alter the enteric flora impacting compound bioavailability (Periti et al., 1992). Therefore, the concurrent administration of antibiotics with test compounds should be carefully considered.

Parasiticides are another class of compounds that can interfere with normal metabolic processes and so can introduce variability into research outcomes. Ivermectin, commonly used as both an anthelmintic and an acaricide, is toxic to certain strains of dogs and mice due to a lack of P-glycoprotein, a member of the adenosine triphosphate (ATP)-binding cassette transporter protein superfamily that is normally present in the blood–brain barrier (Macdonald and Gledhill, 2007). Fenbendazole, a benzimidazole anthelminthic which disrupts parasite tubulin–microtubule equilibrium, is commonly used to treat oxyuriasis in rodents. Fenbendazole interferes with motor function in mice as measured by rotarod, induces select hepatic cytochrome P450 isoforms known to activate procarcinogens, prolongs microglial activation, induces release of striatal dopamine, attenuates the loss of astrocytes, and induces weight loss in F344 rats injected intrastriatally with LPS (Gadad et al., 2010; Hunter et al., 2007; Villar et al., 2007). In addition, several anthelmintics can induce immunomodulatory effects. Ivermectin, levamisole, and thiabendazole are immune potentiators. In one report, Ivermectin activated a tamoxifen-regulated Cre recombinase fusion protein in murine T cells (Corbo-Rodgers et al., 2012). Levamisole stimulates cell-mediated immune responses, enhances the rate of T-lymphocyte differentiation, and increases the activity of effector lymphocytes (Brunner and Muscoplat, 1980; Naylor and Hadden, 2003). In contrast, fenvalerate, oxfendazole, and aminocarb are immune suppressors. Fenbendazole and dieldrin can have both immunostimulatory and immunosuppressive actions depending on experimental conditions and the specific immune function evaluated (Sajid *et al.*, 2006). Fenbendazole has been shown to depress splenic B-cell proliferation, especially in aged mice, by decreasing mRNA and protein expression of a B-lymphocyte transcription factor. Fenbendazole also increases anti-DNA antibody in the (NZB X NZW)F1 model of autoimmunity without altering disease progression and inhibits subcutaneous growth of a human Burkitt lymphoma cell line in SCID mice when coadministered with a vitamin supplement (Cray *et al.*, 2013; Gao *et al.*, 2008; Landin *et al.*, 2009; Villar *et al.*, 2007).

Lastly, as resistance to traditional antibiotics has become more common, a considerable amount of research has been directed toward natural antimicrobial peptides, small cationic peptides with broad antimicrobial activity, such as magainin and indolicidin from frogs and cows, respectively (Kang *et al.*, 2012). As these compounds have moved down the testing 'pipeline', problems with toxicity have occasionally come to light (Kang *et al.*, 2012). As these challenges are overcome, antimicrobial peptides will likely become more commonly used in laboratory animal medicine. Laboratory animal veterinarians and investigators will need to be aware of the physicochemical properties and potential side effects of these compounds.

3. *Pheromones*

Pheromone signals are an important form of communication and are involved in social and sexual behaviors within many animal species (Trotier, 2011). Thus, exposure of laboratory animals to pheromones of members of the same or another species could influence behavior and physiology, and therefore confound research. Compared to insect pheromones, relatively little is known of the chemical nature of mammalian pheromones. Rodents such as mice and rats produce various volatile molecules, including dimethylpyrazine, 2-heptanone, 6-hydroxy-6-methyl-3heptanone, and others, in addition to nonvolatile compounds such as major urinary proteins, steroids, fatty acids, eicosanoids, and peptides, some of which are secreted in the lacrimal and preputial glands (Zhang *et al.*, 2008). These are detected by the vomeronasal organ, an olfactory sensory structure in the brain (Trotier, 2011). In the mouse, the vomeronasal organ expresses as many as 230 distinct receptors (Brennan and Keverne, 2004). Reproductive behavior in rodents is highly responsive to pheromones. For example, aphrodisin, a protein found in the vaginal secretions of hamsters, triggers copulatory behavior in male hamsters (Briand *et al.*, 2004). In mice, major urinary proteins, secreted in large quantities in males, are pheromones which act as a signature allowing female mice to identify individual males (Hurst, 2009). Animal odors from conspecifics or from a different species can also lead to behavioral or physiologic alterations.

Chemical signals released in the urine of male mice enhance aggression in other adult male mice (Lacey *et al.*, 2007) and also inhibit infanticide when sprayed on pups (Mucignat-Caretta *et al.*, 2004). Odors from unfamiliar male mice can even cause primary developmental defects in embryos, including poor development of the trophoblast and inner cell mass, and abnormal overdevelopment of the embryos (Chung *et al.*, 1997). Rodents can also react to pheromones released by conspecifics undergoing stressful procedures. For example, BALB/c mice exposed for 24h to odors from donor mice that were foot-shocked, had suppressed cellular and humoral immune function, and responded with a significant increase in climbing, air sampling, and rearing behaviors (Cocke *et al.*, 1993; Zalaquett and Thiessen, 1991.) In rats, pheromones are released from the perianal region and induce an autonomic stress response, and from the whisker regions where they induce behavioral changes in conspecifics. Handling, blood collection, and injections can elicit their release and can affect nearby animals for as long as 30min (Zalaquett and Thiessen, 1991). Alarm pheromones have also been shown to enhance the acoustic startle response and aggravate stress-induced hyperthermia (Inagaki *et al.*, 2009; Kiyokawa *et al.*, 2004). The impact of alarm pheromones on behavioral test responses in rodents, especially in tests that employ water, should be carefully considered. Rats subjected to the Porsolt forced swim test responded differently based on whether the subjects were tested in clean water or water in which the same or other rats had been previously tested. This response lasted in water aged as long as 8 days and responses were strain- and stock-dependent (Abel and Bilitzke, 1990; Abel, 1991, 1992; Abel and Hannigan, 1992). Lastly, odors derived from ferrets or cats induce anxiogenic responses in rats, including changes in body weight regulation and neuroendocrine responses, thymic involution, and adrenal hyperplasia (Campeau *et al.*, 2008). These and other examples illustrate the potential for pheromones to introduce variability into research involving laboratory animals.

C. Microbial Agents

Despite tremendous progress in pathogen detection and exclusion, unwanted microbes continue to confound research findings with disappointing regularity. In response, the scientific community persists in their efforts to produce, distribute, maintain, and use animals free of microbial pathogens. The effects that microbes can exert on biomedical research are multifaceted. Clinical disease, with its attendant morbidity and mortality, is relatively uncommon but when it occurs can devastate a research project, especially when disease strikes well into a long-term study. More commonly, the effects are insidious. Microbes can induce physiologic changes in the host that complicate the interpretation of results, or of greater concern, can lead to their misinterpretation. Perhaps among the most difficult effects to detect are those induced in genetically altered animal models, many of which have phenotypes that are influenced by the microbial flora with which they are associated. Intelligent use of such animal models requires an improved understanding of the interaction between flora and host.

As the scope of this section is limited, the reader is referred to more extensive reviews on the impact of infectious agents on research (Baker, 2003). The agents included in this section are among those recently reported by large commercial diagnostic laboratories to be commonly identified in mice and rats from pharmaceutical, biotechnology, academic, and governmental institutions in North America and Europe (Prichett-Corning *et al.*, 2009). Mouse and rat pathogens which have been shown to profoundly affect host physiology and therefore confound research are also discussed. As descriptions of these can be found elsewhere in this book, they are not included in the discussion below. Lastly, the value and utility of pathogen-free rodents is not directly addressed but is evident in the descriptions of pathogen effects on the host.

1. Viruses

a. Mouse Hepatitis Virus

The prevalence of MHV infection has declined considerably over the years as pathogen diagnostic methods have improved and investigators have more readily accepted efforts to eliminate the virus from research colonies. In a recent large-scale survey, MHV was detected serologically in 1.57% of samples in North America and 3.25% of samples from Europe (Prichett-Corning *et al.*, 2009). The virus most likely retains a worldwide distribution in spite of its apparent low prevalence. It is highly contagious, contaminates transplantable tumors and cell lines, and has repeatedly demonstrated its ability to alter host physiology and impact research. While MHV is referred to in this chapter as if it were one virus, there are in fact several distinct strains and variants of MHV, each of which displays particular tropisms and effects on the host. Furthermore, the response to MHV infection can be profoundly influenced by the particular host characteristics.

Having the potential to induce both immune stimulation and suppression, MHV can significantly alter the immune system. The effects of MHV in immunocompetent mice, following natural or experimental infection, include thymic involution and apoptosis (Godfraind *et al.*, 1995; Lee *et al.*, 1994); affecting the number and/or activity of macrophage (Belyavskyi *et al.*, 1998; Boorman *et al.*, 1982; Even *et al.*, 1995; Gledhill *et al.*, 1965; Levy *et al.*, 1981; Williams and Di Luzzio, 1980), NK cell (Thompson *et al.*, 2008), or peripheral lymphocyte (de Souza *et al.*, 1991; Even *et al.*, 1995; Gagne *et al.*, 1998; Jolicoeur and Lamontagne, 1995) populations; affecting antibody production (Aparicio *et al.*, 2011; Hooks *et al.*, 1993; Lahmy and Virelizier, 1981; Lardans *et al.*, 1996; Leray *et al.*, 1982; Virelizier *et al.*, 1976) and mucosal immune responsiveness (Casebolt *et al.*, 1987); altering allograft rejection (Cray *et al.*, 1993) and presentation of self-antigen (Smith *et al.*, 2007a) and foreign antigen on dendritic cells (Smith *et al.*, 2007a); altering production of several cytokines (Coutelier *et al.*, 1995; de Souza *et al.*, 1991; Jacques *et al.*, 2009; Li *et al.*, 2010; Pearce *et al.*, 1994; Scott *et al.*, 2008; Zhu *et al.*, 2012); altering the behavior of tumors that induce ascites and expression of cell surface markers on T cells (Fox *et al.*, 1977) and macrophages (Tahara *et al.*, 1993); delaying plasma lactate dehydrogenase elevation after infection (Dillberger *et al.*, 1987); inducing anemia, leukopenia, and thrombocytopenia (Hunstein *et al.*, 1969; Namiki *et al.*, 1977); inducing immune-mediated demyelinization (Houtman and Fleming, 1996); and altering the course or susceptibility of mice to SV and pneumonia virus of mice (PVM) (Carrano *et al.*, 1984), K virus (Tisdale, 1963), and leukoviruses (Manaker *et al.*, 1961) as well as *Mycoplasma* (*Eperythrozoon*) *coccoides* (Lavelle and Bang, 1973), *Salmonella typhimurium* (Fallon *et al.*, 1991), *Trypanosoma cruzi* (Torrecilhas *et al.*, 1999), and *Schistosoma mansoni* (Warren *et al.*, 1969).

Observations have shown that MHV also induces a number of important changes in immunocompromised mouse strains. Importantly, the extent and severity of lesions induced are considerably more severe in immunosuppressed animals (Huang *et al.*, 1996). MHV causes spontaneous differentiation of lymphocytes bearing T-cell markers (Tamura *et al.*, 1978), enhances both the IgM and IgG antibody responses to sheep erythrocytes (Tamura and Fujiwara, 1979), increases the number and/or activity of macrophages (Tamura *et al.*, 1980) and NK cells (Tamura *et al.*, 1981), leads to xenograft rejection (Akimaru *et al.*, 1981), results in hepatosplenic myelopoiesis (Ishida *et al.*, 1978), and induces cytokine production (Pearce *et al.*, 1994).

MHV also modulates a variety of enzyme systems. Hepatic isocitrate dehydrogenase, glucose-6-phosphate dehydrogenase, and aspartate transaminase are all markedly increased during infection, whereas cytochrome P450 microsomal enzymes, including those induced by phenobarbital, NADPH oxidase, aniline hydroxylase, and succinate hydrogenase, are significantly decreased (Budillon *et al.*, 1973; Cacciatore and Antoniello, 1971; Huang *et al.*, 1996; Paradisi *et al.*, 1972; Ruebner and Hirano, 1965). Lastly, MHV-3 alters prothrombinase synthesis (Ding *et al.*, 1998). Other physiologic effects include altering hepatic ferrokinetics (Vacha *et al.*, 1994); modulating the function of endoplasmic reticulum (Bechill *et al.*, 2008) and other cellular organelles (Reggiori *et al.*, 2010);

influencing gene expression (Huang *et al.*, 2007; Wang *et al.*, 2011); affecting the time course of onset of diabetes in NOD mice (Smith *et al.*, 2007b); and altering hepatic regeneration (Carthew, 1981), the number of hepatic sinusoidal fenestrae (Steffan *et al.*, 1995), and the proliferative activity of the bowel (Barthold *et al.*, 1982).

b. Mouse Minute Virus and Rat Minute Virus

The prevalence of mouse minute virus (MMV; also known as minute virus of mice, mice minute virus, murine minute virus) has declined considerably over time and is now uncommon (Prichett-Corning *et al.*, 2009). However, it can still be found as a contaminant of transplantable tumors, cell lines, and virus stocks. Like MHV, differences between strains of MMV and in host genetic makeup result in different host effects. As a parvovirus, the tropism and pathophysiology, and therefore effects of MMV, are generally similar to those of MPV (see below). MMV has a predilection for mitotically active cells and so has its greatest impacts on the hematopoietic system. In fact, the 'immunosuppressive' strain, MMV(i), alters the number and function of all components of the hematopoietic system, including lymphoid, myeloid, erythroid, and megakaryocytic lineages (Lamana *et al.*, 2001; Segovia *et al.*, 2003). The 'prototype' strain, MMV(p), though less well studied, inhibits the growth of intraperitoneally administered Ehrlich ascites tumor cells (Guetta *et al.*, 1986), and can interfere with intracellular signaling (Lachmann *et al.*, 2007). Both strains can induce DNA damage (Adeyemi and Pintel, 2012). Virtually, nothing is known of the physiologic effects of the newly described rat minute virus (RMV)-1 (Wan *et al.*, 2002). However, RMV-1 viruses were detected in the lymphoid tissues of naturally infected rats, suggesting that RMV-1 can infect lymphoid tissues and can have immune-modulating effects on the host (Wan *et al.*, 2002).

c. Murine Norovirus

Based on testing of surveys of samples submitted to laboratory animal diagnostic facilities, murine norovirus (MNV) is currently the most common viral pathogen found in laboratory mice (McInnes *et al.*, 2011; Prichett-Corning *et al.*, 2009). Multiple strains have been identified (Smith *et al.*, 2012), with MNV-1 the most studied. MNV antagonizes the innate immune response to infection by delaying the upregulation of a number of cellular genes activated by the innate pathway (McFadden *et al.*, 2011); downregulates levels of survivin, an apoptosis inhibitor (Bok *et al.*, 2009); and can confound nutritional studies through its effects on intestinal dendritic cells (Paik *et al.*, 2010). It can influence infection with other pathogens. For example, MNV promotes inflammation and lethality in mice secondarily infected with *Escherichia coli* (Kim *et al.*, 2011) and can alter the progression of bacteria-induced

inflammatory bowel disease (Lencioni *et al.*, 2008). MNV alters the duration of shedding of mouse parvovirus (Compton *et al.*, 2010) and mildly influences immune responses to murine cytomegalovirus (Doom *et al.*, 2009), but does not influence immune function in concurrent infection with Friend virus (Ammann *et al.*, 2009), vaccinia virus, or influenza A virus (Hensley *et al.*, 2009).

d. Mouse Parvovirus Type 1 and Rat Parvovirus Type 1

Mouse parvovirus type 1 (MPV-1) and rat parvovirus type 1 (RPV-1) are infrequently reported from laboratory mice and rats, respectively (Prichett-Corning *et al.*, 2009). Although recognized serologically for several years, MPV-1 was first isolated after infecting and interfering with cultures of CD8+, CD4+, and γδ T-cell clones used for studying lymphocyte activation and immunoregulatory mechanisms (McKisic *et al.*, 1993). Since then, few reports have documented the effects of MPV-1 (or MPV-2) infection on host physiology. As noted above for MMV, the parvoviruses have a general tropism for dividing cells and thus affect processes linked to cell division. Most notably, these include processes associated with immune function. In addition to causing lytic infection, MPV-1 was shown to inhibit T-cell proliferation following exposure to IL-2 and antigen, and depress the proliferative response of spleen and lymph node cells from antigen-primed mice (McKisic *et al.*, 1993). MPV-1 accelerates tumor allograft rejection, not by directly infecting the graft but by inducing the 'bystander help' effect (McKisic *et al.*, 1998). RPV-1 is less well characterized and so little is known of its effects on host physiology. It can suppress the development of lymphoid tumors (Jacoby and Ball-Goodrich, 1995).

e. Mouse Rotavirus

Mouse rotavirus, formerly known as epizootic diarrhea of infant mice (EDIM) virus, is uncommonly reported from research animal facilities (Prichett-Corning *et al.*, 2009). Mouse rotavirus has been shown to activate dendritic cells (Lopez-Guerrero *et al.*, 2009) and induce polyclonal B-cell activation (Blutt *et al.*, 2004) in Peyer's patches. Rotavirus infection can alter the course of development of type 1 diabetes (Webster *et al.*, 2013), serve as an initiator in the pathogenesis of experimental biliary atresia through the induction of increased NF-κB and abnormal activation of the osteopontin inflammation pathway (Feng *et al.*, 2011), increase expression Muc2 and modify mucin structure in small intestinal goblet cells (Boshuizen *et al.*, 2005), alter cholesterol and phospholipid content of the intestine (Katyal *et al.*, 2001), increase oxidative stress in the intestine (Sodhi *et al.*, 1996), alter villus microvasculature (Osborne *et al.*, 1991) and gut permeability (Uhnoo *et al.*, 1990), reduce intestinal lactase levels (Collins *et al.*, 1990), and upregulate expression of inducible nitric oxide synthase (iNOS) (Borghan *et al.*, 2007). Rotavirus nonstructural protein NSP4 acts as an enterotoxin to induce diarrhea (Ousingsawat *et al.*, 2011). In addition to these observations, a large volume of literature exists on the effects of rotaviruses of other species on their respective hosts. The reader is advised to consider whether some of these reported effects can also occur in mouse rotavirus infection.

f. Rat Theilovirus

Though moderately uncommon overall, recent surveys indicate that rat theilovirus is among the most common viruses detected in colonies of laboratory rats (Prichett-Corning *et al.*, 2009). Outbred stocks differ in their susceptibility to rat theilovirus (Drake *et al.*, 2008). Essentially nothing is known of its effects on the host. It is likely that rat theilovirus infection can induce similar pathophysiologic alterations noted to occur with other picornaviruses belonging to the genus *Cardiovirus*, including Theiler's murine encephalomyelitis virus (see below).

g. Sendai Virus

Recent surveys of laboratory animals suggest that Sendai virus (SV) has nearly disappeared from laboratory animal facilities (McInnes *et al.*, 2011; Prichett-Corning *et al.*, 2009). In spite of this, its profound effects on host physiology and use as a model of viral pathogenesis in human respiratory disease warrant retention of SV in this text. SV infects both rats and mice, and affects the respiratory system for which it has tropism, but also alters both humoral and cell-mediated immunity. The effects of SV on the immune system are well characterized. SV depresses pulmonary bacterial clearance by altering pulmonary macrophage function (Degre and Glasgow, 1968; Degre and Solberg, 1971). The effects of SV on pulmonary macrophages include altering phagocytosis, inhibiting phagosome–lysosome fusion; decreasing lysosomal enzymes, altering Fc and non-Fc receptor-mediated attachment, and altering the ability to degrade ingested bacteria (Jakab, 1981; Jakab and Warr, 1981). SV inhibits the response of T lymphocytes to mitogens (Garlinghouse and Van Hoosier, 1982; Wainberg and Israel, 1980); causes a lifelong increase in cytotoxic T-cell precursors (Doherty *et al.*, 1994); increases NK-cell cytolytic activity and both the IgM and IgG splenic primary plaque-forming cell responses to sheep erythrocytes (Brownstein and Weir; 1987; Clark *et al.*, 1979); stimulates TNF-α (Yamada *et al.*, 2006), INF-α (Milone and Fitzgerald-Bocarsly, 1998; Payvandi *et al.*, 1998), chemokine and other cytokine (IL-6) expression (Kobayashi *et al.*, 2003); enhances rejection of skin isografts (Streilein *et al.*, 1981); increases the prevalence of spontaneous autoimmune diseases (Kay, 1978, 1979; Kay

et al., 1979); reduces the severity of adjuvant-induced arthritis (Garlinghouse and Van Hoosier, 1978); inhibits the development of leukemia following inoculation of mice with Friend leukemia virus (Wheelock, 1966); and decreases the tumorigenicity of transplantable tumors (Matsuya *et al.*, 1978; Takeyama *et al.*, 1979). Prior or concurrent infection with SV alters the neoplastic response of the respiratory system to carcinogens (Hall *et al.*, 1985; Nettesheim *et al.*, 1974, 1981; Parker, 1980; Peck *et al.*, 1983). In addition, SV infection stimulates the synthesis of the eicosanoid prostaglandin E2 (Kobayashi *et al.*, 2003), induces apoptosis (Bitzer *et al.*, 1999), alters wound healing (Kenyon, 1983), interferes with early embryonic development and fetal growth (Lavilla-Apelo *et al.*, 1992), alters lung microstructure (Wang *et al.*, 2012), and induces cytoplasmic actin remodeling in order to promote efficient virion production (Miazza *et al.*, 2011).

h. Sialodacryoadenitis Virus

Unlike in the past, sialodacryoadenitis virus (SDAV) infection is currently rare in laboratory animal facilities (Prichett-Corning *et al.*, 2009). Infection with SDAV can interfere with research involving the lacrimal and salivary glands; the respiratory, immune, nervous, and ophthalmic systems; and fetal and neonatal development. Effects associated with SDAV infection include degenerative, necrotic, and atrophic alterations in acinar epithelial cells of the lacrimal gland (Wickham *et al.*, 1997); depletion of epidermal growth factor in the salivary glands (Percy *et al.*, 1988); reduction of IL-1 production by alveolar macrophages (Boschert *et al.*, 1988); influx of pulmonary neutrophils and transient increase in pulmonary surfactant protein and chemokine levels (Funk *et al.*, 2009); impairment of olfaction and chemoreception for up to 2 weeks postexposure (Bihun and Percy, 1995); impairment of axonal regeneration (Yu *et al.*, 2011); and ocular megaglobus, hypopyon, and hyphema (Boivin and Theus, 1996). Effects on reproductive development include alteration of estrous cycles (Utsumi *et al.*, 1991), embryonic and neonatal mortality (Utsumi *et al.*, 1991), reduction in food consumption and weight gain (Nunoya *et al.*, 1977), and alteration of growth rates in young rats (Utsumi *et al.*, 1980). Concurrent infection with SDAV can potentiate lesions caused by *Mycobacterium pulmonis* (Schunk *et al.*, 1995).

i. Theiler's Murine Encephalomyelitis Virus

Theiler's murine encephalomyelitis virus (TMEV) is uncommon in laboratory animal facilities (Prichett-Corning *et al.*, 2009). It causes demyelinating myelopathy in aging laboratory mice (Krinke and Zurbriggen, 1997); alteration of seizure susceptibility (Stewart *et al.*, 2010); T cell recruitment (Jin *et al.*, 2011); induction of apoptosis (Stavrou *et al.*, 2011); redistribution of heat shock proteins (Mutsvunguma *et al.*, 2011); axonal loss resulting in electrophysiologic abnormalities and spinal cord atrophy (McGavern *et al.*, 2000); and induction of several chemokines, including lymphotactin, INF-induced protein-10, macrophage inflammatory protein (MIP)-1 beta, monocyte chemoattractant protein-1, and TCA-3 (Mi *et al.*, 2004; Ranschoff *et al.*, 2002), as well as other cytokines such as RANTES, IL-6, and IL-12 (Himeda *et al.*, 2010; Petro, 2005; Rubio *et al.*, 2011; Theil *et al.*, 2000), eicosanoid (Molina-Holgado *et al.*, 2002); and vascular cell adhesion molecule-1 (VCAM-1) (Rubio *et al.*, 2010) expression in the central nervous system and/or elsewhere. In chronic infections TMEV causes a reduction in the number of neuronal progenitor cells and early post-mitotic neurons in chronic infection (Jafari *et al.*, 2012).

2. Bacteria

a. *Citrobacter Rodentium*

Although used experimentally, the prevalence of *Citrobacter rodentium* in laboratory mouse colonies has declined significantly over the years. In fact, it was not detected in several recent surveys conducted on samples from laboratory mouse colonies in various regions of the world (Liang *et al.*, 2009; McInnes *et al.*, 2011; Prichett-Corning *et al.*, 2009). The etiologic agent of transmissible murine colonic hyperplasia has been shown to alter the cytokinetics of the colonic mucosal epithelium (Barthold, 1979); disrupt intestinal cell tight junctions (Guttman *et al.*, 2006); alter intestinal epithelial function (Skinn *et al.*, 2006); alter mucosal enteroendocrine signaling and the enteric nervous system (O'Hara *et al.*, 2006); induce IL-17 and IL-22 (Curtis and Way, 2009; Higgins *et al.*, 1999; Ota *et al.*, 2011) and nuclear factor (NF)-κB (Wang *et al.*, 2006) production; inhibit antigen-specific cytotoxic T-cell activity (Maggio-Price *et al.*, 1998); alter hepatic cytochrome production (Nyagode *et al.*, 2010); induce anxiety-like behavior (Lyte *et al.*, 2006); and promote tumorigenesis (Newman *et al.*, 2001). Concerning the latter, both the susceptibility to colonic neoplasia and the latent period for induction are increased in mice infected with *C. rodentium* and exposed to the carcinogen, 1,2-dimethylhydrazine (Barthold and Beck, 1980). The hyperplastic colonic lesions can also be misinterpreted as preneoplastic, as they resemble focal atypia. *C. rodentium* infection is also associated with increased liver inflammation and hepatitis index scores as well as prominent periportal hepatocellular coagulative necrosis indicative of thrombotic ischemic injury (Raczynski *et al.*, 2012). Lastly, infection with *C. rodentium* can modify immunopathological changes associated with pulmonary *Cryptococcus neoformans* infection (Williams *et al.*, 2006).

b. *Helicobacter* spp.

The importance of the many members of this genus on research is well recognized. The most common and important member, *Helicobacter hepaticus*, has several known effects on host physiology that could alter research studies. In fact, infection of mice with *H. hepaticus* is used as a model system for investigating how intestinal microbiota interact with the host to produce both inflammatory and tolerogenic responses (Fox *et al.*, 2011). The bacterium attained this status following discoveries of its associations with progressive hepatitis, proliferative typhlitis and/or colitis, and with hepatic neoplasia in A-strain mice (Fox *et al.*, 2011; Hailey *et al.*, 2007), including carcinogen-induced neoplasia (Stout *et al.*, 2008). Infection with *H. hepaticus* alters numerous metabolic pathways (Lu *et al.*, 2012). Infection also alters cytokinetics (Nyska *et al.*, 1997); modulates intestinal macrophage responses (Hoffman and Fleming, 2010) as well as other innate (Sterzenbach *et al.*, 2007) and acquired immune responses, including responses to other pathogens (Compton *et al.*, 2003; Gulani *et al.*, 2009); upregulates cell cycle proteins such as cyclin D1, Cdk4, and c-Myc (Ramljak *et al.*, 1998); and produces a cytolethal distending toxin (Liyanage *et al.*, 2010).

Although not as well characterized, *H. bilis* induces similar lesions in immunocompromised mice and rats (Fox *et al.*, 2004; Maggio-Price *et al.*, 2005), including neoplasia (Nguyen *et al.*, 2013). In addition, infection with *H. bilis* has been shown to alter or induce immune responses to other *Helicobacter* spp., as well as to commensal intestinal flora, thereby confounding research on these organisms (Fox, 2007; Lemke *et al.*, 2009). *H. typhlonius*, *H. rodentium*, and other members of the genus infecting mice have been less well studied. It is anticipated that other *Helicobacter* species will be found to induce pathologic changes in immune-deficient mice (Chichlowski *et al.*, 2008).

c. *Mycoplasma Pulmonis*

Unlike in the past, natural infection of laboratory rodents and contamination of transplantable tumor lines with *Mycoplasma pulmonis* are rare (Nicklas *et al.*, 1993; Prichett-Corning *et al.*, 2009). However, when infection does occur, it can significantly impact research in a variety of disciplines. Pulmonary effects of *M. pulmonis* infection include altered ciliary function (Irvani and van As, 1972) which interferes with mucociliary clearance (Cassell *et al.*, 1981); altered respiratory cell kinetics (Wells, 1970); electrogenic ion transport (Lambert *et al.*, 1998); airway innervation (Nohr *et al.*, 1996); surfactant dysfunction (Hickman-Davis *et al.*, 2007); and development of pulmonary lymphatic hyperplasia (Baluk *et al.*, 2005). Changes in pulmonary immune function involve both the number and subpopulation distribution of lymphocytes (Davis *et al.*, 1982). In addition, *M. pulmonis* has been demonstrated to enhance the pulmonary response to carcinogens (Schreiber *et al.*, 1972).

Systemic spread of infection impacts research involving non-pulmonary organs. Infection of the genital

tract alters fecundity, as *M. pulmonis* affects embryo implantation, spermatozoan motility, and fertilization. In a rat model of preterm, premature rupture of membranes in humans, genital infection with *M. pulmonis* increased concentration of matrix metalloproteinases in uterine membranes and amniotic fluid (Peltier *et al.*, 2007). Infection can also accelerate tumor metastasis (Rodríguez-Cuesta *et al.*, 2005) and lead to priapism in CBA mice (Taylor-Robinson and Furr, 2005).

The effects of *M. pulmonis* on the immune system include increased expression of proinflammatory genes in the perinatal brain (Burton *et al.*, 2012); increasing NK cell activity (Lai *et al.*, 1987); suppressing humoral antibody response (Aguila *et al.*, 1988b); stimulating the production of substances mitogenic to B and T cells (Proust *et al.*, 1985; Ross *et al.*, 1992); stimulating production of multiple pro-inflammatory cytokines and modulation by the anti-inflammatory cytokine IL-10 (Sun *et al.*, 2006); recruiting and upregulating of major histocompatibility complex (MHC) class II expressing cells (Umemoto *et al.*, 2002); and reducing the incidence and severity of collagen and adjuvant-induced arthritides (Taurog *et al.*, 1984).

d. *Pasteurella Pneumotropica*

The prevalence of infection of laboratory mice, rats, and other rodents with *Pasteurella pneumotropica* is high in the United States and elsewhere (Hayashimoto *et al.*, 2013; McInnes *et al.*, 2011; Prichett-Corning *et al.*, 2009). The organism can be recovered from multiple sites on and within the host. The most common sites include the upper respiratory, intestinal, and urogenital tracts. Infection of immunodeficient rodents leads to abscess formation, weight loss, and other signs of systemic illness, including death (Artwohl *et al.*, 2000; Kawamoto *et al.*, 2011; Matsumiya and Lavoie, 2003), and can interfere with the growth of transplanted human tumors (Carriquiriborde *et al.*, 2006). In immunocompetent mice, *P. pneumotropica* modulates the transcription of multiple cytokine genes including IL-1β, TNF-α, CCL3, CXCL1, and CXCL2 (Patten *et al.*, 2010), and has been associated with otitis media in CBA/J, but not CBA/CaJ mice (McGinn *et al.*, 1992). Lastly, infection of immunocompetent rats has been associated with chronic necrotizing mastitis (Hong and Ediger, 1978).

e. *Pseudomonas Aeruginosa*

A common commensal in many species, as well as an ubiquitous environmental contaminant, *Pseudomonas aeruginosa* is of major importance to immunocompromised subjects and studies employing the use of indwelling catheters and other percutaneously implanted devices. While the organism preferentially colonizes the upper respiratory and lower digestive tracts, hematogenous spread renders all organ systems susceptible.

Further, mouse strains differ in susceptibility to *P. aeruginosa* (Tam *et al.*, 1999). Lastly, various insults to the pulmonary system, such as hypercapnia, increase susceptibility to *P. aeruginosa* infection and pathology (Gates *et al.*, 2013). Taken together, these variables allow for a wide spectrum of research impact caused by *P. aeruginosa*. Effects associated with infection include high mortality following administration of immunosuppressive drugs (Urano and Maejima, 1978), premature death after exposure to lethal radiation (Miller *et al.*, 1960), concurrent viral infection (Hamilton and Overall, 1978; Seki *et al.*, 2004), and cold stress (Halkett *et al.*, 1968); as well as other forms of physiologic stress associated with increased release of glucocorticoids, catecholamines, and neuroendocrine factors (Verbrugghe *et al.*, 2012). Infection also results in chronic inflammation of the airways (dos Santos *et al.*, 2012); fibrosis caused by the exotoxin pyocyanin (Hao *et al.*, 2012; McIntosh *et al.*, 1992); induction of vascular endothelial growth factor synthesis (Martin *et al.*, 2011); increased vascular permeability (Le Berre *et al.*, 2004; Machado *et al.*, 2011); depressed contact sensitivity (Campa *et al.*, 1985); release of macrophage immune modulating molecules (Thomas *et al.*, 2006); thymic atrophy and apoptosis (Wang *et al.*, 1994); modulation of T-cell proliferation through a form of interbacterial communication known as quorum sensing (Skindersoe *et al.*, 2009); T-cell-dependent immune suppression (Hasløv *et al.*, 1992); enhanced cardiac automaticity and depression from hypoxia (Kwiatkowska-Patzer *et al.*, 1993); delayed wound healing (Rico *et al.*, 2002); reduced quantity and function of pulmonary surfactant (Vanderzwan *et al.*, 1998); and altered behavioral and clinical pathologic parameters following experimental wound infection (Bradfield *et al.*, 1992).

3. *Fungi*

a. *Pneumocystis* spp.

Pneumocystis carinii causes a distinctive interstitial pneumonia in immunocompetent rats that had formerly been attributed to 'rat respiratory virus' (Livingston *et al.*, 2011). In addition, in immunocompromised hosts, *P. carinii* alters alveolar capillary permeability (Yoneda and Walzer, 1981); suppresses the function of alveolar macrophages (Lasbury *et al.*, 2004) through alterations in macrophage gene expression (Cheng *et al.*, 2010); increases levels of multiple pro-inflammatory cytokines and chemokines, arachidonic acid and its metabolites, and the transmembrane protein intercellular adhesion molecule 1 (ICAM-1) (Castro *et al.*, 1993; Lipschik *et al.*, 1996; Liu *et al.*, 2007; Perenboom *et al.*, 1996; Pottratz *et al.*, 1998; Rudner *et al.*, 2007; Wang *et al.*, 2007); inhibits cyclin-dependent kinase activity (Limper *et al.*, 1998) and fibrinogen expression in pulmonary epithelium (Simpson-Haidaris *et al.*, 1998); alters pulmonary

guanosine triphosphate-binding proteins (Oz and Hughes, 1997) and the amount and type of surfactant produced (Gaunsbaek *et al.*, 2013); and modifies the uptake of intratracheally administered compounds (Mordelet-Dambrine *et al.*, 1992). Relatively less is known about *P. murina* infections in mice. However, given the genetic and biologic similarities with *P. carinii*, *P. murina* may likewise confound pulmonary research in mice (Aliouat-Denis, *et al.*, 2008).

4. Parasites

a. Pinworms

The prevalence of pinworm infection (oxyuriasis) in laboratory rodents has declined considerably, though infection remains more common in laboratory rats than in laboratory mice (McInnes *et al.*, 2011; Prichett-Corning *et al.*, 2009). Pinworm infection can alter a variety of biological processes. It retards growth in rats (Wagner, 1988), impedes colonic water and electrolyte absorption (Lubcke *et al.*, 1992), accelerates the development of the hepatic monooxygenase system (Mohn and Philipp, 1981), and causes a significant reduction of activity in behavioral studies (McNair and Timmons, 1977). Oxyuriasis also induces significant hematopoietic changes, including increased myelopoiesis and erythropoiesis, and alters reactivity of bone marrow hematopoietic progenitors to IL-17 by inducing sustained phosphorylation of members of three groups of mitogen-activated protein kinases, as well as enhancing expression of inducible nitric oxide synthase (Ilić *et al.*, 2010). Finally, pinworm infection has been shown to influence the immune system and immune responsiveness. For example, infection induces splenic T- and B-cell proliferation (Beattie *et al.*, 1981; Michels *et al.*, 2006; Sato *et al.*, 1995), alters ovalbumin-induced allergic reactions (Michels *et al.*, 2006), terminates self tolerance and enhances neonatal induction of autoimmune disease and memory (Agersborg *et al.*, 2001; Tung *et al.*, 2001), reduces the development of adjuvant-induced arthritis (Pearson and Taylor, 1975), and is associated with the development of lymphomas in nude mice (Baird *et al.*, 1982).

b. Fur Mites

Fur mites are uncommon on laboratory mice and rare on laboratory rats (Prichett-Corning *et al.*, 2009). Infestation with fur mites can cause secondary amyloidosis (Galton, 1963), increased total serum IgE levels (Roble *et al.*, 2012), altered serum immunoglobulin isotype profile (Jungmann *et al.*, 1996a,b; Pochanke *et al.*, 2006), reduced contact sensitivity reaction to oxazolone (Laltoo and Kind, 1979), and development of lymphocytopenia and granulocytosis (Jungmann *et al.*, 1996a,b). The immunologic response to mite infestation is strain-specific, with the inbred mouse strain NC developing an exaggerated clinical and immunologic response compared to BALB/c and C57BL/6 strains (Morita *et al.*, 1999). Finally, infestation with fur mites alters host susceptibility to other pathogens, likely through modulation of Th cell subpopulations (Welter *et al.*, 2007).

D. Stressors

Stress has been aptly defined as "the effect of physical, physiologic, or emotional factors (stressors) that induce an alteration in an animal's homeostasis or adaptive state" (Kitchen *et al.*, 1987). The alterations that result depend on the severity, nature, and duration of the stressor, and can significantly impact experimental findings. Stress results in stimulation of the hypothalamic–pituitary axis (HPA), resulting in release of corticosteroids from the adrenal cortex and catecholamines from the adrenal medulla. Endogenous opioids, released centrally and peripherally, also mediate stress effects. Stress elicits changes in numerous physiologic processes. The response to stress is influenced by a variety of factors, including host sex, age, and genetics.

For laboratory animals, adverse stress can come from a variety of sources. Stress can be a direct result of environmental influences such as those discussed earlier in this chapter. Stress can also result from experimental manipulations. Included in this category are handling, acute and chronic restraint, social housing, food and/or water deprivation, surgical and other physical manipulations or mechanical inconveniences, and transportation. Anxiety is closely related to stress and is one source of stress in laboratory animals. For a comprehensive review of animal models of anxiety, the reader is referred elsewhere (Kumar *et al.*, 2013).

Handling of animals is a stressor resulting in a multitude of changes in physiologic parameters including heart rate, blood pressure, behavior, and blood glucose, prolactin, or corticosterone levels (Meijer *et al.*, 2007; Sharp *et al.*, 2003). Handling of infant animals can influence host physiology through altered glucocorticoid gene expression and reduced HPA responsiveness to stress, changes that persist through life (Meaney *et al.*, 1996). In mice, anxiety can be reduced by use of handling tunnels and other aids (Gouveia and Hurst, 2013). Stress induces physiologic changes in fishes similar to those seen in mammalian species (Khalil *et al.*, 2012).

Acute and chronic restraints are known stressors. Acute restraint increases adrenocorticotrophin releasing hormone and corticosterone secretion in a time of restraint-dependent manner, whereas chronic restraint decreases body weight gain, increases adrenal weight, and promotes endocrine disruption (García-Iglesias *et al.*, 2013). Restraint can also alter host physiology in many ways. For example, stress can alter the host response to pyrogen (Long *et al.*, 1991), suppress growth *in utero* (Burkuš *et al.*, 2013), alter cognition (Thai *et al.*,

2013), exacerbate decreases in spermatogenesis caused by lead toxicity (Priya and Reddy, 2012), alter nociception (Heidari-Oranjaghi *et al.*, 2012) and taste response (Okamoto *et al.*, 2010), alter brain cytokines in a rat strain-dependent manner (Porterfield *et al.*, 2011), alter T-lymphocyte migration and function (Flint *et al.*, 2011), reduce the number of intestinal IgA-producing B cells (Martínez-Carillo *et al.*, 2011), promote tumorigenesis (Feng *et al.*, 2012), impair gastric emptying (Babygirija *et al.*, 2010), reduce sperm motility (Ren *et al.*, 2010), and increase oxidative stress (Crema *et al.*, 2010).

Food and water deprivation, together or separately, are stressors in laboratory rodents where they invoke a range of behavioral and physiologic adjustments (Rowland, 2007). For example, food restriction augments the effects of psychomotor stimulants in mice (Clifford *et al.*, 2011). In food- and water-deprived rats, the motivation to feed is stronger than the motivation to drink (Cabanac, 1985). Food and water restriction are also stressors for larger animals such as livestock. For example, 24-hour feed and water deprivation induce acute-phase protein secretion and performance in feedlot cattle (Marques *et al.*, 2012).

Many laboratory animals are subjected to surgical or other physical manipulations, or are required to wear or bear physical devices such as infusion ports, tethers, chambers, implants, and other mechanical devices. Many manipulations and devices have been shown to induce stress, thereby altering host physiology. For example, tail bleeding (Tuli *et al.*, 1995a) or placement of an arterial catheter (Sundbom *et al.*, 2011) elevates corticosterone levels in mice. Likewise, surgical manipulation induces IL-6 production (Wehner *et al.*, 2005). In addition to surgical manipulation, unalleviated pain accompanying or resulting from surgery is an adverse stressor that greatly affects host physiology, including cardiovascular parameters (Yeh *et al.*, 2012). Even devices as seemingly inocuous as lightweight plastic back buttons used to secure a metal catheter protector can induce stress in rats (Birkhahn *et al.*, 1979).

Transportation and the stress resulting from it have recently received greater attention by the scientific community. Numerous studies have documented the impacts of transportation on a variety of laboratory species (Arts *et al.*, 2012; Browning and Leite-Browning, 2013; Chandurvelan *et al.*, 2012; Lèche *et al.*, 2013; Munsters *et al.*, 2013; Stemkens-Sevens *et al.*, 2009). Alterations attributable to shipment include elevation of plasma glucocorticoid concentrations, heart rate (Capdevila *et al.*, 2007), neutrophilia, and lymphopenia (Bean-Knudsen and Wagner, 1987); hyperglycemia; changes in serum biochemical indices (Shim *et al.*, 2008); reduced splenic NK-cell activity (Aguila *et al.*, 1988a); depressed humoral and cell-mediated responses to sheep red blood cells and thymic atrophy (Landi *et al.*, 1982); depressed

food consumption, weight loss, and reproductive performance (Hayssen, 1998); behavioral alterations; increased susceptibility to disease; and decreased latency and incidence of tumors (Peters and Kelly, 1977; Wallace, 1976). In general, altered immunologic parameters return to baseline within 48h after arrival, although corticosterone levels remained elevated in mice when measured at 48h (Aguila *et al.*, 1988a; Landi *et al.*, 1982; Toth and January, 1990). However, in some nonhuman primates, including *Macaca fascicularis*, the effects of transportation stress on behavioral repertoires can be long term (Honess *et al.*, 2004). Behavioral and reproductive function in rodents can require greater acclimatization before returning to normal. A 96-h acclimatization period was insufficient for mouse behavior to return to normal after transport (Hoorn *et al.*, 2011; Tuli *et al.*, 1995b). Litter production was reduced and the time of pairing-to-first litter was extended in transported deer mice (Hayssen, 1998) and in C57Bl6/J mice, particularly when mice are transported during the prepubertal/adolescent period (Laroche *et al.*, 2009). Transportation-induced changes can be detected following transport for as little as 4h (Toth and January, 1990). Alterations attributed to transportation are detectable even when animals were shipped by environmentally controlled ground transportation (Aguila *et al.*, 1988a; Toth and January, 1990). When comparing air to ground transport, some investigators found either no differences or greater physiologic change induced by air transport (Aguila *et al.*, 1988a; Landi *et al.*, 1982; Toth and January, 1990). A few reports in the literature indicate that in other cases, recovery from air transportation can be more rapid than from ground transportation. In this regard, Shim *et al.* (2009) reported a physiologic return to normalcy in rats within 1 week of transport. The literature suggests that some physiologic parameters might not return to normal for up to several weeks after transportation (Obernier and Baldwin, 2006). Inter-institutional shipment of animals is not the only source of transport stress. Drozdowicz *et al.* (1990) examined the effects of in-house transport in mice and found that moving animals on a cart for 12 min caused an increase in plasma corticosterone, a decrease in circulating white blood cells and lymphocytes, and a reduction in thymic weight. Corticosterone, white blood cell, and lymphocyte counts returned to normal within 4 hours of transport; however, the circadian release of corticosterone remained abnormal for 1 day.

For many species of laboratory animals, stress can arise from a multitude of psychosocial factors, with profound physiologic consequences (Bartolomucci, 2007). While it is readily accepted that a period of acclimation following arrival into a facility results in a more 'normal' and therefore scientifically relevant research animal, it is also recognized that social interactions with humans can create stress. For example, the activities of personnel in animal-holding rooms, including routine husbandry practices such as cage changing, can increase heart rate and blood pressure, and induce additional physiologic changes in rats (Meller *et al.*, 2011; Sharp *et al.*, 2003). Conversely, human interaction ameliorates stress in domesticated animals such as dogs, which is in part why such interactions are important components of the care of dogs used in teaching and research (Shiverdecker *et al.*, 2013). For social animals such as rodents, isolation, whether experienced early (Fone and Porkess, 2008) or later in life, is stressful. Interestingly, social isolation can affect not only the animals that experience it, but also their offspring (Pisu *et al.*, 2013). Even the removal of an individual from an established group can be stressful for the remaining animals (Burman *et al.*, 2008). For newborn animals, maternal separation is also a highly stressful experience with significant physiologic consequences (Renard *et al.*, 2007). Some stress effects caused by maternal separation can even be transferred across generations (van den Wijngaard *et al.*, 2013). Maternal separation not only affects offspring but is also a significant stressor to the dams (Aguggia *et al.*, 2013).

Improvements in laboratory animal housing achieved through the past several decades have greatly contributed to animal health and well-being. However, it must also be recognized that the environment in which laboratory animals are housed can influence stress levels. For example, stocking density, group size, enclosure type and size, type of bedding material, environmental enrichment devices, and so on are known to influence stress levels in laboratory animals (Sakhai *et al.*, 2013). Stocking (or housing) density reflects the number of animals housed per unit space. Increased stocking density has been associated with a variety of biological effects, including declines in reproductive performance (Christian and LeMunyan, 1958; Pivina *et al.*, 2007), altered organ development (Yildiz *et al.*, 2007), increases in aggressive behavior (Welch *et al.*, 1974), altered immune responsiveness (Hosoi *et al.*, 1998; Yildiz *et al.*, 2007), increased susceptibility to infectious disease (Johnson *et al.*, 1963; Plaut *et al.*, 1969), and enhanced diabetogenic response to streptozotocin (Mazelis *et al.*, 1987). In contrast, others have reported that physiologic functions are unchanged in crowded rats, depending on strain and/or sex (Bean *et al.*, 2008). To keep the former reports in perspective, it should be noted that laboratory animal husbandry regulations and guidelines generally preclude the housing of animals, for example, mice, at densities sufficient to induce these physiologic changes (Nicholson *et al.*, 2009). Enclosure type and size can influence stress levels in a variety of laboratory animal species (Garner *et al.*, 2012; Prola *et al.*, 2013). The influence of wire-bottom flooring remains controversial. While some have reported that housing laboratory rats in wire-bottom caging alters heart rate in a manner suggestive of stress, the same

authors noted that locomotor activity decreased on wire-bottom caging (Giral *et al.*, 2011). Reduced locomotor activity is considered an indicator of a relaxed state (Rock *et al*, 1997). Others have reported that rats housed in wire-bottom caging are more physically active and consumed more feed, suggesting that they were less comfortable than rats housed in solid-bottom caging (Rock *et al.*, 1997). The presence, or not, and type of bedding material can influence stress levels in laboratory rodents (Kulesskaya *et al.*, 2011; Rice *et al.*, 2008). In this regard, it is commonly assumed that environmental enrichment appropriate to the species housed reduces stress in laboratory animals (Simpson and Kelly, 2011), though even here, too much of a good thing can lead to significant, lasting changes in behavioral, physical, or immunologic function (Haemisch and Gärtner, 1997; Hutchinson *et al.*, 2012). In fact, whether the environmental enrichment reduces, has no effect, or increases stress depends on many factors, including stocking density, age, sex, strain, duration of enrichment, and the specific form(s) of enrichment employed (Simpson and Kelly, 2011).

References

Abel, E.L., 1991. Gradient of alarm substance in the forced swimming test. Physiol. Behav. 49, 321–323.

Abel, E.L., 1992. Response to alarm substance in different rat strains. Physiol. Behav. 51, 345–347.

Abel, E.L., Bilitzke, P.J., 1990. A possible alarm substance in the forced swimming test. Physiol. Behav. 48, 233–239.

Abel, E.L., Hannigan, J.H., 1992. Effects of chronic forced swimming and exposure to alarm substance: physiological and behavioral consequences. Physiol. Behav. 52 (4), 781–785.

Adams, H.R., 1976. Antibiotic-induced alterations of cardiovascular reactivity. Fed. Proc. Fed. Am. Soc. Exp. Biol. 35, 1148–1150.

Adams, N., Hannah, J.A., Henry, W., 2000. Environmental influences on the failure to drink in inbred rats with an ethanol preference. Physiol. Behav. 69 (4–5), 563–570.

Adams, N., Oldham, T.D., 1996. Seminatural housing increases subsequent ethanol intake in male Maudsley reactive rats. J. Stud. Alcohol. 57, 349–351.

Adeyemi, R.O., Pintel, D.J., 2012. Replication of minute virus of mice in murine cells is facilitated by virally induced depletion of p21. J. Virol. 86, 8328–8332.

Agersborg, S.S., Garza, K.M., Tung, K.S., 2001. Intestinal parasitism terminates self tolerance and enhances neonatal induction of autoimmune disease and memory. Eur. J. Immunol. 31, 851–859.

Aguggia, J.P., Suárez, M.M., Rivarola, M.A., 2013. Early maternal separation: neurobehavioral consequences in mother rats. Behav. Brain Res. 248, 25–31.

Aguila, H.N., Pakes, S.P., Lai, W.C., Lu, Y.S., 1988a. The effect of transportation stress on splenic natural killer cell activity in C57BL/6J mice. Lab. Anim. Sci. 38, 148–151.

Aguila, H.N., Lai, W.C., Lu, Y.S., Pakes, S.P., 1988b. Experimental *Mycoplasma pulmonis* infection of rats suppresses humoral but not cellular immune response. Lab. Anim. Sci. 38, 138–142.

Akimaru, K., Stuhlmiller, G.M., Seigler, H.F., 1981. Influence of mouse hepatitis virus on the growth of human melanoma in the peritoneal cavity of the athymic mouse. J. Surg. Oncol. 17, 327–339.

Algers, B., 1984. A note on behavioural responses of farm animals to ultrasound. Appl. Anim. Behav. Sci. 12, 387–391.

Aliouat-Denis, C.M., Chabé, M., Demanche, C., Aliouat el, M., Viscogliosi, E., Delhaes, L., et al., 2008. Pneumocystis species, co-evolution and pathogenic power. Infect. Genet. Evol. 8, 708–726.

Al-Mousawi, A.M., Kulp, G.A., Branski, L.K., Kraft, R., Mecott, G.A., Williams, F.N., et al., 2010. Impact of anesthesia, analgesia, and euthanasia technique on the inflammatory cytokine profile in a rodent model of severe burn injury. Shock 34, 261–268.

Altholtz, L.Y., La Perle, K.M., Quimby, F.W., 2006. Dose-dependent hypothyroidism in mice induced by commercial trimethoprim-sulfamethoxazole rodent feed. Comp. Med. 56, 395–401.

American Conference of Governmental Industrial Hygienists, 2013. 2013 TLVs and BEIs, seventh ed. ACGIH, Cincinnati, OH.

Ammann, C.G., Messer, R.J., Varvel, K., Debuysscher, B.L., Lacasse, R.A., Pinto, A.K., et al., 2009. Effects of acute and chronic murine norovirus infections on immune responses and recovery from Friend retrovirus infection. J. Virol. 83, 13037–13041.

Anderson, D.W., Pothakos, K., Schneider, J.S., 2012. Sex and rearing condition modify the effects of perinatal lead exposure on learning and memory. Neurotoxicology 33, 985–995.

Anderson, J.D., Cox, C.S., 1967. Microbial survival. In: Gregory, P.H., Monteith, J.L. (Eds.), "Airborne Microbes" 17th Symposium of the Society of General Microbiology. Cambridge University Press, pp. 203–226.

Anisimov, V.N., Baturin, D.A., Popovich, I.G., Zabezhinski, M.A., Manton, K.G., Semenchenko, A.V., et al., 2004. Effect of exposure to light-at-night on life span and spontaneous carcinogenesis in female CBA mice. Int. J. Cancer 111, 475–479.

Anthony, A., 1962. Criteria for acoustics in animal housing. Lab. Anim. Care 13, 340–347.

Anthony, A., Harclerode, J.E., 1959. Noise stress in laboratory rodents. II. Effects of chronic noise exposures on sexual performance and reproductive function of guinea pigs. J. Acoust. Soc. Am. 31, 1437.

Anver, M.R., Cohen, B.J., 1979. Lesions associated with aging. In: Baker, H.J., Lindsey, J.R., Weisbroth, S.H. (Eds.), The Laboratory Rat. Academic Press, New York, pp. 377–399.

Aparicio, J.L., Peña, C., Retegui, L.A., 2011. Autoimmune hepatitis-like disease in C57BL/6 mice infected with mouse hepatitis virus A59. Int. Immunopharmacol. 11, 1591–1598.

Armario, A., Castellanos, J.M., Balasch, J., 1985. Chronic noise stress and insulin secretion in male rats. Physiol. Behav. 34, 359–361.

Armario, A., Lopez-Calderon, A., Jolin, T., Castellanos, J.M., 1986. Sensitivity of anterior pituitary hormones to graded levels of psychological stress. Life Sci. 39, 471–475.

Arts, J.W., Kramer, K., Arndt, S.S., Ohl, F., 2012. The impact of transportation on physiological and behavioral parameters in Wistar rats: implications for acclimatization periods. ILAR J. 53, 82–98.

Artwohl, J.E., Flynn, J.C., Bunte, R.M., Angen, O., Herold, K.C., 2000. Outbreak of Pasteurella pneumotropica in a closed colony of STOCK-Cd28(tm1Mak) mice. Contemp. Top. Lab. Anim. Sci. 39, 39–41.

Asarian, L., Geary, N., 2006. Modulation of appetite by gonadal steroid hormones. Philos. Trans. R. Soc. Lond. B. Biol. Sci. 361, 1251–1263.

Aschoff, J., 1960. Exogenous and endogenous components in circadian rhythms. Cold Spring Harb. Symp. Quant. Biol. 25, 11–28.

Auger, A.P., 2003. Sex differences in the developing brain: crossroads in the phosphorylation of cAMP response element binding protein. J. Neuroendocrinol. 15, 622–627.

Augustsson, H., van de Weerd, H.A., Kruitwagen, C.L., Baumans, V., 2003. Effect of enrichment on variation and results in the light/dark test. Lab. Anim. 37, 328–340.

Augustine, L.M., Fisher, C.D., Lickteig, A.J., Aleksunes, L.M., Slitt, A.L., Cherrington, N.J., 2008. Gender divergent expression of Nqo1 in Sprague Dawley and August Copenhagen x Irish rats. J. Biochem. Mol. Toxicol. 22 (2), 93–100.

Azar, T.A., Sharp, J.L., Lawson, D.M., 2008. Effect of housing rats in dim light or long nights on heart rate. J. Am. Assoc. Lab. Anim. Sci. 47 (4), 25–34.

Azuma, Y., Shinohara, M., Wang, P.L., Suese, Y., Yasuda, H., Ohura, K., 2000. Comparison of inhibitory effects of local anesthetics on immune functions of neutrophils. Int. J. Immunopharmacol. 22, 789–796.

Babygirija, R., Zheng, J., Bülbül, M., Cerjak, D., Ludwig, K., Takahashi, T., 2010. Sustained delayed gastric emptying during repeated restraint stress in oxytocin knockout mice. J. Neuroendocrinol. 22, 1181–1186.

Baer, L.A., Corbin, B., Vasques, M.F., 1997. Effects of the use of filtered microisolator tops on cage microenvironment and growth rate of mice. Lab. Anim. Sci. 47, 327–329.

Baird, S.M., Beattie, G.M., Lannom, R.A., Lipsick, J.S., Jensen, F.C., Kaplan, N.O., 1982. Induction of lymphoma in antigenically stimulated athymic mice. Cancer Res. 42, 198–206.

Baker, D.G., 2003. Natural Pathogens of Laboratory Animals: Their Effects on Research. American Society for Microbiology Press, Washington, DC, 385 pages.

Baker, P.J., 2005. Genetic control of the immune response in pathogenesis. J. Periodontol. 76, 2042–2046.

Balazs, T., Murphy, J.B., Grice, H.C., 1962. The influence of environmental changes on the cardiotoxicity of isoprenaline in rats. J. Pharm. Pharmacol. 14, 750–755.

Baldwin, A.L., Primeau, R.L., Johnson, W.E., 2006. Effect of noise on the morphology of the intestinal mucosa in laboratory rats. J. Am. Assoc. Lab. Anim. Sci. 45 (1), 74–82.

Baldwin, J.D., 1968. The social behavior of the adult male squirrel monkey in a seminatural environment. Folia Primatol. 9, 281–314.

Baldwin, A.L., Bell, I.R., 2007. Effect of noise on microvascular integrity in laboratory rats. J. Am. Assoc. Lab. Anim. Sci. 46 (1), 58–65.

Baluk, P., Tammela, T., Ator, E., Lyubynska, N., Achen, M.G., Hicklin, D.J., et al., 2005. Pathogenesis of persistent lymphatic vessel hyperplasia in chronic airway inflammation. J. Clin. Invest. 115, 247–257.

Banaceur, S., Banasr, S., Sakly, M., Abdelmelek, H., 2013. Whole body exposure to 2.4 GHz WIFI signals: effects on cognitive impairment in adult triple transgenic mouse models of Alzheimer's disease (3xTg-AD). Behav. Brain Res. 240, 197–201.

Bantle, J.A., 1971. Effects of mechanical vibrations on the growth and development of mouse embryos. Aerosp. Med. 42, 1087–1091.

Barlow, S.M., 1972. Teratogenic effects of restraint, cold and audiogenic stress in mice and rats. University of London. PhD thesis.

Barnard, C.J., Behnke, J.M., Sewell, J., 1996. Environmental enrichment, immunocompetence, and resistance to Babesia microti in male mice. Physiol. Behav. 60, 1223–1231.

Barnett, S.A., 1965. Adaptation of mice to cold. Biol. Rev. 40, 5–51.

Barnett, S.A., 1973. Maternal processes in the cold-adaptation of mice. Biol. Rev. 48, 477–508.

Barthold, S.W., 1979. Autoradiographic cytokinetics of colonic mucosal hyperplasia in mice. Cance Res. 39, 24–29.

Barthold, S.W., Beck, D., 1980. Modification of early dimethylhydrazine carcinogenesis by colonic mucosal hyperplasia. Cancer Res. 40, 4451–4455.

Barthold, S.W., Smith, A.L., Lord, P.F.S., Bhatt, P.N., Jacoby, R.O., Main, A.J., 1982. Epizootic coronaviral typhlocolitis in suckling mice. Lab. Anim. Sci. 32, 376–383.

Bartolomucci, A., 2007. Social stress, immune functions and disease in rodents. Front. Neuroendocrinol. 28, 28–49.

Basner, M., Babisch, W., Davis, A., Brink, M., Clark, C., Janssen, S., et al., 2014. Auditory and non-auditory effects of noise on health. Lancet 383, 1325–1332.

Bass, J., 2012. Circadian topology of metabolism. Nature 491, 348–356.

Baumann, L., Holbech, H., Keiter, S., Kinnberg, K.L., Knörr, S., Nagel, T., et al., 2013. The maturity index as a tool to facilitate the interpretation of changes in vitellogenin production and sex ratio in the fish sexual developmenttest. Aquat. Toxicol. 128-129, 34–42.

Baumans, V., Schlingmann, F., Vonck, M., van Lith, H.A., 2002. Individually ventilated cages: beneficial for mice and men? Contemp. Top. Lab. Anim. Sci. 41, 13–19.

Bean, K., Nemelka, K., Canchola, P., Hacker, S., Sturdivant, R.X., Rico, P.J., 2008. Effects of housing density on Long Evans and Fischer 344 rats. Lab. Anim. 37, 421–428.

Bean-Knudsen, D.E., Wagner, J.E., 1987. Effect of shipping stress on clinicopathologic indicators in F344/N rats. Am. J. Vet. Res. 48, 306–308.

Beattie, G.M., Baird, S.M., Lipsick, J.S., Lannom, R.A., Kaplan, N.O., 1981. Induction of T- and B-lymphocyte responses in antigenically stimulated athymic mice. Cancer Res. 41, 2322–2327.

Beaulieu, A., Reebs, S.G., 2009. Effects of bedding material and running wheel surface on paw wounds in male and female Syrian hamsters. Lab. Anim. 43, 85–90.

Bechill, J., Chen, Z., Brewer, J.W., Baker, S.C., 2008. Coronavirus infection modulates the unfolded protein response and mediates sustained translational repression. J. Virol. 82, 4492–4501.

Beilin, B., Martin, F.C., Shavit, Y., Gale, R.P., Liebeskind, J.C., 1989. Suppression of natural killer cell activity by high-dose narcotic anesthesia in rats. Brain Behav. Immun. 3, 129–137.

Bell, R.W., 1974. Ultrasounds in small rodents: arousal produced and arousal producing. Dev. Psychobiol. 7, 39–42.

Bell, R.W., Nitschke, W., Zachman, T.A., 1972. Ultrasounds in three inbred strains of young mice. Behav. Biol. 7, 805–814.

Bellhorn, R.W., 1980. Lighting in the animal environment. Lab. Anim. Sci. 30, 440–450.

Belyavskyi, M., Belyavskaya, E., Levy, G.A., Leibowitz, L., 1998. Cornoavirus MHV-3-induced apoptosis in macrophages. Virology 250, 41–49.

Benderlioglu, Z., Eish, J., Weil, Z.M., Nelson, R.J., 2005. Low temperatures during early development influence subsequent maternal and reproductive function in adult female mice. Physiol. Behav. 87, 416–423.

Bergin, I.L., Taylor, N.S., Nambiar, P.R., Fox, J.G., 2005. Eradication of enteric helicobacters in Mongolian gerbils is complicated by the occurrence of Clostridium difficile enterotoxemia. Comp. Med. 55, 265–268.

Bette, M., Schlimme, S., Mutters, R., Menendez, S., Hoffmann, S., Schulz, S., 2004. Influence of different anaesthetics on proinflammatory cytokine expression in rat spleen. Lab. Anim. 38, 272–279.

Bianchi, S.L., Tran, T., Liu, C., Lin, S., Li, Y., et al., 2008. Brain and behavior changes in 12-month old Tg2576 and nontransgenic mice exposed to anesthetics. Neurobiol. Aging. 29, 1002–1010.

Bielinska, M., Kiiveri, S., Parviainen, H., Mannisto, S., Heikinheimo, M., Wilson, D.B., 2006. Gonadectomy-induced adrenocortical neoplasia in the domestic ferret (Mustela putorius furo) and laboratory mouse. Vet. Pathol. 43, 97–117.

Bihun, C.G., Percy, D.H., 1995. Morphologic changes in the nasal cavity associated with sialodacryoadenitis virus infection in the Wistar rat. Vet. Pathol. 32, 1–10.

Bilotta, J., 2000. Effects of abnormal lighting on the development of zebrafish visual behavior. Behav. Brain Res. 116, 81–87.

Birkhahn, R.H., Long, C.L., Fitkin, D., Blakemore, W.S., 1979. Stress induced by light weight back button used to prepare the rat for continuous intravenous infusion. J. Parenter. Enteral. Nutr. 3, 421–423.

Bitzer, M., Prinz, F., Bauer, M., Spiegel, M., Neubert, W.J., Gregor, M., et al., 1999. Sendai virus infection induces apoptosis through activation of caspase-8 (FLICE) and caspase-3 (CPP32). J. Virol. 73, 702–708.

Blask, D.E., Dauchy, R.T., Sauer, L.A., Krause, J.A., Brainard, G.C., 2002. Light during darkness, melatonin suppression and cancer progression. Neuro. Endocrinol. Lett. Suppl. 2, 52–56.

Blount, B.C., Alwis, K.U., Jain, R.B., Solomon, B.L., Morrow, J.C., Jackson, W.A., 2010. Perchlorate, nitrate, and iodide intake through tap water. Environ. Sci. Technol. 44, 9564–9570.

Blutt, S.E., Crawford, S.E., Warfield, K.L., Lewis, D.E., Estes, M.K., Conner, M.E., 2004. The VP7 outer capsid protein of rotavirus induces polyclonal B-cell activation. J. Virol. 78, 6974–6981.

Boivin, G.P., Theus, S.A., 1996. Ophthalmic lesions in dexamethasone-treated rats naturally infected with sialodacryoadenitis virus while concurrently used for Pneumocystis carinii propagation. Contemp. Top. Lab. Anim. Sci. 35, 73–75.

Bok, K., Prikhodko, V.G., Green, K.Y., Sosnovtsev, S.V., 2009. Apoptosis in murine norovirus-infected RAW264.7 cells is associated with downregulation of survivin. J. Virol. 83, 3647–3656.

Bollinger, T., Bollinger, A., Oster, H., Solbach, W., 2010. Sleep, immunity, and circadian clocks: a mechanistic model. Gerontology 56, 574–580.

Bologne, R., Demoulin, A., Schaaps, J.P., Hustin, J., Lambotte, R., 1983. Influence of ultrasonics on the fecundity of female rats. C. R. Seances Soc. Biol. Fil. 177, 381–387.

Bolon, B., Bonnefoi, M.S., Roberts, K.C., Marshall, M.W., Morgan, K.T., 1991. Toxic interactions in the rat nose: pollutants from soiled bedding and methyl bromide. Toxicol. Pathol. 19, 571–579.

Boorman, G.A., Luster, M.I., Dean, J.H., Cambell, M.L., Lauer, L.A., Talley, F.A., et al., 1982. Peritoneal and macrophage alterations caused by naturally occurring mouse hepatitis virus. Am. J. Pathol. 106, 110–117.

Borghan, M.A., Mori, Y., El-Mahmoudy, A.B., Ito, N., Sugiyama, M., Takewaki, T., et al., 2007. Induction of nitric oxide synthase by rotavirus enterotoxin NSP4: implication for rotavirus pathogenicity. J. Gen. Virol. 88, 2064–2072.

Borovsky, V., Herman, M., Dunphy, G., 1998. CO2 asphyxia increases plasma norepinephrine in rats via sympathetic nerves. Am. J. Physiol. 274, R19–R22.

Borriello, S.P., 1995. Clostridial disease of the gut. Clin. Infect. Dis. 20 (Suppl. 2), S242–S250.

Boschert, K.R., Schoeb, T.R., Chandler, D.B., Dillehay, D.L., 1988. Inhibition of phagocytosis and interleukin-1 production in pulmonary macrophages from rats with sialodacryoadenitis virus infection. J. Leukoc. Biol. 44, 87–92.

Boshuizen, J.A., Reimerink, J.H., Korteland-van Male, A.M., van Ham, V.J., Bouma, J., Gerwig, G.J., et al., 2005. Homeostasis and function of goblet cells during rotavirus infection in mice. Virology 337, 210–221.

Bourke, C.H., Raees, M.Q., Malviya, S., Bradburn, C.A., Binder, E.B., Neigh, G.N., 2013. Glucocorticoid sensitizers Bag1 and Ppid are regulated by adolescent stress in a sex-dependent manner. Psychoneuroendocrinology 38, 84–93.

Bradfield, J.F., Schachtman, T.R., McLaughlin, R.M., Steffen, E.K., 1992. Behavioral and physiologic effects of inapparent wound infection in rats. Lab. Anim. Sci. 42, 572–578.

Brainard, G.C., Richardson, B.A., King, T.S., Matthews, S.A., Reiter, R.J., 1983. The suppression of pineal melatonin content and N-acetyltransferase activity by different light irradiances in the Syrian hamsters: a dose-response relationship. Endocrinology 113, 293–296.

Brainard, G.C., Rollag, M.D., Hanifin, J.P., 1997. Photic regulation of melatonin in humans: ocular and neural signal transduction. J. Biol. Rhythms 12, 537–546.

Brand, J.M., Kirchner, H., Poppe, C., Schmucker, P., 1998. Cytokine release and changes in mononuclear cells in peripheral blood under the influence of general anesthesia. Anaesthesist 47, 379–386.

Brennan, P.A., Keverne, E.B., 2004. Something in the air? new insights into mammalian pheromones. Curr. Biol. 14, R81–R89.

Briand, L., Trotier, D., Pernollet, J.C., 2004. Aphrodisin, an aphrodisiac lipocalin secreted in hamster vaginal secretions. Peptides 25, 1545–1552.

Brockman, R.P., 1981. Effect of xylazine on plasma glucose, glucagon and insulin concentrations in sheep. Res. Vet. Sci. 30, 383–384.

Broderson, J.R., Lindsey, J.R., Crawford, J.E., 1976. The role of environmental ammonia in respiratory mycoplasmosis of rats. Am. J. Pathol. 85, 115–127.

Brodie, D.A., Woodbury, D.M., 1958. Acid-base changes in brain and blood of rats exposed to high concentrations of carbon dioxide. Am. J. Physiol. 192, 91–94.

Brooks, S.P., Lampi, B.J., Bihun, C.G., 1999. The Influence of euthanasia methods on rat liver metabolism. Contemp. Top. Lab. Anim. Sci. 38 (6), 19–24.

Brown, A.M., 1976. Minireview: ultrasound and communication in rodents. Comp. Biochem. Physiol. 53, 313–317.

Brown, E.L., Ullrich, S.E., Pride, M., Kripke, M.L., 2001. The effect of UV irradiation on infection of mice with Borrelia burgdorferi. Photochem. Photobiol. 73, 537–544.

Brown, N.M., Setchell, K.D., 2001. Animal models impacted by phytoestrogens in commercial chow: implications for pathways influenced by hormones. Lab. Invest. 81, 735–747.

Browning Jr., R., Leite-Browning, M.L., 2013. Comparative stress responses to short transport and related events in Hereford and Brahman steers. J. Anim. Sci. 91, 957–969.

Brownstein, D.G., Weir, E.C., 1987. Immunostimulation in mice infected with Sendai virus. Am. J. Vet. Res. 48, 1692–1696.

Bruce, D.L., 1972. Halothane inhibition of phytohemagglutinin-induced transformation of lymphocytes. Anesthesiology 36, 201–205.

Bruce, D.L., 1975. Halothane Inhibition of RNA and protein synthesis of PHA-treated human lymphocytes. Anesthesiology 42, 11–14.

Brunner, C.J., Muscoplat, C.C., 1980. Immunomodulatory effects of levamisole. J. Am. Vet. Med. Assoc. 176, 1159–1162.

Brunner, L.J., Dipiro, J.T., Feldman, S., 1994. Metabolic cage isolation reduces antipyrine clearance in rats. J. Pharm. Pharmacol. 46, 581–584.

Bryan, T.E., Gildersleeve, R.P., 1988. Effects of nonionizing radiation on birds. Comp. Biochem. Physiol. A 89, 511–530.

Buckley, J.P., Smookler, H.H., 1970. Cardiovascular and biochemical effects of chronic intermittent neurogenic stimulation. In: Welch, B.L., Welch, A.S. (Eds.), Physiological Effects of Noise. Plenum Press, New York, pp. 75–84.

Buddaraju, A.K., Van Dyke, R.W., 2003. Effect of animal bedding on rat liver endosome acidification. Comp. Med. 53, 616–621.

Budillon, G., Carella, M., DeMarco, F., Mazzacca, G., 1973. Effect of phenobarbital on MHV-3 viral hepatitis of the mouse. Pathol. Microbiol 39, 461–466.

Burkart, W., Jung, T., Frasch, G., 1999. Damage pattern as a function of radiation quality and other factors. C. R. Acad. Sci. III 322, 89–101.

Burkuš, J., Cikoš, S., Fabian, D., Kubandová, J., Czikková, S., Koppel, J., 2013. Maternal restraint stress negatively influences growth capacity of preimplantation mouse embryos. Gen. Physiol. Biophys. 32, 129–137.

Burman, O., Owen, D., Abouismail, U., Mendl, M., 2008. Removing individual rats affects indicators of welfare in the remaining group members. Physiol. Behav. 93, 89–96.

Burton, A., Kizhner, O., Brown, M.B., Peltier, M.R., 2012. Effect of experimental genital mycoplasmosis on gene expression in the fetal brain. J. Reprod. Immunol. 93, 9–16.

Butler, M.M., Griffey, S.M., Clubb Jr., F.J., Gerrity, L.W., Campbell, W.B., 1990. The effect of euthanasia technique on vascular arachidonic acid metabolism and vascular and intestinal smooth muscle contractility. Lab. Anim. Sci. 40, 277–283.

Cabanac, M., 1985. Influence of food and water deprivation on the behavior of the white rat foraging in a hostile environment. Physiol. Behav. 35, 701–709.

Cacciatore, L., Antoniello, S., 1971. Arginase activity of mouse serum and liver tissue in some conditions of experimental liver damage. Enzymologia 41, 112–120.

Campa, M., De Libero, G., Benedettini, G., Mori, L., Angioni, M.R., Marelli, P., et al., 1985. Polyclonal B cell activators inhibit contact sensitivity to oxazolone in mice by potentiating the production of anti-hapten antibodies that induce T suppressor lymphocytes acting through the release of soluble factors. Int. Arch. Allergy Appl. Immunol. 78, 391–395.

Campeau, S., Nyhuis, T.J., Sasse, S.K., Day, H.E., Masini, C.V., 2008. Acute and chronic effects of ferret odor exposure in Sprague–Dawley rats. Neurosci. Biobehav. Rev. 32, 1277–1286.

Campion, S.N., Cappon, G.D., Chapin, R.E., Jamon, R.T., Winton, T.R., Nowland, W.S., 2012. Isoflurane reduces motile sperm counts in the Sprague–Dawley rat. Drug Chem. Toxicol. 35, 20–24.

Cantor, K.P., 2010. Carcinogens in drinking water: the epidemiologic evidence. Rev. Environ. Health 25, 9–16.

Capdevila, S., Giral, M., Ruiz de la Torre, J.L., Russell, R.J., Kramer, K., 2007. Acclimatization of rats after ground transportation to a new animal facility. Lab. Anim. 41, 255–261.

Caputa, M., Demicka, A., 1995. Warm rearing modifies temperature regulation in rats. J. Physiol. Pharmacol. 46, 195–203.

Carrano, V.A., Barthold, S.W., Beck, D.S., Smith, A.L., 1984. Alteration of viral respiratory infections of mice by prior infection with mouse hepatitis virus. Lab. Anim. Sci. 34, 573–576.

Carriquiriborde, M., Milocco, S.N., Principi, G., Cagliada, P., Carbone, C., 2006. Pasteurella pneumotropica produces regression of human tumors transplanted in immunodeficiency mice. Medicina (B Aires) 66, 242–244.

Carthew, P., 1981. Inhibition of the mitotic response in regenerating mouse liver during viral hepatitis. Infect. Immun. 33, 641–642.

Case, C.P., Plummer, C.J., 1993. Changing the light intensity of the visual environment results in large differences in numbers of synapses and in photoreceptor size in the retina of the young adult rat. Neuroscience 55, 653–666.

Casebolt, D.B., Spalding, D.M., Schoeb, T.R., Lindsey, J.R., 1987. Suppression of immune response induction in Peyer's patch lymphoid cells from mice infected with mouse hepatitis virus. Cell. Immunol. 109, 97–103.

Casellas, J., Medrano, J.F., 2008. Within-generation mutation variance for litter size in inbred mice. Genetics 179, 2147–2155.

Caso, G., McNurlan, M.A., Mileva, I., Zemlyak, A., Mynarcik, D.C., Gelato, M.C., 2013. Peripheral fat loss and decline in adipogenesis in older humans. Metabolism 62, 337–340.

Cassell, G.H., Lindsey, J.R., Davis, J.K., Davidson, M.K., Brown, M.B., Mayo, J.G., 1981. Detection of natural Mycoplasma pulmonis infection in rats and mice by an enzyme-linked immunosorbent assay. Lab. Anim. Sci. 31, 676–682.

Cassidy, J.P., Caulfield, C., Jones, B.R., Worrall, S., Conlon, L., Palmer, A.C., et al., 2007. Leukoencephalomyelopathy in specific pathogen-free cats. Vet. Pathol. 44, 912–916.

Castro, M., Morgenthaler, T.I., Hoffman, O.A., Standing, J.E., Rohrbach, M.S., Limper, A.H., 1993. Pneumocystis carinii induces the release of arachidonic acid and its metabolites from alveolar macrophages. Am. J. Respir. Cell Mol. Biol. 9, 73–81.

Catlin, F.I., 1986. Noise-induced hearing loss. Am. J. Otol. 7, 141–149.

Caulfield, C.D., Cassidy, J.P., Kelly, J.P., 2008. Effects of gamma irradiation and pasteurization on the nutritive composition of commercially available animal diets. J. Am. Assoc. Lab. Anim. Sci. 47 (6), 61–66.

Caulfield, C.D., Kelly, J.P., Jones, B.R., Worrall, S., Conlon, L., Palmer, A.C., et al., 2009. The experimental induction of leukoencephalomyelopathy in cats. Vet. Pathol. 46, 1258–1269.

Celly, C.S., Atwal, O.S., McDonell, W.N., Black, W.D., 1999. Histopathologic alterations induced in the lungs of sheep by use of alpha2-adrenergic receptor agonists. Am. J. Vet. Res. 60, 154–161.

Chance, M.R.A., 1957. The contribution of environment to uniformity. Collected Papers of the Laboratory Animals Bureau 6, 59–73.

Chandurvelan, R., Marsden, I.D., Gaw, S., Glover, C.N., 2012. Field-to-laboratory transport protocol impacts subsequent physiological biomarker response in the marine mussel, *Perna canaliculus*. Comp. Biochem. Physiol. A Mol. Integr. Physiol. 164, 84–90.

Chang, H.Y., Mitzner, W., Watson, J., 2012. Variation in airway responsiveness of male C57BL/6 mice from 5 vendors. J. Am. Assoc. Lab. Anim. Sci. 51, 401–406.

Chang, S.K., Riviere, J.E., 1991. Percutaneous absorption of parathion in vitro in porcine skin: effects of dose, temperature, humidity, and perfusate composition on absorptive flux. Fundam. Appl. Toxicol. 17, 494–504.

Chang, S.K., Brownie, C., Riviere, J.E., 1994. Percutaneous absorption of topical parathion through porcine skin: in vitro studies on the effect of environmental perturbations. J. Vet. Pharmacol. Ther. 17, 434–439.

Chen, K.K., Anderson, R.C., Steldt, F.A., Mills, C.A., 1943. Environmental temperature and drug action in mice. J. Pharmacol. Exp. Ther. 79, 127–132.

Cheng, B.H., Liu, Y., Xuei, X., Liao, C.P., Lu, D., Lasbury, M.E., et al., 2010. Microarray studies on effects of *Pneumocystis carinii* infection on global gene expression in alveolar macrophages. BMC Microbiol. 10, 103.

Cheng, Y.J., Yang, B.C., Liu, M.Y., 2006. Lead increases lipopolysaccharide-induced liver injury through tumor necrosis factor-alpha overexpression by monocytes/macrophages: role of protein kinase C and P42/44 mitogen-activated protein kinase. Environ. Health Perspect. 114, 507–513.

Cherbut, C., Ferre, J.P., Corpet, D.E., Ruckebusch, Y., Delori-Laval, J., 1991. Alterations of intestinal microflora by antibiotics. Effects on fecal excretion, transit time, and colonic motility in rats. Digest Dis. Sci. 36, 1729–1734.

Chichlowski, M., Sharp, J.M., Venderford, D.A., Myles, M.H., Hale, L.P., 2008. *Helicobacter typhlonius* and *Helicobacter rodentium* differentially affect the severity of colon inflammation and inflammation-associated neoplasia in IL10-deficient mice. Comp. Med. 58, 534–541.

Chinn, I.K., Blackburn, C.C., Manley, N.R., Sempowski, G.D., 2012. Changes in primary lymphoid organs with aging. Semin. Immunol. 24, 309–320.

Choi, G.C., McQuinn, J.S., Jennings, B.L., Hassett, D.J., Michaels, S.E., 1994. Effect of population size on humidity and ammonia levels in individually ventilated microisolation rodent caging. Contemp. Top. Lab. Anim. Sci. 33, 77–81.

Christian, J.J., LeMunyan, C.D., 1958. Adverse effects of crowding on lactation and reproduction of mice and two generations of their progeny. Endocrinology 63, 517–529.

Chung, H.J., Reyes, A.B., Watanabe, K., Tomogane, H., Wakasugi, N., 1997. Embryonic abnormality caused by male pheromonal effect in pregnancy block in mice. Biol. Reprod. 57, 312–319.

Cinti, D.L., Lemelin, M.A., Christian, J., 1976. Induction of liver microsomal mixed-function oxidases by volatile hydrocarbons. Biochem. Pharmacol. 25, 100–103.

Clark, E.A., Russell, P.H., Egghart, M., Horton, M.A., 1979. Characteristics and genetic control of NK-cell-mediated cytotoxicity activated by naturally acquired infection in the mouse. Int. J. Cancer 24, 688–699.

Clark Jr., J.A., Myers, P.H., Goelz, M.F., Thigpen, J.E., Forsythe, D.B., 1997. Pica behavior associated with buprenorphine administration in the rat. Lab. Anim. Sci. 47, 300–303.

Clayton, T.A., Baker, D., Lindon, J.C., Everett, J.R., Nicholson, J.K., 2009. Pharmacometabonomic identification of a significant host-microbiome metabolic interaction affecting human drug metabolism. Proc. Natl. Acad. Sci. USA 106, 14728–14733.

Clemente, J.C., Ursell, L.K., Parfrey, L.W., Knight, R., 2012. The impact of the gut microbiota on human health: an integrative view. Cell 148, 1258–1270.

Clifford, S., Zeckler, R.A., Buckman, S., Thompson, J., Hart, N., Wellman, P.J., et al., 2011. Impact of food restriction and cocaine on locomotion in ghrelin- and ghrelin-receptor knockout mice. Addict. Biol. 16, 386–392.

Clough, G., 1982. Environmental effects on animals used in biomedical research. Biol. Rev. 57, 487–523.

Clough, G., Fasham, J.A.L., 1975. A 'silent' fire alarm. Lab. Anim. 9, 193–196.

Cocke, R., Moynihan, J.A., Cohen, N., Grota, L.J., Ader, R., 1993. Exposure to conspecific alarm chemosignals alters immune responses in BALB/c mice. Brain Behav. Immun. 7, 36–46.

Collins, J., Candy, D.C., Starkey, W.G., Spencer, A.J., Osborne, M.P., Stephen, J., 1990. Disaccharidase activities in small intestine of rotavirus-infected suckling mice: a histochemical study. J. Pediatr. Gastroenterol. Nutr. 11, 395–403.

Compton, S.R., Ball-Goodrich, L.J., Zeiss, C.J., Johnson, L.K., Johnson, E.A., Macy, J.D., 2003. Pathogenesis of mouse hepatitis virus infection in gamma interferon-deficient mice is modulated by co-infection with *Helicobacter hepaticus*. Comp. Med 53, 197–206.

Compton, S.R., Paturzo, F.X., Macy, J.D., 2010. Effect of murine norovirus infection on mouse parvovirus infection. J. Am. Assoc. Lab. Anim. Sci. 49, 11–21.

Conney, A.H., Burns, J.J., 1972. Metabolic interactions among environmental chemicals and drugs. Science 178, 576–586.

Coomans, C.P., van den Berg, S.A., Houben, T., van Klinken, J.B., van den Berg, R., Pronk, A.C., et al., 2013. Detrimental effects of constant light exposure and high-fat diet on circadian energy metabolism and insulin sensitivity. FASEB J. 27, 1721–1732.

Cooper, K.E., Ferguson, A.V., Veale, W.L., 1980. Modification of thermoregulatory responses in rabbits reared at elevated environmental temperatures. J. Physiol. (London) 303, 165–172.

Corbo-Rodgers, E., Staub, E.S., Zou, T., Smith, A., Kambayashi, T., Maltzman, J.S., 2012. Oral ivermectin as an unexpected initiator of CreT2-mediated deletion in T cells. Nat. Immunol. 13, 197–198.

Corning, B.F., Lipman, N.S., 1991. A comparison of rodent caging system based on microenvironmental parameters. Lab. Anim. Sci. 41, 498–503.

Corsi, M., Mariconti, P., Calvillo, L., Falchi, M., Tiengo, M., Ferrero, M.E., 1995. Influence of inhalational, neuroleptic and local anaesthesia on lymphocyte subset distribution. Int. J. Tissue React. 17, 211–217.

Coutelier, J.P., Van Broeck, J., Wolf, S.F., 1995. Interleukin-12 gene expression after viral infection in the mouse. J. Virol. 69, 1955–1958.

Crabbe, J.C., Wahlsten, D., Dudek, B.C., 1999. Genetics of mouse behavior: interactions with laboratory environment. Science 284, 1670–1672.

Cray, C., Mateo, M.O., Altman, N.H., 1993. *In vitro* and long-term *in vivo* immune dysfunction after infection of BALB/c mice with mouse hepatitis virus strain A59. Lab. Anim. Sci. 43, 169–174.

Cray, C., Watson, T., Zaias, J., Altman, N.H., 2013. Effect of fenbendazole on an autoimmune mouse model. J. Am. Assoc. Lab. Anim. Sci. 52, 286–289.

Crema, L.M., Diehl, L.A., Aguiar, A.P., Almeida, L., Fontella, F.U., Pettenuzzo, L., et al., 2010. Effects of chronic restraint stress and 17-β-estradiol replacement on oxidative stress in the spinal cord of ovariectomized female rats. Neurochem. Res. 35, 1700–1707.

Crippa, L., Gobbi, A., Ceruti, R.M., Clifford, C.B., Remuzzi, A., Scanziani, E., 2000. Ringtail in suckling Munich Wistar Fromer rats: a histopathologic study. Comp. Med. 50, 536–539.

Crosby, C., Culley, D.J., Baxter, M.G., Yukhananov, R., Crosby, G., 2005. Spatial memory performance 2 weeks after general anesthesia in adult rats. Anesth. Analg. 101, 1389–1392.

Cryan, J.F., Dinan, T.G., 2012. Mind-altering microorganisms: the impact of the gut microbiota on brain and behavior. Nat. Rev. Neurosci. 13, 701–712.

Cuccurazzu, B., Leone, L., Podda, M.V., Piacentini, R., Riccardi, E., Ripoli, C., et al., 2010. Exposure to extremely low-frequency (50 Hz) electromagnetic fields enhances adult hippocampal neurogenesis in C57BL/6 mice. Exp. Neurol. 226, 173–182.

Cudilo, E., Al Naemi, H., Marmorstein, L., Baldwin, A.L., 2007. Knockout mice: is it just genetics? Effect of enriched housing on fibulin-4(+/−) mice. PLoS One 2, e229.

Cullen, B.F., 1974. The effects of halothane and nitrous oxide on phagocytosis and human leukocyte metabolism. Anesth. Analg. 53, 531–536.

Cullen, B.F., Sample, W.F., Chretien, P.B., 1972. The effect of halothane on phytohemagglutinin-induced transformation of human lymphocytes in Vitro. Anesthesiology 36, 206–212.

Cullen, B.F., Duncan, P.G., Ray-Keil, L., 1976. Inhibition of cell-mediated cytotoxicity by halothane and nitrous oxide. Anesthesiology 44, 386–390.

Culley, D.J., Baxter, M., Yukhananov, R., Crosby, G., 2003. The memory effects of general anesthesia persist for weeks in young and aged rats. Anesth. Analg. 96, 1004–1009.

Culley, D.J., Baxter, M.G., Crosby, C.A., Yukhananov, R., Crosby, G., 2004a. Impaired acquisition of spatial memory 2 weeks after isoflurane and isoflurane-nitrous oxide anesthesia in aged rats. Anesth. Analg. 99, 1393–1397.

Culley, D.J., Baxter, M.G., Yukhananov, R., Crosby, G., 2004b. Long-term impairment of acquisition of a spatial memory task following isoflurane-nitrous oxide anesthesia in rats. Anesthesiology 100, 309–314.

Curtis, M.M., Way, S.S., 2009. Interleukin-17 in host defense against bacterial, mycobacterial and fungal pathogens. Immunology 126, 177–185.

Dallman, M.F., Akana, S.F., Bell, M.E., Bhatnagar, S., Choi, S., Chu, A., et al., 1999. Warning! Nearby construction can profoundly affect your experiments. Endocrine 11, 111–113.

Dalvie, D., Xiang, C., Kang, P., Zhou, S., 2013. Interspecies variation in the metabolism of zoniporide by aldehyde oxidase. Xenobiotica 43, 399–408.

Daubeck, J.L., Daughety, M.J., Petty, C., 1974. Lincomycin-induced cardiac arrest: a case report and laboratory investigation. Anesth. Analg. 53, 563–567.

Dauchy, R.T., Sauer, L.A., Blask, D.E., Vaughan, G.M., 1997. Light contamination during the dark phase in "photoperiodically controlled" animal rooms: effect on tumor growth and metabolism in rats. Lab. Anim. Sci. 47, 511–518.

Dauchy, R.T., Blask, D.E., Sauer, L.A., Brainard, G.C., Krause, J.A., 1999. Dim light during darkness stimulates tumor progression by enhancing tumor fatty acid uptake and metabolism. Cancer Lett. 144 (2), 131–136.

Davis, J.A., Greenfield, R.E., Brewer, T.G., 1993. Benzocaine-induced methemoglobinemia attributed to topical application of the anesthetic in several laboratory animal species. Am. J. Vet. Res. 54, 1322–1326.

Davis, J.K., Thorp, R.B., Maddox, P.A., Brown, M.B., Cassell, G.H., 1982. Murine respiratory mycoplasmosis in F344 and LEW rats: evolution of lesions and lung lymphoid cell populations. Infect. Immun. 36, 720–729.

Davis III, R.T., Stabley, J.N., Dominguez II, J.M., Ramsey, M.W., McCullough, D.J., Lesniewski, L.A., et al., 2013. Differential effects of aging and exercise on intra-abdominal adipose arteriolar function and blood flow regulation. J. Appl. Physiol. 114, 808–815.

Degre, M., Glasgow, L.A., 1968. Synergistic effect in viral bacterial infection. I. Combined infection of the respiratory tract in mice with parainfluenza virus and Hemophilus influenza. J. Infect. Dis. 118, 449–462.

Degre, M., Solberg, L.A., 1971. Synergistic effect in viral bacterial infection. III. Histopathologic changes in the trachea of mice following viral and bacterial infection. Acta Pathol. Microbiol. Scand 79, 129–136.

de Magalhães, J.P., 2013. How ageing processes influence cancer. Nat. Rev. Cancer 13, 357–365.

Denda, M., Sato, J., Masuda, Y., Tsuchiya, T., Koyama, J., Kuramoto, M., et al., 1998. Exposure to a dry environment enhances epidermal permeability barrier function. J. Invest. Dermatol. 111, 858–863.

Denkins, Y.M., Kripke, M.L., 1993. Effect of UV irradiation on lethal infection of mice with Candida albicans. Photochem. Photobiol. 57 (2), 266–271.

De Sarro, A., De Sarro, G., 2001. Adverse reactions to fluoroquinolones. an overview on mechanistic aspects. Curr. Med. Chem. 8, 371–384.

de Souza, M.S., Smith, A.L., Bottomly, K., 1991. Infection of BALB/cByJ mice with the JHM strain of mouse hepatitis virus alters in vitro splenic T cell proliferation and cytokine production. Lab. Anim. Sci. 41, 99–105.

Diercks, A.K., Schwab, A., Rittgen, W., Kruspel, A., Heuss, E., Schenkel, J., 2010. Environmental influences on the production of pre-implantation embryos. Theriogenology 73, 1238–1243.

DiGiacoma, R.F., Deeb, B.J., Anderson, R.J., 1992. Hypervitaminosis A and reproductive disorders in rats. Lab. Anim. Sci. 42, 250–254.

Dillberger, J.E., Monroy, P., Altman, N.H., 1987. Delayed increase in plasma lactic dehydrogenase activity in mouse hepatitis virus-infected mice subsequently infected with lactic dehydrogenase virus. Lab. Anim. Sci. 37, 792–794.

Ding, J.W., Ning, W., Liu, M.F., Lai, A., Peltekian, K., Fung, L., et al., 1998. Expression of the fg12 and its protein product (prothrombinase) in tissues during murine hepatitis virus strain-3 (MHV-3) infection. Adv. Exp. Med. Biol. 440, 609–618.

Dispersyn, G., Sage, D., Challet, E., Pain, L., Touitou, Y., 2009. Plasma corticosterone in rats is specifically increased at recovery from propofol anesthesia without concomitant rise of plasma ACTH. Chronobiol. Int. 26, 697–708.

Dobbie, J.W., Smith, M.J.B., 1982. Silicate nephrotoxicity in the experimental animal: the missing factor in analgesic nephropathy. Scottish Med. J 27, 10–16.

Doherty, P.C., Hou, S., Tripp, R.A., 1994. CD8+ T-cell memory to viruses. Curr. Opin. Immunol. 6, 545–552.

Dolinoy, D.C., Weidman, J.R., Waterland, R.A., Jirtle, R.L., 2006. Maternal genistein alters coat color and protects Avy mouse offspring from obesity by modifying the fetal epigenome. Environ. Health Perspect. 114, 567–572.

Domer, D.A., Erickson, R.L., Petty, J.M., Bergdall, V.K., Hickman-Davis, J.M., 2012. Processing and treatment of corncob bedding affects cage-change frequency for C57BL/6 mice. J. Am. Assoc. Lab. Anim. Sci. 51, 162–169.

Donini, L.M., Savina, C., Cannella, C., 2003. Eating habits and appetite control in the elderly: the anorexia of aging. Int. Psychogeriatr. 15, 73–87.

Donnelly, H., Saibaba, P., 1993. Light intensity and the oestrous cycle in albino and normally pigmented mice. Lab. Anim. 27, 385–390.

Doom, C.M., Turula, H.M., Hill, A.B., 2009. Investigation of the impact of the common animal facility contaminant murine norovirus on experimental murine cytomegalovirus infection. Virology 392, 153–161.

Doughty, M.J., Stuart, D., 1995. Quantification of the hemolysis associated with use of T-61 as a euthanasia agent in rabbits – a comparison with Euthanyl (pentobarbital sodium) and the impact on serum hexosaminidase measurements. Can. J. Physiol. Pharmacol. 73, 1274–1280.

dos Santos, G., Kutuzov, M.A., Ridge, K.M., 2012. The inflammasome in lung diseases. Am. J. Physiol. Lung Cell. Mol. Physiol 303, 627–633.

Drake, M.T., Riley, L.K., Livingston, R.S., 2008. Differential susceptibility of SD and CD rats to a novel rat theilovirus. Comp. Med. 58, 458–464.

Drickamer, L.C., 1977. Seasonal variation in litter size, bodyweight and sexual maturation in juvenile female house mice (Mus muculus). Lab. Anim. 11, 159–162.

Drickamer, L.C., 1984. Seasonal variations in acceleration and delay of sexual maturation in female mice by urinary chemosignals. J. Reprod. Fertil. 72, 55–58.

Drickamer, L.C., 1990a. Environmental factors and age of puberty in female house mice. Dev. Psychobiol. 23, 63–73.

Drickamer, L.C., 1990b. Seasonal variation in fertility, fecundity and litter sex ration in laboratory and wild stocks of house mice. Lab. Anim. Sci. 40, 284–288.

Drozdowicz, C.K., Bowman, T.A., Webb, M.L., Lang, C.M., 1990. Effect of in-house transport on murine plasma corticosterone concentration and blood lymphocyte populations. Am. J. Vet. Res. 51, 1841–1846.

Duan, W.P., Sun, Z.W., Li, Q., Li, C.J., Wang, L., Chen, W.Y., et al., 2012. Normal age-related viscoelastic properties of chondrons and chondrocytes isolated from rabbit knee. Chin. Med. J. 125, 2574–2581.

Duke, J.L., Zammit, T.G., Lawson, D.M., 2001. The effects of routine cage-changing on cardiovascular and behavioral parameters in male Sprague–Dawley rats. Contemp. Top. Lab. Anim. Sci. 40, 17–20.

DuMond, F.V., Hutchinson, T.C., 1967. Squirrel monkey reproduction: the fatted male phenomenon and seasonal spermatogenesis. Science 158, 1467–1470.

Duncan, T.E., O'Steen, W.K., 1985. The diurnal susceptibility of rat retinal photoreceptors to light-induced damage. Exp. Eye Res. 41, 497–507.

Dušková, M., Pospíšilová, H., 2011. The role of non-aromatizable testosterone metabolite in metabolic pathways. Physiol. Res. 60, 253–261.

Edwards, G.S., Fox, J.G., Policastro, P., Goff, U., Wolf, M.H., Fine, D.H., 1979. Volatile nitrosamine contamination of laboratory animal diets (letter). Cancer Res. 39, 1857–1858.

Edwards, R.G., McCutcheon, E.P., Knapp, C.F., 1972. Cardiovascular changes produced by brief whole-body vibration of animals. J. Appl. Physiol. 32, 386–390.

Elyasi, S., Khalili, H., Dashti-Khavidaki, S., Mohammadpour, A., 2012. Vancomycin-induced nephrotoxicity: mechanism, incidence, risk factors and special populations. A literature review. Eur. J. Clin. Pharmacol. 68, 1243–1255.

Even, C., Rowland, R.R., Plagemann, P.G., 1995. Mouse hepatitis virus infection of mice causes long-term depletion of lactate dehydrogenase-elevating virus-permissive macrophages and T lymphocyte alterations. Virus Res. 39, 355–364.

Everitt, J.I., Ross, P.W., Davis, T.W., 1988. Urologic syndrome associated with wire caging in AKR mice. Lab. Anim. Sci. 38, 609–611.

Exon, J.H., Koller, L.D., O'Reilly, C.A., Bercz, J.P., 1987. Immunotoxicologic evaluation of chlorine-based drinking water disinfectants, sodium hypochlorite and monochloramine. Toxicology 44, 257–269.

Fadakar, K., Saba, V., Farzampour, S., 2013. Effects of extremely low frequency electromagnetic field (50 Hz) on pentylenetetrazol-induced seizures in mice. Acta Neurol. Belg. 113, 173–177.

Fallon, M.T., Benjamin Jr., W.H., Schoeb, T.R., Briles, D.E., 1991. Mouse hepatitis virus strain UAB infection enhances resistance to Salmonella typhimurium in mice by inducing suppression of bacterial growth. Infect. Immun. 59, 852–856.

Fanning, S.L., Appel, M.Y., Berger, S.A., Korngold, R., Friedman, T.M., 2009. The immunological impact of genetic drift in the B10.BR congenic inbred mouse strain. J. Immunol. 183, 4261–4272.

Fay, R., 1988. Hearing in Vertebrates: A Psychophysics Data Book. Hill Fay Associates, Winnetka, IL.

Feldman, D.B., Gupta, B.N., 1976. Histopathologic changes in laboratory animals resulting from various methods of euthanasia. Lab. Anim. Sci. 26, 218–221.

Felt, S.A., Cowan, A.M., Luong, R., Green, S.L, 2012. Mortality and morbidity in African Clawed Frogs (Xenopus laevis) associated with construction noise and vibrations. J. Am. Assoc. Lab. Anim. Sci. 51, 253–256.

Feng, J., Yang, J., Zheng, S., Qiu, Y., Chai, C., 2011. Silencing of the rotavirus NSP4 protein decreases the incidence of biliary atresia in murine model. PLoS One 6, e23655.

Feng, Z., Liu, L., Zhang, C., Zheng, T., Wang, J., Lin, M., et al., 2012. Chronic restraint stress attenuates p53 function and promotes tumorigenesis. Proc. Natl. Acad. Sci. USA 109, 7013–7018.

Ferguson, D.R., Bailey, M.M., 2013. Reproductive performance of mice in disposable and standard individually ventilated cages. J. Am. Assoc. Lab. Anim. Sci. 52, 228–232.

Fernandes, C., File, S.E., 1993. Beware the builders: construction noise changes [14C]GABA release and uptake from amygdaloid and hippocampal slices in the rat. Neuropharmacology 32, 1333–1336.

Fernandes, G., 2008. Progress in nutritional immunology. Immunol. Res. 40, 244–261.

Fettman, M.J., Valerius, K.D., Ogilvie, G.K., Bedwell, C.L., Richardson, K.L., Walton, J.A., et al., 1999. Effects of dietary cysteine on blood sulfur amino acid, glutathione, and malondialdehyde concentrations in cats. Am. J. Vet. Res. 60, 328–333.

Fidler, I.J., 1977. Depression of macrophages in mice drinking hyperchlorinated water. Nature 270, 735–736.

Fink, G.B., Iturrian, W.B., 1970. Influence of age, auditory conditioning and environmental noise on sound induced seizures and seizure threshold in mice. In: Welch, B.L., Welch, A.S. (Eds.), Physiological Effects of Noise. Plenum Press, New York, pp. 211–226.

Flint, M.S., Budiu, R.A., Teng, P.N., Sun, M., Stolz, D.B., Lang, M., et al., 2011. Restraint stress and stress hormones significantly impact T lymphocyte migration and function through specific alterations of the actin cytoskeleton. Brain Behav. Immun. 25, 1187–1196.

Flynn, R.J., 1959. Studies on the etiology of ringtail of rats. Proc. Anim. Care Panel 9, 155–160.

Fone, K.C., Porkess, M.V., 2008. Behavioural and neurochemical effects of post-weaning social isolation in rodents – relevance to developmental neuropsychiatric disorders. Neurosci. Biobehav. Rev. 32, 1087–1102.

Fonken, L.K., Kitsmiller, E., Smale, L., Nelson, R.J., 2012. Dim nighttime light impairs cognition and provokes depressive-like responses in a diurnal rodent. J. Biol. Rhythms 27, 319–327.

Fonken, L.K., Nelson, R.J., 2013. Dim light at night increases depressive-like responses in male C3H/HeNHsd mice. Behav. Brain Res. 243, 74–78.

Fowell, D.J., Locksley, R.M., 1999. Leishmania major infection of inbred mice: unmasking genetic determinants of infectious diseases. Bioessays 21, 510–518.

Fox, J.G., 2007. Helicobacter bilis: bacterial provocateur orchestrates host immune responses to commensal flora in a model of inflammatory bowel disease. Gut 56, 898–900.

Fox, J.G., Murphy, J.C., Igras, V.E., 1977. Adverse effects of mouse hepatitis virus on ascites myeloma passage in the BALB/c mouse. Lab. Anim. Sci. 27, 173–179.

Fox, J.G., Rogers, A.B., Whary, M.T., Taylor, N.S., Xu, S., Feng, Y., et al., 2004. Helicobacter bilis-associated hepatitis in outbred mice. Comp. Med. 54, 571–577.

Fox, J.G., Ge, Z., Whary, M.T., Horwitz, B.H., 2011. Helicobacter hepaticus infection in mice: models for understanding lower bowel inflammation and cancer. Mucosal Immunol. 4, 22–30.

Frahm, J., Lantow, M., Lupke, M., Weiss, D.G., Simkó, M., 2006. Alteration in cellular functions in mouse macrophages after exposure to 50 Hz magnetic fields. J. Cell. Biochem. 99, 168–177.

Frick, K.M., Stearns, N.A., Pan, J.Y., Berger-Sweeney, J., 2003. Effects of environmental enrichment on spatial memory and neurochemistry in middle-aged mice. Learn. Mem. 10, 187–198.

Friedman, M., Byers, S.O., Brown, A.E., 1967. Plasma lipid responses of rats and rabbits to an auditory stimulus. Am. J. Physiol. 212, 1174–1178.

Fuhrman, G.J., Fuhrman, F.A., 1961. Effects of temperature on the action of drugs. Annu. Rev. Pharmacol. 1, 65–78.

Fuller, J.L., Sjursen Jr., F.H., 1967. Audiogenic seizures in eleven mouse strains. J. Hered. 58, 135–140.

Fullwood, S., Hicks, T.A., Brown, J.C., Norman, R.L., McGlone, J.J., 1998. Floor space needs for laboratory mice: C57BL/6 males in solid-bottom cages with bedding. ILAR J. 39, 29–36.

Funk, C.J., Manzer, R., Miura, T.A., Groshong, S.D., Ito, Y., Travanty, E.A., et al., 2009. Rat respiratory coronavirus infection: replication in airway and alveolar epithelial cells and the innate immune response. J. Gen. Virol. 90, 2956–2964.

Gabory, A., Ferry, L., Fajardy, I., Jouneau, L., Gothié, J.D., Vigé, A., et al., 2012. Maternal diets trigger sex-specific divergent trajectories of gene expression and epigenetic systems in mouse placenta. PLoS One 7, e47986.

Gadad, B.S., Daher, J.P.L., Hutchinson, E.K., Brayton, C.F., Dawson, T.M., Plentnikov, M.V., et al., 2010. Effect of fenbendazole on 3 behavioral tests in male C57BL/6N mice. J. Am. Assoc. Lab. Anim. Sci. 49, 821–825.

Gaertner, D.J., Boschert, K.R., Schoeb, T.R., 1987. Muscle necrosis in Syrian hamsters resulting from intramuscular injections of ketamine and xylazine. Lab. Anim. Sci. 37, 80–83.

Gaestel, M., 2010. Biological monitoring of non-thermal effects of mobile phone radiation: recent approaches and challenges. Biol. Rev. Camb. Philos. Soc. 85, 489–500.

Gagne, S., Thibodeau, L., Lamontagne, L., 1998. Clonal deletion of some V beta[+] T cells in peripheral lymphocytes from C57BL/6 mice infected with MHV3. Adv. Exp. Med. Biol. 440, 485–489.

Galani, R., Jarrard, L.E., Will, B.E., Kelche, C., 1997. Effects of postoperative housing conditions on functional recovery in rats with lesions of the hippocampus, subiculum, or entorhinal cortex. Neurobiol. Learn. Mem. 67, 43–56.

Galloway, J.H., 1968. Antibiotic toxicity in white mice. Lab. Anim. Care 18, 421–425.

Galton, M., 1963. Myobic mange in the mouse leading to skin ulceration and amyloidosis. Am. J. Pathol. 43, 855–865.

Gamble, M.R., Clough, G., 1976. Ammonia build-up in animal boxes and its effect on rat tracheal epithelium. Lab. Anim. 10, 93–104.

Gao, P., Dang, C.V., Watson, J., 2008. Unexpected antitumorigenic effect of fenbendazole when combined with supplementary vitamins. J. Am. Assoc. Lab. Anim. Sci. 47 (6), 37–40.

García-Iglesias, B.B., Mendoza-Garrido, M.E., Gutiérrez-Ospina, G., Rangel-Barajas, C., Noyola-Díaz, M., Terrón, J.A., 2013. Sensitization of restraint-induced corticosterone secretion after chronic restraint in rats: involvement of 5-HT$_7$ receptors. Neuropharmacology 71, 216–227.

Gare, M., Schwabe, D.A., Hettrick, D.A., Kersten, J.R., Warltier, D.C., Pagel, P.S., 2001. Desflurane, sevoflurane, and isoflurane affect left atrial active and passive mechanical properties and impair left atrial-left ventricular coupling in vivo: analysis using pressure volume relations. Anesthesiology 95, 689–698.

Garlinghouse Jr., L.E., Van Hoosier, G.L., 1978. Studies on adjuvant-induced arthritis, tumor transplantability, and serologic response to bovine serum albumin in Sendai virus infected rats. Am. J. Vet. Res. 39, 297–300.

Garlinghouse Jr., L.E., Van Hoosier Jr., G.L., 1982. The suppression of lymphocytic mitogenesis in Sendai virus infected rats. Am. Soc. Microbiol. Abstr. Annu. Meet., 258.

Garner, J.P., Kiess, A.S., Mench, J.A., Newberry, R.C., Hester, P.Y., 2012. The effect of cage and house design on egg production and egg weight of White Leghorn hens: an epidemiological study. Poult. Sci. 91, 1522–1535.

Garssen, J., de Gruijl, F., Mol, D., de Klerk, A., Roholl, P., Van Loveren, H., 2001. UVA exposure affects UVB and cis-urocanic acid-induced systemic suppression of immune responses in Listeria monocytogenes-infected BALB/c mice. Photochem. Photobiol. 73, 432–438.

Garssen, J., van der Molen, R., de Klerk, A., Norval, M., van Loveren, H., 2000. Effects of UV irradiation on skin and nonskin-associated herpes simplex virus infections in rats. Photochem. Photobiol. 72, 645–651.

Gates, K.L., Howell, H.A., Nair, A., Vohwinkel, C.U., Welch, L.C., Beitel, G.J., et al., 2013. Hypercapnia impairs lung neutrophil function and increases mortality in murine *Pseudomonas* pneumonia. Am. J. Respir. Cell Mol. Biol. 49, 821–828.

Gaunsbaek, M.Q., Rasmussen, K.J., Beers, M.F., Atochina-Vasserman, E.N., Hansen, S., 2013. Lung surfactant protein D (SP-D) response and regulation during acute and chronic lung injury. Lung 191 (3), 295–303.

Geber, W.F., 1970. Cardiovascular and teratogenic effects of chronic intermittent noise stress. In: Welch, B.L., Welch, S.A. (Eds.), Physiological Effects of Noise. Plenum Press, New York, pp. 85–90.

Gerber, S.B., Leonard, A., Jacquet, P., 1980. Toxicity, mutagenicity, and teratogenicity of lead. Mutat. Res. 76, 115–141.

Gerdin, A.K., Igosheva, N., Roberson, L.A., Ismail, O., Karp, N., Sanderson, M., et al., 2012. Experimental and husbandry procedures as potential modifiers of the results of phenotyping tests. Physiol. Behav. 106, 602–611.

Gil, A.G., Silvan, G., Illera, M., Illera, J.C., 2004. The effects of anesthesia on the clinical chemistry of New Zealand white rabbits. Contemp. Top. Lab. Anim. Sci. 43 (3), 25–29.

Gilbert, M.E., Kelly, M.E., Samsam, T.E., Goodman, J.H., 2005. Chronic developmental lead exposure reduces neurogenesis in adult rat hippocampus but does not impair spatial learning. Toxicol. Sci. 86, 365–374.

Giral, M., García-Olmo, D.C., Kramer, K., 2011. Effects of wire-bottom caging on heart rate, activity and body temperature in telemetry-implanted rats. Lab. Anim. 45, 247–253.

Gledhill, A.W., Bilbey, D.L.J., Niven, J.S.F., 1965. Effect of certain murine pathogens on phagocytic activity. Br. J. Exp. Pathol. 46, 433–442.

Godfraind, C., Holmes, K.V., Coutelier, J.P., 1995. Thymus involution induced by mouse hepatitis virus A59 in BALB/c mice. J. Virol. 69, 6541–6547.

Goettsch, W., Garssen, J., De Gruijl, F.R., Van Loveren, H., 1994. Effects of UV-B on the resistance against infectious diseases. Toxicol. Lett. 72, 359–363.

Goldfine, I.D., Arieff, A.I., 1979. Rapid inhibition of basal and glucose-stimulated insulin release by xylazine. Endocrinology 105, 920–922.

Gordon, A.H., Hart, P.D., Young, M.R., 1980. Ammonia inhibits phagosome-lysosome fusion in macrophages. Nature 286, 79–80.

Gordon, C.J., Fogelson, L., 1994. Metabolic and thermoregulatory responses of the rat maintained in acrylic or wire-screen cages: implications for pharmacological studies. Physiol. Behav. 56, 73–79.

Gordon, C.J., Lee, K.L., Chen, T.L., Killough, P., Ali, J.S., 1991. Dynamics of Behavioral Thermoregulation in the Rat. Am. J. Physiol. 261, R705–R711.

Gordon, C.J., 2004. Effect of cage bedding on temperature regulation and metabolism of group-housed female mice. Comp. Med. 54 (1), 63–68.

Gos, T., Hauser, R., Krzyzanowsk, M., 2002. Regional distribution of glutamate in the central nervous system of rat terminated by carbon dioxide euthanasia. Lab. Anim. 36, 127–133.

Gould, E.M., 2008. The effect of ketamine/xylazine and carbon dioxide on plasma luteinizing hormone releasing hormone and testosterone concentrations in the male Norway rat. Lab. Anim. 42, 483–488.

Gouveia, K., Hurst, J.L., 2013. Reducing mouse anxiety during handling: effect of experience with handling tunnels. PLoS One 8, e66401.

Goyer, R.A., 1991. Transplacental transfer of cadmium and fetal effects. Fundam. Appl. Toxicol. 16, 22–23.

Greenberg, A.J., Hackett, S.R., Harshman, L.G., Clark, A.G., 2011. Environmental and genetic perturbations reveal different networks of metabolic regulation. Mol. Syst. Biol. 7, 563.

Greenman, D.L., Bryant, P., Kodell, R.L., Sheldon, W., 1982. Influence of cage shelf level on retinal atrophy in mice. Lab. Anim. Sci. 32, 353–356.

Guengerich, F.P., 1995. Influence of nutrients and other dietary materials on cytochrome P-450 enzymes. Am. J. Clin. Nutr. 61, 651S–658S.

Guetta, E., Graziani, Y., Tal, J., 1986. Suppression of Ehrlich ascites tumors in mice by minute virus of mice. J. Natl. Cancer Inst. 76, 1177–1180.

Guha, D., Williams, E.F., Nimitkitpaisan, Y., Bose, S., Dutta, S.N., Pradhan, S.N., 1976. Effects of sound stimulus on gastric secretion and plasma corticosterone level in rats. Res. Commun. Chem. Pathol. Pharmacol. 13, 273–281.

Guillet, R., Wyatt, J., Baggs, R.B., Kellogg, C.K., 1988. Anesthetic-induced corneal lesions in developmentally sensitive rats. Invest. Ophthalmol. Vis. Sci. 29, 949–954.

Gul, A., Celebi, H., Uğraş, S., 2009. The effects of microwave emitted by cellular phones on ovarian follicles in rats. Arch. Gynecol. Obstet. 280, 729–733.

Gulani, J., Norbury, C.C., Bonneau, R.H., Beckwith, C.S., 2009. The effect of *Helicobacter hepaticus* infection on immune responses specific to herpes simplex virus type 1 and characteristics of dendritic cells. Comp. Med. 59, 534–544.

Guttman, J.A., Samji, F.N., Li, Y., Vogl, A.W., Finlay, B.B., 2006. Evidence that tight junctions are disrupted due to intimate bacterial contact and not inflammation during attaching and effacing pathogen infection *in vivo*. Infect. Immun. 74, 6075–6084.

Gwosdow, A.R., Besch, E.L., 1985. In: Hamm Jr., T.E. (Ed.), Effect of Thermal History on the Rat"Human Vibration: Basic Characteristics. Hemisphere Press, Washington, DC, pp. 25–52.

Hackbarth, H., Burow, K., Schimansky, G., 1983. Strain differences in inbred rats: influence of strain and diet on haematological traits. Lab. Anim. 17, 7–12.

Haemisch, A., Gärtner, K., 1997. Effects of cage enrichment on territorial aggression and stress physiology in male laboratory mice. Acta Physiol. Scand. Suppl. 640, 73–76.

Hadlow, W.J., Grimes, E.F., Jay, G.E., 1955. Stilbesterol-contaminated feed and reproductive disturbances in mice. Science 122, 643–644.

Hailey, J.R., Haseman, J.K., Bucher, J.R., Radovsky, A.E., Malarky, D.E., Miller, R.T., et al., 2007. Impact of *Helicobacter hepaticus* infection in B6C3F$_1$ mice from twelve National Toxicology Program two-year carcinogenesis studies. Toxicol. Pathol. 26, 602–611.

Halkett, J.A.E., Davis, A.J., Natsios, G.A., 1968. The effect of cold stress and *Pseudomonas aeruginosa* gavage on the survival of three-week-old Swiss mice. Lab. Anim. Care 18, 94–96.

Hamilton, J.R., Overall Jr., J.C., 1978. Synergistic infection with murine cytomegalovirus and Pseudomonas aeruginosa in mice. J. Infect. Dis. 137 (6), 775–782.

Hanberger, H., Edlund, C., Furebring, M., Giske, G.C., Melhus, A., Nilsson, L.E., Swedish Reference Group for Antibiotics, 2013. Rational use of aminoglycosides – review and recommendations by the Swedish Reference Group for Antibiotics (SRGA). Scand. J. Infect. Dis. 45, 161–175.

Hanson, M.L., Holásková, I., Elliott, M., Brundage, K.M., Schafer, R., Barnett, J.B., 2012. Prenatal cadmium exposure alters postnatal immune cell development and function. Toxicol. Appl. Pharmacol. 261, 196–203.

Hall, W.C., Lubet, R.A., Henry, C.J., Collins Jr., M.J., 1985. Sendai virus disease processes and research complications. In: Hamm Jr., T.E. (Ed.), Complications of Viral and Mycoplasmal Infections in Rodents to Toxicology Research and Testing. Hemisphere Press, Washington, DC, pp. 25–52.

Hall, J.A., Wander, R.C., Gradin, J.L., Shi-Hua, D., Jewell, D.E., 1999. Effect of dietary n-6-to-n-3 fatty acid ratio on complete blood and total white blood cell counts, and T-cell subpopulations in aged dogs. Am. J. Vet. Res. 60, 319–327.

Hall, J.E., White, W.J., Lang, C.M., 1980. Acidification of drinking water: its effects on selected biologic phenomena in male mice. Lab. Anim. Sci. 30, 643–651.

Hao, Y., Kuang, Z., Walling, B.E., Bhatia, S., Sivaguru, M., Chen, Y., et al., 2012. *Pseudomonas aeruginosa* pyocyanin causes airway goblet cell hyperplasia and metaplasia and mucus hypersecretion by inactivating the transcriptional factor FoxA2. Cell Microbiol. 14, 401–415.

Harper, C., Lawrence, C., 2011. The Laboratory Zebrafish. CRC Press, Boca Raton, FL, pp. 254.

Harris, A.W., Basten, A., Gebski, V., Noonan, D., Finnie, J., Bath, M.L., et al., 1998. A test of lymphoma induction by long term-exposure of E mu-Pim 1 transgenic mice to 50 Hz magnetic fields. Radiat. Res. 149, 300–307.

Hart, J.S., 1963. Physiological responses to cold in non-hibernating homeotherms In: Herzfeld, C.M. (Ed.), Temperature: Its Measurement and Control in Science and Industry, vol. 3. Reinhold, New York, pt. 3.

Hasenau, J.J., Baggs, R.B., Kraus, A.L., 1993. Microenvironments in microisolation cages using BALB/c and CD-1 Mice. Contemp. Top. Lab. Anim. Sci. 32, 11–16.

Haseneder, R., Starker, L., Berkmann, J., Kellermann, K., Jungwirth, B., Blobner, M., et al., 2013. Sevoflurane anesthesia improves cognitive performance in mice, but does not influence in vitro long-term potentiation in hippocampus CA1 stratum radiatum. PLoS One 8, e64732.

Hasløv, K., Fomsgaard, A., Takayama, K., Fomsgaard, J.S., Ibsen, P., Fauntleroy, M.B., et al., 1992. Immunosuppressive effects induced by the polysaccharide moiety of some bacterial lipopolysaccharides. Immunology 186, 378–393.

Hathway, G.J., Koch, S., Low, L., Fitzgerald, M., 2009. The changing balance of brainstem-spinal cord modulation of pain processing over the first weeks of rat postnatal life. J. Physiol. 587, 2927–2935.

Hauser Jr., W.E., Remington, J.S., 1982. Effect of antibiotics on the immune response. Am. J. Med. 72, 711–716.

Hautekeete, M.L., 1995. Hepatotoxicity of antibiotics. Acta Gastroenterol. Belg. 58, 290–296.

Hautzinger, G.M., Piacsek, B.E., 1973. Influence of duration, intensity and spectrum of light exposure on sexual maturation of female rats. Fed. Proc. 32, 213.

Hayashimoto, N., Morita, H., Ishida, T., Yasuda, M., Kameda, S., Uchida, R., et al., 2013. Current microbiological status of laboratory mice and rats in experimental facilities in Japan. Exp. Anim. 62, 41–48.

Hayssen, V., 1998. Effect of transatlantic transport on reproduction of agouti and nonagouti deer mice, *Peromyscus maniculatus*. Lab. Anim. 32, 55–64.

Heffner, R., Heffner, H., 1980. Hearing in the elephant (*Elephas maximus*). Science 208, 318–320.

Heidari-Oranjaghi, N., Azhdari-Zarmehri, H., Erami, E., Haghparast, A., 2012. Antagonism of orexin-1 receptors attenuates swim- and restraint stress-induced antinociceptive behaviors in formalin test. Pharmacol. Biochem. Behav. 103, 299–307.

Heindel, J.J., vom Saal, F.S., 2008. Meeting report: batch-to-batch variability in estrogenic activity in commercial animal diets-importance and approaches for laboratory animal research. Environ. Health Perspect. 116, 389–393.

Hemphill, F.E., Kaeberle, M.L., Buck, W.B., 1971. Lead suppression of mouse resistance to *Salmonella typhimurium*. Science 172, 1031–1032.

Hensley, S.E., Pinto, A.K., Hickman, H.D., Kastenmayer, R.J., Bennink, J.R., Virgin, H.W., et al., 2009. Murine norovirus infection has no significant effect on adaptive immunity to vaccinia virus or influenza A virus. J. Virol. 83, 7357–7360.

Hermann, L.M., White, W.J., Lang, C.M., 1982. Prolonged exposure to acid, chlorine, or tetracycline in drinking water: effects on delayed-type hypersensitivity, hemagglutination titers, and reticuloendothelial clearance rates in mice. Lab. Anim. Sci. 32, 603–608.

Hertz-Picciotto, I., Park, H.Y., Dostal, M., Kocan, A., Trnovec, T., Sram, R., 2008. Prenatal exposures to persistent and non-persistent organic compounds and effects on immune system development. Basic Clin. Pharmacol. Toxicol. 102, 146–154.

Hickman-Davis, J.M., Wang, Z., Fierro-Perez, G.A., Chess, P.R., Page, G.P., Matalon, S., et al., 2007. Surfactant dysfunction in SP-A-/- and iNOS-/- mice with mycoplasma infection. Am. J. Respir. Cell Mol. Biol. 36, 103–113.

Higgins, L.M., Frankel, G., Douce, G., Dougan, G., MacDonald, T.T., 1999. *Citrobacter rodentium* infection in mice elicits a mucosal Th1 cytokine response and lesions similar to those in murine inflammatory bowel disease. Infect. Immun. 67, 3031–3039.

Hill, R.A., Boon, W.C., 2009. Estrogens, brain, and behavior: lessons from knockout mouse models. Semin. Reprod. Med. 27, 218–228.

Himeda, T., Okuwa, T., Muraki, Y., Ohara, Y., 2010. Cytokine/chemokine profile in J774 macrophage cells persistently infected with DA strain of Theiler's murine encephalomyelitis virus (TMEV). J. Neurovirol. 16, 219–229.

Hite, M., Hanson, H.M., Bohidar, N.R., Conti, P.A., Mattis, P.A., 1977. Effect of cage size on patterns of activity and health of beagle dogs. Lab. Anim. Sci. 27, 60–64.

Hodgson, E., Kulkarni, A.P., Fabacher, D.L., Robacker, K.M., 1980. Induction of hepatic drug metabolizing enzymes in mammals by pesticides: a review. J. Environ. Sci. Health 15, 723–754.

Hofer, M.A., Shair, H., 1978. Ultrasonic vocalization during social interaction and isolation in 2-week-old rats. Dev. Psychobiol. 11, 495–504.

Hoffman, J.C., 1973. The influence of photoperiods on reproductive functions in female mammals. In: Geiger S.R. (Ed.), Handbook of Physiology, Section 7: Endocrinology, Vol. II. American Physiological Society, Washington, DC, pp. 57–77.

Hoffman, S.M., Fleming, S.D., 2010. Natural *Helicobacter* infection modulates mouse intestinal muscularis macrophage responses. Cell Biochem. Funct. 28, 686–694.

Honess, P.E., Johnson, P.J., Wolfensohn, S.E., 2004. A study of behavioural response of non-human primates to air transport and re-housing. Lab. Anim. 38, 119–132.

Homberger, F.R., Pataki, Z., Thomann, P.E., 1993. Control of *Pseudomonas aeruginosa* infection in mice by chlorine treatment of drinking water. Lab. Anim. Sci. 43, 635–637.

Hong, C.C., Ediger, R.D., 1978. Chronic necrotizing mastitis in rats caused by *Pasteurella pneumotropica*. Lab. Anim. Sci. 28, 317–320.

Hooks, J.J., Percopo, C., Wang, Y., Detrick, B., 1993. Retina and retinal pigment epithelial cell autoantibodies are produced during murine coronavirus retinopathy. J. Immunol. 151, 3381–3389.

Hooper, L.V., Stappenbeck, T.S., Hong, C.V., Gordon, J.I., 2003. Angiogenins: a new class of microbicidal proteins involved in innate immunity. Nat. Immunol. 4, 269–273.

Hoorn, E.J., McCormick, J.A., Ellison, D.H., 2011. High tail-cuff blood pressure in mice 1 week after shipping: the need for longer acclimation. 24, 534–536.

Hori, T., Harakawa, S., Herbas, S.M., Ueta, Y.Y., Inoue, N., Suzuki, H., 2012. Effect of 50 Hz electric field in diacylglycerol acyltransferase mRNA expression level and plasma concentration of triacylglycerol, free fatty acid, phospholipid and total cholesterol. Lipids Health Dis. 11, 68.

Hosoi, J., Tsuchiya, T., Denda, M., Ashida, Y., Takashima, A., Granstein, R.D., et al., 1998. Modification of LC phenotype and suppression of contact hypersensitivity response by stress. J. Cutan. Med. Surg. 3, 79–84.

Houtman, J.J., Fleming, J.O., 1996. Dissociation of demyelination and viral clearance in congenitally immunodeficient mice infected with murine coronavirus JHM. J. Neurovirol. 2, 101–110.

Howard, H.L., McLaughlin-Taylor, E., Hill, R.L., 1990. The effect of mouse euthanasia technique on subsequent lymphocyte proliferation and cell mediated lympholysis assays. Lab. Anim. Sci. 40, 510–514.

Howdeshell, K.L., Peterman, P.H., Judy, B.M., Taylor, J.A., Orazio, C.E., Ruhlen, R.L., et al., 2003. Bisphenol A is released from used polycarbonate animal cages into water at room temperature. Environ. Health Perspect. 111, 1180–1187.

Hsu, W.H., 1988. Yohimbine increases plasma insulin concentrations and reverses xylazine-induced hypoinsulinemia in dogs. Am. J. Vet. Res. 49, 242–244.

Huang, D.S., Emancipator, S.N., Fletcher, D.R., Lamm, M.E., Mazanec, M.B., 1996. Hepatic pathology resulting from mouse hepatitis virus infection in severe combined immunodeficiency mice. Lab. Anim. Sci. 46, 167–173.

Huang, J., Xiao, F., Yu, H., Huang, T., Huang, H., Ning, Q., 2007. Differential gene expression profiles in acute hepatic failure model in mice infected with MHV-3 virus intervened by anti-hepatic failure compound. J. Huazhong Univ. Sci. Technolog. Med. Sci 27, 538–542.

Huerkamp, M.J., Lehner, N.D.M., 1994. Comparative effects of forced-air, individual cage ventilation or an absorbent bedding additive on mouse isolator cage microenvironment. Contemp. Top. Lab. Anim. Sci. 33, 69–72.

Huerkamp, M.J., Dillehay, D.L., Lehner, N.D.M., 1994. Effect of intra-cage ventilation and automatic watering on outbred mouse reproductive performance and weanling growth. Contemp. Top. Lab. Anim. Sci. 33, 58–62.

Hunstein, W., Perings, E., Eggeling, B., Uhl, N., 1969. Panmyelophthisis and viral hepatitis. Experimental study with the MHV-3 mouse hepatitis virus. Acta Haematol. 42, 336–346.

Hunt, P.A., Koehler, K.E., Susiarjo, M., Hodges, C.A., Ilagan, A., Voigt, R.C., et al., 2003. Bisphenol A exposure causes meiotic aneuploidy in the female mouse. Curr. Biol. 13, 546–553.

Hunter, R.L., Choi, D.Y., Kincer, J.F., Cass, W.A., Bing, G., Gash, D.M., 2007. *Fenbendazole* treatment may influence lipopolysaccharide effects in rat brain. Comp. Med. 57, 487–492.

Hurst, J.L., 2009. Female recognition and assessment of males through scent. Behav. Brain Res. 200, 295–303.

Hutchinson, E.K., Avery, A.C., VandeWoude, S., 2012. Environmental enrichment during rearing alters corticosterone levels, thymocyte numbers, and aggression in female BALB/c mice. J. Am. Assoc. Lab. Anim. Sci. 51, 18–24.

Idda, M.L., Kage, E., Lopez-Olmeda, J.F., Mracek, P., Foulkes, N.S., Vallone, D., 2012. Circadian timing of injury-induced cell proliferation in zebrafish. PLoS One 7, e34203.

Inagaki, H., Nakamura, K., Kiyokawa, Y., Kikusui, T., Takeuchi, Y., Mori, Y., 2009. The volatility of an alarm pheromone in male rats. Physiol. Behav. 96 (4–5), 749–752.

Ilić, V., Krstić, A., Katić-Radivojević, S., Jovčić, G., Milenković, P., Bugarski, D., 2010. *Syphacia obvelata* modifies mitogen-activated protein kinases and nitric oxide synthases expression in murine bone marrow cells. Parasitol. Int. 59, 82–88.

Ingelman-Sundberg, M., Zhong, X.B., Hankinson, O., Beedanagari, S., Yu, A.M., Peng, L., et al., 2013. Potential role of epigenetic mechanisms in the regulation of drug metabolism and transport. Drug. Metab. Dispos. 41, 1725–1731.

Ingham, E., Turnbull, L., Kearney, J.N., 1991. The effects of minocycline and tetracycline on the mitotic response of human peripheral blood-lymphocytes. J. Antimicrob. Chemother. 27, 607–617.

Inudo, M., Ishibashi, H., Matsumura, N., Matsuoka, M., Mori, T., Taniyama, S., et al., 2004. Effect of estrogenic activity, and phytoestrogen and organochlorine pesticide contents in an experimental fish diet on reproduction and hepatic vitellogenin production in medaka (*Oryzias latipes*). Comp. Med. 54, 673–680.

Irvani, J., van As, A., 1972. Mucus transport in the tracheobronchial tree of normal and bronchitic rats. J. Pathol. 106, 81–93.

Isensee, J., Ruiz Noppinger, P., 2007. Sexually dimorphic gene expression in mammalian somatic tissue. Gend. Med. 4, S75–S95.

Ishida, T., Tamura, T., Ueda, K., Fujiwara, K., 1978. Hepatosplenic myelosis in the nude mouse naturally infected with mouse hepatitis virus. Jpn. J. Vet. Sci. 40, 739–743.

Istaphanous, G.K., Ward, C.G., Nan, X., Hughes, E.A., McCann, J.C., McAuliffe, J.J., et al., 2013. Characterization and quantification of isoflurane-induced developmental apoptotic cell death in mouse cerebral cortex. Anesth. Analg. 116, 845–854.

Ito, T., Ingalls, T.H., 1981. Sodium pentobarbital-induced mutations in the hamsters. Arch. Environ. Health 36, 316–320.

Izmerov, N.F., 1985. Current problems of nonionizing radiation. Scand. J. Work Environ. Health 11, 223–227.

Jacobsen, K.O., Villa, V., Miner, Venit, L., Whitnall, M.H., 2004. Effects of *anesthesia* and vehicle injection on circulating blood elements in C3H/HeN male mice. Contemp. Top. Lab. Anim. Sci. 43 (5), 8–12.

Jacoby, R.O., Ball-Goodrich, L.J., 1995. Parvovirus infections of mice and rats. Semin. Virol. 6, 329–333.

Jacques, A., Bleau, C., Turbide, C., Beauchemin, N., Lamontagne, L., 2009. Macrophage interleukin-6 and tumour necrosis factor-alpha are induced by coronavirus fixation to Toll-like receptor but not carcinoembryonic cell adhesion antigen 1a. Immunology 128, 181–192.

Jafari, M., Haist, V., Baumgärtner, W., Wagner, S., Stein, V.M., Tipold, A., et al., 2012. Impact of Theiler's virus infection on hippocampal neuronal progenitor cells: differential effects in two mouse strains. Neuropathol. Appl. Neurobiol. 38, 647–664.

Jakab, G.J., 1981. Interactions between Sendai virus and bacterial pathogens in the murine lung: a review. Lab. Anim. Sci. 31, 170–177.

Jakab, G.J., Warr, G.A., 1981. Immune enhanced phagocytic dysfunction in pulmonary macrophages infected with parainfluenza 1 (Sendai) virus. Am. Rev. Respir. Dis. 124, 575–581.

Jans, J.E., Woodside, B., 1987. Effects of litter age, litter size, and ambient temperature on the milk ejection reflex in lactating rats. Dev. Psychobiol. 20, 333–344.

Jansson, J.O., Edén, S., Isaksson, O., 1985. Sexual dimorphism in the control of growth hormone secretion. Endocr. Rev. 6, 128–150.

Jensen, M.M., Rasmussen Jr., A.F., 1970. Audiogenic stress and susceptibility to infection. In: Welch, B.L., Welch, A.S. (Eds.), Physiological Effects of Noise. Plenum Press, New York.

Jensen, M.N., Ritskes-Hoitinga, M., 2007. How isoflavone levels in common rodent diets can interfere with the value of animal models and with experimental results. Lab. Anim. 41, 1–18.

Jevtovic-Todorovic, V., Hartman, R.E., Izumi, Y., Benshoff, N.D., Dikranian, K., Zorumski, C.F., et al., 2003. Early exposure to common anesthetic agents causes widespread neurodegeneration in the developing rat brain and persistent learning deficits. J. Neurosci. 23, 876–882.

Jevtovic-Todorovic, V., Absalom, A.R., Blomgren, K., Brambrink, A., Crosby, G., Culley, D.J., et al., 2013. Anaesthetic neurotoxicity and neuroplasticity: an expert group report and statement based on the BJA Salzburg Seminar. Br. J. Anaesth. 111, 143–151.

Jia, H., Duan, Y., Cao, T., Zhao, B., Lv, F., Yuan, L., 2005. Immediate and long term effects of color Doppler ultrasound on myocardial cell apoptosis of fetal rats. Echocardiography 22, 415–420.

Jimenez-Valera, M., Sampedro, A.A., Moreno, E., Ruiz-Bravo, A., 1995. Modification of immune response in mice by ciprofloxacin. Antimicrob. Agents Chemother. 39, 150–154.

Jin, Y., Shu, L., Sun, L., Liu, W., Fu, Z., 2010. Temperature and photoperiod affect the endocrine disruption effects of ethinylestradiol, nonylphenol and their binary mixture in zebrafish (*Danio rerio*). Comp. Biochem. Physiol. C. Toxicol. Pharmacol 15, 258–263.

Jin, Y.H., Kang, H.S., Mohindru, M., Kim, B.S., 2011. Preferential induction of protective T cell responses to Theiler's virus in resistant (C57BL/6 x SJL)F1 mice. J. Virol. 85, 3033–3040.

Johlin, J.M., 1944. Influence of atmospheric temperature upon reaction of rabbits to insulin. Proc. Soc. Exp. Biol. Med. 55, 122–124.

Johnson, T., Lavender, J.F., Hultin, E., Rasmussen Jr., A.F., 1963. The influence of avoidance-learning stress on resistance to coxsackie B virus in mice. J. Immunol. 91, 569–579.

Jolicoeur, P., Lamontagne, L., 1995. Impairment of bone marrow pre-B and B cells in MHV3 chronically-infected mice. Adv. Exp. Med. Biol. 380, 193–195.

Jori, A., Bianchetti, A., Prestini, P.E., 1969. Effect of essential oils on drug metabolism. Biochem. Pharmacol. 18, 2081–2085.

Ju, Y.H., Doerge, D.R., Allred, K.F., Allred, C.D., Helferich, W.G., 2002. Dietary genistein negates the inhibitory effect of tamoxifen on growth of estrogen-dependent human breast cancer (MCF-7) cells implanted in athymic mice. Cancer Res. 62, 2474–2477.

Jungmann, P., Guenet, J.L., Cazenave, P.A., Coutinho, A., Huerre, M., 1996a. Murine acariasis. I. Pathological and clinical evidence suggesting cutaneous allergy and wasting syndrome in BALB/c mouse. Res. Immunol. 147, 27–38.

Jungmann, P., Freitas, A., Bandeira, A., Nobrega, A., Coutinho, A., Marcos, M.A., et al., 1996b. Murine acariasis. II. Immunological dysfunction and evidence for chronic activation of Th-2 lymphocytes. Scand. J. Immunol. 43, 604–612.

Kacew, S., Dixit, R., Ruben, Z., 1998. Diet and rat strain as factors in nervous system function and influence of confounders. Biomed. Environ. Sci. 11, 203–217.

Kai, T., Bremerich, D.H., Jones, K.A., Warner, D.O., 1998. Drug-specific effects of volatile anesthetics on Ca^{2+} sensitization in airway smooth muscle. Anesth. Analg. 87, 425–429.

Kalenka, A., Hinkelbein, J., Feldmann Jr., R.E., Kuschinsky, W., Waschke, K.F., Maurer, M.H., 2007. The effects of sevoflurane anesthesia on rat brain proteins: a proteomic time-course analysis. Anesth. Analg. 104, 1129–1135.

Kallnik, M., Elvert, R., Ehrhardt, N., Kissling, D., Mahabir, E., Welzl, G., et al., 2007. Impact of IVC housing on emotionality and fear learning in male C3HeB/FeJ and C57BL/6J mice. Mamm. Genome 18, 173–186.

Kalsbeek, A., Yi, C.X., Cailotto, C., la Fleur, S.E., Fliers, E., Buijs, R.M., 2011. Mammalian clock output mechanisms. Essays Biochem. 49, 137–151.

Kang, S.J., Kim, D.H., Mishig-Ochir, T., Lee, B.J., 2012. Antimicrobial peptides: their physicochemical properties and therapeutic application. Arch. Pharm. Res. 35, 409–413.

Kaplan, B.F.L., Sulentic, C.E.W., Holsapple, M.P., Kaminski, N.E., 2013. Toxic responses of the immune system. In: Klassen, C.D. (Ed.), Casarett and Doull's Toxicology, The Basic Science of Poisons, eighth ed. McGraw-Hill Education, New York, pp. 485–545.

Karagöz, I., Biri, A., Babacan, F., Kavutçu, M., 2007. Evaluation of biological effects induced by diagnostic ultrasound in the rat foetal tissues. Mol. Cell Biochem. 217–224.

Karle, E.J., Gehring, F., Deerberg, F., 1980. Acidifying of drinking water and its effect on enamel lesions of rat teeth. Z. Versuchstierkd. 22, 80–88.

Karmarkar, S.W., Bottum, K.M., Tischkau, S.A., 2010. Considerations for the use of anesthetics in neurotoxicity studies. Comp. Med. 60, 256–262.

Katoh, H., Utsu, S., Chen, T.P., Moriwaki, K., 1990. H-2 polymorphisms in outbred strains of mice. Lab. Anim. Sci. 40, 490–494.

Katyal, R., Rana, S., Vaiphei, K., Ojha, S., Singh, V., Singh, K., 2001. Effect of rotavirus infection on lipid composition and glucose uptake in infant mouse intestine. Indian J. Gastroenterol. 20, 18–21.

Katzav, S., Shapiro, J., Segal, S., Feldman, M., 1986. General anesthesia during excision of a mouse tumor accelerates postsurgical growth of metastases by suppression of natural killer cell activity. Isr. J. Med. Sci. 22, 339–345.

Kawamoto, E., Sasaki, H., Okiyama, E., Kanai, T., Ueshiba, H., Ohnishi, N., et al., 2011. Pathogenicity of *Pasteurella pneumotropica* in immunodeficient NOD/ShiJic-scid/Jcl and immunocompetent Crlj:CD1 (ICR) mice. Exp. Anim. 60, 463–470.

Kay, M.M.B., 1978. Long term subclinical effects of parainfluenza (Sendai) infection on immune cells of aging mice. Proc. Soc. Exp. Biol. Med. 158, 326–331.

Kay, M.M.B., 1979. Parainfluenza infection of aged mice results in autoimmune disease. Clin. Immunol. Immunopathol. 12, 301–315.

Kay, M.M.B., Mendoza, J., Hausman, S., Dorsey, B., 1979. Age related changes in the immune system of mice of eight medium and long lived strains and hybrids. II. Short- and long-term effects of natural infection with parainfluenza type 1 virus (Sendai). Mech. Ageing Devel. 11, 347–362.

Kc, P., Haxhiu, M.A., Trouth, C.O., 2002. CO2-induced c-Fos expression in hypothalamic vasopressin containing neurons. Respir. Physiol. 129, 289–296.

Keenan, K.P., Laroque, P., Ballam, G.C., Soper, K.A., Dixit, R., Mattson, B.A., et al., 1996. The effects of diet, ad libitum overfeeding, and moderate dietary restriction on the rodent bioassay: the uncontrolled variable in safety assessment. Toxicol. Pathol. 24, 757–768.

Kelce, W.R., Wilson, E.M., 1997. Environmental antiandrogens: developmental effects, molecular mechanisms, and clinical implications. J. Mol. Med. (Berl) 75 (3), 198–207.

Kelche, C., Dalrymple-Alford, J.C., Will, B., 1988. Housing conditions modulate the effects of intracerebral grafts in rats with brain lesions. Behav. Brain Res. 28, 287–295.

Keller, L.S.F., White, W.J., Snider, M.T., Lang, M.C., 1989. An evaluation of intracage ventilation in three animal caging systems. Lab. Anim. Sci. 39, 237–242.

Kempermann, G., Brandon, E.P., Gage, F.H., 1998. Environmental stimulation of 129/SvJ mice causes increased cell proliferation and neurogenesis in the adult dentate gyrus. Curr. Biol. 8, 939–942.

Kennedy, B.W., Beal, T.S., 1991. Minerals leached into drinking water from rubber stoppers. Lab. Anim. Sci. 41, 233–236.

Kenyon, A.J., 1983. Delayed wound healing in mice associated with viral alteration of macrophages. Am. J. Vet. Res. 44, 652–656.

Khalil, N.A., Hashem, A.M., Ibrahim, A.A., Mousa, M.A., 2012. Effect of stress during handling, seawater acclimation, confinement, and induced spawning on plasma ion levels and somatolactin-expressing cells in mature female *Liza ramada*. J. Exp. Zool. A Ecol. Genet. Physiol. 317, 410–424.

Kharasch, E.D., 1998. Compound A: toxicology and clinical relevance. Anaesthesist 47 (Suppl. 1), S7–S10.

Kim, E.J., Kim, E.S., Covey, E., Kim, J.J., 2010. Social transmission of fear in rats: the role of 22-kHz ultrasonic distress vocalization. PLoS One 5, e15077.

Kim, Y.G., Park, J.H., Reimer, T., Baker, D.P., Kawai, T., Kumar, H., et al., 2011. Viral infection augments Nod1/2 signaling to potentiate lethality associated with secondary bacterial infections. Cell Host Microbe. 16, 496–507.

Kitchen, H., Aronson, A.L., Bittle, J.L., McPherson, C.W., Morton, D.B., Pakes, S.P., et al., 1987. Panel report on the colloquium on recognition and alleviation of animal pain and distress. J. Am. Vet. Med. Assoc. 191, 1186–1191.

Kitchen, A.M., Martin, A.A., 1996. The effects of cage size and complexity on the behaviour of captive common marmosets, Callithrix jacchus jacchus. Lab. Anim. 30 (4), 317–326.

Kittikulsuth, W., Sullivan, J.C., Pollock, D.M., 2013. ET-1 actions in the kidney: evidence for sex differences. Br. J. Pharmacol. 168, 318–326.

Kiyokawa, Y., Kikusui, T., Takeuchi, Y., Mori, Y., 2004. Modulatory role of testosterone in alarm pheromone release by male rats. Horm. Behav. 45 (2), 122–127.

Klein, R.M., 1986. Models for the study of cell proliferation in the developing gastrointestinal tract. J. Pediatr. Gastroenterol. Nutr. 5, 513–517.

Kligerman, A.D., Chapin, R.E., Erexson, G.L., Germolec, D.R., Kwanyuen, P., Yang, R.S., 1993. Analyses of cytogenetic damage in rodents following exposure to simulated groundwater contaminated with pesticides and a fertilizer. Mutat. Res. 300, 125–134.

Kobayashi, N., Bagheri, N., Nedrud, J.G., Strieter, R.M., Tomino, Y., Lamm, M.E., et al., 2003. Differential effects of Sendai virus infection on mediator synthesis by mesangial cells from two mouse strains. Kidney Int. 64, 1675–1684.

Koedrith, P., Kim, H., Weon, J.I., Seo, Y.R., 2013. Toxicogenomic approaches for understanding molecular mechanisms of heavy metal mutagenicity and carcinogenicity. Int. J. Hyg. Environ. Health. 216 (5), 587–598.

Koivusalo, M., Vartiainen, T., 1997. Drinking water chlorination by-products and cancer. Rev. Environ. Health 12, 81–90.

Kokolus, K.M., Capitano, M.L., Lee, C.T., Eng, J.W., Waight, J.D., Hylander, B.L., et al., 2013. Baseline tumor growth and immune control in laboratory mice are significantly influenced by sub-thermoneutral housing temperature. Proc. Natl. Acad. Sci. USA 18 [Epub ahead of print].

Komori, T., Fujiwara, R., Tanida, M., Nomura, J., Yokoyama, M.M., 1995a. Effects of citrus fragrance on immune function and depressive states. Neuroimmunomodulation 2, 174–180.

Komori, T., Fujiwara, R., Tanida, M., Nomura, J., 1995b. Potential antidepressant effects of lemon odor in rats. Eur. Neuropsychopharmacol. 5, 477–480.

Komori, T., Matsumoto, T., Motomura, E., Shiroyama, T., 2006. The sleep-enhancing effect of valerian inhalation and sleep-shortening effect of lemon inhalation. Chem. Senses 8, 731–737.

Kong, S., Zhang, S., Chen, Y., Wang, W., Wang, B., Chen, Q., et al., 2012. Determinants of uterine aging: lessons from rodent models. Sci. China Life Sci. 55, 687–693.

Koppel, J., Kuchar, S., Mozes, S., Petrusova, K., Jasenovec, A., 1982. Changes in blood sugar after administration of xylazine and adrenergic blockers in the rat. Vet. Med. (Praha) 27, 113–118.

Kostomitsopoulos, N., Alexakos, P., Eleni, K., Doulou, A., Paschidis, K., Baumans, V., 2012. The effects of different types of individually ventilated caging systems on growing male mice. Lab. Anim. (NY) 41, 192–197.

Kozul, C.D., Nomikos, A.P., Hampton, T.H., Warnke, L.A., Gosse, J.A., Davey, J.C., et al., 2008. Laboratory diet profoundly alters gene expression and confounds genomic analysis in mouse liver and lung. Chem. Biol. Interact. 173, 129–140.

Kozul-Horvath, C.D., Zandbergen, F., Jackson, B.P., Enelow, R.I., Hamilton, J.W., 2012. Effects of low-dose drinking water arsenic on mouse fetal and postnatal growth and development. PLoS One 7, e38249.

Krinke, G.J., Zurbriggen, A., 1997. Spontaneous demyelinating myelopathy in aging laboratory mice. Exp. Toxicol. Pathol. 49, 501–503.

Krohn, T.C., Hansen, A.K., Dragsted, N., 2003. The impact of low levels of carbon dioxide on rats. Lab. Anim. 37, 94–99.

Krupp, J.J., Levine, J.D., 2010. Biological rhythms: the taste-time continuum. Curr. Biol. 20, R147–R149.

Krzisch, M., Sultan, S., Sandell, J., Demeter, K., Vutskits, L., Toni, N., 2013. Propofol anesthesia impairs the maturation and survival of adult-born hippocampal neurons. Anesthesiology 118, 602–610.

Kufoy, E.A., Pakalnis, V.A., Parks, C.D., Wells, A., Yang, C.H., Fox, A., 1989. Keratoconjunctivitis sicca with associated secondary uveitis elicited in rats after systemic xylazine/ketamine anesthesia. Exp. Eye Res. 49, 861–871.

Kuhnen, G., 1997. The effect of cage size and environmental enrichment on the generation of fever in golden hamster. Ann. N. Y. Acad. Sci. 813, 398–400.

Kuhnen, G., 1998. Reduction of fever by housing in small cages. Lab. Anim. 32, 42–45.

Kuleskaya, N., Rauvala, H., Voikar, V., 2011. Evaluation of social and physical enrichment in modulation of behavioural phenotype in C57BL/6J female mice. PLoS One 6, e24755.

Kumar, V., Bhat, Z.A., Kumar, D., 2013. Animal models of anxiety: a comprehensive review. J. Pharmacol. Toxicol. Methods 68, 175–183.

Kumlin, T., Heikkinen, P., Laitinen, J.T., Juutilainen, J., 2005. Exposure to a 50-hz magnetic field induces a circadian rhythm in 6-hydroxymelatonin sulfate excretion in mice. J. Radiat. Res. 46, 313–318.

Kurima, K., Hertzano, R., Gavrilova, O., Monahan, K., Shpargel, K.B., Nadaraja, G., et al., 2011. A noncoding point mutation of Zeb1 causes multiple developmental malformations and obesity in Twirler mice. PLoS Genet. 7, e1002307.

Kutza, J., Gratz, I., Afshar, M., Murasko, D.M., 1997. The effects of general anesthesia and surgery on basal and interferon stimulated natural killer cell activity of humans. Anesth. Analg. 85, 918–923.

Kurzer, M.S., Xu, X., 1997. Dietary phytoestrogens. Annu. Rev. Nutr. 17, 353–381.

Kwiatkowska-Patzer, B., Patzer, J.A., Heller, L.J., 1993. *Pseudomonas aeruginosa* exotoxin A enhances automaticity and potentiates hypoxic depression of isolated rat hearts. Proc. Soc. Exp. Biol. Med. 202, 377–383.

Lacey, J.C., Beynon, R.J., Hurst, J.L., 2007. The importance of exposure to other male scents in determining competitive behaviour among inbred male mice. Appl. Anim. Behav. Sci. 104, 130–142.

Lachmann, S., Bär, S., Rommelaere, J., Nüesch, J.P., 2007. Parvovirus interference with intracellular signalling: mechanism of PKCη activation in MVM-infected A9 fibroblasts. Cell. Microbiol. 10, 755–769.

Lagutchik, M.S., Mundie, T.G., Martin, D.G., 1992. Methemoglobinemia induced by benzocaine-based topically administered anesthetic in eight sheep. J. Am. Vet. Med. Assoc. 201, 1407–1410.

Lahmy, C., Virelizier, J.L., 1981. Prostaglandins as probable mediators of the suppression of antibody production by mouse hepatitis virus infection. Ann. Immunol. 132, 101–105.

Lai, H., Carino, M.A., Ushijima, I., 1998. Acute exposure to a 60 Hz magnetic field affects rats' water-maze performance. Bioelectromagnetics 19, 117–122.

Lai, H., 2004. Interaction of microwaves and a temporally incoherent magnetic field on spatial learning in the rat. Physiol. Behav. 82, 785–789.

Lai, W.C., Pakes, S.P., Lu, Y.S., Brayton, C.F., 1987. *Mycoplasma pulmonis* infection augments natural killer cell activity in mice. Lab. Anim. Sci. 37, 299–303.

Lakshman, M., Xu, L., Ananthanarayanan, V., Cooper, J., Takimoto, C.H., Helenowski, I., et al., 2008. Dietary genistein inhibits metastasis of human prostate cancer in mice. Cancer Res. 68, 2024–2032.

Laltoo, H., Kind, L.S., 1979. Reduction in contact sensitivity reactions to oxazolone in mite-infested mice. Infect. Immun. 26, 30–35.

Lamana, M.L., Albella, B., Bueren, J.A., Segovia, J.C., 2001. *In vitro* and *in vivo* susceptibility of mouse megakaryocytic progenitors to strain i of parvovirus minute virus of mice. Exp. Hematol. 29, 1303–1309.

Lambert, L.C., Trummell, H.Q., Singh, A., Cassell, G.H., Bridges, R.J., 1998. *Mycoplasma pulmonis* inhibits electrogenic ion transport across murine epithelial cell monolayers. Infect. Immun. 66, 272–279.

Landi, M.S., Kreider, J.W., Lang, C.M., Bullock, L.P., 1982. Effects of shipping on the immune function in mice. Am. J. Vet. Res. 43, 1654–1657.

Landin, A.M., Frasca, D., Zaias, J., Van der Put, E., Riley, R.L., Altman, N.H., et al., 2009. Effects of fenbendazole on the murine humoral immune system. J. Am. Assoc. Lab. Anim. Sci. 48 (3), 251–257.

Lanum, J., 1978. The damaging effects of light on the retina. Empirical findings, theoretical and practical implications. Surv. Ophthalmol. 22, 221–249.

Lardans, V., Godfraind, C., van der Logt, J.T., Heesen, W.A., Gonzalez, M.D., Coutelier, J.P., 1996. Polyclonal B lymphocyte activation induced by mouse hepatitis virus A59 infection. J. Gen. Virol. 77, 1005–1009.

Laroche, J., Gasbarro, L., Herman, J.P., Blaustein, J.D., 2009. Reduced behavioral response to gonadal hormones in mice shipped during the peripubertal/adolescent period. Endocrinology 150, 2351–2358.

Larsen, M.G., Baatrup, E., 2010. Functional behavior and reproduction in androgenic sex reversed zebrafish (*Danio rerio*). Environ. Toxicol. Chem. 29, 1828–1833.

Larsen, M.G., Bilberg, K., Baatrup, E., 2009. Reversibility of estrogenic sex changes in zebrafish (Danio rerio). Environ. Toxicol. Chem. 28 (8), 1783–1785.

Lasbury, M.E., Lin, P., Tschang, D., Durant, P.J., Lee, C.H., 2004. Effect of bronchoalveolar lavage fluid from *Pneumocystis carinii*-infected hosts on phagocytic activity of alveolar macrophages. Infect. Immun. 72, 2140–2147.

La Vail, M.M., 1976. Survival of some photoceptor cells in albino rats following long-term exposure to continuous light. Invest. Ophthalmol. 15, 64–72.

Lavelle, G.C., Bang, F.B., 1973. Differential growth of MHV (PRI) and MHV (C3H) in genetically resistant C3H mice rendered susceptible by eperythrozoon infection. Arch. Gesamte Virusforsch. 41, 175–184.

Lavilla-Apelo, C., Kida, H., Kanagawa, H., 1992. The effect of experimental infection of mouse preimplantation embryos with paramyxovirus Sendai. J. Vet. Med. Sci. 54, 335–340.

Le Berre, R., Faure, K., Fauvel, H., Viget, N.B., Ader, F., Prangère, T., et al., 2004. Apoptosis inhibition in *P. aeruginosa*-induced lung injury influences lung fluid balance. Intensive Care Med. 30, 1204–1211.

Lèche, A., Della Costa, N.S., Hansen, C., Navarro, J.L., Marin, R.H., Martella, M.B., 2013. Corticosterone stress response of Greater Rhea (*Rhea americana*) during short-term road transport. Poult. Sci. 92, 60–63.

Lee, J.F., Liao, P.M., Tseng, D.H., Wen, P.T., 1998. Behavior of organic polymers in drinking water purification. Chemosphere 37, 1045–1061.

Lee, S.K., Youn, H.Y., Hasegawa, A., Nakayama, H., Goto, N., 1994. Apoptotic changes in the thymus of mice infected with mouse hepatitis virus, MHV-2. J. Vet. Med. Sci. 56, 879–882.

Lee, T.M., McClintock, M.K., 1986. Female rats in a laboratory display seasonal variation in fecundity. J. Reprod. Fertil. 77, 51–59.

Legates, T.A., Dunn, D., Weber, E.T., 2009. Accelerated re-entrainment to advanced light cycles in BALB/cJ mice. Physiol. Behav. 98, 427–432.

Lemke, L.B., Ge, Z., Whary, M.T., Feng, Y., Rogers, A.B., Muthupalani, S., et al., 2009. Concurrent *Helicobacter bilis* infection in C57BL/6 mice attenuates proinflammatory *H. pylori*-induced gastric pathology. Infect. Immun. 77, 2147–2158.

Lencioni, K.C., Seamons, A., Treuting, P.M., Maggio-Price, L., Brabb, T., 2008. Murine norovirus: an intercurrent variable in a mouse model of bacteria-induced inflammatory bowel disease. Comp. Med. 58, 522–533.

Lephart, E.D., West, T.W., Weber, K.S., Rhees, R.W., Setchell, K.D., Adlercreutz, H., et al., 2002. Neurobehavioral effects of dietary soy phytoestrogens. Neurotoxicol. Teratol. 24, 5–16.

Leray, D., Dupuy, C., Dupuy, J.M., 1982. Immunopathology of mouse hepatitis virus type 3 infection. IV. MHV3-induced immunodepression. Clin. Immunol. Immunopathol. 23, 539–547.

Levy, G.A., Leibowitz, J.L., Edington, T.S., 1981. Induction of monocyte procoagulant activity by murine hepatitis virus type 3 parallels disease susceptibility in mice. J. Exp. Med. 154, 1150–1163.

Levy, J., 2000. The effects of antibiotic use on gastrointestinal function. Am. J. Gastroenterol. 95, S8–S10.

Leys, L.J., McGaraughty, S., Radek, R.J., 2012. Rats housed on corncob bedding show less slow-wave sleep. J. Am. Assoc. Lab. Anim. Sci. 51, 764–768.

Li, Y., Liu, Y., Jiang, Z., Guan, J., Yi, G., Cheng, S., et al., 2009. Behavioral change related to Wenchuan devastating earthquake in mice. Bioelectromagnetics 30, 613–620.

Li, J., Liu, Y., Zhang, X., 2010. Murine coronavirus induces type I interferon in oligodendrocytes through recognition by RIG-I and MDA5. J. Virol. 84, 6472–6482.

Liang, C.-T., Shih, A., Chang, Y.-H., Liu, C.-W., Lee, Y.-T., Hsieh, W.-C., et al., 2009. Microbial contaminations of laboratory mice and rats in Taiwan from 2004-2007. J. Am. Assoc. Lab. Anim. Sci. 48, 381–386.

Lieggi, C.C., Artwohl, J.E., Leszczynski, J.K., Rodriguez, N.A., Fickbohm, B.L., Fortman, J.D., 2005. Efficacy and safety of stored and newly prepared tribromoethanol in ICR mice. Contemp. Top. Lab. Anim. Sci. 44 (1), 17–22.

Limper, A.H., Edens, M., Anders, R.A., Leof, E.B., 1998. *Pneumocystis carinii* inhibits cyclin-dependent kinase activity in lung epithelial cells. J. Clin. Invest. 101, 1148–1155.

Lindsey, J.R., Conner, M.W., Baker, H.J., 1978. Physical, chemical and microbial factor affecting biologic response "Symposium on Laboratory Animal Housing" (Inst. Lab. Anim. Resour.). Natl. Acad. Sci.-Natl. Resour. Counc. Washington, DC, pp. 37–43.

Line, S.W., Morgan, K.N., Markowitz, H., Strong, S., 1989. Influence of cage size on heart rate and behavior in rhesus monkeys. Am. J. Vet. Res. 50, 1523–1526.

Lipman, N.S., 1999. Isolator rodent caging systems (state of the art): a critical review. Contemp. Top. Lab. Anim. Sci. 38, 9–17.

Lipschik, G.Y., Treml, J.F., Moore, S.D., 1996. *Pneumocystis carinii* glycoprotein A stimulates interleukin-8 production and inflammatory cell activation in alveolar macrophages and cultured monocytes. J. Eukaryot. Microbiol. 43, 16S–17S.

Lipsky, M.M., Skinner, M., Oconnell, C., 1993. Effects of chloroform and bromodichloromethane on DNA synthesis in male F344 rat kidney. Environ. Health Perspect. 101 (Suppl. 5), 249–252.

Liu, K.Q., Yin, W.D., Xue, G.P., Zhang, J.S., 2007. Study on the changes of soluble intercellular adhesion molecule-1 level in sera of rats infected with *Pneumocystis carinii*. Zhongguo Ji Sheng Chong Xue Yu Ji Sheng Chong Bing Za Zhi 25 27–31, 35.

Livingston, R.S., Besch-Williford, C.L., Myles, M.H., Franklin, C.L., Crim, M.J., Riley, L.K., 2011. *Pneumocystis carinii* infection causes lung lesions historically attributed to rat respiratory virus. Comp. Med. 61, 45–59.

Liyanage, N.P., Manthey, K.C., Dassanayake, R.P., Kuszynski, C.A., Oakley, G.G., Duhamel, G.E., 2010. *Helicobacter hepaticus* cytolethal distending toxin causes cell death in intestinal epithelial cells via mitochondrial apoptotic pathway. Helicobacter 15, 98–107.

Lockett, M.F., 1970. Effects of sound on endocrine function and electrolyte excretion. In: Welch, B.L., Welch, A.S. (Eds.), Physiological Effects of Noise. Plenum Press, New York, pp. 21–42.

Logge, W., Kingham, J., Karl, T., 2013. Behavioural consequences of IVC cages on male and female C57BL/6J mice. Neuroscience 237, 285–293.

Loh, D.H., Navarro, J., Hagopian, A., Wang, L.M., Deboer, T., Colwell, C.S., 2010. Rapid changes in the light/dark cycle disrupt memory of conditioned fear in mice. PLoS One 5, e12546.

Lohmiller, J.J., Lipman, N.S., 1998. Silicon crystals in water of autoclaved glass bottles. Contemp. Top. Lab. Anim. Sci. 37, 62–65.

Long, N.C., Morimoto, A., Nakamori, T., Murakami, N., 1991. The effect of physical restraint on IL-lbeta- and LPS-induced fever. Physiol. Behav. 50, 625–628.

Longstreth, J., de Gruijl, F.R., Kripke, M.L., Abseck, S., Arnold, F., Slaper, H.I., et al., 1998. Health risks. J. Photochem. Photobiol. B. 46, 20–39.

Lopez, G.U., Gerba, C.P., Tamimi, A.H., Kitajima, M., Maxwell, S.L., Rose, J.B., 2013. Appl. Environ. Microbiol. 79, 5728–5734.

Lopez-Guerrero, D.V., Meza-Perez, S., Ramirez-Pliego, O., Santana-Calderon, M.A., Espino-Solis, P., Gutierrez-Xicotencatl, L., et al., 2009. Rotavirus infection activates dendritic cells from Peyer's patches in adult mice. J. Virol. 84, 1856–1866.

López-Olmeda, J.F., Tartaglione, E.V., de la Iglesia, H.O., Sánchez-Vázquez, F.J., 2010. Feeding entrainment of food-anticipatory activity and per1 expression in the brain and liver of zebrafish under different lighting and feeding conditions. Chronobiol. Int. 27, 1380–1400.

Lu, K., Knutson, C.G., Wishnok, J.S., Fox, J.G., Tannenbaum, S.R., 2012. Serum metabolomics in a *Helicobacter hepaticus* mouse model of inflammatory bowel disease reveal important changes in the microbiome, serum peptides, and intermediary metabolism. J. Proteome Res. 11, 4916–4926.

Lubcke, R., Hutcheson, F.A., Barbezat, G.O., 1992. Impaired intestinal electrolyte transport in rats infested with the common parasite *Syphacia muris*. Dig. Dis. Sci. 37, 60–64.

Lukacinova, A., Benacka, R., Sedlakova, E., Lovasova, E., Nistiar, F., 2012. Multigenerational lifetime low-dose exposure to heavy metals on selected reproductive parameters in rats. J. Environ. Sci. Health A Tox. Hazard Subst. Environ. Eng. 47, 1280–1287.

Lynch, M.A., Brodt, M.D., Silva, M.J., 2010. Skeletal effects of whole-body vibration in adult and aged mice. J. Orthop. Res. 28 (2), 241–247.

Lyte, M., Li, W., Opitz, N., Gaykema, R.P., Goehler, L.E., 2006. Induction of anxiety-like behavior in mice during the initial stages of infection with the agent of murine colonic hyperplasia *Citrobacter rodentium*. Physiol. Behav. 89, 350–357.

Macdonald, N., Gledhill, A., 2007. Potential impact of ABCB1 (p-glycoprotein) polymorphisms on avermectin toxicity in humans. Arch. Toxicol. 81, 553–563.

MacMillian, R., 2009. Human vibration basic characteristics: occupational health and safety practitioner. In: Guo, J. (Ed.), Worksafe, Western Perth (Australia), pp. 10–16.

Machado, G.B., de Oliveira, A.V., Saliba, A.M., de Lima, C.D., Suassuna, J.H., Plotkowski, M.C., 2011. *Pseudomonas aeruginosa* toxin ExoU induces a PAF-dependent impairment of alveolar fibrin turnover secondary to enhanced activation of coagulation and increased expression of plasminogen activator inhibitor-1 in the course of mice pneumosepsis. Respir. Res. 12, 104.

MacPhail, R.C., Brooks, J., Hunter, D.L., Padnos, B., Irons, T.D., Padilla, S., 2009. Locomotion in larval zebrafish: influence of time of day, lighting and ethanol. Neurotoxicology 30 (1), 52–58.

Maggio-Price, L., Nicholson, K.L., Kline, K.M., Birkebak, T., Suzuki, I., Wilson, D.L., et al., 1998. Diminished reproduction, failure to thrive, and altered immunologic function in a colony of T-cell receptor transgenic mice: possible role of *Citrobacter rodentium*. Lab. Anim. Sci. 48, 145–155.

Maggio-Price, L., Bielefeldt-Ohmann, H., Treuting, P., Iritani, B.M., Zeng, W., Nicks, A., et al., 2005. Dual infection with *Helicobacter bilis* and *Helicobacter hepaticus* in p-glycoprotein-deficient mdr1a-/- mice results in colitis that progresses to dysplasia. Am. J. Pathol. 166, 1793–1806.

Malberg, J.E., Seiden, L.S., 1998. Small changes in ambient temperature cause large changes in 3,4-methylenedioxymethamphetamine (MDMA)-induced serotonin neurotoxicity and core body temperature in the rat. J. Neurosci. 18, 5086–5094.

Malenke, J.R., Magnanou, E., Thomas, K., Dearing, M.D., 2012. Cytochrome P450 2B diversity and dietary novelty in the herbivorous, desert woodrat (*Neotoma lepida*). PLoS One 7, e41510.

Manaker, R.A., Piczak, C.W., Miller, A.A., Stanton, M.F., 1961. A hepatitis virus complicating studies with mouse leukemia. J. Natl. Cancer Inst. 27, 29–45.

Mani, S.K., Reyna, A.M., Alejandro, M.A., Crowley, J., Markaverich, B.M., 2005. Disruption of male sexual behavior in rats by tetrahydrofurandiols (THF-diols). Steroids 70, 750–754.

Marashi, V., Barnekow, A., Sachser, N., 2004. Effects of environmental enrichment on males of a docile inbred strain of mice. Physiol. Behav. 82, 765–776.

Markaverich, B.M., Alejandro, M.A., Markaverich, D., Zitzow, L., Casajuna, N., Camarao, N., et al., 2002a. Identification of an endocrine disrupting agent from corn with mitogenic activity. Biochem. Biophys. Res. Commun. 291, 692–700.

Markaverich, B., Mani, S., Alejandro, M.A., Mitchell, A., Markaverich, D., Brown, T., et al., 2002b. A novel endocrine-disrupting agent in corn with mitogenic activity in human breast and prostatic cancer cells. Environ. Health Perspect. 110, 169–177.

Markovic, S.N., Murasko, D.M., 1990. Anesthesia inhibits poly I: C induced stimulation of natural killer cell cytotoxicity in mice. Clin. Immunol. Immunopathol. 56, 202–209.

Markovic, S.N., Murasko, D.M., 1991. Inhibition of induction of natural killer activity in mice by general anesthesia (Avertin): role of interferon. Clin. Immunol. Immunopathol. 60, 181–189.

Markovic, S.N., Murasko, D.M., 1993. Anesthesia inhibits interferon-induced natural killer cell cytotoxicity via induction of CD8+ suppressor cells. Cell. Immunol. 151, 474–480.

Markovic, S.N., Knight, P.R., Murasko, D.M., 1993. Inhibition of interferon stimulation of natural killer cell activity in mice anesthetized with halothane or isoflurane. Anesthesiology 78, 700–706.

Marques, J.M., Olsson, I.A., 2007. The effect of preweaning and postweaning housing on the behaviour of the laboratory mouse (Mus musculus). Lab. Anim. 41, 92–102.

Marques, R.S., Cooke, R.F., Francisco, C.L., Bohnert, D.W., 2012. Effects of twenty-four hour transport or twenty-four hour feed and water deprivation on physiologic and performance responses of feeder cattle. J. Anim. Sci. 90, 5040–5046.

Martin, C., Thévenot, G., Danel, S., Chapron, J., Tazi, A., Macey, J., et al., 2011. *Pseudomonas aeruginosa* induces vascular endothelial growth factor synthesis in airway epithelium *in vitro* and *in vivo*. Eur. Respir. J. 38, 939–946.

Martin, G.M., 2011. The biology of aging: 1985–2010 and beyond. FASEB J. 25, 3756–3762.

Martínez-Carrillo, B.E., Godinez-Victoria, M., Jarillo-Luna, A., Oros-Pantoja, R., Abarca-Rojano, E., Rivera-Aguilar, V., et al., 2011. Repeated restraint stress reduces the number of IgA-producing cells in Peyer's patches. Neuroimmunomodulation 18, 131–141.

Maślanka, T., Jaroszewski, J.J., Chrostowska, M., 2004. Pathogenesis of quinolone-induced arthropathy: a review of hypotheses. Pol. J. Vet. Sci. 7, 323–331.

Masoro, E.J., 1992. Aging and proliferative homeostasis: modulation by food restriction in rodents. Lab. Anim. Sci. 42, 132–137.

Matos-Cruz, V., Blasic, J., Nickle, B., Robinson, P.R., Hattar, S., Halpern, M.E., 2011. Unexpected diversity and photoperiod dependence of the zebrafish melanopsin system. PLoS One 6, e25111.

Matsumiya, L.C., Lavoie, C., 2003. An outbreak of *Pasteurella pneumotropica* in genetically modified mice: treatment and elimination. Contemp. Top. Lab. Anim. Sci. 42, 26–28.

Matsuya, Y., Kusano, T., Endo, S., Takahashi, N., Yamane, I., 1978. Reduced tumorigenicity by addition *in vitro* of Sendai virus. Eur. J. Cancer 14, 837–850.

Mayeux, P., Dupepe, L., Dunn, K., Balsamo, J., Domer, J., 1995. Massive fungal contamination in animal care facilities traced to bedding supply. Appl. Environ. Microbiol. 61, 2297–2301.

Mazelis, A.G., Albert, D., Crisa, C., Fiore, H., Parasaram, D., Franklin, B., et al., 1987. Relationship of stressful housing conditions to the onset of diabetes mellitus induced by multiple, sub-diabetogenic doses of streptozotocin in mice. Diabetes Res. 6, 195–200.

Mazze, R.I., Cousins, M.J., Kosek, J.C., 1973. Strain differences in metabolism and susceptibility to the nephrotoxic effects of methoxyflurane in rats. J. Pharmacol. Exp. Ther. 184, 481–488.

McCullough, K.C., Summerfield, A., 2005. Basic concepts of immune response and defense development. ILAR J. 46, 230–240.

McFadden, N., Bailey, D., Carrara, G., Benson, A., Chaudhry, Y., Shortland, A., et al., 2011. Norovirus regulation of the innate immune response and apoptosis occurs via the product of the alternative open reading frame 4. PLoS Pathog. 7, e1002413.

McGavern, D.B., Murray, P.D., Rivera-Quinones, C., Schmelzer, J.D., Low, P.A., Rodriguez, M., 2000. Axonal loss results in spinal cord atrophy, electrophysiological abnormalities and neurological deficits following demyelination in a chronic inflammatory model of multiple sclerosis. Brain 123, 519–531.

McGinn, M.D., Bean-Knudsen, D., Ermel, R.W., 1992. Incidence of otitis media in CBA/J and CBA/CaJ mice. Hear. Res. 59, 1–6.

McGlone, J.J., Anderson, D.L., Norman, R.L., 2001. Floor space needs for laboratory mice: BALB/cJ males or females in solid-bottom cages with bedding. Contemp. Top. Lab. Anim. Sci. 40 (3), 21–25.

McInnes, E.F., Rasmussen, L., Fung, P., Auld, A.M., Alvarez, L., Lawrence, D.A., et al., 2011. Prevalence of viral, bacterial and parasitological diseases in rats and mice used in research environments in Australasia over a 5-y period. Lab. Anim. 40, 341–350.

McIntosh, J.C., Simecka, J.W., Ross, S.E., Davis, J.K., Miller, E.J., Cassell, G.H., 1992. Infection-induced airway fibrosis in two rat strains with differential susceptibility. Infect. Immun. 60, 2936–2942.

McKisic, M.D., Lancki, D.W., Otto, G., Padrid, P., Snook, S., Cronin II, D.C., et al., 1993. Identification and propagation of a putative immunosuppressive orphan parvovirus in cloned T cells. J. Immunol. 150, 419–428.

McKisic, M.D., Macy Jr., J.D., Delano, M.L., Jacoby, R.O., Paturzo, F.X., Smith, A.L., 1998. Mouse parvovirus infection potentiates allogeneic skin graft rejection and induces syngeneic graft rejection. Transplantation 65, 1436–1446.

McNair, D.M., Timmons, E.H., 1977. Effects of *Aspiculuris tetraptera* and *Syphacia obvelata* on exploratory behavior of an inbred mouse strain. Lab. Anim. Sci. 27, 38–42.

Meaney, M.J., Diorio, J., Francis, D., Widdowson, J., LaPlante, P., Caldji, C., et al., 1996. Early environmental regulation of forebrain glucocorticoid receptor gene expression: implications for adrenocortical responses to stress. Dev. Neurosci. 18, 49–72.

Meijer, M.K., Sommer, R., Spruijt, B.M., van Zutphen, L.F., Baumans, V., 2007. Influence of environmental enrichment and handling on the acute stress response in individually housed mice. Lab. Anim. 41, 161–173.

Meinl, W., Sczesny, S., Brigelius-Flohé, R., Blaut, M., Glatt, H., 2009. Impact of gut microbiota on intestinal and hepatic levels of phase 2 xenobiotic-metabolizing enzymes in the rat. Drug Metab. Dispos. 37, 1179–1186.

Meller, A., Kasanen, I., Ruksenas, O., Apanaviciene, N., Baturaite, Z., Voipio, H.M., et al., 2011. Refining cage change routines: comparison of cardiovascular responses to three different ways of cage change in rats. Lab. Anim. 45, 167–173.

Memarzadeh, F., Harrison, P.C., Riskowski, G.L., Henze, T., 2004. Comparison of environment and mice in static and mechanically ventilated isolator cages with different air velocities and ventilation designs. Contemp. Top. Lab. Anim. Sci. 43 (1), 14–20.

Menaker, M., Eskin, A., 1966. Entrainment of circadian rhythms by sound in *Passer domesticus*. Science 154, 1579–1581.

Mendoza, S.P., Lowe, E.L., Davidson, J.M., Levine, S., 1978. Annual cyclicity in the squirrel monkey (*Saimiri sciureus*): the relationship between testosterone, fatting, and sexual behavior. Horm. Behav. 11, 295–303.

Mercier, F.J., Denjean, A., 1996. Guinea-pig tracheal responsiveness *in vitro* following general anaesthesia with halothane. Eur. Respir. J. 9, 1451–1455.

Metcalf, J.F., Wilson, G.B., 1987. Use of mitogen-induced lymphocyte transformation to assess toxicity of aminoglycosides. J. Environ. Pathol. Toxicol. Oncol. 7, 27–37.

Meyer, L.M., Löfgren, S., Holz, F.G., Wegener, A., Söderberg, P., 2013. Bilateral cataract induced by unilateral UVR-B exposure –

evidence for an inflammatory response. Acta Ophthalmol. 91, 236–242.

Mi, W., Belyavskyi, M., Johnson, R.R., Sieve, A.N., Storts, R., Meagher, M.W., et al., 2004. Alterations in chemokine expression following Theiler's virus infection and restraint stress. J. Neuroimmunol. 151, 103–115.

Miazza, V., Mottet-Osman, G., Startchick, S., Chaponnier, C., Roux, L., 2011. Sendai virus induced cytoplasmic actin remodeling correlates with efficient virus particle production. Virology 410, 7–16.

Michels, C., Goyal, P., Nieuwenhuizen, N., Brombacher, F., 2006. Infection with *Syphacia obvelata* (pinworm) induces protective Th2 immune responses and influences ovalbumin-induced allergic reactions. Infect. Immun. 74, 5926–5932.

Mihara, T., Kikuchi, T., Kamiya, Y., Koga, M., Uchimoto, K., Kurahashi, K., et al., 2012. Day or night administration of ketamine and pentobarbital differentially affect circadian rhythms of pineal melatonin secretion and locomotor activity in rats. Anesth. Analg. 115, 805–813.

Miller, C.P., Hammond, C.W., Anderle, S.K., 1960. Studies on susceptibility to infection following ionizing radiation. V. Comparison of intraperitoneal and intravenous challenge at intervals following different doses of x-radiation. J. Exp. Med. 111, 773–784.

Miller, G.F., Barnard, D.E., Woodward, R.A., Flynn, B.M., Bulte, J.W., 1997. Hepatic hemosiderosis in common marmosets, *Callithrix jacchus*: effect of diet on incidence and severity. Lab. Anim. Sci. 47, 138–142.

Milligan, S.R., Sales, G.D., Khirynkh, K., 1993. Sound levels in rooms housing laboratory animals: an uncontrolled daily variable. Physiol. Behav. 53, 1067–1076.

Milone, M.C., Fitzgerald-Bocarsly, P., 1998. The mannose receptor mediates induction of IFN-alpha in peripheral blood dendritic cells by enveloped RNA and DNA viruses. J. Immunol. 161, 2391–2399.

Mineur, Y.S., Crusio, W.E., 2009. Behavioral effects of ventilated microenvironment housing in three inbred mouse strains. Physiol. Behav. 97, 334–340.

Mitsushima, D., Takase, K., Takahashi, T., Kimura, F., 2009. Activational and organisational effects of gonadal steroids on sex-specific acetylcholine release in the dorsal hippocampus. J. Neuroendocrinol. 21, 400–405.

Mizuno, S., Ishida, A., 1982. Selective enhancement of the cytotoxicity of the bleomycin derivative, peplomycin, by local anesthetics alone and combined with hyperthermia. Cancer Res. 42, 4726–4729.

Modric, S., Martinez, M., 2011. Patient variation in veterinary medicine-part II – influence of physiological variables. J. Vet. Pharmacol. Ther. 34, 209–223.

Mohn, G., Philipp, E.M., 1981. Effects of *Syphacia muris* and the anthelmintic fenbendazole on the microsomal monooxygenase system in mouse liver. Lab. Anim. 15, 89–95.

Molano, A., Huang, Z., Marko, M.G., Azzi, A., Wu, D., Wang, E., et al., 2012. Age-dependent changes in the sphingolipid composition of mouse CD4+ T cell membranes and immune synapses implicate glucosylceramides in age-related T cell dysfunction. PLoS One 7, e47650.

Molina-Holgado, E., Arevalo-Martin, A., Ortiz, S., Vela, J.M., Guaza, C., 2002. Theiler's virus infection induces the expression of cyclooxygenase-2 in murine astrocytes: inhibition by the anti-inflammatory cytokines interleukin-4 and interleukin-10. Neurosci. Lett. 324, 237–241.

Montenegro, M.A., Palomino, H., Palomino, H.M., 1995. The influence of earthquake induced stress on human facial clefting and its simulation in mice. Arch. Oral. Biol. 40, 33–37.

Morales, S.V.M., Llopis, G.A., Tejerizo, P.M.L., Ferrandiz, F.J., 1993. Concentration on nitrates in drinking water and its relationship with bladder cancer. J. Environ. Pathol. Toxicol. Oncol. 12, 229–236.

Mordelet-Dambrine, M., Danel, C., Farinotti, R., Urzua, G., Barritault, L., Huchon, G.J., 1992. Influence of *Pneumocystis carinii* pneumonia

on serum and tissue concentrations of pentamidine administered to rats by tracheal injections. Am. Rev. Respir. Dis. 146, 735–739.

Morita, E., Kaneko, S., Hiragun, T., Shindo, H., Tanaka, T., Furukawa, T., et al., 1999. Fur mites induce dermatitis associated with IgE hyperproduction in an inbred strain of mice, NC/Kuj. J. Dermatol. Sci. 19, 37–43.

Morris, C.J., Aeschbach, D., Scheer, F.A., 2012. Circadian system, sleep and endocrinology. Mol. Cell. Endocrinol. 349, 91–104.

Morris, R.D., Audet, A.M., Angelillo, I.F., Chalmers, T.C., Mosteller, F., 1992. Chlorination, chlorination by-products, and cancer: a meta-analysis. Am. J. Public Health 82, 955–964.

Morseth, S.L., Dengerink, H.A., Wright, J.W., 1985. Effect of impulse noise on water consumption and blood pressure in the female rat. Physiol. Behav. 34, 1013–1016.

Moudgil, G.C., 1986. Update on Anaesthesia and the Immune Response. Can. Anaesth. Soc. J 33, 554–560.

Mrosovsky, N., 1988. Phase response curve for social entrainment. J. Comp. Physiol. 162, 35–46.

Mucignat-Caretta, C., Cavaggioni, A., Caretta, A., 2004. Male urinary chemosignals differentially affect aggressive behavior in male mice. J. Chem. Ecol. 30, 777–791.

Mulder, J.B., 1971. Animal behavior and electromagnetic energy waves. Lab. Anim. Sci. 21, 389–393.

Munsters, C.C., de Gooijer, J.W., van den Broek, J., van Oldruitenborgh-Oosterbaan, M.M., 2013. Heart rate, heart rate variability and behaviour of horses during air transport. Vet. Rec. 172, 15.

Mutsvunguma, L.Z., Moetlhoa, B., Edkins, A.L., Luke, G.A., Blatch, G.L., Knox, C., 2011. Theiler's murine encephalomyelitis virus infection induces a redistribution of heat shock proteins 70 and 90 in BHK-21 cells, and is inhibited by novobiocin and geldanamycin. Cell Stress Chaperones. 16, 505–515.

Namiki, M., Takayama, H., Fujiwara, K., 1977. Viral growth in splenic megakaryocytes of mice experimentally infected with mouse hepatitis virus MHV-2. Jpn. J. Exp. Med. 47, 41–48.

National Research Council, 2011. Guide for the Care and Use of Laboratory Animals. National Academy of Sciences, Washington, DC.

National Toxicology Program, 1997. Effect of dietary restriction on toxicology and carcinogenesis studies in F344/N rats and B6C3F1 mice. Natl. Toxicol. Program Tech. Rep. Ser 460, 1–414.

Natusch, C., Schwarting, R.K., 2010. Using bedding in a test environment critically affects 50-kHz ultrasonic vocalizations in laboratory rats. Pharmacol. Biochem. Behav. 96, 251–259.

Naylor, P.H., Hadden, J.W., 2003. T cell targeted immune enhancement yields effective T cell adjuvants. Int. Immunopharmacol. 3, 1205–1215.

Nelson, J.B., 1960. The problems of disease and quality in laboratory animals. J. Med. Educ. 35, 34–43.

Nelson, R.J., Zucker, I., 1987. Spontaneous testicular recrudescence of Syrian hamsters: role of stimulatory photoperiods. Physiol. Behav. 39, 616–617.

Nettesheim, P., Schreiber, H., Cresia, D.A., Richter, C.B., 1974. Respiratory infections in the pathogenesis of lung cancer. Recent Results Cancer Res. 44, 138–157.

Nettesheim, P., Topping, D.C., Jambasi, R., 1981. Host and environmental factors enhancing carcinogenesis in the respiratory tract. Ann. Rev. Pharmacol. Toxicol. 21, 133–163.

Newberne, P.M., McConnell, R.G., 1980. Dietary nutrients and contaminants in laboratory animal experimentation. J. Environ. Pathol. Toxicol. 4, 105–122.

Newberne, P.M., Weigert, J., Kula, N., 1979. Effects of dietary fat on hepatic mixed-function oxidases and hepatocellular carcinoma induced by aflatoxin B1 in rats. Cancer Res. 39, 3986–3991.

Newman, J.V., Kosaka, T., Sheppard, B.J., Fox, J.G., Schauer, D.B., 2001. Bacterial infection promotes colon tumorigenesis in $Apc^{Min/+}$ mice. J. Infect. Dis. 184, 227–230.

Newton, W.M., 1978. Environmental impact on laboratory animals. Adv. Vet. Sci. Comp. Med. 22, 1–28.

Nguyen, D.D., Muthupalani, S., Goettel, J.A., Eston, M.A., Mobley, M., Taylor, N.S., et al., 2013. Colitis and colon cancer in WASP-deficient mice require *Helicobacter* species. Inflamm. Bowel Dis. 19, 2041–2050.

Nichelmann, M., Tzschentke, B., 2002. Ontogeny of thermoregulation in precocial birds. Comp. Biochem. Physiol. A Mol. Integr. Physiol. 131, 751–763.

Nicholson, A., Malcolm, R.D., Russ, P.L., Cough, K., Touma, C., Palme, R., et al., 2009. The response of C57BL/6J and BALB/cJ mice to increased housing density. J. Am. Assoc. Lab. Anim. Sci. 48, 740–753.

Nicklas, W., Kraft, V., Meyer, B., 1993. Contamination of transplantable tumors, cell lines, and monoclonal antibodies with rodent viruses. Lab. Anim. Sci. 43, 296–300.

Nittby, H., Grafström, G., Eberhardt, J.L., Malmgren, L., Brun, A., Persson, B.R., et al., 2008. Radiofrequency and extremely low-frequency electromagnetic field effects on the blood-brain barrier. Electromagn. Biol. Med. 27, 103–126.

Nitzki, F., Kruger, A., Reifenberg, K., Wojnowski, L., Hahn, H., 2007. Identification of a genetic contamination in a commercial mouse strain using two panels of polymorphic markers. Lab. Anim. 41, 218–228.

Njaa, L.R., Utne, F., Braeckkan, O.R., 1957. Effect of relative humidity on rat breeding and ringtail. Nature (London) 180, 290–291.

Noell, W.K., Albrecht, R., 1971. Irreversible effects of visible light on the retina: role of vitamin A. Science 172, 76–80.

Nohr, D., Buob, A., Gartner, K., Weihe, E., 1996. Changes in pulmonary calcitonin gene-related peptide and protein gene product 9.5 innervation in rats infected with *Mycoplasma pulmonis*. Cell Tissue Res. 283, 215–219.

Norton, J.N., Kinard, W.L., Reynolds, R.P., 2011. Comparative vibration levels perceived among species in a laboratory animal facility. J. Am. Assoc. Lab. Anim. Sci. 50, 653–659.

Nossaman, B.C., Amouzadeh, H.R., Sangiah, S., 1990. Effects of chloramphenicol, cimetidine and phenobarbital on and tolerance to xylazine-ketamine anesthesia in dogs. Vet. Hum. Toxicol. 32, 216–219.

Noti, J.D., Blachere, F.M., McMillen, C.M., Lindsley, W.G., Kashon, M.L., Slaughter, D.R., et al., 2013. High humidity leads to loss of infectious influenza virus from simulated coughs. PLoS One 8 (2), e57485.

Nugent, B.M., Tobet, S.A., Lara, H.E., Lucion, A.B., Wilson, M.E., Recabarren, S.E., et al., 2012. Hormonal programming across the lifespan. Horm. Metab. Res. 44, 577–586.

Nunamaker, E.A., Otto, K.J., Artwohl, J.E., Fortman, J.D., 2013. Leaching of heavy metals from water bottle components into the drinking water of rodents. J. Am. Assoc. Lab. Anim. Sci. 52, 22–27.

Nunoya, T., Itabashi, M., Kudow, S., Hayashi, M., Tajima, M., 1977. An epizootic outbreak of sialodacryoadenitis in rats. Jpn. J. Vet. Sci. 39, 445–450.

Nyagode, B.A., Lee, C.M., Morgan, E.T., 2010. Modulation of hepatic cytochrome P450s by *Citrobacter rodentium* infection in interleukin-6- and interferon-γ-null mice. J. Pharmacol. Exp. Ther. 335, 480–488.

Nyska, A., Maronpot, R.R., Eldridge, S.R., Haseman, J.K., Hailey, J.R., 1997. Alteration in cell kinetics in control B6C3F$_1$ mice infected with *Helicobacter hepaticus*. Toxicol. Pathol. 25, 591–596.

Obernier, J.A., Baldwin, R.L., 2006. Establishing an appropriate period of acclimatization following transportation of laboratory animals. ILAR J. 47, 364–369.

Odum, J., Tinwell, H., Jones, K., Van Miller, J.P., Joiner, R.L., Tobin, G., et al., 2001. Effect of rodent diets on the sexual development of the rat. Toxicol. Sci. 61, 115–127.

O'Hara, A.M., Shanahan, F., 2006. The gut flora as a forgotten organ. EMBO Rep. 7, 688–693.

O'Hara, J.R., Skinn, A.C., MacNaughton, W.K., Sherman, P.M., Sharkey, K.A., 2006. Consequences of *Citrobacter rodentium* infection on enteroendocrine cells and the enteric nervous system in the mouse colon. Cell. Microbiol. 8, 646–660.

Oishi, K., 2009. Disrupted light-dark cycle induces obesity with hyperglycemia in genetically intact animals. Neuro. Endocrinol. Lett. 30, 458–461.

Oishi, K., Itoh, N., 2013. Disrupted daily light–dark cycle induces the expression of hepatic gluconeogenic regulatory genes and hyperglycemia with glucose intolerance in mice. Biochem. Biophys. Res. Commun. 432, 111–115.

Okamoto, A., Miyoshi, M., Imoto, T., Ryoke, K., Watanabe, T., 2010. Chronic restraint stress in rats suppresses sweet and umami taste responses and lingual expression of T1R3 mRNA. Neurosci. Lett. 486, 211–214.

Olmstead, A.W., Lindberg-Livingston, A., Degitz, S.J., 2010. Genotyping sex in the amphibian, *Xenopus* (*Silurana*) *tropicalis*, for endocrine disruptor bioassays. Aquat. Toxicol. 98, 60–66.

Olovson, S.G., 1986. Diet and breeding performance in cats. Lab. Anim. 20, 221–230.

Olsson, I.A., Sherwin, C.M., 2006. Behaviour of laboratory mice in different housing conditions when allowed to self-administer an anxiolytic. Lab. Anim. 40, 392–399.

Organisciak, D.T., Darrow, R.M., Barsalou, L., Kutty, R.K., Wiggert, B., 2003. Susceptibility to retinal light damage in transgenic rats with rhodopsin mutations. Invest. Ophthalmol. Vis. Sci. 44, 486–492.

Orr, S.L., Le, D., Long, J.M., Sobieszczuk, P., Ma, B., Tian, H., et al., 2013. A phenotype survey of 36 mutant mouse strains with gene-targeted defects in glycosyltransferases or glycan-binding proteins. Glycobiology 23, 363–380.

Osborne, M.P., Haddon, S.J., Worton, K.J., Spencer, A.J., Starkey, W.G., Thornber, D., et al., 1991. Rotavirus-induced changes in the microcirculation of intestinal villi of neonatal mice in relation to the induction and persistence of diarrhea. J. Pediatr. Gastroenterol. Nutr. 12, 111–120.

O'Steen, W.K., Anderson, K.V., 1972. Photoreceptor degeneration after exposure of rats to incandescent illumination. Z. Zellforsch. Mikrosk. Anat. 127, 306–313.

O'Steen, W.K., Shear, C.R., Anderson, K.V., 1973. Retinal damage after prolonged exposure to visible light. A light and electron microscopic study. Am. J. Anat. 134, 5–22.

Ota, N., Wong, K., Valdez, P.A., Zheng, Y., Crellin, N.K., Diehl, L., et al., 2011. IL-22 bridges the lymphotoxin pathway with the maintenance of colonic lymphoid structures during infection with *Citrobacter rodentium*. Nat. Immunol. 12, 941–948.

Otleş, S., Cağindi, O., 2010. Health importance of arsenic in drinking water and food. Environ. Geochem. Health. 32, 367–371.

Ousingsawat, J., Mirza, M., Tian, Y., Roussa, E., Schreiber, R., Cook, D.I., et al., 2011. Rotavirus toxin NSP4 induces diarrhea by activation of TMEM16A and inhibition of Na+ absorption. Pflugers Arch. 461, 579–589.

Overton, J.M., 2010. Phenotyping small animals as models for the human metabolic syndrome: thermoneutrality matters. Int. J. Obes. (Lond) 34 (Suppl. 2), S53–S58.

Oyama, T., 1973. Endocrine responses to anesthetic agents. Brit. J. Anaesth. 45, 276–281.

Oz, H.S., Hughes, W.T., 1997. *Pneumocystis carinii* infection alters GTP-binding proteins in the lung. J. Parasitol. 83, 679–685.

Paik, J., Fierce, Y., Drivdahl, R., Treuting, P.M., Seamons, A., Brabb, T., et al., 2010. Effects of murine norovirus infection on a mouse model of diet-induced obesity and insulin resistance. Comp. Med. 60, 189–195.

Pakes, S.P., Lu, Y.S., Meunier, P.C., 1984. Factors that complicate animal research. In: Fox, J.G., Cohen, B.J., Loew, F.M. (Eds.), Laboratory Animal Medicine. Academic Press, Orlando, FL, pp. 649–665.

Panemangalore, M., Bebe, F.N., 2005. Interaction between pesticides and essential metal copper increases the accumulation of copper in the kidneys of rats. Biol. Trace. Elem. Res. 108 (1–3), 169–184.

Paradisi, F., Graziano, L., Maio, G., 1972. Histochemistry of glutamic-oxaloacetic transaminase in mouse liver during MHV3 infection. Experimentia 28, 551–552.

Pardon, M.C., Sarmad, S., Rattray, I., Bates, T.E., Scullion, G.A., Marsden, C.A., et al., 2009. Repeated novel cage exposure-induced improvement of early Alzheimer's-like cognitive and amyloid changes in TASTPM mice is unrelated to changes in brain endocannabinoids levels. Neurobiol. Aging. 30, 1099–1113.

Parker, J.C., 1980. The possibilities and limitations of virus control in laboratory animals. In: Spiegel, A., Erichsen, S., Solleveld, H.A. (Eds.), Animal Quality and Models in Research. Gustav Fischer Verlag, New York, pp. 161–172.

Parkinson, A.W., Ogilvie, B.W., Buckley, D.B., Kazmi, F., Czerwinski, M., Parkinson, O., 2013. Biotransformation of xenobiotics. In: Klaasen, C.D. (Ed.), Casarett and Doull's Toxicology, the Basic Science of Poisons, eighth ed. McGraw-Hill Education, New York, pp. 161–295.

Patten Jr., C.C., Myles, M.H., Franklin, C.L., Livingston, R.S., 2010. Perturbations in cytokine gene expression after inoculation of C57BL/6 mice with *Pasteurella pneumotropica*. Comp. Med. 60, 18–24.

Payne, J.K., 2011. Altered circadian rhythms and cancer-related fatigue outcomes. Integr. Cancer Ther. 10, 221–233.

Payvandi, F., Amrute, S., Fitzgerald-Bocarsly, P., 1998. Exogenous and endogenous IL-10 regulate IFN-alpha production by peripheral blood mononuclear cells in response to viral stimulation. J. Immunol. 160, 5861–5868.

Pearce, B.D., Hobbs, M.V., McGraw, T.S., Buchmeier, M.J., 1994. Cytokine induction during T-cell-mediated clearance of mouse hepatitis virus from neurons *in vivo*. J. Virol. 68, 5483–5495.

Pearson, D.J., Taylor, G., 1975. The influence of the nematode *Syphacia obvelata* on adjuvant arthritis in rats. Immunology 29, 391–396.

Pecaut, M.J., Smith, A.L., Jones, T.A., Gridley, D.S., 2000. Modification of immunologic and hematologic variables by method of CO_2 euthanasia. Comp. Med. 50, 595–602.

Peck, R.M., Eaton, G.J., Peck, E.B., Litwin, S., 1983. Influence of Sendai virus on carcinogenesis in strain A mice. Lab. Anim. Sci. 33, 154–156.

Peltier, M.R., Barncy, B.M., Brown, M.B., 2007. Effect of experimental genital mycoplasmosis on production of matrix metalloproteinases in membranes and amniotic fluid of Sprague–Dawley rats. Am. J. Reprod. Immunol. 57, 116–121.

Percy, D.H., Hayes, M.A., Kocal, T.E., Wojcinski, Z.W., 1988. Depletion of salivary gland epidermal growth factor by sialodacryoadenitis virus infection in the Wistar rat. Vet. Pathol. 25, 183–192.

Perenboom, R.M., Beckers, P., Van Der Meer, J.W., Van Schijndel, A.C., Oyen, W.J., Corstens, F.H., et al., 1996. Pro-inflammatory cytokines in lung and blood during steroid-induced *Pneumocystis carinii* pneumonia in rats. J. Leukoc. Biol. 60, 710–715.

Periti, P., Mazzei, T., Mini, E., Novelli, A., 1992. Pharmacokinetic drug interactions of macrolides. Clin. Pharmacokinet. 23, 106–131.

Perkins, S.E., Lipman, N.S., 1995. Characterization and qualification of microenvironmental contaminants in isolator cages with a variety of contact beddings. Contemp. Top. Lab. Anim. Sci. 34, 93–98.

Perkins, S.E., Lipman, N.S., 1996. Evaluation of microenvironmental conditions and noise generation in three individually ventilated rodent caging systems and static isolator cages. Contemp. Top. Lab. Anim. Sci. 35, 61–65.

Perremans, S., Randall, J.M., Rombouts, G., Decuypere, E., Geers, R., 2001. Effect of whole body vibration in the vertical axis on cortisol and adrenocorticotropic hormone levels in piglets. J. Anim. Sci. 79, 975–981.

Peters, L., Kelly, H., 1977. Influence of stress and stress hormones on transplantability of a non-immunogenic syngeneic mouse tumor. Cancer 39, 1482–1488.

Peterson, E.A., 1980. Noise in the animal environment. Lab. Anim Sci. 30, 422–439.

Petro, T.M., 2005. Disparate expression of IL-12 by SJL/J and B10.S macrophages during Theiler's virus infection is associated with activity of TLR7 and mitogen-activated protein kinases. Microbes Infect. 7, 224–232.

Pettinger, W.A., Tanaka, K., Keeton, K., Campbell, W.B., Brooks, S.N., 1975. Renin Release, an Artifact of Anesthesia and its Implications in Rats (38597). Proc. Soc. Exper. Biol. Med. 148, 625–630.

Phillips, J.B., Youmans, P.W., Muheim, R., Sloan, K.A., Landler, L., Painter, M.S., et al., 2013. Rapid learning of magnetic compass direction by C57BL/6 mice in a 4-armed 'plus' water maze. PLoS One 8, e73112.

Pierson, M., Liebman, S.L., 1992. Noise exposure-induced audiogenic seizure susceptibility in sprague–dawley rats. Epilepsy Res. 13, 35–42.

Pisu, M.G., Garau, A., Olla, P., Biggio, F., Utzeri, C., Dore, R., et al., 2013. Altered stress responsiveness and hypothalamic-pituitary-adrenal axis function in male rat offspring of socially isolated parents. J. Neurochem. 126, 493–502.

Pivina, S.G., Shamolina, T.S., Akulova, V.K., Ordian, N.E., 2007. Sensitiveness to social stress in female rats with alteration of the pituitary-adrenal axis stress reactivity. Ross. Fiziol. Zh. Im. I. M. Sechenova. 93, 1319–1325.

Plaut, S.M., Alder, R., Friedman, S.B., Ritterson, A.L., 1969. Social factors and resistance to malaria in the mouse: effects of group vs. individual housing on resistance to *Plasmodium berghei* infection. Psychosom. Med. 31, 536–540.

Pochanke, V., Hatak, S., Hengartner, H., Zinkernagel, R.M., McCoy, K.D., 2006. Induction of IgE and allergic-type responses in fur mite-infested mice. Eur. J. Immunol. 36, 2434–2445.

Poole, T.B., Morgan, M.D.R., 1976. Social and territorial behavior of laboratory mice (*Mus musculus L.*) in small complex areas. Anim. Behav. 24, 476–480.

Popovich, I.G., Zabezhinski, M.A., Panchenko, A.V., Piskunova, T.S., Semenchenko, A.V., Tyndyk, M.L., et al., 2013. Exposure to light at night accelerates aging and spontaneous uterine carcinogenesis in female 129/Sv mice. Cell Cycle 12, 1785–1790.

Popper, C.W., Chiueh, C.C., Kopin, I.J., 1977. Plasma catecholamine concentrations in unanesthetized rats during sleep, wakefulness, immobilization and after decapitation. J. Pharmacol. Exp. Ther. 202 (1), 144–148.

Port, C.D., Garvin, P.J., Ganote, C.E., Sawyer, D.C., 1978. Pathologic changes induced by an euthanasia agent. Lab. Anim. Sci. 28, 4481.

Porter, G., Lane-Petter, W., Horne, M., 1963. Effects of strong light on breeding mice. J. Anim. Tech. Assoc. 14, 117–119.

Porterfield, V.M., Zimomra, Z.R., Caldwell, E.A., Camp, R.M., Gabella, K.M., Johnson, J.D., 2011. Rat strain differences in restraint stress-induced brain cytokines. Neuroscience 188, 48–54.

Portfors, C.V., 2007. Types and functions of ultrasonic vocalizations in laboratory rats and mice. J. Am. Assoc. Lab. Anim. Sci. 46 (1), 28–34.

Potgieter, F.J., Wilke, P.I., van Jaarsveld, H., Alberts, D.W., 1996. The in vivo effect of different bedding materials on the antioxidant levels of rat heart, lung and liver tissue. J. S. Afr. Vet. Assoc. 67 (1), 27–30.

Pottratz, S.T., Reese, S., Sheldon, J.L., 1998. *Pneumocystis carinii* induces interleukin 6 production by an alveolar epithelial cell line. Eur. J. Clin. Invest. 28, 424–429.

Prichett-Corning, K.R., Cosentino, J., Clifford, C.B., 2009. Contemporary prevalence of infectious agents in laboratory mice and rats. Lab. Anim. 43, 165–173.

Prien, T., Traber, D.L., Linares, H.A., Davenport, S.L., 1988. Haemolysis and artifactual lung damage induced by an euthanasia agent. Lab. Anim. 22 (2), 170–172.

Priya, P.H., Reddy, P.S., 2012. Effect of restraint stress on lead-induced male reproductive toxicity in rats. J. Exp. Zool. A Ecol. Genet. Physiol. 317, 455–465.

Procaccini, C., Jirillo, E., Matarese, G., 2012. Leptin as an immunomodulator. Mol. Aspects Med. 33, 35–45.

Prola, L., Cornale, P., Renna, M., Macchi, E., Perona, G., Mimosi, A., 2013. Effect of breed, cage type, and reproductive phase on fecal corticosterone levels in doe rabbits. J. Appl. Anim. Welf. Sci. 16, 140–149.

Proust, J.J., Bucholz, M.A., Nordin, A.A., 1985. A "lymphokine-like" soluble product that induces proliferation and maturation of B cells appears in the serum-free supernatant of a T cell hybridoma as a consequence of mycoplasmal contamination. J. Immunol. 134, 390–396.

Pucak, G.J., Lee, C.S., Zaino, A.S., 1977. Effects of prolonged high temperature on testicular development and fertility in the male rat. Lab. Anim. Sci. 27, 76–77.

Puig, N.R., Ferrero, P., Bay, M.L., Hidalgo, G., Valenti, J., Amerio, N., et al., 2002. Effects of sevoflurane general anesthesia: immunological studies in mice. Int. Immunopharmacol. 2, 95–104.

Pye, A., 1973. The destructive effect of intense pure tones on the cochleae of mammals. In: Taylor, A. (Ed.), Disorders of Aural Function. Academic Press, London, pp. 89–96.

Rabat, A., 2007. Extra-auditory effects of noise in laboratory animals: the relationship between noise and sleep. J. Am. Assoc. Lab. Anim. Sci. 46, 35–41.

Rabat, A., Bouyer, J.J., Aran, J.M., Courtiere, A., Mayo, W., Le Moal, M., 2004. Deleterious effects of an environmental noise on sleep and contribution of its physical components in a rat model. Brain Res. 1009, 88–97.

Raczynski, A.R., Muthupalani, S., Schlieper, K., Fox, J.G., Tannenbaum, S.R., Schauer, D.B., 2012. Enteric infection with Citrobacter rodentium induces coagulative liver necrosis and hepatic inflammation prior to peak infection and colonic disease. PLoS One 7, e33099.

Raff, H., Bruder, E.D., Cullinan, W.E., Ziegler, D.R., Cohen, E.P., 2011. Effect of animal facility construction on basal hypothalamic-pituitary-adrenal and renin-aldosterone activity in the rat. Endocrinology 152, 1218–1221.

Ramljak, D., Jones, A.B., Diwan, B.A., Perantoni, A.O., Hochadel, J.F., Anderson, L.M., 1998. Epidermal growth factor and transforming growth factor-alpha-associated overexpression of cyclin D1, Cdk4, and c-Myc during hepatocarcinogenesis in Helicobacter hepaticus-infected A/JCr mice. Cancer Res. 58, 3590–3597.

Rammes, G., Starker, L.K., Haseneder, R., Berkmann, J., Plack, A., Zieglgänsberger, W., et al., 2009. Isoflurane anaesthesia reversibly improves cognitive function and long-term potentiation (LTP) via an up-regulation in NMDA receptor 2B subunitexpression. Neuropharmacology 56, 626–636.

Ramsey, K.A., Larcombe, A.N., Sly, P.D., Zosky, G.R., 2013. In utero exposure to low dose arsenic via drinking water impairs early life lung mechanics in mice. BMC Pharmacol. Toxicol. 14, 13.

Ranschoff, R.M., Wei, T., Pavelko, K.D., Lee, J.C., Murray, P.D., Rodriquez, M., 2002. Chemokine expression the central nervous system of mice with a viral disease resembling multiple sclerosis: roles of CD4[+] and CD8[+] T cells and viral persistence. J. Virol. 76, 2217–2224.

Rao, G.N., Ney, E., Herbert, R.A., 1997. Influence of diet on mammary cancer in transgenic mice bearing an oncogene expressed in mammary tissue. Breast Cancer Res. Treat. 45, 149–158.

Rasmussen, S., Glickman, G., Norinsky, R., Quimby, F.W., Tolwani, R.J., 2009. Construction noise decreases reproductive efficiency in mice. J. Am. Assoc. Lab. Anim. Sci. 48, 363–370.

Reeb, C., Jones, R., Bearg, D., Bedigan, H., Myers, D., Paigen, B., 1998. Microenvironment in ventilated animal cages with differing ventilation rates, mice populations, and frequency of bedding changes. Contemp. Top. Lab. Anim. Sci. 37 (2), 43–49.

Reeb-Whitaker, C.K., Paigen, B., Beamer, W.G., Bronson, R.T., Churchill, G.A., Schweitzer, I.B., et al., 2001. The impact of reduced frequency of cage changes on the health of mice housed in ventilated cages. Lab. Anim. 35 (1), 58–73.

Reggiori, F., Monastyrska, I., Verheije, M.H., Cali, T., Ulasli, M., Bianchi, S., et al., 2010. Coronaviruses hijack the LC3-I-positive EDEMosomes, ER-derived vesicles exporting short-lived ERAD regulators, for replication. Cell Host Microbe. 7, 500–508.

Reichle, F.M., Conzen, P.F., 2003. Halogenated inhalational anaesthetics. Best Pract. Res. Clin. Anaesthesiol. 17, 29–46.

Reid, W.C., Carmichael, K.P., Srinivas, S., Bryant, J.L., 1999. Pathologic changes associated with use of tribromoethanol (avertin) in the Sprague Dawley rat. Lab. Anim. Sci. 46, 665–667.

Ren, L., Li, X., Weng, Q., Trisomboon, H., Yamamoto, T., Pan, L., et al., 2010. Effects of acute restraint stress on sperm motility and secretion of pituitary, adrenocortical and gonadal hormones in adult male rats. J. Vet. Med. Sci. 72, 1501–1506.

Renard, G.M., Rivarola, M.A., Suárez, M.M., 2007. Sexual dimorphism in rats: effects of early maternal separation and variable chronic stress on pituitary-adrenal axis and behavior. Int. J. Dev. Neurosci. 25, 373–379.

Repacholi, M.H., 1997. Radiofrequency field exposure and cancer: what do the laboratory studies suggest? Environ. Health Perspect. 105, 1565–1568.

Repacholi, M.H., Basten, A., Gebski, V., Noonan, D., Finnie, J., Harris, A.W., 1997. Lymphomas in E mu-Pim 1 transgenic mice exposed to pulsed 900 MHZ electromagnetic fields. Radiat. Res. 147, 631–640.

Rex, A., Kolbasenko, A., Bert, B., Fink, H., 2007. Choosing the right wild type: behavioral and neurochemical differences between 2 populations of Sprague–Dawley rats from the same source but maintained at different sites. J. Am. Assoc. Lab. Anim. Sci. 46, 13–20.

Reynolds, K.A., Mena, K.D., Gerba, C.P., 2008. Risk of waterborne illness via drinking water in the United States. Rev. Environ. Contam. Toxicol. 192, 117–158.

Rice, C.J., Sandman, C.A., Lenjavi, M.R., Baram, T.Z., 2008. A novel mouse model for acute and long-lasting consequences of early life stress. Endocrinology 149, 4892–4900.

Rice, S.A., Fish, K.J., 1987. Anesthetic considerations for drug metabolism studies in laboratory animals. Lab. Anim. Sci. 37, 520.

Richardson, S.D., Plewa, M.J., Wagner, E.D., Schoeny, R., Demarini, D.M., 2007. Occurrence, genotoxicity, and carcinogenicity of regulated and emerging disinfection by products in drinking water: a review and roadmap for research. Mutat. Res. 636 (1–3), 178–242.

Richter, C., 1968. Inherent twenty-four hour and lunar clocks of a primate-the squirrel monkey. Commun. Behav. Biol. 1, 305–322.

Richter, S.H., Zeuch, B., Riva, M.A., Gass, P., Vollmayr, B., 2013. Environmental enrichment ameliorates depressive-like symptoms in young rats bred for learned helplessness. Behav. Brain Res. 252, 287–292.

Rico, R.M., Ripamonti, R., Burns, A.L., Gamelli, R.L., DiPietro, L.A., 2002. The effect of sepsis on wound healing. J. Surg. Res. 102, 193–197.

Ritter, L., Solomon, K., Sibley, P., Hall, K., Keen, P., Mattu, G., et al., 2002. Sources, pathways, and relative risks of contaminants in surface water and groundwater: a perspective prepared for the Walkerton inquiry. J. Toxicol. Environ. Health A 65, 1–142.

Robacker, K.M., Kulkarni, A.P., Hodgson, E., 1981. Pesticide induced changes in the mouse hepatic microsomal cytochrome P-450-dependent monooxygenase system and other enzymes. J. Environ. Sci. Health 16, 529–545.

Roble, G.S., Boteler, W., Riedel, E., Lipman, N.S., 2012. Total IgE as a serodiagnostic marker to aid murine fur mite detection. J. Am. Assoc. Lab. Anim. Sci. 51, 199–208.

Rock, F.M., Landi, M.S., Hughes, H.C., Gagnon, R.C., 1997. Effects of caging type and group size on selected physiologic variables in rats. Contemp. Top. Lab. Anim. Sci. 36, 69–72.

Rodríguez-Cuesta, J., Vidal-Vanaclocha, F., Mendoza, L., Valcárcel, M., Gallot, N., Martínez de Tejada, G., 2005. Effect of asymptomatic natural infections due to common mouse pathogens on the metastatic progression of B16 murine melanoma in C57BL/6 mice. Clin. Exp. Metastasis 22, 549–558.

Rogers, A.B., Theve, E.J., Feng, Y., Fry, R.C., Taghizadeh, K., Clapp, K.M., et al., 2007. Hepatocellular carcinoma associated with liver-gender disruption in male mice. Cancer Res. 67, 11536–11546.

Romanovsky, A.A., Ivanov, A.I., Shimansky, Y.P., 2002. Selected Contribution: ambient temperature for experiments in rats: a new method for determining the zone of thermal neutrality. J. Appl. Physiol. 92, 2667–2679.

Ronis, M.J., Badger, T.M., Shema, S.J., Roberson, P.K., Shaikh, F., 1998a. Effects on pubertal growth and reproduction in rats exposed to lead perinatally or continuously throughout development. J. Toxicol. Environ. Health 53, 327–341.

Ronis, M.J., Gandy, J., Badger, T., 1998b. Endocrine mechanisms underlying reproductive toxicity in the developing rat chronically exposed to dietary lead. J. Toxicol. Environ. Health 54, 77–99.

Ross, S.A., 2010. Evidence for the relationship between diet and cancer. Exp. Oncol. 32, 137–142.

Ross, S.E., Simecka, J.W., Gambill, G.P., Davis, J.K., Cassell, G.H., 1992. Mycoplasma pulmonis possesses a novel chemoattractant for B lymphocytes. Infect. Immun. 60, 669–674.

Rosenbaum, M.D., VandeWoude, S., Johnson, T.E., 2009. Effects of cage-change frequency and bedding volume on mice and their microenvironment. J. Am. Assoc. Lab. Anim. Sci. 48, 763–773.

Rosenfeld, C.S., Roberts, R.M., 2004. Maternal diet and other factors affecting offspring sex ratio: a review. Biol. Reprod. 71, 1063–1070.

Rosenfeld, C.S., Grimm, K.M., Livingston, K.A., Brokman, A.M., Lamberson, W.E., Roberts, R.M., 2003. Striking variation in the sex ratio of pups born to mice according to whether maternal diet is high in fat or carbohydrate. Proc. Natl. Acad. Sci. USA 100, 4628–4632.

Rothkötter, H.J., Sowa, E., Pabst, R., 2002. The pig as a model of developmental immunology. Hum. Exp. Toxicol. 21, 533–536.

Rought, S.E., Yau, P.M., Chuang, L.F., Doi, R.H., Chuang, R.Y., 1999. Effect of the chlorinated hydrocarbons heptachlor, chlordane, and toxaphene on retinoblastoma tumor suppressor in human lymphocytes. Toxicol. Lett. 104, 127–135.

Rowland, N.E., 2007. Food or fluid restriction in common laboratory animals: balancing welfare considerations with scientific inquiry. Comp. Med. 57, 149–160.

Royals, M.A., Getzy, D.M., VandeWoude, S., 1999. High fungal spore load in corncob bedding associated with fungal-enduced rhinitis in two rats. Contemp. Top Lab. Anim. Sci. 38, 64–66.

Rubin, C.T., Capilla, E., Luu, Y.K., Busa, B., Crawford, H., Nolan, D.J., et al., 2007. Adipogenesis is inhibited by brief, daily exposure to high frequency, extremely low-magnitude mechanical signals. Proc. Natl. Acad. Sci. USA 104, 17879–17884.

Rubio, N., Cerciat, M., Unkila, M., Garcia-Segura, L.M., Arevalo, M.A., 2011. An in vitro experimental model of neuroinflammation: the induction of interleukin-6 in murine astrocytes infected with Theiler's murine encephalomyelitis virus, and its inhibition by oestrogenic receptor modulators. Immunology 133, 360–369.

Rubio, N., Sanz-Rodriguez, F., Arevalo, M.A., 2010. Up-regulation of the vascular cell adhesion molecule-1 (VCAM-1) induced by Theiler's murine encephalomyelitis virus infection of murine brain astrocytes. Cell. Commun. Adhes. 17, 57–68.

Rudner, X.L., Happel, K.I., Young, E.A., Shellito, J.E., 2007. Interleukin-23 (IL-23)-IL-17 cytokine axis in murine Pneumocystis carinii infection. Infect. Immun. 75, 3055–3061.

Ruebner, B.H., Hirano, T., 1965. Viral hepatitis in mice. Changes in oxidative enzymes and phosphatases after murine hepatitis virus (MHV-3) infection. Lab. Invest. 14, 157–168.

Rutten, A.A., de Groot, A.P., 1992. Comparison of cereal-based diet with purified diet by short term feeding studies in rats, mice and hamsters, with emphasis on toxicity characteristics. Food Chem. Toxicol. 30, 601–610.

Saibaba, P., Sales, G.D., Stodulski, G., Hau, J., 1996. Behaviour of rats in their home cages: daytime variations and effects of routine husbandry procedures analysed by time sampling techniques. Lab. Anim. 30, 13–21.

Sajid, M.S., Iqbal, Z., Muhammad, G., Iqbal, M.U., 2006. Immunomodulatory effect of various anti-parasitics: a review. Parasitology 132, 301–313.

Sakhai, S.A., Preslik, J., Francis, D.D., 2013. Influence of housing variables on the development of stress-sensitive behaviors in the rat. Physiol. Behav. 120C, 156–163.

Sakurai, A., Atkins, C.M., Alonso, O.F., Bramlett, H.M., Dietrich, W.D., 2012. Mild Hyperthermia worsens the neuropathological damage associated with mild traumatic brain injury in rats. J. Neurotrauma. 29, 313–321.

Sales, G., Pye, J.D., 1974. Ultrasonic Communications by Animals. Chapman and Hall, London.

Sales, G.D., 1991. The effect of 22 kHz calls and artificial 38 kHz signals on activity in rats. Behav. Process. 24, 83–93.

Sales, G.D., Smith, J.D., 1980. Ultrasonic behavior and mother-infant interactions in rodents. In: Smotherman, W., Bell, R.W. (Eds.), Maternal Influences and Early Behaviour. Spectrum Press Inc., New York, pp. 105–133.

Sales, G.D., Wilson, K.J., Spencer, K.E., Milligan, S.R., 1988. Environmental ultrasound in laboratories and animal houses: a possible cause for concern in the welfare and use of laboratory animals. Lab. Anim. 22, 369–375.

Saltarelli, C.G., Coppola, C.P., 1979. Influence of visible light on organ weights of mice. Lab. Anim. Sci. 29, 319–322.

Samy, T.S., Knöferl, M.W., Zheng, R., Schwacha, M.G., Bland, K.I., Chaudry, I.H., 2001. Divergent immune responses in male and female mice after trauma-hemorrhage: dimorphic alterations in T lymphocyte steroidogenic enzyme activities. Endocrinology 142, 3519–3529.

Sánchez-Vázquez, F.J., Terry, M.I., Felizardo, V.O., Vera, L.M., 2011. Daily rhythms of toxicity and effectiveness of anesthetics (MS222 and eugenol) in zebrafish (Danio rerio). Chronobiol. Int. 28, 109–117.

Sanford, A.N., Clark, S.E., Talham, G., Sidelsky, M.G., Coffin, S.E., 2002. Influence of bedding type on mucosal immune responses. Comp. Med 52, 429–432.

Santos, M.M., Micael, J., Carvalho, A.P., Morabito, R., Booy, P., Massanisso, P., et al., 2006. Estrogens counteract the masculinizing effect of tributyltin in zebrafish. Comp. Biochem. Physiol. C. Toxicol. Pharmacol. 142, 151–155.

Sanyal, S., Hawkins, R.K., 1986. Development and degeneration of retina in rds mutant mice: effects of light on the rate of degeneration in albino and pigmented homozygous and heterozygous mutant and normal mice. Vision Res. 26, 1177–1185.

Sanz, P., Rodriguez-Vicente, M.C., Villar, P., Repetto, M., 1988. Uncontrollable atmospheric conditions which can affect animal experimentation. Vet. Hum. Toxicol. 30, 452–454.

Sato, J., Denda, M., Ashida, Y., Koyama, J., 1998. Loss of water from the stratum corneum induces epidermal DNA synthesis in hairless mice. Arch. Dermatol. Res. 290, 634–637.

Sato, J., Denda, M., Chang, S., Elias, P.M., Feingold, K.R., 2002. Abrupt decreases in environmental humidity induce abnormalities in permeability barrier homeostasis. J. Invest. Dermatol. 119, 900–904.

Sato, K., Ooi, H.K., Nonaka, N., Oku, Y., Kamiya, M., 1995. Antibody production in *Syphacia obvelata* infected mice. J. Parasitol. 81, 559–562.

Sato, W., Enzan, K., Mitsuhata, H., Mazaki, Y., Kayaba, M., Suzuki, M., 1996. Effect of sevoflurane on release of TNF-alpha and IL-1 beta from human monocytes. Masui 45, 309–312.

Sawada, T., Kosaka, T., 1981. Morphological recovery in the polycystic ovaries of persistent estrus rats induced by continuous illumination (author's transl). Jikken. Dobutsu. 30, 487–490.

Schecter, A.J., Olson, J., Papke, O., 1996. Exposure of laboratory animals to polychlorinated dibenzodioxins and polychlorinated dibenzofurans from commercial rodent chow. Chemosphere 32, 501–508.

Schmid, P., Horejsi, R.C., Mlekusch, W., Paletta, B., 1989. The influence of noise stress on plasma epinephrine and its binding to plasma protein in the rat. Biomed. Biochim. Acta 48 (7), 453–456.

Schoeb, T.R., Davidson, M.K., Lindsey, J.R., 1982. Intracage ammonia promotes growth of *Mycoplasma pulmonis* in the respiratory tract of rats. Infect. Immun. 38, 212–217.

Schreiber, H., Nettesheim, P., Lijinsky, W., Richter, C.B., Walburg Jr., H.E., 1972. Induction of lung cancer in germ free, specific pathogen free, and infected rats by N-nitroso-heptamethyleneimine: enhancement of respiratory infection. J. Natl. Cancer Inst. 4, 1107–1114.

Schunk, M.K., Percy, D.H., Rosendal, S., 1995. Effect of time of exposure to rat coronavirus and *Mycoplasma pulmonis* on respiratory tract lesions in the Wistar rat. Can. J. Vet. Res. 59, 60–66.

Scott, E.P., Branigan, P.J., Del Vecchio, A.M., Weiss, S.R., 2008. Chemokine expression during mouse-hepatitis-virus-induced encephalitis: contributions of the spike and background genes. J. Neurovirol. 14, 5–16.

Segovia, J.C., Guenechea, J.M., Bueren, J.A., Almendral, J.M., 2003. Parvovirus infection suppresses long-term repopulating hematopoietic stem cells. J. Virol. 77, 8495–8503.

Seki, M., Higashiyama, Y., Tomono, K., Yanagihara, K., Ohno, H., Kaneko, Y., et al., 2004. Acute infection with influenza virus enhances susceptibility to fatal pneumonia following *Streptococcus pneumoniae* infection in mice with chronic pulmonary colonization with *Pseudomonas aeruginosa*. Clin. Exp. Immunol. 137, 35–40.

Sengupta, M., Bishayi, B., 2002. Effect of lead and arsenic on murine macrophage response. Drug Chem. Toxicol. 25 (4), 459–472.

Selgrade, M.K., Repacholi, M.H., Koren, H.S., 1997. Ultraviolet radiation-induced immune modulation: potential consequences for infectious, allergic, and autoimmune disease. Environ. Health Perspect. 105, 332–334.

Semple-Rowland, S.L., Dawson, W.W., 1987a. Cyclic light intensity threshold for retinal damage in albino rats raised under 6 lux. Exp. Eye Res. 44, 643–661.

Semple-Rowland, S.L., Dawson, W.W., 1987b. Retinal cyclic light damage threshold for albino rats. Lab. Anim. Sci. 37, 289–298.

Seyfried, T.N., Todorova, M.T., Poderycki, M.J., 1999. Experimental models of multifactorial epilepsies: the EL mouse and mice susceptible to audiogenic seizures. Adv. Neurol. 79, 279–290.

Sfakianakisi, D.G., Lerisi, I., Mylonas, C.C., Kentouri, M., 2012. Temperature during early life determines sex in zebrafish, *Danio rerio* (Hamilton, 1822). J. Biol. Res.-Thessaloniki 17, 68–73.

Shang, H.T., Wei, H., Yue, B.F., Xu, P., 2008. Microsatellite analysis in Wistar and Sprague-Darley outbred rats. Fen. Zi Xi Bao Sheng Wu Xue Bao 41, 28–34.

Shapiro, R., 1980. Chemical contamination of drinking water: what it is and where it comes from. Lab. Anim. 9, 45–51.

Shapiro, J., Jersky, J., Katzav, S., Feldman, M., Segal, S., 1981. Anesthetic drugs accelerate the progression of postoperative metastases of mouse tumors. J. Clin. Invest. 68, 678–685.

Sharon, I.M., Feller, R.P., Burney, S.W., 1971. The effects of lights of different spectra on caries incidence in the golden hamster. Arch. Oral Biol. 16, 1427–1432.

Sharp, J., Zammit, T., Azar, T., Lawson, D., 2003. Stress-like responses to common procedures in individually and group-housed female rats. Contemp. Top. Lab. Anim. Sci. 42, 9–18.

Sharp, J.L., Zammit, T.G., Azar, T.A., Lawson, D.M., 2002. Stress-like responses to common procedures in male rats housed alone or with other rats. Contemp. Top. Lab. Anim. Sci. 41, 8–14.

Shaw, P.J., Ganey, P.E., Roth, R.A., 2010. Idiosyncratic drug-induced liver injury and the role of inflammatory stress with an emphasis on an animal model of trovafloxacin hepatotoxicity. Toxicol. Sci. 118, 7–18.

Shear, C.R., O'Steen, W.K., Anderson, K.V., 1973. Effects of short-term low intensity light on the albino rat retina. An electron microscopic study. Am. J. Anat. 138, 127–132.

Shen, J.X., Xu, Z.M., Yu, Z.L., Wang, S., Zheng, D.Z., Fan, S.C., 2011. Ultrasonic frogs show extraordinary sex differences in auditory frequency sensitivity. Nat. Commun. 14, 342.

Shenaeva, T.A., 1990. Effects of vibration and noise on the reproductive function in experimental animals. Gig. Tr. Prof. Zabol. 9, 16–21.

Shim, S., Lee, S., Kim, C., Kim, B., Jee, S., Lee, S., et al., 2009. Effects of air transportation cause physiological and biochemical changes indicative of stress leading to regulation of chaperone expression levels and corticosterone concentration. Exp. Anim. 58, 11–17.

Shim, S.B., Lee, S.H., Kim, C.K., Kim, B.G., Kim, Y.K., Jee, S.W., et al., 2008. The effects of long-duration, low-temperature ground transportation on physiological and biochemical indicators of stress in mice. Lab. Anim. 37, 121–126.

Shirakami, G., Magaribuchi, T., Shingu, K., Saito, Y., O'higashi, T., Nakao, K., et al., 1995. Effects of anesthesia and surgery on plasma endothelin levels. Anesth. Analg. 80, 449–453.

Shiverdecker, M.D., Schiml, P.A., Hennessy, M.B., 2013. Human interaction moderates plasma cortisol and behavioral responses of dogs to shelter housing. Physiol. Behav. 109, 75–79.

Siegel, M.A., Jensen, R.A., 1986. The effects of naloxone and cage size on social play and activity in isolated young rats. Behav. Neural. Biol. 45, 155–168.

Silverman, J., Adams, J.D., 1983. N-nitrosamines in laboratory animal feed and bedding. Lab. Anim. Sci. 33, 161–164.

Silverman, J., Bays, D.W., Baker, S.P., 2009. Ammonia and carbon dioxide concentrations in disposable and reusable static mouse cages. Lab. Anim. (NY) 38, 16–23.

Simpson, J., Kelly, J.P., 2011. The impact of environmental enrichment in laboratory rat behavioural and neurochemical aspects. Behav. Brain Res. 222, 246–264.

Simpson-Haidaris, P.J., Courtney, M.A., Wright, T.W., Goss, R., Harmsen, A., Gigliotti, F., 1998. Induction of fibrinogen expression in the lung epithelium during *Pneumocystis carinii* pneumonia. Infect. Immun. 66, 4431–4439.

Singh, R.R., Jefferies, A.J., Lankadeva, Y.R., Lombardo, P., Schneider-Kolsky, M., Hilliard, L., et al., 2012. Increased cardiovascular and renal risk is associated with low nephron endowment in aged females: an ovine model of fetal unilateral nephrectomy. PLoS One 7, e42400.

Skindersoe, M.E., Zeuthen, L.H., Brix, S., Fink, L.N., Lazenby, J., Whittall, C., et al., 2009. *Pseudomonas aeruginosa* quorum-sensing signal molecules interfere with dendritic cell-induced T-cell proliferation. FEMS Immunol. Med. Microbiol. 55, 335–345.

Skinn, A.C., Vergnolle, N., Zamuner, S.R., Wallace, J.L., Cellars, L., MacNaughton, W.K., et al., 2006. *Citrobacter rodentium* infection causes iNOS-independent intestinal epithelial dysfunction in mice. Can. J. Physiol. Pharmacol. 84, 1301–1312.

Skinner, K.M., Manikkam, M., Guerrero-Bosagna, C., 2011. Epigenetic transgenerational actions of endocrine disruptors. Reprod. Toxicol. 31, 337–343.

Sloan, R.C., Rosenbaum, M., O'Rourke, D., Oppelt, K., Frasier, C.R., Waston, C.A., et al., 2011. High doses of ketamine-xylazine anesthesia reduce cardiac ischemia reperfusion injury in guinea pigs. J. Am. Assoc. Lab. Anim. Sci. 50, 349–354.

Smiler, K.L., Stein, S., Hrapkiewicz, K.L., Hiben, J.R., 1990. Tissue response to intramuscular and intraperitoneal injections of ketamine and xylazine in rats. Lab. Anim. Sci. 40, 60–64.

Smith, A.L., Mabus, S.L., Muir, C., Woo, Y., 2005. Effects of housing density and cage floor space on three strains of young adult inbred mice. Comp. Med. 55, 368–376.

Smith, C.M., Gill, M.B., May, J.S., Stevenson, P.G., 2007a. Murine gammaherpesvirus-68 inhibits antigen presentation by dendritic cells. PLoS One 2, 1048.

Smith, D.B., McFadden, N., Blundell, R.J., Meredith, A., Simmonds, P., 2012. Diversity of murine norovirus in wild-rodent populations: species-specific associations suggest an ancient divergence. J. Gen. Virol. 93, 259–266.

Smith, E., Stockwell, J.D., Schweitzer, I., Langley, S.H., Smith, A.L., 2004. Evaluation of cage micro-environment of mice housed on various types of bedding materials. Contemp. Top. Lab. Anim. Sci. 43 (4), 12–17.

Smith, K.A., Efstathiou, S., Cooke, A., 2007b. Murine gammaherpesvirus-68 infection alters self-antigen presentation and type 1 diabetes onset in NOD mice. J. Immunol. 179, 7325–7333.

Snedeker, S.M., Hay, A.G., 2012. Do interactions between gut ecology and environmental chemicals contribute to obesity and diabetes? Environ. Health Perspect. 120, 332–339.

Spalding, J.F., Archuleta, R.F., Holland, L.M., 1969a. Influence of the visible colour spectrum on activity in mice. Lab. Anim. Care 19, 50–54.

Spalding, J.F., Holland, L.M., Tietjen, G.L., 1969b. Sex ratio of progeny from mice reared under various colour lighting conditions. Lab. Anim. Care 19, 602–604.

Spindler, S.R., 2005. Rapid and reversible induction of the longevity, anticancer and genomic effects of caloric restriction. Mech. Ageing Dev. 126, 960–966.

Sodhi, C.P., Katyal, R., Rana, S.V., Attri, S., Singh, V., 1996. Study of oxidative-stress in rotavirus infected infant mice. Indian J. Med. Res. 104, 245–249.

Stavinoha, W.B., 1993. Use of microwaves for rapid fixation of tissues in vivo. Scanning 15, 115–117.

Stavrou, S., Ghadge, G., Roos, R.P., 2011. Apoptotic and antiapoptotic activity of L protein of Theiler's murine encephalomyelitis virus. J. Virol. 85, 7177–7185.

Steffan, A.M., Pereira, C.A., Bingen, A., Valle, M., Martin, J.P., Koehren, F., et al., 1995. Mouse hepatitis virus type 3 infection provokes a decrease in the number of sunusoidal endothelial cell fenestrae both in vivo and in vitro. Hepatology 22, 395–401.

Stemkens-Sevens, S., van Berkel, K., de Greeuw, I., Snoeijer, B., Kramer, K., 2009. The use of radiotelemetry to assess the time needed to acclimatize guineapigs following several hours of ground transport. Lab. Anim. 43, 78–84.

Stenvers, D.J., Jonkers, C.F., Fliers, E., Bisschop, P.H., Kalsbeek, A., 2012. Nutrition and the circadian timing system. Prog. Brain Res. 199, 359–376.

Sterzenbach, T., Lee, S.K., Brenneke, B., von Goetz, F., Schauer, D.B., Fox, J.G., et al., 2007. Inhibitory effect of enterohepatic Helicobacter hepaticus on innate immune responses of mouse intestinal epithelial cells. Infect. Immun. 75, 2717–2728.

Stevens, J.C., Banks, G.T., Festing, M.F., Fisher, E.M., 2007. Quiet mutations in inbred strains of mice. Trends. Mol. Med. 13, 512–519.

Stewart, K.A., Wilcox, K.S., Fujinami, R.S., White, H.S., 2010. Theiler's virus infection chronically alters seizure susceptibility. Epilepsia 51, 1418–1428.

Stott, W.T., Kan, H.L., McFadden, L.G., Sparrow, B.R., Gollapudi, B.B., 2004. Effect of strain and diet upon constitutive and chemically induced activities of several xenobiotic-metabolizing enzymes in rats. Regul. Toxicol. Pharmacol. 39, 325–333.

Stout, M.D., Kissling, G.E., Suárez, F.A., Malarkey, D.E., Herbert, R.A., Bucher, J.R., 2008. Influence of Helicobacter hepaticus infection on the chronic toxicity and carcinogenicity of triethanolamine in B6C3F1 mice. Toxicol. Pathol. 36, 783–794.

Streilein, J.W., Shadduck, J.A., Pakes, S.P., 1981. Effects of splenectomy and Sendai virus infection on rejection of male skin isografts by pathogen free C57BL/6 female mice. Transplantation 32, 34–37.

Stroud, F.C., Appt, S.E., Wilson, M.E., Franke, A.A., Adams, M.R., Kaplan, J.R., 2006. Concentrations of isoflavones in macaques consuming standard laboratory monkey diet. J. Am. Assoc. Lab. Anim. Sci. 45 (4), 20–23.

Stubbs, R.J., 1999. Peripheral signals affecting food intake. Nutrition 15, 614–625.

Stuhlman, R.A., Wagner, J.E., 1971. Ringtail in Mystromys albicaudatis: a case report. Lab. Anim. Sci. 21, 585–587.

Stutler, S.A., Johnson, E.W., Still, K.R., Schaeffer, D.J., Hess, R.A., Arfsten, D.P., 2007. Effect of method of euthanasia on sperm motility of mature Sprague–Dawley rats. Assoc. Lab. Anim. Sci. 46 (2), 13–20.

Summa, K.C., Vitaterna, M.H., Turek, F.W., 2012. Environmental perturbation of the circadian clock disrupts pregnancy in the mouse. PLoS One 7, e37668.

Sun, X., Jones, H.P., Hodge, L.M., Simecka, J.W., 2006. Cytokine and chemokine transcription profile during Mycoplasma pulmonis infection in susceptible and resistant strains of mice: macrophage inflammatory protein 1beta (CCL4) and monocyte chemoattractant protein 2 (CCL8) and accumulation of CCR5+ Th cells. Infect. Immun. 74, 5943–5954.

Sundbom, R., Jacobsen, K.R., Kalliokoski, O., Hau, J., Abelson, K.S., 2011. Post-operative corticosterone levels in plasma and feces of mice subjected to permanent catheterization and automated blood sampling. In Vivo 25, 335–342.

Surbeck, H., 1995. Determination of natural radionuclides in drinking water: a tentative protocol. Sci. Total Environ. 173–174, 91–109.

Suzuki, T., Bramlett, H.M., Ruenes, G., Dietrich, W.D., 2004. The effects of early post traumatic hyperthermia in female and ovariectomized rats. J. Neurotrauma. 21, 842–853.

Svobodová, A.R., Galandáková, A., Sianská, J., Doležal, D., Ulrichová, J., Vostálová, J., 2011. Acute exposure to solar simulated ultraviolet radiation affects oxidative stress-related biomarkers in skin, liver and blood of hairless mice. Biol. Pharm. Bull. 34, 471–479.

Swarm, R.L., Roberts, G.K., Levy, A.C., Hines, L.R., 1973. Observations on the thyroid gland in rats following the administration of sulfamethoxazole and trimethoprim. Toxicol. Appl. Pharmacol. 24, 351–363.

Székely, M., Mercer, J.B., 1999. Thermosensitivity changes in cold-adapted rats. J. Therm. Biol. 24, 369–371.

Szymusiak, R., Satinoff, E., 1981. Maximal REM sleep time defines a narrower thermoneutral zone than does minimal metabolic rate. Physiol. Behav. 26, 687–690.

Tabuchi, K., Nishimura, B., Nakamagoe, M., Hayashi, K., Nakayama, M., Hara, A., 2011. Ototoxicity: mechanisms of cochlear impairment and its prevention. Curr. Med. Chem. 18, 4866–4871.

Taets, C., Aref, S., Rayburn, A.L., 1998. The clastogenic potential of triazine herbicide combinations found in potable water supplies. Environ. Health Perspect. 106, 197–201.

Tahara, S., Bergmann, C., Nelson, G., Anthony, T., Dietlin, S., Kyuwa, S., et al., 1993. Effects of mouse hepatitis virus infection on host cell metabolism. Adv. Exp. Med. Biol. 342, 111–116.

Takeyama, H., Kawashima, K., Yamada, K., Ito, Y., 1979. Induction of tumor resistance in mice by L1210 leukemia cells persistently infected with HVJ (Sendai virus). Gann 70, 493–501.

Tam, M., Snipes, G.J., Stevenson, M.M., 1999. Characterization of chronic brochopulmonary Pseudomonas aeruginosa infection in resistant and susceptible inbred mouse strains. Microb. Pathog. 20, 710–719.

Tamura, H., Ohgami, N., Yajima, I., Iida, M., Ohgami, K., Fujii, N., et al., 2012. Chronic exposure to low frequency noise at moderate levels causes impaired balance in mice. PLoS One 7, e39807.

Tamura, T., Fujiwara, K., 1979. IgM and IgG response to sheep red blood cells in mouse hepatitis virus infected nude mice. Microbiol. Immunol. 23, 177–183.

Tamura, T., Machii, K., Ueda, K., Fujiwara, K., 1978. Modification of immune response in nude mice infected with mouse hepatitis virus. Microbiol. Immunol. 22, 557–564.

Tamura, T., Sakaguchi, A., Kai, C., Fujiwara, K., 1980. Enhanced phagocytic activity of macrophages in mouse hepatitis virus infected nude mice. Microbiol. Immunol. 24, 243–247.

Tamura, T., Sakaguchi, A., Ishida, T., Fujiwara, K., 1981. Effect of mouse hepatitis virus infection on natural killer cell activity in nude mice. Microbiol. Immunol. 25, 1363–1368.

Taniguchi, T., Yamamoto, K., 2005. Anti-inflammatory effects of intravenous anesthetics on endotoxemia. Mini Rev. Med. Chem. 5, 241–245.

Targowski, S.P., Klucinski, W., Babiker, S., Nonnecke, B.J., 1984. Effect of ammonia on *in vivo* and *in vitro* immune responses. Infect. Immun. 43, 289–293.

Taurog, J.D., Leary, S.L., Cremer, M.A., Mahowald, M.L., Sandberg, G.P., Manning, P.J., 1984. Infection with *Mycoplasma pulmonis* modulates adjuvant and collagen-induced arthritis in Lewis rats. Arthritis Rheum. 27, 943–946.

Taylor-Robinson, D., Furr, P.M., 2005. *Mycoplasma*-enhanced priapism in mice. Int. J. STD AIDS 16, 383–385.

Thaete, L.G., Levin, S.I., Dudley, A.T., 2013. Impact of anaesthetics and analgesics on fetal growth in the mouse. Lab. Anim. 47, 175–183.

Thai, C.A., Zhang, Y., Howland, J.G., 2013. Effects of acute restraint stress on set-shifting and reversal learning in male rats. Cogn. Affect. Behav. Neurosci. 13, 164–173.

Thangavel, C., Dhir, R.N., Volgin, D.V., Shapiro, B.H., 2007. Sex-dependent expression of CYP2C11 in spleen, thymus and bone marrow regulated by growth hormone. Biochem. Pharmacol. 74, 1476–1484.

Theil, D.J., Tsunoda, I., Libbey, J.E., Derfuss, T.J., Fujinanami, R.S., 2000. Alterations in cytokine but not chemokine mRNA expression during three distinct Theiler's virus infections. J. Neuroimmunol. 104, 22–30.

Thigpen, J.E., Li, L.A., Richter, C.B., Lebetkin, E.H., Jameson, C.W., 1987. The mouse bioassay for the detection of estrogenic activity in rodent diets: II. Comparative estrogenic activity of purified, certified and standard open closed formula rodent diets. Lab. Anim. Sci. 37, 602–605.

Thigpen, J.E., Setchell, K.D.R., Ahlmark, K.B., Locklear, J., Spahr, T., Caviness, G.F., et al., 1999. Phytoestrogen content of purified open- and closed-formula laboratory animal diets. Lab. Anim. Sci. 49, 530–536.

Thigpen, J.E., Setchell, K.D.R., Haseman, J.K., Saunders, H.E., Caviness, G.F., Kissling, G.E., et al., 2007. Variations in phytoestrogen content between different mill dates of the same diet produces significant differences in the time of vaginal opening in CD1 mice and F344 rats but not in CD Sprague–Dawley rats. Environ. Health Perspect. 115, 1717–1726.

Thigpen, J.E., Setchell, K.D., Padilla-Banks, E., Haseman, J.K., Saunders, H.E., Caviness, G.F., et al., 2007. Variations in phytoestrogen content between different mill dates of the same diet produces significant differences in the time of vaginal opening in CD-1 mice and F344 rats but not in CD Sprague-Dawley rats. Environ. Health Perspect. 115 (12), 1717–1726.

Thigpen, J.E., Setchell, K.D., Kissling, G.E., Locklear, J., Caviness, G.F., Whiteside, T., et al., 2013. The estrogenic content of rodent diets, bedding, cages, and water bottles and its effect on bisphenol A studies. J. Am. Assoc. Lab. Anim. Sci. 52, 130–141.

Thomas, G.L., Böhner, C.M., Williams, H.E., Walsh, C.M., Ladlow, M., Welch, M., et al., 2006. Immunomodulatory effects of *Pseudomonas aeruginosa* quorum sensing small molecule probes on mammalian macrophages. Mol. Biosyst. 2, 132–137.

Thomas, M.A., Klaper, R.D., 2012. Psychoactive pharmaceuticals induce fish gene expression profiles associated with human idiopathic autism. PLoS One 7, e32917.

Thompson, J.S., Brown, S.A., Khurdayan, V., Zeynalzadedan, A., Sullivan, P.G., Scheff, S.W., 2002. Early effects of tribromoethanol, ketamine/xylazine, pentobarbitol, and isoflurane anesthesia on hepatic and lymphoid tissue in ICR mice. Comp. Med. 52, 63–67.

Thompson, R.C., Petrik, J., Nash, A.A., Dutia, B.M., 2008. Expansion and activation of NK cell populations in a gammaherpesvirus infection. Scand. J. Immunol. 67, 489–495.

Tisdale, W.A., 1963. Potentiating effect of K-virus on mouse hepatitis virus (MHV-S) in weanling mice. Proc. Soc. Exp. Biol. Med. 114, 774–777.

Tolo, K.J., Erichsen, S., 1969. Acidified drinking water and dental enamel in rats. Z. Versuchstierkd 11, 229–233.

Torrecilhas, A.C., Faquim-Mauro, E., Da Silva, A.V., Abrahamsohn, I.A., 1999. Interference of natural mouse hepatitis virus infection with cytokine production and susceptibility to *Trypanosoma cruzi*. Immunology 96, 381–388.

Torronen, R., Karenlampi, S., Pelkonen, K., 1994. Hepa-1 enzyme induction assay as an *in vitro* indicator of the CYP1A1-inducing potencies of laboratory rodent diets *in vivo*. Life Sci. 55, 1945–1954.

Toth, L.A., January, B., 1990. Physiological stabilization of rabbits after shipping. Lab. Anim. Sci. 40, 384–387.

Traslavina, R.P., King, E.J., Loar, A.S., Riedel, E.R., Garvey, M.S., Ricart-Arbona, R., et al., 2010. Euthanasia by CO_2 inhalation affects potassium levels in mice. J. Am. Assoc. Lab. Anim. Sci. 49, 316–322.

Trotier, D., 2011. Vomeronasal organ and human pheromones. Eur. Ann. Otorhinolaryngol. Head Neck Dis. 128, 184–190.

Trumbo, P.R., 2010. Perchlorate consumption, iodine status, and thyroid function. Nutr. Rev. 68, 62–66.

Tsai, P.P., Pachowsky, U., Stelzer, H.D., Hackbarth, H., 2002. Impact of environmental enrichment in mice. 1: effect of housing conditions on body weight, organ weights and haematology in different strains. Lab. Anim. 36, 411–419.

Tsai, P.P., Stelzer, H.D., Hedrich, H.J., Hackbarth, H., 2003. Are the effects of different enrichment designs on the physiology and behaviour of DBA/2 mice consistent? Lab. Anim. 37, 314–327.

Tu, H., Diberadinis, L.J., Lipman, N.S., 1997. Determination of air distribution, exchange, velocity, and leakage in three individually ventilated rodent caging systems. Contemp. Top. Lab. Anim. Sci. 36, 69–73.

Tudoric, N., Coon, R.L., Kampine, J.P., Bosnjak, Z.J., 1995. Effects of halothane and isoflurane on antigen-and leukotriene-D4-induced constriction of guinea pig trachea. Acta Anaesthesiol. Scand. 39, 1111–1116.

Tuli, J.S., Smith, J.A., Morton, D.B., 1995a. Corticosterone, adrenal, and spleen weight in mice after tail bleeding, and its effect on nearby animals. Lab. Anim. 29, 90–95.

Tuli, J.S., Smith, J.A., Morton, D.B., 1995b. Stress measurements in mice after transportation. Lab. Anim. 29, 132–138.

Tung, K.S., Agersborg, S.S., Alard, P., Garza, K.M., Lou, Y.H., 2001. Regulatory T-cell, endogenous antigen and neonatal environment in the prevention and induction of autoimmune disease. Immunol. Rev. 182, 135–148.

Turner, P.V., Albassam, M.A., 2005. Susceptibility of rats to corneal lesions after injectable anesthesia. Comp. Med. 55, 175–182.

Twaddle, N.C., Churchwell, M.I., McDaniel, L.P., Doerge, D.R., 2004. Autoclave sterilization produces acrylamide in rodent diets: implications for toxicity testing. J. Agric. Food Chem. 52, 4344–4349.

Tzvetkov, D., 1993. Effect of vibrations on the organism-possibilities for development of non-specific diseases and their prognostication. Cent. Eur. J. Public Health 1, 10–15.

Uhnoo, I.S., Freihorst, J., Riepenhoff-Talty, M., Fisher, J.E., Ogra, P.L., 1990. Effect of rotavirus infection and malnutrition on uptake of a dietary antigen in the intestine. Pediatr. Res. 27, 153–160.

Umemoto, E.Y., Brokaw, J.J., Dupuis, M., McDonald, D.M., 2002. Rapid changes in shape and number of MHC class II expressing cells in rat airways after *Mycoplasma pulmonis* infection. Cell. Immunol. 220, 107–115.

Unüvar, T., Büyükgebiz, A., 2012. Fetal and neonatal endocrine disruptors. J. Clin. Res. Pediatr. Endocrinol. 4, 51–60.

Uran, S.L., Aon-Bertolino, M.L., Caceres, L.G., Capani, F., Guelman, L.R., 2012. Rat hippocampal alterations could underlie behavioral abnormalities induced by exposure to moderate noise levels. Brain Res. 1471, 1–12.

Urano, T., Maejima, K., 1978. Provocation of pseudomoniasis with cyclophosphamide in mice. Lab. Anim. 12, 159–161.

U.S. Nuclear Regulatory Commission (USNRC), 1996. Regulatory Guide: Instruction Concerning Risks from Occupational Radiation Exposure. Regulatory Guide No. 8.29. U.S. G. P. O., Washington, DC.

U.S. Nuclear Regulatory Commission (USNRC), 1999. Regulatory Guide: Instruction Concerning Prenatal Radiation Exposure. Regulatory Guide No. 8.13. U.S. G. P. O., Washington, DC.

Ushakov, I.B., Soloshenko, N.V., Kozlovskiĭ, A.P., 1983. Resonance frequencies of vibration in rats. Kosm. Biol. Aviakosm. Med. 17 (6), 65–68.

Utsumi, K., Ishikawa, T., Maeda, T., Shimizu, S., Tatsumi, H., Fujiwara, K., 1980. Infectious sialodacryoadenitis and rat breeding. Lab. Anim. 14, 303–307.

Utsumi, K., Maeda, K., Yokota, Y., Fukugawa, S., Fujiwara, K., 1991. Reproductive disorders in female rats infected with sialodacryoadenitis virus. Jikken Dobutsu 40, 361–365.

Vacha, J., Znojil, V., Pospisil, M., Hola, J., Pipalova, I., 1994. Microcytic anemia and changes in ferrokinetics as late after-effects of glucan administration in murine hepatitis virus-infected C57BL/10ScSnPh mice. Int. J. Immunopharmacol. 16, 51–60.

Vaickus, L.J., Bouchard, J., Kim, J., Natarajan, S., Remick, D.G., 2010. Inbred and outbred mice have equivalent variability in a cockroach allergen-induced model of asthma. Comp. Med 60, 420–426.

Van Winkle, T.J., Balk, M.W., 1986. Spontaneous corneal opacities in laboratory mice. Lab. Anim. Sci. 36, 248–255.

van den Wijngaard, R.M., Stanisor, O.I., van Diest, S.A., Welting, O., Wouters, M.M., Cailotto, C., et al., 2013. Susceptibility to stress induced visceral hypersensitivity in maternally separated rats is transferred across generations. Neurogastroenterol. Motil 25(12), e780–790.

van der Veen, J., Poort, Y., Birchfield, D.J., 1972. Effect of relative humidity on experimental transmission of Sendai virus in mice. Proc. Soc. Exp. Biol. Med. 140, 1437–1440.

Van Loo, P.L., Mol, J.A., Koolhaas, J.M., Van Zutphen, B.F., Baumans, V., 2001. Modulation of aggression in male mice: influence of group size and cage size. Physiol. Behav. 72, 675–683.

Vanderzwan, J., McCaig, L., Mehta, S., Joseph, M., Whitsett, J., McCormack, D.G., et al., 1998. Characterizing alterations in the pulmonary surfactant system in a rat model of *Pseudomonas aeruginosa* pneumonia. Eur. Respir. J. 12, 1388–1396.

Vandenberg, L.N., Pennarola, B.W., Levin, M., 2011. Low frequency vibrations disrupt left right patterning in the xenopus embryo. PLoS One 6, e23306.

Vandenberg, L.N., Stevenson, C., Levin, M., 2012. Low frequency vibrations induce malformations in two aquatic species in a frequency-, waveform-, and direction-specific manner. PLoS One 7, e51473.

van't Land, B., Schijf, M.A., Martin, R., Garssen, J., van Bleek, G.M., 2011. Influencing mucosal homeostasis and immune responsiveness: the impact of nutrition and pharmaceuticals. Eur. J. Pharmacol. 668, S101–S107.

Vaughan, D.K., Nemke, J.L., Fliesler, S.J., Darrow, R.M., Organisciak, D.T., 2002. Evidence for a circadian rhythm of susceptibility to retinal light damage. Photochem. Photobiol. 75, 547–553.

Verbrugghe, E., Boyen, F., Gaastra, W., Bekhuis, L., Leyman, B., Van Parys, A., et al., 2012. The complex interplay between stress and bacterial infections in animals. Vet. Microbiol. 155, 115–127.

Vessel, E.S., Lang, C.M., White, W.J., Passanati, G.T., Hill, R.N., Clemens, T.L., et al., 1976. Environmental and genetic factors affecting the response of laboratory animals to drugs. Fed. Proc. Fed. Am. Soc. Exp. Biol. 35, 1125–1132.

Villar, D., Cray, C., Zaias, J., Altman, N.H., 2007. Biologic effects of fenbendazole in rats and mice: a review. J. Am. Assoc. Lab. Anim. Sci. 46 (6), 8–15.

Virelizier, J.L., Virelizier, A.M., Allison, A.C., 1976. The role of circulating interferon in the modifications of the immune responsiveness to mouse hepatitis virus (MHV-3). J. Immunol. 117, 748–753.

Vogelweid, C.M., Zapien, K.A., Honigford, M.J., Li, L., Li, H., Marshall, H., 2011. Effects of a 28-day cage-change interval on intracage ammonia levels, nasal histology, and perceived welfare of CD1 mice. J. Am. Assoc. Lab. Anim. Sci. 50, 868–878.

Wade, A.E., Holl, J.E., Hilliard, C.C., Molton, E., Greene, F.E., 1968. Alteration of drug metabolism in rats and mice by an environment of cedarwood. Pharmacology 1, 317–328.

Wagner, M., 1988. The effect of infection with the pinworm *(Syphacia muris)* on rat growth. Lab. Anim. Sci. 38, 476–478.

Wahlsten, D., Metten, P., Phillips, T.J., Boehm, S.L., Burkhart-Kasch, S., Dorow, J., et al., 2003. Different data from different labs: lessons from studies of gene environment interaction. J. Neurobiol. 54, 283–311.

Wahlsten, D., Bachmanov, A., Finn, D.A., Crabbe, J.C., 2006. Stability of inbred mouse strain differences in behavior and brain size between laboratories and across decades. Proc. Natl. Acad. Sci. USA 103, 16364–16369.

Wainberg, M.A., Israel, E., 1980. Viral inhibition of lymphocyte mitogenesis. I. Evidence for the nonspecificity of the effect. J. Immunol. 124, 64–70.

Waldemarson, A.H., Hedenqvist, P., Salomonsson, A.C., Häggblom, P., 2005. Mycotoxins in laboratory rodent feed. Lab. Anim. 39, 230–235.

Walker, E.A., Castegnaro, M., Griciute, L., 1979. N-Nitrosamines in the diet of experimental animals. Cancer Lett. 6, 175–178.

Wallace, M.E., 1976. Effects of stress due to deprivation and transport in different genotypes of house mouse. Lab. Anim. 10, 335–347.

Walzer, P.D., Kim, C.K., Linke, J., Pogue, C.L., Huerkamp, M.J., Chrisp, C.E., et al., 1989. Outbreaks of *Pneumocystis carinii* pneumonia in colonies of immunodeficient mice. Infect. Immun. 57, 62–70.

Wan, C.-H., Söderlund-Venermo, M., Pintel, D., Riley, L.K., 2002. Molecular characterization of three newly recognized rat parvoviruses. J. Gen. Virol. 83, 2075–2083.

Wang, G., Chen, G., Zheng, D., Cheng, G., Tang, H., 2011. PLP2 of mouse hepatitis virus A59 (MHV-A59) targets TBK1 to negatively regulate cellular type I interferon signaling pathway. PLoS One 18, e17192.

Wang, J., Gigliotti, F., Bhagwat, S.P., Maggirwar, S.B., Wright, T.W., 2007. *Pneumocystis* stimulates MCP-1 production by alveolar epithelial cells through a JNK-dependent mechanism. Am. J. Physiol. Lung Cell. Mol. Physiol. 292, 1495–1505.

Wang, S.D., Huang, K.J., Lin, Y.S., Lei, H.Y., 1994. Sepsis-induced apoptosis of the thymocytes in mice. J. Immunol. 152, 5014–5021.

Wang, W., Nguyen, N.M., Agapov, E., Holtzman, M.J., Woods, J.C., 2012. Monitoring in vivo changes in lung microstructure with ^{3}He MRI in Sendai virus-infected mice. J. Appl. Physiol. 112, 1593–1599.

Wang, Y., Xiang, G.S., Kourouma, F., Umar, S., 2006. *Citrobacter rodentium*-induced NF-kappaB activation in hyperproliferating colonic epithelia: role of p65 (Ser536) phosphorylation. Br. J. Pharmacol. 148, 814–824.

Warren, K.S., Rosenthal, M.S., Domingo, E.O., 1969. Mouse hepatitis virus (MHV3) infection in chronic murine *schistosomiasis mansoni*. Bull. N. Y. Acad. Med. 45, 211–224.

Wasserman, D.E., 1987. Human Aspects of Occupational Vibration, Advances in Human Factors Factors/Ergonomics, Vol. 8. Elsevier, New York.

Watts, G., 2011. Something in the water. BMJ 343, d7236.

Webster, N.L., Zufferey, C., Pane, J.A., Coulson, B.S., 2013. Alteration of the thymic T cell repertoire by rotavirus infection is associated with delayed type 1 diabetes development in non-obese diabetic mice. PLoS One 8, e59182.

Wehner, S., Schwarz, N.T., Hundsdoerfer, R., Hierholzer, C., Tweardy, D.J., Billiar, T.R., et al., 2005. Induction of IL-6 within the rodent intestinal muscularis after intestinal surgical stress. Surgery 137, 436–446.

Weihe, W.H., 1965. Temperature and humidity climatograms for rats and mice. Lab. Anim. Care 15, 18–28.

Weihe, W.H., 1971. The significance of the physical environment for the health and state of adaptation of laboratory animals. Defining the Laboratory Animal. National Academy of Sciences, Washington, DC, pp. 353–378.

Weihe, W.H., 1973. The effect of temperature on the action of drugs. In: Lomax, P., Schonbaum, E. (Eds.), The Pharmacology of Thermoregulation. Karger, Basel, Germany.

Weihe, W.H., 1976. Influence of light on animals. In: McSheehy, T. (Ed.), Control of the Animal House Environment Lab. Anim. Ltd, London, pp. 63–76. Lab. Anim. Handbook No. 7.

Weihe, W.H., Brezowsky, H., Schwarzenbach, F.R., 1961. Der Nachweiz einer Wirkung des Klimas und Wetters auf das Wachstum der Ratte. Pflugers Archiv fur die gesamte Physiologie des Menschen und der Tiere 273, 514–527.

Weihe, W.H., Schidlow, J., Strittmatter, J., 1969. The effect of light intensity on the breeding and development of rats and golden hamsters. Int. J. Biometeorol. 13, 69–79.

Weiss, B., Stern, S., Cernichiari, E., Gelein, R., 2005. Methylmercury con-tamination of laboratory animal diets. Environ. Health Perspect. 113, 1120–1122.

Welch, B.L., Brown, D.G., Welch, A.S., Lin, D.C., 1974. Isolation, restrictive confinement, or crowding of rats for one year. I. Weight, nucleic acids, and protein of brain regions. Brain Res. 75, 71–84.

Wells, A.B., 1970. The kinetics of cell proliferation in the tracheobronchial epithelia of rats with and without chronic respiratory disease. Cell Tissue Kinet. 3, 185–206.

Welter, A., Mineo, J.R., de Oliveira Silva, D.A., Lourenço, E.V., Vieira Ferro, E.A., Roque-Barreira, M.C., et al., 2007. BALB/c mice resistant to *Toxoplasma gondii* infection proved to be highly susceptible when previously infected with *Myocoptes musculinus* fur mites. Int. J. Exp. Pathol. 88, 325–335.

Wenger, K.H., Freeman, J.D., Fulzele, S., Immel, D.M., Powell, B.D., Molitor, P., et al., 2010. Effect of whole body vibration on bone properties in aging mice. Bone 47, 746–755.

Westmark, C.J., Westmark, P.R., Malter, J.S., 2013. Soy-based diet exacerbates seizures in mouse models of neurological disease. J. Alzheimers Dis. 33, 797–805.

Wheelock, E.F., 1966. The effects of nontumor viruses on virus-induced leukemia in mice: reciprocal interference between Sendai virus and Friend leukemia virus in DBA/2 mice. Proc. Natl. Acad. Sci. USA 55, 774–780.

White, N.R., Barfield, R.J., 1987. Role of the ultrasonic vocalization of the female rat (*Rattus norvegicus*) in sexual behavior. J. Comp. Psychol. 101, 73–81.

Whiteside, T.E., Thigpen, J.E., Kissling, G.E., Grant, M.G., Forsythe, D., 2010. Endotoxin, coliform, and dust levels in various types of rodent bedding. J. Am. Assoc. Lab. Anim. Sci. 49, 184–189.

Wickham, L.A., Huang, Z., Lambert, R.W., Sullivan, D.A., 1997. Effect of sialodacryoadenitis virus exposure on acinar epithelial cells from the rat lacrimal gland. Ocul. Immunol. Inflamm. 5, 181–195.

Wightman, S.R., Mann, P.C., Wagner, J.E., 1980. Dihydrostreptomycin toxicity in the Mongolian gerbil. Meriones Unguiculatus. Lab. Anim. Sci. 30, 71–75.

Wilkening, G.M., Sutton, C.H., 1990. Health effects of nonionizing radiation. Med. Clin. North Am. 74, 489–507.

Williams, A.E., Edwards, L., Hussell, T., 2006. Colonic bacterial infection abrogates eosinophilic pulmonary disease. J. Infect. Dis. 193, 223–230.

Williams, D.I., 1971. Maze exploration in the rat under different levels of illumination. Anim. Behav. 19, 365–367.

Williams, D.L., Di Luzzio, N.R., 1980. Glucan-induced modification of murine viral hepatitis. Science 108, 67–69.

Williams-Blangero, S., 1993. Research-oriented genetic management of non-human primate colonies. Lab. Anim. Sci. 43, 535–540.

Wilson, L.M., Baldwin, A.L., 1999. Environmental stress causes mast cell degranulation, endothelial and epithelial changes, and edema in the rat intestinal mucosa. Microcirculation 6, 189–198.

Win-Shwe, T.T., Nakajima, D., Ahmed, S., Fujimaki, H., 2013. Impairment of novel object recognition in adulthood after neonatal exposure to diazinon. Arch. Toxicol. 87, 753–762.

Wise, A., 1982. Interaction of diet and toxicity – The future role of purified diet in toxicological research. Arch. Toxicol. 50, 287–299.

Wogan, G.N., 1968. Aflatoxin risks and control measures. Fed. Proc. Fed. Am. Soc. Exp. Biol. 27, 932–938.

Wogan, G.N., Kensler, T.W., Groopman, J.D., 2012. Present and future directions of translational research on aflatoxin and hepatocellular carcinoma. A review. Food Addit. Contam. Part A Chem. Anal Control Expo. Risk Assess. 29, 249–257.

Wolstenholme, G.E.W., O'Connor, M., 1967. Effects of External Stimuli on Reproduction. Ciba Foundation Study No. 26. J. & A. Churchill, London.

Wolstenholme, T.J., Rissman, F.E., Connelly, J.J., 2011. The role of bisphenol A in shaping the brain, epigenome and behavior. Horm. Behav. 59, 296–305.

Woodbury, D.M., Rollins, L.T., Gardner, M.D., Hirschi, W.L., Hogan, J.R., Rallison, M.L., et al., 1958. Effects of carbon dioxide on brain excitability and electrolytes. Am. J. Physiol. 192 (1), 79–90.

Wright, J.F., Seibold, H.R., 1958. Estrogen contamination of pelleted feed for laboratory animals. Effects on guinea pig production. J. Am. Vet. Med. Assoc. 132, 258–261.

Wurtman, R.J., 1975. The effects of light on man and other mammals. Ann. Rev. Physiol. 37, 467–483.

Xie, L., Jacobson, J.M., Choi, E.S., Busa, B., Donahue, L.R., Miller, L.M., et al., 2006. Low-level mechanical vibrations can influence bone resorption and bone formation in the growing skeleton. Bone 39, 1059–1066.

Xu, X.L., Pan, C., Hu, J.X., Liu, X.T., Li, Y.F., Wang, H., et al., 2012. Effects of isoflurane inhalation on the male reproductive system in rats. Environ. Toxicol. Pharmacol. 34, 688–693.

Yagil, R., Etzion, Z., Berlyne, G.M., 1976. Changes in rat milk quantity and quality due to variations in litter size and high ambient temperature. Lab. Anim. Sci. 26, 33–37.

Yang, C.S., Brady, J.F., Hong, J.Y., 1992. Dietary effects on cytochromes P450, xenobiotic metabolism, and toxicity. FASEB J. 6, 737–744.

Yajima, M., Matsumoto, M., Harada, M., Hara, H., Yajima, T., 2013. Effects of constant light during perinatal periods on the behavioral and neuronal development of mice with or without dietary lutein. Biomed. Res. 34, 197–204.

Yamada, H., Le, Q.T., Kousaka, A., Higashi, Y., Tsukane, M., Kido, H., 2006. Sendai virus infection up-regulates trypsin I and matrix metalloproteinase-9, triggering viral multiplication and matrix degradation in rat lungs and lung L2 cells. Arch. Virol. 151, 2529–2537.

Yamaguchi, N., Sonoyama, K., Kikuchi, H., Nagura, T., Aritsuka, T., Kawabata, J., 2005. Gastric colonization of *Candida albicans* differs in mice fed commercial and purified diets. J. Nutr. 135, 109–115.

Yan, J.G., Agresti, M., Bruce, T., Yan, Y.H., Granlund, A., Matloub, H.S., 2007. Effects of cellular phone emissions on sperm motility in rats. Fertil. Steril. 88, 957–964.

Yasenkov, R., Deboer, T., 2012. Circadian modulation of sleep in rodents. Prog. Brain Res. 199, 203–218.

Yeh, Y.C., Sun, W.Z., Ko, W.J., Chan, W.S., Fan, S.Z., Tsai, J.C., et al., 2012. Dexmedetomidine prevents alterations of intestinal microcirculation that are induced by surgical stress and pain in a novel rat model. Anesth. Analg. 115, 46–53.

Yildiz, A., Hayirli, A., Okumus, Z., Kaynar, O., Kisa, F., 2007. Physiological profile of juvenile rats: effects of cage size and cage density. Lab. Anim. 36, 28–38.

Yoneda, K., Walzer, P.D., 1981. Mechanism of pulmonary alveolar injury in experimental *Pneumocystis carinii* pneumonia in the rat. Br. J. Exp. Pathol. 62, 339–346.

York, J.M., McDaniel, A.W., Blevins, N.A., Guillet, R.R., Allison, S.O., Cengel, K.A., et al., 2012. Individually ventilated cages cause chronic low-grade hypoxia impacting mice hematologically and behaviorally. Brain Behav. Immun. 26, 951–958.

Yu, V.M., Mackinnon, S.E., Hunter, D.A., Brenner, M.J., 2011. Effect of sialodacryoadenitis virus infection on axonal regeneration. Microsurgery 31, 458–464.

Zalaquett, C., Thiessen, D., 1991. The effects of odors from stressed mice on conspecific behavior. Physiol. Behav. 50, 221–227.

Zanger, U.M., Schwab, M., 2013. Cytochrome P450 enzymes in drug metabolism: regulation of gene expression, enzyme activities, and impact of genetic variation. Pharmacol. Ther. 138, 103–141.

Zaretsky, D.V., Molosh, A.I., Zaretskaia, M.V., Rusyniak, D.E., DiMicco, J.A., 2010. Increase in plasma ACTH induced by urethane is not a consequence of hyperosmolality. Neurosci. Lett. 479, 10–12.

Zee, P.C., Attarian, H., Videnovic, A., 2013. Circadian rhythm abnormalities. Continuum (Minneap. Minn.) 19, 132–147.

Zeller, W., Meier, G., Burki, K., Panoussis, B., 1998. Adverse effects of tribromoethanol as used in the production of transgenic mice. Lab. Anim. 32, 407–413.

Zhang, J.X., Liu, Y.J., Zhang, J.H., Sun, L., 2008. Dual role of preputial gland secretion and its major components in sex recognition of mice. Physiol. Behav. 95, 388–394.

Zhang, X.P., List, W.F., 1996. Effects of halothane, isoflurane and sevoflurane on calcium-related contraction in porcine coronary arteries. Acta Anaesthesiol. Scand. 40, 815–819.

Zhang, B.L., Zannou, E., Sannajust, F., 2000. Effects of photoperiod reduction on rat circadian rhythms of BP, heart rate, and locomotor activity. Am. J. Physiol. Regul. Integr. Comp. Physiol. 279 (1), R169–R178.

Zheng, H., Dong, Y., Xu, Z., Crosby, G., Culley, D.J., Zhang, Y., et al., 2013. Sevoflurane anesthesia in pregnant mice induces neurotoxicity in fetal and offspring mice. Anesthesiology 118, 516–526.

Zheng, W., Shen, H., Blaner, W.S., Zhao, Q., Ren, X., Graziano, J.H., 1996. Chronic lead exposure alters transthyretin concentration in rat cerebrospinal fluid: the role of the choroid plexus. Toxicol. Appl. Pharmacol. 139, 445–450.

Zhu, L., Chen, T., Lu, Y., Wu, D., Luo, X., Ning, Q., 2012. Contribution of IL-17 to mouse hepatitis virus strain 3-induced acute liver failure. J. Huazhong Univ. Sci. Technolog. Med. Sci 32, 552–556.

Zondek, B., Tamari, I., 1967. Effects of auditory stimuli on reproduction. In: Wolstenholme, G.E.W., O'Connor, M. (Eds.), Effects of External Stimuli on Reproduction Ciba Foundation Study Group, no. 26 J. & A. Churchill Ltd., London, pp. 4–19.

Zurita, E., Chagoyen, M., Cantero, M., Alonso, R., González-Neira, A., López-Jiménez, A., et al., 2011. Genetic polymorphisms among C57BL/6 mouse inbred strains. Transgenic Res. 20, 481–489.

CHAPTER

34

Animal Models in Biomedical Research

Kirk J. Maurer, DVM, PhD, ACLAM[a] and
Fred W. Quimby, VMD, PhD, ACLAM[b]

[a]Center For Comparative Medicine and Research, Dartmouth College Lebanon, NH, USA
[b]Rockefeller University, New Durham, NH, USA

OUTLINE

I. INTRODUCTION

Animal models have been used to contribute to scientific discovery throughout the millenna. This chapter will focus on a general description of animal models and will highlight the contribution of animals to scientific discovery utilizing historical advancements as well as key recent advancements. Although, in general, animal models can span the phylogenetic tree, the chapter presented herein will focus its attention on the use of vertebrate animals in research.

II. WHAT IS AN ANIMAL MODEL?

A. Types of Models

1. Introduction

There are many types of models used in biomedical research, e.g., *in vitro* assay, computer simulation, mathematical models, and animal models. Vertebrate animals represent only a fraction of the models used, yet they have been responsible for critical research advancements (National Research Council, 1985). Invertebrate models have made a profound impact in the areas of neurobiology, genetics, and development and include the nematode *Caenorhabditis elegans*, protozoa, cockroaches, sea urchins, the fruit fly *Drosophila melanogaster*, *Aplysia*, and squid, among others. The sea urchin, for instance, contributed to the discovery of meiosis, events associated with fertilization, discovery of cell sorting by differential adhesion, basic control of cell cycling, and cytokinesis (National Research Council, 1985). Similar lists can be prepared for insects, squid, and other marine invertebrates. These invertebrate models have been previously reviewed and are not the major focus of this discussion (National Research Council, 1985; Woodhead, 1989; Huber *et al.*, 1990; Jasny and Koshland, 1990).

A model serves as a surrogate and is not necessarily identical to the subject being modeled (National

Laboratory Animal Medicine, Third Edition
DOI: http://dx.doi.org/10.1016/B978-0-12-409527-4.00034-1

Research Council, 1998; Scarpelli, 1997). In this chapter it is assumed that the human biological system is the subject being modeled; however, many of the advances made through studies of animal models have been applicable to animals other than humans. Conceptually, animals may model analogous processes (relating one structure or process to another) or homologous processes (reflecting counterpart genetic sequences). Prior to the rapid advancement of genomic sequencing and genomic manipulation, many animal models were selected as phenotypic analogs of human processes and conditions insofar as the human condition appeared similar even though the underlying genetic homology may or may not have been identical. To date, the primary driver of homologous modeling has been the genetically manipulated mouse. The rapid advancement of genetic manipulation in other species will likely result in an expansion of homologous modeling in these other species.

Another useful concept in modeling concerns one-to-one modeling *versus* many-to-many modeling. In one-to-one modeling a model is sought that generally demonstrates a similar phenotype to that which is being modeled. Examples of one-to-one modeling include many infectious diseases and both spontaneous and induced monogenetic diseases. Many-to-many modeling results from analysis of a process in an organism or organisms where each component feature of that process is evaluated at several hierarchical levels, e.g., system, organ, tissue, cell, and subcellular levels (National Research Council, 1985; Office of Technology Assessment, 1986). The understanding that many of the most common diseases such as cancer and obesity are complex, often polygenic, with multiple interacting environmental influences has made the use of many-to-many modeling more common. The advent of high-throughput techniques such as sequencing, transcriptomics and proteomics has facilitated this process. Often, many-to-many modeling requires the use of multiple model systems including computational modeling, *in vitro* modeling, *in vivo* modeling, and population-based studies in humans. Importantly, each has its own relative strengths and weaknesses and each may be used to continuously refine a hypothesis or group of hypotheses.

In this context it is important to note that despite the many different factors modifying the evolutionary history of humans and other animals, comparative genomics demonstrate that there remains an impressive degree of genetic conservation between commonly utilized research species and humans.

2. Spontaneous and Induced Animal Models

Animal models can be classified as spontaneous or induced. Spontaneous models may be represented by normal animals with phenotypic similarity to those of humans or by abnormal members of a species that arise through spontaneous mutation(s). In contrast, animals submitted to surgical, genetic, chemical, or other manipulation resulting in an alteration to their normal physiologic state are induced models. The single largest category of induced models are those which arise through intentional genetic manipulation. Occasionally, investigators will refer to another category of animal model, the so-called negative model. This is an animal that fails to develop or is protected from developing a particular phenotype.

Some of the best-characterized spontaneous models are those with naturally occurring mutations that lead to disorders similar to those in man. Among the best-known spontaneous models are the Gunn rat (hereditary hyperbilirubinemia), piebald lethal and lethal spotting strains of mice (aganglionic megacolon), nonobese diabetic mouse and BB Wistar rats (type 1 diabetes mellitus), New Zealand Black and New Zealand White mice and their hybrids (autoimmune disease), nude mice (DiGeorge syndrome), SCID mice (severe combined immunodeficiency), Watanabe rabbits (hypercholesterolemia), Brattleboro rats (neurogenic diabetes insipidus), obese chickens (autoimmune thyroiditis), spontaneously hypertensive rats (SHR-primary hypertension), dogs and mice with Duchenne X-linked muscular dystrophy, dogs with hemophilia A and B, swine with hyper-low-density lipoproteinemia and malignant hyperthermia, mink with Chediak–Higashi syndrome, cats with achalasia, gerbils with epilepsy, cattle with ichthyosis congenita and hyperkeratosis, and sheep with Dubin–Johnson syndrome (Andrews *et al.*, 1979). A significant limitation of spontaneous models is that their development or occurrence is quite often unpredictable and often relies upon chance.

A unique and compelling subset of spontaneous animal models are veterinary clinical patients as models of disease treatment. Recently, new cancer treatments including novel chemotherapeutics have been evaluated in dogs that presented with spontaneous tumors (Peterson *et al.*, 2010). These models are intriguing because they have the potential to directly benefit the animals in which the drugs and treatments are being tested and to eventually benefit human patients. Further, unlike other commonly utilized species (i.e., inbred mice) the spontaneous tumors which develop in these veterinary patients may more faithfully recapitulate the heterogeneity of human tumors.

Induced models have been used to unravel some of the most important concepts in physiology and medicine. Surgical models contributed greatly to the understanding of brain plasticity, (Florence *et al.*, 1998; Jones and Pons, 1998; Merzenich, 1998), organ transplantation; coronary bypass surgery; balloon angioplasty; replacement of heart valves; development of cardiac pacemakers; the discovery of insulin; fluid therapy and other treatments for shock, liver failure, and gallstones; and surgical resection of the intestines, including the technique of colostomy (Council on Scientific Affairs, 1989; Bay et al., 1995; Quimby, 1994a, 1995). Additional useful models have been induced by diet or administration of drugs or chemicals. Alloxan and streptozotocin have been used to study insulin-dependent diabetes because, when injected, these chemicals selectively destroy the beta cells of the islets of Langerhans (Golob et al., 1970; Sisson and Plotz, 1967). More recently, chemical mutagenesis approaches have been utilized as a tool to conduct forward mutagenesis screening in mice and zebrafish (Becker et al., 2006). Diet-induced models have been responsible for discovery of most vitamins and the necessity for trace minerals as nutrients, as well as for exploration of the pathogenesis of many diseases. Observations of chickens with beriberi (thiamin deficiency) resulted in a cure for humans (and animals) and led to the discovery of vitamins (Eijkman, 1965). In fact, dietary manipulations in the chicken alone have contributed to our knowledge of rickets (Kwan et al., 1989), vitamin A deficiency (Bang et al., 1972), vitamin B_6 deficiency (Masse et al., 1989), zinc deficiency (O'Dell et al., 1990), Friedreich's ataxia (van Gelder and Belanger, 1988), fetal alcohol syndrome (Means et al., 1988), and atherosclerosis (Kottke and Subbiah, 1978; Kritchevsky, 1974).

Often complex induced models are used by combining multiple experimental manipulations. An excellent example is the humanized severe combined immunodeficient (*hu-SCID*) mouse, where a natural mutation in the *RAG1* gene prevents T- or B-cell antigen receptor rearrangements, resulting in a severe combined immunodeficiency. When this mouse is injected with human lymphocytes or stem cells, it adopts the immune system of humans (Carballido et al., 2000). Injection of this reconstituted mouse with HIV-1 virus leads to viral propagation and a small-animal model for the assessment of anti-HIV drugs (Mosier, 1996). More recently the NSG (NOD, SCID, IL2 receptor knockout) mouse has been utilized to create 'humanized' mice. Specifically, these already immunodeficient mice are exposed to myeloablative irradiation and then reconstituted with human stem cells, generally hCD34+ human hematopoietic stem cells. These mice can then be utilized to study a variety of human infectious and immunological diseases (Zhang et al., 2010). A promising new model has been developed for personalized cancer treatment. In general these rely on transplanting tissue biopsies from patients with tumors into a variety of immunodeficient mice and testing various treatment modalities to determine which treatment might be most efficacious for that patient's specific tumor (Hidalgo et al., 2011). The results of these studies are promising insofar as drug susceptibility identified in orthotopically transplanted

mice seems to faithfully reflect susceptibility noted in the human patients (Hidalgo et al., 2011).

Another recent induced model involves manipulation of the host microbiota and the understanding of the critical role that the microbiota plays in a variety of diseases (Ukhanova et al., 2012; Garrett et al., 2010; Gordon, 2005; Backhed et al., 2005; Hooper et al., 2002). The mouse, and in particular the gnotobiotic mouse, have largely been responsible for our understanding of this process. In a series of elegant studies it was demonstrated that the microbiome of mice is critical for the development of diet-induced obesity and that this phenotype can be altered by altering the microbiome (Turnbaugh et al., 2008; Backhed et al., 2007; Turnbaugh et al., 2006). Likewise, other studies have demonstrated that the microbiome plays roles in a variety of diverse diseases (Fremont-Rahl et al., 2013; Greer et al., 2013; Hansen et al., 2013; Karlsson et al., 2013; Kostic et al., 2013; Mathis and Benoist, 2012; Schwabe and Jobin, 2013). One thing that differs between these induced models and many others described within this chapter is that the inducing factor in these models is not an exogenous source (e.g., toxin, pathogen, surgery) but is something that is entirely indigenous to the animal. The ability of the microbiome to impact a broad range of host processes invariably leads to the realization that the ability to replicate certain phenotypes or studies may be impacted by the microbiome. That is to say, study variability at different institutions and perhaps even among different rooms and mouse colonies at the same institutions may be impacted by unknown variations in the microbiome of the research subject.

Animals have, of course, served as models of toxicology and drug safety for a very long time. The use of animal models in drug safety, pharmacology, and toxicity testing are an important component of preclinical studies involving these products. Traditional rodent models of toxicology studies include the B6C3F1 hybrid mouse and the Fisher F344 rat which have been characterized extensively to describe their spontaneous histological lesions as reference points in toxicological studies (Ward et al., 1979, Goodman et al., 1979). Larger animal models including dogs, various nonhuman primates and swine have also been utilized in toxicological and drug safety research (Gad, 2007).

3. Genetically Manipulated Animals

Due to the close homology of the mouse genome to the human genome direct manipulation of the mouse genome has produced a great number of animal models that robustly mimic the intended human disease phenotype. The techniques utilized to create knockout and transgenic mice are covered in more detail in other chapters in this text and are extensively detailed in other texts; however, we will briefly detail some historical and common methods used to generate these induced models here (Behringer et al., 2013, Pluck and Klasen, 2009).

a. Chemical Mutagenesis

When the drug N-nitroso-N-ethylurea (ENU) is injected into male mice, single base pair mutations are created in the germ cells. By breeding progeny and backcrossing mice, homozygotes for the mutated allele are obtained. Genes in mouse embryonic stem cells (ESCs) can be mutated by use of ENU. Many useful models of human disease have been so created in mice, including models for phenylketonuria (mutated phenylalanine hydroxylase gene), α-thalassemia (α-globin), β-thalassemia (β-globin), osteopetrosis (carbonic anhydrase II), glucose-6-phosphate deficiency, tetrahydrobiopterin-deficient hyperphenylalaninemia (GTP-cyclohydrolase I), Duchenne muscular dystrophy (dystrophin), triose-phosphate isomerase deficiency, adenomatous intestinal polyposis coli, hypersarcosinemia (sarcosine dehydrogenase), erythropoietic protoporphyria (ferrochelatase), and glutathionuria (γ-glutamytranspeptidase) (Herweijer et al., 1997).

Zebrafish, *Danio rerio*, have been used extensively for studies in development because their embryos are transparent, each clutch contains 50–100 embryos, and the fish are amenable to large-scale mutagenesis using compounds like ENU (Driever and Fishman, 1996). Distinct genes have different mutability rates; however, ENU is reported to induce genetic mutations at average induction rates of 1 in 1000. This estimate serves as the basis for large-scale genomic screens (Nusslein-Volhard, 1994).

A limitation of ENU mutagenesis is that mutations occur relatively randomly. Once a phenotype is established, in order to determine which gene was mutated to produce the phenotype, chromosomal mapping and large-scale sequencing were necessary. Until very recently, large-scale rapid automated sequencing was for the most part unavailable or available as a very limited and expensive resource. More recently, the cost and availability of automated high-throughput sequencing has made sequencing and data analysis of mice and zebrafish created by these forward genetic screens more reasonable.

b. Irradiation

Irradiation was used as a germline mutagen dating back to the early 1920s. X-rays have been shown to cause small chromosomal deletions in mouse spermatogonia, postmeiotic germ cells, and oocytes (Takahashi et al., 1994). Examples of radiation-induced models in wide use include the beige mouse (*bg*), dominant cataract (*Cat-2t*), and cleidocranial dysplasia (Roths et al., 1999). Because X-rays often produce large deletions, this technique has significant practical limitations due to low recovery rate of mutant mice.

c. Transgenics and Targeted Mutations

The first method of transgenic manipulation was described by Gordon and Ruddle (1981) and involved direct insertion of cloned genetic material into the pronucleus of a fertilized mouse egg. This method is relatively straight-forward but is limited in that the site of integration is fairly random. Around the same time, mouse ESC lines were first produced and maintained in culture (Martin, 1981). This discovery allowed investigators to insert genes by targeted homologous recombination, using vectors that contain selectable markers. As a result, ESCs with a targeted mutation can be microinjected into a developing mouse embryo which is then implanted into pseudopregnant recipient mothers. Offspring are chimeras because they contain cells of both cultured ESC origin and embryo origin. With molecular screening and appropriate matings, eventually founders that have germline expression of the mutation are produced.

These technologies can be utilized to create gain of function and loss of function mutants and combinations of the two. Through the use of tissue-specific promoters or enhancers and receptors whose transcription can be controlled by exogenous drugs and chemicals, gene expression can be altered so that it occurs in a tissue specific or temporally regulated fashion. A common example of this is created by flanking the gene of interest with *loxP* sequences (so called 'floxed' genes/mice), which are targets for bacteriophage Cre recombinase. Crossing floxed mice to mice expressing Cre recombinase under control of desired promoter results in tissue-specific exon excision and ablation of gene function (Gordon, 1997; Nagy and Rossant, 1996). Alternatively, Cre can be exogenously provided by viral or other vectors which can be administered to specific anatomic sites (brain, lungs, liver, etc.) by direct injection or through viral tissue targeting (van der Neut, 1997). Insertion of a tetracycline element into this system allows genes to be turned off or on in response to tetracycline administration (Utomo et al., 1999). Another example is creating a fusion between Cre under the control of a tissue-specific promoter which is turned on in response to a mutated steroid ligand-binding domain. Cre expression is driven by administering tamoxifen or other similar synthetic steroids to the mice (Schwenk et al., 1998).

The use of the Cre-lox system has proven so valuable to research that there are any number of commercially available Cre-expressing strains of mice under the control of a number of tissue-specific promoters or chemical mediators which can be purchased from commercial vendors and bred directly to 'floxed' mice. Examples include Cre being driven from the albumin promoter (liver), actin promoter (muscle), and CD8 promoters (T-lymphocyte) A complete list of available strains can be found at The Jackson Laboratory Cre repository website (http://jaxmice.jax.org/list/xprs_creRT1801.html).

Another modification of the standard microinjection method for producing transgenic mice is one in which large multilocus segments of human DNA were transferred into the mouse pronucleus in the form of yeast artificial chromosomes (YACs). The entire β-globin multigene locus (248 kb) was cloned into yeast, and once integrated, this locus could be mutated at precise points by homologous recombination. After transferring YACs and mutated YACs into mice, the full developmental expression of epsilon, gamma, beta, and delta genes was observed since the YAC also contained the human locus control region that interacts with structural genes to ensure that the correct globin is produced at the proper time and place during development (Peterson et al., 1998; Porcu et al., 1997). These YAC transgenic mice are free of the restrictions inherent in single-gene cloned DNA, e.g., the genomic organization is not disrupted around the structural gene; thus, higher levels of transcription and developmental regulation of gene expression can be studied.

The mouse embryo has proven relatively easy to genetically manipulate when compared to some other mammalian genomes. If one examines the relative availability of other genetically engineered mammals it is evident that these techniques have not always readily translated to other species. The limiting factors of these techniques are the fairly low frequency of recombinational events. This low frequency, 1 in 10^4–10^7, for targeted mutation, necessitates the use of large numbers of implantable embryos or the use of ESCs and selectable markers, techniques which may not be readily available for all species (Templeton et al., 1997). Recently however several technologies have allowed for more efficient creation of non-mouse transgenic/knockout animals.

The first of these techniques is lentivirus-mediated transgenic manipulation; briefly, this involves the use of modified lentiviral vectors to deliver exogenous nucleic acid. This technique takes advantage of the natural ability of lentiviruses to integrate into the host genome. There are several advantages to this in comparison to standard pronuclear injection for the creation of transgenic animals. First, the process is not technically demanding, additionally when compared to standard pronuclear injection the amount of progeny bearing the transgene are very high (Park, 2007). The ability to create a higher percentage of progeny expressing the transgene has allowed this technique to be used in a variety of mammalian and avian species because far fewer embryos are needed (Park, 2007).

Another technique is the use of zinc-finger nucleases (ZFN) (Le Provost et al., 2010; Carroll, 2011a,b). These enzymes are targetable recombinases that can be used to induce homologous recombination or removal of a portion of the genome. ZFN contain separate DNA binding and cleavage domains and, unlike standard knockout techniques, rely upon the normal double-strand break repair process of the host (Carroll, 2011a,b). ZFN DNA binding is governed by a distinct three nucleotide sequence; however, not all nucleotide sequences and their corresponding ZFN have been identified (Wei et al., 2013). An advantage of the use of ZFN is that they are far more efficient when compared to standard strategies and efficiencies of around 10% are reported (Carroll, 2011a,b). This high efficiency means the manipulation can be conducted without the use of ESCs and can be done directly in the zygote or embryo (Carroll, 2011a,b). To date, a variety of genetically modified species have been created using this technique and it is important to realize that ZFN is still in its relative infancy meaning the likelihood of even more broad application is quite probable.

The TALEN (transcription activator-like effector nuclease) technique is similar to the ZFN technique insofar as it relies upon a nuclease. TALEN however utilizes TAL (transcription activator-like) effector elements (TALEs). These elements are produced by bacteria and used to modulate transcription of the host genome in a way that benefits the pathogen by binding to host DNA and activating transcription (Doyle et al., 2013). TALEs have the advantage of being able to be engineered to bind to targeted areas of the genome. DNA binding specificity of TALEs was demonstrated to be mediated by two amino acids in the TALE protein that correspond directly with the nucleic acid sequence of the target site (Moscou and Bogdanove, 2009). This is a distinct advantage over ZFN technology because it means that synthetic TALEs can be generated with direct specificity. By further coupling this TALE to a nuclease (TALEN) you can generate DNA cleavage in a site-specific fashion (Bogdanove and Voytas, 2011). To date this technique has proven highly efficient in organisms as diverse as plants and large agricultural animals (Wei et al., 2013).

The final, and most recent, technique is called CRISPR. In bacteria, a CRISPR (clustered regularly interspaced short palindromic repeat) locus is a DNA sequence containing direct nucleic acid repeats with intervening nucleic acid regions called spacers (Wei et al., 2013). Bacteria can incorporate foreign nucleic acids into CRISPR regions of their own genome (Bhaya et al., 2011; Ishino et al., 1987). The bacteria then transcribe this region of DNA and with the help of CRISPR-associated (Cas) nucleases the small transcribed RNA molecules target invading foreign nucleic acid for cleavage (Bhaya et al., 2011). In this manner, bacteria effectively utilize invading viral genomes against themselves in a primitive adaptive immune response (IR). The transcribed CRISPR RNA (crRNA) targets nucleic acid of invading pathogens by direct 'Watson–Crick' base paring and Cas proteins cleave the invader (Reeks et al., 2013).

Genetic manipulation in eukaryotes can therefore be accomplished by generating crRNA molecules against specific genomic regions. The technique is in its infancy but efficiencies of over 90% have been reported in mice and the technique has been used in other species as well (Pennisi, 2013; Sung *et al.*, 2014). Indeed the highly effective nature of this technique has led many to speculate that it could be used to treat or reverse human genetic conditions, but enthusiasm may need to be tempered by findings that there are a high degree of off-target modifications in human cells (Schwank *et al.*, 2013; Fu *et al.*, 2013) Regardless of the long-term capability of the technique to treat human diseases the high efficiency of the technique likely means that it will be used for a greater array of vertebrates in the future.

B. Principles of Model Selection and the 'Ideal' Animal Model

Various authors have attempted to define the 'ideal' animal model. Features such as (a) similarity to the process being mimicked, (b) ease of handling, (c) ability to produce large litters, (d) economy of maintenance, (e) ability to sample blood and tissues sequentially in the same individual, (f) defined genetic composition, and (g) defined disease status are commonly mentioned (Dodds and Abelseth, 1980; Leader and Padgett, 1980). Perhaps the most important single feature of the model is how closely it resembles the original human condition or process. Shapiro uses the term 'validation' as a formal testing of the hypothesis that significant similarities exist between the model and the modeled (Shapiro, 1998). He argues that to be valid, the animal model should be productive of new insights into and effective treatments for the human condition being modeled.

The National Research Council (NRC) recommended some criteria for models to be financially supported (National Research Council, 1998). Among the criteria listed were that the model (1) is appropriate for its intended use(s) (a specific disease model faithfully mimics the human disease and a model system is appropriate for the human system being modeled); (2) can be developed, maintained, and provided at reasonable cost in relation to the perceived or potential scientific values that will accrue from it; (3) is of value for more than one limited kind of research; (4) is reproducible and reliable, so results can be confirmed; and (5) is reasonably available and accessible. These seem to be prudent criteria to follow when a funding organization seeks the greatest benefit within the confines of a finite budget and when an investigator is seeking the best model to utilize. These recommendations also fulfill most of the criteria of an 'ideal' model.

III. NATURE OF RESEARCH

A. Hypothesis Testing and Serendipity

1. The Progressive and Winding Route to Discovery

Francis Bacon (1620) proposed a process of scientific discovery based on a collection of observations, followed by a systematic evaluation of these observaiotns in an effort to demonstrate their truthfulness. Bacon's requirement for elimination of all those inessential conditions (which are not always associated with the phenomenon under study) was, in the end, unachievable, and the process of choosing facts was found to depend on individual judgment. However, Bacon did set the tenets for what would become the method of hypothesis testing.

Arguably, the foundation for sorting fact from fiction in scientific investigations is based on hypothesis testing (a particularly weak aspect of Bacon's philosophy). Although it is never possible to directly prove a hypothesis by experimentation, but rather to disprove one (or more) alternative (null) hypotheses; history has documented the steady (although sometimes slow) progress toward understanding the scientific world. Additionally, observations made during the testing of one hypothesis often have lead investigators in an altogether different direction. One may argue, and rightfully so, that hypothesis testing is an inefficient mechanism for discovery; however, this paradigm of generating a hypothesis based on known facts and designing experiments to disprove the hypothesis generally produces meaningful and reproducible results.

Using coronary bypass surgery as an example demonstrates just how long and often how circuitous the road to medical discovery can be. The earliest studies that contributed to the first successful bypass surgery in the 1970s go back to 1628 when Harvey described the circulation of frogs and reptiles; then in 1667, Hooke hypothesized (and later demonstrated) that pulmonary blood, flowing through lungs distended with air, could maintain the life of animals. These early observations had no impact on medicine until centuries later, primarily because other technologies necessary for successful application of extracorporeal oxygenation in humans, including antisepsis, anticoagulants, blood groups, anesthesia, etc., had not yet been discovered. Dogs played a critical role during this process of discovery, and between 1700 and 1970 contributed knowledge on the differential pressures in the heart; measurements of cardiac output, cardiopulmonary function, and pulmonary capillary pressure; and development of heart chamber catheterization techniques, heart–lung pumps, angiography, indirect revascularization, direct autographs, saphenous vein grafts, balloon catheters, and floating catheters

(Comroe and Dripps, 1974). While examining the history behind the 10 most important clinical advances in cardiopulmonary medicine and surgery, Comroe and Dripps (1976) selected 529 key articles (articles that had an important effect on the direction of research) in order to determine how these critical discoveries came about (Comroe and Dripps, 1976). They found that 41% of these articles reported work that had no relation to the disease it later helped to prevent, treat, or alleviate. This phenomenon probably contributes to the observation that few basic science discoveries, including those conducted using animals, are cited in seminal papers describing a clinical breakthrough.

The idea that major clinical breakthroughs required a long history of basic science discoveries, often involving animals, and often being conducted by individuals who were unaware of the ultimate application of this knowledge, continues to be true today. Rodolfo Llinás after reflecting on 47 years of research aimed at elucidating the nature of neurotransmission, much of it accomplished using the giant axons of squid, states: "In the end, our complete understanding of this process (synaptic transmission) will manifest itself not as a simple insight, but rather as an ungainly reconstruction of parallel events more numerous than elegant" (Llinás et al., 1999).

Both Bacon and Mill, who followed him, believed it was the responsibility of scientists to find the "necessary and sufficient conditions" that describe phenomena. That exhaustive lists of circumstances had to be examined in the search of what was necessary and sufficient never concerned these philosophers (Bacon, 1990; Mill, 1974). Both saw virtue in this process. The scientific method practiced today evolved from the principles of Bacon and Mill and was refined by the middle of the 19th century. The method provides principles and procedures to be used in the pursuit of knowledge and incorporates the recognition of a problem with the accumulation of data through observation and experimentation (empiricism) and the formulation and testing of hypotheses (Poincare, 1905). The method attempts to exclude the imposition of individual values, unsubstantiated generalizations, and deferments to higher authority as mechanisms for seeking the truth. It also subscribes to basing hypotheses only on the facts at hand and then rigorously testing hypotheses under various conditions. Hypotheses that appear to be true today may and indeed are frequently disproved or modified in the future as new conditions are imposed upon them and new technologies employed in the collection of data.

Although great discoveries in biology and medicine have depended on the application of these principles, progress is still often slow. As hypotheses are proven incorrect either slightly or greatly, alternative hypotheses

are sought and tested. Unexpected experimental results require careful consideration; and often the reasoned explanation of this data contributes information critical for the formulation of an alternative hypothesis.

In the mid-1970s, a series of breeding experiments was conducted to test the hypothesis that systemic lupus erythematosus (SLE) resulted from a mutation passed between individuals through simple Mendelian inheritance. Dogs that spontaneously developed SLE were bred and their progeny tested (Lewis and Schwartz, 1971). Surprisingly, no offspring in three generations of inbreeding developed SLE, but over half the offspring developed other autoimmune diseases, including lymphocytic thyroiditis, Sjögrens syndrome, rheumatoid arthritis, and juvenile (type 1) diabetes (Quimby et al., 1979). After careful reexamination of the data, it was hypothesized that multiple, independently segregating genes were involved in the predisposition to autoimmunity and furthermore, that certain genes (class 1) would affect a key component in the immune system common to several autoimmune disorders, with other genes (class 2) acting to modify the expression of class 1 genes, producing a variety of different phenotypes (autoimmune disease syndromes) (Quimby and Schwartz, 1980). Data collected over the next 15 years, using techniques unavailable in the 1970s, have generally upheld this hypothesis and elucidated genetic mechanisms unimaginable at the time (Datta, 2000).

2. Taking Advantage of Unexpected Findings

Serendipity also contributes to important discoveries. In 1889, a laboratory assistant noticed a large number of flies swarming about the urine of a depancreatized dog and brought it to the attention of VonMering and Minkowski. Minkowski discovered, on analysis, that the urine contained high concentrations of sugar. This chance observation helped VonMering and Minkowski discover that the pancreas had multiple functions, one being to regulate blood glucose (Comroe, 1977).

In the late 1800s, Christiaan Eijkman was sent to the Dutch Indies to study the cause of beriberi, a severe polyneuritis affecting residents of Java. While conducting studies, Eijkman noticed that chickens housed near the laboratory developed a similar disease. He tried and failed to transfer the illness from sick to healthy birds; however, shortly thereafter the disorder in chickens spontaneously cleared. Eijkman questioned a laboratory keeper about food provided to the chickens and discovered that for economy, the attendant had previously switched from the regular chicken feed to boiled polished rice, which he obtained from the hospital kitchen. Several months later the practice of providing boiled rice to the chickens was discontinued, which correlated with disease recovery in the birds. This chance observation led Eijkman to conduct feed trials demonstrating that a factor missing in polished rice caused beriberi and that the disease could be cured by eating unpolished rice. These studies led to the discovery of the vitamin thiamin, and were the first to show that disease could be caused by the absence of something rather than the presence of something, e.g., bacteria or toxins (Eijkman, 1965).

These examples reinforce the necessity for making careful observations, investigating unexpected findings, and designing careful follow-up experiments. Eijkman was awarded the Nobel Prize in Medicine in 1929, and Banting and Macleod received the Nobel Prize in 1923 for their discovery of insulin, made possible by the previous observations of VonMering and Minkowski (Leader and Stark, 1987). The issue of serendipity involving laboratory animals in biomedical research was extensively reviewed in a dedicated issue of the *ILAR Journal* (vol 46[4], 2005).

B. Breakthroughs in Technology: Paradigm Shifts

In *The Structure of Scientific Revolutions*, Kuhn (1970) makes a case for scientific communities sharing certain paradigms (Kuhn, 1970). Scientific communities consist of practitioners of a scientific specialty that share similar educations, literatures, communications, and techniques and as a result, frequently have similar viewpoints, goals, and a relative unanimity of judgment. Kuhn believes that science is not an objective progression toward the truth but rather a series of peaceful interludes, heavily influenced by the paradigms (call them theories) shared by the members of a scientific community and interrupted, on occasion, by intellectually violent revolutions that are associated with great gains in new knowledge. Revolutions are a change involving a certain sort of reconstruction of group (community) commitments. They usually are preceded by crisis (from within or outside the community) experienced by the community that undergoes revolution.

Kuhn explains that scientific communities share a disciplinary matrix composed of symbolic generalizations (expressions, displayed without question or dissent by group members), beliefs in particular models, shared values, and exemplars (those concrete problem solutions that all students of the community learn during their training). This disciplinary matrix is what provides the glue that keeps members of the community thinking (problem solving) alike. However, it is also what prevents members from taking high-stake chances and proposing new rules that counter prevailing opinion. Precisely when two members of a community disagree on a theory or principle because they realize that the paradigm no longer provides a sufficient basis for proof

is the debate likely to continue in the form it inevitably takes during scientific revolutions. What happens during revolutions is that the similarity sets established by exemplars and other components of the disciplinary matrix can no longer neatly classify objects into similar groups. An example is the grouping of sun, moon, Mars, and Earth before and after Copernicus, where a convert to the new astronomy must now say (on seeing the moon), "I once took the moon to be a planet, but I was mistaken." As a result of the revolution, scientists with a new paradigm see differently than they did in the past and apply different rules, tools, and techniques to solve problems in the future (Kuhn, 1970).

In the previous edition of this chapter, the author predicted that we were on the verge of just such a paradigm shift in biology. The prediction was that the integration of computation into biology would transform or revolutionize the biological field. This prediction has indeed been prescient. We are now in just such a revolution in biology, a biological revolution that is driven largely by advances in computation. In the past, biological studies were often limited by the ability of the observer to assimilate and analyze data. That is to say, studies were confined because individuals were only able to analyze a finite, relatively small amount of information. Now, large data sets can be analyzed by computer programs which can be used on virtually even the simplest home computer. There are numerous examples of this in the literature today including the widespread use of RNA/cDNA microarrays, high-throughput sequencing, metabolomics and high-throughput drug screening (Kim *et al.*, 2013; Carrico *et al.*, 2013; O'Brien *et al.*, 2012; Rodriguez and Gutierrez-de-Teran, 2013; Henson *et al.*, 2012; Tian *et al.*, 2012; Garcia-Reyero and Perkins, 2011; Koyuturk, 2010; Laird, 2010; Yen *et al.*, 2009; Dalby, 2007; Kleppe *et al.*, 2006; Zhang and Zhang, 2006; Hennig, 2004; Capecchi *et al.*, 2004; Kim, 2002; Varfolomeev *et al.*, 2002; Gerlai, 2002). It is indeed, amazing to consider that merely decades ago it took teams of scientists and a massive input of federal funding to complete the human genome project, whereas today an individual consumer can get their personalized genome sequenced and analyzed (Li-Pook-Than and Snyder, 2013). Of course there are other contributors to this biological revolution aside from computational analysis. Specifically automation, microfluidics and engineering processes have all contributed to this rapid progression.

Aside from analyzing large data sets, computation allows for the generation of *de novo* prediction. That is, computer programs can and are being used to generate new hypotheses. Examples of this type of work are the prediction of three-dimensional protein structure, protein function, and protein–protein interaction based upon amino acid sequence and other input data (Patronov and Doytchinova, 2013; Demel *et al.*, 2008;

Breitling *et al.*, 2008; Schrattenholz and Soskic, 2008; Zhao *et al.*, 2008, Ecker *et al.*, 2008). Indeed there are numerous commercially available software packages that are capable of doing this. An offshoot of this is novel protein design or computationally assisted protein design and modification. That is, using programs to generate modified proteins or chemicals with specific user input characteristics (e.g., altered receptor binding) or capabilities (Patronov and Doytchinova, 2013; Mak *et al.*, 2013; Shublaq *et al.*, 2013).

Indeed, the appearance of computational biology has led to the necessity of completely new methods to analyze data for patterns or trends. That is to say, classical statistical analysis used for decades by biologists often fail to capture the complexity of the large data sets analyzed. For example, if one were to analyze the transcriptional profile of cells or a mouse under several treatment paradigms and then merely determine which genes were expressed at statistically significant levels under these conditions there would invariably be a relatively large and somewhat unmanageable data set. The question then becomes, what do these changes tell us about the system being analyzed and are the individual gene changes truly meaningful. Other analyses therefore may be more beneficial in understanding the system. Various algorithms may be used to classify expression patterns and two commonly used approaches are unsupervised learning and supervised learning schemes (Allison *et al.*, 2006). Unsupervised learning is relatively free of user input whereas supervised learning relies on user input to guide the algorithm. Unsupervised has the advantage of being free of user input bias but also may fail to capture differences which result from sample variability as opposed to true population differences (Allison *et al.*, 2006).

There are other techniques in their scientific infancy today including RNA sequencing which will undoubtedly provide even greater data sets (Wang *et al.*, 2009). RNA sequencing provides transcriptional profile data similar to microarrays but provides greater data discovery power on several levels. First, the expression levels appear to be more precise compared to microarray data (Wang *et al.*, 2009). Additionally, RNA sequencing does not rely upon the known or presumed coding sequence of the organism being examined (Wang *et al.*, 2009). That is, microarrays utilize 'known' cDNA targets and therefore novel or altered transcripts will be missed (Wang *et al.*, 2009). An additional benefit is that relatively large quantities of RNA are required for microarray analysis whereas smaller amounts are needed for RNA sequencing (Wang *et al.*, 2009). There remain some challenges with RNA sequencing including the necessity to assemble the transcriptome, a step which is not necessary in arrays; however, it would appear the advantages of RNA sequencing will soon make this the gold standard in transcriptional profiling.

Another relatively new technique is ChIP Seq (chromatin immunoprecipitation sequencing). This technique is a highthrouput method to determine DNA:protein interactions in which cells are fixed to crosslink proteins to the chromosome and then immunoprecipitated with antibodies specific to the protein of interest (Landt *et al.*, 2012). If the protein has bound to any chromosomal regions this DNA will be co-immunoprecipitated as well. High-throughput DNA sequencing is then conducted to determine genomic regions that are being bound by the protein (Landt *et al.*, 2012). The obvious implication is that the protein is interacting in some fashion with the DNA sequence obtained. Data analysis, of course, relies upon computational assembly and annotation of the sequence and then identifying the chromosomal region/gene it is associated with.

It appears therefore that this is truly a transformative time in the biological sciences. Automation and radical advancements in computation make even the most complex of data sets capable of being analyzed. Perhaps unexpected but nevertheless true is that current finding, based on DNA sequence analysis with comparisons between animals and man, that predictions can be made in a comprehensive, unbiased, hypothesis-free manner (Lander, 2011).

IV. HISTORY OF ANIMAL USE IN BIOMEDICAL RESEARCH

A. Early History

Humans have a history of close interaction with animals that extends back over 20,000 years (with the domestication of poultry in China) and includes the domestication of buffalo, cattle, sheep, and dogs between 6,000 and 10,000 years ago. The earliest written records of animal experimentation date to 2000 BC when Babylonians and Assyrians documented surgery and medications for humans and animals.

True scientific inquiry began in the intellectually liberal climate of ancient Greece where the teachings of Aristotle, Plato, and Hippocrates symbolized a move to understand natural phenomena without resorting to mysticism or demonology. In this environment, philosophy was conceived and wisdom was admired. Early animal experimentation was conducted in 304 BC by the anatomist Erasistratos, who demonstrated the relationship between food intake and weight gain in birds. In the second century AD, the physician Galen used a variety of animals to show that arteries contained blood and not air, as believed by his contemporaries. During this period, physicians carried out careful anatomic dissections, and on the basis of the comparative anatomy of animals and humans, accumulated a remarkable list of achievements, including a description of embryonic development; the establishment of the importance of the umbilical cord for fetal survival; and the recognition of the relationship between the optic nerves, which arise from the eyes, and the brain.

The Greeks, and later the Romans, developed schools of higher learning (including medical schools), created museums, and documented their findings in libraries. Physicians from this period recognized that fever aided the healing process, recognized the inherited nature of certain disorders and classified them, and practiced intubation to prevent suffocation and ligation and excision for the treatment of hemorrhoids. This brief period of scientific inquiry in Europe gave way to the Middle Ages, a 1200-year period characterized by war, religious persecution, and unsavory politics. During the Middle Ages until the Rennaisance, the writings of ancient Greece and Rome remained the final word on science and medicine.

Medical education was revived in 10th-century Salerno, Italy, but because of a prohibition on human dissection that lasted into the 13th century, animals were substituted for humans as models in the instruction of anatomy. Because no investigations took place, virtually no new discoveries in medicine were made. Imagine how handicapped these medieval physicians must have been. They still did not know that the filling of lungs with air was necessary for life, that the body was composed of many cells organized into tissues, that blood circulated and the heart served as its pump, and that blood traverses from arteries to veins in tissues via capillaries; these facts were revealed by Hook in 1667, Swammerdam in 1667, Van Leeuwenhoek in 1680, Harvey in 1628, Malpighi in 1687, and Pecquet in 1651, respectively, each using animals to demonstrate these basic principles. In part, this return to the process of scientific discovery was built on the foundations established by Francis Bacon, a foundation based on collecting facts, developing hypotheses, and attempting to disprove them via experimentation.

The pace of biomedical research increased during the 1700s as Priestley discovered that the life-promoting constituent of air was oxygen. Scientists such as Von Haller, Spallanzani, Trembly, and Stevens, each using animals, discovered the relationship between nerve impulses and muscle contraction, recorded cell division, and associated the process of digestion with the secretions of the stomach. Hales made the first recording of blood pressure in a horse in 1733, Crawford measured the metabolic heat of an animal using water calorimetry in 1788, and Beddoes successfully performed pneumotherapy in animals in 1795 (although it was not until 1917 that Haldane would introduce modern oxygen therapy for humans). By 1815, Laennec had perfected the stethoscope, using animals. Despite these dramatic gains in medical knowledge, physicians were still not aware of the germ theory of disease (and of course could not avoid, prevent, or treat infections) (Quimby, 1994a).

B. From Pasteur to the Genomic Era

In the 1860s, the French scientist Louis Pasteur discovered that microscopic particles, which he called vibrions (i.e., bacteria), were a cause of a fatal disease in silkworms. When he eliminated the vibrions, silkworms grew free of disease; the first demonstration of the germ theory of disease. In 1877, Pasteur turned his attention to two animal diseases, anthrax in sheep and cholera in chickens. In each disease he isolated the causative agent, reduced its virulence by exposure to high temperature, and showed that on injection the attenuated organism imparted protection against the disease. Pasteur referred to this process as vaccination (from Latin *vacca*, 'cow') in homage to the English surgeon Edward Jenner, who discovered that injection of matter from cowpox lesions into humans protected them against smallpox. Pasteur went on to develop the first vaccine against rabies, in which the virus was attenuated by passage through rabbits. This vaccine was shown to impart protection in dogs and later in humans.

Pasteur's work with microscopic organisms as agents of disease quickly led to two other important discoveries. John Lister, having read of Pasteur's discovery, hypothesized that these microorganisms were responsible for wound infections. He impregnated cloth with an antiseptic of carbolic acid and showed that when used as a wound dressing, the antiseptic prevented infection and gangrene. This led to the generalized use of antiseptics before surgery and sterilization of surgical instruments. In 1876, Robert Koch would demonstrate a technique for growing bacteria outside of an animal (*in vitro*) in pure culture. This would reduce the number of animals required to conduct research on infectious agents, and it allowed Koch to establish postulates for definitively associating a specific agent with a specific disease. Using these postulates, Koch discovered the cause of tuberculosis, *Mycobacterium tuberculosis*, and he developed tuberculin used to identify infected animals and people. Between 1840 and 1850, Long and Morton demonstrated the usefulness of ether as a general anesthetic first in animals and later in humans.

1. Contributions to Inheritance

The second half of the 19th century began a new era in biology and medicine. In addition to such medical developments as vaccination, testing for tuberculosis, anesthesia, and blood transfusion, each of which depended on animal experimentation, two other events changed the direction of biological science forever. In 1859, the English naturalist Charles Darwin published *On the Origin of Species*, in which he hypothesized that all life evolves by selection of traits that give one species an advantage over others. Around the same time, the Austrian monk Gregor Mendel used peas to demonstrate that specific traits are inherited in a predictable fashion. Nearly half a century later, the English biologist William Bateson reached the same conclusion by selectively breeding chickens and reported his result, as Mendel's work was being generally recognized.

Mendel proposed two laws of heredity: first, that two different hereditary characters, after being combined in one generation, will again segregate in the next; and second, that hereditary characteristics assort in new daughter cells independently (Sourkes, 1966). Unfortunately, Bateson's investigations with chickens did not always give the numerical results of two independent pairs of characters. This led Sutton and Bovery, at the turn of the century, to conclude that the threadlike intracellular structures seen duplicating and separating into daughter cells carried the hereditary characters. Later Thomas Hunt Morgan, using cytogenetics and selected breeding in fruit flies, clearly demonstrated the phenomenon of genetic linkage (Morgan, 1928). Others went on the verify these observations in plants and animals.

During the first half of the 20th century, revelations concerning the discovery of nucleic acids by Kossel, using salmon sperm and human leukocytes (Sourkes, 1966); the structure of nucleotides by P. A. Levine; and the structure of DNA by Watson, Crick, Wilkins, and Franklin depended on advances in chemistry and X-ray crystallography (Watson and Crick, 1953). In fact, it was the application of X-ray diffraction techniques that finally allowed scientists to deduce the double helical structure of DNA. When Watson and Crick saw Franklin's photographs, it galvanized them into action; by building models of the nucleotides and hypothesizing the points for hydrogen bonding between purines and pyrimidines, they quickly assembled the three-dimensional structure of DNA. Their insight into how the diffraction pattern correlated with helical symmetry allowed for a practical solution to a very complex and, until then, elusive problem. They reinforced the meaning of the term 'great science,' as expressed by Lisa Jardine, "Great science depends on remaining grounded in the real" (Jardine, 1999).

There were 50 years between the isolation of 'nuclein' in leukocytes by Kossel and the discovery of the double-helical structure of DNA, which recognized that the pattern of purine and pyrimidine coupling contained the code for heritability. Likewise, there were 50 years between the hypothesis by Garrod in 1902 that family members with alkaptonuria had inherited a deficiency in a particular enzyme that metabolizes homogentisic acid and Beadle and Tatum's proof, using *Neurospora*, that indeed X-ray-induced genetic mutations affected the production of specific enzymes (Lederberg and Tatum, 1953). To a certain extent, these latter studies

depended on the demonstration that bacteria (and other lower organisms) in fact contained genetic information that controlled protein synthesis in a manner similar to that in eukaryotes (Lwoff, 1953). This breakthrough provided the fuel for the revolution in molecular genetics, which included the biological synthesis of deoxyribonucleic acid (Kornberg *et al.*, 1959) and the genetic regulation of protein synthesis (Jacob and Monod, 1961). It is indeed worth noting that the initial observations on heredity predated these initial molecular genetic discoveries by approximately a century. This rate of scientific discovery would be considered glacial in the context of the current rate of scientific discovery but was instrumental nevertheless. For their achievements in genetics and molecular biology, the following scientists have won the Nobel Prize: Thomas Morgan; Albrecht Kossel; George Beadle, Edward Tatum, and Joshua Lederberg; James Watson, Francis Crick, and Maurice Wilkins; Andre Lwoff, Francois Jacob, and Jacques Monod; and Severo Ochoa and Arthur Kornberg.

2. Progress in the Field of Immunology

a. Origins

There may be no field which greater illustrates the contribution of vertebrate animal research to biomedical discovery then the field of immunology. The section herein attempts to use immunology as an illustrative example demonstrating the contributions of animal models to scientific discovery.

The concept of adaptive immunity, developing protection after exposure to an infectious agent or poison, dates back to at least 430 BC when Thucydides writes of the plague of Athens, "Yet it was with those who had recovered from the disease that the sick and dying found most compassion. These knew what it was from experience and had now no fear themselves; for the same man was never attacked twice—never at least fatally" (Thucydides, 1934). Despite this early recognition, the association of disease with infectious agents was missing. During the 1200s, the Black Death in Europe and the East was attributed to a conjunction of Mars, Saturn, and Jupiter; and later in the fifteenth century the appearance of syphilis in Europe was attributed to another conjunction of the same planets (Silverstein, 1989). It was not until the end of the nineteenth century that studies using animals allowed investigators such as Pasteur, Koch, Ehrlich, von Behring, and Metchnikoff to demonstrate the phenomenon of acquired immunity, the association between infectious agent and disease, the principles of vaccination, and the treatment of diphtheria (and tetanus) with antitoxins.

b. Pioneers of Humoral Immunity

Emil von Behring (1854–1917) was a student of Robert Koch and went on to demonstrate that animals (guinea pigs, rabbits) vaccinated with diphtheria or tetanus organisms developed immunity to infection and to the detrimental effects of their toxins. In two manuscripts published 1890, he describes how he produced antitoxins to diphtheria and tetanus and how cell-free serum from immune animals protected nonimmune animals after passive transfer. Within 1 year the first human was successfully treated for diphtheria, and soon after, serum treatment came into general use. The death rate from diphtheria fell from 35% to 5%, and among those with laryngeal involvement, from 90% to 15%. Von Behring was awarded the Nobel Prize in 1901 (Sourkes, 1966).

Another student of Koch was Paul Ehrlich, who by studying antisera made in animals (particularly guinea pigs) developed a standardized test in 1897 to quantitate toxins and antitoxin. In doing so Ehrlich postulated the unique stereochemical relationship between active sites on antibody and antigen and introduced the concepts of antibody affinity and of functional domains on antibody molecules. Finally, he postulated that antibody formation was the cellular response to the binding of antigen to its surface receptors. He was awarded the Nobel Prize in 1908 along with Elie Metchnikoff (who discovered the antibacterial properties of phagocytes in a variety of animals) (Sourkes, 1966).

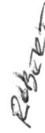

The mentor of both von Behring and Ehrlich, Robert Koch, made many contributions, particularly in the new field of bacteriology; however, he also developed tuberculin and devised the standard tuberculin skin test, which was one of the first demonstrations of cellular immunity (Silverstein, 1989). He was awarded a Nobel Prize in 1905.

In the mix with a group of scientists primarily devoted to the humoral theory of immunity, Elie Metchnikoff proposed a cellular theory of immunity. This was based on his observations of starfish phagocytic cells and their activity in the presence of bacteria. Furthermore, Metchnikoff theorized that immune activation produced a substance that heightened the activity of phagocytes. The work of Pasteur, Koch, Ehrlich, and von Behring all implicated humoral factors as protective in immunity, and the debate between humoral and cellular theories began. It did not help matters that during this debate, which lasted nearly two decades, the discoveries of bacterial agglutination (by Max von Gruber and Hurbert Durham), anaphylaxis (by Paul Portier and Charles Richet), the arthus phenomenon (by Maurice Arthus), and serum sickness (by Clemens von Pirquet and Bela Schick) all supported the humoral theory (and all involved animal research). Subsequently, the Nobel Prize would also be given to Charles Richet for his discovery of anaphylaxis, using dogs, and Jules Bordet for his discovery of complement, using guinea pigs (Bordet, 1909).

Many years passed between Richet's discovery of anaphylaxis and Bovet's discovery of histamine as a major mediator of that phenomenon. Bovet developed an *ex vivo* assay based on exposing strips of sensitized animal uterine tissue to antigen. Later he developed antihistamines for the treatment of asthma and atopy, based on the concept that synthetic molecules that resemble a metabolite of an active agent, e.g., histamine, may block or antagonize the effects of the active compound. Daniel Bovet was awarded the Nobel Prize in 1957 (Sourkes, 1966).

In retrospect, the arguments against a cellular theory seem antiquated, with the discovery of complement receptors on phagocytic cells, the role of complement as an opsonin for phagocytosis by Wright and Douglas, and even Koch's demonstration of the cellular infiltration at the site of a tuberculin reaction. Unfortunately, Metchnikoff was a lone voice in the cellularist doctrine, and in the end most early investigators of the 20th century turned to investigations involving antibody. For nearly 50 years the important area of cellular immunity and the role of lymphocytes in immunity were placed on the back burner. This is an excellent example of Kuhn's contention that scientific communities tend to reinforce the familiar and reject hypotheses that are more controversial and require taking risks (Kuhn, 1970).

During the next 30 years, investigators would study how immunologic (antibody) specificity was expressed and its biological implications (precipitation, agglutination, hemolysis, allergy), how immunologic specificity is structurally determined, and how the information for immunologic specificity is encoded. Major contributions were made by many, but perhaps none had a more profound effect on immunology (and especially medicine) than Karl Landsteiner. Landsteiner studied the phenomenon of red cell agglutination in humans and nonhuman primates. He discovered the ABO blood group and the isoagglutinins associated with them. He later discovered the MN and Rh factor blood groups. The consequences of this work allowed for proper typing of blood for transfusions. Although the MNP group is important primarily in forensic medicine, knowledge of the Rh factor and the antibody therapy developed from it has dramatically reduced the incompatibility disease known as erythroblastosis fetalis (hemolytic disease of the newborn) (Landsteiner, 1945). Other major contributions made by Landsteiner include the demonstration of the first antitissue antibodies (antisperm), description of the first autoimmune disease – paroxysmal cold hemoglobinuria (with Donath in 1904) – the phenomenon of hapten inhibition, and the ability to passively transfer delayed hypersensitivity (with Merrill Chase in 1942). Landsteiner was one of the first to show that poliomyelitis and syphilis could be induced in nonhuman primates. Landsteiner was awarded the Nobel Prize in 1930.

Other advances in immunology that centered primarily on antibodies and their function include the work of Tiselius and Kabat, classifying antibodies as high molecular weight gamma (γ-) globulins; and the work of Porter and Edelman, using myeloma proteins of humans and mice, as well as guinea pig immunoglobulin, to demonstrate the basic structure of antibodies through selective chain cleavage with enzymes. This allowed for primary amino acid sequencing of antibodies, with the resulting acknowledgment of constant and variable regions, repeating domains, and sites for secondary biological activities, e.g., complement fixation (Silverstein, 1989).

Once the structure of antibodies was known, many investigators began a search for the molecular (genetic) basis for proteins with constant and hypervariable regions. Calculations of the amount of DNA required to generate antibodies with all the diversity seen in animals and humans at times exceeded the size of the genome; therefore in 1965, Dreyer and Bennett proposed the existence of multiple variable region genes that could combine with the constant region gene to produce a unique isotype. Tonegawa and colleagues first discovered the presence of the constant region locus, plus multiple variable and joining region genes, which assemble such that a single variable region gene and a single joining region gene combine with the constant region gene to produce a unique light chain. With the assistance of Leroy Hood, Tonegawa later found a fourth gene cluster, called diversity, which contributed a single gene to form the longer heavy chain of immunoglobulin. This important work not only demonstrated how the enormous diversity of antibodies could be encoded in a compact segment of DNA, but also opened the doors to those searching for the elusive T-cell receptor. For their contributions, Porter and Edelman were awarded the Nobel Prize in 1972, and Tonegawa received the award in 1987.

Two other groups made contributions involving antibodies that would revolutionize many areas of the biological sciences. For their contribution of the radioimmunoassay, a technique requiring specific antibodies made in animals (usually rabbits and goats), Rosalyn Yalow, Roger Guillemin, and Andrew Schally won the Nobel Prize in 1977. In 1984, the Nobel Prize was awarded to Cesar Milstein and Georges Kohler for their contribution of monoclonal antibodies and the hybridoma technique. These two assays, and the enzyme-linked immunosorbent assay (ELISA) that followed, revolutionized the detection of specific antigens in tissues and biological fluids and serve today as the basis for disease diagnosis. Monoclonal antibodies have a multitude of purposes, from disease diagnosis to the purification of proteins and therapy for cancer (Dickman, 1998).

c. Pioneers of Cellular Immunity

World War II stimulated research to improve the survivability of grafted tissues, particularly skin for wound victims. Peter Medawar was interested in tissue grafting and was the first to document that second grafts

from the same donor to recipient were rejected more quickly than the first graft, whereas a third-party graft was not. This finding supported the view of immunologic specificity and the secondary response. He and colleagues Brent and Billingham established the field of transplantation biology. When Ray Owen documented that dizygotic cattle twins, which were red cell chimeras, were unable to reject each other's organs, the Australian physician MacFarlane Burnet proposed that immunologic responses arise late in animal development and that during early development, cells of the immune system would catalog available antigens as self (and thus not respond to them). Later in development, the introduction of new antigens would be considered nonself or foreign and elicit an IR (Burnet, 1959). This hypothesis was tested by Medawar and colleagues who exposed neonates to antigens of another strain and then transplanted skin between these inbred strains as adults. They confirmed that early antigen exposure prevented the immune system from recognizing the antigen later as foreign; they called this acquired immunological tolerance (Billingham *et al.*, 1953). These observations were among the first to be made in the new field of transplantation. They paved the way for characterizing the IRs typical of rejection (which are primarily cellular in allograft rejection), the antigens that elicited these responses, and mechanisms for suppressing the response (such as acquired tolerance and immunosuppressive drugs). MacFarlane Burnet and Peter Medawar shared the Nobel Prize for Medicine in 1960.

In the 1950s and 1960s, George Snell and Peter Gorer discovered the genetic locus in mice important in allograft (between individuals of the same species) rejection. The work of many who followed refined the information concerning this very complex locus, the major histocompatibility locus (MHC). However, this feat occurred because George Snell had the inventiveness to inbreed mice, thus generating strains (identical twins) and congenic lines that differed between one another by only a single gene. From this point onward, inbred strains and lines of mice would be the animal model of choice for those studying immunogenetics. They allowed for many of the studies in oncology, transplantation, and molecular biology. Among those who used inbred strains to study the MHC was Baruj Benacerraf of Harvard University. He studied the loci in mice that determined the IR to synthetic polypeptides and named them IR genes. It was later shown that the IR region fell into the MHC class 1 region – a locus that controlled the intercommunication between various immunocytes. Jean Dausset, a French immunologist, discovered that the human leukocyte antigen (HLA) system in humans controlled graft rejection. These HLA antigens were later found to be encoded in the MHC. Benacerraf, Snell, and Dausset shared the Nobel Prize in 1980. Later, inbred strains of rats, rabbits, and guinea pigs would be available to aid future studies, and histocompatibility typing was extended to many species of animals.

Also during the 1960s, Jacques Miller described the role of the thymus in immunity, the origin of the T cell, which would later be found to mediate graft rejection, modulate antibody synthesis, and directly participate in the eradication of infectious agents and cancer (Miller, 1961). By 1966, Claman, Chaperon, and Triplett, as well as Mitchell and Miller, had described T-cell subsets that discriminated between the types of T cells that assisted B cells in antibody production (helper cells) and those with direct cytotoxic activity. In 1970, Gershon and Kondo described suppressor T cells, which modified the activity of other lymphocytes. Now the availability of monoclonal antibodies was allowing scientists to detect surface markers on lymphocytes that could be used to distinguish functional subpopulations of lymphocytes. Availability of inbred strains also allowed investigators to evaluate immune mechanisms by passive transfer of subpopulations of cells between individuals. Early in these investigations, Peter Doherty and Rolf Zinkernagel discovered that certain IRs were MHC-restricted, that is, the lymphocytes of one MHC type could not recognize foreign antigens presented by cells of another MHC type. This led to the discovery that antigen-presenting cells express foreign peptides together with MHC proteins on their surface. Cells presenting MHC II molecules stimulated CD4+ cells, and those presenting antigen together with MHC I molecules stimulated CD8+ cells. These discoveries explained how different cells of the immune system were selected to attack a particular foreign invader and would aid in the understanding of intrathymic education of newly developing T cells to become tolerant to self-antigens (Zinkernagel and Doherty, 1997). For their achievements, Doherty and Zinkernagel were awarded the Nobel Prize in 1996.

First described by Flanagan in 1966, the nude mouse occurred as a spontaneous mutation in which there is developmental failure of the thymic anlage, resulting in a mouse devoid of circulating functional T cells (Flanagan, 1966). The *scid* mouse was described in 1983 by Bosma *et al.*, and due to a mutation in *rag1* gene encoding recombinase activity, this mouse failed to rearrange immunoglobulin or T-cell receptor genes and thus developed a combined (T- and B-cell) immunodeficiency (Bosma *et al.*, 1983). Use of these mice has greatly assisted in unraveling the cellular basis of immunity including the role of secreted cytokines and mechanisms of immune tolerance (Carballido *et al.*, 2000).

d. Transplantation Biology

The reader must now be brought back to the 1960s and the pioneer work of George Snell, to pick up where Peter Medawar, of graft-rejection fame, left off. Several

factors came together during this period to make the allografting of organs successful. First, the preservation and tissue typing of the donor organs were critical. Next, surgical manipulation of organs to allow prompt reestablishment of the blood supply was necessary. Finally, a mechanism of suppressing the cellular IR was essential.

Woodruff, a transplant surgeon in Edinburgh enthralled by the experiment of Medawar and colleagues, found a pair of dizygotic twins who shared each other's red cell types. He hypothesized that they had shared placental circulation and found, after cross-skin grafting them successfully, that humans, like cattle and mice, could develop acquired immunologic tolerance (Woodruff and Lennox, 1959).

During the first half of the 20th century, Carres, Quinby, Dempster, and Simonsen each attempted renal autografts and allografts in nonimmunosuppressed dogs. Although autografts remained functional for longer periods than allografts, all transplants ceased to function due to lack of innervation, lymphatics, or both. It was the many investigations conducted by Joseph Murray during the early 1950s that resulted in a surgical technique that would leave autografted kidneys in dogs completely functional after 2 years (Murray *et al.*, 1963). However, allografts were still quickly rejected. Lawrence was the first to liken the allograft rejection response to delayed hypersensitivity reactions (Lawrence, 1959).

Attempts to suppress immune rejection with steroids, anticoagulants, or both, failed. Following trials in mice and rabbits (Main and Prehn, 1955), a protocol involving total body irradiation followed by bone marrow transplantation and kidney transplantation achieved variable success in human kidney graft recipients (Main and Prehn, 1955). In 1959, Schwartz and Dameshek reported on the ability of 6-mercaptopurine (6-MP) to prevent rabbits from producing an antihuman serum albumin antibody response (Schwartz and Dameshek, 1959). Calne (1960) in London used 6-MP to suppress the rejection of allografted canine kidneys with success, although the drug itself was toxic (Calne, 1960). Calne then urged G. H. Hitchings and G. B. Elion of Burroughs Wellcome Laboratories to become collaborators. New Wellcome drugs greatly improved allograft survival, with dogs surviving normally for years. Hitchings and Elion had developed the imidazole derivative of 6-MP, known as Imuran (azathioprine). This became the mainstay of transplant surgeons for the next 20 years (Murray, 1992).

Following investigations in dogs, orthotopic liver allografts were performed in humans by Moore and Starzl. In 1960, Lower and Shumway developed a surgical technique for transplant of the heart in dogs. This was followed in 1970 by successful heart transplantation in man. Later achievements included transplantation of the bone marrow, pancreas, and portions of the intestinal tract.

The advent of reagents to histocompatibility-type donors and recipients reduced the immunologic barrier between them and led to more appropriate selection of grafts, with a resultant increase in functional longevity of the graft. Also, improved drugs, such as cyclosporin A, rapamycin, and FK506, targeted specific cellular events necessary for initiating the rejection process, causing fewer side effects and leaving the host must less immunologically compromised (Carpenter, 2000). The drug mycophenolate mofetil, under clinical trials when this chapter was first written, is now in widespread clinical use as an anti-rejection and immunosuppressant drug. In addition, monoclonal anti-CD3 antibodies have been used to prevent acute rejection since the early 1980s (Ortho Multicenter Transplant Study Group, 1985). Starzl demonstrated early that kidney rejection in dogs treated with azathioprine could be reversed 88% of the time by injection with steroids (Marchioro et al., 1964). Similar rates were published for humans undergoing the same therapy. It was also shown that delayed hypersensitivity skin tests that were positive in the donor but not the recipient crossed over to the recipient about 77% of the time following a kidney transplant (Starzl et al., 1993). Microchimerism involving the survival of donor leukocytes in the body of the recipient following transplantation was proven using polymerase chain reaction (PCR) and persisted up to 29 years following transplantation (Starzl et al., 1993). The movement of donor leukocytes out of the transplanted graft into immune compartments of the host had been demonstrated in animal models (Qian et al., 1994). It had also been shown that long-standing peripheral tolerance could be achieved in mice made chimeras by neonatal infusion of donor leukocytes (Silvers et al., 1975). These observations fostered the notion that for completely successful organ engraftment, four interrelated phenomena must occur in close temporal sequence: clonal deletion of the recipient immune (antigraft) response, clonal deletion of the donor's leukocyte response, maintenance of clonal exhaustion, and reduction in the immunogenicity of the transplanted organ over time (Starzl and Zinkernagel, 1998).

For some time it has been known that acute allograft rejection is mediated by CD4$^+$ and CD8$^+$ cells. The former are activated by binding foreign antigen in association with MHC class II molecules – in this case, on the donated graft. For proper activation, costimulatory signals mediated via CD28 on T cells and B7 on antigen-presenting cells plus CD40 present on antigen-presenting cells binding CD40L on T cells must be engaged. Once activated, CD4 lymphocytes produce many cytokines that act in an autocrine fashion to stimulate more CD4 cells and a paracrine fashion to activate CD8 cells. Many of these cytokines, such as tumor necrosis factor (TNF), may be liberated by activated CD4 cells within the graft, causing rejection even without the cytotoxic effects of

CD8 cells. These immune mechanisms were largely discovered through research on mice and rats (Sayegh and Turka, 1998).

Investigators demonstrated that blocking the costimulatory pathways for T cells in allografted animals (rodents and nonhuman primates) greatly prolongs graft survival and ablates the acute rejection phenomenon (Kirk et al., 1999). Although prevention of T-cell activation and cytokine release can explain acute graft survival, it does not really explain the long-term survival of grafts observed by Starzl in microchimeric animal and human transplant recipients. One explanation comes from the studies of Li and Wells, where peripheral allograft tolerance was established in mice by a combination of costimulatory blockade and the use of rapamycin. In this study, mice received an MHC-incompatible cardiac transplant plus monoclonal antibodies against CD40L (CD154) plus CTLAIg (which blocks CD28). In this case, heart grafts survived rejection, but skin grafts were rejected. When rapamycin is added to the regimen, permanent engraftment is seen for both heart and skin; however, if cyclosporin A (CsA) is substituted for rapamycin, neither graft survives rejection. The inclusion of CsA thus antagonized the tolerizing effects of both costimulatory blockade and rapamycin. Using cell labeling studies, these investigators found that costimulatory blockade alone inhibited proliferation of alloreactive T cells in vivo while allowing cell cycle-dependent T-cell apoptosis of proliferating T cells. Addition of rapamycin resulted in massive apoptosis of alloreactive T cells, but addition of CsA abolished T-cell proliferation and apoptosis. Subsequent studies demonstrated that the combination of blockade plus rapamycin did not induce tolerance in IL-2 or in bcl-XL transgenics. In both instances, these transgenic mice failed to be induced into T-cell apoptosis. Activation-induced cell death (by apoptosis) occurs when primed cells are repetitively activated by antigen and requires previous exposure to IL-2. Unlike CsA, rapamycin does not block IL-2 production, and it does not block antigen priming for apoptosis. The authors conclude that stable peripheral tolerance can be induced as long as alloreactive T cells are suppressed from initial cytokine production and eliminated by apoptosis (Li et al., 1999; Wells et al., 1999).

Recent data demonstrates that antigen presentation to host T-cells occurs primarily by donor dendritic cells (Ruiz et al., 2013). Dendritic cells were first identified in the late 19th century but their critical role in controlling adaptive IRs was only recently elucidated (Steinman and Banchereau, 2007; Banchereau and Steinman, 1998). Dendritic cells are critical for a variety of adaptive immune processes including T-cell activation, antigen presentation, and importantly in the context of transplant biology inducing immune tolerance (Steinman and Banchereau, 2007). Tolerogenic dendritic cells exist in a variety of organs and immature dendritic cells can be induced to become tolerogenic by a variety of exogenous stimuli including pharmacological and cytokine exposure (Maldonado and von Andrian, 2010). Several studies using rodent models have demonstrated that induction of donor dendritic cells into tolerogenic dendritic cells is an effective strategy for prolonging graft survival (Lutz et al., 2000; Turnquist et al., 2007; van Kooten and Gelderman, 2011; van Kooten et al., 2011). These tolerogenic dendritic cells induce T-regulatory cell populations in recipient animals (Turnquist et al., 2007). More recently Ezzelarab and colleagues extended these rodent studies into nonhuman primates. They induced donor blood monocytes into regulatory dendritic cells and performed kidney transplants using rhesus macaques. Recipients that received donor regulatory dendritic cells along with standard immunosuppressive therapy demonstrated an approximately three-fold increase in graft survival time compared to those which only received standard immunosuppressive therapy (Ezzelarab et al., 2013). Monkeys receiving dendritic cells displayed an increase proportion of regulatory T cells to memory T cells (Ezzelarab et al., 2013).

For their achievements in transplantation biology, Joseph Murray and E. Donnall Thomas were awarded the Nobel Prize in 1990. For their accomplishments in the field of pharmacology (including the development of drugs to treat high blood pressure and gastric ulcer, and immunosuppressant and antiviral drugs) Sir James Black, Gertrude Elion, and George Hitchings were awarded the Nobel Prize in 1988. For his work in elucidating the critical role of dendritic cells in the adaptive IR Ralph Steinman won the Nobel Prize in 2011.

e. Vaccinology

Intimately associated with advances in immunology were advances in vaccinology. Following in the footsteps of Jenner, Pasteur, and Bouquet, Calmette, and Guerin (BCG vaccine), Max Theiler was able to develop a mouse protection assay for yellow fever virus and attenuated viral strains in mice and chickens. Efficacy for these attenuated strains was demonstrated in monkeys and ultimately led to the first vaccine in the 1930s. Theiler was awarded a Nobel Prize in 1951 for his efforts (Strode, 1951). During the second half of the 20th century, vaccines were developed and utilized to protect against diphtheria and pertussis (in the 1940s), poliomyelitis (in the 1950s), rubella or German measles (in the 1960s), pneumococcal, meningococcal diseases, measles, and mumps (in the 1970s), hepatitis A and B and *Haemophilus influenzae* (in the 1980s), and varicella or chicken pox and Lyme disease (in the 1990s). This history of vaccine development depended heavily on the use of animals, especially nonhuman primates (Hilleman, 1998).

Despite this record and the hundreds of millions of human lives saved through vaccination, a safe, effective vaccine against HIV has been elusive. The goal of HIV vaccination has been to induce complete immunity (i.e., elimination of the virus). The induction of sterile immunity through neutralizing antibodies has been elusive (Burton et al., 2004). More recently, based upon data generated from SIV-infected macaques, there has been a shift in emphasis to develop vaccines which induce a greater T-cell response (Schmitz et al., 1999; Sekaly, 2008). Initial attempts to promote this response involved the use of recombinant adenoviral vectors but these efforts regrettably did not prove particularly beneficial when used clinically (Sekaly, 2008). More recently, efforts have been made to alter the IR through immunoregulation using dendritic cells. This approach was first tested in SIV-infected macaques and proved efficacious in reducing viral load (Lu et al., 2003). Recently a similar approach was attempted in humans (Garcia et al., 2013). In the human vaccine trial, patients were immunized with autologous dendritic cells which were treated with heat-inactivated autologous HIV (Garcia et al., 2013). Patients undergoing this regime demonstrated decreased viral load and increased viral specific T-cell responses (Garcia et al., 2013). Similar dendritic cell vaccine approaches are now being evaluated for the treatment of cancers (Palucka et al., 2013; Palucka and Banchereau, 2013a,b).

A familiar infectious foe throughout history is the influenza virus. One of the critical factors in influenza pathogenesis and vaccination strategy is the ability of the virus to become genetically altered by both genetic shift and genetic drift (Webster et al., 1992). Genetic shift refers to the agent's ability to make a wholesale change in its chromosomal makeup whereas genetic drift refers to the ability of the agent to undergo more minor point mutations within its own chromosomes (Webster et al., 1992). Based upon this rapid mutability it is therefore no small feat to develop a vaccine which is effective against the virus (Nichol and Treanor, 2006). There are a variety of animal models including mice, ferrets and rhesus macaques which assist in testing the safety and efficacy of influenza virus vaccines prior to use in humans (van der Laan et al., 2008). The majority of influenza vaccines induce immunity to the hemagglutinin and neuraminidase proteins which are the major surface glycoproteins of the virus (Collin et al., 2009). When the virus undergoes a genetic shift of either of these two major surface antigens there is a greater likelihood of a pandemic outbreak because immunity is lacking (Collin et al., 2009). The most recent global pandemic occurred in 2009 when the H1N1 strain of influenza was identified in humans (Collin et al., 2009; Peiris et al., 2009) The challenge, of course, is that when these new strains emerge it will take time to develop effective vaccine strategies against them.

An alternative approach proposed by some is to produce vaccines against more conserved portions of these proteins (Ekiert *et al.*, 2009). This approach has indeed proven effective when tested in both mice and ferret challenge models of influenza and holds promise for future human broad-spectrum influenza immunization (Wei *et al.*, 2010). In this study a DNA-based approach was utilized and animals were immunized with plasmid vectors encoding hemagglutinin and neuraminidase genes from recent outbreaks followed by boosting with standard seasonal flu vaccine. Following this strategy mice and ferrets challenged with divergent influenza strains demonstrated cross-protection against these strains (Wei *et al.*, 2010).

The majority of cervical cancers are the result of infection with two strains of human papillomavirus (HPV 16 and HPV 18) which is the most common sexually transmitted disease in the United States (Markowitz *et al.*, 2007; Schiffman, 2007; Schiffman *et al.*, 2007). There is a quadravalent vaccine which protects against the two strains of HPV most commonly associated with cervical cancer (HPV 16 and 18) and the two most common strains associated with genital warts (HPV 6 and 11) (Markowitz *et al.*, 2007). There were, of course, many steps involved in the development of these vaccines. Critically for this review, the immunogenicity of the vaccine was tested in mice, African green monkeys, and chimpanzees (Mach *et al.*, 2006; Palker *et al.*, 2001; Shi *et al.*, 2007). Subsequent efficacy studies in humans validated the preclinical data obtained in animals and demonstrated effective immunization against all four strains of virus that lasted as long as 5 years (Shi *et al.*, 2007; Villa *et al.*, 2005).

f. Asthma and the Role of Innate Immunity

Much has been learned about allergic reactions since the discoveries by Richet and Bovet. The molecular pathogenesis of early and late responses, characterized by biphasic reactions mediated by IgE; release of various mediators, and the influx of different populations of cells, has been studied primarily in rats and mice (including knockouts) (Matsuoka *et al.*, 2000). Recently, it has become clear that pattern recognition receptors (PRRs) play a strong role in promoting asthma (Bezemer *et al.*, 2012). PRRs are a group of proteins that are capable of recognizing certain molecular or cellular patterns, pathogen-associated molecular patterns (PAMPS), which are indicative of pathogens. The most well-known of these PRRs are the Toll-like receptors (TLR) which are so named because of their structural similarity to the Toll protein of *Drosophila* which was initially described as a critical developmental gene in *Drosophila* but was later shown to be important in protection from fungal infection (Lemaitre *et al.*, 1996). TLRs have been subsequently identified and characterized in a variety of species with 10 functional TLRs being characterized in humans and 13 in mice (Savva and Roger, 2013). Some of the seminal work characterizing the function of TLR molecules was done using spontaneously arising animal models. Specifically, in substrains of C3H/HeJ and C57BL/10 which were resistant to the effects of systemic LPS administration, it was shown that these phenotypes mapped to the mouse *Tlr4* gene and that in LPS nonresponsive substrains the *Tlr4* gene was mutated (Poltorak *et al.*, 1998a,b). Subsequent studies on TLR4 have demonstrated that in addition to LPS it binds to other PAMPS and the other TLR molecules bind to diverse pathogen molecules including lipotechoic acid (TLR2), flagellin (TLR5 and TLR11), and single-stranded RNA (TLR 7 and TLR8) (Savva and Roger, 2013). The primary role of TLR molecules it seems is to therefore recognize molecular patterns which are not native to the host and through complex signaling pathways induce an IR (Savva and Roger, 2013). As one might imagine, the airways receive a variety of exogenous stimuli from the environment and data generated in animal models has demonstrated that TLR-driven immunoactivation is a critical component of asthma and mast cell activation (Bezemer *et al.*, 2012; Hammad *et al.*, 2009; McCurdy *et al.*, 2001; Zaidi *et al.*, 2006). Likewise TLR modulation has proven effective in ameliorating some animal models of asthma (Bezemer *et al.*, 2012; Fuchs and Braun, 2008; Fuchs *et al.*, 2010). In particular immunomodulation of TLR9 which recognizes CpG DNA motifs has proven efficacious in animal models and has shown promise in human trials (Beeh *et al.*, 2013; Hayashi and Raz, 2006). An important benefit of TLR9 immunotherapy seems to be that it functions regardless of the inciting antigen (Hayashi and Raz, 2006).

C. Genomics, Comparative Genomics, and the Microbiome

1. Introduction

At the time when the previous version of this chapter was written, the first draft of the human genome had not yet been published nor had any other vertebrate genome. Progress made in the intervening 12 years has been nothing but remarkable. Prior to 2001 several complete genomes had been sequenced but the methods were laborious and expensive, primarily utilizing the Sanger method for DNA sequencing (Sanger *et al.*, 1977). Whole-genome sequences were published for 38 bacteria; one yeast; two invertebrates: the nematode, *Caenorhabditis elegans* and the fruit fly, *Drosophila melanogaster*; and one plant, *Arabidopsis thaliana* (Lander, 2011). After 2001 a large number of animal and plant genomes were published in rapid succession primarily due to improvements in sequencing methodology. In 2002 the mouse genome was published (Mouse Genome Sequencing Consortium, 2002) followed by the rat (Gibbs et al., 2004), dog (Lindblad-Toh et al., 2005), and chimpanzee (The Chimpanzee Sequencing and Analysis Consortium, 2005). In addition the final sequences of the human genome was published in the mid-2000s (International Human Genome Sequencing Consortium, 2004) allowing for direct comparison of the human with several other mammalian genomes. Today there are annotated and published genome-wide sequences for over 65 animals including fish, reptiles, birds, mammals, insects, and worms. There are also over 60 mammalian deep coverage genome assemblies and 40 nonmammalian deep coverage genome assemblies which may be combined with 29 mammal and 46 vertebrate alignments and conservation data sets (Meyer et al., 2013) and utilized for comparative genomics research (Alfoldi and Lindblad-Toh, 2013).

Today it is thought that the human genome contains approximately 21,000 protein-coding genes (PCGs) which make up only 1.2% of the sequences found in the genome (Lander, 2011). While much of the noncoding sequence was once thought to have little to no function, it has now been estimated that greater than 80% of the noncoding sequence are involved with at least one cellular process, and this percentage may be closer to 100% when the activities of all cells in the human body are taken into account (The ENCODE Project Consortium, 2012). Conserved noncoding elements (CNEs) are now a focus of research in comparative genomics, since their transcription products appear to influence a variety of important cellular processes (see subsequent sections).

Of the 21,000 PCGs, it is estimated that close to 100,000 proteins are generated due to alternative splicing events (Pan et al., 2008). When post-translational modification is taken into account the number of proteins increases by multitudes (Grune and Sebela, 2013). Therefore, with most of the 2.7 billion nucleotides in the human genome controlling the production of hundreds of thousands of different transcripts and proteins, how much do we actually know about the function of these molecules? The answer is surprisingly little. In fact the presumed function of many of the human PCGs is still not known or predicted from sequence analysis alone. The best understood model, the mouse, has about 22,000 PCG and is 99% orthologous to humans (please refer to Section IV, C, 2 below for a more detailed description of orthologous genes). This model, through targeted mutations, has been used extensively to assess mammalian gene function providing knowledge to conserved processes (White et al., 2013). At the time of this writing, partial phenotypes are described for about 8200 genes in mice (see below) (Schofield et al., 2012). The function of most noncoding sequences remains unknown in both humans and mice.

2. Sequence Comparison Among Human and Animal Genomes

a. Similarity Among Species

Orthologs are genes which evolved from a common ancestral gene by speciation that usually have retained a similar function in different species. Paralogs are genes related by duplication within the genome and often they acquire a new function. After publishing the first draft sequence it was reported that the mouse, Mus musculus, genome was comparable in size and structure to the human genome and that 99% of mouse genes have human orthologs (Mouse Genome Sequencing Consortium, 2002). Having last shared a common ancestor 75 million years ago, and with the human genome filled with more repeat sequences, it was a surprise that over 90% of the mouse genome could be lined up with a region in the human sequence; these conserved long stretches of nucleotides are called conserved synteny. About 5% of the entire mouse genome was conserved with man and since PCGs account for approximately 1.5%, much of the conservation occurred in non-coding elements. Expansion of genes has also occurred in the mouse especially in genes for reproduction, immunity and olfaction (Mouse Genome Sequencing Consortium, 2002).

The rat, Rattus norvegicus, sequence was published in 2004 and 89–90% of rat genes possessed a single ortholog in the human genome. The proportion of orthologs between rat and mice are between 86 and 94% (Gibbs et al., 2004). Some genes in the rat, but not the mouse, arose through expansion of gene families and include genes for pheromones, immunity, chemosensation, detoxification, or proteolysis (Gibbs et al., 2004).

The publication of the chimpanzee, Pan troglodytes, genome in 2005 allowed for the direct comparison of the human genome with its closest living relative (The Chimpanzee Sequencing and Analysis Consortium, 2005). Sequence divergence at orthologous sites was found to be no more than 1.2%. Gene loss, which was expected to be increased as a result of human-specific lineage, was found to be no greater than gene loss in the chimpanzee or either of the two other great apes studied (Kim et al., 2010). There was a noticeable difference in the rate of transposable element insertions between chimpanzee and humans; short interspersed elements (SINEs) were three-fold more active in humans whereas chimpanzees have acquired two new families of retroviral elements. Orthologous proteins are conserved between the two species with 29% remaining identical and the typical ortholog differing by only two amino acids, one per lineage. Analysis of patterns of human diversity relative to hominid divergence identifies several loci as potential candidates for strong selective sweeps in recent human history (more details on this are provided below) (Maricic *et al.*, 2013). A selective sweep is a reduction or elimination of variation among nucleotides in the DNA neighboring a mutation as a result of strong positive natural selection for the mutation (Maricic *et al.*, 2013).

The sequence of the dog, *Canis familaris*, was published in 2005 based on the complete sequence of a boxer breed dog with a compendium of single nucleotide polymorphisms (SNPs) derived from the partial sequences of 11 other breeds (Lindblad-Toh *et al.*, 2005). The initial sequence identified 19,300 predicted genes with 13,816 genes having 1:1:1 orthology between human and mouse genomes. When 4950 gene sets were studied as defined by such criteria as biological function, cellular localization, and co-expression, deviations between the three lineages were small; however, there was greater relative variation between human and mouse and dog-mouse comparisons than in human–dog comparisons (Lindblad-Toh *et al.*, 2005).

The zebrafish, *Danio rerio*, genome was sequenced and published in 2013 and contained many surprising features (Howe *et al.*, 2013). Zebrafish arose from a common ancestor over 340 million years ago and, compared to other vertebrates studied to date, this ancestor underwent an additional round of whole-genome duplication called the teleost-specific duplication (TSD) (Howe *et al.*, 2013). Gene duplicates which evolved from this process are called ohnologues. Expression profiles of these TSD genes show that they demonstrate tissue-preferred expression and are temporally restricted to late stage embryos and early larvae (Yang *et al.*, 2013). The zebrafish genome contains 26,206 PCG, the most of any sequenced vertebrate they have a higher number of species-specific genes than do humans, mice, or chickens (Howe *et al.*, 2013). Sixty-nine percent of zebrafish genes have at least one human ortholog. In humans 47% of the genes have a 1:1 orthologous relationship with zebrafish. Many other human genes have at least two orthologs in zebrafish, the average being 2.28 zebrafish genes per human gene; this probably reflects the TSD. In contrast to humans, zebrafish contain few type I retrotransposable elements, few pseudogenes and greater type II retrotransposable elements. Zebrafish also possess a chromosome (no. 4) which contains species-specific genes and genes which influence sex determination (Howe *et al.*, 2013).

Based on currently available genomes there are now databases which characterize orthology between species. For example, Evola is a database containing orthologs from 14 vertebrate species compared to human genes (Matsuya *et al.*, 2008). Ortholog identification is based on computer analysis of similar genomic and amino acid sequences. This database also features a comparison of alternative splicing variants from human and vertebrate orthologs. The orthologs are also manually curated with molecular evolutionary analysis through a comparison

TABLE 34.1 Number of Orthologs Provided by Evola

Species	Common name	Genes[a]	Human genes[b]
Homo sapiens	Human	22,768	–
Pan troglodytes	Chimpanzee	16,368	15,615
Pongo abelii	Orangutan	16,613	16,972
Macaca mulatta	Rhesus macaque	17,355	17,659
Mus musculus	Mouse	17,492	17,795
Rattus norvegicus	Rat	15,944	16,316
Canis familiaris	Dog	16,414	16,875
Equus ferus caballus	Horse	15,689	16,250
Bos Taurus	Cow	15,688	16,030
Monodelphis domestica	Opossum	15,680	16,039
Gallus gallus domesticus	Chicken	11,405	11,984
Danio rerio	Zebrafish	14,009	13,291
Oryzias latipes	Medaka	11,736	11,829
Tetraodon nigroviridis	Tetraodon	11,654	11,579
Takifugu rubripes	Fugu	12,509	12,414

Derived from the Evola website (H-InvDB 7.5 released September 2010).
[a]*Number of gene orthologous to human.*
[b]*Owing to lineage-specific duplication or loss the numbers are usually different, e.g., 15,570 mouse genes are orthologous to 14,574 human genes; and 22,768 human genes have at least one ortholog among the other 14 species (see Matsuya et al., 2008).*

between the species tree and the gene tree. Table 34.1 lists the number of genes in each of 14 species which have orthologs with a human gene.

b. Animal Genomes Inform Us of the Structure and Function of the Human Genome

i. DEFINING CONSERVATION/CONSTRAINT WITHIN THE HUMAN GENOME There is a tacit assumption that when the DNA sequence remains unchanged between species, especially evolutionary distant species, that these conserved sequences provide a critical function. There are various ways to define conserved sequences and for the most part they first involve aligning the appropriate sequence between the two species being compared. This is much easier to do with PCG than for noncoding elements, since one can scan the genome looking for open reading frames (ORF). Computer programs can be used to search for PCGs based upon well-known and conserved features; however, regulatory elements are much harder to define.

ii. EVOLUTIONARY CONSERVATION INVOLVING VERTEBRATES AND INVERTEBRATES Vertebrates share many orthologous genes with invertebrates. In genera as distant as *Drosophila* and *Mus* there is a high degree of homology in protein sequence and in sequential patterns of expression for genes involved with embryonic development (Wagner *et al.*, 2005). Conservation of some of these regulatory processes dates back to a common ancestor occurring greater than 550 million years ago (Wagner *et al.*, 2005). Clarke and colleagues describe developmental enhancers shared between humans and invertebrates which show no evidence of innovation for over 2 billion years (Clarke *et al.*, 2012).

iii. EVOLUTIONARY CONSERVATION AMONG VERTEBRATES

As might be expected, humans have many PCGs which are not found in invertebrates but are shared among vertebrates including genes encoding the major histocompatibility complex (MHC), antibodies, T-cell receptors, cell signaling molecules, molecules that participate in blood clotting, and many mediators of apoptosis. Aside from coding regions of the genome, vertebrates demonstrate many conserved non-coding regions. When comparing the genome sequences of humans, mice, and rats over 500 ultraconserved non-coding elements (200 bases or more which are perfectly matched) were discovered. Highly CNEs (HCNEs) numbered in the tens of thousands and traced back in evolution to an ancestor common between both humans and fish (Siepel *et al.*, 2005). Large-scale screens in transgenic mice showed that HCNE are transcriptional enhancers associated with embryogenesis (Lander, 2011). Eighty percent of all HCNE in humans are shared with marsupials, 30% are shared with birds and none are maintained in fish; giving rise to the notion that the evolution of species, among vertebrates, depended largely on regulatory sequences rather than proteins (Lander, 2011).

iv. EVOLUTIONARY CONSERVATION AMONG MAMMALS

In an effort to identify protein coding regions in humans, 21,895 putative PCG in the human genome were compared with syntenic regions of the mouse and dog genomes. Orthologs were identified for 18,866 human PCG and paralogs were identified for many others. The remaining 2787 putative PCGs (called orphan genes) were compared to an expanded panel of diverse mammalian genomes and other nonhuman primate genomes using the codon substitution frequency (CSF) score. None of the orphan genes showed conservation to the expanded panel of genomes including in chimpanzees. Aside from demonstrating a tremendous amount of conservation among mammalian PCGs this led Clamp and colleagues to conclude there was no evidence through species conservation to support inclusion of these orphan genes and the revised number of human PCGs was reduced to 19,200 (Clamp *et al.*, 2007).

As described above, there is a great deal of orthology between mammalian genomes (Matsuya *et al.*, 2008). There are many examples of conservation of both coding

and noncoding elements among mammals and many examples demonstrating that deleting these conserved regions results in the mutant having a significant loss of function (Nobrega and Pennacchio, 2004; Visel *et al.*, 2010). However, there are also examples where deleting an ultraconserved element from the mouse genome resulted in no detectable change in the mutant mouse suggesting that ultraconservation alone does not imply necessity (Ahituv *et al.*, 2007).

v. DIFFERENCES BETWEEN PLACENTAL AND NONPLACENTAL MAMMALS

There is strong conservation among placental mammals' PCGs with two-thirds of all PCG having 1:1 orthologs in other species. When CNEs and PCGs were examined between placental and non-plancental mammals (marsupials), at least 20% of placental CNEs were not represented in marsupials whereas only 1% of the placental PCGs were not represented (Mikkelsen *et al.*, 2007). These findings suggest that while most PCGs are conserved throughout the mammalian lineage, about 20% of CNE have arisen since the divergence of marsupials and placental mammals about 180 million years ago.

vi. DIFFERENCES BETWEEN HUMANS AND NHP

When comparing nucleotide sequences at orthologous sites humans differ from chimpanzees by only 1.2% (The Chimpanzee Sequencing and Analysis Consortium, 2005), which is much less than the divergence between two random fruit flies of the same species (Begun *et al.*, 2007). However, when all forms of variability are taken into account chimpanzees differ from humans by 5% (Britten, 2002). Much of the variation occurs in DNA regions encoding regulatory RNAs (Wall, 2013).

Some of the mechanisms reported to be responsible for human lineage-specific traits include accelerated amino acid substitutions (Enard *et al.*, 2002), human-specific protein isoforms produced by novel splice sites in the human genome (Kim and Hahn, 2012), formation of novel transcript variants by DNA insertion (Kim and Hahn, 2012), inactivation of long-established genes (Hahn *et al.*, 2007), and the *de novo* origin of PCGs from non-coding sequences (Knowles and McLysaght, 2009).

An example of the power of using NHPs in comparative genomics is illustrated by studies of the *FOXP2* gene (a forkhead class transcription factor). Mutations in the *FOXP2* gene in humans are associated with deficiencies in spoken language and grammatical impairments (Enard *et al.*, 2002). The *FOXP2* gene is highly conserved among mammals with just one non-synonymous (amino acid changing) mutation separating the gene found in mice and chimpanzees (Enard *et al.*, 2002). However, humans differ from chimpanzees by having two non-synonymous mutations and no synonymous mutations which was significantly different from the expected mutation rate

LANGUAGES
SPEAKING

(Wall, 2013). Comparing the genomes of humans, chimpanzees, and orangutans showed a recent selective sweep in this gene in humans. These findings are consistent with the hypothesis that the non-synonymous mutations in this gene and subsequent positive selection are partially responsible for the orofacial movement control which allows us to speak (Enard *et al.*, 2002). Supporting this, the genomes of Neanderthals and Denisovans also contain these two non-synonymous mutations suggesting positive selection in the human lineage (Reich *et al.*, 2010, 2011; Krause *et al.*, 2007). Further examination of the human gene found a mutation in a transcription factor binding site in intron 8 of the *FOXP2* gene which increases expression. Once again this change is a recent positive selection since they were not found in the Neanderthal genome (Maricic *et al.*, 2013).

vii. DIFFERENCES AMONG HUMANS While the DNA sequence in any two individuals is 99.5% the same, this last 0.5% makes a tremendous difference, especially in disease susceptibility. PCGs that have no variation in the population are said to be non-polymorphic, e.g., a single allele. In many instances a gene has several different sequences and therefore there are multiple alleles. SNPs are changes in a single nucleotide in the DNA sequence. It has been estimated that there are 10–30 million SNPs in the human population comprising 90% of all sequence variation. Sets of SNPs residing on the same chromosome are inherited in blocks. The pattern of SNPs in a block is called a haplotype. There is an international effort to map all the human haplotypes called the International HapMap Consortium (https://hapmap.ncbi.nlm.nih.gov/). This publically available data set can be used to rapidly screen genomes using SNPs to find regions where genes are associated with different diseases. Screens are based on the notion that there are higher frequencies of the contributing genetic components in a group of people with a specific disease or response to an agent. HapMap screening has been successful for identifying patients with a specific illness, with a certain response to a medication or vaccine, with a specific response to an environmental agent, and with a specific response to an infectious disease. Once an investigation finds a chromosome region which has different haplotype distributions in groups with and without the disease, the region is studied in more detail to find which variants in which genes contribute to the disease or response.

Unlike simple Mendelian diseases, which are usually due to a rare mutation in a gene, common genetic variants may play a role in complex diseases (Reich and Lander, 2001). Common variants are defined as having an allele frequency of greater than 1%. HapMap has been successful at mapping multiple loci for complex traits but finding the proper affected and control populations to study these complex diseases required another undertaking. Genome-wide association studies (GWAS) use the HapMap methodologies to look for associations between complex diseases or quantitative traits (like atherosclerosis, macular degeneration, rheumatoid arthritis, Crohn's disease, high blood pressure) and genetic loci. While several landmark studies have been published which elucidated disease pathogenesis, including one identifying genes in the complement pathway associated with age-related macular degeneration (Haines *et al.*, 2005), other studies involving type 2 diabetes (Voight *et al.*, 2010), Crohn's disease (Franke *et al.*, 2010), and elevated LDL levels (Teslovich *et al.*, 2010) often had results which explained only a small proportion of the heritability of the disorder (Lander, 2011).

Approximately 88% of the traits or disease associated loci identified in GWAS studies are located within introns or are intergenic (Hindorff *et al.*, 2009). Many of the human SNPs associated with a disease appear to be conserved especially among mammals, thus a haplotype containing many SNPs may be submitted to review using a comparative approach using existing mammalian databases. Focusing on the conserved SNPs should then serve as the first tier for functional characterization (Alfoldi and Lindblad-Toh, 2013). An example of this approach involves a variant of the gene *SORT1* (sortilin) in humans which was associated with elevated blood lipid levels in human GWAS (Teslovich *et al.*, 2010). Rapid development of a transgenic mouse showed that the variant created a novel transcription factor binding site which, in mice, altered plasma LDL levels (Musunuru *et al.*, 2010). This gene defined a previously unknown regulatory pathway for LDL (Lander, 2011).

Another use of animal models in human GWAS comes from the work of Kitsios and colleagues who juxtaposed human GWAS-discovered loci with mouse models (Kitsios *et al.*, 2010). Of 293 human associations evaluated they identified 51 comparable phenotypes in mice. A total of 27 orthologous genes were found to be associated with the same phenotype in humans and mice. In a gene-centric approach they found a knockout model for 60% of these genes. The knockouts for 35% of these orthologs displayed pre- or postnatal lethality, and for the remaining non-lethal orthologs the same organ system was involved in mice and humans. This study highlights the wealth of available information from mouse models for human GWAS (Kitsios *et al.*, 2010).

3. Epigenetics/Epigenomics

While DNA sequences are in part responsible for gene expression and phenotype, additional non-genomic regulatory networks impart stability and plasticity to genome output, modifying phenotype independent of the genetic blueprint (Levenson and Sweatt, 2006; Mandrioli, 2004). Two common and well-characterized epigenetic mechanisms include covalent modification of histones or DNA molecules primarily by methylation. Histone modification is a highly conserved, universal regulatory mechanism shared by eukaryotic organisms from yeast to man (Levenson and Sweatt, 2006; Mandrioli, 2004). The modification of core histones is complex and involves lysine, arginine, and serine residues in the N-terminal flexible tail regions. Modifications include methylation, acetylation, phosphorylation, ubiquitination, and ADP ribosylation and involve many histone modification enzymes (Li, 2002; Niculescu, 2012). Histone acetylation and deacetylation have been shown to determine the transcriptional activity of the chromatin. DNA methylation is less conserved but common among higher eukaryotic organisms (Li, 2002). DNA methylation of cytosines (mC) is a stable covalent modification that persists in post-mitotic cells throughout their lifetime, defining their cellular identity (Lister et al., 2013). Most methylation in adult mammals takes place where cytosine and guanine nucleotides sit next to each other on a DNA molecule. Cytosine can also be methylated at sites where it does not sit next to guanine but in most regions of the body this non-CG methylation is seldom observed in differentiated cells (Turek-Plewa and Jagodzinski, 2005; Richardson, 2002; Antequera and Bird, 1999).

One of the earliest examples of the role of epigenetics and gene regulation arose from a series of observations made with the agouti locus in mice. Duhl and his colleagues found that among the offspring of inbred agouti parents were littermates which varied in coat color and size despite the fact that they were genetically identical (Duhl et al., 1994a,b). These littermates could have brown coats and normal size, yellow coats and obesity, or have a mottled coat color and have a body size in between the extremes (Adams, 2008).

The agouti gene encodes a protein which binds to the melanocortin receptor. Binding of the protein to the receptor blocks those cells from making the brown pigment, melanin. When the agouti gene is 'on' (actively transcribed) the receptor is blocked and the resultant mice are yellow (Duhl et al., 1994a,b). A similar receptor was described in the brain and associated with feeding behavior and body weight set point (Lu et al., 1994). Later it was discovered that the tipping point for the agouti gene being turned 'on' or 'off' was controlled by the state of DNA methylation (Wolff et al., 1998; Michaud et al., 1994). DNA methylation can take place throughout life but is particularly important during embryonic development. Three active cytosine methyltransferases, Dnmt1, Dnmt3a, and Dnmt3b have been identified in mammals. While Dnmt1 is ubiquitously expressed and is a maintenance methyltransferase, Dnmt3a and Dnmt3b are regulated during development and are required to initiate de novo methylation and establish new methylation patterns (Bestor, 1992; Bestor et al., 1992). By providing a diet rich in methyl donating nutrients to pregnant yellow obese mice, Dolinoy et al. observed that the offspring were mostly brown and non-obese. The availability of methyl groups to developing fetal mice allowed for the methylation of their DNA (including cytosines in the agouti gene) and placed the gene in the 'off' – no transcription – mode. Thus the individual's adult health was markedly influenced by early prenatal factors (Dolinoy et al., 2006).

An extreme example of the role of prenatal nutrition on DNA methylation and subsequent adult phenotype is seen in the development of the queen honeybee. Genetically, queens are identical to workers. Larval honeybees developing in the comb are destined to become a queen if the comb cup, containing the larvae, is filled with royal jelly, a complex protein-rich substance secreted from the glands on the head of the worker bees. In the presence of royal jelly the larva develops functional ovaries and a larger abdomen for egg-laying, that is, it becomes a queen. In the absence of royal jelly the larva develop into sterile workers. Scientists determined that the royal jelly silences a key gene, Dnmt3, which codes for an enzyme involved in genome-wide gene silencing. When Dnmt3 is active in the bee larvae, they become workers but when the jelly turns Dnmt3 off, genes jump into action producing the queen (Kucharski et al., 2008).

Recently Lister reported on the first comparative epigenome methylation maps involving the neurons of the frontal cortices of mice and humans (Lister et al., 2013). In their studies, Lister found that the neuronal cells in the frontal cortex of infant mice lacked non-CG methylation, however, these modifications rapidly developed as they aged and their brains developed. This group also found similar methylation taking place in the human brain especially during the first 2 years of life coinciding with the period of rapid synaptogenesis. Non-CG methylation of genes in the same subject was associated with lower gene expression. The high degree of correlation of non-CG methylation in humans and mice suggest the phenomenon is both conserved and may be responsible for fine tuning of the transcriptome in these cells (Lister et al., 2013). The influence of stress and social environment on epigenetics in rodents has been recently reviewed (Gudsnuk and Champagne, 2012) as has the impact of nutrition on epigenetics in nonhuman primates (Niculescu, 2012).

Another regulatory network that occurs independently of protein coding regions of the genome are the regulatory networks of small RNA molecules. Small non-coding RNA elements play a variety of unique regulatory roles in vertebrates and invertebrates alike (Dogini et al., 2014). The origins and roles of small non-coding RNAs have been recently reviewed and are beyond the scope of the current chapter (Cook and Blelloch, 2013). Small interfering RNA (siRNA) molecules, one class of small non-coding RNAs, serve as a classic example of how animal models paved the way to further advances in genomics. Endogenous siRNAs were first described in nematodes and for a long time they alone among animals were known to have an endogenous siRNA pathway (Okamura and Lai, 2008). However, in 2008, endogenous siRNAs inhibitory pathways were described in both the fruit fly (Kawamura et al., 2008) and in mice (Tam et al., 2008). siRNAs are a class of double-stranded RNAs which are 20–25 bp in length and best known to interfere with the expression of specific genes with complementary nucleotide sequences, although other known activities deal with antiviral mechanisms and the shaping of chromatin structure (Dogini et al., 2014). From the initial observations about the inhibitory action of siRNAs, various investigators pursued the idea of using synthetic siRNAs to target specific mRNA and downregulate or silence their translation into protein, thus abolishing their ultimate function (Elbashir et al., 2001). Improvements in the synthesis and delivery of siRNAs have resulted in creating cultures of mammalian cells with stable knockdown of target transcripts and animal models of human diseases such as leptin receptor deficiency and Parkinson's Disease (Brummelkamp et al., 2002; Hommel et al., 2003), and there is still much interest in using siRNA in human therapeutics (Sindhu et al., 2012).

4. Phenotypic Characterization and Disease Modelling

a. Ontology

In order to better compare genes with similar structure and function between species, a system of vocabularies and classifications that cover several domains of cellular and molecular biology has been created called Gene Ontology (GO) (Harris et al., 2004). This collaborative effort addressed two aspects of information integration: providing consistent descriptors for gene products in different databases and standardizing classifications for sequences and sequence features. Started originally using three model databases: FlyBase (Drosophila), Saccharomyces Genome Database (SGD), and Mouse Genome Informatics (MGI) project, GO has now been extended to several of the world's major databases for plant, animal, and microbial genomes. Within this annotation are several characterizations: Molecular Function, which describes activities such as catalytic and binding activities at the molecular level; Biological Process, which describes biological goals accomplished by one or more ordered assemblies of molecular functions; Cellular component, which describes locations at the levels of subcellular structures and molecular complexes.

High-level processes such as cell death may have both subtypes (apoptosis) and subprocesses (apoptotic chromosome condensation). All this information is combined with Sequence Ontology (SO) which permits the classification and standard representation of sequence features. These large sets of annotations, made using automated methods, cover both model organisms and man.

b. The Phenome

In order to maximize experimental data obtained from model organisms we need rich genotype–phenotype annotations. Unfortunately, until recently, there was no way to make these comparisons on a large scale. Going back through the literature to make associations between gene function and phenotype had proven limited. For example, in hypothesis-driven studies involving animal models only the phenotype of interest to the investigator may be evaluated or reported. Likewise, clinical studies in humans suffer from descriptions relevant to the clinical condition without completely describing the phenotype. Frequently, both types of studies fail to document frequency and co-occurrence of specific phenotype aspects of disease: time, prognosis, molecular features, and therapeutic responsiveness. No common language was capable of capturing the phenotypic changes described in each of these situations in the past literature. Yet there are compelling reasons for developing such an annotation. The following example should illustrate this point. Until recently it was thought that the screening of targeted mutations in mice would not demonstrate clear phenotypes for many genes, yet when Tang and colleagues systematically measured the phenotypic changes in multiple-organ systems in 472 mutants for transmembrane and secreted proteins, they found that 89% of the mice showed a phenotype in at least one organ system and 57% in two or more organ systems. Systematic phenotyping was based on 85 assays spanning immunology, metabolism, cardiology, oncology, growth, ophthalmology, neurology, pathology, reproduction, viability, and embryonic lethality (Tang et al., 2010).

The development of the Mammalian Phenotype Ontology (MPO) in 2004 provided the first formal ontology for the description of mammalian phenotypes. Adopted by the Mouse Genome Informatics (MGI) group, with manual curation, it establishes the mouse as the best phenotypically characterized vertebrate. Recently there has been a commitment of the online Mendelian Inheritance of Man (OMIM) to cross-reference the human phenotype ontology (HPO), elements of morphologic terms, International Classification of Diseases (ICD), and the MPO. This should standardize the structure of clinical synopses and make them available to search and analyze. It is clear that such developments will improve the richness and accuracy of phenotype–disease descriptions with concomitant improvements in the power of informatics to detect similarities between related diseases and subtypes within apparent uniform conditions (Schofield et al., 2011).

c. Collaborative Attempts to Identify Gene Function in the Mouse Through Genotype-Driven Targeted Gene Knockouts

Several collaborative efforts involving investigators from multiple institutions have been created for either the generation of mutant mouse ESC clones or for generating mice from these clones and submitting them to phenotyping cores. The ultimate goal of phenotyping is to assign a function to each gene (Sung et al., 2012).

i. CENTERS PRODUCING GENE TARGETED MOUSE ESC Two large centers dedicated to the production of mutated mouse embryonic stem cells are the International Knockout Mouse Consortium (IKMC) and the Sanger Institute Mouse Genetics Project (MGP). The IKMC is a collaborative program involving the Knockout Mouse Project (KOMP), the European Conditional Mouse Mutagenesis Program (EUCOMM), the North American Conditional Mouse Mutagenesis Project (NorCOMM), and the Texas A&M Institute for Genomic Medicine (TIGM). With the exception of the TIGM, all other members are producing targeted mutations on C57BL6/N ESCs using the knockout first allele method (Sung et al., 2012). The Sanger MGP also makes mice carrying knockout first conditional-ready alleles using the EUCOMM/KOMP-CDS ES cell collection. Both make their ESC available to the public and to Phenotyping Centers like the International Mouse Phenotyping Consortium (IMPC) and the European Mouse Disease Clinic (EUMODIC) for microinjection and mouse phenotyping. It is the responsibility of the MGP and the IKMC to perform the molecular characterization of their mutant mouse strains. Such characterization has been recently published (Ryder et al., 2013). At the time of this writing the EUCOMM/KOMP-CDS ESC clone collection consisted of targeted clones for 12,350 genes, estimated to be 56% of the 22,147 concensus coding sequences for genes present in Ensembl (Ryder et al., 2013; Pruitt et al., 2009).

ii. CENTERS PHENOTYPING MUTANT MICE It is the goal of the IMPC Project to phenotype knockouts for every PCG in the mouse genome by 2021 (Abbott, 2010). Another large phenotyping Center is the EUMODIC which brought together four European mouse groups, the MRC at Harwell (UK), the German mouse clinic in Munich, the Institut Clinique de la Souris (ICS) in France and the Wellcome Trust Sanger Institute (MGP). Several other worldwide centers for mouse phenotyping are making major contributions and are listed by Ayadi

and colleagues (Ayadi et al., 2012). The web portal for all information arising from the IMPC (www.mousephenome.org) provides the biomedical community with unified access to mutant mice and the collection of mouse phenotyping data plus all the standardized protocols followed during phenotyping. Mouse clinics worldwide must submit data according to strict protocols and then the data is manually collated and evaluated for quality control. All data is annotated with biomedical ontologies and integrated with other resources to provide insights into mammalian gene function and human disease. A summary of legacy data submitted by the MGP and EuroPhenome has been recently published (Koscielny et al., 2014).

A recent publication reports the results of the evaluating 489 mutant lines for viability and fertility and 250 lines for adult phenotype out of a total of 900 line produced by MGP (White et al., 2013). The MGP web portal is www.sanger.ac.uk/mouseportal/ and details of the protocols for standardized phenotyping may be found. In the MGP study the 250 lines which completed the adult phenotype screen included genes on all chromosomes except Y and in 34 of these lines no functional information had ever been published. The data reported here included 59 orthologs of human disease genes of which 27 exhibited phenotypes broadly similar to the human disease. However, many additional phenotypes were detected in the mouse mutants suggesting that additional features may also occur in human patients. Interestingly a large portion of the genes underlying recessive disorders are homozygous lethal in mice.

The initial report from the EUMODIC was recently published and summarized the results of analyzing 799 mouse lines with a comprehensive set of physiological and behavioral paradigms (Ayadi et al., 2012). All the data are now available on the EuroPhenome database www.europhenome.org and the mouse lines are available through the European Mutant Mouse Archive (EMMA) and the MGP. Essentially this first publication looked at the same set of mouse lines as the MGP paper and drew the same conclusions. Both had at least one phenotype score for 80% of the lines, 57% of the lines were viable, 13% sub-viable , 30% embryonic lethal, and 7% displayed fertility impairments.

The results of these centers are also reported to the Mouse Gene Informatics website at www.infomatics.jax.org, which now has information on the function of over 7300 mouse genes. The Mouse ENCODE project is a consortium with the goal to enhance the value of the human ENCODE project through relative comparative studies, give access to cell types, tissues, and developmental time points unavailable in humans, and provide a general resource to inform and accelerate research in mouse genomics and disease modeling with human translational potential. One major focus of mouse ENCODE is to identify comprehensively transcriptional regulatory elements in the mouse genome, providing a valuable resource for the understanding the genetic circuitry that controls animal development and lineage specification (www.mouseencode.org).

Despite all these advances in correlating mouse phenotype with that found in man, a recent report by Seok and colleagues cautions investigators when selecting murine models for certain complex human inflammatory diseases to carefully document the transcriptional networks triggered by each insult/agent (Seok et al., 2013).

iii. DEFINING GENE FUNCTION AND DISEASE MODELLING IN SPECIES OTHER THAN MICE The Rat Genome Database (www.rdg.mcw.edu) was created to provide a platform for researchers interested in linking genomic variations to phenotypes in rats. Quantitative Trait Loci (QTL) form the core datasets allowing researchers to identify loci harboring genes associated with disease (Nigam et al., 2013). The resource allows for the cross-species analyses of syntenic regions on the mouse, rat, and human genomes in order to identify regions for further study in all three species. Currently the database holds over 1900 rat QTLs with details about the animals and methods used to determine the QTL. It also houses over 1900 human QTLs and over 4000 mouse QTLs. Multiple ontologies are used to standardize phenotypes, traits, diseases, and experimental methods.

Zebrafish have also been widely used in mutagenesis screening assays (Haffter and Nusslein-Volhard, 1996) which have helped identify many genes essential to the specification of cells types, organ systems, and body axes in vertebrates (Talbot et al., 1995) as well as genes associated with human disease (Lieschke and Currie, 2007; Roscioli et al., 2012).

Closely associated with humans from an environmental standpoint, the dog, which occurs in over 400 modern breeds, is prone to a variety of genetic diseases including cancer, heart disease, deafness, blindness, cataracts, epilepsy, osteoarthritis, and autoimmune diseases. Extensive genealogies are available for most registered breeds. Researchers from 12 European countries are collaborating with veterinarians and breeders to collect DNA from large cohorts of dogs suffering from a range of carefully selected diseases of relevance to human health. The project named LUPA employs a high-density SNP array for the evaluation of mutations associated with disease. Mutations for four monogenic diseases have been identified and several complex diseases have been mapped with fine mapping underway. It is predicted that these analyses will lead to a better understanding of the molecular mechanisms underlying complex disease in both dog and man (Lequarre et al., 2011).

Resources available for pursuing studies using non-human primates in biomedical research include draft sequences for the chimpanzee, cynomolgus monkey, gorilla, orangutan, Aye-aye, and rhesus macaque with partial sequences available from common marmoset, white-cheeked gibbon, African green monkey, Olive baboon, Mouse lemur, Sooty mangabey, pigtail macaque, and Sifaka (Norgren, 2013). In addition mapping of QTL harboring genes for various metabolic processes has proceeded in both rhesus and baboons. There are also 21 species of NHP that are the target of transcriptome projects (Norgren, 2013). These resources have been used to aid in the characterization of numerous human disorders, especially complex disorders, and certain infectious diseases.

Baboons have many anatomic, physiologic, and genetic similarities with man and have been used widely in the study of complex diseases. The availability of a whole-genome baboon linkage map and the ability to use many high-throughput tools created for human samples, such as gene arrays and DNA methylation assays, allow investigators to collect high-quality genetic, genomic, and epigenomic data (Cox et al., 2013). At the Southwest National Primate Research Center, a major focus of research is mapping genes that affect risk factors for atherosclerosis, hypertension, osteoporosis, obesity, and diabetes, and the relating of these genes to human disease. Over 2400 baboons over seven generations have been genotyped with over 290 microsatellite markers and phenotyped for hundreds of quantitative traits. Their research into risk factors in cardiovascular disease (CVD) was designed to investigate diet-by-gene interactions and showed that a substantial proportion of variation in the host to clinically relevant biomarkers of lipid and lipoprotein metabolism was due to genes (Cox et al., 2013). The major thrust of the current research is to localize, identify, and functionally characterize genes responsible for the detected effects. Studies by Rainwater and colleagues showed dietary effects on a pleiotropic network of genes underlying lipoprotein metabolism and inflammation (Rainwater et al., 2010). Another study looked at transcriptional profiles for over 15,000 genes in the peripheral blood mononuclear cells of 500 pedigreed baboons to find pleiotropic QTL influencing networks of co-expressed genes mediating Th1 and Th2 IRs implicated in the inflammatory component of atherogenesis (Vinson et al., 2011). Preliminary transcriptome studies conducted in baboons fed a high-fat, high-sugar diet showed that variation in some genes in response to diet is epigenetically regulated by promoter CpG methylation and /or microRNA targeting (Cox et al., 2013).

Rhesus macaques, *Macaca mulatta*, have been widely used in biomedical and pharmaceutical research based on their physiologic similarity to humans; diseases, especially complex diseases, with similar pathology to man; and their ready availability especially through the National Primate Centers. Since completing the draft sequence of its genome, it has been shown that rhesus macaques share synteny for 89% of the human genes and have 93% mean sequence identity with the human genome (Rhesus Macaque Genome Sequencing and Analysis Consortium, 2007). The US National Primate Centers have large managed breeding programs for rhesus macaques controlling for many environmental variables including nutrition. Because of their relatively early onset of maturity and extended life span, there are frequently successive generations of rhesus macaques available for sampling together with multiple-year pedigree information providing substantial analytical power in genetic studies. Through use of extended rhesus macaque pedigrees, significant heritability has been documented for certain quantitative risk factors of cardiovascular and metabolic diseases (Vinson et al., 2013). The Indian-origin rhesus macaque is thought to be the best model for HIV vaccine testing in part due to the similarity of orthologous genes (to human) encoding proteins regulating immunity including HLA proteins (Shen et al., 2013; Wiseman et al., 2013). In addition, several mutations occurring in rhesus genes, orthologous to human genes, have resulted in similar disease phenotypes in rhesus macaques (Rogers, 2013).

5. The Microbiome

a. Introduction

Beginning in the early 1980s scientists have been interrogating various environments in order to elucidate the breadth of microbial populations in them. Early investigations studied 16S rRNA gene sequences, which are phylogenetically conserved among bacteria, to document microbial species. Today metagenomic studies sequence microbial communities *en mass* (Nelson, 2013). One of the first attempts to conduct such a survey was conducted on samples of sea water from the Sargasso Sea and generated over one billion bp of non-redundant sequences which were thought to represent over 1800 species (Venter et al., 2004). Since this time, similar metagenomic studies have taken place on different anatomical locations in animals and humans. The Human Microbiome Project characterized the microbiome of 242 clinically healthy volunteers from 15–18 anatomic sites (Human Microbiome Project Consortium, 2012). It is now clear that a human's microbiota contains about 100-trillion cells or at least 10-times the number of human cells which comprise the body (Fritz et al., 2013). With microbial cells occupying niches in the skin, oral cavity, nasal cavity, conjunctiva, ear, and gastrointestinal system, it is easy to see why they play a beneficial role in immune development and homeostasis, food digestion, metabolism, and even angiogenesis (Fritz et al., 2013).

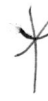

However, there can be negative consequences associated with certain microbiomes or with perturbations in the microbial inhabitants. Pflughoeft and Versalovic have recently reviewed the evidence suggesting that shifts in the structure of the microbial community are linked to such human diseases as inflammatory bowel disease, diabetes mellitus, obesity, CVD, and cancer (Pflughoeft and Versalovic, 2012). Animal models have played an important role in demonstrating the pathogenetic mechanisms involved in many of these diseases and more.

b. Microbiomes Contribution to Health and Disease

In 2002 Ownby and colleagues demonstrated that children raised in households with dogs were protected from subsequent development of allergies and asthma (Ownby et al., 2002). Subsequent studies in mice exposed to dog-associated house dust showed distinct changes in their gut microbial flora (it became restructured with *Lactobacillus johnsonii*) and they developed resistance to experimentally induced allergy (Fujimura et al., 2013). Furthermore, supplementation of wild-type mice with *L. johnsonii* protected them against both airway allergen challenge or infection with respiratory syncytial virus (Fujimura et al., 2013). This GI microbiome modification resulted in down regulation of the Th2 limb of the immune system. Other studies have shown that specific bacteria in the gut microbiome, such as *Clostridium* clades IV and XIV, dramatically alter the IR (Atarashi et al., 2011).

Evidence is accumulating to support the concept of bidirectional signaling between the gastrointestinal tract and the brain which is regulated at the neural, hormonal, and immunological levels. Neurological symptoms and psychological stress are associated with gastrointestinal disorders such as inflammatory bowel disease and irritable bowel syndrome (Rhee et al., 2009; Mawdsley and Rampton, 2005). Animal models have been used extensively to probe the relationship between GI tract microbiome and mental health (Cryan and O'Mahony, 2011; Desbonnet et al., 2013). One example of how animal models are contributing to our knowledge of the gut microbiome–brain axis is shown in studies on autism. Autism spectrum disorder (ASD) appears to be a complex disease, with both genetic and environmental inputs. It has been known for years that pregnant mothers exposed to severe viral infections have an increased risk of giving birth to a child with autism. Masmaniam and colleagues drawing from these observations examined a mouse model of autism where pregnant mothers are immunologically activated by injection of poly I:C (a double-stranded RNA analog; TLR3 agonist) (Hsiao et al., 2013). Their offspring exhibit core communicative, social, and stereotypic behaviors relevant to ASD as well as a common ASD cerebellar neuropathologic change. These offspring also have defects in intestinal integrity (increased intestinal permeability) and alterations in commensal microbiota. By transplanting the bacterium, *Bacteriodes fragillus*, known to restore normalcy in mouse models of colitis and reduce neuroinflammation in mouse models of multiple sclerosis, the investigators found that the gut leakiness was corrected and the main behavioral symptoms improved. Furthermore this group investigated which chemicals were found in the blood of mice with leaky intestines compared to normal mice and found one compound, 4-ethylphenylsulphate (4EPS), was present in the blood of ASD mice at 46-times higher concentration than in controls. Injection of 4EPS into wild-type mice reproduced autism-like behaviors (Hsiao *et al.*, 2013). Taken together, the results suggest a gut microbiome–brain connection in this mouse model of ASD and identify a potential probiotic therapy for human ASD.

The worldwide epidemic of obesity has stimulated efforts to identify environmental and host factors which affect energy balance. Gordon and colleagues examined the gut microbiomes of genetically obese mice and their lean littermates as well as obese and lean human volunteers. They found that the relative abundance of two dominant divisions (phylum) of bacteria, Bacteroidetes and Firmicutes, were altered in the cecum of genetically obese mice; Bacteroidetes was 50% lower and Firmicutes was higher by a corresponding degree. These changes were division-wide and not attributable to diet or food intake. Similar relative changes in these two divisions of bacteria were seen in the distal gut of obese and lean humans and the relative abundance of Bacteroidetes increases in obese individuals as they lose weight, with the increase correlating with weight loss rather than caloric intake. Using biochemical analyses and transplantation of the obese mouse microbiome into germ-free wild-type mice, these investigators were able to show that the microbiome increased capacity to harvest energy from the diet and resulted in increased total body fat phenotype. These studies identify the gut microbiota as an additional contributing factor in the pathophysiology of obesity (Turnbaugh *et al.*, 2006). Later this group transplanted the gut microbiome from a single human into germ-free C57BL/6 mice and observed a stable, multigenerational colonization while mice were maintained on the standard plant polysaccharide-rich diet. However, when these mice were switched to a high fat/high sugar 'Western' diet, the structure of the microbiota shifted within a single day and changed the metabolic pathways in the microbiome and altered microbiome gene expression. Humanized mice on a 'Western' diet had increased adiposity and this trait was transmissible via microbiome transplantation (Turnbaugh *et al.*, 2009). Recently these investigators transplanted fecal microbiota from human adult female twins discordant for obesity into germ-free mice. Such reconstituted mice

expressed a phenotype characteristic of the type of microbiome transplanted. When mice with the obese microbiomes (OB) were house with mice containing the lean microbiome, the OB mice failed to develop increase body mass and obesity-associated metabolic phenotype. This rescue correlated with invasion of specific members of Bacteroidetes from the lean microbiota into the OB microbiota and was diet-dependent (Ridaura *et al.*, 2013). The findings reveal a transmissible, rapid, and modifiable effect of diet-by-microbiota interaction.

Given the association between type 2 diabetes, diet, and obesity it would seem natural to extend the studies cited above with diabetes in animal models. Cani and colleagues previously demonstrated that blood LPS was elevated in people who ate high-fat diets thus causing metabolic endotoxemia which they believed led to the low-grade inflammation typically associated with type 2 diabetes. In order to make the correlation between these metabolic changes, gut microbiota, and disease, they treated mice with oral antibiotics to induce changes in the gut microbiome. They found that antibiotics did profoundly change the level of cecal LPS in high-fat-fed or genetically obese mice. Furthermore this treatment reduced metabolic endotoxemia, and reduced: glucose intolerance, body weight gain, fat mass development, and oxidative stress in these mice (Cani *et al.*, 2008). Cani and colleagues also showed that the absence of the receptor for LPS, CD 14, in genetically obese and diabetic prone mice mimicked the metabolic and inflammatory effects seen with antibiotic treatment. Caricilli and colleagues decided to pursue this idea by investigating the role of a receptor critical in innate immunity, Toll-like receptor-2 (TLR2). They showed that germ-free mice deficient in TLR2 were protected from diet-induced insulin resistance. Looking to see if this insulin-sensitive phenotype could be modified by the gut microbiome, they exposed the germ-free mice to mice carrying a conventional microbiome and applied a variety of metabolic analyses and metagenomics to answer this question. These conventionalized TLR2 KO mice went on to show increased LPS absorption, low-grade inflammation, insulin resistance, glucose intolerance, and obesity. These changes coincided with alterations in the gut microbiome characterized by three-fold increases in Firmicutes and a slight increase in Bacteroidetes compared with control wild-type mice. These changes could be transferred to wild-type mice by transplantation of the microbiota from TLR2 KO mice and this was reversed by treatment of the wild-type mice with antibiotics (Caricilli *et al.*, 2011). At the molecular level these conventionalized TLR2 KOs had activation of the TLR4 pathway but not the TLR2 pathway during the course of insulin resistance. Taken together the results suggest that an interaction between the innate immune system and the gut microbiome may determine the insulin sensitivity of an animal and that the TLRs may play different roles in this process in animals and man.

6. Host–Vector–Parasite Genomics

In an effort to better understand the interplay between the human genes and the infectious agents which afflict them, investigators have made an effort to sequence the whole genomes of most human (and many animal) infectious agents as well as the genomes of the transmission vectors. Perhaps the best example comes from studies of malaria. Malaria is probably the most important parasitic diseases in the world causing up to 500 million new cases and 2.7 million deaths annually mostly occurring in sub-Saharan Africa. With the goal to better understand the molecular basis for growth, replication, infection, transmission and resistance in both the primary parasite, *Plasmodium falciparum*, and its primary vector, *Anopheles gambiae*, international consortia were established to sequence the genomes of these two organisms and document gene expression patterns associated with the life cycles of each.

In 2002 the International *Anopheles gambiae* Genome Project published the first whole-genome sequence for this mosquito (Holt *et al.*, 2002). Results from this and subsequent studies have demonstrated the enzyme families which play a part in the catabolism of xenobiotics and made available SNPs for these genes which allowed the monitoring of the frequency and spread of insecticide resistance alleles. The initial work also identified elements of the innate immune system including the IR to the parasite (Cohuet *et al.*, 2008; Wondji *et al.*, 2007). In 2006 Riehle and colleagues discovered a single genetic control region (called the parasite-resistant island) which controlled *Plasmodium* infection of Anopheles in the wild (Riehle *et al.*, 2006). Li and colleagues, using this information, screened thousands of genomes from infected or non-infected mosquitoes and identified 347 non-synonymous SNPs within genes from Anopheles in malaria endemic regions. Direct association studies found three naturally occurring genetic variations in each of three genes and knockdown assays demonstrated the products of each gene. These SNPs are now being used to develop tools for malaria control in endemic areas (Li *et al.*, 2013).

Around the same time that the Anopheles genome was published, the international group sequencing the whole genome of *Plasmodium falciparum* published their findings (Gardner *et al.*, 2002). Among their many findings the group described the genome of the apicoplast, a relic plasmid, homologous to the chloroplast in plants. This apicoplast arose through secondary endosymbiosis in which the ancestor of all apicomplexans engulfed a eukaryotic alga. The processes controlled by this organelle are essential for the parasite's life including: synthesis of fatty acids, isoprenoids, and heme. Several of

these metabolic pathways are distinct from host (human) pathways and may be the parasite-specific targets for drug development (Gardner *et al.*, 2002).

The group also demonstrated many parasite secretory pathways including those in which parasite-derived proteins are exported to and modify the host erythrocyte. These mechanisms are important because they are responsible for many of the most severe complications in the human disease. In addition the group discussed the parasite's genetic mechanisms for immune evasion and pathogenesis. Because of this work hundreds of new potential targets for vaccination were discovered, many of which are now under development or being tested in the field (Schwartz *et al.*, 2012). One of the greatest drawbacks to advancing vaccine research has been the lack of optimal animal models; IRs in rodents and nonhuman primates have not proved to be reliable indicators of efficacy in the field. In this respect efforts to evaluate malaria vaccine in humanized mice containing human bone marrow (and erythrocytes) and human liver are promising (Arnold *et al.*, 2011; Legrand *et al.*, 2009).

As part of a more comprehensive effort, VectorBase was established by the National Institute of Allergy and Infectious Disease and dedicated to the genomics of invertebrate vectors of human disease. The data base now carries the sequences of over 48 arachnids, gastropods, and insects (www.vectorbase.org).

7. Conclusion

Comparative genomics has achieved more in defining PCGs (which make up about 1.2% of the genome) than noncoding elements, which likely contain more than 50% of the function of the genome. Due to a tremendous international effort, animal models, particularly targeted mutant mice, have provided a functional basis for many PCGs. Mammalian models have a high degree of conservation in the noncoding sequences and should continue to define the function for those, primarily regulatory, elements. Identification of common variants associated with risk for developing complex diseases and traits will be elucidated by further studies in man and NHPs. Once identified, mutant mice will reveal the function of many of these disease genes. The finding of rare variants for human disease will require further progress in sequencing technology since tens of thousands of people, carefully selected into control and affected groups, will be required to elucidate these rare variants. Finally, the availability of mouse lines containing conditional mutations with reporters for every PCG will be indispensable for further investigations which probe the fine specificity of biochemical networks and changes in those networks resulting from environmental interrogation. These models should be expanded to include conserved NCE and together they will determine the products of transcription and translation, including splice variants, many of which will become targets for new drug discovery.

There is no better way to describe the power of comparative genomics then a quote from Alfoldi and Lindblad-Toh, "the use of comparative genomics, enabled by the human genome sequence and the technological advances catalyzed by its generation, has brought a wealth of insights into vertebrate genome evolution, increased our understanding of the human genome, and now offers the potential to decipher human evolution and disease and the inevitable link between the two" (Alfoldi and Lindblad-Toh, 2013).

D. Animals as Recipients of Animal Research

Because humans and nonhuman animals share common physiologic responses, many of the advances sought for humans through the use of animal models also benefit animals themselves. It is beyond the scope of this chapter to completely examine the direct benefits of animal research to animals; however, we hope to use a broad-brush illustrated with both classical and more modern examples to try to impart current and potential future benefits of animal research to animals.

Humans and other vertebrates are susceptible to a large number of infectious diseases, and many disease agents infect both animals and humans. These are called zoonotic agents and are frequently passed between humans and other animals. Certain of these zoonotic diseases are prevented by vaccination in humans and animals, including rabies, anthrax, tetanus, and Lyme disease (Quimby, 1994b).

Since the adoption of the Nuremberg Code in the 1950s, humans have been protected by first testing the safety of new drugs and medical devices in nonhuman animals (Spicker et al., 1988). As a result, an enormous amount of data is known on the safety and pharmacokinetics of these drugs in various animal species. It is therefore not surprising that many drugs designed for human use, such as antibiotics, tranquilizers, steroids, sulfonamides, anesthetics, analgesics, chemotherapeutics, anticoagulants, antiparasitics, antiepileptics, and antihistamines, are all commonly used in veterinary practice (Quimby, 1998). Many surgical techniques intended for humans were first perfected in animals and subsequently used to treat animal disorders. Included among these techniques are repair of spinal cord, hip replacement, fracture repair, repair of congenital heart defects, treatment for burns, and organ transplantation.

Nonhuman animals, particularly dogs, develop a variety of autoimmune and hematologic conditions that are identical to the human counterparts, and as a result, these animals benefit from blood transfusions, immunosuppressant therapy, purified blood components, and hormones, much like humans with the same disorders

(National Research Council, 1994). These same animals benefit from both diagnostic procedures and, in some instances, surgical intervention originally designed for humans.

Pet animals are the beneficiaries of advances in biomedical imaging, and veterinary practitioners utilize X-ray machines, computed tomography, ultrasonography, and fiber-optic endoscopy for animal disease diagnosis.

Knowledge of artificial insemination, semen evaluation and storage, egg incubation, and behavioral adaptation were employed in the successful captive breeding and reintroduction of the eastern peregrine falcon, which has now been removed from the endangered species list. Similarly, assisted-reproduction techniques are being examined and used to help restore populations of animals threatened with extinction (Swanson, 2012; Mahesh et al., 2011; Ganan et al., 2009; Swanson et al., 2007; Luvoni, 2000; Goodrowe et al., 2000).

In the future it seems likely that comparative genomics will provide beneficial data and treatments for a variety of animal problems. A notable example exists in species conservation efforts. Specifically, studies of the genomes of wild populations will assist in identifying those which are genetically distinct and elevate them in preservation efforts (Wall et al., 2013; Bowden et al., 2012). To date such studies have helped to identify the Sumatran orangutan as a separate species (Xu and Arnason, 1996) as well as a fourth subspecies of chimpanzee (Bowden et al., 2012).

Recent genome sequencing of DNA from a permafrost-preserved bone from an ancestral horse dating from 560–780,000 years ago allowed comparison of the genomes of it with modern horses, donkeys, a late Pleistocene horse, and a Przewalski's horse (Orlando et al., 2013). Analysis suggest that the Equus lineage, giving rise to all contemporary horses, donkeys and zebras, occurred about 4 million years ago and that Prezewalski's horses and domestic horse population diverged about 38–72,000 years ago with no evidence for recent admixtures between the two. This provides evidence that the Prezewalski's horses represent the last surviving wild horse population and are worthy of conservation efforts.

Additionally, comparative genomic approaches may also aid in food and fiber production which ultimately benefits animals through more economical animal use and better nutritional support. For example, while most of the genes for metabolism are conserved with other mammals, five metabolism genes in cattle are deleted or highly diverged, and seven are present in duplicate compared to humans implying that these genes are critical or unique to cattle nutrition (Seo et al., 2013). Additionally, transcriptomics data has been collected under differing conditions of nutrition, lactation and growth and will aid in linking the genome of cattle to optimal nutrition and metabolism (Khan *et al.*, 2013).

In conclusion, the sharing of diagnostic methods, preventives, drugs, surgical techniques, medical devices, and biomethodological techniques between humans and other animals adds credence to the "One, health, One medicine" concept (Frank, 2008).

E. Perspectives on the Present State of Animal Research

Throughout this chapter we have attempted to highlight critical historical achievements that utilized animal research and to point out recent progress made using animal models. Of course, it would be impossible to recite, in any meaningful way, all the incredible accomplishments in biology and medicine that occurred during the 20th and early 21st centuries, using animal models. A former surgeon general of the United States has stated that every major achievement in medicine during this century has depended in some fashion on animal research. Over two-thirds of all Nobel Prizes in Physiology and Medicine have been awarded to scientists who used vertebrate animals to accomplish their goals (Leader and Stark, 1987). In a survey of living Nobel laureates, 97% responded that animal experiments have been vital to the discovery and development of many advances in physiology and medicine, and 92% felt strongly that animal experiments are still crucial to the investigation and development of many medical treatments (Seriously Ill for Medical Research (SIMR), 1998).

The 20th century and early 21st century saw an explosion of activity in every area of the biological sciences. Virtually all modern medical treatments and devices, including most that are now taken for granted, were developed through animal research. Advances in the science of cell biology, ecology, developmental biology, respiratory physiology, cardiovascular physiology, endocrinology, biochemistry, bacteriology, virology, parasitology, psychology, ethology, neurobiology, and nutrition and metabolism have enriched and supported the medical disciplines of cardiology, dermatology, surgery, orthopedics, pediatrics, anesthesiology, pharmacology, microbiology, psychiatry, neurology, dentistry, hematology, medical genetics, and women's health. Although this chapter is extensive, it only touches the surface of the use of animal models in scientific discovery. If the reader wishes to explore the topic further, reviews documenting the progress of various aspects of biomedical science and technology have been highlighted through this chapter and additional resources are available (Bergen, 2007; Bliss, 1982; Boverhof *et al.*, 2011; Byrne, 2010; Comroe and Dripps, 1976; Jacobs and Hatfield, 2013; Lombard *et al.*, 2007; Robert and Cohen, 2011; Sourkes, 1966; Weisse, 1991; Michell, 2005; Fox, 2007).

References

Abbott, A., 2010. Mouse project to find each gene's role. Nature 465, 410.

Adams, J.U., 2008. Obesity, epigenetics, and gene regulation. Nat. Educ. 1, 128.

Ahituv, N., Zhu, Y., Visel, A., Holt, A., Afzal, V., Pennacchio, L.A., et al., 2007. Deletion of ultraconserved elements yields viable mice. PLoS Biol. 5, e234.

Alfoldi, J., Lindblad-Toh, K., 2013. Comparative genomics as a tool to understand evolution and disease. Genome Res. 23, 1063–1068.

Allison, D.B., Cui, X., Page, G.P., Sabripour, M., 2006. Microarray data analysis: from disarray to consolidation and consensus. Nat. Rev. Genet. 7, 55–65.

Andrews, E.J., Ward, B.C., Altman, N.H., 1979. Spontaneous Animal Models of Human Disease. Academic Press, New York.

Antequera, F., Bird, A., 1999. CpG islands as genomic footprints of promoters that are associated with replication origins. Curr. Biol. 9, R661–R667.

Arnold, L., Tyagi, R.K., Meija, P., Swetman, C., Gleeson, J., Perignon, J.L., et al., 2011. Further improvements of the P. falciparum humanized mouse model. PLoS One 6, e18045.

Atarashi, K., Tanoue, T., Shima, T., Imaoka, A., Kuwahara, T., Momose, Y., et al., 2011. Induction of colonic regulatory T cells by indigenous Clostridium species. Science 331, 337–341.

Ayadi, A., Birling, M.C., Bottomley, J., Bussell, J., Fuchs, H., Fray, M., et al., 2012. Mouse large-scale phenotyping initiatives: overview of the European Mouse Disease Clinic (EUMODIC) and of the wellcome trust sanger institute mouse genetics project. Mamm. Genome 23, 600–610.

Backhed, F., Ley, R.E., Sonnenburg, J.L., Peterson, D.A., Gordon, J.I., 2005. Host–bacterial mutualism in the human intestine. Science 307, 1915–1920.

Backhed, F., Manchester, J.K., Semenkovich, C.F., Gordon, J.I., 2007. Mechanisms underlying the resistance to diet-induced obesity in germ-free mice. Proc. Natl. Acad. Sci. USA 104, 979–984.

Bacon, F., 1990. Novum Organum: aphorisms, concerning the Interpretation of Nature and the Kingdom of Man. Encyclopaedia Britannica, Chicago, IL.

Banchereau, J., Steinman, R.M., 1998. Dendritic cells and the control of immunity. Nature 392, 245–252.

Bang, B.G., Bang, F.B., Foard, M.A., 1972. Lymphocyte depression induced in chickens on diets deficient in vitamin A and other components. Am. J. Pathol. 68, 147–162.

Bay, A., Carbone, L., Frank, W., Quimby, F., 1995. Swine. CRC Press, Boca Raton, Florida.

Becker, S., De Angelis, M.H., Beckers, J., 2006. Use of chemical mutagenesis in mouse embryonic stem cells. Methods Mol. Biol. 329, 397–407.

Beeh, K.M., Kanniess, F., Wagner, F., Schilder, C., Naudts, I., Hammann-Haenni, A., et al., 2013. The novel TLR-9 agonist QbG10 shows clinical efficacy in persistent allergic asthma. J. Allergy. Clin. Immunol. 131, 866–874.

Begun, D.J., Holloway, A.K., Stevens, K., Hillier, L.W., Poh, Y.P., Hahn, M.W., et al., 2007. Population genomics: whole-genome analysis of polymorphism and divergence in Drosophila simulans. PLoS Biol. 5, e310.

Behringer, R., Gertsenstein, M., Nagy, K., Nagy, A., 2013. Manipulating the Mouse Embryo: A Laboratory Manual. Cold Spring Harbor Laboratory Press, Cold Spring Harbor, NY.

Bergen, W.G., 2007. Contribution of research with farm animals to protein metabolism concepts: a historical perspective. J. Nutr. 137, 706–710.

Bestor, T.H., 1992. Activation of mammalian DNA methyltransferase by cleavage of a Zn binding regulatory domain. EMBO J. 11, 2611–2617.

Bestor, T.H., Gundersen, G., Kolsto, A.B., Prydz, H., 1992. CpG islands in mammalian gene promoters are inherently resistant to de novo methylation. Genet. Anal. Tech. Appl. 9, 48–53.

Bezemer, G.F., Sagar, S., Van Bergenhenegouwen, J., Georgiou, N.A., Garssen, J., Kraneveld, A.D., et al., 2012. Dual role of Toll-like receptors in asthma and chronic obstructive pulmonary disease. Pharmacol. Rev. 64, 337–358.

Bhaya, D., Davison, M., Barrangou, R., 2011. CRISPR-Cas systems in bacteria and archaea: versatile small RNAs for adaptive defense and regulation. Annu. Rev. Genet. 45, 273–297.

Billingham, R.E., Brent, L., Medawar, P.B., 1953. Actively acquired tolerance of foreign cells. Nature 172, 603–606.

Bliss, M., 1982. Banting's, Best's, and Collip's accounts of the discovery of insulin. Bull. Hist. Med. 56, 554–568.

Bogdanove, A.J., Voytas, D.F., 2011. TAL effectors: customizable proteins for DNA targeting. Science 333, 1843–1846.

Bordet, J., 1909. Studies In Immunity. Wiley, New York.

Bosma, G.C., Custer, R.P., Bosma, M.J., 1983. A severe combined immunodeficiency mutation in the mouse. Nature 301, 527–530.

Boverhof, D.R., Chamberlain, M.P., Elcombe, C.R., Gonzalez, F.J., Heflich, R.H., Hernandez, L.G., et al., 2011. Transgenic animal models in toxicology: historical perspectives and future outlook. Toxicol. Sci. 121, 207–233.

Bowden, R., Macfie, T.S., Myers, S., Hellenthal, G., Nerrienet, E., Bontrop, R.E., et al., 2012. Genomic tools for evolution and conservation in the chimpanzee: pan troglodytes elliotti is a genetically distinct population. PLoS Genet. 8, e1002504.

Breitling, R., Gilbert, D., Heiner, M., Orton, R., 2008. A structured approach for the engineering of biochemical network models, illustrated for signalling pathways. Brief Bioinform 9, 404–421.

Britten, R.J., 2002. Divergence between samples of chimpanzee and human DNA sequences is 5%, counting indels. Proc. Natl. Acad. Sci. USA 99, 13633–13635.

Brummelkamp, T.R., Bernards, R., Agami, R., 2002. A system for stable expression of short interfering RNAs in mammalian cells. Science 296, 550–553.

Burnet, F.M., 1959. The Clonal Selection Theory of Acquired Immunity. Cambridge University Press, London.

Burton, D.R., Desrosiers, R.C., Doms, R.W., Koff, W.C., Kwong, P.D., Moore, J.P., et al., 2004. HIV vaccine design and the neutralizing antibody problem. Nat. Immunol. 5, 233–236.

Byrne, H.M., 2010. Dissecting cancer through mathematics: from the cell to the animal model. Nat. Rev. Cancer 10, 221–230.

Calne, R.Y., 1960. The rejection of renal homografts. Inhibition in dogs by 6-mercaptopurine. Lancet 1, 417–418.

Cani, P.D., Bibiloni, R., Knauf, C., Waget, A., Neyrinck, A.M., Delzenne, N.M., et al., 2008. Changes in gut microbiota control metabolic endotoxemia-induced inflammation in high-fat diet-induced obesity and diabetes in mice. Diabetes 57, 1470–1481.

Capecchi, B., Serruto, D., Adu-Bobie, J., Rappuoli, R., Pizza, M., 2004. The genome revolution in vaccine research. Curr. Issues Mol. Biol. 6, 17–27.

Carballido, J.M., Namikawa, R., Carballido-Perrig, N., Antonenko, S., Roncarolo, M.G., De Vries, J.E., et al., 2000. Generation of primary antigen-specific human T- and B-cell responses in immunocompetent SCID-hu mice. Nat. Med. 6, 103–106.

Caricilli, A.M., Picardi, P.K., De Abreu, L.L., Ueno, M., Prada, P.O., Ropelle, E.R., et al., 2011. Gut microbiota is a key modulator of insulin resistance in TLR 2 knockout mice. PLoS Biol. 9, e1001212.

Carpenter, C.B., 2000. Improving the success of organ transplantation. N. Engl. J. Med. 342, 647–648.

Carrico, J.A., Sabat, A.J., Friedrich, A.W., Ramirez, M., Markers, E.S.G.F.E., 2013. Bioinformatics in bacterial molecular epidemiology and public health: databases, tools and the next-generation sequencing revolution. Euro. Surveill. 18, 20382.

Carroll, D., 2011a. Genome engineering with zinc-finger nucleases. Genetics 188, 773–782.

Carroll, D., 2011b. Zinc-finger nucleases: a panoramic view. Curr. Gene Ther. 11, 2–10.

Clamp, M., Fry, B., Kamal, M., Xie, X., Cuff, J., Lin, M.F., et al., 2007. Distinguishing protein-coding and noncoding genes in the human genome. Proc. Natl. Acad. Sci. USA 104, 19428–19433.

Clarke, S.L., Vandermeer, J.E., Wenger, A.M., Schaar, B.T., Ahituv, N., Bejerano, G., 2012. Human developmental enhancers conserved between deuterostomes and protostomes. PLoS Genet. 8, e1002852.

Cohuet, A., Krishnakumar, S., Simard, F., Morlais, I., Koutsos, A., Fontenille, D., et al., 2008. SNP discovery and molecular evolution in Anopheles gambiae, with special emphasis on innate immune system. BMC Genomics 9, 227.

Collin, N., De Radigues, X., World Health Organization, H1n1 Vaccine Task Force, 2009. Vaccine production capacity for seasonal and pandemic (H1N1) 2009 influenza. Vaccine 27, 5184–5186.

Comroe, J.H., 1977. Man-Cans. (Conclusion). The body plethysmograph (body box). Am. Rev. Respir. Dis. 116, 1091–1099.

Comroe, J.H., Dripps, R.D., 1974. Ben Franklin and open heart surgery. Circ. Res. 35, 661–669.

Comroe, J.H., Dripps, R.D., 1976. Scientific basis for the support of biomedical science. Science 192, 105–111.

Cook, M.S., Blelloch, R., 2013. Small RNAs in germline development. Curr. Top. Dev. Biol. 102, 159–205.

Council on Scientific Affairs, 1989. Animals in research. JAMA 261, 3602–3606.

Cox, L.A., Comuzzie, A.G., Havill, L.M., Karere, G.M., Spradling, K.D., Mahaney, M.C., et al., 2013. Baboons as a model to study genetics and epigenetics of human disease. ILAR J. 54, 106–121.

Cryan, J.F., O'mahony, S.M., 2011. The microbiome–gut–brain axis: from bowel to behavior. Neurogastroenterol. Motil. 23, 187–192.

Dalby, P.A., 2007. Engineering enzymes for biocatalysis. Recent Pat. Biotechnol. 1, 1–9.

Datta, S.K., 2000. Positive selection for autoimmunity. Nat. Med. 6, 259–261.

Demel, M.A., Schwaha, R., Kramer, O., Ettmayer, P., Haaksma, E.E., Ecker, G.F., 2008. In silico prediction of substrate properties for ABC-multidrug transporters. Expert Opin. Drug Metab. Toxicol. 4, 1167–1180.

Desbonnet, L., Clarke, G., Shanahan, F., Dinan, T.G., Cryan, J.F., 2013. Microbiota is essential for social development in the mouse. Mol. Psychiatry.

Dickman, S., 1998. Antibodies stage a comeback in cancer treatment. Science 280, 1196–1197.

Dodds, W.J., Abelseth, M.K., 1980. Criteria for selecting the animal to meet the research need. Lab. Anim. Sci. 30, 460–465.

Dogini, D.B., Pascoal, V.D., Avansini, S.H., Vieira, A.S., Pereira, T.C., Lopes-Cendes, I., 2014. The new world of RNAs. Genet. Mol. Biol. 37, 285–293.

Dolinoy, D.C., Weidman, J.R., Waterland, R.A., Jirtle, R.L., 2006. Maternal genistein alters coat color and protects Avy mouse offspring from obesity by modifying the fetal epigenome. Environ. Health Perspect. 114, 567–572.

Doyle, E.L., Stoddard, B.L., Voytas, D.F., Bogdanove, A.J., 2013. TAL effectors: highly adaptable phytobacterial virulence factors and readily engineered DNA-targeting proteins. Trends Cell Biol. 23, 390–398.

Driever, W., Fishman, M.C., 1996. The zebrafish: heritable disorders in transparent embryos. J. Clin. Invest. 97, 1788–1794.

Duhl, D.M., Stevens, M.E., Vrieling, H., Saxon, P.J., Miller, M.W., Epstein, C.J., et al., 1994a. Pleiotropic effects of the mouse lethal yellow (Ay) mutation explained by deletion of a maternally expressed gene and the simultaneous production of agouti fusion RNAs. Development 120, 1695–1708.

Duhl, D.M., Vrieling, H., Miller, K.A., Wolff, G.L., Barsh, G.S., 1994b. Neomorphic agouti mutations in obese yellow mice. Nat. Genet. 8, 59–65.

Ecker, G.F., Stockner, T., Chiba, P., 2008. Computational models for prediction of interactions with ABC-transporters. Drug Discov. Today 13, 311–317.

Eijkman, C., 1965. Antineuritic Vitamin and Beri-Beri. Elsevier, Amsterdam, the Netherlands.

Ekiert, D.C., Bhabha, G., Elsliger, M.A., Friesen, R.H., Jongeneelen, M., Throsby, M., et al., 2009. Antibody recognition of a highly conserved influenza virus epitope. Science 324, 246–251.

Elbashir, S.M., Harborth, J., Lendeckel, W., Yalcin, A., Weber, K., Tuschl, T., 2001. Duplexes of 21-nucleotide RNAs mediate RNA interference in cultured mammalian cells. Nature 411, 494–498.

Enard, W., Przeworski, M., Fisher, S.E., Lai, C.S., Wiebe, V., Kitano, T., et al., 2002. Molecular evolution of FOXP2, a gene involved in speech and language. Nature 418, 869–872.

Ezzelarab, M.B., Zahorchak, A.F., Lu, L., Morelli, A.E., Chalasani, G., Demetris, A.J., et al., 2013. Regulatory dendritic cell infusion prolongs kidney allograft survival in nonhuman primates. Am. J. Transplant. 13, 1989–2005.

Flanagan, S.P., 1966. 'Nude,' a new hairless gene with pleiotropic effects in the mouse. Genet. Res. 8, 295–309.

Florence, S.L., Taub, H.B., Kaas, J.H., 1998. Large-scale sprouting of cortical connections after peripheral injury in adult macaque monkeys. Science 282, 1117–1121.

Fox, J.G., 2007. The Mouse in Biomedical Research. Academic Press, Amsterdam, the Netherlands; New York.

Frank, D., 2008. One world, one health, one medicine. Can. Vet. J. 49, 1063–1065.

Franke, A., Mcgovern, D.P., Barrett, J.C., Wang, K., Radford-Smith, G.L., Ahmad, T., et al., 2010. Genome-wide meta-analysis increases to 71 the number of confirmed Crohn's disease susceptibility loci. Nat. Genet. 42, 1118–1125.

Fremont-Rahl, J.J., Ge, Z., Umana, C., Whary, M.T., Taylor, N.S., Muthupalani, S., et al., 2013. An analysis of the role of the indigenous microbiota in cholesterol gallstone pathogenesis. PLoS One 8, e70657.

Fritz, J.V., Desai, M.S., Shah, P., Schneider, J.G., Wilmes, P., 2013. From meta-omics to causality: experimental models for human microbiome research. Microbiome 1, 1–14.

Fu, Y., Foden, J.A., Khayter, C., Maeder, M.L., Reyon, D., Joung, J.K., et al., 2013. High-frequency off-target mutagenesis induced by CRISPR-Cas nucleases in human cells. Nat. Biotechnol. 31, 822–826.

Fuchs, B., Braun, A., 2008. Modulation of asthma and allergy by addressing toll-like receptor 2. J. Occup. Med. Toxicol. 3 (Suppl. 1), S5.

Fuchs, B., Knothe, S., Rochlitzer, S., Nassimi, M., Greweling, M., Lauenstein, H.D., et al., 2010. A Toll-like receptor 2/6 agonist reduces allergic airway inflammation in chronic respiratory sensitisation to Timothy grass pollen antigens. Int. Arch. Allergy Immunol. 152, 131–139.

Fujimura, K.E., Demoor, T., Rauch, M., Faruqi, A.A., Jang, S., Johnson, C.C., et al., 2013. House dust exposure mediates gut microbiome Lactobacillus enrichment and airway immune defense against allergens and virus infection. Proc. Natl. Acad. Sci. 111 (2).

Gad, S.C., 2007. Animal Models in Toxicology. CRC Press, Boca Raton, FL.

Ganan, N., Gonzalez, R., Garde, J.J., Martinez, F., Vargas, A., Gomendio, M., et al., 2009. Assessment of semen quality, sperm cryopreservation and heterologous IVF in the critically endangered Iberian lynx (Lynx pardinus). Reprod. Fertil. Dev. 21, 848–859.

Garcia, F., Climent, N., Guardo, A.C., Gil, C., Leon, A., Autran, B., et al., 2013. A dendritic cell-based vaccine elicits T cell responses associated with control of HIV-1 replication. Sci. Transl. Med. 5 166ra2.

Garcia-Reyero, N., Perkins, E.J., 2011. Systems biology: leading the revolution in ecotoxicology. Environ Toxicol Chem 30, 265–273.

Gardner, M.J., Hall, N., Fung, E., White, O., Berriman, M., Hyman, R.W., et al., 2002. Genome sequence of the human malaria parasite Plasmodium falciparum. Nature 419, 498–511.

Garrett, W.S., Gordon, J.I., Glimcher, L.H., 2010. Homeostasis and inflammation in the intestine. Cell 140, 859–870.

Gerlai, R., 2002. Phenomics: fiction or the future? Trends Neurosci. 25, 506–509.

Gibbs, R.A., Weinstock, G.M., Metzker, M.L., Muzny, D.M., Sodergren, E.J., Scherer, S., et al., 2004. Genome sequence of the Brown Norway rat yields insights into mammalian evolution. Nature 428, 493–521.

Golob, E.K., Rishi, S., Becker, K.L., Moore, C., 1970. Streptozotocin diabetes in pregnant and nonpregnant rats. Metabolism 19, 1014–1019.

Goodman, D.G., Ward, J.M., Squire, R.A., Chu, K.C., Linhart, M.S., 1979. Neoplastic and nonneoplastic lesions in aging F344 rats. Toxicol. Appl. Pharmacol. 48, 237–248.

Goodrowe, K.L., Walker, S.L., Ryckman, D.P., Mastromonaco, G.F., Hay, M.A., Bateman, H.L., et al., 2000. Piecing together the puzzle of carnivore reproduction. Anim. Reprod. Sci. 60–61, 389–403.

Gordon, J.I., 2005. A genomic view of our symbiosis with members of the gut microbiota. J. Pediatr. Gastroenterol. Nutr. 40 (Suppl. 1), S28.

Gordon, J.W., 1997. Transgenic Animal Models of Disease. Harwood Academic Publishers, Amsterdam, the Netherlands.

Gordon, J.W., Ruddle, F.H., 1981. Integration and stable germ line transmission of genes injected into mouse pronuclei. Science 214, 1244–1246.

Greer, R.L., Morgun, A., Shulzhenko, N., 2013. Bridging immunity and lipid metabolism by gut microbiota. J. Allergy Clin. Immunol. 132, 253–262. quiz 263.

Grune, T., Sebela, M., 2013. Special issue on "protein modification." J. Proteomics 92, 1.

Gudsnuk, K., Champagne, F.A., 2012. Epigenetic influence of stress and the social environment. ILAR J. 53, 279–288.

Haffter, P., Nusslein-Volhard, C., 1996. Large scale genetics in a small vertebrate, the zebrafish. Int. J. Dev. Biol. 40, 221–227.

Hahn, Y., Jeong, S., Lee, B., 2007. Inactivation of MOXD2 and S100A15A by exon deletion during human evolution. Mol. Biol. Evol. 24, 2203–2212.

Haines, J.L., Hauser, M.A., Schmidt, S., Scott, W.K., Olson, L.M., Gallins, P., et al., 2005. Complement factor H variant increases the risk of age-related macular degeneration. Science 308, 419–421.

Hammad, H., Chieppa, M., Perros, F., Willart, M.A., Germain, R.N., Lambrecht, B.N., 2009. House dust mite allergen induces asthma via Toll-like receptor 4 triggering of airway structural cells. Nat. Med. 15, 410–416.

Hansen, C.H., Metzdorff, S.B., Hansen, A.K., 2013. Customizing laboratory mice by modifying gut microbiota and host immunity in an early "window of opportunity." Gut Microbes 4, 241–245.

Harris, M.A., Clark, J., Ireland, A., Lomax, J., Ashburner, M., Foulger, R., et al., 2004. The Gene Ontology (GO) database and informatics resource. Nucleic Acids Res. 32, D258–D261.

Hayashi, T., Raz, E., 2006. TLR9-based immunotherapy for allergic disease. Am. J. Med. 119, 897.e1–897.e6.

Hennig, W., 2004. The revolution of the biology of the genome. Cell Res. 14, 1–7.

Henson, J., Tischler, G., Ning, Z., 2012. Next-generation sequencing and large genome assemblies. Pharmacogenomics 13, 901–915.

Herweijer, H., Harding, C.O., Hagstrom, J.E., Wolff, J., 1997. Animal models in gene therapy. Harwood Academic Publishers, Amsterdam, the Netherlands.

Hidalgo, M., Bruckheimer, E., Rajeshkumar, N.V., Garrido-Laguna, I., De Oliveira, E., Rubio-Viqueira, B., et al., 2011. A pilot clinical study of treatment guided by personalized tumorgrafts in patients with advanced cancer. Mol. Cancer Ther. 10, 1311–1316.

Hilleman, M.R., 1998. Six decades of vaccine development—a personal history. Nat. Med. 4, 507–514.

Hindorff, L.A., Sethupathy, P., Junkins, H.A., Ramos, E.M., Mehta, J.P., Collins, F.S., et al., 2009. Potential etiologic and functional implications of genome-wide association loci for human diseases and traits. Proc. Natl. Acad. Sci. USA 106, 9362–9367.

Holt, R.A., Subramanian, G.M., Halpern, A., Sutton, G.G., Charlab, R., Nusskern, D.R., et al., 2002. The genome sequence of the malaria mosquito *Anopheles gambiae*. Science 298, 129–149.

Hommel, J.D., Sears, R.M., Georgescu, D., Simmons, D.L., Dileone, R.J., 2003. Local gene knockdown in the brain using viral-mediated RNA interference. Nat. Med. 9, 1539–1544.

Hooper, L.V., Midtvedt, T., Gordon, J.I., 2002. How host–microbial interactions shape the nutrient environment of the mammalian intestine. Annu. Rev. Nutr. 22, 283–307.

Howe, K., Clark, M.D., Torroja, C.F., Torrance, J., Berthelot, C., Muffato, M., et al., 2013. The zebrafish reference genome sequence and its relationship to the human genome. Nature 496, 498–503.

Hsiao, E.Y., Mcbride, S.W., Hsien, S., Sharon, G., Hyde, E.R., Mccue, T., et al., 2013. Microbiota modulate behavioral and physiological abnormalities associated with neurodevelopmental disorders. Cell 155, 1451–1463.

Huber, I., Masler, E.P., Rao, B.R., 1990. Cockroaches as Models for Neurobiology: Applications in Biomedical Research. CRC Press, Boca Raton, FL.

Human Microbiome Project Consortium, 2012. Structure, function and diversity of the healthy human microbiome. Nature 486, 207–214.

International Human Genome Sequencing Consortium, 2004. Finishing the euchromatic sequence of the human genome. Nature 431, 931–945.

Ishino, Y., Shinagawa, H., Makino, K., Amemura, M., Nakata, A., 1987. Nucleotide sequence of the iap gene, responsible for alkaline phosphatase isozyme conversion in Escherichia coli, and identification of the gene product. J. Bacteriol. 169, 5429–5433.

Jacob, F., Monod, J., 1961. Genetic regulatory mechanisms in the synthesis of proteins. J. Mol. Biol. 3, 318–356.

Jacobs, A.C., Hatfield, K.P., 2013. History of chronic toxicity and animal carcinogenicity studies for pharmaceuticals. Vet. Pathol. 50, 324–333.

Jardine, L., 1999. Ingenious Pursuits: Building the Scientific Revolution. Nan A. Talese Doubleday, New York.

Jasny, B., Koshland Jr, D.E., 1990. Biological Systems: Papers from Science, 1988–1989. American Association for the Advancement of Science, Washington, DC.

Jones, E.G., Pons, T.P., 1998. Thalamic and brainstem contributions to large-scale plasticity of primate somatosensory cortex. Science 282, 1121–1125.

Karlsson, F., Tremaroli, V., Nielsen, J., Backhed, F., 2013. Assessing the human gut microbiota in metabolic diseases. Diabetes 62, 3341–3349.

Kawamura, Y., Saito, K., Kin, T., Ono, Y., Asai, K., Sunohara, T., et al., 2008. Drosophila endogenous small RNAs bind to Argonaute 2 in somatic cells. Nature 453, 793–797.

Khan, M.J., Hosseini, A., Burrell, S., Rocco, S.M., Mcnamara, J.P., Loor, J.J., 2013. Change in subcutaneous adipose tissue metabolism and gene network expression during the transition period in dairy cows, including differences due to sire genetic merit. J. Dairy Sci. 96, 2171–2182.

Kim, D.S., Hahn, Y., 2012. Human-specific protein isoforms produced by novel splice sites in the human genome after the human–chimpanzee divergence. BMC Bioinformatics 13, 299.

Kim, H.L., Igawa, T., Kawashima, A., Satta, Y., Takahata, N., 2010. Divergence, demography and gene loss along the human lineage. Philos Trans. R. Soc. Lond. B Biol. Sci. 365, 2451–2457.

Kim, J.H., 2002. Bioinformatics and genomic medicine. Genet. Med. 4, 62S–65S.

Kim, M., Lee, K.H., Yoon, S.W., Kim, B.S., Chun, J., Yi, H., 2013. Analytical tools and databases for metagenomics in the next-generation sequencing era. Genomics Inform. 11, 102–113.

Kirk, A.D., Burkly, L.C., Batty, D.S., Baumgartner, R.E., Berning, J.D., Buchanan, K., et al., 1999. Treatment with humanized monoclonal antibody against CD154 prevents acute renal allograft rejection in nonhuman primates. Nat. Med. 5, 686–693.

Kitsios, G.D., Tangri, N., Castaldi, P.J., Ioannidis, J.P., 2010. Laboratory mouse models for the human genome-wide associations. PLoS One 5, e13782.

Kleppe, R., Kjarland, E., Selheim, F., 2006. Proteomic and computational methods in systems modeling of cellular signaling. Curr. Pharm. Biotechnol. 7, 135–145.

Knowles, D.G., Mclysaght, A., 2009. Recent de novo origin of human protein-coding genes. Genome Res. 19, 1752–1759.

Kornberg, A., Zimmerman, S.B., Kornberg, S.R., Josse, J., 1959. Enzymatic Synthesis of Deoxyribonucleic Acid. Influence of Bacteriophage T2 on the Synthetic Pathway in Host Cells. Proc. Natl. Acad. Sci. USA 45, 772–785.

Koscielny, G., Yaikhom, G., Iyer, V., Meehan, T.F., Morgan, H., Atienza-Herrero, J., 2014. The International Mouse Phenotyping Consortium Web Portal, a unified point of access for knockout mice and related phenotyping data. Nucleic Acids Res. 42, D802–D809.

Kostic, A.D., Howitt, M.R., Garrett, W.S., 2013. Exploring host–microbiota interactions in animal models and humans. Genes. Dev. 27, 701–718.

Kottke, B.A., Subbiah, M.T., 1978. Pathogenesis of atherosclerosis. Concepts based on animal models. Mayo Clin. Proc. 53, 35–48.

Koyuturk, M., 2010. Algorithmic and analytical methods in network biology. Wiley Interdiscip. Rev. Syst. Biol. Med. 2, 277–292.

Krause, J., Lalueza-Fox, C., Orlando, L., Enard, W., Green, R.E., Burbano, H.A., et al., 2007. The derived FOXP2 variant of modern humans was shared with Neandertals. Curr. Biol. 17, 1908–1912.

Kritchevsky, D., 1974. Laboratory models for atherosclerosis. Adv. Drug Res. 9, 41–53.

Kucharski, R., Maleszka, J., Foret, S., Maleszka, R., 2008. Nutritional control of reproductive status in honeybees via DNA methylation. Science 319, 1827–1830.

Kuhn, T.S., 1970. The Structure of Scientific Revolutions. University of Chicago Press, Chicago, IL.

Kwan, A.P., Dickson, I.R., Freemont, A.J., Grant, M.E., 1989. Comparative studies of type X collagen expression in normal and rachitic chicken epiphyseal cartilage. J. Cell Biol. 109, 1849–1856.

Laird, P.W., 2010. Principles and challenges of genomewide DNA methylation analysis. Nat. Rev. Genet. 11, 191–203.

Lander, E.S., 2011. Initial impact of the sequencing of the human genome. Nature 470, 187–197.

Landsteiner, K., 1945. Specificity of Serological Reactions. Dover, New York.

Landt, S.G., Marinov, G.K., Kundaje, A., Kheradpour, P., Pauli, F., Batzoglou, S., et al., 2012. ChIP-seq guidelines and practices of the ENCODE and modENCODE consortia. Genome Res. 22, 1813–1831.

Lawrence, H.S., 1959. Homograft sensitivity. An expression of the immunologic origins and consequences of individuality. Physiol. Rev. 39, 811–859.

Leader, R.W., Padgett, G.A., 1980. The genesis and validation of animal models. Am. J. Pathol. 101, 11–16.

Leader, R.W., Stark, D., 1987. The importance of animals in biomedical research. Perspect. Biol. Med. 30, 470–485.

Lederberg, J., Tatum, E.L., 1953. Sex in bacteria; genetic studies, 1945–1952. Science 118, 169–175.

Legrand, N., Ploss, A., Balling, R., Becker, P.D., Borsotti, C., Brezillon, N., et al., 2009. Humanized mice for modeling human infectious disease: challenges, progress, and outlook. Cell Host. Microbe. 6, 5–9.

Lemaitre, B., Nicolas, E., Michaut, L., Reichhart, J.M., Hoffmann, J.A., 1996. The dorsoventral regulatory gene cassette spatzle/Toll/cactus controls the potent antifungal response in Drosophila adults. Cell 86, 973–983.

Le Provost, F., Lillico, S., Passet, B., Young, R., Whitelaw, B., Vilotte, J.L., 2010. Zinc finger nuclease technology heralds a new era in mammalian transgenesis. Trends Biotechnol. 28, 134–141.

Lequarre, A.S., Andersson, L., Andre, C., Fredholm, M., Hitte, C., Leeb, T., et al., 2011. LUPA: a European initiative taking advantage of the canine genome architecture for unravelling complex disorders in both human and dogs. Vet. J. 189, 155–159.

Levenson, J.M., Sweatt, J.D., 2006. Epigenetic mechanisms: a common theme in vertebrate and invertebrate memory formation. Cell Mol. Life Sci. 63, 1009–1016.

Lewis, R.M., Schwartz, R.S., 1971. Canine systemic lupus erythematosus. Genetic analysis of an established breeding colony. J. Exp. Med. 134, 417–438.

Li-Pook-Than, J., Snyder, M., 2013. iPOP goes the world: integrated personalized Omics profiling and the road toward improved health care. Chem. Biol. 20, 660–666.

Li, E., 2002. Chromatin modification and epigenetic reprogramming in mammalian development. Nat. Rev. Genet. 3, 662–673.

Li, J., Wang, X., Zhang, G., Githure, J.I., Yan, G., James, A.A., 2013. Genome-block expression-assisted association studies discover malaria resistance genes in Anopheles gambiae. Proc. Natl. Acad. Sci. USA 110, 20675–20680.

Li, Y., Li, X.C., Zheng, X.X., Wells, A.D., Turka, L.A., Strom, T.B., 1999. Blocking both signal 1 and signal 2 of T-cell activation prevents apoptosis of alloreactive T cells and induction of peripheral allograft tolerance. Nat. Med. 5, 1298–1302.

Lieschke, G.J., Currie, P.D., 2007. Animal models of human disease: zebrafish swim into view. Nat. Rev. Genet. 8, 353–367.

Lindblad-Toh, K., Wade, C.M., Mikkelsen, T.S., Karlsson, E.K., Jaffe, D.B., Kamal, M., et al., 2005. Genome sequence, comparative analysis and haplotype structure of the domestic dog. Nature 438, 803–819.

Lister, R., Mukamel, E.A., Nery, J.R., Urich, M., Puddifoot, C.A., Johnson, N.D., et al., 2013. Global epigenomic reconfiguration during mammalian brain development. Science 341, 1237905.

Llinás, R.R., Ribary, U., Jeanmonod, D., Kronberg, E., Mitra, P.P., 1999. Thalamocortical dysrhythmia: a neurological and neuropsychiatric syndrome characterized by magnetoencephalography. Proc. Natl. Acad. Sci. USA 96, 15222–15227.

Lombard, M., Pastoret, P.P., Moulin, A.M., 2007. A brief history of vaccines and vaccination. Rev. Sci. Tech. 26, 29–48.

Lu, D., Willard, D., Patel, I.R., Kadwell, S., Overton, L., Kost, T., et al., 1994. Agouti protein is an antagonist of the melanocyte-stimulating-hormone receptor. Nature 371, 799–802.

Lu, W., Wu, X., Lu, Y., Guo, W., Andrieu, J.M., 2003. Therapeutic dendritic-cell vaccine for simian AIDS. Nat. Med. 9, 27–32.

Lutz, M.B., Suri, R.M., Niimi, M., Ogilvie, A.L., Kukutsch, N.A., Rossner, S., et al., 2000. Immature dendritic cells generated with low doses of GM-CSF in the absence of IL-4 are maturation resistant and prolong allograft survival in vivo. Eur. J. Immunol. 30, 1813–1822.

Luvoni, G.C., 2000. Current progress on assisted reproduction in dogs and cats: in vitro embryo production. Reprod. Nutr. Dev. 40, 505–512.

Lwoff, A., 1953. Lysogeny. Bacteriol. Rev. 17, 269–337.

Mach, H., Volkin, D.B., Troutman, R.D., Wang, B., Luo, Z., Jansen, K.U., et al., 2006. Disassembly and reassembly of yeast-derived recombinant human papillomavirus virus-like particles (HPV VLPs). J. Pharm. Sci. 95, 2195–2206.

Mahesh, Y., Rao, B.S., Suman, K., Lakshmikantan, U., Charan, K.V., Gibence, H.R., et al., 2011. In vitro maturation and fertilization in the Nilgai (Boselaphus tragocamelus) using oocytes and spermatozoa recovered post-mortem from animals that had died because of foot and mouth disease outbreak. Reprod. Domest. Anim. 46, 832–839.

Main, J.M., Prehn, R.T., 1955. Successful skin homografts after the administration of high dosage X radiation and homologous bone marrow. J. Natl. Cancer Inst. 15, 1023–1029.

Mak, L., Liggi, S., Tan, L., Kusonmano, K., Rollinger, J.M., Koutsoukas, A., et al., 2013. Anti-cancer drug development: computational strategies to identify and target proteins involved in cancer metabolism. Curr. Pharm. Des. 19, 532–577.

Maldonado, R.A., Von Andrian, U.H., 2010. How tolerogenic dendritic cells induce regulatory T cells. Adv. Immunol. 108, 111–165.

Mandrioli, M., 2004. Epigenetic tinkering and evolution: is there any continuity in the role of cytosine methylation from invertebrates to vertebrates? Cell Mol. Life Sci. 61, 2425–2427.

Marchioro, T.L., Axtell, H.K., Lavia, M.F., Waddell, W.R., Starzl, T.E., 1964. The role of adrenocortical steroids in reversing established homograft rejection. Surgery 55, 412–417.

Maricic, T., Gunther, V., Georgiev, O., Gehre, S., Curlin, M., Schreiweis, C., et al., 2013. A recent evolutionary change affects a regulatory element in the human FOXP2 gene. Mol. Biol. Evol. 30, 844–852.

Markowitz, L.E., Dunne, E.F., Saraiya, M., Lawson, H.W., Chesson, H., Unger, E.R., Centers For Disease, C., Prevention & Advisory Committee on Immunization, P., 2007. Quadrivalent human papillomavirus vaccine: recommendations of the Advisory Committee on Immunization Practices (ACIP). MMWR Recomm. Rep 56, 1–24.

Martin, G.R., 1981. Isolation of a pluripotent cell line from early mouse embryos cultured in medium conditioned by teratocarcinoma stem cells. Proc. Natl. Acad. Sci. USA 78, 7634–7638.

Masse, P., Vuilleumier, J.P., Weiser, H., 1989. Pyridoxine status as assessed by the concentration of B6-aldehyde vitamers. Int. J. Vitam. Nutr. Res. 59, 344–352.

Mathis, D., Benoist, C., 2012. The influence of the microbiota on type-1 diabetes: on the threshold of a leap forward in our understanding. Immunol. Rev. 245, 239–249.

Matsuoka, T., Hirata, M., Tanaka, H., Takahashi, Y., Murata, T., Kabashima, K., et al., 2000. Prostaglandin D2 as a mediator of allergic asthma. Science 287, 2013–2017.

Matsuya, A., Sakate, R., Kawahara, Y., Koyanagi, K.O., Sato, Y., Fujii, Y., et al., 2008. Evola: Ortholog database of all human genes in H-InvDB with manual curation of phylogenetic trees. Nucleic Acids Res. 36, D787–D792.

Mawdsley, J.E., Rampton, D.S., 2005. Psychological stress in IBD: new insights into pathogenic and therapeutic implications. Gut 54, 1481–1491.

Mccurdy, J.D., Lin, T.J., Marshall, J.S., 2001. Toll-like receptor 4-mediated activation of murine mast cells. J. Leukoc. Biol. 70, 977–984.

Means, L.W., Burnette, M.A., Pennington, S.N., 1988. The effect of embryonic ethanol exposure on detour learning in the chick. Alcohol 5, 305–308.

Merzenich, M., 1998. Long-term change of mind. Science 282, 1062–1063.

Meyer, L.R., Zweig, A.S., Hinrichs, A.S., Karolchik, D., Kuhn, R.M., Wong, M., et al., 2013. The UCSC Genome Browser database: extensions and updates 2013. Nucleic Acids Res. 41, D64–D69.

Michaud, E.J., Van Vugt, M.J., Bultman, S.J., Sweet, H.O., Davisson, M.T., Woychik, R.P., 1994. Differential expression of a new dominant agouti allele (Aiapy) is correlated with methylation state and is influenced by parental lineage. Genes Dev. 8, 1463–1472.

Michell, A.R., 2005. Comparative clinical science: the medicine of the future. Vet. J. 170, 153–162.

Mikkelsen, T.S., Wakefield, M.J., Aken, B., Amemiya, C.T., Chang, J.L., Duke, S., et al., 2007. Genome of the marsupial Monodelphis domestica reveals innovation in non-coding sequences. Nature 447, 167–177.

Mill, J.S., 1974. A System of Logic, Ratiocinative and Inductive Being a Connected View of the Principles of Evidence and the Methods of Scientific Investigation. Univ. of Toronto Press, Toronto, Canada.

Miller, J.F., 1961. Immunological function of the thymus. Lancet 2, 748–749.

Morgan, T.H., 1928. The Theory of the Gene. Yale Univ. Press, New Haven, CT.

Moscou, M.J., Bogdanove, A.J., 2009. A simple cipher governs DNA recognition by TAL effectors. Science 326, 1501.

Mosier, D.E., 1996. Small animal models for acquired immune deficiency syndrome (AIDS) research. Lab. Anim. Sci. 46, 257–265.

Mouse Genome Sequencing Consortium, 2002. Initial sequencing and comparative analysis of the mouse genome. Nature 420, 520–562.

Murray, J.E., 1992. Human organ transplantation: background and consequences. Science 256, 1411–1416.

Murray, J.E., Merrill, J.P., Harrison, J.H., Wilson, R.E., Dammin, G.J., 1963. Prolonged survival of human–kidney homografts by immunosuppressive drug therapy. N. Engl. J. Med. 268, 1315–1323.

Musunuru, K., Strong, A., Frank-Kamenetsky, M., Lee, N.E., Ahfeldt, T., Sachs, K.V., et al., 2010. From noncoding variant to phenotype via SORT1 at the 1p13 cholesterol locus. Nature 466, 714–719.

Nagy, A., Rossant, J., 1996. Targeted mutagenesis: analysis of phenotype without germ line transmission. J. Clin. Invest. 97, 1360–1365.

National Research Council, 1985. Models for Biomedical Research. National Academy Press, Washington, DC.

National Research Council, 1994. Laboratory Animal Management: Dogs. National Academy Press, Washington, DC.

National Research Council, 1998. Biomedical Models and Resources: Current Needs and Future Opportunities. National Academy Press, Washington, DC.

Nelson, K.E., 2013. Microbiomes. Microb Ecol 65, 916–919.

Nichol, K.L., Treanor, J.J., 2006. Vaccines for seasonal and pandemic influenza. J. Infect. Dis. 194 (Suppl. 2), S111–S118.

Niculescu, M.D., 2012. Nutritional epigenetics. ILAR J 53, 270–278.

Nigam, R., Laulederkind, S.J., Hayman, G.T., Smith, J.R., Wang, S.J., Lowry, T.F., et al., 2013. Rat genome database: a unique resource for rat, human, and mouse quantitative trait locus data. Physiol. Genomics 45, 809–816.

Nobrega, M.A., Pennacchio, L.A., 2004. Comparative genomic analysis as a tool for biological discovery. J. Physiol. 554, 31–39.

Norgren Jr., R.B., 2013. Improving genome assemblies and annotations for nonhuman primates. ILAR J. 54, 144–153.

Nusslein-Volhard, C., 1994. Of flies and fishes. Science 266, 572–574.

O'brien, M.A., Costin, B.N., Miles, M.F., 2012. Using genome-wide expression profiling to define gene networks relevant to the study of complex traits: from RNA integrity to network topology. Int. Rev. Neurobiol. 104, 91–133.

O'dell, B.L., Conley-Harrison, J., Browning, J.D., Besch-Williford, C., Hempe, J.M., Savage, J.E., 1990. Zinc deficiency and peripheral neuropathy in chicks. Proc. Soc. Exp. Biol. Med. 194, 1–4.

Office of Technology Assessment, 1986. Alternatives to Animal Use in Research, Testing, and Education.

Okamura, K., Lai, E.C., 2008. Endogenous small interfering RNAs in animals. Nat. Rev. Mol. Cell Biol. 9, 673–678.

Orlando, L., Ginolhac, A., Zhang, G., Froese, D., Albrechtsen, A., Stiller, M., et al., 2013. Recalibrating Equus evolution using the genome sequence of an early Middle Pleistocene horse. Nature 499, 74–78.

Ortho Multicenter Transplant Study Group, 1985. A randomized clinical trial of OKT3 monoclonal antibody for acute rejection of cadaveric renal transplants. N. Engl. J. Med. 313, 337–342.

Ownby, D.R., Johnson, C.C., Peterson, E.L., 2002. Exposure to dogs and cats in the first year of life and risk of allergic sensitization at 6 to 7 years of age. JAMA 288, 963–972.

Palker, T.J., Monteiro, J.M., Martin, M.M., Kakareka, C., Smith, J.F., Cook, J.C., et al., 2001. Antibody, cytokine and cytotoxic T lymphocyte responses in chimpanzees immunized with human papillomavirus virus-like particles. Vaccine 19, 3733–3743.

Palucka, K., Banchereau, J., 2013a. Dendritic-cell-based therapeutic cancer vaccines. Immunity 39, 38–48.

Palucka, K., Banchereau, J., 2013b. Human dendritic cell subsets in vaccination. Curr. Opin. Immunol. 25, 396–402.

Palucka, K., Coussens, L.M., O'shaughnessy, J., 2013. Dendritic cells, inflammation, and breast cancer. Cancer J. 19, 511–516.

Pan, Q., Shai, O., Lee, L.J., Frey, B.J., Blencowe, B.J., 2008. Deep surveying of alternative splicing complexity in the human transcriptome by high-throughput sequencing. Nat. Genet. 40, 1413–1415.

Park, F., 2007. Lentiviral vectors: are they the future of animal transgenesis? Physiol. Genomics 31, 159–173.

Patronov, A., Doytchinova, I., 2013. T-cell epitope vaccine design by immunoinformatics. Open Biol. 3, 120139.

Peiris, J.S., Poon, L.L., Guan, Y., 2009. Emergence of a novel swine-origin influenza A virus (S-OIV) H1N1 virus in humans. J. Clin. Virol. 45, 169–173.

Pennisi, E., 2013. The CRISPR craze. Science 341, 833–836.

Peterson, K.R., Navas, P.A., Stamatoyannopoulos, G., 1998. beta-YAC transgenic mice for studying LCR function. Ann. N. Y. Acad. Sci. 850, 28–37.

Peterson, Q.P., Hsu, D.C., Novotny, C.J., West, D.C., Kim, D., Schmit, J.M., et al., 2010. Discovery and canine preclinical assessment of a nontoxic procaspase-3-activating compound. Cancer Res. 70, 7232–7241.

Pflughoeft, K.J., Versalovic, J., 2012. Human microbiome in health and disease. Annu. Rev. Pathol. 7, 99–122.

Pluck, A., Klasen, C., 2009. Generation of chimeras by microinjection. Methods Mol. Biol. 561, 199–217.

Poincare, H., 1905. Science and Hypothesis. Walter Scott Publ. Co., London.

Poltorak, A., He, X., Smirnova, I., Liu, M.Y., Van Huffel, C., Du, X., et al., 1998a. Defective LPS signaling in C3H/HeJ and C57BL/10ScCr mice: mutations in Tlr4 gene. Science 282, 2085–2088.

Poltorak, A., Smirnova, I., He, X., Liu, M.Y., Van Huffel, C., Mcnally, O., et al., 1998b. Genetic and physical mapping of the Lps locus: identification of the toll-4 receptor as a candidate gene in the critical region. Blood Cells Mol. Dis. 24, 340–355.

Porcu, S., Kitamura, M., Witkowska, E., Zhang, Z., Mutero, A., Lin, C., et al., 1997. The human beta globin locus introduced by YAC transfer exhibits a specific and reproducible pattern of developmental regulation in transgenic mice. Blood 90, 4602–4609.

Pruitt, K.D., Tatusova, T., Klimke, W., Maglott, D.R., 2009. NCBI Reference Sequences: current status, policy and new initiatives. Nucleic Acids Res. 37, D32–D36.

Qian, S., Demetris, A.J., Murase, N., Rao, A.S., Fung, J.J., Starzl, T.E., 1994. Murine liver allograft transplantation: tolerance and donor cell chimerism. Hepatology 19, 916–924.

Quimby, F.W., 1994a. Armadillos to Zebra Fish: Animals in the Service of Medicine. Encyclopaedia Britannica, Chicago, IL.

Quimby, F.W., 1994b. Twenty-five years of progress in laboratory animal science. Lab. Anim. 28, 158–171.

Quimby, F.W., 1995. The role of attending veterinarians in laboratory animal welfare. J. Am. Vet. Med. Assoc. 206, 461–465.

Quimby, F.W., 1998. Benefits to veterinary medicine from animal research. Appl. Anim. Behav. Sci. 59, 183–192.

Quimby, F.W., Schwartz, R.S., 1980. Etiopathogenesis of Systemic Lupus Erythematosus. Raven Press, New York.

Quimby, F.W., Schwartz, R.S., Poskitt, T., Lewis, R.M., 1979. A disorder of dogs resembling Sjogren's syndrome. Clin. Immunol. Immunopathol. 12, 471–476.

Rainwater, D.L., Vandeberg, J.L., Mahaney, M.C., 2010. Effects of diet on genetic regulation of lipoprotein metabolism in baboons. Atherosclerosis 213, 499–504.

Reeks, J., Naismith, J.H., White, M.F., 2013. CRISPR interference: a structural perspective. Biochem. J. 453, 155–166.

Reich, D., Green, R.E., Kircher, M., Krause, J., Patterson, N., Durand, E.Y., et al., 2010. Genetic history of an archaic hominin group from Denisova Cave in Siberia. Nature 468, 1053–1060.

Reich, D., Patterson, N., Kircher, M., Delfin, F., Nandineni, M.R., Pugach, I., et al., 2011. Denisova admixture and the first modern human dispersals into Southeast Asia and Oceania. Am. J. Hum. Genet. 89, 516–528.

Reich, D.E., Lander, E.S., 2001. On the allelic spectrum of human disease. Trends Genet. 17, 502–510.

Rhee, S.H., Pothoulakis, C., Mayer, E.A., 2009. Principles and clinical implications of the brain–gut–enteric microbiota axis. Nat. Rev. Gastroenterol. Hepatol. 6, 306–314.

Rhesus Macaque Genome Sequencing and Analysis Consortium, 2007. Evolutionary and biomedical insights from the rhesus macaque genome. Science 316, 222–234.

Richardson, B.C., 2002. Role of DNA methylation in the regulation of cell function: autoimmunity, aging and cancer. J. Nutr. 132, 2401S–2405S.

Ridaura, V.K., Faith, J.J., Rey, F.E., Cheng, J., Duncan, A.E., Kau, A.L., et al., 2013. Gut microbiota from twins discordant for obesity modulate metabolism in mice. Science 341, 1241214-1–1241214-10.

Riehle, M.M., Markianos, K., Niare, O., Xu, J., Li, J., Toure, A.M., et al., 2006. Natural malaria infection in Anopheles gambiae is regulated by a single genomic control region. Science 312, 577–579.

Robert, J., Cohen, N., 2011. The genus Xenopus as a multispecies model for evolutionary and comparative immunobiology of the 21st century. Dev. Comp. Immunol. 35, 916–923.

Rodriguez, D., Gutierrez-De-Teran, H., 2013. Computational approaches for ligand discovery and design in class-A G protein-coupled receptors. Curr. Pharm. Des. 19, 2216–2236.

Rogers, J., 2013. In transition: primate genomics at a time of rapid change. ILAR J. 54, 224–233.

Roscioli, T., Kamsteeg, E.J., Buysse, K., Maystadt, I., Van Reeuwijk, J., Van Den Elzen, C., et al., 2012. Mutations in ISPD cause Walker–Warburg syndrome and defective glycosylation of alpha-dystroglycan. Nat. Genet. 44, 581–585.

Roths, J.B., Foxworth, W.B., Mcarthur, M.J., Montgomery, C.A., Kier, A.B., 1999. Spontaneous and engineered mutant mice as models for experimental and comparative pathology: history, comparison, and developmental technology. Lab. Anim. Sci. 49, 12–34.

Ruiz, P., Maldonado, P., Hidalgo, Y., Gleisner, A., Sauma, D., Silva, C., et al., 2013. Transplant tolerance: new insights and strategies for long-term allograft acceptance. Clin. Dev. Immunol. 2013, 210506.

Ryder, E., Gleeson, D., Sethi, D., Vyas, S., Miklejewska, E., Dalvi, P., et al., 2013. Molecular characterization of mutant mouse strains generated from the EUCOMM/KOMP-CSD ES cell resource. Mamm. Genome 24, 286–294.

Sanger, F., Air, G.M., Barrell, B.G., Brown, N.L., Coulson, A.R., Fiddes, C.A., et al., 1977. Nucleotide sequence of bacteriophage phi X174 DNA. Nature 265, 687–695.

Savva, A., Roger, T., 2013. Targeting toll-like receptors: promising therapeutic strategies for the management of sepsis-associated pathology and infectious diseases. Front. Immunol. 4, 387.

Sayegh, M.H., Turka, L.A., 1998. The role of T-cell costimulatory activation pathways in transplant rejection. N. Engl. J. Med. 338, 1813–1821.

Scarpelli, D.G., 1997. Animal Models of Disease: Utility and Limitations. Harwood Academic Publ, Amsterdam, the Netherlands.

Schiffman, M., 2007. Integration of human papillomavirus vaccination, cytology, and human papillomavirus testing. Cancer 111, 145–153.

Schiffman, M., Castle, P.E., Jeronimo, J., Rodriguez, A.C., Wacholder, S., 2007. Human papillomavirus and cervical cancer. Lancet 370, 890–907.

Schmitz, J.E., Kuroda, M.J., Santra, S., Sasseville, V.G., Simon, M.A., Lifton, M.A., et al., 1999. Control of viremia in simian immunodeficiency virus infection by CD8+ lymphocytes. Science 283, 857–860.

Schofield, P.N., Dubus, P., Klein, L., Moore, M., Mckerlie, C., Ward, J.M., et al., 2011. Pathology of the laboratory mouse: an International Workshop on Challenges for High Throuput Phenotyping. Toxicol. Pathol. 39, 559–562.

Schofield, P.N., Hoehndorf, R., Gkoutos, G.V., 2012. Mouse genetic and phenotypic resources for human genetics. Hum. Mutat. 33, 826–836.

Schrattenholz, A., Soskic, V., 2008. What does systems biology mean for drug development? Curr. Med. Chem. 15, 1520–1528.

Schwabe, R.F., Jobin, C., 2013. The microbiome and cancer. Nat. Rev. Cancer 13, 800–812.

Schwank, G., Koo, B.K., Sasselli, V., Dekkers, J.F., Heo, I., Demircan, T., et al., 2013. Functional repair of CFTR by CRISPR/Cas9 in intestinal stem cell organoids of cystic fibrosis patients. Cell Stem Cell 13, 653–658.

Schwartz, L., Brown, G.V., Genton, B., Moorthy, V.S., 2012. A review of malaria vaccine clinical projects based on the WHO rainbow table. Malar. J. 11, 11.

Schwartz, R.S., Dameshek, W., 1959. Drug-induced immunologic tolerance. Nature 183, 1682–1683.

Schwenk, F., Kuhn, R., Angrand, P.O., Rajewsky, K., Stewart, A.F., 1998. Temporally and spatially regulated somatic mutagenesis in mice. Nucleic Acids Res. 26, 1427–1432.

Sekaly, R.P., 2008. The failed HIV Merck vaccine study: a step back or a launching point for future vaccine development? J. Exp. Med. 205, 7–12.

Seo, S., Larkin, D.M., Loor, J.J., 2013. Cattle genomics and its implications for future nutritional strategies for dairy cattle. Animal 7 (Suppl. 1), 172–183.

Seok, J., Warren, H.S., Cuenca, A.G., Mindrinos, M.N., Baker, H.V., Xu, W., Inflammation & Host Response to Injury, Large Scale Collaborative Research Program, 2013. Genomic responses in mouse models poorly mimic human inflammatory diseases. Proc. Natl. Acad. Sci. USA 110, 3507–3512.

Seriously Ill for Medical Research (SIMR), 1998. Centenary Survey of Nobel Laureates in Physiology or Medicine. SIMR, Dunstable, United Kingdom.

Shapiro, K.J., 1998. Looking at animal models: both sides of the debate. Lab. Anim. 27, 26–29.

Shen, S., Pyo, C.W., Vu, Q., Wang, R., Geraghty, D.E., 2013. The essential detail: the genetics and genomics of the primate immune response. ILAR J. 54, 181–195.

Shi, L., Sings, H.L., Bryan, J.T., Wang, B., Wang, Y., Mach, H., et al., 2007. GARDASIL: prophylactic human papillomavirus vaccine development—from bench top to bed-side. Clin. Pharmacol. Ther. 81, 259–264.

Shublaq, N., Sansom, C., Coveney, P.V., 2013. Patient-specific modelling in drug design, development and selection including its role in clinical decision-making. Chem. Biol. Drug Des. 81, 5–12.

Siepel, A., Bejerano, G., Pedersen, J.S., Hinrichs, A.S., Hou, M., Rosenbloom, K., et al., 2005. Evolutionarily conserved elements in vertebrate, insect, worm, and yeast genomes. Genome Res. 15, 1034–1050.

Silvers, W.K., Elkins, W.L., Quimby, F.W., 1975. Cellular basis of tolerance in neonatally induced mouse chimeras. J. Exp. Med. 142, 1312–1315.

Silverstein, A.M., 1989. A History of Immunology. Academic Press, San Diego, CA.

Sindhu, A., Arora, P., Chaudhury, A., 2012. Illuminating the gateway of gene silencing: perspective of RNA interference technology in clinical therapeutics. Mol. Biotechnol. 51, 289–302.

Sisson, J.A., Plotz, E.J., 1967. Effect of alloxan diabetes on maternal and fetal serum lipids in the rabbit. Exp. Mol. Pathol. 6, 274–281.

Sourkes, T.L., 1966. Nobel Prize Winners in Medicine and Physiology 1901–1965. Abelard–Schuman, London.

Spicker, S.F., Alon, I., Devries, A., Engelhardt, H.T.T., 1988. The Use of Human Beings in Research. Kluwer Academic Publishers, Dordrecht, the Netherlands.

Starzl, T.E., Zinkernagel, R.M., 1998. Antigen localization and migration in immunity and tolerance. N. Engl. J. Med. 339, 1905–1913.

Starzl, T.E., Demetris, A.J., Trucco, M., Murase, N., Ricordi, C., Ildstad, S., et al., 1993. Cell migration and chimerism after whole-organ transplantation: the basis of graft acceptance. Hepatology 17, 1127–1152.

Steinman, R.M., Banchereau, J., 2007. Taking dendritic cells into medicine. Nature 449, 419–426.

Strode, G.K., 1951. Yellow Fever. McGraw-Hill, New York.

Sung, Y.H., Baek, I.J., Seong, J.K., Kim, J.S., Lee, H.W., 2012. Mouse genetics: catalogue and scissors. BMB Rep. 45, 686–692.

Sung, Y.H., Kim, J.M., Kim, H.T., Lee, J., Jeon, J., Jin, Y., et al., 2014. Highly efficient gene knockout in mice and zebrafish with RNA-guided endonucleases. Genome Res. 24, 125–131.

Swanson, W.F., 2012. Laparoscopic oviductal embryo transfer and artificial insemination in felids—challenges, strategies and successes. Reprod. Domest. Anim. 47 (Suppl 6), 136–140.

Swanson, W.F., Magarey, G.M., Herrick, J.R., 2007. Sperm cryopreservation in endangered felids: developing linkage of in situ–ex situ populations. Soc. Reprod. Fertil. Suppl. 65, 417–432.

Takahashi, J.S., Pinto, L.H., Vitaterna, M.H., 1994. Forward and reverse genetic approaches to behavior in the mouse. Science 264, 1724–1733.

Talbot, W.S., Trevarrow, B., Halpern, M.E., Melby, A.E., Farr, G., Postlethwait, J.H., et al., 1995. A homeobox gene essential for zebrafish notochord development. Nature 378, 150–157.

Tam, O.H., Aravin, A.A., Stein, P., Girard, A., Murchison, E.P., Cheloufi, S., et al., 2008. Pseudogene-derived small interfering RNAs regulate gene expression in mouse oocytes. Nature 453, 534–538.

Tang, T., Li, L., Tang, J., Li, Y., Lin, W.Y., Martin, F., et al., 2010. A mouse knockout library for secreted and transmembrane proteins. Nat. Biotechnol. 28, 749–755.

The Chimpanzee Sequencing And Analysis Consortium, 2005. Initial sequence of the chimpanzee genome and comparison with the human genome. Nature 437, 69–87.

The ENCODE Project Consortium, 2012. An integrated encyclopedia of DNA elements in the human genome. Nature 489, 57–74.

Templeton, N.S., Roberts, D.D., Safer, B., 1997. Efficient gene targeting in mouse embryonic stem cells. Gene Ther. 4, 700–709.

Teslovich, T.M., Musunuru, K., Smith, A.V., Edmondson, A.C., Stylianou, I.M., Koseki, M., et al., 2010. Biological, clinical and population relevance of 95 loci for blood lipids. Nature 466, 707–713.

Thucydides, 1934. The Peloponnesian War. Modern Library, New York.

Tian, Q., Price, N.D., Hood, L., 2012. Systems cancer medicine: towards realization of predictive, preventive, personalized and participatory (P4) medicine. J Intern Med 271, 111–121.

Turek-Plewa, J., Jagodzinski, P.P., 2005. The role of mammalian DNA methyltransferases in the regulation of gene expression. Cell Mol. Biol. Lett. 10, 631–647.

Turnbaugh, P.J., Ley, R.E., Mahowald, M.A., Magrini, V., Mardis, E.R., Gordon, J.I., 2006. An obesity-associated gut microbiome with increased capacity for energy harvest. Nature 444, 1027–1031.

Turnbaugh, P.J., Backhed, F., Fulton, L., Gordon, J.I., 2008. Diet-induced obesity is linked to marked but reversible alterations in the mouse distal gut microbiome. Cell Host. Microbe. 3, 213–223.

Turnbaugh, P.J., Hamady, M., Yatsunenko, T., Cantarel, B.L., Duncan, A., Ley, R.E., et al., 2009. A core gut microbiome in obese and lean twins. Nature 457, 480–484.

Turnquist, H.R., Raimondi, G., Zahorchak, A.F., Fischer, R.T., Wang, Z., Thomson, A.W., 2007. Rapamycin-conditioned dendritic cells are poor stimulators of allogeneic CD4+ T cells, but enrich for antigen-specific Foxp3+ T regulatory cells and promote organ transplant tolerance. J. Immunol. 178, 7018–7031.

Ukhanova, M., Culpepper, T., Baer, D., Gordon, D., Kanahori, S., Valentine, J., et al., 2012. Gut microbiota correlates with energy gain from dietary fibre and appears to be associated with acute and chronic intestinal diseases. Clin. Microbiol. Infect. 18 (Suppl 4), 62–66.

Utomo, A.R., Nikitin, A.Y., Lee, W.H., 1999. Temporal, spatial, and cell type-specific control of Cre-mediated DNA recombination in transgenic mice. Nat. Biotechnol. 17, 1091–1096.

Van Der Laan, J.W., Herberts, C., Lambkin-Williams, R., Boyers, A., Mann, A.J., Oxford, J., 2008. Animal models in influenza vaccine testing. Expert Rev. Vaccines 7, 783–793.

Van Der Neut, R., 1997. Targeted gene disruption: applications in neurobiology. J. Neurosci. Methods 71, 19–27.

Van Gelder, N.M., Belanger, F., 1988. Embryonic exposure to high taurine: a possible nutritional contribution to Friedreich's ataxia. J. Neurosci. Res. 20, 383–389.

Van Kooten, C., Gelderman, K.A., 2011. In vitro-generated DC with tolerogenic functions: perspectives for in vivo cellular therapy. Methods Mol. Biol. 677, 149–159.

Van Kooten, C., Lombardi, G., Gelderman, K.A., Sagoo, P., Buckland, M., Lechler, R., et al., 2011. Dendritic cells as a tool to induce transplantation tolerance: obstacles and opportunities. Transplantation 91, 2–7.

Varfolomeev, S.D., Uporov, I.V., Fedorov, E.V., 2002. Bioinformatics and molecular modeling in chemical enzymology. Active sites of hydrolases. Biochemistry (Mosc) 67, 1099–1108.

Venter, J.C., Remington, K., Heidelberg, J.F., Halpern, A.L., Rusch, D., Eisen, J.A., et al., 2004. Environmental genome shotgun sequencing of the Sargasso Sea. Science 304, 66–74.

Villa, L.L., Costa, R.L., Petta, C.A., Andrade, R.P., Ault, K.A., Giuliano, A.R., et al., 2005. Prophylactic quadrivalent human papillomavirus (types 6, 11, 16, and 18) L1 virus-like particle vaccine in young women: a randomised double-blind placebo-controlled multicentre phase II efficacy trial. Lancet Oncol. 6, 271–278.

Vinson, A., Curran, J.E., Johnson, M.P., Dyer, T.D., Moses, E.K., Blangero, J., et al., 2011. Genetical genomics of Th1 and Th2 immune response in a baboon model of atherosclerosis risk factors. Atherosclerosis 217, 387–394.

Vinson, A., Prongay, K., Ferguson, B., 2013. The value of extended pedigrees for next-generation analysis of complex disease in the rhesus macaque. ILAR J. 54, 91–105.

Visel, A., Zhu, Y., May, D., Afzal, V., Gong, E., Attanasio, C., et al., 2010. Targeted deletion of the 9p21 non-coding coronary artery disease risk interval in mice. Nature 464, 409–412.

Voight, B.F., Scott, L.J., Steinthorsdottir, V., Morris, A.P., Dina, C., Welch, R.P., et al., 2010. Twelve type 2 diabetes susceptibility loci identified through large-scale association analysis. Nat. Genet 42, 579–589.

Wagner, R.A., Tabibiazar, R., Liao, A., Quertermous, T., 2005. Genome-wide expression dynamics during mouse embryonic development reveal similarities to Drosophila development. Dev. Biol. 288, 595–611.

Wall, J.D., 2013. Great ape genomics. ILAR J. 54, 82–90.

Wall, J.D., Kim, S.K., Luca, F., Carbone, L., Mootnick, A.R., De Jong, P.J., et al., 2013. Incomplete lineage sorting is common in extant gibbon genera. PLoS One 8, e53682.

Wang, Z., Gerstein, M., Snyder, M., 2009. RNA-Seq: a revolutionary tool for transcriptomics. Nat. Rev. Genet. 10, 57–63.

Ward, J.M., Goodman, D.G., Squire, R.A., Chu, K.C., Linhart, M.S., 1979. Neoplastic and nonneoplastic lesions in aging (C57BL/6N x C3H/HeN)F1 (B6C3F1) mice. J. Natl. Cancer Inst. 63, 849–854.

Watson, J.D., Crick, F.H., 1953. Molecular structure of nucleic acids; a structure for deoxyribose nucleic acid. Nature 171, 737–738.

Webster, R.G., Bean, W.J., Gorman, O.T., Chambers, T.M., Kawaoka, Y., 1992. Evolution and ecology of influenza A viruses. Microbiol. Rev. 56, 152–179.

Wei, C., Liu, J., Yu, Z., Zhang, B., Gao, G., Jiao, R., 2013. TALEN or Cas9 – rapid, efficient and specific choices for genome modifications. J. Genet. Genomics 40, 281–289.

Wei, C.J., Boyington, J.C., Mctamney, P.M., Kong, W.P., Pearce, M.B., Xu, L., et al., 2010. Induction of broadly neutralizing H1N1 influenza antibodies by vaccination. Science 329, 1060–1064.

Weisse, A.B., 1991. Into the heart. Hosp. Pract. (Off Ed) 26, 149–152.

Wells, A.D., Li, X.C., Li, Y., Walsh, M.C., Zheng, X.X., Wu, Z., et al., 1999. Requirement for T-cell apoptosis in the induction of peripheral transplantation tolerance. Nat. Med. 5, 1303–1307.

White, J.K., Gerdin, A.K., Karp, N.A., Ryder, E., Buljan, M., Bussell, J.N., et al., 2013. Genome-wide generation and systematic phenotyping of knockout mice reveals new roles for many genes. Cell 154, 452–464.

Wiseman, R.W., Karl, J.A., Bohn, P.S., Nimityongskul, F.A., Starrett, G.J., O'Connor, D.H., 2013. Haplessly hoping: macaque major histocompatibility complex made easy. ILAR J. 54, 196–210.

Wolff, G.L., Kodell, R.L., Moore, S.R., Cooney, C.A., 1998. Maternal epigenetics and methyl supplements affect agouti gene expression in Avy/a mice. FASEB J. 12, 949–957.

Wondji, C.S., Morgan, J., Coetzee, M., Hunt, R.H., Steen, K., Black, W.C.T., et al., 2007. Mapping a quantitative trait locus (QTL) conferring pyrethroid resistance in the African malaria vector Anopheles funestus. BMC Genomics 8, 34.

Woodhead, A.D., 1989. Nonmammalian Animal Models for Biomedical Research. CRC Press, Boca Raton, FL.

Woodruff, M.F., Lennox, B., 1959. Reciprocal skin grafts in a pair of twins showing blood chimaerism. Lancet 2, 476–478.

Xu, X., Arnason, U., 1996. The mitochondrial DNA molecule of Sumatran orangutan and a molecular proposal for two (Bornean and Sumatran) species of orangutan. J. Mol. Evol. 43, 431–437.

Yang, H., Zhou, Y., Gu, J., Xie, S., Xu, Y., Zhu, G., et al., 2013. Deep mRNA sequencing analysis to capture the transcriptome landscape of zebrafish embryos and larvae. PLoS One 8, e64058.

Yen, M.R., Choi, J., Saier Jr., M.H., 2009. Bioinformatic analyses of transmembrane transport: novel software for deducing protein phylogeny, topology, and evolution. J Mol. Microbiol. Biotechnol. 17, 163–176.

Zaidi, A.K., Thangam, E.R., Ali, H., 2006. Distinct roles of Ca^{2+} mobilization and G protein usage on regulation of Toll-like receptor function in human and murine mast cells. Immunology 119, 412–420.

Zhang, L., Meissner, E., Chen, J., Su, L., 2010. Current humanized mouse models for studying human immunology and HIV-1 immuno-pathogenesis. Sci. China Life Sci. 53, 195–203.

Zhang, R., Zhang, C.T., 2006. The impact of comparative genomics on infectious disease research. Microbes Infect. 8, 1613–1622.

Zhao, X.M., Chen, L., Aihara, K., 2008. Protein function prediction with high-throughput data. Amino Acids 35, 517–530.

Zinkernagel, R.M., Doherty, P.C., 1997. The discovery of MHC restriction. Immunol. Today 18, 14–17.

35

Research in Laboratory Animal and Comparative Medicine

J. Mark Cline, DVM, PhD, DACVP and
Thomas B. Clarkson, DVM, DACLAM

Pathology/Comparative Medicine, Wake Forest School of Medicine, Winston-Salem, NC, USA

OUTLINE

I. INTRODUCTION

The importance of the research component of programs in laboratory animal and comparative medicine (CM) has been discussed actively for more than half a century (Clarkson, 1961a, b). At no time, however, have the discussions been more timely or of greater importance to how laboratory animal medicine (LAM) will interface with academic medicine in the future. Programs in laboratory animal and CM are at a major crossroad in their evolution with some uncertainty about whether they will become increasingly regulatory/service oriented or whether balance will be maintained between the service aspects and the traditional commitments of teaching and research. In this chapter we emphasize the importance of the research component as necessary for the LAM specialist to be viewed as a fellow scientist rather than support staff, and to provide a continuing scientific basis to the field.

The most productive research approaches in laboratory animal and CM have been those in which the individuals have capitalized on their clinical backgrounds and combined that skill with investigative skills in developing research directions. For convenience, those research activities can be divided into two main categories: those studies involving diseases of the common laboratory animals and their well-being we refer to as laboratory animal research, and those involving the animal models of human disease as CM research.

LAM and CM are integral to the success of biomedical research. Our profession contributes to all aspects of the field, from basic studies of molecular pathogenesis to clinical practice, population medicine, and epidemiology (Fig. 35.1). These aspects overlap to form a 'translational continuum' in which research and clinical practice each inform the other. The LAM specialist has a duty to participate in disease discovery and model characterization,

Laboratory Animal Medicine, Third Edition
DOI: http://dx.doi.org/10.1016/B978-0-12-409527-4.00035-3

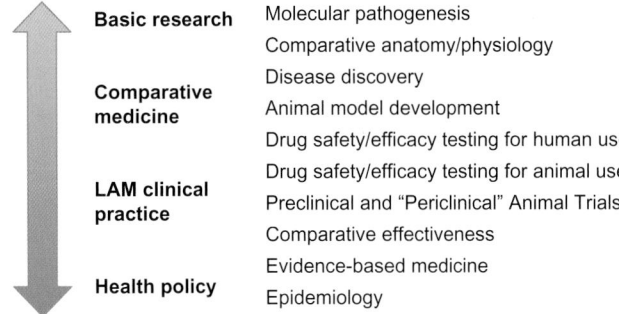

Basic research	Molecular pathogenesis
	Comparative anatomy/physiology
Comparative medicine	Disease discovery
	Animal model development
	Drug safety/efficacy testing for human use
LAM clinical practice	Drug safety/efficacy testing for animal use
	Preclinical and "Periclinical" Animal Trials
	Comparative effectiveness
	Evidence-based medicine
Health policy	Epidemiology

FIGURE 35.1　The translational research continuum.

to disseminate knowledge of normal species biology, and to prevent misinterpretation of research findings. A clinician–scientist mentality is uniquely valuable, and conversely, it is folly to separate clinical laboratory animal medicine from the context of the research. A collaborative approach not only facilitates the proper interpretation of research findings, but also enables the use of research data to inform clinical care. In this regard, communication across disciplines is critical. In particular, publication of clinical observations and research findings is essential to this approach and to the practice of evidence-based medicine. Strategic specialization and demonstration of expertise is accomplished by publication, providing the individual LAM practitioner with a competitive advantage in the job market. Finally, the LAM specialist is often expected to be competent in interpreting and assessing the value of research for those outside the field; integration into the research process enables more effective and credible communication and advocacy with colleagues, administration, and the public.

II. PRINCIPLES OF EXPERIMENTATION

A. Descriptive Studies

Most scientists think of research as being hypothesis-driven. However, the importance to biomedical research and laboratory animal medicine of descriptive studies, clinical case reports, and case series reports cannot be overstated. In working with the 30+ commonly used laboratory animal species, and the hundreds of strains and genetic modifications of mice and rats, it would be the height of hubris to imagine that all of the relevant physiologic characteristics and disease states are known. The evidence points toward the opposite conclusion; that there is much remaining to be discovered about even 'well-known' species. For example, mitochondrial DNA sequencing of rhesus and cynomolgus macaques has revealed a surprising degree of geographic variability in gene sequence in which "Approximately equal amounts of genetic diversity are due to differences

among animals in the same regional population, different regional populations, and different species" (Smith et al., 2007). This intraspecies genetic variability exceeds that of human beings, and for cynomolgus monkeys specifically the intraspecies variability is even more striking (Kanthaswamy et al., 2013). Similarly, recent large-scale transcriptomic studies of mice have uncovered both conserved and divergent patterns of inflammatory responses when compared to human beings (Shay et al., 2013). Depending on the analytic approach to the data, one may uncover differences (Seok et al., 2013) or similarities (Takao and Miyakawa, 2014). These observations indicate that at the most fundamental level we still have much to learn about the best use of animals in research. A deep understanding of species and strain differences is needed, as well as a mechanistically sound approach to the experimental question at hand. The recent explosion of publicly available animal and human gene expression datasets such as the Gene Expression Omnibus (http://www.ncbi.nlm.nih.gov/geo/) (Barrett et al., 2006) has created boundless opportunities for discovery and hypothesis generation; however, most of these data are not yet rooted in phenotypic data or clinical outcomes. These genetic data bring to the field a golden opportunity, and also a scientific and ethical obligation to the LAM clinician scientist, to publish everyday clinical observations, to move anecdotal information into the realm of peer-reviewed data, and to practice evidence-based medicine.

As our understanding of molecular mechanisms of disease grows, the variety and subtlety of potential effects require current scientific fluency. Influences on disease susceptibility and experimental outcomes now include epigenetic imprinting of behavioral characteristics by early life experience of individual animals (Szyf, 2013), and post-transcriptional regulation of gene expression by microRNAs (Gurtan and Sharp, 2013). Future discoveries will continue to push the field toward convergence of clinical and basic knowledge, and deeper understanding of gene–environment interactions.

Disease discovery in laboratory animals continues daily; for example, over a few short years, the putative cause of chronic interstitial pneumonia in rats has progressed from 'unknown' to 'rat respiratory virus' to *Pneumocystis carinii* (Livingston et al., 2011). This type of ongoing intellectual ferment and examination of evidence is necessary to prevent the ossification of anecdotal 'common knowledge' into erroneous dogma.

B. Hypothesis-Driven Research

As in all biomedical research disciplines, the process of discovery in LAM/CM, research follows a cycle. The research cycle (Fig. 35.2) begins with a concept or early hypothesis, which is first explored by a literature review. The literature review allows the investigator

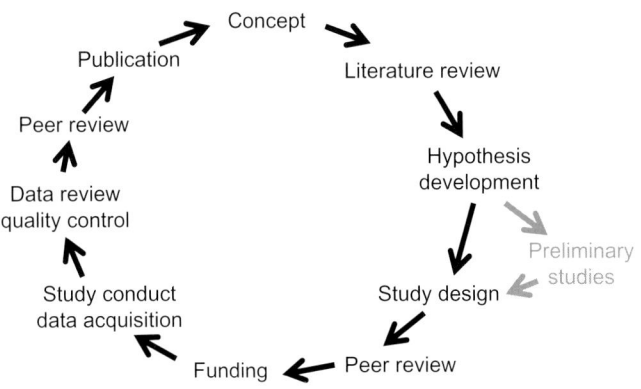

FIGURE 35.2   The research cycle.

first to discover whether his or her research question has already been answered, and second, to refine their concept into a relevant and testable hypothesis in the context of current knowledge. The importance of finding and reading the original peer-reviewed scientific literature cannot be overemphasized; reliance on review articles or web resources leads to misinterpretation. The hypothesis is then developed further through discussions with colleagues and advice from experts in the field. If the nature of the research question is very novel, critical data may be lacking. In this case, preliminary studies may be required in order to determine the feasibility of the work and to generate data that can be used for estimates of statistical power and to minimize numbers of subsequent experimental subjects. Design of a more definitive study proceeds from this process. The study design is best produced by creation of a draft for informal review by colleagues, which often produces surprising and useful changes in the plan. The study design should include considerations of sample size, statistical power, blinding of observations, and plans for data management and contingencies requiring changes in the plan (Landis *et al.*, 2012).

The next step in carrying out the research plan is external peer review, which typically occurs as part of the search for funding. The peer review process conducted by the National Institutes of Health provides the most common model, consisting of (1) receipt of the application; (2) assignment to the most appropriate categorical institute and study section for peer review; (3) anonymous peer review by one to three study section members who are recognized experts in the field; (4) discussion by all members of the study section group; (5) priority scoring by the study section; (6) preliminary feedback to the applicant; (7) secondary review by an expert council for subject matter balance across the portfolio of research projects funded by the institute; and (8) if successful, a notice of grant award.

The execution of the research plan is the next step, which in the case of animal work requires pre-study

institutional animal care and use committee (IACUC) approval, discussed in detail in Chapter 2. This process requires a third phase of peer review, in addition to the preparatory and funding-related review steps, and often helps to illuminate practical and ethical considerations, as well as providing an additional formalized literature review which may further refine the plan. Conduct of studies under the guiding principles of replacement, reduction, and refinement (Russell and Burch, 1959) have the advantage not only of minimizing unnecessary animal use, but of promoting parsimonious study design.

Conduct of a research project requires careful planning and quality control. A widely applied standard for quality assurance in laboratory work involving animals is that of *Good Laboratory Practices* (GLP) (Code of Federal Regulations 21:1:58, 2013). Most study designs do not fit the GLP model, which was designed as a highly formalized and structured mechanism to guide the conduct of drug approval and chemical safety studies for approval by the Food and Drug Administration, in the context of work done by contract research organizations. Nonetheless, much can be gained by adopting elements of GLP practice; the use of standard operating procedures, and documentation of all study activities and any changes in the study plan are essential to success. Flexibility is also required, and a willingness to believe one's own data. Unexpected consequences are part of the experimental process; to quote Isaac Asimov, "The most exciting phrase to hear in science, the one that heralds new discoveries, is not 'Eureka' but 'That's funny….' " Thus, documentation and recognition of both clearly relevant and possibly irrelevant events is critical. The importance of a given finding may not be recognized until years after the original observation.

Publication of expected and unexpected research findings is essential. Unpublished work cannot be critically peer-reviewed or referred to by one's colleagues, and essentially 'did not happen' as far as the scientific community is concerned. The anonymous peer review process provided by biomedical journals is a final quality-control check before the public dissemination of data, and should be a welcome part of the process. Negative findings should also be published; although there is an understandable bias in the scientific literature toward publication of expected findings (Tsilidis *et al.*, 2013), the advancement of biomedical knowledge is not served by withholding disappointing information.

III. ROLE OF THE LABORATORY ANIMAL SPECIALIST IN RESEARCH

The majority of American College of Laboratory Animal Medicine (ACLAM) diplomates working in the

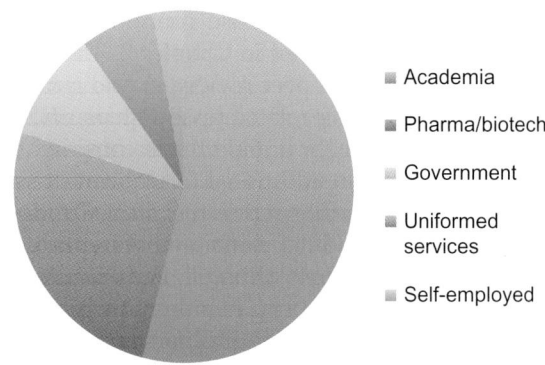

FIGURE 35.3   Employment of ACLAM diplomates.

TABLE 35.1   Experimental Outcomes in Drug Development

Phase	Experimental outcomes
Early development	Mechanism of action Biodistribution Pharmacokinetics
Preclinical animal testing	Safety – acute and chronic toxicity – dose limiting organ toxicity – maximum tolerated dose – no adverse effect level – class-specific effects (e.g., endocrine disruptor effects) Efficacy – biomarker validation – definitive tissue or disease outcomes
Post-approval	Effects of long-term exposure Population-specific effects Identification of secondary/novel mechanisms Exploration of adverse events

field (54%) are employed in academia, with fewer (26%) in industry, 10% in non-military government positions, and 7% in the uniformed services; the remaining 3% are self-employed (ACLAM, 2013; Fig. 35.3). Accordingly, this chapter focuses primarily on academic and industrial research, although the principles discussed apply to all.

In the competitive environment of biomedical research, the most successful investigators form multidisciplinary teams. In the academic medical or veterinary school environment, opportunities abound for collaborative research. The ability to work peacefully and productively with diverse teams is essential. LAM specialists often serve as clinician–scientist collaborators or veterinary consultants as members of a research team, but should not shy away from the role of principal investigator. The increasing emphasis on translational research approaches in recent years makes a comparative perspective uniquely valuable and competitive for funding.

In all research roles the LAM investigator should be cognizant not only of the unique expertise and perspective they bring to the field, but also of the limitations of their expertise. For example, although most LAM investigators are familiar with biostatistics, power calculations, and the use of informatics tools, the expertise of a biostatistician is almost always required in order to plan and interpret high quality research. Similarly, consultation with a pathologist is necessary when tissue evaluations are needed; the perils of 'do it yourself pathology' are myriad, and include such embarrassing consequences as the identification of normal structures as neoplasms (Cardiff et al., 2008; Ince et al., 2008). Diagnostic services of clinical pathology and anatomic pathology support for LAM/CM research are increasingly outsourced, which discourages exploratory work. Decision-making in this regard should not be made solely on the basis of cost. On-site expertise is essential to a healthy research environment.

In the industrial/pharmaceutical setting the focus of research is generally product development for human use. Thus familiarity with the drug approval standards and procedures required by the Food and Drug Administration have become an essential part of the LAM investigator's skill set. In contrast to most hypothesis-driven research, familiarity with GLP standards (Code of Federal Regulations, 1978; WHO, 2009) is often required in this setting. Research opportunities typically fall into three phases, relating to the life cycle of drugs and devices: (1) early development, which is exploratory and provides preliminary evidence of usefulness; (2) preclinical new drug/device testing in preparation for regulatory approval, which provides definitive evidence in a highly structured and regulated context; and (3) post-approval studies conducted after the drug or device is on the market. In each of these phases studies may address mechanism of action, efficacy, safety, or all three (Table 35.1). Publications of product-related findings made in the context of this development path are intensely scrutinized during the regulatory approval phase. However, publication of clinical findings benefits both the field and the sponsor. Furthermore, publications of 'background' findings in control, untreated animals are possible, and provide invaluable data for the placement of experimental findings in the context of the natural disease spectrum or what would otherwise be considered within normal variation for the species, strain, or phenotype.

An additional requirement for research expertise with particular relevance for governmental and regulatory veterinarians is the need to ground policy decisions in mechanistic understanding. This need is highlighted by the FDA Animal Rule (Code of Federal Regulations, 2002; 2012) for approval of new drugs or biological products "when human efficacy studies are neither ethical

TABLE 35.2　Opportunities, Needs, and Strategies for Training in LAM/CM Research

Career stage	Needs	Typical mechanism for support
Undergraduate	Basic understanding of laboratory animal medicine and research	Didactic training in selected institutions with LAM training programs (e.g., NCA&T) *Ad hoc* fellowships, employment, or volunteer work in research laboratories
DVM	Understanding of laboratory animal medicine and research at the professional level Practical experience in the conduct of research	Didactic veterinary training Short-term research fellowships (e.g., NIH T35 programs) Combined DVM/PhD programs
Post-DVM (primarily research)	Advanced training in: 　Translational research strategies 　Biostatistics 　Disease pathophysiology 　Graduate degree qualifications (MS or PhD) 　Development of grant-writing skills 　IACUC training	Research fellowships (e.g., NIH T32 programs)
Post-DVM (primarily clinical)	LAM clinical residency training Publication for board eligibility Development of collaborative research skills IACUC training	LAM residency including structured research training
Junior faculty	Transition from training to independent research in an academic setting IACUC experience	NIH K01, K08, K99 mechanisms
Junior LAM researcher, non-academic	Understanding of project-oriented procedures for clinical care and data collection IACUC experience	Employer-provided training
Mid-career faculty	Updated understanding of developments in LAM/CM research Development of mentorship and leadership skills	K26 Mid-career Award in Mouse Pathobiology Research Sponsored sabbatical Continuing education through courses and workshops

nor feasible," including treatments to prevent or mitigate lethal or permanently disabling injury caused by chemical, biological, radiological, or nuclear agents. Application of this standard requires that:

1. There is a reasonably well-understood pathophysiological mechanism of the toxicity of the (chemical, biological, radiological, or nuclear) substance and its prevention or substantial reduction by the product;
2. The effect is demonstrated in more than one animal species expected to react with a response predictive for human beings, unless the effect is demonstrated in a single animal species that represents a sufficiently well-characterized animal model for predicting the response in human subjects;
3. The animal study endpoint is clearly related to the desired benefit for human patients, generally the enhancement of survival or prevention of major morbidity; and
4. The data or information on the pharmacokinetics and pharmacodynamics of the product or other relevant data or information, in animals and human beings, allows selection of an effective dose in human beings (Code of Federal Regulations, 2002, 2013).

Clearly, any work meeting these standards requires in-depth comparative knowledge of species biology and pathophysiology, and a translational approach to human–animal comparisons.

IV. RESEARCH TRAINING

Research training is a required part of residency training for LAM residents. Such training should, at a minimum, provide research experience sufficient to (1) give LAM residents a working knowledge of how biomedical research operates and thereby 'demystify' the research and publication process; (2) familiarize LAM residents with specific research projects and the research culture; and (3) provide research opportunities and mentorship for writing a first-author research paper, in order to meet the publication requirement for board certification by the ACLAM.

Elements of training should include:

1. Identification of a research mentor, with mutual commitment of time for regular (e.g., weekly) research strategy meetings.
2. Protected 'off call' time for research.

3. 'Embedding' of the resident within a home laboratory to allow active participation in research laboratory meetings, project planning, data analysis, and interpretation.
4. Development of a specific single research project.
5. Creation of a research advisory committee.
6. Structured training in the 'survival skills' needed for a future in biomedical research, including:
   * Scientific writing
   * The publication process
   * Research ethics
   * IACUC/Use of animals
   * Biostatistics
   * The NIH grant review process
   * Opportunities for graduate work

Other research training opportunities abound in the field of LAM/CM, in no small measure due to the natural proximity of the field to biomedical research of many types. Structured training in LAM/CM research is advisable for individuals at all career stages, from exploratory short-term experiences for students, to mid-career awards designed to allow freedom from clinical duties for exploration of research training. Typical training needs and mechanisms for different career stages are summarized in Table 35.2, as well as federally funded opportunities to support training activities. Because specific funding mechanisms change over time, it is also important to develop a familiarity with the process of identifying new opportunities.

V. SUMMARY

Research in Comparative Medicine and Laboratory Animal Medicine is a core element of training in LAM (ACLAM, 2013), and is critical to the continued relevance of the profession in biomedical research. A scholarly approach to clinical care, and active participation in collaborative research, are strategies which can be implemented in most academic, industrial, or governmental settings. Opportunities for research training and collaboration are available. The LAM profession has an ethical obligation to prevent the misinterpretation of study findings, and much to contribute to the understanding of spontaneous animal diseases and the implications of biomedical research for translation to human disease.

Acknowledgment

ACLAM demographics courtesy of Dr. Mel Balk.

References

ACLAM 2013. Role Delineation Document. <http://www.aclam.org/Content/files/files/Public/Active/Role_Delineation_Document-2013-08.pdf>.

Barrett, T., Edgar, R., 2006. Gene expression omnibus: microarray data storage, submission, retrieval, and analysis. Methods Enzymol. 411, 352–369. PubMed PMID: 16939800.

Cardiff, R.D., Ward, J.M., Barthold, S.W., 2008 Jann. "One medicine—one pathology": are veterinary and human pathology prepared? Lab Invest. 88 (1), 18–26. PubMed PMID: 18040269.

Clarkson, T.B., 1961a. Laboratory animal medicine and the medical schools. J. Med. Educ. 36, 1329–1330.

Clarkson, T.B., 1961b. Graduate and professional training in laboratory animal medicine. Fed. Proc. 20, 915–916.

Code of Federal Regulations Title 21 Part 58, revised April 2013. <http://www.accessdata.fda.gov/scripts/cdrh/cfdocs/cfcfr/CFRSearch.cfm?CFRPart=58>.

Code of Federal Regulations, Title 21, Chapter 1, Volume 5, Part 314, Section 610. Final Rule, May 23, 2002; Revised April 1, 2013. <http://www.accessdata.fda.gov/scripts/cdrh/cfdocs/cfcfr/cfrsearch.cfm?cfrpart=314&showfr=1&subpartnode=21:5.0.1.1.4.9>.

Gurtan, A.M., Sharp, P.A., 2013 Oct 9. The role of miRNAs in regulating gene expression networks. J. Mol. Biol. 425 (19), 3582–3600. http://dx.doi.org/10.1016/j.jmb.2013.03.007. Epub 2013 Mar 13. Review. PubMed PMID: 23500488; PubMed Central PMCID: PMC3757117.

Ince, T.A., Ward, J.M., Valli, V.E., Sgroi, D., Nikitin, A.Y., Loda, M., et al., 2008 Sepp. Do-it-yourself (DIY) pathology. Nat. Biotechnol. 26 (9), 978–979. discussion 979. http://dx.doi.org/10.1038/nbt0908-978. PubMed PMID: 18779800.

Kanthaswamy, S., Ng, J., Satkoski Trask, J., George, D.A., Kou, A.J., Hoffman, L.N., et al., 2013 Junn. The genetic composition of populations of cynomolgus macaques (Macaca fascicularis) used in biomedical research. J. Med. Primatol. 42 (3), 120–131. PMID: 23480663; PubMed Central PMCID: PMC3651788.

Landis, S.C., Amara, S.G., Asadullah, K., Austin, C.P., Blumenstein, R., Bradley, E.W., et al., 2012 October 11. A call for transparent reporting to optimize the predictive value of preclinical research. Nature 490 (7419), 187–191. PubMed PMID: 23060188; PubMed Central PMCID: PMC3511845.

Livingston, R.S., Besch-Williford, C.L., Myles, M.H., Franklin, C.L., Crim, M.J., Riley, L.K., 2011 February. Pneumocystis carinii infection causes lung lesions historically attributed to rat respiratory virus. Comp. Med. 61 (1), 45–59. PubMed PMID: 21819681; PubMed Central PMCID: PMC3060427.

Russell, W.M.S., Burch, R.L., 1959. The Principles of Humane Experimental Technique. Methuen, London, UK, pp. xiv + 238. <http://altweb.jhsph.edu/pubs/books/humane_exp/het-toc>.

Seok, J., Warren, H.S., Cuenca, A.G., Mindrinos, M.N., Baker, H.V., Xu, W., Inflammation and Host Response to Injury, Large Scale Collaborative Research Program, 2013 Feb 26. Genomic responses in mouse models poorly mimic human inflammatory diseases. Proc. Natl. Acad. Sci. USA 110 (9), 3507–3512. PubMed PMID: 23401516; PubMed Central PMCID: PMC3587220.

Shay, T., Jojic, V., Zuk, O., Rothamel, K., Puyraimond-Zemmour, D., Feng, T., et al., 2013 February 19. ImmGen Consortium. Conservation and divergence in the transcriptional programs of the human and mouse immune systems. Proc. Natl. Acad. Sci. USA 110 (8), 2946–2951. http://dx.doi.org/10.1073/pnas.1222738110. PubMed PMID: 23382184; PubMed Central PMCID: PMC3581886.

Smith, D.G., McDonough, J.W., George, D.A., 2007 Febb. Mitochondrial DNA variation within and among regional populations of longtail macaques (Macaca fascicularis) in relation to other species of the fascicularis group of macaques. Am. J. Primatol. 69 (2), 182–198. PubMed PMID: 17177314.

Szyf, M., 2013 Jul 20. DNA methylation, behavior and early life adversity. J. Genet. Genomics 40 (7), 331–338. http://dx.doi.org/10.1016/j.jgg.2013.06.004. Epub 2013 Jun 25. PMID: 23876773.

Takao, K., Miyakawa, T., 2014 August 4. Genomic responses in mouse models greatly mimic human inflammatory diseases. Proc. Natl. Acad. Sci. USA pii: 201401965. [Epub ahead of print] PMID: 25092317.

Tsilidis, K.K., Panagiotou, O.A., Sena, E.S., Aretouli, E., Evangelou, E., Howells, D.W., et al., 2013 July. Evaluation of excess significance bias in animal studies of neurological diseases. PLoS Biol. 11 (7), e1001609. PubMed PMID: 23874156; PubMed Central PMCID: PMC3712913.

World Health Organization on behalf of the Special Programme for Research and Training in Tropical Diseases. Handbook: Good laboratory practice (GLP): quality practices for regulated non-clinical research and development. 2nd ed. Accessed at <http://www.who.int/tdr/publications/documents/glp-handbook.pdf>.

36

Design and Management of Research Facilities

Neil S. Lipman, VMD[a] and Steven L. Leary, DVM, DACLAM[b]

[a]Center of Comparative Medicine and Pathology, Memorial Sloan Kettering Cancer Center and the Weil Cornell Medical College, New York, NY, USA [b]Veterinary Affairs, Division of Comparative Medicine, Washington University School of Medicine, St. Louis, MO, USA

I. INTRODUCTION

Reliable research results depend on controlling as many variables as possible. One of the many ways the laboratory animal specialist contributes to research control of animal-related variables is through design of the animal housing facility. Control of genetic variables is primarily a matter of biology, but control of other variables is dependent to a significant degree on the design and management of the research animal facility (Hessler, 1999). Biosecurity (defined as all measures taken to detect, prevent, contain, and eradicate adventitious

Laboratory Animal Medicine, Third Edition
DOI: http://dx.doi.org/10.1016/B978-0-12-409527-4.00036-5

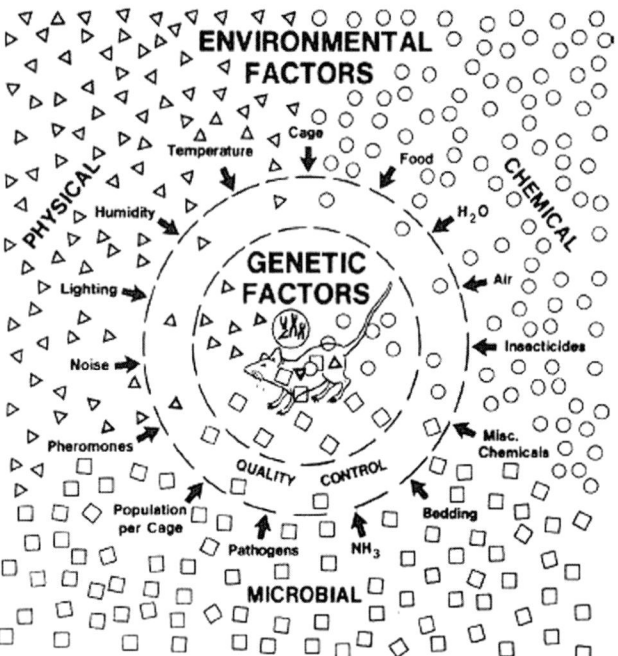

FIGURE 36.1   Conceptual view of the laboratory animal, illustrating how its biology is not only determined by genetic factors, but is also influenced by environmental factors, which may in turn influence experimental data derived from the animals. *From Lindsey* et al. (1978).

infections) is also critical, as infectious agents are well recognized to perturb the animal's physiology and biologic responses, potentially affecting research results. Environmental variables, including genetic, microbial, chemical, and physical, are illustrated in Fig. 36.1. This chapter considers the salient design features of contemporary research animal facilities that effectively control environmental variables and allow for the maintenance of high-quality animal care and use standards while minimizing operational costs. The chapter also includes an overview of macro- and microenvironmental conditions and monitoring, operational considerations, housing systems, and select equipment employed and materials routinely used in animal care facilities.

Planning and designing a research animal housing facility (or vivarium) is an intense, creative process and is most definitely not 'one size fits all'. Of primary consideration are the program requirements: how the facility will be used, what species will be housed, and what research will be supported. The design must effectively support the facility's research activities. For example, facilities housing commercial rodent production (Foster *et al.*, 1963), safety testing (Balk, 1980), and basic biomedical research clearly have different programmatic requirements. However, in spite of the many possible differences, the general requirements have evolved to become well defined, having been the subject of numerous publications and symposia starting from the early days of organized laboratory animal

science and medicine (Brewer, 1952; Brewer and Penfold, 1961; Thorp, 1960; Dolowy, 1961; Runkle, 1964a,b; Jonas, 1965; ILAR, 1978; Hare and O'Donoghue, 1968; Lang and Harrell, 1969, 1972; Simmonds, 1973; Poiley, 1974; Goldstein, 1978; Lang, 1981, 1983; Otis and Foster, 1983; Hessler and Moreland, 1984; Veterans Administration, 1993; Ruys, 1991b; CCAC, 1993; Hessler *et al.*, 1999; Rahija, 1999). References could include the Guide for the Care and Use of Laboratory Animals (ILAR, 2011); the Guide for the Care and Use of Agricultural Animals in Agricultural Research and Teaching, third edition (Federation of Animal Science Societies, 2010); Biosafety in Microbiological and Biomedical Laboratories, fifth edition (CDC-NIH, 2009); the Animal Welfare Act (Code of Federal Regulations, 1993); the Good Laboratory Practices Act (Code of Federal Regulations, 2004); and state and local codes (NABR, 1991). See Hessler (1999) for a review of the developmental history of laboratory animal facilities.

The latest version of the Guide for the Care and Use of Laboratory Animals (eighth edition), hereafter referred to as the Guide, provides considerable information relevant to the design and construction of vivaria as well as an extensive bibliography (ILAR, 2011). Additional sources of valuable, but somewhat dated, general information include the symposium proceedings published in *Laboratory Animal Housing* (ILAR, 1978), the *Handbook of Facilities Planning*, Volume 2 *Laboratory Animal Facilities* (Ruys, 1991a), and *Laboratory Animal Management Rodents* (ILAR, 1996). The National Institutes of Health Design Requirements Manual for Biomedical Laboratories and Animal Research Facilities (DRM) (2008), to which institutions receiving federal support for construction and renovation of animal facilities must adhere, provide more current and useful information pertaining to programming and planning, as well as specific design criteria. The American Society for Heating, Refrigerating, and Air Conditioning Engineers (ASHRAE) publications, including the ASHRAE Handbook-HVAC Applications (2003) and Fundamentals (2001), provide valuable information pertaining to vivarium heating, ventilation, and air-conditioning (HVAC) system design, including animal heat load and psychometric data. Additionally, several recently published American College of Laboratory Animal Medicine (ACLAM) texts are dedicated to or have sections on the topic (Hessler and Lehner, 2009; Fox *et al.*, 2007).

II. FACILITY PLANNING AND DESIGN

A. Goals and Objectives

Although goals and objectives for individual animal research facilities will include differences, there are some common features. Design and construction features and operational protocol philosophy should meet all applicable codes and regulations. Whenever possible, management considerations should be consistent with design criteria. The ability to manage a facility efficiently is, to a large extent, reliant on the design of the facility. Management procedures may be able to compensate for poor design, but often at a high operational cost. Cost-effective design features, combined with appropriate architectural and engineering technology, should be incorporated to facilitate efficient management and minimize facility maintenance. Life cycle cost should be compared with the initial cost to provide true value engineering.

The facility plan, especially as it relates to the movement of materials – for example, clean and soiled caging, animals and personnel – is of critical importance as the plan directly affects operational efficiency and therefore costs. Facility design should be as flexible as possible to accommodate changing research objectives and species utilization while balancing the objectives of cost-effective construction and efficient facility management. Sufficient animal procedure space should be provided to reduce or eliminate the need to work with animals outside of the facility. In rodent housing, the procedure space should be either in or immediately adjacent to the animal housing rooms. Uninterrupted maintenance of the animal's physical environment is essential. Maintenance of relative air pressures in containment and barrier facilities is especially critical. This will require redundancy in the heating, ventilating, and air conditioning (HVAC) systems and sufficient emergency power generating capacity to maintain normal operation of the animal facility.

To provide effective security, controlled access utilizing automated technology should be provided at all key points of entry to the facility and to areas and rooms within the facility as required to facilitate management of the facility. A safe, efficient, and healthy working environment should be provided for animal care personnel. Amenities that make for a quality work environment and enhance the recruitment and retention of staff should be provided. Such amenities include ergonomic and allergen control considerations, adequate locker and shower facilities, break rooms, and training facilities.

B. Location and Arrangement

Site selection and intra-building location are both extremely important considerations when situating the facility. Ideally, the facility should be in close proximity to investigative staff and laboratories whose activities are supported. Siting should be carefully scrutinized in areas subject to natural disasters such as hurricanes, tornadoes, floods and earthquakes (Schub, 2002; Takeshita et al., 1997; Vogelweid et al., 2005). Ground or below-ground facilities may be inadvisable in areas with an elevated water table or that may be subject to flooding. A

site-specific risk analysis may be warranted in disaster-prone areas (Vogelweid et al., 2003). Increasing concern with respect to bioterrorism as well as the security provisions mandated by select agent use should also influence site selection. Transportation, even short distances within a building, may affect select research studies (Drozdowicz et al., 1990). Local environmental factors should also be considered. As an example, episodic vibration generated by nearby passing subway trains may result in sufficient vibration to have an impact on breeding in a basement vivarium.

In general, single-story centralized facilities with direct access to ground-level transportation are operationally most efficient (Jonas, 1978). Although other concepts, including multistory facilities, are feasible and commonly utilized, the more the configuration differs from a single-story plan with direct transportation access, the less efficient it is to operate. Multistory facilities should be provided with at least two dedicated elevators allowing separate transportation of clean and soiled materials and provide redundancy.

The impact of location on HVAC system design and operation is also important. Consideration must be given to the location of system intake and exhaust with respect to each other and the surrounding environment. Uptake of automobile and equipment exhaust into intake manifolds may be problematic, especially in urban settings. Animal odors in the exhaust can adversely affect the surrounding environment. Air intake and exhaust should be physically separated to ensure that exhaust is not entrained into the system. Exhaust should be downstream of prevailing winds, if situated in close proximity to the intake. Giving consideration to facility location with respect to external heating and cooling loads can have a dramatic impact on recurring utility costs as well. The facility location must also take into account the need for HVAC system redundancy as well as access to emergency electrical power to ensure that critical systems, particularly those controlling environmental parameters, remain operational.

Intrabuilding location directly affects operations and therefore operational costs. Material movement, especially in facilities maintaining large rodent populations, must be given high consideration when selecting location. Whenever possible, the facility should be located in close proximity to a loading dock at a site that minimizes the requirement to move supplies considerable distances. Automated systems that facilitate material transfer within the building, such as those providing bedding delivery and removal, make location selection with respect to supply access and waste disposal less critical.

C. Programming

Programming, the decision-making phase that defines the scope of the building project, is often the most challenging and important part of the facility development process. Programming is the owner's/user's opportunity to exchange ideas with the facility designers/architects (Cole, 1991) as well as avoid possible design pitfalls and flaws before they become reality. The final product of the programming phase is a program document describing in detail what research will be housed in the facility and its support requirements. A key component of this document is the space allocation summary, a list of all square footage requirements. From this, animal holding room dimensions can be calculated (space allocations per the Guide; by the number of racks or cages for rodents and per animal for larger species). It is possible to base the size of the proposed animal facility on the historical experience of the institution planning the facility by calculating the ratio of the existing animal facility space to the wet laboratory space or existing animal facility space to the number of biomedical research faculty/staff scientists (Cole and Hessler, 1991; Tyson and Corey, 1999). When programming a facility for a new or expanding research program, historical animal usage per investigator/laboratory or surveying peer programs may also provide valuable insight.

It is important to consider projected changes in the research program as a whole that could affect the need for animal facility space. One way of addressing this issue is to engage the institution's master planning entity to establish a policy whereby any new building with biomedical laboratory space is required to set aside approximately 15% of its total assignable square footage for animal facility space.

Patterns for circulating supplies and personnel should be scrutinized when developing facilities designs. Several corridor systems, including single, dual, and multiple, each with inherent advantages and disadvantages, can be utilized (Fig. 36.2) (Hessler, 1991a). The systems differ with respect to movement of clean and soiled materials as well as personnel with respect to the cagewash area. The provision of separate corridors for circulation of clean and soiled materials, in a dual- or multiple-corridor system, was commonplace in animal facilities designed prior to the development and implementation of isolator caging systems and ventilated cabinets for cage changing and animal manipulation. In contrast, both clean and soiled materials and personnel utilize the same corridor in a single-corridor system. Although this is more efficient with respect to space utilization, the potential for cross-contamination is increased when using a single-corridor as compared to a dual-corridor system. Cross-contamination must be addressed operationally in a single-corridor layout.

Holding rooms and procedure labs can be organized in distinct ways with respect to the corridor(s) that serve them. Rooms can be accessed directly from the corridor, or they can be organized in a suite in which multiple

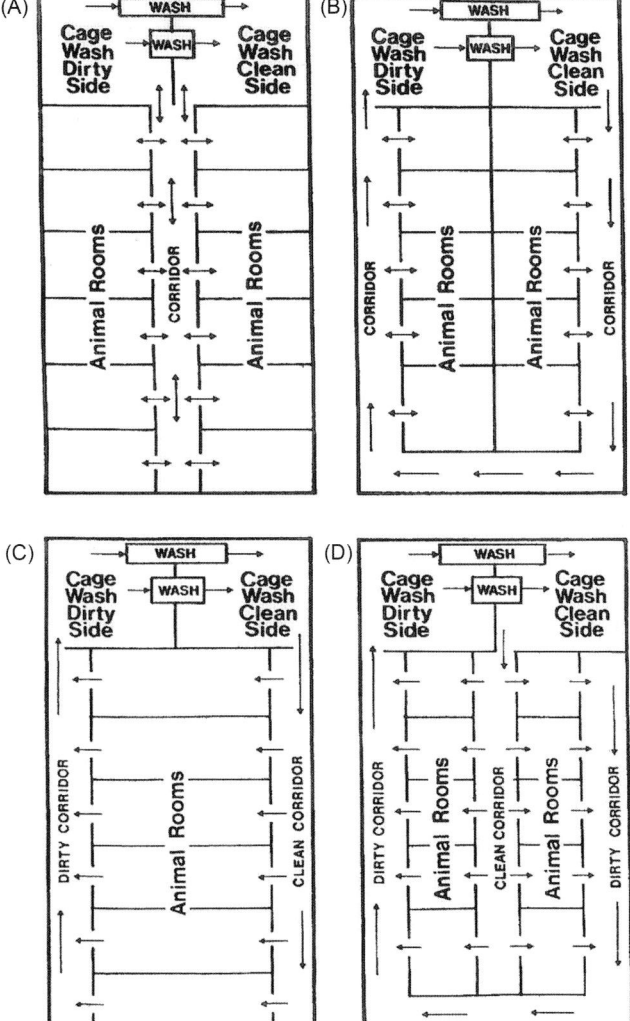

FIGURE 36.2 Four types of circulation patterns, focusing around the cage wash areas: (A) Single-corridor bidirectional pattern; (B) single-corridor unidirectional pattern; (C) dual-corridor pattern with relatively large animal holding rooms; and (D) dual-corridor pattern with relatively small animal holding rooms. All four are drawn within the same footprint to illustrate the relative 'cost' of the different circulation patterns in terms of the percentage of the footprint devoted to corridors (A = 17%; B = 32%; C = 26%; and D = 44%), and the number and size of animal rooms. The actual percentages serve only to accent the significance of choosing a circulation pattern and do not necessarily apply to a particular plan. *From Hessler and Leary (2002).*

rooms are clustered around an anteroom or short corridor accessed from the principal service corridor. A suite usually consists of several holding rooms and one to several procedure laboratories serving the holding rooms within the suite.

A considerable amount of waste material, including soiled bedding, general trash, and animal carcasses, is generated in animal facilities. Waste storage space and the waste disposal transport path require careful consideration. Direct access to ground-level transportation is the most efficient way to remove waste without transporting it through areas outside the animal facility. The most efficient location for waste storage and/or mobile waste storage containers is usually adjacent to the loading dock.

D. Animal Housing Areas

Animal Housing areas may be programmatically divided into categories such as conventional housing, quarantine, biocontainment, and barrier. Each category may be represented in a conventional animal housing area by using special equipment and management procedures or may be a physically distinct area of the animal facility or in some cases, separate facilities. The facility plan is strongly influenced by the procedures to be implemented to ensure the biosecurity of the animals housed within the facility. There are a variety of operational philosophies that can be employed to meet this goal, each of which will influence the layout. Fundamental questions to be addressed before initiating design include whether the facility will operate as a barrier, and, if so, at what level and stringency. The term 'barrier' is used widely in laboratory animal management and operations, but has a variety of connotations. Therefore, it is essential to define the meaning in the context of operational decisions. Decisions include movement of animals, personnel, and materials; housing systems utilized; and the desired animal health status to be maintained. A barrier, both physical and operational, is established around the animals to prevent introduction of unwanted adventitious agents that may adversely affect research, or alternatively, may be used to ensure containment when using hazardous agents. A barrier can be established at the cage, room, suite, and/or facility level. The use of a cage-level barrier is least restrictive with respect to the facility floor plan, except that the holding room must be large enough to accommodate a biological safety cabinet (BSC) typically used for cage changing and animal manipulation.

Following is a description of a generic animal room and functional descriptions of the various categories of animal housing spaces, some or all of which may be required for any given facility.

1. Rodents

The ideal animal room shape, size, and features will depend to a large degree on the intended use of the room. Modular room sizes of approximately 11 ft × 22 ft are often designed and drawn by the building grid size. If the intended use is unknown, a work-around strategy is in order. One might design a generic animal room suitable for housing any of the common laboratory animal species for any type of study. Unfortunately, this strategy tends to be expensive – in terms of both construction and

management costs – and tends to result in animal rooms marginally adequate for some species, too labor intensive to maintain others, but ideal for none. For many animal facility planners, the answer is to separate animal rooms into two types, one for species that require large quantities of water for routine daily sanitation or housing (e.g., aquatic species, dogs, pigs, and nonhuman primates) and those that do not (e.g., rodents and rabbits). However, it may be advisable, especially for facilities supporting changeable research programs, to construct a subset of rooms with the flexibility to accommodate both types.

Because stationary cabinets and other stationary equipment impede sanitation and provide harborage for vermin, animal housing rooms should not contain any fixed casework other than a sink, and even that could be mobile.

a. Conventional Housing

Conventional animal housing areas can be considered anything not specifically designed to be used for one of the following categories.

i. BARRIER As discussed previously, the term 'barrier' or 'barrier facility' refers to facilities and management practices designed to isolate animals from infectious agents. Barrier facility most often refers to a facility used to produce and/or maintain rodents. From the design perspective, a barrier may be a specialized area within a research animal facility or the entire animal housing portion of the facility. The concept of barrier facilities evolved from the animal production industry's interest in maintaining specific pathogen-free (SPF) animals (Foster *et al.*, 1963). However, it became apparent that research facilities required barriers for in-house production of unique rodents and for maintaining disease-free animals for study (Trentin *et al.*, 1966 a,b; Brick *et al.*, 1969; Simmons *et al.*, 1967; Christie *et al.*, 1968). Since the advent of immunosuppressed and genetically engineered rodent models (GEMs), barriers have come to be considered an essential component of most research animal facilities.

Barriers are managed at various levels of microbiological control. The highest level requires facilities designed, equipped, and managed to provide for one or more double-door, pass-through autoclaves through which all sterilized cages and most supplies enter the facility, and vestibules with interlocking doors used to introduce packaged sterile supplies by chemically sanitizing the exterior of the package in the vestibule. Animals can be introduced into the containment facility through the vestibule by sanitizing the exterior of the shipping container or alternatively, by unpacking in and transferring animals through a pass-through BSC located at the barrier's perimeter. A pass-through port

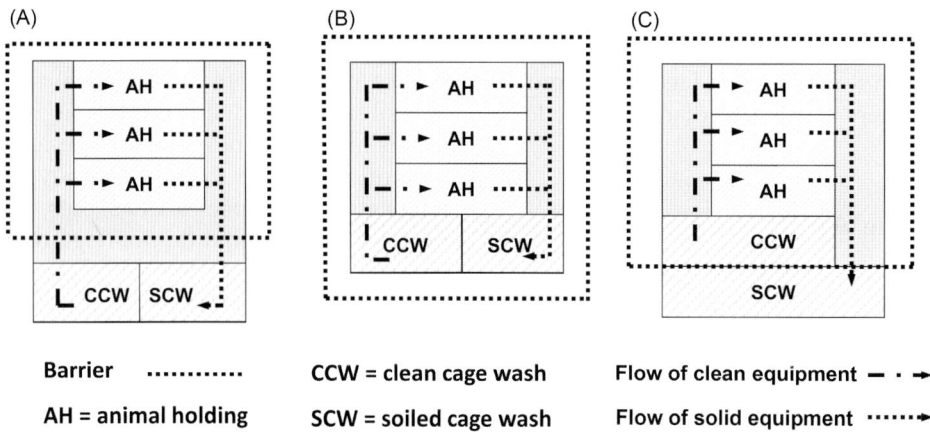

FIGURE 36.3 Schematic representations of the location of 'clean' and 'soiled' cage wash with respect to the barrier. (A) Outside the barrier; (B) within the barrier; and (C) 'soiled' cage wash outside the barrier and the 'clean' cage wash within the barrier. *From Lipman (2007).*

used with strong disinfectants or sterilants can be used to introduce sterile items packaged in watertight containers. Before entering, personnel may be required to shower and change clothes or to wear sterile outer garments over street clothes or uniforms, and to wear head and shoe covers, face mask, and gloves. Air showers are sometimes used at the entrance to barrier facilities.

Depending on the intended use of the barrier, space for laboratories, animal procedures, laboratories for generating and cryopreserving genetically engineered rodents as well as space for specialized imaging and/or irradiation equipment may be required. Large rodent barriers may include a cage sanitation facility inside the barrier, in which case all cages may not need to be autoclaved unless a disease outbreak occurs (Fig. 36.3).

A research rodent barrier may contain a quarantine area (distinct from quarantine used for importing animals from institutions other than commercial rodent breeding facilities) if the genetically engineered rodent generating facility quarantines recipient dams until the young are weaned and the mother's health status is determined. Animal cubicles are often useful for this purpose, even if the animals are housed in isolator cages.

A 'barrier' can be created in conventional animal housing rooms by using various types of cages and equipment, including micro-isolator caging systems, mass air displacement racks with high-efficiency particulate air (HEPA) filters, and flexible-film isolators of the type used for maintaining germfree animals.

The size of the holding room dictates the number of cages maintained. Large rooms are more efficient; however, they may be problematic to manage, as they require the presence of husbandry personnel to change cages for long periods, interfering with research personnel access. Large rooms may accommodate a second biosafety cabinet, relieving competition for hood space between husbandry and research personnel. There is no ideal room

size, but many research facilities prefer rooms with a capacity for 500–800 cages. At this size, when utilizing high-density ventilated caging systems, a rule of thumb is that each cage will require ~0.5 ft^2 of floor space. Therefore, holding rooms will be approximately 250–400 ft^2. Two commonly utilized room configurations for rack installation are illustrated in Fig. 36.4. The library style configuration is more efficient with respect to cage capacity; however, it limits personnel access during cage changing and is less productive, as racks must be relocated for cage changing or cages must be moved on a cart between the rack and the changing station. Racks are typically positioned to provide ~2.5–4.0 ft of space between them. The internal room corridor style is less efficient with respect to capacity but is easier to service, as the equipment and materials used for cage changing are situated and moved within the internal corridors. With this layout, cages can be changed without relocating racks. However, equipment costs are higher, as this layout requires a greater number of single-sided racks, which normally carry a cost premium. Carousel-style rodent cage racks (Fig. 36.5) have come into favor as they allow for extremely high density as the cages can be rotated for access.

ii. ANIMAL CUBICLES Animal cubicles provide maximum flexibility for animal isolation within minimal space by dividing animal rooms into multiple small spaces, typically each large enough to hold one or two cage racks. Dolowy (1961) was the first to describe the concept. Animal cubicles have been variously identified as Illinois cubicles, because those described by Dolowy were at the University of Illinois at Chicago; modified Horsfall cubicles, after isolators first described by Horsfall and Bauer (1940); and animal cubicles. The most common cubicle sizes are approximately 4 ft deep × 6 ft wide (Fig. 36.6), although larger cubicles (e.g., 7 ft × 7 ft)

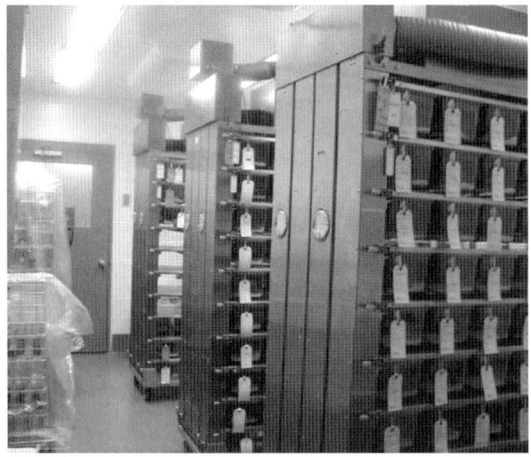
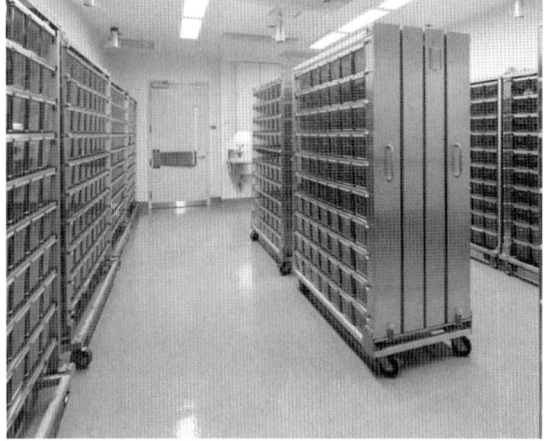

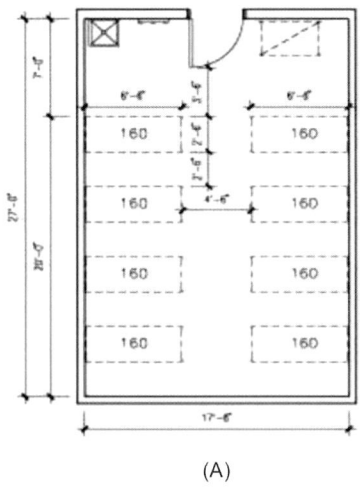
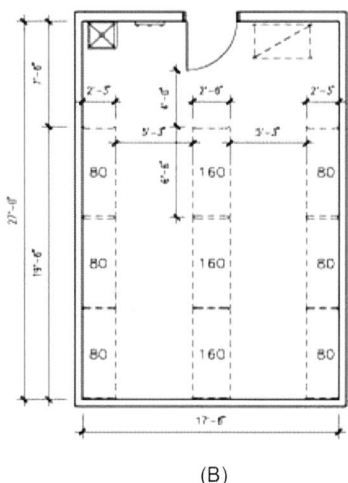

(A) (B)

FIGURE 36.4   Two commonly utilized room configurations for rack installation. (A) The *library style* configuration is more efficient; however, it limits personnel access during cage changing and is less productive as racks must be relocated for cage changing. (B) The *internal room corridor style* is less efficient with respect to capacity but is easier to service, as the equipment and materials used for cage changing are located and moved within the internal corridors. Room schematic courtesy of CUH2A. *From Lipman (2007)*.

that can hold two racks and/or in which a person could perform simple tasks with the doors closed are useful. Typically, animal cubicles are used to house smaller animals in cages on mobile cage racks. The animal cubicle concept has been expanded into 'large-animal cubicles' for housing larger species typically housed in large cages or floor pens (Hessler, 1991b, 1993). Cubicles help to solve the problem of what to do when a facility has plenty of animal housing space but too few spaces to provide the necessary separation of species, source, microbiological status, project, and experimental hazards.

Most cubicle rooms are designed with the air pressure in the service aisle between the cubicles positive to the cubicles. Even so, when a cubicle door is opened, air from that cubicle enters the aisle and then other cubicles in the room. It is therefore reasonable to question the effectiveness of animal cubicles for controlling airborne contaminants. One published study utilizing tracer gas

(White *et al.*, 1983) demonstrated that cubicles housing open cages do not effectively prevent airborne infectious agents from spreading between cubicles in the same room.

Animal cubicles can be built in place or commercially prefabricated. Prefabricated cubicles typically come complete with lighting and internal ventilation, with and without HEPA filtration and the ability to switch between positive and negative relative air pressures. There are many options regarding architectural and engineering features for animal cubicles and animal cubicle rooms. Many of the options along with pros and cons have been described in detail (Hessler and Moreland, 1984; Ruys, 1988; Hessler, 1991b, 1993; Curry *et al.*, 1998).

2. Nonhuman Primates

Nonhuman primates are sometimes housed in conventional animal rooms adjacent to rooms housing other

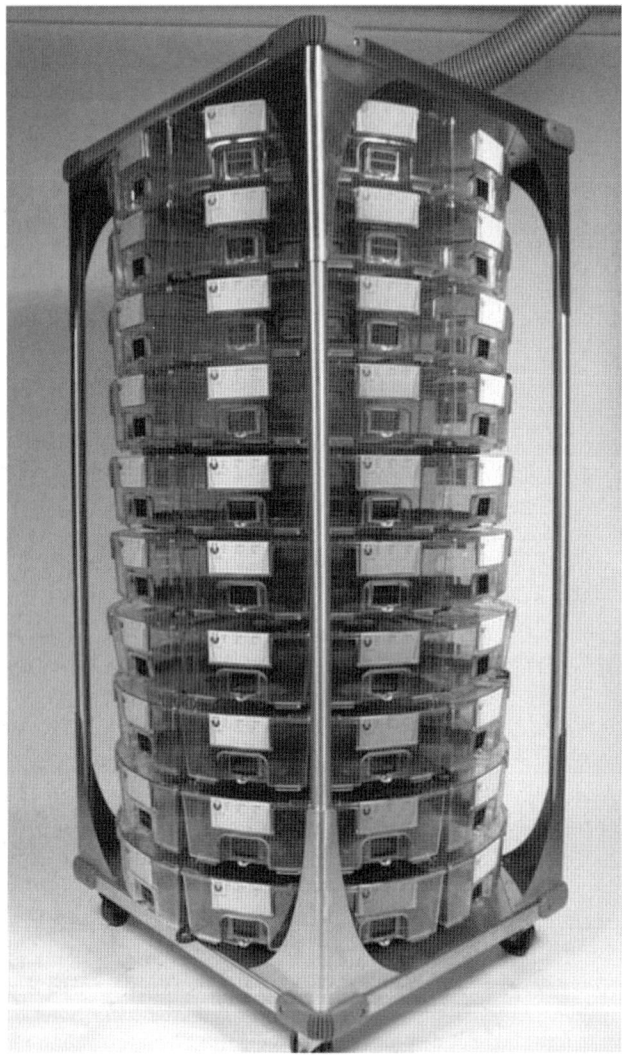

FIGURE 36.5 A carousel-style rodent rack. *Reproduced courtesy of Animal Care Systems, Inc.*

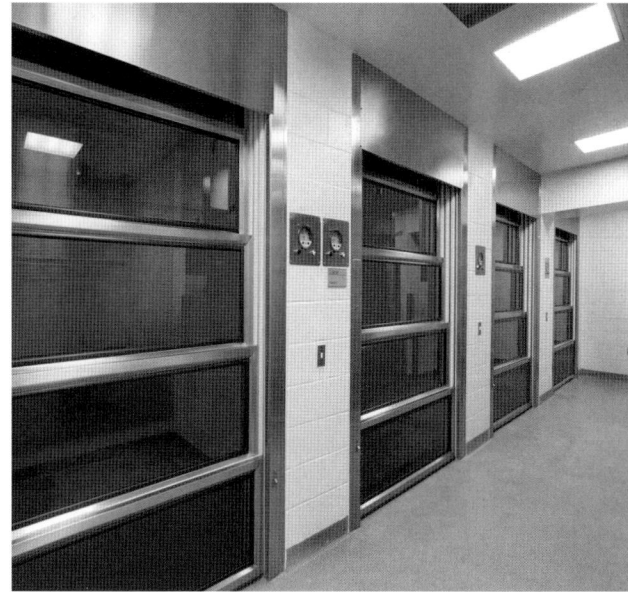

FIGURE 36.6 Animal holding room containing seven cubicles (four shown) with vertically telescoping doors. Mounted adjacent to each cubicle is a magnehelic gauge reflecting the differential pressure between the cubicle and the holding room. Glazing in door panels is tinted red.

laboratory animals. However, because of their relatively 'dirty' microbial status as compared with laboratory rodents, their potential for carrying zoonotic diseases, and the high level of noise they generate, the ideal arrangement is to house nonhuman primates in an isolated area under ABSL-2 standards.

Rooms housing nonhuman primates must be arranged and located to avoid the necessity of transporting animals, cages, or equipment through corridors or on elevators outside the animal facility. The objective is to avoid exposing individuals who do not have an occupational requirement to be exposed to nonhuman primate-associated diseases. Special features for a nonhuman primate housing area or room may include additional security and an entry vestibule that would prevent any animal escaping from its primary enclosure from escaping from the room. Lights and any other fixtures in the animal room must be designed and secured so that animals free

in the room cannot damage them and so that they do not impede capturing the animals. Trough drain systems and hose bibs for spraying down cages are commonly included.

3. Canines and Small Agricultural Mammals

As with nonhuman primates, the ideal housing area for canines and small agricultural mammals (e.g., swine, sheep) is one isolated from other animal housing and human occupancy, because these animals also have a relatively 'dirty' microbial status and generate high noise levels. The zoonotic disease concern, though present, is not as great as with nonhuman primates. The exception is Q fever in sheep, which in certain situations should be maintained under ABSL-2 standards. Animal procedure space should be provided in this area. Because these animals are commonly used as surgical research models, they should be housed near the surgical suite. Rooms may be provided for postoperative recovery and intensive care of surgical patients. Frequently, these species are housed in mobile double-tiered cages, mobile single-tiered pens, or fixed pens. Although dry bedding systems can be used to house these species, it would be unwise to plan a facility to house these species without floor drains. The location of the floor drain is critical to efficient cleaning. Ideally, it should be in an open floor trough located against the sidewalls of the room so that the cages or pens back up to the drain trough. Trap or rim flushing drains are recommended to aid in solid excrement evacuation. If pens are used, the trough should be outside the pens, leaving a minimum 18-inch access aisle between the pens and the wall, with the drain trough in the floor of the trough. The room floor should be sloped at a minimum of $3/16$ inch per foot from a crown in the center of the room to the floor trough on each side of the room. The bottom of the trough should slope a minimum of ¼ inch to the foot toward a 6-inch-diameter drain with a trap flush. There could also be a water source at the high points of the floor of the trough, controlled with the same valve that controls the flow of water to the drain trap flush. Hose bibs or reels for pen and floor cleaning can be included.

E. Support Areas

Functionally, animal facilities are divided into animal housing space and support space. The ratio of support space to animal housing space varies considerably from facility to facility, depending on the programmatic requirements, but typically ranges between 30:70 and 70:30. In general, the smaller the facility the higher the percentage of space devoted to support.

1. Administrative/Training Suite

Managing an animal facility is an increasingly complex business that requires the coordinated effort of a variety of staff. This is best facilitated by providing office and appropriate support space in a well-designed suite located adjacent to animal housing areas, but outside the security perimeter so as to allow administrative and training personnel access to offices without also granting animal facility access. Office space is required for professional, management, supervisory, training, and clerical staff, along with space for office equipment, storage of office supplies, conferencing, training, and storing library and training materials. The type and amount of office space needs to be justified based on activity levels. Animal technician supervisor offices may be scattered throughout animal housing areas, depending on the size of the facility. Office space for veterinary technicians may be located in the facility or adjacent to laboratory space or the surgery suite.

a. Diagnostic Laboratory and Necropsy

It is both efficient and convenient for diagnostic laboratory space to be immediately adjacent to or a part of the administrative/training suite. A necropsy room is required in most facilities for use by both the veterinary and investigative staff. Ideally, this should be located in a relatively isolated area adjacent to refrigerated space used for storing animal carcasses.

2. Aseptic Surgery

In accordance with accepted standards (ILAR, 2011), major survival surgical procedures on non-rodent mammalian species must be conducted in facilities designed and managed for that purpose. Therefore, most facilities housing non-rodent mammalian species will require a surgical suite. The design of the surgery facility will depend on the species and the number and complexity of procedures likely to be performed. Consider the placement of the surgery suite in relation to the housing area for the species to be used. In addition to operating rooms, the surgery suite should include areas or rooms for preparation and storage of sterile supplies, surgeon preparation, animal preparation, postsurgical recovery, and perhaps equipment and supply storage. Ideally, these would be separate rooms. However, if this is not possible, activities in the room where surgery is performed must be limited only to those required for the conduct of the procedure and 'clean' and 'dirty' activities must be separated. (See also Hessler, 1991a).

In general, standards for conducting survival surgical procedures on rodents are less stringent, but aseptic procedures are still required. Therefore, it may be desirable to include a separate room for rodent major survival surgeries if a large number of these procedures are anticipated (ILAR, 2011). This room would not necessarily need to be a part of the surgery suite or be necessarily dedicated to this purpose, but it should be designed with a limited area that may be readily sanitized prior to use for surgery. These surgeries may also be performed in a BSC to separate them from the general room environment and further limit the area to be disinfected. Cunliffe-Beamer (1993) and Brown (1994) describe surgical facilities and management procedures for rodents.

3. Procedure Laboratories

Laboratories in which various research procedures are conducted on animals have become an essential component of a modern vivarium. Many facilities have established policies restricting the return of animals from research laboratories outside the vivarium because of the risk to biosecurity. Although minor procedures may be performed within the holding room (usually in a ventilated cabinet or BSC), complex procedures such as surgery should be conducted in a separate location. Depending on the nature and volume of research activity and concerns regarding the potential for cross-contamination in shared laboratories, facilities may contain as many as one procedure laboratory for every animal holding room, or, more commonly, one procedure room for every four to eight holding rooms. The total number of procedure rooms will be dictated by the scope and activity of the institution's research program. Ideally, the procedure room should be situated in close proximity to the holding room(s) it serves. Procedure laboratories can vary in size from as small as 60–80 ft² to more than 200 ft². The size should be based on proposed activities and necessary equipment. It is desirable to include an equal number of small (~80 ft²) and medium-sized (~150 ft²) procedure laboratories in rodent facilities serving multidisciplinary research programs, although the number and size should be dictated by the research program.

Procedure laboratories should be equipped with a sink and may also include the following features or equipment depending on planned usage: high-intensity lighting (e.g., wall- or ceiling-mounted examination or surgical lighting); laboratory and/or medical gases and services such as vacuum, carbon dioxide, oxygen, and/or medical-grade air; a point exhaust system for waste anesthetic gas scavenging; a refrigerator; sufficient electrical outlets for equipment; and a BSC, ventilated cabinet and/or chemical hood. Casework is a nice feature to include in procedure laboratories; it provides a work surface and storage space. The downside is that casework can be difficult to keep clean and has an unfortunate tendency to become a repository for unused items. These concerns usually can be overcome by careful planning and judicious use of the space. Fig. 36.7 is a photograph of a typical rodent procedure laboratory.

Procedure laboratories are suitable places in which to conduct rodent surgical procedures. Depending on user preference and/or the specific surgical procedure, surgery may be conducted at a bench with kneeholes, a retractable work surface or on a surgical table. (See also Brown, 1994; Cunliffe-Beamer, 1993.)

4. Animal Receiving

The animal receiving area should be designed and operated to minimize the contamination of incoming rodents. The importance of crate decontamination was demonstrated when numerous outbreaks with SDAV in rats were attributed to surface contamination of shipping crates originating in a surgical unit of a commercial vendor (F. Wolf personal communication, 2005). It is becoming common to provide an animal receiving suite with a pass-through feature adjacent to the barrier holding space (Fig. 36.8) The suite consists of two distinct areas separated by a pass-through Class II Type A2 BSC. Filtered shipping crates containing rodents are received and surfaces decontaminated for processing in the 'soiled' receiving area, placed in the BSC and decontaminated a second time before the crate is opened. A technician in the 'clean' receiving area subsequently removes the animals from the crate, usually using disinfectant-treated forceps, placing them into a clean cage, which is then taken into the holding room. The suite is used similarly (but in reverse) to prepare rodents for shipment to other intramural facilities as well as other institutions. When the receiving area is a single room, shipping crates are brought into the room, surface-decontaminated (unless this was done on or near the loading dock) then unpacked in a cage change

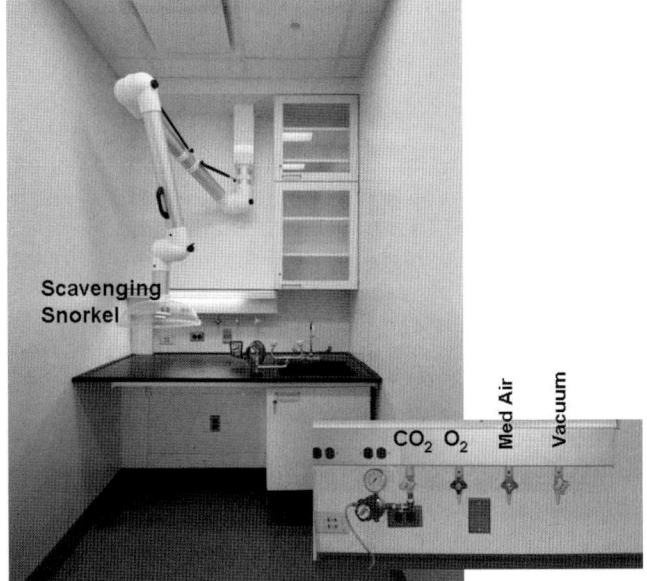

FIGURE 36.7 A typical rodent procedure laboratory containing a scavenging snorkel arm, sink, various gases for anesthesia (O_2 and medical air) and euthanasia (CO_2), and vacuum. A kneehole in the casework is for seated bench work. *From Lipman (2009).*

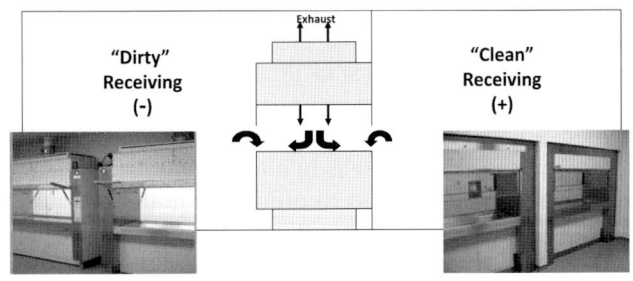

FIGURE 36.8 Elevation of a rodent receiving area separated into soiled and clean areas equipped with pass-through Class II BSCs (inset photos) interposed between the two areas. The clean area is positive pressure with respect to the soiled area. The BSC provides product (animal) protection by bathing the work surface with vertical laminar-flow, HEPA-filtered air and personnel protection by drawing in room air at each sash. The exterior surfaces of a shipping crate would be decontaminated upon receipt at the loading dock or arrival in the dirty receiving area, the crate placed and opened within the BSC, mice transferred into clean caging, and the cage removed into the clean area. *Inset photos courtesy of Nuaire, Inc.*

station, mass air displacement unit or BSC, or taken to the holding room for unpacking.

The receiving area is usually equipped with a computer workstation and printer to record incoming animals and generate cage identification cards. To avoid cross-contamination, rodents may be received into quarantine at a location distinct from that of animals arriving from closed colonies.

Unless the facility uses exclusively rodents, consideration may be given to design features of the animal

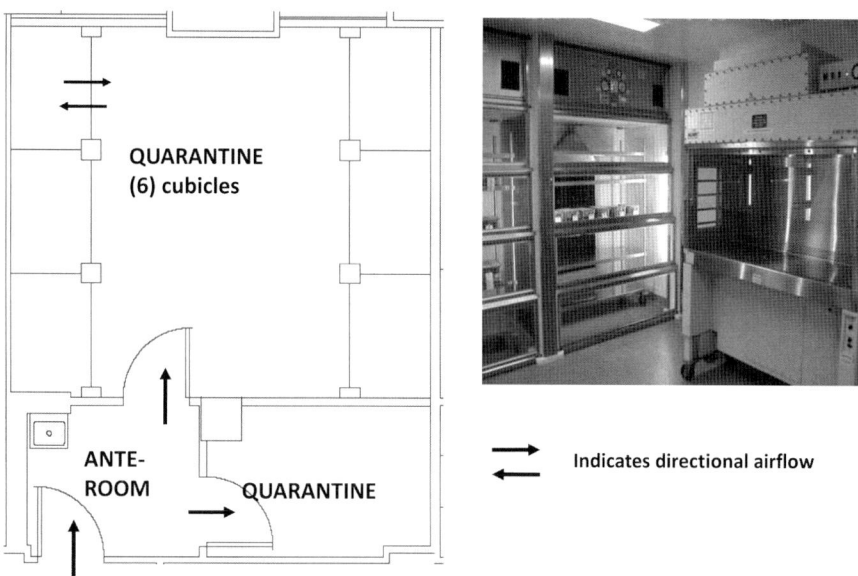

FIGURE 36.9   A schematic drawing of a two-holding room quarantine suite, one of which contains six cubicles, and a photograph of the cubicle-containing holding room with a Class II BSC. The suite also contains an anteroom where PPE is stored and donned. Arrows detail directional air flow. Cubicles can be individually set to operate at either positive or negative pressure. *From Lipman (2007).*

receiving area that assist with larger animals, such as a scale and holding pen to separate animals for weighing.

5. *General*

Other areas required to support animal facility operations include a break room or lounge, locker rooms, housekeeping closets, feed and bedding storage, general facility storage, and caging/equipment maintenance and repair. The design criteria, finishes, and functions of these areas have been reviewed (Hessler and Leary, 2002; Ruys, 1991a). In general, these areas are similar regardless of the species housed.

F. Specialized Facilities

1. *Quarantine*

Quarantine is a combination of physical space, housing system, and procedures to ensure containment and isolation of animals imported from sources identified as posing potential risks to existing colony health. Ideally – but not necessarily – separated physically from the principal colony holding areas, quarantine can be a distinct facility, a suite within a larger facility, or simply a room designated for the purpose. Standards developed for biologic hazard containment at BSL-2 are useful guidelines for rodent quarantine facilities and practices (CDC-NIH, 2009). Rehg and Toth (1998), Otto and Tolwani (2002), and Lipman and Homberger (2003) have described effective quarantine programs. Whatever form the quarantine area takes, it must ensure protection

of product (imported animals) until their microbiologic status meets established criteria. A schematic drawing of a two-room quarantine suite, one of which contains cubicles, is provided in Fig. 36.9.

For rodents, primary or cage-level containment is desirable for quarantine; therefore, static or ventilated isolator cage housing is frequently employed in conjunction with a Class II BSC (preferred) or a ventilated change station for animal manipulation and changing. Secondary levels of containment are also provided. These secondary levels may include the use of cubicles, mass air displacement units such as a flexible-wall, vertical-flow, and/or a holding room or suite of rooms isolated physically from the facility. If the quarantine area is situated in a larger facility, an airlock is strongly recommended, as is maintenance of the quarantine housing areas at negative air pressure to the rest of the facility. PPE (discussed later in this chapter) donned prior to entering the airlock is required for all personnel entering quarantine. Access to a steam sterilizer is desirable as it permits caging and other equipment to be decontaminated before subsequent processing. This can be integrated into the quarantine area or placed at a remote location. Items taken to a remotely sited sterilizer are bagged or otherwise contained so that the surface of the bag or container may be chemically decontaminated upon exiting the quarantine area.

Open cages maintained within a gnotobiotic isolator also offer excellent protection. These isolators are more labor- and material-intensive to operate, but they are particularly valuable for housing animals known to harbor infectious agents and as the animals are not removed from the isolator until quarantine is complete require less stringent facility containment. Another caging option, single-use, disposable caging, completely eliminates the likelihood of transporting adventitious agents but may be cost prohibitive and a less environmentally sound choice (Giuliano, 2012).

2. Hazardous Agent Containment

Research animals are frequently employed in studies in which hazardous chemicals, biologic agents, and/or radionuclides are administered. Certain engineering features are applicable to all hazards. These include the physical isolation of the hazardous animals and waste; room surfaces that are monolithic, sealed, and easily sanitized and do not promote the accumulation of dust; the use of BSCs or chemical hoods appropriate to the hazard and experiment; increased room air exchange rates to dilute environmental contaminants; establishment of directional airflow by configuring supply diffusers and exhaust registers to draw hazards away from human occupants; and the creation of room air pressure differentials to ensure that areas containing hazards have a negative pressure to surrounding spaces. Various resources are available to assist in the determination of appropriate facility and equipment engineering features and practices to maintain a safe environment (Adelberg et al., 1989; CDC-NIH, 2009; Commission on Physical Sciences, Mathematics and Applications, 1995; Evans, Lesnaw (1999); DiBerardinis, 1999; Liberman, 1995; Ruys, 1991b). Many of the facility features described for quarantine are applicable to and appropriate for hazardous agent containment. However, containment and associated safeguards are frequently more stringent.

Biological hazards are classified according to BSLs 1 through 4, with each level dictating specific engineering features and safety practices (CDC-NIH, 2009). Animal studies with BSL-2 agents are relatively common and have become more so with the use of viral vectors for gene therapy studies (Webber and William, 1999; Evans and Lesnaw, 1999). The demand for studies with BSL-3 agents is less common, although many facilities could benefit by having an animal BSL 3 (ABSL-3) facility. Studies with ABSL-2 agents can be conducted in animal rooms using appropriate equipment and ABSL-2 practices, but they are more efficiently and consistently conducted at a higher level of safety in an ABSL-2 facility. In addition, an ABSL-2 facility is highly desirable for quarantine of rodents infected with overt and/or adventitious agents or of unknown health status. Detailed descriptions of ABSL animal facilities and practices are given in other texts (Barkley, 1979; Barkley and Richardson, 1984; Richmond, 1991, 1996; Hessler, 1995; White, 1996; Hessler et al., 1999; King et al., 1999).

The standard design features and practices incorporated into most animal facilities meet BSL-1 standards. The complexity of design and operational practice increases as the biosafety level increases. Additional engineering features may include the use of air locks, pass-through showers and pass-through sterilizers; the provision of additional physical containment devices such as cubicles, HEPA filtration on the exhaust, comprehensive, computer-based environmental monitoring systems and automated HVAC controls; and the provision of redundancy and emergency power to all critical mechanical systems.

The containment of volatile hazards such as hazardous chemicals or select radioisotopes is more complex than containing particulates, as volatile compounds pass through HEPA filters and may not be captured by other types of filter media such as activated carbon. Chemical hoods (personnel protection only) or 100% exhaust BSCs (Class II Type B2[1]) (personnel and product protection), both of which are connected to the building's exhaust system, are useful for cage changing and hazard administration when volatility is a concern. Although specialized supplemental containment equipment that captures cage effluent can be utilized in association with static isolator cages, it is easier to house cages in areas with high air change rates (>50 complete air changes per hour) while also providing directional airflow such that fresh supply air is delivered to the area occupied by personnel and is drawn away over the animals' cages into the exhaust system. For example, a 4 ft × 6 ft cubicle with a linear ceiling diffuser at the front of the cubicle and horizontal slot exhaust at several levels along the back wall, in front of which the cage rack is placed, is useful for studies employing hazardous volatile chemicals. Supplemental PPE may also be necessary to ensure personnel protection.

The decontamination of caging and the disposal of contaminated waste, such as bedding, are of preeminent concern when either or both are presumed to be hazardous. Bedding should be autoclaved prior to dumping and caging should be decontaminated prior to subsequent handling. Sterilization of caging components prior to processing is useful when hazards are heat-labile, such as with most biologic hazards. Although some hazardous chemicals are heat labile, most require chemical deactivation or must be disposed of as an active compound (Fox et al., 1980). Disposable polystyrene or polyethelene cages are useful for highly hazardous chemicals that cannot be easily deactivated. Cage and waste are disposed of as hazardous waste. Class II BSCs and chemical

---

[1] The quantity of volatile chemical used within a Class II Type B2 BSC may be limited as the chemical may degrade the HEPA filter.

hoods can be purchased with a variety of features useful for animal studies employing hazards, including a pass-through door in the wall of the cabinet, permitting the placement of caging directly into a biohazard bag without removal from the cabinet (BSC); a solid waste disposal system integrated into the work surface of the cabinet (BSC); and/or a small cup sink for disposal of liquid waste (chemical hood). The routine use of a Class I BSC designed for bedding disposal in soiled cage wash, beneficial for dust, allergen, and contamination control, is highly recommended when handling cages with hazardous agents, even after decontamination.

The administration of radionuclides to animals mandates adherence to Nuclear Regulatory Commission standards (Code of Federal Regulations, 1999). The standards require institutions using radionuclides to be licensed and to ensure that radiation exposures for all personnel are as low as reasonably achievable (ALARA) through implementation of an appropriate radiation safety protection program. When using radioisotopes *in vivo*, consideration must be given to the specific radioisotope administered, in particular its half-life, energy, and biologic activity, and the amount administered; the protection of personnel exposed to radioactive animals and waste; and the disposal of radioisotope-contaminated materials, including carcasses.

The half-life of the radionuclide has a significant impact on the procedures to be employed for waste disposal and on cage handling. Allowing carcasses and waste to decay for 10 half-lives permits the disposal of these materials into nonradioactive waste streams. Therefore, the administration of radioisotopes with short half-lives permits contaminated materials to be held on-site for decay and subsequently disposed of as nonradioactive waste. Carcasses are held frozen, and caging and bedding are stored until they can be safely processed. Prior to release of carcasses, caging, or bedding, radioisotope activity levels are confirmed with an appropriate device or technique, such as a Geiger counter or surface wipes, by appropriately trained personnel. Animals, caging, and waste contaminated with radioisotopes with long half-lives need to be disposed of at appropriate waste sites by licensed individuals. Although disposable cages are used, more commonly cages are emptied, bedding is processed for off-site disposal, and cages are hand-cleaned with a radioactivity decontaminant until activity is no longer detectable. Cages are then processed through mechanical washers.

Special consideration should be given to the use of mechanical washers for sanitizing caging and related equipment when used with hazardous agents. Because some mechanical washers recirculate wash water or rinse water, hazardous contaminants may accumulate and contaminate other equipment washed in the unit

(Lipman, 1995). Under these circumstances, wash water and/or rinse water should be dumped after the hazardous material has been processed. Many cage/rack washers can be programmed so that waste water is dumped at the end of each cycle, and/or so that there are additional rinse cycles.

3. Necropsy

The inclusion of a room or suite dedicated to necropsy is beneficial in facilities conducting *postmortem* evaluations on animals. Although procedure laboratories are suitable and usually sufficient for necropsying small numbers of rodents, a dedicated, well-designed space for necropsy may be needed if large numbers of rodents or larger species are necropsied. Necropsy should contain a freestanding autopsy table, benchtop workstations, or both for performing gross dissections, conducting perfusions, and trimming tissues. A freestanding table, which provides access on three of four sides, is desirable when larger species need to be accommodated. Because tissue fixatives such as formalin are volatile and hazardous, tables and workstations should be down and/or backdraft, to draw vapors and low level aerosols away from the prosector. Downdraft tables or workstations should provide capture 12 inches above the work surface, while backdraft stations should provide directional air flow over the entire work surface. They should have an integral sink to collect fluids and permit easy washdown. The room should include a BSC, if rodents to be necropsied are infected with BSL-2 or greater agents, or a chemical hood, if they are exposed to hazardous volatile chemicals.

4. Imaging

Technologic advances and demands in various disciplines have resulted in the development and/or adaptation of a host of noninvasive imaging technologies for use in animals, permitting the study of sequential temporal events in the same animal or group of animals. Magnetic resonance imaging (MRI), magnetic resonance spectroscopy (MRS), positron emission tomography (PET), single-photon emission computed tomography (SPECT), ultrasonography, optical imaging techniques, electron paramagnetic resonance imaging, and X-ray computed tomography (CT) are some of the imaging devices currently available for use (Allport and Weissleder, 2001; Benveniste and Blackband, 2002; Budinger *et al.*, 1999; Chatziioannou, 2002; Contag and Bachmann, 2002; Foster *et al.*, 2000; Paulus *et al.*, 2000; Ritman, 2002; Wirrwar *et al.*, 2001). Many facilities using or creating animal models in oncology, neurobiology, developmental biology, gene therapy, immunology, and a variety of other disciplines are becoming highly reliant on imaging technology (Allport and Weissleder, 2001; Benveniste and Blackband, 2002; Budinger *et al.*, 1999;

Chatziioannou, 2002; Paulus *et al.*, 2000). Many institutions are developing multimodality imaging cores because of the high cost of equipment acquisition and maintenance, the need for highly trained personnel to maintain and operate the equipment as well as to acquire and interpret images, and the provision of the necessary infrastructure for storing and distributing large volumes of data. Whether to incorporate the imaging core into an animal facility or have it stand-alone in a separate location is an institutional decision that has important consequences. In either situation, attention must be given to biosecurity, as animals in direct contact with equipment components may act as fomites for disease transmission, and some of the equipment is difficult to sanitize and used by more than one group of investigators.

Integrating the core into the animal facility alleviates concerns relating to transport to and from the site. Although biosecurity concerns are challenging because of personnel and equipment maintenance and repair issues, they are lessened if the core operates within the confines of a barrier along with housing and related support areas. However, this arrangement may not be acceptable at some institutions as animals from various housing sites or even other institutions may need to be imaged. Stand-alone facilities may require additional support spaces, such as procedure laboratories and, potentially, quarantine and/or housing space. In either case, carefully conceived and detailed operational procedures should be established to reduce the likelihood of cross-contamination between individual animals and groups of animals.

The physical layout of the facility will be determined, to some degree, by the imaging modalities supported and the size of the animals that are imaged. Equipment may need to be housed side by side or in adjacent spaces, as equipment producing functional images often need to be co-registered with anatomic images, e.g., PET scanners placed in proximity to MR scanners or CT units, although many multimodality imaging instruments are now available. It is frequently desirable to cluster radioisotopic imaging modalities together, away from those employing non-radioisotopic methods. A radiopharmacy, within or in close proximity to the facility, is necessary to support radioisotopic-based imaging, as the radioactive compounds used are short-lived (hours) or ultra-short-lived (minutes). Although commonly utilized positron-emitting radioisotopes such as F18 (T1/2 = 110 min) are available commercially, immediate access to a cyclotron may be necessary to support studies using ultra-short-lived (<30 min) radiolabeled substances such as O15 or C11, or longer lived radioisotopes such as I90 or C11, which are not available commercially. Procedure space for the administration of tracers, holding rooms for 'hot' animals held for decay, and dedicated freezers for holding radioactive carcasses may also be needed.

Physical requirements are minimal for non-radioisotopic imaging equipment such as CT, SPECT, ultrasound, or optical. Radiation-emitting units (irradiators) for rodents are self-shielded and do not require further shielding. MR scanners, however, require special attention because of their weight, dimensions, ventilation requirements, the fringe field generated (especially from unshielded magnets), the heat load generated, and the potential need for a separate area to support electronics and console. Additional consideration must be given to the structure and composition of the building: the scanner location must support the high floor loads associated with the weight of the magnet and shielding, and the room must be well ventilated and should be provided with redundant ventilation systems to avoid the potential for asphyxiation of personnel and animals associated with cryogen boil-off. Depending on the magnet's design and the size of the fringe field, the room's walls may require steel shielding to contain the stray field so that it does not interfere with other operations or pose safety concerns. Similarly, copper shielding may be required to eliminate interfering radiofrequency energy. The impact of ferrous elements of the building's structure or its components on field homogeneity must also be considered, especially when they are not static, e.g., in the case of the movement of elevators with steel components, the location should allow for the future removal and replacement of the magnet, be vibration free, and provide the considerable cooling required to offset heat generated by the scanner's electronics. However, small, plug-in rodent MR units are available that can be more easily accommodated into an existing space.

5. Aquatics

Increasing numbers of aquatic species, namely fish and frogs, are becoming commonplace in many research animal facilities. While many of the facility issues related to their terrestrial counterparts apply, some do not and there are additional considerations when designing and building facilities to support aquatic animals. There are publications available on this topic (DeTolla *et al.*, 1995; Browne *et al.*, 2007; Diggs and Parker, 2009; Alworth and Vasquez, 2009; Green, 2010; Harper and Lawrence, 2011). When designing facilities for aquatics, special consideration must be given to water spills, leakage (small or catastrophic failure), and condensation, as well as floor and point loads as water is extremely heavy and housing systems, depending on the size, can hold thousands of gallons. Ideally, aquatic facilities, especially those with systems containing large quantities of water, should be located on the lowest level of the building to avoid damage of other areas should an uncontained leak occur.

Whereas for terrestrial species providing appropriately conditioned fresh air is paramount, the provision and maintenance of suitable quality water at an appropriate temperature is essential and differs by species for aquatic animals. They are housed in systems ranging from the small and simple, e.g., static aquaria, to large highly complex recirculating systems. As a result, the holding rooms that contain these systems vary considerably in size. The precision and level at which macroenvironmental temperature needs to be controlled and maintained is dependent on whether the temperature at which the water must be maintained is dependent on macroenvironmental conditions or controlled by an independent water heating or chilling system. If the former, depending on the species and the design and specifications of the HVAC system, supplemental heating or chilling may be required. Special attention to lighting may be necessary as some species require or benefit from full-spectrum lamps. The life support system, depending on the species maintained, the system type and size, and the manufacturer, can be a component of the rack, contained within a housing or console, mounted on a skid, or installed as components within the housing or a designated equipment room. The latter is preferred to contain noise, vibration, and heat load for large systems. Redundancy for key system components, e.g., water distribution pumps, should be provided for large systems.

Large life support systems are highly energy dependent and may require multiple electrical outlets of varying voltage and amperage. Outlets at risk for water exposure should be ground fault interrupted (GFI) or connected to a GFI circuit. All essential system components should be provided emergency power to ensure uninterrupted service. As loss of water flow and maintenance of appropriate water conditions are essential to ensure the health and welfare of the animals, a device which monitors key system components, including water distribution and select water conditions, should be installed. The device should notify staff by telephone, page, or email when parameters fall outside of an acceptable range. Access to a reliable water source of appropriate chemistry and composition is essential. Depending on the species maintained, this may be native or treated well, surface or municipal water, or water filtered by reverse osmosis. Distilled and deionized water should be avoided or run over a column or filter which replaces lost ionic constituents.

Aquatic holding rooms and ancillary support spaces should be constructed from materials impervious to water and that are corrosion resistant. Flooring should be slip resistant, be sloped to drains, and contain floor sinks, drains, or troughs sized to handle housing system effluent, spills, or containment failures. Ideally, exposed components of gasketed lighting fixtures, supply diffusers and exhaust registers, and other room components manufactured from metal should be stainless steel. Casework when provided should be manufactured from epoxy, stainless steel, or laminate. Depending on the

species, the number of animals maintained, and the nature of the research supported, the holding room(s) may be a component of a suite that may include areas for diet preparation, especially when using live feed, laboratory space for embryo, larval or adult screening and/or manipulation, and a separate room and housing system to quarantine incoming animals.

G. Cage Sanitation and Sterilization

Although the terms *sanitation, cleaning, disinfection,* and *sterilization* may seem to be used interchangeably, they are distinct entities; thus, a brief definition of each may be helpful at this point. *Cleaning* refers to the removal of organic and nonorganic debris adhering to surfaces. *Disinfection* (heat or chemical) reduces but may not eliminate microorganisms from surfaces; it also may not produce the same level of reduction depending on the organisms and the forms of organisms present (e.g., vegetative bacteria versus bacterial spores). *Sanitation* is a combination of cleaning and disinfection. *Sterilization* eliminates all life forms, which is impossible to demonstrate; however, the term is used to indicate a high level of disinfection and as a process should be validated on a regular basis using appropriate test measures.

The operation of this area is critical, especially in facilities maintaining large numbers of rodents. Although facilities can be decentralized, transporting cages and related equipment between a housing facility and cage sanitation and processing area in another building or location, this arrangement is undesirable, as it is inefficient and labor-intensive. In addition, the risk of colony exposure to adventitious agents may be increased, as there is a potential for contamination of material during transport; however, this risk can be managed and minimized through operational processes. The determining factor for providing a dedicated cage sanitation area is the size of the population to be supported. There is no set rule; the decision is based on the amount of mechanical washing activity needed to support the program, the availability and proximity of another cage sanitation area for support, the ease by which the equipment can be moved back and forth, and the risk of equipment and facility contamination during transport.

The separation of clean and soiled activity within the area is critical. Recognizing that clean materials are distributed throughout the facility, contamination of clean supplies can have a significant impact on a large number of animals. To avoid cross-contamination, the cage wash area is divided into clean and soiled sections, separated by a wall or bulkhead containing mechanical sanitizing equipment such as a tunnel washer and/or a double-door, pass-through cage/rack washer, and may, depending on operational decisions, include a double-door, pass-through steam sterilizer (i.e., autoclave).

Separation allows the creation of an air pressure differential gradient, such that the clean section is maintained positive with respect to the soiled section, and air containing potential contaminants flows along the gradient. Doors on pass-through equipment should ideally be interlocked to ensure that both doors cannot be opened simultaneously, disrupting the air pressure differential.

The cage wash area is sized to accommodate the fixed equipment to be provided, the mobile equipment that circulates, the personnel assigned to the area, and the activities conducted for all species housed. Because a considerable amount of equipment moves through the cage wash, the space required to accommodate racks, carts, and supplies awaiting sanitation and processing for both clean and soiled materials needs to be determined. This determination requires knowing the frequency of washing required for each equipment item, the footprint of the equipment (large items such as cage racks) or the carts on which they are contained (small items such as shoebox cages, wire bar lids, and water bottles), and the number of hours per day and days per week that the cage wash area will operate. The ability to accommodate the materials that will be serviced in a single day, as well as the space needed for processing, is recommended. The clean area also frequently serves as storage and therefore must be sized accordingly. Dividing the clean area into two sections is preferred so that cage processing and storage is separated from the hot, moisture-laden environment of the cage wash area.

The type, size, and number of mechanical equipment items installed in the area is dependent on population size, species housed, equipment throughput, types of caging systems utilized, and planned operational hours and processes. Facilities processing large volumes of materials may consider purchasing equipment to automate select processes. Details pertaining to automation are described later in this chapter. Mechanical equipment should be installed such that the serviceable section of the equipment is situated in and serviced from the soiled section or installed within a mechanical space, located between the clean and soiled sections, accessible from the latter. Provision of a mechanical space has the added benefit of containing and exhausting the considerable heat load generated from the equipment, and the space can be used to store bulk chemicals used in the washers. Alternatively, chemicals can be stored remotely and piped to the equipment (the remote location is often the loading dock area). Installation of exhaust canopies over the load and unload side of the washing equipment and sterilizer is recommended to contain and exhaust steam effluent escaping from the equipment. Provision of a pit underneath the cage/rack washer and large sterilizer, accommodating the washer's sump and sterilizer chamber, permits preferred floor loading of equipment. In addition, the provision of a separate, grate-covered, shallow (3–4 inches) pit with a drain on the clean side, immediately adjacent to the cage/rack washer and approximately the size of the washer's footprint, is useful to collect water runoff while unloading sanitized equipment.

Both cage wash sections should be equipped with floor drains sufficient to support wet sanitation. Drains, minimally 4 inches in diameter (6 inches preferred), should be sited to avoid accumulation of standing water. Alternatively, cage wash can be equipped with perimeter grate-covered trenches with drains. As modest volumes of contact bedding may end up in the drains, trap or rim flushing drains (possibly with basket strainers) should be considered. Sinks (double sinks in a large cage wash facility), with associated integrated work surfaces, are recommended for both clean and dirty cage wash. Sinks are useful for soaking, washing, and/or rinsing small equipment items. Other items for consideration include hose bibs or reels for wash-down of large equipment, if the equipment is too large for the available mechanical washers, and the room; recoil and rack flushing stations in the clean area if automatic watering is used; a partially enclosed wash-down station in the soiled area for sanitizing large equipment items, especially if a cage/rack washer is not provided; and a Class 1 BSC or automated down-draft waste disposal system for cage dumping, to contain aerosolized bedding particles and waste generated during cage handling in the soiled section.

Because the environment within the cage wash is hostile, floors, walls, and ceilings must be able to withstand a hot, moisture-laden environment and exposure to a variety of chemicals, as well as the frequent movement of considerable heavy equipment. Floors should be slip- and impact-resistant and monolithic, consisting of seamless troweled or broadcast chemical and heat-resistant polymer composites, usually epoxy aggregate, or methyl methacrylate polymer flooring or ceramic tile with epoxy grout. Walls should be constructed of sealed and epoxy-coated cement masonry units (CMUs) or moisture and impact-resistant cement wallboard. Solid ceilings constructed of epoxy-coated gypsum board with aluminum or stainless steel access panels for mechanical service, or a suspended lay-in ceiling consisting of a rust-resistant aluminum or fiberglass grid and solid vinyl-coated acoustical or fiberglass panels, should be used; gasketed lock-in panels are available that permit high-pressure washing. In facilities with sprinkler systems, heads in close proximity to heat-generating equipment should be of the high-temperature type.

1. Equipment

Care of laboratory animals at the level required by contemporary research is an equipment-intensive and equipment-dependent enterprise. Planning a research animal facility requires careful consideration and detailed knowledge of all major equipment to be used in the facility, both fixed and mobile.

a. Cage/Rack Washers

Proper sanitation and equipment sterilization helps maintain adequate control of the research animal's microbial environment. Hand-washing cages and reliance on chemical disinfectants for sanitation cannot be recommended, even for small facilities (Vesell *et al.*, 1973, 1976; Thibert, 1980) as it is labor-intensive, increases the potential for leaving unacceptable chemical residues on the cages, and exposes personnel to chemical hazards. If the decision is made to hand-washing cages, standard operating procedures (SOPs) must be implemented and followed, personnel trained, and strict process controls maintained. Sanitation is better achieved by using mechanical washers and water at temperatures in excess of 82.2°C (180°F) (ILAR, 2011). The 82.2°C (180°F) standard was first published by the National Sanitation Foundation, which set standards for commercial dishwashers (National Science Foundation, 1953). In fact, sanitation can be achieved at temperatures lower than 82.2°C by using longer exposure times, e.g., 1 s at 82.2°C (180°F), 15 s at 71.6°C (161°F), and 30 min at 61.7°C (143°F) (Wardrip *et al.*, 1994). Control systems on contemporary washers monitor water temperature and will not allow the equipment to start or complete a cycle unless the temperature reaches 82.2°C or greater. Sometimes washers are set up such that only the final rinse temperature is 82.2°C or greater. Two basic types of washers are commonly used: cage/rack washers and tunnel washers, also called belt or conveyor washers. Ruys (1991a) provides a detailed description of each type along with utility requirements. In a cage/rack washer, soiled equipment is placed in a chamber and sprayed with high pressure on all sides with large volumes of hot water through a series of selected detergent/rinse cycles, after which it is removed, cleaned, and sanitized. Cage/rack washers come in a variety of chamber sizes. Cabinet washers are the smallest, with a typical chamber size of 122 cm (48 inches) wide × 79 cm (31 inches) high × 86 cm (34 inches) long (Fig. 36.10). Typically, the bottom of the wash chamber is several feet off the floor. Cabinet washers are suitable for cleaning relatively small numbers of cages and water bottles that can be lifted into the chamber. Cage/rack washers are typically pit-mounted so that the floor of the washing chamber is level with the room floor and cage racks may be easily rolled into the chamber (Fig. 36.11). Chamber sizes vary from those that hold only a single cage rack to those that hold many cage racks at a time. Double-door pass-through washers are preferred to allow for separation of soiled and clean cages. Water may be fresh for each cycle, except for the final rinse water, which is saved and used as the pre-rinse water for the next load. An option for storing water between

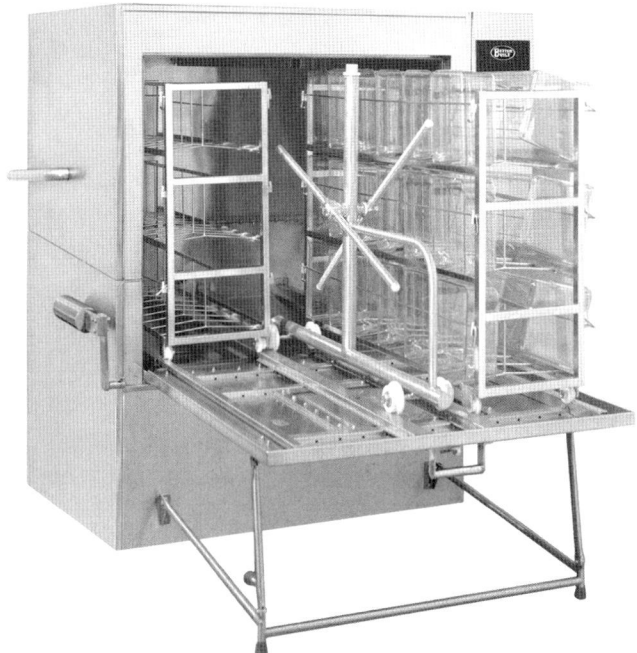

FIGURE 36.10 Cabinet washer with door ajar. Washer equipped with racks and center header to accommodate the maximum number of shoebox cages. *Courtesy of Northwestern Systems Corporation.*

loads is to have side tanks. For example, one side tank can store alkaline detergent wash water; the other can store acid-treated wash water. Older models used electromechanical timers to control cycles, but most newer cage/rack washers are controlled digitally with microprocessors that offer greater flexibility by allowing for a variety of preprogrammed wash and rinse cycles using less water, depending on the type of equipment being cleaned and sanitized.

For facilities supporting sizable numbers of aquatic animals, the installation of a specialized cabinet washer, which, by nature of its spray nozzle configuration and the chemistry of the agents added to during the wash cycle, removes biofilm on the surface of tanks and other system components without the need for labor-intensive hand washing, may be considered.

In the other commonly used type, the tunnel washer (Fig. 36.12 illustrates the load end of a tunnel washer), items to be cleaned and sanitized are placed on a conveyor that moves through a tunnel divided into sections, e.g., pre-rinse, detergent wash, rinse, and final rinse. These come in a variety of sizes; however, a typical tunnel washer has a conveyor about waist high and an opening anywhere from 76–107 cm (30–42 inches) wide × 91 cm (36 inches) high × ~4.6 m (15 ft) long. In addition, it is common to have extensions on the load and unload ends. These could add 46 cm (18 inches) or more on both ends, and a dryer section and bedding dispenser could each add another 1.8 –2.4 m (6–8 ft). It is also useful to

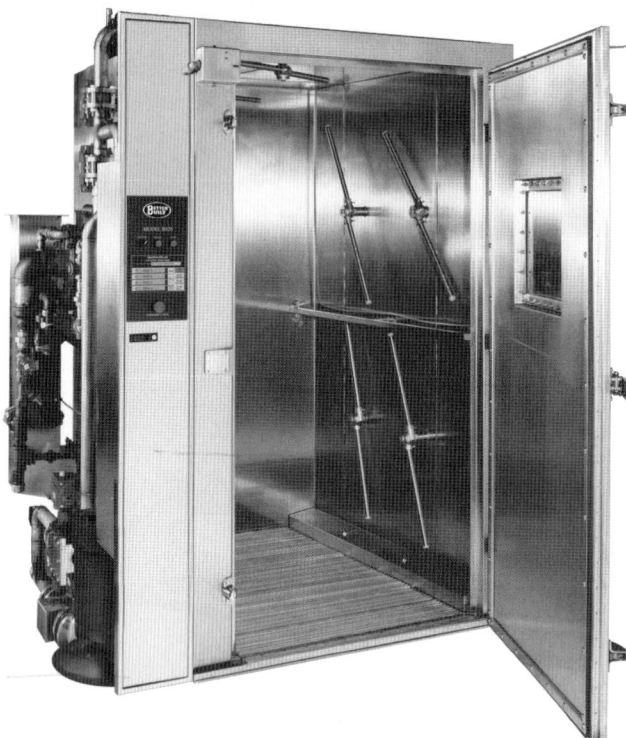

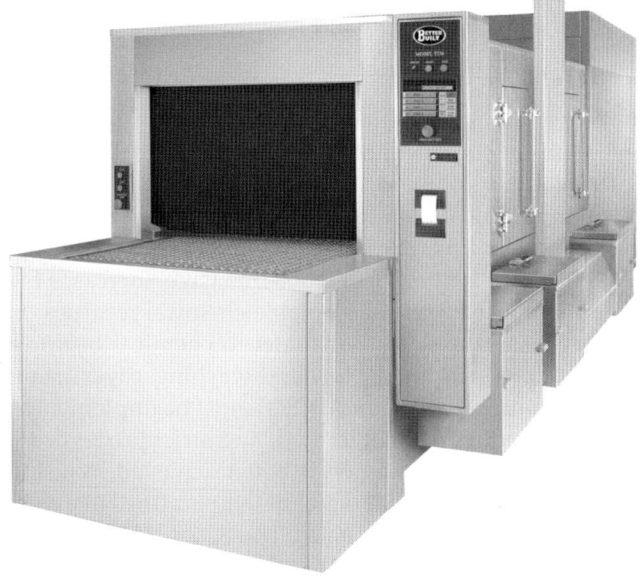

FIGURE 36.12 Load end of a tunnel washer. *Courtesy of Northwestern Systems Corporation.*

FIGURE 36.11 Single-door, pit-mounted, rack washer with door ajar. Note the rotating spray arms on the wall and ceiling of the washer. *Courtesy of Northwestern Systems Corporation.*

have a 3 m (10 ft) or longer roller conveyor to collect cages at the end of the conveyor belt. The width and speed of the conveyor determine the washing capacity: the longer the washing tunnel, the faster the conveyor belt can run with the same amount of exposure time in each section. Tunnel washers are especially useful for sanitizing plastic shoebox rodent cages, cage waste collection pans, water bottles, and other small equipment. Water is usually recirculated: the recirculating rinse water is used for pre-rinse, which is discarded, and the final rinse water flows into the recirculating rinse water to freshen it.

Indexing tunnel washers have separated wash and rinse sections. The conveyor stops to expose the load for a certain amount of time in each section. Tunnel washers used in combination with robots for loading and unloading the conveyor are frequently programmed to index wash.

b. Bedding Disposal

Moving soiled bedding from the cage to a final disposal location is a major logistical and labor-intensive challenge. The most common method is to dump the bedding from the cage to a container, move the container to a larger container outside the animal facility, and move it from there to its final disposal location, usually a landfill or an incinerator. The only significant improvement in this basic method has been the use of

special bedding disposal cabinets (Rake, 1979). These cabinets use mass air movement to draw the soiled bedding dust away from the person dumping the bedding, directing the air first through a gross filter, then through a HEPA filter before discharging it back into the room. This provides a safer work environment for personnel and is especially useful, even essential, for dumping bedding from cages containing known carcinogens or toxic chemicals.

The most efficient method of bedding disposal – if local codes allow – is the use of bedding disposal systems designed to process the bedding into small particulate, then discharge it directly into the sanitary sewer system. These systems come in grinder and hammer types with a hopper for processed material and an auger to move the material through the system. Drain line blockage can be avoided by properly sizing the drains and by directing water from the tunnel washers by a short run of drain coming from the disposal unit to this equipment.

Vacuum systems are commonly used to deliver soiled bedding, either directly from the cage or from a hopper, to a receptacle. From there, it is transported by an auger into an incinerator or dumped directly into a bulk disposal receptacle outside the facility. One very common type of vacuum waste removal uses a short auger at the bottom of a hopper connected to a vacuum system run by a centrifugal separator that allows the bedding to be pulled into a vacuum stream and blown over long distances to larger receptacles such as dumpsters. Either vacuum system must have well-placed clean outs to deal with clogging that may be associated with overly wet bedding or large bedding types (such as shavings).

A less commonly used bedding disposal method, first introduced into research animal facilities in the late 1980s, involves transporting the bedding from a hopper in the cage sanitation area to a bulk disposal receptacle outside the building in a slurry of water. The slurry system separates the water from the bedding at the disposal end and recirculates the water to transport more bedding.

c. Bedding Dispensers

Many different types of mechanical bedding dispensing strategies have been tried, typically ones that fill one or two shoebox rodent cages at a time, but have not been widely accepted, perhaps because of the initial cost, or because they are not significantly faster or more convenient than the old reliable handheld-scoop method. Mechanical dispensers do, however, place a uniform amount of bedding in each cage and help decrease employee repetitive stress injuries, which may mitigate the initial automation cost. For facilities with a large number of bedded rodent cages, bedding dispensers attached to the tunnel washer have been widely used (Fig. 36.13). These have a conveyor in line with, but at a lower level than, the tunnel washer conveyor so that cages fall onto the dispenser conveyor. A mechanical cage rotating device is also available. As the cages fall, they are flipped over and filled with bedding as the conveyor takes them through the dispenser. Even with the most dust-free bedding, this type of dispenser generates a significant amount of dust, much of which can be collected with a vacuum attached to the dispenser. If this type of dispenser is to be used, it is important that the clean side of the cage sanitation area, where the dispenser will be located, be separated from the clean cage storage area to contain the dust to an area as small and as easily cleaned as possible.

d. Sterilization Equipment

Autoclaves that utilize steam under pressure are routinely used in research animal facilities to disinfect cages and supplies required for housing rodents in isolators and/or under barrier conditions, equipment and supplies contaminated with infectious biohazardous agents, and surgical instruments and supplies. Equipment and supplies in the autoclave chamber are exposed to temperatures ranging from 121°C to 132°C (250–270°F). In very small research animal facilities, a single autoclave may be sufficient, but typically more than one will be required. In large facilities, a separate autoclave may be required for each sterilization function. Barrier and biocontainment facilities often require bulk autoclaves that hold from one to four racks of cages. High-vacuum autoclaves are highly recommended because they significantly improve sterilization effectiveness and efficiency compared to gravity autoclaves. Bulk autoclaves usually

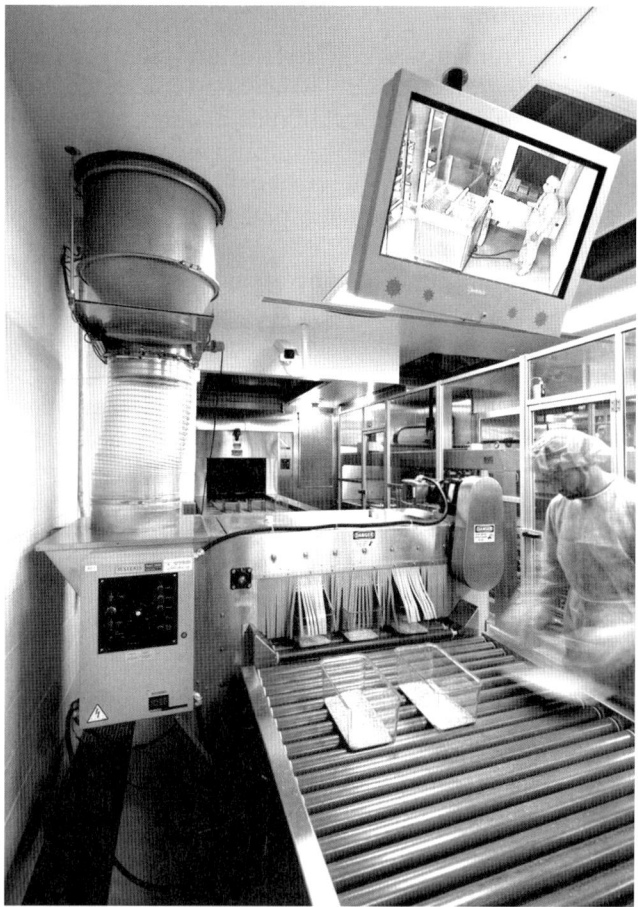

FIGURE 36.13 In-line bedding dispenser positioned at the unload end of a tunnel washer. Bedding is delivered to the dispenser via a pneumatic system from a remote location. Video monitor (above dispenser) receives a video feed from a camera on the load side of the washer.

include hinged or sliding doors, the choice of which will depend on the physical layout of the area where the autoclave is to be installed. Clean steam (i.e., steam to which no chemical rust inhibitors have been added) should be considered for autoclaves used to sterilize animal cages, feed, and bedding to avoid exposing animals to chemical additives typically found in boiler-generated steam.

Ethylene oxide sterilization is rarely required for animal husbandry support but is frequently required for experimental surgery program support. Ethylene oxide is carcinogenic and highly explosive when mixed with air; therefore, detailed safety requirements governing the installation of ethylene oxide sterilization equipment have been established. Its use in some applications is being discontinued in favor of newer technology. Hydrogen peroxide or gaseous chlorine dioxide released in sealed chambers is now being used for sterilization of cages and other hard surface items.

2. Automation

Robotic tunnel washing systems are highly capital-intensive and practical only when large volumes of caging must be processed. Additional advantages include improvement of personnel health and welfare, primarily through the reduction of personnel activities that pose ergonomic hazards with the potential of resulting in repetitive motion injury.

The future portends an increasing use of automated systems for rodent handling and housing, as the number of animals maintained by many institutions continues to increase.

Certain components of rodent husbandry have been automated for years; however, the past decade has seen a marked expansion in the number and complexity of mechanized activities, especially in cage washing. Bedding dispensers on or in association with tunnel washers distribute contact bedding into plastic microisolator cages. The dispenser flips the cage over and fills it with a predetermined quantity of bedding. The system can be further automated by distributing bedding to the dispenser through a vacuum system from a location remote to the unit, preferably in close proximity to the loading dock. Also available are hand-operated dispensers, into which cages are placed and filled. This dispenser type is employed with articulating robotic cage washing systems.

Water bottles are frequently processed in stainlesssteel wire baskets, permitting bulk handling of up to 20–25 bottles. Bottle fillers, which can be fitted with a proportioner to acidify, chlorinate, or dispense an additive, are available to bulk-fill bottles within a basket (Fig. 36.14) as are automated uncapping and capping systems that employ air pressure to both dislodge and reapply an integrated cap with sipper tube or a robotic grip mechanism to apply and remove a screw cap. Fully integrated systems that include an uncapper, bottle washer, filler, and capper (Fig. 36.15) are also available.

Articulating robots (also called foundry robots) can be used with a tunnel washer (Fig. 36.16). On the soiled side of the cage wash, the robot's gripper picks up the uppermost row of soiled cages, which have been nested on specially designed pallets. The robot then dumps the cages and places them on the tunnel washer belt. After washing, the robot on the clean side collects the cages from the washer belt, inserts them into an automated bedding dispenser, then removes and stacks the bedded cages onto pallets. Earlier articulating robot installations required the use of an indexed tunnel washer, which has a lower throughput than a continuous belt washer; however, newer systems are available for use with continuous belt-driven washers. Gantry systems, which employ overhead rails or floor-mounted rail systems, have been developed to support functions similar to those of articulating robots. The cage handling components move along rails above or beside each end of the tunnel washer, performing required functions. These systems can be utilized with continuous belt washers, as they employ optical sensing technology to detect cage location and reposition the cages as they exit the clean side of the washer.

H. Security

The value of research animals combined with the increasingly militant activities of those opposing the

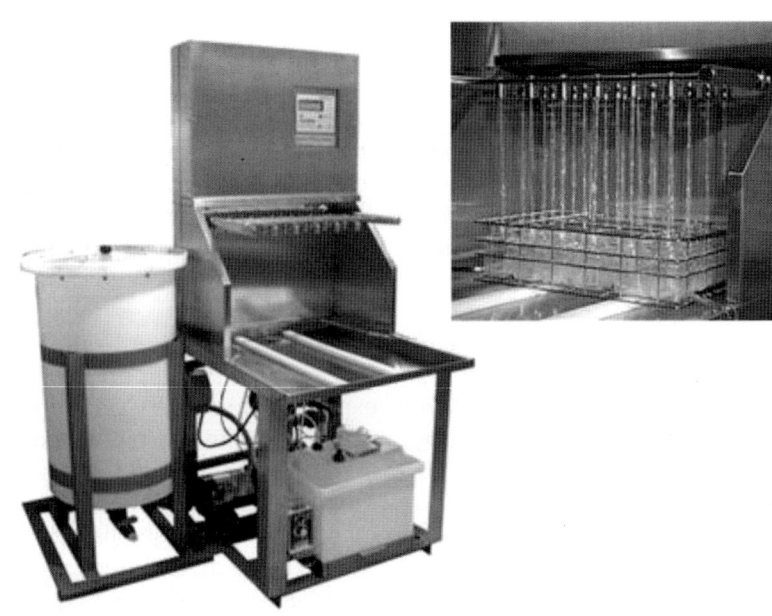

FIGURE 36.14　Bottle filler equipped with a proportioner. *Courtesy of Edstrom Industries, Inc.*

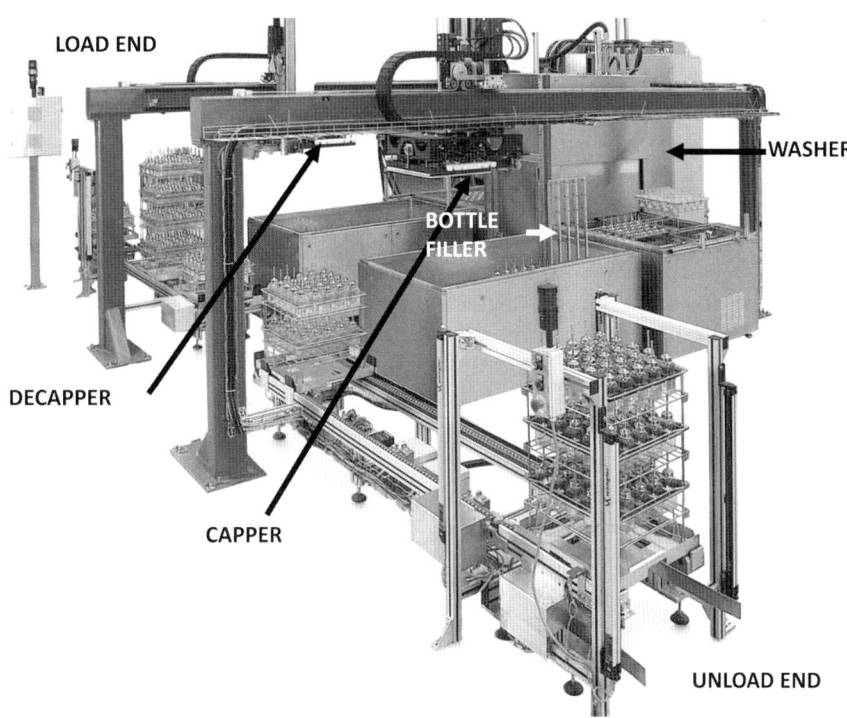

LOAD END

DECAPPER

CAPPER

BOTTLE FILLER

WASHER

UNLOAD END

FIGURE 36.15 Automated rodent bottle handling system. Stacked bottle baskets are loaded onto a conveyor for processing by a gantry-mounted robotic head which will pick up an individual basket, remove the integral sipper tubes/caps from the bottles by pressurizing bottles with air, flip the basket emptying the bottles, and load the bottles and sipper tubes onto a conveyor for washing within an integrated bottle washer. After completion of the washing cycle, another gantry-mounted robotic head collects the sanitized basket with bottles, flips the basket, fills the bottles with water, recaps the bottles, and stacks the baskets for collection from the clean side conveyor. *Courtesy of Tecniplast USA.*

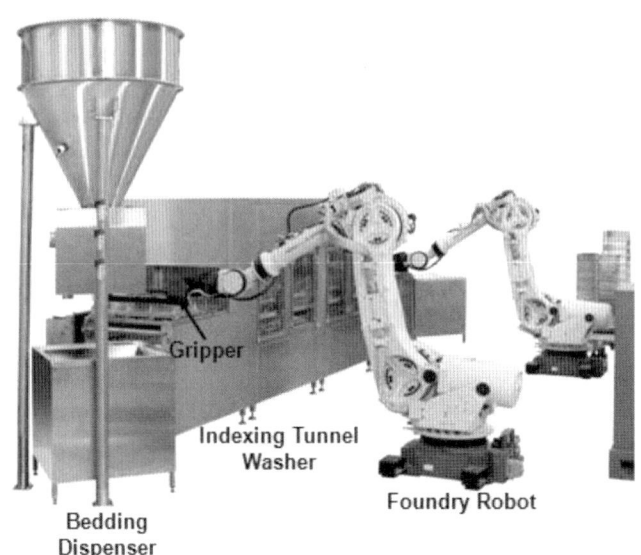

Gripper

Indexing Tunnel Washer

Foundry Robot

Bedding Dispenser

FIGURE 36.16 Image of a tunnel washer served by two foundry robots. The clean side of the tunnel washer with bedding dispenser is seen in the foreground. The clean side robot is collecting three shoebox cages from the washer with its gripper. The robot will turn the cages over, present the cages to the bedding dispenser for filling, and will stack the cages on a pallet. The soiled side robot will collect cages from a pallet, dump the cages, and load them onto the tunnel washer. *Courtesy of Tecniplast USA.*

use of animals in research and safety testing makes a security program a requirement for every animal facility. At a minimum, access to the facility at every entry point should be controlled. Ideally, a multilayered system should be employed, utilizing both external and internal access controls (Mortell, 2010). Cameras with high-quality, wide-angle optics placed at critical locations can be useful as activities can be recorded and reviewed later as necessary. Consideration may be given to security systems that use biometrics (e.g., thumb, palm, or retinal scan; voice recognition) especially for controlling access to areas in which hazardous agents are employed.

Inside the facility, access to animal holding rooms should be limited for the protection of personnel and animal health, as well as research protection. Due to the large number of individuals who require access and the relatively high personnel turnover rate keyed locks and PIN cypher locks are difficult to monitor and control in large research institutions. An automated, microprocessor-controlled system managed by a centralized computer with a user-friendly interface such as a card key or proximity card system allows users to be easily added to or deleted from a database. Additionally, these systems leave an electronic trail (time/date stamp) that is easily traceable if necessary.

I. Commissioning and Validation

Some of the most important aspects of planning, building, and opening a new facility involve commissioning and validation. This is a detailed process that is best facilitated by experienced professionals independent of the architectural and engineering firms and the institution. Commissioning involves challenging, verifying, and documenting the building structure, utilities, systems, and equipment before routine operation is authorized. Validation involves establishing documented evidence that provides a high degree of assurance that a specific test process consistently produces results at predetermined specifications and quality attributes. Detailed protocols should be prepared and tested for every aspect of the facility to document critical component functions as intended. This may include 'open cage' housing of animals in the facility for a period of time to test for pathogenic infections. Recently, environmental sampling of surfaces using PCR technology has become available and has a much greater chance of detecting the presence of DNA or RNA associated with such agents.

III. ENVIRONMENTAL CONTROL AND MONITORING

The provision of a stable environment for the conduct of research is essential to ensure the integrity of the animals and the results obtained. The environment to which animals are exposed must be considered from two perspectives, the *macroenvironment* (MaE) of the room in which the animals are housed and the *microenvironment* (MiE) in the cage with which the animals have direct and prolonged contact. The ME can be vastly different depending upon the species, strain, and number of animals housed, the caging system and bedding employed, and the macroenvironmental conditions (Serrano, 1971; Corning and Lipman, 1991; Hasenau et al., 1993; Perkins and Lipman, 1996; Reeb et al., 1997, 1998). For example, there can be marked differences between the MaE and the MiE when rodents are housed in static isolator cages while, in general, there are minimal differences for large animals housed in pens or open cages.

Extensive effort is devoted to maintaining the temperature, relative humidity (RH), and air quality to which animals are exposed. Guidelines have been established for these parameters (ILAR, 2011). Alterations and fluctuations of environmental conditions are well recognized to influence results in a variety of disciplines.

A. Macroenvironment

The HVAC system is the single most expensive component of a modern vivarium, in both initial acquisition and life cycle costs. Life cycle costs include capital, e.g., acquisition and installation, and operating costs. The system must provide adequate ventilation to provide sufficient oxygen, dilute and remove contaminants, precisely control temperature and humidity, and allow air pressure differentials to be maintained with respect to the environment and created between adjoining spaces. Kowalski et al. (2002) have reviewed the concept of HVAC engineering design and air treatment technology on airborne disease control. Animal facility HVAC systems are commonly usually of the single-duct, constant volume reheat (CVR) type. CVR systems used in vivaria draw in 100% fresh air, then filter, heat or cool, and humidify it before distributing it within the facility. Conditioned air delivered to individual rooms at a constant temperature and humidity is then reheated to the desired temperature at the room level based on the setting of the room's thermostat or more commonly with automated systems, the building automation system/building management system (BAS/BMS). Variable air volume (VAV) systems with reheat are also utilized in animal facilities, as they provide some energy savings as ventilation rates can be tailored to maintain desired environmental conditions. However, energy savings in vivarium VAV systems are frequently less than those attained in other types of installations, as vivarium systems are designed and operated to maintain a minimum number of air changes per hour (ACH), frequently at least 10. ACH are increased above the minimum set point depending on the cooling or heat load. HVAC systems are sized to account for filter loading or the increase in static pressure across system filters which results from debris accumulation. The latest technology employs demand control ventilation systems that monitor select macroenvironmental conditions, e.g., particulate levels and the concentration of organic compounds, and when they fall outside of an established range, interface with the HVAC system to alter room ventilation rates.

Principal HVAC system components include the air handling unit, containing supply fans, various filters, heating and cooling coils, and a humidification manifold; supply distribution ducts; terminal supply devices, each with a reheat coil; supply diffusers; exhaust registers; terminal exhaust devices; exhaust ducts; and exhaust fans. Depending on outside air temperature, incoming air is heated or cooled at the air handling unit before distribution within the facility. The air exiting the air handling unit (discharge temperature) is typically between 55°F and 60°F and reheated by the terminal reheat device, independent of outside air temperature. Grumman (1986) has prepared a useful reference manual that describes HVAC systems and the constituent components.

Intake air is filtered at the air handler. Vivarium air handlers are usually equipped with final particulate filters providing between 85% and 95% dust spot efficiency

(ASHRAE 2008). Prefilters, providing 15–30% efficiency, and sometimes bag filters, providing 60–85% efficiency, are employed to extend the life of the final filter. Depending on the location, particulate filters may be supplemented with activated carbon filters to remove volatile contaminants. However, activated carbon filters have limitations in that their retention capabilities vary by substance, it is challenging to determine when they are fully loaded, and moisture can substantially reduce their useful life. In certain applications, e.g., high-level barriers, operating rooms, or containment suites, HEPA filtration may be desirable on air supply and/or exhaust (Kowalski *et al.*, 2002). HEPA filters are at least 99.97% efficient filtering 0.3-μm-diameter particles. They are more effective capturing particles smaller and larger than 0.3 μm. HEPA filters rely on three mechanisms to achieve their stated efficiency – interception, impaction, and diffusion. As the principal barrier is most frequently implemented at the cage level for rodents when ventilated caging systems are used, HEPA filtration is often included on the supply blowers to supplement the filtration provided by the HVAC system. HEPA filters are also employed in animal changing stations or BSCs utilized for cage changing and animal manipulation.

HVAC system redundancy providing additional capacity beyond that required for normal operations is critical to ensuring environmental conditions are maintained when system components require maintenance, repair, or replacement, or as a result of total system failure. This is achieved by providing additional capacity in critical system components, often by dividing the systems into parallel units with separate air handlers, chillers, heat sources, and control systems. There are many approaches to providing redundancy. The most common being $N + 1$ redundancy in which critical components have at least one independent backup. Another option is cross-connection with other lower priority sources whose support can be sacrificed in times of need.

Providing emergency power to maintain all essential vivarium services, the most critical being life safety (human) and the HVAC system is essential. Ensuring adequate ventilation and MaE temperature control in the event of power loss is necessary to sustain animal life and minimize the impact of MaE fluctuation on the animals. In larger facilities, it is often necessary to prioritize HVAC support to animal holding and other critical areas. This may be accompanied by a reduction of ventilation rates; however, HVAC support must be sufficient to prevent exposure of animals to temperature extremes. Ventilated caging, aquatic life support, environmental monitoring, and security systems should also be served by emergency power.

Modern animal facility HVAC systems employ pressure independent terminal supply and exhaust devices to maintain constant supply or exhaust air volumes,

independent of fluctuations occurring in room or duct pressure. These devices ensure that appropriate room air pressure differentials are maintained. Two general types of terminal devices are available: (1) devices that measure airflow using an in-line sensor which feedback to a control device to maintain a constant volume of air. The control device is either a motorized butterfly damper or, alternatively, pneumatically inflatable/deflatable vanes; and (2) mechanical venturi-type air valves, commonly referred to as Phoenix valves. These devices are set to consistently supply or exhaust a preset airflow rate to create a differential pressure between the area being ventilated and the contiguous space, most likely the corridor serving the area. Positive space pressure is achieved by supplying more air to the space than is exhausted, and *vice versa*, to create a negative pressure differential. Air moves along a pressure gradient in an attempt to establish neutral pressure. In positively ventilated spaces, excess air flows out of the space to the adjoining negative pressure space. The directional movement of air decreases the likelihood of particulates that might serve as fomites, or infectious agents or volatile chemicals used within the space, entering or exiting. The velocity of the air into or out of the space and the static pressure differential between the two spaces are dependent upon the integrity of the space, the number of access points (i.e., doors and access panels) into the space, the volume of air supplied to the room, and the difference between supply and exhaust air volumes. Leaky rooms with numerous openings from which air can escape attain lower static differential pressures and lower airflows than those that are more tightly sealed. It is important to recognize that both features are lost whenever the door to the room is ajar. The static pressure differential is maintained at between 0.02 inches and 0.08 inches of water column (WC). Higher static pressures are desirable for quarantine and hazardous use areas. If static pressure differentials become excessive, e.g., $\pm$ 0.25 inches WC, it may be extremely difficult to open or close doors. There are two methods used to maintain differential air pressures in a modern HVAC system: (1) *volumetric flow tracking*, whereby the BAS/BMS adjusts the terminal devices to maintain a set differential in supply and exhaust air volumes, or (2) *direct pressure control*, in which pressure sensors in the space provide data to the BAS/BMS which subsequently adjusts the terminal devices to maintain the desired pressure.

Although the *Guide* permits selective recirculation of air, this is rarely done (ILAR, 2011). Holding room ventilation rates are based upon several factors, the most important being heat load. The heat loads generated by various species of animals are available (ASHRAE, 2003). In holding rooms with high-density rodent housing, the animals are by far the most significant heat source. These holding rooms are commonly ventilated with 100% fresh air at 10–20 ACH. Rates exceeding 100 ACH may be utilized in rooms or cubicles housing animals exposed to hazardous agents, especially volatile agents where dilution is important for hazard control. Air velocities should not exceed 0.25 m/s at an elevation of 1.8 M, especially when not using filter tops (National Institutes of Health design policy and guidelines, 2003). Other heat load sources commonly encountered in animal facilities include the sun, lighting, personnel, and equipment.

1. Temperature

Provision of MaE temperature within a specified and narrow range is essential. Temperature is the single most important environmental parameter to be controlled, as excursions outside of established ranges and fluctuations can cause clinical signs or death, and/or influence experimental results (reviewed in Chapter 29). It is well recognized that some species, especially rats and mice, have limited capability to thermoregulate, especially when they are exposed to elevated temperatures. Although they can increase perfusion to peripheral tissues, in particular their tail and pinnae, and increase their respiratory rate and wet their fur with saliva, which leads to evaporative heat loss, MaE temperatures potentially as low as 80°F can result in mortality, depending on an animal's genetic background, its age, and/or the experimental procedures to which it has been subjected.

Temperature set point selection in animal holding rooms is a compromise between the temperature most comfortable for personnel and that preferred by the animals. Personnel often prefer lower room temperatures, especially when donning PPE commonly worn in barrier facilities, compared with the higher temperatures preferred by animals (Gordon, 1998). Mice and rats prefer higher temperatures when they are singly housed and the selected temperature is affected by the bedding material used and the availability of nesting material. Animal holding room temperature set points are typically 72–74°F. It is recommended that rooms housing hairless rodent strains, such as nude mice and rats, be maintained at 78–82°F (Gullino et al., 1976). Alternatively, or in addition, the provision of nesting material permits rodents to thermoregulate. Modern, properly designed HVAC systems should be capable of maintaining room temperature within ± 2°F of the set point. Some species, most notably rabbits, prefer lower ambient temperatures and rabbit holding rooms are preferably maintained at 66–68°F. Depending on the number of holding rooms required to accommodate rabbits and the HVAC system design, most notably the discharge temperature of the air handler, terminal cold water coils or supplemental room chillers may be needed to maintain the desired temperature.

Although select MiE conditions can differ dramatically from those in the MaE, temperature differences observed in both static and ventilated isolator cages are biologically insignificant for most studies; they vary by only a few degrees, as plastic polymers used in caging are conductive to heat and present a large surface area for heat exchange, and blowers used in ventilated caging systems generate relatively small heat loads, especially when compared with the animals themselves (Corning and Lipman, 1991; Hasenau et al., 1993; Perkins and Lipman, 1996). Further, the modest increase in MiE temperature is closer to that preferred by mice, and reflects the stability of MaE temperature control (Gordon, 1998).

2. Relative Humidity

Maintaining stable air moisture content is extremely challenging, especially in temperate regions where seasonal and daily excursions in RH can be dramatic. Humidity control is achieved by adding moisture to the supply air stream when ambient humidity is below the desirable level, or removing excess moisture when it exceeds it. Both processes can be challenging. Humidification is achieved by either injecting steam or atomizing water into the supply air stream (Grumman, 1986). A humidistat (more than one can be used) monitors moisture content and feeds back to the steam injector or atomizer to control the amount of moisture added to the system. Humidification systems can be installed by zone or room. Zone systems are preferred for most holding facilities, as individual room humidity control is unnecessary and the systems are maintenance-intensive. However, some species, such as select non-human primate species, e.g., *Macaca fasicularis*, require higher levels of air humidification to ensure their clinical health and therefore individual room or supplemental room humidification may be necessary (Van de Woude and Luzarraga, 1991). Consideration must be given to the duct distribution pattern downstream of the humidifier to reduce the likelihood of condensation within the ducts, and to the location of the humidifier with respect to heating and cooling coils in the air handling unit as well as chemical additives in the steam and water used for humidification. Dehumidification is achieved by lowering the temperature of the supply air as it passes over a cooling coil in the air handler. As the temperature of the air decreases, depending on its moisture content and the temperature of the coil, its dew point is exceeded resulting in moisture condensation. The air when reheated as it is supplied to the room will contain less moisture and therefore a lower RH.

3. Lighting

Light intensity and periodicity are of critical importance to a host of physiologic and behavioral processes, most notably reproductive function (Brainard et al., 1997;

Cherry, 1987; Drickamer, 1977, 1982, 1984, 1990a,b). The standard source of lighting in animal rooms is lighting from recessed or surface-mounted fluorescent ceiling fixtures with water-resistant or watertight, gasketed lenses. High-efficiency light-emitting diode lamps are replacing fluorescent lamps in some facilities; however, the lamps and fixtures are currently more expensive requiring a careful cost analysis. An appropriately designed and operating system is critical.

The effect of light intensity and duration of exposure on retinal degeneration in albino rodents is also well recognized (Weihe, 1976). Intracage light intensity may differ as much as 80-fold in transparent plastic cages from the top to the bottom of a rack when illumination is provided by ceiling fixtures, and differences in phototoxic retinopathy among animals in the same room have been attributed to rack position (Weihe et al., 1969; Greenman et al., 1982). In small areas, such as cubicles, vertical installation of lighting fixtures in the corners of the area is preferred in order to obtain better distribution of light within the space. Current recommendations for light intensity at the cage level are between 130 and 325 lux, unless animals were raised at extremely low levels (6 lux), in which case lower levels may be required (Semple-Rowland, 1987a,b; ILAR, 2011). Illumination at 325 lux is considered adequate for providing routine animal care (Bellhorn, 1980).

A 12-h light:12-h dark (L:D) cycle is most commonly used for most species. However, longer photoperiods (14:10) are preferred by some laboratories for breeding rodents and zebrafish (Mulder, 1971; Harper and Lawrence, 2011). Periodicity is controlled by either a mechanical or an electronic timer, one dedicated timer per room, or the BAS/BMS. Of the three mechanisms, mechanical timers are the most likely to malfunction. Although continuous dark cycles are unlikely to go undetected, the provision of continuous illumination for varying periods may go unnoticed unless they are monitored. Continuous lighting has an overstimulating effect on reproduction, leading to cessation of cycling, permanent vaginal cornification, and development of excess ovarian follicles (Hoffman, 1973; Weihe, 1976). Exposure to as little as 0.2 lux of light during the dark phase of the cycle can reset the circadian rhythm and potentially have an impact on tumor models (Brainard et al., 1983; Dauchy et al., 1997). For that reason, red lamps may be used for lighting during the dark phase, when dark cycle light exposure is problematic. Red lamps are utilized to provide sufficient lighting for human observation of mice during the dark phase when using reverse light cycles that allow the nocturnal (dark) phase of the light cycle to coincide with the human workday. The use of sodium lamps, which emit light at 589 and 589.6 nm, have been promoted in lieu of red lights (McLennan and Taylor-Jeffs, 2004). The emission spectra of sodium

lamps are not detectable to mice but provide excellent visual acuity to humans. Care must also be taken to ensure that task lighting and lamps within cage changing stations or BSCs do not remain on during the dark phase. In addition, coated (red-tint) glass which filters light of the wavelengths detectable by rodents is recommended for use in rodent room door glazing to prevent stray light from the corridor serving the room from disturbing the animals. Mice and rats cannot see light from the low (650 nm red) end of the visible spectrum. Full spectrum lamps, i.e., lamps that emit wavelengths resembling natural daylight, are desirable for select species, e.g., specific amphibians, although they are not routinely employed for all species. When using these lamps, attention must be given to the fixture's lens/diffuser as some will inhibit transmission of UV spectra.

The spectral quality of the lamps selected for use in the vivarium must also be considered, as it may directly influence the ability of personnel to perform particular animal-related activities, such as examining the vulva for signs of estrus or checking plugs; it also has an impact on electrical consumption and may influence the well-being of staff. There is no preferred color. In addition, lamp color selection may differ depending on the specific area to be illuminated. Marshall (1991) has concisely reviewed this topic as it relates to animal facility lighting.

Rodent holding rooms are provided with two-level illumination during the light phase of the cycle: low-intensity lighting when personnel are not present and high-intensity lighting when personnel are attending to the animals. Control can be accomplished in a variety of ways. Most commonly, distinct lamps in multiple-lamp fixtures are controlled separately. For example, 50% of the lamps could be controlled by a timer set to provide the established light cycle, whereas the remaining lamps are controlled by an occupancy sensor or manually activated timer that turns on the remaining lamps when personnel are in the room. The device controlling the second lamp set is equipped with a time-out feature that automatically turns off the lamps after a prescribed interval. Three lamp fixtures can also be employed, a setup in which two of the lamps are controlled as just described while the remaining lamp, a red bulb, is activated only during the dark phase of the cycle. Indicator lamps and/or the provision of light detection by the environmental monitoring system should be provided to ensure lights do not remain on for an extended period of time during the dark phase of the lighting cycle without detection.

4. Noise

The impact of noise on both the physiology and the behavior of laboratory mice is well recognized (Peterson, 1980; reviewed in Chapter 29). The hearing range of animals may be distinctly different from that of humans,

e.g., as many rodents can detect and communicate using ultrasound (>20 kHz), their peak audible range is higher compared with that of humans, and they are incapable of hearing low-frequency sounds (<0.2 KHz (rat); <1 kHz (mouse)) that are audible to humans (Clough and Fasham, 1975; Heffner and Heffner, 2007). The ability of sound to induce audiogenic seizures, especially in susceptible mouse strains such as AKR, BALB/c, CBA, C57, and DBA/2, has been well documented and, in some strains, is age dependent (Clough, 1982). The FVB strain used extensively in transgenic production was shown to develop an often lethal epileptic syndrome that can be induced by noise (Goelz et al., 1998). Of greatest concern is the production of ultrasound, which is audible to some species but undetectable to humans, within the animal facility. Human activity within animal rooms has been shown to generate ultrasound, as can running water and equipment such as cage washers, video display terminals, and oscilloscopes (Sales et al., 1988; Milligan et al., 1993). The increasing and common use of ventilated caging systems, as well as laminar flow and BSCs within animal holding rooms, heightens concerns regarding noise generation in both the MaE and the MiE (Perkins and Lipman, 1996). Fire alarm annunciators produce noise that may disturb animals. An annunciator that produces sound below the auditory threshold of mice has been developed (Clough and Fasham, 1975).

Anthony (1962) recommended that noise in animal facilities not exceed 85 dB, a level equivalent to the current 8-h time-weighted average (TWA) established for human occupational exposure (American Conference of Governmental Industrial Hygienists, 2004). Designing and operating rodent holding rooms at or below the noise criteria (NC)-40 level has been recommended (Pekrul, 1991). The NIH's Design Requirements Manual for Biomedical Laboratories and Animal Research Facilities recommends that animal holding rooms not exceed NC-45 (National Institutes of Health 2008). An NC level, based upon the response of humans to noise, defines the highest sound level permissible for each of eight octave bands, which divide the audible noise spectrum into equal ranges. Rodent holding rooms should be situated away from those housing noise-generating species and equipment. If separation is not possible, creating a buffer zone by interposing rooms or spaces containing noise-insensitive activities or using sound-isolating partitions can be considered. Washable panels containing acoustic absorbing materials are also available.

5. Environmental Monitoring

An automated environmental monitoring system is highly desirable to monitor select parameters within animal holding rooms and other critical vivarium locations. BAS/BMS providers offer monitoring as a system component. Alternatively, stand-alone, independent systems are also available. Although a variety of environmental parameters, including temperature, humidity, supply and exhaust air volumes, room pressure differentials, and light periodicity and intensity, can be monitored, the authors recommend minimally monitoring temperature and light periodicity/intensity in each and RH in a representative number of animal holding rooms, in particular rooms housing species sensitive to low RH. Modest excursions in temperature may significantly alter experimental results or even result in morbidity, while malfunctioning lighting can quickly impair breeding or alter a host of physiologic parameters (reviewed in Chapter 29). In addition, systems can monitor various other functions, including equipment such as ventilated cage rack blowers, electrical power, and/or HVAC components. Environmental monitoring can be integrated into the security system.

Ideally, the monitoring system should be fully automated and should alert facility personnel by local and/or remote alarm, telephone, e-mail, and/or pager when environmental conditions fall outside of established ranges. Alarms should escalate with increasing deviation in the monitored condition and re-alarm at fixed intervals if the condition does not return to its pre-alarm level. When temperature monitoring is provided as a component of the BAS/BMS, the authors recommend installation of a redundant thermostat, independent of the device controlling the reheat coil, to be used for monitoring. This is to avoid a situation in which a single malfunctioning thermostat, serving both control and monitoring functions, leads to abnormal room temperatures while indicating that the new 'abnormal' temperature is at or near the set point. The second thermostat is used to activate an alarm, or, alternatively, a prescribed difference in temperature between the two devices is used to generate an alarm signal. Importantly, the reheat coil should fail closed to prevent room overheating, which is generally more problematic than low room temperatures for most laboratory animal species.

Other areas for monitoring consideration include aquatic life support system components such as pumps and filters as well as select water quality conditions, e.g., temperature, conductivity, and dissolved gasses; feed storage for temperature; and cage wash and areas used for containment for air pressure differential to ensure contagion and hazard control.

B. Microenvironment

The MiE or physical environment to which the animal is directly and continuously exposed has become more important than the MaE especially for rodents since the advent and widespread implementation of microisolator cages for rodent housing during the past 20 years.

Although MaE conditions clearly influence the MiE, conditions at the cage level are influenced by a host of additional factors, including the animals, the caging system employed, and the use and type of contact bedding (Serrano, 1971; Corning and Lipman, 1991; Hasenau et al., 1993; Choi et al. 1994; Perkins and Lipman, 1995, 1996; Reeb et al. 1997, 1998). The MiE in cages is often significantly different from that found in the MaE (Serrano, 1971; Corning and Lipman, 1991; Hasenau et al., 1993; Perkins and Lipman, 1995, 1996). These differences, especially in static microisolator (MI) caging systems, have driven, to a considerable degree, the transition to ventilated caging systems.

The modern filter top consisting of a plastic frame and a filter insert, employed to prevent particulate transfer to and from the cage, reducing contagion transmission as well as containing allergenic proteins, also serves as a significant barrier to air, gas, and moisture exchange (Keller et al., 1989; Sakaguchi et al., 1990; Perkins and Lipman, 1995,1996). MiE moisture content, as well as ammonia and carbon dioxide concentrations, may be significantly higher than that found in the MaE in static MI cages (Serrano, 1971; Corning and Lipman, 1991; Hasenau et al., 1993; Choi et al., 1994; Perkins and Lipman, 1995). The more effective the filter top is as a barrier to particulates, the greater the impact on MiE conditions (Serrano, 1971; Corning and Lipman, 1991). MiE RH may be up to 38% greater than MaE RH, and this difference is most pronounced when cages are housed at lower MaE RH in static MI cages (Corning and Lipman, 1991; Hasenau et al., 1993; Choi et al., 1994). The principal impact of higher MiE RH is on MiE ammonia (NH_3) concentration. The higher the MaE RH, the higher the MiE RH, and subsequently the earlier MiE NH_3 is detectable after cage change. The peak concentration of NH_3 attained is also higher with elevated MaE RH. NH_3 may exceed 350 ppm within 7 days in static MI cages, depending on the bedding used and the MaE RH (Corning and Lipman, 1991).

NH_3 is formed by urease-producing bacteria or bedding containing heat-labile urealytic and urease-activating enzymes, which convert urea into NH_3 (Gale and Smith, 1981). NH_3 accumulation is not a concern when housing axenic or gnotobiotic animals with flora devoid of urease-producing bacteria on autoclaved bedding. There appears to be a critical MaE RH threshold, which is bedding-dependent, above which NH_3 accumulates to a marked level within 7 days in a static MI cage. For pine shavings, the level appears to be ~50% MaE RH, whereas for corncob bedding it appears to be significantly higher, ~70% MaE RH (Lipman and Perkins, 1995; Lipman, 1999). MiE NH_3 concentrations may exceed, by as much as 14-fold, limits (25 ppm 8-h TWA) established by the American Conference of Governmental Industrial Hygienists (2004) for human exposure in the workplace.

Physiologic alterations and interference with research are possible at NH_3 concentrations observed in static isolator cages (Broderson et al., 1976; Gordon et al., 1980; Schoeb et al., 1982; Walzer et al., 1989; Manninen et al., 1998). Humane concerns have also been raised, as NH_3 is a mucous membrane irritant (Lipman, 1992). There is no standard for acceptable MiE NH_3 concentrations in mouse cages. The *Guide* does not provide specific recommendations for acceptable levels of NH_3 (ILAR, 2011). However, the Institute of Laboratory Animal Resources (ILAR) document *Laboratory Animal Management: Rodents* states that "inspired air should contain no more than 25 ppm of NH_3" (Lang et al., 1977). A concentration less than the ACGIH 8-h TWA may be appropriate, as laboratory mice reside in their cages for 24 h a day, 7 days per week, and subtle effects may influence research results (Lipman, 1992). Others have argued that concentrations established for humans are irrelevant and perhaps too low, since wild mice live in burrows in which they may be exposed to high NH_3 concentrations (Reeb-Whitaker et al., 2001). In comparing NH_3 tolerance among species, mice tolerate an intermediate range between humans, which are NH_3 intolerant, and more tolerant species such as bats (Studier et al., 1967; Kapeghian et al., 1982; Reeb-Whitaker et al., 2001). It is interesting to note that the response of mice to ammonia is strain-dependent (Barrows et al., 1978; Tomas et al., 1985).

MiE carbon dioxide (CO_2) concentrations are also markedly elevated in static MI cages, although the biological significance of the elevation is unclear. MiE CO_2 concentrations have been reported which are up to 4000 ppm higher than those measured in the MaE when using static isolators (Lipman and Corning, 1991). Although these concentrations do not exceed the ACGIH exposure limits of 5000 ppm established as an 8-h TWA (American Conference of Governmental Industrial Hygienists, 2004), CO_2 is a respiratory and cardiovascular stimulant and acts as an asphyxiant by displacing oxygen.

Other MiE contaminants have also been detected. An uncharacterized pollutant was suspected while evaluating the effects of inhaled methyl bromide in rats housed in suspended wire-mesh caging, whereas sulfur dioxide and acetic acid, presumably off-gassed from corncob bedding and methane and hydrogen sulfide, were all detected in isolator cages (Bolon et al., 1991; Huerkamp and Lehner, 1994a, 1994b; Perkins and Lipman, 1995).

Although MiE temperatures tend to be elevated in MI cages and increase with additional cage occupants and the use of ventilated caging systems that employ a heat-generating supply blower, the increases observed are modest (~1–2°F) and are not presumed to be of biological significance (Corning and Lipman, 1991; Hasenau et al., 1993; Lipman, 1992).

IV. HOUSING AND EQUIPMENT

A. Materials

Consideration for animal comfort and adequate sanitation are paramount in the design of housing systems and selection of fabrication materials. Resistance to degradation from animal waste and chemicals used for sanitation and disinfection is critical to the longevity of equipment and surfaces. Stainless steel (304 or 316) is by far the most common metal, although aluminum is occasionally used in metal cage and rack construction. The difference between 304 and 316 stainless steel is based on the amount of chromium and nickel in the alloy; molybdenum is added to 316 stainless steel to increase its corrosion resistance. While galvanized steel has and occasionally continues to be used in select applications, e.g., when chain-link fencing is used in pen or run construction, elevated zinc levels and alopecia and achromotrichia have been reported in nonhuman primates housed in galvanized cages (Obeck, 1978). Thermoplastics are used widely in animal housing systems especially for rodents and aquatic species. A variety of plastic polymers are used including polycarbonate (Lexan® or Macrolon®), polyphthalate carbonate (high-temperature polycarbonate), polyetherimide (Ultem®), polysulfone (Udel®), and polyphenyl-sulfone (Radel R®). Each polymer differs with respect to resistance to deterioration from chemical and heat exposure, impact strength, and cost. Polyethylene terephthalate (PET) plastic is commonly used to produce disposable caging. Recently, concerns have been raised in relation to several plastic polymers including polycarbonate, polyphthalate carbonate, and polysulfone, which are used in cage construction. A constituent of these polymers, bisphenol A (BPA), may be released from cages and bottles made of these polymers that is either an un-polymerized constituent or as a result of their degradation (Koehler et al., 2003). Degradation is most likely to occur as a result of hydrolysis at high temperatures; however, Howdeshell et al. (2003) have observed that as polycarbonate cages age there is a marked increase of BPA leaching at room temperatures.

Thermoplastic, in combination with stainless steel, is now commonly used in rabbit and guinea pig caging, where the bottom of the cage, referred to as the sleeve and the component with which the animal has direct and constant contact, is manufactured from plastic and is perforated, while the upper sections of the cage, the door, and the rack from which the cages are suspended over a waste collection pan that is often lined with absorbent paper or bedding material, are usually manufactured from stainless steel. This plastic provides greater warmth and comfort as well as preferred acoustical properties, whereas the metal provides for ease of sanitation and durability.

Expanded metal, metal bars, and wire have long been used as flooring material for housing dogs, swine, sheep, and goats. Polyvinyl chloride-coated expanded metal, molded plastic mesh and fiberglass-slatted flooring have replaced bare metal floors to ensure animal comfort. Coated aluminum is preferred to steel as it is lower in weight and easier to handle (Mench and Krulisch, 1990). Dogs and cats cannot be housed on wire less than or equal to ⅛ inch diameter unless it is plastic or fiberglass coated (USDA-APHIS (U.S. Department of Agriculture, Animal and Plant Health Inspection Service), 1998). The size of the openings or space between slats should be appropriate for the species housed. Openings of ½ inch are recommended for hoofed species (Casebolt, 2009). Small openings are recommended to prevent entrapment of dog toes. Interdigital cysts in beagles were shown to be associated with flat-bar polyvinyl chloride-coated as compared with flat-bar-uncoated stainless steel or diamond-shaped expanded metal polyvinyl chloride-coated floors (Kovacs et al., 2005). When housing directly on monolithic floors with or without contact bedding, flooring should have sufficient texture to provide adequate footing. Texture is most commonly created by adding various amounts of sand or an equivalent material to the flooring's surface coat.

B. Caging, Housing Systems, and Specialized Equipment

There are a wide variety of fixed and mobile housing systems available to house terrestrial and aquatic laboratory animals. For terrestrial species, the pen is the most common fixed cage type utilized in which the animals are housed directly on the floor, with or without contact bedding, or on a raised floor. With special appropriate modifications, floor pens are suitable for housing dogs, cats, livestock, rabbits, nonhuman primates, and adult chickens, as examples. Pen sizes vary based on the species and numbers of animals housed but typically measure between 0.9 and 1.8m (3–6ft) deep by 1.8–3.6m (6–12ft) wide. They are usually cleaned in situ, although modular and collapsible pens are available that permit disassembly/collapse and transport to cage wash for sanitization in a mechanical washer. Systems that house aquatic species containing multiple tanks or aquaria are typically fixed as they require hard-plumbed connections.

Most housing systems consist of multiple cages (tanks) suspended from or sitting on the shelves of a mobile (fixed) rack. Cages for some species are sometimes constructed as an integrated nonremovable part of the rack. For planning, racks typically measure approximately 0.6m (2ft) deep by 1.5–1.8m (5–6ft) wide, and up to 2.3m (7.5ft) high. Exceptions are dog and nonhuman primate cages that may be up to 0.9m (3ft) deep with similar width and height. Additional information on housing systems for various non-rodent species is available (Hessler and Lehner, 2009).

1. Rodent Housing Systems

Rodents are most commonly housed on various types of contact bedding in thermoplastic shoebox cages. Alternatively, wire bottom cages suspended over a litter pan have been used historically for rodents employed in toxicology, although there has been a shift away from these types of systems because of animal welfare concerns as these cages may cause foot lesions and, when given the choice, rodents prefer solid bottom cages with bedding (Blom et al., 1996; Manser et al., 1995, 1996).

a. Static MI Cages

The evolution of rodent caging systems escalated rapidly during the past two decades of the twentieth century. In the early 1980s, a pioneering new filter top design was introduced (Sedlacek et al., 1981). Although filter tops had been available and used for several decades after Lisbeth Kraft first demonstrated the effectiveness of isolator caging for the control of epidemic diarrhea of infant mice, these early designs had shortcomings (Kraft, 1958; Kraft et al., 1964; Serrano, 1971). The Sedlacek-designed static MI cage was marketed commercially and was widely implemented within the United States. Its introduction occurred as conventional rodents were being replaced by SPF animals and irreplaceable genetically engineered mouse colonies were rapidly expanding. Although the cage was highly effective for disease control and containment, it became quickly apparent that MiE conditions within the cage declined rapidly after cage change. While poor MiE air quality was a concern with earlier filter lid designs, air quality was inferior in the Sedlacek-designed MI cage (Lipman and Corning, 1991; Hasenau et al., 1993). Shortly after the introduction of this new static MI cage, a second commercial static MI cage was made available with greater filter surface area. No substantial differences in MiE air quality were observed when comparing the two systems (Lipman and Corning, 1991). The reasons were clear, as smoke and tracer gas studies had demonstrated that air exchange in static MI cages occurs primarily at the cage–lid interface, not at the filter, and air exchange rates in static MI cages were markedly reduced, compared with open cages (Keller et al., 1989).

Static MI cages, despite their disadvantages, have an important role in rodent housing. They are useful for studies in which containment at the cage level is desirable (Bhatt and Jacoby, 1983). Static MIs also retain allergenic proteins within the cage, reducing their levels in the MaE (Sakaguchi et al., 1990). Static MIs can be placed in a secondary enclosure such as a negative flow mass air displacement unit (MADU), a BSC, or a chemical hood for an additional level of containment. When used for hazardous agent containment, static MIs should be opened, and the contaminated animals and cage contents handled, within an appropriate BSC or chemical hood, depending on the hazard employed.

There are four principal ways of affecting poor MiE air quality, notably the accumulation of intracage NH_3 in static MIs: (1) change cages at sufficient frequencies (Corning and Lipman, 1991); (2) utilize a contact bedding with better performance characteristics (Perkins and Lipman, 1995; Smith et al., 2004); (3) reduce MaE RH levels (Corning and Lipman, 1991); and/or (4) increase MaE temperature without altering the moisture content in the air, thereby decreasing MiE RH (Memarzadeh, 1998). Nevertheless, static MIs can influence the biology of the animals housed within. As an example, Baer et al. (1997) observed that the growth rate of mice housed in static MIs for 1-week periods was significantly greater than for those housed in cages without a lid.

b. Ventilated Caging Systems

Concerns regarding poor MiE air quality in static MIs, while at the same time the demand for mouse housing was burgeoning in the 1980s and 1990s, served as major stimuli for the development of and transition to individually ventilated caging (IVC) systems from static MIs. IVCs offer numerous advantages over static systems in addition to dramatically improving MiE air quality (Keller et al., 1983; Wu et al., 1985; Lipman, 1992; Iwarsson and Noren, 1992; Choi et al., 1994; Huerkamp and Lehner, 1994a, 1994b; Yoshida and Tajima, 1995; Perkins and Lipman, 1996). The concentration of both intracage NH_3 and CO_2 is considerably lower in IVCs when compared with static MIs maintained under the same MaE conditions. Further, the day on which NH_3 is first detected is delayed in IVCs. Not only is the intracage air quality improved, the variability in MiE air quality observed among static MIs housed in the same MaE is reduced or eliminated in IVCs (Perkins and Lipman, 1996). As less NH_3 is generated in ventilated cages, air quality is improved for personnel working in animal holding rooms and cage wash. In most facilities, IVC changing is delayed to weekly or even longer, depending on the strains of mice housed, their experimental use, housing density, and institutional perspective (Reeb et al., 1998). In contrast to static MIs, which may require twice-weekly changing, a weekly or longer cage change interval translates to considerable labor savings. In addition to the time-saved changing and sanitizing cages, the quantity of bedding used is also reduced and the longevity of cage components, especially those made of thermoplastic and autoclaved, is also increased, resulting in substantial operational savings.

Another significant advantage of IVCs is the opportunity to markedly increase stocking density when they are employed. In contrast to static MIs housed on a shelf rack, IVCs can house up to 100% more animals, depending on the systems compared, while occupying the same footprint. IVCs can markedly increase housing capacity, permitting institutions to substantially decrease space dedicated to animal housing or house considerably more animals in the space available. As the MiE air volume is considerably smaller than that of the MaE, the MiE can be ventilated at higher rates using less supply air than is needed to ventilate the MaE. This feature, along with the capability of exhausting IVC rack effluent, which contains a considerable component of the thermal load generated by the animals, directly into the building's HVAC system, allows for the potential of using lower air exchange rates to ventilate mouse holding rooms (Lipman, 1993; Clough et al., 1995).

IVCs can also provide, depending on the specific system used, an additional protective barrier to animals housed within the cage (Cunliffe-Beamer and Les, 1983; Lipman et al., 1993). Systems pressurizing the cage with HEPA-filtered supply air provide cage occupants with an additional level of protection from contamination. The effectiveness of IVCs has been demonstrated experimentally using MHV (Lipman et al., 1993).

Although the available IVCs have the common goal of improving intracage ventilation and, therefore, MiE conditions, manufacturers have approached this goal using a variety of design concepts. IVCs have been characterized into two principal classes on the basis on their operating design: (1) intracage supply/perimeter capture and (2) intracage supply/intracage exhaust systems (Lipman, 1999). The latter group can be further divided into direct, indirect, and combination subtypes, depending on whether the supply or exhaust air passes through a filter, at the level of the cage, before entering or exiting the cage. Fig. 36.17A–F provides schematic representations of the various systems.

i. INTRACAGE SUPPLY/PERIMETER CAPTURE
HEPA-filtered air is supplied directly at the level of the cage, resulting in its pressurization. Cage-effluent escapes primarily at the filter top/shoebox cage interface and is captured at the interface and also in the filter by a three-sided U-shaped channel or a canopy. These systems can be operated only in the positive pressure mode. Select independent experimental evaluations have been published on this system type (Choi et al., 1994; Huerkamp and Lehner, 1994a, 1994b; Huerkamp et al., 1994; Perkins and Lipman, 1996; Tu et al., 1997).

ii. INTRACAGE SUPPLY/INTRACAGE EXHAUST (DIRECT)
Air is supplied directly to the cage lid or bottom and exhausted directly from the lid or from a plenum beneath the cage. Many of these systems can be operated in either positive or negative pressure mode by altering the quantity of supply and exhaust air by adjusting blower speed. Independent evaluations of this system type have been published (Hoglund and Renstrom, 2001; Renstrom et al., 2001; Baumans et al., 2002).

iii. INTRACAGE SUPPLY/INTRACAGE EXHAUST (INDIRECT)
These provide supply air and remove exhaust, through a filter in the cage lid which resides directly below a positive and negative plenum or duct. Supply air passes under pressure from the plenum or duct through the filter into the cage, while the reverse occurs for exhaust. Systems can be operated in either a positive or a negative pressure mode by altering the position of dampers manually or electronically altering the quantity of supply and exhaust air by adjusting blower speed and/or the pressure drop across control valves situated in the supply and exhaust ducts. Independent evaluations of this system type have been published (Perkins and Lipman, 1996; Huerkamp and Lehner, 1994a, 1994b; Clough et al., 1995; Tu et al., 1997; Reeb et al., 1998; Hoglund and Renstrom, 2001; Reeb-Whitaker et al., 2001; Renstrom et al., 2001).

iv. INTRACAGE SUPPLY/INTRACAGE EXHAUST (COMBINATION)
A valve(s) on the isolator top is actuated when the cage is placed on the rack and closed when the cage is removed. The valve, which is placed on the supply, provides direct inflow of air, circumventing the filter in the lid, maintaining intracage positive pressure.

IVCs can be integrated into facilities through a variety of methods. Depending on whether the supply air is provided directly from the building's HVAC system, or exhaust is evacuated directly into the system, energy cost reduction may be achieved. Methods of integrating IVCs into facilities have been reviewed (Lipman, 1993; Phoenix Controls Corporation, 2003). Further, the HVAC system can be used to provide supply and exhaust air to the IVC, eliminating the need for independent supply and exhaust blowers; however, this method of installation should be approached with caution because of its complexity.

As the effluent from IVCs may be HEPA-filtered before release into the room or, alternatively, directed into the building's HVAC system, the concentration of allergenic particulate to which personnel are exposed in the MaE may be reduced with particular IVC designs. Murine urinary allergens were orders of magnitude lower in two IVCs, operated at both positive and negative intracage pressure, when compared with open cages (Renstrom et al., 2001). In another study, bacteria, detected using settle plates, were reduced 99% and 94% in comparison with open cages when one IVC was operated in either positive or negative mode, respectively (Clough et al., 1995).

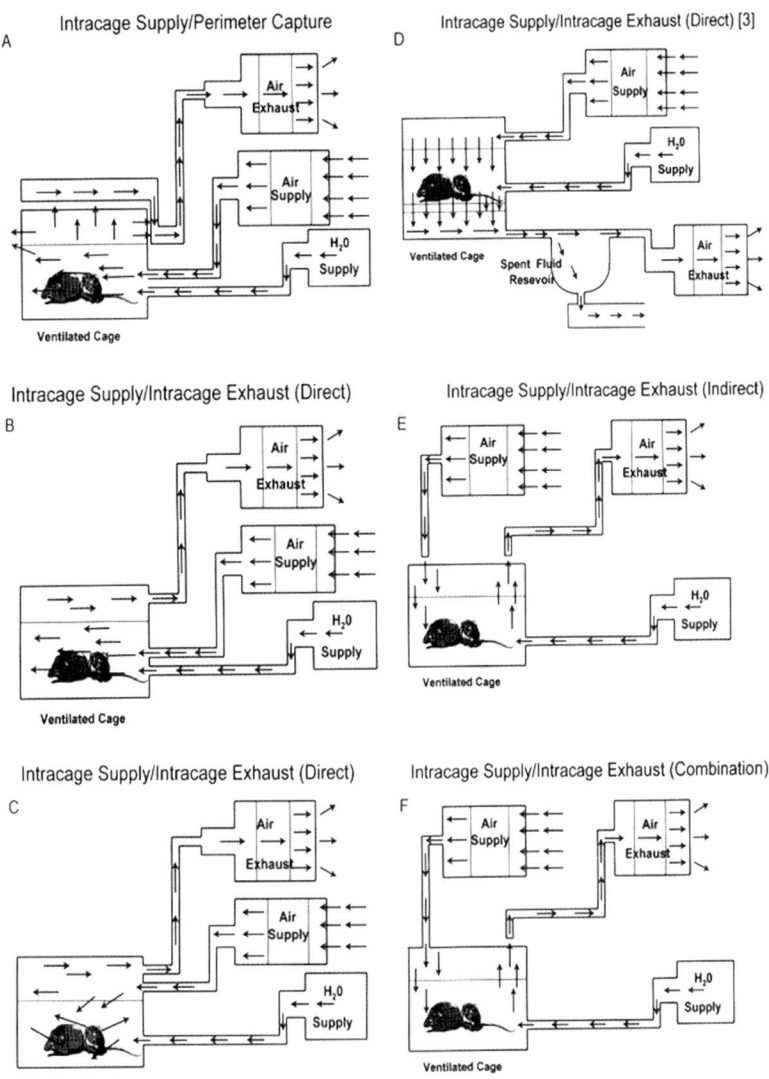

FIGURE 36.17 Schematic representations of types of commercially available ventilated caging systems. Notice that all systems are shown with automatic watering. Vectors representing air flow are shown for illustrative purposes only and do not necessarily reflect air flow patterns within the cage. *From Lipman (1999).*

This feature may not be offered by all IVCs, as several systems operate by pressurizing the cage, attempting to capture cage effluent after it escapes from the cage. Leakage of cage effluent into the MaE has been detected with these systems using a tracer gas (Tu *et al.*, 1997).

Although IVCs provide significant advantages, there are important considerations when selecting or using these systems. The user must clearly understand the operating principles of the system they use. Specific systems differ with respect to the method of introduction and quantity of air supplied to each cage. The ideal intracage ventilation rate for IVCs is unknown and is likely dependent on numerous factors, including species, strain or stock housed, cage population, bedding, and the specific IVC used. An ideal rate in one situation may be insufficient or excessive in another. The criteria used to select intracage

ventilation rates should be based on performance standards. As an example, Reeb-Whitaker *et al.* (2001) evaluated ventilation rates and cage change frequency with respect to breeding performance, weanling weight and growth, plasma corticosterone levels, and pathology in C57BL/6J mice, and determined that ventilating cages at 60 ACH and changing every 14 days were ideal. Another study conducted by the same group concluded that intracage ventilation rates should be increased from 60 to 100 ACH when housing breeding trios and pups *in lieu* of adult males if the same changing frequency and intracage NH_3 concentrations are to be maintained (Reeb *et al.*, 1998). Unless determined otherwise, the authors recommend that ventilation rates be established in IVCs so that, prior to cage change, MiE NH_3 and CO_2 are <25 and 5000 ppm, respectively, and temperature and RH fall within the limits prescribed in the *Guide* (ILAR, 2011). Further, intracage air speed, at locations that cage occupants would expect to encounter, should be ≤50 linear feet per minute (lfpm), a rate considered to be still air in human environments and unlikely to cause appreciable physiologic effect in most species (Clough, 1987; American Society of Heating, Refrigerating, and Air-Conditioning Engineers, Inc., 2001).

There are considerable differences in IVC ventilation rates, based on the manufacturer, the system type, and even the age of the system. Excessive intracage ventilation, especially when air is supplied at the level of the cage, may lead to chilling and dehydration, especially in neonates and hairless mutants. The speed of air to which animals are exposed affects the rate at which heat and moisture are removed from an animal. Air at 20°C moving at 60 lfpm has a cooling effect of approximately 7°C (Weihe, 1971). It may be necessary to increase MiE temperature when housing animals in IVCs with high intracage air velocities, when housing neonates, hairless mutants, or single animals, or when contact bedding is unavailable or is a type that does not provide the animal with the ability to nest. Pheromone dilution may also be problematic when breeding particular *Mus* species, stocks, or strains (Lipman, 1999). Huerkamp *et al.* (1994) have demonstrated a negative synergistic effect between ventilated cages and the use of automatic watering systems leading to increased mouse pup mortality. Further, they demonstrated that pups reared in IVCs were smaller than those reared in static MIs and attributed the change to intracage ventilation. Using preference testing with BALB/c mice, Baumans *et al.* (2002) concluded that the mice avoid cages with high intracage ventilation rates (up to 100 ACH), but the use of nesting material counteracted this avoidance. Ventilation rates can be adjusted in most IVCs by adjusting exhaust and/or supply fan speeds or dampers.

Additional considerations when utilizing and selecting IVCs include heat load, exhaust release, noise generation, power requirements and failure, vibration, blower maintenance and calibration, and sanitation. As IVCs enable users to increase stocking significantly, the heat load generated by the animals may be considerable. The heat load generated by the supply and exhaust blowers when combined with the animals' thermal load, especially in holding rooms with marginal temperature control, may exceed the HVAC system's cooling capacity. Frequently, this issue can be resolved by directly venting the IVC exhaust into the building's HVAC system rather than exhausting directly into the holding room, since much of the thermal load is contained within the exhaust effluent.

It is prudent to place IVCs with dedicated blowers on circuits served by emergency electrical generators, because the design of many IVCs does not provide the capability for passive ventilation in cases of power failure. If IVCs are supplied and/or exhausted by the central HVAC system or by blower units that serve multiple units, emergency power should be provided to ensure these systems remain operational during power loss. In fact, some systems employ solid tops, without filters, and attach firmly to the cage below with a gasket and/or clips. It may be critical in certain installations to ensure that exhaust and supply blower operation are interconnected functionally, such that if one fails, the other is automatically disabled. Most systems are available with warning lights, magnehelic gauges, and audible and/or voltage alarms that require either active or passive monitoring by facility staff. Some IVCs provide for remote monitoring and alarms through the BAS/BMS or security system.

Noise generated by IVC exhaust and/or supply blowers is a consideration that depends on the system type and the number of IVCs maintained per holding room. Blowers may also generate low-level vibration. IVCs with blowers attached directly to the rack are more likely to generate vibration at the cage level. System manufacturers have taken some or all of the steps to reduce or eliminate intracage vibration and noise, including (1) placing rack-mounted blower housings on rubber and/or spring-loaded mounts; (2) housing blowers on a rack/shelf separate from the caging; (3) using flexible plastic hose connectors between the rack air distribution system and the blowers; (4) using the building's HVAC system to provide supply and exhaust air; and/or (5) using low-voltage blowers. The potential impact of noise and vibration is reviewed in Chapter 29.

Because IVCs have extensive air distribution systems, they are considerably more difficult to sanitize than a standard shelf rack. In general, blowers, shelves, and/or access panels must be removed and/or opened before placing an IVC in a rack washer. Access to all plenums and ducts on the cage rack may not be possible with every system. Extensive washing by hand is frequently required, as the air distribution system may not be sanitized adequately in a rack washer because of limited access to the washer spray. There is no consensus on the sanitation frequency for IVCs. Systems are broken down and sanitized annually at the author's (NSL) institution, unless there is a change in the animals' health status or special circumstances dictate more frequent sanitation. Pre-filters, if supplied on IVCs, frequently require changing or cleaning more frequently than final filters, depending on the specific system and the bedding used. The blower units must be disassembled for cleaning, since specific components, including the fan motor and the HEPA filter, cannot be sanitized with liquid. If sanitation of these components is required, gaseous agents may be used. Although it is labor-intensive, IVCs can be decontaminated *in situ* by bagging the entire unit or isolating the holding room and sterilizing using gas sterilants such as paraformaldehyde, gaseous chlorine dioxide, or vaporized hydrogen peroxide with the unit operational. Chemical and/or biological indicators can be employed to validate efficacy. Blowers from select IVCs may need periodic calibration to ensure the supply and exhaust air volumes meet specifications. Because of the difficulty in sanitizing IVCs and the potential for unfiltered cage effluent to be released from some systems, considerable thought must be given to their use before housing animals that are infected with or exposed to hazardous agents. The release of unfiltered cage effluent into the MaE, which has been demonstrated with some systems, raises an additional concern when utilizing hazardous agents (Tu *et al.*, 1997).

2. Isolators

A greater understanding of the influence of bacterial flora on physiology and disease has led to the recent reemergence of gnotobiology at many biomedical research centers. Since the development of the first rigid stainless steel isolator by Reynier for the production and maintenance of gnotobiotic animals, isolators have been and continue to be an important husbandry resource, as they can be used for a variety of purposes including maintaining gnotobiotic animals.

Modern isolators are either of the flexible type, manufactured of polyvinyl chloride or polyurethane, or semirigid, a combination of both rigid (polypropylene) and flexible plastics (Fig. 36.18). They provide complete physical separation between the animals housed within and the surrounding environment, and are used for containment as well as for providing an extremely high level of animal protection. Although, historically, isolator supply and exhaust air was filtered through fiberglass floss media, modern units employ HEPA filters. In research facilities, isolators can be used for biohazard containment as well as for maintaining axenic, gnotobiotic, adventitious agent-contaminated, and/or immunocompromised mouse lines or stocks. The principal disadvantage of using isolators is that they are operationally and space intensive.

3. Mass Air Displacement Units Including Changing Stations and BSC

Various types of equipment employing HEPA-filtered, laminar flow, mass air displacement (MAD) were developed in the late 1970s for animal holding and subsequently for cage changing and animal manipulation. Although many MAD housing designs have been made obsolete by IVC, a number of commercial systems are available and have applications today in specialized settings. MAD units designed for cage changing and animal manipulation have become the standard of rodent husbandry throughout the United States.

MAD, or clean room, technology originated from industries requiring dust-free environments for manufacturing. During the 1970s, the technology was adapted for use in animal research facilities. MAD units are

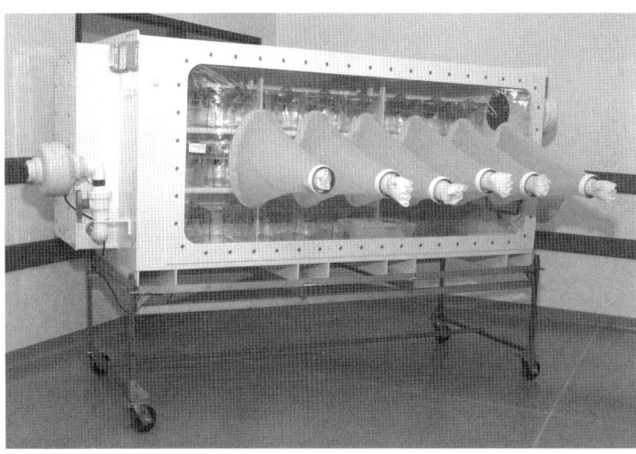

FIGURE 36.18 Semirigid isolator containing both rigid (polypropylene) and flexible (polyurethane) plastics. *Reproduced courtesy of Charles River Laboratories, Inc.*

available to operate in either a positive or a negative mode, providing either product (animal) or personnel (containment) protection, respectively. Operated in a positive mode, a fan supplies large quantities of HEPA-filtered air into a plenum and subsequently through a perforated panel, creating unidirectional laminar airflow bathing the materials to be protected. Although the airflow pattern is laminar at the source, it is disrupted by objects in its path and the pattern is lost as the air moves farther away from the source. Units developed for animal research typically are of the Class 100 type. Class 100 air is defined in the Federal Standard No. 209E as filtered air that contains no more than (100) 0.5-μm particles or larger per cubic foot of air (Code of Federal Regulations, 1992). Negative flow units provide containment as they draw large quantities of air over animals, HEPA-filtering the exhaust effluent before its release into the environment. A further distinguishing feature is whether the air moves vertically, i.e., whether it is delivered/collected from above the cage, or horizontally, in which case it is delivered/collected across the cage.

MAD units include fixed or portable, solid or flexible wall, cubicles or rooms. Using these units, barrier-level animal holding rooms can be established in large open spaces in which environmental control can be simplified and construction costs reduced. Fig. 36.19 provides an example of a facility employing multiple portable, positive flow, flexible wall, vertical flow, MAD rooms for mouse holding and breeding. Similarly, negative flow, portable, MAD cubicles can be set up to segregate shipments or, if operated in a negative pressure mode, can be used for biocontainment. MAD units can be used to create air locks within established hard-walled rooms or to collect aerosols during waste dumping.

Mobile, positive flow, MAD units, known more commonly as cage change or animal transfer stations, are

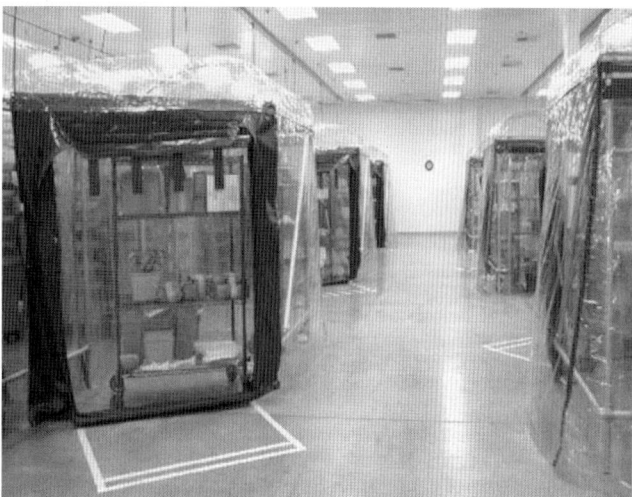

FIGURE 36.19 Multiple portable, positive flow/pressure, flexible wall, vertical flow, MAD rooms for mouse holding and breeding. *Courtesy of Taconic Farms, Inc.*

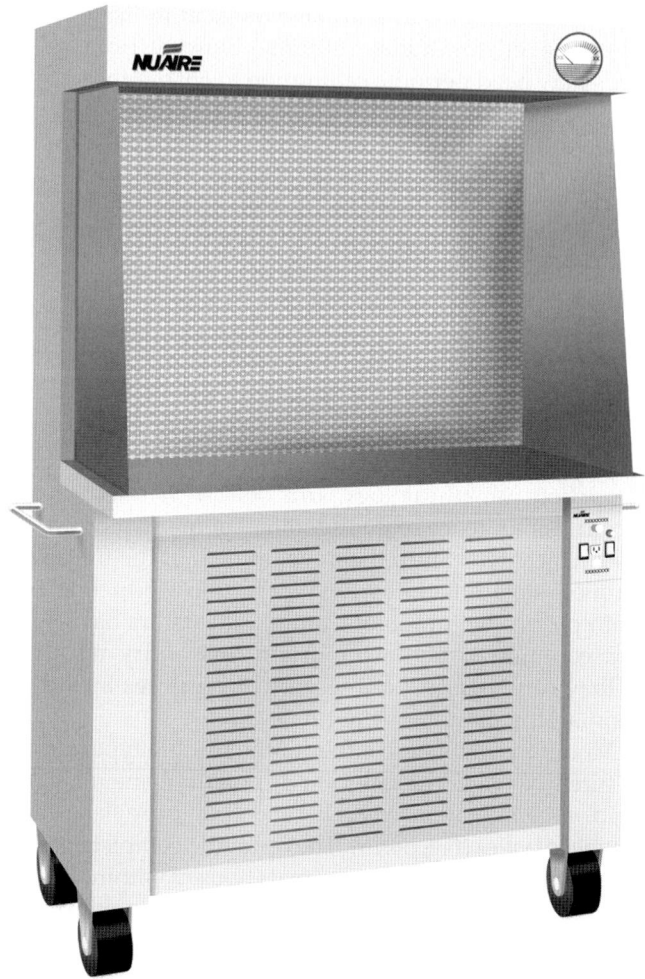

FIGURE 36.20 Portable horizontal flow MAD unit for cage change and animal manipulation. *Courtesy of Nuaire, Inc.*

available to perform cage changing and manipulate animals. In the authors' opinion, vertical flow units, most of which attempt to capture and subsequently filter effluent before release, are preferred to horizontal units, which release larger quantities of particulate into the MaE. Horizontal units are typically tissue culture hoods that have been adapted for use in the animal facility (Fig. 36.20). Horizontal units have ergonomic advantages, because of their large, open work area, and can be purchased so that they are height-adjustable. The newest changing station designs are based on vertical flow and are open for access on either two or three sides. These units can be used by more than one person simultaneously, are height-adjustable, and have a perforated work surface to capture (some) effluent that is HEPA-filtered before release (Fig. 36.21). Some facilities operate change stations continuously to filter room air, reducing particulates. Note that cage changing techniques must be adapted to the unit type, horizontal or vertical, as the direction of airflow dictates the preferred plane and manner in which clean and soiled materials are handled. Changing stations that provide only product protection should never be used with biological hazards.

Although there is no prescribed regulatory requirement for assessing the function of MAD units, a professional certifier should be retained to confirm that filtration meets the Class 100 standard. At the authors' institutions, MAD equipment is tested and certified at least annually.

BSCs are frequently used in the vivarium. They are classified as Class I, II, or III (CDC-NIH, 2009), based on their operational design. Class I cabinets provide personnel protection only. Their use in animal facilities is limited to bedding dump stations, as previously

discussed. Class II cabinets provide both product and personnel protection, and are used for animal and material handling when BSL-2 and BSL-3 agents are used. There are two types (A and B) of Class II BSCs. Air is recirculated in a Type A cabinet and may be released into the MaE or connected to the building's exhaust through a thimble connection. Many facilities use Class II, Type A cabinets for routine cage changing, because of concerns relating to allergens. Type A cabinets have been adapted for cage changing and animal manipulation by increasing the sash height to allow movement of MIs into and out of the cabinet without disturbing the lid, and may be mobile, height-adjustable, and equipped with a variety of options, including pass-through waste disposal ports and feed, water, and cage delivery systems.

Type B cabinets have a 100-lfpm face velocity and negative pressure plenums, and are hard-ducted to the building's exhaust system, making them suitable for use with toxic chemicals and radionuclides. Type B2, or 100% exhaust, cabinets do not recirculate air and therefore are

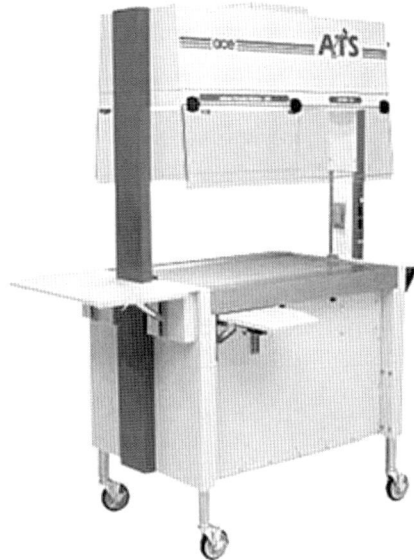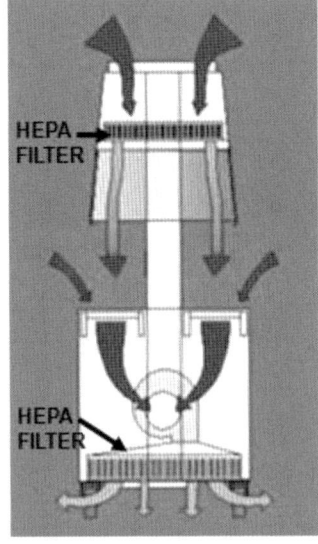

FIGURE 36.21   Vertical flow changing station (left). HEPA-filtered laminar flow air is supplied above the station's work surface; much of the air is captured and is HEPA-filtered before release into the room (right). *Courtesy of Allentown Caging Co., Inc.*

preferred when using highly toxic volatile chemicals, although the quantity of chemical used may need to be limited to avoid degradation of the HEPA filter. When used for the containment of hazardous agents, Class I and II cabinets must be certified to meet National Sanitation Foundation (NSF) International standard 49 upon installation, whenever they are moved, and at least annually (National Sanitation Foundation, 2002). Mobile units that are used for cage changing and animal handling but not for hazardous agent containment should be certified at least annually. Units used for hazardous agent control should be certified each time they are moved.

The use of Class III cabinets, which provide the highest level of containment suitable for organisms requiring BSL-3 and BSL-4 organisms, is highly specialized and beyond the scope of this chapter.

It is important to recognize that both MAD units and BSCs have limitations in that the airflow dynamics that provide either or both product and personnel protection can be easily overwhelmed by the operator's movements when using the unit, air currents in the surrounding area, e.g., those generated by the HVAC system, room door operation, or personnel/equipment moving by the unit, or placement of equipment within the unit's work space.

4. Aquatic Systems

Increasingly, biomedical research programs are utilizing larger numbers of aquatic species, notably zebrafish (*Danio rerio*) and frogs (*Xenopus* sp.), as animal models. Housing systems range from the simple, static tanks and/or aquaria in which water is replaced manually, to complex large high-density recirculating systems supporting hundreds to thousands of tanks. The latter are supported by mechanical systems that recirculate water after treatment to all the tanks on the system. These systems are often supplied with reverse osmosis or filtered municipal water, to ensure the water is free of chemicals, such as chorine or chloramines, which are toxic to many aquatic species, various impurities, and potential biological contaminants such as bacteria and parasites which may cause inapparent or clinical disease. System components include pumps to move water, mechanical and biological filters to remove/neutralize particulate and biological waste, high-energy UV lamps or ozone units for disinfection, heaters/chillers, dosing equipment to measure and maintain appropriate water conditions, as well as various probes to measure temperature, pH, conductivity, total dissolved gasses, and dissolved oxygen. In larger systems, redundancy is provided for all critical components. As some aquatic species require or prefer live feed during select developmental stages (e.g. *Artemia* sp., rotifers, or paramecium) and equipment must be available to rear and/or maintain these dietary components.

V. MATERIALS

A. Feed

The provision of high-quality feed is essential to meet the animal's physiologic needs, specifically growth, maintenance, and reproduction. Most laboratory diets are made from natural ingredients, nutritionally complete, formulated from processed whole grain and commodities and subjected to limited refinement. They are typically produced by pelleting or extrusion. Feed in pelleted form allows the most efficient delivery and the highest energy content per unit due to its density and is the form typically fed to rodents and rabbits. Pelleting, which subjects feed constituents to heat and pressure, also reduces bacterial and fungal loads that may be found in unprocessed ingredients (Halls and Tallentire, 1978). Extrusion generates a biscuit which is less dense with a lower energy content per unit. Extruded diets are less hard than pellets making it preferable for some species or rodent strains. Feed may also be purchased in powdered meal form, permitting the provision of additives to the diet after formulation. However, meal diets tend to cake, and much of the feed can go to waste.

Formulations of natural-ingredient rodent diets differ principally with respect to protein and fat concentration. High-fat (up to 11%) diets are used in research facilities to support rodent breeding because the higher energy content meets the demands of gestation and lactation. However, the accumulation of intraabdominal fat, which may occur with the chronic use of high-fat diet, may shorten the animal's reproductive life span.

Most natural diets are 'closed' formula, meaning the individual components of the diet are not specified, although guaranteed analysis is provided. This allows the diet's ingredients to change in association with commodity prices. Although less commonly utilized, 'open' formula diets, such as NIH-07, are manufactured in accordance with an established known ingredient formulation. As the potential complicating role of dietary phytoestrogens, namely the isoflavones diadzein and genistein, are recognized as a complicating variable in some studies, feed manufacturers are producing diets that avoid protein sources known to contain isoflavones such as soybean meal and alfalfa (Allred *et al.*, 2001; Ju *et al.*, 2001, 2002; Thigpen *et al.*, 2001, 2002, 2003).

Purified diets, such as AIN-76, are formulated from refined ingredients. These are useful when altering the nutritional content of the animal's diet or when compounding with additives. Chemically defined diets are formulated with chemically pure compounds and are utilized when altering a specific nutritional dietary component.

Autoclavable diets, formulated to be sterilized prior to provision, are enriched with heat-labile nutrients, including thiamin, vitamins A and E, pantothenic acid, pyridoxine, and B12, whose concentrations are reduced during autoclaving. Autoclavable diets may also be coated with silicon dioxide in soybean oil to reduce the likelihood of pellet clumping and adherence, which occurs as a result of pellet swelling during steam sterilization. To avoid clumping post autoclaving, feed may be decanted into bags with additional space to accommodate swelling

or it may be sterilized on trays at a depth of ~3 inches. Sterilization cycles must be developed and verified to ensure feed sterility. Pulsed vacuum sterilization is preferred to ensure adequate steam penetration when autoclaving feed in the manufacturer's original packing materials (bag). Feed subject to excessive sterilization may be depleted of essential nutrients and the protein quality may be reduced, but more likely it may become too hard, a result of the polymerization of select feed constituents, for some strains (Ford, 1987). Nutritional analysis of feed post sterilization, using a validated (for sterility) autoclave cycle, is recommended on a regular basis.

Gamma-irradiated diets have become commonplace and have replaced the use of autoclaved diets in a variety of settings, as they require less processing after receipt and are not subject to the effects of heat and temperature that result from autoclaving. Most feed producers subject irradiated diet to between 10 and 40 Kgrey (1–4 Mrad) by exposing the bags to a cobalt source. As feed bags are palletized and then irradiated, exposure differs, depending on a specific bag's location within the load. Although irradiated feed is not purported to be sterile, bacterial (cells and spores) and fungal loads are markedly reduced to less than 100 bacteria or fungi per gram of feed (Cover and Belcher, 1992). This is in contrast to standard diets whose bacterial loads fluctuate seasonally and can reach levels as high as 500,000 total bacteria per gram of feed. Irradiation is purported to be ineffective against some viruses (MPV, for example) as the exposure dose is insufficient. (W. Shek, personal communication, 2004). However, at the author's (NSL) institution implementation of using only gamma-irradiated rodent feed prevented seasonal recurrence of MPV infections in mice. Irradiated feed is available in a variety of packaging. Bulk feed can be purchased in 25-pound multi-ply packaging. The outer paper packaging, which is exposed to contaminants during shipping and storage, can be sprayed with a disinfectant solution and/or carefully removed to reveal a sterile inner plastic bag. The sealed inner plastic bag also permits decontamination with a liquid or spray disinfectant, if necessary. Irradiated diet can also be obtained in small, watertight, vacuum-sealed plastic bags for use in isolators, change stations, or BSCs. Penetration of the plastic is easily noticed as the vacuum seal is lost and the bag inflates. The use of vaporized hydrogen peroxide as a method to decontaminate the external surface of feed bags, even those with an inner plastic bag, must be carefully considered, as the hydrogen peroxide gas may penetrate the feed (author's (NSL) personal communication, 2005). Subjecting irradiated feed bags to an extremely short 'flash' autoclave cycle has been employed as a method for surface decontamination prior to relocation of feed into a rodent barrier (Thurlow *et al.*, 2007).

A variety of 'off-the-shelf' specialty rodent feeds are commercially available and are commonly employed. Examples include feed containing the anthelmintic fenbendazole, as well as several antibiotics including trimethoprim/sulfamethoxazole and doxycycline. Fenbendazole feed is commonly employed to treat mice for nematodes, namely *Syphacia* and *Aspiculuris* spp. Trimethoprim/sulfamethoxazole-compounded feed is used to control pneumocystosis in immunodeficient mouse strains, and doxycycline-containing feed is used to induce or inhibit transcription in conditional transgenic mice that contain components of the tetracycline transactivator system (Coghlan *et al.*, 1993; Lewandoski, 2001; Ryding *et al.*, 2001). Compounded feed, manufactured in special plants, is typically pelleted using distinct dyes, permitting the pellets to be differentiated from standard diets. Feed can also be pigmented using food coloring. Specialty compounded diets are also commonly employed. For example, feed compounded with vitamin E is used to treat ulcerative dermatitis in C57BL/6 mice and genetically engineered mice on a B6 background (Lawson *et al.*, 2005). Various soft and/or moist diets are also commercially available. They are used at weaning to ease the transition from lactation to a pelleted diet; postsurgery to hasten recovery; to improve nutrition of animals subject to the effects of experimental manipulation; for select mutants, such as those with dental deformities that have difficulty ingesting hard, pelleted feed; for animals having difficulty ambulating; and during shipping.

Certified diets are available to meet the requirements of the Food and Drug Administration (FDA)'s Good Laboratory Practice standards, requiring periodic feed analysis for environmental contaminants that may interfere with research studies (Code of Federal Regulations, 2004). Feed samples are analyzed and certified to contain not more than the established maximum level of environmental contaminants, including heavy metals, chlorinated hydrocarbons, organophosphates, and aflatoxins. The shelf life of most commercial diet is limited to 180 days postmilling, as prescribed in the *Guide* (ILAR, 2011). Specialty diets may have a shorter shelf life. Guinea pig and nonhuman primate feed must be used within 3 months of the milling date because of the vitamin C requirement of these species and the labile nature of vitamin C in the feed unless the diet contains stabilized vitamin C.

Consideration must be given to the transportation and storage of diets during distribution, as they may have been subject to elevated environmental temperatures and nutritional degradation. Feed should be maintained under cool and dry conditions. Natural-ingredient diets should be stored at temperatures less than 70°F and relative humidity less than 50%. Exposure of feed to elevated temperatures induces rancidity in which unsaturated fats and lipids are oxidized and convened into hydroperoxides, which subsequently break down into volatile aldehydes, esters, alcohols, ketones, and hydrocarbons, giving the feed a disagreeable odor and taste. Storage of all feed at 4°C (39°F) offers the advantage of significantly retarding the degeneration of nutritional quality to the point of not changing significantly even after 6 months (Fullerton *et al.*, 1982), and it has the added benefit of assisting with vermin control.

B. Bedding

A variety of materials are utilized as both contact and noncontact bedding for laboratory animals. Selection is based on a variety of factors, the two most important being animal comfort and least interference with the experimental manipulation. Other considerations include cost, availability, absorbency, ease of handling, transportation, storage, packaging, dry and wet product weight and disposability; can the product be easily sterilized, and/or irradiated; what are the levels of contaminants (e.g., bacteria, fungi, toxins, vermin, etc.); is the product helpful in controlling ammonia accumulation; and what is the amount of associated dust.

Most animal bedding is manufactured from plant material (e.g., wood, cotton, or corncob) subjected to varying degrees of processing. Minimally processed wood is the most commonly used contact bedding for mice. Soft- or hardwood, devoid of bark, is chopped, shredded, or shaved, then heated at temperatures up to 1200°F to reduce the bacterial and moisture content. Hardwood bedding is manufactured from aspen, beech, maple, and/or birch. Softwoods such as pine or cedar are avoided as the volatile aromatic amines that give these materials their pleasant aroma alter hepatic microsomal enzyme concentrations and therefore xenobiotic processing (Ferguson, 1966; Vessel, 1966). Most wood bedding, especially shredded or shaved products, has excellent rodent nest-building characteristics (Blom *et al.*, 1996).

Corncob bedding – produced from the woody-ring portion of the cob by processing with a hammermill and a roller mill then dried – is available in several pellet sizes. One-eighth inch or a mixture of ⅛ inch and ¼ inch is commonly used for mice, whereas the larger pellet is used for rats and larger rodent species. Corncob is excellent at inhibiting the accumulation of ammonia, and therefore is preferred when using static microisolator caging (Perkins and Lipman, 1995). The results of a recent study indicate that a new type of processed corncob bedding is comparable to autoclaved corncob in controlling intracage ammonia levels (Domer *et al.*, 2012). Corncob can be abrasive and has been associated with foot lesions in highly immunocompromised mouse strains (author's (NSL) personal communication, 2005). Off-gassing of acetic acid has also been observed, presumably from the decay of residual organic matter (Perkins and Lipman, 1995). The density of corncob limits nest building, and therefore, it is frequently supplemented with nesting material or mixed with other bedding types. Autoclaving or purchasing irradiated product is recommended as the porosity of corncob can lead to mold growth in unsterilized or nonirradiated product underneath the sipper tube, where spillover occurs.

A variety of processed wood products, e.g., cellulose, both virgin and recycled, are available for use as both contact and noncontact bedding. Products differ in absorbency, color, shape, and size. They may also be blended with other products, such as corncob. Cellulose products are more expensive than wood and have good nest-building characteristics.

Mice exhibit a preference for large fibrous materials that they can manipulate and use to build a nest (Blom et al., 1996; Van de Weerd et al., 1997a). Nesting material is frequently provided to supplement contact bedding, as preference studies have demonstrated considerable value and it is considered the premier method of providing environmental enrichment for mice (Van de Weerd, 1996; Van de Weerd et al., 1997a). The provision of nesting material has been associated with the reduction of intermale aggression, stress, and food consumption (Olsson and Dahlborn, 2002; Van Loo et al., 2003, 2004). Adequate amounts of nesting material also can relieve thermal stress (Gaskill et al., 2012). A study evaluating the impact of different nesting materials, aspen wood, wool, and paper towel, on reproduction, conducted using three inbred mouse strains, demonstrated no differences attributed to the specific nesting material utilized (Eskola and Kaliste-Korhonen, 1999). A variety of commercial nesting products are available, the most common in the United States being compressed virgin cotton fiber, which is provided in scored sheets that can be separated into ~1-inch squares. Mice dissociate the fibers, using the material to build a nest. The quantity of nesting material should be limited, as an excess may result in cage flooding if the material comes in direct contact with the water bottle, wicking water into the cage. The use of cotton nesting material should be scrutinized in nude or hairless strains lacking eyelashes, as some nesting material composed of compressed cotton fibers has been found in the conjunctival sac, inducing conjunctivitis (Bazille et al., 2001). Toilet tissue (unscented), paper towels, gauze, cotton batting, and processed corn husk have also been utilized as nesting material (Armstrong et al., 1998; Sherwin, 1997; Van de Weerd et al., 1997a).

Certified bedding, in which levels of specific toxic environmental contaminants are measured and determined to not exceed maximum concentrations, are available for use in studies that must meet GLP standards.

A variety of products, most manufactured from cellulose, are available for use as noncontact bedding. Noncontact bedding includes plastic backed absorbent paper and cardboard. Products are available in precut sheets, formed trays, and roll stock. Material used for noncontact bedding can be impregnated with antibiotics to inhibit bacterial growth and the subsequent ammonia production.

C. Water

The reliable provision of high-quality drinking water is essential for animal welfare and scientific integrity. Drinking water varies considerably from region to region, sometimes even from municipality to municipality, with respect to its quality and the concentrations of its constituents. Depending on area geology, the use of surface or well water, proximity to industrial, agricultural, or urban centers, and type of treatment, the water consumed is subject to considerable variation and may be contaminated by pesticides, heavy metals, radionuclides, endocrine disrupters, pharmaceuticals, and other compounds that may produce significant effects that may have a direct impact on research studies (Cantor, 1997; Garcia, 1998; Surbeck, 1995). Municipal water authorities routinely analyze water quality and contaminants in compliance with the Safe Drinking Water Act, overseen by the Environmental Protection Agency (EPA). The results of these analyses should be obtained and reviewed regularly by research facility management, especially when subsequent water treatment is not undertaken. Further analysis of 'point-of-use' samples may be warranted in research buildings with older plumbing systems, from automated water bottle filling stations, and/or automatic watering systems if experimental studies could be affected by discrete changes in water quality and/or constituents or when conducting preclinical laboratory studies under GLPs (Code of Federal Regulations, 2004). GLPs require routine periodic water analysis to ensure that contaminants that may reasonably expected to be present and capable of interfering with the study are not found at levels above those specified in the protocol.

There are a variety of options with respect to the processing of drinking water, ranging from using municipal water without further purification to using reverse osmosis water. Some facilities subject municipal water to filtration to remove particulates ($\geq 5\,\mu m$) and activated carbon to reduce the concentration of contaminants such as organic compounds. Reverse osmosis (RO) is the water purification system employed most often when higher quality water is desirable. RO employs an ultrafiltration membrane, through which water flows under pressure. Up to 99% of inorganic compounds, dissolved ions, organic compounds including toxins and pyrogens, heavy metals, and microorganisms are removed in the filtrate. RO membranes require regular replacement, as they 'foul' as a result of the accumulation of organic material on the membrane. Fouled membranes support bacterial growth, increasing the likelihood of contamination. Membranes are also subject to scale accumulation which favors fouling if used to purify hard water.

UV energy can also be utilized to disinfect water and reduce total organic carbon (reviewed in Edstrom Industries, 2003a). UV disinfection is most often used to supplement another water treatment process method, such as RO purification. UV disinfection involves flowing water around a low-pressure mercury lamp, contained within a UV transparent sleeve, which emits bactericidal UV rays at 254 nm. The bactericidal effectiveness of UV radiation is dependent on dosage, a product of intensity and exposure length. Contaminants, particularly iron, humic and fulvic acids, and suspended solids, reduce the transmission of UV light. UV lamp intensity decays with use, and therefore, lamps must be replaced when they emit light at $<30,000\,\mu w\text{-}s/cm^2$, the minimum intensity adequate to destroy microorganisms. Glass tubes surrounding lamps should be checked and cleaned regularly, and a UV light meter should be used to determine whether lamp replacement is necessary. Although not as commonly employed as UV light, ozone, which oxidizes microorganisms and organic contaminants, can also be used to disinfect water. Ozone disinfection requires an ozone generator as well as a system to diffuse the ozone into the water (Paraskeva and Graham, 2002). The latter two methods are also employed to disinfect recirculating water in aquatic systems while RO treated water is used commonly when initially filling the system as well as for daily water exchange.

Water can be sterilized with steam to destroy vegetative bacteria, bacterial spores, fungi, and viruses. Autoclaving will effectively destroy microorganisms; however, if endotoxins from gram-negative bacteria and other contaminants were present before sterilization they will remain following autoclaving.

Additives are commonly provided in rodent drinking water, the most common being hydrochloric acid or chlorine, both of which are added to reduce bacterial growth in the water reservoir (bottle or bag) and/or water distribution system (automatic watering). Sulfuric acid and tetracycline have also been employed (Hall et al., 1980: Hermann et al., 1982). Water is acidified to attain a pH between 2.5 and 3.0. Solutions with a pH below 3.0 are bactericidal against *Pseudomonas aeruginosa* and other gram-negative eubacteria (Tanner and Samantha, 1992). Although the use of a pH as low as 2.0 has been reported for mice, this has been associated with a reduction in weight gain and water consumption, lower splenic weights, a reduced spleen/body weight ratio, and a reduction in the number of bacterial species

in the terminal ileum (Hall et al., 1980; Hermann et al., 1982). Acidified water is corrosive and should be used only with corrosion-resistant materials such as plastic polymers or Type 316 stainless steel. Grades of stainless without molybdenum (e.g., grade 304), brass, and copper are corroded by acidified water. Automatic proportioners equipped with pH analyzers are available for delivery of acidified water. Acidified water is temporally stable when provided in a noncorrosive system. Autoclavable carboys can be used for individual racks (Tallent, 2012).

Chlorine is also utilized to reduce bacterial and viral contamination in mouse drinking water and, when using automatic watering systems, to control bacterial growth and biofilm accumulation in water distribution systems. Chlorine is added in the form of sodium hypochlorite. It is most effective when the pH of water is between 5 and 7 where HOCl is the predominant form (Edstrom Industries, 2003b). The optimal concentration of chlorine in rodent drinking water has not been determined; however, recommended concentrations in the literature range from 0.5 to 10 ppm (Beck, 1963; Brewer, 1972; Bywater and Kellett, 1977; Homberger et al. 1993). Coliforms and *P. aeruginosa* can be cultured from tap water when the concentration of chlorine falls below 1 ppm (Bywater and Kellett, 1977; McPherson, 1963). *P. aeruginosa* is among the most chlorine-tolerant of the enteric bacteria and is commonly associated with opportunistic infections in immunocompromised rodents. Homberger et al. (1993) determined that adding 6–8 ppm chlorine in drinking water provided in water bottles changed weekly was the ideal concentration to eliminate *P. aeruginosa* and reduce carriage of the organism in infected mice. Although water was also supplemented with chlorine at 10 ppm, this level of supplementation was ineffective, presumably because poor palatability reduced water consumption; however, McPherson (1963) reported elevated consumption of water at pH 12.

The concentration of chlorine dissipates over time as it is off-gassed, especially when water delivery/distribution allows for considerable contact with air, and it reacts with organic matter and other oxidizable contaminants in the water and distribution system. This is particularly problematic when using automatic watering systems that may have considerable distribution networks coated with bacteria-generated biofilm, which oxidizes chlorine. Automatic watering systems can be supplemented with chlorine continuously using an automatic proportioner, ensuring that at least 2 ppm of chlorine is attained at the point of consumption farthest from the chlorine source. Chlorine also dissipates in water bottles. A ~3-ppm decrease in chlorine concentration was observed in water bottles during a 7-day period, although other authors have reported greater dissipation (Homberger et al., 1993; McPherson, 1963). The amount of chlorine supplementation is highly dependent on water quality, with high-quality water generated by RO requiring less chlorine to attain the desired concentration, as RO water contains considerably less organic material and other contaminants. When analyzing a sample for chlorine, the sample should be evaluated immediately after collection as the chorine will dissipate rapidly, especially if the sample is exposed to oxidizing sunlight and/or is agitated and exposed to air.

Supplementation with chlorine at or below 10 ppm is regarded as safe, because there have been no significant effects noted on reproduction or immune function; however, supplementation with chlorine at higher levels may have adverse effects (Les, 1968; Hermann et al., 1982). Fidler (1977) reported decreased in vitro activity of peritoneal macrophages when drinking water was chlorinated at 24–30 ppm. Chlorination of water containing organic matter results in the formation of by-products such as trihalomethanes, some of which, e.g., chloroform, may be cytotoxic, mutagenic, and/or carcinogenic (Lee et al., 1998; Lipsky et al., 1993; Morris et al., 1992; Pilotto, 1995). Therefore, chlorination of RO-treated water, which has fewer organic contaminants, is preferred. Chlorination by-products may be present without on-site chlorination, as many municipal water supplies use chlorine as a disinfectant. Although RO treatment will remove some by-products, small-molecular-weight compounds may pass through the RO membrane and are best removed by absorption using activated carbon.

Chlorine is used at significantly higher concentrations (up to 50 ppm) to disinfect the components of automatic watering systems, including room and rack distribution piping, manifolds, and lixits. Chlorine should not be added to drinking water below pH 5.0 in automatic watering systems, as chlorine will be present as a gas, which may cause swelling of the silicon seals found in drinking water lixits (Edstrom Industries, 2003b).

Other drinking water additives have become commonplace, especially in facilities using genetically engineered and/or mutant mice. Antibiotics may be added to the drinking water to treat and/or prevent bacterial infections, such as Pneumocystis carinii pneumonia, especially in rodents with immunosuppressed phenotypes, and to prevent opportunistic infections in animals subject to whole-body lethal irradiation for bone marrow transplant (Brook et al., 2004; Walzer et al., 1989). Doxycycline or tetracycline or other additives such as zinc in the form of zinc sulfate (Rafferty et al., 1992), may be added to induce or inhibit transcription in conditional transgenic mice. The frequency of change-out of antibiotic-treated water must be considered, as the activity of the antibiotic, once diluted in water, may be less than the frequency of drinking water replacement or may be subject to bacterial and fungal growth as some orally administered anti-infectives are supplemented

with sugar/flavor enhancers, which support the growth of microorganisms, to increase palatability. Finally, the solubility of some antibiotics is poor, requiring periodic bottle agitation. Anthelmintics, such as piperazine and ivermectin, have also been administered via the drinking water to treat murine pinworms (Lipman et al., 1994). Coloring additive-containing drinking water with food dyes is recommended when the additive is otherwise undetectable.

Water may be provided to animals in bottles or disposable bags, or via an automatic system. Depending on the method employed, the provision of drinking water can be one of the most time- and labor-intensive components of husbandry. Whichever delivery system is chosen should be consistent from dam to weaned pups (Gordon and Wyatt, 2011).

Provision of water in bottles has been and continues to be the mainstay of water delivery. Bottles may be manufactured from glass or thermoplastics, with polycarbonate and polysulfone being the most common plastic employed. Bottles provided to rodents may be 'corked' with a rubber stopper and stainless steel sipper tube, 'capped' with an integrated stainless steel cap and sipper tube, or drilled and corked or capped. Bottles with sipper tubes can be placed in a depression slot within the wire bar lid on top of the cage or, alternatively, installed external to the cage, on the cage front. External bottles can be replaced without removing the cage, and if utilizing a filter top, without removing the top. This is of particular advantage if ventilated cages are being used and there is a decreased cage change frequency. External bottles can be easily replaced, although internal large reservoir bottles (>16 ounces) have also been employed in this setting. The principal problem with bottle use is episodic cage flooding, due to an incorrectly seated stopper or cap, defective stopper or cap, or damage to the bottle (usually cracks, especially in aged plastic bottles). Leaky bottles may lead to animal deaths, particularly of neonates, especially when large-capacity bottles are used. Plastic bottles have replaced glass bottles in many facilities because of the weight and safety concerns associated with bottle shattering and glass shards. However, recent studies have identified water contamination with BPA, a constituent monomer found in a number of thermoplastics. BPA is polymerized to produce the desired product under heat and pressure. BPA has estrogenic activity, and leaching into the water may be a significant problem with aged plastic bottles, particularly those made from polycarbonates (Howdeshell et al. 2003; Hunt et al. 2003). It is unclear whether bottles made from polysulfone pose the same risks. Constituents of glass may also leach into drinking water. Lohmiller and Lipman (1998) observed significant elevations of silicon in water when glass bottles used for rodents were filled with untreated municipal water and autoclaved. Although borosilicate (Pyrex) glass would prevent this occurrence, bottles suitable for rodents are available only in milk glass, which degrades when subjected to high temperatures.

Bottle stoppers are available in a variety of materials. The most commonly used in animal facilities, because of price, are siliconized (black) rubber or synthetic (green) neoprene. Neoprene stoppers are resistant to degradation from repetitive autoclaving. Stoppers contain a variety of minerals, including zinc, copper, magnesium, and iron, which can leach into the water, depending on the water processing employed (Kennedy and Beal, 1991).

Several manufacturers have developed systems that use disposable sealed plastic bags with either a disposable or a reusable lixit to deliver water to the cage (Fig. 36.22). The bags, which may be sterile, can be prepared and filled in clean cage wash or at the room in a cage change station.

The provision of drinking water was one of the earliest husbandry activities to be automated. Automatic watering systems have been refined in the past 30 years and are used extensively today. Although problems of cage flooding when used for rodents still persist, the water delivery valve or lixit design has been refined, greatly reducing the likelihood of such events. Prior problems such as leaky valves, small rodents perching on and activating the valve stem, and animals packing bedding in the valve's orifice, all of which could lead to flooding, have been addressed through redesign. Function can be further improved with recalibration and preventive maintenance (Gonzalez et al., 2011). The valve can also be installed so that if a leak occurs, water collects outside the cage. Fig. 36.23 contains a diagram of a typical drinking valve utilized for rodents.

Valve sanitation presents considerable challenges, especially when sterilization is desirable for operational or animal health reasons. Cages are available with integral valves with quick disconnect (QD) fittings, permitting valves to be sanitized with the cage. However, considerable care must be taken during cage replacement to ensure that the QD fitting has been properly engaged; some valves require priming, and bedding and other small particulates can lodge in the components during washing. Alternatively, the valve may remain on the rack and be sanitized *in situ* in a mechanical washer with the rack or it may be cleaned manually. The valve may also be fitted with a QD, permitting removal and sanitation independent of the rack and cage.

Automatic watering systems require other components, including a pressure-reducing device delivering water at the low pressure (as low as ~3 psi for rodents) required for valve function, as well as room and rack distribution systems. The pressure-reducing device is frequently equipped to detect and control a substantial leak to avoid flooding. Equipment is also available to

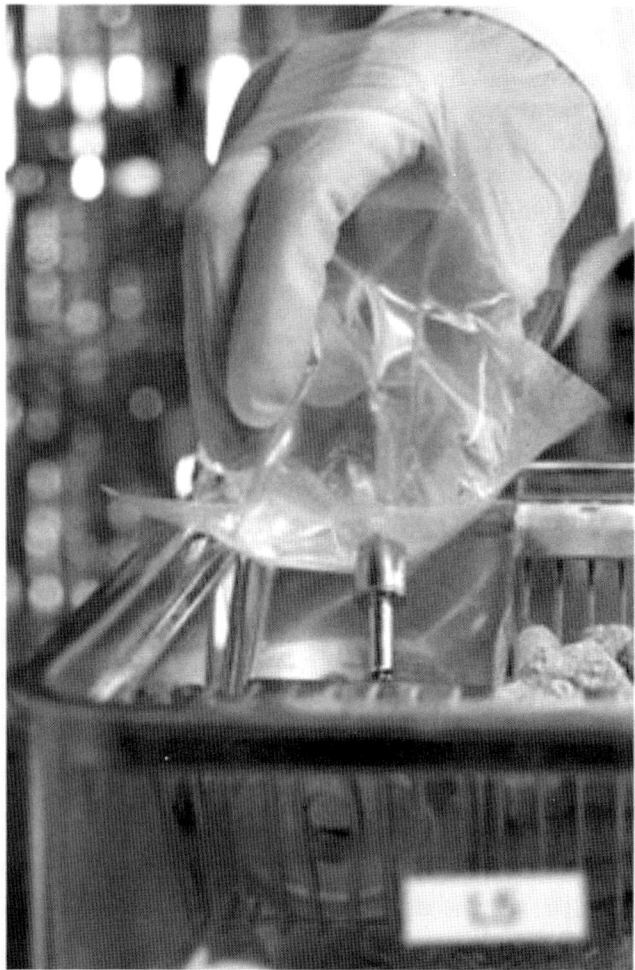

FIGURE 36.22   A disposable sealed plastic bag with drinking valve for provision of water. *Courtesy of Edstrom Industries, Inc.*

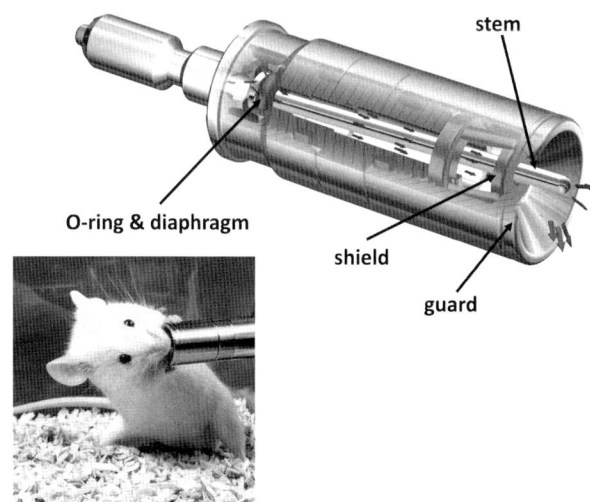

FIGURE 36.23   Schematic of a rodent drinking valve. The mouse manually deflects the stem which allows water to pass around the O-ring and diaphragm. The shield prevents bedding from entering the valve and the guard protects the stem from accidental movement. *Courtesy of Edstrom Industries, Inc.*

filter and to proportion an additive, to acidify, or to chlorinate the water before delivery, as well as to flush the room and/or rack distribution systems with high-pressure water, on a preplanned schedule, to prevent the accumulation of bacteria within the distribution pipe's lumen. Reducing or eliminating bacterial growth within the distribution system remains a considerable problem, especially with bacteria such as *Pseudomonas* spp., which produce a protective biofilm on the luminal surface. Biofilms protect bacteria from shear with high-pressure flushes or chemical additives. Avoiding dead ends in the distribution system and employing a comprehensive sanitation program are essential to control bacterial growth. Rack washers can be equipped with a system to flush the rack distribution system during washing, and automated flushing units, which employ a sanitizing agent such as sodium hypochlorite, are frequently used after the rack is removed from a mechanical washer. Rack sterilization is most effective (Costello *et al.*, 1998).

Although automatic watering systems are effective in reducing operational costs, they are capital-intensive especially when providing water to thousands of rodent cages. The premium paid for the housing rack with a distribution system and valves is the principal cost. In addition, these systems do not permit easy delivery of drinking water additives to individual cages, which may be needed when using conditional mutants whose transgenes are frequently activated or suppressed by water additives such as antibiotics.

D. Chemicals

A variety of chemicals are routinely employed in the daily operation of a vivarium. By far, the most common are a host of detergents, acids, and/or disinfectants used to sanitize the physical plant, as well as the caging and related equipment. Detailed information on the types, applications, and effectiveness of these agents is beyond the scope of this chapter. Detailed information is available in reference texts and review articles, as well as from chemical manufacturers and suppliers (Block, 2001; Favero, 1990; Kahrs, 1995). The selection of appropriate chemical agents for specific functions should be based on sound judgment and tailored to the needs of the program. Disinfectants, with or without detergents, active against a broad spectrum of microorganisms, are used in holding areas, procedure laboratories, and cage wash to sanitize hard surfaces because of the scope of potential microbes that may be present in these areas. Supplementation or substitution with narrow-spectrum agents may be desirable in areas used for containment, quarantine, or isolation where specific agents needing control may be identified. Rotation of disinfectants has been shown to be effective in preventing the development of resistant microorganisms (Conner and Eckman,

1992). The ideal disinfectant is broad spectrum; stable; not adversely affected by salts, organic material, pH, or the mineral content of the water used as a diluent; and, not aromatic, corrosive, toxic, or irritating.

Quaternary ammonium compounds are the most commonly employed broad-spectrum hard surface disinfectants employed in animal research facilities. They are mild cationic chemicals effective against vegetative cells, have good wetting properties, and have considerable inherent detergent activity; however, they are not compatible with soaps and are inactivated by organic material. Surfaces should be thoroughly rinsed and free of soap residue and debris before a quaternary ammonium disinfectant is applied.

The halogens, which include chlorine, iodine, and bromine, have been widely used as disinfectants. Chlorine is effective against all microorganisms including bacterial spores. Organic materials reduce the effectiveness of chlorine disinfectants, requiring surfaces and materials to be cleaned prior to application. Sodium hypochlorite, which can be prepared from household bleach, is ideal for use as a virucide and a hard surface disinfectant. However, chlorine dioxide-based products have become more popular, as they are more selective and are effective over a wider pH range, and their speed of kill is more rapid than sodium hypochlorite. Unlike chlorine found in sodium hypochlorite, chlorine dioxide remains a true gas dissolved in solution. Chlorine dioxide is also more effective in penetrating and dispersing a biofilm, and therefore, bacteria are much slower to reestablish (Mayack *et al.*, 1984). As with sodium hypochlorite, strong aqueous solutions of chlorine dioxide will release gaseous chlorine dioxide, which can be noxious to personnel. The microbicidal efficacy of chlorine dioxide and sodium hypochlorite decreases as temperature decreases. As an example, LeChevallier (1997) found that reducing the temperature from 20°C to 10°C reduced the disinfection effectiveness of chlorine dioxide on *Cryptosporidium* spp. by 40%.

In research facilities, liquid chlorine dioxide is prepared by combining solutions of hydroxyacetic acid and sodium chlorite, or adding a tablet containing sodium chlorite and sodium dichloroisocyanurate, to water. Once prepared, chlorine dioxide solutions have a limited shelf life. The shelf life is 2 weeks or less depending on the concentration and specific product. Chlorine dioxide has also been demonstrated to be useful as a fumigant. It can be generated as a gas at room temperature and remains gaseous under moderate conditions. It can absorb and remains biocidal in surface moisture. Although it must be applied at a RH greater than 60%, excessive humidity does not alter effectiveness. Precautions must be taken with all chlorine-based products, as they are corrosive and can cause skin irritation, although chlorine dioxide is less corrosive and irritating than sodium hypochlorite

(Block, 2001). Iodophors, which contain iodine complexed with an organic solubilizing agent, are stable, relatively odor- and stain-free, and have broad-spectrum antimicrobial properties. They are employed by some institutions to disinfect forceps used for small animal handling.

The alcohols, usually prepared in 70–80% aqueous solutions, have limited usefulness within an animal research facility. They are slow in their germicidal action and are not effective against certain viruses and spores. The bactericidal action of isopropyl alcohol is slightly greater than ethanol (Block, 2001). Synthetic phenols, which are similar to the original compound phenol but lack certain of its undesirable characteristics, are also commonly used as hard surface disinfectants (Block, 2001). They are effective germicides against vegetative bacterial cells and tubercle bacilli. Synthetic phenols are compatible with detergents, making the detergent–disinfectant combination ideal for general sanitation purposes. Skin contact should be avoided, as phenolics are extremely irritating and should never be used to sanitize equipment coming in direct contact with animals.

Peracetic acid (PA) is sometimes used as a disinfectant when maintaining gnotobiotic isolators. PA is usually dispersed as a spray, as the solution is sporicidal in the vapor phase as well as the liquid phase and thus will kill organisms suspended in the air and on surfaces that escape wetting (Block, 2001). Gloves and eye and respiratory protection must be worn when using this agent. Preferably, PA should be handled with gloves in a suitable ventilated cabinet.

The use of vaporized hydrogen peroxide (VHP) is increasing in biomedical research facilities. VHP, a low-temperature sterilant, is created by a mechanical 'generator' and is used to decontaminate sealed enclosures such as a room or materials contained within a sealed enclosure, such as BSCs (Block, 2001). Hydrogen peroxide vapor is compatible with most materials and can be safely used to decontaminate electronic and electrical devices. VHP decomposes into water and oxygen, leaving no hazardous by-products. It is active in the vapor phase and its effectiveness is dependent on environmental moisture.

Various types of chemicals are employed in mechanical cage/rack and tunnel washers, namely alkaline and acid detergents, organic and inorganic acids, and neutralizers. The selection of a specific chemical or chemicals is based on the nature of the soil to be removed; the nature of the water used for washing, e.g., hard or soft; and the regulatory requirement that waste water effluent be neutral pH. Although chemicals can and are frequently utilized to facilitate removal of organic matter and scale as well as to disinfect in mechanical washers, rodent caging can be adequately sanitized in a mechanical washer, using heated water, without chemicals (author's (NSL)

unpublished results, 2005). Thermal death of microorganisms is achieved through the combined effects of temperature and the length of time that the specific temperature is maintained. This characteristic is called the cumulative heat factor (Fuchs, 1951). An equivalent cumulative heat factor can be attained by exposing microorganisms to higher temperatures for shorter times, as opposed to lower temperatures for a longer time period (Wardrip *et al.*, 1994). Thermal death is due principally to heat dissipated from the heated water impinging on the microorganism, rather than to the dissipation of heat from the object being washed (Small, 1983). Therefore, adequate contact with the heated water stream is essential for adequate disinfection. Exposure to water at temperatures in excess of 168°F should adequately kill vegetative bacteria in seconds (Wardrip *et al.*, 2000).

As chemicals and/or their residue may adversely affect the animals, as well as the stability and longevity of thermoplastics from which rodent caging is produced, many facilities opt not to use chemicals in their mechanical washers. Many of the thermoplastics will absorb moisture under the conditions to which they are exposed in the research facility. Chemical-containing moisture or residue remaining after washing, especially at elevated temperatures, hastens the destruction of the plastic, decreasing its longevity and causing the release of biologically active components such as BPA (Koehler *et al.*, 2003). Plastic degradation is of particular concern if the caging is autoclaved and the steam utilized contains chemicals, such as amines, that are used to prevent corrosion in steam lines and boilers. Chipps *et al.* (2012) have recently identified a process that removed residues from and improved the longevity of plastic caging.

When chemicals are utilized in mechanical washers, their provision is automated. In cage/rack washers, they are added during the appropriate phase of the wash cycle following signaling by a microprocessor or programmed logic controller, and are maintained, as in a tunnel washer, at the appropriate steady-state concentration in the wash tank by measuring conductivity using a conductivity probe. Increasing the detergent concentration lowers the electrical resistance of the solution; an increase in resistance is the signal to add additional chemical, until the desired resistance is achieved.

VI. OPERATIONAL ISSUES

There are a host of operational decisions to be considered when managing and overseeing an animal research facility to ensure that the facility operates according to and meets established goals. Several were considered previously with respect to facility design and floor plan. For most facilities, the overarching goal is to ensure that the animals' health status and the environmental conditions to which they are exposed remain stable, permitting collection of reliable experimental data. Operational decisions made with respect to material flow, including clean and soiled caging/equipment, animals, and personnel, are paramount. Ideally, these decisions are considered during facility design such that layout and operations work harmoniously. However, it is not uncommon, especially in older facilities, to find that the facility plan is not ideal for the intended style of operation. Under these circumstances, the operational procedures established are of overriding importance.

As operational workflow is critical, the establishment of written SOPs outlining every routine procedure conducted in the facility is strongly recommended. SOPs relevant to equipment should include routine validation and documentation of performance. They should be critiqued by veterinary, management, and technical staff prior to implementation. They are also a valuable tool for staff training. They should be identified, using a standard naming convention, in a manner that facilitates access by staff. As procedures are subject to change, a mechanism for regular SOP review and revision should be established. Adherence to SOPs is critical, especially for facilities conducting studies that must adhere to Good Laboratory Practice standards (Code of Federal Regulations, 2004).

Critical decisions, with respect to research facility operations, include (1) the level of exclusion; (2) the transport of clean and soiled caging and materials; (3) the flow of service, technical, and investigative personnel; (4) animal receipt and transport; and (5) the use of PPE.

A. Level of Exclusion

The *level of exclusion* refers to the level at which a physical/operational barrier is created between the animal and the environment. The barrier can be placed at the level of the cage, room, and/or facility. Since the development and refinement of the microisolator cage and the ventilated cabinet for cage changing and animal manipulation, most research facilities have elected to establish the barrier at the cage level for rodents. The MI cage creates a physical barrier between the animal and the environment, which contains fomites that potentially carry infectious agents. The physical barrier can be further enhanced by providing a protective barrier, by positively pressurizing the cage, when utilizing ventilated caging (Lipman *et al.*, 1993). The risk of infectious disease exposure is greatest when the cage is opened for changing or when the animals contained within are manipulated. Risk can be minimized by conducting procedures utilizing well-formulated techniques within a ventilated cabinet, such as a change station or BSC. Both units provide product (animal) protection by bathing animals in laminar flow, HEPA-filtered air, and

preventing ingress of air from outside of the cabinet. As personnel contact with animals is limited to arm/hand exposure within the ventilated cabinet, the use of PPE is often limited to hand and arm covering.

Room-level exclusion utilizes 'open' caging, i.e., cages without a filter top, and benchtop changing and animal manipulation, although room- and cage-level exclusion practices can be combined to further reduce the risk of contamination. Exclusion at the room level requires more extensive use of PPE to ensure that personnel, who have direct contact with the animals, do not act as fomites for disease transmission between animals in the same or different animal holding rooms. Room pressurization is also utilized to limit the spread of infectious agents transmitted via aerosols between rooms (Kowalski *et al.*, 2002). Animal holding rooms are usually maintained at positive pressure with respect to the corridor that serves them. Facility- and room-level exclusions are similar, except that the barrier is implemented at the level of the facility or a subsection of the facility.

B. Material Transport

The flow of clean and soiled caging and ancillary materials from and to the cage wash facility and animal holding rooms is a key operational issue that is heavily influenced by floor plan. Some designs provide distinct corridors to separate these activities; however, the use of dual-corridor facilities has become less common as the space utilization efficiency is decreased with this layout, animal facility construction and operational costs have escalated, and the use of SPF animals has become commonplace. The handling and transportation of cages from clean cage wash (CCW) is of critical importance, as the bulk of materials originate from this area and are distributed throughout the facility. An operational failure resulting in material contamination in CCW is likely to be widely disseminated. Key operational decisions pertaining to CCW include personnel entry and exiting procedures, the selection of and use of uniforms and PPE, the entry of expendable materials such as bedding and feed, and the monitoring and validation of washing and sterilization equipment performance.

Similarly, soiled cage wash (SCW) is the repository of all returning and potentially contaminated equipment. Therefore, procedures that ensure adequate containment are necessary, as the potential for contamination resulting from an infectious disease outbreak is omnipresent, and caging from contaminated animals is commonly processed along with cages from 'clean' colonies. As with CCW, personnel entry and exiting procedures and the selection of and use of uniforms and PPE are also of considerable importance in SCW. As large volumes of waste are generated, methods for its disposal must also be established. In single-corridor facilities, the use of reusable or disposable equipment covers during transport is highly recommended, to reduce the likelihood of cross-contamination during the transport of both clean and soiled equipment. Reusable covers should be sanitized before being reused, e.g., in a washing machine or cage/rack washer.

Whether to steam sterilize soiled materials before processing in SCW or before leaving CCW for distribution to animal holding rooms is a fundamental operational issue pertaining to rodent husbandry. Soiled material sterilization is limited to situations when a known contaminant is present. There are as many proponents who favor the routine use of clean material sterilization as there are those who rely solely on sanitation provided by properly functioning mechanical washing equipment. Few would argue that sterilization of contact bedding materials is not worthwhile, because of the high risk of contamination during processing and storage, unless similarly treated by the vendor prior to delivery and appropriate posttreatment handling.

C. Personnel Flow

Procedures should be established for facility access and intra-facility movement of animal resource, investigative, and service personnel. Apart from the significant risk associated with the inadvertent introduction of contaminated research animals, the incursion of wild or feral animals or other pests, and/or the introduction of contaminated supplies, staff serving as fomites can pose a risk to SPF rodent colonies. This risk is markedly enhanced when staff have access to both contaminated and SPF colonies and can be reduced in varying degrees utilizing workflow that restricts personnel to either 'clean' or 'dirty' colonies, requiring clean colony access to proceed before accessing dirty colonies on the same day, restricting work with a single colony on the same day, and/or the use of water or air showers and donning PPE before accessing colonies of differing health status. Particular attention should be paid to institutional and contract service personnel, as they frequently need to access several facilities serving a single institution or multiple institutions in a single day. Procedures for intra-facility personnel movement should also be established. As discussed above for CCW and SCW personnel, a clear delineation in workflow is also necessary for staff providing direct animal care. In dual-corridor facilities, clean corridor access is often limited to clean cage wash personnel, who use the corridor to distribute clean materials to animal holding rooms. The soiled corridor is used by animal care staff providing direct animal care as well as service personnel. Although the authors' preference is to have research personnel use the soiled corridor to avoid contact between clean equipment and research personnel who come in direct contact with animals, some facilities use the clean corridor for research personnel to access animal holding rooms and procedure laboratories.

D. Animal Receipt and Transport

The introduction of animals into the research facility from external sources poses, in the authors' opinion, the single greatest risk of introducing unwanted infectious agents. Facility management must be discriminating when selecting commercial suppliers to provide animals for research, teaching, and testing. Current and historical colony health profiles should be carefully scrutinized to determine the animals' appropriateness for housing in the intended facility, as well as their suitability for research use. In addition, shipping materials and transport methods should be assessed. Whenever possible, suppliers with dedicated means of conveyance should be selected, as the risk of contamination increases when using a common carrier, which may simultaneously transport animals of differing health status, from numerous sources, using a variety of shipping materials. The question of whether to isolate and quarantine incoming animals of desirable health quality from commercial suppliers is complex and is dictated by a variety of issues, including the animals' intended use, their value, the ease of replacing existing colonies if an infectious outbreak would result, the risk that the animals harbor a zoonotic agent, the availability of space, confidence in the supplier based on historical record of maintaining biosecurity, and transportation methods used to deliver the animals to the facility. If quarantine is implemented, the length and scope of testing must be determined. Rehg and Toth (1988) have reviewed the issues associated with rodent quarantine.

As the production of unique genetically engineered rodents has become commonplace, mice and rats are now frequently transferred among noncommercial suppliers such as academic and commercial research institutions. These colonies are frequently 'open,' in that there may be repetitive introductions of new animals from commercial and noncommercial sources and they are frequently accessed by a large number of staff. Therefore, the risk of adventitious agent introduction is significantly enhanced in 'open' colonies as compared to the 'closed' colonies maintained by commercial suppliers. Under most circumstances, institutions typically quarantine or rederive rodents from open colonies. Detailed discussion of the issues associated with importing mice from open colonies and descriptions of importation programs has been described (Rehg and Toth, 1988; Durfee and Faith, 1999; Otto and Tolwani, 2002; Lipman and Homberger, 2003). Common program features include receiving rodents in an area separate from that used for receiving rodents from commercial suppliers, maintaining the animals in distinct rooms or facilities spatially separate from established colonies for a specified time, restricting access to essential personnel, and testing for select adventitious agents. Because of the low sensitivity of diagnostic techniques for endo- and ectoparasites, some institutions routinely treat all incoming animals from noncommercial sources with anthelminthics, although the use of molecular diagnostics may mitigate this need.

The receipt of animals should take place in a suitable area by trained personnel using appropriate techniques. There are two principal methods used for receiving rodents and rabbits: (1) uncrating in a dedicated centralized receiving area(s) or (2) uncrating within the room in which they will subsequently be housed. There are advantages and disadvantages of each method, and institutions may use both, depending on the research facility and source of animals. As animal receiving is associated with considerable risk with respect to cross-contamination with adventitious agents, development of and adherence to stringent operational procedures is essential. The use of a dedicated receiving area permits the centralization of receiving and the assignment of dedicated personnel. As many research institutions utilize computerized animal facility management systems, which require the entry of receiving information into a database, centralized receiving areas are often equipped with computer workstation(s) facilitating data entry. Ventilated cabinets are often employed for uncrating rodents. Class II BSCs are preferred, as the cabinet provides both product (animal) and personnel (environment) protection. In newer facilities, receiving is often situated at the perimeter of the research facility. A pass-through BSC is employed, allowing crated animals to be placed within the BSC from one side and caged animals removed, into the holding area or barrier, on the other. The major disadvantage of a dedicated receiving area is the potential for dissemination of an infectious agent if a contaminated shipment is received and appropriate procedures are not followed. The risk is high, as multiple shipments from various vendors are frequently processed within a limited time frame and animals may be distributed from receiving into various colonies. Alternatively, animals can be uncrated in the housing room. This method of receipt is frequently employed when receiving rodents into quarantine from open colonies, to avoid handling potentially contaminated animals in the same area as those obtained from commercial vendors. Animals can be uncrated by either dedicated receiving personnel or the animal care staff member assigned to service the room in which they will be housed. If dedicated personnel are assigned, they frequently enter multiple rooms on a single day. The enhanced risk of cross-contamination associated with the use of dedicated personnel requires implementation of appropriate safeguards.

Both methods require careful adherence to well-defined operational procedures, including careful inspection of shipping materials for defects before uncrating; thorough disinfection of the cabinet and shipping crate with a suitable hard surface disinfectant before unpacking, and with respect to the cabinet, between crates, ensuring sufficient contact time; equipping personnel with appropriate PPE, especially for the hands and forearms; repeatedly using an appropriate hand sanitizing agent; and using a disinfected implement such as a forceps to relocate animals from the shipping crate to their housing cage ensuring adequate contact time before reuse between crates.

E. Personal Protective Equipment

PPE is employed for a variety of functions. Its options include shoe covers, hair bonnets, a variety of face masks and respirators, laboratory coats, jumpsuits, sleeves, and gloves. Some items are available as disposables, and consideration should be given to their use, as PPE can serve as fomites for disease transmission. However, costs for disposable items can be significant in larger facilities. PPE is employed to protect the animals from exposure to adventitious agents, to protect personnel from environmental or experimental hazards, or both. In most research facilities, the majority of PPE is employed to protect animals from contamination. For this function, the minimal recommended PPE would consist of a laboratory coat and gloves. These garments cover the forearms and hands, the body parts most likely to have direct animal contact. In addition, they serve to protect the handler from sensitizing allergens found on the animals' fur and in their urine. Additional PPE may be desirable, especially when handling animals on the open bench as opposed to a ventilated cabinet. Hair bonnets prevent particulates found in the hair from being shed onto the animals or the work surface on which they are handled; they also reduce the potential of hair contamination from environmental particulates. Face masks and respirators contain droplet nuclei that may contain problematic bacteria, especially when utilizing immunocompromised models, and, if they are of the appropriate type and are properly fitted as required by the Occupational Safety and Health Administration (OSHA), they can reduce exposure to inhalational allergens and hazardous particulates. The use of shoe covers is controversial. Although donning shoe covers, using an appropriate technique, should reduce the potential for introducing environmental contaminants into the space in which they are worn, or alternatively, reduce the potential of cross-contamination when worn in contaminated areas and removed immediately upon exiting, there is limited objective data evaluating their effectiveness. The authors' concern regarding shoe cover use is that inappropriate placement may lead the wearer to touch the soles or tops of the shoes, contaminating the hands, which are likely to have direct contact with the animals and/or their caging, and a recent study demonstrated that shoe covers did not enhance and may actually compromise biosecurity (Hickman-Davis et al., 2012).

Gloves are the most important piece of PPE employed in an animal research facility, as they are essential for protecting the wearer from various animal and environmental hazards and, if properly donned and used, cross-contamination. Although there are a host of glove types available, latex, nitrile, and vinyl are the most commonly utilized in the vivarium. While natural latex is inexpensive and provides an excellent skin barrier, irritant dermatitis, delayed hypersensitivity (Type IV allergy), and immediate hypersensitivity (Type I allergy) reactions are common among workers who routinely wear latex gloves. Estimates indicate that approximately 8–12% of health care workers regularly exposed to latex are sensitized (Katelaris et al., 1996; Kelly et al. 1996; Liss et al., 1997; Ownby et al., 1996; Sussman and Beezhold, 1995). Powdered latex gloves pose a greater risk, in that the cornstarch powder used binds the latex protein, permitting the antigen to reach the skin more easily while also increasing the amount of free latex liberated (Beezhold et al., 1994; Patterson, 1995). In addition, the latex containing powder is aerosolized when the gloves are donned and removed, serving as a significant source of aerosolized latex protein, which can be inhaled. It is important to note that there can be significant differences in the amount of latex protein released, based upon the glove manufacturer (Swanson et al., 1994; Turjanmaa et al., 1988).

Although latex gloves are suitable for many applications, they are not impervious to all chemicals. Nitrile gloves are frequently more suitable for applications involving hazardous chemicals, although suitability for the specific chemical must be verified. Vinyl gloves, while not providing the tactile qualities of latex, may be suitable for many applications.

F. Environmental Enrichment

Increasing attention is being placed on enriching the environment in which animals are housed. "The primary aim of environmental enrichment is to enhance animal well-being by providing animals with sensory and motor stimulation, through structures and resources that facilitate the expression of species-typical behaviors and promote psychological well-being through physical exercise, manipulative activities, and cognitive challenges according to species-specific characteristics" (ILAR, 2011). While environmental enrichment for large animal species was commonplace, only recently have facilities routinely provided additional items to enrich the environment of mouse and rat cages. Large animal enrichment typically includes structural additions to the cage or pen such as perches, ladders, visual barriers, and resting boards. Additionally, dependent on the species and housing system used, supplementary materials including nesting materials, running wheels, dust boxes, shelters, hides, manipulatable and/or chewable objects, and artificial plants may be provided as enrichment dependent on species.

Strategies for providing environmental enrichment to rodents as well as their effects have been recently reviewed (Hutchinson et al., 2005). In addition to the costs associated with the purchase, sanitation, and handling of supplemental materials, which can be significant, especially for rodents as colony sizes can exceed tens of thousands of cages, concerns pertaining to interindividual variation, study repeatability, and the impact on behavioral and physiological responses, which could potentially alter research results, have been raised. Studies have shown that cage enrichment has no effect on individual variability in most behavioral tests, which are more sensitive to environmental perturbations than physiological parameters, and did not increase the risk of collecting conflicting data in replicate experiments (Van de Weerd et al., 2002; Wolfer et al., 2004). However, enrichment has been shown to increase body weight, alter food consumption, and affect immunological parameters, although these findings have been inconsistently observed (Kingston and Hoffman-Goetz, 1996; Van de Weerd et al., 1997b, 2002; Augustsson et al., 2003; Marashi et al., 2004). Various enrichment methods have been proposed, including the provision of nesting material, objects that increase the complexity of the cage or which animals can gnaw, structures in which animals can hide and/or nest, and running wheels. The provision of nesting material is, to date, the only consistently recommended enrichment method for mice and rats (Blom et al., 1992; Van de Weerd et al., 1996, 1997a,b, 1998; Olsson and Dahlborn, 2002). Laboratory rodents will build a nest if they are provided with suitable material (Brain, 1992). Nesting materials used include paper towel, crinkled paper strips, toilet tissue (unscented), processed corn husk, wood wool, gauze cotton batting, and compressed virgin cotton fibers (Sherwin, 1997; Van de Weerd et al., 1997a; Armstrong et al., 1998). Female mice build nests for their offspring, whereas nonbreeding female and male mice may build nests for temperature control, shelter from external disturbances, isolation from conspecifics, and/or excessive light intensity (Brain, 1992; Sherwin, 1997; Van de Weerd et al., 1997a). Nesting material has been shown to decrease aggression in group-housed male mice and has been suggested as a means for compensating for social contact deprivation when housing males singly (Van Loo et al., 2003, 2004).

G. Personnel Training

The foundation of a sound management program is staffing with adequately trained personnel provided with the appropriate resources to carry out their responsibilities in a safe and comfortable environment. Providing training for personnel caring for and using laboratory animals is not only sound management and an ethical imperative, but also a regulatory requirement. The ILAR (1991) publication "Education and Training in the Care and Use of Laboratory Animals: A Guide for Developing Institutional Programs" provides guidelines and resources needed to coordinate and implement a regulatory compliant training program. In addition, the American Association for Laboratory Animal Science (AALAS) offers education programs and materials for training animal care technicians and managers, and administers programs that certifies knowledge at three levels for technical staff, Assistant Laboratory Animal Technician (ALAT), Laboratory Animal Technician (LAT), and Laboratory Animal Technologist (LATG), as well as a program for certifying management personnel, Certified Manager Animal Resources (CMAR), administered in conjunction with the Institute for Certified Professional Managers (ICPM). The AALAS has also established a Technician Certification Registry that allows certified technical staff to demonstrate that they maintain current knowledge. Technicians who participate in the registry and meet its requirements are recognized with the prefix 'R' before their certification designation, e.g., RLAT. Documenting and recognizing achievement is a strong motivator for personnel to gain knowledge and competence. Many institutions have linked AALAS certification to promotion as an additional motivator, and it assists the institution to demonstrate it as appropriately trained and experienced staff, and also establishes the basis for a developmental career ladder.

Institutions commonly administer additional and often institution-specific training programs to both animal care personnel and animal users. These programs frequently include didactic and hands-on sessions on a range of topics often supplemented with written and online resources. The AALAS's Learning Library provides online learning materials for education and training which are often incorporated by member institutions into their training program. In addition, many allied organizations whose mission is focused on laboratory animal welfare and use, as well as various commercial enterprises, offer web-based, written, and classroom training *gratis* or for a fee.

Training is also a critical and mandatory component of an occupational health and safety program. Its scope should be consistent with and tailored to the risks associated with the hazards present in the animal facility. The National Academy of Sciences publication "Occupational Health and Safety in the Care and Use of Research Animals" is an excellent resource (ILAR, 2007).

Ultimately, the IACUC is responsible for ensuring that all personnel who support or use animals in research, teaching, or testing are adequately trained, and provides resources to aid institutions in meeting these requirements (ILAR, 2011).

H. Disaster Planning and Management

Emergency preparedness is an integral, essential and mandated component of an animal care and use program. Animal facilities are critically dependent upon infrastructure and personnel to ensure maintenance of environmental conditions, operate essential systems, and provide animal care. A written disaster plan should be developed in concert with animal facility management, veterinary staff, institutional safety personnel, the institutional official, investigative staff, and facilities maintenance and engineering personnel with the support and input of senior institutional leadership. The plan should be developed in consideration of geographical risks. Local emergency personnel and law enforcement should be provided a copy of the plan for review and integration into a broader areawide plan when the scope of the disaster is local or regional (Vogelweid, 1998). The plan should identify leadership, essential personnel, procedures, and communication strategies to be employed under conditions that disrupt routine operations. Examples include utility failures; physical damage to the animal facility as a result of extreme weather, earthquake, terrorism, fire, and/or flood; personnel shortages resulting from weather, contagious disease, or transportation interruptions; exposure to hazardous agents and materials; and other risks as determined by a thorough assessment. Minimally, the plan should ensure the welfare of animals and personnel. It should include strategies for animal relocation or, if not possible, euthanasia. As many genetically engineered animals are irreplaceable, consideration should be given to proactively cryopreserving germplasm and/or establishing a system to triage breeding stock to prevent loss of irreplaceable resources. The plan should be reviewed and revised regularly, ideally no less than annually, to ensure it reflects current risks, practices, and processes.

VII. CONCLUSIONS

The sophistication, complexity, and size of research facilities that support the use of research animals continue to escalate. Technological enhancements pervade all aspects of animal research facility design, operations, and equipment. As a result, the laboratory animal specialist and research facility management must have a thorough knowledge and keep abreast of a broad array of topics. The maintenance of research animals in a comfortable, stress-free, controlled environment, which is essential to contemporary biomedical research, requires appropriate facilities as well as sound management. Each must complement the other. In addition to providing a stable macroenvironment that minimizes physiological perturbations which may confound research results, animal research facilities must be designed and operated with optimal productivity and efficiency, while ensuring the health status of the animals is maintained. The better the facility is designed to incorporate sound management and efficient animal care, the lower the cost of animal care and the more likely environmental variables will be adequately controlled ensuring that reproducible and reliable data is generated, which in turn reduces the number of animals required to achieve the desired research goals.

References

Adelberg, E., Austrian, R., Bachrach, H.L., 1989. Biosafety in the Laboratory. National Academies Press, Washington DC.

Allred, C., Allred, K., Young, H., et al., 2001. Soy diets containing varying amounts of genistein stimulate growth of estrogen dependent (MCF-7) tumors in a dose-dependent manner. Cancer Res. 61, 5045–5050.

Allport, J., Weissleder, R., 2001. In vivo imaging of gene and cell therapies. Exp. Hematol. 29, 1237–1246.

Alworth, L.C., Vasquez, V.M., 2009. A novel system for individually housing bullfrogs. Lab. Anim. 38, 329–333.

American Conference of Governmental Industrial Hygienists, 2004. Threshold Limit Values for Chemical Substances and Physical Agents and Biological Indices. ACGIH, Cincinnati, OH.

American Society of Heating, Refrigerating, and Air-Conditioning Engineers, Inc., 2001. 2001 ASHRAE Handbook Fundamentals. American Society of Heating, Refrigerating, and Air-Conditioning Engineers, Inc., Atlanta, GA.

American Society of Heating, Refrigerating, and Air-Conditioning Engineers, Inc., 2003. 2003 ASHRAE Handbook Heating, Ventilating, and Air Conditioning Applications. American Society of Heating, Refrigerating, and Air-Conditioning Engineers, Inc., Atlanta, GA.

Anthony, A., 1962. Criteria for acoustics in animal housing. Lab. Anim. Care 13, 340–347.

Armstrong, K., Clark, T., Peterson, M., 1998. Use of corn-husk nesting material to reduce aggression in caged mice. Contemp. Top. Lab. Anim. Sci. 37, 64–66.

Augustsson, H., VandeWeerd, H., Kruitwagen, C., et al., 2003. Effect of enrichment on variation and results in the light/dark test. Lab. Anim. 37, 328–340.

Baer, L.A., Corbin, B., Vasques, M.F., 1997. Effects of the use of filtered microisolator tops on cage microenvironment and growth rate of mice. Lab. Anim. Sci. 47, 327–329.

Balk, M., 1980. Animal-facility design criteria for toxicological testing laboratory. Pharm. Technol. 4, 59–64.

Barkley, W.E., 1979. Abilities and limitations of architectural and engineering features in controlling biohazards in animal facilities. In: Institute of Laboratory Animal Resources, Symposium on Laboratory Animal Housing. National Academy of Sciences, National Research Council, Washington, DC, pp. 158–163.

Barkley, W.E., Richardson, J.H., 1984. Control of biohazards associated with the use of experimental animals. In: Fox, J.G., Cohen, B.J., Loew, F.M. (Eds.), Laboratory Animal Medicine. Academic Press, Orlando, FL, pp. 595–602.

Barrows, C.S., Alaire, Y., Stock, M., 1978. Sensory irritation and incapacitation evoked by thermal decomposition products of polymers and comparison with known sensory irritants. Arch. Environ. Health 33, 79–88.

Baumans, V., Schlingmann, F., Vonck, M., et al., 2002. Individually ventilated cages: beneficial for mice and men? Contemp. Top. Lab. Anim. Sci. 41, 13–19.

Bhatt, P.N., Jacoby, R.O., 1983. An inexpensive containment laboratory for mousepox research [abstr]. Lab. Anim. Sci. 33, 495.

Bazille, P., Walden, S., Koniar, B., et al., 2001. Commercial cotton nesting material as a predisposing factor for conjunctivitis in athymic nude mice. Lab. Anim. 30, 40–42.

Beck, R., 1963. The control of Pseudomonas aeruginosa in a mouse breeding colony by the use of chlorine in the drinking water. Lab. Anim. Care 13, 41–45.

Beezhold, D., Kostyal, D., Wiseman, J., 1994. The transfer of protein allergens from latex gloves: a study of influencing factors. AORN J. 59, 605–613.

Bellhorn, R., 1980. Lighting in the animal environment. Lab. Anim. Sci. 30, 440–450.

Benveniste, H., Blackband, S., 2002. MR microscopy and high resolution small animal MRI: applications in neuroscience research. Prog. Neurobiol. 67, 393–420.

Block, S. (Ed.), 2001. Disinfection, Sterilization, and Preservation, fifth ed. Lippincott Williams & Wilkins, Philadelphia, PA.

Blom, H., vanVorstenbosch, C., Baumans, V., Hoogervorst, M.J.C., Beynen, A.C., van Zutphen, L.F.M., et al., 1992. Description and validation of a preference test system to evaluate housing conditions for laboratory mice. Appl. Anim. Behav. Sci. 35, 67–82.

Blom, H.J.M., Van Tintelen, G., Van, V., 1996. Preferences of mice and rats for types of bedding material. Lab. Anim. 30, 234–244.

Bolon, B., Bonnefoi, M.S., Roberts, K.C., 1991. Toxic interactions in the rat nose: pollutants from soiled bedding and methyl bromide. Toxicol. Pathol. 19, 571–579.

Brain, P., 1992. Understanding the behaviours of feral species may facilitate design of optimal living conditions for common laboratory rodents. Anim. Technol. 43, 99–105.

Brainard, G., Rollag, M., Hanifin, J., 1997. Photic regulation of melatonin in humans: ocular and neural signal transduction. J. Biol. Rhythms 12, 537–546.

Brewer, N., 1972. Sterilization, antiseptics, and detergents. In: Collins, G.R. (Ed.), Syllabus for the laboratory animal technologist. American Association for Laboratory Animal Science (AALAS) Pub. No. 72-2. Joliet, IL. pp. 93–103.

Brewer, N.R., 1952. Some problems in animal quarter construction in urban areas. Proc. Anim. Care Panel 3, 64–69.

Brewer, N.R., Penfold, T.W., 1961. Thoughts concerning the design of animal quarters. Proc. Anim. Care Panel 11, 4–18.

Brick, J.O., Newell, R.F., Doherty, D.G., 1969. A barrier system for breeding and experimental rodent colony; description and operation. Lab. Anim. Care 19, 92–97.

Broderson, J.R., Lindsey, J.R., Crawford, J.E., 1976. The role of environmental ammonia in respiratory irritant gasses. Am. J. Pathol. 85, 115–127.

Brook, I., Elliot, T., Ledney, G., et al., 2004. Management of post-irradiation infection: lessons learned from animal models. Mil. Med. 169, 194–197.

Brown, M.J., 1994. Aseptic surgery for rodents. In: Niemi, S., Venable, J.S. (Eds.), Rodents and Rabbits: Current Research Issues. Scientist Center for Animal Welfare, Bethesda, MD, pp. 67–72.

Browne, R.K., Odum, R.A., Herman, T., Zippel, K., 2007. Facility design and associated services for the study of amphibians. ILAR J. 48 (3), 188–202.

Budinger, T., Benaron, D., Koretsky, A., 1999. Imaging transgenic animals. Annu. Rev. Biomed. Eng. 1, 611–648.

Bywater, J., Kellett, B., 1977. Inhibition of bacteria in mouse drinking water by chlorination. Lab. Anim. 11, 215–217.

Cantor, K., 1997. Drinking water and cancer. Cancer Causes Control 8, 292–308.

Casebolt, D.B., 2009. Facilities for dogs, swine, sheep, goats and miscellaneous species. In: Hessler, J.R., Lehner, N.D.M. (Eds.), Planning and Designing Research Animal Facilities. Academic Press, London, pp. 313–321.

CCAC (Canadian Council on Animal Care), 1993. Approaches to the Design and Development of Cost-Effective Laboratory Animal Facilities. 1993. Canadian Council on Animal Care (CCAC) proceedings. Ottawa, Ontario, Canada: CCAC. 273 pp.

CDC-NIH (Center for Disease Control-National Institues of Health), 2009. Biosafety in Microbiological and Biomedical Laboratories, fifth ed. U.S. Department of Health and Human Services, Public Health Service, Centers for Disease Control and Prevention, and National Institutes of Health, U.S. Government Printing Office, Washington, DC.

Chatziioannou, A., 2002. PET scanners dedicated to molecular imaging of small animal models. Mol. Imaging Biol. 4, 47–63.

Cherry, J.A., 1987. The effect of photoperiod on development of sexual behavior in fertility in golden hamsters. Physiol. Behav. 39, 521–552.

Chipps, J., Bergdall, V.K., Hanson, N., Hadziselimovic, D., 2012. Increasing the usable lifespan of clouded rodent caging via implementation of a novel cage wash sanitation process. J. Am. Assoc. Lab. Anim. Sci. 51, 637.

Choi, G., McQuinn, J.S., Jennings, B.L., 1994. Effect of population size on humidity and ammonia levels in individually ventilated microisolation rodent caging. Contemp. Top. Lab. Anim. Sci. 33, 77–81.

Christie, R.J., Williams, F.P., Whitney, J.R., Johnson, D.J., 1968. Techniques used in the establishment and maintenance of a barrier mouse breeding colony. Lab. Anim. Care 18, 544–549.

Clough, G., 1982. Environmental effects on animals used in biomedical research. Biol. Rev. 57, 487–523.

Clough, G., Fasham, J., 1975. A "silent" fire alarm. Lab. Anim. 9, 193–196.

Clough, G., Wallace, J., Gamble, M.R., 1995. A positive, individually ventilated caging system: a local barrier system to protect both animals and personnel. Lab. Anim. 29, 139–151.

Code of Federal Regulations, 1992. Airborne Particulate Cleanliness Classes in Cleanrooms and Clean Zones. FED-STD-209e Institute of Environmental Sciences, Mount Prospect, IL.

Code of Federal Regulations, 1993. Animals and Animal Products, 9 CFR §1.1–§4.1.

Code of Federal Regulations, 1999. Standards for Protection Against Radiation, 10 C.F.R. §20.1001–20.2402.

Code of Federal Regulations, 2004. Good Laboratory Practice Regulations, 21 C.F.R. §58.1–58.219.

Coghlan, L., Lee, D., Psencik, B., et al., 1993. Practical and effective eradication of pinworms (Syphacia muris) in rats by use of fenbendazole. Lab. Anim. Sci. 43, 481–487.

Cole, M.N., 1991. Laboratory animal facility planning In: Ruys, T. (Ed.), Handbook of Facilities Planning, vol. 2 Van Nostrand Reinhold, New York, pp. 199–214. "Laboratory animal facilities".

Cole, M.N., Hessler, J.R., 1991. Space standards In: Ruys, T. (Ed.), Handbook of Facilities Planning, vol. 2. Van Nostrand Reinhold, New York, pp. 67–75. "Laboratory animal facilities".

Commission on Physical Sciences, Mathematics and Applications, 1995. Prudent practices in the laboratory: handling and disposal of chemicals. National Academies Press, Washington, DC.

Conner, D., Eckman, M., 1992. Rotation of phenolic disinfectants. Pharm. Tech. 148–160.

Contag, C., Bachmann, M., 2002. Advances in in vivo bioluminescence imaging of gene expression. Annu. Rev. Biomed. Eng. 4, 235–260.

Corning, B., Lipman, N., 1991. A comparison of rodent caging system based on microenvironmental parameters. Lab. Anim. Sci. 41, 498–503.

Costello, T., Watkins, L., Straign, M., Bean, W., Toth, L., Rehg, J., et al., 1998. Effectiveness of rack sanitation procedures for elimination of bacteria from automatic watering manifolds. Contemp. Top. Lab. Anim. Sci. 37, 50–51.

Cover, C., Belcher, L., 1992. Effect of an irradiated rodent diet on growth and food consumption: a comparative study. Contemp. Top. Lab. Anim. Sci. 31, 13–17.

Cunliffe-Beamer, T.L., 1993. Applying principles of aseptic surgery to rodents. AWIC Newslett. 4, 3–6.

Cunliffe-Beamer, T.L., Les, E.P., 1983. Effectiveness of pressurized individually ventilated (PIV) cages in reducing transmission of pneumonia virus of mice (PVM) [abstr]. Lab. Anim. Sci. 33, 495.

Curry, G., Hughes, H.C., Loseby, D., Reynolds, S., et al., 1998. Advances in cubicle design using computational fluid dynamics as a design tool. Lab. Anim. 32, 117–127.

Dauchy, R., Sauer, L., Blask, D., Vaughn, G.M., 1997. Light contamination during the dark phase in "photoperiodically controlled" animal rooms: effect on tumor growth and metabolism in rats. Lab. Anim. Sci. 47, 511–518.

DeTolla, L.J., Sriniva, S., Whitaker, B.R., Andrews, C., Hecker, B., Kane, A.S., 1995. Guidelines for the care and use of fish in research. ILAR J. 37, 159–172.

DiBerardinis, L.J., 1999. Handbook of Occupational Safety and Health. John Wiley & Sons Inc., New York.

Diggs, H.E., Parker, J.M., 2009. Aquatic Facilities. In: Hessler, J.R., Lehner, N. D. M. (Eds.), Planning and Designing Research Animal Facilities. Academic Press, London, UK, pp. 323–331.

Dolowy, W.C., 1961. Medical research laboratory of the University of Illinois. Proc. Anim. Care Panel 11, 267–290.

Domer, D.A., Erickson, R.L., Petty, J.M., Bergdall, V.K., Hickman-Davis, J.M., 2012. Processing and treatment of corncob bedding affects cage-change frequency for C57BL/6 mice. J. Am. Assoc. Lab. Anim. Sci. 51, 162–169.

Drickamer, L., 1977. Seasonal variation in litter size, body weight, and sexual maturation in juvenile female house mice. Lab. Anim. 11, 159–162.

Drickamer, L., 1982. Acceleration and delay of sexual maturation in female mice via chemosignals: circadian rhythm effects. Biol. Reprod. 27, 596–601.

Drickamer, L., 1984. Seasonal variations in acceleration and delay of sexual maturation in female mice by urinary chemosignals. J. Reprod. Fertil. 72, 55–58.

Drickamer, L., 1990a. Environmental factors and age of puberty in female house mice. Dev. Psychobiol. 23, 63–73.

Drickamer, L., 1990b. Seasonal variation in fertility, fecundity, and litter sex ratios in laboratory and wild stocks of house mice. Lab. Anim. Sci. 40, 284–288.

Drozdowicz, C.K., Bowman, T.A., Webb, M.L., Lang, C.M., 1990. Effect of in-house transport on murine plasma corticosterone concentration and blood lymphocyte populations. Am. J. Vet. Res. 51, 1841–1846.

Durfee, W., Faith, R., 1999. Biological security: quarantine and testing policies for protecting transgenic colonies. Lab. Anim. 28, 45–48.

Edstrom Industries, 2003a. Ultraviolet Disinfection. Edstrom Industries, Waterford, WI.

Edstrom Industries, 2003b. Chlorination of Drinking Water. Edstrom Industries, Waterford, WI.

Eskola, S., Kaliste-Korhonen, E., 1999. Nesting material and number of females per cage: effects on mouse productivity in BALB/c, C57BL/6J, DBA/2 and NIH/S mice. Lab. Anim. 33, 122–128.

Evans, M.E., Lesnaw, J.A., 1999. Infection control in gene therapy. Infect. Control Hosp. Epidmemiol. 20(8), 568–576.

Federation of Animal Science Societies, 2010. Guide for the Care and Use of Agricultural Animals in Research and Teaching. Third Edition. Champaign, IL.

Favero, M., 1990. Sterilization and disinfection strategies used in hospitals. In: Cundy, K. (Ed.), Infection Control: Dilemmas and Practical Solutions. Plenum Press, New York, pp. 63–68.

Ferguson, H., 1966. Effect of red cedar chip bedding on hexobarbital and pentobarbital sleep time. J. Pharm. Sci. 55, 1142–1148.

Fidler, I., 1977. Depression of macrophages in mice drinking hyperchlorinated water. Nature 270, 735–736.

Ford, D., 1987. Nutrition and feeding. In: Poole, T.B. (Ed.), The UFAW Handbook on the Care and Management of Laboratory Animals, sixth ed. Longman Scientific & Technical, Essex, England.

Foster, F., Pavlin, C., Harasiewicz, K., Christopher, D.A., Turnbull, D.H., et al., 2000. Advances in ultrasound biomicroscopy. Ultrasound Med. Biol. 26, 1–27.

Foster, H.L., Foster, S.J., Pfau, E.S., 1963. The large scale production of caesarean originated, barrier-sustained mice. Lab. Anim. Care 13, 23–25.

Fox, J., Donahue, P., Essigmann, J., 1980. Efficacy of inactivation of representative chemical carcinogens utilizing commercial alkaline and acidic cage wash compounds. J. Environ. Pathol. Toxicol. 4, 97–106.

Fox, J.G., Barthold, S.W., Davisson, M.T., Newcomer, C.E., Quimby, F.W., Smith, A.L., 2007. The Mouse in Biomedical Research, second ed. Academic Press, Burlington, MA.

Fuchs, A., 1951. Bacterial Value of Dishwashing Machine Sprays. U.S. Public Health Serv, Washington, DC.

Fullerton, F.R., Greenman, D.L., Kendall, D.C., 1982. Effectgs of storage conditions on nutritional qualities of semipurified (AIJN–76) and natural ingredient (NIH–07) diets. J. Nutr. 12, 567–573.

Gale, G.R., Smith, A.B., 1981. Ureolytic and urease-activating properties of commercial laboratory animal bedding. Lab. Anim. Sci. 31, 56–59.

Garcia, T., 1998. Pharmaceutical drugs appearing in Europe's drinking water. <http://www.envirolink.org>.

Gaskill, B.N., Gordon, C.J., Pajor, E.A., Lucas, J.R., Davis, J.K., Garner, J.P., 2012. Heat or insulation: behavioral titration of mouse preference for warmth or access to a nest. PLoS One 3, e32799.

Giuliano, G. (2012). Decision on durable or disposable plastic caging systems. <http://www.alnmag.com>.

Goelz, M, Mahler, J., Harry, J., Myers, P., Clarck, J., Thigpen, J.E., et al., 1998. Neuropathologic findings associated with seizures in FVB mice. Lab. Anim. Sci. 48, 34–37.

Goldstein, S.J., 1978. A theory of architecture: the orchestration of information "Symposium on Laboratory Animal Housing" (Institute of Laboratory animal Resources). National Academy of Sciences – National Research Council, Washington, DC, pp. 16–24.

Gonzalez, D.M., Graciano, S.J., Karlstad, J., Leblanc, M., Clark, T., Holmes, S., et al., 2011. Failure and life cycle evaluation of watering valves. J. Am. Assoc. Lab. Anim. Sci. 50, 713–718.

Gordon, C., 1998. Behavioral thermoregulatory responses of single- and group-housed mice. Physiol. Behav. 65, 255–262.

Gordon, A., Wyatt, J., 2011. The water delivery system affects the rate of weight gain in C57BL/6J mice during the first week after weaning. J. Am. Assoc. Lab. Anim. Sci. 50, 37–40.

Gordon, A.H., Hart, P.D., Young, M.R., 1980. Ammonia inhibits phagosome-lysosome fusion in macrophages. Nature 286, 79–80.

Green, S.L., 2010. The Laboratory *Xenopus sp.* The Laboratory Animal Pocket Reference Series. CRC Press, Taylor & Francis Group, Boca Raton, FL, p. 156.

Greenman, D., Bryant, P., Kodell, R., et al., 1982. Influence of cage shelf level on retinal atrophy in mice. Lab. Anim. Sci. 32, 353–356.

Grumman, D.L., 1986. Air-Handling Systems Ready Reference Manual. McGraw-Hill, New York, p. 170.

Gullino, P., Ediger, R., Giovanella, B., Merchant, B., Outzen, H.C.J., Reed, N.D., et al., 1976. Guide for the care and use of the nude (thymus-deficient) mouse in biomedical research. ILAR News 19, 3–20.

Hall, J., White, W.J., Lang, C.M., 1980. Acidification of drinking water: its effects on selected biologic phenomena in male mice. Lab. Anim. Sci. 30, 643–651.

Halls, N., Tallentire, A., 1978. Effects of processing and gamma irradiation on the microbiological contaminants of a laboratory animal diet. Lab. Anim. 12, 5–10.

Hare, R., O'Donoghue, P.N. (Eds.), 1968. Laboratory Animal Symposia: The Design and Function of Laboratory Animal Houses. Laboratory Animals Ltd., Ashrod Kent, England.

Harper, C., Lawrence, C., 2011. The Laboratory Zebrafish. CRC Press. Boca Raton, FL, p. 188.

Hasenau, J., Baggs, R., Kraus, A., 1993. Microenvironments in microisolation cages using BALB/c and CD-1 mice. Contemp. Top. Lab. Anim. Sci. 32, 11–16.

Heffner, H.E., Heffner, R.S., 2007. Hearing ranges of laboratory animals. J. Am. Assoc. Lab. Anim. Sci. 46, 11–13.

Hermann, L., White, W.J., Lang, C.M., 1982. Prolonged exposure to acid, chlorine, or tetracycline in drinking water: effects on delayed-type hypersensitivity, hemagglutination titers, and reticuloendothelial clearance rates in mice. Lab. Anim. Sci. 32, 603–608.

Hessler, J.R., 1991a. Single versus dual-corridor systems: advantages, limitations, and alternatives for effective contamination control In: Ruys, T. (Ed.), Handbook of Facilities Planning, vol. 2. Van Nostrand Reinhold, New York, pp. 59–67. "Laboratory Animal Facilities".

Hessler, J.R., 1991b. Animal cubicles. In: Ruys, T. (Ed.), Handbook of Facilities Planning, vol. 2. Van Nostrand Reinhold, New York, pp. 135–154. "Laboratory Animal Facilities".

Hessler, J.R., 1993. Animal cubicles: questions, anwers, options, opinions. Lab. Anim. 22, 21–32.

Hessler, J.R., 1995. Methods of biocontainment. In: Bayne, K.A.L., Greene, M., Prentice, M.E.D. (Eds.), Current Issues and New Frontiers in Animal Research Scientists. Center for Animal Welfare, Greenbelt, MD, pp. 61–58.

Hessler, J.R., 1999. The history of environmental improvements in laboratory animal science: caging systems, equipment, and facility design. In: McPherson, C.W., Mattingly, S.F. (Eds.), 50 Years of Laboratory Animal Science. Sheridan Books, Memphis, TN, pp. 92–120.

Hessler, J., Leary, S., 2002. Design and management of animal facilities. In: Fox, J., Anderson, L. (Eds.), Laboratory Animal Medicine, second ed. Academic Press, New York, pp. 909–953.

Hessler, J.R., Lehner, N.D.M., 2009. Planning and Designing Research Animal Facilities. Academic Press, London.

Hessler, J.R., Moreland, A.F., 1984. Design and management of animal facilities. In: Fox, G., Cohen, B.J., Lowe, F.M. (Eds.), Laboratory Animal Medicine. Academic Press, Orlando, FL, pp. 505–526.

Hessler, J.R., Broderson, R., King, C., 1999. Animal research facilities and equipment. In: Richmond, J.Y. (Ed.), Anthology of Biosafety 1. Perspectives on Laboratory Design. American Biological Safety Association, Mundelein, IL, pp. 191–217.

Hickman-Davis, J.M., Nicolaus, M.L., Petty, J.M., Harrison, D.M., Bergdall, V.K., 2012. Effectiveness of shoe covers for bioexclusion within an animal facility. J. Am. Assoc. Lab. Anim. Sci. 51, 181–188.

Hoffman, J.C, 1973. The influence of photoperiods on reproductive functions in female mammals. In: Greep, R.O. and Astwood, E.B. (Eds.) Handbook of Physiology, Endocrinology II, Part I, Section 7. American Physiological Society. Washington, DC, pp. 57–77.

Hoglund, A., Renstrom, A., 2001. Evaluation of individually ventilated cage systems for laboratory rodents: cage environment and animal health aspects. Lab. Anim. 35, 51–57.

Homberger, F., Pataki, Z., Thomann, P., 1993. Control of *Pseudomonas aeruginosa* infection in mice by chlorine treatment of drinking water. Lab. Anim. Sci. 43, 635–637.

Horsfall, F.L., Bauer, J.H., 1940. Individual isolation of infected animals in a single room. J. Bacteriol. 40, 569–580.

Howdeshell, K.L., Peterman, P.H., Judy, B.M., et al., 2003. Bisphenol A is released from used polycarbonate animal cages into water at room temperature. Environ. Health Perspect. 111, 1180–1187.

Huerkamp, M.J., Lehner, N.D.M., 1994a. Comparative effects of forced-air, individual cage ventilation or an absorbent bedding additive on mouse isolator cage microenvironment. Contemp. Top. Lab. Anim. Sci. 33, 58–61.

Huerkamp, M.J., Dillehay, D., Lehner, N., 1994b. Effect of intracage ventilation and automatic watering on outbred mouse reproductive performance and weanling growth. Contemp. Top. Lab. Animal. Sci. 33, 58–62.

Hutchinson, E., Avery, A., VandeWoude, S., 2005. Environmental enrichment for laboratory rodents. ILAR J. 46, 148–161.

Hunt, P.A., Koehler, K.E., Susiarjo, M., et al., 2003. Bisphenol A exposure causes meiotic aneuploidy in the female mouse. Cur. Bio. 13, 546–553.

ILAR (Institute of Laboratory Animal Resources), 1978. Laboratory Animal Housing. Institute of Laboratory Animal Resources, Commission on Life Sciences, National Research Council, National Academies Press, Washington, DC.

ILAR, 1991. Education and Training in the Care and Use of Laboratory Animals: A Guide for Developing Institutional Programs. Institute of Laboratory Animal Resources, Commission on Life Sciences, National Research Council, National Academies Press, Washington, DC.

ILAR (Institute of Laboratory Animal Resources), 1996. Laboratory Animal Management: Rodents. Institute of Laboratory Animal Resources, Commission on Life Sciences, National Research Council, National Academy Press, Washington, DC.

ILAR, 2007. Occupational Health and Safety in the Care and Use of Research Animals. The National Academies Press, Washington, DC, National Research Council.

ILAR (Institute of Laboratory Animal Resources), 2011. Guide for the Care and Use of Laboratory Animals, eighth ed. Institute of Laboratory Animal Resources, Commission on Life Sciences, National Research Council, National Academies Press, Washington, DC.

Iwarsson, K., Noren, L., 1992. Comparison of microenvironmental conditions in standard versus forced-air ventilated rodent filter-top cages. Scand. J. Lab. Anim. Sci. 19, 167–173.

Jonas, A.M., 1978. Centralized versus dispersed animal care facilities. In: Laboratory animal housing: Proceedings of a symposium held at Hunt Valley, Maryland, September 22–23, 1976. Institute of Laboratory Animal Resources, Commission on Life Sciences, National Research Council, National Academy of Sciences. National Academy Press. Washington, DC, pp. 11–15.

Jonas, A.M., 1965. Laboratory animal facilities. J. Am. Vet. Med. Assoc. 146, 600–606.

Ju, Y., Allred, C., Allred, K., Karko, K.L., Doerge, D.R., Helferich, W.G., et al., 2001. Physiological concentrations of dietary genistein dose-dependently stimulate growth of estrogen-dependent human breast cancer (MCF-7) tumors implanted in athymic nude mice. J. Nutr. 131, 2957–2962.

Ju, Y., Doerge, D., Allred, K., Allred, C.D., Helferich, W.G., et al., 2002. Dietary genistein negates the inhibitory effect of tamoxifen on growth of estrogen-dependent human breast cancer (MCF-7) cells implanted in athymic mice. Cancer Res. 62, 2474–2477.

Kahrs, R., 1995. General disinfection guidelines. Rev. Sci. Tech. 14, 105–163.

Kapeghian, J.C., Mincer, H.H., Jones, A.B., Verlangieri, A.J., Waters, I.W., et al., 1982. Acute inhalation toxicity of ammonia in mice. Bull. Environ. Contam. Toxicol. 29, 371–378.

Katelaris, C., Widmer, R., Lazarus, R., 1996. Prevalence of latex allergy in a dental school. Med. J. Aust. 164, 711–714.

Keller, G.L., Mattingly, S., Knapke, F., 1983. A forced air individually ventilated caging system for rodents. Lab. Anim. Sci. 33, 580–582.

Keller, L.S., White, W.J., Snider, M.T., 1989. An evaluation of intracage ventilation in three animal caging systems. Lab. Anim. Sci. 39, 237–242.

Kelly, K., Sussman, G., Fink, J., 1996. Stop the sensitization. J. Allergy Clin. Immunol. 98, 857–858.

Kennedy, B., Beal, T., 1991. Minerals leached into drinking water from rubber stoppers. Lab. Anim. Sci. 41, 233–236.

King, C., Hessler, J.R., Broderson, R., 1999. Small animal research facilities management. In: Richmond, J.Y. (Ed.), Anthology of Biosafety 1. Perspectives on Laboratory Design American Biological Safety Association, Mundelein, IL, pp. 219–231.

Kingston, S., Hoffman-Goetz, L., 1996. Effect of environmental enrichment and housing density on immune system reactivity to acute exercise stress. Physiol. Behav. 60, 145–150.

Koehler, K.E., Voigt, R.C., Thomas, S., et al., 2003. When disaster strikes: rethinking caging materials. Lab. Anim. 32, 24–27.

Kovacs, M.S., McKiernan, S., Potter, D.M., Chilappagari, S., 2005. An epidemiological study of interdigital cysts in a research Beagle colony. Contemp. Top. Lab. Anim. Sci. 44, 17–21.

Kowalski, W., Bahnfleth, W., Carey, D., 2002. Engineering control of airborne disease transmission in animal laboratories. Contemp. Top. Lab. Anim. Sci. 41, 9–17.

Kraft, L.M., 1958. Observations on the control and natural history of epidemic diarrhea of infant mice (EDIM). Yale J. Biol. Med. 31, 121–137.

Kraft, L.M., Pardy, R.F., Pardy, S.A., 1964. Practical control of diarrheal disease in a commercial colony. Lab. Anim. Care 14, 16.

Lang, C.M., 1981. Special design considerations for animal facilities. In: Fox D.G. (Ed.), Proceedings of the National Cancer Institute Symposium on Design of Biomedical Research Facilities, Cancer Research Safety Monograph, vol. 4, National Institute of Health Publications. No. 81–2305, Bethesda, MD, pp. 117–127.

Lang, C.M., 1983. Design and management of research facilities for mice In: Foster, H.L. Small, J.D. Fox, J.G. (Eds.), The Mouse in Biomedical Research, vol. 3. Academic Press, New York, pp. 37–50.

Lang, C.M., Harrell, B.T., 1969. An ideal animal resource facility. Am. Inst. Archit. J. 52, 57–61.

Lang, C.M., Harrell, B.T., 1972. Guidelines for a quality program of laboratory animal medicine in a medical school. J. Med. Educ. 47, 267–271.

Lang, C.M., Altman, N.H., Brennan, P.C., et al., 1977. Laboratory animal management: rodents. ILAR News 20, 5–15.

Lawson, G.W., Sato, A., Fairbanks, L.A., Lawson, P.T., 2005. Vitamin E as treatment for ulcerative dermatitis in C57BL/6 mice and strains with C57BL/6 background. Contemp. Top Lab. Anim. Sci. 44, 18–21.

LeChevallier, M., 1997. Chlorine dioxide for control of Cryptosporidium and disinfection byproducts. In "Proceedings 1996 Water Quality Technology Conference; Pt II". Boston, MA, AWWA, p. 11.

Lee, J., Liao, P., Tseng, D., Wen, P.T., et al., 1998. Behavior of organic polymers in drinking water purification. Chemosphere 37, 1045–1061.

Les, E.P., 1968. Effect of acidified chlorinated water on reproduction in C3H/HEJ and C57BL/6J mice. Lab. Anim. Care 18, 210–213.

Lewandoski, M., 2001. Conditional control of gene expression in the mouse. Nat. Rev. Genet. 2, 743–755.

Liberman, D. (Ed.), 1995. Biohazards Management Handbook. Marcel Dekker Inc., New York.

Lindsey, J.R., Conner, M.W., Baker, H.J., 1978. Physical, chemical and microbial factors affecting biologic response. Laboratory Animal Housing. Institute of Laboratory Animal Resources, Commission on Life Sciences, National Research Council, National Academies Press, Washington, DC.

Lipman, N.S., 1992. Microenvironmental conditions in isolator cages: an important research variable. Lab. Anim. 21, 23–27.

Lipman, N.S., 1993. Strategies for architectural integration of ventilated caging systems. Contemp. Top. Lab. Anim. Sci. 32, 7–12.

Lipman, N.S., 1999. Isolator rodent caging systems (state of the art): a critical view. Contemp. Top. Lab. Anim. Sci. 38, 9–17.

Lipman, N.S., 2007. Design and management of research facilities for mice. In: Fox, J.G., Barthold, S.W. (Eds.), The Mouse in Biomedical Research, second ed. Academic Press, Burlington, MA.

Lipman, N.S., 2009. Rodent facilities and caging systems. In: Hessler, J.R., Lehner, N.D.M. (Eds.), Planning and Designing Research Animal Facilities. Academic Press, London.

Lipman, N.S., Perkins, S.E., 2002. Factors that may influence animal research. In: Fox, J., Anderson, L. (Eds.), Laboratory Animal Medicine, second ed. Academic Press, New York, pp. 1143–1165.

Lipman, N.S., Homberger, F., 2003. Rodent quality assurance testing: use of sentinel animal systems. Lab. Anim. 32, 32–39.

Lipman, N.S., Dalton, S., Stuart, A., Arruda, K., et al., 1994. Eradication of pinworms (*Syphacia obvelata*) from a large mouse breeding colony by combination oral anthelmintic therapy. Lab. Anim. Sci. 44, 517–520.

Lipsky, M., Skinner, M., O'Connell, C., 1993. Effects of chloroform and bromodichloromethane on DNA synthesis in male F344 rat kidney. Environ. Health. Perspect. 101 (Suppl. 5), 249–252.

Liss, G., Sussman, G., Deal, K., Brown, S., Cividino, M., Siu, S., et al., 1997. Latex allergy: epidemiological study of 1351 hospital workers. Occup. Environ. Med. 54, 335–342.

Lohmiller, J., Lipman, N.S., 1998. Silicon crystals in water of autoclaved glass bottles. Contemp. Top. Lab. Anim. Sci. 37, 62–65.

Manninen, A.S., Antilla, S., Savolainen, H., 1998. Rat metabolic adaptation to ammonia inhalation. Proc. Soc. Biol. Med. 187, 278–281.

Manser, C.E., Morris, H., Broom, D.M., 1995. An investigation into the effects of solid grid cage flooring on the welfare of laboratory rats. Lab. Anim. 29, 353–363.

Manser, C.E., Elliot, H., Morris, T.H., et al., 1996. The use of a novel operant test to determine the strength of preference for flooring in laboratory rats. Lab. Anim. 30, 1–6.

Marashi, V., Barnekow, A., Sachser, N., 2004. Effects of environmental enrichment on males of a docile inbred strain of mice. Physiol. Behav. 82, 765–776.

Marshall, R., 1991. Electrical systems In: Ruys, T. (Ed.), Handbook of Facilities Planning, vol. 2. Van Nostrand Reinhold, New York, pp. 342–350.

Mayack, L.A., Soracco, R.J., Wilde, E.W., et al., 1984. Comparative effectiveness of chlorine and chlorine dioxide regimes for biofouling control. Water Res. 18, 593–594.

McLennan, I., Taylor-Jeffs, J., 2004. The use of sodium lamps to brightly illuminate mouse houses during the dark phases. Lab. Anim. 38, 384–392.

McPherson, C.W., 1963. Reduction of and coliform bacteria in mouse drinking water following treatment with hydrochloride acid or chlorine. Lab. Anim. Care 13, 737–744.

Memarzadeh, F., 1998. Ventilation Design Handbook on Animal Research Facilities Using Static Microisolators. National Institutes of Health, Office of the Director, Bethesda, MD.

Mench, J.A., Krulisch, L. (Eds.), 1990. Canine Research Environment. Scientists Center for Animal Welfare, Bethesda, MD.

Milligan, S., Sales, G., Khirynkh, K., 1993. Sound levels in rooms housing laboratory animals: an uncontrolled daily variable. Physiol. Behav. 53, 1067–1076.

Morris, R., Audet, A., Angelillo, I., Chambers, T.C., Mosteller, F., et al., 1992. Chlorination, chlorination by-products, and cancer: a meta-analysis. Am. J. Public Health 82, 955–964.

Mulder, J., 1971. Animal behavior and electromagnetic energy waves. Lab. Anim. Sci. 21, 389–393.

NABR (National Association for Biomedical Research), 1991. State Laws Concerning the Use of Animals in Research. NABR, Washington, DC.

National Institutes of Health design policy and guidelines, 2003. <http://orf.od.nih.gov/policy/despolicy-index.htm>.

National Institutes of Health, Design Requirements Manual for Biomedical Laboratories and Animal Research Facilities, 2008. <http://orf.od.nih.gov/PoliciesAndGuidelines/Biomedicaland AnimalResearchFacilitiesDesignPoliciesandGuidelines/Pages/ DesignRequirements ManualPDF.aspx>.

National Sanitation Foundation, 2002. Standard 49 Class II (laminar flow) biohazard cabinetry. NSF International, Ann Arbor, MI.

National Science Foundation, May 1953. NS Standard No. 3 for Commercial Spray Type Dishwashing Machines. NSF International, Ann Arbor, MI, amended April 1965 and November 1977.

Obeck, D.K., 1978. Galvanized caging as a potential factor in the development of the "fading infant" or "white monkey" syndrome. Lab. Anim. Sci. 28, 698–704.

Olsson, I., Dahlborn, K., 2002. Improving housing conditions for laboratory mice: a review of "environmental enrichment". Lab. Anim. 36, 243–270.

Otis, A.P., Foster, H.L., 1983. Management and design of breeding facilities In: Foster, H.L., Small, J.D., Fox, J.G. (Eds.), Laboratory Mouse in Biomedical Research, vol. 3. Academic Press, New York, p. 20.

Otto, G., Tolwani, R., 2002. Use of microisolator caging in a risk-based mouse import and quarantine program: a retrospective study. Contemp. Top. Lab. Anim. Sci. 41, 20–27.

Ownby, D., Ownby, H., McCullough, J., et al., 1996. The prevalence of anti-latex IgE antibodies in 1000 volunteer blood donors. J. Allergy Clin. Immunol. 97, 1188–1192.

Paraskeva, P., Graham, N.J., 2002. Ozonation of municipal wastewater effluents. Water Environ. Res. 74, 569–581.

Patterson, P., 1995. Allergy issues complicate buying decision for gloves. OR Manager 11, 8–14, 19.

Paulus, M., Gleason, S., Kennel, S., et al., 2000. High resolution x-ray computed tomography: an emerging tool for small animal cancer research. Neoplasia 2, 62–70.

Pekrul, D., 1991. Noise control. In: Ruys, T. (Ed.), Handbook of Facilities Planning, vol. 2. Van Nostrand Reinhold, New York, pp. 166–173.

Perkins, S., Lipman, N., 1996. Evaluation of microenvironmental conditions and noise generation in three individually ventilated rodent caging systems and static isolator cages. Contemp. Top. Lab. Anim. Sci. 35, 61–65.

Perkins, S.E., Lipman, N.S., 1995. Characterization and qualification of microenvironmental contaminants in isolator cages with a variety of contact bedding. Contemp. Top. Lab. Anim. Sci. 34, 93–98.

Peterson, E., 1980. Noise and laboratory animals. Lab. Anim. Sci. 30, 422–439.

Phoenix Controls Corporation, 2003. Vivarium Sourcebook, third ed. Phoenix Controls Corporation, United States, p. 76.

Pilotto, L., 1995. Disinfection of drinking water, disinfection by-products, and cancer: what about Australia? Aust. J. Public Health 19, 89–93.

Poiley, S.M., 1974. Housing requirement – general considerations. In: Melby Jr., E.C., Altman, N.H. (Eds.), Handbook of Laboratory Animal Science, vol. 1. CRC Press, Cleveland, OH, pp. 21–60.

Rafferty, J., Fan, C., Potter, P.M., Watson, A.J., Cawkwell, L., O'Connor, P.J., et al., 1992. Tissue-specific expression and induction of human O6-alkylguanine-DNA alkyltransferase in transgenic mice. Mol. Carcinog. 6, 26–31.

Rahija, R.J., 1999. Animal facility design. Occup. Med. 14, 407–422.

Rake, B.W., 1979. Microbiological evaluation of biological safety cabinet modified for bedding disposal. Lab. Anim. Sci. 29, 625–632.

Reeb, C., Jones, R., Bearg, D., 1997. Impact of room ventilation rates on mouse cage ventilation and microenvironment. Contemp. Top. Lab. Anim. Sci. 36, 74–79.

Reeb, C., Jones, R., Bearg, D., 1998. Microenvironment in ventilated animal cages with differing ventilation rates, mice populations, and frequency of bedding changes. Contemp. Top. Lab. Anim. Sci. 37, 43–49.

Reeb-Whitaker, C.K., Paigen, B., Beamer, W.G., et al., 2001. The impact of reduced frequency of cage changes on the health of mice housed in ventilated cages. Lab. Anim. 35, 58–73.

Rehg, J., Toth, L., 1988. Rodent quarantine programs: purpose, principles, and practice. Lab. Anim. Sci. 30, 323–329.

Renstrom, A., Bjoring, G., Hoglund, A., 2001. Evaluation of individually ventilated cage systems for laboratory rodents: occupational health aspects. Lab. Anim. 35, 42–50.

Richmond, J.Y., 1991. Hazard reduction in animal research facilities. Lab. Anim. 20, 23–29.

Richmond, J.Y., 1996. Animal biosafety levels 1–4: an overview. In: Richmond J.Y. (Ed.), Proceedings of the Fourth National Symposium on Biosafety: Working Safely with Animals, Atlanta, GA, Centers for Disease Control, pp. 5–8.

Ritman, E., 2002. Molecular imaging in small animals – roles of micro-CT. J. Cell Biochem. Suppl. 39, 116–124.

Runkel, R.S., 1964a. Laboratory animal housing – Part I. Am. Inst. Architects. 41, 55–59.

Runkel, R.S., 1964b. Laboratory animal housing – Part I. Am. Inst. Architects. 41, 77–80.

Ruys, T., 1988. Isolation cubicles: space and cost analysis. Lab. Anim. 17 25–23.

Ruys, T., 1991a. Cage, rack, and tunnel washer. In: Ruys, T. (Ed.), Handbook of Facilities Planning, vol. 2. Van Nostrand Reinhold, New York, pp. 267–279. Laboratory Animal Facilities.

Ruys, T. (Editor). 1991b. Handbook of Facilities Planning, Volume 2: Laboratory Animal Facilities. Van Nostrand Reinhold. New York, pp. 267–279.

Ruys, T., 1991b. Handbook of facilities planning In: Ruys, T. (Ed.), Laboratory Animal Facilities, vol. 2 Van Nostrand Reinhold, New York, pp. 267–279.

Ryding, A., Sharp, M., Mullins, J., 2001. Conditional transgenic technologies. J. Endocrinol. 171, 1–14.

Sakaguchi, M., Inouye, S., Miyazawa, H., 1990. Evaluation of countermeasures for reduction of mouse airborne allergens. Lab. Anim. Sci. 40, 613–615.

Sales, G., Wilson, K., Spencer, K., Milligan, S.R., et al., 1988. Environmental ultrasound in laboratories and animal houses: a possible cause for concern in the welfare and use of laboratory animals. Lab. Anim. 22, 369–375.

Schoeb, T.R., Davidson, M.K., Lindsey, J.R., 1982. Intracage ammonia promotes growth of *Mycoplasma pulmonis* in the respiratory tract of rats. Infect. Immun. 38, 212–217.

Schub, T., 2002. The year of the flood: tropical storm Allison's impact on the Texas Medical Center. Lab. Anim. (NY) 31, 34–39.

Sedlacek, R.S., Orcutt, R.P., Suit, H.D., 1981. A flexible barrier at cage level for existing colonies: production and maintenance of a limited stable anaerobic flora in a closed inbred mouse colony. In: Sasaki, S. (Ed.), Recent Advances in Germ Free Research. Tokai University Press, Tokyo, Japan, pp. 56–69.

Semple-Rowland, S., Dawson, W., 1987a. Cyclic light intensity threshold for retinal damage in albino rats raised under 6 LUX. Exp. Eye Res. 44, 643–661.

Semple-Rowland, S., Dawson, W., 1987b. Retinal cyclic light damage threshold for albino rats. Lab. Anim. Sci. 37, 289–298.

Serrano, L., 1971. Carbon dioxide and ammonia in mouse cages: effect of cage covers, population and activity. Lab. Anim. Sci. 21, 680–684.

Sherwin, C., 1997. Observations on the prevalence of nest-building in non-breeding TO strain mice and their use of two nesting materials. Lab. Anim. 31, 125–132.

Simmonds, R.C., 1973. Selected topics in laboratory animal medicine – the design of laboratory animal homes. Aeromed. Rev. 7–73, 1–45.

Simmons, M.L., Wynn, L.P.I., Choat, E.E., 1967. A facility design for production of pathogen free, inbred mice. ASHRAE J. 9, 27–31.

Small, J.D., 1983. Environment and equipment monitoring In: Foster, H., Small, J.D. (Eds.), The Mouse in Biomedical Research, vol. 3. Academic Press, New York, pp. 83–101.

Smith, E., Stockwell, J.D., Schweitzer, I., Langley, S.H., Smith, A.L., 2004. Evaluation of cage micro-environment of mice housed on various types of bedding materials. Contemp. Top. Lab. Anim. Sci. 43, 12–17.

Studier, E., Beck, L., Lindeborge, R.G., 1967. Tolerance and initial metabolic response to ammonia intoxication in selected bats and rodents. J. Mammal. 48, 564–572.

Surbeck, H., 1995. Determination of natural radionuclides in drinking water: a tentative protocol. Sci. Total. Environ. 173–174, 91–109.

Sussman, G.L., Beezhold, D.H., 1995. Allergy to latex rubber. Ann. Intern. Med. 122, 43–46.

Swanson, M., Bubak, M., Hunt, L., Yunginger, J.W., Warner, M.A., Reed, C.E., et al., 1994. Quantification of occupational latex aeroallergens in a medical center. J. Allergy Clin. Immunol. 94, 445–451.

Takeshita, M., Kanayama, T., Suma, M., Hiohara, T., et al., 1997. Earthquake damage to a laboratory animal facility. Vet. Med. Sci. 59, 63–65.

Tallent, B., 2012. A novel approach to provide acidified water to an entire rodent rack using the unit's automatic watering system. J. Am. Assoc. Lab. Anim. Sci. 51, 667.

Tanner, R., Samantha, J., 1992. Rapid bactericidal effect of low pH against *Pseudomonas aeruginosa*. J. Ind. Microbiol. 10, 111–117.

Thibert, P., 1980. Control of microbial contamination in the use of laboratory rodents. Lab. Anim. Sci. 30, 339–348.

Thigpen, J., Locklear, J., Haseman, J., Saunders, H., Grant, M.F., Forsythe, D.B., et al., 2001. Effects of the dietary phytoestrogens daidzein and genistein on the incidence of vulvar carcinomas in 129/J mice. Cancer Detect. Prev. 25, 527–532.

Thigpen, J., Haseman, J., Saunders, H., Locklear, J., Caviness, G., Grant, M., et al., 2002. Dietary factors affecting uterine weights of immature CD-1 mice used in uterotrophic bioassays. Cancer Detect. Prev. 26, 381–393.

Thigpen, J., Haseman, J., Saunders, H., Setchell, K.D., Grant, M.G., Forsyth, D.B., et al., 2003. Dietary phytoestrogens accelerate the time of vaginal opening in immature CD-1 mice. Comp. Med. 53, 477–485.

Thorp, W.T.S., 1960. The design of animal quarters: a symposium on laboratory animals–their care and their facilities. J. Med. Educ. 35, 4–14.

Thurlow, R., Arriola, R., Stoll, C.E., Lipman, N.S., 2007. Evaluation of a flash disinfection process for surface decontamination of gamma-irradiated feed packaging. J. Am. Lab. Anim. Sci. 46, 46–49.

Tomas, T., Oliskiewicz, W., Czerczak, S., Sokal, J., et al., 1985. Decrease in the respiration rate in mice as an indicator of the irritating effects of chemical substances on the upper respiratory tract. Med. Pr. 36, 295–302.

Trentin, J.L., Van Hoosier, Jr., G.L., Shields, J., Stephens, K., Stenback, W.A., Parker, J.C., 1966a. Limiting the viral spectrum of the laboratory mouse. Natl. Cancer. Inst. Monogr. 10, 147–160.

Trentin, J.L., Van Hoosier, Jr., G.L., Shields, J., Stephens, K., Stenback, W.A., Parker, J.C., 1966b. Establishment of a caesarean-derived, gnotobiote foster nursed inbred mouse colony with observations on the control of Pseudomonas. Lab. Anim. Care. 16, 109–118.

Tu, H., Diberadinis, L.J., Lipman, N.S., 1997. Determination of air distribution, exchange, velocity, and leakage in three individually ventilated rodent caging systems. Contemp. Top. Lab. Animal. Sci. 36, 69–73.

Turjanmaa, K., Laurila, K., Makinen-Kikjunen, S., Reunala, T., et al., 1988. Rubber contact urticaria. Contact Derm. 19, 362–367.

Tyson, K.W., Corey, M.A., 1999. Facility design: forecasting space requirements. Lab. Anim. 28, 28–31.

USDA-APHIS (U.S. Department of Agriculture, Animal and Plant Health Inspection Service), 1998. Wire flooring and temperature standards amendment. Anim. Care. Q. Rep. (Winter 1997/Spring 1998), 3.

Van de Weerd, H., 1996. Environmental Enrichment for Laboratory Mice: Preferences and Consequences. Print Partners Ipskamp.

Van de Weerd, H., Van Loo, P., Van Zutphen, L., Koolhaas, J.M., Baumans, V., et al., 1997a. Preferences for nesting material as environmental enrichment for laboratory mice. Lab Anim. 31, 133–143.

Van de Weerd, H., Van Loo, P., Van Zutphen, L., Koolhaas, J.M., Baumans, V., et al., 1997b. Nesting material as environmental enrichment has no adverse effects on behavior and physiology of laboratory mice. Physiol. Behav. 62, 1019–1028.

Van de Weerd, H., Van Loo, P., Van Zutphen, L., Koolhaas, J.M., Baumans, V., et al., 1998. Strength of preference for nesting material as environmental enrichment for laboratory mice. Appl. Anim. Behav. Sci. 55, 369–382.

Van de Weerd, H., Aarsen, E., Mulder, A., Kruitwagen, C.L., Hendriksen, C.F., Baumans, V., et al., 2002. Effects of environmental enrichment for mice: variation in experimental results. J. Appl. Anim. Welf. Sci. 5, 87–109.

Van de Woude, S.J., Luzarraga, M.B., 1991. The role of Branhamella catarrhalis in the "bloody nose syndrome" of cynomolgus macaques. Lab. Anim. Sci. 41, 401–406.

Van Loo, P., Van Zutphen, L., Baumans, V., 2003. Male management: coping with aggression problems in male laboratory mice. Lab. Anim. 37, 300–313.

Van Loo, P.L., Van de Weerd, H.A., Van Zutphen, L.F., Baumans, V., et al., 2004. Preference for social contact versus environmental enrichment in male laboratory animals. Lab. Anim. 38, 178–188.

Vessel, E., 1966. Induction of drug-metabolizing enzymes in liver microsomes of rats and mice by softwood bedding. Science 157, 1057–1058.

Vesell, E.S., Lang, C.M., White, W.J., Passananti, G.T., Tripp, S.L., et al., 1973. Hepatic drug metabolism in rats: impairment in a dirty environment. Science 179, 896–897.

Vesell, E.S., Lang, C.M., White, W.J., Passananti, G.T., Hill, R.N., Clemens, T.L., et al., 1976. Environmental and genetic factors affecting theresponse of laboratory animals to drugs. Fed. Proc., Fed. Am. Soc. Exp. Biol. 35, 1125–1132.

Veterans Administration, 1993. Veterinary Medical Unit (VMU). VA Design Guide. Department of Veterans Affairs, Veterans Health Administration, Office of Construction Management., Office of Architecture and Engineering, Standards Service, Washington, DC.

Vogelweid, C.M., 1998. Developing emergency management plans for university laboratory animal programs and facilities. Contemp. Top. Lab. Anim. Sci. 37, 52–56.

Vogelweid, C., Hill, J., Shea, R., Truby, S.J., Schantz, L.D., et al., 2003. Using site assessment and risk analysis to plan and build disaster-resistant programs and facilities. Lab. Anim. (NY) 32, 40–44.

Vogelweid, C., Hill, J., Shea, R., Johnson, D.B., et al., 2005. Earthquakes and building design: a primer for the laboratory animal professional. Lab. Anim. (NY) 34 (7), 35–42.

Walzer, P.D., Kim, C.K., Linke, M.J., Pogue, C.L., Huerkamp, M.J., Chrisp, C.E., et al., 1989. Outbreaks of Pneumocystis carinii pneumonia in colonies of immunodeficient mice. Infect. Immun. 57, 62–70.

Wardrip, C., Artwohl, J., Mennett, B., 1994. A review of the role of temperature versus time in an effective cage sanitation program. Contemp. Top. Lab. Anim. Sci. 33, 66–68.

Wardrip, C., Artwohl, J., Oswald, J., Bennett, B.T., et al., 2000. Verification of bacterial killing effects of cage wash time and temperature combinations using standard penicylinder methods. Contemp. Top. Lab. Anim. Sci. 39, 9–12.

Webber, D.J., William, A.R., 1999. Gene therapy: a new challenge for infection control. Infect. Control Hosp. Epidemiol. 20, 530–532.

Weihe, W.H., Schidlow, J., Strittmatter, J., 1969. The effect of light intensity on the breeding and development of rats and golden hamsters. Int. J. Biometeorol. 13 (1), 69–79.

Weihe, W.H., 1971. The significance of the physical environment for the health and state of adaptation of laboratory animals. In: Defining the Laboratory Animal, Proceedings of the IVth Symposium, International Committee on Laboratory Animals and the Institute of Laboratory Animal Resources, National Research Council, National Academy of Sciences, Washington, DC. pp. 353-378.

Weihe, W., 1976. Influence of light on animals In: McSheehy, T. (Ed.), Control of the Animal House Environment, vol. 7. Laboratory Animal Ltd., London, pp. 63–76.

White, W.J., Hughes, H.C., Singh, S.B., Lang, C.M., et al., 1983. Evaluation of a cubicle containment system in preventing gaseous and particulate air-borne cross-contamination. Lab. Anim. Sci. 33, 571–576.

White, W.J., 1996. Special containment devices for research animals. In: Richmond, J.Y. (Ed.), Proceeding of the Fourth National Symposium on Biosafety: Working Safely with Research Animals, Atlanta, GA, CDC, pp. 109–112.

Wirrwar, A., Schramm, N., Vosberg, H., Muller-Gartner, H.W., 2001. High resolution SPECT in small animal research. Rev. Neurosci. 12, 187–193.

Wolfer, D., Litvin, O., Morf, S., Nitsch, R.M., Lipp, H.P., Wurbel, H., et al., 2004. Laboratory animal welfare: cage enrichment and mouse behaviour. Nature 432, 821–822.

Wu, D., Joiner, G.N., Mcfarland, A., 1985. A forced-air ventilation system for rodent caging. Lab. Anim. Sci. 35, 499–504.

Yoshida, K.M., Tajima, M., 1995. Invention of forced-air-ventilated microisolation cage and rack system-environment within cages: temperature and ammonia concentration. Exp. Anim. 43, 703–710.

CHAPTER

37

Program Management

Steven M. Niemi, DVM, DACLAM

Harvard University Faculty of Arts and Sciences, Cambridge, MA, USA

OUTLINE

I. INTRODUCTION AND DEFINITIONS

The intent of this chapter is to consider the components of managing work and managing personnel in the context of laboratory animal care. Laboratory animal care is broadly defined in this chapter to encompass the overlapping elements of husbandry, clinical and preventive laboratory animal veterinary medicine, and regulatory oversight. This is an appropriate subject for this textbook for at least two reasons. First, few, if any, programs of animal care are performed entirely by one person and so an assembly of individual tasks with individual responsibility is required (a process of organization intended to accomplish a task or larger objective, otherwise known as management). Second, effective management of animal care is becoming more important than ever, in light of increasing constraints on funding for biomedical research and preclinical testing amid rising costs, growing regulatory burdens (National

Science Board, 2014; Thulin *et al.*, 2014), and tepid public support (Gallup, 2013).

Is the practice of management 'science' or is it 'art?' Can it be learned, tested, and evaluated in an objective and reproducible manner, or is it an innate skill that relies on subjective judgment and is mastered only after much trial and error? The complicated answer is to this simple yet essential question is 'yes.' And as if that is not murky enough, there are many and occasionally conflicting descriptions of purportedly successful management styles and tactics. One has only to peruse the business section of an actual or virtual bookstore or plug in management phrases to an online search engine to be easily overwhelmed by the variety of approaches to this subject.

This chapter will differ from others in this textbook in that it will not provide a comprehensive or necessarily balanced review of the management literature, even when confined to lab animal care. Nevertheless, there are some

Laboratory Animal Medicine, Third Edition
DOI: http://dx.doi.org/10.1016/B978-0-12-409527-4.00037-7

1599

basic lessons for managing work and people that remain true, based on collective experience as well as collective (but not necessarily conventional) wisdom.[1] The focus of this chapter is two-fold: (1) to address underserved topics in lab animal management that are important for success; and (2) to encourage the reader to explore management challenges and solutions described for other industries simply because many of those insights for getting work done well can be easily applied to our field. For an overview of lab animal management, the reader is referred to more comprehensive and introductory publications (Sukow et al., 2002; Silverman, 2008). In addition, there are organizations dedicated to managing lab animal care that are also recommended for general information on this subject (www.aalas.org, www.lama-online.org).

We begin with fundamental concepts such as a straightforward definition of management. One definition developed by this author over many years is *matching the needs of the organization with the needs of the employee.*[2] One may also define management by paraphrasing Ricardo Haussman, who wrote that "Manufacturing is order, intelligently applied" (Haussmann, 2013). The same can be said for successfully managing a program of lab animal care (abbreviated as 'program' for the remainder of this chapter). The basic responsibility of management in any enterprise is "to make people capable of joint performance through common goals, common values, the right structure, and the training and development they need to perform and to respond to change" (Drucker, 2001). With respect to the program, the purpose of organization is to ensure work is done effectively, efficiently, safely, and in compliance with current regulations, accreditation standards (if applicable), and institutional policies. Thus, we arrive at the first management task for the program: to state the purpose for which it exists and what it intends to achieve, i.e., what is its mission?

II. MISSION AND STRATEGY: WHERE IT ALL STARTS

Articulating the program's purpose in a mission or vision statement is often a good place to start. The statement should be short and clear, and speak to all who rely on successful management of the program. Such stakeholders include researchers and educators (animal users), vivarium staff, the institution in which the program is located, governmental regulators and the public on whose behalf those regulators work, and the animals themselves. The mission statement can be a single statement or sentence, a brief paragraph, or a list of purposes or objectives. An example of a simple yet comprehensive mission statement for the program is provided below:

- To provide reliable, affordable, and responsive laboratory animal care and research services in pursuit of scientific knowledge and medical breakthroughs
- To avoid or minimize pain and distress in animals under our care
- To maintain a fulfilling, respectful, and safe workplace[3]

Getting from the program's mission to how it is structured, measured, and financed to serve that mission requires a strategy, specifically one that addresses the expectations of the various stakeholders while considering the potential impact of extramural trends and influences. In order to communicate the strategy to stakeholders and provide an organized reference for retrospective analysis, a strategic plan is recommended, preferably written by the program's director (NB: a related exercise, the business plan, is conventionally generated for stand-alone enterprises rather than operating subsidiaries like most programs and contains most of the same components). The plan should be no more than 20 single-spaced pages, including figures and tables, and cover the next three fiscal years. Any strategy intended for a longer time frame becomes increasingly tenuous in the outer years, while a shorter interval often cannot reflect the consequences of recent or current changes.

The plan should begin with a strategic assessment that considers the current state of the program and what internal and external drivers may require it to change. This assessment can include projections in lab animal use at the institution, such as species mix and new animal models; internal or external funding and supply costs, including impacts on animal census, staffing, and space; regulatory and accreditation requirements; risks of natural or man-made interruptions to the program; etc. A simple yet comprehensive tool for this purpose is known as a 'S-W-O-T' analysis, an acronym comprising evaluations of an organization's current Strengths, Weaknesses, Opportunities and Threats (Collis, 2005). Many sources

1. The perspectives and opinions of the author may not reflect those of other contributors to this textbook, its editors, the American College of Laboratory Animal Medicine or the publisher.
2. This definition may confuse by appearing to focus solely on the human element while ignoring other basic facets of management, such as marketing, sales, finance, operations, regulations, etc. But because every component of management involves persons doing something on behalf of the organization, the emphasis on the employee or other human agent is justified.
3. Reprinted with permission, Massachusetts General Hospital Center for Comparative Medicine, Boston, MA.

of information may be tapped for this section, including goals or budget guidelines from central/corporate leadership, investigator/faculty surveys on shifts in research and funding, career development needs and aspirations from animal care staff, pending changes in the regulatory landscape, and pursuit of accreditation or reaccreditation. Next, the plan should describe how the program will respond to those anticipated changes while maintaining or strengthening its core competencies, and establish key action items needed to achieve those goals. The plan should end with target milestones and projected financial results. The final product should answer the following questions: what comprises success for the program, what do we need to accomplish in order to succeed, what will it cost, and how will we know if we get there?

The person(s) to whom the program reports should formally review and approve the plan before it is implemented and shared with program staff and other interested parties, such as animal users and IACUC leadership. The plan should also be considered and labeled 'CONFIDENTIAL,' especially if it describes institution-wide strategic ambitions or initiatives or unconventional approaches to animal care that require piloting and thorough analysis before full-scale implementation (see Section V below). Once the strategic plan is launched, an easy means and schedule for tracking progress toward the plan's objectives is recommended. Targets and timelines should be specific and quantified to facilitate measuring if and by how much the program is either 'on plan' or not. Such assessments should be shared with the same persons and groups that received the original plan. In addition, a well-written strategic plan can be an effective tool for communications and outreach to stakeholders as well recruiting outstanding candidates for one's program.

Are financial metrics the only ones that matter? They are certainly easily understood and just as easily available for comparing past performance *versus* future goals. But relying on financial budgets and forecasts alone may lead employees not to pay attention to other measurements just as critical for success. For example, improving the safety of the workplace may be a necessary strategic goal, to be measured by reducing the number of lapses or potential hazards identified during semiannual IACUC inspections. The plan could target actual or percent reductions in occupational safety findings over the plan's time course. Program leadership would then initiate additional training, discussion groups, mock inspections and audits against Standard Operating Procedures (SOPs) and other management activities while tracking progress toward that goal. One helpful management tool for tracking progress toward strategic goals besides finance alone is known as the 'balanced scorecard,' developed by Robert Kaplan and popularized in many versions since (Kaplan and Norton, 2005). Typically divided into four

quadrants, the balanced scorecard begins with a financial perspective, but provides space for three other equally important categories considered indispensable for a unit's success. These are Customer Perspective, Internal Processes, and Organizational Innovation and Learning. The author's prior program used the balanced scorecard for tracking various non-financial goals considered strategically important. Examples include "Improve operability of sanitation equipment to 97%" (Internal Processes), "Complete training of 100% of animal care staff before they work unsupervised" (Organizational Innovation and Learning), "Reduce customer dissatisfaction to less than 25% regarding animal pen/cage conditions" (Customer Perspective), and "Complete ≥85% of all departmental annual performance reviews within 20 business days of an employee's official review date" (Internal Processes).

The frequency for issuing new strategic plans depends on the size and complexity of the program as well as the diversity and intensity of external influences on the program. In situations involving major changes, such as significant program expansion or retraction or adding large numbers of a new species, the plan may require revision on a yearly basis. Or if there are no major, unanticipated changes, the plan may remain a useful document until the end of its intended time frame draws near. Regardless of how often a plan may be revised or replaced, it should be reviewed at least annually to determine if the original strategy drivers still apply and if the resultant goals still represent the best options to pursue.

III. MANAGING PEOPLE

A program providing lab animal care can be considered a business that delivers a service, in this case ensuring that animals retain their scientific or educational value while simultaneously ensuring those same animals are not subjected to unnecessary pain or distress from such care. Unlike manufacturing a product sold to customers that does not create value until it is used by those customers, a service creates value only at the time it is performed by the employee. That is why employees are the most important asset in any service enterprise, whether it be banking, insurance, parcel delivery, retail sales, education, or lab animal care. In order to succeed, the service business must have employees who are knowledgeable, dedicated, reliable, customer-focused, and team-oriented. Much of the management literature already available in the field of lab animal care deals with standard themes for managing employees, such as training, communication, team building, rewarding superior performers, and handling difficult employees. So the remainder of this section will cover complementary elements for managing staff effectively.

One must start by returning to the definition of management given in the Introduction above: *matching the needs of the organization with the needs of the employee*. This helps to remind the manager that all employees are also individuals with their own lives, concerns, and personal plans that may fall outside the workplace but nevertheless can influence their performance if both entities' needs do not match. The best feeling any manager can get is when he or she corrects an imbalance between the organization's needs and the employee's needs so both the organization and the employee of previous concern return to a mutually productive relationship. Of course, such outcomes are not always possible and terminating a problem employee may be the only option left. But it has been the experience and observations of the author that when an employee is struggling to succeed in his or her job, those struggles are usually not his/her fault but a result of inadequate training, insufficient resources (e.g., equipment, time, money) or a mismatch between the employee's core competencies and the assigned task. For example, someone in sales who is not comfortable approaching strangers or someone in accounting who is not detail-oriented are more likely to encounter difficulties than others innately better suited for those roles. This conclusion does not dismiss the value of training and preparation for handling those responsibilities well, but sometimes an initial mismatch is hard to overcome. Thus, a responsible manager feels obligated to explore multiple ways to reverse an employee's decline, either through more training or better support. An imaginative manager feels stimulated by the challenge of finding or creating a different role more compatible with that employee's inherent attributes, if possible. By contrast and only in a small minority of cases is the employee neither truly interested nor competent in serving the needs of the organization. In both of those cases, the sooner the employee is removed, the better, rather than subjecting him or her and the rest of the workforce to continued disruptions and mistakes.

The cycle of employment usually begins with recruitment. Given the critical value of employees in a program, one should aim to attract the best applicants possible. Thus, job listings and advertisements should include not only the activities and responsibilities involved, but also describe (credibly) the stature and positive culture of the program and parent institution, as well as employee opportunities for development and advancement. When identifying promising candidates from the applicant pool, it pays to ignore the erroneous label of someone being 'over-qualified.' The enlightened manager is always searching for new employees that have more training and experience than needed for the immediate job; such new hires usually require less on-boarding supervision and time before working independently and can help advance the program toward its strategic

goals or in response to changing needs. Once finalists are selected, usually in concert with the institution's human resources department, they are invited for interviews. It is useful to have all levels of the program staff represented in these interviews, especially subordinates who report to the position being filled. Advance training in interviewing may be useful for staff not knowledgeable or experienced in this activity, if for no other reason than to be instructed on inappropriate or unallowable questions one may ask a candidate (Anthony, 2011). In addition, junior or inexperienced workers are often more comfortable conducting a group interview session rather than going one-on-one with a stranger. If the available position is at a high level or routinely interacts with stakeholders outside the program, then those groups should be added to the interview schedule. Remember that this is also a two-way assessment, with the candidate sizing up the program and institution while being evaluated as a future employee at the same time. So it behooves the program to make sure vivaria are neat and clean before giving the candidate a tour, and that specific interests the candidate may have are highlighted during his or her visit, with honest answers provided to direct questions so the candidate has no misconceptions about the position or program. In other words, the program is in just as active a selling mode as the candidate. And it never hurts to follow up the visit with a thank you note and an offer to answer any new questions, to be coordinated with Human Resources so both inside parties are on the same page and deliver the same messages.

The mechanics of hiring a candidate are usually the purview of Human Resources. However, there may be details that require more decisions by program leadership, including adjustments to the original compensation package, starting date, additional perquisites, and reporting lines within the program. In cases involving a highly prized candidate, one may be tempted to exceed budgeted compensation and other expenses as well as accede to special requests or demands. Rather than cave in to those temptations, it is better to realize that no single individual is so important or irreplaceable that the organization cannot succeed without him or her. This is especially true in a team-based environment where everyone else rightly expects equal treatment and equal compensation for equal work. Consequently, the entire workforce will be watching to see how an obviously attractive candidate is courted and compare that treatment to theirs. In a truly fair and transparent culture, the newest and longest-term employees are managed in an identical manner even though their respective responsibilities may differ.

A program should have a defined system for teaching and training new employees as well as current employees assigned to new tasks. The trainee should be given sufficient time and guidance to master those tasks, to be validated by successfully performing them during a competency assessment before approval is granted. Just as importantly, trainers should be trained in effective training methods and be able to perform the same tasks under the same competency assessment. It is useful to document which employees have received training on which tasks and passed the respective assessments. This comes in handy during performance review and goal-setting sessions (see below) as well as providing managers a means of identifying skill gaps in the program's responsibilities and strategic goals.

Once employees are hired and trained, it is incumbent on program leadership to enhance the investment in such important human assets by developing good workers further and retaining them in the program. A convenient mechanism for meeting these management objectives is an annual employee performance review and plan. Usually required at larger institutions and linked to annual operating budgets, performance reviews, and plans also provide critical feedback from the workforce to program leadership and higher if performed correctly. A good performance review and planning process starts with '360-degree' input from co-workers at various levels of the organization and possibly others if helpful (e.g., animal users, IACUC staff, vendors). This author has found simple and free-ranging questionnaires to be more informative to both parties than survey forms that require the submitter to score an employee's attributes on a numerical scale assigned to specific topics. An effective 360-degree survey is as simple as four questions:

1. What does (employee name) do well and where has he/she shown improvement over the past year?
2. Where can (employee name) further improve in his/her current role?
3. What can I (the employee's supervisor) do to make it easier for (employee name) to succeed?
4. Additional comments?

Questionnaires are both distributed and received in confidence, optimally coming back a week or two before the first of two meetings between the supervisor and employee. That allows the supervisor enough time to review, transcribe, and assemble questionnaire feedback while at the same time eliminating or anonymizing responses that either are inappropriate or identify the source. The original 360-degree responses are then deleted and not included in the employee's file. The compiled 360-degree input is then given to the employee the day before the meeting to review and digest.

The performance review and plan should consist of two meetings, the first being substantive but off-the-record, and the second confirmatory and *pro forma*. This approach allows for an initial and informal conversation of 45–60 min to review the following four topics provided to the employee in advance of the meeting. First, how well has the employee met the needs of the organization over the past 12 months ("what have you done for us?")? This question addresses past performance, including progress toward last year's goals and documenting any mitigating circumstances if those goals were not met (NB: good goal writing will be described later in this section). Also note the question is framed so the beneficiary is a collective rather than personal identity, so one is not asking "what have you done for me?" but rather for the entire program and its parent institution.

For this topic, the compiled 360-degree input is helpful in identifying strong and weak areas of performance to both parties from others closely involved in the employee's work. Often, an evaluation form requires the supervisor to quantify the employee's performance, resulting in an overall score that can be easily compared across the entire institution. Regardless of how narrow or wide a scale of numbers is involved, the value of the employee's final score merits further discussion. The simplest arrangement is a scale of 1 to 3, with 2 corresponding to doing a good job and being a good employee, 1 being worse than 2 and 3 being better than 2 (readers can expand or adapt this to their respective institutions' scales).

Most employees will perform their jobs well but rarely go above and beyond what is expected or required of them; on a scale of 1 to 3, they earned a score of 2 along with praise and thanks for doing so. An expression of gratitude is important in this situation for framing reasonable expectations. It also helps avoid score 'inflation' and the misimpression that only a score of 3 is good while a score of 2 is mediocre and therefore deflating. In a well-managed program there may be a small percentage of employees who consistently exceed expectations and are obviously able to handle much more than currently assigned, justifying a performance score of 3. These employees should be formally recognized as such, even while their achievements likely are well known to the rest of the workforce. In a well-managed program that provides sufficient training and resources and is able to match individual employee talents with good fitting roles, there should be only a small percentage of employees who perform poorly, and deserve a score of 1. The inferior performance of these employees is also likely well known to most if not all co-workers. If the supervisor and employee have an honest relationship and conduct more frequent conversations about work and performance than only at the time of the annual review, observations and conclusions discussed in this meeting should be merely confirmations rather than surprises.

Regardless of how many '3's' and '1's' are identified, those scores should be considered temporary by both the employee and the program. For superior performers, it is an opportunity to raise the bar and expand or change the role of those employees to do more or different work over the next 12 months, thereby taking advantage of their talents and providing them new challenges and responsibilities more likely to incentivize them stay rather than leave. In doing so, they would be expected to attain a performance score of 2 in their new role at the next annual performance evaluation. If they continue to earn 3's, then either they were not stretched enough, the supervisor was not willing to score their performances accurately, the program did not have sufficient flexibility or money, or managers were not sufficiently creative to challenge those employees enough. Similarly, poor performers should be managed so their score of 1 is temporary, to be elevated to a 2 by the time of the next annual performance review, either via fair but persistent corrective oversight or a change in responsibilities that better match those employees' capabilities. In both outlier categories (3's and 1's), the program should closely coordinate and document changes in individual employee roles with the institution's human resources department.

One must appreciate that resolving the performance of those scoring 1's is more urgent than those scoring 3's. Poor performance is a serious drag on the entire program's productivity and morale, and an understandable threat to program leadership's credibility the longer inferior performance is tolerated. As stated above, the cause of poor performance should be thoroughly explored because it is often (but not always) a result of circumstances that can be rectified with more training, resources, or redirection. If the manager is uncomfortable discussing negative reviews and outcomes with a poor performer, there are many courses and publications about how to do this in a humane yet resolute manner, often provided by the institution's human resources department. The author has found value in coaching supervisors by rehearsing the performance review conversation in advance of the actual meeting with the employee, with the program's director playing the role of the problem employee, sometimes with someone from the human resources department participating in those rehearsals. Confronting the director (playing the problem employee) with negative performance issues as a supportive and confidential rehearsal can help alleviate the supervisor's discomfort and hesitation in raising such issues with the employee. These sessions provide useful mentoring of the supervisor in so-called 'soft' skills and help ensure the supervisor has the correct script and confidence to deliver the message properly. As with other formal conversations with a problem employee besides the annual performance review that involve disciplinary actions, at least one additional person representing the institution besides the supervisor should be present as a witness; this is usually someone

from the human resources department. In situations in which the employee belongs to a labor union, that employee may have a contractual right to have someone from the union present at those meetings as his or her advocate and to ensure fairness and objectivity.

The second topic in this first of two performance review/plan meetings between supervisor and employee is also retrospective and considers how well the organization met the needs of the employee over the past 12 months ("what have we done for you?"). This question addresses past performance of the program and parent institution, including how well the supervisor is guiding the employee's work as well as facilitating the employee's personal and career development goals established last year. Those needs and goals may involve more flexible or different work hours due to changed family obligations, official lab animal technician certification, pursuit of an educational degree, a career switch to a new field, or impending retirement. Presuming the employee has been earnest in his or her pursuit of those needs and goals, how well the supervisor and the rest of program leadership have helped speaks volumes to the entire workforce about how committed the program is willing to invest in its employees and their welfare and how appreciative it is of their contributions.

The third topic is how the employee will meet the needs of the organization for the next 12 months ("what will you do for us?"). This involves setting performance goals and can be a source of mutual frustration and likely failure if not done properly. Good goals are reasonable, objective, finite, quantified, accompanied by timelines, and limited only to performance issues or new assignments that are of greatest concern or opportunity (Anon: *Writing SMART Results Expectations*). Depending on the institution, these goals may be proposed by the employee, the supervisor, or both, to be reviewed as drafts in this first meeting. A useful approach is to include no more than three goals for the upcoming year. By contrast, bad goals are vague, open-ended and relative, such as 'try harder,' 'do better' or 'show improvement in (one's attitude, attendance, teamwork, productivity, etc.),' and too numerous. Every goal should be as detailed as possible, allowing both parties to define the assignment easily. In addition, every goal should include numerical elements, allowing both parties to measure progress easily.

For example, rather than tell an employee to be more involved in team activities, establish a three-part goal over the next 12 months for the employee to (1) attend at least nine of 12 monthly team meetings (and remain for the entire duration of the meeting unless excused in advance by the supervisor); (2) chair two of those team meetings; (3) present three team project proposals for consideration at those meetings, with the employee's participation to be documented by an assigned person (e.g., the employee, the supervisor, the meeting chair).

Reviewing project proposals prior to the meeting gives both parties another opportunity to engage constructively and keeps this goal active instead of conveniently forgotten or ignored. Another example of bad *versus* good goals: rather than saying the employee needs to get more work done, assign the employee to maintain a daily diary of tasks assigned and tasks completed, including the number of units/task, such as the number of cages changed, and allow space in the diary for additional comments by the employee. This goal should include a regularly scheduled meeting with the supervisor to review the diary together and identify elements that may require better guidance or more resources needed from the program, or highlight unacceptable performance; the more frequent the meetings, the more effective the supervision and more likely the employee will improve or face disciplinary action sooner.

The fourth and final topic for this first meeting involves how the organization will meet the needs of the employee over the next 12 months ("what will we do for you?"). Identical to setting goals for employee performance, these goals for personal and career development should be appropriate, measureable and few in number. If a valued and trustworthy employee wants to take courses toward certification or a degree that are only given during the work day and if the program can accommodate that employee's absence during that class, then a development goal could combine allowances for specified absences for this purpose and requirements for makeup work that also occurs during the regular workweek so as not to trigger overtime or violate the institution's defined workweek. If the employee belongs to a labor union and if the collective bargaining agreement already provides time off for classes that qualify, then this development goal should specify the reason for this absence.

Another useful development goal involves grooming employees for possible (but not promised) promotion after they received training for that new role. This is also valuable for developing a 'bench' of reserves ready to step up and fill a vacancy in a management or technical specialty position when those slots become available. In these cases, the employee targeted as having potential and who presumably wishes to advance would be given an annual development goal of attending at least one regional or national meeting in the relevant field, to be followed by a proposal to program leadership describing an improvement initiative or addressing a strategic goal. Or the employee may be challenged to research a particular topic of mutual interest in depth during regular work hours, including interviews with thought leaders in that field, and similarly devise an improvement project for consideration. If the grooming involves management, then the employee may be offered time during regular work hours to shadow another manager and meet with him or her on a regular basis to compare notes and absorb some wisdom. Managers who serve as mentors in cases like these should have pride in the program, an engaging personality, an appreciation of the investment required for mentoring and enthusiasm for developing junior employees to assume higher roles. In order to optimize the likelihood of success to develop employees in this regard, the program is obligated to provide adequate time and possibly funds rather than burden the employee with more tasks and expect him or her to succeed in spite of the added workload. As part of their training, it may be fruitful to involve mentees in an evaluation of what work actually needs supervision and how supervision may be restructured for better productivity at all levels (Kuntz *et al.*, 2004).

After these four topics are addressed in the first meeting, the supervisor then fits the salient points of the discussion into the institution's performance review/plan format, shares that with the employee as a draft to ensure what is written accurately depicts what was discussed and agreed to. After any necessary adjustments, the second meeting is scheduled within a week after the first, to review and sign the final version of the official document, and should take no more than 10 minutes.

The employment cycle ends when the employee leaves. That departure may be for positive reasons such as enrolling full-time in graduate or professional school, or accepting a job elsewhere at a higher level or for more pay, or for negative reasons such as cost-cutting, poor performance, or the employee's frustration with the workplace reaching its limit. Regardless of the reason for leaving, it pays to remain on good terms if possible because the lab animal care community is a small one and the departing employee will be a source of opinion about the program, whether intentionally or not. In addition, it is important to capture the employee's impressions of the program while they are still fresh and when appropriate. A useful tool for this purpose is the exit interview, conducted either by program leadership or a human resources representative. The interview can include a questionnaire as well as a conversation, but regardless of the format, it is important to ask the employee to describe the attributes and deficits of the program, including details. The exit interview can then be valuable in identifying and correcting management lapses for the remaining employees and other stakeholders.

IV. MANAGING MONEY

Financial budgets should be recognized as firm performance goals for program leadership and critical tools for program management. The parent institution has included the program's revenues and expenses in its larger, comprehensive monetary projections for the applicable period of time, usually the institution's fiscal year. Therefore, program leadership should realize it is imperative not to stray from these projections, especially to avoid larger deficits, unless there is an unanticipated and significant development and with the knowledge and approval of the institution.

Budgets come in two complementary versions. One is the operating budget in which all revenues and expenses apply only to a single fiscal year and are not extended to other, future years. The other is the capital budget, involving only large expenses that are amortized (buildings and land) or depreciated (equipment) so the acquisition cost is spread over more than one fiscal year. The cost threshold defining what is a capital expense (e.g., starting at $5000) and how many years' capital expenses are to be distributed are determined by the institution's finance policies and in accordance with conventional accounting practices. We will begin with operating budgets because they are usually more controlled by the program itself, and then turn to capital budgets later. Operating budgets include expected revenues, direct (operating) costs (expenses), and indirect (non-operating) costs (expenses). Each will be discussed separately below.

A. Revenues

It is important to appreciate that no program, at least in the United States and to the knowledge of the author, is either profitable or breakeven if *all* applicable costs are included. Thus, every program is subsidized to some extent for costs not covered by external revenues. In industry and some non-profit institutions, there are no revenues from outside sources so all costs are paid for by internal funds. For other non-profits and academic institutions, cost recovery usually involves *per diem* charges for husbandry and veterinary services. It is helpful for a program to specify for animal users and program staff what is and what is not included in the *per diem* service package. A sample distinction is provided in Table 37.1 (NB: for research expenses charged to a federal grant or contract, the content of the *per diem* service package and the price at which *per diem* services are charged are determined, in part, by federal policy and subject to government audit [National Center for Research Resources Office of Science Policy and Public Liaison, 2000; ILAR/ NRC, 2000]. Academic institutions receiving US government grants or contracts are subjected to strict rules and the reader is advised to review those in depth with his/ her respective research finance administrators; (U.S. Office of Management and Budget, 2004, 2013.)

A common complaint by academic investigators is the high price of their *per diems* when compared to colleagues at other institutions who are charged less. What is not appreciated or conveniently forgotten is that

TABLE 37.1 Sample Components of *Per Diem* Charges

INCLUDED

- Animal model and protocol/amendment consultation
- Training in routine animal procedures (e.g., handling, restraint, injections, sample collection, anesthesia, post-operative care)
- Routine husbandry (includes separating animals for pregnancy and weaning; includes changing biohazard and toxic chemical cages; excludes changing cages with radioactive isotopes)
- Routine environmental enrichment (special enrichment provision TBD)
- Animal and special diet procurement from approved vendors
- Coordination of animal shipments imported from unapproved sources
- Coordination of animal shipments exported to other research institutions
- Colony health assessment program, including surveillance and vendor monitoring
- Isolation and elimination of colony infection threats
- Daily and emergency animal health assessment, diagnosis, communication, resolution
- Veterinary care not protocol-related (includes diagnostic necropsies, laboratory tests)
- Compressed CO_2 gas and chambers supplied for euthanasia
- Animal facility and equipment maintenance

NOT INCLUDED[a]

- Pathogen-screening assays for animals imported from non-approved vendors or sources
- Special husbandry (e.g., providing special feed or water per the protocol)
- Breeding colony management
- Rodent rederivation and embryo/sperm cryopreservation
- Shipping off-campus and transport containers
- Research activities (e.g., injections, sample collection, anesthesia, post-operative care)
- Research-related veterinary treatments (e.g., trimming teeth of breeder mice afflicted with malocclusion)
- Euthanasia for research/culling purposes

[a]*Costs to be borne by the investigator or available from the program at an additional charge; prices available on request.*

most programs' *costs* in the United States are roughly the same, even when geographical differences are taken into account. That is because there are only a limited number of ways lab animals can be maintained in good quality and on a large scale, especially in bigger programs. The difference in the *price* (*per diem* rate) for those animal care services is, therefore, more likely due to differing subsidies between academic institutions; better endowed, more generous or more ambitious entities are able or willing to underwrite a larger portion of animal care costs and charge investigators less *versus* those that must or choose to charge users for a bigger share of the costs. Thus, the *per diem* rate schedule can represent an amalgam of political, financial and regulatory realities.

Per diem fees and ancillary charges in the operating budget should be based on credible animal or cage census projections and realistic demand for non-husbandry services and products. Research grants and contracts specifically engaging program personnel can also be included, but should be separate from core service activities in order to allow easier management of both without confusion. In institutions relying on *per diem* charges for partial cost recovery, *per diem* rates should be established for several years into the future so animal users can include price increases (or decreases!) in their grant budgets. As goes for any price projections, those future *per diem* rates should include the caveat that they may change to reflect unplanned events and provide the program and institution some financial flexibility.

B. Direct Expenses

Direct expenses should encompass everything involved in providing core husbandry and veterinary services by the program that is purchased by or otherwise charged to the program. Common categories of direct expenses include labor (further divided into salaries, wages, benefits, overtime, temporary staff), materials and supplies (e.g., feed, bedding, environmental enrichment devices, sanitizing chemicals, personal protective equipment), and a catchall sometimes labeled 'other direct expenses,' the contents of which are usually defined by the institution and can include software, commercial lab fees for health surveillance and diagnostic assays, consultants, preventive maintenance contracts for equipment, professional and technical society memberships, seminars and travel, to mention a few. Institutions usually have assigned categories for each type of revenue and expense in operating budgets, and it behooves program leadership to become fluent in those categories for optimal financial management. Sometimes line items can be aggregated or condensed for easier viewing and for sharing financials with subordinates, and should be discussed with the institution's accounting department if deemed helpful.

C. Indirect Expenses

These expenses usually pertain to institution-wide costs assigned to multiple departments and other entities on a *pro rata* basis, often as a percentage of total square feet. Examples include central administration or corporate expenses, energy consumption, taxes (if applicable), and aggregate amortization and depreciation expenses for that year. Sometimes these costs are applied as a percentage of revenues, direct expenses or a combination of both to the program's operating budget, to make sure they are transparently applied in a consistent fashion to this and other units within the institution. In other cases, indirect expenses are not listed in a program's operating budget, but still should be recognized as legitimate costs

for conducting the program's business and opportunities for the program to reduce those costs. For example, vivaria likely consume more energy than other units, given the large energy demands for maintaining lab animal environments in narrower ranges than for workers in laboratories or offices. If the program realizes significant energy savings through conservation initiatives, those savings may be distributed across the entire institution rather than credited back to the program (doing the right thing financially does not always yield obvious financial advantages but one's contributions should be communicated to higher levels nevertheless).

Capital budgets, by definition, involve large expenditures and institutions usually have a limit on how much they are willing to invest on expensive items. Thus, capital purchases are usually approved only after all units in the institution have submitted their requests to a centralized, senior-level review. To optimize the chances for the most important requests to get the most attention, the program's capital requests should be prioritized according to the category of need involved. One suggested approach to prioritizing capital needs starts with facility and equipment improvements or acquisitions focused on occupational safety, to be followed (in declining order) by animal welfare, regulatory compliance, accreditation, and ending with productivity/efficiency. Pressure from animal users to increase housing capacity by expanding vivarium space or purchasing additional caging may influence capital budgeting decisions.

The operating budget, once finalized, should be frequently compared against actual operating revenues and expenses as they occur, in combination with anticipated changes in financial activity over the remainder of the fiscal year. This exercise can be done monthly, every two months or quarterly, and includes a year-to-date report of past revenues and expenses as well as a forecast of revenue and spending through the end of the fiscal year. The adept manager will combine these reports with other inputs (e.g., census trends, pricing elasticity, current or upcoming staff vacancies, productivity gains, less expensive vendors) to shape future spending and hiring so the budget target is still likely to be met. One metric that should be scrutinized regularly is census (occupancy) as a percentage of available or budgeted capacity. Vivarium space is expensive to maintain, even when empty. Just like other businesses with high fixed costs and profit margins largely driven by occupancy rates, such as hotels and airlines, changes in census are major determinants of financial performance. This is especially true for academic programs dependent on *per diem* charges for partial cost recovery and even more so for commercial contract research organizations that are entirely dependent on study contracts to cover all costs plus a profit.

One useful tactic to help stay on track of one's budget is to have more rather than fewer employees engaged in following financial data and participating in financial matters, with the obvious exception of individual and perhaps aggregated compensation figures. Workers closest to the actual work are often the first to see opportunities for new revenues or savings. Inviting their feedback on financial options also helps accelerate their operational knowledge of the program and builds closer ties among all levels of employees. Excluding salaries and wages, all other components of operating and capital budgets and forecasts are appropriate for sharing with all program staff. Before such inclusion is expanded, employees should be trained in the financial specifics of the program and related reports; this is easier than one may expect because employees usually manage their own budgets at home too. Often called 'open book management,' this concept was popularized by Jack Stack who used it to rescue a failing industrial parts manufacturing business (Rhodes and Amend, 1986) and then expanded it with detailed advice for managers in all fields (Stack, 2013). Including more employees in financial management should not be misinterpreted as automatically giving authority to more employees to make financial decisions. That remains the ultimate responsibility of program leadership. But how that responsibility may be shared or delegated depends on the culture and the capabilities of the organization.

One final note for this section: readers knowledgeable in accounting will recognize that this discussion has focused solely on components of the income statement, also known as the profit and loss statement. The other two fundamental accounting documents that portray an organization's financial performance, i.e., the balance sheet and cash flow statement, are just as important but will not be mentioned further only because they are the domain of other units in an organization and rarely, if ever, involve program leadership.

V. MANAGING OPERATIONS

Now that the program's mission, strategy, people and finances have been covered, it is time to focus on the actual work performed. This is known as operations and involves everything done in the program pertaining to lab animal care. Components include receipt and housing of incoming animals, feeding, watering, cage and vivarium sanitation, clinical and preventive veterinary care, taking census, ordering supplies, billing for services, training program employees and animal users, conducting meetings, maintaining occupational health programs, and preparing regulatory and accreditation documents, just to mention a few. Many familiar publications, starting with the federal Animal Welfare Act (United Stated Government, 2013a) and the ILAR Guide (2011), and other chapters in this textbook specify what

animal care tasks must or should be done in the vivarium. But those directives do not specify *how* those activities must be conducted, thereby providing flexibility and an opportunity for creativity to motivated managers. To avoid repeating the obvious to an informed readership, this section will focus on two related aspects of 'how' involving operations that merit additional comment: quality and continuous improvement.

Advances in the management of lab animal care are hindered by two basic realities. First, no program has to compete for customers, unlike most businesses. In most industries, customers can choose from more than one provider and make their selections based on reliability, convenience, price, brand status, etc. Such options rarely, if ever, exist to animal users. They usually have no choice but to entrust their animals to their institution's internal program, regardless of the quality of care provided. There is strong quantitative evidence for perhaps an intuitive correlation between better management and better organizational performance, driven, in large part, by the demands of competition. In the absence of competition, poor management is not penalized and thus not motivated to do better. Conversely, strong competition may present organizations with existential threats, requiring management to do better in order to avoid failure or elimination (Collins, 2001; Bloom and Van Reenen, 2007).

Second, and as stated earlier, no program is financially profitable or even breaks even when all costs for animal care are included. Instead, every program enjoys a financial safety net of sorts that ensures it will not run out of cash or be shut down due to financial troubles (this is distinguished from the financial state of the parent institution). This financial cushion stifles the voice of the customer even further because the entity that pays for lab animal facilities and capital equipment and also subsidizes the animal care operating budget (i.e., the institution) is not the ultimate user/beneficiary of those animal care services.

This combined freedom from financial self-sustainability and lack of competition encourages management practices that rely on regulatory and accreditation standards as indirect and potentially weak surrogates for quality and innovation. Conventionally, program management has been judged to be sufficient, if not superlative, as long as compliance and accreditation are maintained and not much more. If the incentive to improve and innovate is not strong or persistent, then improvement and innovation will not occur in a significant or continuous fashion. This circumstance does not apply to commercial firms that sell equipment, supplies, and animals to programs. Their business environment is highly competitive, resulting in the many advances we enjoy today such as pathogen-free animals shipped in protective containers, consistently high-quality feed and bedding, automatic watering systems, rodent cage changing stations providing purified, laminar-flow air, and rodent cages that are microbiologically secure and individually ventilated. One may reasonably argue that compliance and accreditation were responsible for many of those advances and have proved worthy frameworks for adequate veterinary care and other definers of good quality. That was certainly true when animal colonies were afflicted with recurring natural infections, primary and secondary enclosures lacked reliable environmental controls and animal models were cheaper and simpler (e.g., lethal endpoints). Most of those threats to good animal welfare and good science have been reduced or eliminated, and the field has become comfortable with equating rare mishaps, such as rodent deaths from flooded cages, with reasonably attainable quality.

But science does not stand still. Today an animal user is more likely to be interested in subtle endpoints (e.g., changes detected at cellular and molecular levels), accompanied by reports of subtle husbandry influences on a wide variety of models, such as the effect of environmental enrichment devices on neurodegenerative diseases (Wood et al., 2010; Lazarov et al., 2005) and cancer (Cao et al., 2010), gut microflora on behavior (Bravo et al., 2011) and immunity (Ivanov et al., 2009), ambient temperature on cancer (Kokolus et al., 2013) and cardiovascular physiology (Swoap et al., 2004), or social housing on neural networks (Sallet et al., 2011) and wound healing (Vitalo et al., 2012). The more we discover how these and other animal care variables can affect research results, the wider the concept of acceptable quality becomes. Going forward, programs will be expected to deliver an expanded selection of husbandry combinations, in addition to avoiding mistakes, before it can be considered a good-quality service provider.

Just as important, earlier times of abundant basic and applied biomedical research funding are being replaced by an increasingly constrained economic landscape in developed countries, forcing both non-profit and for-profit scientific enterprises to scale back, possibly for decades to come. This is occurring at the same time that less developed countries are expanding their biomedical research capacities at lower operating costs. While the United States continues to outspend other nations on non-profit and for-profit biomedical research and development, that spending declined by $12 billion (adjusted for inflation) between 2007 and 2012. By contrast, China's spending increased $6.4 billion over the same period (Chakma et al., 2014). Some of those newcomers still have a long way to go but it is only a matter of when, not if, many life science institutions in emerging economies become globally competitive. When more countries and institutions vigorously compete for limited life sciences funding and talent, their respective animal care programs must follow suit or be will replaced with other business models, such as mergers and outsourcing.

The reader may ask what do these trends of expanding scientific demands and heightened global competition have to do with operations? The response is that they create more pressure and incentive than ever before for management innovations in how work gets done in the vivarium. This pressure is best represented by the following question: what can the program do better for less money? How can quality be improved, in terms of both fewer errors and more husbandry flexibility, at less cost? Part of the answer requires one to define and measure quality; without those, it is difficult to convincingly compare a program's prior quality to today's or future quallity. Unfortunately, no established definition and metrics of quality exist in lab animal care at this time (regulatory compliance and accreditation are not sufficient, as stated above). But one can start by targeting errors and reducing their incidence. That is because rework as a result of mistakes is expensive, burdening a program already pressured to conserve expenses with additional costs to repair or replace what was damaged or lost due to worker or machine error. And eliminating mistakes is a relatively cheap way simultaneously to improve quality plus reduce costs over time.

For example, one can log the occurrence of flooded rodent cages or rodent deaths from flooded cages as a percentage of total rodents or inhabited cages for a defined period of time. After changes are implemented in how cages and watering systems are maintained or monitored, one can observe if the incidence of flooding or deaths drops and by how much. Similarly, one could track accidental injuries of any species arising from caging or husbandry practices, before and after changes were instituted to reduce those injuries. Another example, this time involving occupational safety, is to compare the number of human exposures from macaque bites and scratches that require first aid and medical follow-up to the total number of human–macaque interactions over the same time period. That exposure (error) rate would then be tracked going forward as management changes are implemented in how handlers are trained and how macaques are handled. An important maxim inferred in these examples is the necessity for quantifying results before and after changes are made in a process, often stated as "if you can't measure it, you can't manage it."

The above discussion and examples involve the same approach to measuring and improving quality, albeit much less sophisticated, as provided by six-sigma and statistical process control (SPC) principles and tools. Six-sigma refers to a goal of less than four errors per every million possible chances for that error to occur, and offers a structured approach to problem solving and piloting corrective options (Pyzdek and Keller, 2009). SPC allows any activity to be precisely measured for error rate averages and ranges before and after management changes in that activity (Keller, 2011). Both management tools have proven invaluable in many industries, from manufacturing (Chopra, 2004; Boepple, 2013) to utility companies (Hart et al., 1988) to healthcare (Chao and Courtney, 2012), and recently to lab animal care (Fitzhugh, 2012; Winnicker, 2012). The reader is encouraged to explore the many publications and websites devoted to six-sigma and SPC descriptions and applications, and to experiment with their use in the vivarium. Categories of operations activities appropriate for establishing and tracking error rates can start with workplace safety, followed by animal welfare, user satisfaction and regulatory compliance, in that order. This is not intended to suggest compliance is of low importance but, instead, to liberate one's thinking without engineering standards clouding one's imagination. In other words, one may discover a better-quality management tactic from leading companies in other industries without being distracted by the fact that these are other industries. One can then consider implementation in lab animal care perhaps via a novel performance standard (Klein and Bayne, 2007) as encouraged by U.S. regulators and guidance documents (ARENA-OLAW, 2002).

The other part of the answer to the question of how can one improve operations quality while reducing costs invokes what is known as 'lean' management. This field of management is devoted to identifying and eliminating unnecessary work, thereby reducing total costs or allowing limited capital to be redirected to other, more necessary activities without requiring more funds. The key word here is 'unnecessary,' defined as anything that does not provide value to the customer (Womack and Jones, 2003). An enlightening lean exercise is to scrutinize every operations task while asking if it truly is valuable to the animal user or animal; an easy-to-remember categorization of wasteful activities is provided in Table 37.2. As a result of such an exercise, some established (and expensive) practices may not make sense and invite changes. For example, why is water heated to 180°F to wash rodent cages if those cages will be autoclave-sterilized prior to reuse? The hot water engineering

TABLE 37.2   Types of Wasteful Work[a]

D efects
O ver-production
W aiting
N eglected Employee Creativity
T ransportation
I nventory Excess
M otion
E xtra Processing

[a]Reprinted with permission, The Murli Group, Mystic, CT (www.themurligroup.com).

standard is a holdover from earlier days before rodent cage sterilization post-washing became routine, and the hot water is no longer necessary for sanitation purposes.

Similarly, why should a rodent cage be changed every two weeks (per the conventional engineering standard) if it does not need to be changed at that time? A cage housing one or two adult mice will take longer to reach a soiled threshold than a cage housing five adult mice, as determined by bedding appearance, moisture and ammonia levels. In addition, it has been shown that fewer disturbances, such as cage changing, can improve the survivability of mouse pups (Reeb-Whitaker et al., 2001). A management experiment at the author's former program revealed that up to 30% of mouse cages did not need changing at a 2-week interval; for a large program such as this one, delaying or eliminating 30% of mouse cage changes represented major potential savings in labor and supplies as well as less disturbance for the mice. Not only did animal users not object, they participated in establishing visual thresholds for when a cage needed changing (Brandolini et al., 2009). On a related note, because certain parts of a rodent cage do not get as dirty as quickly as other parts, why not wash those cleaner parts later and conserve labor, water, chemicals and washing capacity in the meantime? One study found that rodent isolation cage tops could go as long as 6 months between washes, compared to cage bottoms (Schondelmeyer et al., 2006).

Let us turn our attention to capital equipment and infrastructure, such as facility surfaces and air handling systems. There are two basic approaches to keeping these in good working order: either wait until something breaks and then have it repaired or replaced, or perform preventive maintenance so items are inspected on a regular schedule and parts are changed, also on a regular schedule. It is intuitive that one saves time and money over the long run by employing preventive rather than reactive maintenance. But the same question raised above for changing rodent cages can be applied to preventive maintenance of capital equipment and facilities, i.e., why replace (change) equipment and parts before they actually need replacing? How much time and money may be wasted when a perfectly good machine or part is exchanged for a new one if no exchange is necessary at that time? Recent advances in capital equipment and facilities maintenance have combined electronic sensors, wireless communication and software into a better approach, known as 'condition-based maintenance' (CBM) or 'predictive maintenance' (Levitt, 2009). In this approach, machines are constantly monitored by 'smart' sensors that identify when a component is nearing the end of its reliability. Those sensors transmit their findings to the responsible party so maintenance can be performed before that component fails. If the component is functioning normally, with no detection of fatigue or pending failure, no maintenance is scheduled and money is saved. Currently, no such (CBM) systems are popular yet in our field but it makes sense to adapt this lean approach to animal care facilities and equipment given their high costs.

Other questionable and expensive activities abound in many vivaria today, based on historical needs or practice standards that may no longer make sense, such as excessive personal protective equipment in barrier rodent colonies that use self-contained caging. Another conventional practice worth challenging is the lengthy sentinel surveillance program for quarantining and treating mice imported from non-commercial sources, *versus* swabbing those mice on arrival for polymerase chain reaction assays to detect excluded pathogens (and eliminating the need for sentinels) (Henderson *et al.*, 2013). A useful management metaphor for identifying possible waste or unnecessary activities is 'friction,' a label applied to processes that require more time than seems reasonable, such as the number of steps required to log on to a computer. For example, why does anyone need to sign a credit card slip when making a purchase when few merchants verify the signature anymore (Pogue, 2012)? In the same sense, what processes in the vivarium involve waiting for something to get done? Can those processes be revised to reduce or eliminate wait times?

Lean management goes hand in hand with six-sigma since reducing errors and eliminating unnecessary work are usually tightly linked in many operational tasks. Thus, one often hears of 'lean sigma,' a blending of two related goals often using identical tools, and extended forward in time under the philosophy of continuous improvement. Combining these three elements has been most prominently expounded by the Toyota Motor Company in what has become known as Toyota Production Systems (TPS) and embraced in almost every industry. One illuminating aspect of a continuous improvement philosophy practiced by Toyota and others is avoiding the term, 'solution,' instead using the term 'countermeasure' when improving a process. That is because 'solution' may imply finality and avoid re-examining that process later to consider even more improvements. By contrast, 'countermeasure' is intended to serve as a placeholder of sorts and to encourage further analysis and modification (thus, a journey of continuous improvement is never completed). TPS principles have been distilled into 14 points provided in Appendix 1 for the reader to study (Liker, 2004). While these may seem simple or obvious, their introduction and sustained use may be initially unsettling to programs with top-down or opaque management cultures. Yet the benefits can be significant in terms of programmatic gains in quality and efficiency as well as employee inclusion and empowerment.[4]

Lean management, six sigma and TPS tools are becoming more popular in our field and to great effect for many operational tasks (Kahn and Umrysh, 2008; Kelly, 2011; Britz, 2004; Cosgrove, 2012; Tummala and Granowski, 2014; Bassuk and Washington, 2014). The reader is advised to become acquainted with those tools and their applications, including value stream maps, takt time, root cause analysis, kaizen events, 5-S, 5 Why's, just-in-time inventory controls such as kan-ban cards, and more. A fictional primer on lean management principles is recommended as an excellent starting point (Goldratt *et al.*, 2004).

One simple example of applying continuous improvement in vivarium operations involves written instructions for performing work. How a given task is executed is usually described and defined by a SOP. The original purpose of SOPs was to ensure that all workers doing the same work were trained and retrained on how that work should be done, in the hope of standardizing output and avoiding mistakes. The problem with SOPs is that they have evolved into lengthy and arcane descriptions, either printed in massive tomes or maintained in bottomless computer databases. That may facilitate regulatory audits to confirm that pertinent SOP's exist and are reviewed and updated regularly (e.g., US Food and Drug Administration Good Laboratory Practices: United States Government, 2013b). But the value of those SOP's as effective and efficient training tools is lost. Ideally, written instructions should be brief, plainly written and easily accessed for quick reference during training or if needed later; instructions for performing complex tasks can be separated into smaller and more digestible segments. One-page SOPs, including photographs and displayed at the biosafety hood, cage washer, autoclave, stockroom, etc., have been demonstrated to be more effective than conventional SOPs (Gibbons and Jarrell, 2006). Alternatively, one could access those same SOPs via a smartphone application ('app') while learning or performing the corresponding task. In both cases, master versions of all SOPs can still be maintained in a central archive and indexed for easy retrieval, audit and modification in a tightly controlled process. These simplified SOPs therefore remain wholly compatible with regulatory requirements and accreditation expectations.

Some final advice for improving operational tasks pertains to pilot assessments. When making a change to an existing process, presumably for the better, it is recommended to perform at least one trial evaluation of that change before applying it across the entire program. What may seem conceptually obvious and logical on paper or in conversation sometimes yields less convincing results when actually tried in the vivarium, or is more difficult to implement even though the ultimate benefits are still likely. Thus, one is encouraged to test an operational change while controlling for other variables,

---

4. Numerous examples of lean and TPS benefits in vivarium management are available at www.virtualvivarium.com.

identical to a scientific experiment, on a small scale first. Then analyze the resultant data, preferably with thresholds for statistical significance, and obtain feedback from the employees performing the trial. If the results confirm the original hypothesis, one may either confirm that change as the new normal or repeat the experiment as many times as deemed necessary. If possible, it is helpful to have dedicated cages, pens, racks, or other pertinent equipment available for such trials. One could even conduct those trials initially without any animals in those enclosures, especially if there is a chance animal welfare may be compromised, such as changing how automatic watering valves are set or serviced or adjusting the volume of emergency alarms in or near animal housing rooms. And testing alternatives to eliminating unnecessary work can employ metrics as simple as comparing the number of steps or measuring the distance animal care personnel walk to perform a task, via the current process *versus* a candidate countermeasure.

All of these considerations underscore the value of extensive planning and testing, another tenet of lean and six-sigma management and TPS. The cycle of Plan-Do-Check-Act (known as 'PDCA') places the most emphasis on its first three steps, in which 'Do' refers to piloting, before the fourth step of changing a task on a large scale ('Act') is done. An excellent PDCA management tool was developed by Toyota and is known as the A3 report, so named because the entire description of an improvement trial must fit on one side of a single sheet of paper 420 × 297 mm in size and labeled as 'A3' (an international standard and functionally comparable to 11 × 17 inches in the United States) and still be easily read. Just like other TPS tools, this approach was designed to avoid waste, primarily time. It forces the writer to economize thoughts and words while still conveying all salient information to the reader (Sobek and Smalley, 2008). The A3 form and underlying philosophy have been used successfully to evaluate and implement process improvements in program management, such as standardizing weekend and holiday animal health checks (Bassuk and Washington, 2013).

VI. CONCLUDING REMARKS

The underlying motivation for writing this chapter was threefold: (1) to highlight the value of adept management as defined in the broadest terms; (2) to identify new drivers of change that will impact program performance; and (3) to introduce proven management methods from other industries that will enable programs to flourish in the midst of those changes. Going forward, both established and aspiring program managers at all levels need to expand their business knowledge and skills in order to sustain their value to the various stakeholders in lab animal husbandry and medicine. Because managing

employees and processes is a universal endeavor that cuts across many industries, continuing education in this regard is often most informative by familiarizing oneself with companies recognized in the business press as 'most admired'(Colvin, 2013), and studying companies that have overcome obstacles or implemented a better way of doing business (Hammond, 2002). Managing can be an exciting and rewarding activity, especially in as dynamic and challenging field as ours. Those who choose to step up and continue in this occupation are to be appreciated and supported with just as much investment in their career development as others who choose technical and professional roles.

APPENDIX 1. EXECUTIVE SUMMARY OF THE 14 TOYOTA WAY PRINCIPLES (REPRINTED WITH PERMISSION, McGRAW-HILL EDUCATION HOLDINGS, LLC, PHILADELPHIA, PA)

Section I: Long-Term Philosophy

Principle 1. Base your management decisions on a long-term philosophy, even at the expense of short-term financial goals.

- Have a philosophical sense of purpose that supersedes any short-term decision making. Work, grow, and align the whole organization toward a common purpose that is bigger than making money. Understand your place in the history of the company and work to bring the company to the next level. Your philosophical mission is the foundation for all the other principles.
- Generate value for the customer, society, and the economy—it is your starting point. Evaluate every function in the company in terms of its ability to achieve this.
- Be responsible. Strive to decide your own fate. Act with self-reliance and trust in your own abilities. Accept responsibility for your conduct and maintain and improve the skills that enable you to produce added value.

Section II: The Right Process Will Produce the Right Results

Principle 2. Create a continuous process flow to bring problems to the surface.

- Redesign work processes to achieve high value-added, continuous flow. Strive to cut back to zero the amount of time that any work project is sitting idle or waiting for someone to work on it.

- Create flow to move material and information fast as well as to link processes and people together so that problems surface right away.
- Make flow evident throughout your organizational culture. It is the key to a true continuous improvement process and to developing people.

Principle 3. Use 'pull' systems to avoid overproduction.

- Provide your downline customers in the production process with what they want, when they want it, and in the amount they want. Material replenishment initiated by consumption is the basic principle of just-in-time.
- Minimize your work in process and warehousing of inventory by stocking small amounts of each product and frequently restocking based on what the customer actually takes away.
- Be responsive to the day-by-day shifts in customer demand rather than relying on computer schedules and systems to track wasteful inventory.

Principle 4. Level out the workload (*heijunka*). (Work like the tortoise, not the hare.)

- Eliminating waste is just one-third of the equation for making lean successful. Eliminating overburden to people and equipment and eliminating unevenness in the production schedule are just as important – yet generally not understood at companies attempting to implement lean principles.
- Work to level out the workload of all manufacturing and service processes as an alternative to the stop/ start approach of working on projects in batches that is typical at most companies.

Principle 5. Build a culture of stopping to fix problems, to get quality right the first time.

- Quality for the customer drives your value proposition.
- Use all the modern quality assurance methods available.
- Build into your equipment the capability of detecting problems and stopping itself. Develop a visual system to alert team or project leaders that a machine or process needs assistance. *Jidoka* (machines with human intelligence) is the foundation for 'building in' quality.
- Build into your organization support systems to quickly solve problems and put in place countermeasures.
- Build into your culture the philosophy of stopping or slowing down to get quality right the first time to enhance productivity in the long run.

Principle 6. Standardized tasks and processes are the foundation for continuous improvement and employee empowerment.

- Use stable, repeatable methods everywhere to maintain the predictability, regular timing, and regular output of your processes. It is the foundation for flow and pull.
- Capture the accumulated learning about a process up to a point in time by standardizing today's best practices. Allow creative and individual expression to improve upon the standard; then incorporate it into the new standard so that when a person moves on you can hand off the learning to the next person.

Principle 7. Use visual control so no problems are hidden.

- Use simple visual indicators to help people determine immediately whether they are in a standard condition or deviating from it.
- Avoid using a computer screen when it moves the worker's focus away from the workplace.
- Design simple visual systems at the place where the work is done, to support flow and pull.
- Reduce your reports to one piece of paper whenever possible, even for your most important financial decisions.

Principle 8. Use only reliable, thoroughly tested technology that serves your people and processes.

- Use technology to support people, not to replace people. Often it is best to work out a process manually before adding technology to support the process.
- New technology is often unreliable and difficult to standardize and therefore endangers 'flow.' A proven process that works generally takes precedence over new and untested technology.
- Conduct actual tests before adopting new technology in business processes, manufacturing systems, or products.
- Reject or modify technologies that conflict with your culture or that might disrupt stability, reliability, and predictability.
- Nevertheless, encourage your people to consider new technologies when looking into new approaches to work. Quickly implement a thoroughly considered technology if it has been proven in trials and it can improve flow in your processes.

Section III: Add Value to the Organization by Developing Your People

Principle 9. Grow leaders who thoroughly understand the work, live the philosophy, and teach it to others.

- Grow leaders from within, rather than buying them from outside the organization.

- Do not view the leader's job as simply accomplishing tasks and having good people skills. Leaders must be role models of the company's philosophy and way of doing business.
- A good leader must understand the daily work in great detail so he or she can be the best teacher of your company's philosophy.

Principle 10. Develop exceptional people and teams who follow your company's philosophy.

- Create a strong, stable culture in which company values and beliefs are widely shared and lived out over a period of many years.

- Train exceptional individuals and teams to work within the corporate philosophy to achieve exceptional results. Work very hard to reinforce the culture continually.
- Use cross-functional teams to improve quality and productivity and enhance flow by solving difficult technical problems. Empowerment occurs when people use the company's tools to improve the company.
- Make an ongoing effort to teach individuals how to work together as teams toward common goals. Teamwork is something that has to be learned.

Principle 11. Respect your extended network of partners and suppliers by challenging them and helping them improve.

- Have respect for your partners and suppliers and treat them as an extension of your business.
- Challenge your outside business partners to grow and develop. It shows that you value them. Set challenging targets and assist your partners in achieving them.

Section IV: Continuously Solving Root Problems Drives Organizational Learning

Principle 12. Go and see for yourself to thoroughly understand the situation (*genchi genbutsu*).

- Solve problems and improve processes by going to the source and personally observing and verifying data rather than theorizing on the basis of what other people or the computer screen tell you.
- Think and speak based on personally verified data.
- Even high-level managers and executives should go and see things for themselves, so they will have more than a superficial understanding of the situation.

Principle 13. Make decisions slowly by consensus, thoroughly considering all options; implement decisions rapidly (*nemawashi*).

- Do not pick a single direction and go down that one path until you have thoroughly considered alternatives. When you have picked, move quickly and continuously down the path.
- *Nemawashi* is the process of discussing problems and potential solutions with all of those affected, to collect their ideas and get agreement on a path forward. This consensus process, though time-consuming, helps broaden the search for solutions, and once a decision is made, the stage is set for rapid implementation.

Principle 14. Become a learning organization through relentless reflection (*hansei*) and continuous improvement (*kaizen*).

- Once you have established a stable process, use continuous improvement tools to determine the root cause of inefficiencies and apply effective countermeasures.
- Design processes that require almost no inventory. This will make wasted time and resources visible for all to see. Once waste is exposed, have employees use a continuous improvement process (kaizen) to eliminate it.
- Protect the organizational knowledge base by developing stable personnel, slow promotion, and very careful succession systems.

References

Anon. Writing SMART Results Expectations. <http://www.ncdhhs.gov/humanresources/pms/pm/smart.pdf>.

Anthony, J., 2011. Don't ask a job applicant these questions. <http://www.microsoft.com/business/en-us/resources/management/recruiting-staffing/dont-ask-a-job-applicant-these-questions.aspx>.

ARENA-OLAW Institutional Animal Care and Use Committee Guidebook, second ed, 2002 (also available at <http://grants.nih.gov/grants/olaw/GuideBook.pdf>).

Bassuk, J.A., Washington, I.M., 2013. The A3 problem solving report: a 10-step scientific method to execute performance improvements in an academic research vivarium. PLoS One 8, e76833.

Bassuk, J.A., Washington, I.M., 2014. Iterative development of visual control systems in a research vivarium. PLoS One 9, e90076.

Bloom, N., Van Reenen, J., 2007. Measuring and explaining management practices across firms and countries. Quart. J. Econom. 122, 1351–1408.

Boepple, J., 2013. Samsung Electronics: Using Affinity Diagrams and Pareto Charts. Harvard Business School Press, Boston, MA, Number KEL738.

Brandolini, J., Gentile, S., Pina, F., Jarrell, D.M., 2009. Standardizing the definition of a "dirty" soiled rodent cage. J. Amer. Assoc. Lab. Anim. Sci. 48, 541.

Bravo, J.A., Forsythe, P., Chew, M.V., et al., 2011. Ingestion of Lactobacillus strain regulates emotional behavior and central GABA receptor expression in a mouse via the vagus nerve. Proc. Natl. Acad. Sci. USA 108, 16050–16055.

Britz, W.R., 2004. Lean for lab animal managers. Anim. Lab. News 3(3), May/June.

Cao, L., Liu, X., Lin, E.J., et al., 2010. Environmental and genetic activation of a brain-adipocyte bdnf/leptin axis causes cancer remission and inhibition. Cell 142, 52–64.

Chakma, J., Sun, G.H., Steinberg, J.D., Sammut, S.M., Jagsi, R., 2014. Asia's ascent—global trends in biomedical R&D expenditures. N. Engl. J. Med. 370, 3–6.

Chao, R., Courtney, T., 2012. Arcadia Medical Center (B). Harvard Business School Press., Number UV6041.

Chopra, S., 2004. Six Sigma Quality at Flyrock Tires. Harvard Business School Press, Boston, MA, Number KEL028.

Collins, J., 2001. Good to Great: Why Some Companies Make the Leap… And Others Don't. HarperCollins, New York.

Collis, D.J., 2005. Strategy: Create and Implement the Best Strategy for Your Business. Harvard Business Press Books, Boston, MA.

Colvin, G., 2013. The World's Most Admired Companies: Built for Brilliance. Fortune. <http://money.cnn.com/2013/02/28/news/companies/most-admired-companies.pr.fortune/index.html?iid=wma_sp_lead>.

Cosgrove, C., 2012. An overview of lean management in lab animal facilities. Anim. Lab. News November/December.

Drucker, P.F., 2001. The Essential Drucker. Harper, New York.

Fitzhugh, D.C., 2012. Untangling and improving the IACUC protocol review process using lean six sigma methodology. Presentation, AALAS 63rd National Meeting, Minneapolis, MN, November 8.

Gallup poll, 2013. "Perceived moral acceptability of medical testing using animals, by age", June 3; <http://www.gallup.com>.

Gibbons, C., Jarrell, D., 2006. The one-page standard operating procedure (SOP) as a tool for successful standardization adopted from the Toyota Production System (TPS) approach. J. Amer. Assoc. Lab. Anim. Sci. 45, 81.

Goldratt, E.M., Cox, J., Whitford, D., 2004. The Goal: A Process of Ongoing Improvement, third ed. North River Press, Great Barrington, MA.

Hammond, J.S., 2002. Learning by the Case Method (Revised). Harvard Business School Press, Boston, MA, Number 9-376-241.

Hart, C.W.L., Maher, D., Montelongo, M., 1988. Florida Power Light Quality Improvement (QI) Story Exercise (A). Harvard Business School Press, Boston, MA, Number 689041.

Haussmann, R., 2013. How to make the next big thing. Sci. Amer. 308, 37.

Henderson, K.S., Perkins, C.L., Havens, R.B., et al., 2013. Efficacy of direct detection of pathogens in naturally infected mice by using a high-density PCR array. J. Amer. Assoc. Lab. Anim. Sci. 52, 763–772.

Institute for Laboratory Animal Research, National Research Council, 2000. Strategies That Influence Cost Containment in Animal Research Facilities. National Academies Press, Washington, DC (also available at <http://www.nap.edu/catalog.php?record_id=10006>).

Institute for Laboratory Animal Research, National Research Council, 2011. Guide for the Care and Use of Laboratory Animals, eighth ed. National Academies Press, Washington, DC (also available at <http://www.nap.edu/catalog.php?record_id=12910>).

Ivanov, I.I., Atarashi, K., Manel, N., et al., 2009. Induction of intestinal Th17 cells by segmented filamentous bacteria. Cell 139, 485–498.

Kahn, N., Umrysh, B.M., 2008. Improving animal research facility operations through the application of lean principles. Inst. Lab. Anim. Res. (ILAR) e-J. 49, e15–e22.

Kaplan, R.S., Norton, D.P., 2005. The best of HBR 1992. The balanced scorecard – measures that drive performance. Harvard Bus. Rev. July/August.

Keller, P., 2011. Statistical Process Control Demystified. McGraw-Hill, New York.

Kelly, H., 2011. Lean in the lab: a primer. ALN World July/August.

Klein, H.J., Bayne, K.A., 2007. Establishing a culture of care, conscience, and responsibility: addressing the improvement of scientific discovery and animal welfare through science-based performance standards. Inst. Lab. Anim. Res. J. 48 (1), 3–11.

Kokolus, K.M., Capitano, M.L., Lee, C.T., et al., 2013. Baseline tumor growth and immune control in laboratory mice are significantly influenced by subthermoneutral housing temperature. Proc. Natl. Acad. Sci. USA 110, 20176–20181.

Kuntz, M.J., Lefrancois, J.P., Yergey, N.S., Klein, H.J., Goldberg, J., Laird, S., 2004. Increasing supervisory effectiveness in a laboratory animal facility. J. Amer. Assoc. Lab. Anim. Sci. 43, 50–53.

Lazarov, O., Robinson, J., Tang, Y.P., et al., 2005. Environmental enrichment reduces Abeta levels and amyloid deposition in transgenic mice. Cell 120, 701–713.

Levitt, J., 2009. The Handbook of Maintenance Management, second ed. Industrial Press, New York.

Liker, J., 2004. The Toyota Way: 14 Management Principles from the World's Greatest Manufacturer. McGraw-Hill, New York.

National Center for Research Resources Office of Science Policy and Public Liaison, 2000. Cost Analysis and Rate Setting Manual for Animal Research Facilities. NIH Publication., No. 00-2006, Bethesda, MD (also available at <http://grants.nih.gov/grants/policy/air/rate_setting_manual_2000.pdf>).

National Science Board, 2014. Reducing Investigators' Administrative Workload for Federally Funded Research. National Science Foundation, Arlington, TX.

Pogue, D., 2012. Technology's friction problem. Sci. Amer. 307, 28.

Pyzdek, T., Keller, P., 2009. The Six Sigma Handbook, third ed. McGraw-Hill, New York.

Reeb-Whitaker, C.K., Paigen, B., Beamer, W.G., et al., 2001. The impact of reduced frequency of cage changes on the health of mice housed in ventilated cages. Lab. Anim. 35 (1), 58–73.

Rhodes, L., Amend, P., 1986. The turnaround – How a dying division of International Harvester became one of America's most competitive small companies. Inc., 42–48. August.

Sallet, J., Mars, R.B., Noonan, M.P., et al., 2011. Social network size affects neural circuits in macaques. Science 334, 697–700.

Schondelmeyer, C.W., Dillehay, D.L., Webb, S.K., Huerkamp, M.J., Mook, D.M., Pullium, J.K., 2006. Investigation of appropriate sanitization frequency for rodent caging accessories: evidence supporting less-frequent cleaning. J. Amer. Assoc. Lab. Anim. Sci. 45, 40–43.

Silverman, J., 2008. Managing the Laboratory Animal Facility, second ed. CRC Press, Boca Raton, FL.

Sobek, D.K., Smalley, A., 2008. Understanding A3 Thinking: a Critical Component of Toyota's PDCA Management System. Taylor & Francis Group, New York.

Stack, J., 2013. The Great Game of Business, Expanded and Updated: The Only Sensible Way to Run a Company. Crown Publishing/Random House, New York.

Sukow, M.A., Douglas, F.A., Weichbrod, R.H. (Eds.), 2002. Management of Laboratory Animal Care and Use Programs CRC Press, Boca Raton, FL.

Swoap, S.J., Overton, J.M., Garber, G., 2004. Effect of ambient temperature on cardiovascular parameters in rats and mice: a comparative approach. Amer. J. Physiol. Regul. Integr. Comp. Physiol. 287, R391–R396.

Thulin, J.D., Bradfield, J.F., Bergdall, V.K., et al., 2014. The cost of self-imposed regulatory burden in animal research. FASEB J.

published online before print April 30, 2014, <http://dx.doi.org/10.1096/fj.14-254094>.

Tummala, S., Granowski, J.A., 2014. Lean concepts for vivarium operational excellence. Lab. Anim. Sci. Prof. 2 (1), 26–30.

U.S. Office of Management and Budget, 2004. Circular A-21 (Cost Principles for Educational Institutions). Revised May 10, 2004; <http://www.whitehouse.gov/omb/circulars_a021_2004/>.

U.S. Office of Management and Budget, 2013. Circular A-133 (Audits of State, Local Governments, and Non-Profit Organizations), <http://www.whitehouse.gov/omb/circulars/a133_compliance_supplement_2013>.

United States Government, 2013a. Code of Federal Regulations Title 9, Chapter I – Animal and Plant Health Inspection Service, Department of Agriculture, Subchapter A – Animal Welfare, Part 3 – Standards (also available at <http://www.aphis.usda.gov/animal_welfare/downloads/Animal%20Care%20Blue%20Book%20-%202013%20-%20FINAL.pdf>).

United States Government, 2013b. Code of Federal Regulations Title 21, Title 21 – Food And Drugs, Chapter I – Food And Drug Administration, Department of Health And Human Services, Subchapter A, Part 58 Good Laboratory Practice for Nonclinical Laboratory Studies, Subpart E, Section 58.81, Standard Operating Procedures (also available at <http://www.gpo.gov/fdsys/granule/CFR-1999-title21-vol1/CFR-1999-title21-vol1-part58/content-detail.html>).

Vitalo, A.G., Gorantla, S., Fricchione, J.G., et al., 2012. Environmental enrichment with nesting material accelerates wound healing in isolation-reared rats. Behav. Brain Res. 226, 606–612.

Winnicker, C., 2012. New frontiers in workforce development; enhancing animal care and welfare utilizing lean six sigma techniques. Presentation, AALAS 63rd National Meeting, Minneapolis, MN, November 5.

Womack, J.P., Jones, D.T., 2003. Lean Thinking: Banish Waste and Create Wealth in Your Corporation, Revised and Updated. Free Press, New York.

Wood, N.I., Carta, V., Milde, S., et al., 2010. Responses to environmental enrichment differ with sex and genotype in a transgenic mouse model of Huntington's Disease. PLoS One 5, e9077.

CHAPTER

38

Laboratory Animal Behavior

Kathryn A.L. Bayne, MS, PhD, DVM, DACLAM, DACAW, CAAB[a], Bonnie V. Beaver, DVM, MS, DSc (hon), DPNAP, DACVB, DACAW[b], Joy A. Mench, DPhil[c] and Christina Winnicker, DVM, MPH, DACLAM[d]

[a]AAALAC International, Corporate Dr., Suite #203, Frederick, MD, USA [b]Department of Small Animal Clinical Sciences, College of Veterinary Medicine, Texas A&M University, College Station, TX, USA [c]Department of Animal Science and Center for Animal Welfare, University of California, Davis, CA, USA [d]Enrichment & Behavioral Medicine, Department of Animal Welfare, Charles River Laboratories, Wilmington, MA, USA

OUTLINE

I. INTRODUCTION

The study of laboratory animal behavior has increased steadily over the last decade, with expanding emphasis on a variety of commonly used species. In the United States, this trend was initially focused on species for which there was a regulatory requirement to consider normalizing behavior, specifically the U.S. Department of Agriculture's requirement to promote the psychological well-being of nonhuman primates as reflected in the 1991 Animal Welfare Regulations (AWRs). With the advent of the seventh edition of the *Guide* (NRC, 1996),

Laboratory Animal Medicine, Third Edition
DOI: http://dx.doi.org/10.1016/B978-0-12-409527-4.00038-9

more emphasis was placed on addressing the structural, social, and activity elements in all laboratory animals' cage or pen environments in what was referred to as a 'behavioral management program.' The implication that environmental enrichment is a *de facto* means of normalizing laboratory animal behavior is evidenced by the discussion of this topic as one component of the microenvironment (i.e., cage) for all laboratory species in the eighth edition of the *Guide* (NRC, 2011). The 2011 *Guide* also devoted an entire section to 'Behavioral and Social Management,' highlighting the importance of motor, cognitive, and social activity; the social environment, noting that single housing of social species should be the exception; and procedural habituation and training of animals.

Scientists should be concerned about the behavioral state of animals kept in laboratories, not only for ethical reasons but for reasons of science, as behavioral abnormalities may be accompanied by physiological or immunological variations from the norm, thereby potentially confounding research data. For example, it has been made clear that the central nervous system has a significant direct effect on the immune system independent of corticosteroids (Dantzer and Kelley, 1989; Kingston and Hoffman-Goetz, 1996). Moreover, there is a wealth of literature on the effects of enriched and impoverished environments on behavior, showing that the complexity of the environment affects brain development, memory, learning ability, problem solving, and social interactions with humans and other animals (for a review of the effects of enrichment on mice, see Bayne and Wurbel, 2012). Enriched environments can also mitigate the effects of undernutrition and old age; promote recovery from brain trauma; and alter drug responses, tumor latency, LD_{50}, and the development of disease (see, e.g., Chance, 1957; DePass *et al.*, 1986; Renner and Rosenzweig, 1987; Claassen, 1994; Kempermann *et al.*, 1997; Kerr *et al.*, 2010; de Sousa *et al.*, 2011).

As society's concern for animal welfare in general and laboratory animal welfare in particular has gained momentum, the linkage between welfare and behavior has become more widely recognized. Three important methodologies have been used to help determine what animals require, and each has its own advantages and limitations (Mason *et al.*, 1998; Dawkins, 1990). The first is simply to observe what animals do and to prepare an ethogram of those behaviors based on frequency, duration, and the time at which they perform those behaviors. One can then compare time budgets in different environments, with perhaps the natural species ethogram being the 'gold standard' (e.g., Lawlor, 1984; Stauffacher, 1997a; Poole, 1992, 1998), though Shepherdson (1998) has argued that while using the behavior of wild animals as a benchmark for evaluating captive animal behavior has been cited since Hediger (1969), the natural behavior of many species is still unknown or incompletely

known. This approach can also be used to determine whether and how animals interact with the captive environment and the objects in that environment, such as furniture and toys (Mench, 1994). Also with this type of approach, one can measure physiological variables or use psychometric tests (such as the open field test for anxiety) and subsequently determine how the results vary from those obtained in other environments (see Broom and Johnson, 1993; Cooper and Hendrie, 1994). The disadvantage of this approach is that the standard for what is 'normal' may be subjectively biased by the observer's knowledge and personal experience.

The second approach is to offer animals a choice of environments or aspects of an environment to see which they prefer to spend their time in, referred to as preference testing. This is a long-standing experimental technique going back to the work of Craig (1918). In preference tests, animals have free access to different choices, and the amount of time spent with each choice is measured. However, the results should be treated cautiously (Duncan, 1978; Dawkins, 1990; Fraser, 1996) as animals may not indicate what is in their long-term best interests and can choose only from the environments offered by the experimenter. Also, an animal's choice may vary with experience.

The third method to assess animal needs builds on preference testing by determining how hard the animal will work to reach a certain environment and comparing this effort with other behaviors, thereby testing the *strength* of its preferences. Animals will continue to work hard for essentials like food and water but make less effort for different substrates, environments, or social interactions. In this manner it may be possible to rank the relative importance of various activities in the behavioral repertoire to separate needs from wants from luxuries (see Dawkins, 1990, 1992). Limitations to this test are based on the inherent variability in the stimuli used to test the animals and in making equivalent comparisons between them.

Behavior problems encountered in captive animals can be classified broadly and simply as 'qualitative' or 'quantitative' aberrant expressions of behavior (Erwin and Deni, 1979). This classification scheme implies either that species-typical behavior is modified in the amount expressed, such as an excessive amount of time spent in the behavior or the absence of the behavior, or that the behavior itself has been modified such that it is expressed in response to an atypical stimulus or is directed to an inappropriate target. In either case, a mismatch between the response and the stimulus is evident (Bayne, 1996). Fox (1968) has stated that a behavior that initially began as a means for the animal to adapt to the conditions that elicited the behavioral change frequently becomes maladaptive and can "become emancipated or released independent of the original... stimuli." Crockett (1998) includes altered activity cycles in the list of behavioral measures that may reflect inadequate well-being.

The effects of stereotypies on health and well-being are less clear-cut than for many other kinds of abnormal behaviors, such as self-biting (Mason, 1991; Lawrence and Rushen, 1993; Mench and Mason, 1997). To some extent the ambiguous definition for a stereotyped behavior (one that is repetitive, unvarying, and non-goal oriented) may be applied to some normal behaviors (e.g., walking) for which the goal is simply not known (Fraser, 2008). Also, there is conflicting evidence as to whether the performance of stereotypic behavior results from stress or actually reduces stress levels (Ladewig et al., 1993), potentially serving as a coping mechanism through sensorimotor stimulation (Mason and Latham, 2004) or arousal reduction (Novak et al., 2013). Stereotypies are a heterogeneous category of behaviors that can include a variety of locomotor, postural, or gestural patterns. Their development can be influenced by a number of factors, such as neurological predispositions, exposure to stressors, impoverished environmental conditions, and frustration of the motivation to perform particular behaviors. Once they are established, the expression of stereotypies can be difficult to stop. Since there is general agreement that stereotypies indicate that the animal's environment is or has been inadequate in some way, a better approach is to minimize the potential or prevent the development of stereotypies by providing opportunities for the expression of species-typical behaviors (Duncan et al., 1993). For a broader perspective on environmental factors likely to impinge on animal welfare and science, see Clough (1982), Rose (1994), and Fraser (2008).

In recent years, increased emphasis has been placed on providing social enrichment (e.g., social housing) to social species of animals used in research, testing, and education. For example, AAALAC International states that it considers social housing to be the default method of housing unless otherwise justified based on social incompatibility resulting from inappropriate behavior, veterinary concerns regarding animal well-being, or scientific necessity approved by the IACUC (http://www.aaalac.org/accreditation/positionstatements.cfm#social). The *Guide* (NRC, 2011) advises that an understanding of the species-typical social behavior is essential to determining if the laboratory animal should be housed singly, in a pair, or in a group. One long-standing framework for categorizing the social unit is based on the amount of male integration into the unit (Eisenberg et al., 1972), with the social units being thusly identified as: solitary, bi-parental family; single-male harems; age-graded male troops; and multi-male troops. However, the laboratory environment poses certain challenges in meeting this objective and thus an innovative approach is necessary. Obstacles to overcome include the inability for some animals to remove themselves from an aggressive animal in the cage; the housing of animals by sex, which can result in atypical forced social interactions (e.g., all male groups of B57 mice); breeding paradigms that specify how animals are housed (e.g., trio breeding); and cage designs that limit the expression of species-typical social behaviors.

The goals of enrichment are to decrease the incidence of abnormal behaviors and to increase the diversity of normal behaviors expressed. The evaluation of any enrichment can be carried out in any of the three ways described above (Bayne et al., 1992c; Beaver, 1989; Benn, 1995; Hart, 1994; Markowitz and Gavazzi, 1995; Newberry, 1995; Poole, 1998; Scharmann, 1991; Stauffacher, 1997a). However, it has to be remembered that simply changing an animal's behavior pattern does not necessarily mean the change is for the better. It may simply result in one stereotypic behavior being substituted for another. Therefore, a basic understanding of the species-typical behavior of the animal and an ongoing program to evaluate the effects of an enrichment program are key to improving the behavioral well-being of laboratory animals. This chapter will review some fundamental behaviors of the more common laboratory animals and link these to environmental enrichments that can improve animal well-being and provide a more refined animal model for research.

II. RODENTS

In recent years, the importance of understanding and managing the behavior of laboratory animals has become a significant focus for vivarium management and regulators alike. The 8th edition of the *Guide* (NRC, 2011) emphasizes the understanding of the behavioral repertoire of the species that staff work with in order to facilitate species appropriate behaviors and identify abnormal behaviors requiring intervention. The European Directive (Animals Used for Scientific Purposes: Directive 2010/63/EU) follows up on the European Convention (ETS 123) with even stricter guidelines on the behavioral care of animals used for experimental and other scientific purposes. Thus, the understanding of the normal behavioral repertoire of the species we house becomes important in order to develop training for staff and a behaviorally relevant environmental enrichment program. Rodents have been kept in captivity for at least a century and some species far longer. Despite this, they retain many of their natural characteristics and instincts that evolved in their wild ancestors, as evidenced from studies of their behaviors when they are placed in more 'natural' habitats (e.g., Boice, 1977). This may generate ideas about how to modify their environments to suit them better and so reduce any adverse effects they may feel (Brain, 1992). However, the fact that there are several hundred strains of rodents (specifically, rats and mice, both inbred and outbred) raises the question of whether the environmental requirements are the same for all strains. This section will review the normal behavior of the most common laboratory rodents (mice, rats, hamsters, gerbils, and guinea pigs) and rabbits.

A. Mice

Mice are a highly adaptable species, though their position as a prey species marks much of their behavioral repertoire. In order to avoid predations they are nocturnal, with crepuscular peaks of activity and avoidance of open and brightly lit spaces (Southern, 1954; Rowe, 1981; Ward, 1981; Gray, 1991; Gordon *et al.*, 1998; Jennings *et al.*, 1998). In the wild, mice forage for nesting material and limited food resources and will wander significant distances in order to do so (DeLong, 1967; Macdonald *et al.*, 2000). While the requirement to wander in search of limited resources is obviously unnecessary in the laboratory environment, mice retain the behavioral drive to forage, and this behavioral need can be fulfilled by the provision of scattered food, treats such as sunflower seeds, or nesting material provided either as floor scatter or in various packages that require searching, digging, and processing to obtain and use the nesting material (see Figure 38.1A, B, and C).

The social structure of mice is complex, being composed of familiar groups containing a dominant male, one or more females, and their sub-adult offspring (Crowcroft, 1973; Latham and Mason, 2004). Territory size is generally based on resources and has been reported to range from 1–80,000 square meters (Young *et al.*, 1950; Southern, 1954; Chambers *et al.*, 2000). All adults within a territory will defend it (Crowcroft, 1973). Mice use olfactory cues, rather than sight or sound, to establish a hierarchy. Urinary cues, as well as scent deposited from the plantar glands on the feet, define territory boundaries and runways (König, 2012). Disturbing the cage environment, by cleaning for example, can therefore precipitate a bout of fighting while scent marking is carried out and the order reestablished (Hurst *et al.*, 1993). Blom *et al.* (1993) found that while NMRI mice preferred clean to soiled cages that had not been cleaned for 4–6 days, 2-day soiled cages were preferred to clean ones. This may have implications for routine husbandry of animals and would be interesting to reevaluate in ventilated cages.

Aggression has been shown to be influenced by strain, age, and prior encounters. Generally mice become more territorial, more aggressive, and more infanticidal as the population density increases (Crowcroft, 1973; Latham and Mason, 2004). However, both larger groups and larger cage sizes have been associated with an increase in social instability and subsequent increase in aggression

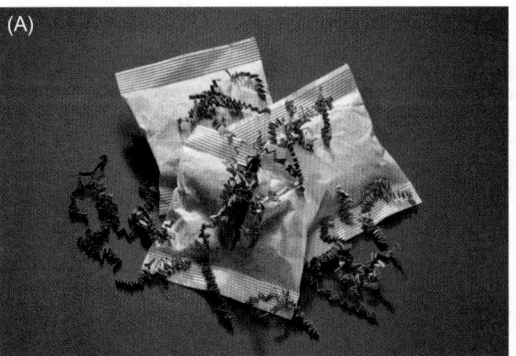
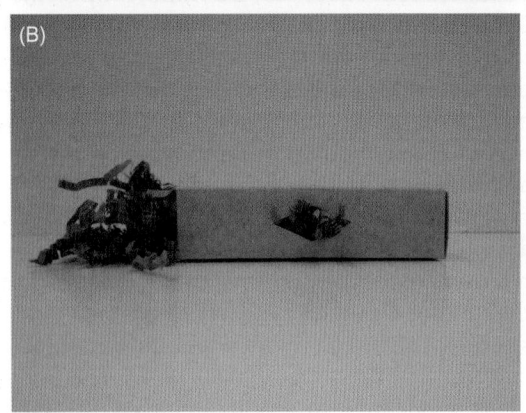
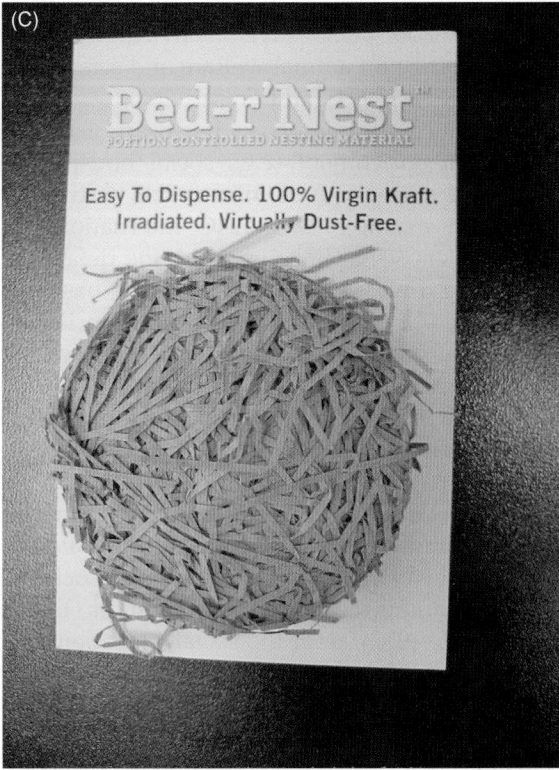

FIGURE 38.1   Examples of commercially available nesting material delivery packages. (A) EnviroPak Courtesy of WF Fisher and Son 2013; (B) Nesting Foraging Box Charles River 2012; (C) Nesting Material: Anderson.

(Poole and Morgan, 1973; Van Loo and Mol, 2001). Cage complexity can also influence aggression: shelters have been shown to induce aggression (Howerton *et al.*, 2008), as they provide a 'choke point' or ambush site where mice need to express territorial behavior and a valued resource to defend. The provision of clustered resources in a previously unenriched cage has also been shown to increase aggression in C57BL/6J mice, but the provision of these same enrichments in a more dispersed distribution did not (Akre *et al.*, 2011). Early life experience also appears to have some influence on later life aggression patterns in mice. One study by Kikusui *et al.* (2004) demonstrated that early weaned Balb/c mice, that is mice weaned at 14 days as opposed to 21, showed increased anxiety when measured by elevated plus maze and increased conspecific aggression upon regrouping after isolation. Increased anxiety and aggression were also caused by brief periods of maternal separation and thermal stress in neonatal pups (Hohmann *et al.*, 2013) and increased aggression has been observed in mice raised without enrichment (Hutchinson *et al.*, 2012). Thus, neonatal handling and weaning paradigms appear to affect later aggressive tendencies.

Participation in aggressive encounters can affect levels of pituitary hormones, including the reproductive gonadotropins (animals may become infertile), adrenocorticotropic hormones (ACTH), as well as catecholamine levels in the adrenal medulla (Brain, 1990). Corticosterone levels can be higher in defeated subordinate mice, especially when they are kept in noncomplex conditions, such as bedded polycarbonate cages (Durschlag and Stauffacher, 1996), but can also be higher in dominant animals with a large territory to defend (Bishop and Chevins, 1989). In addition, immune function has been shown to decrease with an increase in the number of attacks received (Barnard *et al.*, 1996).

Ways shown to successfully reduce aggression include housing mice together before puberty is reached, using more docile strains, and replacing conspecifics as soon as possible if they have to be separated, since even the removal of an animal for 24h can increase the level of aggression on its return (Babcock and Graham-Goodwin, 1997). It has also been shown that complete cage change (changing the cage and the substrate) (Gray and Hurst, 1995), the provision of new or destructible enrichment (Ambrose and Morton, 2000), and the provision of nesting material (Armstrong *et al.*, 1998) also decreased aggression, suggesting that decreasing the familiarity of the environment while providing flexible avenues for escape can decrease aggression in socially housed mice. In addition to providing nesting material, the transfer of nesting material has been shown to decrease subsequent aggression whereas the transfer of dirty bedding has been shown to increase aggression and is not recommended (Van Loo *et al.*, 2000).

Considerable work has recently been done to look at what sorts of environments and substrates mice choose and how hard they will work to access them. The traditional housing system for rodents has been wire-bottom cages, but these are increasingly being replaced, when appropriate, with solid-bottom cages. This raises the question of what sort of bedding material is appropriate and liked by the animals. Given a choice, mice avoid wire-bottom cages, preferring solid-bottom cages with shredded filter paper (Blom *et al.*, 1993, 1996), which they will work hard to obtain (Roper, 1973). When a cage was constructed as half mesh and half solid, the mice used the mesh half more as a latrine and rested in the solid part, a tendency confirmed in later studies where mice in enriched cages urinated in certain locations, unlike animals kept in standard conditions (Van de Weerd *et al.*, 1996).

Mice behaviorally thermoregulate, burrowing to escape heat and building nests for warmth (Crowcroft, 1973; Latham and Mason, 2004; Gaskill *et al.*, 2012). Providing nesting material in the laboratory environment allows mice an occupational enrichment as well as the ability to behaviorally thermoregulate. This can be quite valuable, as it has been shown that typical room temperatures of 20–22°C cause cold stress in mice (Gordon *et al.*, 1998; Gaskill *et al.*, 2009, 2011b, 2012). The cooler ambient temperatures likely allow us to house mice at laboratory densities, however. In the wild, fighting to establish a territory is mitigated in colder seasons, as huddling is used as a thermoregulatory strategy and nests are shared with non-territory holders in the colder months (Crowcroft, 1973; Greenberg, 1972). This theory is further supported by the fact that increasing the ambient laboratory temperature to even 25°C induces aggression (Greenberg, 1972). Nesting material has also been shown to be a preferred enrichment (Van de Weerd *et al.*, 1998), as well as a valued resource that they are willing to work to obtain (Roper, 1973).

When providing nesting material for mice, it is important that the proper substrate be provided in order to fully elicit nest building behavior in the laboratory setting (Hess *et al.*, 2008). While strain differences have been documented in nest building ability and quality (Lee and Wong, 1970; Lee, 1973), the type of material appears to also be influential on the quality of the resulting nest. Crinkled paper nesting material has shown in multiple studies to be structurally appropriate for mice of multiple strains to build a good quality nest. Nest quality has been compared to the 'dome-shaped, complex, multilayered nests' built by wild mice (Hess *et al.*, 2008; Gaskill *et al.*, 2011c). Furthermore, in rank order, mice preferred shredded filter paper to wood chips to sawdust, and there were no strain differences in these preferences between BALB/c and C57BL/6 mice. Blom *et al.* (1996) attributed the preference for the paper to the higher irritancy of fine sawdust particles, but mice were also able to manipulate the paper and build nests, which might have contributed to their preference. When nesting materials were specifically tested, it was found that paper was preferred to wood products (i.e., paper tissues, towels, and strips to wood wool or shavings), and combinations of nesting materials were preferred. Other materials, such as compressed cotton and facial tissues can be used by mice to build nests, however these materials are not without issue. Highly compressed cotton has shown difficult for 'poor nest building' strains (e.g., C57BL/6, DBA, C3H) to build with (Lee, 1972; Hess et al., 2008) and the dust or fibers have been associated with eye lesions in nudes (Bazille et al., 2001) and injuries to mouse pups (Rowson and Michaels, 1980).

Sherwin (1996) found that mice were prepared to work as hard, within the imposed cost of having to traverse 30 cm of shallow water, to reach a running wheel, deep sawdust (6–7 cm), a conspecific (unfamiliar male of the same strain), or increased space or shelter (plastic cup), as for food. The author interpreted these findings to indicate that the animals place a value on all of these items.

Structural enrichments increase cage complexity, which has been shown to improve learning, memory, and brain physiology (Kempermann et al., 1997; Morgan and Tromborg, 2007; Arai et al., 2009), immune function (Kingston and Hoffman-Goetz, 1996) and reduce tumor growth (Cao et al., 2010). However, the use of plastic shelters has been associated with increased aggression (Howerton et al., 2008; Swetter et al., 2011) and disruption of social hierarchies (Barnard et al., 1996), and so should be implemented with caution. Any enrichment to reduce aggression has to be carefully designed, as simply providing objects that mice can occupy may increase the amount of territory to defend and so promote aggression (Haemisch et al., 1994). However, if adequate space is provided in addition to shelters, the degree of injury may be reduced by allowing the opportunity for submissive posturing rather than overt fighting (Durschlag and Stauffacher, 1996). These affects are likely strain and/or sex dependent, making this enrichment strategy most appropriate for groups of females or individually housed mice.

Considering that mice have not been shown to have a play drive, it is unlikely that manipulanda or other objects intended for play interactions are of any enrichment value. The burying behavior observed with balls or marbles is considered to be fear avoidance (Deacon, 2006) and it is reasonable to extrapolate that the interaction with any other 'toy'-like object is similar avoidance behavior.

Mice kept in traditional cages may gnaw on the cage wire, jump and circle around the tops of cages, chew, and dig (e.g., Tuli, 1993; Würbel et al., 1996; Hobbs et al., 1997). Stereotypic behaviors, such as bar mouthing, jumping, circling, and flipping have been associated with abnormal brain function (Garner et al., 2011). Significant differences between strains in the kinds of behaviors expressed have been observed. For example, nude mutants jump more than the parent wild-type strain (Zur: ICR), which in turn, gnaw more; and DBA/2 mice exhibit more eating, grooming, and exploring than do CD-1 or B6CBAF$_1$/J strains (Hobbs et al., 1997). Some behaviors may be modified through the provision of nesting materials (Gross et al., 2011), and empty water bottles and tunnels can be used as resting areas (Ward, 1981; Hobbs et al., 1997). Würbel and colleagues (1998) also found that providing a cardboard tube significantly reduced wire gnawing in ICR mice. The tube provided shelter, resulting in increased resting periods, which probably indicated a feeling of security. In another study, mice (BALB/c and Crl:NMRI strains) kept in an enriched environment (polyvinyl chloride [PVC] tube, nesting material, and a metal grid) did more climbing and eating than the controls kept in standard caging; but there were strain differences in that BALB/c mice spent more time than NMRI climbing and moving about, but NMRI spent more time resting and grooming (Van de Weerd et al., 1996).

Barbering (hair nibbling and whisker chewing) is observed in mice, and usually manifests as an area of hair loss over the upper back (shoulder and neck) as well as the whisker bed. (Hauschka, 1952; Long, 1972; Thornberg et al., 1973; Litterst, 1974). While previously believed to be a social dominance behavior (Sarna et al., 2000), barbering has been induced by dietary interventions associated with an increase in serotonin (Dufour et al., 2010), alleviated by anti-oxidant treatments (Vieira et al., 2012) and has been validated as a model of trichotillomania, or compulsive hair-pulling (Garner et al., 2004). Thus, it appears that barbering has a primary neurologic etiology, similar to a compulsive disorder observed in people.

While well-conceived and designed environmental enrichment certainly improves the welfare of animals, there has been debate on the effect of enrichment on study parameters and standardization. Some of this debate has come from the inconsistent use of the term enrichment: any environmental accoutrement should not be considered enriching if it is not biologically relevant, shows no welfare benefit, or worse has welfare consequences. As we learn more about the behavioral repertoire of the species with which we work, particularly rodents, our ability to design and deliver truly beneficial enrichments will continue to improve. It is the opinion of the author that we will find there is no 'one size fits all' solution, even for a particular species, given the different needs and preferences of the different sexes, ages, and strains of animals under our care. While there are concerns that environmental enrichment may increase variance through decreased standardization, at least one study has shown this not to be the case (Wolfer *et al.*, 2004). On the contrary, strict standardization may adversely affect external validity, and at least one author suggests that environmental enrichment could be judiciously applied to combat this issue (Wurbel and Garner, 2007).

B. Rats

Considered crepuscular or nocturnal, rats are observed to be active both day and night (Calhoun, 1962) and show a range of natural active behaviors, such as exploration, inquisitiveness, digging, aggression, rearing, climbing, and jump/pounce/roll/wrestle/hold behaviors, etc., in play, with a well-defined circadian rhythm (Blanchard *et al.*, 1975; Flannelly and Lore, 1977; Silverman, 1978; Cowan, 1983; Weihe, 1987; Blanchard *et al.*, 1988; Lore and Schultz, 1989; Batchelor, 1994). Choice tests have confirmed that they are inquisitive about novel environments (e.g., Hughes, 1968). Activity and habitat have adapted as the species spread from Asia to inhabit the world, alongside human migration (Yoshida, 1980).

Rats build elaborate burrow systems. Burrow tunnels average only 7.5 cm in height connecting multiple chambers (Meehan, 1984) with entrances located near vertical walls or under horizontal surfaces to provide protected cover for entry/exit (Calhoun, 1962). Blom *et al.* (1995) determined on the basis of preference tests that females preferred cages with low heights (80 mm as opposed to heights of 320 mm; time spent in each was 29.9% compared to 19.2%), and males preferred the lowest height (38.6% in 80 mm) but also spent considerable time in higher cages (25.3% in 320 mm). Wild rats build nests within the burrow (Barnett, 1963) and both male and female laboratory rats will build nests (Boice, 1977; Blom *et al.*, 1996; Jegstrup *et al.*, 2005). Long fiber nesting materials are preferred over shavings or tissue, and were not observed to be eaten (Manser *et al.*, 1998a; Van Loo and Baumans, 2004). While the motivation to nest build varies by strain, state (e.g., pregnancy) (Meehan, 1984) and temperature (Barnett, 1963), it is a motivated behavior and may fulfill the behavioral need to burrow somewhat.

Rats live in colonies of hundreds of animals, consisting of males, females, and their sub-adult offspring (Hurst *et al.*, 1996; Hurst *et al.*, 1997; Patterson-Kane *et al.*, 2002). The rat's social structure is generally a dominance hierarchy (Calhoun, 1962), however at higher population densities it becomes despotic, with one rat dominant and the others subordinate (Lott, 1984; Hurst *et al.*, 1996). Young rats spend time playing, and if prevented from doing so at critical developmental ages, abnormal sexual, social, and aggressive behaviors develop (Vanderschuren *et al.*, 1997). As play interactions are focused on the head and scruff, rather than the flank or

sex organs, it is likely that play behavior aids in the later development of mating behaviors rather than aggressive or dominant interactions (Pellis and Pellis, 1987). This supposition is further supported by the fact that playing rat pups emit a 50 kHz vocalization, associated with a positive affective state, suggesting that the interaction is a pleasurable one (Vanderschuren *et al.*, 1997). It is well known among caretakers and pet owners that when rats are kept in isolation, they tend to become more aggressive and may exhibit increased susceptibility to disease (Wiberg and Grice, 1963; Baer, 1991). Wiberg and Grice (1963) observed that not only did the rats become more intractable, but their adrenal and thyroid glands increased in weight, their spleen and thymus decreased in weight, and their tolerance to chemical toxicity decreased, as shown by a reduced LD_{50}. Damon *et al.* (1986) showed that the LD_{50} was also reduced if animals were not acclimated to a new environment, such as a metabolic cage, and acclimation has been shown to stabilize urinary excretion of steroids (Gomez-Sanchez and Gomez-Sanchez, 1991). Such noticeable effects are evident even after a few days and can be affected by overcrowding as well as isolation, resulting in increased corticosterone levels (Capel *et al.*, 1980a, b; Holson *et al.*, 1991). Brain and Benton (1979) have argued that it is not easy to determine whether these effects are truly due to isolation, as the variance could also be due to factors such as individual responses, strain, sex, and previous housing conditions. Work by Hurst *et al.* (1998) examining social sexual strategies suggests that the effects of social isolation may be different for males and females. Single housing of females had much less effect on time budgeting and corticosteroid levels than for males, e.g., tail chasing was less for females than males, but escape behaviors such as bar chewing were higher. Rose (1993) concludes that there is abundant evidence that individual housing of rats produces significant behavioral changes that impair physical and psychological fitness for research. The wealth of literature on the effects on behavior of enriched and impoverished environments has also shown substantial effects on brain development, including morphological and physiological aspects, synapse density, memory, learning ability, problem solving, brain responses to undernutrition and old age, recovery from brain trauma, and altered corticosterone levels (e.g., see Renner and Rosenzweig, 1987; Claassen, 1994; Kempermann *et al.*, 1997; Hurst *et al.*, 1998). Chromodacryorrhea, the red staining due to porphyrin secretions from the Harderian gland around the eye, is a sign of stress (Buzzell, 1996) and has been validated as a quantifiable measure of such (Mason *et al.*, 2004). At least one study's results (Segovia *et al.*, 2008) suggest that, at least in the aged rat, environmental enrichment did not significantly change the effects of stress reducing working memory performance.

Laboratory rats are less aggressive toward humans, more curious and less fearful of novel objects, and are more easily handled than their wild counterparts, suggesting some degree of 'domestication' (Barnett, 1963). 'Gentling,' or frequent gentle handling, has been used to increase the handleability of the rat. Both gentle human contact and 'tickling,' or the simulation of play behaviors with a rat using your hand, have both been shown to be rewarding, and the latter has even decreased the stress from repeated IP injection (Davis and Perusse, 1988; Cloutier et al., 2010).

The type of flooring preferred by rats is coincident with their long-term health, as solid floors are preferred to grid floors (Van de Weerd et al., 1996), and it is generally observed that grid floors are associated with superficial foot lesions leading to ulceration, inflammation, pain, and swelling (Kohn and Barthold, 1984). Preference testing can be difficult in a species as adaptive as the rat (Sorensen et al., 2005).

Regardless of previous experience of flooring type, rats spend more time resting on solid floors compared with the wire floors (88%:12%), but wire floors are nearly equally used during the rats' active period (55%:45%) and for defecation and urination. Furthermore, a comparison of rats kept on the two types of flooring revealed no differences in weight gain, food or water consumption, ease of handling, and many physiological parameters, including immune function and catecholamine, testosterone, and corticosteroid levels (Manser, 1992; Nagel and Stauffacher, 1994; Manser et al., 1995; Van de Weerd et al., 1996; Stauffacher, 1997b). Therefore, there would seem to be no reason not to use solid-bottom cages given the increased potential for animal well-being. Moreover, rats will work (by lifting a weighted barrier) as hard to reach solid-bottom floors as they will to reach a novel environment (Manser et al., 1996).

Solid-bottom cages require bedding, and choice tests have shown that rats prefer cages with wood shavings and paper bedding to those with sawdust (Blom et al., 1996; Van de Weerd et al., 1996). Paper bedding may also be more acceptable in toxicological studies. Blom et al. (1993, 1996) showed that rats preferred materials with large fibrous particles, that were manipulable, and that may produce ultrasound by particles rubbing against each other (see also Manser et al., 1998a).

For a social species like the rat, housing with conspecifics is the most complex and behaviorally relevant enrichment strategy. Rats in captivity are social: they are often found lying together or grooming conspecifics, and are easily handled (Barnett, 1963) and should be socially housed in captivity. Socially housed rats show reduced stereotypic behaviors (Hurst et al., 1997, 1998).

Nesting material is a good enrichment for rats, as both males and females will build nests. Long-fiber nesting materials are preferred over other nesting substrates (Manser et al., 1998a) and strain-specific preferences in material and method of provision of the material have been documented (Jegstrup et al., 2005). Shelters, however, may be preferred over nesting material (Manser et al., 1998b; Patterson-Kane et al., 2001) and should be considered in addition to nesting material, as rats will preferentially move nesting material into the shelter when given the opportunity (Manser et al., 1998b). Other structural complexities, such as climbing platforms, were preferred over a standard cage but not over nesting materials, indicating that while there may be some value to climbing structures, it is not of highest value (Bradshaw and Poling, 1991). Play objects are likely of little to no enrichment value, as rats have not been shown to play with objects. As rats do easily acclimate to human handling and research procedures, an acclimation and handling program would be recommended.

C. Hamsters

Native to the dry, rocky, resource-deprived plains of western Asia, hamsters are naturally active at night. Leaving their burrows to search out resources, they forage for food, stuff it into their cheek pouches, and carry it back to their burrow for hoarding (Whittaker, 2010). The ability to hoard is a strongly driven behavior in hamsters (Guerra and Ades, 2002) and both food and nesting material will be hoarded. Allowing access to both food and nesting material that can be easily obtained and carried, such as providing these items on the cage floor, can fulfill this behavioral need.

Hamsters build burrows, and provided appropriate substrate, will do so in captivity. In captivity, hamsters show a preference for solid-bottom caging over wire-bottom caging (Arnold and Estep, 1994) perhaps due to the ability to accommodate natural digging, burrowing, and nest-building behaviors in this style of caging. Provided with deep enough bedding, hamsters will burrow to a depth similar to that of natural burrows (Gattermann et al., 2001; Hauzenberger et al., 2006). Each burrow consists of two tunnels off of the nest chamber: a toilet chamber and a food storage chamber (Gattermann et al., 2001). Hamsters will also make use of shelters, tunnels, and nest boxes (McClure and Thomson, 1992; Arnold and Estep, 1994; Veillette and Reebs, 2011), perhaps fulfilling the behavioral need for a burrow. In addition, both male and female hamsters will build nests when provided nesting material, and prefer used nesting material even when new material is readily available (Richards, 1969; Veillette and Reebs, 2010).

Hamsters are a solitary animal, marking territory and resources with scent from urine, feces, or scent gland secretions (Johnston et al., 1993). Hamsters are fiercely territorial, defending their territories against intruders. Females are larger and more aggressive than males (Grelk et al., 1974; Kuhnen, 2002). Agonistic encounters consist of dominance displays responded to with submissive and retreat behaviors by the subordinate animal (Lerwill and Makings, 1971). In spite of being a solitary species, hamsters are frequently successfully group housed in the laboratory. Socially housed hamsters spend more time in contact than not, suggesting a value to social interaction (Arnold and Estep, 1990). Prior experience with social housing may play a role in this social housing tolerance. Socially raised male hamsters showed submissive behaviors at closer distances than ones raised in isolation (Huang and Hazlett, 1974). Since laboratory hamsters are raised in social environments, they have generally adapted to a social housing environment.

Common abnormal behaviors observed in hamsters include gnawing of cage bars and lids, and may be either boredom or escape related (Arnold and Estep, 1994; Hauzenberger *et al.*, 2006). Both wire gnawing and stereotypic wheel-running have been shown to be reduced by the provision of deep bedding suitable for burrowing (Hauzenberger *et al.*, 2006).

Based on occupation times, hamsters have been shown to prefer solid-bottom cages with bedding, regardless of their age or sex (Arnold and Estep, 1994). Providing hamsters with enough bedding material to burrow in would be ideal, though a shelter may also provide security if deep enough bedding for burrowing cannot be provided (Hauzenberger *et al.*, 2006). Nesting material and food, provided inside the cage to allow for foraging, processing, and hoarding behaviors, would also be enriching for hamsters. Since hamsters are generally raised socially in the laboratory environment, they have developed some tolerance for social housing paradigms. While caution should be exercised when attempting social housing of this species, in a well-managed behavioral husbandry program it likely should be attempted.

D. Gerbils

Gerbils are native to the steppes of Asia, in desert habitats. Like hamsters, gerbils are from a naturally resource-poor area. Thus, also like hamsters, gerbils forage for food and carry it for hoarding to their burrows (Ågren *et al.*, 1989a, b). In captivity, feeding gerbils on the floor or from J-feeders allows them to exhibit this foraging and hoarding behavior, and has been shown to result in increased weight gain (Mulder *et al.*, 2010).

Unlike hamsters, gerbils are a social, not solitary, species, and live in multi-male, multi-female groups. Territories are marked via scent from the ventral marking gland, chin sebaceous glands, feces, and urine. Consisting of both above ground territory and an underground burrow system, the familial territory is defended by both males and females. Gerbils remain in their familial territory until expelled around the time of maturity, generally by the dominant female (Scheibler *et al.*, 2005).

Gerbils dig and live in complex burrow systems. The behavioral drive to dig a burrow is strong, and in captivity stereotypic digging behavior is observed (Wiedenmayer, 1997). This behavior was not alleviated by the provision of a sand substrate (Pettijohn and Barkes, 1978) but was by the provision of a tunnel with a blind end or burrow chamber (Wiedenmayer, 1997; Waiblinger and Koenig, 2007). The alleviation of the digging behavior by the provision of a burrow-containing tunnel structure suggests that the stereotypy is a result of frustrated burrow building behavior when not provided with either the structure itself or an appropriate burrowing substrate out of which such a burrow can be constructed. Thus, the drive to build a burrow is likely strongly motivated and should be accommodated in the captive environment.

Grooming spreads saliva and Harderian gland secretions over the pelt and may be a form of behavioral thermoregulation. The saliva acts to cool the gerbil while the Harderian glands protect against wetness and cold when the temperature drops (Thiessen, 1988).

While abnormal bar chewing is observed in gerbils (Moons *et al.*, 2012), stereotypic digging is the most common abnormal behavior of gerbils described (Wiedenmayer, 1997). This behavior is believed to be frustrated attempts to build a burrow, and the provision of substrate suitable for burrow construction or a bent tunnel structure has been shown to decrease the abnormal behavior (Wiedenmayer, 1997). It should be noted that substrate suitable for digging but not structurally sound enough to build a burrow in did not alleviate the behavior (Pettijohn and Barkes, 1978; Wiedenmayer, 1997).

Bedding suitable for burrowing and/or burrow chambers with an L-shaped entrance (Waiblinger, 2002) would be valuable enrichments for the gerbil's environment. A sand bath may also be of value, as gerbils will sand bathe given the opportunity (Eisenberg, 1967). Sand bathing is a behavior common to all desert dwelling rodents, and is important to the health of the pelage of these rodents. The provision of food inside the cage or on the cage floor, to allow foraging behavior and hoarding, is also recommended.

E. Guinea Pigs

Guinea pigs were domesticated between 6000 and 3000 years ago as a food source and sacrificial offering in Peru (Anderson, 1987). They are crepuscular animals (active at dawn and dusk) but unlike other rodents, appear not to build burrows. When faced with a threat, guinea pigs either freeze or stampede, and stampeding can result in injury, particularly in the young or in pregnant females (North, 1999).

Guinea pigs are a social animal. Manning and colleagues (1984) found that guinea pigs like to lie beside each other. Social dominance in guinea pigs has been reported as both linear and triangular (Kunkel and Kunkel, 1964; Rood, 1972; Coulon, 1975), and they generally live in family groups. It appears that space and the age and size of the group influence these hierarchal structures. Domesticated guinea pigs exhibit even more sociopositive behaviors than their wild counterparts (Kunzl and Sachser, 1999) and as such form social groups more easily; fighting generally does not occur among groups of related or unrelated males raised without females, or groups of non-breeding females. Since they are social animals that like to be in contact with conspecifics, guinea pigs should be kept in groups wherever possible. In addition to conspecific socialization, frequent gentle handling of guinea pigs will condition them to being manipulated.

Guinea pigs have a large, complex vocal repertoire. In agonistic interactions, the subordinate male is observed to purr to appease the dominant male. The same purr is used by dominant males toward females or offspring. Thus, each call can have multiple meanings or uses based on context. Berryman (1976) recorded the structure and duration of guinea pig vocalizations and found that 11 distinct calls could be identified, ranging from chuts and chutters to whirs and tweets.

White et al. (1990) suggested that guinea pigs did not utilize the whole of the cage area; however, Scharmann (1991) found that when the cage was enriched through the addition of hay and straw, then they burrowed and hid in it. As guinea pigs are rather timid animals, they like cage or pen furniture that enables them to hide, such as boxes or plastic pipes (Noonan, 1994; Meyer, 1995). Walters and colleagues (2012) found that the provision of a hut decreased fecal cortisol in pair-housed male guinea pigs, suggesting that shelter improves welfare and decreases stress. Open housing space with shelters or other environmental complexity meets the behavioral needs of guinea pigs through providing them with sheltered areas to escape from aggressive encounters and retreat from the view of potential threats. It is therefore reasonable to surmise that shelter, whether in the form of hay or other furniture, both increases the space utilization of the cage and provides the security of a sheltered area. PVC pipes, cardboard or wood shelters, plastic huts, straw, or bedding can all fulfill this need. Solid flooring with bedding substrate is recommended. One study found that bedding preference, for wood shavings *versus* shredded paper, varied depending on time of day (Kawakami et al., 2003).

Scharmann (1991) observed that guinea pigs spent some time chewing on the bars and hoppers of the cage. This behavior could be stopped by adding pieces of wood, which gave the guinea pigs something else to gnaw on. Whether this simply displaces one type of oral stereotypy with another is not clear. In captivity, guinea pigs have also been observed to chew hair and ears of

their conspecifics. The provision of hay has been shown to decrease hair loss (Gerold et al., 1997) and chewing rings of PVC pipe and decreasing stocking density have a similar mitigating effect.

III. RABBITS

Rabbits are a prey species that live in underground burrows composed of hundreds of animals, called warrens. While rabbits naturally live in large groups, they're not necessarily closely grouped: in a free-living population under study, the distance between individual does averages about 1 ft, and was up to 3 ft between a dominant and secondary buck (Lockley, 1961). In spite of being a seemingly social species in wild populations, social housing in captivity has proven challenging for rabbits. A review of group-housed does for farm production revealed increased rates of injury and mortality as well as increased cortisol levels compared to individually housed does suggesting chronic stress (Szendro and McNitt, 2012). A study of genetically hyperlipidemic rabbits, however, showed that rabbits housed either alone or in unstable social environments displayed physiologic parameters associated with chronic stress (Noller et al., 2013). While rabbits may be a 'social' species, clearly successfully socially housing them is not straightforward. Rabbits live in social groups when the benefits (such as predation avoidance) outweigh the costs of living socially (like social stress and resource competition). As an example, Held et al. (1995) found that rabbits chose a solitary pen when it contained desired resources like straw, boxes, or ledges, and chose the social pen only when the solitary choice was smaller and barren in comparison. In general, social housing is more successful if immature animals are used. Groups of female rabbits can be formed, and the hierarchy established remains relatively stable if the group dynamic is held stable (Noller et al., 2013). Groups of male rabbits may also be established, although the bucks are typically castrated (Podberscek et al., 1991b; Raje and Stewart, 1997). It should also be noted that there are reports of strain differences in aggressive behavior, which may influence the success of group housing rabbits (e.g., Dutch rabbits are more aggressive than New Zealand Whites) (Morton, 1993). Group-housed rabbits may be provided climbing structures, wood shavings, or other appropriate floor covering to encourage foraging; and tunnels, buckets, barrels, or boxes for escape and hiding behaviors. Introducing rabbits in a larger, complex space may help facilitate pairing or grouping success. The results of a study by Valuska and Mench (2013) suggest that not only do does introduced in a larger enclosure show higher levels of affiliative and lower levels of aggressive behavior than does introduced in a smaller enclosure, but the does that were exposed first to unfamiliar does in the large enclosure were less aggressive toward future introductions even in smaller enclosures. In other words, the experience of meeting the unfamiliar doe in the larger enclosure tempered their response to meeting unfamiliar does later on. The opposite effect was seen in does that were first introduced to unfamiliar does in the smaller enclosure, suggesting that prior experience and first introductions in a large enclosure may be vital to longer term success in social housing. Adding objects such as visual blocks and platforms allows subordinates to escape dominants, and give the rabbits something other than the newly introduced conspecific to explore. Another method applied to help group formation is to sedate the animals and either place them in close proximity or actually chin rub them on each other in order to confer a familiar scent. Love and Hammond (1991) found that using this method then placing the rabbits in a clean pen resulted in some chasing that settled within 24 h. Groups that are introduced at a young age appear to have better success as a stable social group than those that are introduced later. In one research institution's experience, groups that have more disruption from experimental protocol manipulations were more likely to become socially unstable and fight (J. Wyatt, personal communication).

Plexiglas panels have also been used to separate male rabbits but still give them visual contact with conspecifics. Rabbits pair-housed in this way showed significant changes in circadian rhythms, resting diurnally with periods of activity at dawn and dusk and maintenance behaviors such as feeding and grooming nocturnally, compared to non-socially housed rabbits that predominantly rested irrelevant of time of day (Lofgren et al., 2010).

The expression of chasing, jumping, gamboling, rearing, and other behaviors requiring space for their performance is facilitated in group-housing conditions that are adequately enriched and in which the animals have established compatible relationships. It may not always be possible to determine the rank relationship between dyads of rabbits (Turner et al., 1997). However, social hierarchies for groups of mature does may be stable for long periods of time (e.g., 30 months as reported by Turner et al., 1997) with no differences detected between high- and low-ranking animals in several immunocompetence measures. Hence, the authors proposed that group housing may be an appropriate means of maintaining antibody-producing animals. Similarly, Whary et al. (1993) determined no significant difference in growth rate, humoral immunity, delayed-type hypersensitivity response, adrenal gland weight, or circulating corticosterone level between group-housed and single-caged does. The authors did observe a higher feed intake and lower lymphocyte count in group-housed rabbits.

As there was no significant difference in growth rate despite the higher food consumption level, the authors postulated a better feed-conversion to body-weight rate. Also, since the significantly lower white blood cell count occurred during only 1 week of observation and did not reflect a typical stress profile (leukocytosis and increased corticosterone level), it was not considered of biological relevance.

Abnormal behaviors observed in rabbits housed in the laboratory include bar chewing (Morton, 1993; Raje and Stewart, 1997), which can result in broken teeth; excessive grooming leading to denuded areas and possible gastrointestinal problems; and psychogenic polydipsia with secondary polyuria (Potter and Borkowski, 1998). Several other stereotypes have been described, such as head swaying or weaving, vertical sliding of the nose between cage bars, pushing on cage parts with the head, pawing or digging at the cage floor or food hopper, and rapid circling (Morton, 1993). Circling behavior can be expressed in two normal contexts: (1) an aggressive encounter; or (2) courtship (Morton, 1993). Excessive passive behavior, manifested as sitting in a hunched posture for a prolonged period of time or sitting with the head lowered in the cage corner, is also described as undesirable stereotyped behavior (Morton, 1993). These authors further describe individually housed animals as exhibiting increased inactivity, increased lying down, and incomplete behavior patterns or movements, as compared to group-housed rabbits. This observation has also been noted by Podberscek et al. (1991b), who identified more 'maintenance' behaviors in caged rabbits and more comfort behaviors (e.g., grooming) in penned rabbits. Although the incidence of abnormal behaviors is reduced in group-housed rabbits (Morton, 1993), aggression between animals is of sufficient concern (especially between bucks) to warrant careful consideration of the appropriate method of housing selected.

Rabbits given the choice between three different cage heights (20, 30, and 40 cm) preferred the lowest cage height during resting periods, but had no significant preference between the cage heights during active periods (Princz et al., 2005). Additionally, rabbits in pens showed more comfort behaviors and less resting or idle behaviors, and no stereotypic behaviors compared to rabbits housed in cages (Podberscek et al., 1991b), suggesting some welfare benefits to pen caging. Verga et al. (2007) is an excellent review of environmental effects on rabbits housed in groups and the reader is encouraged to refer there for further information.

Environmental enrichment techniques that appear to be the most successful for rabbits are those that provide the animals with the opportunity to express a greater range of species-typical behaviors. For example, objects on which rabbits can chew are very desirable. Rabbits naturally spend up to 70% of their daily time budget foraging, and are physiologically evolved to graze on low caloric density foodstuffs. Thus, they are 'hardwired' to continually forage and graze, so hay or some other roughage makes for an excellent occupational enrichment. A variety of objects are available, including plastic toys, Nylabones®, Gumaknots®, empty cardboard boxes, and food items to gnaw on (e.g., Bunny Blocks®). Soda cans, wiffle balls, sections of PVC pipe, balls, and suspended metallic items (e.g., washers) have been used to encourage nudging, playing, and investigation behaviors. Objects are frequently suspended in the cage to induce postures akin to the natural rearing position of rabbits. Rabbits are, however, capable of destroying cage objects made of plastic or thin metal and ingesting the material. Therefore, for reasons of health of the animal and scientific objectives, sturdy objects that have been assessed for safety and durability are recommended.

Handling kits in the first days of life reduces fear of humans (Pongracz and Altbacker, 2003), and rabbits are readily trainable and can be easily acclimated to human handling, research procedures, and equipment, particularly when handled at young ages (Wyly et al., 1975; Pongracz and Altbacker, 2001; Csatádi et al., 2005; Swennes et al., 2011). One research facility uses audio cues (e.g., a knock on the door) to signal room entry and visual cues (e.g., colored signs) to indicate certain procedures to allow the rabbits to anticipate common procedures and alleviate stress in the animals. Even at older ages, acclimation to handling and procedures increases observable tameness in laboratory rabbits (Swennes et al., 2011), and should be part of a behavioral husbandry program for rabbits.

IV. LABORATORY DOGS AND CATS

During a long association with humans, dogs and cats have had many roles, from companion, to hunter, to laboratory animal. The behavioral changes necessary for each of these roles have developed in dogs for over 12,000 years and approximately 3,000 years for cats (Beaver, 2003; Beaver, 2009), yet humans have not always done a good job at recognizing the relevance of behavior to each specific role. In the case of laboratory dogs and cats, the validity of data gathered may be called into question because of behavioral factors, including environmental stress and caretaker interactions (Beaver, 1989; Benn, 1995).

A. Social Behavior

Socialization of puppies and kittens is particularly important for those housed as laboratory animals because of the need to interact with conspecifics and human caretakers. For puppies, the socialization period is generally accepted to be from 3–12 weeks of age (Scott and Fuller, 1965), with reinforcement of socialization needing to be an ongoing process to prevent behavioral regression (Boxall et al., 2004). The feline socialization period is a little less certain than it is for puppies. It is generally thought to begin at about 3 weeks of age, after the eyes and ears open and end between 7 and 9 weeks of age (Beaver, 2003; Karsh and Turner, 1988). Dogs are social animals and would normally spend about three-fourths of their time close to other pack members (Beaver, 1981; Fox and Bekoff, 1975). This strong tendency for social interaction means that individually housed dogs will spend as much time as possible interacting with other dogs when released into an exercise area together (Campbell, et al., 1988). Dogs penned in chain link runs will lie next to one another, touching through the fence. When resting areas are specifically provided in runs, it is best to determine where the dog wants to rest so that the bench or mat can be appropriately placed. Dogs that are group housed interact with each other and investigate the pen floor more, so activity levels for these dogs are usually higher (Hubrecht et al., 1992, 1993; Hite et al., 1977).

Once socialized to humans, dogs have a strong predisposition to interact with humans (Serpell, 2011). In research facilities, dog interactions with humans have been shown to be an important source of enrichment and stimulation and even preferred over dog–dog interactions (Hubrecht, 1993; Meunier et al., 2012). Studies have shown that petting and gentle handling can decrease stress responses in dogs (Hennessy et al., 1998; Lynch and Gantt, 1968). Many institutions now include human interactions as part of the daily routine for the dogs (Loveridge, 1998).

For group-housed dogs, it is desirable to maintain stable groups. The introduction of new members or removal of one from an established pack means that social orders must be readjusted. The most significant switch would be combining dogs for the creation of a completely new group. Dominance mounting, ear sniffing, and communicative posturing are evident for several days while individuals determine what their social position is in the new pack. This can be stressful to some individuals and may affect data.

Cats are often housed in groups, even though their social behavior can be strained by forced interactions. With abundant horizontal and vertical space, food stations, and resting spots, cats can seek their own comfort level with conspecifics. Individual cats may interact regularly with one or two close associates, several within the group, or remain primarily to themselves. Group-housed cats will spend about 85% of their resting time alone (Podberscek et al., 1991a), but most individuals will spend time around other cats, usually specific ones. Studies by Barry and Crowell-Davis (1999) have shown that pet house cats will maintain a distance of 1–3 m from each other most of the time, so even in home environments cats are not necessarily close. The introduction of new cats into a group is likely to be disruptive, so this should be done gradually, with a long period for the social adjustments being allowed before any research trials begin. It is also important to keep in mind that when a cat has been removed from a group, even for a few hours, if it brings back a strange odor, severe aggression toward it may occur. This can be significant and last long enough so as to prevent the cat from ever rejoining the group.

Human interaction is also an important component of social behavior for cats in that the more time that was spent handling cats, the more outgoing, friendly, and confident they became (Overall and Dyer, 2005). When the cats rush up to greet people entering the area or room, even leaving their toys, the value of social interactions with humans becomes obvious (National Health and Medical Research Council for the Australian Government, 2008).

B. Activity Levels and Housing

Activity levels of dogs housed in cages or runs have been reported, but studies are somewhat difficult to compare. In cages of approximately 1 m × 1 m × 1 m, the average dog travels 55 m/h but only spends 8% of its time in motion (Hughes et al., 1989). It will also spend 12.7% sitting, and 6.6% of the time lying (Hite et al., 1977). Beagles housed in runs of approximately 1.25 m × 2.5 m spend 69% of their time lying or sleeping, compared to 74% of the time when the same dogs are caged instead (Neamand et al., 1975). The actual 24-h time distribution of activities of beagles housed individually in runs includes (Beaver, 2009):

Grooming: 20 min, 1.4% of 24 h
Sitting: 63 min, 4.4% of 24 h
Standing: 83 min, 5.8% of 24 h
Walking: 278 min, 19.3% of 24 h
Lying in sternal recumbency: 200 min, 13.9% of 24 h
Lying in lateral recumbency: 263 min, 18.3% of 24 h
Lying in sternal and lateral recumbency: 529 min, 36.7% of 24 h
Lying on the back: 4 min, 0.3% of 24 h

Meunier and colleagues (2012) compared time budgets in the first and second 15 min of 30-min exercise sessions of laboratory beagles exercised as a group in a large area. On average the dogs engaged in active behaviors for greater than 90% of the time during the first 15 min and greater than 75% of the time during the second 15 min in three different exercise scenarios. Activity levels will increase when people are present, even without significant direct interaction (Campbell

et al., 1988; Hughes et al., 1989). Physiological parameters cannot differentiate between dogs under long term confinement, those that have access to daily exercise periods, and those given forced exercise on treadmills (Clark et al., 1991; Tipton et al., 1974; Newton, 1972). While dogs housed in larger cages or runs are more active, data suggests that there are limits in the activity to cage size ratio (Hetts et al., 1992). Studies vary as to whether socially isolated dogs were more or less active (Hetts et al., 1992; Hubrecht et al., 1992), but socially isolated dogs do become highly aroused in response to the presence of humans. Individually housed dogs also exhibited an increased frequency of barking, stereotypic behaviors, and aggressive behaviors (Hubrecht et al., 1992; Mertens and Unshelm, 1991).

Noise levels tended to follow activity patterns. In kennels, the barking follows a diurnal pattern but can remain relatively high throughout the day (Sales et al., 1997). Noise levels reached 80–95 dB when dogs were barking or humans cleaning (Milligan et al., 1993), and levels regularly exceeded 100 dB and often reached 125 dB when dogs were barking in response to humans (Sales et al., 1997). Noise measurements as a result of barking can be significantly reduced by using kennels that provide more visual and social opportunities for the dogs (Meunier unpublished data, 2012).

Activity levels during cage confinement have not been reported for cats. In general, they rest more than dogs when confined to cages. When kept as a group in a cat room, they still have personal space requirements but will spend time exploring. When given the chance, cats have been found to spend 61% of their time on shelves off the floor, and 68% of the running is done on shelves. A laboratory cat's preferred location for sleeping (89% of the time) and for sitting (48%) is above the floor (Podberscek et al., 1991a). Colony cats will spend up to 16 h a day resting (Podberscek et al., 1991a).

During a 24-h period, the typical laboratory cat will divide its time into behaviors of maintenance (36%), comfort (30%), locomotion (24.5%), marking and investigation (4%), vocalization (2%), play (2%), and agonistic behavior 1%); with overall activity levels highest in the morning when caretakers arrive and for approximately 30 min before and after, and levels lowest in the afternoons. Maintenance behaviors include feeding and resting, while comfort behaviors relate to body care, such as grooming and stretching. Allogrooming and close-proximity resting are the most common social behaviors shown between cats and make up much of the 30% time spent on comfort behaviors (Podberscek et al., 1991a). The less obvious function for allogrooming, but probably more significant one, is that it can be a way of redirecting potential aggression (Van den Bos, 1998). Groomers tend to be higher ranking cats (Van den Bos, 1998), rather than the other way around.

C. Behavior Abnormalities

1. Stereotypies

Studies have shown that while activity levels do not vary greatly between individually housed and group-housed dogs, the type of activity might. For example, solitary dogs showed more repetitive locomotor behaviors (Hubrecht *et al.*, 1992; Mertens and Unshelm, 1991). The development of stereotypic activity patterns is dependent on a number of factors besides how the animal is kept. Genetics, social factors, dietary energy, individual stress level, and environmental conditions may contribute to the development of these atypical activities (Fox, 1965). Stereotypic pacing is one of the more common problems, expressed by the dog walking back and forth along the front of a cage or run. Usually the animal will throw its head up as it comes to the end of its left-to-right or right-to-left motion. Continuous circling is another stereotypy dogs can show.

The development of stereotypies is thought to represent a coping mechanism by the animal. Interpretation of experimental results must take into consideration whether or not endorphins or stress hormones could have an effect. Prevention of a problem behavior is usually easier than dealing with it after it is well developed. Appropriate enrichment can increase the complexity of behavior shown and help prevent undesirable behaviors from the beginning (Hubrecht, 1993).

2. Psychogenic Stress Responses

Several behaviors of dogs and cats are associated with events that are apparently stressful to the animal. In clinical behavioral medicine, they are so pathognomonic that stress intervention is initiated even if a specific stressor cannot be identified. Acral lick dermatitis (lick granulomas) in dogs and psychogenic alopecia in cats are the result of a normal behavior shown in excess. The condition in cats is more common in individually housed cats, and will often disappear if that cat is placed with at least one other compatible cage mate (DeLuca and Kranda, 1992). Psychogenic polydipsia may first be noticed as polyuria. Urine spraying of vertical surfaces is a feline marking behavior associated with the invasion of territory or a perceived stress within that territory. Abrupt changes in cat litter type can result in 50% of the cats refusing to use the litter box and an increased incidence in spraying. Half of the cats will begin to use the new litter within a week, but that still leaves 25% that eliminate outside the box (Beaver, 2003).

Environmental enrichment has been successfully used to reduce the incidence of psychogenic stress responses (Beaver, 1981, 1989; Benn, 1995; Markowitz and Gavazzi, 1995). Group housing for dogs, elimination of new additions to group-housed cats, increased human contacts, play toys, social interaction time for individually housed dogs, obedience lessons for dogs, trick learning, cage puzzles to earn treats or food, visually interesting activities in the room of cages, individual hiding areas like boxes or resting shelves for cats, food choices, and prey chasing simulation for cats are but a few ideas.

3. Excessive Vocalization

Laboratory dogs often bark excessively, and cats can show a similar problem with their meows. Some research facilities use debarking surgery. This may control the noise, but it does not address the behavioral aspects of the problem. The vocalizations and simultaneous increases in activity are usually associated with the sounds of humans entering the kennel/cage area. Eventually the behaviors are reinforced by the human feeding or interacting with the cat or dog. The undesired behavior has just been rewarded. To prevent reinforcing undesired behaviors management needs to look at alternatives such as group housing, kennel design, people around much of the time, triggering noises played most of the time so they lose their influence, and rewarding quiet behaviors instead of noisy ones.

D. Other Behaviors of Laboratory Dogs and Cats

There are many other behaviors commonly shown by laboratory animals that are uncommon in pet counterparts. These are usually associated with the environment rather than with abnormal behaviors. Cats often lie in the litter box, usually after it has been cleaned. Both dogs and cats may play in or tip water bowls or food bowls. They apparently create their own games with things that move. Scratching posts for cats allow them to express a normal behavior which may reduce their need to perform other foot-oriented behaviors.

V. NONHUMAN PRIMATES

In the United States, ensuring the expression of appropriate nonhuman primate behavior in the laboratory has been the subject of increased interest and attention since regulatory language published by the U.S. Department of Agriculture calling for an 'environment to promote the psychological well-being of nonhuman primates' (AWRs) sparked several years of intensive research effort focused on identifying environmental factors that would improve the mental/behavioral health of primates used in research. Extensive bibliographies have subsequently been published (http://www.nal.usda.gov/awic/pubs/Primates2009/; http://grants.nih.gov/grants/olaw/Enrichment_for_Nonhuman_Primates.pdf; http://awionline.org/lab_animals/biblio/index.html), which deal exclusively with this topic.

A. Types of Behavior Problems

A number of theories have been advanced to explain the spontaneous occurrence of abnormal behavior in nonhuman primates, including genetics, boredom, frustration, redirected aggression, disease, and neurological developmental abnormality. Although the occurrence of developmentally induced abnormal behavior is well documented in nonhuman primates (Harlow and Harlow, 1962; Mitchell, 1968; Sackett, 1965), many of the other possible etiologies of aberrant behavior tend to be supported mostly by anecdotal evidence. In general, however, the consensus appears to be that if the abnormal behavior is not due to a genetic tendency and is not developmentally induced (e.g., isolation rearing), then a lack of the appropriate level of stimulation (cognitive, social, etc.) is considered key to the manifestation of aberrant behavior. Rommeck *et al.* (2009) have stated that nursery rearing "is the single most important risk factor" in the development of abnormal behavior. Their research has demonstrated that different types of pair-housing of infant macaques can mitigate the expression of different types of abnormal behavior.

While it could be argued that inappropriate environmental stimulation is a causative factor, it may simply be correlative. For example, it is unclear if a reduction in the amount of time spent in food processing (compared to the free-ranging state) may cause increased oral behavior in a primate, e.g., oral exploration of the environment, such as cage licking, polydipsia, uriposia (urine drinking), masturbation, or self-biting, due to an appetitive drive that is not satisfied, or if the occurrence of these behaviors simply may be correlated with a reduction in feeding behaviors because of the increased time available to the animal to engage in these activities. The expression of abnormal behavior displayed by the nonhuman primate may also depend in part on the housing of the animal. For example, macaques may pace around the perimeter of a cage or large enclosure, but a combination of stereotypic pacing and somersaulting may be more likely to occur in a smaller-sized cage. Recently, Vandeleest *et al.* (2011) have determined that rhesus monkeys that lived more of their lives indoors, were singly housed for most of their lives and had experienced more anesthetic and blood draw procedures were more likely to exhibit motor stereotypy. In a review of the records of 4000 rhesus monkeys, Gottlieb *et al.* (2013a) determined that numerous factors can impact the expression of stereotypic motor behaviors. Specifically, they found that males exhibit stereotypic motor behaviors and self-biting more often than females, as did indoor-reared animals as compared to outdoor-reared animals and these behaviors were positively correlated with the number of pair separations animals experienced or housing in the bottom cages on a rack or near the room entrance.

Conversely, these behaviors decreased with the amount of time the animals lived outdoors. The authors also noted that motor stereotypies decreased with age, and the frequency of room moves and number of projects the animal participated in positively predicted motor stereotypy.

The literature on captive primate behavior is replete with examples of manifestations of atypical captive animal behavior. Although the significance of the expression of atypical behaviors is highly variable, a rating scale has been developed for rhesus monkeys, which ranks behaviors according to how detrimental they are to the animal (Bayne and Novak, 1998).

B. Effects of Behavior Problems on Research

Nonhuman primates are used in a variety of research endeavors, including cancer, heart disease, neurological disorders, AIDS research, vision, nutrition, reproduction, and dental research. A disturbance in the normal physiology or behavior of these animal models can have far-reaching effects on the advancement of science in these and other areas of study. Primates living in captive conditions can manifest abnormal immunological, hormonal, cardiovascular, and behavioral parameters.

C. Environmental Enrichment

Many abnormal behavior patterns can become highly entrenched, with their elimination described in only limited instances of intense remediation programs (O'Neill, 1989). Reduction (but not elimination) of some aberrant behaviors has been achieved by employing specific environmental-enrichment techniques targeted to particular behaviors (Bayne *et al.*, 1991). For example, primates that engage in excessive grooming may benefit from a grooming board constructed of artificial shearling to deflect some of the grooming activity to another object (Bayne *et al.*, 1991). A primate that engages in self-biting may redirect this behavior to a Kong® toy. Animals that exhibit excessive repetitive locomotion may be distracted from this activity by offering a suitably appealing food item in a foraging device (Bayne *et al.*, 1992c). Although some consideration should be given to implementing enrichment techniques that can help resolve specific abnormalities detected in the animal, the optimum enrichment program should, in general, encompass a diversity of approaches to increasing the complexity of the animal's home environment. However, not all enrichments are equal in reducing the expression of abnormal behaviors. For example, Gottlieb and McCowan (2011) determined that while three different types of foraging devices enhanced the expression of foraging behavior in rhesus monkeys, even beyond the time of availability of the forging device, the devices had varying impacts on the expression of stereotypic behavior. Specifically, in their study one foraging device actually increased the expression of motor stereotypy. Such an example underscores the importance of ensuring that the enrichment device is evaluated not only for increasing the animal's time spent in species-typical behaviors, but also for the expression of abnormal behaviors which might increase within the time budget.

1. Enclosure Size, Design, and Furnishings

The size, design, and complexity of the primary enclosure can profoundly impact the well-being of the primate occupant. Although current regulations and guidelines vary slightly in the precise floor space and vertical height recommended (AWRs, NRC, 2011, European Directive 2010/63/EU), the goal of providing the animal with sufficient space to engage in some degree of species-typical locomotion and postures is common among them. To that end, primate cages should accommodate the increased cage height necessary for arboreal species. Indeed, the adequacy of caging that does not accommodate tail length of perched animals has been questioned (Poole, 1991). The eighth edition of the *Guide* (NRC, 2011) accordingly addresses this point, "...the ability to stand or to perch with adequate vertical space to keep their body, including their tail, above the cage floor can improve their well-being...." Similarly, the amount of floor space provided to the caged primate has received considerable attention. Initially, the sentiment was propounded that more floor space was automatically 'better' for the animal. Subsequent research, however, did not consistently substantiate that claim (e.g., Bayne and McCully, 1989; Line *et al.*, 1991a). Although in some species more floor space reduced the occurrence of stereotypic behavior (Paulk *et al.*, 1977; Boot *et al.*, 1985), in other cases the provision of more vertical height had the same result (Watson and Shively, 1996). And, the *Guide* (NRC, 2011) also captured this point, "Consideration of floor area alone may not be sufficient in determining adequate cage size; with some species, cage volume and spatial arrangement may be of greater importance." Sometimes, simply moving the animal from the lower-tiered cage to the upper tier can influence the behavior of the animal (Scott, 1991). Unfortunately, some reports of improved well-being ostensibly resulting from increased cage space are confounded by the concurrent provision of cage complexities (e.g., Kitchen and Martin, 1996).

Cage design has evolved dramatically from the 'turkey cage' style common in the 1960s and 1970s to modular units with removable walls and floors, and walls with colored pictures (e.g., Erwin and Landon, 1992). Cage additions, such as tunnels, have been suggested as a way to modify the cage environment to provide the animals with additional cage space, access to different views in the holding room, and closer proximity to other animals (Rumbaugh *et al.*, 1991). Access to large exercise cages has also been proposed as another means of offering variety from the primary enclosure, an opportunity to engage in social interactions and for the expression of greater locomotion concomitant with a reduction in stereotypic behavior (Bryant *et al.*, 1988; Griffis *et al.*, 2013; Wolff and Ruppert, 1991; Kessel-Davenport and Brent, 1994). Cages have been modified to include visual barriers (Reinhardt *et al.*, 1991a; Reinhardt and Reinhardt, 1991), windows, and 'grooming contact bars' (Crockett *et al.*, 1997) to give primates more control over their social environment.

A variety of cage furnishings have also been described. These typically provide the animal with greater opportunity to express a range of postural adjustments. Many cage furnishings are more easily incorporated into the group-housing enclosure simply due to the size constraints of the single-cage environment. However, additions to cage enclosures that have been reported include swings (Bayne *et al.*, 1989), ladders, perches (Watson, 1991; Williams *et al.*, 1988), shelves, tunnels, Primahedrons, and nest boxes (Scott, 1991). Both synthetic and natural materials have been used successfully (e.g., branches, rope, and PVC). The size and complexity of the cage furnishings will depend on the space available in the enclosure. Frequently, a simple metal bar is incorporated into the squeeze-back apparatus of the single cage as a perch. However, telephone poles and entire trees have also been provided as perches and climbing structures to captive primates in large outdoor enclosures (Maki and Bloomsmith, 1989). In group-housing enclosures, shelves are typically mounted at staggered heights to minimize hierarchically based aggression between animals. Complex pathways have been created for group-housed callitrichids, using rope as artificial vines (Snowdon and Savage, 1991). The importance of perching to captive primates is underscored by the observation that it is frequently the most-used enrichment device in a variety of 'nonnutritive'/nonsocial enrichments (Bayne *et al.*, 1994; Reinhardt, 1994a). Perches allow primates to choose between different elevations in the cage and may provide a sense of increased security as a consequence of the animal being off the cage floor. Verandas also can also serve as an area for species like macaques to sit and rest as well as expanding visual opportunities.

Cage furnishings such as tunnels the animals can run through, sit in, or sit on have additional value, as they provide a 'visual break' that can arrest an aggressive chase sequence. They also can provide shy animals with a place that is out of sight to other animals and personnel. Some primates (e.g., marmosets) use elbow-shaped PVC pipes or sealed wooden boxes for denning/nesting purposes. In large enclosures, concrete culverts have been used as tunnels.

Pools of water have been provided to primates housed in larger enclosures. Although sanitation and animal safety concerns must be addressed, such pools have been implemented successfully with juvenile macaques (e.g., National Institutes of Health), providing the animals with the opportunity to swim, splash, and 'fish' for objects in the pool. Toddler play pools and horse troughs are among the containers that have been adapted for use in primate housing.

2. Food Strategies

In free-ranging conditions, foraging behaviors of nonhuman primates can occupy from 7–65% of the diurnal activity budget (Milton, 1980; Herbers, 1981; Strier, 1987; Malik and Southwick, 1988; Marriott, 1988). Indeed, it has been described as the "single most time-consuming behavior" during some seasons of the year (Malik and Southwick, 1988).

Increasing the amount of time primates spend engaged in forage-like activities (searching patterns, food processing, and consumption) can be accomplished by: (1) hiding the food and requiring the animal to search for it (Anderson and Chamove, 1984; Boccia, 1989; Scott, 1991); (2) requiring the animal to solve a puzzle or task to access the food (Rosenblum and Smiley, 1984; Line and Houghton, 1987; Gust et al., 1988; Bloom and Cook, 1989; Scott, 1991); (3) providing food that requires processing time (Bloomsmith, 1992; Smith et al., 1989); or (4) reducing the size of the food item so that the time spent in obtaining an appreciable quantity of food is extended (Bayne et al., 1991, 1992c). Many of these approaches also promote the animal's expression of cognitive skills (such as problem solving) and fine-tuned motor skills.

The diet of the animal can be broadened by the inclusion of food treats. The density, flavor, shape, and color of the treat are dimensions that can introduce variety into an otherwise monotonous diet. However, as recommended in the *Guide* (NRC, 2011), the diet should be nutritionally balanced; therefore, the provision of treats should be done judiciously. Any reduction in the well-being of the animal by engendering obesity through excessive food-treat provisioning is strongly discouraged. As with any other enrichment technique, the health and well-being of the animal and common sense should prevail.

3. Manipulanda

Increasing the complexity of the cage environment by providing 'toys' has been widely implemented. Although the inclusion of objects for primates to manipulate is a provision of the AWRs, the actual benefit to the animal of including manipulanda in the cage may be inconsistent (Bayne et al., 1992a). The species, sex, and age of the animal and type of toy can influence the animal's response to the item (Crockett et al., 1989; O'Neill, 1988; Line et al.,

1991b; Weld et al., 1991). A criticism of the use of simple toys as enrichment devices is based on the finding that the animals' interest in them wanes quickly, although 'use' of the toys tends to stabilize at a low level (e.g., Bloomsmith et al., 1990; Bayne, 1989; Line and Morgan, 1991). It has been suggested that perhaps a schedule of toy removal and reintroduction would prolong the animals' interest and use of the objects (Crockett et al., 1989; Paquette and Prescott, 1988), and indeed toy rotation seems to be the prevalent approach used in most facilities. Manipulanda that are commercially manufactured and fabricated in-house are typically used. There is some preliminary evidence to suggest that among a variety of rubber and plastic objects presented, balls are manipulated the least by some monkeys, while a wishbone-shaped toy was most favored (Weld et al., 1991). Thus, early judgments on the success of a toy as enrichment should be avoided until a variety of objects have been evaluated in the context of each facility.

Other enrichment techniques that generally come under the category of manipulanda are mirrors and grooming boards. Although studies evaluating mirror viewing have tended to be rather short-term, the pattern of initial high use progressing to a low rate of use seems to be consistent (Collinge, 1989; O'Neill-Wagner et al., 1997). However, use appears to vary among individuals, with some retaining frequent use of mirrors, while other individual animals lose interest rapidly. This further underscores the need to evaluate enrichment for the individual animal. In chimpanzees, mirror use actually resulted in an increase in agonistic behavior and a decrease in affiliative behavior (Lambeth and Bloomsmith, 1992). Grooming boards made of artificial shearling have been shown to reduce stereotypical behavior in macaques (rhesus and cynomolgus) and baboons (Bayne et al., 1991; Lam et al., 1991; Pyle et al., 1996). The devices encouraged both grooming and foraging behavior in the primates.

D. Social Behavior

Despite the inherent diversity of members of the order Primate, most species used in the research environment live in social units. In free-ranging conditions, these social units may be composed of monogamous pairs (e.g., owl monkeys), groups that are highly structured (e.g., baboons), groups that are less cohesive in their membership (e.g., squirrel monkey troops have been described as an 'aggregate,' or readily 'subdivided' into smaller groups; see Rosenblum and Coe, 1977; Thorington, 1968), or groups that are organized along matrilines (e.g., rhesus monkeys). It is this basic social nature of nonhuman primates that has engendered the approach that the 'best' method of providing environmental stimulation is another animal (e.g., Love, 1995).

Although concerns about animal health and safety, personnel safety, accessibility to specific animals, variability in research data, and cost have been factors that have discouraged widespread implementation of social housing, regulatory requirements, federal policy, and accreditation standards essentially describe the default means of housing as a social environment, with any deviation from this necessitating a justification based on the health and well-being of the animal or a research requirement (AWRs, AAALAC International). More important, however, studies have shown that singly housed primates manifest greater abnormal behavior than do socially housed animals (e.g., Bayne et al., 1992b); higher levels of self-grooming and lower levels of activity (Eaton et al., 1994); and higher 'tension-related' behaviors (Baker, 1996). Fundamental to successful social housing is knowledge of the species' natural behavior, inclusive of its social organization (DiVincenti and Wyatt, 2011).

Reports on the success of social housing of laboratory primates vary. Line et al. (1990b) reported the death of one female, hospitalization of one male, and injuries to eight other animals out of 13 aged rhesus monkeys in the period after grouping. Jensen et al. (1980) reported a mortality rate of 11% in bonnet macaques due to injury over a 3-month period following group formation and 9% mortality in rhesus monkeys over the first 6 months following group formation. Conversely, Kaplan et al. (1980) were able to reduce mortality resulting from fighting by identifying ongoing social disruption (removal of some animals from the group with the introduction of new animals) and then modifying management practices. Bayne et al. (1995) reviewed the injury records for three research facilities housing rhesus macaques and cynomolgus monkeys. They determined that 12% of the records evaluated for group-housed monkeys involved a wounding incident. The authors concluded that group-housed females acquired wounds and required wound management more frequently than group-housed males, and that group-housed animals that were wounded were likely to be injured again, although most wounds required only minor treatment. McCully et al. (1992) similarly reported only minor wounding among 30 adult rhesus monkeys housed in groups of three to eight animals (five groups of adult males and one group of adult and subadult females with one adult male). A number of factors can influence the success of group formation, such as species, rearing experience, group size (e.g., Erwin, 1979; McIntyre and Petto, 1993), and method of group formation (Bernstein and Mason, 1962).

The formation of pairs of primates, while also having some risk associated with it, appears to be more practical in the laboratory environment and more readily achieved than group housing, though Doyle et al. (2008) have presented persuasive data that the stress of pair-formation in socially experienced adult male macaques

can be minimal when properly managed. Recent data (Baker et al., 2012) have demonstrated that isosexual pair housing of adult rhesus monkeys led to a reduction in abnormal behavior as well as anxiety-related behaviors, based on serum cortisol measurements and behavioral observations. For cynomolgus monkeys, compatible female–female pairs have been described by Line et al. (1990a) and Crockett et al. (1994). However, formation of compatible male–female and familiar male–male pairs using cages equipped with grooming-contact bars has also been described (Crockett et al., 1997). Other successful pairs described in the literature include female baboons (Jerome and Szostak, 1987), male bonnet macaques (Coe and Rosenblum, 1984), adult male and adult female rhesus monkeys (e.g., Reinhardt, 1988, 1994b), and male and female stumptail macaques (Reinhardt, 1994c).

The extent to which social housing influences the physiology of the research primate has not been fully evaluated; however, there is evidence that some parameters are modified. Coe (1991) determined that natural killer cell activity decreased following the introduction of females into the housing area in which both dominant and subordinate male rhesus monkeys were pair-housed. He further demonstrated that the testosterone levels in the dominant partner of pair-housed male squirrel monkeys were consistently higher than those of the subordinate partner (Coe, 1991). Gonzalez et al. (1982) reported that plasma cortisol levels were lower in pair-housed female squirrel monkeys than in individually or group-housed females. They further reported that increases in cortisol levels following a stressor (handling and anesthesia) were smaller in pair-housed females. Capitanio (1998) has described a higher mortality in simian immunodeficiency virus (SIV)-infected macaques that were exposed to unstable social affiliations shortly after inoculation of the virus. He suggests that both the hypothalamic-pituitary-adrenal and the sympathetic-adrenal-medullary systems are influenced by social instability-induced stress. Coelho et al. (1991) found that baboons given visual, tactile, and auditory contact between wire-mesh walls with a familiar companion had lower blood pressure than when they were housed alone or with unfamiliar animals. This 'social buffering,' or amelioration of a stress response due to the presence of a compatible social partner, has also been well-documented in macaques (e.g., Gust et al., 1994, 1996; Gilbert and Baker, 2011, and for a review see Kikusui et al., 2006). Reinhardt et al. (1988) found that the body weights of female rhesus monkeys that were pair-housed did not vary significantly in the first month following pair housing as compared to baseline weights, although subordinate animals did exhibit a significant weight gain in the second month following pair housing. Reinhardt et al. (1991b) further demonstrated that there was no significant difference in the mean serum cortisol level between the dominant and subordinate partners of rhesus monkey pairs. Stanton *et al.* (1985) similarly identified a 'social buffering' in squirrel monkeys, wherein cortisol secretion in response to a fear-inducing stimulus was highest in individually housed animals, was attenuated somewhat by the presence of a single cagemate, and was at baseline level when the monkeys were housed with several other squirrel monkeys.

Through these early lessons in forming pairs and groups of nonhuman primates, much has been learned and social housing methods have vastly improved. As our knowledge about appropriate methods to provide social housing of nonhuman primates increased, so too did the philosophical tone in the *Guide* (NRC, 2011) become biased toward social housing, stating that "Single housing should be the exception…." Of note, AAALAC International, which uses the *Guide* in its assessments of animal care and use programs has taken an even stronger stance, stating in one of its very few Position Statements that "Social housing will be considered by AAALAC International as the default method of housing unless otherwise justified based on social incompatibility resulting from inappropriate behavior, veterinary concerns regarding animal well-being, or scientific necessity approved by the IACUC (or comparable oversight body)." AAALAC offers this further guidance, "When necessary, single housing of social animals should be limited to the minimum period necessary and, where possible, visual, auditory, olfactory and, depending on the species, protected tactile contact with compatible conspecifics should be provided."

E. Novelty and Predictability

Many environmental enrichment programs depend to a large degree on the provision of manipulanda (toys) to the primates. More than one study has shown, however, that the animals' interest in the toy, while initially high, declines rapidly (Millar *et al.*, 1988). Some programs have attempted to circumvent this response by rotating the types of objects provided to the animals with the goal of sustaining a higher interest in them (e.g., National Institutes of Health, 1991). However, species differences (Fragaszy and Mason, 1978) and age differences (Millar *et al.*, 1988) in responses of primates to novel objects have been described. For example, titi monkeys responded to a novel object with distress and arousal, while squirrel monkeys did not; and older callitrichid offspring generally contacted novel objects first and for longer periods than either parents or younger offspring.

The objects to be used in an enrichment program should be chosen based on not only their sanitizability and their safety, but also on their relative efficacy. Sambrook and Buchanan-Smith (1996) determined that guenons who showed an interest in novel objects preferred those that were responsive (made a noise when manipulated) and showed no preference for visually complex objects over visually simplistic objects.

Predictability in an animal's environment is often linked to the animal having some control over certain environmental elements. Indeed, Fragaszy and Adams-Curtis (1991) propose that having control over the environment is more important to the animal than novelty. In some species, animals are less stressed if they can predict when an unpleasant stimulus is going to occur or when they can control its occurrence with their behavior (Shepherdson, 1998). For example, Gottlieb *et al.* (2013b) have shown that conducting a routine husbandry activity, such as feeding and enrichment distribution, on a predictable schedule reduces the expression of motor stereotypies and displacement behaviors in rhesus monkeys. It should be noted, however, that Novak and Drewson (1989) suggest that too much predictability in the environment may be 'boring' for animals. Chamove and Moodie (1990) have demonstrated that novelty can stimulate exploratory behavior and elicit arousal behavior that has beneficial effects. However, novelty can also be a stressor; therefore, an enrichment plan that incorporates novelty should be evaluated carefully.

F. Personnel Interactions

The potential impact of personnel on research animal well-being is quite significant (Jennings and Prescott, 2009). Animal care staff should be trained in the general behavior of the species for which they provide care. In particular, they should be cognizant of simple facial and postural signals that communicate messages to the primates (e.g., a direct stare is interpreted as an aggressive behavior by macaques, and a yawn may be interpreted as an open-mouth threat). Although few objective studies have been conducted on the effect of positive personnel interaction with laboratory primates, Bayne *et al.* (1993) observed that increasing personnel time with primates in bouts of 2 min, three times a week (while distributing food treats), resulted in a significant reduction of certain undesirable behaviors (e.g., repetitive locomotion and other stereotypic behaviors) and increase in some positive behaviors (e.g., grooming).

O'Neill (1989) suggested that stability in personnel is very important, and that certain characteristics, such as patience and kindness, are essential, while Wolfle (1996) stated that staff should be carefully selected and should be "caring and compassionate." Choosing personnel with suitable characteristics for work with research animals can start as early as the initial interview (Mandrell, 1996) by assessing the individual's attitude toward animals in general and animal research in particular. Mandrell (1996) suggested that personnel in leadership roles should set the example for animal treatment by demonstrating a "genuine caring attitude."

However, primates may be aggressive to personnel providing routine care, and such a situation can become stressful for both the animal and individual involved. Positive reinforcement training has been used to increase cooperation in a variety of animal species, including laboratory primates (e.g., Shapiro et al., 2003). This technique has also been shown to be successful at reducing the level of aggression directed to staff primarily through a desensitization and behavioral shaping program (Minier et al., 2011). Such a program can be highly enriching for both the nonhuman primates and their caregivers.

The increased interactions between staff and the primates in their care resulting from time spent providing enrichment or positive reinforcement training can lead to very strong attachments for the animals on the part of the staff. This caring attitude can only enhance the overall quality of life for the animals, but can be challenging for the employee when certain work assignments (euthanasia being the most extreme example) have to be fulfilled. In such a case, the procedure may need to be conducted by another staff member. The trade-off is well worthwhile, however, as routine duties are more enriching for the animal care staff as they engage in designing enrichment methodologies and learn more about the animals in their care (Roberts, 1989).

VI. FARM ANIMALS

Farm animal behavior has been studied extensively, both because behavior influences production traits and because of the increasing concern about the welfare of intensively farmed animals. There are now many books on farm animal behavior written primarily for application to the commercial production situation, but which also provide information useful for structuring behavioral environments in the laboratory setting. Some of these provide overviews of the behavior of domesticated animals in general (e.g., Broom and Fraser, 2007; Price, 2008; Jensen, 2009; Houpt, 2010; Ekesbo, 2011), while others focus on specific farm animal species (e.g., cattle: Phillips, 2010; poultry: Appleby et al., 2004; horses: Mills and McDonnell, 2005 and McGreevy, 2012; sheep: Lynch et al., 1992). There is also an increasing number of books focusing on farm animal welfare from a broad perspective, but which also contain significant information about behavioral management, behavioral problems, and human–animal interactions (e.g., general: Appleby et al., 2011; cattle: Rushen et al., 2007; horses: Waran, 2007; sheep: Dwyer, 2008; pigs: Marchant-Forde, 2009).

Farm animals have been domesticated and selected for desirable production traits for thousands of years. Indirectly, they have also been selected for their behavioral adaptability to a range of social and physical environments. Nevertheless, farm animals can and do display behavioral problems in agricultural and laboratory settings. Domestication and selection have resulted largely in quantitative rather than qualitative changes in behavior (Price, 2002). Although the frequency and intensity of expression of particular behaviors have been changed, the repertoire of behavior is generally strikingly similar to that characteristic of ancestral species. More 'naturalistic' environments can therefore be helpful in minimizing some behavioral problems. However, genetic factors should not be overlooked, since some behavioral problems arise primarily as a consequence of selection for production traits while others are exacerbated by such selection (Grandin and Deesing, 2013). For example, commercial turkeys selected for high growth rates can no longer mate naturally, not because mating behavior has been changed by selection but because the size and breast conformation of the male makes mating physically impossible. Some genetic stocks of animals may show exaggerated fear responses or be particularly difficult to handle, both of which can lead to problems during interactions between animals and personnel in the laboratory. Genetically engineered farm animals may also have special behavioral problems and needs (Mench, 1999).

A. Types of Behavior Problems

A variety of behavior problems can be observed in farm animals (Broom and Fraser, 2007). These include stereotypic behaviors, aberrant or problematical social behaviors, apathy or lethargy, hyperactivity, and excessive fearfulness. Abnormal behaviors include locomotor stereotypies such as weaving, pacing, and route-tracing; and oral behaviors such as wool-eating by sheep, feather pecking and cannibalism by poultry, bar biting by pigs, tongue rolling by cattle, and wind-sucking by horses (see Table 38.1).

Some abnormal behaviors can result in injury or death to the animal or to the animal's conspecifics. For example, calves may groom themselves excessively and ingest large quantities of hair, which accumulates in the rumen and clogs the rumen openings. Excessive ingestion of wood or litter by farm animals can also lead to impaction in the digestive tract. Behaviors that cause injury to other animals include cannibalism of her young by a parturient sow (sow savaging); feather pecking (allopecking) and cannibalism by poultry; anal massage, belly nosing, and tail biting by pigs; sucking of another animal's ears, navel, scrotum, prepuce, or udder by cattle; and wool eating by confined sheep. Other abnormal or problematical social behaviors include excessively frequent or severe aggression (directed either toward other animals or humans), sexual dysfunction, and poor

TABLE 38.1   Behavioral Problems and Environmental Enrichment for Farm Animals

Farm animal	Behavioral problems[a]		Environmental enrichment[b]			
	Self or environment directed	Other-directed	Manipulanda and occupational	Physical (enclosures and furnishings)	Sensory	Food strategies
Cattle	Head-rubbing; eye rolling; tongue rolling; excessive coat licking; pica	Inter-sucking	Exercise; grooming devices		Olfactory enrichment	Pasture; adequate roughage
Horses	Pacing; weaving; tail-rubbing; pawing; stall-kicking; head bobbing; wind-sucking; crib biting; pica		Exercise; 'toys' (e.g., balls, hanging objects)	Paddock or pasture access	Pheromones; music (?)	Forage (esp. straw); food balls
Sheep and Goats	Wool eating; biting non-nutritive items (e.g., slats)	Wool eating	Foraging/chewing items	Climbing structures (goats)		Feed supplement devices
Poultry	Pacing; head-shaking; stereotyped pecking	Feather pecking; cannibalism	Novel objects; foraging materials	Nestboxes (for egg-laying birds); perches; substrate for dustbathing; swimming water; cover; novel objects	Video; odors	Food variety
Swine	Sham chewing; bar or tether biting; pica	Cannibalism; anal massage; tail-biting; belly-nosing	Malleable materials (e.g., soil, straw, peat, branches); hanging ropes or other hanging objects (chains, hoses); nesting material	Subdivision of space; visual barriers; bedding; wallows or cooling devices (e.g., showers)	Odors; tactile stimulation of snout mouth	Food rewards; hidden food treats; forage; chewable but inedible substrates

[a]From Broom and Fraser (2007).
[b]From FASS (2010).

maternal behavior. Behavior problems that cause injury are typically dealt with in agricultural production settings by permanently altering the animals, for example, by beak-trimming poultry, tail-docking pigs, and dehorning cattle.

Although there has been a great deal of research on many of these problems, in many cases the etiology, and hence the remedy, is still unclear. Feather pecking and cannibalism in poultry and other captive birds are examples of common and persistent behavioral abnormalities that have multifactorial causes (reviewed by Newberry, 2004 and Rodenburg et al., 2013). Feather pecking is the pecking and pulling at the feathers of another bird; cannibalism is the pecking and tearing of the skin and underlying tissues of another bird. Feather pecking ranges from allopreening and gentle feather pecking, apparently normal behaviors that cause little or no feather damage, to severe feather pecking and pulling. In addition, there are two types of cannibalism, the first involving skin damage that occurs as a result of feather pecking and the other involving pecks directed to the cloaca (vent pecking), typically ensuing when the cloaca is everted during egg-laying. Cloacal cannibalism often causes the death of the cannibalized bird.

Factors that influence the development and incidence of feather pecking and cannibalism include light intensity, position of the enclosure in the building, housing system, genetics, group size, type and availability of food, housing density, fearfulness, and exposure to stressors. Of particular importance is the absence of litter material that can be used for foraging, exploration, and dustbathing. Food deficiencies can also be a trigger, with dietary fiber perhaps playing a particularly important role in feather pecking. Feather-peckers often ingest the feathers that they eat and also prefer higher-fiber diets when given a choice (Kalmendal and Bessei, 2012).

Ingesting feathers may be important for digestive function if the diet is too low in fiber, since ingested feathers have been shown to speed up food passage in the same way that fiber does (Harlander-Matauschek *et al.*, 2006).

In other cases the etiology of a particular problem is more straightforward. Young piglets may manipulate the belly of other piglets, using their snout in the same way that they would use their snout to massage the udder of the sow. Belly nosing occurs when piglets are weaned earlier than the normal weaning age of 8–12 weeks, which is a common practice in commercial production where piglets can be weaned as early as 1–2 weeks of age (Widowski *et al.*, 2008). Belly nosing can have negative effects on both the recipient and performer of the behavior: the ventral surface of the piglet being belly-nosed can become inflamed (Broom and Fraser, 2007), and piglets that belly-nose spend less time at the feeder and have poorer growth rates (Widowski *et al.*, 2008).

B. Effect of Behavior Problems on Research

As alluded to above, many behavior problems have demonstrated consequences for the animal's health and well-being, and thus can negatively affect research. For example, even in the absence of cannibalism, having feathers pulled out by another bird is painful for chickens (Gentle and Hunter, 1990), and the resulting poorer plumage condition impairs thermoregulation (Tauson and Svensson, 1980). Wool-bitten sheep may develop skin lesions and are also more susceptible to helminth parasites, suggesting that they are immunocompromised (Lynch *et al.*, 1992).

Even when animals are not displaying behavioral problems, providing opportunities for the performance of natural behaviors can promote health and physiological normality. An example is the provision of either nutritive or nonnutritive artificial teats to weaned calves. Not only does this decrease cross-sucking and abnormal licking of the pen bars (Haley *et al.*, 1998), but the calves show increased secretion of insulin and digestive enzymes when they are allowed to suckle shortly after receiving a milk meal (de Passillé *et al.*, 1993). Calves that are able to suck milk from artificial teats rather than drink it from a bucket also show signs of reduced sympathetic activation and are calmer (Vessier *et al.*, 2002). Other effects of increasing behavioral opportunities for farm animals are discussed in the sections that follow.

C. Environmental Enrichment

Environmental enrichment strategies for farm animals have been recently reviewed by Mench *et al.* (2010) in the FASS *Guide for the Care and Use of Agricultural Animals* (and see Table 38.1). This publication provides detailed information and references about current research on the use and effectiveness of a variety of enrichments for pigs, horses, cattle, poultry, and swine. Thus, only a general overview will be provided here.

1. Enclosure Size and Furnishings

Farm animals can be kept in a variety of different types of enclosures in the laboratory setting, ranging in size from small cages or pens to extensive outdoor paddocks. The appropriate enclosure type and size will depend on a variety of factors, including the age, sex, and reproductive status of the animal; the type of research; the social environment; and in more extensive enclosures, the terrain and hence availability and distribution of resources such as food, water, cover, and shade (NRC, 2011; FASS, 2010). Some types of enclosure furnishings discussed in this section may be practical only in certain types of enclosures.

When furnishings are provided, consideration should be given to their placement and size, the materials from which they are made, and their potential to have both positive and negative effects on welfare. Perches for fowl are an example of furnishings that have both benefits and drawbacks (see review in Mench *et al.*, 2010). Fowl are highly motivated to perch and will use perches extensively, particularly at night. Perches allow subordinates to seek refuge from other birds and can minimize cannibalistic pecking, as well as decrease fearfulness. Perches can also improve musculoskeletal strength, particularly in the legs and wings, because they promote exercise. On the other hand, perches can contribute to the development of a painful foot problem, bumblefoot, and are associated with keelbone deviations in laying hens. Many factors can affect the use of perches and the incidences of these kinds of problems, including the strain or breed of bird, the perch diameter and shape, the perch material and particularly the ability to maintain cleanliness of the perch surface, and perch height and placement.

Enclosure furnishings are less critical for livestock than poultry. However, it is important that feeders, waterers, and flooring surfaces or walking areas for farm animals be designed to accommodate natural feeding, drinking, and movement patterns. Poor flooring surfaces are major contributors to injury and lameness (Webb and Nilsson, 1983), and badly designed feeders can also cause injury (Taylor, 1995). For caged or crated animals, enclosure design can also be critical. Tauson (1985) found that laying-hen cages with certain floor slopes, bar orientations, cage-locking devices, and bar spacing caused birds to become trapped and injured during feeding and other behaviors.

2. Food Strategies

Except when kept on pasture, farm animals are typically fed formulated, concentrated feeds. Farm animals can certainly self-select nutritious diets, but providing food variety is not commonly used as a means of behavioral enrichment for farm animals, except that poultry may be given supplemental oyster shell and grit and livestock may be given salt blocks and hay.

Chickens and pigs are omnivores and would normally spend a large part of their day foraging for diverse types of food (Stolba and Wood-Gush, 1989; Dawkins, 1989). Ruminants similarly spend a large part of their day grazing and selectively ingest particular types of plants. Many oral and locomotor-type behavior problems in farm animals seem to be associated, at least in part, with the lack of foraging opportunities due to the feeding of concentrated feeds, or with the use of feed restriction to control body weight (Kyriazakis and Tolkamp, 2011; Bergeron et al., 2008).

3. Manipulanda

Farm animals manipulate objects primarily with their mouths, beaks, muzzles, or snouts; so behaviors directed toward manipulanda may be closely related to foraging and feeding behaviors, as well as to some social behaviors, like biting. The effects of manipulanda on behavior and performance traits have been evaluated primarily for pigs and chickens (Mench et al., 2010), mainly in the context of reducing abnormal oral behaviors. Providing manipulanda can be beneficial in this regard, but does not always result in improvements in welfare. For example, sows may simply redirect oral stereotypies like bar biting, which seem to be caused by feed restriction rather than confinement, to hanging manipulanda (Terlouw et al., 1991) and even to rocks if the sows are housed outdoors (Dailey and McGlone, 1997).

In general, manipulanda are only effective as long-term enrichment stimuli if they have biological relevance to the animal (Newberry, 1995). Pigs will root in an earth-filled trough initially, but this behavior diminishes with time (Appleby and Wood-Gush, 1988). Straw that is renewed daily elicits sustained interest, however, probably because of the combination of novelty and palatability (Fraser et al., 1991). In addition, chickens seem to habituate quickly to some manipulanda and stop interacting with them (Gao et al., 1994; Sherwin, 1993). Rotation of enrichments objects can help to sustain interest (Trickett et al., 2009).

One type of manipulable object, bedding, can stimulate many behaviors. The effects of straw bedding on pig welfare are reviewed by Tuyttens (2005). Pigs provided with straw have a more diverse behavioral repertoire, and manipulate the straw for foraging and nest-building. Straw provides a more comfortable lying surface than concrete, reduces loading on the hooves compared to concrete, and can contribute to thermal comfort under cold conditions. Pigs given straw may also perform fewer abnormal oral behaviors like tail-biting. Bedding

is also used by chickens for nest building and dust-bathing. Dustbathing regulates the amount of lipids on the feathers and reduces feather damage (Van Liere and Bokma, 1987; Nørgaard-Nielsen et al., 1993). Maintaining good hygienic conditions is a concern when bedding is provided, and for this reason bedding can also be associated with negative effects on welfare, including by increasing the incidence of certain health problems in pigs (Tuyttens, 2005) and causing foot and hock burns or footpad infections in chickens, which can contribute to lameness (Lay et al., 2011).

D. Social Behavior

In natural environments, feral farm animals (and their nondomestic ancestors) live in small or moderate-sized groups. The basic social unit in these groups comprises adult females and their offspring. Males typically associate with the female group during the breeding season, but during the nonbreeding season either are usually relatively solitary or form small bachelor groups. However, animals farmed commercially are now kept in groups that may differ significantly from this pattern, for example, single-sex or single-age groups that may be considerably larger or smaller than the feral norm. Farm animals are generally tolerant of a range of social conditions, but behavioral problems may arise under certain circumstances. These problems include excessive aggression or dominance-related problems, poor parenting, sexual dysfunction, and abnormal behaviors that lead to injury of other animals or that result, at least in part, from being housed in social isolation or deprived of maternal stimulation. These problems are more common in confined farm animals and can be exacerbated by many nonsocial factors, such as floor, feeder, and waterer space; enclosure configuration, including lack of 'escape' areas for subordinate animals; and lack of general environmental stimulation.

Social behavior in farm animals has been studied extensively, and because of the many different types of social environments in which farm animals may be housed in the laboratory, it is beyond the scope of this chapter to discuss social housing at length. Detailed information about the social behavior and behavioral problems of each species of farm animal, as well as possible remedies for problems, can be found in Gonyou and Keeling (2001). Social stressors can negatively impact farm animals' health status by causing them to become immunocompromised, thus increasing their susceptibility to disease (Proudfoot et al., 2012). Regardless, providing adequate social stimulation is important for farm animal well-being, and appropriate social companionship can have stress-buffering effects (Rault, 2012). Therefore, whenever possible farm animals should be housed in compatible social groups or at least be provided with visual, auditory and/or olfactory contact with conspecifics. Details about housing and management of social groups of cattle, swine, horses, sheep and goats, and poultry can be found in Federation of Animal Science Societies (2010).

E. Novelty, Predictability, and Exploration

Having some degree of predictability is important for farm animals. For example, Carlstead (1986) found that pigs that were fed at unpredictable intervals were more aggressive than pigs that were given a reliable signal (e.g., a bell) when food was about to be delivered. Similarly, lambs exposed to a sudden event (the appearance of a plastic panel) had a lower heart rate and reduced startle responses if they could predict the event due to an environmental cue, or if the event occurred at regular intervals (Greiveldinger et al., 2007).

However, lack of environmental challenge associated with highly predictable environments that lack novel stimuli has been implicated as a major cause of apathy and boredom in confined animals (Špinka and Wemelsfelder, 2011). Novelty may be attractive to farm animals because it enables them to gain information about their environment, that is, it serves an exploratory function (Mench, 1998). Hens placed in an enclosure that contains abundant resources still spend a proportion of their time exploring an empty tunnel attached to their enclosure (Nicol and Guilford, 1991). Pigs will similarly explore a pen adjacent to their home pen (Wood-Gush et al., 1990), particularly if it contains a novel object (Wood-Gush and Vestergaard, 1991). Exploratory behaviors are decreased when animals experience stress; for example, diseased calves are less likely to engage in non-nutritive exploratory visits to an automated milk feeder than healthy calves, although they visit as often to drink as healthy calves (Svensson and Jensen, 2007). Play behavior can also be considered to be a form of exploration and is similarly reduced when animals experience stress (Boissy et al., 2007). There is growing evidence that providing novelty, as well as opportunities for exploration and anticipation of valued rewards, can contribute to promoting positive mental states in animals (Boissy et al., 2007).

However, as Wemelsfelder (1993) points out, it is not enough for animals simply to be exposed to novelty – they must also be allowed to interact with it in some biologically meaningful way. Newberry (1999) found that chickens would readily and repeatedly enter pens adjacent to their home pen. They strongly preferred an adjacent pen containing the same resources as those in the home pen (food, water, heat, and wood shavings), but adjacent pens that contained either frequently changed novel objects or supplemental resources (peat moss, a bale of straw, and an elevated platform) were also used. Empty adjacent pens were least preferred. In addition to interacting with novel stimuli, animals should also be able to avoid them if they so choose. If animals cannot control their exposure to a novel stimulus, it may cause fear instead of eliciting exploration (e.g., Murphy, 1977). Rearing conditions are important with respect to an animal's response to novelty and predictability. Chicks raised in visually complex environments, for example, show less fear of novelty than chicks raised in visually plain environments (Broom, 1969).

Farm animals may also benefit from being exposed to structured cognitive challenges, which can increase engagement with the environment (Manteuffel et al. 2009). An example is the performance of positively motivated instrumental behaviors (Manteuffel et al., 2009), which can stimulate anticipatory behaviors and learning. As an example, pigs trained to discriminate acoustic signals to perform an operant task in order to receive a food reward showed changes in autonomic nervous system responses consistent with increased arousal and positive emotional responses (Zebunke et al., 2011). Providing pigs with opportunities to perform this task in their home pens also had other benefits, promoting better wound healing (Ernst et al., 2006) and increased activity, reduced fear, and decreased abnormal behavior (Puppe et al., 2007). It is important that operant devices not cause so much challenge that they result in animals becoming frustrated to the extent that their welfare is reduced (Lindberg and Nicol, 1994).

F. Personnel Interactions

Large farm animals can be dangerous to humans. An understanding of farm animal behavior is critical to appropriate handling. Using specialized equipment (e.g., squeeze chutes) or handling aids (e.g., flags) can also be helpful when large livestock have to be restrained or moved. Principles of livestock handling to minimize injury and stress to both animals and humans are discussed in Grandin (2007). Poultry can also cause injuries to humans by pecking or scratching, and handling seems to be particularly stressful for them because of their general fear of humans (Duncan, 1992). Poultry should be handled gently in an upright position, with their wings restrained, to minimize distress and struggling (Kannan and Mench, 1996; Mench and Blatchford, 2013), and laying hens should be removed from their enclosures particularly carefully because of their bone fragility (Knowles and Wilkins, 1998).

Farm animal–personnel interactions, and especially the critical importance of the attitudes and behaviors of caretakers toward farm animals in ensuring good animal welfare, are discussed in detail in Hemsworth and Coleman (2011). Negative interactions with humans have been shown to have many undesirable effects on the behavior and physiology of farm animals (Hemsworth and Coleman, 2011; Waiblinger *et al.*, 2006; Rushen and de Passillé, 2010). Not only does negative handling increase fearfulness, it can also result in reduced reproductive success and growth, acute and chronic stress, decreased immunocompetence, increased aggression toward humans, and increased handling difficulty. Conversely, socializing farm animals via regular, gentle handling can have beneficial effects, decreasing fearfulness and in some cases improving physiological functioning. Even fairly brief visual contact with humans without handling can decrease fear responses, at least in chickens (Jones, 1996).

VII. CONCLUSIONS

A sound understanding of the species-appropriate behavior of the variety of animals used in biomedical research is essential to ensuring proper animal care and promoting quality animal health and welfare. When these factors are optimized, the quality of the data generated is clearly enhanced. Thus, it is incumbent on the laboratory animal medicine and science community to embed information about laboratory animal behavior into institutional training programs and to ensure that care and use decisions take into consideration the animals' behavior.

References

Ågren, G., Zhou, Q., Zhong, W., 1989a. Ecology and social behaviour of Mongolian gerbils, *Meriones unguiculatus*, at Xilinhot, Inner Mongolia, China. Anim. Behav. 37 (1), 11–27.

Ågren, G., Zhou, Q., Zhong, W., 1989b. Territoriality, cooperation and resource priority: hoarding in the Mongolian gerbil. *Meriones unguiculatus*. Anim. Behav. 37 (1), 28–32.

Akre, A.K., Bakken, M., Hovland, A.L., Palme, R., Mason, G., 2011. Clustered environmental enrichments induce more aggression and stereotypic behaviour than do dispersed enrichments in female mice. Appl. Anim. Behav. Sci. 131, 145–152.

Ambrose, N., Morton, D.B., 2000. The use of cage enrichment to reduce male mouse aggression. J. Appl. Anim. Welf. Sci. 3 (2), 117–125.

Anderson, J.R., Chamove, A.S., 1984. Allowing captive primates to forage Standards in Laboratory Animal Management, Symposium Proceedings, Part 2. Universities Federation for Animal Welfare, Potters Bar, United Kingdom, pp. 253–256.

Anderson, L., 1987. Guinea pig husbandry and medicine. Vet. Clin. North Am. Small Anim. Pract. 17 (5), 1045–1060.

Appleby, M.C., Wood-Gush, D.G.M., 1988. Effect of earth as an additional stimulus on the behaviour of confined pigs. Behav. Process. 17, 83–91.

Appleby, M.C., Mench, J.A., Hughes, B.O., 2004. Poultry Production Systems: Behaviour, Management, and Welfare. CAB International, Wallingford, Oxon, United Kingdom.

Appleby, M.C., Mench, J.A., Olsson, I.A.S., Hughes, B.O., 2011. Animal Welfare, second ed. CAB International, Wallingford, Oxon, United Kingdom.

Arai, J.A., Li, S., Hartley, D.M., Feig, L.A., 2009. Transgenerational rescue of a genetic defect in long-term potentiation and memory formation by Juvenile enrichment. J. Neurosci. 29 (5), 1496–1502.

Armstrong, K.R., Clark, T.R., Peterson, M.R., 1998. Use of cornhusk nesting material to reduce aggression in cages mice. Contemp. Top. Lab. Anim. Sci. 37 (4), 64–66.

Arnold, C.E., Estep, D.Q., 1990. Effects of housing on social preference and behaviour in male golden hamsters (*Mesocricetus auratus*). Appl. Anim. Behav. Sci. 27 (3), 253–261.

Arnold, C.E., Estep, D.Q., 1994. Laboratory caging preferences in golden-hamsters (*Mesocricetus auratus*). Lab. Anim. 28 (3), 232–238.

Babcock, A.M., Graham-Goodwin, H., 1997. Importance of preoperative training and maze difficulty in task performance following hippocampal damage in the gerbil. Brain Res. Bull. 42 (6), 415–419.

Baer, H., 1991. Long-term isolation stress and its effects on drug responses in rodents. Lab. Anim. Sci. (21), 341–349.

Baker, K.C., 1996. Chimpanzees in single cages and small social groups: effects of housing on behavior. Contemp. Top. Lab. Anim. Sci. 35, 71–74.

Baker, K.C., Bloomsmith, M.A., Oettinger, B., Neu, K., Griffis, C., Schoof, V., et al., 2012. Benefits of pair housing are consistent across a diverse population of rhesus macaques. Appl. Anim. Behav. 137 (3–4), 148–156.

Barnard, C.J., Behnke, J.M., Sewell, J., 1996. Environmental enrichment, immunocompetence, and resistance to *Babesia microti* in male mice. Physiol. Behav. 60 (5), 1223–1231.

Barnett, S.A., 1963. The Rat: A Study in Behavior. University of Chicago Press, IL.

Barry, K.J., Crowell-Davis, S.L., 1999. Gender differences in the social behavior of the neutered indoor-only domestic cat. Appl. Anim. Behav. Sci. 64, 193–211.

Batchelor, G.R., 1994. The rest/activity rhythm of the laboratory rat housed under different systems. Anim. Technol. 45, 181–187.

Bayne, K., 1989. Nylon balls re-visited. Lab. Prim. Newsl. 28, 5–6.

Bayne, K., 1996. Normal and abnormal behaviors of laboratory animals: what do they mean? Lab. Anim. 25, 21–24.

Bayne, K., McCully, C., 1989. The effect of cage size on the behavior of individually housed rhesus monkeys. Lab. Anim. 18, 25–28.

Bayne, K., Novak, M., 1998. Behavioral disorders. In: Bennett, B.T., Abee, C.R., Henrickson, R. (Eds.), Nonhuman Primates in Biomedical Research: Diseases. Academic Press, New York, pp. 485–500.

Bayne, K., Wurbel, H., 2012. Mouse enrichment. In: Hedrich, H. (Ed.), The Laboratory Mouse, second ed. Elsevier, New York, pp. 545–564.

Bayne, K., Suomi, S., Brown, B., 1989. A new monkey swing. Lab. Prim. Newsl. 28, 16–17.

Bayne, K., Mainzer, H., Dexter, S., Campbell, G., Yamada, F., Suomi, S., 1991. The reduction of abnormal behaviors in individually housed rhesus monkeys (*Macaca mulatta*) with a foraging/grooming board. Amer. J. Primatol. 23, 23–35.

Bayne, K., Hurst, J., Dexter, S., 1992a. Evaluation of the preference to and behavioral effects of an enriched environment on male rhesus monkeys. Lab. Anim. Sci. 42, 38–45.

Bayne, K., Dexter, S., Suomi, S., 1992b. A preliminary survey of the incidence of abnormal behavior in rhesus monkeys (*Macaca mulatta*) relative to housing condition. Lab. Anim. 21, 38–46.

Bayne, K., Dexter, S., Mainzer, H., McCully, C., Campbell, G., Yamada, F., 1992c. The use of artificial turf as a foraging substrate for individually housed rhesus monkeys (*Macaca mulatta*). Anim. Welf. 1, 39–53.

Bayne, K., Dexter, S., Strange, G., 1993. The effect of food treat provisioning and human interaction on the behavioral well-being of rhesus monkeys (*Macaca mulatta*). Contemp. Top. Lab. Anim. Sci. 32, 6–9.

Bayne, K., Strange, G.M., Dexter, S.L., 1994. Influence of food enrichment on cage side preference. Lab. Anim. Sci. 44, 624–629.

Bayne, K., Haines, M., Dexter, S., Woodman, D., Evans, C., 1995. Nonhuman primate wounding prevalence: a retrospective analysis. Lab. Anim. 24, 40–44.

Bazille, P.G., Walden, S.D., Koniar, B.L., Gunther, R., 2001. Commercial cotton nesting material as a predisposing factor for conjunctivitis in athymic nude mice. Lab. Anim. 30 (5), 40–42.

Beaver, B.V., 1981. Behavioral considerations for laboratory dogs and cats. Compend. Cont. Edu. 2, 212–215.

Beaver, B.V., 1989. Environmental enrichment for laboratory animals. ILAR News 31, 5–11.

Beaver, B.V., 2003. Feline Behavior: A Guide for Veterinarians, second ed. Saunders, St. Louis, MO.

Beaver, B.V., 2009. Canine Behavior: Insights and Answers, second ed. Saunders, St. Louis, MO.

Benn, D.M., 1995. Innovations in research animal care. J. Am. Vet. Med. Assoc. 206, 465–468.

Bergeron, R., Badnell-Waters, A.J., Lambton, S., Mason, G., 2008. Stereotypic oral behavior in captive ungulates: foraging, diet, and gastrointestinal function. In: Mason, G., Rushen, J. (Eds.), Stereotypic Animal Behaviour: Fundamentals and Applications to Welfare CAB International, Wallingford, United Kingdom, pp. 19–57.

Bernstein, I.S., Mason, W.A., 1962. Group formation by rhesus monkeys. Anim. Behav. 11, 28–31.

Berryman, J.C., 1976. Guinea-pig vocalizations – their structure, causation and function. Zeitschrift Fur Tierpsychologie – J. Comparat. Ethol. 41 (1), 80–106.

Bishop, M.L., Chevins, P.F.D., 1989. Territory Formation by Mice under Laboratory Conditions: Welfare Considerations. UFAW, Wheat-Hampstead, United Kingdom.

Blanchard, R.J., Fukunaga, K., Blanchard, D.C., Kelley, M.J., 1975. Conspecific aggression in the laboratory rat. J. Comp. Physiol. Psychol. 89 (10), 1204–1209.

Blanchard, R.J., Flannelly, K.J., Blanchard, D.C., 1988. Life-span studies of dominance and aggression in established colonies of laboratory rats. Physiol. Behav. 43 (1), 1–7.

Blom, H.J.M., Baumans, V., Van Vorstenbosch, C.J.A.H.V., Van Zutphen, L.F.M., Beynen, A.C., 1993. Preference tests with rodents to assess housing conditions. Anim. Welf. 2, 81–87.

Blom, H.J.M., Van Tintelen, G., Baumans, V., Van Den Broek, J., Beynen, A.C., 1995. Development and application of a preference test system to evaluate housing conditions for laboratory rats. Appl. Anim. Behav. Sci. 43, 279–290.

Blom, H.J.M., Van Tintelen, G., Van Vorstenbosch, C.J.A.H.V., Baumans, V., Beynen, A.C., 1996. Preferences of mice and rats for types of bedding material. Lab. Anim. 30, 234–244.

Bloom, K.R., Cook, M., 1989. Environmental enrichment: behavioral responses of rhesus to puzzle feeders. Lab. Anim. 18, 25–31.

Bloomsmith, M., 1992. Environmental enrichment research to promote the well-being of chimpanzees. In: Erwin, J., Landon, J.G. (Eds.), Chimpanzee Conservation and Public Health: Environments for the Future. Diagnon/Bioqual, Rockville, MD, pp. 155–163.

Bloomsmith, M.A., Finlay, T.W., Merhalski, J.J., Maple, T.L., 1990. Rigid plastic balls as enrichment for captive chimpanzees. Lab. Anim. Sci. 40, 319–322.

Boccia, M.L., 1989. Preliminary report on the use of a natural foraging task to reduce aggression and stereotypies in socially housed pigtail macaques. Lab. Primate. Newsl. 28, 3–4.

Boice, R., 1977. Burrows of wild and albino rats – effects of domestication, outdoor raising, age, experience, and maternal state. J. Comp. Physiol. Psychol. 91 (3), 649–661.

Boissy, A., Manteuffel, G., Jensen, M.B., Moe, R.O., Spruijt, B., Keeling, L.J., et al., 2007. Assessment of positive emotions in animals to improve their welfare. Physiol. Behav. 92, 375–397.

Boot, R., Leussink, A.B., Vlug, R.F., 1985. Influence of housing conditions on pregnancy outcome in cynomolgus monkeys (Macaca fascicularis). Lab. Anim. Sci. 19, 42–47.

Boxall, J., Heath, S., Bate, S., Brautigam, J., 2004. Modern concepts of socialisation for dogs: implications for their behaviour, welfare and use in scientific procedures. Alt. Lab. Anim. 32 (Suppl. 2), 81–93.

Bradshaw, A.L., Poling, A., 1991. Choice by rats for enriched versus standard home cages: plastic pipes, wood platforms, wood chips, and paper towels as enrichment items. J. Exper. Anal. Behav. 55, 245–250.

Brain, P.F., 1990. Stress in agonistic contexts in rodents. In: Dantzer, R., Zayan, R. (Eds.), Stress in Domestic Animals. Kluwer Academic Publ., Dordrecht, The Netherlands, pp. 73–85.

Brain, P.F., 1992. Understanding the behaviours of feral species may facilitate design of optimal living conditions for common laboratory rodents. Anim. Technol. 43, 99–105.

Brain, P.F., Benton, D., 1979. The interpretation of physiological correlates of differential housing in laboratory rats. Life Sci. 24, 99–116.

Broom, D.M., 1969. Effects of visual complexity during rearing on chicks—reactions to environmental change. Anim. Behav. 17, 773–780.

Broom, D.M., Fraser, A.F., 2007. Domestic Animal Behaviour and Welfare, fourth ed. CAB International, Wallingford, United Kingdom.

Broom, D.M., Johnson, K.G., 1993. Stress and Animal Welfare. Chapman & Hall, London, United Kingdom.

Bryant, C.E., Rupniak, N.M.J., Iversen, S.D., 1988. Effects of different environmental enrichment devices on cage stereotypies and autoaggression in captive cynomolgus monkeys. J. Med. Primatol. 17, 257–269.

Buzzell, G.R., 1996. The harderian gland: perspectives. Microscopy Res. Tech. 34, 2–5.

Calhoun, J.B., 1962. The Ecology and Sociology of the Norway Rat. U.S. Department of Health, Education, and Welfare, Bethesda, MD.

Campbell, S.A., Hughes, H.C., Griffin, H.E., Landi, M.S., Mallon, F.M., 1988. Some effects of limited exercise on purpose-bred beagles. Am. J. Vet. Res. 49, 1298–1301.

Cao, L., Liu, X., Lin, E.-J.D., Wang, C., Choi, E.Y., Riban, V., et al., 2010. Environmental and genetic activation of a brain-adipocyte BDNF/Leptin axis causes cancer remission and inhibition. Cell 142, 52–64.

Capel, I.D., Jenner, M., Pinnock, M.H., Dorrell, H.M., Williams, D.C., 1980a. The effect of isolation stress on some hepatic drug and carcinogen metabolising enzymes in rats. J. Environ. Pathol. Toxicol. 4 (2–3), 337–344.

Capel, I.D., Jenner, M., Pinnock, M.H., Dorrell, H.M., Williams, D.C., 1980b. The effect of overcrowding stress on carcinogen-metabolizing enzymes of the rat. Environ. Res. 23 (1), 162–169.

Capitanio, J., 1998. Social experience and immune system measures in laboratory-housed macaques: implications for management and research. ILAR J. 39, 12–20.

Carlstead, K., 1986. Predictability of feeding: its effect on agonistic behaviour and growth in grower pigs. Appl. Anim. Behav. Sci. 16, 25–38.

Chambers, L.C., Singleton, G.R., Krebs, C.J., 2000. Movements and social organisation of wild house mice (Mus domesticus) in the wheatlands of northwestern Australia. J. Mammol. 81, 59–69.

Chamove, A.S., Moodie, E.M., 1990. Are alarming events good for captive monkeys. Appl. Anim. Behav. Sci. 27, 169–176.

Chance, M.R.A., 1957. Mammalian behaviour studies in medical research. Lancet 270, 678–690.

Claassen, V., 1994. Neglected Factors in Pharmacology and Neuroscience Research: Biopharmaceutics, Animal Characteristics, Maintenance, Testing Conditions (Techniques in the Behavioral and Neural Sciences), Book 12. Elsevier, Amsterdam, The Netherlands.

Clark, J.D., Calpin, J.P., Armstrong, R.B., 1991. Influence of type of enclosure on exercise fitness of dogs. Am. J. Vet. Res. 52, 1024–1028.

Clough, G., 1982. Environmental effects on animals used in biomedical research. Biol. Rev. 57, 487–523.

Cloutier, S., Wahl, K., Newberry, R., 2010. Playful handling mitigates the stressfulness of injections in laboratory rats, AALAS Meeting Official Program, 167 (Abstract), Atlanta, GA.

Coe, C.L., 1991. Is social housing of primates always the optimal choice?. In: Novak, M.A., Petto, A.J. (Eds.), Through the Looking Glass: Issues of Psychological Well-Being in Captive Nonhuman

Primates. American Psychological Assoc., Washington, DC, pp. 78–92.

Coe, C.L., Rosenblum, L.A., 1984. Male dominance in the bonnet macaque: a malleable relationship. In: Barchas, P.R., Mendoza, S.P. (Eds.), Social Cohesion. Essays toward a Sociophysiological Perspective. Greenwood Press, Westport, CT, pp. 31–64.

Coelho, A.M., Carey, K.D., Shade, R.E., 1991. Assessing the effects of social environment on blood pressure and heart rates of baboons. Am. J. Primatol. 23, 257–267.

Collinge, N., 1989. Mirror reactions in a zoo colony of cebus monkeys. Zoo Biol. 8, 89–98.

Cooper, S.J., Hendrie, C.A., 1994. Ethology and Psychopharmacology. John Wiley & Sons, New York.

Coulon, J., 1975. Etude de la hierarchie sociale chez le cobaye domestique. Behaviour 53, 183–199.

Cowan, P.E., 1983. Exploration in small mammals: ethology and ecology. In: Archer, J., Birke, L.J.A. (Eds.), Exploration in Animals and Humans Van Nostrand Reinhold, United Kingdom, pp. 147–175.

Craig, W., 1918. Appetites and aversions as constituents of instincts. Biol. Bull. 34, 91–107.

Crockett, C.M., 1998. Psychological well–being of captive nonhuman primates: lessons from laboratory studies. In: Shepherson, D.J., Mellen, J.D., Hutchins, M. (Eds.), Second Nature: Environmental Enrichment for Captive Animals. Smithsonian Institution Press, Washington, DC, pp. 129–152.

Crockett, C.M., Bielitzky, J., Carey, A., Velez, A., 1989. Kong toys as enrichment devices for singly-caged macaques. Lab. Primate Newsl. 28, 21–22.

Crockett, C.M., Bowers, D.M., Bowden, D.M., Sackett, G.P., 1994. Sex differences in compatibility of pair-housed adult longtailed macaques. Am. J. Primatol. 32, 73–94.

Crockett, C., Bellanca, R.U., Bowers, C.L., Bowden, D.M., 1997. Grooming-contact bars provide social contact for individually caged laboratory macaques. Contemp. Top. Lab. Anim. Sci. 36, 53–60.

Crowcroft, P., 1973. Mice All Over. Chicago Zoological Society, Chicago, IL.

Csatádi, K., Kustos, K., Eiben, C.S., Bilko, A., Altbäcker, V., 2005. Even minimal human contact linked to nursing reduces fear responses toward humans in rabbits. Appl. Anim. Behav. Sci. 95, 123–128.

Dailey, J.W., McGlone, J.J., 1997. Oral/nasal/facial and other behaviors of sows kept individually outdoors on pasture, soil or indoors in gestation crates. Appl. Anim. Behav. Sci. 52, 25–43.

Damon, E.G., Eidson, A.F., Hobbs, C.H., Hahn, F.F., 1986. Effect of acclimation on nephrotoxic response of rats to uranium. Lab. Anim. Sci. 36, 24–27.

Dantzer, R., Kelley, K.W., 1989. Stress and immunity: an integrated view of relationships between the brain and the immune system. Life Sci. 44, 1995–2008.

Davis, H., Perusse, R., 1988. Human-based social interaction can reward a rat's behavior. Learn. Behav. 16 (1), 89–92.

Dawkins, M.S., 1989. Time budgets in red junglefowl as a baseline for the assessment of welfare in domestic fowl. Appl. Anim. Behav. Sci. 24, 77–80.

Dawkins, M.S., 1990. From an animal's point of view: motivation, fitness, and animal welfare. Behav. Brain Sci. 13, 1–61.

Dawkins, M.S., 1992. Animal Suffering: The Science of Animal Welfare, second ed. Chapman & Hall, London.

Deacon, R.M.J., 2006. Digging and marble burying in mice: simple methods for *in vivo* identification of biological impacts. Nat. Protocols 1 (1), 122–124.

DeLong, K.T., 1967. Population ecology of feral house mice. Ecology 48 (4), 611–634.

DeLuca, A.M., Kranda, K.C., 1992. Environmental enrichment. Lab. Anim. 21, 38–44.

DePass, L.R., Weil, C.S., Ballantyne, B., Lewis, S.C., Losco, P.E., Reid, J.B., et al., 1986. Influence of housing conditions for mice on the results of a dermal oncogenicity assay. Fundam. Appl. Toxicol. 7, 601–608.

de Passillé, A.M.B., Christopherson, R., Rushen, J., 1993. Nonnutritive sucking by the calf and postprandial secretion of insulin, CCK, and gastrin. Physiol. Behav. 54, 1069–1073.

DeSousa, A.A., Reis, R., Bento-Torres, J., Trevia, N., de Almeida Lins, N.A., Passos, A., et al., 2011. Influence of enriched environment on viral encephalitis outcomes: behavioral and neuropathological changes in albino Swiss mice. PLoS One 6 (1), e15597.

DiVincenti Jr., L., Wyatt, J.D., 2011. Pair housing of macaques in research facilities: a science-based review of benefits and risks. J. Am. Assoc. Lab. Anim. Sci. 50 (6), 856–863.

Doyle, L.A., Baker, K.C., Cox, L.D., 2008. Physiological and behavioral effects of social introduction on adult male rhesus macaques. Am. J. Primatol. 70 (6), 542–550.

Dufour, B.D., Adeola, O., Cheng, H.W., Donkin, S.S., Klein, J.D., Pajor, E.A., et al., 2010. Nutritional up-regulation of serotonin paradoxically induces compulsive behavior. Nutr. Neurosci. 13 (6), 256–264.

Duncan, I.J.H., 1978. The interpretation of preference tests in animal behaviour. Appl. Anim. Ethol. 4, 197–200.

Duncan, I.J.H., 1992. The effect of the researcher on the behaviour of poultry. In: Davis, H., Balfour, D. (Eds.), The Inevitable Bond. Cambridge University Press, Cambridge, pp. 285–294.

Duncan, I.J.H., Rushen, J., Lawrence, A.B., 1993. Conclusions and implications for animal welfare. In: Lawrence, A.B., Rushen, J. (Eds.), Stereotypic Animal Behaviour. Fundamentals and Applications to Welfare CAB International, Wallingford, United Kingdom, pp. 193–206.

Durschlag, M., Stauffacher, M., 1996. Effects of environmental enrichment on agonistic interactions and endocrine states in male Zur:ICR mice Second World Congress on Alternatives and Animal Use in the Life Sciences. Frame, Nottingham, England.

Dwyer, C., 2008. The Welfare of Sheep. Springer, Dodrecht, The Netherlands.

Eaton, G.G., Kelley, S.T., Axthelm, M.K., Iliff-Sizemore, S.A., 1994. Psychological well-being in paired adult female rhesus (*Macaca mulatta*). Am. J. Primatol. 33, 89–99.

Eisenberg, J.F., 1967. A comparative study in rodent ethology with emphasis on social behavior, I. Proc. U S Natl. Mus. 122 (3597), 1–50.

Eisenberg, J.F., Muckenhirn, N.A., Kuehn, R.E., 1972. The relation between ecology and social structure in primates. Science 176, 863–874.

Ekesbo, I., 2011. Farm Animal Behaviour: Characteristics for Assessment of Health and Welfare. CAB International, Wallingford, United Kingdom.

Ernst, K., Tuchscherer, M., Kanitz, E., Puppe, B., Manteuffel, G., 2006. Effects of attention and rewarded activity on immune parameters and wound healing in pigs. Physiol. Behav. 89, 448–456.

Erwin, J., 1979. Aggression in captive macaques: interaction of social and spatial factors. In: Erwin, J., Maple, T., Mitchell, G. (Eds.), Captivity and Behavior: Primates in Laboratories, Breeding Colonies, and Zoos. Van Nostrand Reinhold, New York, pp. 139–171.

Erwin, J., Deni, R., 1979. Strangers in a strange land: abnormal behavior or abnormal environments? In: Erwin, J., Maple, T., Mitchell, G. (Eds.), Captivity and Behavior: Primates in Laboratories, Breeding Colonies, and Zoos. Van Nostrand Reinhold, New York, pp. 1–28.

Erwin, J., Landon, J.G., 1992. Spacious biocontainment suites for chimpanzees in infectious disease research. In: Erwin, J., Landon, J.G. (Eds.), Chimpanzee Conservation and Public Health: Environments for the Future Diagnon/Bioqual, Rockville, MD, pp. 65–69.

European Directive, Annex III, Guidelines for Accommodation and Care of Animals, 2010. Council Directive 2010/63/EU on the approximation of laws, regulations, and administrative provisions of the member states regarding the protection of animals used for other scientific purposes. Off. J. Eur. Union L 276, 33–79.

Federation of Animal Science Societies (FASS), 2010. Guide for the Care and Use of Agricultural Animals in Research and Teaching. Savoy, IL.

Flannelly, K.L., Lore, R., 1977. Observations of the subterranean activity of domesticated and wild rats (Rattus norvegicus): a descriptive study. Physiol. Rec. 27, 315–329.

Fox, M.W., 1965. Environmental factors influencing stereotyped and allelomimetic behavior in animals. Lab. Anim. Care 15, 363–370.

Fox, M.W., 1968. Introduction: the concepts of normal and abnormal behavior. In: Fox, M. (Ed.), Abnormal Behavior in Animals. Saunders, London, pp. 1–5.

Fox, M.W., Bekoff, M., 1975. The behaviour of dogs. In: Hafez, E.S.E. (Ed.), The Behaviour of Domestic Animals. Willliams and Wilkins Co., Baltimore, MD, pp. 370.

Fragaszy, D.M., Adams-Curtis, L.E., 1991. Environmental challenges in groups of capuchins. In: Box, H.O. (Ed.), Primate Responses to Environmental Change Chapman & Hall, London, pp. 239–264.

Fragaszy, D.M., Mason, W.A., 1978. Response to novelty in Saimiri and Callicebus: influence of social context. Primates 19, 311–331.

Fraser, D., 1996. Preference and motivational testing to improve animal well-being. Lab. Anim. 25, 27–31.

Fraser, D., 2008. Understanding Animal Welfare: The Science in its Cultural Context. Wiley-Blackwell, United Kingdom.

Fraser, D., Phillips, P.A., Thompson, B.K., Tennessen, T., 1991. Effect of straw on the behavior of growing pigs. Appl. Anim. Behav. Sci. 30, 307–318.

Gao, W., Feddes, J.J.R., Robinson, F.E., Cook, H., 1994. Effects of stocking density on the incidence of usage of enrichment devices by White Leghorn hens. J. Appl. Poult. Res. 3, 336–341.

Garner, J.P., Weisker, S.M., Dufour, B., Mench, J.A., 2004. Barbering (fur and whisker trimming) by laboratory mice as a model of human trichotillomania and obsessive-compulsive spectrum disorders. Comp. Med. 54 (2), 216–224.

Garner, J.P., Thogerson, C.M., Dufour, B.D., Würbel, H., Murray, J.D., Mench, J.A., 2011. Reverse-translational biomarker validation of abnormal repetitive behaviors in mice: an illustration of the 4P's modeling approach. Behav. Brain Res. 219 (2), 189–196.

Gaskill, B.N., Rohr, S.A., Pajor, E.A., Lucas, J.R., Garner, J.P., 2009. Some like it hot: mouse temperature preferences in laboratory housing. Appl. Anim. Behav. Sci. 116, 279–285.

Gaskill, B.N., Winnicker, C.L., Garner, J.P., et al., 2011a. Energy reallocation to breeding performance through improved behavioral thermoregulation. J. Am. Assoc. Lab. Anim. Sci. 50 (5), 741.

Gaskill, B.N., Rohr, S.A., Pajor, E.A., Lucas, J.R., Garner, J.P., 2011b. Working with what you've got: changes in thermal preference and behavior in mice with or without nesting material. J. Therm. Biol. 36, 1193–1199.

Gaskill, B.N., Winnicker, C., Garner, J.P., Pritchett-Corning, K.R., 2011c. The naked truth: breeding performance in outbred and inbred strains of nude mice with and without nesting material. J. Am. Assoc. Lab. Anim. Sci. 50 (5), 741.

Gaskill, B.N., Gordon, C.J., Pajor, E.A., Lucas, J.R., Davis, J.K., Garner, J.P., 2012. Heat or insulation: behavioral titration of mouse preference for warmth or access to a nest. PLoS One 7 (3), e32799. http://dx.doi.org/10.1371/journal.pone.0032799.

Gattermann, R., Fritzsche, P., Neumann, K., Al-Hussein, I., Kayser, A., Abiad, M., et al., 2001. Notes on the current distribution and the ecology of wild golden hamsters (Mesocricetus auratus). J. Zool. 254 (3), 359–365.

Gentle, M.J., Hunter, L.N., 1990. Physiological and behavioural responses associated with feather removal in Gallus gallus var. domesticus. Res. Vet. Sci. 50, 95–101.

Gerold, S., Huisinga, E., Iglauer, F., Kurzawa, A., Morankic, A., Reimers, S., 1997. Influence of feeding hay on the alopecia of breeding guinea pigs. Zentrale Veterinarmed A 44 (6), 341–348.

Gilbert, M.H., Baker, K.C., 2011. Social buffering in adult male rhesus macaques (Macaca mulatta): effects of stressful events in single versus pair housing. J. Med. Primatol. 40 (2), 71–78.

Gomez-Sanchez, E.P., Gomez-Sanchez, C.E., 1991. 19-Nordeoxy corticosterone, aldosterone, and corticosterone excretion in sequential urine samples from male and female rats. Steroids 56 (8), 451–454.

Gonyou, H.W., Keeling, L.J. (Eds.), 2001. Social Behaviour in Domestic Animals. CAB International, Wallingford, United Kingdom.

Gonzalez, C.A., Coe, C.L., Levine, S., 1982. Cortisol responses under different housing conditions in female squirrel monkeys. Psychoneuroendocrin 7, 209–216.

Gordon, C.J., Becker, P., Ali, J.S., 1998. Behavioral thermoregulatory responses of single- and group-housed mice. Physiol. Behav. 65 (2), 255–262.

Gottlieb, D., McCowan, B., 2011. Assessment of the efficacy of three types of foraging enrichment for rhesus macaques (Macaca mulatta). J. Am. Assoc. Lab. An. Sci. 50, 1–7.

Gottlieb, D., Capitanio, J., McCowan, B., 2013a. Risk factors for stereotypy and self-abusive behavior in rhesus macaques (Macaca mulatta); animal's history, current environment, and personality. Am. J. Primatol. 75, 995–1008.

Gottlieb, D., Coleman, K., McCowan, B., 2013b. The effects of predictability in daily husbandry routines on captive rhesus macaques (Macaca mulatta). Appl. Anim. Behav. Sci. 143, 117–127.

Grandin, T. (Ed.), 2007. Livestock Handling and Transport, third ed. CAB International, Wallingford, United Kingdom.

Grandin, T., Deesing, M.J., 2013. Genetics and the Behavior of Domestic Animals, second ed. Academic Press, San Diego, CA.

Gray, J.A., 1991. The Psychology of Fear and Stress. Cambridge University Press, Cambridge.

Gray, S., Hurst, J.L., 1995. The effects of cage cleaning on aggression within groups of male laboratory mice. Anim. Behav. 49, 821–826.

Greenberg, G., 1972. The effects of ambient temperature and population density on aggression in two inbred strains of mice, Mus musculus. Behaviour 42, 119–130.

Greiveldinger, L., Vessier, I., Boissy, A., 2007. Emotional experience in sheep: predictability of a sudden event lowers subsequent emotional responses. Physiol. Behav. 92, 675–683.

Grelk, D.F., Papson, B.A., Cole, J.E., Rowe, F.A., 1974. The influence of caging conditions and hormone treatments on fighting in male and female hamsters. Hormones Behav. 5 (4), 355–366.

Griffis, D.M., Martin, A.L., Perlman, J.E., Bloomsmith, M.A., 2013. Play caging benefits the behavior of singly housed laboratory rhesus macaques (Macaca mulatta). J. Am. Assoc. Lab. Anim. Sci. 52 (5), 534–540.

Gross, A.N.-M., Engel, A.K.J., Würbel, H., 2011. Simply a nest? Effects of different enrichments on stereotypic and anxiety-related behaviour in mice. Appl. Anim. Behav. Sci. 134, 239–245.

Guerra, R.F., Ades, C., 2002. An analysis of travel costs on transport of load and nest building in golden hamster. Behav. Process. 57 (1), 7–28.

Gust, D.A., Swenson, R.B., Smith, M.B., Sikes, J., 1988. An apparatus and procedure for studying the choice component of foraging in a captive group of chimpanzees. Primates 29, 139–143.

Gust, D.A., Gordon, T.P., Brodie, A.R., McClure, H.M., 1994. Effect of a preferred companion in modulating stress in adult female rhesus monkeys. Physiol. Behav. 55, 681–684.

Gust, D.A., Gordon, T.P., Brodie, A.R., McClure, H.M., 1996. Effect of companions in modulating stress associated with new group formation in juvenile rhesus macaques. Physiol. Behav. 59, 941–945.

Haemisch, A., Voss, T., Gärtner, K., 1994. Effects of environmental enrichment on aggressive behaviour, dominance hierarchies, and endocrine state in male DBA/2J mice. Physiol. Behav. 56 (5), 1041–1048.

Haley, D.B., Rushen, J., Duncan, I.J.H., Widowski, T.M., de Passillé, A.-M., 1998. Effects of resistance to milk flow and the provision of hay on nonnutritive suckling by dairy calves. J. Dairy Sci. 81 2165–2127.

Harlander-Matauschek, A., Piepho, H.P., Bessei, W., 2006. The effect of feather eating on feed passage in laying hens. Poult. Sci. 85, 21–25.

Harlow, H.F., Harlow, M.K., 1962. The effects of rearing conditions on behavior. Bull. Menninger Clin. 26, 213–224.

Hart, L.A., 1994. Opportunities for environmental enrichment in the laboratory. Lab. Anim. 23, 24–27.

Hauschka, T.S., 1952. Whisker eating mice. J. Hered. 43, 77–80.

Hauzenberger, A.R., Gebhardt-Henrich, S.G., Steiger, A., 2006. The influence of bedding depth on behaviour in golden hamsters (*Mesocricetus auratus*). Appl. Anim. Behav. Sci. 100, 280–294.

Hediger, H., 1969. The Psychology and Behaviour of Animals in Zoos and Circuses. Dover Publications, Inc., New York.

Held, S.D.E., Turner, R.J., Wootton, R.J., 1995. Choices of laboratory rabbits for individual or group-housing. Appl. Anim. Behav. Sci. 46, 81–91.

Hemsworth, P.B., Coleman, G.J., 2011. Human–Livestock Interactions. The Stockperson and the Productivity and Welfare of Intensively Farmed Animals, second ed. CAB International, Wallingford, United Kingdom.

Hennessy, M.B., Williams, M.T., Miller, D.D., Douglas, C.W., Voith, V.L., 1998. Influence of male and female petters on plasma cortisol and behaviour: can human interaction reduce the stress of dogs in a public animal shelter? Appl. Anim. Behav. Sci. 61, 63–77.

Herbers, J.M., 1981. Time resources and laziness in animals. Oecologia 49, 252–262.

Hess, S.E., Rohr, S., Dufour, B.D., Gaskill, B.N., Pajor, E.A., Garner, J.P., 2008. Home improvement: C57BL/6J mice given more naturalistic nesting materials build better nests. J. Am. Assoc. Lab. Anim. Sci. 47 (6), 25–31.

Hetts, S., Clark, J.D., Calpin, J.P., Arnold, C.E., Mateo, J.M., 1992. Influence of housing conditions on beagle behavior. Appl. Anim. Behav. Sci. 34, 137–155.

Hite, M., Hanson, H.M., Bohidar, N.R., Conti, P.A., Mattis, P.A., 1977. Effect of cage size on patterns of activity and health of beagle dogs. Lab. Anim. Sci. 27, 60–64.

Hobbs, B.A., Kozubal, W., Nebiar, F.F., 1997. Evaluation of objects for environmental enrichment of mice. Contemp. Top. 36, 69–71.

Hohmann, C.F., Hodges, A., Beard, N., Aneni, J., 2013. Effects of brief stress exposure during early postnatal development in balb/CByJ mice: I. Behavioral characterization. Dev. Psychobiol 55 (3), 283–293.

Holson, R.R., Scallet, A.C., Ali, S.F., Turner, B.B., 1991. 'Isolation stress' revisited: isolation-rearing effects depend on animal care methods. Physiol. Behav. 49 (6), 1107–1118.

Houpt, K.A., 2010. Domestic Animal Behavior for Veterinarians and Animal Scientists, fifth ed. Blackwell, Ames, IA.

Howerton, C., Garner, J., Mench, J.A., 2008. Effects of a running wheel-igloo enrichment on aggression, hierarchy linearity, and stereotypy in group-housed male CD-1 (ICR) mice. Appl. Anim. Behav. Sci. 115 (1), 90–103.

Huang, D., Hazlett, B.A., 1974. Submissive distance in Golden-Hamster *Mesocricetus auratus*. Anim. Behav. 22 (2), 467–472.

Hubrecht, R.C., 1993. A comparison of social and environmental enrichment methods for laboratory housed dogs. Appl. Anim. Behav. Sci. 37, 345–361.

Hubrecht, R.C., Serpell, J.A., Poole, T.B., 1992. Correlates of pen size and housing conditions on the behaviour of kenneled dogs. Appl. Anim. Behav. Sci. 34, 365–383.

Hughes, H.C., Campbell, S., Kenney, C., 1989. The effects of cage size and pair housing on exercise of beagle dogs. Lab. Anim. Sci. 39, 302–305.

Hughes, R., 1968. Behaviour of male and female rats with free choice of two environments differing in novelty. Anim. Behav. 16, 92–96.

Hurst, J.L., Fang, J., Barnard, C., 1993. The role of substrate odours in maintaining social tolerance between male house mice, *Mus musculus domesticus*. Anim. Behav. 45 (5), 997–1006.

Hurst, J.L., Barnard, C.J., Hare, R., Wheeldon, E.B., West, C.D., 1996. Housing and welfare in laboratory rats: time-budgeting and pathophysiology in single-sex groups. Anim. Behav. 52, 335–360.

Hurst, J.L., Barnard, C.J., Nevison, C.M., West, C.D., 1997. Housing and welfare in laboratory rats: welfare implications of isolation and social contact among caged males. Anim. Welf. 6 (4), 329–347.

Hurst, J.L., Barnard, C.J., Nevison, C.M., West, C.D., 1998. Housing and welfare in laboratory rats: the welfare implications of social isolation and social contact among females. Anim. Welf. 7 (2), 121–136.

Hutchinson, E.K., Avery, A.C., Vandewoude, S., 2012. Environmental enrichment during rearing alters corticosterone levels, thymocyte numbers, and aggression in female BALB/c mice. J. Am. Assoc. Lab. Anim. Sci. 51 (1), 18–24.

Jegstrup, I.M., Vestergaard, R., Vach, W., Ritskes-Hoitinga, M., 2005. Nest-building behaviour in male rats from three inbred strains: BN/HsdCpb, BDIX/OrlIco and LEW/Mol. Anim. Welf. 14 (2), 149–156.

Jennings, M., Batchelor, G.R., Brain, P.F., Dick, A., Elliott, H., Francis, R.J., et al., 1998. Refining rodent husbandry: the mouse – report of the rodent refinement working party. Lab. Anim. 32 (3), 233–259.

Jennings, M., Prescott, M.J., (eds.) 2009. Refinements in husbandry, care and common procedures for non-human primates. Ninth report of the BVAAWF/FRAME/RSPCA/UFAW Joint Working Group on Refinement. Lab. Anim. 43 (Suppl. 1) S1:1–S1:47.

Jensen, P. (Ed.), 2009. The Ethology of Domestic Animals. CAB International, Wallingford, United Kingdom.

Jensen, G.D., Blanton, F.L., Gribble, D.H., 1980. Older monkeys' (*Macaca radiata*) response to new group formation: behavior, reproduction, and mortality. Exp. Gerontol. 15, 399–406.

Jerome, C.P., Szostak, L., 1987. Environmental enrichment for adult, female baboons (*Papio anubis*). Lab. Anim. Sci. 37, 508–509.

Johnston, R.E., Derzie, A., Chiang, G., Jernigan, P., Lee, H.-C., 1993. Individual scent signatures in golden hamsters: evidence for specialization of function. Anim. Behav. 45 (6), 1061–1070.

Jones, R.B., 1996. Fear and adaptability in poultry: insights, implications, and imperatives. World Poult. Sci. J. 52, 131–174.

Kalmendal, R., Bessei, W., 2012. The preference for high-fiber feed in laying hens divergently selected on feather pecking. Poult. Sci. 91, 1785–1789.

Kannan, G., Mench, J.A., 1996. Influence of different handling methods and crating periods on plasma corticosterone concentrations in broilers. Br. Poult. Sci. 37, 21–31.

Kaplan, J.R., Manning, P., Zucker, E., 1980. Reduction of mortality due to fighting in a colony of rhesus monkeys (*Macaca mulatta*). Lab. Anim. Sci. 30, 565–570.

Karsh, E.B., Turner, D.C., 1988. The human–cat relationship. In: Turner, D.C., Bateson, P. (Eds.), The Domestic Cat: The Biology of its Behaviour. Cambridge University Press, New York, pp. 159–177.

Kawakami, K., Takeuchi, T., Yamaguchi, S., Ago, A., Nomura, M., Gonda, T., et al., 2003. Preference of guinea pigs for bedding materials: wood shavings versus paper cutting sheet. Exp. Anim. 52 (1), 11–15.

Kempermann, G., Kuhn, H.G., Gage, F.H., 1997. More hippocampal neurons in adult mice living in an enriched environment. Nature 386 (6624), 493–495.

Kerr, B., Silva, P.A., Walz, K., Young, J.I., 2010. Unconventional transcriptional response to environmental enrichment in a mouse model of Rett syndrome. PLoS One 5, e11534.

Kessel-Davenport, A.L., Brent, L., 1994. Effects of an enriched exercise cage on the behaviors of singly housed baboons (Papio sp.). Am. J. Primatol. 33, 220.

Kikusui, T., Takeuchi, Y., Mori, Y., 2004. Early weaning induces anxiety and aggression in adult mice. Physiol. Behav. 81 (1), 37–42.

Kikusui, T., Winslow, J.T., Mori, Y., 2006. Social buffering: relief from stress and anxiety. Phil. Trans. R. Soc. B 361, 2215–2228.

Kingston, S.G., Hoffman-Goetz, L., 1996. Effect of environmental enrichment and housing density on immune system reactivity to acute exercise stress. Physiol. Behav. 60, 145–150.

Kitchen, A.M., Martin, A.A., 1996. The effects of cage size and complexity on the behaviour of captive common marmosets, Callithrix jacchus jacchus. Lab. Anim. 30, 317–326.

Knowles, T.G., Wilkins, L.J., 1998. The problem of broken bones during the handling of laying hens – a review. Poult. Sci. 77 1798–1793.

Kohn, D.F., Barthold, S.W., 1984. Biology and diseases of rats. In: Fox, J.G., Cohen, B.J., Loew, F.M. (Eds.), Laboratory Animal Medicine. Academic Press, New York, pp. 91–122.

König, B., 2012. The behaviour of the house mouse. In: Hedrich, H.J. (Ed.), The Laboratory Mouse. Academic Press, New York, pp. 367–381.

Kuhnen, G., 2002. Comfortable quarters for hamsters in research institutions. In: Reinhardt, V., Reinhardt, A. (Eds.), Comfortable Quarters for Laboratory Animals. Animal Welfare Institute, Washington, DC, pp. 33–37.

Kunkel, P., Kunkel, I., 1964. Beitrage zue Thologie des Hausmeerschweinchens, Cavia Porcellus. Bull. Ecol. Soc. Am., 52–54.

Kunzl, C., Sachser, N., 1999. The behavioral endocrinology of domestication: a comparison between the domestic guinea pig (Cavia aperea f. porcellus) and its wild ancestor, the cavy (Cavia aperea). Horm. Behav. 35, 28–37.

Kyriazakis, I., Tollcamp, B., 2011. Hunger and thirst. In: Appleby, M.C., Mench, J.A., Olsson, I.A.S., Hughes, B.O. (Eds.), Animal Welfare, second ed. CAB International, Wallingford, United Kingdom, pp. 44–63.

Ladewig, J., de Passillé, A.M., Rushen, J., Schouten, W., Terlouw, E.M.C., Von Borell, E., 1993. Stress and the physiological correlates of stereotypic behavior. In: Lawrence, A.B., Rushen, J. (Eds.), Stereotypic Animal Behaviour. Fundamentals and Applications to Welfare. CAB International, Wallingford, United Kingdom, pp. 97–118.

Lam, K., Rupniak, N.M.J., Iversen, S.D., 1991. Use of a grooming and foraging substrate to reduce cage stereotypies in macaques. J. Med. Primatol. 20, 104–109.

Lambeth, S.P., Bloomsmith, M.A., 1992. Mirror as enrichment for captive chimpanzees (Pan troglodytes). Lab. Anim. Sci. 42, 261–266.

Latham, N., Mason, G., 2004. From house mouse to mouse house: the behavioural biology of free-living Mus musculus and its implications in the laboratory. Appl. Anim. Behav. Sci. 86 (3–4), 261–289.

Lawlor, M.M., 1984. Behavioural approaches to rodent management. in: Standards in Laboratory Animal Management, Proceedings of a LASA/UFAW Symposium. Universities Federation for Animal Welfare, Potters Bar, United Kingdom, pp. 40–49.

Lawrence, A.B., Rushen, J. (Eds.), 1993. Stereotypic Animal Behaviour. Fundamentals and Applications to Welfare. CAB International, Wallingford, Oxon, United Kingdom.

Lay, D.C., Fulton, R.M., Hester, P.Y., Karcher, D.M., Kjaer, J.B., Mench, J.A., et al., 2011. Hen welfare in different housing systems. Poult. Sci. 90, 278–294.

Lee, C.T., 1972. Development of nest-building behavior in inbred mice. J. Gen. Psychol. 87, 13.

Lee, C.T., 1973. Genetic analysis of nest building behavior in laboratory mice (Mus-musculus). Behav. Genet. 3 (3), 247–256.

Lee, C.T., Wong, P.T.P., 1970. Temperature effect and strain differences in the nest-building behavior of inbred mice. Psychonom. Sci. 20 (1), 9.

Lerwill, C.J., Makings, P., 1971. Agonistic behavior of golden-hamster Mesocricetus auratus (Waterhouse). Anim. Behav. 19 (4), 714–721.

Lindberg, A.C., Nicol, C.J., 1994. An evaluation of the effect of operant feeders on welfare of hens maintained on litter. Appl. Anim. Behav. Sci. 41, 211–227.

Line, S.W., Houghton, P., 1987. Influence of an environmental enrichment device on general behavior and appetite in rhesus macaques. Lab. Anim. Sci. 37, 508.

Line, S.W., Morgan, K.N., 1991. The effects of two novel objects on the behavior of singly caged adult rhesus macaques. Lab. Anim. Sci. 41, 365–369.

Line, S.W., Morgan, K.N., Markowitz, H., Roberts, J., Riddell, M., 1990a. Behavioral responses of female long-tailed macaques (Macaca fascicularis) to pair formation. Lab. Prim. News 29, 1–5.

Line, S.W., Morgan, K.N., Roberts, J.A., Markowitz, H., 1990b. Preliminary comments on resocialization of aged macaques. Lab. Prim. News 29, 8–12.

Line, S.W., Markowitz, H., Morgan, K.N., Strong, S., 1991a. Effects of cage size and environmental enrichment on behavioral and physiological responses of rhesus macaques to the stress of daily events. In: Novak, M.A., Petto, A.J. (Eds.), Through the Looking Glass: Issues of Psychological Well-Being in Captive Nonhuman Primates. American Psychological Association, Washington, DC, pp. 160–179.

Line, S.W., Morgan, K.N., Markowitz, H., 1991b. Simple toys do not alter the behavior of aged rhesus monkeys. Zoo Biol. 10, 473–484.

Litterst, C.I., 1974. Mechanically self-induced muzzle alopecia in lab mice. Lab. Anim. Sci. 24, 806–809.

Lockley, R.M., 1961. Social structure and stress in the rabbit warren. J. Anim. Ethol. 30 (2), 385–423.

Lofgren, J.L., Wong, C., Hayward, A., Karas, A.Z., Morales, S., Quintana, P., et al., 2010. Innovative social rabbit housing. J. Am. Assoc. Lab. Anim. Sci. 49 (5) 659–659.

Long, S.Y., 1972. Hair-nibbling and whisker-trimming as indicators of social hierarchy in mice. Anim. Behav. 20, 10–12.

Lore, R.K., Schultz, L.A., 1989. The ecology of wild rats: applications in the laboratory In: Blanchard, R.J. Brain, D.C. Blanchard, S. Parmigiani, S. (Eds.), Ethoexperimental Approaches to the Study of Behavior, vol. 48. Kluwer Academic Publishing, Dordrecht, The Netherlands, pp. 607–622.

Lott, D.F., 1984. Intraspecific variation in the social systems of wild vertebrates. Behaviour 88 (3/4), 266–325.

Love, J., Hammond, K., 1991. Group-housing rabbits. Lab Anim. 20 (8), 37–43.

Love, J.A., 1995. Implementation of innovative housing for laboratory animals. In: Johnston, N.E. (Ed.), Proceedings of the Animals in Science Conference: Perspectives on Their Use, Care, and Welfare. Monash University Press, Melbourne, Australia, p. 168.

Loveridge, G.G., 1998. Environmentally enriched dog housing. Appl. Anim. Behav. Sci. 59, 101.

Lynch, J.J., Gantt, W., 1968. The heart rate component of the social reflex in dogs: the conditional effect of petting and person. Conditioned Reflex 3, 69–80.

Lynch, J.J., Hinch, G.N., Adams, D.B., 1992. The Behaviour of Sheep. CAB International, Wallingford, United Kingdom.

Macdonald, D.W., Tew, T.E., Todd, I.A., Garner, J.P., Johnson, P.J., 2000. Arable habitat use by wood mice (*Apodemus sylvaticus*). 3. A farm-scale experiment on the effects of crop rotation. J. Zool. 250, 313–320.

Maki, S., Bloomsmith, M.A., 1989. Uprooted trees facilitate the psychological well-being of captive chimpanzees. Zoo Biol. 8, 79–87.

Malik, I., Southwick, C.H., 1988. Feeding behavior and activity patterns of rhesus monkeys (*Macaca mulatta*) at Tughlaqabad, India. In: Fa, J.E., Southwick, C.H. (Eds.), Ecology and Behavior of Food-Enhanced Primate Groups. Alan R. Liss, New York, pp. 95–111.

Mandrell, T.D., 1996. Personnel considerations: Hiring, training, attitudes. In: Krulisch, L., Mayer, S., Simmonds, R.C. (Eds.), The Human/Research Animal Relationship Scientists. Center for Animal Welfare, Greenbelt, MD, pp. 99–104.

Manning, P.J., Wagner, J.E., et al., 1984. Biology and diseases of guinea pigs. In: Fox, J.G., Cohen, B.J., Loew, F.M. (Eds.), Laboratory Animal Medicine. Academic Press, New York. pp. 149–181.

Manser, C., 1992. The Assessment of Stress in Laboratory Animals. RSPCA, Horsham, United Kingdom.

Manser, C.E., Morris, T.H., Broom, D.M., 1995. An investigation into the effects of solid or grid cage flooring on the welfare of laboratory rats. Lab. Anims. 29, 353–365.

Manser, C.E., Elliott, H., Morris, T.H., Broom, D.M., 1996. The use of a novel operant test to determine the strength of preference for flooring in laboratory rats. Lab. Anims. 30, 1–6.

Manser, C.E., Broom, D.M., Overend, P., Morris, T.H., 1998a. Investigations into the preference of laboratory rats for nest-boxes and nesting materials. Lab. Anims. 32, 23–35.

Manser, C.E., Broom, D.M., Overend, P., Morris, T.H., 1998b. Operant studies to determine the strength of preference in laboratory rats for nest-boxes and nesting materials. Lab. Anims. 32 (1), 36–41.

Manteuffel, G., Langbein, J., Puppe, B., 2009. Increasing farm animal welfare by positively motivated instrumental behavior. Appl. Anim. Behav. Sci. 118, 191–198.

Marchant-Forde, J., 2009. The Welfare of Pigs. Springer, Dodrecht, The Netherlands.

Markowitz, H., Gavazzi, A., 1995. Eleven principles for improving the quality of captive animal life. Lab. Anim. 24, 30–33.

Marriott, B.M., 1988. Time budgets of rhesus monkeys (*Macaca mulatta*) in a forest habitat in Nepal and on Cayo Santiago. In: Fa, J.E., Southwick, C.H. (Eds.), Ecology and Behavior of Food-Enhanced Primate Groups. Alan R. Liss, New York, pp. 125–149.

Mason, G., Latham, N., 2004. Can't stop, won't stoop: is stereotypy a reliable welfare indicator? Anim. Welf. 13, S57–S69.

Mason, G., McFarland, D.M., Garner, J., 1998. A demanding task using economic techniques to assess animal priorities. Anim. Behav. 55, 1071–1075.

Mason, G.J., 1991. Stereotypies: a critical review. Anim. Behav. 41, 1015–1037.

Mason, G.J., Wilson, D., Hampton, C., Würbel, H., 2004. Non-invasively assessing disturbance and stress in laboratory rats by scoring chromodacryorrhoea. ATLA 32 (S1), 153–159.

McClure, D.E., Thomson, J.L., 1992. Cage enrichment for hamsters housed in suspended wire cages. Contemp. Top. Lab. Anim. Sci. 31, 33.

McCully, C.L., Godwin, K.S., Brown, P., Mandrell, T., Bayne, K., Southers, J., et al., 1992. A social housing strategy for rhesus monkeys used frequently in biomedical research. Contemp. Top. Lab. Anim. Sci. 31, 33–34.

McGreevy, P., 2012. Equine Behavior: A Guide for Veterinarians and Equine Scientists. Saunders, Philadelphia, PA.

McIntyre, D., Petto, A.J., 1993. Effect of group size on behavior of group-housed female rhesus macaques (*Macaca mulatta*). Lab. Prim. Newsl. 32, 1–4.

Meehan, A.P., 1984. Rats and Mice: Their Biology and Control. Brown Knight and Truscott Ltd., Tonbridge, Kent, United Kingdom.

Mench, J.A., 1994. Environmental enrichment and exploration. Lab. Anim. 23, 38–41.

Mench, J.A., 1988. The development of aggressive behavior in male broiler chicks: a comparison with laying-type males and the effects of feed restriction. Appl. Anim. Behav. Sci. 21, 233–242.

Mench, J.A., 1998. Environmental enrichment and the importance of exploratory behavior. In: Shepherdson, D.J., Mellen, J.D., Hutchins, M. (Eds.), Second Nature: Environmental Enrichment for Captive Animals. Smithsonian Institution Press, Washington, DC, pp. 30–46.

Mench, J.A., 1999. Ethics, animal welfare, and transgenic farm animals. In: Murray, J.D., Anderson, G.B., Oberbauer, A.M., McGloughlin, M.M. (Eds.), Transgenic Animals in Agriculture. CAB International, Wallingford, United Kingdom, pp. 251–268.

Mench, J.A., Blatchford, R.A., 2013. Birds as laboratory animals. In: Bayne, K., Turner, P.V. (Eds.), Laboratory Animal Welfare. Elsevier, San Diego, CA, pp. 279–297.

Mench, J.A., Mason, G.J., 1997. Behaviour. In: Appleby, M.C., Hughes, B.O. (Eds.), Animal Welfare. CAB International, Wallingford, United Kingdom, pp. 127–143.

Mench, J., Newberry, R., Millman, S., Tucker, C., Katz, L., 2010. Environmental enrichment Guide for the Care and Use of Agricultural Animals in Research and Teaching. FASS, Savoy, IL, pp. 30–43.

Mertens, P.A., Unshelm, J., 1991. Effects of group and individual housing on the behavior of kenneled dogs in animal shelters. Anthrozoos 9, 40–51.

Meunier, L.D., Gilmore, K.M., Watson, E.S., Merkt, J.E., 2012. Evaluation of Canine Behaviors and Time Budgets during Three Different Exercise Scenarios [Abstract]. American Association of Laboratory Animal Science meeting, Minneapolis, MN.

Meyer, D., 1995. Environmental enrichment: creating a happy environment in the animal house. In: Johnston, N. (Ed.), Animals in Science. Monash University Press, Melbourne, Australia, pp. 257–262.

Millar, S.K., Evans, S., Chamove, A.S., 1988. Older offspring contact novel objects soonest in callitrichid families. Biol. Behav. 13, 82–96.

Milligan, S.R., Sales, G.D., Khirnykh, K., 1993. Sound levels in rooms housing laboratory animals: an uncontrolled daily variable. Physiol. Behav. 53, 1067–1075.

Mills, D.S., McDonnell, S.M., 2005. The Domestic Horse: The Origins, Development, and Management of its Behaviour. Cambridge University Press, Cambridge, United Kingdom.

Milton, K., 1980. The Foraging Strategies of Howler Monkeys: A Study in Primate Economics. Columbia University Press, New York.

Minier, D.E., Tatum, L., Gottlieb, D.H., Cameron, A., McCowan, B., 2011. Human-directed contra-aggression training using positive reinforcement with single and multiple trainers for indoor-housed rhesus macaques. J. Appl. Anim. Behav. Sci. 132, 178–186.

Mitchell, G., 1968. Persistent behavior pathology in rhesus monkeys following early social isolation. Folia Primatol. 8, 132–147.

Moons, C.P.H., Breugelmans, S., Cassiman, N., Kalmar, I.D., Peremans, K., Hermans, K., et al., 2012. The effect of different working definitions on behavioral research involving stereotypies in Mongolian gerbils (*Meriones unguiculatus*). J. Am. Assoc. Lab. Anim. Sci. 51 (2), 170–176.

Morgan, K.N., Tromborg, C.T., 2007. Sources of stress in captivity. Appl. Anim. Behav. Sci. 102 (3–4), 262–302.

Morton, D.B., 1993. Refinements in rabbit husbandry: second report of the BVAAWF/FRAME/RSPCA/UFAW joint working group on refinement. Lab. Anim. 27, 301–329.

Mulder, G.B., Pritchett-Corning, K.R., Gramlich, M.A., Crocker, A.E., 2010. Method of feed presentation affects the growth of Mongolian gerbils (*Meriones unguiculatus*). J. Am. Assoc. Lab. Anim. Sci. 49 (1), 36–39.

Murphy, L.B., 1977. Responses of domestic fowl to novel food and objects. Appl. Anim. Ethol. 3, 335–349.

Nagel, R., Stauffacher, M., 1994. Ethologische Grundlagen zur Beurteilung der Tiergerechtheit der Haltung von Ratten in Vollgitterkafigen. Tierlaboratorium 17, 119–132.

National Health and Medical Research Council, Australian Government, 2008. Guidelines to Promote the Wellbeing of Animals Used for Scientific Purposes: The Assessment and Alleviation of Pain and Distress in Research Animals. <www.nhmrc.gov.au/guidelines/publications/ea18>.

National Institutes of Health (NIH), 1991. Nonhuman Primate Intramural Management Plan. National Institutes of Health, Bethesda, MA.

National Research Council (NRC), 1996. Guide for the Care and Use of Laboratory Animals. National Academy Press, Washington, DC.

National Research Council (NRC), 2011. Guide for the Care and Use of Laboratory Animals. National Academy Press, Washington, DC.

Neamand, J., Sweeny, W.T., Creamer, A.A., Conti, P.A., 1975. Cage activity in the laboratory beagle: a preliminary study to evaluate a method of comparing cage size to physical activity. Lab. Anim. Sci. 25, 180–183.

Newberry, R.C., 1995. Environmental enrichment: increasing the biological relevance of captive environments. Appl. Anim. Behav. Sci. 44, 229–243.

Newberry, R.C., 1999. Why chickens cross the road: exploratory behaviour in young domestic fowl. Appl. Anim. Behav. Sci. 63, 311–321.

Newton, W.M., 1972. An evaluation of the effects of various degrees of long-term confinement on adult beagle dogs. Lab. Anim. Sci. 22, 860–864.

Nicol, C.J., Guilford, T., 1991. Exploratory activity as a measure of motivation in deprived hens. Anim. Behav. 41, 333–341.

Noller, C.M., Szeto, A., Mendez, A.J., Llabre, M.M., Gonzales, J.A., Rossetti, M.A., et al., 2013. The influence of social environment on endocrine, cardiovascular and tissue responses in the rabbit. Inter. J. Psychophysiol. 88 (3), 282–288.

Noonan, D., 1994. The guinea-pig (Cavia porcellus). ANZCCART News 7 Insert.

Nørgaard-Nielsen, G., Vestergaard, K., Simonsen, H.B., 1993. Effects of rearing experience and stimulus enrichment on feather damage in laying hens. Appl. Anim. Behav. Sci. 38, 345–352.

North, D., 1999. The guinea pig. In: Poole, T.B. (Ed.), The UFAW Handbook on the Care and Management of Laboratory Animals, seventh ed. Blackwell Science, Oxford, UK, pp. 367–388.

Novak, M., Drewson, K.H., 1989. Enriching the lives of captive primates: issues and problems. In: Segal, E. (Ed.), Housing, Care, and Psychological Well-being of Captive and Laboratory Primates. Noyes Publications, Park Ridge, NJ, pp. 161–182.

Novak, M.A., Hamel, A.F., Kelly, B.J., Dettmer, A.M., Meyer, J.S., 2013. Stress, the HPA axis and nonhuman primate well-being: a review. Appl. Anim. Behav. Sci. 143 (2), 135–149.

O'Neill, P., 1988. Developing effective social and environment enrichment strategies for macaques in captive groups. Lab. Anim. 17, 23–26.

O'Neill, P., 1989. A room with a view for captive primates: issues, goals, related research, and strategies. In: Segal, E. (Ed.), Housing, Care, and Psychological Well-being of Captive and Laboratory Primates. Noyes Publications, Park Ridge, NJ, pp. 135–160.

O'Neill-Wagner, P.L., Wright, A.C., Weed, J.L., 1997. Curious response of three monkey species to mirrors. AZAA Regional Conf. Proc., pp. 95–101.

Overall, K.L., Dyer, K., 2005. Enrichment strategies for laboratory animals from the viewpoint of clinical veterinary behavioral medicine: emphasis on cats and dogs. ILAR J. 46, 202–216.

Paquette, D., Prescott, J., 1988. Use of novel objects to enhance environments of captive chimpanzees. Zoo Biol. 7, 15–23.

Patterson-Kane, E.C., Harper, D.N., Hunt, M., 2001. The cage preferences of laboratory rats. Lab. Anim. 35 (1), 74–79.

Patterson-Kane, E.G., Hunt, M., Harper, D., 2002. Rats demand social contact. Anim. Welf. 11 (3), 327–332.

Paulk, H.H., Dienske, H., Ribbens, L.G., 1977. Abnormal behavior in relation to cage size in rhesus monkeys. J. Abnorm. Psychol. 86, 87–92.

Pellis, S.M., Pellis, V.C., 1987. Play-fighting differs from serious fighting in both target of attack and tactics of fighting in the laboratory rat Rattus norvegicus. Aggressive Behav. 13 (4), 227–242.

Pettijohn, T.F., Barkes, B.M., 1978. Surface choice and behavior in adult Mongolian gerbils. Psychol. Rec. 28, 299–303.

Phillips, C.J.C., 2010. Cattle Behaviour and Welfare. Blackwell, Oxford, United Kingdom.

Podberscek, A.L., Blackshaw, J.K., Beattie, A.W., 1991a. The behavior of laboratory colony cats and their reactions to familiar and unfamiliar person. Appl. Anim. Behav. Sci. 31, 119–130.

Podberscek, A.L., Blackshaw, J.K., Beattie, A.W., 1991b. The behaviour of group penned and individually caged laboratory rabbits. Appl. Anim. Behav. Sci. 28, 353–363.

Pongracz, P., Altbacker, V., 2001. Human handling might interfere with conspecific recognition in the European Rabbit (Oryctolagus cuniculus). Develop. Psychobiol. 39 (1), 53–62.

Pongracz, P., Altbacker, V., 2003. Arousal, but not nursing, is necessary to elicit a decreased fear reaction toward humans in rabbit (Oryctolagus cuniculus) pups. Develop. Psychobiol. 43 (3), 192–199.

Poole, T.B., 1991. Criteria for the provision of captive environments. In: Box, H.O. (Ed.), Primate Responses to Environmental Change. Chapman & Hall, London, pp. 357–374.

Poole, T.B., 1992. The nature and evolution of behavioural needs in mammals. Anim. Welf. 1, 203–220.

Poole, T.B., 1998. Meeting a mammal's psychological needs: basic principles. In: Shepherson, D.J., Mellen, J.D., Hutchins, M. (Eds.), Second Nature: Environmental Enrichment for Captive Animals. Smithsonian Institution Press, Washington, DC, pp. 1–12.

Poole, T.B., Morgan, H.D.R., 1973. Differences in aggressive behaviour between male mice (Mus musculus L.) in colonies of different sizes. Anim. Behav. 21 (4), 788–795.

Potter, M.P., Borkowski, G.L., 1998. Apparent psychogenic polydipsia and secondary polyuria in laboratory-housed New Zealand white rabbits. Contemp. Top. Lab. Anim. Sci. 37 (6), 87–89.

Price, E.O., 2002. Animal Domestication and Behavior. CAB International, Wallingford, United Kingdom.

Price, E.O., 2008. Principles and Applications of Domestic Animal Behavior. CAB International, Wallingford, United Kingdom.

Princz, Z., Szendrõ, Z.S., Radnai, I., Biró-Németh, E., Orova, Z., 2005. Free choice of rabbits among cages with different height. Proc. 17th Hungarian Conf. Rabbit Production, Kaposvar, World Rabbit Sci. 14, 16.

Proudfoot, K.L., Weary, D.M., von Keyserlingk, M.A.G., 2012. Linking the social environment to illness in farm animals. Appl. Anim. Behav. Sci. 138, 203–215.

Puppe, B., Ernst, K., Schön, P.C., Manteuffel, G., 2007. Cognitive enrichment affects behavioural reactivity in domestic pig. Appl. Anim. Behav. Sci. 105, 75–86.

Pyle, D.A., Bennett, A.L., Zarcone, T.J., Turkkan, J.S., 1996. Use of two food foraging devices by singly housed baboons. Lab. Prim. Newsl. 35, 10–15.

Raje, S., Stewart, K.L., 1997. Group housing for male New Zealand white rabbits. Lab. Anim. 26 (4), 36–38.

Rault, J.-L., 2012. Friends with benefits: social support and its relevance for farm animal welfare. Appl. Anim. Behav. Sci. 136, 1–14.

Reinhardt, V., 1988. Preliminary comments on pairing unfamiliar adult rhesus monkeys for the purpose of environmental enrichment. Lab. Prim. Newsl. 27, 1–3.

Reinhardt, V., 1994a. Comparing the effectiveness of PVC swings versus PVC perches as environmental enrichment objects for caged female rhesus macaques. Lab. Prim. Newsl. 30, 5–6.

Reinhardt, V., 1994b. Continuous pair-housing of caged Macaca mulatta: risk evaluation. Lab. Prim. Newsl. 33, 1–4.

Reinhardt, V., 1994c. Social enrichment for previously single-caged stumptail macaques. Anim. Technol. 5, 37–41.

Reinhardt, V., Reinhardt, A., 1991. Impact of a privacy panel on the behavior of caged female rhesus monkeys living in pairs. J. Exp. Anim. Sci. 34, 55–58.

Reinhardt, V., Reinhardt, A., 1998. Environmental Enrichment for Non-Human Primates: An Annotated Bibliography for Animal Care Personnel, second ed. Animal Welfare Institute, Washington, DC.

Reinhardt, V., Cowley, D., Eisele, S., Vertein, R., Houser, W.D., 1988. Pairing compatible female rhesus monkeys for the purpose of cage enrichment has no negative impact on body weight. Lab. Prim. News 27, 13–15.

Reinhardt, V., Pape, R., Zweifel, D., 1991a. Multifunctional cage for macaques housed in pairs or in small groups. AALAS Bull. 30, 14–15.

Reinhardt, V., Cowley, D., Eisele, S., 1991b. Serum cortisol concentrations of single-housed and isosexually pair-housed adult rhesus macaques. J. Exp. Anim. Sci. 34, 73–76.

Renner, M.J., Rosenzweig, M.R., 1987. Enriched and Impoverished Environments. Effects on Brain and Behavior. Springer-Verlag, New York.

Richards, M.P., 1969. Effects of oestrogen and progesterone on nest building in golden hamster. Anim. Behav. 17, 356–361.

Roberts, J.A., 1989. Environmental enrichment, providing psychological well-being for people and primates. Am. J. Primatol. (Suppl. 1), 25–30.

Rodenburg, T.B., van Krimpen, M.M., de Jong, I.C., de Haas, E.N., Kops, M.S., Reidstra, B.J., et al., 2013. The prevention and control of feather pecking in laying hens: identifying the underlying principles. World's Poult. Sci. J. 69, 361–373.

Rommeck, I., Gottlieb, D., Strand, S., McCowan, B., 2009. The effects of four nursery-rearing strategies on the development of self-directed behavior in laboratory-housed rhesus macaques (*Macaca mulatta*). J. Am. Assoc. Lab. Anim. Sci. 408, 395–401.

Rood, J.P., 1972. Ethological and behavioural comparison of three genera of Argentine cavies. Anim. Behav. Monogr. 5, 1–83.

Roper, T.J., 1973. Nesting material as a reinforcer for female mice. Anim. Behav. 21, 733–740.

Rose, M., 1993. Social behaviour of rats and mice – individuals and groups. ANZCCART News 6, 10–11.

Rose, M.A., 1994. Environmental factors likely to impact on an animal's well-being: an overview. in: Improving the Well-Being of Animals in the Research Environment, Proceedings conference in Glen Osmond Australia: ANZCCART, pp. 99–116.

Rosenblum, L.A., Coe, C.L., 1977. The influence of social structure on squirrel monkey socialization. In: Chevalier-Skolnikoff, S., Poirier, F.E. (Eds.), Primate Bio-Social Development: Biological, Social, and Ecological Determinants. Garland Publishing, New York, pp. 479–499.

Rosenblum, L.A., Smiley, J., 1984. Therapeutic effects of an imposed foraging task in disturbed monkeys. J. Child Psychol. Psychiatry 25, 485–497.

Rowe, F., 1981. Wild house mouse biology and control. In: Berry, R.J. (Ed.), Biology of the House Mouse. Academic Press, London, pp. 575–590.

Rowson, K.E.K., Michaels, L., 1980. Injury to young mice caused by cottonwool used as nesting material. Lab. Anim. 14 (3), 187. –187.

Rumbaugh, D.M., Washburn, D., Savage-Rumbaugh, E.S., 1991. On the care of captive chimpanzees: methods of enrichment. In: Segal, E. (Ed.), Housing, Care, and Psychological Wellbeing of Captive and Laboratory Primates. Noyes Publications, New Jersey, pp. 357–375.

Rushen, J., de Passillé, A.M., von Keyserlingk, M.A.G., Weary, D.M., 2007. The Welfare of Cattle. Springer, Dodrecht, The Netherlands.

Sackett, G.P., 1965. Effects of rearing conditions upon monkeys (*M. mulatta*). Child Dev. 36, 855–868.

Sales, G., Hubrecht, R., Peyvandi, A., Milligan, S., Shield, B., 1997. Noise in dog kenneling: is barking a welfare problem for dogs? Appl. Anim. Behav. Sci. 52, 321–329.

Sambrook, T.D., Buchanan-Smith, H.M., 1996. What makes novel objects enriching? A comparison of the qualities of control and complexity. Lab. Prim. Newsl. 35, 1–4.

Sarna, J.R., Dyck, R.H., Whishaw, I.Q., 2000. The Dalila effect: C57BL6 mice barber whiskers by plucking. Behav. Brain Res. 108, 39–45.

Scharmann, W., 1991. Improved housing of mice, rats and guinea-pigs: a contribution to the refinement of animal experiments. ATLA 19, 108–114.

Scheibler, E., Weinandy, R., Gattermann, R., 2005. Intra-family aggression modulates physiological features of the Mongolian gerbil *Meriones unguiculatus*. Acta Zool. Sin. 51 (6), 989–997.

Scott, L., 1991. Environmental enrichment for single housed common marmosets. In: Box, H.O. (Ed.), Primate Responses to Environmental Change. Chapman & Hall, London, pp. 265–274.

Scott, J.P., Fuller, J.L., 1965. Genetics and the Social Behavior of the Dog. University of Chicago Press, Illinois.

Segovia, G., Del Arco, A., de Blas, M., Garrido, P., Mora, F., 2008. Effects of an enriched environment on the release of dopamine in the prefrontal cortex produced by stress and on working memory during aging in the awake rat. Behav. Brain Res. 187 (2), 304–311.

Serpell, J., 2011. Why dogs are different. In: Proceedings of the CAAT Workshop on Critical Evaluation of the Use of Dogs in Biomedical Research and Testing, Baltimore, MD.

Shapiro, S.J., Bloomsmith, M.A., Laule, G.E., 2003. Positive reinforcement training as a technique to alter nonhuman primate behavior: quantitative assessments of effectiveness. J. Appl. Anim. Welf. Sci. 6, 175–187.

Shepherdson, D.J., 1998. Tracing the path of environmental enrichment in zoos. In: Shepherson, D.J., Mellen, J.D., Hutchins, M. (Eds.), Second Nature: Environmental Enrichment for Captive Animals. Smithsonian Institution Press, Washington, DC, pp. 1–12.

Sherwin, C.M., 1993. The pecking behaviour of laying hens provided with a simple motorized pecking device. Br. Poult. Sci. 34, 235–240.

Sherwin, C.M., 1996. Laboratory mice persist in gaining access to resources: a method of assessing the importance of environmental features. Appl. Anim. Behav. Sci. 48, 203–214.

Silverman, A.P., 1978. Animal Behaviour in the Laboratory. Chapman & Hall, London.

Smith, A., Lindburg, D.G., Vehrencamp, S., 1989. Effect of food preparation on feeding behavior of lion-tailed macaques. Zoo Biol. 8, 57–65.

Snowdon, C.T., Savage, A., 1991. Psychological well-being of captive primates: general considerations and examples from callitrichids. In: Segal, E. (Ed.), Housing, Care, and Psychological Wellbeing of Captive and Laboratory Primates. Noyes Publications, New Jersey, pp. 75–88.

Sørensen, D.B., Krohn, T., Hansen, H.N., Ottesen, J.L., Hansen, A.K., 2005. An ethological approach to housing requirements of golden hamsters, Mongolian gerbils and fat sand rats in the laboratory – a review. Appl. Anim. Behav. Sci. 94 (3–4), 181–195.

Southern, H.N., 1954. House Mice. Oxford University Press, London.

Špinka, M., Wemelsfelder, F., 2011. Environmental challenge and animal agency. In: Appleby, M.C., Mench, J.A., Olsson, I.A.S., Hughes, B.O. (Eds.), Animal Welfare. CAB International, Wallingford, United Kingdom, pp. 27–43.

Spoolder, H.A.M., Burbridge, J.A., Edwards, S.A., Simmins, P.H., Lawrence, A.B., 1995. Provision of straw as a foraging substrate reduces the development of excessive chain and bar manipulation in food restricted sows. Appl. Anim. Behav. Sci. 43, 249–262.

Stanton, M.E., Patterson, J.M., Levine, S., 1985. Social influences on conditioned cortisol secretion in the squirrel monkey. Psychoneuroendocrinology 10, 125–134.

Stauffacher, M., 1997a. Housing requirements: what ethology can tell us. In: Van Zutphen, L.F.M., Balls, M. (Eds.), Animal Alternatives, Welfare and Ethics Elsevier, Amsterdam, The Netherlands, pp. 179–186.

Stauffacher, M., 1997b. Comparative studies on housing conditions. Proceedings of the Sixth FELASA Symposium, London, Royal Society of Medicine Press, Ltd.

Stolba, A., Wood-Gush, D.G.M., 1989. The behaviour of pigs in a semi-natural environment. Anim. Prod. 48, 419–425.

Strier, K.B., 1987. Activity budgets of woolly spider monkeys or muriquis (Brachyteles arachnoides). Am. J. Primatol. 13, 385–395.

Svensson, C., Jensen, M.B., 2007. Short communication: identification of diseased calves by use of data from automatic milk feeders. J. Dairy Sci. 90, 994–997.

Swennes, A.G., Alworth, L.C., Harvey, S.B., Jones, C.A., King, C.S., Crowell-Davis, S.L., 2011. Human handling promotes compliant behavior in adult laboratory rabbits. JAALAS 50 (1), 41–45.

Swetter, B.J., Karpiak, C.P., Canon, J.T., 2011. Separating the effects of shelter from additional cage enhancements for group-housed BALB/cJ mice. Neurosci. Lett. 495 (3), 205–209.

Szendro, Z., McNitt, J.I., 2012. Housing of rabbit does: group and individual systems: a review. Livestock Science 150 (1–3), 1–10.

Tauson, R., 1985. Mortality in laying hens caused by differences in cage design. Acta Agric. Scand. 35, 165–174.

Tauson, R., Svensson, S.A., 1980. Influence of plumage condition on the hen's feed requirement. Swedish J. Agric. Res. 10, 35–39.

Taylor, I.A., 1995. Designing equipment around behavior Animal Behavior and the Design of Livestock and Poultry Systems. Plant and Life Sciences Publishing (formerly Northeast Regional Agricultural Engineering Service), Ithaca, NY.

Terlouw, E.M.C., Lawrence, A.B., Illius, A.W., 1991. Influences of feeding level and physical restriction on development of stereotypies in sows. Anim. Behav. 42, 981–991.

Thiessen, D.D., 1988. Body temperature and grooming in the Mongolian gerbil. Ann. NY Acad. Sci. 525, 27–39.

Thorington Jr., R.W., 1968. Observations of squirrel monkeys in a Colombian forest. In: Rosenblum, L.A., Cooper, R.W. (Eds.), The Squirrel Monkey. Academic Press, New York, pp. 69–85.

Thornberg, L.P., Stowe, H.D., Pick, J.R., 1973. The pathogenesis of the alopecia due to hair-chewing in mice. Lab. Anim. Sci. 23, 843–850.

Tipton, C.M., Carey, R.A., Eastin, W.C., Erickson, H.H., 1974. A submaximal test for dogs: evaluation of effects of training, detraining, and cage confinement. J. Appl. Physiol. 37, 271–275.

Trickett, S.L., Guy, J.H., Edwards, S.A., 2009. The role of novelty in environmental enrichment for the weaned pig. Appl. Anim. Behav. Sci. 116, 45–51.

Tuli, J.S. 1993. Stress and parasitic infection in laboratory mice. PhD thesis, University of Birmingham.

Turner, R.J., Held, S.D., Hirst, J.E., Billinghurst, G., Wootton, R.J., 1997. An immunological assessment of group-housed rabbits. Lab. Anim. 31, 362–372.

Tuyttens, F.A.M., 2005. The importance of straw for pig and cattle welfare: a review. Appl. Anim. Behav. Sci. 92, 261–282.

U.S. Department of Agriculture, 1991. Title 9, CFR Part 3, Animal Welfare; Standards; Final Rule. Fed. Reg., Vol. 56, No. 32, February 15.

Valuska, A., Mench, J., 2013. Size does matter: the effect of enclosure size on aggression and affiliation between female New Zealand White rabbits during mixing. Appl. Anim. Behav. Sci. 149, 72–76.

Vandeleest, J.J., McCowan, B., Capitanio, J.P., 2011. Early rearing interacts with temperament and housing to influence the risk for motor stereotypy in rhesus monkeys (Macaca mulatta). Appl. Anim. Behav. Sci. 132, 81–89.

Van den Bos, R., 1998. The function of allogrooming in domestic cats (Felis silvestris catus): a study in a group of cats living in confinement. J. Ethol. 16, 1–13.

Vanderschuren, L., Niesink, R.J.M., Van Pee, J.M., 1997. The neurobiology of social play behavior in rats. Neurosci. Biobehav. Rev. 21 (3), 309–326.

Van de Weerd, H.A., Van den Broek, F.A.R., Baumans, V., 1996. Preference for different types of flooring in two rat strains. Appl. Anim. Behav. Sci. 46, 251–261.

Van de Weerd, H.A., van Loo, P.L.P., van Zutphen, L.F.M., Koohaas, J.M., Baumans, V., 1998. Strength of preference for nesting material as environmental enrichment for laboratory mice. Appl. Anim. Behav. Sci. 55, 369–382.

Van Liere, D.W., Bokma, S., 1987. Short-term feather maintenance as a function of dust-bathing in laying hens. Appl. Anim. Behav. Sci. 18, 197–204.

Van Loo, P.L.P., Mol, J.A., 2001. Modulation of aggression in male mice: influence of group size and cage size. Physiol. Behav. 72 (5), 675–683.

Van Loo, P.L.P., Baumans, V., 2004. The importance of learning young: the use of nesting material in laboratory rats. Lab. Anim. 38 (1), 17–24.

Van Loo, P.L.P., Kruitwagen, C.L.J.J., van Zutphen, L.F.M., Koolhaas, J.M., Baumans, V., 2000. Modulation of aggression in male mice: influence of cage cleaning and scent marks. Anim. Welf. 9, 281–295.

Veillette, M., Reebs, S.G., 2010. Preference of Syrian hamsters to nest in old versus new bedding. Appl. Anim. Behav. Sci. 125 (3–4), 189–194.

Veillette, M., Reebs, S.G., 2011. Shelter choice by Syrian hamsters (Mesocricetus auratus) in the laboratory. Anim. Welf. 20 (4), 603–611.

Verga, M., Luzi, F., Carenzi, C., 2007. Effects of husbandry and management systems on physiology and behaviour of farmed and laboratory rabbits. Horm. Behav. 52 (1), 122–129.

Vessier, I., de Passilé, A.-M.B., Després, G., Rushen, J., Charpentier, I., Ramirez de la Fe, A.R., et al., 2002. Does nutritive and non-nutritive suckling reduce other oral behaviours and stimulate rest in calves? J. Anim. Sci. 80, 2574–2587.

Vieira, G., Lossie, A.C., Ajuwon, K., Garner, P., 2012. Is hair and feather pulling a disease of oxidative stress? Paper presented at the Trichotillomania Learning Center 19th Annual National Conference, Trichotillomania and Related Body Focused Repetitive Behaviors. Chicago, IL.

Waiblinger, E., 2002. Comfortable quarters for gerbils in research institutions. In: Reinhardt, V., Reinhardt, A. (Eds.), Comfortable Quarters for Laboratory Animals Animal Welfare Institute, Washington, DC, pp. 18–25.

Waiblinger, E., Koenig, B., 2007. Housing and husbandry conditions affect stereotypic behaviour in laboratory gerbils. Altex-Alternativen Zu Tierexperimenten 24, 67–69.

Waiblinger, S., Boivin, X., Pederson, V., Tosi, M.-V., Janszak, A.M., Visser, E.K., et al., 2006. Assessing the human–animal relationship in farmed species: a critical review. Appl. Anim. Behav. Sci. 101, 185–242.

Walters, S.L., Torres-Urbano, C.J., et al., 2012. The impact of huts on physiological stress: a refinement in post-transport housing of male guineapigs (Cavia porcellus). Lab. Anim. 46 (3), 220–224.

Waran, N., 2007. The Welfare of Horses. Springer, Dodrecht, The Netherlands.

Ward, R.J., 1981. Diet and nutrition. In: Berry, R.J. (Ed.), Biology of the House Mouse Academic press inc, London, pp. 255–266.

Watson, D.S.B., 1991. A built-in perch for primate squeeze cages. Lab. Anim. Sci. 41, 378–379.

Watson, S.L., Shively, C.A., 1996. Effects of cage configuration on behavior in cynomolgus macaques. International Primatological Society/American Society of Primatologist Congress Abstracts.

Webb, N.G., Nilsson, C., 1983. Flooring and injury – an overview. In: Baxter, S.H., Baxter, M.R., McCormack, J.A.C. (Eds.), Farm Animal Housing and Welfare. Curr. Top. Vet. Med. Anim. Sci. 24, pp. 226–261.

Weihe, W., 1987. The laboratory rat. In: Poole, T.B. (Ed.), Handbook on the Care and Management of Laboratory Animals Longman Science and Technical, Harlow, United Kingdom.

Weld, K., Metz, B., Erwin, J., 1991. Environmental enrichment for *Macaca fascicularis:* effects of shape and substance of manipulable objects. Am. J. Primatol. 24, 139.

Wemelsfelder, F., 1993. The concept of animal boredom and its relationship to stereotyped behaviour. In: Lawrence, A.B., Rushen, J. (Eds.), Stereotypic Animal Behaviour. Fundamentals and Applications to Welfare. CAB International, Wallingford, United Kingdom, pp. 65–95.

Whary, M., Peper, R., et al., 1993. The effects of group housing on the research use of the laboratory rabbit. Lab. Anim. 27, 330–341.

White, W., 1990. The effect of cage space and environmental factors. In: Guttman, H.N. (Ed.), Guidelines for the Well-Being of Rodents in Research Scientists Center for Animal Welfare, Greenbelt, Maryland, pp. 29–44.

Whittaker, D., 2010. The UFAW Handbook on The Care and Management of Laboratory and Other Research Animals; The Syrian hamster. Wiley-Blackwell.

Wiberg, G., Grice, H.C., 1963. Long-term isolation stress in rats. Science 142 (3591), 507.

Wiedenmayer, C., 1997. Causation of the ontogenetic development of stereotypic digging in gerbils. Anim. Behav. 53, 461–470.

Wiedenmayer, C., 1997. Stereotypies resulting from a deviation in the ontogenetic development of gerbils. Behav. Processes 39 (3), 215–221.

Widowski, T.M., Torrey, S., Bench, C., Gonyou, H.W., 2008. Development of ingestive behavior and the relationship to belly-nosing in early-weaned piglets. Appl. Anim. Behav. Sci. 110, 109–127.

Williams, L.E., Abee, C.R., Barnes, S.R., Ricker, R.B., 1988. Cage design and configuration for an arboreal species of primate. Lab. Anim. Sci. 38, 289–291.

Wolff, A., Ruppert, G., 1991. A practical assessment of a non-human primate exercise program. Lab. Anim. 20, 36–39.

Wolfer, D.P., Litvin, O., et al., 2004. Laboratory animal welfare: cage enrichment and mouse behaviour. Nature 432, 821–822.

Wolfle, T., 1996. How different species affect the relationship. In: Krulisch, L., Mayer, S., Simmonds, R.C. (Eds.), The Human/Research Animal Relationship. Scientists Center for Animal Welfare, Greenbelt, MD, pp. 85–90.

Wood-Gush, D.G.M., Vestergaard, K., 1991. The seeking of novelty and its relation to play. Anim. Behav. 42, 599–606.

Wood-Gush, D.G.M., Vestergaard, K., Petersen, V., 1990. The significance of motivation and environment in the development of exploration in pigs. Biol. Behav. 15, 39–52.

Würbel, H. J. Garner 2007. Refinement of rodent research through environmental enrichment and systematic randomization. National Centre for the Replacement, Refinement and Reduction of Animals in Research #9.

Würbel, H., Chapman, R., Rutland, C., 1998. Effect of feed and environmental enrichment on development of stereotypic wire-gnawing in laboratory mice. Appl. Anim. Behav. Sci. 60 (1), 69–81.

Wurbel, H., Stauffacher, M., Von Holst, D., 1996. Stereotypies in laboratory mice- quantitative and qualitative description of the otogeny of "wire chewing" and jumping in Zur:ICR and Zur:ICR nu -mice. Ethology 102, 371–385.

Wyly, M.V., Denenberg, V.H., et al., 1975. Handling rabbits in infancy: in search of a critical period. Dev. Psychobiol. 8 (2), 179–186.

Yoshida, T.H., 1980. Cytogenetics of the Black Rat. University of Tokyo Press, Tokyo.

Young, H., Strecker, R., et al., 1950. Localisation of activity in two indoor populations of house mice, Mus musculus. Journal of Mammology 31, 403–410.

Zebunke, M., Langbein, J., Manteuffel, G., Puppe, B., 2011. Autonomic reactions indicating positive affect during acoustic reward learning in domestic pigs. Anim. Behav. 81, 481–489.

CHAPTER

39

Animal Welfare

Marilyn J. Brown, DVM, MS, DACLAM, DECLAM[a] and Christina Winnicker, DVM, MPH, DACLAM[b]

[a]Global Animal Welfare, Department of Animal Welfare, Charles River Laboratories, Wilmington, MA, USA [b]Enrichment & Behavioral Medicine, Department of Animal Welfare, Charles River Laboratories, Wilmington, MA, USA

I. INTRODUCTION

The term 'animal welfare,' in both the lay and scientific community, is often used to refer to a concept. In this context, positive animal welfare may be substituted with the term 'well-being.' Animal welfare serves as a cornerstone, or foundation, for laboratory animal medicine and the use of animals in research. 'Animal welfare' also refers to a measurable state in an animal which may be related to the adequacy of an animal's ability to cope with its environment. Animal welfare is a branch of science which looks at these measurable states in almost all areas of our interaction with animals – agriculture, entertainment, companionship, research, and others. This chapter will highlight the significant emphasis on animal welfare in the field of laboratory animal science and medicine, beginning with some of the history, philosophies, ethics and events which have shaped the impact of animal welfare on the use of animals in research. Laws and regulations will only be briefly mentioned as they are covered elsewhere in this book; however, guidelines and principles, such as the 3Rs, will be covered in more detail. Using examples of reduction and refinement, strategies for optimizing laboratory animal welfare in general and

Laboratory Animal Medicine, Third Edition
DOI: http://dx.doi.org/10.1016/B978-0-12-409527-4.00039-0

in several specific areas of research will be discussed. Animal welfare as a science, measuring the animal's perception of their state of well-being and going beyond just physiologic measurement of health and production, will be discussed, with particular focus on the use of behavioral monitoring to measure welfare.

II. ANIMAL WELFARE AS A KEY COMPONENT IN RESEARCH, TEACHING, AND TESTING USING ANIMALS

A discussion of animal welfare should begin with defining the term. There are many definitions of animal welfare and only a few are provided here to highlight the similarities and also some of the nuanced differences. The reader is referred to the American College of Animal Welfare (ACAW) website (http://www.acaw.org/animal_welfare_principles.html) and the various references in this chapter for additional definitions. Many of the definitions and principles of animal welfare focus upon how animal welfare is influenced by humans and thus may be looked upon as what we 'owe' animals.

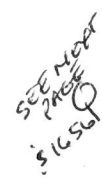

> Welfare is a broad term which includes the many elements that contribute to an animal's quality of life, including those referred to in the 'five freedoms' (freedom from hunger, thirst and malnutrition; freedom from fear and distress; freedom from physical and thermal discomfort; freedom from pain, injury and disease; and freedom to express normal patterns of behaviour). (*OIE Animal Welfare Guidelines, 2005*)

> ...animal welfare is concerned with assuring humane treatment of animals; maintaining good health, minimizing negative states such as pain, enhancing positive states, and giving animals freedom to behave in ways that are natural to that species. (*Gilbert et al., 2012*)

> Animal Welfare ... "is the degree of pleasure that an animal obtains from performing a behavior or obtaining a valued resource, rather than the amount of suffering caused by the inability to perform the behaviour or the absence of the resource. (*Appleby et al., 2011*)

Signs of the growing recognition of the importance of animal welfare are the inclusion of animal welfare as a strategic imperative for the American Veterinary Medical Association (AVMA) for the second consecutive planning period, creation of a Division of Animal Welfare within the AVMA, and a standing Animal Welfare Committee of the AVMA. Although the concept of animal welfare is not new to the field of veterinary medicine, the increased focus on animal welfare can be demonstrated in the newly created American College of Animal Welfare (ACAW) incorporated in 2010 and recognized by the AVMA in 2012. Many readers of this book will be veterinarians so it is apt to begin the discussion

of animal welfare with reference to the AVMA Animal Welfare Principles. (Although the AVMA is the largest veterinary medical association, it should be noted that they are by no means the only veterinary association to have principles and guidelines pertaining to animal welfare so readers are encouraged to look at guidelines from their own professional associations.) The AVMA Animal Welfare Principles state:

- The responsible use of animals for human purposes, such as companionship, food, fiber, recreation, work, education, exhibition, and research conducted for the benefit of both humans and animals, is consistent with the Veterinarian's Oath.
- Decisions regarding animal care, use, and welfare shall be made by balancing scientific knowledge and professional judgment with consideration of ethical and societal values
- Animals must be provided with water, food, proper handling, health care, and an environment appropriate to their care and use, with thoughtful consideration for their species-typical biology and behavior.
- Animals should be cared for in ways that minimize fear, pain, stress, and suffering.
- Procedures related to animal housing, management, care, and use should be continuously evaluated, and when indicated, refined, or replaced.
- Conservation and management of animal populations should be humane, socially responsible, and scientifically prudent.
- Animals shall be treated with respect and dignity throughout their lives and, when necessary, provided a humane death.
- The veterinary profession shall continually strive to improve animal health and welfare through scientific research, education, collaboration, advocacy, and the development of legislation and regulations (https://www.avma.org/KB/Policies/Pages/AVMA-Animal-Welfare-Principles.aspx Accessed May 11, 2015).

Animal welfare, as a key component in research, teaching and testing involving animals, can be found in the very title of the primary law impacting animal research in the United States – The Animal *Welfare* Act (AWA) and the subsequent Animal *Welfare* Regulations which provide details for implementation of the AWA. Research supported by Public Health Service funds, must comply with the Office of Laboratory Animal *Welfare* (OLAW). Researchers and Institutional Animal Care and Use Committees (IACUCs) are urged to use resources provided by the Animal *Welfare* Information Center of the National Agriculture Library to search for alternatives during the planning and execution of their studies. In *The Guide for the Care and Use of Laboratory Animals*, the word 'welfare' occurs 178 times and 'well-being' occurs 68 times (NRC, 2011). Organizations providing support to the research industry include groups such as the Laboratory Animal *Welfare* Exchange (LAWTE); Scientist Center for Animal *Welfare* (SCAW); United Federation for Animal *Welfare* (UFAW), to name just a few. Clearly, welfare is an important consideration of veterinary medicine as a whole, but particularly in the areas of research, teaching and testing.

Animal welfare is a key component in research, teaching and testing involving animals, but how did we get here?

III. ANIMAL WELFARE – A HISTORICAL AND PHILOSOPHICAL PERSPECTIVE

Our relationship with animals began when man only hunted animals for food and clothing or feared animals for man's safety. It has evolved into domestication of animals for many human uses including food and clothing, transportation, companionship, entertainment and research. We moved away from humans as the 'shepherds' or stewards over animals during the industrial revolutions where populations moved from rural to urban settings. Organizations such as the British Society for the Protection of Animals (1866) and the American Humane Association (1874) were formed as society became increasingly concerned about animal welfare (Patterson-Kane and Golab, 2013). At the same time, shelters for stray animals were also being established. The impetus for these developments was concern for horses and later dogs and cats. The first legislation which represented a concern for animals in research was the Cruelty to Animals Act (1876) in Great Britain. This legislation licensed researchers using animals with a focus on painful research and the use of anesthesia. Only three prosecutions resulted from this Act (Patterson-Kane and Golab, 2013).

The period after World War II saw an awakening in awareness of, and concern for, animal welfare in the research setting. Within the research community, organizations such as the American Association for Laboratory Animal Science (AALAS) was formed in 1950 followed closely by the American College of Laboratory Animal Medicine (ACLAM) in 1958 and the American Association for the Accreditation of Laboratory Animal Care (AAALAC) in 1965. These organizations had a common goal of providing better care for animals used in research, teaching and testing through better facilities and development of formal qualifications for those involved in laboratory animal science and medicine. Another key event impacting laboratory animal welfare included the publication of the first *Guide for the Care and Use of Laboratory Animals* in 1963 (hereafter referred to as the *Guide*). For the public, two pivotal events raised concerns about animals used in research, particularly how pets could be acquired by random source animal dealers and how these animals were kept in some situations. The first was an article in

Sports Illustrated in 1965 which highlighted the story of Pepper, a dog that was stolen from a home and who ended up in a research laboratory (Phinizy, 1965). The other was in *Life* Magazine in 1966 where poor conditions at vendor were exposed (Wayman, 1966). The public outcry led to the passing of the first Animal Welfare Act in the United States in 1966. Concurrently, in agriculture, public concern for animal welfare increased after the publication of Animal Machines by Ruth Harrison in 1964 highlighting the plight of agricultural animals in postindustrial farming (Harrison, 1964). Later the Brambell Report (Brambell, 1965) described guidelines, referred to as the Five Freedoms, in response to concerns about the welfare of agricultural animals in the United Kingdom. These guidelines are also applicable to laboratory animals and will be elaborated upon later in this chapter.

Although animal research oversight committees had been in place at some institutions, the requirement for such committees only became mandatory in 1979 (Patterson-Kane and Golab, 2013). With subsequent revisions of the AWA in 1985, 1990, 2002, 2007, and 2008, passage of the Health Research Extension Act of 1985 and subsequent Public Health Service Policy on Humane Care and Use of Laboratory Animals, as well as revisions of the *Guide* in 1978, 1985, 1996, and most recently in 2011, the scope and functions of the animal welfare oversight committee, called the Institutional Animal Care and Use Committee (IACUC) in the United States, has continued to be defined and expanded. The *Guide* defines the animal care and use program as comprised of "all activities conducted by and at an institution that have a direct impact on the well-being of animals…" and places the responsibility for the oversight of the program in the hands of the IACUC (NRC, 2011).

While it is not the purpose of this chapter to focus on philosophy and ethics, some mention of philosophies such as the moral standing of animals and basic ethical theories helps to put animal welfare into a philosophical context. Readers interested in exploring this further, might seek additional references listed (Mill, 1863; Frey, 1988; Regan and Singer, 1989; Tannenbaum, 1991; Carruthers, 1992; Cohen and Regan, 2001; Olsson *et al.*, 2011; Rollin, 2011; Gilbert *et al.*, 2012; Brown, 2013). The moral status of animals has been considered by some as "the key question in veterinary ethics" (Rollin, 2011). The question of the moral status of animals is not the same as the question if animals matter (Carruthers, 1992). Carruthers says "common sense morality" indicates that animals have partial moral standing because their lives and experiences have direct moral significance, but much less than humans. Criteria for ascribing moral status can use a 'uni-criterial approach' which uses a key property of life such as capacity to feel pain, language, ability to reason, or personhood. Alternatively, a 'multi-criterial approach' where more than one valid criterion and more than one type of moral status with different types imposing obligations on moral agents can be used (Hill, 1992; Warren, 1997).

Ethical or moral theories provide a framework for reaching decisions when faced with an ethical or moral dilemma (Brown, 2013). Some useful qualities of an adequate theory include: universal validity (ability to apply it in all similar circumstances and by all comparable individuals), evident to reason, ease of determination if theory applies to a given situation, provision of a basis for moral motivation and the ability to provide guidance in the face of needed decisions. Ethical theories generally fall into two major categories, deontological, which are based upon the idea of right and wrong or teleological, which are consequential, by evaluating the results of actions. Deontological theories vary based upon what is considered right or wrong and often deal with concepts of duty and moral obligation. Utilitarianism is the most prominent of the teleological theories. Utilitarianism seeks to provide the greatest good (or least harm) to the greatest number of individuals. Challenges with this theory include determination of who 'counts' as an individual (the question of moral standing) and balance of the theory with commonly held beliefs about the 'rights' of an individual – the principle of equal consideration protects lives, liberty and well-being of individuals only if it maximizes overall utility. Utilitarianism has been used to both support the use of animals in research (Russow, 1990) and to conclude a vast majority of animal research is immoral (Singer, 1975). The harm:benefit analysis of a proposed study by an IACUC is an example of a utilitarian calculation in which the moral significance of humans is usually considered greater than that of animals. A well known exception to this approach is the concept of 'speciesism,' first proposed by Ryder in 1975 (Ryder, 1975) but popularized by Singer in 1975 (Singer, 1975).

Finally, as we look at how some historical events have impact upon views about animal welfare, it is also important to note other cultural influences that impact on how society views animal welfare and our obligations toward animals. Today, many people have grown up around pets and often pets are referred to as 'members of the family.' Spending on pets is reported to be in the billions of dollars each year as estimated by the American Pet Products Association (http://www.americanpetproducts.org/press_industrytrends.asp). Of the people who refused to relocate during Hurricane Katrina in New Orleans, 44% gave their reason for refusing relocation as wanting to stay near their pet. Disney studios made a mouse an American icon – who can say they have not heard of Mickey Mouse? Animals have been 'humanized' in TV and film – Mr. Ed, the talking horse of the 1950s; the animals in Charlotte's web in 1972; Stuart Little in 1991; and a rat as the star of a popular film, Ratatouille in 2007.

Concern about animal welfare is not just based upon anthropomorphic images in the media. As science helps us better understand both animal behavior and physiology and as discussions of animals' emotional/mental states and feelings become more mainstream, concern for animal welfare will likely continue to grow. The laboratory animal science community have the opportunity to be leaders in optimizing animal welfare.

IV. GUIDELINES AND PRINCIPLES

As mentioned earlier, in 1965 a committee was convened in London to look at concerns with the welfare of agricultural animals. This committee developed guidelines referred to as the Five Freedoms which include: (1) Freedom from Hunger and Thirst – by ready access to fresh water and a diet to maintain full health and vigor; (2) Freedom from Discomfort – by providing an appropriate environment including shelter and a comfortable resting area; (3) Freedom from Pain, Injury, or Disease – by prevention or rapid diagnosis and treatment; (4) Freedom to Express Normal Behavior – by providing sufficient space, proper facilities and company of the animal's own kind; (5) Freedom from Fear and Distress – by ensuring conditions and treatment which avoid mental suffering (Brambell, 1965).

Between 1982 and 1984, international interdisciplinary consultations were undertaken by the Council for International Organizations of Medical Sciences (CIOMS) to create the International Guiding Principles for Biomedical Research Involving Animals (CIOMS, 1985). These principles were fully endorsed by the European Medical Research Councils (EMRC) and World Health Organization Advisory Committee on Medical Research in 1984 and served as a foundation for the US National Institutes of Health, US Interagency Research Animal Committee (IRAC), and the US Government Principles for the Utilization and Care of Vertebrate Animals used in Testing, Research, and Training in 1985 (Table 39.1). The CIOMS Principles were revised in 2013 and are found in Table 39.2. Both sets of Principles can be found in the 2011 edition of the Guide (NRC, 2011) and the IRAC Principles can also be found on the cover of the PHS Policy (OLAW, 2002).

Although the principles and guidelines listed above had significant impact on animal welfare in the laboratory, perhaps the simplest and the one with greatest impact on animal research today is the Three Rs of Russell and Burch (Russell and Burch, 1959). The CIOMS Principles previously mentioned include reference to the 3Rs. The Statement of Task to the revision committee of the latest Guide begins with "The use of laboratory animals for biomedical research, testing and education is guided by the principles of the 3Rs..." (NRC, 2011). The term 'the three (3) Rs' or the word alternatives, replacement,

TABLE 39.1 IRAC US Government Principles for the Utilization and Care of Vertebrate Animals Used in Testing, Research, and Training

The development of knowledge necessary for the improvement of the health and well-being of humans as well as other animals requires in vivo experimentation with a wide variety of animal species. Whenever U.S. Government agencies develop requirements for testing, research, or training procedures involving the use of vertebrate animals, the following principles shall be considered; and whenever these agencies actually perform or sponsor such procedures, the responsible Institutional Official shall ensure that these principles are adhered to:

I. The transportation, care, and use of animals should be in accordance with the *Animal Welfare Act* (7 U.S.C. 2131 *et. seq.*) and other applicable Federal laws, guidelines, and policies.

II. Procedures involving animals should be designed and performed with due consideration of their relevance to human or animal health, the advancement of knowledge, or the good of society.

III. The animals selected for a procedure should be of an appropriate species and quality and the minimum number required to obtain valid results. Methods such as mathematical models, computer simulation, and in vitro biological systems should be considered.

IV. Proper use of animals, including the avoidance or minimization of discomfort, distress, and pain when consistent with sound scientific practices, is imperative. Unless the contrary is established, investigators should consider that procedures that cause pain or distress in human beings may cause pain or distress in other animals.

V. Procedures with animals that may cause more than momentary or slight pain or distress should be performed with appropriate sedation, analgesia, or anesthesia. Surgical or other painful procedures should not be performed on unanesthetized animals paralyzed by chemical agents.

VI. Animals that would otherwise suffer severe or chronic pain or distress that cannot be relieved should be painlessly killed at the end of the procedure or, if appropriate, during the procedure.

VII. The living conditions of animals should be appropriate for their species and contribute to their health and comfort. Normally, the housing, feeding, and care of all animals used for biomedical purposes must be directed by a veterinarian or other scientist trained and experienced in the proper care, handling, and use of the species being maintained or studied. In any case, veterinary care shall be provided as indicated.

VIII. Investigators and other personnel shall be appropriately qualified and experienced for conducting procedures on living animals. Adequate arrangements shall be made for their in-service training, including the proper and humane care and use of laboratory animals.

IX. Where exceptions are required in relation to the provisions of these Principles, the decisions should not rest with the investigators directly concerned but should be made, with due regard to Principle II, by an appropriate review group such as an institutional animal care and use committee. Such exceptions should not be made solely for the purposes of teaching or demonstration.

IRAC (1985).

reduction or refinement is found 131 times in the *Guide* (NRC, 2011). The AWA refers to the concept of the 3Rs and alternatives throughout the Regulations (CFR, rev. 1998). Likewise, the EU Directive states "The care and use of live animals for scientific purposes is governed by internationally established principles of replacement, reduction and refinement…" (Anonymous, 2010). These three words, or the words 3Rs or alternatives are found 90 times in the EU Directive. Inclusion of the concept of the 3Rs in multinational laws, regulations and guidelines has given these concepts significant influence over how global animal research is conducted today.

The 3Rs are a common theme in the *Guide* which states "Throughout the *Guide*, scientists and institutions are encouraged to give careful and deliberate thought to the decision to use animals taking into consideration the contribution that such use will make to new knowledge, ethical concerns, and the availability of alternatives to animal use. A practical strategy for decision making, [is] the "Three Rs" (Replacement, Reduction, and Refinement) approach…" (NRC, 2011).

The concept of the 3Rs is also infused in US regulations covering research using animals. Although the US

Animal Welfare Act (AWA) regulations do not include the word 'alternatives' in its section of definitions, the term is used several times in the regulations themselves (Brown and Smiler, 2012). For example, in the section on IACUC review of protocols the regulations state protocols must indicate that (i) Procedures involving animals will avoid or minimize discomfort, distress, and pain to the animals; (ii) The principle investigator has considered alternatives to procedures that may cause more than momentary or slight pain or distress to the animals, and has provided a written narrative description of the methods and sources, e.g. The Animal Welfare Information Center, used to determine that alternatives were not available (AWA [Animal Welfare Act], 1990). The focus of USDA inspectors on adherence to this section of the regulations can be appreciated when looking at the USDA Research Facility Inspection Guide which instructs inspectors several times to evaluate institutional compliance in this area (USDA, 2009). In addition, the requirement for a search for alternatives is the subject of an Animal Care Policy – Policy 12 (APHIS, 2000). Strategies to enhance search efficiency using a search filter for PubMed have been published (Hooijmans *et al.*,

TABLE 39.2   International Guiding Principles for Biomedical Research Involving Animals   *CIOMS   2013*

The following principles should be used for the international scientific community to guide the responsible use of vertebrate animals in scientific and/or educational activities.

I. The advancement of scientific knowledge is important for improvement of human and animal health and welfare, conservation of the environment, and the good of society. Animals play a vital role in these scientific activities and good animal welfare is integral to achieving scientific and educational goals. Decisions regarding the welfare care and use of animals should be guided by scientific knowledge and professional judgment, reflect ethical and societal values and consider the potential benefits and the impact on the well-being of the animals involved.

II. The use of animals for scientific and/or educational purposes is a privilege that carries with it moral obligations and responsibilities for institutions and individuals to ensure the welfare of these animals to the greatest extent possible. This is best achieved in an institution with a culture of care and conscience in which individuals working with animals willingly, deliberately, and consistently act in an ethical, humane and compliant way. Institutions and individuals using animals have an obligation to demonstrate respect for animals, to be responsible and accountable for their decisions and actions pertaining to animal welfare, care and use, and to ensure that the highest standards of scientific integrity prevail.

III. Animal should be used only when necessary and only when their use is scientifically and ethically justified. The principles of the Three Rs – Replacement, Reduction and Refinement – should be incorporated into the design and conduct of scientific and/or educational activities that involve animals. Scientifically sound results and avoidance of; unnecessary duplication of animal-based experimental design. When no alternative methods, such as mathematical models, computer simulation, in vitro biological systems, or other non-animals (adjunct) approaches are available to replace the use of live animals, the minimum number of animals should be used to achieve the scientific or educational goals. Cost and convenience must not take precedence over these principles.

IV. Animals selected for the activity should be suitable for the purpose and of an appropriate species and genetic background to ensure scientific validity and reproducibility. The nutritional, microbiological, and general health status as well as the physiological and behavioral characteristics of the animals should be appropriate to the planned use as determined by scientific and veterinary medical experts and/or the scientific literature.

V. The health and welfare of animals should be primary considerations in decisions regarding the program of veterinary medical care to include animal acquisition and/or production, transportation, husbandry and management, housing, restraint and final disposition of animals, whether euthanasia, rehoming or release. Measures should be taken to ensure that the animal's environment and management are appropriate for the species and contribute the animal's well-being.

VI. The welfare, care and use of animals should be under the supervision of a veterinarian or scientists trained and experienced in the health, welfare, proper handling, and use of the species being maintained or studied. L The individual or team responsible for animal welfare, care and use should be involved in the development and maintenance of all aspects of the program. Animal health and welfare should be continuously monitored and assessed with measures to ensure that indicators of potential suffering are promptly detected and managed. Appropriate veterinary care should always be available and provided as necessary by a veterinarian.

VII. Investigators should assume that procedures that would cause pain or distress in human beings cause pain or distress in animals, unless there is evidence to the contrary. Thus, there is a moral imperative to prevent or minimize stress, distress, discomfort and pain in animals, consistent with sound scientific or veterinary medical practice. Taking into account the research and educational, goals, more than momentary or minimal pain and/or distress in animals should be managed by refinement of experimental techniques and/or appropriate sedation, analgesia, anesthesia, non-pharmacologic interventions, and/or other palliative measures developed in consultation with a qualified veterinarian or scientist. Surgical or other painful procedures should not be performed on unanesthetized animals. *— to REDUCE, MODERATE INTENSITY OF*

supposedly not shown as VII
VIII. Endpoints and timely interventions should be established for both humane and experimental reasons. Humane endpoints and/or interventions should be established before animal use begins, should be assessed throughout the course of the study, and should be applied as early as possible to prevent, ameliorate, or minimize unnecessary and/or unintended pain and/or distress. Animals that would otherwise suffer severe or chronic pain, distress or discomfort that cannot be relieved and is not part of the experimental design, should be removed from the study and/or euthanized using a procedure appropriate for the species and condition of the animal.

IX. It is the responsibility of the institution to ensure that personnel responsible for the welfare, care and use of animals are appropriately qualified and competent through training and experience for the procedures they perform. Adequate opportunities should be provided for on-going training and education in the humane and responsible treatment of animals. Institutions also are responsible for supervision of personnel to ensure proficiency and the use of appropriate procedures.

X. While implementation of these Principles may vary from country to country according to cultural, economic, religious and social factors, a system of animal use oversight that verifies commitment to the Principles should be implemented in each country. This system should include a mechanism for authorization (such as licensing or registering of institutions, scientist and/or projects) and oversight which may be assessed at the institutional, regional, and/or national level. The oversight framework should encompass both ethical review of animal use as well as considerations related to animal welfare and care. It should promote a harm benefit analysis for animal use, balancing the benefits derived from the research or educational activity with the potential for pain and/or distress experienced by the animal. Accurate records should be maintained to document a system of sound program management, research oversight, and adequate veterinary care.

2010a). A "Gold Standard Publication Checklist" has been proposed to help fully integrate the 3Rs into systematic reviews of the literature (Hooijmans *et al.*, 2010b).

In the section on personnel qualifications, the AWA says that the institution should ensure adequate training and qualifications and that this is fulfilled in part through the provision of training and instruction on the "concept, availability, and use of research or testing methods that limit the use of animals [Reduction] or minimize animal distress [Refinement]" (AWA [Animal Welfare Act], 1990). The AWA further indicates that research staff should be trained on the "utilization of services (e.g., National Agriculture Library of Medicine) available to find information:… (ii) On alternatives to the use of live animals in research [Replacement];…" (AWA [Animal Welfare Act], 1990).

In addition to the specific references above, the AWA regulations also refer to the use of anesthetics, analgesics and sedatives, the availability of appropriate veterinary care, the use of appropriate housing; and timely, appropriate euthanasia – all of which demonstrate the concept of 'refinement' (Brown and Smiler, 2012).

The PHS Policy contains similar language regarding minimizing discomfort, distress, pain, use of appropriate anesthesia, and the use of humane endpoints – all examples of refinement. In addition, the PHS Policy refers to the IRAC Principles, requiring institutions receiving PHS funds to use the *Guide* as a basis for their animal care and use programs.

National and international agencies and organizations such as the Interagency Coordinating Committee on the Validation of Alternative Methods (ICCVAM) (http://iccvam.niehs.nih.gov/), the European Centre for the Validation of Alternative Methods (ECVAM) (http://ecvam.jrc.ec.europa.eu/), and the National Centre for the Replacement, Refinement and Reduction of Animals in Research (NC3Rs) (http://www.nc3rs.org.uk/) are charged with helping to find and promote the use of alternatives (Brown and Smiler, 2012).

With so much 'official' emphasis on the 3Rs, why is there a perception that the concept is not being adequately implemented in practice? It has been suggested that scientists and IACUCs do not fully understand the concepts of the 3Rs (Graham, 2002; Schuppli and Fraser, 2005). In addition to incomplete understanding of the concepts, factors believed to negatively influence the full implementation of the 3Rs included a belief that the scientists themselves would implement the 3Rs; funding agencies reviewed the use of the 3Rs when reviewing proposals; sample size, rather than study design, was the important criteria for reduction; and focusing upon potential harm from procedures without considering potential distress from husbandry and housing was appropriate. Although such conclusions were based upon very small groups (4 and 3 IACUCs, respectively),

these are troubling observations and indicate the need for greater emphasis on the 3Rs in training programs for scientists and IACUCs (Brown and Smiler, 2012). Others suggest that the extent of the 3Rs implementation is "substantially underestimated" due to the lack of recognition by the scientist or protocol review committee that a proposed procedure will result in a 3Rs outcome (Mellor *et al.*, 2007).

It would be disingenuous to imply that, although well established, the concept of the 3Rs is universally accepted. In an article titled *Time to Abandon the Three Rs*, Derbyshire wrote that the 3Rs "draw attention away from the value of experimentation and toward the importance of animal welfare" (Derbyshire, 2006). Although the article supports the concept of reducing animal stress for the sake of science, this article clearly does not recognize the opportunity to balance between facilitating science and, at the same time, applying the 3Rs.

A. Replacement

Replacement refers to methods that avoid using animals. The term includes absolute replacements (i.e., replacing animals with inanimate systems such as computer programs) as well as relative replacements (i.e., replacing animals, such as vertebrates, with animals that are lower on the phylogenic scale) (NRC, 2011). Relative replacement may be controversial to some people as it implies 'speciesism' (Singer, 1975). Like many of the ethical considerations relating to animal use, this concept can also be considered on a continuum. Society, in general, often differentiates between humans and non human animals. However, when we consider the animal world, different opinions exist about our obligations to some species *versus* others. For example, nonhuman primates and animals commonly kept as pets such as horses, dogs, and cats seem to be considered differently than rats and mice, which are considered differently from fruit flies, worms, and so on. This is consistent with what Patterson-Kane terms the ethics of care. This philosophy "honors the human–animal bond as a morally significant and ethically acceptable attachment that creates a duty to care for and protect a specific animal regardless of the objective status of the animal" (Patterson-Kane and Golab, 2013).

Development of fully validated and accepted replacement alternatives can be a frustratingly slow process, but scientists and regulatory agencies must ensure that products are non hazardous (or appropriately labeled if hazardous). However, there are significant examples of successful replacement of live animals (Brown and Smiler, 2012). Perhaps one of the most criticized uses of animals for toxicity testing is the Draize test in rabbits. This test was developed to determine ocular toxicity caused by products and chemicals. Ocular toxicity tests represent one of the four most commonly conducted product safety tests (ICCVAM, 2010). The 3Rs were implemented by the development of validated and accepted replacements for screening products – the bovine corneal opacity and permeability test using an isolated cow eye or an isolated chicken eye (both by-products of the meat industry), and the cytosensor microphysiometer. One refinement, a balanced preemptive pain-management plan for rabbit Draize tests which still are required, has also been validated and accepted (ICCVAM, 2010).

A second example of implementation of the 3Rs involves the replacement of rabbits in the rabbit pyrogen test by using an *in vitro* Limulus Ameobecyte Lysate (LAL) Test. In this safety test, blood of horseshoe crabs is collected and the animals are returned, unharmed, back to the ocean. A component of the horseshoe crab's blood reacts with bacterial endotoxin or lipopolysacchride, a membrane component of gram-negative bacteria, allowing detection of bacterial contamination. Previous tests required the injection of drugs, biologics, medical devices, or raw materials into rabbits to look for a febrile response to indicate contamination with endotoxins. Now the majority of these products are chemically tested using LAL instead of being injected into rabbits (Brown and Smiler, 2012).

B. Reduction

"*Reduction* includes strategies for obtaining comparable levels of information from the use of fewer animals or for maximizing the information obtained from any given number of animals (without increasing pain or distress) to ultimately require fewer animals to acquire the same scientific information. This approach relies on an analysis of experimental design, applications of newer technologies, the use of appropriate statistical methods, and control of environmentally related variability in animal housing and study areas" (NRC, 2011).

Strategies to reduce the numbers of animals needed include improved experimental design, by formulation of a good experimental question and logical development of a hypothesis (Frey, 2014), appropriate statistical design of a study (Dell *et al.*, 2002), and improved selection of an animal model, including selection of animals with the most appropriate health and genetic status. Control of the genetic status is an advantage of using rats and mice. The use of inbred strains of rats and mice allows scientists to control and investigate genetic variation, and to evaluate responses to treatments on specific areas of interest (Festing, 2004). The use of animals without confounding disease or genetic variation results in less variation and requires fewer animals to determine a treatment effect.

Individuals involved with study design, study review, or as a member of the research team have the ethical imperative to ensure studies use the minimum numbers of animals necessary to achieve the scientific objective. Scientists should design studies with particular attention to methodology, statistics and choice of model. Veterinarians and facility staff should collaborate to minimize non-experimental variables in animal care. IACUCs should be diligent during review of the protocol, semiannual program and facility evaluations, and review of post approval monitoring to ensure that the appropriate number of animals have been used. Having a statistician on the IACUC is one strategy that may be helpful (Brown and Smiler, 2012).

C. Refinement

"*Refinement* refers to modifications of husbandry or experimental procedures to enhance animal well-being and to minimize or eliminate pain and distress" (NRC, 2011). In the authors' opinion, refinement is commonly employed by scientists in ongoing efforts to improve their science – better animal welfare leading to better-quality science, particularly in cases where the impacts of animal distress would be a confounding variable. Many scientists do not recognize this as utilization of 'alternatives,' even though it clearly falls within the 3Rs (Mellor *et al.*, 2007). However, this is also an area where scientists, veterinarians and IACUCs can make significant strides to enhance animal welfare (Brown and Smiler, 2012). Use of less invasive procedures (e.g,. the use of a blood pressure cuff *versus* a catheter) is one method of refining a study. However, there are also situations where an invasive procedure, such as implantation of telemetry, can result in much less stressful data collection (Stephens *et al.*, 2002). Other general refinements utilized in experimental procedures include microsampling to decrease the amount of blood needed (which also leads to a reduction of the animals needed) and imaging which allows non-invasive collection of data over time, rather than euthanizing animals at multiple time-points to follow progression of a disease. Examples of other refinements which would often be most influenced by the laboratory animal medicine professional would be more accurate recognition of pain and the use of analgesics and supportive care, implementation of humane endpoints and enhanced housing and husbandry. These will be discussed in more detail as we review strategies to optimize animal welfare.

V. STRATEGIES TO OPTIMIZE ANIMAL WELFARE

Refinement and reduction are two key areas where the laboratory animal professional can optimize animal welfare. Strategies which can aid in optimizing animal welfare include: input into experimental design to minimize the number of animals that need to be used and facilitating sharing of animal resources when possible; recognition of signs of pain, distress, and other negative welfare states; pharmacologic and non-pharmacologic interventions to minimize pain, distress, and other negative welfare states; pre-study agreement on humane endpoints and providing input during research actively modify those endpoints if needed; acclimatizing animals to potentially painful or distressful situations; and training animals to cooperate in experimental procedures and provision of appropriate environmental enrichment.

Carbone and Garnett, in a chapter on Ethical Issues in Anesthesia and Analgesia in Laboratory Animals state, "… the prime ethical concerns in laboratory animal welfare are what animals consciously experience: their pain, distress, fear, boredom, happiness and psychological well being" (Carbone and Garnett, 2008). The emotional dimension of pain, a characteristic of suffering, requires pain pathways to extend to higher levels of the cortex which has been reported as being unique to humans and some other primates (such as apes) (Nuffield Council on Bioethics, 2005). "However, the absence of analogous structures cannot necessarily be taken to mean that they [animals] are incapable of experiencing pain, suffering or distress or any other higher order states of conscious experience" (Nuffield Council on Bioethics, 2005).

"Fundamental to the relief of pain in animals is the ability to recognize its clinical signs in specific species" (NRC, 2011). Thus it is imperative that a program of animal care and use includes adequate training of all personnel with animal responsibilities. It has been suggested that some animals (particularly prey species) may try to mask pain to avoid displaying abnormal activity and increasing their risk of predation (Roughan and Flecknell, 2000). In addition, many of these animals are most active during the dark cycle, when observations are more difficult. Since clinical indices of pain may be very subtle, it is important to be able to recognize a departure from normal behavior and appearance (Table 39.3) (NRC, 2003). A short list of general signs and measurements includes: animals vigorously seeking to escape;

changes in biological characteristics such as food and water consumption and body weight; blood levels of hormones and glucose; adrenal gland mass; and species-specific appearance, posture, and behavior (Moberg, 1985, 2000). Behavioral indicators of pain in mice and rats have also been described (Flecknell, 1999; Roughan and Flecknell, 2000, 2001, 2003; Karas, 2003; Kohn et al., 2007). Guidelines for the assessment and management of pain in rodents and rabbits have been published by the ACLAM (ACLAM, 2006).

The potential for pain-relieving medications to interfere with research objectives/results should be considered. Many studies have been carried out investigating analgesic effect on a wide variety of parameters (e.g., litter size, body weight, behavior, and hemodynamic parameters) (Lamon et al., 2008; Valentim et al., 2008; McBrier, et al., 2009; Bourque et al., 2010; Goulding et al., 2010). Instead of assuming that analgesics cannot be given, literature searches should be conducted to determine if studies have been done validating the effect on the variables of concern, and investigators should be required to provide scientific justification for withholding analgesia. If data does not exist, consideration should be given for conducting and publishing an appropriate study to indicate which analgesics are, or are not, a viable scientific option for future experiments. In addition to considering the potential impact of pain-relieving drugs on research, the impact of not relieving pain must also be considered as such states can result in adverse physiologic and behavioral consequences such as weight loss, compromised immune function, and tumor progression (NRC, 2009). It has been suggested that administering analgesics to both control and test animals is a way to ensure appropriate comparisons (Stokes and Marsman, 2014). If it is determined that a study must involve unrelieved pain, there should be well defined criteria for removal of an animal from study and clearly defined procedures for how such decisions will be made (Stokes and Marsman, 2014). There is a growing understanding in neurology of the similarities of emotional pain, such as the pain of social separation,

TABLE 39.3 Indicators of Pain in Several Common Laboratory Animals

Species	General behavior	Appearance	Other
Rodents	Decreased activity; excessive licking and scratching; self-mutilation; may be unusually aggressive; abnormal locomotion (stumbling, falling); writhing; does not make nest; hiding	Piloerection; rough/stained haircoat; abnormal stance or arched back; porphyrin staining (rats)	Rapid, shallow respiration; decreased food/water consumption; tremors
Rabbit	Head pressing; teeth grinding; may become more aggressive; increased vocalizations; excessive licking and scratching; reluctant to locomote	Excessive salivation; hunched posture	Rapid, shallow respiration; decreased food/water consumption

NRC (2003).

No single observation is sufficiently reliable to indicate pain; rather several signs, taken in the context of the animal's situation should be evaluated. The signs of pain may vary with the type of procedure (e.g., orthopedic versus abdominal pain).

to physical pain (Panksepp *et al.*, 1997; Kross *et al.*, 2011; McMillan, 2014). In the past, the alleviation of pain has been limited to the alleviation of physical pain. As our understanding of emotional pain increases, the quantification and alleviation of distress from emotional pain will also increase.

Defining distress in animals has proven to be a difficult task. The ILAR Committee on the Recognition and Alleviation of Distress in Laboratory Animals stated "However, the absence of analogous structures cannot necessarily be taken to mean that they [animals] are incapable of experiencing pain, suffering or distress or any other higher order states of conscious experience" (NRC, 2008).

STRESS DEFN

Stress has been defined as "the biological response an animal exhibits in an attempt to cope with threats to its homeostasis" (Stokes, 2000). This response can involve immunologic, metabolic, autonomic, neuroendocrine, and behavioral changes (Moberg, 2000; Moberg and Mench, 2000). The type, pattern, and level of the response depend upon the strength, severity, intensity, and duration of the stressor(s). The aversive state of distress results when an animal is unable to adapt to the stressor(s). By limiting the frequency, strength, severity, intensity, and/or duration of the stressor(s), it may be possible to limit the level of distress in the animal. One method is to reduce the cumulative stress an animal experiences (e.g., allowing recovery or adaptation to a given stressful situation before adding additional stressors) or refining practices and procedures to make the individual stressors less severe or shorter (Brown and Smiler, 2012).

Non-pharmacological approaches to minimizing pain and distress should also be considered. Interventions should allow the animal to maintain good hydration and nutritional status and may include moistening food, provision of food and water in a more readily accessible location, supplemental food and liquid which may be more highly palatable, or provision of parenteral fluids and/or nutrition. Making the animal as physically comfortable as possible, by providing additional bedding or nesting material, removing items from the cage which may cause injury in the animal's debilitated state, and adding or removing social partners as appropriate can also be strategies to improve welfare.

Humane endpoints are a refinement of experimental endpoints that result in more severe animal pain and distress. Scientific or experimental endpoints are defined as occurring when the objectives of the study have been reached. Humane endpoints occur at the point at which pain or distress is prevented, terminated, or relieved in an experimental animal, and are used to reduce the severity and/or duration of an animal's pain and/or distress (Stokes and Marsman, 2014). The scientific and humane endpoints can occur at the same time, in other words, the scientific endpoint occurs prior to the development of pain or distress. Studies that may result in severe or chronic pain or significant alterations in the animal's ability to maintain normal physiology, or adequately respond to stressors, should contain descriptions of appropriate humane endpoints or provide science-based justification as to why a particular, accepted humane endpoint cannot be employed (Brown and Smiler, 2012). Veterinary consultation must occur when pain or distress is beyond the level anticipated in the protocol description or when interventional control is not possible (NRC, 2011). Most of the ethical principles guiding humane animal research mention the use of humane endpoints, (Bankowski, 1985; Council for International Organizations of Medical Sciences (CIOMS), 1985; IRAC, 1985) and clinical signs, physiologic parameters, biochemical measurements and other parameters that can potentially serve as early biomarkers for such endpoints (Stokes, 2002; Stokes and Marsman, 2014). Stokes provides an overview and reviews specific situations where endpoints are utilized (Stokes, 2000, 2002).

The need, criteria and timing for humane endpoints should be part of pre-study planning which is best done as a research team of scientists, technicians, and veterinarians (CCAC, 1998; OECD, 2000; NCR, 2003). Because endpoints are an important element of IACUC protocol review, it is essential that a protocol contains all appropriate information regarding the criteria for humane endpoints, observation schedules and training of personnel to adequately observe for the agreed upon criteria. Approved pilot studies may be useful for gathering this information if it is not known at the time of protocol submission. In addition, the criteria and other details may need to be modified when unexpected adverse events occur. The IACUC should be notified when this happens and the protocol amended as needed (Brown and Smiler, 2012).

Development of criteria for humane endpoints may be general and applicable to any study, such as when an institution adopts standards or policies that cover situations when study specific endpoints have not been determined. These documents often appear as Standard Operating Procedures (SOPs) or guidelines, and may be developed and instituted by the IACUC, the veterinary staff, the institutional administration, or any collaboration of the above. The policies should encompass generic clinical or behavioral conditions that potentially are associated with pain and distress, and should be widely recognized and accepted by the research staff (Brown and Smiler, 2012). General clinical signs which may be monitored include: weight loss, inability to ambulate adequately to obtain food and/or water, and body condition scores (Figure 39.1) (Hickman and Swan, 2010). Anorexia, or lack of appetite, is a significant observation since parenteral supplementation in rodents is not commonly used. In some cases in these species, clinical observations are only obvious when advanced illness,

BC 1
Rat is emaciated
- Segmentation of vertebral column prominent if not visible.
- Little or no flesh cover over dorsal pelvis. Pins prominent if not visible.
- Segmentation of caudal vertebrae prominent.

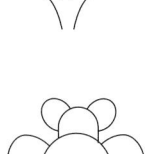

BC 2
Rat is under conditioned
- Segmentation of vertebral column prominent.
- Thin flesh cover over dorsal pelvis, little subcutaneous fat. Pins easily palpable.
- Thin flesh cover over caudal vertebrae, segmentation palpable with slight pressure.

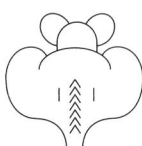

BC 3
Rat is well-conditioned
- Segmentation of vertebral column easily palpable.
- Moderate subcutaneous fat store over pelvis. Pins easily palpable with slight pressure.
- Moderate fat store around tail base, caudal vertebrae may be palpable but not segmented.

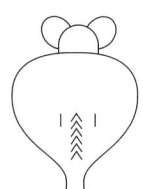

BC 4
Rat is overconditioned
- Segmentation of vertebral column palpable with slight pressure.
- Thick subcutaneous fat store over dorsal pelvis. Pins of pelvis palpable with firm pressure.
- Thick fat store over tail base, caudal vertebrae not palpable.

BC 5
Rat is obese
- Segmentation of vertebral column palpable with slight pressure; may be a continuous column.
- Thick subcutaneous fat store over dorsal pelvis. Pins of pelvis palpable with firm pressure.
- Thick fat store over tail base, caudal vertebrae not palpable.

FIGURE 39.1 Body condition scoring scale for the rat. *From Hickman and Swan (2010).*

toxicity, or impending death (e.g., a moribund state) are reached (Toth, 2000). Toth described various clinical signs indicative of the moribund state including impaired ambulation which prevents animals from reaching food or water; excessive weight loss and extreme emaciation; lack of physical and mental alertness; difficult labored breathing; and inability to remain upright (Toth, 2000). It is important to note that using the moribund state as an endpoint does not eliminate pain and distress that an animal experiences progressing to that state (Stokes and Marsman, 2014). Ongoing refinements, using objective data-based criteria, that is predictive of impending death avoids animals being found dead and allows for collection of tissues and other biological specimens that may otherwise be wasted (Stokes and Marsman, 2014).

In some cases, humane endpoints may be developed for a specific type of study (Montgomery, 1987; Olfert, 1996; Dennis, 2000; Olfert and Godson, 2000; Sass, 2000; Workman *et al.*, 2010) or a specific individual study (Hickman and Swan, 2010; Singh *et al.*, 2010). The use of scoring systems has been described and usually utilizes multiple observations which, in total, identify the humane endpoint (Lloyd and Wolfensohn, 1998; Morton, 2000, 2003; Medina, 2004). Other systematic approaches have also been described (Morton, 2000; Medina, 2004). There are excellent references available in the *Guide* that review the establishment and use of humane endpoints to avoid death as an end point (NRC, 2011).

To be prepared for situations when unanticipated clinical observations of pain and distress may occur, the institution should have sufficient veterinary oversight in place to advise when alleviation of negative consequences from experimental procedures should be addressed. This may result in animals receiving veterinary medical care, dosing holidays, removal from the experiment, or euthanasia to best align with the scientific objectives of the research. These decisions are ideally made through a collaborative discussion including animal care, scientific and veterinary staff. However, in cases where the animals are significantly compromised, the veterinarian is obligated to take whatever actions are necessary for animal welfare (AWA [Animal Welfare Act], 1990; OECD, 2000). When multiple animals receiving the same treatment exhibit severe adverse effects, consideration should be given to adjusting the endpoint in the remaining animals, stopping the study and restoring the health of the animals, or to euthanizing an entire treatment group if experimental objectives can no longer be achieved.

Euthanasia means 'good death.' It is important to consider in discussions about laboratory animal welfare because a majority of laboratory animals are euthanized (Carbone, 2014). Euthanasia is often one of the only remaining options to implement humane endpoints – when death best meets the animal's needs. Carbone has identified three key areas where animal welfare issues are related to euthanasia: "decisions about when and whether to euthanize an animal; potential animal pain and distress in the minutes to hours preceding the euthanasia process; and pain and distress of the euthanasia process itself" (Carbone, 2014). Of the criteria for judging euthanasia methods, Carbone identifies the following as having the greatest impact on animal welfare: ability to induce loss of consciousness and death with a minimum of pain and distress; time required to induce loss of consciousness; reliability; irreversibility; compatibility with species, age, and health status; and ability to maintain equipment in proper working order (Carbone, 2014). Different euthanasia methods score higher or lower than others in each of these criteria so one method may be the best in some circumstances but completely inappropriate in others. In the US, the definitive guide on euthanasia is the AVMA Guidelines for the Euthanasia of Animals (AVMA Panel on Euthanasia, 2013) which was the result of two years of work by a group of veterinary and non-veterinary scientists, using a multidisciplinary approach. Methods are listed as acceptable, acceptable with conditions, or unacceptable. Those listed as acceptable with conditions are considered to be equivalent to those listed as acceptable when all criteria for their application have been met (Carbone, 2014).

There are three main reasons a decision may be made to euthanize an animal. As previously mentioned, an animal may be euthanized for humane reasons. Animals may also be euthanized as an integral part of the study to collect tissues and samples, or animals may be euthanized as a default because there is no present or planned future use for the animal. It is this third reason which presents the greatest concern for animal welfare. Although philosophical debate exists about whether death is, in fact, a harm to animals and if they have insufficient cognition and self-awareness of their future (Cigman, 1989; Regan, 1989; DeGrazia, 1996; Kaldewaig, 2008; Harman, 2011; Carbone, 2014), reuse or rehoming should be a considered as an alternative to euthanasia where practical and legal (Carbone, 2014).

In the situation where euthanasia is being performed for humane reasons, prompt action is necessary. This can be facilitated by clear understanding of the criteria needed to make the decision to terminate the animal's life and a well-defined delineation of personnel responsibilities. Alternatively, there may be situations where euthanasia is not urgent. In these cases, husbandry considerations such as presence of food, water, bedding, and housing with compatible conspecifics remain important considerations, as well as euthanizing in the home cage of the animal when possible. Care should also be taken to use the minimal amount of restraint necessary to ensure that the animal and operator are both safe and secure.

Although the general principles of euthanasia apply internationally, the actual accepted methods of euthanasia may differ in various reports and regulations (Anonymous, 2010; AVMA Panel on Euthanasia, 2013). It is beyond the scope of this chapter to provide a review of the significant body of literature on the subject, so it is necessary for laboratory animal professionals and IACUCs to develop a mechanism to remain current regarding new developments in euthanasia methods and how they impact animal welfare. Research on euthanasia is complex, making it difficult for any single study to be able to compare or rank various techniques scientifically. Studies look at behavioral observations, physiology (neurophysiology and stress endocrinology), and even extrapolate from the experiences of human volunteers. "No single study can compare and rank different techniques which complicates evidence based euthanasia updates" (Carbone, 2014), but as a procedure which will be performed on a vast majority of laboratory animals, researchers must continuously review the literature for best welfare recommendations.

Acclimatization, or the process by which an animal can adjust to a gradual change in their environment, can also be a refinement technique. The gradual acclimatization of animals to procedures, particularly procedures that may be distressful, allows the animal to become familiarized with the procedure. Predictability reduces stress and distress, and has even been shown to decrease perceived pain in both animals and humans (Bolles and Fanselow, 1980; Carlsson et al., 2006). Operant conditioning can be used to train animals in techniques that elicit voluntary cooperation to research procedures. While the training of dogs to sit for exams and nonhuman primates to extend an arm or leg for blood collection which are the most common examples, all species can be trained to cooperate in the laboratory. Hurst and West developed a method of handling mice with either an open hand or in a tunnel structure instead of the common tail-base method of restraint. Studies found that the mice were less anxious in the elevated plus maze test, and they displayed increased voluntary interaction with the handler (Hurst and West, 2010).

The ability to express normal patterns of behavior is also a refinement to standard laboratory housing, as well as one of the Five Freedoms. The ability of an animal to display a normal behavioral repertoire frequently requires either the provision of some substrate (e.g., appropriate nesting material) or complex environment (e.g., visual blocks for socially housed nonhuman primates). Understanding what substrates or environmental complexities an animal desires requires an understanding of their natural behavioral repertoire, behavioral motivations, and the complexities of their social structures and interactions, as well as an appreciation for how their natural behavioral repertoire may have been shifted due to domestication.

VI. EXAMPLES OF CHALLENGING RESEARCH AND OPPORTUNITIES FOR ANIMAL WELFARE OPTIMIZATION

A. Genetically Altered Research Models

The use of genetically altered (GA) animals has seen a 10-fold increase in the past decade. This increased use is driven by many factors such as the desire to study gene function and to create new models of disease (Medina and Hawkins, 2014). The use of GA animals offers some unique opportunities to enhance animal welfare and the 3Rs since careful phenotyping can reveal early indicators of disease that may replace the need to develop more serious clinical disease (Brown and Murray, 2006). At the same time animal welfare concerns exist with the creation, maintenance and use of GA animals (Brown and Murray, 2006; Wells *et al.*, 2006; NRC, 2011). When lines are created, there are significant numbers of animals that do not have the genes of interest and are used for other purposes or euthanized. To determine if the animal has incorporated the desired genetic modification, the animal must be tissue typed, usually by taking blood, ear, or tail tissue (Hamann *et al.*, 2010; Ravine and Suthers, 2012; Bonaparte *et al.*, 2013). In addition to expressing the desired phenotype under study, unforeseen traits may be expressed, thus making close monitoring of the colony a critical concern (Rose, 2011). Using a harmonized list of Mouse Welfare Terms (http://mousewelfareterms. org) can help to ensure that animals are monitored and described in a consistent manner. Creation and use of a mouse passport, a document that describes phenotype, husbandry considerations, and special needs, can help reduce the welfare impact of transport and acclimatization to new facilities if they include details of husbandry refinements that can alleviate welfare problems. To maximize the use of created lines, sharing of established lines of interest is encouraged using searchable databases for registering GA lines such as International Mouse Strain Resource (http://www.findmice.org). Creation of GA lines is a time-consuming and expensive process, both in terms of resources and appropriate animal care. Once a line is created, cryopreserving GA lines can minimize the numbers of mice which must be maintained (Medina and Hawkins, 2014). An additional discussion of animal welfare concerns in the use of GA lines can be found in *The Ethics of Research Involving Animals* by the Nuffield Council on Bioethics (Nuffield Council on Bioethics, 2005).

B. Cancer Research

The use of animals continues to be essential to understand the fundamental mechanisms of malignancy and to discover improved methods to prevent, diagnose, and treat cancer. An excellent summary of standards and recommendations for animal care and use in cancer research will serve as a basis for this section (Workman *et al.*, 2010). The recommendations include study design, statistics, and pilot studies; choice of tumor models (e.g., genetically engineered, orthotopic, and metastatic); therapy (including drugs and radiation); imaging humane endpoints (including tumor burden and site); and publication of best practice.

As with other examples of studies with animal welfare challenges, when designing studies with unknown tumors, pilot tumor growth studies using small numbers of animals can establish patterns of local and metastatic growth. They also highlight adverse effects associated with tumor progression, allowing the development of observation and treatment strategies and identification of humane endpoints (Brown and Smiler, 2012). For metastatic models, pilot experiments should define the extent and time course of dissemination to internal organs if such information is not already available. Early endpoints reduce non-specific systemic effects and may increase the precision of the results obtained (Workman *et al.*, 2010).

Aseptic technique, anesthetics and post-implantation analgesia are recommended for the subcutaneous implantation of tumor material. For injection of cell suspensions, the minimum number of cells in the smallest volume should be used, consistent with the properties of the tumor. Implantation of tumor material into the muscle requires special justification as it is more likely to affect mobility and cause pain. The choice of site for solid tumors will influence the maximum acceptable tumor load and the appropriate humane endpoints. Sites such as the footpad, tail, eye, or bone are likely to be painful or distressing and require special justification and earlier endpoints. Footpad injection, which has been traditionally used to potentiate lymphatic dissemination, is unacceptable without exceptional scientific justification and should then only involve a single paw (Workman *et al.*, 2010). Similarly, tumors that metastasize to sensitive sites need great care (Workman *et al.*, 2010). If brain tumors can be justified, body weight loss is reportedly a sensitive endpoint (Redgate *et al.*, 1991) and MRI or bioluminescent imaging (BLI) techniques can be very useful (van Furth *et al.*, 2003; Ragel *et al.*, 2008; McCann *et al.*, 2009). Tumor size and burden is an important consideration in determining endpoints. When procedures are used to improve tumor take rate, for example, moderate doses of whole-body irradiation, the added potential impact on animal welfare should be considered.

The use of biomarkers, imaging, and measurement of circulating tumor cells can facilitate humane endpoints in these studies (Glinskii *et al.*, 2003; Komatsubara *et al.*, 2005). Intravital microscopic imaging uses a wide variety of optical imaging techniques, often incorporating fluorescent or bioluminescent genetic reporters or markers, including nanoparticles (Hoffman, 2005). This type of imaging has particular animal welfare issues because it involves surgery to provide optical clarity and visualization on a microscope stage or using fiber-optic light guides (Weissleder and Pittet, 2008). Surgical implantation of 'window' chambers for tumor implantation enables imaging to be performed over days to weeks (Dewhirst *et al.*, 1987; Lehr *et al.*, 1993; Brown *et al.*, 2001; Reyes-Aldasoro *et al.*, 2008). Here, general anesthesia is only essential for the initial surgery and imaging may be performed with restrained animals. Acclimation to restraint techniques should be used to decrease stress associated with restraint and positive reinforcement training techniques to elicit animal cooperation with the restraint techniques should be implemented wherever possible. Strict aseptic technique and good post-operative care and analgesia are essential (Richardson and Flecknell, 2005; Flecknell, 2008).

C. Neuroscience and Behavioral Research

While data collection in behavioral research is observational, the study design frequently requires the denial of some behavior in order to measure the motivation for it, or motivate animals to perform tasks. Many behavioral research protocols, for example, require feed or water restriction in order to motivate animals to perform tasks (Toth and Gardiner, 2000). The deprivation of food and water is considered to be a procedure that may cause pain and distress (APHIS, 1997), and the use of a highly preferred food or the least restriction necessary is encouraged (NRC, 2011). Specific strategies can be employed, however, to decrease the potential distress associated with food and water restriction when it is necessary for the study. Animals should be acclimated to the restriction regime, and feeding or watering protocols should take into account both potential nutritional imbalances and the timing of natural feeding behaviors and incorporate strategies accordingly to accommodate both. A well-defined monitoring program should be in place, to document and have defined endpoints or intervention strategies for criteria such as body weight, food and water intake, general physical appearance and activity, and hydration status (Brown and Smiler, 2012).

Neurobehavioral measurements may require invasive devices or long-term tethering or other restrictions in order to gain the required data measurements. If learned behavior is going to be required of the animal, conditioning or training should be carried out prior to the surgery in order to preemptively eliminate animals that will not train from being surgical candidates (NRC, 2003). For protocols or procedures that will require restricted movement or the tolerance of a long-term, indwelling device, animals need to be acclimated to the restraint or device, the restraint should be of the minimum duration necessary to achieve the scientific endpoints, and procedures need to be scientifically justified (Brown and Smiler, 2012).

Animal models of neurodegenerative, neural trauma, or psychoses can in and of themselves cause detriment to the animals' welfare, but may be necessary in order to study the condition. The confirmation of sterile technique if surgeries are to be performed is vital. It is also critical to anticipate and plan for the supportive care of the created condition or surgical complications. Supportive care measures such as easier access to food or water for neurologically impaired animals, the addition of additional or softer bedding for animals where ambulation or activity is affected, and the development of humane endpoints can also improve welfare in these models (Brown and Smiler, 2012).

Neuroscience and behavioral testing are likely the most vulnerable research paradigms to being confounded by many of the refinements previously discussed. Efforts to decrease anxiety, through environmental enrichment or behavioral management techniques like acclimation, could adversely affect results, and yet, the behavioral research paradigms that measure anxiety (e.g., the light–dark box, elevated plus maze, open-field testing, and forced swim test) must, by design, induce anxiety. In general, aversive stimuli are only acceptable when well tolerated by the animal and produce neither maladaptive behaviors (Brown and Smiler, 2012) nor excessive escape–avoidance activity (NRC, 2003). A delicate balance between the welfare of the animals in these types of research and the value of the research question to be answered by the work is often needed.

VII. SCIENCE OF ANIMAL WELFARE

A. Introduction

Taking the assumption that using animals in research has a negative impact on their welfare, implementation of replacement and reduction strategies of the 3Rs, such as those described previously, are obvious improvements in animal welfare. This leaves the third R, refinement, as the remaining strategy we can take to improve animal welfare. The aforementioned reduction of pain and distress strategies and the implementation of humane endpoints are clear examples of refinements. For more subtle refinements, scientific evaluation of the procedure is required to determine whether the refinements are actually improving welfare. While examples of research have shown how animal welfare has been improved with certain refinements, there is certainly much more to be learned about the welfare state of the animals in our care and how to accurately assess whether the behavioral management and environmental enrichment programs we are providing are indeed supporting good welfare. Our aim is to help the reader to understand the science of animal welfare, including objective measures that can be used to assess welfare, as well as to stimulate you to think about what you might do to add to the body of information to increase the proper objective evaluation of refinements made that are intended to improve animal welfare.

Historically, the improvement of animal welfare via refinement concentrated on the reduction of negative welfare states. Examples would include: the recognition of pain via vigilant monitoring (particularly in prey species) (Roughan and Flecknell, 2006; Langford, 2010; Keating et al., 2012), the judicious use of anesthesia, analgesia, and supportive care measures, and the development of humane endpoints where pain and distress can be prevented, relieved, or minimized. For prey species, simply being moved or handled can be a stressor (Gartner *et al.*, 1980; Burn *et al.*, 2006). As previously described, habituation to handling, particularly when paired with positive reinforcement (Jezierski and Konecka, 1996; Csatadi *et al.*, 2005; Meijer *et al.*, 2006) or prefaced by being put into a positive affective state (Cloutier and Newberry, 2009) can decrease the distress associated with common research handling.

Operant conditioning and complex environments with ethologically relevant environmental enrichment provide animals with choice and control and are likely to provide a positive welfare state for the animals and not just alleviate the negative. Some enrichment, such as 'tickling' in rats (Cloutier and Newberry, 2008; Cloutier *et al.*, 2010) has been shown to induce a positive effective state. With improved understanding of behavior and refined welfare assessments, it is the opinion of the authors that the provision of good animal welfare will go beyond just the alleviation of the negative, and be the promotion of positive experiences, as suggested by Weary (Weary, 2011).

B. Modern Animal Welfare Science

By the mid-20th century, the disciplines of ethology and neuroscience were starting to garner widespread acceptance in the scientific community, and were contributing to our understanding of the animal experience. The appendix to the Brambell Report proposed various ways to research stress, pain, discomfort, fear, and other aspects of welfare, tying animal behavior to welfare for the first time. The period shortly after World War II was dominated by efforts in animal protection, like the Animal Welfare Act, rather than assessment of animal welfare. The scientific discipline through the 1970s and 1980s consisted of developments in ethology (the study of behavior) and the understanding of behavioral motivations. Preference testing measured how hard an animal would work to obtain a resource, and comparisons of the behavior of free-living and captive animals were used to measure what was 'good' for animals: behaviors that they naturally displayed or were motivated to work for. By the mid 1980s, the definition of welfare included behavioral and biological needs that were being measured in these ways, and the reader is referred to further works referenced for detail (Dawkins, 1980; Broom, 1988, 2009; Duncan, 1993, 1996; Fraser, 1999). Animal welfare as a scientific discipline developed around 1990. The discipline, however, stands on the shoulders of aforementioned decades of work in the veterinary, behavioral, nutritional, physiological, and other animal-based sciences. The difference is this animal welfare as an independent discipline is focused

on the measurement of the animal's perception in addition to their physical state and behavior. In other words, animal welfare is measurable and therefore a scientific discipline in its own right. Debate continues between those that supported welfare as a purely emotional state (Dawkins, 1980, 1990; Sandoe and Simonsen, 1992), and those who tend to present welfare as a purely physical state of health and normal physiological function. The current position is that welfare involves aspects of all three areas: the contribution of physical state, including health and physiology, the behaviors, and the emotional state of the animal.

The mental state of the animal cannot be directly measured like the physiology and behavior, so it has to be inferred through the other two measures. Cortisol is frequently used to measure stress and/or welfare states of animals, but its measurement alone is not analogous to measuring stress, in that both eustress and distress can elevate cortisol, and that cortisol can be decreased in situations of chronic stress (Moberg and Mench, 2000). A constellation of such measures, such as body weight and food consumption; general clinical signs such as hunched posture, and rough hair coat; and behavior, assessed together, frequently is the best overall measure of welfare. As the measurement of objective physiologic parameters and observation of clinical signs are better covered in standard veterinary texts on the various species, we will discuss the observation and quantification of behavior as it relates to the measurement of welfare in more detail.

C. Assessing Animal Welfare

1. Behavior Assessment

The study and understanding of a species' natural behavior can predict its reaction to different stimuli and give an indication of the state of the animal in captivity. However, most animals can, and do adapt their behavior to the environment and situation, some differences may just illustrate the adaptability of the animal and be no reflection of welfare, so comparisons between wild or free-living animal behavior, or 'naturalness,' has been criticized as a measure of animal welfare (Dawkins, 2008). Domestication does not always change behavior; it may instead change behavior quantitatively not qualitatively. For example, domesticated guinea pigs show higher levels of sociopositive behavior than their wild cavy counterparts (Sachser *et al.*, 2004).

An ethogram, or a list of observable behaviors, is an integral tool to measuring behavior. In order to be most useful, the behaviors in an ethogram should be meaningful, both to the paradigm being measured and the species being observed; in other words, as non-subjective as possible. Clear, well-described, non-overlapping, unambiguous definitions of the behaviors listed in the ethogram that have been discussed and agreed upon by all observers ensure better behavioral observation and assessment accuracy.

Continuous recording of behaviors allows for the documentation of the occurrence and duration of every behavior, and true calculations of frequency, duration, latency, sequence, as well as true time budgets. It's also almost prohibitively time consuming, unless you're a behaviorist, a grad student, or a naturalist. In most laboratory animal settings, interval scanning is the most useful and common method of recording behavior. As a general rule, frequent behaviors can have long intervals between observations; quick or infrequent behaviors need to have shorter intervals. For rare behaviors, a one–zero or yes–no technique of recording during focal scan sessions, or watching behaviors for a defined period of time and documenting whether or not the behavior occurred in that interval, may be most useful. For further instruction on data collection methods, the reader is referred to works by Martin and Bateson or Altmann for further detail (Altmann, 1974; Martin and Bateson, 2004) and to Beaver and Bayne (Beaver and Bayne, 2014) for an excellent overview of further resources.

In order to use behavior to indicate the state of the animal, however, the ethogram must contain not just the behaviors of the animal but also the temporal, environmental and social context in which the behavior is occurring (Appleby *et al.*, 2011). The first question you can answer with behavioral observation is "what do they do." Because you can never actually know the "why" a behavior is done, the context can provide the all-important clues. Any one set of behavioral responses rarely indicates reduced welfare, though changes in the frequencies of individual and social behaviors or the suppression of behaviors can suggest that there are welfare problems. For example, play or exploratory behavior decreases with decreased welfare (Arnsten *et al.*, 1985; Krachun *et al.*, 2010) and may thus be "luxuries" that are dispensed with during periods of stress. Behavior that occurs out of context may also indicate disturbance. A thorough understanding of the natural behavioral repertoire of the species being evaluated is vital to putting welfare states into context.

2. Avoidance and Anxiety

Over the years, a variety of tests have been developed to equate or quantify the amount of avoidance and relate it to the animals' level of anxiety based on fearful reactions or situational avoidance. Examples of these assessments include the light/dark box test, where a rodent is allowed choice between a brightly lit section and a darkened section of an environment. Based on a rodent's instinct as a prey species to avoid open, lit, exposed places, an animal that spends a greater amount of time in that area is interpreted to be 'less anxious.' Likewise, the open-field or elevated plus maze are designed to assess the animals' willingness to enter an open area as a measure of anxiety. The issue with these types of tests is that they are measuring 'state' anxiety, or anxiety induced by a particular situation, in a particular time and place. Welfare, however, requires more a measure of 'trait' anxiety, an assessment of the animals' general being over time, which does not vary from moment to moment but reflects the *mental* state, as opposed to the *physical* state that the animal is in. The usefulness, shortcomings, and suggestions for refinements of these types of tests are more thoroughly covered in works by Bourin and Rodgers (Rodgers, 1997; Rodgers *et al.*, 1997; Bourin *et al.*, 2007), and the reader is referenced to those sources for further detail.

3. Preference Testing

Observing an animal's preference can give us an indication of what might improve an animal's welfare. This testing paradigm can be set up in a few slightly different ways. One is to set up a complex environment with multiple options and measure where or with what the animal spends its time. A simpler setup is to allow the animal to choose between two options, with all other variables held constant. Interpretation of preference testing is fraught with complexity, however, as it can be influenced by the state of the animal (e.g., swine chose bedded or bare floors based on room temperature [Fraser, 1985]) or previous experience (e.g., rodents made better nests with materials with which they had prior exposure [Van Loo and Baumans, 2004]). It must also be understood that animals may not always choose what is best for them, so choice tests alone may not be adequate in determining what is best for the animal and its welfare. As an example, rabbits have evolved to graze on low-caloric-density forage material but when provided with high-calorie or free-choice high-quality food, they will eat to obesity. In addition, choice testing does not infer any sort of importance to the resource or environment chosen. Using two choices only tells which of the two choices is preferred, even if neither is particularly good for the animal. Another consideration is that just because an animal spends a long period of time performing a particular behavior or interacting with a particular enrichment, does not necessarily mean that item holds high value or is very important for welfare. For instance, a diabetic will likely spend a large portion of their day doing things other than insulin injection, however they would work very hard to get to the insulin should its access be restricted, due to its importance to their welfare.

4. Consumer Demand

In order to better assess the strength of a preference, testing paradigms that infer a cost to the access of the enrichment can quantify the preference. Some sort of barrier, such as a weighted door (Ågren *et al.*, 1989) or longer distance (Guerra and Ades, 2002) can be placed between the animal and the desired resource. The weight can be sequentially increased to determine the 'cost' that the animal will endure for access to the resource. Alternatively, the preference for a resource can be compared to another known desired or aversive resource, giving each a relative value.

5. Cognitive Bias Assessment

Cognitive bias measures of animals' emotional or 'affective' state by measuring the way that an animal perceives incoming information and responds to it. This concept for animals is based on work that shows that people in negative emotional states will show increased attention to negative stimuli and are more likely to make pessimistic interpretations of ambiguous situations. These paradigms have been applied to animals in attempts to assess their cognitive bias. Harding trained rats to press a lever to either receive a food reward when one tone was heard or avoid a negative (white noise) stimulus when a different tone was heard. When the rats were placed in an environment of chronic stress (constant unpredictable disturbances in their housing conditions) the rats responded to ambiguous tones as though they expected the negative stimulus more often than rats in a non-stressful environment (Harding *et al.*, 2004). Conversely, a different researcher found that rats raised in enriched environments were more likely to expect a positive reward (Brydges *et al.*, 2011). While this kind of work is still in its relative infancy, it is possible that with further refinements of this type of testing, it might be possible to assess the emotional state of our animals more directly or to make general statements on the types of environmental enrichments or behavioral management strategies that positively or negatively affect the laboratory animal species.

6. Coming Together

While preference, consumer demand, and cognitive bias testing may seem to be advanced techniques for the everyday application in the assessment of laboratory animal welfare, they have the potential to forward our efforts to support animal welfare in the laboratory environment. Their application displays an opportunity for collaborative work on applying science to refine procedures in the laboratory for the benefit the animals. While the authors acknowledge that there are real challenges of resources and practicality, we hope that we have illuminated areas where these disciplines can bring together the concept of animal welfare with the science of animal welfare to develop practical and scientifically sound methods to measure the welfare of animals under our care.

VIII. CONCLUSION AND SUMMARY

The science, study and philosophical concept of animal welfare have been the culmination of an ethical journey. Starting with philosophy and based on our relationship with animals, progressing through a series of ethical questions and obligations that directed the development of laws, regulations, and guidelines to ensure our moral obligations in looking after animal welfare, the current field in which we now scientifically assess and support strategies to measure an animals' welfare has come to be. Whenever possible, subjective data should be used to develop assessment parameters, husbandry and enrichment conditions, and to determine humane endpoints. There is a moral obligation to ensure good welfare for all animals, including those in the laboratory setting. The challenge is to meld the philosophy and the science into a practical application that positively affects the animal's welfare. While we acknowledge that the sheer numbers of animals (in particular rodents), economic constraints and resource availability are real challenges to our ability to develop and implement welfare supportive programs, we would purport that these are not insurmountable obstacles. The provision of good welfare is not a static program: as the science in this field continues to progress, our understanding and abilities will grow, and occasional review of the entire program, with adjustments as indicated, will be essential.

References

ACLAM, 2006. Guidelines for the Assessment and Management of Pain in Rodents and Rabbits 2011.

Ågren, G., Zhou, Q., et al., 1989. Territoriality, cooperation and resource priority: hoarding in the Mongolian gerbil, *Meriones unguiculatus*. Anim. Behav. 37, 28–32.

Altmann, J., 1974. Observational study of behavior: sampling methods. Behaviour 49 (3/4), 227–267.

Anonymous, 2010. Directive 2010/63/UE of the European Parliament and of the Council of 22 September 2010 on the protection of animals used for scientific purposes. Off. J. Eur. Union L 276, 33–79.

APHIS, 1997. Painful Procedures. APHIS Policy #11. U. S. D. o. A. Animal and Plant Health Inspection Service.

APHIS, 2000. Consideration of Alternatives to Painful/Distressful Procedures. APHIS Policy #12. U. S. D. o. A. Animal and Plant Health Inspection Service.

Appleby, M., Mench, J.A. (Eds.), 2011. Animal Welfare. CABI, Oxfordshire UK.

Arnsten, A.F.T., Berridge, C., et al., 1985. Stress produces opioid-like effects on investigatory behavior. Pharmacol. Biochem. Behav. 22 (5), 803–809.

AVMA Panel on Euthanasia, 2013. AVMA Guidelines for Euthanasia of Animals: 2013 Edition.

AWA [Animal Welfare Act], 1990. Animal Welfare Act. PL (Public Law) 89-544. 2011.

Bankowski, Z., 1985. CIOMS international guiding principles for biomedical research involving animals. <http://cioms.ch/publications/guidelines/1985_texts_of_guidelines.htm> (accessed 11.05.15.).

Beaver, B., Bayne, K., 2014. Animal welfare assessment considerations.. In: Bayne, K., Turner, P. (Eds.), Laboratory Animal Welfare. Elsevier, Amsterdam, the Netherlands, pp. 29–38.

Bolles, R.C., Fanselow, M.S., 1980. A perceptual-defensive-recuperative model of fear and pain. Behav. Brain Sci. 3 (2), 291–301.

Bonaparte, D., Cinelli, P., Douni, E., et al., 2013. FELASA guidelines for the refinement of methods for genotyping genetically-modified rodents: a report of the Federation of European Laboratory Animal Science Associations Working Group. Lab. Anim. 47 (3), 134–145.

Bourin, M., Petit-Demouliere, B., et al., 2007. Animal models of anxiety in mice. Fundam. Clin. Pharamacol. 21, 567–574.

Bourque, S.L., Adams, M.A., et al., 2010. Comparison of buprenorphine and meloxicam for postsurgical analgesia in rats: effects on body weight, locomotor activity, and hemodynamic parameters. J. Am. Assoc. Lab. Anim. Sci. 49 (5), 617–622.

Brambell, R., 1965. Report of he Technical Committee to Enquire into the Welfare of Animals Kept under Intensive Livestock Husbandry Systems. H. M. s. S. Office, London, p. 85.

Broom, D.M., 1988. The scientific assessment of animal-welfare. Appl. Anim. Behav. Sci. 20 (1-2), 5–19.

Broom, D.M., 2009. A history of animal welfare science. Acta Biotheor. 59 (2), 121–137.

Brown, E.B., Campbell, R.B., et al., 2001. In vivo measurement of gene expression, angiogenesis and physiological function in tumors using multiphoton laser scanning microscopy. Nat. Med. 7 (7), 864–868.

Brown, M., 2013. Ethics and animal welfare. In: Bayne, T. (Ed.), Laboratory Animal Welfare. Elsevier, New York, pp. 7–14.

Brown, M.J., Murray, K.A., 2006. Phenotyping of genetically engineered mice: humane, ethical, environmental, and husbandry issues. ILAR J. 47 (2), 118–123.

Brown, M.J., Smiler, K., 2012. Ethical, regulatory and non-regulatory considerations. In: Suckow, M.A., Stevens, K.A., Wilson, R.P. (Eds.), The Laboratory Rabbit, Guinea Pig, Hamster, and Other Rodents. Elsevier, Amsterdam, the Netherlands, pp. 3–31.

Brydges, N.M., Leach, M., et al., 2011. Environmental enrichment induces optimistic cognitive bias in rats. Anim. Behav. 81, 169–175.

Burn, C.C., Peters, A., et al., 2006. Long-term effects of cage-cleaning frequency and bedding type on laboratory rat health, welfare, and handleability: a cross-laboratory study. Lab. Anim. 40, 353–370.

Carbone, L., 2014. Euthanasia and laboratory animal welfare. In: Bayne, K., Turner, P.V. (Eds.), Laboratory Animal Welfare. Elsevier, Amsterdam, the Netherlands, pp. 157–169.

Carbone, L., Garnett, N., 2008. Ethical issues in anesthesia and analgesia in laboratory animals. In: Fish, R., Brown, M., Danneman, P., Karas, A. (Eds.), Anesthesia and Analgesia in Laboratory Animals. Elsevier, London, UK, pp. 561–568.

Carlsson, K., Anderson, J., et al., 2006. Predicatbility modulates the affective and sensory-discriminative neural processing of pain. Neuroimage 32 (4), 1804–1814.

Carruthers, P., 1992. The Animals Issue Moral Theory in Practice. Cambridge University Press, Cambridge.

CCAC, 1998. Guidelines in: Choosing an Appropriate Endpoint in Experiments using Animals for Research, Teaching and Testing. Canadian Council on Animal Care, Ottawa, Canada.

CFR, rev, 1998. USDA Regulations. 9. U. S. D. o. A. Animal and Plant Health Inspection Service. Office of Federal Register, Washington, DC.

Cigman, R., 1989. Why death does not harm animals. In: Regan, T., Singer, P. (Eds.), Animal Rights and Human Obligations. Prentice Hall, Englewood Cliffs, NJ, pp. 150–152.

Cloutier, S., Newberry, R.C., 2008. Use of a conditioning technique to reduce stress associated with repeated intra-peritoneal injections in laboratory rats. Appl. Anim. Behav. Sci. 112, 158–173.

Cloutier, S., Newberry, R.C., 2009. Tickled pink: playful handling as social enrichment for laboratory rats. AWI Quarterly (Spring), 24–25.

Cloutier, S., Wahl, K., et al., 2010. Playful Handling Mitigates the Stressfulness of Injections in Laboratory Rats. AALAS, Atlanta, GA.

Cohen, C., Regan, T., 2001. The Animal Rights Debate. Rowman & Littlefield, Lanham, MD.

Council for International Organizations of Medical Sciences (CIOMS), 1985. CIOMS International Guiding Principles for Biomedical Research Involving Animals. 2(ii).

Csatadi, K., Kustos, K., et al., 2005. Even minimal human contact linked to nursing reduces fear responses toward humans in rabbits. Appl. Anim. Behav. Sci. 95, 123–128.

Dawkins, M., 2008. The science of animal suffering. Ethology 114 (10), 937–945.

Dawkins, M.S., 1990. From an animal's point of view – Motivation, Fitness, and Animal-Welfare. Behav. Brain Sci. 13 (1), 1–61.

Dawkins, M.S., 1980. Animal Suffering: The Science of Animal Welfare. Chapman & Hall, London, UK.

DeGrazia, D., 1996. Taking Animals Seriously. Cambridge University Press, Cambridge.

Dell, R.B., Holleran, S., et al., 2002. Sample size determination. ILAR J. 43 (4), 207–213.

Dennis Jr., M.B., 2000. Humane endpoints for genetically engineered animal models. ILAR J. 41 (2), 94–98.

Derbyshire, S.W.G., 2006. Time to abandon the three Rs. Scientist 20 (2), 14–17.

Dewhirst, M.W., Gustafson, C., et al., 1987. Temporal effects of 5.0 Gy radiation in healing subcutaneous microvasculature of a dorsal flap window chamber. Radiat. Res. 112 (3), 581–591.

Duncan, I.J.H., 1993. Welfare is to do with what animals feel. J. Agric. Environ. Ethics 6 (Suppl. 2), 8–14.

Duncan, I.J.H., 1996. Animal welfare defined in terms of feelings. Acta Agri. Scand. A Anim. Sci. 0 (Suppl. 27), 29–35.

Festing, M.F., 2004. The choice of animal model and reduction. Altern. Lab. Anim. 32 (Suppl. 2), 59–64.

Flecknell, P., 2008. Analgesia from a veterinary perspective. Br. J. Anaesth. 101 (1), 121–124.

Flecknell, P.A., 1999. Pain – assessment, alleviation and avoidance in laboratory animals. ANZCCART News 12 (4), 1–6.

Fraser, D., 1985. Selection of bedded and unbedded areas by pigs in relation to environmental temperature and behavior. Appl. Anim. Behav. Sci. 14 (2), 117–126.

Fraser, D., 1999. Animal ethics and animal welfare science: bridging the two cultures. Appl. Anim. Behav. Sci. 65 (3), 171–189.

Frey, D., 2014. Experimental design: reduction and refinement in studies using animals. In: Bayne, K., Turner, P.V. (Eds.), Laboratory Animal Welfare. Elsevier, Amsterdam, the Netherlands, pp. 95–113.

Frey, R.G., 1988. Moral standing, the value of lives, and speciesism. Between Species 4 (3), 191–201.

Gartner, K., Buttner, D., et al., 1980. Stress response of rats to handling and experimental procedures. Lab. Anim. 14 (3), 267–274.

Gilbert, S., Kaebnick, G., Murray, T., 2012. Animal Research Ethics: Evolving Views and Practices. A Hastings Center Special Report, The Hastings Center.

Glinskii, A.B., Smith, B.A., et al., 2003. Viable circulating metastatic cells produced in orthotopic but not ectopic prostate cancer models. Cancer Res. 63 (14), 4239–4243.

Goulding, D.R., Myers, P.H., et al., 2010. The effects of perioperative analgesia on litter size in Crl:CD1(ICR) mice undergoing embryo transfer. J. Am. Assoc. Lab. Anim. Sci. 49 (4), 423–426.

Graham, K., 2002. A study of three IACUCs and their views of scientific merit and alternatives. J. Appl. Anim. Welf Sci. 5 (1), 75–81.

Guerra, R.F., Ades, C., 2002. An analysis of travel costs on transport of load and nest building in golden hamster. Behav. Proces. 57 (1), 7–28.

Hamann, M., Lange, N., Kuschka, J., Richter, A., 2010. Non-invasive genotyping of transgenic mice: comparison of different commercial kits and required amounts. ALTEX 27 (3), 185–190.

Harding, E., Paul, E., et al., 2004. Animal behaviour: cognitive bias and affective state. Nature 427 (6972) 312-312.

Harman, E., 2011. The moral significance of animal pain and animal death. In: Beauchamp, T.L., Frey, R.G. (Eds.), The Oxford Handbook of Animal Ethics. Oxford University Press, Oxford, pp. 126–137.

Harrison, R., 1964. Animal Machines: The New Factory Farming Industry, V. Stuart.

Hickman, D.L., Swan, M., 2010. Use of a body condition score technique to assess health status in a rat model of polycystic kidney disease. J. Am. Assoc. Lab. Anim. Sci. 49 (2), 155–159.

Hill, T.E., 1992. Kantian pluralism. Ethics 10 (4), 346.

Hoffman, R.M., 2005. The multiple uses of fluorescent proteins to visualize cancer in vivo. Nat. Rev. Cancer 5 (10), 796–806.

Hooijmans, C.R., Leenaars, M., et al., 2010a. A gold standard publication checklist to improve the quality of animal studies, to fully integrate the three Rs, and to make systematic reviews more feasible. Altern. Lab. Anim. 38 (2), 167–182.

Hooijmans, C.R., Tillema, A., et al., 2010b. Enhancing search efficiency by means of a search filter for finding all studies on animal experimentation in PubMed. Lab. Anim. 44 (3), 170–175.

Hurst, J.L., West, R.S., 2010. Taming anxiety in laboratory mice. Nat. Meth. 7 (10), 825–826.

ICCVAM, 2010. NICEATM-ICCVAM Test Method Evaluations – Ocular Toxicity. NICEATM-ICCVAM, Washington, DC, 2011.

IRAC, 1985. U.S. Government Principles for Utilization and Care of Vertebrate Animals Used in Testing, Research, and Training. F. Register. Office of Science and Technology Policy, Washington, DC.

Jezierski, T.A., Konecka, A.M., 1996. Handling and rearing results in young rabbits. Appl. Anim. Behav. Sci. 46, 243–250.

Kaldewaig, F., 2008. Animals and the harm of death. In: Amstrong, S.J., Botzler, R.G. (Eds.), The Animal Ethics Reader. Routledge, London, pp. 59–62.

Karas, A., 2003. Measuring Pain and Detection of Pain in Various Species. Excerpted from the Syllabus for Pain Medicine – A Course for Veterinary Technicians. Becker College and Tufts University School of Veterinary Medicine.

Keating, S.C.J., Thomas, A.A., et al., 2012. Evaluation of EMLA Cream for preventing pain during tattooing of rabbits: changes in physiological, behavioural and facial expression responses. PLoS One 7 (9), e44437.

Kohn, D.F., Martin, T.E., et al., 2007. Guidelines for the assessment and mangement of pain in rodents and rabbits. JAALAS 46 (2), 97–108.

Komatsubara, H., Umeda, M., et al., 2005. Detection of cancer cells in the peripheral blood and lung of mice after transplantation of human adenoid cystic carcinoma. Kobe J. Med. Sci. 51 (5-6), 67–72.

Krachun, C., Rushen, J., et al., 2010. Play behaviour in dairy calves is reduced by weaning and by a low energy intake. Appl. Anim. Behav. Sci. 122 (2-4), 71–76.

Kross, E., Berman, M.G., et al., 2011. Social rejection shares somatosensory representations with physical pain. PNAS 108 (15), 6270–6275.

Lamon, T.K., Browder, E.J., et al., 2008. Adverse effects of incorporating ketoprofen into established rodent studies. J. Am. Assoc. Lab. Anim. Sci. 47 (4), 20–24.

Langford, D.J., 2010. Coding of facial expressions of pain in the laboratory mouse. Nat. Methods 7 (6), 447–449.

Lehr, H.A., Leunig, M., et al., 1993. Dorsal skinfold chamber technique for intravital microscopy in nude mice. Am. J. Pathol. 143 (4), 1055–1062.

Lloyd, M.H., Wolfensohn, S.E., 1998. Practical use of distress scoring systems in the application of humane end points Humane Endpoints in Animal Experiments for Biomedical Research. Zeist, The Netherlands.

Martin, P., Bateson, P., 2004. Measuring Behavior: An Introductory Guide. Cambridge University Press, Cambridge.

McBrier, N.M., Neuberger, T., et al., 2009. Magnetic resonance imaging of acute injury in rats and the effects of buprenorphine on limb volume. J. Am. Assoc. Lab. Anim. Sci. 48 (2), 147–151.

McCann, C.M., Waterman, P., et al., 2009. Combined magnetic resonance and fluorescence imaging of the living mouse brain reveals glioma response to chemotherapy. Neuroimage 45 (2), 360–369.

McMillan, F., 2014. Emotional pain: why it can matter more to animals than physical pain. World Congress 9, Prague, Czech Republic.

Medina, L.V., 2004. How to balance humane endpoints, scientific data collection, and appropriate veterinary interventions in animal studies. Contemp. Top. 43 (5), 56–62.

Medina, L.V., Hawkins, P., 2014. Contemporary Issues in Laboratory Animal Welfare. In: Bayne, K., Turner, P.V. (Eds.), Laboratory Animal Welfare. Elsevier, Amsterdam, the Netherlands.

Meijer, M.K., Kramer, K., et al., 2006. The effect of routine experimental procedures on physiological parameters in mice kept under different husbandry conditions. Anim. Welfare 15 (1), 31–38.

Mellor, D.J., Schofield, J.C., et al., 2007. Underreporting of the three Rs deployment that occurs during the planning of protocols that precedes their submission to animal ethics committees. AATEX 14 (Special issue), 785–788.

Mill, J.S., 1863. Utilitarianism. Parker, Son and Bourn, London.

Moberg, G.P., 1985. Biological response to stress: key to assessment of animal well-being. In: Moberg, G.P. (Ed.), Animal Stress. American Physiological Society, Bethesda, MD, pp. 27–49.

Moberg, G.P., 2000. Biological responses to stress. In: Moberg, G.P., Mench, J.A. (Eds.), Biology of Animal Stress: Implications for Animal Welfare. CAB International, Oxon, pp. 1–21.

Moberg, G.P., Mench, J.A., 2000. The Biology of Animal Stress: Basic Principles and Implications for Animal Welfare. CAL International, Wallingford, Oxon, U.K.

Montgomery Jr., C.A., 1987. Control of animal pain and distress in cancer and toxicologic research. J. Am. Vet. Med. Assoc. 191 (10), 1277–1281.

Morton, D., 2003. Implementing Assessment Techniques for Pain Management and Humane Endpoints. Pain Management and Humane Endpoints, Washington, DC.

Morton, D.B., 2000. A systematic approach for establishing humane endpoints. ILAR J. 41 (2), 80–86.

NRC, 2003. Guidelines for the Care and Use of Mammals in Neuroscience and Behavioral Research. National Academy Press, Washington, DC.

NRC, 2008. Recognition and Alleviation of Distress in Laboratory Animals. National Academies Press, Washington, DC.

NRC, 2009. Recognition and Alleviation of Pain in Laboratory Animals. National Academies Press, Washington, DC.

NRC, 2011. Guide for the Care and Use of Laboratory Animals. National Academies Press, Washington, DC.

Nuffield Council on Bioethics, 2005. The Ethics of Research Involving Animals. Nuffield Council on Bioethics, London, 1, p. 335.

OECD, 2000. Guidance Document on the Recognition, Assessment, and Use of Clinical Signs as Humane Endpoints for Experimental Animals used in Safety Evaluation. Series on Testing and Assessment. Paris, Environmental Health and Safety Publilcations, Series on Testing and Assessment, No. 19: 3–39.

OIE Animal Welfare Guidelines, 2005. Terrestrial Animal Health Code, Section: Animal Welfare, Chapter 7. http://www.oie.int/en/international-standard-setting/terrestrial-code/access-online/ Accessed May 10, 2015.

OLAW, 2002. Public Health Service Policy on Humane Care and Use of Laboratory Animals. National Institute of Health.

Olfert, E., 1996. Considerations for defining an acceptable endpoint in toxicological experiments. Lab. Anim. 25, 38–43.

Olfert, E.D., Godson, D.L., 2000. Humane endpoints for infectious disease animal models. ILAR J. 41 (2), 99–104.

Olsson, I.A., Robinson, P., et al., 2011. Ethics of animal research In: Hau, J. Shapiro, S.J. (Eds.), Handbook of Laboratory Animal Science, CRC Press, Boca Raton, FL, pp. 21–37.

Panksepp, J., Nelson, E., et al., 1997. Brain systems for the mediation of social separation-distress and social-reward. Ann. NY Acad. Sci. (807), 78–100.

Patterson-Kane, E., Golab, G.C., 2013. History, Philosophies and concepts, of animal welfare. In: Bayne, K., Turner, P.V. (Eds.), Laboratory Animal Welfare. Elsevier, Amsterdam, the Netherlands, pp. 1–6.

Phinizy, C., 1965. The lost pets that stray into labs. Sports Illust., 36–49.

Ragel, B.T., Elam, I.L., et al., 2008. A novel model of intracranial meningioma in mice using luciferase-expressing meningioma cells. Laboratory investigation. J. Neurosurg. 108 (2), 304–310.

Ravine, D., Suthers, G., 2012. Quality standards adn samples in genetic testing. J. Clin. Pathol. 65 (5), 389–393.

Redgate, E.S., Deutsch, M., et al., 1991. Time of death of CNS tumor-bearing rats can be reliably predicted by body weight-loss patterns. Lab. Anim. Sci. 41 (3), 269–273.

Regan, T., 1989. Why death does not harm animals. In: Regan, T., Singer, P. (Eds.), Animal Rights and Human Obligations. Prentice Hall, Englewood Cliffs, NJ, pp. 153–157.

Regan, T., Singer, P., 1989. Animal Rights and Human Obligations. Prentice Hall, Englewood Cliffs, NJ.

Reyes-Aldasoro, C.C., Wilson, I., et al., 2008. Estimation of apparent tumor vascular permeability from multiphoton fluorescence microscopic images of P22 rat sarcomas in vivo. Microcirculation 15 (1), 65–79.

Richardson, C.A., Flecknell, P.A., 2005. Anaesthesia and post-operative analgesia following experimental surgery in laboratory rodents: are we making progress? Altern. Lab. Anim. 33 (2), 119–127.

Rodgers, R.J., 1997. Animal models of 'anxiety': where next? Behav. Pharmacol. 8 (6-7), 477–496. discussion 497-504.

Rodgers, R.J., Cao, B.J., et al., 1997. Animal models of anxiety: an ethological perspective. Braz. J. Med. Biol. Res. 30 (3), 289–304.

Rollin, B.E., 2011. Putting the Horse befoe Descartes. Temple University Press, Philadelphia, PA.

Rose, M., 2011. Humane endpoints and genetically modified animal models: opportunities and challenges Proceedings of the November 2008 International Workshop "Animal Research in a Global Environment." National Academies Press, Washington DC.

Roughan, J.V., Flecknell, P.A., 2000. Effects of surgery and analgesic administration on spontaneous behaviour in singly housed rats. Res. Vet. Sci. 69 (3), 283–288.

Roughan, J.V., Flecknell, P.A., 2001. Behavioural effects of laparotomy and analgesic effects of ketoprofen and carprofen in rats. Pain 90 (1-2), 65–74.

Roughan, J.V., Flecknell, P.A., 2003. Evaluation of a short duration behaviour-based post-operative pain scoring system in rats. Eur. J. Pain 7 (5), 397–406.

Roughan, J.V., Flecknell, P.A., 2006. Training in behaviour-based post-operative pain scoring in rats: an evaluation based on improved recognition of analgesic requirements. Appl. Anim. Behav. Sci. 96, 327–342.

Russell, W.M.S., Burch, R.L., 1959. The Principles of Humane Experimental Technique. W.M.S. Russell, London.

Russow, L.M., 1990. Animals, science, and ethics – Section I. Ethical theory and the moral status of animals. Hastings Cent. Rep. 20 (3), S4–S7.

Ryder, R., 1975. Victims of Science: The Use of Animals in Research. Davis-Poynter, London.

Sachser, N., Kunzl, C., et al., 2004. The welfare of laboratory guinea pigs. Welfare Lab. Anim. 2, 181–209.

Sandoe, P., Simonsen, H.B., 1992. Assessing animal welfare: Where does science end and philosophy begin? Anim. Welfare 1 (4), 257–267.

Sass, N., 2000. Humane endpoints and acute toxicity testing. ILAR J. 41 (2), 114–123.

Schuppli, C.A., Fraser, D., 2005. The interpretation and application of the three Rs by animal ethics committee members. Altern. Lab. Anim. 33 (5), 487–500.

Singer, P., 1975. Animal Liberation – A New Ethics for our Treatment of Animals. Avon Books, New York.

Singh, P.K., Patil, C.R., et al., 2010. Zinc disc implantation model of urinary bladder calculi and humane endpoints. Lab. Anim. 44 (3), 226–230.

Stephens, M.L., Conlee, K., et al., 2002. Possibilities for refinement and reduction: future improvements within regulatory testing. ILAR J. 43 (Suppl.), S74–S79.

Stokes, W.S., 2000. Reducing unrelieved pain and distress in laboratory animals using humane endpoints. Ilar J. 41 (2), 59–61.

Stokes, W.S., 2002. Humane endpoints for laboratory animals used in regulatory testing. ILAR J. 43 (Suppl.), S31–S38.

Stokes, W.S., Marsman, D.S., 2014. Animal Welfare Considerations in Biomedical Research and Testing. In: Bayne, K., Turner, P.V. (Eds.), Laboratory Animal Welfare. Elsevier, Amsterdam, the Netherlands, pp. 115–140.

Tannenbaum, J., 1991. Ethics and animal welfare: the inextricable connection. J. Am. Vet. Med. Assoc. 198 (8), 1360–1376.

Toth, L.A., 2000. Defining the moribund condition as an experimental endpoint for animal research. ILAR J. 41 (2), 72–79.

Toth, L.A., Gardiner, T.W., 2000. Food and water restriction protocols: physiological and behavioral considerations. Contemp. Top Lab. Anim. Sci. 39 (6), 9–17.

USDA, 2009. USDA Research Facility Inspection Guide. USDA-APHIS, Washington, DC, 2011.

Valentim, A.M., Alves, H.C., et al., 2008. The effects of depth of isoflurane anesthesia on the performance of mice in a simple spatial learning task. J. Am. Assoc. Lab. Anim. Sci. 47 (3), 16–19.

van Furth, W.R., Laughlin, S., et al., 2003. Imaging of murine brain tumors using a 1.5 Tesla clinical MRI system. Can J. Neurol. Sci. 30 (4), 326–332.

Van Loo, R.L.R., Baumans, V., 2004. The importance of learning young: the use of nesting material in laboratory rats. Lab. Anim. 38 (1), 17–24.

Warren, M.A., 1997. Moral Status: Obligations to Persons and Other Living Things. Clarendon Press, Oxford.

Wayman, S., 1966. Concentration Camps for dogs. Life Mag 60, 25–28.

Weary, D.M., 2011. A Good Life for Laboratory Animals – How Far Must Refinement Go? ALTEX Proceedings, 8th World Congress Alternatives. Springer, Montreal, Canada.

Weissleder, R., Pittet, M.J., 2008. Imaging in the era of molecular oncology. Nature 452 (7187), 580–589.

Wells, D.J., Playle, L.C., et al., 2006. Assessing the welfare of genetically altered mice. Lab. Anim. 40 (2), 111–114.

Workman, P., Aboagye, E.O., et al., 2010. Guidelines for the welfare and use of animals in cancer research. Br. J. Cancer 102 (11), 1555–1577.

Index

Herpes simplex virus 1, 397
Herpes virus (HV), 397, 987–988
  infections, 77, 431
    MCMV, 77–78
    MTV, 78
Herpes Virus of Marmots (HVM), 366
Herpesvirus simiae. See Macacine herpesvirus
  1 (McHV-1)
Heterocephalus glaber. See Naked mole rats
Heterophil. *See* Pseudoeosinophil
HEV. *See* Hepatitis E virus (HEV)
HF. *See* Heart failure (HF)
HFRS. *See* Hemorrhagic fever with renal
  syndrome (HFRS)
HFUS systems. *See* High-frequency
  ultrasound systems (HFUS systems)
HGG. *See* Hypergammaglobulinemia (HGG)
HI. *See* Hyperinsulinemia (HI)
Hibernation, 215, 357
High-density lipoproteins (HDL), 895
High-efficiency particulate air (HEPA), 54,
  463–464, 473, 1269, 1300–1301, 1548,
  1554, 1564–1565
High-frequency ultrasound systems (HFUS
  systems), 1244
Highly conserved noncoding elements
  (HCNE), 1516
Highly pathogenic avian influenza (HPAI
  H5N1), 39
Hirsutism. *See* Tremor
Histocompatibility complex, 45
Histophilus Somni (H. Somni), 648
Histoplasma capsulatum (H. capsulatum), 399
Histoplasmosis, 862–863
HIV. *See* Human immunodeficiency virus (HIV)
HLA system. *See* Human lymphocyte
  antigen system (HLA system)
HM. *See* Health monitoring (HM)
HME system. *See* Hepatic microsomal
  enzyme system (HME system)
hMG. *See* human menopausal gonadotropin
  (hMG)
Hog cholera. *See* Classical swine fever (CSF)
'Holstein–Friesian', 624
Homologous recombination (HR), 51
  in ES cells, 1424, 1425f
Homologous repair (HR), 1424–1425
Homology directed repair (HDR), 1424–1425
Hookworms, 527–528
Host–vector–parasite genomics, 1524
'House mouse' clade, 44, 84
Housing system, 1570–1577
  aquatic system, 1577
  density, 1023
  and equipment
    caging system, 1570–1577
    materials, 1570
    specialized equipment, 1570–1577
  ferrets, 578–579, 579t
  isolators, 1575
  Japanese quail, 1094–1095
  MAD, 1575–1577
  rodent housing system, 1571
    static MI cages, 1571
    ventilated caging system, 1571–1575
  semi-rigid isolator, 1575f

Housing-related issues, 1452–1453
HPA. *See* Hypothalamic–pituitary axis (HPA)
HPAI H5N1. *See* Highly pathogenic avian
  influenza (HPAI H5N1)
HPO. *See* Human phenotype ontology
  (HPO)
HPS. *See* Hantavirus pulmonary syndrome
  (HPS)
HR. *See* Homologous recombination (HR);
  Homologous repair (HR)
HS. *See* Heat shock (HS)
HSV. *See* Herpes simplex virus (HSV)
HTLV. *See* Human T-cell lymphotrophic
  virus (HTLV)
hu-SCID. See humanized severe combined
  immunodeficient (*hu-SCID*)
human chorionic gonadotropin (hCG), 165,
  585–586, 606
Human cutaneous mycobacteriosis, 1041,
  1338
Human cytomegalovirus (HCMV), 1372
Human ergonomics, 1064–1065
Human genome, 1513–1514
  PCG, 1514
  sequence comparison among human and
    animal genomes
    animal genomes, 1515–1517
    collaborative attempts to identifying
      gene function, 1520–1522
    epigenetics/epigenomics, 1517–1519
    ontology, 1519
    orthologs providing by Evola, 1515t
    phenome, 1519–1520
    similarity among species, 1514–1515
Human herpes virus 1. *See* Herpes simplex
  virus 1
Human immunodeficiency virus (HIV), 1077,
  1372
  HIV-1, 1329
  HIV-2, 1329
  vaccination, 1512
Human interaction, 1629
Human lymphocyte antigen system (HLA
  system), 628, 1509–1510
human menopausal gonadotropin (hMG),
  255
Human microbiota, 1289
Human phenotype ontology (HPO),
  1519–1520
Human T-cell lymphotrophic virus (HTLV),
  875–877, 1331
  HTLV-1, 658, 1374
Humane endpoints, 1662
humanized severe combined
  immunodeficient (*hu-SCID*), 1499
Humidification system, 1566
Humidity control, 1566
Humoral immunity pioneers, 1507–1509
HUS. *See* Hemolytic uremic syndrome (HUS)
Husbandry
  amphibians, 934–939
  cane mice, 310
  chinchillas, 388–389
  cotton rats, 312
  deer mice, 307–308
  degus, 327–328

  dogs, 513
  ferrets, 578–579
  gerbils and jirds, 317–318
  grasshopper mice, 305
  ground squirrels, 291
  guinea pig, 249
  kangaroo rats, 300
  laboratory woodchuck, 353–356
  mice, 53–57
  multimammate rats, 325–326
  naked mole rats, 330
  pack rats, 302
  pocket gophers, 298–299
  prairie dogs, 294
  rabbits, 421
  rats, 152–153
  reptiles, 969–974
  rice rats, 309
  ruminants, 626–627
  swine, 696–699
  Syrian hamster, 218–219
  voles, 323
  white-tailed rats, 315
  Xenopus laevis, 945–946
  zebra finches, 1115–1119
HV. *See* Herpes virus (HV)
HVAC system. *See* Heating, ventilation,
  and air conditioning system (HVAC
  system)
HVM. *See* Herpes Virus of Marmots (HVM)
Hybrid imaging methods, 1245
Hydatid cyst disease. *See* Echinococcosis
Hydatid disease, 317
Hydrocephalus, 194, 445–446
Hydrometra, 450
Hydronephrosis, 193
Hydropericardium syndrome, 1102
Hydrophobia. *See* Rabies
Hymenolepis (rodentolepis) nana infestation,
  123–124
Hymenolepis diminuta (H. diminuta). See
  Rodentolepis nana (*R. nana*)
Hymenolepis nana (H. nana). See Rodentolepis
  nana (*R. nana*)
Hyperacute rejection (HAR), 706–707
Hyperammonemia, 607
Hypercholesterolemia, 448
Hyperestrogenism, 606–607
Hypergammaglobulinemia (HGG), 597
Hyperglobulinemia, 894
Hyperinsulinemia (HI), 895
Hyperlipidemia, 448
Hyperplasia of gland of nictitating
  membrane, 548–549
Hyperthermia, 896
Hypertrophic cardiomyopathy (HCM),
  210–211
Hypnosis, 1155
Hypocalcemia, 682–683
Hypoglycemia, 895–896
Hypomagnesemic tetany, 683
Hypophysectomy, 1233
Hypothalamic–pituitary axis (HPA), 1468
Hypothermia, 896
Hypothyroidism, 529–531, 607
Hypovitaminosis A, 1001